KU-627-854
369 0136457

Infectious Diseases of the Fetus and Newborn Infant

Infectious Diseases of the Fetus and Newborn Infant

Sixth Edition

Jack S. Remington, MD
Professor, Department of Medicine
Division of Infectious Diseases and Geographical Medicine
Stanford University School of Medicine
Stanford, California

Chairman, Department of Immunology and Infectious Diseases
Research Institute, Palo Alto Medical Foundation
Palo Alto, California

Jerome O. Klein, MD
Professor of Pediatrics
Boston University School of Medicine
Maxwell Finland Laboratory for Infectious Diseases
Boston Medical Center
Boston, Massachusetts

Christopher B. Wilson, MD
Professor and Chair
Department of Immunology
Professor of Pediatrics
University of Washington School of Medicine
Seattle, Washington

Carol J. Baker, MD
Professor of Pediatrics
Professor of Molecular Virology and Microbiology
Head, Section of Infectious Diseases
Baylor College of Medicine
Texas Children's Hospital Foundation
Chair in Pediatric Infectious Diseases
Houston, Texas

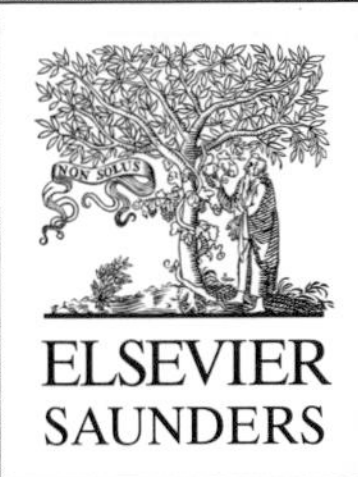

ELSEVIER
SAUNDERS

1600 John F. Kennedy Blvd.
Suite 1800
Philadelphia, PA 19103-2899

INFECTIOUS DISEASES OF THE FETUS AND NEWBORN INFANT ISBN 0-7216-0537-0

Notice

Knowledge and best practice in this field are constantly changing. As new research and experience broaden our knowledge, changes in practice, treatment, and drug therapy may become necessary or appropriate. Readers are advised to check the most current information provided (i) on procedures featured or (ii) by the manufacturer of each product to be administered, to verify the recommended dose or formula, the method and duration of administration, and contraindications. It is the responsibility of practitioners, relying on their own experience and knowledge of the patient, to make diagnoses, to determine dosages and the best treatment for each individual patient, and to take all appropriate safety precautions. To the fullest extent of the law, neither the Publisher nor the Editors assume any liability for any injury and/or damage to persons or property arising out of or related to any use of the material contained in this book.

The Publisher

Library of Congress Cataloging-in-Publication Data

Infectious diseases of the fetus and newborn infant / [edited by] Jack S. Remington …
[et al.]—6th ed.
p. ; cm.
Includes bibliographical references and index.
ISBN 0-7216-0537-0
1. Communicable diseases in newborn infants. 2. Communicable diseases in pregnancy—Complications. 3. Fetus—Diseases. 4. Neonatal infections. I. Remington, Jack S., 1931-
[DNLM: 1. Communicable Diseases—Infant, Newborn. 2. Fetal Diseases. 3. Infant, Newborn, Diseases. WC 100 I42 2006]
RJ275.I54 2006
618.92¢01—dc22

2004051422

Acquisitions Editor: Todd Hummel
Developmental Editor: Jennifer Ehlers
Publishing Services Manager: Frank Polizzano
Project Manager: Lee Ann Draud
Design Coordinator: Ellen Zanolle

Printed in the United States of America

Last digit is the print number: 9 8 7 6 5 4 3 2 1

To my sister, Jill

J.S.R.

To those most dear to us:

Linda, Andrea, Bennett, Adam, Zachary, Alex, Evan, and Dana

J.O.K.

Sherryl, Alyssa and Bryan, Amelia and Floyd, and Helen

C.B.W.

My parents, Jack and Jane; Marcie, Morven, Susan, Laura, and Tom

C.J.B.

And to the mentors, colleagues, fellows, and students who have enriched our academic and personal lives, and to the physicians and the women and infants with infectious diseases for whom they care

Silence

The gentle silence of the dandelion seed
floating on
a wisp of warm air

of the violet
opening
to the morning sun

of the motion of
the butterfly's wings
as it sucks the nectar
of a cherry blossom

The silence is broken
by the cries
of all of the infants destroyed
and the anguish of their mothers
whose tears cannot reverse
what the organism has wrought

The quiet silence of the womb
harboring an unborn child
awaiting its first breath
of deserved normality

Not the sad silence
of deafness
or
of retardation
or
of blindness
Nor of the sad silence
of the grave

How can we silence the sad silence?

Jack (2005)

CONTRIBUTORS

Stuart P. Adler, MD
Professor and Division Chair, Department of Pediatrics, Division of Infectious Diseases, Virginia Commonwealth University School of Medicine, Medical College of Virginia Campus, Richmond, Virginia
Human Parvovirus Infections

Charles A. Alford, Jr., MD
Professor Emeritus of Pediatrics, University of Alabama School of Medicine, University of Alabama at Birmingham, Birmingham, Alabama
Rubella

Ann M. Arvin, MD
Lucille Salter Packard Professor of Pediatrics and Professor of Microbiology and Immunology, Stanford University School of Medicine, Stanford, California
Herpes Simplex Virus Infections

Carol J. Baker, MD
Professor of Pediatrics and Professor of Molecular Virology and Microbiology; Head, Section of Infectious Diseases, Baylor College of Medicine; Texas Children's Hospital Foundation Chair in Pediatric Infectious Diseases, Houston, Texas
Current Concepts of Infections of the Fetus and Newborn Infant; Bacterial Sepsis and Meningitis; Group B Streptococcal Infections; Syphilis; Pneumocystis *and Other Less Common Fungal Infections*

Elizabeth D. Barnett, MD
Associate Professor of Pediatrics, Boston University School of Medicine; Maxwell Finland Laboratory for Infectious Diseases, Boston Medical Center, Boston, Massachusetts
Bacterial Infections of the Respiratory Tract

Catherine M. Bendel, MD
Associate Professor of Pediatrics and Director, Neonatal-Perinatal Medicine Fellowship Program, University of Minnesota Medical School, Minneapolis, Minnesota
Candidiasis

Robert Bortolussi, MD, FRCPC
Professor of Pediatrics and Associate Professor of Microbiology and Immunology, Dalhousie University Faculty of Medicine; Chief of Research IWK Health Centre, Halifax, Nova Scotia, Canada
Listeriosis

John S. Bradley, MD
Associate Professor of Pediatrics, University of California, San Diego, School of Medicine, La Jolla; Director, Division of Infectious Diseases, Children's Hospital of San Diego, San Diego, California
Hepatitis

William Britt, MD
Professor, Department of Pediatrics and Infectious Disease, University of Alabama at Birmingham School of Medicine, Birmingham, Alabama
Cytomegalovirus Infections

James D. Cherry, MD, MSc
Professor of Pediatrics, David Geffen School of Medicine at UCLA; Member, Division of Infectious Diseases, Mattel Children's Hospital at UCLA, Los Angeles, California
Enterovirus and Parechovirus Infections

Thomas G. Cleary, MD
Professor, University of Texas School of Public Health; Attending Physician, Hermann Hospital, Houston, Texas
Microorganisms Responsible for Neonatal Diarrhea

Louis Z. Cooper, MD
Professor Emeritus of Pediatrics, Columbia University College of Physicians and Surgeons, New York, New York
Rubella

Carl T. D'Angio, MD
Associate Professor of Pediatrics, University of Rochester School of Medicine and Dentistry; Attending Neonatologist, Golisano Children's Hospital at Strong, Rochester, New York
Laboratory Aids for Diagnosis of Neonatal Sepsis

Toni Darville, MD
Professor of Pediatrics and Immunology/Microbiology, University of Arkansas Medical Sciences; Attending Physician, Arkansas Children's Hospital, Little Rock, Arkansas
Chlamydia *Infections*

Jill K. Davies, MD
Assistant Professor, Department of Obstetrics and Gynecology, University of Colorado Health Sciences Center, Denver, Colorado
Obstetric Factors Associated with Infections in the Fetus and Newborn Infant

Georges Desmonts, MD
Chief (retired), Laboratoire de Sérologie Néonatale et de Recherche sur la Toxoplasmose, Institut de Puériculture, Paris, France
Toxoplasmosis

Morven S. Edwards, MD
Professor of Pediatrics, Section of Infectious Diseases, Baylor College of Medicine; Attending Physician, Texas Children's Hospital, Houston, Texas
Group B Streptococcal Infections

Joanne E. Embree, MD, FRCPC
Head and Professor, Department of Medical Microbiology, University of Manitoba Faculty of Medicine; Professor, Department of Pediatrics and Child Health, and Head, Section of Pediatric Infectious Disease, Winnipeg Regional Health Authority, Winnipeg, Manitoba, Canada
Gonococcal Infections

Roberto P. Garofalo, MD
Professor of Pediatrics, University of Texas Medical Branch at Galveston; Child Health Center, Galveston, Texas
Human Milk

Michael A. Gerber, MD
Professor of Pediatrics, University of Cincinnati College of Medicine; Attending Pediatrician, Cincinnati Children's Hospital Medical Center, Cincinnati, Ohio
Lyme Disease

Anne A. Gershon, MD
Professor of Pediatrics, Columbia University College of Physicians and Surgeons; Director, Division of Pediatric Infectious Diseases, Columbia University Medical Center, New York, New York
Chickenpox, Measles, and Mumps

Ronald S. Gibbs, MD
Department of Obstetrics and Gynecology, University of Colorado Health Sciences Center, Denver, Colorado
Obstetric Factors Associated with Infections in the Fetus and Newborn Infant

Kathleen M. Gutierrez, MD
Assistant Professor, Department of Pediatrics, Stanford University School of Medicine, Stanford, California
Herpes Simplex Virus Infections

R. Doug Hardy, MD
Assistant Professor of Pediatrics and Internal Medicine, University of Texas Southwestern Medical Center; Attending Physician, Children's Medical Center Dallas and Parkland Hospital, Dallas, Texas
Mycoplasmal Infections

Joan A. Heath, BSN, RN
Manager, Infection Control Program, Children's Hospital and Regional Medical Center, Seattle, Washington
Infections Acquired in the Nursery: Epidemiology and Control

David Ingall, MD
Professor Emeritus, Departments of Pediatrics and Obstetrics and Gynecology, Northwestern University Medical School, Chicago; Chairman Emeritus, Department of Pediatrics, Evanston Northwestern Health Care, Evanston, Illinois
Syphilis

Jerome O. Klein, MD
Professor of Pediatrics, Boston University School of Medicine; Maxwell Finland Laboratory of Infectious Diseases, Boston Medical Center, Boston, Massachusetts
Current Concepts of Infections of the Fetus and Newborn Infant; Bacterial Sepsis and Meningitis; Bacterial Infections of the Respiratory Tract; Bacterial Infections of the Urinary Tract

William C. Koch, MD
Associate Professor, Department of Pediatrics, Virginia Commonwealth University School of Medicine, Medical College of Virginia Campus, Richmond, Virginia
Human Parvovirus Infections

David B. Lewis, MD
Associate Professor of Pediatrics, Division of Immunology and Transplantation Biology, Stanford University School of Medicine, Stanford; Attending Physician, Lucile Salter Packard Children's Hospital at Stanford, Palo Alto, California
Developmental Immunology and Role of Host Defenses in Fetal and Neonatal Susceptibility to Infection

Sarah S. Long, MD
Professor of Pediatrics, Drexel University College of Medicine; Chief, Section of Infectious Diseases, St. Christopher's Hospital for Children, Philadelphia, Pennsylvania
Bacterial Infections of the Urinary Tract

Timothy L. Mailman, MD
Assistant Professor of Pediatrics, Division of Infectious Diseases, Dalhousie University Faculty of Medicine; Director of Microbiology, IWK Health Centre, Halifax, Nova Scotia, Canada
Listeriosis

Yvonne A. Maldonado, MD
Associate Professor, Department of Pediatrics and Department of Health Research and Policy, Stanford University School of Medicine, Stanford; Attending Physician, Lucile Salter Packard Children's Hospital at Stanford, Palo Alto, California
Acquired Immunodeficiency Syndrome in the Infant; Less Common Viral Infections; Less Common Protozoan and Helminth Infections; Pneumocystis *and Other Less Common Fungal Infections*

George H. McCracken, Jr., MD
Department of Pediatrics, University of Texas Southwestern Medical School, Dallas, Texas
Clinical Pharmacology of Antibacterial Agents

Rima McLeod, MD
Jules and Doris Stein RPB Professor, University of Chicago, Division of Biological Sciences, Pritzker School of Medicine; Attending Physician, University of Chicago Hospitals, Michael Reese Hospital and Medical Center, Chicago, Illinois
Toxoplasmosis

Julia A. McMillan, MD
Professor, Department of Pediatrics, Division of Infectious Diseases, Johns Hopkins University School of Medicine; Attending Physician, Johns Hopkins Hospital, Baltimore, Maryland
Smallpox and Vaccinia

Michael J. Miller, MD
Professor of Pediatrics, Oregon Health Sciences University School of Medicine, Portland, Oregon
Pneumocystis *and Other Less Common Fungal Infections*

James P. Nataro, MD, PhD
Professor of Pediatrics, Medicine, Microbiology, and Biochemistry, Center for Vaccine Development, University of Maryland School of Medicine, Baltimore, Maryland
Microorganisms Responsible for Neonatal Diarrhea

Victor Nizet, MD
Associate Professor of Pediatrics, Division of Infectious Diseases, University of California, San Diego, School of Medicine, La Jolla; Attending Physician, Children's Hospital and Health Center, San Diego, California
Group B Streptococcal Infections

Pearay L. Ogra, MD
Professor, Department of Pediatrics, Division of Infectious Diseases, State University of New York at Buffalo, School of Medicine and Biomedical Sciences; Attending Physician, Women and Children's Hospital of Buffalo, Buffalo, New York
Human Milk

Rachel C. Orscheln, MD
Instructor and Fellow, Pediatric Infectious Diseases, Washington University in St. Louis School of Medicine; Attending Physician, St. Louis Children's Hospital, St. Louis, Missouri
Staphylococcal Infections

Miguel L. O'Ryan, MD
Professor, Microbiology and Mycology Program, Institute of Biomedical Sciences, Faculty of Medicine, University of Chile, Santiago, Chile
Microorganisms Responsible for Neonatal Diarrhea

Gary D. Overturf, MD
Professor of Pediatrics and Pathology, University of New Mexico School of Medicine; Director, Pediatric Infectious Diseases, Children's Hospital of New Mexico, Albuquerque, New Mexico
Bacterial Infections of the Bones and Joints; Focal Bacterial Infections

Debra L. Palazzi, MD
Assistant Professor of Pediatrics, Baylor College of Medicine; Attending Physician, Texas Children's Hospital, Ben Taub General Hospital, and Woman's Hospital of Texas, Houston, Texas
Bacterial Sepsis and Meningitis

Octavio Ramilo, MD
Professor of Pediatrics, University of Texas Southwestern Medical Center; Attending Physician, Children's Medical Center Dallas and Parkland Hospital, Dallas, Texas
Mycoplasmal Infections

David K. Rassin, PhD
Professor of Pediatrics, University of Texas Medical Branch at Galveston; Child Health Center, Galveston, Texas
Human Milk

Jack S. Remington, MD
Professor of Medicine, Division of Infectious Diseases and Geographic Medicine, Stanford University School of Medicine, Stanford; Marcus A. Krupp Research Chair and Chairman, Department of Immunology and Infectious Diseases, Research Institute, Palo Alto Medical Foundation, Palo Alto, California
Current Concepts of Infections of the Fetus and Newborn Infant; Toxoplasmosis

Xavier Sáez-Llorens, MD
Professor of Pediatrics, University of Panama School of Medicine; Vice-Chairman and Head of Infectious Diseases, Hospital del Niño, Panama City, Panama
Clinical Pharmacology of Antibacterial Agents

Joseph W. St. Geme III, MD
Professor of Pediatrics and Molecular Microbiology, Washington University in St. Louis School of Medicine; Attending Physician, Pediatrics and Pediatric Infectious Diseases, St. Louis Children's Hospital, St. Louis, Missouri
Staphylococcal Infections

Pablo J. Sanchez, MD
Professor of Pediatrics, Divisions of Neonatal-Perinatal Medicine and Pediatric Infectious Diseases, University of Texas Southwestern Medical School; Attending Physician, Parkland Health and Hospital System and Children's Medical Center Dallas, Dallas, Texas
Syphilis

Eugene D. Shapiro, MD
Professor of Pediatrics, Epidemiology, and Investigative Medicine, Yale University School of Medicine; Attending Pediatrician, Children's Hospital at Yale–New Haven, New Haven, Connecticut
Lyme Disease

Henry R. Shinefield, MD
Clinical Professor of Pediatrics and Dermatology, University of California, San Francisco, School of Medicine; Co-Director, Vaccine Study Center, Kaiser Permanente Medical Group, San Francisco, California
Staphylococcal Infections

Sergio Stagno, MD
Professor and Chairman, Department of Pediatrics, University of Alabama at Birmingham School of Medicine; Physician-in-Chief, Children's Hospital of Alabama, Birmingham, Alabama
Cytomegalovirus Infections

Jeffrey R. Starke, MD
Professor and Vice-Chairman, Department of Pediatrics, Baylor College of Medicine; Chief of Pediatrics, Ben Taub General Hospital, Houston, Texas
Tuberculosis

Barbara J. Stoll, MD
Chair, Department of Pediatrics, Emory University School of Medicine; President and CEO, Emory Children's Center; Medical Director, Children's Healthcare of Atlanta, Atlanta, Georgia
Neonatal Infections: A Global Perspective

Philippe Thulliez, MD
Chief, Laboratoire d'Immunoanalyses et Recherche sur la Toxoplasmose, Institut de Puériculture, Paris, France
Toxoplasmosis

Geoffrey A. Weinberg, MD
Associate Professor, Department of Pediatrics, Division of Infectious Diseases, University of Rochester School of Medicine and Dentistry; Director, Pediatric HIV Program, Golisano Children's Hospital at Strong, Rochester, New York
Laboratory Aids for Diagnosis of Neonatal Sepsis

Richard J. Whitley, MD
Professor, Department of Medicine, University of Alabama at Birmingham, Birmingham, Alabama
Herpes Simplex Virus Infections

Christopher B. Wilson, MD
Professor and Chair, Department of Immunology, and Professor of Pediatrics (Infectious Diseases), University of Washington School of Medicine; Attending Physician, Children's Hospital and Regional Medical Center, Seattle, Washington
Current Concepts of Infections of the Fetus and Newborn Infant; Developmental Immunology and Role of Host Defenses in Fetal and Neonatal Susceptibility to Infection

Danielle M. Zerr, MD, MPH
Assistant Professor, Department of Pediatrics, University of Washington School of Medicine; Chair, Infection Control, Children's Hospital and Regional Medical Center, Seattle, Washington
Infections Acquired in the Nursery: Epidemiology and Control

PREFACE

Major advances in biology and medicine made during the past several decades have contributed greatly to our understanding of infections that affect the fetus and newborn. As the medical, social, and economic impact of these infections becomes more fully appreciated, the time is again appropriate for an intensive summation of existing information on this subject. Our goal for the sixth edition of this text is to provide a complete, critical, and contemporary review of this information. We have directed the book to all students of medicine interested in the care and well-being of children and hope to include among our readers medical students, practicing physicians, microbiologists, and health care workers. We believe the text to be of particular importance for obstetricians and physicians who are responsible for the pregnant woman and her developing fetus; pediatricians and family doctors who care for newborn infants; and primary care physicians, neurologists, audiologists, ophthalmologists, psychologists, and other specialists who are responsible for children who suffer the sequelae of infections acquired in utero or during the first month of life.

The scope of this book encompasses infections of the fetus and newborn, including those acquired in utero, during the delivery process, and in the early months of life. When appropriate, sequelae of these infections that affect older children and adults are included as well. Infection in the adult is described when pertinent to the developing fetus and newborn infant. Each chapter includes a review of the history, microbiology, epidemiology, pathogenesis and pathology, clinical signs and symptoms, diagnosis, prognosis, treatment, and prevention of the infection. The length of the chapters varies considerably. In some instances, this variation is related to the available fund of knowledge on the subject; in others (e.g., the chapters on toxoplasmosis, neonatal diarrhea, varicella, measles, and mumps), the length of the chapter is related to the fact that no recent comprehensive reviews of these subjects are available.

The first, second, third, fourth, and fifth editions of this text were published in 1976, 1983, 1990, 1995, and 2001, respectively. As of this writing, in the spring of 2005, it is most interesting to observe the changes that have occurred in the interval since publication of the last edition. New authors provide fresh perspectives. Major revisions of most chapters suggest the importance of new information about infections of the fetus and newborn infant.

Each of the authors of the different chapters is a recognized authority in the field and has made significant contributions to our understanding of infections in the fetus and newborn infant. Most of these authors are individuals whose major investigative efforts on this subject have taken place during the past 25 years. Almost all were supported, in part or totally, during their training period and subsequently, by funds obtained from the National Institutes of Health or from private agencies such as March of Dimes. It is clear that the major advances of this period would not have been possible without these funding mechanisms and the freedom given to the investigators to pursue programs of their own choosing. Thus, the advances present in this text are also a testimony to the trustees of agencies and the legislators and other federal officials who provided unencumbered research funds from the 1960s to the present day.

We were Fellows at the Thorndike Memorial Laboratory (Harvard Medical Unit, Boston City Hospital) in the early 1960s. Although subsequently we worked in separate areas of investigation on the two coasts, one of us as an internist and the other as a pediatrician, we maintained close contact, and, because of a mutual interest in infections of the fetus and newborn infant and their long-term effects, we joined our efforts to develop this text. For this edition, we are proud to have added, as Associate Editors, Carol J. Baker and Christopher B. Wilson. Carol trained in infectious diseases in Boston with J.O.K. and Maxwell Finland, and Chris trained in immunology and infectious diseases in Palo Alto with J.S.R. Carol has become a world-recognized expert in all aspects of group B streptococcal infections and is the Texas Children's Hospital Foundation Chair in Pediatric Infectious Diseases in Houston. Chris has become a prominent developmental immunologist and is now Chair of the Department of Immunology at the University of Washington School of Medicine. We look to Carol and Chris to help us maintain the quality and value of this text for many editions to come.

We are indebted to our teachers and associates and especially to the one individual who had a dominant influence in our training, Dr. Maxwell Finland. We deeply appreciate the example he set, his wise counsel, and his interest in and support of our investigative programs. We also wish to express our appreciation to Todd Hummel, Jennifer Ehlers, Lee Ann Draud, and the staff of Elsevier, Inc., for guiding this project to a successful conclusion; to Ms. Nancy Ahonen and Robin Schroeder for secretarial assistance; and to Ms. Trisha Mitchell for her editorial assistance.

Jack S. Remington
Jerome O. Klein

We are pleased to have joined Jack and Jerry in editing this book, which since its inception has been a unique resource for physicians caring for the mother, fetus, and newborn infant. We are also grateful for the investigators working in the field, who have improved life for mother and infant, and for the chapter authors, who bring their comprehensive understanding of their topics to enlighten readers.

Carol J. Baker
Christopher B. Wilson

CONTENTS

Section I

GENERAL INFORMATION

Chapter 1

CURRENT CONCEPTS OF INFECTIONS OF THE FETUS AND NEWBORN INFANT

Jerome O. Klein • Carol J. Baker • Jack S. Remington • Christopher B. Wilson

OVERVIEW

Current concepts of pathogenesis, microbiology, diagnosis, and management of infections of the fetus and newborn infant are briefly reviewed in this chapter. Also in this first section of the book are chapters providing a global perspective on fetal and neonatal infections and chapters addressing obstetric factors, immunity, host defenses and the role of human breast milk in fetal and neonatal infections. Chapters containing detailed information about specific bacterial, viral, protozoan, helminth, and fungal infections follow. This edition concludes with chapters addressing nosocomial infections and the diagnosis and therapy of infections in the fetus and neonate.

A number of changes have occurred in epidemiology, diagnosis, prevention, and management of infectious diseases of the fetus and newborn infant since publication of the last edition of this book. Some of these changes are noted in Table 1-1 and are discussed in this and the relevant chapters.

Substantial progress has taken place to reduce the burden of infectious diseases in the fetus and newborn infant. The incidence of early-onset group B streptococcal disease has been reduced by aggressive use of intrapartum chemoprophylaxis and, in particular, by the culture-based chemoprophylaxis strategy now recommended for universal use in the United States; vertical transmission of human immunodeficiency virus (HIV) has been reduced by identification of the infected mother with subsequent treatment, including the use of brief regimens that are practical for use in countries with high prevalence but limited resources; there has been a commitment of resources by government agencies and philanthropies, such as the Bill and Melinda Gates Foundation, to combat global infectious diseases in mothers and children; use of polymerase chain reaction (PCR) techniques in etiologic diagnosis has expanded, permitting more rapid and specific identification of microbial pathogens; and in the United States, national legislation on postpartum length of hospital stay has been enacted to prevent insurers from restricting insurance coverage for hospitalization to fewer than 48 hours after vaginal deliveries or 96 hours after cesarean deliveries.

Setbacks in initiatives to reduce the global burden of infectious disease in the fetus and newborn infant include the continuing increase in the prevalence of HIV infection in many developing countries, particularly among women; the lack of finances to provide effective treatment for these women and their newborn infants; and in the United States, the increase in antimicrobial resistance among nosocomial pathogens, as well as in incidence of invasive fungal infections among infants of extremely low birth weight.

Use of the Internet has grown further, allowing access to information hitherto unavailable to physicians or parents. The physician may obtain current information about diseases and management and various guidelines for diagnosis and treatment. The interested parent who has access to the Internet can explore a variety of Internet sites that present a vast array of information and, unfortunately, misinformation. As an example of the latter, a case of neonatal tetanus was associated with the use of cosmetic facial clay (Indian Healing Clay) as a dressing on an umbilical cord stump. The product had been publicized as a healing salve by midwives on an Internet site on "cordcare."[1] Because much of the information on the Internet is from commercial sources and parties with varying interests and expertise, the physician should assist the interested parent and patient in finding Internet sites of value. A selected list of Internet sites pertinent to infectious diseases of the fetus and newborn infant is provided in Table 1-2.

Vital statistics relevant to infectious disease risk in neonates in the United States for 2001 are listed in Table 1-3.[2] Of importance are the disparities in birth weight, prenatal care, and neonatal mortality among different racial and ethnic groups.

The number of infectious diseases in fetuses and newborn infants must be extrapolated from selected studies (see chapters on diseases). Approximately 1% of newborn infants excrete cytomegalovirus (CMV), greater than 4% of infants are born to mothers infected with *Chlamydia trachomatis*, and bacterial sepsis develops in 1 to 4 infants per 1000 live births. Since the institution of intrapartum chemoprophylaxis in the United States, the number of infants with early-onset group B streptococcal disease has declined, with reduction in incidence from approximately 1.5 cases to 0.4 case per 1000 live births, and is expected to decline further with the universal adoption of the culture-based strategy.[3] In the United States, the use of maternal highly active antiretroviral treatment (HAART) and peripartum chemoprophylaxis has led to a reduction in the rate of mother-to-child transmission of HIV from approximately 25% of infants born to mothers who received no treatment to 2%; less complex but practical regimens of intrapartum prophylaxis have helped to reduce the rate of transmission in the developing world.[4] Among sexually transmitted diseases, the rate of congenital syphilis declined substantially in the United States to 13.4 per 100,000 live births in 2000, and although rates remain higher in the South, only two states have rates greater than 40 per 100,000 live births.[5] Immunization has virtually eliminated congenital rubella syndrome in newborn infants of mothers who were themselves born in the United States, but cases continue to occur in infants of foreign-born mothers; 24 of 26 infants with congenital rubella born between 1997 and 1999 were born to foreign-born mothers, and 21 of these were born to Hispanic mothers.[6]

Table 1–1 Recent Changes in Epidemiology and Management of Infectious Diseases of the Fetus and Newborn Infant
Epidemiology
Increased viability of very low birth weight infants at risk for invasive infectious diseases
Increased number of multiple births (offten of very low birth weight) due to successful techniques for management of infertility
Global perspective of vertically transmitted infectious diseases
Early discharge from the nursery mandated by insurance programs reversed by legislation to ensure adequate observation for infants at risk for sepsis
Diagnosis
Polymerase chain reaction assay for diagnosis of infection in mother, fetus, and neonate
Decreased use of fetal blood sampling and chorionic villus sampling for diagnosis of infectious diseases
Prevention
Intrapartum antibiotic prophylaxis to prevent early-onset group B streptococcal infection widely implemented
Antiretroviral therapy in pregnancy to prevent transmission of human immunodeficiency virus (HIV) to fetus
Treatment
Antiretroviral therapy in mother to treat HIV infection in fetus
Antitoxoplasmosis therapy in mother to treat infection in fetus
Spread within nurseries of multiple antibiotic-resistant bacterial pathogens
Increased use of vancomycin for β-lactam-resistant gram-positive infections
Increased use of acyclovir for infants with suspected herpes simplex infection

Infection acquired in utero can result in resorption of the embryo, abortion, stillbirth, malformation, intrauterine growth retardation, prematurity, and the untoward sequelae of chronic postnatal infection. Infection acquired during the birth process or soon after birth may result in severe systemic disease that leads to death or persistent postnatal infection. Both in utero infection and infection acquired during the birth process may lead to late-onset disease. The infection may not be apparent at birth but may manifest with signs of disease weeks, months, or years later, as exemplified by the chorioretinitis of *Toxoplasma gondii* infection, the hearing loss of rubella, and the immunologic defects that result from HIV infection. The immediate as well as the long-term effects of these infections constitute a major problem throughout the world.

INFECTIONS OF THE FETUS

Pathogenesis

Pregnant women not only are exposed to the infections prevalent in the community but also are likely to reside with young children or to associate with groups of young children,

Table 1–2 Selected Internet Sites of Value for Physicians Interested in Infectious Diseases of the Fetus and Newborn Infant

Agency for Health Care Policy and Research	http://www.ahcpr.gov
American Academy of Pediatrics	http://www.aap.org
American College of Obstetricians and Gynecologists	http://www.acog.org
Centers for Disease Control and Prevention	http://www.cdc.gov
Food and Drug Administration	http://www.fda.gov
Immunization Action Coalition	http://www.immunize.org
Information on AIDS Trials	http://www.actis.org
Morbidity and Mortality Weekly Report	http://www.cdc.gov/epo/mmwr/mmwr.html
National Center for Health Statistics	http://www.cdc.gov/nchs
Pediatric Infectious Diseases and selected bibliography[a]	http://www.pedid.uthscsa.edu

[a]Described in Jenson HB, Baltimore RS. A World Wide Web selected bibliography for pediatric infectious diseases. Clin Infect Dis 28:395–398, 1999.

Table 1–3 Vital Statistics Relevant to Newborn Health in the United States in 2002

		Racial/Ethnic Origin of Mother		
Feature	***All Births***	***Non-Hispanic White***	***Non-Hispanic Black***	***Hispanic***
Live births[a]	4.022	2.298	0.578	0.877
Birth weight				
<2500 g	7.9%	7.0%	13.5%	6.7%
<1500 g	1.4%	1.2%	3.1%	1.2%
First-trimester Prenatal care	84.1%	89.0%	76.0%	77.4%
Multiple births[b]	33.0	37.3	35.7	21.5
Neonatal (<28 days) Mortality rate[b]				
All birth weights	4.7	3.9	9.5	3.8[c]
<2500 g	48.6	—	—	—
<1500 g	220.3	—	—	—

[a]m = 10^6.
[b]per 1000 live births.
[c]Data for 2000-2002 average annual rate/1000 live births.
From: Martin JA, Kochanek KD, Strobino DM, et al. Annual Summary of Vital Statistics—2003. Pediatrics 115:619–634, 2005.

which represents a significant additional factor in exposure to infectious disease. The vast majority of infections in the pregnant woman affect the upper respiratory and gastrointestinal tracts and either resolve spontaneously without therapy or are readily treated with antimicrobial agents. Such infections usually remain localized and have no effect on the developing fetus. The infecting organism may invade the bloodstream, however, and subsequently infect the placenta and fetus.

Successful pregnancy is a unique example of immunologic tolerance—the mother must be tolerant of her allogeneic fetus (and vice versa). The basis for maternal-fetal tolerance is incompletely understood, but is known to reflect both local modifications of host defenses at the maternal-fetal interface and more global changes in immunologic competence in the mother. Specific factors acting locally in the placenta include indoleamine 2,3-dioxygenase, which suppresses cell-mediated immunity by catabolizing the essential amino acid tryptophan, and regulatory proteins that prevent complement activation.[7,8] As pregnancy progresses, a general shift from T_H1-type cell-mediated immunity to T_H2-type responses also occurs in the mother, although this description probably constitutes an overly simplistic view of more complex immunoregulatory changes.[9,10] Nonetheless, because T_H1-type cell-mediated immunity is important in host defense against intracellular pathogens, the T_H2 bias established during normal gestation may compromise successful immunity against organisms such as *T. gondii*. In addition, it has been proposed that a strong curative T_H1 response against an organism may overcome the protective T_H2 cytokines at the maternal-fetal interface, resulting in fetal loss.

Transplacental spread after maternal infection and invasion of the bloodstream is the usual route by which the fetus becomes infected. Uncommonly, the fetus may be infected by extension of infection in adjacent tissues and organs, including the peritoneum and the genitalia, during parturition, or as a result of invasive methods for the diagnosis and therapy of fetal disorders, such as the use of monitors, sampling of fetal blood, and intrauterine transfusion.

The microorganisms of concern are listed in Table 1-4 and include those identified in the acronym TORCH: ***To****xoplasma gondii*, **r**ubella virus, **C**MV, and **h**erpes simplex virus (HSV) (as a point of historical interest, the O in TORCH originally stood for "**o**ther infections/pathogens," reflecting an early appreciation of this possibility). A new acronym is needed to include the other well-described causes of in utero infection: syphilis, enteroviruses, varicella-zoster virus (VZV), HIV, Lyme disease (*Borrelia burgdorferi*), and parvovirus. In certain geographic areas, *Plasmodium* and *Trypanosoma cruzi* are responsible for in utero infections. TORCHES CLAP (see Table 1-4) is an inclusive acronym. THE BAC PORCH is easily remembered but relies on an idealized spelling for the word *back*. CHAST LOVER includes a truncated spelling of the word *chaste*.[11] CHEAP TORCHES has been suggested to include congenital and perinatal infections; it includes an H for hepatitis B and C and an E for everything else that is sexually transmitted (gonorrhea and *Chlamydia*, *Ureaplasma*, and papillomavirus infections) but ignores Lyme disease.[12] Because no clear successor to TORCH has been devised, other acronyms are still welcome. New pathogens are being discovered, however, so it is unlikely that any acronym will be "permanent."

Table 1–4 Suggested Acronym for the Microorganisms Responsible for Infection of the Fetus

To	*Toxoplasma gondii*
R	Rubella virus
C	Cytomegalovirus
H	Herpes simplex virus
E	Enteroviruses
S	Syphilis (*Treponema pallidum*)
C	Chickenpox (varicella-zoster virus)
L	Lyme disease (*Borrelia burgdorferi*)
A	AIDS (human immunodeficiency virus)
P	Parvovirus B19

AIDS, acquired immunodeficiency syndrome.

Case reports indicate that other organisms are unusual causes of infections transmitted by the pregnant woman to her fetus, including *Brucella melitensis*,[13] *Coxiella burnetii* (Q fever),[14] *Babesia microti* (babesiosis),[15] human T lymphotropic virus types I and II (although the main route of transmission of these viruses is through breast-feeding),[16,17] hepatitis G and TT viruses,[18,19] human herpesvirus 6,[20,21] and dengue.[22]

Before rupture of fetal membranes, organisms in the genital tract may invade the amniotic fluid and produce infection of the fetus. These organisms can invade the fetus through microscopic defects in the membranes, particularly in devitalized areas overlying the cervical os. It also is possible that microorganisms gain access to the fetus from descending infection through the fallopian tubes in women with salpingitis or peritonitis, or from direct extension of an infection in the uterus, such as myometrial abscess or cellulitis. Available evidence, however, does not suggest that transtubal or transmyometrial passage of microbial agents is a significant route of fetal infection.

Invasive techniques that have been developed for in utero diagnosis and therapy are potential sources of infection for the fetus. Abscesses have been observed in infants who had scalp punctures for fetal blood sampling or electrocardiographic electrodes clipped on their scalps. Osteomyelitis of the skull and streptococcal sepsis have followed local infection at the site of a fetal monitoring electrode[23]; HSV infections at the fetal scalp electrode site also have been reported. Intrauterine transfusion for severe erythroblastosis diagnosed in utero also has resulted in infection of the fetus: In one case, CMV infection reportedly resulted from intrauterine transfusion[24]; in another instance, contamination of donor blood with a gram-negative coccobacillus, *Acinetobacter calcoaceticus*, led to an acute placentitis and subsequent fetal bacteremia.[25]

Fetal infection in the absence of rupture of internal membranes usually occurs by the transplacental route after invasion of the maternal bloodstream. Microorganisms in the blood may be carried within white blood cells or attached to erythrocytes, or they may be present independent of cellular elements.

Microbial Invasion of the Maternal Bloodstream

The potential consequences of invasion of the mother's bloodstream by microorganisms or their products (Fig. 1-1) include (1) placental infection without infection of the fetus, (2) fetal infection without infection of the placenta, (3) absence of both fetal and placental infection, and (4) infection of both placenta and fetus.

PLACENTAL INFECTION WITHOUT INFECTION OF THE FETUS

After reaching the intervillous spaces on the maternal side of the placenta, organisms can remain localized in the placenta without affecting the fetus. Evidence that placentitis does occur independently of fetal involvement has been demonstrated after maternal tuberculosis, syphilis, malaria, coccidioidomycosis, and CMV, rubella virus, and mumps vaccine virus infection. The reasons for the lack of spread to the fetus after the placental infection has been established are unknown. Defenses of the fetus that may operate after infection of the placenta include the villous trophoblast, placental macrophages, and locally produced immune factors such as antibodies and cytokines.

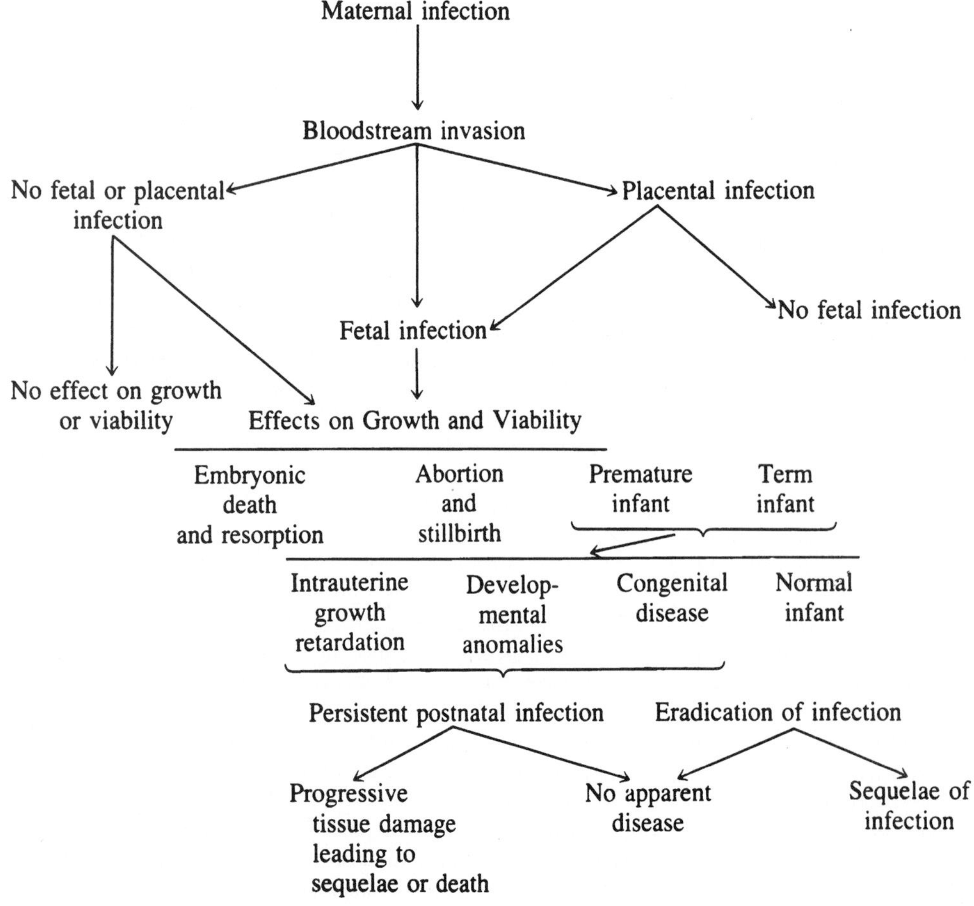

Figure 1–1 Pathogenesis of hematogenous transplacental infections.

FETAL INFECTION WITHOUT INFECTION OF THE PLACENTA

Microorganisms may traverse the chorionic villi directly through pinocytosis, placental leaks, or diapedesis of infected maternal leukocytes and erythrocytes. Careful histologic studies, however, usually reveal areas of placentitis sufficient to serve as a source of fetal infection.

ABSENCE OF FETAL AND PLACENTAL INFECTION

Invasion of the bloodstream by microorganisms is not uncommon in pregnant women, yet in most cases neither fetal nor placental infection results. Bacteremia may accompany abscesses or cellulitis, bacterial pneumonia, pyelonephritis, appendicitis, endocarditis, or other pyogenic infections; nevertheless, placental or fetal infection as a consequence of such bacteremias is rare. In most cases, the fetus probably is protected through efficient clearance of microbes by the maternal reticuloendothelial system and circulating leukocytes.

A number of bacterial diseases of the pregnant woman, including typhoid fever, pneumonia, sepsis caused by gram-negative bacteria, and urinary tract infections, may affect the developing fetus without direct microbial invasion of the placenta or fetal tissues. Similarly, protozoal infection in the mother, such as malaria, and systemic viral infections, including varicella, variola, and measles, also may affect the fetus indirectly. Fever, anoxia, circulating toxins, or metabolic derangements in the mother during these infections can affect the pregnancy—abortion, stillbirth, and premature delivery are among the possible results.

The effect of microbial toxins on the developing fetus is uncertain. The fetus may be adversely affected by toxic shock in the mother due to *Staphylococcus aureus* or *Streptococcus pyogenes* infection. Botulism in pregnant women has not been associated with disease in the infant.[26,27] A unique case of Guillain-Barré syndrome in mother and child shows that infection-induced antibody-mediated autoimmune disease in the mother may be transmitted to her infant. In this case, the disease was diagnosed in the mother during week 29 of pregnancy. A healthy infant was delivered per vagina at 38 weeks of gestation, while the mother was quadriplegic and on respiratory support. On day 12 of life, however, flaccid paralysis of all limbs, with absence of deep tendon reflexes, developed in the infant, and cerebrospinal fluid examination revealed increased protein concentration without white blood cells.[28] The delay in onset of paralysis in the infant appeared to reflect the fact that the transplacentally transferred blocking antibodies were specifically directed at epitopes of the mature but not the fetal neuromuscular junction. The infant improved following administration of intravenous immune globulin (IGIV).[29]

The association of maternal urinary tract infection with premature delivery and low birth weight is a well-studied example of a maternal infection that adversely affects growth and development of the fetus, even though there is no evidence of fetal or placental infection. Asymptomatic bacteriuria in pregnancy has been linked to an excess in the number of low-birth-weight infants.[30,31] In one early study, when the bacteriuria was eliminated by appropriate antibiotic therapy, the incidence of pyelonephritis was lower in the women who received treatment than in the women who did not, and the rate of premature and low-birth-weight infants was the same among the women in the treatment group as among nonbacteriuric women.[32] A recent meta-analysis concluded that antibiotic treatment is effective in reducing the risk of pyelonephritis in pregnancy and also appears to reduce risk for preterm delivery, although the evidence supporting this latter conclusion is not as strong.[33] The basis for the premature delivery and low birth weight of infants of bacteriuric women remains obscure.[34]

INFECTION OF PLACENTA AND FETUS

Microbes may be disseminated from the infected placenta to the fetal bloodstream through infected emboli of necrotic chorionic tissues or through direct extension of placental infection to the fetal membranes, with secondary amniotic fluid infection and aspiration by the fetus.

Infection of the Embryo and Fetus

Hematogenous transplacental spread may result in death and resorption of the embryo, abortion and stillbirth of the fetus, and live birth of a premature or term infant who may or may not be healthy. The effects of fetal infection may appear in the live-born infant as low birth weight (resulting from intrauterine growth retardation), developmental anomalies, congenital disease, or none of these. Infection acquired in utero may persist after birth and cause significant abnormalities in growth and development that may be apparent soon after birth or may not be recognized for months or years. The variability of the effects of fetal infection is emphasized by reports of biovular twin pregnancies that produced one severely damaged infant and another with minimal or no detectable abnormalities.[35-40]

Embryonic Death and Resorption. A variety of organisms may infect the pregnant woman in the first few weeks of gestation and produce death and resorption of the embryo. Because loss of the embryo usually occurs before the woman realizes she is pregnant or seeks medical attention, it is difficult to estimate the incidence of this outcome for any single infectious agent. The incidence of early pregnancy loss after implantation from all causes has been estimated to be 31%. The proportion of cases of loss due to infection is unknown.[41]

Abortion and Stillbirth. The earliest recognizable effects of fetal infection are seen after the sixth to eighth week of pregnancy and include abortion and stillbirth. Intrauterine death may result from overwhelming fetal infection, or the microorganisms may interfere with organogenesis to such an extent that the development of functions necessary for continued viability is interrupted. The precise mechanisms responsible for early spontaneous termination of pregnancy are unknown; in many cases, it is difficult to ascertain whether fetal death caused or resulted from the expulsion of the fetus.

A number of modifying factors probably determine the ultimate outcome of intrauterine infection; these include virulence or tissue tropism of the microorganisms, stage of pregnancy, associated placental damage, and severity of the maternal illness. Primary infection is likely to have a more important effect on the fetus than recurrent infection.[42] For example, recurrence of CMV infection is less severe than primary infection. Available studies do not distinguish between the direct effect of the microorganisms on the developing fetus and the possibility of an indirect effect attributable to illness or poor health of the mother.

Table 1–5 Effects of Transplacental Fetal Infection on the Fetus and Newborn Infant

Organisms or Disease	Prematurity	Intrauterine Growth Retardation/Low Birth Weight	Developmental Anomalies	Congenital Disease	Persistent Postnatal Infection
Viruses					
Rubella virus	–	+	+	+	+
Cytomegalovirus	+	+	+	+	+
Herpes simplex	+	–	–	+	+
Varicella-zoster virus	–	(+)	+	+	+
Mumps virus	–	–	–	(+)	–
Rubeola virus	+	–	–	+	–
Vaccinia virus	–	–	–	+	–
Smallpox virus	+	–	–	+	–
Coxsackieviruses B	–	–	(+)	+	–
Echoviruses	–	–	–	–	–
Polioviruses	–	–	–	+	–
Influenza virus	–	–	–	–	–
Hepatitis B virus	+	–	–	+	+
Human immunodeficiency virus	(+)	(+)	(+)	+	+
Lymphocytic choriomeningitis virus	–	–	–	+	–
Parvovirus	–	–	–	+	–
Bacteria					
Treponema pallidum	+	–	–	+	+
Mycobacterium tuberculosis	+	–	–	+	+
Listeria monocytogenes	+	–	–	+	–
Campylobacter fetus	+	–	–	+	–
Salmonella typhosa	+	–	–	+	–
Borrelia burgdorferi	–	–	–	+	–
Protozoa					
Toxoplasma gondii	+	+	–	+	+
Plasmodium	(+)	+	–	+	+
Trypanosoma cruzi	+	+	–	+	–

+, evidence for effect; –, no evidence for effect; (+), association of effect with infection has been suggested and is under consideration.

Prematurity. *Prematurity* is defined as the birth of a viable infant before week 37 of gestation. Premature birth may result from almost any agent capable of establishing fetal infection during the last trimester of pregnancy. Those microorganisms commonly responsible for stillbirth and abortion also are implicated as significant causes of prematurity (Table 1-5).

Previous studies have demonstrated that women in premature labor in whom results of amniotic fluid cultures for bacteria are positive have elevated levels of multiple proinflammatory cytokines in their amniotic fluid.[43-48] In many patients with elevated levels of interleukin-6 (IL-6), results of amniotic fluid culture were negative. Premature births are invariably observed, however, in women in premature labor in whom results of amniotic fluid culture are positive and who also have elevated amniotic fluid levels of IL-6. To further clarify the role of measurement of levels of IL-6 in amniotic fluid, Hitti and colleagues[44] amplified bacterial 16S recombinant RNA (rRNA) encoding DNA by PCR to detect amniotic fluid infection in women in premature labor whose membranes were intact. PCR assay detected bacterial infection in significantly more patients in whom results of amniotic fluid cultures were negative but IL-6 levels were elevated. These data suggest that as many as 33% of women in premature labor in whom results of amniotic fluid culture are negative but IL-6 amniotic fluid levels are elevated have amniotic fluid infection. The investigators concluded that the association between amniotic fluid infection and premature labor may be underestimated on the basis of amniotic fluid cultures. They further suggested that use of the broad-spectrum bacterial 16S rDNA PCR assay may be useful for diagnosis of infected amniotic fluid. In any case, elevated levels of amniotic fluid IL-6 are clearly associated with an increased risk of preterm delivery, even in cases in which cultures and PCR assay have failed to detect infection.[49] Although this finding is likely to reflect infection undetected by either technique, it remains possible that factors other than infection contribute to preterm labor and elevated amniotic fluid IL-6.

Intrauterine Growth Retardation and Low Birth Weight. Infection of the fetus may result in birth of an infant who is small for gestational age (SGA). Although low birth weight and "small for date" infants are associated with many maternal infections, evidence for a causal relationship is only sufficient for congenital rubella, VZV infection, toxoplasmosis, and CMV infection.

The organs of infants dying with congenital rubella syndrome or CMV infection contain a decreased number of morphologically normal cells.[50,51] By contrast, in small-for-dates infants whose growth deficit is due to noninfectious causes such as maternal toxemia or placental abnormalities, the parenchymal cells are normal in number but have a reduced amount of cytoplasm, presumably because of fetal malnutrition.[52,53]

Developmental Anomalies and Teratogenesis. CMV, rubella virus, and VZV cause developmental anomalies in the human fetus. Coxsackieviruses B3 and B4 have been associated with congenital heart disease. The pathogenetic mechanisms responsible for the fetal abnormalities produced by most infectious agents remain obscure. Histologic studies of abortuses and congenitally infected infants have suggested, however, that the ultimate mode of action of some viruses rests in their ability to cause cell death, alterations in cell growth, or chromosomal damage. Lesions resulting from the inflammatory processes caused by the microorganisms must be distinguished from defects that arise from a direct effect of the organisms on the growth of cells and tissues in the developing embryo or fetus. Inflammation and tissue destruction, rather than teratogenic activity, appear to be responsible for the widespread structural abnormalities characteristic of congenital syphilis, transplacental HSV and VZV infection, and toxoplasmosis. Infants with congenital toxoplasmosis may have microcephaly, hydrocephalus, or microphthalmia, but these manifestations usually result from an intense necrotizing process containing numerous organisms and are more appropriately defined as lesions of congenital infection rather than as effects of teratogenic activity of the organism.

Some mycoplasmas[54] and viruses[55,56] produce chromosomal damage in circulating human lymphocytes or in human cells in tissue culture. The relationship of these changes in structure to the production of congenital abnormalities in the fetus is unknown.

Congenital Disease. Clinical evidence of intrauterine infections may be present at birth or may manifest soon thereafter or years later. The signs result from tissue damage or secondary physiologic changes caused by the invading organisms. The clinical manifestations in the newborn infant of infection acquired in utero or at delivery are given in Table 1-6. In infants with congenital rubella, toxoplasmosis, syphilis, or congenital CMV, HSV, or enterovirus infection, signs of widely disseminated infection may be evident during the neonatal period. Such signs include jaundice, hepatosplenomegaly, and pneumonia, each of which reflects lesions caused by microbial invasion and proliferation rather than by defects in organogenesis. These signs of congenital infection are not detected until the neonatal period, although the pathologic processes responsible for their occurrence have been progressing for weeks or months before delivery. In some infants, the constellation of signs is sufficient to suggest the likely congenital infection (Table 1-7). In other infants, the signs are transient and self-limited and resolve as neonatal defense mechanisms control the spread of the microbial agent and tissue destruction. If damage is severe and widespread at the time of delivery, the infant is likely to die.

It is frequently difficult to determine whether the infection in the newborn infant was acquired in utero, during the delivery process, or post partum. If the onset of clinical signs after birth occurs within the minimal incubation period for the disease (e.g., 3 days for enteroviruses, 10 days for VZV and rubella viruses), it is likely that the infection was acquired before delivery. The interval between exposure to malaria in the mother and congenital malaria in the infant can be prolonged; one case of congenital malaria resulting from *Plasmodium malariae* occurred in the United States in an infant born 25 years after the infant's mother had emigrated from China.[57] Children infected with HIV perinatally can be diagnosed by 6 months of age using the DNA (or RNA) PCR method, which has largely replaced other approaches for viral detection.[58] A variable fraction (less than half) of perinatally infected children are infected with HIV in utero, depending on the setting and maternal treatment.[59] Virus-negative infants who later become virus-positive may have been infected at or shortly before delivery.

Healthy Infants. A majority of newborn infants infected in utero by rubella virus, *T. gondii*, CMV, HIV, or *Treponema pallidum* have no signs of congenital disease. Fetal infection by a limited inoculum of organisms or with a strain of low virulence or minimal potential for pathology may be responsible for this low incidence of clinical disease in infected infants. Alternatively, gestational age may be the most important factor in determining the ultimate consequences of prenatal infection. When congenital rubella and toxoplasmosis are acquired during the last trimester of pregnancy, the incidence of clinical disease in the infected infants is lower than when microbial invasion occurs during the first or second trimester. Congenital syphilis results from exposure during the second or third but not the first trimester.

Absence of clinically apparent disease in the newborn may be misleading. Careful observation of infected but healthy-appearing children over the course of months or years often reveals defects that were not apparent at birth. The failure to recognize such defects early in life may be due to the inability to test young infants for the functions involved. Hearing defects identified years after birth may be the only manifestation of congenital rubella. Significant sensorineural deafness and other central nervous system deficiencies have afflicted children with congenital CMV infection who were considered to be normal during the neonatal period. Delayed recognition of other manifestations of in utero infection, including failure to thrive, visual defects, and minimal to severe brain dysfunction (including motor, learning, language, and behavioral disorders), can follow toxoplasmosis, rubella, and CMV infections. Infants infected with HIV usually are asymptomatic at birth and for the first few months of life. The median age for onset of signs of congenital HIV infection is approximately 3 years, but many children remain asymptomatic for more than 5 years. Failure to thrive, persistent diarrhea, recurrent suppurative infections, and diseases associated with opportunistic infections that occur weeks to months or years after birth are signs of perinatal infection related to HIV. Of particular concern is the report by Wilson and colleagues[49] that found stigmata of congenital *T. gondii* infection, including chorioretinitis and blindness, in almost all 24 children at follow-up evaluations; the children had serologic evidence of infection but were without apparent signs of disease at birth and did not receive treatment or received inadequate treatment.

Because abnormalities may become obvious only as the child develops and reaches or fails to reach appropriate physiologic or developmental milestones, it is of utmost importance to give careful and thorough follow-up examin-

Table 1–6 Clinical Manifestations of Neonatal Infection Acquired in Utero or at Delivery

	Microorganism						
Clinical Sign	**Rubella Virus**	**Cytomegalovirus**	***Toxoplasma gondii***	**Herpes Simplex Virus**	***Treponema pallidum***	**Enteroviruses**	**Group B *Streptococcus* or *Escherichia coli***
Hepatosplenomegaly	+	+	+	+	+	+	–
Jaundice	+	+	+	+	+	+	+
Adenopathy	+	–	–	–	+	+	–
Pneumonitis	+	+	+	+	+	+	+
Lesions of Skin or Mucous Membranes							
Petechiae or purpura	+	+	+	+	+	+	+
Vesicles	–	–	–	+ +	–	–	–
Maculopapular exanthems	–	–	+	+	+ +	+	–
Lesions of Nervous System							
Meningoencephalitis	+	+	+	+	+	+	+
Microcephaly	–	+ +	+	+	–	–	–
Hydrocephalus	+	+	+ +	+	–	–	–
Intracranial calcifications	–	+ +	+ +	–	–	–	–
Paralysis	–	–	–	–	–	+ +	–
Hearing deficits	+	+	–	–	–	–	–
Lesions of Heart							
Myocarditis	+	–	+	+	–	+ +	–
Congenital defects	+ +	–	–	–	–	–	–
Bone lesions	+ +	–	+	–	+ +	–	–
Eye Lesions							
Glaucoma	+ +	–	–	–	+	–	–
Chorioretinitis or retinopathy	+ +	+	+ +	+	+	–	–
Cataracts	+ +	–	+	+	–	–	–
Optic atrophy	–	+	+	–	–	–	–
Microphthalmia	+	–	+	–	–	–	–
Uveitis	–	–	+	–	+	–	–
Conjunctivitis or keratoconjunctivitis	–	–	–	+ +	–	+	–

–, either not present or rare in infected infants; +, occurs in infants with infection; + +, has special diagnostic significance for this infection.

Table 1–7 Syndromes in the Neonate Caused by Congenital Infections

Microorganism	Signs
Toxoplasma gondii	Hydrocephalus, diffuse intracranial calcification, chorioretinitis
Rubella virus	Cardiac defects, sensorineural hearing loss, cataracts; microcephaly, "blueberry muffin" skin lesions, hepatomegaly, interstitial pneumonitis, myocarditis, disturbances in bone growth, intrauterine growth retardation
Cytomegalovirus	Microcephaly, periventricular calcifications, jaundice, petechiae or purpura, hepatosplenomegaly, intrauterine growth retardation
Herpes simplex virus	Skin vesicles or scarring, eye scarring, microcephaly or hydranencephaly; vesicular skin rash, keratoconjunctivitis, meningoencephalitis; sepsis with hepatic failure
Treponema pallidum	Bullous, macular, or eczematous skin lesions involving the palms and soles; rhinorrhea; dactylitis and other signs of osteochondritis and periostitis; hepatosplenomegaly; lymphadenopathy
Varicella-zoster virus	Limb hypoplasia, cicatricial skin lesions, ocular abnormalities, cortical atrophy
Parvovirus B19	Nonimmune hydrops fetalis
Human immunodeficiency virus	Severe thrush, failure to thrive, recurrent bacterial infections, calcification of the basal ganglia

ations to infants born to women known to be infected during pregnancy.

Persistent Postnatal Infection. Microbial agents may continue to survive and replicate in tissues for months or years after in utero infection. Rubella virus and CMV have been isolated from various body fluids and tissues over long periods of time from children with abnormalities at birth, as well as from those who appeared healthy. In some congenital infections, including rubella, toxoplasmosis, syphilis, tuberculosis, malaria, and CMV, HSV, and HIV infection, progressive tissue destruction has been demonstrated. Recurrent eye and skin infections can occur as a result of HSV infection acquired in utero or at the time of delivery. A progressive encephalitis has occurred with congenital rubella infection.[60,61] The clinical manifestations of congenital infection in these children had been stable for many years when deterioration of motor and mental functions occurred at ages 11 to 14 years. Rubella virus was isolated from the brain biopsy specimen of a 12-year-old child. Fetal parvovirus B19 infection can persist for months after birth with persistent anemia due to suppressed hematopoiesis.[62]

The mechanisms responsible for maintaining or terminating chronic fetal and postnatal infections are only partially understood. Humoral immune responses, as determined by measurement of either fetal immunoglobulin M (IgM) antibodies or specific IgG antibodies that develop in the neonatal period, appear to be intact in almost all infants (see Chapter 4). The importance of cell-mediated immunity, cytokines, complement, and other host defense mechanisms remains to be defined. The evidence is insufficient at present to support a causal relation between deficiencies in any one of these factors and persistent postnatal infection. It is noteworthy that all of the diseases associated with persistent postnatal infection—with the exception of rubella but including syphilis, tuberculosis, malaria, toxoplasmosis, hepatitis, and CMV, HSV, VZV, and HIV infections—also can produce prolonged and, in certain instances, lifelong infection when acquired later in life.

Efficiency of Transmission of Microorganisms from Mother to Fetus

The efficiency of transmission from the infected, immunocompetent mother to the fetus varies among microbial agents and also can vary with the trimester of pregnancy. In utero transmission of rubella virus and *T. gondii* occurs primarily as a result of primary infection, whereas in utero transmission of CMV, HIV, and *T. pallidum* can occur in consecutive pregnancies. The risk of congenital rubella infection in fetuses of mothers with symptomatic rubella was high in the first trimester (90% before 11 weeks of gestation), declined to a low of 25% at 23 to 26 weeks, and then rose to 67% after 31 weeks. Infection in the first 11 weeks of gestation was uniformly teratogenic, whereas no birth defects occurred in infants infected after 16 weeks of gestation.[63] By contrast, the frequency of stillbirth and clinical and subclinical congenital *T. gondii* infection among offspring of women who acquired *T. gondii* infection during pregnancy was least in the first trimester (14%), increased in the second trimester (29%), and was highest in the third trimester (59%).[64]

Congenital CMV infection results from primary and recurrent infections. On the basis of studies in Birmingham, Alabama, and other centers, Whitley and Stagno and their colleagues[65,66] estimate that 1% to 4% of women have primary infection during pregnancy, that 40% of these women transmit the infection to the fetus, and that 5% to 15% of the infants have signs of CMV disease. Congenital infection due to recurrent CMV infection occurs in 0.5% to 1% of livebirths, but less than 1% of the infected infants have clinically apparent congenital disease.

The transmission rate of HIV infection from the infected mother who received no treatment to the fetus is estimated to be about 25%, but the data are insufficient to identify efficiency of transmission by trimester. Risk of transmission does not appear to be greater in mothers who acquire primary infection during pregnancy than mothers who were infected before they became pregnant.[67]

Diagnosis of Infection in the Pregnant Woman

Clinical Diagnosis

Symptomatic or Clinical Infection. In many instances, the diagnosis of infection in the pregnant woman and congenital infection in the newborn infant can be suspected on the basis of clinical signs or symptoms. Careful examination can be sufficient to suggest a specific diagnosis, particularly when typical clinical findings are accompanied by a well-documented history of exposure (see Tables 1-6 and 1-7).

Asymptomatic or Subclinical Infection. Many infectious diseases with serious consequences for the fetus are difficult or impossible to diagnose in the mother solely on clinical grounds. Asymptomatic or subclinical infections may be caused by rubella virus, CMV, *T. gondii*, *T. pallidum*, HSV, and HIV. The vast majority of women infected during pregnancy with these organisms have no apparent signs of disease; only 50% of women infected with rubella virus have a rash, and although occasional cases of CMV mononucleosis are recognized, these make up a very small proportion of women who acquire primary CMV infection during pregnancy. Similarly, the number of women with clinical manifestations of toxoplasmosis is less than 10%, and few women have systemic illness associated with primary HSV infection. The genital lesions associated with HSV infection and syphilis often are not recognized.

Recurrent and Chronic Infection. Some microorganisms can infect a susceptible person more than once, and when such reinfections occur in a pregnant woman, the organism can affect the fetus. These reinfections generally are associated with waning host immunity, but low levels of circulating antibodies may be detectable. Such specific antibodies would be expected to provide some protection against hematogenous spread and transplacental infection. Fetal disease, however, has followed reexposure of immune mothers to vaccinia,[68] variola,[69] and rubella[70] viruses.

In addition, an agent that causes infection capable of persisting in the mother as a chronic asymptomatic infection could infect the fetus long after the initial infection had occurred. Such delayed infection is common for congenital CMV and HIV infections, which have been observed in infants from consecutive pregnancies of the same mother. Reports of infection of the fetus as a result of chronic infection of the mother have been cited in cases of malaria[71] syphilis,[72] hepatitis,[73] herpes zoster[40] and herpes simplex,[74] and *T. gondii* infection.[75] In the case of *T. gondii*, congenital transmission from the chronically infected woman occurs almost solely when the woman is immunocompromised during pregnancy.

Preconceptional Infection. The occurrence of acute infection immediately before conception may result in infection of the fetus, and the association may go unrecognized. Congenital rubella has occurred in the fetus in cases in which the mother was infected 3 weeks to 3 months before conception. A prolonged viremia or persistence of virus in the maternal tissues may be responsible for infection of the embryo or fetus. The same has occurred rarely in cases of maternal infection with *T. gondii*.[76]

Isolation and Identification of the Infectious Agents

General Approach. Diagnostic tests for microorganisms or infectious diseases are part of routine obstetric care; special care is warranted for selected patients who are known or suspected to be exposed to the infectious agent or have clinical signs of the infectious disease. A list of diagnostic tests and the types of intervention that may be required if a diagnosis is made is provided in Table 1-8. The specific interventions for each disease are provided in subsequent chapters.

The most direct mode of diagnosis is isolation of the microbial agent from tissues and body fluids such as blood, cerebrospinal fluid, or urine. Isolation of the agent must be considered with knowledge of its epidemiology and natural history in the host. For example, isolation of an enterovirus from feces during the summer months may represent colonization rather than significant infection that might result in hematogenous spread to the fetus. Isolation of an enterovirus from a body fluid in which it is never present under normal circumstances or identification of a significant rise in antibody titer would be necessary to define an acute infectious process.

Tests for the presence of hepatitis B virus surface antigen (HBsAg) should be performed in all pregnant women. The Centers for Disease Control and Prevention (CDC) has estimated that 16,500 births occur each year in the United States to women who are positive for HBsAg. Infants born to mothers who are positive for this antigen have up to a 90% chance of acquiring perinatal hepatitis B virus infection. If infection is identified soon after birth, use of hepatitis B immune globulin combined with hepatitis B vaccine is an effective mode of prevention of infection. For these reasons, the Advisory Committee on Immunization Practices of the U.S. Public Health Service[77] and the American Academy of Pediatrics[78] recommend universal screening of all pregnant women for HBsAg.

Because the amniotic fluid contains viruses or bacteria shed from the placenta, skin, urine, or tracheal fluid of the infected fetus, this fluid, which can be obtained earlier during gestation and with somewhat less risk than with fetal blood sampling, also may be used to detect the infecting organism by culture, antigen detection test, or PCR assay. Amniocentesis and the analysis of desquamated fetal cells in the amniotic fluid have been used for the early diagnosis of genetic disorders for some time. The seminal publication in 1983 by Daffos and colleagues,[79] in which fetal blood sampling for prenatal diagnosis was first described, provided a method for diagnosing a variety of infections in the fetus that previously could be diagnosed only after birth. Their methods were widely adopted and have contributed significantly both to our understanding of the immune response of the fetus to a variety of pathogens, including rubella virus, VZV, CMV, and *T. gondii*,[80-83] and to a more objective approach to treatment of infection in the fetus before birth.

Fetal blood sampling and amniocentesis are performed under ultrasound guidance. The method is not free of risk; amniocentesis alone carries a risk of fetal injury or death as high as 1%,[47,84] and fetal blood sampling, a risk of approximately 1.4%.[85] Amniotic fluid may be examined for the presence of the infecting organism or its antigens, DNA, or RNA. Fetal blood can be examined for the same parameters, as well as to detect antibodies formed by the fetus against the pathogen (e.g., IgA or IgM antibodies that do not normally

Table 1–8 Management of Infections in the Pregnant Woman[a]

Microorganism or Disease	Diagnostic Test	Time of Test			Intervention[a]
		First Visit	*Third Trimester*	*At Delivery*	
Routine Care					
Mycobacterium tuberculosis	Tuberculin skin test	+			Therapy
Gonorrhea	Culture or antigen	+	+		Therapy
Hepatitis B	Serology	+			H BIG[b]
Chlamydia	Antigen	+	+		Therapy
Syphilis	Serology	+	+	+[c]	Therapy
Rubella	Serology	+			Postpartum vaccine
Group B *Streptococcus*	Culture		+		Intrapartum prophylaxis
Herpes simplex	Examination	+	+	+	Cesarean section
	Culture				Therapy
Special Care if Exposed or with Clinical Signs					
Human immunodeficiency virus (HIV)	Serology	+			Therapy
Parvovirus	Ultrasound				Intrauterine transfusion
	Serology				
Toxoplasmosis	Serology				Therapy
	Polymerase chain reaction (PCR) assay				
	Culture (amniotic fluid, fetal blood)				
Varicella-zoster virus	Serology, cytology				Therapy

[a]See appropriate chapters.
[b]Hepatitis B immune globulin only in women with high-risk factors, and hepatitis B vaccine for neonate.
[c]At delivery in areas with high prevalence of infection.
Modified from table prepared by Riley L, Fetter S, Geller D, Boston City Hospital and Boston University School of Medicine.

cross the placental barrier). Fetal blood sampling usually is performed during or after week 18 of gestation.

The fetus that is diagnosed as being infected with a specific pathogen or that is at high risk for infection (e.g., the fetus of a nonimmune woman who acquires her infection with *T. gondii* or rubella virus during pregnancy) may be followed by ultrasound examination to detect abnormalities such as dilation of the cerebral ventricles.

Isolation, Culture, and Polymerase Chain Reaction Assay. Isolation of CMV and rubella virus[86] and demonstration of HBsAG[87] from amniotic fluid obtained by amniocentesis have been reported. The PCR technique has proved to be both sensitive and specific for diagnosis of many infections in the pregnant woman, fetus, and newborn. Thus, detection of the DNA/RNA of an organism has, in many instances, replaced the necessity for its isolation to make a definitive diagnosis. The PCR method decreases the time to diagnosis and increases the sensitivity for diagnosis of many of these infectious agents, as exemplified by the prenatal diagnosis of infections caused by parvovirus,[88,89] CMV,[90-92] *T. gondii*,[93,94] and rubella virus.[95,96] As with all diagnostic testing, however, caution is required in interpreting the results of prenatal PCR testing. The sensitivity of PCR results on amniotic fluid is uncertain. For example, a negative result on amniotic fluid PCR assay occurs in up to one third of cases of congenital toxoplasmosis,[94,96] and in infants with congenital rubella, results of amniotic fluid PCR assay can be negative while those for fetal blood are positive. Combined diagnostic approaches in which PCR is used in concert with fetal serology and other diagnostic modalities (e.g., serial fetal ultrasonography) to test amniotic fluid and fetal blood may offer the greatest sensitivity and predictive power in cases in which congenital infection is suspected and this information is important in management decisions.[94,97] Also, false-positive detection of viral DNA has been observed at frequencies as high as 5% in fluids obtained for genetic testing when congenital fetal infection was not suspected or documented.

Cytologic and Histologic Diagnosis. Review of cytologic preparations and tissue sections may provide a presumptive diagnosis of certain infections. For example, cervicovaginal smears or cell scrapings from the base of vesicles are valuable in diagnosing VZV and HSV infections. Typical changes include multinucleated giant cells and intranuclear inclusions. These morphologic approaches, however, have largely been replaced by more specific testing methods to detect VZV, HSV, and CMV infection using direct immunofluorescence techniques or immunoperoxidase staining. The diagnosis of acute toxoplasmosis can be made from the characteristic histologic changes in lymph nodes or by demonstration of the tachyzoite in tissue specimens obtained by biopsy of infected tissues or at autopsy.

Detailed descriptions of the changes associated with infections of the placenta are presented in a monograph by Fox.[98] Examination of the placental parenchyma, the membranes, and the cord may provide valuable information leading to diagnosis of the infection and identification of the mode of transmission to the fetus (in utero or ascending infection).

Serologic Diagnosis. The serologic diagnosis of infection in the pregnant woman most often requires demonstration of a significant rise in antibody titer against the suspected agent. Ideally, the physician should have available information about the patient's serologic status at the onset of pregnancy to identify women who are unprotected against *T. pallidum*, *T. gondii*, and rubella virus or who are infected with hepatitis B virus or HIV. This valuable procedure has already been adopted by many obstetricians.

Difficulties in interpretation of serologic test results seldom arise when patients are seen shortly after exposure or at the onset of symptoms. In certain infections (e.g., rubella, toxoplasmosis), however, a relatively rapid increase in antibody levels may preclude the demonstration of a significant rise in titer in patients who are tested more than 7 days after the onset of the suspected illness. A diagnosis may be obtained in these circumstances through the measurement of antibodies that rise more slowly over a period of several weeks. Demonstration of IgA and IgE antibodies (in addition to the more conventional use of tests for IgG and IgM antibodies) is useful in the early diagnosis of infection in the pregnant woman, fetus, and newborn and should serve as an impetus to commercial firms to make these methods more widely available for use by health care providers. The same pertains to IgG avidity tests. For example, the latter have proved accurate in ruling out recently acquired infection with *T. gondii*,[99] cytomegalovirus,[100,101] and rubella virus.[102,103] At present, these tests require special techniques and are not performed routinely by most laboratories, so local or state health departments should be consulted for further information regarding their availability.

Use of Skin Tests. Routine skin tests for diagnosis of tuberculosis should be considered a part of prenatal care. Tuberculin skin tests can be administered to the mother without risk to the fetus.

Universal Screening

Prenatal care in the United States includes routine screening for serologic evidence of syphilis and rubella; culture or antigen evidence of *Chlamydia trachomatis*, group B *Streptococcus*, or hepatitis B virus infection; screening for urinary tract infection; and skin testing for tuberculosis. The demonstration that treatment of the HIV-infected mother significantly reduces the transmission of the virus to the fetus has led to recommendations by some authorities for universal HIV screening for all pregnant women in the United States. Current CDC guidelines support voluntary HIV testing under conditions that simplify consent procedures while preserving a woman's right to refuse testing if she does not think it is in her best interest.[104]

Pregnant women with known HIV infection should be monitored and given appropriate treatment to enhance mother and fetal well-being and to prevent maternal-to-fetal transmission. Pregnant women should be examined carefully for the presence of HIV-related infections including gonorrhea, syphilis, and *C. trachomatis* infection. Baseline antibody titers should be obtained for those opportunistic infections, such as *T. gondii*, which are observed commonly in HIV-infected women and which may be transmitted to their fetuses. More detailed information on management of an HIV-infected pregnant woman and her infant is given in Chapter 21.

Diagnosis of Infection in the Newborn Infant

Infants with congenital infection due to rubella virus, CMV, HSV, *T. gondii*, or *T. pallidum* may present similarly with one or more of the following abnormalities: purpura, jaundice, hepatosplenomegaly, pneumonitis, and meningoencephalitis. Some findings have specific diagnostic significance (see Tables 1-5 and 1-6).

In certain congenital infections, the organism may be isolated from tissues and body fluids. Infants may excrete CMV and rubella virus in the urine for weeks to months after birth. *T. pallidum* may be found in the cerebrospinal fluid, in nasal secretions, and in the skin lesions of syphilis. Results of HIV culture or PCR assay are positive at birth in approximately 30% to 50% of congenitally infected infants, but results are positive in nearly 100% of infected infants by 4 to 6 months of life.

Serologic tests are available through state or commercial laboratories for the TORCH group of microorganisms (*T. gondii*, *T. pallidum*, rubella virus, CMV, and HSV) and for certain other congenitally acquired infections. To distinguish passively transferred maternal IgG antibody from antibody synthesized by the neonate in response to infection in utero, it is necessary to obtain two blood specimens from the infant. Because the half-life of IgG is approximately 3 days, the first sample is obtained soon after birth, and the second sample should be obtained at least two half-lives or approximately 6 weeks after the first specimen.

IgA, IgE, and IgM antibodies do not cross the placenta. Antigen-specific IgA, IgE, and IgM antibodies in the infant's blood provides evidence of current infection, but few commercial laboratories employ reliable assays for these antibodies for the purpose of identifying congenital infections, as described in a Public Health Advisory from the Food and Drug Administration outlining the limitations of *Toxoplasma* IgM commercial test kits.

Although most congenital infections occur as a single entity, many HIV-infected mothers are co-infected with other infectious agents that may be transmitted to the newborn. The neonate born to an HIV-infected mother should be considered at risk for other sexually transmitted infections such as syphilis, gonorrhea, and *C. trachomatis* infection. In addition, co-infection has been documented for CMV.[105,106]

Prevention and Management of Infection in the Pregnant Woman

Prevention of Infection

Pregnant women should avoid contact with persons with communicable diseases, particularly if the women are known to be seronegative (e.g., for CMV) or have no prior history of the disease (e.g., with VZV). In some cases, specific measures can be taken. The pregnant woman should avoid intercourse with her sexual partner if he has a vesicular lesion on the penis that may be due to HSV or if he is known or suspected to be infected with HIV. Pregnant women should avoid eating raw or undercooked lamb, pork, and beef, because such products sometimes contain *T. gondii*. They also should avoid contact with cat feces, or objects or materials contaminated with cat feces, because these are highly infectious if they harbor oocysts of *T. gondii* (see Chapter 31). Pregnant women should not eat unpasteurized dairy products (including all soft cheeses), prepared meats (hot dogs, deli meat, and paté), and undercooked poultry, because such foods often contain *Listeria monocytogenes* (see Chapter 14).

Immunization

Routine immunization schedules for infants and children with currently available live vaccines, including measles, poliomyelitis, mumps, and rubella, should confer protection against these infections throughout the childbearing years.

Public health authorities and obstetricians generally agree that immunization during pregnancy poses only theoretical risks to the developing fetus. Nevertheless, pregnant women should receive a vaccine only when the vaccine is unlikely to cause harm, the risk for disease exposure is high, and the infection would pose a significant risk to the mother (e.g., influenza) or fetus (e.g., tetanus).[107] The following considerations are of importance with regard to immunization of the pregnant woman.

- The only vaccines routinely recommended for administration during pregnancy in the United States, when indicated for either primary or booster immunization, are those for tetanus, diphtheria, and influenza.[108] Such vaccines are inactivated. Inactivated vaccines, including typhoid fever vaccine, are not considered hazardous to the pregnant woman or her fetus and often can be of major benefit when indicated. An example is the use of tetanus toxoid vaccines in areas of the world in which infection in the newborn from unsterile delivery and cord care carries a significant risk of fatal outcome. In the United States, pregnant women are at increased risk for influenza-like illness that requires hospitalization when compared with nonpregnant women of similar age. For this reason, routine immunization of pregnant women at the onset of the influenza season is recommended by the Advisory Committee on Infectious Diseases of the CDC.[108] In women at increased risk for certain serious bacterial infections, such as invasive pneumococcal or meningococcal disease (e.g., those with sickle cell disease or HIV infection), immunization should precede pregnancy if at all possible. If immunization has not occurred before pregnancy and the risk is significant (e.g., with a meningococcal outbreak in the community), the women should be vaccinated.
- Pregnancy is a contraindication to administration of all live vaccines, except when susceptibility and exposure are highly probable and the disease to be prevented constitutes a greater threat to the woman and her fetus than a possible adverse effect of the vaccine. For example, yellow fever vaccine is indicated for pregnant women who are at substantial risk for imminent exposure to infection (such as with international travel). A report of IgM antibodies to yellow fever in the infant of a woman immunized during pregnancy suggests that transplacental transmission of the yellow fever vaccine virus does occur, although the incidence of congenital infection is unknown.[109]
- Varicella vaccine should not be administered to pregnant women, because the possible effects on fetal development are unknown. When postpubertal females are immunized, pregnancy should be avoided for at least 2 months following immunization.
- Because several weeks can elapse before pregnancy is evident, caution and selectivity are indicated in administering a live virus vaccine to any woman of childbearing age. The demonstration of prolonged virus shedding after immunization with live virus vaccine suggests that pregnancy should be avoided when possible for 2 to 3 months subsequent to the administration of any live immunizing agent.
- The risk to the mother or fetus from immunization of members of her immediate family or other intimate contacts is uncertain. The use of attenuated measles, rubella, mumps, and varicella vaccines rarely results in dissemination of these viruses to susceptible subjects in the immediate environment, but household spread of attenuated polioviruses through contact with recently vaccinated, susceptible individuals in the family is common. From March 1995 through March 2003, 509 pregnant women whose pregnancy outcomes are known were inadvertently given varicella vaccine (VARIVAX Pregnancy Registry). No offspring had congenital varicella, and the rate of congenital anomalies was no greater than that in the general population. Furthermore, presence of a pregnant woman in the household is not a contraindication to varicella immunization of a child in that household, and varicella-susceptible women should be vaccinated post partum.

Use of Immune Globulin

Human immune serum globulin administered after exposure to rubella, varicella, measles, or hepatitis A virus may modify clinical signs and symptoms of the disease but has not proved to be consistently effective in preventing disease, and presumably viremia, in susceptible persons. Human immune serum globulin is of undetermined value in protecting the fetus of a susceptible woman against infection with these viruses. Its use after maternal exposure to rubella virus should be limited to women to whom therapeutic abortion is unacceptable, in the event of documented infection during pregnancy.

Antimicrobial Therapy

Almost without exception, antimicrobial agents administered systemically to the mother pass to the fetus. Management of pregnant women with acute infections amenable to therapy should be the same as that of nonpregnant patients but with attention paid to the possible effects on the fetus of the antimicrobial drug. Pregnant women with recently acquired acute toxoplasmosis, Lyme disease, and syphilis should undergo treatment as outlined in the specific chapters devoted to those topics. Women who are colonized with *C. trachomatis* or group B streptococci may receive treatment under selected circumstances, considered in the next section.

The landmark study of Connor and colleagues demonstrated reduction of maternal-infant transmission of HIV from 25.5% to 8.3% using zidovudine in women who had peripheral $CD4^+$ T lymphocyte counts of more than 200 cells per μL and were mildly symptomatic.[110] The currently recommended treatment regimen in the United States is oral zidovudine administered to pregnant women beginning at

14 to 34 weeks of gestation and continuing throughout pregnancy, intravenous zidovudine during labor and delivery, and oral zidovudine to the newborn for the first 6 weeks of life (see Chapter 21). This complex and costly regimen is not feasible for resource-limited countries, but recent studies in Uganda using one dose of nevirapine administered to the mother in labor and a single dose to the neonate before discharge provide a model.[111]

INFECTIONS ACQUIRED BY THE NEWBORN INFANT DURING BIRTH

Pathogenesis

The developing fetus is protected from the microbial flora of the maternal genital tract. Initial colonization of the newborn and of the placenta usually occurs after rupture of maternal membranes. If delivery is delayed after membranes rupture, the vaginal microflora can ascend and in some cases produce inflammation of fetal membranes, umbilical cord, and placenta. Fetal infection also can result from aspiration of infected amniotic fluid. Some viruses are present in the genital secretions (HSV, CMV, hepatitis B virus, or HIV) or blood (hepatitis B or C virus or HIV). If delivery follows shortly after rupture of the membranes, the infant can be colonized during passage through the birth canal. A variety of microorganisms may be present in the maternal birth canal, as summarized in Table 1-8; included are gram-positive cocci (staphylococci and streptococci), gram-negative cocci (*Neisseria meningitidis* [rarely] and *Neisseria gonorrhoeae*), gram-negative enteric bacilli (*Escherichia coli*, *Proteus* species, *Klebsiella* species, *Pseudomonas* species, *Salmonella*, and *Shigella*), anaerobic bacteria, viruses (CMV, HSV, rubella virus, and HIV), fungi (predominantly *Candida albicans*), *C. trachomatis*, mycoplasmas, and protozoa (*Trichomonas vaginalis* and *T. gondii*). As indicated in Table 1-8, some of these organisms are significantly associated with disease in the newborn infant, whereas others affect the neonate rarely, if at all.

The newborn initially is colonized on the skin, mucosal surfaces, including the nasopharynx, oropharynx, conjunctivae, umbilical cord, and external genitalia, and the gastrointestinal tract (from swallowing of infected amniotic fluid or vaginal secretions). In most infants, the organisms proliferate at these sites without causing illness. A few infants become infected by direct extension from the sites of colonization (e.g., otitis media from nasopharyngeal colonization). Alternatively, invasion of the bloodstream can ensue, with subsequent dissemination of infection. The umbilical cord was a particularly common portal of entry for systemic infection before local disinfection methods became routine. This site was common because the devitalized tissues are an excellent medium for bacterial growth and because the thrombosed umbilical vessels provide direct access to the bloodstream. Microorganisms also can infect abrasions or skin wounds. Today the most frequent sources for bloodstream invasion are the lung from aspirated infected amniotic fluid or vaginal contents and the gastrointestinal tract from transmigration of microbial flora across the gut wall.

Infants in whom bacterial sepsis develops often have certain risk factors not evident in infants in whom significant infections do not develop. Among these factors are preterm delivery at a gestational age less than 37 weeks, low birth weight, prolonged rupture of maternal membranes, maternal intra-amniotic infection, traumatic delivery, and fetal anoxia. Relative immaturity of the immune system is considered to be one factor in increased risk of infection during the neonatal period. The role of host defenses in neonatal infection is discussed in detail in Chapter 4.

Preterm birth is the single most significant risk factor for infections acquired just before or during delivery of the infant or in the nursery. The increasing number of extremely and very low birth weight infants has continued to heighten concern for infection as a cause of morbidity and mortality. Furthermore, various modalities for treatment of infertility have continued to increase the number of multiple-birth pregnancies, and a gestational age of less than 28 weeks is not uncommon following various modalities for treatment of infertility. A recent summary of 6215 very low birth weight neonates (birth weight of 401 to 1500 g) from the National Institute of Child Health and Human Development Neonatal Research Network reported that 21% had one or more episodes of blood culture–proven late-onset sepsis.[112] Infection rate was inversely correlated with birth weight and gestational age, and infected infants had a significantly prolonged mean hospital stay (79 days) compared with uninfected infants (60 days). Also, infants with late-onset sepsis were significantly more likely to die than uninfected infants (18% versus 7%), especially if they were infected with gram-negative organisms (36%) or fungi (32%).[112]

The value of certain defense mechanisms remains controversial. Vernix caseosa has no specific antibacterial properties, but retention of vernix probably is of value because it provides a protective barrier to the skin. Breast milk influences the composition of the fecal flora by suppression of *E. coli* and other gram-negative enteric bacilli and encouragement of growth of lactobacilli. In addition, breast milk contains secretory IgA, lysozymes, white blood cells, and lactoferrin (an iron-binding protein that significantly inhibits the growth of *E. coli* and other microorganisms); however, the importance of these constituents for colonization and systemic infection in the neonate acquired at or shortly after birth is uncertain (see Chapter 5).

The virulence of the invading microorganism also must be considered as a factor in the pathogenesis of neonatal sepsis. Certain phage types of *S. aureus* (types 80 and 81) were responsible for most cases of disease in the staphylococcal pandemic of the 1950s. Phage group 2 *S. aureus* strains have been responsible for the staphylococcal scalded skin syndrome sometimes seen in neonates (toxic epidermal necrolysis). Other evidence suggests that the K1 capsular antigens of *E. coli* and type III strains of group B *Streptococcus* possess virulence properties that account for their propensity to cause invasion of the blood-brain barrier during bacteremia when compared with non-K1 and non–type III strains.

Microbiology

The agents responsible for early-onset (before 72 hours) neonatal sepsis are those found in the maternal birth canal.[113,114] Most of these organisms are considered to be saprophytic, but on occasion they can be responsible for maternal infection and its sequelae, including endometritis and puerperal fever. A review of the microbial flora of the adult female genital

Table 1–9 Association of Neonatal Disease with Microorganisms Present in the Maternal Birth Canal

	Association with Neonatal Disease		
Microorganism	***Significant***	***Uncommon***	***Rare or None***
Bacteria			
Lactobacillus			+
Staphylococcus epidermidis			+
Staphylococcus aureus		+	
Alpha-hemolytic streptococci		+	
Group A streptococci	+		
Group B streptococci	+		
Enterococcus	+		
Escherichia coli	+		
Proteus species		+	
Klebsiella species		+	
Pseudomonas species		+	
Salmonella species		+	
Shigella species		+	
Alkaligenes faecalis		+	
Neisseria meningitidis		+	
Neisseria gonorrhoeae	+		
Haemophilus influenzae		+	
Haemophilus parainfluenzae		+	
Gardnerella vaginalis			+
Listeria monocytogenes	+		
Vibrio fetus		+	
Corynebacterium			+
Bacillus subtilis			+
Anaerobic Bacteria[113]			
Bacteroides		+	
Peptostreptococcus			+
Veillonella			+
Clostridium species		+	
Bifidobacterium			+
Eubacterium			+
Mycobacterium tuberculosis			+
Viruses			
Cytomegalovirus	+		
Herpes simplex virus	+		
Rubella virus			+
Hepatitis B virus	+		
Human papillomavirus			+
Lymphocytic choriomeningitis virus			+
Human immunodeficiency virus		+	
Fungi			
Candida albicans	+		
Candida glabrata			+
Coccidioides immitis		+	
Saccharomyces			+
Chlamydiaceae			
Chlamydia trachomatis	+		
Mycoplasmataceae			
Mycoplasma hominis		+	
Ureaplasma urealyticum		+	
Protozoa			
Toxoplasma gondii		+	
Trichomonas vaginalis		+	

tract and its association with neonatal infection and disease is presented in Table 1-9.

Before the introduction of the sulfonamides and penicillin in the 1940s, gram-positive cocci, particularly group A streptococci, were responsible for most cases of neonatal sepsis. After the introduction of antimicrobial agents, gram-negative enterics, in particular *E. coli*, were the predominant causes of serious bacterial infections of the newborn. An increase in serious neonatal infection caused by group B streptococci was noted in the early 1970s, and currently, group B streptococci and *E. coli* continue to be the most frequent causative agents for early-onset neonatal sepsis and for late-onset sepsis in term infants. By contrast, late-onset (after 7 days) sepsis in preterm neonates remaining in the neonatal intensive care unit for weeks or months have sepsis caused by commensal organisms (e.g., coagulase-negative staphylococci and *Enterococcus*) as well as by organisms acquired from the mother and from the nursery environment. The bacteria responsible for neonatal sepsis are discussed in Chapter 6.

Mycoplasmas, anaerobic bacteria, and viruses (including HSV, hepatitis B virus, CMV, and HIV) that colonize the maternal genital tract also are acquired during birth.

Diagnosis

Review of the maternal record provides important clues for diagnosis of infection in the neonate. Signs of illness during pregnancy, exposure to sexual partners with transmissible infections, and results of cultures (e.g., for *C. trachomatis*, *N. gonorrhoeae*, or group B streptococci), serologic tests (e.g., for HIV infection, rubella, hepatitis B and C, or syphilis), and tuberculin skin tests or chest radiographs should be identified in the pregnancy record. The delivery chart should be checked for peripartum events that indicate risk of sepsis in the neonate, including premature rupture of membranes, prolonged duration (longer than 18 hours) of rupture of membranes, evidence of fetal distress and fever or other signs of maternal infection such as bloody diarrhea, respiratory or gastrointestinal signs (i.e., enterovirus), indications of large concentrations of pathogens in the genitalia (as reflected in bacteriuria due to group B streptococci), and evidence of invasive bacterial infections in prior pregnancies.

The clinical diagnosis of systemic infection in the newborn can be difficult. The initial signs of infection may be subtle and nonspecific. Not only are the signs of infectious and noninfectious processes similar, but also the signs of in utero infection are indistinguishable from those of infections acquired either during the birth process or subsequently, during the first few days of life. Respiratory distress, lethargy, irritability, poor feeding, jaundice, emesis, and diarrhea are associated with a variety of infectious and noninfectious causes.

Some clinical manifestations of neonatal sepsis, such as hepatomegaly, jaundice, pneumonitis, purpura, and meningitis, are common to many of the infections that are acquired in utero or during delivery. Certain signs, however, are related to specific infections (see Tables 1-6 and 1-7). Many signs of congenital infection are not evident at birth: hepatitis B infection should be considered in the infant with onset of jaundice and hepatosplenomegaly between 1 and 6 months of age; CMV infection acquired at or soon after delivery is associated with an afebrile protracted pneumonitis; enterovirus infection should be considered in the infant with acute cerebrospinal fluid pleocytosis in the first months of life. Most infants with congenital HIV infection do not have signs of disease during the first months of life. Uncommonly, signs may be present at birth. Srugo and colleagues[115] described an infant with signs of meningoencephalitis at 6 hours of life; HIV was isolated from cerebrospinal fluid.

Most early-onset bacterial infections are nonfocal except in the circumstance of respiratory distress at or shortly after birth, in which the chest radiograph reveals pneumonia. Focal infections are frequent with late-onset neonatal sepsis and include otitis media, pneumonia, soft tissue infections, urinary tract infections, septic arthritis, osteomyelitis, and peritonitis. Bacterial meningitis is of particular concern because of the substantial mortality rate and the significant morbidity in survivors. Few infants have overt meningeal signs, and a high index of suspicion and examination of the cerebrospinal fluid are required for early diagnosis.

Routine laboratory methods now available are of limited assistance in the diagnosis of systemic infections in the newborn infant. In bacterial sepsis, the total white blood cell count is variable and supports a diagnosis of bacterial sepsis only if it is high (more than 30,000 cells per mm^3) or very low (fewer than 5000 cells per mm^3). Immunoglobulin is produced by the fetus and newborn infant in response to infection. Increased levels of IgM have been measured in the serum of newborns with infections (i.e., syphilis, rubella, cytomegalic inclusion disease, toxoplasmosis, and malaria) acquired transplacentally. Increased levels of IgM also result from postnatally acquired bacterial infections. Not all infected infants, however, have increased levels of serum IgM, and some infants who do have elevated concentrations of total IgM are apparently uninfected. Thus, identification of increased levels of total IgM in the newborn is suggestive of an infectious process acquired before or shortly after birth, but this finding is not specific and is of limited assistance in diagnosis and management.

Because inflammation of the placenta and umbilical cord may accompany peripartum sepsis, pathologic examination of sections of these tissues may assist in the diagnosis of infection in the newborn. Of note, however, histologic evidence of inflammation also is noted in the absence of evidence of neonatal sepsis. In the immediate postnatal period, gastric aspirate, pharyngeal mucus, or fluid from the external ear canal has been used to delineate exposure to potential pathogens but are not useful in the diagnosis of neonatal sepsis.

Isolation of microorganisms from a usually sterile site, such as blood, cerebrospinal fluid, or skin vesicle fluid, or from a suppurative lesion or a sterilely obtained sample of urine, remains the only valid method of diagnosing systemic infection. Aspiration of any focus of infection in a critically ill infant (e.g., needle aspiration of middle ear fluid in an infant with otitis media or from the joint or metaphysis of an infant with osteoarthritis) should be performed to determine the etiologic agent. In very low birth weight infants, commensal microorganisms, such as coagulase-negative staphylococci, *Enterococcus*, or *Candida*, isolated from a usually sterile body site should be considered pathogens until proven otherwise. Culture of infectious agents from the nose, throat, skin, umbilicus, or stool indicates colonization; these agents may include the pathogens that are responsible for the disease but in themselves do not establish the presence of active systemic infection.

PCR assay to detect the nucleic acid of a variety of important pathogens including viruses and *Pneumocystis jiroveci*, enzyme immunoassay for *T. gondii*, and electron microscopy to identify CMV and rotaviruses are useful new tests available for diagnosis. When appropriate, serologic studies should be performed to ascertain the presence of in utero or postnatal infection. Serologic tests are available through local or state laboratories for HIV, rubella, parvovirus B19, *T. gondii*, and *T. pallidum*. For some of these infections (e.g., rubella), the serologic assay measures IgG. To distinguish passively transferred maternal antibody from antibody derived from infection in the neonate, it is necessary to obtain two blood specimens from the infant. Because the half-life of IgG is estimated to be 23 days, the first sample is obtained soon after birth, and the second sample should be obtained at least two half-lives or approximately 6 weeks after the first specimen. Measurement of IgM antibody provides evidence of current infection in the neonate, but none of these assays has proven reliability at present.

Management

Successful management of neonatal bacterial sepsis depends on a high index of suspicion based on maternal history and infant signs, prompt initiation of appropriate antimicrobial therapy while diagnostic tests are performed, and meticulous supportive measures. If the physician considers that a newborn may have bacterial infection, culture specimens should be obtained and treatment with antimicrobial agents active against the probable pathogens should be initiated immediately. In general, initial therapy must include agents active against gram-positive cocci, particularly group B and other streptococci, and gram-negative enteric bacilli. Ampicillin is the preferred agent with effectiveness against gram-positive cocci and *L. monocytogenes*. The choice of therapy for gram-negative infections depends on the current pattern of antimicrobial susceptibility in the local community. Most experts prefer ampicillin and gentamicin as agents for therapy for early-onset presumptive sepsis, with the addition of cefotaxime for presumptive bacterial meningitis.[116] Intrapartum antimicrobial therapy results in concentrations of drug in the blood of the newborn infant that can suppress growth of group B streptococci and possibly other susceptible organisms in blood obtained for culture. The requirement for more than one blood specimen for the microbiologic diagnosis of early-onset sepsis places a substantial burden on the clinician.

An algorithm has been prepared to guide empirical management of neonates born to mothers who received intrapartum antimicrobial prophylaxis for prevention of early-onset group B streptococcal infection.[117] These infants may be divided into three management groups:

1. Neonates who have signs of sepsis or those whose mothers are colonized with group B streptococci and have chorioamnionitis should receive a full diagnostic evaluation with institution of empirical treatment.
2. Term neonates who appear healthy and whose mothers received penicillin, ampicillin, or cefazolin 4 or more hours before delivery do not require further evaluation or treatment.
3. Healthy-appearing term neonates whose mothers received prophylaxis less than 4 hours before delivery and neonates born at less than 35 weeks of gestation whose mothers received prophylaxis of any duration before delivery should be observed for 48 hours or longer and should receive a limited evaluation, including white blood cell count and differential and culture of blood.[117]

Infants in the first two categories are readily identified, but assignment of infants to the third category often is problematic because of the vague end points. Recent recommendations for prevention and treatment of early-onset group B streptococcal infection are discussed in Chapter 13.

The choice of antibacterial drugs should be reviewed when results of cultures and susceptibility tests become available. The clinician should be sure to select drugs that have been studied for appropriate dose, interval of dosing, and safety in neonates, especially very low birth weight infants, and that have the narrowest antimicrobial spectrum that would be effective (see Chapter 37). The duration of therapy depends on the initial response to the appropriate antibiotics but should be 10 days in most infants with sepsis, pneumonia, or minimal or absent focal infection; the *minimal* duration of therapy for uncomplicated meningitis caused by group B streptococci or *L. monocytogenes* is 14 days and for gram-negative enteric bacilli is 21 days.[117]

The clinical pharmacology of antibiotics administered to the newborn infant is unique and cannot be extrapolated from the data on absorption, excretion, and toxicity in the adult. The safety of new antimicrobial agents is a particular concern because toxic effects may not be detected until several years later (see Chapter 37).

Development of resistance of microbial pathogens to antimicrobial agents is a constant concern. Group B streptococci remain uniformly susceptible to penicillins and cephalosporins, but many isolates now are resistant to erythromycin and clindamycin.[118,119] The one or two doses of a penicillin or cephalosporin administered as part of a peripartum prophylactic regimen for prevention of group B streptococcal infection in the neonate would not be expected to significantly affect the genital flora, but surveillance for alteration in the flora and antibiotic susceptibility should be maintained. Because the nursery is a small, closed community, development of resistance is a greater concern with nosocomial infections than with infections acquired in utero or at delivery.

Despite the use of appropriate antimicrobial agents and optimal supportive therapy, mortality from neonatal sepsis remains substantial. With the hope of improving survival and decreasing the severity of sequelae in survivors, investigators have turned their attention to studies of adjunctive modes of treatment that provide supplements for the demonstrated deficits in the host defenses of the infected neonate. These therapies include use of standard hyperimmune immunoglobulins, leukocyte growth factors, and monoclonal antibody preparations that are pathogen specific.

Antiviral therapies are available for treatment for newborns infected with HSV (acyclovir), VZV (acyclovir), and HIV. Acyclovir and zidovudine are well tolerated in the pregnant woman. Because early use of acyclovir for herpes simplex infections in neonates has been associated with improved outcome, physicians may choose to begin therapy for presumptive disease due to HSV and reevaluate therapy when results of cultures and PCR assay are known and more information is available about the clinical course.

The results of phase II and III trials examining safety, pharmacodynamics, and efficacy of ganciclovir treatment of symptomatic congenital CMV infection have been reported.[120,121] The phase II trial established the safe dose of ganciclovir in infants and demonstrated an antiviral effect with suppression of viruria.[120] Neutropenia (63%), thrombocytopenia, and altered hepatic enzymes were noted in a majority of the infants. Nearly half of the infants required dosage adjustments because of severe neutropenia. The phase III randomized, controlled trial of intravenous ganciclovir for 6 weeks in 100 infants with central nervous system CMV involvement at birth demonstrated hearing improvement or maintained hearing in 84% of infants who received ganciclovir, compared with 41% of control infants (see Chapter 23).[121]

Prevention

Immunoprophylaxis

Immune globulins may be valuable for prevention of certain infections that occur during the neonatal period. Zoster immune globulin is effective in the prevention or the attenuation of neonatal varicella, but its manufacture has been discontinued (as of 2005). Hepatitis B immune globulin is effective for the interruption of perinatal transmission of hepatitis B virus carrier state, especially when combined with immunization with hepatitis B vaccine. Intravenous immune globulin (IGIV) reduced the number of late-onset infections, particularly those caused by coagulase-negative staphylococci, in low-birth-weight premature infants in one multicenter, randomized controlled study[121] but not in another.[122] Currently, pathogen-specific hyperimmune globulins or monoclonal antibody preparations for staphylococci (see Chapter 17) are under investigation.

Universal immunization of infants with hepatitis B vaccine has been recommended by the American Academy of Pediatrics since 1992.[123] Prior selective strategies of vaccination in high-risk populations and serologic screening of all pregnant women for HB_sAg had little impact on control of hepatitis B infections or their sequelae, and public health authorities believe that infant immunization offers the most feasible approach to protection of all persons and eventual elimination of the disease. Infants born to HB_sAg-positive women should receive hepatitis B immune globulin at or shortly after birth and should be immunized at birth. Further improvement in this prevention strategy may be achieved if a universal birth dose of hepatitis B vaccine is recommended, thereby allowing intervention for those infants whose maternal records are incorrect or not available before hospital discharge

Chemoprophylaxis

Antimicrobial agents capable of crossing biologic membranes can achieve concentrations of drug in the fetus comparable with concentrations in other well-vascularized tissues after administration to the mother. Prevention of group B streptococcal infection in the newborn by administration of ampicillin to the mother was demonstrated by Boyer and colleagues[124] and other investigators as early as 1983 (see Chapter 13). A prevention strategy was recommended for use by the American Academy of Pediatrics in 1992.[125] These guidelines were revised in 1997, and current recommendations from the CDC are endorsed by the American Academy of Pediatrics, the American College of Obstetricians and Gynecologists, and the American Academy of Family Physicians. Current recommendations are for universal culture screening of all pregnant women at 35 to 37 weeks of gestation and for administration of intravenous penicillin during labor.[3] Concentrations of drug are achieved in the fetus that are more than 30% of the concentrations in the blood of the mother,[126] and bactericidal concentrations against group B streptococci are achieved in amniotic fluid 3 hours after a maternal dose (see Chapters 13 and 37). Parenteral antimicrobial therapy administered to the mother in labor is essentially treating the fetus earlier in the course of the intrapartum infection. If the fetus has been infected, the regimen is treatment, not prophylaxis, and for some infected fetuses the treatment administered in utero will be insufficient to prevent early-onset group B streptococcal disease.[128] Although the prophylactic regimen has decreased the incidence of early-onset group B streptococcal disease (by more than 80% in a Pittsburgh survey[127]), the regimen has had no impact on the incidence of late-onset disease.[3]

Other modes of chemoprophylaxis administered to the neonate are the use of ophthalmic drops or ointments for prevention of gonococcal ophthalmia and the administration of zidovudine to infants born to HIV-infected mothers. Administration of antibacterial agents to infants with minimal or ambiguous clinical signs is therapy for presumed sepsis and should not be considered prophylaxis.

INFECTIONS OF THE NEWBORN INFANT IN THE FIRST MONTH OF LIFE

When fever or other signs of systemic infection occur in the first weeks or months of life, appropriate management requires consideration of the various sources of infection. Five types of such infection based on source can be recognized: (1) congenital infections with onset in utero; (2) infections acquired during the birth process from the maternal genital tract; (3) infections acquired in the nursery; (4) infections acquired in the household after discharge from the nursery; and (5) infection that suggests an anatomic defect, underlying immunologic disease or metabolic abnormality.

Pathogenesis and Microbiology

Congenital Infections

Signs of congenital infection may not appear for weeks, months, or years following birth. Diagnosis and management are discussed in the disease chapters.

Infections Acquired during Delivery

Although maternal intrapartum prophylaxis has reduced the incidence of early-onset group B streptococcal disease, the regimen has not altered the incidence of late-onset disease,[3] with signs occurring from 6 to 89 days of life, and in very low birth weight infants up to 6 months of age. The pathogenesis of late-onset group B streptococcal disease remains obscure, but it is likely that even when vertical transmission from the mother at birth is prevented, exposure to either the mother (in whom colonization resumes after delivery) and other colonized family members or caregivers can serve as a source for colonization through direct contact. Why sepsis develops without warning in an infant who has no risk factors for sepsis and was well for days to weeks remains a mystery. This concern also is relevant in infants who acquire late-onset disease due to *E. coli* and *L. monocytogenes*.

Nursery-Acquired Infections

After arrival in the nursery, the newborn may become infected by various pathways involving either human carriers or contaminated materials and equipment.

Human sources in the hospital include personnel, mothers, and other infants. The methods of transmission may include the following:

- *Droplet spread* from the respiratory tract of adults or other newborn infants. Outbreaks of respiratory virus infections in prolonged-stay nurseries are frequent; viruses present include influenza, respiratory syncytial, and parainfluenza viruses.[128] Methods for identification and control are provided in Chapter 35.
- *Carriage* of the microorganism on the hands of hospital personnel. A study has suggested that the hands may be not only a means of transmission but also a significant reservoir of bacteria.[129]
- *Suppurative lesions.* Although spread of staphylococcal and streptococcal infections to infants or mothers may be associated with asymptomatic carriers, the most serious outbreaks have been caused by a member of the medical or nursing staff with a significant lesion.
- *Human milk.* CMV, HIV, HSV, human T cell lymphotropic virus type I (HTLV-I),[130] HTLV-II,[131] and HB_sAg have been identified in mother's milk and may be transmitted to the neonate by this route. CMV-infected milk from banks can be dangerous for infants without passively transferred maternal antibody.

  The role of breast milk in transmission of HIV is of concern because of the importance of breast-feeding in providing nutrition and immunologic protection in the first year of life. Breast milk has been documented to be the likely source of HIV infection in neonates whose mothers were transfused with HIV-infected blood after delivery or in whom disease developed post partum through sexual contact.[132] These acute infections need to be differentiated from the usual event in which the mother is infected throughout pregnancy. Infection during the acute period occurs before development of antibody and may be a time when breast milk has a high titer of transmissible virus. Because of the importance of breast-feeding in the nutrition of infants in developing countries, the World Health Organization (WHO) first recommended that women in developing countries be encouraged to breast-feed even if they were known to be infected with HIV.[133] By contrast, in the United States and Western Europe, HIV-infected mothers were discouraged from breast-feeding because other forms of nutrition were available.[134] In July 1998, the United Nations changed its position and issued recommendations to discourage women infected with HIV from breast-feeding. The statement recognized that many infants were infected by the breast milk of HIV-infected mothers. The recommendation also noted that in some cultures, women may become stigmatized for not breast-feeding, and that in some places, alternatives such as formula are unaffordable or unsafe. The number of congenitally infected infants in developing countries that have no resources for prevention in pregnancy has reached alarming proportions: 70% of women at a prenatal clinic in Zimbabwe and 30% of women in urban areas in six African countries were infected. The United Nations survey indicated that by the year 2000, breast-feeding would be responsible for more than one third (greater than 200,000) of children newly infected with HIV unless some attempts were made to limit this route of transmission.[135]

  Infection of breast milk by bacterial pathogens such as *S. aureus*, group B streptococci, *L. monocytogenes*,[136] and *Salmonella* species can result in neonatal disease. Bacteria that are components of skin flora, including *Staphylococcus epidermidis* and α-hemolytic streptococci, frequently are cultured from freshly expressed human milk and are unlikely to be of importance in the breast-fed infant. If these bacteria are allowed to multiply in banked breast milk, infection of the neonate is possible in theory, but no substantive data have been presented to suggest that this is an important problem.

Other possible sources of infection in the nursery include the following:

- *Blood products.* Blood used for replacement or exchange transfusion in neonates should be determined to be safe by techniques of proven efficacy, including tests for hepatitis B antigen, hepatitis C, HIV antibody, CMV antibody, and *Plasmodium* species in malaria-endemic areas.
- *Equipment* has been implicated in common-source nursery outbreaks. The most frequent factors in transmission of infection in such instances have been contaminated solutions used in nebulization equipment, room humidifiers, and bathing solutions. Several gram-negative bacteria, including *Pseudomonas aeruginosa*, *Serratia marcescens*, and *Flavobacterium*, have been so troublesome in the past that they have been termed "water bugs" because of their ability to multiply in aqueous environments at room temperature. In the past decade, few solution- or equipment-related outbreaks due to these organisms have been reported, because of the scrupulous infection control practices that are enforced in most intensive care nurseries.
- *Catheterization* of the umbilical vein and artery has been associated with sepsis, umbilical cellulitis, and abscess formation, but again, careful hygienic practices with insertion of these devices make these complications rare. Intravenous alimentation using central venous catheters has been lifesaving for some infants but also is associated with increased risk for catheter-related bacteremia or fungemia.
- *Parenteral feeding* with lipid emulsions has been associated with neonatal sepsis due to coagulase-negative staphylococci and *Candida* species. Strains of staphylococci isolated from infected ventricular shunts or intravascular catheters produce a slime or glycocalyx that promotes adherence and growth of colonies on the surfaces and into the walls of synthetic polymers used in the manufacture of catheters. The slime layer also protects the bacteria against the action of antibiotics and phagocytosis. The introduction of lipid emulsion through the venous catheter provides nutrients for growth of the bacteria and fungi.[137]

Hand hygiene remains the single most important element in the control of the spread of infectious diseases in the nursery. Hand hygiene measures should be implemented before and after every patient contact. Surveys of hospital employees indicate that rigorous adherence to hand hygiene, although the most simple of infection control techniques, is still lacking in most institutions. A study by Brown and colleagues in a Denver neonatal intensive care unit indicated that compliance with appropriate hand-washing techniques was low for both medical and nursing personnel.[138] Compliance was monitored using a direct observation technique; of 252 observed encounters of nurses, physicians, and respiratory therapists with babies, 25% of the personnel broke contact with the infant by touching self (69%) or touching another baby (4%), and 25% did not wash before patient contact.

Waterless, alcohol-based hand hygiene products have been introduced into nurseries recently. Their ease of application and requirement for less time than hand washing in achieving reduction of microorganisms should increase adherence with hand hygiene recommendations. According to recent surveys, waterless soap products have gained rapid acceptance by nursery personnel including physicians.

Early discharge at 24 or 48 hours was a common practice several years ago as hospitals and third-party payers have attempted to reduce costs of health care. Study of a cohort of more than 300,000 births in Washington documented that newborns discharged home early (before 30 hours after birth) were at increased risk for rehospitalization during the first month of life; the leading causes were jaundice, dehydration, and sepsis, with onset within 7 days after discharge. Among 1253 infants who were rehospitalized within the first month of life, sepsis was the cause in 55 cases (4.4%) who were discharged early, contrasted with 42 (3.4%) who were discharged late.[139] These and other reports, combined with corrective legislation in a number of states, have led to recommendations that newborns remain hospitalized at least 48 hours after vaginal birth and 72 hours after cesarean section delivery.

Prevention of disease in the first months of life may be accomplished by immunization of the mother with passive transfer of protective antibody to the neonate. Immunization of women in the childbearing years or during pregnancy is of proven value in prevention of neonatal tetanus but also has been considered for prevention of invasive disease in the first months of life. Maternal immunization with polysaccharide and conjugate *Haemophilus influenzae* type b vaccines has provided protective levels of antibody to the infant[140] and therefore may be considered for prevention of invasive pneumococcal infection in young infants, especially in resource-limited countries, where disease often occurs during the first few months of life.[141] Immunization of the mother during pregnancy is likely to be protective for other diseases in the neonate due to encapsulated organisms, including group B streptococci, [142] pneumococci, and meningococci, and has been considered for prevention of infection due to respiratory syncytial virus[143] and *Bordetella pertussis*.[144]

Community-Acquired Infections

The newborn infant is susceptible to many of the infectious agents that colonize other members of the household and caregivers. The physician should consider illnesses in these contacts before discharging the infant from the hospital. If signs of an infectious disease develop after 15 to 30 days of life in an infant who was well when discharged from the nursery and whose gestation and delivery did not involve significant risk factors, the infection probably was acquired from a household or community contact. A careful history of illness in family members can suggest the source of the infant's disease (e.g., respiratory viruses, skin infections, a prolonged illness with coughing).

An infant also can be a source of infection for household contacts. The infant with congenital rubella syndrome can shed virus for many months and is a significant source of infection for susceptible close contacts. The same is true for the infant with the vesicular lesions of herpes simplex or the syphilitic infant with rhinitis or skin rash. Suppurative lesions related to *S. aureus* in a household member can expose an infant to a virulent strain that causes disseminated infection.

Infections That Indicate Underlying Abnormalities

Infection may serve as the first clue for identification of an underlying anatomic, metabolic, or immune system abnormality. Infants with galactosemia, iron overload, chronic granulomatous disease, and leukocyte adhesion defects are susceptible to certain invasive gram-negative infections. Genitourinary infection in the first months of life can point to an anatomic or a physiologic defect of the urinary tract. Similarly, otitis media in the first month of life may be an indication of a midline defect of the palate or of a eustachian tube dysfunction. Meningitis caused by non-neonatal pathogens (e.g., coagulase-negative staphylococci) can be a clue to the presence of a dermoid sinus tract to the intradural space. In infants with underlying humoral immune defects, systemic infections may not develop until passively acquired maternal antibody has dissipated. Because the half-life of IgG is about 3 weeks, such infections are likely to occur after 3 months of age.

Epidemiology

Nursery-acquired nosocomial infections can become epidemic, and a common source may be identified by simple epidemiologic investigation. Organisms that frequently are the cause of nursery epidemics include *S. aureus*, group A streptococci, enteroviruses, respiratory viruses, rotavirus, and gram-negative bacilli. Infections attributed to gram-negative bacilli often are caused by multiple antimicrobial drug–resistant strains, especially extended-spectrum β-lactamase (ESBL)–producing *E. coli* and *Klebsiella* species in nurseries where use of third-generation cephalosporins is extensive.

The most complete documentation of nursery-acquired infection was developed during the worldwide pandemic of *S. aureus* disease in the 1950s. A variety of preventive measures were attempted, including environmental manipulations, hexachlorophene bathing, and systemic antibiotics. For unknown reasons, the pandemic began to subside about 1963. These factors are discussed further in Chapter 17.

Epidemic diarrhea in the newborn infant that is associated with infection with *E. coli*, *Salmonella*, and other agents is discussed in Chapter 20. In addition, several viruses have been implicated in nursery outbreaks of gastrointestinal and respiratory diseases. They include rotaviruses, various enteroviruses (see Chapters 20 and 30), respiratory syncytial virus, parainfluenza virus, influenza virus, and adenoviruses.

Health care workers can expose neonates to or acquire an infection from neonates. Studies of the carriage of staphylococci and streptococci usually note a significant incidence in personnel. In some cases, the infections are acquired from the infants. Studies of the shedding of rubella virus and CMV in the urine and saliva of infants with congenital infections indicate that these materials are infectious for susceptible adults working in the nursery, but appropriate hand hygiene prevents transmission. Infection control is discussed in Chapter 35.

Each hospital should have an infection control program for personnel. Serologic screening of female hospital personnel for rubella antibodies should be performed at the time of employment. Vaccination is advised for nonpregnant women who are seronegative. Health care workers in nurseries should undergo serologic testing for varicella if they have no history of prior infection and should be vaccinated if they are seronegative. All hospital employees should receive the hepatitis B vaccine series and should be tested annually with a tuberculin skin test.

Diagnosis and Management

The diagnosis and management of infection acquired by the infant in the nursery or at home are similar to those of infection acquired during delivery. The management of late-onset bacterial infections is discussed in Chapters 6, 13, 14, and 17.

REFERENCES

1. U.S. Food and Drug Administration Medical Bulletin Summer:4, 1998.
2. Arias E, MacDorman MF, Strobino DM, Guyer B. Annual summary of vital statistics—2002. Pediatrics 112:1215-1230, 2003.
3. Schrag S, Gorwitz R, Fultz-Butts K, Schuchat A. Prevention of perinatal group B streptococcal disease. Revised guidelines from CDC. MMWR Recomm Rep 51:1-22, 2002.
4. Sullivan JL. Prevention of mother-to-child transmission of HIV—what next? J Acquir Immune Defic Syndr 34(Suppl 1):S67-S72, 2003.
5. Congenital syphilis—United States, 2000. MMWR Morb Mortal Wkly Rep 50:573-577, 2001.
6. Control and prevention of rubella: evaluation and management of suspected outbreaks, rubella in pregnant women, and surveillance for congenital rubella syndrome. MMWR Recomm Rep 50:1-23, 2001.
7. Mellor AL, Chandler P, Lee GK, et al. Indoleamine 2,3-dioxygenase, immunosuppression and pregnancy. J Reprod Immunol 57:143-150, 2002.
8. Xu C, Mao D, Holers VM, et al. A critical role for murine complement regulator crry in fetomaternal tolerance. Science 287:498-501, 2000.
9. Gaunt G, Ramin K. Immunological tolerance of the human fetus. Am J Perinatol 18:299-312, 2001.
10. Chaouat G, Zourbas S, Ostojic S, et al. A brief review of recent data on some cytokine expressions at the materno-foetal interface which might challenge the classical T_H1/T_H2 dichotomy. J Reprod Immunol 53:241-256, 2002.
11. Ronel DN, Klein JO, Ware KG. New acronym needed for congenital infections. Pediatr Infect Dis J 14:921, 1995.
12. Ford-Jones EL, Kellner JD. "CHEAP TORCHES": an acronym for congenital and perinatal infections. Pediatr Infect Dis J 14:638-640, 1995.
13. Chheda S, Lopez SM, Sanderson EP. Congenital brucellosis in a premature infant. Pediatr Infect Dis J 16:81-83, 1997.
14. Stein A, Raoult D. Q fever during pregnancy: a public health problem in southern France. Clin Infect Dis 27:592-596, 1998.
15. New DL, Quinn JB, Qureshi MZ, et al. Vertically transmitted babesiosis. J Pediatr 131:163-164, 1997.
16. Fujino T, Nagata Y. HTLV-I transmission from mother to child. J Reprod Immunol 47:197-206, 2000.
17. Van Dyke RB, Heneine W, Perrin ME, et al. Mother-to-child transmission of human T-lymphotropic virus type II. J Pediatr 127: 924-928, 1995.
18. Schroter M, Polywka S, Zollner B, et al. Detection of TT virus DNA and GB virus type C/hepatitis G virus RNA in serum and breast milk: determination of mother-to-child transmission. J Clin Microbiol 38:745-747, 2000.
19. Feucht HH, Zollner B, Polywka S, et al. Vertical transmission of hepatitis G. Lancet 347:615-616, 1996.
20. Adams O, Krempe C, Kogler G, et al. 1998. Congenital infections with human herpesvirus 6. J Infect Dis 178:544-546.
21. Lanari M, Papa I, Venturi V, et al. Congenital infection with human herpesvirus 6 variant B associated with neonatal seizures and poor neurological outcome. J Med Virol 70:628-632, 2003.
22. Chye JK, Lim CT, Ng KB, et al. Vertical transmission of dengue. Clin Infect Dis 25:1374-1377, 1997.
23. Overturf GD, Balfour G. Osteomyelitis and sepsis: severe complications of fetal monitoring. Pediatrics 55:244-247, 1975.
24. King-Lewis PA, Gardner SD. Congenital cytomegalic inclusion disease following intrauterine transfusion. BMJ 2:603-605, 1969.
25. Scott JM, Henderson A. Acute villous inflammation in the placenta following intrauterine transfusion. J Clin Pathol 25:872-875, 1972.
26. St Clair EH, DiLiberti JH, O'Brien ML. Observations of an infant born to a mother with botulism. Letter to the editor. J Pediatr 87:658, 1975.
27. Robin L, Herman D, Redett R. Botulism in pregnant women. N Engl J Med 335:823-824, 1996.
28. Luijckx GJ, Vles J, de Baets M, et al. Guillain-Barré syndrome in mother and newborn child. Lancet 349:27, 1997.
29. Buchwald B, de Baets M, Luijckx GJ, et al. Neonatal Guillain-Barré syndrome: blocking antibodies transmitted from mother to child. Neurology 53:1246-1253, 1999.
30. Naeye RL. Causes of the excessive rates of perinatal mortality and prematurity in pregnancies complicated by maternal urinary-tract infections. N Engl J Med 300:819-823, 1979.
31. Savage WE, Hajj SN, Kass EH. Demographic and prognostic characteristics of bacteriuria in pregnancy. Medicine (Baltimore) 46:385-407, 1967.
32. Norden CW, Kass EH. Bacteriuria of pregnancy—a critical appraisal. Annu Rev Med 19:431-470, 1968.
33. Smaill F. Antibiotics for asymptomatic bacteriuria in pregnancy. Cochrane Database Syst Rev CD000490, 2001.
34. Millar LK, Cox SM. Urinary tract infections complicating pregnancy. Infect Dis Clin North Am 11:13-26, 1997.
35. Shearer WT, Schreiner RL, Marshall RE, et al. Cytomegalovirus infection in a newborn dizygous twin. J Pediatr 81:1161-1165, 1972.
36. Stokes JH, Beerman H. Modern Clinical Syphilology: Diagnosis, Treatment, Case Study. Philadelphia, WB Saunders, 1968.
37. Ray CG, Wedgwood RJ. Neonatal listeriosis. Six case reports and a review of the literature. Pediatrics 34:378-392, 1964.
38. Marsden JP, Greenfield CRM. Inherited smallpox. Arch Dis Child 9:309, 1934.
39. Forrester RM, Lees VT, Watson GH. Rubella syndrome: escape of a twin. BMJ 5500:1403, 1966.
40. Feldman GV. Herpes zoster neonatorum. Arch Dis Child 27:126-127, 1952.
41. Wilcox AJ, Weinberg CR, O'Connor JF, et al. Incidence of early loss of pregnancy. N Engl J Med 319:189-194, 1988.
42. Brabin BJ. Epidemiology of infection in pregnancy. Rev Infect Dis 7:579-603, 1985.
43. Hillier SL, Witkin SS, Krohn MA, et al. The relationship of amniotic fluid cytokines and preterm delivery, amniotic fluid infection, histologic chorioamnionitis, and chorioamnion infection. Obstet Gynecol 81:941-948, 1993.
44. Hitti J, Riley DE, Krohn MA, et al. Broad-spectrum bacterial rDNA polymerase chain reaction assay for detecting amniotic fluid infection among women in premature labor. Clin Infect Dis 24:1228-1232, 1997.
45. Romero R, Yoon BH, Mazor et al. The diagnostic and prognostic value of amniotic fluid white blood cell count, glucose, interleukin-6, and Gram stain in patients with preterm labor and intact membranes. Am J Obstet Gynecol 169:805-816, 1993.
46. Romero R, Yoon BH, Mazor M, et al. A comparative study of the diagnostic performance of amniotic fluid glucose, white blood cell count, interleukin-6, and Gram stain in the detection of microbial invasion in patients with preterm premature rupture of membranes. Am J Obstet Gynecol 169:839-851, 1993.

47. Roper EC, Konje JC, De Chazal RC, et al. Genetic amniocentesis: gestation-specific pregnancy outcome and comparison of outcome following early and traditional amniocentesis. Prenat Diagn 19: 803-807, 1999.
48. Jacobsson B, Mattsby-Baltzer I, Andersch B, et al. Microbial invasion and cytokine response in amniotic fluid in a Swedish population of women in preterm labor. Acta Obstet Gynecol Scand 82:120-128, 2003.
49. El-Bastawissi AY, Williams MA, Riley DE, et al. Amniotic fluid interleukin-6 and preterm delivery: a review. Obstet Gynecol 95: 1056-1064, 2000.
50. Naeye RL, Blanc W. Pathogenesis of congenital rubella. JAMA 194: 1277-1283, 1965.
51. Naeye RL. Cytomegalic inclusion disease. The fetal disorder. Am J Clin Pathol 47:738-744, 1967.
52. Naeye RL, Kelly JA. Judgment of fetal age. 3. The pathologist's evaluation. Pediatr Clin North Am 13:849-862, 1966.
53. Naeye RL. Infants of prolonged gestation. A necropsy study. Arch Pathol 84:37-41, 1967.
54. Allison AC, Paton GR. Chromosomal abnormalities in human diploid cells infected with mycoplasma and their possible relevance to the aetiology of Down's syndrome (mongolism). Lancet 2:1229-1230, 1966.
55. Nichols WW. The role of viruses in the etiology of chromosomal abnormalities. Am J Hum Genet 18:81-92, 1966.
56. Nusbacher J, Hirschhorn K, Cooper LZ. Chromosomal abnormalities in congenital rubella. N Engl J Med 276:1409-1413, 1967.
57. Congenital malaria in children of refugees—Washington, Massachusetts, Kentucky. MMWR Morb Mortal Wkly Rep 30:53-55, 1981.
58. Nesheim S, Palumbo P, Sullivan K, et al. Quantitative RNA testing for diagnosis of HIV-infected infants. J Acquir Immune Defic Syndr 32: 192-195, 2003.
59. Balasubramanian R, Lagakos SW. Estimation of the timing of perinatal transmission of HIV. Biometrics 57:1048-1058, 2001.
60. Townsend JJ, Baringer JR, Wolinsky JS, et al. Progressive rubella panencephalitis. Late onset after congenital rubella. N Engl J Med 292: 990-993, 1975.
61. Weil ML, Itabashi H, Cremer NE, et al. Chronic progressive panencephalitis due to rubella virus simulating subacute sclerosing panencephalitis. N Engl J Med 292:994-998, 1975.
62. Donders GG, Van Lierde S, Van Elsacker-Niele AM, et al. Survival after intrauterine parvovirus B19 infection with persistence in early infancy: a two-year follow-up. Pediatr Infect Dis J 13:234-236, 1994.
63. Miller E, Cradock-Watson JE, Pollock TM. Consequences of confirmed maternal rubella at successive stages of pregnancy. Lancet 2:781-784, 1982.
64. Desmonts G, Couvreur J. Congenital toxoplasmosis: a prospective study of the offspring of 542 women who acquired toxoplasmosis during pregnancy. Pathophysiology of congenital disease. *In* Thalhammer O, Baumgarten K, Pollack A (eds). Perinatal Medicine, Sixth European Congress. Stuttgart: Georg Thieme, 1979, pp 51-60.
65. Fowler KB, Stagno S, Pass RF, et al. The outcome of congenital cytomegalovirus infection in relation to maternal antibody status. N Engl J Med 326:663-667, 1992.
66. Stagno S, Whitley RJ. Herpesvirus infections of pregnancy. Part I: Cytomegalovirus and Epstein-Barr virus infections. N Engl J Med 313:1270-1274, 1985.
67. Roongpisuthipong A, Siriwasin W, Simonds RJ, et al. HIV seroconversion during pregnancy and risk for mother-to-infant transmission. J Acquir Immune Defic Syndr 26:348-351, 2001.
68. Green DM, Reid SM, Rhaney K. Generalised vaccinia in the human foetus. Lancet 1:1296-1298, 1966.
69. Sharma R, Jagdev DK. Congenital smallpox. Scand J Infect Dis 3: 245-247, 1971.
70. Eilard T, Strannegard O. Rubella reinfection in pregnancy followed by transmission to the fetus. J Infect Dis 129:594-596, 1974.
71. Harvey B, Remington JS, Sulzer AJ. IgM malaria antibodies in a case of congenital malaria in the United States. Lancet 1:333-335, 1969.
72. Nelson NA, Struve VR. Prevention of congenital syphilis by treatment of syphilis in pregnancy. JAMA 161:869-872, 1956.
73. Zuckerman AJ, Taylor PE. Persistence of the serum hepatitis (SH-Australia) antigen for many years. Nature 223:81-82, 1969.
74. Nahmias AJ, Alford CA, Korones SB. Infection of the newborn with herpesvirus hominis. Adv Pediatr 17:185-226, 1970.
75. Desmonts G, Couvreur J, Thulliez P. [Congenital toxoplasmosis. 5 cases of mother-to-child transmission of pre-pregnancy infection.] Presse Med 19:1445-1449, 1990.
76. Vogel N, Kirisits M, Michael E, et al. Congenital toxoplasmosis transmitted from an immunologically competent mother infected before conception. Clin Infect Dis 23:1055-1060, 1996.
77. Hepatitis B virus: a comprehensive strategy for eliminating transmission in the United States through universal childhood vaccination. Recommendations of the Immunization Practices Advisory Committee (ACIP). MMWR Recomm Rep 40:1-25, 1991.
78. Pickering LK (ed). Red Book: Report of the Committee on Infectious Diseases. Elk Grove Village, Ill, American Academy of Pediatrics, 2003.
79. Daffos F, Capella-Pavlovsky M, Forestier F. Fetal blood sampling via the umbilical cord using a needle guided by ultrasound. Report of 66 cases. Prenat Diagn 3:271-277, 1983.
80. Daffos F, Forestier F, Grangeot-Keros L, et al. Prenatal diagnosis of congenital rubella. Lancet 2:1-3, 1984.
81. Daffos F, Forestier F, Capella-Pavlovsky M, et al. Prenatal management of 746 pregnancies at risk for congenital toxoplasmosis. N Engl J Med 318:271-275, 1988.
82. Hohlfeld P, Vial Y, Maillard-Brignon C, et al. Cytomegalovirus fetal infection: prenatal diagnosis. Obstet Gynecol 78:615-618, 1991.
83. Grangeot-Keros L, Pillot J, Daffos F et al. Prenatal and postnatal production of IgM and IgA antibodies to rubella virus studied by antibody capture immunoassay. J Infect Dis 158:138-143, 1988.
84. Hanson FW, Happ RL, Tennant FR, et al. Ultrasonography-guided early amniocentesis in singleton pregnancies. Am J Obstet Gynecol 162: 1376-1381, 1990.
85. Ghidini A, Sepulveda W, Lockwood CJ, et al. Complications of fetal blood sampling. Am J Obstet Gynecol 168:1339-1344, 1993.
86. Skvorc-Ranko R, Lavoie H, St-Denis P, et al. Intrauterine diagnosis of cytomegalovirus and rubella infections by amniocentesis. CMAJ 145:649-654, 1991.
87. Papaevangelou G, Kremastinou T, Prevedourakis C, et al. Hepatitis B antigen and antibody in maternal blood, cord blood, and amniotic fluid. Arch Dis Child 49:936-939, 1974.
88. Torok TJ, Wang QY, Gary GW Jr, et al. Prenatal diagnosis of intrauterine infection with parvovirus B19 by the polymerase chain reaction technique. Clin Infect Dis 14:149-155, 1992.
89. Wattre P, Dewilde A, Subtil D, et al. A clinical and epidemiological study of human parvovirus B19 infection in fetal hydrops using PCR Southern blot hybridization and chemiluminescence detection. J Med Virol 54:140-144, 1998.
90. Lazzarotto T, Varani S, Guerra B, et al. Prenatal indicators of congenital cytomegalovirus infection. J Pediatr 137:90-95, 2000.
91. Lazzarotto T, Gabrielli L, Foschini MP, et al. Congenital cytomegalovirus infection in twin pregnancies: viral load in the amniotic fluid and pregnancy outcome. Pediatrics 112:153-157, 2003.
92. Revello MG, Sarasini A, Zavattoni M, et al. Improved prenatal diagnosis of congenital human cytomegalovirus infection by a modified nested polymerase chain reaction. J Med Virol 56:99-103, 1998.
93. Hohlfeld P, Daffos F, Costa JM, et al. Prenatal diagnosis of congenital toxoplasmosis with a polymerase-chain-reaction test on amniotic fluid. N Engl J Med 331:695-699, 1994.
94. Romand S, Wallon M, Franck J, et al. Prenatal diagnosis using polymerase chain reaction on amniotic fluid for congenital toxoplasmosis. Obstet Gynecol 97:296-300, 2001.
95. Bosma TJ, Corbett KM, Eckstein MB, et al. Use of PCR for prenatal and postnatal diagnosis of congenital rubella. J Clin Microbiol 33:2881-2887, 1995.
96. Gay-Andrieu F, Marty P, Pialat J, et al. Fetal toxoplasmosis and negative amniocentesis: necessity of an ultrasound follow-up. Prenat Diagn 23:558-560, 2003.
97. Enders G, Bader U, Lindemann L, et al. Prenatal diagnosis of congenital cytomegalovirus infection in 189 pregnancies with known outcome. Prenat Diagn 21:362-377, 2001.
98. Fox H. Pathology of the Placenta. Philadelphia, WB Saunders, 1978.
99. Liesenfeld O, Montoya JG, Kinney S, et al. Effect of testing for IgG avidity in the diagnosis of *Toxoplasma gondii* infection in pregnant women: experience in a U.S. reference laboratory. J Infect Dis 183: 1248-1253, 2001.
100. Nigro G, Anceschi MM, Cosmi EV. Clinical manifestations and abnormal laboratory findings in pregnant women with primary cytomegalovirus infection. Br J Obstet Gynecol 110:572-577, 2003.
101. Revello MG, Gerna G. Diagnosis and management of human cytomegalovirus infection in the mother, fetus, and newborn infant. Clin Microbiol Rev 15:680-715, 2002.

102. Tang JW, Aarons E, Hesketh LM, et al. Prenatal diagnosis of congenital rubella infection in the second trimester of pregnancy. Prenat Diagn 23:509-512, 2003.
103. Gutierrez J, Rodriguez MJ, De Ory F, et al. Reliability of low-avidity IgG and of IgA in the diagnosis of primary infection by rubella virus with adaptation of a commercial test. J Clin Lab Anal 13:1-4, 1999.
104. Revised recommendations for HIV screening of pregnant women. MMWR Recomm Rep 50:63-85, 2001 (quiz CE61-19a62–CE66-19a62).
105. Mussi-Pinhata MM, Yamamoto AY, Figueiredo LT, et al. Congenital and perinatal cytomegalovirus infection in infants born to mothers infected with human immunodeficiency virus. J Pediatr 132:285-290, 1998.
106. Thomas DL, Villano SA, Riester KA, et al. Perinatal transmission of hepatitis C virus from human immunodeficiency virus type 1-infected mothers. Women and Infants Transmission Study. J Infect Dis 177: 1480-1488, 1998.
107. Immunization during pregnancy. ACOG Technical Bulletin, vol. 64. Washington, DC, American College of Obstetrics and Gynecology, 1982.
108. Centers for Disease Control and Prevention. Prevention and control of influenza. Recommendations of the Advisory Committee on Immunization Practices. MMWR Recomm Rep 50(RR-4):1-44, 2001.
109. Tsai TF, Paul R, Lynberg MC, Letson GW. Congenital yellow fever virus infection after immunization in pregnancy (see comments). J Infect Dis 168:1520-1523, 1993.
110. Connor EM, Sperling RS, Gelber R, et al. Reduction of maternal-infant transmission of human immunodeficiency virus type 1 with zidovudine treatment. Pediatric AIDS Clinical Trials Group Protocol 076 Study Group. N Engl J Med 331:1173-1180, 1994.
111. Jackson JB, Musoke P, Fleming T, et al. Intrapartum and neonatal single-dose nevirapine compared with zidovudine for prevention of mother-to-child transmission of HIV-1 in Kampala, Uganda: HIVNET 012 randomised trial. Lancet 354:795-802, 2003.
112. Stoll BJ, Hansen N, Fanaroff AA, et al. Late-onset sepsis in very low birth weight neonates: the experience of the NICHD neonatal research network. Pediatrics 110:285-291, 2002.
113. Rosebury T. Microorganisms Indigenous to Man. New York, McGraw-Hill, 1962.
114. Gorbach SL, Menda KB, Thadepalli H, Keith L. Anaerobic microflora of the cervix in healthy women. Am J Obstet Gynecol 117:1053-1055, 1973.
115. Srugo I, Wittek AE, Israele V, Brunell PA. Meningoencephalitis in a neonate congenitally infected with human immunodeficiency virus type 1. J Pediatr 120:93-95, 1992.
116. Edwards MS, Baker CJ. Bacterial infections in the neonate. *In* Long SS, Pickering LK, Prober CG (eds). Principles and Practice of Pediatric Infectious Diseases. Philadelphia, Churchill Livingstone, 2002.
117. Fernandez M, Hickman ME, Baker CJ. Antimicrobial susceptibilities of group B streptococci isolated between 1992 and 1996 from patients with bacteremia or meningitis. Antimicrob Agents Chemother 42:1517-1519, 1998.
118. Biedenbach DJ, Stephen JM, Jones RN. Antimicrobial susceptibility profile among β-haemolytic *Streptococcus* spp. Collected in SENTRY antimicrobial surveillance program—North America, 2001. Diagn Microb Infect Dis 46:291-294, 2003.
119. Whitley RJ, Cloud G, Gruber W, et al. Ganciclovir treatment of symptomatic congenital cytomegalovirus infection: results of a phase II study. National Institute of Allergy and Infectious Diseases Collaborative Antiviral Study Group. J Infect Dis 175:1080-1086, 1997.
120. Kimberlin DW, Lin CY, Sanchez PJ, et al. Effect of ganciclovir therapy on hearing in symptomatic congenital cytomegalovirus disease involving the central nervous system: a randomized, controlled trial. J Pediatr 98:16-25, 2003.
121. Baker CJ, Melish ME, Hall RT, et al. Intravenous immune globulin for the prevention of nosocomial infection in low-birth-weight neonates. The Multicenter Group for the Study of Immune Globulin in Neonates. N Engl J Med 327:213-219, 1992 (see comments).
122. Fanaroff AA, Korones SB, Wright LB, et al. A controlled trial of intravenous immune globulin to reduce nosocomial infections in very-low-birth-weight infants. N Engl J Med 330:1107-1113, 1994.
123. American Academy of Pediatrics Committee on Infectious Diseases. Universal hepatitis B immunization. Pediatrics 89:795-800, 1992.
124. Boyer KM, Gadzala CA, Burd LI, et al. Selective intrapartum chemoprophylaxis of neonatal group B streptococcal early-onset disease. I. Epidemiologic rationale. J Infect Dis 148:795-801, 1983.
125. American Academy of Pediatrics Committee on Infectious Diseases and Committee on Fetus and Newborn. Guidelines for prevention of group B streptococcal (GBS) infection by chemoprophylaxis. Pediatrics 90:775-778, 1992.
126. MacAulay MA, Abou-Sabe M, Charles D. Placental transfer of ampicillin. Am J Obstet Gynecol 96:943-950, 1966.
127. Brozanski BS, Jones JG, Krohn MA, et al. Effect of a screening-based prevention policy on prevalence of early-onset group B streptococcal sepsis. Obstet Gynecol 95:496-501, 2000.
128. Moisiuk SE, Robson D, Klass L, et al. Outbreak of parainfluenza virus type 3 in an intermediate care neonatal nursery. Pediatr Infect Dis J 17:49-53, 1998.
129. Knittle MA, Eitzman DV, Baer H. Role of hand contamination of personnel in the epidemiology of gram-negative nosocomial infections. J Pediatr 86:433-437, 1975.
130. Nagamine M, Nakashima Y, Uemura S, et al. DNA amplification of human T lymphotropic virus type I (HTLV-I) proviral DNA in breast milk of HTLV-I carriers. Letter to the editor. J Infect Dis 164: 1024-1025, 1991.
131. Heneine W, Woods T, Green D, et al. Detection of HTLV-II in breastmilk of HTLV-II infected mothers. Letter to the editor. Lancet 340:1157-1158, 1992.
132. Dunn DT, Newell ML, Ades AE, Peckham CS. Risk of human immunodeficiency virus type 1 transmission through breastfeeding (see comments). Lancet 340:585-588, 1992.
133. World Health Organization. Breast feeding/breast milk and human immunodeficiency virus (HIV). Wkly Epidemiol Rec 33:245, 1987.
134. American Academy of Pediatrics Work Group on Breastfeeding. Breastfeeding and the use of human milk. Pediatrics 100:1035-1039, 1997.
135. Altman LK. AIDS brings a shift on breast-feeding. The New York Times, 1998, pp 1 and 6.
136. Svabic-Vlahovic M, Pantic D, Pavicic M, Bryner JH. Transmission of *Listeria monocytogenes* from mother's milk to her baby and to puppies. Letter to the editor. Lancet 2:1201, 1988.
137. Klein JO. From harmless commensal to invasive pathogen—coagulase-negative staphylococci. N Engl J Med 323:339-340, 1990 (editorial; comment).
138. Brown J, Froese-Fretz A, Luckey D, Todd JK. High rate of hand contamination and low rate of hand washing before infant contact in a neonatal intensive care unit. Pediatr Infect Dis J 15:908-910, 1996.
139. Liu LL, Clemens CJ, Shay DK, et al. The safety of newborn early discharge. The Washington State experience. JAMA 278:293-298, 1997 (see comments) [published erratum appears in JAMA 278:2067, 1997].
140. Englund JA, Glezen WP. Maternal immunization with *Haemophilus influenzae* type b vaccines in different populations. Vaccine 21: 3455-3459, 2003.
141. Lehmann D, Pomat WS, Riley ID, et al. Studies of maternal immunization with pneumococcal polysaccharide vaccine in Papua New Guinea. Vaccine 21:3446-3450, 2003.
142. Baker CJ, Rench MA, McInnes P. Immunization of pregnant women with group B streptococcal type III capsular polysaccharide–tetanus toxoid conjugate vaccine. Vaccine 21:3469-3472, 2003.
143. Munoz FM, Piedra PA, Glezen WP. Safety and immunogenicity of respiratory syncytial virus purified fusion protein-2 vaccine in pregnant women. Vaccine 21:3465-3467, 2003.
144. Healy CM, Munoz FM, Rench MA, et al. Prevalence of pertussis antibodies in maternal delivery, cord and infant serum. J Infect Dis 190:335-340, 2004.

Chapter 2

NEONATAL INFECTIONS: A GLOBAL PERSPECTIVE

Barbara J. Stoll

One of the greatest challenges to global public health is to eliminate the gaps between rich and poor countries in health care resources, in access to preventive and curative services, and in health outcomes. Although infant mortality has declined by more than 50% since 1955,[1] neonatal mortality has changed little in some of the world's poorest countries. Worldwide, neonatal mortality accounts for a substantial proportion of deaths of both infants and children younger than 5 years.[1-3] The World Health Organization (WHO) estimates that more than 4 million neonates die each year and that 98% of these deaths occur in developing countries.[2,3] Causes of neonatal mortality, especially in developing countries, are difficult to ascertain, partly because many of these deaths occur at home, unattended by medical personnel, and partly because critically ill neonates often present with nondiagnostic signs and symptoms of disease. Infectious diseases, birth asphyxia, and complications of prematurity are thought to be the major causes of neonatal death worldwide.[2-5]

Although access to sophisticated technology is limited in developing countries, neonatal mortality related to infection could be substantially reduced by simple, known interventions before and during pregnancy, labor, and delivery; in the immediate postpartum period; and in the early days of life.[2,3,5,6] The global burden of infectious diseases in the newborn, direct and indirect causes of neonatal mortality attributed to infection, specific infections of relevance in developing countries, and strategies to reduce both the incidence of neonatal infection and morbidity and mortality in infants who do become infected are reviewed in this chapter.

BACKGROUND AND GENERAL CONSIDERATIONS

Infection as a Cause of Neonatal Death: Hospital- and Community-Based Studies

In developing countries, where most births and neonatal deaths occur at home and are not attended by doctors or other trained health care workers, deaths are underreported and information on cause of death is often incomplete. Accurate data on causes of death are useful for many reasons. Such data are important for providers of primary care, for investigators as they design interventions for prevention and treatment, for local and national health administrators, and for decision makers who implement and evaluate health care programs.

To evaluate the impact of infection as a cause of neonatal death, hospital- and community-based studies from developing countries (in Africa, Asia, the Indian subcontinent, the Pacific, the Middle East, and the Americas) that report neonatal mortality rates and present data on infection as a cause of death were reviewed. Neonatal deaths are defined as deaths among liveborn infants during the first 28 days of life, and the neonatal mortality rate (NMR) is reported per 1000 livebirths.[7] Early neonatal deaths are those that occur in the first week of life, and late neonatal deaths are those that occur between 8 and 28 days of life. Infections associated with neonatal death in these studies included bacterial sepsis and meningitis, respiratory infection, neonatal tetanus, omphalitis, and diarrhea.

Twenty-nine hospital-based studies published from 1980 onward were reviewed.[5,8-36] Epidemiologic studies varied in size, ranging from approximately 1000 to more than 100,000 livebirths and approximately 50 to 800 neonatal deaths. Data on infection as a cause of early neonatal death were presented in 17 of 29 studies; infection was associated with 7% to 54% of early neonatal deaths in these studies. Five studies reported data on infection as a cause of late neonatal death: 30% to 73% of these late deaths were associated with infection. Eighteen of the 29 studies presented data on infection as a cause of neonatal deaths overall (birth to 28 days). In these studies, infection was associated with 4% to 56% of all neonatal deaths.

Thirty-six community-based studies were reviewed.[37-74] Total population in each study ranged from several thousand to 60 million people, number of births ranged from under 1000 to more than 1 million, and number of neonatal deaths ranged from 7 to approximately 7000. Thirteen of the 36 studies presented data on infection as a cause of early neonatal death: 0% to 45% of early neonatal deaths were associated with infection. Seven community studies reported numbers of infections responsible for late neonatal deaths: 44% to 100% of late neonatal deaths were associated with infection. Thirty-one of the 36 studies presented data on infection as a cause of all neonatal deaths. Infection was associated with 8% to 85% of all deaths in these studies.

It is well known that neonatal deaths in developing countries are underreported and that infection as a cause of death is underestimated because of imprecision in diagnosis. Remarkably few published studies worldwide present detailed surveillance data on numbers of births and neonatal deaths and on probable causes of death. Although hospital-based studies are important for accurately determining causes of morbidity and mortality, they do not always reflect what is happening in the community. Carefully conducted community studies are needed. Furthermore, in many parts of the developing world, neonatal deaths are underestimated owing to inadequate vital registration, especially of home births. If a child dies before the birth has been reported, there is a good chance that neither the birth nor the death will be recorded. If we estimate that 30% to 40% of neonatal deaths are associated with infections and use the WHO 2001 estimate of 4,035,000 neonatal deaths per year in the less developed regions of the world,[3] we can estimate that infection is responsible for between 1.2 and 1.6 million neonatal deaths per year, or between 3300 and 4500 deaths per day in the less developed countries of the world.

Incidence of Neonatal Sepsis and Meningitis and Associated Mortality

Hospital-based studies from developing countries were reviewed to determine the incidence of neonatal sepsis and meningitis, the case-fatality rates (CFRs) associated with these infections, and the spectrum of bacterial pathogens in different regions of the world. Cases reported occurred among infants born in hospitals, as well as those referred from home or other health facilities. Fifty-three studies[11,75-126] from developing countries, published between 1980 and 2000, were reviewed to evaluate neonatal sepsis and meningitis in different geographic regions. Forty of these studies are primarily reports of neonatal sepsis, and 16 studies present data on bacterial meningitis. The vast majority of studies do not distinguish among maternally acquired, community-acquired, and nosocomial infections. Table 2-1 summarizes data by region.

In all regions, sepsis was responsible for a substantial burden of disease, with high CFRs reported in the vast majority of studies. Overall, incidence of neonatal sepsis ranged from 2 to 21 per 1000 livebirths (average 6 per 1000 livebirths), with CFRs of 1% to 69%. Of note, only two studies reported CFRs under 10%, whereas a majority of the studies reported sepsis CFRs above 30%. Fewer studies on neonatal meningitis were available from which to present incidence and CFRs by region. The incidence of neonatal meningitis ranged from 0.33 to 2.8 per 1000 livebirths (average 1 per 1000 livebirths), with CFRs ranging from 13% to 59% in these reports. Using these hospital-based rates and recent United Nations estimates of approximately 132,787,000 births per year in the less developed countries of the world,[127] we estimate that approximately 800,000 cases of neonatal sepsis and 130,000 cases of neonatal meningitis occur in developing

Table 2–1 Incidence and Case Fatality Rate (CFR) for Sepsis and Meningitis from Hospital-Based Studies in Developing Countries

Region	Incidence of Sepsis (case[s] per 1000 live births)	CFR (%)	Incidence of meningitis (case[s] per 1000 live births)	CFR (%)
India/Pakistan/Southeast Asia/Pacific	2.4-16	2-69	—	45
Sub-Saharan Africa	6-21	27-56	0.7-1.9	18-59
Middle East/North Africa	1.8-12	13-45	0.33-1.5	16-32
Americas/Caribbean	2-9	1-31	0.4-2.8	13-35

Data updated from Stoll BJ. The global impact of neonatal infection. Clin Perinatol 24:1, 1997.

Table 2–2 Organisms Associated with Sepsis and Meningitis in Developing Countries

	Organisms Associated with Sepsis		Organisms Associated with Meningitis	
Region	*% Gram-Negative*	*% GBS*	*% Gram-Negative*	*% GBS*
India/Pakistan/Southeast Asia/Pacific	21-85	0-5	22-100	0-15
Sub-Saharan Africa	16-68	0-30	22-77	0-61
Middle East/North Africa	25-98	0-24	20-87	0-70
Americas/Caribbean	31-71	2-37	33-63	3-56

GBS, group B streptococcus.
Data updated from Stoll BJ. The global impact of neonatal infection. Clin Perinatol 24:1, 1997.

countries each year. Because the vast majority of neonates in developing countries are born at home and because many lack access to medical care if they become ill, these numbers are undoubtedly a gross underestimate of the true numbers of these infections. The high CFRs for both sepsis and meningitis (compared with those in developed countries) suggest that early detection and improved management of infected neonates would reduce mortality.

Bacterial Pathogens Associated with Infections in Different Geographic Regions

Historical reviews from developed countries have demonstrated that the predominant organisms responsible for neonatal infections change over time.[128,129] Prospective microbiologic surveillance is therefore important to guide empirical therapy, to identify new agents of importance for neonates, to recognize epidemics, and to monitor changes over time. Moreover, the organisms associated with neonatal infection are different in different geographic areas, reinforcing the need for local microbiologic surveillance. In areas where blood cultures in sick neonates cannot be performed, knowledge of the bacterial flora of the maternal genital tract may serve as a surrogate marker for organisms causing early-onset neonatal sepsis, meningitis, and pneumonia. The vast majority of studies on the causes of neonatal sepsis and meningitis are hospital reviews that include data on infants born in hospitals as well as those transferred from home or other facilities. Sixty-five studies published between 1980 and 2003 were reviewed to determine the spectrum of bacterial pathogens responsible for neonatal sepsis and meningitis in developing countries and to compare these pathogens with the organisms prevalent in the developed world.* In most of these studies, it is difficult to determine whether infections were of maternal origin or were hospital or community acquired. Also, the infants' ages at the time of infection are not always specified. The studies vary in the detail with which culture methods are presented. It is therefore difficult to judge the quality and reliability of the microbiologic data presented.

Fifty-four studies present data on bacterial sepsis.† The spectrum of organisms presented in these studies does indeed differ from what is known from developed countries. Although the group B streptococcus (GBS) remains the most important bacterial pathogen associated with early-onset neonatal sepsis in many developed countries,[150] studies from developing countries present a different picture (Table 2-2). The most striking finding from the 23 studies from India, Pakistan, Asia, and the Pacific is the low rate of GBS sepsis.* Half of these studies, summarizing data from more than 1000 patients with positive blood cultures, report no isolates of GBS, and the other studies report 67 cases among 4525 infected neonates (1.5%). Gram-negative organisms were isolated significantly more frequently than gram-positive organisms, with *Klebsiella* being the most frequently isolated pathogen in half of the studies. Fourteen studies present data from sub-Saharan Africa.† Again, group B streptococci were uncommon, isolated in only 8% of the 1529 patients with bacteremia. However, in three studies, group B streptococci were the most common agents found.[9,11,90] In half of the studies, *Staphylococcus aureus* was the most frequently isolated agent.

Overall, there was an almost equal distribution of gram-negative and gram-positive infections. Among 11 of 12 studies from the Middle East or North Africa,‡ GBS infection also was uncommon (48 of 1216 [4%]), with only one study reporting group B streptococci in a substantial number of infected neonates (25 of 106 [24%]).[93] Gram-negative organisms were somewhat more likely to be associated with sepsis in these studies. The five studies from the Americas[98,118,135,138,139] present a varying range of gram-negative and gram-positive pathogens. The two largest of these studies, from Mexico[138] and Panama,[98] identified only 18 of 804 (2%) infants with GBS, whereas a study from the French West Indies reported 40 of 107 (37%) septic neonates infected with GBS.[106]

Table 2-2 summarizes data from 19 studies of bacterial meningitis in developing countries.§ Among 721 culture-confirmed cases, 470 (65%) were caused by gram-negative pathogens. Group B streptococci were uncommon in a majority of the studies.

World Health Organization Young Infant Study

A multicenter project to determine the bacterial etiology and clinical signs of serious infections in infants younger than 90

*See references 9, 11, 75-78, 80-88, 90-112, 114, 115, 118, 120-123, 130-149.
†See references 9, 11, 77, 78, 81, 82, 84, 86, 90-95, 97-100,102-112, 114, 115, 118, 120-122, 130-133, 135-149.

*See references 81, 82, 84, 92, 95, 97, 99, 106, 108, 109, 111, 112, 114, 129, 132, 140-144.
†See references 9, 11, 77, 90, 100, 104, 105, 110, 115, 130, 136, 137, 145, 148.
‡See references 86, 91, 93, 94, 102, 103, 107, 120-122, 133, 146.
§See references 75, 76, 80, 83, 85, 87, 88, 93, 96, 98, 101, 115, 121-124, 134, 140, 143.

days was sponsored by WHO and conducted between 1990 and 1992 in four developing countries: Ethiopia, The Gambia, Papua New Guinea, and the Philippines.[115,143,144,151-155] This is the largest prospective study to date of early infant infections in developing countries. In the four different countries, 2453 sick young infants had blood cultures performed and 507 had lumbar punctures. Seven percent (167 of 2453 cases) of all blood cultures were positive: 10% in The Gambia, 9% in Ethiopia, 5% in Papua New Guinea, and 4% in the Philippines. Eight percent (40 of 507) of all cerebrospinal fluid cultures were positive. As might have been predicted, clinical symptoms were not helpful in distinguishing among infections caused by different pathogens. Overall, 30% of infants with positive blood cultures died. Serious infection was most common in the first week of life, with a majority of the deaths occurring in infants younger than 1 week of age.

A total of 1673 infants were evaluated in the first 4 weeks of life. Of these patients, 5% had positive blood cultures; 57% had gram-positive organisms, and 43% had gram-negative organisms. The most frequently isolated organisms were *S. aureus* (23%), *Streptococcus pyogenes* (20%), *Escherichia coli* (18%), and *Streptococcus pneumoniae* (10%). The virtual absence of GBS in this large study in four countries is striking (present in only 2 of 84 positive blood cultures). Nineteen patients had neonatal meningitis (11 had bacteremia as well); 63% of these were due to gram-negative organisms and 37% to gram-positive organisms. The most frequent isolates were *S. pneumoniae* (in 5 of 19 [26%]) and *E. coli* (in 4 of 19 [21%]). Only one neonate had GBS meningitis. Of interest, *S. pneumoniae* was the most frequent organism isolated in the second and third months of life, accounting for 30% (25 of 83) of all positive blood cultures and 55% (12 of 22) of all positive cerebrospinal fluid cultures. An important conclusion of this study is that the pneumococcus must be considered in any case of serious infection in a young infant in a developing country, particularly if signs of meningitis are present.

Group B Streptococcal Infections

It is unclear why neonates in some developing countries are rarely infected with GBS. The most important risk factor for invasive GBS disease in the neonate is exposure to the organism via the mother's genital tract. Other known risk factors include young maternal age, preterm birth, prolonged rupture of the membranes, maternal chorioamnionitis, exposure to a high inoculum of a virulent GBS strain, and a low maternal serum concentration of antibody to the capsular polysaccharide of the colonizing GBS strain.[156] In the United States, differences in GBS colonization rates have been identified among women of different ethnic groups that appear to correlate with infection in newborns. In an attempt to understand the low rates of invasive GBS disease reported among neonates in many developing countries, Stoll and Schuchat[157] reviewed 34 studies published between 1980 and 1998 that evaluated GBS colonization rates in women. These studies reported culture results from 7730 women, with an overall colonization rate of 12.7%. Studies that used culture methods that were judged to be appropriate found significantly higher colonization rates than those that used inadequate methods (675 of 3801 women [17.8%] versus 308 of 3929 [7.8%]). When analyses were restricted to studies with adequate methods, the prevalence of colonization by region was Middle East/North Africa, 22%; Asia/Pacific, 19%; sub-Saharan Africa, 19%; India/Pakistan, 12%; and Americas, 14%.

The distribution of GBS serotypes varied among studies. GBS serotype III, the most frequently identified invasive serotype in the West, was identified in all studies reviewed and was the most frequently identified serotype in one half of the studies. Serotype V, which has only recently been recognized as a cause of invasive disease in developed countries,[158] was identified in studies from Peru[159] and The Gambia.[160] Monitoring serotype distribution is important because candidate GBS vaccines are considered for areas with high rates of disease.

With estimated colonization rates among women in developing countries as high as 18%, higher rates of invasive neonatal disease than have been reported would be expected. Low rates of invasive GBS disease in some developing countries may be explained by less virulent strains, by genetic differences in susceptibility to disease, by as-yet unidentified beneficial cultural practices, or by high concentrations of transplacentally acquired protective antibody in serum (i.e., a mother may be colonized yet have protective concentrations of type-specific GBS antibody).

Hospital-based surveillance in developing countries may be insensitive at detecting sepsis in very young infants. In developing countries, where most deliveries occur at home, infants with early-onset sepsis often get sick and die at home or are taken to local health care facilities, where a diagnosis of possible sepsis may be missed, or where blood cultures cannot be performed. In this setting there may be underdiagnosis of infection by early-onset pathogens, including GBS. In the WHO Young Infant Study,[151] 1673 infants were evaluated in the first month of life; only 2 had cultures positive for GBS. The absence of GBS in this study cannot be explained by the evaluation of insufficient numbers of sick neonates (360 of the1673 infants were younger than 1 week of age).

Increasing evidence suggests that heavy colonization with GBS increases the risk of delivering a preterm low-birth-weight (LBW) infant.[161] Population differences in the prevalence of heavy GBS colonization have been reported in the United States, where African Americans have a significantly higher risk of heavy colonization. If heavy colonization is more prevalent among women in developing countries and results in an increase in numbers of preterm LBW infants, GBS-related morbidity may appear as illness and death related to prematurity. By contrast, heavy colonization could increase maternal type-specific GBS antibody concentrations, resulting in lower risk of neonatal disease. Further studies in developing countries are needed to explore these important issues.

Antibiotic Therapy

Studies of bacterial etiology have implications for presumptive antibiotic therapy of bacterial infection in neonates. Currently, the drugs most frequently used to treat suspected severe neonatal infections, in both developed and developing countries, are a combination of penicillin or ampicillin and an aminoglycoside (usually gentamicin).[162] Antibiotic therapy must be tailored to the specific microbiologic needs of a particular geographic region based on local surveillance data, especially if blood cultures are not performed and cannot be used to guide therapy. In addition, issues related to drug supply, availability, quality, and cost must be addressed. The problem of antibiotic resistance is now recognized to be a global problem, and the emergence of antibiotic-resistant pathogens is particularly alarming in developing countries. Although the extent of the problem is unknown, hospital-based studies on the bacterial etiology of neonatal sepsis and reports of nosocomial outbreaks from a variety of countries demonstrate that antibiotic resistance is a problem among neonates in developing countries.[122,145,163-165] The widespread availability of antibiotics and their indiscriminate and inappropriate use contribute to this problem. The possibility of resistance must be considered in infants who deteriorate despite recommended antibiotic therapy.

ACUTE RESPIRATORY INFECTIONS

The WHO estimated in 1994 that almost 800,000 deaths due to acute respiratory infections (ARIs) occur in neonates in developing countries each year.[4,166] Among young infants, most of these deaths are due to pneumonia, bronchiolitis, or laryngotracheitis. Pneumonia in neonates, like neonatal sepsis, may be of early or late onset (either acquired during birth from organisms that colonize or infect the maternal genital tract or acquired later from organisms in the hospital, home, or community). Although only a few studies of the bacteriology of neonatal pneumonia have been performed, the findings suggest that organisms causing disease are similar to those that cause neonatal sepsis.[167,168] The role of viruses in neonatal pneumonia, especially in developing countries, remains unclear. Recent studies from developed countries suggest that viruses, including respiratory syncytial virus, parainfluenza viruses, adenoviruses, and influenza viruses, contribute to respiratory morbidity and mortality, especially during epidemic periods.[169,170]

In a review of the magnitude of ARI mortality in developing countries, Garenne and co-workers[166] estimated that 21% of all ARI deaths in children younger than age 5 years occur in the neonatal period (1254 of 6041 ARI deaths in 12 countries). In a carefully conducted community study published in 1993, Bang and associates[171] determined that 66% of ARI deaths in the first year of life occurred in the neonatal period.

It is difficult to determine the incidence of neonatal ARI in developing countries because many sick neonates are never referred for medical care. In a large community study of ARI in Bangladeshi children, the highest incidence of ARI was in children younger than 5 months of age.[172] In the study by Bang and associates,[171] there were 64 cases of pneumonia among 3100 children (incidence of 21 per 1000), but this finding underestimates the true incidence because it was known that many neonates were never brought for care. The risk of pneumonia and of ARI-related death increases in infants who are of low birth weight and/or malnourished and in those who are not breast-fed.[173,174] In a study of LBW infants in India,[175] in which infants were visited weekly and mothers queried about disease, there were 61 episodes of moderate to severe ARI among 211 LBW infants and 125 episodes among 448 normal-weight infants. Although 33% episodes occurred in LBW infants, 79% of the deaths occurred in this weight group.

Tuberculosis

Tuberculosis (TB) remains a major global public health threat and has become the biggest killer of young women worldwide, with an estimated 1 million deaths occurring annually among women of childbearing age (15 to 44 years). The vast majority of infections and deaths due to TB occur in developing countries. TB during pregnancy may have adverse consequences for mother and baby, including increased risk of miscarriage, prematurity, low birth weight, and neonatal death.[176-179] Adverse perinatal outcomes are increased in mothers who have late diagnosis or incomplete or irregular therapy.[177] Ideally, diagnosis and treatment of TB in women should occur before pregnancy. The lung remains the most common site of infection; however, the prevalence of extrapulmonary TB is increasing. A 1999 study from India reviewed the outcomes of 33 pregnancies complicated by extrapulmonary TB.[180] Extrapulmonary TB confined to the lymph nodes had no adverse effect on maternal or fetal outcome. Disease at other sites (skeleton, intestines, kidney, meninges, endometrium), however, was associated with increased maternal disability and reduced fetal growth. Although congenital TB is rare, the fetus may become infected by hematogenous spread in a woman with placentitis, by swallowing or aspirating infected amniotic fluid, or by direct contact with an infected cervix at the time of delivery.[173] The most common route of infection of the neonate, however, is through airborne transmission of *Mycobacterium tuberculosis* from an infected untreated mother to her infant. Infected newborns are at particularly high risk of developing severe disease, including fulminant septic shock with disseminated intravascular coagulation and respiratory failure.[176,181]

The resurgence of TB and the increased risk of TB among those who are infected with the human immunodeficiency virus (HIV) are well known. In areas where HIV is endemic, TB rates are rising. In a 1999 study from Zambia, TB was the major nonobstetric cause of maternal death, and 92% of women with TB-related deaths were co-infected with HIV.[182] In a 1997 report from South Africa,[183] 11 neonates with culture-confirmed perinatal TB were described, 6 of whom had congenital TB. Six mothers were HIV positive, and three of their infants also were HIV infected; one infant died. Pregnant women who are co-infected with HIV may be at increased risk for placental or genital TB, resulting in an increased risk of transmission to the fetus.[183,184] In areas of the world where both TB and HIV are endemic, there must be a high index of suspicion for both diseases in the mother and the neonate.

Home-Based Neonatal Care

Several studies have evaluated community-based care for acute respiratory illness to identify sick neonates in a timely fashion and to provide treatment in their own homes. Datta and colleagues[175] implemented a program of ARI control at the primary health care level and demonstrated that improved detection and treatment could reduce mortality among LBW infants (weighing less than 2500 g). Interventions involved training primary health care workers and treating moderate to severe ARI with oral penicillin (125 mg twice a day for 5 days) using a "decision and action" classification. They compared numbers of episodes of ARI and CFRs among LBW infants in intervention and control villages. The ARI-specific mortality rate was 30 deaths per 1000 livebirths in the intervention area, versus 71 per 1000 livebirths in the control area (6/199 versus 15/211, respectively).

In a similar study of the feasibility of managing neonatal pneumonia in the community, Bang and colleagues[171] demonstrated reduction in ARI mortality in 1993 with a primary health care program. Community interventions used by this group included extensive health education of possible caregivers (traditional birth attendants, paramedics, and village health workers) and specific case management—continued breast-feeding and oral co-trimoxazole syrup for 7 days. Community-based management of pneumonia had a significant impact in reducing pneumonia-associated mortality. In the intervention area, the neonatal mortality rate from all causes was 64 per 1000 children and the pneumonia-specific mortality rate was 17 per 1000 versus 84 per 1000 and 29 per 1000, respectively, in control villages, representing a 24% reduction in mortality overall and a 40% reduction in pneumonia-specific mortality in the intervention villages. The CFR for neonatal pneumonia in the Bang study was 15% (10 of 65 died) in the intervention area, lower than what has been reported from hospital-based studies in India,[167] suggesting that cases managed in the community are diagnosed and treated earlier than are hospitalized cases.

Both of these intervention studies identified cultural barriers to care, including noncompliance with referral and medication use. Bhandari and associates[185] studied 2007 infants (aged 0 to 2 months) at two urban slum clinics in Delhi, India. Because of severe illness, hospital admission was advised for 273 (14%) of these infants, including 104 patients with ARI. Only 24% of families of sick infants and 20% of families of those with ARI complied with recommendations for hospitalization. The other infants were treated as outpatients and at home (with no deaths in the ARI group). These data suggest that improved community or domiciliary management of sick newborns may be the only way to improve outcome in some settings.

In a 1999 study, Bang and colleagues[39] implemented a comprehensive program of home-based neonatal care in a remote rural area of India. Trained female village health care workers identified pregnant women, visited them in their homes during the pregnancy, attended the delivery (along with traditional birth attendants), observed the neonate at birth and resuscitated the infant if necessary (using a simple resuscitation device), and visited the mother and baby in the home on days 1, 3, 5, 7, 14, 21, and 28 and any other time if called by the family. These health care workers were specifically trained to encourage mothers to breast-feed in the first hour after birth, to maintain a normal body temperature in the newborn by keeping the home warm and using clothing appropriately, and to identify severe illnesses including clinical sepsis, pneumonia, or meningitis. Criteria used to diagnose presumed sepsis, pneumonia, or meningitis in the infant included presence of normal crying at birth followed by development of a weak or abnormal cry; initial presence of normal sucking followed by cessation of sucking; onset of drowsiness or unconsciousness; skin temperature above 99° F or below 95° F; pus on the skin or umbilicus; diarrhea, persistent vomiting, or abdominal distention; grunting or severe retractions; and a respiratory rate of 60 or more per minute in a quiet baby. If the presumptive diagnosis was sepsis, pneumonia, or meningitis, the parents were advised to take the infant to the clinic or hospital. If parents were unwilling to have the child hospitalized, home-based care was offered. This care included antibiotics (intramuscular gentamicin [5 mg twice daily for 10 days for preterm newborns or those with birth weights less than 2500 g or 7.5 mg twice daily for 7 days for term newborns or those with birth weights greater than 2500 g] and oral co-trimoxazole [sulfamethoxazole 200 mg and trimethoprim 40 mg/5 mL] 1.25 mL twice daily for 7 days), support to maintain a normal temperature and to promote breast-feeding, and very close follow-up with home visits twice a day for 7 to 10 days. Investigators compared health outcomes in 39 intervention and 47 control villages that had similar population characteristics and baseline mortality rates (1993 to 1995). Specific home-based neonatal care was studied in the intervention villages in 1995 to 1998. The vast majority of births in the intervention villages occurred at home (95%), and 43% of the neonates had low birth weights (less than 2500 g). Very few neonates in the intervention villages were hospitalized for a severe illness (less than 1% during study period). In this study, the CFR for severe neonatal illness declined from 16.6% before the intervention to 2.8% after the intervention ($P < .05$). Moreover, early neonatal mortality, overall neonatal mortality, and infant mortality rates all declined significantly in the intervention villages (50% reduction, 62% reduction, and 46% reduction, respectively). Of interest, mortality was reduced at all birth weights (less than 1500 g, 1500 to 1999 g, 2000 to 2499 g, and 2500 g or greater). This comprehensive home-based system for neonatal care was accepted by families and was successful in reducing mortality.

The strategy of home-based neonatal care currently is being studied in other settings and other areas of the world, where referral to hospital for the sick neonate may not be acceptable to families or even possible.

SEXUALLY TRANSMITTED DISEASES

It is estimated that over 333 million new cases of the four major curable sexually transmitted diseases (STDs)—syphilis, gonorrhea, chlamydial infection, and *Trichomonas* infection—occur worldwide each year, the vast majority in developing countries.[186] The largest number of new infections occur in South and Southeast Asia, followed by sub-Saharan Africa and then Latin America and the Caribbean. STDs rank among the leading causes of morbidity worldwide, a burden borne disproportionately by women of reproductive age. Because STDs in pregnant women often are asymptomatic, women may receive delayed or no treatment.[187] Most STDs are easily transmitted from mother to child during pregnancy or delivery.[188] The burden of neonatal disease in developing countries is difficult to estimate. Adverse pregnancy outcomes associated with untreated STDs include miscarriage, preterm delivery, intrauterine growth restriction, congenital infections, and maternal, fetal, and neonatal mortality.[188,189] Neonatal HIV infection is discussed later.

Worldwide there are approximately 7 million new cases of syphilis per year among women of childbearing age.[186] Rates of congenital syphilis parallel rates in women of reproductive age. Studies from developing countries published between 1993 and 2000 have found seroprevalence rates of syphilis that are significantly higher than those found in developed countries.[190-192] Untreated syphilis during pregnancy increases the risk of late fetal death, low birth weight, preterm delivery, and severe neonatal disease.[190,193] Data from a demonstration project in Zambia indicated that syphilis was the most significant cause of adverse pregnancy outcome among women attending antenatal clinics.[194] A prospective study of congenital syphilis in a Papua New Guinea hospital published in 2000 found that the infection was responsible for 6% of admissions and 22% of all neonatal deaths.[195]

Syphilis is transmitted from an infected mother to the fetus largely via transplacental infection, and rarely by contact with an infectious genital lesion during delivery. Active infection with syphilis in pregnant women is estimated to result in fetal or infant death or disability for 50% to 80% percent of affected pregnancies.[196] A majority of the infants born to mothers with untreated syphilis are asymptomatic at birth, but without treatment, clinical manifestations of disease may develop months to years after birth. Symptoms of early congenital syphilis include intrauterine growth restriction, anemia, thrombocytopenia, jaundice, and heptosplenomegaly.[197] The most devastating complications of untreated or late congenital syphilis are neurologic manifestations that include mental retardation, hydrocephalus, cranial nerve palsies, and seizures. With adequate treatment for infected mothers, syphilis is a preventable cause of neonatal morbidity and death.

Neonates delivered vaginally to mothers with untreated gonorrhea are at great risk of developing gonococcal conjunctivitis, which, if left untreated, can lead to blindness. Rarely, disseminated gonococcal infection develops in neonates. Similarly, chlamydial infections occur in approximately two thirds of infants born by vaginal delivery to infected mothers.[188] *Chlamydia* can cause conjunctivitis and/or pneumonia, which may not be evident until the infant is several weeks old. (See later section on ophthalmia neonatorum.)

The control of STDs in pregnancy is a public health priority, especially in developing countries where rates of infection are high. Because STDs and chorioamnionitis have been associated with increased rates of mother-to-infant transmission of HIV, a community randomized trial of STD control for HIV infection prevention (antibiotics once in pregnancy) was conducted in the Rakai district of Uganda between 1994 and 1998.[198] Although antibiotic treatment did not reduce maternal HIV acquisition or perinatal HIV transmission, pregnancy outcome was improved, with decreased rates of neonatal death, low birth weight, and preterm delivery. Before presumptive therapy can be undertaken on a large scale, it must be studied further. Several countries have initiated STD control programs. The goals are to reduce STD transmission rates; to promote early diagnosis and appropriate treatment to prevent complications; and to reduce the risk of HIV infection. A special emphasis on women is needed.[199]

HUMAN IMMUNODEFICIENCY VIRUS INFECTION

The Joint United Nations Programme on HIV/AIDS (UNAIDS) and the WHO estimate that in 2003 more than 40 million people worldwide are infected with HIV and that approximately 5 million new infections occur each year.[200] Most HIV infections occur in the developing world; more than 90% of those infected live in sub-Saharan Africa, Asia, Latin America, or the Caribbean. Women are particularly vulnerable to HIV infection. Worldwide approximately 50% of cases occur in women and more than 600,000 children are infected with HIV each year, mostly by maternal-to-child transmission either in utero, at the time of delivery, or through breast-feeding.[200,201]

Because HIV increases deaths among young adults—both male and female—the acquired immunodeficiency syndrome (AIDS) epidemic has resulted in a generation of AIDS orphans. It is estimated that by the year 2010, more than 20 million children younger than 15 years of age will have been orphaned by AIDS, the vast majority in sub-Saharan Africa.[202] It is well known that maternal mortality increases neonatal and infant deaths, independent of HIV infection. Global estimates for the number of people living with HIV infection/AIDS, the number newly infected in 2003, and total AIDS deaths in 2003 are presented in Table 2-3.

Transmission

There is great disparity between developed and developing countries in mother-to-child transmission of HIV.[200,201,203] In the era of antiretroviral therapy and obstetric interventions, including increased rates of scheduled cesarean section, transmission rates as low as 2% have been reported for Europe and North America.[204-209] By contrast, rates remain high (21% to 48%) among breast-feeding infants born to HIV-infected mothers in developing countries, in the absence of antiretroviral therapy.[210-213] This disparity is due primarily to differences in access to antiretroviral drugs (to reduce transmission) and to differences in breast-feeding practices. Other factors that may influence transmission rates in developing countries include co-infection with other STDs[214]; poor nutritional and/or immunologic status of the mother[215]; micronutrient deficiencies, particularly vitamin A deficiency[216]; maternal anemia[212,213]; specific obstetric factors including placental abruption, premature or prolonged rupture of the membranes, chorioamnionitis, obstetrical procedures, and mode of delivery[212,213,217-222]; virulence of the infecting HIV strain; viral phenotype and genotype; antiviral drug resistance[223]; viral load; and advanced maternal disease.[224]

Breast-Feeding and Human Immunodeficiency Virus

HIV is present in breast milk, and postnatal transmission by means of breast-feeding is an important mode of transmission in developing countries.[225-233] A review of published studies evaluated transmission risk among mothers who were infected prenatally and postnatally.[227] Based on five studies in which the mother had been infected prenatally (as is most often the case), the additional risk of HIV trans-

Table 2–3 **Regional HIV/AIDS Statistics and Features, End of 2003**[a]

Region	Adults and Children Living with HIV/AIDS	Adults and Children Newly Infected with HIV	Adult Prevalence (%)[b]	Adult and Child Deaths Due to AIDS
Sub-Saharan Africa	25.0-28.2 million	3.0-3.4 million	7.5-8.5	2.2-2.4 million
North Africa and Middle East	470,000-730,000	43,000-67,000	0.2-0.4	35,000-50,000
South and South-east Asia	4.6-8.2 million	610,000-1.1 million	0.4-0.8	330,000-590,000
East Asia and Pacific	700,000-1.3 million	150,000-270,000	0.1-0.1	32,000-58,000
Latin America	1.3-1.9 million	120,000-180,000	0.5-0.7	49,000-70,000
Caribbean	350,000-590,000	45,000-80,000	1.9-3.1	30,000-50,000
Eastern Europe and Central Asia	1.2-1.8 million	180,000-280,000	0.5-0.9	23,000-37,000
Western Europe	520,000-680,000	30,000-40,000	0.3-0.3	2,600-3,400
North America	790,000-1.2 million	36,000-54,000	0.5-0.7	12,000-18,000
Australia and New Zealand	12,000-18,000	700-1,000	0.1-0.1	<100
Total	40 million (34-46 million)	5 million (4.2-5.8 million)	1.1 (0.9-1.3)	3 million (2.5-3.5 million)

[a]The ranges around the estimates in this table define the boundaries within which the actual numbers lie, based on the best available information. These ranges are more precise than those of previous years, and work is under way to increase even further the precision of the estimates that will be published mid-2004.

[b]The proportion of adults (15 to 49 years of age) living with HIV/AIDS in 2003, using 2003 population numbers.

AIDS, acquired immunodeficiency syndrome; HIV, human immunodeficiency virus [infection].

Data from AIDS Epidemic Update 2003, Geneva, WHO, UNAIDS, 2003.

mission with breast-feeding (above the in utero and delivery risks) was estimated to be 14% (95% confidence interval [CI] 7% to 22%). By contrast, when the mother developed her primary infection after birth of her infant, transmission risk increased substantially—estimated from four studies to be 29% (95% CI 16% to 42%). Worldwide, WHO estimated in 1998 that between one third and one half of all HIV-infected infants acquire infection postnatally from breast-feeding.[233]

Gaps remain in the understanding of how HIV is transmitted to the infant through breast-feeding. Although extended breast-feeding accounts for approximately 40% of infant HIV infections worldwide, most breast-fed infants remain uninfected despite prolonged breast-feeding and repeated exposure to HIV.[225] Mechanisms associated with transmission through breast milk or by breast-feeding, as well as factors related to protection, remain unclear. The risk of postnatal transmission increases as duration of breast-feeding increases.[233,234-239] Therefore, prolonged breast-feeding may be an important risk factor for transmission. A 2001 study from South Africa[240] compared HIV transmission rates in exclusively breast-fed, mixed-fed, and never-breast-fed (formula-fed) infants to assess whether the pattern of breast-feeding has an impact on early mother-to-infant transmission of HIV. Of 529 infants followed prospectively, 150 never breast-fed, 118 were exclusively breast-fed, and 261 received breast milk and other foods in the first 3 months of life. Transmission rates by day 1, which reflect in utero transmission, did not differ among groups (approximately 6%). Excluding those who were HIV positive on day 1, the proportion of infants infected at 3, 6, and 15 months of age did not differ significantly in those who never received breast milk (18%, 19%, 19%) versus those who were exclusively breast-fed (6%, 19%, 25%). The infection rate was significantly higher, however, in the group of infants who were partially breast-fed and received mixed feedings (24%, 26%, 36%; $P = .01$). This study suggests that exclusive breast-feeding and early weaning may reduce postnatal HIV transmission.

Other factors that might influence the infectivity of breast milk and breast-feeding include the concentration of cell-free or cell-associated HIV in breast milk; viral strain; the presence or absence of HIV-specific antibodies, particularly secretory immunoglobulin A (IgA) or IgM, or cytotoxic T cells in breast milk, lactoferrin, lysozymes, and other factors with specific antiviral activity; and the presence of mastitis with or without overt nipple cracks and bleeding.[225,226,241,242] Furthermore, infant susceptibility to infection through breast-feeding might be affected by stomach pH, oral ulceration, gastroenteritis, prematurity or low birth weight, nutritional status, and the presence of mucosal (salivary, gastrointestinal) or serum anti-HIV antibodies or cytotoxic T lymphocytes.[225,230,241] Further studies are needed to better define risk factors for HIV transmission by breast-feeding and interventions to reduce risk.

Although breast-feeding by HIV-positive mothers is discouraged in Europe and North America, where safe and affordable alternatives to breast milk are available, the issue of breast-feeding and HIV is much more complicated in developing countries, where breast-feeding has proven benefits and where artificial feeding has known risks. Benefits of breast-feeding include decreased risk of diarrhea and other infectious diseases, improved nutritional status, and decreased infant mortality[243] (see later section on breast-feeding).

In 1998, UNAIDS, WHO, and the United Nations Children's Fund (UNICEF) issued a joint policy statement on HIV and infant feeding to help decision makers in different countries develop their own policies regarding feeding practices in the context of HIV infection.[233] The statement addresses several issues: the human rights perspective, prevention of HIV infection in women, the health of mothers and children, and elements for establishing a policy on HIV status and infant feeding. As a general principle, the document supports breast-feeding. Furthermore, the statement encourages access to voluntary and confidential HIV testing for both women and men of reproductive age, as well as education regarding the implications of their HIV status for the health and welfare of their children. Because mothers may wish to keep their HIV status confidential, the statement acknowledges that women must be empowered to make decisions regarding infant feeding and supported to carry out their decision:

> This should include efforts to promote a hygienic environment, essentially clean water and sanitation, that will minimize health risks when a breast milk substitute is used. When children born to women living with HIV can be ensured uninterrupted access to nutritionally adequate breast milk substitutes that are safely prepared and fed to them, they are at less risk of illness and death if they are not breast-fed. However, when these conditions are not fulfilled, in particular in an environment where infectious diseases and malnutrition are the primary causes of death during infancy, artificial feeding substantially increases children's risk of illness and death.[233]

Several issues are implicit in this document. Breast-feeding has been actively promoted for many years to improve child survival. Discouraging breast-feeding is contrary to these policies, and alternatives to breast-feeding may be socially unacceptable in certain settings as well as potentially unsafe. The risks of breast-feeding in the context of maternal HIV infection must be explained in a clear, supportive, and non-judgmental manner. Moreover, universal access to voluntary HIV testing, although a clear human right, has broad social as well as financial implications.[244] Women may feel coerced into being tested, rather than undertaking a truly voluntary decision. There is a stigma to being infected with HIV, which in some settings may lead to spousal rejection or abuse, loss of friends and family support networks, and loss of jobs or livelihood. Programs to reduce breast-feeding or limit its duration among HIV-infected women (thereby decreasing transmission to their infants) must not reduce breast-feeding among women who are uninfected as well and must ensure that safe and affordable (maybe even free) breast milk substitutes are readily available. Although scientists have attempted, through mathematical modeling, to define levels of HIV seroprevalence and non–HIV-related child mortality at which breast-feeding might be either discouraged or promoted, there are no simple solutions to this very complicated issue.[245,246] A possible decline in breast-feeding in developing countries could have grave consequences. Exclusive breastfeeding for 6 months followed by rapid weaning has been proposed to reduce postnatal transmission of HIV. Other proposed strategies include antiretroviral propylaxis of mother and infant throughout the period of breast-feeding, caloric and micronutrient supplements for the breast-feeding mother, and measures to reduce breast milk stasis and mastitis.[225]

Prevention of Human Immunodeficiency Virus Infection in Developing Countries

Primary prevention of HIV infection among women of childbearing age is the most successful but most difficult way to prevent the infection of infants. Improving the social status of women, education of both men and women, ensuring access to information about HIV infection and its prevention, promotion of safer sex through condom use, social marketing of condoms, and treatment of other STDs that increase the risk of HIV transmission are potential strategies that have been successful at reducing infection.[199,201]

Prevention of Transmission from an Infected Mother to Her Infant

Antiretroviral Strategies

With over 600,000 infants infected perinatally each year worldwide, prevention strategies are urgently needed. In 1994, a clinical trial performed in the United States and France (Pediatric AIDS Clinical Trials Group [ACTG] Protocol 076)[204] demonstrated that zidovudine (AZT) (100 mg five times per day) administered orally to HIV-infected pregnant women with no prior treatment with antiretroviral drugs during pregnancy, beginning at 14 to 34 weeks of gestation and continuing throughout pregnancy, and then intravenously during labor (2 mg/kg over 1 hour followed by 1 mg/kg per hour until delivery), and orally to the newborn for the first 6 weeks of life (2 mg/kg every 6 hours) reduced perinatal transmission by 67.5%, from 25.5% (95% CI 18.4% to 32.5%) to 8.3% (95% CI 3.9% to 12.8%). The regimen was recommended as standard care in the United States and quickly became common practice.[247] However, because of feasibility issues and high costs, this regimen is unavailable to the vast majority of HIV-infected pregnant women in developing countries. In many such countries, women receive limited or no prenatal care; intravenous dosing may be unsafe, impractical, or impossible; and women either give birth at home or come to a hospital or clinic only when they are already in labor. Thus, newer, simpler, less expensive methods to reduce mother-to-infant transmission of HIV are needed for the majority of women and children in the world.

A number of modified AZT trials were published between 1999 and 2000.[248-251] These trials evaluated a shorter prenatal course, oral rather than intravenous dosing in labor, a shorter newborn course, or no AZT to the neonate. In a joint U.S. Centers for Disease Control and Prevention (CDC) and Thai Ministry of Public Health trial, 397 asymptomatic Thai women were randomized to receive either placebo or AZT in the last month of pregnancy (300-mg tablets; one tablet orally twice daily from 36 weeks until labor, one tablet at the onset of labor, and one tablet every 3 hours until delivery). Infants did not receive AZT and were not breast-fed (infant formula was provided free for 18 months). Transmission was reduced 50%, from 18.9% (95% CI 13.2% to 24.2%) in the placebo group to 9.4% (95% CI 5.2% to 13.5%) in the AZT group.[248]

The Thai trial, although highly effective, did not address the issue of whether short-course AZT would be effective in a more symptomatic population, and one in which breast-feeding is the norm. In Côte d'Ivoire, as in the rest of Africa, most HIV-infected women are counseled to breast-feed their infants because of high infant mortality without breast-feeding, the cost of infant formula, and the stigma associated with alternative feeding regimens. A trial using the Thai treatment regimen was performed in Côte d'Ivoire among a cohort of pregnant women who breast-fed their infants from birth.[249] In the Côte d'Ivoire trial, transmission was reduced from 21.7% in the placebo group ($n = 140$) to 12.2% in the treatment group ($n = 140$) at 1 month (44% reduction) and from 24.9% to 15.7% at 3 months (37% reduction). To further investigate the efficacy of this regimen in breast-feeding women, the results of similar studies performed in Burkina Faso and Côte d'Ivoire were combined.[250] At 6 months of age, the probability of HIV infection was 18.0% in the AZT group ($n = 192$) versus 27.5% in the placebo group

($n = 197$), a 38% reduction of early vertical transmission of HIV, despite breast-feeding. The Perinatal HIV Prevention Trial (PHPT) compared several different AZT regimens using the same doses as in the Thai trial just described.[251] They compared a "long-long regimen" started at 28 weeks of gestation, with 6 weeks of treatment for the infant; a "short-short regimen" started at 35 weeks of gestation, with 3 days of treatment for the infant; a "long-short regimen"; and a "short-long regimen." Transmission rates for the short-short group were significantly higher, and that regimen was stopped. The regimens in the other arms had equivalent efficacy (6.5%, 4.7%, 8.6%), although in utero transmission rates were lower in the groups with longer maternal therapy.

With the introduction of two- and three-drug combination therapy to reduce viral load in people with AIDS, investigators began to study AZT in combination with other drugs for use in pregnancy in developing countries (in the late 1990s). The PETRA (*Pe*rinatal *Tra*nsmission) trial performed in South Africa, Uganda, and Tanzania studied four regimens: regimen A, AZT plus lamivudine (3TC) starting at 36 weeks of gestation followed by oral intrapartum dosing and 7 days of postpartum dosing of mother and infant; regimen B, without the postpartum dosing; regimen C, intrapartum AZT alone; and regimen D, placebo. At 6 weeks, regimens A and B were effective at reducing transmission (5.7% and 8.9% versus 14.2% and 15.3%, for the four regimens, respectively). Benefits diminished considerably by 18 months, however, when transmission rates were 15%, 18%, 20%, and 22%.[252]

Nevirapine is a non-nucleoside reverse transcriptase inhibitor that has potent antiviral activity, is rapidly absorbed orally, and passes quickly through the placenta. The safety and efficacy of short-course nevirapine versus AZT given to women during labor and to neonates in the first week of life were evaluated in the HIV Network for Prevention (HIVNET) 012 trial conducted in Uganda between 1997 and 1999.[253] Six hundred twenty-six HIV-infected women (313 in each group) were randomly assigned to receive single-dose nevirapine (200 mg orally at onset of labor and 2 mg/kg to their babies within 72 hours of birth) or AZT (600 mg orally at onset of labor and 300 mg every 3 hours until delivery; and 4 mg/kg orally twice a day to babies for 7 days after birth). Almost all infants were breast-fed from birth (98.8%), and 95.6% were still breast-feeding at 14 to 16 weeks. The HIV transmission rates in the nevirapine and the AZT groups were 8.2% and 10.4%, respectively, at birth (P = not significant [NS]), 11.9% and 21.3% at 6 to 8 weeks ($P = .0027$), and 13.1% and 25.1% at 14 to 16 weeks of age ($P = .0006$). When nevirapine and AZT were both started at the onset of labor, nevirapine reduced HIV transmission by almost 50% in a breast-feeding population. Of note, the 25.1% transmission rate in the AZT group was higher than that reported in the AZT trials from Côte d'Ivoire,[249,250] but the drug was started at 36 weeks (not at the onset of labor) in those studies. Although nevirapine appeared to be safe, long-term follow-up evaluation of infants is needed. A study at 11 public hospitals in Saharan Africa (1999 to 2000) compared single-dose nevirapine with a combination of AZT and 3TC (SAINT).[254] New HIV infections were detected in 5.7% (95% CI 3.7 to 7.8) and 3.6% (95% CI 2.0 to 5.3) in the nevirapine and the AZT/3TC groups, respectively (Table 2-4). Concerns have been raised about the possible emergence of resistance mutations following the use of intrapartum regimens of nevirapine.[254a]

In many areas of the developing world, women present late in labor with unknown HIV status. A study from Malawi published in 2003 demonstrated that postexposure prophylaxis can offer protection against HIV infection to babies who missed opportunities for prenatal and intrapartum prophylaxis.[255] Combination therapy with single-dose nevirapine plus AZT for 1 week was superior to nevirapine alone (rate of new infections at 6 to 8 weeks was 7.7% versus 12.1%; $P = .03$). A pilot public health program in the Cameroon confirmed the efficacy of single-dose nevirapine given to HIV-infected women during labor and to the child within 72 hours of birth for reducing mother-to-child transmission.[256] This study demonstrated that antiretroviral therapy can be used outside of clinical trials, in real-life settings in developing countries, to successfully lower the rate of mother-to-child transmission.

Antiretroviral therapy requires the identification of HIV-infected women early enough in pregnancy to allow them access to therapy; therefore, a system for voluntary, confidential HIV counseling and testing must be in place. Furthermore, women must understand the implications of HIV infection, the drug intervention, and the possibility that even with antiviral therapy they might transmit infection to their infants. Interventions to reduce mother-to-child transmission of HIV, especially the administration of antiretroviral drugs and the avoidance of breast-feeding, make it difficult for HIV-positive women to keep their infection status private. If women fear stigmatization, discrimination, and even violence if they are identified as HIV infected, they will be unable or reluctant to take advantage of strategies to reduce transmission to their infants. Providing voluntary counseling and testing, antiviral drugs, and alternatives to breast-feeding to reduce maternal-to-child HIV transmission has potential wider benefits for society, including improvement in the quality of health care services for mothers and children, and opportunities to address primary prevention of HIV; care for HIV-infected men, women, and children; support for HIV orphans; and discriminatory societal attitudes.

Several demonstration projects to reduce mother-to-child transmission of HIV were initiated in the late 1990s in selected low-income countries, including Botswana, Burkina Faso, Cambodia, Côte d'Ivoire, Honduras, Rwanda, Tanzania, Thailand, Uganda, Zambia, and Zimbabwe.[257] These projects provide early access to adequate antenatal care; voluntary and confidential counseling and HIV testing for women and their partners; antiretroviral drugs during pregnancy and delivery for HIV-positive women; improved care during labor and delivery; counseling for HIV-positive women explaining a range of choices for infant feeding; and support for HIV-positive women who choose not to breast-feed. UNICEF is working with governments and infant formula companies to identify ways of providing safe and affordable alternatives to breast milk. At the same time, UNICEF, WHO, and UNAIDS continue to promote breast-feeding as the best feeding method for mothers who are HIV negative or who do not know their HIV status.

Other Strategies

Cesarean Section. Meta-analyses of North American and European studies performed in the late 1990s found that elective cesarean section reduced the risk of mother-to-child transmission of HIV by more than 50%.[218,219] However

Table 2–4 Studies of Antiretroviral Therapy during Pregnancy from the Developing Countries

Study, Year (Location)	Treatment Arms	Administration: Antepartum, by Week of Gestation: *Mid*	*Late*	*Intrapartum*	*Postpartum, by Neonatal Age*	Transmission Rates (%)	Reduction, (%) [Time of Ascertainment]	*P* Value
PACTG 076,[204] 1994	Zidovudine	14-34 (median, 26)			6 wk	8.3	67	.001
	Placebo					25.5		
Shaffer et al,[248] 1999	Zidovudine					9.4	50	.008
(Thailand)	Placebo		36			18.9		
Wiktor et al,[249] 1999	Zidovudine					12.2	44 [1 mo]	.05
(Ivory Coast)	Placebo		36			21.7		
Dabis et al,[250] 1999	Zidovudine					16.8	37 [3 mo]	.04
(Ivory Coast and Burkina Faso)	Placebo		36		1 wk[a]	25.1		
PETRA,[252] 2002	Zidovudine + lamivudine					7.8	52 [6 wk]	.001
A	Placebo		36		1 wk	16.5		
B	Zidovudine + lamivudine					10.8	38 [6 wk]	.02
	Placebo				1 wk	16.5		
C	Zidovudine + lamivudine					15.7	5 [6 wk]	.82
	Placebo					16.5		
Guay et al,[253] 1999	Nevirapine				3 days	11.9	44 [2 mo]	.003
(Uganda)	Zidovudine				1 wk	21.3		
PHPT—Lallemant et al,[251] 2000 (Thailand)[c]								
Long-long	Zidovudine	28			6 wk	6.5	Referent	
Long-short	Zidovudine	28			3 days	4.7	28	.86
Short-long	Zidovudine		35		6 wk	8.6	0	.15
Short-short	Zidovudine		35		3 days	10.5	0	.004
SAINT—Moodley et al,[254] 2003	Zidovudine + lamivudine				1 wk	10.2	23 [8 wk]	>.10
(South Africa)	Nevirapine				3 days	13.3		

[a]Treatment was given to the mother for 1 week post partum.
[b]A, B, and C refer to the three arms of the PETRA study.
[c]The PHPT was a four-arm study of long (starting at 28 weeks) and short (starting at 35 weeks) maternal treatment, and long (continuing until week 6) and short (continuing until 3 days) neonatal treatment. The short-short arm of the PHPT study was found in an interim analysis to result in higher transmission rates compared with the long-long arm, and this regimen was dropped from the study.
PACTG, Pediatric AIDS Clinical Trials Group; PETRA, Perinatal Transmission study; PHPT, Perinatal HIV Prevention Trial; SAINT, South African Intrapartum Nevirapine Trial.
Data updated from Kourtis A, Bulterys M, Nesheim S, et al. Understanding the timing of HIV transmission from mother to infant. JAMA 285:709, 2001.

Table 2–5 Actions to Reduce Mother-to-Child Transmission of HIV

Pre- and Perinatal Transmission
Expand access to PMCT interventions while improving the quality/efficacy of the strategy
Develop strategies to lower the cost of new diagnostic tools for HIV infection in infancy in the appropriate settings
Trials to answer questions concerning nevirapine resistance—alternative agents? novel strategies?
Study innovative strategies to deliver interventions to women who do not have access to HIV testing or antenatal care
Postnatal Transmission
Integration of basic science studies on postnatal transmission within clinical research (collection of samples)
Define standardized and agreed-upon methodologic tools for postnatal transmission studies
Investigate new approaches to make implementation easier—e.g., early diagnosis of HIV infection in infants
Pediatric Infection
Development of affordable and reliable tests/repository of samples for evaluation of new technologies for early HIV diagnosis of children in resource-limited settings
Development and evaluation of pediatric HIV/AIDS diagnostic algorithms
Surveillance of ARV resistance (development of affordable and reliable tests) and adherence
Cross-Cutting Actions
Better coordination of funding sources
Optimize partnerships between researchers
Link HIV prevention programmes with PMTCT
Increase number of providers of PMTCT, taking into account regional context
Early communication with all stakeholders
Social and cultural studies including studies on culturally appropriate counseling should be part of clinical research protocols
Implementation of PMTCT programs should be in the context of household care/treatment and of sustainability by countries; care of children should be linked with that of the mother/family (prevention and care), and continuity of this care and coordination is critical
Research should support the foregoing principles and be relevant to the host country

AIDS, acquired immunodeficiency syndrome; ARV, AIDS-related virus; HIV, human immunodeficiency virus; PMCT, xxxxx; PMTCT, xxxxx.
From Menu E, Scarlatti G, Barré-Sinoussi F, et al. Mother-to-child transmission of HIV: developing integration of healthcare programmes with clinical, social and basic research studies. Report of the International Workshop held at Cobe Marina Lodge, Kasane, Botswana, 21-25 January 2003. Acta Pediatr 92:1343, 2003.

cesarean section is appropriate for reducing perinatal transmission of HIV only if it can be performed in a well-staffed and well-equipped facility in which risks to mother and baby are low.[258]

Vaginal Lavage. Use of vaginal microbicides during labor and delivery to reduce the amount of HIV the neonate comes in contact with during delivery, and cleaning the infant's skin immediately after delivery, have been studied. To date, efficacy has not been demonstrated, but additional research is under way.[259]

Additional Interventions. It has been suggested that a package of interventions to reduce mother-to-child transmission of HIV should be implemented, including the following[260]:

- Expansion and strengthening of family planning and information and services, as well as HIV prevention activities
- Early access to quality antenatal care from trained health workers
- Voluntary counseling and HIV testing for women and their partners
- Provision of antiretroviral medication to prevent HIV transmission from seropositive women to their babies
- Improved care during labor, delivery, and the post-partum period
- Counseling for HIV-positive women on infant feeding choices, with replacement feeding made available when needed and support for women in all of their feeding practices

An international workshop identified specific actions that need to be taken by the global community to reduce mother-to-child HIV transmission (Table 2-5).[261]

Human Immunodeficiency Virus and Child Survival

Although there have been tremendous gains in child survival over the past 3 decades, with reductions worldwide in deaths due to diarrhea, pneumonia, and vaccine-preventable diseases, the AIDS epidemic threatens to undermine this dramatic trend.[262] In parts of the developing world, AIDS has already had a negative impact on child survival; in sub-Saharan Africa, AIDS has become a leading cause of death among infants and children (Table 2-6). Moreover, there is a complex link between increasing mortality of children under 5 years old and high rates of HIV prevalence in adults, related to both mother-to-child transmission of HIV and the compromised ability of parents who are ill themselves to care for young children.[263]

NEONATAL TETANUS

More is known about neonatal tetanus than about any other newborn infection occurring in developing countries. There is a vast published literature on neonatal tetanus. Neonatal tetanus traditionally has been an underreported "silent" illness. Because it attacks newborns in the poorest countries of the world in the first few days of life while they are still confined to home, because of a high and rapid CFR (85%

Table 2–6 Percentage of Infant Deaths Due to AIDS: Projections for the Year 2010

Country	U.S. Bureau of the Census[a]	U.N. Population Divisions[b]
Botswana	61	35
Zimbabwe	58	27
Kenya	41	12
Zambia	40	17
Rwanda	31	6
Uganda	31	10
Malawi	30	9
Tanzania	29	6
Burkina Faso	27	6
Côte d'Ivoire	26	8
Central African Republic	23	6
Lesotho	20	5
Burundi	18	3
Cameroon	18	3
Congo	16	11
Brazil	13	0
Congo, Democratic Republic	10	3
Haiti	7	7
Thailand	5	7

[a]Data from U.S. Bureau of the Census. The Demographic Impacts of HIV/AIDS: Perspectives from the World Population Profile, 1996.
[b]Data from U.N. Population Division, World Population Prospects: the 1996 Revision, 1997.
AIDS, acquired immunodeficiency syndrome.

Table 2–7 Tetanus Toll: Estimated Neonatal Deaths[a]

Country	Deaths
India	48,600
Nigeria	34,600
Pakistan	21,600
Ethiopia	13,400
Bangladesh	10,400
Congo, Democratic Republic	10,000
Somalia	8,800
China	8,600
Afghanistan	4,200
Indonesia	4,100
Niger	3,600
Mozambique	3,000
Nepal	3,000
Angola	2,700
Chad	2,500
Mali	2,400
Senegal	2,300
Yemen	2,300
Sudan	2,200
Ghana	2,000
Burkina Faso	1,600
Cambodia	1,500
Cameroon	1,500
Côte d'Ivoire	1,100
Liberia	600
Mauritania	200
Guinea-Bissau	100
Total	196,900

[a]The numbers of deaths in the table are estimated, as most neonatal deaths occur at home, before the baby reaches 2 weeks of age, and neither the birth nor the death is reported.
Data from The Progress of Nations 2000. New York, UNICEF, 2000.

untreated),[264] and because of poor access to medical care, the disease may go unrecognized.[265-267] Retrospective community surveys of neonatal tetanus have been conducted since the late 1970s to determine burden of disease and mortality rates.[268] The surveillance case definition of neonatal tetanus is relatively straightforward—that is, the ability of a newborn to suck at birth and for the first few days of life, followed by inability to suck starting between 3 and 10 days of age, spasms, stiffness, convulsions, and death. Using this definition and the verbal autopsy technique, country surveys have estimated the magnitude of the problem worldwide.

In 2000, WHO estimated that approximately 200,000 deaths per year are still caused by neonatal tetanus.[267] The vast majority of cases and deaths occur in a limited number of countries. Eighty percent deaths worldwide occur in only eight countries—India, Nigeria, Pakistan, Ethiopia, Bangladesh, the Democratic Republic of Congo, Somalia, and China (Table 2-7).[265,266] In view of the significant disease burden, WHO and UNICEF have called for the elimination (defined as fewer than 1 case per 1000 livebirths) of neonatal tetanus by the year 2005. To date, 104 of 161 developing countries have achieved elimination of neonatal tetanus.[266]

Neonatal tetanus is a completely preventable disease. It can be prevented by immunizing the mother before or during pregnancy and/or by ensuring a clean delivery, clean cutting of the umbilical cord, and proper care of the cord in the days after birth. Clean delivery practices have additional benefits—prevention of other maternal and neonatal infections, in addition to tetanus. Tetanus threatens mothers as well as babies, and tetanus-related mortality is a complication of both induced abortion and childbirth in unimmunized women.[269] Immunization of women with at least three doses of tetanus toxoid vaccine provides complete prevention against both maternal and neonatal tetanus. The global elimination of maternal tetanus has recently been added to the elimination goals.

OMPHALITIS

In developed countries, aseptic delivery techniques and cord care have decreased the occurrence of umbilical infection, or omphalitis. Furthermore, prompt diagnosis and antimicrobial therapy have decreased morbidity and mortality if omphalitis develops. Omphalitis continues to be a problem, however, in developing countries, where hygienic cord care practices are not universal.[270] The necrotic tissue of the umbilical cord is an excellent medium for bacterial growth. The umbilical stump is rapidly colonized by bacteria from the maternal genital tract and from the environment. This colonized necrotic tissue, in close proximity to umbilical vessels, provides microbial pathogens with direct access to the bloodstream. It is not surprising that umbilical infection is common in developing countries, with the triad of home births, unsterile cutting of the cord, and unhygienic cord care after birth. Omphalitis may remain a localized infection or may spread to the abdominal wall, the peritoneum, the umbilical or portal vessels, or the liver. Infants who present with abdominal wall cellulitis or necrotizing fasciitis have a high incidence of associated bacteremia (often polymicrobial) and a high mortality rate.[270-272]

There are only a limited number of recent studies on umbilical infection from developing countries.[45,68,273-276] Overall, incidence of omphalitis in these studies ranged from 2 to 54 per 1000 livebirths, with the CFR ranging from 0% to 15%. Guvenc and associates[275] identified 88 newborns with omphalitis at a university hospital in eastern Turkey over a 2-year period. These included 54 patients with local symptoms only and 34 with systemic symptoms. The overall CFR was 15%, but all deaths occurred among patients with systemic signs, with a CFR of 38% in this group. Gram-positive organisms were isolated from 68% of umbilical cultures, gram-negative organisms were isolated from 60%, and multiple organisms were cultured in 28% of patients. Airede[273] studied 33 Nigerian neonates with omphalitis. The incidence of omphalitis was 2 per 1000 livebirths, and the prevalence was 16 per 1000 hospital admissions. There were no deaths in this series. Aerobic bacteria were isolated from 70%, and anaerobic bacteria were isolated from 30%. Sixty percent of the aerobic isolates were gram-positive organisms, and polymicrobial isolates were common. Three studies from India were identified that present data on omphalitis or umbilical sepsis. Singhal and associates[68] reported that umbilical sepsis developed in 28 of 920 live-born infants (30 per 1000), and two of these infants died (CFR 7%). Four percent of all neonatal deaths in this study were attributed to umbilical sepsis. Bhardwaj and Hasan[45] reported that developed umbilical sepsis developed in11 of 204 live-born infants(54 per 1000); there were no deaths in this group. Faridi and colleagues[274] studied 182 Indian neonates with omphalitis, including 104 hospital-born and 78 home-delivered infants. The incidence of omphalitis in the hospital-born group was 24 per 1000 livebirths. Overall, gram-negative organisms were isolated more frequently than gram-positive organisms (57% versus 43%), but *S. aureus* was the single most frequent isolate (28%). In one report from Turkey, 85 neonates with bacteriologically proven omphalitis were evaluated.[276] *S. aureus* and *E. coli* were the most frequent organisms isolated. Overall CFR was 13%, with no difference between term and preterm infants. In a study from Papua New Guinea published in 1999, umbilical cultures were performed in 116 young infants with signs suggestive of omphalitis. The most frequently isolated organisms were group A β-hemolytic streptococci (44%), *S. aureus* (39%), *Klebsiella* (17%), *E. coli* (17%), and *Proteus mirabilis* (16%).[143] In infants with both omphalitis and bacteremia, the same organism may be cultured from both umbilicus and blood. In the Papua New Guinea study cited earlier, newborns with sepsis and omphalitis had *S. aureus*, group A β-hemolytic streptococci, and *Klebsiella pneumoniae* each isolated from both sites.

The method of caring for the umbilical cord after birth affects both bacterial colonization and time to cord separation.[277,278] It is generally agreed that application of antimicrobial agents to the umbilical cord reduces bacterial colonization. The effect of such agents on reducing infection is less clear.[278] During a study of pregnancy in a rural area of Papua New Guinea, Garner and colleagues[279] detected a high prevalence of neonatal fever and umbilical infection, which were associated with the subsequent development of neonatal sepsis. They designed an intervention program for umbilical cord care that included maternal health education and umbilical care packs containing acriflavine spirit and new razor blades. Neonatal sepsis was significantly less frequent in the intervention group (1 case perof 67 versus 8 of 64; $P = .02$). This study, published in 1994, documented the importance of umbilical infection in the etiology of neonatal sepsis in the setting of a rural developing country and demonstrated that a simple cord care intervention could reduce infectious morbidity.

DIARRHEA

It is generally agreed that diarrheal episodes are more common in infants older than 6 months than in those who are younger.[280,281] It is thought that the high prevalence of breast-feeding in the first month of life, the fact that most of the world's children are born at home rather than in the hospital, and the relative segregation of infants for a period of time after birth are factors that protect the newborn from diarrhea. Mortality from diarrhea is thought to be greatest in the first year of life.

Numerous studies published in the 1980s and 1990s have investigated the epidemiology of diarrhea in hospital and community settings and the role of breast milk and breast-feeding in protection against disease.[282-288] Clemens and colleagues followed a cohort of 198 breast-fed Egyptian neonates for the first 6 months of life.[288] Neonates for whom breast-feeding was initiated within the first 3 days of life, when breast milk contains colostrum (early group; $n = 151$), had a 26% lower rate of diarrhea during the first 6 months of life than that in infants who started breast-feeding later (late group; $n = 47$) (early versus late: 6.4 episodes versus 9.0 episodes per child-year; $P < .05$). Huilan and associates[282] studied the agents associated with diarrhea in children from birth to 35 months of age from five hospitals in China, India, Mexico, Myanmar, and Pakistan. A total of 3640 cases of diarrhea were studied, 28% of which occurred in infants younger than 6 months of age. Data on the detection of rotavirus, enterotoxigenic *E. coli*, and *Campylobacter* were provided by age. Five percent of isolates of these agents (17 of 323) were from neonates (birth to 29 days). Black and colleagues[284] performed community studies of diarrheal epidemiology and etiology in a periurban community in Peru. The incidence of diarrhea was 9.8 episodes per child in the first year of life and did not differ significantly by month of age (0.64 to 1.0 episode per child-month) from that in infants having diarrhea from birth. Mahmud and colleagues[285] prospectively followed a cohort of 1476 Pakistani newborns from four different communities. Eighteen percent of infants evaluated in the first month of life (180 of 1028) had diarrhea.

Although most infants in developing countries are born at home, those born in hospitals are at risk for nosocomial diarrheal infections. Aye and co-workers[287] studied diarrheal morbidity in neonates born at the largest maternity hospital in Rangoon, Myanmar. Diarrhea was a significant problem, with rates of 7 cases per 1000 livebirths for infants born vaginally and 50 per 1000 for infants delivered by cesarean section. These differences were attributed to the following: infants born by cesarean section remain hospitalized longer, are handled more by staff and less by their own mothers, and are less likely to be exclusively breast-fed.

Rotavirus is one of the most important causes of diarrhea among infants and children worldwide, occurring most commonly in infants aged 3 months to 2 years. In developing countries, an estimated 800,000 children die of rotavirus diarrhea each year, and infections occur earlier in infancy.[289,290] There are few reports of rotavirus infection in newborns.[291] It appears that in most cases, neonatal infection is asymptomatic, and that neonatal infection may protect against severe diarrhea in subsequent infections.[292,293] Neonates are generally infected with unusual rotavirus strains that may be less virulent and may serve as natural immunogens.[294] The rate of infection among neonates may be more common than was previously thought. Cicirello and associates[294] screened 169 newborns at six hospitals in Delhi, India, and found a rotavirus prevalence of 26%. Prevalence increased directly with length of hospital stay. The high prevalence of neonatal infections in Delhi (and perhaps in other developing country settings) could lead to priming of the immune system and have implications for vaccine efficacy.

Several of the community-based studies reviewed earlier present data on diarrhea as a cause of neonatal death.[46,49,52,54,56-59,68,69] In these studies, diarrhea was responsible for 1% to 12% of all neonatal deaths. In 9 of the 10 studies, 70 of 2673 neonatal deaths (3%) were attributed to diarrhea. Whereas diarrhea is more common in infants after 6 months of age, it is clearly a problem, in terms of both morbidity and mortality, for neonates in developing countries. The WHO estimates that there are 4,035,000 neonatal deaths per year in the less developed regions of the world.[3] If 3% of all neonatal deaths are due to diarrhea, approximately 120,000 neonatal deaths per year are associated with diarrhea.

OPHTHALMIA NEONATORUM

Ophthalmia neonatorum, defined as purulent conjunctivitis in the first 28 days of life, remains a common problem in many developing countries. The risk of infection in the neonate is directly related to the prevalence of maternal infection and the frequency of ocular prophylaxis. Infants born in areas of the world with high rates of STDs are at greatest risk. Data on incidence and bacteriologic spectrum from specific countries are limited. Although a wide array of agents are cultured from infants with ophthalmia neonatorum,[293-298] *Neisseria gonorrhoeae* (the gonococcus) and *Chlamydia trachomatis* are the most important etiologic agents from a global perspective.[298-303] The pathogenesis of infection is similar for these two agents: Infection is acquired from an infected mother during passage through the birth canal or through an ascending route. Infection due to one etiologic agent cannot be distinguished from infection due to the other by clinical examination; both produce a purulent conjunctivitis. However, gonococcal ophthalmia may appear earlier and is more severe than chlamydial conjunctivitis. Untreated gonococcal conjunctivitis may lead to corneal scarring and blindness, whereas the risk of severe ocular damage is low with chlamydial infection. Without ocular prophylaxis, ophthalmia neonatorum will develop in 30% to 42% of infants born to mothers with untreated *N. gonorrhoeae* infection,[299,300,302] and in approximately 30% of infants exposed to *Chlamydia*.[300]

Strategies to prevent or ameliorate ocular morbidity related to ophthalmia neonatorum include (1) primary prevention of STDs; (2) antenatal screening for and treatment of STDs (particularly gonorrhea and *Chlamydia* infection); (3) eye prophylaxis at birth; and (4) early diagnosis and treatment of ophthalmia neonatorum.[302] For developing countries, eye prophylaxis soon after birth is the most cost-effective and feasible strategy. Eye prophylaxis is used primarily to prevent gonococcal ophthalmia. Primary prevention of STDs in developing countries is limited, although promotion of condom use has been successful in reducing STDs in some countries.[304,305] Screening women at prenatal and STD clinics and treatment based on a syndromic approach (i.e., treat for possible infections in all women with vaginal discharge without laboratory confirmation) is cost-effective but may lead to overtreatment of uninfected women and missed cases. Because primary infection with both *N. gonorrhoeae* and *Chlamydia* is usually asymptomatic, pregnant women need to be specifically screened for STDs to ensure early diagnosis and treatment of the mother before delivery of her neonate.

Eye prophylaxis consists of cleaning the eyelids and instilling an antimicrobial agent into the eyes as soon after birth as possible. The agent should be placed directly into the conjunctival sac (using clean hands), and the eyes should not be flushed after instillation. Infants born both vaginally and by cesarean section should receive prophylaxis. Although no agent is 100% effective at preventing disease, the use of 1% silver nitrate solution (introduced by Credé in 1881)[306] dramatically reduced the incidence of ophthalmia neonatorum. This inexpensive agent is still widely used in many parts of the world and is the most successful prophylactic antimicrobial agent in history. The major problems with silver nitrate are that it may cause chemical conjunctivitis in up to 50% of infants and that it has limited antimicrobial activity against *Chlamydia*.[301,307,308] In developing countries in which heat and improper storage may be a problem, evaporation and concentration are particular concerns. Although 1% tetracycline and 0.5% erythromycin ointments are commonly used in developed countries, and are as effective as silver nitrate for the prevention of gonococcal conjunctivitis, these agents are more expensive and unavailable in many parts of the world. Moreover, silver nitrate appears to be a better prophylactic agent in areas where penicillinase-producing *N. gonorrhoeae* (PPNG) is a problem.[309]

The ideal prophylactic agent for developing countries would have a broad antimicrobial spectrum and also be available and affordable. Povidone-iodine is an inexpensive, nontoxic topical agent that is potentially widely available in developing countries. Preliminary studies suggest that it may be useful in preventing ophthalmia neonatorum. A prospective masked, controlled trial of ocular prophylaxis using 2.5% povidone-iodine solution, 1% silver nitrate solution, or 0.5% erythromycin ointment was conducted in Kenya.[310] Of 3117 neonates randomized to receive a study drug, 13.1% in the povidone-iodine group versus 15.2% of those who received erythromycin and 17.5% in the silver nitrate group developed infectious conjunctivitis ($P < .01$). The high rates of infection in this group despite ocular prophylaxis are striking. Although there was no significant difference among agents in prevention of gonococcal ophthalmia (1% or less for each agent), povidone-iodine was more effective than either other agent in preventing chlamydial conjunctivitis. A 2003 study by the same group compared prophylaxis with one drop and with two drops of the povidone-iodine solution instilled in both eyes at birth in 719 Kenyan neonates. No cases of *N. gonorrhoeae* infection were identified. Double application did not change the rates of infection with *C. trachomatis* (4.2% and 3.9%).[311] Although the antimicrobial spectrum of povidone-iodine is wider than that of other topical agents[312] and antibacterial resistance has not been demonstrated,[313] published data on the efficacy of povidone-iodine against PPNG are not yet available. Of note, 2.5% povidone-iodine might also be useful as an antimicrobial agent for cord care—of relevance in the prevention of omphalitis (see earlier). Further studies of the safety and efficacy of this agent are particularly important for its use in developing countries.

The frequency of ocular prophylaxis in developing countries is unknown. In consideration of the high rates of STDs among pregnant women in many developing countries, eye prophylaxis is an important blindness prevention strategy. For infants born at home, a single dose of antimicrobial agent for ocular prophylaxis could be added to traditional birth attendant or home delivery kits. The strategy of ocular prophylaxis is more cost-effective than early diagnosis and appropriate treatment. Furthermore, in areas of the world in which access to medical care is limited and effective drugs are scarce or unavailable, it may be the only viable strategy.

No prevention strategy is 100% effective. Even with prophylaxis, 5% to 10% of infants will develop ophthalmia. All infants with ophthalmia must be given appropriate treatment—even if they received prophylaxis at birth. A single dose of either ceftriaxone (25 to 50 mg/kg intravenously [IV] or intramuscularly [IM], not to exceed 125 mg) or cefotaxime (100 mg/kg, IV or IM) is effective therapy for gonococcal ophthalmia caused by both PPNG and non-PPNG strains.[309] Gentamicin and kanamycin also have been shown to be effective therapeutic agents and may be more readily available in some settings. Rarely, gonococcal infection acquired at birth may become disseminated, resulting in arthritis, septicemia, and even meningitis. Neonates with disseminated gonococcal disease require systemic therapy with ceftriaxone (25 to 50 mg/kg once daily) or cefotaxime (25 mg/kg IM or IV twice daily) for 7 days (arthritis, sepsis) or 10 to 14 days (meningitis). If a lumbar puncture cannot be performed (and meningitis cannot be ruled out) in an infant with evidence of dissemination, the longer period of therapy should be chosen.[309] Infants with chlamydial conjunctivitis should receive a 2-week course of oral erythromycin (50 mg/kg per day in four divided doses). After the immediate neonatal period, oral sulfonamides may be used.[309]

Intraocular instillation of human milk or colostrum has been used as a traditional remedy for ophthalmia neonatorum in some developing countries. An interesting 1996 study from Nigeria demonstrated that colostrum (but not mature milk) resulted in in vitro inhibition of growth of *S. aureus* and a variety of coliform organisms.[314] A similar study compared in vitro activity of colostrum to that of povidone-iodine and confirmed that colostrum inhibited growth of *N. gonorrhoeae* as well as *S. aureus*.[315] Although an unorthodox prophylactic or therapeutic agent, colostrum or human milk deserves further study, especially for rural areas with limited access to health care facilities.

MALARIA

From a global perspective, malaria is one of the most important infectious diseases. More than 40% of the world's population live in areas with malaria risk. The WHO estimates that 300 to 500 million cases occur annually, with 1.5 to 3 million deaths. More than half of all malaria deaths occur in children younger than 5 years of age.[316] The disease is mainly confined to poorer tropical areas of Africa, Asia, and Latin America. Countries in sub-Saharan Africa account for more than 90% of malaria cases. Each year approximately 24 million African women become pregnant in malaria-endemic areas and are at risk for malaria during pregnancy.[317] Four species of the malaria parasite infect humans: *Plasmodium falciparum*, *Plasmodium vivax*, *Plasmodium ovale*, and *Plasmodium malariae*. *P. falciparum* is responsible for the most severe form of disease and is the predominant parasite in tropical Africa, Southeast Asia, the Amazon area, and the Pacific. Groups at greatest risk for severe disease and death are young nonimmune children, pregnant women (especially primigravidas), and nonimmune adults.[318]

Malaria in Pregnancy

Preexisting levels of immunity determine susceptibility to infection and severity of disease.[317-321] In areas of high endemicity or high stable transmission, where there are high levels of protective immunity, the effects of malaria on the mother and fetus are less severe than in areas where malaria transmission is low or unstable (i.e., sporadic, periodic). It is unclear why pregnant women (even with preexisting immunity) are at increased risk for malaria. Severe maternal complications (cerebral malaria, pulmonary edema, renal failure) occur most commonly in women with little or no immunity and are most frequent with infections due to *P. falciparum*. Severe malaria may result in pregnancy-related maternal death.

Malaria parasitemia is more common, and the parasite burden is higher in pregnant than in nonpregnant women.[319,320] This increase in both prevalence and density of parasitemia is highest in primiparous women and decreases with increasing parity.[320] The parasite burden is highest in the second trimester and decreases with increasing gestation.[321-323] The most important effects of malaria on pregnant women are severe anemia[319] and placental infection.[317-321,324,325] The prevalence of anemia can be as high as 78%, and anemia is more common and more severe in primigravidas.[325] A 1999 study highlighted the importance of *P. vivax* infection (as well as the much more studied *P. falciparum*) as a cause of pregnancy-related morbidity, including anemia.[326]

Perinatal Outcome

Perinatal outcome is directly related to placental malaria. Malaria is associated with an increase in spontaneous abortions, stillbirths, preterm delivery, and intrauterine growth restriction, particularly in areas where malaria is acquired by nonimmune women.[321,327,328] Reported rates of fetal loss range from 9% to 50%.[320] The uteroplacental vascular space is thought to be a relatively protected site for parasite sequestration and replication.[324,329] Placental malaria is

Table 2–8 **Countries Reporting Chloroquine-Resistant Malaria**

Sub-Saharan Africa		Middle East and North Africa	
Angola	Liberia	Iran	Sudan
Benin	Madagascar	Oman	Yemen
Botswana	Malawi	**Central Asia**	
Burkina Faso	Mali	Afghanistan	
Burundi	Mauritania	**East/South Asia and Pacific**	
Cameroon	Mozambique	Bangladesh	Nepal
Central African Republic	Namibia	Cambodia[a]	Pakistan
Chad	Niger	China	Papua New Guinea
Congo	Nigeria	India	Philippines
Congo, Democratic Republic	Rwanda	Indonesia	Sri Lanka
Côte d'Ivoire	Senegal	Lao Rep.	Thailand[a]
Eritrea	Sierra Leone	Malaysia	Viet Nam
Ethiopia	Somalia	Myanmar[a]	
Gabon	South Africa	**Americas**	
The Gambia	Tanzania	Bolivia	Panama
Ghana	Togo	Brazil[a]	Paraguay
Guinea	Uganda	Colombia	Peru
Guinea-Bissau	Zambia	Ecuador	Venezuela
Kenya	Zimbabwe		

[a]*Plasmodium falciparum* has widespread resistance to more than one drug.
Data from World Health Organization. International Travel and Health—Vaccination Requirements and Health Advice. Geneva, World Health Organization, 1997; and from The Progress of Nations 1997. New York, UNICEF, 1997.

characterized by the presence of parasites and leukocytes in the intervillous space, pigment within macrophages, proliferation of cytotrophoblasts, and thickening of the trophoblastic basement membrane.[325] Placental infection may alter the function of the placenta, reducing oxygen and nutrient transport and resulting in intrauterine growth retardation, and may allow the passage of infected red blood cells to the fetus, resulting in congenital infection. In primigravidas living in endemic areas, placental malaria occurs in 16% to 63% of women, whereas in multigravidas, the prevalence is much lower at 12% to 33%.[319,320]

The most profound effect of placental malaria is the reduction of birth weight.[321,330,331] Both *P. falciparum* and *P. vivax* infection during pregnancy are associated with a reduction in birth weight.[326] Steketee and associates[330] have estimated that in highly endemic settings, placental malaria may account for approximately 13% of cases of low birth weight secondary to intrauterine growth retardation. In Africa, malaria is thought to be an important contributor to low birth weight in the almost 3.5 million LBW infants born annually.[332] Of importance, malaria is one of the few preventable causes of low birth weight. Because low birth weight is a major determinant of neonatal and infant mortality in developing countries, malaria may indirectly increase mortality by increasing low birth weight.[333] An important benefit of malaria prevention programs will be a reduction of low birth weight and low birth weight–associated infant mortality.[334]

Congenital Malaria

Transplacental infection of the fetus also may occur. It is relatively rare in populations with prior immunity (0.1% to 1.5%)[319] but more common in nonimmune mothers. It is thought that the low rate of fetal infection concomitant with a high incidence of placental infection is due in part to protection from transplacental maternal antibodies.[335,336]

The clinical characteristics of neonates with congenital malaria (i.e., malaria parasitemia on peripheral blood smear) include fever, respiratory distress, pallor, anemia, hepatomegaly, jaundice, and diarrhea. There is a high mortality rate with congenital infection.[337] The global burden of disease related to congenital malaria is unknown.

Prevention and Treatment of Malaria

Pregnant women living in malaria-endemic areas need access to services that can provide prompt, safe, and effective treatment for malaria. Chloroquine, the safest, cheapest, most widely available antimalarial drug, has been the agent of choice for the prevention and treatment of malaria in pregnancy.[338] However, in all areas where *P. falciparum* is prevalent, the parasite is at least partially resistant to chloroquine (Table 2-8).[316] There are a limited number of safe and effective antimalarials available for use in pregnancy. For a drug to be considered safe, it must be safe for the mother, safe for the fetus, and ideally also safe for the breast-feeding infant.[339] New drug development has been impeded by the fact that pregnant women have been excluded from drug development programs because of the justified fear of risks to the fetus.[340]

A 2002 systematic review of prevention versus therapy in pregnant women examined studies on the effectiveness of prompt therapy for malaria infection, prophylaxis with antimalarial drugs to prevent infection, and reduced exposure to mosquito-borne infection by using insecticide-treated bednets.[341] Chemoprophylaxis is associated with reduced maternal disease, including anemia and placental infection. One study found that the incidence of placental malaria is reduced by prophylaxis, even when chloroquine is used in areas with chloroquine-resistant malaria.[342] In addition, prophylaxis has been found to have a positive effect on birth weight and risk of preterm delivery.[343]

Table 2–9 Estimated Global Burden of Disease—Major Neonatal Infections

Infection	Estimated No. of Cases	Estimated Case-Fatality Rate (%)	Estimated No. of Deaths
Neonatal sepsis	800,000	40	320,000
Neonatal meningitis	130,000	40	52,000
Neonatal tetanus	240,000	85	200,000
Acute respiratory infection	2,650,000	30	800,000
Diarrhea	25,000,000	0.6	150,000
Human immunodeficiency virus infection	600,000	?[a]	?[a]
Total	29,420,000		1,522,000

[a]Data unavailable: Most HIV-related deaths occur after the neonatal period.
Data updated from Stoll BJ. The global impact of neonatal infection. Clin Perinatol 24:1997.

A major problem with both chemoprophylaxis and prompt therapy for known or suspected infection is that it is often difficult to deliver services to pregnant women, especially those who live in areas remote from health centers. Intermittent presumptive therapy involves two or three doses of a safe and effective antimalarial given to women in malaria-endemic areas with the presumption that they are at high risk to be infected. Recent studies from Africa have demonstrated that intermittent preventive treatment (IPT) can reduce the incidence of malaria and its adverse consequences.[344,345] These interventions are particularly important and cost-effective in pregnancy.[343,346] In 2000, the WHO recommended IPT with sulfadoxine-pyrimethamine in malaria-endemic areas where *P. falciparum* is resistant to chloroquine and sensitive to sulfadoxine-pyrimethamine.[347] This drug is effective in a single dose, is not bitter, and is relatively well tolerated. In areas where malaria transmission is lower and *P. vivax* as well as *P. falciparum* is a problem, finding an appropriate drug regimen is more difficult.[348]

Other Malaria Control Measures

Although the benefits of antimalarial chemoprophylaxis have been established, poor compliance[349] and increasing drug resistance have led to trials of alternative prevention strategies. Use of insecticide-treated bed nets has been successful in reducing childhood morbidity and mortality in malaria-endemic areas.[350-352] The effects of bed nets on malaria in pregnancy have been inconsistent, however. A study in Tanzania found a significant reduction in parasitemia and anemia.[353] A study from the Thai-Myanmar border found a significant reduction in maternal anemia, with only a marginal effect on peripheral parasitemia[354]; a study from The Gambia found a reduction in severe anemia in the dry season and fewer preterm deliveries in the rainy season,[355] but studies from Ghana[356] and Kenya[357] showed no significant impact of insecticide-impregnated bed nets on malaria-associated morbidity in pregnant women, including anemia and low birth weight. Given the number of pregnant women living in malarious areas, research on non–drug control strategies are needed for this high-risk group. The use of social marketing has increased bed net use. An additional benefit of bed net use is protection of the neonate, who almost always sleeps with the mother in this setting.[353]

Studies published in 2003 have shown an association between malaria and HIV in pregnancy with an increase in the risk of maternal malaria and of placental malaria in HIV-positive mothers.[358-360] Furthermore, co-infection with malaria and HIV infection in pregnancy has been shown to increase mother-to-child transmission of HIV[360] and both perinatal and early infant mortality.[361]

GLOBAL BURDEN OF INFECTIOUS DISEASES AMONG NEWBORNS

Table 2-9 summarizes estimates of the global burden for the most important neonatal infections. These estimates are based on the review of studies presented earlier and selected WHO and United Nations documents.[5,7,127,266] In summary, of the estimated 132,787,000 children born in developing countries each year, more than 20% (or almost 30 million children) develop a neonatal infection and more than 1,500,000 infants die of infection in the neonatal period each year.

DIRECT AND INDIRECT CAUSES OF NEONATAL DEATH RELATED TO INFECTION

The immediate or direct medical causes of neonatal death related to infection include sepsis, meningitis, omphalitis, neonatal tetanus, pneumonia, TB, diarrhea, malaria, and HIV infection/AIDS. There are, however, a vast array of indirect causes for many of the infectious deaths in developing countries (Table 2-10). These contributory factors have social as well as medical roots. Sociocultural factors include poverty (not just of individuals but of governments as well), illiteracy, low social status of women, lack of political power (for women and children) and lack of will in those who have power, gender discrimination (for both mother and neonate), harmful traditional or cultural practices, poor hygiene, lack of clean water and sanitation, the cultural belief that a sick newborn is doomed to die (and is, moreover, replaceable), the family's inability to recognize danger signs in the newborn, inadequate access to high-quality medical care (either because it is unavailable or because of the lack of transport for emergency care) or the lack of supplies or appropriate

Table 2–10 **Direct and Indirect Causes of Neonatal Death Related to Infections in Less Developed Countries**

Direct Causes of Death	Indirect Causes of Death
Medical	**Sociocultural**
Sepsis	Poverty
Meningitis	Illiteracy
Omphalitis with sepsis	Low social status of women
Tetanus	Lack of potential power
Pneumonia	Gender discrimination (for mother and newborn)
Tuberculosis	Harmful traditional practices
Diarrhea	Poor hygiene
Malaria	Lack of clean water and sanitation
HIV infection/AIDS	Cultural belief that a sick newborn is doomed to die
	Inability to recognize danger signs in sick newborn
	Poor care-seeking behavior
	Inadequate access to high-quality medical care
	Lack of transport for emergency care
	Lack of appropriate drugs
	Maternal death
	Medical
	Poor maternal health
	Untreated maternal infections including sexually transmitted diseases, urinary tract infection, chorioamnionitis
	Failure to fully immunize mother against tetanus
	Inappropriate management of labor and delivery
	Unsanitary cutting and care of umbilical cord
	Failure to promote early and exclusive breast-feeding (HIV dilemma noted)
	Prematurity/low birth weight

AIDS, acquired immunodeficiency syndrome; HIV; human immunodeficiency virus.
Data updated from Stoll BJ. The global impact of neonatal infection. Clin Perinatol 24:1, 1997.

drugs, and maternal death.[2,3,362,363] Medical factors that may also contribute to an infectious neonatal death include poor maternal health, untreated maternal infections (including STDs, urinary tract infection, and chorioamnionitis), failure to fully immunize the mother against tetanus, inappropriate management of labor and delivery, unsanitary cutting and care of the umbilical cord, failure to promote early and exclusive breast-feeding, and prematurity and/or low birth weight.[2-4,364,365] To promote change, families must know enough to identify illness and must want and be able to seek care. Health care workers (of all levels) must know what to do and must have the resources to support needed therapy. Moreover, better maternal care—both preventive and curative—is preventive medicine for the newborn.

With the scientific knowledge currently available, it is possible to address the medical causes of infectious death and to make a significant impact on mortality. It is far harder to address the sociocultural factors that, in some settings, make a medical approach to preventing and treating these diseases impossible. Coordinated activities are needed to bring about change that is sustainable by countries on their own, over the long haul. This will involve a multidisciplinary approach—bringing together people with different interests, from different backgrounds, different agencies, different government ministries—to seek solutions to problems and to implement change at the local level. Finally, it will involve the global acknowledgment that this is the right thing to do (i.e., a moral imperative) and, therefore, the long-term commitment of substantial funding to help provide needed services to poor countries. The challenge for the next decade is to link science and medicine with social solutions through a global commitment to long-term, long-lasting change so that improvements in both maternal and newborn health can be achieved and sustained.

STRATEGIES TO LIMIT INFECTION IN THE NEONATE AND TO REDUCE INFECTION-ASSOCIATED MORTALITY

Strategies to prevent or reduce neonatal infections, and to reduce morbidity and mortality in those newborns in whom infection develops, involve putting into practice what is known and inventing creative ways to make these interventions workable in a developing country context. Use of simple, cost-effective technologies that are potentially available at the village or district hospital level could have a major impact in reducing morbidity and mortality related to neonatal infection. Moreover, public health, medical, and social interventions all have a role to play in reducing the global burden of neonatal infection. Several potential interventions are reviewed here (Table 2-11).

Maternal Immunization to Prevent Neonatal Disease

There is growing interest in the possibility of using maternal immunization to protect neonates and very young infants from infection through passively acquired transplacental or breast milk antibodies, or both.[366,367] Immunization of pregnant women with tetanus toxoid has dramatically reduced cases of neonatal tetanus and is the classic example of maternal

Table 2–11 Interventions to Reduce Neonatal Infections or to Reduce Infection-Associated Mortality in Developing Countries

Antenatal Care
Tetanus immunization
Maternal immunization with new vaccines in the future (e.g., group B streptococci, *Haemophilus influenzae* type b, pneumococcus)
Primary prevention of sexually transmitted disease, including HIV infection, through maternal education and safer sex using condoms
Diagnosis and treatment of sexually transmitted diseases, urinary tract infection, malaria, tuberculosis, other infections
Plan clean and safe delivery
Intrapartum/Delivery Care
Prevent prolonged labor
Optimal management of complications, including fever, premature rupture of membranes, puerperal sepsis
Clean delivery
Clean cutting of umbilical cord/optimal cord care
Breast-feeding
Promote early and exclusive breast-feeding (HIV dilemma noted)
Gender Issues
Promote gender equality
Encourage education of girls
Interventions to Decrease Low Birth Weight and/or Prematurity
Delay childbearing in young adolescents
Promote maternal education
Improve maternal nutrition: caloric supplementation before and during pregnancy
Reduce tobacco use
Diagnose and treat sexually transmitted diseases
Malaria prophylaxis and treatment
Limit maternal work load during pregnancy
Maternal support to decrease stress/anxiety
Community-Based Interventions
Train birth attendants to identify problems in the newborn, treat simple problems, refer newborns with serious illness
Promote and support breast-feeding (HIV dilemma noted)
Maternal education regarding personal and domestic hygiene, newborn care, childhood immunization
Home-based diagnosis and treatment of newborn infections
Early Identification and Improved Treatment of Neonates with Infection
Integrated approach to the sick young infant (WHO/UNICEF)
Improve newborn care at all levels: home, village, health center, district hospital, referral hospital
Neonatal Immunization
Bacillus Calmette-Guérin, hepatitis B, other new vaccines (e.g., rotavirus)

HIV, human immunodeficiency virus; UNICEF, United Nations Children's Fund; WHO, World Health Organization.
Data updated from Stoll BJ. The global impact of neonatal infection. Clin Perinatol 24:1, 1997.

immunization and subsequent passive immunization to protect the newborn. Because most IgG antibody is transported across the placenta in the last 4 to 6 weeks of pregnancy, maternal immunization to prevent neonatal disease through transplacental antibodies is most promising for term newborns, who will have adequate antibody levels at birth. By contrast, this strategy will be less successful for preterm infants because of insufficient passage of maternal antibodies. Boosting breast milk antibodies by immunizing the mother is a potential strategy for reducing infection in both term and preterm infants. Vaccines being currently developed or field tested to reduce or prevent neonatal infection by passive immunization include vaccines against GBS, *S. pneumoniae*, and *Haemophilus influenzae*.[368-377]

Because most neonatal GBS disease—especially the most severe—occurs in the first hours of life, maternal immunization to provide passive protection to the neonate is a potentially important strategy. A problem with GBS vaccines has been poor immunogenicity. Studies performed in the last decade have focused on the immunogenicity of polysaccharide-protein conjugate vaccines and suggest that conjugate vaccines may be highly effective in pregnant women.[369] Published data suggest that candidate GBS polysaccharide–tetanus toxoid conjugates are safe in adults and elicit antibody levels above what is likely to be passively protective for neonates.[370,371] Multivalent vaccines, which could provide protection against multiple GBS serotypes, are particularly promising.[372]

Pneumococcal polysaccharide vaccines have been administered safely to pregnant women.[373,374] One study from Bangladesh reported that pneumococcal vaccination during pregnancy increased type-specific IgG serum antibody in both mother and infant.[373] Cord blood levels of antibody were about half those of the mother, with IgG1 subclass antibodies preferentially transferred to the infant. The estimated antibody half-life in the infant was 35 days. Immunization increased breast milk antibody as well. However, in a study of the 23-valent pneumococcal vaccine given to women before pregnancy, neither mothers nor infants had significantly elevated pneumococcus-specific antibody at delivery.[375] If passive immunization does not interfere with active immunization of young infants, vaccination of pregnant women could potentially be used to prevent pneumococcal disease in early infancy. The recent finding from the WHO Young Infant Study that *S. pneumoniae* is an important cause of sepsis and meningitis in young infants[151] supports the continued investigation of maternal immunization with pneumococcal vaccines as a prevention strategy for developing countries.

In developed countries, invasive disease resulting from *H. influenzae* type b (HIB) has been almost completely eliminated by the use of HIB conjugate vaccines.[378] However, in many parts of the world, HIB remains an important cause of life-threatening infections in infancy, particularly pneumonia and meningitis. Although HIB infection is rare in the neonatal period, approximately 40% of cases of HIB disease in developing countries occur in infants younger than 6 months of age.[379,380] Both neonatal and maternal immunization strategies are being explored to target populations in which HIB infections occur in young infants.[367,376,377] A study from The Gambia[376] showed that maternal immunization with HIB polysaccharide–tetanus protein conjugate vaccine increased both maternal and neonatal antibody concentrations. At 2 months of age, 60% of infants of vaccinated mothers had antibody concentrations considered to be protective. Similar results were found in a study of native American women immunized with HIB conjugate vaccines before pregnancy. Significant antibody elevations were detected at birth in infants born to these women.[375]

Additional studies of the safety, efficacy, and effectiveness of immunizing pregnant women with specific vaccines are needed. They must address issues of safety to the mother, fetus, and young infant. Furthermore, they must assess protection against specific diseases (e.g., sepsis, pneumonia, meningitis) as well as protection against all causes of neonatal and infant mortality. The subsequent response of the infant to active immunization also must be evaluated, to ensure that passive immunization does not interfere with the infant's ability to mount an immune response. Therefore, in developing countries, studies must be carried out in settings in which it is possible to maintain surveillance throughout infancy.

Neonatal Immunization

Protection of young infants against vaccine-preventable diseases requires vaccines that are immunogenic in early life.[381] A number of vaccines are currently given to newborns or young infants: bacillus Calmette-Guérin (BCG), hepatitis B, polio, diphtheria, tetanus, pertussis, and HIB. The BCG vaccine, developed early in this century, is a live attenuated strain of *Mycobacterium bovis*. The WHO promotes the use of BCG in newborns to prevent TB, and this vaccine is widely used in developing countries in which TB is a common and potentially lethal disease. Although approximately 3 billion doses have been given, the efficacy of this vaccine is still debated. Vaccine efficacy in many prospective trials and case-control studies of vaccine use at all ages ranges from possibly harmful to 90% protective.[382] One meta-analysis of BCG studies in newborns and infants concluded that the vaccine was effective and reduced infection in children by more than 50%.[383] BCG reduced the risk of pulmonary TB, TB meningitis, disseminated TB, and death from TB. Factors that may explain the variability of responses to BCG vaccination in different studies and populations include use of a wide variety of vaccine preparations, regional differences in environmental flora that may alter vaccine response, and population differences.[367] The safety of BCG in immunocompromised patients (e.g., those with HIV infection) is unclear.

Hepatitis B vaccination of newborns has proved that neonatal immunization can prevent neonatal infections and their sequelae.[384] Studies from both developed and developing countries have shown that hepatitis B vaccine administered in the immediate newborn period can significantly reduce the rate of neonatal infection and the development of a chronic hepatitis B surface antigen (HB_sAg) carrier state.[385] The efficacy of vaccine alone (without hepatitis B immune globulin [H-BIG]) has allowed developing countries that cannot screen pregnant women and do not have H-BIG to make a major impact in reducing the infection of newborns. Recently, the WHO recommended that all countries add hepatitis B vaccine to their routine childhood immunization programs.[386] In addition, studies of neonatal immunization with polio vaccine, HIB conjugate vaccines, and pneumococcal conjugate vaccines suggest some protection with neonatal vaccination that might reduce but not eliminate disease.[367]

Rotavirus diarrhea is a major killer of young infants in developing countries, causing approximately 800,000 childhood deaths per year. The development of a live oral quadrivalent rhesus rotavirus vaccine, which has been shown to be highly effective in young infants, particularly at preventing severe disease, is exciting and potentially very important.[387] Additional studies in developing countries are needed before rotavirus vaccines can be added to routine childhood vaccination programs. The quadrivalent rhesus rotavirus vaccine, highly effective in preventing severe disease in Venezuelan children,[388] has never been tested in African or Asian children. Factors that might influence efficacy in developing countries include younger age at infection, potentially larger viral inoculum, presence of different or unusual strains of rotavirus, and poorer nutritional status.[289] Unlike children in developed countries, those in developing countries experience most severe episodes of rotavirus diarrhea in the first year of life. Vaccines will need to be delivered early—perhaps at birth. Further studies on the safety and efficacy of rotavirus vaccine in neonates are needed.[294,387]

With the global problem of increasing antibiotic resistance, maternal and neonatal immunization have become even more important strategies to pursue. In developing countries, issues of vaccine cost, availability, and efficacy in the field are particularly pressing and are major barriers to the use of vaccines that are known to be safe and effective in developed countries. Efforts to reduce vaccine cost by studying lower doses of vaccine and use of single-dose vials for multiple-dose use are promising.[389] Ultimately, the reduction of vaccine cost is in the hands of vaccine manufacturers.

Antenatal Care and Prevention of Neonatal Infection

The care and general well-being of the mother are inextricably linked to the health of her newborn. Antenatal care can play an important role in the prevention or reduction of neonatal infections.[390] Both preventive and curative interventions directed toward the mother can have beneficial effects on the fetus or newborn or both. Tetanus immunization of the pregnant woman is an essential component of any developing country's antenatal care program and, as discussed earlier, will prevent neonatal tetanus.[365,391] The diagnosis and treatment of STDs—especially syphilis, gonorrhea, and chlamydial infection—can have a significant impact on neonatal morbidity and mortality.[186,188] In areas of the world in which syphilis is endemic, congenital syphilis may be a major cause of neonatal morbidity and mortality.[392] Antenatal treatment of gonorrhea and chlamydial infection can prevent neonatal infection with these agents—ophthalmia neonatorum (for gonorrhea and chlamydial infection), disseminated gonorrhea, and neonatal respiratory disease (for chlamydial infection).[186,188] Moreover, STDs and maternal urinary tract infection increase the mother's risk of puerperal sepsis, with its associated increased risk of neonatal sepsis. In malaria-endemic areas, treatment of maternal malaria can have an impact on newborn health, particularly through a reduction in the incidence of low birth weight.[393]

Antenatal care also is an important setting for maternal education regarding danger signs during pregnancy, labor, and delivery—especially maternal fever, prolonged or premature rupture of the membranes, and prolonged labor—and danger signs to watch for in the newborn. Moreover, it is the time and place for the mother to plan where and by whom she will be delivered and for the health care worker to stress the importance of a clean delivery, preferably with a trained skilled birth attendant.

Intrapartum and Delivery Care and Prevention of Neonatal Infection

It is universally recognized that poor aseptic techniques during labor and delivery, including performing procedures with unclean hands and unclean instruments and unhygienic cutting of the umbilical cord, are major risk factors for both maternal and neonatal infections.[390] It is essential to promote safe and hygienic practices at every level of the health care system where women deliver (i.e., home, health center, district or referral hospital). Proper management of labor and delivery can have a significant impact on the prevention of neonatal infection. It is important to emphasize the need for clean hands, clean perineum, clean delivery surface, clean instruments, clean cord care, use of an appropriate clean delivery kit, avoidance of harmful traditional practices, prevention of unnecessary vaginal examinations, prevention of prolonged labor, and optimal management of pregnancy complications including prolonged rupture of the membranes, maternal fever, and chorioamnionitis/puerperal sepsis.[5]

If the mother does develop a puerperal infection, the newborn requires special attention and should be treated for presumed sepsis.[390] Prolonged rupture of the membranes, maternal fever during labor, and chorioamnionitis are particular risk factors for early-onset neonatal sepsis and pneumonia in both developed and developing countries.[394-396] Ideally, high-risk infants who are born at home should be referred to the nearest health care facility for observation and antibiotic therapy. In practice, this may be either impossible or unacceptable to the family, and ways to deliver care to the mother and the newborn in the home must be developed and evaluated. The traditional birth attendant or other health care worker who attends the birth has a critical role to play in the early health of the newborn.

Breast-Feeding

The promotion of early and exclusive breast-feeding is one of the most important interventions for the maintenance of newborn health and the promotion of optimal growth and development.[5] Breast-feeding is especially important in developing countries, where safe alternatives to breast milk are often unavailable or too expensive. Moreover, poor hygiene and a lack of clean water and clean feeding utensils make artificial formula an important vehicle for the transmission of infection. Breast milk has many unique anti-infective factors, including secretory IgA antibodies, lysozyme, and lactoferrin. In addition, breast milk is rich in receptor analogues for certain epithelial structures that microorganisms need for attachment to host tissues, an initial step in infection.[397] Many studies performed in the 1980s and 1990s have shown that breast-feeding reduces the risk of infectious diseases, including neonatal sepsis, diarrhea, and possibly respiratory tract infection.[283,398-402] Moreover, there is evidence that breast-feeding protects against infection-related neonatal and infant mortality.[403-406]

The HIV epidemic has raised questions about the safety of breast-feeding in areas in which there is a high prevalence of HIV infection among lactating women.[225-233,241,407] HIV may be transmitted through breast-feeding. A major question for any setting is whether the benefits of breast-feeding outweigh the risk of postnatal transmission of HIV through breast milk.[407] For many areas of the world, where infectious diseases, especially diarrheal diseases, are a primary cause of infant death, breast-feeding, even when the mother is HIV infected, remains the safest mode of infant feeding. Countries with high and low reported rates of exclusive breast-feeding are listed in Table 2-12.[316]

Table 2–12 Breast-Feeding Rates in Developing Countries[a,b]

Exclusive Breast-Feeding Rates of 10% or Less		Exclusive Breast-Feeding Rates of 50% or More	
Country	*%*	*Country*	*%*
Niger	1	Rwanda	90
Nigeria	2	Burundi	89
Angola	3	Ethiopia	74
Côte d'Ivoire	3	Tanzania	73
Haiti	3	Uganda	70
Central African Republic	4	Egypt	68
		Eritrea	65
Thailand	4	China	64
Cameroon	7	Mauritania	60
Paraguay	7	Bangladesh	54
Maldives	8	Turkmenistan	54
Senegal	9	Bolivia	53
Dominican Republic	10	Iran	53
Togo	10	India	51
Trinidad/Tobago	10	Guatemala	50

[a]Breast-feeding in infants younger than 4 months of age.
[b]Data from DHS MICS and other nationwide surveys, 1987-1996.
From The Progress of Nations 1997. New York, UNICEF, 1997.

Maternal Education and Socioeconomic Status

Maternal education, literacy, and overall socioeconomic status are powerful influences on the health of both mother and newborn.[408-411] Education of girls must be promoted and expanded so that women of reproductive age know enough to seek preventive services, understand the implications of danger signs during labor and delivery and in their newborns, and recognize that they must obtain referral care for obstetric or newborn complications, or both. Improvements in education and socioeconomic status are obviously linked. They may affect child health by allowing the mother a greater voice in the family with greater decision-making power, making her better informed about domestic hygiene, disease prevention, or disease recognition, or enhancing her ability to seek medical attention outside the home and to comply with medical advice.

Low Birth Weight and Prematurity

Low birth weight (2500 g or less) constitutes a major public health problem. Worldwide, approximately 90% of LBW infants are born in developing countries.[412] Low birth weight is caused by impaired fetal growth, shortened gestation, or a combination of both. In developing countries, low birth weight is caused more frequently by intrauterine growth retardation than by prematurity.[332,412] Data suggest that both preterm and LBW infants are at increased risk for infection and infection-related mortality.[413-415] Therefore, strategies to reduce the frequency of low birth weight and prematurity could have a measurable impact on neonatal infection. Potential interventions to improve intrauterine growth or to lengthen gestation, or both, include delaying childbearing in adolescents, improved maternal education, caloric supplementation before and during pregnancy, general improvements in nutrition, malaria prophylaxis or treatment, treatment of STDs and other maternal infections, efforts to reduce tobacco use, improved water and sanitation, limitation of maternal work during pregnancy, and general improvement in socioeconomic conditions.[332]

Community-Based Interventions

In parts of the world in which a majority of births occur at home, primary health care at the village level will need to put added emphasis on care of the newborn. The birth attendant is responsible for observation of the newborn at and after birth and deciding that the newborn is healthy and ready to be "discharged" to the care of the mother. It is important to link postpartum care of the mother with surveillance and care of the newborn. The postpartum visit should be used to detect and treat the sick newborn as well as to evaluate the mother. Birth attendants need to be trained to identify problems in the newborn, to treat simple problems (e.g., skin infections), and to refer those that are potentially life-threatening (e.g., suspected sepsis). Moreover, they should provide all new mothers with breast-feeding support and give advice regarding personal hygiene/cleanliness and other prevention strategies such as immunization. Improvement in domestic hygiene should be encouraged, including sanitary disposal of wastes, use of clean water, and hand washing, so that the newborn enters a clean home and is less likely to encounter pathogenic organisms. In some settings, families will refuse to take even a sick newborn to a hospital, and care will need to be brought into the village or home. Community interventions need to be designed and modified to meet the needs of mothers and newborns in different settings in different countries and need further evaluation.

Early Identification and Improved Treatment of Neonates with Infection

If untreated, infections in newborns can rapidly become severe and life-threatening. Therefore, early identification and appropriate treatment of newborns with infection are critical to survival. In developing countries, where access to care may be limited, diagnosis and treatment are particularly difficult. It is important to recognize maternal and neonatal factors that increase risk of infection in the newborn. These include maternal infections during pregnancy (STDs, urinary tract infection, others), premature or prolonged rupture of membranes, prolonged labor, fever during labor, unhygienic obstetric practices or cord care, poor hand-washing practices, low birth weight/prematurity, artificial feeding, and generally unhygienic living conditions.[2-4]

In areas without sophisticated technology and the diagnostic help of laboratory tests and x-ray studies, treatment decisions must be made on the basis of the history and findings on physical examination. In the WHO Young Infant Study, clinical predictors of neonatal sepsis were studied in more than 3000 sick infants younger than 2 months of age in Ethiopia, The Gambia, Papua New Guinea, and the Philippines.[416] In multivariable analysis, 14 signs were independent predictors of severe disease: reduced feeding ability, absence of spontaneous movement, temperature greater than 38° C, drowsiness or unconsciousness, a history of a feeding problem or change in activity, state of agitation, the presence of lower chest indrawing (retractions), respiratory rate greater than 60, grunting, cyanosis, a history of convulsions, a bulging fontanel, and slow digital capillary refill. The presence of any one of these signs had a sensitivity for severe disease (sepsis, meningitis, hypoxemia, or radiologically proven pneumonia) of 87% and a specificity of 54%.

Mothers, birth attendants, and other health care workers and family members must be educated so that they can identify danger signs in the newborn and understand that prompt and appropriate therapy may make the difference between life and death. The positive deviance (PD) approach involves investigating children (in this case newborns) with healthy outcomes despite adverse conditions, identifying model practices among successful families, and designing an intervention to transfer these behaviors to other mothers and families. Save the Children has studied the PD approach in newborns in Pakistan. In-depth interviews were conducted to identify common behaviors among parents of surviving asphyxiated newborns, thriving LBW babies, surviving newborns who demonstrated danger signs, and normal newborns. PD families had better maternal care, better routine and special newborn care, and better care-seeking behavior.[417] A study from Sri Lanka, a developing country with relatively low neonatal and infant mortality rates, identified a high level of care-seeking behavior among mothers, particularly for illnesses with acute, high-risk danger signs.[418]

An integrated approach to the sick child, including the young infant, has been developed by the WHO and

UNICEF.[419] This strategy promotes prompt recognition of disease, appropriate therapy using standardized case management, referral of serious cases, and prevention through improved nutrition (breast-feeding of the neonate), and immunization. This approach stresses diagnosis using simple clinical signs that can be taught to health care workers at all levels. The health care worker assesses the child by questioning the mother and examining the child, classifies the illness as serious or not, and determines if the infant needs urgent treatment and referral, specific treatment and advice, or only simple advice and home management. Importance of breast-feeding is stressed, and follow-up instructions are given. All young infants are checked for specific danger signs that equate with need for emergency care and urgent referral. Because the signs of serious bacterial infection in the newborn are not easily recognized, every young infant with danger signs is given treatment for a possible bacterial infection. All newborns with suspected severe infection receive antibiotics as soon as possible and are then referred for hospitalization. In situations where referral is impossible or unacceptable to the family, community-based interventions must be designed, implemented, and evaluated.

CONCLUSION

The 1996 World Health Report[420] highlights the global importance of infectious diseases, especially among young children, and stresses the impact of new or emerging diseases. Neonatal infections are old diseases. Furthermore, each infection-related death should be considered a potentially preventable death. What is needed is a new recognition that they are important causes of morbidity and mortality and that simple interventions are available that can have a significant impact on reducing the incidence of both infection and death related to infection in developing countries.

REFERENCES

1. World Health Report 1998. Geneva, World Health Organization, 1998.
2. Bale JR, Stoll BJ, Lucas AO (eds). Improving Birth Outcomes: Meeting the Challenge in the Developing World. Washington, DC, Institute of Medicine, The National Academy Press, 2003.
3. The State of the World's Newborns: A Report from Saving Newborn Lives. Washington, DC, Save the Children, 2001.
4. Mother-baby package: Implementing safe motherhood in countries. WHO/FHE/MSM/94. 11.
5. Stoll BJ. The global impact of neonatal infection. Clin Perinatol 24:1–21, 1997.
6. Stoll BJ, Measham AR. Children can't wait: improving the future for some of the world's poorest infants. J Pediatr 139:729–733, 2001.
7. World Health Organization. Perinatal Mortality: A Listing of Available Information. Geneva, World Health Organization, 1996.
8. Adeyokunnu AA, Taiwo O, Antia AU. Childhood mortality among 22,255 consecutive admissions in the University College Hospital, Ibadan. Niger J Paediatr 7:7–15, 1980.
9. English M, Ngama M, Musumba C. Causes and outcome of young infant admissions to a Kenyan district hospital. Arch Dis Child 88:438–443, 2003.
10. Agarwal VK, Gupta SC, Chowdhary SR, et al. Some observations on perinatal mortality. Indian Pediatr 19:233–238, 1982.
11. Aiken CGA. The causes of perinatal mortality in Bulawayo, Zimbabwe. Cent Afr J Med 38:263–281, 1992.
12. Baja-Panlilio H, Cabigas-Resurreccion J, Matanguihan AT, et al. Perinatal morbidity and mortality in the Philippines. Asia-Oceania J Obstet Gynaecol 12:331–339, 1986.
13. Boo NY, Nasri NM, Cheong SK, et al. A 2-year study of neonatal mortality in a large Malaysian Hospital. Singapore Med J 32:142–147, 1991.
14. Chaturvedi P, Potdar S. Change in neonatal care pattern and neonatal mortality in a rural medical college. Indian Pediatr 25:171–178, 1988.
15. Dawodu AH, Umran KA, Faraidy AA. Neonatal vital statistics: a 5-year review in Saudi Arabia. Ann Trop Paediatr 8:187–192, 1988.
16. Dommisse J. The causes of perinatal deaths in the Greater Cape Town area: a 12-month survey. S Afr Med J 80:270–275, 1991.
17. Dutta D, Bhattacharya MK, Bhattacharya SK, et al. Influence of admission weight on neonatal mortality amongst hospitalised neonates in Calcutta. J Indian Med Assoc 90:308–309, 1992.
18. Geetha T, Chenoy R, Stevens D, et al. A multicentre study of perinatal mortality in Nepal. Paediatr Perinat Epidemiol 9:74–89, 1995.
19. Gupta PK, Gupta AP. Perinatal mortality. Indian Pediatr 22:201–205, 1985.
20. Horpaopan S, Ratrisawasdi V, Vichitpahanakarn P, et al. Perinatal mortality at Children's and Rajvithi Hospitals in 1983-1987. J Med Assoc Thai 72:376–381, 1989.
21. Hotrakitya S, Tejavej A, Siripoonya P. Early neonatal mortality and causes of death in Ramathibodi Hospital: 1981-1990. J Med Assoc Thai 76:119–129, 1993.
22. Kazimoto TPK. Review of perinatal mortality at Muhimbili maternity block. J Gynecol East Cent Afr 1:105–108, 1982.
23. Maouris P. Reducing perinatal mortality in Vila Central Hospital, Vanuatu. P N G Med J 37:178–180, 1994.
24. Njokanma OF, Olanrewaju DM. A study of neonatal deaths at the Ogun State University Teaching Hospital, Sagamu, Nigeria. J Trop Med Hyg 98:155–160, 1995.
25. Njokanma OF, Sule-Odu AO, Akesode FA. Perinatal mortality at the Ogun State University Teaching Hospital, Sagamu, Nigeria. J Trop Pediatr 40:78–81, 1994.
26. Okolo AA, Omene JA. Trends in neonatal mortality in Benin City, Nigeria. Int J Gynaecol Obstet 23:191–195, 1985.
27. Oyedeji GA, Olamijulo SK, Joiner KT. Experience at Wesley: 1,391 consecutive admissions into the neonatal unit (Hurford Ward). J Trop Pediatr 29:206–212, 1983.
28. Panja S, Bhattacharyya I, Das Gupta M. Low birth weight infants—study of mortality. Indian Pediatr 21:201–205, 1984.
29. Pengsa K, Taksaphan S. Perinatal mortality at Srinagarind Hospital. J Med Assoc Thai 70:667–672, 1987.
30. Pradeep M, Rajan L, Sudevan P. Perinatal mortality—a hospital based study. Indian Pediatr 32:1091–1094, 1995
31. Sangamnerkar M, Sutaria UD, Shrotri AN. Pattern of neonatal mortality in a government teaching institute. Asia-Oceania J Obstet Gynaecol 14:219–225, 1988.
32. Santhanakrishnan BR, Gopal S, Jayam S. Perinatal mortality in a referral teaching hospital in Madras city. Indian J Pediatr 53:359–363, 1986.
33. Singh M. Hospital-based data on perinatal and neonatal mortality in India. Indian Pediatr 23:579–584, 1986.
34. Singh M, Deorari AK, Khajuria RC, et al. Perinatal and neonatal mortality in a hospital. Indian J Med Res 94:1–5, 1991.
35. Siripoonya P, Tejavej A, Boonpasat Y. Early neonatal mortality at Ramathibodi Hospital: 1969-1978. J Med Assoc Thai 64:546–549, 1981.
36. Vince JD. Neonatal care in perspective: results of neonatal care at Port Moresby. Papua New Guinea Med J 30:127–134, 1987.
37. Alam N. Repeated neonatal deaths in families with special reference to causes of death. Paediatr Perinat Epidemiolo 13:78–88, 1999.
38. Bang AT, Bang RA, Sontakke PG, and the SEARCH team. Management of childhood pneumonia by traditional birth attendants. Bull World Health Organ 72:897–905, 1994.
39. Bang AT, Bang RA, Baitule SB, et al. Effect of home-based neonatal care and management of sepsis on neonatal mortality: field trial in rural India. Lancet 354:1955–1961, 1999.
40. Barros FC, Victora CG, Vaughan JP, et al. Perinatal mortality in southern Brazil: a population-based study of 7392 births. Bull World Health Organ 65:95–104, 1987.
41. Bartlett AV, Paz de Bocaletti ME. Intrapartum and neonatal mortality in a traditional indigenous community in rural Guatemala. Acta Paediatr Scand 80:288–296, 1991.
42. Bartlett AV, Paz de Bocaletti ME, Bocaletti MA. Neonatal and early postneonatal morbidity and mortality in a rural Guatemalan community: the importance of infectious diseases and their management. Pediatr Infect Dis J. 10:752–757, 1991.

43. Ben-Li L, Dao-zhong Z, Hong-qi T, et al. Perinatal mortality rate in 11 Jiangsu cities. Chin Med J 98:157–160, 1985.
44. Bendib A, Dekkar N, Lamdjadani N. Facteurs associés á la mortalité juvénile, infantile et néonatale. Arch Fr Pediatr 50:741–747, 1993.
45. Bhardwaj N, Hasan SB. High perinatal and neonatal mortality in rural India. J R Soc Health 113:60–63, 1993.
46. Bhatia S. Patterns and causes of neonatal and postneonatal mortality in rural Bangladesh. Stud Fam Plann 20:136–146, 1989.
47. Bourne DE, Rip MR, Woods DL. Characteristics of infant mortality in the RSA 1929-1983: II. Causes of death among white and coloured infants. S Afr Med J 73:230–232, 1988.
48. Choudhary SR, Jayaswal ON. Infant and early childhood mortality in urban slums under ICDS scheme-a prospective study. Indian Pediatr 26:544–549, 1989.
49. De Francisco A, Hall AJ, Armstrong Schellenberg JRM, et al. The pattern of infant and childhood mortality in Upper River Division, The Gambia. Ann Trop Paediatr 13:345–352, 1993.
50. Fauveau V, Wojtyniak B, Mostafa G, et al. Perinatal mortality in Matlab, Bangladesh: a community-based study. Int J Epidemiol 19:606–612, 1990.
51. Fonseka P, Wijewardene K, Harendra de Silva DG, et al. Neonatal and post-neonatal mortality in the Galle district. Ceylon Med J 39:82–85, 1994.
52. Garg SK, Mishra VN, Singh JV, et al. Neonatal mortality in Meerut district. Indian J Med Sci 47:222–225, 1993.
53. Greenwood AM, Greenwood BM, Bradley AK, et al. A prospective survey of the outcome of pregnancy in a rural area of The Gambia. Bull World Health Organ 65:635–643, 1987.
54. Islam MS, Rahaman MM, Aziz KMS, et al. Infant mortality in rural Bangladesh: an analysis of causes during neonatal and postneonatal periods. J Trop Pediatr 28:294–298, 1982.
55. Jalil F, Lindblad BS, Hanson LA, et al. Early child health in Lahore, Pakistan: IX. Perinatal events. Acta Paediatr 390(Suppl):95–107, 1993.
56. Kandeh BS. Causes of infant and early childhood deaths in Sierra Leone. Soc Sci Med 23:297–303, 1986.
57. Khan SR, Jalil F, Zaman S, et al. Early child health in Lahore, Pakistan: X. Mortality. Acta Paediatr 390(Suppl):109–177, 1993.
58. Knobel RH, Yang WS, Ho MS. Urban-rural and regional differences in infant mortality in Taiwan. Soc Sci Med 39:815–822, 1994.
59. Kumar V, Datta N, Saini SS. Infant mortality in a rural community development block in Haryana. Indian J Pediatr 49:795–802, 1982.
60. Leach A, McArdle TF, Banya S, et al. Neonatal mortality in a rural area of The Gambia. Ann Trop Paediatr 19:33–43, 1999.
61. Marsh D, Majid N, Rasmussen Z, et al. Cause-specific child mortality in a mountainous community in Pakistan by verbal autopsy. J Pak Med Assoc 11:226–229, 1993.
62. Mohamed TA. Registration of births' and infants' deaths in demo village in Fayoum governorate. J Egypt Public Health Assoc 65:207–220, 1990.
63. Moir JS, Garner PA, Heywood PF, et al. Mortality in a rural area of Madang Province, Papua New Guinea. Ann Trop Med Parasitol 83:305–319, 1989.
64. Rahman S, Nessa F. Neonatal mortality patterns in rural Bangladesh. J Trop Pediatr 35:199–202, 1989.
65. Rip MR, Bourne DE, Woods DL. Characteristics of infant mortality in the RSA 1929-1983: I. Components of the white and coloured infant mortality rate. S Afr Med J 73:227–229, 1988.
66. Shah U, Pratinidhi AK, Bhatlawande PV. Perinatal mortality in rural India: intervention through primary health care: II. Neonatal mortality. J Epidemiol Commun Health 38:138–142, 1984.
67. Singhal PK, Mathur GP, Mathur S, et al. Perinatal mortality: in ICDS urban slum area. Indian Pediatr 23:339–343, 1986.
68. Singhal PK, Mathur GP, Mathur S, et al. Neonatal morbidity and mortality in ICDS urban slums. Indian Pediatr 27:485–488, 1990.
69. Sivagnanasundram C, Sivarajah N, Wijayaratnam A. Infant deaths in a health unit area of Northern Sri Lanka. J Trop Med Hyg 88:401–406, 1985.
70. Soudarssanane MB, Srinivasa DK, Narayan KA, et al. Infant mortality in Pondicherry—an analysis of a cohort of 8185 births. Indian Pediatr 29:1379–1384, 1992.
71. Taha TE, Gray RH, Abdelwahab MM. Determinants of neonatal mortality in central Sudan. Ann Trop Paediatr 13:359–364, 1993.
72. Thora S, Awadhiya S, Chansoriya M, et al. Perinatal and infant mortality in urban slums under I.C.D.S. scheme. Indian Pediatr 23:595–598, 1986.
73. Urrutia JJ, Sosa R, Kennell JH, et al. Prevalence of maternal and neonatal infections in a developing country: possible low-cost preventive measures. *In* Perinatal Infections, vol 77. Amsterdam, Ciba Foundation Symposium, 1980, pp 171–186.
74. Woodruff AW, Adamson EA, El-Suni A, et al. Infants in Juba, Southern Sudan: the first six months of life. Lancet 2:262–264, 1983.
75. Adhikari M, Coovadia YM, Singh D. A 4-year study of neonatal meningitis: clinical and microbiological findings. J Trop Pediatr 41:81–85, 1995.
76. Airede AI. Neonatal bacterial meningitis in the middle belt of Nigeria. Dev Med Child Neurol 35:424–430, 1993.
77. Airede AK. Neonatal septicaemia in an African city of high altitude. J Trop Pediatr 38:189–191, 1992.
78. Das PK, Basu K, Chakraborty P, et al. Clinical and bacteriological profile of neonatal infections in metropolitan city based medical college nursery. J Indian Med Assoc 97:3–5, 1999.
79. Kuruvilla KA, Pillai S, Jesudason M, et al. Bacterial profile of sepsis in a neonatal unit in south India. Indian Pediatr 35:851–858, 1998.
80. Ali Z. Neonatal meningitis: a 3-year retrospective study at the Mount Hope Women's Hospital, Trinidad, West Indies. J Trop Pediatr 41:109–111, 1995.
81. Bhutta ZA, Naqvi SH, Muzaffar T, et al. Neonatal sepsis in Pakistan: presentation and pathogens. Acta Paediatr Scand 80:596–601, 1991.
82. Boo NY, Chor CY. Six year trend of neonatal septicaemia in a large Malaysian maternity hospital. J Paediatr Child Health 30:23–27, 1994.
83. Chotpitayasunondh T. Bacterial meningitis in children: etiology and clinical features, an 11-year review of 618 cases. Southeast Asian J Trop Med Public Health 25:107–115, 1994.
84. Chugh K, Aggarwal BB, Kaul VK, et al. Bacteriological profile of neonatal septicemia. Indian J Pediatr 55:961–965, 1988.
85. Coovadia YM, Mayosi B, Adhikari M, et al. Hospital-acquired neonatal bacterial meningitis: the impacts of cefotaxime usage on mortality and of amikacin usage on incidence. Ann Trop Paediatr 9:233–239, 1989.
86. Daoud AS, Abuekteish F, Obeidat A, et al. The changing face of neonatal septicaemia. Ann Trop Paediatr 15:93–96, 1995.
87. Dawodu AH, Ashiru JO. The changing pattern of causative bacterial organisms in neonatal meningitis. Niger J Paediatr 10:1–5, 1983.
88. Elzouki AY, Vesikari T. First international conference on infections in children in Arab countries. Pediatr Infect Dis J 4:527–531, 1985.
89. Gupta PK, Murali MV, Faridi MM, et al. Clinical profile of *Klebsiella* septicemia in neonates. Indian J Pediatr 60:565–572, 1993.
90. Haffejee IE, Bhana RH, Coovadia YM, et al. Neonatal group B streptococcal infections in Indian (Asian) babies in South Africa. J Infect 22:225–231, 1991.
91. Haque KN, Chagia AH, Shaheed MM. Half a decade of neonatal sepsis, Riyadh, Saudi Arabia. J Trop Pediatr 36:20–23, 1990.
92. Khatua SP, Das AK, Chatterjee BD, et al. Neonatal septicemia. Indian J Pediatr 53:509–514, 1986.
93. Koutouby A, Habibullah J. Neonatal sepsis in Dubai, United Arab Emirates. J Trop Pediatr 41:177–180, 1995.
94. Kuruvilla AC. Neonatal septicaemia in Kuwait. J Kwt Med Assoc 14:225–231, 1980.
95. Lim NL, Wong YH, Boo NY, et al. Bacteraemic infections in a neonatal intensive care unit-a nine-month survey. Med J Malaysia 50:59–63, 1995.
96. Longe AC, Omene JA, Okolo AA. Neonatal meningitis in Nigerian infants. Acta Paediatr Scand 73:477–481, 1984.
97. Mondal GP, Raghavan M, Vishnu BB, et al. Neonatal septicaemia among inborn and outborn babies in a referral hospital. Indian J Pediatr 58:529–533, 1991.
98. Moreno MT, Vargas S, Poveda R, et al. Neonatal sepsis and meningitis in a developing Latin American country. Pediatr Infect Dis J 13:516–520, 1994.
99. Namdeo UK, Singh HP, Rajput VJ, et al. Bacteriological profile of neonatal septicemia. Indian Pediatr 24:53–56, 1987.
100. Nathoo KJ, Mason PR, Chimbira THK, and the Puerperal Sepsis Study Group. Neonatal septicaemia in Harare Hospital: aetiology and risk factors. Cent Afr J Med 36:150–156, 1990.
101. Nathoo KJ, Pazvakavamba I, Chidede OS, et al. Neonatal meningitis in Harare, Zimbabwe: a 2-year review. Ann Trop Paediatr 11:11–15, 1991.
102. Ohlsson A, Bailey T, Takieddine F. Changing etiology and outcome of neonatal septicemia in Riyadh, Saudi Arabia. Acta Paediatr Scand 75:540–544, 1986.
103. Ohlsson A, Serenius F. Neonatal septicemia in Riyadh, Saudi Arabia. Acta Paediatr Scand 70:825–829, 1981.
104. Okolo AA, Omene JA. Changing pattern of neonatal septicaemia in an African city. Ann Trop Paediatr 5:123–126, 1985.

105. Owa JA, Olusanya O. Neonatal bacteraemia in Wesley Guild Hospital, Ilesha, Nigeria. Ann Trop Paediatr 8:80–84, 1988.
106. Prasertsom W, Ratrisawadi V, Thanasophon Y, et al. Early versus late onset neonatal septicemia at Children's Hospital. J Med Assoc Thai 73:106–109, 1990.
107. Rajab A, DeLouvois J. Survey of infection in babies at the Khoula Hospital, Oman. Ann Trop Paediatr 10:39–43, 1990.
108. Sharma PP, Halder D, Dutta AK, et al. Bacteriological profile of neonatal septicemia. Indian Pediatr 24:1011–1017, 1987.
109. Sinha N, Deb A, Mukherjee AK. Septicemia in neonates and early infancy. Indian J Pediatr 53:249–256, 1986.
110. Tafari N, Ljungh-Wadstrom A. Consequences of amniotic fluid infection: early neonatal septicaemia. *In* Perinatal Infections, vol 77. Amsterdam, Ciba Foundation Symposium, 1980, pp 55–67.
111. Yardi D, Gaikwad S, Deodhar L. Incidence, mortality and bacteriological profile of septicemia in pediatric patients. Indian J Pediatr 51:173–176, 1984.
112. Saxena S, Anand NK, Saini L, et al. Bacterial infections among home delivered neonates: clinical picture and bacteriological profile. Indian Pediatr 17:17–24, 1980.
113. Wong NACS, Hunt LP, Marlow N. Risk factors for developing neonatal septicaemia at a Malaysian Hospital. J Trop Pediatr 43:54–58, 1997.
114. Bhutta ZA, Yusuf K. Neonatal sepsis in Karachi: factors determining outcome and mortality. J Trop Pediatr 43:65–70, 1997.
115. Muhe L, Tilahun M, Lulseged S, et al. Etiology of pneumonia, sepsis, and meningitis in young infants below 3 months of age in Ethiopia. Pediatr Infect Dis J Suppl 18:S56–S61, 1999.
116. Ghiorghis B. Neonatal sepsis in Addis Ababa, Ethiopia: a review of 151 bacteremic neonates. Ethiopian Med J 35:169–176, 1997.
117. Kago I, Wouafo Ndayo M, Tchokoteu PF, et al. Neonatal septicemia and meningitis caused by gram-negative bacilli in Yaonde: clinical, bacteriological and prognostic aspects. Bull Soc Pathol Exot 84:573–581, 1991.
118. Robillard PY, Nabeth P, Hulsey TC, et al. Neonatal bacterial septicemia in a tropical area: four-year experience in Guadeloupe (French West Indies). Acta Paediatr 82:687–689, 1993.
119. Rodriguez CJ, Fraga JM, Garcia Riestra C, et al. Neonatal sepsis: epidemiologic indicators and relation to birth weight and length of hospitalization time. Anal Español Pediatr 48:401–408, 1998.
120. Dawodu A, Al Umran K, Twum-Danso K. A case control study of neonatal sepsis: experience from Saudi Arabia. J Trop Pediatr 43:84–88, 1997.
121. Greenberg D, Shinwell ES, Yagupsky P. A prospective study of neonatal sepsis and meningitis in Southern Israel. Pediatr Infect Dis J 16:768–773, 1997.
122. Leibovitz E, Flidel-Rimon O, Juster-Reicher A, et al. Sepsis at a neonatal intensive care unit: a four-year retrospective study (1989-1992). Isr J Med Sci 33:734–738, 1997.
123. Daoud AS, Al-Sheyyab M, Abu-Ekteish F, et al. Neonatal meningitis in Northern Jordan. J Trop Pediatr 42:267–270, 1996.
124. Campagne G, Djibo S, Schuchat A, et al. Epidemiology of bacterial meningitis in Niamey, Niger, 1981-1996. Bull World Health Organ 77:499–508, 1999.
125. Nel E. Neonatal meningitis: mortality, cerebrospinal fluid, and microbiological findings. J Trop Pediatr 46:237–239, 2000.
126. Gebremariam A. Neonatal meningitis in Addis Ababa: a 10-year review. Ann Trop Paediatr 18:279–283, 1998.
127. The State of the World's Children 2004. New York, UNICEF, 2004.
128. Bennett R, Eriksson M, Melen B, et al. Changes in the incidence and spectrum of neonatal septicemia during a fifteen-year period. Acta Paediatr Scand 74:687–690, 1985.
129. Gladstone IM, Ehrenkranz RA, Edberg SC, et al. A ten-year review of neonatal sepsis and comparison with the previous fifty-year experience. Pediatr Infect Dis J 9:819–825, 1990.
130. Antia-Obong OE, Utsalo SJ. Bacterial agents in neonatal septicaemia in Calabar, Nigeria: review of 100 cases. Trop Doct 21:169–170, 1991.
131. Bhatia BD, Chugh SP, Narang P, et al. Bacterial flora in mothers and babies with reference to causative agent in neonatal septicemia. Indian Pediatr 26:455–459, 1989.
132. Chaturvedi P, Agrawal M, Narang P. Analysis of blood-culture isolates from neonates of a rural hospital. Indian Pediatr 26:460–465, 1989.
133. El Rifai MR. A study of 214 neonates with infection in the Maternity and Children's Hospital of Riyadh, Saudi Arabia. Ann Trop Paediatr 2:119–122, 1982.
134. Liebowitz LD, Koornhof HJ, Barrett M, et al. Bacterial meningitis in Johannesburg-1980-1982. S Afr Med J 66:677–679, 1984.
135. MacFarlane DE. Neonatal group B streptococcal septicaemia in a developing country. Acta Paediatr Scand 76:470–473, 1987.
136. Musoke RN, Malenga GJ. Bacterial infections in neonates at the Kenyatta Hospital nursery. A prospective study. East Afr Med J 61:909–916, 1984.
137. Nathoo KJ, Mason PR, Gwanzure L, et al. Severe Klebsiella infection as a cause of mortality in neonates in Harare, Zimbabwe: evidence from postmortem blood cultures. Pediatr Infect Dis J 12:840–844, 1993.
138. Solorzano-Santos F, Diaz-Ramos RD, Arredondo-Garcia JL. Diseases caused by group B Streptococcus in Mexico. Letter. Pediatr Infect Dis J 9:66, 1990.
139. St. John MA, Lewis DB, Archer E. Current problems of neonatal septicaemia in Barbados. West Indian Med J 35(Suppl):16, 1986.
140. Rao PS, Baliga M, Shivananda PG. Bacteriology of neonatal septicaemia in a rural referral hospital in South India. J Trop Pediatr 39:230–233, 1993.
141. Monga K, Fernandez A, Deodhar L. Changing bacteriological patterns in neonatal septicaemia. Indian J Pediatr 53:505–508, 1986.
142. Pruekprasert P, Chongsuvivatwong V, Patamasucon P. Factors influencing case-fatality rate of septicemic children. Southeast Asian J Trop Med Public Health 25:678–683, 1994.
143. Lehmann D, Michael A, Omena M, et al. The bacterial and viral etiology of severe infection in children aged less than three months in the highlands of Papua New Guinea. Pediatr Infect Dis J Suppl 18:S42–S49, 1999.
144. Gatchalian SR, Quiambao BP, Morelos AMR, et al. Bacterial and viral aetiology of serious infections in very young Filipino infants. Pediatr Infect Dis J Suppl 18:S50–S55, 1999.
145. Ako-Nai AK, Adejuyigbe EA, Ajayi FM, et al. The bacteriology of neonatal septicaemia in Ile-Ife, Nigeria. J Trop Pediatr 45:146–151, 1999.
146. Asindi AA, Bilal NE, Fatinni YA, et al. Neonatal septicemia. Saudi Med J 20:942–946, 1999.
147. Bhakoo ON. Neonatal bacterial infections in Chandigarh: a decade of experience. Indian J Pediatr 47:419–424, 1980.
148. Cisse MF, Sow AI, Ba M, et al. Bacteriology of neonatal septicemia in Dakar. Press Med 21:413–416, 1992.
149. Khatoon S, Khatun M. Clinical and bacteriological profile of neonatal septicaemia and their outcome. Bangladesh J Child Health 17:48–53, 1993.
150. Moore MR, Schrag SJ, Schuchat A. Effects of intrapartum antimicrobial prophylaxis for prevention of group-B-streptococcal disease on the incidence and ecology of early-onset neonatal sepsis. Lancet 3:201–213, 2003.
151. WHO Young Infant Study Group. The bacterial etiology of serious infections in young infants in developing countries—results of a multicenter study. Pediatr Infect Dis J Suppl 18:S17–S22, 1999.
152. Mulholland EK, Ogunlesi OO, Adegbola RA, et al. Etiology of serious infections in young Gambian infants. Pediatr Infect Dis J Suppl 18:S35–S41, 1999.
153. WHO Young Infants Study Group. Clinical prediction of serious bacterial infections in young infants in developing countries. Pediatr Infect Dis J Suppl 18:S23–S31, 1999.
154. Lehmann D, Sanders RC, Marjen B, et al. High rates of Chlamydia trachomatis infections in young Papua New Guinean infants. Pediatr Infect Dis J Suppl 18:S62–S69, 1999.
155. WHO Young Infants Study Group. Conclusions from the WHO multicenter study of serious infections in young infants. Pediatr Infect Dis J Suppl 18:S32–S34, 1999.
156. Centers for Disease Control and Prevention. Prevention of perinatal group B streptococcal disease. Revised Guidelines from CDC. MMWR Morb Mortal Wkly Rep 51:1–22, 2002.
157. Stoll BJ, Schuchat A. Maternal carriage of group B streptococci in developing countries. Pediatr Infect Dis J 17:499–503, 1998.
158. Blumberg HM, Stephens DS, Modansky M, et al. Invasive group B streptococcal disease: the emergence of serotype V. J Infect Dis 173:365–373, 1996.
159. Collins TS, Calderon M, Gilman RH, et al. Group B streptococcal colonization in a developing country: its association with sexually transmitted disease and socioeconomic factors. Am J Trop Med 59:633-636, 1998.
160. Suara RO, Adegbola RA, Baker CJ, et al. Carriage of group B streptococci in pregnant Gambian mothers and their infants. J Infect Dis 70:1316–1319, 1994.
161. Regan JA, Klebanoff MA, Nugent RP, et al, for the VIP Study Group. Colonization with group B streptococci in pregnancy and adverse outcome. Am J Obstet Gynecol 174:1354–1360, 1996.

162. Klein JO. Bacterial sepsis and meningitis. In Remington JS, Klein JO (eds). Infectious Diseases of the Fetus and Newborn Infant, 5th ed. Philadelphia, WB Saunders, 2000, pp 943-998.
163. Duke T, Michael A. Increase in sepsis due to multi-resistant enteric gram-negative bacilli in Papua New Guinea. Lancet 353:2210–2211, 1999.
164. Bhutta ZA. Enterobacter sepsis in a newborn—a growing problem in Karachi. J Hosp Infect 34:211–216, 1996.
165. Musoke RN, Revathi G. 2000 emergence of multidrug-resistant gram-negative organisms in a neonatal unit and the therapeutic implications. J Trop Pediatr 46:86–91.
166. Garenne M, Ronsmans C, Campbell H. The magnitude of mortality from acute respiratory infections in children under 5 years in developing countries. World Health Stat Q 45:180–191, 1992.
167. Misra S, Bhakoo ON, Ayyagiri A, et al. Clinical and bacteriological profile of neonatal pneumonia. Indian J Med Res 93:366–370, 1991.
168. Patwari AK, Bisht S, Srinjvasari A, et al. Aetiology of pneumonia in hospitalized children. J Trop Pediatr 42:15–19, 1996.
169. Monto AS, Lehmann. Acute respiratory infections (ARI) in children: prospects for prevention. Vaccine 16:1582–1588, 1998.
170. Ploin D, Liberas S, Thouvenot D, et al. Influenza burden in children newborn to eleven months of age in a pediatric emergency department during the peak of an influenza epidemic. Pediatr Infect Dis J 22:S218–222, 2003.
171. Bang AT, Bang RA, Morankar VP, et al. Pneumonia in neonates: can it be managed in the community? Arch Dis Child 68:550–556, 1993.
172. Zaman K, Baqui AH, Yunas M, et al. Acute respiration infections in children: a community-based longitudinal study in rural Bangladesh. J Trop Pediatr 43:133–137, 1997.
173. Victora CG, Kirkwood BR, Ashworth A, et al. Potential interventions for the prevention of childhood pneumonia in developing countries: improving nutrition. Am J Clin Nutr 70:309–320, 1999.
174. Arifeen S, Black RE, Antelman G, et al. Exclusive breastfeeding reduces acute respiratory infection and diarrhea deaths among infants in Dhaka slums. Pediatrics 108:e67, 2001.
175. Datta N, Kumar V, Kumar L, et al. Application of case management to the control of acute respiratory infections in low-birth-weight infants: a feasibility study. Bull World Health Organ 65:77–82, 1987.
176. Starke JR. Tuberculosis: an old disease but a new threat to the mother, fetus, and neonate. Clin Perinatol 24:107–127, 1997.
177. Jana N, Vasishta K, Jindal SK, et al. Perinatal outcome in pregnancies complicated by pulmonary tuberculosis. Int J Gynecol Obstet 44:119–124, 1994.
178. Figueroa-Damián R, Arredondo-García JL. Neonatal outcome of children born to women with tuberculosis. Arch Med Res 32:66–69, 2001.
179. Smith KC. Congenital tuberculosis: a rare manifestation of a common infection. Curr Opin Infect Dis 15:269–274, 2002.
180. Jana N, Vasishta K, Saha SC, et al. Obstetrical outcomes among women with extrapulmonary tuberculosis. N Engl J Med 341:645–649, 1999.
181. Mazade MA, Evans EM, Starke JR, et al. Congenital tuberculosis presenting as sepsis syndrome: case report and review of the literature. Pediatr Infect Dis J 20:439–442, 2001.
182. Ahmed Y, Mwaba P, Chintu C, et al. A study of maternal mortality at the University Teaching Hospital, Lusaka, Zambia: the emergence of tuberculosis as a major non-obstetric cause of maternal death. Intl J Tuberc Lung Dis 3:675–680, 1999.
183. Adhikari M, Pillay T, Pillay D. Tuberculosis in the newborn: an emerging disease. Pediatr Infect Dis J 16:1108–1112, 1997.
184. Cantwell MF, Shehab ZM, Costello AM, et al. Brief report: congenital tuberculosis. N Engl J Med 330:1051–1054, 1994.
185. Bhandari N, Bahl R, Bhatnagar V, et al. Treating sick young infants in urban slum setting. Lancet 347:1774–1775, 1996.
186. Gerbase AC, Rowley JT, Mertens TE. Global epidemiology of sexually transmitted diseases. Lancet 351(suppl III):2–4, 1998.
187. Sturm AW, Wilkinson D, Ndovela N, et al. Pregnant women as a reservoir of undetected sexually transmitted diseases in rural South Africa: implications for disease control. Am J Public Health 88:1243–1245, 1998.
188. Moodley P, Sturm AW. Sexually transmitted infections, adverse pregnancy outcome and neonatal infection. Semin Neonatol 5:255–269, 2000.
189. Goldenberg RL, Andrews WW, Yuan AC, et al. Sexually transmitted diseases and adverse outcomes of pregnancy. Clin Perinatol 24:23–41, 1997.
190. McDermott J, Steketee R, Larsen S, et al. Syphilis-associated perinatal and infant mortality in rural Malawi. Bull World Health Organ 71:773–780, 1993.
191. Rotchford K, Lombard C, Zuma K, et al. Impact on perinatal mortality of missed opportunities to treat maternal syphilis in rural South Africa: baseline results from a clinic randomized control trial. Trop Med Int Health 5:800–804, 2000.
192. Lindstrand A, Bergström S, Bugalho A, et al. Perinatal transmission of parturient syphilis in Mozambique. Int J STD AIDS 7:378–379, 1996.
193. Lumbiganon P, Piaggio G, Villar J, et al. The epidemiology of syphilis in pregnancy. Int J STD AIDS 13:486–494, 2002.
194. Hira SK, Bhat GJ, Chikamata DM, et al. Syphilis intervention in pregnancy: Zambian demonstration project. Genitourinary Med 66:159–164, 1990.
195. Frank D, Duke T. Congenital syphilis at Goroka Base Hospital: incidence, clinical features and risk factors for mortality. P N G Med J 43:121–126, 2000.
196. Gloyd S, Chai S, Mercer MA. Antenatal syphilis in sub-Saharan Africa: missed opportunities for mortality reduction. Health Policy Planning 16:29–34, 2001.
197. Stoll BJ. Congenital syphilis: evaluation and management of neonates born to mothers with reactive serologic tests for syphilis. Pediatr Infect Dis J 13:845–853, 1994.
198. Gary RH, Wabwire-Mangen F, Kigozi G, et al. Randomized trial of presumptive sexually transmitted disease therapy during pregnancy in Rakai, Uganda. Am J Obstet Gynecol 185:1209–1217, 2001.
199. Brabin L. Clinical management and prevention of sexually transmitted diseases: a review focusing on women. Acta Tropica 75:53–70, 2000.
200. AIDS Epidemic Update 2003. Geneva, WHO, UNAIDS, 2003.
201. McIntyre J. HIV in Pregnancy: A Review. WHO/CHS/RHR/99.15, 1999.
202. Africa's Orphaned Generations. New York, UNICEF, 2003.
203. Coovadia HM, Rollins NC. Current controversies in the perinatal transmission of HIV in developing countries. Semin Neonatol 4:193–200, 1999.
204. Connor EM, Sperling RS, Gelber R, et al. Reduction of maternal-infant transmission of human immunodeficiency virus type 1 with zidovudine treatment. N Engl J Med 331:1173–1180, 1994.
205. Cooper ER, Nugent RP, Diaz C, et al. After AIDS clinical trial 076: the changing pattern of zidovudine use during pregnancy, and the subsequent reduction in the vertical transmission of human immunodeficiency virus in a cohort of infected women and their infants. Women and Infants Transmission Study Group. J Infect Dis 174:1207–1211, 1996.
206. Simonds RJ, Steketee R, Nesheim S, et al. Impact of zidovudine use on risk and risk factors for perinatal transmission of HIV. Perinatal AIDS Collaborative Transmission Studies. AIDS 12:301–308, 1998.
207. Mandelbrot L, Landreau-Mascaro A, Rekacewicz C, et al. Lamivudine-zidovudine combination for prevention of maternal-infant transmission of HIV-1. J Am Med Assoc 285:2083–2093, 2001.
208. The Working Group on Mother-to-Child Transmission of HIV. Rates of mother-to-child transmission of HIV-1 in Africa, America, and Europe: results from 13 perinatal studies. J Acquir Immune Defic Syndr Hum Retrovirol 8:506–510, 1995.
209. Kourtis A, Bulterys M, Nesheim S, et al. Understanding the timing of HIV transmission from mother to infant. JAMA 285:709–712, 2001.
210. Brocklehurst P. Interventions for reducing the risk of mother-to-child transmission of HIV infection. Cochrane Database Syst Rev 3, 2003.
211. De Cock KM, Fowler MG, Mercier E, et al. Prevention of mother-to-child HIV transmission in resource-poor countries: translating research into policy and practice. JAMA 283:1175–1182, 2000.
212. St. Louis ME, Kamenga M, Brown C, et al. Risk for perinatal HIV-1 transmission according to maternal immunologic, virologic, and placental factors. JAMA 269:2853–2859, 1993.
213. Bobat R, Coovadia H, Coutsoudis A, et al. Determinants of mother-to-child transmission of human immunodeficiency virus type 1 infection in a cohort from Durban, South Africa. Pediatr Infect Dis J 15:604–610, 1996.
214. Mandelbrot L, Mayaux MJ, Bongain A, et al. Obstetrics: obstetric factors and mother-to-child transmission of human immunodeficiency virus type 1: the French perinatal cohorts. Am J Obstet Gynecol 175:661–667, 1996.
215. Landers DV. Nutrition and immune function: II. Maternal factors influencing transmission. J Nutr 126:2637s–2640s, 1996.
216. Semba RD. Overview of the potential role of vitamin A in mother-to-child transmission of HIV-1. Acta Paediatr Suppl 421:107–112, 1997.

217. The International Perinatal HIV Group. Duration of ruptured membranes and vertical transmission of HIV-1: a meta-analysis from 15 prospective cohort studies. AIDS 15:357–368, 2001.
218. The International Perinatal HIV Group. The mode of delivery and the risk of vertical transmission of human immunodeficiency virus type 1—a meta-analysis of 15 prospective cohort studies. N Engl J Med 340:977–987, 1999.
219. Read JS, Newell M-L. Cesarean delivery for prevention of mother-to-child transmission of HIV. Cochrane Database Syst Rev 3, 2003.
220. Landesman SH, Kalish LA, Burns DN, et al. Obstetrical factors and the transmission of human immunodeficiency virus type 1 from mother to child. N Engl J Med 334:1617–1623, 1996.
221. Newell ML, Dunn DT, Peckham CS, et al, for the European Collaborative Study. Caesarean section and risk of vertical transmission of HIV-1 infection. Lancet 343:1464–1467, 1994.
222. The European Mode of Delivery Collaboration. Elective caesarean-section versus vaginal delivery in prevention of vertical HIV-1 transmission: a randomised clinical trial. Lancet 353:1035–1039, 1999.
223. Fowler MG, Mofenson L, McConnell M. The interface of perinatal HIV prevention, antiretroviral drug resistance, and antiretroviral treatment: what do we really know? JAIDS 34:308–311, 2003.
224. Abrams EJ, Wiener J, Carter R, et al. Maternal health factors and early pediatric antiretroviral therapy influence the rate of perinatal HIV-1 disease progression in children. AIDS 17:867–877, 2003.
225. Kourtis AP, Butera S, Ibegbu C, et al. Breast milk and HIV-1: vector of transmission or vehicle of protection. Lancet 3:786–793, 2003.
226. Tess BH, Rodrigues LC, Newell ML, et al. Breastfeeding, genetic, obstetric and other risk factors associated with mother-to-child transmission of HIV-1 in Sao Paulo State, Brazil. AIDS 12:513–520, 1998.
227. Dunn DT, Newell ML, Ades AE, et al. Risk of human immunodeficiency virus type 1 transmission through breastfeeding. Lancet 340:585–588, 1992.
228. Bertolli J, St. Louis ME, Simonds RJ, et al. Estimating the timing of mother-to-child transmission of human immunodeficiency virus in a breastfeeding population in Kinshasa, Zaire. J Infect Dis 174:722–726, 1996.
229. Ekpini ER, Wiktor SZ, Satten GA, et al. Late postnatal mother-to-child transmission of HIV-1 in Abidjan, Côte d'Ivoire. Lancet 349:1054–1059, 1997.
230. Kreiss J. Breastfeeding and vertical transmission of HIV-1. Acta Paediatr Suppl 421:113–117, 1997.
231. Fowler MG, Newell ML. Breast-feeding and HIV-1 transmission in resource-limited settings. JAIDS 30:230–239, 2002.
232. Bobat R, Moodley D, Coutsoudis A, et al. Breastfeeding by HIV-1 infected women and outcome in their infants: a cohort study from Durban, South Africa. AIDS 11:1627–1633, 1997.
233. World Health Organization/UNAIDS. HIV and Infant Feeding: A Policy Statement Developed Collaboratively by UNAIDS, WHO, and UNICEF. Geneva, WHO, UNAIDS, 1998, pp 20–21.
234. de Martino M, Pier-Angelo T, Tozzi AE, et al. HIV-1 transmission through breast-milk: appraisal of risk according to duration of feeding. AIDS 6:991–997, 1992.
235. Miotti PG, Taha TET, Kumwenda NI, et al. HIV transmission through breastfeeding: a study in Malawi. JAMA 282:744–749, 1999.
236. Nduati R, John G, Mbori-Ngacha D, et al. Effect of breastfeeding and formula feeding on transmission of HIV-1: a randomized clinical trial. JAMA 283:1167–1174, 2000.
237. Fawzi W, Msamanga G, Spiegelman D, et al. Transmission of HIV-1 through breastfeeding among women in Dar es Salaam, Tanzania. JAIDS 31:331–338, 2002.
238. Richardson BA, John-Stewart GC, Hughes JP, et al. Breast-milk infectivity in human immunodeficiency virus type 1-infected mothers. JID 187:736–740, 2003.
239. Leroy V, Newell ML, Dabis F, et al. International multicentre pooled analysis of late postnatal mother-to-child transmission of HIV-1 infection. Lancet 352:597–600, 1998.
240. Coutsoudis A, Pillay K, Kuhn L, et al. Method of feeding and transmission of HIV-1 from mothers to children by 15 months of age: prospective cohort study from Durban, South Africa. AIDS 15:379–387, 2001.
241. Van de Perre P. Postnatal transmission of human immunodeficiency virus type 1: the breastfeeding dilemma. Am J Obstet Gynecol 173:483–487, 1995.
242. Semba RD, Kumwenda N, Hoover DR, et al. Human immunodeficiency virus load in breast milk, mastitis, and mother-to-child transmission of human immunodeficiency virus type 1. J Infect Dis 180:93–98, 1999.
243. Coutsoudis A, Rollins N. Breast-feeding and HIV transmission: the jury is still out. J Pediatr Gastroenterol Nutr 36:434–442, 2003.
244. Abdool-Karim Q, Abdool-Karim SS, Coovadia HM, et al. Informed consent for HIV testing in a South African hospital: is it truly informed and truly voluntary? Am J Public Health 88:637–640, 1998.
245. Del Fante P, Jenniskens F, Lush L, et al. HIV, breastfeeding and under-5 mortality: modelling the impact of policy decisions for or against breastfeeding. J Trop Med Hyg 96:203–211, 1993.
246. Kuhn L, Stein Z. Infant survival, HIV infection, and feeding alternatives in less-developed countries. Am J Public Health 87:926–931, 1997.
247. Centers for Disease Control and Prevention. Public Health Service Task Force recommendations for the use of antiretroviral drugs in pregnant women infected with HIV-1 for maternal health and for reducing perinatal HIV-1 transmission in the United States. MMWR Morb Mortal Wkly Rep 47(rr-2):1–30, 1998.
248. Shaffer N, Chuachoowong R, Mock P, et al. Short-course zidovudine for perinatal HIV-1 transmission in Bangkok, Thailand: a randomised controlled trial. Lancet 353:773–780, 1999.
249. Wiktor SZ, Ekpini E, Karon JM, et al. Short-course oral zidovudine for prevention of mother-to-child transmission of HIV-1 in Abidjan, Côte d'Ivoire: a randomised trial. Lancet 353:781–785, 1999.
250. Dabis F, Msellati P, Meda N, et al. 6-Month efficacy, tolerance, and acceptability of a short regimen of oral zidovudine to reduce transmission of HIV in breastfed children in Côte d'Ivoire and Burkina Faso: a double-blind placebo-controlled multicentre trial. Lancet 353:786–792, 1999.
251. Lallemant M, Jourdain G, Le Coeur S, et al. A trial of shortened zidovudine regimens to prevent mother-to-child transmission of human immunodeficiency virus type 1. N Engl J Med 343:982–991, 2000.
252. Petra Study Team. Efficacy of three short-course regimens of zidovudine and lamivudine in preventing early and late transmission of HIV-1 from mother to child in Tanzania, South Africa, and Uganda (Petra study): a randomised, double-blind, placebo-controlled trial. Lancet 359:1178–1186, 2002.
253. Guay LA, Musoke P, Fleming T, et al. Intrapartum and neonatal single-dose nevirapine compared with zidovudine for prevention of mother-to-child transmission of HIV-1 in Kampala, Uganda: HIVNET 012 randomised trial. Lancet 354:795–802, 1999.
254. Moodley D, Moodley J, Coovadia H, et al. A multicenter randomized controlled trial of nevirapine versus a combination of zidovudine and lamivudine to reduce intrapartum and early postpartum mother-to-child transmission of human immunodeficiency virus type 1. J Infect Dis 187:725–735, 2003.
254a. Jourdain G, Ngo-Giang-Huong N, Le Coeur S, et al. Intrapartum exposure to nevirapine and subsequent maternal responses to nevirapine-based antiretroviral therapy. N Engl J Med 351:229–240, 2004.
255. Taha TE, Kumwenda NI, Gibbons A, et al. Short postexposure prophylaxis in newborn babies to reduce mother-to-child transmission of HIV-1: NVAZ randomised clinical trial. Lancet 362:1171–1177, 2003.
256. Ayouba A, Tene G, Cunin P, et al. Low rate of mother-to-child transmission of HIV-1 after nevirapine intervention in a pilot public health program in Yaoundé, Cameroon. 34:274–280, 2003.
257. World Health Organization. New initiative to reduce HIV transmission from mother-to-child in low-income countries. WHO/UNAIDS press release, June 1998.
258. Read JS. Cesarean section delivery to prevent vertical transmission of human immunodeficiency virus type 1. Associated risks and other considerations. Ann N Y Acad Sci 918:115–121, 2000.
259. Mandelbrot L, Msellati P, Meda N, et al. 15 month follow up of African children following vaginal cleansing with benzalkonium chloride of their HIV infected mothers during late pregnancy and delivery. Sex Transm Infect 78:267–270, 2002.
260. Pilot P, Coll-Seck A. Preventing mother-to-child transmission of HIV in Africa. Bull World Health Organ 77:869–870, 1999.
261. Menu E, Scarlatti G, Barré-Sinoussi F, et al. Mother-to-child transmission of HIV: developing integration of healthcare programmes with clinical, social and basic research studies. Report of the International Workshop held at Chobe Marina Lodge, Kasane, Botswana, 21-25 January 2003. Acta Paediatr 92:1343–1348, 2003.
262. Bennett JV, Rogers MF. Child survival and perinatal infections with human immunodeficiency virus. Am J Dis Child 145:1242–1247, 1991.

263. Adetunji J. Trends in under-5 mortality rates and the HIV/AIDS epidemic. Bull World Health Organ 78:1200–1206, 2000.
264. Stroh G, Aye KU, Thaung U, et al. Measurement of mortality from neonatal tetanus in Burma. Bull World Health Organ 65:309–316, 1987.
265. World Health Organization. Maternal and neonatal tetanus elimination by 2005. Strategies for achieving and maintaining elimination. www.who.int/vaccines-documents, 2000.
266. The Progress of Nations 2000. New York: UNICEF, 2000
267. World Health Organization, UNICEF, World Bank. State of the World's Vaccines and Immunization. Geneva: World Health Organization, 2002.
268. Galazka A, Stroh G. Neonatal tetanus: guidelines on the community-based survey on neonatal tetanus mortality. WHO/EPI/GEN/86/8. Geneva, World Health Organization, 1995.
269. Rochat R, Akhter HH. Tetanus and pregnancy-related mortality in Bangladesh. Lancet 354:565, 1999.
270. Cushing AH. Omphalitis: a review. Pediatr Infect Dis J 4:282–285, 1985.
271. Samuel M, Freeman NV, Vaishnav A, et al. Necrotizing fasciitis: a serious complication of omphalitis in neonates. J Pediatr Surg 29:1414–1416, 1994.
272. Sawin RS, Schaller RT, Tapper D, et al. Early recognition of neonatal abdominal wall necrotizing fasciitis. Am J Surg 167:481–484, 1994.
273. Airede AI. Pathogens in neonatal omphalitis. J Trop Pediatr 38:129–131, 1992.
274. Faridi MM, Rattan A, Ahmad SH. Omphalitis neonatorum. J Indian Med Assoc 91:283–285, 1993.
275. Guvenc H, Guvenc M, Yenioglu H, et al. Neonatal omphalitis is still common in eastern Turkey. Scand J Infect Dis 23:613–616, 1991.
276. Guvenc H, Aygun AD, Yasar F, et al. Omphalitis in term and preterm appropriate for gestational age and small for gestational age infants. J Trop Pediatr 43:368–372, 1997.
277. Baley JE, Fanaroff AA. Neonatal infections: I. Infection related to nursery care practices. *In* Sinclair JC, Bracken MB (eds). Effective Care of the Newborn Infant. New York, Oxford University Press, 1992, pp 454–476.
278. Rush J, Chalmers I, Enkin M. Care of the new mother and baby. *In* Chalmers I, Enkin M, Keirse MJNC (eds). Effective Care in Pregnancy and Childbirth, vol 2. New York, Oxford University Press, 1989, pp 1333–1346.
279. Garner P, Lai D, Baea M, et al. Avoiding neonatal death: an intervention study of umbilical cord care. J Trop Pediatr 40:24–28, 1994.
280. Bern C, Martines J, de Zoysa I, et al. The magnitude of the global problem of diarrhoeal disease: a ten-year update. Bull World Health Organ 70:705–714, 1992.
281. Snyder JD, Merson MH. The magnitude of the global problem of acute diarrhoeal disease: a review of active surveillance data. Bull World Health Organ 60:605–613, 1982.
282. Huilan S, Zhen LG, Mathan MM, et al. Etiology of acute diarrhoea among children in developing countries: a multicentre study in five countries. Bull World Health Organ 89:s49–s55, 1991.
283. de Zoysa I, Rea M, Martines J. Why promote breastfeeding in diarrhoeal disease control programmes? Health Pol Plan 6:371–379, 1991.
284. Black RE, Lopez de Romana G, Brown KH, et al. Incidence and etiology of infantile diarrhea and major routes of transmission in Huascar, Peru. Am J Epidemiol 129:785–799, 1989.
285. Mahmud A, Jalil F, Karlberg J, et al. Early child health in Lahore, Pakistan: VII. Diarrhoea. Acta Paediatr Suppl 390:79–85, 1993.
286. Stoll BJ, Glass RI, Huq MI, et al. Surveillance of patients attending a diarrhoeal disease hospital in Bangladesh. BMJ 285:1185–1188, 1982.
287. Aye DT, Sack DA, Wachsmuth IK, et al. Neonatal diarrhea at a maternity hospital in Rangoon. Am J Public Health 81:480–481, 1991.
288. Clemens J, Elyazeed RA, Rao M, et al. Early initiation of breastfeeding and the risk of infant diarrhea in rural Egypt. Pediatrics 104:e3, 1999.
289. Parashar UD, Bresee JS, Gentsch JR, et al. Rotavirus Emerg Infect Dis 4:1–10, 1998.
290. Espinoza F, Paniagua M, Hallander H, et al. Rotavirus infections in young Nicaraguan children. Pediatr Infect Dis J 16:564–571, 1997.
291. Haffejee IE. The epidemiology of rotavirus infections: a global perspective. J Pediatr Gastroenterol Nutr 20:275–286, 1995.
292. Bishop RF, Barnes GL, Cipriani E, et al. Clinical immunity after neonatal rotavirus infection: a prospective longitudinal study in young children. N Engl J Med 309:72–76, 1983.
293. Bhan MK, Lew JF, Sazawal S, et al. Protection conferred by neonatal rotavirus infection against subsequent diarrhea. J Infect Dis 168:282–287, 1993.
294. Cicirello HG, Das BK, Gupta A, et al. High prevalence of rotavirus infection among neonates born at hospitals in Delhi, India: predisposition of newborns for infection with unusual rotavirus. Pediatr Infect Dis J 13:720–724, 1994.
295. Nsanze H, Dawodu A, Usmani A, et al. Ophthalmia neonatorum in the United Arab Emirates. Ann Trop Paediatr 16:27–32, 1996.
296. Verma M, Chhatwal J, Varughese PV. Neonatal conjunctivitis: a profile. Indian Pediatr 31:1357–1361, 1994.
297. Pandey KK, Bhat BV, Kanungo R, et al. Clinico-bacteriological study of neonatal conjunctivitis. Indian J Pediatr 57:527–531, 1990.
298. Sergiwa A, Pratt BC, Eren E, et al. Ophthalmia neonatorum in Bangkok: the significance of Chlamydia trachomatis. Ann Trop Paediatr 13:233–236, 1993.
299. Galega FP, Heymann DL, Nasah BT. Gonococcal ophthalmia neonatorum: the case for prophylaxis in tropical Africa. Bull World Health Organ 62:95–98, 1984.
300. Laga M, Plummer FA, Nzanze H, et al. Epidemiology of ophthalmia neonatorum in Kenya. Lancet 2:1145–1148, 1986.
301. Laga M, Plummer FA, Piot P, et al. Prophylaxis of gonococcal and chlamydial ophthalmia neonatorum: a comparison of silver nitrate and tetracycline. N Engl J Med 318:653–657, 1988.
302. Laga M, Meheus A, Piot P. Epidemiology and control of gonococcal ophthalmia neonatorum. Bull World Health Organ 67:471–478, 1989.
303. Fransen L, Nsanze H, Klauss V, et al. Ophthalmia neonatorum in Nairobi, Kenya. The roles of *Neisseria gonorrhoeae* and *Chlamydia trachomatis.* J Infect Dis 153:862–869, 1986.
304. Hanenberg RS, Rojanapithayakorn W, Kunasol P, et al. Impact of Thailand's HIV-control programme as indicated by the decline of sexually transmitted diseases. Lancet 344:243–246, 1994.
305. Nelson KE, Celentano DD, Eiumtrakol S, et al. Changes in sexual behavior and decline in HIV infection among young men in Thailand. N Engl J Med 335:297–303, 1996.
306. Credé KSF. Die Verhütung der Augenentzündung der Neugeborenen. Arch Gynekol 17:50–53, 1881.
307. Hammerschlag MR, Cummings C, Roblin PM, et al. Efficacy of neonatal ocular prophylaxis for the prevention of chlamydial and gonococcal conjunctivitis. N Engl J Med 320:769–772, 1989.
308. Zanoni D, Isenberg SJ, Apt L. A comparison of silver nitrate with erythromycin for prophylaxis against ophthalmia neonatorum. Clin Pediatr 31:295–298, 1992.
309. American Academy of Pediatrics. 2000 Red Book: Report of the Committee on Infectious Diseases, 25th ed. Chicago, American Academy of Pediatrics, 2000.
310. Isenberg SJ, Apt L, Wood M. A controlled trial of povidone-iodine as prophylaxis against ophthalmia neonatorum. N Engl J Med 332:562–566, 1995.
311. Isenberg SJ, Apt L, Del Signore M, et al. A double application approach to ophthalmia neonatorum prophylaxis. Br J Ophthalmol 87:1449–1452, 2003.
312. Benevento WJ, Murray P, Reed CA, et al. The sensitivity of Neisseria gonorrhoeae, Chlamydia trachomatis, and herpes simplex type II to disinfection with povidone-iodine. Am J Ophthalmol 109:329–333, 1990.
313. Hounag ET, Gilmore OJA, Reid C, et al. Absence of bacterial resistance to povidone iodine. J Clin Pathol 29:752–755, 1976.
314. Ibhanesebhor SE, Otobo ES. In vitro activity of human milk against the causative organisms of ophthalmia neonatorum in Benin City, Nigeria. J Trop Pediatr 42:327–329, 1996.
315. Zeligs BJ, MacDowell-Carneiro AL, Pati S, et al. Antimicrobial studies of two alternative prophylactic regimens used in developing countries against ophthalmia neonatorum: human colostrum and providone-iodine. Pediatr Res 45:758, 1999.
316. The Progress of the Nations 1997. New York, UNICEF, 1997.
317. Steketee RW, Wirima JJ, Slutsker L, et al. The problem of malaria and malaria control in pregnancy in sub-Saharan Africa. Am J Trop Med Hyg 55:2–7, 1996.
318. Shulman CE, Dorman EK. Importance and prevention of malaria in pregnancy. Trans R Soc Trop Med Hyg 97:30–35, 2003.
319. Brabin BJ. An analysis of malaria in pregnancy in Africa. Bull World Health Organ 61:1005–1016, 1983.
320. McGregor IA. Epidemiology, malaria, and pregnancy. Am J Trop Med Hyg 33:517–525, 1984.
321. Nosten F, ter Kuile F, Maelankirri L, et al. Malaria during pregnancy in an area of unstable endemicity. Trans R Soc Trop Med Hyg 85:424–429, 1991.

322. Gilles HM, Lawson JB, Sibelas M, et al. Malaria, anaemia and pregnancy. Ann Trop Med Parasitol 63:245–263, 1969.
323. Egwunyenga OA, Ajayi JA, Duhlinska-Popova DD. Malaria in pregnancy in Nigerians: seasonality and relationship to splenomegaly and anaemia. Indian J Malariol 34:17–24, 1997.
324. McGregor IA, Wilson ME, Billewicz WZ. Malaria infection of the placenta in The Gambia, West Africa; its incidence and relationship to stillbirth, birthweight and placental weight. Trans R Soc Trop Med Hyg 77:232–244, 1983.
325. Matteelli A, Caligaris S, Castelli F, et al. The placenta and malaria. Ann Trop Med Parasitol 91:803–810, 1997.
326. Nosten F, McGready R, Simpson A, et al. Effects of *Plasmodium vivax* malaria in pregnancy. Lancet 354:546–549, 1999.
327. Okoko BJ, Ota MO, Yamuah LK, et al. Influence of placental malaria infection on fetal outcome in the Gambia: twenty years after Ian Mcgregor. J Health Popul Nutr 20:4–11, 2002.
328. Okoko BJ, Enwere G, Ota MOC. The epidemiology and consequences of maternal malaria: a review of immunological basis. Acta Tropica 87:193–205, 2003.
329. Galbraith RM, Fox H, Hsi B, et al. The human maternal-foetal relationship in malaria: II. Histological, ultrastructural and immunopathological studies of the placenta. Trans R Soc Trop Med Hyg 74:61–72, 1980.
330. Steketee RW, Wirima JJ, Hightower AW, et al. The effect of malaria and malaria prevention in pregnancy on offspring birthweight, prematurity, and intrauterine growth retardation in rural Malawi. Am J Trop Med Hyg 55:33–41, 1996.
331. Bouvier P, Breslow N, Doumbo O, et al. Seasonality, malaria, and impact of prophylaxis in a West African village: II. Effect on birthweight. Am J Trop Med Hyg 56:384–389, 1997.
332. Kramer MS. Determinants of low birth weight: methodological assessment and metaanalysis. Bull World Health Organ 65:663–737, 1987.
333. Luxemburger C, McGready R, Kham A, et al. Effects of malaria during pregnancy on infant mortality in an area of low malaria transmission. Am J Epidemiol 154:459–465, 2001.
334. Greenwood AM, Armstrong JRM, Byass P, et al. Malaria chemoprophylaxis, birth weight and child survival. Trans R Soc Trop Med Hyg 86:483–485, 1992.
335. Nguyen-Dinh P, Steketee RW, Greenberg AE, et al. Rapid spontaneous post-partum clearance of Plasmodium falciparum parasitemia in African women. Lancet 2:751–752, 1988.
336. Chizzolini C, Trottein R, Bernard FX, et al. Isotypic analysis, antigen specificity, and inhibitory function of maternally transmitted Plasmodium falciparum-specific antibodies in Gabonese newborns. Am J Trop Med Hyg 45:57–64, 1991.
337. Ibhanesebhor SE. Clinical characteristics of neonatal malaria. J Trop Pediatr 41:330–333, 1995.
338. Wolfe MS, Cordero JF. Safety of chloroquine in chemosuppression of malaria during pregnancy. BMJ 290:1466–1467, 1985.
339. Newman RD, Parise ME, Slutsker L, et al. Safety, efficacy and determinants of effectiveness of antimalarial drugs during pregnancy: implications for prevention programmes in Plasmodium falciparum-endemic sub-Saharan Africa. Trop Med Int Health 8:488–506, 2003.
340. Nosten F, McGready R, Looareesuwan S, et al. Editorial: maternal malaria: time for action. Trop Med Int Health 8:485–487, 2003.
341. Garner P, Gulmezoglu AM. Prevention versus treatment for malaria in pregnant women. Cochrane Database Syst Rev (Issue 3), 2002.
342. Cot M, Roisin A, Barro D, et al. Effect of chloroquine chemoprophylaxis during pregnancy on birthweight: results of a randomized trial. Am J Trop Med Hyg 46:21–27, 1992.
343. Steketee RW, Nahlen BL, Parise ME, et al. The burden of malaria in pregnancy in malaria-endemic areas. Am J Trop Med Hyg 64(1-2 suppl):28–35, 2001.
344. Schultz LJ, Steketee RW, Chitsulo L, et al. Evaluation of maternal practices, efficacy, and cost-effectiveness of alternative antimalarial regimens for use in pregnancy: chloroquine and sulfadoxine-pyrimethamine. Am J Trop Med Hyg 55(1 suppl):87–94, 1996.
345. Shulman CE, Dorman EK, Cutts F, et al. Intermitten sulphadoxine-pyrimethamine to prevent severe anaemia secondary to malaria in pregnancy: a randomised placebo-controlled trial. Lancet 353:632–636, 1999.
346. Goodman CA, Coleman PG, Mills AJ. The cost-effectiveness of antenatal malaria prevention in sub-Saharan Africa. Am J Trop Med Hyg 64(1-2 suppl):45–56, 2001.
347. WHO Expert Committee on Malaria. WHO Tech Rep Ser 892:i–v, 1–74, 2000.
348. Steketee RW. Malaria prevention in pregnancy: when will the prevention programme respond to the science. J Health Popul Nutr 20:1–3, 2002.
349. Heyman DL, Steketee RW, Wirima JJ, et al. Antenatal chloroquine prophylaxis in Malawi: chloroquine resistance, compliance, protective efficacy and cost. Trans R Soc Trop Med Hyg 84:496–498, 1990.
350. Alonso PL, Lindsay SW, Armstrong JRM, et al. The effect of insecticide-treated bed nets on mortality of Gambian children. Lancet 337:1499–1502, 1991.
351. Nevill CG, Some ES, Mung'ala VO, et al. Insecticide-treated bednets reduce mortality and severe morbidity from malaria among children on the Kenyan Coast. Trop Med Intern Health 1:139–146, 1996.
352. Binka FN, Kubaaje A, Adjuik M, et al. Impact of permethrin-impregnated bednets on child mortality in Kassena-Nankana district, Ghana: a randomized controlled trial. Trop Med Intern Health 1:147–154, 1996.
353. Marchant T, Schellenberg JA, Edgar T, et al. Socially marketed insecticide-treated nets improve malaria and anaemia in pregnancy in southern Tanzania. Trop Med Int Health 7:149–158, 2002.
354. Dolan G, ter-Kuile FO, Jacovtot V, et al. Bednets for the prevention of malaria and anaemia in pregnancy. Trans R Soc Trop Med Hyg 87:620–626, 1993.
355. D'Alessandro U, Langerock P, Bennett S, et al. The impact of a national impregnated bednet programme on the outcome of pregnancy in primigravidae in The Gambia. Trans R Soc Trop Med Hyg 90:487–492, 1996.
356. Browne EN, Maude GH, Binka FN. The impact of insecticide-treated bednets on malaria and anaemia in pregnancy in Kassena-Nankana district, Ghana: a randomized controlled trial. Trop Med Int Health 6:667–676, 2001.
357. Shulman CE, Dorman EK, Talisuna AO, et al. A community randomized controlled trial of insecticide-treated bednets for the prevention of malaria and anaemia among primigravid women on the Kenyan coast. Trop Med Intern Health 3:197–204, 1998.
358. Ladner J, Leroy V, Karita E, et al. Malaria, HIV and pregnancy. AIDS 17:275–276, 2003.
359. van Eijk AM, Ayisi JG, Ter Kuile FO, et al. HIV increase the risk of malaria in women of all gravidities in Kisumu, Kenya. AIDS 17:595–603, 2003.
360. Brahmbhatt H, Kigozi G, Wabwire-Mangen F, et al. The effects of placental malaria on mother-to-child HIV transmission in Rakai, Uganda. AIDS 17:2539–2541, 2003.
361. Ticconi C, Mapfumo M, Dorrucci M, et al. Effect of maternal HIV and malaria infection on pregnancy and perinatal outcome in Zimbabwe. J Acquir Immune Defic Syndr 34:289–294, 2003.
362 The World's Women 1995: Trends and Statistics. Social Statistics and Indicators. New York, United Nations Publication, 1995.
363. Tomasevski K: Women and Human Rights. Atlantic Highlands, NJ, Zed Books, 1993.
364. Maternal and perinatal infections: a practical guide: report of a WHO consultation. WHO/MCH/91.10. Geneva, World Health Organization, 1991.
365. Maternal care for the reduction of perinatal and neonatal mortality. Geneva, World Health Organization, 1986.
366. Vicari M, Englund J, Glezen P, et al (eds). Protection of newborns through maternal immunization. Vaccine 21:3352–3502, 2003.
367. Fischer GW, Ottolini MG, Mond JJ. Prospects for vaccines during pregnancy and in the newborn period. Clin Perinatol 24:231–249, 1997.
368. Baker C, Rench M, Edwards M, et al. Immunization of pregnant women with a polysaccharide vaccine of group B streptococcus. N Engl J Med 319:1180–1185, 1988.
369. Baker CJ, Edwards MS. Group B streptococcal conjugate vaccines. 88:375–378, 2003.
370. Lin F-YC, Philips JB III, Azimi PH, et al. Level of maternal antibody required to protect neonates against early-onset disease caused by group B streptococcus type Ia: a multicenter seroepidemiology study. J Infect Dis 184:1022–1028, 2001.
371. Baker CJ, Rench MA, McInnes P. Immunization of pregnant women with group B streptococcal type III capsular polysaccharide-tetanus toxoid conjugate vaccine. Vaccine 21(24):3468-3472, 2003.
372. Baker CJ, Rench MA, Fernandez M, et al. Safety and immunogenicity of a bivalent group B streptococcal conjugate vaccine for serotypes II and III. J Infect Dis 188:66–73, 2003.

373. Shahid NS, Steinhoff MC, Hoque SS, et al. Serum, breast milk, and infant antibody after maternal immunisation with pneumococcal vaccine. Lancet 346:1252–1257, 1995.
374. O'Dempsey TJD, McArdle T, Ceesay SJ, et al. Immunization with a pneumococcal capsular polysaccharide vaccine during pregnancy. Vaccine 14:963–970, 1996.
375. Santosham M, Englund JA, McInnes P, et al. Safety and antibody persistence following Haemophilus influenzae type b conjugate or pneumococcal polysaccharide vaccines given before pregnancy in women of childbearing age and their infants. Pediatr Infect Dis J 20:931–940, 2001.
376. Mulholland K, Suara RO, Siber G, et al. Maternal immunization with Haemophilus influenzae type b polysaccharide-tetanus protein conjugate vaccine in The Gambia. JAMA 275:1182–1188, 1996.
377. Englund JA, Glezen WP, Thompson C, et al. Haemophilus influenzae type b-specific antibody in infants after maternal immunization. Pediatr Infect Dis J 16:1122–1130, 1997.
378 Bisgard KM, Kao A, Leake J, et al. Haemophilus influenzae invasive disease in the United States, 1994-1995: near disappearance of a vaccine-preventable childhood disease. Emerg Infect Dis 4:229–237, 1998.
379. Bijlmer HA. Epidemiology of Haemophilus influenzae invasive disease in developing countries and intervention strategies. *In* Ellis RW, Granoff DM (eds). Development and Uses of Haemophilus b Conjugate Vaccines. New York, Marcel Dekker, 1994, pp 247–264.
380. Funkhouser A, Steinhoff MD, Ward J. Haemophilus influenzae disease and immunization in developing countries. Rev Infect Dis 13(Suppl 6):S542–S554, 1991.
381. Marchant A, Newport M. Prevention of infectious diseases by neonatal and early infantile immunization: prospects for the new millennium. Curr Opin Infect Dis 13:241–246, 2000.
382. Smith PG. Case-control studies of the efficacy of BCG against tuberculosis. *In* International Union Against Tuberculosis (ed). Proceedings of the XXVIth IUAT World Conference on Tuberculosis and Respiratory Diseases, Singapore. Japan, Professional Postgraduate Services International, 1987, pp 73–79.
383. Colditz GA, Berkey CS, Mosteller F, et al. The efficacy of bacillus Calmette-Guérin vaccination of newborns and infants in the prevention of tuberculosis: meta-analyses of the published literature. Pediatrics 96:29–35, 1995.
384. Delage G, Remy-Prince S, Montplaisir S. Combined active-passive immunization against the hepatitis B virus: five-year follow-up of children born to hepatitis B surface antigen-positive mothers. Pediatr Infect Dis J 12:126–130, 1993.
385. Andre FE, Zuckerman AJ. Review: Protective efficacy of hepatitis B vaccines in neonates. J Med Virol 44:144–151, 1994.
386. World Health Organization. Expanded programme on immunization: Global advisory group. Wkly Epidemiol Rec 3:11–16, 1992.
387. Glass RI, Bresee JS, Parashar U, et al. Rotavirus vaccines at the threshold. Nat Med 3:1324–1325, 1997.
388. Perez-Schael I, Guntinas MJ, Perez M, et al. Efficacy of the rhesus rotavirus-based quadrivalent vaccine in infants and young children in Venezuela. N Engl J Med 337:1181–1187, 1997.
389. Lagos R, Valenzuela MT, Levine OS, et al. Economisation of vaccination against Haemophilus influenzae type b: a randomised trial of immunogenicity of fractional-dose and two-dose regimens. Lancet 351:1472–1476, 1998.
390. World Health Organization. The Prevention and Management of Puerperal Infections. Geneva, World Health Organization, 1992.
391. World Health Organization. The global elimination of neonatal tetanus: progress to date. Bull World Health Organ 72:155–164, 1994.
392. Walker DG, Walker GJ. Forgotten but not gone: the continuing scourge of congenital syphilis. Lancet Infect Dis 2:432–436, 2002.
393. Kuate DB. Epidemiology and control of infant and early childhood malaria: a competing risks analysis. Int J Epidemiol 24:204–217, 1995.
394. Airede AI. Prolonged rupture of membranes and neonatal outcome in a developing country. Ann Trop Paediatr 12:283–288, 1992.
395. Asindi AA, Omene JA. Prolonged rupture of membrane and neonatal morbidity. East Afr Med J 57:707–711, 1980.
396. Raghavan M, Mondal GP, Vishnu BB, et al. Perinatal risk factors in neonatal infections. Indian J Pediatr 59:335–340, 1992.
397. Hanson LA, Hahn-Zoric M, Berndes M, et al. Breast feeding: overview and breast milk immunology. Acta Paediatr Jpn 36:557–561, 1994.
398. Ashraf RN, Jalil F, Zaman S, et al. Breast feeding and protection against neonatal sepsis in a high risk population. Arch Dis Child 66:488–490, 1991.
399. Brown KH, Black RE, Lopez de Romana G, et al. Infant-feeding practices and their relationship with diarrheal and other diseases in Huascar (Lima), Peru. Pediatrics 83:31–40, 1989.
400. Feachem G, Koblinsky MA. Interventions for the control of diarrhoeal diseases among young children: promotion of breast-feeding. Bull World Health Organ 62:271–291, 1984.
401. Glezen WP. Epidemiological perspective of breastfeeding and acute respiratory illnesses in infants. *In* Mestecky J (ed). Immunology of Milk and the Neonate. New York, Plenum Press, 1991, pp 235–240.
402. Narayanan I, Murthy NS, Prakash K, et al. Randomised controlled trial of effect of raw and holder pasteurised human milk and of formula supplements on incidence of neonatal infection. Lancet 2:1111–1113, 1984.
403. Habicht JP, DaVanzo J, Butz XVP. Does breastfeeding really save lives, or are apparent benefits due to biases? Am J Epidemiol 123:279–290, 1986.
404. Srivastava SP, Sharma VK, Jha SP. Mortality patterns in breast versus artificially fed term babies in early infancy: a longitudinal study. Indian Pediatr 31:1393–1396, 1994.
405. Victora CG, Smith PG, Vaughan JP, et al. Infant feeding and deaths due to diarrhea: a case-control study. Am J Epidemiol 129:1032–1041, 1989.
406. Victora CG, Vaughan JP, Lombardi C, et al. Evidence for protection by breast-feeding against infant deaths from infectious diseases in Brazil. Lancet 11:319–322, 1987.
407. Brahmbhatt H, Gray RH. Child mortality associated with reasons for non-breastfeeding and weaning: is breastfeeding best for HIV-positive mothers? AIDS 17:879–885, 2003.
408. Bicego GT, Boerma JT. Maternal education and child survival: a comparative study of survey data from 17 countries. Soc Sci Med 36:1207–1227, 1993.
409. Victora CG, Huttly SRA, Barros FC, et al. Maternal education in relation to early and late child health outcomes: findings from a Brazilian cohort study. Soc Sci Med 34:899–905, 1992.
410. World Development Report 1993: Investing in Health. New York, Oxford University Press, 1993.
411. van Ginneken JK, Lob-Levyt J, Gove S. Potential interventions for preventing pneumonia among young children in developing countries: promoting maternal education. Trop Med Intern Health 1:283–294, 1996.
412. Villar J, Belizan JM. The relative contribution of prematurity and fetal growth retardation to low birth weight in developing and developed societies. Am J Obstet Gynecol 143:793–798, 1982.
413. Stoll BJ, Hansen N, Fanaroff AA, et al. Late-onset sepsis in very low birth weight neonates: the experience of the NICHD Neonatal Research Network. Pediatrics 110:285–291, 2002.
414. Victora CG, Barros FC, Vaughan JP, et al. Birthweight and infant mortality: a longitudinal study of 5914 Brazilian children. Int J Epidemiol 16:239–245, 1987.
415. Victora CG, Smith PG, Vaughan JP, et al. Influence of birth weight on mortality from infectious diseases: a case-control study. Pediatrics 81:807–811, 1988.
416. Weber MW, Carlin JB, Gatchalian S, et al. Predictors of neonatal sepsis in developing countries. Pediatr Infect Dis J 22:711–717, 2003.
417. Marsh DR, sternin M, Khadduri R, et al. Identification of model newborn care practices through a positive deviance inquiry to guide behavior-change interventions in Haripur, Pakistan. Food Nutr Bull 23:109–118, 2002.
418. Amarasiri de Silva MW, Wijekoon A, Hornik R, et al. Care seeking in Sri Lanka: one possible explanation for low childhood mortality. Soc Sci Med 53:1363–1372, 2001.
419. World Health Organization. Integrated management of the sick child. Bull World Health Organ 73:435–740, 1995.
420. World Health Organization. World Health Report 1996: Fighting Disease, Fostering Development. Geneva, World Health Organization, 1996.

Chapter 3

OBSTETRIC FACTORS ASSOCIATED WITH INFECTIONS IN THE FETUS AND NEWBORN INFANT

Jill K. Davies • Ronald S. Gibbs

Early-onset neonatal infection often has its origin in utero. Thus, risk factors for neonatal sepsis include prematurity, premature rupture of the membranes (PROM), and maternal fever during labor (which may be caused by clinical intra-amniotic infection). This chapter focuses on these major obstetric conditions. Included in addition to these three "classic" topics is a discussion of new information indicating that intrauterine exposure to bacteria is linked to major neonatal sequelae, including cerebral palsy, bronchopulmonary dysplasia (BPD), and respiratory distress syndrome (RDS).

INTRA-AMNIOTIC INFECTION

Clinically evident intrauterine infection during the latter half of pregnancy develops in 1% to 10% of pregnant women and leads to increased maternal morbidity as well as perinatal mortality and morbidity. In general, the diagnosis is clinically based on the presence of fever and other signs and symptoms, such as maternal or fetal tachycardia, uterine tenderness, foul odor of the amniotic fluid, and maternal leukocytosis. Although not invariably present, rupture of the membranes or labor also occurs in most cases. Some prospective reports have noted higher rates (4.2% to 10.5%)[1-3] than in older retrospective studies (1% to 2%).[4] A number of terms have been applied to this infection, including *chorioamnionitis*, *intrapartum infection*, *amniotic fluid infection*, and *intra-amniotic infection* (IAI). We use the last designation to distinguish this clinical syndrome from bacterial colonization of amniotic fluid (also referred to as "microbial invasion of the amniotic cavity") and from histologic inflammation of the placenta (i.e., histologic chorioamnionitis).

Pathogenesis

Before labor and membrane rupture, amniotic fluid is nearly always sterile. With the onset of labor or with membrane rupture, bacteria from the lower genital tract usually enter the amniotic cavity. This ascending route is the most common pathway for development of IAI.[4] In 1988, Romero and co-workers described four stages of ascending intrauterine infection (Fig. 3-1). Shifts in vaginal or cervical flora and the presence of pathologic bacteria in the cervix represent stage I. Bacterial vaginosis may also be classified as stage I. In stage II, bacteria ascend from the vagina/cervix into the decidua, the specialized endometrium of pregnancy. The inflammatory response here allows organisms to invade the amnion and chorion leading to chorioamnionitis. In stage III, bacteria invade chorionic vessels (choriovasculitis) and migrate through to the amnion into the amniotic cavity to cause IAI. Once in the amniotic cavity, bacteria may gain access to the fetus through several potential mechanisms, culminating in stage IV; fetal bacteremia, sepsis, and pneumonia may result.[5]

Occasional instances of documented IAI in the absence of rupture of membranes or labor support a presumed hematogenous or transplacental route of infection. Fulminant IAI without labor and without rupture of membranes may be caused by *Listeria monocytogenes*.[6-10] Maternal sepsis due to this organism often manifests as maternal flulike illness and may result in death of the fetus. In an outbreak caused by "Mexican-style" cheese contaminated with *Listeria*, several maternal deaths occurred.[11] Other virulent organisms, such

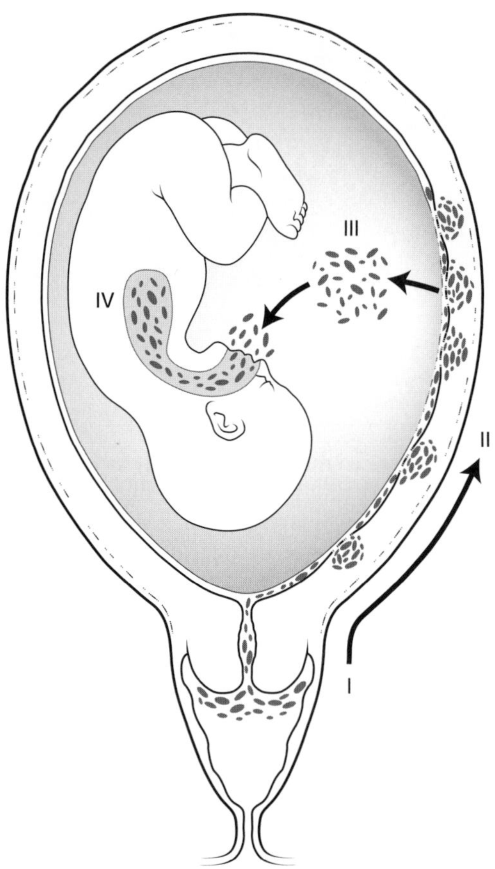

Figure 3–1 The stages of ascending infection. (From Romero R, Mazor M. Infection and preterm labor: pathways for intrauterine infections. Clin Obstet Gynecol 31:558, 1988.)

as group A streptococci, also have been the cause of transplacental infection.[12] IAI may develop less commonly as a consequence of obstetric procedures such as cervical cerclage, diagnostic amniocentesis, cordocentesis (percutaneous umbilical cord blood sampling), or intrauterine transfusion. The absolute risk is small with all of these procedures: IAI develops in 2% to 8% of patients after cerclage,[13-16] in less than 1% of patients after amniocentesis,[17] and in 5% of patients after intrauterine transfusion.[18] Higher risks are encountered, however, when cerclage is performed when the cervix is dilated and effaced.

Two large studies of risk factors for IAI identified characteristics of labor as the major risk factors by logistic regression analysis. These features included low parity, increased number of vaginal examinations in labor, as well as increased duration of labor, membrane rupture, and internal fetal monitoring.[3,4] More recently, risk factors for IAI have been stratified for term versus preterm pregnancies.[19] For patients at term with IAI, the study investigators observed, by logistic regression analysis, that the independent risk factors were membrane rupture for longer than 12 hours (odds ratio [OR] 5.81), internal fetal monitoring (OR 2.01), and more than four vaginal examinations in labor (OR 3.07). For preterm pregnancies, these three risk factors were again identified as being independently associated with IAI, but with differing ORs. Specifically, in the preterm pregnancies, membrane rupture for longer than 12 hours was associated with an OR of 2.49; for internal fetal monitoring, the OR was 1.42; and for more than four examinations, the OR was 1.59. One interpretation of these data regarding risk factors among preterm pregnancies is that there was some other risk factor not detected in this survey. Additionally, meconium staining of the amniotic fluid has been associated with an increased risk of chorioamnionitis (4.3% versus 2.1%).[20] Prior spontaneous and elective abortion (at less than 20 weeks) in the immediately preceding pregnancy has also been associated with development of IAI in the subsequent pregnancy (OR 4.3 and 4.0, respectively).[21]

In 1996, a multivariable analysis demonstrated quantitatively the importance of chorioamnionitis in neonatal sepsis.[22] The OR for neonatal sepsis accompanying clinical chorioamnionitis was 25, whereas for preterm delivery, membrane rupture for longer than 12 hours, endometritis, and group B streptococcal colonization, the ORs all were less than 5. Epidural anesthesia has been associated with fever in labor (independent of infection).[23] This knowledge must be considered in determining the etiology of fever in a patient who has an epidural anesthetic in place.

Although Naeye had reported an association between recent coitus and development of chorioamnionitis defined by histologic study,[24] further analysis of the same population refuted this association.[25] Other studies have not demonstrated any relationship between coitus and PROM, premature birth, or perinatal death.[26]

Microbiology

The cause of IAI is often polymicrobial. Gibbs and colleagues reported a microbiologic case-control study of amniotic fluid from 52 patients with clinical IAI.[27] The following organisms were found in the amniotic fluid from patients with IAI: *Bacteroides* species, 25%; group B streptococci, 12%; other aerobic streptococci, 13%; *Escherichia coli,* 10%; other aerobic gram-negative rods, 10%; *Clostridium* species, 9%; *Peptococcus* species, 7%; and *Fusobacterium* species, 6%. The mean number of bacterial isolates in patients with IAI was 2.2. For the 52 patients with clinical IAI, aerobes and anaerobes were isolated from 48%; aerobes only from 38%; anaerobes alone from 8%; and no aerobes or anaerobes from 6%. Cultures of amniotic fluid from patients with IAI were more likely to have more than 10^2 colony-forming units (CFUs) of any isolate per milliliter, any number of high-virulence isolates, and more than 10^2 CFUs/mL of high-virulence isolates. Only 8% of these cultures from control patients had 10^2 CFUs/mL or more of high-virulence isolates. The isolation rate of low-virulence organisms, such as lactobacilli, diphtheroids, and *Staphylococcus epidermidis,* was similar in both the IAI and the control groups. In smaller studies, a similar spectrum of organisms was reported.[13,28] *Neisseria gonorrhoeae* was not isolated in any of these studies, but it appears to be an infrequent cause of amnionitis.[29,30]

A role for genital mycoplasmas has been suggested by case reports describing their isolation from amniotic fluid of clinically infected patients and by epidemiologic studies showing an association between the isolation of *Mycoplasma hominis* or *Ureaplasma* and placental inflammation.[31,32] Unfortunately, these latter studies did not demonstrate correlation of isolation of genital mycoplasmas with clinical infection in the mother or neonate. In a controlled study of

IAI, Blanco and co-workers reported that 35% of cultures of amniotic fluid from patients with IAI yielded *M. hominis,* whereas only 8% of matched control cultures showed *M. hominis* ($P < .001$).[33] *Ureaplasma urealyticum* was isolated from amniotic fluid from 50% of the infected and uninfected patients. In a subsequent study, Gibbs and colleagues found *M. hominis* in the blood of 2% of women with IAI and reported a serologic response in 85% of women with IAI who also had *M. hominis* in the amniotic fluid.[34] This rate of serologic response was significantly higher than that in asymptomatic control women or in infected women without *M. hominis* in the amniotic fluid ($P < .001$).[34] Cultures of blood and serologic results did not clarify the role of *U. urealyticum.* Thus, the pathogenic potential of *M. hominis* is high in IAI, but the pathogenic status of *U. urealyticum* is unclear in this infection.

Data related to the role of *Chlamydia trachomatis* in infections of amniotic fluid are in conflict. Martin and co-workers prospectively studied perinatal mortality in women whose pregnancies were complicated by antepartum maternal chlamydial infections.[35] Two of the six fetal deaths in the *Chlamydia*-positive group were associated with chorioamnionitis compared with one of eight in the control group. Wager and colleagues showed that the rate of occurrence of intrapartum fever was higher in patients with antepartum *C. trachomatis* infection (9%) than in patients without *C. trachomatis* isolated from the cervix (1%).[36] The data are interesting but must be interpreted with caution because of the limited number of patients and because the control group may not have been sufficiently similar to the infected group. Furthermore, *C. trachomatis* has not been isolated from amniotic cells or placental membranes of patients with IAI.[37,38] In a preliminary study, no difference was found in the rate of serologic response to *C. trachomatis* in women with IAI compared with that in asymptomatic women.[39]

In a large prospective study, Sperling and colleagues reported amniotic fluid culture results from 408 cases of IAI. The most commonly isolated organisms were *U. urealyticum* (47%), *M. hominis* (31%), *Prevotella bivia* (29%), *Gardnerella vaginalis* (24%), group B streptococci (15%), anaerobic streptococci (9%), *E. coli* (8%), *Fusobacterium* species (6%), enterococci (5%), and other aerobic gram-negative rods (5%).[40] A summary of representative data for five microbiologic studies is given in Table 3-1. Because of differences among these studies in microbiologic and collection techniques and in reporting format for isolates, Table 3-2 is meant to show broad, overall results.

Evidence has shown that maternal bacterial vaginosis is causally linked to IAI.[41] The evidence may be categorized as follows: (1) the microorganisms in bacterial vaginosis and in chorioamnionitis are similar; (2) bacterial vaginosis is

Table 3–1 Microbes Isolated in Amniotic Fluid from Cases of Intra-amniotic Infection: A Summary of Studies

Microbe	Representative % Isolated
Genital Mycoplasmas	
Ureaplasma urealyticum	47-50
Mycoplasma hominis	31-35
Anaerobes	
Prevotella bivia	11-29
Peptostreptococcus	7-33
Fusobacterium species	6-7
Aerobes	
Group B streptococci	12-19
Enterococci	5-11
Escherichia coli	8-12, 55
Other aerobic gram-negative rods	5-10
Gardnerella vaginalis	24

Data from references 13, 27, 28, 33, and 40. See text.

Table 3–2 Comparative Studies of Intrapartum versus Postpartum Maternal Antibiotic Therapy in Treatment of Intra-amniotic Infection

Author, Year	Design/Setting	No. of Patients	Maternal Intrapartum Antibiotic Regimen	Benefits of Intrapartum Treatment
Sperling et al,[73] 1987	Retrospective/pubic teaching hospital in San Antonio, Texas	257	Penicillin G plus gentamicin IV	NNS reduced from 19.6% in postpartum treatment group to 2.8% in intrapartum treatment group ($P = .001$)
Gilstrap et al,[75] 1988	Retrospective/public teaching hospital in Dallas, Texas	273	Varied[a]	NNS reduced from 5.7% in postpartum treatment group to 1.5% in intrapartum treatment group ($P = .06$); group B streptococcal bacteremia reduced from 5.7% to 0% ($P = .004$)
Gibbs et al,[74] 1988	Randomized clinical trial/ same as Sperling (1987)	45	Ampicillin plus gentamicin IV	NNS reduced from 21% to 0%; maternal morbidity also decreased ($P = .05$)

[a]Antibiotic regimens noted as 47% received ampicillin or penicillin in combination with gentamicin and clindamycin; 22%, ampicillin or penicillin with gentamicin; 20%, cefoxitin; and 11%, other antibiotics.

IV, intravenously; NNS, neonatal sepsis confirmed by blood culture.

associated with the isolation of organisms in the chorioamnion; and (3) bacterial vaginosis is associated with development of clinical chorioamnionitis in selected populations.[42-44] It has been demonstrated that treatment of bacterial vaginosis in high risk populations prenatally decreases the risk of chorioamnionitis and other pregnancy outcomes.[47] However, in the large Maternal Fetal Medicine Units Network trial, screening and treatment did not lead to benefit either in the overall patient population or in the secondary analysis of women with prior preterm birth.[48] Subsequently, an American College of Obstetricians and Gynecologists (ACOG) Practice Bulletin on assessment of risk factors for preterm birth advocated that screening and treating of either high- or low-risk women would not be expected to reduce the overall rate of preterm birth.[49] However, in select populations of high-risk women such as those with prior preterm birth and bacterial vaginosis early in pregnancy, we still recommend treatment of those women.

Amniotic fluid cultures from cases of intra-amniotic infection accompanying a low-birth-weight infant are more likely to contain the anaerobic organism *Fusobacterium* (21.6% versus only 3.8% in non–low-birth-weight cases, $P < .001$) and *P. bivia* (46% versus 28%, $P = .035$). There were no significant differences, however, in the isolation rates of group B streptococci, *E. coli*, other aerobes, or genital mycoplasmas between cases from low-birth-weight and non–low-birth-weight infants.[40]

Bloodstream isolates from newborns in 408 cases of IAI were reported as follows: *E. coli*, 5 cases; group B streptococci, 4 cases; *Staphylococcus aureus*, 2 cases; enterococci, 2 cases; other streptococci, 3 cases; and 1 case each for *Enterobacter* species, *Haemophilus influenzae*, *Haemophilus parainfluenzae*, and microaerophilic streptococci.[40] Thus, of 20 isolates, group B streptococci and *E. coli* accounted for 45% of isolates, even though these organisms were present in the amniotic fluid of just 20% of cases.

The role of viruses in causing IAI is less well delineated. Yankowitz and associates evaluated fluid from 77 midtrimester genetic amniocentesis by polymerase chain reaction (PCR) assay for the presence of adenovirus, enterovirus, respiratory syncytial virus (RSV), Epstein-Barr virus (EBV), parvovirus, cytomegalovirus (CMV), and herpes simplex virus (HSV). Six samples were positive (three adenovirus, one parvovirus, one CMV, and one enterovirus), and two resulted in pregnancy loss, one at 21 weeks (adenovirus) and one at 26 weeks (CMV).[50]

Diagnosis

Diagnosis of IAI requires a high index of suspicion because the clinical signs and symptoms may be subtle. Moreover, usual laboratory indicators of infection, such as positive stains for organisms or leukocytes and positive culture results, are found more frequently than is clinically evident infection. Microorganisms are easily grown in culture from the amniotic fluid or chorioamniotic membranes using standard techniques. Cassell and colleagues demonstrated positive cultures from the chorioamniotic space twice as frequently as from the intra-amniotic space (20% versus 9%), lending further support to the theory that microorganisms ascend from the vagina through the chorioamniotic space to gain access to the amniotic cavity and then the fetus.[51]

The rate of positive amniotic fluid cultures for microorganisms is higher with preterm PROM (32.4%) than with preterm labor with intact membranes (12.8%).[52]

Rates of IAI are probably underestimated with preterm PROM, because severe oligohydramnios may preclude sampling success. Additionally, women in labor on hospital admission generally are not sampled but have been shown to have higher rates of microbial invasion of the amniotic cavity at (39%) than those in women not in labor (25%). When they do enter labor, the risk of microbial invasion of the amniotic cavity is still higher at 75%.[53]

Clinical diagnosis of IAI usually is based on maternal fever, maternal or fetal tachycardia, uterine tenderness, foul odor of amniotic fluid, and leukocytosis. Other causes of fever in the parturient patient include epidural analgesia, concurrent infection of the urinary tract or other organ systems and perhaps dehydration, illicit drug use and other rare conditions. The differential diagnosis of fetal tachycardia consists of prematurity, medications, arrhythmias, and hypoxia, whereas for maternal tachycardia other possible causes are drugs, hypotension, dehydration, and anxiety as well as intrinsic cardiac conditions, hypothyroidism, as well as pulmonary embolism. In general, the most common clinical and laboratory criteria for diagnosis of IAI are fever, leukocytosis, and ruptured membranes; fetal tachycardia and maternal tachycardia are noted in a variable percentage of cases.[1,45,46] Foul-smelling amniotic fluid and uterine tenderness, although more specific signs, occur in a minority of the cases. Bacteremia occurs in less than 10% of cases. Because peripheral blood leukocytosis is common during normal labor, this result does not always indicate infection. As a predictor of IAI, leukocytosis (white blood cell counts greater than 12,000/mm^3) had a sensitivity of 67%, specificity of 86%, positive predictive value of 82%, and negative predictive value of 72%.[54]

Direct examination of the amniotic fluid may provide important diagnostic information. Samples can be collected transvaginally by aspiration of an intrauterine pressure catheter, by needle aspiration of the forewaters, or by amniocentesis. Outside of research protocols, transabdominal amniocentesis is the most common technique.

There is a significant association between detecting white blood cells or bacteria in a stain of uncentrifuged amniotic fluid and clinical infection.[27,55] In a case-control study, white blood cells were seen on smear in 67% of cases of IAI and in only 12% of controls ($P = .001$). Bacteria were seen on smear in 81% of cases of IAI and in 29% of controls ($P < .001$).[27] With suspected IAI, detection of bacteria or white blood cells on a smear of uncentrifuged fluid supports the diagnosis, but there are frequent false-positive and false-negative results.

Several other recent tests of amniotic fluid have been evaluated as predictors of IAI. In a small case-control study, Hoskins and co-workers found that the leukocyte esterase test showed excellent performance (91% sensitivity, 95% specificity, and 95% positive and 91% negative predictive values) when the clinical diagnosis of chorioamnionitis was used as the gold standard.[54] Low concentrations of amniotic fluid glucose (variably reported at less than 10 to 20 mg/dL) are strongly associated with positive amniotic fluid culture and less strongly associated with clinical IAI.[56-58]

Recently, attention has been directed to proinflammatory cytokines as markers of IAI. During the course of intrauterine infection, bacteria reach the decidua, stimulating a maternal inflammatory response. Once bacteria gain access to the amniotic cavity and the fetus, the fetal inflammatory response can be activated.

Interleukin-6 (IL-6) is an immunostimulatory cytokine and a key mediator of fetal host response to infection. Several lines of investigation indicate that IL-6 may be the future diagnostic test of choice. For example, elevated levels of IL-6 in the amniotic fluid have been a more sensitive rapid test for the detection of microbial invasion of the amniotic cavity than amniotic fluid glucose, amniotic fluid Gram stain, or amniotic fluid white blood cell count. Amniotic fluid IL-6 levels have also been shown to be increased with positive cultures of either the amniotic fluid or the amniochorion.[59] Elevation of IL-6 levels in the amniotic fluid also is a very sensitive indicator of acute histologic chorioamnionitis and the identification of neonates at risk for significant morbidity and mortality.[60] Maternal serum IL-6 levels also have been reported to be elevated when preterm labor is associated with intrauterine infection.[61] Finally, fetal production of IL-6 (as determined by cordocentesis) is an independent risk factor for the occurrence of severe neonatal morbidity, including sepsis and pneumonia.[62,63] Additional areas of research currently include cervicovaginal production of cytokines.

PCR, a molecular biologic technique that amplifies the signal of small amounts of DNA, is likely to change the future of diagnosis of IAI. Several studies have evaluated amniotic fluid samples using PCR techniques. PCR assay has a higher sensitivity than that of culture for detection of microorganisms in the amniotic fluid, particularly in patients whose amniotic fluid is culture negative but other markers indicate evidence of an inflammatory response.[59,64-67]

Chronic Intra-amniotic Infection

Increasing evidence is accumulating to suggest that IAI also may exist as a chronic condition. Several studies have performed microbiologic studies of midtrimester genetic amniocentesis fluid. Risk of adverse pregnancy outcome is increased when patients are asymptomatic but have positive results on such studies at midtrimester amniocentesis, compared with patients with culture-negative fluid.[59] Similarly, amniotic fluid IL-6 concentrations were found to be significantly higher in patients experiencing a loss following midtrimester amniocentesis than in those patients delivering at term.[68,69]

Emerging evidence also suggests that chronic inflammation may also be present in maternal serum. Goldenberg and colleagues recently showed elevated granulocyte colony-stimulating factor (G-CSF) at 24 and 28 weeks in women subsequently delivering prematurely.[70]

These data then beg the question of whether infection could be present before conception. The documented increased risk of recurrent preterm birth would lend credence to this hypothesis, but studies have not yet proved this hypothesis.[71,72]

Management and Short-Term Outcome

Traditionally, the effectiveness of management has been viewed in terms of short-term maternal and neonatal outcomes, including maternal sepsis, neonatal sepsis, pneumonia, meningitis, and perinatal death. This section discusses the management principles of these short-term outcomes.

In the past, there was debate regarding timing of antibiotic administration, but it has now become standard to begin treatment during labor, as soon as possible after the maternal diagnosis of IAI is made. Three studies, including a randomized clinical trial, have demonstrated benefits from intrapartum antibiotic therapy compared with immediate postpartum treatment (see Table 3-2).[73-75] In a large, nonrandomized allocation of intrapartum versus immediate postpartum treatment, the former treatment was associated with a significant decrease in neonatal bacteremia (2.8% versus 19.6%; $P < .001$) and a reduction in neonatal death from sepsis (0.9% versus 4.3%; $P = .07$).[73] Another large study showed an overall reduction in neonatal sepsis ($P = .06$), especially bacteremia due to group B streptococci (0% versus 4.7%; $P = .004$), with use of intrapartum treatment.[75] Then, in a randomized clinical trial, Gibbs and associates demonstrated that intrapartum treatment provided both maternal benefits (decreased hospital stay, lower mean temperature post partum) and neonatal benefits (decrease in sepsis: 0% versus 21%, $P = .03$, and decreased hospital stay). In this study, neonatal treatment was identical and consisted of intravenous ampicillin and gentamicin begun within 1 to 2 hours of birth and continued for at least 72 hours. If bacteremia or neonatal pneumonia was diagnosed, antibiotics were continued for 10 days.[74]

Pharmacokinetic studies[76] done during early pregnancy show that ampicillin concentrations in maternal and fetal sera are comparable 60 to 90 minutes after administration (Fig. 3-2). Penicillin G levels in fetal serum are one third of the maternal levels 120 minutes after administration.[77] In addition, ampicillin has some activity against *E. coli*. Accordingly, ampicillin is preferable to penicillin G for treatment of IAI. When used in combination with an aminoglycoside, ampicillin should be administered first, because it has the broader antimicrobial spectrum. In late pregnancy, gentamicin also crosses the placenta rapidly, but peak fetal levels may be low, especially if maternal levels are subtherapeutic.[78] An initial gentamicin dose of at least 1.5 to 2.0 mg/kg followed by 1.0 to 1.5 mg/kg every 8 hours is indicated because of the potential for unfavorable gentamicin kinetics. As an alternative, a newer penicillin or cephalosporin with excellent activity against aerobic gram-negative bacteria might be used. However, there is little published experience with these other antibiotics in IAI. Levels of ampicillin and aminoglycosides in amniotic fluid usually are below fetal serum levels, and peak concentrations in amniotic fluid may be attained only after 2 to 6 hours.[76-78] The kinetics of newer penicillin and cephamycin antibiotics have not been studied extensively in pregnancy.

The duration of maternal treatment post partum in cases of chorioamnionitis is debatable. One randomized trial compared single-dose versus multidose postpartum treatment of mothers and reported that single-dose treatment was accompanied by a shorter time to discharge (33 hours in the single-dose group versus 57 hours in the multidose group; $P = .001$).[79] However, the single-dose group had a nearly threefold increase in failure of therapy, but this did not achieve statistical significance (11% in the single-dose treatment group versus 3.7% in the multidose group; $P = .27$).

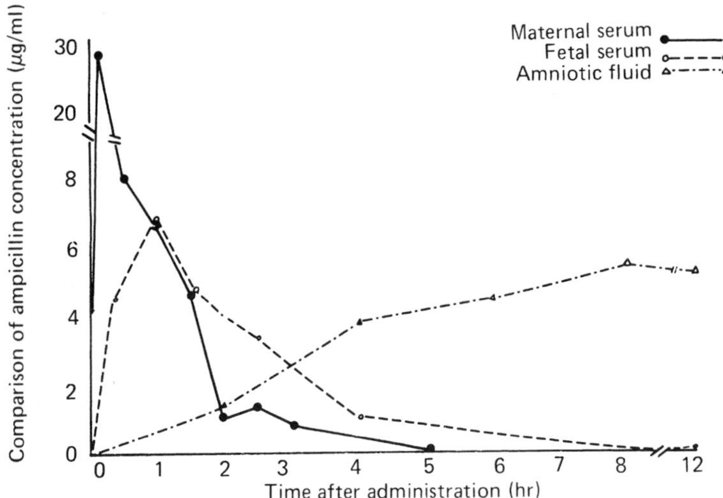

Figure 3–2 Ampicillin levels achieved with systemic administration to the mother. (From Bray RE, Boe RW, Johnson WL. Transfer of ampicillin into fetus and amniotic fluid from maternal plasma in late pregnancy. Am J Obstet Gynecol 96:938, 1966.)

Turnquist and associates also studied postpartum antibiotic therapy given when IAI was present, but only when cesarean section was performed. All patients received one dose of preoperative intravenous gentamicin and clindamycin. Patients were then randomized to receive no further antibiotics or to continue clindamycin plus gentamicin and had received ampicillin intravenously every 6 hours after a diagnosis of IAI was made. Our preference is to administer antibiotics for 24 hours or more after resolution of fever.

With regard to timing of delivery, short-term outcome is excellent without the use of arbitrary time limits.[1,80,81] Cesarean delivery usually is reserved for standard obstetric indications, not for IAI itself. In nearly all cases, delivery occurred within 8 hours after diagnosis of IAI (mean interval was 3 to 5 hours). No critical interval from diagnosis of amnionitis to delivery could be identified. Yet nearly in all of these cases the pregnancy was at or near term. Rates of cesarean section are two to three times higher among patients with IAI than in the general population, owing to patient selection (most cases occur in women with dystocia already diagnosed) and a poor response to oxytocin.[82,83] There is no demonstrated advantage of the extraperitoneal caesarean technique over the transperitoneal technique in decreasing maternal complications of IAI.[84-87]

In the past, we used a combination of an intravenous penicillin and intravenous gentamicin as soon as the diagnosis was made and cultures had been obtained.[1,46] Several studies have reported good results with similar regimens.[80] When a cesarean section is necessary, clindamycin should be added post partum to these antibiotics because of the importance of anaerobes in post–cesarean section infection and the high failure rate (20%) with therapy with penicillin-gentamicin after cesarean section for IAI.[4] Other initial regimens with cefoxitin alone or ampicillin plus a newer cephalosporin may be equally effective, but no comparative trials have been performed.

Since 1979, retrospective studies have shown a vastly improved perinatal outcome compared with that reported in earlier studies. Gibbs and colleagues reported a retrospective study of 171 patients with IAI in whom therapy (with penicillin G and kanamycin) usually was begun at the time of diagnosis.[4] The mean gestational age of the neonate was 37.7 weeks. There were no maternal deaths, and bacteremia was found in only 2.3% of mothers. Among women with IAI, the rate of cesarean delivery was increased approximately threefold to 35%, mainly because of dystocia. In all mothers the outcome was good. There was only one episode of septic shock, with no pelvic abscesses or maternal deaths. Similar results were reported from Los Angeles County Hospital.[45]

Gibbs and colleagues found that when IAI is present, the perinatal mortality rate (140 per 1000 births) was approximately seven times the overall perinatal mortality rate for infants weighing more than 499 g (which was 18.2 per 1000 births).[4] Yet none of the perinatal deaths was clearly attributable to infection; of live-born infants weighing more than 1000 g, none died of infection. In the study by Koh and co-workers, the perinatal mortality rate was lower (28.1 per 1000 births), which probably reflected the higher mean gestational age (39.3 weeks).[45] There were no intrapartum fetal deaths and only four neonatal deaths. Again, no deaths were due to infection. Neither perinatal nor maternal complications correlated with more prolonged diagnosis-to-delivery intervals. Because patients who underwent cesarean section had more complicated courses, it was concluded that cesarean section should be reserved for patients with standard obstetric indications for this procedure in addition to IAI.

Yoder and colleagues later provided a prospective, case-control study of 67 neonates with microbiologically confirmed IAI at term.[46] There was only one perinatal death, which was unrelated to infection. Cerebrospinal fluid culture results were negative for all 49 infants tested, and there was no clinical evidence of meningitis. Findings on chest radiographs were interpreted as possible pneumonia in 20% of patients and as unequivocal pneumonia in only 4%. Neonatal bacteremia was documented in 8%. There was no significant difference in the frequency of low Apgar scores between the IAI and control groups.

Two other retrospective studies have been confirmatory. In 1984, Looff and Hager reported the outcomes of 104 pregnancies with clinical chorioamnionitis.[80] The mean gestational age was 36 weeks. The perinatal mortality rate was 123 per 1000 births. Nearly all of the excess mortality

Table 3–3 **Perinatal Outcome in Preterm Amnionitis (Intra-amniotic Infection)**

	Amnionitis[a]		Control[a]	
Measure (%)	*Reference[88] (N = 47)*	*Reference[89] (N = 92)*	*Reference[88] (N = 204)*	*Reference[89] (N = 606)*
Perinatal death	13	25	3[b]	6[b]
Respiratory distress syndrome	34	62	16[b]	35[b]
Total infections	17	28	7[b]	11[b]
Intraventricular hemorrhage	NR	56	NR[b]	22[b]

[a]At centers reporting these results, there were active referral services. In these series of consecutive patients with preterm premature rupture of membranes, those with amnionitis are compared with those without.
[b]Rates are significantly lower than for amnionitis group in corresponding study.
NR, not reported.

was attributed to prematurity rather than to sepsis. These authors also reported an increase in the cesarean delivery rate (26%). In 1985, Hauth and co-workers reviewed data for 103 pregnancies with clinical chorioamnionitis at term.[81] The mean interval from diagnosis of amnionitis to delivery was 3.1 hours, which confirmed the absence of a critical interval for delivery. In this study, the overall perinatal mortality rate was 9.7 per 1000 births and the cesarean delivery rate was 42%.

Neonates born prematurely have a higher frequency of complications if their mothers have IAI. Garite and Freeman noted that the perinatal death rate was significantly higher in 47 preterm neonates with IAI than in 204 neonates with similar birth weights but without IAI.[88] The group with IAI also had a significantly higher percentage (13% versus 3%; $P < .05$) with RDS and total infection. A larger but similar comparative study of 92 patients with chorioamnionitis and 606 controls of similar gestational age also demonstrated significant increases in mortality, RDS, intraventricular hemorrhage (IVH), and clinically diagnosed sepsis in the group with chorioamnionitis (Table 3-3).[89] When Sperling and associates stratified outcomes in cases of IAI by birth weight, cases leading to low birth weight were associated with more frequent maternal bacteremia (13.5% versus 4.9%; $P = .06$), early-onset neonatal sepsis (16.2% versus 4.1%; $P = .005$), and neonatal death from sepsis (10.8% versus 0; $P < .001$).[40]

In a retrospective, case-control study, Ferguson and co-workers reported neonatal outcome after chorioamnionitis.[90] Seventy percent of newborns weighed less than 2500 g. In 116 matched pairs, the authors found more deaths (20% versus 11%), more sepsis (6% versus 2%), and more asphyxia (27% versus 16%) in the group with chorioamnionitis. None of these differences, however, achieved statistical significance.

Choriamnionitis has been previously a maternal infection. Increasing evidence indicates that the fetus is primarily involved in the inflammatory response leading to premature delivery. The fetal inflammatory response syndrome (FIRS), well described by Yoon and co-authors, characterizes preterm PROM and spontaneous preterm labor, with a systemic pro-inflammatory cytokine response resulting in earlier delivery and with an increased risk of complications.[91] Additionally, these investigators show an association between the fetal inflammatory cascade and fetal white matter damage.[92] It remains unclear, however, whether cytokines mediate this damage or directly cause the damage, or if infection itself is responsible for the damage. Cytokines also can be stimulated by a number of noninfectious insults such as hypoxia, reperfusion injury, and toxins.[93]

Long-Term Outcome

Hardt and colleagues studied long-term outcomes in preterm infants (weighing less than 2000 g) born after a pregnancy with chorioamnionitis and found a significantly lower mental development index (Bayley's score) for these infants than noted for preterm control infants (104 ± 18 versus 112 ± 14; $P = .017$).[94] Morales reported 1-year follow-up of preterm infants born after pregancy with chorioamnionitis and of control infants. He did not observe differences in mental and physical development, but adjustments were made for IVH and RDS, both of which were more frequent in the amnionitis group.[89]

Intriguing new information strongly suggests that intrauterine exposure to bacteria is associated with long-term serious neonatal complications, including cerebral palsy or its histologic precursor, periventricular leukomalacia (PVL), as well as major pulmonary problems of bronchopulmonary dysplasia (BPD) and RDS. The unifying hypothesis states that intrauterine exposure of the fetus to infection leads to abnormal fetal production of proinflammatory cytokines. This leads in turn to fetal cellular damage in the brain, lung, and potentially other organs. This FIRS has been likened to the systemic inflammatory response syndrome (SIRS) in adults. The evidence linking infection to cerebral palsy may be summarized as follows:

1. Intrauterine exposure to maternal or placental infection is associated with an increased risk of cerebral palsy both in preterm and term infants.[95,96]
2. Clinical chorioamnionitis in very low birth weight infants is significantly associated with an increase in PVL ($P = .001$).[97]
3. The levels of inflammatory cytokines are increased in the amniotic fluid of infants with white matter lesions (PVL), and there is overexpression of these cytokines in neonatal brain with PVL.[98]
4. Experimental intrauterine infection in rabbits leads to brain white matter lesions.[99]
5. Marked inflammation of the fetal side of the placenta is associated with adverse neurologic outcomes. Coexisting evidence of infection and thrombosis, particularly on the

fetal side of the placenta, is associated with a heightened risk of cerebral palsy or neurologic impairment in term and preterm infants. Additionally, histologic funisitis is associated with an increased risk of subsequent cerebral palsy (OR 5.5, 95% confidence interval [CI] 1.2 to 24.5).[97,100,101] This risk underscores the importance of sending placentas for gross and microscopic examination in the setting of IAI.

The association between IAI and cerebral palsy differs for the term infant and the preterm infant. A recent review article nicely outlines the controversies in this area, including the associations among microbiologic, clinical, and histologic chorioamnionitis.[102] Additionally, emerging evidence points to genetic predispositions to inflammation and thrombosis; cytokine polymorphisms also may be linked to cerebral palsy.[93]

In addition to cellular and tissue damage in the fetal brain, an overexuberant cytokine response induced by bacteria may damage other fetal tissues, such as the lung, contributing to RDS and BPD.[103] In support of this hypothesis, a case-control study of infants with and without RDS was conducted. Those with RDS were significantly more likely to have elevated levels of amniotic fluid tumor necrosis factor (TNF)-α, a positive culture of the amniotic fluid, and severe histologic chorioamnionitis ($P < .05$ for each association). Elevated amniotic fluid IL-6 levels were also twice as common in the group with RDS, but this association did not achieve statistical significance. Furthermore, preterm fetuses with elevated cord blood IL-6 concentrations (greater than 11 pg/mL) were more likely to develop RDS (64% versus 24%; $P < .005$) than were those without elevated cord IL-6 levels. Rates of occurrence of BPD also were increased (11% versus 5%), but the observed difference was not statistically significant.[62] Curley and associates found elevated matrix metalloproteinase-9 (MMP-9) concentration in bronchoalveolar lavage fluid in preterm neonates with pregnancies complicated by chorioamnionitis compared with age-matched uninfected controls. These investigators hypothesize that increased MMP levels in the lung cause destruction of the extracellular matrix, breaking down type IV collagen in the basement membrane and leading to the failure of alveolarization and to fibrosis components of chronic lung disease.[104]

More recently, genetic predisposition toward exuberant host response to tissue injury has been described. Proinflammatory cytokine polymorphisms such as TNF-α 308 relate to bacterial endotoxin and an increased risk of preterm delivery.[105-107]

In summary, IAI has a significant adverse effect on mother and neonate, but vigorous antibiotic therapy and reasonably prompt delivery result in an excellent short-term prognosis, especially for the mother and the term neonate. With the combination of prematurity and amnionitis, serious sequelae are more likely for the neonate. Newly developing information suggests that intrauterine infection is linked to major neonatal long-term complications. A complex interplay of cytokine genotype may contribute to long-term complications as well.

Conclusion

The unanswered question remains: Why does IAI develop in some patients and not in others? Investigations of maternal and fetal genotypes for pro-inflammatory markers, among others, as well as study of mucosal immunity and host response, may help to answer this important question, as well as clarifying when neonatal damage will occur. It is not until we understand the answers to these questions that satisfactory therapeutic approaches can be developed.

Table 3–4 Proposed Prevention Strategies for Clinical Intra-amniotic Infection

Prompt management of dystocia
Induction of labor with premature rupture of membranes at term
Antibiotic prophylaxis with preterm premature rupture of membranes
Antibiotic prophylaxis with preterm labor, but with intact membranes
Antibiotic prophylaxis for group B streptococcal infection
Prenatal treatment of bacterial vaginosis
Chlorhexidine vaginal irrigations in labor
Infection control measures

Prevention

As categorized in Table 3-4, numerous approaches have been proposed for the prevention of IAI. Among these, prompt management of dystocia has been shown to decrease chorioamnionitis, as well as to shorten labor and reduce the cesarean section rate.[108] Similarly, induction in women with PROM at term most likely results in fewer maternal infections than may occur with expectant management.[109] Antibiotic prophylaxis for patients with preterm PROM decreases chorioamnionitis as well as other complications.[110,111] Treatment for bacterial vaginosis in high-risk women decreases incidence of preterm birth. Antibiotic prophylaxis for patients in preterm labor (but with intact membranes) does not appear to decrease frequency of chorioamnionitis.[112] Intrapartum prophylaxis for the prevention of neonatal group B streptococcal sepsis is now a national standard in known group B streptococci–colonized parturients or those in at-risk categories. It is presumed that this approach also decreases chorioamnionitis, but there are no definitive data to support this. Prenatal treatment of bacterial vaginosis in low-risk women, chlorhexidine vaginal washes in labor, and specific infection control measures have not been demonstrated to be effective.[19,113-115]

INFECTION AS A CAUSE OF PRETERM BIRTH

Preterm birth is the leading perinatal problem in the United States. Infants born before week 37 of gestation account for approximately 11% of births but for 60% to 80% of all perinatal deaths.[116-118] In most cases, the underlying cause of premature labor is not evident. Evidence from many sources points to a relationship between preterm birth and genitourinary tract infections (Table 3-5).[119,120] Infection leading to preterm birth may arise in the lower genital tract, the urinary tract, or a more remote site such as the lung or periodontal tissues.[121]

Table 3-5 Evidence for Relationship between Preterm Births and Subclinical Genitourinary Tract Infection

- The incidence of histologic chorioamnionitis is increased after preterm birth.
- The incidence of clinical infection is increased after preterm birth in both mother and neonate.
- Some lower genital tract microbes or infections are associated with an increased risk of preterm birth.
- There are biochemical mechanisms linking prematurity and infection.
- Infection and inflammation cause cytokine release and prostaglandin production.
- Bacteria and bacterial products induce preterm delivery in animal models.
- Amniotic fluid tests for bacteria are positive in some patients in premature labor.
- Some antibiotic trials have shown a decrease in numbers of preterm births.

Histologic Chorioamnionitis and Prematurity

Over the past 3 decades, one of the most consistent observations is that placentas in premature births are more likely to demonstrate evidence of inflammation (i.e., histologic chorioamnionitis) (Fig. 3-3). In a series of 3500 consecutive placentas, Driscoll found infiltrates of polymorphonuclear cells in 11%.[122] Clinically evident infection developed in only a few of the women in this study, but the likelihood of neonatal sepsis and death was increased.[123]

An association has been established between histologic chorioamnionitis and chorioamnion infection (defined as a positive culture).[123] Odds ratios (ORs) have been reported from 2.8 to 14, this relationship being stronger among preterm deliveries than among term deliveries. Overall, the organisms found in the chorioamnion are similar to those found in the amniotic fluid in cases of clinical IAI. This array of organisms supports an ascending route for chorioamnion infection in most cases.

Although it is not certain how histologic chorioamnionitis and membrane infection cause preterm delivery or preterm PROM, studies suggest that they lead to weakening of the membranes (as evidenced by lower bursting tension, less work to rupture, and less elasticity[124] in vitro) and to production of prostaglandins by the amnion.[125,126]

Clinical Infection and Prematurity

Both premature infants and women who previously gave birth to premature infants are more likely to develop clinically evident infection.[127] In a large study of more than 9500 deliveries, confirmatory evidence has shown that chorioamnionitis, endometritis, and neonatal infection all were significantly increased in preterm pregnancies, even after correcting for the presence of PROM.[128] These observations suggest that subclinical infection led to the labor and that infection became clinically evident after delivery. Some investigators argue that there is no causal relationship but that infection develops more frequently in premature infants because, for example, they are compromised hosts or because they have more invasive monitoring in the nursery.

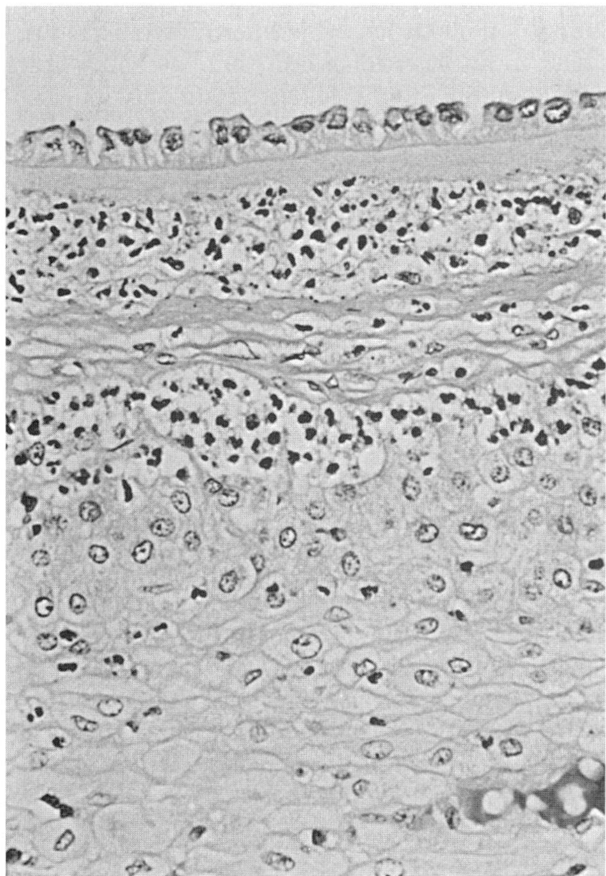

Figure 3-3 Infiltrates of polymorphonuclear cells are seen in the fetal membranes. Inflammation of the placenta and membranes has been consistently observed more often after preterm births than after term births.

Association of Lower Genital Tract Organisms or Infections with Prematurity

Premature birth has been associated with isolation of several organisms from the maternal lower genital tract and with subclinical infections, as listed in Table 3-6. Lower genital tract colonization with *U. urealyticum* is not associated with preterm birth. Similarly, cervical infection with *C. trachomatis* is not associated with preterm birth. However, other lower genital tract or urinary infections, including those due to *N. gonorrhoeae* and *Trichomonas vaginalis* and bacteriuria, are associated with preterm birth. Bacterial vaginosis, characterized by high concentrations of anaerobes, *Gardnerella vaginalis*, and genital mycoplasmas, with a corresponding decrease in the normal vaginal lactobacilli, has been consistently associated with premature birth.

Maternal genital tract colonization with group B streptococci may lead to neonatal sepsis, especially when birth occurs prematurely or when the membranes have been ruptured for prolonged intervals. In addition, an association between colonization of the cervix with these organisms and premature birth has been found by Regan and co-workers.[129] These investigators noted delivery at less than 32 weeks in 1.8% of the total population but in 5.4% of women colonized with group B streptococci ($P < .005$). PROM also occurred significantly more often in the colonized group

Table 3–6 Association of Lower Genitourinary Tract Infections with Preterm Birth

Infection	Odds Ratio for Preterm Birth (95% confidence Interval)
Ureaplasma urealyticum	1.0 (0.8-1.2)[a]
Chlamydia trachomatis	0.7 (0.36-1.37)[b,c]
Neisseria gonorrhoeae	5.31 (1.57-17.9)[d]
Trichomonas vaginalis	1.3 (1.1-1.4)[e]
Bacterial vaginosis	2.19 (1.54-3.12)[f]
Bacteriuria	1.64 (1.35-1.78)[g]

[a]Data from Carey JC, Blackwelder WC, Nugent RP, et al. Antepartum cultures for *Ureaplasma urealyticum* are not useful in predicting pregnancy outcome. Am J Obstet Gynecol 1991; 164:728.
[b]Data from Sweet RL, Landers DV, Walker C, et al. *Chlamydia trachomatis* infection and pregnancy outcome. Am J Obstet Gynecol 156:824, 1987.
[c]Data from Harrison HR, Alexander ER, Weinstein L, et al. Cervical *Chlamydia trachomatis* and mycoplasmal infections in pregnancy. JAMA 250:1721, 1983.
[d]Data from Elliott B, Brunham RC, Laga M, et al. Maternal gonococcal infection as a preventable risk factor for low birth weight. J Infect Dis 161:531, 1990.
[e]Data from Cotch MF, Pastorek JG, Nugent RP, et al. *Trichomonas vaginalis* associated with low birth weight and preterm delivery. Sex Transm Dis 24:353, 1997.
[f]Data from Leitich H, Bodner-Adler B, Brunbauer M, et al. Bacterial vaginosis as a risk factor for preterm delivery: a meta-analysis. Am J Obstet Gynecol 189:139, 2003.
[g]Romero R, Oyarzun E, Mazor M, et al. Meta-analysis of the relationship between asymptomatic bacteriuria and preterm delivery/low birth weight. Obstet Gynecol 73:567, 1989.

(15.3% versus 8.1%; $P < .005$). Of six studies evaluating the association between group B streptococci genital colonization and preterm labor or delivery, five found no association.[120] In contrast with the conflicting data regarding group B streptococcal genital colonization, group B streptococcal bacteriuria has been consistently associated with preterm delivery, and treatment of this bacteriuria resulted in a marked reduction in prematurity (37.5% in the placebo group versus 5.4% in the treatment group).[130-132] Current recommendations for prevention of perinatal group B streptococcal infection from the Centers for Disease Control and Prevention (CDC) are for intrapartum treatment only, with the exception of group B streptococcal bacteriuria, which should be treated antepartum. The CDC recommend adoption of universal screening. The *universal screening approach* involves screening women at 35 to 37 weeks of gestation with proper collection and culture techniques, followed by intrapartum treatment for all women with positive cultures.[133]

Untreated acute pyelonephritis has been found to be consistently associated with a 30% risk of preterm labor and delivery. A meta-analysis[134] showed that women with asymptomatic bacteriuria had a 60% higher rate of low birth weight (95% CI 1.4 to 1.9) and a 90% higher rate of preterm delivery (95% CI 1.3 to 1.9).

Amniotic Fluid Cultures in Preterm Labor

Among patients with signs and symptoms of preterm labor, the probability of finding a positive result on tests for bacteria depends on several factors. These factors are the specimen tested, the population under investigation, and the technique used for microbial detection. Thus, when standard culture techniques have been used for the amniotic fluid of patients clinically defined as being in preterm labor, the likelihood of positive cultures ranges from 0% to 25%. Yet with culture of the amniotic fluid of patients in preterm labor who deliver a preterm infant within 72 hours of the amniocentesis, the likelihood of a positive result has been 22%. With use of more sensitive assays such as PCR assay, the probability of finding bacteria in the amniotic fluid of patients in preterm labor has been as high as 30% to 55%.[135-139] Because bacteria are likely to be present in the amniotic membranes before appearing in the amniotic fluid, the rate of positive cultures of the membranes for patients in preterm labor has been 32% to 61%. Histologic evidence of chorioamnion infection is extremely common, being found in approximately 80% of placentas after the birth of an infant weighing 1000 g or less.

Biochemical Links of Prematurity and Infection

The widely accepted working hypothesis is that bacteria ascending into the uterine cavity are able to directly stimulate cytokine activity. IL-1, IL-6, and TNF-α, the proinflammatory cytokines, have been shown to be produced by the fetal membranes, decidua, and myometrium. Patients with elevated levels of these cytokines in the amniotic fluid have shorter amniocentesis-to-delivery intervals than those for patients without elevated cytokine levels. Levels also are elevated when preterm labor is associated with IAI.[140] In addition, elevated amniotic fluid IL-6 levels have been found to prospectively identify those fetuses destined for significant neonatal morbidity and mortality.[141] Similarly, Gomez and associates demonstrated that elevated fetal plasma levels of IL-6 in patients with preterm PROM, but not in labor, had a higher rate of delivery within 48 hours compared with those who delivered more than 48 hours after cordocentesis. These important findings suggest a fetal inflammatory cytokine response triggers spontaneous preterm delivery.[142]

Immunomodulatory cytokines such as IL-1 receptor antagonist (IL-1ra), IL-10, and transforming growth factor (TGF)-β play a regulatory role in the cytokine response, allowing for a downregulation of this response. IL-1ra has been shown in humans to increase in response to IAI.[143] Similarly, IL-10 inhibits IL-1β–induced preterm labor in a rhesus model.[144]

Animal models have been used to evaluate cytokine-mediated initiation of preterm birth. Romero and colleagues demonstrated that systemic administration of IL-1 induced preterm birth in a murine model.[145] Similarly, Kaga and co-workers gave low-dose lipopolysaccharide (LPS) intraperitoneally to preterm mice, causing preterm delivery.[146] Again in the murine model, others demonstrated preterm birth after intrauterine inoculation of *E. coli*.

Other investigators have used inoculation of live bacteria to study the infection–cytokine–preterm birth pathway. For example, in rabbits, we found that intrauterine inoculation of *E. coli*, *Fusobacterium* species, or group B streptococci led to rapid induction of labor at 70% gestation with an accompanying increase in histologic infiltrate and elaboration of TNF-α into the amniotic fluid. More recently, using our rabbit model, we demonstrated that intrauterine inoculation

Table 3–7 **Randomized Trial of Erythromycin for Treatment of Vaginal *Ureaplasma urealyticum* Infection in Pregnancy**

Outcome	Treatment Group *Erythromycin (N = 605)*	*Placebo (N = 576)*	P *Value*
Birth weight (g, mean ± SD)	3302 ± 557	3326 ± 558	NS
Birth weight <2500 g (%)	7	6	NS
Gestational age at delivery ≥36 wk (%)	8.6	8.2	NS
Premature rupture of membranes at ≥36 wk (%)	2.5	2.5	NS
Stillbirth (%)	0.5	0.5	NS
Neonatal death (%)	0.2	0	NS

NS, not significant; SD, standard deviation.

of the anaerobe *P. bivia* at 70% gestation led to establishment of a "chronic" infection in 64% of animals, with preterm birth occurring in 33%.[147] Also using a rhesus monkey model, Gravett and colleagues inoculated group B streptococci at 78% gestation and found resulting increases in amniotic fluid cytokines and prostaglandins followed by a progressive cervical dilatation.[148]

Antibiotic Trials

These treatment trials may be categorized into three general types as follows: (1) antibiotics given during prenatal care to patients at increased risk of preterm delivery; (2) antibiotics given adjunctively with tocolytics to women in preterm labor; and (3) antibiotics given to women with preterm PROM but not yet in labor.

In the prototype of the first category of antibiotic trial, Kass and colleagues[149] and McCormack and associates[150] noted a reduction in the percentage of low-birth-weight infants delivered of women who received oral erythromycin for 6 weeks in the third trimester, compared with those delivered of women who were given a placebo. Of note, these results were not confirmed in a National Institutes of Health–sponsored, multi-institutional study. More than 1100 women with genital *U. urealyticum* were randomized to receive placebo or erythromycin beginning at 26 to 28 weeks of gestation and continuing until 35 weeks. Here, no improvement was detected in any outcome measure (Table 3-7). Two retrospective, nonrandomized studies have reported reductions in PROM, low birth weight, and preterm labor through antenatal treatment of *C. trachomatis* infection.[151,152] However, the only randomized treatment trial for *C. trachomatis* infection in pregnancy led to conflicting results.[152a]

Treatment with metronidazole should be offered to women who have symptomatic *T. vaginalis* infection in pregnancy in order to relieve maternal symptoms.[153] Metronidazole is safe for use in the first trimester of pregnancy.[154] Yet when pregnant women with asymptomatic *T. vaginalis* infection at 24 to 29 weeks of gestation were randomized to receive treatment with either metronidazole or placebo, rates of delivery at less than 37 weeks and at less than 37 weeks due to preterm labor were both increased in the group given metronidazole (relative risk 1.8 [95% CI 1.2 to 2.7] for delivery at less than 37 weeks and relative risk 3.0 [95% CI 1.5 to 5.9] for delivery at less than 37 weeks due to preterm labor).[155]

Table 3–8 **Risk of Selected Adverse Outcomes with Use of Antibiotics in Preterm Labor with Intact Membranes**

Outcome	Relative Risk[a] (95% CI)
Preterm birth	0.99 (0.92-1.05)
Delivery within 48 hours	1.04 (0.89-1.23)
Perinatal mortality	1.22 (0.88-1.70)
Neonatal death	1.52 (0.99-2.34)

[a]A relative risk (RR) less than 1.0 favors antibiotics, and an RR greater than 1.0 favors controls. The RR is statistically significant if the 95% CI (confidence interval) excludes 1.0.

From King J, Flenady V. Prophylactic antibiotics for inhibiting preterm labour with intact membranes. Cochrane Database Syst Rev (1), 2003.

Because of the consistent association of bacterial vaginosis with preterm birth, several treatment trials have been carried out in pregnancy. A recent meta-analysis reported no significant reduction in preterm delivery when women with bacterial vaginosis were given antibiotic therapy as part of their prenatal care. Similarly, there is no significant reduction in preterm labor with treatment for bacterial vaginosis in women with previous preterm birth or in women at low risk for preterm birth. Of major importance, however, in the subset of women with both previous preterm birth and treatment for at least 7 days with an oral regimen, there was a significant reduction in preterm delivery (OR 0.42, 95% CI 0.27 to 0.67). Whether vaginal treatment of bacterial vaginosis is effective in preventing preterm birth is unclear. In the meta-analysis, no benefit was obtained by vaginal treatment.[156] Yet, in a recent trial of a 3-day course of clindamycin cream beginning at less than 20 weeks, a decreased incidence of preterm birth was observed (4% preterm birth in the antibiotic group versus 10% in the placebo group; $P < .03$).[157]

Among women in preterm labor with intact membranes, there have been several studies and recent meta-analyses. For example, the ORACLE II study demonstrated no delay in delivery or no improvement in a composite outcome that included neonatal death, chronic lung disease, or cerebral anomaly.[158] In the Cochrane meta-analysis, a total of 7428 women in 11 trials were assessed. As shown in Table 3-8, the use of antibiotics did not decrease preterm birth delivery within 48 hours or perinatal mortality. Of interest, the relative risk for neonatal death in the antibiotic treatment group was 1.52 (95% CI 0.99 to 2.34). There was a significant reduction in postpartum intrauterine infection with use of antibiotics, but this reduction was not seen as sufficient justification for widespread use of antibiotics in preterm labor. In a subanalysis, the reviewers looked at trials employing antibiotics that were active against anaerobes (i.e., metronidazole or clindamycin). Here there were significant benefits in delivery within 7 days and in neonatal intensive care unit (NICU) admissions. However, these benefits were not accompanied by significant reductions in major end points such as preterm birth, perinatal mortality, or neonatal sepsis.

Among patients with preterm PROM, again there have been several large trials. In 2003, the Cochrane Library updated its meta-analysis of these trials. In 13 trials comprising 6000 patients, antibiotics in this clinical setting had consistent benefits. Among women exposed to antibiotics, delivery within 48 hours, or within 7 days, or development of chorioamnionitis was less likely. Their neonates were less likely to have infection or sepsis. See Table 3-9.

Table 3–9 Risk of Selected Adverse Outcomes with Use of Antibiotics for Preterm Premature Rupture of Membranes

Outcome	Relative Risk[a] (95% CI)
Delivery within 48 hours	0.71 (0.58-0.87)
Delivery within 7 days	0.8 (0.71-0.9)
Chorioamnionitis	0.57 (0.37-0.86)
Neonatal infection	0.68 (0.53-0.87)
Abnormalities on cerebral ultrasound examination	0.82 (0.68-0.98)

[a]A relative risk (RR) less than 1.0 favors antibiotics, and an RR greater than 1.0 favors controls. The RR is statistically significant if the 95% CI (confidence interval) excludes 1.0.

Data from reference 27.

Lack of consistent findings in these antibiotic trials raises the question of why antibiotics have been effective in so few clinical situations. One likely explanation is that a true effective antibiotic may be "diluted out" by inclusion in the trials of patients in whom premature labor is not due to infection, for example, patients in preterm labor at 34 to 37 weeks. Another likely explanation is that once clinical signs and symptoms of preterm labor begin, the complex biochemical reactions have progressed too far to be stopped by antibiotic therapy alone.

Widespread use of antibiotics for the purpose of prolonging a premature pregnancy raises concerns regarding selection of resistant organisms and masking of infection. To date, evidence of selection pressure has been limited mainly to very low birth weight infants.[159] Concerns over masking infection is now of great concern, especially in view of recent evidence that intrauterine exposure to bacteria is associated with long-term adverse neonatal outcomes including cerebral palsy and PVL.[160,161]

For reasons other than prevention of preterm birth, detection and treatment of *N. gonorrhoeae*, *C. trachomatis*, and bacteriuria are appropriate. Our recommendations for use of antibiotics to prevent preterm birth are summarized in Table 3-10. However, future research is urgently needed to identify markers in women who are in preterm labor as a

Table 3–10 Consensus on Use of Antibiotics to Prevent Preterm Birth

Opinion	Comment
During Prenatal Care	
1. Treat *Neisseria gonorrhoeae* and *Chlamydia trachomatis* infection.	Screening and treatment of these two sexually transmitted organisms should follow standard recommendations to prevent spread to sexual partner(s) and the newborn. Published nonrandomized trials show improved pregnancy outcome with treatment.
2. Treat bacteriuria, including group B streptococcal bacteriuria.	Screening and treatment for bacteriuria is a standard practice to prevent pyelonephritis. A meta-analysis concluded that bacteriuria is directly associated with preterm birth.
3. Screen for and treat bacterial vaginosis in patients at high risk for preterm birth. In these high-risk women, treat with an oral metronidazole for 1 week or more.	A meta-analysis has shown benefit in women with high-risk pregnancies with this treatment.
4. Treat symptomatic *Trichomonas vaginalis* infection to relieve maternal symptoms, but do not screen for or treat asymptomatic trichomoniasis.	This opinion is based on randomized trials in asymptomatic infected women.
5. Do not treat *Ureaplasma urealyticum* genital colonization.	One double-blind treatment trial that corrected for confounding infections showed no benefit.
6. Do not treat group B streptococcal genital colonization.	One double-blind treatment trial showed no benefit.
With Preterm Labor and Intact Membranes	
1. Give group B streptococcal prophylaxis to prevent neonatal sepsis.	As recommended by the Centers for Disease Control and Prevention and the American College of Obstetricians and Gynecologists.
2. Do not give antibiotics routinely to prolong pregnancy.	Meta-analyses concluded that antibiotics gave no neonatal benefit, overall.
With Preterm Premature Rupture of Membranes	
1. Give group B streptococcal prophylaxis to prevent neonatal sepsis.	As recommended by the Centers for Disease Control and Prevention and the American College of Obstetricians and Gynecologists.
2. Give additional antibiotics in pregnancies at 24 to 32 weeks.	Meta-analyses concluded that there was substantial benefit to the neonate.

result of infection, in whom intervention with antibiotics or other novel therapies is most likely to be of benefit. In addition, detection of women genetically predisposed to infection-induced preterm birth is important. For example, some investigators have identified associations between polymorphisms in the cytokine gene complexes, including that for TNF-α, and preterm PROM or spontaneous preterm birth.[162-165]

PREMATURE RUPTURE OF MEMBRANES

PROM is a common but poorly understood problem. Because there is little understanding of its etiology, management has been largely empirical, and obstetricians have been sharply divided over what constitutes the best approach to care. Indeed, the problem is complex. Gestational age and demographic factors influence the outcome with PROM. Therapeutic modalities added within the past 2 decades include corticosteroids, tocolytics, and more potent antibiotics, but their place in therapy remains controversial. Of major importance is the marked improvement in survival of low-birth-weight infants. This chapter emphasizes developments since 1970. The literature has been reviewed periodically.[166-169]

Definition

Lack of standard, clear terminology has hindered understanding of PROM. Most authors define PROM as rupture at any time before the onset of contractions, but *premature* also carries the connotation of preterm pregnancy. To avoid confusion, we reserve *preterm* to refer to rupture occurring at a gestational age less than 37 weeks. Others using the expression "prolonged rupture of the membranes" have used the same acronym, PROM.

The *latent period* is defined as the time from membrane rupture to onset of contractions. It is to be distinguished from the *latent phase*, which designates the phase of labor that precedes the active phase. "Conservative" or "expectant" management refers to the period of watchful waiting when IAI has been at least clinically excluded in the setting of PROM.

In addition to IAI, terms used to describe maternal or perinatal infections during labor include *fever in labor*, *intrapartum fever*, *chorioamnionitis*, *amnionitis*, and *intrauterine infection*. In most reports, clinical criteria used for these diagnoses include fever, uterine irritability or tenderness, leukocytosis, and purulent cervical discharge. After delivery, maternal uterine infection is referred to as *endometritis*, *endomyometritis*, or *metritis*. These clinical diagnoses usually are based on fever and uterine tenderness. In few studies, however, were presumed maternal infections confirmed by blood or genital tract cultures.

For neonates, the most common term used to report infection is *neonatal sepsis*, but some authors use a positive blood or cerebrospinal fluid culture result, whereas others use clinical signs of sepsis without bacteriologic confirmation.

Incidence

In several reports, the incidence of PROM has ranged from 3% to 7% of total deliveries,[170,171] whereas PROM related to preterm birth has occurred in approximately 1% of all pregnancies.[7-9] In some referral centers, however, preterm PROM accounted for 30% of all preterm births.[175]

Etiology

Several clinical variables have been associated with PROM,[173,176] including cervical incompetence, cervical operations and lacerations, multiple pregnancies, polyhydramnios, antepartum hemorrhage, and heavy smoking. In most instances, however, none of these clinical variables are present. No association has been found between the frequency of PROM and maternal age, parity, maternal weight, fetal weight and position, maternal trauma, or type of work.[166,178]

Physical properties of membranes that rupture prematurely also have been investigated. Studies of the collagen content of amnion in patients with PROM have led to conflicting results, perhaps because of important differences in methodology. Of interest, patients with Ehlers-Danlos syndrome, a hereditary defect in collagen synthesis, are at increased risk of preterm PROM. Other reports have shown that membranes from women with PROM are thinner than membranes from women without PROM.[178] Using in vitro techniques to measure rupturing pressure, investigators have found that the membranes from patients with PROM withstand either the same or higher pressure before bursting than do membranes from women without PROM.[179-181] Such observations have suggested a local defect at the site of rupture, rather than a diffuse weakening, in membranes that rupture before labor. These studies of physical properties should be interpreted with caution because of differences in measuring techniques, possible deterioration of membrane preparations, and need for proper controls. In addition to being a possible cause of premature labor, subclinical infection may be a cause of PROM (see previous section). Acute inflammation of the placental membranes is twice as common when membranes rupture within 4 hours before labor than when they rupture after the onset of labor, which suggests that this "infection" may be the cause of PROM.[177] Supporting this hypothesis, increases in amniotic fluid matrix metalloproteases (MMP-1, -8, and -9) as well as decreases in matrix metalloprotease (MMP-1 and -2) inhibitors have been demonstrated in women experiencing preterm PROM.[182,183]

Several reports have suggested a relationship among coitus, histologic inflammation, and PROM. In additional analyses, two successive singleton pregnancies in each of 5230 women (10,460 pregnancies) were considered.[184] Preterm PROM occurred in only 2% of 773 pregnancies when there was no recent coitus and histologic chorioamnionitis, but it occurred in 23% of 96 pregnancies when both of these features were present. However, a causal role of coitus or infection was not established, because there may have been other factors that were not considered. Evaluation of successive pregnancies would not necessarily have eliminated these confounding variables. In the South African black population, the rates of histologic chorioamnionitis and PROM were increased when coitus had occurred within the last 7 days. Use of a condom during coitus resulted in less placental inflammation. In addition, PROM occurred more often ($P < .01$) when there had been male orgasm during coitus.[185] Because organisms may attach to sperm, it has been hypothesized that sperm carry organisms into the endocervix or uterus.

Further evidence is provided by bacteriologic studies. Patients with PROM before term or with prolonged membrane rupture are more likely to have anaerobes in the endocervical cultures than are women without PROM at term.[186,187] These observations may be interpreted as showing that subclinical anaerobic "infection" leads to PROM. The increased presence of anaerobes in cervical cultures, however, may reflect hormonal or other influences at different stages of gestation.

Investigations of risk factors for preterm PROM are likely to provide insight into the etiology of this condition. In the largest case-control study, Harger and colleagues reported 341 cases and 253 controls.[188] Only three independent variables were associated with preterm PROM in a logistic regression analysis. These were previous preterm delivery (OR 2.5, 95% CI 1.4 to 2.5), uterine bleeding in pregnancy, and cigarette smoking. The OR accompanying bleeding increased with bleeding in late pregnancy and with the number of trimesters in which bleeding occurred (OR for first-trimester bleeding 2.4, 95% CI 1.5 to 3.9; OR for third-trimester bleeding 6.5, 95% CI 1.9 to 23; OR for bleeding in more than one trimester 7.4, 95% CI 2.2 to 26). For cigarette smoking, the OR was higher for those who continued smoking (2.1, 95% CI 1.4 to 3.1) than for those who stopped (1.6, 95% CI 0.8 to 3.3). Because previous preterm pregnancy is a historical feature and little can be done to prevent bleeding in pregnancy, this study provides additional reason to encourage all patients, especially women of reproductive age, to stop smoking.

In the vast majority of cases, the specific etiology of preterm PROM remains unknown.

Diagnosis

In most cases, PROM is readily diagnosed by history, physical findings, and simple laboratory tests such as determination of pH (Nitrazine [phenaphthazine] test [Bristol-Myers Squibb, Princeton, NJ]) or detection of ferning. Although these tests are accurate in approximately 90% of cases, they yield false-positive and false-negative results, especially in women with small amounts of amniotic fluid in the vagina. Other biochemical and histochemical tests and intra-amniotic injection of various dyes have been suggested, but they have not gained wide acceptance. Ultrasound examination also has been used as a diagnostic technique, because finding oligohydramnios suggests PROM. Oligohydramnios, however, has many additional causes.

Natural History

The onset of regular uterine contractions occurs within 24 hours after membrane rupture in 80% to 90% of term patients.[1] The latent period exceeds 24 hours in 19% of patients at term and exceeds 48 hours in 12.5%.[188,189] Only 3.6% of term patients do not begin labor within 7 days.[188]

Before term, latent periods are longer among patients with PROM. Confirming earlier studies, more recent investigations have shown latent periods of 24 hours in 57% to 83%,[189,190] of 72 hours in 15% to 26%,[172,191,192] and of 7 days in 19% to 41% of patients.[172,189] There is an inverse relationship between gestational age and the proportion of patients with latent periods of 3 days.[191] There is also an inverse relationship between advancing gestation and a decreased risk of chorioamnionitis. One third of women with pregnancies between 25 and 32 weeks of gestation had latent periods of 3 days, whereas for pregnancies between 33 and 34 and between 35 and 36 weeks, the values were 16% and 4.5%, respectively. In 53 cases of PROM at 16 to 25 weeks (mean, 22.6 weeks), the median length of time from PROM to delivery was 6 days (range, 1 to 87 days; mean, 17 days).[193] In a population-based study of 267 cases of PROM before 34 weeks, fully 76% of women were already in labor at the time of admission, and an additional 5% had an indicated delivery. Only 19% were candidates for expectant management, and of these women, 60% went into labor within 48 hours.[194] Thus, the natural history of PROM reveals that labor usually develops within a few days.

In a minority of the cases of PROM, the membranes can "reseal," especially with rupture of membranes after amniocentesis. With expectant management, 2.8% to 13% may anticipate the cessation of leakage of amniotic fluid.[195,196]

Complications

Analysis of complications described in recent studies is complex because of differences in study design. Table 3-11, however, attempts to summarize complications observed in studies with more than 100 infants. Direct comparisons of data from one study to another require extreme caution. The wide-ranging differences are attributable to major differences in populations at risk, gestational age, definitions, and management.

The most common complication among cases with PROM before 37 weeks is RDS, which is found in 10% to 40% of neonates. (A small number of studies have reported RDS in as many as 60% to 80% of newborns.) Neonatal sepsis was documented in less than 10%, whereas amnionitis (based on clinical criteria only) occurred in 4% to 60%.[197] Endometritis developed in 3% to 29% of patients in most reports, but it is not clear whether patients with amnionitis are included in the endometritis category. In selected groups,

Table 3–11 Complications in Newborns after Premature Rupture of Membranes[a]

Complication	Rate (%)
Perinatal mortality, overall	0-43
Term	0-2.5
All preterm	2-43
1000-1500 g	29
1501-2500 g	7
RDS, all preterm	10-42
1000-1500 g	42
1501-2500 g	7
Infection	
Amnionitis	4-33
Maternal (overall)	3-29
Endometritis	3-29
Neonatal sepsis	0-7
Neonatal overall (including clinically diagnosed sepsis)	3-281

[a]Studies with more than 100 infants.
RDS, respiratory distress syndrome.

such as women who undergo cesarean section after PROM, endometritis occurs in up to 70% of patients.

When latent periods in preterm pregnancies are prolonged, pulmonary hypoplasia is an additional neonatal complication. When rupture of membranes occurs before 19 weeks, the incidence of pulmonary hypoplasia has been reported as 60%.[198] In cases where PROM occurred before 26 weeks and with long intervals (e.g., more than 5 weeks) between rupture and delivery, Nimrod and colleagues noted a 27% incidence of pulmonary hypoplasia.[200] Other studies demonstrate a lower incidence of pulmonary hypoplasia.[199] Pulmonary hypoplasia is rare if PROM occurs after 26 weeks of gestation.[201] In addition, pulmonary hypoplasia is poorly predicted antenatally by ultrasound examination.[202] Ultrasound estimates of interval fetal lung growth include lung length, chest circumference, chest circumference–abdominal circumference ratio, or chest circumference–femur length ratio. An additional 20% of neonates had fetal skeletal deformities as a result of compression. Nonskeletal restriction deformities of prolonged intrauterine crowding similar to features of Potter's syndrome include abnormal facies with low-set ears and epicanthal folds. Limbs may be malpositioned and flattened.[203]

Low Apgar scores, less than 7 at 5 minutes of life, are noted in 15% to 64% of live-born infants.[204-207] This complication is most common among very low birth weight infants. Other complications of PROM, especially in the preterm pregnancy, include malpresentation, cord prolapse, and congenital anomalies. In view of the long list of potential hazards, it is not surprising that premature infants surviving after PROM often are subject to prolonged hospitalization.

Perinatal mortality depends mainly on gestational age. The wide variation in results in Table 3-11 for preterm infants reflects different groupings of gestational ages. It is not certain whether infants with PROM have higher mortality than that for infants of the same gestational age without PROM.

Causes of perinatal death may be determined by examining data from four large series (Table 3-12).[208-210] Two of these studies included stillbirths; two studies excluded them. Overall, RDS was the leading cause of death. Deaths were presumed to be due to hypoxia when there was an antepartum or intrapartum death of a very small infant. In both frequency and severity, RDS was a greater threat than infection to the preterm fetus.

Table 3–12 Primary Causes of Death among Preterm Infants Born with Premature Rupture of Membranes

Cause	% of Perinatal Deaths[a]
RDS	29-70
Infection	3-19
Congenital anomaly	9-27
Asphyxia-anoxia	5-46[b]
Others[c]	9-27

[a]Overall perinatal mortality was 13% to 24%.
[b]Includes stillbirths with birth weight between 500 and 1000 g.
[c]Includes atelectasis, erythroblastosis fetalis, intracranial hemorrhage, and necrotizing enterocolitis.
RDS, respiratory distress syndrome.
Data from references 149, 179, 180, and Romero R, Kadar N, Hobbins JC. Infection and labor. Am J Obstet Gynecol 157:815, 1987.

Maternal mortality as a complication of PROM is rare. Studies document only one maternal death (related to chorioamnionitis, severe toxemia, and cardiorespiratory arrest) in more than 3000 women with PROM.[211] Case reports of maternal death from sepsis complicating PROM appear sporadically.[212]

Approach to Diagnosis of Infection

Because of the frequency and potential severity of maternal and fetal infections after PROM, various tests have been studied as predictors of infection. One review critically appraised eight tests and found no test to be ideal.[213] Several authors have evaluated the use of amniocentesis and microscopic examination of amniotic fluid for the presence of bacteria. This approach is limited, however, because amniotic fluid is available in only half of the patients. Clinical infection is more common in women with positive smears or cultures, but 20% to 30% of these women or their newborns had no clinical evidence of infection.[214-217] In addition, amniocentesis may potentially be accompanied by trauma, bleeding, initiation of labor, or introduction of infection, although Yeast and co-authors reported no increase in onset of labor and no trauma in their retrospective series.[218] Table 3-13 summarizes the diagnostic and prognostic value of several tests of amniotic fluid.[219]

Because the value of amniocentesis in patients with preterm PROM has not been determined precisely, most practitioners do not employ this test routinely for several reasons. Most patients with PROM and positive amniotic fluid culture results are in labor within 48 hours, and culture results often are delayed and available after the fact. Because at least some patients have positive culture results with no clinical evidence of infection, there is concern regarding unnecessary delivery of preterm infants. Finally, it has not been demonstrated that clinical decisions based on data from amniocentesis lead to an improved perinatal outcome. Feinstein and colleagues evaluated 73 patients with preterm PROM who underwent amniocentesis.[220] When the Gram stain or culture result was positive, delivery was accomplished. Results were compared with those of 73 matched patients from a historical group. Compared with controls, patients managed by amniocentesis had less clinically diagnosed amnionitis (7% versus 20%; $P < .05$) and fewer low Apgar scores for their infants at 5 minutes (3% versus 12%; $P < .05$). There were, however, no significant differences in rates of overall infection (22% versus 30%), "possible neonatal sepsis" (12% versus 14%), or perinatal deaths (1% versus 3%). Although there were apparent advantages to management by amniocentesis, historically controlled studies have serious limitations, and no significant decreases in overall infection of perinatal mortality were found. In a small comparative study of expectant management versus the use of amniocentesis, Cotton and colleagues reported a significantly shorter neonatal hospital stay in the amniocentesis group ($P < .01$), but more than 25% of patients were excluded because no amniotic fluid pocket was seen.[221] Also, there were no significant differences in rates of maternal infection, neonatal sepsis, or neonatal death. Ohlsson and Wang found Gram

Table 3–13 Diagnostic Values of Amniotic Fluid Testing in Detection of Positive Amniotic Fluid Culture in Patients with Preterm Labor and Intact Membranes

Diagnostic Index	Sensitivity	Specificity	Positive Predictive Value	Negative Predictive Value
Gram stain	7/11 (63.64%)	108/109 (99.08%)	7/8 (87.50%)	108/112 (96.43%)
IL-6 (≥11.30 ng/mL)	11/11 (100.0%)	90/109 (82.57%)	11/30 (36.67%)	90/90 (100.0%)
WBC count (≥50 cells/mm³)	7/11 (63.64%)	103/109 (94.50%)	7/13 (53.85%)	103/107 (96.26%)
Glucose (≤14 mg/dL)	9/11 (81.82%)	80/109 (81.65%)	9/29 (31.03%)	89/91 (97.80%)
Gram stain plus WBC count (≥50 cells/mm³)	10/11 (90.91%)	102/109 (93.58%)	10/17 (58.82%)	102/103 (99.03%)
Gram stain plus glucose (≤14 mg/dL)	10/11 (90.91%)	88/109 (80.73%)	10/31 (32.26%)	88/89 (98.88%)
Gram stain plus IL-6 (>11.30 ng/mL)	11/11 (100.0%)	89/109 (81.65%)	11/31 (35.48%)	89/89 (100.0%)
Gram stain plus glucose (≤14 mg/dL) plus WBC count (≥50 cells/mm³)	10/11 (90.91%)	85/109 (77.98%)	10/34 (29.41%)	85/86 (98.84%)
Gram stain plus WBC count (≥50 cells/mm³) plus IL-6 (≥11.30 ng/mL)	11/11 (100.0%)	87/109 (79.82%)	11/33 (33.33%)	87/87 (100.0%)
Gram stain plus glucose (≤14 mg/dL) plus IL-6 (≥11.30 ng/mL)	11/11 (100.0%)	78/109 (71.56%)	11/42 (26.19%)	78/78 (100.0%)
Gram stain plus WBC count (≥50 cells/mm³) plus IL-6 (≥11.30 ng/ml) plus glucose (≤14 mg/dL)	11/11 (100.0%)	76/109 (69.72%)	11/44 (25.00%)	76/76 (100.0%)

IL-6, interleukin-6; WBC, white blood cell.

Data from Romero R, Yoon BH, Mazor M, Gomez R, et al. The diagnostic and prognostic value of amniotic fluid white blood cell count, glucose, interleukin-6, and Gram stain in patients with preterm labor and intact membranes. Am J Obstet Gynecol 169:805, 1993.

stain and culture of amniotic fluid to have a modest positive predictive value for clinical chorioamnionitis.[214] Thus, clear evidence for the widespread use of amniocentesis in PROM is not available. In view of the more recent information regarding the association of cerebral palsy and infection, these issues should be reinvestigated in a controlled fashion.

Noninvasive procedures such as measuring the level of maternal serum C-reactive protein and amniotic fluid volume have also been suggested as predictors of infection. Several groups have evaluated C-reactive protein as such a predictor.[222-226] An elevated level of C-reactive protein in serum from patients with PROM has a modest positive predictive value for histologic amnionitis (40% to 96%), but its predictive value for clinically evident infection is poor (10% to 45%). The value of a normal level of C-reactive protein for predicting absence of clinical chorioamnionitis is better (80% to 97%). In view of the low predictive value of a positive test, a decision to attempt delivery based solely on an elevated C-reactive protein level does not appear wise.

Women who have PROM with oligohydramnios appear to be at increased risk for clinically evident infection, but the positive predictive value is modest (33% to 47%). In 1985, Gonik and co-workers noted that "amnionitis" developed in 8 (47%) of 17 patients with no pocket of amniotic fluid larger than 1 by 1 cm on ultrasound examination, whereas amnionitis developed in 3 (14%) of 22 patients with adequate pockets (i.e., larger than 1 by 1 cm) ($P < .05$).[227] To improve the predictability of these tests, Vintzileos and colleagues used a biophysical profile that included amniotic fluid volume, fetal movement and tone, fetal respirations, and a nonstress test.[228] However, positive predictive value of the biophysical profile has been variable (31% to 60% for clinical chorioamnionitis and 31% to 47% for neonatal sepsis).[214]

Treatment of Preterm Premature Rupture of Membranes before Fetal Viability

Because fetal viability is nil throughout nearly all of the second trimester, the traditionally recommended approach to PROM in this period of gestation has been to induce labor. However, retrospective reports have provided pertinent data on expectant management for PROM before fetal viability.[229-233] As expected, the latent period is relatively long (mean, 12 to 19 days; median, 6 to 7 days). Although in these reports, maternal clinically evident infections were common (amnionitis in 35% to 59% and endometritis in 13% to 17%), none of these infections were serious, but maternal death from sepsis has been reported.[234] Of note, there was an appreciable neonatal survival rate of 13% to 50%, depending on gestational age at membrane rupture and duration of the latent period. In cases with PROM at less than 23 weeks, the perinatal survival rate was 13% to 47%; whereas with PROM at 24 to 26 weeks, it was 50%.[232,233] The incidence of stillbirths is higher (15%) with midtrimester preterm PROM than with later preterm PROM (1%). The incidence of lethal pulmonary hypoplasia is 50% when membrane rupture occurs before 19 weeks.[235] Accordingly, with appropriate counseling, expectant management may be offered even in the second trimester for selected cases of PROM (Table 3-14). As neonatal survival in the periviable periods continues to improve, the numbers of infants afflicted by moderate to severe disabilities remains substantial.[236] These concerns should be clearly communicated to the mother before delivery. As discussed subsequently, a plan for group B streptococcal surveillance and treatment also would be indicated.

Investigational Treatment Measures

Highly experimental protocols are investigating the possibility of extrinsic materials to promote resealing of the amniotic membranes.[237] This idea stems from the use of a blood patch

Table 3–14 Summary of Management Plans for Premature Rupture of Membranes

Management	
In Second Trimester (<26-28 wk)	
A. Induction	
B. Expectant management	Retrospective works show high maternal infection rate but 13% to 50% neonatal survival
In Early Third Trimester (26-34 wk)	
A. Tocolytics to delay delivery	Randomized trials show no important benefits
B. Corticosteroids to accelerate lung maturity	CDC consensus statement recommends use between 24 and 32 wk
C. Antibiotics for prophylaxis of neonatal group B streptococcal infection	Efficiency established in randomized trial
D. Antibiotics to prolong latent period	Risk-benefit ratio unresolved; limit to randomized trials; optimal duration of antibiotics unresolved
E. Expectant management	Approach followed most commonly; if premature rupture of membranes occurs >32 wk, randomized trials show no neonatal benefit to expectant management
At or Near Term (>35 wk)	
A. Early induction, within 12-24 hr	
B. Late induction, after approximately 24 hr	
C. Expectant management until labor or infection develop	Recent evidence supports both option A and option C
D. Prostaglandin E_1 and E_2 preparations to ripen cervix/induce labor	Randomized trials and historical data support safety and efficacy

CDC, Centers for Disease Control and Prevention.

for treatment of spinal headache.[238] An aggressive interventional protocol for early midtrimester PROM using gelatin sponge for cervical plugging in patients with spontaneous or iatrogenic preterm PROM at less than 22 weeks with significant oligohydramnios (maximal vertical pocket less than 1.5 cm) evaluated transabdominal or transcervical placement of the gelatin sponge. This measure was in addition to broad-spectrum antibiotic therapy and cervical cerclage. Eight of 15 women undergoing the procedure reached a late enough stage in gestation to allow fetal viability, and 30% of infants survived to hospital discharge. Three of the surviving infants had talipes equinovarus, and two had bilateral hip dysplasia and torticollis. Quintero and colleagues[239] introduced an "amniopatch" consisting of autologous or heterologous platelets and cryoprecipitate through a 22-gauge needle intra-amniotically into seven patients with preterm PROM 16 to 24 weeks following fetoscopy or genetic amniocentesis and reported a fetal survival rate of 42.8% (three of seven). Of the remaining patients, two had unexplained fetal death, one miscarried, and a fourth had an underlying bladder outlet obstruction that prevented resealing of membranes. With spontaneous rupture of membranes, 0 of 12 patients have had resealing of their membranes.[238] The investigators speculate that with spontaneous rupture of membranes, rupture sites are larger, are located over the internal cervical os, are less amenable to patching, and are more susceptible to ascending infection and weakening of the lower portion of the membranes by proinflammatory agents.

To address the larger defect with spontaneous preterm PROM, Quintero and colleagues have investigated the use of an "amnio graft," achieved by laser-welding the amniotic membranes using Gore-Tex materials and a collagen-based graft material (Biosis), as well as combined use with a fibrin glue, with variable success in both animal models and selected patients.[238-240] Use of a fibrin sealant was associated with a 53.8% survival rate when the sealant was placed transcervically. In their study, mean gestational age at rupture of membranes was 19 weeks 4 days; at treatment, 20 weeks 5 days; and at delivery, 27 weeks 4 days, with a mean latency of 48 days from initial rupture to delivery. Additional research in this area is necessary to establish the safety and efficacy of this modality.

Treatment of Preterm Premature Rupture of Membranes in Early Third Trimester

It is at the gestational age interval of 24 to 34 weeks that management is most controversial. Yet new information has become available, and sophisticated meta-analyses have been performed. Controversial components of therapy, including corticosteroids, tocolytics, and antibiotics, are reviewed here. Specific situations such as HSV and HIV infection and cerclage coexisting with PROM are reviewed later in the chapter (see Table 3-14).

Corticosteroids

Many investigators have used corticosteroids in at least some patients with PROM.[241-243] In some studies, the investigators found evidence for an increased rate of maternal postpartum infection after administration of corticosteroids. The infections occurred mainly after vaginal delivery and were mild. Of still greater concern is the observation of some investigators that the rate of neonatal sepsis was increased when corticosteroids were used. However, most studies have not found this association.

Some studies reported significant (or nearly significant) decreases in the occurrence of RDS, but others found no significant decrease when corticosteroids were used in patients with PROM.[244-253] There are major difficulties in interpreting these studies. In some of the more rigorously designed studies of corticosteroid use, the numbers of patients with PROM were small. Thus, real differences may have been missed (a beta error). In most studies, there were at least small decreases in the incidence of RDS in the corticosteroid group. A relatively wide range of gestational ages was studied. The minimum number of weeks of gestation for entry into a study ranged from 25 to 32, and the maximum ranged from 32 to 37. Because an equal effect of corticosteroids on the rate of RDS is unlikely at all gestational age intervals, real differences may have been missed in some intervals, because data for these intervals were combined with data for other gestational ages. Finally, experiments measuring the surfactant-inducing potency of corticosteroids suggest differences in the efficacy of various corticosteroid preparations and various dosages.

Several studies, including three meta-analyses, have attempted to resolve the confusion.[254-256] Unfortunately, the authors reached differing conclusions. Ohlsson concluded that in preterm PROM, corticosteroid treatment "cannot presently be recommended to prevent RDS ... outside a randomized controlled trial.[254] The reasons underlying this conclusion are that the evidence that it decreases RDS is weak and its use increases the incidence of endometritis and may increase neonatal infections." On the other hand, Crowley and associates concluded that corticosteroids were effective in preventing RDS after preterm PROM (OR 0.44, 95% CI 0.32 to 0.60) and that they were not associated with a significant increase in perinatal infection (OR 0.84, 95% CI 0.57 to 1.23) or neonatal infection (OR 1.61, 95% CI 0.9 to 3.0).[255] Lovett and colleagues, in a prospective, double-blind trial of treatment for preterm PROM, did use corticosteroids in all patients. They also found significant decreases in mortality, sepsis, and RDS rates, as well as increased birth weight, when corticosteroids and antibiotics were given compared with use of corticosteroids alone. In addition, Lewis and co-workers investigated use of ampicillin-sulbactam in preterm PROM and then randomized patients to receive weekly corticosteroids versus placebo between 24 and 34 weeks. They found a decrease in RDS (44% versus 18%; $P = .03$ or .29, 95% CI 0.10% to 0.82%) in the corticosteroid treatment group with no increase in maternal or neonatal infection complications.[256] Lee's group also evaluated use of weekly steroids in a randomized double-blind trial in women at 24 to 32 weeks with preterm PROM, compared with only a single course of steroids. Although the investigators found no differences in the overall composite neonatal morbidity between the groups (34.2% versus 41.8%), they did find an increased rate of chorioamnionitis in the weekly-course group (49.4% versus 31.7%; $P = .04$). Of note, in the group with gestational age at delivery of 24 to 27 weeks, there was a significant reduction in RDS from 100% in the single-course group to 26.5% ($P = .001$) in the weekly-course group.[257]

Leitich and associates concluded that corticosteroids appear to diminish the beneficial effects of antibiotics in the treatment of preterm PROM. This was based on the results of their meta-analysis of five randomized trials of antibiotics and preterm PROM in which corticosteroids were used, which they compared with those of their previous meta-analysis of preterm PROM without corticosteroids. They found nonsignificant differences in mortality, sepsis, RDS, IVH, and necrotizing enterocolitis when both antibiotics and corticosteroids were used. By contrast, when antibiotics but not corticosteroids were used, they found a significant decrease in chorioamnionitis (OR 0.37, $P = .0001$), postpartum endometritis (OR 0.47, $P = .03$), neonatal sepsis (OR 0.27, $P = .002$), and IVH (OR 0.48, $P = .02$).[258]

The National Institutes of Health (NIH) Consensus Development Panel in 1995 recommended that corticosteroids be given in the absence of IAI to women with preterm PROM at less than 30 to 32 weeks of gestation because the benefits of corticosteroids may outweigh the risk at this gestational age, particularly with IVH. Because the number of patients receiving corticosteroids with PROM at more than 32 weeks of gestation was small, the consensus panel chose to restrict its recommendation to less than 32 weeks of gestation. Recommended dosing includes betamethasone 12 mg intramuscularly every 24 hours for two doses or dexamethasone 6 mg every 12 hours for four doses. The consensus panel reconvened in 2000 and reconfirmed their original recommendations. Repeat dosing of steroids was not recommended outside of randomized trials. Guinn and colleagues found no decrease in neonatal morbidity with serial weekly courses of betamethasone compared with single course therapy.[259]

Antibiotics

Patients with preterm PROM are candidates for prophylaxis against group B streptococci.[260-262] In addition, one innovative report noted use of combination antibiotics in an asymptomatic patient with preterm PROM because of bacterial colonization of the amniotic fluid, which was detected by amniocentesis. A second amniocentesis 48 hours after therapy revealed a sterile culture.[263]

Some studies of preterm pregnancies have found an increased rate of amnionitis to be associated with an increasing length of the latent period,[205,208,264] whereas others[207] have not. In patients with preterm PROM, digital vaginal examination should be avoided until labor develops, although transvaginal or transperineal ultrasound can be safely used to assess cervical length without increasing the risk of infection.[265] Some studies noted that prolonged ROM decreased the incidence of RDS,[210,211] others noted no significant effect.[207-209,242,245,266,267] These discrepancies may be explained by differences in experimental design (such as grouping of various gestational ages and using different sample sizes) or in definitions of clinical complications.

Antibiotics of several classes have been found to prolong pregnancy in the setting of preterm PROM. Two large multicenter clinical trials with different approaches had adequate power to evaluate the utility of antibiotics in the setting of preterm PROM. Mercer and Arheart[268] evaluated the use of antibiotics in PROM with a meta-analysis. They evaluated such outcomes as length of latency, chorioamnionitis, postpartum infection, neonatal survival, neonatal sepsis, RDS, IVH, and necrotizing enterocolitis. Several classes of antibiotics were used, including penicillins and cephalosporins, although few studies used either tocolytics or corticosteroids. Benefits of antibiotics in this analysis included a significant reduction in chorioamnionitis, IVH, and confirmed neonatal sepsis. There was a significant decrease in the number of women delivering within 1 week of membrane rupture (OR 0.56, CI 0.41 to 0.76), but no significant differences were seen in necrotizing enterocolitis, RDS, or mortality. The evidence currently supports use of antibiotics in preterm PROM to prolong latency and to decrease maternal and neonatal infectious complications, but further studies to select the preferred agent have yet to be performed.

The Maternal Fetal Medicine Units Network of the National Institutes of Child Health and Development (NICHD) conducted a large, multicenter trial of antibiotics after PROM but also did not use tocolytics or corticosteroids. Patients with preterm PROM at between 24 and 32 weeks were included. Patients were randomized to receive aggressive intravenous antibiotic therapy consisting of ampicillin (2 g intravenously [IV] every 6 hours) and erythromycin (250 mg IV every 6 hours) for the first 48 hours, followed by 5 days of oral therapy of amoxicillin (250 mg every 8 hours) and enteric coated erythromycin (333 mg orally every 8 hours) or placebo. Antibiotic treatment resulted in prolongation of pregnancy. Twice (50%) as many patients in the antibiotic treatment group remained pregnant after 7 days and 21 days composite neonatal morbidity was reduced in the antibiotic treatment group from 53% to 44% ($P < .05$). In addition, individual neonatal comorbid conditions occurred less often in the antibiotic treatment group: RDS (40.5% versus 48.7%), stage 3/4 necrotizing enterocolitis (2.3% versus 5.8%), patent ductus arteriosus (PDA) (11.7% versus 20.2%), BPD (13.0% versus 20.5%) ($P < .05$ for each). Occurrence rates for specific infections including neonatal group B streptococci–associated sepsis (0% versus 1.5%), overall neonatal sepsis (8.4% versus 15.6%), and pneumonia (2.9% versus 7.0%) all were significantly less ($P < .05$) in the antibiotic treatment group.

The second large trial was the multicenter, multiarm ORACLE trial of oral antibiotics in women with preterm PROM at less than 37 weeks. Over 4000 patients were randomized to receive oral erythromycin, amoxicillin–clavulanic acid, both, or placebo for up to 10 days. All of the antibiotic regimens prolonged pregnancy compared with placebo. Amoxicillin–clavulanic acid, however, increased the risk for neonatal necrotizing enterocolitis (1.9% versus 0.5%; $P = .001$), and this regimen is now advised against. The investigators demonstrated a significant decrease in perinatal morbidity, RDS, and necrotizing enterocolitis with use of ampicillin and erythromycin.[269]

Egarter and associates found in a meta-analysis of seven published studies a 68% reduction of neonatal sepsis and a 50% decreased risk of IVH in infants born to mothers receiving antibiotics after preterm PROM. They did not, however, find any significant differences in either RDS or neonatal mortality.[270]

The Cochrane Library has reviewed antibiotic use in preterm PROM in more than 6000 women in 19 trials. This meta-analysis also found that antibiotic use in preterm PROM was associated with an increased latent period at 48 hours and 7 days and reduction in major neonatal comorbid conditions or indicators such as neonatal infection, surfactant use, oxygen therapy, and abnormalities on head ultrasound examination prior to hospital discharge. Of interest, there was an increased risk of necrotizing enterocolitis in the two trials involving 2492 babies in which co-amoxiclav was administered to the mother (relative risk 4.6, 95% CI 1.98 to 10.72). Another included trial in the meta-analysis compared erythromycin to co-amoxiclav; the investigators found fewer deliveries at 48 hours in the co-amoxiclav group but no difference at 7 days. However, they also found a decrease in necrotizing enterocolitis when erythromycin rather than co-amoxiclav was used (relative risk 0.46, 95% CI 0.23 to 0.94).[271] Thus, they recommended that co-amoxiclav should be avoided in the setting of preterm PROM.

Owing to concerns of emergence of resistant organisms, another question involves duration of antibiotic therapy in preterm PROM. Two recent small trials have evaluated this question. Segel and assocites compared 3 days and 7 days of ampicillin in patients at 24 to 33 weeks with preterm PROM. In their 48 patients, there was no difference in 7-day latency as well as no difference in rates of chorioamnionitis, postpartum endometritis, and neonatal morbidity and mortality.[272] Lewis and colleagues studied 3 days versus 7 days of ampicillin-sulbactam (3 g IV every 8 hours) and similarly found no difference in outcomes between groups.[273] Both of these studies are small, so the final answer to this important question remains unanswered. We use 7 days of antibiotics, usually ampicillin and erythromycin, following the dosing from the NICHD trial.

Tocolytics and Development of Respiratory Distress Syndrome

Older studies suggested a decrease in the rate of RDS with use of beta-adrenergic drugs, but in the National Collaborative Study, use of tocolytics in patients with ruptured membranes increased the likelihood of RDS by about 350%.[274] In addition, two small randomized controlled trials have assessed use of tocolytics in the presence of PROM.[275,276] Neither found any significant increase in time to delivery or in birth weight or any decrease in RDS or neonatal hospital stay. These studies, however, did not use antibiotics or corticosteroids. Tocolytics have been shown to prolong pregnancy by about 48 hours in patients with intact membranes, but their efficacy with preterm PROM remains debatable. In the patient with preterm PROM and no contractions, tocolytics need not be given. In the patient with preterm PROM and contractions, IAI should be ruled out before consideration of tocolytics. Tocolytics could be considered in the early third trimester to maximize impact of antenatal corticosteroids (48-hour delay) on neonatal morbidity and mortality. Interested readers are referred to a recent review of this subject.[277]

Determination of Fetal Lung Maturity

Some clinicians determine the status of fetal pulmonary maturity and proceed with delivery if the lungs are mature. Amniotic fluid may be collected by amniocentesis or from the posterior vagina. Either presence of phosphatidylglycerol or a lecithin-to-sphingomyelin ratio higher than 2 in amniotic fluid has been reported to be a good predictor of pulmonary maturity. In a series of patients with PROM before 36 weeks, Brame and MacKenna determined whether phosphatidylglycerol was present in the vaginal pool and delivered patients when there was presence of phosphatidylglycerol, spontaneous labor, or evidence of sepsis.[278] Of 214 patients, 47 had phosphatidylglycerol present initially and were delivered. Of the remaining 167, 36 (21%) were subsequently found to have phosphatidylglycerol and were induced or delivered by cesarean section. Evidence of maternal infection developed in 8 (5%) and spontaneous labor developed in 123 (74%) of the 167 patients. Phosphatidylglycerol in amniotic fluid from the vagina reliably predicted fetal lung maturity; however, its absence did not necessarily mean that RDS would develop. Of 131 patients who did not show phosphatidylglycerol in the vaginal pool in any sample, 82 (62%) were delivered of infants who had no RDS. Lewis and colleagues also showed the presence of a mature Amniostat-FLM (Hana Biologies, Irvine, Calif) in a vaginal pool sample from 18% of 201 patients, and none developed RDS.

Intentional Preterm Induction in the Mid-Third Trimester

Even with PROM, delivery of a premature infant simply because the lungs show biochemical maturity may be questioned in view of other potential hazards of prematurity and the potential difficulties of the induction.

Two papers have examined this controversial issue. With respect to the new information regarding the association among preterm PROM, chorioamnionitis, and subsequent development of cerebral palsy, the use of intentional mid-third-trimester induction is receiving increased attention.

Mercer and colleagues compared expectant management and immediate induction in 93 pregnancies complicated by PROM between 32 and 36 weeks 6 days, when mature fetal lung profiles were documented. They found significant prolongation of latent period and of maternal hospitalization, as well as increased neonatal length of stay, and increased antimicrobial use in the expectant management group despite no increase in documented neonatal sepsis. Thus, they concluded that in women with preterm PROM at 32 through 36 weeks with a mature fetal lung profile, immediate induction of labor reduces the duration of hospitalization in both mother and neonates.[279] Cox and Leveno similarly studied pregnancies complicated by preterm PROM at 30 to 34 weeks of gestation. Consenting patients were randomly assigned to one of two groups: expectant management versus immediate induction. Corticosteroids, tocolytics, and antibiotics were not used in either group. Fetal lung profiles were not determined. The investigators found a significant increase in the incidence of chorioamnionitis and antepartum hospitalization in the expectant management group. In addition, they found no clinically significant differences in birth weight or frequency of IVH, necrotizing enterocolitis, neonatal sepsis, RDS, or perinatal death. They concluded that there were no clinically significant neonatal advantages to expectant management of ruptured membranes and decreased antepartum hospitalization in those women managed with immediate induction.[280]

Fetal Surveillance

Owing to concerns regarding cord compression and cord prolapse as well as the development of intrauterine and fetal infection, daily fetal monitoring in the setting of preterm PROM has been studied. Vintzileos and colleagues demonstrated that infection developed when the nonstress test became nonreactive 78% of the time, compared with only 14% when the nonstress test remained reactive.[281] Similarly, the biophysical profile score of 6 or less also predicted perinatal infection.[282] As a result, we recommend daily monitoring with nonstress tests. If the nonstress test is nonreactive, further workup with biophysical profile should be performed. Because there are currently no large studies evaluating outpatient management of preterm PROM, we recommend hospitalization until delivery.

Conclusion

Despite availability of recent data and sophisticated meta-analyses, we believe the evidence supports the use of expectant management in the absence of IAI and in the absence of documented fetal lung maturity in the third trimester until 34 completed weeks. If expectant management is chosen, corticosteroids to enhance fetal organ maturation should be given until 32 weeks. In addition, broad-spectrum antibiotics consisting of ampicillin and erythromycin should be administered for 7 days. Bacterial vaginosis should also be treated if present. In general, tocolytics should be avoided. Daily fetal surveillance is also recommended. Appropriate group B streptococcal prophylaxis in this high-risk group is strongly encouraged during labor. From a cost-effectiveness standpoint, Grable and co-workers looked at PPROM between 32 and 36 weeks. Using their decision analysis based on 1996 cost data, they weighed the costs of maternal hospitalization, latency, infection, and minor/major neonatal morbidity versus that of immediate induction. They found that it is most effective to delay delivery by 1 week between 32 and 34 weeks and to induce at presentation at or after 35 weeks.[283,284]

Recurrence

Recurrence of PPROM in a subsequent pregnancy following an index pregnancy complicated by PPROM has been estimated to be 13.5% to 44%. In Lee and colleagues' population-based case-control study, there was an odds ratio of 20.6 for recurrent PPROM and 3.6 for recurrent preterm birth. However, the estimated gestational age of index preterm PROM is poorly predictive of subsequent timing of recurrent events. The other two studies had higher recurrence of risks but probably included transferred patients, so that the study populations constituted a more select group.[285-288]

Prevention

Because preterm PROM often is accompanied by both maternal and neonatal adverse events, prevention of preterm PROM is desirable. Prediction of preterm PROM was evaluated in a large prospective trial, the Preterm Prediction Study,[288] sponsored by the NICHD Maternal Fetal Medicine Units Network. Prior preterm birth and preterm birth secondary to preterm PROM were associated with subsequent preterm birth. In nulliparas, preterm PROM is associated with medical complications, work in pregnancy, symptomatic contractions, bacterial vaginosis, and low body mass index. In multiparas, associated risk factors included prior preterm PROM, prior preterm birth due to preterm labor, and low body mass index. In both nulliparas and multiparas, a cervix found to be shorter than 25 mm by endovaginal ultrasound examination was associated with preterm PROM. A positive fetal fibronectin also was predictive of preterm PROM in both nulliparas (16.7%) and multiparas (25%). Multiparas with a prior history of preterm birth, a short cervix, and a positive fetal fibronectin had a 31-fold higher risk of PROM and delivery before

35 weeks compared with women without these risk factors (25% versus 0.8%; $P = .001$).[289]

Special Situations

Cerclage and Preterm Premature Rupture of Membranes

Classic obstetric dogma has suggested immediate removal of the cervical cerclage stitch when preterm PROM occurs. Risks associated with the retained stitch include maternal infection from bacterial proliferation emanating from the foreign body and cervical lacerations consequent to progression of labor despite the retained stitch. Small retrospective studies have shown conflicting results.

Currently, there are not enough data in the literature to recommend removal or retention of the suture. If there is no evidence of IAI or preterm labor in very premature gestations, one could consider leaving the stitch in during corticosteroid administration while there is uterine quiescence. After corticosteroids are maximized after 48 hours, then the stitch might be removed.[290-294]

Preterm Premature Rupture of Membranes and Herpes Simplex Virus

In a retrospective review from 1986 to 1996 of 29 patients with preterm PROM and a history of recurrent genital herpes, there were no cases of neonatal herpes. However, the 95% CI suggests that the risk of vertical transmission could be as high as 10%. The mean estimated gestational age at membrane rupture was 27.7 weeks. Mean estimated gestational age at maternal herpetic lesion development was 28.7 weeks. With continued expected management, mean estimated gestational age at delivery was 30.6 weeks in the study group. Of the 29 patients, 13 (45%) were delivered by cesarean section. Additionally, although delivery was performed for obstetric indication only, 8 of 13 patients undergoing cesarean section had active lesions as the only or a secondary indication for cesarean section. In this study, risk of neonatal death from complications of prematurity was 10%. Risk of major neonatal morbidity was 41%. The risks of major morbidity and mortality would have been considerably higher had there been iatrogenic delivery at the time of development of their herpetic lesion. Thus, it appears prudent when there is a history of recurrent HSV infection to continue expectant management in the significantly preterm gestation. In the setting of primary herpes (or nonprimary first episode), with the higher viral loads that entails, early delivery theoretically may prevent vertical transmission, but this has not been specifically studied. Only 8 of the patients in this study received acyclovir treatment. Thus, use of acyclovir for symptomatic outbreaks would theoretically reduce the risk of transmission, as well as decreasing the number of cesarean sections performed for presence of active lesions at the time of delivery.[295] Additionally, Scott and associates have demonstrated a decreased cesarean section rate in term patients with a history of recurrent HSV infection.[296]

Human Immunodeficiency Virus and Preterm Premature Rupture of Membranes

There are no specific data regarding the subset of patients with preterm PROM who are seropositive for HIV. With highly active antiretroviral therapy (HAART) and a low viral load, expectant management of preterm PROM after clinical exclusion of IAI might be considered, because the complications of prematurity with gestational age of less than 32 weeks, and certainly less than 28 weeks, are significant. With continued HAART, the risk of vertical transmission should remain low. The physician should discuss and document potential risks and benefits with the mother regarding the possibility of vertical transmission or neonatal morbidity and mortality. Intravenous infusion of zidovudine should be initiated at admission, if the antiretroviral regimen permits, because latency can be unpredictively short in many patients with preterm PROM.[297] If, after a period of observation and no evidence of spontaneous preterm labor, intravenous zidovudine may be discontinued and oral HAART continued.

Treatment of Term Premature Rupture of Membranes

Approximately 8% of pregnant women at term experience PROM, although contractions commence spontaneously within 24 hours of membrane rupture in 80% to 90% of patients.[197] After greater than 24 hours elapses following membrane rupture at term, the incidence of neonatal infection is approximately 1%, but this risk increases to 3% to 5% when clinical chorioamnionitis is diagnosed.[298] For many years, the practice in most institutions had been to induce labor in term patients within approximately 12 hours of PROM, primarily because of concerns about development of chorioamnionitis and neonatal infectious complications. More recently, three studies have demonstrated that in most patients, expectant management can be safely applied (see Table 3-14). The designs of these three reports were different.

Kappy and associates reported a retrospective review in a private population.[299] Duff and colleagues performed a randomized study in indigent patients with unfavorable cervix characteristics (less than 2 cm dilated, less than 80% effaced) and with no complications of pregnancy (e.g., toxemia, diabetes, previous cesarean section, malpresentation, meconium-stained fluid).[300] In the patients assigned to the induction group, initiation of induction generally was at 12 hours after rupture of membranes. The excess cesarean deliveries in the induction group were for failed induction. In the induction group, there was a higher probability of IAI. In the study by Conway and colleagues, all patients were observed until the morning after admission.[301] Induction of labor was then undertaken if the patient was not in labor.

Wagner and co-workers provided yet another variant by comparing early induction (at 6 hours after PROM) to late induction (at 24 hours after PROM).[302] In their population at a Kaiser Permanente hospital, the results favored early induction by shortening maternal hospital stay and decreasing neonatal sepsis evaluations. Recent work also has evaluated use of oral and vaginal prostaglandin preparations (prostaglandins E_1 and E_2) to ripen the cervix or induce labor after PROM at term. These preparations appear to be effective in shortening labor without increasing maternal or neonatal infection.[303-305]

Hannah and colleagues evaluated four management schemes in women with PROM at term: (1) immediate induction with oxytocin, (2) immediate induction with vaginal prostaglandin E_2, (3) expectant management for up to 4 days followed by oxytocin induction, and (4) expectant management followed by prostaglandin E_2 induction. Although no differences in cesarean section rates or frequency of neonatal sepsis were found, an increase in chorioamnionitis was noted in the expectant management groups, and all deaths not caused by congenital anomalies occurred in the expectant management group. Of note, patient satisfaction was higher in the immediate induction group. A secondary analysis demonstrated five variables as independent predictors of neonatal sepsis: clinical chorioamnionitis (OR 5.89), presence of group B streptococci (OR 3.08), seven to eight vaginal examinations (OR 2.37), duration of ruptured membranes 24 to 48 hours (OR 1.97), greater than 48 hours from membrane rupture to active labor (OR 2.25), and maternal antibiotics before delivery (OR 1.63).[306]

We endorse immediate induction with oxytocin in women with PROM at term if the condition of the cervix is favorable and the patient is willing. If the condition of the cervix is unfavorable, induction with appropriate doses of prostaglandins may be used before use of oxytocin. Intrapartum antibiotic prophylaxis against group B streptococci should be used according to the 2002 guidelines,[260] which emphasize universal screening of all gravidas at 35 to 37 weeks. All seropositive women should receive intravenous antibiotics in labor. Changes in the 2002 recommendations over the previous guidelines also include antibiotic guidelines for those with high- and low-risk penicillin allergy, as well as checking antibiotic sensitivities due to emerging antibiotic resistance, particularly resistance of erythromycin and clindamycin to group B streptococci.

REFERENCES

1. Gibbs RS, Duff P. Progress in pathogenesis and management of clinical intra-amniotic infection. Am J Obstet Gynecol 164:1317, 1991.
2. Newton ER, Prihoda TJ, Gibbs RS. Logistic regression analysis of risk factors for intra-amniotic infection. Obstet Gynecol 73:571, 1989.
3. Soper DE, Mayhall CG, Dalton HP. Risk factors for intra-amniotic infection: a prospective epidemiologic study. Am J Obstet Gynecol 161:562, 1989.
4. Gibbs RS, Castillo MS, Rodgers PJ. Management of acute chorioamnionitis. Am J Obstet Gynecol 136:709, 1980.
5. Romero R, Espinoza J, Chaiworapongsa T, Kalache K. Infection and prematurity and the role of preventive strategies. Sem Neonatol 7:259, 2002.
6. Halliday HL, Hirata T. Perinatal listeriosis: a review of twelve patients. Am J Obstet Gynecol 133:405, 1979.
7. Shackleford PG. Listeria revisited. Am J Dis Child 131:391, 1977.
8. Fleming AD, Ehrlich DW, Miller NA, et al. Successful treatment of maternal septicemia due to *Listeria monocytogenes* at 26 weeks' gestation. Obstet Gynecol 66:52S, 1985.
9. Petrilli ES, D'Ablaing G, Ledger WJ. *Listeria monocytogenes* chorioamnionitis: diagnosis by transabdominal amniocentesis. Obstet Gynecol 55:5S, 1980.
10. Boucher M, Yonekura ML. Perinatal listeriosis (early-onset): correlation of antenatal manifestations and neonatal outcome. Obstet Gynecol 68:593, 1986.
11. Listeriosis outbreak associated with Mexican-style cheese—California. MMWR Morb Mortal Wkly Rep 34:357, 1985.
12. Monif GRG. Antenatal group A streptococcal infection. Am J Obstet Gynecol 123:213, 1975.
13. Charles D, Edwards WR. Infectious complications of cervical cerclage. Am J Obstet Gynecol 141:1065, 1981.
14. Kuhn RJP, Pepperell RJ. Cervical ligation: a review of 242 pregnancies. Aust N Z J Obstet Gynaecol 17:79, 1977.
15. Aarnoudse JG, Huisjes HJ. Complications of cerclage. Acta Obstet Gynecol Scand 58:255, 1979.
16. Harger JH. Comparison of success and morbidity in cervical cerclage procedures. Obstet Gynecol 56:543, 1980.
17. Burnett RG, Anderson WR. The hazards of amniocentesis. J Iowa Med Soc 58:133, 1968.
18. Queenan JT. Modern Management of the Rh Problem, 2nd ed. Hagerstown, Md, Harper & Row, 1977, p 180.
19. Soper DJ, Mayhall CG, Froggatt JW. Characterization and control of intra-amniotic infection in an urban teaching hospital. Am J Obstet Gynecol 175:304, 1996.
20. Tran SH, Caughey AB, Musci TJ. Meconium-stained amniotic fluid is associated with puerperal infections. Am J Obstet Gynecol 189:746, 2003.
21. Krohn MJ, Germain M, Muhlemann K, Hickok D. Prior pregnancy outcome and the risk of intra amniotic infection in the following pregnancy. Am J Obstet Gynecol 178:381, 1998.
22. Yancey MK, Duff P, Kubilis P, et al. Risk factors for neonatal sepsis. Obstet Gynecol 87:188, 1996.
23. Herbst A, Wolner-Hanssen P, Ingemarsson I. Risk factors for fever in labor. Obstet Gynecol 86:790, 1995.
24. Naeye RL. Coitus and associated amniotic-fluid infections. N Engl J Med 301:1198, 1979.
25. Klebanoff MA, Nugent RP, Rhoads GG. Coitus during pregnancy: is it safe? Lancet 2:914, 1984.
26. Mills JL, Harlap S, Harley EE. Should coitus late in pregnancy be discouraged? Lancet 2:136, 1981.
27. Gibbs RS, Blanco JD, St. Clair PJ, et al. Quantitative bacteriology of amniotic fluid from patients with clinical intra-amniotic infection at term. J Infect Dis 145:1, 1982.
28. Gravett MG, Eschenbach DA, Speigel-Brown CA, et al. Rapid diagnosis of amniotic fluid infection by gas-liquid chromatography. N Engl J Med 306:725, 1982.
29. Nickerson CW. Gonorrhea amnionitis. Obstet Gynecol 42:815, 1973.
30. Handsfield HH, Hodson WA, Holmes KK. Neonatal gonococcal infection: I. Orogastric contamination with *Neisseria gonorrhoeae.* JAMA 225:697, 1973.
31. Brunnel PA, Dische RM, Walker MB. *Mycoplasma,* amnionitis, and respiratory distress syndrome. JAMA 207:2097, 1969.
32. Shurin PA, Alpert S, Rosner B, et al. Chorioamnionitis and colonization of the newborn infant with genital mycoplasmas. N Engl J Med 293:5, 1975.
33. Blanco JD, Gibbs RS, Malherbe H, et al. A controlled study of genital mycoplasmas in amniotic fluid from patients with intra-amniotic infection. J Infect Dis 147:650, 1983.
34. Gibbs RS, Cassell GH, Davis JK, et al. Further studies on genital mycoplasmas in intra-amniotic infection: blood cultures and serologic response. Am J Obstet Gynecol 154:717, 1986.
35. Martin DH, Koustsky L, Eschenbach DA, et al. Prematurity and perinatal mortality in pregnancies complicated by maternal *Chlamydia trachomatis* infections. JAMA 247:1585, 1982.
36. Wager GP, Martin DH, Koustsky L, et al. Puerperal infectious morbidity: relationship to route of delivery and to antepartum *Chlamydia trachomatis* infection. Am J Obstet Gynecol 138:1028, 1980.
37. Pankuch GA, Applebaum PC, Lorenz RP, et al. Placental microbiology and histology and the pathogenesis of chorioamnionitis. Obstet Gynecol 64:803, 1984.
38. Dong Y, Ramzy I, Kagan-Hallet SK, et al. A microbiologic clinical study of placental inflammation at term. Obstet Gynecol 70:175, 1987.
39. Gibbs RS, Schachter JS. Chlamydial serology in patients with intra-amniotic infection and controls. Sex Transm Dis 14:213, 1987.
40. Sperling RS, Newton E, Gibbs RS. Intra-amniotic infection in low birth weight infants. J Infect Dis 157:113, 1988.
41. Gibbs RS. Chorioamnionitis and bacterial baginosis. Am J Obstet Gynecol 169:460, 1993.
42. Silver HM, Sperling RS, St. Clair PJ, et al. Evidence relating bacterial vaginosis to intra-amniotic infection. Am J Obstet Gynecol 161:808, 1989.
43. Gravett MG, Nelson HP, DeRouen T, et al. Independent associations of bacterial vaginosis and *Chlamydia trachomatis* infection with adverse pregnancy outcome. JAMA 256:1899, 1986.
44. Newton ER, Piper J, Peairs W. Bacterial vaginosis and intra-amniotic infection. Am J Obstet Gynecol 176:672, 1997.
45. Koh KS, Chan FH, Monfared AH, et al. The changing perinatal and maternal outcome in chorioamnionitis. Obstet Gynecol 53:730, 1979.

46. Yoder RP, Gibbs RS, Blanco JD, et al. A prospective, controlled study of maternal and perinatal outcome after intra-amniotic infection at term. Am J Obstet Gynecol 145:695, 1983.
47. McDonald H, Brocklehurst P, Parsons J, Vigneswaran R. Antibiotics for treating bacterial vaginosis in pregnancy. Cochrane Database Syst Rev CD00262(13), 2003.
48. Carey JC, Klebanoff MA, Hauth JC, et al. Metronidazole to prevent preterm delivery in pregnant women with asymptomatic bacterial vaginosis. N Engl J Med 342:534, 2000.
49. ACOG Practice Bulletin No. 31. Assessment of Risk Factors for Preterm Birth. Washington, DC, American College of Obstetricians and Gynecologists, 2001.
50. Yankowitz J, Weiner CP, Henderson J, Grant S, Towbin JA. Outcome of low risk pregnancies with evidence of intraamniotic viral infection detected by PCR on amniotic fluid obtained at second trimester genetic amniocentesis. J Soc Gynecol Invest 3:132A, 1996.
51. Cassell G, Andrews W, Hauth J, et al. Isolation of microorganisms from the chorioamnion is twice that from amniotic fluid at cesarean delivery in women with intact membranes. Am J Obstet Gynecol 168:424, 1993.
52. Goncalves LF, Chairworapongsa T, Romero R. Intrauterine infection and prematurity. Mental retardation and developmental diabilities. Intrauter Infect Prematurity 8:3, 2002.
53. Romero R, Quintero R, Oyarzun E, et al. Intraamniotic infection and the onset of labor in preterm premature rupture of the membranes. Am J Obstet Gynecol 159:661, 1988.
54. Hoskins IA, Johnson TRB, Winkel CA. Leukocyte esterase activity in human amniotic fluid for the rapid detection of chorioamnionitis. Am J Obstet Gynecol 157:730, 1987.
55. Miller JM, Pupkin MJ, Hill GB. Bacterial colonization of amniotic fluid from intact fetal membranes. Am J Obstet Gynecol 136:796, 1980.
56. Romero R, Jimenez C, Lohda A, et al. Amniotic fluid glucose concentration: a rapid and simple method for the detection of intra-amniotic infection in preterm labor. Am J Obstet Gynecol 163:968, 1990.
57. Kirshon B, Rosenfeld B, Mari G, et al. Amniotic fluid glucose and intra-amniotic infection. Am J Obstet Gynecol 164:818, 1991.
58. Kiltz R, Burke M, Porreco R. Amniotic fluid glucose concentration as a marker for intra-amniotic infection. Obstet Gynecol 78:619, 1991.
59. Andrews WW, Hauth JC, Goldenberg RL, et al. Amniotic fluid interleukin-6: correlation with upper genital tract microbial colonization and gestational age in women delivered after spontaneous labor versus indicated delivery. Am J Obstet Gynecol 173:606, 1995.
60. Yoon BH, Romero R, Kim CH, et al. Amniotic fluid interleukin-6: a sensitive test for antenatal diagnosis of acute inflammatory lesions of preterm placenta and prediction of perinatal morbidity. Am J Obstet Gynecol 172:960, 1995.
61. Greig PC, Murtha AP, Jimmerson CJ, et al. Maternal serum interleukin-6 during pregnancy and during term and preterm labor. Obstet Gynecol 90:465, 1997.
62. Gomez R, Romero R, Ghezzi F, et al. The fetal inflammatory response syndrome. Am J Obstet Gynecol 179:194, 1998.
63. Gomez R, Ghezzi F, Romero R, et al. Premature labor and intra-amniotic infection. Clin Perinatol 22:281, 1995.
64. Hitti J, Riley DE, Krohn MA, et al. Broad spectrum bacterial rDNA polymerase chain reaction assay for detecting amniotic fluid infection in women in preterm labor. Clin Infect Dis 24:1228, 1997.
65. Oyarzun E, Yamamoto M, Kato S, et al. Specific detection of 16 micro-organisms in amniotic fluid by polymerase chain reaction and its correlation with preterm delivery occurrence. Am J Obstet Gynecol 179:1115, 1998.
66. Markenson GR, Martin RK, Tillotson-Criss M, et al. The use of the polymerase chain reaction to detect bacteria in amniotic fluid in pregnancies complicated by preterm labor. Am J Obstet Gynecol 177:1471, 1997.
67. Goncalves LF, Chairworapongsa T, Romero R. Intrauterine infection and prematurity. Mental retardation and developmental disabilities. Intrauter Infect Prematurity 8:3, 2002.
68. Romero R, Munoz H, Gomez R, et al. Two-thirds of spontaneous abortion/fetal deaths after genetic amniocentesis are the results of pre-existing subclinical inflammatory process of the amniotic cavity. Am J Obstet Gynecol 172:261, 1995.
69. Wenstrom KD, Andrews WW, Tamura T, et al. Elevated amniotic fluid interleukin-6 levels at genetic amniocentesis predict subsequent pregnancy loss. Am J Obstet Gynecol 175:830, 1996.
70. Goldenberg RL, Andrews WW, Mercer BM, et al. The Preterm Prediction study: granulocyte colony-stimulating factor and spontaneous preterm birth. Am J Obstet Gynecol 182:625, 2000.
71. Goldenberg RL, Hauth JC, Andrews WW. Intrauterine infection and preterm delivery. N Engl J Med 342:1500, 2000.
72. Andrews WW, Goldenberg R, Hauth J, et al. Interconceptional antibiotics to prevent spontaneous preterm birth (SPTB): a randomized trial. Am J Obstet Gynecol 2003;189:S57 (abstract).
73. Sperling RS, Ramamurthy RS, Gibbs RS. A comparison of intrapartum versus immediate postpartum treatment of intra-amniotic infection. Obstet Gynecol 70:861, 1987.
74. Gibbs RS, Dinsmoor MJ, Newton ER, et al. A randomized trial of intrapartum vs immediate postpartum treatment of women with IAI. Obstet Gynecol 72:823, 1988.
75. Gilstrap LC, Laveno KJ, Cox SM, et al. Intrapartum treatment of acute chorioamnionitis: impact on neonatal sepsis. Am J Obstet Gynecol 159:579, 1988.
76. Bray RE, Boe RW, Johnson WL. Transfer of ampicillin into fetus and amniotic fluid from maternal plasma in late pregnancy. Am J Obstet Gynecol 96:938, 1966.
77. Charles D. Dynamics of antibiotic transfer from mother to fetus. Semin Perinatol 1:89, 1977.
78. Weinstein AJ, Gibbs RS, Gallagher M. Placental transfer of clindamycin and gentamicin. Am J Obstet Gynecol 124:688, 1976.
79. Chapman SJ, Owen J. Randomized trial of single-dose versus multiple-dose cefotetan for the postpartum treatment of intrapartum chorioamnionitis. Am J Obstet Gynecol 177:831, 1997.
80. Looff JD, Hager WD. Management of chorioamnionitis. Surg Gynecol Obstet 158:161, 1984.
81. Hauth JC, Gilstrap LC, Hankins GDV, et al. Term maternal and neonatal complications of acute chorioamnionitis. Obstet Gynecol 66:59, 1985.
82. Duff P, Sanders R, Gibbs RS. The course of labor in term patients with chorioamnionitis. Am J Obstet Gynecol 147:391, 1983.
83. Silver RK, Gibbs RS, Castillo M. Effect of amniotic fluid bacteria on the course of labor in nulliparous women at term. Obstet Gynecol 68:587, 1986.
84. Perkins RP. The merits of extraperitoneal cesarean section: a continuing experience. J Reprod Med 19:154, 1977.
85. Hanson H. Revival of the extraperitoneal cesarean section. Am J Obstet Gynecol 130:102, 1978.
86. Imig JR, Perkins RP. Extraperitoneal cesarean section: a new need for old skills: a preliminary report. Am J Obstet Gynecol 125:51, 1976.
87. Yonekura ML, Wallace R, Eglinton WR. Amnionitis-optimal operative management: extraperitoneal cesarean section vs low cervical transperitoneal cesarean section. Third Annual Meeting of the Society of Perinatal Obstetricians, San Antonio, January 1983 (abstract 24A).
88. Garite TJ, Freeman RK. Chorioamnionitis in the preterm gestation. Obstet Gynecol 59:539, 1982.
89. Morales WJ. The effect of chorioamnionitis on the developmental outcome of preterm infants at one year. Obstet Gynecol 70:183, 1987.
90. Ferguson MG, Rhodes PG, Morrison JC, et al. Clinical amniotic fluid infection and its effect on the neonate. Am J Obstet Gynecol 151:1058, 1985.
91. Yoon BH, Romero R, Park JS, et al. The relationship among inflammatory lesions of the umbilical cord (funisitis), umbilical cord plasma interleukin 6 concentration, amniotic fluid infection, and neonatal sepsis. Am J Obstet Gynecol 183:1124, 2000.
92. Yoon BH, Jun JK, Romero R, et al. Amniotic fluid inflammatory cytokines (interleukin-6, interleukin-1beta, and tumor necrosis factor-alpha), neonatal brain white matter lesions, and cerebral palsy. Am J Obstet Gynecol 177:19, 1997.
93. Gibson CS, MacLennan AH, Goldwater PN, Dekker GA. Antenatal causes of cerebral palsy: associations between inherited thrombophilias, viral and bacterial infection, and inherited susceptibility to infection. Obstet Gynecol Surv 58:209, 2003.
94. Hardt NS, Kostenbauder M, Ogburn M, et al. Influence of chorioamnionitis on long-term prognosis in low birth weight infants. Obstet Gynecol 65:5, 1985.
95. Murphy DJ, Seller S, MacKenzie IZ, et al. Case-control study of antenatal and intrapartum risk factors for cerebral palsy in very preterm singleton babies. Lancet 346:1449, 1995.
96. Grether JK, Nelson KB. Maternal infection and cerebral palsy in infants of normal birth weight. JAMA 278:207, 1997.
97. Alexander JM, Gilstrap LC, Cox SM, et al. Clinical chorioamnionitis and the prognosis for very low birth weight infants. Obstet Gynecol 91:725, 1998.

98. Yoon BH, Romero R, Kim CJ, et al. High expression of tumor necrosis factor-alpha and interleukin-6 in periventricular leukomalacia. Am J Obstet Gynecol 177:406, 1997.
99. Yoon BH, Kim CJ, Romer R, et al. Experimentally induced intrauterine infection causes fetal brain white matter lesions in rabbits. Am J Obstet Gynecol 177:797, 1997.
100. Redline RW, O'Riordan A. Placental lesions associated with cerebral palsy and neurologic impairment following term birth. Arch Pathol Lab Med 124:1785, 2000.
101. Redline RW, Wilson-Costello D, Borawshi E, et al. Placental lesions associated with neurologic impairment and cerebral palsy in very low birth weight infants. Arch Pathol Lab Med 122:1091, 1998.
102. Willoughby RE Jr, Nelson KB. Choriamnionitis and brain injury. Clin Perinatol 29:603, 2002.
103. Hitti J, Krohn MA, Patton DL, et al. Amniotic fluid tumor necrosis factor-β and the risk of respiratory distress syndrome among preterm infants. Am J Obstet Gynecol 177:50, 1997.
104. Curley AE, Sweet DG, Thornton C, et al. Chorioamnionitis and increased neonatal lavage fluid matrix metalloproteinase 9 levels: implications for antenatal origins of chronic lung disease. Am J Obstet Gynecol 188:871, 2003.
105. Roberts AK, Monzon-Bordonalsa F, Van Deerlin PG, et al. Association of polymorphism within the promoter of the tumor necrosis factor alpha gene with increased risk of preterm premature rupture of membranes. Am J Obstet Gynecol 180:1297, 1999.
106. Gene MR, Gerber S, Nesih M, Witkin SS. Polymorphism in the interleukin-1 gene complex and spontaneous preterm delivery. Am J Obstet Gynecol 187:157, 2002.
107. Ferrand PE, Parry S, Sammel M, et al. A polymorphism in the matrix metalloproteinase-9 promoter is associated with increased risk of preterm premature rupture of membranes in African Americans. Mol Hum Reprod 8:494, 2002.
108. Lopez-Zeno JA, Peaceman AM, Adashek JA, et al. A controlled trial of a program for the active management of labor. N Engl J Med 326:450, 1992.
109. Mozurkewich EL, Wolf FM. Premature rupture of membranes at term: a meta-analysis of three management schemes. Obstet Gynecol 89:1035, 1997.
110. Mercer BM, Arheart KL. Antimicrobial therapy in expectant management of preterm premature rupture of the membranes. Lancet 346:1271, 1995.
111. Mercer BM, Miodovnik M, Thurnau GR, et al. Antibiotic therapy for reduction of infant morbidity after preterm premature rupture of the membranes. JAMA 278:989, 1997.
112. Egarter C, Leitich H, Husslein P, et al. Adjunctive antibiotic treatment in preterm labor and neonatal morbidity: a meta-analysis. Obstet Gynecol 88:303, 1996.
113. Eschenbach DA, Duff P, McGregor JA, et al. 2% Clindamycin vaginal cream treatment of bacterial vaginosis in pregnancy. Annual Meeting of the Infectious Diseases Society for Obstetrics and Gynecology, 1993 (abstract).
114. Rouse DJ, Hauth JC, Andrews WW, et al. Chlorhexidine vaginal irrigation for the prevention of peripartal infection: a placebo-controlled randomized clinical trial. Am J Obstet Gynecol 176:617, 1997.
115. Sweeten KM, Erikse NL, Blanco JD. Chlorhexidine versus sterile water vaginal wash during labor to prevent peripartum infection. Am J Obstet Gynecol 176:426, 1997.
116. Brans YW, Escobedo MB, Hayashsi RH, et al. Perinatal mortality in a large perinatal center: five-year review of 31,000 births. Am J Obstet Gynecol 148:284, 1984.
117. National Center for Health Statistics. Advance report of final natality statistics, 1980. Mon Vital Stat Rep 31, 1982.
118. Hamilton BE, Martin JA, Sutton PD. Births: Preliminary data for 2002. Natl Vital Stat Rep 51:1, 2003.
119. Minkoff H. Prematurity: infection as an etiologic factor. Obstet Gynecol 62:137, 1983.
120. Gibbs RS, Romero R, Hillier SL, et al. A review of premature birth and subclinical infection. Am J Obstet Gynecol 166:1515, 1992.
121. Gibbs RS. The relationship between infections and adverse pregnancy outcomes: an overview. Ann Periodontol 6:153, 2001.
122. Driscoll SG. The placenta and membranes. *In* Charles D, Finlands M (eds). Obstetrical and Perinatal Infections. Philadelphia, Lea & Febiger, 1973, p. 532.
123. Russell P. Inflammatory lesions of the human placenta: I. Clinical significance of acute chorioamnionitis. Am J Diagn Gynecol Obstet 1:127, 1979.
124. Schoonmaker JN, Lawellin DW, Lunt B, et al. Bacteria and inflammatory cells reduce chorioamniotic membrane integrity and tensile strength. Obstet Gynecol 74:590, 1989.
125. Bernal A, Hansell DJ, Khont TY, et al. Prostaglandin E production by the fetal membranes in unexplained preterm labour and preterm labour associated with chorioamnionitis. Br J Obstet Gynaecol 96:1133, 1989.
126. Lamont RF, Anthony F, Myatt L, et al. Production of prostaglandin E_2 by human amnion in vitro in response to addition of media conditioned by microorganisms associated with chorioamnionitis and preterm labor. Am J Obstet Gynecol 162:819, 1990.
127. Daikoku NH, Kaltzeider F, Johnson TR, et al. Premature rupture of membranes and preterm labor: neonatal infection and perinatal mortality risks. Obstet Gynecol 58:417, 1981.
128. Seo K, McGregor JA, French JA. Preterm birth is associated with increased risk of maternal and neonatal infection. Obstet Gynecol 79:75, 1992.
129. Regan JA, Chao S, James LS. Premature rupture of membranes, preterm delivery, and group B streptococcal colonization of mothers. Am J Obstet Gynecol 141:184, 1981.
130. Moller M, Thomsen AC, Borch K, et al. Rupture of fetal membranes and premature delivery associated with group B streptococci in urine of pregnant women. Lancet 2:69, 1989.
131. White CP, Wilkins EGL, Roberts C, et al. Premature delivery and group B streptococcal bacteriuria. Lancet 2:586, 1984.
132. Thomsen AC, Morup L, Hansen KB. Antibiotic elimination of group B streptococci in urine in prevention of preterm labour. Lancet 1:591, 1987.
133. U.S. Department of Health and Human Services. Prevention of perinatal group B streptococcal disease: a public health perspective. Morbid Mortal Wkly Rep 45(RR7):1, 1996.
134. Romero R, Mazor M. Infection and preterm labor. Clin Obstet Gynecol 31:553, 1988.
135. Gibbs RS, Romero R, Hillier SL, et al. A review of premature birth and subclinical infection. Am J Obstet Gynecol 166:1515, 1992.
136. Romero R, Sirtori M, Oyarzun E, et al. Infection and labor V. Prevalence, microbiology, and clinical significance of intraamniotic infection in women with preterm labor and intact membranes. Am J Obstet Gynecol 161:817, 1989.
137. Hitti J, Riley DE, Krohn MA, et al. Broad-spectrum bacterial rDNA polymerase chain reaction assay for detecting amniotic fluid infection among women in premature labor. Clin Infect Dis 24:1228, 1997.
138. Oyarzun E, Yamamoto M, Kato S, et al. Specific detection of 16 micro-organisms in amniotic fluid by polymerase chain reaction and its correlation with preterm delivery occurrence. Am J Obstet Gynecol 179:1115, 1998.
139. Markenson GR, Martin RK, Tillotson-Criss M, et al. The use of the polymerase chain reaction to detect bacteria in amniotic fluid in pregnancies complicated by preterm labor. Am J Obstet Gynecol 177:1471, 1997.
140. Gomez R, Ghezzi F, Romero R, et al. Premature labor and intra-amniotic infection. Clin Perinatol 22:281, 1995.
141. Yoon BH, Romero R, Kim CH, et al. Amniotic fluid interleukin-6: a sensitive test for antenatal diagnosis of acute inflammatory lesions of preterm placenta and prediction of perinatal morbidity. Am J Obstet Gynecol 172:960, 1995.
142. Gomez R, Romero R, Ghezzi F, et al. The fetal inflammatory response syndrome. Am J Obstet Gynecol 179:194, 1998.
143. Fidel PL Jr, Romero R, Ramirez M, et al. Interleukin-1 receptor antagonist (IL-1ra) production by human amnion, chorion, and decidua. Am J Reprod Immun 32:1, 1994.
144. Gravett MG. Interleukin-10 (IL-10) inhibits interleukin-1β (IL-1β) induced preterm labor in Rhesus monkeys. Annual Meeting of the Infectious Diseases Society for Obstetrics and Gynecology, 1998 (abstract).
145. Romero R, Mazor M, Tartokovsky B. Systemic administration of interleukin-1 induces parturition in mice. Am J Obstet Gynecol 165:969, 1991.
146. Kaga N, Katsuki Y, Obsta M, et al. Repeated administration of low dose lipopolysaccharide induces preterm delivery in mice: a model for human preterm parturition and for assessment of the therapeutic ability of the drugs against preterm delivery. Am J Obstet Gynecol 174:754, 1996.
147. Gibbs RS, McDuffie RS Jr, Kunze M, et al. Experimental intrauterine infection with *Prevotella bivia* in New Zealand white rabbits. Am J Obstet Gynecol 190:1082, 2004.

148. Gravett MG, Witkin SS, Haluska GJ, et al. Obstetrics: an experimental model for intraamniotic infection and preterm labor in rhesus monkeys. Am J Obstet Gynecol 171:1660, 1994.
149. Kass EH, McCormack WM, Lin JS, et al. Genital mycoplasmas as a cause of excess premature delivery. Trans Assoc Am Physicians 94:261, 1981.
150. McCormack WM, Rosner B, Lee Y, et al. Effect on birth weight of erythromycin treatment of pregnant women. Obstet Gynecol 69:202, 1987.
151. Cohen J, Valle JC, Calkins BM. Improved pregnancy outcome following successful treatment of chlamydial infection. JAMA 263:3160, 1990.
152. Ryan GM Jr, Abdella TN, McNeely SG, et al. *Chlamydia trachomatis* infection in pregnancy and effect of treatment on outcome. Am J Obstet Gynecol 162:34, 1990.
152a. Marten DH, Eschenbach DA, Cotch MF, et al. Double-blind placebo-controlled treatment trial of *Chlamydia trachomatis* endocervical infections in pregnant women. Infect Dis Obstet Gynecol 5:10-17, 1997.
153. Centers for Disease Control and Prevention. Sexually transmitted diseases treatment guidelines 2002. MMWR Recomm Rep 51(RR-6), 2002.
154. Burton P, Taddio A, Ariburno O, et al. Fetus-placenta-newborn: safety of metronidazole in pregnancy: a meta-analysis. Am J Obstet Gynecol 172:525, 1995.
155. Klebanoff MA, Carey JC, Hauth JC, et al. Failure of metronidazole to prevent preterm delivery among pregnant women with asymptomatic *Trichomonas vaginalis* infection. N Engl J Med 345:487, 2001.
156. Leitich H, Brunbauer M, Bodner-Adler B, et al. Antibiotic treatment of bacterial vaginosis in pregnancy: a meta-analysis. Am J Obstet Gynecol 188:752, 2003.
157. Lamont RF, Duncan SL, Mandal D, et al. Intravaginal clindamycin to reduce preterm birth in women with abnormal genital tract flora. Obstet Gynecol 101:516, 2003.
158. Kenyon SL, Taylor DJ, Tarnow-Mordi W, et al. Broad-spectrum antibiotics for spontaneous preterm labour: the ORACLE II randomized trial. Lancet 357:989, 2001.
159. Stoll BJ, Hansen N, Fanaroff AA, et al. Changes in pathogens causing early-onset sepsis in very-low-birth-weight infants. N Engl J Med 347:240, 2002.
160. Hitti J, Krohn MA, Patton DL, et al. Amniotic fluid tumor necrosis factor-alpha and the risk of respiratory distress syndrome among preterm infants. Am J Obstet Gynecol 177:50, 1997.
161. Grether JK, Nelson KB. Maternal infection and cerebral palsy in infants of normal birth weight. JAMA 278:207, 1997.
162. Roberts AK, Monzon-Bordonaba F, Van Deerlin PG, et al. Association of polymorphism within the promoter of the tumor necrosis factor alpha gene with increased risk of preterm premature rupture of the fetal membranes. Am J Obstet Gynecol 180:1297, 1999.
163. Genc MR, Gerber S, Nesin M, et al. Polymorphism in the interleukin-1 gene complex and spontaneous preterm delivery. Am J Obstet Gynecol 187:157, 2002.
164. Ferrand PE, Parry S, Sammel M, et al. A polymorphism in the matrix metalloproteinase-9 promoter is associated with increased risk of preterm premature rupture of membranes in African Americans. Mol Hum Reprod 8:494, 2002.
165. Dizon-Townson DS, Major H, Varner M, et al. A promoter mutation that increases transcription of the tumor necrosis factor-alpha gene is not associated with preterm delivery. Am J Obstet Gynecol 177:810, 1997.
166 Gunn GC, Mishell DR, Morton DG. Premature rupture of the fetal membranes: a review. Am J Obstet Gynecol 106:469, 1970.
167. Gibbs RS, Blanco JD. Premature rupture of the membranes. Obstet Gynecol 60:671, 1982.
168. Garite TJ. Premature rupture of the membranes: the enigma of the obstetrician. Am J Obstet Gynecol 151:1001, 1985.
169. ACOG Practice Bulletin No. 1. Washington, DC, American College of Obstetricians and Gynecologists, June 1998.
170. Bada HS, Alojipan LC, Andrews BF. Premature rupture of membranes and its effect on the newborn. Pediatr Clin North Am 24:491, 1977.
171. Fayez JA, Hasan AA, Jonas HS, et al. Management of premature rupture of the membranes. Obstet Gynecol 52:17, 1978.
172. Christensen KK, Christensen P, Ingemarsson L, et al. A study of complications in preterm deliveries after prolonged premature rupture of the membranes. Obstet Gynecol 48:670, 1976.
173. Evaldson G, Lagrelius A, Winiarski J. Premature rupture of the membranes. Acta Obstet Gynecol Scand 59:385, 1980.
174. Graham RJ, Gilstrap LC III, Lauth JC, et al. Conservative management of patients with premature rupture of fetal membranes. Obstet Gynecol 59:607, 1982.
175. Arias R, Tomich P. Etiology and outcome of low birth weight and preterm infants. Obstet Gynecol 60:277, 1982.
176. Eggers TR, Doyle LW, Pepperell RJ. Premature rupture of the membranes. Med J Aust 1:209, 1979.
177. Naeye RL, Peters EC. Causes and consequences of premature rupture of membranes. Lancet 1:192, 1980.
178. Artal R, Sokol RJ, Newman M, et al. The mechanical properties of prematurely and non-prematurely ruptured membranes, methods, and preliminary results. Am J Obstet Gynecol 125:655, 1976.
179. Parry-Jones E, Priya S. A study of the elasticity and tension of fetal membranes and of the relation of the area of the gestational sac to the area of the uterine cavity. Br J Obstet Gynecol 83:205, 1976.
180. Al-Zaid NS. Bursting pressure and collagen content of fetal membranes and their relation to premature rupture of the membranes. Br J Obstet Gynecol 87:227, 1980.
181. Lavery JP, Miller CE. Deformation and creep in the human chorio-amniotic sac. Am J Gynecol 134:366, 1979.
182. Vadillo-Ortega F, Hernandez A, Bonzalez-Avila G, et al. Increased matrix metallo-proteinase activity and reduced tissue inhibitor of metalloproteinase-1 levels in amniotic fluid from pregnancies complicated by preterm rupture of membranes. Am J Obstet Gynecol 174:1321, 1996.
183. Maymon E, Romero R, Pacora P, et al. Human neutrophil collagenase (matrix metalloproteinase 8) in preterm premature rupture of the membranes and intrauterine infection. Am J Obstet Gynecol 183:94, 2000.
184. Naeye RI. Factors that predispose to premature rupture of the fetal membranes. Obstet Gynecol 60:93, 1982.
185. Naeye RL, Ross S. Coitus and chorioamnionitis: a prospective study. Early Hum Dev 6:91, 1982.
186. Creatsas G, Pavlatos M, Lolis D, et al. Bacterial contamination of the cervix and premature rupture of the membranes. Am J Obstet Gynecol 139:522, 1981.
187. DelBene VE, Moore E, Rogers M, et al. Bacterial flora of patients with prematurely ruptured membranes. South Med J 70:950, 1977.
188. Harger JH, Hsing AW, Tuomala RE, et al. Risk factors for preterm premature rupture of fetal membranes: a multicenter case-control study. Am J Obstet Gynecol 163:130, 1990.
189. Kappy KA, Cetrulo CL, Knuppel RA, et al. Premature rupture of the membranes at term: a comparison of induced and spontaneous labors. J Reprod Med 27:29, 1982.
190. Kappy KA, Cetrulo CL, Knuppel RA, et al. Premature rupture of the membranes: a conservative approach. Am J Obstet Gynecol 134:655, 1979.
191. Nochimson DJ, Petrie RH, Shah BL, et al. Comparisons of conservation and dynamic management of premature rupture of membranes/premature labor syndrome: new approaches to the delivery of infants which may minimize the need for intensive care. Clin Perinatol 7:17, 1979.
192. Johnson JW, Daikoku NH, Niebyl JR, et al. Premature rupture of the membranes and prolonged latency. Obstet Gynecol 57:574, 1981.
193. Miller JM Jr, Brazy JE, Gall SA, et al. Premature rupture of the membranes: maternal and neonatal infectious morbidity related to betamethasone and antibiotic therapy. J Reprod Med 25:173, 1980.
194. Taylor J, Garite TJ. Premature rupture of membranes before fetal viability. Obstet Gynecol 64:615, 1984.
195. Cox SM, Williams ML, Leveno KJ. The natural history of preterm ruptured membranes: what to expect of expectant management. Obstet Gynecol 71:558, 1988.
196. Johnson JWC, Egerman RS, Moorehead J. Cases with ruptured membranes that "reseal." Am J Obstet Gynecol 163:1024, 1990.
197. Mercer BM. Management of premature preterm rupture of membranes before 26 weeks' gestation. Obstet Gynecol Clin North Am 19:339, 1992.
198. Mercer BM. Premature rupture of membranes. ACOG Practice Bulletin, 1998.
199. Rotschild A, Ling EW, Puterman ML, Farquharson D. Neonatal outcome after prolonged preterm rupture of the membranes. Am J Obstet Gynecol 162:46, 1990.
200. Nimrod C, Varela-Gittings F, Machin G, et al. The effect of very prolonged membrane rupture on fetal development. Am J Obstet Gynecol 148:540, 1984.

201. Vergani P, Ghidini A, Locatelli A, et al. Risk factors for pulmonary hypoplasia in second trimester PROM. Am J Obstet Gynecol 170:1359, 1994.
202. Rotschild A, Lind EW, Puterman ML, et al. Neonatal outcome after prolonged preterm rupture of membranes. Am J Obstet Gynecol 162:46, 1990.
203. Lauria MR, Gonik B, Romero R. Pulmonary hypoplasia: pathogenesis, diagnosis, and antenatal prediction. Obstet Gynecol 86:466, 1995.
204. Mercer BM. Preterm premature rupture of membranes. Obstet Gynecol 101:178, 2003.
205. Fayez JA, Hasan AA, Jonas HS, et al. Management of premature rupture of the membranes. Obstet Gynecol 52:17, 1978.
206. Evaldson G, Lagrelius A, Winiarski J. Premature rupture of the membranes. Acta Obstet Gynecol Scand 59:385, 1980.
207. Perkins RP. The neonatal significance of selected perinatal events among infants of low birth weight: II. The influence of ruptured membranes. Am J Obstet Gynecol 142:7, 1982.
208. Schreiber J, Benedetti T. Conservative management of preterm premature rupture of the fetal membranes in a low socioeconomic population. Am J Obstet Gynecol 136:92, 1980.
209. Bada HS, Alojipan LC, Andrews BF. Premature rupture of membranes and its effect on the newborn. Pediatr Clin North Am 24:491, 1977.
210. Eggers TR, Doyle LW, Pepperell RJ. Premature rupture of the membranes. Med J Aust 1979;1:209.
211. Berkowitz RL, Kantor RD, Beck FJ, et al. The relationship between premature rupture of the membranes and the respiratory distress syndrome: an update and plan of management. Am J Obstet Gynecol 131:503, 1978.
212. Daikoku NH, Kaltreider F, Khouzami VA, et al. Premature rupture of membranes and spontaneous preterm labor: maternal endometritis risks. Obstet Gynecol 59:13, 1982.
213. Jewett JF. Committee on maternal welfare: prolonged rupture of the membranes. N Engl J Med 292:752, 1975.
214. Ohlsson A, Wang E. An analysis of antenatal tests to detect infection in preterm premature rupture of the membranes. Am J Obstet Gynecol 162:809, 1990.
215. Garite TJ, Freeman RK, Linzey EM, et al. The use of amniocentesis in patients with premature rupture of membranes. Obstet Gynecol 54:226, 1979.
216. Zlatnik FJ, Cruikshank DP, Petzold CR, et al. Amniocentesis in the identification of inapparent infection in preterm patients with premature rupture of the membranes. J Reprod Med 29:656, 1984.
217. Vintzileos AM, Campbell WA, Nochimson DJ, et al. Qualitative amniotic fluid volume versus amniocentesis in predicting infection in preterm premature rupture of the membranes. Obstet Gynecol 67:579, 1986.
218. Yeast JD, Garite TJ, Dorchester W. The risks of amniocentesis in the management of premature rupture of the membranes. Am J Obstet Gynecol 149:505, 1984.
219. Romero R, Yoon BH, Mazor M, et al. The diagnostic and prognostic value of amniotic fluid white blood cell count, glucose, interleukin-6, and Gram stain in patients with preterm labor and intact membranes. Am J Obstet Gynecol 169:805, 1993.
220. Feinstein SJ, Vintzileos AM, Lodeiro JG, et al. Amniocentesis with premature rupture of membranes. Obstet Gynecol 68:147, 1986.
221. Cotton DB, Gonik B, Bottoms SF. Conservative versus aggressive management of prematerm rupture of membranes: a randomized trial of amniocentesis. Am J Perinatol 1:322, 1984.
222. Evans MI, Hajj SN, Devoe LD, et al. C-reactive protein as a predictor of infectious morbidity with premature rupture of membranes. Am J Obstet Gynecol 138:648, 1980.
223. Farb HF, Arnesen M, Geistler P, et al. C-reactive protein with premature rupture of membranes and premature labor. Obstet Gynecol 62:49, 1983.
224. Hawrylyshyn P, Bernstein P, Milligan JE, et al. Premature rupture of membranes: the role of C-reactive protein in the prediction of chorioamnionitis. Am J Obstet Gynecol 147:240, 1983.
225. Guinn D, Atkinson MW, Sullivan L, et al. Single vs weekly courses of antenatal corticosteroids for women at risk of preterm delivery: a randomized controlled trial. JAMA 286:1581, 2001.
226. Romem Y, Artal R. C-reactive protein as a predictor for chorioamnionitis in cases of premature rupture of the membranes. Am J Obstet Gynecol 150:546, 1984.
227. Gonik B, Bottoms SF, Cotton DB. Amniotic fluid volume as a risk factor in preterm premature rupture of the membranes. Obstet Gynecol 65:456, 1985.
228. Vintzileos AM, Campbell WA, Nochimson DJ, et al. The fetal biophysical profile in patients with premature rupture of the membranes—an early predictor of fetal infection. Am J Obstet Gynecol 152:510, 1985.
229. Beydoun SN, Yasin SY. Premature rupture of the membranes before 28 weeks: conservative management. Am J Obstet Gynecol 155:471, 1986.
230. Taylor J, Garite TJ. Premature rupture of membranes before fetal viability. Obstet Gynecol 64:615, 1984.
231. Major CA, Kitzmiller JL. Perinatal survival with expectant management of midtrimester rupture of membranes. Am J Obstet Gynecol 163:838, 1990.
232. Moretti M, Sibai BM. Maternal and perinatal outcome of expectant management of premature rupture of membranes in the midtrimester. Am J Obstet Gynecol 159:390, 1988.
233. Dinsmoor MJ, Bachman R, Haney E, et al. Outcomes after expectant management of extremely preterm premature rupture of the membranes. Am J Obstet Gynecol 190:183, 2004.
234. Moretti M, Sibai B. Maternal and perinatal outcome of expectant management of premature rupture of the membranes in the midtrimester. Am J Obstet Gynecol 159:390, 1988.
235. Rotschild A, Ling EW, Puterman ML. Neonatal outcome after prolonged preterm rupture of membranes. Am J Obstet Gynecol 162:46, 1990.
236. American Academy of Pediatrics. Perinatal care at the threshold of viability. Pediatrics 96:974, 1995.
237. O'Brien JM, Barton J, Milligan DA. An aggressive interventional protocol for early midtrimester premature rupture of the membranes using gelatin sponge for cervical plugging. Am J Obstet Gynecol 187:1143, 2002.
238. Quintero RA. Treatment of previable premature ruptured membranes. Clin Perinatol 30:573, 2003.
239. Quintero RA, Morales WJ, Allen M, et al. Treatment of iatrogenic previable premature rupture of membranes with intra-amniotic injection of platelets and cryoprecipitate (amniopatch); preliminary experience. Am J Obstet Gynecol 181:744, 1999.
240. Scissione AC, Manley JS, Pollock M, et al. Intracervical fibrin sealants: a potential treatment for early preterum premature rupture of membranes. Am J Obstet Gynecol 184:368, 20013.
241. Liggins GC. Prenatal glucocorticoid treatment: prevention of respiratory distress syndrome: lung maturation and prevention of hyaline membrane disease. Report of the 70th Ross Conference on Pediatric Research. Columbus, Ohio, Ross Laboratories, 1976, p 97.
242. Block MF, Klin OR, Crosby WM. Antenatal glucocorticoid therapy for the prevention of respiratory distress syndrome in the premature infant. Obstet Gynecol 50:186, 1977.
243. Morrison JC, Whybrew WD, Bucovaz ET, et al. Injection of corticosteroids into mothers to prevent neonatal respiratory distress syndrome. Am J Obstet Gynecol 131:358, 1978.
244. Taeusch HW, Frigoletto F, Kitzmiller J, et al. Risk of respiratory distress syndrome after prenatal dexamethasone treatment. Pediatrics 63:64, 1979.
245. Papageorgiou AN, Desgranges MF, Masson M, et al. The antenatal use of betamethasone in the prevention of respiratory distress syndrome: a controlled double-blind study. Pediatrics 63:73, 1979.
246. Collaborative Group on Antenatal Steroid Therapy. Effect of antenatal dexamethasone administration on the prevention of respiratory distress syndrome. Am J Obstet Gynecol 141:276, 1981.
247. Garite TJ, Freeman RK, Linzey EM, et al. Prospective randomized study of corticosteroids in the management of premature rupture of the membranes and the premature gestation. Am J Obstet Gynecol 141:508, 1981.
248. Barrett JM, Boehm FH. Comparison of aggressive and conservative management of premature rupture of fetal membranes. Am J Obstet Gynecol 144:12, 1982.
249. Schmidt PL, Sims ME, Strassner HT, et al. Effect of antepartum glucocorticoid administration upon neonatal respiratory distress syndrome and perinatal infection. Am J Obstet Gynecol 148:178, 1984.
250. Iams JDE, Talbert ML, Barrows H, et al. Management of preterm prematurely ruptured membranes: a prospective randomized comparison of observation versus use of steroids and timed delivery. Am J Obstet Gynecol 151:32, 1985.
251. Simpson GF, Harbert GM Jr. Uses of β-methasone in management of preterm gestation with premature rupture of membranes. Obstet Gynecol 66:168, 1985.
252. Nelson LH, Meis PJ, Hatjis CG, et al. Premature rupture of membranes: a prospective, randomized evaluation of steroids, latent phase, and expectant management. Obstet Gynecol 66:55, 1985.

253. Morales WJ, Diebel ND, Lazar AJ, et al. The effect of antenatal dexamethasone administration on the prevention of respiratory distress syndrome in preterm gestations with premature rupture of membranes. Am J Obstet Gynecol 154:591, 1986.
254. Ohlsson A. Treatments of preterm premature rupture of the membranes: a meta-analysis. Am J Obstet Gynecol 160:890, 1989.
255. Crowley PA. Antenatal corticosteroid therapy: a meta-analysis of the randomized trials, 1972 to 1994. Am J Obstet Gynecol 173:322, 1995.
256. Lewis DF, Brody K, Edwards MS, et al. Preterm premature ruptured membranes: a randomized trial of steroids after treatment with antibiotics. Obstet Gynecol 88:801, 1996.
257. Lee MJ, Davies J, Guinn D, et al. Single versus weekly courses of antenatal steroids in preterm premature rupture of membranes. Obstet Gynecol 103:274, 2004.
258. Leitich H, Egarter C, Reisenberger K, et al. Concomitant use of glucocorticoids: a comparison of two meta-analysis on antibiotic treatment in PROM. Am J Obstet Gynecol 178:899, 1998.
259. Guinn D, Davies J, and the Betamethasone Study Group. Multicenter randomized trial of single versus weekly courses of antenatal corticosteroids (ACS). Presented by D. Guinn at the Society for Maternal-Fetal Medicine 2001 Annual Meeting. Am J Obstet Gynecol 184:S6, 2001.
260. U.S. Department of Health and Human Services. Prevention of perinatal group B streptococcal disease: revised guidelines from CDC. MMWR Morbid Mortal Wkly Rep 51(RR11):1, 2002.
261. Minkoff H, Mead P. An obstetric approach to the prevention of early-onset group B beta-hemolytic streptococcal sepsis. Am J Obstet Gynecol 154:973, 1986.
262. Boyer KM, Gotoff SP. Prevention of early-onset neonatal group B streptococcal disease with selective intrapartum chemoprophylaxis. N Engl J Med 314:1665, 1986.
263. Romero R, Scioscia AL, Edberg SC, et al. Use of parenteral antibiotic therapy to eradicate bacterial colonization of amniotic fluid in premature rupture of membranes. Obstet Gynecol 67:15S, 1986.
264. Thibeault DW, Emmanouilides GC. Prolonged rupture of fetal membranes and decreased frequency of respiratory distress syndrome and patent ductus arteriosus in preterm infants. Am J Obstet Gynecol 129:43, 1977.
265. Schutte MF, Treffess PE, Kloostrerman GJ, et al. Management of premature rupture of membranes: the risk of vaginal examination to the infant. Am J Obstet Gynecol 146:395, 1983.
266. Christensen KK, Christensen P, Ingemarsson L, et al. A study of complications in preterm deliveries after prolonged premature rupture of the membranes. Obstet Gynecol 48:670, 1976.
267. Jones MD Jr, Burd LI, Bowes WA Jr, et al. Failure of association of premature rupture of membranes with respiratory-distress syndrome. N Engl J Med 292:1253, 1975.
268. Mercer BM, Arheart KL. Antimicrobial therapy in expectant management of preterm premature rupture of the membranes. Lancet 346:1271, 1995.
269. Mercer BM, Miodovnik M, Thurnau GR, et al. Antibiotic therapy for reduction of infant morbidity after preterm premature rupture of the membranes. JAMA 278:989, 1997.
270. Egarter C, Leitich H, Karas H, et al. Antibiotic treatment in PPROM and neonatal morbidity: a meta-analysis. Am J Obstet Gynecol 174:589, 1996.
271. Kenyon S, Boulvain M, Neilson J. Antibiotics for preterm rupture of membranes. Cochrane Database Syst Rev CD001058(2), 2003.
272. Segel SY, Miles AM, Clothier B, et al. Duration of antibiotic therapy after preterm premature rupture of fetal membranes. Am J Obstet Gynecol 189:799, 2003.
273. Lewis DF, Adair CD, Robichan AG, et al. Antibiotic therapy in preterm premature rupture of membranes: are seven days necessary? A preliminary, randomized clinical trial. Am J Obstet Gynecol 188:1413, 2003.
274. Curet LB, Rao AV, Zachman RD, et al. Association between ruptured membranes, tocolytic therapy, and respiratory distress syndrome. Am J Obstet Gynecol 148:263, 1984.
275. Garite TJ, Keegan KA, Freeman RK, et al. A randomized trial of ritodrine tocolysis versus expectant management in patients with premature rupture of membranes at 25 to 30 weeks of gestation. Am J Obstet Gynecol 157:388, 1987.
276. Weiner CP, Renk K, Klugman M. The therapeutic efficacy and cost effectiveness of aggressive tocolysis for premature labor associated with premature rupture of the membranes. Am J Obstet Gynecol 159:216, 1988.
277. Fontenot MT, Lewis DF. Tocolytic therapy and preterm premature rupture of membranes. Clin Perinatol 28:787, 2001.
278. Brame RG, MacKenna J. Vaginal pool phospholipids in management of premature rupture of membranes. Am J Obstet Gynecol 145:992, 1983.
279. Mercer BM, Crocker LG, Boe NM, et al. Induction versus expectant management in premature rupture of the membranes with mature amniotic fluid at 32 to 36 weeks: a randomized trial. Am J Obstet Gynecol 169:775, 1993.
280. Cox SM, Leveno KJ. Intentional delivery versus expectant management with preterm ruptured membranes at 30 to 34 weeks' gestation. Obstet Gynecol 86:875, 1995.
281. Vintzileos AM, Campbell WA, Nochimson DJ, et al. The use of the nonstress test in patients with premature rupture of membranes. Am J Obstet Gynecol 155:149, 1986.
282. Hanley ML, Vintzileos AM. Biophysical testing in premature rupture of the membranes. Semin Perinatol 20:418, 1996.
283. Grable IA. Cost effectiveness of induction after preterm premature rupture of membranes. Am J Obstet Gynecol 187:1153, 2002.
284. Naef RW, Allbert JR, Ross EL, et al. Premature rupture of membranes at 34 to 37 weeks' gestation: aggressive versus conservative management. Am J Obstet Gynecol 178:126, 1998.
285. Lee T, Carpenter MW, Heber WW, Silver HM. Preterm premature rupture of membranes: risks of recurrent complications in the next pregnancy among a population-based sample of gravid women. Am J Obstet Gynecol 188:209, 2003.
286. Naeye RL. Factors that predispose to premature rupture of the fetal membranes. Obstet Gynecol 60:93, 1982.
287. Asrat T, Lewis DF, Garite TJ, et al. Rate of recurrence of preterm premature rupture of membranes in consecutive pregnancies. Am J Obstet Gynecol 165:1111, 1991.
288. Mercer BM, Goldenberg RL, Moawad AH, et al. The Preterm Prediction Study: effect of gestational age and cause of preterm birth on subsequent obstetric outcome. Am J Obstet Gynecol 181:1216, 1999.
289. Mercer BM, Goldenberg RL, Meis PJ, et al. The Preterm Prediction Study: prediction of preterm premature rupture of membranes through clinical findings and ancillary testing. The National Institute of Child Health and Human Development Maternal-Fetal Medicine Units Network. Am J Obstet Gynecol 183:738, 2000.
290. Blickstein J, Katz Z, Lancet M, Molgimer BM. The outcome of pregnancies complicated by preterm rupture of membranes with and without cerclage. Int J Obstet Gynecol 28:237, 1989.
291. Yeast JD, Garite TR. The role of cervical cerclage in the management of preterm premature rupture of the membranes. Am J Obstet Gynecol 158:106, 1988.
292. Ludmir, Bader J, Chen L, et al. Poor perinatal outcome associated with retained cerclage in patients with premature rupture of membranes. Obstet Gynecol 84:823, 1994.
293. Jenkins TM, Berghella V, Shlossman PA, et al. Timing of cerclage removal after preterm premature rupture of membranes: maternal and neonatal outcomes. Am J Obstet Gynecol 183:847, 2000.
294. McElrath TF, Norwitz ER, Leiberman ES, Heffner LI. Preinatal outcome after preterm premature rupture of membranes with in situ cervical cerclage. Am J Obstet Gynecol 187:1147, 2002.
295. Carol A, Major CA, Towers CV, et al. Expectant management of preterm premature rupture of membranes complicated by active recurrent genital herpes. Am J Obstet Gynecol 188:155, 2003.
296. Scott LL, Sanchez PJ, Jackson GL, et al. Acyclovir suppression to prevent cesarean delivery after first-episode genital herpes. Obstet Gynecol 87:69, 1996.
297. Watts DH. Management of human immunodeficiency virus infection in pregnancy. N Engl J Med 346:1879, 2002.
298. Gerdes JS. Clinicopathologic approach to the diagnosis of neonatal sepsis. Clin Perinatol 18:361, 1991.
299. Kappy KA, Cetrulo CL, Knuppel RA, et al. Premature rupture of the membranes at term: a comparison of induced and spontaneous labors. J Reprod Med 27:29, 1982.
300. Duff WP, Huff RW, Gibbs RS. Management of the term patient who has premature rupture of the membranes and a cervix unfavorable for induction. Obstet Gynecol 63:697, 1984.
301. Conway DI, Prendiville WJ, Morris A, et al. Management of spontaneous rupture of the membranes in the absence of labor in primigravid women at term. Am J Obstet Gynecol 150:947, 1984.
302. Wagner MV, Chin VP, Peters CJ, et al. A comparison of early and delayed induction of labor with spontaneous rupture of membranes at term. Obstet Gynecol 74:93, 1989.

303. Meikle SF, Bissell ME, Freedman WL, et al. A retrospective review of the efficacy and safety of PGE_2 with premature rupture of the membranes at term. Obstet Gynecol 80:76, 1992.
304. Mahmood TA, Dick MJ, Smith NC, et al. Role of prostaglandin in the management of prelabour rupture of the membranes at term. Br J Obstet Gynaecol 99:112,1992.
305. Ray DA, Garite TJ. Prostaglandin E_2 for induction in patients with premature rupture of membranes at term. Am J Obstet Gynecol 166:836, 1992.
306. Seaward PGR, Hannah ME, Myhr TL, et al. International multicenter Term PROM Study: evaluation of predictors of neonatal infection in infants born to patients with premature rupture of membranes at term. Am J Obstet Gynecol 179:635, 1998.

Chapter 4

DEVELOPMENTAL IMMUNOLOGY AND ROLE OF HOST DEFENSES IN FETAL AND NEONATAL SUSCEPTIBILITY TO INFECTION

David B. Lewis • Christopher B. Wilson

The human fetus and neonate, particularly the premature neonate, are unduly susceptible to a wide variety of microbes. This susceptibility results from limitations of both innate and adaptive (antigen-specific) immunity, and from limitations in processes through which the innate immune system facilitates and directs the development of protective antigen-specific immunity. This chapter focuses on the ontogeny of the cellular and humoral components of the immune system and their function in the human fetus, neonate, and young infant. Antigen-specific immunity is discussed first, followed by innate mechanisms of host defense. The relationship between deficiencies in immune function in the neonate and fetus and their increased susceptibility to bacterial, viral, and protozoal infections are examined, followed by a brief review of current and potential applications of immunotherapy as therapeutic adjuncts or for the prevention of these infections.

The immune system is composed of hematopoietic cells, including lymphocytes, mononuclear phagocytes, myeloid and lymphoid dendritic cells (DCs), and granulocytes; certain nonhematopoietic cells, such as follicular DCs and thymic epithelial cells; and humoral factors, such as cytokines (Tables 4-1 and 4-2) and complement components. The mature hematopoietic cells of mammals are derived from pluripotent hematopoietic stem cells (HSCs). HSCs are generated during ontogeny from embryonic para-aortic tissue (the splanchnopleure), fetal liver, and bone marrow.[1] The yolk sac, which is extraembryonic, is a major site of nonlymphoid hematopoiesis starting at about the third week of embryonic development and is supplanted by the fetal liver at 8 weeks of gestation and, finally, by the bone marrow after 5 months of gestation. HSCs are found in the para-aortic tissue region by day 27 of human gestation, and cells with blood-forming potential in vitro have been identified in this region as early as day 19 of development.[2] Hematopoiesis by the fetal liver and bone marrow is established by seeding of these sites with circulating HSCs derived from para-aortic tissue.[3] All major lineages of hematopoietic cells that are part of the immune system are present in the human by the beginning of the second trimester. Their ontogeny from HSCs is discussed in separate sections of this chapter.

Table 4–1 Major Human Cytokines and TNF Family Ligands: Structure, Cognate Receptors, and Receptor-Mediated Signal Transduction Pathways

Cytokine Family	Members	Structure	Cognate Receptor Family	Proximal Signal Transduction Pathway(s)
IL-1	IL-1α, IL-1β, IL-18 (IL-1γ), and IL-1 receptor antagonist	β-Trefoil, monomers; processed and secreted	IL-1 receptor	IRAK; JNK
Hematopoietin	IL-2–IL-7, IL-9–IL3, IL-15, IL-17, IL-19, IL-29, CSFs, oncostatin-M, and IFNs (α, β, γ, and others); class II subfamily consists of IL-10, IL-19, IL-20, IL-22, IL-24, IL-26, and IFNs	Four α-helical; monomers except for IL-5 and IFNs (homodimers) and IL-12, IL-23, and IL-27 (heterodimers); secreted	Hematopoietin receptors	JAK tyrosine kinases/STAT, Src and Syk tyrosine kinases
TNF ligand	TNF-α, lymphotoxin-α, -β, CD27L, CD30L, CD40L, OX40L, TRAIL, and others	β-Jellyroll; homotrimers; type II membrane proteins and secreted	TNF receptor family	TRAFs and proteins mediating apoptosis
TGF-β	TGF-β1, -β2, -β3, bone morphogenetic proteins	Cysteine knot; processed and secreted	TGF-β receptors type 1 and type 2 heterodimers (intrinsic serine threonine kinases)	Smad proteins
Chemokines		Three-stranded β-sheet; all but fractalkine are secreted	Seven membrane-spanning domains	G protein–mediated
CXC ligand subfamily	CXCL1-14, CXCL16		CXCR1–CXCR6	
CC ligand subfamily	CCL1-5, CCL7, CCL8, CCL11, CCL13-CCL28		CCR1–CCR10	
C ligand subfamily	XCL1 (lymphotactin), XCL2 (SCM-1β)		XCR1	
CX3C ligand subfamily	CX3CL (fractalkine)		CX3CR1	

CSF, colony-stimulating factors; IFN, interferon; IL, interleukin; IRAK, IL-1 receptor–associated serine/threonine kinase; JNK, c-Jun N-terminal kinase; STAT, signal transducer and activator of transcription; TGF, transforming growth factor; TNF, tumor necrosis factor; TRAFs, TNF-α receptor–associated factors; TRAIL, TNF-related apoptosis–inducing ligand.

T LYMPHOCYTES AND ANTIGEN PRESENTATION

Overview

T lymphocytes, which are commonly referred to as T cells, are so named because the vast majority originate in the thymus. Along with B lymphocytes (B cells), which develop in the bone marrow, T cells comprise the adaptive or antigen-specific immune system. T lymphocytes play a central role in antigen-specific immunity because they directly mediate cellular immune responses and play a critical role in facilitating antigen-specific humoral immune responses by B cells.

Most T cells recognize antigen in the form of peptides bound to major histocompatibility complex (MHC) molecules on antigen-presenting cells (APCs). Antigen-specific T cell receptors (TCRs) are heterodimeric molecules composed of either α and β chains (αβ-TCRs) (Fig. 4-1) or γ and δ chains (γδ-TCRs).[4] The amino-terminal portion of each of these chains is variable and is involved in antigen recognition. As discussed later, the highly variable nature of this portion of the TCR is generated, in large part, as a result of TCR gene rearrangement of variable (V), diversity (D), and joining (J) segments. By contrast, the carboxy-terminal region of each of the four TCR chains is monomorphic or constant. The TCR on the cell surface is invariably associated with the nonpolymorphic complex of CD3 proteins, which include CD3-γ, -δ, -ε, and -ζ (see Fig. 4-1).[5,6] The cytoplasmic domains of proteins of the CD3 complex include 10 immunoreceptor tyrosine-based activation motifs (ITAMs), which serve as docking sites for intracellular tyrosine kinases that transduce activation signals to the interior of the cell after the TCR has been engaged by antigen.[6]

Nearly all T cells that bear an αβ-TCR, hereafter referred to as αβ T cells, also express on their surface the CD4 or CD8 co-receptors in a mutually exclusive manner. The CD4 co-receptor is expressed as a monomeric or homo-oligomeric complex.[7] The CD8 co-receptor may consist either of CD8-α/CD8-β heterodimers or CD8-α/CD8-α homodimers.[8] The αβ T cells mainly express CD8-α/CD8-β heterodimers; a subset of T cells with γδ-TCRs, hereafter referred to as γδ

Table 4–2 Immunoregulatory Effects of Select Cytokines, Chemokines, and TNF Ligand Family Proteins and Their Production by Human Neonatal Cells

Cytokine	Principal Cell Source	Major Biologic Effects	Production by Neonatal versus Adult Cells	Reference(s)
IL-1α, IL-1-β	Many cell types; Mϕ are a major source	Fever, inflammatory response, cofactor in T and B cell growth	MNCs: normal after LPS treatment; ?reduced in premature	1080, 1405
IL-2	T cells	T > B cell growth, increased cytotoxicity by T and NK cells, increased cytokine production and sensitivity to apoptosis by T cells, growth and survival of regulatory T cells	T cells: normal with most polyclonal stimuli; neonatal < adult after CD3 mAb treatment	326, 342, 343
IL-3	T cells	Growth of early hematopoietic precursors (also known as multi-CSF)	T cells: neonatal and adult naïve < adult memory MNCs: neonatal < adult	342, 1406, 1407
IL-4	T cells, mast cells, basophils, eosinophils	Required for IgE synthesis; enhances B cell growth and MHC class II expression; promotes T cell growth and T_H2 differentiation, mast cell growth factor; enhances endothelial VCAM-1 expression	T cells: Neonatal and adult naïve < adult memory	342, 343
IL-5	T cells, NK cells, mast cells, basophils, eosinophils	Eosinophil growth, differentiation, and survival	T cells: neonatal and adult naïve < adult memory	342
IL-6	Mϕ, fibroblasts, T cells	Hepatic acute-phase protein synthesis, fever, T and B cell growth and differentiation	T cells: neonatal < adult naive < adult memory MNC: term normal to slightly reduced; premature ~25% of adult Mϕ: neonatal < adult after RSV infection Whole blood: neonatal = adult	1408-1412
IL-7	Stromal cells of bone marrow and thymus	Essential thymocyte growth factor	Not known	
IL-8 (CXCL8)	Mϕ, endothelial cells, fibroblasts, epithelial cells, T cells	Chemotaxis and activation of neutrophils	MNCs: neonatal < adult or normal in different studies using LPS stimulation; preterm < term Mϕ: decreased after GBS incubation Whole blood: neonatal = adult	1082, 1083, 1408, 1413
IL-9	T cells, mast cells	T cell and mast cell growth factor	Not known	
IL-10	Mϕ, T, cells, B cells, NK cells, B cells, NK cells, keratinocyes, eosinophils	Inhibits cytokine production by T cells and mononuclear cell inflammatory function; promotes B cell growth and isotype switching, NK cell cytotoxicity	T cells: neonatal and adult naïve < adult memory MNC: neonatal < adult (lectin or LPS) Mϕ: neonatal < adult Whole blood: neonatal = adult	346, 731, 1088, 1408
IL-11	Marrow stromal cells, fibroblasts	Hematopoietic precursor growth, acute-phase reactants by hepatocytes	Fibroblasts: neonatal > adult	1414

continued

Table 4–2 Immunoregulatory Effects of Select Cytokines, Chemokines, and TNF Ligand Family Proteins and Their Production by Human Neonatal Cells—cont'd

Cytokine	Principal Cell Source	Major Biologic Effects	Production by Neonatal versus Adult Cells	Reference(s)
IL-12	Dendritic cells, Mϕ	Enhances T_H1 differentiation, T cell growth, T cell and NK cell cytotoxicity; induces IFN-γ secretion by T cells and NK cells; enhances B cell response to TI antigens	MNCs: neonatal and young children < adult or normal after LPS in different studies; normal in response to *S. aureus* DC: neonatal < adult in response to LPS or pertussis toxin	69, 73, 85-88, 911, 1415, 1416
IL-13	T cells, mast cells, basophils, eosinophils	Very similar to those of IL-4, with possible exception of lacking direct T cell effects and greater effect on goblet cells of lung	T cells: neonatal and adult naïve $CD4^+$ < adult memory $CD4^+$ Neonatal $CD8^+$ > adult $CD8^+$	358, 1417
IL-15	Epithelial cells, bone marrow stromal cells, activated monocytes	Enhances NK cell development, growth, survival, cytotoxicity, and cytokine production; T cell chemoattractant and growth factor	MNC: neonatal < adult after LPS stimulation	891
IL-17	T cells	Enhances T cell proliferation; proinflammatory cytokine release by macrophages	Not known	
IL-18	Macrophages, hepatic Kupffer cells, intestinal and skin epithelia	Promotes T_H1 differentiation; production of IL-2 and GM-CSF by T cells, and IFN-γ by T cells, NK cells, and B cells; T cell– and NK cell–mediated cytotoxicity, DC recruitment	MNCs: neonatal 65% of adult in response to group B streptococci	1093
IL-21	T cells	Enhances proliferation of B cells, naive T cells; NK cell differentiation and cytotoxicity	Not known	
IL-23	Dendritic cells, Mϕ	Similar effects to those of IL-12	Not known	
IL-25	T_H2 cells, mast cells	Promotes T_H2 cytokine secretion by T cells and APCs (?Mϕ)	Not known	
IL-27	Dendritic cells, Mϕ	Promotes responsiveness of T cells to IL-12; inhibits T_H2 differentiation	Not known	
IFN-α	Dendritic cells, Mϕ	Inhibits viral replication; increases MHC class I expression and NK cell cytotoxicity	MNCs: normal to some stimuli but reduced to most stimuli, including HSV, parainfluenza virus, unmethylated CpG DNA and poly (I:C), particularly in premature	69, 82, 83, 84, 1091, 1418
IFN-β	Fibroblasts, epithelial cells, dendritic cells	Same as for IFN-α	MNC: normal	82
IFN-γ	T cells, NK cells, eosinophils (?), IL-18–stimulated B cells	Same as for IFN-α and -β; also activates Mϕ, increases MHC class II and antigen presentation molecules, inhibits IgE production, enhances B cell response to TI antigens, promotes T_H1 differentiation	T cells: neonatal and adult naïve < adult memory; neonatal < adult naïve with allostimulation NK cells: normal after HSV and IL-2 stimulation MNCs: neonatal < adult after IL-12 and IL-15 treatment	86, 326, 343, 356, 891, 924, 1415, 1419

continued

Table 4–2 Immunoregulatory Effects of Select Cytokines, Chemokines, and TNF Ligand Family Proteins and Their Production by Human Neonatal Cells—cont'd

Cytokine	Principal Cell Source	Major Biologic Effects	Production by Neonatal versus Adult Cells	Reference(s)
TNF-α	Mϕ, T cells, and NK cells	Fever and inflammatory response effects similar to IL-1, shock, hemorrhagic necrosis of tumors, and increased VCAM-1 expression on endothelium; induces catabolic state	T cells: neonatal < adult MNCs: neonatal < adult after IL-15 or LPS treatment Mϕ: neonatal < adult after RSV infection; preterm < adult after LPS treatment Whole blood: neonatal = adult	348, 891, 1080, 1408, 1412, 1420
CD40 ligand (CD154)	T cells, lower amounts by B cells and DCs	B cell growth factor; promotes isotype switching, promotes IL-12 production by dendritic cells, activates Mϕ	T cells: neonatal < adult naïve after calcium ionophore and phorbol ester; neonatal ≤ adult or adult naïve after CD3 mAb and allostimulation	356, 362, 364, 376-379
Fas ligand	Activated T cells, NK cells retina, testicular epithelium	Induces apoptosis of cells expressing Fas, including effector B and T cells	T cells: neonatal < adult after CD3 and CD28 mAbs	362
Flt-3 ligand	Bone marrow stromal cells	Potent DC growth factor; promotes growth of myeloid and lymphoid progenitor cells in conjunction with other cytokines	Unknown	
G-CSF	Mϕ, fibroblasts, epithelial cells	Growth of granulocyte precursors	MNCs: neonate normal or slightly < than adults Mϕ: term similar and preterm < adult	344, 962, 1421
GM-CSF	Mϕ, endothelial cells, T cells	Growth of granulocyte-Mϕ precursors and dendritic cells, enhances granulocyte-Mϕ function and B cell antibody production	T cells: neonatal < adult MNC: neonatal < adult Mϕ: normal after LPS stimulation	342, 344, 1421, 1422
CCL3 (MIP-1α)	Mϕ, T cells	Mϕ chemoattractant; T cell activator	MNCs: neonatal < adult	1083
CCL5 (RANTES)	Mϕ, T cells, fibroblasts, epithelial cells	Mϕ and memory T cell chemoattractant; enhances T cell activation; blocks HIV co-receptor	T cells: neonatal < adult	357
TGF-β	Mϕ, T cells, fibroblasts, epithelial cells, others	Inhibits Mϕ activation; inhibits T_H1 T cell responses	MNCs: neonate < adult	1083

APC, antigen-presenting cell; CSF, colony-stimulating factor; DC = dendritic cell; G-CSF, granulocyte colony-stimulating factor; GM-CSF, granulocyte-macrophage colony-stimulating factor; GBS, group B streptocci; HIV, human immunodeficiency virus; HSV, herpes simplex virus; IFN, interferon; IgE, immunoglobulin E; IL, interleukin; LPS, lipopolysaccharide; Mϕ, mononuclear phagocytes; mAb, monoclonal antibody; MHC, major histocompatbility complex; MIP-1α, macrophage inflammatory protein-1α; MNCs, circulating mononuclear cells; NK, natural killer; RSV, respiratory syncytial virus; *S. aureus*, *Staphylococcus aureus*; TGF, transforming growth factor; TI, T cell–independent; TNF, tumor necrosis factor; VCAM-1, vascular cell adhesion molecule-1.

T cells, express CD8-α/CD8-α homodimers. Those αβ T cells expressing CD4 or CD8 are commonly referred to as $CD4^+$ or $CD8^+$ T cells, respectively. Nearly all αβ T cells recognize protein antigens in the form of peptide fragments bound to classic MHC molecules—peptide–MHC class I complexes in the case of $CD8^+$ T cells and peptide–MHC class II molecules in the case of $CD4^+$ T cells. Thus, antigen processing—the generation of peptide fragments from protein antigens—and antigen presentation—the display of peptide-MHC complexes on the surface of cells—play an essential role in enabling T cells to recognize and respond to microbes.

Certain types of cells express MHC class I molecules and also constitutively express MHC class II molecules, which endows them with enhanced capacity to present antigenic peptides to T cells. Such cells commonly are referred to as APCs and include DCs, mononuclear phagocytes, and B lymphocytes. DCs express particularly high amounts of MHC class I and class II molecules, as well as other proteins

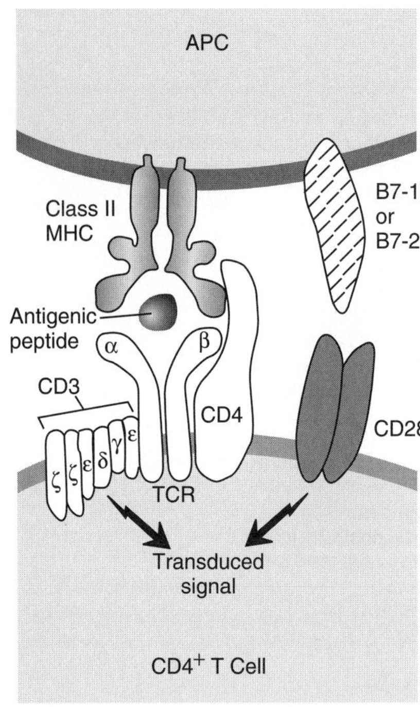

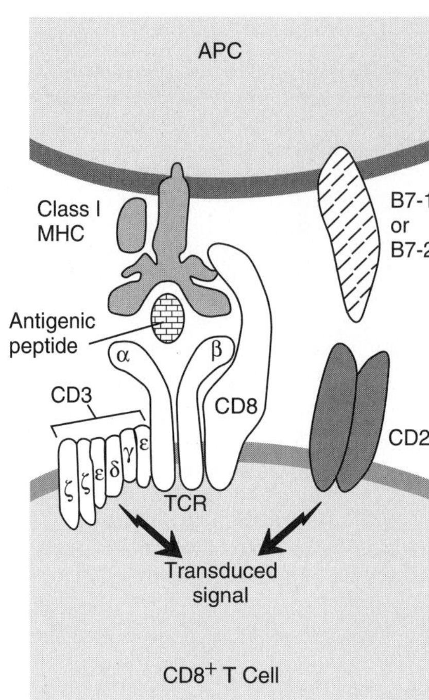

Figure 4–1 T cell recognition of antigen and activation. The αβ T cell receptor (αβ-TCR) recognizes antigen presented by the antigen-presenting cell (APC) in the form of antigenic peptides bound to major histocompatibility complex (MHC) molecules on the APC surface. Most $CD4^+$ T cells recognize peptides bound to MHC class II, whereas most $CD8^+$ T cells recognize peptides bound to MHC class I. This MHC restriction is the result of a thymic selection process, and is due in part to an intrinsic affinity of the CD4 and CD8 molecules for the MHC class II and class I molecules, respectively. Once antigen is recognized, the CD3 protein complex, which is invariably associated with the αβ-TCR, acts as a docking site for tyrosine kinases that transmit activating intracellular signals. Interaction of the T cell CD28 molecule with either CD80 (B7-1) or CD86 (B7-2) provides an important co-stimulatory signal to the T cell, leading to complete activation, rather than partial activation or functional inactivation (anergy).

that allow them to effectively take up and present antigen to naïve $CD4^+$ and $CD8^+$ T cells, allowing them to play a critical role in the initiation of primary antigen-specific T cell responses.[9] Thus, DCs, which are part of the innate immune system, are a critical link between innate immunity and the induction of antigen-specific T cell–mediated immunity.

In contrast with αβ T cells, a majority of γδ T cells appear to recognize either stress-induced, nonclassic MHC molecules themselves or nonpeptide antigens, such as host- or pathogen-derived lipid-containing molecules, bound to these nonclassic MHC molecules.

Basic Aspects of Antigen Presentation

Antigen Presentation by Class I Major Histocompatibility Complex Molecules

Three major types of MHC class I heavy chains exist in humans: the human leukocyte antigens HLA-A, -B, and -C, which are encoded by three genes clustered on chromosome 6, in a region known as the MHC locus. Classic MHC class I molecules consist of a polymorphic α or heavy chain, which is associated with a monomorphic light chain, β_2-microglobulin. MHC molecules have a special cleft or groove for presenting antigenic peptides (Fig. 4-2; see also Fig. 4-1). In MHC class I molecules, this cleft is formed by the α1 and α2 domains of the heavy chain. Peptides bound to MHC class I are preferentially recognized by the $CD8^+$ subset rather than the by $CD4^+$ subset of αβ T cells. This specificity is due, at least in part, to an affinity of the CD8 molecule for the α3 domain of the heavy chain, which is distinct from the portion of the heavy chain involved in binding peptide.

Most peptides bound to MHC class I molecules are derived from proteins synthesized de novo within host cells (see Fig. 4-2). The bulk of these peptides are derived from recently translated proteins rather than as a result of turnover of stable proteins, thereby minimizing any delay in detecting pathogen-derived peptides that may result from recent infection.[10] In uninfected cells, these peptides are derived from host proteins; that is, they are self-peptides. Recently synthesized host proteins that are targeted for degradation, for example, because of misfolding or defective post-translational modification, are a major source of self-peptides that bind to MHC class I. After intracellular infection, such as with a virus, peptides derived from viral proteins endogenously synthesized within the cell bind to and are presented by MHC class I. Antigenic peptides are derived predominantly by enzymatic cleavage of proteins in the cytoplasm by a specialized organelle called the proteasome. A specific peptide transporter or pump, the transporter associated with antigen processing (TAP), then shuttles peptides formed in the cytoplasm to the endoplasmic reticulum, where peptides are able to bind to recently synthesized MHC class I molecules. Peptide binding stabilizes the association of the heavy chain with β_2-microglobulin in this compartment and allows the complex to transit to the cell surface.

Peptides bound to MHC class I molecules in vivo typically are 8 to 10 amino acids in length. The peptide-binding groove is closed at both ends so that larger peptides cannot be accommodated. For a given MHC allele, certain positions (anchor residues) within the peptide can be encoded only by specific amino acids for effective binding to the cleft. Amino acid residues at other, more variable positions point out of the cleft and are recognized by the TCR (epitope residues). The antigen recognition process clearly imposes significant restrictions on the ability of peptides from a particular protein to be immunogenic, because the peptide must both bind to the MHC molecule and be recognized by the TCR.

These constraints on peptide immunogenicity are offset by the availability of the three different types of MHC class I molecules (HLA-A, -B, and -C), each of which is highly polymorphic. The human HLA-A, -B, and -C heavy chain genes

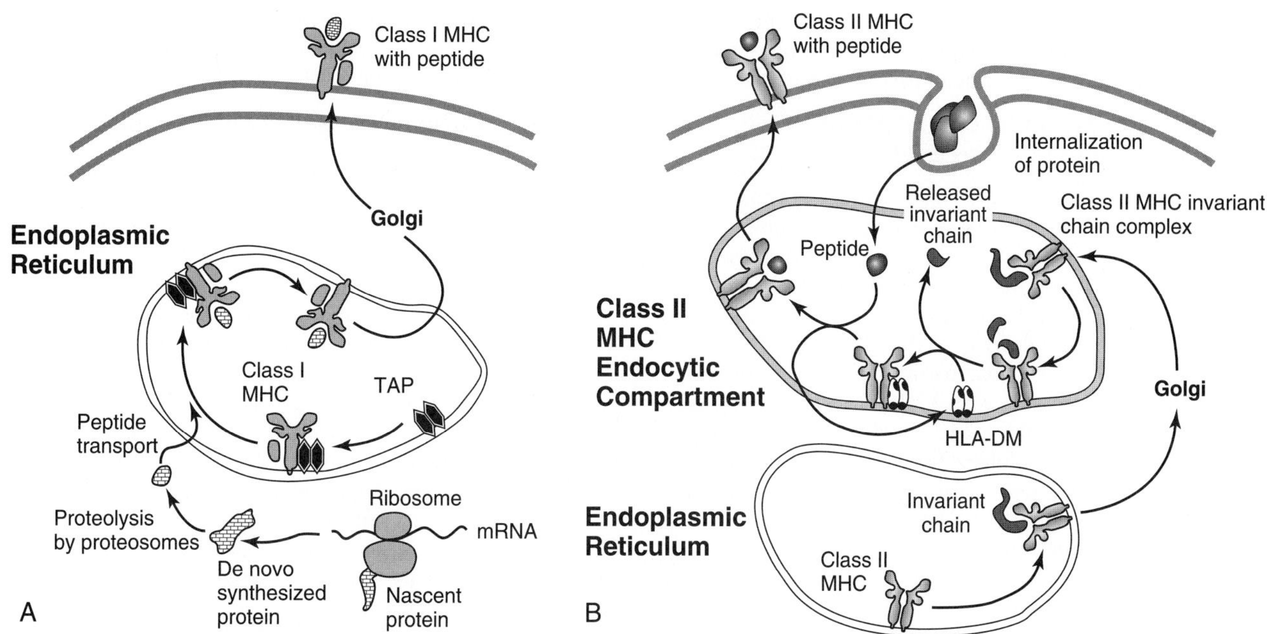

Figure 4–2 Intracellular pathways of antigen presentation. **A,** Foreign peptides that bind to major histocompatibility complex (MHC) class I are derived predominantly from cytoplasmic proteins synthesized de novo within the cell. Viral proteins entering cells following fusion of an enveloped virus with the cell membrane may also enter this pathway. Dendritic cells are particularly efficient at taking up proteins for the MHC class I pathway by micro- or macropinocytosis. These cells also can transfer proteins taken up as part of necrotic or apoptotic debris into the MHC class I pathway, a process known as cross-presentation. Cytoplasmic proteins are degraded by proteasomes into peptides, which then enter into the endoplasmic reticulum via the TAP ("transporter associated with antigen processing") system. Peptide binding by de novo synthesized MHC class I takes place within the endoplasmic reticulum. **B,** Foreign peptides that bind to MHC class II are mainly derived from either internalization proteins found in the extracellular space or that are components of cell membrane. The invariant chain binds to recently synthesized MHC class II and prevents peptide binding until a specialized cellular compartment for MHC class II peptide loading is reached. In this compartment, the invariant chain is proteolytically cleaved and released and peptides derived from internalized proteins may now bind to MHC class II. The human leukocyte antigen (HLA)-DM molecule facilitates the loading of peptide within this compartment. In dendritic cells, proteins that enter into the MHC class II antigen presentation pathway can be transferred to the MHC class I pathway by cross-presentation.

have at least 303, 558, and 150 different molecularly defined alleles, respectively,[11] with the greatest degree of polymorphism found in the region encoding the antigenic cleft.[12] MHC polymorphism ensures that at the individual and population levels, MHC molecules are able to bind and present a wide variety of peptides to T cells. It has been proposed that populations in which the MHC alleles are less polymorphic, such as Native Americans, may be at greater risk for certain infections owing to limitations in the diversity of antigenic peptides that can be presented.[13]

MHC class I molecules and the cell components required for peptide generation, transport, and MHC class I binding are virtually ubiquitous in the cells of vertebrates. The advantage to the host is that cytotoxic $CD8^+$ T cells can then recognize and lyse cells infected with intracellular pathogens in most tissues. Adult neuronal cells are one of the few cell types that constitutively lack MHC class I.[14] Because neurons are predominantly postmitotic cells, lack of MHC class I molecules may help to limit immune-mediated destruction of a cell type with a limited capacity to be replaced. MHC class I molecules are expressed by some populations of fetal neuronal cells, however, and this expression appears to play a role in neuronal development that is distinct from antigen presentation.[15] MHC class I HLA-A, -B, and -C molecules also are absent from the trophoblast of the human placenta, which may serve to limit the recognition of fetal-derived trophoblast cells as foreign by maternal T cells. The abundance of MHC class I molecules is increased by exposure to interferons (IFNs), which also can induce the expression of modest amounts of MHC class I molecules on cell types that normally lack expression, including neuronal cells.

DCs appear to be unique in their ability to present antigenic peptides on MHC class I molecules by an additional pathway, known as cross-presentation, in which extracellular proteins that are taken up as large particles (phagocytosis), as small particles (macropinocytosis), or in soluble form (micropinocytosis) are then transferred from endocytic vesicles to the cytoplasm and subsequently loaded onto MHC class I molecules through TAP.[16] Phagocytosis of apoptotic cells or blebs from apoptotic cells appears to be a particularly efficient source of antigens for cross-presentation.[16] Cross-presentation is enhanced by exposure of DCs to IFN-α and IFN-β, which together constitute type I IFN, and are typically produced at high levels during viral infections.[17] Cross-presentation is essential for the induction of primary $CD8^+$ T cell responses directed toward antigens of pathogens that do not directly infect APCs (e.g., most viruses) and therefore cannot be directly loaded into the MHC class I pathway. Other viruses, such as those of the herpesvirus family, can directly infect APCs but also disrupt conventional MHC class I antigen presentation (discussed in more detail later on). In this situation, the cross-presentation pathway may allow peptides derived from viral proteins taken up by the cell to reach the TAP transporter before the expression of virally encoded gene products that disrupt antigen presentation.[18]

Antigen Presentation by Class II Major Histocompatibility Complex Molecules

In MHC class II molecules, an α and a β chain each contribute to the formation of the groove in which antigenic peptides bind (see Fig. 4-2).[19] MHC class II–peptide complexes are recognized primarily by αβ T cells of the $CD4^+$ but not by the $CD8^+$ subset. This is due, at least in part, to an affinity of the CD4 molecule for a domain of the MHC class II β chain distinct from the region that forms part of the peptide-binding groove. In contrast with MHC class I, peptides that bind to MHC class II proteins are derived mostly from phagocytosis or endocytosis of soluble or membrane-bound proteins (see Fig. 4-2). In the absence of foreign proteins, a majority of peptides bound to MHC class II molecules are self-peptides derived from proteins found either on the cell surface or secreted by the cell. Newly synthesized MHC class II molecules associate in the endoplasmic reticulum with a protein called the invariant chain, which impedes their binding of endogenous peptides in this compartment. The loading of exogenously derived peptides and the removal of invariant chain from MHC class II are facilitated by HLA-DM (see Fig. 4-2), a nonpolymorphic heterodimeric protein that is encoded in the MHC locus.[19] Peptide loading appears to occur in a late endocytic compartment or compartments, which have been called CIIV or MIIC (class II vesicles or MHC class II compartment),[20] effectively separating peptides binding to MHC class I and to MHC class II into two separate pools. Unlike the MHC class I cleft, the MHC class II cleft is open at both ends, allowing the binding of larger peptides. Most MHC class II peptides are from 14 to 18 amino acids in length, although they can be substantially longer.

As with MHC class I molecules, the genes that encode the α and β chains of the three major types of human MHC class II molecules—HLA-DR, -DP, and -DQ—are located on chromosome 6 and are highly polymorphic, particularly in the region encoding the peptide-binding cleft.[21] In humans and primates, HLA-DR allelic diversity is mediated solely by the HLA-DR β chain, because the HLA-DR α chain is monomorphic. HLA-DRβ protein is encoded mainly at the *DRB1* locus, for which there are 362 known molecular alleles.[11] Some HLA-DRβ proteins may be encoded by less polymorphic loci, such *DRB3*, that are closely linked to *DRB1*. The HLA-DPα, -DPβ, -DQα, and -DQβ gene loci are highly polymorphic, consisting of 20, 107, 25, and 56 known molecular alleles, respectively.[11] HLA-DR is expressed at substantially higher levels than HLA-DP or HLA-DQ, which probably accounts for its predominance as the restricting MHC class II type for many $CD4^+$ T cell immune responses.

The distribution of MHC class II in uninflamed tissues is much more restricted than MHC class I,[22] with constitutive MHC class II mainly limited to APCs, such as DCs, mononuclear phagocytes, and B cells. Limiting MHC class II expression in most situations to these cell types makes teleologic sense, because the major function of these professional APCs is to process foreign antigen for recognition by $CD4^+$ T cells. Other cell types can be induced to express MHC class II and, in some cases, present antigen to $CD4^+$ T cells, as a consequence of tissue inflammation or exposure to cytokines, particularly IFN-γ but also tumor necrosis factor-α (TNF-α) or granulocyte-macrophage colony-stimulating factor (GM-CSF) (see Tables 4-1 and 4-2).

Nonclassic Antigen-Presentation Molecules

HLA-E. HLA-E is a nonclassic and nonpolymorphic MHC molecule similar to conventional MHC class I in its dependency on the TAP transporter for peptide loading and in its obligate association with β_2-microglobulin.[23] In contrast with conventional MHC class I, HLA-E preferentially binds hydrophobic peptides derived from the amino-terminal leader sequences of most alleles of HLA-A, -B, and -C.[24] Low levels of HLA-E surface expression can be detected on most cell types,[25] consistent with the nearly ubiquitous distribution of HLA-A, -B, and -C and the TAP system. The principal role for HLA-E is to interact with the CD94-containing receptors on natural killer (NK) lymphocytes and to regulate their function (see later section on NK cell inhibitory receptors). HLA-E messenger RNA (mRNA) is detectable in human fetal liver early during the second trimester.[26]

HLA-G. HLA-G, which is expressed at high levels by human cytotrophoblasts and macrophages within the maternal uterine wall, has limited polymorphism but otherwise is quite similar to MHC class I in its association with β_2-microglobulin and structure. HLA-G occurs as either an integral membrane protein or a secreted isoform.[27] Cytolytic activity by NK cells normally is limited by engagement of inhibitory receptors, many of which recognize MHC class I. Because trophoblast cells lack expression of most conventional MHC class I molecules, the surface expression of HLA-G, which is particularly high during the first trimester of pregnancy, may limit their lysis by maternal or fetal NK cells.

HLA-G engages CD94-NKG2A, the same inhibitory receptor utilized by HLA-E for inhibiting NK cell–mediated cytotoxicity.[28] In addition, membrane-bound HLA-G engages inhibitory receptors expressed on T cells, including p49, immunoglobulin-like transcript (ILT)-2, and ILT-4; this may account for the ability of HLA-G to inhibit the proliferation of adult T cells in response to allogeneic stimuli.[29] Because HLA-G also is expressed by cells found outside the placenta (e.g., circulating adult monocytes after treatment with IFN-γ),[30] it also may regulate the later phases of the T cell immune response.

Soluble HLA-G is present at relatively high levels in the serum of pregnant women and in lower amounts in cord blood and in the peripheral blood of nonparous women and men.[27] The in vivo function of soluble HLA-G remains unclear, but it may inhibit immune responses. Consistent with this proposed function, soluble HLA-G can induce Fas (CD95)-dependent apoptosis of activated $CD8^+$ T cells, apparently by engaging CD8 and increasing surface expression of Fas ligand (CD95L).[31]

MICA and MICB. MHC class I–related chains A and B (MICA and MICB), the genes for which also are found at the MHC locus, have limited but clear homology with conventional MHC class I molecules.[32,33] In contrast with conventional MHC class I, however, they lack a binding site for CD8, are not associated with β_2-microglobulin, and do not appear to be involved with the presentation of peptide antigens. Instead, these molecules are expressed on stressed intestinal epithelial cells, such as those experiencing heat shock, and are recognized by γδ T cells that bear Vδ1-containing γδ-TCR. MICA and MICB also may be induced on other cell types in response to infection with viruses, such as those of the herpesvirus group. MICA and MICB are ligands for NKG2D found on most NK cells, and on some $CD8^+$ T cells and γδ T cells, which can either activate or act in concert with TCR-mediated signals to activate these cells.[34,35]

CD1. The human CD1 locus includes four nonpolymorphic genes, CD1a through CD1d.[36,37] CD1 molecules associate with β_2-microglobulin but have limited structural homology with either MHC class I or MHC class II proteins. In humans, they are expressed mainly on APCs, including DCs.[9] CD1b efficiently binds and presents highly hydrophobic lipoglycan molecules of mycobacteria, such as lipoarabinomannans, mycolic acid, and glucose monomycolate, and some self-lipids, such as G_{M1} ganglioside.[36,37]

Mycobacterial lipoglycans undergo processing and loading onto CD1b in an endosomal compartment that is similar or identical to the compartment where peptides are loaded onto MHC class II molecules. Subsets of $CD8^+$ T cells and of the rare $CD4^-CD8^-$ αβ T cells respond to microbial lipids on CD1b and CD1c molecules, and a subset of γδ T cells recognizes as-yet uncharacterized antigens on CD1c molecules.[36]

CD1d, the only member of the human CD1 cluster that also is expressed in the mouse, appears to be specialized for the presentation of hydrophobic nonpeptide molecules, such as endogenous lipids or glycolipid molecules. As in the case of CD1b, loading of antigens onto CD1d is apparently accomplished in a "late" endosomal compartment similar or identical to the compartment where peptides are loaded onto MHC class II molecules. A unique subset of αβ T cells, which are autoreactive to CD1d in vitro, are commonly referred to as NK T cells (see later on); NK T cells are mainly $CD4^-$ and $CD8^-$ and express a canonical TCR α chain (Vα24JαQ).

Dendritic Cells

DCs, the sentinels of the immune system, are bone marrow–derived cells that in their mature form display characteristic cytoplasmic protrusions or dendrites. DCs in the circulation and tissues are heterogeneous with regard to their surface phenotype and functional attributes, and the precursor-product relationship of these subsets with each other and with other cell types remains controversial.[9] A common feature of DCs is the absence of most or all cell surface molecules that characterize other bone marrow–derived cell lineages (that is, they lack lineage markers), including molecules typically expressed on T cells (with the exception of a low level of expression of CD4), B cells, NK cells, and granulocytes. By contrast, DCs do express MHC class II, and mature DCs express much greater amounts of MHC class II (and MHC class I) than any other cell type. Thus, DCs are lineage marker–negative (Lin^-), MHC class II–positive, mononuclear cells of hematopoietic origin.

As described later on, DCs are poised to respond rapidly to microbial invasion by secretion of cytokines and presentation of microbial antigens to T cells, which leads to T cell activation and functional differentiation. It also is clear that DCs modulate the function of B cells and NK cells and, in steady-state conditions that prevail in uninfected persons, play a central role in maintaining a state of tolerance to self-antigens by presenting them to T cells in the absence of accessory signals required for T cell activation; these functions are not discussed further.[38]

DC1 (Myeloid Subset of) Dendritic Cells. In this chapter, $CD11c^+$ DCs are collectively referred to as DC1 cells or myeloid DCs.[39] DCs in the skin include Langerhans cells, which express CD1a and Birbeck granules but lack expression of the factor XIIIa coagulation factor, and interstitial cells of the dermis, which conversely lack Birbeck granules and are factor XIIIa positive. Both express CD11c and ILT-1.[9,40] Interstitial DC1 cells are found in essentially all tissues and are highly effective in uptake of antigen in soluble or particulate form.[41]

DC1 cells in uninflamed tissues are said to be immature because they express only moderate levels of MHC class I and class II molecules on their surface. Immature DC1 cells also are found in the blood—probably in transit to the tissues—but in small numbers (0.2% to 0.4% of peripheral blood mononuclear cells [PBMCs]) relative to monocytes (approximately 10% of PBMCs), a cell type from which DC1 cells can be derived.[42] After exposure of immature DC1 cells to inflammatory stimuli, further antigen uptake ceases, and maturation ensues in which antigenic peptides derived from previously internalized particles are displayed on their cell surface in the groove of MHC class I and class II molecules, which are now expressed in great abundance on the cell surface.

Exposure of immature DCs to inflammatory stimuli results in their migration from the tissues to the T cell–dependent areas of secondary lymphoid organs, such as the lymph nodes and spleen. The migration of leukocytes, including DCs, is mediated by a combinatorial and multistep process determined by the pattern of expression on the cell surface of adhesion molecules and chemokine receptors and by the local patterns and gradients of adhesion molecule and chemokine receptor ligands in tissues (see Tables 4-1 and 4-2). Chemokines constitute a cytokine superfamily with more than 50 members known at present, most of which are secreted and of relatively low molecular weight.[43,44] Chemokines are produced by a large number of cell types and selectively attract various leukocyte populations, which bear the appropriate G protein–linked chemokine receptors. They can be divided into four families according to their pattern of amino-terminal cysteine residues: CC, CXC, C, and CX3C (X represents a noncysteine amino acid between the cysteines). A nomenclature for the chemokines and their receptors has been adopted, in which the family is first given (e.g., CC), followed by L for ligand (the chemokines itself) and a number or followed by R (for receptor) and a number. Functionally, chemokines also can be defined by their principal function—in homeostatic or inflammatory cell migration—and by the subsets of cells on which they act.[45] Maturing DCs increase surface expression of the CCR7 chemokine receptor and decrease expression of most other chemokine receptors. This results in the migration of these cells through lymphatics to T cell–rich areas of secondary lymphoid organs that express the CCR7 ligands CCL19 and CCL21.[46]

DC1 cell maturation and migration can be triggered by a variety of stimuli, including pathogen-derived products that are recognized through Toll-like receptors (TLRs) (Table 4-3),[47]

Table 4–3 Human Toll-like Receptors (TLRs)

Toll-like Receptor	Ligand	Site of Interaction with Ligand	Signal Transduction/Effector Molecules
TLR-1	Heterodimerizes with TLR-2	Cell surface	MyD88-dependent induction of cytokines
TLR-2	Peptidoglycan and lipoteichoic acid of gram-positive bacteria, mycoplasmal and meningococcal lipopeptides, mycobacterial lipoarabinomannan, *Neisseria* porins, and others; recognition of some ligands is dependent on heterodimerization with TLR-1 or TLR-6	Cell surface	MyD88-dependent induction of cytokines
TLR-3	Double-stranded RNA (viruses)	Endosome	TRIF-dependent induction of type I IFN and cytokines
TLR-4	LPS, RSV (?fibronectin)	Cell surface	MyD88- and TRIF-dependent induction of cytokines; TRIF-dependent induction of type I IFN
TLR-5	Flagellin	Cell surface	MyD88-induced cytokines
TLR-6	Heterodimerizes with TLR-2	Cell surface	MyD88-dependent induction of cytokines
TLR-7	Imidazoquinoline drugs, single-stranded RNA molecules (viruses)	Endosome	MyD88-dependent induction of type I IFN and cytokines
TLR-8	Imidazoquinoline drugs, single-stranded RNA molecules (viruses)	Endosome	MyD88-dependent induction of type I IFN and cytokines
TLR-9	Unmethylated CpG DNA (bacteria and viruses)	Endosome	MyD88-dependent induction of cytokines and type I IFN
TLR-10	Unknown	Unknown	Unknown

IFN, interferon; LPS, lipopolysaccharide; RSV, respiratory syncytial virus.

by endogenous cytokines, such as interleukin (IL)-1, TNF-α, and GM-CSF (see Tables 4-1 and 4-2), and by engagement of CD40 on the DC surface by CD40 ligand (CD154), a molecule that is expressed at particularly high levels by activated $CD4^+$ T cells (Table 4-4). Thus, the function and localization of DC1 cells are highly plastic and rapidly modulated either by direct recognition of microbes or their products, by cytokines produced by neighboring DCs and other cells of the innate system, or by products of T cells to which they present antigens.

The TLR family of transmembrane proteins recognizes microbial structures that, for the most part, are essential for the proper function of microbes that express them. These microbial structures are relatively invariant and are not present in normal mammalian cells (see Table 4-3). For this reason, recognition of these "pathogen-associated molecular patterns" by TLRs provides infallible evidence for microbial invasion alerting the innate immune system to respond appropriately.[48] To date, 10 different TLRs have been identified in humans,[47] with distinct recognition specificities and patterns of expression, and both shared and unique downstream response pathways (see Table 4-3). For example, TLR-2, along with TLR-1 and TLR-6, recognizes bacterial lipopeptides, peptidoglycan and lipoteichoic acid on the surface of gram-positive bacteria, fungal surface structures, and cytomegalovirus (CMV); TLR-3 recognizes viral double-stranded RNA, a component of the life cycle of many viruses, and a synthetic mimic of double-stranded RNA, poly(I:C); TLR-4 recognizes lipopolysaccharide (LPS) from gram-negative bacteria and a protein encoded by respiratory syncytial virus (RSV); TLR-5 recognizes bacterial flagellin; TLR-7 and TLR-8 recognize single-stranded RNA, a characteristic of RNA viruses, such as influenza virus[49,50]; TLR-9 recognizes DNA from bacteria, which contain unmethylated CpG dinucleotide residues (CpG DNA)[47] and from DNA viruses, such as herpes simplex virus (HSV), in which these CpG residues also are unmethylated.[51,52] Because TLR-9 does not recognize DNA containing methylated CpG residues, which predominate in human DNA, this receptor serves as a means to distinguish host from pathogen-related DNA. Signals from each of these TLRs induce maturation and migration of DCs, but the patterns of cytokine production induced vary both with the TLR that is being activated and with the cell type on which the TLR is expressed (see Table 4-3).[39,53] Notably, DC1 cells express TLRs that recognize bacterial, fungal, and protozoal cell surface structures but do not express TLR-9. Consequently, DC1 cells are not activated in response to unmethylated CpG DNA, a potent inducer of IFN-α production by another DC population, pre-DC2 cells. DC1 cells express TLR-3, however, and signal through TLR-3 to induce type I IFN.

Mature DC1 cells express high levels of peptide-MHC complexes and molecules that act as co-stimulatory signals for T cell activation, such as CD80 (B7-1) and CD86 (B7-2), and consequently are highly efficient for presenting antigen in a manner that leads to the activation of naïve $CD4^+$ and $CD8^+$ T cells (see Fig. 4-1 and Table 4-4).[9] DCs not only play a critical role in T cell activation but also influence the quality of the T cell response that ensues by directing the differentiation of naïve $CD4^+$ T cells into T helper I (T_HI) (capable of producing IFN-γ but not IL-4, IL-5, or IL-13) or T_H2 (capable of producing IL-4, IL-5, or IL-13 but not IFN-γ) effector T cells (see later sections on differentiation and homeostasis of activated T cells). For example, the production by DCs of IL-12, a heterodimeric cytokine consisting of a p35 and a p40 chain, or of type I IFN skews differentiation toward the T_H1 pathway.[54-56]

Table 4–4 Selected Pairs of Surface Molecules Involved in T Cell–Antigen-Presenting Cell (APC) Interactions

T Cell Surface Molecule	T Cell Distribution	Corresponding Ligand(s) on APCs	APC Distribution
CD2	Most T cells; higher on memory cells, lower on adult naïve and neonatal T cells	LFA-3 (CD58), CD59	Leukocytes
CD4	Subset of $\alpha\beta$ T cells with predominantly helper activity	MHC class II β chain	Dendritic cells, Mϕ, B cells, others (see text)
CD5	All T cells	CD72	B cells, Mϕ
CD8	Subset of $\alpha\beta$ T cells with predominantly cytotoxic activity	MHC glass I heavy chain	Ubiquitous
LFA-1 (CD11a/CD18)	All T cells; higher on memory cells, lower on adult naïve and neonatal T cells	ICAM-1 (CD54) ICAM-2 (CD102) ICAM-3 (CD50)	Leukocytes (ICAM-3 > ICAM-1,-2) and endothelium (ICAM-1, ICAM-2); most ICAM-1 expression requires activation
CD28	Most $CD4^+$ T cells, subset of $CD8^+$ T cells	CD80 (B7-1) CD86 (B7-2)	Dendritic cells, Mϕ, activated B cells
ICOS	Effector and memory T cells; not on resting naive cells	B7RP-1 (B7h)	B cells, Mϕ, dendritic cells, endothelial cells
VLA-4 (CD49d/CD29)	All T cells; higher on memory cells, lower on adult naïve and neonatal T cells	VCAM-1 (CD106)	Activated or inflamed endothelium (increased by TNF, IL-1, IL-4)
ICAM-1 (CD54)	All T cells; higher on memory cells, lower on adult virgin and neonatal T cells	LFA-1 (CD11a/CD18)	Leukocytes
TLA-4 (CD152)	Activated T cells	CD80 CD86	Dendritic cells, Mϕ, activated B cells, activated T cells
CD40 ligand (CD154)	Activated $CD4^+$ T cells; lower on neonatal $CD4^+$ T cells	CD40	Dendritic cells, Mϕ, B cells, thymic epithelial cells
PD-1	Activated $CD4^+$ and $CD8^+$ T cells	PD-L1, PD-L2	Dendritic cells, Mϕ, B cells, regulatory T cells

CTLA-4, cytotoxic T lymphocyte antigen-4; ICAM, intercellular adhesion molecule; ICOS, inducibe co-stimulator; IL, interleukin; LFA, leukocyte function antigen; Mϕ, mononuclear phagocytes; MHC, major histocompatibility complex; PD, programmed death [molecule]; VCAM, vascular all adhesion molecule; VLA-4, very late antigen-4.

DC2 (Plasmacytoid) Subset of Dendritic Cells. DC2 cells and their immediate precursors, pre-DC2 cells, appear to constitute a cell lineage distinct from DC1-lineage cells. Human DC2-lineage cells have a characteristic surface phenotype with high expression of the IL-3 receptor (CD123), low expression of CD4, and lack of CD11c and ILT-1.[40] Pre-DC2 cells, also referred to as plasmacytoid DCs, are found in the blood and secondary lymphoid organs, particularly in inflamed lymph nodes.[40,53] The difference in their pattern of localization from that of immature DC1 cells is due to differences in expression of chemokine receptors.[40] In contrast with immature DC1 cells, pre-DC2 cells have a limited capacity for antigen uptake and presentation.[40] Pre-DC2 and DC2 cells also differ from DC1-lineage cells by a capacity to produce large amounts of IFN-α and IL-12 in response to unmethylated CpG DNA, such as is contained in the HSV genome, and to RNA viruses, such as influenza virus,[40,57-59] and by their lack of response to LPS or peptidoglycan. The difference in responsiveness of immature DC1 and DC2 cells to different microbes and microbial structures parallels differences in TLR expression—pre-DC2 and immature DC2 cells express TLR-7 and TLR-9, whereas immature DC1 cells express TLR-1, -2, -3, -4, -5, and -6 (see Table 4-3). Studies indicate that pre-DC2 cells use TLR-9 to recognize HSV through its unmethylated genomic CpG DNA.[51,52] Single-stranded RNA contained in RNA viruses, such as influenza virus, activates pre-DC2 cells through TLR-7 or TLR-8, or both.[50] Activated pre-DC2 cells secrete high levels of type I IFN, which probably plays an important role in early innate antiviral immunity by inducing a systemic antiviral state.

As with immature DC1 cells, activation of pre-DC2 cells by TLR, cytokines, or CD40 ligand also results in their maturation, including acquisition of the cytoplasmic protrusions characteristic of DCs, upregulation of CCR7 and migration to T cell–rich areas of lymph nodes, and an increased capacity to present antigen to naïve T cells. Although pre-DC2 cells cultured in IL-3 alone (to maintain viability in vitro) induce naïve neonatal T cells to produce a mixture of IFN-γ and IL-10, the addition of CD40 ligand or influenza virus leads to the differentiation of naïve neonatal T cells into T_H1 cells that produce IFN-γ but not IL-10 or IL-4.[40] The strong T_H1 polarization requires the production by DC2 cells of IFN-α in response to influenza virus, and IFN-α and IL-12 in response to CD40 ligand[40]; the response to CD40 ligand may involve additional mediators because, in the absence of T cells, CD40 ligand induces little or no IL-12 and IFN-α production by pre-DC2 cells.[60] Nonetheless, pre-DC2 cells activated through TLR-7 and TLR-9 probably act locally in the lymphoid tissues to favor the development of T_H1 cells and to enhance local adaptive immune responses,[61] in addition to their role in innate antiviral defense.

Antigen Presentation in the Fetus and Neonate

As discussed later, antigen-specific T cell responses in the fetus, neonate, and young infant are reduced or delayed compared with responses in the adult. These reduced or delayed responses may reflect differences intrinsic to neonatal T cells, limitations of neonatal APC function, or both. Because DCs appear to play an essential role in antigen presentation to naïve T cells as part of primary immune responses, and because virtually all T cells in the fetus and neonate are naïve (as discussed more fully in the section on T cell development and function in the fetus and neonate), differences in the numbers and functions of neonatal DCs would be expected to have important effects on T cell responses in the fetus and neonate. Accordingly, the following discussion first considers general aspects of MHC expression in the fetus and neonate and then focuses on DCs, followed by antigen presentation by other cell types.

Major Histocompatibility Complex Molecule Expression in the Fetus and Neonate

The expression of MHC class I and class II molecules by fetal tissues is evident by 12 weeks of gestation,[62,63] and all of the major APCs, including mononuclear phagocytes, B cells, and DCs,[64] are present by this time. Fetal tissues are vigorously rejected after transplantation into non–MHC-matched hosts, indicating that surface MHC expression is sufficient to initiate an allogeneic response, probably by host cytotoxic $CD8^+$ T cells. This vigorous allogeneic response does not exclude subtle deficiencies in antigen presentation in the fetus and neonate, particularly under conditions that more stringently test APC function (e.g., during infection with herpesviruses that inhibit peptide loading of MHC class I).[65] MHC class I expression on neonatal lymphocytes is lower than on adult cells.[66] The amount of MHC class II expressed per cell by neonatal monocytes or B cells is similar to or greater than that expressed by adult cells,[66] but a greater fraction of neonatal monocytes lack HLA-DR surface expression.[67]

Circulating Neonatal Dendritic Cells

Although most DCs are found in the tissues, small numbers, consisting of immature DC1 and pre-DC2 cells and representing approximately 0.5% of circulating blood mononuclear cells, are found in the blood. Information regarding blood DCs in the human neonate comes from phenotypic analyses and very limited functional studies, inferences regarding their function based on studies using mixed blood mononuclear cells or whole blood assays, and phenotypic and functional studies on DCs derived by culturing blood monocytes in vitro. In the neonatal circulation, DCs with a pre-DC2 surface phenotype ($Lin^-HLA\text{-}DR^{mid}CD11c^-CD33^-CD123^{hi}$) predominate in cord blood and early infancy, constituting about 75% of the total $Lin^-HLA\text{-}DR^+$ DCs,[68] and approximately 0.75% of total blood mononuclear cells.[69] The relative increase in pre-DC2 cells in neonates and infants[70] may reflect an increased proportion of less differentiated $CD11c^-CD123^{mid}$ cells in cord blood.[71] The remaining 25% of DCs have an $HLA\text{-}DR^{hi}CD11c^+CD33^+CD123^{lo}$ surface phenotype that is similar to the phenotype of circulating adult DC1 cells, except that CD83 expression is absent.[68] After the neonatal period, the numbers of DC2-lineage cells appear to decline with increasing postnatal age, whereas the numbers of DC1 cells do not. The biologic significance of the predominance of DC2-lineage cells in the neonatal circulation is uncertain, but this predominance may reflect a high rate of the colonization of lymphoid tissue, which is undergoing rapid expansion at this age.

Expression of MHC class II (HLA-DR) and co-stimulatory molecules on neonatal and on adult blood DC1 and pre-DC2 cells is similar.[69,72] Stimulation with LPS (a TLR-4 ligand) and poly(I:C) (a TLR-3 ligand) was shown to increase the expression of HLA-DR and CD86 on DC1 cells to a similar extent, but CD40 and CD80 increased less in neonatal than in adult DC1 cells.[72] Stimulation with unmethylated CpG DNA (a TLR-9 ligand) increased the expression of HLA-DR on pre-DC2 cells to a similar extent, but CD40, CD80, and CD86 increased less in neonatal than in adult pre-DC2 cells. Also, stimulation with pertussis toxin enhanced HLA-DR, CD80, and CD86 expression on adult DC1 cells (pre-DC2 cells do not respond to pertussis toxin) but not on neonatal DCs.[73] It should be noted that each of the studies from which the findings described in this paragraph were derived originated from one group of investigators, and the results have not yet been confirmed by others.

The first studies to directly test the ability of cord blood DCs to activate T cells was done before the availability of markers that allow them to be isolated relatively rapidly and in high purity. In these studies, cells cultured overnight in vitro were substantially less effective than adult cells in activating allogeneic T cell proliferation.[74,75] This decreased activity was associated with reduced levels of expression of HLA-DR and the adhesion molecule ICAM-1[74] (see Table 4-4). In the more recent studies cited in the previous paragraph, however, in which expression of HLA-DR was evaluated on uncultured DCs, HLA-DR expression on neonatal and on adult DC1 and pre-DC2 cells did not differ significantly. The lower level of HLA-DR expression by neonatal DCs in the earlier studies by Hunt and colleagues probably reflects the overnight culture or the predominance of pre-DC2 cells in neonatal blood, which express lower levels of HLA-DR than do DC1 cells.[40,68] DC2-lineage cells are highly prone to die during culture in vitro, and the use of an overnight protocol for cell isolation may adversely affect cord blood DCs, in which pre-DC2 cells are predominant.

Although more recent studies found that circulating DCs from cord blood can allogeneically stimulate cord blood T cells in vitro,[68,76,77] their efficiency was not compared with that of adult DCs. Virtually all of the allostimulatory activity of cord blood DCs is mediated by the DC1 subset rather than by the pre-DC2 subset,[68] raising the possibility that neonatal DC1 cells are functionally normal on a cell-by-cell basis. It should be noted that activation of allogeneic T cells does not require uptake, processing, and presentation of exogenous antigens and is not as stringent a test of APC function as is activation of foreign antigen–specific T cells. A direct comparison of DC1 lineage cells from the neonate and the adult is necessary to define the adequacy of neonatal myeloid DC antigen presentation. Like pre-DC2 cells from the tonsils of older children,[78,79] cord blood pre-DC2 cells are ineffective at uptake of either protein or peptide antigens.[77] It is unclear whether maturation of pre-DC2 cells in the neonate (e.g., by exposure to viruses) results in a similar increase in capacity for antigen presentation that is observed with adult pre-DC2 cells.

DCs also can influence whether naïve $CD4^+$ T cells differentiate into producers of mainly T_H2 cytokines, mainly T_H1 cytokines, or a mixture of both (also referred to as a T_H0

cytokine profile), with the outcome dependent on the type of DCs and the conditions used for activation.[39,53,80,81] For example, antigen presentation by pre-DC2 cells favors the differentiation of naïve T cells into T_H2 cells, unless these cells have been activated by viruses or unmethylated CpG DNA, which causes them to release IFN-α or IL-12 and, in turn, drives potent T_H1 polarization.[81] The predominance of pre-DC2 cells in the fetus and neonate may account for the tendency toward T_H2 skewing of immune responses to environmental allergens and the limited response to intracellular pathogens in these age groups, the maintenance of fetal-maternal tolerance during pregnancy, and the lower risk of graft-versus-host disease following cord blood transplantation.

In addition to the predominance of pre-DC2 cells in the neonatal circulation, the ability of neonatal DCs to produce type I IFN and IL-12 also appears to be somewhat diminished compared with that of DCs from adults. With specific exceptions noted later on, the relevant studies have been done with total blood mononuclear cells or whole blood, rather than purified DCs. Because DCs are the dominant source of IFN-α and IL-12 produced in response to the stimuli employed, it is likely that the findings reflect production by DCs. In an early study, type I IFN production by neonatal blood mononuclear cells was equivalent to that of adult cells for a variety of inducers, including HSV and other viruses.[82] Other studies, however, have found that type I IFN production and the frequency of IFN-α–producing cells in response to HSV were diminished compared with those in adults, particularly for prematurely born infants.[83] Similar results were obtained for blood cells stimulated with parainfluenza viruses[84] and unmethylated DNA.[69] It is likely that the decreased production of type I IFN by neonatal blood cells in response to viruses or unmethylated CpG DNA reflects decreased production by DC2-lineage cells signaling through TLR-9, but this decrease has been shown directly only for the response to unmethylated CpG DNA.[69] Neonatal blood cells also produce less IFN-α in response to poly(I:C), which activates DC1 cells through TLR-3.[72] Overall, these more recent studies suggest that neonatal DC1- and DC2-type cells produce approximately 0% to 30% as much type I IFN as that produced by adult cells. The production of bioactive IL-12, a heterodimer of p35 and p40, also appears to be reduced in response to LPS but not to all stimuli. For example, neonatal and adult blood mononuclear cells stimulated with *Staphylococcus aureus*, or other gram-positive and gram-negative bacterial cells produce equivalent amounts of IL-12.[85-88]

Neonatal Monocyte-Derived Dendritic Cells

Mature DCs can differentiate in vitro from a variety of precursor cells, including blood monocytes, pre-DC2 cells, $CD34^+$ myelomonocytic cells, and even granulocytes, depending on the cytokines and culture conditions employed. Although both adult peripheral and cord blood monocytes cultured with GM-CSF and IL-4 give rise to immature DCs similar to the DC1 lineage,[89-91] monocyte-derived DCs from cord blood express less HLA-DR, CD1a, and co-stimulatory molecules (CD40 and CD80) than are expressed by adult cells. Consistent with these reductions in HLA-DR and co-stimulatory molecule expression, monocyte-derived DCs from cord blood have decreased allostimulatory activity for T cells compared with that of adult monocyte-derived DCs.[90-93]

Cord blood monocyte-derived DCs also have a low capacity to produce IL-12 in response to LPS, engagement of CD40, or treatment with double-stranded RNA [poly(I:C)]; this is apparently due to a selective decrease in mRNA expression of the IL-12 (p35) chain component.[93] Reduced IL-12 expression may account for decreased production of IFN-γ by adult $CD4^+$ T cells after allogeneic stimulation by cord blood–derived DCs compared with production after stimulation by adult monocyte–derived DCs.

These findings using monocyte-derived DCs provide an explanation for limitations in T_H1 immunity, such as delayed-type hypersensitivity skin reactions and antigen-specific $CD4^+$ T cell IFN-γ production, which are discussed later on. The relevance of these findings obtained with monocyte-derived DCs is supported by observations in mice suggesting that myeloid DCs can directly differentiate from monocytes when these undergo transendothelial trafficking.[94,95] It remains unclear, however, if the differentiation of monocytes into DCs following high doses of exogenous cytokines faithfully mimics DC differentiation from less mature precursors in vivo. A rigorous comparison of the gene and protein expression profiles and function of monocyte-derived DCs with freshly isolated highly purified DC populations may help clarify this issue.

Fetal Tissue Dendritic Cells

Our knowledge of tissue DCs in the human fetus and neonate is limited. Epidermal Langerhans cells and dermal DCs are found in fetal skin by 16 weeks of gestation,[96] and immature DC1-lineage cells are found in the interstitium of solid organs by this age. Cells with the features of pre-DC2 cells are found in fetal lymph nodes between 19 and 21 weeks of gestation[78]; they have an immature phenotype and are not recent emigrants from inflamed tissues.

Antigen Presentation by Neonatal Monocytes and B Cells

APC function of monocytes and B cells from human neonates has not been characterized in great detail. MHC class II–mediated antigen presentation by monocytes appears to be intact, since neonatal and adult monocytes are similarly effective in presenting soluble protein antigens or alloantigens to induce T cell proliferation,[97,98] a response that is mainly MHC class II dependent. One report suggested that a substantial fraction of MHC class II molecules on neonatal but not adult B cells are "empty"—that is, they lack peptides in the binding groove.[99] Accordingly, neonatal B cells may be functionally limited as APCs.

Basic Aspects of T Cell Development and Function

Prothymocytes and Major Thymocyte Subsets

With the exception of a subset of the T cells found in the gut and perhaps the liver,[100-102] most αβ T cells develop from immature progenitor cells within the unique microenvironment of the thymus. The thymus arises from the ventral portions of the third and fourth pharyngeal pouches. Both ectoderm and mesoderm contribute to the formation of this tissue. The human thymus does not have a population of self-replenishing stem cells and therefore probably requires a continual input of thymocyte progenitor cells (prothymocytes) to maintain thymocytopoiesis, as is true for the mouse.[103] The human prothymocyte probably is a lymphoid cell that lacks TCR α or TCR β chains and expresses CD3 molecules in its cytoplasm and the CD7 protein on its surface, with little or no expression of CD4 or CD8. CD7 also is found on mature T cells and NK cells, suggesting a close relationship between these two cell types.[104]

The precursor-product relationship between the prothymocyte and other immature lymphocyte progenitor cells remains controversial, as does the extent to which the prothymocyte is committed to the T cell or NK cell lineages before thymic entry.[105] Prothymocytes may be derived from the common lymphocyte progenitor (CLP) cell, which is capable of giving rise to the T, B, and NK cell lineage when exposed to appropriate environmental cues. Cells with the properties suggestive of CLPs, based on in vitro differentiation assays, are found in cord blood and have a $CD34^+CD38^-CD7^+$ surface phenotype.[106,107] Nonetheless, a study in the mouse has found striking differences between bone marrow CLPs and the most immature lymphocyte populations found in the thymus, suggesting that prothymocytes could have a CLP-independent source.[108]

The prothymocyte probably enters the thymus through postcapillary venules located near the corticomedullary junction (Fig. 4-3).[109] This process may depend on expression of the CD44 and α_6 integrin molecules by the prothymocyte.[105] Human prothymocytes may retain the ability to differentiate into the NK cell lineage even after entering the thymus,[104] which is consistent with later occurrence of the split between T cell and the NK cell lineages than between the T cell and the B cell lineages. The engagement of Notch 1 on the prothymocyte cell surface by ligands expressed by thymic epithelial cells, such as a Delta-1,[110] appears to be a key event in promoting T-lineage cell differentiation.

Intrathymic cellular progeny of the prothymocyte give rise to the three major subsets of thymocytes characteristic of the postnatal thymus. These subsets are named according to their pattern of surface expression of CD4 and CD8 and are further characterized by their surface expression of αβ-TCR–CD3 complexes. Thymocytes can be classified as double-negative ($CD4^-CD8^-$), which express little or no CD4 or CD8 (hence, double-negative) or αβ-TCR–CD3 and are direct products of the prothymocyte; double-positive ($CD4^{hi}CD8^{hi}$) which express medium levels of αβ-TCR–CD3 and are derived from double-negative cells; and single-positive ($CD4^{hi}CD8^-$ and $CD4^-CD8^{hi}$), which express high levels of αβ-TCR–CD3 and are derived from double-positive cells. In humans, there is also an intermediate stage between double-negative and double-positive thymocytes that is characterized by a $CD4^{lo}CD8^-CD3^-$ surface phenotype.[111] The double-negative progeny of the prothymocyte undergo cell division and progressive differentiation as they move outward in the cortex toward the subcapsular region. These cells then reverse course and move from the outer to the inner cortex as double-positive thymocytes. Finally, double-positive cells become single-positive thymocytes in the medulla, which probably exit the thymus through blood vessels located in the medulla.

Intrathymic Generation of T Cell Receptor Diversity

T (and B) lymphocytes undergo a unique developmental event, the generation of a highly diverse repertoire of antigen receptors through DNA recombination, a process referred to as V(D)J recombination. This diversity is generated through the random rearrangement and juxtaposition into a single exon of variable (V), diversity (D), and joining (J) segments to form in each cell a unique TCR α and TCR β gene sequence.[4] The unrearranged human TCR β chain gene spans 685 kilobases of DNA on human chromosome 7 and contains 46 potentially functional V gene segments located upstream of two constant (C) regions, each associated with one D and six J segments (Fig. 4-4).[112] The human TCR α chain gene locus on chromosome 14 contains 54 V segments and 61 J segments that can potentially be used for TCR α gene rearrangement.[112]

V(D)J recombination is a highly ordered process and is controlled at multiple levels.[113-115] The restriction of the process of V(D)J recombination to cells of the T and B lymphocyte lineage results from the unique expression in their precursors of two recombination-activating genes, *RAG1* and *RAG2*. Recombination of the TCR genes is further restricted to cells of the T lymphocyte rather than B lymphocyte lineage by mechanisms (e.g., histone acetylation) that allow RAG access to the TCR genes only in T cell progenitors. The RAG proteins are critically involved in the initiation of the recombination process—they recognize and cleave conserved sequences flanking each V, D, and J segment. Other proteins, including a high-molecular-weight DNA-dependent protein kinase and its associated Ku70 and Ku80 proteins, DNA ligase IV and its associated XRCC4 protein, and Artemis, then perform nonhomologous DNA end-joining of the cleaved V(D)J segments. Unlike RAG proteins, these other proteins involved in nonhomologous DNA end-joining are expressed in most cells and are involved in repair of double-stranded DNA breaks.[116] Genetic deficiency of any of the proteins involved in the rearrangement process results in a form of severe combined immunodeficiency (SCID), because T cell and B cell development depend on the surface expression of rearranged TCR and immunoglobulin genes, respectively. Human SCID due to genetic immunodeficiency of RAG-1, RAG-2, and Artemis is well documented.[117]

The complementarity-determining regions (CDRs) of the TCR and immunoglobulin molecules are those that are involved in forming the three-dimensional structure that binds with antigen. The V segments encode the CDR1 and CDR2 regions for both TCR chains. The CDR3 region, where the distal portion of the V segment joins the (D)J segment, is a particularly important source of αβ-TCR diversity for peptide-MHC recognition,[118] and is the center of the antigen-binding site for peptide-MHC complexes. CDR3 (also known as junctional) diversity is achieved by multiple mechanisms. These mechanisms include (1) the addition of one or two nucleotides that are palindromic to the end of the cut gene segment (termed P-nucleotides); these nucleotides are added as part of the process of asymmetrical repairing of "hairpin" ends (the two strands of DNA are joined at the ends) that are generated by RAG endonuclease activity[119]; (2) the activity of terminal deoxytransferase (TdT), which randomly adds nucleotides (called N-nucleotides) to the ends of segments undergoing rearrangement; TdT addition is a particularly

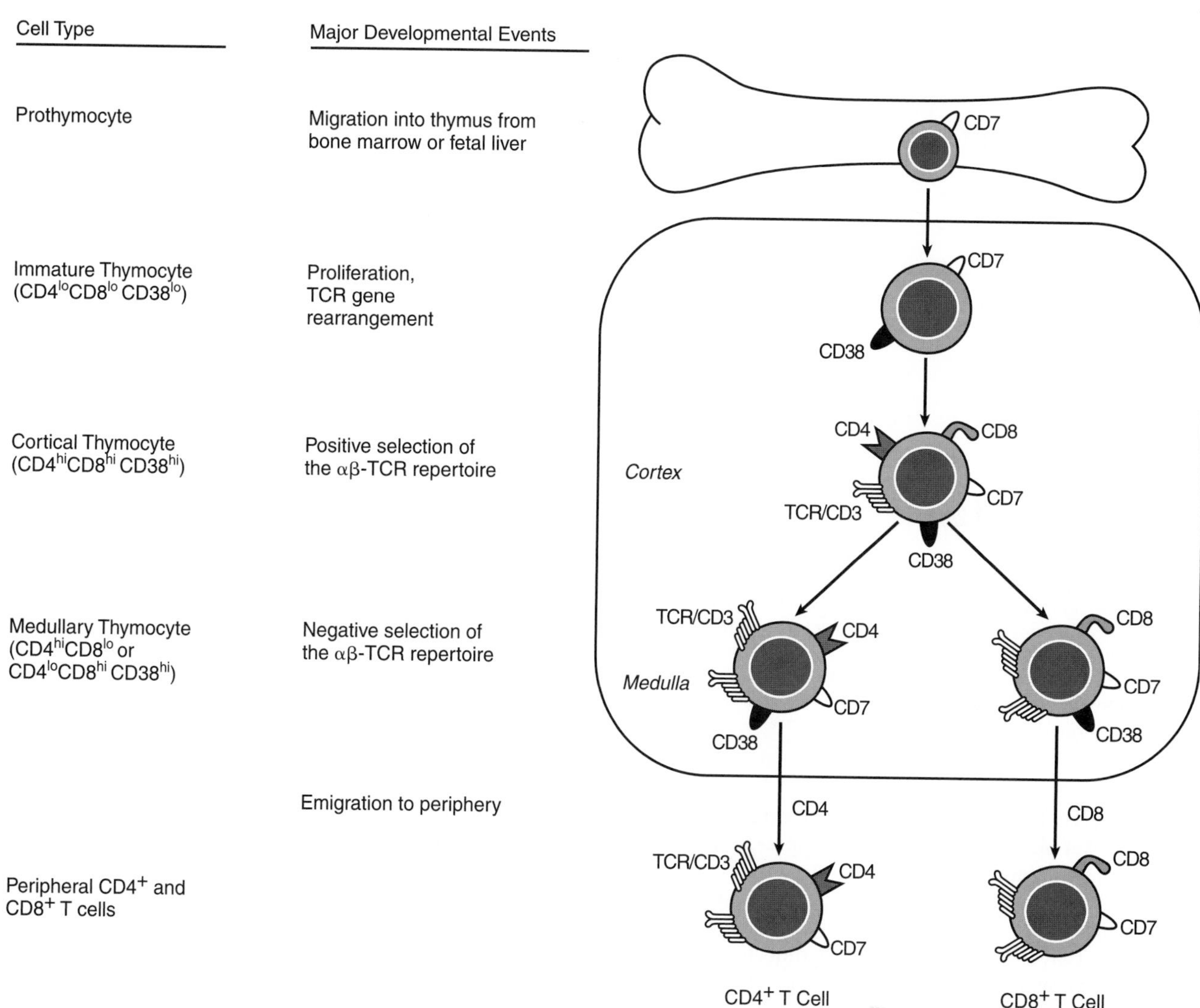

Figure 4–3 Putative stages of human αβ T cell receptor–positive (αβ-TCR$^+$) thymocyte development. Prothymocytes from the bone marrow or fetal liver, which express CD7, enter the thymus via vessels at the junction between the thymic cortex and medulla. They differentiate to progressively more mature αβ-TCR$^+$ thymocytes, defined by their pattern of expression of the αβ-TCR–CD3 complex, CD4, CD8, and CD38. TCR α and TCR β chain genes are rearranged in the outer cortex. Positive selection occurs mainly in the central thymic cortex by interaction with thymic epithelial cells, and negative selection occurs mainly in the medulla by interaction with thymic dendritic cells. Following these selection processes, medullary thymocytes emigrate into the circulation and colonize the peripheral lymphoid organs as CD4$^+$ and CD8$^+$ T cells with high levels of the αβ-TCR–CD3 complex. These recent thymic emigrants (RTEs) also contain signal joint T cell receptor excision circles (TRECs), which are a circular product of TCR gene rearrangement. Most RTEs probably lack CD38 surface expression. By contrast, in neonates, most peripheral T cells retain surface expression of CD38 and have high amounts of TREC compared with adult peripheral T cells.

important mechanism for diversity generation because every three additional nucleotides encodes a potential codon, potentially increasing repertoire diversity by a factor of 20; and (3) exonuclease activity that results in a variable loss of nucleotide residues, as part of the DNA repair process.

Together, the mechanisms for generating diversity can theoretically result in as many as 1×10^{15} types of αβ-TCR. In reality, the final repertoire of naïve T cells in the adult human circulation is on average a total of 1×10^6 different TCR β chains, each pairing on average with at least 25 different TCR α chains.[120] This results in a maximum of about 1×10^8 different combinations of TCR α and TCR β chains for the naïve T cell αβ-TCR repertoire. Because in young adults the body has approximately 2×10^{11} CD4$^+$ T cells and 1×10^{11} CD8$^+$ T cells,[121,122] of which about 50% belong to the naïve subset, the average clonal size for a naïve T cell is approximately 500 to 1000.[120,123]

RAG expression commences in double-negative thymocytes, and because the TCR β gene is the first to become accessible to RAG proteins, it is the first to undergo rearrangement (a small fraction of double-negative cells may undergo TCR γ and TCR δ gene rearrangement, and this is discussed in more detail in the section on γδ T cells). The TCR α gene is not accessible and does not rearrange at this stage. The TCR β chain D segment first rearranges to a downstream J segment, with the deletion of intervening DNA. This is followed by rearrangement of a V segment to the DJ segment, resulting in a contiguous (VDJ) β chain gene segment, which is joined to the constant (C) region segment by mRNA splicing. If a VDJ segment lacks premature translation stop

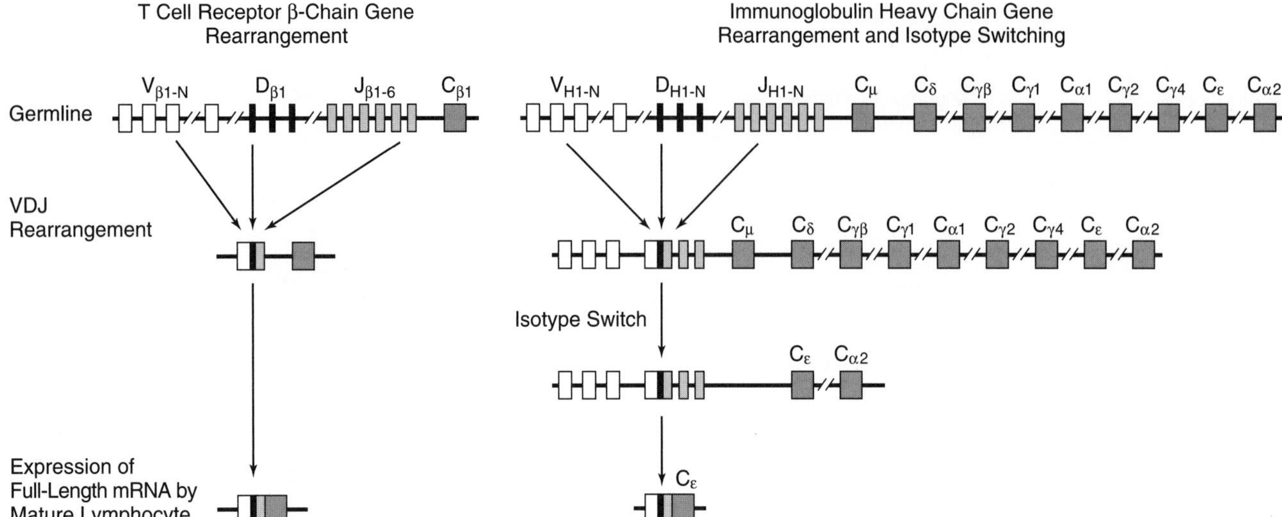

Figure 4–4 The T cell receptor (TCR) and immunoglobulin genes are formed by rearrangement in immature lymphocytes. The TCR β chain gene and the immunoglobulin heavy chain genes are shown as examples. A similar process is involved with rearrangement of the TCR α, γ, and δ chain genes, and with the immunoglobulin light chain genes. Rearrangement involves the joining of dispersed segments of variable (V), diversity (D), and joining (J) gene segments with the deletion of intervening DNA. This allows expression of a full-length mRNA transcript that can be translated into a functional protein, provided that there are no premature translational stop codons. Immunoglobulin heavy chain genes undergo an additional rearrangement called isotype switching, in which the constant (C) region segment is changed without alteration of the antigen combining site formed by the V, D, and J segments. The isotype switch from IgM to IgE is shown.

codons, the TCR β chain protein may be expressed on the thymocyte surface in association with a pre-TCR α chain protein (pre-Tα) and some of the CD3 complex proteins. This pre-Tα complex is capable of triggering many or most of the signals that are characteristic of engagement of the mature αβ-TCR[124] and instructs the thymocyte to increase its surface expression of CD4 and CD8, to start rearrangement of the TCR α chain gene, and to stop rearrangement of the other TCR β chain allele. This inhibition of TCR β chain gene rearrangement results in allelic exclusion, so that greater than 99% of αβ T cells express only a single type of TCR β chain gene.[125]

Rearrangement of the TCR α chain gene then occurs at the double-positive stage and involves the joining of V segments directly to J segments, without intervening D segments. If successful, this leads to the expression of a TCR αβ heterodimer on the cell surface in association with CD3 proteins to form the TCR-CD3 complex. Allelic exclusion is ineffective for the TCR α chain gene, and it is estimated that as many as one third of peripheral human αβ T cells may express two types of TCR α chains.[126] RAG protein expression normally ceases in cortical thymocytes, limiting gene rearrangement to early thymocyte development.

Thymocyte Selection and Maturation of Double-Positive to Single-Positive Thymocytes

Positive Selection. Thymocytes that have successfully rearranged and express αβ-TCRs have a $CD4^{hi}CD8^{hi}$ surface phenotype (see Fig. 4-3) undergo a selective process that tests the appropriateness of their TCR specificity, known as positive selection. Positive selection requires that the αβ-TCR recognize self-peptides bound to MHC molecules displayed on epithelial cells of the thymic cortex.[127,128] The αβ-TCR interacts not only with the MHC-associated peptide but also with regions of the MHC that form the groove,[129] for which it has an intrinsic affinity.[130] This recognition of both portions of the MHC groove and peptide presumably applies to positive selection in the thymus as well as to the recognition of foreign antigen by peripheral αβ T cells. If the TCR has sufficient but not too high affinity for self-peptide–MHC complexes, the thymocyte receives a signal allowing its survival. If this signal is absent or weak, the thymocyte dies by apoptosis as a result of activation of caspases, a family of intracellular cysteine proteases. Too strong a signal also does not result in effective positive selection. Positive selection also is influenced by interactions between MHC molecules and the CD4 and CD8 molecules. As mentioned previously, MHC class I and class II molecules have constant domains located outside of their peptide-binding grooves that have affinity for CD8 and CD4, respectively. As a result of these interactions, most $CD4^{hi}CD8^-$ thymocytes (and their peripheral $CD4^+$ T cell descendants) recognize peptides bound to MHC class II molecules, and most $CD4^-CD8^{hi}$ T cells (and peripheral $CD8^+$ T cells) recognize peptides bound to MHC class I molecules (see Fig. 4-3). Positive selection also extinguishes *RAG* gene expression, terminating further TCR-α rearrangement.

Negative Selection. Positively selected $CD4^{hi}CD8^-$ and $CD4^-CD8^{hi}$ thymocytes enter the medulla, where they undergo a second selection process called negative selection, in which they are eliminated by apoptosis if their TCR has too high an affinity for self-peptide–MHC complexes expressed on medullary DCs.[128] Negative selection helps eliminate αβ T cells with TCRs that could pose a risk of autoimmune reactions and is an important influence on the final TCR repertoire.[131] Thymic epithelial cells found in the medulla express a diverse array of self-antigens (e.g., insulin, myelin basic protein) that help in this elimination.[132] A transcription factor encoded by the autoimmune regulator (*AIRE*) gene enhances the expression of self-antigen by thymic epithelial cells.[133] As a net result of either the failure to productively rearrange the TCR α or TCR β chain gene, the lack of positive selection, or the occurrence of negative selection, only about 2% to 3% of the progeny of hematopoietic lymphoid precursors that enter the thymus emerge as mature single-positive thymocytes.[134]

Impact of Thymocyte Selection on Self-MHC Restriction and MHC Alloreactivity. Because the region forming the peptide-binding groove of MHC molecules is highly polymorphic in the human population (see section on basic aspects of antigen presentation), a result of positive selection is that T cells have a strong preference for recognizing a particular foreign peptide bound to self-MHC, rather than to the MHC of an unrelated person. On the other hand, the fact that TCR has intrinsic affinity for MHC molecules[130] accounts for the ability of an APC bearing foreign MHC molecules to activate a substantial proportion (up to several percent) of T cells—the allogeneic response. In the allogeneic response, T cells are activated by novel antigen specificities that are thought to result from the combination of a foreign MHC with multiple self-peptides.[129,135] Because these self-peptide–foreign MHC specificities are not expressed in the thymus, T cells capable of recognizing them have not been eliminated by the negative selection process in the medulla.

Thymocyte Growth and Differentiation Factors

The factors within the thymic microenvironment that are essential for thymocyte development include key cytokines produced by thymic epithelial cells, such as IL-7. Persons lacking a functional IL-7 receptor, owing to a genetic deficiency of either the IL-7 receptor α chain[136] or the common γ chain (γc) cytokine receptor (CD132) with which the α chain associates,[117] have abortive thymocyte development and lack mature αβ T cells. A similar phenotype is observed with genetic deficiency of the JAK-3 tyrosine kinase, which is associated with the cytoplasmic domain of the γc cytokine receptor and delivers activation signals to the interior of the cell.[137] B cell development is spared in these human genetic immunodeficiencies.

Thymocyte Postselection Maturation

$CD4^{hi}CD8^-$ and $CD4^-CD8^{hi}$ thymocytes are the most mature αβ T-lineage cell population in the thymus and predominate in the thymic medulla. Many of the functional differences between peripheral $CD4^+$ and $CD8^+$ T cells appear to be established during the later stages of thymic maturation, presumably as a result of differentiation induced by positive selection: Mature $CD4^{hi}CD8^-$ thymocytes, like peripheral $CD4^+$ T cells, are enriched in cells that can secrete certain cytokines, such as IL-2, and in providing help for B cells in producing immunoglobulin.[138] $CD4^-CD8^{hi}$ thymocytes, like peripheral $CD8^+$ T cells, are relatively limited in their ability to produce IL-2 but, once primed by antigen, are effective in mediating cytotoxic activity.[139]

Thymocyte Emigration and Homing to Secondary Lymphoid Tissue

Mature $CD4^{hi}CD8^-$ and $CD4^-CD8^{hi}$ single-positive thymocytes enter into the circulation as antigenically naïve $CD4^+$ and $CD8^+$ αβ T cells, respectively. These circulating T cells preferentially home to the secondary lymphoid tissue (see Fig. 4-3),[140] as antigenically naïve $CD4^+$ and $CD8^+$ T cells, respectively. Secondary lymphoid tissue consists of the lymph nodes, spleen, and mucosa-associated lymphoid tissue (MALT). Development of lymph nodes and Peyer's patches in mice is dependent on signaling by members of the TNF cytokine gene family through the lymphotoxin-β (LT-β) receptor (see Table 4-1).[141]

As described for DCs, the migration of mature thymocytes into the circulation and their entry into the peripheral lymphoid organs are determined in part by the pattern of expression on the cell surface of chemokine receptors and by the local patterns and gradients of chemokine receptor ligands in tissues (see Table 4-1). Departure of naïve T cells from the thymus and entry into the secondary lymphoid tissues coincide with and are mediated in part by a change in the expression of chemokine receptors on their surface.[43,45] As they enter the medulla, mature single-positive thymocytes begin to lose expression of CCR9 and to gain expression of CCR7. As explained later on, this alteration allows them to leave the thymic medulla, where chemokines binding to CCR9 (TECK, CCL25) are found, and enter the secondary lymphoid tissues, where chemokines that bind to CCR7 are found.

Adhesion molecules and their ligands also play an important role in leukocyte trafficking, including thymic emigration and entry to peripheral lymphoid tissue. Two major families of adhesion molecules govern leukocyte migration: the selectins and the integrins. The three selectins are L-selectin (CD62L), which is constitutively expressed on many types of leukocytes, including naïve and certain subsets of memory T cells, and E-selectin (CD62E) and P-selectin (CD62P), both of which are expressed on activated vascular endothelium; P-selectin also is expressed on activated platelets.[142,143] Selectins bind to multivalent carbohydrate ligands, which are displayed on specific protein or lipid backbones on the cell surface.

The other major adhesion molecules are the integrins, which are heterodimers composed of different combinations of α and β chains. All T cells express $\alpha_1\beta_2$ integrin, also known as leukocyte function antigen (LFA)-1, and subsets of T cells express other integrins, including $\alpha_4\beta_1$ (very late antigen-4 [VLA-4]) and $\alpha_4\beta_7$. Integrins bind to members of the immunoglobulin superfamily: LFA-1 binds to intercellular cell adhesion molecules ICAM-1, -2, and -3, and VLA-4 binds to vascular cell adhesion molecule-1 (VCAM-1), which is induced on activated endothelial cells. Mucosal addressin cell adhesion molecule-1 (MAdCAM-1), expressed on endothelial cells in the gut, is a ligand for L-selectin and for the $\alpha_4\beta_7$ integrin. Many integrins also bind to components of the extracellular matrix, which is thought to contribute to leukocyte migration in the tissues after cells migrate across the vascular endothelium.

The initial interaction of leukocytes with the vascular endothelium is mediated by selectins and their ligands.[142,143] This low-affinity, high-valency interaction is facilitated by the display of selectins on the tips of microvilli, where they are positioned to sample the endothelial surface. If ligand is displayed, leukocytes are induced to roll along the endothelium, which allows them to survey for the presence of chemokines. In the case of naïve T cells, surface expression

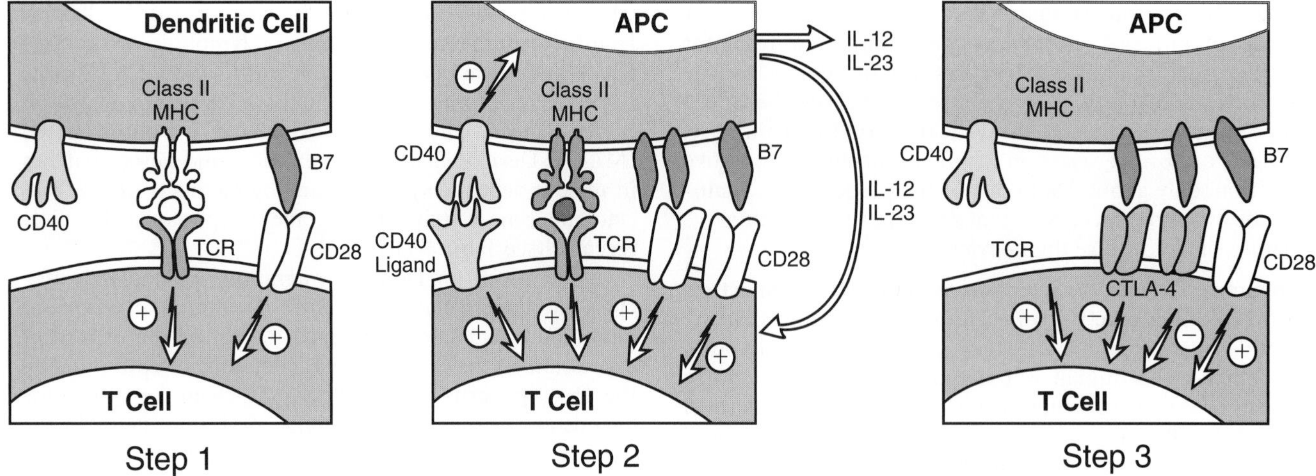

Figure 4–5 T cell–antigen-presenting cell (APC) interactions early during the immune response to peptide antigens. A major histocompatibility complex (MHC) class II–restricted response by CD4⁺ T cells is shown as an example. Dendritic cells are probably the most important APCs for antigenically naïve T cells and constitutively express CD80 or CD86 (B7 molecules), CD40, and MHC class II molecules on their cell surface. Engagement of αβ T cell receptor (αβ-TCR) on the $CD4^+$ T cell by antigenic peptides bound to MHC molecules on the DC, in conjunction with co-stimulation by B7 (CD80/CD86) interactions with CD28 interactions, leads to T cell activation (*Step 1*). The activated T cell expresses CD40 ligand (CD154) on its surface, which engages CD40 on the dendritic cell; this increases B7 expression on the dendritic cell, enhancing T cell co-stimulation (*Step 2*). CD40 engagement also activates the dendritic cell to produce cytokines, such as interleukin (IL)-12. IL-12, in turn, promotes the proliferation and differentiation of T cells into T_H1-type effector cells that produce high levels of interferon (IFN)-γ and low or undetectable amounts of IL-4. Cytotoxic T lymphocyte antigen-4 (CTLA-4) (i.e., CD152) is expressed on the T cells during the later stages of T cell activation. Engagement of CTLA-4 by B7 molecules on the APC delivers negative signals that help terminate T cell activation (*Step 3*).

of L-selectin allows them to bind to the peripheral lymph node addressin, which is expressed on the surface of the specialized high endothelium of the postcapillary venules (HEV) in the peripheral lymph nodes, Peyer's patches, and tonsils.[140]

Tethered to the surface of the HEV is the chemokine, CCL21, which binds to CCR7 on the surface of naïve T cells. CCL21, and another CCR7 ligand, CCL19, are produced by stromal cells and perhaps some APCs in the lymph node. The engagement of CCR7 on naïve T cells by CCL21 triggers signals leading to an increase in the affinity of LFA-1, allowing the naïve T cells to bind avidly to the LFA-1 ligands ICAM-1 and ICAM-2 on the vascular endothelium. This stops T cell rolling, allowing the T cell to undergo diapedesis across the endothelium and to enter the T cell zones of the lymph node. There CCL19 is produced by DCs, resulting in the juxtaposition of naïve T cells and DCs.

Naïve T Cell Recirculation and Homeostasis

If naïve T cells encounter DCs presenting cognate peptide-MHC complexes, they stop migrating and remain in the lymph node. If they do not encounter such DCs, they migrate through the lymph node to the efferent lymph and thereby return to the bloodstream. Thus, naïve T cells continually circulate between the blood and secondary lymphoid tissues, allowing them the opportunity to continuously sample APCs for their cognate antigen. Because they regulate this homeostatic recirculation of naïve T cells, CCL19 and CCL21 are referred to as homeostatic chemokines.

Studies in mice indicate that the survival of naïve T cells in the periphery is dependent on two major exogenous factors. The first is continuous interaction with self-peptide–MHC complexes,[144] which appears to be particularly important for the survival of the antigenically naïve $CD8^+$ T cell population.[145,146] Whether this survival signal is analogous to positive selection in the thymus in its requirements for a diverse self-peptide repertoire remains unclear. The second major factor appears to be signals provided through the γc component of cytokine receptors—in the absence of γc, naïve T cells appear to survive for fewer than 5 days.[147] It appears that the role of γc in naïve T cell survival is primarily if not solely to transduce signals in response to IL-7 through the IL-7Rα–γc receptor complex.[148] By contrast, once naïve T cells are activated in response to cognate peptide-MHC complexes, homeostasis is maintained by different mechanisms, which are discussed next.

T Cell Activation

The TCR-CD3 complex is linked to an intricate and highly interconnected complex of kinases, phosphatases, and adapter molecules that transduce signals in response to engagement of the TCR and, in αβ T cells, the appropriate CD4 or CD8 co-receptor by cognate peptide-MHC complexes (Fig. 4-5; see also Fig. 4-1). It is thought that lipid rafts play a critical role in facilitating the assembly of signaling complexes at specific regions of the plasma membrane; these complexes in turn recruit adapters and signal-transducing proteins.[149] A proximal event is activation of tyrosine kinases followed by events that lead to elevation of the T cell free intracellular calcium concentration ($[Ca^{2+}]_i$). An increased calcium concentration in turn leads to the activation of calcineurin and the translocation of nuclear factor of activated T cells (NFAT) transcription factors from the cytosol to the nucleus. Concurrent activation of the extracellular signal-regulated kinase/mitogen-activated protein kinase (ERK/MAPK) pathway enhances activation of other transcription factors, including activator protein-1/activating transcription factor (AP-1/ATF). Collectively, these transcription factors induce the transcription of genes encoding key proteins for activation, such as cytokines, cell cycle regulators, and, in cytotoxic T cells, proteins involved in killing other cells, such as perforins. The expression of more than 100 genes is altered as a result of the activation process.[150,151]

T Cell Activation versus Anergy. For full T cell activation that leads to cytokine production and commitment of the cell to proliferate, signaling through the trimolecular αβ-TCR–peptide–MHC complex and through accessory or co-stimulatory signaling pathways must exceed a specific threshold. The nature and magnitude of the signal transmitted through the αβ-TCR–CD3 complex are a function of the affinity of the TCR for the peptide-MHC complex and the duration of their interaction.[152,153] Low-affinity interactions that do not trigger full T cell activation may lead to a state of long-term unresponsiveness to subsequent stimulation, which is referred to as anergy. Anergy is thought to contribute to the maintenance of tolerance by mature T cells to certain self-antigens—in particular, those that are not expressed in the thymus in sufficient abundance to induce negative selection.

From in vitro experiments, it has been estimated that naïve $CD4^+$ T cells require sustained αβ-TCR signaling for 20 to 24 hours to become activated. Surprisingly, studies suggest that a much shorter period of αβ-TCR–peptide–MHC interaction is required to activate naïve $CD8^+$ T cells—as little as 2 hours is sufficient for cells to commit to proliferation.[154,155] As with naïve $CD4^+$ T cells, however, cell division does not commence for approximately 24 hours after the initiation of signaling. The basis for this difference between naïve $CD4^+$ and $CD8^+$ T cells is not known. In any case, optimal signals provided through αβ-TCR–peptide–MHC interactions generally are not sufficient to fully activate either naïve $CD4^+$ or $CD8^+$ T cells—additional co-stimulatory signals play an important role in allowing naïve T cells to commit to cytokine production and proliferation. By contrast, memory T cells have a lower activation threshold, are less dependent on these co-stimulatory signals, and can commit to proliferate following engagement of their αβ-TCR for as little as 1 hour.[152,156]

Facilitation of T Cell Activation by Co-stimulatory Interactions. Although signals transmitted by the CD3 complex in response to engagement of the αβ-TCR by peptide-MHC complexes on APCs are necessary for T cell activation, many authorities argue that these signals, commonly referred to collectively as signal 1, rarely are sufficient for full activation of naïve T cells under most physiologic conditions. Rather, it appears that the immune system has evolved a strategy by which to "tune down" the response of naïve T cells relative to that of memory T cells, thereby rendering naïve T cells dependent on secondary co-stimulatory signals (signal 2) provided by other molecular interactions between APCs and T cells. Signal 2 alone does not lead to T cell activation but acts in concert with signal 1 provided through αβ-TCR–CD3 to facilitate full T cell activation rather than anergy. Co-stimulatory signals (signal 2) appear to be particularly important if the abundance and duration of antigenic peptide–MHC complexes are limiting.

The best-characterized co-stimulatory signal is provided by the engagement of CD28 on the T cell with CD80 (B7-1) or CD86 (B7-2) on APCs (see Table 4-4).[157,158] CD80 and CD86 are related proteins belonging to the immunoglobulin superfamily, which are expressed at low levels on immature DCs, mononuclear phagocytes, and B cells. The expression of both CD80 and CD86 can be induced on APCs by a variety of factors such as LPS exposure, B cell receptor cross-linking, and CD40 signaling (see Fig. 4-5). Thus, APCs primed by these factors, and, in particular, mature DCs, express high levels of CD80 and CD86.

CD80 and CD86 both bind to CD28, which is constitutively expressed on T cells. Signaling through CD28 lowers the strength or duration of TCR signaling needed to fully activate T cells, which is particularly important for naïve T cells, in which the threshold for full activation is high compared with that for memory and effector T cells.[156,159] The Human Genome Project has contributed to the identification of a family of related co-stimulatory molecules that collectively constitute the B7 superfamily.[158] These co-stimulatory molecules may play a role in selective enhancement of certain types of T cell responses. For example, B7-H3 appears to favor the production of IFN-γ, at least in humans, whereas B7-related protein-1 (B7RP-1) and its receptor on T cells (the inducible co-stimulator [ICOS]) favor the production of IL-4 and B cell help.[158] Other members of the family, such as PD-1 ("programmed death-1"), may act to dampen the T cell response by inducing T cell apoptosis.

Activated T cells express on their surface CD40 ligand, a member of the TNF ligand family (see Tables 4-1 and 4-4), which engages the CD40 molecule on B cells, DCs, and mononuclear phagocytes.[160-162] CD40 engagement by CD40 ligand induces the expression of CD80 and CD86 on these APCs. As mentioned previously, CD40 engagement also may induce DCs to produce IL-12, IL-23, and other cytokines (see Fig. 4-5) and to express increased levels of CD80 and CD86, which modulate the development and function of effector T cells, as described later on. Interactions between CD40 and CD40 ligand appear to play an important role in vivo in the expansion of $CD4^+$ T cells during a primary immune response but may be less critical for expansion of $CD8^+$ T cells.[163,164] TNF-α and TRANCE (also known as RANK ligand) are additional members of the TNF ligand family that are expressed on activated T cells and that also can stimulate APC function. Thus, activation-induced expression of TNF ligand family members on naïve T cells can amplify the primary immune responses by priming the function of APCs.

Differentiation and Homeostasis of Activated T Cells

When naïve $CD4^+$ T cells first encounter foreign peptide–MHC complexes during a primary immune response, they extinguish expression of LKLF, a transcription factor that maintains naïve T cells in a resting state,[165,166] and produce a limited number of cytokines, including IL-2 in robust amounts and CD40 ligand in modest amounts (Fig. 4-6). They also are induced to express high-affinity IL-2 receptor complexes composed of the IL-2R α and β chains and γc.

Engagement of the IL-2 receptor complex by IL-2, acting as both an autocrine and a paracrine growth factor, triggers T cells to undergo multiple rounds of proliferation, thereby expanding the numbers of antigen-specific T cells, and to differentiate into effector T cells (see Fig. 4-6).[153,167,168] They also express on their surface CD69 and Fas molecules[169] and downregulate expression of Bcl-2, an intracellular protein that protects against apoptosis.[170] Downregulation of Bcl-2

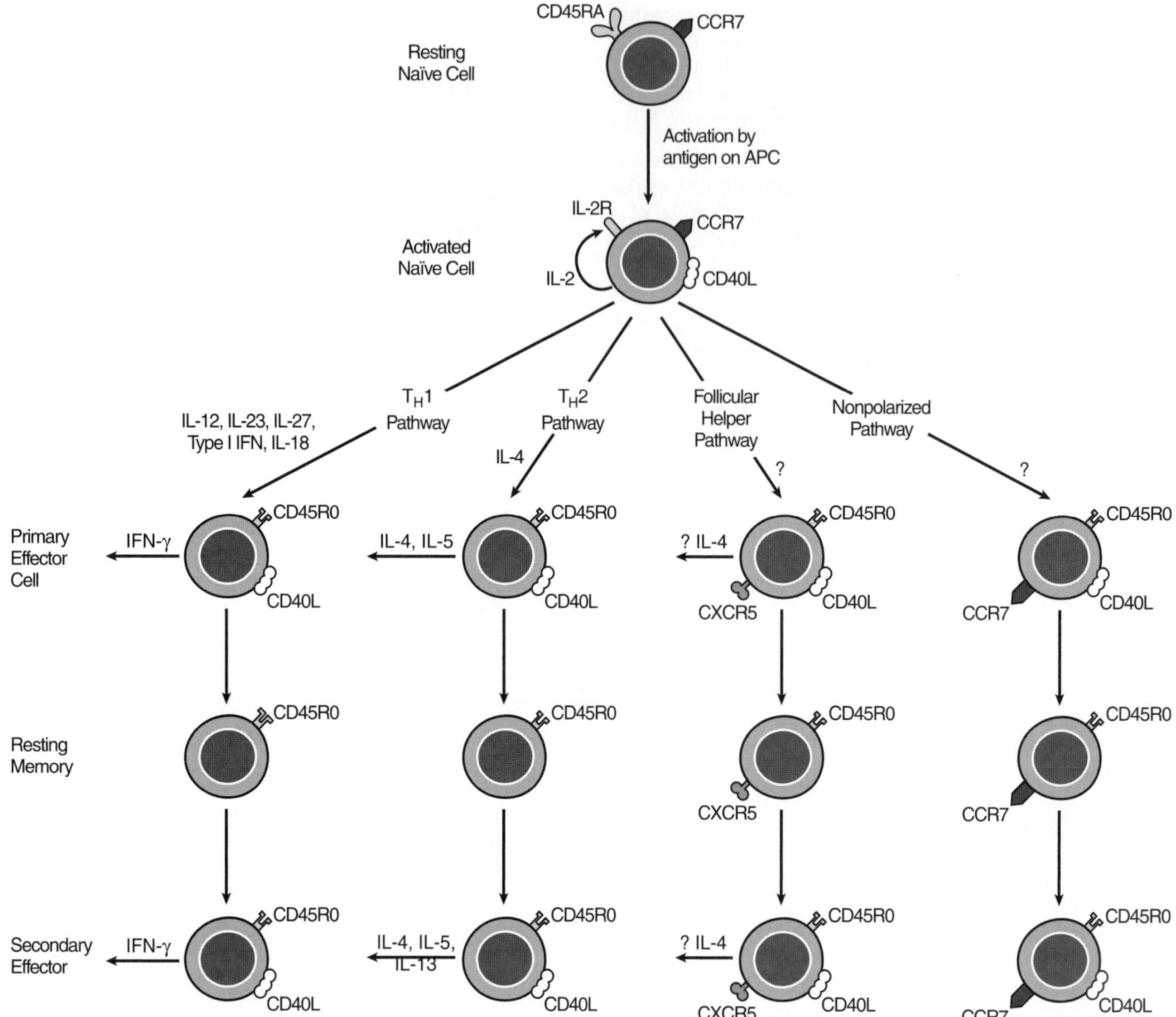

Figure 4–6 Differentiation of antigenically naïve CD4⁺ T cells into T_H1, T_H2, unpolarized, and T follicular helper effector and memory T cells. Antigenically naïve CD4⁺ T cells express high levels of the CD45RA isoform of the CD45 surface protein tyrosine phosphatase. They are activated by antigen presented by antigen-presenting cells (APCs) to express CD40 ligand and interleukin (IL)-2 and to undergo clonal expansion and differentiation, which is accompanied by expression of the CD45RO isoform and loss of the CD45RA isoform. Most effector cells die by apoptosis, but a small fraction of these cells persist as memory cells which express high levels of CD45RO. Exposure of expanding effector cells to IL-12 family cytokines, IL-18, and intereron (IFN)-γ favors their differentiation into T_H1 effector cells that secrete IFN-γ, whereas exposure to IL-4 favors their differentiation into T_H2 effector cells that secrete IL-4, IL-5, and IL-13. Many memory cells are nonpolarized and do not express either T_H1 or T_H2 cytokines. They may be enriched for cells that continue to express the CCR7 chemokine receptor, which favors their recirculation between the blood and the lymph nodes and spleen. T follicular helper cells, which express high levels of CXCR5, move into B cell follicle areas, where they express CD40 ligand and provide help for B cell responses. The signals that promote the accumulation of memory T follicular helper cells and their capacity to produce cytokines are poorly understood. Memory cells rechallenged with antigen undergo rapid clonal expansion into secondary effector cells that mediate the same functions as the initial memory population. Most secondary effector cells eventually die by apoptosis.

sensitizes these cells to apoptosis, which is countered by signals through the IL-2 receptor complex; this makes effector T cells dependent for their survival on IL-2 (or other cytokines that signal through the γc cytokine receptor) to induce the expression of Bcl-xL, which, like Bcl-2, inhibits apoptosis.[171] Thus, when concentrations of IL-2 become limiting, effector T cell attrition occurs, dampening the immune response. Conversely, IL-2 signals may sensitize T cells to Fas-mediated activation-induced cell death. Thus, the role of IL-2 in the expansion, survival, or death of effector T cells is determined by a balance between prosurvival and proapoptotic effects of IL-2.

In this regard, it is notable that studies suggest that antigen-induced proliferation of murine $CD4^+$ T cells in vivo, in striking contrast with findings in vitro, does not require signals through the IL-2 receptor or other receptor complexes that contain γc[147]; whether this also is true for $CD8^+$ T cells and in humans is not known. Alhough these results do not exclude a role for IL-2 in antigen-induced proliferation of $CD4^+$ T cells, they reinforce the observation that the dominant effect observed in humans with IL-2 receptor α chain deficiency is autoimmunity.[171,172] The basis for this effect is not certain, but it may reflect defects in activation-induced cell death mediated by Fas–Fas ligand interactions, and defects in regulatory T cells (see later section).[173]

Regardless of the role of IL-2 and IL-2 receptors in the initial proliferation of naïve T cells, proliferation leads to an expansion in the numbers of the responding T cell population. This increase is a key feature of antigen-specific immunity. In the absence of prior exposure, the frequency of T lymphocytes capable of recognizing and responding to that antigen is small, generally less than 1:100,000, but in response to infection can increase to greater than 1:20 for $CD8^+$ T cells and greater than 1:1000 for $CD4^+$ T cells in less than a week.[174] Furthermore, the phenotype and function of these cells are permanently changed from those characteristic of naïve T cells to those associated with memory or effector T cells.

T_H1 and T_H2 $CD4^+$ T Cells. The functions of effector T cells, particularly those of the $CD4^+$ subset, are mediated in large part by the multiple additional cytokines they produce that are not produced by naïve T cells. Most of these cytokines are secreted, although some (e.g., some members of the TNF ligand family) may be predominantly expressed on the T cell surface. These cytokines include IL-3, IL-4, IL-5, IL-9, IL-10, IL-13, IL-17, IL-21, interferon-γ (IFN-γ), GM-CSF, CD40 ligand, TNF-α, and Fas ligand.[175,176] Table 4-2 summarizes the major immunomodulatory effects of T cell–derived cytokines and of cytokines produced by other cell types that act on T cells. Some key effects of cytokines in T cell proliferation, differentiation, and effector function, and in B cell, NK cell, and mononuclear phagocyte function, are discussed later on.

Two major types of $CD4^+$ effector T cells, T_H1 and T_H2, initially were described in mice, and similar profiles of polarized cytokine expression subsequently have been confirmed in other species, including humans.[177-180] IFN-γ is the signature cytokine produced by T_H1 effector cells, which also produce substantial amounts of IL-2, lymphotoxin-α, and TNF-α, but little or no IL-4, IL-5, and IL-13. By contrast, IL-4 is the signature cytokine of T_H2 cells, which also produce IL-5, IL-9, and IL-13, but little or no IFN-γ or IL-2.

More overlap or variability in patterns of cytokine production may be present in humans than in mice. Cells producing effector cytokines of both types are commonly referred to as T_H0 cells, which often are seen following vaccination with protein antigens or following viral infections, such as influenza virus or CMV.[181,182] Generation of T_H0 cells in vitro seems to be favored by the presence of large amounts of IL-2 in the absence of cytokines that polarize differentiation toward either T_H1 or T_H2 effector cells.[179,183,184] An alternative possibility is that T_H0 cells have undergone less proliferation and differentiation and for this reason have not yet become committed T_H1 or T_H2 cells.[46,156] In addition to their differing cytokine profiles, T_H1 and T_H2 cells also differ in chemokine receptor and cell adhesion molecule expression.[43,45,140,185,186] This may allow T_H1 and T_H2 cells to differentially localize to particular tissues—for example, T_H2 cells often are found in the mucosa.

Regulation of T_H1 versus T_H2 Differentiation. Factors contributing to the generation of T_H1 versus T_H2 cells include the strength of the activating signals, nature and abundance of co-stimulatory molecules on APCs, and the cytokine milieu, with the last playing the dominant role.[177,179,183] T_H1 effector development is favored by the exposure of $CD4^+$ T cells during their initial activation to high levels of IL-12, IL-18, IL-23, and IL-27 produced by APCs and to IFN-γ produced by NK cells and other T cells (see Fig. 4-6). In humans but not in mice, IFN-α also is a potent inducer of T_H1 cells.[177,178] Chemokines also may affect T_H1 versus T_H2 differentiation.[187] The importance of these cytokines in the development of robust T_H1 responses and of IFN-γ in human host defense is demonstrated by the increased susceptibility of patients with genetic defects in IL-12, IL-12 receptors, IFN-γ receptors, or signal transducer and transcriptional activator-1 (STAT-1), which transduces IFN-γ receptor–derived signals, to infection with intracellular pathogens, particularly mycobacteria and *Salmonella*.[188]

T_H2 development is favored when $CD4^+$ T cells initially are activated in the presence of IL-4 or in the absence of IL-12, IL-18, IL-23, IL-27, IFN-α, or IFN-γ (see Fig. 4-6), or both. The source of IL-4 in a primary $CD4^+$ T cell response leading to the generation of T_H2 cells is uncertain. It is possible that in the absence of cytokines favoring T_H1 development, the low levels of IL-4 produced by naïve T cells are sufficient,[184] but NK T cells, mast cells, basophils, and eosinophils also produce IL-4 and may contribute in some situations. High levels of co-stimulation through CD86[189] and the engagement of OX40 on the T cell by OX40 ligand, a member of the TNF ligand superfamily expressed by B cells, also may favor T_H2 rather than T_H1 $CD4^+$ T cell development.[190]

Evidence in the mouse suggests that the development and propagation of T_H1 and T_H2 T cells not only are influenced by these exogenous factors but are determined by the expression within $CD4^+$ T cells of opposing transcription factors that dictate T_H1 versus T_H2 development.[177,178] GATA-binding protein–3 appears to be a master regulator of T_H2 T cell development.[191] The expression of GATA-3 is sufficient to override the other influences described earlier, and to reinforce its own expression through a positive feedback loop. Conversely, T-bet induces the development of T_H1 cells, and many of the T_H1-promoting cytokines, such as IFN-γ, may induce T-bet expression in recently activated naïve $CD4^+$ T cells.[192]

T Cell Help for Antibody Production

T cells play a crucial role in the regulation of B cell proliferation, immunoglobulin class switching, affinity maturation, and memory B cell generation in response to proteins or protein conjugates. The enhancement of B cell responses is commonly referred to as T cell help. This process is critically dependent on the recognition through the αβ-TCR of cognate peptide-MHC complexes on B cells, and on multiple contact-dependent interactions (see Fig. 4-5) between members of the TNF ligand–TNF receptor families (see Table 4-1) and the CD28-B7 families (see Table 4-4). Recently activated $CD4^+$ T cells that express CXCR5 migrate to B cell follicles and likely provide key help for antibody production (Table 4-5). CXCR5 is the receptor for CXCL13 (BCA-1), a chemokine produced by stromal cells of the B cell follicle. The function of these follicular $CXCR5^{hi}$ $CD4^+$ T cells, also

Table 4–5 Neonatal Passive Immunity: Placental Passage of Maternal Antibodies

Good Passive Transfer (IgG)	Poor Passive Transfer	No Passive Transfer[a]
Tetanus antitoxin	*B. pertussis* Ab	*Salmonella* somatic (O) Ab
Diphtheria antitoxin	*Shigella flexneri* Ab	*Escherichia coli* H and O Abs
Bordetella pertussis agglutinin	*Streptococcus* Mg Ab	Heterophile Ab
Antistreptolysin Ab		Wassermann Ab
Antistaphylolysin Ab		Natural (anti-A, anti-B) isoagglutinins
Poliomyelitis Ab		Rh saline (complete) agglutinins
Measles-mumps-rubella Ab		Reaginic Ab (IgE)
Herpes simplex Ab		
Haemophilus influenzae Ab (see text)		
Group B streptococcal aB		
Salmonella flagellar (H) Ab		
Rh incomplete (Coombs') Ab		
Immune (anti-A, anti-B) isoagglutinins		
VDRL Ab		
Long-acting thyroid stimulator		
Antinuclear Ab (ANA)		

[a]Mostly IgM.

Ab, antibody; IgE, IgG, immunoglobulins E, G; VDRL, Venereal Disease Research Laboratory [text].

Adapted from Miller ME, Stiehm ER. Immunology and resistance to infection. *In* Remington JS, Klein JO (eds). Infectious Diseases of the Fetus and Newborn Infant, 2nd ed. Philadelphia, WB Saunders, 1983, with permission.

known as T follicular helper cells,[193,194] is discussed in more detail in the section on naïve B cell activation, clonal expansion, immune selection, and T cell help.

The importance of cognate T cell help is clearly illustrated by the phenotype of patients with X-linked hyper–immunoglobulin M (hyper-IgM) syndrome, who have genetic defects in the expression of CD40 ligand.[195] In affected individuals, the marked paucity of immunoglobulin isotypes other than IgM and inability to generate memory B cell responses indicate that these responses critically depend on the engagement of CD40 on B cells by CD40 ligand on T cells. Engagement of CD40 on B cells in conjunction with other signals provided by cytokines, such as IL-4 and IL-21, markedly enhances immunoglobulin production and class switching and B cell survival. OX-40 ligand–OX40 and TNF-α–TNF-α receptor interactions also contribute.[196]

The interaction of CD28 on T cells with CD80 and CD86 on B cells also is important, because inhibition of this interaction markedly impedes T cell–dependent antibody responses, similar to the effects observed in the absence of CD40 signaling.[87,157] Activated and memory $CD4^+$ T cells also express ICOS, a ligand for B7RP-1, which is constitutively expressed on B cells and a variety of other cell types.[158] ICOS co-stimulates the T cell response, and inhibition of ICOS–B7RP-1 interactions impedes the production of IgG and the development of T_H2 responses in mice. The identification of ICOS deficiency as a cause of hypogammaglobulinemia and poor antibody responses to vaccination[197] supports the importance of ICOS-B7RP interactions in humans. Other interactions, such as that between LFA-1 and CD54 (ICAM-1), may enhance T cell–dependent B cell responses,[198] an idea supported by the finding that humans with CD18 deficiency, which is a component of the LFA-1 integrin, have depressed antibody responses after immunization.[199]

Soluble cytokines produced by activated T cells influence the type of immunoglobulin produced by B cells. Experiments in mice in which the IL-2, IL-4, IL-5, or IFN-γ gene or, in some cases, their specific receptors and associated STAT signaling molecules have been disrupted by gene targeting suggest that these cytokines are important for the proper regulation of B cell immunoglobulin isotype expression. For example, inactivation of the IL-4 gene, components of the high-affinity IL-4 receptor, or the STAT-6 protein involved in IL-4 receptor signal transduction results in a greater than 90% decrease in IgE production, whereas the production of other antibody isotypes is largely unperturbed.[200]

Effector T Cell Migration to Relevant Tissues

Once effector T cells have acquired the ability to mediate protective functions, they must migrate to the appropriate tissues for them to be useful. To do so, effector cells also acquire patterns of chemokine receptors and cell adhesion molecules that facilitate entry into inflamed or infected tissues (see Table 4-4).[43,45,201,202] Effector T cells no longer express CCR7, so they are no longer attracted by the homeostatic chemokines produced in the T cell zone of lymphoid tissues (CCL19 and CCL21). The T follicular helper subset of effector $CD4^+$ T cells, which expresses high levels of CXCR5, migrates to B cell follicles, which express CXCL13, the only ligand for this chemokine receptor. By contrast, most T_H1, T_H2, and CD8 effector T cells leave the lymphoid tissues and migrate to extralymphoid target organs. This migration results from the reduction in expression of the lymph node–homing receptor L-selectin and increased or de novo expression of other adhesion molecules that facilitate entry into other tissues, including LFA-1, VLA-4 and, in the case of cells that migrate to the skin, cutaneous lymphocyte antigen (CLA), or, in the case of cells that migrate to the gut, the $\alpha_4\beta_7$ integrin.[140,186] T_H1 cells (and effector $CD8^+$ cells that produce IFN-γ) express CCR5, the chemokine receptor for CCL3 (macrophage inflammatory protein-1α [MIP-1α]), CCL4 (MIP-1β), and CCL5 (RANTES), and CXCR3, the chemokine receptor for CXCL9 (monokine induced by gamma interferon [MIG], CXCL10 (interferon-γ–inducible protein 10 [IP-10]), and CXCL11 (interferon-inducible T-cell α chemoattractant). The former chemokines (CCL3, CCL4, and CCL5) characteristically are produced in inflamed tissues, and the last three (CCL9, CCL10, and CCL11) are specifically produced in response to IFN-γ. These chemokines also are found at sites of effective cell-mediated immune responses, including delayed-type hypersensitivity (DTH) reactions, to which they attract not only T_H1 $CD4^+$ T cells and effector $CD8^+$ T cells but also DCs and monocytes. Conversely, T_H2 T cells uniquely express a receptor for prostaglandin D, CRTH2,[203] and preferentially express CCR2, CCR3, and CCR8, which are receptors for CCL13 (monocyte chemoattractant protein-4 [MCP-4], CCL11, CCL14, and CCL26 (eotaxins 1, 2, and 3), and CCL1 (inflammatory cytokine-309), respectively. These chemokines characteristically are found at sites of allergic responses. As some of their names suggest, these chemokines also attract eosinophils, thus helping to orchestrate concerted T_H2-dependent responses.

Termination of the T Cell Effector Response

To prevent excessive immune responses, active mechanisms for terminating the T cell response operate on multiple levels. CD45 is a protein tyrosine phosphatase that promotes T cell activation by counteracting the phosphorylation of tyrosine residues that inhibit the function of tyrosine kinases involved in T cell activation, such as Lck. Because dimerization of CD45 impedes its phosphatase activity, it is possible that the preferential expression of the low-molecular-weight CD45RO isoform on effector $CD4^+$ T cells may facilitate CD45 dimerization and thereby attenuate the immune response.[204] T cell activation is also limited by the engagement of cytotoxic T lymphocyte antigen-4 (CTLA-4) (i.e., CD152) on the T cell by CD80 and CD86 on the APC. CTLA-4 is expressed mainly on the T cell surface during the later stages of activation. In mice genetically deficient in CTLA-4, a fatal autoimmune syndrome develops that is mediated by $CD4^+$ T cells.[205] How CTLA-4 acts to terminate T cell activation is controversial. Engagement of this molecule has been variously reported to activate inhibitory signaling pathways in the T cell and to induce T cell anergy, apoptosis, and the secretion of antiproliferative cytokines, such as transforming growth factor (TGF)-β.[206] It also is possible that CTLA-4 does not act primarily within conventional antigen-specific $CD4^+$ T cells, but acts mainly within the regulatory T cell subset to facilitate their ability to suppress the function of other T cells (see section on regulatory T cells). A controversial mechanism involves the engagement of CD80 and CD86 on the T cell by CTLA-4 of the regulatory T cell, generating a negative signal that suppresses T cell activation. Similarly, the engagement of the B7 family member PD-1 on activated T cells by its B7 family ligands PDL1 (B7-H1) and PDL2, expressed on APCs (see Table 4-4) and in certain tissues, dampens the effector T cell response.[158]

In addition to attenuating the generation of effector T cells, most effector T cells generated during a robust immune response to infection are eliminated by apoptosis. Evidently, such elimination is achieved by multiple mechanisms. A major mechanism is active induction of apoptosis through death receptors of the TNF ligand gene family and in particular, by Fas ligand. Fas ligand and its receptor, Fas, both are expressed by activated effector T cells (see Table 4-2). Furthermore, at the same time at which IL-2 transduces signals driving the proliferation of activated, effector T cells, it sensitizes them to Fas-induced apoptosis by reducing the expression of molecules that block death signals downstream of Fas.[7,207,208] Other members of the TNF receptor and TNF ligand family also may participate in this process—for example, TNF-α may help to trigger apoptosis by effector $CD8^+$ T cells. Effector $CD8^+$ T cell expansion is limited by perforin and IFN-γ produced by these cells, although the mechanism by which this is mediated is not known.[209]

In addition to these active mechanisms for the induction of apoptosis, T cell activation terminates the expression of the anti-apoptotic Bcl-2 protein. This renders effector T cells dependent on the expression of the related Bcl family member, Bcl-xL, expression of which is driven by cytokines, in particular, cytokines signaling through γc, such as IL-2, IL-7, and IL-15.[171,210] Thus, as the immune response evolves and the availability of these cytokines becomes limiting, apoptosis of effector T cells ensues, owing to a passive, death-by-neglect mechanism.

Memory T Cells

Characteristics and Origins of Memory T Cells. Although greater than 90% of antigen-specific effector T cells generated during a robust primary immune response die, a fraction persist as memory T cells. Memory T cells account for the enhanced secondary T cell response to subsequent challenge—this reflects both the substantially greater frequency of antigen-specific memory T cells (approximately 1:100 to 1:10,000) than that of antigen-specific T cells in a naïve host (approximately 1:100,000 for most antigens), and the enhanced functions of memory compared with those of naïve T cells.[164,211-213] Memory T cells retain many of the functions of the effector T cells that characterized the immune response from which the memory T cells arose. These functions include a lowered threshold for activation and the ability to produce more rapidly the effector cytokines that characterized the effector T cell response from which they arose, that is, T_H1 or T_H2.[156] Turnover of memory T cells occurs slowly, but more rapidly than that of naïve T cells, and memory T cells appear to persist for decades in the absence of further contact with foreign antigenic peptide–MHC complexes.[212]

Our understanding of the key determinants of the genesis of memory T cells remains incomplete. It has been proposed that memory T cells are derived, perhaps stochastically, from a small subset of effector T cells that survive and persist.[212,213] This suggestion is consistent with the estimation that human memory T cells arise from naïve T cell precursors after an average of 14 cell divisions.[214] Alternatively, memory T cells may differentiate directly from naïve T cells rather than through an effector T cell intermediate,[215] or may arise from those T cells that do not proliferate or differentiate to the same extent as for cells that acquire full effector function, or effector T cells that subsequently undergo apoptosis.[156,212] Co-stimulatory interactions, including those between CD28 and CD80 (and CD86) and between CD40 ligand and CD40, seem to play a role in the generation of memory T cells,[174] and humans genetically deficient in CD40 ligand have reduced $CD4^+$ T cell recall responses to previously administered protein vaccines.[216]

Most human memory $CD4^+$ T cells can be distinguished from naïve cells by their surface expression of the CD45RO rather than the CD45RA isoform of CD45 (see Fig. 4-6). In addition, memory and effector T cells typically express higher levels of adhesion molecules, such as the VLA-4 β_1 integrin, than levels observed on naïve T cells (see Table 4-4).[217] About 40% of circulating adult CD4$^+$ T cells have this CD45RA^{lo}CD45RO^{hi} (VLA-4^{hi}) memory/effector surface phenotype. Another 10% to 15% of circulating CD4$^+$ T cells have a CD45RA^{mid}CD45RO^{mid} surface phenotype and memory/effector-like function,[218] but their relationship to CD45RO^{hi} T cells remains unclear. In contrast with memory/effector T cells, most naïve CD4$^+$ T cells have a CD5RA^{hi}-CD45RO^{lo} surface phenotype,[219] although a minority of these CD45RA^{hi} T cells may be revertants from either CD45RO^{hi} or CD45RO^{mid} cells.[217] Such revertants may be more prominent in certain immunopathologic contexts, such as following allogeneic hematopoietic cell transplantation.[220]

Activation and propagation of CD45RA^{hi}CD45RO^{lo} CD4$^+$ T cells in vitro result in their acquisition of memory/effector cell-like features, including a lower threshold for activation, a CD45RA^{lo}CD45RO^{hi} phenotype, an enhanced ability to produce effector cytokines (e.g., IFN-γ, IL-4), and an increased ability to provide help for B cell antibody production.[217,221] These findings support the notion that CD45RA^{hi} T cells are precursors of CD45RO^{hi} T cells, and that this differentiation occurs following T cell activation, and, in addition, are consistent with the observation that the CD45RA^{lo}CD45RO^{hi} cell subset consists mainly of memory T cells that respond to recall antigens.

Memory CD8$^+$ T cells are similar to those of the CD4$^+$ subset in expressing a CD45RA^{lo}CD45RO^{hi} surface phenotype and in possessing an enhanced capacity to produce multiple cytokines compared with that in their naïve precursors.[218,222] In addition, unlike with memory CD4$^+$ T cells, a substantial subset of these CD45RO^{hi} CD8$^+$ T cells express CD11b, CD57, and killer inhibitory receptors (KIRs).[223] KIRs bind self-HLA-A, -B, or -C alleles and deliver an inhibitory signal into the cell. KIRs are expressed at high levels on most or all human NK lymphocytes. The importance of KIR expression by CD8$^+$ T cells remains unclear, but KIRs are hypothesized to regulate effector function, such as cytotoxicity, by raising the threshold for activation by antigenic peptide–MHC complexes. Human effector CD8$^+$ T cells also can be distinguished from circulating naïve CD8$^+$ T cells by surface phenotype: Most human CD8$^+$ effector cells have a CD45RA^{hi}CD27$^-$CD28$^-$ surface phenotype and a high capacity to mediate cytotoxicity and to produce T$_H$1-type effector cytokines, including TNF-α and IFN-γ.[218,222,224] By contrast, naïve CD8$^+$ T cells have a CD45RA^{hi}CD27$^+$CD28$^+$ surface phenotype and a limited ability to mediate cytotoxicity and to secrete these cytokines.

Localization and Homeostasis of Memory T Cells. The localization of memory T cells correlates with and probably is determined by differential expression of adhesion molecules and chemokine receptors. Studies suggest the existence of distinct central (lymphoid homing) and effector (tissue homing) memory T cell populations.[43,156,201] Central memory T cells express on their surface the CCR7 receptor and high levels of L-selectin, the lymph node homing receptor. By contrast, effector memory T cells lack CCR7 and express low levels of L-selectin. In humans, the generation of T$_{H1}$ effector memory CD4$^+$ T cells appears to require intact receptor signaling for IL-12 and IL-23.[225] Central memory T cells demonstrate delayed or limited production of effector cytokines, whereas effector memory T cells rapidly produce these cytokines, including in response to cognate antigen for the TCR.[226] Studies in the mouse also support this notion and suggest that a substantial subset of memory T cells are present in tissues, including the lung, liver, and gut, where they are poised to mediate rapid protection against rechallenge. The central memory subset, found in lymph nodes, is thought to provide a backup and potentially longer-lived reservoir of memory cells. The central memory pool may be a larger fraction of the memory pool for CD4$^+$ than for CD8$^+$ T cells.[43] The specific tissues to (or through) which memory T cells migrate also appear to be determined by the pattern of chemokine receptors and adhesion molecules they express. Those found in the skin express the CLA adhesin and chemokine receptors CCR4 and CCR10, whereas those in the small intestine express the $\alpha_4\beta_7$ integrin and CCR9.[43,45,140,186]

The cellular and molecular interactions that are involved in the generation and maintenance of memory T cells remain incompletely understood. Turnover of memory T cells appears to be much more frequent than that of naïve T cells, suggesting that the process is a dynamic one.[212] Unlike with naïve T cells, the maintenance of memory T cells appears not to require continued contact with self-peptide–MHC complexes. For memory CD8$^+$ T cells, IL-7 and IL-15 appear to be critical for their maintenance.[146,148,212] IL-7 also may be required to promote the transition of effector CD4$^+$ T cells to memory cells.[227] What sustains established memory CD4$^+$ T cells is not known, but neither these nor other cytokines that signal through the γc cytokine receptor chain appear to be required.

Activation of Memory T Cells. When memory T cells re-encounter antigenic peptide–MHC complexes ("recall antigen") as part of the secondary response, they are activated and undergo expansion and differentiation into a secondary effector population (see Fig. 4-6). The secondary immune response to recall antigen is typically more rapid and robust than the primary response to an antigen that has never been encountered previously. This difference is due both to the greater frequency of antigen-specific memory T cells than of naïve T cells with TCRs that recognize the same antigens and to the enhanced function of these memory T cells and their secondary effector progeny.[156,212,213] For example, individual secondary effectors generated from memory CD8$^+$ T cells may express both perforin and effector cytokines, whereas primary effectors generated from naïve CD8$^+$ T cells may express either perforin or cytokines, but not both.

Regulatory T Cells

The phenomenon of T cell–mediated immune suppression—dominant inhibition of the response of one subset of T cells by another—was observed many years ago, and the cells mediating the inhibition were referred to as suppressor T cells.[228] Their nature and even existence remained uncertain, however, until the mid-1990s, when studies by Sakaguchi and colleagues in the mouse and Roncarolo and associates in humans provided evidence that a subset of CD4$^+$ T cells were involved in the active suppression of autoimmunity.[229-231] These regulatory or suppressor T cells are found within the small fraction of circulating human $CD4^+$ T cells that are $CD25^+$. Although not all cells of this phenotype mediate suppression, many do. CD25 is the IL-2 receptor α chain, which, in conjunction with the IL-2 receptor β chain, and the γc cytokine receptor, comprises the high-affinity IL-2 receptor. Regulatory $CD4^+CD25^+$ T cells appear to depend on IL-2 and high-affinity IL-2 receptors for their generation and maintenance.

Regulatory T cells are generated in the thymus during the normal process of positive and negative selection and can also be induced by activation of naïve peripheral $CD4^+$ T cells in the presence of certain cytokines, including IL-10 and type I IFN.[232] Suppression requires activation through the αβ-TCR (e.g., antigenic peptide–MHC), but thereafter, regulatory T cell–mediated suppression is not antigen specific. Different mechanisms of inhibition have been described, including the production of IL-10, TGF-β, or CTLA-4 (the last has been proposed to downregulate T cell responses by engaging their surface CD80 and CD86 molecules, resulting in a negative intracellular signal). In vitro studies suggest that contact-dependent inhibition of the activation of other T cells through an APC-independent process is a major mechanism by which regulatory T cells mediate suppression, although the molecular basis for this inhibition is not known.

Natural Killer T Cells

A small population of circulating human T cells express αβ-TCR but lack expression of both CD4 and CD8 and also express NKR-P1A, the human orthologue of the mouse NK1.1 protein. These features, as well as others, such as CD56 and CD57 surface expression and a developmental dependence on the cytokine IL-15,[233] also are characteristic of NK cells, a non–T cell lymphocyte population. For this reason, these T cells frequently are referred to as NK T cells or natural T cells.

Similar to murine T cells expressing NK1.1, human NK T cells have a restricted repertoire of αβ-TCR (TCR α chains containing the Vα24JαQ segments in association with TCR-β chains containing Vβ11 segments)[234-236] and mainly recognize antigens presented by the nonclassic MHC molecule, CD1d, rather than by MHC class I or class II molecules. The CD1d-restricted antigens that can be recognized by NK T cells include certain lipid molecules, such as α-galactosylceramide,[203,237] as well as certain hydrophobic peptides. Murine studies indicate that NK T cells may be derived from $CD4^{hi}CD8^{hi}$ double-positive thymocytes by the interaction of their αβ-TCR with CD1d; the nature of CD1d-associated ligands in this selection process is unclear.[105]

NK T cells have the ability to secrete high levels of IL-4 and IFN-γ and to express Fas ligand and the TNF-related apoptosis–inducing ligand (TRAIL) on their cell surface on primary stimulation, a capacity not observed with most antigenically naïve αβ T cells.[203,238] The physiologic role of NK T cells remains controversial. Although these cells may contribute to host defense against certain infections, murine studies suggest that NK T cells are negative regulators of certain T cell–mediated immune responses, particularly those involved in autoimmune disease[239] and in graft-versus-host disease following hematopoietic cell transplantation.[240] The regulatory function of NK T cells on autoimmune disease may be relevant in humans, because a decreased number of NK T cells may predispose affected persons to the development of insulin-dependent diabetes mellitus.[241]

T Cell Development and Function in the Fetus and Neonate

Thymic Ontogeny

The fetal liver at 6 to 8 weeks of gestation contains $CD34^+$ lymphoid cells that appear to include prothymocytes, because these lymphoid cells can undergo in vitro differentiation into T-lineage cells.[1,242] Initial colonization of the fetal thymus by prothymocytes, which probably come from the fetal liver, occurs at approximately 8.5 weeks of gestation.[243] Thymocytes expressing proteins that are characteristic of T-lineage cells, including CD4, CD8, and the αβ-TCR–CD3 complex, are found shortly after the initial colonization at 8.5 weeks of gestation.[243] By 12 weeks of gestation, the pattern of expression of a number of other proteins expressed by thymocytes, such as CD2, CD5, CD38, and the CD45 isoforms, matches that in the postnatal thymus. Concurrently, a clear architectural separation between the thymic cortex and medulla is evident,[244] with Hassall's corpuscles observable in the thymic medulla shortly thereafter.[245] By 14 weeks of gestation, the three major human thymocyte subsets (double-negative, double-positive, and mature single-positive) characteristic of the postnatal thymus are found (see Fig. 4-3). Fetal thymocyte expression of the chemokine receptors CXCR4 and CCR5, which also are co-receptors for entry of human immunodeficiency virus (HIV)-1, has been found by 18 to 23 weeks of gestation[246] and is likely to be present earlier.

Medullary DCs in the fetus but not in the adult express high levels of CD80,[247] a ligand for CD28 and CTLA-4. CTLA-4 is expressed not only at the late stages of activation of mature T cells but also by thymocytes.[248] Murine experiments suggest that both CD80 and CD86 participate in negative selection by interaction with CD28; CTLA-4 engagement in this context appears to prevent negative selection. By contrast, some in vitro experiments using human cells suggest that a CD80–CTLA-4 interaction could enhance the process of negative selection,[248] but an in vivo role of CD80 in human fetal thymocyte development remains uncertain. The ICOS co-stimulatory molecule also is prominently expressed by the thymus as early as 17 weeks of gestation.[249] The role of ICOS in human thymocyte development is unclear, because it is not known if B7RP-1, the only identified ligand of ICOS,[250] also is expressed in this tissue. Studies in mice and humans with ICOS deficiency suggest that ICOS is not required for normal thymocyte development.[197,251]

Thymic cellularity increases dramatically during the second and third trimesters of fetal gestation. Transient thymic involution, mainly the loss of cortical double-positive ($CD4^{hi}CD8^{hi}$) thymocytes, which is evident within 1 day after birth, probably begins at the end of the third trimester.[252] This involution may be a consequence of the elevation in circulating levels of glucocorticoids that occurs during the third trimester before delivery. Thymic recovery is evident by 1 month following delivery and is paralleled by a sharp decline in glucocorticoid levels within hours after birth.[252] This transient involution is followed by a resumption of increased thymic cellularity, with peak thymus size attained at about age 10 years. When complete thymectomy is performed during the first year of life, subsequent circulating numbers of $CD4^+$ and $CD8^+$ T cells are decreased, indicating the importance of postnatal production of thymocytes for maintenance of the peripheral T cell compartment.[253]

After puberty, the thymus involutes, with the gradual replacement of the cortex and medulla by fat. Single-positive thymocytes within the medulla are relatively spared during the involutionary process, in comparison with double-positive thymocytes in the cortex.[254] Nevertheless, the thymus of adults remains active[255] and is capable of increasing its output of antigenically naïve T cells in response to severe T cell lymphopenia (e.g., following intense cytoablative chemotherapy[256] or treatment with highly active combination antiretroviral therapy for HIV infection[257]). The mechanisms by which increased thymocytopoiesis is triggered by severe lymphopenia is unclear but may include the increased production of IL-7.[258]

Fetal and Neonatal T Cell Receptor Repertoire

The generation of the αβ-TCR repertoire by the process of V(D)J recombination of the TCR α and TCR β genes probably occurs within a few days after colonization of the thymus by prothymocytes. The usage of D and J segments in rearrangement of the TCR β chain gene in the thymus at approximately 8 weeks of gestation is less diverse than at 11 to 13 weeks of gestation or subsequently.[259,260] This restriction is not explained by an effect of positive or negative selection in the thymus, because it applies to D-to-J rearrangements, which are not expressed on the immature thymocyte cell surface.[259,261] The CDR3 region of the TCR β chain transcripts is reduced in length and sequence diversity in the human fetal thymus between 8 and 15 weeks of gestation, probably owing to decreased amounts of the TdT enzyme, which performs N-nucleotide addition during V(D)J recombination.[259-262] TdT activity and CDR3 length both are increased by the second trimester,[259-261] and Vβ and Vα segment usage in the thymus and peripheral lymphoid organs is diverse.[260,261,263,264] The αβ-TCR repertoire of cord blood T cells that is expressed on the cell surface is characterized by a diversity of TCR β usage and CDR3 length that is similar to that of antigenically naïve T cells in adults and infants, indicating that the functional preimmune repertoire is fully formed by birth.[265-267]

Because the CDR3 region of the TCR chains is a major determinant of antigen specificity,[118] decreased CDR3 diversity, in conjunction with restricted usage of V(D)J segments, theoretically could limit recognition of foreign antigens by the fetal αβ-TCR repertoire, particularly during the first trimester. The effects of any potential "holes" in the αβ-TCR repertoire of the human fetus from limitations in CDR3 are likely to be subtle, however, particularly after the second trimester, when V segment usage is diverse. This is suggested by the fact that the T cell response to immunization and viral challenge generally is normal in mice that are completely deficient in TdT as a result of selective gene targeting.[268]

Repertoire analysis using CDR3 spectratyping suggests that there is greater oligoclonal expansion of αβ T cells during the third trimester, particularly after 28 weeks of gestation, than in adults, and that these oligoclonal expansions involve a variety of different Vβ segment families.[269] Whether this oligoclonal expansion is antigen driven, such as by a response to maternally derived immunoglobulins (e.g., immunoglobulin idiotypes),[269] or is a form of homeostatic proliferation is unknown.

Positive selection of thymocytes appears to be an important influence on the αβ-TCR repertoire during human fetal and neonatal development. This influence can be assessed by determining if the frequency of preimmune (antigenically naïve) αβ T cells, such as those predominantly found in the healthy neonate, expressing a particular V segment is skewed toward either $CD4^+$ or $CD8^+$ T cells. Such skewing suggests that these particular V segments have been positively selected primarily by MHC class II or class I molecules, respectively. Analysis of neonatal T cells found that Vα12.1 segments were expressed at a higher frequency by $CD8^+$ T cells, whereas Vβ6.7, Vβ8, and Vβ12 segments were expressed at a higher frequency by $CD4^+$ T cells.[270-272] This skewing also is evident in the frequency with which these V segments are expressed by $CD4^{hi}CD8^-$ thymocytes versus $CD4^-CD8^{hi}$ thymocytes in the infant.[273] Skewing also occurs when human fetal liver is used as a source of stem cells to reconstitute human fetal thymic development in SCID mice.[264]

T Cell Receptor Excision Circles

T cell receptor excision circles (TRECs) are generated during TCR gene rearrangement of thymocytes. TRECs appear to persist for long periods in T-lineage cells that are not proliferating, and the TREC content of peripheral T cells has been used clinically to assess thymic output. Although TRECs are generated at each rearrangement step of the TCR α and TCR β chain genes, those generated during Vα to Jα joining, and which contain TCR δ gene locus, have been the most frequently employed for human studies. Among human thymocyte subsets, the highest levels of TCR δ locus–containing TRECs are in $CD4^{hi}CD8^{hi}CD3^-$ double-positive thymocytes (approximately 150 TRECs per 100 cells), suggesting that both TCR α chain gene alleles commonly undergo rearrangement.[274] TREC levels progressively decline as double-positive cells acquire high levels of the αβ-TCR–CD3 complex, in all likelihood reflecting mitosis that results from successful positive selection.[274]

Consistent with this model, the TREC content of adult antigenically naïve T cells is significantly higher than that of memory T cells, which have undergone marked clonal expansion. TREC levels in unfractionated T cells or purified naïve T cell populations have been used to monitor the recovery of thymic output and T cell reconstitution in various clinical situations. These studies, however, have generally assumed that naïve T cells have not undergone mitosis as a result of post-thymic, antigen-independent mechanisms, such as homeostatic proliferation.[275] In fact, such homeostatic proliferation of naïve peripheral T cells may occur in humans in cases of peripheral T cell destruction, such as HIV-1 infection, resulting in decreased TREC content and a potential underestimate of thymic output.[276]

Ontogeny of T Cell Surface Phenotype

Circulating T cells are detectable as early as 12.5 weeks of gestation, demonstrating the emigration of mature T-lineage cells from the thymus.[277] By 14 weeks of gestation, $CD4^+$ and $CD8^+$ T cells are found in the fetal liver and spleen, and $CD4^+$ T cells are detectable in lymph nodes.[278] The percentage of T cells in the fetal or premature circulation gradually increases during the second and third trimesters of pregnancy through approximately 6 months of age,[279] followed by a gradual decline to adult levels during childhood.[280] The ratio of $CD4^+$ to $CD8^+$ T cells in the circulation is relatively high during fetal life (about 3.5) and gradually declines with age.[280] The levels of expression of the αβ-TCR, CD3, CD4, CD5, CD8, and CD28 proteins on fetal and neonatal αβ T cells are similar to those in adult T cells (D. Lewis, unpublished data, 2000).[98,281,282]

CD31. CD31, also known as platelet endothelial cell adhesion molecule-1 (PECAM-1), is expressed in large amounts on most adult peripheral $CD4^+$ T cells that have a naïve ($CD45RA^{hi}$) surface phenotype but is absent or decreased on most memory $CD4^+$ T cells. With aging, the fraction of adult $CD45RA^{hi}$ $CD4^+$ T cells that are $CD31^{lo}$ gradually increases, and these cells have a very low TREC content relative to with that of the $CD31^{hi}$ $CD45RA^{hi}$ subset of $CD4^+$ T cells.[283] These $CD31^{lo}$ naïve $CD4^+$ T cells do not appear to contain CD45RO cells that have reverted to a CD45RA surface phenotype, because they lack the capacity to express cytokines characteristic of memory/effector cells, such as IFN-γ, and do not share any cell surface phenotype markers with $CD45RO^{hi}$ memory $CD4^+$ T cells. These findings suggest that $CD31^{lo}$ naïve $CD4^+$ T cells are derived from $CD31^{hi}$ naïve $CD4^+$ T cells by a process of homeostatic proliferation in the periphery, and that $CD31^{hi}CD45RA^{hi}$ T cells have more recently emigrated from the thymus than have $CD31^{lo}$ cells.

Most neonatal $CD45RA^{hi}$ T cells are $CD31^{hi}$, but approximately 10% to 20% have been reported to be $CD31^{lo}$.[283,284] Neonatal $CD45RA^{hi}$ $CD4^+$ T cells tend to have a modestly higher TREC content than that of adult $CD45RA^{hi}$ $CD4^+$ T cells, suggesting that TREC content may gradually decline in peripheral naïve $CD4^+$ T cells with time.[283] It is unclear if the neonatal $CD31^{lo}$ subset of naïve $CD4^+$ T cells has low levels of TREC similar to that found in adult $CD31^{lo}$ naïve $CD4^+$ T cells. Such low levels would suggest that these $CD31^{lo}$ naïve $CD4^+$ T cells in the fetal and neonatal circulation have proliferated or are currently in the process of proliferating, a possibility that is supported by one study[123] (see section on fetal and neonatal thymic output and peripheral T cell homeostasis). Alternatively, a finding of high TREC content in $CD31^{lo}$ naïve $CD4^+$ T cells of the neonate would suggest that this population may be an immature population that gives rise to $CD31^{hi}$ naïve $CD4^+$ T cells.

CD38. CD38 is an ectoenzyme that generates cyclic adenosine diphosphate (ADP)-ribose, a metabolite that induces intracellular calcium mobilization. It is expressed on most thymocytes, some activated peripheral blood T cells and B cells, plasma cells, and DCs. Unlike adult naïve T cells, virtually all peripheral fetal and neonatal T cells express the CD38 molecule,[285-288] suggesting that peripheral T cells in the fetus and neonate may represent a thymocyte-like immature transitional population. In contrast with circulating T cells, a significant fraction of T cells in the fetal spleen between 14 and 20 weeks of gestation lack CD38 expression,[289] indicating that CD38 may be downregulated on entry into secondary lymphoid tissue. Neonatal $CD4^+$ T cells lose expression of CD38 after in vitro culture with IL-7 for 10 days,[290] which implies that this cytokine promotes further maturation independently of engagement of the αβ-TCR–CD3 complex. The precursor-product relationship between $CD38^+$ and $CD38^-$ peripheral naïve T cells in humans is unclear.

The role of CD38 in the function of human T cells and other cell types also is unknown. In mice, CD38 is required for chemokine-mediated migration of mature DCs into secondary lymphoid tissue, and as a consequence, CD38 deficiency impairs humoral immunity to T cell–dependent antigens. Of interest, mice, in contrast with humans, have relatively low levels of thymocyte expression of CD38, and CD38 deficiency in these animals does not have a clear impact on thymocyte development or intrinsic T cell function.

CD45 Isoforms. Circulating T cells in the term and preterm (22 to 30 weeks of gestation) neonate and in the second- and third-trimester fetus predominantly express a $CD45RA^{hi}$-$CD45RO^{lo}$ surface phenotype,[288,291,292] which also is found on antigenically naïve T cells of adults. About 30% of circulating T cells of the term neonate are $CD45RA^{lo}CD45RO^{lo}$,[293] a surface phenotype that is rare or absent in circulating adult T cells. Because these $CD45RA^{lo}CD45RO^{lo}$ T cells are functionally similar to neonatal $CD45RA^{hi}CD45RO^{lo}$ T cells, and become $CD45RA^{mid}CD45RO^{lo}$ T cells when incubated in vitro with fibroblasts,[293] they appear to be immature thymocyte-like cells rather than naïve cells that have been activated in vivo to express the CD45RO isoform.

Most studies have found that the healthy neonate and the late-gestation fetus lack circulating $CD45RO^{hi}$ T cells, consistent with their limited exposure to foreign antigens. A lack of surface expression of other memory/effector markers, such as β_1 integrins (e.g., VLA-4), and, in the case of $CD8^+$ T cells, KIR[294] and CD11b,[295,296] also is consistent with an antigenically naïve population predominating in the healthy neonate.

A postnatal precursor-product relationship between $CD45RA^{hi}CD45RO^{lo}$ and $CD45RA^{lo}CD45RO^{hi}$ T cells is suggested by the fact that the proportion of αβ T cells with a memory/effector phenotype and the capacity of circulating T cells to produce cytokines, such as IFN-γ, both gradually increase, whereas the proportion of antigenically naïve T cells decreases, with increasing postnatal age.[280,297] These increases in the ability to produce cytokines and expression of the $CD45RO^{hi}$ phenotype presumably are due to cumulative antigenic exposure and T cell activation, leading to the generation of memory T cells from antigenically naïve T cells.

In premature or term neonates who are stressed, a portion of circulating T-lineage cells are $CD3^{lo}$ and co-express CD1, CD4, and CD8,[285] a phenotype characteristic of immature thymocytes of the cortex.[298] It is likely that stress results in the premature release of cortical thymocytes into the circulation, but the immunologic consequences of this release are unclear.

Fetal and Neonatal Thymic Output and Peripheral T Cell Homeostasis

Phenotype of Recent Thymic Emigrants. Recent thymic emigrants (RTEs) have been variously defined as peripheral T cells that have emigrated from the thymus within 2 weeks to several months. Some authorities have even considered circulating naïve T cells in the term neonate to be synonymous with RTEs.[290] This population, however, is likely to contain substantial numbers of thymic emigrants (and their extrathymically generated descendants) that exited the thymus more than 6 months earlier. RTEs would be expected to be enriched for TRECc compared with other naïve CD4$^+$ T cells that have been out in the periphery for longer periods of time, because these older cells would have had a greater opportunity to undergo antigen-independent (spontaneous) proliferation.

Based on the criterion of TREC enrichment, the expression of CD103 ($\alpha_E\beta_7$ integrin) by circulating naïve CD45RA^{hi} CD8$^+$ T cells[299] is a potential marker for CD8$^+$ T-lineage RTEs. Consistent with the high activity of thymus during the last trimester, between 6% and 20% of circulating neonatal naïve CD8$^+$ T cells are CD103$^+$, whereas substantially lower numbers of these cells are found in the adult circulation.[300] As discussed earlier, CD31 also identifies adult naïve CD45RA^{hi} CD4$^+$ T cells that have higher levels of TREC than the CD31$^-$ fraction of this cell population. This finding suggests that CD31 loss may occur with some form of antigen-independent proliferation of naïve CD4$^+$ T cells, and that RTEs of the CD4$^+$ T lineage are likely to be CD31^{hi}. However, because about 90% of neonatal and greater than 80% of adult naïve CD4$^+$ T cells are CD31^{hi}, only a small fraction of these CD31^{hi} cells are likely to be RTEs, if "recent" is defined as weeks to months. CCR9 expression also has recently been found to be greater on CD45RA^{hi} CD4$^+$ T cells in the newborn and infant than in older persons, suggesting that this could also enrich for CD4$^+$ T-lineage cell RTEs.[301] These circulating CCR9$^+$ cells have not been analyzed for their TREC content, however. The development of additional markers for RTEs, particularly of the CD4$^+$ T cell lineage, and additional studies of TREC content for naïve T cell populations identified using these markers may allow a more accurate assessment of thymic output at various ages of fetal and postnatal life.

Spontaneous Naïve Peripheral T Cell Proliferation. Naïve T cells may undergo proliferation by processes that are distinct from those of full activation by cognate antigen and appropriate co-stimulation, and such proliferative processes may make a significant contribution to expansion of the peripheral T cell pool during development. Based on flow cytometric analysis of expression of the Ki67 antigen, a significantly higher fraction of naïve (CD45RO^{lo}) CD4$^+$ and CD8$^+$ T cells in the third-trimester fetus and the term neonate are spontaneously in cell cycle than the fraction of adult naïve T cells.[123] The highest levels are observed at 26 weeks of gestation, and these gradually decline with gestational age. Even at term, however, the frequencies reported for naïve CD4$^+$ and CD8$^+$ T cells—approximately 1.4% and 3.2%, respectively—are sevenfold those of adult naïve T cells and are substantially higher than those observed for adult CD45RO^{hi} T cells.[123] These results are supported by other in vitro assays of mitosis, such as the incorporation of radioactive tritiated (^{3}H)-thymidine or the loss of fluorescence after labeling cell membranes with carboxyfluorescein succinimidyl ester (CFSE) (D. Lewis, unpublished data, 2003).

Although the mechanism underlying this proliferation of human fetal and neonatal naïve T cells is unclear, it differs from that in rodent models of homeostatic proliferation, including in the neonatal mouse,[302] in that the proliferation occurs in the absence of peripheral lymphopenia. As discussed next, one potential explanation for this increased spontaneous proliferation is an increased sensitivity of fetal and neonatal T cells to cytokines, such as IL-7 and IL-15. It will be of interest in future studies to determine if spontaneously proliferating naïve T cells in fetus and neonate have a diverse TCR repertoire (as would be predicted by a model of generalized increased sensitivity to cytokines) and whether they can be distinguished from noncycling cells by other markers, such as those that are induced during naïve T cell proliferation in the setting of peripheral lymphopenia, and by reduced TREC content.

Antigen-Independent Naïve T Cell Proliferation in Response to IL-7 and IL-15. Murine studies show that the homeostatic proliferation in the lymphopenic host and survival of naïve CD4$^+$ and CD8$^+$ T cells depends on IL-7.[148,258,303,304] Since human neonatal naïve CD4$^+$ T cells are capable of higher levels of polyclonal cell proliferation than adult naïve CD4$^+$ T cells in response to IL-7,[123,305-307] it is plausible that IL-7–dependent proliferation could account for the high rate of spontaneous CD4$^+$ T cell proliferation in the human fetus and neonate, and contribute to the normal and rapid expansion of the peripheral CD4$^+$ T cell compartment at this age. The increased IL-7 proliferative response is associated with increased expression of the IL-7 receptor α chain component by neonatal naïve CD4$^+$ T cells compared with adult naïve CD4$^+$ T cells,[305-307] although surface expression of the other component of the IL-7 receptor, the γc cytokine receptor was actually decreased on neonatal naïve CD4$^+$ T cells compared with that on adult naïve cells in one study.[307]

Murine studies indicate that positive selection results in a dramatic upregulation of both the IL-7 receptor α chain and the γc cytokine receptor on CD4– and CD8–single-positive thymocytes.[308] In vitro thymic organ culture experiments suggest that IL-7 plays a key role in the postselection expansion of the single-positive thymocyte population by a mechanism that does not involve $\alpha\beta$-TCR engagement.[308] Therefore, it is plausible that this increased ability to proliferate in response to IL-7 might particularly be a feature of RTEs, and that the naïve neonatal CD4$^+$ T cell compartment is enriched in cells with these properties.[306] Another possibility, not mutually exclusive, is that neonatal naïve CD4$^+$ T cells may retain thymocyte features, such as a proapoptotic tendency and high levels of IL-7 receptor expression, for substantially longer periods of time following thymic emigration than is the case with adult naïve CD4$^+$ T cells. In support of this "maturational" arrest model is the observation that virtually all neonatal T cells and thymocytes express high levels of CD38, whereas this marker is virtually absent from adult naïve T cells.

Whether IL-7 not only contributes to extrathymic expansion of naïve CD4$^+$ T cells but also influences their maturation remains unclear. IL-7 treatment of neonatal naïve CD4$^+$ T cells for relatively long periods (7 or 14 days) does not decrease expression of CD45RA or L-selectin and does not increase the expression of CD45RO.[290,305,309,310] The extent to which IL-7 treatment, alone, of neonatal naïve CD4$^+$ T cells results in acquisition of a phenotype with selective features of both naïve and memory/effector cells remains contentious: Results are conflicting regarding whether IL-7 treatment increases surface expression of CD11a, a memory/effector cell marker; the activation-dependent proteins CD25 and CD40 ligand; or the capacity of neonatal CD4$^+$ T cells to produce T_H1 and T_H2 cytokines.[290,305]

In contrast with IL-7, IL-15 is not required for naïve T cell survival and has its most important effects on the CD8$^+$

rather than the $CD4^+$ subset of effector/memory T cells.[311] These findings do not, however, eliminate a possible role for IL-15 in naïve T cell expansion in certain contexts, such as in the fetus and neonate. Consistent with this possible role, neonatal naïve $CD8^+$ T cells are more responsive to treatment with a combination of IL-7 and IL-15 than is the analogous adult cell population, as indicated by loss of CFSE staining with culture after in vitro labeling.[123] Whether this enhanced effect is related to increased levels of IL-15 receptors on neonatal T cells is unknown. Also unclear are the effects of treatment with this combination of cytokines on neonatal naïve $CD8^+$ T cell phenotype and function.

Fetal Extrathymic T Cell Differentiation

The human fetal liver contains rearranged VDJ transcripts of the TCR β chain as early as 7.5 weeks of gestation, and pre-Tα transcripts can be found as early 6 weeks of gestation.[312,313] This raises the possibility that extrathymic differentiation of αβ-TCR–bearing T cells could occur in the fetal liver before such differentiation in the thymus. In the adult liver, $CD4^{hi}CD8^-$ and $CD4^-CD8^-$ T cells with characteristics distinct from those of NK T cells (which also may have, in part, an extrathymic origin) have been described in conjunction with detection of transcripts for pre-Tα and the RAG genes. Thus, it is possible that some liver T cells may be generated in situ even in adults.

Extrathymic differentiation of αβ T cells may occur in the fetal intestine, because the lamina propria of the fetal intestine contains $CD3^-CD7^+$ lymphocytes expressing pre-Tα transcripts as early as 12 to 14 weeks of gestation, and these cells have the capacity to differentiate into αβ T cells.[314] Although it is unclear if these $CD3^-CD7^+$ precursors cells have a thymic or other origin, the Vβ repertoire of αβ T-lineage cells in the fetal intestine differs substantially from that of contemporaneous fetal αβ T-lineage cells found in the circulation, suggesting their independent origin.[314] Extrathymic intestinal T cell development has been clearly shown to occur in mice in specialized structures of the small intestine (cryptopatches), but no analogous structures containing immature lymphocytes have been observed in humans.[315] In humans, the lamina propria and epithelium of the jejunum are potential sites of extrathymic T cell development in adults, in that immature lymphocytes with markers indicative of T-lineage commitment ($CD2^+CD7^+CD3^-$) are found at these sites. These cells co-localize with transcripts for pre-Tα and the RAG-1 gene,[316] consistent with this tissue being a site of T cell differentiation.

Fetal and Neonatal T Cell Function

In Vitro Assays of T Cell Activation. Before presenting results of studies in which fetal and neonatal versus adult T cell activation and function have been compared, we shall consider some limitations of prior in vitro studies of human T cells. As discussed in detail earlier, naïve T cell activation follows engagement of the αβ-TCR–CD3 complex by cognate peptide antigen presented on MHC molecules on the APC, most typically a DC. Full activation usually requires additional co-stimulatory interactions, such as engagement of CD28 on the T cell by CD80 or by CD86 on the APC (see Figs. 4-1 and 4-5), although many others may also play a role, depending on the in vivo context. In many earlier studies of human T cells, the cells were polyclonally activated with mitogenic lectins, such as phytohemagglutinin (PHA), concanavalin A (Con A), or pokeweed mitogen (PWM). These mitogens appear to cross-link surface molecules involved in T cell activation, such as CD3 or CD28, and probably many others, as well as surface molecules on APCs. Their precise mode of molecular action is not known, however. In the last 2 decades, monoclonal antibodies (mAbs) with defined specificity for surface proteins also have been used as polyclonal T cell activators. MAbs reactive with the CD3-ε protein are used, alone or in conjunction with anti-CD28 mAb. Anti-CD28 mAb is used to mimic the co-stimulatory effect of engagement of CD28 by CD80 or CD86. Neither mitogenic lectins nor mAbs, however, fully mimic the intracellular signal transduction events that occur after physiologic activation of T cells by APCs presenting antigen peptides. For example, the effects on T cell intracellular signaling following engagement of CD28 by mAb differs substantially from that observed following engagement by CD80 and CD86, the physiologic ligands.[317] Depending on the experimental conditions, the epitope recognized, and the form of the mAb (e.g., bivalent versus monovalent, with or without Fc domains), mAbs to a surface molecule may act as either agonists or antagonists of that molecule's function.

Furthermore, most studies comparing neonatal versus adult T cell activation have used unfractionated T cells or unpurified circulating mononuclear cells. Memory T cells, however, generally have more robust signaling and activation-induced gene expression than are seen in naïve T cells, including responses induced by anti-CD3 mAb or by antigenic peptide–MHC complexes.[318-322] Naïve T cells also seem to be particularly dependent on co-stimulation through engagement of CD28, whereas memory T cells are less so and may use a variety of other co-stimulatory pathways.[323] Therefore, studies in which neonatal T cells were compared with naïve T cells from adults are more likely to indicate bona fide ontogenetically related differences in activation or effector function than are studies with unpurified cells.

Fetal T Cell Function. A minority but substantial proportion of T cells in the second trimester fetal spleen are $CD45RA^{lo}$-$CD45RO^{hi}$, a T cell population that is absent from the spleen of young infants.[292] These fetal $CD45RO^{hi}$ T cells express high levels of CD25 (IL-2 receptor α chain) and proliferate with IL-2, suggesting that they have recently been activated and undergone expansion.[292] In contrast with adult $CD45RO^{hi}$ T cells, however, these fetal spleen $CD45RO^{hi}$ T cells express low surface levels of CD2 and LFA-1 and proliferate poorly after activation with either anti-CD2 or anti-CD3 mAb, suggesting that they are not fully functional.[292] Their αβ-TCR repertoire is diverse, suggesting that these T cells are expanding in a non–antigen-specific manner. Such antigen-independent expansion can occur in cases where the number of niches for T cells in the peripheral lymphoid tissue is large relative to the number of T cells (e.g., following adoptive transfer of T cells into lymphopenic recipients).[146] It also is plausible that this may be the case in the rapidly growing fetus, particularly early in gestation. Whether these fetal spleen $CD45RO^{hi}$ T cells contribute to the postnatal T cell compartment, however, is unknown.

Mucosal T cells are present in the fetal intestine by 15 to 16 weeks of gestation, and these cells have the capacity to secrete substantial amounts of IFN-γ after treatment with anti-CD3 mAb in combination with exogenous IFN-α.[324] IFN-α directs differentiation of naïve CD4+ T cells, including those of the neonate, toward a T_H1 effector cytokine profile dominated by production of IFN-γ and not IL-4, IL-5, or IL-13.[56] A similar mechanism may occur in these fetal explant cultures. Although it is not clear what T cell type is the major source of IFN-γ in this tissue, these observations suggest the possibility that a similar T_H1 skewing of T cell responses might occur in cases of fetal viral infection involving the intestine in which type I IFN (IFN-α/β) is induced.

Neonatal T Cell Proliferation and IL-2 Production and Responsiveness after Activation in Vitro. Most studies have found that in response to stimulation in vitro with mitogenic lectins, bacterial superantigens, or allogeneic cells proliferation, as assessed by incorporation of ^{3}H-thymidine, and IL-2 production by circulating neonatal T cells and by adult T cells is similar.[265,325-331] This argues that the limitations in proximal signal transduction for neonatal T cells may not be of functional consequence, at least for cytokine production and initial DNA synthesis in response to strong stimuli.

In general, neonatal T cells, nearly all of which are naïve, and antigenically naïve (CD45RA^{hi}) adult T cells do not proliferate as well or produce as much IL-2 as unfractionated adult T cells after activation by anti-CD2 or anti-CD3 mAb.[221,332-335] These differences might be attributable, at least in part, to the presence of large numbers of memory T cells in the adult but not the neonatal T cell populations, which, as discussed earlier, are more responsive to anti-CD2 or anti-CD3 mAb stimulation.

Studies in which antigenically naïve CD45RA^{hi} CD4+ T cells from neonates and adults were directly compared also have found decreased responses by neonatal cells, however. For example, compared with adult naïve CD4+ T cells, neonatal naïve CD4+ T cells produced less IL-2 mRNA and expressed fewer high-affinity IL-2 receptors in response to stimulation with anti-CD2 mAb.[336-338] These differences were abrogated when phorbol ester, which bypasses proximal signaling pathways, was included,[336] suggesting that the capacity to express IL-2 and high-affinity receptors is not absolutely limited for neonatal cells, but signals leading to their induction may not be transmitted efficiently. Similarly, the production of IL-2 by neonatal naïve CD4+ T cells is reduced compared with that by adult CD45RA^{hi} CD4+ T cells after allogeneic stimulation with adult monocyte-derived DCs (D. Lewis, unpublished data, 2004), again arguing that neonatal cells may be intrinsically limited in their ability to be physiologically activated for IL-2 production.

The ability of activated T cells to efficiently divide in response to IL-2 depends on the expression of high-affinity IL-2 receptors, which consists of CD25 (IL-2 receptor α chain), β chain (shared with the IL-15 receptor), and the γc cytokine receptor (shared with multiple other cytokine receptors). In contrast with IL-2 production, neonatal T cells appear to express similar or higher amounts of CD25 after stimulation with anti-CD3 mAb.[326] This finding is consistent with the signal transduction pathways leading to the induction of CD25 being distinct from those involved in IL-2 production, and with neonatal T cells have a relatively selective limitation in signals required for cytokine production, rather than a generalized limitation acting at an early step of the activation cascade. Basal expression of the γc cytokine receptor by neonatal T cells is lower than that by either adult CD45RA^{hi} or CD45RO^{hi} T cells.[339] The importance of this finding is unclear, because activated neonatal T cells proliferate in response to exogenous IL-2 as well as or better than adult T cells, as indicated by ^{3}H-thymidine incorporation.[326] Radioactive thymidine incorporation assays, however, do not provide mitotic information at the single cell level and examine only DNA synthesis and not actual cell proliferation. The application of recently developed techniques, such as cell membrane staining with CFSE,[340] which allows an assessment of the mitotic history of individual cells, should be helpful in better defining the replicative potential of neonatal T cells.

Two in vitro studies suggest that neonatal T cells may be less able to differentiate into effector cells in response to neoantigen (see section on neonatal T cell co-stimulation and anergy). One study, using limiting dilution techniques and circulating mononuclear cells from CMV-nonimmune donors, found that the frequency of neonatal T cells proliferating in response to whole inactivated CMV antigen was significantly less than that of adult T cells.[97] A pitfall of this study is that it used a complex antigen preparation, and one to which the T cells of adults might have previously been primed by infections other than CMV. Another study[341] found that neonatal mononuclear cells had decreased antigen-specific T cell proliferation and IL-2 production in response to a protein neoantigen, keyhole limpet hemocyanin, compared with those in adult cells. Although these results require confirmation, they are consistent with the more limited ability of neonatal naïve CD4+ T cells to produce IL-2 in response to allogeneic DCs than that of adult naïve cells (D. Lewis, unpublished data, 2004).

Neonatal T Cell Cytokine and Chemokine Production. In contrast with IL-2, the production of most other cytokines or their cognate mRNAs by unfractionated neonatal T cells or the CD4+ T cell subset appears to be reduced in response to multiple stimuli, including anti-CD3 mAb mitogen, or pharmacologic agents (e.g., the combination of calcium ionophore and phorbol ester) compared with that in adult T cells. For most cytokines (IL-3, IL-4, IL-5, IL-6, IL-10, IL-13, IFN-γ, and GM-CSF), this is a marked reduction[326,342-347]; for a few, such as TNF-α,[348] the reduction is modest. As with neonatal T cells, naïve T cells from adults have a reduced capacity to produce most of these cytokines compared with that of adult memory/effector T cells,[347,349,350] although adult naïve T cells may produce substantial amounts of IL-13.[351] The low capacity of neonatal T cells to produce IFN-γ and IL-4 is due to an almost complete absence of IFN-γ and IL-4 mRNA–expressing cells,[343] which is paralleled by a lack of cells expressing detectable levels of these cytokines following polyclonal activation and analysis by flow cytometry after intracellular staining.[352-355]

These results suggest that part of the deficiency in cytokine production by neonatal T cells is due to the fact that almost all neonatal T cells are naïve. But are naïve neonatal T cells equivalent to adult naïve T cells in cytokine production? We have found that highly purified naïve CD4+ T cells from neonates have a reduced capacity to produce IFN-γ in vitro compared with that of adult naïve CD4+ T cells following stimulation with the same pool of monocyte-derived DCs from multiple unrelated blood donors.[356] This finding strongly suggests that the capacity of neonatal naïve $CD4^+$ T cells to produce IFN-γ is intrinsically more limited, even when a potent, physiologic APC population is used for antigen presentation.

Cytokine production by neonatal $CD8^+$ T cells has not been as well characterized as for the $CD4^+$ T cell subset. The lack of a memory ($CD45RO^{hi}$) $CD8^+$ T cell subset in the neonate appears to account for reduced production of the chemokine RANTES (CCL5) by neonatal T cells compared with that by adult cells.[357] A striking result, which needs to be confirmed, is that neonatal naïve $CD8^+$ T cells produce substantially more IL-13, which is characteristic of T_H2 immune responses, than that produced by analogous adult cells after stimulation with anti-CD3 and anti-CD28 mAbs and exogenous IL-2.[358] It will be of interest to determine if this unusual cytokine profile also applies to antigen-specific immune responses mediated by neonatal $CD8^+$ T cells, such as to viral pathogens.

Neonatal T cells have been intensively studied for their cytokine secretion phenotype, but relatively little is known regarding the postnatal ontogeny of T cell cytokine production during the first year of life. A study using PHA as a stimulus found that the capacity of peripheral blood lymphocytes obtained from newborns was similar to umbilical vein cord blood in having a low capacity to produce IFN-γ, IL-4, and IL-10.[359] The capacity of peripheral blood lymphocytes to produce all three of these cytokines gradually increased during the first year of life,[359] consistent with the acquisition of increased cytokine production as a result of the progressive acquisition of memory T cells resulting from exposure to foreign antigens.

Mechanisms for Decreased Cytokine Production in Neonatal T Cell. Secretion of most cytokines by T cells requires de novo transcription and translation of the cytokine gene. Cytokine induction by T cells is a complex process involving multiple signal transduction pathways that become active following engagement of the αβ-TCR–CD3 complex and co-stimulatory molecules,[204,360] which culminates in the intranuclear accumulation of transcription factors required for cytokine gene expression, including members of the NFAT, nuclear factor-κB (NF-κB)/Rel, and AP-1 (fos/jun) families.[361] For many cytokine genes, a key event leading to de novo gene transcription is an activation-induced increase in the concentration of free intracellular calcium ($[Ca^{2+}]_i$), which is required for NFAT nuclear location and transcriptional activity.[361]

Certain studies comparing adult and neonatal T cells or $CD4^+$ T cells have suggested that neonatal T cells have substantial limitations in proximal signal transduction events that are required for the expression of cytokine genes and other activation-dependent molecules, such as CD40 ligand and Fas ligand. These limitations include a generalized decrease in the overall level of activation-induced tyrosine phosphorylation of intracellular proteins compared with that in unfractionated adult T cells,[335] decreased activation-induced phosphorylation of CD3-ε, decreased phosphorylation and enzyme activity of the Lck and ZAP-70 tyrosine kinases and the ERK2, JNK, and p38 kinases,[362] and reduced basal and activation-induced levels of phospholipase C isoenzymes.[363] It remains unclear if these reported deficiencies in proximal signal transduction events apply specifically to neonatal naïve T cells but not to adult naïve T cells, because these studies did not fractionate adult T cells into naïve and memory subsets. One study has found that highly purified neonatal naïve $CD4^+$ T cells have a substantially reduced increase in $[Ca^{2+}]_i$ following anti-CD3 mAb cross-linkage, compared with that observed in identically treated adult naïve cells.[364] Although the mechanism for this reduced calcium response remains to be defined, it is plausible that this reduction may account, in part, for reduced neonatal T cell expression of genes positively regulated by NFAT, such as secreted cytokines and, as discussed later on, CD40 ligand.

Reduced IL-4 and IFN-γ mRNA expression by polyclonally activated neonatal $CD4^+$ and $CD8^+$ T cells compared with that observed in adult T cells is due primarily to reduced transcription of these cytokine genes. These differences in cytokine mRNA expression do not appear to solely reflect differences in proximal signal transduction, because they have been observed not only following activation through the αβ-TCR–CD3 complex[342] but also after activation with ionomycin and phorbol myristate acetate (PMA),[343] which bypass proximal signal transduction events. IFN-γ and IL-4 are expressed mainly by memory/effector T cell populations, rather than by the naïve T cell populations[349]; thus, the reduced expression of these cytokines by neonatal T cells can be accounted for by the lack of memory/effector cells in the circulating neonatal T cell population. For many genes, including the IFN-γ gene, DNA methylation of the locus represses transcription by decreasing the ability of transcriptional activator proteins to bind to regulatory elements, such as promoters and enhancers.[365,366] Thus, reduced expression of IFN-γ by neonatal T cells may also result in part from greater methylation of DNA in the IFN-γ gene locus in neonatal and adult naïve T cells than in adult memory T cells.[367,368]

In addition to decreased cytokine gene transcription, decreased cytokine mRNA stability also may play a role for reduced cytokine production by neonatal T cells. For example, decreased IL-3 production by neonatal T cells appears to be due mainly to reduced IL-3 mRNA stability, rather than to decreased gene transcription.[345] The mechanism for this reduced mRNA stability remains unclear. Decreased mRNA stability also has been observed for other cytokines after stimulation of cord blood mononuclear cells,[369] but whether this also holds for purified neonatal T cells has not been addressed.

Cytokine Production by Neonatal T Cells after Short-Term In Vitro Differentiation. The generation of effector T cells from naïve precursors in response to antigen in vivo can be mimicked by in vitro stimulation, such as by engagement of the αβ-TCR–CD3 complex in conjunction with accessory cells (non–T cells contained in PBMCs) and exogenous cytokines.[370] Neonatal T cells, if polyclonally activated under conditions that favor repeated cell division (strong activation stimuli in common with the provision of exogenous IL-2), resemble antigenically naïve adult T cells in efficiently acquiring the characteristics of effector cells. These characteristics include a $CD45RA^{lo}CD45RO^{hi}$ surface phenotype, an enhanced ability to be activated by anti-CD2 or anti-CD3 mAb, and an increased capacity to produce cytokines (e.g., IL-4, IFN-γ).[221,329,342,371]

The signals that are involved in determining whether T cells become producers of IFN-γ or IL-4 is discussed later in more detail in the section on differentiation and homeostasis of activated T cells.

Although neonatal $CD4^+$ T cells can be effectively primed for expression of effector cytokines by strong mitogenic stimuli, their capacity to differentiate into T_H1 effector cells under more physiologic conditions may be more limited: Neonatal naïve $CD4^+$ T cells stimulated with allogeneic DCs were found to have decreased frequency of IFN-γ^+ cells, based on intracellular cytokine staining, compared with that observed in adult naïve $CD4^+$ T cells in response to short-term (i.e., 24 to 48 hours' duration) stimulation by allogeneic DCs.[356]

This decreased expression of IFN-γ by neonatal $CD4^+$ T cells activated under these more physiologic conditions of DC-mediated allogeneic stimulation probably is due to several factors. First, neonatal $CD4^+$ T cells are less effective than adult naïve cells at inducing the co-cultured DCs to produce IL-12, a key cytokine for promoting IFN-γ production.[356] Second, neonatal naïve $CD4^+$ T cells have decreased expression of CD40 ligand (discussed in more detail later on), which is important in the acquisition of antigen-specific $CD4^+$ T cells with T_H1 immune function.[216] Third, neonatal $CD4^+$ T cells have decreased expression of certain transcription factors, such as the NFATc2 protein, that may play a role in the induction of IFN-γ gene transcription as well as IL-2 and CD40 ligand expression.[347,372,373] Fourth, the greater methylation of DNA of the IFN-γ genetic locus in neonatal T cells than in adult naïve T cells may also contribute to a reduced and delayed acquisition of IFN-γ production following activation in vitro.[368] Together, these mechanisms intrinsic to the T cell, as well as immaturity of DC function (see section on antigen presentation in the fetus and neonate), may account for the delayed acquisition of IFN-γ production by antigen-specific $CD4^+$ T cells after infection in the neonatal period (see section on antigen-specific T cell function in the fetus and neonate).

Fetal and Neonatal T Cell Expression of Tumor Necrosis Factor Ligand Family Members

CD40 Ligand. CD40 ligand (CD154), a member of the TNF ligand family, is expressed at high levels on the cell surface by activated but not by resting $CD4^+$ T cells. CD40 ligand engages CD40, a molecule expressed by APCs—including DCs, mononuclear phagocytes, and B cells—and, perhaps, by $CD8^+$ T cells. The CD40 ligand–CD40 interaction is essential for many events in adaptive immunity, including the generation of memory $CD4^+$ T cells of the T_H1 type (capable of producing IFN-γ but not IL-4), memory B cells, and immunoglobulin isotype switching.[374]

Durandy and colleagues[375] reported that a substantial proportion of circulating fetal T cells between 19 and 31 weeks of gestation expressed CD40 ligand in vitro in response to polyclonal activation. Whether fetal T cells that can express CD40 ligand have a distinct surface phenotype, such as evidence of prior in vivo activation[292] or spontaneous cell proliferation[123] from those lacking this capacity is unclear. By contrast, T cells from later-gestational-age fetuses and from neonates have a much more limited capacity to produce CD40 ligand after activation with calcium ionophore and phorbol ester.[375-378]

Expression of CD40 ligand by activated neonatal $CD4^+$ T cells remains reduced for at least 10 days postnatally, but is almost equal to adult cells by 3 to 4 weeks after birth[375] (D. Lewis, unpublished data, 2000). In most of these studies, activated neonatal $CD4^+$ T cells of cord blood expressed markedly lower amounts of CD40 ligand surface protein and mRNA than either adult $CD45RA^{hi}$ or $CD45RO^{hi}$ $CD4^+$ T cells.[377-379] Thus, decreased CD40 ligand expression may not be due to the lack of a memory/effector population in the neonatal T cell compartment, but may represent a true developmental limitation in cytokine production.

Decreased CD40 ligand production by neonatal T cells also has been documented in the mouse,[380] suggesting that it may be a feature of RTEs. Consistent with this idea, human $CD4^{hi}CD8^-$ thymocytes, the immediate precursors of antigenically naïve $CD4^+$ T cells, also have a low capacity to express CD40 ligand.[378,381] As with most T cell–derived cytokines characteristic of effector cells, when neonatal T cells are strongly activated in vitro into an effector-like T cell population, they acquire a markedly increased capacity to produce CD40 ligand on restimulation, demonstrating that this reduction is not a fixed phenotypic feature.[375,378]

In view of the importance of CD40 ligand in multiple aspects of the immune response,[374] limitations in CD40 ligand production could contribute to decreased antigen-specific immunity mediated by T_H1 effector cells and B cells in the neonate. A potential limitation of the initial studies showing a relative deficiency of CD40 ligand expression by neonatal T cells is that they used calcium ionophore and phorbol ester for stimulation, a combination that maximizes the production of CD40 ligand but may not accurately mimic physiologic T cell activation. Reduced CD40 ligand surface expression by purified neonatal naïve $CD4^+$ T cells compared with that observed in adult naïve $CD4^+$ T cells also has been observed after stimulation with a variety of stimuli that engage the αβ-TCR–CD3 complex, bacterial superantigen (which engages the Vβ segment of the TCR β chain), anti-Vβ mAbs, and anti-CD3 mAbs, either alone or in combination with anti-CD28 mAb,[364] suggesting that this reduction is likely to be applicable to physiologic T cell activation. Similar results have been independently obtained for anti-CD3 and anti-CD28 mAb stimulation using unfractionated neonatal and adult T cells.[362] Other studies, however, have found equivalent levels of CD40 ligand expression by neonatal and adult T cells using anti-CD3 mAb stimulation,[382,383] suggesting that the particular in vitro conditions used (e.g., the particular anti-CD3 mAb and cell culture conditions) may influence the outcome of the assay.

The ability of neonatal and adult T cells to produce CD40 ligand in response to allogeneic stimulation, a condition that should closely mimic T cell activation through the recognition of foreign peptide–MHC complexes, has also been studied. Neonatal $CD4^+$ T cells stimulated allogeneically can express some CD40 ligand and induce IL-12 production by DCs after 3 days of culture, but the ability of adult T cells to do so was not evaluated.[384] Another study found that CD40 ligand expression by neonatal T cells was similar to that by adult T cells after 5 days of allogeneic stimulation with irradiated adult monocyte-derived DCs.[385] By contrast, other studies[356] found that CD40 ligand expression by purified neonatal naïve $CD4^+$ T cells was substantially less than in adult naïve $CD4^+$ T cells after 24 to 48 hours of stimulation. This reduced

CD40 ligand production was accompanied by reduced IL-12 production (by monocyte-derived DCs) and IL-2 and IFN-γ production (by naïve $CD4^+$ T cells). Together, these findings suggest that CD40 ligand surface expression initially may be more limited for neonatal naïve $CD4^+$ T cells, but that with continued priming, at least in vitro, this can be overcome.

Thus, the differentiation of neonatal naïve $CD4^+$ T cells into T_H1 effector cells by CD40 ligand– and IL-12–dependent processes may be limited during the early stages of T cell differentiation.

Other Tumor Necrosis Factor Family Ligands. Fas ligand, another member of the TNF ligand family, plays a key role in inducing apoptotic cell death on target cells that express Fas on the surface. Fas ligand may trigger the apoptosis of any cell type that expresses Fas and in so doing eliminate intracellular pathogens, such as viruses. A more prominent role of the Fas ligand–Fas interaction, at least in humans, is to eliminate previously activated lymphocytes and prevent autoimmune disease.[386] Thus, human Fas deficiency is associated with antibody-mediated autoimmunity rather than defects in viral clearance.

Neonatal T cells have decreased Fas ligand expression after anti-CD3 and anti-CD28 mAb stimulation compared with that in adult cells.[362] Whether neonatal T cells have a decreased level of Fas expression as well remains to be determined. Iwama and colleagues[387] reported that circulating levels of Fas ligand are elevated in newborns, but the cellular source of this protein and its functional significance are unclear. The role of Fas–Fas ligand interactions in regulating apoptosis of neonatal T cells is discussed in the section on neonatal T cell apoptosis.

Neonatal T Cell Co-stimulation and Anergy

Neonatal T cells produce IL-2 and proliferate as well as do adult T cells in response to the combination of anti-CD3 mAb and mouse APCs expressing human CD80 or CD86, indicating that CD28-mediated signaling is intact.[281] This finding also is supported by a study showing that anti-CD28 mAb treatment of neonatal T cells markedly augments their ability to produce IL-2 and proliferate in response to anti-CD2 mAb.[337,338]

Superantigens activate T cells by binding to a portion of the TCR β chain outside of the peptide antigen recognition site but otherwise mimic activation by peptide–MHC complexes in most respects. Neonatal T cells differ from adult $CD45RA^{hi}$ T cells in their tendency to become anergic rather than competent for increased cytokine secretion following priming with bacterial superantigen bound to MHC class II–transfected murine fibroblasts.[330] This anergic tendency is developmentally regulated, because $CD4^{hi}CD8^-$ thymocytes, the immediate precursors of antigenically naïve $CD4^+$ T cells, also are prone to anergy when treated under these conditions.[388] Consistent with this anergic tendency, newborns with toxic shock syndrome–like exanthematous disease, in which the Vβ2-bearing T cell population is markedly expanded in vivo by the superantigen TSST-1, have a greater fraction of anergic Vβ2-bearing T cells than is found in adults with TSST-1–mediated toxic shock syndrome.[389]

Some studies also have found that neonatal but not adult $CD4^+$ T cells primed by alloantigen, in the form of Epstein-Barr virus (EBV)-transformed human B cells, become nonresponsive to restimulation by alloantigen or by a combination of anti-CD3 and anti-CD28 mAbs.[390,391] Preliminary studies implicate a lack of Ras signaling as the basis for this reduced responsiveness.[391] Together, these results, taken with those using bacterial superantigen, suggest that neonatal and, presumably, fetal T cells have a greater tendency to become anergic, particularly under conditions in which production of inflammatory mediators or co-stimulation (e.g., by CD40, CD80, or CD86 on the APC) may be limited.

ICOS is a CD28 homologue that interacts with B7RP-1, a B7 family molecule expressed on both APCs and nonhematopoietic cells.[250] ICOS is not expressed by naïve T cells but is detectable at the later stages of naïve T cell activation, and is constitutively expressed by established effector and memory T cells.[250] Although murine studies initially indicated that the ICOS–B7RP-1 interaction is important for the activation of T_H2 rather than T_H1 effector cells, more recent investigations also have implicated ICOS co-stimulation in T_H1-predominant immunopathology.[392,393] The expression of ICOS and B7RP-1 by neonatal cells has not been reported.

Fetal and Neonatal Effector $CD4^+$ T Cell Generation In Vitro

Activated neonatal $CD4^+$ T cells can be differentiated in vitro into either T_H1- or T_H2-like effector cells by incubation for several days to weeks with IL-12 and anti-IL-4 antibody or with IL-4 and anti-IL-12 antibody, respectively.[56,284,394,395] In most cases, IL-2 is added after the initial activation phase to promote survival and expansion of the effector cells. Treatment of neonatal T cells with IL-4 and anti-IL-12 upregulates GATA-3,[396] which acts as a master transcription factor promoting T_H2 effector generation. Treatment of neonatal $CD4^+$ T cells with the combination of IL-12 and anti-IL-4 mAb probably also is effective at inducing T-bet, a master transcriptional regulator promoting T_H1 effector generation. These studies also indicate that neonatal T cells express functional receptors for IL-4 and IL-12, including the activation-induced IL-12 receptor β_2 subunit.[56] Mature single-positive ($CD4^{hi}CD8^-$ or $CD4^-CD8^{hi}$) fetal thymocytes obtained as early as 16 weeks of gestation can be also differentiated into either T_H1 or T_H2 effector cells by such cytokine treatment,[397] indicating that the capacity to acquire a polarized cytokine profile is established relatively early in fetal life.

Purified naïve ($CD45RA^{hi}$) neonatal T cells proliferate substantially more in response to IL-4 than do analogous adult cells,[398] suggesting a way by which neonatal T cells might be more prone to become T_H2 effectors. Studies by Delespesse and associates[284] also suggest that neonatal and adult $CD45RA^{hi}$ $CD4^+$ T cells may differ in their tendency to become T_H2-like effector cells under certain conditions in vitro; when these cells were primed using a combination of anti-CD3 mAb, a fibroblast cell line expressing low amounts of the CD80 co-stimulatory molecule, and exogenous IL-12, production of IL-4 by neonatal $CD4^+$ T cells was enhanced compared with that by adult cells. Moreover, these investigators found that the neonatal effector T cells generated had a substantially lower capacity to produce IFN-γ than adult cells, and these differences persisted even when endogenous IL-4 was blocked with an anti–IL-4 receptor antibody.[399] This tendency of neonatal $CD4^+$ T cells to develop a T_H2- or T_H0-like cytokine profile may not necessarily apply to more physiologic conditions of stimuli, however, because no IL-4 production by neonatal naïve CD4+ T cells was detected in response to allogeneic DC stimulation (D. Lewis, unpublished data, 2004).

Fetal and Neonatal T Cell Chemokine Receptor Expression

The differential expression of chemokine receptors by T cells is important in their selective trafficking either to sites where naïve T cells may potentially encounter antigen for the first time, such as the spleen and lymph nodes, or to inflamed tissues for effector functions.[400] CCR7 expression by naïve T cells allows these cells to recirculate between the blood and uninflamed lymphoid organs, which constitutively express the two major ligands for CCR7: CCL19 and CCL21. Naïve T cells in the adult express CCR1, CCR7, and CXCR4 on their surface and have low to undetectable levels of CCR5. The role served by CCR1 and CXCR4 expression on naïve T cells is unclear, and CCR1 may be nonfunctional in this cell type.[401] Neonatal naïve T cells have a phenotype similar to those of adult naïve cells, except that they lack CCR1 surface expression, and unlike adult naïve T cells, they do not increase CXCR3 expression, nor do they decrease CCR7 expression, after activation by means of anti-CD3 and anti-CD28 mAbs.[282,402] The CCR7 expressed on neonatal T cells is functional and mediates chemotaxis of these cells in response to CCL19 and CCL21.[403] These results suggest that activated neonatal T cells may be limited in their capacity to traffic to nonlymphoid tissue sites of inflammation and, instead, may continue to recirculate between the blood and peripheral lymphoid organs.

CCR5 recognizes a number of chemokines that are produced at high levels by leukocytes at sites of inflammation, including CCL2 (MIP-1α), CCL4 (MIP-1β), and CCL5 (RANTES), and is an important chemokine receptor for the entry of T cells into inflamed or infected tissues. Neonatal T cells can increase their surface expression of CCR5 by treatment with either mitogen or IL-2.[404] The observation that CCR5 is expressed by fetal mesenteric lymph node T cells during the second trimester of pregnancy[246] suggests that this CCR5 can be upregulated in vivo by a mechanism that does not involve antigenic stimulation. CCR5 expression on CD4+ T cells gradually increases after birth, in parallel with the appearance of memory cells, suggesting that this process occurs in vivo as part of memory cell generation.[405]

As discussed earlier, neonatal naïve CD4+ T cells also have the capacity to acquire expression of chemokines characteristic of T_H1 or T_H2 effectors following their differentiation in a polarized cytokine milieu (IL-12 and anti-IL-4 for T_H1 and IL-4 and anti-IL-12 for T_H2). The T_H1 effectors generated in vitro tend to express CXCR3, CCR5, and CX3CR1, whereas T_H2 effectors tend to express CCR4 and, to a lesser extent, CCR3.[400,406,407] Studies of freshly isolated memory CD4+ T cells suggest that expression of CXCR3 and CCR4 may be more accurate predictors of cells with T_H1 and T_H2 cytokine profiles, respectively.[408,409] In many cases, a combination of chemokine receptors—for example, CXCR3 and CCR5 for the T_H1 cytokine producers—may be the most predictive of highly polarized patterns of cytokine production by memory T cells.[409]

Early Postnatal Ontogeny of Memory T Cell Subsets In Vivo

Memory T cells are heterogeneous in their expression of CCR7. $CCR7^{hi}$ T cells (central memory cells) appear to preferentially recirculate between the secondary lymph nodes and blood, have limited effector function, and may serve as a reservoir for the generation of additional memory cells. The $CCR7^{lo}$ cell population (effector memory cells) is enriched in memory cells that can rapidly induce effector functions, such as IFN-γ or IL-4 production or cytotoxin expression. The $CCR7^{lo}$ cell subset also is enriched in the expression of other chemokine receptors, which facilitates these cells preferential entry into inflamed or infected tissues.[400] It has been proposed that central memory cells are intermediates between naïve T cells and effector memory T cells,[410] but this concept remains highly controversial. A study of the TCR repertoire of human CD8+ T cells suggests that most effector memory cells are not derived from central memory precursor,[411] but it is unclear if this also applies to the peripheral CD4+ T cells.

The memory CD4+ T cell subset in infants and young children has a significantly higher ratio of central memory to effector memory CD4+ T cells than that observed in adults.[226] The frequency of effector memory CD4+ T cells that can produce IFN-γ and the amount of IFN-γ produced per cell in response to bacterial superantigen, however, are similar in the blood of infants and young children and in that of adults.[226] This finding indicates that effector memory cells generated during infancy are functionally similar to those of adults. It is likely that the greater proportion of central memory cells also applies to memory CD4+ T cell responses that occur in the first few months of life, but this remains to be shown. The mechanism responsible for the greater fraction of central memory cells in infants and children is unclear. One possibility is that the decreased proportion of effector memory CD4 T cells may reflect reduced activity of IL-12/IL-23–dependent T_H1 pathway, because effector memory CD4+ T cells are markedly reduced in IL-12Rβ1 deficiency, which ablates IL-12 and IL-23 signaling.[225]

Fetal and Neonatal T Cell–Mediated Cytotoxicity

T cell–mediated cytotoxicity involves two major pathways of killing of cellular targets either through the secretion of the perforin and granzyme cytotoxins or through the engagement of Fas by Fas ligand (Fig. 4-7). The recent and growing use of cord blood for hematopoietic cell transplantation, and the finding that its use is associated with reduced graft-versus-host disease compared with that seen with adult bone marrow, have led to great interest in the capacity of neonatal T cells to mediate cytotoxicity and to potentiate graft rejection.

Early studies mostly used unfractionated mononuclear cells as a source of killer cells in a variety of non–antigen-specific assays, such as lectin-mediated cytotoxicity or redirected cytotoxicity using anti-CD3 mAb. Reduced cytotoxicity was observed with lectin-activated cord blood lymphocytes, particularly if purified T cells were used.[412-414] T cells also can be sensitized in vitro for cytotoxicity using allogeneic stimulator cells followed by testing for cytotoxic activity against allogeneic target cells. Using this approach, most studies have found that neonatal T cells are moderately less effective than adult T cells as cytotoxic effector cells.[415-418,419] As with the acquisition of T_H1 effector function by neonatal

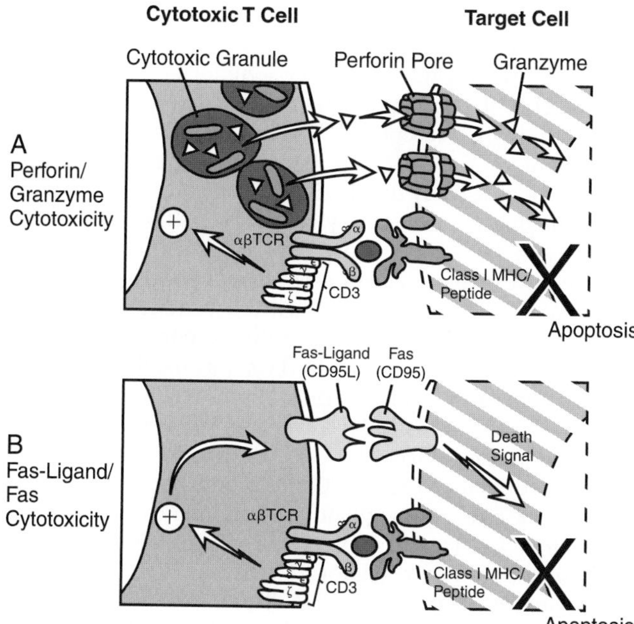

Figure 4–7 Two major mechanisms of antigen-specific major histocompatibility complex (MHC) class I–restricted T cell–mediated cytotoxicity. Engagement of αβ T cell receptor (αβ-TCR) of CD8+ T cells by antigenic peptides bound to major histocompatibility complex (MHC) class I molecules on the target cell leads to T cell activation and target cell death. **A,** Cytotoxicity may occur by the extracellular release of the contents of cytotoxic granules from the T cell, including perforins, granzymes, and other cytotoxins, such as granulysin. Perforins introduce pores by which granzymes can enter into the target cell, leading to the triggering of apoptosis and cell death. **B,** Activation of T cells results in their surface expression of Fas ligand, which engages Fas on the target cell, resulting in the delivery of death signal culminating in apoptosis. Other related molecules, such as TRAIL (TNF-related apoptosis-inducing ligand), may play a role in cytotoxicity.

CD4+ T cells, more substantial defects in T cell–mediated cytotoxicity by neonatal T cells after allogeneic priming is observed when no exogenous cytokines, such as IL-2,[420,421] are added, suggesting that this decreased cytolytic activity might be physiologically significant in vivo. The mechanism for reduced neonatal T cell–mediated cytotoxicity remains poorly understood. Two studies have found that only a low percentage of neonatal CD8+ T cells constitutively express perforin, whereas approximately 30% of adult CD8+ T cells contain this protein.[422,423] By contrast, another study found that approximately 30% of neonatal T cells expressed perforin, a frequency that was similar to that for adult T cells.[424]

Effector and memory CD8+ T cells kill more efficiently than antigenically naïve T cells after stimulation with lectin or anti-CD3 mAb[425] or after allogeneic sensitization.[218,426,427] Thus, the apparent deficiency of neonatal cytotoxic T lymphocyte (CTL) activity after in vitro activation or priming may in some part reflect the absence among neonatal CD8+ T cells of effector and memory cells, as identified by their expression of CD45RO or by their lack of CD27 and CD28, or by both.[428]

The capacity of fetal T cells to mediate cytotoxicity has until recently not received as much scrutiny, despite its relevance to the development of fetal therapy using HSCs. CD8+ T cells bearing αβ-TCRs can be cloned as polyclonal lines from human fetal liver by 16 weeks of gestation.[312,313] These CD8+ T cell lines have proliferative activity in response to allogeneic stimulation,[312,313] but their reactivity toward HLA antigens and their cytolytic activity are not known. More compelling is a study documenting robust fetal effector CD8+ T cell responses, including clonal expansion, IFN-γ production, and perforin expression, in response to congenital CMV infection[429] (see section on T cell response to congenital infection). This finding demonstrates that the capacity to generate a functional CD8+ T cell effector population in vivo is established in utero, at least under conditions of chronic stimulation.

Neonatal T Cell Apoptosis

The elimination of effector T cells by apoptosis is important for lymphocyte homeostasis, with a failure of this process resulting in autoimmunity and severe immunopathology, such as hemophagocytosis. This process can be studied using effector T cells that are generated in vitro from naïve precursors either by acutely withdrawing exogenous cytokines, such as IL-2, used in effector generation, or by reactivating the effector cells (e.g., using anti-CD3 mAb). IL-2, in particular, not only promotes the clonal expansion of T cells but also makes effector T cells vulnerable to apoptosis following its withdrawal. This susceptibility of effector T cells to apoptosis compared with naïve T cells is due to decreased expression of Bcl-2 and upregulation of Fas and the p55 (type I) and p75 (type II) TNF-α receptors (TNFRs).[430] Engagement of Fas or TNFRs by their cognate ligands results in the rapid induction of effector cell apoptosis. Effector B cells are similarly prone to the induction of apoptotic cell death by these pathways. Together, these observations may account for the tendency of mice with genetic disruptions of either IL-2 or its specific receptor components (CD25 [IL-2 receptor α chain], IL-2 receptor β chain, and the γc cytokine receptor) to develop abnormal expansions of T lymphocyte populations. In mice with compromised IL-2 production or IL-2 receptor signaling, reduced regulatory T cell function also may contribute to such T cell expansion (see section on regulatory T cells of the neonate).

Circulating mononuclear cells from cord blood, including naïve CD4+ T cells, are more prone than those from the adult circulation to undergo spontaneous apoptosis in vitro.[290,306,309,431,432] The mechanism does not involve Fas engagement, because Fas levels are low to undetectable on freshly isolated neonatal lymphocytes, including CD4+ and CD8+ T cells.[432-436] This finding is consistent with limitation of expression mainly to memory/effector cells, which are largely absent in the neonatal circulation.[435] The Bcl-2 family of intracellular proteins includes members that either prevent or promote apoptosis by their effects on mitochondrial integrity. The increased tendency of neonatal naïve CD4 and unfractionated T cells to undergo apoptosis may be related to their expression of a lower ratio of Bcl-2 (anti-apoptotic) to Bax (pro-apoptotic) protein compared with that in adult T cells.[306,437] Neonatal naïve T cells have a more marked decrease than adult T cells in expression of Bcl-2 and Bcl-XL (also antiapoptotic) following 7 days in culture without exogenous cytokines.[309] Treatment of neonatal naïve CD4+ T cells with IL-7 can block spontaneous apoptosis,[290,309,310] and this effect is accompanied by increased expression of Bcl-2 and Bcl-XL.[290,309] The tendency for neonatal T cells to spontaneously undergo apoptosis can also be blocked by incubation with insulin-like growth factor-1 (IGF-1), although the mechanism is unclear.[432] The circulating levels of soluble Fas, soluble TNF, and soluble p55 TNFR increase in the first several days after birth,[438] and it has been proposed that the apoptotic tendency of neonatal lymphocytes may be downregulated in the immediate postnatal period by these factors.

Although neonatal T cells have an increased tendency to undergo spontaneous apoptosis, their activation in vitro (priming) may render them less prone than adults cells to undergo apoptosis by Fas ligand or TNF-α engagement, probably because they express less Fas, p55 TNFR, TNFR-associated death domain (TRADD), and caspase-3 molecules that are involved in this process.[437,439] By contrast, restimulation of primed neonatal T cells using anti-CD3 mAb induces greater apoptosis than occurs with use of similarly treated adult T cells; this anti-CD3 mAb–induced pathway in neonatal cells appears to be Fas independent.[437] These results suggest a mechanism by which the clonal expansion of neonatal T cells might be limited following activation through the αβ-TCR–CD3 complex, and the means to counteract this apoptotic tendency, such as administration of IL-2, other exogenous γc cytokine receptor–utilizing cytokines, or IGF-1.[432] It remains unclear, however, whether adult naïve T cells primed under the same conditions as for neonatal T cells retain the tendency of unfractionated adult T cells for greater Fas- and p55 TNFR–mediated apoptosis and reduced anti-CD3 mAb-mediated apoptosis.

Neonatal circulating mononuclear cells, probably including T cells, also are more prone than adult mononuclear cells to undergo apoptosis after engagement of MHC class I achieved by mAb treatment,[431] apparently by a mechanism independent of Fas–Fas ligand interactions. The physiologic importance of the spontaneous and MHC class I–induced apoptotic pathways for fetal lymphocytes is unclear. It is plausible that an increased tendency of fetal T lymphocytes to undergo apoptosis after engagement of MHC class I might be a mechanism to maintain tolerance against noninherited maternal alloantigens.

Regulatory T Cells of the Neonate

$CD4^+CD25^+$ regulatory T cells appear to play an important role in peripheral tolerance to autoantigens,[440] transplantation antigens,[441] and antigens derived from normal endogenous bacterial flora of the gut.[442] The importance of this regulatory T cell population in humans in preventing autoimmune enteritis and endocrine disease is clearly illustrated by the immune dysregulation, polyendocrinopathy, enteropathy, and X-linked inheritance (IPEX) syndrome. This disorder is the first recognized example in humans of a single-gene deficiency that appears to result in a selective defect of regulatory T cells, rather than those that are involved with effector function. The syndrome is due to defects in the gene encoding FoxP3, a member of the forkhead protein family of transcription factors. FoxP3 is expressed by $CD4^+$ T cells, with particularly high levels contained in the $CD4^+CD25^+$ subset of T cells, which include cells with regulatory (immunosuppressive) function. FoxP3-deficient mice also lack regulatory T cells, whereas enforced expression of Fox3P in naïve murine $CD4^+$ T cells confers a regulatory phenotype,[443] suggesting that this transcription factor may act as the key factor for the induction and possibly function of regulatory $CD4^+$ T cells.

Murine studies indicate that the accumulation of peripheral $CD4^+CD25^+$ T cells requires IL-2 and the components of the high-affinity IL-2 receptor.[444] The high-affinity IL-2 receptor consists of CD25 (IL-2R α chain), the IL-2R β chain (CD122), which also is used by the IL-15 receptor, and the γc cytokine receptor that also is used by receptors for IL-4, IL-7, IL-9, IL-15, and IL-21.[445,446] How $CD4^+CD25^+$ T cells regulate autoreactive or alloreactive T cells remains poorly understood. In vitro studies suggest that cell-cell contact is required. Studies have implicated TGF-β (either secreted or regulatory T cell–associated), IL-10, and CTLA-4 as mediating the inhibitory effects of regulatory cells, but the relative importance of these mechanisms is controversial.[444] It also is unclear if these inhibitory effects in vivo are mainly indirect (e.g., through regulatory T cell–APC interactions) or occur through regulatory T cell–nonregulatory T cell interactions after the regulatory T cell has first interacted with an APC[444] (see also previous section on regulatory T cells).

About 5% of circulating $CD4^+$ T cells in neonates, infants, and young children express high levels of CD45RA and CD25 and contain CD45RO transcripts.[447] This T cell subset may be a transitional population between antigenically naïve and memory/effector T cells, although its antigen specificity has not been reported. These cells have some surface phenotypic similarities to a population of $CD4^+CD25^+$ regulatory T cells described in the circulation of adult humans and in mice. Both murine and human studies have shown that $CD4^+CD25^+$ regulatory T cells can inhibit the activation of non-$CD25^+$ T cells in vitro.[442,448-450] In a recent study, however, only adult but not neonatal $CD4^+CD25^+$ T cells were capable of suppressing T cell responses to self-antigen.[451] Additional characterization of the function of neonatal $CD4^+CD25^+$ T cells and their expression of markers characteristic of regulatory cells, such as FoxP3, will be of interest.

Natural Killer T Cells of the Neonate

As discussed earlier (see section on NK T cells), NK T cells are distinct from most αβ T cells in their restricted αβ-TCR repertoire and their recognition of antigens presented by the nonclassic MHC molecules, CD1d. Murine studies suggest that NK T cells may contribute to host defense in certain infections, promote airway hyperreactivity in allergen-induced asthma,[452] and regulate immunopathology (as in autoimmunity and graft-versus-host disease),[453] but the immunologic role of human NK T cells remains poorly defined, as do the ligands recognized by their TCRs. Only small numbers of NK T cells (less than 1.0% of circulating T cells) are present in the neonatal circulation, but these subsequently increase with aging.[454] This finding suggests that NK T cells may undergo postnatal expansion, for example, in relation to exposure to a ubiquitous antigen presented by CD1d molecules, or that their production by the thymus or at extrathymic sites occurs mainly postnatally. Neonatal NK T cells are similar to adult NK T cells in having a memory/effector-like cell surface phenotype, including expression of CD25, the CD45RO isoform, and a low level of expression of L-selectin.[455,456] In the case of murine NK T cells, many of these activation phenotypic features are found on NK T cells during intrathymic development, indicating that these are a result of differentiation rather than prior antigenic stimulation in the periphery before birth.

The neonatal NK T cell population can be expanded in vitro using a combination of anti-CD3 and anti-CD28 mAbs, PHA, IL-2, and IL-7.[457] Although neonatal NK T cells have a surface phenotype similar to that of adult NK T cells, they produce only limited amounts of IL-4 or IFN-γ on primary stimulation, indicating functional immaturity.[455] This decreased capacity may be due to mechanisms similar to those for the reduced IFN-γ production by neonatal $CD4^+$ T cells, such as decreased levels of the NFATc2 transcription factor or increased methylation of the IFN-γ genetic locus.

Following in vitro expansion, neonatal NK T cells produce higher levels of IL-4 and lower amounts of IFN-γ than those produced by similarly treated adult NK T cells.[457] The cytokine profile of neonatal NK T cells demonstrates greater plasticity than that of adult NK T cells: Expansion of the neonatal NK T cell population and priming using either DC1 or DC2 cells in conjunction with PHA, IL-2, and IL-7 result in an IL-4–predominant or an IFN-γ–predominant cytokine expression profile, respectively. By contrast, similarly treated adult NK T cells retain their ability to produce both cytokines,[457] suggesting a loss of plasticity of NK T cells toward T_H1 versus T_H2 polarization after birth. Polarization of neonatal NK T cells toward IL-4 but not IFN-γ secretion might be potentially useful in the treatment of graft-versus-host disease and autoimmune diseases by adoptive transfer.[240,241]

The capacity of cytokine-derived neonatal NK T cells and those directly isolated from the infant to mediate cytotoxicity has not been reported. Neonatal $CD56^+$ T cells constitutively express less perforin than do adult cells.[423] Because the $CD56^+$ T cell population is highly enriched in CD1d-restricted NK T cells, NK T cell cytotoxicity probably is limited at birth and gradually increases with age. Culturing of neonatal NK T cells in vitro for several weeks results in acquisition of potent cytotoxic activity against a variety of tumor cell targets,[458] indicating that developmental limitations can be overcome following expansion and differentiation.

Gamma-Delta T Cells

Phenotype and Function

Gamma-delta T cells, which express a TCR heterodimer consisting of a gamma (γ) and a delta (δ) chain in association with the CD3 complex proteins, are rarer than αβ T cells in most tissues. A major exception is the intestinal epithelium, where they predominate.[459] Although some γδ-TCRs can recognize conventional peptide antigens presented by MHC, most directly recognize three-dimensional nonprotein or protein structures. The antigen-combining site of the γδ-TCR shares some structural features with that of immunoglobulin molecules,[460] which is consistent with preferential recognition of three-dimensional structures by both of these receptors.

Human γδ T cells expressing the Vγ2Vδ2 receptors can proliferate and secrete cytokines after recognition of isopentenyl and prenyl phosphates derived from mycobacteria[461,462] or of alkylamines derived from many species of bacteria, including important neonatal pathogens such as *Listeria* and *Escherichia coli*.[459,463-465] Human γδ T cells express NKG2D, which recognizes the MHC class I–like molecule MICA.[466,467] This NKG2D–MICA interaction enhances the antigen-dependent effector function of Vγ2Vδ2 γδ T cells.[468] Such enhancement in vivo may be a consequence of the induction of MICA on APCs by mycobacteria and other pathogens.[468]

This in vitro activation of γδ T cells probably is relevant in vivo, because increased numbers are found in the skin lesions of patients with leprosy and in the blood of patients with malaria[459,463] and acute herpesvirus infections.[469,470] Resident γδ T cells of the murine skin can produce epithelium-specific growth factors that may help maintain epithelial integrity during stress.[471] The observation that MICA is expressed on heat shock–stressed epithelial cells, and, presumably, in stressed or infected epithelium in vivo, is consistent with a similar role for human γδ T cells.

Gamma-delta T cells also may have important immunosurveillance function for malignancy, because murine cutaneous γδ T cells can kill skin carcinoma cells by a mechanism that involves engagement of NKG2D by Rae-1 and H60, which have homology with human MICA.[472] Murine studies also suggest that γδ T cells may help decrease inflammatory responses to pathogens, such as *Listeria*, by killing activated macrophages by cell-mediated cytotoxicity.[473]

Most activated γδ T cells express high levels of perforin, serine esterases, and granulysin and are capable of cytotoxicity against tumor cells and other cell targets, such as infected cells.[474] Gamma-delta T cells also can secrete a variety of cytokines in vitro, including TNF-α, IFN-γ, and IL-4,[459,463] as well as chemokines that may help recruit inflammatory cells to the tissues. Cytokine production can be potently activated by products from live bacteria, such as isobutylamine[475] and by type I IFN or by agents that potently induce it, such as oligonucleotides containing unmethylated CpG motifs.[476]

Murine studies suggest that these cells are critical for mucosal immunity. Mice lacking γδ T cells have markedly decreased numbers of intestinal IgA plasma cells and demonstrate decreased IgA production after oral immunization with foreign protein and adjuvant.[477] Murine γδ T cells also may contribute to defense of the host against intracellular pathogens, including HSV, *Listeria*, and *Mycobacterium tuberculosis*, particularly if αβ T cell function is compromised.[478-480] Human Vγ2Vδ2 γδ T cells following adoptive transfer into SCID mice can mediate rapid and potent antibacterial activity against both gram-positive and gram-negative bacteria, with protection associated with the production of IFN-γ.[481]

Only about 2% to 5% of T-lineage cells of the thymus and peripheral blood express γδ-TCR in most persons.[482] Unlike in most αβ T cells, whose development requires an intact thymus, a significant proportion of γδ T cells can develop by a thymic-independent pathway, and normal numbers of γδ T cells are found in cases of complete thymic aplasia.[482] This may be explained, at least in part, by the differentiation of γδ T cells directly from primitive lymphohematopoietic precursor cells found in the small intestine, as has been demonstrated in the mouse.[483]

Ontogeny of Gamma-Delta T Cell Receptor Gene Rearrangement

The human TCR γ and δ chain genes undergo a programmed rearrangement of dispersed segments analogous to that of the TCR α and TCR β chain genes. The TCR γ, TCR δ, and TCR β gene loci of immature double-negative cells appear to undergo rearrangement in the thymus at the same time.[484] If the TCR γ and TCR δ gene rearrangements are productive, this may somehow suppress TCR β chain rearrangement. Alternatively, if the TCR β chain gene is productively rearranged, this may suppress TCR γ and TCR δ rearrangement. Signals through the pre-TCR complex that includes the TCR β chain may be involved in this suppression, although this suggestion is controversial.[484] Unlike with αβ T cells, the development of γδ T cells occurs normally in the absence of a pre-TCR complex.[485] Most γδ T cells lack surface expression of either CD4 or the CD8 β chain, suggesting that they may not undergo the process of positive selection that is obligatory for αβ T cells.[486] Whether γδ cells undergo negative selection is unclear.[487]

Rearranged TCR δ genes are first expressed extrathymically in the liver and primitive gut between 6 and 9 weeks of gestation.[488,489] Rearrangement of the human TCR γ and TCR δ genes in the fetal thymus begins shortly after its colonization with lymphoid cells, with TCR δ protein detectable by 9.5 weeks of gestation.[243] Gamma-delta T cells comprise about 10% of the circulating T cell compartment at 16 weeks, a percentage that gradually declines to less than 3% by term.[291,490]

Although there is potential for the formation of a highly diverse γδ-TCR repertoire, peripheral γδ T cells use only a small number of V segments, which vary with age and with tissue location. These can be divided into two major groups, Vγ2Vδ2 cells and Vδ1 cells, in which a Vδ1-bearing TCR δ chain predominantly pairs with a TCR γ chain using a Vγ segment other than Vγ1. Most γδ-TCR$^+$ thymocytes in the first trimester of fetal life express Vδ2 segments. This is followed by γδ-TCR$^+$ thymocytes that express Vδ1, which predominate at least through infancy in the thymus. Most circulating fetal and neonatal γδ T cells also are Vδ1 bearing, with only about 10% bearing Vδ2,[454] and these Vδ1 cells constitute the predominant γδ T cell population of the small intestinal epithelium after birth. In contrast with the early-gestation fetal thymus and the fetal and neonatal circulation, Vδ2 T cells predominate in the fetal liver and spleen early during the second trimester[491,492] and appear before γδ TCR$^+$ thymocytes,[243,493] suggesting that they are produced extrathymically by the fetal liver.

As indicated by TCR spectratyping, the TCR δ chains utilizing either Vδ1 or Vδ2 segments usually are oligoclonal at birth.[494,495] Because this oligoclonality also is characteristic of the adult γδ T cell repertoire, this is not due to postnatal clonal expansion but reflects an intrinsic feature of this cell lineage. By age 6 months, γδ T cells bearing Vγ2 Vδ2 segments become predominant and remain so during adulthood,[496] probably because of their preferential expansion in response to ubiquitous antigen(s), such as endogenous bacterial flora.[464]

Ontogeny of Gamma-Delta T Cell Function

Although neonatal γδ T cells proliferate in vitro in response to mycobacterial lipid antigens,[497] they express lower levels of serine esterases than do adult γδ T cells, suggesting they are less effective cytotoxic cells.[498] Gamma-delta T cell clones derived from cord blood also have a markedly reduced capacity to mediate cytotoxicity against tumor cell extracts.[490] Because these neonatal clones also have lower CD45RO surface expression than that observed in the adult clones, their reduced activity may reflect their antigenic naïveté. In contrast with freshly isolated neonatal γδ T cells, activation and propagation of these fetal and neonatal γδ T cells in culture (e.g., with exogenous IL-2) do not enhance their function. The function of fetal liver γδ T cells remains unclear, although one report suggests that they have cytotoxic reactivity against maternal MHC class I[493] and thereby may prevent engraftment of maternal T cells.

Antigen-Specific T Cell Function in the Fetus and Neonate

Delayed Cutaneous Hypersensitivity, Graft Rejection, and Graft-versus-Host Disease

Skin test reactivity to cell-free antigens assesses a form of DTH that requires the function of antigen-specific CD4$^+$ T cells. Skin test reactivity to common antigens such as *Candida*, streptokinase-streptodornase, and tetanus toxoid usually is not detectable in neonates.[499-501] Absence of such reactivity reflects a lack of antigen-specific sensitization, because in vitro T cell reactivity (e.g., cellular proliferation by peripheral blood mononuclear cells) to these antigens also is absent. When leukocytes, and presumably antigen-specific CD4$^+$ T cells, from sensitized adults are adoptively transferred to neonates, children, or adults, however, only neonates fail to respond to antigen-specific skin tests.[502] As discussed later on, this finding indicates that the neonate may be deficient in other components of the immune system required for DTH, such as APCs or producers of inflammatory chemokines or cytokines. Such deficiencies may account, at least in part, for diminished skin reactivity in the neonate after specific sensitization or after intradermal injection with T cell mitogens.[503,504] Diminished skin reactivity to intradermally administered antigens persists postnatally up to 1 year of age.[505]

Neonates, including those born prematurely, are capable of rejecting foreign tissues, such as skin grafts, although the this rejection may be delayed compared with adults.[506] Experiments using human–SCID mouse chimeras also suggest that second trimester human fetal T cells are capable of becoming cytotoxic effector T cells in response to foreign antigens, and in rejecting solid tissue allografts.[507] Clinical transplantation of fetal blood from one unaffected fraternal twin to another with β-thalassemia did not result in marrow engraftment, despite a sharing of similar MHC haplotypes; instead, there was a postnatal recipient cytotoxic T cell response against donor leukocytes.[508] A T cell response to alloantigens can also be detected in newborns following in utero irradiated red blood cell transfusions from unrelated donors; these neonates have a significantly greater percentage of CD45RO^{hi} T cells than is seen in healthy controls.[509,510] Thus, fetal T cells appear similar to neonatal T cells in being able to mediate allogeneic responses in vivo, including graft rejection.

Another indication that neonatal T cells can mediate allogeneic responses is the fact that blood transfusions rarely induce graft-versus-host disease in the neonate. Rare cases of persistence of donor lymphocytes and of graft-versus-host disease have developed following intrauterine transfusion in the last trimester as well as in transfused premature neonates, however.[511-514] Because the infusion of fresh leukocytes induces partial tolerance to skin grafts,[506] tolerance for transfused lymphocytes might occur by a similar mechanism, predisposing the fetus or neonate to graft-versus-host disease. Together, these observations suggest a partial immaturity in T cell and inflammatory mechanisms required for DTH and for graft rejection.

T Cell Reactivity to Environmental Antigens

Specific antigen reactivity theoretically can develop in the fetus by exposure to antigens transferred from the mother, by transfer of specific cellular immunity from maternal lymphocytes, or by infection of the fetus itself.[515] Several studies suggest that fetal T cells have become primed to environmental or dietary protein allergens as a result of maternal exposure and transfer to the fetus.[516-518] A criticism of these studies is that the antigen-specific proliferation is low compared with the basal proliferation of cord blood mononuclear cells. In addition, many of these studies used antigen extracts rather than defined recombinant proteins or peptides, and these may have nonspecific stimulatory effects.

Prenatal sensitization has been assessed by incorporation of ^{3}H-thymidine by cord blood mononuclear cells, as well as antigen-induced cytokine production, as determined using either reverse transcriptase–polymerase chain reaction (PCR) assay for cytokine transcripts (IL-4, IL-5, IL-9, and IFN-γ), cell culture supernatant cytokine enzyme-linked immunosorbent assays (ELISAs) (for IL-5, IL-10, and IL-13),[519-521] and a cell-based cytokine ELISA for IL-4 and IFN-γ.[522] In some studies, the production of IL-10 in these cultures is high relative to that of the classic T_H2 cytokines (IL-4, IL-5, IL-9, and IL-13). IFN-γ production was 100-fold higher than IL-4 production, a ratio that is still reduced compared with that in adult cells. This cytokine profile has been interpreted as a T_H2-biased response or a regulatory T cell (IL-10–dominant) response. Whether T_H2 priming of fetal T cells to environmental antigens is a risk factor for the postnatal development of atopic disease remains controversial. Its frequent occurrence suggests that priming per se may be a normal outcome of fetal exposure to such antigens.[519,520]

Prenatal priming of T cells by environmental allergens can be demonstrated as early as 20 weeks of gestation, based on their proliferative responses to seasonal allergens.[523] These responses are weak, however, and the cytokine profile was not reported. In one study, protein allergen–specific T cell proliferation detected at birth was more common when allergen exposure occurred in the first or second trimester rather than in the third trimester.[518] This finding could reflect decreased maternal-fetal transport of antigen during late pregnancy or an intrinsic capacity of early- and late-gestation fetal T cells to be primed.

Fetal T Cell Sensitization to Maternally Adminstered Vaccines and Maternally Derived Antigens

In contrast with protein allergens, antigen-specific fetal T cell priming to vaccines has not been documented, such as following maternal vaccination during the last trimester of pregnancy with tetanus toxoid or inactivated influenzavirus A or B.[524] Absence of such priming suggests that fetal sensitization to foreign proteins may be relatively inefficient, particularly when exposure is temporally limited. Whether this reflects relatively inefficient maternal-fetal transfer of protein antigens or intrinsic limitations of the fetus for antigen presentation and T cell priming, or both, is unclear. Even if it is assumed that the capacity for fetal T cells to be primed by foreign antigens is similar to that of antigenically naïve adult T cells, the immune response to maternally derived foreign vaccine proteins by fetal T cells would be expected to be poor compared with the maternal response, because the antigen probably would enter into the fetal circulation with little if any accompanying activation of the innate response required for efficient T cell activation.

Growing evidence, however, suggests that fetal T cell sensitization can occur in cases of antigen exposure due to chronic infection of the mother with parasites or viruses: Parasite (schistosomal, filarial, and plasmodial) antigen-specific cytokine production by peripheral blood lymphocytes, probably of T cell origin, was detectable at birth in infants without congenital infection who were born to infected mothers.[525,526] Of interest, this apparent T cell immunity persisted for at least 1 year after birth in the absence of postnatal infection with parasites and was associated with downregulation of *Mycobacterium bovis* Calmette-Guérin (bacille Calmette-Guérin [BCG])-specific IFN-γ production following neonatal administration of BCG vaccine.[525] These results suggest that fetal exposure to parasitic antigens without infection can downregulate subsequent postnatal T_H1 responses to unrelated antigens. HIV peptide–specific IL-2 production by cord blood $CD4^+$ T cells also has been reported in uninfected infants born to HIV-infected mothers, suggesting that fetal T cell sensitization can occur in cases of chronic viral infection of the mother without congenital infection.[527]

Maternal Transfer of T Cell Immunity to the Fetus

The literature contains many reports of cord blood lymphocyte proliferation or cytokine production in response to antigens that the fetus is presumed not to have encountered. These antigen responses have been attributed to passive transfer of T cell immunity from the mother. For example, in studies in which in vitro reactivity of lymphocytes was studied between birth and the first week of life, specific reactivity to tuberculin purified protein derivative (PPD),[528,529] *Mycobacterium leprae*,[530] measles,[531] and rubella[532] was observed. Infants with pathogen or vaccine reactive lymphocytes usually constituted a minority (less than 20%) of those born to mothers without evidence of active infection, however, and the data were interpreted as evidence for the transfer of maternal cellular immunity.[532,533] Responses usually are weak and may represent laboratory artifacts rather than true sensitization. It also is important to consider that mycobacterial products, such as PPD or *M. leprae* extracts, can activate γδ T cells in the absence of specific prior sensitization. Lipoglycan antigens bound to CD1 may mediate these responses. In vitro reactivity of neonatal T cells to extracts of gram-negative bacteria or *S. aureus* also has been reported.[534-536] Some of these stimuli may act as mitogens or superantigens, however, rather than as MHC-restricted peptide antigens. T cells, including those from the neonate, are effectively activated by superantigens of *S. aureus* and other bacteria.[265,329]

Although maternal-to-fetal transfer of leukocytes occurs, their number in the fetus is very low (usually <0.1%)[537]; accordingly, detectable antigen-specific cellular immunity by conventional assays is unlikely. Thus, reports of neonatal T cell responses as a result of transfer of maternal immunity should remain suspect unless the T cell population is identified and its antigen specificity and MHC restriction are demonstrated.

T Cell Response to Congenital Infection

CD4⁺ T Cells. Pathogen-specific T cell proliferative responses and cytokine responses (IL-2 and IFN-γ) in infants and children with congenital infection (e.g., with *Treponema pallidum*, CMV, varicella-zoster virus [VZV], or *Toxoplasma*) are markedly decreased compared with such responses in infants and children with postnatal infection, or are absent entirely.[538-543] These assays mainly detected $CD4^+$ T cell responses, because antigen preparations (e.g., whole cell lysates of virally infected cells) and APC populations (e.g., peripheral blood monocytes and B cells as the predominant APCs with few DCs) were used that favor activation of MHC class II–restricted rather than class I–restricted responses. These reduced $CD4^+$ T cell responses are particularly true with first- or second-trimester infections. With severe infections in the first trimester, a direct deleterious effect on T cell development is possible. T cells from infants and children with congenital toxoplasmosis, however, retain the ability to respond to alloantigen, mitogen, and, in one case, tetanus toxoid.[543] A more recent study by King and colleagues[526] has examined adaptive immune responses to *Plasmodium falciparum* antigens using cord blood from neonates in an area of Kenya with a high rate of maternal-to-fetal malarial transmission. These investigators found that malaria antigen–induced $CD4^+$ T cell cytokine production (IFN-γ, IL-4, and IL-13) was detectable in these neonates, but not in samples from North American neonates.[526] Thus, the limited ability of the fetus to mount $CD4^+$ T cell responses to pathogen-derived antigens is not absolute, and dual T_H1- and T_H2-type immune responses can develop after some congenital infections or fetal exposure to pathogenic antigens from the mother.

The reduced $CD4^+$ T cell responses seen in many types of congenital infection may be the result of antigen-specific unresponsiveness (e.g., anergy, deletion, or ignorance—the failure of the $CD4^+$ T cell to be initially activated by antigen). As discussed earlier, it is unlikely that a decreased TCR repertoire limits these immune responses, particularly after the second trimester onward. Decreased responses do not occur to all pathogens: In one study, 10-year-old children congenitally infected with mumps had DTHs to mumps antigen, indicating persistence of mumps-specific memory/effector T cells.[544]

CD8⁺ T Cells. $CD8^+$ T cell responses to congenital infections appear to be relatively robust, which is in marked contrast with those of $CD4^+$ T cells. In congenital CMV infection, high frequencies of CMV-specific $CD8^+$ T cells were detectable by staining with CMV peptide–MHC class I tetramers, and these cells demonstrated perforin expression, cytolytic activity, and the capacity to produce cytokines, such as IFN-γ, similar to those of chronically infected adults.[429] Similarly, in HIV-1 infection, an expansion of HIV-specific cytotoxic T cells was detected at birth, indicating that fetal T cells were activated by viral antigens.[545] In another case of in utero HIV infection, HIV-specific T cell–mediated cytotoxicity was detected at age 4 months and persisted for several years despite a high HIV viral load.[546] Congenital infection with *Trypanosoma cruzi* also results in a marked expansion of $CD8^+$ T cells over $CD4^+$ T cells, with evidence of oligoclonality of the TCR repertoire, indicating that this is antigen driven.[547] These $CD8^+$ T cells are enriched in markers for activation (HLA-DR^{hi}), memory ($CD45RO^{hi}$), and end-stage effector cells ($CD28^-$), and for cytotoxicity ($perforin^+$), and have markedly greater capacity to produce IFN-γ and TNF-α than is seen in $CD8^+$ T cells from uninfected newborns; in comparison with $CD8^+$ T cells, $CD4^+$ T cells in these congenitally infected newborns appear to have undergone much less clonal expansion and acquisition of effector function.[547] Congenital infection with viruses or *Toxoplasma* during the second and third trimesters may result in the appearance of $CD45RO^{hi}$ memory T cells and an inverse ratio of $CD4^+$ to $CD8^+$ T cells,[548-550] findings that also suggest that fetal $CD8^+$ T cells are activated and expanded in response to serious infection. These alterations in CD45RO expression by T cells in congenital infection may persist at least through early infancy.[551,552]

T Cell Response to Postnatal Infections and Vaccination

CD4⁺ T Cells. Postnatal infection with HSV results in antigen-specific proliferation and cytokine (IL-2 and IFN-γ) production by $CD4^+$ T cells. These responses are substantially delayed, however, compared with those in adults with primary HSV infection.[553,554] It is unclear at what postnatal age the kinetics of this response becomes similar to that in adults. Recent studies of CMV-specific $CD4^+$ T cell immunity (expression of IL-2, IFN-γ, and CD40 ligand) in older infants and young children with primary infection found substantially reduced responses compared with those in adults with infection of similar duration.[226] This reduced $CD4^+$ T cell response was associated with persistent shedding of the virus into secretions.[226] It is likely that reduced CMV-specific $CD4^+$ T cell responses also apply to the neonate and young infant with perinatal or postnatally acquired infection, who also persistently shed the virus for several years following acquisition. Of interest, as in congenital CMV infection,[429] older infants and young children with primary CMV infection had robust CMV-specific $CD8^+$ T cell responses similar to those in adults.[226,555]

Infants between 6 and 12 months of age also demonstrate lower IL-2 production in response to tetanus toxoid than that observed in older children and adults.[327] This finding suggests that either antigen-specific memory $CD4^+$ T cell generation or function is decreased during early infancy. Whether this reflects limitations in antigen processing, T cell activation and co-stimulation, or proliferation and differentiation remains unclear.

In contrast with postnatally acquired herpesvirus infections or inactivated vaccine antigens, BCG vaccination at birth versus 2 months or 4 months of age was equally effective in inducing $CD4^+$ T cell proliferative and IFN-γ responses to PPD, extracellular *M. tuberculosis* antigens, and an *M. tuberculosis* intracellular extract.[93,556] The responses were robust not only at 2 months following immunization but also at 1 year of age, and no skewing toward T_H2 cytokine production was noted,[556] even by PPD-specific CD4+ T cell clones.[93] Thus, early postnatal administration of BCG vaccine does not result in decreased vaccine-specific T_H1 responses, tolerance, or T_H2 skewing. How these responses compare with those in older children and adult vaccinees is not known. Early BCG vaccination also may influence antigen-specific responses to unrelated vaccine antigens. BCG given at birth increased T_H1- and T_H2-specific responses and antibody titers to hepatitis B surface antigen (HBsAg) given simultaneously.[557] BCG given at birth did not enhance the T_H1 response to tetanus toxoid given at 2 months of age but did increase the T_H2 response (IL-13 production). It is likely that BCG vaccination may accelerate DC maturation, so that these cells can augment either T_H1 or T_H2 responses.

The T cell–specific response to oral poliovirus vaccine (OPV), another live vaccine, suggests a decreased T_H1 response. Neonates given OPV at birth and at 1, 2, and 3 months of age demonstrate lower OPV-specific CD4+ T cell proliferation and IFN-γ production and have fewer IFN-γ–positive cells compared with adults who were immunized as children but not recently reimmunized.[558] By contrast, their antibody titers were higher than those in adults, suggesting that CD4+ T cell help for B cells is not impaired. It is plausible that OPV may be less effective at inducing a T_H1 response than BCG in neonates and young infants because of its limited replication, site of inoculation, or ability to stimulate APCs in a manner conducive to T_H1 immunity, relative to BCG, which induces persistent infection in the recipient.

Although neonates and young infants have been suggested to have skewing of CD4+ T cell responses toward a T_H2 cytokine profile, this may be an oversimplification. For example, the tetanus toxoid–specific response following vaccination indicates that both T_H1 (IFN-γ) and T_H2 (IL-5 and IL-13) memory responses occur, particularly following the third vaccine dose at 6 months of age.[182] The tetanus toxoid–specific T_H1 response may transiently decrease by 12 months of age, whereas T_H2 responses are not affected.[182]

CD8+ T Cells. As discussed, CD8+ T cell responses to CMV infection acquired in utero[429] or during infancy and early childhood[555] are robust, and it is likely that this also applies for infection acquired perinatally or during the early infancy. Cytotoxic responses to HIV in perinatally infected infants suggest that CD8+ T cells capable of mediating cytotoxicity have undergone clonal expansion in vivo as early as 4 months of age.[559] Their cytotoxicity may be reduced and delayed in appearance compared with that in adults, however.[560] There is also decreased HIV-specific CD8+ T cell production of IFN-γ by young infants after perinatal HIV infection,[561] and an inability to generate HIV-specific cytotoxic T cells following highly active antiretroviral therapy (HAART).[562] When evaluated beyond infancy, cytolytic activity directed to HIV envelope proteins was commonly detected, but cytolytic activity directed against gag or pol proteins was rarely detected,[545] suggesting that the antigenic repertoire of cytotoxic CD8+ T cells was less diverse than in adults.

HIV-1 infection may inhibit antigen-specific immunity by depleting circulating DCs,[563] impairing antigen presentation,[564] decreasing thymic T cell output,[565] and promoting T cell apoptosis.[566] In addition, maintenance of HIV-specific CD8+ T cells with effector function depends on HIV-specific CD4+ T cells and may be selectively and severely impaired by the virus. Regardless of the precise mechanism, the suppressive effects of HIV-1 on cytotoxic responses may be relatively specific for HIV-1, because HIV-infected infants who lack HIV-specific cytotoxic T cells may maintain cytolytic T cells against EBV and CMV.[561,562] Surprisingly, some of the inhibitory effects of HIV-1 infection also may occur in HIV-exposed but uninfected infants born to HIV-infected mothers.[565,567]

In one older study, RSV-specific cytotoxicity was more pronounced and frequent in infants 6 to 24 months of age than in younger infants.[568] These results, which need to be repeated using more current assays, suggest that the CD8+ T cell response to RSV gradually increases with postnatal age. Murine studies indicate that RSV infection suppresses CD8+ T cell–mediated effector activity (IFN-γ production and cytolytic activity) and that only transient memory CD8+ T cell responses occur following infection.[569] Longitudinal studies of CD8+ T cell immunity to RSV in children and adults following primary and secondary infection will be of interest to determine if this immunoevasive mechanism applies to humans.

Summary

T cell function in the fetus and neonate is impaired compared with that in adults. Diminished functions include T cell participation in cutaneous DTH and, as also discussed in the next section, T cell help for B cell differentiation. Selectively decreased cytokine production by fetal and neonatal T cells, such as decreased IFN-γ secretion and expression of CD40 ligand, may contribute to these deficits. The repertoire of αβ-TCR probably is adequate, except in early gestation. Following fetal or neonatal infection, the acquisition of CD4+ T cell antigen-specific responses typically is delayed. In vitro studies suggest that deficiencies of DC function and activation and differentiation of antigenically naïve CD4+ T cells into memory/effector T cells may be contributory. In contrast with diminished CD4+ T cell function, CD8+ T cell–mediated cytotoxicity and cytokine production in response to strong chronic stimuli, such as congenital CMV infection or allogeneic cells, appear to be intact in the fetus and neonate. The mother does not transfer T cell–specific immunity to the fetus. T cell sensitization may occur during fetal life to environmental allergens, but such sensitization must be confirmed.

B CELLS AND IMMUNOGLOBULIN

Basic Aspects of B Cells and Immunoglobulin Production

Overview

Mature B cells are lymphocytes that are identifiable by their surface expression of immunoglobulin. Immunoglobulin, which is synonymous with antibody, is a heterotetrameric protein consisting of two identical heavy chains and two identical light chains linked by disulfide bonds (Fig. 4-8).[570] As with the TCR, the amino-terminal portion of the antibody chains is highly variable as a consequence of the assembly of V, D, and J gene segments (heavy chain) or V and J segments (light chain) to a monomorphic constant (C) region. Antibody molecules are distinct from the αβ-TCR, however, in

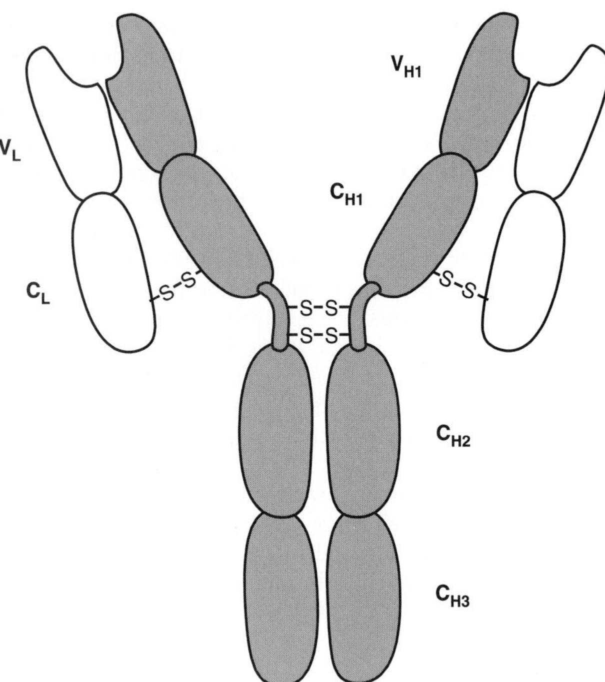

Figure 4–8 Structure of an immunoglobulin molecule. The immunoglobulin molecule consists of two heavy chains (*dark shading*) and two light chains (*unshaded*) linked together by disulfide bonds. The antigen-combining site is formed by amino-terminal region of the heavy and light chains contained in the VH and VL domains of the heavy and light chains, respectively. For IgG, IgD, and IgA, the constant region C_{H3} domain of the heavy chain encodes isotype or subclass specificity, which determines the ability of the immunoglobulin to fix complement, bind to Fc receptors, and be actively transported from the mother to the fetus during gestation. IgM and IgE (*not shown*) are structurally similar except that they contain an additional C_{H4} domain conferring these properties, and they lack a hinge region.

that they typically recognize antigens found on intact proteins or other molecules, such as complex carbohydrates. Thus, the B cell recognition of antigen is typically highly sensitive to its three-dimensional structure.

B cells are activated to proliferate and differentiate into antibody-secreting cells after surface immunoglobulin (sIg) binds antigen. The sIg molecule is invariably associated with the nonpolymorphic membrane proteins, Ig-α (CD79a) and Ig-β (CD79b), which, in conjunction with sIg, constitute the B cell receptor (BCR). Ig-α and Ig-β, which are structural and functional homologues of the CD3 complex proteins, are expressed as disulfide-linked heterodimers and contain ITAM motifs in their cytoplasmic tails. As in T cells, these ITAMs act as docking sites for signaling molecules, such as the Lyn and Syk tyrosine kinases.

For B cells to be activated effectively and to produce antibody against protein antigens requires help from T cells in most cases. This help is in the form of soluble cytokines, such as IL-4 and IL-21,[571] and of cell surface–associated signals, such as CD40 ligand, which is transiently expressed on the surface of activated CD4+ T cells. The engagement of CD40, which is constitutively expressed by the B cell, also is instrumental in inducing B cells to undergo immunoglobulin isotype switching, for example, from IgM to IgE (see Fig. 4-4). In isotype switching, the C region at the carboxy terminus of the immunoglobulin heavy chain gene is replaced with another isotype-specific segment, but the antigen-combining site at the amino terminus is preserved. In cases in which the antigen has multiple and identical surface determinants (e.g., complex polysaccharides, certain viral proteins with repetitive motifs) and multiple sIgs are cross-linked, antigen binding alone may be sufficient to induce B cell activation without cognate (direct cell-cell interaction) help from T cells. In this case, other signals derived from non–T cells, such as cytokines, or from microorganisms, such as bacterial lipoproteins or bacteria-derived DNA containing unmethylated CpG motifs, may enhance antibody responses.[572]

As with T cells, B cells receive additional regulatory signals from the engagement of surface molecules other than the BCR that act as either co-stimulatory or inhibitory molecules. Of the co-stimulatory molecules, a complex consisting of CD19, CD21, and CD81 is best defined.[573] CD21, also known as complement receptor 2, binds the CD3d fragment of the C3 complement component. CD19 and CD81 transmit intracellular activation signals after complement binding to CD21. Gene disruption experiments indicate that expression of both CD19 and CD21 by B cells is essential for production of antibody to protein antigens.[574] Mice lacking complement receptor 2 (of which CD21 is one component) also have a reduced ability to respond to low doses of polysaccharide antigens, which may account for the increased susceptibility to infection with *Streptococcus pneumoniae* in these animals.[575]

The activation of B cells by BCR engagement and co-stimulation is counterbalanced by a number of surface molecules on the B cell that transmit inhibitory intracellular signals. For example, B cell activation is suppressed when a surface receptor for the Fc (fragment crystallizable) portion of IgG, FcγRIIB, is engaged concurrently with the BCR by antigen-IgG complexes.[576] This serves as a negative feedback mechanism mediated by immunoreceptor tyrosine-based inhibitory motif (ITIM) motifs to limit antibody production; for example, gene knockout mice lacking FcγRIIB have substantially increased levels of circulating antibody after immunization.[577]

In addition to their secretion of antibodies, mature B cells express MHC class II and also may participate in antigen processing and presentation to CD4+ T cells. Memory B cells are probably more effective than antigenically naïve B cells, because they constitutively express higher surface levels of CD80 or CD86 molecules that provide co-stimulatory signals to T cells. Interactions between ICOS on the T cell and B7RP-1 (B7h or ICOS ligand) on the B cells may also be essential.[197] The preferential source of protein for antigenic peptides presented to T cells by B cells probably is sIg-protein complexes internalized from the cell surface. The internalized proteins are degraded to peptides that can then be presented back on the B cell surface bound to MHC class II molecules. Because the sIg-antigen interaction is of high affinity, B cell antigen presentation theoretically permits CD4+ T cells to be activated at relatively low concentrations of antigen. Depending on the particular antigen, however, experimental conditions and nature of the responding T cell (naïve or memory), the presentation of protein antigen by resting (antigenically naïve) B cells can result in either CD4+ T cell activation, apoptosis, or antigen-specific tolerance. The observation that CD4+ T cell T_H1 immunity is intact in patient with X-linked agammaglobulinemia suggests that B cells do not play a central role in MHC class II antigen presentation.[578] DCs are likely to be more important than B cells for presenting protein antigens to $CD4^+$ T cells in vivo, particularly in an infectious or inflammatory context.

Immunoglobulin Structure and the Genetic Basis for Immunoglobulin Diversity

The amino-terminal region of each pair of heavy and light chains is variable; together these form the antigen-binding fragment (Fab) portion of immunoglobulin, which contains the antigen-binding site (see Fig. 4-8). As with the TCR, the variable region of each chain can be subdivided into three hypervariable CDR1, CDR2, and CDR3 regions, and four intervening, less variable framework regions. The three-dimensional folding of the antibody molecules results in the approximation of the three CDR regions into a contiguous antigen recognition site, with CDR3 located at the center and the CDR1 and CDR2 regions forming the outer border of the site.[579] The carboxy-terminal portion of the heavy and light chain genes is monomorphic or constant (i.e., is a C region) and consists of three constant heavy (CH) domains and one constant light (CL) domain, respectively (see Fig. 4-8). The heavy chains also have a hinge region at which the two halves are joined by disulfide bonds. The heavy chain C region is the Fc portion of immunoglobulin and contains sites that determine complement fixation, placental transport, and binding to leukocyte Fc receptors. The portion of the heavy chain C region encoded by the last exon of heavy chain gene defines antibody isotype or isotype subclass, of which there are nine in humans: IgM, IgD, IgG_1, IgG_2, IgG_3, IgG_4, IgA_1, IgA_2, and IgE. Light chains comprise two types, kappa and lambda, each containing a distinct type of C region.

The heavy chain and kappa and lambda light chains are synthesized independently from genes located on human chromosomes 14, 2, and 22, respectively. Analogous to the β chain of the TCR, the heavy immunoglobulin chain is encoded by V, D, J, and C regions. Approximately 38 to 46 functional V segments and 23 different D segments are dispersed over 1100 kilobases (kb) of DNA upstream of the JC region.[112] There are six different J segments located near the C region. Antibody gene rearrangement is required to bring the V, D, and J regions together to form a single exon that is juxtaposed to the C region so that the gene can be expressed (see Fig. 4-4). The same recombinase enzyme complex required for TCR gene rearrangement, including the RAG-1 and RAG-2 proteins, mediates this process. The assembly of the light chain genes from multiple potential segments is similar, except that D segments are not used. The human kappa light chain gene locus consists of 30 to 35 functional V segments, 5 J segments, and a single C segment, and the human lambda light chain gene locus encodes 29 to 33 functional V segments and 4 to 5 functional J segments, with each J associated with its own C segment.[112] As in the TCR chains, the CDR1 and CDR2 regions of the antigen-combining site are encoded entirely by the V segments, and the CDR3 is encoded at the junction of the V, D, and J segments.

As with the TCR genes, antibody diversity is generated by the juxtaposition of various combinations of V, D, and J segments and the imprecision in the joining process itself: Nucleotides at junctions may be removed by exonucleolytic activity or, alternatively, added by the TdT enzyme or as P nucleotides. Finally, in the case of the heavy chain gene, D-to-D joining can occur, and D segments also can rearrange by inversion or deletion.[580] Together, these mechanisms permit a theoretical immunoglobulin repertoire of more than 10^{12} specificities to be generated from fewer than 10^3 somatic gene segments. For reasons that are not clear, however, immunoglobulin heavy chain V segment usage by immature pre-B cells and antigenically naïve B cells appears to be dominated by relatively few segments.[581,582] Thus, actual immunoglobulin diversity is less than would be predicted if segment usage were completely random. As in the case of the TCR genes, the CDR3 region appears to be the most important source of diversity.

The rearrangement process maximizes the generation of diversity at the expense of precision. Consequently, a majority of pre-B cells fail to produce a functional immunoglobulin molecule, do not mature, and subsequently die. The inefficiency of generating productive rearrangements for both heavy and light chains is offset by the high rate of proliferation of immature pro- and pre-B cells. Still further diversification is possible later in B cell differentiation by processes known as somatic mutation and receptor editing, which are described later on.

B Cell Maturation and Pre-immune Selection

Pro-B Cell and Pre-B Cell Maturation. The pro-B cell is the most immature cell type that is known to be committed to differentiate along the B lineage. It is thought to be derived from a less mature lymphocyte progenitor that retains the capacity for differentiation into the major lymphocyte lineages. B cell differentiation may be a default pathway that occurs in the absence of Notch 1 signaling,[583] which promotes T-lineage cell development. Human pro-B cells have a $CD10^{hi}CD19^-CD34^{hi}$ surface phenotype. They also express the RAG and TdT proteins and undergo D-to-J and then V-to-DJ immunoglobulin heavy chain gene rearrangements. D-to-J heavy chain gene rearrangements also may occur in immature lymphocytes that are not committed to the B lineage, but V-to-DJ rearrangement may be a characteristic feature of committed B-lineage cells. In cases in which the immunoglobulin heavy chain is productively rearranged, it is expressed cytoplasmically and on the B-lineage cell surface as part of the pre-BCR complex, which consists of a surrogate light chain (a VpreB and a λ5/14.1 segment[584,585]) in association with Ig-α–Ig-β heterodimers. Expression of the pre-BCR complex defines the pre-B cell stage, and pre-B cells have a $CD10^{hi}CD19^{hi}CD34^-$ surface phenotype. Pro-B cells and pre-B cells of the adult are found only in the bone marrow. In the fetus, these cells are found in the liver and omentum and in smaller numbers in the lung and kidney.[586]

The heavy chain gene usually rearranges first, initially with a joining of a D segment to a J segment.[587] Rearrangement results in the excision of intervening DNA as signal joint circles (analogous to the TRECs generated during TCR gene rearrangement) so that the heavy chain gene segments can be transcribed as a single unit. If the D-to-J segment is productively rearranged, its transcripts are translated into DJC heavy chain protein. If a nonproductive D-to-J rearrangement occurs, a second attempt at productive D-to-J rearrangement usually is made by the heavy chain gene on the other chromosome 14. D-to-J heavy chain gene rearrangement and protein expression are followed by the joining of a V segment to the D-to-J segment. Productive V(D)J rearrangement results in the expression of full-length heavy chain protein in the cytoplasm. In humans, the first easily recognized pre-B cells are those that contain cytoplasmic IgM heavy chains but no light chains or sIg.

The expression of the pre-BCR by the pre-B cell blocks rearrangement of the other heavy chain gene allele (allelic exclusion) and results in proliferation of the pre-B cell for four to five divisions,[588] with concurrent downregulation of RAG and TdT activity. The human pro-B cell to pre-B cell transition is dependent on the ability to form a functional pre-BCR complex and is blocked by mutations in the Cμ segment of the heavy chain gene, Ig-α, the cytoplasmic Btk tyrosine kinase, and the B cell linker (BLNK) cytoplasmic adapter protein.[589] The requirement for Ig-α–Ig-β, Btk, and BLNK probably is attributable to their role in pre-BCR signal transduction.[589,590] No known ligand for pre-BCR has been defined, and much of its extracellular domain of heavy chain is dispensable for its function,[591] suggesting that it may have ligand-independent basal signaling function. After cell proliferation, the pre-B cell exits from cycling, upregulates RAG and TdT activity, and promotes immunoglobulin light chain rearrangement.[592] In some pre-B cells, productive light chain rearrangements can occur in the absence of productive heavy chain rearrangements, at least in the fetal bone marrow, suggesting that heavy chain gene rearrangement is not obligatory for light chain rearrangement.[587]

After the expression of the pre-BCR, a similar process of gene rearrangement subsequently occurs to assemble light chain genes from V and J segments. Allelic exclusion also usually acts at the light chain level, so that only a single type of light chain is produced. Kappa light chain gene rearrangement usually occurs first, and if neither kappa chain gene rearrangement is productive, this apparently permits lambda chain gene rearrangement to proceed.[593] Approximately 60% of human immunoglobulin molecules utilize kappa light chains, and the remainder use lambda light chains.[594] If rearrangement and expression of a complete kappa or lambda light chain subsequently occur, a functional immunoglobulin molecule is assembled and expressed as sIg. The end result of allelic exclusion is that a B cell usually synthesizes only a single immunoglobulin protein, although each cell has the genetic information to produce two heavy chains and four light chains. Compared with that of the heavy chain, allelic exclusion of immunoglobulin light chains is relatively "leaky" such that 0.2% to 0.5% of circulating B cells express both a kappa and a lambda light chain in their surface IgM.[595]

Transitional B Cells and Surface Ig–Mediated Selection. The initial expression of sIg by B-lineage cells is in the form of both the IgM and IgD isotypes. This is the result of alternative mRNA splicing of the exons of the heavy chain gene that encode isotype specificity. In human adults, these $IgM^{hi}IgD^{hi}$ transitional B cells are distinct from pre-B cells in their lack of CD10 expression[596] and are the immediate precursors of B cell emigrants from the bone marrow. Murine studies indicate that after these transitional B cells emigrate from the bone marrow, they undergo further maturation in peripheral lymphoid organs, such as the spleen, to become fully mature naïve B cells.

Transitional B cells are similar to thymocytes in that they undergo negative and positive selection processes based on sIg complex signaling before becoming mature naïve cells that are activated in the periphery by foreign antigens. Evidence for positive and negative selection of B cells in human adults comes from comparisons of the immunoglobulin repertoire of pre-B and transitional B cells versus that of mature naïve B cells.[597]

Positive selection of immature transitional B cells likely occurs in the bone marrow as well as in the periphery (see later) and requires an intact BCR complex and presumably involves either some interaction of the antigen-combining site of the BCR with self-molecules[598] or basal signaling by the BCR complex, or both.[599] In contrast with positive selection of thymocytes, which involves mainly cortical epithelial cells that present self-peptides, B cell positive selection is a poorly understood process.

Murine experiments, such as utilizing B cells expressing self-reactive transgenic sIg, have shown that negative selection can either eliminate (clonal deletion) or inactivate (clonal anergy) or change the Ig specificity (receptor editing) of potentially autoreactive antigenically naïve B cells in the bone marrow.[600,601] Clonal deletion may be favored when developing B cells encounter self-antigen displayed on cell membranes, and clonal anergy may be favored when these B cells encounter soluble self-antigen.[600] Receptor editing of the rearranged immunoglobulin chain genes occurs through secondary V-to-J light chain gene rearrangements. This involves V segments located 5′ and J segments that are located 3′ to the current VJ rearrangement. Replacement of V heavy chain gene segments with previously unrearranged upstream V segments in mature B cells also is possible, but this is a rare form of editing. As suggested by mouse studies, only 10% of naïve B cells produced in the bone marrow may leave the periphery to colonize peripheral lymphoid organs as a result of these negative selection processes. Receptor editing may be the predominant mechanism for B cell tolerance in the bone marrow.[602]

Maturation of Transitional B Cells into Naïve B Cells. Transitional B cells of the murine spleen initially localize to the outer periarteriolar sheaths. The maturation of transitional B cells also requires engagement of the B-cell activating factor (BAFF) receptor with BAFF, a TNF ligand family member.[603,604] BCR-derived and other signal transduction events involved in positive selection also may determine whether these cells will become antigenically naïve follicular B cells, marginal zone B cells, or B-1 B cells, each of which has a distinct phenotype, location, and function in immunity. A critical parameter in determining the fate of transitional B cells is apparently BCR signal strength.[605,606] Similar fate decisions may occur among human transitional B cells, but information on the cellular and molecular events involved is limited. Follicular B cells include most of those that are those involved in adaptive immune responses to T-dependent antigens, such as proteins, and are the predominant naïve B cell subset of cells in the circulation or secondary lymphoid tissue. The following discussion of B cell activation and differentiation by foreign antigen applies to follicular B cells, unless noted otherwise. Marginal zone and B-1 B cells, which have distinct roles from follicular B cells in immunity, are discussed in separate sections later on.

The commitment to a follicular B cell fate results in upregulation of CXCR5. This chemokine receptor recognizes

CXCL13, a chemokine produced within the follicles that promotes the entry of the B cell into the follicle.[607] In some cases, negative selection of transitional B cells may occur by a process of follicular exclusion, in which they fail to upregulate CXCR5.[600] CXCR5 upregulation and follicular entry coincide with the acquisition of mature B cell functions, including a decreased tendency to undergo apoptosis after BCR engagement, an increased responsiveness to T cell help (e.g., CD40 ligand and soluble cytokines), increased expression of CD86, and maturation of intracellular signaling in response to BCR engagement.

Naïve B Cell Activation, Clonal Expansion, Immune Selection, and T Cell Help

Mature antigenically naïve B cells of the follicular subset that survive positive and negative selection are $IgM^{hi}IgD^{hi}CD27^{lo/-}$.[608] They also express CXCR4 and CXCR5, which promotes their recirculation between the follicles of the peripheral lymphoid organs, including the spleen, lymph nodes, and Peyer's patches, which express the chemokine ligands for these receptors, and the blood and lymph.[609] The encounter of naïve B cells of the follicle with antigen recognized by the sIg triggers their activation and proliferation under appropriate conditions. This may initially involve the formation of immune synapse with an APC, such as a DC, analogous to that formed as part of initial naïve T cell activation.[610] As with naïve T cells, activation of naïve B cells by BCR engagement has a relatively high signal threshold compared with that of memory cells,[611] a feature that may prevent inappropriate activation by low-affinity self-antigens. In the case of protein antigens, this is followed by antigen internalization and entry into the MHC class II antigen presentation pathway.[612] Activation also increases B cell expression of CCR7, which promotes B cell movement toward the outer border of the T cell zone,[613] and of OX40 ligand,[614] which can provide T cell co-stimulation.

In T cell–dependent activation, antigenically naïve $CD4^+$ T cells probably are first activated by DCs independently of B cells in the periarteriolar lymphoid sheath region of the spleen and the paracortical region of the lymph nodes. $CD4^+$ T cells that are activated by DCs bearing antigenic peptide–MHC class II complexes and CD80-CD86 co-stimulatory molecules express CD40 ligand, OX40, ICOS, and CXCR5.[615,616] These activated $CD4^+$ T cells may either leave the lymphoid organ to become effector or memory T cells or become $CD4^+$ T cells specialized to provide help to B cells.[617] $CD4^+$ T cells destined to leave the lymphoid organ and to enter sites of tissue inflammation and participate in inflammatory responses (e.g., T_H1 cytokine secretion) are P-selectin^{hi}, CXCR3$^+$, and CXCR5$^-$.

By contrast, $CD4^+$ T cells that are retained in the lymph node and that eventually enter the follicle as T follicular helper cells are P-selectin$^-$ and CXCR3$^-$ but express CXCR5. This CXCR5 expression promotes movement of these $CD4^+$ T cells to the outer border of the T cell zone, to contact antigen-activated B cells at the edge of the follicular zone (also known as the mantle region).[618] Here, $CD4^+$ T cell activation is reinforced by recognition of antigenic peptides displayed on MHC class II molecules of the B cell, and the interaction of CD40 ligand and OX40 on the T cell with CD40 and OX40 ligand on the B cell enhances B cell activation. OX40 engagement of the $CD4^+$ T cell also promotes its differentiation into an effector cell producing T_H2 rather than T_H1 cytokines and promotes upregulation or retention of expression of CXCR5. These CXCR5^{hi} $CD4^+$ T cells then enter into the follicle, where they provide help to B cells as T follicular helper cells.[193,194] T follicular helper cells are CD57^{hi}[619] and provide B cell help by expressing CD40 ligand, secreting cytokines such as IL-4[620] and, probably, IL-21,[571] and providing ICOS-dependent B cell co-stimulation.[621]

During the initial immune response, most antigenically naïve follicular B cells are derived from clones expressing antibody variable regions with relatively low affinity for antigen. As in the case of the TCR, activation through the BCR is also not necessarily an all-or-none phenomenon. For example, high-affinity binding to IgM of the BCR may allow B cell proliferation to occur in the absence of any T cell help, whereas lower-affinity binding may result in proliferation only in the presence of additional T cell–derived signals.[622]

Antigen-specific B cells proliferate strongly within the B cell follicle, leading to the formation of germinal centers. The more avidly the B cell binds antigen, the stronger is the stimulus to proliferate. The major source of antigen for triggering the extensive B cell proliferation of the germinal center may be provided by antigen complexed with antibody bound to Fc receptors on follicular DCs, although this point is controversial.[623] The follicular DC is a nonhematopoietic cell type that appears to have the unusual capacity to bind antigen-antibody complexes for long periods on their cell surface.

Immunoglobulin variants are generated among germinal center B cells by the process of somatic hypermutation, in which immunoglobulin genes accumulate apparently random point mutations within productively rearranged V, D, and J segments. These variants undergo a selection process favoring B cells that bear sIg with high affinity for antigen. Such high-affinity immunoglobulin provides high levels of BCR signaling, favoring germinal center B cell survival rather than a default pathway of apoptosis. Somatic hypermutation requires an activation-induced cytidine deaminase (AID), which is expressed only by germinal center B cells.[624] It remains unclear how the effects of the mutator are focused on the variable region of immunoglobulin and its immediate flanking sequences. The peak of somatic mutation is approximately 10 to 12 days after immunization with a protein antigen.[625] Although some light chain receptor editing may occur in human germinal centers, it does not appear to be an important influence on shaping the final immunoglobulin repertoire after somatic hypermutation takes place.[626]

Germinal center B cells that receive appropriate survival signals leave the germinal center to persist as memory B cells, which are CD27^{hi}.[608] The engagement of CD40 on germinal center B cells by CD40 ligand on T cells is absolutely required for memory B cell generation but may not be involved in initial germinal center B cell proliferation.[627] Efficient memory B cell generation requires the binding by CD21 on B cells of C3 complement components, such as C3d, apparently derived from the classic complement pathway.[628] Once a memory B cell is generated, further somatic mutation of its immunoglobulin genes apparently does not occur.[629] Memory B cells enter the recirculating lymphocyte pool, where they preferentially colonize the skin and mucosa, sites that are likely to have direct contact with antigen, as well as the marginal zone of the spleen, where they are poised to respond to blood-borne antigens. Once memory B cells are generated, they appear to persist indefinitely even in the absence of any subsequent exposure to the inciting antigen.[630-632]

Generation of Plasma Cells and the Molecular Basis for Immunoglobulin Secretion

Some activated B cells become plasmablasts and migrate to extrafollicular regions of the lymph node or spleen, where they become short-lived plasma cells that mainly produce IgM. Differentiation of these plasma cells does not require and may be inhibited by the CD40 ligand–CD40 interaction.[633] This accounts for relatively normal or increased IgM responses in patients with genetic deficiency of CD40 ligand. In the absence of CD40 engagement, germinal center B cells that have survived the selection process probably differentiate by a default pathway to become long-lived plasma cells, which can persist in the spleen and bone marrow for at least a year.[634] In mice, long-lived plasma cells are distinguishable from short-lived plasma cells by their lack of MHC class II expression.[634] Plasma cells are concentrated in peripheral lymphoid tissue, liver, and bone marrow, as well as in lymphoid tissue of the gastrointestinal and respiratory tracts.

The membrane-bound form of immunoglobulin is slightly longer than the secreted form and contains a carboxy-terminal region that anchors the molecule in the cell membrane. The secretory form of immunoglobulin lacks this membrane-anchoring segment as a result of a change in splicing of the heavy chain mRNA. Maturation of B cells into plasma cells is associated with a marked increase in their capacity to secrete immunoglobulin and with loss of sIg expression. Plasma cells rather than mature B cells account for most of the secreted antibody during both primary and secondary immune responses. Human memory B cells can differentiate into plasma cells in response to antigen-independent mechanisms, such as exposure to oligonucleotides containing unmethylated CpG DNA (a ligand for TLR-9) or activated T cells.[632] Such polyclonal activation of memory B cells has been proposed to maintain levels of specific antibody for a lifetime once a memory B cell response has been generated.

Switching of Immunoglobulin Isotype and Class

Human B cells produce five isotypes of antibody: IgM, IgD, IgG, IgA, and IgE. The IgG and IgA isotypes can be, respectively, divided into the IgA_1 and IgA_2 and the IgG_1, IgG_2, IgG_3, and IgG4 subclasses. During their process of differentiation into plasma cells, B cells are able to change from IgM to other antibody isotypes without changing antigen specificity (see Fig. 4-4). With the exception of IgD expression, this switching usually involves isotype recombination, the genetic replacement of the IgM-specific portion of the constant region (C_μ) of the heavy chain with a new isotype-specific gene segment. As in V(D)J recombination, the intervening DNA is excised as a large circle. Isotype recombination is mediated by switch regions that are positioned immediately upstream of each of the isotype-specific C regions, with the exception of IgD. Successive multiple isotype switching by a single B cell also can occur, for example, IgM to IgA to IgG to IgE.[635]

Genetic studies of the hyper-IgM syndrome, in which there is a generalized block in isotype switching from IgM to other isotypes, have revealed that the process requires interactions between CD40 ligand on the T cell and CD40 on the B cell, the AID gene product (which also is required for somatic hypermutation), and the uracil *N*-glycolyase (UNG) enzyme.[624] Mutations in all of these genes have been identified in persons with the hyper-IgM syndrome, but the precise function of AID and UNG in this process remains unclear. Secreted cytokines derived from T cells or other cell types play an important role in promoting or inhibiting switching to a specific isotype. For example, IL-4 or IL-13 is absolutely required for isotype switching to IgE, a process that can be inhibited by the presence of IFN-γ.[636] Cytokine-induced switching to a particular isotype segment strongly correlates with the cytokine-inducing transcription that is initiated immediately upstream of this region. In some instances, hormones also may play a role in isotype switching. For example, vasoactive intestinal peptide in conjunction with CD40 engagement can induce human B cells to produce high levels of IgA_1 and IgA_2.[637]

During a primary immune response, isotype switching by B cells appears to occur shortly after these cells enter into the follicle.[638] These B cells may have received the requisite T cell–derived signals (i.e., cytokines and CD40 ligand) during their interaction with T cells at the border between the follicle and T cell zones. Switch recombination after primary immunization is evident in peripheral lymphoid tissue 4 days after immunization with protein antigen and peaks between 10 and 18 days.[639] Switch recombination also is triggered during memory B cell responses, is detectable within 24 hours of secondary immunization, and peaks between 3 and 4 days.[639] Most memory B cells or plasma cells switch to another isotype by gene rearrangement, and somatic mutations are most common in antibodies other than IgM. Some adult B cells express surface IgM but not IgD or other isotypes, however; these cells appear to consist of memory B cells that have not undergone isotype switching but are somatically mutated.[640] Somatic hypermutation also occurs in IgM^+ B cells from patients with CD40 ligand deficiency.[641] Finally, isotype switching and memory B cell generation without somatic hypermutation occur in mice lacking Bcl-6, a mutation that results in the absence of germinal centers.[642] Thus, isotype switching and somatic hypermutation can occur independently in at least some contexts.

Regulation of B Cell Proliferation and Differentiation

B cell activation and differentiation are subject to regulation at multiple steps by cell-cell contact and soluble factors, as well as by intracellular signaling molecules and transcription factors. Such regulation may be specific for particular stages of B cell development. For example, Btk, a tyrosine kinase expressed by B-lineage cells, plays a role in cell activation after engagement of the pre-BCR or BCR complexes. Functional mutations in Btk result in the syndrome of X-linked agammaglobulinemia, in which B cell development is arrested at a pre-B cell stage.[643] BAFF, a TNF ligand family member, which is produced by mononuclear phagocytes and DCs, is important for B-lineage cell survival and proliferation at later stages, such as the transitional and mature B cells.[644] By contrast, the engagement of CD40 by CD40 ligand is not required for B cell development but is essential for the generation of memory B cells from mature antigenically naïve B cells.[195] Cytokines, such as TNF-α, and chemokines, such as CXCL12 (SDF-1), that are expressed in the bone marrow microenvironment appear to be important for long-term plasma cell survival.[645] As previously discussed, most cytokines secreted by T cells, such as IL-2, IL-4, and IFN-γ, are not essential for B cell development but are important regulators of B cell isotype.[636]

Finally, particular transcription factors or combination of these play key roles in regulating virtually all of the steps of B-lineage cell differentiation. For example, the Pax-5 transcription factor acts as both a transcriptional activator of many genes involved in B cell development and as a transcriptional repressor of inappropriate non–B cell lineage genes.[646] In the case of plasma cell differentiation, the B lymphocyte-induced maturation protein-1 (BLIMP-1) transcription factor inhibits the activity of Pax5 and promotes a gene expression program that favors plasmablast differentiation and antibody secretion.[647]

Marginal Zone B Cells of the Spleen

Spleen marginal zone memory B cells can be distinguished from antigenically naïve B cells by their high levels of surface expression of CD148, a protein tyrosine phosphatase, and CD27.[648] The human spleen has distinct anatomic sites that may play specialized roles in the production of antibody against blood-derived particulate antigens and purified repetitive carbohydrate antigens. Important examples of such carbohydrate antigens are the capsular polysaccharides of pathogenic bacteria, such as *S. pneumoniae*, *Neisseria meningitidis*, and *Haemophilus influenzae*. Antigens and leukocytes enter the spleen through vascular sinusoids located in the red pulp that are in proximity to the marginal zone area. The white pulp area contains periarteriolar sheaths of lymphocytes, mainly T cells, as well as periarteriolar follicles, which are mainly B cells. These, in turn, are surrounded by a microanatomic site known as the marginal zone that contains loose clusters of B cells, DCs, macrophages, and some $CD4^+$ T cells.[649]

Marginal zone B cells have unique phenotypic and functional properties that may be important in their response to blood-borne particulate antigens and to polysaccharide antigens. Murine and human marginal zone B cells of the spleen have similar $IgM^{hi}IgD^{-/lo}CD21^{hi}$ surface phenotypes[650] and include naïve and memory B cell subsets.[651-653] Compared with naïve follicular B cells, marginal zone B cells express lower levels of IgD and CD23 and higher levels of CD21. Marginal zone B cells, along with B-1 B cells, which are discussed later on, are important sources of early IgM response to blood-borne antigens, such as those associated with the surface of circulating bacteria.[654] The high levels of CD21 expression by marginal zone B cells may facilitate their binding of C3d-coated blood-borne antigens, such as encapsulated bacteria.[575] In addition, marginal zone B cells are more readily activated by non-BCR signals, such as LPS, and more rapidly become effector cells than naïve follicular B cells after activation.[655] This enhanced reactivity may be important in their being able to respond to purified polysaccharide antigens in the absence of T cell signals. Marginal zone B cells also appear "poised" to differentiate into plasmablasts because of their constitutive expression of the BLIMP-1 transcription factor, which acts as a master transcriptional regulator promoting plasma cell differentiation.[647]

Splenic B cells of the marginal zone have been implicated as the key population in mediating responses to blood-borne particulate antigens. These particulate antigens may be taken up immature DCs in the blood and transported to the spleen, where they interact with marginal zone B cells to rapidly induce IgM-secreting plasmablasts.[654,656] Splenic marginal zone B cells also may be required for the generation of antibody responses to purified polysaccharide antigens. As discussed later on, this immune response does not require T cell help (see section on development of B cell capacity to respond to T cell–dependent [TD] and T cell–independent [TI] antigens). Immunization with TI antigens before human splenectomy maintains the capacity of the immune system to respond to these antigens subsequently.[657] This finding suggests that the activation of splenic B cells recognizing polysaccharide antigens may result in their migration and persistence in other lymphoid organs. The pathways by which capsular polysaccharide antigens reach the marginal zone are unknown, and the role that marginal zone DCs or macrophages play in activating marginal zone B cells to produce antibody to purified polysaccharides remains poorly understood.

How human marginal zone B cells differentiate from naïve precursors also remains poorly understood. In mice, transitional B cells of the spleen appear to give rise to naïve marginal zone cells in cases in which BCR signaling is relatively weak. Transitional B cells that express low levels of CD1d have been proposed as the immediate precursors of murine marginal zone B cells, which are $CD1^{hi}$,[606] but whether human marginal zone B cells are $CD1^{hi}$ remains unclear. Murine marginal zone B cells express relatively high levels of the LFA-1 and VLA-4 integrins. These integrins are involved in retaining these B cells in the marginal zone compartment by binding to their respective ligands—ICAM-1 and VCAM-1.[658]

The origin of marginal zone B cells that participate in the response to polysaccharide antigens also remains controversial. Naïve marginal zone B cells are relatively sessile, which had suggested that this population would be the major contributor to polysaccharide antigen responses in vivo. A recent study, however, suggests that naïve follicular B cells in the circulation can enter the marginal zone and acquire a marginal zone phenotype and respond to purified polysaccharide immunization in the absence of T cell help.[659] These findings, which require confirmation, raise the possibility that the splenic microenvironment may induce B cells with a follicular phenotype to acquire the characteristics and immunologic function of marginal zone B cells.

B-1 and B-2 Cells

B cells that express CD5 and that have low levels of surface expression of CD45RA appear to represent a distinct B cell subset that has been termed B-1. The B-1 subset can be further divided into B-1a cells, in which CD5 is expressed on the cell surface, and B-1b cells, in which CD5 expression is limited to the RNA level.[660] B cells that lack CD5 mRNA or protein expression and that are $CD45RA^{hi}$ compose the B-2 lineage; they include most of the peripheral B cells in the adult, as well as most marginal zone B cells of the spleen. In mice, B-1 cells are restricted largely to the peritoneal and pleural cavities; this compartmentalization suggests a specialized function.[654] By contrast, human B-1a cells are more widely distributed in the circulation and in the follicular mantle regions of the tonsil, spleen, and other lymphoid tissue.[650]

In mice, naïve B-1 cells and marginal zone B cells both are important contributors to the early production of IgM in response to blood-borne particulate antigens and to other T-independent antigens. Murine B-1 cells and marginal zone B cells also share other features that are distinct from follicular B cells, such as expression of CD9, a high level of effectiveness as APCs for T cells in vitro, an enhanced capacity to be activated by LPS or CD40 engagement, and an ability to rapidly enter the cell cycle after activation.[654] It is possible that these common features are involved in the rapid onset of immune responses mediated by B-1 and marginal zone B cells. In contrast with mice, however, most human B-1 cells have an $IgM^{hi}IgD^{hi}CD21^{lo}CD23^{hi}$ surface phenotype that is distinct from that of human splenic marginal zone B cells, which are predominantly $IgM^{hi}IgD^{lo/-}CD21^{hi}CD23^{-}$.[650] These phenotypic differences, along with those in cell distribution, raise the possibility that the B-1 cells in humans may have immunologic roles distinct from those of murine B-1 cells and marginal zone B cells.

B-1 and B-2 cells appear to be subject to different positive and negative influences of the preimmune (i.e., before exposure to foreign antigen) immunoglobulin repertoire.[661,662] B-1 cells have a tendency to produce antibodies that are mainly of the IgM isotype and that are polyreactive; that is, individual antibodies typically are of low affinity but are able to react with multiple unrelated antigens. In contrast with B-1 cells, B-2 cells typically produce high-affinity antibodies that usually are monoreactive, bind only a single antigen or highly related antigens,[663] and often are of isotypes other than IgM.[664,665] B-1 cells are commonly reactive with both self-antigens, such as DNA, and foreign antigens, such as viral proteins or bacteria-derived products, such as phosphorylcholine. In mice, strong BCR signals during transitional B cell maturation favor differentiation into B-1 cells over other cell fates, and this may account for the tendency of these cells to be polyreactive. The expression on B-1a cells of CD5, which probably serves as a negative regulator of BCR signaling, may help protect autoreactive B-1a cells from negative selection and apoptosis.[654] Murine B-1 cells also may be relatively resistant, compared with B-2 cells, to the induction of Fas expression after CD40 engagement, and to Fas-mediated apoptosis.[654]

In the adult human, somatic hypermutation of immunoglobulin molecules is common for both B-1 and B-2 cells. This finding suggests that both cell types in humans are subject to an antigen-driven selection process after activation[662,666] and that activated B-1 cells tend to become memory cells that have not undergone isotype switching.[667] Whether B-1 cells are derived from a separate lineage or are induced to differentiate from a common precursor that is shared with B-2 cells[668] remains controversial.

As discussed later, B-1 cells predominate during early fetal development. These cells have been proposed to play a role in regulation and development of the immune system in early ontogeny, perhaps in the induction of tolerance to self-antigens, or in host defense, by provision of polyreactive IgM antibodies that are pathogen reactive.

Ontogeny of B Cells and Immunoglobulins

B Cell Development and Immunoglobulin Isotype Expression

Conventional B Cells. Pre-B cells are first detected in the human fetal liver and omentum by 8 weeks of gestation and in the fetal bone marrow by 13 weeks of gestation.[669,670] Between 18 and 22 weeks of gestation, pro- or pre-B cells also can be detected in the liver, lung, and kidney.[586] These fetal organs also express the CXCL12 (SDF-1) chemokine, which serves as a critical chemoattractant for B cell precursors expressing the CXCR4 chemokine receptor.[671] These findings raise the possibility that B cell lymphopoiesis may occur in these organs in situ at this stage of fetal development.

By mid-gestation, the bone marrow is the predominant site of pre-B cell development.[672] B cell lymphopoiesis occurs solely in the bone marrow after 30 weeks of gestation and for the remainder of life.[586] The neonatal circulation contains higher levels of $CD34^{+}CD38^{-}$ progenitor cells that are capable of differentiating into B cells than are found in the bone marrow compartment of children or adults.[673] The concentration of B cells in the circulation is higher during the second and third trimesters than at birth and further declines by adulthood.[287,674] B cells expressing surface IgM are present by 10 weeks of gestation.[669] Unlike IgM^{+} adult B cells in the peripheral lymphoid organs, most of which also express surface IgD, fetal B cells at this stage express IgM without IgD.[669,675] Such $IgM^{+}IgD^{-}$ B cells constitute a transitory stage between pre-B cells and mature $IgM^{+}IgD^{+}$ B cells, and it is at this stage that the CD21 surface molecule is expressed.

Murine studies have shown that exposure of transitional $IgM^{+}IgD^{-}$ B cells to antigens, including those found in the adult bone marrow, results in clonal anergy rather than activation.[676] The susceptibility of transitional $IgM^{+}IgD^{-}$ cells to clonal anergy maintains B cell tolerance to soluble self-antigens present at high concentrations. Thus, antigen exposure in utero may induce B cell tolerance rather than an antibody response and may account for the observation that early congenital infection sometimes results in pathogen-specific defects in immunoglobulin production. In some cases, such as congenital mumps, these defects may occur despite normal T cell responses, such as DTH,[544] suggesting a direct inhibitory effect on antigen-specific B cell function.

Between 8 and 11 weeks of gestation, transcripts for IgA and IgG can be detected in the liver,[677] followed shortly by the appearance of B cells bearing sIg of the IgA, IgG, and IgD isotypes. By 16 weeks of gestation, fetal bone marrow B cells expressing sIg of all heavy chain isotypes are detectable.[678] The stimulus for isotype switching during fetal development remains unclear, because in the adult, isotype switching typically occurs in response to B cell activation by foreign protein antigens. The frequency of B cells in tissues rapidly increases, so that by 22 weeks of gestation, the proportion of B cells in the spleen, blood, and bone marrow is similar to that in the adult.[675,669]

Neonatal B cells have increased surface levels of IgM compared with those for adult B cells; these differences persist for several years.[679,680] In a flow cytometric study in which nonspecific binding was carefully excluded, neonatal B cells expressing surface IgG or IgA were below the limit of detectability (i.e., less than 1% of circulating B cells).[681] True germinal centers in the spleen and lymph nodes are absent during fetal life but appear during the first months after postnatal antigenic stimulation.[682]

B-1 Cells. Another distinct feature of fetal and neonatal B cells is the high frequency of CD5 expression, indicating that they belong to the B-1a subset.[683] More than 40% of B cells in the fetal spleen, omentum, and circulation at mid-gestation are $CD5^+$,[664,665,684] but lesser numbers are found in the fetal liver and bone marrow.[684] $CD5^+$ B cells also are present in the neonatal circulation[280] and gradually decline with postnatal age.[664,685,686] Like adult B-1a cells, the fetal and newborn B-1a cells express IgM antibodies that are polyreactive, including reactivity with self-antigens, such as DNA.[663-665,687]

Although $CD5^+$ B cells may help to regulate the immune system in early ontogeny, including the induction of tolerance to self-antigens, they lack most surface markers characteristic of previously activated B cells.[664] The extent to which human $CD5^+$ and $CD5^-$ B cells represent distinct lineages remains contentious. For example, activation using a combination of antibody to IgM, engagement of CD40, and exogenous IL-4 results in the loss of CD5 expression by both neonatal and adult $CD5^+$ cells,[680] raising the possibility of a precursor-product relationship between $CD5^+$ and $CD5^-$ B cells.

B-1 cells constitute the major source of the low amounts of circulating "natural" IgM present at birth produced in the absence of antigenic stimulation. Murine studies have defined a role for natural IgM: Mice in which secretory but not surface IgM was eliminated by gene targeting had decreased primary responses to T cell–dependent antigens[688] and an increased susceptibility to acute peritonitis from endogenous bacteria due to a lack of natural IgM antibodies.[689] Although natural IgM antibodies are of low affinity, they can activate complement, which may allow antigenically naïve B cells to become activated as a result of receiving of co-stimulation via CD21 (complement receptor 2). Natural IgM does not appear to play a role in enhancing the response to polysaccharide antigens, at least in mice.[688-690]

Development of the Immunoglobulin Repertoire

V(D)J Segment Usage. The primary or preimmune immunoglobulin repertoire, which consists of all antibodies that can be expressed before encounter with antigen, is determined by the number of different B cell clones with distinct antigen specificity. This preimmune immunoglobulin repertoire is limited during the initial stages of B cell development in the fetus in comparison with that in the adult. In the early to mid-gestation human fetus, the set of V segments used to generate the heavy chain gene is smaller than in the adult.[691,692] The V segments are scattered throughout the heavy chain gene locus.[693] Differences in the usage of particular heavy chain D and J segments between the first and second trimesters and term also have been identified.[580] These developmental differences are intrinsic rather than the result of environmental influences, because they occur in immature B cell precursors lacking a pre-BCR complex.

By the third trimester, the V and D segment heavy chain gene repertoire of peripheral B cells appears to be similar to that of the adult, although there may be overrepresentation of certain segments, such as DH7-27.[694] Certain heavy chain V segments expressed in adult B cells are not found in neonatal B cells,[695,696] but it is unlikely that this limits the neonatal humoral immune response. Other V segments, such as V_{H3}, are present at a greater frequency in the preimmune Ig repertoire.[696,697] This increased representation may confer on antibody molecules the ability to bind protein A of *S. aureus*, thus providing some intrinsic protection during the perinatal period.

Role of CDR3 Length and Terminal Deoxytransferase. The length of the CDR3 region of the immunoglobulin heavy chain, which is formed at the junction of the V segment with the D and J segments, is shorter in the mid-gestation fetus than at birth[698] or in adulthood, including in pre-B cells.[699] This is due, in part, to decreased TdT, which is responsible for N-nucleotide additions. This decreased TdT expression is an intrinsic property of neonatal $CD34^+$ precursor cells not yet committed to the B lineage, because in vitro differentiation of B-lineage cells from neonatal $CD34^+$ cells results in lower amounts of TdT than are present in similar cells generated from adult $CD34^+$ cells.[700]

Up to 25% of heavy chain CDR3 regions in fetal B cells lack N additions, and in the remaining, the size of the N-nucleotide additions is smaller than for neonatal or adult CDR3 regions. The CDR3 region is the most hypervariable portion of immunoglobulins, and a short CDR3 region significantly reduces the diversity of the fetal immunoglobulin repertoire.[695] The CDR3 region of the heavy chain gene remains relatively short at the beginning of the third trimester and gradually increases in length until birth.[137,694,701,702]

Because the CDR3 region is at the center of the antigen-binding pocket of the antibody,[579] reduced CDR3 diversity could limit the efficiency of the antibody response. A complete lack of amino-terminal additions would be predicted to result in antibodies with combining sites that are relatively flat and potentially inefficient at combining with antigen.[580] The importance of shortened CDR3 regions by themselves in limiting antibody responses is doubtful, however, because gene knockout mice lacking TdT produce normal antibody responses following immunization or infection.[268] Although a combination of lack of TdT and limitations in V and D usage could limit the ability of the fetal B cells to recognize a full spectrum of foreign antigens, particularly before mid-gestation, such a "hole in the repertoire" has not been documented.

In mice, premature expression of TdT during fetal development achieved by transgenesis appears to be detrimental in adulthood by preventing the appearance of certain antibody specificities, such as with antibodies that are reactive with phosphorylcholine.[703] This perturbation results in the increased susceptibility of mice to *S. pneumoniae*, which contains phosphorylcholine as a cell wall component, and suggests that a lack of TdT expression during early ontogeny may be important for normal repertoire formation.

An analysis of productive and nonproductive lambda light chain gene repertoire of the human fetal spleen at 18 weeks of gestation found evidence indicating positive selection, receptor editing (an indication that developing B cells are encountering self-antigens that mediate negative selection), and expansion of B cells expressing specific light chains.[704] Similar findings apply to the kappa light chain repertoire of cord blood B cells.[705] Together, these findings suggest that the preimmune fetal immunoglobulin repertoire is significantly shaped by self-antigens.

Somatic Hypermutation. Although most neonatal and fetal immunoglobulin heavy chain gene variable regions appear not to have undergone somatic mutation,[696,698] the relevant studies examined heavy chain transcripts for IgM, an isotype in which somatic mutation is uncommon in the adult, except in IgM^+IgD^- memory B cells.[706,707] By contrast, somatic mutations are detectable in some neonatal B cells expressing IgG or IgA transcripts.[702] Among neonatal B cells that bear somatic mutations, the mutational frequency per length of DNA is similar to that of adult B cells. Together, these observations indicate that somatic hypermutation occurs normally by birth in the B cell compartment.

Neonatal B Cell Surface Phenotype

In adults, CD10 expression ceases at the antigenically naïve B cell stage. By contrast, most fetal bone marrow and spleen B cells express CD10.[683,708] $CD10^+$ B cells may constitute an immature transitional population but are functionally mature as indicated by their ability to undergo isotype switching. Small numbers of $CD10^+$ B cells are found at birth and these gradually decline during infancy.[709]

Increased expression of CD38 on neonatal B cells also has been observed.[679,680] Unfractionated neonatal B cells, a majority of which are $CD5^+$, and adult naïve B cells have similar levels of surface IgD, CD19, CD21, CD22, CD23, CD40, CD44, CD80, CD81, and CD86.[679,680,710-713] Expression of the CCR6 and CXCR5 chemokine receptors is similar by both cell types,[714,715] but neonatal B cells may have modestly lower levels of CCR7 than those observed in adult cells.[715] Rijkers and colleagues[716] reported that neonatal B cells also have reduced CD21 expression, possibly accounted for by an increased percentage of $CD21^-$ cells in the neonatal $CD5^-$ B cell subset.[711] Surface expression of the FcγRII receptor (CD32) is reduced on neonatal B cells,[679,717] possibly rendering them less subject to the inhibitory effect of antigen-antibody complexes.

Neonatal $CD5^-$ B cells have reduced expression of several adhesion molecules, including CD11a, CD44, CD54 (ICAM-1), and L-selectin.[715,718] A similar reduction is found in the $CD5^-$ B cells of adult patients during the first 3 months after either autologous or heterologous bone marrow transplantation but resolves by 14 months after transplantation.[718]

Circulating neonatal B cells have lower levels of MHC class II than those observed for adult splenic B cells and, unlike adult cells, an inability to increase intracellular calcium after engagement of MHC class II by mAb.[719] Moreover, because neonatal B cells proliferate as well as or better than adult splenic B cells after MHC class II engagement,[719] these alterations in signaling appear unlikely to compromise neonatal B cell function. A more recent finding[720] is absence of significant differences in MHC class II expression by circulating fetal B cells of the third trimester of pregnancy and in that by adult cells.

Cerutti and colleagues[721] reported that circulating neonatal B cells, of which approximately 90% were of the B-1a subset, expressed CD28, which typically is found on T cells and not on B cells. Neonatal B cells also expressed substantially more CD27 and CD80 than do adult spleen B cells, in which greater than 95% of the cells are of the B-2 subset. Whether this unusual neonatal surface phenotype also applies to the adult B-1a subset was not determined. What role CD28 on B cells plays in the immune response in vivo also is unclear. Nonetheless, the presence of CD80 and CD27, markers for adult memory B cells, suggest that some circulating neonatal B-1a cells have undergone activation in vivo.

Fetal and Neonatal T Cell–Dependent Immunoglobulin Production and Isotype Switching

Early in vitro studies of neonatal immunoglobulin production utilized PWM, a polyclonal activator of both T and B cells. In this system, immunoglobulin production was low compared with that in adults, and mixing experiments suggested that neonatal T cells acted as suppressors of immunoglobulin production by either adult or neonatal B cells. Further fractionation of the T cell populations in this assay suggested that in the absence of memory/effector T cells, antigenically naïve ($CD45RA^{hi}CD45RO^{lo}$) $CD4^+$ T cells of either the neonate or the adult acted as suppressors of antibody production.[221] The relevance of the suppression to neonatal B cell responses in vivo remains unclear, however. In any case, priming of neonatal or adult antigenically naïve $CD4^+$ T cells in vitro resulted in their acquisition of a $CD45RA^{lo}CD45RO^{hi}$ phenotype and, concurrently, an ability to enhance rather than suppress PWM-induced immunoglobulin production.[221] This increased capacity for B cell help probably reflects the fact that priming of naïve T cells induces enhanced expression of CD40 ligand and cytokines needed for T cell–dependent help for B cell responses.

When B cells are activated by exogenous cytokines (e.g., IL-4, IL-10, or cytokine-containing supernatants from activated T cells) and a cellular source of CD40 ligand (e.g., CD40 ligand expressing fibroblasts) or EBV infection, neonatal B cell production of IgM, IgG_1, IgG_2, IgG_3, IgG_4, and IgE is similar to that in adult antigenically naïve B cells.[378,722-724] Isotype switching is associated with cell division, and neonatal and adult B cells demonstrate a similar acquisition of switching starting after the third cell division.[725] Pre-B cells have the capacity for isotype switching even during fetal ontogeny: For example, isotype switching and IgE and IgG_4 production by fetal B and pre-B cells at 12 weeks of gestation can be induced in vitro.[683,726-728] IgA_1 and IgA_2 are produced in similar amounts by antigenically naïve fetal and adult B cells on stimulation with anti-CD40 antibody and vasoactive intestinal peptide hormone. Fetal pre-B cells also can synthesize IgA under these conditions.[637] When human fetal or neonatal B cells develop in, or are adoptively transferred into, SCID mice, they are capable of isotype switching and immunoglobulin production if appropriate T cell–derived signals are present.[507,729,730]

Other studies, however, suggest that isotype switching and antibody production by fetal and neonatal B cells is limited compared with these processes in antigenically naïve (IgM^+IgD^+) adult B cells. Durandy and colleagues[379] found that IgM, IgG, and IgE production by fetal B cells at midgestation was substantially lower than that of neonatal or adult B cells, suggesting an intrinsic hyporesponsiveness to CD40 or cytokine receptor engagement, or both. Neonatal B cells produce substantially less IgA than do adult naïve B cells in the presence of adult T cells stimulated by anti-CD3 mAb (as a source of CD40 ligand) and exogenous cytokines, such as IL-10.[731] These limitations of fetal and neonatal isotype switching and antibody production probably reflect intrinsic limitations of B cell function, particularly when T cell help may be limited. Such limited production is not due to decreased activation or proliferation, because neonatal B cells proliferate normally in response to engagement of CD40 or surface IgM, or both.[680]

Neonatal T cells activated for a few hours and histologically fixed provide less help for neonatal B cell immunoglobulin production and isotype switching than do similarly treated adult T cells.[378] Because the help provided by these fixed T cells probably is through CD40 ligand, reduced expression of CD40 ligand (or similar activation-induced molecules) by naïve neonatal T cells in the first few hours after activation may limit fetal and neonatal B cell immune responses. Whether decreased neonatal DC function also contributes to diminished B cell responses has not been determined.

IgM and IgG synthesis are detected as early as 12 weeks of gestation in fetal organ cultures.[732] Immunoglobulin-secreting plasma cells are detectable by week 15 of gestation, and those secreting IgG and IgA by 20 and 30 weeks of gestation, respectively.[733] In general, neonatal B cells can differentiate into IgM-secreting plasma cells as efficiently as adult cells. Splawski and Lipsky[734] found that T cell–dependent immunoglobulin production by neonatal $CD5^+$ and $CD5^-$ B cells is more readily inhibited by agents that raise intracellular cyclic adenosine monophosphate (cAMP), such as prostaglandin E_2 (PGE_2).

Development of B Cell Capacity to Respond to T Cell–Dependent and T Cell–Independent Antigens

Definition of T-Dependent and T-Independent Antigens. The chronology of the response to different antigens differs, depending on the need for cognate T cell help (Table 4-6). Largely on the basis of findings on murine studies, antigens can be divided into those dependent on a functional thymus and cognate help (direct cell-cell interactions) provided by mature αβ T cells (T-dependent antigens) and those partially or completely independent of T cell help (T-independent antigens). The T-independent (TI) antigens can be further divided into TI type I and TI type II, in accordance with their dependence on cytokines produced by T cells (or other cells).

Most proteins are T-dependent antigens requiring cognate T cell–B cell interaction for production of antibodies (other than small amounts of IgM). The antibody response to T-dependent antigens is characterized by the generation of memory B cells with somatically mutated, high-affinity immunoglobulin and the potential for isotype switching.

TI type I antigens are those that bind to B cells and directly activate them in vitro to produce antibody without T cells or exogenous cytokines. In the human, one such TI type I antigen is fixed *Brucella abortus*. TI type II antigens are mostly polysaccharides with multiple identical subunits, and certain proteins that contain multiple determinants of identical or similar antigenic specificity. Responses to these antigens are enhanced in vitro and in vivo by a variety of cytokines, including IL-6, IL-12, IFN-γ, and GM-CSF.[735-738] NK cells, T cells, or macrophages may provide these cytokines. TI type II responses also are enhanced by bacterially derived LPS, lipoproteins, porin proteins, or unmethylated CpG DNA.[737,739,740] This enhancement probably occurs primarily by engagement of TLR on B cells.[572] The response to TI type II antigens is characterized by the lack of B cell memory or somatic hypermutation and is restricted largely to the IgM and IgG_2 isotypes.[716]

Response to T-Dependent Antigens. The capacity of the neonate to respond to T-dependent antigens is well established at birth (see Table 4-6) and is only modestly reduced in comparison with the response in the adult. Any of several mechanisms, alone or in combination, may be responsible for this modest reduction: decreased DC interactions or function with $CD4^+$ T cells or B cells; limitations in $CD4^+$ T cell activation and expansion into a T helper/effector cell population; impaired cognate interactions between $CD4^+$ T cells and B cells; or an intrinsic B cell defect. Another possibility is that T-dependent antigens preferentially upregulate CD22, which raises the threshold for B cell activation, on neonatal compared with adult B cells.[711]

Most studies of the neonatal immune response to T-dependent antigens have not evaluated antibody affinity, a reflection of somatic mutation, or isotype expression. Such responses might be limited early in the immune response because of decreased CD40 ligand expression by $CD4^+$ T cells.[364,376-379] Studies are needed to determine if reductions in CD40 ligand expression by antigen-specific T cells also occurs in response to neonatal vaccination, and, if so, whether such reduced expression correlates with reduced memory B cell development, decreased isotype switching, and somatic hypermutation.

Table 4–6 Hierarchy of Antibody Responsiveness to Different Antigens

Species	Type of Antigen	Examples of Antigen	Age at Onset of Antibody Response
Mouse	T cell–dependent	TNP–KLH	Birth
	T cell–independent type I	TNP–*Brucella abortus*	Birth
	T cell–independent type II	TNP-Ficoll	Delayed (2-3 wk of age)
Human	T cell–dependent	Tetanus toxoid, HbsAg, *Haemophilus influenzae* conjugate vaccine, bacteriophage φX174	Birth
	T cell–independent type I	TNP–*B. abortus*	Birth
	T cell–independent type II	Bacterial capsular polysaccharides (*H. influenza* type b, *Neisseria meningitidis, Streptococcus pneumoniae,* GBS)	Delayed (6–24 mo of age)

GBS, group B streptococci, HbsAgs, hepatitis B surface antigen; KLH, keyhole limpet hemocyanin; TNP, trinitrophenol.

Response to T-Independent Antigens. Antibody production by human neonatal B cells to a TI type I antigen in vitro (*B. abortus*) is only modestly reduced[741] (see Table 4-6). This reduction may reflect a decreased ability of antigen-activated B cells to proliferate rather than a decreased precursor frequency of antigen-specific clones.[741]

In humans and mice, the response to TI type II antigens is the last to appear chronologically (see Table 4-6). This helps to account for the neonate's susceptibility to infection with encapsulated bacteria, such as group B streptococci,[742,743] and the poor response to polysaccharide antigens, such as the unconjugated capsular polysaccharides of *H. influenzae* type b, meningococci, and pneumococci, until approximately 2 to 3 years of age. The poor response in children younger than 2 years of age is associated with their lack of circulating memory ($CD27^{hi}$) B cells that express IgM and have not undergone isotype switching.[744] The reduction or absence of these IgM memory B cells in adult patients after splenectomy suggests that they may depend on the spleen microenvironment for their generation or long-term survival. Whether the decreased responses to TI type II antigens during early childhood reflects an intrinsic B cell immaturity or decreased function of other cells such as APCs of the spleen, or both, remains unclear.

Decreased expression of CD21 on neonatal B cells has been proposed as a possible mechanism for limitations in TI type II response in the neonate. CD19 is expressed in association with CD21, the type 2 complement receptor, and serves to transduce B cell–activating signals when CD21 is engaged by C3 complement components, thereby inducing polysaccharide-reactive B cells to proliferate in vivo. Genetic disruption experiments in mice support the idea that the type 2 complement receptor, which includes CD21 and CD35 in mice, is important for TI type II antibody responses to pathogens, such as *S. pneumoniae.*[575] In vitro studies of human splenic tissue suggest that TI type II antigens activate complement and bind C3, and then localize to the marginal zone splenic B cells expressing type 2 complement receptors.[716] Incubation of human splenic tissue with pneumococcal polysaccharides and complement results in preferential binding of the polysaccharide and C3, presumably as a complex, to $CD21^+$ B cells of this area of the spleen.[745] Rijkers and colleagues[716] and Griffioen and associates[746] found lower CD21 expression on neonatal B cells than on adult B cells.[746] This group of investigators[747] also found that the response to bacterial polysaccharides (at approximately 2 to 3 years of age) correlates with the appearance of B cells expressing CD21 in the marginal zone region of the spleen.

These observations argue for an intrinsic immaturity in B cell responsiveness to TI type II antigens. Decreased expression of CD21 by neonatal B cells has not been confirmed by others, however.[679,713] Alternative mechanisms, such as limitations in APC populations of the splenic marginal zone, also have not been excluded.

Human neonatal B cells demonstrate a marked decrease in CD22 expression following engagement of IgM, a stimulus used to mimic a TI type II antigen.[711] Because CD22 is a negative regulator of B cell activation, however, this finding does not readily explain the diminished response, unless it results in hyperresponsive neonatal B cells prone to apoptosis.

Dextran-conjugated anti-immunoglobulin mAbs have been used to mimic the events in TI type II antibody responses in vitro.[737] Human neonatal B cells respond to this stimulus as well as adult B cells, suggesting that the lack of the neonatal TI type II response is not due to an intrinsic limitation of B cell function.[748] B cells that respond to dextran-conjugated anti-immunoglobulin mAbs, however, may be functionally distinct from B cells that respond to polysaccharides or other TI type II antigens.

Murine neonatal B cells are able to proliferate in response to the TI type II antigen trinitrophenol (TNP)-Ficoll, or to the polyclonal stimulus goat–anti-murine IgM, if CpG-containing oligonucleotides with unmethylated cytosine residues are present[740]; such unmethylated CpG DNA is known to activate these cells through TLR-9.[749] CpG oligonucleotides also induce human cord blood and adult peripheral blood B cells to respond similarly in terms of cell proliferation, the production of chemokines (CCL3 [MIP-1α] and CCL4 [MIP-1β]), and upregulation of CD86 and MHC class II expression.[715] Thus, neonatal B cells appear to have an intact TLR-9–mediated B cell activation pathway.

Specific Antibody Response by the Fetus to Maternal Immunization and Congenital Infection

Response to Fetal Immunization in Animal Models. Early studies by Silverstein and colleagues of the antibody response of fetal sheep and rhesus monkeys to immunization with foreign proteins were conceptually important in establishing two major features of the ontogeny of B cell immune competence for T cell–dependent antigens in larger mammals. First, immune competence for T cell–dependent antigens is established early during fetal ontogeny: Primary immunization of fetal rhesus monkeys between 103 and 127 days of gestation (out of a total of 160 days) with sheep red blood cells (SRBCs), a T cell–dependent antigen, results in the formation of SRBC-reactive B cells in the spleen; reimmunization 3 weeks later results in a rapid antibody response utilizing IgG.[750] In fetal sheep, the antibody response to bacteriophage φX174 occurs as early as 40 days after conception,[751] and again, isotype switching is evident during the fetal response. Together, these findings suggest that B cell response to protein antigens, including isotype switching and probably memory cell generation, are functional during fetal life. Second, these responses occur in a predictable, stepwise fashion for particular antigens. For example, in fetal sheep, the antibody response to keyhole limpet hemocyanin and lymphocytic choriomeningitis virus are first detectable at about 80 and 120 days, respectively, after conception.[751] These differences in the responsiveness to particular antigens are not explained by limitations in the repertoires of surface Ig or αβ-TCRs, because it is known that a diverse repertoire is established early in ontogeny.

No correlation exists between the physical or chemical characteristics of particular antigens and their immunogenicity during ontogeny. For example, bacteriophage φX174 and bacteriophage T4 both are particulate antigens that should interact in a similar manner. In fetal sheep, however, bacteriophage T4 becomes immunogenic 60 days after φX174 does so. Baboon fetuses immunized with HBsAg vaccine have a robust IgG antibody response, and this response is boosted by postnatal immunization.[752]

Response to Maternal Immunization. In studies by one group of investigators, antibody responses by the human fetus may occur following maternal immunization with tetanus toxoid during the third trimester but not earlier, as shown by the presence of IgM tetanus antibodies at birth.[753,754] Whether tetanus-specific IgG responses at birth were reduced, as suggested by reports of reduced $CD4^+$ T cell responses to tetanus vaccine in young infants,[327] remains unclear. Infants with tetanus-specific antibodies at birth had enhanced secondary antibody responses following tetanus immunization, indicating that fetal antigen exposure was a priming event rather than a tolerizing one.[753] By contrast, Englund and associates[524] were unable to demonstrate neonatal tetanus toxoid–specific IgM antibody or T cell proliferation following maternal tetanus toxoid vaccination in the third trimester. Similarly, no fetal response to maternal immunization with inactivated trivalent influenza vaccine was noted.[524] If a fetal antibody response to maternal vaccination with polysaccharide-protein conjugate vaccines occurred, such vaccines could be used during pregnancy to ensure that protective antibody levels were present at birth.

Response to Intrauterine Infection. Specific antibody may be present at birth to agents of intrauterine infection, including rubella virus, CMV, HSV, VZV, and *Toxoplasma gondii* and often can be used to diagnose congenital infection. Not all fetuses have an antibody response to intrauterine infection, however; specific IgM antibody was undetectable in 34% of infants with congenital rubella,[755] 19% to 33% of infants with congenital *Toxoplasma* infection,[756,757] and 11% of infants with congenital CMV infection.[758] When congenital infection is severe during the first or second trimester, antibody production may be delayed until late childhood.[542] This delay may reflect a lack of T cell help, because antigen-specific T cell responses often are reduced in parallel with B cell responses.

Congenital *Toxoplasma* infection may lead to detectable IgE and IgA anti-*Toxoplasma* antibodies at birth or during early infancy.[759] Similarly, filaria- or schistosome-specific IgE is present in the sera of most newborns following maternal filiariasis or schistosomiasis.[760] Thus, T cell–dependent isotype switching and immunoglobulin production occurs during fetal life, at least for certain pathogens. In fact, with some infectious agents, such as *Toxoplasma*, IgA or IgE antibodies may be more sensitive than IgM antibodies for diagnosis of congenital infection. The titers of IgA and IgE anti-*Toxoplasma* antibodies may be lower at 20 to 30 weeks of gestation than after birth,[761-763] however, indicating that their production is delayed in the context of congenital infection.

Specific Antibody Responses by the Neonate and Young Infant to Protein Antigens

Immunization of neonates usually elicits a protective response to protein antigens, including tetanus and diphtheria toxoids,[764] OPV,[765] *Salmonella* flagellar antigen,[742,743] bacteriophage φX174,[766] and HBsAg (with hepatitis B vaccine).[767] The response to some vaccines, however, may be less vigorous in the neonate than in older children or adults. A diminished primary response to recombinant hepatitis B vaccine has been noted in term neonates lacking maternally derived HBsAg antibody, compared with that in unimmunized children and adults.[767,768] The ultimate anti-HBsAg titers achieved in neonates after secondary and tertiary immunizations are similar to those in older children, indicating that neonatal immunization does not result in tolerance.[767] If initial immunization is delayed until 1 month of age, the antibody response to primary hepatitis B vaccination is increased and nearly equivalent to that in older children, suggesting that the developmental limitations responsible for reduced antibody responses are transient.[767,769] Similarly, 2-week-old infants immunized with a single dose of diphtheria or tetanus toxoid demonstrated delayed production of specific antibody compared with that in older infants; by 2 months of age, their response was similar to that of 6-month-old infants,[770] suggesting rapid maturation of T-dependent responses. The switch from IgM to IgG also may be delayed following neonatal vaccination for some (e.g., *Salmonella* H vaccine[743]) but not all (e.g., bacteriophage φX174[766]) antigens. Immunization of infants born to HIV-infected mothers with recombinant HIV-1 gp120 vaccine in MF59 adjuvant, beginning at birth, also resulted in high antibody titers, indicating that early postnatal vaccination is not tolerigenic.[771]

Unlike with other vaccines, in newborns given whole-cell pertussis vaccination, not only may they demonstrate a poor initial antibody response, but their subsequent antibody response to certain antigenic components, such as pertussis toxin, may be less than in infants initially immunized at 1 month of age or older,[772-774] suggesting low-level tolerance. Whole-cell pertussis vaccine immunization of premature infants (born at 28 to 36 weeks of gestation) at 2 months of age elicited responses similar to those in 2-month-old term infants,[765] indicating that this putative tolerigenic period wanes rapidly and is relatively independent of gestational age. This low-level tolerance appears to be restricted to whole-cell pertussis vaccine, because an inhibitory effect has not been observed following administration of diphtheria or tetanus toxoid[764] or hepatitis B vaccine given within 48 hours of birth.[767] Administration of OPV at birth enhanced rather than inhibited the response to subsequent immunization, also indicating that immunization through the mucosal route does not produce tolerance.[775]

The antibody response to measles vaccine given at 6 months of age is significantly less than when the vaccine is given at 9 or at 12 months of age, even when the inhibitory effect of maternal antibody is controlled for.[776] This decreased response is not due to a lack of measles-specific T cells, because measles antigen–specific T cell proliferation and IL-12 and IFN-γ proliferation were similar in the three age groups.[776-778] The basis for this reduced response is not known.

Specific Antibody Responses by the Term Neonate to Polysaccharide and Polysaccharide-Protein Conjugates

In contrast with the response to protein antigens, the newborn's response to polysaccharide antigens is absent or severely blunted, as demonstrated by an inability to mount an antibody response to unconjugated *H. influenzae* type b polysaccharide vaccine or to group B streptococcal capsular antigens after infection. The response to some polysaccharide antigens can be demonstrated by 6 months of age, but the response to vaccination with *H. influenzae* or *N. meningitidis* type C, or to most pneumococcal polysaccharides, is poor until approximately 18 to 24 months.[779] This inability to respond to polysaccharides and other TI type II antigens is not clearly understood but evidently is not due to a lack of the appropriate antibody repertoire, at least for *H. influenzae*.[780] The delayed postnatal appearance of marginal zone B cells in the spleen has been proposed to account for this delayed response (see section on development of B cell capacity to respond to T cell–dependent and T cell–independent antigens), although this suggestion remains controversial.

Covalent conjugation of *H. influenzae* capsular polysaccharide to a protein carrier renders it immunogenic in infants as young as 2 months of age and primes for an enhanced antibody response to unconjugated vaccine given at 12 months of age. Because the response to the unconjugated vaccine usually is poor at this age, the conjugate vaccine is thought to have induced polysaccharide-specific B cell memory.[781] Similarly, the administration of a single dose of *H. influenzae* type b polysaccharide–tetanus toxoid conjugate to term neonates as early as a few days of age may enhance the antibody response to unconjugated *H. influenzae* type b polysaccharide vaccine at 4 months of age.[782] This enhanced response is weak, however, and does not occur when the neonate is primed with tetanus toxoid followed by immunization with conjugate vaccine at 2 months of age.[783]

Coupling of the *H. influenzae* type b polysaccharide to a protein carrier converts a TI type II antigen to a T-dependent antigen.[784] This is accompanied by an enhanced magnitude and higher-avidity antibody response on subsequent boosting, presumably resulting from T-dependent memory B cell generation and somatic hypermutation. The early interactions between T cells and B cells in response to such carbohydrate-protein conjugate vaccines are summarized in Figure 4-9. Conjugation of *H. influenzae* type b polysaccharide to tetanus or diphtheria toxoid does not change the repertoire of the antibodies produced from that of the free polysaccharide.[780,781] The neonatal response to conjugate vaccines now mimics the response to other T-dependent antigens. Vaccination with protein–capsular polysaccharide conjugate vaccines containing polysaccharides of *S. pneumoniae* (types 4, 6B, 9V, 14, 18C, 19F, and 23F)[785-787] and *N. meningitidis* (types A and C)[788] is immunogenic in infants as young as 2 months of age and primes them for subsequent memory responses.

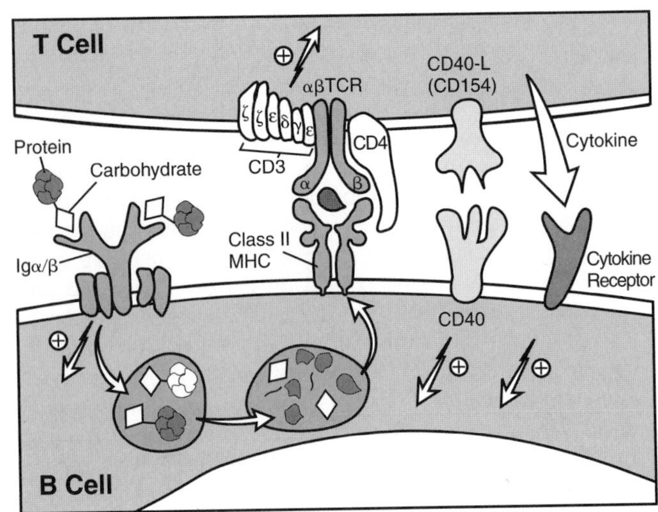

Figure 4–9 Interactions between B cells and T cell in the response to vaccines consisting of purified carbohydrate (e.g., bacterial capsular polysaccharide) covalently linked to protein carrier. The carbohydrate moiety of the conjugate is bound by surface immunoglobulin (sIg) on B cells, resulting in the internalization of the conjugate. Peptides derived from the protein moiety of the conjugate are presented by major histocompatibility complex (MHC) class II on the B cell, resulting in the activation of the T cell and expression of CD40 ligand. Engagement of CD40 on the B cell by CD40 ligand, in conjunction with cytokines secreted by the T cell, results in carbohydrate-specific B cell proliferation, immunoglobulin isotype switching, secretion of antibody, and memory B cell generation.

Antibody Responses by the Premature Infant to Immunization

Preterm neonates of 24 weeks of gestation or greater produce antibody to protein antigens such as diphtheria toxoid, diphtheria-pertussis-tetanus vaccine, and oral and inactivated poliovirus vaccines as well as do term neonates, when the vaccines are administered at 2, 4, and 6 months of age.[765,789-791] The antibody response in premature infants to multiple doses of hepatitis B vaccine, initially administered at birth, are clearly reduced compared with that in term infants.[792] These titers are substantially increased if immunization of the premature is delayed until 5 weeks of age, indicating the importance of postnatal age rather than of a particular body weight.[793]

The antibody levels after three doses of *H. influenzae*–type capsular polysaccharide–tetanus conjugate vaccine are significantly less in premature infants than in term infants, however, when vaccination is begun at 2 months of age.[794] This reduced antibody response is particularly true in premature infants with chronic lung disease,[795] in whom it may result in part from glucocorticoid treatment. As in term infants, the response of premature infants to polysaccharide antigens remains diminished during the first 2 years of life.

Maternally Derived Immunoglobulin G Antibody

The mechanism by which IgG is transferred to the fetus is only incompletely understood but depends on the recognition of maternal IgG through its Fc domain. IgG is internalized by the trophoblast, possibly by pinocytosis.[796] The next step in transport involves the FcRn, an intracellular IgG receptor that is a unique β_2-microglobulin–associated nonpolymorphic member of the MHC class I family.[797] FcRn lacks a functional peptide-binding groove and, instead, uses a different region of the molecule for binding IgG through its Fc domain. IgG bound to FcRn receptor undergoes transcytosis across the syncytiotrophoblast, followed by its release into the interstitium in the vicinity of endothelial cells surrounding fetal villous vessels.[798] How IgG is internalized and transported across the endothelium of fetal villous vessels is unclear, because these cells express only low or undetectable amounts of FcRn.[796] In addition to the syncytiotrophoblast, FcRn is widely expressed by nonplacental tissues, where it binds to pinocytosed IgG and recycles it to the circulation. This recycling system accounts for the very long half-life of IgG.

Maternal IgG and FcRn expression can be detected in placental syncytiotrophoblasts during the first trimester,[797] but transport does not occur, because circulating fetal concentrations of IgG remain below 100 mg/dL until about 17 weeks. The maternally derived placental cytotrophoblast, which is found between the syncytiotrophoblast and the fetal endothelium during the first trimester, may act as a barrier to IgG transport. This cytotrophoblast layer becomes

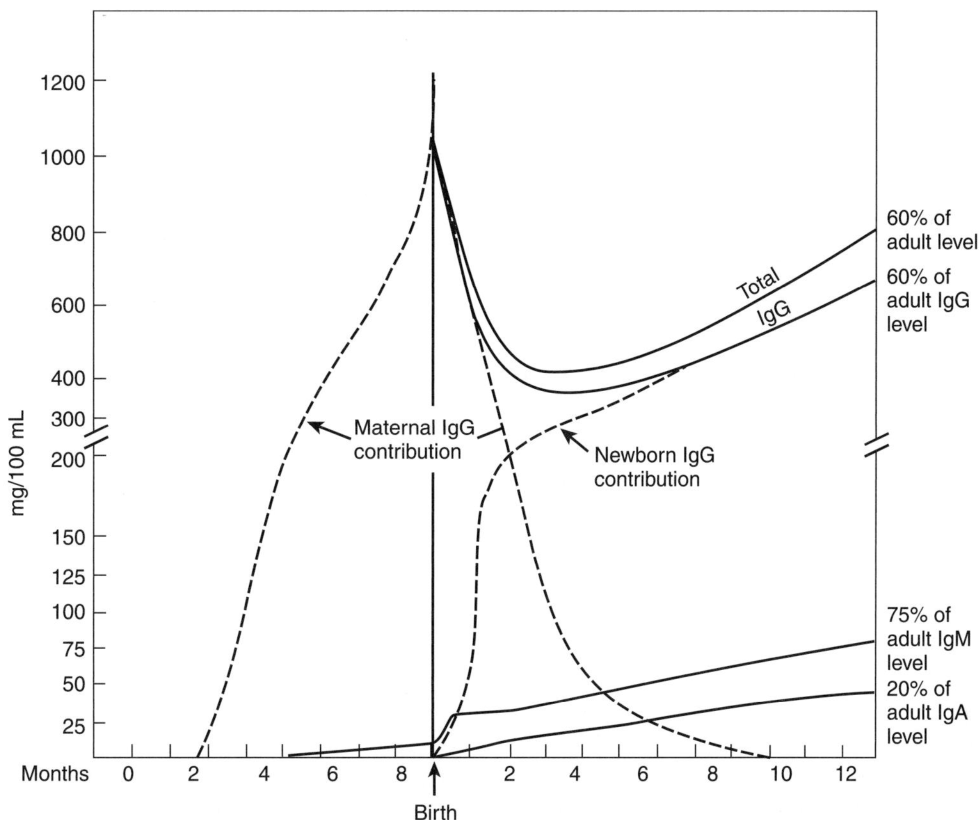

Figure 4–10 Immunoglobulin (IgG, IgM, and IgA) levels in the fetus and in the infant the first year of life. The IgG of the fetus and newborn infant is solely of maternal origin. The maternal IgG disappears by age 9 months, by which time endogenous synthesis of IgG by the infant is well established. The IgM and IgA of the neonate are entirely endogenously synthesized because maternal IgM and IgA do not cross the placenta. (Data from Saxon A, Stiehm ER. The B-lymphocyte system. *In* Stiehm ER [ed]. Immunologic Disorders in Infants and Children, 3rd ed. Philadelphia, WB Saunders, 1989, pp 40-67.)

discontinuous as the villous surface area expands during the second trimester.[797]

IgG is detectable in the fetus by 17 weeks of gestation, after which circulating concentrations of IgG in the fetus rise steadily, reaching half of the term serum concentration by about 30 weeks, and equaling that of the mother by about 38 weeks.[799,800] In some instances, fetal IgG concentrations may exceed those of the mother,[801] which is associated with the IgG concentration within the syncytiotrophoblast prior to its release into the fetal interstitial space.[802]

The fetus synthesizes little IgG, so that the concentration in utero reflects almost solely maternally derived antibody (Fig. 4-10).[803] Accordingly, the degree of prematurity is reflected in proportionately lower neonatal IgG concentrations. The IgG_2 concentration in cord blood relative to that in maternal blood is low at birth, particularly in preterm infants, whereas the overall fetal-to-maternal ratio is usually near 1.0 for the other IgG subclasses.[804-806] The low IgG_2 concentration appears to reflect a relatively low affinity of the receptor involved in the IgG trophoblastic uptake for IgG_2. IgM, IgA, IgD, and IgE do not cross the placenta. Evidence for transamniotic transfer of IgG to the fetus also is lacking.[802]

Placental Transfer of Specific Antibodies

The fetus receives IgG antibodies against antigens to which the mother has been exposed by infection or vaccination (see Table 4-5). For example, in mothers immunized with *H. influenzae* type b capsular polysaccharide antigen at 34 to 36 weeks of gestation, concentrations of anticapsular antibody are high and result in protective antibody levels in her infant for approximately the first 4 months of life. In the absence of recent immunization or natural exposure, the maternal antibody IgG antibody titer may be too low to be protective to the neonate. Protection of the infant may be absent even if the mother is protected, because she has memory B cells and can mount a rapid recall antibody response on infectious challenge. In addition, if maternal antibodies are primarily IgM antibodies directed against gram-negative pathogens, such as *E. coli* and *Salmonella*,[742,743] the fetus will not be protected because IgM does not traverse the placenta. Finally, premature infants may not receive sufficient amounts of IgG for protection, because the bulk of maternal IgG is transferred to the fetus after 34 weeks of gestation,[807] thereby accounting for the greater susceptibility of premature compared with term neonates to certain infections, such as with VZV.[808]

Inhibition of Neonatal Antibody Responses by Maternal Antibodies. Maternal antibody also may inhibit the production by the fetus or newborn of antibodies of the same specificity. This inhibition varies with the maternal antibody titer and with the type and amount of antigen. Maternal anti-

Table 4–7 Levels of Immunoglobulins in Sera of Normal Subjects, by Age[a]

	IgG		IgM		IgA		Total Immunoglobulins	
Age	*mg/dL*	*Percentage of Adult Level*	*mg/dL*	*Percentage of Adult Level*	*mg/dL*	*Percentage of Adult Level*	*mg/dL*	*Percentage of Adult Level*
Newborn	1031 ± 200[b]	89 ± 17	11 ± 5	11 ± 5	2 ± 3	1 ± 2	1044 ± 201	67 ± 13
1–3 mo	430 ± 119	37 ± 10	30 ± 11	30 ± 11	21 ± 13	11 ± 7	418 ± 127	31 ± 9
4–6 mo	427 ± 186	37 ± 16	43 ± 17	43 ± 17	28 ± 18	14 ± 9	498 ± 204	32 ± 13
7–12 mo	661 ± 219	58 ± 19	54 ± 23	55 ± 23	37 ± 18	19 ± 9	752 ± 242	48 ± 15
13–24 mo	762 ± 209	66 ± 18	58± 23	59 ± 23	50 ± 24	25 ± 12	870 ± 258	56 ± 16
25–36 mo	892 ± 183	77 ± 16	61 ± 19	62 ± 19	71 ± 37	36 ± 19	1024 ± 205	65 ± 14
3–5 yr	929 ± 228	80 ± 20	56 ± 18	57 ± 18	93 ± 27	47 ± 14	1078 ± 245	69 ± 17
6–8 yr	923 ± 256	80 ± 22	65 ± 25	66 ± 25	124 ± 45	62 ± 23	1112 ± 293	71 ± 20
9–11 yr	1124 ± 235	97 ± 20	79 ± 33	80 ± 33	131 ± 60	66 ± 30	1334 ± 254	85 ±17
12–16 yr	946 ± 124	82 ± 11	59 ± 20	60 ± 20	148 ± 63	74 ± 32	1153 ± 169	74 ± 12
Adult	1158 ± 305	100 ± 26	99 ± 27	100 ± 27	200 ± 61	100 ± 31	1457 ± 353	100 ± 24

[a]The values were derived from measurements made for 296 normal children and 30 adults. Levels were determined by the radial diffusion technique, using specific rabbit antisera to human immunoglobulins.
[b]One standard deviation.
Adapted with permission from Stiehm ER, Fudenberg HH. Serum levels of immune globulins in health and disease: a survey. Pediatrics 37:715, 1966.

body markedly inhibits the response to measles and rubella vaccine, but not mumps vaccine[809]; this is the reason for delaying measles-mumps-rubella (MMR) vaccine until at least 12 months of age. Inhibition of the response to these live-attenuated viral vaccines may result in part from reduced replication of vaccine virus in the recipient.

Maternal antibodies also may inhibit the neonatal response to nonreplicating vaccines such as whole-cell pertussis vaccine,[774] diphtheria toxoid,[810] *Salmonella* flagellar antigen,[743] and inactivated poliovirus vaccine.[811] Maternal antibody may bind to and mask the immunogenic epitope, preventing it from binding to surface Ig and activating antigen-specific B cells. In addition, the formation of antigen–maternal IgG antibody complexes can inhibit activation of B cells via surface Ig by simultaneous engagement of the inhibitory FcγRII receptor by the IgG component of the complex. Alternatively, maternal antibody may lead to the rapid clearance of vaccine antigen and decreased immunogenicity. Finally, for certain antibodies, such as anti-HbsAg, neither maternal antibodies nor hepatitis B immune globulin administration has a substantial inhibitory effect on the newborns immune response to hepatitis B vaccination.

Immunoglobulin Synthesis by the Fetus and Neonate

Imunnoglobulin G

IgG is the predominant immunoglobulin isotype at all ages (Table 4-7).[812] In adults, IgG_1 is the predominant subclass, accounting for approximately 70% of total IgG; IgG_2, IgG_3, and IgG_4 account for approximately 20%, 7%, and 3% of the total, respectively.[813] Passively derived maternal IgG is the source of virtually all of the IgG subclasses detected in the normal fetus and neonate. Because the IgG plasma half-life is about 21 days, these maternally derived levels fall rapidly after birth. IgG synthesized by the neonate and that derived from the mother are approximately equal when the neonate reaches 2 months of age; by 10 to 12 months of age, the IgG is nearly all derived from synthesis by the infant. As a consequence of the fall in passively derived IgG and increased synthesis of IgG, values reach a nadir of approximately 400 mg/dL in term infants at 3 to 4 months of age and rise thereafter (see Table 4-7 and Fig. 4-10). The premature infant has lower IgG concentrations at birth, which reach a nadir at 3 months of age; mean IgG values of 82 and 104 mg/dL are observed in infants born at 25 to 28 and 29 to 32 weeks of gestation, respectively.

By 1 year, the total IgG concentration is approximately 60% of that in adults. IgG_3 and IgG_1 subclasses reach adult concentrations by 8 years, whereas IgG_2 and IgG_4 do so by 10 and 12 years of age, respectively.[814] As discussed earlier, maternal IgG may inhibit certain postnatal antibody responses by binding to FcγRII receptors and by rapidly clearing or masking potential antigens. The slow onset of IgG synthesis in the neonate, however, is predominantly an intrinsic limitation of the neonate, rather than of maternal antibody; indeed, a similar pattern of IgG development was observed in a neonate born to a mother with untreated agammaglobulinemia.[815]

The slow rise in IgG_2 concentrations parallels the poor antibody response to bacterial polysaccharide antigens (e.g., *H. influenzae* polyribosyl ribitol phosphate [PRP]), antibodies, which are predominantly IgG_2.[816] Of interest, the postpartum order in which adult levels of isotype expression are achieved closely parallels the order of the heavy chain gene segments that encode these isotypes. Thus, postnatal regulation of isotype switching is mediated in part at the heavy chain gene locus (e.g., its chromatin configuration may be developmentally regulated).

Although passive maternal antibody plays an important role in protection, it limits the value of immunoglobulin and antibody levels in the diagnosis of immunodeficiency or infection in the young infant.

Immunoglobulin M

IgM is the only isotype besides IgG that binds and activates complement, requiring only a single IgM molecule for activation. IgM increases from a mean of 6 mg/dL in premature infants born at less than 28 weeks of gestation to 11 mg/dL at term,[817,818] which is approximately 8% of the maternal IgM level. This IgM, which is likely to be preimmune (i.e., not the result of a B cell response to foreign antigens), is enriched for polyreactive antibodies produced by B-1 cells. Murine studies suggest that such natural IgM plays an important role in innate defense against infection, allowing time for the initiation of antigen-specific B cell response; it also enhances antigen-specific B cell responses through its ability to fix complement and thereby co-stimulate B cell activation through complement receptor 2 (CD21).[688-690] Some of the human neonatal IgM is monomeric and therefore nonfunctional, however, as opposed to its usual pentameric functional form.[819,820]

Postnatal IgM concentrations rise rapidly for the first month and then more gradually thereafter, presumably in response to antigenic stimulation (see Fig. 4-10 and Table 4-7). By 1 year of age, values are approximately 60% of those in adults. The postnatal rise is similar in premature and in term infants.[819] Elevated (greater than 20 mg/dL) IgM concentrations in cord blood suggest possible intrauterine infections,[821] but many infants with congenital infections have normal cord blood IgM levels.[758]

Immunoglobulin A

IgA does not cross the placenta, and its concentration in cord blood usually is 0.1 to 5.0 mg/dL, approximately 0.5% of the levels in maternal sera.[818] Concentrations are similar in term and in premature neonates,[817] and both IgA_1 and IgA_2 are present.

At birth, the frequency of IgA_1- and IgA_2-bearing B cells is equivalent. Subsequently, a preferential expansion of the IgA_1-bearing cell population occurs, presumably as a result of postnatal exposure to environmental antigens.[822] Concentrations in serum increase to 20% of those in adults by 1 year of age and rise progressively through adolescence (see Table 4-7). Increased cord blood IgA concentrations are observed in some infants with congenital infection.[821] Elevated IgA is common in young infants infected by vertical transmission with HIV. IgA has a relatively short half-life in plasma of approximately 5 days. Secretory IgA is present in substantial amounts in the saliva by 10 days after birth.[823]

Immunoglobulin D

IgD is detectable by sensitive techniques in serum from cord blood in term and premature infants.[817,824] Mean serum levels at birth are approximately 0.05 mg/dL[818] and increase during the first year of life. Circulating IgD has no clear functional role. The immune response of mice in which IgD expression has been eliminated by gene targeting appears to be normal. On the other hand, surface IgD can replace surface IgM in B cell function in the mouse. Together, these results suggest that the functions of IgM and IgD are largely redundant.

Immunoglobulin E

Although IgE synthesis by the fetus is detectable as early as 11 weeks, concentrations of IgE in cord blood are typically low, with a mean of approximately 0.5% of that of maternal levels.[818] This IgE is of fetal origin, and concentrations are higher in infants born at 40 to 42 weeks of gestation than in those born at 37 to 39 weeks.[818] The rate of postnatal increase varies and is greater in infants predisposed to allergic disease or greater environmental exposure to allergens.[825,826] The concentration of IgE at birth appears to have limited predictive value for later development of atopic disease.[827]

Summary

The neonate is partially protected from infection by passive maternal IgG antibody, predominantly transferred during the latter third of pregnancy. Fetal IgG concentrations are equal to or higher than maternal concentrations after 34 weeks of gestation. The inability of the neonate to produce antibodies in response to polysaccharides, particularly bacterial capsular polysaccharides, limits resistance to bacterial pathogens to which the mother has little or no IgG antibody. The basis for this defect remains unclear, but it may reflect an intrinsic limitation of B function or a deficiency in the anatomic microenvironment required for B cells to become activated and differentiate into plasma cells. By contrast, the neonatal IgM response to most protein antigens is intact and only slightly limited for IgG responses to certain vaccines. Nevertheless, a clear difference between neonates and older infants has been observed in the magnitude of the antibody response to most protein neoantigens, but this difference rapidly resolves following birth. A limited antibody response of premature infants to immunization with protein antigens occurs during the first month of life but not subsequently. Thus, chronologic (i.e., postnatal) age is more of a determinant of antibody responses to T-dependent antigens than is gestational age. Isotype expression by B cells after immunization with T-dependent antigens is limited by altered T cell function, such as reduced CD40 ligand production, and intrinsic limitations of B cell maturation and function. These limitations are exaggerated in the fetus.

NATURAL KILLER CELLS

Basic Aspects of Natural Killer Cells and Their Function

Overview

NK cells are large granular lymphocytes with cytotoxic function that do not rearrange either the TCR or immunoglobulin genes and therefore lack surface expression of TCR-CD3 and sIg. Virtually all circulating human NK cells in the adult express the NKp30 and NKp46 natural cytotoxicity receptors that appear to be NK cell specific.[828,829] Most adult NK cells also express proteins that are not unique to the NK cell lineage and are found on T cells or other cell types. These proteins include killer inhibitory receptors (KIRs), CD94-NKG2 family members, NKG2D, and 2B4, which are involved in either negative (KIR and CD94-NKG2A) or positive (NKG2D and 2B4) regulation of natural cytotoxicity. Most adult NK cells also express CD2, CD16, CD56, and CD161 (NKR-P1A) molecules,[829-831] and approximately 50% express CD57.[830] CD16 is a component of the FcγRIIIB receptor, which is activated by binding IgG coated on target cells. CD2 and CD57 may be involved in NK cell adhesion to either target cells or endothelium. Although the function of CD56 in NK cells is unclear, it has been used as a marker to differentiate subpopulations of NK cells (see later).[832] The function of CD161 is unclear. Finally, most or all NK cells express proteins involved in the intracellular propagation of activation signals, including CD3-ξ, FcεR1γ, and DNAX-activation protein (DAP) 10 and DAP-12.[833] NK cells are produced mainly in the bone marrow and appear to be derived from a common T cell and NK cell precursor cell (see later).

NK cells are functionally defined by their ability to lyse virally infected or tumor target cells in a non–MHC-restricted manner that does not require prior sensitization.[834] NK cells preferentially recognize and kill cells with reduced or absent expression of MHC self–class I expression (natural cytotoxicity). This is in contrast with cytotoxic T cells, which are triggered to lyse targets following the recognition of foreign antigenic peptides bound to self-MHC (MHC-restricted cytotoxicity) or self-peptides bound to foreign MHC (allogeneic cytotoxicity). This property also endows NK cells with the capacity to reject bone marrow grafts from persons lacking recipient MHC alleles even if they do not express foreign MHC alleles. This phenomenon is known as hybrid resistance and may be important in the immunology of the rejection of nonautologous hematopoietic cell grafts. Donor NK cells may also facilitate donor cell engraftment and a graft-versus-leukemia effect when mismatched hematopoietic cell transplants are given to leukemia patients.[835] NK cells also have the ability to kill target cells that are coated with IgG antibodies, a process known as antibody-dependent cellular cytotoxicity (ADCC). ADCC requires the recognition of IgG bound to the target cell by the NK cell FcγRIIIB receptor (CD16).[836]

NK cells are particularly important in the early containment of viral infections, especially with pathogens that may initially avoid control by adaptive immune mechanisms. Viral infection of host cells by those of the herpesvirus group, including HSV, CMV, and VZV, and some adenoviruses leads to decreased surface expression of MHC class I molecules, which is discussed in more detail under "Viruses" in the section on host defense against specific classes of neonatal pathogens. Viral protein–mediated decreases in expression of MHC class I may limit the ability of $CD8^+$ T cells to lyse virally infected cells, and to clonally expand from naïve precursors. These virus-mediated effects may be particularly important during early infection, when $CD8^+$ T cells with appropriate antigen specificity are present at a low frequency. By contrast, decreased MHC class I expression facilitates recognition and lysis by NK cells. The importance of NK cells in the initial control of human herpesvirus infections is suggested by the observation that persons with selective deficiency of NK cells or of their function are prone to severe infection with HSV, CMV, and VZV (D. Lewis and C. Wilson, unpublished observations, 1992).[837,838]

Natural Killer Cell Development

The bone marrow is assumed to be the major site for postnatal NK cell production. $CD34^+$ cells lacking markers for mature cell lineages (Lin^-) and expressing CD7 or CD38 are found in the adult bone marrow and the neonatal or adult circulation and appear to be enriched for NK cell progenitors.[839,840] Committed NK cell precursors in mice are identified by their expression of the IL-2Rβ chain, an obligatory component of functional receptors for both IL-2 and IL-15. Murine NK cell precursors appear to require Flt3 ligand or c-kit ligand, or both, for their differentiation from HSCs, but not cytokines that utilize the γc cytokine receptor.[840] In humans, culture of $CD34^+$ HSCs with Flt3 ligand or c-Kit ligand results in the induction of IL-2Rβ chain expression and increased levels of CD34 on the cell surface. These $CD34^{hi}$IL-$2R\beta^{hi}$ cells, which lack CD7 and CD56 and other NK cell markers, appear to be committed NK cell precursors, because their subsequent culture with IL-15 results in acquisition of most features of mature NK cells, including expression of CD56, KIR, and NKG2A, as well as natural cytotoxicity and the capacity for cytokine and chemokine production.[841]

Various immature precursor populations in the bone marrow and circulation, such as $CD34^+CD7^+Lin^-$ cells can differentiate into NK cells, thymocytes or lymphoid DCs, depending on the culture conditions employed, suggesting the existence of a common T/NK/lymphoid DC progenitor.[842,843] A close relationship of NK cells to T lymphocytes is also suggested by the transient cytoplasmic expression of the CD3-ε and CD3-δ components by unactivated human fetal liver NK cells.[830,844] The precise point at which there is an irreversible commitment to NK cell lineage development in vivo remains unclear.

In vitro studies suggest a NK lineage cell developmental sequence in which NKR-P1A expression is acquired early. A small population of $CD3^-CD7^+CD16^-CD56^-NKR^-P1A^+$ lymphocytes in the neonatal and adult circulation suggests that this cell type constitutes a normal intermediate stage in NK cell development.[845] This cell surface phenotype may be followed by acquisition of NKp30, NKp46, 2B4, and NKG2D expression, based on the phenotype of reconstituting NK cells that appear in bone marrow transplant recipients[846] and in vitro differentiation studies.[847] At the later stages, NK cells acquire surface expression of KIR, CD94-NKG2A, CD2, CD16, and CD56 and the capacity for natural cytotoxicity and cytokine production.[839,843,845,847]

IL-15 is particularly important for directing uncommitted lymphocyte precursors to differentiate into the NK cell lineage[848] and for promoting the survival of mature NK cells.[849] NK cells are absent from mice that are genetically deficient in IL-15, components of the IL-15 receptor, or IRF-1 transcription factor, which is required for IL-15 production.[850] The major source of IL-15 for NK cell development probably is stromal fibroblasts of the bone marrow. IL-15 signaling can occur by its binding to a trimeric complex consisting of the IL-15 receptor α chain, the IL-2 receptor β chain and the γc chain. In addition, IL-15 bound to IL-15 receptor α chains on one cell can activate another cell that expresses only IL-2 receptor β and γc chains but not IL-15 receptor α chain. This dependence on IL-15 signaling probably accounts for the absence of NK cells as well as T cells in X-linked SCID, which is due to a genetic deficiency of γc cytokine receptor chain.[117] IL-7, which also uses the γc chain for its signaling, is not required for human NK cell development, because patients with IL-7 receptor α chain deficiency lack T cells but have normal numbers of NK cells.[117] IL-21, a recently identified cytokine produced by activated $CD4^+$ T cells that also uses a γc-containing receptor,[446] can promote human NK cell development in vitro.[851] It is unclear, however, if IL-21 is produced within the human bone marrow microenvironment in vivo, where it could influence NK cell development.

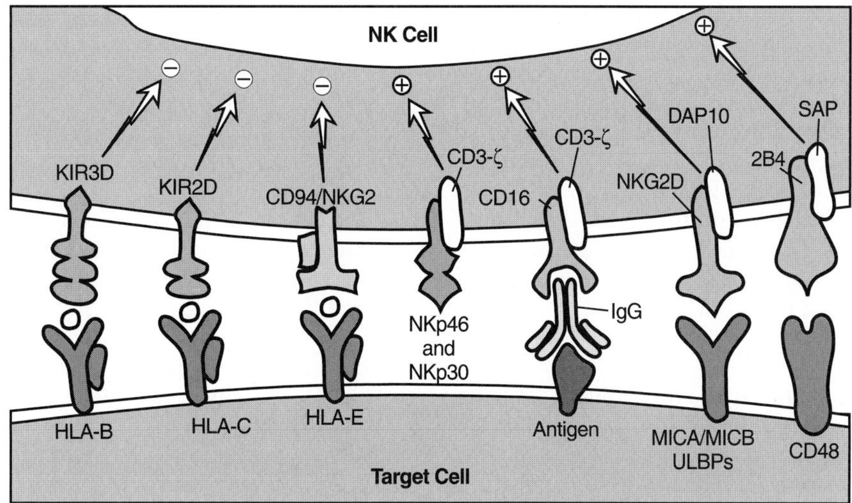

Figure 4–11 Positive and negative regulation of natural killer (NK) cell cytotoxicity by receptor-ligand interactions. NK cell cytotoxicity is inhibited by engagement of killer inhibitory receptors (KIRs) by major histocompatibility complex (MHC) class I molecules, such as human leukocyte antigens HLA-B and HLA-C. In addition, NK cells are inhibited when the CD94-NKG2 complex, a member of the C-type lectin family, on the NK cell is engaged by HLA-E. HLA-E binds hydrophobic leader peptides derived from HLA-A, -B, and -C molecules and requires these for its surface expression. Thus, HLA-E surface expression on a potential target cell indicates the overall production of conventional MHC class I molecules. These inhibitory influences on NK cell cytotoxicity are overcome if viral infection of the target cell results in decreased MHC class I and HLA-E levels. NK cell cytotoxicity is positively regulated by the engagement of NKG2D, which interacts with MICA, MICB, and ULBPs; 2B4, which interacts with CD48; and natural cytotoxicity receptors, such as NKp30 and NKp46, for which the ligands on the target cell are unknown. CD16 is an Fc receptor for immunoglobulin G (IgG) and mediates antibody-dependent cellular cytotoxicity against cells coated with antibody (e.g., against viral proteins found on the cell surface). Positive receptors mediate their intracellular signals through associated CD3-ζ, FcεR1, DAP10, or DAP12 proteins. MICA and MICB, MHC class I–related chains A and B; ULBPs, UL16 (a cytomegalovirus protein)-binding proteins.

Natural Killer Cell Inhibitory Receptors

NK cell cytotoxicity is regulated by a complex array of inhibitory and activating receptor-ligand interactions with target cells (Fig. 4-11). NK cells are inhibited overall by recognition of MHC class I, or segments derived from them, that are expressed on nontransformed, uninfected cells. Binding of the NK cell to MHC class I is presumed to provide a net inhibitory signal that predominates over activating signals. Infection of the host target cell can downregulate inhibitory ligands, such as MHC class I, and upregulate other molecules promoting NK cell–mediated cytotoxicity, such as LFA-3 and MICA and MICB. How these multiple signals are appropriately integrated to regulate cytotoxicity remains unclear. Two major families of MHC class I receptors exist in humans: KIRs and the CD94-containing C-type lectins.[852,853] The major inhibitory receptor of the CD94 family consists of a heterodimer of CD94 and NKG2 A, each of which is encoded by a single nonpolymorphic gene. CD85j (ILT 2), a member of the immunoglobulin-like transcript family, also is expressed on NK cells and can bind to both MHC class I and nonclassic MHC, such as HLA-G.[854] Because its role in regulating NK cell cytotoxicity is not well defined, however, it is not discussed further.

KIRs vary in size depending on whether they contain two (KIR2D) or three (KIR3D) extracellular immunoglobulin-like domains, and whether they have long or short cytoplasmic domains. The long cytoplasmic domain contains an ITIM, which is tyrosine phosphorylated following KIR engagement; this recruits protein tyrosine phosphatases that inhibit NK cell activation and cytotoxicity.[855] KIR with short cytoplasmic motifs also are known as killer-activated receptors (KARs) and provide activating rather than inhibitory signals. KIRs and KARs are encoded in a tight gene cluster, forming haplotypes that are inherited in codominant fashion. Persons may inherit haplotypes that contain up to 11 KIR genes, whereas others may have a haplotype lacking any functional inhibitory KIRs (i.e., those KIRs with cytoplasmic ITIM).[856] Further complexity is due to the possibility of multiple alleles at KIR loci.[852] Most human KIRs recognize either HLA-B or HLA-C alleles, although one has been identified that recognizes certain alleles of HLA-A.[852] Particular KIRs often recognize closely related MHC class I alleles. Although KIR binding may be influenced by particular peptides that are bound to the MHC class I groove, this typically has a relatively subtle impact.

These potential limitations in KIR recognition of self–MHC class I alleles, which could theoretically lead to NK cell autoreactivity, may be overcome by CD94–NKG2 A. Consistent with this idea, an analysis of multiple NK cell clones from normal human donors found that the minority of NK cells that lacked all KIR with ITIM motifs invariably expressed CD94–NKG2 A.[857] Like KIRs with long cytoplasmic tails, the NKG2 A protein also has a cytoplasmic ITIM that mediates

NK cell inhibition. The external domains of CD94 and NKG2 A are both C-type lectins that are structurally distinct from KIR, however, and the CD94–NKG2 A complex recognizes HLA-E rather than classic HLA molecules. HLA-E preferentially binds nine–amino acid hydrophobic peptides derived from the leader sequences of HLA-A, -B, and -C molecules.[24] Because HLA-E requires these leader sequences for its intracellular assembly, stability, and transport, the amount of HLA-E on the cell surface is an indication of the overall levels of conventional MHC class I molecules that are expressed by the potential target cell.[858]

Natural Killer Cell Adhesion

Most resting NK cells are found in the circulation and spleen. The small population of circulating NK cells that are $CD16^{low/-}$ and $CD56^{+}$ may be specialized in the surveillance of solid organs, including the maternal decidua.[859] As for cytotoxic T cells, target cell recognition can be divided into a binding phase and an effector phase of either NK cell triggering or inactivation. A number of NK cell–target cell interactions may be utilized for binding (e.g., CD2-CD58, CD27-CD70, β_2 integrin–ICAM, CD44–MAdCAM-1[860]), and some of these interactions may also play a role in triggering NK cell activation.

Natural Killer Cell–Activating Receptors and Cytotoxicity

NKp30, NKp44, and NKp46 are natural cytotoxicity receptors that are members of the immunoglobulin superfamily. NKp30 and NKp46 are expressed on resting NK cells, but NKp44 is expressed only after treatment of NK cells with cytokines, such as IL-2. NKp30 and NKp46 use homo- or heterotrimers of CD3-ζ or the FcεR1γ chains, or both, which contain ITAMs, to transmit their intracellular signals (see Fig. 4-11). NKp46 uses DAP-12, another ITAM-containing protein, for this purpose. All of these receptors appear to activate intracellular tyrosine kinases, such as Zap-70 and Syk.[833] The ligands that are used by these receptors for killing tumor cells or cells infected with herpesviruses remain unclear. NKp44 and NKp46 have been reported to be able to trigger NK cell cytotoxicity through their recognition of influenza virus hemagglutinin and Sendai (parainfluenza family) virus hemagglutinin-neuraminidase.[861] The importance of such NK cell recognition in influenza infection in vivo is unknown, however, and may be limited by the ability of NK cells to reach the respiratory epithelial cell, the major cell type that is productively infected.

NKG2 D is an activating receptor on NK cells as well as on certain T cell populations. Engagement of NKG2 D triggers activation of the phosphatidylinositol (PI) 3-kinase pathway by the NKG2 D–associated DAP 10 adapter protein (see Fig. 4-11).[833] NKG2 D recognizes MICA and MICB, which are nonclassic MHC molecules that are expressed on stressed or infected cells,[862] as well as UL16-binding proteins (ULBPs). ULPBs are a group of GPI-linked MHC class I–like molecules expressed on many cell types that were first identified and named based on their ability to bind to the human CMV UL16 viral protein. In CMV infection, the secretion of UL16 probably limits NK cell– and T cell–mediated activation by binding to ULBPs on the potential activating target cell surface. Little is known of how ULBP expression is regulated during infection in vivo.

The proteins 2B4 (CD244) and NTBA are members of the SLAM protein family and are expressed on most NK cells.[863] The first, 2B4, binds to CD48, a protein that is expressed by B cells and T cells; the ligand for NTBA remains unclear. Both 2B4 and NTBA engagement triggers NK cell activation through SLAM-associated protein (SAP), an intracellular adapter protein. The X-linked lymphoproliferative syndrome is due to genetic deficiency of SAP and results in severe, often life-threatening infection from primary EBV infection, with a high associated risk for the development of lymphoma or chronic hypogammaglobulinemia.[863] SAP deficiency allows alternative molecules, the SH2-domain–containing phosphatases (SHPs), to bind the cytoplasmic tails of 2B4 and NTBA. This results in inhibition of NK cell function rather than merely the loss of activating function, a mechanism that may contribute to the severity and sequelae of EBV infection in these patients. In human NK cells, the activating signals involve DAP-10.[864]

Certain members of the MHC class I KIR and CD94 receptor families also are candidates to contribute to NK cell activation. These activating KIRs, such as KIR2DS, also are referred to as KARs. KARs retain the characteristic extracellular immunoglobulin-like domains of KIRs but have short cytoplasmic tails that lack ITIMs and, instead, associate with DAP 12.[833] Similarly, the NKG2 C component of the CD94–NKG2 C heterodimeric receptor lacks an ITIM and activates NK cells by its association with DAP 12.[865] The KARs and the CD94-containing C-type lectin receptors have identical or very similar ligand specificity as their respective inhibitory forms. How NK cells integrate the effects on natural cytotoxicity of activating forms of the KIR family or C-type lectin receptors that recognize the same or similar ligands as their inhibitory counterparts remains unclear.

As with T cells, NK cell–mediated cytotoxicity involves the release of perforin and granzymes from pre-formed cytotoxic granules. NK cell–mediated cytotoxicity also may be mediated by Fas ligand[866] or TRAIL[867] expressed on the activated NK cell surface. Fas ligand–mediated cytotoxicity appears to occur mainly following treatment of NK cells with stimulatory cytokines, such as IL-2, or during ADCC, rather than during natural cytotoxicity (see section on ADCC). Most mouse studies suggest that Fas ligand–mediated cytotoxicity in NK cells is of minor or no importance compared with perforin/granzyme-dependent cytotoxicity in the control of viral infections.[868] Fas–Fas ligand interactions also may not be essential for human NK cell control of viral infections: Persons with the autoimmune lymphoproliferative syndrome (ALPS), in which there is dominant-negative inhibition of Fas, do not experience an increased severity of herpesvirus infections, such as with CMV.[869]

Antibody-Dependent Cellular Cytotoxicity

In addition to natural cytotoxicity, NK cell–mediated ADCC is triggered when IgG bound to target cells engages the FcγRIIIA receptor on the NK cell.[836] The FcγRIIIA receptor, which is also found on macrophages and a small subset of T cells, consists of the CD16 molecule, which binds IgG via its Fc domain, and its associated homo- or heterotrimers of CD3-ζ or the FcεR1γ chain, or both.[833] Because of the relative ease with which ADCC can be triggered experimentally, substantially more is known of the events in activation and effector function than for natural cytotoxicity. As in the case of T cell activation, FcγRIIIA engagement appears to sequentially activate tyrosine kinases of the Src and Syk families, followed by downstream signals, that include increased $[Ca^{2+}]_i$ and activation of Rho, Ras, p38 mitogen–activated protein kinase, and extracellular signal-regulated kinases.[833] In contrast with natural cytotoxicity, in which perforin/granzyme-dependent mechanisms appear to be predominant, ADCC appears to utilize both perforin/granzyme- and Fas ligand–dependent cytotoxic mechanisms.[870]

Natural Killer Cell Cytokine Responsiveness and Dependence

NK cell proliferation and cytotoxicity are enhanced in vitro by cytokines produced by T cells (IL-2, IFN-γ), APCs (IL-1, IL-10, IL-12, IL-18, and IFN-α), and nonhematopoietic cells such as bone marrow mesenchymal cells (IL-15, stem cell factor, and Flt3 ligand) and fibroblasts (IFN-β). Certain CC chemokines, such as monocyte chemotactic protein-1 CCL2 (monocyte chemotactic protein [MCP]-1), CCL3 (MIP-1α), and CCL4 (MIP-1β), also may enhance NK cell function. IL-15, which appears critical for the development of NK cells in the bone marrow, also promotes the survival of mature NK cells[849] and, like IL-12, increases the expression of perforin and granzymes.[871] NK cell cytotoxicity in vivo is modestly decreased in mice genetically deficient in IFN-γ,[872] IL-12,[873] or IL-18,[874] and markedly depressed in combined IL-12 and IL-18 deficiency. These findings suggest that IL-12 and IL-18 largely act in a nonredundant fashion to help maintain NK cell cytotoxicity in vivo, and this maintenance is mediated, at least in part, by the induction of IFN-γ by these cytokines. The role of the recently identified members of the IL-12 family—that is, IL-23 and IL-27[875]—in regulating NK cell function in vivo remains unclear.

When NK cells are primed by cytokine exposure or are triggered in vitro for ADCC, they also become prone to apoptosis in the absence of exogenous cytokine exposure. Apoptosis of primed NK cells can occur in vitro after engagement of their surface CD2, CD16, or CD94 molecules.[876] Analogous to effector T cell populations, this tendency for NK effector cells to undergo apoptosis may help limit total NK cell numbers and avoid abnormal lymphoproliferation. The extent to which NK cell apoptosis occurs in vivo, particularly following natural cytotoxicity, is unknown.

Natural Killer Cell Cytokine and Chemokine Production

NK cells are also important producers of IFN-γ and TNF-α in the early phase of the immune response to viruses, and IFN-γ may promote the development of CD4 T cells into T_H1 effector cells. NK cell–mediated IFN-γ production may be induced by the ligation of surface β_1 integrins on the NK cell surface,[877] as well as by the cytokines IL-1, IL-12, and IL-18,[878] which are produced by DCs and mononuclear phagocytes. The combination of IL-12 and IL-15 also potently induces NK cells to produce the CC chemokine MIP-1α (CCL-3),[879] which may help chemoattract other types of mononuclear cells to sites of infection, where NK cell–mediated lysis takes place. NK cells from HIV-infected persons also are able to produce a variety of CC chemokines, including MIP-1α, MIP-1β, and RANTES in response to treatment with IL-2 alone; these chemokines may help prevent HIV infection of T cells and mononuclear phagocytes by acting as antagonists of the HIV co-receptor. NK cells also can be triggered to produce a similar array of cytokines during ADCC in vitro, but the role of such ADCC-derived cytokines in regulating immune responses in vivo remains poorly defined.

Some of the cytokine-dependent mechanisms by which NK cells, T cells, and APCs may influence each other's function, such as in response to infection with viruses and other intracellular pathogens, are summarized in Figure 4-12. In addition, studies in mice indicate that cytokines produced by NK cells, such as IFN-γ, also may allow the B cells to respond to TI-type antigens, such as purified polysaccharides and certain protein antigens with repetitive B cell epitopes.[880] Human NK cells also have been shown to produce T_H2 cytokines such as IL-5 and IL-13, but the importance of these in regulating immune function in vivo remains unclear.

Peripheral Natural Killer Cell Subsets

Mature NK cells found outside of the bone marrow can be further subdivided into $CD56^{hi}$ and $CD56^{lo}$ populations that demonstrate low and high levels, respectively, of CD16 surface expression.[881] $CD56^{hi}$ cells usually are only a minority of mature NK cells in the circulation but express CCR7 and L-selectin and predominate in lymph node tissue. Compared with $CD56^{lo}$ cells, $CD56^{hi}$ cells have a limited capacity to carry out either natural cytotoxicity or ADCC. By contrast, $CD56^{lo}$ NK cells have a much more limited capacity to produce cytokines and chemokines than that observed for the $CD56^{hi}$

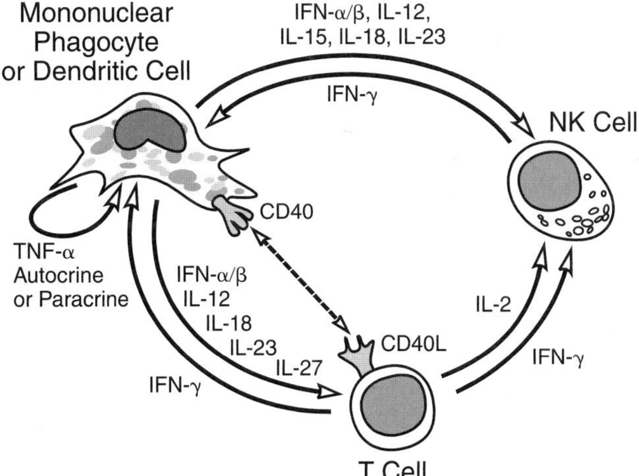

Figure 4–12 Cytokines link innate and antigen-specific immune mechanisms against intracellular pathogens. Activation of T cells by antigen-presenting cells, such as dendritic cells and mononuclear phagocytes, results in the expression of CD40 ligand and the secretion of cytokines, such as interkeukin (IL)-2 and interferon (IFN)-γ. Mononuclear phagocytes are activated by IFN-γ and the engagement of CD40 with increased microbicidal activity. Mononuclear phagocytes produce tumor necrosis factor (TNF)-α, which enhances their microbicidal activity in a paracrine or autocrine manner. Mononuclear phagocytes also secrete the cytokines IFN-α/β, IL-12, IL-15, IL-18, IL-23, and IL-27. These cytokines promote T_H1 effector cell differentiation and most also promote natural killer (NK) cell activation. IL-15 (*not shown*) also is particularly important for the generation of effector and memory $CD8^+$ T cells. NK cell activation is further augmented by IL-2 and possibly by IL-21, which are produced by $CD4^+$ T cells. Activated NK cells in turn secrete IFN-γ, which further enhances mononuclear phagocyte activation and T_H1 effector cell differentiation.

subset.[882] These features suggest that the CD56^{hi} subset could regulate lymph node T cells and DCs through cytokine secretion. The precursor-product relationship between CD56^{lo} and CD56^{hi} NK cells and the mechanisms by which they are generated in vivo (e.g., CD56^{hi} cells have been proposed as terminal effector cells)[883] remain controversial.

Natural Killer Cells of the Maternal Decidua and Their Regulation by Human Leukocyte Antigen G

The maternal decidua contains a prominent population of NK cells, and these cells may help contribute to the maintenance of pregnancy. NK cells belonging to the CD56^{hi} subset (high capacity for cytokine production and low capacity for cytotoxicity) predominate. Murine studies suggest that NK cell–derived cytokines, such as IFN-γ, may play a role in helping remodel the spiral arteries of the placenta. Although the NK cell populations of the decidua have a low capacity for cytotoxicity, their presence in a tissue lacking expression of conventional MHC class I molecules could potentially contribute to placental damage and fetal rejection. The expression by trophoblast of HLA-G (see section on nonclassic antigen presentation molecules), which is at particularly high levels during the first trimester of pregnancy, has been hypothesized to engage inhibitory receptors on maternal NK cells of the decidual or circulation in order to limit such damage. HLA-G–mediated inhibition of NK cell cytotoxicity may involve engagement of CD94–NKG2 A, certain KIRs, CD85j (ILT2), or as-yet uncharacterized receptors.[884]

Natural Killer Cell Development and Function in the Fetus and Neonate

Fetal and Neonatal Natural Killer Cell Development and Surface Phenotype

The development of human NK cells precedes that of αβ T cells during ontogeny, demonstrating their thymic independence. The fetal liver produces NK cells as early as 6 weeks of gestation, which become increasingly abundant during the second trimester.[830] CD34$^+$CD38$^+$Lin$^-$ cells of the second trimester fetal liver give rise to NK-like cells rather than T-lineage cells after culture in vitro with the cytokines IL-7, IL-15, and Flt-3 ligand,[885] suggesting that the fetal liver is the main site of development of NK cells rather than extrathymic T cells. In the murine fetal thymus, NK cells appear prior to αβ-TCR$^+$ thymocytes.[886] A similar sequence of events applies in humans, but the immunologic importance of thymus-derived NK cells remains unclear. The bone marrow is the major site for NK cell production from late gestation onward.

The precise developmental sequence of NK cell maturation in the bone marrow remains poorly understood. CD34$^+$Lin$^-$ cells expressing CD7 or CD38 are found in the adult bone marrow and the neonatal or adult circulation and appear to be enriched for NK cell progenitors.[104,839] In vitro treatment of these progenitor cells with cytokines or stromal cells, or both, results in the appearance of CD56$^+$ cells with NK cell features, including natural cytotoxicity and CD94 surface expression.[887,888]

Studies using in vitro cultures of single neonatal CD34$^+$Lin$^-$ blood cells suggest that during differentiation the commitment to NK lineage is made first, followed by the acquisition of inhibitory receptors.[889] CD34$^+$ cells with these or similar characteristics in the thymus also can differentiate into thymocytes or lymphoid DCs, depending on the culture conditions, suggesting the existence of a common T/NK/lymphoid DC.[842]

IL-15 appears to be critical for directing less committed lymphocyte precursors into the NK lineage,[848,890] and for promoting the survival of mature NK cells.[849] Neonatal mononuclear cells produce less IL-15 than do adult cells after LPS stimulation.[891] It is unlikely, however, that this applies to IL-15–producing cells at major sites of NK cell development, such as the fetal bone marrow and fetal liver, because NK cells are present in greatest numbers in the circulation during the second trimester of fetal development,[892] and their number in the neonatal circulation (approximately 15% of total lymphocytes) is typically the same as or greater than in adults.[830] These observations suggest that developing NK lineage cells in fetus and neonate have normal IL-15 responsiveness.

In contrast with adult NK cells, most fetal liver NK cells express the CD3-ε and CD3-δ components associated with the TCR and lack CD16 surface expression[830]: Virtually all fetal and neonatal NK cells lack expression of CD57.[893,894] The surface expression of CD7, CD16, CD18, CD44, and the KIR (p70 or NKB1) by circulating neonatal and adult NK cells is similar.[893,894] The fraction of fetal and neonatal NK cells that express CD2 or CD56, however, is reduced by about 30% to 50%, compared with that in the adult.[830,831,893,895] Fetal NK cells, unlike adult NK cells, also may frequently express CD28, but it is unclear if they respond to engagement by CD80 or CD86, the ligands of CD28.

Fetal and Neonatal Natural Killer Cell–Mediated Cytotoxicity

The cytolytic function of NK cells increases progressively during fetal life to reach values approximately 50% (a range of 15% to 60% in various studies) of those in adult cells at term, as determined in assays using tumor cell targets, such as the K562 erythroleukemia cell line, and either unpurified[414,896-901] or NK cell–enriched preparations.[830,893,897,899,902-904] Reduced cytotoxic activity by neonatal NK cells has been observed in studies using cord blood from vaginal or cesarean section deliveries or peripheral blood obtained 2 to 4 days after birth.[905] Full function is not achieved until the age of at least 9 to 12 months. Cytolytic function is also markedly reduced by bacterial sepsis in neonates.[905] NK cells from the premature infant also have reduced cytotoxic function compared with those of the term neonate.[830,906] The reduced cytolytic activity appears to reflect primarily diminished postbinding cytotoxic activity and diminished recycling to kill multiple targets. This reduction of cytolytic activity parallels the reduced number of CD56$^+$ NK cells—when only CD56$^+$ neonatal NK cells are studied, their cytolytic activity is usually similar to that in adult NK cells.[830,903] This finding might not seem consistent with the notion that in adults, the CD56^{lo} NK cells are more cytolytic than the CD56^{hi} subset.[882] Many neonatal NK cells, however, have much lower or undetectable levels of CD56 compared with those in the adult CD56^{lo} NK cell subset, suggesting that they are less mature than this adult cell population.

Whether neonatal NK cells have decreased cytolytic activity compared with that of adult cells depends in part on the target cell used. For example, NK cells from term neonates were found to have similar cytotoxic activity as adult cells against non-K562 tumors. Decreased cytotoxic activity by neonatal NK cells compared with adult cells also is consistently observed with HSV-infected[830,907,908] and CMV-infected target cells.[909] By contrast, both neonatal and adult NK cells have equivalent cytotoxic activity against HIV-1–infected cells.[906,910] These results suggest that ligands on the target cell or its intrinsic sensitivity to induction of apoptosis may influence fetal and neonatal NK cell function. The mechanisms of these pathogen-related differences remain unclear, but may contribute to the severity of neonatal HSV infection.

Paralleling the reduction in natural cytotoxic activity of neonatal cells, ADCC of neonatal mononuclear cells is approximately 50% of that of adult mononuclear cells, including against HSV-infected targets.[906] In contrast with natural cytotoxicity, decreased ADCC mediated by purified neonatal NK cells appears to be caused in part by an adhesion defect in the presence of antibody.[894]

As they do for adult NK cells, cytokines such as IL-2, IL-12, IL-15, IFN-α, IFN-β, and IFN-γ can augment the cytolytic activity of neonatal NK cells within a few hours.[893,894,911,912] Consistent with the ability of IL-2 and IFN-γ to augment their cytolytic activity, neonatal NK cells express on their surface receptors for IL-2 and IFN-γ in numbers that are equal to or greater than those of adult NK cells.[913] Neonatal NK cells are less responsive to activation by the combination of IL-12 and IL-15 than are adult NK cells, however, as indicated by the induction of CD69 surface expression.[914,915]

Circulating neonatal NK cells have increased natural cytotoxic activity and ADCC activity on incubation from 18 hours to 3 weeks with IL-2, IL-12, IL-15, or IL-18 or combinations, which leads to their differentiation into lymphokine-activated killer (LAK) cells.[66,419,441,895,906,908,912,914-920] Neonatal LAK cells often have cytotoxic activity equivalent to that of adult LAK cells, suggesting that neonatal NK cells have a normal capacity to be primed by exogenous cytokines.

The generation of neonatal LAK cells from NK cells also increases their surface expression of CD56 as a result of differentiation of $CD56^-$ NK cells into $CD56^+$ LAK cells, rather than expansion from the preexisting neonatal $CD56^+$ NK population.[917,921] This finding suggests that the neonatal $CD56^-$ NK cell population is a phenotypically and functionally immature NK cell subset that gives rise to a mature $CD56^+$ population.

The mechanisms responsible for decreased NK cell–mediated cytotoxicity in the neonate are undefined. Soluble MHC class I is present at a 10-fold greater concentration in cord serum than that in adult serum; the greater concentration could contribute to decreased neonatal NK cytotoxicity, perhaps by engaging KIRs.[908] Exposure to levels of soluble MHC class I present in cord blood has only a modest inhibitory effect on NK cytotoxicity in vitro,[908] however, so this is unlikely to be a major factor. Cell-mediated suppression also has been proposed, although this effect has not been shown in mixing experiments.[922] Nor is decreased neonatal NK cell–mediated cytotoxicity due to decreased binding to target cells,[908] or to decreased levels of intracellular perforin or granzyme B.[917]

Treatment of neonatal NK cells, including the $CD56^-$ subset, with ionomycin and PMA enhances natural cytotoxicity to levels present in adult NK cells.[917] This increase is blocked by inhibitors of granule exocytosis, indicating that decreased release of granules containing perforin and granzyme may contribute to reduced neonatal NK cytotoxicity. Finally, decreased neonatal NK cytotoxicity is not determined at the level of the HSC or later precursor cells of the NK cell lineage: Donor-derived NK cells appear early following cord blood transplantation, with good cytotoxicity effected through the perforin/granzyme and Fas–Fas ligand cytotoxic pathways.[923]

Cytokine Production by Neonatal Natural Killer Cells

Neonatal NK cells produce IFN-γ as effectively as adult NK cells in response to exogenous IL-2 and HSV[924] or to polyclonal stimulation with ionomycin and PMA.[354] IL-12–induced production of IFN-γ by neonatal mononuclear cells (most likely NK cells) may be reduced compared with that in adult cells.[85,911] Purified neonatal NK cells, however, produce substantially more IFN-γ than adult NK cells after stimulation with the combination of IL-12 and IL-18.[924a] Fewer neonatal NK cells express TNF-α than do adult NK cells following ionomycin and PMA stimulation.[354] The production of other cytokines by neonatal NK cells, particularly with physiologic stimuli, is not known.

Natural Killer Cells in Congenital Infection

Congenital viral or *Toxoplasma* infection during the second trimester may increase the number of circulating NK cells.[892] Elevation of number of NK cells can persist until birth, accompanied by decreased NK cell expression of the CD45RA isoform and increased expression of the CD45RO isoform of the CD45 tyrosine phosphatase.[551] This $CD45RA^{lo}CD45RO^{hi}$ phenotype suggests in vivo activation, similar to that in NK cells incubated in vitro with IL-2 or tumor cell targets.[925]

Summary

Although NK cells appear early during gestation and are present in normal numbers by mid- to late gestation, approximately 50% of these cells at birth are $CD56^-$. This surface phenotype is a marker for NK cell immaturity, but the relationship between $CD56^-$ and $CD56^+$ cells is unclear. Neonatal NK cells have decreased cytotoxicity to several target cells, including virus-infected target cells, compared with adult NK cells, most of which are $CD56^+$. Neonatal NK cell cytotoxicity can be augmented by incubation with cytokines in vitro, suggesting a potential immunotherapeutic strategy.

PHAGOCYTES

Origin and Differentiation of Phagocytes

Phagocytes are derived from a common precursor myeloid stem cell, which often is referred to as the colony-forming unit–granulocyte-monocyte (CFU-GM) (Fig. 4-13). The formation of myeloid stem cells from pluripotent HSCs and further differentiation of the myeloid precursor into mature granulocytes and monocytes are governed by (1) stromal

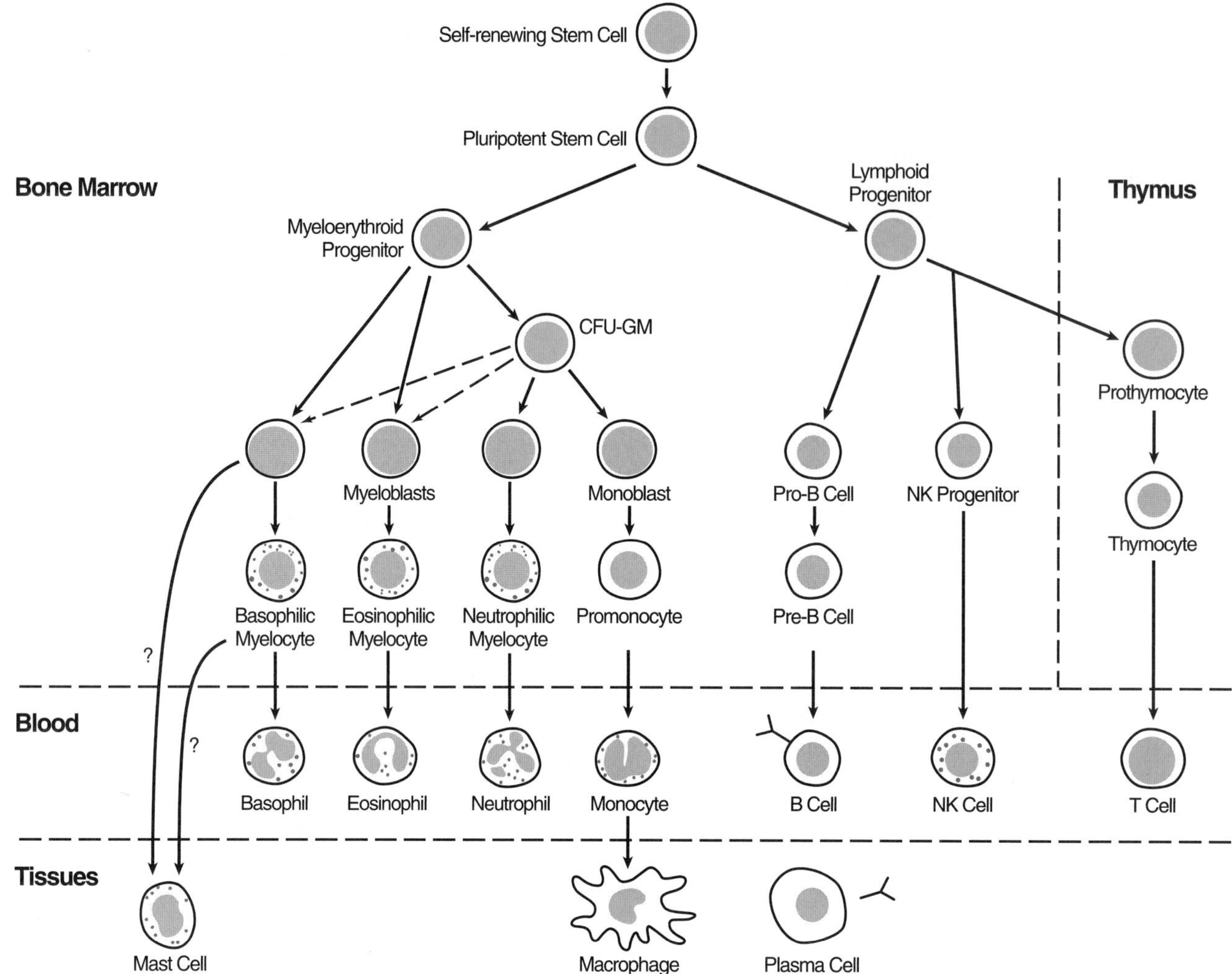

Figure 4–13 Myeloid and lymphoid differentiation and tissue compartments in which they occur. CFU-GM, colony-forming unit–granulocyte-macrophage.

cells present in the bone marrow environment and the cell-cell contacts between these cells and hematopoietic progenitors and (2) soluble colony-stimulating factors (CSFs) and other cytokines produced by these and other cells (see Table 4-2).[926,927] Factors that act primarily on early HSCs include stem cell factor (also known as steel factor or c-Kit ligand) and Flt-3 ligand. The response to these factors is enhanced by granulocyte colony-stimulating factor (G-CSF) and thrombopoietin, hematopoietic growth factors originally identified by their ability to enhance the production of neutrophils and platelets, respectively, and by IL-1, IL-3, and IL-6. Other factors act later and are more specific for given myeloid lineages: GM-CSF acts to increase the production of neutrophils, eosinophils, and monocytes; G-CSF acts to increase neutrophil production; macrophage colony-stimulating factor (M-CSF) acts to increase monocyte production; and IL-5 enhances eosinophil production.

The precise role of these mediators in normal steady-state hematopoiesis is becoming clearer, primarily as a result of studies in mice with targeted disruptions of the relevant genes. Genetic defects in the production of biologically active stem cell factor or its receptor c-Kit lead to mast cell deficiency and severe anemia, with less severe defects in granulocytopoiesis and in formation of megakaryocytes,[928] whereas deficiency of Flt-3 ligand has no overt effect except on B cell progenitors. Deficiency for both Flt-3 ligand and c-Kit has a more severe phenotype than for either alone, indicating partial redundancy in their function. Deficient production of M-CSF is associated with some diminution in macrophage numbers and a marked deficiency in maturation of osteoclasts (presumably from monocyte precursors), which results in a form of osteopetrosis.[929] Mice with a targeted disruption of G-CSF or its receptor and humans with mutations in the G-CSF receptor are neutropenic (although they do not completely lack neutrophils) and have fewer multi-lineage hematopoietic progenitor cells.[927] By contrast, in mice, GM-CSF deficiency causes pulmonary alveolar proteinosis but does not affect the numbers of neutrophils, monocytes, or eosinophils, whereas IL-5 deficiency results in an inability to increase the numbers of eosinophils in response to parasites or allergens. Thus, hematopoietic growth factors appear to play complex and, in some cases, partially overlapping roles in normal steady-state production of myeloid cells.

In response to an infectious or inflammatory stimulus, CSF production is increased. Under these conditions, concentrations sufficient to enhance growth and differentiation of myeloid cells are produced and are believed to play an important role in the enhanced marrow production and release of granulocytes and monocytes that are observed. Similarly, when given exogenously, these factors enhance production of the indicated cell lineages.[930]

Neutrophilic Polymorphonuclear Leukocytes

Origin and Derivation of Neutrophils in the Mature Host

Polymorphonuclear leukocytes or granulocytes are derived from CFU-GM. Neutrophilic granulocytes are the principal cells of interest in relation to defense against pyogenic pathogens. This section specifically addresses these cells. The first identifiable committed granulocyte precursor is the myeloblast, which sequentially matures into myelocytes, metamyelocytes, bands, and mature neutrophilic granulocytes or polymorphonuclear leukocytes. Myelocytes and more mature neutrophilic granulocytes cannot replicate and constitute the postmitotic neutrophilic storage pool.[931] Mature neutrophils enter the circulation, where they remain for 8 to 10 hours and are distributed equally and dynamically between circulating cells and those adherent to the vascular endothelium.[931] After leaving the circulation, neutrophils normally do not recirculate, and after about 24 hours in tissues, they die.

The postmitotic neutrophil storage pool is an important reserve, because these cells can be rapidly released into the circulation in response to inflammation. Furthermore, increased production of stem cells in response to inflammation requires approximately 5 to 7 days before it can contribute to increased neutrophil output. Accelerated maturation or replication from nonstem cells in the mitotic compartment may enhance this neutrophil output somewhat. Nevertheless, the storage pool size is a critical determinant of the host's capacity to increase neutrophil output in response to infection.

As indicated, the control of granulocyte production and release is regulated by CSFs or hematopoietic growth factors. Neutrophil production is specifically favored by G-CSF but also is facilitated by the more broadly acting IL-3 and GM-CSF. These factors enhance the proliferation of neutrophil precursors by driving progenitor cells to enter the cell cycle and, in the case of G-CSF, biasing progenitors capable of differentiating into granulocytes or monocytes into the neutrophil differentiation pathway. Granulocyte production also appears to be under potential negative regulation by prostaglandins and iron-containing proteins such as lactoferrin.[927,931] These negative regulators are produced by granulocytes and monocytes, suggesting that mature cells may self-regulate production. Release of neutrophils from the marrow may be enhanced in part by cytokines, including IL-1 and TNF-α, in response to infection or inflammation.[926]

Migration to Sites of Infection

After release from the bone marrow into the blood, neutrophils circulate until they are called on to enter the tissues at sites of infection or injury. Neutrophils adhere selectively to endothelium in inflamed tissues but not in normal tissues. The adhesion and subsequent migration of neutrophils through blood vessels and into the tissues are governed by cell adhesins expressed on the neutrophil and on the vascular endothelium and by specific chemotactic factors.

Adhesion

The adhesion molecules that are known to play a central role in neutrophil adherence are derived from one of three families of cell surface glycoproteins: the selectins, the integrins, and certain members of the immunoglobulin gene superfamily.[932,933]

The selectins are named by the cell types in which they are primarily expressed: L-selectin by leukocytes, E-selectin by endothelial cells, and P-selectin by platelets and endothelial cells. Selectins are named for their ability to bind to specific types of carbohydrates that are selectively expressed on different tissues; binding is mediated through a lectin-like domain found in all family members. L-selectin is constitutively expressed on leukocytes and appears to bind to tissue- or inflammation-specific carbohydrate-containing ligands on endothelial cells. E-selectin and P-selectin are expressed only on activated, not resting, endothelial cells or platelets. E- and P-selectin bind to sialylated glycoproteins on the surface of leukocytes, including P-selectin glycoprotein ligand-1 (PSGL-1). L-selectin binds to glycoproteins (including CD34 and MAdCAM-1) and to glycolipids that are expressed on vascular endothelial cells in specific tissues.

The integrins are a large family of heterodimeric proteins composed of an α and a β chain. Integrins expressing a β_2 (CD18) chain, which associates on the plasma membrane with one of four α (CD11) chains, are found only on leukocytes. The β_2 integrins play a critical role in neutrophil function, because unlike other types of leukocytes, neutrophils do not express other integrins in substantial amounts. The β_2 integrins (also known as leukocyte integrins) are constitutively expressed on neutrophils, but both their abundance and their avidity for their endothelial ligands are increased after activation of neutrophils—for example, in response to chemotactic factors. LFA-1 (CD11a-CD18) and Mac-1 (CD11b-CD18) appear to play the predominant role in leukocyte–endothelial cell interactions, whereas CD11c-CD18 plays a lesser role and CD11d-CD18 participates in leukocyte-leukocyte interactions. The endothelial ligands for LFA-1 are members of the immunoglobulin-like family and include ICAM-1 and ICAM-2. Both are constitutively expressed on endothelium, but ICAM-1 expression is increased markedly by exposure to inflammatory mediators, including IL-1, TNF-α, and LPS.

These adhesion molecules and chemotactic factors act in a coordinated fashion to allow neutrophil recruitment into tissues in response to infection or injury. In response to injury or inflammatory cytokines, P-selectin is transferred from endothelial or platelet stores to the surface of the endothelium of capillaries or postcapillary venules within minutes. This mechanism allows neutrophils in the blood to adhere in a low-avidity fashion, which results in rolling of these cells along the vessel walls. This step is transient and reversible unless a second, high-avidity interaction is triggered. If, at the time of the low-avidity binding, neutrophils also encounter chemotactic factors (discussed later) released from the tissues or from the endothelium itself, they rapidly upregulate the avidity of the LFA-1 and Mac-1 integrins and translocate additional LFA-1 and Mac-1 from specific granules to the neutrophil cell surface. This process enhances binding to ICAM-1 and ICAM-2 on endothelial cells. The high-avidity interaction of these integrins with ICAMs, in the presence of a gradient of chemotactic factors from the tissue to the blood vessel, appears to trigger the migration of neutrophils across the endothelium and into the tissues. Over a matter of several hours, the intensity of this response can be further upregulated by the de novo expression of E-selectin and increased expression of ICAM-1 on endothelium in response to mediators (e.g., platelet-activating factor [PAF], TNF-α) produced at the site of infection or injury.

The profound importance of integrin- and selectin-mediated leukocyte adhesion processes in the normal inflammatory response is illustrated by the genetic leukocyte adhesion deficiency syndromes.[934] Deficiency of the common β_2 integrin chain results in the absence on the plasma membrane of all β_2 integrins. This results in inability of leukocytes to exit the bloodstream and reach sites of infection and injury in the tissues. Affected patients are profoundly susceptible to infections with pathogenic and nonpathogenic bacteria, have poor tissue healing, and commonly die in the first years of life. Such patients not uncommonly present in early infancy with delayed separation of the umbilical cord, omphalitis, and severe bacterial infection without pus formation. A related syndrome—leukocyte adhesion deficiency syndrome type II—is due to a defect in synthesis of the carbohydrate selectin ligands. This disorder results in a similar defect in neutrophil function and predisposition to infection but also is associated with more general problems related to defects in proper glycosylation of proteins. Studies of mice deficient in specific selectins indicate that P-selectin and E-selectin play partially redundant roles, and that L-selectin acts in concert with either of these two selectins and their ligands to facilitate neutrophil recruitment to sites of inflammation.

Chemotaxis

Chemotaxis is important for focusing the delivery of leukocytes to the site of infection or injury. Random movement of leukocytes, even if accelerated by stimuli, would be inefficient. Sensing of chemotactic gradients is achieved through cell surface receptors for specific chemotactic factors. A number of receptors for specific chemotactic factors have been molecularly cloned and are related by their common structure. This is consistent with their interaction with heterotrimeric G proteins, which serve to transduce the signal from these receptors. Chemotactic agents may be derived directly from bacterial components or surrogates, such as *N*-formylated Met-Leu-Phe (fMLP) peptide; from activated complement, such as C5a; and from host cell lipids, such as leukotriene B_4 (LTB_4) and PAF. These chemotactic agents are produced within minutes, because they are derived from preexisting microbial or host components.[935] In addition, a large family of chemotactic cytokines (chemokines) are synthesized by macrophages and other cells within hours (see Tables 4-1 and 4-2).[43,936,937] Chemokines may be displayed on the luminal side of the vascular endothelium through binding to proteoglycans and appear to play an important role in the maintenance and evolution of the inflammatory response.

The receptors for chemotactic agents are located on the cell surface, and additional stores are present in cytoplasmic granules. On exposure to low concentrations of chemotactic agents, the cells express additional receptors on the plasma membrane; some of these are of higher affinity and increase the ability of the cell to sense the chemotactic agent.[938] The cells also sense the spatial gradient of chemotactic agents; a difference of as little as 0.1% can be detected. The cells then orient so that they are flattened at the end toward the highest concentration (the lamellipodium) and have a thin tail (the uropod) at the opposite end. This polarization of the cell requires an intact cytoskeleton network and a fluid cell membrane. The polarized cell contains increased numbers of receptors for chemotactic agents and for IgG at the flattened lamellipodium. Chemotactic agents engaged to receptors on the neutrophil lamellipodium trigger a local and selective release of granules, which contain a pool of the β_2 integrins, including Mac-1. Adhesion to the endothelium is thereby augmented at this point of contact, and translocation between endothelial cells is facilitated. Neutrophils may then attach to and ultimately pass through the basement membrane to reach the tissues. PECAM-1 (CD31), which is expressed on both neutrophils and endothelial cells, and components of the extracellular matrix (e.g., fibronectin and laminin) contribute at this stage.[939] Release of digestive enzymes from lysosomes also may facilitate movement of neutrophils through the endothelium and tissues. Neutrophils must undergo considerable deformation to allow diapedesis through the endothelium. Migration through the tissues also is likely to be facilitated by the reversible adhesion and de-adhesion between ligands on the neutrophil surface, including the integrins, with components of the extracellular matrix, such as fibronectin and collagen.

Phagocytosis and Killing

Phagocytosis by neutrophils occurs in two phases: recognition and ingestion.[940] The recognition phase usually involves binding of opsonized bacteria to specific receptors on the cell surface. Opsonin-independent surface phagocytosis also may occur but is less efficient, particularly for encapsulated organisms. Opsonization, a process whereby immunoglobulin, complement, or certain other host-derived proteins, or all three, are bound to the surface of the organism, is discussed later in this chapter. Neutrophils contain specific receptors for the Fc portion of the IgG molecule (Fcγ receptors) and receptors for two different forms of the activated third component of complement.[576] C3b is bound by CR1, and C3bi by CR3 and CR4; CR3 and CR4, respectively, are the CD11b-CD18 and CD11c-CD18 integrins described previously.[941] Opsonized bacteria bind and cross-link Fcγ and C3b-C3bi receptors, and this cross-linkage transmits a signal for ingestion and, in the case of Fcγ receptors, for the activation of the cell's microbicidal mechanisms. Signal transduction from these receptors is not fully elucidated but appears to involve a series of intracellular events, including increases in $[Ca^{2+}]_i$ and activation of tyrosine kinases, serine/threonine protein kinases (including protein kinase C), phospholipase A_2, and small guanosine triphosphate (GTP)-binding proteins.

Once ingested, microbes are exposed to a variety of potent microbicidal products. Oxygen-dependent microbicidal mechanisms are of central importance, as illustrated by the severe compromise in defenses against a wide range of pyogenic pathogens (with the exception of catalase-negative bacteria) observed in children with a genetic defect in this system.[942] This disorder—chronic granulomatous disease—results from a defect in one of four intracellular proteins that together form the phagocyte oxidase. This oxidase consists of two plasma membrane–associated and two cytosolic components. In response to activation of the cell—for example, during receptor-mediated phagocytosis—these four components are assembled in the plasma membrane into an enzymatic complex that transfers an electron to the oxygen molecule. This forms superoxide anion, which has weak microbicidal activity and is a precursor for more toxic compounds, including hydrogen peroxide and hydroxyl radicals. The assembly of the oxidase in the plasma membrane allows these products to be secreted into the nascent or fully formed phagocytic vacuole, where their activity can be focused on the microbe. The activity of hydrogen peroxide also can be augmented by myeloperoxidase, a protein stored in neutrophil granules, which are discharged into the phagocytic vacuole.

In addition to myeloperoxidase, the neutrophil contains other granule proteins with potent microbicidal activity. These mediate oxygen-independent killing. Many of these are relatively small, cationic proteins with direct microbicidal activity, including the defensins, elastase, cathepsin G, and a protein that binds selectively to gram-negative lipopolysaccharide, bactericidal permeability-increasing (BPI) protein.[658,943,944]

Production of Inflammatory Mediators by Neutrophils

Neutrophils produce leukotrienes, primarily LTB_4, PAF, and certain cytokines that facilitate the inflammatory response. These include IL-1,[945] TNF-α,[946] and members of the CXC chemokine family, such as IL-8 (CXCL8).[43,936] Thus, in addition to playing a direct role in microbicidal killing, neutrophils may modulate the inflammatory response.

Neutrophils in the Fetus and Neonate

Neutrophil Production and Release

Neutrophil precursors are detected first in the yolk sac and then in the liver, spleen, and bone marrow, appearing somewhat later than macrophage precursors.[947,948] Mature neutrophils are first detected by 14 to 16 weeks of gestation. The numbers of circulating neutrophil precursors (CFU-GMs) are 10- to 20-fold higher in the fetus and neonate than in the adult, and neonatal bone marrow also contains an abundance of neutrophil precursors.[947,949] The rate of proliferation of circulating neutrophil precursors in the human neonate appears to be near maximal,[947,950] however, suggesting that the capacity to increase the numbers of CFU-GMs in response to infection may be limited. In contrast with the numbers of CFU-GMs, in the mid-gestation human fetus, the numbers of postmitotic neutrophils in the fetal liver and bone marrow are markedly lower than in term newborns and adults.[951] Furthermore, at this stage of gestation, neutrophils constitute less than 10% of circulating leukocytes, rising to values of 50% to 60% at term.

Within hours of birth, the numbers of circulating neutrophils increase sharply in term and preterm neonates.[952,953] One study of healthy term neonates reported absolute neutrophil counts at 4 hours of 9.5×10^3 to $21.5 \times 10^3/mm^3$ (10th to 90th percentile) and an immature-to-mature neutrophil ratio of 0.05 to 0.27.[954] The number of neutrophils normally peaks shortly thereafter, whereas the fraction of neutrophils that are immature (bands and less mature forms) remains constant at about 15% (Fig. 4-14). Values may be influenced by a number of factors. Most important is the response to sepsis. Septic infants may have normal or increased neutrophil counts. Sepsis and other perinatal complications, including maternal hypertension, periventricular hemorrhage, and severe asphyxia, can cause neutropenia, however, and severe or fatal sepsis often is associated with persistent neutropenia, particularly in preterm neonates.[947,955,956] Neutropenia may be associated with increased margination of circulating neutrophils, which occurs early in response to infection.[931] Neutropenia that is sustained, however, often reflects depletion of the neonate's, particularly the premature

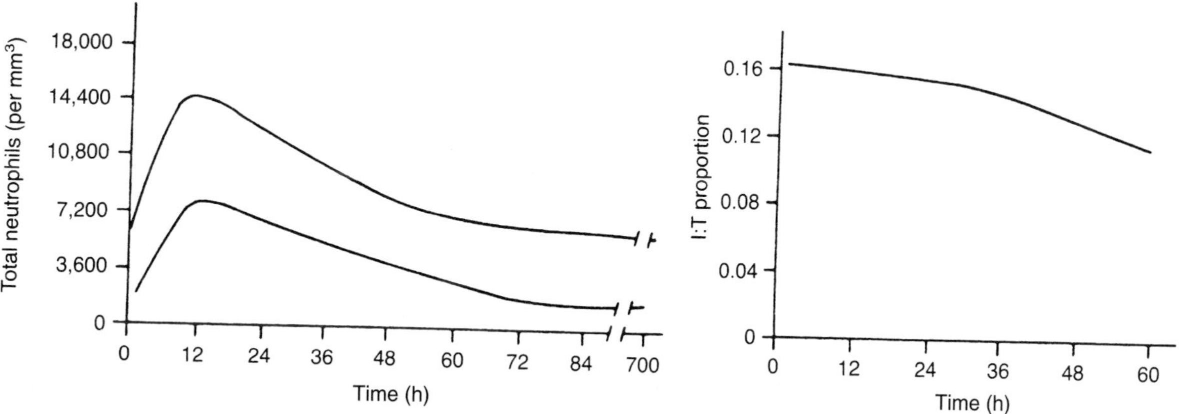

Figure 4–14 Change in total number of neutrophils (*left*) and in ratio of immature to total neutrophils (I:T, *right*) in the neonate. (Data from Manroe BL, Weinberg AG, Rosenfeld CR, et al. The neonatal blood count in health and disease. I. Reference values for neutrophilic cells. J Pediatr 95:89-98, 1979.)

neonate's, limited postmitotic neutrophil storage pool. Accordingly, septic neutropenic neonates in whom the neutrophil storage pool is depleted are more likely to die than are those with normal neutrophil storage pools.[956] Leukemoid reactions also are observed at a frequency of approximately 1% in term neonates in the absence of infection or other definable cause. Such reactions appear to reflect increased marrow production of neutrophils and are not consistently associated with increased G-CSF concentrations.[957]

As discussed earlier, CSFs, particularly G-CSF, are important for neutrophil production, survival, and optimal function. Mononuclear cells and monocytes from mid-gestation fetuses and premature neonates generally produce less G-CSF and GM-CSF after stimulation in vitro than do similar cell populations from adults, whereas cells from term neonates produce amounts that are similar to or modestly less than those of adults (see Table 4-4). In contrast with these findings, circulating G-CSF levels in healthy infants are highest in the first hours after birth, and levels in premature neonates are generally higher than in term neonates.[958-960] Levels decline rapidly in the neonatal period and subsequently decline more slowly with aging. One study reported a direct correlation between circulating levels of G-CSF and the blood absolute neutrophil count, although this finding has not been confirmed in other studies.[958,959] Plasma G-CSF levels tend to be elevated in infected mature and premature neonates,[960] although some studies have found considerable overlap with the levels of those who are uninfected.[961] In one report, G-CSF levels in neutropenic neonates without sepsis were not elevated above normal, whereas levels in neutropenic adults undergoing chemotherapy were markedly increased.[962] Although the cause of neutropenia in these neonates was not described, these observations raise the possibility that deficient G-CSF production might be a contributory factor to neutropenia in some neonates.

Overall, the available data suggest that the most critical deficiency in phagocyte defenses in the fetus and neonate, particularly the premature neonate, is their limited ability to accelerate neutrophil production in response to infection. This age-specific limitation appears to result in large part from a limited neutrophil storage pool, and perhaps a more limited ability to increase neutrophil production in response to infection. This limitation in neutrophil production is not clearly due to a deficiency in the production of G-CSF in vivo, although such deficiency may be a factor in some cases. As discussed under "Colony-Stimulating Factors" in the section on adjunctive therapy of pyogenic infections, trials of G-CSF or GM-CSF have been undertaken to determine whether this form of intervention can ameliorate these deficits in neutrophil production.

Migration to Sites of Infection

In addition to defects in neutrophil production in response to infection, a substantial body of evidence suggests that the ability of neonatal neutrophils to migrate from the blood into sites of infection and inflammation may be reduced or delayed.[963] In human neonates, the early inflammatory response in the skin often contains a larger number of eosinophils than in adults, and the transition from a neutrophilic to a mononuclear cell–dominated response is delayed. Similarly, the influx of neutrophils into the peritoneal cavity in response to fMLP, group B streptococci, or *E. coli* was markedly reduced in neonatal rats compared with that in adult rats[964]; this occurred in spite of greater release of marrow neutrophil stores in neonates than in adults. This diminished delivery of neutrophils may result in part from defects in adhesion and chemotaxis.

Adhesion of neonatal neutrophils under resting conditions is normal or at most modestly impaired, whereas adhesion of activated cells is deficient.[965,966] Adhesion of neonatal neutrophils to activated endothelium under conditions of flow similar to those found in capillaries or postcapillary venules is variable but on average only 40% to 45% of that observed with adult neutrophils.[967,968] This decreased adhesion appears to reflect, at least in part, a deficiency in the abundance of L-selectin and ability to shed this protein from the surface of neonatal neutrophils and decreased binding of these cells to P-selectin.[967-969] Many studies[967,968,970] find that resting neonatal and adult neutrophils have similar amounts of the β_2 integrins Mac-1 (CD11b-CD18) and LFA-1 (CD11a-CD18) on their plasma membrane. Neutrophils from term and, in particular, preterm neonates, however, have a reduced ability to upregulate expression of these integrins after exposure to chemotactic agents, which is due in part to reduced intracellular stores of these molecules in their granules. This reduced capacity for integrin upregulation is associated with a parallel decrease in adhesion to activated endothelium or purified ICAM-1.[971] Two studies, however, have concluded that expression of Mac-1 and LFA-1 is not reduced on resting or stimulated neonatal neutrophils, and that diminished expression observed in other studies may be an artifact of the methods used to purify neutrophils.[969,972] Nonetheless, the preponderance of data suggests that a deficit in adhesion underlies in part the diminished ability of neonatal neutrophils to migrate through endothelium into tissues.[967,971]

In nearly all studies in which neutrophil migration has been examined in vitro, chemotaxis of neonatal neutrophils was less than that of adult neutrophils (Table 4-8). When compared directly, chemotaxis of neonatal peripheral blood neutrophils seems to be more impaired than that of cord blood neutrophils.[973] Some studies have found that chemotaxis remains less than that of adult cells until the infant reaches at least 1 to 2 years of age, whereas others have suggested more rapid maturation.[973,974] The response of neonatal neutrophils to a variety of chemotactic factors, including fMLP, LTB_4, PAF, and IL-8, is reduced.[975-977] Neutrophil chemotaxis in premature infants is at least as impaired as that of term neonates. Most[963] but not all[978] studies have found that the number and affinity of receptors for fMLP are similar in adult and in neonatal neutrophils, whereas receptors for C5a may be reduced.[979] Thus, decreased chemotaxis probably is due in large part to an event downstream of binding of the chemotaxin to its specific receptor, such as the increases in $[Ca^{2+}]_i$ and inositol phospholipid generation and the change in cell membrane potential within the neutrophil.[980,981] An additional factor may be the reduced deformability of neonatal neutrophils, particularly immature granulocytes, which may limit their ability to enter the tissues after binding to the vascular endothelium.[966] This defect appears to reflect a diminished capacity of neonatal neutrophils to reorganize their cytoskeleton in response to stimulation, rather than altered amounts of tubulin or actin.[963]

Table 4–8 Chemotaxis of Neonatal Granulocytes

Cell Source	Assay	Stimulus	Percentage of Adult Response	Comment	Reference
Cord blood	3-μm Nucleopore filter	EAS	79	Normal random motility	973
Peripheral blood	Agarose	ZAS	27	Low until 2 yr of age	974
Cord blood, peripheral blood	3-μm Nucleopore filter	EAS	125 53	Still low at 6 mo of age; normal chemokinesis	1051
Cord blood	Agarose	ZAS	≤30	More severe with lower concentration of ZAS	982
Peripheral blood	5-μm cellulose filter, whole blood	ZAS	79	Ill neonates = 62%	1423
Cord blood	Cellulose filter, 3, 5, or 8 μm	Casein	37-60	Normal random motility, normal chemokinesis	1424
Cord blood	Agarose 3-μm cellulose	EAS	60-80 <15	Normal random motility	1425
Peripheral blood	5-μm cellulose filter	ZAS	88		1426
Peripheral blood	Cellulose filter	ZAS	~50	Equal to adult by 2 wk response	1427
Cord blood	Agarose	fMLP	70	Low until 1 yr of age	976

EAS, endotoxin-activated serum; fMLP = *N*-formylated Met-Leu-Phe peptide (bacterial surrogate); ZAS, zymosan-activated serum.

Because chemotaxis by neonatal neutrophils is relatively more impaired at low than at high concentrations of chemotactic factors,[982] decreased generation of chemotactic factors in neonatal serum[973,982] may compound the intrinsic chemotactic deficits of neonatal neutrophils. The generation of other chemotactic agents, such as LTB_4, by neonatal neutrophils appears to be normal, however.[983] Finally, not all changes in response to chemotactic factors are abnormal in neonatal neutrophils: Upregulation of the type 1 complement receptor (CR1) is normal or at most slightly impaired.[972,984]

Phagocytosis and Killing of Bacteria by Neonatal Neutrophils

Under optimal in vitro conditions, neutrophils from healthy human term and preterm neonates bind and ingest gram-positive and gram-negative bacteria as well as or only slightly less efficiently than do cells from adults.[963,985,986] Levels of opsonins, including IgG, and of complement are reduced in serum from neonates, in particular preterm neonates. Consistent with this finding, phagocytosis of bacteria by neutrophils from preterm but not term neonates is reduced compared with that observed for cells from adults when assayed in whole blood.[987-989] This deficiency appears to be due primarily to differences in plasma components rather than to differences between neutrophils.[987] Neutrophils from preterm neonates, however, also have reduced numbers of receptors for IgG—FcγRIII (CD16)—and for complement—C3bi (CD11b-CD18, also known as Mac-1), compared with neutrophils from term neonates and adults.[972,989,990] Neutrophils from preterm neonates also express less of the LPS co-receptor CD14 and are less able to upregulate CD11b and to secrete elastase in response to LPS.[991]

When concentrations of opsonins are limited,[992] neutrophils from term neonates ingest bacteria less efficiently than those from adults. The basis for this decreased efficiency is unknown, because FcγRII, FcγRIII, CR1, and CR3 expression is similar.[989] Decreased upregulation of the C3bi receptor, which is the β_2 integrin Mac-1, by neonatal neutrophils in response to chemotactic factor or LPS priming may play a role.[993,994]

Killing of ingested gram-positive and gram-negative bacteria and *Candida* organisms by neutrophils from healthy neonates has been normal in most studies.[963,986] Variable and usually mildly decreased bactericidal activity has been noted against *Pseudomonas aeruginosa*,[995] *S. aureus*,[996] and certain strains of group B streptococci, however.[997-999] Deficits in killing by neonatal neutrophils were found to be more apparent at high ratios of bacteria to neutrophils.[1000] Microbicidal activity of neutrophils from sick or stressed neonates (most of whom were born prematurely and had sepsis, respiratory impairment, hyperbilirubinemia, premature rupture of membranes, or hypoglycemia) is more clearly reduced[1001,1002] despite normal[1002] or only variably decreased[1001] phagocytosis. It should be noted, however, that neutrophils from adults with similar illnesses also may have diminished microbicidal activity.[1001] Whether neonatal neutrophils are more severely compromised by illness than those of comparable adults remains to be determined.

Studies to elucidate the mechanisms for differences in microbicidal activity of human neonatal neutrophils have focused on the generation of microbicidal toxic oxygen metabolites.[963,986] In most studies, generation of superoxide anion by human neonatal and fetal neutrophils has been similar to that observed in adult cells. Similarly, neutrophils from term and preterm neonates generate hydrogen peroxide at least as efficiently as cells from adults. By contrast, production of the toxic hydroxyl radical and chemiluminescence (an index of oxygen radical production) may be decreased.[1003] Group B streptococci are highly susceptible to killing by hydroxyl radical but relatively resistant to the action of superoxide anion and hydrogen peroxide.[1004] Thus, if generation of hydroxyl radical by neutrophils from some neonates is deficient, this may contribute to a defect in microbicidal activity for a clinically important pathogen.

Oxygen-independent microbicidal mechanisms of neonatal neutrophils remain poorly characterized. Their ability to release the lysosomal enzymes lysozyme and β-glucuronidase appears to be intact.[963,986] Their content of specific granules and the release of specific granule contents (e.g., lactoferrin) on activation appear to be reduced, however. Compared with adult neutrophils, neonatal neutrophils are deficient in BPI, a cationic antimicrobial protein with activity against gram-negative bacteria that is present in primary granules, despite comparable amounts of myeloperoxidase and defensins.[1005]

Effects of Immunomodulators

After systemic treatment with G-CSF and GM-CSF, expression of CR3 (CD11b-CD18) on neonatal neutrophil increases.[950] Studies performed in vitro indicate that IFN-γ and GM-CSF enhance the chemotactic response of neonatal neutrophils.[950,1006] At higher concentrations, however, GM-CSF inhibits chemotaxis; such concentrations are associated with enhancement of oxygen radical production.[1007] The methylxanthine pentoxifylline exhibits a biphasic enhancement of chemotaxis by neonatal neutrophils.[963] None of these agents causes full normalization of chemotaxis compared with that in adult cells. Of potential concern, indomethacin, which is used clinically to facilitate ductal closure in premature neonates, impairs chemotaxis of cells from term and preterm neonates.[1008] Clinical trials of immunomodulators are discussed in the section on adjunctive therapy of pyogenic infections.

Eosinophilic Granulocytes

In adults and older children, eosinophils represent a small percentage of the circulating granulocytes. Their numbers are increased in allergic states, parasitic (particularly metazoal) infections, and in certain autoimmune or malignant disease states. In the fetus and neonate, eosinophils commonly represent a sizable fraction of the total number of circulating granulocytes. At 18 to 30 weeks of gestation, total granulocytes represent only about 10% of total circulating leukocytes, whereas eosinophils constitute 10% to 20% of total granulocytes.[1009] Similarly, in premature neonates, the numbers of eosinophils are increased relative to those in term neonates, often reaching values of 1500 to 3000 cells per mm^3 and representing up to one third of total granulocytes in the first month of life.[1010,1011] The postnatal increase of eosinophils lags behind that of neutrophils, peaking at the third to fourth week of postnatal life. A relative increase in the abundance of eosinophils in inflammatory exudates is seen in neonates, paralleling their greater numbers in the circulation.[968] In addition to prematurity, certain conditions have been associated with a relatively greater degree of eosinophilia; these include Rh disease, total parenteral nutrition, and transfusions.[1010] In contrast with conditions such as allergic and parasitic diseases, neonatal eosinophilia is not associated with increased amounts of circulating IgE.[1011] The basis or the significance of the eosinophilic tendency of the neonate is not known. Certain of the functional deficits observed in neonatal neutrophils, such as the diminished expression of adhesion molecules important in leukocyte migration into tissues, have been observed in neonatal eosinophils.[968]

Mononuclear Phagocytes

Origin and Differentiation in the Adult

Blood monocytes are derived from bone marrow precursors (monoblasts and promonocytes), which in turn are the precursors of tissue macrophages. Together, monocytes and tissue macrophages are referred to as mononuclear phagocytes. These cells have multiple functions, including the clearance of dead host cells, phagocytosis of microbes, presentation of antigen to T cells, secretion of inflammatory mediators, and cell-mediated cytotoxicity.

Under steady-state conditions, monocytes are released from the bone marrow within 24 hours and circulate in the blood for 1 to 3 days before moving to the tissues.[1012] Once they have left the blood, monocytes do not recirculate but differentiate into macrophages, which are present in all tissues. Monocytes lose granule myeloperoxidase as they differentiate into tissue macrophages. Other changes depend on the local tissue conditions. For example, monocytes and peritoneal macrophages rely primarily on anaerobic glycolysis, whereas alveolar (lung) macrophages utilize aerobic cytochrome oxidation as well.[1013,1014] The functions of macrophages are readily modulated by cytokines, and macrophages can fuse to form multinucleated giant cells. The estimated life span of macrophages in the tissues is 4 to 12 weeks, and they are capable of limited replication in situ.[1013,1014]

Migration to Sites of Infection: Adherence, Chemotaxis, and Delayed Hypersensitivity Reactions

Like neutrophils, mononuclear phagocytes express the adhesion molecules L-selectin and β_2 integrins. These cells, unlike neutrophils, also express substantial amounts of the $\alpha_4\beta_1$ integrin (VLA-4).[1015,1016] Expression of VLA-4 allows monocytes, unlike neutrophils, to adhere efficiently to endothelium expressing VCAM-1, the ligand for VLA-4. VCAM-1 is a member of the immunoglobulin gene superfamily, which is expressed only on endothelial cells that have been activated by exposure to cytokines or bacterial products such as LPS. The avidity of VLA-4 for VCAM-1 is low in the absence of activation, but activation of monocytes by chemotactic factors enhances avidity, allowing firm adhesion and presumably transendothelial migration.[1016] VLA-4 allows monocytes to enter tissues in states in which there is little or no neutrophilic inflammation, such as DTHs. The expression of VLA-4 also may account for the capacity of monocytes but not neutrophils to enter tissues in patients with the type I leukocyte adhesion deficiency syndrome, who lack β_2 integrin expression due to a genetic deficiency of CD18 (discussed previously).

Like that in neutrophils, monocyte chemotaxis is induced by bacterial products, such as fMLP, and by activated complement components, PAF, and LTB_4. Chemokines (see Tables 4-1 and 4-2) that are chemotactic for neutrophils, however, are not generally chemotactic for monocytes, and vice versa—neutrophils are most responsive to certain CXC chemokines, such as CXCL8 (IL-8), while monocytes respond to CC chemokines, such as CCL2 (MCP-1).[43,937]

The acute inflammatory response induced by a transient irritant (e.g., dermal abrasion) is characterized by an initial infiltration of neutrophils that is followed within 6 to 12 hours by the influx of mononuclear phagocytes.[1012] The orchestration of this sequential influx of leukocytes appears to be governed by the temporal order in which specific chemokines and endothelial adhesins are expressed and by the slower migration rate of monocytes versus neutrophils. Cutaneous DTH responses are characterized by an influx of mononuclear phagocytes and lymphocytes. This response reaches maximum at 24 to 72 hours after antigen infiltration.

Experimental evidence in mice and humans undergoing DTHs suggests that this process is governed, at least in part, by cytokines. These include IL-1, TNF-α, and chemokines, which are produced by DCs, epithelial cells, and mast cells, and IL-2 and IFN-γ, which are produced by effector T cells infiltrating the subcutaneous tissues.[937,1017] The expression of these cytokines and the induction by IFN-γ of MHC class II antigen reach their maximum before the peak influx of cells and induration, consistent with a role in causation.

Antimicrobial Properties of Monocytes and Macrophages

Although neutrophils ingest and kill pyogenic bacteria more efficiently, resident macrophages are the initial line of phagocyte defense against microbial invasion in the tissues. When the microbial insult is modest, these cells may be sufficient to clear the microbes. If they are not, mononuclear phagocytes then direct the recruitment of circulating neutrophils and monocytes through the production of inflammatory mediators and cytokines. Monocytes and macrophages express each of the three Fcγ receptors for IgG[576]; Fcα receptors for IgA[1018]; CR1 and CR3 receptors for C3b and C3bi, respectively[1019]; and CD14, multiple TLRs, and receptors that allow them to phagocytose unopsonized unencapsulated bacteria, yeasts, certain viruses, and effete cells, such as mannose-fucose, β-glucan, and scavenger receptors.[47,940,1020] Phagocytosis is greatly facilitated when the microbe or particle is coated with immunoglobulin, complement, or both (i.e., opsonization, discussed later).

Phagocytosis of particles and subsequent microbicidal mechanisms of mononuclear phagocytes parallel those of neutrophils in most respects. Mononuclear phagocytes generate reactive oxygen metabolites, but in lesser amounts than are produced by neutrophils. Circulating monocytes but not tissue macrophages contain myeloperoxidase, which facilitates the microbicidal activity of hydrogen peroxide. The expression of microbicidal granule proteins differs somewhat in mononuclear phagocytes versus neutrophils; for example, human mononuclear phagocytes express β-defensins but not the α-defensins, which are expressed at high levels by neutrophils.[1021] Several unique mechanisms of antimicrobial activity are mediated primarily by activated macrophages, as discussed later on.

The microbicidal activity of resident tissue macrophages is relatively modest. This limited activity may be important in allowing macrophages to remove dead or damaged host cells and small numbers of microbes without excessively damaging tissues through release of microbicidal materials, which also are toxic to host cells. Macrophage microbicidal and proinflammatory functions are enhanced in a process commonly referred to as macrophage activation, discussed next.[986,1022]

Mononuclear Phagocyte Activation

Macrophage activation results from the integration of signals emanating from TLRs following their engagement by microbial structures or molecules released by necrotic host cells (see section on DCs), cytokines derived from other cells, including IFN-γ and, to a more limited extent, TNF-α or GM-CSF, activated complement components, and immune complexes, and by the engagement of CD40 on macrophages by CD40 ligand on activated CD4⁺ T cells.[1022,1023] Cytokines produced by activated macrophages, including TNF-α, GM-CSF, IL-12 family of cytokines, IL-15, and IL-18, can further amplify macrophage activation through autocrine or paracrine mechanisms, as described in more detail later.

The increased antimicrobial activity of activated macrophages results in part from increased expression of FcγRI, enhanced phagocytic activity, and increased production of reactive oxygen metabolites in response to phagocytic or other stimuli. Other antimicrobial mechanisms induced by activation of these cells include the catabolism of tryptophan by indoleamine 2,3-dioxygenase, scavenging of iron, and production of nitric oxide and its metabolites by the inducible nitric oxide synthase (iNOS). The last is a major mechanism by which activated murine macrophages inhibit or kill a variety of intracellular pathogens. Expression of iNOS by human macrophages is less consistently observed and less robust than that noted for murine macrophages, and the role of nitric oxide in the antimicrobial activity of human macrophages is uncertain.[1024]

Activation of macrophages plays a critical role in defense against infection with intracellular bacterial and protozoal pathogens that replicate within phagocytic vacuoles of resting macrophages. Support for this notion comes from studies in humans and mice with genetic deficiencies in proteins that participate in macrophage activation. Humans with genetic deficiencies involving the IFN-γ receptor, IL-12, the IL-12 receptor, or STAT-1 (a signaling molecule downstream of the IFN-γ receptor) suffer unduly from infections with *Mycobacteria* spp. and *Salmonella* spp.[1025] Similarly, mice deficient in these cytokines or their receptors are much more susceptible to these infections and to infections with other intracellular pathogens, including *T. gondii*. Deficiency of TNF-α or its receptors also impairs defenses to certain of these pathogens, including *L. monocytogenes* and mycobacteria.[1026] Patients with the X-linked hyper-IgM syndrome, which is due to a defect in CD40 ligand, have defects in antibody production that result from the importance of CD40 ligand in T cell–mediated help for B cell responses (see section on T cell help for antibody production).[195] In addition, these patients are predisposed to disease due to *Pneumocystis jiroveci* and *Cryptosporidium parvum*. Mice with CD40 ligand deficiency also are at greater risk for infection with *P. jiroveci* but, unlike those with IFN-γ, IL-12, or TNF-α deficiency, are not more susceptible to infection with *L. monocytogenes*.[161] These findings suggest that secreted cytokine- and CD40 ligand–mediated macrophage activation may play, at least in part, distinct roles in host defense.

Regulation of the Immune and Inflammatory Responses by Cytokines Produced by Mononuclear Phagocytes

In addition to the induction of increased antimicrobial activity, mononuclear phagocytes produce a number of cytokines when activated by ligand binding to TLRs and by engagement of CD40, cytokines, activated complement components, immune complexes, or other mediators.[1022,1023] These mononuclear phagocyte-derived cytokines contribute to the systemic response to infection, including the induction of fever and the acute-phase response, and play important local roles in the regulation of inflammation (see Table 4-2).[1027,1028] IL-1, TNF-α, IL-6, and IFH-α/β (also known as type I IFN) induce fever by stimulating vascular endothelial cells in the hypothalamic area to produce PGE_2. PGE_2 acts in turn on cells within the anterior hypothalamus to cause fever, which accounts for the antipyretic effect of drugs that inhibit prostaglandin synthesis. Fever may have a beneficial role in host resistance to infection by inhibiting the growth of certain microorganisms and by enhancing host immune responses.[1029] TNF-α, IL-1, and IL-6 act on the liver to induce the acute-phase response, which is associated with decreased albumin synthesis and increased synthesis of complement components C3 and factor B, haptoglobin, fibrinogen, C-reactive protein, and other proteins. G-, GM-, and M-CSF enhance the production of their respective target cell populations, increasing the numbers of phagocytes available. At the sites of infection or injury, TNF-α and IL-1 increase endothelial cell expression of adhesion molecules, including E- and P-selectin, ICAM-1, and VCAM-1; increase endothelial cell procoagulant activity; and enhance neutrophil adhesiveness by upregulating β_2 integrin expression.[932,939] CXC chemokines enhance the avidity of neutrophil β_2 integrins for ICAM-1 and attract neutrophils into the inflammatory-infectious focus; CC chemokines play a similar role in attracting mononuclear phagocytes and lymphocytes.[43,936] These and additional factors contribute to edema, redness, and leukocyte infiltration, which characterize inflammation.

Mononuclear phagocytes (and DCs) are important sources of IFN-α/β, IL-12, IL-15, and IL-18.[42,53,1022,1030,1031] These cytokines enhance NK cell lytic function and production of IFN-γ and facilitate the development of effector T_H1 and $CD8^+$ T cells, which play a critical role in control of infection with intracellular bacterial, protozoal, and viral pathogens and inhibit the development of T_H2 T cells.[89,179] IFN-α/β also directly inhibits viral replication in host cells,[1032,1033] as do IFN-γ and TNF-α.[1034] IFN-γ enhances the capacity of macrophages to produce IL-12 and TNF-α and inhibits IL-10 production, thereby amplifying its own production and T_H1 T cell responses.[89,1035]

The production of cytokines by mononuclear phagocytes normally is restricted temporally and anatomically to cells in contact with microbial products, antigen-stimulated T cells, or other agonists (discussed previously) found at sites of infection or secondary lymphoid organs draining these sites. When produced in excess, however, these cytokines are injurious.[1036,1037] When excess production of proinflammatory cytokines occurs systemically, septic shock and disseminated intravascular coagulation may ensue, underscoring the importance of closely regulated and anatomically restricted production of proinflammatory mediators.

Tight control of inflammation normally is achieved by a combination of positive and negative feedback regulation. For example, TNF-α, IL-1, and microbial products that induce their production also cause macrophages to produce cytokines that attenuate inflammation, including IL-10,[1038] TGF-β,[1039] and the IL-1 receptor antagonist.[945] The production of these anti-inflammatory cytokines also is enhanced by exposure of macrophages to cytokines produced by T_H2 T cells, including IL-4, IL-10, IL-13, and TGF-β. By contrast, cytokines produced by T_H1 T cells, particularly IFN-γ, attenuate the production of IL-10.

Activated mononuclear phagocytes also secrete a number of noncytokine products that are potentially important in host defense mechanisms. These include complement components, fibronectin, and lysozyme.[1040]

Mononuclear Phagocytes in the Fetus and Neonate

Macrophages are detectable as early as 4 weeks of fetal life in the yolk sac and are found shortly thereafter in the liver and then in the bone marrow.[1041] The capacity of the fetus and the neonate to produce monocytes, as indicated by development of macrophage colonies when fetal liver or neonatal bone marrow or blood is grown in culture, is at least as great as that of adults.[1042] The numbers of monocytes per volume of blood in neonates are equal to or greater than those in adults.[1043]

The numbers of tissue macrophages in human neonates are less well characterized. Limited data in humans, which are consistent with data in various animal species, suggest that the lung contains few macrophages until shortly before term.[1044] Postnatally, the numbers of lung macrophages increase to adult levels by 24 to 48 hours in healthy monkeys.[1045] The blood of premature neonates contains increased numbers of pitted erythrocytes or erythrocytes containing Howell-Jolly bodies.[1046] Because these abnormal erythrocytes normally are removed by splenic and perhaps liver macrophages, the numbers or function, or both, of these macrophages may be reduced in the fetus and premature infant.

Migration to Sites of Infection and Delayed Hypersensitivity

The influx of monocytes into sites of inflammation is delayed and attenuated in neonates compared with that observed in adults.[1047,1048] Similarly, cutaneous DTH, which depends on an influx of monocytes and lymphocytes into the site, is diminished in neonates.[502,506,1049] This is true even when antigen-specific T cell responses are evident in vitro, suggesting that decreased migration of monocytes and lymphocytes into the tissues is responsible for the poor response in neonates. These differences may result from decreased generation of chemotactic factors, such as CC chemokines, or decreased chemotaxis of neonatal monocytes, or both.

Whether neonatal monocyte chemotaxis is impaired is unclear. In all but one of the studies[1050] in which cord blood chemotaxis and adult monocyte chemotaxis were compared, no difference was found. In the two studies in which peripheral blood rather than cord blood was used,[973,1051] however, chemotaxis of neonatal cells was less than that of adult cells and remained less until the child reached 6 to 10 years of age.[974] The basis for reduced chemotaxis is unknown.

Data regarding adhesion molecules on monocytes from neonates are limited to two conflicting reports. One study reported increased amounts of the β_2 integrin Mac-1 (CD11b-CD18) on resting and activated neonatal monocytes,[972] whereas the other found expression to be modestly lower.[1052]

The capacity of fetal and neonatal macrophages to process and present antigen to T cells was discussed previously in the section on antigen presentation by neonatal monocytes and B cells.

Activity of Monocytes and Macrophages against Pyogenic Pathogens

Monocytes from human neonates ingest and kill *S. aureus*, *E. coli*, and group B streptococci as well as do monocytes from adults.[997,1050,1053-1055] The ability of neonatal monocyte-derived macrophages (monocytes cultured in vitro) to phagocytose bacteria or other particles through receptors for mannose-fucose, IgG, complement, and opsonin-independent pathways appears not to differ from that of similarly prepared cells from adults. The production of microbicidal oxygen metabolites by neonatal and adult monocytes also is similar.[1054,1056-1059]

Neonatal and adult monocyte-derived macrophages phagocytose but do not efficiently kill *Candida* and group B streptococci. Incubation with IFN-γ or GM-CSF activates adult macrophages, allowing them to kill these organisms.[1060-1062] By contrast, GM-CSF but not IFN-γ activates neonatal macrophages to produce superoxide anion and to kill these organisms. The lack of response to IFN-γ by neonatal macrophages was associated with normal binding to but decreased signaling downstream of IFN-γ receptors. The poor response of neonatal macrophages to IFN-γ may be compounded by the diminished production of this cytokine by neonatal NK and T cells, as described in previous sections.

Neonatal tissue macrophages are difficult to obtain, and few studies of their microbicidal activity have been performed. Macrophages obtained from aspirated bronchial fluid of neonates were less effective at killing the yeast form of *Candida* than were bronchoalveolar macrophages from adults.[1063] To our knowledge, this result has not been reproduced, and the decreased effectiveness could reflect differences in the source of cells, rather than representing a true difference between neonates and adults. Nonetheless, similar studies with alveolar macrophages from newborn and particularly premature newborn monkeys, rabbits, and rats also showed reduced phagocytic or microbicidal activity, or both.[1064-1069]

Activity of Monocytes and Macrophages against Intracellular Pathogens

Control of infection with obligatory or facultative (i.e., capable of) intracellular pathogens is mediated by factors that limit entry into cells, inhibit intracellular replication, induce microbial killing or dormancy within cells, or lyse infected cells prior to microbial replication. Neonatal monocytes ingest and kill *T. gondii*[1070,1071] and *L. monocytogenes* (C. Wilson, unpublished data, 1980). In contrast with the results with *Candida* and group B streptococci noted earlier, both monocyte-derived and placental macrophages from human neonates are activated by IFN-γ to kill or restrict the growth of *Toxoplasma* as effectively as cells from adults.[1062]

Neonatal monocytes, monocyte-derived macrophages, and fetal macrophages are not more permissive than adult cells for replication of HSV.[1072,1073] Monocytes and macrophages also can inhibit viral replication by lysing virus-infected cells in either the absence or the presence of antibody.[1074] Monocytes from neonates may be slightly less cytotoxic than those from adults in the absence of antibody, but they are equivalent in the presence of antibody.[1074,1075]

Exogenous IFN-γ induces resistance to *L. monocytogenes* infection in neonatal rats and to HSV infection in neonatal mice.[1076,1077] This finding suggests that in these species, the antimicrobial activity of host macrophages (and other host cells mediating resistance to these microbes) can be enhanced sufficiently to be protective, given the provision of this cytokine. This also implies that the deficit in production of IFN-γ and certain other cytokines (e.g., TNF-α) that facilitate resistance to these microbes may be an important factor in the neonate's increased susceptibility, which is discussed later.

Cytokine and Inflammatory Mediator Production by Mononuclear Phagocytes from the Fetus and Neonate

Monocytes and macrophages are stimulated to produce G-, GM-, and M-CSF and the proinflammatory cytokines IL-1, TNF-α, IL-6, and IL-8 by a number of mediators. These mediators include LPS, which activates cells through the TLR-4–MD2 receptor complex[47,1020]; group B streptococci, which activate cells through TLR-2 plus TLR-6 and through an as-yet undefined TLR or TLR-related receptor[1078]; and IL-1,[1079] which activates cells through the type I IL-1 receptor. In response to these stimuli, neonatal monocytes and blood mononuclear cells produce these cytokines in variable amounts, ranging from approximately 25% to 75% of the amounts produced by adult cells (summarized in Table 4-2). TNF-α production by monocyte-derived and tissue (placental) macrophages from term neonates is reduced to a greater extent than occurs with blood monocytes and appears to be upregulated less by IFN-γ than in cells from adults.[1080] In some studies, however, production of G-CSF, IL-1β, and IL-6 by neonatal monocytes was similar to that in adult cells,[88,344,962,1080-1084] and in other studies, production of IL-1α, IL-6, and IL-8 by whole blood, which probably reflected production predominantly by monocytes, was greater than in adult cells.[354,1085] Monocytes from preterm neonates produce less TNF-α, G-CSF, and IL-8 in response to LPS than those from term neonates and adults. Collectively, these findings suggest that neonatal monocytes and macrophages have a variable and relatively subtle deficiency in the production of proinflammatory cytokines compared with that in adult cells.

Reduced production of proinflammatory mediators by neonatal monocytes and blood mononuclear cells appears to be balanced in most contexts by a comparable reduction in the generation of the anti-inflammatory cytokines, IL-10 and TGF-β.[1083,1086-1088] This may not be the case in certain pathologic contexts, however. Alveolar macrophages from preterm neonates with hyaline membrane disease produce less IL-10 in vivo relative to TNF-α than alveolar macrophages from term neonates.[1089,1090] This imbalance may be a factor in the development of inflammatory lung disease.

The production by neonatal monocytes of IFN-α/β, IL-12, IL-15, and IL-18 also appears to be modestly reduced. These cytokines inhibit viral replication and enhance NK, T_H1, and $CD8^+$ T cell differentiation and function, so these deficiencies collectively could impede defenses against viral and nonviral intracellular pathogens. In earlier studies, production of IFN-α/β by neonatal mononuclear cells and monocytes was normal in response to a variety of inducers including HSV and other viruses.[82,1091] As noted earlier in the section on circulating neonatal DCs, however, more recent studies using whole blood or blood mononuclear cells have found that HSV-induced IFN-α/β production and the fraction of cells that produced IFN-α/β in response to HSV were diminished compared with those in adults, particularly for prematurely born infants.[83] Neonatal blood cells also produced less IFN-α/β when stimulated with parainfluenza viruses.[69,72,84] Overall, these more recent studies suggest that neonatal cells produce approximately 10% to 30% as much IFN-α/β as produced by adult cells. It is likely that the decreased production of IFN-α/β by neonatal blood cells in response to viruses or unmethylated CpG DNA reflects predominantly decreased production by DC2 cells rather than monocytes, but this association has been shown directly only for the response to unmethylated DNA.[72] One group of investigators reported that the production of IL-12 and IL-15 by blood mononuclear cells (which probably reflected production by monocytes) from term neonates after stimulation with LPS was approximately 25% of that by cells from adults.[369,891] Joyner and colleagues and La Pine and associates also reported that neonatal blood mononuclear cells produced less IL-12 and IL-18, although the reduction in IL-18 was modest (approximately 65% of the amounts produced by cells from adults).[1092,1093] Other investigators, however, have reported that neonatal and adult blood mononuclear cells stimulated with *S. aureus*, other gram-positive and gram-negative bacterial cells, produce equivalent amounts of IL-12.[86,88] Nonetheless, the results of studies with blood mononuclear cells and DCs from neonates suggest that in response to most stimuli, cells from neonates produce less IL-12 and IFN-α/β than those from adults.

When bioassays are used collectively to measure chemokines that are chemotactic for monocytes, no differences in production by neonatal and adult cell preparations are observed.[1053,1054] This does not exclude deficits in production of individual chemokines, however. Indeed, cord blood mononuclear cells produced only approximately 25% as much of the CC chemokine CCL3 (MIP-1α) as that from adult cells.[1083] The extent to which these assays reflect chemokine production by monocytes is not known.

The basis for lower production of cytokines by neonatal monocytes and macrophages in response to microbial products that signal through TLRs is incompletely understood. Yan and colleagues reported that neonatal monocytes have reduced amounts of MyD88, an intracellular adapter protein that is essential for proinflammatory cytokine production downstream of TLR.[1094] Because MyD88 also is an adapter downstream of the IL-1 and IL-18 receptors,[1079] reduced expression of MyD88 by neonatal monocytes also could explain reduced responses to IL-1. These investigators also reported that the expression of TLR-4 and CD14 was similar on neonatal and on adult monocytes, and neonatal monocytes failed to upregulate the expression of these molecules in response to LPS, which may reflect impaired LPS signaling due to reduced expression of MyD88. To our knowledge, the expression of other TLR has not been directly assessed in neonatal monocytes. Others report that unstimulated neonatal monocytes express similar or slightly reduced amounts of CD14, a co-receptor for LPS and certain other microbial structures that trigger monocyte cytokine production through TLR-4 and some other TLRs.[92,1081,1095] Compared with blood from healthy adults, neonatal blood contains lower amounts of soluble CD14, but similar amounts of soluble LPS-binding protein (LBP), and the concentrations of both rise in response to infection, as they do in adults.[1096] Like CD14, LBP is important in the activation of TLR-4 by LPS. The reduced amounts of soluble CD14 may account for the earlier observation that neonatal cord blood contains lower amounts of a soluble protein(s) that facilitates the response of monocytes to LPS.[1081]

Overall, the foregoing results indicate neonatal monocytes, macrophages, and mixed blood mononuclear cells commonly produce lesser amounts of many cytokines, chemokines, and IFN-α/β in response to activation by microbial ligands or other proinflammatory cytokines. The molecular basis for these differences is incompletely understood; such differences may reflect a general reduction in signaling in response to these mediators and more selective deficits in the induction of specific cytokines, such as the p35 subunit of IL-12.[93]

Engagement of CD40 on mononuclear phagocytes by CD40 on activated T cells also is an important pathway for the induction of macrophage activation and cytokine production. Because the expression of CD40 ligand on activated neonatal T cells may be diminished (see earlier), macrophage activation through this pathway may be compromised in neonates. This pathway would be further compromised if CD40 expression on neonatal monocytes or macrophages was reduced. Data on this point are conflicting, however, with one group reporting comparable expression[1097] and another group reporting reduced expression.[1098]

Summary

The most clearly defined, clinically important deficits in neonatal phagocytic defenses are the diminished neutrophil storage pool and the reduced ability of neonatal neutrophils to migrate from the blood to sites of infection. Phagocytosis and killing by neonatal neutrophils are largely intact but are compromised when opsonins are limiting or the bacterial density is high. These deficits are greater in preterm neonates. Blood monocytes from neonates are normal in number and similar to adult monocytes in phagocytic and microbicidal activity. By contrast, migration of neonatal monocytes into sites of inflammation or DTH is reduced. Tissue macrophages from neonatal animals have reduced phagocytic and microbicidal activity, and this also may be the case in humans. The capacity of mononuclear phagocytes to produce both pro- and anti-inflammatory cytokines may be modestly reduced in term neonates and further reduced in premature neonates. These modest deficiencies may be compounded by a concomitant deficiency in production of IFN-γ by neonatal T cells and NK cells and by impaired responsiveness of neonatal mononuclear phagocytes to IFN-γ.

HUMORAL MEDIATORS OF INFLAMMATION AND OPSONIZATION

A wide range of humoral factors participate in the response to infection and inflammation.[839-841] Some of these factors normally are present in plasma, including complement components, mannan-binding lectin (MBL), fibronectin, coagulation factors, and components of the kinin system. Others, such as products of arachidonic acid metabolism (the prostaglandins, PAF, and leukotrienes), endorphins, amines (including histamine, catecholamines, and serotonin), and lysosomal enzymes, are produced and released from leukocytes, endothelial cells, and other cells. Studies in animal models have implicated some of these mediators in the unfavorable response of neonatal animals to infection[1099,1100]

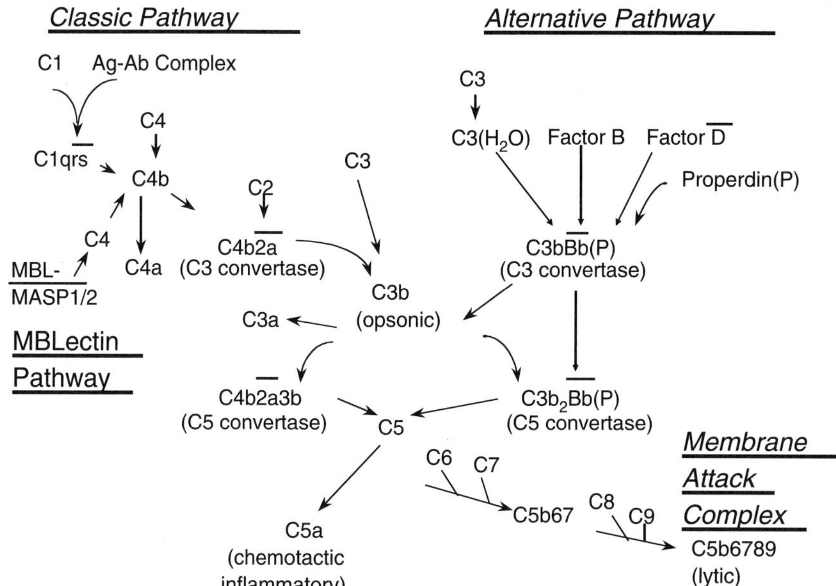

Figure 4–15 Complement activation. The classic and mannan-binding lectin (MBL) pathways of activation intersect with the alternative pathway at C3. The MBL pathway of activation (*not shown*) is identical to the classic pathway starting with the cleavage of C4. Once C3 is activated, this is followed by activation of the terminal components, which generate the membrane attack complex (C5b6789). Enzymatically active proteases, which serve to cleave and activate subsequent components, are shown with an overbar.

and suggest the possibility that therapy directed toward modulating production of the mediators may be beneficial. A better understanding of the relative role of these mediators in particular clinical situations, such as septic shock, will be required, however, to develop rational approaches to modulate their production or actions.

Complement

The complement system is composed of serum proteins that can be activated sequentially in an orderly cascade. The complement cascade can be activated through one of three pathways—the classic, MBL, and alternative pathways, each of which leads to the generation of activated C3, C3 and C5 convertases, and the membrane attack complex. Reviews of the complement system are available.[1101]

Classic and Mannan-Binding Lectin Pathways

Activation of the classic pathway is initiated when antibodies capable of engaging C1q to their Fc portion (IgM, IgG_1, IgG_2, and IgG_3 in humans) complex with microbial (or other) antigens. The formation of complexes alters the conformation of IgM and juxtaposes two IgG molecules, which creates an appropriate binding site for C1q. This is followed by the sequential binding of C1r and C1s to C1q. C1s can then cleave C4 followed by C2, and the larger fragments of these bind covalently to the surface of the microbe or particle, forming the classic pathway C3 convertase (C2aC4b). C3 convertase cleaves C3, thereby liberating C3b, which binds to the microbe or particle, and C3a, which is released into the fluid phase.

MBL activates the complement cascade in a similar manner. When MBL engages the surface of a microbe, its confirmation is altered, creating a binding site for MASP1 and MASP2, which are the functional equivalents of C1r and C1s. These in turn cleave C4 and C2, and their larger fragments bind to the surface of the microbe or particle, forming the classic pathway C3 convertase. C-reactive protein, a host-derived acute-phase protein that binds to structures on the surface of certain bacteria, particularly *S. pneumoniae*, also may substitute for antibody in the activation of the classic pathway.[1028,1102]

Alternative Pathway

The alternative pathway is phylogenetically older and constitutively active. Although it is facilitated by the F(ab′)2 portion of antibody, antibody is not required for its activation. The continuous but inefficient hydrolysis of C3 in solution creates a binding site for factor B. This complex is in turn cleaved by factor D, generating C3b and Bb. If C3b and Bb bind to a microorganism, they form a more efficient system, which binds and activates additional C3 molecules, depositing C3b on the microbe and liberating C3a into the fluid phase. This interaction is facilitated by factor P (properdin) and inhibited by alternative pathway factors H and I. The classic pathway, by creating particle-bound C3b, also can activate the alternative pathway, thereby amplifying complement activation (Fig. 4-15). This amplification step may be particularly important in the presence of small amounts of antibody.

Bacteria vary in their capacity to activate the alternative pathway, which is determined by their ability to bind C3b and to protect the complex of C3b and Bb from the inhibitory effects of factors H and I. Sialic acid, a component of many bacterial polysaccharide capsules, including those of group B streptococci and *E. coli* K1, favors factor H binding. Thus, many virulent pathogens are protected from the alternative pathway by their capsules, although this protection may vary from strain to strain. Antibody is needed for efficient opsonization of such organisms.

Terminal Components and Membrane Attack Complex

Bound C3b, C4b, and C2a together form the C5 convertase, which cleaves C5. The smaller fragment, C5a, is released into solution. The larger fragment, C5b, binds to the surface of the microbe and triggers the recruitment of the terminal components, C6 to C9, which together form the membrane attack complex.

Biologic Consequences of Complement Activation

Binding of C3b on the microbial surface facilitates microbial killing or removal, through the interaction of C3b with CR1 receptors on phagocytes. C3b also is cleaved to C3bi, which binds to the CR3 receptor (Mac-1, Cd11b-CD18) and CR4 receptor (CD11c-CD18). C3bi receptors are β_2 integrins, which are present on neutrophils, macrophages, and certain other cell types and also play a role in cell adhesion, as noted in previous sections of this chapter. Along with IgG antibody, which binds to Fcγ receptors on phagocytes, C3b and C3bi promote phagocytosis and killing of bacteria and fungi.

C3b also is a key component of the C5a convertase, which leads to the cleavage of C5, release of C5a into the fluid phase, binding of C5b on the microbial surface, and formation of the membrane attack complex. This complex can be assembled only in lipid-containing cell membranes, which include the outer membrane of gram-negative bacteria and the plasma membrane of infected host cells. Once assembled in the membrane, this complex may lyse the cell. Such lysis appears to be a central defense mechanism against meningococci and systemic gonococcal infection. Certain gram-negative organisms have mechanisms to impede complement-mediated lysis, and gram-positive bacteria are intrinsically resistant to complement-mediated lysis because they do not have an outer membrane. As a result, in contrast with the important role of complement-mediated opsonization, complement-mediated lysis may play a limited role in defense against common neonatal bacterial pathogens.

The soluble fragment of C5, C5a, and, to a more limited degree, C3a and C4a cause vasodilatation and increase vascular permeability. C5a also is a potent chemotactic factor for neutrophils, monocytes, and eosinophils. It stimulates these cells to degranulate, adhere to endothelium, and release leukotrienes, which themselves are potent mediators of inflammation.

In addition to these roles for complement in innate immunity, complement facilitates B cell responses to T cell–dependent antigens. As discussed in the section on B cells and immunoglobulin, C3d bound to antigen complexed with antibody (produced as part of the initial B cell response) amplifies the antibody response by simultaneous engagement of the C3d receptor (CD21) along with the B cell antigen receptor.[574] C3d also may facilitate B cell responses by enhancing the retention of antigen-antibody complexes on follicular DCs. Mice that are genetically deficient in C3, C4, or the complement receptors for C3b and C3d have diminished antibody responses to immunization with protein antigens.[574]

Complement Biosynthesis

The hepatocyte appears to be the principal cell type that synthesizes complement components.[732,1101] Macrophages synthesize complement proteins, except those complement components that form the terminal membrane attack complex. Other cell types, including fibroblasts, may produce certain complement proteins.

Complement in the Fetus and Neonate

Little, if any, maternal complement is transferred to the fetus. Fetal synthesis of complement components can be detected in tissues as early as 6 to 14 weeks of gestation, depending on the specific complement component and tissue examined.[732,1103]

Table 4–9 Summary of Published Complement Levels in Neonates[a]

Complement Component	Mean % of Adult Levels	
	Term Neonate	*Preterm Neonate*
CH_{50}	56-90 (5)[b]	45–71 (4)
AP_{50}	49-65 (4)	40-55 (3)
Clq	61-90 (4)	27-58 (3)
C4	60-100 (5)	42-91 (4)
C2	76-100 (3)	67-96 (2)
C3	60-100 (5)	39-78 (4)
C5	73-75 (2)	67 (1)
C6	47-56 (2)	36 (1)
C7	67-92 (2)	72 (1)
C8	20-36 (2)	29 (1)
C9	<20-52 (3)	<20-41 (2)
B	35-64 (4)	36-50 (4)
P	33-71 (6)	16-65 (3)
H	61 (1)	—
C3bi	55 (1)	—

[a]Number of studies.
[b]Data from the review of Johnston RB, Stroud RM. Complement and host defense against infection. J Pediatr 90:169–179, 1977; from Notarangelo LD, Chirico G, Chiara A, et al. Activity of classical and alternative pathways of complement in preterm and small-for-gestational-age infants. Pediatr Res 18:281-285, 1984; from Davis CA, Vallota EH, Forristal J. Serum complement levels in infancy: age-related changes. Pediatr Res 13:1043-1046, 1979; from Lassiter HA, Watson SW, Sefring ML, Tanner JE. Complement factor 9 deficiency in serum of human neonates. J Infect Dis 166:53-57, 1992; from Wolach B, Dolfin T, Regev R, et al. The development of the complement system after 28 weeks' gestation. Acta Paediatr 86:523-527, 1997; Zilow G, Bruessau J, Hauck W, Zilow EP. Quantitation of complement component C9 deficiency in term and preterm neonates. Clin Exp Immunol 97:52-59, 1994, with permission.

Table 4-9 summarizes published reports on classic pathway complement activity (CH_{50}) and alternative pathway complement activity (AP_{50}) and individual complement components in neonates. Substantial interindividual variability is seen, and in many term neonates, values of individual complement components or of CH_{50} or AP_{50} are within the adult range. Alternative pathway activity (AP_{50}) and alternative pathway components (B, P) are more consistently decreased than are classic pathway (CH_{50}) activity and components.

A clear deficiency has been identified in the amount of the terminal complement component C9, which is important for lytic activity against serum-sensitive, gram-negative microbes, and this deficiency correlates with poor killing of gram-negative bacteria by serum from neonates. The C9 deficiency in neonatal serum appears to be a more important factor in the inefficient killing of *E. coli* K1 than the deficiency in antigen-specific IgG antibodies.[1104] A functional deficiency of C3, which is deposited on microbes but is not efficiently cross-linked, may contribute to decreased opsonic activity.[1105]

Preterm infants demonstrate a greater and more consistent decrease in both classic and alternative pathway complement activity and concentrations of individual complement components.[1106] Mature but small-for-gestational-age infants have CH_{50} and AP_{50} values similar to those for healthy term infants.[1107] The concentration of most complement proteins increases postnatally and reach adult values by 6 to 18 months of age.[1108]

C-Reactive Protein

C-reactive protein can activate the classic complement pathway when bound to certain gram-positive bacteria. It does not cross the placenta. Term and preterm neonates can produce C-reactive protein as well as adults.[1109] Serum concentrations may be higher in healthy neonates than in healthy adults.

Mannan-Binding Lectin

With rare exception, glycoproteins containing terminal mannose sugars are not found on extracellular proteins in mammals, because they are modified in the endoplasmic reticulum before transport through the Golgi complex. By contrast, terminal mannose, fucose, glucose, and *N*-acetyl glucosamine are found on the surfaces of gram-positive and gram-negative bacteria, mycobacteria, yeasts, and certain viruses and parasites.[1110,1111]

Tissue macrophages contain mannose-fucose receptors, which bind to microbes with surface mannose-fucose–containing carbohydrate polymers and thereby are activated for phagocytosis and killing. By contrast, neutrophils and blood monocytes lack mannose-fucose receptors. The liver, however, produces a homologous secreted protein, MBL, which also is referred to as mannose-binding protein. MBL can bind to microbes with surface mannose or fucose and facilitate phagocytosis and killing by neutrophils and monocytes.[1110,1111]

MBL is a member of a family of structurally homologous proteins known as collectins.[1111] MBL is a calcium-dependent lectin that circulates as an 18-mer composed of 3 to 6 identical homotrimeric structural units. MBL is homologous to C1q and can bind to Clq receptors on mononuclear phagocytes. It also activates complement, thereby opsonizing the microbe for phagocytosis and killing by neutrophils and monocytes. It is an acute-phase protein, so the concentration of MBL increases in inflammation. Engagement of MBL is impeded by capsular polysaccharides of most virulent gram-negative pathogens.

Approximately 5% to 7% of the general population is deficient in MBL as a result of a polymorphism in codon 54.[1110,1111] Although some persons with this deficiency may experience increased numbers of infections, most do not, suggesting that MBL plays an auxiliary role in host defense. The concentration of MBL in the blood of term neonates is similar to that in adults. Values in preterm neonates are approximately 50% lower,[1112] but whether this reduction contributes to their increased risk for infection is not known. Infants with lower levels of MBL in cord blood were noted to have higher rates of admission, particularly for viral infections, in the first year of life in one study.[1113]

Surfactant Apoproteins

Surfactant apoproteins A and D also are members of the collectin family. They are synthesized by the type 2 alveolar epithelial cells and Clara cells in the lung epithelium, and by certain extrapulmonary cell types.[1111,1114] Like MBL, surfactant apoprotein A binds to mannose-glucose polymers found on the surface of gram-positive and gram-negative bacteria, mycobacteria, and yeasts. Mice deficient in surfactant apoprotein A are much more susceptible to pulmonary infection with group B streptococci, *H. influenzae*, RSV, and *P. aeruginosa*. By contrast, mice deficient in surfactant apoprotein D appear to clear microbes normally. Thus, surfactant deficiency may be one factor in the greater risk of the preterm neonate for pulmonary infections.

Lipopolysaccharide-Binding Protein

LBP is produced by the liver, and production is increased as part of the acute-phase response. LBP facilitates binding of LPS to CD14 and presumably thereafter to TLR-4.[47,1023] LBP and CD14 together lower by several orders of magnitude the concentration of LPS needed to prime or activate macrophages through TLR-4 and promote binding of gram-negative bacteria by these cells. Neonatal blood and adult blood contain similar amounts of LBP, and the concentration rises further in response to infection.[1096]

Fibronectin

Fibronectin is a ubiquitous glycoprotein, which exists in two forms—circulating and tissue. The liver synthesizes most of the fibronectin found in the plasma, whereas fibroblasts, endothelial cells and other cell types synthesize tissue fibronectin. Fibronectin enhances the initial adherence of neutrophils and monocytes to endothelium.[1115] Fibronectin also has opsonic properties,[1116,1117] although compared with antibody or complement, it plays a minor role. It also may have a direct phagocytosis-enhancing effect on monocytes and stimulated neutrophils.[861] Fragments of fibronectin also are chemotactic for monocytes. Fibronectin may also activate mononuclear phagocytes and DCs through TLR-4.[1118]

Plasma fibronectin concentrations are low in neonates, particularly in prematures.[1119,1120] Concentrations may be further reduced in sepsis, birth asphyxia, or respiratory distress syndrome. Plasma fibronectin concentrations reach the lower limit of normal for adults by 1 year of age.[1121]

Opsonic Activity

Measurement of opsonic activity tests the ability of serum to enhance the phagocytosis (or phagocytosis and killing) of a particular organism or particle. Some organisms are effective activators of the alternative pathway, whereas others require antibody to activate complement. Thus, depending on the organism or particle tested, opsonic activity reflects specific antibody, MBL, C-reactive protein, classic or alternative complement pathway activity, or combinations of these. Accordingly, it is not surprising that the efficiency with which neonatal sera opsonize organisms is quite variable. For example, although opsonization of *S. aureus* was normal in neonatal sera in all studies,[992,1122,1123] opsonization of group B streptococci,[1122,1124] *S. pneumoniae*,[1123] *E. coli*,[1122,1125] and other gram-negative rods[1122,1125] was decreased against some strains and in some studies but not in others.

Neonatal sera generally are less able to opsonize organisms in the absence of antibody. This difference is compatible with deficits in the function of the alternative and MBL pathways,[1126-1128] and with the moderate reduction in alternative pathway components. This difference is not due to a reduced ability of neonatal sera to initiate complement activation through the alternative pathway.[1129] Neonatal sera also are less able to opsonize some strains of group B streptococci in a classic pathway–dependent but antibody-independent manner, which may reflect deficits in classic pathway activation through C-reactive protein or activation of the MBL pathway.[1124,1130] The deficit in antibody-independent opsonization is accentuated in sera from premature neonates and may be further impaired by the depletion of complement components in septic neonates.

Chemotactic Factor Generation

Complement activation also generates fluid-phase components with chemotactic activity for neutrophils and monocytes, most of which is due to C5a.[1131] Sera from term neonates generate less chemotactic activity than adult sera, and this diminished activity reflects a defect in complement activation rather than antibody.[973,1051,1131] It is likely that the differences found in these studies using sera from term neonates would be greater if sera from preterm neonates were tested, but this remains to be determined. These in vitro observations notwithstanding, preterm and term neonates do generate substantial amounts of activated complement products in response to infection in vivo.[1132]

Summary

Compared with adults, neonates have moderately diminished alternative complement pathway activity, slightly diminished classic complement pathway activity, and decreased abundance of some terminal complement components. Fibronectin and MBL concentrations are also slightly lower. Consistent with these findings, neonatal sera are less effective than adult sera in antibody-independent opsonization and in opsonization when concentrations of antibody are limiting. Generation of complement-derived chemotactic activity also is moderately diminished. These differences are greater in preterm than in term neonates. Preterm neonates also may have compromised lung defenses as a result of reduced abundance of surfactant apoprotein A. These deficiencies, in concert with phagocyte deficits described earlier, may contribute to delayed inflammatory responses and impaired bacterial clearance in neonates.

HOST DEFENSE AGAINST SPECIFIC CLASSES OF NEONATAL PATHOGENS

For the purposes of understanding host defenses required for protection, microbes can be broadly classified as extracellular pathogens, which include pyogenic bacteria, such as group B streptococci, and fungi, such as *Candida albicans* and intracellular pathogens. Intracellular pathogens can be further divided into those that replicate in the cytosol of host cells, which include viruses and *L. monocytogenes*, and those that replicate within phagocytic vacuoles, such as *T. gondii*. This section discusses host defenses to each type of pathogen, using group B streptococci, HSV, and *T. gondii* as examples. Differences in immune function that predispose the neonate to infection are discussed, as are potential avenues for immunologic intervention. Additional details regarding the virulence determinants of specific microbes and relevant aspects of host defense are provided in the chapters on the specific organisms.

Pyogenic Bacteria: Group B Streptococci

Overview of Host Defense Mechanisms

Infection of the neonate with group B streptococci (i.e., "GBS") in most cases results from aspiration of infected amniotic or vaginal fluid, followed by adherence to and subsequent invasion through the respiratory mucosa. Initial colonization is influenced by the organism's ability to adhere to mucosal epithelial cells. Physical disruption of the mucosal epithelium may not be required for tissue invasion, because group B streptococci can enter into the cytoplasm of cultured respiratory epithelial cells by an actin microfilament–dependent process.[1133] Specific secretory IgA antibody and fibronectin may decrease bacterial adherence to the mucosa. Epithelial cells in the skin, tongue, and airways express β-defensins, which are potent antimicrobial peptides.[1134] β-Defensins are active against group B streptococci, as they are against group A streptococci in the skin,[1135] and constitute an important local defense mechanism.[1136,1137]

Once group B streptococci cross the mucosal epithelium and enters the tissues, phagocytes and opsonins become the critical elements of defense. Antibody and complement opsonize the bacteria for phagocytosis and killing by neutrophils and macrophages, but like all gram-positive bacteria, these organisms are resistant to lysis by complement. Strains of *E. coli* and other gram-negative bacteria that are lysed by antibody and complement are nonpathogenic in more mature hosts but may cause invasive infections in neonates.[1104] Group B streptococci and strains of *E. coli* that cause serious neonatal infections possess type-specific polysaccharide capsules, which impede or block antibody-independent activation of the alternative and MBL complement pathways.[1124,1130,1138] Consistent with this notion, there is an inverse correlation between the degree of encapsulation and the deposition of C3b on type III group B streptococci through the alternative pathway,[1139] although some studies have not found an effect of capsule on complement deposition.[1140]

Efficient complement activation leading to deposition of C3b and C3bi on the bacterial surface is dependent on type-specific anticapsular IgM or IgG antibody.[1141] Consistent with these findings, susceptibility to infection with type III group B streptococci is essentially limited to infants lacking type-specific antibody (see Chapter 13). Complement also plays an important role. In animal models, complement components C3 and C4 are required for protection before the development of type-specific antibodies, suggesting that antibody-independent activation of the C4 complement component by the MBL pathway is involved, whereas C3 but not C4 is required once type-specific antibodies are produced.[1142] C3 also is needed for optimal synthesis of group B streptococcal type-specific antibodies in animal models.[1143] IgG-coated and, in the lung, surfactant apoprotein A–coated bacteria are ingested by phagocytes, and ingestion is augmented by C3b and C3bi. Neutrophils and activated macrophages phagocytose IgM- and C3b-coated bacteria through the C3b and C3bi receptors, although this is less efficient than phagocytosis of IgG- and C3b-coated bacteria.[1101] In the presence of antibody and complement, fibronectin facilitates binding and phagocytosis of group B streptococci and facilitates protection in neonatal rats.[1144,1145]

Small numbers of group B streptococci may be cleared by resident lung macrophages.[1065] If the bacteria are not cleared, neutrophils and monocytes are recruited to the site of infection by chemotactic factors, including fMLP, C5a, LTB_4, PAF, and chemokines (e.g., CXCL8).[1146] Many strains of group B streptococci contain an enzyme, C5a-ase, which degrades C5a. This enzyme appears to degrade human but not murine C5 and, consistent with this notion, impedes bacterial clearance in C5-deficient mice reconstituted with human C5 protein.[1147] In addition to recruitment of neutrophils from the circulation, release of the mature neutrophil storage pool and upregulation of neutrophil production by the bone marrow may be required to provide sufficient numbers of neutrophils to contain the infection.

Entry of neutrophils and monocytes into tissues is dependent on the upregulation of adhesion molecules on the lung vascular endothelium by inflammatory mediators and cytokines. Entry also is dependent on chemotactic factor–induced increases in the abundance and avidity of integrins on neutrophils and monocytes. Collectively, these events allow these cells to bind firmly to and migrate between vascular endothelial cells.[932] After entering the tissues, these phagocytes are drawn to the sites of infection because they contain the highest concentrations of chemotactic factors. Chemotactic factors also prime neutrophils and macrophages to more efficiently ingest and kill group B streptococci in situ.[963,986]

Ingested bacteria are exposed to a variety of potentially microbicidal products (discussed earlier). Although streptococci generate hydrogen peroxide, it appears that phagocytes must generate reactive oxygen metabolites to kill group B streptococci efficiently. Non–oxygen-dependent microbicidal factors, including acid, elastase, cathepsin G, and cationic proteins, also contribute to killing of bacteria by neutrophils.[658] IL-12 facilitates IFN-γ production, and both cytokines enhance the resistance of neonatal rats to group B streptococcal infection.[1148,1149] The mechanism by which IFN-γ enhances resistance is not known but may involve enhanced phagocyte microbicidal activity. Whether IFN-γ contributes to protection in humans is not known.

In cases in which group B streptococci overwhelms neonatal defenses, septic shock may result and is the most frequent cause of death resulting from systemic infection due to group B streptococci in neonates. Septic shock results from systemic overproduction of inflammatory mediators, including TNF-α, IL-1, and IL-6, by phagocytes and other host cells.[1027,1037] Both encapsulated and unencapsulated type III group B streptococci induce production of these cytokines by human monocytes in vitro,[1150] and exogenous fibronectin synergizes with these organisms in this induction.[1151] A soluble factor from group B streptococci induces inflammatory mediator production by signaling through TLR-2 plus TLR-6; other components of group B streptococci induce these mediators through an as-yet undefined TLR or TLR-related receptor.[1078] Neutralization of TNF-α enhances survival in animal models,[1152] even when begun 12 hours after inoculation with these organisms.[1153] Similarly, administration of IL-10, which inhibits production of TNF-α and other proinflammatory cytokines, enhances survival in animals.[1154] These findings have not been reproduced in humans, however. In fact, treatment of sepsis with a soluble TNF-α antagonist led to increased mortality in adults,[1155] and similar studies have not been undertaken in neonates.

Neonatal Defenses

With rare exceptions,[1156] neonatal group B streptococcal infection occurs only in infants who do not receive protective amounts of group B streptococcal type-specific antibodies from their mothers.[1141,1157] Although the concentrations of group B streptococcal type-specific IgG antibodies in cord sera are usually slightly less than in maternal sera at term, term neonates born to mothers with protective concentrations of IgG antibodies generally are protected. In infants born before 34 weeks of gestation, the amounts of group B streptococcal type-specific antibodies often are markedly less than in the mother[1158]; accordingly, preterm neonates may not be protected even though their mothers' serum contains protective amounts of IgG antibodies.

Production of type-specific antibodies by infected neonates is unlikely to contribute to protection. Infected neonates commonly do not make detectable type-specific antibodies during the first month after infection, although a few transiently synthesize IgM but not IgG antibodies.[1159] By 3 months of postnatal age, sera from uninfected neonates and from those who had previous type III group B streptococcal infection usually contain type III group B streptococcus–specific IgM antibodies.[1160,1161] It is not clear, however, that these antibodies require the exposure of normal infants to type III group B streptococci; they could develop naturally or result from a cross-reactive immune response to another source of antigens to which the infant is exposed postnatally.

In the absence of type-specific antibodies, subtle but cumulative deficits in a number of other host defense mechanisms probably contribute to the neonate's susceptibility to group B streptococci. Type III group B streptococci efficiently adhere to mucosal epithelial cells of neonates, particularly ill neonates.[1162,1163] Neonates also lack secretory IgA and, compared with older children, have reduced amounts of fibronectin in their secretions. Reduced amounts of surfactant apoprotein A in the lungs of preterm neonates, a paucity of alveolar macrophages in the lungs of term and particularly preterm neonates before birth, and diminished phagocytosis and killing of bacteria by these cells may facilitate invasion through the respiratory tract. Limitations in the generation of chemotactic factors or deficits in the chemotactic responses of neonatal neutrophils, or both, may result in delayed recruitment of neutrophils to sites of infection. Once they reach sites of infection, neonatal neutrophils may kill bacteria less efficiently because of limited amounts of opsonins, because the local bacterial density has reached high levels, or because the microbicidal activity of neutrophils is decreased in certain neonates. Rapidly progressive infection can deplete the limited marrow neutrophil reserve to compound the problem.

Although the lack of type-specific antibodies and a multitude of subtle deficits in neonatal defenses together predispose to the development of invasive group B streptococcal disease, why does disease develop in less than 10% of infants who both lack type-specific antibodies and are born to colonized mothers?[1164] At present, the answer to this question is incomplete. Among neonates who lack type-specific antibodies, the risk for development of group B streptococcal disease appears to be greater in those born to mothers with high-density genital tract colonization or group B streptococcal amnionitis and also may vary with the virulence of the strain. It also is likely that the variations in host defense between different persons contribute, such as differences in antibody-independent complement activation, and that these deficits are greater in more premature neonates.[1165]

Overview of Immunologic Interventions for Neonatal Group B Streptococcal Sepsis

As summarized in the preceding section, the principal host defense deficits that predispose the neonate to infections with group B streptococci and other pyogenic pathogens appear to be a deficiency of opsonins, particularly protective antibodies, and a limited capacity to increase neutrophil production and mobilize neutrophils to sites of infection. Attempts have been made to address both of these deficits through immunologic interventions. Evidence is currently insufficient, however, to support the routine use of any form of immunologic intervention for prevention or adjunctive therapy of bacterial or fungal infections in the neonate.

Prevention

Selective intrapartum chemoprophylaxis with penicillin or ampicillin clearly has reduced the rate of early-onset disease due to group B streptococci. The efficacy of this form of intervention is likely to be increased by the exclusive use of the risk factor–based approach (see Chapter 13). Even so, chemoprophylaxis cannot prevent all neonatal disease. A more appealing strategy would be to ensure that mothers have adequate amounts of IgG anti–group B streptococcal antibodies to protect their infants passively. Initial results of immunization of pregnant women with purified group B streptococcal polysaccharide were limited by a relatively low response rate of 60%. These limitations may be circumvented, however, by the development of group B streptococcal capsular polysaccharide–protein conjugate vaccines. Studies show that 80% to 93% of adults immunized with type Ia, Ib, II, III, and V capsular polysaccharide–protein conjugate vaccines respond with approximately fourfold titer rises, with geometric mean titers ranging from 2.7 μg/mL for type III to 18.3 μg/mL for type Ia.[1141] If these results can be reproduced, an equally immunogenic multivalent vaccine can be compounded, and issues related to maternal immunization can be addressed, this would provide an attractive approach to the prevention of group B streptococcal disease in neonates.

Before 1993, five major randomized, controlled trials evaluated the efficacy of intravenous immunoglobulin (IVIG) for the prevention of nosocomial or late-onset pyogenic infections in premature neonates, a group at increased risk of infection.[1166] Of these five studies, only one showed a statistically significant reduction in the frequency of infections,[1167] and none showed a reduction in mortality rate or length of hospital stay. A 1997 meta-analysis of 12 randomized controlled trials, which included 4933 infants, showed a slight but statistically significant reduction in the incidence of sepsis ($P < .02$).[1168] The most recent meta-analysis by the Cochrane collaboration in 2001, which included 19 randomized controlled trials with a total of 4986 infants, found a 3% reduction in sepsis ($P = .02$).[1169] It should be noted that the stringency with which sepsis was defined in these studies varied. Perhaps more important, IVIG prophylaxis had no effect on mortality rates. Similarly, a recent multicenter randomized, controlled trial in premature neonates at increased risk due to total IgG concentrations less than 400 mg/dL found no significant reduction in sepsis or other tangible benefit of IVIG prophylaxis. Thus, the authors of the two meta-analyses and other reviews[1168-1170] concluded that IVIG is not indicated for routine prophylaxis in preterm and low-birth-weight neonates, because there is no effect on long-term outcome and the small apparent decrease in the rate of sepsis is not sufficient to justify the cost and potential risks associated with its use.

Recombinant G-CSF and GM-CSF augment granulocyte production and function in neonatal animals and provide some protection against challenge with pyogenic bacteria, including group B streptococci, in these neonatal animal models.[950,1170,1171] These findings prompted clinical trials to determine if administration of recombinant G-CSF or GM-CSF to human neonates would result in increased levels of circulating neutrophils and protect at-risk neonates from sepsis. Three randomized trials of prophylaxis with recombinant GM-CSF and one comparative observational study of prophylaxis with recombinant G-CSF have been conducted.[950,1170,1172] These studies have shown that both G-CSF and GM-CSF increase circulating neutrophil counts and appear to be well tolerated. A meta-analysis of the studies with GM-CSF showed no reduction in mortality rates, however.[1172] The small, nonrandomized observational study found that prophylactic administration of recombinant G-CSF to neutropenic low-birth-weight infants born to mothers with preeclampsia led to a reduction in proven bacterial infections in these patients.[1173] No randomized, controlled trials with G-CSF have been conducted, however, so its utility as a prophylactic agent is essentially untested. Thus, the available evidence does not support the prophylactic use of G-CSF or GM-CSF in neonates.

Adjunctive Therapy of Pyogenic Infections

PASSIVE ANTIBODY

In three early studies, each of which evaluated a different population of patients, and two of which used a different preparation of IVIG, whereas the third study used a preparation of mixed immune globulins, concluded that the administration of IVIG as adjunctive therapy of neonatal sepsis reduced mortality.[1166,1174] Because of the small numbers of neonates studied, lack of concurrent controls, or absence of a prospective design, these studies did not provide sufficient information to form firm conclusions regarding efficacy; evidence of IVIG toxicity was not observed, however, in these and in two other prospective, controlled studies.[1175-1177] In the study by Weisman and co-workers,[1175,1176] all premature neonates were randomly assigned to receive IVIG selected for high titers of antibody to group B streptococci or albumin placebo within 12 hours of birth. Although no efficacy for prevention of late-onset infection was found, IVIG may have been beneficial among the 31 patients with early-onset sepsis, which was most commonly due to group B streptococci. Among these 31, 5 of 16 placebo recipients but none of 14 IVIG-treated recipients died within the first 7 days of life. Two late deaths occurred in the IVIG group, however, so that survival at 8 weeks of age did not differ significantly from that in the control group, although the trend still favored the IVIG group. The treatment arm of the study was terminated early, because the monitoring group concluded that the prophylactic arm of the trial did not show efficacy of IVIG. Another study performed in Saudi Arabia suggested benefit from therapeutic administration of an IgM-containing immunoglobulin preparation not available in the United States, but this study did not include a randomized control group.[1178]

These studies have been followed by a number of relatively small but prospective clinical trials of adjunctive IVIG therapy for neonatal sepsis. These small studies were conducted in a variety of different countries with differing risks for infection, management approaches, and preparations of IVIG. The Cochrane collaboration performed a meta-analysis of 13 such randomized control trials from seven countries involving neonates with suspected or proved invasive bacterial or fungal infections.[1169] In the six trials (with 318 subjects) that included neonates with clinically suspected infection, IVIG had a marginal effect on mortality rate (relative risk 0.63; 95% confidence interval 0.41% to1.00%, $P = .05$). In the seven trials (with 262 subjects) that evaluated outcome only in neonates subsequently proved to have invasive infections, mortality also was marginally reduced by IVIG (relative risk 0.51; 95% confidence interval 0.31% to 0.98%, $P = .04$). The authors concluded that the marginal statistical significance and the variability in study design and quality do not allow firm conclusions to be made at the present time.[1169] We agree with their conclusions. Although additional prospective, placebo-controlled studies of adjunct therapy with IVIG in septic neonates are indicated, the current evidence is insufficient to support routine use.

An alternative to the use of IVIG might be the use of hyperimmune immunoglobulin or mAb preparations. Hyperimmune group B streptococcal IVIG administered before infectious challenge significantly reduced the mortality rate among newborn rhesus monkeys infected with these organisms by the intragastric route; however, the control group in this experiment received neither conventional IVIG nor antibiotic therapy.[1179] Although preliminary studies with hyperimmune group B streptococcal IVIG suggested that it is well tolerated by neonates with suspected neonatal sepsis,[1179] no reports of its efficacy in a controlled trial have been published. Similarly, although a human mAb directed against the group B streptococcal–specific carbohydrate has been developed, provided protection in neonatal rats, and was shown to be safe in neonatal macaques,[1180,1181] it has not been tested in human clinical trials. Polyclonal human antibodies and humanized mAbs directed against components of staphylococci, including coagulase-negative staphylococci, have been developed but have not yet been evaluated clinically.

NEUTROPHIL TRANSFUSIONS

Neutrophil transfusions enhance survival rate in certain animal models of neonatal sepsis, but the clinical efficacy of neutrophil transfusion in septic human neonates is uncertain. Three of five controlled studies showed statistically significant improvement in the survival rate for neonates receiving granulocyte transfusions compared with that for infants not receiving this therapy.[1170] Nonetheless, small sample sizes and differences in entry criteria for treatment and control groups, in methods of neutrophil preparation, in numbers of neutrophils per transfusion, in numbers of transfusions, and in bacterial pathogens causing disease preclude a meaningful meta-analysis of these studies. Although neutrophil storage pool depletion has been used as a selection criterion for neonates for whom transfusion may be beneficial, the difficulty in ascertainment of neutrophil storage pool size in clinical practice and the failure of this parameter to predict outcome in some studies make this measure an imperfect criterion in clinical practice. The utility of neutrophil transfusions is further compromised by the difficulty in obtaining these cells in a timely fashion and the potential complications of transfusions, including the risk of infection. For these reasons, neutrophil transfusions cannot be recommended as routine therapy for neonates with suspected or proven sepsis.

COLONY-STIMULATING FACTORS

Another approach to augmenting neutrophil numbers, function, or both is the administration of recombinant G-CSF or GM-CSF. Administration of both G-CSF and GM-CSF has shown benefit as adjunctive therapy for established pyogenic infections in experimental animals. In initial studies, administration of G-CSF to human neonates ranging in gestational age from 26 to 40 weeks with presumed early-onset sepsis significantly increased the numbers of circulating neutrophils, bone marrow neutrophil storage pool size, and neutrophil expression of CR3 receptors (CD11b-CD18) without short- or long-term adverse effects.[1182-1184] Subsequent studies have addressed therapeutic efficacy and safety, and two groups of investigators recently have published meta-analyses of these therapeutic trials in suspected or proven neonatal sepsis. The most comprehensive of these came from the Cochrane collaboration in 2003, which analyzed all causes of mortality in 257 infants with suspected sepsis from 7 randomized clinical trials.[1172] Survival was not improved by adjunctive treatment with G-CSF or GM-CSF; G-CSF was used in most of these studies. On the other hand, a subset analysis from three of these studies that included 97 infants with neutropenia (absolute neutrophil count less than $1700/mm^3$) showed an apparent reduction in mortality (relative risk = 0.34; 95% confidence interval 0.12% to 0.92%). In an earlier meta-analysis of five studies involving 73 neonates who received G-CSF and 82 controls by Bernstein and colleagues, the mortality rate was significantly reduced ($P < .05$), but if data from two nonrandomized trials were excluded, there was no significant difference (observed risk 0.43; 95% confidence interval 0.14% to1.23%, $P = .13$).[1185] No significant adverse effects of G-CSF adjunct therapy were noted in these studies, and one long-term follow-up study also found no adverse effects. Thus, as with the meta-analyses of adjunct therapy of neonatal sepsis with IVIG, data regarding the use of G-CSF for adjunctive therapy of neonatal sepsis indicate that it is safe and might be useful in some situations. Nonetheless, evidence is currently insufficient to support the routine use of G-CSF or GM-CSF as adjunctive therapy in septic neonates.

Summary

Substantial advances have occurred in our understanding of factors that compromise the neonate's defenses against bacterial infections. As a result of this information, a number of clinical trials have evaluated the use of IVIG, G-CSF, or GM-CSF for the prophylaxis or adjunctive treatment of neonatal infections. The results from these studies have been disappointing or inconclusive. To date, there is no established role for these or any other form of immunologic therapies in the prevention or treatment of bacterial or fungal infections in human neonates. The existing data probably are sufficient to conclude that the prophylactic use of IVIG is not cost-effective and that such use of GM-CSF is not beneficial. Conversely, randomized clinical trials to test the potential benefit of IVIG in septic neonates or G-CSF in clinically septic neonates with neutropenia, or combinations of these agents, as adjunctive therapeutic agents for the treatment of neonatal sepsis may be indicated.

Viruses

Overview of Host Defense Mechanisms

Effective viral host defense mechanisms of vertebrates typically are dependent on a combination of innate and adaptive immune mechanisms that are highly interlinked. Because viruses replicate intracellularly, innate and adaptive mechanisms that control or block infection within cells, such as NK cells and CD8+ T cells, respectively, and prevent spread of virus from cell to cell are the most critical for effective host defense. Antibody and complement also may modify viral expression, especially by preventing spread of virus into the central nervous system (CNS), but in most tissues the cellular immune response is critical for control of viral replication and the elimination of virally infected cells. This section focuses on host defenses operative against HSV-1 and HSV-2, both of which cause strikingly more severe primary disease in the neonate than in the immunocompetent adult.[1186] The immune responses to other viruses, such as CMV, HIV-1, and enteroviruses, are included where relevant. HSV-1 and HSV-2 mostly are collectively referred to here as HSV, because these two viruses are very closely related and, in most instances, have very similar pathogenic properties. The following discussion is based in large part on data from in vivo studies using HSV in mice and in vitro studies using human cells.

HSV is an enveloped virus with a large DNA genome that is contained within an inner core lined by capsid protein. The inner capsid is surrounded by a loose collection of proteins called the tegument. The production of HSV progeny results in the irreversible destruction of the host cell, resulting in viral release. Despite this lytic effect, a substantial proportion of both primary HSV-1 and HSV-2 infections are asymptomatic.[1187] Following recovery from acute infection, HSV persists for life in humans, owing to a latent state established in neurons, such as those of the trigeminal ganglion. In cells containing latent virus, the viral genome is in a circular configuration and associated with host-derived histone proteins.

Innate Antiviral Immunity

The antiviral immune response generally can be divided into two phases. The first is an early, nonspecific phase (typically the first 5 to 7 days in HSV infection) involving innate immune mechanisms. This is followed by a later, antigen-specific phase involving adaptive immunity mediated by T and B cells and their products.[1188] The early phase is critical, because infection either may be successfully contained or, alternatively, may disseminate throughout the host. An overview of the role that interferons, cytokines, and chemokines, and the innate immune cells that produce them, play in the control of HSV follows. Immunity by gamma-delta T cells, which appears to play an early and non–antigen-specific role in the response to HSV, is included here as an innate immune mechanism.

Type I Interferons. Type I IFN consists of IFN-α (encoded by multiple highly homologous and clustered genes) and IFN-β, which utilize a common type I IFN receptor that is widely expressed. IFN-β is made mainly by nonhematopoietic cell types, such as fibroblasts, in response to viral infection, whereas IFN-α is produced in particularly high levels by plasmacytoid DCs of the DC2 cell lineage.[57,59] HSV triggers high levels of type I IFN secretion by plasmacytoid DCs in a TLR-9–dependent fashion.[51] The HSV double-stranded DNA genome is unmethylated at CpG dinucleotide residues, and DNA containing these unmethylated residues is a TLR-9 ligand.[749] The secretion of high levels of IFN-α by DC2 cells results in a systemic antiviral state and enhances local adaptive immune responses, as result of the exposure of secondary lymphoid tissue to this cytokine.[61]

The type I IFN receptor mediates its effects by JAK tyrosine kinase–dependent phosphorylation of STAT-1 and STAT-2. STAT-1, STAT-2, and IRF-9 form a heterotrimeric complex that binds to IFN-stimulated response elements (ISREs) of genomic DNA and influences the gene transcription.[1189] STAT-1 also can homodimerize and bind to GASs ("gamma-interferon–activating sequences"), which induce a distinct set of genes from those utilizing ISREs.[1032] Because these STAT-1 homodimers (but not other STATs) and GAS-regulated genes are activated when IFN-γ binds to its specific receptor,[1032] type I IFN may potentially induce genes that are characteristic of IFN-γ responses, but not vice versa. However, for antiviral host defense in humans, including to HSV, only the ISRE genes appear to be critical.[1190,1191]

Substantial amounts of type I IFN are found in the tissues of HSV-infected animals and humans.[1192,1193] Although HSV efficiently induces type I IFN production, the virus is relatively resistant to its antiviral effects. This relative resistance may account for the limited effectiveness of type I IFN in treating recurrences of established HSV infections, such as of the eye. The resistance may be due in part to ability of the HSV ICP34.5 protein to prevent shutting off of host cell protein synthesis by type I IFN.[1194] HSV infection of certain cell types also may inhibit type I IFN–mediated activation of the JAK/STAT pathway.[1195] In contrast with the resistance to type I IFN alone, HSV may be controlled effectively in mice by a combination of type I IFN and IFN-γ.[1196] Whether this synergy between type I IFN and IFN-γ applies to human infection remains unclear.

IFN-γ. IFN-γ is produced by NK cells and γδ T cells, which are components of the early innate immune response to HSV, as well as by CD4+ and CD8+ T cells that appear later during the adaptive immune response. The effect on HSV infection of genetic disruption of IFN-γ or the IFN-γ receptor, or of IFN-γ neutralization in wild-type mice, has varied, depending on the model and dose of virus employed. In general, IFN-γ is important in the initial containment of disease following primary infection at most sites, such as the vagina, footpad, skin, and cornea, rather than in maintaining latency.[1197-1202] In survivors of infection, the lack of IFN-γ also was associated with increased viral load in the eye or trigeminal ganglion basally[1197] and after reactivation by ultraviolet (UV) irradiation[1202] or hyperthermia.[1203] Of interest, greater severity of HSV disease after corneal infection also was observed in mice lacking the IFN-γ receptor than in those lacking the IFN-γ ligand,[1204,1205] which raises the possibility of an as-yet unidentified additional ligand for the IFN-γ receptor that contributes to host defense, although this finding also may reflect technical rather than meaningful biologic differences.

IL-1 Family Cytokines. IL-1 is induced at sites of HSV infection, such as the cornea, and may contribute to pathogenic inflammation.[1206] IL-1α administered to neonatal mice can enhance survival,[1207] but the role of endogenously produced IL-1 in the control of HSV infections is unclear. In mice, the administration of IL-18, another IL-1 family member, provides substantial protection against systemic HSV infection by a mechanism dependent mainly on IFN-γ but not on NK cells.[1208] Mice lacking IL-18 also are more vulnerable to intravaginal challenge with HSV.[1209]

IL-12 Family. The IL-12, IL-23, and IL-27 family of cytokines have multiple potentially important antiviral host effects, including promoting NK cell cytotoxicity, $CD4^+$ and $CD8^+$ T cell proliferation and differentiation (i.e., to T_H1 cells and CTL, respectively), and IFN-γ production by mature NK cells and T cells.[1210] These cytokines, in conjunction with type I IFN, also favor T_H1 differentiation from naïve $CD4^+$ T cell precursors in humans.[56] This synergy may account for the predominance of IFN-γ–producing virus-specific $CD4^+$ and $CD8^+$ T cells in most viral infections, such as with herpesviruses.[1211] IL-12 is produced by DCs, including those of the DC2 lineage, and mononuclear phagocytes infected with HSV infection in vitro,[1212] and IL-23 transcripts have been detected in the neuronal ganglia of HSV-infected mice.[1213] Although HSV infection of myeloid DCs also can downregulate IL-12 production in vitro,[1214] these infected cells may induce neighboring uninfected cells to produce IL-12. HSV-infected epithelial cells also appear to secrete factors that result in the induction of IL-12 by inflammatory leukocytes.[1215] Mice lacking both IL-12 and IL-23 are more susceptible to HSV infection,[1209] but it is unclear if these cytokines are important for control of HSV infection in humans. In fact, patients with a genetic deficiency that abrogates both IL-12 and IL-23 signaling do not seem prone to more severe infection with HSV or other viruses.[225,1191] In certain contexts, IL-12 and IL-23 may have a deleterious impact on the outcome of infection by contributing to inflammatory damage, such as in cases of established HSV keratitis.[1216]

IL-15. IL-15, which has a key role in NK cell development and $CD8^+$ T cell immunity, also is a potent activator of NK cells for enhanced cytotoxicity against most herpesviruses, including HSV.[1217] Exposure of human PBMCs to HSV also upregulates NK cell cytotoxicity by an IL-15–dependent mechanism.[1218] In mice, serum levels of IL-15 can be detected, peaking at approximately 3 days after HSV inoculation,[1219] suggesting a role in innate immunity. Studies in mice given IL-15,[1219] or in which IL-15 or a component of its receptor has been genetically disrupted,[1220] support the importance of this cytokine in the control of systemic HSV infection.

Chemokines. HSV infection induces the secretion of a number of CXC and CC chemokines by leukocytes and epithelial cells that are important in leukocyte recruitment and maintenance of inflammation. These chemokines may have either beneficial or deleterious effects for a given site of infection. For example, in HSV keratitis, CCL3 (MIP-1α) contributes to inflammatory disease but does not influence viral replication,[1221] whereas CXCL8 (IL-8), a potent neutrophil chemoattractant, may be helpful in viral control.[1222] The CXC chemokine CXCL10 (MIG), when produced in the cornea, may be detrimental by causing an influx of mononuclear phagocytes that can spread HSV to the other parts of the eye.[1172] Chemokines also may skew the outcome of the adaptive immune response to viral infection. For example, CCL2 (MCP-1) in the cerebrospinal fluid of mice infected with HSV-2 may reduce survival by skewing $CD4^+$ T cell immunity toward a T_H2 rather than a T_H1 antiviral response.[1223] HSV-1 infection of mice induces high levels of intracerebral CCL2 in a TLR-2–dependent manner; TLR-2 deficiency is associated with improved survival,[1224] but it is unclear to what extent this improvement is due to reduced expression of CCL2 or other chemokines. Elevated cerebrospinal fluid levels of the CC chemokines CCL2, CCL3α, and CCL5 (RANTES), and of CXCL8, also have been documented in cases of human HSV encephalitis,[1225] suggesting their role in CNS inflammation. CNS mononuclear phagocytes, such as macrophages or microglial cells, are likely sources of at least a portion of these chemokines, as supported by the capacity of these cell types to produce chemokines on infection with HSV in vitro.[1226,1227]

Mononuclear Phagocytes. Macrophages are likely to play an important role in the early and local containment of HSV infection by their secretion of cytokines and, at least in mice, by the expression of iNOS. In mice, early infection containment appears to involve mainly macrophages, which produce TNF-α, and γδ T cells, which produce IFN-γ.[1228] Systemic depletion of mononuclear phagocytes or γδ T cells, or of the cytokines these cells produce, increases HSV-1 replication in the cornea[1229] and associated ganglia.[480,1228] HSV infection of mononuclear phagocytes also synergizes with IFN-γ for promoting iNOS expression,[1230] which may be detrimental (keratitis)[1231] or beneficial (pneumonia[1232] and encephalitis[1233]), depending on the site of infection. HSV can directly infect mononuclear phagocytes in vitro, but the resultant infection usually is nonpermissive and does not result in viral replication. Such nonreplicative infection may result in apoptosis,[1234] which could limit antiviral immune mechanisms, such as cytokine production.

Myeloid Dendritic Cells. The in vivo role of DCs in the control of HSV is poorly understood. In the murine HSV-2 vaginal infection model, submucosal DCs but not other APC populations (e.g., B cells or macrophages) may be key for viral antigen presentation to T cells in the draining lymph nodes.[1235] As discussed previously (see section on neonatal monocyte-derived DCs), culturing blood monocytes with IL-4 and GM-CSF result in their acquiring features of immature DCs, and these cells can be induced to acquire features of mature DCs using proinflammatory stimuli, such as TNF-α. HSV can efficiently infect both mature and immature monocyte-derived DCs[1236,1237] and is able to replicate in immature but not mature monocyte-derived DCs. HSV infection of monocyte-derived DCs also decreases expression of key co-stimulatory molecules and adhesion molecules,[1238] and of markers indicative of their maturity, such as CD83[1239]; this decrease is associated with a decreased capacity of these cells to activate T cells in vitro.[1240] Finally, HSV infection of purified DCs from adult humans stimulates them to secrete IFN-α and IL-1, but not to secrete IL-12 or to express increased amounts of CD80 or CD86.[1241] These findings suggest that DCs are not effectively activated by HSV infection and may be direct cellular targets of HSV-mediated immunosuppression. Mouse models have not demonstrated detectable in vivo infection of DCs after either infection of the footpad[1242] or vagina,[1235] however, raising the issue of how frequently these cells are infected in vivo in humans.

Natural Killer Cells. NK cells provide a particularly important restraint on viral replication and dissemination before the appearance of adaptive immunity, as shown by the severity of primary infections with herpesviruses, including HSV, CMV, and VZV in patients with a selective lack of NK cells.[837] Although the initial disease is severe, NK cell–deficient patients are able to eventually clear virus, presumably by T cell–mediated immunity[837] (D. Lewis and C. Wilson, unpublished data, 1990). Similarly, if NK cells in mice are eliminated using a specific antiserum given concurrently with HSV, the viral titers in internal organs and the mortality rate both are markedly increased; however, this treatment has no significant effect if started 5 days after viral challenge.[1243] NK cells accumulate at sites of viral inoculation, and depletion of these cells by specific antiserum results in local spread of the infection.[1244] Murine CMV studies suggest that NK cell–derived IFN-γ may be more important than cytolytic activity for this early protection.[1245] IFN-γ may act directly on some cell types, such as hepatocytes, to limit viral replication by a noncytolytic mechanism, as has been observed for other viruses, such as hepatitis B virus.[1246-1248] IFN-γ also increases MHC expression (both class I and class II), which facilitates antigen presentation to $CD4^+$ and $CD8^+$ T cells. The presence of NK cell–derived IFN-γ during the early phases of naïve T cell activation also may increase expression of the T-bet transcription factor and may favor T cell differentiation into T_H1 cells.[1249]

Gamma-Delta T Cells. Gamma-delta T cells, particularly those bearing Vγ2Vδ2 TCR (based on the current nomenclature), obtained from HSV-seropositive donors can lyse HSV-infected cells in a non–MHC-restricted manner.[490] They are discussed as part of the innate immune response because of evidence in mice that they appear early at sites of HSV infection in conjunction with mononuclear phagocytes. The ligands on the target cells that activates these T cells remain to be defined but probably are host-derived molecules, because such T cell activation also is observed with viruses that are not closely related to HSV, such as vaccinia virus.

Adaptive Antiviral Immune Mechanisms

Adaptive immune responses mediated by HSV antigen–specific T cells and B cells are first detected 5 to 7 days after the onset of primary HSV infection in adult humans, with the peak response achieved at approximately 2 to 3 weeks after infection.[554,1250,1251] Antigen-specific immunity does not eradicate infection (i.e., achieve sterile immunity) but rather terminates active viral replication and the acute infection. T cells play the critical role in resolution of active HSV infection and the maintenance of viral latency.[1252,1253] The general importance of T cells in the control of human HSV and other herpesvirus infections is indicated by the increased susceptibility of persons with quantitative (e.g., purine nucleoside phosphorylase deficiency and late HIV infection) or qualitative (e.g., Wiskott-Aldrich syndrome) T cell and antigen presentation defects. Mouse studies suggest that both $CD4^+$ and $CD8^+$ T cells and IFN-γ contribute to HSV clearance,[1254] and that $CD4^+$ T cells may be more important than $CD8^+$ T cells in the control of HSV infections of the skin and peripheral nervous system.[1255] The relative importance of $CD4^+$ and $CD8^+$ T cells in HSV infections in humans, including at particular sites, is uncertain, however. Of importance, B cells do appear to be able to provide protection in the absence of T cells.[1200,1251,1255]

$CD4^+$ T Cells. $CD4^+$ T cells may help control HSV infection by inhibiting viral replication through the production of IFN-γ, TNF-α, and CD40 ligand.[1199,1256] The IFN-γ–mediated increase in expression of the molecules involved in MHC class I antigen presentation also may help override the inhibition of MHC class I antigen presentation by HSV (see later). CD40 ligand expression by $CD4^+$ T cells also is essential for HSV-specific antibody production by B cells and antibody isotype switching, and for the ability of $CD4^+$ T cells to become long-term memory T cells, including those of the T_H1 subset.[1257] Genetic or antibody disruption of CD40 ligand–CD40 interactions in mice results in increased CNS infection and paralysis compared with that in wild-type mice after footpad inoculation with HSV, and in reductions in $CD4^+$ but not $CD8^+$ T cell responses.[163] In rare patients with CD40 deficiency, production of IFN-α by plasmacytoid DCs is decreased in response to HSV infection in vitro,[1258] which strongly supports the idea that CD40 engagement contributes to human antiviral immunity. $CD4^+$ T cells also promote the generation and survival of anti-HSV effector $CD8^+$ T cells in mice,[1254,1259,1260] but the precise mechanism remains unclear. Production of IL-2 by $CD4^+$ T cells also may contribute to the expansion and differentiation of effector $CD8^+$ T cells.

HSV-specific $CD4^+$ T cells in humans have been identified in the circulation[1261] and from sites of recurrent infection in the skin,[1262,1263] cervix,[1264] cornea,[1265] and retina.[1265] These $CD4^+$ T cells recognize peptide epitopes from a variety of HSV proteins, including those of the envelope, tegument, and capsid.[1211,1264] As suggested by murine studies,[163,1266] the development of HSV-specific $CD4^+$ T cell immunity critically depends on an intact CD28-CD80 or CD86 co-stimulatory pathway. The HSV-specific circulating $CD4^+$ T cell response of humans is characterized by a predominant T_H1 cytokine profile,[1267] consistent with the ability of the virus to induce type I IFN, IL-12, and IL-23 at sites of infection, as discussed earlier. HSV infection also may promote T_H1 immunity by inducing T cells at early stages of activation to produce osteopontin, which helps maintain IL-12 production by APCs and inhibits IL-10 production, thereby favoring a T_H1 adaptive immune response.[1268]

Finally, cytotoxic $CD4^+$ T cells may directly lyse HSV-infected cells that express viral peptides on MHC class II molecules. Such cytotoxic $CD4^+$ T cells frequently have been isolated from the circulation of HSV-infected persons after expansion in vitro and appear to compose about 30% of the cytotoxic T cells in HSV infection in mice.[1262,1269] The actual frequency of these HSV-specific cytotoxic $CD4^+$ T cells in the human circulation is unknown. Human $CD4^+$ cytotoxic cells can recognize peptides derived from viral glycoproteins found in the HSV lipid envelope,[1252,1270,1271] such as gB, gC, and gD,[1272] and it is likely that these viral glycoproteins enter into the MHC class II antigen-processing endocytic pathway after first fusing with the host cell membrane. Human $CD4^+$ T cell cytolytic activity probably is mediated mainly by the perforin/granzyme pathway.[777] Potential target cells include not only professional MHC class II–bearing APCs (e.g., mononuclear phagocytes, B cells, DCs) but many other cell types that can express MHC class II and, in most cases, present antigen after their exposure to IFN-γ, GM-CSF, or TNF-α. Substantial $CD8^+$ T cell responses to HSV are generated in humans, however, and HSV-specific $CD8^+$ T cells compose a prominent part of the viral response in tissues, such as the skin and cervix; these findings raise questions about how important $CD4^+$ T cell–mediated cytotoxicity is in the local control of infection.

$CD8^+$ T Cells. The efficient clearance of most viral infections depends on $CD8^+$ T cell–mediated cytotoxicity, in which infected target cells are induced to undergo apoptosis by the secretion of perforin and granzymes or the engagement of Fas by Fas ligand (see Fig. 4-7). Direct evidence for the importance of $CD8^+$ T cells in the control of herpesvirus infections in humans comes from studies showing that the adoptive transfer of donor-derived $CD8^+$ T cells against CMV or EBV provides protection of hematopoietic cell transplant recipients from primary infection with these viruses.[1273,1274] In animal models, $CD8^+$ T cells also appear key in resolving HSV lytic infection of neuronal ganglia during primary infection,[1275] and in preventing reactivation of virus from latency in sensory neurons, possibly by an IFN-γ–dependent mechanism.[1276] Direct recognition of infected ganglion cells by $CD8^+$ T cells is likely, because HSV infection induces detectable MHC class I expression by sensory neurons.[1277] Noncytolytic mechanisms,[1278] such as IFN-γ production[1276] or the secretion of granzyme A,[1279] may be key for $CD8^+$ T cells to maintain latency and to prevent viral spread. Cytolytic mechanisms, such as the perforin/granzyme system, may not be necessary for control of HSV infection at particular tissue sites, such as the cornea, and instead contribute to inflammatory disease.[1280] $CD8^+$ T cells with high levels of direct cytolytic activity are found at sites of focal temporal lobe lesions in mice with experimental HSV encephalitis,[1281] and such cytolytic activity might well contribute to neuronal destruction as part of viral clearance.

In adults with chronic infection, HSV-specific $CD8^+$ T cells that can lyse HSV-infected targets are found mainly at sites of local recurrence of virus, such as the skin adjacent to the genital tract, the cervix,[1253,1262,1264,1269,1282] and cornea.[1283] By contrast, HSV-specific $CD8^+$ T cells are not detectable in the circulation with use of standard techniques, such as intracellular cytokine staining after stimulation with whole HSV,[1261] but can be expanded in vitro from the blood of HSV-immune donors.[1284,1285] The human $CD8^+$ T cell response appears to be dominated by HSV proteins that are internal structural components of the virion, such as those of the tegument and nucleocapsid, or that are rapidly induced on viral entry, such as proteins encoded by immediate-early genes.[1286,1287] These proteins apparently can be processed into peptides and presented on MHC class I molecules before the inhibitory effects of certain viral proteins, which are discussed later on. Viral glycoproteins of the HSV lipid envelope do not appear to be important antigens for MHC class I–restricted responses, perhaps because they fuse with the host cell membrane and do not enter in the cytoplasm in substantial amounts.[1288] The $CD8^+$ T cell immune response to primary HSV infection infections has not been characterized.

Viral Inhibition of Antigen Presentation and Effect on the T Cell Immune Response. In view of the importance of MHC class I antigen presentation in antiviral control, it is not surprising that many herpesviruses, including HSV and CMV, have accumulated multiple gene products to inhibit MHC class I antigen presentation.[1289] Inhibition of the MHC class I pathway limits not only $CD8^+$ T cell–mediated cytotoxicity but also the generation of CTL from naïve CD8 T cells, although the presence of HSV-specific $CD8^+$ T cells at sites of infection shows that this inhibition is overcome, at least eventually. Human CMV also encodes proteins that inhibit MHC class II antigen presentation (reviewed by Mocarski[1290]). Although specific proteins in HSV that inhibit MHC class II antigen presentation have not been identified, they may well exist: Infection of mice with virulent HSV strains results in CNS lesions in which MHC class II expression remains intracellular, thereby avoiding any chance of detection by $CD4^+$ T cells.[1291]

Two HSV proteins, the viral host shutoff protein and the ICP47 immediate-early protein, are particularly important for the inhibition of the MHC class I pathway. The viral host shutoff protein is required for viral pathogenicity[1242] and increases destruction of cellular mRNA and decreases host cell protein synthesis, including MHC class I molecules.[1288] This down regulation of MHC class I limits $CD8^+$ T cell–mediated cytotoxicity of HSV-infected target cells, such as fibroblasts and keratinocytes.[1292] The ICP47 protein binds to the TAP transporter and prevents the loading of peptides onto MHC class I molecules and the transport of MHC class I molecules to the cell surface.[1288,1293-1296]

The importance of selective inhibition of MHC class I antigen presentation in the pathogenicity of HSV and CMV has not yet been formally tested in vivo, but of note, NK cells and HSV antigen–specific $CD4^+$ T cells are detected earlier than antigen-specific $CD8^+$ T cells in lesions of adult humans with recurrent HSV-2 disease.[1262] IFN-γ produced by infiltrating NK and $CD4^+$ T cells may help override the inhibitory effects of ICP47 on MHC class I expression,[1288,1297] thereby allowing the subsequent eradication of virus by $CD8^+$ T cells, which increase in lesions around the time of viral clearance.[1253,1262] This model is supported by the observation that patients with selective CD4+ lymphopenia, such as HIV infection, have a lower frequency of circulating HSV antigen–specific CD8+ CTL precursors and more frequent and severe recurrences of genital disease.[1282] Once HSV-specific CD8+ T cells arrive at local sites of infection, such as the cervix, they may persist,[1264] providing relative resistance to reinfection.

The ability to address the role of CD4+ versus CD8+ T cells in the control of primary HSV infection using murine models is partly compromised by the fact that HSV ICP47 inhibits murine TAP poorly,[1295] which may explain the greater ease with which anti-HSV CD8+ cytolytic T cells have been detected in mice compared with humans.[1252,1253,1262,1298-1300] This species difference also raises a concern that murine models may not faithfully replicate the role of a particular mechanism for the control of the virus in humans. Many HSV gene products are dispensable in vitro, suggesting an in vivo role that has yet to be defined, such as immunoevasion or immunomodulation. We currently lack a complete knowledge of HSV-encoded immunoevasive functions, and of any differences between humans and mice in such functions. This point is important to keep in mind when applying the results of murine models to human HSV disease.

Chemotactic and Homing Receptor Expression by Viral Antigen–Specific T Cells. In established HSV infection, most recurrences of viral replication occur in keratinocytes found at epithelial sites, such as the skin and genitourinary mucosa. During these recurrences, virus-specific CD4+ T cells and NK cells may infiltrate the sites by 48 hours after the appearance of lesions. Infiltration by these cells is followed several days later by the appearance of virus-specific CD8+ T cells, which is associated with viral clearance.[1262] Consistent with the importance of CD8+ T cell immunity at these local sites of replication, a majority of CD8+ T cells that recognize a particular HSV peptide, as assessed by staining with viral peptide-MHC class I tetramers, express CLA,[1263] an adhesion molecule that is involved in homing of T cells to skin and other tissues that contain keratinocytes. It is likely that HSV-specific T cells that enter other sites of viral replication, such as the CNS during HSV encephalitis, utilize a distinct combination of homing and chemotactic receptors to achieve selective trafficking. Based on studies of other neutrotropic viruses, the expression of CCR2 and CCR5 by CD8+ T cells may be important for entry into the CNS.[1301] Other chemokine and homing receptor combinations are likely to be involved in trafficking of HSV-specific T cells to the liver and gastrointestinal tract in cases of disseminated disease.

B Cells, Antibody, Antibody-Dependent Cellular Cytotoxicity, and Complement

Although preexisting antibody (e.g., that induced by vaccination) can prevent certain viral infections, antibody probably plays a relatively limited role in the control of viral infections that are established. This limitation probably also applies to human herpesvirus infections, because patients with X-linked agammaglobulinemia, who lack mature B cells and antibody production, generally are not more susceptible to these pathogens. Nonetheless, antibody may serve an auxiliary role in HSV host defense, particularly when cellular components of the response are deficient, such as in the human neonate. Antibody also may be important for prevention of dissemination of viral infections to the CNS, as has been well documented in agammaglobulinemic or hypogammaglobulinemic patients, who can develop paralytic poliomyelitis or severe chronic encephalitis with echoviruses or coxsackieviruses.[1302]

In contrast with these observations regarding human HSV disease, murine models suggest a more important role of B cells and antibody in host defense. In the cutaneous HSV model, mice lacking B cells as a result of selective gene targeting have been reported to be markedly more susceptible to infection and to have impaired T_H1 responses.[1303] This finding of decreased T_H1 responses is particularly surprising in view of the normal or even increased T_H1 immunity seen in humans with X-linked agammaglobulinemia.[578] B cell–deficient mice also have more local inflammation and viremia than are seen in wild-type mice following intravaginal challenge with attenuated strains.[1304] Of interest, serum from nonimmune wild-type mice transferred into B cell–deficient mice was found to decrease vaginal HSV shedding, suggesting that natural antibody may inhibit viral replication.[1304] Whether such antibody activity is found in the human circulation is unknown.

Human HSV infection results in the induction of antibodies against a diverse set of HSV proteins, including the surface glycoproteins involved in cell attachment and entry.[1305] The production of most HSV-specific antibodies by B cells is T cell dependent. If antibody is passively acquired, as in the case of maternal-to-fetal transfer, humoral immunity may exist independently of T cell immunity. Enveloped viruses, including HSV, can be lysed by antibody and complement in vitro, but lysis is unlikely to be an important mechanism in vivo because of the high concentrations of antibody required.[1306] Under relatively physiologic conditions, IgG and alternative pathway complement components can coat the surfaces of some viruses, including HSV, thereby effectively neutralizing their infectivity, possibly by preventing their attachment or fusion with cell membranes.[1306,1307] Antibodies also can react with viral proteins found on the surface of infected cells, and IgG and complement components can lyse in vitro human cells infected with a number of different viruses, including HSV. The importance of complement in viral host defense in humans is uncertain, however, because serious viral infection is not a feature seen in patients with severe inherited complement deficiency[1308] or in animals made acutely hypocomplementemic.[1309] The apparent limited impact of antibody and complement on HSV infection in humans may reflect viral immunoevasion mechanisms that hamper antibody effector functions. For example, the HSV gC protein is an inhibitor of the complement cascade, especially through the alternative pathway,[1310] and acts by directly binding C3.[1311] The gE-gI heterodimer also binds the Fc portion of antibody molecules and ablates their neutralization activity.[1312] It is possible that these or other HSV-encoded inhibitory mechanisms that block viral neutralization may not be as effective in mice as in humans, analogous with ICP47 inhibition of TAP. Thus, species-specific difference in host-virus interactions might also contribute to the strikingly different roles of B cells in control of HSV in humans versus mice.

A potentially more effective system for the elimination of virus-infected cells by specific antibody is by ADCC, with

NK cells probably being the most efficient ADCC effector cells.[1313] As discussed previously (see section on ADCC), the specificity of cytotoxicity is due to the specific recognition by antibody of viral antigens present on the infected cell surface. In vitro ADCC requires relatively low concentrations of antibody and occurs rapidly (within hours),[1314] making it less likely that the virus will have had sufficient time to produce infectious particles. ADCC mediated by all types of effector cells is upregulated by cytokines, such as IFN-γ, type I IFN, IL-12, and IL-15.[1315-1317] In vitro ADCC activity correlates in some cases with protection against serious viral infections in humans and in animal models, but it remains uncertain to what extent this protection is due to ADCC occurring in vivo.

Neonatal Defenses

HSV infection is severe in term infants infected at the time of parturition, as well as in the uncommon cases when it is acquired in utero. Characteristically, HSV infection in neonates spreads rapidly to produce either disseminated or CNS disease. Enteroviral infections also are severe and may be fatal when acquired in the perinatal period, and, like HSV infections, have a propensity to produce disseminated or CNS disease. Another similarity between HSV and enteroviral infections is that infection acquired after the neonatal period (after age 4 weeks) is typically effectively controlled, suggesting that common developmental limitations in antiviral immunity are responsible. Deficiencies in the function of neonatal NK cells and DCs probably are important contributors to poor early control of infection by the innate immune response. Neonates also may develop critical antigen-specific T cell responses to the virus too slowly to prevent the virus from producing irreparable tissue injury or death. The following discussion focuses mainly on limitations in cellular innate and adaptive antiviral immune mechanisms of the neonate, because these are the best characterized. Neonatal DC function is discussed in the context of the role of this cell as the key APC for naïve T cell activation.

Innate Immunity: Cytokine Production. Relatively little is known concerning the innate immune response during primary HSV infection in neonates. In an early study, type I IFN production by neonatal lymphocytes and monocytes was equivalent to that in adult cells for a variety of inducers, including HSV and other viruses.[82] A more recent study,[83] however, found that type I IFN production by PBMCs and the frequency of IFN-α–producing cells (assayed by the ELISPOT technique) in response to fixed HSV were diminished compared with that in adults, particularly for prematurely born infants. It is likely that the major cell type that produces type I IFN in this assay is the plasmacytoid DC (DC2), and that IFN secretion is TLR-9 dependent, but direct comparisons of type I IFN production by neonatal and adult plasmacytoid DCs have not been reported. There are also no studies in which neonatal and adult myeloid DCs have been evaluated for their function in response to HSV.

The in vitro production of other cytokines by cells of the innate immune system that might play a role in enhancing NK cell and T_H1 T cell responses may be decreased in neonates. For example, IL-12 and IL-15 production by mononuclear cells (presumably mainly by monocytes) from term neonates after stimulation with LPS was approximately 25% of that by adult cells.[85,891] Whether such cytokines are produced in amounts sufficient to limit NK cell or T cell immunity in neonates with HSV infection is not known. Of note, such reduced responses are highly stimulus dependent. For example, neonatal and adult blood mononuclear cells stimulated with *S. aureus* produce equivalent amounts of IL-12,[85-87,891] and only slightly less IL-18 is produced by adult cells in response to group B streptococci.[1093] Freshly isolated neonatal and adult monocytes also express similar low levels of CD40,[1097] but whether they have similar capacity to produce cytokines in response to CD40 ligand engagement remains unclear. The capacity of neonatal mononuclear phagocytes to produce more recently identified cytokines of the IL-12 family, such as IL-23 and IL-27, is unknown.

Natural Killer Cells. As discussed earlier in the section on fetal and neonatal NK cell–mediated cytotoxicity, fetal and neonatal NK cells have reduced cytotoxic activity compared with those of adults, including against HSV-infected[830,907,908] or CMV-infected target cells.[909] Paralleling the reduction in natural cytotoxic activity of neonatal cells, ADCC of neonatal mononuclear cells is approximately 50% of that of adult mononuclear cells, including against HSV-infected targets.[906] Decreased ADCC mediated by purified neonatal NK cells appears to be caused in part by an adhesion defect in the presence of antibody.[894] Whether differences exist between the neonate and the adult for cytokine-primed NK cell cytotoxicity against targets infected with HSV or other herpesviruses is unclear. Cytokine production by NK cells is another potentially important mechanism of host defense against HSV. Neonatal NK cells produce IFN-γ as effectively as adult NK cells in response to exogenous IL-2 and HSV[924] or to polyclonal stimulation with ionomycin and PMA.[354] The adequacy of neonatal NK cell production of these and other cytokines in response to physiologic stimulation (e.g., with HSV-infected cell targets in the absence of exogenous cytokines) is not known.

Regardless of the precise mechanism, reduced NK cell cytolytic activity may be an important contributor to the pathogenesis of neonatal HSV infection. In a murine model, the age-related maturation of NK cell function parallels the development of resistance to HSV,[1076,1188] and neonatal mice, which, like human neonates, are more susceptible to HSV infection, can be protected by adoptive transfer of human blood mononuclear cells from adults but not from neonates. Addition of IL-2 augments protection mediated by cells from adults but not by cells from neonates, and protection is dependent on IFN-γ production by the transferred cells. The failure of human neonatal cells to transfer resistance in this model also can be corrected by the addition of IFN-γ, a cytokine produced poorly by neonatal $CD4^+$ T cells, as discussed later on. This finding suggests that lack of IFN-γ production may be one important difference between adult and neonatal cells. Whether deficits in NK cell IFN-γ production and cytotoxicity may contribute to the failure of neonatal mononuclear cells to confer protection in this model is uncertain. It also is important to point out that the role of IFN-γ in controlling HSV infections in humans is uncertain, because severe HSV infection has not been reported as a major complication of patients with deficiency of IFN-γ receptors. The potential limitations of these murine models, which also apply to those that include the adoptive transfer of human cells, have been discussed erlier in the section on viral inhibition of antigen presentation and effect on the T cell immune response.

Of importance, no studies have directly compared NK cell function against HSV targets in neonates versus adults with primary HSV infection, including after treatment with various immunostimulatory cytokines. Nor have there been measurements of systemic or cell-associated levels of cytokines that could be useful for augmenting NK cell function in this infection. It is also unknown if neonatal NK cell activity is reduced against enteroviruses.

Adaptive Immunity: Antigen Presentation

In addition to its well-known inhibition of MHC class I antigen presentation, HSV infection of neonatal monocytes,[1318] monocyte-derived DCs,[1236] or B cells[1319] can block the ability of these cells to activate $CD4^+$ T cells. As discussed previously, however, the extent to which HSV directly infects DCs and other APCs in vivo remains unclear.

$CD4^+$ T Cells. In two studies in which T cell responses in neonates and adults with primary HSV infection were compared,[553,554] HSV-specific proliferation of peripheral blood mononuclear cells and production of IFN-γ and TNF-α were markedly diminished and delayed in the neonates compared with these measures in the adults. The neonates did not achieve adult levels of these responses for 3 to 6 weeks after clinical presentation, whereas the adults developed robust responses within 1 week. In both studies, HSV antigen-specific responses by peripheral blood mononuclear cells used viral antigen preparations that are processed mainly by the MHC class II rather than the class I pathway, mainly assaying $CD4^+$ T cell function. Other reports indicate that antigen-specific $CD4^+$ T cell responses commonly are slow to develop in neonates infected perinatally or in utero with CMV.[539] Delayed $CD4^+$ T cell responses to primary CMV infection also have been observed for older infants and young children compared with such responses in adults,[226] suggesting that limitations in developing $CD4^+$ T cell responses to at least some herpesviruses may continue beyond the neonatal period. Because, as discussed above, $CD4^+$ T cells provide multiple effector functions that may be critical for the resolution of HSV infection—including direct antiviral cytokine production and help for $CD8^+$ T cells and B cells—this marked lag in development of HSV-specific $CD4^+$ T cell responses in neonates could be an important contributor to the tendency of neonatal HSV infection to disseminate and to cause prolonged disease.

The basis for the delayed development of HSV antigen-specific $CD4^+$ T cells in neonates is not known; the delay could reflect limitations intrinsic to these cells or limitations in APC function. For example, because immature DCs are primed for efficient antigen presentation by engagement of their CD40 molecule by CD40 ligand expressed by activated T cells, or by exposure to microbes or inflammatory cytokines induced by microbes, lack of prior exposure to microbes, which occurs in a cumulative manner after birth, might contribute to the increased susceptibility of the neonate to infection with HSV. A recent study showing reduced basal DC function in adult mice lacking functional TLR-4 supports the idea that postnatal exposure to microbial products may contribute to the maturation of DC function.[1320]

Intrinsic limitations in $CD4^+$ T cell function might also contribute to the reduced and delayed HSV-specific $CD4^+$ T cell immune response. Neonatal naïve $CD4^+$ T cells have a substantially reduced capacity to express CD40 ligand compared with adult naïve $CD4^+$ T cells after activation in vitro with allogeneic DCs, a condition that should closely mimic physiologic activation by foreign antigen.[356] The importance of CD40 ligand–CD40 interactions in the accumulation of memory $CD4^+$ T cells with T_H1 activity has already been mentioned.[1257] Compared with analogous adult cells, neonatal naïve $CD4^+$ T cells also have decreased capacity to generate key intracellular signals after activation, such as elevation of $[Ca^{2+}]_i$,[364] reduced expression of certain transcription factors involved in cytokine production,[372,373] and greater methylation of certain cytokine genes.[368] These mechanisms may contribute to the tendency of activated neonatal $CD4^+$ T cells to become anergic rather than develop into effector cells,[330,388,389] and to the delay in the appearance of IFN-γ production by antigen-specific $CD4^+$ T cells following infection with HSV (and CMV) in the neonatal period.

Neonates also have been reported to have a lower frequency of precursor T cells capable of responding to HSV and CMV.[1321] This finding is unlikely to be due to a limitation in the diversity of the αβ-TCR repertoire,[265-267] however, and is more likely to be an artifact of in vitro culture conditions that may favor the survival of adult rather than neonatal T cells.

$CD8^+$ T Cells. There are, to the best of our knowledge, no published studies of antigen-specific cytotoxic T cell responses in the fetus, neonate, or young infant in response to HSV. This lack reflects, in part, the technical difficulties of performing classic cytotoxicity assays, which require HLA-matched or autologous virally infected target cells. This limitation might be overcome by newer approaches, such as flow cytometric detection of intracellular perforin in viral antigen-specific $CD8^+$ T cells identified using HSV peptide–class I HLA tetramers.

As discussed in detail in the section on T cell response to congenital infection, a recent study of congenital CMV infection using CMV peptide–HLA-A2 tetramers found a robust response in the fetus, neonate, and young infant in terms of both frequency of $CD8^+$ T cells and their function.[429] Although this finding suggests that strong stimulation, particularly if persistent, may induce virus-specific $CD8^+$ T cell responses in the fetus, it does not exclude a potential lag in the appearance of $CD8^+$ T cells in the fetus or perinatally infected infant compared with adults with primary CMV. Evidence from perinatal HIV-1 infection also suggests such a lag in the appearance of $CD8^+$ T cell–mediated cytotoxicity and cytokine production, recognizing a diverse repertoire of viral antigens compared with that in adults with primary HIV-1 infection.[560-562] A caveat is that this delay may be attributable to the immunosuppressive properties of HIV-1, rather than a deficit specific to neonates. The potential for a general lag in $CD8^+$ T cell immunity also is suggested by older studies that have found that naïve $CD8^+$ T cells of the fetus and neonate generate less CTL activity than analogous adult cells after activation and culture in vitro (see section on fetal and neonatal T cell–mediated cytotoxicity). As indicated by the data on HSV-specific $CD4^+$ T cell responses, even a lag of days to weeks in the development of HSV-specific CD8$^+$ T cell immunity after primary infection would likely be a major contributor to the morbidity of this infection in neonates.

T Cell Chemotactic and Homing Receptor Expression. Human neonatal naïve T cells differ from those of adults in that they do not increase CXCR3 expression and decrease CCR7 expression after activation by anti-CD3 and anti-CD28 monoclonal antibodies.[282,402] CXCR3 facilitates T cell trafficking to inflamed tissues that have been exposed to IFN-γ, whereas CCR7 mediates entry into lymphoid tissues in response to the CCL19 and CCL21 chemokines.[403] These findings suggest that activated neonatal T cells may be limited in their capacity to traffic to nonlymphoid sites of inflammation, such as sites of HSV infection.

B Cells, Antibody, Antibody-Dependent Cellular Cytotoxicity, and Complement. Neonates have a modestly reduced antibody response, particularly for IgG, than older infants to most protein neoantigens, whereas IgM responses are similar. These decreased responses and isotype switching may be due, at least in part, to decreased expression of CD40 ligand by neonatal naïve CD4$^+$ T cells during their initial interaction with APCs.[356,364] Although these limitations in antibody response to T cell–dependent antigens may resolve by early infancy, they probably apply to HSV-specific antibodies made in response to neonatal HSV infection. Thus, assuming that HSV-specific antibody that is neutralizing or involved in ADCC contributes to the control of primary HSV infection in humans, it is possible that limitations in isotype switching from IgM to IgG or a slower rate of somatic hypermutation of IgG responses could contribute to the severity of neonatal infection.

The neonate also is partially protected from infection by passive maternal IgG antibody, transferred predominantly during the latter third of pregnancy. Fetal IgG concentrations are equal to or higher than maternal concentrations after 34 weeks of gestation, reflecting active transport mechanisms. In newborns with gestational age less than 38 weeks, a greater fraction of this maternally derived HSV-specific IgG may enter into the CNS,[1322] reflecting a generally less effective blood-brain barrier. The risk of transmission of HSV from mother to infant in cases of primary or initial maternal infection is much higher (approximately 35%) than in cases of recurrent maternal infection. This difference may reflect, in part, lesser amounts of virus in the maternal genital tract in recurrent infection but also may be due to protection by passively acquired HSV type-specific antibody, particularly to glycoprotein G.[1323] Kohl and colleagues[1324] also have shown that of HSV-infected infants, those with greater concentrations of ADCC antibody had less severe disease. In otherwise healthy adults and older children with primary HSV infection, who by definition lack antibody to HSV, however, severe disease does not develop, as it does in neonates with primary infection. This finding indicates that the deficits intrinsic to the neonate are the important factors predisposing to severe infection. Nevertheless, passively acquired antibody may play a role in decreasing transmission or ameliorating disease severity.

Adjunctive Therapy of Herpesvirus Infections

The foregoing studies raise the possibility that neonates could be passively protected by administration of antibody to HSV, particularly antibody that would facilitate ADCC. In vitro studies also suggest that polyclonal antibodies or mAbs could potentially be protective by directly blocking HSV transmission from neurons to epithelial cells.[1325] Passive antibody can even provide substantial protection from a low-inoculum HSV challenge in the absence of both type I IFN signaling and T and B cells, by IL-12- and IFN-γ–dependent mechanisms,[1326] at least in mice. Human mAb, murine mAb that have been humanized, or specific hyperimmunoglobulin could potentially be employed for this purpose. The phage display technique recently has been used to select human mAb with an ability to effectively neutralize either HSV-1 or HSV-2 at a relatively low concentration in vitro,[1327] but it remains to be seen if these or related antibodies will be efficacious in limiting the extent of primary HSV infection in humans. The unique capacity of IFN-γ to endow human neonatal blood mononuclear cells with the ability to protect neonatal mice from infection suggests that exogenous IFN-γ also may be a potentially useful means to enhance the human neonate's resistance to HSV. In the experimental models described by Kohl,[1188] however, passive immunotherapy must be given before or at the time of infection. This requirement raises the concern that such therapy, if administered once infection is established, may be less effective, at least in controlling virally induced tissue damage. In addition, unanticipated fatal toxicity from administration of IL-12 to adult cancer patients[1328] indicates caution in the use of exogenous cytokine therapy in the seriously ill neonate. It should be emphasized again that there is as yet no direct evidence that the initial innate immune response of the neonate to HSV infection is deficient in terms of cytokine production (e.g., for IL-12, TNF-α, and IFN-γ) derived from cells other than T cells.

Facilitating the more rapid development of antigen-specific CD4$^+$ and CD8$^+$ T cells with appropriate effector function might be a more physiologic approach, allowing these cells and the cytokines they produce to properly localize to the sites of infection. Further elucidation of the cellular and molecular mechanisms that underlie the lag in the development of antigen-specific immunity in the neonate in response to HSV may help in devising therapies to overcome these limitations in host defenses. Neonatal CD4$^+$ T cells, if polyclonally activated under conditions that favor repeated cell division (strong activation stimuli in common with the provision of exogenous IL-2), are similar to naïve adult T cells in efficiently acquiring the characteristics of effector cells, including the capacity to produce cytokines, such as IFN-γ and TNF-α.[342] This finding suggests that such approaches applied in vivo (e.g., IL-2 immunotherapy) might similarly enhance neonatal T cell clonal expansion and differentiation.

Herpes Simplex Virus Vaccines

HSV-2 vaccines employing recombinant glycoproteins, such as glycoproteins B and D in combination,[1199,1329] or glycoprotein D alone,[1330] with various adjuvants have had limited efficacy in preventing infection in persons who are HSV-2 seronegative, and in providing substantial clinical benefit to those who are already HSV-2 infected. Although these vaccines have induced high levels of IgG antibodies against the glycoprotein immunogens, these antibodies may not efficiently mediate ADCC.[1331] Thus, if ADCC is important in preventing maternal-to-neonatal HSV transmission, these vaccines are not unlikely to be beneficial in reducing neonatal HSV disease.[1332] Further efforts to develop a vaccine that will prevent or at least ameliorate disease in adults and in neonates are indicated. Following the failure of the recombinant glycoprotein vaccines, a number of other strategies are being considered, including replication-defective HSV vaccines (e.g., using gD-deficient HSV viruses that can undergo only one round of productive infection or other viruses that encode HSV proteins).[1211,1333] It also will be important to define which immunologic parameters most closely correlate with reduced disease and with reduced viral shedding in adults as well as in children, to help focus on the appropriate goals of vaccination.

Nonviral Intracellular Pathogens

Overview of Host Defense Mechanisms

In addition to viruses, certain nonviral intracellular pathogens can replicate within cells and cause severe fetal or neonatal infection. These include *Salmonella* spp., *L. monocytogenes*, and *M. tuberculosis*, which are facultative intracellular pathogens, and *T. gondii* (hereafter referred to as *Toxoplasma*) and *Chlamydia trachomatis*, which are obligate intracellular pathogens. Unlike pyogenic bacteria, for which phagocytosis usually results in death, phagocytosis for these pathogens is a means of entry into an intracellular haven. Each of these pathogens readily infects tissue macrophages of the reticuloendothelial system. In addition, *Toxoplasma* can infect virtually any nucleated mammalian cell type, and this nonspecificity has important consequences for the pathogenesis of toxoplasmosis. The following discussion of host defense mechanisms focuses primarily on *Toxoplasma*. Relevant information from studies of *L. monocytogenes* and the protozoan *Leishmania major*, an extensively studied obligate intracellular pathogen in rodents, is included.

During acute toxoplasmosis in humans, the replicating form, the tachyzoite, is found both extracellularly and intracellularly. A 30-kDa tachyzoite surface protein, P30, appears to be involved in the initial attachment of *Toxoplasma* to host cells.[1334] Antibodies frequently are made against this protein after infection and constitute a basis for serodiagnosis.[1334,1335] Intracellular *Toxoplasma* organisms are found principally in specialized parasitophorous vacuoles, which are derived from the host cell membrane but lack the features normally associated with phagocytic or endocytic vacuoles.[1336] These vacuoles, from which lysosomal components and host plasma membrane proteins are excluded, allow the free exchange of nutrients with the host cell cytoplasm, facilitating parasite replication.[1337] Cellular invasion by tachyzoites occurs without generating a respiratory burst in human macrophages[1338] or activating microbicidal nitric oxide production in murine macrophages.[1339] In response to adverse intracellular conditions that slow its replication,[1340] the tachyzoite is somehow induced to convert into a less metabolically active form, the bradyzoite. Bradyzoites can persist in many tissues for years or decades in the form of cysts. As discussed later, limiting chronic *Toxoplasma* infection to this quiescent state depends on antigen-specific cellular immunity; acquired T cell immunodeficiency, such as pharmacologic immunosuppression or HIV infection, may allow bradyzoites to reconvert to tachyzoites that resume invasive infection.

Murine studies suggest that the control of acute infection by *Toxoplasma* and other nonviral intracellular pathogens, such as *L. monocytogenes* and *L. major*, involves an initial innate response involving DCs, NK cells, and mononuclear phagocytes, followed by an antigen-specific response in which T cell immunity is critical.[1341-1343] αβ T cells are particularly important for the chronic maintenance of *Toxoplasma* organisms in a quiescent state within infected host cells. The distinctiveness of the early innate response compared with the later antigen-specific response in mice is demonstrated by the observation that genetic susceptibility of common laboratory strains to acute *Toxoplasma* infection does not correlate with susceptibility to chronic infection.[1344]

A model for how cytokines link the activity of innate and antigen-specific immune mechanisms (see Fig. 4-12) in acute toxoplasmosis and during infection with other nonviral intracellular pathogens is described next. This model is based largely on studies in mice utilizing spontaneously occurring or genetically manipulated immunodeficient strains, antibody treatment, or both to deplete particular cell types or to neutralize cytokine and cytokine receptors: *Toxoplasma* tachyzoites, or products they secrete, induce DCs or mononuclear phagocytes to produce cytokines, including IL-1, IL-12, IL-15, IL-18, and TNF-α.[1345-1349] These cytokines, in conjunction with *Toxoplasma* organism–derived products, induce NK cells to produce IFN-γ; NK cell–derived IFN-γ, in turn, increases toxoplasmacidal activity within mononuclear phagocytes, helping limit the initial extent of infection.[1343, 1345, 1350] IFN-γ, IL-12, IL-18, and TNF-α produced by innate (i.e., NK cells, DCs, and monocytes) rather than antigen-specific (i.e., T cells) mechanisms appear essential for the initial control of acute infection.[1345,1349,1350] IFN-γ produced by NK cells, in conjunction with IL-12 and IL-18 produced by mononuclear phagocytes and DCs, also favors the differentiation of antigen-specific $CD4^+$ T cells into T_H1 effector T cells that secrete large amounts of IFN-γ. T_H1 effector T cells, in turn, produce IFN-γ that contains the parasite during the late phase of acute infection and helps limit the spread of infection in tissues should *Toxoplasma* cysts reactivate into tachyzoites. T cells, the IFN-γ they produce, and IL-12, IL-15, and IL-23 produced by non–T cells that sustain T_H1 responses all appear to be essential for the lifelong control of reactivation, as shown from studies in chronically infected mice.[1342,1343,1347,1348,1351]

Although the foregoing model as outlined emphasizes the role of proinflammatory and T_H1-type cytokines in controlling *Toxoplasma* infection, it is important to note that *Toxoplasma* actively inhibits this process in several ways. *Toxoplasma* inhibits signaling pathways involved in the induction of IL-12 and TNF-α, including nuclear translocation of NF-κB and STAT-1.[1352] This inhibition may account for the observation that infection of human mononuclear phagocytes and DCs with *Toxoplasma* induces very little IL-12, whereas the production of IL-12 can be markedly upregulated by engagement of CD40 on these cells by CD40 ligand on activated T cells.[1352-1354] Inhibition of IL-12 and TNF-α production by *Toxoplasma* may allow it to evade initial activation of protective immunity or may be an important mechanism by which the organism avoids inducing an excessive and potentially lethal inflammatory response to the infection.[1352,1355] Consistent with the latter possibility, in mice *Toxoplasma* counters the induction of proinflammatory cytokines by inducing the anti-inflammatory cytokine IL-10. This capability is biologically important, because mice that are genetically deficient in IL-10 generate excessive amounts of IL-12, TNF-α, and IFN-γ in response to acute *Toxoplasma* infection and die with inflammatory liver necrosis.[1356]

Some cytokines may mediate both positive and negative roles in the immune response to *Toxoplasma* organisms. For example, IL-4 production occurs relatively late in primary murine toxoplasmosis and, in this context, may enhance, rather than inhibit, the differentiation of protective IFN-γ–producing T_H1 effector T cells.[1357] With *Leishmania* infection in certain mouse strains, IL-4 that is produced early inhibits T_H1 effector T cell generation.[179] By contrast, IL-4 produced during the chronic phase of murine infection appears to inhibit the host's ability to control *Toxoplasma* cyst replication within the CNS.[1358] These observations emphasize the importance of the temporal sequence of cytokine expression for appropriate immunoregulation.

Innate Immunity

Natural Killer Cells. Most murine studies support a role for NK cells as a link between the initial innate response and the development of antigen-specific immunity to *Toxoplasma*: NK cell depletion or neutralization of NK cell–derived IFN-γ prevents the development of a protective immune response after vaccination with attenuated *Toxoplasma* in mice that have $CD4^+$ T cells but are genetically deficient in $CD8^+$ αβ T cells and NK T cells.[1359] This pathway may be less important in the fully immunocompetent host, however, because experiments with wild-type mice depleted of NK cells have yielded conflicting results regarding whether NK cells are important for the control of early primary *Toxoplasma* infection.[1360]

Cytokines produced by nonlymphoid cells during the early phase of toxoplasmosis may play a critical role in the early control of infection by multiple mechanisms, including the stimulation of NK cells and NK T cells to produce IFN-γ, enhancement of T_H1 effector cell generation, and activation of mononuclear phagocyte microbicidal activity. Although mononuclear phagocytes are a potent source of cytokines, such as IL-12, when incubated in vitro with *Toxoplasma* organisms or their products, DCs also are a major source of IL-12 in the early response to *Toxoplasma* in vivo.[1354] This finding suggests that mononuclear phagocytes may act downstream of DCs in the innate phase of the immune response to infection.

Mononuclear Phagocytes. The critical role of macrophages in resistance to intracellular nonviral pathogens was first demonstrated in animal studies of *L. monocytogenes* in which depletion of macrophages increased susceptibility.[1361] In the first days of infection, the rate at which monocytes are recruited to the site of infection and the microbicidal activity of these cells correlate with the control of *Toxoplasma* in animals.[1362] As discussed in the section on mononuclear phagocytes, monocyte entry into infected tissues requires the coordinated interaction of selectins, integrins (particularly those of the $β_1$ group), and CC chemokine receptors on the monocyte with counterligands on the endothelium and extracellular matrix. Transcripts for CCL3 (MIP-1α) are present in the CNS of SCID mice with *Toxoplasma* encephalitis, suggesting that CCL3 attracts mononuclear phagocytes in vivo.[1350] Infection of human monocytes by *Toxoplasma* tachyzoites also results in the induction of CD80 and increased expression of CD86.[1353] The increased expression of these co-stimulatory molecules may enhance proliferation and IFN-γ production by T cells early in *Toxoplasma* infection and may assist in the differentiation of T_H1 effector cells from naïve T cells.[1353]

In general, the microbicidal activity of human monocytes against *Toxoplasma* is greater than that of macrophages.[1363,1364] In vitro studies with mononuclear phagocytes or microglial cells, which are mononuclear phagocytes of the CNS, demonstrate that both oxidative and nonoxidative mechanisms are involved in limiting intracellular *Toxoplasma* replication. The ability of human monocytes to kill *Toxoplasma* organisms in the absence of exogenous cytokines depends mainly on oxidative mechanisms,[1363] whereas human macrophages, including those from lung alveoli and peritoneum, kill *Toxoplasma* by a nonoxidative mechanism.[1365,1366] Phagocytosis and killing of *Toxoplasma* by monocyte-derived human macrophages are substantially reduced when these cells are infected in vitro with HIV-1. This effect appears to be due to the induction of PGE_2 by HIV-1, a mechanism that could contribute to the reactivation of *Toxoplasma* observed in HIV-1–infected patients.[1367]

Cytokines are critical regulators of mononuclear phagocyte activity. IFN-γ produced by activated T cells or NK cells is the most important activator of macrophages for toxoplasmacidal activity.[1343,1350] In vitro studies have demonstrated that macrophages first primed by treatment with IFN-γ can be triggered for toxoplasmacidal activity by incubation with TNF-α; treatment with IFN-γ alone is ineffective.[1368] IFN-γ is able to induce toxoplasmacidal activity in monocytes or monocyte-derived macrophages from patients with chronic granulomatous disease, confirming the existence of cytokine-dependent, nonoxidative killing.[1363] One such mechanism is the induction of the enzyme indoleamine 2,3-dioxygenase, which catalyzes the first step in tryptophan degradation and deprives replicating *Toxoplasma* of this essential nutrient.[1369,1370] Indoleamine 2,3-dioxygenase is induced by IFN-γ in human and murine cells, and the failure of IFN-γ–deficient mice to upregulate its expression in response to *Toxoplasma* infection has been correlated with their markedly greater susceptibility.[1371] The relative importance of indoleamine 2,3-dioxygenase in the control of *Toxoplasma* in vivo remains to be shown, however.

Experiments with gene knockout mice lacking iNOS indicate that this enzyme is required for the control of persistent *Toxoplasma* infection in rodents.[1342] Pharmacologic blockade of iNOS activity also results in exacerbation of chronic infection in mice. As discussed in the section on mononuclear phagocytes, iNOS is a nitric oxide–producing enzyme expressed mainly by mononuclear phagocytes. In murine toxoplasmosis, the induction of iNOS appears to be dependent on the production of IFN-γ and TNF-α, both of which can directly activate mononuclear phagocytes for increased iNOS expression.[1342] The mechanism by which iNOS mediates an antitoxoplasmal effect in vivo remains unclear. In most cytokine-activated human mononuclear phagocyte populations, iNOS activity has been low or undetectable, with the exception of alveolar macrophages from patients with tuberculosis, and the importance of iNOS in limiting *Toxoplasma* or other intracellular pathogens in humans remains unclear.[1024]

Adaptive Immunity

Alpha-Beta T Cells. The importance of T lymphocytes in protection of humans from *Toxoplasma* infection is suggested by the marked increase in the incidence of severe infection in HIV-1–infected patients who have quantitative and qualitative $CD4^+$ T cell deficiency. This critical role for T cells in controlling toxoplasmosis is supported by the marked susceptibility of rodents with genetic T cell immunodeficiencies (e.g., nude or SCID rodents), and by the ability of splenocytes or T cells from immune animals to transfer resistance adoptively to susceptible recipients.[1350,1351] The importance of $CD4^+$ and $CD8^+$ T cells in protection depends on the phase of infection. In acute infection, $CD8^+$ T cells appear to be more protective than $CD4^+$ T cells, although both subsets afford some protection to unvaccinated rodents.[1372] $CD4^+$ and $CD8^+$ T cells both are necessary to limit the extent of CNS infection in the brain,[1373] and $CD4^+$ T cells are required for the development of long-term protective immunity.[1374] By contrast, once protective immunity has developed, $CD4^+$ or $CD8^+$ T cells can independently limit acute reactivation of chronic *Toxoplasma* infection—this protection requires the secretion of IFN-γ.[1375]

Studies with perforin knockout mice suggest that the perforin/granzyme cytotoxicity mechanism is more important in the control of chronic toxoplasmosis, particularly in the brain, than in the control of acute infection.[1376] Such cytotoxicity is more likely to be mediated by T cells than by NK cells, although this preferential effect remains to be shown. Human $CD4^+$ and $CD8^+$ T cells can lyse *Toxoplasma*-infected cells,[1377] and in the case of $CD4^+$ T cells, this cytotoxicity is MHC class II restricted.[1378] Whether lysis results in the intracellular death of *Toxoplasma* organisms is unclear, however; if it does not, whether any released viable tachyzoites are cleared by mononuclear phagocytes or through direct lysis by antibody and complement, or both, also remains unclear. If such released tachyzoites were able to infect new cellular targets, such cytotoxicity might be detrimental to the host. *Toxoplasma* also may inhibit lysis of infected cells by NK and T cells, limiting the efficacy of cell-mediated cytotoxic mechanisms.[603]

The production of IFN-γ and other cytokines by T_H1 effector and memory T cells, which have undergone clonal expansion from naïve precursors, is essential for the control of acute toxoplasmosis and to prevent reactivation of chronic infection.[1341,1343] This also is true for protection against other intracellular bacterial and protozoal pathogens that survive and replicate within phagocytic vacuoles, such as *Salmonella* spp. and *M. tuberculosis*. An additional novel pathway for inducing IFN-γ production by naïve $CD45RA^{hi}CD45RO^{lo}$ αβ T cells has been identified for *Toxoplasma*. Cells with this phenotype obtained from *Toxoplasma*-seronegative donors, including neonates, produce IFN-γ and proliferate in response to autologous monocytes infected with *Toxoplasma* tachyzoites.[1353] This response appears to utilize MHC class II antigen presentation and is dependent on the upregulation of CD80 and CD86 molecules and the production of IL-12 by infected monocytes, which in turn are dependent on the engagement of CD40 on APCs by CD40 ligand on activated T cells. This response does not have the restricted Vβ repertoire characteristic of responses to a superantigen, but whether an antigenic peptide or nonprotein antigen is involved remains unclear. Notably, this response is not observed with dead parasites or with low concentrations of parasites, both of which are sufficient to activate memory T cells in seropositive persons. Thus, the activation of naïve T cells is likely to occur only when large numbers of infected mononuclear phagocytes or DCs are present in the T cell zones of secondary lymphoid tissues, as might be the case early in an acute infection or in immunocompromised patients. It not known whether this type of response occurs in vivo in infected humans or mice.

Gamma-Delta T Cells. Gamma-delta T cells, mainly those encoding Vγ2Vδ2 TCRs, are increased in the circulation of children with postnatally acquired primary toxoplasmosis.[1379,1380] These cells are predominantly $CD45RA^{lo}$-$CD45RO^{hi}$, suggesting that they have been activated in vivo.[1380] This expansion appears to be a direct effect of *Toxoplasma* organisms on this cell population, because Vγ2Vδ2-bearing T cells, when incubated with peripheral blood mononuclear cells that have internalized killed parasites, are activated to secrete cytokines (IL-2, IFN-δ, and TNF-α) and to proliferate.[1381] Of interest, lysis of *Toxoplasma*-infected cells by these Vγ2Vδ2 T cells occurs in an MHC-unrestricted manner and does not require previous infection of the donor by *Toxoplasma*.[1381]

The role of γδ T cells in host defense against *Toxoplasma* remains controversial. *Toxoplasma* infection induces increased numbers of γδ T cells in the spleen and peritoneum, and mice depleted of γδ T cells by mAb treatment die more rapidly than controls when challenged with high numbers of *Toxoplasma* bradyzoites.[1382] Gamma-delta T cells also undergo expansion in mice lacking αβ T cells, and the transfer of γδ T cells into mice lacking $CD4^+$ and $CD8^+$ T cells, NK T cells, and NK cells affords protection.[1383] These γδ T cells produce IFN-γ and lyse autologous *Toxoplasma*-infected macrophages. It is unclear whether γδ T cells improve the outcome of infection in these systems by the secretion of cytokines, cell-mediated cytotoxicity, or other mechanisms. In contrast with these studies, Sayles and colleagues,[1384] using a lower inoculum of bradyzoites, found no evidence either for the in vivo expansion of γδ T cells in wild-type mice or for any deleterious effects of γδ T cell depletion.

B Cells and Antibody. In contrast with *L. monocytogenes*, in which antibodies appear to contribute minimally to host resistance to infection,[1361,1385] antibodies probably make some contribution to defense against *Toxoplasma*. Mice that cannot mount an antibody response are slightly more susceptible to late death from *Toxoplasma* infection than are normal mice, and antiserum from convalescent animals has only a slight protective effect.[1386] Antibody and complement lyse extracellular *Toxoplasma*, and this effect is the basis of the Sabin-Feldman dye assay for anti-*Toxoplasma* antibodies. Antibody-coated *Toxoplasma* organisms also are killed by resting mouse and human macrophages, probably through Fc receptor–mediated entry into an intracellular vacuole that, unlike the parasitophorous vacuole, fuses with lysosomes.[1387] Antibody alone provides minimal protection in adult and newborn mice, but it enhances protection by activated macrophages.[1388] T cell–deficient mice are much more susceptible than are antibody-deficient animals, however, and are not protected by antibody. The fact that *Toxoplasma* encephalitis in adult patients with acquired immunodeficiency syndrome (AIDS) typically develops by recrudescence of latent infection despite the presence of preexisting anti-*Toxoplasma* antibodies[1389] underscores the importance of T cells rather than B cells in the control of chronic infection with this pathogen.

Fetal and Neonatal Defenses

Information regarding initial aspects of the immune response by the human fetus and neonate to *Toxoplasma* is limited. Neonatal monocytes can ingest and kill *Toxoplasma*[1070,1071] and *L. monocytogenes* (C. Wilson, unpublished data, 1980), and monocyte-derived and placental macrophages from human neonates are activated by IFN-γ to kill or restrict the growth of *Toxoplasma* as effectively as are cells from adults.[1070,1390]

Nonetheless, it is likely that other limitations in responses by mononuclear phagocytes, and limitations in the response by NK cells and T cells, contribute to the increased susceptibility of the human fetus to *Toxoplasma* infection. Limitations in cytokine production, particularly IFN-γ, TNF-α, and IL-12, would be expected to be deleterious. Studies in neonatal rodents, which are highly susceptible to infection with *L. monocytogenes*, support the idea that reduced cytokine production or responsiveness may limit neonatal immunity. In neonatal mice and rats, administration of recombinant IFN-γ before or at the time of infection protects from acute infection and allows the development of protective immunity.[1077,1391] In adult animals, TNF-α, or agents that induce TNF-α, enhance resistance, whereas this effect is not observed in neonates. Co-administration of suboptimal doses of IFN-γ and TNF-α protects neonatal rats. Acquisition of resistance to infection correlates with acquisition of adult competence for TNF-α production[1077] and also is likely to correlate with competence for IFN-γ production, but whether it does so has not been evaluated. During fetal *Toxoplasma* infection, the ability of NK cells to produce IFN-γ and TNF-α and of mononuclear phagocytes to produce TNF-α and other proinflammatory cytokines is unknown.

Toxoplasma, like many congenital viral pathogens, such as CMV, is much more likely to produce severe untoward infection when the mother acquires primary infection early in pregnancy. The most severely damaged infants are likely to have acquired infection during the first trimester, when their numbers of T cells and their αβ-TCR repertoire for antigen recognition are limited compared with those of the fetus in the latter half of gestation. Nonetheless, αβ-TCR repertoire limitations are unlikely to be an important mechanism in most cases of fetal toxoplasmosis, because severe sequelae may result in infants infected during mid- to late gestation, and in most infants infected at any time during gestation, sequelae ultimately develop. Similarly, *L. cytogenes* infection occurring in infants in the latter part of gestation usually is severe. This line of evidence suggests that mechanisms acting to contain *Toxoplasma* and *L. monocytogenes* infection are still immature in late gestation and at term relative to those of older persons.

Toxoplasma-specific memory CD4$^+$ T cell responses, which are evident in response to low concentrations of soluble antigen, often are delayed in their appearance in congenital toxoplasmosis and may not be detectable until weeks or months after birth. McLeod and colleagues found that lymphocyte proliferation in response to *Toxoplasma* antigens, which primarily detects responses by CD4$^+$ T cells, was below the limit of detection in 11 of 25 congenitally infected infants younger than 1 year of age.[543] The most severely affected infants were more likely to have undetectable or low antigen-specific T cell responses. Furthermore, when memory T cells were first detected by lymphocyte proliferation assays in congenitally infected children, their capacity to produce IL-2 and IFN-γ often was less than that of memory T cells from adults with postnatal *Toxoplasma* infection.[543] Fatoohi and colleagues also found that anti-*Toxoplasma* T cell responses (determined using a different and less standardized assay) were lower in eight congenitally infected infants younger than 1 year of age than in persons with acquired *Toxoplasma* infection and congenitally infected children studied when they were older than 1 year of age.[1392] Nonetheless, anti-*Toxoplasma* T cell responses were detectable in most of the congenitally infants younger than 1 year of age by this assay. Why Peyron and colleagues detected responses in a larger fraction of infants than those studied by McLeod and associates is unknown. The larger number might merely reflect differences in experimental technique or differences in their patient populations, or both.

McLeod and colleagues[543] evaluated a referral population in which the children were more severely affected, did not receive early treatment and were born to mothers who did not receive treatment, whereas early treatment and less severe disease were typical for the children studied by Peyron and associates.[1392] Together, these data suggest that antigen-specific CD4$^+$ T cell responses may develop more slowly or be diminished in congenitally infected infants, particularly those with more severe disease, compared with such responses in older patients. No published information is available regarding antigen-specific CD8$^+$ T cell responses in neonates with congenital *Toxoplasma* infection.

A similar impairment, lag, or both in the development of antigen-specific CD4$^+$ T cell responses has been observed in infants with congenital infection due to *T. pallidum*, CMV, VZV, or rubella virus[538-542,1393,1394] and, as discussed earlier, in neonates infected postnatally with HSV.[553,554] Similarly, Tu and colleagues found that antigen-specific CD4$^+$ T cell responses may be low in infants and young children with postnatally acquired CMV infection until active viral replication ceases, whereas antigen-specific CD8$^+$ T cell responses are detectable much earlier.[226] Whether the initial poor CD4$^+$ T cell response, lag in its appearance, or both are due to (1) failure of antigen presentation sufficient to induce activation of naïve antigen-specific T cells (immunologic ignorance), (2) limited proliferation of activated antigen-specific T cells, (3) sequestration of antigen-specific effector T cells at sites of infection, or (4) the induction of anergy (long-term unresponsiveness) or deletion of antigen-specific T cells, as has been observed with in vitro priming of neonatal T cells with alloantigens[391] or superantigens,[330] or to some combination of these mechanisms, is not known. Regardless of the precise mechanisms, these findings suggest that infection of the immunologically immature fetus may in some cases lead to complete or partial antigen-specific unresponsiveness that may persist for some time after birth.

At least some neonates and young infants with congenital *Toxoplasma* infection demonstrate increased expansion of the Vγ2Vδ2-bearing γδ T cell population, most of which express a CD45RA^{lo}CD45RO^{hi} surface phenotype, indicating prior activation in vivo.[552] An analysis of a very limited number of patients has found that the γδ T cell population in the congenitally infected neonate demonstrate a poor proliferative response to stimulation by peripheral blood mononuclear cells infected with viable or irradiated *Toxoplasma* organisms.[552] Other functions, such as the secretion of cytokines by these cells, were not assessed, however, and rigorous age-matched controls were not employed. These results, which need to be confirmed, raise the possibility of an anergic state in γδ T cells in infants with congenital toxoplasmosis.

As noted, naïve CD45RA^{hi}CD45RO^{lo} CD4^{+} T cells from donors who have not been infected with *Toxoplasma* can proliferate in response to autologous *Toxoplasma*-infected mononuclear cells.[1353] CD4^{+} T cells from neonates, however, proliferate less well in response to autologous *Toxoplasma*-infected mononuclear cells than do phenotypically naïve CD4^{+} T cells from adults. As noted previously, the relevance of this novel in vitro response to protection against infection in vivo remains to be defined.

Although the foregoing results suggest that multiple aspects of cell-mediated immunity against *Toxoplasma* organisms are compromised in the human fetus and neonate, particularly in early gestation, antigen-specific antibody responses to *Toxoplasma* are commonly detectable (see Chapter 31 for more details). For example, antibodies to the P30 *Toxoplasma* antigen are frequently detectable in the fetus and neonate after congenital infection and are useful for serodiagnosis. Anti-P30 IgA antibodies are found in most neonates after congenital infection, whereas anti-P30 IgM antibodies are found in a minority.[1335,1395] *Toxoplasma*-specific IgE antibodies also are frequently present within the first 2 months of life in congenitally infected infants.[1396] Anti-P30 IgA and IgE antibodies are not unique to the fetus and neonate but also are common in older persons with acquired toxoplasmosis. Together, these results suggest that isotype switching of antibodies from IgM to the IgA and IgE isotypes can occur in utero, particularly in the face of continuing antigenic stimulation. Because IL-4 or IL-13 produced by CD4^{+} T cells is likely to be required for the production of protein antigen-specific IgE antibodies, these results also suggest that the CD4^{+} T cell response to *Toxoplasma* organisms in the fetus may include the production of these cytokines.

Implications for Immunologic Intervention

The findings in human neonates, in concert with the results of studies in rodents, suggest that correction of the deficits in NK cell function, cytokine production, and T cell responses could facilitate treatment of infections with intracellular pathogens, such as *Toxoplasma*. Several limitations are apparent, however. For example, treatment of neonatal rats with IFN-γ or IFN-α after establishment of infection with *L. monocytogenes* is not effective, whereas concomitant therapy or pretreatment is effective.[1397] These findings are perhaps not surprising in view of the evidence that IFN-γ is important only in the early phase of this infection. In the case of congenital infection with *Toxoplasma*, therapy would need to be initiated and maintained in utero, when maternal infection is often asymptomatic, and there is no obvious way by which this could be safely targeted to the fetus. In fact, data in mouse models suggest that increased production of IFN-γ during maternal infection may contribute to fetal loss as a result of maternal rejection of the fetus as a foreign allograft.[1398] After birth, it may be possible to provide exogenous IFN-γ (or perhaps TNF-α, IL-12, or IL-15), but the same caveats noted for treatment in cases of viral infection would apply. If studies in other patient populations (e.g., those with HIV infection) provide evidence that IFN-γ, TNF-α, IL-12, or IL-15 alone or in some combination can contribute to resolution of established infections, their use in conjunction with antimicrobial therapy for the treatment of neonates with congenital toxoplasmosis might be considered. Alternatively, approaches that seek to modify the deficit in development of antigen-specific effector T cells may prove to be more effective.

A live-attenuated *Toxoplasma* vaccine has been developed for veterinary use in sheep.[1399] Although this vaccine reduces the rate of abortion due to *Toxoplasma* infection of pregnant dams, it does not prevent transmission of infection from mother to fetus. Live *Toxoplasma* vaccines in humans that result in latent infection are not desirable, because they pose the risk of reactivation and dissemination in the immunocompromised person. Immunization with certain recombinant *Toxoplasma* proteins, with DNA vaccines in which such proteins are encoded, and with these in combination with various adjuvants or recombinant cytokines has been tried in rodents.[1347] For example, immunization with the immunodominant tachyzoite surface antigen SAG-1 induces protection in adult mice, but its ability to reduce the risk of mother-to-pup transmission resulting in congenital infection is inconsistent.[1400,1401] No vaccine is likely to be available in the near future for the prevention of congenital *Toxoplasma* infection.

IMMUNOPROPHYLAXIS IN THE NEONATE

Passive Immunization

There is currently no established use for IVIG in the immunoprophylaxis or adjunctive treatment of infection in the neonate. Intramuscular immune globulin (0.02 mL/kg) is indicated for prophylaxis of exposure to hepatitis A, as soon as possible after exposure.[1402] Immune globulin (0.25 mL/kg) may also be given to prevent or modify measles in neonates when the mother has active infection. Specific human hyperimmune globulin preparations are indicated in some situations. Hyperimmune hepatitis B immune globulin (HBIG) is indicated in conjunction with hepatitis B vaccine in infants born to mothers who are hepatitis B surface antigen positive. HBIG is given at a dose of 0.5 mL at a site different from that used for vaccine administration. Both HBIG and hepatitis B vaccine should be given as soon as possible, preferably within 12 hours after birth.[1402] Infants with neonatal tetanus or at risk for it may be given tetanus immune globulin. Precise dosages for treatment in this age group are not established; in older persons, generally a dose of 3000 to 6000 U is given, whereas dosages of 500 U may be effective for the neonate.[1402]

Varicella-zoster immune globulin (VZIG), which is given intramuscularly, is available from local distribution centers and is indicated (in a dose of 125 units [1.25 mL]) for the prophylaxis of infection in those cases in which clinical maternal chickenpox develops between 5 days before and 48 hours after the time of delivery.[1402] Infants born to mothers who have hypogammaglobulinemia may benefit from prophylactic administration of immune globulin in cases in which mothers have not received adequate immune globulin replacement therapy near term and when IgG levels in the neonate are documented to be low or are likely to be so.

Palivizumab (Synagis) is a humanized monoclonal antibody to RSV, which is indicated for the prevention of RSV infection in high-risk infants and children. High-risk groups include children with chronic lung disease or hemodynamically significant heart disease, or who were born at less than 32 weeks of gestation; those born at 32 to 35 weeks should receive treatment only if there are additional risk factors. Palivizumab is administered intramuscularly in a dose of 15 mg/kg monthly.[1403] A hyperimmune RSV immune globulin (RespiGam) also is available for use but is less convenient and should not be used in those with hemodynamically significant heart disease; it is given intravenously at a dose of 15 mL/kg monthly.

Active Immunization

The rationale for and against immunization in the neonatal period is described more fully in the sections on B cells and immunoglobulin and on T cell reactivity to specific antigens. The only vaccines commonly administered to neonates are hepatitis B, BCG, and live oral poliovirus vaccine (OPV) vaccines. In the United States, hepatitis B vaccine is recommended for neonates, but the other two vaccines are not used. Although neonatal immunization is preferred, hepatitis B vaccination also may be started at 2 months of age unless the neonate may have been exposed to the virus during delivery, in which case vaccination and treatment with HBIG within 12 hours of birth are indicated.[1403] Most other vaccines that induce T cell–dependent antibody responses, such as whole-cell or acellular pertussis, *H. influenzae* type b polysaccharide–protein conjugate, diphtheria-tetanus, and inactivated poliovirus vaccine, are routinely begun at approximately age 2 months.[1403] Premature or small-for-gestational-age infants also may be immunized with these vaccines at this age. Although immunization at birth is attractive from a public health point of view, there is concern that responses to some vaccines may be lower (with diphtheria vaccine) or that long-term responses may be reduced (with whole-cell pertussis vaccine)[773] compared with immunization given at age 2 months. Nonetheless, the potential benefits of neonatal vaccination, particularly in the developing world, are such that further studies in this area are warranted.

Recognition of Primary Immunodeficiency in the Neonate

Recognition of primary immunodeficiency in the neonate often is possible. Several syndromes have characteristic clinical findings that permit early diagnosis—for example, thrombocytopenia with low mean platelet volume in Wiskott-Aldrich syndrome; hypocalcemia, unusual facies, and congenital heart disease in DiGeorge and velocardiofacial syndromes; and skeletal dwarfism in cartilage-hair hypoplasia. Other affected children may present with laboratory abnormalities in the neonatal period that are suggestive of the diagnosis, such as marked elevations of IgE level in some patients with hyperimmunoglobulin E syndrome, and elevated IgE and hypereosinophilia in patients with Omenn's syndrome, which is a form of SCID due to partial RAG deficiency. Patients with leukocyte adhesion defect (LAD) due to CD18 deficiency may have omphalitis or other soft tissue infection and late (after 3 weeks of age) separation of the umbilical cord. The diagnosis of CD18 deficiency can readily be made by flow cytometric analysis of leukocytes. Delayed cord separation as an isolated clinical finding rarely is due to LAD; therefore, a complete blood count may be useful in such a situation—children with LAD commonly have persistent leukocytosis due to elevated numbers of neutrophils even when they are clinically uninfected. Chronic granulomatous disease may manifest in the neonatal period and should be considered in a term neonate who experiences severe bacterial infection with catalase-positive bacteria or with fungi and who does not have other risk factors for these. Patients with SCID may present with severe or recalcitrant mucocutaneous candidiasis, protracted diarrhea, *P. jiroveci* pneumonia, severe eczema, or any combination of these symptoms. SCID is often associated with lymphopenia. A family history of immunodeficiency or early, unexplained death is suggestive. HIV infection, particularly when congenitally acquired, should always be considered in the differential diagnosis in neonates who appear to have SCID, particularly if lymphadenopathy or splenomegaly is present. In general, unusually severe, recalcitrant, or recurrent infections, especially if due to organisms of low virulence and without other predisposing factors (such as extreme prematurity, multiple courses of empirical antibiotic therapy, multiple catheters, or other aspects of prolonged intensive care) should prompt consideration of primary immunodeficiency.

Normal term neonates lack cutaneous delayed-type hypersensitivity responses to antigens, have IgG values similar to those of their mother, and have little or no circulating IgM and IgA. Thus, these common screening tests for immunodeficiency in older children are of little value in the neonate. Depending on the presenting features, useful tests might include (1) chest radiograph or computed tomography for thymus size (useful only if secondary causes of thymic involution, e.g., stress, can be excluded); (2) a total lymphocyte count, which is helpful when low (fewer than 1500 lymphocytes per mm^3), although a normal count does not exclude immunodeficiency; (3) enumeration of T, B, and NK cell numbers by flow cytometry; (4) analysis of lymphocyte proliferation to mitogens, superantigens, anti-CD3 plus anti-CD28 mAbs, or allogeneic cells; (5) assessment of lymphocyte effector responses, including cytotoxicity and lymphokine release; (6) staining for CD11a, CD11b, and CD18 when leukocyte adhesion deficiency is strongly suspected; and (7) tests to screen for defects in the neutrophil oxidative burst, the cause of chronic granulomatous disease, which include an analysis of neutrophil hydrogen peroxide generation by flow cytometry (e.g., dihydrorhodamine test) and the nitroblue tetrazolium (NBT) test. More detailed discussion of the evaluation of neonates for primary immunodeficiency is available.[1404] Early, aggressive antimicrobial therapy, appropriate isolation, and early specific treatment of the immunologic disorder (e.g., IVIG for SCID and B cell immunodeficiency) are indicated whenever possible.

REFERENCES

1. Tavian M, Robin C, Coulombel L, et al. The human embryo, but not its yolk sac, generates lympho-myeloid stem cells: mapping multipotent hematopoietic cell fate in intraembryonic mesoderm. Immunity 15:487-495, 2001.
2. Peault B, Tavian M. Hematopoietic stem cell emergence in the human embryo and fetus. Ann N Y Acad Sci 996:132-140, 2003.
3. Aiuti A, Tavian M, Cipponi A, et al. Expression of CXCR4, the receptor for stromal cell–derived factor-1 on fetal and adult human lympho-hematopoietic progenitors. Eur J Immunol 29:1823-1831, 1999.
4. Glusman G, Rowen L, Lee I, et al. Comparative genomics of the human and mouse T cell receptor loci. Immunity 15:337-349, 2001.
5. Kane LP, Lin J, Weiss A. Signal transduction by the TCR for antigen. Curr Opin Immunol 12:242-249, 2000.
6. Pitcher LA, van Oers NS. T-cell receptor signal transmission: who gives an ITAM? Trends Immunol 24:554-560, 2003.
7. Algeciras-Schimnich A, Griffith TS, Lynch DH, et al. Cell cycle–dependent regulation of FLIP levels and susceptibility to Fas-mediated apoptosis. J Immunol 162:5205-5211, 1999.
8. Devine L, Kavathas PB. Molecular analysis of protein interactions mediating the function of the cell surface protein CD8. Immunol Res 19:201-210, 1999.
9. Banchereau J, Briere F, Caux C, et al. Immunobiology of dendritic cells. Annu Rev Immunol 18:767-811, 2000.
10. Yewdell JW, Reits E, Neefjes J. Making sense of mass destruction: quantitating MHC class I antigen presentation. Nat Rev Immunol 3:952-961, 2003.
11. Anthony Nolan website. Accessed June 2004. (http:/www.anthonynolan.org.uk/HIG/lists)
12. Mason PM, Parham P. HLA class I region sequences, 1998. Tissue Antigens 51:417-466, 1998.
13. Black FL. Why did they die? Science 258:1739-1740, 1992.
14. Griffin DE, Levine B, Tyor WR, et al. The immune response in viral encephalitis. Semin Immunol 4:111-119, 1992.
15. Huh GS, Boulanger LM, Du H, et al. Functional requirement for class I MHC in CNS development and plasticity. Science 290:2155-2159, 2000.
16. Larsson M, Fonteneau JF, Bhardwaj N. Dendritic cells resurrect antigens from dead cells. Trends Immunol 22:141-148, 2001.
17. Le Bon A, Etchart N, Rossmann C, et al. Cross-priming of CD8$^+$ T cells stimulated by virus-induced type I interferon. Nat Immunol 4:1009-1015, 2003.
18. Arrode G, Boccaccio C, Lule J, et al. Incoming human cytomegalovirus pp65 (UL83) contained in apoptotic infected fibroblasts is cross-presented to CD8(+) T cells by dendritic cells. J Virol 74:10018-10024, 2000.
19. Bryant PW, Lennon-Dumenil AM, Fiebiger E, et al. Proteolysis and antigen presentation by MHC class II molecules. Adv Immunol 80:71-114, 2002.
20. Neefjes J. CIIV, MIIC and other compartments for MHC class II loading. Eur J Immunol 29:1421-1425, 1999.
21. Marsh S. HLA class II region sequences. Tissue Antigens 51:467-507, 1998.
22. Daar AS, Fuggle SV, Fabre JW, et al. The detailed distribution of HLA-A, B, C antigens in normal human organs. Transplantation 38:287-292, 1984.
23. Poznansky MC, Olszak IT, Foxall RB, et al. Tissue source dictates lineage outcome of human fetal CD34(+)CD38(–) cells. Exp Hematol 29:766-774, 2001.
24. O'Callaghan CA. Natural killer cell surveillance of intracellular antigen processing pathways mediated by recognition of HLA-E and Qa-1b by CD94/NKG2 receptors. Microbes Infect 2:371-380, 2000.
25. Braud VM, Allan DS, Wilson D, et al. TAP- and tapasin-dependent HLA-E surface expression correlates with the binding of an MHC class I leader peptide. Curr Biol 8:1-10, 1998.
26. Houlihan JM, Biro PA, Fergar-Payne A, et al. Evidence for the expression of non–HLA-A, -B, -C class I genes in the human fetal liver. J Immunol 149:668-675, 1992.
27. Hunt JS, Jadhav L, Chu W, et al. Soluble HLA-G circulates in maternal blood during pregnancy. Am J Obstet Gynecol 183:682-688, 2000.
28. Carosella ED, Paul P, Moreau P, et al. HLA-G and HLA-E: fundamental and pathophysiological aspects. Immunol Today 21:532-534, 2000.
29. Riteau B, Menier C, Khalil-Daher I, et al. HLA-G inhibits the allogeneic proliferative response. J Reprod Immunol 43:203-211, 1999.
30. Yang Y, Chu W, Geraghty DE, et al. Expression of HLA-G in human mononuclear phagocytes and selective induction by IFN-gamma. J Immunol 156:4224-4231, 1996.
31. Fournel S, Aguerre-Girr M, Huc X, et al. Cutting edge: soluble HLA-G1 triggers CD95/CD95 ligand-mediated apoptosis in activated CD8$^+$ cells by interacting with CD8. J Immunol 164:6100-6104, 2000.
32. Steinle A, Groh V, Spies T. Diversification, expression, and gamma delta T cell recognition of evolutionarily distant members of the MIC family of major histocompatibility complex class I-related molecules. Proc Natl Acad Sci U S A 95:12510-12515, 1998.
33. Li P, Willie ST, Bauer S, et al. Crystal structure of the MHC class I homolog MIC-A, a gammadelta T cell ligand. Immunity 10:577-584, 1999.
34. Groh V, Rhinehart R, Randolph-Habecker J, et al. Costimulation of CD8alphabeta T cells by NKG2D via engagement by MIC induced on virus-infected cells. Nat Immunol 2:255-260, 2001.
35. Jamieson AM, Diefenbach A, McMahon CW, et al. The role of the NKG2D immunoreceptor in immune cell activation and natural killing. Immunity 17:19-29, 2002.
36. Jayawardena-Wolf J, Bendelac A. CD1 and lipid antigens: intracellular pathways for antigen presentation. Curr Opin Immunol 13:109-113, 2001.
37. Porcelli SA, Segelke BW, Sugita M, et al. The CD1 family of lipid antigen-presenting molecules. Immunology Today 19:362-368, 1998.
38. Steinman RM, Hawiger D, Nussenzweig MC. Tolerogenic dendritic cells. Annu Rev Immunol 21:685-711, 2003.
39. Liu YJ. Dendritic cell subsets and lineages, and their functions in innate and adaptive immunity. Cell 106:259-262, 2001.
40. Cella M, Jarrossay D, Facchetti F, et al. Plasmacytoid monocytes migrate to inflamed lymph nodes and produce large amounts of type I interferon. Nat Med 5:919-923, 1999.
41. Mellman I, Steinman RM. Dendritic cells: specialized and regulated antigen processing machines. Cell 106:255-258, 2001.
42. Liu YJ, Kanzler H, Soumelis V, et al. Dendritic cell lineage, plasticity and cross-regulation. Nat Immunol 2:585-589, 2001.
43. Mackay CR. Chemokines: immunology's high impact factors. Nat Immunol 2:95-101, 2001.
44. Rossi D, Zlotnik A. The biology of chemokines and their receptors. Annu Rev Immunol 18:217-242, 2000.
45. Moser B, Loetscher P. Lymphocyte traffic control by chemokines. Nat Immunol 2:123-128, 2001.
46. Lanzavecchia A, Sallusto F. Regulation of T cell immunity by dendritic cells. Cell 106:263-266, 2001.
47. Takeda K, Kaisho T, Akira S. Toll-like receptors. Annu Rev Immunol 21:335-376, 2003.
48. Janeway CA Jr, Medzhitov R. Innate immune recognition. Annu Rev Immunol 20:197-216, 2002.
49. Diebold SS, Kaisho T, Hemmi H, et al. Innate antiviral responses by means of TLR7-mediated recognition of single-stranded RNA. Science 303:1529-1531, 2004.
50. Lund JM, Alexopoulou L, Sato A, et al. Recognition of single-stranded RNA viruses by Toll-like receptor 7. Proc Natl Acad Sci U S A 101:5598-5603, 2004.
51. Lund J, Sato A, Akira S, et al. Toll-like receptor 9-mediated recognition of Herpes simplex virus-2 by plasmacytoid dendritic cells. J Exp Med 198:513-520, 2003.
52. Krug A, Luker GD, Barchet W, et al. Herpes simplex virus type 1 activates murine natural interferon-producing cells through toll-like receptor 9. Blood 103:1433-1437, 2004.
53. Palucka K, Banchereau J. How dendritic cells and microbes interact to elicit or subvert protective immune responses. Curr Opin Immunol 14:420-431, 2002.
54. Farrar JD, Murphy KM. Type I interferons and T helper development. Immunol Today 21:484-489, 2000.
55. Parronchi P, Mohapatra S, Sampognaro S, et al. Effects of interferon-alpha on cytokine profile, T cell receptor repertoire and peptide reactivity of human allergen-specific T cells. Eur J Immunol 26: 697-703, 1996.
56. Rogge L, Barberis ML, Biffi M, et al. Selective expression of an interleukin-12 receptor component by human T helper 1 cells. J Exp Med 185:825-831, 1997.
57. Siegal FP, Kadowaki N, Shodell M, et al. The nature of the principal type 1 interferon-producing cells in human blood. Science 284: 1835-1837, 1999.

58. Kadowaki N, Liu YJ. Natural type I interferon-producing cells as a link between innate and adaptive immunity. Hum Immunol 63: 1126-1132, 2002.
59. Bauer M, Redecke V, Ellwart JW, et al. Bacterial CpG-DNA triggers activation and maturation of human $CD11c^-$, $CD123^+$ dendritic cells. J Immunol 166:5000-5007, 2001.
60. Jarrossay D, Napolitani G, Colonna M, et al. Specialization and complementarity in microbial molecule recognition by human myeloid and plasmacytoid dendritic cells. Eur J Immunol 31:3388-3393, 2001.
61. Le Bon A, Schiavoni G, D'Agostino G, et al. Type i interferons potently enhance humoral immunity and can promote isotype switching by stimulating dendritic cells in vivo. Immunity 14:461-470, 2001.
62. Hofman FM, Danilovs JA, Taylor CR. HLA-DR (Ia)-positive dendritic-like cells in human fetal nonlymphoid tissues. Transplantation 37:590-594, 1984.
63. Oliver AM, Thomson AW, Sewell HF, et al. Major histocompatibility complex (MHC) class II antigen (HLA-DR, DQ, and DP) expression in human fetal endocrine organs and gut. Scand J Immunol 27:731-737, 1988.
64. Fossum S. The life history of dendritic leukocytes (DL). Curr Top Pathol 79:101-124, 1989.
65. Vossen MT, Westerhout EM, Soderberg-Naucler C, et al. Viral immune evasion: a masterpiece of evolution. Immunogenetics 54:527-542, 2002.
66. Keever CA, Abu HM, Graf W, et al. Characterization of the allore-activity and anti-leukemia reactivity of cord blood mononuclear cells. Bone Marrow Transplant 15:407-419, 1995.
67. Kanakoudi-Tsakalidou F, Debonera F, Drossou-Agakidou V, et al. Flow cytometric measurement of HLA-DR expression on circulating monocytes in healthy and sick neonates using monocyte negative selection. Clin Exp Immunol 123:402-407, 2001.
68. Borras FE, Matthews NC, Lowdell MW, et al. Identification of both myeloid $CD11c^+$ and lymphoid $CD11c^-$ dendritic cell subsets in cord blood. Br J Haematol 113:925-931, 2001.
69. De Wit D, Olislagers V, Goriely S, et al. Blood plasmacytoid dendritic cell responses to CpG oligodeoxynucleotides are impaired in human newborns. Blood 103:1030-1032, 2004.
70. Teig N, Moses D, Gieseler S, et al. Age-related changes in human blood dendritic cell subpopulations. Scand J Immunol 55:453-457, 2002.
71. Hagendorens MM, Ebo DG, Schuerwegh AJ, et al. Differences in circulating dendritic cell subtypes in cord blood and peripheral blood of healthy and allergic children. Clin Exp Allergy 33:633-639, 2003.
72. De Wit D, Tonon S, Olislagers V, et al. Impaired responses to toll-like receptor 4 and toll-like receptor 3 ligands in human cord blood. J Autoimmun 21:277-281, 2003.
73. Tonon S, Goriely S, Aksoy E, et al. Bordetella pertussis toxin induces the release of inflammatory cytokines and dendritic cell activation in whole blood: impaired responses in human newborns. Eur J Immunol 32:3118-3125, 2002.
74. Hunt DW, Huppertz HI, Jiang HJ, et al. Studies of human cord blood dendritic cells: evidence for functional immaturity. Blood 84: 4333-4343, 1994.
75. Petty RE, Hunt DW. Neonatal dendritic cells. Vaccine 16:1378-1382, 1998.
76. Sorg RV, Kogler G, Wernet P. Functional competence of dendritic cells in human umbilical cord blood. Bone Marrow Transplant 22 Suppl 1:S52-54, 1998.
77. Sorg RV, Kogler G, Wernet P. Identification of cord blood dendritic cells as an immature CD11c- population. Blood 93:2302-2307, 1999.
78. Olweus J, BitMansour A, Warnke R, et al. Dendritic cell ontogeny: a human dendritic cell lineage of. Proc Natl Acad Sci U S A 94: 12551-12556, 1997.
79. Grouard G, Rissoan MC, Filgueira L, et al. The enigmatic plasma-cytoid T cells develop into dendritic cells with interleukin (IL)-3 and CD40-ligand. J Exp Med 185:1101-1111, 1997.
80. Rissoan MC, Soumelis V, Kadowaki N, et al. Reciprocal control of T helper cell and dendritic cell differentiation. Science 283:1183-1186, 1999.
81. Cella M, Facchetti F, Lanzavecchia A, et al. Plasmacytoid dendritic cells activated by influenza virus and CD40L drive a potent T_H1 polarization. Nat Immunol 1:305-310, 2000.
82. Ray CG. The ontogeny of interferon production by human leukocytes. Journal Of Pediatrics 76:94-98, 1970.
83. Cederblad B, Riesenfeld T, Alm GV. Deficient herpes simplex virus–induced interferon-alpha production by blood leukocytes of preterm and term newborn infants. Pediatr Res 27:7-10, 1990.
84. Neustock P, Kruse A, Bein G, et al. Failure to detect type 1 interferon production in human umbilical cord vein endothelial cells after viral exposure. J Interferon Cytokine Res 15:129-135, 1995.
85. Lee S, Suen Y, Chang L, et al. Descreased interleukin-12 (IL-12) from activated cord blood versus adult peripheral blood mononuclear cells and upregulation of interferon-gamma, natural killer, and lymphokine-activated killer activity by IL-12 in cord blood mononuclear cells. Blood 88:645-654, 1996.
86. Scott ME, Kubin M, Kohl S. High level interleukin-12 production, but diminished interferon-gamma production, by cord blood mononuclear cells. Pediatric Research 41:547-553, 1997.
87. Perez-Melgosa M, Ochs HD, Linsley PS, et al. Carrier-mediated enhancement of cognate T cell help: the basis for enhanced immunogenicity of meningococcal outer membrane protein poly-saccharide conjugate vaccine. Eur J Immunol 31:2373-2381, 2001.
88. Karlsson H, Hessle C, Rudin A. Innate immune responses of human neonatal cells to bacteria from the normal gastrointestinal flora. Infect Immun 70:6688-6696, 2002.
89. Moser M, Murphy KM. Dendritic cell regulation of T_H1-T_H2 development. Nat Immunol 1:199-205, 2000.
90. Zheng Z, Takahashi M, Narita M, et al. Generation of dendritic cells from adherent cells of cord blood with granulocyte-macrophage colony-stimulating factor, interleukin-4, and tumor necrosis factor-alpha. J Hematother Stem Cell Res 9:453-464, 2000.
91. Liu E, Tu W, Law HK, et al. Decreased yield, phenotypic expression and function of immature monocyte-derived dendritic cells in cord blood. Br J Haematol 113:240-246, 2001.
92. Liu E, Tu W, Law HK, et al. Changes of CD14 and CD1a expression in response to IL-4 and granulocyte-macrophage colony-stimulating factor are different in cord blood and adult blood monocytes. Pediatr Res 50:184-189, 2001.
93. Goriely S, Vincart B, Stordeur P, et al. Deficient IL-12(p35) gene expression by dendritic cells derived from neonatal monocytes. J Immunol 166:2141-2146, 2001.
94. Randolph GJ, Beaulieu S, Lebecque S, et al. Differentiation of mono-cytes into dendritic cells in a model of transendothelial trafficking. Science 282:480-483, 1998.
95. Randolph GJ, Inaba K, Robbiani DF, et al. Differentiation of phago-cytic monocytes into lymph node dendritic cells in vivo. Immunity 11:753-761, 1999.
96. Drijkoningen M, De Wolf-Peeters C, Van der Steen K, et al. Epidermal Langerhans' cells and dermal dendritic cells in human fetal and neonatal skin: an immunohistochemical study. Pediatr Dermatol 4:11-17, 1987.
97. Chilmonczyk BA, Levin MJ, McDuffy R, et al. Characterization of the human newborn response to herpesvirus antigen. J Immunol 134:4184-4188, 1985.
98. Sanchez MJ, Muench MO, Roncarolo MG, et al. Identification of a common T/natural killer cell progenitor in human fetal thymus. J Exp Med 180:569-576, 1994.
99. Garban F, Ericson M, Roucard C, et al. Detection of empty HLA class II molecules on cord blood B cells. Blood 87:3970-3976, 1996.
100. Dejbakhsh-Jones S, Jerabek L, Weissman IL, et al. Extrathymic maturation of alpha beta T cells from hemopoietic stem cells. J Immunol 155:3338-3344, 1995.
101. Ohteki T, Okuyama R, Seki S, et al. Age-dependent increase of extrathymic T cells in the liver and their appearance in the periphery of older mice. J Immunol 149:1562-1570, 1992.
102. Ohteki T, Wilson A, Verbeek S, et al. Selectively impaired develop-ment of intestinal T cell receptor gamma $delta^+$ cells and liver $CD4^+$ $NK1^+$ T cell receptor alpha $beta^+$ cells in T cell factor-1-deficient mice. Eur J Immunol 26:351-355, 1996.
103. Donskoy E, Goldschneider I. Thymocytopoiesis is maintained by blood-borne precursors throughout postnatal life. A study in parabiotic mice. J Immunol 148:1604-1612, 1992.
104. Blom B, Res PC, Spits H. T cell precursors in man and mice. Crit Rev Immunol 18:371-388, 1998.
105. Pear WS, Tu L, Stein PL. Lineage choices in the developing thymus: choosing the T and NKT pathways. Curr Opin Immunol 16:167-173, 2004.
106. Verhasselt B, Kerre T, Naessens E, et al. Thymic repopulation by CD34(+) human cord blood cells after expansion in stroma-free culture. Blood 94:3644-3652, 1999.

107. Hao QL, Zhu J, Price MA, et al. Identification of a novel, human multilymphoid progenitor in cord blood. Blood 97:3683-3690, 2001.
108. Allman D, Sambandam A, Kim S, et al. Thymopoiesis independent of common lymphoid progenitors. Nat Immunol 4:168-174, 2003.
109. Petrie HT. Cell migration and the control of post-natal T-cell lymphopoiesis in the thymus. Nat Rev Immunol 3:859-866, 2003.
110. Jaleco AC, Neves H, Hooijberg E, et al. Differential effects of Notch ligands Delta-1 and Jagged-1 in human lymphoid differentiation. J Exp Med 194:991-1002, 2001.
111. Kraft DL, Weissman IL, Waller EK. Differentiation of CD3$^-$4$^-$8$^-$human fetal thymocytes in vivo: characterization of a CD3$^-$4$^+$8$^-$ intermediate. J Exp Med 178:265-277, 1993.
112. imgt.cines.fr. Accessed June, 2004. (http://imgt.cines.fr/textes/IMG Trepertoire/LocusGenes/tabgenes/human/geneNumber.html)
113. Agrawal A, Eastman QM, Schatz DG. Transposition mediated by RAG1 and RAG2 and its implications for the evolution of the immune system. Nature 394:744-751, 1998.
114. Gellert M. A new view of V(D)J recombination. Genes Cells 1: 269-275, 1996.
115. Hiom K, Gellert M. Assembly of a 12/23 paired signal complex: a critical control point in V(D)J recombination. Mol Cell 1:1011-1019, 1998.
116. Lieber MR, Ma Y, Pannicke U, et al. Mechanism and regulation of human non-homologous DNA end-joining. Nat Rev Mol Cell Biol 4:712-720, 2003.
117. Kalman L, Lindegren ML, Kobrynski L, et al. Mutations in genes required for T-cell development: IL7R, CD45, IL2RG, JAK3, RAG1, RAG2, ARTEMIS, and ADA and severe combined immunodeficiency: HuGE review. Genet Med 6:16-26, 2004.
118. Davis MM, Lyons DS, Altman JD, et al. T cell receptor biochemistry, repertoire selection and general features of TCR and Ig structure. Ciba Found Symp 204:94-100, discussion 100-104, 1997.
119. Lewis SM. P nucleotides, hairpin DNA and V(D)J joining: making the connection. Semin Immunol 6:131-141, 1994.
120. Arstila TP, Casrouge A, Baron V, et al. A direct estimate of the human alphabeta T cell receptor diversity. Science 286:958-961, 1999.
121. Haase AT. Population biology of HIV-1 infection: viral and CD4$^+$ T cell demographics and dynamics in lymphatic tissues. Annu Rev Immunol 17:625-656, 1999.
122. Westermann J, Pabst R. Distribution of lymphocyte subsets and natural killer cells in the human body. Clin Investig 70:539-544, 1992.
123. Schonland SO, Zimmer JK, Lopez-Benitez CM, et al. Homeostatic control of T-cell generation in neonates. Blood 102:1428-1434, 2003.
124. von Boehmer H, Aifantis I, Gounari F, et al. Thymic selection revisited: how essential is it? Immunol Rev 191:62-78, 2003.
125. Padovan E, Giachino C, Cella M, et al. Normal T lymphocytes can express two different T cell receptor beta chains: implications for the mechanism of allelic exclusion. J.Exp.Med. 181:1587-1591, 1995.
126. Padovan E, Casorati G, Dellabona P, et al. Expression of two T cell receptor alpha chains: dual receptor T cells. Science 262:422-424, 1993.
127. Barton G, Rudensky A. Requirement for diverse, low-abundance peptides in positive selection of T cells. Science 283:67-70, 1999.
128. Starr TK, Jameson SC, Hogquist KA. Positive and negative selection of T cells. Annu Rev Immunol 21:139-176, 2003.
129. Housset D, Malissen B. What do TCR-pMHC crystal structures teach us about MHC restriction and alloreactivity? Trends Immunol 24:429-437, 2003.
130. Zerrahn J, Held W, Raulet DH. The MHC reactivity of the T cell repertoire prior to positive and negative selection. Cell 88:627-636, 1997.
131. van Meerwijk JP, Marguerat S, Lees RK, et al. Quantitative impact of thymic clonal deletion on the T cell repertoire. J Exp Med 185: 377-383, 1997.
132. Derbinski J, Schulte A, Kyewski B, et al. Promiscuous gene expression in medullary thymic epithelial cells mirrors the peripheral self. Nat Immunol 2:1032-1039, 2001.
133. Venanzi ES, Benoist C, Mathis D. Good riddance: thymocyte clonal deletion prevents autoimmunity. Curr Opin Immunol 16:197-202, 2004.
134. Jameson SC, Bevan MJ. T-cell selection. Curr Opin Immunol 10: 214-219, 1998.
135. Sherman L. The molecular basis of allorecognition. Annu Rev Immunol 11:385-402, 1993.
136. Puel A, Ziegler SF, Buckley RH, et al. Defective IL7R expression in T(−) B(+)NK(+) severe combined immunodeficiency. Nat Genet 20: 394-397, 1998.
137. Villa A, Sobacchi C, Notarangelo LD, et al. V(D)J recombination defects in lymphocytes due to RAG mutations: severe immunodeficiency with a spectrum of clinical presentations. Blood 97:81-88, 2001.
138. Ceredig R, Dialynas DP, Fitch FW, et al. Precursors of T cell growth factor producing cells in the thymus: ontogeny, frequency, and quantitative recovery in a subpopulation of phenotypically mature thymocytes defined by monoclonal antibody GK-1.5. J Exp Med 158:1654-1671, 1983.
139. Ceredig R, Glasebrook AL, MacDonald HR. Phenotypic and functional properties of murine thymocytes. I. Precursors of cytolytic T lymphocytes and interleukin 2-producing cells are all contained within a subpopulation of "mature" thymocytes as analyzed by monoclonal antibodies and flow microfluorometry. J Exp Med 155:358-379, 1982.
140. Campbell JJ, Butcher EC. Chemokines in tissue-specific and microenvironment-specific lymphocyte homing. Curr Opin Immunol 12:336-341, 2000.
141. Nishikawa S, Honda K, Vieira P, et al. Organogenesis of peripheral lymphoid organs. Immunol Rev 195:72-80, 2003.
142. Butcher EC, Picker LJ. Lymphocyte homing and homeostasis. Science 272:60-66, 1996.
143. Springer TA. Traffic signals on endothelium for lymphocyte recirculation and leukocyte emigration. Annu Rev Physiol 57:827-872, 1995.
144. Tanchot C, Rosado MM, Agenes F, et al. Lymphocyte homeostasis. Semin Immunol 9:331-337, 1997.
145. Markiewicz MA, Brown I, Gajewski TF. Death of peripheral CD8$^+$ T cells in the absence of MHC class I is Fas-dependent and not blocked by Bcl-xL. Eur J Immunol 33:2917-2926, 2003.
146. Surh CD, Sprent J. Regulation of naïve and memory T-cell homeostasis. Microbes Infect 4:51-56, 2002.
147. Lantz O, Grandjean I, Matzinger P, et al. Gamma chain required for naïve CD4$^+$ T cell survival but not for antigen proliferation. Nat Immunol 1:54-58, 2000.
148. Schluns KS, Kieper WC, Jameson SC, et al. Interleukin-7 mediates the homeostasis of naïve and memory CD8 T cells in vivo. Nat Immunol 1:426-432, 2000.
149. Latour S, Veillette A. Proximal protein tyrosine kinases in immunoreceptor signaling. Curr Opin Immunol 13:299-306, 2001.
150. Alizadeh AA, Eisen MB, Davis RE, et al. Distinct types of diffuse large B-cell lymphoma identified by gene expression profiling. Nature 403:503-511, 2000.
151. Feske S, Giltnane J, Dolmetsch R, et al. Gene regulation mediated by calcium signals in T lymphocytes. Nat Immunol 2:316-324, 2001.
152. Lanzavecchia A, Sallusto F. The instructive role of dendritic cells on T cell responses: lineages, plasticity and kinetics. Curr Opin Immunol 13:291-298, 2001.
153. Jelley-Gibbs DM, Lepak NM, Yen M, et al. Two distinct stages in the transition from naïve CD4 T cells to effectors, early antigen-dependent and late cytokine-driven expansion and differentiation. J Immunol 165:5017-5026, 2000.
154. Kaech SM, Ahmed R. Memory CD8$^+$ T cell differentiation: initial antigen encounter triggers a developmental program in naïve cells. Nat Immunol 2:415-422, 2001.
155. van Stipdonk MJ, Lemmens EE, Schoenberger SP. Naïve CTLs require a single brief period of antigenic stimulation for clonal expansion and differentiation. Nat Immunol 2:423-429, 2001.
156. Lanzavecchia A, Sallusto F. Progressive differentiation and selection of the fittest in the immune response. Nat Rev Immunol 2:982-987, 2002.
157. Lenschow DJ, Walunas TL, Bluestone JA. CD28/B7 system of T cell costimulation. Ann Rev Immunol 14:233-258, 1996.
158. Coyle AJ, Gutierrez-Ramos JC. The expanding B7 superfamily: increasing complexity in costimulatory signals regulating T cell function. Nat Immunol 2:203-209, 2001.
159. Margulies DH. TCR avidity: it's not how strong you make it, it's how you make it strong. Nat Immunol 2:669-670, 2001.
160. Lanzavecchia A, Sallusto F. Antigen decoding by T lymphocytes: from synapses to fate determination. Nat Immunol 2:487-492, 2001.
161. Grewal IS, Flavell RA. CD40 and CD154 in cell-mediated immunity. Annu Rev Immunol 16:111-135, 1998.
162. Foy TM, Aruffo A, Bajorath J, et al. Immune regulation by CD40 and its ligand GP39. Annu Rev Immunol 14:591-617, 1996.

163. Edelmann KH, Wilson CB. Role of CD28/CD80-86 and CD40/CD154 costimulatory interactions in host defense to primary herpes simplex virus infection. J Virol 75:612-621, 2001.
164. Whitmire JK, Ahmed R. Costimulation in antiviral immunity: differential requirements for CD4(+) and CD8(+) T cell responses. Curr Opin Immunol 12:448-455, 2000.
165. Kuo CT, Leiden JM. Transcriptional regulation of T lymphocyte development and function. Annu Rev Immunol 17:149-187, 1999.
166. Buckley AF, Kuo CT, Leiden JM. Transcription factor LKLF is sufficient to program T cell quiescence via a c-Myc–dependent pathway. Nat Immunol 2:698-704, 2001.
167. Dubey C, Croft M, Swain SL. naïve and effector CD4 T cells differ in their requirements for T cell receptor versus costimulatory signals. J Immunol 157:3280-3289, 1996.
168. Reiner SL, Seder RA. Dealing from the evolutionary pawnshop: how lymphocytes make decisions. Immunity 11:1-10, 1999.
169. Miyawaki T, Uehara T, Nibu R, et al. Differential expression of apoptosis-related Fas antigen on lymphocyte subpopulations in human peripheral blood. J Immunol 149:3753-3758, 1992.
170. Akbar AN, Borthwick N, Salmon M, et al. The significance of low bcl-2 expression by CD45RO T cells in normal individuals and patients with acute viral infections. The role of apoptosis in T cell memory. J Exp Med 178:427-438, 1993.
171. Nelson BH, Willerford DM. Biology of the interleukin-2 receptor. Adv Immunol 70:1-81, 1998.
172. Roifman CM. Human IL-2 receptor alpha chain deficiency. Pediatr Res 48:6-11, 2000.
173. Suzuki H, Zhou YW, Kato M, et al. Normal regulatory alpha/beta T cells effectively eliminate abnormally activated T cells lacking the interleukin 2 receptor beta in vivo. J Exp Med 190:1561-1572, 1999.
174. Kaech SM, Wherry EJ, Ahmed R. Effector and memory T-cell differentiation: implications for vaccine development. Nat Rev Immunol 2:251-262, 2002.
175. Spellberg B, Edwards JE Jr. Type 1/Type 2 immunity in infectious diseases. Clin Infect Dis 32:76-102, 2001.
176. Liles WC, Van Voorhis WC. Review: nomenclature and biologic significance of cytokines involved in inflammation and the host immune response. J Infect Dis 172:1573-1580, 1995.
177. Glimcher LH. Lineage commitment in lymphocytes: controlling the immune response. J Clin Invest 108:s25-s30, 2001.
178. Asnagli H, Murphy KM. Stability and commitment in T helper cell development. Curr Opin Immunol 13:242-247, 2001.
179. Fearon DT, Locksley RM. The instructive role of innate immunity in the acquired immune response. Science 272:50-53, 1996.
180. Romagnani S. The Th1/Th2 paradigm. Immunol Today 18:263-266, 1997.
181. Toellner KM, Luther SA, Sze DM, et al. T helper 1 (Th1) and Th2 characteristics start to develop during T cell priming and are associated with an immediate ability to induce immunoglobulin class switching. J Exp Med 187:1193-1204, 1998.
182. Rowe J, Macaubas C, Monger T, et al. Heterogeneity in diphtheria-tetanus-acellular pertussis vaccine-specific cellular immunity during infancy: relationship to variations in the kinetics of postnatal maturation of systemic Th1 function. J Infect Dis 184:80-88, 2001.
183. O'Garra A. Cytokines induce the development of functionally heterogeneous T helper cell subsets. Immunity 8:275-283, 1998.
184. Grogan JL, Mohrs M, Harmon B, et al. Early transcription and silencing of cytokine genes underlie polarization of T helper cell subsets. Immunity 14:205-215, 2001.
185. Kim CH, Rott L, Kunkel EJ, et al. Rules of chemokine receptor association with T cell polarization in vivo. J Clin Invest 108:1331-1339, 2001.
186. Campbell DJ, Kim CH, Butcher EC. Chemokines in the systemic organization of immunity. Immunol Rev 195:58-71, 2003.
187. Luther SA, Cyster JG. Chemokines as regulators of T cell differentiation. Nat Immunol 2:102-107, 2001.
188. Ottenhoff TH, De Boer T, van Dissel JT, et al. Human deficiencies in type-1 cytokine receptors reveal the essential role of type-1 cytokines in immunity to intracellular bacteria. Adv Exp Med Biol 531:279-294, 2003.
189. Schweitzer AN Sharpe AH. Studies using antigen-presenting cells lacking expression of both B7-1 (CD80) and B7-2 (CD86) show distinct requirements for B7 molecules during priming versus restimulation of Th2 but not Th1 cytokine production. J Immunol 161:2762-2771, 1998.
190. Flynn S, Toellner KM, Raykundalia C, et al. CD4 T cell cytokine differentiation: the B cell activation molecule, OX40 ligand, instructs CD4 T cells to express interleukin 4 and upregulates expression of the chemokine receptor, Blr-1. J Exp Med 188:297-304, 1998.
191. Zheng W, Flavell RA. The transcription factor GATA-3 is necessary and sufficient for Th2 cytokine gene expression in CD4 T cells. Cell 89:587-596, 1997.
192. Szabo SJ, Sullivan BM, Peng SL, et al. Molecular mechanisms regulating Th1 immune responses. Annu Rev Immunol 21:713-758, 2003.
193. Breitfeld D, Ohl L, Kremmer E, et al. Follicular B helper T cells express CXC chemokine receptor 5, localize to B cell follicles, and support immunoglobulin production. J Exp Med 192:1545-1552, 2000.
194. Schaerli P, Willimann K, Lang AB, et al. CXC chemokine receptor 5 expression defines follicular homing T cells with B cell helper function. J Exp Med 192:1553-1562, 2000.
195. Ramesh N, Geha RS, Notarangelo LD. CD40 ligand and the hyper-IgM syndrome. *In* Ochs HD, Smith CIE, Puck JM (eds). Primary Immunodeficiency Diseases: A Molecular and Genetic Approach. New York, Oxford University Press, 1999, pp 233-249.
196. Watts TH, DeBenedette MA. T cell co-stimulatory molecules other than CD28. Curr Opin Immunol 11:286-293, 1999.
197. Grimbacher B, Hutloff A, Schlesier M, et al. Homozygous loss of ICOS is associated with adult-onset common variable immunodeficiency. Nat Immunol 4:261-268, 2003.
198. Bromley SK, Iaboni A, Davis SJ, et al. The immunological synapse and CD28-CD80 interactions. Nat Immunol 2:1159-1166, 2001.
199. Ochs HD, Nonoyama S, Farrington ML, et al. The role of adhesion molecules in the regulation of antibody responses. Semin Hematol 30:72-79, 1993.
200. Takeda K, Tanaka T, Shi W, et al. Essential role of Stat6 in IL-4 signalling. Nature 380:627-630, 1996.
201. Masopust D, Vezys V, Marzo AL, et al. Preferential localization of effector memory cells in nonlymphoid tissue. Science 291:2413-2417, 2001.
202. Jenkins MK, Khoruts A, Ingulli E, et al. In vivo activation of antigen-specific CD4 T cells. Annu Rev Immunol 19:23-45, 2001.
203. Nieda M, Nicol A, Koezuka Y, et al. TRAIL expression by activated human CD4(+)V alpha 24 NK T cells induces in vitro and in vivo apoptosis of human acute myeloid leukemia cells. Blood 97: 2067-2074, 2001.
204. Hermiston ML, Xu Z, Majeti R, et al. Reciprocal regulation of lymphocyte activation by tyrosine kinases and phosphatases. J Clin Invest 109:9-14, 2002.
205. Chambers CA, Allison JP. Costimulatory regulation of T cell function. Curr Opin Cell Biol 11:203-210, 1999.
206. Greenwald RJ, Boussiotis VA, Lorsbach RB, et al. CTLA-4 regulates induction of anergy in vivo. Immunity 14:145-155, 2001.
207. Van Parijs L, Abbas AK. Homeostasis and self-tolerance in the immune system: turning lymphocytes off. Science 280:243-248, 1998.
208. Siegel RM, Chan FK, Chun HJ, et al. The multifaceted role of Fas signaling in immune cell homeostasis and autoimmunity. Nat Immunol 1:469-474, 2000.
209. Badovinac VP, Tvinnereim AR, Harty JT. Regulation of antigen-specific $CD8^+$ T cell homeostasis by perforin and interferon-gamma. Science 290:1354-1358, 2000.
210. Hofmann SR, Ettinger R, Zhou YJ, et al. Cytokines and their role in lymphoid development, differentiation and homeostasis. Curr Opin Allergy Clin Immunol 2:495-506, 2002.
211. Ahmed R, Gray D. Immunological memory and protective immunity: understanding their relation. Science 272:54-60, 1996.
212. Sprent J, Surh CD. Generation and maintenance of memory T cells. Curr Opin Immunol 13:248-254, 2001.
213. Hu H, Huston G, Duso D, et al. CD4(+) T cell effectors can become memory cells with high efficiency and without further division. Nat Immunol 2:705-710, 2001.
214. Weng NP, Levine BL, June CH, et al. Human naïve and memory T lymphocytes differ in telomeric length and replicative potential. Proc Natl Acad Sci U S A 92:11091-11094, 1995.
215. Liu Y, Wenger RH, Zhao M, et al. Distinct costimulatory molecules are required for the induction of effector and memory cytotoxic T lymphocytes. J Exp Med 185:251-262, 1997.
216. Ameratunga R, Lederman HM, Sullivan KE, et al. Defective antigen-induced lymphocyte proliferation in the X-linked hyper-IgM syndrome. J Pediatr 131:147-150, 1997.

217. Sanders ME, Makgoba MW, Sharrow SO, et al. Human memory T lymphocytes express increased levels of three cell adhesion molecules (LFA-3, CD2, and LFA-1) and three other molecules (UCHL1, CDw29, and Pgp-1) and have enhanced IFN-gamma production. J Immunol 140:1401-1407, 1988.
218. Hamann D, Baars PA, Rep MH, et al. Phenotypic and functional separation of memory and effector human CD8+ T cells. J Exp Med 186:1407-1418, 1997.
219. Young JL, Ramage JM, Gaston JS, et al. In vitro responses of human CD45RObrightRA- and CD45RO-RAbright T cell subsets and their relationship to memory and naïve T cells. Eur J Immunol 27: 2383-2390, 1997.
220. Fallen PR, Duarte RF, McGreavey L, et al. Identification of non-naïve CD4+CD45RA+ T cell subsets in adult allogeneic haematopoietic cell transplant recipients. Bone Marrow Transplant 32:609-616, 2003.
221. Clement LT. Isoforms of the CD45 common leukocyte antigen family: markers for human T-cell differentiation. J Clin Immunol 12:1-10, 1992.
222. Hamann D, Kostense S, Wolthers KC, et al. Evidence that human CD8+CD45RA+CD27- cells are induced by antigen and evolve through extensive rounds of division. Int Immunol 11:1027-1033, 1999.
223. McMahon CW, Raulet DH. Expression and function of NK cell receptors in CD8+ T cells. Curr Opin Immunol 13:465-470, 2001.
224. Champagne P, Ogg GS, King AS, et al. Skewed maturation of memory HIV-specific CD8 T lymphocytes. Nature 410:106-111, 2001.
225. Cleary AM, Tu W, Enright A, et al. Impaired accumulation and function of memory CD4 T cells in human IL-12 receptor beta 1 deficiency. J Immunol 170:597-603, 2003.
226. Tu W, Chen S, Sharp M, et al. Persistent and selective deficiency of CD4+ T cell immunity to cytomegalovirus in immunocompetent young children. J Immunol 172:3260-3267, 2004.
227. Li J, Huston G, Swain SL. IL-7 promotes the transition of CD4 effectors to persistent memory cells. J Exp Med 198:1807-1815, 2003.
228. Damle NK, Engleman EG. Antigen-specific suppressor T lymphocytes in man. Clin Immunol Immunopathol 53:S17-24, 1989.
229. Shevach EM, Piccirillo CA, Thornton AM, et al. Control of T cell activation by CD4+CD25+ suppressor T cells. Novartis Found Symp 252:24-36, discussion 36-44, 106-114, 2003.
230. Sakaguchi S. Naturally arising CD4+ regulatory T cells for immunologic self-tolerance and negative control of immune responses. Annu Rev Immunol 22:531-562, 2004.
231. Battaglia M, Roncarolo MG. The role of cytokines (and not only) in inducing and expanding T regulatory type 1 cells. Transplantation 77:S16-S18, 2004.
232. Levings MK, Sangregorio R, Galbiati F, et al. IFN-alpha and IL-10 induce the differentiation of human type 1 T regulatory cells. J Immunol 166:5530-5539, 2001.
233. Ohteki T, Ho S, Suzuki H, et al. Role for IL-15/IL-15 receptor beta-chain in natural killer 1.1+ T cell receptor-alpha beta+ cell development. J Immunol 159:5931-5935, 1997.
234. Porcelli S, Yockey CE, Brenner MB, et al. Analysis of T cell antigen receptor (TCR) expression by human peripheral blood CD4-8- alpha/beta T cells demonstrates preferential use of several V beta genes and an invariant TCR alpha chain. J Exp Med 178:1-16, 1993.
235. Lantz O, Bendelac A. An invariant T cell receptor alpha chain is used by a unique subset of major histocompatibility complex class I-specific CD4+ and CD4-8- T cells in mice and humans. J Exp Med 180:1097-1106, 1994.
236. Dellabona P, Padovan E, Casorati G, et al. An invariant V alpha 24-J alpha Q/V beta 11 T cell receptor is expressed in all individuals by clonally expanded CD4-8- T cells. J Exp Med 180:1171-1176, 1994.
237. Kawano T, Tanaka Y, Shimizu E, et al. A novel recognition motif of human NKT antigen receptor for a glycolipid ligand. Int Immunol 11:881-887, 1999.
238. Godfrey DI, Hammond KJ, Poulton LD, et al. NKT cells: facts, functions and fallacies. Immunol Today 21:573-583, 2000.
239. Wilson SB, Kent SC, Patton KT, et al. Extreme Th1 bias of invariant Valpha24JalphaQ T cells in type 1 diabetes. Nature 391:177-181, 1998.
240. Zeng D, Lewis D, Dejbakhsh-Jones S, et al. Bone marrow NK1.1(−) and NK1.1(+) T cells reciprocally regulate acute graft versus host disease. J Exp Med 189:1073-1081, 1999.
241. Bach JF. Non-Th2 regulatory T-cell control of Th1 autoimmunity. Scand J Immunol 54:21-29, 2001.
242. Poggi A, Demarest JF, Costa P, et al. Expression of a wide T cell receptor V beta repertoire in human T lymphocytes derived in vitro from embryonic liver cell precursors. Eur J Immunol 24:2258-2261, 1994.
243. Haynes BF, Heinly CS. Early human T cell development: analysis of the human thymus at the time of initial entry of hematopoietic stem cells into the fetal thymic microenvironment. J Exp Med 181: 1445-1458, 1995.
244. Horst E, Meijer CJ, Duijvestijn AM, et al. The ontogeny of human lymphocyte recirculation: high endothelial cell antigen (HECA-452) and CD44 homing receptor expression in the development of the immune system. Eur J Immunol 20:1483-1489, 1990.
245. Gilhus NE, Matre R, Tonder O. Hassall's corpuscles in the thymus of fetuses, infants and children: immunological and histochemical aspects. Thymus 7:123-135, 1985.
246. Kitchen SG, Zack JA. Distribution of the human immunodeficiency virus coreceptors CXCR4 and CCR5 in fetal lymphoid organs: implications for pathogenesis in utero. AIDS Res Hum Retroviruses 15:143-148, 1999.
247. Vandenberghe P, Delabie J, de-Boer M, et al. In situ expression of B7/BB1 on antigen-presenting cells and activated B cells: an immunohistochemical study. Int Immunol 5:317-321, 1993.
248. Cilio CM, Daws MR, Malashicheva A, et al. Cytotoxic T lymphocyte antigen 4 is induced in the thymus upon in vivo activation and its blockade prevents anti–CD3-mediated depletion of thymocytes. J Exp Med 188:1239-1246, 1998.
249. Beier KC, Hutloff A, Dittrich AM, et al. Induction, binding specificity and function of human ICOS. Eur J Immunol 30:3707-3717, 2000.
250. Sharpe AH, Freeman GJ. The B7-CD28 superfamily. Nat Rev Immunol 2:116-126, 2002.
251. Dong C, Juedes AE, Temann UA, et al. ICOS co-stimulatory receptor is essential for T-cell activation and function. Nature 409:97-101, 2001.
252. Varas A, Jimenez E, Sacedon R, et al. Analysis of the human neonatal thymus: evidence for a transient thymic involution. J Immunol 164:6260-6267, 2000.
253. Ramos SB, Garcia AB, Viana SR, et al. Phenotypic and functional evaluation of natural killer cells in thymectomized children. Clin Immunol Immunopathol 81:277-281, 1996.
254. Baroni CD, Valtieri M, Stoppacciaro A, et al. The human thymus in ageing: histologic involution paralleled by increased mitogen response and by enrichment of OKT3+ lymphocytes. Immunology 50:519-528, 1983.
255. Poulin JF, Viswanathan MN, Harris JM, et al. Direct evidence for thymic function in adult humans. J Exp Med 190:479-486, 1999.
256. Mackall CL, Fleisher TA, Brown MR, et al. Age, thymopoiesis, and CD4+ T-lymphocyte regeneration after intensive chemotherapy. N Engl J Med 332:143-149, 1995.
257. Douek D, McFarland R, Keiser P, et al. Changes in thymic function with age and during the treatment of HIV infection. Nature 396: 690-695, 1998.
258. Fry TJ, Mackall CL. Interleukin-7: master regulator of peripheral T-cell homeostasis? Trends Immunol 22:564-571, 2001.
259. George JF Jr, Schroeder HW Jr. Developmental regulation of D beta reading frame and junctional diversity in T cell receptor-beta transcripts from human thymus. J Immunol 148:1230-1239, 1992.
260. Raaphorst FM, van Bergen J, van den Bergh RL, et al. Usage of *TCRAV* and *TCRBV* gene families in human fetal and adult TCR rearrangements. Immunogenetics 39:343-350, 1994.
261. Raaphorst FM, Kaijzel EL, Van Tol MJ, et al. Non-random employment of V beta 6 and J beta gene elements and conserved amino acid usage profiles in CDR3 regions of human fetal and adult TCR beta chain rearrangements. Int Immunol 6:1-9, 1994.
262. Bonati A, Zanelli P, Ferrari S, et al. T-cell receptor beta-chain gene rearrangement and expression during human thymic ontogenesis. Blood 79:1472-1483, 1992.
263. Doherty PJ, Roifman CM, Pan SH, et al. Expression of the human T cell receptor V beta repertoire. Mol Immunol 28:607-612, 1991.
264. Vandekerckhove BA, Baccala R, Jones D, et al. Thymic selection of the human T cell receptor V beta repertoire in SCID-hu mice. J Exp Med 176:1619-1624, 1992.
265. Garderet L, Dulphy N, Douay C, et al. The umbilical cord blood alphabeta T-cell repertoire: characteristics of a polyclonal and naïve but completely formed repertoire. Blood 91:340-346, 1998.
266. Kou ZC, Puhr JS, Rojas M, et al. T-cell receptor Vbeta repertoire CDR3 length diversity differs within CD45RA and CD45RO T-cell subsets in healthy and human immunodeficiency virus-infected children. Clin Diagn Lab Immunol 7:953-959, 2000.

267. van den Beemd R, Boor PP, van Lochem EG, et al. Flow cytometric analysis of the Vbeta repertoire in healthy controls. Cytometry 40: 336-345, 2000.
268. Gilfillan S, Bachmann M, Trembleau S, et al. Efficient immune responses in mice lacking N-region diversity. Eur J Immunol 25:3115-3122, 1995.
269. Schelonka RL, Raaphorst FM, Infante D, et al. T cell receptor repertoire diversity and clonal expansion in human neonates. Pediatr Res 43:396-402, 1998.
270. Grunewald J, Janson CH, Wigzell H. Biased expression of individual T cell receptor V gene segments in $CD4^+$ and $CD8^+$ human peripheral blood T lymphocytes. Eur J Immunol 21:819-822, 1991.
271. DerSimonian H, Band H, Brenner MB. Increased frequency of T cell receptor V alpha 12.1 expression on $CD8^+$ T cells: evidence that V alpha participates in shaping the peripheral T cell repertoire. J Exp Med 174:639-648, 1991.
272. Cossarizza A, Kahan M, Ortolani C, et al. Preferential expression of V beta 6.7 domain on human peripheral $CD4^+$ T cells. Implication for positive selection of T cells in man. Eur J Immunol 21:1571-1574, 1991.
273. Grunewald J, Shankar N, Wigzell H, et al. An analysis of alpha/beta TCR V gene expression in the human thymus. Int Immunol 3: 699-702, 1991.
274. Okamoto Y, Douek DC, McFarland RD, et al. Effects of exogenous interleukin-7 on human thymus function. Blood 99:2851-2858, 2002.
275. Hazenberg MD, Verschuren MC, Hamann D, et al. T cell receptor excision circles as markers for recent thymic emigrants: basic aspects, technical approach, and guidelines for interpretation. J Mol Med 79:631-640, 2001.
276. Hazenberg MD, Hamann D, Schuitemaker H, et al. T cell depletion in HIV-1 infection: how $CD4^+$ T cells go out of stock. Nat Immunol 1:285-289, 2000.
277. Pahal GS, Jauniaux E, Kinnon C, et al. Normal development of human fetal hematopoiesis between eight and seventeen weeks' gestation. Am J Obstet Gynecol 183:1029-1034, 2000.
278. Asano S, Akaike Y, Muramatsu T, et al. Immunohistologic detection of the primary follicle (PF) in human fetal and newborn lymph node anlages. Pathol Res Pract 189:921-927, 1993.
279. Settmacher U, Volk HD, Jahn S, et al. Characterization of human lymphocytes separated from fetal liver and spleen at different stages of ontogeny. Immunobiology 182:256-265, 1991.
280. Hannet I, Erkeller YF, Lydyard P, et al. Developmental and maturational changes in human blood lymphocyte subpopulations. Immunol Today 13:215, 218, 1992. [See comments.]
281. Cayabyab M, Phillips JH, Lanier LL. CD40 preferentially costimulates activation of $CD4^+$ T lymphocytes. J Immunol 152:1523-1531, 1994.
282. Sato K, Kawasaki H, Nagayama H, et al. Chemokine receptor expressions and responsiveness of cord blood T cells. J Immunol 166:1659-1666, 2001.
283. Kimmig S, Przybylski GK, Schmidt CA, et al. Two subsets of naïve T helper cells with distinct T cell receptor excision circle content in human adult peripheral blood. J Exp Med 195:789-794, 2002.
284. Delespesse G, Yang LP, Ohshima Y, et al. Maturation of human neonatal $CD4^+$ and $CD8^+$ T lymphocytes into Th1/Th2 effectors. Vaccine 16:1415-1419, 1998.
285. Wilson M, Rosen FS, Schlossman SF, et al. Ontogeny of human T and B lymphocytes during stressed and normal gestation: phenotypic analysis of umbilical cord lymphocytes from term and preterm infants. Clin Immunol Immunopathol 37:1-12, 1985.
286. Comans-Bitter WM, de Groot R, van den Beemd R, et al. Immunophenotyping of blood lymphocytes in childhood. Reference values for lymphocyte subpopulations. J Pediatr 130:388-393, 1997.
287. Carballido JM, Namikawa R, Carballido-Perrig N, et al. Generation of primary antigen-specific human T- and B-cell responses in immunocompetent SCID-hu mice. Nat Med 6:103-106, 2000.
288. Tsegaye A, Wolday D, Otto S, et al. Immunophenotyping of blood lymphocytes at birth, during childhood, and during adulthood in HIV-1–uninfected Ethiopians. Clin Immunol 109:338-346, 2003.
289. Asma GE, Van den Bergh RL, Vossen JM. Use of monoclonal antibodies in a study of the development of T lymphocytes in the human fetus. Clin Exp Immunol 53:429-436, 1983.
290. Hassan J, Reen DJ. IL-7 promotes the survival and maturation but not differentiation of human post-thymic $CD4^+$ T cells. Eur J Immunol 28:3057-3065, 1998.
291. Peakman M, Buggins AG, Nicolaides KH, et al. Analysis of lymphocyte phenotypes in cord blood from early gestation fetuses. Clin Exp Immunol 90:345-350, 1992.
292. Byrne JA, Stankovic AK, Cooper MD. A novel subpopulation of primed T cells in the human fetus. J Immunol 152:3098-3106, 1994.
293. Bofill M, Akbar AN, Salmon M, et al. Immature CD45RA(low) RO(low) T cells in the human cord blood. I. Antecedents of $CD45RA^+$ unprimed T cells. J Immunol 152:5613-5623, 1994.
294. D'Andrea A, Lanier LL. Killer cell inhibitory receptor expression by T cells. Curr Top Microbiol Immunol 230:25-39, 1998.
295. Azuma M, Cayabyab M, Phillips JH, et al. Requirements for CD28-dependent T cell–mediated cytotoxicity. J Immunol 150:2091-2101, 1993.
296. Azuma M, Phillips JH, Lanier LL. $CD28^-$ T lymphocytes. Antigenic and functional properties. J Immunol 150:1147-1159, 1993.
297. Frenkel L, Bryson YJ. Ontogeny of phytohemagglutinin-induced gamma interferon by leukocytes of healthy infants and children: evidence for decreased production in infants younger than 2 months of age. J Pediatr 111:97-100, 1987.
298. Lanier LL, Allison JP, Phillips JH. Correlation of cell surface antigen expression on human thymocytes by multi-color flow cytometric analysis: implications for differentiation. J Immunol 137:2501-2507, 1986.
299. McFarland RD, Douek DC, Koup RA, et al. Identification of a human recent thymic emigrant phenotype. Proc Natl Acad Sci U S A 97:4215-4220, 2000.
300. Evans JT, Okamoto Y, Douek DC, et al. Thymocyte differentiation from lentivirus-marked CD34(+) cells in infant and adult human thymus. J Immunol Methods 245:31-43, 2000.
301. Olaussen RW, Farstad IN, Brandtzaeg P, et al. Age-related changes in $CCR9^+$ circulating lymphocytes: are $CCR9^+$ naïve T cells recent thymic emigrants? Scand J Immunol 54:435-439, 2001.
302. Min B, McHugh R, Sempowski GD, et al. Neonates support lymphopenia-induced proliferation. Immunity 18:131-140, 2003.
303. Marrack P, Bender J, Hildeman D, et al. Homeostasis of alpha beta TCR^+ T cells. Nat Immunol 1:107-111, 2000.
304. Vivien L, Benoist C, Mathis D. T lymphocytes need IL-7 but not IL-4 or IL-6 to survive in vivo. Int Immunol 13:763-768, 2001.
305. Fukui T, Katamura K, Abe N, et al. IL-7 induces proliferation, variable cytokine-producing ability and IL- 2 responsiveness in naïve $CD4^+$ T-cells from human cord blood. Immunol Lett 59: 21-28, 1997.
306. Hassan J, Reen DJ. Human recent thymic emigrants—identification, expansion, and survival characteristics. J Immunol 167:1970-1976, 2001.
307. Dardalhon V, Jaleco S, Kinet S, et al. IL-7 differentially regulates cell cycle progression and HIV-1–based vector infection in neonatal and adult $CD4^+$ T cells. Proc Natl Acad Sci U S A 98:9277-9282, 2001.
308. Hare KJ, Jenkinson EJ, Anderson G. An essential role for the IL-7 receptor during intrathymic expansion of the positively selected neonatal T cell repertoire. J Immunol 165:2410-2414, 2000.
309. Soares MV, Borthwick NJ, Maini MK, et al. IL-7–dependent extrathymic expansion of $CD45RA^+$ T cells enables preservation of a naïve repertoire. J Immunol 161:5909-5917, 1998.
310. Webb LM, Foxwell BM, Feldmann M. Putative role for interleukin-7 in the maintenance of the recirculating naïve $CD4^+$ T-cell pool. Immunology 98:400-405, 1999.
311. Jameson SC. Maintaining the norm: T-cell homeostasis. Nat Rev Immunol 2:547-556, 2002.
312. Renda MC, Fecarotta E, Dieli F, et al. Evidence of alloreactive T lymphocytes in fetal liver: implications for fetal hematopoietic stem cell transplantation. Bone Marrow Transplant 25:135-141, 2000.
313. Renda MC, Fecarotta E, Maggio A, et al. In utero fetal liver hematopoietic stem cell transplantation: is there a role for alloreactive T lymphocytes. Blood 96:1608-1609, 2000.
314. Howie D, Spencer J, DeLord D, et al. Extrathymic T cell differentiation in the human intestine early in life. J Immunol 161:5862-5872, 1998.
315. Moghaddami M, Cummins A, Mayrhofer G. Lymphocyte-filled villi: comparison with other lymphoid aggregations in the mucosa of the human small intestine. Gastroenterology 115:1414-1425, 1998.
316. Bas A, Hammarstrom SG, Hammarstrom ML. Extrathymic TCR gene rearrangement in human small intestine: identification of new splice forms of recombination activating gene-1 mRNA with selective tissue expression. J Immunol 171:3359-3371, 2003.

317. Yang Y, Nunes FA, Berencsi K, et al. Inactivation of E2a in recombinant adenoviruses improves the prospect for gene therapy in cystic fibrosis. Nat Genet 7:362-369, 1994.
318. Sanders ME, Makgoba MW, June CH, et al. Enhanced responsiveness of human memory T cells to CD2- and CD3 receptor–mediated activation. Eur J Immunol 19:803-808, 1989.
319. Horgan KJ, Van Seventer GA, Shimizu Y, et al. Hyporesponsiveness of "naïve" ($CD45RA^+$) human T cells to multiple receptor-mediated stimuli but augmentation of responses by co-stimuli. Eur J Immunol 20:1111-1118, 1990.
320. Kimachi K, Croft M, Grey HM. The minimal number of antigen–major histocompatibility complex class II complexes required for activation of naïve and primed T cells. Eur J Immunol 27:3310-3317, 1997.
321. Zaitseva MB, Lee S, Rabin RL, et al. CXCR4 and CCR5 on human thymocytes: biological function and role in HIV-1 infection. J Immunol 161:3103-3113, 1998.
322. Liu K, Li Y, Prabhu V, et al. Augmentation in expression of activation-induced genes differentiates memory from naïve $CD4^+$ T cells and is a molecular mechanism for enhanced cellular response of memory $CD4^+$ T cells. J Immunol 166:7335-7344, 2001.
323. Woodside DG, Long DA, McIntyre BW. Intracellular analysis of interleukin-2 induction provides direct evidence at the single cell level of differential coactivation requirements for $CD45RA^+$ and $CD45RO^+$ T cell subsets. J Interferon Cytokine Res 19:769-779, 1999.
324. Monteleone G, Pender SL, Wathen NC, et al. Interferon-alpha drives T cell-mediated immunopathology in the intestine. Eur J Immunol 31:2247-2255, 2001.
325. Pittard WB 3rd, Miller K, Sorensen RU. Normal lymphocyte responses to mitogens in term and premature neonates following normal and abnormal intrauterine growth. Clin Immunol Immunopathol 30:178-187, 1984.
326. Wilson CB, Westall J, Johnston L, et al. Decreased production of interferon-gamma by human neonatal cells. Intrinsic and regulatory deficiencies. J Clin Invest 77:860-867, 1986.
327. Clerici M, DePalma L, Roilides E, et al. Analysis of T helper and antigen-presenting cell functions in cord blood and peripheral blood leukocytes from healthy children of different ages. J Clin Invest 91:2829-2836, 1993.
328. Caux C, Massacrier C, Vanbervliet B, et al. Interleukin 10 inhibits T cell alloreaction induced by human dendritic cells. Int Immunol 6:1177-1185, 1994.
329. Hayward A, Cosyns M. Proliferative and cytokine responses by human newborn T cells stimulated with staphylococcal enterotoxin B. Pediatr Res 35:293-298, 1994.
330. Takahashi N, Imanishi K, Nishida H, et al. Evidence for immunologic immaturity of cord blood T cells. Cord blood T cells are susceptible to tolerance induction to in vitro stimulation with a superantigen. J Immunol 155:5213-5219, 1995.
331. Trivedi HN, HayGlass KT, Gangur V, et al. Analysis of neonatal T cell and antigen presenting cell functions. Hum Immunol 57:69-79, 1997.
332. Gerli R, Bertotto A, Crupi S, et al. Activation of cord T lymphocytes. I. Evidence for a defective T cell mitogenesis induced through the CD2 molecule. J Immunol 142:2583-2589, 1989.
333. Splawski JB, Jelinek DF, Lipsky PE. Delineation of the functional capacity of human neonatal lymphocytes. J Clin Invest 87:545-553, 1991.
334. Splawski JB, Lipsky PE. Cytokine regulation of immunoglobulin secretion by neonatal lymphocytes. J Clin Invest 88:967-977, 1991.
335. Ansart-Pirenne H, Soulimani N, Tartour E, et al. Defective *IL2* gene expression in newborn is accompanied with impaired tyrosine-phosphorylation in T cells. Pediatr Res 45:409-413, 1999.
336. Hassan J, O'Neill S, O'Neill LA, et al. Signalling via CD28 of human naïve neonatal T lymphocytes. Clin Exp Immunol 102:192-198, 1995.
337. Hassan J, Rainsford E, Reen DJ. Linkage of protein kinase C-beta activation and intracellular interleukin-2 accumulation in human naïve CD4 T cells. Immunology 92:465-471, 1997.
338. Hassan J, Reen DJ. Cord blood $CD4^+CD45RA^+$ T cells achieve a lower magnitude of activation when compared with their adult counterparts. Immunology 90:397-401, 1997.
339. Saito S, Morii T, Umekage H, et al. Expression of the interleukin-2 receptor gamma chain on cord blood mononuclear cells. Blood 87:3344-3350, 1996.
340. Lyons AB. Analysing cell division in vivo and in vitro using flow cytometric measurement of CFSE dye dilution. J Immunol Methods 243:147-154, 2000.
341. Hassan J, Reen DJ. Reduced primary antigen-specific T-cell precursor frequencies in neonates is associated with deficient interleukin-2 production. Immunology 87:604-608, 1996.
342. Ehlers S, Smith KA. Differentiation of T cell lymphokine gene expression: the in vitro acquisition of T cell memory. J Exp Med 173:25-36, 1991.
343. Lewis DB, Yu CC, Meyer J, et al. Cellular and molecular mechanisms for reduced interleukin 4 and interferon-gamma production by neonatal T cells. J Clin Invest 87:194-202, 1991.
344. English BK, Hammond WP, Lewis DB, et al. Decreased granulocyte-macrophage colony-stimulating factor production by human neonatal blood mononuclear cells and T cells. Pediatr Res 31:211-216, 1992.
345. Lee SM, Knoppel E, van de Ven C, et al. Transcriptional rates of granulocyte-macrophage colony-stimulating factor, granulocyte colony-stimulating factor, interleukin-3, and macrophage colony-stimulating factor genes in activated cord versus adult mononuclear cells: alteration in cytokine expression may be secondary to post-transcriptional instability. Pediatr Res 34:560-564, 1993.
346. Chheda S, Palkowetz KH, Garofalo R, et al. Decreased interleukin-10 production by neonatal monocytes and T cells: relationship to decreased production and expression of tumor necrosis factor-alpha and its receptors. Pediatr Res 40:475-483, 1996.
347. Dolganov G, Bort S, Lovett M, et al. Coexpression of the interleukin-13 and interleukin-4 genes correlates with their physical linkage in the cytokine gene cluster on human chromosome 5q23-31. Blood 87:3316-3326, 1996.
348. English BK, Burchett SK, English JD, et al. Production of lymphotoxin and tumor necrosis factor by human neonatal mononuclear cells. Pediatr Res 24:717-722, 1988.
349. Lewis DB, Prickett KS, Larsen A, et al. Restricted production of interleukin 4 by activated human T cells. Proc Natl Acad Sci U S A 85:9743-9747, 1988.
350. Salmon M, Kitas GD Bacon PA. Production of lymphokine mRNA by $CD45R^+$ and $CD45R^-$ helper T cells from human peripheral blood and by human $CD4^+$ T cell clones. J Immunol 143:907-912, 1989.
351. Jung T, Wijdenes J, Neumann C, et al. Interleukin-13 is produced by activated human $CD45RA^+$ and $CD45RO^+$ T cells: modulation by interleukin-4 and interleukin-12. Eur J Immunol 26:571-577, 1996.
352. Chalmers IM, Janossy G, Contreras M, et al. Intracellular cytokine profile of cord and adult blood lymphocytes. Blood 92:11-18, 1998.
353. Krampera M, Vinante F, Tavecchia L, et al. Progressive polarization towards a T helper/cytotoxic type-1 cytokine pattern during age-dependent maturation of the immune response inversely correlates with CD30 cell expression and serum concentration. Clin Exp Immunol 117:291-297, 1999.
354. Krampera M, Tavecchia L, Benedetti F, et al. Intracellular cytokine profile of cord blood T- and NK-cells and monocytes. Haematologica 85:675-679, 2000.
355. Schatt S, Holzgreve W, Hahn S. Stimulated cord blood lymphocytes have a low percentage of Th1 and Th2 cytokine secreting T cells although their activation is similar to adult controls. Immunol Lett 77:1-2, 2001.
356. Chen L, Jullien P, Stepick-Biek P, Lewis DB. Neonatal naïve CD4 T cells have a decreased capacity to express CD40-ligand (CD154) and to induce dendritic cell IL-12 production after allogeneic stimulation. Abstract 309. Federation of Clinical Immunology Socieities (FOCIS) Annual Meeting, Boston, 2001, p 45.
357. Hariharan D, Ho W, Cutilli J, et al. C-C chemokine profile of cord blood mononuclear cells: RANTES production. Blood 95:715-718, 2000.
358. Ribeiro-do-Couto LM, Boeije LC, Kroon JS, et al. High IL-13 production by human neonatal T cells: neonate immune system regulator? Eur J Immunol 31:3394-3402, 2001.
359. Vigano A, Esposito S, Arienti D, et al. Differential development of type 1 and type 2 cytokines and beta-chemokines in the ontogeny of healthy newborns. Biol Neonate 75:1-8, 1999.
360. Nel AE. T-cell activation through the antigen receptor. Part 1: Signaling components, signaling pathways, and signal integration at the T-cell antigen receptor synapse. J Allergy Clin Immunol 109: 758-770, 2002.
361. Rao A, Avni O. Molecular aspects of T-cell differentiation. Br Med Bull 56:969-984, 2000.
362. Sato K, Nagayama H, Takahashi TA. Aberrant CD3- and CD28-mediated signaling events in cord blood. J Immunol 162:4464-4471, 1999.

363. Miscia S, Di Baldassarre A, Sabatino G, et al. Inefficient phospholipase C activation and reduced Lck expression characterize the signaling defect of umbilical cord T lymphocytes. J Immunol 163:2416-2424, 1999.
364. Jullien P, Cron RQ, Dabbagh K, et al. Decreased CD154 expression by neonatal CD4+ T cells is due to limitations in both proximal and distal events of T cell activation. Int Immunol 15:1461-1472, 2003.
365. Dialynas DP, Lee MJ, Gold DP, et al. Preconditioning with fetal cord blood facilitates engraftment of primary childhood T-cell acute lymphoblastic leukemia in immunodeficient mice. Blood 97: 3218-3225, 2001.
366. Fitzpatrick DR, Wilson CB. Methylation and demethylation in the regulation of genes, cells, and responses in the immune system. Clin Immunol 109:37-45, 2003.
367. Melvin AJ, McGurn ME, Bort SJ, et al. Hypomethylation of the interferon-gamma gene correlates with its expression by primary T-lineage cells. Eur J Immunol 25:426-430, 1995.
368. White GP, Watt PM, Holt BJ, et al. Differential patterns of methylation of the IFN-gamma promoter at CpG and non-CpG sites underlie differences in IFN-gamma gene expression between human neonatal and adult CD45RO- T cells. J Immunol 168:2820-2827, 2002.
369. Suen Y, Lee SM, Qian J, et al. Dysregulation of lymphokine production in the neonate and its impact on neonatal cell mediated immunity. Vaccine 16:1369-1377, 1998.
370. Swain SL, Bradley LM, Croft M, et al. Helper T-cell subsets: phenotype, function and the role of lymphokines in regulating their development. Immunol Rev 123:115-144, 1991.
371. Pirenne H, Aujard Y, Eljaafari A, et al. Comparison of T cell functional changes during childhood with the ontogeny of CDw29 and CD45RA expression on CD4+ T cells. Pediatr Res 32:81-86, 1992.
372. Kadereit S, Mohammad SF, Miller RE, et al. Reduced NFAT1 protein expression in human umbilical cord blood T lymphocytes. Blood 94:3101-3107, 1999.
373. Kiani A, Garcia-Cozar FJ, Habermann I, et al. Regulation of interferon-gamma gene expression by nuclear factor of activated T cells. Blood 98:1480-1488, 2001.
374. Schonbeck U, Libby P. The CD40/CD154 receptor/ligand dyad. Cell Mol Life Sci 58:4-43, 2001.
375. Durandy A, De-Saint-Basile G, Lisowska GB, et al. Undetectable CD40 ligand expression on T cells and low B cell responses to CD40 binding agonists in human newborns. J Immunol 154:1560-1568, 1995.
376. Brugnoni D, Airo P, Graf D, et al. Ineffective expression of CD40 ligand on cord blood T cells may contribute to poor immunoglobulin production in the newborn. Eur J Immunol 24:1919-1924, 1994.
377. Fuleihan R, Ahern D, Geha RS. Decreased expression of the ligand for CD40 in newborn lymphocytes. Eur J Immunol 24:1925-1928, 1994.
378. Nonoyama S, Penix LA, Edwards CP, et al. Diminished expression of CD40 ligand by activated neonatal T cells. J Clin Invest 95:66-75, 1995.
379. Durandy A, De Saint BG, Lisowska-Grospierre B, et al. Undetectable CD40 ligand expression on T cells and low B cell. J Immunol 154: 1560-1568, 1995.
380. Flamand V, Donckier V, Demoor FX, et al. CD40 ligation prevents neonatal induction of transplantation tolerance. J Immunol 160: 4666-4669, 1998.
381. Fuleihan R, Ahern D, Geha RS. CD40 ligand expression is developmentally regulated in human thymocytes. Clin Immunol Immunopathol 76:52-58, 1995.
382. Splawski JB, Nishioka J, Nishioka Y, et al. CD40 ligand is expressed and functional on activated neonatal T cells. J Immunol 156:119-127, 1996.
383. Reen DJ. Activation and functional capacity of human neonatal CD4 T-cells. Vaccine 16:1401-1408, 1998.
384. Ohshima Y, Delespesse G. T cell–derived IL-4 and dendritic cell–derived IL-12 regulate the lymphokine-producing phenotype of alloantigen-primed naïve human CD4 T cells. J Immunol 158: 629-636, 1997.
385. Matthews NC, Wadhwa M, Bird C, et al. Sustained expression of CD154 (CD40L) and proinflammatory cytokine production by alloantigen-stimulated umbilical cord blood T cells. J Immunol 164:6206-6212, 2000.
386. Lenardo MJ. Molecular regulation of T lymphocyte homeostasis in the healthy and diseased immune system. Immunol Res 27:387-398, 2003.
387. Iwama H, Akutsu H, Kuretake S, et al. Serum concentrations of soluble Fas antigen and soluble Fas ligand in mother and newborn. Arch Gynecol Obstet 263:108-110, 2000.
388. Imanishi K, Seo K, Kato H, et al. Post-thymic maturation of migrating human thymic single-positive T cells: thymic CD1a-CD4+ T cells are more susceptible to anergy induction by toxic shock syndrome toxin-1 than cord blood CD4+ T cells. J Immunol 160: 112-119, 1998.
389. Takahashi N, Kato H, Imanishi K, et al. Immunopathophysiological aspects of an emerging neonatal infectious disease induced by a bacterial superantigen. J Clin Invest 106:1409-1415, 2000.
390. Risdon G, Gaddy J, Horie M, et al. Alloantigen priming induces a state of unresponsiveness in human umbilical cord blood T cells. Proc Natl Acad Sci U S A 92:2413-2417, 1995.
391. Porcu P, Gaddy J, Broxmeyer HE. Alloantigen-induced unresponsiveness in cord blood T lymphocytes is associated with defective activation of Ras. Proc Natl Acad Sci U S A 95:4538-4543, 1998.
392. Sporici RA, Beswick RL, von Allmen C, et al. ICOS ligand costimulation is required for T-cell encephalitogenicity. Clin Immunol 100: 277-288, 2001.
393. Rottman JB, Smith T, Tonra JR, et al. The costimulatory molecule ICOS plays an important role in the immunopathogenesis of EAE. Nat Immunol 2:605-611, 2001.
394. Demeure CE, Wu CY, Shu U, et al. In vitro maturation of human neonatal CD4 T lymphocytes II. Cytokines present at priming modulate the development of lymphokine production. J Immunol 152:4775-4782, 1994.
395. Sornasse T, Larenas PV, Davis KA, et al. Differentiation and stability of T helper 1 and 2 cells derived from naïve human neonatal CD4+ T cells, analyzed at the single-cell level. J Exp Med 184:473-483, 1996.
396. Macaubas C, Holt PG. Regulation of cytokine production in T-cell responses to inhalant allergen:GATA-3 expression distinguishes between Th1- and Th2-polarized immunity. Int Arch Allergy Immunol 124:176-179, 2001.
397. Yamaguchi E, de Vries J, Yssel H. Differentiation of human single-positive fetal thymocytes in vitro into IL-4– and/or IFN-gamma–producing CD4+ and CD8+ T cells. Int Immunol 11:593-603, 1999.
398. Early E, Reen D. Antigen-independent responsiveness to interleukin-4 demonstrates differential regulation of newborn human T cells. Eur J Immunol 26:2885-2889, 1996.
399. Bullens DM, Rafiq K, Kasran A, et al. naïve human T cells can be a source of IL-4 during primary immune responses. Clin Exp Immunol 118:384-391, 1999.
400. Langenkamp A, Messi M, Lanzavecchia A, et al. Kinetics of dendritic cell activation: impact on priming of T_H1, T_H2 and nonpolarized T cells. Nat Immunol 1:311-316, 2000.
401. Sato K, Kawasaki H, Morimoto C, et al. An abortive ligand-induced activation of CCR1-mediated downstream signaling event and a deficiency of CCR5 expression are associated with the hyporesponsiveness of human naïve CD4+ T cells to CCL3 and CCL5. J Immunol 168:6263-6272, 2002.
402. Berkowitz RD, Beckerman KP, Schall TJ, et al. CXCR4 and CCR5 expression delineates targets for HIV-1 disruption of T cell differentiation. J Immunol 161:3702-3710, 1998.
403. Christopherson Kn, Brahmi Z, Hromas R. Regulation of naïve fetal T-cell migration by the chemokines Exodus-2 and Exodus-3. Immunol Lett 69:269-273, 1999.
404. Mo H, Monard S, Pollack H, et al. Expression patterns of the HIV type 1 coreceptors CCR5 and cells and monocytes from cord and adult blood. AIDS Res Hum Retroviruses 14:607-617, 1998.
405. Auewarakul P, Sangsiriwut K, Pattanapanyasat K, et al. Age-dependent expression of the HIV-1 coreceptor CCR5 on CD4+ lymphocytes in children. J Acquir Immune Defic Syndr 24:285-287, 2000.
406. Bonecchi R, Bianchi G, Bordignon PP, et al. Differential expression of chemokine receptors and chemotactic responsiveness of type 1 T helper cells (Th1s) and Th2s. J Exp Med 187:129-134, 1998.
407. Fraticelli P, Sironi M, Bianchi G, et al. Fractalkine (CX3CL1) as an amplification circuit of polarized Th1 responses. J Clin Invest 107: 1173-1181, 2001.
408. Chipeta J, Komada Y, Zhang XL, et al. Neonatal (cord blood) T cells can competently raise type 1 and 2 immune responses upon polyclonal activation. Cell Immunol 205:110-119, 2000.
409. Tokimasa S, Ohta H, Sawada A, et al. Lack of the Polycomb-group gene rae28 causes maturation arrest at the early B-cell developmental stage. Exp Hematol 29:93-103, 2001.

410. Sallusto F, Lenig D, Forster R, et al. Two subsets of memory T lymphocytes with distinct homing potentials and effector functions. Nature 401:708-712, 1999.
411. Baron V, Bouneaud C, Cumano A, et al. The repertoires of circulating human CD8(+) central and effector memory T cell subsets are largely distinct. Immunity 18:193-204, 2003.
412. Campbell AC, Waller C, Wood J, et al. Lymphocyte subpopulations in the blood of newborn infants. Clin Exp Immunol 18:469-482, 1974.
413. Andersson U, Bird AG, Britton BS, et al. Humoral and cellular immunity in humans studied at the cell level from birth to two years of age. Immunol Rev 57:1-38, 1981.
414. Lubens RG, Gard SE, Soderberg-Warner M, et al. Lectin-dependent T-lymphocyte and natural killer cytotoxic deficiencies in human newborns. Cell Immunol 74:40-53, 1982.
415. Rayfield LS, Brent L, Rodeck CH. Development of cell-mediated lympholysis in human foetal blood lymphocytes. Clin Exp Immunol 42:561-570, 1980.
416. Granberg C, Hirvonen T. Cell-mediated lympholysis by fetal and neonatal lymphocytes in sheep and man. Cell Immunol 51:13-22, 1980.
417. Risdon G, Gaddy J, Broxmeyer HE. Allogeneic responses of human umbilical cord blood. Blood Cells 20:566-570, 1994.
418. Risdon G, Gaddy J, Stehman FB, et al. Proliferative and cytotoxic responses of human cord blood T lymphocytes following allogeneic stimulation. Cell Immunol 154:14-24, 1994.
419. Harris DT. In vitro and in vivo assessment of the graft-versus-leukemia activity of cord blood. Bone Marrow Transplant 15:17-23, 1995.
420. Barbey C, Irion O, Helg C, et al. Characterisation of the cytotoxic alloresponse of cord blood. Bone Marrow Transplant 22(Suppl 1): S26-S30, 1998.
421. Slavcev A, Striz I, Ivaskova E, et al. Alloresponses of cord blood cells in primary mixed lymphocyte cultures. Hum Immunol 63:155-163, 2002.
422. Berthou C, Legros MS, Soulié A, et al. Cord blood T lymphocytes lack constitutive perforin expression in contrast to adult peripheral blood T lymphocytes. Blood 85:1540-1546, 1995.
423. Kogawa K, Lee SM, Villanueva J, et al. Perforin expression in cytotoxic lymphocytes from patients with hemophagocytic lymphohistiocytosis and their family members. Blood 99:61-66, 2002.
424. Rukavina D, Laskarin G, Rubesa G, et al. Age-related decline of perforin expression in human cytotoxic T lymphocytes and natural killer cells. Blood 92:2410-2420, 1998.
425. de-Jong R, Brouwer M, Miedema F, et al. Human CD8+ T lymphocytes can be divided into $CD45RA^+$ and $CD45RO^+$ cells with different requirements for activation and differentiation. J Immunol 146: 2088-2094, 1991.
426. Akbar AN, Salmon M, Ivory K, et al. Human $CD4^+CD45RO^+$ and $CD4^+CD45RA^+$ T cells synergize in response to alloantigens. Eur J Immunol 21:2517-2522, 1991.
427. Mescher MF. Molecular interactions in the activation of effector and precursor cytotoxic T lymphocytes. Immunol Rev 146:177-210, 1995.
428. Appay V, Dunbar PR, Callan M, et al. Memory $CD8^+$ T cells vary in differentiation phenotype in different persistent virus infections. Nat Med 8:379-385, 2002.
429. Marchant A, Appay V, Van Der Sande M, et al. Mature CD8(+) T lymphocyte response to viral infection during fetal life. J Clin Invest 111:1747-1755, 2003.
430. Penninger JM, Kroemer G. Molecular and cellular mechanisms of T lymphocyte apoptosis. Adv Immunol 68:51-144, 1998.
431. El Ghalbzouri A, Drenou B, Blancheteau V, et al. An in vitro model of allogeneic stimulation of cord blood: induction of Fas independent apoptosis. Hum Immunol 60:598-607, 1999.
432. Tu W, Cheung PT, Lau YL. Insulin-like growth factor 1 promotes cord blood T cell maturation and inhibits its spontaneous and phytohemagglutinin-induced apoptosis through different mechanisms. J Immunol 165:1331-1336, 2000.
433. Suda T, Hashimoto H, Tanaka M, et al. Membrane Fas ligand kills human peripheral blood T lymphocytes, and soluble Fas ligand blocks the killing. J Exp Med 186:2045-2050, 1997.
434. Drenou B, Choqueux C, El Ghalbzouri A, et al. Characterisation of the roles of CD95 and CD95 ligand in cord blood. Bone Marrow Transplant 22(Suppl 1):S44-S47, 1998.
435. Potestio M, Pawelec G, Di Lorenzo G, et al. Age-related changes in the expression of CD95 (APO1/FAS) on blood lymphocytes. Exp Gerontol 34:659-673, 1999.
436. Kuntz TB, Christensen RD, Stegner J, et al. Fas and Fas ligand expression in maternal blood and in umbilical cord blood in preeclampsia. Pediatr Res 50:743-749, 2001.
437. Aggarwal S, Gupta A, Nagata S, et al. Programmed cell death (apoptosis) in cord blood lymphocytes. J Clin Immunol 17:63-73, 1997.
438. Malamitsi-Puchner A, Sarandakou A, Tziotis J, et al. Evidence for a suppression of apoptosis in early postnatal life. Acta Obstet Gynecol Scand 80:994-997, 2001.
439. Aggarwal S, Gollapudi S, Yel L, et al. TNF-alpha-induced apoptosis in neonatal lymphocytes: TNFRp55 expression and downstream pathways of apoptosis. Genes Immun 1:271-279, 2000.
440. Chatenoud L, Salomon B, Bluestone JA. Suppressor T cells—they're back and critical for regulation of autoimmunity! Immunol Rev 182:149-163, 2001.
441. Sakaguchi S, Sakaguchi N, Shimizu J, et al. Immunologic tolerance maintained by $CD25^+CD4^+$ regulatory T cells: their common role in controlling autoimmunity, tumor immunity, and transplantation tolerance. Immunol Rev 182:18-32, 2001.
442. Singh B, Read S, Asseman C, et al. Control of intestinal inflammation by regulatory T cells. Immunol Rev 182:190-200, 2001.
443. Hori S, Nomura T, Sakaguchi S. Control of regulatory T cell development by the transcription factor Foxp3. Science 299:1057-1061, 2003.
444. Gavin M, Rudensky A. Control of immune homeostasis by naturally arising regulatory $CD4^+$ T cells. Curr Opin Immunol 15:690-696, 2003.
445. Leonard WJ. Role of Jak kinases and STATs in cytokine signal transduction. Int J Hematol 73:271-277, 2001.
446. Habib T, Nelson A, Kaushansky K. IL-21: a novel IL-2-family lymphokine that modulates B, T, and natural killer cell responses. J Allergy Clin Immunol 112:1033-1045, 2003.
447. Kanegane H, Miyawaki T, Kato K, et al. A novel subpopulation of $CD45RA^+CD4^+$ T cells expressing IL-2 receptor alpha-chain (CD25) and having a functionally transitional nature into memory cells. Int Immunol 3:1349-1356, 1991.
448. Ng WF, Duggan PJ, Ponchel F, et al. Human CD4(+)CD25(+) cells: a naturally occurring population of regulatory T cells. Blood 98: 2736-2744, 2001.
449. Baecher-Allan C, Brown JA, Freeman GJ, et al. $CD4^+CD25^{high}$ regulatory cells in human peripheral blood. J Immunol 167: 1245-1253, 2001.
450. Taams LS, Smith J, Rustin MH, et al. Human anergic/suppressive CD4(+)CD25(+) T cells: a highly differentiated and apoptosis-prone population. Eur J Immunol 31:1122-1131, 2001.
451. Wing K, Lindgren S, Kollberg G, et al. CD4 T cell activation by myelin oligodendrocyte glycoprotein is suppressed by adult but not cord blood $CD25^+$ T cells. Eur J Immunol 33:579-587, 2003.
452. Akbari O, Stock P, DeKruyff RH, et al. Role of regulatory T cells in allergy and asthma. Curr Opin Immunol 15:627-633, 2003.
453. Kronenberg M, Gapin L. The unconventional lifestyle of NKT cells. Nat Rev Immunol 2:557-568, 2002.
454. Musha N, Yoshida Y, Sugahara S, et al. Expansion of $CD56^+$ NK T and gamma delta T cells from cord blood of human neonates. Clin Exp Immunol 113:220-228, 1998.
455. D'Andrea A, Goux D, De Lalla C, et al. Neonatal invariant $Valpha24^+$ NKT lymphocytes are activated memory cells. Eur J Immunol 30:1544-1550, 2000.
456. van Der Vliet HJ, Nishi N, de Gruijl TD, et al. Human natural killer T cells acquire a memory-activated phenotype before birth. Blood 95:2440-2442, 2000.
457. Kadowaki N, Antonenko S, Ho S, et al. Distinct cytokine profiles of neonatal natural killer T cells after expansion with subsets of dendritic cells. J Exp Med 193:1221-1226, 2001.
458. Gansuvd B, Hagihara M, Yu Y, et al. Human umbilical cord blood NK T cells kill tumors by multiple cytotoxic mechanisms. Hum Immunol 63:164-175, 2002.
459. Kaufmann SH. Gamma/delta and other unconventional T lymphocytes: what do they see and what do they do? Proc Natl Acad Sci U S A 93:2272-2279, 1996.
460. Li H, Lebedeva MI, Llera AS, et al. Structure of the Vdelta domain of a human gammadelta T-cell antigen receptor. Nature 391:502-506, 1998.
461. Tanaka Y, Morita CT, Nieves E, et al. Natural and synthetic non-peptide antigens recognized by human gamma delta T cells. Nature 375:155-158, 1995.

462. Garcia VE, Sieling PA, Gong J, et al. Single-cell cytokine analysis of gamma delta T cell responses to nonpeptide mycobacterial antigens. J Immunol 159:1328-1335, 1997.
463. Kabelitz D. Function and specificity of human gamma/delta-positive T cells. Crit Rev Immunol 11:281-303, 1992.
464. Kolenko V, Bloom T, Rayman P, et al. Inhibition of NF-kappa B activity in human T lymphocytes induces caspase-dependent apoptosis without detectable activation of caspase-1 and -3. J Immunol 163:590-598, 1999.
465. Feurle J, Espinosa E, Eckstein S, et al. *Escherichia coli* produces phosphoantigens activating human gamma delta T cells. J Biol Chem 277:148-154, 2002.
466. Groh V, Steinle A, Bauer S, et al. Recognition of stress-induced MHC molecules by intestinal epithelial gammadelta T cells. Science 279: 1737-1740, 1998.
467. Ghaffari-Tabrizi N, Bauer B, Villunger A, et al. Protein kinase Ctheta, a selective upstream regulator of promoter activation in Jurkat T cells. Eur J Immunol 29:132-142, 1999.
468. Das H, Groh V, Kuijl C, et al. MICA engagement by human Vgamma2Vdelta2 T cells enhances their antigen-dependent effector function. Immunity 15:83-93, 2001.
469. De Paoli P, Gennari D, Martelli P, et al. Gamma delta T cell receptor-bearing lymphocytes during Epstein-Barr virus infection. J Infect Dis 161:1013-1016, 1990.
470. Dechanet J, Merville P, Lim A, et al. Implication of gammadelta T cells in the human immune response to cytomegalovirus. J Clin Invest 103:1437-1449, 1999.
471. Witherden DA, Rieder SE, Boismenu R, et al. A role for epithelial gamma delta T cells in tissue repair. Springer Semin Immunopathol 22:265-281, 2000.
472. Girardi M, Oppenheim DE, Steele CR, et al. Regulation of cutaneous malignancy by gammadelta T cells. Science 294:605-609, 2001.
473. Egan PJ, Carding SR. Downmodulation of the inflammatory response to bacterial infection by gammadelta T cells cytotoxic for activated macrophages. J Exp Med 191:2145-2158, 2000.
474. Dieli F, Troye-Blomberg M, Farouk SE, et al. Biology of gammadelta T cells in tuberculosis and malaria. Curr Mol Med 1:437-446, 2001.
475. Wang L, Das H, Kamath A, et al. Human V gamma 2V delta 2 T cells produce IFN-gamma and TNF-alpha with an on/off/on cycling pattern in response to live bacterial products. J Immunol 167: 6195-6201, 2001.
476. Rothenfusser S, Hornung V, Krug A, et al. Distinct CpG oligonucleotide sequences activate human gamma delta T cells via interferon-alpha/-beta. Eur J Immunol 31:3525-3534, 2001.
477. Fujihashi K, McGhee JR, Kweon MN, et al. gamma/delta T cell-deficient mice have impaired mucosal immunoglobulin A responses. J Exp Med 183:1929-1935, 1996.
478. Ladel CH, Blum C, Dreher A, et al. Protective role of gamma/delta T cells and alpha/beta T cells in tuberculosis. Eur J Immunol 25: 2877-2881, 1995.
479. Ladel CH, Blum C, Kaufmann SH. Control of natural killer cell-mediated innate resistance against the intracellular pathogen Listeria monocytogenes by gamma/delta T lymphocytes. Infect Immun 64:1744-1749, 1996.
480. Sciammas R, Kodukula P, Tang Q, et al. T cell receptor-gamma/delta cells protect mice from herpes simplex virus type 1-induced lethal encephalitis. J Exp Med 185:1969-1975, 1997.
481. Wang L, Kamath A, Das H, et al. Antibacterial effect of human V gamma 2V delta 2 T cells in vivo. J Clin Invest 108:1349-1357, 2001.
482. Borst J, Vroom TM, Bos JD, et al. Tissue distribution and repertoire selection of human gamma delta T cells: comparison with the murine system. Curr Top Microbiol Immunol 173:41-46, 1991.
483. Saito H, Kanamori Y, Takemori T, et al. Generation of intestinal T cells from progenitors residing in gut cryptopatches. Science 280:275-278, 1998.
484. MacDonald HR, Radtke F, Wilson A. T cell fate specification and alphabeta/gammadelta lineage commitment. Curr Opin Immunol 13:219-224, 2001.
485. Saint-Ruf C, Panigada M, Azogui O, et al. Different initiation of pre-TCR and gammadeltaTCR signalling. Nature 406:524-527, 2000.
486. Bigby M, Markowitz JS, Bleicher PA, et al. Most gamma delta T cells develop normally in the absence of MHC class II molecules. J Immunol 151:4465-4475, 1993.
487. Chien YH, Jores R, Crowley MP. Recognition by gamma/delta T cells. Annu Rev Immunol 14:511-532, 1996.
488. McVay LD, Jaswal SS, Kennedy C, et al. The generation of human gammadelta T cell repertoires during fetal development. J Immunol 160:5851-5860, 1998.
489. McVay LD, Carding SR. Generation of human gammadelta T-cell repertoires. Crit Rev Immunol 19:431-460, 1999.
490. Bukowski JF, Morita CT, Brenner MB. Recognition and destruction of virus-infected cells by human gamma delta CTL. J Immunol 153: 5133-5140, 1994.
491. Erbach GT, Semple JP, Osathanondh R, et al. Phenotypic characteristics of lymphoid populations of middle gestation human fetal liver, spleen and thymus. J Reprod Immunol 25:81-88, 1993.
492. Wucherpfennig KW, Liao YJ, Prendergast M, et al. Human fetal liver gamma/delta T cells predominantly use unusual rearrangements of the T cell receptor delta and gamma loci expressed on both $CD4^+CD8^-$ and $CD4^-CD8^-$ gamma/delta T cells. J Exp Med 177: 425-432, 1993.
493. Miyagawa Y, Matsuoka T, Baba A, et al. Fetal liver T cell receptor gamma/delta$^+$ T cells as cytotoxic T lymphocytes specific for maternal alloantigens. J Exp Med 176:1-7, 1992.
494. Beldjord K, Beldjord C, Macintyre E, et al. Peripheral selection of V delta 1^+ cells with restricted T cell receptor delta gene junctional repertoire in the peripheral blood of healthy donors. J Exp Med 178:121-127, 1993.
495. Shen J, Andrews DM, Pandolfi F, et al. Oligoclonality of Vdelta1 and Vdelta2 cells in human peripheral blood mononuclear cells: TCR selection is not altered by stimulation with gram-negative bacteria. J Immunol 160:3048-3055, 1998.
496. Parker CM, Groh V, Band H, et al. Evidence for extrathymic changes in the T cell receptor gamma/delta repertoire. J Exp Med 171: 1597-1612, 1990.
497. Tsuyuguchi I, Kawasumi H, Ueta C, et al. Increase of T-cell receptor gamma/delta-bearing T cells in cord blood of newborn babies obtained by in vitro stimulation with mycobacterial cord factor. Infect Immun 59:3053-3059, 1991.
498. Smith MD, Worman C, Yuksel F, et al. T gamma delta-cell subsets in cord and adult blood. Scand J Immunol 32:491-495, 1990.
499. Steele RW, Suttle DE, LeMaster PC, et al. Screening for cell-mediated immunity in children. Am J Dis Child 130:1218-1221, 1976.
500. Munoz AI, Limbert D. Skin reactivity to *Candida* and streptokinase-streptodornase antigens in normal pediatric subjects: influence of age and acute illness. J Pediatr 91:565-568, 1977.
501. Franz ML, Carella JA, Galant SP. Cutaneous delayed hypersensitivity in a healthy pediatric population: diagnostic value of diptheria-tetanus toxoids. J Pediatr 88:975-977, 1976.
502. Warwick W, Good RA, Smith RT. Failure of passive transfer of delayed hypersensitivity in the newborn human infant. J Lab Clin Med 56:139-147, 1960.
503. Uhr JW, Dancis J, Neumann CG. Delayed-type hypersensitivity in premature neonatal humans. Nature 187:1130-1131, 1960.
504. Bonforte RJ, Topilsky M, Siltzbach LE, et al. Phytohemagglutinin skin test: a possible in vivo measure of cell-mediated immunity. J Pediatr 81:775-780, 1972.
505. Kniker WT, Lesourd BM, McBryde JL, et al. Cell-mediated immunity assessed by Multitest CMI skin testing in infants and preschool children. Am J Dis Child 139:840-845, 1985.
506. Fowler R Jr, Schubert WK, West CD. Acquired partial tolerance to homologous skin grafts in the human infant at birth. Ann N Y Acad Sci 87:403-428, 1960.
507. Rouleau M, Namikawa R, Antonenko S, et al. Antigen-specific cytotoxic T cells mediate human fetal pancreas allograft rejection in SCID-hu mice. J Immunol 157:5710-5720, 1996.
508. Orlandi F, Giambona A, Messana F, et al. Evidence of induced non-tolerance in HLA-identical twins with hemoglobinopathy after in utero fetal transplantation. Bone Marrow Transplant 18:637-639, 1996.
509. Vietor HE, Bolk J, Vreugdenhil GR, et al. Alterations in cord blood leukocyte subsets of patients with severe hemolytic disease after intrauterine transfusion therapy. J Pediatr 130:718-724, 1997.
510. Vietor HE, Hawes GE, van den Oever C, et al. Intrauterine transfusions affect fetal T-cell immunity. Blood 90:2492-2501, 1997.
511. Naiman JL, Punnett HH, Lischner HW, et al. Possible graft-versus-host reaction after intrauterine transfusion for Rh erythroblastosis fetalis. N Engl J Med 281:697-701, 1969.
512. Parkman R, Mosier D, Umansky I, et al. Graft-versus-host disease after intrauterine and exchange transfusions for hemolytic disease of the newborn. N Engl J Med 290:359-363, 1974.

513. Berger RS, Dixon SL. Fulminant transfusion-associated graft-versus-host disease in a premature infant. J Am Acad Dermatol 20:945-950, 1989.
514. Flidel O, Barak Y, Lifschitz-Mercer B, et al. Graft versus host disease in extremely low birth weight neonate. Pediatrics 89:689-690, 1992.
515. Field EJ, Caspary EA. Is maternal lymphocyte sensitisation passed to the child? Lancet 2:337-342, 1971.
516. Szepfalusi Z, Nentwich I, Gerstmayr M, et al. Prenatal allergen contact with milk proteins. Clin Exp Allergy 27:28-35, 1997.
517. Prescott S, Macaubas C, Yabuhara A, et al. Developing patterns of T cell memory to environmental allergens during the first two years of life. Int Arch Allergy Immunol 113:75-79, 1997.
518. Van-Duren-Schmidt K, Pichler J, Ebner C, et al. Prenatal contact with inhalant allergens. Pediatr Res 41:128-131, 1997.
519. Prescott S, Macaubas C, Holt B, et al. Transplacental priming of the human immune system to environmental allergens: universal skewing of initial T cell responses toward the Th2 cytokine profile. J Immunol 160:4730-4737, 1998.
520. Prescott SL, Macaubas C, Smallacombe T, et al. Reciprocal age-related patterns of allergen-specific T-cell immunity in normal vs. atopic infants. Clin Exp Allergy 28(Suppl 5):39-44, discussion 50-31, 1998.
521. Miller RL, Chew GL, Bell CA, et al. Prenatal exposure, maternal sensitization, and sensitization in utero to indoor allergens in an inner-city cohort. Am J Respir Crit Care Med 164:995-1001, 2001.
522. Devereux G, Hall AM, Barker RN. Measurement of T-helper cytokines secreted by cord blood in response to allergens. J Immunol Methods 234:13-22, 2000.
523. Szepfalusi Z, Pichler J, Elsasser S, et al. Transplacental priming of the human immune system with environmental allergens can occur early in gestation. J Allergy Clin Immunol 106:530-536, 2000.
524. Englund JA, Mbawuike IN, Hammill H, et al. Maternal immunization with influenza or tetanus toxoid vaccine for passive antibody protection in young infants. J Infect Dis 168:647-656, 1993.
525. Malhotra I, Mungai P, Wamachi A, et al. Helminth- and bacillus Calmette-Guérin–induced immunity in children sensitized in utero to filariasis and schistosomiasis. J Immunol 162:6843-6848, 1999.
526. King CL, Malhotra I, Wamachi A, et al. Acquired immune responses to *Plasmodium falciparum* merozoite surface protein-1 in the human fetus. J Immunol 168:356-364, 2002.
527. Kuhn L, Coutsoudis A, Moodley D, et al. T-helper cell responses to HIV envelope peptides in cord blood: against intrapartum and breast-feeding transmission. AIDS 15:1-9, 2001.
528. Schlesinger JJ, Covelli HD. Evidence for transmission of lymphocyte responses to tuberculin by breast-feeding. Lancet 2:529-532, 1977.
529. Shiratsuchi H, Tsuyuguchi I. Tuberculin purified protein derivative–reactive T cells in cord blood lymphocytes. Infect Immun 33:651-657, 1981.
530. Barnetson RS, Bjune G, Duncan ME. Evidence for a soluble lymphocyte factor in the transplacental transmission of T-lymphocyte responses to *Mycobacterium leprae*. Nature 260:150-151, 1976.
531. Gallagher MR, Welliver R, Yamanaka T, et al. Cell-mediated immune responsiveness to measles. Its occurrence as a result of naturally acquired or vaccine-induced infection and in infants of immune mothers. Am J Dis Child 135:48-51, 1981.
532. Thong YH, Hurtado RC, Rola-Pleszczynski M, et al. Transplacental transmission of cell-mediated immunity. Letter to the editor. Lancet 1:1286-1287, 1974.
533. Leikin S, Oppenheim JJ. Differences in transformation of adult and newborn lymphocytes stimulated by antigen, antibody, and antigen-antibody complexes. Cell Immunol 1:468-475, 1970.
534. Brody JI, Oski FA, Wallach EE. Neonatal lymphocyte reactivity as an indicator of intrauterine bacterial contact. Lancet 1:1396-1398, 1968.
535. Ivanyi L, Lehner T. Interdependence of in vitro responsiveness of cord and maternal blood lymphocytes to antigens from oral bacteria. Clin Exp Immunol 30:252-258, 1977.
536. Rubin HR, Sorensen RU, Polmar SH. Lymphocyte responses of human neonates to bacterial antigens. Cell Immunol 57:307-315, 1981.
537. Lo Y, Lo E, Watson N, et al. Two-way traffic between mother and fetus: biologic and clinical implications. Blood 88:4390-4395, 1996.
538. Friedmann PS. Cell-mediated immunological reactivity in neonates and infants with congenital syphilis. Clin Exp Immunol 30:271-276, 1977.
539. Starr SE, Tolpin MD, Friedman HM, et al. Impaired cellular immunity to cytomegalovirus in congenitally infected children and their mothers. J Infect Dis 140:500-505, 1979.
540. Pass RF, Stagno S, Britt WJ, et al. Specific cell-mediated immunity and the natural history of congenital infection with cytomegalovirus. J Infect Dis 148:953-961, 1983.
541. Buimovici-Klein E, Cooper LZ. Cell-mediated immune response in rubella infections. Rev Infect Dis 7(Suppl 1):S123-S128, 1985.
542. Paryani SG, Arvin AM. Intrauterine infection with varicella-zoster virus after maternal varicella. N Engl J Med 314:1542-1546, 1986.
543. McLeod R, Mack DG, Boyer K, et al. Phenotypes and functions of lymphocytes in congenital toxoplasmosis. J Lab Clin Med 116: 623-635, 1990.
544. Aase JM, Noren GR, Reddy DV, et al. Mumps-virus infection in pregnant women and the immunologic response of their offspring. N Engl J Med 286:1379-1382, 1972.
545. Luzuriaga K, Holmes D, Hereema A, et al. HIV-1-specific cytotoxic T lymphocyte responses in the first year of life. J Immunol 154: 433-443, 1995.
546. Brander C, Goulder PJ, Luzuriaga K, et al. Persistent HIV-1–specific CTL clonal expansion despite high viral burden post in utero HIV-1 infection. J Immunol 162:4796-4800, 1999.
547. Hermann E, Truyens C, Alonso-Vega C, et al. Human fetuses are able to mount an adultlike CD8 T-cell response. Blood 100:2153-2158, 2002.
548. Hohlfeld P, Forestier F, Marion S, et al. *Toxoplasma gondii* infection during pregnancy: T lymphocyte subpopulations in mothers and fetuses. Pediatr Infect Dis J 9:878-881, 1990.
549. Thilaganathan B, Carroll SG, Plachouras N, et al. Fetal immunological and haematological changes in intrauterine infection. Br J Obstet Gynaecol. 101:418-421, 1994.
550. Bruning T, Daiminger A, Enders G. Diagnostic value of CD45RO expression on circulating T lymphocytes of fetuses and newborn infants with pre-, peri- or early post-natal infections. Clin Exp Immunol 107:306-311, 1997.
551. Michie C, Scott A, Cheesbrough J, et al. Streptococcal toxic shock–like syndrome: evidence of superantigen activity and its effects on T lymphocyte subsets in vivo. Clin Exp Immunol 98:140-144, 1994.
552. Hara T, Ohashi S, Yamashita Y, et al. Human V delta 2^+ gamma delta T-cell tolerance to foreign antigens of *Toxoplasma gondii*. Proc Natl Acad Sci U S A 93:5136-5140, 1996.
553. Sullender WM, Miller JL, Yasukawa LL, et al. Humoral and cell-mediated immunity in neonates with herpes simplex virus infection. J Infect Dis 155:28-37, 1987.
554. Burchett SK, Corey L, Mohan KM, et al. Diminished interferon-gamma and lymphocyte proliferation in neonatal and postpartum primary herpes simplex virus infection. J Infect Dis 165:813-818, 1992.
555. Gibson L, Piccinini G, Lilleri D, et al. Human cytomegalovirus proteins pp65 and immediate early protein 1 are common targets for CD8(+) T cell responses in children with congenital or postnatal human cytomegalovirus infection. J Immunol 172:2256-2264, 2004.
556. Marchant A, Goetghebuer T, Ota MO, et al. Newborns develop a Th1-type immune response to *Mycobacterium bovis* bacillus Calmette-Guérin vaccination. J Immunol 163:2249-2255, 1999.
557. Ota MO, Vekemans J, Schlegel-Haueter SE, et al. Influence of *Mycobacterium bovis* bacillus Calmette-Guérin on antibody and cytokine responses to human neonatal vaccination. J Immunol 168:919-925, 2002.
558. Vekemans J, Ota MO, Wang EC, et al. T cell responses to vaccines in infants: defective IFNgamma production after oral polio vaccination. Clin Exp Immunol 127:495-498, 2002.
559. Riviere Y, Buseyne F. Cytotoxic T lymphocytes generation capacity in early life with particular reference to HIV. Vaccine 16:1420-1422, 1998.
560. Pikora CA, Sullivan JL, Panicali D, et al. Early HIV-1 envelope-specific cytotoxic T lymphocyte responses in vertically infected infants. J Exp Med 185:1153-1161, 1997.
561. Park AY, Scott P. IL-12: keeping cell-mediated immunity alive. Scand J Immunol 53:529-532, 2001.
562. Luzuriaga K, McManus M, Catalina M, et al. Early therapy of vertical human immunodeficiency virus type 1 (HIV-1) infection: control of viral replication and absence of persistent HIV-1–specific immune responses. J Virol 74:6984-6991, 2000.
563. Pacanowski J, Kahi S, Baillet M, et al. Reduced blood $CD123^+$ (lymphoid) and $CD11c^+$ (myeloid) dendritic cell numbers in primary HIV-1 infection. Blood 98:3016-3021, 2001.
564. Stumptner-Cuvelette P, Morchoisne S, Dugast M, et al. HIV-1 Nef impairs MHC class II antigen presentation and surface expression. Proc Natl Acad Sci U S A 98:12144-12149, 2001.

565. Nielsen SD, Jeppesen DL, Kolte L, et al. Impaired progenitor cell function in HIV-negative infants of HIV-positive mothers results in decreased thymic output and low CD4 counts. Blood 98:398-404, 2001.
566. Badley AD, Pilon AA, Landay A, et al. Mechanisms of HIV-associated lymphocyte apoptosis. Blood 96:2951-2964, 2000.
567. Chougnet C, Kovacs A, Baker R, et al. Influence of human immunodeficiency virus--infected maternal environment on development of infant interleukin-12 production. J Infect Dis 181:1590-1597, 2000.
568. Chiba Y, Higashidate Y, Suga K, et al. Development of cell-mediated cytotoxic immunity to respiratory syncytial virus in human infants following naturally acquired infection. J Med Virol 28:133-139, 1989.
569. Chang J, Braciale TJ. Respiratory syncytial virus infection suppresses lung $CD8^+$ T-cell effector activity and peripheral $CD8^+$ T-cell memory in the respiratory tract. Nat Med 8:54-60, 2002.
570. Rajewsky K. Clonal selection and learning in the antibody system. Nature 381:751-758, 1996.
571. Ozaki K, Spolski R, Feng CG, et al. A critical role for IL-21 in regulating immunoglobulin production. Science 298:1630-1634, 2002.
572. Vos Q, Lees A, Wu ZQ, et al. B-cell activation by T-cell-independent type 2 antigens as an integral part of the humoral immune response to pathogenic microorganisms. Immunol Rev 176:154-170, 2000.
573. Poe JC, Hasegawa M, Tedder TF. CD19, CD21, and CD22: multifaceted response regulators of B lymphocyte signal transduction. Int Rev Immunol 20:739-762, 2001.
574. Fearon DT, Carroll MC. Regulation of B lymphocyte responses to foreign and self-antigens by the CD19/CD21 complex. Annu Rev Immunol 18:393-422, 2000.
575. Haas KM, Hasegawa M, Steeber DA, et al. Complement receptors CD21/35 link innate and protective immunity during *Streptococcus pneumoniae* infection by regulating IgG3 antibody responses. Immunity 17:713-723, 2002.
576. Ravetch JV, Bolland S. IgG Fc receptors. Annu Rev Immunol 19: 275-290, 2001.
577. Takai T, Ono M, Hikida M, et al. Augmented humoral and anaphylactic responses in Fc gamma RII-deficient mice. Nature 379:346-349, 1996.
578. Vekemans J, Amedei A, Ota MO, et al. Neonatal bacillus Calmette-Guérin vaccination induces adult-like IFN-gamma production by $CD4^+$ T lymphocytes. Eur J Immunol 31:1531-1535, 2001.
579. Padlan EA. Anatomy of the antibody molecule. Mol Immunol 31: 169-217, 1994.
580. Schroeder HW Jr, Ippolito GC, Shiokawa S. Regulation of the antibody repertoire through control of HCDR3 diversity. Vaccine 16: 1383-1390, 1998.
581. Stewart AK, Huang C, Stollar BD, et al. High-frequency representation of a single VH gene in the expressed human B cell repertoire. J Exp Med 177:1227, 1993.
582. Kraj P, Rao SP, Glas AM, et al. The human heavy chain Ig V region gene repertoire is biased at all stages of B cell ontogeny, including early pre-B cells. J Immunol 158:5824-5832, 1997.
583. Hardy RR. B-cell commitment: deciding on the players. Curr Opin Immunol 15:158-165, 2003.
584. Martensson IL, Rolink A, Melchers F, et al. The pre-B cell receptor and its role in proliferation and Ig heavy chain allelic exclusion. Semin Immunol 14:335-342, 2002.
585. Minegishi Y, Coustan-Smith E, Wang YH, et al. Mutations in the human lambda5/14.1 gene result in B cell deficiency and agammaglobulinemia. J Exp Med 187:71-77, 1998.
586. Nunez C, Nishimoto N, Gartland GL, et al. B cells are generated throughout life in humans. J Immunol 156:866-872, 1996.
587. Kubagawa H, Cooper MD, Carroll AJ, et al. Light-chain gene expression before heavy-chain gene rearrangement in pre-B cells transformed by Epstein-Barr virus. Proc Natl Acad Sci U S A 86:2356-2360, 1989.
588. Hoffmann R, Melchers F. A genomic view of lymphocyte development. Curr Opin Immunol 15:239-245, 2003.
589. Conley ME. Genes required for B cell development. J Clin Invest 112:1636-1638, 2003.
590. Kouro T, Nagata K, Takaki S, et al. Bruton's tyrosine kinase is required for signaling the CD79b-mediated pro-B to pre-B cell transition. Int Immunol 13:485-493, 2001.
591. Muljo SA, Schlissel MS. The variable, C(H)1, C(H)2 and C(H)3 domains of Ig heavy chain are dispensable for pre-BCR function in transgenic mice. Int Immunol 14:577-584, 2002.
592. Jung D, Alt FW. Unraveling V(D)J recombination; insights into gene regulation. Cell 116:299-311, 2004.
593. Brauninger A, Goossens T, Rajewsky K, et al. Regulation of immunoglobulin light chain gene rearrangements during early B cell development in the human. Eur J Immunol 31:3631-3637, 2001.
594. Blomberg BB, Glozak MA, Donohoe ME. Regulation of human lambda light chain gene expression. Ann N Y Acad Sci 764:84-98, 1995.
595. Giachino C, Padovan E, Lanzavecchia A. $Kappa^+lambda^+$ dual receptor B cells are present in the human peripheral repertoire. J Exp Med 181:1245-1250, 1995.
596. Carsetti R, Rosado MM, Wardmann H. Peripheral development of B cells in mouse and man. Immunol Rev 197:179-191, 2004.
597. Brezinschek HP, Brezinschek RI, Lipsky PE. Analysis of the heavy chain repertoire of human peripheral B cells using single-cell polymerase chain reaction. J Immunol 155:190-202, 1995.
598. Wang H, Clarke SH. Positive selection focuses the VH12 B-cell repertoire towards a single B1 specificity with survival function. Immunol Rev 197:51-59, 2004.
599. Fuentes-Panana EM, Bannish G, Monroe JG. Basal B-cell receptor signaling in B lymphocytes: mechanisms of regulation and role in positive selection, differentiation, and peripheral survival. Immunol Rev 197:26-40, 2004.
600. Healy JI, Goodnow CC. Positive versus negative signaling by lymphocyte antigen receptors. Annu Rev Immunol 16:645-670, 1998.
601. Ait-Azzouzene D, Skog P, Retter M, et al. Tolerance-induced receptor selection: scope, sensitivity, locus specificity, and relationship to lymphocyte-positive selection. Immunol Rev 197:219-230, 2004.
602. Halverson R, Torres RM, Pelanda R. Receptor editing is the main mechanism of B cell tolerance toward membrane antigens. Nat Immunol 5:645-650, 2004.
603. Goebel S, Gross U, Luder CG. Inhibition of host cell apoptosis by *Toxoplasma gondii* is accompanied by reduced activation of the caspase cascade and alterations of poly(ADP-ribose) polymerase expression. J Cell Sci 114:3495-3505, 2001.
604. Waldschmidt TJ, Noelle RJ. Immunology. Long live the mature B cell—a baffling mystery resolved. Science 293:2012-2013, 2001.
605. Casola S, Otipoby KL, Alimzhanov M, et al. B cell receptor signal strength determines B cell fate. Nat Immunol 5:317-327, 2004.
606. Pillai S, Cariappa A, Moran ST. Positive selection and lineage commitment during peripheral B-lymphocyte development. Immunol Rev 197:206-218, 2004.
607. Chung JB, Silverman M, Monroe JG. Transitional B cells: step by step towards immune competence. Trends Immunol 24:343-349, 2003.
608. Klein U, Rajewsky K, Kuppers R. Human immunoglobulin $(Ig)M^+IgD^+$ peripheral blood B cells expressing the CD27 cell surface antigen carry somatically mutated variable region genes: CD27 as a general marker for somatically mutated (memory) B cells. J Exp Med 188:1679-1689, 1998.
609. Okada T, Ngo VN, Ekland EH, et al. Chemokine requirements for B cell entry to lymph nodes and Peyer's patches. J Exp Med 196: 65-75, 2002.
610. Batista FD, Iber D, Neuberger MS. B cells acquire antigen from target cells after synapse formation. Nature 411:489-494, 2001.
611. Feldhahn N, Schwering I, Lee S, et al. Silencing of B cell receptor signals in human naïve B cells. J Exp Med 196:1291-1305, 2002.
612. Clark MR, Massenburg D, Siemasko K, et al. B-cell antigen receptor signaling requirements for targeting antigen to the MHC class II presentation pathway. Curr Opin Immunol 16:382-387, 2004.
613. Reif K, Ekland EH, Ohl L, et al. Balanced responsiveness to chemoattractants from adjacent zones determines B-cell position. Nature 416:94-99, 2002.
614. Croft M. Co-stimulatory members of the TNFR family: keys to effective T-cell immunity? Nat Rev Immunol 3:609-620, 2003.
615. McHeyzer-Williams MG. B cells as effectors. Curr Opin Immunol 15:354-361, 2003.
616. Langenkamp A, Nagata K, Murphy K, et al. Kinetics and expression patterns of chemokine receptors in human $CD4^+$ T lymphocytes primed by myeloid or plasmacytoid dendritic cells. Eur J Immunol 33:474-482, 2003.
617. Campbell DJ, Kim CH, Butcher EC. Separable effector T cell populations specialized for B cell help or tissue inflammation. Nat Immunol 2:876-881, 2001.
618. Garside P, Ingulli E, Merica RR, et al. Visualization of specific B and T lymphocyte interactions in the lymph node. Science 281:96-99, 1998.

619. Kim CH, Rott LS, Clark-Lewis I, et al. Subspecialization of CXCR5$^+$ T cells: B helper activity is focused in a germinal center-localized subset of CXCR5$^+$ T cells. J Exp Med 193:1373-1381, 2001.
620. Johansson-Lindbom B, Ingvarsson S, Borrebaeck CA. Germinal centers regulate human Th2 development. J Immunol 171:1657-1666, 2003.
621. Mak TW, Shahinian A, Yoshinaga SK, et al. Costimulation through the inducible costimulator ligand is essential for both T helper and B cell functions in T cell–dependent B cell responses. Nat Immunol 4:765-772, 2003.
622. Kouskoff V, Famiglietti S, Lacaud G, et al. Antigens varying in affinity for the B cell receptor induce differential B lymphocyte responses. J Exp Med 188:1453-1464, 1998.
623. Haberman AM, Shlomchik MJ. Reassessing the function of immune-complex retention by follicular dendritic cells. Nat Rev Immunol 3:757-764, 2003.
624. de Villartay JP, Fischer A, Durandy A. The mechanisms of immune diversification and their disorders. Nat Rev Immunol 3:962-972, 2003.
625. Jacob J, Kelsoe G, Rajewsky K, et al. Intraclonal generation of antibody mutants in germinal centres. Nature 354:389-392, 1991.
626. Goossens T, Brauninger A, Klein U, et al. Receptor revision plays no major role in shaping the receptor repertoire of human memory B cells after the onset of somatic hypermutation. Eur J Immunol 31: 3638-3648, 2001.
627. Gray D, Dullforce P, Jainandunsing S. Memory B cell development but not germinal center formation is impaired by in vivo blockade of CD40–CD40 ligand interaction. J Exp Med 180:141-155, 1994.
628. Carroll MC. The role of complement and complement receptors in induction and regulation of immunity. Annu Rev Immunol 16: 545-568, 1998.
629. McHeyzer-Williams MG, Nossal GJ, Lalor PA. Molecular characterization of single memory B cells. Nature 350:502-505, 1991.
630. Crotty S, Felgner P, Davies H, et al. Cutting edge: long-term B cell memory in humans after smallpox vaccination. J Immunol 171: 4969-4973, 2003.
631. Bernasconi NL, Traggiai E, Lanzavecchia A. Maintenance of serological memory by polyclonal activation of human memory B cells. Science 298:2199-2202, 2002.
632. Maruyama M, Lam KP, Rajewsky K. Memory B-cell persistence is independent of persisting immunizing antigen. Nature 407:636-642, 2000.
633. Shapiro-Shelef M, Calame K. Plasma cell differentiation and multiple myeloma. Curr Opin Immunol 16:226-234, 2004.
634. Slifka MK, Ahmed R. Long-lived plasma cells: a mechanism for maintaining persistent antibody production. Curr Opin Immunol 10:252-258, 1998.
635. Zhang K, Mills FC, Saxon A. Switch circles from IL-4–directed epsilon class switching from human B lymphocytes. Evidence for direct, sequential, and multiple step sequential switch from mu to epsilon Ig heavy chain gene. J Immunol 152:3427-3435, 1994.
636. Coffman RL, Lebman DA, Rothman P. Mechanism and regulation of immunoglobulin isotype switching. Adv Immunol 54:229-270, 1993.
637. Kimata H, Fujimoto M. Induction of IgA1 and IgA2 production in immature human fetal B cells and pre-B cells by vasoactive intestinal peptide. Blood 85:2098-2104, 1995.
638. Pape KA, Kouskoff V, Nemazee D, et al. Visualization of the genesis and fate of isotype-switched B cells during a primary immune response. J Exp Med 197:1677-1687, 2003.
639. Toellner KM, Gulbranson JA, Taylor DR, et al. Immunoglobulin switch transcript production in vivo related to the site and time of antigen-specific B cell activation. J Exp Med 183:2303-2312, 1996.
640. Ochs HD, Winkelstein J. Disorders of the B-cell system. *In* Stiehm ER (ed). Immunologic Disorders in Infants and Children. Philadelphia, WB Saunders, 1996, pp 296-338.
641. Weller S, Faili A, Garcia C, et al. CD40-CD40L independent Ig gene hypermutation suggests a second B cell diversification pathway in humans. Proc Natl Acad Sci U S A 98:1166-1170, 2001.
642. Toyama H, Okada S, Hatano M, et al. Memory B cells without somatic hypermutation are generated from Bcl6-deficient B cells. Immunity 17:329-339, 2002.
643. Khan WN. Regulation of B lymphocyte development and activation by Bruton's tyrosine kinase. Immunol Res 23:147-156, 2001.
644. Mackay F, Schneider P, Rennert P, et al. BAFF and APRIL: a tutorial on B cell survival. Annu Rev Immunol 21:231-264, 2003.
645. Cassese G, Arce S, Hauser AE, et al. Plasma cell survival is mediated by synergistic effects of cytokines and adhesion-dependent signals. J Immunol 171:1684-1690, 2003.
646. Bartholdy B, Matthias P. Transcriptional control of B cell development and function. Gene 327:1-23, 2004.
647. Calame KL, Lin KI, Tunyaplin C. Regulatory mechanisms that determine the development and function of plasma cells. Annu Rev Immunol 21:205-230, 2003.
648. Tangye SG, Liu YJ, Aversa G, et al. Identification of functional human splenic memory B cells by expression of CD148 and CD27. J Exp Med 188:1691-1703, 1998.
649. Timens W, Poppema S. Lymphocyte compartments in human spleen. An immunohistologic study in normal spleens and uninvolved spleens in Hodgkin's disease. Am J Pathol 120:443-454, 1985.
650. Dono M, Zupo S, Colombo M, et al. The human marginal zone B cell. Ann N Y Acad Sci 987:117-124, 2003.
651. Spencer J, Perry ME, Dunn-Walters DK. Human marginal-zone B cells. Immunol Today 19:421-426, 1998.
652. Dunn-Walters DK, Isaacson PG, Spencer J. Analysis of mutations in immunoglobulin heavy chain variable region genes of microdissected marginal zone (MGZ) B cells suggests that the MGZ of human spleen is a reservoir of memory B cells. J Exp Med 182:559-566, 1995.
653. Tierens A, Delabie J, Michiels L, et al. Marginal-zone B cells in the human lymph node and spleen show somatic hypermutations and display clonal expansion. Blood 93:226-234, 1999.
654. Martin F, Kearney JF. B1 cells: similarities and differences with other B cell subsets. Curr Opin Immunol 13:195-201, 2001.
655. Oliver AM, Martin F, Kearney JF. IgM^{high}CD21^{high} lymphocytes enriched in the splenic marginal zone generate effector cells more rapidly than the bulk of follicular B cells. J Immunol 162:7198-7207, 1999.
656. Balazs M, Martin F, Zhou T, et al. Blood dendritic cells interact with splenic marginal zone B cells to initiate T-independent immune responses. Immunity 17:341-352, 2002.
657. Amlot PL, Hayes AE. Impaired human antibody response to the thymus-independent antigen, DNP-Ficoll, after splenectomy. Implications for post-splenectomy infections. Lancet 1:1008-1011, 1985.
658. Reeves EP, Lu H, Jacobs HL, et al. Killing activity of neutrophils is mediated through activation of proteases by K^+ flux. Nature 416: 291-297, 2002.
659. Vinuesa CG, Sze DM, Cook MC, et al. Recirculating and germinal center B cells differentiate into cells responsive to polysaccharide antigens. Eur J Immunol 33:297-305, 2003.
660. Kasaian MT, Ikematsu H, Casali P. Identification and analysis of a novel human surface CD5– B lymphocyte subset producing natural antibodies. J Immunol 148:2690-2702, 1992.
661. Brezinschek HP, Foster SJ, Brezinschek RI, et al. Analysis of the human VH gene repertoire. Differential effects of selection and somatic hypermutation on human peripheral CD5(+)/IgM$^+$ and CD5(−)/IgM$^+$ B cells. J Clin Invest 99:2488-2501, 1997.
662. Dorner T, Brezinschek HP, Foster SJ, et al. Comparable impact of mutational and selective influences in shaping the expressed repertoire of peripheral IgM$^+$/CD5$^-$ and IgM$^+$/CD5$^+$ B cells. Eur J Immunol 28:657-668, 1998.
663. Chen ZJ, Wheeler CJ, Shi W, et al. Polyreactive antigen-binding B cells are the predominant cell type in the newborn B cell repertoire. Eur J Immunol 28:989-994, 1998.
664. Bhat NM, Kantor AB, Bieber MM, et al. The ontogeny and functional characteristics of human B-1 CD5$^+$ B cells. Int Immunol 4:243-252, 1992.
665. Kipps TJ, Robbins BA, Carson DA. Uniform high frequency expression of autoantibody-associated crossreactive idiotypes in the primary B cell follicles of human fetal spleen. J Exp Med 171:189-196, 1990.
666. Schettino EW, Chai SK, Kasaian MT, et al. VHDJH gene sequences and antigen reactivity of monoclonal antibodies produced by human B-1 cells: evidence for somatic selection. J Immunol 158:2477-2489, 1997.
667. Klein U, Kuppers R, Rajewsky K. Evidence for a large compartment of IgM-expressing memory B cells in humans. Blood 89:1288-1298, 1997.
668. Nash PB, Purner MB, Leon RP, et al. *Toxoplasma gondii*–infected cells are resistant to multiple inducers of apoptosis. J Immunol 160: 1824-1830, 1998.
669. Gathings WE, Lawton AR, Cooper MD. Immunofluorescent studies of the development of pre-B cells, B lymphocytes and immunoglobulin isotype diversity in humans. Eur J Immunol 7:804-810, 1977.

670. Solvason N, Chen X, Shu F, et al. The fetal omentum in mice and humans. A site enriched for precursors of CD5 B cells early in development. Ann N Y Acad Sci 65:10-20, 1992.
671. Coulomb-L'Hermin A, Amara A, Schiff C, et al. Stromal cell–derived factor 1 (SDF-1) and antenatal human B cell lymphopoiesis: expression of SDF-1 by mesothelial cells and plate epithelial cells. Proc Natl Acad Sci U S A 96:8585-8590, 1999.
672. Nishimoto N, Kubagawa H, Ohno T, et al. Normal pre-B cells express a receptor complex of mu heavy chains and surrogate light-chain proteins. Proc Natl Acad Sci U S A 88:6284-6288, 1991.
673. Arakawa-Hoyt J, Dao MA, Thiemann F, et al. The number and generative capacity of human B lymphocyte progenitors, measured in vitro and in vivo, is higher in umbilical cord blood than in adult or pediatric bone marrow. Bone Marrow Transplant 24:1167-1176, 1999.
674. Schultz C, Reiss I, Bucsky P, et al. Maturational changes of lymphocyte surface antigens in human blood: comparison between fetuses, neonates and adults. Biol Neonate 78:77-82, 2000.
675. Gupta S, Pahwa R, O'Reilly R, et al. Ontogeny of lymphocyte sub-populations in human fetal liver. Proc Natl Acad Sci U S A 73:919-922, 1976.
676. Metcalf ES, Klinman NR. In vitro tolerance induction of neonatal murine B cells. J Exp Med 143:1327-1340, 1976.
677. Baskin B, Islam KB, Smith CI. Characterization of the CDR3 region of rearranged alpha heavy chain genes in human fetal liver. Clin Exp Immunol 112:44-47, 1998.
678. Dosch HM, Lam P, Hui MF, et al. Concerted generation of Ig isotype diversity in human fetal bone marrow. J Immunol 143:2464-2469, 1989.
679. Macardle PJ, Weedon H, Fusco M, et al. The antigen receptor complex on cord B lymphocytes. Immunology 90:376-382, 1997.
680. Gagro A, McCloskey N, Challa A, et al. CD5-positive and CD5-negative human B cells converge to an indistinguishable population on signalling through B-cell receptors and CD40. Immunology 101:201-209, 2000.
681. Wedgwood JF, Weinberger BI, Hatam L, et al. Umbilical cord blood lacks circulating B lymphocytes expressing surface IgG or IgA. Clin Immunol Immunopathol 84:276-282, 1997.
682. Zheng B, Kelsoe G, Han S. Somatic diversification of antibody responses. J Clin Immunol 16:1-11, 1996.
683. Punnonen J, Aversa GG, Vandekerckhove B, et al. Induction of isotype switching and Ig production by $CD5^+$ and $CD10^+$ human fetal B cells. J Immunol 148:3398-3404, 1992.
684. Antin JH, Emerson SG, Martin P, et al. Leu-1^+ ($CD5^+$) B cells. A major lymphoid subpopulation in human fetal spleen: phenotypic and functional studies. J Immunol 136:505-510, 1986.
685. Griffiths CS, Patterson JA, Berger CL, et al. Characterization of immature T cell subpopulations in neonatal blood. Blood 64: 296-300, 1984.
686. Small TN, Keever C, Collins N, et al. Characterization of B cells in severe combined immunodeficiency disease. Hum Immunol 25: 181-193, 1989.
687. Lydyard PM, Quartey PR, Broker B, et al. The antibody repertoire of early human B cells. I. High frequency of autoreactivity and poly-reactivity. Scand J Immunol 31:33-43, 1990.
688. Ehrenstein MR, O'Keefe TL, Davies SL, et al. Targeted gene disruption reveals a role for natural secretory IgM in the maturation of the primary immune response. Proc Natl Acad Sci U S A 95: 10089-10093, 1998.
689. Boes M, Prodeus A, Schmidt T, et al. A critical role of natural immunoglobulin M in immediate defense against systemic bacterial infection. J Exp Med 188:2381-2386, 1998.
690. Boes M, Esau C, Fischer MB, et al. Enhanced B-1 cell development, but impaired IgG antibody responses in mice deficient in secreted IgM. J Immunol 160:4776-4787, 1998.
691. Schroeder HJ, Hillson JL, Perlmutter RM. Early restriction of the human antibody repertoire. Science 238:791-793, 1987.
692. Cuisinier AM, Guigou V, Boubli L, et al. Preferential expression of VH5 and VH6 immunoglobulin genes in early human B-cell ontogeny. Scand J Immunol 30:493-497, 1989.
693. Schutte ME, Ebeling SB, Akkermans-Koolhaas KE, et al. Deletion mapping of Ig VH gene segments expressed in human CD5 B cell lines. JH proximity is not the sole determinant of the restricted fetal VH gene repertoire. J Immunol 149:3953-3960, 1992.
694. Zemlin M, Schelonka RL, Bauer K, et al. Regulation and chance in the ontogeny of B and T cell antigen receptor repertoires. Immunol Res 26:265-278, 2002.
695. Sanz I. Multiple mechanisms participate in the generation of diversity of human H chain CDR3 regions. J Immunol 147: 1720-1729, 1991.
696. Mortari F, Newton JA, Wang JY, et al. The human cord blood antibody repertoire. Frequent usage of the VH7 gene family. Eur J Immunol 22:241-245, 1992.
697. Silverman GJ, Sasano M, Wormsley SB. Age-associated changes in binding of human B lymphocytes to a VH3-restricted unconventional bacterial antigen. J Immunol 151:5840-5855, 1993.
698. Raaphorst FM, Timmers E, Kenter MJ, et al. Restricted utilization of germ-line VH3 genes and short diverse third complementarity-determining regions CDR3 in human fetal B lymphocyte immunoglobulin heavy chain rearrangements. Eur J Immunol 22:247-251, 1992.
699. Raaphorst FM, Raman CS, Tami J, et al. Human Ig heavy chain CDR3 regions in adult bone marrow pre-B cells display an adult phenotype of diversity: evidence for structural selection of DH amino acid sequences. Int Immunol 9:1503-1515, 1997.
700. Hirose Y, Kiyoi H, Itoh K, et al. B-cell precursors differentiated from cord blood $CD34^+$ cells are more immature than those derived from granulocyte colony-stimulating factor–mobilized peripheral blood $CD34^+$ cells. Immunology 104:410-417, 2001.
701. Cuisinier AM, Fumoux F, Moinier D, et al. Rapid expansion of human immunoglobulin repertoire VH, V kappa, V lambda expressed in early fetal bone marrow. New Biol 2:689-699, 1990.
702. Mortari F, Wang JY, Schroeder HJ. Human cord blood antibody repertoire. Mixed population of VH gene segments and CDR3 distribution in the expressed C alpha and C gamma repertoires. J Immunol 150:1348-1357, 1993.
703. Benedict CL, Kearney JF. Increased junctional diversity in fetal B cells results in a loss of protective anti-phosphorylcholine antibodies in adult mice. Immunity 10:607-617, 1999.
704. Lee J, Monson NL, Lipsky PE. The V lambda J lambda repertoire in human fetal spleen: evidence for positive selection and extensive receptor editing. J Immunol 165:6322-6333, 2000.
705. Girschick HJ, Lipsky PE. The kappa gene repertoire of human neonatal B cells. Mol Immunol 38:1113-1127, 2002.
706. van Es JH, Meyling FH, Logtenberg T. High frequency of somatically mutated IgM molecules in the human adult blood B cell repertoire. Eur J Immunol 22:2761-2764, 1992.
707. Nicholson IC, Brisco MJ, Zola H. Memory B lymphocytes in human tonsil do not express surface IgD. J Immunol 154:1105-1113, 1995.
708. LeBien TW, Wormann B, Villablanca JG, et al. Multiparameter flow cytometric analysis of human fetal bone marrow B cells. Leukemia 4:354-358, 1990.
709. Calado RT, Garcia AB, Falcao RP. Age-related changes of immuno-phenotypically immature lymphocytes in normal human peripheral blood. Cytometry 38:133-137, 1999.
710. Elliott SR, Macardle PJ, Roberton DM, et al. Expression of the costimulator molecules, CD80, CD86, CD28, and CD152, on lymphocytes from neonates and young children. Hum Immunol 60:1039-1048, 1999.
711. Viemann D, Schlenke P, Hammers HJ, et al. Differential expression of the B cell–restricted molecule CD22 B lymphocytes depending upon antigen stimulation. Eur J Immunol 30:550-559, 2000.
712. Elliott SR, Roberton DM, Zola H, et al. Expression of the costimulator molecules, CD40 and CD154, on lymphocytes from neonates and young children. Hum Immunol 61:378-388, 2000.
713. Thornton CA, Holloway JA, Warner JO. Expression of CD21 and CD23 during human fetal development. Pediatr Res 52:245-250, 2002.
714. Krzysiek R, Lefevre EA, Bernard J, et al. Regulation of CCR6 chemokine receptor expression and responsiveness to macrophage inflammatory protein-3alpha/CCL20 in human B cells. Blood 96:2338-2345, 2000.
715. Tasker L, Marshall-Clarke S. Functional responses of human neonatal B lymphocytes to antigen receptor cross-linking and CpG DNA. Clin Exp Immunol 134:409-419, 2003.
716. Rijkers GT, Sanders EA, Breukels MA, et al. Infant B cell responses to polysaccharide determinants. Vaccine 16:1396-1400, 1998.
717. Jessup CF, Ridings J, Ho A, et al. The Fc receptor for IgG (Fc gamma RII; CD32) on human neonatal B lymphocytes. Hum Immunol 62:679-685, 2001.
718. Parra C, Rold'an E, Brieva JA. Deficient expression of adhesion molecules by human $CD5^-$ B lymphocytes both after bone marrow transplantation and during normal ontogeny. Blood 88:1733-1740, 1996.

719. Garban F, Truman JP, Lord J, et al. Signal transduction via human leucocyte antigen class II molecules distinguishes between cord blood, normal, and malignant adult B lymphocytes. Exp Hematol 26:874-884, 1998.
720. Jones CA, Holloway JA, Warner JO. Phenotype of fetal monocytes and B lymphocytes during the third trimester of pregnancy. J Reprod Immunol 56:45-60, 2002.
721. Cerutti A, Trentin L, Zambello R, et al. The CD5/CD72 receptor system is coexpressed with several functionally relevant counterstructures on human B cells and delivers a critical signaling activity. J Immunol 157:1854-1862, 1996.
722. Banchereau J, Briere F, Liu YJ, et al. Molecular control of B lymphocyte growth and differentiation. Stem Cells (Dayt) 12:278-288, 1994.
723. Servet DC, Bridon JM, Djossou O, et al. Delayed IgG2 humoral response in infants is not due to intrinsic T or B cell defects. Int Immunol 8:1495-1502, 1996.
724. Gudmundsson KO, Thorsteinsson L, Gudmundsson S, et al. Immunoglobulin-secreting cells in cord blood: effects of Epstein-Barr virus and interleukin-4. Scand J Immunol 50:21-24, 1999.
725. Tangye SG, Ferguson A, Avery DT, et al. Isotype switching by human B cells is division-associated and regulated by cytokines. J Immunol 169:4298-4306, 2002.
726. Punnonen J, Aversa G, de-Vries J-E. Human pre-B cells differentiate into Ig-secreting plasma cells in the presence of interleukin-4 and activated $CD4^+$ T cells or their membranes. Blood 82:2781-2789, 1993.
727. Punnonen J, de Vries JE. IL-13 induces proliferation, Ig isotype switching, and Ig synthesis by immature human fetal B cells. J Immunol 152:1094-1102, 1994.
728. Punnonen J, Cocks BG, de Vries JE. IL-4 induces germ-line IgE heavy chain gene transcription in human fetal pre-B cells. Evidence for differential expression of functional IL-4 and IL-13 receptors during B cell ontogeny. J Immunol 155:4248-4254, 1995.
729. Ueno Y, Ichihara T, Hasui M, et al. T-cell-dependent production of IgG by human cord blood B cells in reconstituted SCID mice. Scand J Immunol 35:415-419, 1992.
730. Vandekerckhove BA, Jones D, Punnonen J, et al. Human Ig production and isotype switching in severe combined immunodeficient-human mice. J Immunol 151:128-137, 1993.
731. Splawski J, Yamamoto K, Lipsky P. Deficient interleukin-10 production by neonatal T cells does not expalin their ineffectiveness at promoting neonatal B cell differentiation. Eur J Immunol 28:4248-4256, 1998.
732. Gitlin D, Biasucci A. Development of gamma G, gamma A, gamma M, beta IC-beta IA, Ca 1 esterase inhibitor, ceruloplasmin, transferrin, hemopexin, haptoglobin, fibrinogen, plasminogen, alpha 1-antitrypsin, orosomucoid, beta-lipoprotein, alpha 2-macroglobulin, and prealbumin in the human conceptus. J Clin Invest 48:1433-1446, 1969.
733. Gathings WE, Kubagawa H, Cooper MD. A distinctive pattern of B cell immaturity in perinatal humans. Immunol Rev 57:107-126, 1981.
734. Splawski JB, Lipsky PE. Prostaglandin E_2 inhibits T cell–dependent Ig secretion by neonatal but not adult lymphocytes. J Immunol 152:5259-5267, 1994.
735. Ambrosino DM, Delaney NR, Shamberger RC. Human polysaccharide-specific B cells are responsive to pokeweed mitogen and IL-6. J Immunol 144:1221-1226, 1990.
736. Peeters CC, Tenbergen-Meekes AM, Heijnen CJ, et al. Interferon-gamma and interleukin-6 augment the human in vitro antibody response to the *Haemophilus influenzae* type b polysaccharide. J Infect Dis 165(Suppl 1):S161-S162, 1992.
737. Snapper CM, Mond JJ. A model for induction of T cell-independent humoral immunity in response to polysaccharide antigens. J Immunol 157:2229-2233, 1996.
738. Buchanan RM, Arulanandam BP, Metzger DW. IL-12 enhances antibody responses to T-independent polysaccharide vaccines in the absence of T and NK cells. J Immunol 161:5525-5533, 1998.
739. Snapper CM, Rosas FR, Jin L, et al. Bacterial lipoproteins may substitute for cytokines in the humoral immune response to T cell–independent type II antigens. J Immunol 155:5582-5589, 1995.
740. Chelvarajan RL, Raithatha R, Venkataraman C, et al. CpG oligodeoxynucleotides overcome the unresponsiveness of neonatal B cells to stimulation with the thymus-independent stimuli anti-IgM and TNP-Ficoll. Eur J Immunol 29:2808-2818, 1999.
741. Golding B, Muchmore AV, Blaese RM. Newborn and Wiskott-Aldrich patient B cells can be activated by TNP-*Brucella abortus*: evidence that TNP-*Brucella abortus* behaves as a T-independent type 1 antigen in humans. J Immunol 133:2966-2971, 1984.
742. Fink C, Miller WE Jr, Dorward B, Lospalluto J. The formation of macroglobulin antibodies II. Studies on neonatal infants and older children. J Clin Invest 41:1422-1428, 1962.
743. Smith R, Eitzman DV. The development of the immune response. Pediatrics 33:163-183, 1964.
744. Kruetzmann S, Rosado MM, Weber H, et al. Human immunoglobulin M memory B cells controlling *Streptococcus pneumoniae* infections are generated in the spleen. J Exp Med 197:939-945, 2003.
745. Peset-Llopis MJ, Harms G, Hardonk MJ, et al. Human immune response to pneumococcal polysaccharides: complement-mediated localization preferentially on CD21-positive splenic marginal zone B cells and follicular dendritic cells. J Allergy Clin Immunol 97: 1015-1024, 1996.
746. Griffioen AW, Toebes EA, Zegers BJ, et al. Role of CR2 in the human adult and neonatal in vitro antibody response to type 4 pneumococcal polysaccharide. Cell Immunol 143:11-22, 1992.
747. Timens W, Rozeboom T, Poppema S. Fetal and neonatal development of human spleen: an immunohistological study. Immunology 60:603-609, 1987.
748. Halista SM, Johnson-Robbins LA, El-Mohandes AE, et al. Characterization of early activation events in cord blood B cells after stimulation with T cell–independent activators. Pediatr Res 43:496-503, 1998.
749. Kaisho T, Akira S. Toll-like receptors as adjuvant receptors. Biochim Biophys Acta 1589:1-13, 2002.
750. Silverstein AM, Prendergast RA, Parshall CJ Jr. Cellular kinetics of the antibody response by the fetal rhesus monkey. J Immunol 104:269-271, 1970.
751. Silverstein A. Ontogeny of the immune response: a perspective. *In* Cooper MD, Dayton DH (eds). Development of Host Defenses. New York, Raven Press, 1977, pp 1-10.
752. Watts AM, Stanley JR, Shearer MH, et al. Fetal immunization of baboons induces a fetal-specific antibody response. Nat Med 5: 427-430, 1999.
753. Gill TJ, Repetti CF, Metlay LA, et al. Transplacental immunization of the human fetus to tetanus by immunization of the mother. J Clin Invest 72:987-996, 1983.
754. Vanderbeeken Y, Sarfati M, Bose R, et al. In utero immunization of the fetus to tetanus by maternal vaccination during pregnancy. Am J Reprod Immunol Microbiol 8:39-42, 1985.
755. Enders G. Serologic test combinations for safe detection of rubella infections. Rev Infect Dis 7(Suppl 1):S113-S122, 1985.
756. Naot Y, Desmonts G, Remington JS. IgM enzyme-linked immunosorbent assay test for the diagnosis of congenital *Toxoplasma* infection. J Pediatr 98:32-36, 1981.
757. Chumpitazi BF, Boussaid A, Pelloux H, et al. Diagnosis of congenital toxoplasmosis by immunoblotting and relationship with other methods. J Clin Microbiol 33:1479-1485, 1995.
758. Griffiths PD, Stagno S, Pass RF, et al. Congenital cytomegalovirus infection: diagnostic and prognostic significance of the detection of specific immunoglobulin M antibodies in cord serum. Pediatrics 69:544-549, 1982.
759. Pinon JM, Toubas D, Marx C, et al. Detection of specific immunoglobulin E in patients with toxoplasmosis. J Clin Microbiol 28: 1739-1743, 1990.
760. King CL, Malhotra I, Mungai P, et al. B cell sensitization to helminthic infection develops in utero in humans. J Immunol 160:3578-3584, 1998.
761. Desmonts G, Daffos F, Forestier F, et al. Prenatal diagnosis of congenital toxoplasmosis. Lancet 1:500-504, 1985.
762. Stepick-Biek P, Thulliez P, Araujo FG, et al. IgA antibodies for diagnosis of acute congenital and acquired toxoplasmosis. J Infect Dis 162:270-273, 1990.
763. Decoster A, Darcy F, Caron A, et al. Anti-P30 IgA antibodies as prenatal markers of congenital toxoplasma infection. Clin Exp Immunol 87:310-315, 1992.
764. Dengrove J, Lee EJ, Heiner DC, et al. IgG and IgG subclass specific antibody responses to diphtheria and tetanus toxoids in newborns and infants given DTP immunization. Pediatr Res 20:735-739, 1986.
765. Smolen P, Bland R, Heiligenstein E, et al. Antibody response to oral polio vaccine in premature infants. J Pediatr 103:917-919, 1983.
766. Uhr J, Dancis J, Franklin E, et al. The antibody response to bacteriophage in newborn premature infants. J Clin Invest 41:1509-1513, 1962.
767. West DJ. Clinical experience with hepatitis B vaccines. Am J Infect Control 17:172-180, 1989.

768. Lee SS, Lo YC, Young BW, et al. A reduced dose approach to hepatitis B vaccination for low-risk newborns and preschool children. Vaccine 13:373-376, 1995.
769. Greenberg DP. Pediatric experience with recombinant hepatitis B vaccines and relevant safety and immunogenicity studies. Pediatr Infect Dis J 12:438-445, 1993.
770. Dancis J, Osborn JJ, Kunz HW. Studies of the immunology of the newborn infant. IV. Antibody formation in the premature infant. Pediatrics 12:151-157, 1953.
771. McFarland EJ, Borkowsky W, Fenton T, et al. Human immunodeficiency virus type 1 (HIV-1) gp120-specific antibodies in neonates receiving an HIV-1 recombinant gp120 vaccine. J Infect Dis 184:1331-1335, 2001.
772. Peterson J. Immunization in the young infant. Response to combined vaccines: I-IV. Am J Dis Child. 81:484-491, 1951.
773. Provenzano R, Wetterow LH, Sullivan CL. Immunization and antibody response in the newborn infant. I. Pertussis inoculation within twenty-four hours of birth. N Engl J Med 273:959-965, 1965.
774. Baraff LJ, Leake RD, Burstyn DG, et al. Immunologic response to early and routine DTP immunization in infants. Pediatrics 73:37-42, 1984.
775. Schoub BD, Johnson S, McAnerney J, et al. Monovalent neonatal polio immunization—a strategy for the developing world. J Infect Dis 157:836-839, 1988.
776. Gans HA, Arvin AM, Galinus J, et al. Deficiency of the humoral immune response to measles vaccine in infants immunized at age 6 months. JAMA 280:527-532, 1998.
777. Gans HA, Maldonado Y, Yasukawa LL, et al. IL-12, IFN-gamma, and T cell proliferation to measles in immunized infants. J Immunol 162:5569-5575, 1999.
778. Gans H, Yasukawa L, Rinki M, et al. Immune responses to measles and mumps vaccination of infants at 6, 9, and 12 months. J Infect Dis 184:817-826, 2001.
779. Smith DH, Peter G, Ingram DL, et al. Responses of children immunized with the capsular polysaccharide of *Hemophilus influenzae*, type b. Pediatrics 52:637-644, 1973.
780. Adderson EE, Shackelford PG, Quinn A, Carroll WL. Restricted Ig H chain V gene usage in the human antibody response to *Haemophilus influenzae* type b capsular polysaccharide. J Immunol 147:1667-1674, 1991.
781. Granoff DM, Holmes SJ, Osterholm MT, et al. Induction of immunologic memory in infants primed with *Haemophilus influenzae* type b conjugate vaccines. J Infect Dis 168:663-671, 1993.
782. Eskola J, Kayhty H. Early immunization with conjugate vaccines. Vaccine 16:1433-1438, 1998.
783. Lieberman JM, Greenberg DP, Wong VK, et al. Effect of neonatal immunization with diphtheria and tetanus toxoids on antibody responses to *Haemophilus influenzae* type b conjugate vaccines. J Pediatr 126:198-205, 1995.
784. Schlesinger Y, Granoff DM. Avidity and bactericidal activity of antibody elicited by different *Haemophilus influenzae* type b conjugate vaccines. The Vaccine Study Group. JAMA 267:1489-1494, 1992.
785. Siber G. Pneumococcal disease: prospects for a new generation of vaccines. Science 265:1385-1387, 1994.
786. Anderson EL, Kennedy DJ, Geldmacher KM, et al. Immunogenicity of heptavalent pneumococcal conjugate vaccine in infants. J Pediatr 128:649-653, 1996.
787. Daum RS, Hogerman D, Rennels MB, et al. Infant immunization with pneumococcal CRM197 vaccines: effect of saccharide size on immunogenicity and interactions with simultaneously administered vaccines. J Infect Dis 176:445-455, 1997.
788. Fairley CK, Begg N, Borrow R, et al. Conjugate meningococcal serogroup A and C vaccine: reactogenicity and immunogenicity in United Kingdom infants. J Infect Dis 174:1360-1363, 1996.
789. Bernbaum JC, Daft A, Anolik R, et al. Response of preterm infants to diphtheria-tetanus-pertussis immunizations. J Pediatr 107:184-188, 1985.
790. Koblin BA, Townsend TR, Muanoz A, et al. Response of preterm infants to diphtheria-tetanus-pertussis vaccine. Pediatr Infect Dis J 7:704-711, 1988.
791. Adenyi-Jones SC, Faden H, Ferdon MB, et al. Systemic and local immune responses to enhanced-potency inactivated poliovirus vaccine in premature and term infants. J Pediatr 120:686-689, 1992.
792. Lau YL, Tam AY, Ng KW, et al. Response of preterm infants to hepatitis B vaccine. J Pediatr 121:962-965, 1992.
793. Kim SC, Chung EK, Hodinka RL, et al. Immunogenicity of hepatitis B vaccine in preterm infants. Pediatrics 99:534-536, 1997.
794. Greenberg DP, Vadheim CM, Partridge S, et al. Immunogenicity of *Haemophilus influenzae* type b tetanus toxoid conjugate vaccine in young infants. The Kaiser-UCLA Vaccine Study Group. J Infect Dis 170:76-81, 1994.
795. Washburn LK, O'Shea TM, Gillis DC, et al. Response to *Haemophilus influenzae* type b conjugate vaccine in chronically ill premature infants. J Pediatr 123:791-794, 1993.
796. Leach JL, Sedmak DD, Osborne JM, et al. Isolation from human placenta of the IgG transporter, FcRn, and localization to the syncytiotrophoblast: implications for maternal-fetal antibody transport. J Immunol 157:3317-3322, 1996.
797. Simister NE. Human placental Fc receptors and the trapping of immune complexes. Vaccine 16:1451-1455, 1998.
798. Story CM, Mikulska JE, Simister NE. A major histocompatibility complex class I–like Fc receptor cloned from human placenta: possible role in transfer of immunoglobulin G from mother to fetus. J Exp Med 180:2377-2381, 1994.
799. Kohler PF, Farr RS. Elevation of cord over maternal IgG immunoglobulin: evidence for an active placental IgG transport. Nature 210: 1070-1071, 1966.
800. Gusdon JP Jr. Fetal and maternal immunoglobulin levels during pregnancy. Am J Obstet Gynecol 103:895-900, 1969.
801. Pitcher-Wilmott RW, Hindocha P, Wood CB. The placental transfer of IgG subclasses in human pregnancy. Clin Exp Immunol 41:303-308, 1980.
802. Landor M. Maternal-fetal transfer of immunoglobulins. Ann. Allergy Asthma Immunol 74:279-283, 1995.
803. Martensson L, Fudenberg HH. Gm genes and gamma G-globulin synthesis in the human fetus. J Immunol 94:514-520, 1965.
804. Hay FC, Hull MG, Torrigiani G. The transfer of human IgG subclasses from mother to foetus. Clin Exp Immunol 9:355-358, 1971.
805. Oxelius VA, Svenningsen NW. IgG subclass concentrations in preterm neonates. Acta Paediatr Scand 73:626-630, 1984.
806. Malek A, Sager R, Schneider H. Maternal-fetal transport of immunoglobulin G and its subclasses during the third trimester of human pregnancy. Am J Reprod Immunol 32:8-14, 1994.
807. Morell A, Sidiropoulos D, Herrmann U, et al. IgG subclasses and antibodies to group B streptococci, pneumococci, and tetanus toxoid in preterm neonates after intravenous infusion of immunoglobulin to the mothers. Pediatr Res 20:933-936, 1986.
808. Linder N, Waintraub I, Smetana Z, et al. Placental transfer and decay of varicella-zoster virus antibodies in preterm infants. J Pediatr 137: 85-89, 2000.
809. Sato H, Albrecht P, Reynolds DW, et al. Transfer of measles, mumps, and rubella antibodies from mother to infant. Its effect on measles, mumps, and rubella immunization. Am J Dis Children 133: 1240-1243, 1979.
810. Vahlquist B. Response of infants to diphtheria immunization. Lancet 1:16-18, 1949.
811. Perkins F, Yetts R, Gaisford W. Response of infants to a third dose of poliomyelitis vaccine given 10 to 12 months after primary immunization. BMJ 1:680-682, 1959.
812. Stiehm ER, Fudenberg HH. Serum levels of immune globulins in health and disease: a survey. Pediatrics 37:715-727, 1966.
813. Lee SI, Heiner DC, Wara D. Development of serum IgG subclass levels in children. Monogr Allergy 19:108-121, 1986.
814. Ochs HD, Wedgwood RJ. IgG subclass deficiencies. Annu Rev Med 38:325-340, 1987.
815. Kobayashi RH, Hyman CJ, Stiehm ER. Immunologic maturation in an infant born to a mother with agammaglobulinemia. Am J Dis Child 134:942-944, 1980.
816. Granoff DM, Shackelford PG, Pandey JP, et al. Antibody responses to *Haemophilus influenzae* type b polysaccharide vaccine in relation to Km 1 and G2m 23 immunoglobulin allotypes. J Infect Dis 154: 257-264, 1986.
817. Cederqvist LL, Ewool LC, Litwin SD. The effect of fetal age, birth weight, and sex on cord blood immunoglobulin values. Am J Obstet Gyn 131:520-525, 1978.
818. Avrech OM, Samra Z, Lazarovich Z, et al. Efficacy of the placental barrier for immunoglobulins: correlations between maternal, paternal and fetal immunoglobulin levels. Int Arch Allergy Immunol 103: 160-165, 1994.
819. Allansmith M, McClellan BH, Butterworth M, et al. The development of immunoglobulin levels in man. J Pediatr 72:276-290, 1968.

820. Perchalski JE, Clem LW, Small PJ. 7S gamma-M immunoglobulins in normal human cord serum. Am J Med Sci 256:107-111, 1968.
821. Alford CJ, Stagno S, Reynolds DW. Diagnosis of chronic perinatal infections. Am J Dis Child 129:455-463, 1975.
822. Conley ME, Kearney JF, Lawton AR, et al. Differentiation of human B cells expressing the IgA subclasses as demonstrated by monoclonal hybridoma antibodies. J Immunol 125:2311-2316, 1980.
823. Seidel BM, Schulze B, Kiess W, et al. Determination of secretory IgA and albumin in saliva of newborn infants. Biol Neonate 78:186-190, 2000.
824. Josephs SH, Buckley RH. Serum IgD concentrations in normal infants, children, and adults and in patients with elevated IgE. J Pediatr 96:417-420, 1980.
825. Bazaral M, Orgel HA, Hamburger RN. IgE levels in normal infants and mothers and an inheritance hypothesis. J Immunol 107:794-801, 1971.
826. Young M, Geha RS. Ontogeny and control of human IgE synthesis. Clin Immunol Allergy 5:339-349, 1985.
827. Edenharter G, Bergmann RL, Bergmann KE, et al. Cord blood-IgE as risk factor and predictor for atopic diseases. Clin Exp Allergy 28: 671-678, 1998.
828. Sivori S, Vitale M, Morelli L, et al. P46, a novel natural killer cell–specific surface molecule that mediates cell activation. J Exp Med 186:1129-1136, 1997.
829. Biassoni R, Cantoni C, Marras D, et al. Human natural killer cell receptors: insights into their molecular function and structure. J Cell Mol Med 7:376-387, 2003.
830. Phillips JH, Hori T, Nagler A, et al. Ontogeny of human natural killer NK cells: fetal NK cells mediate cytolytic function and express cytoplasmic CD3 epsilon,delta proteins. J Exp Med 175:1055-1066, 1992.
831. Nakazawa T, Agematsu K, Yabuhara A. Later development of Fas ligand-mediated cytotoxicity as compared with granule-mediated cytotoxicity during the maturation of natural killer cells. Immunology 92:180-187, 1997.
832. Cooper MA, Fehniger TA, Caligiuri MA. The biology of human natural killer-cell subsets. Trends Immunol 22:633-640, 2001.
833. Lanier LL. Natural killer cell receptor signaling. Curr Opin Immunol 15:308-314, 2003.
834. Lanier LL. On guard—activating NK cell receptors. Nat Immunol 2:23-27, 2001.
835. Ruggeri L, Capanni M, Urbani E, et al. Effectiveness of donor natural killer cell alloreactivity in mismatched hematopoietic transplants. Science 295:2097-2100, 2002.
836. Perussia B. Fc receptors on natural killer cells. Curr Top Microbiol Immunol 230:63-88, 1998.
837. Biron CA, Byron KS, Sullivan JL. Severe herpesvirus infections in an adolescent without natural killer cells. N Engl J Med 320:1731-1735, 1989.
838. Orange JS, Fassett MS, Koopman LA, et al. Viral evasion of natural killer cells. Nat Immunol 3:1006-1012, 2002.
839. Miller JS, Alley KA, McGlave P. Differentiation of natural killer (NK) cells from human primitive marrow progenitors in a stroma-based long-term culture system: identification of a $CD34^{+}7^{+}$ NK progenitor. Blood 83:2594-2601, 1994.
840. Colucci F, Caligiuri MA, Di Santo JP. What does it take to make a natural killer? Nat Rev Immunol 3:413-425, 2003.
841. Yu H, Hanes M, Chrisp CE, et al. Microbial pathogenesis in cystic fibrosis: pulmonary clearance of mucoid *Pseudomonas aeruginosa* and inflammation in a mouse model of repeated respiratory challenge. Infect Immun 66:280-288, 1998.
842. Marquez C, Trigueros C, Franco JM, et al. Identification of a common developmental pathway for thymic natural killer cells and dendritic cells. Blood 91:2760-2771, 1998.
843. Poggi A, Costa P, Morelli L, et al. Expression of human NKRP1A by $CD34^{+}$ immature thymocytes: NKRP1A-mediated regulation of proliferation and cytolytic activity. Eur J Immunol 26:1266-1272, 1996.
844. Hori T, Phillips JH, Duncan B, et al. Human fetal liver-derived $CD7^{+}CD2^{low}CD3^{-}CD56^{-}$ clones that express CD3 gamma, delta, and epsilon and proliferate in response to interleukin-2 (IL-2), IL-3, IL-4, or IL-7: implications for the relationship between T and natural killer cells. Blood 80:1270-1278, 1992.
845. Bennett IM, Zatsepina O, Zamai L, et al. Definition of a natural killer $NKR^{-}P1A^{+}/CD56^{-}/CD16^{-}$ functionally immature human NK cell subset that differentiates in vitro in the presence of interleukin 12. J Exp Med 184:1845-1856, 1996.
846. Vitale C, Chiossone L, Morreale G, et al. Analysis of the activating receptors and cytolytic function of human natural killer cells undergoing in vivo differentiation after allogeneic bone marrow transplantation. Eur J Immunol 34:455-460, 2004.
847. Sivori S, Falco M, Marcenaro E, et al. Early expression of triggering receptors and regulatory role of 2B4 in human natural killer cell precursors undergoing in vitro differentiation. Proc Natl Acad Sci U S A 99:4526-4531, 2002.
848. Mingari MC, Vitale C, Cantoni C, et al. Interleukin-15–induced maturation of human natural killer cells from early thymic precursors: selective expression of CD94/NKG2-A as the only HLA class I–specific inhibitory receptor. Eur J Immunol 27:1374-1380, 1997.
849. Carson WE, Fehniger TA, Haldar S, et al. A potential role for interleukin-15 in the regulation of human natural killer cell survival. J Clin Invest 99:937-943, 1997.
850. Lodolce JP, Boone DL, Chai S, et al. IL-15 receptor maintains lymphoid homeostasis by supporting lymphocyte homing and proliferation. Immunity 9:669-676, 1998.
851. Sivori S, Cantoni C, Parolini S, et al. IL-21 induces both rapid maturation of human $CD34^{+}$ cell precursors towards NK cells and acquisition of surface killer Ig-like receptors. Eur J Immunol 33: 3439-3447, 2003.
852. Vilches C, Parham P. KIR: diverse, rapidly evolving receptors of innate and adaptive immunity. Annu Rev Immunol 20:217-251, 2002.
853. Natarajan K, Dimasi N, Wang J, et al. Structure and function of natural killer cell receptors: multiple molecular solutions to self, nonself discrimination. Annu Rev Immunol 20:853-885, 2002.
854. Colonna M, Nakajima H, Cella M. Inhibitory and activating receptors involved in immune surveillance by human NK and myeloid cells. J Leukoc Biol 66:718-722, 1999.
855. McVicar DW, Burshtyn DN. Intracellular signaling by the killer immunoglobulin-like receptors and Ly49. Sci STKE 2001:RE1, 2001.
856. Uhrberg M, Parham P, Wernet P. Definition of gene content for nine common group B haplotypes of the Caucasoid population: KIR haplotypes contain between seven and eleven KIR genes. Immunogenetics 54:221-229, 2002.
857. Valiante NM, Uhrberg M, Shilling HG, et al. Functionally and structurally distinct NK cell receptor repertoires in the peripheral blood of two human donors. Immunity 7:739-751, 1997.
858. Lanier LL. NK cell receptors. Annu Rev Immunol 16:359-393, 1998.
859. Croy BA, Esadeg S, Chantakru S, et al. Update on pathways regulating the activation of uterine natural killer cells, their interactions with decidual spiral arteries and homing of their precursors to the uterus. J Reprod Immunol 59:175-191, 2003.
860. Helander TS, Timonen T. Adhesion in NK cell function. Curr Top Microbiol Immunol 230:89-99, 1998.
861. Arnon TI, Achdout H, Lieberman N, et al. The mechanisms controlling the recognition of tumor- and virus-infected cells by NKp46. Blood 103:664-672, 2004.
862. Wu J, Chalupny NJ, Manley TJ, et al. Intracellular retention of the MHC class I–related chain B ligand of NKG2D by the human cytomegalovirus UL16 glycoprotein. J Immunol 170:4196-4200, 2003.
863. Engel P, Eck MJ, Terhorst C. The SAP and SLAM families in immune responses and X-linked lymphoproliferative disease. Nat Rev Immunol 3:813-821, 2003.
864. Snyder MR, Weyand CM, Goronzy JJ. The double life of NK receptors: stimulation or co-stimulation? Trends Immunol 25:25-32, 2004.
865. Carretero M, Llano M, Navarro F, et al. Mitogen-activated protein kinase activity is involved in effector functions triggered by the CD94/NKG2-C NK receptor specific for HLA-E. Eur J Immunol 30:2842-2848, 2000.
866. Oshimi Y, Oda S, Honda Y, et al. Involvement of Fas ligand and Fas-mediated pathway in the cytotoxicity of human natural killer cells. J Immunol 157:2909-2915, 1996.
867. Zamai L, Ahmad M, Bennett I, et al. Natural killer (NK) cell-mediated cytotoxicity: differential use of TRAIL and Fas ligand my immature and mature primary human NK cells. J Exp Med 188:2375-2380, 1998.
868. Van-den-Broek MF, Kagi D, Hengartner H. Effector pathways of natural killer cells. Curr Top Microbiol Immunol 230:123-131, 1998.
869. Arkwright PD, Rieux-Laucat F, Le Deist F, et al. Cytomegalovirus infection in infants with autoimmune lymphoproliferative syndrome (ALPS). Clin Exp Immunol 121:353-357, 2000.

870. Eischen CM, Schilling JD, Lynch DH, et al. Fc receptor-induced expression of Fas ligand on activated NK cells facilitates cell-mediated cytotoxicity and subsequent autocrine NK cell apoptosis. J Immunol 156:2693-2699, 1996.
871. Salvucci O, Mami-Chouaib F, Moreau JL, et al. Differential regulation of interleukin-12– and interleukin-15–induced natural killer cell activation by interleukin-4. Eur J Immunol 26:2736-2741, 1996.
872. Dalton DK, Pitts-Meek S, Keshav S, et al. Multiple defects of immune cell function in mice with disrupted interferon-gamma genes. Science 259:1739-1742, 1993.
873. Magram J, Sfarra J, Connaughton S, et al. IL-12–deficient mice are defective but not devoid of type 1 cytokine responses. Ann N Y Acad Sci 795:60-70, 1996.
874. Takeda K, Tsutsui H, Yoshimoto T, et al. Defective NK cell activity and Th1 response in IL-18–deficient mice. Immunity 8:383-390, 1998.
875. Trinchieri G, Pflanz S, Kastelein RA. The IL-12 family of heterodimeric cytokines: new players in the regulation of T cell responses. Immunity 19:641-644, 2003.
876. Ida H, Anderson P. Activation-induced NK cell death triggered by CD2 stimulation. Eur J Immunol 28:1292-1300, 1998.
877. Mainiero F, Gismondi A, Soriani A, et al. Integrin-mediated ras-extracellular regulated kinase (ERK) signaling regulates interferon gamma production in human natural killer cells. J Exp Med 188: 1267-1275, 1998.
878. Hunter CA, Chizzonite R, Remington JS. IL-1 beta is required for IL-12 to induce production of IFN-gamma by NK cells. A role for IL-1 beta in the T cell–independent mechanism of resistance against intracellular pathogens. J Immunol 155:4347-4354, 1995.
879. Bluman EM, Bartynski KJ, Avalos BR, et al. Human natural killer cells produce abundant macrophage inflammatory protein-1 alpha in response to monocyte-derived cytokines. J Clin Invest 97: 2722-2727, 1996.
880. Tay CH, Szomolanyi-Tsuda E, Welsh RM. Control of infections by NK cells. Curr Top Microbiol Immunol 230:193-220, 1998.
881. Cooper MA, Fehniger TA, Turner SC, et al. Human natural killer cells: a unique innate immunoregulatory role for the CD56(bright) subset. Blood 97:3146-3151, 2001.
882. Jacobs R, Hintzen G, Kemper A, et al. CD56bright cells differ in their KIR repertoire and cytotoxic features from CD56dim NK cells. Eur J Immunol 31:3121-3127, 2001.
883. Loza MJ, Perussia B. The IL-12 signature: NK cell terminal $CD56^{+}$high stage and effector functions. J Immunol 172:88-96, 2004.
884. Pazmany L, Mandelboim O, Vales-Gomez M, et al. Human leucocyte antigen-G and its recognition by natural killer cells. J Reprod Immunol 43:127-137, 1999.
885. Jaleco AC, Blom B, Res P, et al. Fetal liver contains committed NK progenitors, but is not a site for development of $CD34^{+}$ cells into T cells. J Immunol 159:694-702, 1997.
886. Carlyle JR, Michie AM, Cho SK, et al. Natural killer cell development and function precede alpha beta T cell differentiation in mouse fetal thymic ontogeny. J Immunol 160:744-753, 1998.
887. Mrozek E, Anderson P, Caligiuri MA. Role of interleukin-15 in the development of human $CD56^{+}$ natural killer cells from $CD34^{+}$ hematopoietic progenitor cells. Blood 87:2632-2640, 1996.
888. Carayol G, Robin C, Bourhis JH, et al. NK cells differentiated from bone marrow, cord blood and peripheral blood stem cells exhibit similar phenotype and functions. Eur J Immunol 28:1991-2002, 1998.
889. Miller JS, McCullar V. Human natural killer cells with polyclonal lectin and immunoglobulinlike receptors develop from single hematopoietic stem cells with preferential expression of NKG2A and KIR2DL2/L3/S2. Blood 98:705-713, 2001.
890. Miller JS. The biology of natural killer cells in cancer, infection, and pregnancy. Exp Hematol 29:1157-1168, 2001.
891. Qian JX, Lee SM, Suen Y, et al. Decreased interleukin-15 from activated cord versus adult peripheral blood mononuclear cells and the effect of interleukin-15 in upregulating antitumor immune activity and cytokine production in cord blood. Blood 90:3106-3117, 1997.
892. Thilaganathan B, Abbas A, Nicolaides KH. Fetal blood natural killer cells in human pregnancy. Fetal Diagn Ther 8:149-153, 1993.
893. Bradstock KF, Luxford C, Grimsley PG. Functional and phenotypic assessment of neonatal human leucocytes expressing natural killer cell–associated antigens. Immunol Cell Biol 71:535-542, 1993.
894. Kohl S, Sigouroudinia M, Engleman EG. Adhesion defects of antibody-mediated target cell binding of neonatal natural killer cells. Pediatr Res 46:755-759, 1999.
895. Gaddy J, Risdon G, Broxmeyer HE. Cord blood natural killer cells are functionally and phenotypically immature but readily respond to interleukin-2 and interleukin-12. J Interferon Cytokine Res 15: 527-536, 1995.
896. Toivanen P, Uksila J, Leino A, et al. Development of mitogen responding T cells and natural killer cells in the human fetus. Immunol Rev 57:89-105, 1981.
897. Tarkkanen J, Saksela E. Umbilical-cord-blood-derived suppressor cells of the human natural killer cell activity are inhibited by interferon. Scand J Immunol 15:149-157, 1982.
898. Ueno Y, Miyawaki T, Seki H, et al. Differential effects of recombinant human interferon-gamma and interleukin 2 on natural killer cell activity of peripheral blood in early human development. J Immunol 135:180-184, 1985.
899. Seki H, Ueno Y, Taga K, et al. Mode of in vitro augmentation of natural killer cell activity by recombinant human interleukin 2: a comparative study of $Leu\text{-}11^{+}$ and $Leu\text{-}11^{-}$ cell populations in cord blood and adult peripheral blood. J Immunol 135:2351-2356, 1985.
900. Baley JE, Schacter BZ. Mechanisms of diminished natural killer cell activity in pregnant women and neonates. J Immunol 134:302-3048, 1985.
901. Nair MP, Schwartz SA, Menon M. Association of decreased natural and antibody-dependent cellular cytotoxicity and production of natural killer cytotoxic factor and interferon in neonates. Cell Immunol 94:159-171, 1985.
902. Kaplan J, Shope TC, Bollinger RO, et al. Human newborns are deficient in natural killer activity. J Clin Immunol 2:350-355, 1982.
903. Sancho L, de la Hera A, Casas J, et al. Two different maturational stages of natural killer lymphocytes in human newborn infants. J Pediatr 119:446-454, 1991.
904. McDonald T, Sneed J, Valenski WR, et al. Natural killer cell activity in very low birth weight infants. Pediatr Res 31:376-380, 1992.
905. Georgeson GD, Szony BJ, Streitman K, et al. Natural killer cell cytotoxicity is deficient in newborns with sepsis and recurrent infections. Eur J Pediatr 160:478-482, 2001.
906. Merrill JD, Sigaroudinia M, Kohl S. Characterization of natural killer and antibody-dependent cellular cytotoxicity of preterm infants against human immunodeficiency virus–infected cells. Pediatr Res 40:498-503, 1996.
907. Cicuttini FM, Martin M, Petrie HT, et al. A novel population of natural killer progenitor cells isolated from human umbilical cord blood. J Immunol 151:29-37, 1993.
908. Webb BJ, Bochan MR, Montel A, et al. The lack of NK cytotoxicity associated with fresh HUCB may be due to the presence of soluble HLA in the serum. Cell Immunol 159:246-261, 1994.
909. Harrison CJ, Waner JL. Natural killer cell activity in infants and children excreting cytomegalovirus. J Infect Dis 151:301-307, 1985.
910. Jenkins M, Mills J, Kohl S. Natural killer cytotoxicity and antibody-dependent cellular cytotoxicity of human immunodeficiency virus–infected cells by leukocytes from human neonates and adults. Pediatr Res 33:469-474, 1993.
911. Lau AS, Sigaroudinia M, Yeung MC, et al. Interleukin-12 induces interferon-γ expression and natural killer cytotoxicity in cord blood mononuclear cells. Pediatr Res 39:150-155, 1996.
912. Nguyen QH, Roberts RL, Ank BJ, et al. Interleukin (IL)-15 enhances antibody-dependent cellular cytotoxicity and natural killer activity in neonatal cells. Cell Immunol 185:83-92, 1998.
913. Han P, Hodge G, Story C, et al. Phenotypic analysis of functional T-lymphocyte subtypes and natural killer cells in human cord blood: relevance to umbilical cord blood transplantation. Br J Haematol 89:733-740, 1995.
914. Lin SJ, Chao HC, Kuo ML. The effect of interleukin-12 and interleukin-15 on CD69 expression of T-lymphocytes and natural killer cells from umbilical cord blood. Biol Neonate 78:181-185, 2000.
915. Lin SJ, Yan DC. ICAM-1 (CD54) expression on T lymphocytes and natural killer cells from umbilical cord blood: regulation with interleukin-12 and interleukin-15. Cytokines Cell Mol Ther 6:161-164, 2000.
916. Umemoto M, Azuma E, Hirayama M, et al. Two cytotoxic pathways of natural killer cells in human cord blood: implications in cord blood transplantation. Br J Haematol 98:1037-1040, 1997.
917. Gaddy J, Broxmeyer HE. Cord blood $CD16^{+}56^{-}$ cells with low lytic activity are possible precursors of mature natural killer cells. Cell Immunol 180:132-142, 1997.

918. Condiotti R, Nagler A. Effect of interleukin-12 on antitumor activity of human umbilical cord blood and bone marrow cytotoxic cells. Exp Hematol 26:571-579, 1998.
919. Lin SJ, Yang MH, Chao HC, et al. Effect of interleukin-15 and Flt3-ligand on natural killer cell expansion and activation: umbilical cord vs. adult peripheral blood mononuclear cells. Pediatr Allergy Immunol 11:168-174, 2000.
920. Condiotti R, Zakai YB, Barak V, et al. Ex vivo expansion of CD56$^+$ cytotoxic cells from human umbilical cord blood. Exp Hematol 29: 104-113, 2001.
921. Malygin AM, Timonen T. Non-major histocompatibility complex–restricted killer cells in human cord blood: generation and cytotoxic activity in recombinant interleukin-2–supplemented cultures. Immunology 79:506-508, 1993.
922. Dominguez E, Madrigal JA, Layrisse Z, et al. Fetal natural killer cell function is suppressed. Immunology 94:109-114, 1998.
923. Brahmi Z, Hommel-Berrey G, Smith F, et al. NK cells recover early and mediate cytotoxicity via perforin/granzyme and Fas/FasL pathways in umbilical cord blood recipients. Hum Immunol 62:782-790, 2001.
924. Hayward AR, Herberger M, Saunders D. Herpes simplex virus–stimulated interferon-γ production by newborn mononuclear cells. Pediatr Res 20:398-401, 1986.
924a. NomuraA, Takada H, Tin CH, et al. Functional analysis of cord blood natural killer cells and T cells: a distinctive interleukin-18 response. Exp Hematol 29:1169-1176, 2001.
925. Braakman E, Sturm E, Vijverberg K, et al. Expression of CD45 isoforms by fresh and activated human gamma delta T lymphocytes and natural killer cells. Int Immunol 3:691-697, 1991.
926. Furman WL, Crist WM. Biology and clinical applications of hemopoietins in pediatric practice. Pediatrics 90:716-728, 1992.
927. Metcalf D. Cellular hematopoiesis in the twentieth century. Semin Hematol 36:5-12, 1999.
928. Zsebo KM, Williams DA, Geissler EN, et al. Stem cell factor is encoded at the Sl locus of the mouse and is the ligand for the c-kit tyrosine kinase receptor. Cell 63:213-224, 1990.
929. Wiktor-Jedrzejczak W, Bartocci A, Ferrante AJ, et al. Total absence of colony-stimulating factor 1 in the macrophage-deficient osteopetrotic op/op mouse. Proc Natl Acad Sci U S A 87:4828-4832, 1990.
930. Dale DC. Colony-stimulating factors for the management of neutropenia in cancer patients. Drugs 62(Suppl 1):1-15, 2002.
931. Walker RI, Willemze R. Neutrophil kinetics and the regulation of granulopoiesis. Rev Infect Dis 2:282-292, 1980.
932. Springer TA. Traffic signals for lymphocyte recirculation and leukocyte emigration: the multistep paradigm. Cell 76:301-314, 1994.
933. Liu L, Kubes P. Molecular mechanisms of leukocyte recruitment: organ-specific mechanisms of action. Thromb Haemost 89:213-220, 2003.
934. Bunting M, Harris ES, McIntyre TM, et al. Leukocyte adhesion deficiency syndromes: adhesion and tethering defects involving beta 2 integrins and selectin ligands. Curr Opin Hematol 9:30-35, 2002.
935. Harvath L. Neutrophil chemotactic factors. EXS 59:35-52, 1991.
936. Luster AD. Chemokines—chemotactic cytokines that mediate inflammation. N Engl J Med 338:436-445, 1998.
937. Luster AD. The role of chemokines in linking innate and adaptive immunity. Curr Opin Immunol 14:129-135, 2002.
938. Haribabu B, Richardson RM, Verghese MW, et al. Function and regulation of chemoattractant receptors. Immunol Res 22:271-279, 2000.
939. Ley K. Molecular mechanisms of leukocyte recruitment in the inflammatory process. Cardiovasc Res 32:733-742, 1996.
940. Underhill DM, Ozinsky A. Phagocytosis of microbes: complexity in action. Annu Rev Immunol 20:825-852, 2002.
941. Brown EJ. Complement receptors, adhesion, and phagocytosis. Infect Agents Dis 1:63-70, 1992.
942. Segal BH, Leto TL, Gallin JI, et al. Genetic, biochemical, and clinical features of chronic granulomatous disease. Medicine (Baltimore) 79:170-200, 2000.
943. Levy O. Antibiotic proteins of polymorphonuclear leukocytes. Eur J Haematol 56:263-277, 1996.
944. Yang D, Chertov O, Oppenheim JJ. Participation of mammalian defensins and cathelicidins in anti-microbial immunity: receptors and activities of human defensins and cathelicidin (LL-37). J Leukoc Biol 69:691-697, 2001.
945. Dinarello CA. Interleukin-1. Cytokine Growth Factor Rev 8:253-265, 1997.
946. Vassalli P. The pathophysiology of tumor necrosis factors. Annu Rev Immmunol 10:411-452, 1992.
947. Christensen RD. Hematopoiesis in the fetus and neonate. Pediatr Res 26:531-535, 1989.
948. Playfair J, Wolfendale M, Kay H. The leucocytes of peripheral blood in the human foetus. Br J Haematol 9:336-344, 1963.
949. Ohls RK, Li Y, Abdel-Mageed A, et al. Neutrophil pool sizes and granulocyte colony-stimulating factor production in human mid-trimester fetuses. Pediatri Res 37:806-811, 1995.
950. Banerjea MC, Speer CP. The current role of colony-stimulating factors in prevention and treatment of neonatal sepsis. Semin Neonatol 7:335-349, 2002.
951. Laver J, Duncan E, Abboud M, et al. High levels of granulocyte and granulocyte-macrophage colony-stimulating factors in cord blood of normal full-term neonates. J Pediatr 116:627-632, 1990.
952. Mouzinho A, Rosenfeld CR, Sanchez PJ, et al. Revised reference ranges for circulating neutrophils in very-low-birth-weight neonates. Pediatrics 94:76-82, 1994.
953. Manroe BL, Weinberg AG, Rosenfeld CR, et al. The neonatal blood count in health and disease. I. Reference values for neutrophilic cells. J Pediatr 95:89-98, 1979.
954. Schelonka RL, Yoder BA, des Jardins SE, et al. Peripheral leukocyte count and leukocyte indexes in healthy newborn term infants. J Pediatr 125:603-606, 1994.
955. Engle WD, Rosenfeld CR, Mouzinho A, et al. Circulating neutrophils in septic preterm neonates: comparison of two reference ranges. Pediatrics 99:E10, 1997.
956. Christensen RD, Calhoun DA, Rimsza LM. A practical approach to evaluating and treating neutropenia in the neonatal intensive care unit. Clin Perinatol 27:577-601, 2000.
957. Calhoun DA, Kirk JF, Christensen RD. Incidence, significance, and kinetic mechanism responsible for leukemoid reactions in patients in the neonatal intensive care unit: a prospective evaluation. J Pediatr 129:403-409, 1996.
958. Ishiguro A, Inoue K, Nakahata T, et al. Reference intervals for serum granulocyte colony-stimulating factor levels in children. J Pediatr 128:208-212, 1996.
959. Wilimas JA, Wall JE, Fairclough DL, et al. A longitudinal study of granulocyte colony-stimulating factor levels and neutrophil counts in newborn infants. J Pediatr Hematol Oncol 17:176-179, 1995.
960. Gessler P, Kirchmann N, Kientsch-Engel R, et al. Serum concentrations of granulocyte colony-stimulating factor in healthy term and preterm neonates and in those with various diseases including bacterial infections. Blood 82:3177-3182, 1993.
961. Kennon C, Overturf G, Bessman S, et al. Granulocyte colony-stimulating factor as a marker for bacterial infection in neonates. J Pediatr 128:765-769, 1996.
962. Schibler KR, Liechty KW, White WL, et al. Production of granulocyte colony-stimulating factor in vitro by monocytes from preterm and term neonates. Blood 82:2478-2484, 1993.
963. Hill HR. Biochemical, structural, and functional abnormalities of polymorphonuclear leukocytes in the neonate. Pediatr Res 22: 375-382, 1987.
964. Schuit KE, Homisch L. Inefficient in vivo neutrophil migration in neonatal rats. J Leuk Biol 35:583-586, 1984.
965. Anderson DC, Hughes BJ, Smith CW. Abnormal mobility of neonatal polymorphonuclear leukocytes. Relationship to impaired redistribution of surface adhesion sites by chemotactic factor or colchicine. J Clin Invest 68:863-874, 1981.
966. Anderson DC, Hughes BJ, Wible LJ, et al. Impaired motility of neonatal PMN leukocytes: relationship to abnormalities of cell orientation and assembly of microtubules in chemotactic gradients. J Leuk Biol 36:1-15, 1984.
967. Anderson DC, Abbassi O, Kishimoto TK, et al. Diminished lectin-, epidermal growth factor-, complement binding domain-cell adhesion molecule-1 on neonatal neutrophils underlies their impaired CD18-independent adhesion to endothelial cells in vitro. J Immunol 146:3372-3379, 1991.
968. Smith JB, Kunjummen RD, Kishimoto TK, et al. Expression and regulation of L-selectin on eosinophils from human adults and neonates. Pediatr Res 32:465-471, 1992.
969. Rebuck N, Gibson A, Finn A. Neutrophil adhesion molecules in term and premature infants: normal or enhanced leucocyte integrins but defective L-selectin expression and shedding. Clin Exp Immunol 101:183-189, 1995.

970. McEvoy LT, Zakem-Cloud H, Tosi MF. Total cell content of CR3 (CD11b/CD18) and LFA-1 (CD11a/CD18) in neonatal neutrophils: relationship to gestational age. Blood 87:3929-3933, 1996.
971. Anderson DC, Rothlein R, Marlin SD, et al. Impaired transendothelial migration by neonatal neutrophils: abnormalities of Mac-1 CD11b/CD18-dependent adherence reactions. Blood 76:2613-2621, 1990.
972. Adinolfi M, Cheetham M, Lee T, et al. Ontogeny of human complement receptors CR1 and CR3: expression of these molecules on monocytes and neutrophils from maternal, newborn and fetal samples. Eur J Immunol 18:565-569, 1988.
973. Pahwa SG, Pahwa R, Grimes E, et al. Cellular and humoral components of monocyte and neutrophil chemotaxis in cord blood. Pediatr Res 11:677-680, 1977.
974. Klein RB, Fischer TJ, Gard SE, et al. Decreased mononuclear and polymorphonuclear chemotaxis in human newborns, infants, and young children. Pediatrics 60:467-472, 1977.
975. Dos Santos C, Davidson D. Neutrophil chemotaxis to leukotriene B_4 in vitro is decreased for the human neonate. Pediatr Res 33:242-246, 1993.
976. Yasui K, Masuda M, Tsuno T, et al. An increase in polymorphonuclear leucocyte chemotaxis accompanied by a change in the membrane fluidity with age during childhood. Clin Exp Immunol 81:156-159, 1990.
977. Tan ND, Davidson D. Comparative differences and combined effects of interleukin-8, leukotriene B_4, and platelet-activating factor on neutrophil chemotaxis of the newborn. Pediatr Res 38:11-16, 1995.
978. Nunoi H, Endo F, Chikazawa S, et al. Chemotactic receptor of cord blood granulocytes to the synthesized chemotactic peptide *N*-formyl-methionyl-leucyl-phenylalanine. Pediatr Res 17:57-60, 1983.
979. Nybo M, Sorensen O, Leslie R, et al. Reduced expression of C5a receptors on neutrophils from cord blood. Arch Dis Child 78: 129-132, 1998.
980. Sacchi F, Hill HR. Defective membrane potential changes in neutrophils from human neonates. J Exp Med 160:1247-1252, 1984.
981. Santoro P, Agosti V, Viggiano D, et al. Impaired D-myo-inositol 1,4,5-triphosphate generation from cord blood polymorphonuclear leukocytes. Pediatr Res 38:564-567, 1995.
982. Boner A, Zeligs BJ, Bellanti JA. Chemotactic responses of various differentiational stages of neutrophils from human cord and adult blood. Infect Immun 35:921-928, 1982.
983. Kikawa Y, Shigematsu Y, Sudo M. Leukotriene B_4 biosynthesis in polymorphonuclear leukocytes from blood of umbilical cord, infants, children, and adults. Pediatr Res 20:402-406, 1986.
984. Bruce MC, Baley JE, Medvik KA, et al. Impaired surface membrane expression of C3bi but not C3b receptors on neonatal neutrophils. Pediatr Res 21:306-311, 1987.
985. Bektas S, Goetze B, Speer CP. Decreased adherence, chemotaxis and phagocytic activities of neutrophils from preterm neonates. Acta Paediatr Scand 79:1031-1038, 1990.
986. Johnston RB Jr. Function and cell biology of neutrophils and mononuclear phagocytes in the newborn infant. Vaccine 16:1363-1368, 1998.
987. Fujiwara T, Kobayashi T, Takaya J, et al. Plasma effects on phagocytic activity and hydrogen peroxide production by polymorphonuclear leukocytes in neonates. Clin Immunol Immunopathol 85:67-72, 1997.
988. Falconer AE, Carr R, Edwards SW. Impaired neutrophil phagocytosis in preterm neonates: lack of correlation with expression of immunoglobulin or complement receptors. Biol Neonate 68:264-269, 1995.
989. Falconer AE, Carr R, Edwards SW. Neutrophils from preterm neonates and adults show similar cell surface receptor expression: analysis using a whole blood assay. Biol Neonate 67:26-33, 1995.
990. Payne NR, Fleit HB. Extremely low birth weight infants have lower Fc gamma RIII (CD 16) plasma levels and their PMN produce less Fc gamma RIII compared to adults. Biol Neonate 69:235-242, 1996.
991. Henneke P, Osmers I, Bauer K, et al. Impaired CD14-dependent and independent response of polymorphonuclear leukocytes in preterm infants. J Perinat Med 31:176-183, 2003.
992. Miller ME. Phagocyte function in the neonate: selected aspects. Pediatrics 64:709-712, 1979.
993. Jones DH, Schmalstieg FC, Dempsey K, et al. Subcellular distribution and mobilization of MAC-1 CD11b/CD18 in neonatal neutrophils. Blood 75:488-498, 1990.
994. Qing G, Rajaraman K, Bortolussi R. Diminished priming of neonatal polymorphonuclear leukocytes by lipopolysaccharide is associated with reduced CD14 expression. Infect Immun 63:248-252, 1995.
995. Cocchi P, Marianelli L. Phagocytosis and intracellular killing of *Pseudomonas aeruginosa* in premature infants. Helv Paediatr Acta 22:110-118, 1967.
996. Coen R, Grush O, Kauder E. Studies of bactericidal activity and metabolism of the leukocyte in full-term neonates. J Pediatr 75: 400-406, 1969.
997. Becker ID, Robinson OM, Bazaan TS, et al. Bactericidal capacity of newborn phagocytes against group B beta-hemolytic streptococci. Infect Immun 34:535-539, 1981.
998. Stroobant J, Harris MC, Cody CS, et al. Diminished bactericidal capacity for group B streptococcus in neutrophils from "stressed" and healthy neonates. Pediatr Res 18:634-637, 1984.
999. Shigeoka AO, Charette RP, Wyman ML, et al. Defective oxidative metabolic responses of neutrophils from stressed neonates. J Pediatr 98:392-398, 1981.
1000. Mills EL, Thompson T, Bjeorkstaen B, et al. The chemiluminescence response and bactericidal activity of polymorphonuclear neutrophils from newborns and their mothers. Pediatrics 63:429-434, 1979.
1001. Wright WC Jr, Ank BJ, Herbert J, et al. Decreased bactericidal activity of leukocytes of stressed newborn infants. Pediatrics 56:579-584, 1975.
1002. Shigeoka AO, Santos JI, Hill HR. Functional analysis of neutrophil granulocytes from healthy, infected, and stressed neonates. J Pediatr 95:454-460, 1979.
1003. Ambruso DR, Altenburger KM, Johnston RB Jr. Defective oxidative metabolism in newborn neutrophils: discrepancy between superoxide anion and hydroxyl radical generation. Pediatrics 64:722-725, 1979.
1004. Wilson CB, Weaver WM. Comparative susceptibility of group B streptococci and *Staphylococcus aureus* to killing by oxygen metabolites. J Infect Dis 152:323-329, 1985.
1005. Levy O, Martin S, Eichenwald E, et al. Impaired innate immunity in the newborn: newborn neutrophils are deficient in bactericidal/permeability-increasing protein. Pediatrics 104:1327-1333, 1999.
1006. Hill HR, Augustine NH, Jaffe HS. Human recombinant interferon gamma enhances neonatal polymorphonuclear leukocyte activation and movement, and increases free intracellular calcium. J Exp Med 173:767-770, 1991.
1007. Cairo MS, van de Ven C, Toy C, et al. Recombinant human granulocyte-macrophage colony-stimulating factor primes neonatal granulocytes for enhanced oxidative metabolism and chemotaxis. Pediatr Res 26:395-399, 1989.
1008. Kamran S, Usmani SS, Wapnir RA, et al. In vitro effect of indomethacin on polymorphonuclear leukocyte function in preterm infants. Pediatr Res 33:32-35, 1993.
1009. Forestier F, Daffos F, Galactaeros F, et al. Hematological values of 163 normal fetuses between 18 and 30 weeks of gestation. Pediatr Res 20:342-346, 1986.
1010. Bhat AM, Scanlon JW. The pattern of eosinophilia in premature infants. A prospective study in premature infants using the absolute eosinophil count. J Pediatr 98:612, 1981.
1011. Rothberg AD, Cohn RJ, Argent AC, et al. Eosinophilia in premature neonates. Phase 2 of a biphasic granulopoietic response. S Afr Med J 64:539-541, 1983.
1012. van Furth R, Raeburn JA, van Zwet TL. Characteristics of human mononuclear phagocytes. Blood 54:485-500, 1979.
1013. Hocking WG, Golde DW. The pulmonary-alveolar macrophage (first of two parts). N Engl J Med 301:580-587, 1979.
1014. Hocking WG, Golde DW. The pulmonary-alveolar macrophage (second of two parts). N Engl J Med 301:639-645, 1979.
1015. Butcher EC. Leukocyte–endothelial cell recognition: three or more steps to specificity and diversity. Cell 67:1033-1036, 1991.
1016. Hemler ME. VLA proteins in the integrin family: structures, functions, and their role on leukocytes. Annu Rev Immunol 8:365-400, 1990.
1017. Orme IM, Cooper AM. Cytokine/chemokine cascades in immunity to tuberculosis. Immunol Today 20:307-312, 1999.
1018. Monteiro RC, Van De Winkel JG. IgA Fc receptors. Annu Rev Immunol 21:177-204, 2003.
1019. Sengelov H. Complement receptors in neutrophils. Crit Rev Immunol 15:107-131, 1995.
1020. Underhill DM. Toll-like receptors: networking for success. Eur J Immunol 33:1767-1775, 2003.

1021. Duits LA, Ravensbergen B, Rademaker M, et al. Expression of beta-defensin 1 and 2 mRNA by human monocytes, macrophages and dendritic cells. Immunology 106:517-525, 2002.
1022. Gordon S. Alternative activation of macrophages. Nat Rev Immunol 3:23-35, 2003.
1023. Aderem A. Role of Toll-like receptors in inflammatory response in macrophages. Crit Care Med 29:S16-18, 2001.
1024. Nathan C, Shiloh MU. Reactive oxygen and nitrogen intermediates in the relationship between mammalian hosts and microbial pathogens. Proc Natl Acad Sci U S A 97:8841-8848, 2000.
1025. Casanova JL, Abel L. The human model: a genetic dissection of immunity to infection in natural conditions. Nat Rev Immunol 4:55-66, 2004.
1026. Ottenhoff TH, Verreck FA, Lichtenauer-Kaligis EG, et al. Genetics, cytokines and human infectious disease: lessons from weakly pathogenic mycobacteria and salmonellae. Nat Genet 32:97-105, 2002.
1027. Glauser MP. Pathophysiologic basis of sepsis: considerations for future strategies of intervention. Crit Care Med 28:S4-S8, 2000.
1028. Gabay C, Kushner I. Acute-phase proteins and other systemic responses to inflammation. N Engl J Med 340:448-454, 1999.
1029. Dinarello CA, Cannon JG, Wolff SM. New concepts on the pathogenesis of fever. Rev Infect Dis 10:168-189, 1988.
1030. Eckmann L, Kagnoff MF. Cytokines in host defense against *Salmonella*. Microbes Infect 3:1191-1200, 2001.
1031. Doherty TM. T-cell regulation of macrophage function. Curr Opin Immunol 7:400-404, 1995.
1032. Katze MG, He Y, Gale M Jr. Viruses and interferon: a fight for supremacy. Nat Rev Immunol 2:675-687, 2002.
1033. Taniguchi T, Takaoka A. The interferon-alpha/beta system in antiviral responses: a multimodal machinery of gene regulation by the IRF family of transcription factors. Curr Opin Immunol 14:111-116, 2002.
1034. Boehm U, Klamp T, Groot M, et al. Cellular responses to interferon-gamma. Annu Rev Immunol 15:749-795, 1997.
1035. Murphy KM, Reiner SL. The lineage decisions of helper T cells. Nat Rev Immunol 2:933-944, 2002.
1036. Calandra T, Bochud PY, Heumann D. Cytokines in septic shock. Curr Clin Top Infect Dis 22:1-23, 2002.
1037. Cross AS, Opal SM. A new paradigm for the treatment of sepsis: is it time to consider combination therapy? Ann Intern Med 138:502-505, 2003.
1038. Moore KW, de Waal Malefyt R, Coffman RL, et al. Interleukin-10 and the interleukin-10 receptor. Annu Rev Immunol 19:683-765, 2001.
1039. Letterio JJ, Roberts AB. Regulation of immune responses by TGF-beta. Annu Rev Immunol 16:137-161, 1998.
1040. Nathan CF. Secretory products of macrophages. J Clin Invest 79: 319-326, 1987.
1041. Kelemen E, Jaanossa M. Macrophages are the first differentiated blood cells formed in human embryonic liver. Exp Hematol 8: 996-1000, 1980.
1042. Ueno Y, Koizumi S, Yamagami M, et al. Characterization of hemopoietic stem cells CFUc in cord blood. Exp Hematol 9:716-722, 1981.
1043. Weinberg AG, Rosenfeld CR, Manroe BL, et al. Neonatal blood cell count in health and disease. II. Values for lymphocytes, monocytes, and eosinophils. J Pediatr 106:462-466, 1985.
1044. Alenghat E, Esterly JR. Alveolar macrophages in perinatal infants. Pediatrics 74:221-223, 1984.
1045. Jacobs RF, Wilson CB, Smith AL, et al. Age-dependent effects of aminobutyryl muramyl dipeptide on alveolar macrophage function in infant and adult *Macaca* monkeys. Am Rev Resp Dis 128:862-867, 1983.
1046. Freedman R, Johnston D, Mahoney M, et al. Development of splenic reticuloendothelial function in neonates. J Pediatr 96:466-468, 1980.
1047. Sheldon W, Caldwell J. The mononuclear cell phase of inflammation in the newborn. Bull Johns Hopkins Hosp 112:258-269, 1963.
1048. Bullock JD, Robertson AF, Bedenbender JG, et al. Inflammatory response in the neonate re-examined. Pediatrics 44:58-61, 1969.
1049. Smith S, Jacobs RF, Wilson CB. The immunobiology of childhood tuberculosis: a window on the ontogeny of cellular immunity. J Pediatr 131:16-26, 1997.
1050. Weston WL, Carson BS, Barkin RM, et al. Monocyte-macrophage function in the newborn. Am J Dis Child 131:1241-1242, 1977.
1051. Raghunathan R, Miller ME, Everett S, et al. Phagocyte chemotaxis in the perinatal period. J Clin Immunol 2:242-245, 1982.
1052. Marwitz PA, Van Arkel-Vigna E, Rijkers GT, et al. Expression and modulation of cell surface determinants on human adult and neonatal monocytes. Clin Exp Immunol 72:260-266, 1988.
1053. Dretschmer RR, Stewardson RB, Papierniak CK, et al. Chemotactic and bactericidal capacities of human newborn monocytes. J Immunol 117:1303-1307, 1976.
1054. Hawes CS, Kemp AS, Jones WR. In vitro parameters of cell-mediated immunity in the human neonate. Clin Immunol Immunopathol 17:530-536, 1980.
1055. Orlowski JP, Sieger L, Anthony BF. Bactericidal capacity of monocytes of newborn infants. J Pediatr 89:797-801, 1976.
1056. Speer CP, Ambruso DR, Grimsley J, et al. Oxidative metabolism in cord blood monocytes and monocyte-derived macrophages. Infect Immun 50:919-921, 1985.
1057. Speer CP, Wieland M, Ulbrich R, et al. Phagocytic activities in neonatal monocytes. Eur J Pediatr 145:418-421, 1986.
1058. Speer CP, Gahr M, Wieland M, et al. Phagocytosis-associated functions in neonatal monocyte-derived macrophages. Pediatr Res 24:213-216, 1988.
1059. Conly ME, Speert DP. Human neonatal monocyte–derived macrophages and neutrophils exhibit normal nonopsonic and opsonic receptor–mediated phagocytosis and superoxide anion production. Biol Neonate 60:361-366, 1991.
1060. Marodi L. Deficient interferon-gamma receptor–mediated signaling in neonatal macrophages. Acta Paediatr Suppl 91:117-119, 2002.
1061. Marodi L, Kaposzta R, Nemes E. Survival of group B streptococcus type III in mononuclear phagocytes: differential regulation of bacterial killing in cord macrophages by human recombinant gamma interferon and granulocyte-macrophage colony-stimulating factor. Infect Immun 68:2167-2170, 2000.
1062. Marodi L, Kaposzta R, Campbell DE, et al. Candidacidal mechanisms in the human neonate. Impaired IFN-gamma activation of macrophages in newborn infants. J Immunol 153:5643-5649, 1994.
1063. D'Ambola JB, Sherman MP, Tashkin DP, et al. Human and rabbit newborn lung macrophages have reduced anti-*Candida* activity. Pediatr Res 24:285-290, 1988.
1064. Ganz T, Sherman MP, Selsted ME, et al. Newborn rabbit alveolar macrophages are deficient in two microbicidal cationic peptides, MCP-1 and MCP-2. Am Rev Resp Dis 132:901-904, 1985.
1065. Martin TR, Ruzinski JT, Rubens CE, et al. The effect of type-specific polysaccharide capsule on the clearance of group B streptococci from the lungs of infant and adult rats. J Infect Dis 165:306-314, 1992.
1066. Bellanti JA, Nerurkar LS, Zeligs BJ. Host defenses in the fetus and neonate: studies of the alveolar macrophage during maturation. Pediatrics 64:726-739, 1979.
1067. Coonrod JD, Jarrells MC, Bridges RB. Impaired pulmonary clearance of pneumococci in neonatal rats. Pediatr Res 22:736-742, 1987.
1068. Sherman MP, Johnson JT, Rothlein R, et al. Role of pulmonary phagocytes in host defense against group B streptococci in preterm versus term rabbit lung. J Infect Dis 166:818-826, 1992.
1069. Kurland G, Cheung AT, Miller ME, et al. The ontogeny of pulmonary defenses: alveolar macrophage function in neonatal and juvenile rhesus monkeys. Pediatr Res 23:293-297, 1988.
1070. Wilson CB, Haas JE. Cellular defenses against *Toxoplasma gondii* in newborns. J Clin Invest 73:1606-1616, 1984.
1071. Berman JD, Johnson WD Jr. Monocyte function in human neonates. Infect Immun 19:898-902, 1978.
1072. Plaeger-Marshall S, Ank BJ, Altenburger KM, et al. Replication of herpes simplex virus in blood monocytes and placental macrophages from human neonates. Pediatr Res 26:135-139, 1989.
1073. Mintz L, Drew WL, Hoo R, et al. Age-dependent resistance of human alveolar macrophages to herpes simplex virus. Infect Immun 28:417-420, 1980.
1074. Kohl S. Herpes simplex virus immunology: problems, progress, and promises. J Infect Dis 152:435-440, 1985.
1075. Milgrom H, Shore SL. Assessment of monocyte function in the normal newborn infant by antibody-dependent cellular cytotoxicity. J Pediatr 91:612-614, 1977.
1076. Kohl S. Protection against murine neonatal herpes simplex virus infection by lymphokine-treated human leukocytes. J Immunol 144:307-312, 1990.
1077. Bortolussi R, Rajaraman K, Serushago B. Role of tumor necrosis factor-alpha and interferon-gamma in newborn host defense against *Listeria monocytogenes* infection. Pediatr Res 32:460-464, 1992.

1078. Henneke P, Takeuchi O, Malley R, et al. Cellular activation, phagocytosis, and bactericidal activity against group B streptococcus involve parallel myeloid differentiation factor 88-dependent and independent signaling pathways. J Immunol 169:3970-3977, 2002.
1079. O'Neill LA. Signal transduction pathways activated by the IL-1 receptor/toll-like receptor superfamily. Curr Top Microbiol Immunol 270:47-61, 2002.
1080. Burchett SK, Weaver WM, Westall JA, et al. Regulation of tumor necrosis factor/cachectin and IL-1 secretion in human mononuclear phagocytes. J Immunol 140:3473-3481, 1988.
1081. Cohen L, Haziot A, Shen DR, et al. CD14-independent responses to LPS require a serum factor that is absent from neonates. J Immunol 155:5337-5342, 1995.
1082. Rowen JL, Smith CW, Edwards MS. Group B streptococci elicit leukotriene B_4 and interleukin-8 from human monocytes: neonates exhibit a diminished response. J Infect Dis 172:420-426, 1995.
1083. Chang M, Suen Y, Lee SM, et al. Transforming growth factor-beta 1, macrophage inflammatory protein-1 alpha, and interleukin-8 gene expression is lower in stimulated human neonatal compared with adult mononuclear cells. Blood 84:118-124, 1994.
1084. Sautois B, Fillet G, Beguin Y. Comparative cytokine production by in vitro stimulated mononucleated cells from cord blood and adult blood. Exp Hematol 25:103-108, 1997.
1085. Hebra A, Kramer R, Johnson JT, et al. Detection of intracellular tumor necrosis factor alpha in stimulated fetal cells. J Surg Res 82:300-304, 1999.
1086. Chheda S, Palkowetz KH, Garofalo R, et al. Decreased interleukin-10 production by neonatal monocytes and T cells: relationship to decreased production and expression of tumor necrosis factor-alpha and its receptors. Pediatr Res 40:475-483, 1996.
1087. Kotiranta-Ainamo A, Rautonen J, Rautonen N. Imbalanced cytokine secretion in newborns. Biol Neonate 85:55-60, 2004.
1088. Kotiranta-Ainamo A, Rautonen J, Rautonen N. Interleukin-10 production by cord blood mononuclear cells. Pediatr Res 41:110-113, 1997.
1089. Jones CA, Cayabyab RG, Kwong KY, et al. Undetectable interleukin (IL)-10 and persistent IL-8 expression early in hyaline membrane disease: a possible developmental basis for the predisposition to chronic lung inflammation in preterm newborns. Pediatr Res 39: 966-975, 1996.
1090. Blahnik MJ, Ramanathan R, Riley CR, et al. Lipopolysaccharide-induced tumor necrosis factor-alpha and IL-10 production by lung macrophages from preterm and term neonates. Pediatr Res 50: 726-731, 2001.
1091. Kohl S, Harmon MW. Human neonatal leukocyte interferon production and natural killer cytotoxicity in response to herpes simplex virus. J Interferon Res 3:461-463, 1983.
1092. Joyner JL, Augustine NH, Taylor KA, et al. Effects of group B streptococci on cord and adult mononuclear cell interleukin-12 and interferon-gamma mRNA accumulation and protein secretion. J Infect Dis 182:974-977, 2000.
1093. La Pine TR, Joyner JL, Augustine NH, et al. Defective production of IL-18 and IL-12 by cord blood mononuclear cells influences the T helper-1 interferon gamma response to group B streptococci. Pediatr Res 54:276-281, 2003.
1094. Yan SR, Qing G, Byers DM, et al. Role of MyD88 in diminished tumor necrosis factor alpha production by newborn mononuclear cells in response to lipopolysaccharide. Infect Immun 72:1223-1229, 2004.
1095. Kampalath B, Cleveland RP, Kass L. Reduced CD4 and HLA-DR expression in neonatal monocytes. Clin Immunol Immunopathol 87:93-100, 1998.
1096. Berner R, Furll B, Stelter F, et al. Elevated levels of lipopolysaccharide-binding protein and soluble CD14 in plasma in neonatal early-onset sepsis. Clin Diagn Lab Immunol 9:440-445, 2002.
1097. Varis I, Deneys V, Mazzon A, et al. Expression of HLA-DR, CAM and co-stimulatory molecules on cord blood monocytes. Eur J Haematol 66:107-114, 2001.
1098. Sorg RV, Andres S, Kogler G, et al. Phenotypic and functional comparison of monocytes from cord blood and granulocyte colony-stimulating factor-mobilized apheresis products. Exp Hematol 29:1289-1294, 2001.
1099. Hemming VG, O'Brien WF, Fischer GW, et al. Studies of short-term pulmonary and peripheral vascular responses induced in oophorectomized sheep by the infusion of a group B streptococcal extract. Pediatri Res 18:266-269, 1984.
1100. O'Brien WF, Golden SM, Bibro MC, et al. Short-term responses in neonatal lambs after infusion of group B streptococcal extract. Obstet Gynecol 65:802-806, 1985.
1101. Janeway CA, Travers P, Walport M, et al. Immunobiology. New York, Garland Publishing, 2001.
1102. Szalai AJ, Agrawal A, Greenhough TJ, et al. C-reactive protein: structural biology and host defense function. Clin Chem Lab Med 37:265-270, 1999.
1103. Kohler PF. Maturation of the human complement system. I. Onset time and sites of fetal C1q, C4, C3, and C5 synthesis. J Clin Invest 52:671-677, 1973.
1104. Lassiter HA, Watson SW, Seifring ML, et al. Complement factor 9 deficiency in serum of human neonates. J Infect Dis 166:53-57, 1992.
1105. Zach TL, Hostetter MK. Biochemical abnormalities of the third component of complement in neonates. Pediatr Res 26:116-120, 1989.
1106. Johnston RB Jr, Altenburger KM, Atkinson AW Jr, et al. Complement in the newborn infant. Pediatrics 64:781-786, 1979.
1107. Notarangelo LD, Chirico G, Chiara A, et al. Activity of classical and alternative pathways of complement in preterm and small for gestational age infants. Pediatr Res 18:281-285, 1984.
1108. Davis CA, Vallota EH, Forristal J. Serum complement levels in infancy: age related changes. Pediatri Res 13:1043-1046, 1979.
1109. Ainbender E, Cabatu EE, Guzman DM, et al. Serum C-reactive protein and problems of newborn infants. J Pediatr 101:438-440, 1982.
1110. Eisen DP, Minchinton RM. Impact of mannose-binding lectin on susceptibility to infectious diseases. Clin Infect Dis 37:1496-1505, 2003.
1111. Holmskov U, Thiel S, Jensenius JC. Collections and ficolins: humoral lectins of the innate immune defense. Annu Rev Immunol 21:547-578, 2003.
1112. Lau YL, Chan SY, Turner MW, et al. Mannose-binding protein in preterm infants: developmental profile and clinical significance. Clin Exp Immunol 102:649-654, 1995.
1113. Kielgast S, Thiel S, Henriksen TB, et al. Umbilical cord mannan-binding lectin and infections in early childhood. Scand J Immunol 57:167-172, 2003.
1114. McCormack FX, Whitsett JA. The pulmonary collectins, SP-A and SP-D, orchestrate innate immunity in the lung. J Clin Invest 109: 707-712, 2002.
1115. Marino JA, Pensky J, Culp LA, et al. Fibronectin mediates chemotactic factor-stimulated neutrophil substrate adhesion. J Lab Clin Med 105:725-730, 1985.
1116. Proctor RA. The staphylococcal fibronectin receptor: evidence for its importance in invasive infections. Rev Infect Dis 9(Suppl 4): S335-S340, 1987.
1117. Proctor RA. Fibronectin: an enhancer of phagocyte function. Rev Infect Dis 9(Suppl 4):S412-S419, 1987.
1118. Okamura Y, Watari M, Jerud ES, et al. The extra domain A of fibronectin activates Toll-like receptor 4. J Biol Chem 276: 10229-10233, 2001.
1119. Barnard DR, Arthur MM. Fibronectin cold insoluble globulin in the neonate. J Pediatr 102:453-455, 1983.
1120. Gerdes JS, Yoder MC, Douglas SD, et al. Decreased plasma fibronectin in neonatal sepsis. Pediatrics 72:877-881, 1983.
1121. McCafferty MH, Lepow M, Saba TM. Normal fibronectin levels as a function of age in the pediatric population. Pediatr Res 17:482-485, 1983.
1122. Dossett JH, Williams RC Jr, Quie PG. Studies on interaction of bacteria, serum factors and polymorphonuclear leukocytes in mothers and newborns. Pediatrics 44:49-57, 1969.
1123. Geelen SP, Fleer A, Bezemer AC, et al. Deficiencies in opsonic defense to pneumococci in the human newborn despite adequate levels of complement and specific IgG antibodies. Pediatr Res 27: 514-518, 1990.
1124. Edwards MS, Buffone GJ, Fuselier PA, et al. Deficient classical complement pathway activity in newborn sera. Pediatr Res 17: 685-688, 1983.
1125. Winkelstein JA, Kurlandsky LE, Swift AJ. Defective activation of the third component of complement in the sera of newborn infants. Pediatr Res 13:1093-1096, 1979.
1126. Mills EL, Bjorksten B, Quie PG. Deficient alternative complement pathway activity in newborn sera. Pediatr Res 13:1341-1344, 1979.
1127. Kobayashi Y Usui T. Opsonic activity of cord serum—an evaluation based on determination of oxygen consumption by leukocytes. Pediatr Res 16:243-246, 1982.

1128. Marodi L, Leijh PC, Braat A, et al. Opsonic activity of cord blood sera against various species of microorganism. Pediatr Res 19:433-436, 1985.
1129. Adamkin D, Stitzel A, Urmson J, et al. Activity of the alternative pathway of complement in the newborn infant. J Pediatr 93: 604-608, 1978.
1130. Eads ME, Levy NJ, Kasper DL, et al. Antibody-independent activation of C1 by type Ia group B streptococci. J Infect Dis 146:665-672, 1982.
1131. Anderson DC, Hughes BJ, Edwards MS, et al. Impaired chemotaxigenesis by type III group B streptococci in neonatal sera: relationship to diminished concentration of specific anticapsular antibody and abnormalities of serum complement. Pediatr Res 17:496-502, 1983.
1132. Zilow EP, Hauck W, Linderkamp O, et al. Alternative pathway activation of the complement system in preterm infants with early onset infection. Pediatr Res 41:334-339, 1997.
1133. Rubens CE, Smith S, Hulse M, et al. Respiratory epithelial cell invasion by group B streptococci. Infect Immun 60:5157-5163, 1992.
1134. Bals R. Epithelial antimicrobial peptides in host defense against infection. Respir Res 1:141-150, 2000.
1135. Gallo RL, Nizet V. Endogenous production of antimicrobial peptides in innate immunity and human disease. Curr Allergy Asthma Rep 3:402-409, 2003.
1136. Nizet V, Ohtake T, Lauth X, et al. Innate antimicrobial peptide protects the skin from invasive bacterial infection. Nature 414: 454-457, 2001.
1137. Poyart C, Pellegrini E, Marceau M, et al. Attenuated virulence of *Streptococcus agalactiae* deficient in D-alanyl-lipoteichoic acid is due to an increased susceptibility to defensins and phagocytic cells. Mol Microbiol 49:1615-1625, 2003.
1138. Pluschke G Achtman M. Degree of antibody-independent activation of the classical complement pathway by K1 *Escherichia coli* differs with O antigen type and correlates with virulence of meningitis in newborns. Infect Immun 43:684-692, 1984.
1139. Marques MB, Kasper DL, Pangburn MK, et al. Prevention of C3 deposition by capsular polysaccharide is a virulence mechanism of type III group B streptococci. Infect Immun 60:3986-3993, 1992.
1140. Campbell JR, Baker CJ, Edwards MS. Deposition and degradation of C3 on type III group B streptococci. Infect Immun 59:1978-1983, 1991.
1141. Baker CJ, Edwards MS. Group B streptococcal conjugate vaccines. Arch Dis Child 88:375-378, 2003.
1142. Wessels MR, Butko P, Ma M, et al. Studies of group B streptococcal infection in mice deficient in complement component C3 or C4 demonstrate an essential role for complement in both innate and acquired immunity. Proc Natl Acad Sci U S A 92:11490-11494, 1995.
1143. Pozdnyakova O, Guttormsen HK, Lalani FN, et al. Impaired antibody response to group B streptococcal type III capsular polysaccharide in C3- and complement receptor 2–deficient mice. J Immunol 170:84-90, 2003.
1144. Hill HR, Shigeoka AO, Augustine NH, et al. Fibronectin enhances the opsonic and protective activity of monoclonal and polyclonal antibody against group B streptococci. J Exp Med 159:1618-1628, 1984.
1145. Jacobs RF, Kiel DP, Sanders ML, et al. Phagocytosis of type III group B streptococci by neonatal monocytes: enhancement by fibronectin and gammaglobulin. J Infect Dis 152:695-700, 1985.
1146. Matsukawa A, Lukacs NW, Hogaboam CM, et al. III. Chemokines and other mediators, 8. Chemokines and their receptors in cell-mediated immune responses in the lung. Microsc Res Tech 53: 298-306, 2001.
1147. Bohnsack JF, Widjaja K, Ghazizadeh S, et al. A role for C5 and C5a-ase in the acute neutrophil response to group B streptococcal infections. J Infect Dis 175:847-855, 1997.
1148. Cusumano V, Mancuso G, Genovese F, et al. Neonatal hypersusceptibility to endotoxin correlates with increased tumor necrosis factor production in mice. J Infect Dis 176:168-176, 1997.
1149. Mancuso G, Cusumano V, Genovese F, et al. Role of interleukin 12 in experimental neonatal sepsis caused by group B streptococci. Infect Immun 65:3731-3735, 1997.
1150. Williams PA, Bohnsack JF, Augustine NH, et al. Production of tumor necrosis factor by human cells in vitro and in vivo, induced by group B streptococci. J Pediatr 123:292-300, 1993.
1151. Peat EB, Augustine NH, Drummond WK, et al. Effects of fibronectin and group B streptococci on tumour necrosis factor-α production by human culture-derived macrophages. Immunol. 841995.
1152. Teti G, Mancuso G, Tomasello F. Cytokine appearance and effects of anti-tumor necrosis factor alpha antibodies in a neonatal rat model of group B streptococcal infection. Infect Immun 61:227-235, 1993.
1153. Givner LB, Gray L, O'Shea TM. Antibodies to tumor necrosis factor-alpha: use as adjunctive therapy in established group B streptococcal disease in newborn rats. Pediatr Res 38:551-554, 1995.
1154. Cusumano V, Genovese F, Mancuso G, et al. Interleukin-10 protects neonatal mice from lethal group B streptococcal infection. Infect Immun 64:2850-2852, 1996.
1155. Fisher CJ Jr, Agosti JM, Opal SM, et al. Treatment of septic shock with the tumor necrosis factor receptor:Fc fusion protein. The Soluble TNF Receptor Sepsis Study Group. N Engl J Med 334:1697-1702, 1996.
1156. Hemming VG, Hall RT, Rhodes PG, et al. Assessment of group B streptococcal opsonins in human and rabbit serum by neutrophil chemiluminescence. J Clin Invest 58:1379-1387, 1976.
1157. Lin FY, Philips JB 3rd, Azimi PH, et al. Level of maternal antibody required to protect neonates against early-onset disease caused by group B streptococcus type Ia: a multicenter, seroepidemiology study. J Infect Dis 184:1022-1028, 2001.
1158. Christensen KK, Christensen P, Duc G, et al. Correlation between serum antibody-levels against group B streptococci and gestational age in newborns. Eur J Pediatr 142:86-88, 1984.
1159. Baker CJ, Edwards MS Kasper DL. Role of antibody to native type III polysaccharide of group B streptococcus in infant infection. Pediatrics 68:544-549, 1981.
1160. Edwards MS, Hall MA, Rench MA, et al. Patterns of immune response among survivors of group B streptococcal meningitis. J Infect Dis 161:65-70, 1990.
1161. Boyer KM, Klegerman ME, Gotoff SP. Development of IgM antibody to group B Streptococcus type III in human infants. J Infect Dis 165:1049-1055, 1992.
1162. Nealon TJ, Mattingly SJ. Role of cellular lipoteichoic acids in mediating adherence of serotype III strains of group B streptococci to human embryonic, fetal, and adult epithelial cells. Infect Immun 43:523-530, 1984.
1163. Broughton RA, Baker CJ. Role of adherence in the pathogenesis of neonatal group B streptococcal infection. Infect Immun 39:837-843, 1983.
1164. Anthony BF, Concepcion NF, Wass CA, et al. Immunoglobulin G and M composition of naturally occurring antibody to type III group B streptococci. Infect Immun 46:98-104, 1984.
1165. Kallman J, Schollin J, Schalen C, et al. Impaired phagocytosis and opsonisation towards group B streptococci in preterm neonates. Arch Dis Child Fetal Neonatal Ed 78:F46-50, 1998.
1166. Hill HR. Intravenous immunoglobulin use in the neonate: role in prophylaxis and therapy of infection. Pediatr Infect Dis J 12:549-558, 1993.
1167. Baker CJ, Melish ME, Hall RT, et al. Intravenous immune globulin for the prevention of nosocomial infection in low-birth-weight neonates. The Multicenter Group for the Study of Immune Globulin in Neonates. N Engl J Med 327:213-219, 1992.
1168. Jenson HB, Pollock BH. Meta-analyses of the effectiveness of intravenous immune globulin for prevention and treatment of neonatal sepsis. Pediatrics 99:E2, 1997.
1169. Ohlsson A, Lacy JB. Intravenous immunoglobulin for preventing infection in preterm and/or low-birth-weight infants. Cochrane Database Syst Rev CD000361, 2001.
1170. Suri M, Harrison L, Van de Ven C, et al. Immunotherapy in the prophylaxis and treatment of neonatal sepsis. Curr Opin Pediatr 15:155-160, 2003.
1171. La Gamma EF, De Castro MH. What is the rationale for the use of granulocyte and granulocyte-macrophage colony-stimulating factors in the neonatal intensive care unit? Acta Paediatr Suppl 91:109-116, 2002.
1172. Carr R, Modi N, Dore C. G-CSF and GM-CSF for treating or preventing neonatal infections. Cochrane Database Syst Rev CD003066, 2003.
1173. Kocherlakota P, La Gamma EF. Preliminary report: rhG-CSF may reduce the incidence of neonatal sepsis in prolonged preeclampsia-associated neutropenia. Pediatrics 102:1107-1111, 1998.
1174. Friedman CA, Wender DF, Temple DM, et al. Intravenous gamma globulin as adjunct therapy for severe group B streptococcal disease in the newborn. Am J Perinatol 7:1-4, 1990.
1175. Weisman LE, Stoll BJ, Kueser TJ, et al. Intravenous immune globulin therapy for early-onset sepsis in premature neonates. J Pediatr 121: 434-443, 1992.

1176. Weisman LE, Stoll BJ, Kueser TJ, et al. Intravenous immune globulin prophylaxis of late-onset sepsis in premature neonates. J Pediatr 125:922-930, 1994.
1177. Christensen RD, Brown MS, Hall DC, et al. Effect on neutrophil kinetics and serum opsonic capacity of intravenous administration of immune globulin to neonates with clinical signs of early-onset sepsis. J Pediatr 118:606-614, 1991.
1178. Haque KN, Remo C, Bahakim H. Comparison of two types of intravenous immunoglobulins in the treatment of neonatal sepsis. Clin Exp Immunol 101:328-333, 1995.
1179. Fischer GW, Weisman LE, Hemming VG. Directed immune globulin for the prevention or treatment of neonatal group B streptococcal infections: a review. Clin Immunol Immunopathol 62:92-97, 1992.
1180. Hill HR, Gonzales LA, Knappe WA, et al. Comparative protective activity of human monoclonal and hyperimmune polyclonal antibody against group B streptococci. J Infect Dis 163:792-798, 1991.
1181. Raff HV, Bradley C, Brady W, et al. Comparison of functional activities between IgG1 and IgM class-switched human monoclonal antibodies reactive with group B streptococci or *Escherichia coli* K1. J Infect Dis 163:346-354, 1991.
1182. Rosenthal J, Healey T, Ellis R, et al. A two-year follow-up of neonates with presumed sepsis treated with recombinant human granulocyte colony-stimulating factor during the first week of life. J Pediatr 128:135-137, 1996.
1183. Gillan ER, Christensen RD, Suen Y, et al. A randomized, placebo-controlled trial of recombinant human granulocytes colony stimulatoring facor administration in newborn infants with presumed sepsis: significant induction of peripheral and bone marrow neutrophilia. Blood 84:1427-1433, 1994.
1184. Drossou-Agakidou V, Kanakoudi-Tsakalidou F, Sarafidis K, et al. Administration of recombinant human granulocyte-colony stimulating factor to septic neonates induces neutrophilia and enhances the neutrophil respiratory burst and beta$_2$ integrin expression. Results of a randomized controlled trial. Eur J Pediatr 157:583-588, 1998.
1185. Bernstein HM, Pollock BH, Calhoun DA, et al. Administration of recombinant granulocyte colony-stimulating factor to neonates with septicemia: A meta-analysis. J Pediatr 138:917-920, 2001.
1186. Kimberlin DW. Neonatal herpes simplex infection. Clin Microbiol Rev 17:1-13, 2004.
1187. Langenberg AG, Corey L, Ashley RL, et al. A prospective study of new infections with herpes simplex virus type 1 and type 2. Chiron HSV Vaccine Study Group. N Engl J Med 341:1432-1438, 1999.
1188. Kohl S. The neonatal human's immune response to herpes simplex virus infection: a critical review. Pediatr Infect Dis J 8:67-74, 1989.
1189. Grandvaux N, tenOever BR, Servant MJ, et al. The interferon antiviral response: from viral invasion to evasion. Curr Opin Infect Dis 15:259-267, 2002.
1190. Dupuis S, Dargemont C, Fieschi C, et al. Impairment of mycobacterial but not viral immunity by a germline human STAT1 mutation. Science 293:300-303, 2001.
1191. Dupuis S, Jouanguy E, Al-Hajjar S, et al. Impaired response to interferon-alpha/beta and lethal viral disease in human STAT1 deficiency. Nat Genet 33:388-391, 2003.
1192. Lebon P, Ponsot G, Aicardi J. Early intrathecal synthesis of interferon in herpes encephalitis. Biomedicine 31:267-271, 1979.
1193. Zawatzky R, Engler H, Kirchner H. Experimental infection of inbred mice with herpes simplex virus. III. Comparison between newborn and adult C57BL/6 mice. J Gen Virol 60:25-29, 1982.
1194. Leib DA, Harrison TE, Laslo KM, et al. Interferons regulate the phenotype of wild-type and mutant herpes simplex viruses in vivo. J Exp Med 189:663-672, 1999.
1195. Yokota S, Yokosawa N, Kubota T, et al. Herpes simplex virus type 1 suppresses the interferon signaling pathway by inhibiting phosphorylation of STATs and janus kinases during an early infection stage. Virology 286:119-124, 2001.
1196. Sainz B Jr, Halford WP. Alpha/beta interferon and gamma interferon synergize to inhibit the replication of herpes simplex virus type 1. J Virol 76:11541-11550, 2002.
1197. Lekstrom-Himes JA, LeBlanc RA, Pesnicak L, et al. Gamma interferon impedes the establishment of herpes simplex virus type 1 latent infection but has no impact on its maintenance or reactivation in mice. J Virol 74:6680-6683, 2000.
1198. Yu Z, Manickan E, Rouse BT. Role of interferon-gamma in immunity to herpes simplex virus. J Leukoc Biol 60:528-532, 1996.
1199. Holterman A-X, Rogers K, Edelmann K, et al. An important role for MHC class-restricted T cells, and limited role for interferon-γ, in protection of mice against lethal herpes simplex virus infection. J Virol 731999.
1200. Milligan GN, Bernstein DI. Interferon-gamma enhances resolution of herpes simplex virus type 2 infection of the murine genital tract. Virology 229:259-268, 1997.
1201. Bouley DM, Kanangat S, Wire W, et al. Characterization of herpes simplex virus type-1 infection and herpetic stromal keratitis development in IFN-gamma knockout mice. J Immunol 155: 3964-3971, 1995.
1202. Minami M, Kita M, Yan XQ, et al. Role of IFN-gamma and tumor necrosis factor-alpha in herpes simplex virus type 1 infection. J Interferon Cytokine Res 22:671-676, 2002.
1203. Cantin E, Tanamachi B, Openshaw H. Role for gamma interferon in control of herpes simplex virus type 1 reactivation. J Virol 73: 3418-3423, 1999.
1204. Cantin E, Tanamachi B, Openshaw H, et al. Gamma interferon (IFN-gamma) receptor null-mutant mice are more susceptible to herpes simplex virus type 1 infection than IFN-gamma ligand null-mutant mice. J Virol 73:5196-5200, 1999.
1205. Han X, Lundberg P, Tanamachi B, et al. Gender influences herpes simplex virus type 1 infection in normal and gamma interferon-mutant mice. J Virol 75:3048-3052, 2001.
1206. Keadle TL, Usui N, Laycock KA, et al. IL-1 and TNF-alpha are important factors in the pathogenesis of murine recurrent herpetic stromal keratitis. Invest Ophthalmol Vis Sci 41:96-102, 2000.
1207. Berkowitz C, Becker Y. Recombinant interleukin-1 alpha, interleukin-2 and M-CSF-1 enhance the survival of newborn C57BL/6 mice inoculated intraperitoneally with a lethal dose of herpes simplex virus-1. Arch Virol 124:83-93, 1992.
1208. Fujioka N, Akazawa R, Ohashi K, et al. Interleukin-18 protects mice against acute herpes simplex virus type 1 infection. J Virol 73: 2401-2409, 1999.
1209. Harandi AM, Svennerholm B, Holmgren J, et al. Interleukin-12 (IL-12) and IL-18 are important in innate defense against genital herpes simplex virus type 2 infection in mice but are not required for the development of acquired gamma interferon–mediated protective immunity. J Virol 75:6705-6709, 2001.
1210. Trinchieri G. Interleukin-12 and the regulation of innate resistance and adaptive immunity. Nat Rev Immunol 3:133-146, 2003.
1211. Koelle DM, Corey L. Recent progress in herpes simplex virus immunobiology and vaccine research. Clin Microbiol Rev 16:96-113, 2003.
1212. Malmgaard L, Paludan SR, Mogensen SC, et al. Herpes simplex virus type 2 induces secretion of IL-12 by macrophages through a mechanism involving NF-kappaB. J Gen Virol 81:3011-3020, 2000.
1213. Broberg EK, Setala N, Eralinna JP, et al. Herpes simplex virus type 1 infection induces upregulation of interleukin-23 (p19) mRNA expression in trigeminal ganglia of BALB/c mice. J Interferon Cytokine Res 22:641-651, 2002.
1214. Pollara G, Speidel K, Samady L, et al. Herpes simplex virus infection of dendritic cells: balance among activation, inhibition, and immunity. J Infect Dis 187:165-178, 2003.
1215. Kumaraguru U, Rouse BT. The IL-12 response to herpes simplex virus is mainly a paracrine response of reactive inflammatory cells. J Leukoc Biol 72:564-570, 2002.
1216. Osorio Y, Wechsler SL, Nesburn AB, et al. Reduced severity of HSV-1–induced corneal scarring in IL-12–deficient mice. Virus Res 90: 317-326, 2002.
1217. Gosselin J, Tomolu A, Gallo RC, et al. Interleukin-15 as an activator of natural killer cell-mediated antiviral response. Blood 94:4210-4219, 1999.
1218. Fawaz LM, Sharif-Askari E, Menezes J. Up-regulation of NK cytotoxic activity via IL-15 induction by different viruses: a comparative study. J Immunol 163:4473-4480, 1999.
1219. Tsunobuchi H, Nishimura H, Goshima F, et al. Memory-type CD8$^+$ T cells protect IL-2 receptor alpha–deficient mice from systemic infection with herpes simplex virus type 2. J Immunol 165: 4552-4560, 2000.
1220. Ashkar AA, Rosenthal KL. Interleukin-15 and natural killer and NKT cells play a critical role in innate protection against genital herpes simplex virus type 2 infection. J Virol 77:10168-10171, 2003.
1221. Tumpey TM, Cheng H, Cook DN, et al. Absence of macrophage inflammatory protein-1alpha prevents the development of blinding herpes stromal keratitis. J Virol 72:3705-3710, 1998.

1222. Banerjee K, Biswas PS, Kim B, et al. CXCR2–/– mice show enhanced susceptibility to herpetic stromal keratitis: a role for IL-6-induced neovascularization. J Immunol 172:1237-1245, 2004.
1223. Nakajima H, Kobayashi M, Pollard RB, et al. Monocyte chemoattractant protein-1 enhances HSV-induced encephalomyelitis by stimulating Th2 responses. J Leukoc Biol 70:374-380, 2001.
1224. Kurt-Jones EA, Chan M, Zhou S, et al. Herpes simplex virus 1 interaction with Toll-like receptor 2 contributes to lethal encephalitis. Proc Natl Acad Sci U S A 101:1315-1320, 2004.
1225. Rosler A, Pohl M, Braune HJ, et al. Time course of chemokines in the cerebrospinal fluid and serum during herpes simplex type 1 encephalitis. J Neurol Sci 157:82-89, 1998.
1226. Lokensgard JR, Cheeran MC, Hu S, et al. Glial cell responses to herpesvirus infections: role in defense and immunopathogenesis. J Infect Dis 186(Suppl 2):S171-S179, 2002.
1227. Melchjorsen J, Pedersen FS, Mogensen SC, et al. Herpes simplex virus selectively induces expression of the CC chemokine RANTES/CCL5 in macrophages through a mechanism dependent on PKR and ICP0. J Virol 76:2780-2788, 2002.
1228. Kodukula P, Liu T, Rooijen NV, et al. Macrophage control of herpes simplex virus type 1 replication in the peripheral nervous system. J Immunol 162:2895-2905, 1999.
1229. Cheng H, Tumpey TM, Staats HF, et al. Role of macrophages in restricting herpes simplex virus type 1 growth after ocular infection. Invest Ophthalmol Vis Sci 41:1402-1409, 2000.
1230. Baskin H, Ellermann-Eriksen S, Lovmand J, et al. Herpes simplex virus type 2 synergizes with interferon-gamma in the induction of nitric oxide production in mouse macrophages through autocrine secretion of tumour necrosis factor-alpha. J Gen Virol 78:195-203, 1997.
1231. MacLean A, Wei XQ, Huang FP, et al. Mice lacking inducible nitric-oxide synthase are more susceptible to herpes simplex virus infection despite enhanced Th1 cell responses. J Gen Virol 79:825-830, 1998.
1232. Adler H, Beland JL, Del-Pan NC, et al. Suppression of herpes simplex virus type 1 (HSV-1)-induced pneumonia in mice by inhibition of inducible nitric oxide synthase (iNOS, NOS2). J Exp Med 185:1533-1540, 1997.
1233. Fujii S, Akaike T, Maeda H. Role of nitric oxide in pathogenesis of herpes simplex virus encephalitis in rats. Virology 256:203-212, 1999.
1234. Fleck M, Mountz JD, Hsu HC, et al. Herpes simplex virus type 2 infection induced apoptosis in peritoneal macrophages independent of Fas and tumor necrosis factor-receptor signaling. Viral Immunol 12:263-275, 1999.
1235. Zhao X, Deak E, Soderberg K, et al. Vaginal submucosal dendritic cells, but not Langerhans cells, induce protective Th1 responses to herpes simplex virus-2. J Exp Med 197:153-162, 2003.
1236. Salio M, Cella M, Suter M, et al. Inhibition of dendritic cell maturation by herpes simplex virus. Eur J Immunol 29:3245-3253, 1999.
1237. Samady L, Costigliola E, MacCormac L, et al. Deletion of the virion host shutoff protein (vhs) from herpes simplex virus (HSV) relieves the viral block to dendritic cell activation: potential of vhs(–) HSV vectors for dendritic cell–mediated immunotherapy. J Virol 77: 3768-3776, 2003.
1238. Mikloska Z, Bosnjak L, Cunningham AL. Immature monocyte-derived dendritic cells are productively infected with herpes simplex virus type 1. J Virol 75:5958-5964, 2001.
1239. Kruse M, Rosorius O, Kratzer F, et al. Inhibition of CD83 cell surface expression during dendritic cell maturation by interference with nuclear export of CD83 mRNA. J Exp Med 191:1581-1590, 2000.
1240. Kruse M, Rosorius O, Kratzer F, et al. Mature dendritic cells infected with herpes simplex virus type 1 exhibit inhibited T-cell stimulatory capacity. J Virol 74:7127-7136, 2000.
1241. Ghanekar S, Zheng L, Logar A, et al. Cytokine expression by human peripheral blood dendritic cells stimulated in vitro with HIV-1 and herpes simplex virus. J Immunol 157:4028-4036, 1996.
1242. Mueller SN, Jones CM, Smith CM, et al. Rapid cytotoxic T lymphocyte activation occurs in the draining lymph nodes after cutaneous herpes simplex virus infection as a result of early antigen presentation and not the presence of virus. J Exp Med 195:651-656, 2002.
1243. Habu S, Akamatsu K, Tamaoki N, et al. In vivo significance of NK cell on resistance against virus (HSV-1) infections in mice. J Immunol 133:2743-2747, 1984.
1244. Tanigawa M, Bigger JE, Kanter MY, et al. Natural killer cells prevent direct anterior-to-posterior spread of herpes simplex virus type 1 in the eye. Invest Ophthalmol Vis Sci 41:132-137, 2000.
1245. Orange JS, Wang B, Terhorst C, et al. Requirement for natural killer cell–produced interferon gamma in defense against murine cytomegalovirus infection and enhancement of this defense pathway by interleukin 12 administration. J Exp Med 182:1045-1056, 1995.
1246. Thimme R, Oldach D, Chang KM, et al. Determinants of viral clearance and persistence during acute hepatitis C virus infection. J Exp Med 194:1395-1406, 2001.
1247. Thimme R, Wieland S, Steiger C, et al. CD8(+) T cells mediate viral clearance and disease pathogenesis during acute hepatitis B virus infection. J Virol 77:68-76, 2003.
1248. Biermer M, Puro R, Schneider RJ. Tumor necrosis factor alpha inhibition of hepatitis B virus replication involves disruption of capsid Integrity through activation of NF-kappaB. J Virol 77:4033-4042, 2003.
1249. Ho IC, Glimcher LH. Transcription: tantalizing times for T cells. Cell 109(Suppl):S109-S120, 2002.
1250. Lafferty WE, Brewer LA, Corey L. Alteration of lymphocyte transformation response to herpes simplex virus infection by acyclovir therapy. Antimicrob Agents Chemother 26:887-891, 1984.
1251. Whitley RJ. Herpes simplex virus. *In* Fields BN, Knipe DM, Howley PM (eds). Fields Virology, vol 2. Philadelphia, Lippincott-Raven, 1996, pp 2297-2342.
1252. Schmid DS, Rouse BT. The role of T cell immunity in control of herpes simplex virus. Curr Top Microbiol Immunol 179:57-74, 1992.
1253. Posavad CM, Koelle DM, Corey L. Tipping the scales of herpes simplex virus reactivation: the important responses are local. Nat Med 4:381-382, 1998.
1254. Smith PM, Wolcott RM, Chervenak R, et al. Control of acute cutaneous herpes simplex virus infection: T cell–mediated viral clearance is dependent upon interferon-gamma (IFN-gamma). Virology 202: 76-88, 1994.
1255. Manickan E, Rouse BT. Roles of different T-cell subsets in control of herpes simplex virus infection determined by using T-cell deficient mouse-models. J Virol 69:8178-8179, 1995.
1256. Ruby J, Bluethemann H, Aguet M, et al. CD40 ligand has potent antiviral activity. Nat Med 1:437-441, 1995.
1257. Jain A, Atkinson TP, Lipsky PE, et al. Defects of T-cell effector function and post-thymic maturation in X-linked hyper-IgM syndrome. J Clin Invest 103:1151-1158, 1999.
1258. Fontana S, Moratto D, Mangal S, et al. Functional defects of dendritic cells in patients with CD40 deficiency. Blood 102:4099-4106, 2003.
1259. Mercadal CM, Martin S, Rouse BT. Apparent requirement for $CD4^+$ T cells in primary anti-herpes simplex virus cytotoxic T-lymphocyte induction can be overcome by optimal antigen presentation. Viral Immunology 4:177-186, 1991.
1260. Stohlman SA, Bergmann CC, Lin MT, et al. CTL effector function within the central nervous system requires $CD4^+$ T cells. J Immunol 160:2896-2904, 1998.
1261. Asanuma H, Sharp M, Maecker HT, et al. Frequencies of memory T cells specific for varicella-zoster virus, herpes simplex virus, and cytomegalovirus by intracellular detection of cytokine expression. J Infect Dis 181:859-866, 2000.
1262. Koelle DM, Posavad CM, Barnum GR, et al. Clearance of HSV-2 from recurrent genital lesions correlates with infiltration of HSV-specific cytotoxic T lymphocytes. J Clin Invest 101:1500-1508, 1998.
1263. Koelle DM, Liu Z, McClurkan CM, et al. Expression of cutaneous lymphocyte-associated antigen by CD8(+) T cells specific for a skin-tropic virus. J Clin Invest 110:537-548, 2002.
1264. Koelle DM, Schomogyi M, Corey L. Antigen-specific T cells localize to the uterine cervix in women with genital herpes simplex virus type 2 infection. J Infect Dis 182:662-670, 2000.
1265. Verjans GM, Dings ME, McLauchlan J, et al. Intraocular T cells of patients with herpes simplex virus (HSV)-induced acute retinal necrosis recognize HSV tegument proteins VP11/12 and VP13/14. J Infect Dis 182:923-927, 2000.
1266. Thebeau LG, Morrison LA. Mechanism of reduced T-cell effector functions and class-switched antibody responses to herpes simplex virus type 2 in the absence of B7 costimulation. J Virol 77:2426-2435, 2003.
1267. Carmack MA, Yasukawa LL, Chang SY, et al. T cell recognition and cytokine production elicited by common and type-specific glycoproteins of herpes simplex virus type 1 and type 2. J Infect Dis 174: 899-906, 1996.
1268. Ashkar S, Weber GF, Panoutsakopoulou V, et al. Eta-1 (osteopontin): an early component of type-1 (cell-mediated) immunity. Science 287:860-864, 2000.

1269. Koelle DM, Abbo H, Peck A, et al. Direct recovery of herpes simplex virus (HSV)-specific T lymphocyte clones from recurrent genital HSV-2 lesions. J Infect Dis 169:956-961, 1994.
1270. Schmid DS, Mawle AC. T cell responses to herpes simplex viruses in humans. Rev Infect Dis 13(Suppl 11):946-949, 1991.
1271. Yasukawa M, Zarling JM. Human cytotoxic T cell clones directed against herpes simplex virus-infected cells. III. Analysis of viral glycoproteins recognized by CTL clones by using recombinant herpes simplex viruses. J Immunol 134:2679-2682, 1985.
1272. Mikloska Z, Cunningham AL. Herpes simplex virus type 1 glycoproteins gB, gC and gD are major targets for CD4 T-lymphocyte cytotoxicity in HLA-DR expressing human epidermal keratinocytes. J Gen Virol 79:353-361, 1998.
1273. Walter EA, Greenberg PD, Gilbert MJ, et al. Reconstitution of cellular immunity against cytomegalovirus in recipients of allogeneic bone marrow by transfer of T-cell clones from the donor. N Engl J Med 333:1038-1044, 1995.
1274. Gahn B, Hunt G, Rooney CM, et al. Immunotherapy to reconstitute immunity to DNA viruses. Semin Hematol 39:41-47, 2002.
1275. Speck P, Simmons A. Precipitous clearance of herpes simplex virus antigens from the peripheral nervous systems of experimentally infected C57BL/10 mice. J Gen Virol 79:561-564, 1998.
1276. Liu T, Khanna KM, Carriere BN, et al. Gamma interferon can prevent herpes simplex virus type 1 reactivation from latency in sensory neurons. J Virol 75:11178-11184, 2001.
1277. Pereira RA, Simmons A. Cell surface expression of H2 antigens on primary sensory neurons in response to acute but not latent herpes simplex virus infection in vivo. J Virol 73:6484-6489, 1999.
1278. Martz E, Gamble SR. How do CTL control virus infections? Evidence for prelytic halt of herpes simplex. Viral Immunol 5:81-91, 1992.
1279. Pereira RA, Simon MM, Simmons A. Granzyme A, a noncytolytic component of CD8(+) cell granules, restricts the spread of herpes simplex virus in the peripheral nervous systems of experimentally infected mice. J Virol 74:1029-1032, 2000.
1280. Chang E, Galle L, Maggs D, et al. Pathogenesis of herpes simplex virus type 1–induced corneal inflammation in perforin-deficient mice. J Virol 74:11832-11840, 2000.
1281. Hudson SJ, Streilein JW. Functional cytotoxic T cells are associated with focal lesions in the brains of SJL mice with experimental herpes simplex encephalitis. J Immunol 152:5540-5547, 1994.
1282. Posavad CM, Koelle DM, Shaughnessy MF, et al. Severe genital herpes infections in HIV-infected individuals with impaired herpes simplex virus–specific $CD8^+$ cytotoxic T lymphocyte responses. Proc Natl Acad Sci U S A 94:10289-10294, 1997.
1283. Maertzdorf J, Verjans GM, Remeijer L, et al. Restricted T cell receptor beta-chain variable region protein use by cornea-derived $CD4^+$ and $CD8^+$ herpes simplex virus–specific T cells in patients with herpetic stromal keratitis. J Infect Dis 187:550-558, 2003.
1284. Torpey DJD, Lindsley MD, Rinaldo CR Jr. HLA-restricted lysis of herpes simplex virus–infected monocytes and macrophages mediated by $CD4^+$ and $CD8^+$ T lymphocytes. J Immunol 142:1325-1332, 1989.
1285. Tigges MA, Koelle D, Hartog K, et al. Human $CD8^+$ herpes simplex virus–specific cytotoxic T-lymphocyte clones recognize diverse virion protein antigens. J Virol 66:1622-1634, 1992.
1286. Mikloska Z, Ruckholdt M, Ghadiminejad I, et al. Monophosphoryl lipid A and QS21 increase CD8 T lymphocyte cytotoxicity to herpes simplex virus–2 infected cell proteins 4 and 27 through IFN-gamma and IL-12 production. J Immunol 164:5167-5176, 2000.
1287. Koelle DM, Chen HB, Gavin MA, et al. CD8 CTL from genital herpes simplex lesions: recognition of viral tegument and immediate early proteins and lysis of infected cutaneous cells. J Immunol 166:4049-4058, 2001.
1288. Tigges MA, Leng S, Johnson DC, et al. Human herpes simplex virus (HSV)-specific $CD8^+$ CTL clones recognize HSV-2–infected fibroblasts after treatment with IFN-gamma or when virion host shutoff functions are disabled. J Immunol 156:3901-3910, 1996.
1289. Lorenzo ME, Ploegh HL, Tirabassi RS. Viral immune evasion strategies and the underlying cell biology. Semin Immunol 13:1-9, 2001.
1290. Mocarski ES Jr. Immunomodulation by cytomegaloviruses: manipulative strategies beyond evasion. Trends Microbiol 10:332-339, 2002.
1291. Lewandowski GA, Lo D, Bloom FE. Interference with major histocompatibility complex class II–restricted antigen presentation in the brain by herpes simplex virus type 1: a possible mechanism of evasion of the immune response. Proc Natl Acad Sci U S A 90:2005-2009, 1993.
1292. Koelle DM, Tigges MA, Burke RL, et al. Herpes simplex virus infection of human fibroblasts and keratinocytes inhibits recognition by cloned $CD8^+$ cytotoxic T lymphocytes. J Clin Invest 91: 961-968, 1993.
1293. Ahn K, Meyer TH, Uebel S, et al. Molecular mechanism and species specificity of TAP inhibition by herpes simplex virus ICP47. EMBO J 15:3247-3255, 1996.
1294. Hill A, Jugovic P, York I, et al. Herpes simplex virus turns off the TAP to evade host immunity. Nature 375:411-415, 1995.
1295. Tomazin R, van Schoot NE, Goldsmith K, et al. Herpes simplex virus type 2 ICP47 inhibits human TAP but not mouse TAP. J Virol 72: 2560-2563, 1998.
1296. Bauer D, Tampe R. Herpes viral proteins blocking the transporter associated with antigen processing TAP—from genes to function and structure. Curr Top Microbiol Immunol 269:87-99, 2002.
1297. Mikloska Z, Kesson AM, Penfold MET, et al. Herpes simplex virus protein targets for CD4 and CD8 lymphocyte cytotoxicity in cultured epidermal keratinocytes treated with interferon-gamma. J Infect Dis 173:7-17, 1996.
1298. Simmons A, Tscharke D, Speck P. The role of immune mechanisms in control of herpes simplex virus infection of the peripheral nervous system. Curr Top Microbiol Immunol 179:31-56, 1992.
1299. Bonneau RH, Salvucci LA, Johnson DC, et al. Epitope specificity of H-2Kb-restricted, HSV-1-, and HSV-2-cross-reactive cytotoxic T lymphocyte clones. Virology 195:62-70, 1993.
1300. Cose SC, Kelly JM, Carbone FR. Characterization of a diverse primary herpes simplex virus type 1 gB-specific cytotoxic T-cell response showing a preferential Vbeta bias. J Virol 69:5849-5852, 1995.
1301. Nansen A, Marker O, Bartholdy C, et al. $CCR2^+$ and $CCR5^+CD8^+$ T cells increase during viral infection and migrate to sites of infection. Eur J Immunol 30:1797-1806, 2000.
1302. Sanna PP, Burton DR. Role of antibodies in controlling viral disease: lessons from experiments of nature and gene knockouts. J Virol 74:9813-9817, 2000.
1303. Deshpande SP, Kumaraguru U, Rouse BT. Dual role of B cells in mediating innate and acquired immunity to herpes simplex virus infections. Cell Immunol 202:79-87, 2000.
1304. Harandi AM, Svennerholm B, Holmgren J, et al. Differential roles of B cells and IFN-gamma-secreting CD4(+) T cells in innate and adaptive immune control of genital herpes simplex virus type 2 infection in mice. J Gen Virol 82:845-853, 2001.
1305. Westra DF, Verjans GM, Osterhaus AD, et al. Natural infection with herpes simplex virus type 1 (HSV-1) induces humoral and T cell responses to the HSV-1 glycoprotein H:L complex. J Gen Virol 81: 2011-2015, 2000.
1306. Frank MM. The complement system in host defense and inflammation. Rev Infect Dis 1:483-501, 1979.
1307. Gollins SW, Porterfield JS. A new mechanism for the neutralization of enveloped viruses by antiviral antibody. Nature 321:244-246, 1986.
1308. Figueroa JE, Densen P. Infectious diseases associated with complement deficiencies. Clin Microbiol Rev 4:359-395, 1991.
1309. McKendall RR. IgG-mediated viral clearance in experimental infection with herpes simplex virus type 1: role for neutralization and Fc-dependent functions but not C′ cytolysis and C5 chemotaxis. J Infect Dis 151:464-470, 1985.
1310. Fries LF, Friedman HM, Cohen GH, et al. Glycoprotein C of herpes simplex virus 1 is an inhibitor of the complement cascade. J Immunol 137:1636-1641, 1986.
1311. Lubinski J, Wang L, Mastellos D, et al. In vivo role of complement-interacting domains of herpes simplex virus type 1 glycoprotein gC. J Exp Med 190:1637-1646, 1999.
1312. Johnson DC, Hill AB. Herpesvirus evasion of the immune system. Curr Top Microbiol Immunol 232:149-177, 1998.
1313. Kohl S, Starr SE, Oleske JM, et al. Human monocyte-macrophage–mediated antibody-dependent cytotoxicity to herpes simplex virus–infected cells. J Immunol 118:729-735, 1977.
1314. Shore SL, Melewicz FM, Milgrom H, et al. Antibody-dependent cell-mediated cytotoxicity to target cells infected with herpes simplex viruses. Adv Exp Med Biol 73 Pt B:217-227, 1976.
1315. Petroni KC, Shen L, Guyre PM. Modulation of human polymorphonuclear leukocyte IgG Fc receptors and Fc receptor–mediated functions by IFN-γ and glucocorticoids. J Immunol 140:3467-3472, 1988.
1316. Lin SJ, Roberts RL, Ank BJ, et al. Effect of interleukin (IL)-12 and IL-15 on activated natural killer (ANK) and antibody-dependent cellular cytotoxicity (ADCC) in HIV infection. J Clin Immunol 18:335-345, 1998.

1317. Poaty-Mavoungou V, Toure FS, Tevi-Benissan C, et al. Enhancement of natural killer cell activation and antibody-dependent cellular cytotoxicity by interferon-alpha and interleukin-12 in vaginal mucosae Sivmac251-infected *Macaca fascicularis*. Viral Immunol 15:197-212, 2002.
1318. Hayward AR, Read GS, Cosyns M. Herpes simplex virus interferes with monocyte accessory cell function. J Immunol 150:190-196, 1993.
1319. Barcy S, Corey L. Herpes simplex inhibits the capacity of lymphoblastoid B cell lines to stimulate $CD4^+$ T cells. J Immunol 166: 6242-6249, 2001.
1320. Dabbagh K, Dahl ME, Stepick-Biek P, et al. Toll-like receptor 4 is required for optimal development of Th2 immune responses: role of dendritic cells. J Immunol 168:4524-4530, 2002.
1321. Hayward AR, Herberger MJ, Groothuis J, et al. Specific immunity after congenital or neonatal infection with cytomegalovirus or herpes simplex virus. J Immunol 133:2469-2473, 1984.
1322. Osuga T, Morishima T, Hanada N, et al. Transfer of specific IgG and IgG subclasses to herpes simplex virus across the blood-brain barrier and placenta in preterm and term newborns. Acta Paediatr 81:792-796, 1992.
1323. Ashley RL, Dalessio J, Burchett S, et al. Herpes simplex virus-2 (HSV-2) type-specific antibody correlates of protection in infants exposed to HSV-2 at birth. J Clin Invest 90:511-514, 1992.
1324. Kohl S, West MS, Prober CG, et al. Neonatal antibody-dependent cellular cytotoxic antibody levels are associated with the clinical presentation of neonatal herpes simplex virus infection. J Infect Dis 160:770-776, 1989.
1325. Mikloska Z, Sanna PP, Cunningham AL. Neutralizing antibodies inhibit axonal spread of herpes simplex virus type 1 to epidermal cells in vitro. J Virol 73:5934-5944, 1999.
1326. Vollstedt S, Franchini M, Alber G, et al. Interleukin-12– and gamma interferon–dependent innate immunity are essential and sufficient for long-term survival of passively immunized mice infected with herpes simplex virus type 1. J Virol 75:9596-9600, 2001.
1327. Burioni R, Williamson RA, Sanna PP, et al. Recombinant human Fab to glycoprotein D neutralizes infectivity and prevents cell-to-cell transmission of herpes simplex viruses 1 and 2 in vitro. Proc Natl Acad Sci U S A 91:355-359, 1994.
1328. Cohen J. IL-12 deaths: explanation and a puzzle. Science 270:908, 1995.
1329. Straus SE, Wald A, Kost RG, et al. Immunotherapy of recurrent genital herpes with recombinant herpes simplex virus type 2 glycoproteins D and B: results of a placebo-controlled vaccine trial. J Infect Dis 176:1129-1134, 1997.
1330. Stanberry LR, Spruance SL, Cunningham AL, et al. Glycoprotein-D-adjuvant vaccine to prevent genital herpes. N Engl J Med 347: 1652-1661, 2002.
1331. Kohl S, Charlebois ED, Sigouroudinia M, et al. Limited antibody-dependent cellular cytotoxicity antibody response induced by a herpes simplex virus type 2 subunit vaccine. J Infect Dis 181:335-339, 2000.
1332. Straus SE, Corey L, Burke RL, et al. Placebo-controlled trial of vaccination with recombinant glycoprotein D of herpes simplex virus type 2 for immunotherapy of genital herpes. Lancet 343:1460-1463, 1994.
1333. Whitley RJ, Roizman B. Herpes simplex viruses: is a vaccine tenable? J Clin Invest 110:145-151, 2002.
1334. Mineo JR, McLeod R, Mack D, et al. Antibodies to *Toxoplasma gondii* major surface protein SAG-1, P30 inhibit infection of host cells and are produced in murine intestine after peroral infection. J Immunol 150:3951-3964, 1993.
1335. Decoster A. Detection of IgA anti-P30 SAG1 antibodies in acquired and congenital toxoplasmosis. Curr Top Microbiol Immunol 219:199-207, 1996.
1336. Sibley LD. *Toxoplasma gondii*: perfecting an intracellular life style. Traffic 4:581-586, 2003.
1337. Schwab JC, Beckers CJ, Joiner KA. The parasitophorous vacuole membrane surrounding intracellular *Toxoplasma gondii* functions as a molecular sieve. Proc Natl Acad Sci U S A 91:509-513, 1994.
1338. Wilson CB, Tsai V, Remington JS. Failure to trigger the oxidative metabolic burst by normal macrophages: possible mechanism for survival of intracellular pathogens. J Exp Med 151:328-346, 1980.
1339. Adams LB, Hibbs JB Jr, Taintor RR, et al. Microbiostatic effect of murine-activated macrophages for *Toxoplasma gondii*. Role for synthesis of inorganic nitrogen oxides from L-arginine. J Immunol 144:2725-2729, 1990.
1340. Bohne W, Heesemann J, Gross U. Reduced replication of *Toxoplasma gondii* is necessary for induction of bradyzoite-specific antigens: a possible role for nitric oxide in triggering stage conversion. Infect Immun 62:1761-1767, 1994.
1341. Alexander J, Hunter CA. Immunoregulation during toxoplasmosis. Chem Immunol 70:81-102, 1998.
1342. Yap GS, Sher A. Cell-mediated immunity to *Toxoplasma gondii*: initiation, regulation and effector function. Immunobiology 201: 240-247, 1999.
1343. Sher A, Collazzo C, Scanga C, et al. Induction and regulation of IL-12–dependent host resistance to *Toxoplasma gondii*. Immunol Res 27:521-528, 2003.
1344. Suzuki Y, Orellana MA, Wong SY, et al. Susceptibility to chronic infection with *Toxoplasma gondii* does not correlate with susceptibility to acute infection in mice. Infect Immun 61:2284-2288, 1993.
1345. Gazzinelli RT, Amichay D, Sharton-Kersten T, et al. Role of macrophage-derived cytokines in the induction and regulation of cell-mediated immunity to *Toxoplasma gondii*. Curr Top Microbiol Immunol 219:127-139, 1996.
1346. Pelloux H, Ambroise-Thomas P. Cytokine production by human cells after *Toxoplasma gondii* infection. Curr Top Microbiol Immunol 219:155-163, 1996.
1347. Khan IA, Casciotti L. IL-15 prolongs the duration of $CD8^+$ T cell–mediated immunity in mice infected with a vaccine strain of *Toxoplasma gondii*. J Immunol 163:4503-4509, 1999.
1348. Khan IA, Moretto M, Wei XQ, et al. Treatment with soluble interleukin-15Ralpha exacerbates intracellular parasitic infection by blocking the development of memory $CD8^+$ T cell response. J Exp Med 195:1463-1470, 2002.
1349. Cai G, Kastelein R, Hunter CA. Interleukin-18 (IL-18) enhances innate IL-12-mediated resistance to *Toxoplasma gondii*. Infect Immun 68:6932-6938, 2000.
1350. Hunter CA, Suzuki Y, Subauste CS, et al. Cells and cytokines in resistance to *Toxoplasma gondii*. Curr Top Microbiol Immunol 219: 113-125, 1996.
1351. Denkers EY, Gazzinelli RT. Regulation and function of T-cell-mediated immunity during *Toxoplasma gondii* infection. Clin Microbiol Rev 11:569-588, 1998.
1352. Denkers EY, Kim L, Butcher BA. In the belly of the beast: subversion of macrophage proinflammatory signalling cascades during *Toxoplasma gondii* infection. Cell Microbiol 5:75-83, 2003.
1353. Subauste CS. CD154 and type-1 cytokine response: from hyper IgM syndrome to human immunodeficiency virus infection. J Infect Dis 185(Suppl 1):S83-S89, 2002.
1354. Scott P, Hunter CA. Dendritic cells and immunity to leishmaniasis and toxoplasmosis. Curr Opin Immunol 14:466-470, 2002.
1355. Sacks D, Sher A. Evasion of innate immunity by parasitic protozoa. Nat Immunol 3:1041-1047, 2002.
1356. Gazzinelli RT, Wysocka M, Hieny S, et al. In the absence of endogenous IL-10, mice acutely infected with *Toxoplasma gondii* succumb to a lethal immune response dependent on $CD4^+$ T cells and accompanied by overproduction of IL-12, IFN-gamma and TNF-alpha. J Immunol 157:798-805, 1996.
1357. Suzuki Y, Yang Q, Yang S, et al. IL-4 is protective against development of toxoplasmic encephalitis. J Immunol 157:2564-2569, 1996.
1358. Roberts CW, Ferguson DJ, Jebbari H, et al. Different roles for interleukin-4 during the course of *Toxoplasma gondii* infection. Infect Immun 64:897-904, 1996.
1359. Denkers EY, Gazzinelli RT, Martin D, et al. Emergence of $NK1.1^+$ cells as effectors of IFN-gamma dependent immunity to *Toxoplasma gondii* in MHC class I–deficient mice. J Exp Med 178:1465-1472, 1993.
1360. Shirahata T, Yamashita T, Ohta C, et al. $CD8^+$ T lymphocytes are the major cell population involved in the early gamma interferon response and resistance to acute primary *Toxoplasma gondii* infection in mice. Microbiol Immunol 38:789-796, 1994.
1361. Unanue ER. Macrophages, NK cells and neutrophils in the cytokine loop of *Listeria* resistance. Res Immunol 147:499-505, 1996.
1362. McLeod R, Estes RG, Mack DG, et al. Immune response of mice to ingested *Toxoplasma gondii*: a model of toxoplasma infection acquired by ingestion. J Infect Dis 149:234-244, 1984.
1363. Murray HW, Rubin BY, Carriero SM, et al. Human mononuclear phagocyte antiprotozoal mechanisms: oxygen-dependent vs oxygen-independent activity against intracellular *Toxoplasma gondii*. J Immunol 134:1982-1988, 1985.

1364. Wilson CB, Remington JS. Activity of human blood leukocytes against *Toxoplasma gondii*. J Infect Dis 140:890-895, 1979.
1365. Catterall JR, Black CM, Leventhal JP, et al. Nonoxidative microbicidal activity in normal human alveolar and peritoneal macrophages. Infect Immun 55:1635-1640, 1987.
1366. Catterall JR, Sharma SD, Remington JS. Oxygen-independent killing by alveolar macrophages. J Exp Med 163:1113-1131, 1986.
1367. Biggs BA, Hewish M, Kent S, et al. HIV-1 infection of human macrophages impairs phagocytosis and killing of *Toxoplasma gondii*. J Immunol 154:6132-6139, 1995.
1368. Sibley LD, Adams LB, Fukutomi Y, et al. Tumor necrosis factor-alpha triggers antitoxoplasmal activity of IFN-gamma primed macrophages. J Immunol 147:2340-2345, 1991.
1369. Thomas SM, Garrity LF, Brandt CR, et al. IFN-gamma-mediated antimicrobial response. Indoleamine 2,3-dioxygenase–deficient mutant host cells no longer inhibit intracellular *Chlamydia* spp. or *Toxoplasma* growth. J Immunol 150:5529-5534, 1993.
1370. Dai W, Pan H, Kwok O, et al. Human indoleamine 2,3-dioxygenase inhibits *Toxoplasma gondii* growth in fibroblast cells. J Interferon Res 14:313-317, 1994.
1371. Silva NM, Rodrigues CV, Santoro MM, et al. Expression of indoleamine 2,3-dioxygenase, tryptophan degradation, and kynurenine formation during in vivo infection with *Toxoplasma gondii*: induction by endogenous gamma interferon and requirement of interferon regulatory factor 1. Infect Immun 70:859-868, 2002.
1372. Suzuki Y, Orellana MA, Schreiber RD, et al. Interferon-gamma: the major mediator of resistance against *Toxoplasma gondii*. Science 240:516-518, 1988.
1373. Brown CR, McLeod R. Class I MHC genes and $CD8^+$ T cells determine cyst number in *Toxoplasma gondii* infection. J Immunol 145:3438-3441, 1990.
1374. Araujo FG. Depletion of $L3T4^+CD4^+$ T lymphocytes prevents development of resistance to *Toxoplasma gondii* in mice. Infect Immun 59:1614-1619, 1991.
1375. Gazzinelli R, Xu Y, Hieny S, et al. Simultaneous depletion of $CD4^+$ and $CD8^+$ T lymphocytes is required to reactivate chronic infection with *Toxoplasma gondii*. J Immunol 149:175-180, 1992.
1376. Denkers EY, Sher A. Role of natural killer and $NK1^+$ T-cells in regulating cell-mediated immunity during *Toxoplasma gondii* infection. Biochem Soc Trans 25:699-703, 1997.
1377. Montoya JG, Lowe KE, Clayberger C, et al. Human $CD4^+$ and $CD8^+$ T lymphocytes are both cytotoxic to *Toxoplasma gondii*–infected cells. Infect Immun 64:176-181, 1996.
1378. Curiel TJ, Krug EC, Purner MB, et al. Cloned human $CD4^+$ cytotoxic T lymphocytes specific for *Toxoplasma gondii* lyse tachyzoite-infected target cells. J Immunol 151:2024-2031, 1993.
1379. Scalise F, Gerli R, Castellucci G, et al. Lymphocytes bearing the gamma delta T-cell receptor in acute toxoplasmosis. Immunology 76:668-670, 1992.
1380. De Paoli P, Basaglia G, Gennari D, et al. Phenotypic profile and functional characteristics of human gamma and delta T cells during acute toxoplasmosis. J Clin Microbiol 30:729-731, 1992.
1381. Subauste CS, Chung JY, Do D, et al. Preferential activation and expansion of human peripheral blood gamma delta T cells in response to *Toxoplasma gondii* in vitro and their cytokine production and cytotoxic activity against *T. gondii*–infected cells. J Clin Invest 96:610-619, 1995.
1382. Hisaeda H, Nagasawa H, Maeda K, et al. Gamma delta T cells play an important role in hsp65 expression and in acquiring protective immune responses against infection with *Toxoplasma gondii*. J Immunol 155:244-251, 1995.
1383. Kasper LH, Matsuura T, Fonseka S, et al. Induction of gamma delta T cells during acute murine infection with *Toxoplasma gondii*. J Immunol 157:5521-5527, 1996.
1384. Sayles PC, Rakhmilevich AL, Johnson LL. Gamma delta T cells and acute primary *Toxoplasma gondii* infection in mice. J Infect Dis 171: 249-252, 1995.
1385. Edelson BT, Unanue ER. Immunity to *Listeria* infection. Curr Opin Immunol 12:425-431, 2000.
1386. Frenkel JK, Taylor DW. Toxoplasmosis in immunoglobulin M–suppressed mice. Infect Immun 38:360-367, 1982.
1387. Joiner KA, Fuhrman SA, Miettinen HM, et al. *Toxoplasma gondii*: fusion competence of parasitophorous vacuoles in Fc receptor-transfected fibroblasts. Science 249:641-646, 1990.
1388. Eisenhauer P, Mack DG, McLeod R. Prevention of peroral and congenital acquisition of *Toxoplasma gondii* by antibody and activated macrophages. Infect Immun 56:83-87, 1988.
1389. Luft BJ, Brooks RG, Conley FK, et al. Toxoplasmic encephalitis in patients with acquired immune deficiency syndrome. JAMA 252: 913-917, 1984.
1390. Wilson CB. Congenital nonbacterial infections: diagnosis, treatment and prevention. Perinatol Neonatol 9:9, 1985.
1391. Chen Y, Nakane A, Minagawa T. Recombinant murine gamma interferon induces enhanced resistance to *Listeria monocytogenes* infection in neonatal mice. Infect Immun 57:2345-2349, 1989.
1392. Fatoohi AF, Cozon GJ, Wallon M, et al. Cellular immunity to *Toxoplasma gondii* in congenitally infected newborns and immunocompetent infected hosts. Eur J Clin Microbiol Infect Dis 22: 181-184, 2003.
1393. Hayashi N, Kimura H, Morishima T, et al. Flow cytometric analysis of cytomegalovirus-specific cell-mediated immunity in the congenital infection. J Med Virol 71:251-258, 2003.
1394. Cauda R, Prasthofer EF, Grossi CE, et al. Congenital cytomegalovirus: immunological alterations. J Med Virol 23:41-49, 1987.
1395. Huskinson J, Thulliez P, Remington JS. *Toxoplasma* antigens recognized by human immunoglobulin A antibodies. J Clin Microbiol 28:2632-2636, 1990.
1396. Wong SY, Hajdu MP, Ramirez R, et al. Role of specific immunoglobulin E in diagnosis of acute toxoplasma infection and toxoplasmosis. J Clin Microbiol 31:2952-2959, 1993.
1397. Bortolussi R, Burbridge S, Durnford P, et al. Neonatal *Listeria monocytogenes* infection is refractory to interferon. Pediatr Res 29:400-402, 1991.
1398. Krishnan L, Guilbert LJ, Wegmann TG, et al. T helper 1 response against *Leishmania major* in pregnant C57BL/6 mice increases implantation failure and fetal resorptions. Correlation with increased IFN-gamma and TNF and reduced IL-10 production by placental cells. J Immunol 156:653-662, 1996.
1399. Buxton D, Innes EA. A commercial vaccine for ovine toxoplasmosis. Parasitology 110(Suppl 6):S11-S16, 1995.
1400. Letscher-Bru V, Pfaff AW, Abou-Bacar A, et al. Vaccination with *Toxoplasma gondii* SAG-1 protein is protective against congenital toxoplasmosis in BALB/c mice but not in CBA/J mice. Infect Immun 71:6615-6619, 2003.
1401. Couper KN, Nielsen HV, Petersen E, et al. DNA vaccination with the immunodominant tachyzoite surface antigen (SAG-1) protects against adult acquired *Toxoplasma gondii* infection but does not prevent maternofoetal transmission. Vaccine 21:2813-2820, 2003.
1402. Pickering LK (ed). Red Book: Report of the Committee on Infectious Diseases, 26th ed. Elk Grove Village, Ill, American Academy of Pediatrics, 2003.
1403. Diseases CoI. Revised indications for the use of palivizumab and respiratory syncytial virus immune globulin intravenous for the prevention of respiratory syncytial virus infections. Pediatrics 112:1442-1446, 2003.
1404. Stiehm ER, Ochs HD, Winkelstein JA. Immunologic Disorders in Infants and Children. Philadelphia, Saunders, 2004.
1405. Bortolussi R, Issekutz T, Burbridge S, et al. Neonatal host defense mechanisms against *Listeria monocytogenes* infection: the role of lipopolysaccharides and interferons. Pediatr Res 25:311-315, 1989.
1406. Bessler H, Straussberg R, Gurary N, et al. Effect of dexamethasone on IL-2 and IL-3 production by mononuclear cells in neonates and adults. Arch Dis Child Fetal Neonatal Ed 75:F197-F201, 1996.
1407. Cairo MS, Suen Y, Knoppel E, et al. Decreased G-CSF and IL-3 production and gene expression from mononuclear cells of newborn infants. Pediatr Res 31:574-578, 1992.
1408. Seghaye MC, Heyl W, Grabitz RG, et al. The production of pro- and anti-inflammatory cytokines in neonates assessed by stimulated whole cord blood culture and by plasma levels at birth. Biol Neonate 73:220-227, 1998.
1409. Yachie A, Takano N, Ohta K, et al. Defective production of interleukin-6 in very small premature infants in response to bacterial pathogens. Infect Immun 60:749-753, 1992.
1410. Liechty KW, Koenig JM, Mitchell MD, et al. Production of interleukin-6 by fetal and maternal cells in vivo during intra-amniotic infection and in vitro after stimulation with interleukin-1. Pediatr Res 29:1-4, 1991.
1411. Schibler KR, Liechty KW, White WL, et al. Defective production of interleukin-6 by monocytes: a possible mechanism underlying

several host defense deficiencies of neonates. Pediatr Res 31:18-21, 1992.
1412. Matsuda K, Tsutsumi H, Sone S, et al. Characteristics of IL-6 and TNF-alpha production by respiratory syncytial virus–infected macrophages in the neonate. J Med Virol 48:199-203, 1996.
1413. Taniguchi T, Matsuzaki N, Shimoya K, et al. Fetal mononuclear cells show a comparable capacity with maternal mononuclear cells to produce IL-8 in response to lipopolysaccharide in chorioamnionitis. J Reprod Immunol 23:1-12, 1993.
1414. Suen Y, Chang M, Lee SM, et al. Regulation of interleukin-11 protein and mRNA expression in neonatal and adult fibroblasts and endothelial cells. Blood 84:4125-4134, 1994.
1415. Lee SM, Suen Y, Chang L, et al. Decreased interleukin-12 (IL-12) from activated cord versus adult peripheral blood mononuclear cells and upregulation of interferon-gamma, natural killer, and lymphokine-activated killer activity by IL-12 in cord blood mononuclear cells. Blood 88:945-954, 1996.
1416. Upham JW, Lee PT, Holt BJ, et al. Development of interleukin-12–producing capacity throughout childhood. Infect Immun 70: 6583-6588, 2002.
1417. Dolganov G, Bort S, Lovett M, et al. Coexpression of the interleukin-13 and interleukin-4 genes correlates with their physical linkage in the cytokine gene cluster on human chromosome 5q23-31. Blood 87:3316-3326, 1996.
1418. Handzel ZT, Levin S, Dolphin Z, et al. Immune competence of newborn lymphocytes. Pediatrics 65:491-496, 1980.
1419. Lewis DB, Larsen A, Wilson CB. Reduced interferon-gamma mRNA levels in human neonates. Evidence for an intrinsic T cell deficiency independent of other genes involved in T cell activation. J Exp Med 163:1018-1023, 1986.
1420. Weatherstone KB, Rich EA. Tumor necrosis factor/cachectin and interleukin-1 secretion by cord blood monocytes from premature and term neonates. Pediatr Res 25:342-346, 1989.
1421. Cairo MS, Suen Y, Knoppel E, et al. Decreased stimulated GM-CSF production and GM-CSF gene expression but normal numbers of GM-CSF receptors in human term newborns compared with adults. Pediatr Res 30:362-367, 1991.
1422. Buzby JS, Lee SM, Van Winkle P, et al. Increased granulocyte-macrophage colony-stimulating factor mRNA instability in cord versus adult mononuclear cells is translation-dependent and associated with increased levels of A + U-rich element binding factor. Blood 88:2889-2897, 1996.
1423. Krause PJ, Maderazo EG, Scroggs M. Abnormalities of neutrophil adherence in newborns. Pediatrics 69:184-187, 1982.
1424. Fontan G, Lorente F, Garcia R, et al. In vitro human neutrophil movement in umbilical cord blood. Clin Immunol Immunopathol 20:224-230, 1981.
1425. Tono-Oka T, Nakayama M, Uehara H, et al. Characteristics of impaired chemotactic function in cord blood leukocytes. Pediatr Res 13:148-151, 1979.
1426. Usmani S, Schlessel J, Sia C, et al. Polymorphonuclear leukocyte function the preterm neonate. Pediatrics 87:675-679, 1991.
1427. Eisenfeld L, Krause P, Herson V, et al. Longitudinal study of neutrophil adherence and motility. J Pediatr 117:926-929, 1990.

Chapter 5

HUMAN MILK*

Pearay L. Ogra • David K. Rassin • Roberto P. Garofalo

Mother's milk delivered naturally through breast-feeding has been the sole source of infant nutrition in mammalian species for millions of years. Since human beings learned to domesticate cattle about 10,000 years ago, nonhuman mammalian milk also has been used to supplement or replace maternal milk in the human infant. The development and widespread use of commercially prepared infant formula products have been phenomena of the 20th century and notably of the past 6 decades. Additional information acquired during the last several years has reinforced existing concepts on the role of breast-feeding in protecting the infant against infections, in providing an ideal source of infant nutrition, in modulating infectious immune responses, and in suppressing the evolution of neoplasms and autoimmune disease later in life.[1]

Over the past few decades, the immune responses on intestinal and respiratory mucosal surfaces to local infections have been intensely studied. These investigations have led to the development of concepts of immunity on mucosal surfaces of gastrointestinal, respiratory, and genitourinary tracts and identification of mucosa-associated lymphoid tissue (MALT) and local mechanisms of defense that are distinct from the internal (systemic) immune system.

This chapter reviews existing information on major aspects of the physiologic, nutritional, immunologic, and anti-infective components of the products of lactation. Also discussed is the most recent evidence on the contribution of human milk to the development of immunologic integrity in the infant and its influence on the outcome of infections and other host-antigen interactions in the neonate.

PHYSIOLOGY OF LACTATION

Developmental Anatomy of the Mammary Gland

The rudimentary mammary tissue undergoes several developmental changes during morphogenesis and lactogenesis: In the 4-mm human embryo, the breast tissue appears as a tiny mammary band on the chest wall[2,3]; by the 7-mm embryonic stage, the mammary band develops into the mammary line, along which eventually develops the true mammary anlage; by the 12-mm stage, a primitive epithelial nodule develops; by the 30-mm stage, the primitive mammary bud appears. These initial phases of development take place in both genders (Table 5-1). Further development in the male, however, appears to be limited by androgenic or other male-associated substances.[4,5] Castration in male rat embryos early in gestation leads to female breast development, whereas ovariectomy in the female does not alter the course of development of the mammary anlage. Toward the end of pregnancy, initial phases of fetal mammary differentiation seem to occur under the influence of placental and transplacentally acquired maternal hormones, with transient development of the excretory and lactiferous ductular systems. Such growth, differentiation, and secretory activities are transient and regress soon after birth.[5,6]

At thelarche, and later on at menarche, true mammary growth and development begin in association with rapidly increasing levels of estrogens, progesterone, growth hormone, insulin, adrenocorticosteroids, and prolactin.[6,7] Estrogens appear to be important for the growth and development of the ductular system, and progestins, for lobuloalveolar development (see Table 5-1). Final differentiation of the breast associated with growth and proliferation of the acinar lobes and alveoli continues to be influenced by the levels of estrogen and progesterone. Other peptide hormones, such as prolactin, insulin, and placental chorionic somatomammotropin, appear to be far more important for the subsequent induction and maintenance of lactation (see Table 5-1).

It appears that prolactin secretion from the pituitary gland is under neural control and that the increasing innervation of the breast observed throughout pregnancy is regulated by estrogens.[7] Intense neural input in virgin and parturient but not in currently pregnant mammals has been shown to result in lactation. For example, lactation in goats can be induced by milking maneuvers. Adoptive breast-feeding also is well documented in primitive human societies. Sudden and permanent cessation of suckling can result in the termination of milk secretion and involution of the breast to the prepregnant state as the concentrations of prolactin decline. Estrogen and progesterone also may amplify the direct effects of prolactin or may induce additional receptors for this peptide hormone on appropriate target tissues in the breast.

*This chapter is dedicated to Lars A. Hansen, MD, PhD, the discoverer of sIgA in human milk, the father of modern "mother's milk feeding practices," and a remarkable human being.

Table 5–1 Possible Endocrine Factors in Growth of Human Female Mammary Glands

Clinical State	Growth Characteristics	Maturational Hormones
Prenatal	Rudimentary	None
Infancy	Rudimentary	None
Puberty	Growth and budding of milk ducts	Growth hormone, prolactin-estrogen, adrenocortical steroids, prolactin (high doses)
Pregnancy	Growth of acinar lobules and alveoli	Estrogen, progesterone, prolactin, growth hormone, adrenocortical steroids
Parturition	Alveolar growth	Prolactin, adrenocortical steroids
Lactational growth of tissue	None	None
Secretory products	Casein, α-lactalbumin	Prolactin, insulin, adrenocortical steroids

Endocrine Control of Mammary Gland Function

Breast tissue is responsive to hormones, even as a rudimentary structure, as illustrated by the secretion of "witch's milk" by both male and female newborns in response to exposure to maternal secretion of placental lactogen, estrogens, and progesterone.[3] The secretion of this early milk ceases after exposure to maternal hormones has waned. Sexual differentiation, marked by puberty, is the next major stage in mammary development. As pointed out earlier, androgens inhibit the development of mammary tissue in the male, whereas the development of mammary tissue in the female is dependent on estrogen, progesterone, and pituitary hormones.[8] The postpubertal mammary gland undergoes cyclical changes in response to the release of hormones that takes place during the menstrual cycle. The last stage of development occurs during menopause, when the decline in estrogen secretion results in some atrophy of mammary tissue.

During the menstrual cycle, the mammary gland responds to the sequential release of estrogen and progesterone with a hyperplasia of the ductal system that continues through the secretory phase and declines with the onset of menstruation. The concentration of prolactin modestly increases during the follicular stage of the menstrual cycle but remains constant during the secretory phase.[9] Prolactin secretion appears to be held in readiness for the induction and maintenance of lactation.

Initiation and Maintenance of Lactation. Pregnancy is marked by profound hormonal changes reflecting major secretory contributions from the placenta, the hypothalamus, and the pituitary gland, with contributions from a number of other endocrine glands (e.g., the pancreas, thyroid, and parathyroid). Increased estrogen and progesterone levels during pregnancy stimulate secretion of prolactin from the pituitary, whereas placental lactogen appears to inhibit the release of a prolactin-inhibiting factor from the hypothalamus. Prolactin, lactogen, estrogen, and progesterone all aid in preparing the mammary gland for lactation. Initially in gestation, an increased growth of ductule and alveolobular tissue occurs in response to estrogen and progesterone. In the beginning of the second trimester, secretory material begins to appear in the luminal cells. By the middle of the second trimester, mammary development has proceeded sufficiently to permit lactation to occur should parturition take place.

Once the infant is delivered, a major regulatory factor, the placenta, is lost, and new regulatory factors including the maternal-infant interaction and neuroendocrine regulation are gained for control of lactation. Loss of placental hormone secretion results in an endocrine hypothalamic stimulation of prolactin release from the anterior pituitary gland, as well as neural stimulation of oxytocin from the posterior pituitary. The stimulation of the nipple by suckling activates a neural pathway that results in release of both prolactin and oxytocin. Prolactin is responsible for stimulating milk production, whereas oxytocin stimulates milk ejection (the combination is known as the *let-down reflex*). Oxytocin also stimulates uterine contractions, which the mother may feel while she is breast-feeding; this response helps to restore the uterus to prepregnancy tone.

Milk production and ejection are thus dependent on the complex interaction of stimulation by the infant's suckling, neural reflex of the hypothalamus to such stimulation, release of hormones from the anterior and posterior pituitary, and response of the mammary gland to these hormones to complete the cycle.

Milk Secretion. Milk is produced as the result of synthetic mechanisms within the mammary gland, as well as the transport of components from blood. Milk-specific proteins are synthesized in the mammary secretory cells, packaged in secretory vesicles, and exocytosed into the alveolar lumen. Lactose is secreted into the milk in a similar manner, whereas many monovalent ions, such as sodium, potassium, and chloride, are dependent on active transport systems based on sodium-potassium adenosine triphosphatases (Na^+, K^+-ATPases). In some situations, the mammary epithelium, which may behave as a "mammary barrier" between interstitial fluid derived from blood and the milk because of the lack of space between these cells, may "leak," permitting direct diffusion of components into the milk. This barrier results in the formation of different pools or compartments of milk components within the mammary gland and is responsible for maintaining gradients of these components from the blood to the milk.

Lipid droplets can be observed within the secretory cells of the mammary gland and are surrounded by a milk fat globule membrane. These fat droplets appear to fuse with the apical membrane of the secretory cells and then to be either exocytosed or "pinched off" into the milk.[8] Some whole cells also are found in milk, including leukocytes, macrophages, lymphocytes, and broken or shed mammary epithelial cells. The mechanisms by which these cells enter the milk are complex and include, among others, specific cellular receptor-mediated homing of antigen sensitized lymphocytes.

As the structure of the mammary gland is compartmentalized, so is that of the milk. The gross composition of milk consists of cytoplasm encased by cellular membranes in milk fat globule membranes (fat compartments made up of fat droplets), a soluble compartment containing water-soluble constituents, a casein-micelle compartment containing acid-precipitable proteins with calcium and lactose, and a cellular compartment. The relative amounts of these components change during the course of lactation, generally with less fat and more protein in early lactation than in late lactation. Thus, the infant consumes a dynamic complex solution that has physical properties permitting unique separation of different functional constituents from one another, presumably in forms that best support growth and development.

Lactation Performance. Successful lactation performance depends on continued effective contributions from the neural, endocrine, and maternal-infant interactions that were initiated at the time of delivery. The part of this complex behavior most liable to inhibition is the mother-child interaction. An early attachment of the infant to the breast is mandatory to begin stimulation of the neural pathways essential to maintaining prolactin and oxytocin release.

A healthy newborn infant placed between the mother's breasts will locate a nipple and begin to suck spontaneously within the first hour of birth.[10] This rapid attachment to the mother may reflect olfactory stimuli from the breast received by the infant at birth.[11] Frequent feedings are necessary for the mother to maintain an appropriate level of milk production for the infant's proper growth and development. Programs to support lactation performance must emphasize proper maternal-infant bonding, relaxation of the mother, support for the mother, technical assistance to initiate breast-feeding properly and to cope with problems, and reduction of environmental hindrances. Such hindrances may include lack of rooming-in in the hospital, use of extra formula feeds, and lack of convenient day care for working mothers.

Lactation ceases when suckling stops; therefore, any behavior that reduces the amount of suckling by the infant initiates weaning or the end of lactation. Introduction of water in bottles or of 1 or 2 bottles of formula a day may begin the weaning process regardless of the time after parturition but can be most damaging to the process when the mother-infant dyad is first establishing lactation.

Secretory Products of Lactation: Nutritional Components of Human Colostrum and Milk

Colostrum and milk contain a rich diversity of nutrients, including electrolytes, vitamins, minerals, and trace metals; nitrogenous products; enzymes; and immunologically specific cellular and soluble products. The distribution and relative content of various nutritional substances found in human milk are presented in Table 5-2. The chemical composition often exhibits considerable variation among lactating women and in the same woman at different times of lactation,[12] as well as between samples obtained from mothers of low-birth-weight infants and from mothers of full-term infants.[13,14] Mature milk contains the following average amounts of major chemical constituents per deciliter: total solids, 11.3 g; fat, 3.0 g; protein, 0.9 g; whey protein nitrogen, 760 mg; casein nitrogen, 410 mg; α-lactalbumin, 150 mg; serum albumin, 50 mg; lactose, 7.2 g; lactoferrin, 150 mg; and lysozyme, 50 mg. Human milk contains relatively low amounts of vitamins D and E (see Table 5-2) and little or no β-lactoglobulin (the major whey protein in bovine milk). The fat globule membrane appears to have a high content of oleic acid, linoleic acid, phosphatidylpeptides, and inositol.[15] In addition, a binding ligand that promotes absorption of zinc has been identified in human milk.[16,17] Temporal studies have indicated that concentrations of many

Table 5–2 Distribution of Secretory Products in Human Colostrum and Milk[a]

Water 86%-87.5%; Total Solids 11.5 g
Nutritional Components
Lactose 6.9-7.2 g
Fat 3.0-4.4 g
Protein 0.9-1.03 g
α-Lactalbumin 150-170 mg
β-Lactoglobulin trace
Serum albumin 50 mg
Electrolytes, Minerals, Trace Metals
Sodium 15-17.5 mg
Potassium 51-55 mg
Calcium 32-43 mg
Phosphorus 14-15 mg
Chloride 38-40 mg
Magnesium 3 mg
Iron 0.03 mg
Zinc 0.17 mg
Copper 15-105 μg
Iodine 4.5 μg
Manganese 1.5-2.4 μg
Fluoride 5-25 μg
Selenium 1.8-3.2 μg
Boron 8-10 μg
Nitrogen Products Total 0.15-2 g
Whey protein nitrogen 75-78 mg
Casein protein nitrogen 38-41 mg
Nonprotein nitrogen 25% of total nitrogen
Urea 0.027 g
Creatinine 0.021 g
Glucosamine 0.112 g
Vitamins
C 4.5-5.5 mg
Thiamine (B_1) 12-15 μg
Niacin 183.7 μg
B_6 11-14 μg
B_{12} <0.05 μg
Biotin 0.6-0.9 μg
Folic acid 4.1-5.2 μg
Choline 8-9 mg
Inositol 40-46 mg
Pantothenic acid 200-240 μg
A (retinol) 54-56 μg
D <0.42 IU
E 0.56 μg
K 1.5 μg

[a]Estimates based on amount per deciliter.

chemical components, especially nitrogen, calcium, and sodium, decrease significantly as the duration of lactation increases.[18,19] Several components, however, have been found to change in concentration as a function of water content, because their total daily output appears to be remarkably constant, at least during the first 8 weeks of lactation.[20,21]

Milk production progresses through three distinct phases, characterized by the secretion of colostrum, transitional (early) milk, and mature milk. Colostrum comprises lactational products detected just before and for the first 3 to 4 days of lactation. It consists of yellowish, thick fluid, with a mean energy value of greater than 66 kilocalories (kcal)/dL, and contains high concentrations of immunoglobulin, protein, fat, fat-soluble vitamins, and ash. Transitional milk usually is observed between days 5 and 14 of lactation, and mature milk is found thereafter. The concentrations of many nutritional components decline as milk production progresses to synthesis of mature milk. The content of fat-soluble vitamins and proteins decreases as the water content of milk increases. Conversely, levels of lactose, fat, and water-soluble vitamins and total caloric content have been shown to increase as lactation matures.[22,23]

As the result of several manufacturing errors, the nutrient composition of infant formulas has been legislated,[24] resulting in the paradoxical situation that human milk may not always meet the recommended standards for some nutrients, whereas infant formulas may exceed the recommendation. Human milk nutrient composition varies with time of lactation (colostrum versus early milk versus mature milk) and, to some extent, maternal nutritional status. The appropriate amounts of each nutrient must be considered within these constraints.

Minerals. The mineral content of human milk is low relative to that of infant formulas and very low compared with that of cow's milk, from which most formulas are prepared, so that although human milk is sufficient to support growth and development, it also represents a fairly low solute load to the developing kidney. The levels of major minerals tend to decline during lactation, with the exception of that of magnesium, but with considerable variability among women tested.[25] Sodium, potassium, chloride, calcium, zinc, and phosphorus all appear to be more bioavailable in human milk than in infant formulas, reflecting their lower concentrations in human milk. Iron is readily bioavailable to the infant from human milk but may have to be supplemented later in lactation.[26,27] Preterm infants fed human milk may need supplements of calcium and sodium.[28]

Vitamins. Human milk contains sufficient vitamins to maintain infant growth and development, with the caveat that water-soluble vitamins are particularly dependent on maternal intake of these nutrients.[29] The preterm infant may require supplements of vitamins D, E, and K when fed human milk.[30,31] The low content of vitamin D in human milk has been related to the development of rickets in a few breast-fed infants, as discussed later.[32] Vitamin D deficiency may be a particular problem in breast-fed infants who are not exposed to at least 30 minutes of sunshine per week.[33]

Carbohydrates and Energy. Lactose is the primary sugar found in human milk and usually is the carbohydrate chosen for the preparation of commercial formulas. Lactose supplies approximately half the energy (of a total 67 kcal/dL) taken in by the infant from human milk. Lactose (a disaccharide of glucose and galactose) also may be important to the neonate as a carrier of galactose, which may be more readily incorporated into gangliosides in the central nervous system than galactose derived from glucose in the neonate.[34] Also, glycogen may be synthesized more efficiently from galactose than from glucose in the neonate because of the relatively low activity of glucokinase in early development.[35] Human milk also contains other sugars, including glucose and galactose and more than 100 different oligosaccharides.[36] These oligosaccharides may have protective functions for the infant, especially with respect to their ability to bind to gastrointestinal pathogens.[37]

Lipids. Fats provide almost half of the calories in human milk, primarily in the form of triacylglycerols (triglycerides).[38] These lipids are supplied in the form of fat globules enclosed in plasma membranes derived from the mammary epithelial cells.[39] The essential fatty acid, linoleic acid, supplies about 10% of the calories derived from the lipid fraction. The triacylglycerols serve as precursors for prostaglandins, steroids, and phospholipids and as carriers for fat-soluble vitamins. The lipid profiles of human milk differ dramatically from those of commercial formulas, and despite considerable adaptation of such formulas, human milk lipids are absorbed more efficiently by the infant.

Cholesterol, an important lipid constituent of human milk (12 mg/dL), usually is found in only trace amounts in commercial formulas. It has been suggested that cholesterol may be an essential nutrient for the neonate.[40] A lack of cholesterol in early development may result in turning on of cholesterol-synthetic mechanisms that are difficult to turn off later in life, influencing induction of hypercholesterolemia.[41] Some studies suggest that breast-feeding of the neonate is associated with lowered adult serum cholesterol levels and reduced deaths from ischemic heart disease.[42]

Recently, interest has increased in the role that long-chain polyunsaturated fatty acids (LC-PUFAs) may play in human milk, especially docosahexaenoic acid (DHA) and arachidonic acid (AA). These LC-PUFAs are not found in unsupplemented infant formulas but are present in human milk. They are structural components of brain and retinal membranes and thus may be important for both cognitive and visual development. In addition, they may have a role in preventing atopy.[43] Numerous studies have found that infants fed formula without DHA or AA have reduced red blood cell amounts of these fatty acids[44,45]; however, findings in visual and cognitive functional studies in term infants have been inconsistent.[46,47] These studies have been complicated by the finding of slower growth in some preterm infants fed LC-PUFA–supplemented formulas.[48] The inconsistent findings in supplemented formula–fed babies may reflect the difficulty in determining the optimal amounts of DHA to AA, and their precursors linoleic and linolenic acids, in such supplemented formulas. Thus, these lipids appear to be best delivered from human milk.

Protein and Nonprotein Nitrogen. The exact protein content of mature human milk is variable but falls close to 1.0 g/dL, in contrast with that of infant formulas, which usually contain 1.5 g/dL; the milk from mothers who deliver preterm infants may have slightly more protein.[49] The nutritionally available protein may be even less than 1.0 g/dL—as low as 0.8 g/dL—as a result of the proportion of proteins that is utilized for non-nutritional purposes. In addition, human milk contains a considerably greater percentage of nonprotein nitrogen (25% of the total nitrogen) when compared with formulas (5% of the total nitrogen).[50]

Human milk protein is primarily whey predominant (acid-soluble protein), whereas formulas prepared from bovine milk classically reflect the 18% whey–82% casein protein composition in that species. The whey-to-casein protein ratio in humans may change during lactation, with the whey component ranging from 90% (early milk) to 60% (mature milk) to 50% (late milk).[51] Formulas for preterm infants have been reconstituted from bovine milk to provide 60% whey and 40% casein proteins; all of the major formulas for term infants in the United States are now bovine whey protein–predominant preparations, in an attempt to make them closer to human milk in composition. These differences in protein quality are reflected by differences in the plasma and urine amino acid responses of infants fed human milk or formulas that are casein protein predominant or whey protein predominant.[52-54] In general, however, term infants do not respond with the dramatic differences seen in preterm infants when fed formulas with different protein quality.[55-58]

The nonprotein nitrogen component of human milk contains a variety of compounds that may be of importance to the development of the neonate: polyamines, nucleotides, creatinine, urea, free amino acids, carnitine, and taurine.[59] The significance of the presence of these components is not always clear, but when they are not fed, as in the case of infant formulas that contain little taurine[52] or of soy formulas that contain little carnitine,[60] apparent deficiencies that may influence the development of the infant occur. Taurine is important for bile salt conjugation, as well as for support of appropriate development of the brain and retina,[40] whereas carnitine appears to be important for appropriate fatty acid metabolism.[61]

Nucleotides, in particular, appear to bridge the gap between the nutritional and the immunologic roles of human milk components. Human milk contains a majority of these compounds in the form of polymeric nucleotides or nucleic acids,[62,63] whereas formulas contain nucleotides (when they are supplemented) only in the monomeric forms (Table 5-3). Nucleotides appear to enhance intestinal development, promote iron absorption, and modify lipid metabolism in their nutritional role.[64] On the other hand, these compounds perform an immunologic function by promoting killer cell cytotoxicity and interleukin-2 (IL-2) production by stimulated mononuclear cells from infants either breast-fed or fed nucleotide-supplemented formulas.[65] Nucleotide supplementation also has been reported to reduce the number of episodes of infant diarrhea in a group of lower-socioeconomic-status infants in Chile, in a manner analogous to that for protection afforded by human milk.[66] In 1998 it was reported that nucleotide-supplemented formulas promote the immune response of infants to *Haemophilus influenzae* type b polysaccharide immunization at 7 months of age, and a similar response was observed for diphtheria immunization.[67] Infants fed human milk for more than 6 months demonstrated a similar response and also exhibited an enhanced titer response to oral polio vaccine; this latter response was not observed in the nucleotide-supplemented formula–fed group.[67] Thus, nucleotides are emerging as both nutritional and immunologic components of human milk.

Table 5–3 Nucleotides in Human Milk and Supplemented Formula

	Human Milk[a]	Human Milk[b] (%)	Formula[a]
Nucleic acid	48	42	4
Nucleotides	36	52	81
Nucleotides	8	7	15
Total (μmol/L)	402	163	141

[a]See ref. 62.
[b]See ref. 63.

Nutritional Proteins. As noted, the nutritional proteins in human milk are classified as either whey (acid-soluble) or casein (acid-precipitable). Within these two classes of proteins, several specific proteins are responsible for supporting the nutritional needs of the infant.

Human casein is made up primarily of β- and κ-casein, although the actual distribution of these two proteins is not clear.[68] By contrast, bovine milk contains α_{s1}- and α_{s2}-casein (neither of which is found in human milk), in addition to β- and κ-casein.[69] These two human milk casein proteins appear to account for approximately 30% of the protein found in human milk, in contrast with the earlier calculation of 40% (the amount commonly used to prepare reconstituted, so-called humanized formulas from bovine milk, which normally contains 82% casein proteins).

The whey protein fraction contains all of the proposed functional proteins in human milk (immunoglobulins, lysozyme, lactoferrin, enzymes, cytokines, peptide hormones), in addition to the major nutritional protein, α-lactalbumin. The whey proteins make up approximately 70% of human milk proteins, in contrast with 18% in bovine milk. Whereas α-lactalbumin is the major whey protein in human milk, β-lactoglobulin is the major whey protein in bovine milk (and is not found in human milk).[50] A consistent fraction of human milk whey protein is made up of serum albumin. Its source remains unclear; some evidence indicates that it may be synthesized in the mammary gland.[70] Most of the serum albumin, however, probably is synthesized outside the mammary gland.

Thus, milk proteins are characterized by their site of synthesis, as well as being species specific. Therefore, proteins such as α-lactalbumin and β-lactoglobulin are species and organ specific, whereas proteins such as serum albumin are species specific but not organ specific.[71] The net result of these differences in proteins utilized for nutrition by the neonate is that different amounts of amino acids are ingested by the neonate, depending on the source of milk; even reconstitution of the whey and casein classes of proteins from one species in a ratio similar to that of another species does not result in an identical amino acid intake. These differences are reflected in plasma amino acid profiles of infants fed commercial milks versus human milk, regardless of the ratios of reconstitution.[54]

Bioactive Proteins and Peptides. Whereas a major proportion of human milk protein is composed of the nutritional proteins just described, a significant number of the remaining proteins subserve a variety of functions, either other than or in addition to the nutritional support of the neonate. These proteins include carrier proteins, enzymes, hormones, growth factors, immunoglobulins, and cytokines (the latter two are discussed later under "Resistance to Infection"). Whether these proteins are still functional once they have been ingested by the neonate has not always been established, but it is clear that human milk supplies a mixture that is potentially far more complex than just nutritional substrate.

Carrier Proteins. A number of nutrients are supplied to the neonate bound to proteins found in human milk. This binding may play an important role in making these nutrients bioavailable. Lactoferrin is an iron-binding protein (a property that also may play a role in its bacteriostatic action) that is apparently absorbed intact by the infant.[72] Lactoferrin may be important in the improved absorption of iron by the infant from human milk compared with that from cow's milk preparations, which contain little lactoferrin.[26] Lactoferrin also may bind other minerals, including zinc and manganese, although the preferred mineral form appears to be the ferric ion.

A number of other proteins appear to be important as carriers of vitamins and hormones. Folate-binding, vitamin B_{12}–binding, and vitamin D–binding proteins all have been identified in human milk. These proteins appear to have some resistance to proteolysis, especially when they are saturated with the appropriate vitamin ligand.[73] Serum albumin acts as a carrier of a number of ligands, whereas α-lactalbumin acts as a carrier for calcium. Finally, proteins that bind thyroid hormone and corticosteroids have been reported to be present in human milk,[74,75] although serum albumin may in part fulfill this function.

Enzymes. The activity of more than 30 enzymes has been detected in human milk.[76] Most of these enzymes appear to originate from the blood, with a few originating from secretory epithelial cells of the mammary gland. Little is known about the role of these enzymes, other than lysozyme and the lipases, in human milk. The enzymes found in human milk range from ATPases to antioxidant enzymes, such as catalase, to phosphatases and glycolytic enzymes. Although these enzymes have important roles in normal body metabolism, it is not clear how many of them either function in the milk itself or survive ingestion by the infant to function in the neonate.

Lysozyme appears to have a part in the antibacterial function of human milk, whereas the lipases have a more nutrient-related role in modulating fat metabolism for the neonate. Two lipases have been identified in human milk, a lipoprotein lipase and a bile salt–stimulated lipase.[77] Lipoprotein lipase appears to be involved in determining the pattern of lipids found in human milk by regulating uptake into milk at the level of the mammary gland. Human milk bile salt–stimulated lipase is an acid-stable protein that compensates for the low activity of lipases secreted into the digestive tract during early development.[78] Thus, these two enzymes regulate both the amount and the pattern of lipid that appears in milk as well as the extremely efficient absorption of lipid by the infant. Human milk lipid is absorbed much more readily than lipid from commercial milk formulas despite the many adaptations that have been made to improve absorption, illustrating the effective mechanisms supported by the lipases.

Hormones and Growth Factors. Both peptide and steroid hormones, as well as growth factors, have been identified in trace amounts in human milk, although as with most of the enzymes, it is not clear to what degree they function in the neonate to whom they have been supplied. As discussed previously, binding proteins for corticosteroids and thyroxine have been identified in milk and, by extrapolation from observations of other milk components, may play a role in making these bioactive compounds more readily available to the infant.

Among the hormones identified in human milk are insulin, oxytocin, calcitonin, and prolactin. Most of these hormones appear to be absorbed by the infant, but their role in in vivo function remains unclear.[79] Breast-fed infants appear to have a different endocrine response from that of formula-fed infants, presumably reflecting the intake of hormones from human milk.[80] The advantages or disadvantages to the infant of these responses, however, are unknown.

Human milk also contains a rich mixture of growth factors, including epidermal growth factor (EGF) and nerve growth factor.[81] In addition, a variety of gastrointestinal peptides have been identified in human milk. Presumably, the supply of these various factors to the infant through the milk compensates for their possible deficiency in the infant during early development.

The composition of human milk provides a complex and complete nutritional substrate to the neonate. Human milk supplies not only individual nutrients but also enzymes involved in metabolism, carriers to improve absorption, and hormones that may regulate metabolic rates. Commercial formulas have not yet been developed to the point that they can provide an analogous complete nutritional system.

RESISTANCE TO INFECTION

Component Mechanisms of Defense: Origin and Distribution

Fresh human milk contains a wealth of components that provide specific, as well as nonspecific, defenses against infectious agents and environmental macromolecules (Table 5-4). These component factors include cells, such as T and B lymphocytes, polymorphonuclear neutrophils (PMNs) (i.e., polymorphonuclear leukocytes), and macrophages; soluble products, especially immunoglobulins; secretory immunoglobulin A (sIgA); immunomodulatory cytokines and cytokine receptors; components of the complement system; several carrier proteins; enzymes; and a number of endocrine hormones or hormone-like substances. Additional soluble factors that are active against streptococci, staphylococci, and tumor viruses also have been identified.[22] Other soluble milk factors with potential implications in host defense include the bifidus factor, which promotes growth of bifidobacteria, and an EGF, which promotes growth of mucosal epithelium and maturation of intestinal brush border. The developmental characteristics of sIgA have been studied more extensively than those of other components.[82-84]

On the basis of available information, it is clear that a majority of IgA-producing cells observed in milk have their origin in the precursor immunocompetent cells in the gut-associated lymphoid tissue (GALT) and bronchus-associated

Table 5–4 Immunologically and Pharmacologically Active Components and Hormones Observed in Human Colostrum and Milk

Soluble	Cellular	Hormones and Hormone-like Substances
Immunologically Specific	**Immunologically Specific**	Epidermal growth factors
Immunoglobulin sIgA (11S), 7S IgA, IgG, IgM, IgE, IgD, secretory component	T lymphocytes	Prostaglandins
	B lymphocytes	Neurotensin
T Cell Products	**Accessory Cells**	Relaxin
Histocompatibility Antigens	Neutrophils	Somatostatin
Nonspecific Factors	Macrophages	Bombesin
Complement	Epithelial cells	Gonadotropins
Chemotactic factors		Ovarian steroids
Properdin		Thyroid-releasing hormone
Interferon		Thyroid-stimulating hormone
α-Fetoprotein		Thyroxine and triiodothyronine
Bifidus factor		Adrenocorticotropin
Antistaphylococcal factor(s)		Corticosteroids
Antiadherence substances		Prolactin
Epidermal growth factor		Erythropoietin
Folate uptake enhancer		Insulin
Antiviral factors(s)		
Migration inhibition factor		
Carrier Proteins		
Lactoferrin		
Transferrin		
B_{12}-binding protein		
Corticoid-binding protein		
Enzymes		
Lysozyme		
Lipoprotein lipase		
Leukocyte enzymes		

Table 5–5 Specific Antibody or Cell-Mediated Immunologic Reactivity in Human Colostrum and Milk

Bacteria	Viruses	Other
Escherichia coli (O + K antigens and enterotoxin)	Rotavirus	*Candida albicans*
Salmonella	Rubella virus	*Giardia* species
Shigella species	Poliovirus types 1, 2, 3	*Entamoeba histolytica*
Vibrio cholerae	Echoviruses	Food proteins
Bacteroides fragilis	Coxsackieviruses A and B	
Streptococcus pneumoniae	Respiratory syncytial virus[a]	
Bordetella pertussis	Cytomegalovirus[a]	
Clostridium tetani and *Clostridium difficile*	Influenza A virus	
Corynebacterium diphtheriae	Herpes simplex virus type 1	
Streptococcus mutans	Arboviruses	
Haemophilus influenzae type B	Semliki Forest virus	
Mycobacterium tuberculosis[a]	Ross River virus	
	Japanese B virus	
	Dengue virus	
	Human immunodeficiency virus	
	Hepatitis A and B viruses	

[a]Evidence of reactivity for both antibody and cellular immunity.

lymphoid tissue (BALT). Exposure of IgA precursor B lymphocytes in the GALT or BALT to microbial and dietary antigens in the mucosal lumen is an important prerequisite for their initial activation and proliferation. Such antigen-sensitized cells eventually are transported through the systemic circulation to other mucosal surfaces, including the mammary glands and, as plasma cells, initiate the synthesis of immunoglobulin against specific antigens previously experienced in the mucosa of the respiratory or alimentary tract.[82,83] It has been proposed that T cells observed in the milk also may be derived from GALT and BALT in a manner similar to that of IgA-producing cells. Little or no information is available regarding the site of origin of other cellular or soluble immunologic components normally present in human milk. Specific antibody and cellular immune reactivity against many respiratory and enteric bacterial and viral pathogens and ingested food proteins also are present in human breast milk (Table 5-5).

Soluble Products

Immunoglobulin A. As observed in other peripheral mucosal sites, the major class of immunoglobulin in human colostrum and milk is the 11S sIgA. Other isotypes—namely, 7S IgA, IgG, IgM, IgD, and IgE—also are present. The IgA exists as a dimer of two 7S IgA molecules linked together by a polypeptide chain, the J-chain, and is associated with a nonimmunoglobulin protein referred to as the secretory component. The sIgA protein constitutes about 75% of the total nitrogen content of human milk. The IgA dimers produced by plasma cells at the basal surface of the mammary epithelium are transported to specialized columnar epithelial cells, where they acquire the secretory component before their discharge into the alveolar spaces.[83,84]

Sequential quantitation of class-specific immunoglobulin in human colostrum and milk has demonstrated that the highest levels of sIgA and IgM are present during the first few days of lactation (Fig. 5-1). Levels of IgA are 4 to 5 times greater than those of IgM, 20 to 30 times greater than those of IgG, and 5 to 6 times greater than those of serum IgA.[84] As lactation progresses, IgA declines to levels that range from 20 to 27 mg per gram of protein, and IgM levels decline to 3.5 to 4.1 mg/g. IgG levels do not show any significant change during early and late lactation and usually are maintained in the range of 1.4 to 4.9 mg/g (see Fig. 5-1). Although a dramatic and rapid decline in milk IgA and IgM occurs during the first week of life, this decrease is more than balanced by an increase in the volume of milk produced as the process of lactation becomes established (see Fig. 5-1).

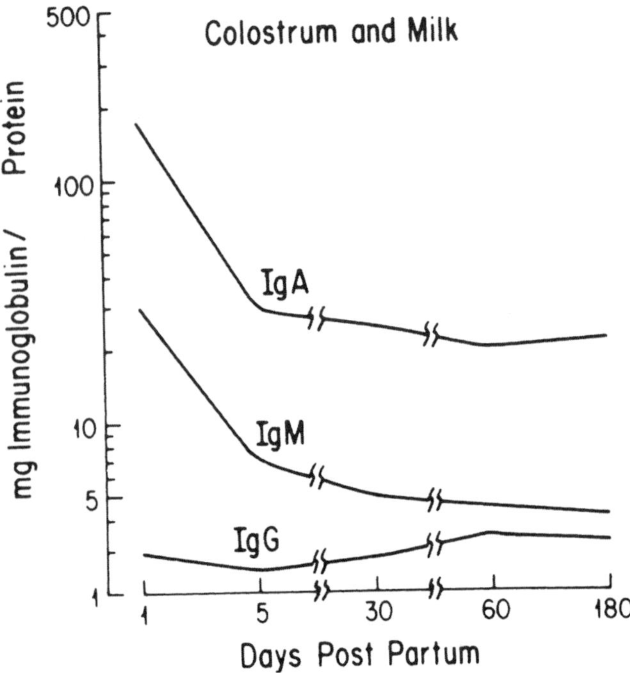

Figure 5–1 Comparison of the mean levels of IgG, IgA, and IgM in colostrum and milk at different intervals after the onset of lactation in mothers who were breast-feeding. (Data from Ogra SS, Ogra PL. Immunologic aspects of human colostrum and milk. II. Characteristics of lymphocyte reactivity and distribution of E-rosette forming cells at different times after the onset of lactation. J Pediatr 92:550-555, 1978.)

IgA antibodies found in milk possess specificity for infectious agents endemic to or pathogenic for the intestinal and respiratory tracts (see Table 5-4). These antibodies may be present in the milk in the absence of specific circulating IgA. In a study in which pregnant women were given oral feedings of *Escherichia coli* 083, development of IgA antibody in human milk was evident in the absence of detectable serum antibody-specific responses.[85] In another study, investigators have observed similar responses in animal models using intrabronchial immunization with *Streptococcus pneumoniae*. These and other studies[86-89] have strongly supported the concept of a bronchomammary, as well as an enteromammary, axis of immunologic reactivity in the breast.

Despite the elegance of studies that have defined the mechanisms of IgA cell trafficking from GALT and BALT to the mammary glands, it is clear that the actual number of B cells or IgA plasma cells in the mammary glands is sparse. At the same time, colostrum and milk may contain large amounts of IgA (as much as 11 g in colostrum and as much as 1 to 3 g per day in later milk), as shown in Table 5-6. The reasons underlying the apparent disparity between the content of immunoglobulin-producing cells and concentrations of immunoglobulin are not known. It may be related to the unique hormonal environment of the mammary glands. The hormones that have been consistently observed in human milk are listed in Table 5-4.

The effect of pregnancy- and lactation-related hormones on regulation of immunologic reactivity present in the resting and lactating breast has been examined.[90] In a study on immunoglobulin production in the nonlactating human breast, several interesting findings were noted.[91] Few mononuclear cells were present in the nonlactating breast of nulliparous and of parous women, although IgA-containing cells predominated. Synthesis of IgA appeared to be slightly increased in the parous women. IgA was found in the mammary tissues during the proliferative stage of the menstrual cycle in the nulliparous women and during the luteal phase in the parous women. The number of IgA-producing cells in the nonlactating breast was observed to increase with parity. These findings suggest that the immunologic makeup of the nonlactating, as well as the lactating, breast may be significantly influenced by the hormonal milieu. In another study of virgin mice given exogenously administered hormones,[92] an extended exposure to estrogen, progesterone, and prolactin was necessary for maximal increments in IgA-producing plasma cells in the breast. Similarly, castrated males exposed to these hormones became moderately receptive to mammary gland homing of cells specific for IgA synthesis. As would be expected, testosterone eliminated female breast receptivity to these cells. These studies suggest the existence of a hormonally determined homing mechanism in the mammary gland for class-specific, immunoglobulin-producing cells.

More recent studies have proposed another possible influence of lactational hormones on immunocompetent cells. In limited observations, combinations of prolactin with estrogen and progesterone (in concentrations observed normally at the beginning of parturition) appeared to have an amplifying effect on the synthesis and secretion of IgA from peripheral blood lymphocytes.[93] This observation raises the possibility that the high levels of sIgA observed in colostrum and milk may be the result of selective, hormonally mediated proliferation of antigen-sensitized IgA cells in the peripheral blood. The immunoglobulin could acquire secretory component during its passage through the mammary epithelium and eventually appear in the colostrum or milk as mature sIgA. Although the appearance of sIga antibody in milk characteristically follows antigenic exposure in the GALT or BALT, the precise nature of the IgA content in milk appears to be determined by a variety of other factors operating in the mucosal lymphoid tissue. These include the regulatory T cell network in the GALT and possibly in the BALT,[94] the nature of antigens (soluble proteins versus particulate microbial agents),[95] and the route of primary versus secondary antigenic exposure.[96]

It has been estimated that the breast-fed infant may consistently receive an amount of about 1 g of IgA each day. Approximately $\frac{1}{100}$ of this amount each day is IgM and IgG.[97,98] The estimates of lactational immunoglobulin delivered to the breast-fed infant at different periods of lactation are presented in Table 5-6. Most ingested IgA is eliminated in the feces, although up to 10% may be absorbed from the intestine into the circulation within the first 18 to 24 hours after birth. Approximately 70% to 75% of ingested milk IgA survives passage through the gut and is excreted in the feces.[99] Feces of breast-fed infants contain functional antibodies present in the ingested milk.[100] Other studies also support the finding of prolonged survival of milk IgA in the gastrointestinal tract. Infants fed human milk have demonstrated the presence of all immunoglobulin classes in the feces. Fecal IgA content was three to four times greater than that of IgM after human milk feeding. Comparative studies on survival of human milk IgA and bovine IgG in the neonatal intestinal tract have suggested that the fecal content of IgA may be 14 to 20 times greater after human milk feeding than that of bovine IgG after feeding of bovine immune globulin.[101]

Direct information about the role of milk IgA in antimicrobial defense is available in several studies. Secretory IgA interferes with bacterial adherence to cell surfaces.[102] Colostrum and milk can inhibit the activity of *E. coli* and *Vibrio cholerae* enterotoxins in experimental settings.[103] The antitoxic activity of human milk appears to correlate well with its IgA content but not with its IgM and IgG content. Precoating of *V. cholerae* with specific sIgA protects infant mice from disease.[104] Similar results have been obtained by using specific purified milk sIgA in preventing *E. coli*– and *Shigella dysenteriae*–induced disease in rabbits.[105] Less definite, but suggestive, is a study conducted with human milk feeding relative to the intestinal implantation of orally administered live poliovirus vaccine.[106] This study found that breast-feeding may reduce the degree of seroconversion for poliovirus antibody in the vaccinated infants. Because antipolio IgA is present in human milk and colostrum, the investigators concluded that specific IgA may bind poliovirus and influence viral replication in the intestinal mucosa. Extensive experience with oral polio immunization worldwide, however, has not found an association between breast-feeding and live vaccine failures. Other studies have clearly shown that the magnitude of poliovirus replication in the intestine is determined by the presence and level of preexisting sIgA antibody. With high levels of intestinal IgA antibody, little or no replication of vaccine virus was observed in the gut. With lower levels, varying degrees of viral replication could be demonstrated.[107]

Indirect evidence, obtained from a more clinical perspective, suggests a protective role for milk against a variety of mucosal infections. Breast-feeding has been strongly implicated in supporting gastrointestinal homeostasis in the neonate and in establishing normal gut flora. Observations have shown the absence of diarrheal disease in breast-fed infants, even in the face of contamination of the fed milk with *E. coli* and *Shigella* species.[108] A preventive and therapeutic role for breast-feeding also has been suggested in nursery outbreaks of such disease due to enteropathogenic strains of *E. coli*[109] and diarrhea associated with rotavirus.[110] Breast-feeding plays an inhibitory role in the appearance of *E. coli* O83 agglutinins found in the feces of colonized infants. A decrease in the incidence of neonatal sepsis, specifically that associated with gram-negative bacilli and *E. coli* K1 serotypes, also has been linked to breast-feeding.[111,112] Milk IgA, possibly by limiting ingestion of foreign antigens by the neonate, or by binding of foreign proteins with specific antibodies to prevent absorption, or by both processes, may decrease the incidence of atopic-allergic diseases.[113-115] The frequency of IgE skin test–positive results has been described as being lower among breast-fed infants, possibly because of decreased exposure to cow's milk proteins or presence of maternal blocking antibodies.[116] Indirect epidemiologic data suggest that breast-feeding is protective against certain respiratory bacterial and viral infections.[117,118] Whereas the epidemiologic studies strongly support a protective role of breast-feeding, it is not possible in these studies to dissect the relative contribution of sIgA from that of other soluble or cellular components present in colostrum and milk.

Table 5–6 Level of Immunoglobulins in Colostrum and Milk and Estimates of Delivery of Lactational Immunoglobulins to the Breast-Feeding Neonate[a]

	Percentage of Total Proteins Represented by Immunoglobulin			Output of Immunoglobulin (mg/24 hr)		
Day Post Partum	*IgG*	*IgM*	*IgA*	*IgG*	*IgM*	*IgA*
1	7	3	80	80	120	11,000
3	10	45	45	50	40	2000
7	1-2	4	20	25	10	1000
7-28	1-2	2	10-15	10	10	1000
<50	1-2	0.5-1	10-15	10	10	1000

[a]Estimates based on the available data for total immunoglobulin and daily protein synthesis (see references 6, 83, 84).

Immunoglobulin G and Immunoglobulin M. Normal neonates exhibit characteristic paucity or lack of IgA during the first 7 to 10 days after birth. At that time, the presence of IgM and IgG in milk may be important to compensate for immunologic functions not present in the mucosal sites. For example, both IgG and IgM participate in complement fixation and specific bactericidal activity, functions not associated with IgA. Studies carried out after oral feeding of immune serum globulin (mostly IgG) have suggested that IgG may survive in the gastrointestinal tract of low-birth-weight infants.[119] Thus, other immunoglobulin isotypes in milk also may be able to serve as effective substitutes for IgA in the neonates of IgA-deficient mothers in prevention of infection with enteric or respiratory pathogens.

Immunoglobulin E and Immunoglobulin D. Studies on the distribution and role of IgE or IgD in colostrum and milk are few. Normal cord blood contains little or no IgE or IgD. The highest IgE concentrations observed in normal neonates usually are less than 5 ng/mL. Investigations have failed to demonstrate local synthesis of IgE in the breast.[120-122] Although IgE may be detected in up to 40% of colostrum and milk samples, the concentrations are extremely low, and many samples of colostrum and milk contain no IgE activity when paired samples of serum contain high IgE levels. On the other hand, IgD has been detected in most colostrum and milk samples. It has been suggested that nursing women with high serum IgD levels are more likely to have high IgD concentrations in their milk. The possibility of some local production of both IgE and IgD cannot be ruled out.[122]

Cellular Elements

Human colostrum and milk contain lymphocytes, monocytes-macrophages, neutrophils, and epithelial cells.[123] Early colostrum contains the highest concentration of cells, approximately 1×10^6 to 3×10^6 cells per mL. By the end of the first week of lactation, cell concentration is of the order of 10^5 cells per mL. Total cell numbers delivered to the newborn throughout lactation may, however, remain constant when adjustments are made for the increase in volume of milk produced.[124] The two major cell populations in human milk are difficult to distinguish by common staining methods because of the large number of intracytoplasmic inclusions, neutrophils, and macrophages. More accurate estimates made by flow cytometry analysis suggest that the relative percentages of neutrophils, macrophages, and lymphocytes in early milk samples are approximately 80%, 15%, and 4%, respectively.[125,126] The remaining cells are present in smaller amounts, especially in the absence of active suckling, engorgement, or local breast infection.

Macrophages. Histochemically, the milk macrophage differs from the blood monocyte in demonstrating decreased peroxidase staining, with increased lysosomes and significant amounts of immunoglobulin, especially IgA, in the cytoplasm.[127-129] The intracellular immunoglobulin in macrophages represents up to 10% of milk IgA.[130] Kinetic studies on the release of IgA by human milk macrophages suggest that immunoglobulin release by macrophages, unlike that by other phagocytic cells, is a time-dependent phenomenon and is not significantly influenced by the use of secretagogues or stimulants, such as phorbol myristate acetate.[130] Active phagocytosis, however, is associated with significant increase in release of IgA.[131] In other studies, milk macrophages have been found to be efficient in release of superoxide anions after in vitro stimulation with phorbol myristate acetate.[132,133] Milk macrophages have the capacity to be primed by appropriate stimulation for greater release of superoxide anions.[133] It has been shown that milk macrophages obtained from preterm-delivered lactating mothers have a significantly higher phagocytic index than that for the macrophages in term milk. The bactericidal activity appears to be similar in pre- and full-term milk macrophages, however.[132] In neutrophils, milk macrophages appear to be activated, as demonstrated by the increased expression of CD11b and decreased expression of L-selectin.[125]

The precise functions of macrophages in colostrum or milk have not been fully explored. These cells have been suggested as potential transport vehicles for IgA.[128,129] Milk macrophages possess phagocytic activity against *Staphylococcus aureus*, *E. coli*, and *Candida albicans*, with possible cytocidal activity against the first two organisms.[134] Milk macrophages participate in antibody-dependent, cell-mediated cytotoxicity for herpes simplex virus type 1–infected cells.[135] Infection of milk macrophages by respiratory syncytial virus results in the production of the pro-inflammatory cytokines IL-1β, IL-6, and tumor necrosis factor-α (TNF-α).[136] These cells also are involved in a variety of other biosynthetic and excretory activities, including production of lactoferrin, lysozyme,[137] components of complement,[138] properdin factor B, epithelial growth factor(s), and T lymphocyte–suppressive factor(s).[82] Milk macrophages also have been suggested to be important in regulation of T cell function.[139,140]

Lymphocytes. Milk contains a small number of lymphocytes, 80% of which are T cells and 4% to 6% of which are B cells.[126] The small number of B cells reflects the sessile nature of these cells, which enter the lamina propria of the mammary gland to transform into plasma cells. Although several investigators have been unable to show in vitro antibody synthesis by milk lymphocytes, studies performed with colostral B cells transformed by Epstein-Barr virus have shown production of IgG, as well as J-chain–containing IgM and IgA.[141] A small population of $CD16^+$ natural killer (NK) cells also can be identified in most milk samples but cannot be accurately quantitated.[126] In functional studies, however, colostral cells exhibit NK cytotoxicity, which is enhanced by interferon and IL-2. Colostral cells also elicit antibody- and lectin-dependent cellular cytotoxic responses. The NK, as well as the antibody- and lectin-dependent, responses in colostral cells, however, have been observed to be significantly lower than those of autologous peripheral blood cells. Reduced cellular cytotoxicity of colostral cells also has been observed against virus-infected targets and certain bacteria. In fact, with several specific virus-infected targets, colostrum and milk cells conspicuously lack cellular cytotoxicity when compared with autologous peripheral blood cells. There is also an apparent exclusion of cytolytic T cells in the milk that are specific for certain human leukocyte antigen (HLA) phenotypes.[142,143]

A majority of T lymphocytes in colostrum and milk are mature $CD3^+$ cells. Both $CD4^+$ (helper) and $CD8^+$ (cytotoxic and suppressor) populations are present in human milk, with a proportion of $CD8^+$ T cells higher than that found in human blood (Table 5-7). The $CD4^+/CD8^+$ ratio in milk is

Table 5–7 Lymphocyte Subpopulations in Human Milk and Autologous Blood[a]

Lymphocyte Subpopulation	Human Milk	Blood
CD3+[b]	83 ± 11	75 ± 7
CD3+ CD4+[b]	36 ± 13	44 ± 6
CD3+ CD8+[b]	43 ± 12	27 ± 4
CD4+/CD8+[c]	0.88 ± 0.35	1.70 ± 0.45
CD19+[b]	6 ± 4	14 ± 5

[a]Expressed as mean ± standard deviation (SD).
[b]Expressed as percentage of total lymphocytes.
[c]Ratio of CD3+/CD4+ to CD3+/CD8+ lymphocytes.
Adapted from Wirt DP, Adkins LT, Palkowetz KH, et al. Activated-memory T lymphocytes in human milk. Cytometry 13:282-290, 1992.

significantly lower than that observed in peripheral blood and is not due to an increase of CD8+ cells in the peripheral blood of women during the postpartum period. Colostral and milk T lymphocytes manifest in vitro proliferative responses on stimulation with a number of mitogens and antigens. Several studies have shown a selectivity in lymphocyte stimulation responses in colostral and milk lymphocytes to various antigens when compared with peripheral blood lymphocyte responses.[124,144] Antigens such as rubella virus stimulate T lymphocytes in secretory sites and milk, as well as in systemic sites.[124] By contrast, *E. coli* K1 antigen whose exposure is limited to mucosal sites produces stimulation of lymphoproliferative responses only in milk lymphocytes. These findings support the concept of select T cell populations in the mammary gland.

In addition to antigen selectivity, a general hyporesponsiveness to mitogenic stimulation of milk lymphocytes relative to peripheral blood lymphocytes has been observed.[124,140] The decreased reactivity of milk lymphocytes to phytohemagglutinin (PHA) may be partly the result of a relative deficiency of certain populations of T cells in milk. Macrophage–T cell interactions also have been postulated as being responsible for this relative hyporesponsiveness,[84] although it is not known whether the effects are the result of decreased helper or increased suppressor function. Recent studies have shown that milk lymphocytes exhibit reduced responses to allogeneic cells but display good ability to stimulate alloreactivity.[142] Treatment of milk lymphocytes with monoclonal antibodies cytotoxic for T lymphocytes or with anti-HLA class II antigen–specific monoclonal antibodies has resulted in a substantial reduction in in vitro proliferative responses to bacterial antigens. It appears that, in general, the T cell proliferative responses to PHA and tetanus toxoid in breast-fed infants are significantly higher than those in bottle-fed infants, possibly secondary to the presence of maternally derived cell growth factors and other lymphokines present in human milk.[140,145]

Virtually all CD4+ and CD8+ T cells in milk bear the CD45 isoform CD45RO that is associated with immunologic memory.[126,146] In addition, the proportion of T cells that display other phenotypic markers of activation, including CD25 (IL-2R) and HLA-DR, is much greater than that in blood.[126,147] Consistent with their memory phenotype, T cells in human milk produce interferon-γ (IFN-γ).[146] Furthermore, a significantly greater number of CD4+ T cells in colostrum express the CD40 ligand (CD40L) compared with autologous or heterologous blood T cells.[148] Cognate interaction between the CD40L on T cells and the CD40 on B cells is a necessary step for antibody production in vivo and is congenitally deficient in the newborn. The function of these memory T cells in the recipient human infant is currently unknown, however. Mucous membrane sites in the alimentary or respiratory tract, or both, of the recipient infant would seem to be potential entry sites for human milk leukocytes. Of considerable interest, very small numbers of memory T cells are detected in blood in infancy.[149] Thus, it is possible that maternal memory T cells in milk compensate for the developmental delay in their production in the infant. In this regard, the proportion of T lymphocytes bearing the T cell receptor-$\gamma\delta$ (TCR-$\gamma\delta$) is approximately two times greater in colostrum than in blood.[150,151] Human TCR-$\gamma\delta^+$ cells populate organized lymphoid tissues and represent half of the intraepithelial lymphocytes in the gut.[152] Thus, the intestinal epithelia may have a selective affinity for TCR-$\gamma\delta^+$ cells and provide a favorable environment for maternal T cells in milk to be transferred to the breast-fed infant. Evidence from experimental animal studies indicates that milk lymphocytes enter tissues of the neonate,[153-156] but this has not been demonstrated in humans. In addition, the possible transfer of histocompatibility antigens and T cells to the neonate through breast-feeding has been examined by determining the fate of skin grafts in suckling rats fed by allogeneic mothers.[157] Such foster feeding of milk may result not only in increased allogeneic graft survival but also in development of "runting" syndrome, possibly as a result of a graft-versus-host–type reaction in the breast-fed animal. Effects of the transfer may be related to dosage of ingested allogeneic cells, in that increasing cell numbers transferred may prolong skin graft survival but may also increase the likelihood of a graft-versus-host reaction. Of note, the suckling rat gut has a higher degree of permeability to whole proteins than that characteristic of the human intestine. Furthermore, clinical experience in immunodeficient neonates has never supported the development of graft-versus-host reaction–like disease in the breast-fed human infant. In humans, possible transfer of maternal T cell reactivity to tuberculin protein from the mother to the neonate through the process of breast-feeding has been observed.[99,158,159] The implications of these observations are that maternal cellular products or soluble mediators of cellular reactivity may be transferred passively to the neonate through breast-feeding. Admittedly, however, the occurrence of such phenomena in humans has not been studied carefully. Thus, it must be emphasized that at present, evidence to suggest any T cell–mediated immunologic risks associated with breast-feeding in humans is lacking. On the other hand, it is still unknown whether milk T cells, either TCR-$\alpha\beta^+$ or TCR-$\gamma\delta^+$, play a role in the transfer of adoptive immunoprotection to the recipient infant.

Neutrophils. Milk contains large numbers of neutrophils. Although the absolute counts in actively nursing mothers exhibit considerable variability between different samples, highest numbers are generally observed during the first 3 to 4 days of lactation. The numbers of neutrophils decrease significantly after 3 to 4 weeks of lactation, and only rare neutrophils are observed in samples collected after 60 to 80 days post partum. Leukocytes in human milk appear to be metabolically activated. Indeed, although the neutrophils are phagocytic and produce toxic oxygen radicals, they do not respond well to chemoattractants by increasing their adherence, polarity, or directed migration in in vitro systems.[160] This diminished response was found to be due to prior activation in that the neutrophils in milk displayed a phenotypic pattern that is typical of activated neutrophils. The expression of CD11b, the α chain subunit of Mac-1, was increased, and the expression of L-selectin was decreased.[125]

Epithelial Cells. On the basis of their anatomic distribution, epithelial cells in the human mammary gland can be classified into two main types: myoepithelial and luminal. Epithelial cells of both types, however, appear to be more heterogeneous on histologic and physicochemical testing.[142,161,162] They include secretory cells, which contain abundant rough endoplasmic reticulum, lipid droplets, and Golgi apparatus. The secretory cells appear to produce casein micelle. The squamous epithelial cells usually are seen in the regions of the cutaneous junction of the nipples, especially near the galactophores. The ductal or luminal cells, which exist in clusters, have many short microvilli, tight junctions, and remnants of desmosomes.[161,162] Studies using monoclonal antibodies have shown that in rodents, as many as 10 different types of epithelial cells in the adult mammary glands may exist. These cell types probably represent various stages of differentiation of mammary gland epithelium. These include, in the mammary end buds, the distinct cell types of the tip and the main compartment peripheral cell types I and II and, in alveoli as well as in the ducts of the mammary glands, the luminal cell types I and II and myoepithelial cells.[161] It is not known, however, whether similar epithelial cell differentiation occurs in the human mammary gland.

In human milk, relatively few epithelial cells are observed in the early phases of lactation. Most epithelial cells appear after 2 to 3 weeks and are seen in appreciable numbers, even as long as 180 to 200 days after the onset of lactation. With the possible exception of the synthesis of secretory component and casein and possibly other products, with which secretory epithelial cells have been associated in the stroma of the mammary gland, the role of epithelial cells in the milk remains to be defined.

Possible Functional Roles for Cellular Elements. The information reviewed thus far provides strong evidence for the existence of a number of dynamic cellular reactions in the mammary gland, colostrum, and milk. Unfortunately, the specific functional role, collectively or individually, for the epithelial cells, monocytes, neutrophils, or lymphocytes in the mammary gland or the milk remains to be defined. In view of the high degree of selectivity and the differences in the quantitative and functional distribution of cellular elements, it is suggested that the mammary gland, like mucosal surfaces, may function somewhat partitioned from the cellular elements in peripheral blood, in a manner similar to that for other peripheral sites (such as the genital tract) of the common mucosal system. It is, however, not known whether the characteristic proportions of macrophages, T lymphocytes, other cytotoxic cells, or epithelial cells are designed for any specific functions localized to the mammary gland in the lactating mother or to epithelium or lumen of the intestinal or respiratory mucosa of the breast-feeding infant, or both. The observations on the transfer of delayed hypersensitivity reactions in human neonates and of graft-versus-host reactivity in the rat raise the possibility that milk cells may function as important vehicles in transfer of maternal immunity to neonates. The potential beneficial and harmful roles of such cell-mediated transfer through the mucosal routes, however, need to be investigated further. The paucity of NK and other cytotoxic cells in the colostrum may have a role for the breast-feeding neonate, especially in influencing the antigen processing and uptake of replicating microorganisms and their immune response at systemic or mucosal levels or both. Although colostral cells await further elucidation of their function in the mammary glands and the suckling neonate, it is likely that their presence in the milk represents a highly selective phenomenon and not a mere contamination with peripheral blood cells.

Other Possible Defense Factors

Human colostrum and milk contain all components of the complement system. Active production of C3 has been reported in vitro in breast milk cell cultures.[163,164] Interferon,[165] migration inhibition factor,[158] and α-fetoprotein[148] also are present in human milk, although their roles have not yet been fully elucidated (see Table 5-4).

Iron-binding proteins present in colostrum and milk, such as lactoferrin,[166] have bacteriostatic activity in vitro against *E. coli*, *S. aureus*, and *C. albicans*.[137] Some evidence suggests enhanced bactericidal activity of lactoferrin in association with IgA. Lysozyme and bifidus factor (a collection of glycosamides that promote growth of *Lactobacillus* and bifidobacterial species, whose growth in turn inhibits growth of enteric gram-negative aerobic bacilli) may function as ancillary inhibitors of gut and skin pathogens. Antistaphylococcal factors appear to be active against experimental staphylococcal infections and may be important for local mammary gland protection.[166,167] Of particular interest is the demonstration of certain oligosaccharides that prevent attachment of *S. pneumoniae* to human epithelial cells[168] and of high-molecular-weight substances that inhibit virulence of enterotoxins of Enterobacteriaceae organisms (see Table 5-4).

Nonimmunoglobulin antiviral factors have been demonstrated in lipid and aqueous phases of human milk. These factors have shown activity against influenza A and B viruses, herpes simplex virus, Semliki Forest virus, Japanese B encephalitis virus, rubella virus, rhinovirus, and rotavirus (see Table 5-4). The milk-associated antiviral factors have been shown to have inhibitory functions only in vitro. Their in vivo role in neonatal and maternal infections remains to be elucidated. Recent studies also have demonstrated the presence of other substances in human milk that promote growth and maturation of intestinal epithelial tissue[169] and uptake of folate by the intestinal cells.[170]

Several recent studies have generated interest in the potential role of nonantibody proteins, bile salt lipases, whey proteins, and trace metals present in human milk in the control of enteric infections.[171-174] Several species of gram-positive and gram-negative bacteria frequently can be killed by incubation with human milk whey but not commercial infant formula.[171] The mechanisms responsible for such antibacterial activity are not known. The synergistic interaction among IgA, lactoferrin, and iron has been suggested to play a role in such defense.[171-172]

Concentrations of free fatty acid and possibly monoglycerides seem to increase during storage of milk because of spontaneous lipolysis generated by lipoprotein lipase.[175,176] Antibody-independent antiparasitic effect of stored, but not fresh, human milk against *Giardia lamblia* or *Entamoeba histolytica* has been attributed to such free fatty acids.[177] In additional studies conducted in vitro, bile salt–stimulated lipase, the major lipase in human milk, has been found to cause hydrolysis of milk triglycerides. It remains to be seen whether free fatty acids induce significant in vivo protection in the intestine against intestinal parasites. On the other hand, bile salts themselves may stimulate the growth of *G. lamblia*.[173]

Nonantibody proteins, several carrier proteins, and cellular enzyme proteins are present in milk in high concentrations. Concentrations of lysozyme range from 30 to 50 mg/100 mL in early colostrum to 5 to 10 mg/100 mL in late milk. The susceptibility of an organism to lysozyme depends on the availability of the peptidoglycan substrate. In certain situations in which the peptidoglycan may be blocked by lipoproteins, the organisms are relatively resistant to lysozymes.[173,174]

DIRECT-ACTING ANTIMICROBIAL AGENTS

General Features. The defense agents in human milk, although biochemically diverse, share certain features: (1) They usually are common to mucosal sites. (2) They are adapted to resist digestion in the gastrointestinal tract of the recipient infant. (3) They protect by noninflammatory mechanisms. (4) They act synergistically with each other or with factors produced by the infant. (5) Most components of the immune system in human milk are produced throughout lactation and during gradual weaning, but (6) there is often an inverse relationship between the production of these factors in the mammary gland and their production by the infant during the same time frames of lactation and postnatal development. Indeed, as lactation proceeds, the concentration of many factors in human milk declines. Concomitantly, the mucosal production of these factors rises in the developing infant. It is unclear whether the inverse relationship between these processes is due to feedback mechanisms or whether the processes are independent.

Carbohydrate Components. Human milk contains several oligosaccharides and glycoconjugates, including monosialogangliosides that are receptor analogues for heat-labile toxins produced by *V. cholerae* and *E. coli*[178]; fucose-containing oligosaccharides that inhibit the hemagglutinin activity of the classic strain of *V. cholerae*[179]; fucosylated oligosaccharides that protect against heat-stable enterotoxin of *E. coli*[180]; mannose-containing high-molecular-weight glycoproteins that block the binding of the El Tor strain of *V. cholerae*[178]; and glycoproteins and glycolipids that interfere with the binding of colonization factor (CFA/II) fimbriae on enterotoxigenic *E. coli*.[181] The inhibition of toxin binding is associated with acidic glycolipids containing sialic acid (gangliosides). Although the quantities of total gangliosides in human and in bovine milk are similar, the relative frequencies of each type of ganglioside in milk from these two species are distinct. More than 50 types of monosialylated oligosaccharides have been identified in human milk, and new types are still being recognized.[182] Monosialoganglioside 3 constitutes about 74% of total gangliosides in human milk, but the percentage is much lower in bovine milk.[183,184] Also, the level of the enterotoxin receptor ganglioside G_{M1} is 10 times greater in human than in bovine milk.[184] This difference may be of clinical importance because G_{M1} inhibits enterotoxins of *E. coli* and *V. cholerae*.[185] It also is of interest that intact human milk fat globules, as well as the mucin from the membranes of these structures, inhibit the binding of S-fimbriated *E. coli* to human buccal epithelial cells.[186]

Oligosaccharides in human milk also interfere with the attachment of *H. influenzae* and *S. pneumoniae*.[187] In this regard, *N*-acetylglucosamine (G1cNAc) (1-3)Gal-disaccharide subunits block the attachment of *S. pneumoniae* to respiratory epithelium. Moreover, recent evidence indicates that human milk interferes with the binding of human immunodeficiency virus (HIV) envelope antigen gp120 to CD4 molecules on T cells.[188] Some evidence from animal models suggests that the oligosaccharides and glycoconjugates in human milk protect in vivo,[189-191] but relevant clinical data are scarce.[192]

In addition to the direct antimicrobial effects of the carbohydrates in human milk, nitrogen-containing oligosaccharides in human milk are growth promoters for *Lactobacillus bifidus* var. *pennsylvanicus*,[193] glycoproteins, and glycopeptides.[194,195] The bifidus growth promoter activity associated with caseins may reside in the oligosaccharide moiety of those complex molecules.[196] It appears that these factors are responsible to a great extent for the predominance of *Lactobacillus* species in the bacterial flora of the large intestine of the breast-fed infant. These bacteria produce large amounts of acetic acid, which aids in suppressing the multiplication of enteropathogens. It also has been reported that *Lactobacillus* species strain GG aids in the recovery from acute rotavirus infections[197] and may enhance the formation of circulating cells that produce specific antibodies of the IgG, IgA, and IgM isotypes, as well as serum levels of those antibodies.[198]

Generation of Antiviral, Antiparasitic Lipids from Substrata in Human Milk. Human milk supplies defense agents from fat as it is partially digested in the recipient's alimentary tract. Fatty acids and monoglycerides produced from milk fats by bile salt–stimulated lipase or lipoprotein lipase in human milk,[199] lingual/gastric lipase from the recipient from birth,[200] or pancreatic lipase after a few weeks of age are able to disrupt enveloped viruses.[201-205] These antiviral lipids may aid in preventing coronavirus infections of the intestinal tract[206] and also may defend against intestinal parasites such as *G. lamblia* and *E. histolytica*.[207,208]

Proteins. The principal proteins in human milk that have direct antimicrobial properties include the following.

α-Lactalbumin. α-Lactalbumin is a major component of the milk proteins and may possess some important functions of immunologic defense. This protein appears as large complexes of several α-lactalbumin molecules, which can induce apoptosis in transformed embryonic and lymphoid cell lines. A lower number of such aggregated α-lactalbumin molecules binding oleic acid as a co-factor can induce cytolysis of several types of malignant cells. Such preparations of *h*uman α-lactalbumin *m*ade *l*ethal to *t*umor cells (HAMLET) are highly effective in inducing apoptosis. The antitumor cytolytic activity with HAMLET also has been observed against large numbers of human tumors.

Lactoferrin. Lactoferrin, the dominant whey protein in human milk, is a single-chain glycoprotein with two globular lobes, both of which display a site that binds ferric iron.[209] More than 90% of the lactoferrin in human milk is in the form of apolactoferrin (i.e., it does not contain ferric iron),[210] which competes with siderophilic bacteria and fungi for ferric iron[211-215] and thus disrupts the proliferation of these microbial pathogens. The epithelial growth–promoting activities of lactoferrin in human milk also may aid in the defense of the recipient infant.[216] The mean concentration of lactoferrin in human colostrum is between 5 and 6 mg/mL.[217] As the volume of milk production increases, the concentration falls to about 1 mg/mL at 2 to 3 months of lactation.[218,219]

Because of its resistance to proteolysis,[220-222] the excretion of lactoferrin in stool is higher in human milk–fed than in cow's milk–fed infants.[72,223-225] The mean intake of milk lactoferrin per day in healthy breast-fed, full-term infants is about 260 mg/kg at 1 month of lactation and 125 mg/kg by 4 months.[223] The quantity of lactoferrin excreted in the stools of low-birth-weight infants fed human milk is approximately 185 times that in stools of infants fed a cow's milk formula.[226] That estimate, however, may be too high because of the presence of immunoreactive fragments of lactoferrin in the stools of human milk–fed infants.[227]

In addition, a significant increment in the urinary excretion of intact and fragmented lactoferrin occurs as a result of human milk feedings.[227-229] Recent stable isotope studies suggest that the increments in urinary lactoferrin and its fragments are principally from ingested human milk lactoferrin.[230]

Lysozyme. Relatively high concentrations of lysozyme single-chain protein are present in human milk.[218,219,231-235] This 15-kDa agent lyses susceptible bacteria by hydrolyzing β-1,4 linkages between *N*-acetylmuramic acid and 2-acetylamino-2-deoxy-D-glucose residues in cell walls.[236] Lysozyme is relatively resistant to digestion by trypsin or denaturation due to acid. The mean concentration of lysozyme is about 70 μg/mL in colostrum,[218] about 20 μg/mL at 1 month of lactation, and 250 μg/mL by 6 months.[219] The approximate mean daily intake of milk lysozyme in healthy, full-term, completely breast-fed infants is 3 to 4 mg/kg at 1 month of lactation and 6 mg/kg by 4 months.[223]

Few studies have been conducted to examine the fate of human milk lysozyme ingested by the infant. The amount of lysozyme excreted in the stools of low-birth-weight infants fed human milk is approximately eight times that found in the stools of infants fed a cow's milk formula,[226] but the urinary excretion of this protein does not increase as a result of human milk feedings.

Fibronectin. Fibronectin, a high-molecular-weight protein that facilitates the uptake of many types of particulates by mononuclear phagocytic cells, is present in human milk (mean concentration in colostrum, 13.4 mg/L).[237] The in vivo effects and fate of this broad-spectrum opsonin in human milk are not known.

Complement Components. The components of the classical and alternative pathways of complement are present in human milk, but the concentrations of these components, except C3, are exceptionally low.[163,164]

ANTI-INFLAMMATORY AGENTS

Although a direct anti-inflammatory effect of human milk has not been demonstrated in vivo, a number of clinical observations suggest that breast-feeding protects the recipient infant from injury to the intestinal or respiratory mucosa.[238,239] This protection may be due in part to the more rapid elimination or neutralization of microbial pathogens in the lumen of the gastrointestinal tract by specific or broad-spectrum defense agents from human milk, but other features of human milk suggest that this is not the sole explanation. Phlogistic agents and the systems that give rise to them are poorly represented in human milk.[240] By contrast, human milk contains a host of anti-inflammatory agents,[241] including a heterogeneous group of growth factors with cytoprotective and trophic activity for the mucosal epithelium, antioxidants, antiproteases, cytokines and cytokine receptors and antagonists, and other bioactive agents that inhibit inflammatory mediators or block the selected activation of leukocytes. Like the antimicrobial factors, some of these factors are well adapted to operate in the hostile environment of the recipient's alimentary tract.

Growth factors in human milk include EGF,[169,242] the transforming growth factors TGF-α[243] and TGF-β,[244] lactoferrin,[216] mammary gland–derived growth factor,[245] and polyamines.[246,247] These and a host of hormones,[248] including insulin-like growth factor (IGF), vascular endothelial growth factor (VEGF), growth hormone–releasing factor (GHF), hepatocyte growth factor (HGF), prolactin, leptin, and cortisol,[249] may affect the growth and maturation of epithelial barriers, limit the penetration of pathogenic microorganisms and free antigens, and prevent allergic sensitization. Corticosterone, a glucocorticoid that is present in high concentrations in rat milk, speeds gut closure in the neonatal rat.[250] Although macromolecular absorption does not appear to be as marked in the human neonate,[251-253] the function of the mucosal barrier system in early infancy is important to host defense, and this system may be affected by factors in human milk. In this regard, the maturation of the intestinal tract as measured by mucosal mass, DNA, and protein content of the small intestinal tract appears to be influenced by milk, particularly early milk secretions.[254]

Antioxidant activity in colostrum has been shown to be associated with an ascorbate compound and uric acid.[255] In addition, two other antioxidants present in human milk, α-tocopherol[256,257] and β-carotene,[257] are absorbed into the circulation by the recipient gastrointestinal mucosa. Serum vitamin E concentrations rise in breast-fed infants from a mean of 0.3 mg/mL at birth to approximately 0.9 mg/mL on the fourth day of life.[256]

The pleiotropic cytokine IL-10, a potent suppresser of macrophage, T cell, and NK cell function, has been demonstrated at very high concentrations in samples of human milk collected during the first 80 hours of lactation.[258] IL-10 is present not only in the aqueous phase of the milk but also in the lipid layer. Its bioactive properties were confirmed by the finding that human milk samples inhibited blood lymphocyte proliferation and that this property was greatly reduced by treatment with anti-IL-10 antibody. Of interest, mice with a targeted disruption in the IL-10 gene, when raised under conventional housing conditions, spontaneously develop a generalized enterocolitis that becomes apparent at the age of 4 to 8 weeks (time of weaning).[259] These observations suggest that IL-10 in human milk may play a critical role in the homeostasis of the immature intestinal barrier by regulating aberrant immune responses to foreign antigens. Soluble receptors and cytokine receptor antagonists also are potent anti-inflammatory agents. Human colostrum and mature milk have been shown to contain biologically active levels of IL-1 receptor antagonist (IL-1Ra) and soluble TNF-α receptors I and II (sTNF-αRI and sTNF-αRII).[260] The in vivo relevance of these observations also has been confirmed in a chemically induced colitis model of rats. Animals with colitis fed human milk had significantly lower neutrophilic inflammation than animals fed either chow or infant formula.[261] Similar "protective" effects were seen in rats with colitis fed an infant formula supplemented with IL-1Ra,[261] suggesting that this anti-inflammatory agent present in milk may contribute to the broad protection against different injuries provided by human milk feeding.

The presence in human milk of platelet-activating factor acetylhydrolase (PAF-AH), the enzyme that catalyzes the degradation and inactivation of PAF, is intriguing.[262] Indeed, elevated serum concentrations of PAF have been found in rat and human neonates with necrotizing enterocolitis (NEC), whereas the concentrations of PAF-AH were found to be significantly lower than in control (unaffected) neonates.[263,264] It also is of interest that serum concentrations of PAF-AH at birth are below those in adults and then gradually rise.[265] The enzyme is actively transferred from the mucosal to the serosal fluid in intestine of neonatal rats, particularly in the earliest postnatal period.[266] Other anti-inflammatory factors present in human milk include an IgE-binding factor, related antigenically to the FcεRII (the lower-affinity receptor for IgE), that suppresses the in vitro synthesis of human IgE,[267] and the glycophosphoinositol-containing molecule protectin (CD59) that inhibits insertion of the complement membrane attack complex (MAC) to cell targets.[268] The in vivo fate and effects of these anti-inflammatory factors in human milk are still poorly understood.

MODULATORS OF THE IMMUNE SYSTEM

Several seemingly unrelated types of observations suggest that breast-feeding modulates the development of the immune system of the recipient infant:

- Both prospective and retrospective epidemiologic studies have shown that breast-fed infants are at less risk for development of certain chronic immunologically mediated disorders later in childhood, including allergic diseases,[269] Crohn's disease,[270] ulcerative colitis,[271] insulin-dependent diabetes mellitus,[272] and some lymphomas.[273]
- Humoral and cellular immune responses to specific antigens (i.e., vaccines) given during the first year of life appear to develop differently in breast-fed and in formula-fed infants. Several studies have reported increased serum antibody titers to *H. influenzae* type b polysaccharide,[274] oral poliovirus,[275] tetanus,[276] and diphtheria toxoid[277] immunizations in breast-fed infants. In regard to cell-mediated immunity, breast-fed infants given bacille Calmette-Guérin (BCG) vaccine either at birth or later show a significantly higher lymphocyte transformation response to purified protein derivative (PPD) than that in infants who were never breast-fed.[277] Moreover, maternal renal allografts survive better in persons who were breast-fed than in those who were not.[278-280] In this respect, the in vitro allogeneic responses between the blood lymphocytes of mothers (stimulating cells) and their infants (responding cells), as measured by an analysis of the frequencies of cytotoxic T lymphocyte (CTL) precursors directed against HLA alloantigens (CTL allorepertoire), are low in breast-fed infants.[281]
- Increased levels of certain immune factors in breast-fed infants, which could not be explained simply by passive transfer of those substances, also suggest an immunomodulatory activity of human milk. Breast-fed infants produce higher blood levels of interferon in response to respiratory syncytial virus infection.[282] It also was found that the increments in blood levels of fibronectin that were achieved by breast-feeding could not be due to the amounts of that protein in human milk.[237] In addition, it was found that human milk feeding led to a more rapid development in the appearance of sIgA in external secretions,[226,228,229,276,283] some of which, such as urine, are far removed anatomically from the route of ingestion.[228,229]

These and other observations suggest that the ability of human milk to modulate the development of the infant's own mucosal and systemic immune systems may be associated with immunoregulatory factors present in colostrum and in more mature milk. Several different types of immunomodulatory agents can be identified in human milk.[241] Among the numerous substances with proven or potential ability to modulate the infant immune response are prolactin,[284] α-tocopherol,[256] lactoferrin,[285] nucleotides,[67] anti-idiotypic sIgA,[286] and cytokines.[287] It is evident that many of these factors in milk have other primary biologic functions, as in the case of hormones or growth factors, and that their potential as immune regulatory agents overlaps with their antimicrobial or anti-inflammatory properties.[241]

Cytokines in Human Milk. In the 1990s, several cytokines, chemokines, and growth factors that mediate the effector phases of natural and specific immunity were discovered in human milk. These include IL-1β, IL-6, IL-7, IL-10, IL-12, IL-8, growth-related peptide-α (GRO-α), monocyte chemotactic protein-1 (MCP-1), granulocyte colony-stimulating factor (G-CSF), macrophage colony-stimulating factor (M-CSF), and TGF-β (Table 5-8). Human milk displays a number of cytokine-characteristic biologic activities, including the stimulation of growth, differentiation of immunoglobulin production by B cells,[288-290] enhancement of thymocyte proliferation,[291] inhibition of IL-2 production by T cells,[292] and suppression of IgE production.[267] IL-1β[293] and TNF-α[294] were the first two cytokines quantified in human milk. In colostrum, TNF-α is present mainly in fractions of molecular weight between 80 and 195 kDa, probably bound to its soluble receptors.[260] Milk TNF-α is secreted both by milk macrophages[294,295] and by the mammary epithelium.[296] IL-6 was first demonstrated in human milk by a specific bioassay.[297] In this study, anti-IL-6–neutralizing antibodies

Table 5–8 Cytokines, Chemokines, and Colony-Stimulating Factors in Human Milk

Cytokines	Chemokines	Colony-Stimulating Factors
IL-1β	IL-8	G-CSF
IL-6	GRO-α	M-CSF
IL-7		
IL-8		
IL-10	MCP-1	GM-CSF
IL-16[a]		TGF-β
IFN-γ	RANTES	
TNF-α	Eotaxin[a]	

G-CSF, granulocyte colony-stimulating factor; GM-CSF, granulocyte-macrophage colony-stimulating factor; GRO-α, growth-related peptide-α; IL, interleukin; MCP-1, monocyte chemotactic protein-1; M-CSF, monocyte colony-stimulating factor; RANTES, regulated upon activation, normal T cell expressed and secreted; TGF-β, transforming growth factor-β; TNF-α, tumor necrosis factor-α.

inhibited IgA production by colostrum mononuclear cells, suggesting that IL-6 may be involved in the production of IgA in the mammary gland. The presence of IL-6 in milk also has been demonstrated by immunoassays.[294,296,298,299] In like manner, IL-6 is localized in high-molecular-weight fractions of human milk.[298] The association of IL-6 with its own receptor has not been studied in milk, although the expression of IL-6 receptor by the mammary epithelium[296] and in secreted form in the milk[260] may explain the high molecular weight of this cytokine in human milk. The expression of IL-6 messenger ribonucleic acid (mRNA) and protein in milk cells and in the mammary gland epithelium suggests that both milk mononuclear cells and the mammary gland are likely major sources of this cytokine.[295,296,300] The presence of IFN-γ in human milk also has been reported,[151,296,299] although some investigators have found significant levels of IFN-γ only in milk samples obtained from mothers whose infants had been delivered by cesarean section. The significance of this observation is not clear at present. IFN-γ bioactivity as well as its association with specific subsets of milk T cells also remains to be determined.[151] (The presence and possible function of IL-10 in human milk are discussed in the section "Anti-inflammatory Agents.")

Chemokines are a novel class of small cytokines with discrete target cell selectivity that are able to recruit and activate different populations of leukocytes.[301] Two major subfamilies, the CXC and the CC chemokines, are defined by the splicing of the conserved cysteine residues, which are separated by either one amino acid (CXC chemokines) or adjacent amino acids (CC chemokines). IL-8 and GRO-α belong to the CXC family and are mainly chemotactic factors for neutrophils. On the other hand, CC chemokines, which include MCP-1, macrophage inflammatory protein-1α (MIP-1α), and RANTES (*r*egulated upon *a*ctivation, *n*ormal *T* cell *e*xpressed and *s*ecreted), are chemotactic factors for monocytes, basophils and eosinophils, and T lymphocytes.[302] The presence of both CXC and CC chemokines has been described in human milk (see Table 5-8). IL-8 concentration was first determined in a small group of milk samples by Basolo and colleagues.[296] These investigators identified the expression and secretion of IL-8 by mammary epithelial cells, although milk cells also appear to produce this chemokine.[295,300] Another member of the CXC chemokine found in human milk is GRO-α, along with the two CC chemokines MCP-1 and RANTES.[300] Expression of MCP-1 and, to a lesser extent, RANTES mRNA was confirmed in studies of milk cells.[300] Recently, high levels of the CC chemokine eotaxin, a potent and specific chemotactic factor for eosinophils and subtype 2 helper T cells (T_H2), also have been demonstrated in human milk.[303]

Colony-stimulating factors—highly specific protein factors that regulate cell proliferation and differentiation in the process of hematopoiesis—were discovered relatively recently in human milk. Although colony-stimulating activity was demonstrated in milk in 1983,[304] G-CSF, M-CSF, and granulocyte-macrophage colony-stimulating factor (GM-CSF) were not specifically identified and measured in human milk until the 1990s.[151,305-307] The concentrations of M-CSF in particular appear to be 10- to 100-fold those in serum, and M-CSF evidently is produced by epithelial cells of the ducts and alveoli of the mammary gland under the regulatory activity of female sex hormones.[306]

Although it is tempting to speculate that cytokines present in milk may be able to interact with mucosal tissues in the respiratory and alimentary tracts of the recipient infant, the functional expression of specific receptors for cytokines on epithelial or lymphoid cells in the airway and gastrointestinal mucosa has not been fully explored.[241] A receptor-independent mechanism of cytokine uptake by the gastrointestinal mucosa during the neonatal period has not been demonstrated to date.

Milk and Altered Pregnancy

Several investigators have examined the effects of prematurity, early weaning, galactorrhea, and maternal malnutrition on the process of lactation. The immunologic aspects of these studies have focused largely on evaluation of the total content of sIgA and specific antibody activity. As described previously, the mammary secretions of nonlactating breast contain sIgA, although the amount appears to be much lower than in the lactating breast.[308] Mammary secretions of patients with galactorrhea appear to contain sIgA in concentrations similar to those of normal postpartum colostrum.[309] Although malnutrition has been associated with reduced secretory antibody response in other external secretions, maternal malnutrition does not seem to affect the total sIgA concentration or antimicrobial-specific antibody activity in the milk.[310]

The nutritional as well as immunologic composition of milk from mothers of premature infants appears to be significantly different from that of milk from mothers of infants born at term.[14,219,311,312] Comparative studies conducted during the first 12 weeks of lactation suggest that the mean concentrations of lactoferrin and lysozyme are higher in preterm than in term milk. Secretory IgA is the predominant immunoglobulin in preterm as well as in term milk, although the sIgA concentration appears to be significantly higher in preterm milk collected during the first 8 to 12 weeks of lactation. Secretory IgA antibody activity against certain organisms (*E. coli* somatic antigen) in the preterm milk was observed to be somewhat less than, or at best similar to, that found in term milk. In addition, the number of lymphocytes and macrophages in milk appears to be lower at 2 weeks but significantly higher at 12 weeks in milk from mothers with preterm (born at 34 to 38 weeks of gestational age) infants than in milk from those with full-term infants.[311] The authors of these investigations have proposed that some of the observed changes may reflect the lower volume of milk produced by mothers delivered of preterm infants. The possibility remains that changes in the immunologic profile of preterm milk may be a consequence of inadequate stimulation by the preterm infant, alterations in the maternal hormonal milieu, or other factors underlying premature delivery itself.

BENEFITS AND RISKS OF HUMAN MILK

Benefits

Gastrointestinal Homeostasis and Prevention of Diarrhea

Development of mucosal integrity in the gut appears to depend on maturation of the mucosal tissue itself and the establishment of a normal gut flora. The former represents an anatomic and enzymatic blockage to invasion of microorganisms and antigens, and the latter, an inhibition of colonization by pathogenic bacteria. Although permeability of the neonatal gut to immunoglobulin is rather short-lived or incompletely developed, unprotected or damaged neonatal gut is permeable to a host of other proteins and macromolecules for several weeks or longer. Large milk protein peptides and bovine serum albumin have been shown to enter the circulation and produce a circulating antibody response. The inflamed or ischemic gut is even more porous to both antigens and pathogens. A variety of proven and presumed mechanisms for the role of both IgA and the normal flora have been proposed to compensate for these temporary inadequacies. Evidence for gut-trophic substances in humans is still preliminary. Ample epidemiologic evidence exists for a positive effect of breast-feeding in establishing the normal gut flora. Most compelling are the observations in rural Guatemala of gross contamination of milk by potentially pathogenic aerobic, gram-negative bacilli, including *E. coli* and *Shigella* species, with an absence both of diarrheal illness and of significant numbers of these organisms in the feces of infants during the period of lactation. In addition, the diverse serotypes of aerobic, gram-negative bacilli present in the oropharynx and the gastrointestinal tract of the neonate may serve as a source of antigen to boost the presensitized mammary glands, leading to a further modulation of specific bacterial growth in the mucosa.[313] The precise role of antibody that blocks adherence of these pathogens to the gut and the effects of other factors, such as lactoperoxidase, lactoferrin, lysozyme, and *Bifidobacterium bifidum*, in those situations are undetermined.

Extensive epidemiologic evidence supports the "prophylactic value" of breast-feeding in the prevention or amelioration of diarrheal disease and is summarized in several reviews.[22,82,314,315] Ample experimental animal data on the value of specific colostral antibody in preventing diarrheal illness are available from studies of colostral deprivation. These include colibacteriosis associated with *E. coli* K88 in swine; rotaviral gastroenteritis in cattle, swine, and sheep; and diarrheal illness associated with transmissible gastroenteritis of swine.[316] In humans, cholera is rare in infancy, especially in endemic areas where the prevalence of breast-feeding is high. The experience with an outbreak of cholera in the Persian Gulf lends support to the possibility that the absence of breast-feeding is an important variable in increasing the risk of cholera in infancy.

A few reports have claimed that nursery outbreaks of diarrhea associated with enteropathogenic strains of *E. coli* can be interrupted by use of breast milk. Conflicting data exist regarding prevention of human rotaviral infection and disease. Evaluation of nursery outbreaks of rotaviral disease has suggested that the incidence both of infection and of illness was lower in breast-fed infants, but the incidence of symptoms in formula-fed infants also was very low. Studies carried out in Japan have noted a fivefold decrease in incidence of rotaviral infection among breast-fed infants younger than 6 months of age. It must be emphasized that most rotavirus infections in neonates are asymptomatic, regardless of breast- or bottle-feeding.[317-321] On the basis of careful clinical observations, Bishop and co-workers[322] in Australia first questioned the positive effects of breast-feeding in rotavirus infection. More recent case-control studies of enteric viral infections in breast-fed infants have suggested that breast-feeding may protect infants from hospitalization rather than from infection itself.[323,324] Longitudinal follow-up of a large cohort of infants during a community outbreak of rotavirus has shown that attack rates of rotavirus infection were similar in breast-fed and in bottle-fed infants. The frequency of clinical disease with diarrhea, however, appeared to be significantly lower in breast-fed infants. Of interest, the protection observed in these patients was more a reflection of altered microbial flora from breast-feeding than of specific immunologic protection against rotavirus. Thus, it appears that breast-feeding provides significant protection against diarrheal disease, although the mechanism of such protection remains to be defined.[323,324]

Necrotizing Enterocolitis

NEC is a complex illness of the stressed premature infant, often associated with hypoxia, gut mucosal ischemia, and necrolysis and death.[325,326] Clinical manifestations have, on a few occasions, been associated with bacteremia and invasion by gram-negative bacilli, particularly *Klebsiella pneumoniae*, into the intestinal submucosa. Clinical manifestations include abdominal distention, gastric retention, and bloody diarrhea. Classic radiographic findings include air in the bowel wall (pneumatosis intestinalis), air in the portal system, and free infradiaphragmatic air (signifying perforation). Treatment involves decompression, systemic antibiotics, and, often, surgery.[327-329]

A number of studies have suggested a beneficial role of breast milk in preventing or modifying the development of NEC in high-risk human infants. Some pediatric centers have claimed virtual absence of NEC in breast-fed infants; however, many instances of the failure of milk feeding to prevent human NEC also have been reported. In fact, outbreaks of NEC related to *Klebsiella* and *Salmonella* species secondary to banked human milk feedings have been documented.[127,330,331] In an asphyxiated neonatal rat model of NEC, the entire syndrome could be prevented with feeding of maternal milk. The crucial factor in the milk appeared to be the cells, probably the macrophages.[127] It also is possible that antibody and nonspecific factors play a role, as does establishment of a gut flora. Prophylactic oral administration of immunoglobulin has been found to have a profound influence on the outcome of NEC in well-controlled studies.[331] Penetration of the gut by pathogens and antigens is increased with ischemic damage, and noncellular elements of milk may aid in blockage of this transit.[332]

The role of enteric anaerobic organisms has been seriously considered in the pathogenesis of NEC. Cytolytic toxins of *Clostridium difficile* and other clostridial species have been demonstrated in infants with NEC, often significantly more frequently than in normal infants.[333-336]

Clearly, NEC is a complex disease entity whose pathogenesis and cause remain to be defined. Although breast-feeding may be protective, a number of other factors are clearly related to the mechanism of mucosal injury and the pathogenesis of this syndrome.

Neonatal Sepsis

The incidence of bacteremia among premature infants fed breast milk has been suggested to be significantly lower than that among those receiving formula feedings or no feeding.[337-339] It has been shown that a high percentage of cases of neonatal bacteremia and meningitis caused by gram-negative bacilli are associated with the *E. coli* K1 serotype. Both antibody and compartmentalized cellular reactivity to this serotype have been demonstrated in human colostrum. High colostral antibody titers are associated most often with the colonization by the organism in the maternal gut. Other studies have, however, failed to demonstrate clear evidence of protection against systemic infection in breast-fed infants.[340-342]

Prevention of Atopy and Asthma

One of the most challenging developments in human milk research has been the demonstration in breast-fed infants of a reduced incidence of diseases with auto- or dysregulated immunity, long after the termination of breast-feeding.[269-273] Since the first report in 1936,[343] numerous published studies have addressed the effect of infant feeding on the development of atopic disease and asthma. Beneficial results of breast-feeding as prophylaxis against atopy have been observed in most of the studies; in others, however, beneficial effects were reported only in infants with a genetically determined risk for atopic disease. Finally, no beneficial effect at all or even an increased risk has been suggested in some breast-fed infants. Kramer, in an extensive meta-analysis of 50 studies published before 1986 that focused on infant feeding and atopic disease, has attempted to shed some light on the controversy.[344] Seven of the 13 studies on asthma included in this analysis claimed a protective effect of breast-feeding, whereas 6 claimed no protection. Several serious methodologic drawbacks, however, have been noted in this analysis. In a number of the studies analyzed, early infant feeding history was obtained months or years after the feeding period, ascertainment of the infant feeding history was obtained by interviewers who were aware of the disease outcome, or insufficient duration and exclusivity of breast-feeding were documented; all were confounding variables that considered inappropriate "exposure standards." Nonblind ascertainment of disease outcome was found to be the most common violation of the "outcome standards."

Kramer's analysis also found that failure to control for confounding variables was a common violation in "statistical analysis standards" identified in several studies. Indeed, the effect of infant feeding on subsequent asthma may be confounded by other variables that are associated both with infant feeding and with unique investigational conditions. Factors that seem to have the greatest potential for confounding effects include the family history of atopic disease, socioeconomic status, and parental cigarette smoking. Only 1 of 13 studies on asthma included in the meta-analysis adequately controlled for these confounding factors. Moreover, 3 of the studies that did not demonstrate a protective effect of breast-feeding on asthma had inadequate statistical power. The effect of infant feeding on the severity of outcome and on the age at onset of the disease was virtually ignored in most of the studies.[344]

Although this extensive meta-analysis may suggest some uncertainty about the prophylactic benefit of breast-feeding, two recent studies strongly support a positive effect of breast-feeding on the development of atopic disease and asthma. The first study[269] consisted of prospective, long-term evaluation from infancy until the age of 17 years; the prevalence of atopy was significantly higher in those infants with short-duration (less than 1 month) or no breast-feeding, which increased to a demonstrable difference by the age of 17 years, than in the infants with intermediate-duration (1 to 6 months) or prolonged (longer than 6 months) breast-feeding. The differences in the prevalence of atopy persisted when the groups were divided according to positive or negative atopic heredity. Furthermore, the atopy manifestations in the different infant feeding groups did not remain constant with age. In particular, respiratory allergy, including asthma, increased greatly in prevalence up to the age of 17 years, with a prevalence as high as 64% in the group with short-duration or no breast-feeding.[269] In the second study, a prospective, longitudinal study of the prevalence and risk factors for acute and chronic respiratory illness in childhood, the investigators examined the relationship of infant feeding to recurrent wheezing at age 6 years and the association with lower respiratory tract illnesses associated with wheezing early in life.[345] Children who were never breast-fed had significantly higher rates of recurrent wheezing at 6 years of age. Increasing duration of breast-feeding beyond 1 month was not associated with significantly lower rates of recurrent wheezing. The effect of breast-feeding was apparent for children both with and without wheezing lower respiratory tract illnesses in the first 6 months of life. In contrast with the findings of the first study, however, the effect of breast-feeding was significant only among nonatopic children.[345]

The exact mechanisms by which breast-feeding seems to confer long-lasting protection against allergic sensitization are poorly understood. It is likely, however, that multiple synergistic mechanisms may be responsible for this effect, including (1) maturation of the recipient gastrointestinal and airway mucosa, promoted by growth factors present in human milk[242-244]; (2) inhibition of antigen absorption by milk sIgA[346]; (3) reduced incidence of mucosal infections and consequent sensitization to bystander antigens[347]; (4) changes in the microbial flora of the intestine of breast-fed infants[325]; and (5) direct immunomodulatory activity of human milk components on the recipient infant.[241] A number of earlier and more recent studies have greatly contributed to the understanding of macromolecular transport across the immature gut and its consequences in terms of the generation of circulating antibody or immune complexes, the processes that are blocked predominantly by sIgA, the glycocalyx, and the intestinal enzymes. These mucosal immunologic events have been the basis for the concept of immune exclusion. Immune exclusion is not absolute, however, because uptake of some antigens across the gut may be enhanced rather than blocked by interaction with antibody at the mucosal surface. Beginning with the observations of IgA-deficient patients, it has become clear that the absence of the IgA barrier in the gut is associated with both an increased incidence of circulating antibodies directed against many food antigens and an increased occurrence of atopic-allergic diseases.[346] Some studies have noted complement activation in serum after feeding of bovine milk to children with cow's milk allergy. The neonate is similar in some respects to the IgA-deficient patient,[348] and increased transintestinal uptake of food antigen with consequent circulating antibody formation in the premature infant has been reported.[349] Other studies have suggested that early breast-feeding, even of short duration, is associated with a decreased serum antibody response to cow's milk proteins.[253] Prolonged breast-feeding not only may partially exclude foreign antigens through immune exclusion but may also, because the mother's milk is the infant's sole food, prevent their ingestion.[350] It must, however, be emphasized that intact bovine milk proteins and other food antigens and antibodies have been observed in samples of colostrum and milk.[6]

Other Benefits

As described previously, epidemiologic evidence suggests that bacterial and viral respiratory infections are less frequent and less severe among breast-fed infants in a variety of cultures and socioeconomic settings. Antibodies and immunologic reactivity directed against herpes simplex virus, respiratory syncytial virus, and other infectious agents[86,95,118,351,352] have been quantitated in colostrum and milk. Adoptive experiments in suckling ferrets have shown that protection of the young against respiratory syncytial virus can be transferred in colostrum containing specific antibody. The neonatal ferret gut, however, is quite permeable to macromolecules and permits passage of large quantities of virus-specific IgG. In the absence of either documented antibody or cellular transfer in the human neonate across the mucosa, any mechanisms of protection against respiratory syncytial virus and other respiratory pathogens remain obscure.

Data are lacking in humans regarding passive protection on other mucosal surfaces, such as the eye, ear, or genitourinary tract. Some epidemiologic evidence suggests that recurrence of otitis media with effusion is strongly associated with early bottle-feeding and that breast-feeding may confer protection against otitis media with effusion for the first 3 years of life.[353] Foster feeding–acquired antibody to herpes simplex virus has been found to result in significant protection against reinfection challenge in experimental animal studies.[351]

A number of other benefits have been associated with breast-feeding, including natural contraception during active nursing[354] and protection against sudden infant death syndrome,[355] diabetes,[356] obesity,[357] and high cholesterol level and ischemic heart disease later in life.[42] Of particular recent interest has been the association of breast-feeding with improved intellectual performance in older children. Several studies have demonstrated enhanced cognitive outcome in breast-fed children, although controversy exists regarding the mechanisms by which such improved performance may occur.[358-360] Health benefits for the mother also may be associated with breast-feeding: A reduced incidence of breast cancer has been noted in women who have lactated.[361]

Potential Risks

Noninfectious Risks

Several potentially harmful effects have been associated with breast-feeding. Some provocative data suggest that non-autologous human milk may, under certain conditions, be nutritionally inadequate for the premature infant.[22,23] The concentration of anti-Rhesus factor (anti-Rh) antibodies in milk appears to be too low to pose any threat to the incompatible neonate. Variable concentrations of medicinal products and their metabolites are excreted in colostrum and milk (Table 5-9). Environmental contaminants such as dichlorodiphenyl trichloroethane (DDT), polychlorinated biphenyls (PCBs), and mercury have been demonstrated in high concentrations in human milk.[22,362]

The failure to initiate lactation properly during early breast-feeding may present a risk of dehydration to the infant, because insufficient fluids may be ingested. Inappropriate introduction of bottles and pacifiers also may interfere with proper induction of lactation. Later in lactation, introduction of bottles may induce premature weaning as the result of a reduction in the milk supply.

Although human milk is the optimal form of nutrition for most healthy term infants, some circumstances have been identified in which breast-feeding is contraindicated and some in which continued breast-feeding should be conducted with caution to protect the infant. Infants with inherited metabolic diseases may be best nourished by treatment with alternative forms of nutrition. In particular, neonates with diagnosed galactosemia need to have galactose removed from their diet; in other words, they need to be switched to a milk containing lactose-free carbohydrate (because lactose is a glucose-galactose disaccharide). Infants diagnosed with phenylketonuria may receive some human milk to support their requirement for phenylalanine but often may be better managed by use of specially prepared commercial milks.

Management of hyperbilirubinemia associated with breast-feeding, so-called breast milk jaundice, has been an area of some controversy. The mechanism responsible for this form of jaundice is unknown but has been suggested to reflect inhibitors of glucuronidation, deficiency of related enzymes, excessive lipid breakdown, and insufficient milk intake.[363,364] Recent recommendations suggest that a more laissez-faire approach to this problem is appropriate.[365] Increasing milk

Table 5–9 Drugs in Maternal Circulation Known to Pose Potential Health Problems for the Breast-Feeding Infant

Drugs	Drugs	Environmental Contaminants
Anticoagulants	Autonomic drugs	Dichlorodiphenyl trichloroethane (DDT)
Ethyl biscoumacetate	Atropine	Polybromated biphenyls (PBBs)
Phenindione	Laxatives	Polychlorinated biphenyls (PCBs)
Anticonvulsants	Anthraquinone derivatives	Heptachlor
Mysoline	(Dialose Plus, Dorbane, Doxidon,	Mirex
Phenobarbital	Peri-Colace)	Lead
Phenytoin (diphenylhydantoin)	Aloe	Radioisotopes
Carbamazepine	Calomel	Caffeine
Antidepressants	Cascara	Food proteins
Lithium	Narcotics	Nicotine
Antihypertensives	Heroin	Cadmium
Reserpine	Methadone	Alcohol
Antimetabolites	Oral contraceptives	
Cyclophosphamide	Pain killers	
Methotrexate	Propoxyphene (Darvon)	
Antimicrobials	Sedatives	
Chloramphenicol	Barbiturates	
(Chloromycetin)	Bromides	
Metronidazole (Flagyl)	Chloral hydrate	
Tinidazole	Diazepam (Valium)	
Nalidixic acid	Steroids	
Nitrofurantoin[a]	Prednisone	
Sulfonamides[a]	Prednisolone	
Antithyroid drugs	Miscellaneous	
Iodide	Dihydrotachysterol (DHT)	
Thiouracil	Ergot alkaloids	
Radioactive iodine	Gold thioglucose	

[a]This drug causes problems mainly in infants suffering from the inherited deficiency of glucose-6-phosphate dehydrogenase.
Adapted from Packard VS. Human milk and infant formula. *In* Stewart GE (ed). Food and Science Technology Series. New York, Academic Press, 1982, p 118, with permission.

volume by increasing the number of feedings may be the most appropriate approach to breast milk jaundice; however, severe cases may necessitate phototherapy. Increased intake of fluids in breast-feeding infants appears to be effective in many cases.[366]

Several instances of specific nutrient deficiencies in breast-fed infants have been described, specifically related to lack of vitamin K, vitamin D, vitamin B_{12}, folic acid, vitamin C, and carnitine. In each of these instances, several case reports have appeared warning against deficiencies that have resulted in clinical consequences to the neonate. For example, hemorrhagic disease reported in a few breast-fed infants was successfully treated with vitamin K.[367] These infants did not receive vitamin K at birth. Mothers who practice unusual dietary habits, such as strict vegetarianism, may have reduced levels of vitamin B_{12} and folic acid in their milk, and deficiencies in breast-fed infants of such mothers have been reported.[368,369] Cases of rickets in breast-fed infants have been reported, particularly during winter among infants not exposed to the sun.[32,370] Deficiency of carnitine, a nutrient responsible for modulating fat absorption, also has been reported to result in clinical symptoms in breast-fed infants in mothers ingesting unusual diets.[61,371]

These various clinical expressions of nutrient deficiency in milk are of concern, but they also should be put in the context of nutrient deficiencies observed in formula-fed infants. Clearly, millions of infants in developing countries are at severe risk of malnutrition when they are formula-fed because of the economic stress of supplying sufficient formula. Even in developed countries, large numbers of nutrient deficiencies and associated clinical symptoms have occurred as a result of accidents in the manufacture of formulas.[372] The most notable of these accidents have taught us the effects of early vitamin B_6 deficiency, folic acid deficiency, and chloride deficiency. Formula feeding also has been associated with an increased incidence of diabetes.[373]

Thus, some situations arise in which breast-feeding must be carefully considered as an appropriate feeding modality for the infant. Commercial formulas also represent risks, however. The infant is best served by observant pediatricians and mothers who promptly respond to any clinical signs in the neonate.

Infectious Risks

The presence of microbial contamination in milk is of serious concern. Contaminated milk has been implicated in neonatal infection with *S. aureus*, group B hemolytic streptococci, mycobacteria, and, possibly, *Salmonella* species (Table 5-10). Mastitis and breast abscess have been associated with the presence of bacterial pathogens in human milk. Such inflammation of the breast will often resolve even with continued breast-feeding. Resolution of the inflammation may be related to the presence of antisecretory factor (AF), a factor induced in the milk by enterotoxin-producing bacteria that appears to promote recovery from acute bacterial mastititis. In general, feeding an infant from a breast affected by an abscess is not recommended.[1] Infant feeding on the affected breast may be resumed, however, once the mother

Table 5–10 **Spectrum of Infectious Agents[a] Recovered in Human Milk and Their Possible Role in Infections in the Neonate**

Agent in Milk	Effect on Breast-Fed Neonate[b]		
	Seroconversion	*Replication of Agent with Illness*	*Replication of Agent without Illness*
Rubella virus	++ (25-30)	0	++ (56)
Cytomegalovirus	+	±	++ (58)
Hepatitis B virus	–	?	++
Hepatitis C virus	–	–	–
Varicella-zoster virus	?	?	?
West Nile virus	±	±	±
Herpes simplex virus	–	+	–
Human immunodeficiency virus (HIV)	+	±	++
Tumor viruses	–	–	+
HTLV-1	+	±	+
HTLV-2	+	±	+
Coxiella burnetii	–	–	–
Streptococcus species	–	±	+
Staphylococcus species	–	±	+
Enterotoxin	–	–	–
Mycobacterium species	–	–	–
Salmonella species	–	–	++
Escherichia coli	–	–	+

[a]All agents listed can be rendered noninfectious by heat inactivation at 62.5° C.
[b]+ to ++, modest to strong evidence; ±, presumptive evidence; ?, inconclusive data; –, not known; 0, absent; ( ), percentage of subjects reported.
HTLV, human T-lymphotropic virus.

has received adequate treatment. Furthermore, breast-feeding may continue on the unaffected breast. Mothers with active tuberculosis should refrain from breast-feeding for at least 2 weeks or longer after institution of appropriate treatment if they are considered contagious.[1]

Viral contaminants of maternal origin in the milk include rubella virus, herpes simplex virus, hepatitis B virus (HBV), cytomegalovirus (CMV), HIV-1, human T-lymphotropic virus type 1 (HTLV-1), and, possibly, HTLV-2 (see Table 5-10). For most viruses, although transmission has been documented as evidenced by seroconversion, no serious illness in the neonate, with the possible exception of CMV infection–related illness secondary to breast-feeding, has been reported.[22,314] Occasional reports of possible neonatal herpes simplex virus infection associated with presence of the virus in the mother's milk may just as easily have been caused by an infant-to-mammary gland rather than a mammary gland-to-infant route of inoculation.[374] Both the RNA-dependent DNA polymerase and structural proteins of C-type tumor viruses, possibly related to mouse mammary tumor and Mason-Pfizer viruses, have been identified in human breast tissue and products of lactation.[82] An association between breast-feeding of female infants and the development of breast cancer has been hypothesized in families with a strong history of carcinoma of the breast. Epidemiologic evidence to support such an association is lacking, however. Breast-feeding may in fact be a protective factor relative to maternal risk of such neoplastic disease.[375] Therefore, with adherence to reasonable maternal hygiene and in the absence of intense chemical contamination, generally few proven or well-defined contraindications to natural breast-feeding exist. Current recommendations regarding the transmission of infectious virus in human milk and their implications for the breast-fed infant are summarized next.

Human Immunodeficiency Virus Infection. Recently, serious concern has been voiced regarding the potential risk of the transmission of HIV from infected mothers to their suckling neonates through the process of breast-feeding. The possibility of postnatal transmission of this virus from mother to child has been considered in a large number of infants breast-fed in the United States and in other parts of the world. In some of these infants, breast-feeding has been implicated as one of the major risk factors for acquisition of HIV infection. Since 1985, small but significant numbers of infants with HIV infection possibly acquired through the process of breast-feeding have been reported.[376] In virtually all reported cases, maternal seroconversion for HIV antibody probably occurred after delivery of the infant. More than 50% of these mothers acquired the infection through heterosexual transmission, and about 30% through blood transfusion. Few of the mothers were judged to be intravenous drug users. Although acquisition of HIV infection before delivery cannot be ruled out with certainty, the likely route of transmission in these infants has been presumed to be through breast-feeding. The most convincing observations are based on several maternal-infant pairs in whom maternal seroconversion to HIV antibody occurred 4 months or longer after delivery.[377]

A number of studies have demonstrated HIV in milk.[378-382] The findings include isolation of HIV from milk supernatants collected from symptom-free women and from cellular fractions of maternal milk, recovery of HIV virions in the histiocytes and cell-free extracts of milk by electron microscopy, and detection of viral DNA by polymerase chain

Table 5–11 Comparisons of HIV-I Transmission Rates in Infants Born to HIV-Infected Mothers Relative to Breast- and Bottle-Feeding

	Percentage of Infected Infants	
Country of Study Population	*Breast-Fed (N = 353)*	*Bottle-Fed (N = 108)*
Haiti	25	0
USA	0	29
USA	28	33
Congo	52	0
Zaire	18	25

HIV, human immunodeficiency virus.
Adapted from Ruff AJ, Halsey NA, Coberly J. Breast-feeding and maternal-infant transmission of human immunodeficiency virus type 1. J Pediatr 121:325-329, 1992.

reaction (PCR) assay in greater than 70% of samples from HIV-seropositive lactating women. Limited epidemiologic studies carried out to date, however, have failed to demonstrate the magnitude of risk of HIV infection in breast-fed infants. Cohort studies[383] in different populations have suggested increased, reduced, or similar transmission rates in breast-feeding and in non–breast-feeding (bottle-feeding) infants of seropositive mothers (Table 5-11). Thus, it appears that although precise epidemiologic data are still lacking, a majority of breast-fed infants born to HIV-seropositive mothers remain uninfected despite the presence of HIV DNA in the milk in a high proportion of such mothers. Nevertheless, the risk of acquisition of HIV infection through breast-feeding must not be ignored. On the basis of meta-analysis of available data, it has been estimated that the additional risk of HIV infection through breast-feeding may be as high as 22%.[384] Some studies have suggested that breast-feeding contributes up to a 50% increase in the overall vertical transmission of HIV infection.[385]

Despite the potential risk of HIV infection in infants of HIV-infected breast-feeding mothers, consideration of cessation of breast-feeding must be balanced against other beneficial effects as outlined in this chapter. In a 1990 study, breast-fed HIV-infected children progressed to acquired immunodeficiency syndrome (AIDS) at a slower rate than that noted for bottle-fed children.[386]

Current estimates indicate the overall risk of acquiring HIV infection from breast-feeding to be about 16%. Of all HIV-infected infants, 47% may be infected by means of breast-feeding. Among those breast-fed for 3 months or longer, the rate of infection was estimated to be approximately 21%, and among those breast-fed for 2 months or less, the rate of infection was approximately 13%.[1] It is, however, important to realize that a number of other risk factors contribute to the increased transfer of HIV through breast-feeding. Associated maternal factors include younger age, multiple deliveries, high virus load, lower number of $CD4^+$ lymphocytes, and maternal mastitis. Other risk factors associated with the maternal milk include high viral load in the milk, long duration of breast-feeding, especially mixed formula feeding and breast-feeding, low levels of antiviral factor in the milk (low CTL, sIgA, lactoferrin, lysozyme). Evidence of oral candidiasis in the breast-feeding neonate also appears to be a risk factor for development of breast-feeding–associated HIV infection.[1]

Current recommendations from the American Academy of Pediatrics state that in populations such as that of the United States, in which the risk of death from infectious diseases and malnutrition is low and in which safe and effective alternative sources of feeding are readily available, HIV-infected women should be counseled not to breast-feed their infants nor to donate milk. All pregnant women in the United States should be counseled and encouraged to be tested for HIV infection. Data are not available about the safety of breast-feeding by mothers receiving highly active antiretroviral therapy (HAART).

In geographic areas in which infectious diseases and malnutrition are important causes of death early in life, the feeding decision may be more complex. The World Health Organization (WHO) states that if a mother is infected with HIV, replacement of human milk to decrease the risk of HIV transmission may be preferable to breast-feeding, provided that the risk associated with replacement feeding is less than the potential risk of HIV transmission. Implementation of this suggestion has many obstacles. The WHO policy stresses the need for continued support for breast-feeding by mothers who are HIV negative or of unknown HIV serostatus, improved access to HIV counseling and testing, and government efforts to ensure uninterrupted access to nutritionally adequate human milk substitutes.[1]

Cytomegalovirus Infection. CMV infection is a common perinatal infection. The virus is shed in the milk in about 25% of infected mothers. Although breast-feeding from infected mothers may result in seroconversion in up to 70% of breast-feeding neonates, the infection often is not associated with clinical symptoms of disease. Low-birth-weight infants (born at less than 1500 g), however, may exhibit evidence of clinical disease, with thrombocytopenia, neutropenia, or hepatosplenomegaly seen in 50% of breast-feeding–infected babies. The decision to breast-feed a premature baby by an infected mother should be based on weighing the potential benefits of human milk versus the risk of CMV transmission. [1]

Hepatitis B Virus Infection. Hepatitis B surface antigen (HBsAg) has been detected in milk of HBV-infected mothers. Nevertheless, breast-feeding does not increase the risk of HBV infection among these infants. Infants born to HBV-positive mothers should receive hepatitis B immune globulin (HBIG) and the recommended series of hepatitis B vaccine without any delay in the institution of breast-feeding.[1]

Hepatitis C Virus Infection. The RNA of hepatitis C virus (HCV) and antibody to HCV have been detected in the milk from infected mothers. Transmission by means of breast-feeding, however, has not been documented in anti-HCV–positive, anti-HIV–negative mother. According to current guidelines, HCV infection does not contraindicate breast-feeding.[1]

Rubella. Rubella virus has been recovered from milk after natural as well as vaccine-associated infection. It has not been associated with significant disease in infants, however, although transient seroconversion has been frequently demonstrated. No contraindication to breast-feeding exists in women recently immunized with currently licensed rubella vaccines.

West Nile Virus Infection. The RNA of west Nile virus has been detected in human milk, and seroconversion in breast-feeding infants also has been observed. Although West Nile virus can be transmitted in milk, its extent of transmission in humans remains to be determined. Most infants and children infected with the virus to date have been asymptomatic or have had minimal disease.[1]

Infection Due to Human T-Lymphotropic Viruses 1 and 2. Epidemiologic studies strongly suggest the possibility of mother-to-infant transmission of HTLV-1 by breast-feeding. In the United States, currently it is recommended that HTLV-1–infected women should not breast-feed. On the other hand, the status of maternal-infant transmission of HTLV-2 through the process of breast-feeding has not been well established, and until additional information is available, breast-feeding should not be recommended in seropositive women.[1]

Summary

It is apparent that human colostrum and milk are richly endowed with a wide variety of cellular and soluble components that participate in many nutritional, immunologic, and anti-infective processes of specific benefit to the neonate. The function of the products of lactation and maternal breast-feeding best characterized to date is nutritional support, and modulation and/or compensation for the transient mucosal immune deficiency against infectious and dietary macromolecules in the autologous infant.

In general, it is quite safe for the mother to collect her milk for later feeding or to directly breast-feed her own neonate. Nevertheless, increasing concerns regarding contamination of human milk by infectious agents have resulted in the limited use of either milk banks or wet nursing. Because of the transfer of infectious agents from maternal blood to milk (see Table 5-10), several national advisory committees have recommended that patients who have known transmissible infectious viral or bacterial diseases should not breast-feed.[388]

Other clinical situations in which withholding breast-feeding is appropriate because of high metabolite content in the milk include presence of galactosemia (galactose from lactose), phenylketonuria (phenylalanine), and other amino acid disorders in the infant.

As shown in Tables 5-9 and 5-10, many drugs, infectious agents, and environmental agents can be transferred to the infant in maternal milk. Rather than stopping breast-feeding, a nursing mother should avoid use of any drug unless it is absolutely essential. Many organohalides and fat-soluble environmental products, such as DDT and PCBs, may be present in higher concentrations in human milk.[22] Although not much is known about their risk to the infant, it is generally agreed that unless the degree of exposure in the mother is extremely high, the benefits of breast-feeding outweigh the possible risks associated with environmental contaminants. Caffeine, alcohol, and nicotine also present potential hazards to the infant (see Table 5-9). It is advisable to reduce or preferably discontinue the intake of tobacco, caffeine-containing products, and alcoholic beverages during lactation and nursing.

CURRENT TRENDS IN BREAST-FEEDING

Both international[389] and national[1,390,391] organizations have endorsed breast-feeding as the optimal means of feeding for the healthy term infant. In general, the percentage of mothers initiating breast-feeding in developing countries is 80% or higher and often 90% or more.[392] The health and economic consequences for bottle-fed infants in these countries are severe, however. In the United States, at one point in the early 1970s, the rate of breast-feeding initiation was as low as 25%. This low point was followed by an increase to a high of 61.9% in 1982. After 1982 a slow decline was observed (to 52.2% in 1989), after which a modest increase has been observed since the early 1990s.[393]

The pattern of breast-feeding initiation is accompanied by concomitant changes in maintenance of breast-feeding to 6 months, from 24% (1984) to 18% (1989) to 21.6% (1995).[393,394] These changes took place despite goals set by the U.S. Surgeon General for 75% of infants to be breast-feeding in the first week of life and 35% at 6 months.[395] These goals were reestablished for the year 2000.[396]

Within the United States, a variety of demographic patterns appear to be associated with breast-feeding behavior. Older mothers, mothers with a college education, and higher-income mothers all are more likely to breast-feed. By contrast, black and Hispanic mothers, mothers of lower socioeconomic status who are participants in the Women, Infants, and Children (WIC) program of the U.S. Department of Health and Human Services and mothers who live in the southern regions of the United States are much less likely to breast-feed. The low rate of breast-feeding for mothers enrolled in WIC is of particular concern, as that agency has a specific policy to encourage breast-feeding. Many states, however, now depend on formula manufacturer rebates to fund part of their WIC programs, creating something of a conflict of interest. The disturbing part of the demographic pattern of breast-feeding in the United States is that the infants of lower-socioeconomic-status mothers, who would accrue the greatest health and economic benefits from breast-feeding, are those least likely to be breast-fed.

Although demographic studies indicate who is breast-feeding, they do not explain the behavioral differences among groups of mothers. One of the more complete models designed to explain breast-feeding behavior includes components that address maternal attitudes and family, societal, cultural, and environmental variables.[397] Individual studies have shown that the maternal decision-making process is closely related to the social support and influence that come from the family members surrounding the mother.[398] The husband in particular appears to have a strong positive influence, whereas the mother's mother may have a negative influence on the breast-feeding decision. Social support appears to be different among ethnic groups, as are maternal attitudes; such differences may provide one explanation for differences in breast-feeding behavior among ethnic groups.[399,400]

SUMMARY AND CONCLUSIONS

Clearly, human milk contains a wide variety of soluble and cellular components with a diverse spectrum of biologic functions. The major milk components identified to date exhibit antimicrobial, anti-inflammatory, pro-inflammatory, and/or immunoregulatory functions; cytotoxicity for tumor cells; ability to repair tissue damage; and receptor analogue functions, as well as other metabolic effects. The relative contributions of different milk components to these biologic effects are summarized in Table 5-12.

The bulk of antimicrobial effects are associated with milk immunoglobulin, especially the sIgA isotype, which makes up to 80% of all immunoglobulins in the human body. Clinical observations have demonstrated that milk antibodies protect against a large number of intestinal pathogens such as *Campylobacter*, *Shigella*, *E. coli*, *V. cholerae*, *Giardia*, rotavirus, and respiratory pathogens such as respiratory syncytial virus. The milk antibodies also effectively neutralize toxins and a variety of human viruses. The role of small amounts of IgG and IgM in milk has not been fully examined. Recently, it has been suggested that milk IgG may hydrolyze nucleotides and DNA.[401] In general, milk IgA antibodies induce antimicrobial protection in the absence of any inflammation, a characteristic of other complement-binding immunoglobulins such as IgG and IgM.

Significant numbers of PMNs, macrophages, and epithelial cells are observed in the milk. Their precise function in the milk remains to be determined. It is possible that their primary task is the defense of the mammary gland itself. The lymphocytes present in the milk transfer immunologic information and may offer significant T cell–mediated immunologic defense to the suckling neonate. Breast-fed infants seem to become tolerant to their mothers' HLA, which may have important implications regarding immune responsiveness and allograft rejection.[402]

Lactoferrin, a major milk protein, also may play an important role in antimicrobial defense. It can kill bacteria, fungi, and viruses without causing inflammation. Lactoferrin also has been found to block mechanisms that result in the expression of pro-inflammatory cytokines (TNF-α, IL-6, IL-1β) by inhibiting nuclear transcription factor (NF$\kappa\beta$) activation mechanisms.[403]

Recent observations have suggested that α-lactalbumin may exist in human milk as large complexes binding to oleic acid. Such complexes, referred to as *h*uman α-lactalbumin *m*ade *le*thal to *t*umor cells (HAMLET), induce apoptosis of all malignant cells tested to date. These complexes have remarkably little to no effect on normal cells.[404,405]

Additional recent studies have suggested that milk contains large numbers of cytokines, chemokines, and growth factors. Although their precise role in the milk remains to be determined, some of these may act as signals for recruitment of pro-inflammatory and or immunoregulatory cells to the mucosal sites. TGF-β may be important in downregulating immune response and induction of tolerance, thereby decreasing the risk of allergic disease. IL-7 may promote development of a $\gamma\delta$ T cell population in cryptopatches which are small aggregates of lymphocytes in the intestinal crypts, and in the maintenance of thymus size.[406,407] It also has been shown that increased levels of IL-1β, TNF-α, IL-6, and possibly other cytokines increase the level of leptin, an appetite-regulating hormone that is present in significant quantities in mammary epithelial cells, milk fat globules, and milk.[407,408] Leptin has several immunologic effects, including differentiation and proliferation of hematopoietic cells and regulation of monocyte-macrophage function. It also influences T cell response by enhancing IL-2 and IFN-γ production (for T_H1 cells) and IL-4 and IL-10 production (for T_H2 cells). Leptin is absorbed by the breast-feeding infant[408,409] and may be associated with prevention of obesity observed in breast-fed infants.

Another important recent observation with milk relates to the presence of antisecretory factor (AF). It has been observed in samples of milk, possibly induced by exposure to enterotoxin-producing bacteria.[410] It possesses significant effect on intestinal fluid secretions. The precise function of AF remains to be determined. Preliminary observations, however, suggest that AF may be highly effective in treatment of inflammatory bowel disease.[411,412]

Human milk has been found to possess large quantities of soluble CD14 and soluble Toll-like receptors TLR-2 and TLR-4, important elements for innate immunity.[413,414] CD14 promotes differentiation in expression of B cell function and anti-inflammatory effect of lactoferrin. Intestinal epithelium does not possess CD14, and it is possible that milk CD14 facilitates phagocytosis of organisms that require expression of this ligand. The TLR-2 and TLR-4 bind to a variety of microorganisms and may play an important role in downregulating inflammatory responses in the mucosal sites.

It is beyond the scope of this chapter to explore in any detail the reasons for and possible benefits of the evolution of mammalian life forms. Nevertheless, the passive transfer of the diversity of maternal biologic experiences to the neonate through the process of breast-feeding represents an essential component of the survival mechanism in the mammalian neonate. For millions of years, maternal products of lactation delivered through the process of breast-feeding have been the sole source of nutrition and immunity during the neonatal period and early infancy for all mammals, including the human infant. During the past 150 to 300 years, however, the human societal culture has undergone remarkable changes in rapid succession, which have had a major impact on the basic mechanisms of maternal-neonatal interaction and breast-feeding. Such changes include introduction of sanitation and nonhuman milk and formula feeds for neonatal nutrition, use of antimicrobial agents, introduction of processed foods, and exposure to newer environmental macromolecules and dietary antigens. The introduction of such manmade changes in the neonatal environment has had a profound impact on human homeostatic mechanisms and at the same time allowed new insights into the role of breast-feeding in the developing human neonate.

Comparative analysis of natural (traditional) forms of breast-feeding and artificial feeding modalities of modern times has demonstrated clearly that natural breast-feeding is associated with significant reduction in infant mortality and morbidity, protection against acute infectious diseases (both in the acute phase of the disease and with long-term reexposure), and possible protection against allergic disorders and autoimmune disease, acute and chronic inflammatory disorders, obesity, diabetes mellitus and other metabolic

Table 5–12 Possible Role of Soluble and Cellular Factors Identified in Human Milk

Factor	Antimicrobial	Anti-inflammatory	Pro-inflammatory	Immunoregulatory	Antitumor	Receptor Blockade	Tissue Maturation	Other
Immunoglobulin (sIgA)	+++	++	—	++				++
Other immunoglobulins	+++	+	++	+				
T lymphocyte products	+++	++	++					
PMNs, macrophages	++		+	++				
Lactoferrin	+++	+++						
α-Lactalbumin (HAMLET)		++			+++			
Carbohydrates								
Oligosaccharides	++	++				++		
Glycoconjugates	++	++				++		
Glycolipids								
Lipid and fat globules	++							
Nucleotides	+			++			++	
Defensins	+			+				
Lysozymes	±							
Cytokines, chemokines								
TGF-β		++	++	++(↓)				
IL-10		++	++	++(↓)				
IL-1β		++	++	++(↓)				
TNF-α				++				
IL-6				↑++				
IL-7				(thymus)				
Others				++				
Prostaglandins		++						
Antisecretory factor		+++						++
Leptin[a]				++			++	++
Antiproteases		++						
Growth factors		++		+++				
(TLR-2, TLR-4) CD14		+++		+++				

[a]IL-1β, TNF-α, IL-6 are associated with increased levels of leptin.

HAMLET, *h*uman α-lactalbumin *m*ade *l*ethal to *t*umor cells; IL, interleukin; PMNs, polymorphonuclear neutrophils [leukocytes]; sIgA, secretory immunoglobulin A; TGF, transforming growth factor; TLR, Toll-like receptor; TNF, tumor necrosis factor; + to +++, minimal to moderate effect; —, no effect.

disorders, allograft rejection, and development of a number of malignant conditions in childhood or later in life. Newer evidence suggests a protective role of breast-feeding in modulating many respiratory, intestinal, and urinary tract infections, otitis media, and NEC in the neonate. This information has been recently reviewed by Hanson in an elegant monograph.[415] Despite the overwhelmingly protective role attributed to natural breast-feeding and the evolutionary advantages related to the development of lactation, several infectious agents have acquired, during the course of evolution, the ability to evade immunologic factors in milk and to use milk as the vehicle for maternal-to-infant transmission. The potential for the acquisition of infections such as those due to HIV, HTLV, CMV, and possibly other pathogens highlights potential hazards of breast-feeding in some clinical situations.

Thus, it is reasonable to conclude that the development of lactation, the hallmark of mammalian evolution, is designed to enhance the survival of the neonate of the species, and that breast-feeding may have a remarkable spectrum of immediate and long-term protective functions.

REFERENCES

1. American Academy of Pediatrics. Human milk. *In* Pickering LK (ed). 2003 Red Book: Report of the Committee on Infectious Diseases, 26th ed. Elk Grove Village, Ill, American Academy of Pediatrics, 2003, p 117.
2. Kratochwil K. Experimental analysis of the prenatal development of the mammary gland. *In* Kretchmer N, Rossi E, Sereni F (eds). Milk and Lactation, Modern Problems in Paediatrics, vol 15. Basel, S. Karger, 1975, pp 1-15.
3. Vorherr H. The Breast: Morphology, Physiology and Lactation. New York, Academic Press, 1974.
4. Goldman AS, Shapiro B, Neumann F. Role of testosterone and its metabolites in the differentiation of the mammary gland in rats. Endocrinology 99:1490-1495, 1976.
5. Kleinberg DL, Niemann W, Flamm E. Primate mammary development: effects of hypophysectomy, prolactin inhibition, and growth hormone administration. J Clin Invest 75:1943-1950, 1985.
6. Ogra SS, Ogra PL. Components of immunologic reactivity in human colostrum and milk. *In* Ogra PL, Dayton D (eds). Immunology of Breast Milk. New York, Raven Press, 1979, pp 185-195.
7. Pasteels JL. Control of mammary growth and lactation by the anterior pituitary: an attempt to correlate classic experiments on animals with recent clinical findings. *In* Kretchmer N, Rossi E, Sereni F (eds). Milk and Lactation: Modern Problems in Paediatrics, vol 15. Basel, S. Karger, 1975, pp 80-95.
8. Mepham TB. Physiology of Lactation. Milton Keynes, England, Open University Press, 1987.
9. Frantz AG. Prolactin. N Engl J Med 298:201-207, 1978.
10. Widström AM, Ransjo-Arvisson AB, Christensson K, et al. Gastric suction in healthy newborn infants. Acta Paediatr Scand 76:566-572, 1987.
11. Varendi H, Porter RH, Winberg J. Does the newborn baby find the nipple by smell? Lancet 344:989-990, 1994.
12. Lönnerdal B, Forsum E, Hambraeus L. The protein content of human milk. I. A transversal study of Swedish normal mothers. Nutr Rep Int 13:125-134, 1976.
13. Schanler RJ, Oh W. Composition of breast milk obtained from mothers of premature infants as compared to breast milk obtained from donors. J Pediatr 96:679-681, 1980.
14. Sann L, Bienvenu F, Lahet C. Comparison of the composition of breast milk from mothers of term and preterm infants. Acta Paediatr Scand 70:115-116, 1981.
15. Mata L. Breast-feeding: main promoter of infant health. Am J Clin Nutr 31:2058-2065, 1978.
16. Hurley LS, Lonnerdal B, Stanislowski AG. Zinc citrate, human milk and acrodermatitis enteropathica. Lancet 1:677-678, 1979.
17. Eckhert CD, Sloan MV, Duncan JR. Zinc binding: a difference between human and bovine milk. Science 195:789-790, 1977.
18. Fomon SJ. Infant Nutrition, 2nd ed. Philadelphia, WB Saunders, 1974.
19. Woodruff CW. The science of infant nutrition and the art of infant feeding. JAMA 240:657-661, 1978.
20. Moran R, Vaughn R, Orth DN, et al. Epidermal growth factor concentrations and daily production in breast milk during seven weeks post delivery in mothers of premature infants. Pediatr Res 16:171A, 1982.
21. Moran R, Bonum P, Vaughn R, et al. The concentration and daily output of trace elements, vitamins and carnitine in breast milk from mothers of premature infants for seven postnatal weeks. Pediatr Res 16:172A, 1982.
22. Ogra PL, Greene HL. Human milk and breast-feeding: an update on the state of the art. Pediatr Res 16:266-271, 1982.
23. Greene HL, Courtney ME. Breast-feeding and infant nutrition. *In* Ogra PL (ed). Neonatal Infections: Nutritional and Immunologic Interactions. Orlando, Fla, Grune & Stratton, 1984, pp 265-284.
24. Code of Federal Regulations, Title 21, Pat 107.100. Washington, DC, U.S. Government Printing Office, 1992, p 84.
25. Anderson RR. Variations in major minerals of human milk during the first 5 months of lactation. Nutr Res 12:701-711, 1992.
26. Saarinen UM, Siimes MA, Dallman PR. Iron absorption in infants: high bioavailability of breast milk iron as indicated by extrinsic tag method of iron absorption and by the concentration of serum ferritin. J Pediatr 91:36-39, 1977.
27. McMillan JA, Oski FA, Louire G, et al. Iron absorption from human milk, simulated human milk, and proprietary formulas. Pediatrics 60:896-900, 1977.
28. Fomon S, Ziegler E, Vasquez H. Human milk and the small premature infant. Am J Dis Child 131:463-467, 1977.
29. Gopalan C, Belavady B. Nutrition and lactation. Fed Proc 20(Suppl 7):177-184, 1961.
30. Gorten MK, Cross ER. Iron metabolism in premature infants. II. Prevention of iron deficiency. J Pediatr 64:509-520, 1964.
31. American Academy of Pediatrics Committee on Nutrition. Nutritional needs of low-birth-weight infants. Pediatrics 60:519-530, 1977.
32. O'Connor P. Vitamin D-deficiency rickets in two breast-fed infants who were not receiving vitamin D supplementation. Clin Pediatr 16:361-363, 1977.
33. Specker BL, Valonis B, Hertzberg V, et al. Sunshine exposure and serum 25-hydroxyvitamin D concentrations in exclusively breast-fed infants. J Pediatr 107:372-376, 1985.
34. Moser HW, Karnovsky ML. Studies on the biosynthesis of glycolipids and other lipids of the brain. J Biol Chem 234:1990-1997, 1959.
35. Kliegman RM, Miettinen EL, Morton S. Potential role of galactokinase in neonatal carbohydrate assimilation. Science 220:302-304, 1983.
36. Newburg DS, Neubauer SH. Carbohydrate in milks: analysis, quantities and significance. *In* Jensen RG (ed). Handbook of Milk Composition. San Diego, Academic Press, 1995, pp 273-349.
37. Newburg DS. Do the binding properties of oligosaccharides in milk protect human infants from gastrointestinal bacteria? J Nutr 127: 980S-984S, 1997.
38. Department of Health and Social Security. The composition of mature human milk. Report 12. London, Her Majesty's Stationery Office, 1977.
39. Jensen RG, Ferris AM, Lammi-Keefe CJ. Lipids in human milk and infant formulas. Annu Rev Nutr 12:417-441, 1992.
40. Rassin DK, Räihä NCR, Gaull GE. Protein and taurine nutrition in infants. *In* Lebenthal E (ed). Textbook of Gastroenterology and Nutrition in Infancy. New York, Raven Press, 1981, pp 391-401.
41. Reiser R, Sidelman Z. Control of serum cholesterol homeostasis by cholesterol in the milk of the suckling rat. J Nutr 102:1009-1016, 1972.
42. Fall CHD, Barker DJP, Osmond C, et al. Relation of infant feeding to adult serum cholesterol concentration and death from ischaemic heart disease BMJ 304:801-805, 1992.
43. Galli E, Picardo M, Chini L, et al. Analysis of polyunsaturated fatty acids in newborn seRA: a screening tool for atopic disease. Br J Dermatol 130:752-756, 1994.
44. Innis SM, Auestad N, Siegman JS. Blood lipid docosahexaenoic acid in term gestation infants fed formulas with high docosahexaenoic acid, low eicosapentaenoic acid fish oil. Lipids 31:617-625, 1996.
45. Carlson SE, Ford AJ, Werkman SH, et al. Visual acuity and fatty acid status of term infants fed human milk and formulas with and without docosahexaenoate and arachidonate from egg yolk lecithin. Pediatr Res 39:882-888, 1996.
46. Auestad N, Montalto MB, Hall RT, et al. Visual acuity, erythrocyte fatty acid composition and growth in term infants fed formulas with

long chain polyunsaturated fatty acids for one year. Pediatr Res 41: 1-10, 1997.
47. Birch EE, Hoffman DR, Usuy R, et al. Visual acuity and the essentiality of docosahexaenoic acid and arachidonic acid in the diet of term infants. Pediatr Res 44:201-209, 1998.
48. Carlson SE, Werkman SH, Tolley EA. Effect of long-chain n-3 fatty acid supplementation on visual acuity and growth of preterm infants with and without bronchopulmonary dysplasia. Am J Clin Nutr 63:687-689, 1996.
49. Gross SJ, Geller J, Tomarelli RM. Composition of breast milk from mothers of preterm infants. Pediatrics 68:490-493, 1981.
50. Hambraeus L. Proprietary milk versus human breast milk in infant feeding: a critical appraisal from the nutritional point of view. Pediatr Clin North Am 24:17-36, 1977.
51. Kunz C, Lönnerdal B. Re-evaluation of the whey protein/casein ratio of human milk. Acta Paediatr 81:107-112, 1992.
52. Järvenpää A-L, Räihä NCR, Rassin DK, et al. Milk protein quantity and quality in the term infant. II. Effects on acidic and neutral amino acids. Pediatrics 70:221-230, 1982.
53. Janas LM, Picciano MF, Hatch TF. Indices of protein metabolism in term infants fed human milk, whey-predominant formula, or cow's milk formula. Pediatrics 75:775-784, 1985.
54. Picone TA, Benson JD, Moro G, et al. Growth, serum biochemistries, and amino acids of term infants fed formulas with amino acid and protein concentrations similar to human milk. J Pediatr Gastroenterol Nutr 9:351-360, 1989.
55. Gaull GE, Rassin DK, Räihä NCR, et al. Milk protein quantity and quality in low-birth-weight infants. III. Effects on sulfur-containing amino acids in plasma and urine. J Pediatr 90:348-355, 1977.
56. Rassin DK, Gaull GE, Heinonen K, et al. Milk protein quantity and quality in low-birth-weight infants. II. Effects on selected essential and nonessential amino acids in plasma and urine. Pediatrics 59:407-422, 1977.
57. Rassin DK, Gaull GE, Räihä NCR, et al. Milk protein quantity and quality in low-birth-weight infants. IV. Effects on tyrosine and phenylalanine in plasma and urine. J Pediatr 90:356-360, 1977.
58. Räihä NCR, Heinonen K, Rassin DK, et al. Milk protein quantity and quality in low-birth-weight infants. I. Metabolic responses and effects on growth. Pediatrics 57:659-674 1976.
59. Gaull GE, Jensen RG, Rassin DK, et al. Human milk as food. Adv Perinatal Med 2:47-120, 1982.
60. Novak M, Wieser PB, Buch M, et al. Acetyl-carnitine and free carnitine in body fluids before and after birth. Pediatr Res 13:10-15, 1979.
61. Schmidt-Sommerfeld E, Novak M, Penn D, et al. Carnitine and development of newborn adipose tissue. Pediatr Res 12:660-664, 1978.
62. Thorell L, Sjoberg L-B, Hernell O. Nucleotides in human milk: sources and metabolism by the newborn infant. Pediatr Res 40:845-852, 1996.
63. Leach JL, Baxter JH, Molitor BE, et al. Total potentially available nucleotides of human milk by stage of lactation. Am J Clin Nutr 61:1224-1230, 1995.
64. Uauy R. Dietary nucleotides and requirements in early life. *In* Lebenthal E (ed). Textbook of Gastroenterology and Nutrition in Infancy. New York, Raven Press, 1989, pp 265-280.
65. Carver JD, Pimentel B, Cox WI, et al. Dietary nucleotide effects upon immune function in infants. Pediatrics 88:359-363, 1991.
66. Brunser O, Espinosa J, Araya M, et al. Effect of dietary nucleotide supplementation on diarrhoeal disease in infants. Acta Paediatr 83: 188-191, 1994.
67. Pickering L, Granoff DM, Erickson JR, et al. Modulation of the immune system by human milk and infant formula containing nucleotides. Pediatrics 101:242-249, 1998.
68. Lönnerdal B, Forsum E. Casein content of human milk. Am J Clin Nutr 41:113-120, 1985.
69. Kunz C, Lönnerdal B. Casein micelles and casein subunits in human milk. *In* Atkinson SA, Lönnerdal B (eds). Protein and Non-Protein Nitrogen in Human Milk. Boca Raton, Fla, CRC Press, 1989, pp 9-27.
70. Phillippy BO, McCarthy RD. Multi-origins of milk serum albumin in the lactating goat. Biochim Biophys Acta 584:298-303, 1979.
71. Jenness R. Biosynthesis and composition of milk. J Invest Dermatol 63:109-118, 1974.
72. Spik G, Brunet B, Mazunier-Dehaine C, et al. Characterization and properties of the human and bovine lactoferrins extracted from the faeces of newborn infants. Acta Paediatr Scand 71:979-985, 1982.
73. Trugo NMF, Newport MJ. Vitamin B_{12} absorption in the neonatal piglet. II. Resistance of the vitamin B_{12}–binding protein in cow's milk to proteolysis in vivo. Br J Nutr 54:257-267, 1985.
74. Oberkotter LV, Tenore A, Pasquariello PS, et al. Tyroxine-binding proteins in human breast milk similar to serum thyroxine-binding globulin. J Clin Endocrinol Metab 57:1133-1139, 1983.
75. Payne DW, Peng LH, Pearlman WH. Corticosteroid-binding proteins in human colostrum and milk and rat milk. J Biol Chem 251: 5272-5279, 1976.
76. Blanc B. Biochemical aspects of human milk-comparison with bovine milk. World Rev Nutr Diet 36:1-89, 1981.
77. Olivecrona T, Hernell O. Human milk lipases and their possible role in fat digestion. Pädiät Pädo 11:600-604, 1976.
78. Hamosh M. Lingual and breast milk lipases. Adv Pediatr 29:33-67, 1982.
79. Koldovsky O, Thomburg W. Peptide hormones and hormone-like substances in milk. *In* Atkinson SA, Lönnerdal B (eds). Protein and Non-Protein Nitrogen in Human Milk. Boca Raton, Fla, CRC Press, 1989, pp 53-65.
80. Lucas A, Blackburn AM, Green AA, et al. Breast vs bottle: endocrine responses are different with formula feeding. Lancet 1:1267-1269, 1980.
81. Koldovsky O, Štrbák V. Hormones and growth factors in human milk. *In* Jensen RG (ed). Handbook of Human Milk Composition. San Diego, Academic Press, 1995, pp 428-436.
82. Ogra PL, Losonsky GA. Defense factors in products of lactation. *In* Ogra PL (ed). Neonatal Infections: Nutritional and Immunologic Interactions. Orlando, Fla, Grune & Stratton, 1984, pp 67-68.
83. Losonsky GA, Ogra PL. Mucosal immune system. *In* Ogra PL (ed). Neonatal Infections: Nutritional and Immunologic Interactions. Orlando, Fla, Grune & Stratton, 1984, pp 51-65.
84. Ogra SS, Ogra PL. Immunologic aspects of human colostrum and milk. I. Distribution characteristics and concentrations of immunoglobulins at different times after the onset of lactation. J Pediatr 92: 546-549, 1978.
85. Goldblum RM, Ahlatedt S, Carlson B, et al. Antibody forming cells in human colostrum after oral immunization. Nature 257:797-799, 1975.
86. Fishaut JM, Murphy D, Neifert M, et al. The broncho-mammary axis in the immune response to respiratory syncytial virus. J Pediatr 99:186-191, 1981.
87. Orskov F, Sorenson KB. *Escherichia coli* serogroups in breast-fed and bottle-fed infants. Acta Pathol Microbiol Scand B 83:25-30, 1975.
88. van Genderen J. Diphtheria-antitoxin in Kolostrum und Muttermilch bei Menschen. Z Immunutaetsforsch Allerg Klin Immunol 83:54-59, 1934.
89. Montgomery PC, Rosner BR, Cohn J, et al. The secretory antibody response: anti-DNP antibodies induced by dinitrophenylated type III pneumococcus. Immunol Commun 3:143-156, 1974.
90. Lamm M, Weisz-Carrington P, Roux ME, et al. Mode of induction of an IgA response in the breast and other secretory sites by oral antigen. *In* Ogra PL, Dayton D (eds). Immunology of Breast Milk. New York, Raven Press, 1979, pp 105-114.
91. Drife J, McClelland DB, Pryde A, et al. Immunoglobulin synthesis in the "resting" breast. BMJ 2:503-506, 1976.
92. Weisz-Carrington P, Roux ME, McWilliams M, et al. Hormonal induction of the secretory immune system in the mammary gland. Proc Natl Acad Sci U S A 75:2928-2932, 1978.
93. Cumella JC, Ogra PL. Pregnancy associated hormonal milieu and bronchomammary cell traffic. *In* Hamosh M, Goldman AS (eds). Human Lactation 2. New York, Plenum Publishing, 1986, pp 507-524.
94. Strober, W, Elson CO, Graeff A. Class specific T cell regulation of mucosal immune responses. *In* Strober W, Hanson L, Sell KW (eds). Recent Advances in Mucosal Immunity. New York, Raven Press, 1982, pp 121-130.
95. Peri BA, Theodore CM, Losonsky GA, et al. Antibody content of rabbit milk and serum following inhalation or ingestion of respiratory syncytial virus and bovine serum albumin. Clin Exp Immunol 48: 91-101, 1982.
96. Losonsky GA, Fiskaut JM, Strussenberg JG, et al. Effect of immunization against rubella on lactation products. I. Development and characterization of specific immunologic reactivity in breast milk. J Infect Dis 145:654-660, 1982.
97. McClelland DBL, McGrath J, Samson, RR. Antimicrobial factors in human milk: studies of concentration and transfer to the infant during the early stages of lactation. Acta Paediatr Scand Suppl 271:1-20, 1978.
98. Pitt J. The milk mononuclear phagocyte. Pediatrics 64:745-749, 1979.
99. Ogra SS, Weintraub D, Ogra PL. Immunologic aspects of human colostrum and milk. III. Fate and absorption of cellular and soluble

components in the gastrointestinal tract of the newborn. J Immunol 119:245-248, 1977.
100. Kenny JF, Boesman MI, Michaels RH. Bacterial and viral copro-antibodies in breast-fed infants. Pediatrics 39:201-213, 1967.
101. Haneberg B. Immunoglobulins in feces from infants fed human or bovine milk. Scand J Immunol 3:191-197, 1974.
102. McClelland DBL, Samson RR, Parkin DM, et al. Bacterial agglutination studies with secretory IgA prepared from human gastrointestinal secretions and colostrum. Gut 13:450-458, 1972.
103. Stoliar OA, Pelley RP, Kaniecki-Green E, et al. Secretory IgA against enterotoxins in breast milk. Lancet 1:1258-1261, 1976.
104. Steele EJ, Chicumpa W, Rowley D. Isolation and biological properties of three classes of rabbit antibody in *Vibrio cholerae.* J Infect Dis 130:93-103, 1974.
105. Cantey JR. Prevention of bacterial infections of mucosal surfaces of immune secretory IgA. Adv Exp Med Biol 107:461-470, 1978.
106. Plotkin SA, Katz M, Brown RE, et al. Oral poliovirus vaccination in newborn African infants: the inhibitory effect of breast-feeding. Am J Dis Child 111:27-30, 1966.
107. Ogra PL, Karzon DT. The role of immunoglobulins in the mechanism of mucosal immunity to virus infection. Pediatr Clin North Am 17:385-390, 1970.
108. Mata LJ, Wyatt RG. The uniqueness of human milk: host resistance to infection. Am J Clin Nutr 24:976-986, 1971.
109. Svirsky-Gross S. Pathogenic strains of coli (O;111) among prematures and the cause of human milk in controlling the outbreak of diarrhea. Ann Pediatr (Paris) 190:109-115, 1958.
110. Yolken RH, Wyatt RG, Mata L, et al. Secretory antibody directed against rotavirus in human milk-measurement by means of an ELISA. J Pediatr 93:916-921, 1978.
111. Glode MP, Sutton A, Robbins JB, et al. Neonatal meningitis due to *Escherichia coli* K1. J Infect Dis 136(Suppl):S93-S97, 1977.
112. Ellestad-Sayed J, Coodin FJ, Dilling LA, et al. Breast-feeding protects against infection in Indian infants. Can Med Assoc J 120:295-298, 1979.
113. Chandra RK. Prospective studies on the effect of breast-feeding on incidence of infection and allergy. Acta Paediatr Scand 68:691-694, 1979.
114. Eastham EJ Walker, WA. Adverse effects of milk formula ingestion on the gastrointestinal tract: an update. Gastroenterology 76:365-374, 1979.
115. Soothill JF. Immunodeficiency, allergy and infant feeding. *In* Hambraeus L, Hanson LA, McFarlane H (eds). Food and Immunology: Proceedings of a Symposium Co-sponsored by the Swedish Medical Research Council. Stockholm, Almqvist & Wiksell, 1977, pp 88-91.
116. Stevenson DD, Orgal HA, Hamburger RN. Development of IgE in newborn human infants. J Allergy Clin Immunol 48:61-72, 1971.
117. Downham MAPS, Scott R, Sims DG, et al. Breast-feeding protects against respiratory syncytial virus infections. BMJ 2:274-276, 1976.
118. Scott R, de Landazuri MO, Gardner PS, et al. Human antibody dependent cell–mediated cytotoxicity against target cells infected with respiratory syncytial virus. Clin Exp Immunol 28:19-26, 1977.
119. Blum P, Phelps DL, Ank BJ, et al. Survival of oral human immune serum globulin in the gastrointestinal tract of low birth weight infants. Pediatr Res 15:1256-1260, 1981.
120. Bahna SL, Keller MA, Heiner DC. IgE and IgD in human colostrum and plasma. Pediatr Res 16:604-607, 1982.
121. Keller MA, Heiner, DC, Kidd RM, et al. Local production of IgG4 in human colostrum. J Immunol 130:1654-1657, 1983.
122. Keller MA, Heiner DC, Myers AS, et al. IgD in human colostrum. Pediatr Res 19:122-126, 1985.
123. Smith CW, Goldman AS. The cells of human colostrum. I. In vitro studies of morphology and functions. Pediatr Res 2:103-109, 1968.
124. Ogra SS, Ogra PL. Immunologic aspects of human colostrum and milk. II. Characteristics of lymphocyte reactivity and distribution of E-rosette forming cells at different times after the onset of lactation. J Pediatr 92:550-555, 1978.
125. Keeney SE, Schmalstieg FC, Palkowetz KH, et al. Activated neutrophils and neutrophil activators in human milk: increased expression of CD116 and decreased expression of L-selectin. J Leukocyte Biol 54(2):97-104, 1993.
126. Wirt DP, Adkins LT, Palkowetz KH, et al. Activated-memory T lymphocytes in human milk. Cytometry 13:282-290, 1992.
127. Pitt J, Barlow B, Heird, WC. Protection against experimental necrotizing enterocolitis by maternal milk. I. Role of milk leucocytes. Pediatr Res 11:906-909, 1977.
128. Pittard WB, Bill K. Immunoregulation by breast milk cells. Cell Immunol 42:437-441, 1979.
129. Pittard WB III, Polmar SH, Fanaroff AA. The breast milk macrophage: potential vehicle for immunoglobulin transport. J Reticuloendothel Soc 22:597-603, 1977.
130. Clemente J, Leyva-Cobian F, Hernandez M, et al. Intracellular immunoglobulins in human milk macrophages: ultrastructural localization and factors affecting the kinetics of immunoglobulin release. Int Arch Allergy Appl Immunol 80:291-299, 1986.
131. Weaver EA, Goldblum RM, Davis CP, et al. Enhanced immunoglobulin A release from human colostral cells during phagocytosis. Infect Immun 34:498-502, 1981.
132. Schlesinger L, Munoz C, Arevalo M, et al. Functional capacity of colostral leukocytes from women delivering prematurely. J Pediatr Gastroenterol Nutr 8:89-94, 1989.
133. Cummings NP, Neifert MR, Pabst MJ, et al. Oxidative metabolic response and microbicidal activity of human milk macrophages: effect of lipopolysaccharide and muramyl dipeptide. Infect Immun 49:435-439, 1985.
134. Robinson JE, Harvey BA, Sothill JF. Phagocytosis and killing of bacteria and yeast by human milk after opsonization in aqueous phase of milk. BMJ 1:1443-1445, 1978.
135. Kohl S, Malloy MM, Pickering LK, et al. Human colostral antibody dependent cellular cytotoxicity against herpes simplex virus infected cells mediated by colostral cells. J Clin Lab Immunol 1:221-224, 1978.
136. Sone S, Tsutsumi H, Takeuchi R, et al. Enhanced cytokine production by milk macrophages following infection with respiratory syncytial virus. J Leukoc Biol 61:630-636, 1997.
137. Kirkpatrick CH, Green I, Rich RR, et al. Inhibition of growth of *Candida albicans* by iron-unsaturated lactoferrin: relation to host defense mechanisms in chronic mucocutaneous candidiasis. J Infect Dis 124:539-544, 1971.
138. Murillo GJ, Goldman AS. The cells of human colostrum. II. Synthesis of IgA and B-1C. Pediatr Res 4:71-75, 1970.
139. Diaz-Uanen E, Williams RC Jr. T and B lymphocytes in human colostrum. Clin Immunol Immunopathol 3:248-255, 1974.
140. Oksenberg JR, Persity E, Brautbar C. Cellular immunity in human milk. Am J Reprod Immunol Microbiol 8:125-129, 1985.
141. Hanson LA, Ahlstedt S, Andersson B., et al. Protective factors in milk and development of the immune system. J Pediatr 75:172-175, 1985.
142. Ogra PL, Ogra SS. Cellular aspects of immunologic reactivity in human milk. *In* Hanson LA (ed). Biology of Human Milk. Nestlé Nutrition Workshop Series, vol 15. New York, Raven Press, 1988, pp 171-184.
143. Nair MP, Schwartz SA, Slade HB, et al. Comparison of the cellular cytotoxic activities of colostral lymphocytes and maternal peripheral blood lymphocytes. J Reprod Immunol 7:199-213, 1985.
144. Parmely MJ, Beer AE, Billingham RE. In vitro studies on the T-lymphocyte population of human milk. J Exp Med 144:358-370, 1976.
145. Shinmoto H, Kawakami H, Dosako S, et al. IgA specific helper factor in human colostrum Clin. Exp Immunol 66:223-230, 1986.
146. Bertotto A, Gerli R, Fabietti G, et al. Human breast milk T lymphocytes display the phenotype and functional characteristics of memory T cells. Eur J Immunol 20:1877-1880, 1990.
147. Gibson CE, Eglinton BA, Penttila IA, et al. Phenotype and activation of milk-derived and peripheral blood lymphocytes from normal and coeliac subjects. Immunol Cell Biol 69:387-391, 1991.
148. Bertotto A, Castellucci G, Pradicioni M, et al. CD40 ligand expression on the surface of colostral T cells. Arch Dis Child 74:F135-F136, 1996.
149. Hayward AR, Lee J, Beverley PCL. Ontogeny of expression of UCHL1 antigen on TcR-1$^+$ (CD4/8) and TcR$^+$ T cells. Eur J Immunol 19: 771-773, 1989.
150. Bertotto A, Castellucci G, Fabietti G, et al. Lymphocytes bearing the T cell receptor $\gamma\delta$ in human breast milk. Arch Dis Child 65:1274-1275, 1990.
151. Eglinton BA, Roberton DM, Cummins AG. Phenotype of T cells, their soluble receptor levels, and cytokine profile of human breast milk. Immunol Cell Biol 72:306-313, 1994.
152. Trejdosiewicz LK. Intestinal intraepithelial lymphocytes and lympho-epithelial interactions in the human gastrointestinal mucosa. Immunol Lett 32:13-19, 1992.
153. Head JR, Beer AE, Billingham RE. Significance of the cellular component of the maternal immunologic endowment in milk. Transplant Proc 9:1465-1471, 1977.

154. Jain L, Vidyasagar D, Xanthou M, et al. In vivo distribution of human milk leucocytes after ingestion by newborn baboons. Arch Dis Child 64:930-933, 1989.
155. Schnorr KL, Pearson LD. Intestinal absorption of maternal leukocytes by newborn lambs. J Reprod Immunol 6:329-337, 1984.
156. Weiler IJ, Hickler W, Spenger R. Demonstration that milk cells invade the neonatal mouse. Am J Reprod Immunol 4:95-98, 1983.
157. Beer AE, Billingham RE, Head J. The immunologic significance of the mammary gland. J Invest Dermatol 63:65-74, 1974.
158. Mohr JA, Leu R, Mabry W. Colostral leukocytes. J Surg Oncol 2: 163-167, 1970.
159. Schlesinger JJ, Covelli HD. Evidence for transmission of lymphocyte response to tuberculin by breast-feeding. Lancet 2:529-532, 1977.
160. Thorpe LW, Rudloff HE, Powell LC, et al. Decreased response of human milk leukocytes to chemoattractant peptides. Pediatr Res 20:373-377, 1986.
161. Dulbecco R, Unger M, Armstrong B, et al. Epithelial cell types and their evolution in the rat mammary gland determined by immunological markers. Proc Natl Acad Sci U S A 80:1033-1037, 1983.
162. Allen R, Dulbecco R, Syka P, et al. Developmental regulation of cytokeratins in cells of the rat mammary gland studies with monoclonal antibodies. Proc Natl Acad Sci U S A 81:1203-1207, 1984.
163. Ballow M, Fang F, Good RA, et al. Developmental aspects of complement components in the newborn. Clin Exp Immunol 18:257-266, 1974.
164. Nakajima S, Baba AS, Tamura N. Complement system in human colostrum. Int Arch Allergy Appl Immunol 54:428-433, 1977.
165. Tomasi TB Jr. New areas arising from studies of secretory immunity. Adv Exp Med Biol 107:1-8, 1978.
166. György P. A hitherto unrecognized biochemical difference between human milk and cow's milk. Pediatrics 11:98-108, 1953.
167. György P, Dhanamitta S, Steers E. Protective effects of human milk in experimental staphylococcus infection. Science 137:338-340, 1962.
168. Hanson LA, Ahlstedt S, Anderson B, et al. Mucosal immunity. Ann N Y Acad Sci 409:1-21, 1983.
169. Carpenter G. Epidermal growth factor is a major growth-promoting agent in human milk. Science 210:198-199, 1980.
170. Colman N, Hettiarachchy N, Herbert V. Detection of a milk factor that facilitates folate uptake by intestinal cells. Science 211:1427-1429, 1981.
171. Dolan SA, Boesman-Finkelstein M, Finkelstein RA. Antimicrobial activity of human milk against pediatric pathogens. J Infect Dis 154: 722-725, 1986.
172. Boesman-Finkelstein M, Finkelstein RA. Antimicrobial effects of human milk: inhibitory activity on enteric pathogens. FEMS Microbiol 27:167-174, 1985.
173. Farthing MJG, Keusch GT, Carey MC. Effects of bile and bile salts on growth and membrane lipid uptake by *Giardia lamblia*. J Clin Invest 76:1727-1732, 1985.
174. Reiter B. Role of nonantibody proteins in milk in the protection of the newborn. *In* Williams AF, Baum JD (eds). Human Milk Banking. New York, Nestlé Nutrition, Raven Press, 1984, pp 29-53.
175. Hernell O, Bläckberg L, Olivecrona T. Human milk lipases. *In* Lebenthal E. (ed). Gastroenterology and Nutrition in Infancy. New York, Raven Press, 1981, pp 347-354.
176. Hernell O, Bläckberg L. Lipase and esterase activities in human milk. *In* Jensen RG, Neville MC. (eds). Human Lactation: Milk Components and Methodologies. New York, Plenum Publishing, 1985, pp 267-276.
177. Hernell O, Blackberg L. Antiparasitic factors in human milk. *In* Hanson LA (ed). Biology of Human Milk. Nestlé Nutrition Workshop Series, vol 15. New York, Raven Press, 1988, pp 159-170.
178. Holmgren J, Svennerholm AM, Ahren C. Nonimmunoglobulin fraction of human milk inhibits bacterial adhesion (hemagglutination) and enterotoxin binding of *Escherichia coli* and *Vibrio cholerae*. Infect Immun 33:136-141, 1981.
179. Holmgren J, Svennerholm AM, Lindblad M. Receptor-like glycocompounds in human milk that inhibit classical and *El Tor Vibrio cholerae* cell adhererence (hemagglutination). Infect Immun 39: 147-154, 1983.
180. Newburg DS, Pickering LK, McCluer RH, et al. Fucosylated oligosaccharides of human milk protect suckling mice from heat-stable enterotoxin of *Escherichia coli*. J Infect Dis 162:1075-1080, 1990.
181. Holmgren J, Svennerholm A-M, Lindblad M, et al. Inhibition of bacterial adhesion and toxin binding by glycoconjugate and oligosaccharide receptor analogues in human milk. *In* Goldman AS, Atkinson SA, Hanson LNA (eds). Human Lactation 3: The Effects of Human Milk on the Recipient Infant. New York and London, Plenum Press, 1987, pp 251-259.
182. Grönberg G, Lipniunas P, Lundgren T, et al. Structural analysis of five new monosialylated oligosaccharides from human milk. Arch Biochem Biophys 296:597-610, 1992.
183. Laegreid A, Kolsto Otnaess, AB, Bryn K. Purification of human milk gangliosides by silica gel chromatography and analysis of trifluoroacetate derivatives by gas chromatography. J Chromatogr 377:59-67, 1986.
184. Laegreid A, Kolsto Otnaess AB, Fuglesang J. Human and bovine milk: comparison of ganglioside composition and enterotoxin-inhibitory activity. Pediatr Res 20:416-421, 1986.
185. Laegreid A, Kolsto Otnaess AB. Trace amounts of ganglioside GM1 in human milk inhibit enterotoxins from *Vibrio cholerae* and *Escherichia coli*. Life Sci 40:55-62, 1987.
186. Schroten H, Hanisch FG, Plogmann R, et al. Inhibition of adhesion of S-fimbriated *Escherichia coli* to buccal epithelial cells by human milk fat globule membrane components: a novel aspect of the protective function of mucins in the nonimmunoglobulin fraction. Infect Immun 60:2893-2899, 1992.
187. Andersson B, Porras O, Hanson LA, et al. Inhibition of attachment of *Streptococcus pneumoniae* and *Haemophilus influenzae* by human milk and receptor oligosaccharides. J Infect Dis 153:232-237, 1986.
188. Newburg DS, Viscidi RP, Ruff A, et al. A human milk factor inhibits binding of human immunodeficiency virus to the CD4 receptor. Pediatr Res 31:22-28, 1992.
189. Otnaess AB, Svennerholm AM. Non-immunoglobulin fraction in human milk protects rabbit against enterotoxin-induced intestinal fluid secretion. Infect Immun 35:738-740, 1982.
190. Ashkenazi S, Newburg DS, Cleary TG. The effect of human milk on the adherence of enterohemorrhagic *E. coli* to rabbit intestinal cells. *In* Mesteky J, Blair C, Ogra PL (eds). Immunology of Milk and the Neonate. New York, Plenum Press, 1991, pp 173-177.
191. Cleary TG, Chambers JP, Pickering LK, Protection of suckling mice from the heat-stable enterotoxin of *Escherichia coli* by human milk. J Infect Dis 148:1114-1119, 1983.
192. Glass RL, Svenneholm AM, Stoll BJ, et al. Protection against cholera in breast-fed children by antibodies in breast milk. N Engl J Med 308:1389-1392, 1983.
193. György P, Jeanloz RW, Nicolai H, et al. Undialyzable growth factors for *Lactobacillus bifidus* var. *pennsylvanicus*: protective effect of sialic acid bound to glycoproteins and oligosaccharides against bacterial degradation. Eur J Biochem 43:29-33, 1974.
194. Bezkorovainy A, Grohlich D, Nichols JH. Isolation of a glycopeptide fraction with *Lactobacillus bifidus* subspecies *pennsylvanicus* growth-promoting activity from whole human milk casein. Am J Clin Nutr 32:1428-1432, 1979.
195. Nichols JH, Bezkorovainy A, Paque R. Isolation and characterization of several glycoproteins from human colostrum whey. Biochim Biophys Acta 412:99-108, 1975.
196. Bezkorovainy A, Topouzian N. *Bifidobacterium bifidus* var. *pennsylvanicus* growth promoting activity of human milk casein and its derivates. Int J Biochem 13:585-590, 1981.
197. Isolauri E, Juntanen M, Rautanen T, et al. A human *Lactobacillus* strain (*Lactobacillus* GG) promotes recovery from acute diarrhea in children. Pediatrics 88:90-97, 1991.
198. Kaila M, Isolauir E, Elina S, et al. Enhancement of the circulating antibody secreting cell response in human diarrhea by a human *Lactobacillus* strain. Pediatr Res 32:141-144, 1992.
199. Hamosh M. Enzymes in human milk: their role in nutrient digestion, gastrointestinal function, and nutrient delivery to the newborn infant. *In* Lebenthal E (ed). Textbook of Gastroenterology and Nutrition in Infancy, 2nd ed. New York, Raven Press, pp 121-134.
200. Institute of Medicine (U.S.) Subcommittee on Nutrition During Lactation, et al. Nutrition During Lactation: Summary, Conclusions and Recommendations. Washington, DC, National Academy Press, 1991.
201. Issacs CE, Thormar H, Pessolano T. Membrane-disruptive effect of human milk: inactivation of enveloped viruses. J Infect Dis 154: 966-971, 1986.
202. Stock CC, Francis T Jr. The inactivation of the virus of epidemic influenza by soaps. J Exp Med 71:661-681, 1940.
203. Thormar H, Isaacs CE, Brown HR, et al. Inactivation of enveloped viruses and killing of cells by fatty acids and monoglycerides. Antimicrobiol Agents Chemother 31:27-31, 1987.
204. Welsh JK, Arsenakis M, Coelen RJ, et al. Effect of antiviral lipids, heat, and freezing on the activity of viruses in human milk. J Infect Dis 140:322-328, 1979.

205. Welsh JK, May JT. Anti-infective properties of breast milk. J Pediatr 94:1-9, 1979.
206. Resta S, Luby JP, Rosenfeld CR, et al. Isolation and propagation of a human enteric coronavirus. Science 229:978-981, 1985.
207. Gillin FD, Reiner DS, Wang C-S. Human milk kills parasitic protozoa. Science 221:1290-1292, 1983.
208. Gillin FD, Reiner DS, Gault MJ. Cholate-dependent killing of *Giardia lamblia* by human milk. Infect Immun 47:619-622, 1985.
209. Anderson BF, Baker HM, Dodson EJ, et al. Structure of human lactoferrin at 3.1-resolution. Proc Natl Acad Sci U S A 84:1769-1773, 1987.
210. Fransson G-B, Lonnerdal B. Iron in human milk. J Pediatr 96:380-384, 1980.
211. Arnold RR, Cole MF, McGhee JR. A bactericidal effect for human milk lactoferrin. Science 197:263-265, 1977.
212. Bullen JJ, Rogers HJ, Leigh L. Iron-binding proteins in milk and resistance of *Escherichia coli* infection in infants. BMJ 1:69-75, 1972.
213. Spik G, Cheron A, Montreuil J, et al. Bacteriostasis of a milk-sensitive strain of *Escherichia coli* by immunoglobulins and iron-binding proteins in association. Immunology 35:663-671, 1978.
214. Stephens S, Dolby JM, Montreuil J, et al. Differences in inhibition of the growth of commensal and enteropathogenic strains of *Escherichia coli* by lactoferrin and secretory immunoglobulin A isolated from human milk. Immunology 41:597-603, 1980.
215. Stuart J, Norrel S, Harrington JP. Kinetic effect of human lactoferrin on the growth of *Escherichia coli*. Int J Biochem 16:1043-1047, 1984.
216. Nichols BL, McKee KS, Henry JF, et al. Human lactoferrin stimulates thymidine incorporation into DNA of rat crypt cells. Pediatr Res 21:563-567, 1987.
217. Goldblum RM, Garza CA, Johnson CA, et al. Human milk banking. II. Relative stability of immunologic factors in stored colostrum. Acta Paediatr Scand 71:143-144, 1981.
218. Goldblum RM, Garza CA, Johnson CA, et al. Human milk banking I. Effects of container upon immunologic factors in mature milk. Nutr Res 1:449-459, 1981.
219. Goldman AS, Garza CA, Johnson CA, et al. Immunologic factors in human milk during the first year of lactation. J Pediatr 100:563-567, 1982.
220. Brines RD, Brock JH. The effect of trypsin and chymotrypsin on the in vitro antimicrobial and iron-binding properties of lactoferrin in human milk and bovine colostrum. Biochim Biophys Acta 759: 229-235, 1983.
221. Samson RR, Mirtle C, McClelland DBL. The effect of digestive enzymes on the binding and bacteriostatic properties of lactoferrin and vitamin B_{12} binder in human milk. Acta Paediatr Scand 69:517-523, 1980.
222. Spik G, Montreuil J. Études comparatives de la structure de la tranferrine de la lactotransferrine humaines. Finger-printing des hydrolytes protéasiques des deux glycoproteides. CR Seances Soc Biol Paris 160:94-98, 1996.
223. Butte NF, Goldblum RM, Fehl LM, et al. Daily ingestion of immunologic components in human milk during the first four months of life. Acta Paediatr Scand 73:296-301, 1984.
224. Davidson LA, Lonnerdal B. Lactoferrin and secretory IgA in the feces of exclusively breast-fed infants. Am J Clin Nutr 41:852A, 1985.
225. Davidson LA, Lonnerdal B. The persistence of human milk proteins in the breast-fed infant. Acta Paediatr Scand 76:733-740, 1987.
226. Schanler RJ, Goldblum RM, Garza C, et al. Enhanced fecal excretion of selected immune factors in very low birth weight infants fed fortified human milk. Pediatr Res 20:711-715, 1986.
227. Goldman AS, Garza C, Schanler RJ, et al. Molecular forms of lactoferrin in stool and urine from infants fed human milk. Pediatr Res 27:252-255, 1990.
228. Goldblum RM, Schanler RJ, Garza C, et al. Human milk feeding enhances the urinary excretion of immunologic factors in birth weight infants. Pediatr Res 25:184-188, 1989.
229. Prentice A. Breast-feeding increases concentrations of IgA in infants' urine. Arch Dis Child 62:792-795, 1987.
230. Hutchens TW, Henry JF, Yip T-T, et al. Origin of intact lactoferrin and its DNA-binding fragments found in the urine of human milk-fed preterm infants: evaluation of stable isotopic enrichment. Pediatr Res 29:243-250, 1991.
231. Chandan RC, Shahani KM, Holly RG. Lysozyme content of human milk. Nature (London) 204:76, 1964.
232. Jolles J, Jolles P. Human tear and human milk lysozymes. Biochemistry 6:411-417, 1967.
233. Goldman AS, Garza C, Johnson CA, et al. Immunologic components in human milk during weaning. Acta Paediatr Scand 72:133-134, 1983.
234. Goldman AS, Goldblum RM, Garza C. Immunologic components in human milk during the second year of lactation. Acta Paediatr Scand 72:461-462, 1983.
235. Peitersen B, Bohn L, Anderson H. Quantitative determination of immunoglobulins, lysozyme, and certain electrolytes during a 24-hour period, and in milk from the individual mammary gland. Acta Paediatr Scand 64:709-717, 1975.
236. Chipman DM, Sharon N. Mechanism of lysozyme action. Science 165:454-465, 1969.
237. Friss HE, Rubin LG, Carsons S, et al. Plasma fibronectin concentrations in breast-fed and formula fed neonates. Arch Dis Child 63:528-532, 1988.
238. Cunningham AS, Jelliffe DB, Jelliffe EFP. Breast-feeding and health in the 1980s: a global epidemiologic review. J Pediatr 118:659-666, 1991.
239. Glass RI, Stoll BJ. The protective effect of human milk against diarrhea. Acta Paediatr Scand 351:131-136, 1989.
240. Goldman AS, Thorpe LW, Goldblum RM, et al. Anti-inflammatory properties of human milk. Acta Paediatr Scand 75:689-695, 1986.
241. Garofalo RP, Goldman AS. Expression of functional immunomodulatory and anti-inflammatory factors in human milk. Clin Perinatol 26:361-377, 1999.
242. Klagsbrun M. Human milk stimulates DNA synthesis and cellular proliferation in cultured fibroblasts. Proc Natl Acad Sci U S A 75:5057-5061, 1978.
243. Okada M, Ohmura E, Kamiya Y, et al. Transforming growth factor (TGF)-α in human milk. Life Sci 48:1151-1156, 1991.
244. Saito S, Yoshida M, Ichijo M, et al. Transforming growth factor-beta (TGF-β) in human milk. Clin Exp Immunol 94:220-224, 1993.
245. Kidwell WR, Bano M, Burdette K, et al. Human lactation. Mammary derived growth factors in human milk. *In* Jensen RG, Neville MC (eds). Human Lactation: Milk Components and Methodologies. New York and London, Plenum Press, 1985, pp 209-219.
246. Sanguansermsri J, György P, Zilliken F. Polyamines in human and cow's milk. Am J Clin Nutr 27:859-865, 1974.
247. Romain N, Dandrifosse G, Leusette C, et al. Polyamine concentration in rat milk and food, human milk, and infant formulas. Pediatr Res 32:58-63, 1992.
248. Koldovsky O, Bedrick A, Pollack P, et al. Hormones in milk: their presence and possible physiological significance. *In* Goldman AS, Atkinson SA, Hanson LA (eds). Human Lactation 3: The Effects of Human Milk on the Recipient Infant. New York and London, Plenum Press, 1987, pp 183-193.
249. Kulski JK, Hartmann PE. Milk insulin, GH and TSH: relationship to changes in milk lactose, glucose and protein during lactogenesis in women. Endocrinol Exp 17:317-326, 1983.
250. Teichberg S, Wapnir RA, Moyse J, et al. Development of the neonatal rat small intestinal barrier to nonspecific macromolecular absorption. II. Role of dietary corticosterone. Pediatr Res 32:50-57, 1992.
251. Weaver LT, Walker WA. Uptake of macromolecules in the neonate. *In* Lebenthal E (ed). Human Gastrointestinal Development. New York, Raven Press, 1989, pp 731-748.
252. Axelsson I, Jakobsson I, Lindberg T, et al. Macromolecular absorption in preterm and term infants. Acta Paediatr Scand 78:532-537, 1989.
253. Eastham EJ, Lichauco T, Grady ML, et al. Antigenicity of infant formulas: role of immature intestine on protein permeability. J Pediatr 93:561-564, 1978.
254. Widdowson EM, Colombo VE, Artavanis CA. Changes in the organs of pigs in response to feeding for the first 24 h after birth. II. The digestive tract. Biol Neonate 28:272-281, 1976.
255. Buescher ES, McIlheran SM. Colostral antioxidants: separation and characterization of two activities in human colostrum. J Pediatr Gastroenterol Nutr 14:47-56, 1992.
256. Chappell JE, Francis T, Clandinin MT. Vitamin A and E content of human milk at early stages of lactation. Early Hum Dev 11:157-167, 1985.
257. Ostrea EM Jr, Balun JE, Winkler R, et al. Influence of breast-feeding on the restoration of the low serum concentration of vitamin E and β-carotene in the newborn infant. Am J Obstet Gynecol 154:1014-1017, 1986.
258. Garofalo R, Chheda S, Mei F, et al. Interleukin-10 in human milk. Pediatr Res 37:444-449, 1995.
259. Kühn R, Löhler J, Rennick D, et al. Interleukin-10–deficient mice develop chronic enterocolitis. Cell 25:263-274, 1993.

260. Buescher ES, Malinowska I. Soluble receptors and cytokine antagonists in human milk. Pediatr Res 40:839-844, 1996.
261. Grazioso C, Werner A, Alling D, et al. Anti-inflammatory effects of human milk on chemically induced colitis in rats. Pediatr Res 42: 639-643, 1997.
262. Furukawa M, Narahara H, Johnston JM. The presence of platelet-activating factor acetylhydrolase activity in milk. J Lipid Res 34: 1603-1609, 1993.
263. Caplan MS, Kelly A, Hsueh W. Endotoxin and hypoxia-induced intestinal necrosis in rats: the role of platelet activating factor. Pediatr Res 31:428-434, 1992.
264. Caplan MS, Sun X-M, Hsueh W, et al. The role of platelet activating factor and tumor necrosis factor-alpha in neonatal necrotizing enterocolitis. J Pediatr 116:960-964, 1990.
265. Caplan MM, Hsueh W, Kelly A, et al. Serum PAF acetylhydrolase increases during neonatal maturation. Prostaglandins 39:705-714, 1990.
266. Furukawa M, Frenkel RA, Johnston JM. Absorption of platelet-activating factor acetylhydrolase by rat intestine. Am J Physiol 266: G935-G939, 1994.
267. Sarfati M, Vanderbeeken Y, Rubio-Trujillo M, et al. Presence of IgE suppressor factors in human colostrum. Eur J Immunol 16:1005-1008, 1986.
268. Bjørge L, Jensen TS, Kristoffersen EK, et al. Identification of the complementary regulatory protein CD59 in human colostrum and milk. Am J Reprod Immunol 35:43-50, 1996.
269. Saarinen UM, Kajosaari M. Breast-feeding as prophylaxis against atopic disease: prospective follow-up study until 17 years old. Lancet 346:1065-1069, 1995.
270. Koletzko S, Sherman P, Corey M, et al. Role of infant feeding practices in development of Crohn's disease in childhood. BMJ 298:1617-1618, 1989.
271. Koletzko S, Griffiths A, Corey M, et al. Infant feeding practices and ulcerative colitis in childhood. BMJ 302:1580-1581, 1991.
272. Mayer EJ, Hamman RF, Gay EC, et al. Reduced risk of IDDM among breast-fed children. Diabetes 37:1625-1632, 1988.
273. Davis MK, Savitz DA, Grauford B. Infant feeding in childhood cancer. Lancet 2:365-368, 1988.
274. Pabst HF, Spady DW. Effect of breast-feeding on antibody response to conjugate vaccines. Lancet 336:269-270, 1990.
275. Hahn-Zoric M, Fulconis F, Minoli I, et al. Antibody responses to parenteral and oral vaccines are impaired by conventional and low protein formula as compared to breast-feeding. Acta Paediatr Scand 79:1137-1142, 1990.
276. Stephens S, Kennedy CR, Lakhani PK, et al. In-vivo immune responses of breast- and bottle-fed infants to tetanus toxoid antigen and to normal gut flora. Acta Paediatr Scand 73:426-432, 1984.
277. Pabst HF, Grace M, Godel J, et al. Effect of breast-feeding on immune response to BCG vaccination. Lancet 1:295-297, 1989.
278. Campbell DA Jr, Lorber MI, Sweeton JC, et al. Maternal donor-related transplants: influence of breast-feeding on reactivity to the allograft. Transplant Proc 15:906-909, 1983.
279. Campbell DA Jr, Lorber MI, Sweeton JC, et al. Breast-feeding and maternal-donor renal allografts. Transplantation 37:340-344, 1984.
280. Kois WE, Campbell DA Jr, Lorber MI, et al. Influence of breast-feeding on subsequent reactivity to a related renal allograft. J Surg Res 37:89-93, 1984.
281. Zhang L, van BreeS, van Rood JJ, et al. Influence of breast-feeding on the cytotoxic T cell allorepertoire in man. Transplantation 52:914-916, 1991.
282. Chiba Y, Minagawa T, Miko K, et al. Effect of breast-feeding on responses of systemic interferon and virus-specific lymphocyte transformation in infants with respiratory syncytial virus infection. J Med Virol 21:7-14, 1987.
283. Stephens S. Development of secretory immunity in breast-fed and bottle fed infants. Arch Dis Child 61:263-269, 1986.
284. Gala RR. Prolactin and growth hormone in the regulation of the immune system. Proc Soc Exp Biol Med 198:513-527, 1991.
285. Nuijens JH, van Berkel PH, Schanbacher FL. Structure and biological action of lactoferrin. J Mammary Gland Biol Neoplasia 1:285-295, 1996.
286. Hahn-Zoric M, Carlsson B, Jeansson S, et al. Anti-idiotypic antibodies to polio virus in commercial immunoglobulin preparations, human serum, and milk. Pediatr Res 33:475-480, 1993.
287. Garofalo RP, Goldman AS. Cytokines, chemokines, and colony-stimulating factors in human milk: the 1997 update. Biol Neonate 74:134-142, 1998.
288. Pittard BK III. Differentiation of cord blood lymphocytes into IgA-producing cells in response to breast milk stimulatory factor. Clin Immunol Immunopathol 13:430-434, 1979.
289. Juto P. Human milk stimulates B cell function. Arch Dis Child 60: 610-613, 1985.
290. Julius MH, Janusz M, Lisowski J. A colostral protein that induces the growth and differentiation of resting B lymphocytes. J Immunol 140:1366-1371, 1988.
291. Soder O. Isolation of interleukin-1 from human milk. Int Arch Allergy Appl Immunol 83:19-23, 1987.
292. Hooton JW, Pabst HF, Spady DW, et al. Human colostrum contains an activity that inhibits the production of IL-2. Clin Exp Immunol 86:520-524, 1991.
293. Munoz C, Endres S, van der Meer J, et al. Interleukin-1 beta in human colostrum. Res Immunol 141:501-513, 1990.
294. Rudloff HE, Schmalstieg FC, Mushtaha AA, et al. Tumor necrosis factor-α in human milk. Pediatr Res 31:29-33, 1992.
295. Skansen-Saphir U, Linfors A, Andersson U. Cytokine production in mononuclear cells of human milk studied at the single-cell level. Pediatr Res 34:213-216, 1993.
296. Basolo F, Conaldi PG, Fiore L, et al. Normal breast epithelial cells produce interleukins-6 and 8 together with tumor-necrosis factor: defective IL-6 expression in mammary carcinoma. Int J Cancer 55:926-930, 1993.
297. Saito S, Manuyama M, Kato Y, et al. Detection of IL-6 in human milk and its involvement in IgA production. J Reprod Immunol 20:267-276, 1991.
298. Rudloff HE, Schmalstieg FC, Palkowetz KH, et al. Interleukin-6 in human milk. J Reprod Immunol 23:13-20, 1993.
299. Bocci V, von Bremen K, Corradeschi F, et al. Presence of interferon-α and interleukin-6 in colostrum of normal women. Lymphokine Cytok Res 12:21-24, 1993.
300. Srivastava MD, Srivastava, A, Brouhard B, et al. Cytokines in human milk. Res Commun Mol Pathol Pharmacol 93:263-287, 1996.
301. Oppenheim JJ, Zachariae COC, Mukaida N, et al. Properties of the novel proinflammatory supergene "intercrine" cytokine family. Annu Rev Immunol 9:617-648, 1991.
302. Baggiolini M, Dewald B, Moser B. Interleukin-8 and related chemotactic cytokines—CXC and CC chemokines. Adv Immunol 55:97-179, 1994.
303. Bottcher MF, Jenmalm MC, Bjorksten B. Cytokine, chemokine and secretory IgA levels in human milk in relation to atopic disease and IgA production in infants. Pediatr Allergy Immunol 14:35-41, 2003.
304. Sinha SK, Yunis AA. Isolation of colony stimulating factor from milk. Biochem Biophys Res Commun 114:797-803, 1983.
305. Gilmore WS, McKelvey-Martin VJ, Rutherford S, et al. Human milk contains granulocyte-colony stimulating factor (G-CSF). Eur J Clin Nutr 48:222-224, 1994.
306. Hara T, Irie K, Saito S, et al. Identification of macrophage colony-stimulating factor in human milk and mammary epithelial cells. Pediatr Res 37:437-443, 1995.
307. Gasparoni A, Chirico G, De Amici M, et al. Granulocyte-macrophage colony stimulating factor in human milk. Eur J Pediatr 156:69, 1996.
308. Yap PL, Miller WR, Humeniuk V, et al. Milk protein concentrations in the mammary secretions of non-lactating women. J Reprod Immunol 3:49-58, 1981.
309. Yap PL, Pryde EA, McClelland DB. Milk protein concentrations in galactorrhoeic mammary secretions. J Reprod Immunol 1:347-357, 1980.
310. Carlsson BS, Ahlstedt S, Hanson LA, et al. *Escherichia coli*–O antibody content in milk from healthy Swedish mothers from a very low socioeconomic group of a developing country. Acta Paediatr Scand 65:417-423, 1976.
311. Goldman AS, Garza C, Nichols B, et al. Effects of prematurity on the immunologic system in human milk. J Pediatr 101:901-905, 1982.
312. Gross SJ, Buckley RH, Wakel SS, et al. Elevated IgA concentrations in milk produced by mothers delivered of preterm infants. J Pediatr 99:389-393, 1981.
313. Lodinova R, Jouya V. Antibody production by the mammary gland in mothers after oral colonization of their infants with a nonpathogenic strain *E. coli* 083. Acta Paediatr Scand 66:705-708, 1977.
314. May JT. Antimicrobial properties and microbial contaminants of breast milk—an update. Aust Paediatr J 20:265-269, 1984.
315. The breast-fed infant: a model for performance. Report of the 91st Ross Conference on Pediatric Research. Columbus, Ohio, Ross Laboratories, 1986.

316. Sandine W, Muralidh KS, Elliker PR, et al. Lactic acid bacteria in food and health: a review with special references to enteropathogenic *Escherichia coli* as well as certain enteric diseases and their treatment with antibiotics and lactobacilli. J Milk Food Technol 35:691-702, 1972.
317. Bishop RF, Cameron DJ, Barnes GL, et al. The aetiology of diarrhea in newborn infants. Ciba Found Symp 42:223-236, 1976.
318. Cameron DJ, Bishop RF, Veenstra AA, et al. Noncultivable viruses and neonatal diarrhea: fifteen-month survey in a newborn special care nursery. J Clin Microbiol 8:93-98, 1978.
319. Cameron DJ, Bishop RF, Veenstra AA, et al. Pattern of shedding of two noncultivable viruses in stools of newborn babies. J Med Virol 2:7-13, 1978.
320. Chrystei IL, Totterdell BM, Bonatvala JE. Asymptomatic endemic rotavirus infections in the newborn. Lancet 1:1176-1178, 1978.
321. Murphy AM, Albrey MB, Crewe EB. Rotavirus infections of neonates. Lancet 2:1149-1150, 1977.
322. Bishop RF, Cameron DJ, Veenstra AA, et al. Diarrhea and rotavirus infection associated with differing regimens for postnatal care of newborn babies. J Clin Microbiol 9:525-529, 1979.
323. Duffy LC, Riepenhoff-Talty M, Byers TE, et al. Modulation of rotavirus enteritis during breast-feeding. Am J Dis Child 140:1164-1168, 1986.
324. Duffy LC, Byers TE, Riepenhoff-Taltz M, et al. The effects of infant feeding on rotavirus-induced gastroenteritis: a prospective study. Am J Public Health 76:259-263, 1986.
325. Frantz ID III, L'Heureux P, Engel RR, et al. Necrotizing enterocolitis. J Pediatr 86:259-263, 1975.
326. Bell MJ, Feigen RD, Ternberg JL. Changes in the incidence of necrotizing enterocolitis associated with variation of the gastrointestinal microflora in neonates. Am J Surg 138:629-631, 1979.
327. Book LS, Overall JC, Herbst JJ, et al. Clustering of necrotizing enterocolitis: interruption by infection-control measures. N Engl J Med 297:984-986, 1977.
328. Bunton GL, Durbin GM, McIntosh M, et al. Necrotizing enterocolitis. Arch Dis Child 52:772-777, 1977.
329. Kliegman RM, Pittard WB, Fanaroff AA. Necrotizing enterocolitis in neonates fed human milk. J Pediatr 95:450-453, 1979.
330. Moriartey RR, Finer NN, Cox SF, et al. Necrotizing enterocolitis and human milk. J Pediatr 94:295-296 1979.
331. Eibl MM, Wolf HM, Furnkranz H, et al. Prophylaxis of necrotizing enterocolitis by oral IgA-IgG: review of a clinical study in low birth weight infants and discussion of the pathogenic role of infection. J Clin Immunol 10:72S-77S, 1990.
332. Pitt J. Necrotizing enterocolitis: a model for infection-immunity interaction. *In* Ogra PL (ed). Neonatal Infections: Nutritional and Immunologic Interactions. Orlando, Fla, Grune & Stratton, 1984, pp 173-184.
333. Donta ST, Myers MG. *Clostridium difficile* toxin in asymptomatic neonates. J Pediatr 100:431-434, 1982.
334. Howard FM, Flynn DM, Bradley JM, et al. Outbreak of necrotizing enterocolitis caused by *Clostridium butyricum*. Lancet 2:1099-1102, 1977.
335. Zeissler J, Rossfeld-Sternberg L. Enteritis necroticans due to *Clostridium welchii* type F. BMJ 1:267-269, 1949.
336. Pederson PV, Hansen FH, Halveg AB, et al. Necrotizing enterocolitis of the newborn—is it gas gangrene of the bowel? Lancet 2:715-716, 1976.
337. Weinberg RJ, Tipton G, Klish WJ, et al. Effect of breast-feeding on morbidity in rotavirus gastroenteritis. Pediatrics 74:250-253, 1984.
338. Research Subcommittee of the South-East England Faculty. The influence of breast-feeding on the incidence of infectious illness during the first year of life. Practitioner 209:356-362, 1972.
339. Fallot ME, Boyd JL, Oski FA. Breast-feeding reduces incidence of hospital admissions for infection in infants. Pediatrics 65:1121-1124, 1980.
340. Elger MS, Rausen AR, Silverio J. Breast vs. bottle feeding. Clin Pediatr 23:492-495, 1984.
341. Habicht J-P, DaVanzo J, Butz WP. Does breast-feeding really save lives, or are apparent benefits due to biases? Am J Epidemiol 123:279-290, 1986.
342. Bauchner H, Leventhal JM, Shapiro ED. Studies of breast-feeding and infections. How good is the evidence? JAMA 256:887-892, 1986.
343. Grulee CG, Sanford HN. The influence of breast and artificial feeding on infantile eczema. J Pediatr 9:223-225, 1936.
344. Kramer MS. Does breast-feeding help protect against atopic disease? Biology, methodology, and a golden jubilee of controversy. J Pediatr 112:181-190, 1988.
345. Wright AL, Holberg CJ, Taussig LM, et al. Relationship of infant feeding to recurrent wheezing at age 6 years. Arch Pediatr Adolesc Med 149:758-763, 1995.
346. Hanson LA, Ahlstedt S, Carlsson B, et al. Secretory IgA antibodies against cow's milk proteins in human milk and their possible effect in mixed feeding. Int Arch Allergy Appl Immunol 54:457-462, 1977.
347. Uhnoo IS, Freihort J, Riepenhoff-Talty M, et al. Effect of rotavirus infection and malnutrition on uptake of dietary antigen in the intestine. Pediatr Res 27:153-160, 1990.
348. Brandtzaeg P. The secretory immune system of lactating human mammary glands compared with other exocrine organs. Ann N Y Acad Sci 409:353-382, 1983.
349. Rieger CHL, Rothberg RM. Development of the capacity to produce specific antibody to an ingested food antigen in the premature infant. J Pediatr 87:515-518, 1975.
350. Businco L, Marchetti F, Pellegrini G, et al. Prevention of atopic disease in "at risk newborns" by prolonged breast-feeding. Ann Allergy 51:296-299, 1983.
351. Kohl S, Loo LS. The relative role of transplacental and milk immune transfer in protection against lethal neonatal herpes simplex virus infection in mice. J Infect Dis 149:38-42, 1984.
352. Laegreid A, Kolsto Otnuess AB, Orstorik I, et al. Neutralizing activity in human milk fractions against respiratory syncytial virus. Acta Paediatr Scand 75:696-701, 1986.
353. Saarinen UM. Prolonged breast-feeding as prophylaxis for recurrent otitis media. Acta Paediatr Scand 71:567-571, 1982.
354. Short RV. Breast-feeding. Sci Am 250:35-41, 1984.
355. Gunther M. The neonate's immunity gap, breast-feeding and cot death. Lancet 1:441-442, 1975.
356. Pettitt DJ, Forman MR, Hanson RL, et al. Breast-feeding and incidence of non–insulin-dependent diabetes mellitus in Pima Indians. Lancet 350:166-168, 1997.
357. Kramer MS. Do breast-feeding and delayed introduction of solid foods protect against subsequent obesity? J Pediatr 98:883-887, 1981.
358. Rodgers B. Feeding in infancy and later ability and attainment: a longitudinal study. Dev Med Child Neurol 20:421-426, 1978.
359. Rogan WJ, Gladen BC. Breast-feeding and cognitive development. Early Hum Dev 31:181-193, 1993.
360. Horwood LJ, Fergusson DM. Breast-feeding and later cognitive and academic outcomes. Pediatrics 101:99, 1998.
361. Katsouyani K, Lipworth L, Trichopoulou A, et al. A case-control study of lactation and cancer of breast. Br J Cancer 73:814-818, 1996.
362. Packard VS. Human Milk and Infant Formula. New York, Academic Press, 1982, p 118-119.
363. Lawrence RA. Breast-Feeding: A Guide for the Medical Profession, 2nd ed. St. Louis, CV Mosby, 1985.
364. Arias IM, Gartner LM. Production of unconjugated hyperbilirubinemia in full-term new-born infants following administration of pregnane-3,20-diol. Nature 203:1292-1293, 1966.
365. Newman TB, Maisels ML. Evaluation and treatment of jaundice in the term newborn: a kinder, gentler approach. Pediatrics 89:809-818, 1992.
366. Gartner L. Management of jaundice in the well baby. Pediatrics 89:826-827, 1992.
367. O'Connor ME, Livingston DS, Hannah J, et al. Vitamin K deficiency and breast-feeding. Am J Dis Child 137:601-602, 1983.
368. Zmora E, Gorodescher R, Bar-Ziv J. Multiple nutritional deficiencies in infants from a strict vegetarian commune. Am J Dis Child 133: 141-144, 1979.
369. Nau SB, Stickler GB, Hawort JC. Serum 25-hydroxyvitamin D in infantile rickets. Pediatrics 57:221-225, 1976.
370. Higinbotham MC, Sweetman L, Nyhan WL. A syndrome of methylmalonic aciduria, homocystinuria, megaloblastic anemia and neurologic abnormalities in a vitamin B_{12}–deficient breast-fed infant of a strict vegetarian. N Engl J Med 299:317-323, 1978.
371. Kanaka C, Schütz B, Zuppinger KA. Risks of alternative nutrition in infancy: a case report of severe iodine and carnitine deficiency. Eur J Pediatr 151:786-788, 1992.
372. Anderson SA, Chinn HI, Fisher KD. A background paper on infant formulas. Bethesda, Md, Life Sciences Research Office, FASEB, 1980.
373. Saukkonen T, Virtanen SM, Karppinen M, et al. Childhood Diabetes in Finland Study Group. Significance of cow's milk protein antibodies as risk factor for childhood IDDM: interactions with dietary cow's milk intake and HLA-DQB1 genotype. Diabetologia 41:72-78, 1998.

374. Dunkle LM, Schmidt RR, Connor DM. Neonatal herpes simplex infection possibly acquired via maternal breast milk. Pediatrics 63:250-251, 1979.
375. Vorherr H. Hormonal and biochemical changes of pituitary and breast during pregnancy. Semin Perinatol 3:193-198, 1979.
376. Ziegler JB, Cooper DA, Johnson RO, et al. Postnatal transmission of AIDS-associated retrovirus from mother to infant. Lancet 1:896-898, 1985.
377. Van de Perre P, Simonon A, Msellati P, et al. Postnatal transmission of the human immunodeficiency virus type 1 from mother to infant: a prospective cohort study in Kigali, Rwanda. N Engl J Med 325: 593-598, 1991.
378. Thiry L, Sprecher-Goldberger S, Jonckheer T, et al. Isolation of AIDS virus from cell-free breast milk of three healthy virus carriers. Letter to the editor. Lancet 2:891-892, 1985.
379. Vogt MW, Witt DJ, Craven DE, et al. Isolation of HTLV-III/LAV from cervical secretions of women at risk of AIDS. Letter to the editor. Lancet 1:525-527, 1986.
380. Bucens M, Armstrong J, Stuckey M. Virologic and electron microscopic evidence for postnatal HIV transmission via breast milk. Fourth International Conference on AIDS, Stockholm, 1988 (abstract).
381. Pezzella M, Caprilli F, Cordiali Fei P, et al. The presence of HIV-1 genome in human colostrum from asymptomatic seropositive mothers, vol 6. International Conference on AIDS, 1990, p 165.
382. Ruff A, Coberly J, Farzadegan H, et al. Detection of HIV-1 by PCR in breast milk, vol 7. International Conference on AIDS, 1991, p 300.
383. Ruff AJ, Halsey NA, Coberly J. Breast-feeding and maternal-infant transmission of human immunodeficiency virus type 1. J Pediatr 121:325-329, 1992.
384. Newell M-L, Gray G, Bryson YJ. Prevention of mother-to-child transmission of HIV-1 infection. AIDS 11(Suppl A):S165-S172, 1997.
385. European Collaborative Study. Caesarean section and risk of vertical transmission of HIV-1 infection. Lancet 343:1464-1467, 1994.
386. Tozzi A, Pezzotti P, Greco D. Does breast-feeding delay progression to AIDS in HIV-infected children? AIDS 4:1293-1294, 1990.
387. Gottlieb S. UN amends policy on breast-feeding. BMJ 317:297, 1998.
388. American College of Obstetricians and Gynecologists Committee statement. Breast-feeding. Washington, DC, American College of Obstetricians and Gynecologists, 1985.
389. ESPGAN Committee on Nutrition. Guidelines on infant nutrition. I. Recommendations for the composition of an adapted formula. Acta Paediatr Scand 262(Suppl):1-20, 1977.
390. Nutrition Committee of the Canadian Pediatric Society and the Committee on Nutrition of the American Academy of Pediatrics. Breast-feeding: a commentary in celebration of the International Year of the Child, 1979. Pediatrics 62:591-601, 1978.
391. Ambulatory Pediatric Association. The World Health Organization code of marketing of breastmilk substitutes. Pediatrics 68:432-434, 1981.
392. Kent MM. Breast-Feeding in the Developing World: Current Patterns and Implications for Future Trends. Washington, DC, Population Reference Bureau, 1981.
393. Ryan AS. The resurgence of breast-feeding in the United States. Pediatrics 99:1-5, 1997.
394. Ryan AS, Rush D, Krieger FW, et al. Recent declines in breast-feeding in the United States, 1984 through 1989. Pediatrics 88:719-727, 1988.
395. Report of the Surgeon General's Workshop on Breast-feeding and Human Lactation. Washington, DC, U.S. Department of Health and Human Services, Public Health Service, 1984.
396. Healthy People 2000: National Health Promotion and Disease Prevention Objectives. Washington, DC, U.S. Department of Health and Human Services, Public Health Service, 1990, pp 379-380.
397. Bentovim A. Shame and other anxieties associated with breast-feeding: a systems theory and psychodynamic approach. Ciba Found Symp 45:159-178, 1976.
398. Baranowski T, Bee DE, Rassin DK, et al. Social support, social influence, ethnicity and the breast-feeding decision. Soc Sci Med 17:1599-1611, 1983.
399. Baranowski T, Rassin DK, Richardson CJ, et al. Attitudes toward breast-feeding. J Dev Behav Pediatr 7:367-372, 1986.
400. Baranowski T, Rassin DK, Richardson CJ, et al. Expectancies of infant-feeding methods among mothers in three ethnic groups. Psychol Health 5:59-75, 1990.
401. Semenov DV, Kanyshkova TG, Karotaeva NA, et al. Catalytic nucleotide-hydrolyzing antibodies in milk and serum of clinically healthy human mothers. Med Sci Monit 10:BR23-BR33, 2004.
402. Deroche A, Nepomnaschy I, Torello S, et al. Regulation of parental alloreactivity by reciprocal F_1 hybrids. The role of lactation. J Reprod Immunol 23:235-245, 1993.
403. Togawa J, Nagase H, Tanaka K, et al. Lactoferrin reduces colitis in rats via modulation of the immune system and correction of cytokine imbalance. Am J Physiol Gastrointest Liver Physiol 283:G187-G195, 2002.
404. Svensson M, Hakansson A, Mossberg AK, et al. Conversion of alpha-lactalbumin to a protein inducing apoptosis. Proc Natl Acad Sci U S A 97:4221-4226, 2000.
405. Svanborg C, Agerstam H, Aronson A, et al. HAMLET kills tumor cells by an apoptosis-like mechanism—cellular, molecular, and therapeutic aspects. Adv Cancer Res 88:1-29, 2003.
406. Laky K, Lefrancois L, Freeden-Jeffry U, et al. The role of IL-7 in thymic and extrathymic development of TCR gamma delta cells. J Immunol 161:707-713, 1998.
407. Lopez-Alarcon M, Garza C, Habicht JP, et al. Breastfeeding attenuates reductions in energy intake induced by a mild immunologic stimulus represented by DPTH immunization: possible roles of interleukin-1beta, tumor necrosis factor-alpha and leptin. J Nutr 132:1293-1298, 2002.
408. Savino F, Costamagna M, Prino A, et al. Leptin levels in breast-fed and formula-fed infants. Acta Paediatr 91:897-902, 2002.
409. Lord G. Role of leptin in immunology. Nutr Rev 60:S35-S38, 2002.
410. Bjorck S, Bosaeus I, Ek E, et al. Food induced stimulation of the antisecretory factor can improve symptoms in human inflammatory bowel disease: a study of a concept. Gut 46:824-829, 2000.
411. Lonnroth I, Martinsson K, Lange S. Evidence of protection against diarrhoea in suckling piglets by a hormone-like protein in the sow's milk. Zentralbl Veterinarmed B 35:628-635, 1988.
412. Eriksson A, Shafazand M, Jennische E, et al. Effect of antisecretory factor in ulcerative colitis on histological and laborative outcome: a short period clinical trial. Scand J Gastroenterol 38:1045-1049, 2003.
413. labeta MO, Vidal K, Nores JE, et al. Innate recognition of bacteria in human milk is mediated by a milk-derived highly expressed pattern recognition receptor, soluble CD14. J Exp Med 191:1807-1812, 2000.
414. Vidal K, Labeta MO, Schiffrin EJ, et al. Soluble CD14 in human breast milk and its role in innate immune responses. Acta Odontol Scand 59:330-334, 2001.
415. Hanson LA. Immunobiology of Human Milk: How Breastfeeding Protects Babies. Amarillo, Tex, Pharmasoft Publishing, 2004.

Section II

BACTERIAL INFECTIONS

Chapter 6

BACTERIAL SEPSIS AND MENINGITIS

Debra L. Palazzi • Jerome O. Klein • Carol J. Baker

Bacterial sepsis in the neonate is a clinical syndrome characterized by systemic signs of infection and accompanied by bacteremia in the first month of life. Meningitis in the neonate usually is a sequela of bacteremia and is discussed in this chapter because meningitis and sepsis typically share a common cause and pathogenesis. Infections of the bones, joints, and soft tissues and of the respiratory, genitourinary, and gastrointestinal tracts can be accompanied by bacteremia, but the cause, clinical features, diagnosis, and management of these infections are sufficiently different to warrant separate discussions. Sepsis and meningitis caused by group B *Streptococcus, Staphylococcus aureus, Neisseria gonorrhoeae, Listeria monocytogenes, Salmonella* species, and *Mycobacterium tuberculosis* are described in other chapters.

The two patterns of disease, early-onset and late-onset, have been associated with systemic bacterial infections during the first month of life (Table 6-1). Early-onset disease typically presents as a fulminant, systemic illness during the first 24 hours of life, with most other cases presenting on the second day of life. Infants with early-onset disease can have a history of one or more obstetric complications, including premature or prolonged rupture of maternal membranes, preterm onset of labor, chorioamnionitis, and peripartum maternal fever, and many of the infants are premature or of low birth weight. Bacteria responsible for early-onset disease are acquired hours before delivery from overt or occult rupture of membranes or from the birth canal during delivery. The mortality rate varies from 3% to as high as 50% in some series, especially with gram-negative pathogens. Late-onset disease is variably defined as occurring after 72 hours to 6 days (e.g., group B *Streptococcus*) of life. Very late onset infection due to group B *Streptococcus* (disease in infants older than 3 months) is discussed in Chapter 13. Term infants with late-onset infections can have a history of obstetric complications, but these are less characteristic than in early-onset sepsis or meningitis. Bacteria responsible for late-onset sepsis and meningitis include those acquired from the maternal genital tract and organisms acquired after birth from human contacts or infrequently from contaminated hospital equipment or materials where prolonged intensive care is needed for a neonate. The mortality rate usually is lower than that for early-onset sepsis but can vary between 2% and 40%, with the latter figure typically for very low birth weight (VLBW) infants with gram-negative sepsis. Because different microorganisms are responsible for disease by age at onset, the choice of antimicrobial agents also differs. Some organisms, such as *Escherichia coli,* groups A and B streptococci, and *L. monocytogenes,* can be responsible for early-onset and late-onset infections, whereas others, such as *S. aureus,* coagulase-negative staphylococci, and *Pseudomonas aeruginosa,* rarely cause early-onset and typically are associated with late-onset disease. The survival of VLBW infants with prolonged stays in the neonatal intensive care unit has been accompanied by increased risk for nosocomial or hospital-associated infections and for very late onset disease[1] (see Chapter 35).

Table 6–1 Characteristics of Early-Onset and Late-Onset Neonatal Sepsis

Characteristic	Early-Onset[a]	Late-Onset[b]
Time of onset (days)	0-6	7-90
Complications of pregnancy or delivery	+	±
Source of organism	Mother's genital tract	Mother's genital tract; postnatal environment
Usual clinical presentation	Fulminant	Slowly progressive or fulminant
	Multisystem	Focal
	Pneumonia frequent	Meningitis frequent
Mortality rate (%)	3-50[c]	2-40

[a]Many studies define early-onset sepsis as that which occurs in the first 72 hours of life; others in the first 5 or 6 days of life.
[b]Very small premature infants may have late-onset sepsis beyond 90 days of life.
[c]Higher mortality rates in earlier studies.

BACTERIOLOGY

The changing pattern of organisms responsible for neonatal sepsis is reflected in a series of reports by pediatricians at the Yale–New Haven Hospital covering the period of 1928 to 1999[2-7] (Table 6-2). Before development of the sulfonamides, gram-positive cocci caused most cases of neonatal sepsis. With the introduction of antimicrobial agents, gram-negative enteric bacilli, particularly *E. coli,* became the predominant cause of serious infection in the newborn. *S. aureus* was a major pathogen between 1950 and 1963 but subsequently diminished in importance for reasons that remain unclear. Reports for the periods of 1966 to 1978 and 1979 to 1988 indicate the importance of group B streptococci, *E. coli,* and coagulase-negative staphylococcal (CoNS) species, predominantly *Staphylococcus epidermidis,* in neonatal sepsis. The latest reports also document the problem of sepsis in very premature and low-birth-weight infants who have survived with the aid of sophisticated life-support equipment and advances in neonatal intensive care.

The etiologic pattern of microbial infection observed at Yale Medical Center also has been reported in studies of neonatal sepsis carried out at other centers during the same intervals (Table 6-3). Studies indicate that group B streptococci and gram-negative enteric bacilli, predominantly

Table 6–2 Bacteria Causing Neonatal Sepsis at Yale–New Haven Hospital, 1928-1988

	No. of Cases					
Organism	1928-1932[a]	1933-1943[b]	1944-1957[b]	1958-1965[c]	1966-1978[d]	1979-1988[e]
Beta-hemolytic streptococci	15	18	11	8	86	83
Group A		16	5	0	0	0
Group B		2	4	1	76	64
Group D		0	1	7	9	19
Viridans streptococci						11
Staphylococcus aureus	11	4	8	2	12	14
Staphylococcus epidermidis						36
Streptococcus pneumoniae	2	5	3	2	2	2
Haemophilus species				1	9	9
Escherichia coli	10	11	23	33	76	46
Pseudomonas aeruginosa	1	0	13	11	5	6
Klebsiella and *Enterobacter* species	0	0	0	8	28	25
Others	0	6	4	9	21	38
Total no. of cases	39	44	62	73	239	270
Mortality rate for years	87%	90%	67%	45%	26%	16%

[a]Data from reference 2.
[b]Data from reference 3.
[c]Data from reference 4.
[d]Data from reference 5.
[e]Data from reference 6.

E. coli, were the most frequent pathogens for sepsis, but other organisms were prominent in some centers. *S. aureus* was an important cause of sepsis in the mid-1980s in Finland[20] and East Africa[32] and a more recently significant pathogen in Connecticut[7] and southern Israel[31]; *Streptococcus viridans* was the most frequent isolate from neonatal blood cultures in Philadelphia[14]; *S. epidermidis* was responsible for 53% of cases in Liverpool,[22] and CoNS account for 35% to 48% of all late-onset sepsis in VLBW infants across the United States[17,18] and in Israel[37]; and *Klebsiella* and *Enterobacter* species were the most common bacterial pathogens in Tel Aviv.[30] Sepsis and focal infections in neonates in developing countries are further discussed in Chapter 2.

Table 6–3 Surveys of Neonatal Bacteremia

Country or Region	Site	Year of Publication	Reference
United States	New Haven	1933	2
		1958	3
		1966	4
		1981	5
		1990	6
		2001	7
	New York	1949	8
	Minneapolis	1956	9
	Nashville	1961	10
	Baltimore	1965	11
	Los Angeles	1981	12
	Indianapolis	1982	13
	Philadelphia	1985	14
	Kansas City	1987	15
	Multicenter	1998	16
	Eastern Virginia	2000	17
	Multicenter	2002	18
Canada	Montreal	1985	19
Europe	Finland	1985	20
		1989	21
	Liverpool	1985	22
	Göttingen	1985	23
	Göteborg	1990	24
	London	1981	25
		1991	26
	Mallorca	1993	27
	Denmark	1991	28
	Norway	1998	29
Middle East	Tel Aviv	1983	30
	Beer-Sheva	1997	31
Africa	Nigeria	1984	32
	Ethiopia	1997	33
	South Africa	1998	34
Asia	Hyderabad	1985	35
Australia	South Brisbane	1997	36

The survey of five university hospitals in Finland[20] provides data about the association of the etiologic agent and mortality based on age at onset of sepsis (Table 6-4) and birth weight (Table 6-5). Infants with sepsis onset during the first 24 hours of life and weighing less than 1500 g at birth had the highest mortality rate.

The mortality rates for neonatal sepsis over time are documented in the Yale Medical Center reports. In the pre-antibiotic era, neonatal sepsis usually was fatal. Even with the introduction of penicillins and aminoglycosides in the reports from 1944 to 1965, death resulted from sepsis in most infants. Concurrent with the introduction of neonatal intensive care units and technologic support for cardiorespiratory and metabolic functions beginning in the early 1970s, the mortality rate was reduced to 16%.

The Yale data also provide information about the microorganisms responsible for early-onset and late-onset sepsis (Table 6-6). Group B streptococci were responsible for most early-onset disease. *E. coli* and CoNS were the major pathogens of late-onset disease, with the latter afflicting VLBW infants almost exclusively. A wide variety of gram-positive cocci and gram-negative bacilli caused disease after age 30 days.

Survival of VLBW infants (<1500 g) has been accompanied by an increased risk for invasive, nosocomial, or health care–associated bacterial infection as a cause of morbidity and mortality. The danger of sepsis is documented in a multicenter trial that enrolled 2416 VLBW infants in a study of the efficacy of intravenous immunoglobulin in preventing nosocomial infections.[16] Sixteen percent of the VLBW infants developed septicemia at a median age of 17 days, with an overall mortality rate of 21% and a hospital stay that averaged 98 days; infants without sepsis had an overall mortality rate of 9% and 58-day average length of stay.

Organisms responsible for bacterial meningitis in the newborn are listed in Table 6-7, which summarizes data collected from 1932 to 1997 at neonatal centers in the United States,[38-41,44] The Netherlands,[42] Great Britain,[43,45] and Israel.[31] Gram-negative enteric bacilli and group B streptococci currently are responsible for most cases. Organisms that cause acute bacterial meningitis in older children and adults—*Streptococcus pneumoniae, Neisseria meningitidis,* and non-

Table 6–4 Bacteremia in Finnish Neonates Related to Times of Onset of Signs and Mortality

	Mortality for Onset of Signs at					
	<24 hr		24 hr–7 day		8–20 day	
Organism	*No. Died/Total*	%	*No. Died/Total*	%	*No. Died/Total*	%
Group B streptococci	28/93	30	0/26	0	1/11	0
Escherichia coli	8/26	31	14/45	31	3/10	30
Staphylococcus aureus	3/14	21	7/64	11	1/12	8
Other	15/47	32	9/55	16	4/7	57
Total	54/180	30	30/190	16	9/40	23

Data from Vesikari R, Janas M, Gronroos P, et al. Neonatal septicemia. Arch Dis Child 60:542–546, 1985.

Table 6–5 Bacteremia in Finnish Neonates Related to Birth Weight and Mortality

	Mortality for Onset of Signs at					
	<1500 g		1500-2500 g		>2500 g	
Organism	*No. Died/Total*	%	*No. Died/Total*	%	*No. Died/Total*	%
Group B streptococci	11/15	73	10/36	20	8/79	10
Escherichia coli	11/15	73	8/19	42	6/47	13
Staphylococcus aureus	4/9	44	4/26	15	3/55	5
Other	12/18	67	7/21	33	9/70	13
Total	38/57	67	29/102	28	26/251	10

Data from Vesikari R, Janas M, Gronroos P, et al. Neonatal septicemia. Arch Dis Child 60:542–546, 1985.

Table 6–6 Microbiology of Neonatal Sepsis at Yale–New Haven Hospital, 1979-1988

	No. of Isolates				
	Age When Cultured (days)				
Microorganism	*0-4*	*5-30*	*>30*	*Transported Infants*	*Total*
Staphylococcus aureus	1	4	4	5	14
Coagulase-negative staphylococci	1	10	10	12	33
Group B streptococci	51	4	3	6	64
Enterococcus species	4	7	3	4	18
Viridans streptococci	2	3	2	4	11
Streptococcus pneumoniae	2	0	0	0	2
Listeria monocytogenes	2	0	0	0	2
Escherichia coli	13	17	6	10	46
Klebsiella pneumoniae	0	3	8	7	18
Enterobacter cloacae	1	1	3	2	7
Pseudomonas aeruginosa	0	1	3	2	6
Haemophilus influenzae	7	0	0	1	8
Candida species	0	2	5	4	11
Miscellaneous	9	2	6	10	27
Total	93	54	53	67	267

Data from Gladstone IM, Ehrenkranz RA, Edberg SC, Baltimore RS. A ten-year review of neonatal sepsis and comparison with the previous fifty-year experience. Pediatr Infect Dis J 9:819, 1990.

typeable *Haemophilus influenzae*—are relatively infrequent causes of meningitis in the neonate.[46] A nationwide survey of causative agents of neonatal meningitis in Sweden between 1976 and 1983 indicated a shift from bacterial to viral or unidentified microorganisms, with lower attributable mortality rates.[47]

Group B Streptococci

Group B β-hemolytic streptococci were implicated in human disease shortly after the precipitin-grouping technique was described.[48] Neonatal sepsis caused by this organism was recognized, but only a few sporadic cases were reported.[3,49] For the past 3 decades, group B streptococci have been the most common organisms causing invasive disease in neonates throughout the United States and western Europe (see Chapter 13).

Streptococcus agalactiae, the species designation of group B streptococci, has a characteristic colonial morphology on suitable solid media. The organism produces a mucoid colony with a narrow zone of β-hemolysis on sheep blood agar media. The group B streptococci can be differentiated immunochemically on the basis of their type-specific polysaccharides. Ten capsular types Ia, Ib, II, III, IV, V, IV, VI, VII, and VIII have been characterized, and most invasive human isolates can be classified as one of these types.

Group B streptococci have been isolated from various sites and body fluids, including throat, skin, wounds, exudates, stool, urine, cervix, vagina, blood, joint, pleural or peritoneal fluids, and cerebrospinal fluid (CSF). The organisms frequently are found in the lower gastrointestinal and genital tracts of adult women and men and in the lower gastrointestinal and upper respiratory tracts of newborns. Patterns of early-onset, late-onset, and very late onset disease have been associated with group B streptococci (see Table 6-1). Early-onset disease presents as a multisystem illness with rapid onset typically during the first day or two of life and is frequently characterized by severe respiratory distress. The pathogenesis is presumed to be similar to that of other forms of early-onset sepsis of neonates. Isolates may belong to any

Table 6–7 Bacteria Associated with Neonatal Meningitis in Selected Studies

	No. of Cases of Association								
Organism	Boston (38)[a] 1932-1957 77 Cases	Los Angeles (39) 1963-1968 125 Cases	Houston (40) 1967-1972 51 Cases	Multihospital Survey[b] (41) 1971-1973 131 Cases	The Netherlands (42) 1976-1982 280 Cases	Great Britain (43) 1985-1987 329 Cases	Dallas (44) 1969-1989 257 Cases	Israel (31)[c] 1986-1994 32 Cases	Great Britain (45) 1996-1997 144 Cases
β-hemolytic streptococci (group not stated)	9	12							
β-hemolytic streptococci									
Group A			1	2					
Group B			18	41	68	113	134	6	69
Group D				2	4				1
Staphylococcus epidermidis or coagulase-negative *Staphylococcus*		5		3		9		2	2
Staphylococcus aureus	12	1	3	1	7	4			
Streptococcus pneumoniae	7	4	3	2	6	21	18		8
Listeria monocytogenes		6	5	7	12	21			7
Escherichia coli	25	44	16[d]	50	132	2	42	4	26
Pseudomonas aeruginosa	4	1	2	2	4	3		1	
Klebsiella and *Enterobacter* species	3	13	[d]	3	19	8	10	4	
Proteus species	2	5	[d]	4	5	8	3	2	
Haemophilus species		2	2	3	2	12			1
Neisseria meningitidis	1			1	3	14			6
Salmonella species	2	4		3	3	2	4		1
Miscellaneous	12	28	1	7	15	32	46		23

[a]Numbers in parentheses are reference numbers.
[b]Survey of 16 newborn nurseries participating in neonatal meningitis study of intrathecal gentamicin under the direction of Dr. George McCracken, Jr.
[c]Authors report an additional nine cases of gram-positive and six cases of gram-negative meningitis with organisms not otherwise specified.
[d]Authors report 16 cases related to enteric bacteria, including *E. coli*, *Proteus* species, and *Klebsiella-Enterobacter* group.

of the serotypes of group B streptococci, but types Ia, III, and V predominate. The mortality rate is estimated at 8% but was as high as 50% in the 1970s.[50]

Clinical manifestations of late-onset neonatal sepsis are more insidious than those of early-onset disease, and meningitis is frequently a part of the clinical picture. However, some infants with meningitis have a fulminant onset with rapid progression to centrally mediated apnea. Many of the infants are products of a normal pregnancy and delivery and have no problems in the nursery. It is uncertain whether group B streptococcal infection was acquired at the time of birth and carried until disease developed, was acquired after delivery from the mother or other household contacts, or was acquired from other infants or personnel in the nursery. Nearly 80% of strains belong to serotype III. The mortality rate, estimated at 3%, is lower than that for early-onset disease. With increasing survival of extremely low birth weight (ELBW) (<1000 g) infants, very late onset disease (>89 days) has been described in the past decade.[37]

In addition to sepsis and meningitis, other manifestations of neonatal disease caused by group B streptococci include pneumonia, empyema, facial cellulitis, ethmoiditis, orbital cellulitis, conjunctivitis, necrotizing fasciitis, osteomyelitis, suppurative arthritis, and impetigo. Bacteremia without systemic or focal signs of sepsis can occur. Group B streptococcal infection in pregnant women can result in peripartum infections, including septic abortion, chorioamnionitis, peripartum bacteremia, septic pelvic thrombophlebitis, meningitis, and toxic shock syndrome.[51]

Group A Streptococci

Streptococcal puerperal sepsis has been recognized as a cause of morbidity and mortality among parturient women since the 16th century.[52-56] Neonatal group A streptococcal infection now is reported infrequently[57-68] but can occur rarely in epidemic form in nurseries.[57-61] The reemergence of virulent group A streptococcal infections, including invasive disease and toxic shock syndrome, has been reflected in more case reports of severe disease in the pregnant woman and the newborn.

Group A streptococcal disease in the mother can affect the fetus or newborn in three clinical patterns. Maternal streptococcal bacteremia during pregnancy can lead to in utero infection resulting in fetal loss or stillbirth; the fetus can be affected by transplacentally transmitted group A streptococcal toxins resulting from maternal infection; and acquisition of group A streptococci from the maternal genital tract can cause early-onset neonatal sepsis similar to early-onset group B streptococcal disease. In the first form of disease, previously healthy pregnant women with influenza-like signs and symptoms have been reported. This presentation rapidly progressed to disseminated intravascular coagulopathy and shock; four of five women died; stillbirth or fetal loss occurred in three cases; one neonate developed group A streptococcal sepsis and recovered; and a fifth infant was unaffected.[69-71]

The second manifestation of fetal or neonatal group A streptococcal disease is caused by production of toxins transferred across the placenta to the fetus. Babl and colleagues (personal communication, 1999) described a woman who had bacteremia due to group A *Streptococcus* at term, extensive infection of the placenta, and toxic shock syndrome leading to disseminated intravascular coagulopathy. A severely depressed but uninfected infant was delivered by cesarean section with resulting hypoxic encephalopathy. Presumably, the infant was affected by transplacental passage of streptococcal toxins. The virulence factors produced by group A streptococci that are important in the systemic toxicity characteristic of streptococcal toxic shock syndromes are largely the extracellular toxins, such as pyrogenic exotoxin A, B, and C; mitogenic factor; and streptococcal superantigen. These toxins have the ability to induce cytokine production by monocytes and lymphocytes. The result is T cell proliferation with production of interleukin-2, interferon-γ, and tumor necrosis factor-β.[72-75] It remains unclear whether the immune system of a fetus or neonate is sufficiently mature to respond to superantigens with subsequent cytokine production or whether the effect on the fetus results from cytokines produced on the maternal side of the placenta and passed to the fetal circulation. In the third form of disease, early-onset group A streptococcal infection in the neonate was acquired from maternal genitalia or pharynx and frequently was fatal. A review by Greenberg and colleagues[76] of 15 cases of neonatal sepsis due to group A streptococci reported between 1976 and 1999 identified nine cases of early-onset sepsis (three deaths) and six cases of late-onset sepsis (one death).

In addition to sepsis, meningitis, and toxin-mediated disease in the neonate, focal infections, including cellulitis, omphalitis, Ludwig's angina,[77] pneumonia, and osteomyelitis, have been reported. Because all group A streptococci are susceptible to β-lactam antibiotics, the current strategy for prevention or treatment of infections due to group B streptococci also could apply to infections caused by group A streptococci.

Streptococci Other than Groups A and B

Group C streptococci have been associated with puerperal sepsis, but neonatal sepsis or meningitis related to these organism is rare.[78-80] Group G streptococci are an infrequent cause of neonatal sepsis and pneumonia.[81-85] Maternal intrapartum transmission was the likely source for most cases,[83] and concurrent endometritis and bacteremia in the mother and sepsis in the neonate have been reported.[84] Dyson and Read[83] found very high rates of colonization in neonates born at New York Hospital in a 1-year survey of discharge cultures in 1979; the monthly incidence of cultures of group G streptococci from the nose and umbilicus varied between 41% and 70%. During this period, group B streptococcal colonization was only 1% to 11%.[83] Auckenthaler and colleagues[85] have reviewed group G streptococcal bacteremia, and their review includes invasive disease in newborns.

Enterococcus now is considered taxonomically distinct from group D streptococci and a unique genus. However, much of the earlier literature about neonatal sepsis combined enterococci (i.e., *Streptococcus faecalis* and *Streptococcus faecium*) and nonenterococci (i.e., *Streptococcus bovis* and *Streptococcus mitis*), and because of this historical context, the two groups are combined in this section. Enterococci are differentiated from nonenterococci by their ability to grow in 6.5% NaCl broth and to withstand heating at 60° C for 30 minutes.

In general, *Enterococcus* species are resistant to cephalosporins, are only moderately susceptible to penicillin G and ampicillin, and require the synergistic activity of penicillin at high dosage and an aminoglycoside for maximal bactericidal action; nonenterococcal strains are susceptible to penicillin G, ampicillin, and most cephalosporins. Vancomycin-resistant *Enterococcus* (VRE) has been reported from neonatal intensive care units and raises concerns about the efficacy of antimicrobial agents currently approved for use in neonates.[86] Use of high doses of ampicillin is one option, but other drugs may be suggested by the susceptibility pattern (see Chapter 37). New agents, such as the streptogramin combination of quinupristin and dalfopristin and the oxazolidinone linezolid are effective against VRE infections in adults. However, limited pharmacokinetic data are available to guide use of these agents in neonates.[87]

Most cases of group D streptococcal sepsis in the neonate are caused by *Enterococcus faecalis,* with a smaller number caused by *Enterococcus faecium* and *S. bovis*[88-93]; rare cases due to *S. mitis* have been reported.[94,95] In the 4 years beginning in 1974, 37 neonates with group D streptococcal sepsis (including 30 related to enterococci and 7 to nonenterococcal isolates) occurred among 30,059 deliveries at Parkland Memorial Hospital in Dallas.[88] During this period, group D streptococci were second only to group B streptococci (99 cases) and were more common than *E. coli* (27 cases) as a cause of neonatal sepsis. The clinical presentation in most cases was similar to that of early-onset sepsis of any cause.[90] Among infants with respiratory distress as a prominent sign of infection, the chest radiographs were similar to those demonstrating the hyaline membrane–appearing pattern of group B streptococcal infection. Enterococcal bacteremia during the 10 years beginning January 1977 was reported in 56 neonates from the Jefferson Davis Hospital in Houston, Texas.[96] These 56 infants had the three clinical syndromes: early-onset disease was a mild illness with respiratory distress or diarrhea; late-onset infection often was severe with apnea, bradycardia, shock, and increased requirement for oxygen and mechanical ventilation; many cases were nosocomial.[96] Case series of neonatal sepsis or meningitis, or both, due to group D streptococci (including enterococci) also have been reported from Children's Hospital Medical Center of Cincinnati (13 cases from 1970 to 1976),[97] the Hospital for Sick Children in Toronto (9 cases from 1985 to 1989),[98] and New York Hospital/Cornell Medical Center (138 episodes of enterococcal bacteremia from 1974 to 1993).[86] Group D enterococci also have been recovered from CSF[88,92] and urine[88] of infants with sepsis. Outbreaks of bacteremia and meningitis related to *E. faecium* were reported from the neonatal intensive care units at the Medical College of Virginia[99] and Children's Hospital of Denver.[100]

Viridans streptococci are a heterogeneous group of α-hemolytic and nonhemolytic streptococci that are constituents of the normal flora of the respiratory and gastrointestinal tracts of infants, children, and adults. There are several classification schemata for these streptococci, and they may bear different designations in the literature. Viridans streptococci accounted for 23% of isolates from cultures of blood and CSF obtained from neonates at the Jefferson Davis Hospital, Houston.[101] Only group B streptococci were more common (28%) as a cause of neonatal sepsis. Most infants had early-onset infection with clinical features similar to those of sepsis caused by other pathogens, but 22.6% had no signs of infection. One infant had meningitis. The case-fatality rate was 8.8%. Sepsis related to viridans streptococci also has been reported from Finland,[20] Liverpool,[22] Indianapolis,[13] and Montreal.[19] It is clear from these studies that isolation of viridans streptococci from the blood culture of a neonate suspected to have sepsis cannot be considered a contaminant, as is the case in many other patient populations.

Staphylococcus aureus and *Staphylococcus epidermidis*

S. aureus and CoNS, especially *S. epidermidis*, colonize skin and mucosa. Isolation of *S. aureus* from tissue, blood, or other body fluid usually is clearly associated with disease. Most episodes of sepsis due to *S. aureus* are hospital acquired, and mortality remains high (23% among 216 Swedish neonates with *S. aureus* bacteremia during the years 1967 to 1984), with low birth weight as the most important risk factor.[102] Disease in newborn infants caused by *S. aureus* and CoNS is discussed in Chapter 17.

The apparent increased incidence of CoNS sepsis[13,16-18,37] has been associated with increased survival of VLBW and ELBW infants with developmentally immature immune systems and with the introduction of invasive procedures for maintenance and monitoring of the infants, including long-term vascular access devices. Because CoNS are present on the skin, isolation of these organisms from a single culture of blood can represent skin contamination but also can indicate bloodstream invasion. Collection of two cultures of blood at separate sites can assist in differentiating skin or blood culture bottle contamination from bloodstream invasion in the infant with suspected late-onset sepsis.[103] The significance of a positive blood culture yielding CoNS is discussed in "Microbiologic Techniques."

Many episodes of sepsis caused by CoNS are associated with the use of vascular catheters. *S. epidermidis* and other CoNS species can adhere to and grow on surfaces of synthetic polymers used in the manufacture of catheters. Strains obtained from infected ventricular shunts or intravenous catheters produce a mucoid substance (i.e., slime or glycocalyx) that stimulates adherence of microcolonies to various surfaces in the environment and on epithelial surfaces.[104] In addition to this adhesin function, the slime may protect staphylococci against antibiotics and host defense mechanisms such as opsonophagocytosis. Parenteral nutrition with a lipid emulsion administered through a venous catheter with organisms adherent to the polymer provides nutrients for growth of the bacteria, leading to invasion of the bloodstream when the organisms reach an inoculum of sufficient size.[105]

Three cases of fatal sepsis caused by CoNS occurred in VLBW infants with cytomegalovirus infection. At autopsy, the bacteria were cultured from the blood, spleen, and meninges. These cases suggest that concurrent cytomegalovirus infection may further suppress immune functions in the neonate and lead to increased virulence of the bacterial infection.[106]

Listeria monocytogenes

The prevalence of *L. monocytogenes* in packaged meat, dairy, or other food products and the danger to immunocompromised patients and pregnant women was documented in a 2002 outbreak involving 46 patients in eight states. This outbreak was caused by isolates of *L. monocytogenes* sharing a relatively uncommon pulsed-field gel electrophoresis pattern; the cases included seven deaths of adults and miscarriages or stillbirths in three pregnant women.[107] *Listeria* can be found in unprocessed animal products, including milk, meat, poultry, cheese, ice cream, and processed meats, and on fresh fruits and vegetables. Most people exposed to *L. monocytogenes* do not develop illness, but the pregnant woman can suffer pregnancy loss, and the neonate can develop early or late-onset sepsis and meningitis. Neonatal disease due to *Listeria* is discussed in Chapter 14.

Escherichia coli

Coliform organisms are prevalent in the maternal birth canal, and most infants are colonized in their lower gastrointestinal or respiratory tracts during or just before delivery. The antigenic structure of *E. coli* is complex; members of this species account for more than 145 different somatic (O) antigens, approximately 50 flagellar (H) antigens, and 80 different capsular (K) antigens. Although there is a wide genetic diversity of human commensal isolates of *E. coli*, strains causing neonatal pathology are derived from a limited number of clones.[108]

One of the capsular antigens of *E. coli*, K1, is uniquely associated with neonatal meningitis.[109-111] K1 antigen is an acidic polysaccharide that is immunochemically identical to the capsular antigen of group B *N. meningitidis*. McCracken and co-workers[109] found K1 strains in the blood or CSF of most (65 of 77) neonates with meningitis related to *E. coli*. These strains also were cultured from the blood of some infants (14 of 36) and adults (43 of 301) with sepsis but without meningitis. The K1 capsular antigen was present in 88% of 132 strains from neonates with *E. coli* meningitis reported from The Netherlands.[42] K1 antigen was related to invasive disease and to a more severe outcome. Infants with meningitis caused by K1 strains had significantly higher mortality and morbidity rates than did infants with meningitis caused by non-K1 *E. coli* strains.[110] The severity of disease was directly related to the presence, amount, and persistence of K1 antigen in the CSF. Strains of *E. coli* with K1 antigen were isolated from cultures of stool of 7% to 38% (varying with time and location of the study) of healthy newborns and from approximately 50% of nurses and mothers of the infants.[111,112] The K1 strains have been present in the birth canal of mothers and subsequently in cultures from their newborns, indicating that these newborn infants acquired the organisms vertically from their mothers.[112,113] However, high rates of carriage of K1 strains by nursery personnel indicate that postnatal acquisition of the K1 strains in the nursery also may occur.[111,112]

Pili or fimbriae are filamentous surface appendages that may play a role in the pathogenesis of disease caused by *E. coli*.[114] Pili assist adherence of *E. coli* to epithelial cell surfaces, an initial step in the development of invasive disease. Fimbriated strains of *E. coli* have been associated with infections of the urinary tract in infants (see Chapter 9). The epidemiology of fimbriated *E. coli* and the relationship of these strains to fecal colonization of neonates and development of extraintestinal infections are discussed in a monograph by Tullus.[115]

Klebsiella Species and *Enterobacter* Species

Klebsiella is a genus of Enterobacteriaceae that has emerged as a significant nosocomial pathogen in neonates.[31,44,116,117] The four recognized species include *Klebsiella pneumoniae, Klebsiella oxytoca, Klebsiella terrigena,* and *Klebsiella planticola*. *K. pneumoniae*, the most common human pathogen, and *K. oxytoca* cause neonatal infections of the bloodstream, urinary tract, central nervous system, lung, skin, and soft tissues.[118-120] Previously thought to be a nonpathogenic organism inhabiting soil and water, *K. planticola* has been implicated as a cause of neonatal sepsis.[121,122]

In a 4-year retrospective study from Israel,[123] *Klebsiella* species caused 31% of late-onset neonatal sepsis. Greenberg and colleagues[31] performed an 8-year prospective study of neonatal sepsis and meningitis at Soroka University Medical Center during the years 1986 to 1994; 49 (20%) of 250 cases were caused by *K. pneumoniae*, with a mortality rate of 29%. Risk factors for infection included preterm, VLBW, prolonged rupture of membranes (>24 hours), and cesarean section or instrument delivery.

The reservoirs for transmission of *Klebsiella* infections include the hands of health care workers and the gastrointestinal tracts of hospitalized infants. Multidrug resistance, in the form of extended spectrum β-lactamase production, of *Klebsiella* strains causing neonatal infections and nursery outbreaks has become a substantial problem in some nurseries and is associated with increased morbidity and mortality.[124-126] Enhanced infection control measures and changes in use of routine broad-spectrum antibiotics can reduce the frequency of these serious infections.

Among the *Enterobacter aerogenes* (i.e., *Aerobacter aerogenes*) species, *Enterobacter cloacae, Enterobacter sakazakii,* and *Enterobacter hormaechei* have caused sepsis and a severe form of necrotizing meningitis in neonates.[127-132] *Enterobacter* septicemia was the most common nosocomial infection in neonates at the Ondokuz Mayis University Hospital in Samsun, Turkey, from 1988 to 1992.[133] Willis and Robinson[128] reviewed 17 cases of neonatal meningitis caused by *E. sakazakii*; cerebral abscess or cyst formation developed in 77% of the infants, and 50% of the infants died. Bonadio and colleagues[129] reviewed 30 cases of *E. cloacae* bacteremia in children, including 10 infants younger than 2 months old. Of importance was the high frequency of multidrug resistance among isolates from patients in the neonatal intensive care units that was attributed to routine extended spectrum cephalosporin usage.[134]

In addition to the gastrointestinal tracts of hospitalized infants and hands of health care personnel, sources and modes of transmission of *Enterobacter* infections in the neonate include contaminated infant formula,[135,136] contaminated total parenteral nutrition fluid,[137,138] bladder catheterization devices,[137] and contaminated saline.[139] Effective infection control measures require reinforcement of procedures, including proper hand hygiene, aseptic technique, isolation protocols, and disinfection of environmental surfaces.

Citrobacter Species

Organisms of the genus *Citrobacter* are gram-negative bacilli that are occasional inhabitants of the gastrointestinal tract and are responsible for disease in neonates and debilitated or immunocompromised patients. The genus has undergone frequent changes in nomenclature, making it difficult to relate the types identified in reports of newborn disease over the years. For example, in 1990, *Citrobacter koseri* replaced *Citrobacter diversus*.[140] For the purposes of this chapter, *C. koseri* replaces *C. diversus*, even though the original article may refer to the latter name.

Citrobacter species are responsible for sporadic and epidemic clusters of neonatal sepsis and meningitis, and *C. koseri* is uniquely associated with brain abscesses.[140-148] Neonatal disease can occur as early-onset or late-onset presentations. Outbreaks of *C. koseri* in neonatal intensive care units resulting in sepsis and meningitis, septic arthritis, and skin and soft tissue infections were reviewed by Doran.[140] Other focal infections in neonates due to *Citrobacter* species include bone, pulmonary, and urinary tract infections.[140]

During the period of 1960 to 1980, 74 cases of meningitis caused by *Citrobacter* species were reported to the Centers for Disease Control and Prevention (CDC) of the U.S. Public Health Service.[141] In 1999, Doran reviewed an additional 56 cases of neonatal meningitis due to *Citrobacter* species.[140] Combining results from the two studies, brain abscess developed in 73 (76%) of 96 patients for whom information was available. The pathogenesis of brain abscess caused by *C. koseri* is uncertain; cerebral vasculitis with infarction and bacterial invasion of necrotic tissues is the likely explanation.[146] Persistence of *C. koseri* in the central nervous system is suggested by a case report of recovery of the organism from the CSF during a surgical procedure 4 years after treatment of neonatal meningitis.[145] The mortality rate for meningitis due to *Citrobacter* species was about 30%; most of the infants who survived had some degree of mental retardation. A review of 110 survivors of *Citrobacter* meningitis revealed only 20 infants who were believed to have structurally intact brains and development that was age appropriate.[140]

Citrobacter species usually are resistant to ampicillin and variably susceptible to aminoglycosides. Historically, most infants were treated with a combination of penicillin or cephalosporin plus an aminoglycoside. Surgical drainage has been used in some cases with variable success. Choosing antimicrobial agents with the most advantageous susceptibility pattern and selected surgical drainage appears to be the most promising approach to therapy, but no one regimen has been found to be more successful than another. Plasmid profiles, biotypes, serotypes, and chromosomal restriction endonuclease digests are useful as epidemiologic markers for the study of isolates of *C. koseri*. Morris and colleagues[147] used these markers to investigate an outbreak of six cases of neonatal meningitis caused by *C. koseri* in three Baltimore hospitals between 1983 and 1985. Identification of a specific outer membrane protein associated with strains isolated from CSF but uncommon elsewhere can provide a marker for virulent strains of *C. koseri* according to some investigators.[148]

Serratia marcescens and *Pseudomonas* Species

Like other members of Enterobacteriaceae, *Serratia marcescens* increasingly is associated with hospital-acquired infections among infants in the neonatal intensive care unit.[149-151] Late-onset sepsis has occurred in infants infected from health care equipment,[151-153] the hands of heath care workers,[154] milk bottles,[150] aqueous solutions such as theophylline,[150] hand hygiene washes,[151] and lipid parenteral feeds.[153] The gastrointestinal tracts of hospitalized infants provide a reservoir for transmission and infection.[152]

In a review of neonatal bacteremia and meningitis caused by *S. marcescens* by Campbell and colleagues,[155] 11 (29%) of 38 infants had meningitis as a complication of their bacteremia. Mean gestational age and birth weight were 28 weeks and 1099 g, respectively. All patients required mechanical ventilation, 90% had central venous catheters in situ, 90% had received prior antibiotics, 50% had a prior intraventricular hemorrhage, 40% had a hemodynamically significant patent ductus arteriosis treated medically or surgically, and 20% had necrotizing enterocolitis with perforation. All patients were treated for a minimum of 21 days with combination antimicrobial therapy that included a third-generation cephalosporin or a ureidopenicillin and an aminoglycoside, typically gentamicin. Three of 10 patients died. Four of the seven survivors developed severe hydrocephalus requiring ventriculoperitoneal shunt placement and had poor neurologic outcome. Poor neurologic outcome also was documented in a report of *S. marcescens* brain abscess resulting in multicystic encephalomalacia and severe developmental retardation.[156]

P. aeruginosa usually is a cause of late-onset disease in infants who are presumably infected from their endogenous flora or from equipment, from aqueous solutions, or occasionally from the hands of health care workers. Stevens and colleagues[14] reported nine infants with *Pseudomonas* sepsis, four of whom presented in the first 72 hours of life. In three of these infants, the initial signs were those of respiratory distress, and chest radiographs were consistent with hyaline membrane disease. Noma (i.e., gangrenous lesions of the nose, lips, and mouth) in a neonate has been associated with bacteremia caused by *P. aeruginosa*.[157]

A retrospective review of sepsis in infants admitted over the 10-year period from 1988 through 1997 to the neonatal intensive care unit at Children's Hospital of the King's Daughters in Norfolk, Virginia, identified 825 cases of late-onset sepsis.[17] Infants with *Pseudomonas* sepsis had the highest frequency of clinically fulminant onset (56%), and 20 (56%) of the 36 (56%) infants with *Pseudomonas* sepsis died within 48 hours of blood culture collection.

P. aeruginosa conjunctivitis in the neonate is a danger because it is rapidly destructive to the tissues of the eye and because it may lead to sepsis and meningitis. Shah and Gallagher[158] reviewed the course of 18 infants at Yale–New Haven Hospital newborn intensive care unit who had *P. aeruginosa* isolated from cultures of the conjunctiva during the 10 years beginning in 1986. Five infants developed bacteremia, including three with meningitis, and two infants died.

Salmonella Species

Nontyphi *Salmonella* infection is an uncommon cause of sepsis and meningitis in neonates, but a significant proportion of cases of *Salmonella* meningitis occur in young infants. The CDC observed that approximately one third of 290 *Salmonella* isolates from CSF reported during 1968 to 1979 were from patients younger than 3 months of age, and more than one half were from infants younger than 1 year of age.[159] A 21-year review of gram-negative enteric meningitis in Dallas beginning in 1969 identified *Salmonella* as the cause in 4 of 72 cases.[44] Investigators from Turkey reported seven cases of neonatal meningitis caused by *Salmonella* during the years 1995 to 2001.[160] Two of the five survivors developed communicating hydrocephalus, and one had a subdural empyema.

Reed and Klugman[161] reviewed 10 cases of neonatal typhoid that occurred in a rural African hospital. Six of the infants had early-onset sepsis with acquisition of the organism from the maternal genital tract, and four had late-onset infection with acquisition from a carrier or an environmental source. Two neonates developed meningitis, and three died.

Neisseria meningitidis

Although *N. meningitidis* is a leading cause of bacterial sepsis and meningitis among children and adolescents, it rarely is associated with invasive infection in neonates.[31,45,162] *N. meningitidis* may colonize the female genital tract[163-165] and has been associated with pelvic inflammatory disease.[166] The infant can be infected at delivery by organisms present in the maternal genital tract, or intrauterine infection can result during maternal meningococcemia.[167] Meningococcal sepsis is rare in the neonate, but more than 50 cases (including 13 from the preantibiotic era) have been described.[168-170] Early-onset and late-onset forms[163,164,170] of meningococcal sepsis in neonates have been reported. Purpura similar to that of meningococcemia in older children has been observed in a 15-day-old[171] and a 25-day-old infant.[172]

Shepard and colleagues[170] from the CDC reported 22 neonates with invasive meningococcal disease from a 10-year active, population-based surveillance of 10 states with diverse populations and more than 31 million persons. The average annual incidence was 9 cases per 100,000 people (versus 973.8 per 100,000 for group B *Streptococcus*). Sixteen patients had meningitis, and 6 of these also had meningococcemia. Six patients had early-onset disease. The overall mortality rate was 14%. Ten isolates were serogroup B, four were serogroup C, three were serogroup Y, one was nongroupable, and four were unavailable.

Haemophilus influenzae

Because of the introduction of *H. influenzae* type b conjugate vaccines in 1988, there has been a substantial decrease in the incidence in *H. influenzae* type b disease in infants and children in the United States and many other countries.[173-175] Given the estimated proportion of individuals that are completely immunized, the decrease in *H. influenzae* type b invasive disease has exceeded expectations. The reduction in *H. influenzae* carriage associated with vaccination and the consequent decreased transmission from immunized children to unimmunized infants and children likely explains this effect.[176-178]

Despite increased reporting of invasive infections caused by nontypeable *H. influenzae* in adults and older children,[179-181] such infections in neonates remain uncommon.[182-185] Four clinical syndromes have been associated with neonatal disease caused by *H. influenzae*: sepsis or respiratory distress syndrome; meningitis; soft tissue or joint infection; and otitis media or mastoiditis. The overall mortality rate was 5.5% for 45 cases reviewed by Friesen and Cho[186]; the mortality rate was 90% for 20 infants with a gestation lasting less than 30 weeks. Clinical and epidemiologic characteristics were similar to those of neonatal disease caused by group B streptococci, including early-onset (within 24 hours of birth) and late-onset presentations, signs simulating respiratory distress syndrome, and a high mortality rate. Autopsy of infants with bacteremia related to nontypeable *H. influenzae* and signs of respiratory distress syndrome revealed hyaline membranes with gram-negative coccobacilli within the membranes, similar to findings of hyaline membranes due to group B streptococci.[187] Examination of placentas from mothers of infants with sepsis caused by nontypeable *H. influenzae* revealed acute chorioamnionitis and acute villitis in some.[183] *H. influenzae* also has been responsible for maternal disease, including bacteremia, chorioamnionitis,[188] acute or chronic salpingitis, and tubo-ovarian abscess.[184]

Neonatal sepsis caused by *Haemophilus parainfluenzae*[189-191] and *Haemophilus aphrophilus*[192] has been reported.

Streptococcus pneumoniae

Although pneumococci rarely are isolated from cultures from the cervix or vagina of gynecologic patients or pregnant women, cases of early-onset pneumococcal sepsis in neonates have been reported.[193-198] Bortolussi and colleagues[193] reported five infants with pneumococcal sepsis who had respiratory distress and clinical signs of infection on the first day of life. Three infants died, two within 12 hours of onset. *S. pneumoniae* was isolated from the vaginas of three of the mothers. Radiographic features were consistent with hyaline membrane disease or pneumonia, or both. The clinical features were strikingly similar to those of early-onset group B streptococcal infection, including the association of prolonged interval after rupture of membranes, early-onset respiratory distress, abnormal chest roentgenograms, hypotension, leukopenia, and rapid deterioration. Fatal pneumococcal bacteremia in a mother 4 weeks postpartum, and the same disease and outcome in her healthy term infant who died at 6 weeks of age, suggested an absence of protective antibody in mother and child.[194]

Hoffman and colleagues from the United States Multicenter Pneumococcal Surveillance Group[198] reported 20 cases of neonatal *S. pneumoniae* sepsis or meningitis in a review of 4428 episodes of pneumococcal infection at eight children's hospitals from 1993 to 2001. Ninety percent of the infants were born at term, with a mean age at the onset of infection of 18.1 days. Only two of the mothers had clinically apparent infections at the time of delivery. Eight neonates had meningitis and 12 had bacteremia; four of the bacteremic neonates also had pneumonia. The most common infecting pneumococcal serotypes were 19 (32%), 9 (18%), and 18 (11%). Penicillin and ceftriaxone nonsusceptibility were observed in 21.4% and 3.6% of isolates, respectively. Three deaths (15%) occurred, all within 36 hours of presentation.

Anaerobic Bacteria

Improvements in techniques for isolation and identification of the various genera and species of anaerobic bacteria have provided a better understanding of the anaerobic flora of humans and their role in disease.[199] With the exception of *Clostridium tetani* and *Clostridium botulinum,* all of the anaerobic bacteria belong to the normal flora of humans. Anaerobes are present on the skin, in the mouth, in the intestines, and in the genital tract. They account for the greatest proportion of the bacteria of the stool. All are present in the intestines, and have been isolated from the external genitalia or vagina of pregnant and nonpregnant women.[200-202] Newborns are colonized with these organisms during or just before delivery. A review of the literature on neonatal bacteremia due to anaerobic bacteria by Brook[203] in 1990 included 179 cases, with a mortality rate of 26%. *Bacteroides* and *Clostridium* species were the most common isolates. Predisposing factors for infection included premature rupture of membranes, preterm delivery, and necrotizing enterocolitis.

Anaerobic bacteria have been isolated from the blood of newborns with sepsis,[204-206] from various organs at autopsy,[204] from an infant with an adrenal abscess,[207] from an infant with an infected cephalhematoma,[208] and from infants with necrotizing fasciitis of the scalp associated with placement of a scalp electrode.[209] Feder[210] reviewed meningitis caused by *Bacteroides fragilis*; seven of nine reported cases occurred in neonates.

The incidence of neonatal sepsis caused by anaerobic bacteria remains uncertain, but recent data are available from some surveys that suggest the incidence is low (<5%).[17,31,203] Noel and colleagues[205] identified 29 episodes of anaerobic bacteremia in neonates in the intensive care unit at New York Hospital during 18 years. Chow and co-workers[204] analyzed 59 cases of neonatal sepsis associated with anaerobic pathogens and classified them into four groups: transient bacteremia after premature rupture of membranes and maternal amnionitis; sepsis after postoperative complications; fulminant septicemia (in the case of clostridial infections); and intrauterine death associated with septic abortion. The mortality rate associated with neonatal anaerobic sepsis reported in the literature ranges from 4% to 38%.[204,211,212]

Infections caused by *Clostridium* species can be localized, as in the case of omphalitis,[213] cellulitis, and necrotizing fasciitis,[214] or can manifest as sepsis or meningitis.[215] Disease in neonates has been related to *Clostridium perfringens, Clostridium septicum, Clostridium sordellii, Clostridium butyricum, Clostridium tertium,* and *Clostridium paraputrificum.*[216] The presenting signs usually are similar to those of other forms of bacterial sepsis. Chaney[215] reported a case of bacteremia caused by *C. perfringens* in mother and child in which the neonate had classic features of adult clostridial sepsis, including active hemolysis, hyperbilirubinemia, and hemoglobinuria. Motz and colleagues[217] reviewed five cases of clostridial meningitis due to *C. butyricum* and *C. perfringens.* Clostridial sepsis is accompanied by a high mortality rate.[215]

Neonatal tetanus is caused by the gram-positive anaerobic spore-forming bacillus, *C. tetani.* The organism is present in soil and can be present in human and animal feces. Infection usually occurs after contamination of the umbilical stump. In the United States, tetanus in the newborn is rare.[218] Since 1984, only three cases of neonatal tetanus have been reported.[218-220] The most recent case, reported from Montana in 1998, was an infant born to an unimmunized mother; the parents used a *C. tetani*–contaminated clay powder to accelerate drying of the umbilical cord. The use of this product had been promoted on an Internet site on "cord care" for use by midwives.[221]

In contrast to the United States, most cases of tetanus worldwide occur in neonates. In developing countries, the incidence and mortality of neonatal tetanus remain high.[222-224] Mustafa and colleagues[225] conducted a retrospective neonatal tetanus survey among rural and displaced communities in the East Nile Province in the Sudan and observed that neonatal tetanus was a major cause of neonatal mortality. The incidence in the displaced community was 7.1 cases per 1000 livebirths, more than double that reported from the stable rural community (3.2 per 1000). In both communities, coverage with two doses of tetanus toxoid was about 58%.

The mortality rate for neonatal tetanus in Djakarta in 1982 was 6.9 deaths per 1000 livebirths; in the island provinces of Indonesia, it was 10.7 deaths per 1000 livebirths.[226] The mortality rate for neonates with tetanus in Lima, Peru, was 45% and was not improved with use of intrathecal tetanus antitoxin.[227] However, a meta-analysis of intrathecal therapy in tetanus suggested benefit in adults but not in neonates.[228]

Application of contaminated materials to the umbilical cord is associated with deep-rooted customs and rituals in developing countries. A case-control study to identify risk factors for neonatal tetanus in rural Pakistan identified application of ghee (i.e., clarified butter from the milk of water buffaloes or cows) to the umbilical wound as the single most important risk factor.[229] Although commercial ghee is available in Pakistan, the ghee used in rural areas is made at home from unpasteurized milk. Oudesluys-Murphy[230] observed that application of some materials, including ghee and a stone wrapped in wet cloth, increased the risk of neonatal tetanus among Yoruba women but that other practices of cord care decreased the incidence, including searing of the cord with heat in China during the Ming dynasty and use of a candle flame to scar the cord in Guatemala. Neonatal tetanus is a preventable disease; use of hygienic techniques at delivery and a program of tetanus toxoid immunization of children and young adults, particularly of pregnant women, are effective in eliminating this lethal disease.[230-233]

Commensal Organisms

Species of bacteria and fungi that are normal flora of skin and mucous membranes can invade the bloodstream of neonates under certain circumstances. The bacteria include coagulase-negative *Staphylococcus* species, gram-positive rods other than *Listeria,* gram-negative cocci other than *N. meningitidis* and *N. gonorrhoeae,* and gram-positive anaerobes. The clinical significance of a blood culture positive for a commensal species often is obscure. Interpretation of culture results that identify commensal species and the management of infants with positive cultures are discussed later in "Diagnosis."

Mixed Infections

Multiple organisms frequently are present in brain, liver, or lung abscesses; aspiration in the lung after pneumonia; or pleural empyema but infrequently are found in cultures of the blood or CSF. When several species are found, the significance of each is uncertain because it is possible that one or more of the organisms in a mixed culture is a contaminant.

Bacteremia with more than one organism occurs in patients with immunodeficiency, major congenital abnor-

Table 6–8 **Unusual Pathogens Responsible for Neonatal Sepsis and Meningitis**

Organism	Reference
Achromobacter species	Boukadida et al.,[240] Hearn and Gander,[241] Manjra et al.[242]
Acinetobacter species	Huang et al.,[243] Melamed et al.,[244] Mittal et al.[245]
Aerococcus viridans	Park and Grossman[246]
Bacillus cereus	Tokieda et al.,[247] van der Zwet et al.,[248] Hilliard et al.[249]
Borrelia species	Van Holten et al.,[250] Melkert and Stel[251]
Brucella species	Chheda et al.,[252] Shamo'on and Izzat,[253] Giannacopoulos et al.[254]
Burkholderia cepacia	Kahyaoglu et al.[255]
Campylobacter species	Morooka et al.,[256] Wolfs et al.,[257] Viejo et al.[258]
Capnocytophaga species	Feldman et al.,[259] Edwards et al.,[260] Rosenman et al.[261]
Corynebacterium species	Beckwith et al.,[262] Berner et al.[263]
Edwardsiella tarda	Vohra et al.,[264] Mowbray et al.[265]
Escherichia hermanii	Ginsberg and Daum[266]
Flavobacterium species	Tizer et al.,[267] Chiu et al.,[268] Hoque et al.,[269] Tekerekoglu et al.[270]
Gardnerella vaginalis	Berardi-Grassias et al.,[271] Moran and Payne,[272] Catlin,[273] Amaya et al.[274]
Helicobacter cinaedi	Orlicek et al.[275]
Lactobacillus species	Broughton et al.,[276] Thompson et al.[277]
Leptospira species	Gsell et al.,[278] Lindsay and Luke,[279] Shaked et al.[280]
Leuconostoc species	Hardy et al.,[281] Handwerger et al.,[282] Friedland et al.,[283] Carapetis et al.[284]
Morganella morganii	Rowen and Lopez,[285] Valencia and Piecuch,[286] Casanova-Roman et al.[287]
Pasteurella species	Clapp et al.,[288] Escande et al.,[289] Zaramella et al.,[290] Ahmed et al.[291]
Plesiomonas (or *Aeromonas*) species	Terpeluk et al.,[292] Fujita et al.,[293] Gupta et al.[294]
Proteus mirabilis	Velvis et al.,[295] Hervás et al.,[296] Kassim et al.[297]
Pseudomonas pseudomallei	Lumbiganon et al.,[298] Halder et al.[299]
Pseudomonas testosteroni	Barbaro et al.[300]
Psychrobacter immobilis	Lloyd-Puryear et al.[301]
Shigella sonnei	Ruderman et al.,[302] Rebarber et al.[303]
Stomatococcus mucilaginosus	Langbaum and Eyal[304]
Vibrio cholerae	Bose et al.,[305] Kerketta et al.[306]
Yersinia enterocolitica	Pacifico et al.,[235] Challapalli and Cunningham[307]
Yersinia pestis	White et al.[308]

malities, or contamination of a body fluid with multiple organisms, as is present in peritonitis typically as a sequela of severe necrotizing enterocolitis in the VLBW infant. Neonatal meningitis due to *S. pneumoniae* and *Acinetobacter calcoaceticus*[234] and sepsis due to *P. aeruginosa* and *Yersinia enterocolitica*[235] have been reported. Although included in a series of cases of neonatal sepsis by some investigators, mixed cultures are not identified by most. Mixed infections were reported by Tessin and co-workers[24] in 5% of 231 Swedish neonates, by Vesikari and associates[21] in 4% of 377 Finnish infants, and by Bruun and Paerregaard[28] in 7% of 81 Danish neonates. Faix and Kovarik[236] reviewed the records of 385 specimens of blood or CSF submitted to the microbiology laboratories at the University of Michigan Medical Center for the period of September 1971 to June 1986. More than one organism was present in 38 specimens from 385 infants in the neonatal intensive care unit; 15 (3.9%) infants had multiple pathogens associated with clinical signs of sepsis or meningitis. The mortality was high (60%). Factors predisposing to mixed infection included prolonged rupture of membranes (>24 hours), total parenteral nutrition, necrotizing enterocolitis, presence of an intravascular catheter or ventriculostomy, and entities associated with multiple pathogens, including peritonitis, pseudomembranous colitis, and hepatic necrosis. Chow and colleagues[204] reported polymicrobial bacteremia in eight newborns with anaerobic co-isolates or aerobic and anaerobic organisms in combination. An outbreak of polymicrobial bacteremia caused by *K. pneumoniae* and *E. cloacae* associated with use of a contaminated lipid emulsion was reported by Jarvis and colleagues.[237]

Mixed infections also can include bacteria and viruses or bacteria and fungi, typically *Candida*, in the situation of intravascular central catheter or peritoneal infections associated with bowel perforation. Sferra and Pacini[238] reported mixed viral-bacterial meningitis in five patients, including neonates with CSF isolates of enterovirus and group B *Streptococcus* in a 10-day-old child and enterovirus and *Salmonella* in a 12-day-old child.

Uncommon Bacterial Pathogens

Uncommon bacterial pathogens responsible for neonatal sepsis and meningitis are listed in Table 6-8 with their references, and they are reviewed by Giacoia.[239]

EPIDEMIOLOGY

Incidence of Sepsis and Meningitis

The reported incidence of neonatal sepsis varies from less than 1 to 8.1 cases per 1000 livebirths.[12,24,27,31,116,123,309-312] A 2-year study of 64,858 infants from the Atlanta metropolitan area beginning in January 1982 (Table 6-9) reported an incidence of early-onset group B streptococcal disease of 1.09 per 1000 livebirths and 0.57 per 1000 livebirths for late-onset disease.[310] The increased usage of intrapartum antibiotic prophylaxis for women with group B streptococcal colonization with or without other risk factors associated with neonatal group B streptococcal disease has been associated with a 70% reduction in the incidence of early-onset group B streptococcal sepsis to 0.44 per 1000 livebirths in

Table 6–9 Incidence and Mortality of Group B Streptococcal Disease by Birth Weight, Atlanta 1982-1983

		Early Onset		Late Onset	
Birth Weight	Total Births	*Cases (Deaths)*	*Cases/ 1000*	*Cases (Deaths)*	*Cases/ 1000*
<1500 g	835	5 (1)	5.99	0	0
1500-2499 g	4,380	11 (2)	2.51	6 (0)	1.37
>2500 g	59,303	53 (5)	0.89	23 (0)	0.39

Data from Schuchat A, Oxtoby M, Cochi S, et al. Population-based risk factors for neonatal group B streptococcal disease: Results of a cohort study in metropolitan Atlanta. J Infect Dis 162:672, 1990.

1999, a rate comparable to that of late-onset sepsis[7] (see Chapter 13).

The incidence of meningitis usually is a fraction of the number of neonates with early-onset sepsis. During the 8-year period from 1986 to 1994 at the Soroka University Medical Center in southern Israel, Greenberg and colleagues[31] found incidences of neonatal bacterial sepsis and meningitis of 3.2 cases and 0.5 case per 1000 livebirths, respectively. Certain pathogens that cause bloodstream invasion, such as group B streptococci, *E. coli*, and *L. monocytogenes*, are more likely to be accompanied by meningeal invasion than others (e.g., *S. aureus*). Meningitis is more frequent during the first month of life than in any subsequent period (see Table 6-6).

Characteristics of Infants Who Develop Sepsis

Host susceptibility, socioeconomic factors, obstetric and nursery practices, and the health and nutrition of mothers are important in the pathogenesis of neonatal sepsis and meningitis. Infants who develop sepsis, particularly early-onset disease, usually have a history of one or more risk factors associated with the pregnancy and delivery that significantly increase the risk for neonatal infection. These factors include preterm delivery or low birth weight, premature rupture of membranes (i.e., rupture before the onset of labor), prolonged time of rupture of membranes, maternal peripartum infection, septic or traumatic delivery, and fetal hypoxia.

Birth Weight

The factor associated most significantly with enhanced risk for bacterial sepsis and meningitis in neonates is low birth weight[16,31,313-315] (see Tables 6-5 and 6-9). Infection is the most common cause of death in VLBW infants.[314,315] However, with the exception of infection caused by group B streptococci, it is unusual for a term infant to develop early-onset sepsis after an uneventful pregnancy and delivery. In a study in England and Wales, neonates weighing less than 2000 g at birth acquired meningitis six times more frequently than did infants weighing more than 2000 g.[45] The lower the infant's birth weight, the higher is the incidence of sepsis (see Table 6-5). An Israeli study of 5555 VLBW infants documented the increased risk of late-onset sepsis with decreasing birth weight; late-onset sepsis occurred in 16.8% of neonates with a birth weight of 1250 to 1500 g, 30.6% of neonates weighing 1000 to 1249 g, 46.4% of those weighing 750 to 999 g, and 53% of those weighing less than 750 g at birth.[37] In a study

Table 6–10 Relationship of Attack Rates and Fatalities of Neonatal Group B Streptococcal Early-Onset Disease to Perinatal Characteristics

Characteristic	Attack Rate per 1000 Livebirths	Mortality Rate (%)
Birth weight (g)		
<1000	26	90
1001-1500	8	25
1501-2000	9	29
2001-2500	4	33
>2500	1	3
Rupture of membranes (hr)		
<18	1	20
19-24	6	27
25-48	9	18
>48	11	33
Peak intrapartum temperature (°C)		
<37.5	2	29
>37.5	7	17
Perinatal risk factors		
Present	7.6	33
Absent	0.6	6
Total no. of infants = 32.384	2	26

Data from Boyer KM, Gadzala CA, Burd LI, et al. Selective intrapartum chemoprophylaxis of neonatal group B streptococcal early-onset disease: I. Epidemiologic rationale. J Infect Dis 148:795–801, 1983.

of infants in Atlanta (see Table 6-9), the importance of birth weight was identified as a predisposing factor for development of early-onset and late-onset sepsis. If VLBW infants survived the first days of life, rates of sepsis decreased but remained elevated[310]; 16% of 2416 infants with birth weights of 501 to 1500 g who were enrolled in a study sponsored by the National Institute of Child Health developed sepsis at a median of 17 days of age.[16]

Risk Factors of Infant and Mother

The relative importance of other factors associated with systemic infection in the newborn is more difficult to define. Greenberg and co-workers[31] found that certain conditions were common in their prospective study of 229 infants with sepsis and meningitis: 130 (57%) were premature (<37 weeks' gestation); 64 (28%) were delivered by cesarean section or instrumental delivery; 43 (19%) had an Apgar score of less than 7 at 5 minutes; and 27 (2%) had a prolonged (>24 hours) interval after rupture of maternal membranes. Investigators in Pakistan[316] found that maternal urinary tract infection, maternal fever, vaginal discharge and vaginal examinations during labor were maternal factors significantly associated with neonatal early-onset sepsis, whereas low Apgar scores at birth and the need for endotracheal intubation were significant neonatal risk factors.

Attack rates for early-onset group B streptococcal sepsis in a study from Chicago[317] were affected by birth weight, duration of rupture of membranes, and occurrence of maternal peripartum fever. Infants with one or more of these perinatal risk factors had an attack rate of 8 per 1000 livebirths and a mortality rate of 33%, compared with infants without such risk factors, who had an attack rate of 0.6 per 1000 livebirths and a mortality rate of 6% (Table 6-10).

Table 6–11 **Selected Characteristics of Women,[a] Their Pregnancies, and Newborns in the Collaborative Perinatal Study of the National Institute of Neurological Diseases and Stroke**

Characteristic	Percent with Characteristics	
	White Women	*Black Women*
Premature rupture of membranes: time from rupture to onset of labor		
<8 hr	70.9	56.7
8-23 hr	18.3	21.9
24-48 hr	5.4	11.7
49 + hr	5.4	9.7
Puerperal infection	3.6	4.1
Type of delivery		
Vaginal vertex	91.7	92.4
Vaginal breech	3.3	2.6
Cesarean section	4.9	5.0
Birth weight <2500 g	7.1	13.4
Neutrophilic infiltration of		
Amnion	9.0	7.9
Chorion	13.1	15.6
Umbilical vein	14.6	7.5

[a]Approximately 18,700 white women and 19,800 black women were evaluated. Data from reference 319.

Maternal fever during labor or after delivery suggests a concurrent infectious event in mother and infant, but noninfectious events may be responsible for maternal fever. Use of epidural analgesia for pain relief during labor is associated with increases in maternal temperature. Intrapartum fever of more than 38° C (100.4° F) occurred an average of 6 hours after initiation of the epidural anesthesia in 14.5% of women receiving an epidural anesthetic compared with 1.0% of women not receiving an epidural agent; the rate of fever increased from 7% in women with labors of less than 6 hours to 36% for labors lasting longer than 18 hours. There was no difference in the incidence of neonatal sepsis in the infants born to 1045 women who received epidural analgesia (0.3%) compared with infants born to women who did not have epidural analgesia (0.2%).[318] Fetal core temperature may be elevated during maternal temperature elevation, and increased temperature may be present transiently in the neonate after delivery.

Ethnicity

The Collaborative Perinatal Research Study provides historical information on 38,500 pregnancies[319]; selected data for white and black women are presented in Table 6-11. Black women had a higher rate of premature rupture of membranes lasting more than 24 hours (21.4%) compared with white women (10.8%); black women had a higher rate of puerperal infection (4.1%) compared with white women (3.6%); and more black infants weighed less than 2500 g at birth (13.4%) compared with white infants (7.1%). Recent published data concurs with that observed 30 years ago. The National Center for Health Statistics reports continued disparities between blacks and whites in maternal and infant health indicators.[320] In 1996, significant differences were found between blacks and the general population in terms of neonatal mortality (9.6 versus 4.8 deaths per 1000 livebirths), low birth weight (13% versus 7.4%), and severe complications of pregnancy (23 versus 14 complications per 100 deliveries). A review of the literature from 1966 to 1994 reported significantly increased rates of severe histologic chorioamnionitis, maternal fever during labor, prolonged rupture of membranes and early neonatal mortality from sepsis in blacks compared with whites.[321]

Table 6–12 **Incidence of Fetal and Neonatal Infections by Sex**

Infection	No. of Infants		Ratio of Male to Female
	Male	*Female*	
Intrauterine infections			
Syphilis	118	134	0.89
Tuberculosis	15	14	1.07
Toxoplasmosis	118	103	1.14
Listeriosis	26	37	0.70
Perinatal sepsis			
Gram-negative organisms	82	34	2.41
Gram-positive organisms	58	31	1.87
Perinatal meningitis			
Gram-negative organisms	126	44	2.87
Gram-positive organisms	45	39	1.15

Data based on a review of the literature and study of Johns Hopkins Hospital case records, 1930-1963.[323]

In a study of group B streptococcal disease in infants from the Atlanta metropolitan area,[310] black infants had a higher incidence than nonblack infants of early-onset disease; the risk of late-onset disease was 35 times greater in black than in white infants. Thirty percent of early-onset disease and 92% of late-onset disease could be attributed to black race after controlling for other significant risk factors, such as low birth weight and maternal age younger than 20 years. The increased incidence of group B streptococcal disease in blacks of all ages was observed in a survey by the CDC in selected counties in California, Georgia, and Tennessee and the entire state of Oklahoma. The rate of disease of 13.5 cases per 100,000 blacks was significantly higher than the 4.5 cases per 100,000 whites. In neonates with early-onset infection, 2.7 cases per 1000 livebirths occurred in blacks and 1.3 cases per 1000 livebirths occurred in whites.[322] Maternal factors such as socioeconomic status, nutrition, recently acquired sexually transmitted diseases, or racial differences in maternally acquired protective antibodies may result in the increased risk of group B streptococcal disease among blacks.

Gender

Historical data have suggested that there is a predominance of male neonates affected by sepsis and meningitis but not by in utero infections[323,324] (Table 6-12). This difference partially may reflect the fact that female infants had lower rates of respiratory distress syndrome (i.e., hyaline membrane disease) than did male infants. Torday and colleagues[325] studied fetal pulmonary maturity by determining lecithin-to-sphingomyelin ratios and concentrations of saturated phosphatidylcholine and cortisol in amniotic fluid of fetuses between 28 and 40 weeks' gestation. Female infants had higher indices of pulmonary maturity than did male infants. These data provide a biochemical basis for the increased risk of respiratory distress syndrome in male infants and the possible role of these factors of pulmonary maturation in the development of pulmonary infection. Later studies failed to confirm a significant increased risk for bacterial sepsis and meningitis among male infants.[31,326-328]

Geographic Factors

The cause of neonatal sepsis varies from hospital to hospital and from one community to another. These differences probably reflect characteristics of the population served, including unique cultural features and sexual practices, local obstetric and nursery practices, and patterns of antimicrobial agent usage. The bacteriology of neonatal sepsis and meningitis in western Europe[20-28] (see Table 6-3) and Jamaica[329] is generally similar to that in the United States. In tropical areas, a somewhat different pattern can be observed.[330-332] In Riyadh, Saudi Arabia, from 1980 through 1984, *E. coli*, *Klebsiella*, and *Serratia* species were the dominant causes of neonatal sepsis; group B *Streptococcus* was an infrequent cause.[332] However, later data from this geographic location revealed *E. coli* and CoNS, respectively, were the most common pathogens causing early-onset and late-onset sepsis.[333]

At Obafemi Awolowo University in Nigeria between 1994 and 1995, 59 cases of neonatal septicemia were reported.[330] Gram-positive bacteria were isolated from 60% of cases, with *S. aureus* accounting for 34% and *S. epidermidis* for 8%. *L. monocytogenes*, previously uncommon in this region, accounted for 14% of cases. Of the 40% of neonates with bloodstream infection caused by gram-negative organisms, *P. aeruginosa* was isolated from 25%, *K. pneumoniae* from 14%, and *E. coli* from 7%. Twenty-four bacterial isolates were cultured from CSF; 92% of these were gram-negative enteric bacilli. *P. aeruginosa* (32%), *K. pneumoniae* (23%), *Citrobacter freundii* (23%), and *E. coli* (14%) were most commonly isolated from CSF.

In a prospective survey from 1995 to 1996 of neonatal sepsis in South India,[331] 131 episodes of sepsis occurred among 125 newborn infants. Thirty (24%) infants had early-onset sepsis, and 95 (76%) had late-onset sepsis. *E. coli* and *E. faecalis* were the predominant pathogens in early-onset sepsis, whereas *Klebsiella* species and *E. faecalis* most commonly caused late-onset sepsis. Group B *Streptococcus* accounted for only two cases of early-onset disease. *Klebsiella* also was the most frequent cause of sepsis (43 of 176 positive blood cultures) in the neonatal unit at Chris Hani Baraqwanath Hospital in Johannesburg, South Africa, in the year beginning March 1996.[34] Group B *Streptococcus* was the next most frequent pathogen, accounting for 26 cases, and group A streptococcal sepsis occurred in 12 infants.

The rates and risk factors of maternal and neonatal group B streptococcal (GBS) colonization vary in different communities.[334-336] Amin and colleagues in the United Arab Emirates[334] evaluated 563 pregnant women from similar socioeconomic and ethnic backgrounds and reported a GBS colonization rate of 10.1%. In Athens, Greece, maternal and neonatal colonization rates were 6.6% and 2.4%, respectively, with a vertical transmission rate of 22.5%.[335] Middle-class women followed in the private setting were more frequently colonized with GBS than those followed in a public hospital. No association was found between colonization with GBS and maternal age, nationality, marital status, previous obstetric history, cesarean section, infant birth weight, or preterm birth.

Stoll and Schuchat[336] reviewed data on female genital colonization with GBS from 34 reports in the literature and emphasized the importance of appropriate specimen collection and inoculation into selective (antibiotic containing) broth media in the ascertainment of accurate colonization rates. Analysis of data from studies employing adequate methods revealed regional GBS colonization rates of 12% in India and Pakistan, 19% in Asian and Pacific countries, 19% in sub-Saharan Africa, 22% in the Middle East and North Africa, and 14% in the Americas. A comparison of studies that did and did not use selective broth media revealed significantly higher GBS colonization rates in the populations where selective broth media was employed to assess colonization. Other reasons for varying rates of GBS colonization and disease may include socioeconomic factors or differences in sexual practices, hygiene, or nutrition.

Socioeconomic Factors

The lifestyle pattern of mothers, including cultural practices, housing, nutrition, and level of income, appears to be important in determining infants at risk for infection. The most significant factors enhancing risk for neonatal sepsis are low birth weight and prematurity, and the incidence of these is inversely related to socioeconomic status. Various criteria for determining socioeconomic status have been used, but no completely satisfactory and reproducible standard is available. Maternal education, resources, and access to health care can affect the risk of neonatal sepsis. A CDC report[337] evaluating the awareness of perinatal group B streptococcal infection among women of childbearing age in the United States revealed that women with a high school education or less, women with a household income of less than $25,000, and women reporting black, Asian/Pacific Islander, or other ethnicity had lower awareness of perinatal GBS infections than other women.

Procedures

Most VLBW infants have one or more procedures that place them at risk for infection. Any disruption of the protective capability of the intact skin or mucosa can be associated with infection. In a multicenter study of neonatal intensive care unit patients, increased risk of bacteremia was associated with parenteral nutrition, mechanical ventilation, peripherally inserted central catheters, peripheral venous catheters, and umbilical artery catheters.[338]

Nursery Outbreaks or Epidemics

The nursery is a small community of highly susceptible infants where patients have contact with many adults, including parents, physicians, nurses, respiratory therapists, and diagnostic imaging technicians (see Chapter 35). Siblings may enter the nursery or mothers' hospital suites and represent an additional source of infection. In these circumstances, outbreaks or epidemics of respiratory and gastrointestinal illness, most of which is caused by nonbacterial agents, can occur. Spread of microorganisms to the infant occurs by droplets from the respiratory tracts of parents, nursery personnel, or other infants. Organisms can be transferred from infant to infant by the hands of health care workers. Individuals with open or draining lesions are especially hazardous agents of transmission.

Staphylococcal infection and disease are a concern in many nurseries in the United States (see Chapter 35). Epidemics or outbreaks associated with contamination of nursery equipment and solutions caused by *Proteus* species, *Klebsiella* species, *S. marcescens*, *Pseudomonas* species, and *Flavobacterium* also have been reported. An unusual and unexplained outbreak of early-onset group B streptococcal sepsis with an attack rate of 14 per 1000 livebirths occurred in Kansas City during January through August of 1990.[339]

The availability of molecular techniques to distinguish among bacterial strains provides an important epidemiologic tool in the investigation of nursery outbreaks. Previously, methods to determine strain relatedness relied on antibiotic susceptibility patterns, biochemical profiles, and plasmid or phage analysis.[147,340] More recent techniques permit the discrimination of strains based on bacterial chromosomal polymorphisms. Pulse-field gel electrophoresis, ribotyping, multilocus sequence typing, and polymerase chain reaction–based methods are widely used tools to assign strain identity or relatedness.[341-343]

Antimicrobial agents play a major role in the ecology of the microbial flora in the nursery. Extensive and prolonged use of these drugs eliminates susceptible strains and allows for proliferation of resistant subpopulations of neonatal flora. There is selective pressure toward colonization by microorganisms that are resistant to the antimicrobial agents used in the nurseries and, because of cross-resistance patterns, to similar drugs within an antimicrobial class.

A historical example of the selective pressure of a systemic antimicrobial agent is provided by Gezon and co-workers[58] in their use of benzathine penicillin G to control an outbreak of group A streptococcal disease. All infants entering the nursery during a 3-week period were treated with a single intramuscular dose of penicillin. Before institution of this policy, most strains of *S. aureus* in the nursery were susceptible to penicillin G. One week after initiation of the prophylactic regimen and for the next 2 years, almost all strains of *S. aureus* isolated from newborns in this nursery were resistant to penicillin G.

During a 4-month period in 1997, van der Zwet and colleagues[344] investigated a nosocomial nursery outbreak of gentamicin-resistant *K. pneumoniae* in which 13 neonates became colonized and 3 became infected. Molecular typing of strains revealed clonal similarity of isolates from eight neonates. The nursery outbreak was terminated by the substitution of amikacin for gentamicin in neonates when treatment with an aminoglycoside was believed to be warranted. Development of resistance in gram-negative enteric bacilli also has been documented in an Israeli study after widespread use of aminoglycosides.[345]

Extensive or routine use of third-generation cephalosporins in the nursery, especially for all neonates with suspected sepsis, can lead to more rapid emergence of drug-resistant gram-negative enteric bacilli than occurs with the standard regimen of ampicillin and an aminoglycoside. Investigators in Brazil[124] performed a prospective investigation of extended-spectrum β-lactamase (ESBL)–producing *K. pneumoniae* colonization and infection during the 2-year period from 1997 to 1999 in the neonatal intensive care unit. A significant independent risk factor for colonization was receipt of a cephalosporin and an aminoglycoside. Previous colonization was an independent risk factor for infection. In India, Jain and co-workers[134] concluded that indiscriminate use of third-generation cephalosporins was responsible for the selection of ESBL-producing, multiresistant strains in their neonatal intensive care unit, where ESBL production was detected in 86.6% of *Klebsiella* species, 73.4% of *Enterobacter* species, and 63.6% of *E. coli* strains. Nosocomial infections in the nursery and their epidemiology and management are further discussed in Chapter 35.

Unexplained Changes in the Pattern of Microorganisms in the Nursery

New strains of bacteria may appear in a nursery without changes in invasive procedures or techniques, nursery practices, or antimicrobial use. The cause of the worldwide epidemic of *S. aureus* disease in the 1950s is uncertain, as is the reason for its diminished importance in the late 1960s. The incidence of serious infections caused by group B streptococci increased in the 1970s, and there is no ready explanation for the appearance or persistence of this organism as a major cause of neonatal morbidity and mortality.

PATHOGENESIS

The developing fetus is relatively protected from the microbial flora of the mother. However, procedures disturbing the integrity of the uterine contents, such as amniocentesis,[346] cervical cerclage,[347,348] transcervical chorionic villus sampling,[349] or percutaneous umbilical blood sampling,[346,350] can permit entry of skin or vaginal organisms into the amniotic sac, causing amnionitis and secondary fetal infection.

Initial colonization of the neonate usually takes place after rupture of the maternal membranes.[323,351] In most cases, the infant is colonized with the microflora of the birth canal during delivery. However, if delivery is delayed, vaginal bacteria may ascend the birth canal and, in some cases, produce inflammation of the fetal membranes, umbilical cord, and placenta.[352] Fetal infection can then result from aspiration of infected amniotic fluid,[353] leading to stillbirth, premature delivery, or neonatal sepsis.[346,352,354,355] The organisms most commonly isolated from infected amniotic fluid are group B streptococci, *E. coli* and other enteric bacilli, anaerobic bacteria, and genital mycoplasmas.[346,354]

There are studies reporting that amniotic fluid inhibits the growth of *E. coli* and other bacteria due to the presence of lysozyme, transferrin, immune globulins (IgA and IgG but not IgM), zinc and phosphate, and lipid-rich substances.[355-361] The addition of meconium to amniotic fluid in vitro has resulted in increased growth of *E. coli* and group B streptococci in some studies.[362,363] However, in other in vitro studies of the bacteriostatic activity of amniotic fluid, there is not inhibition of the growth of group B streptococci.[364-366] Further discussion of bacterial inhibition by amniotic fluid is available in Chapter 3.

Infection of the mother at the time of birth, particularly genital infection, can play a significant role in the development of infection in the neonate. Transplacental hematogenous infection during or shortly before delivery (including the period of separation of the placenta) is possible, although it is more likely that the infant is infected just before or during passage through the birth canal. Among reports of concurrent bacteremia in mother and neonate are cases caused by *H. influenzae* type b,[367] *H. parainfluenzae*,[191] *S. pneumoniae*,[368,369] group A *Streptococcus*,[370] *N. meningitidis*,[371] *Citrobacter* species,[372] and *Morganella morgagnii*[373]; and concurrent cases of meningitis have been reported as caused by *S. pneumoniae*,[374] *N. meningitidis*,[371] and group B streptococci.[375] Many neonates are bacteremic at the time of delivery, which indicates that invasive infection occurred antepartum.[376] Infants with signs of sepsis during the first 24 hours of life also have the highest mortality rate.[20] These data suggest the importance of initiating chemoprophylaxis for women with group B streptococcal colonization or other risk factors for invasive disease in the neonate at the time of onset of labor (see Chapter 13).[377]

Microorganisms acquired by the newborn infant just before or during birth colonize the skin and mucosal surfaces, including the conjunctivae, nasopharynx, oropharynx, gastrointestinal tract, umbilical cord, and in the female infant, the external genitalia. Normal skin flora of the newborn includes coagulase-negative staphylococci, diphtheroids, and *E. coli*.[378] In most cases, the microorganisms proliferate at the initial site of attachment without resulting in illness. Occasionally, contiguous areas may be infected by direct extension (e.g., sinusitis and otitis can occasionally occur from upper respiratory tract colonization).

Bacteria can be inoculated into the skin and soft tissue by obstetric forceps, and organisms may infect these tissues if abrasions or congenital defects are present. Scalp abscesses can occur in infants who have electrodes placed during labor for monitoring of heart rate.[379-381] The incidence of this type of infection in the hands of experienced clinicians, however, is generally quite low (0.1% to 5.2%).[382] A 10-year survey of neonatal enterococcal bacteremia detected 6 of 44 infants with scalp abscesses as the probable source of their bacteremia.[380] The investigators were unable from the data available to deduce whether these abscesses were associated with fetal scalp monitoring, intravenous infusion, or other procedures that resulted in loss of the skin barrier.

Transient bacteremia can accompany procedures that traumatize mucosal membranes such as endotracheal suctioning.[383] Invasion of the bloodstream also can follow multiplication of organisms in the upper respiratory tract or other foci. Although the source of bacteremia frequently is inapparent, careful inspection can reveal a focus, such as an infected circumcision site or infection of the umbilical stump, in some neonates. Metastatic foci of infection can follow bacteremia and can involve the lungs, kidney, spleen, bones, or central nervous system.

Most cases of neonatal meningitis result from bacteremia. Fetal meningitis followed by stillbirth[384] or hydrocephalus, presumably because of maternal bacteremia and transplacentally acquired infection, has been described but is exceedingly rare. Although CSF leaks caused by spiral fetal scalp electrodes do occur, no cases of meningitis have been traced to this source.[385-386] After delivery, the meninges can be invaded directly from an infected skin lesion, with spread through the soft tissues and skull sutures and along thrombosed bridging veins,[351] but in most circumstances, bacteria gain access to the brain through the bloodstream to the choroid plexus during the course of sepsis.[384] Infants with developmental defects such as a midline dermal sinus or myelomeningocele are particularly susceptible to invasion of underlying nervous tissue.[44]

Brain abscesses can result from hematogenous spread of microorganisms (i.e., septic emboli) and proliferation in tissue that is devitalized because of anoxia or vasculitis with hemorrhage or infarction. Certain organisms are more likely than others to invade nervous tissue and cause local or widespread necrosis.[44] Most cases of meningitis related to *C. koseri* (formerly *C. diversus*) and *E. sakazakii* are associated with cyst and abscess formation. Other gram-negative bacilli with potential to cause brain abscesses include *Proteus, Pseudomonas, S. marcescens*, and occasionally group B streptococci.[148,155,387-389] Volpe comments that bacteria associated with brain abscesses are those that cause meningitis with severe vasculitis.[390]

Host Factors

Infants with one or more predisposing factors (e.g., low birth weight, premature rupture of membranes, septic or traumatic delivery, fetal hypoxia, maternal peripartum infection) are at increased risk for sepsis. Microbial factors such as inoculum size[391] and virulence properties of the organism[346] undoubtedly are significant. Immature function of phagocytes and decreased inflammatory and immune effector responses are characteristic of very small infants and can contribute to the unique susceptibility of the fetus and newborn (see Chapter 4).

Metabolic factors are likely to be important in increasing risk for sepsis and severity of the disease. Fetal hypoxia and acidosis can impede certain host defense mechanisms or allow localization of organisms in necrotic tissues. Infants with hyperbilirubinemia can suffer impairment of various immune functions, including neutrophil bactericidal activity, antibody response, lymphocyte proliferation, and complement functions (see Chapter 4). The indirect hyperbilirubinemia that commonly occurs with breast-feeding jaundice rarely is associated with neonatal sepsis.[392] Late-onset jaundice and direct hyperbilirubinemia can be the result of an infectious process. Evidence of diffuse hepatocellular damage and bile stasis have been described in such infants.[393,394]

Hypothermia in newborns, generally defined as a rectal temperature equal to or below 35° C (95° F), is associated with a significant increase in the incidence of sepsis, meningitis, pneumonia, and other serious bacterial infections.[395-398] In developing countries, hypothermia is a leading cause of death during the winter. Hypothermia frequently is accompanied by abnormal leukocyte counts, acidosis, and uremia, each of which can interfere with resistance to infection. However, the exact cause of increased morbidity in infants presenting with hypothermia remains poorly understood. In many infants, it is unclear whether hypothermia predisposes to or results from bacterial infection.

Infants with galactosemia have increased susceptibility to sepsis caused by gram-negative enteric bacilli, in particular *E. coli*.[399-401] Among eight infants identified with galactosemia by routine newborn screening in Massachusetts, four had systemic infection caused by *E. coli.*[400] Three of these four infants died of sepsis and meningitis; the fourth infant, who had a urinary tract infection, survived. A survey of state programs in which newborns are screened for galactosemia revealed that among 32 infants detected, 10 had systemic infection, and 9 died of bacteremia. *E. coli* was the infecting organism in nine of the infants, and group D *Streptococcus* was the pathogen in the 10th infant. It appears that galactosemic neonates have an unusual predisposition to severe infection with *E. coli*, and bacterial sepsis is a significant cause of death among these infants. Depressed neutrophil function due to elevated serum galactose levels is postulated to be a possible cause of their predisposition to sepsis.[402,403]

Other inherited metabolic diseases have not been associated with a higher incidence of neonatal bacterial infection. A poorly documented increase in the relative frequency of sepsis has been observed among infants with hereditary fructose intolerance.[404] Infants with methylmalonic acidemia and other inborn errors of branched-chain amino acid metabolism manifest neutropenia as a result of bone marrow suppression by accumulated metabolites; however, no increased incidence of infection has been described in this group of infants.[405,406] Shurin[402] observed that infants became ill when serum galactose levels were high when glucose levels were likely to be low and that susceptibility to infection diminished when dietary control was initiated.

Iron may have an important role in the susceptibility of neonates to infection, but this continues to be controversial. Iron added to serum in vitro enhances the growth of many organisms, including *E. coli*, *Klebsiella* species, *Pseudomonas* species, *Salmonella* species, *L. monocytogenes*, and *S. aureus*. Iron-binding proteins, lactoferrin and transferrin, are present in serum, saliva, and breast milk. However, the newborn has low levels of these proteins.[407] Barry and Reeve[408] demonstrated an increased incidence of sepsis in Polynesian infants who were treated with intramuscular iron. Prophylactic regimens of intramuscular iron dextran were administered to these infants soon after birth because of a high incidence of iron-deficiency anemia. The regimen was shown to be effective in preventing anemia of infancy, but an extraordinary increase in bacterial sepsis occurred. The incidence of sepsis in newborns receiving iron was 17 cases per 1000 livebirths, whereas the incidence of sepsis in infants who did not receive iron was 3 cases per 1000 livebirths; during a comparable period, the rate of sepsis for European infants was 0.6 case per 1000 livebirths. Special features of sepsis in the infants who received iron soon after birth were late-onset, paucity of adverse perinatal factors, and predominance of *E. coli* as the cause of sepsis. During the period studied, *E. coli* was responsible for 26 of 27 cases of sepsis in iron-treated Polynesian infants and for none of three cases of sepsis in the infants who did not receive iron. Results of this study were similar to the experience reported by Farmer[409] for New Zealand infants given intramuscular iron. The incidence of meningitis caused by *E. coli* increased fivefold in infants who received iron and decreased when the use of iron was terminated.

Infection in Twins

Studies have suggested a higher risk for contracting ascending intrauterine infection in the first than the second born of twins.[410,411] Pass and colleagues[412] showed that low-birth-weight twins were at higher risk for group B streptococcal infection than were low-birth-weight singletons; infection developed in 3 of 56 twin births, or 53.5 cases per 1000 livebirths, compared with infections in 7 of 603 singleton births, or 11.6 cases per 1000 livebirths. Edwards and colleagues[413] studied group B streptococcal infection in 12 index cases of multiple gestations. Early-onset disease occurred in both twins in one pair and in one twin in five other pairs; late-onset infection occurred in both infants in two pairs and in one twin in four other pairs. Cases of late-onset group B streptococcal disease in twin pairs occurred closely in time to one another: 19 and 20 days in one set and at 28 and 32 days of age in the other set.

In twins, the presence of virulent organisms in the environment, especially the maternal genital tract; their absence of specific maternal antibodies; and their similar genetic heritage probably contribute to the risk for invasive infection. It seems logical that twins, particularly if monochorionic, should have high rates of simultaneous early-onset infection, but it is particularly intriguing that some cases of late-onset disease occur in twins almost simultaneously. Infections in twins, including disease related to *T. pallidum*, echoviruses 18 and 19, and *Toxoplasma gondii*, are discussed in Chapters 18, 24, and 31, respectively. Neonatal infections in twins have been caused by group A streptococci[414] (case report of streptococcal sepsis in a mother and infant twins) and *Salmonella* species,[415] malaria,[416,417] coccidioidomycosis,[418] cytomegalovirus infection,[419-421] and rubella.[422]

The Umbilical Cord as a Focus of Infection

Historically, the umbilical cord was a particularly common portal of entry for systemic infection in the newborn, and infection by this route can still occur. The devitalized tissue is an excellent medium for bacterial growth, and the recently thrombosed umbilical vessels provide direct access to the bloodstream. Epidemics of erysipelas, staphylococcal disease, tetanus, and gas gangrene of the umbilicus were common in the 19th century. The introduction of simple hygienic measures in cord care resulted in a marked reduction of omphalitis.[423] In 1930, Cruickshank wrote, "in Prague, before antiseptic and aseptic dressing of the cord was introduced, sepsis neonatorum was as common as puerperal sepsis ... after the introduction of cord dressing in the hospital the number of newborn children developing fever sank from 45% to 11.3%."[424,425]

Closure of the umbilical vessels and the subsequent aseptic necrosis of the cord begins soon after the infant takes the first breath; the umbilical arteries contract, the blood flow is interrupted, and the cord tissues, deprived of a blood supply, undergo aseptic necrosis. The umbilical stump acquires a rich flora of microorganisms. Within hours, the umbilical stump is colonized with large numbers of gram-positive cocci, particularly *Staphylococcus* species, and shortly thereafter with fecal organisms.[425,426] These bacteria can invade the open umbilical wound, causing a localized infection with purulent discharge and, as a result of delayed obliteration of the umbilical vessels, bleeding from the umbilical stump. From this site, infection can proceed into the umbilical vessels, along the fascial planes of the abdominal wall, or into the peritoneum[423,425,427,428] (Fig. 6-1).

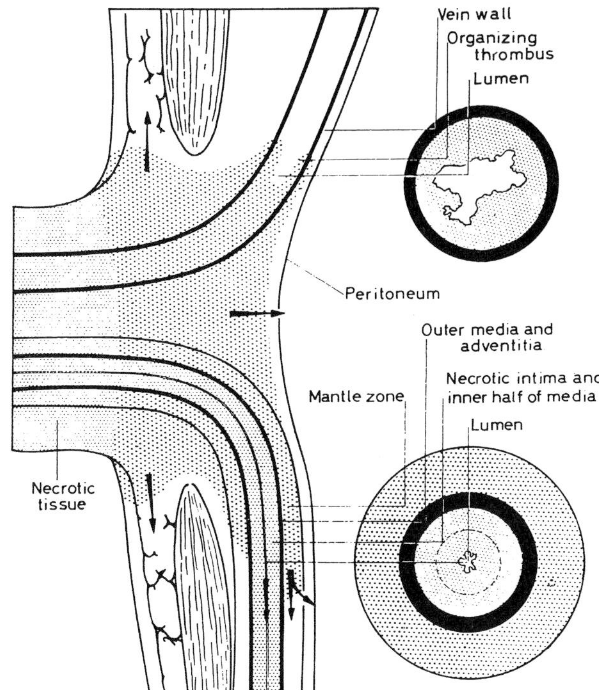

Figure 6–1 After birth, the necrotic tissue of the umbilical stump separates. This provokes some inflammation, which is limited by a fibroblastic reaction extending to the inner margin of the coarsely *stippled area*. The inner half of the media and the intima of the umbilical arteries become necrotic, but this does not stimulate an inflammatory reaction. *Arrows* indicate routes by which infection may spread beyond the granulation tissue barriers. Organisms invading the thrombus in the vein may disseminate by emboli. (From Morison JE. Foetal and Neonatal Pathology, 3rd ed. Washington, DC, Butterworth, 1970.)

Although umbilical discharge or an "oozing" cord is the most common manifestation of omphalitis, periumbilical cellulitis and fasciitis are the conditions most often associated with hospitalization.[427] Infants presenting with fasciitis have a high incidence of bacteremia, intravascular coagulopathy, shock, and death.[427] Septic embolization arising from the infected umbilical vessels is uncommon but can produce metastatic spread to various organs, including the lungs, pancreas, kidneys, and skin.[423] Such emboli can arise from the umbilical arteries and from the umbilical vein, because final closure of the ductus venosus and separation of the portal circulation from the inferior vena cava and the systemic circulation are generally delayed until day 15 to 30 of life.[429]

Complications of omphalitis, now a rare infection in developed countries because of modern umbilical cord care, include a variety of infections such as septic umbilical arteritis,[423,430] suppurative thrombophlebitis of the umbilical or portal veins or the ductus venosus,[430-432] peritonitis,[428,430,431,434] intestinal gangrene,[428] liver abscess, endocarditis, pylephlebitis,[428,435] and subacute necrotizing funisitis.[436] Some of these infections can occur in the absence of signs of omphalitis.[423,430]

Administration of Drugs to the Mother before Delivery

Almost all antimicrobial agents cross the placenta. Antimicrobial drugs administered to the mother at term can alter the initial microflora of the neonate and can complicate the diagnosis of infection in the neonate. Chapter 37 reviews the clinical pharmacology of antimicrobial agents administered to the mother.

Several studies have shown that corticosteroid administration to mothers in preterm labor to enhance pulmonary maturation in the fetus resulted in a significant decrease in the incidence and severity of neonatal respiratory distress syndrome but an increase in maternal infection, particularly endometritis, when compared with placebo.[437] A trend toward increased neonatal infection also was described among infants whose mothers received corticosteroid treatment.[437] Many other investigators have found that corticosteroids administered to the mother at term had no effect on maternal or neonatal infections.[437-439]

Substance abuse during pregnancy can affect immune function in the neonate. Significant abnormalities in T cell function and an apparent increased incidence of infections have been found during the first year of life among infants born to alcohol-addicted[440,441] and heroin-addicted[442,443] mothers. The adverse effects of cocaine and opiates on placental function, fetal growth and development, and prematurity also may predispose to a greater likelihood of neonatal infection.[443,444] Unfortunately, drug abuse is a multifactorial problem; it is virtually impossible to separate the consequences of direct pharmacologic effects on the fetus from those due to inadequate nutrition, lack of prenatal care, and infectious medical complications encountered in addicted pregnant women.[443-445]

Administration of Drugs Other than Antibiotics to the Neonate

Administration of indomethacin to neonates for the closure of a patent ductus arteriosus has been associated with a higher incidence of sepsis and necrotizing enterocolitis in the indomethacin-treated groups compared with infants treated with surgery or other medications.[446-448] The mechanism by which indomethacin predisposes low-birth-weight infants to sepsis is unknown.[448]

O'Shea and colleagues[449] described the outcomes of VLBW (500 to 1250 g) infants given dexamethasone at 15 to 25 days of age for the prevention of chronic lung disease. Among 61 infants treated with tapering doses of dexamethasone for 42 days, there was no increase in the incidence of sepsis or the number of sepsis evaluations in the treatment group when compared with a control population.

A strong association between intravenous lipid administration to newborns and coagulase-negative staphylococcal bacteremia has been confirmed.[105] Although the infants in this study were of low birth weight, ill, and were using non-umbilical central venous catheters for nutrition, administration of lipid emulsion was an independent risk factor for bacteremia. It was postulated that the role of lipid as a growth medium for bacteria, the mechanical blockage of the catheter by deposition of lipid in the lumen, and the effect of lipid emulsions on the function of neutrophils and macrophages each might contribute to the observed increased risk for bacteremia.

The effects of prostaglandins and leukotrienes in the perinatal period have been reviewed by Heymann.[450] Prostaglandin E_1 has been used in the management of congenital malformations for which it is critical to maintain the ductus arteriosus in a dilated position. Adverse effects of prostaglandin E_1 that can be confused with sepsis included temperature elevation, hypotension, and jitteriness.

PATHOLOGY

Infants with severe and rapidly fatal sepsis generally have minimal or no histologic indication of an infectious process.[351,451] Findings typical of bacteremia, such as multiple disseminated abscesses of similar size, purulent vasculitis, and intravascular identification of bacteria, are evident in a minority of infants.[451] Shock accompanying sepsis sometimes causes findings such as periventricular leukomalacia and intraventricular hemorrhage, scattered areas of nonzonal hepatic necrosis, renal medullary hemorrhage, renal cortical or acute tubular necrosis, and adrenal hemorrhage and necrosis. Evidence of disseminated intravascular coagulopathy, manifested by strands of interlacing fibrin in the vessels or by a well-demarcated subarachnoid fibrinous hematoma, also can be present.[384,451] The pathology of infections of the respiratory, genitourinary, and gastrointestinal tracts and focal suppurative diseases is discussed in subsequent chapters.

The pathology of neonatal meningitis[384,452,453] and brain abscess[454,455] is similar to that in the older child and adult. The major features are ventriculitis (including inflammation of the choroid plexus), vasculitis, cerebral edema, infarction, cortical neuronal necrosis, and periventricular leukomalacia; chronic pathologic features include hydrocephalus, multicystic encephalomalacia and porencephaly, and cerebral cortical and white matter atrophy.[456] Significant collections of purulent material can be present in the sulci and subarachnoid space, particularly around the basal cisterns, of infants with meningitis. Because the fontanelles are open, exudative material can collect around the base of the brain without a significant increase in intracranial pressure. Hydrocephalus may result from closure of the aqueduct or the foramina of the fourth ventricle by purulent exudate or by means of inflammatory impairment of CSF resorption through the arachnoid channels.[384,457] Ventriculitis has been described in 20% to 90% of cases[44,384,457] and often is the reason for persistence of bacteria in CSF when obstruction ensues and for a slow clinical recovery.[458] Acute inflammatory cells infiltrate the ependymal and subependymal tissues, causing destruction of the epithelial lining of the ventricles. Hemorrhage, venous thrombosis, and subdural effusions often are present.

Brain abscesses and cysts in the neonate are distinguished by the relatively large size of the lesions and relatively poor capsule formation. They occur most frequently in association with meningitis caused by *C. koseri*, *E. sakazakii*, *S. marcescens*, and *Proteus mirabilis* and usually are located in the cerebrum, involving several lobes.[148,155,387,390] These organisms characteristically give rise to a hemorrhagic meningoencephalitis caused by intense bacterial infiltration of cerebral vessels and surrounding tissues. The resulting vascular occlusion is followed by infarction and widespread necrosis of cerebral tissue with liquefaction and formation of multiple loculated abscesses and cysts.[387,390]

CLINICAL MANIFESTATIONS

Signs of fetal distress can be the earliest indication of infection in neonates with sepsis, beginning at or soon after delivery. Fetal tachycardia in the second stage of labor was evaluated as a sign of infection by Schiano and colleagues.[459] Pneumonia or sepsis occurred in 3 of 8 infants with marked fetal tachycardia (>180 beats per minute), in 7 of 32 infants with mild tachycardia (160 to 179 beats per minute), and in 1 of 167 infants with lower heart rates.

A low Apgar score, suggesting distress at or before delivery, also has been correlated with sepsis in the newborn period. Infants delivered vaginally had a 56-fold higher risk of sepsis when the Apgar score was less than 7 at 5 minutes compared with infants with higher Apgar scores.[460] Among infants with rupture of the amniotic membranes for 24 hours or more, St. Geme and colleagues[352] found a significant increase in the risk for perinatal bacterial infection among those with an Apgar score of less than 6 at 5 minutes but found no association with fetal tachycardia (>160 beats per minute).

The Apgar score is well characterized in term infants but less so in premature infants who have the higher attack rates for sepsis. Because low Apgar scores (<3 at 1 minute, <6 at 5 minutes) were significantly associated with low birth weight and shorter gestation, the use of the score is less valuable as an indicator of sepsis in premature than in term infants.[461]

The earliest signs of sepsis often are subtle and nonspecific. Poor feeding, diminished activity, or just "not looking well" can be the only early evidence that infection is present. More prominent findings are respiratory distress, apnea, lethargy, fever or hypothermia, jaundice, vomiting, diarrhea, and skin manifestations, including petechiae, abscesses, and sclerema.[462]

The nonspecific and subtle nature of the signs of sepsis in newborns is even more problematic in identifying sepsis in the VLBW infant. In a study by Fanaroff and colleagues,[16] the clinical signs of late-onset sepsis in 325 infants weighing 501 to 1500 g at birth included increasing apnea and bradycardia episodes (55%), increasing oxygen requirement (48%), feeding intolerance, abdominal distention or guaiac-positive stools (46%), lethargy and hypotonia (37%), and temperature instability (10%). Unexplained metabolic acidosis (11%) and hypoglycemia (10%) were the most common laboratory indicators of the metabolic derangement accompanying sepsis.

Bonadio and co-workers[463] attempted to determine the most reliable clinical signs of sepsis in more than 200 febrile infants from birth to 8 weeks old. They found that changes in affect, peripheral perfusion, and respiratory status best identified those infants with serious bacterial infection. Alterations in feeding pattern, level of alertness, level of activity, and muscle tone also were present; however, these signs were less sensitive indicators.

Focal infection involving any organ can occur in infants with sepsis, but most often (excluding pneumonia or meningitis), this occurs in neonates with late-onset rather than early-onset disease. Evaluation of infants with suspected bacteremia must include a careful search for primary or secondary foci such as meningitis, pneumonia, urinary tract infection, septic arthritis, osteomyelitis, peritonitis, or soft tissue infection.

Table 6–13 Clinical Signs of Bacterial Sepsis

Clinical Sign	Percent of Infants with Sign
Hyperthermia	51
Hypothermia	15
Respiratory distress	33
Apnea	22
Cyanosis	24
Jaundice	35
Hepatomegaly	33
Lethargy	25
Irritability	16
Anorexia	28
Vomiting	25
Abdominal distention	17
Diarrhea	11

Data from references 3, 4, 10, and 11.

Table 6–14 Clinical Signs of Bacterial Meningitis

Clinical Sign	Percent of Infants with Sign
Hypothermia or fever	62
Lethargy or irritability	52
Anorexia or vomiting	48
Respiratory distress	41
Bulging or full fontanelle	35
Seizures	31
Jaundice	28
Nuchal rigidity	16
Diarrhea	14

Data from references 38, 45, 452, 455, and 471.

Serious bacterial infections are uncommon in neonates without any clinical evidence of illness,[463] even among those with maternal risk factors for infection.[464] Occasionally, bacteremia occurs without clinical signs.[465-467] Albers and associates[465] described the case histories of three infants without signs of illness for whom blood cultures were performed as part of a nursery study involving 131 infants. Blood was obtained from peripheral veins at different times during the first 10 days of life. The same pathogen was isolated repeatedly (i.e., three, three, and two times) from the blood of the three infants even though they remained well. The infants subsequently were treated with appropriate antimicrobial agents. Bacteremia caused by group B streptococci can occur with minimal or no systemic or focal signs,[467-469] and it may be sustained over several days.[470] Most healthy-appearing infants with group B streptococcal bacteremia were born at term and had early-onset (<7 days old) infection. Similarly, among 44 neonates with enterococcal bacteremia, 3 (17%) of 18 with early-onset infection but none with late-onset infection appeared well.[96] The incidence of bacteremia without clinical signs is uncertain because few cultures of blood are performed for infants who show no signs of sepsis.

Table 6-13 lists the common clinical signs of neonatal bacterial sepsis. Clinical signs of neonatal bacterial meningitis are given in Table 6-14. Noninfectious conditions that can present with clinical manifestations similar to those of sepsis are shown in Table 6-15.

Fever and Hypothermia

The temperature of the infant with sepsis may be elevated, depressed, or normal.[468-474] In a multicenter survey of nearly 250 infants with early-onset group B streptococcal bacteremia, approximately 85% had a normal temperature (36° C to 37.2° C [96.8° F to 99° F]) at the time of their admission to the neonatal intensive care unit.[468] In comparing temperatures by gestational age, it was observed that term infants were more likely to have fever than preterm infants (12% versus 1%), whereas preterm infants more frequently had hypothermia (13% versus 3%). Phagocytes of the infant born after an uncomplicated labor can produce adult concentrations of interleukin-1, a potent pyrogen. The phagocytes of infants born after cesarean section have a markedly suppressed ability to produce this pyrogen.[475] In the studies reviewed in Table 6-13, approximately one half of the infants had fever. Hypothermia, which was mentioned in one study, occurred in 15% of the infants.

Fever is variably defined for newborns. A temperature of 38.0° C (100.4° F) measured rectally generally is accepted as the lower limit of the definition of fever. Although some clinical studies indicate that axillary,[476,477] skin-mattress,[476] and infrared tympanic membrane thermometry[477] are accurate and less dangerous than rectal measurements for obtaining core temperature, the reliability of these methods, particularly in febrile infants, has been questioned.[478-481] The current method of choice for determining the presence of fever in neonates is a rectal temperature taken at a depth of 2 to 3 cm past the anal margin. In infants with suspected sepsis without fever, it has been shown that a *difference* between core (rectal) and skin (sole of the foot) temperature of more than 3.5° C can be a more useful indicator of infection than measurement of core temperature alone.[474]

There is no study of temperatures in neonates that is prospective, assesses all infants (febrile and afebrile), includes rectal and axillary temperatures, includes preterm and term infants, and requires positive cultures of blood or other body fluids to define invasive bacterial infection. However, Voora and colleagues[482] observed 100 term infants in Chicago with an axillary or rectal temperature of 37.8° C (100.1° F) or higher during the first 4 days of life, and Osborn and Bolus[483] conducted a retrospective review of 2656 term infants in Los Angeles. Both groups of investigators reported that temperature elevation in healthy term infants was uncommon. Approximately 1% of neonates born at term had at least one episode of fever, measured as 37.8° C (100.1° F) or higher per axilla.[482] Temperature elevation infrequently was associated with systemic infection when a single evaluation occurred. None of 64 infants in these two studies who had a single episode of fever developed clinical evidence of systemic infection (cultures of blood or other body fluids were not obtained). By contrast, temperature elevation that was sustained for more than 1 hour frequently was associated with infection. Of seven infants with sustained fever in the Osborn and Bolus study,[483] five had proven bacterial or viral infections. Of 65 infants reported by Voora and colleagues,[482] 10 had documented systemic bacterial disease. Temperature elevation without other signs of infection was infrequent. Only one

Table 6–15 Differential Diagnosis of Clinical Signs Associated with Neonatal Sepsis and Some Noninfectious Conditions

Respiratory Distress (apnea, cyanosis, costal and sternal retraction, rales, grunting, diminished breath sounds, tachypnea)
Transient tachypnea of the newborn
Respiratory distress syndrome
Atelectasis
Aspiration pneumonia, including meconium aspiration
Pneumothorax
Pneumomediastinum
Central nervous system disease: hypoxia, hemorrhage
Congenital abnormalities, including tracheoesophageal fistula, choanal atresia, diaphragmatic hernia, hypoplastic lungs
Congenital heart disease
Cardiac arrhythmia
Hypothermia (neonatal cold injury)
Hypoglycemia
Neonatal drug withdrawal syndrome
Medication error with inhaled epinephrine

Temperature Abnormality (hyperthermia or hypothermia)
Altered environmental temperature
Disturbance of central nervous system thermoregulatory merchanism, including anoxia, hemorrhage, kernicterus
Hyperthyroidism or hypothyroidism
Neonatal drug withdrawal syndrome
Dehydration
Congenital adrenal hyperplasia
Vaccine reaction

Jaundice
Breast milk jaundice
Blood group incompatibility
Red cell hemolysis, including blood group incompatibility, G6PD deficiency
Resorption of blood from closed space hemorrhage
Gastrointestinal obstruction, including pyloric stenosis
Extrahepatic or intrahepatic biliary tract obstruction
Inborn errors of metabolism, including galactosemia, glycogen storage disease type IV, tyrosinemia, disorders of lipid metabolism, peroxisomal disorders, defective bile acid synthesis (trihydroxycoprostanic acidemia)
Hereditary diseases, including cystic fibrosis, α_1-antitrypsin deficiency, bile excretory defects (Dubin-Johnson, Rotor, Byler, Aagenaes syndrome)
Hypothyroidism
Prolonged parenteral hyperalimentation

Hepatomegaly
Red cell hemolysis, including blood group incompatibility, G6PD deficiency
Infant of a diabetic mother
Inborn errors of metabolism, including galactosemia, glycogen storage disease, organic acidemias, urea cycle disorders, hereditary fructose intolerance, peroxisomal disorders
Biliary atresia
Congestive heart failure
Benign liver tumors, including hemangioma, hamartoma
Malignant liver tumors, including hepatoblastoma, metastatic neuroblastoma, congenital leukemia

Gastrointestinal Abnormalities (anorexia, regurgitation, vomiting, diarrhea, abdominal distention)
Gastrointestinal allergy
Overfeeding, aerophagia
Intestinal obstruction (intraluminal or extrinsic)
Necrotizing enterocolitis
Hypokalemia
Hypercalcemia or hypocalcemia
Hypoglycemia
Inborn errors of metabolism, including galactosemia, urea cycle disorders, organic acidemias
Ileus secondary to pneumonia
Congenital adrenal hyperplasia
Gastric perforation
Neonatal drug withdrawal syndrome

Lethargy
Central nervous system disease, including hemorrhage, hypoxia, or subdural effusion
Congenital heart disease
Neonatal drug withdrawal syndrome
Hypoglycemia
Hypercalcemia
Familial dysautonomia

Seizure Activity (tremors, hyperactivity, muscular twitching)
Hypoxia
Intracranial hemorrhage or kernicterus
Congenital central nervous system malformations
Neonatal drug withdrawal syndrome
Hypoglycemia
Hypocalcemia
Hyponatremia, hypernatremia
Hypomagnesemia
Inborn errors of metabolism, including urea cycle disorders, organic acidemias, galactosemia, glycogen storage disease, peroxisomal disorders
Pyridoxine deficiency

Petechiae and Purpura
Birth trauma
Blood group incompatibility
Neonatal isoimmune thrombocytopenia
Maternal idiopathic thrombocytopenic purpura
Maternal lupus erythematosus
Drugs administered to mother
Giant hemangioma (Kasabach-Merritt syndrome)
Thrombocytopenia with absent radii (TAR) syndrome
Disseminated intravascular coagulopathy
Coagulation factor deficiencies
Congenital leukemia
Child abuse

infant (with cytomegalovirus infection) of the five Los Angeles infants had fever without other signs. Only two infants (with bacteremia caused by *E. coli* or group B *Streptococcus*, respectively) of the 10 Chicago infants with fever and proven bacterial disease had no other signs of infection.

In addition to infection, fever may be caused by an elevation in ambient temperature, dehydration, retained blood or extensive hematoma, and damage to the temperature-regulating mechanisms of the central nervous system. Less common noninfectious causes of fever are hyperthyroidism, cystic fibrosis, familial dysautonomia, and ectodermal dysplasia. When thermoregulatory devices that monitor and modify infant temperature are introduced, the use of fever or hypothermia as a diagnostic sign of sepsis sometimes is impeded.

Respiratory Distress

Signs of respiratory distress, including tachypnea, grunting, flaring of the alae nasi, intercostal retractions, rales, and decreased breath sounds, are common and important findings in the infant suspected of having sepsis. Respiratory distress syndrome and aspiration pneumonia must be considered in the differential diagnosis. Apnea is one of the most specific signs of sepsis but usually occurs in the setting of a fulminant onset or after other nonspecific signs have been present for hours or days. Clinical signs of cardiovascular dysfunction, including tachycardia, arrhythmia, and poor peripheral perfusion, that occur in the absence of congenital heart disease are sensitive and specific signs of sepsis.

Jaundice

Jaundice is present in approximately one third of infants with sepsis and is a common finding in infants with urinary tract infection.[484-487] It can develop suddenly or subacutely and occasionally is the only sign of sepsis. Jaundice usually decreases after institution of appropriate antimicrobial therapy. It occurs in septic infants irrespective of the type of bacterial pathogen.

Organomegaly

The liver edge is palpable in premature infants and can extend to 2 cm below the costal margin in healthy term infants. Ashkenazi and colleagues[488] evaluated liver size in healthy term infants examined within 24 hours of birth and again between 72 and 96 hours. Measurements ranged between 1.6 and 4.0 cm below the costal margin, and there was no significant difference between early and late examinations. Reiff and Osborn[489] suggested that determination of liver span by palpation and percussion is a more reliable technique than identifying the liver projection below the costal margin. Hepatomegaly is a common sign of in utero infections and of some noninfectious conditions such as cardiac failure and metabolic diseases, including galactosemia and glycogen storage disease. Splenomegaly is less common than hepatomegaly and infrequently is mentioned in reports of bacterial sepsis of the newborn.[490]

Lymph nodes infrequently are palpable in newborns unless they are infected with viruses, spirochetes, or protozoa. Bamji and colleagues[491] examined 214 healthy neonates in New York and identified palpable nodes at one or more sites in one third of the infants. Embree and Muriithi[492] examined 66 healthy, term Kenyan neonates during the first 24 hours of life and found palpable axillary nodes (27.7%) but no palpable inguinal nodes. Adenopathy is a sign of congenital infection caused by rubella virus, *T. gondii, T. pallidum,* and enteroviruses. Adenitis can occur in drainage areas involved with bacterial soft tissue infection. Although adenopathy is not an important sign of systemic bacterial infection in neonates, cellulitis-adenitis syndrome, a rare clinical manifestation of late-onset group B streptococcal infection in infants, is a condition in which local inflammation can be the only initial sign of sepsis that can include concurrent meningitis.[493-495]

Gastrointestinal Signs

Gastrointestinal disturbances, including poor feeding, regurgitation or vomiting, large gastric residuals in infants fed by tube, diarrhea, and abdominal distention, are common and significant early signs of sepsis. The first indications of illness can be a change in feeding pattern or lethargy during feedings.

Skin Lesions

A variety of skin lesions can accompany bacteremia, including cellulitis, abscess, petechiae, purpuric lesions, sclerema, erythema multiforme, and ecthyma. These lesions are described in Chapter 10.

Neurologic Signs

The onset of meningitis in the neonate is accompanied by identical signs of illness as observed in infants with sepsis. Meningitis can be heralded by increasing irritability, alteration in consciousness, poor tone, tremors, lip smacking or twitching of facial muscles or an extremity. Seizures were present in 31% of the infants reviewed in Table 6-14, but Volpe[496] identified seizures, in many cases subtle, in 75% of infants with bacterial meningitis. Approximately one half of the seizures were focal, and at their onset, they usually were subtle. Focal signs, including hemiparesis, horizontal deviation of the eyes, and cranial nerve deficits involving the seventh, third, and sixth cranial nerves, in that order of frequency, can be identified.[496] Because cranial sutures in the neonate are open and allow for expansion of the intracranial contents and for increasing head size, a full or bulging fontanelle can be absent.[469,497] The presence of a bulging fontanelle is not related to gestational age. Among 72 newborns with gram-negative enteric bacillary meningitis, a bulging fontanelle was seen in 18% and 17% of term and preterm infants, respectively.[44] Nuchal rigidity, an important sign in older children and adults, is uncommon in neonates.[44]

In addition to the physical findings observed in infants with meningitis, several investigators have reported the occurrence of fluid and electrolyte abnormalities associated with inappropriate antidiuretic hormone secretion, including hyponatremia, decreased urine output, and increased weight gain.[457,460] Occasionally, the onset of meningitis has been followed by a transient or persistent diabetes insipidus.[497]

Early clinical signs of brain abscess in the newborn are subtle and frequently unnoticed by the physician or parent. Presenting signs include those of increased intracranial pressure (e.g., emesis, bulging fontanelle, enlarging head size, separated sutures), focal cerebral signs (e.g., hemiparesis, focal seizures), and acute signs of meningitis. Of six infants with brain abscesses described by Hoffman and colleagues,[454] two were febrile and two had seizures, and five had increased head size.

Other focal infections in the nervous system include pneumococcal endophthalmitis in a neonate with meningitis,[498] pseudomonal endophthalmitis in a premature neonate with late-onset sepsis,[499] and epidural abscess caused by *S. aureus* in 3-week-old,[500] 4-week-old,[501] and 7-week-old infants.[502]

DIAGNOSIS

The diagnosis of systemic infection in the newborn is difficult to establish on the basis of clinical findings alone. A history of one or more risk factors for neonatal sepsis associated with the pregnancy and delivery often is associated with early-onset infection, but there can be no clues before the onset of subtle signs in the term infant who develops late-onset sepsis. The extensive list of conditions that must be considered in the differential diagnosis for the various signs that are associated with sepsis or meningitis and noninfectious conditions is given in Table 6-15. Laboratory tests to assist in the diagnosis of sepsis are discussed in Chapter 36.

Maternal History

Many infants, particularly those born prematurely, who develop systemic infection just before or shortly after delivery, are born to women who have one or more risk features for early-onset sepsis in their infants. These features include preterm labor, premature rupture of the membranes at any time during gestation, prolonged rupture of membranes, chorioamnionitis, prolonged labor, intrauterine scalp electrodes, and traumatic delivery. The following features are identified by the American College of Obstetrics and Gynecology (ACOG) as the basis for identification of women who should receive intrapartum antibiotic prophylaxis to prevent early-onset group B streptococcal disease[503,504]:

1. Antenatal colonization with group B *Streptococcus*
2. Unknown group B streptococcal colonization status

and

a. Preterm labor (less than 37 weeks' gestation)
b. Fever during labor (defined by temperature of 38.0° C [100.4° F] or more)
c. Rupture of membranes for 18 or more hours

3. A urine culture that grows group B *Streptococcus* during the current pregnancy
4. Prior delivery of a neonate with invasive group B streptococcal infection

Microbiologic Techniques

Isolation of microorganisms from a usually sterile site, such as the blood, CSF, urine, other body fluids (e.g., peritoneal, pleural, joint, middle ear), or tissues (e.g., bone marrow, liver, spleen) remains the most valid method of diagnosing bacterial sepsis. Infectious agents cultured from the nose, throat, external auditory canal, skin, umbilicus, or stool indicate colonization and can include organisms that cause sepsis, but isolation of a microorganism from these sites does not establish invasive systemic infection. The limited sensitivity, specificity, and predictive value of body surface cultures in a neonatal intensive care unit was documented using a database of 24,584 cultures from 3371 infants by Evans and colleagues.[505] These investigators strongly discouraged the use of cultures from these sites in diagnosing neonatal sepsis because of their poor correlation with the pathogen in the blood and their expense.

Culture of Blood

Isolation of a pathogenic microorganism from the blood is the only method to establish the diagnosis of neonatal sepsis.

METHODS

Technology has evolved from manually read, broth-based methods to continuously monitored, automated blood culture systems that use enriched media for processing of blood culture specimens. Automated and semiautomated systems for continuous blood culture monitoring are standard in laboratories in the United States.[507-509] Before the widespread use of automated blood-culturing systems, lysis direct plating was the most often employed method of isolating bacteria. Positive cultures were recognized by growth of colonies on agar and provided a rapid means to obtaining quantitative blood culture results from pediatric patients.[510] St. Geme and colleagues[511] used this technique to investigate the distinction of sepsis from contamination in cultures of blood growing coagulase-negative staphylococci.

TIME TO DETECTION OF A POSITIVE BLOOD CULTURE

Bacterial growth is evident in most cultures of blood from neonates within 48 hours.[512,513] With use of conventional culture techniques and subculture at 4 and 14 hours, only 4 of 105 cultures that had positive results (one group B *Streptococcus* and three *S. aureus*) required more than 48 hours of incubation.[512] By use of a radiometric technique (BACTEC 460), 40 of 41 cultures that grew group B *Streptococcus* and 15 of 16 cultures with *E. coli* were identified within 24 hours.[514]

OPTIMAL NUMBER OF CULTURES

The optimal number of cultures to obtain for the diagnosis of bacteremia in the newborn remains uncertain. A single blood culture from an infant with sepsis can be negative, but most studies suggest a sensitivity of 90% or slightly more. Sprunt[515] suggested the use of two blood cultures "not primarily to increase the yield of organisms..." but to "minimize the insecurity and debates over the meaning of the findings." The value of one or of multiple site blood cultures to establish the diagnosis of neonatal sepsis is discussed by Wiswell and Hachey.[516] Two or more blood cultures increase the likelihood of identifying a pathogen in a neonate with sepsis by a few percent, but the need to initiate therapy promptly can make this practice difficult.

OPTIMAL VOLUME OF BLOOD

The optimal volume of blood needed to detect bacteremia in neonates has not been determined. Neal and colleagues[517] evaluated the volume of neonatal blood submitted for culture by physicians who were unaware of the study and found that the mean blood volume per patient was 1.05 mL. Dietzman and co-workers[518] suggested that 0.2 mL of blood was sufficient to detect bacteremia caused by *E. coli*. The relationship between colony counts of *E. coli* from blood cultures from infants with sepsis and meningitis and mortality was evaluated. Meningitis occurred only in neonates with more than 1000 colonies of *E. coli* per milliliter of blood. These data of Dietzman and associates[518] are supported by experimental results indicating that common pediatric pathogens can be reliably recovered from 0.5 mL of blood even when cultured at blood-to-broth ratios of 1:100.[519,520] However, several more recent studies have found that in the circumstance of low inoculum bacteremia (<10 colony-forming units/mL of blood), the collection of only 0.5 mL of blood proved inadequate for the reliable detection of common pathogens.[521-523] It appears that if one blood culture is to be collected before antimicrobial therapy is initiated, a volume of 1 mL or more will ensure the greatest sensitivity.

CULTURES OF BLOOD FROM UMBILICAL VESSELS AND INTRAVASCULAR CATHETERS

Umbilical vessel and intravascular catheters are essential in the care of neonates in the intensive care unit and are preferred blood culture sampling sites.[524-526] Results of cultures of blood obtained from indwelling umbilical or central venous catheters can present ambiguities in interpretation (e.g., contamination versus catheter colonization versus systemic infection). Obtaining blood cultures from a peripheral vessel and catheters in the ill-appearing neonate is useful in the interpretation of results.

DISTINGUISHING CLINICALLY IMPORTANT BACTEREMIA FROM BLOOD CULTURE CONTAMINATION

The increased use of intravascular catheters in neonates has resulted in an increase in the incidence of bacteremia, particularly that caused by coagulase-negative staphylococci (CoNS), and uncertainty regarding the significance of some results. Investigators have considered criteria based on clinical signs and microbiologic factors.

Yale investigators[6] used the following criteria to define the role of commensal organisms in neonatal sepsis: one major clinical sign, such as apnea, bradycardia, core temperature greater than 38.0° C or less than 36.5° C documented at the time the blood culture was obtained plus another blood culture positive for the same organism obtained within 24 hours of the first or an intravascular access device in place before major clinical signs occurred. Some microbiologic features can be useful in differentiating sepsis from contamination:

1. Time to growth in conventional media: The longer the time needed to detect growth (>2 to 3 days), the more likely that skin or intravascular line contamination was present.
2. Number of cultures positive: If peripheral and intravascular catheter specimens are positive, the presence of the organism in the blood is likely; if the catheter specimen alone is positive, intravascular line colonization may have occurred; if multiple cultures from an indwelling vascular catheter are positive or if a single culture is positive and the patient has had a clinical deterioration, a bloodstream infection must be presumed.
3. Organism type: Organisms that are part of skin flora (e.g., diphtheroids, nonhemolytic streptococci, CoNS) suggest contamination in certain cases as described previously, whereas known bacterial pathogens must be considered to be associated with sepsis. Contamination is more likely when multiple species grow in one blood culture bottle, different species grow in two bottles, or only one of several cultures before or during antimicrobial therapy is positive.
4. Clinical signs: If the infant is well without use of antibiotics, growth of a commensal organism from a blood culture is more likely to be a contaminant.

In an attempt to resolve the question of sepsis versus contamination, investigators have used multiple site blood cultures,[516] comparisons of results of cultures of blood and cultures of skin at the venipuncture site,[527] and quantitative blood cultures.[511] These techniques are of investigational interest, but the results do not suggest that any one is of sufficient value to be adopted for clinical practice. Healy and colleagues[528] suggest that isolation of CoNS of the same species or antimicrobial susceptibility from more than one blood culture or from one blood culture obtained from an indwelling catheter or a peripheral vessel and a normally sterile body site represents true infection if the patient is a premature infant with signs of clinical sepsis. At present, management of the sick premature infant, especially the VLBW patient, with a positive blood culture for CoNS requires that the organism be considered a pathogen and managed with appropriate antimicrobial agents. If the infant is well, the microbiologic results given earlier should be considered in the decision to continue or discontinue use of an antimicrobial agent. Another culture of blood should be obtained when the initial culture result is ambiguous.

Buffy-Coat Examination

The rapid diagnosis of bacteremia by identification of microorganisms in the buffy leukocyte layer of centrifuged blood is a method used for many years and has been evaluated for use in newborn infants.[529-535] By using Gram and methylene blue stains of the buffy-coat preparation, immediate and accurate information was obtained for 37 (77%) of 48 bacteremic, clinically septic infants in the four studies.[530-532,534] Positive results were found for gram-positive and gram-negative organisms. In contrast to findings reported for adult populations,[536] there were no false-positive results among almost 200 infants with negative blood cultures. Failure to identify organisms was attributed to extreme neutropenia in several patients.

The large inoculum of microorganisms in the blood of neonates with sepsis most probably explains the excellent sensitivity of leukocyte smears. Smears can be positive with as few as 50 colonies per milliliter of *S. aureus* in the peripheral blood; approximately 50% of neonates with *E. coli* bacteremia have higher concentrations.[518] *Candida* and *S. epidermidis* septicemia in young infants also have been diagnosed by this method.[537-539] Strom[540] reported that bacteria were identified in peripheral blood smears in 17 of 19 infants with septicemia. However, Rodwell and associates[541] were able to identify bacteria in direct blood smears for only 4 of 24 bacteremic neonates. In is likely that the disparity in these results reflects differences in patient populations or distribution of etiologic agents or both. The buffy-coat examination of blood smears has become infrequently used in laboratories since the introduction of automated systems for continuous blood culture monitoring.

Culture of Urine

Infants with sepsis can have a urinary tract origin or a concomitant urinary tract infection. The yield from culture of urine is low in early-onset sepsis and most often reflects metastatic spread to the bladder from the bacteremia, but in late-onset infection, the yield is substantially higher. Visser and Hall[542] found positive cultures of urine in only 1.6% of infants with early-onset sepsis compared with 7.4% of infants with late-onset sepsis. DiGeronimo[543] performed a chart review of 146 clinically septic infants who had cultures of blood and urine. Of 11 infants with positive blood cultures, only one infant with group B *Streptococcus* bacteremia had a positive urine culture. These data suggest that cultures of urine yield very limited information about the source of infection in infants with signs of sepsis before age 7 days. In contrast, it is apparent that urine should be collected for culture from infants with suspected late-onset sepsis before initiation of antimicrobial therapy.

Because of the difficulty in collecting satisfactory clean-voided specimens of urine from the newborn, bladder catheterization or suprapubic needle aspiration of bladder urine frequently is performed. These methods are simple and safe and suprapubic bladder aspiration avoids the ambiguities inherent in urine obtained by other methods.[544-546] If a suprapubic aspirate cannot be performed for technical or medical reasons, catheterization is a satisfactory method of obtaining urine although ambiguous results can occur because of contamination from the urethra, especially in VLBW neonates.

Cultures of Tracheal Aspirates and Pharynx

Because of the association of pneumonia and bacteremia, investigators have sought to determine the risk of sepsis on the basis of colonization of the upper respiratory tract. Lau and Hey[547] found that among ventilated infants who became septic, the same organism usually was present in cultures of tracheal aspirate and blood. However, growth of a bacterial pathogen from a tracheal aspirate culture does not predict which infants will develop sepsis. Similarly, cultures of the pharynx or trachea do not necessarily predict the causative organism in the blood of a neonate with clinical sepsis.[548] Unless the patient has a change in respiratory status documented clinically and radiographically, routine use of cultures from the pharynx or trachea have very limited diagnostic value.

Diagnostic Needle Aspiration and Tissue Biopsy

Direct aspiration of tissues or body fluids through a needle or catheter is used for the diagnosis of a wide variety of infectious and noninfectious diseases.[549] Aspiration of an infectious focus in lung, pleural space, middle ear, pericardium, bones, joints, abscess, and other sites provides immediate and specific information to guide therapy. Biopsy of the liver or bone marrow can assist in diagnosing occult infections, but this rarely is necessary.

Autopsy Microbiology

Two factors must be considered in interpreting bacterial cultures obtained at autopsy: the frequent isolation of organisms usually considered to be nonpathogenic and the difficulty of isolating fastidious organisms such as anaerobic bacteria. To minimize these problems, it is important that specimens be collected with proper aseptic technique and as early as possible after death.

It is a common belief that organisms in the intestinal and respiratory tracts gain access to tissues after death, but it also is possible that bacteremia occurs shortly before death and is not a postmortem phenomenon. Eisenfeld and colleagues[550] identified the same organisms in specimens obtained before and within 2 hours after death. Confusion in the interpretation of results of bacteriologic cultures often is obviated by the review of slides prepared directly from tissues and fluids. If antimicrobial treatment was administered before death, organisms can be observed on a smear even though they are not viable. Pathogens would be expected to be present in significant numbers and accompanied by inflammatory cells, whereas contaminants or organisms that invade tissues after death, if they are seen, would be present in small numbers with no evidence of an inflammatory process.[551,552]

Rapid Techniques for Detection of Bacterial Antigens in Body Fluid Specimens

In the 1970s, the limulus lysate assay for detection of endotoxin produced by gram-negative bacteria based on a gelation reaction between lysates of *Limulus* (horseshoe crab) amebocytes and bacterial endotoxin was investigated for diagnosis of neonatal meningitis with equivocal results.[553-557] Counterimmunoelectrophoresis also was used successfully for detecting the capsular polysaccharide antigens of various pathogenic bacteria, including *S. pneumoniae, N. meningitidis, H. influenzae,* and group B streptococci (see Chapter 13) in CSF, serum, and urine. Less complex and more rapid detection methods have replaced these two assays.

Latex agglutination assays, based on specific agglutination of antibody-coated latex particles by bacterial antigens, has been shown to be helpful in early detection of bacterial antigens in the CSF of patients with acute meningitis. This method of antigen detection now is preferred because of its speed, simplicity, and greater sensitivity for selected organisms. Kits designed to detect cell wall or capsular or cell wall antigen released into body fluids are commercially available. Among the prevalent bacterial pathogens in neonatal infections, only group B *Streptococcus* can be detected by latex agglutination. The sensitivity of latex agglutination methods for identifying infants with group B streptococcal meningitis varies between 73% and 100% for CSF and 75% and 84% for urine.[558] Possible cross-reactions have occurred when concentrated urine was tested. The group B *Streptococcus* cell wall antigen can cross react with those from *S. pneumoniae*, coagulase-negative staphylococci, enterococci, and gram-negative enteric bacteria, including *P. mirabilis* and *E. cloacae*. False-positive results in urine for a positive latex agglutination test for group B *Streptococcus* often were caused by contamination of bag specimens of urine with the streptococci from rectal or vaginal colonization.[559] The poor specificity of group B *Streptococcus* antigen detection methods used with urine led to the Food and Drug Administration recommendation in 1996 that these methods not be employed except for testing of CSF and serum.

Lumbar Puncture and Examination of Cerebrospinal Fluid

Because meningitis can accompany sepsis with no clinical signs to differentiate between bacteremia alone and bacteremia with meningitis, a lumbar puncture should be considered for examination of the CSF in any neonate before initiation of therapy. Up to 15% of infants with sepsis have accompanying meningitis. The overall incidence of bacterial meningitis is less than 1 case per 1000 infants, but the incidence for low-birth-weight (<2500 g) infants or premature infants is several-fold higher than that for term infants. For the diagnosis of some noninfectious central nervous system diseases in neonates (e.g., intracranial hemorrhage), cranial ultrasonography and, occasionally, computed tomography or magnetic resonance imaging are the techniques of choice. For infants with hypoxic-ischemic encephalopathy, lumbar puncture should be considered only for those infants in whom meningitis is a possible diagnosis.

Some investigators suggest that too many healthy term infants have a diagnostic evaluation for sepsis, including lumbar puncture, based solely on maternal risk features and that the lumbar puncture rarely provides clinically useful information. Other investigators have questioned the role of an admission lumbar puncture in the premature infant with respiratory distress and found that the yield of the procedure is very low.[560-562] Of more than 1700 infants with respiratory distress syndrome evaluated for meningitis, bacterial pathogens were identified in the CSF of only 4. Three of the four infants with meningitis were bacteremic with the same pathogen.[560] A large, retrospective study assessed the value of lumbar puncture in the evaluation of suspected sepsis during the first week of life and found that bacteria were isolated from 9 of 728 CSF specimens, but only one infant was believed to have bacterial meningitis.[563] Fielkow and colleagues[564] found no cases of meningitis among 284 healthy-appearing infants who had a lumbar puncture performed because of maternal risk factors, whereas 2.5% of 799 neonates with clinical signs of sepsis had meningitis regardless of maternal risk factors. More recent data regarding the usefulness of lumbar puncture is provided by Wiswell and co-workers.[565] These investigators conclude from their data, collected in the era of maternal intrapartum prophylaxis for the prevention of early-onset group B streptococcal sepsis, that up to 28% of infants with meningitis have sterile blood cultures. In summary, the value of a lumbar puncture has been established for infants with clinical signs of sepsis, but lumbar puncture performed because of maternal risk features in a healthy-appearing neonate is less likely to be useful.

METHOD OF LUMBAR PUNCTURE

Lumbar puncture is more difficult to perform in the neonate than in the older child or adult; traumatic lumbar punctures resulting in blood in the CSF are more frequent, and care must be taken in the infant who is in respiratory distress. Gleason and colleagues[566] suggest that the procedure be performed with the infant in the upright position or, if performed in the flexed position, be modified with neck extension. Pinheiro and associates[567] evaluated the role of locally administered lidocaine before lumbar puncture and found that the local anesthesia decreased the degree of struggling of the infant. However, other investigators have concluded that local anesthesia failed to influence physiologic changes in the neonate undergoing lumbar puncture.[568] Fiser and colleagues[569] suggest that the administration of oxygen before lumbar puncture prevents most hypoxemia resulting from this procedure in infants.

The physician can choose to withhold or delay lumbar puncture in some infants who would be placed at risk for cardiac or respiratory compromise by the procedure. Weisman and colleagues[570] observed that transient hypoxemia occurred during lumbar puncture performed in the lateral position (i.e., left side with hips flexed to place knees to chest) but occurred less frequently when the infant was in a sitting position or modified lateral position (i.e., left side with hips flexed to 90 degrees). Reasons for withholding lumbar puncture in older children, such as signs of increased intracranial pressure, signs of a bleeding disorder, and infection in the area that the needle will traverse to obtain CSF, are less likely to be concerns in the neonate.

Ventricular puncture should be considered in the infant with meningitis who does not respond clinically or microbiologically to antimicrobial therapy because of ventriculitis, especially with obstruction between the ventricles and lumbar CSF. Ventriculitis is diagnosed on the basis of elevated white blood cell count (>100 cells/mm^3) or identification of bacteria by culture, Gram stain, or antigen detection. Ventricular puncture is a potentially hazardous procedure and should be performed only by a physician who is an expert in the technique.

IF A LUMBAR PUNCTURE IS NOT PERFORMED

Is it sufficient to culture only blood and urine for the diagnosis of neonatal bacterial meningitis? Visser and Hall[571] demonstrated that the blood culture was sterile when the CSF yielded a pathogen in 6 (15%) of 39 infants with bacterial meningitis. Franco and colleagues[572] reported that in 26 neonates with bacterial meningitis, only 13 had a positive blood culture. A significant number of infants with meningitis will not have this diagnosis established unless a lumbar puncture is performed.

Ideally, the lumbar puncture should be performed before the initiation of antimicrobial therapy, but there are alternative strategies for infants who may not tolerate the procedure. If the physician believes that lumbar puncture would endanger the infant with presumed sepsis and meningitis, therapy should be initiated after blood (and urine for late-onset illness) is obtained for culture. After the infant is stabilized, lumbar puncture should be performed. Even several days after the start of antibiotic therapy, CSF pleocytosis and abnormal CSF chemistry assays usually should identify the presence or absence of an inflammatory reaction, although CSF culture may be sterile.

EXAMINATION OF CEREBROSPINAL FLUID

The cell content and chemistry of the CSF of healthy newborn infants differ from those of older infants, children, and adults (Table 6-16). The values vary widely during the first weeks of life, and the normal range must be considered in evaluation of CSF in infants suspected to have meningitis.[573-582] The cell content in the CSF of a neonate is higher than that in older infants. Polymorphonuclear leukocytes often are present in the CSF of normal newborns, whereas more than a single polymorphonuclear neutrophil in the CSF of older infants or children should be considered abnormal. Similarly, protein concentration is higher in preterm than in term infants and highest in VLBW infants[582] (Table 6-17). In term infants, the total protein concentration decreases with age, reaching values of healthy older infants (<40 mg/dL) before the third month of life. In low-birth-weight or preterm infants, CSF protein concentrations may not fall within normal values for older infants for several months after birth. CSF glucose levels are lower in neonates than in older infants and can be related to the lower concentrations of glucose observed in blood. Healthy term infants can have blood glucose levels as low as 30 mg/dL, and preterm infants may have levels as low as 20 mg/dL.[582] The physiologic basis for the higher concentration of protein and the increased numbers of white blood cells in the CSF of healthy, uninfected preterm and term infants is unknown. The explanations that have been offered include possible mechanical irritation of the meninges during delivery and an increased permeability of the blood-brain barrier.

In nearly all of the studies of the CSF in newborns, *normal* or *healthy* refers to the absence of clinical manifestations at the time of examination of the CSF. Only the

Table 6–16 Hematologic and Chemical Characteristics of Cerebrospinal Fluid in Healthy Newborns: Results of Selected Studies

Study (year)	No. of Patients	Age (days)	White Blood Cells[a] (mm³)	Neutrophils[a] (mm³)	Glucose[a] (mg/dL)	Protein[a] (mg/dL)
Naidoo[573] (1968)	135	1	12 (0-42)	7 (0-26)	48 (38-64)	73 (40-148)
	20	7	3 (0-9)	2 (0-5)	55 (48-62)	47 (27-65)
Sarff et al.[574] (1976)	87	Most < 7	8.2 ± 7.1 Median 5 (0-32)	61	52 (34-119)	90 (20-170)
Bonadio et al.[575] (1992)	35	0-4 wk	11.0 ± 10.4 Median 8.5	0.4 ± 1.4 Median 0.15	46 ± 10.3	84 ± 45.1
	40	4-8 wk	7.1 ± 9.2 Median 4.5	0.2 ± 0.4 Median 0	46 ± 10.0	59 ± 25.3
Ahmed et al.[576] (1996)	108	0-30	7.3 ± 13.9 Median 4	0.8 ± 6.2 Median 0	51.2 ± 12.9	64.2 ± 24.2

[a]Expressed as mean with range (number in parentheses) or ± standard deviation unless otherwise specified.
Data from Ahmed A, Hickey S, Ehrett S, et al. Cerebrospinal fluid values in the term neonate. Pediatr Infect Dis J 15:298, 1996.

Table 6–17 Hematologic and Chemical Characteristics of Cerebrospinal Fluid in Healthy Very Low Birth Weight Infants

Birth Weight (g)	Age (days)	No. of Samples	Red Blood Cells (mm³) Mean (Range)	White Blood Cells (mm³) Mean (Range)	Polymorphonuclear Leukocytes (%) Mean (Range)	Glucose (mg/dL) Mean (Range)	Protein (mg/dL) Mean (Range)
<1000	0-7	6	335 (0-1780)	3 (1-8)	11 (0-50)	70 (41-89)	162 (115-222)
	8-28	17	1465 (0-19,050)	4 (0-14)	8 (0-66)	68 (33-217)	159 (95-370)
	29-84	15	808 (0-6850)	4 (0-11)	2 (0-36)	49 (29-90)	137 (76-260)
1000-1500	0-7	8	407 (0-2450)	4 (1-10)	4 (0-28)	74 (50-96)	136 (85-176)
	8-28	14	1101 (0-9750)	7 (0-44)	10 (0-60)	59 (39-109)	137 (54-227)
	29-84	11	661 (0-3800)	8 (0-23)	11 (0-48)	47 (31-76)	122 (45-187)

Data from Rodriguez AF, Kaplan SL, Mason EO. Cerebrospinal fluid values in the very low birth weight infant. J Pediatr 116:971, 1990.

study by Ahmed and colleagues[576] included in the definition of *normal* the absence of viral infection defined by lack of evidence of cytopathic effect in five cell lines and negative polymerase chain reaction for enteroviruses. None of the studies included information about the health of the infant after the newborn period. It now is recognized that infants with congenital infections, such as rubella, cytomegalovirus infection, toxoplasmosis, acquired immunodeficiency syndrome, and syphilis, can have no signs of illness during the newborn period. Observations of these infants over the course of months or years can reveal abnormalities that are inapparent at birth. Until more data are available, it would appear prudent to observe carefully infants with white blood cells in excess of 20 per mm³ or a protein level in excess of 100 mg/dL in the CSF and, if clinical signs indicate, to obtain paired serum samples for serologic assays and viral cultures from body fluids or tissues for congenital central nervous system infections (i.e., *T. gondii*, rubella virus, cytomegalovirus, herpes simplex virus, human immunodeficiency virus, and *T. pallidum*).

In newborns with bacterial meningitis, there can be thousands of white blood cells in the CSF, and polymorphonuclear leukocytes predominate early in the course of the disease.[38,574] The number of white blood cells in the CSF can vary greatly in infants with both gram-negative and gram-positive meningitis. The median number of cells per cubic millimeter in the CSF of 98 infants with gram-negative meningitis was more than 2000 (range, 6 to 40,000), whereas the median number of cells per cubic millimeter in 21 infants with group B streptococcal meningitis was less than 100 (range, 8 to >10,000).[574] The concentration of glucose in CSF usually is less than two thirds of the concentration in blood. The concentration of protein can be low (<30 mg/dL) or very high (>1000 mg/dL). CSF parameters observed in the healthy term neonate can overlap with those observed in the infant with meningitis.

A Gram-stain smear of CSF should be examined for bacteria, and appropriate media should be inoculated with the CSF specimen. Sarff and colleagues[574] detected organisms in Gram-stain smears of CSF in 83% of infants with group B streptococcal meningitis and in 78% of those with gram-negative meningitis. After initiation of appropriate antimicrobial therapy, gram-positive bacteria usually clear from the CSF within 36 hours, whereas in some patients with meningitis caused by gram-negative enteric bacilli cultures can remain positive for many days.[581]

Microorganisms can be isolated from CSF that has normal white blood cell and chemistry test values. Visser and Hall[571] reported normal CSF parameters (cell count < 25; protein level < 200 mg/dL) in 6 (15%) of 39 infants with culture-proven meningitis. Subsequent examination of the CSF identified an increase in the number of cells and in the protein level. Presumably, the initial lumbar puncture was performed early in the course of meningitis before an inflammatory response occurred. Other investigators reported isolation of enterovirus[583] and *S. pneumoniae*[584] from the CSF of neonates in the absence of pleocytosis.

Identification of bacteremia without meningitis defined by the absence of pleocytosis or isolation of a pathogen from culture of CSF can be followed by meningeal inflammation on subsequent examinations. Sarman and colleagues[585] identified six infants with gram-negative bacteremia and initial normal CSF who developed evidence of meningeal inflammation 18 to 59 hours after the first examination. Although the investigators suggest that a diagnosis of gram-negative bacteremia in the neonate warrants repeat lumbar puncture to identify the optimal duration of therapy, this recommendation could be broadened to include all infants with bacteremia and initial negative studies of CSF. Dissemination of the organisms from the blood to the meninges can occur after the first lumbar puncture before sterilization of the blood by appropriate antimicrobial therapy occurs. This is especially likely to occur in neonates with intense bacteremia where sterilization by β-lactam agents (i.e., third-generation cephalosporins) is inoculum dependent.

Investigators have sought a sensitive and specific CSF metabolic determinant of bacterial meningitis with little success. Among products that have been evaluated and found to be inadequate to distinguish bacterial meningitis from other neurologic disease (including cerebroventricular hemorrhage and asphyxia) are γ-aminobutyric acid,[586] lactate dehydrogenase,[587] and creatine kinase brain isoenzyme.[588] Cyclic-3′,5′-adenosine monophosphate was elevated in the CSF of neonates with bacterial meningitis compared with the CSF of infants who had nonbacterial meningitis or a control group.[589] Elevated CSF concentrations of C-reactive protein have been reported for infants older than 4 weeks with bacterial meningitis[590,591]; however, the test was found to be of no value in neonates.[591,592] Current investigations of the pro-inflammatory cytokines interleukin-6 and interleukin-8 indicate that there is a cytokine response in the CSF after birth asphyxia and that these assays are not useful in detecting the infant with meningitis.[593,594]

THE TRAUMATIC LUMBAR PUNCTURE

A traumatic lumbar puncture can result in blood in the CSF and can complicate the interpretation of the results for CSF white blood cell count and chemistries. Schwersenski and colleagues[563] found that 13.8% of 712 CSF specimens obtained during the first week of life were bloody and that an additional 14.5% were considered inadequate for testing.

If the total number of white blood cells compared with the number of red blood cells exceeds the value for whole blood, the presence of CSF pleocytosis is suggested. Some investigators have found that the observed white blood cell counts in bloody CSF were lower than would be predicted based on the ratio of white-to-red blood cells in peripheral blood; the white blood cells lyse more rapidly than red blood cells, or the number of white blood cells is decreased for other reasons.[595-598] Several formulas have been used in an attempt to interpret cytologic findings in CSF contaminated by blood.[599-601] However, none of the corrections applied to bloody CSF can be used with confidence for excluding meningitis in the neonate.[602-604]

Protein in CSF usually is elevated after a traumatic lumbar puncture because of the presence of red blood cells. It has been estimated in older children and adults that an increase of 1 mg/dL in CSF protein occurs for every 1000 red blood cells/μL. The concentration of glucose does not appear to be altered by blood from a traumatic lumbar puncture; a low CSF glucose concentration should be considered an important finding even when associated with a traumatic lumbar puncture.

Because a "bloody tap" is difficult to interpret, it can be valuable to repeat the lumbar puncture 24 to 48 hours later. If the results of the second lumbar puncture reveal a normal white blood cell count, bacterial meningitis can be excluded. Even if performed without trauma or apparent bleeding, CSF occasionally can be ambiguous because white blood cells can be elicited by the irritant effect of blood in the CSF.

BRAIN ABSCESS

Brain abscess is a rare entity in the neonate, usually complicating meningitis caused by certain gram-negative bacilli. The CSF in the infant with a brain abscess can demonstrate a pleocytosis of a few hundred cells with a mononuclear predominance and an elevated protein level. Bacteria may not be seen by Gram stain of the CSF if meningitis is not present. Sudden clinical deterioration and the appearance of many cells (>1000 per mm^3), with a majority of polymorphonuclear cells, suggest rupture of the abscess into the CSF.

Laboratory Aids

Laboratory aids in the diagnosis of systemic and focal infection in the neonate include peripheral white blood cell and differential counts, platelet counts, acute-phase reactants, blood chemistries, histopathology of the placenta and umbilical cord, smears of gastric or tracheal aspirates, and diagnostic imaging studies. New assays for diagnosis of early-onset sepsis, including serum concentrations of neutrophil CD 11b,[605] granulocyte colony-stimulating factor,[606] interleukin receptor antagonist,[607] interleukin-6,[607-610] and procalcitonin,[611-613] show promise for increased sensitivity and specificity compared with other laboratory assessments, such as white blood cell count, absolute neutrophil count, and acute-phase reactants. However, pro-inflammatory cytokines, including interleukin-1 and interleukin-6 and tumor necrosis factor-α, have been identified in serum and CSF in infants after perinatal asphyxia, raising doubts about the specificity of some of these markers.[593,594,614,615] Mehr and Doyle[616] review the recent literature on cytokines as aids in the diagnosis of neonatal bacterial sepsis. These assays and procedures are discussed in detail in Chapter 36.

MANAGEMENT

If the maternal history or infant clinical signs suggest the possibility of neonatal sepsis, blood and CSF (all infants) and cultures of urine and other clinically evident focal sites should be collected (all infants with suspected late-onset infection). If respiratory abnormalities are apparent or respiratory status has changed, a radiograph of the chest should be performed. Because the clinical manifestations of sepsis can be subtle, the progression of the disease can be rapid, and the mortality rate remains high when compared with that for older infants with serious bacterial infection, empirical treatment should be initiated promptly. Many infants who have a clinical course typical of bacterial sepsis are treated empirically because of the imperfect sensitivity of a single blood culture in the diagnosis of sepsis.

Choice of Antimicrobial Agents

Initial Therapy for Presumed Sepsis

The choice of antimicrobial agents for the treatment of suspected sepsis is based on knowledge of the prevalent organisms responsible for neonatal sepsis by age of onset and hospital setting as well as on their patterns of antimicrobial susceptibility. Initial therapy for the infant who develops clinical signs of sepsis during the first few days of life (early-onset disease) must include agents active against gram-positive cocci, particularly group B *Streptococcus*, other streptococci, and *L. monocytogenes*, and gram-negative enteric bacilli. Treatment of the infant who becomes septic while in the nursery after age 6 days (late-onset disease) must include therapy for hospital-acquired organisms, such as *S. aureus*, gram-negative enteric bacilli, CoNS (in the VLBW infant), and occasionally *P. aeruginosa*, as well as for maternally acquired etiologic agents.

Group B streptococci continue to demonstrate uniform in vitro susceptibility to penicillins and cephalosporins. In a study of 231 isolates of group B streptococci from patients with invasive infection, all strains were killed by concentrations of penicillin G of less than 0.25 μg/mL.[617] Ampicillin, the penicillinase-resistant penicillins, and third-generation cephalosporins also are active in vitro but aminoglycosides are relatively inactive. In vitro studies[618-620] and experimental animal models of bacteremia,[621,622] however, indicate that the bactericidal activity of ampicillin and penicillin against group B streptococci and *L. monocytogenes* is enhanced by the addition of gentamicin (synergy). Some physicians prefer to continue the combination of ampicillin and gentamicin for 48 to 72 hours, but once group B *Streptococcus* is identified as the etiologic agent, the drug of choice for therapy is penicillin administered intravenously for the remainder of the treatment regimen. There are no clinical data to indicate that continuing an aminoglycoside in combination with a penicillin results in more rapid recovery or improved outcome for infected neonates (see Chapter 13).

Most strains of *S. aureus* that cause disease in neonates produce β-lactamase and are resistant to penicillin G and ampicillin. Many of these organisms are susceptible to the penicillinase-resistant penicillins, such as nafcillin, and to first-generation cephalosporins. Methicillin-resistant staphylococci that are resistant to other penicillinase-resistant penicillins and cephalosporins have been encountered in many nurseries in the United States. Antimicrobial susceptibility patterns must be monitored by surveillance of staphylococcal strains causing infection and disease in each neonatal intensive care unit. Bacterial resistance must be considered whenever staphylococcal disease is suspected or confirmed in a patient, and empirical vancomycin therapy should be initiated until the susceptibility pattern of the organism is known. Virtually all staphylococcal strains isolated from neonates have been susceptible to vancomycin. Synergistic activity is provided by the combination of an aminoglycoside (see Chapter 17). Vancomycin- or glycopeptide-resistant *S. aureus* has been reported from Japan and the United States, but none of these strains has been isolated from neonates.

CoNS can cause systemic infection in VLBW infants and in neonates with or without devices such as an intravascular catheter or a ventriculoperitoneal shunt. Vancomycin is the drug of choice for treatment of serious CoNS infections. If daily cultures from an indwelling device continue to grow CoNS, removal of the foreign material probably will be necessary to cure the infection.

Group D streptococci vary in their susceptibility to penicillins. Nonenterococcal strains, including *S. bovis*, are highly susceptible to penicillin, but *Enterococcus* species are only moderately susceptible to penicillin and highly resistant to cephalosporins. Optimal antimicrobial therapy for neonatal infections caused by *Enterococcus* includes ampicillin or vancomycin in addition to an aminoglycoside, typically gentamicin or tobramycin.

L. monocytogenes is susceptible to penicillin and ampicillin and resistant to cephalosporins. Ampicillin is the preferred agent for treating *L. monocytogenes*, although an aminoglycoside can be continued in combination with ampicillin if the patient has meningitis. Specific management of *L. monocytogenes* infection is discussed in Chapter 14.

The choice of antibiotic therapy for infections caused by gram-negative bacilli depends on the pattern of susceptibility for these isolates in the nursery that cares for the neonate. These patterns vary by hospital or community and by time within the same institution or community. Although isolates from neonates should be monitored to determine the emergence of new strains with unique antimicrobial susceptibility patterns, the general pattern of antibiotic susceptibility in the hospital is a good guide to initial therapy for neonates. The aminoglycosides, including gentamicin, tobramycin, netilmicin, and amikacin, are highly active in vitro against virtually all isolates of *E. coli*, *P. aeruginosa*, and *Enterobacter*, *Klebsiella*, and *Proteus* species.

Role of Third-Generation Cephalosporins

The third-generation cephalosporins, cefotaxime, ceftriaxone, and ceftazidime, possess attractive features for therapy for bacterial sepsis and meningitis in newborns. These features include excellent in vitro activity against group B streptococci and *E. coli* and other gram-negative enteric bacilli. Ceftazidime is highly active in vitro against *P. aeruginosa*. None of the cephalosporins is active against *L. monocytogenes* or *Enterococcus*, and activity against *S. aureus* is variable. These cephalosporins provide concentrations of drug at most sites of infection that greatly exceed the minimum inhibitory concentrations of susceptible pathogens, and there is no dose-related toxicity. Clinical and microbiologic results of studies of sepsis and meningitis in neonates suggest that the third-generation cephalosporins are comparable to the traditional regimens of penicillin and an aminoglycoside (see Chapter 37).[623-626] Because ceftriaxone can displace bilirubin from serum albumin, it is not recommended for use in neonates unless it is the only agent effective against the bacterial pathogen.

The rapid development of resistance of gram-negative enteric bacilli when cefotaxime is used extensively for presumptive therapy for neonatal sepsis suggests that extensive use of third or fourth-generation cephalosporins can lead to rapid emergence of drug-resistant bacteria in nurseries.[627] Empirical use of cefotaxime in neonates should be restricted to those with evidence of meningitis or with gram-negative sepsis. Continued cefotaxime therapy should be limited to those infants with gram-negative meningitis caused by susceptible organisms or those with ampicillin-resistant enteric infections.[628]

Current Practice

The combination of ampicillin and an aminoglycoside, usually gentamicin or tobramycin, is suitable for initial treatment of presumed early-onset neonatal sepsis.[629] If there is a concern for endemic or epidemic staphylococcal infection, typically occurring beyond 6 days of age, the initial treatment of late-onset neonatal sepsis should include vancomycin.

The increasing use of antibiotics, particularly in neonatal intensive care units, can result in alterations in antimicrobial susceptibility patterns of bacteria and can necessitate changes in initial empirical therapy. This alteration of the microbial flora in nurseries where the use of broad-spectrum antimicrobial agents is routine supports recommendations from the CDC for the judicious use of antibiotics. The hospital laboratory must regularly monitor isolates of pathogenic bacteria to assist the physician in choosing the most appropriate therapy. The clinical pharmacology and dosage schedules of the various antimicrobial agents considered for neonatal sepsis are provided in Chapter 37.

Continuation of Therapy When Results of Cultures Are Available

The choice of antimicrobial therapy should be reevaluated when results of cultures and susceptibility tests become available. The duration of therapy depends on the initial response to the appropriate antibiotics but should be 10 days, with sepsis documented by positive culture of blood and minimal or absent focal infection. The usual duration of therapy for infants with meningitis caused by gram-negative enteric bacilli is 21 days. However, in complicated cases of meningitis caused by gram-negative enteric bacilli, group B streptococci, or other pathogens, the duration of therapy is variable and is best determined in consultation with an infectious diseases specialist.

The third-generation cephalosporins cefotaxime, ceftriaxone, and ceftazidime have important theoretical advantages for treatment of sepsis or meningitis compared with therapeutic regimens that include an aminoglycoside. Unlike the aminoglycosides, third-generation cephalosporins are not associated with ototoxicity and nephrotoxicity. However, little toxicity from aminoglycosides occurs when use is brief or, when continued for the duration of therapy, if serum trough levels are maintained at less than 2 μg/mL. Because cephalosporins have no dose-related toxicity, measurements of serum concentrations, obligatory with the use of aminoglycosides beyond 72 hours or in infants with renal insufficiency, are unnecessary. However, routine use of the cephalosporins for presumptive sepsis therapy in neonates often leads to problems with drug-resistant enteric organisms. Extensive use of the third-generation cephalosporins in the nursery could result in the emergence of resistance caused by de-repression of chromosomally mediated β-lactamases.[630] Cefotaxime is preferred to other third-generation cephalosporins for use in neonates because it has been used more extensively[624-626,631] and because it does not affect the binding of bilirubin.[630,632] Ceftazidime in combination with an aminoglycoside should be used in therapy for *P. aeruginosa* meningitis because of its excellent in vitro activity and its good penetration into the CSF. Use of ceftriaxone in the neonate should be determined on a case-by-case basis because of its ability to displace bilirubin from serum albumin and result in biliary sludging.

Management of the Infant Whose Mother Received Intrapartum Antimicrobial Agents

Antimicrobial agents commonly are administered to women in labor who have risk factors associated with sepsis in the fetus, including premature delivery, prolonged rupture of membranes, fever, or other signs of chorioamnionitis or group B streptococcal colonization. Antimicrobial agents cross the placenta and achieve concentrations in fetal tissues that are parallel to concentrations achieved in other well-vascularized organs. Placental transport of antibiotics is discussed in more detail in Chapter 37.

Protocols for prevention of group B streptococcal infection in the newborn by administration of a penicillin to the mother were published in 1992 by ACOG[633] and the American Academy of Pediatrics (AAP).[634] These guidelines were revised in 1996 by the CDC,[635] in 1997 by the AAP,[636] and in 2002 by the CDC,[637] AAP, and ACOG.[504] Recent data suggest that nearly 50% of women receive intrapartum chemoprophylaxis because of the presence of one or more risk factors for neonatal sepsis or because of a positive antenatal screening culture for group B *Streptococcus*.[638]

When ampicillin or penicillin is administered to the mother, drug concentrations are achieved in the fetus that are more than 30% of the concentrations in the blood of the mother.[639] Concentrations of penicillin, ampicillin, and cefazolin that are bactericidal for group B streptococci are achieved in the amniotic fluid approximately 3 hours after completion of a maternal intravenous dose. Parenteral antibiotic therapy administered to a mother with signs of chorioamnionitis in labor essentially is treating the fetus early in the course of the intrapartum infection.[640,641] However, for some infected fetuses, the treatment administered in utero is insufficient to prevent signs of early-onset group B streptococcal disease. Although maternal intrapartum prophylaxis has been associated with a 75% decrease in the incidence of early-onset group B streptococcal disease since 1993,[641,642] the regimen has had no impact on the incidence of late-onset disease.[643]

The various algorithms prepared to guide empirical management of the neonate born to a mother with risk factors for group B streptococcal disease who received intrapartum antimicrobial prophylaxis for prevention of early-onset group B streptococcal disease focus on three clinical scenarios[504,637,644,645]:

1. Infants who have signs of sepsis should receive a full diagnostic evaluation and should be treated, typically with ampicillin and gentamicin, until laboratory studies are available.

2. Infants born at 35 or more weeks' gestation who appear healthy and whose mothers received intrapartum prophylaxis with penicillin, ampicillin, or cefazolin for 4 or more hours before delivery do not have to be evaluated or treated but should be observed in the hospital for 48 hours.

3. Infants who are less than 35 weeks' gestation who appear healthy and whose mothers received penicillin, ampicillin, or cefazolin for less than 4 hours before delivery should receive a limited evaluation, including a blood culture and a complete blood cell count with a differential count, and be observed for 48 hours in the hospital. The same management probably is necessary for infants of any gestation whose mothers received vancomycin for prophylaxis because nothing is known about the amniotic fluid penetration of this drug or its efficacy in preventing early-onset group B streptococcal disease.

The first two clinical scenarios are readily identified, but the third category often leads to controversy regarding optimal management. Recent recommendations for prevention and treatment of early-onset group B streptococcal infection are discussed in detail in Chapter 13.

Management of the infant born to a mother who received an antimicrobial agent within hours of delivery must include consideration of the effect of the drug on cultures obtained from the infant after birth. Intrapartum therapy provides some treatment of the infant in utero, and variable concentrations of drug will be present in the infant's body fluids. If the infant is infected and the bacterial pathogen is susceptible to the drug administered to the mother, cultures of the infant can be sterile despite a clinical course suggesting sepsis.

Treatment of the Infant Whose Bacterial Culture Results Are Negative

Whether or not the mother received antibiotics before delivery, the physician must decide on the subsequent course of therapy for the infant who was treated for presumed sepsis and whose bacterial culture results are negative. If the neonate appears to be well and there is reason to believe that infection was unlikely, treatment can be discontinued at 48 hours. If the clinical condition of the infant remains uncertain and suspicion of an infectious process remains, therapy should be continued as outlined for documented bacterial sepsis unless another diagnosis becomes apparent. Significant bacterial infection can occur without bacteremia. Squire and colleagues[646] found that results of premortem blood cultures were negative in 7 (18%) of 39 infants with unequivocal infection at autopsy. Some infants with significant systemic bacterial infection may not be identified by the usual single blood culture technique. The physician must consider this limitation when determining length of empirical therapy. However, if treatment for infection is deemed necessary, parenteral administration for 10 days is recommended.

Management of the Infant with Catheter-Associated Infection

Investigators in Connecticut found that multiple catheters, low birth weight, low gestational age at birth, and low Apgar scores were significant risk factors for late-onset sepsis.[525] Benjamin and colleagues[526] reported a retrospective study at Duke University from 1995 to 1999 of all neonates who had central venous access. The goal of the Duke study was to evaluate the relationship between central venous catheter removal and outcome in bacteremic neonates. Infants bacteremic with *S. aureus* or a gram-negative rod who had their catheter retained beyond 24 hours had a 10-fold higher rate of infection-related complications than those in whom the central catheter was removed promptly. Compared with neonates who had three or fewer positive intravascular catheter blood cultures for coagulase-negative staphylococci, neonates who had four consecutive positive blood cultures were at significantly increased risk for end-organ damage and death. In neonates with central venous catheter-associated infection, prompt removal of the device is advised unless there is rapid clinical improvement and sterilization of blood cultures after initiation of therapy.

Treatment of Neonatal Meningitis

Because the pathogens responsible for neonatal meningitis are largely the same as those that cause neonatal sepsis, initial therapy and subsequent therapy are similar. Meningitis caused by gram-negative enteric bacilli can pose special management problems. Eradication of the pathogen often is delayed, and serious complications can occur.[44,119,388,631] The persistence of gram-negative bacilli in CSF despite bactericidal levels of the antimicrobial agent led to the evaluation of lumbar intrathecal[647] and intraventricular[648] gentamicin. Mortality and morbidity were not significantly different in infants who received parenteral drug alone or parenteral plus intrathecal therapy.[647] The study of the intraventricular gentamicin was stopped early because of the high mortality in the parenteral plus intraventricular therapy group.[648]

Feigin and colleagues[629] provide a review of the management of meningitis in children, including neonates. Ampicillin or penicillin G, initially with an aminoglycoside, are appropriate antimicrobial agents for treating infection caused by group B streptococci. Cefotaxime has superior in vitro and in vivo bactericidal activity against many microorganisms.[624] Treatment of enteric gram-negative bacillary meningitis should include cefotaxime and an aminoglycoside until results of susceptibility testing are known.

If meningitis develops in a low-birth-weight infant who has been in the nursery for a prolonged period or in a neonate who has received previous courses of antimicrobial therapy for presumed sepsis, alternative empirical antibiotic regimens should be considered. Enterococci and antibiotic-resistant, gram-negative enteric bacilli are potential pathogens in these settings. A combination of vancomycin, an aminoglycoside, and cefotaxime may be appropriate. Ceftazidime in addition to an aminoglycoside should be considered for *P. aeruginosa* meningitis.

Other antibiotics may be necessary for the treatment of highly resistant organisms. Meropenem,[649] ciprofloxacin,[650-652] or trimethoprim-sulfamethoxazole[270,653] can be the only antimicrobial agents active in vitro against bacteria that are highly resistant to broad-spectrum β-lactam antibiotics or aminoglycosides. Some of these drugs require careful monitoring because of toxicity to the newborn (see Chapter 37), and ciprofloxacin has not been approved for use in the United

Table 6–18 Infectious and Noninfectious Causes of Aseptic Meningitis[a] in the Neonate

Cause	Disease
Infectious agent	
Bacteria	Partially treated meningitis
	Parameningeal focus (brain or epidural abscess)
	Tuberculosis
Viruses	Herpes simplex meningoencephalitis
	Cytomegalovirus
	Enteroviruses
	Rubella
	Acquired immunodeficiency syndrome
	Lymphocytic choriomeningitis
	Varicella
Spirochetes	Syphilis
	Lyme disease
Parasites	Toxoplasmosis
	Chagas' disease
Mycoplasma	*Mycoplasma hominis* infection
	Ureaplasma urealyticum infection
Fungi	Candidiasis
	Coccidioidomycosis
	Cryptococcosis
Noninfectious causes	
Trauma	Subarachnoid hemorrhage
	Traumatic lumbar puncture
Malignancy	Teratoma
	Medulloblastoma
	Choroid plexus papilloma and carcinoma

[a]*Aseptic meningitis* is defined as meningitis in the absence of evidence of bacterial pathogen detectable in cerebrospinal fluid by usual laboratory techniques.

States in infants younger than 3 months. Definitive treatment of meningitis caused by gram-negative enteric bacilli should be determined by in vitro susceptibility tests, and assistance from an infectious diseases specialist can be helpful.

If cultures of blood and CSF for bacterial pathogens by usual laboratory techniques are negative in the neonate with meningitis, the differential diagnosis of aseptic meningitis must be reviewed, particularly in view of diagnosing treatable infections (Table 6-18).

Management of the Infant with a Brain Abscess

If purulent foci or abscesses are present, they should be drained. However, some brain abscesses resolve with medical therapy alone.[388,654] Brain abscesses can be polymicrobial or result from organisms that uncommonly cause meningitis such as *Citrobacter,*[141,143] *Enterobacter,*[128] *Proteus,*[388] and *Salmonella* species.[652] Aspiration of the abscess provides identification of the pathogens to guide rational antimicrobial therapy.

Treatment of the Infant with Meningitis Whose Bacterial Culture Results Are Negative

In the absence of a detectable bacterial pathogen, an aggressive diagnostic approach is necessary for the infant with meningitis, defined by CSF pleocytosis and variable changes in the concentration of CSF protein and glucose. The most frequent cause of aseptic or nontuberculous bacterial meningitis in the neonate is prior antimicrobial therapy resulting in negative blood and CSF cultures. Congenital infections need to be excluded. Treatable diseases, such as partially treated bacterial disease, meningoencephalitis due to herpes simplex virus, syphilis, cytomegalovirus, toxoplasmosis, Lyme disease in regions where *Borrelia* is prevalent, tuberculosis, and malignancy, need to be considered in the differential diagnosis. The history of illness and contacts in the mother and family and epidemiologic features, such as animal exposures and recent travel, should be explored. Reexamination of the infant for focal signs of disease, including special techniques such as ophthalmologic examination, and consideration of appropriate diagnostic imaging studies of the long bones, skull, and brain can provide further information in determining the source of infection. Treatment of possible bacterial or nonbacterial causes of aseptic meningitis may be necessary before the results of culture, polymerase chain reaction, or serology tests are available to indicate the diagnosis.

Treatment of Anaerobic Infections

The importance of anaerobic bacteria as a cause of serious neonatal infection is uncertain. *Clostridium, Peptococcus,* and *Peptostreptococcus* are highly sensitive to penicillin G, but *B. fragilis* sp. usually are resistant. If anaerobic organisms are known or suspected to be responsible for infection (as in peritonitis), initiating therapy with a clinically appropriate agent, such as clindamycin, metronidazole, ticarcillin, or piperacillin, is warranted.

Adjunctive Therapies for Treatment of Neonatal Sepsis

Despite appropriate antimicrobial and optimal supportive therapy, mortality rates resulting from neonatal sepsis remain high, especially for the VLBW infant. With the hope of improving survival and decreasing the severity of sequelae in survivors, investigators have considered adjunctive modes of treatment, including granulocyte transfusion, exchange transfusion, and the use of standard intravenous immune globulin or pathogen-specific polyclonal or monoclonal antibody reagents for deficits in neonatal host defenses. These therapies are discussed in further detail in Chapters 4 and 13. Pentoxifylline has been documented to reduce plasma tumor necrosis factor-α concentrations in premature infants with sepsis and to improve survival, but the number of infants treated (five of five survived) and number of controls (one of four survived) was too small to provide more than a suggestion of efficacy.[655] In neutropenic infants with sepsis, the administration of granulocyte colony-stimulating factor and human granulocyte-macrophage colony-stimulating factor have had variable effects on outcome.[656-659] Although the results of selected studies indicate that some of these techniques improved survival, the potential adverse effects (e.g., graft-versus-host reaction, pulmonary leukocyte sequestration) are sufficiently concerning to warrant further study in experimental protocols.

Human immunoglobulin preparations for intravenous administration (IGIV) have been assessed for adjunctive therapy for neonatal sepsis based on the hypothesis that infected infants lack circulating antibodies against bacterial pathogens and that IGIV can provide some antibody for protection. Hill[660] reviewed four clinical trials and reported a mortality rate of 15% (9 of 60) in untreated infants and 3% (2 of 59) in IGIV-treated infants. A meta-analysis of studies of IGIV for the treatment of neonates with sepsis showed a sixfold decrease in the mortality rate in infants who received IGIV in addition to standard therapies.[661] In contrast, Noya[662] concluded that IGIV has not been demonstrated conclusively to be effective in the treatment of neonatal sepsis. A multicenter randomized placebo-controlled trial of IGIV therapy for neonatal sepsis in infants with a birth weight greater than 1000 g showed no difference in mortality between the IGIV-treated and untreated groups.[663]

PROGNOSIS

Before the advent of antibiotics, almost all infants with neonatal sepsis died.[5] Dunham[2] reported that physicians used various treatments, including "erysipelas serum" and transfusions, without altering the course of the disease. The introduction of sulfonamides and penicillin and later introduction of broad-spectrum antibiotics such as chloramphenicol and streptomycin decreased the mortality rate to about 60%.[3,5] During this period, some infants undoubtedly died because of treatment with high dosages of chloramphenicol, which can cause cardiovascular collapse (i.e., gray baby syndrome).

The introduction of the aminoglycosides, first with kanamycin in the early 1960s and gentamicin late in that decade, vastly improved therapy for bacteremia due to gram-negative organisms, the leading cause of sepsis at that time.[664] These therapies, together with an improved understanding of neonatal physiology and advances in life-support systems, combined to result in a steady decrease in neonatal mortality in the United States[664] and in Europe[21,24,665,666] during the period from 1960 to 1985. Mortality rates for sepsis, including infants of all weights and gestational ages, decreased from 40% to 50% in the 1960s[4,664,665,667] to 10% to 20% in the 1970s and 1980s.[20,21,24,468,469,664,666] Population-based surveillance of selected counties in the United States conducted by the CDC from 1993 to 1998 reported 2196 cases of neonatal sepsis due to group B *Streptococcus*, of which 92 (4%) were fatal.[644]

The postnatal age at which infection occurs, once thought to be of prognostic significance, has become less important within the past 2 decades. Fulminant sepsis, with signs of illness present at birth or during the first day of life, has a high mortality rate, varying from 14% to 20%[21,31,330,662] to as high as 70%.[667] However, when infections occurring during the first 24 hours of life, most of which are caused by group B *Streptococcus*, are excluded from the analysis, the percentage of deaths due to early-onset sepsis does not differ significantly from that associated with late-onset infection.[20,21,24,96,469,664,665] Mortality from sepsis is higher for preterm than for term infants in virtually all published studies[7,16,20,21,24,31,468,469] but is approximately the same for all major bacterial pathogens[20,24] (see Tables 6-4 and 6-5).

In recent surveys, the mortality rate for neonatal meningitis has declined from 25%[20,42,666,668] to 10% to 15%.[31,44,45,669,670] This decrease represents a significant improvement from prior years, when studies reported a case-fatality rate of more than 30%.[39,455,647,648,671] Mortality is greater among preterm than term infants.[31,44,45,497,672]

Significant sequelae develop in 17% to 60% of infants who survive neonatal meningitis caused by gram-negative enteric bacilli or group B streptococci.[44,666,668,673-675] These sequelae include mental and motor disabilities, convulsive disorders, hydrocephalus, hearing loss, and abnormal speech patterns. The most extensive experience with the long-term observation of infants who had group B streptococcal meningitis as neonates was reported by Edwards and colleagues.[674] Sixty-one patients were treated between 1974 and 1979, and 21% died. Of the 38 survivors who were available for evaluation at 3 years of age or older, 29% had severe neurologic sequelae, 21% had minor deficits, and 50% were functioning normally. Presenting factors that were associated with death or severe disability included comatose or semicomatose state, decreased perfusion, total peripheral white blood cell count less than 5000/mm^3, absolute neutrophil count less than 1000/mm^3, and CSF protein level greater than 300 mg/dL. A comparable study evaluating 35 newborns over a period of 3 to 18 years demonstrated more favorable outcomes with 60% of survivors considered normal at the time of follow-up compared with sibling controls, 15% with mild to moderate neurologic residua, and 25% with major sequelae.[671] Franco and co-workers[672] reported the results of frequent and extensive neurologic, developmental, and psychometric assessments on a cohort of 10 group B streptococcal meningitis survivors followed for one to 14 years and found that one child had severe central nervous system damage, five children, including one with hydrocephalus, had mild academic or behavioral problems, and four children were normal.

The neurodevelopmental outcomes described for infants with gram-negative bacillary meningitis are similar to those reported for group B streptococcal meningitis. Unhanand and colleagues[44] reported findings from their 21-year experience with gram-negative meningitis at two hospitals in Dallas, Texas. Among 72 patients less than 28 days old at the onset of symptoms, there were 60 survivors, 43 of whom were followed and evaluated for a period of at least 6 months. Neurologic sequelae, occurring alone or in combination, were described in 56% and included hydrocephalus (≈30%), seizure disorder (≈30%), developmental delay (≈30%), cerebral palsy (25%), and hearing loss (15%). Forty-four percent of the survivors were developmentally normal at follow-up. Among infants with gram-negative bacillary meningitis, thrombocytopenia, CSF white blood cell count greater than 2000/mm^3, CSF protein greater than 200 mg/dL, CSF glucose–to–blood glucose ratio of less than 0.5, prolonged (>48 hours) positive CSF cultures, and elevated endotoxin and interleukin-1 concentrations in CSF were indicators of a poor outcome.[44,457,676] Investigators in England and Wales[670] found that independent predictors of adverse outcome 12 hours after admission were the presence of seizures, coma, ventilatory support, and leukopenia.

Computed tomography reveals a high incidence of central nervous system residua among newborns with meningitis. McCracken and colleagues[677] report that, among 44 infants with gram-negative bacillary meningitis, only 30% of computed tomographic scans were considered normal. Hydrocephalus was found in 20% of cases; areas of infarct, cerebritis, diffuse encephalomalacia, or cortical atrophy in 30%; brain abscess in about 20%; and subdural effusions in 7%. Two or more abnormalities were detected in about one third of infants.

The prognosis of brain abscess in the neonate is guarded because about one half of these children die, and sequelae such as hydrocephalus are common among survivors. Of 17 children who had brain abscess during the neonatal period and were followed for at least 2 years, only 4 had normal intellect and were free of seizures.[388] In neonates with brain abscess, the poor outcome probably is caused by destruction of brain parenchyma as a result of hemorrhagic infarcts and necrosis.

PREVENTION

Obstetric Factors

Improvement in the health of pregnant women with increased use of prenatal care facilities has led to lower rates of prematurity. Increased use of antenatal steroids in pregnant women with preterm labor and of surfactant in their infants has resulted in significantly fewer cases of respiratory distress syndrome. More appropriate management of prolonged interval after rupture of maternal membranes, maternal peripartum infections, and fetal distress has improved infant outcome. Because these factors are associated with sepsis in the newborn, improved care of the mother should decrease the incidence of neonatal infection. The development of neonatal intensive care expertise and units with appropriate equipment has resulted in the survival of VLBW infants. Increasingly, obstetric problems are anticipated, and mothers are transferred to medical centers with neonatal intensive care units before delivery.

Chemoprophylaxis

The use of antibiotics to prevent infection can be valuable when they are directed against specific microorganisms for a limited time. In the neonate, the use of silver nitrate eye drops or intramuscular ceftriaxone to prevent gonococcal ophthalmia, vaccination with bacillus Calmette-Guérin (BCG) or prophylactic use of isoniazid to reduce morbidity from tuberculosis in infants who must return to endemic areas, and use of hexachlorophene baths to prevent staphylococcal disease have been recognized as effective modes of chemoprophylaxis. The value of using antimicrobial agents against unknown pathogens in infants believed to be at high risk of infection or undergoing invasive procedures is uncertain. Studies of penicillin administered to the mother during labor for prevention of neonatal disease caused by group B streptococci are reviewed earlier and in Chapter 13.

Baier and colleagues[678] investigated daily administration of vancomycin for the prevention of CoNS bacteremia in low-birth-weight infants. Vancomycin was effective in reducing colonization and bacteremia when added to parenteral nutrition fluids for infants weighing 500 to 1500 g. Infants were randomized to receive vancomycin or no antibiotic for the duration of parenteral nutrition in a study blinded to the investigators. Nine infants in the control group developed bacteremia or fungemia, and one infant in the vancomycin-treated group developed candidemia. All invasive episodes occurred in infants weighing less than 1000 g, and there were no isolates of vancomycin-resistant strains of CoNS. Although the data suggest a beneficial effect for the vancomycin-treated infants, the number of patients studied was too small to verify this conclusion with adequate statistical power and this prophylactic regimen is not recommended.

Maternal Factors

The antiviral and antibacterial activity of human milk has been recognized for many years[679-682] and is discussed extensively in Chapter 5. Evidence that breast-feeding defends against neonatal sepsis and gram-negative meningitis was reported more than 30 years ago from Sweden.[683] Later studies carried out in Pakistan have shown that even partial breast-feeding appears to be protective among neonates in a resource-limited nation with a high neonatal mortality rate from clinical sepsis.[684] Breast-fed infants have a lower incidence of gastroenteritis, respiratory illness, and otitis media than those who are formula fed. A protective effect of breast-feeding against infections of the urinary tract also has been suggested.[685]

Observations that breast-feeding enhances lymphocyte responses to a purified protein derivative (PPD) of *M. tuberculosis* in infants given BCG vaccination at birth indicates that the effects of breast milk are not limited to those of an antibody-mediated mucosal protection.[686] The clinical significance of this increased specific cellular immune response during the first few weeks of life remains to be determined.

Immunoprophylaxis

The immaturity of the neonatal immune system is characterized by decreased levels of antibody against common pathogens; decreased complement activity, especially alternative pathway components; diminished polymorphonuclear leukocyte production, mobilization, and function; diminished T lymphocyte cytokine production to many antigens; and reduced concentrations of plasma and cell surface fibronectin.[660] Recognition of these factors has resulted in attempts at therapeutic intervention aimed specifically at each component of the deficient immune response.

Infants are protected from infection by passively transferred maternal IgG. To enhance the infant's ability to ward off severe infections, immunization of pregnant women and women in the childbearing years has been selectively adopted.[687,688] Programs to immunize pregnant women in resource limited countries with tetanus toxoid have markedly decreased the incidence of neonatal tetanus. Investigational programs for immunization of pregnant women with polysaccharide pneumococcal, *H. influenzae* type b and group B streptococcal vaccines aim to provide infants with protection in the first months of life. Studies of safety and immunogenicity of polysaccharide conjugate vaccines for group B streptococci show promise of a reduction in incidence of late-onset and early-onset disease in newborns.[689] Use of vaccines in pregnant women is discussed in Chapter 1.

Several clinical trials have explored the use of IGIV to correct the antibody deficiency of neonates, particularly very preterm newborns, and thereby reduce the incidence of sepsis. The results of these investigations were reviewed in 1993 by Hill.[660] Two of six studies indicated that IGIV reduced the incidence of late-onset infections, particularly those due to coagulase-negative staphylococci, but did not affect mortality. The remaining four studies failed to demonstrate any effect of IGIV on the incidence of late-onset sepsis, mortality, morbidity, or length of hospital stay. A meta-analysis performed in 1998 by Jenson and Pollack[661] found that prophylactic IGIV was of minimal but demonstrable benefit in preventing sepsis in premature, low-birth-weight infants. A recent prospective, randomized, placebo-controlled, multicenter trial found no effect of prophylactic IGIV on preventing sepsis when administered to neonates who were less than 33 weeks' gestation.[690] The use of hyperimmune IGIV preparations and human monoclonal antibodies to prevent specific infections (e.g., CoNS, *S. aureus*) in high-risk neonates is being explored.

Sidiropoulos and co-workers[691] studied the benefit of low-dose (12 g in 12 hours) or high-dose (24 g daily for 5 days) IGIV given to pregnant women at risk for preterm delivery because of chorioamnionitis. Cord blood IgG levels were doubled in infants older than 32 weeks' gestational age whose mothers received the higher dosage schedule but were unaffected in infants born earlier, suggesting little or no placental transfer of IGIV before the 32nd week of gestation. Among the infants delivered after 32 weeks, 6 (37%) of 16 born to untreated mothers developed clinical, laboratory, or radiologic evidence of infection and required antimicrobial therapy, whereas none of 7 infants born to treated mothers became infected. Although this study suggests that intrauterine fetal prophylaxis can be beneficial in selected cases, widespread use of IGIV for all women having premature onset of labor is not feasible because of timing before delivery, widespread shortages of IGIV, and cost.

The decreased number of circulating polymorphonuclear leukocytes and reduced myeloid reserves in the bone marrow of newborns have been ascribed to impaired production of cytokines, interleukin-3, granulocyte colony-stimulating factor, granulocyte-macrophage colony-stimulating factor, tumor necrosis factor-α, and interferon-γ.[692,693] Considerable experience with in vitro myeloid cell cultures and animal models[694,695] and with human trials[696] suggests that cytokine therapy can be an effective aid in preventing sepsis among newborns with hereditary or acquired congenital neutropenia. Treatment of a small number of infants with early signs of sepsis with pentoxifylline to reduce the concentrations of tumor necrosis factor-α showed promise,[655] but there are no studies that have used pentoxifylline for prevention of sepsis. Similarly, preliminary studies of granulocyte colony-stimulating factor in neonates are inconsistent in demonstrating that absolute neutrophil counts are increased or that the incidence of sepsis is reduced.[656,657,696]

Fibronectins are high-molecular-weight glycoproteins, produced primarily by the liver and endothelial cells, that facilitate cell-to-cell and cell-to-substrate adhesion.[697,698] They are involved in numerous functions, including hemostasis; vascular integrity; tissue repair; T lymphocyte activation; leukocyte migration, adhesion, and phagocytosis; and reticuloendothelial clearance. Plasma fibronectin concentrations in newborns are about one third to one half those of adults, and premature infants have levels significantly lower than those of term infants. These concentrations are further decreased in neonates with perinatal asphyxia, respiratory distress syndrome, and sepsis.[699] Studies in animal models and adults with sepsis suggest that fibronectin administration can be of value in improving host defenses and in reducing the risk of nosocomial infection in neonates.

Decontamination of Fomites

Because contamination of equipment poses a significant infectious challenge for the newborn, disinfection of all materials that are involved in the care of the newborn is an important responsibility of nursery personnel. The basic mechanisms of large pieces of equipment must be cleaned appropriately or replaced because they have been implicated in nursery epidemics. The use of disposable equipment and materials packaged in individual units, such as containers of sterile water for a nebulization apparatus, are important advances in the prevention of infection. The frequency of catheter-associated CoNS sepsis has led to attempts to prevent bacterial colonization of intravascular catheters through use of attachment-resistant polymeric materials, antibiotic impregnation, and immunotherapy directed against adherence factors.[700] These procedures are reviewed in Chapter 35.

Epidemiologic Surveillance

Endemic Infection

Nursery-acquired infections can become apparent days to several months after discharge of the infant. A surveillance system that provides information about infections within the nursery and involves follow-up of infants after discharge should be established. Various techniques can be used for surveillance and are reviewed in Chapter 35.

Epidemic Infection

The medical and nursing staff must be aware of the possibility of outbreaks or epidemics in the nursery. Prevention of disease is based on the level of awareness of personnel. Infection in previously well infants who lack high-risk factors associated with sepsis must be viewed with suspicion. Several cases of infection occurring within a brief period, caused by the same or an unusual pathogen, and occurring in close physical proximity should raise concern about the possibility of a nursery outbreak. Techniques for management of infection outbreaks in nurseries are discussed in Chapter 35.

SEPSIS IN THE NEWBORN RECENTLY DISCHARGED FROM THE HOSPITAL

When fever or other signs of systemic infection occur in the first weeks after the newborn is discharged from the nursery, appropriate management requires consideration of the possible sources of infection. Infection acquired at birth or from a household contact is the most likely cause. Congenital infection can be present with signs of disease that are detected after discharge. Late-onset infection from microorganisms acquired in the nursery can occur weeks or occasionally months after birth. Infection can occur after discharge because of underlying anatomic, physiologic, or metabolic abnormalities.

The newborn is susceptible to infectious agents that colonize or cause disease in other household members. If an infant whose gestation and delivery were uneventful is discharged from the nursery and develops signs of an infectious disease in the first weeks of life, the infection was probably acquired from someone in the infant's environment. Respiratory and gastrointestinal infections are common and can be accompanied by focal disease such as otitis media. A careful history of illnesses in household members can suggest the source of the infant's infection.

Congenital Infection

Signs of congenital infection can appear or be identified after discharge from the nursery. Hearing impairment caused by congenital rubella or cytomegalovirus infection can be noticed by a parent at home. Hydrocephalus with gradually increasing head circumference caused by congenital toxoplasmosis can be apparent only after serial physical examinations. Chorioretinitis, jaundice, or pneumonia can occur as late manifestations of congenital infection. A lumbar puncture may be performed in the course of a sepsis evaluation. CSF pleocytosis and increased protein concentration can be caused by congenital infection and warrant appropriate diagnostic studies.

Late-Onset Disease

Late-onset disease can present after the first week to months after birth as sepsis and meningitis or other focal infections. Group B *Streptococcus* (see Chapter 13) is the most frequent cause of late-onset sepsis in the neonate. Organisms acquired in the nursery also can cause late-onset disease. Skin and soft tissue lesions or other focal infections, including osteomyelitis and pneumonia from *S. aureus,* can occur weeks after birth. The pathogenesis of late-onset sepsis is obscure in many cases. The reason why an organism becomes invasive and causes sepsis or meningitis after colonizing the mucous membranes, skin, or upper respiratory, genitourinary, or gastrointestinal tracts remains obscure. Nosocomially acquired or health care–associated organisms are discussed in further detail in Chapter 35.

Infections in the Household

Infection can be associated with an underlying anatomic defect, physiologic abnormality, or metabolic disease. The infant who fails to thrive or presents with fever can have a urinary tract infection as the first indication of an anatomic abnormality. Infants with lacrimal duct stenosis or choanal atresia can develop focal infection. Sepsis caused by gram-negative enteric bacilli occurs frequently in infants with galactosemia (see "Pathogenesis").

The infected infant can be an important source of infection to family members. In one study in New York,[701] 12.6% of household contacts developed suppurative lesions during the 10-month period after introduction into the home of an infant with a staphylococcal lesion. The incidence of suppurative infections in household contacts of infants without lesions was less than 2%. Damato and co-workers[702] demonstrated colonization of neonates with enteric organisms possessing R factor–mediated resistance to kanamycin and persistence of these strains for more than 12 months after birth. During the period of observation, one third of the household contacts of the infants became colonized with the same strain.

Infections in infants have been associated with bites or licks from household pets. *Pasteurella multocida* is part of the oral flora of dogs, cats, and rodents. Meningitis caused by *P. multocida* was reported in seven infants younger than 2 months.[703] A 5-week-old infant with *P. multocida* meningitis frequently was licked by the family dog, and the organism was identified in cultures of the dog's mouth but not of the parents' throats. *P. multocida* meningitis in a 3-week-old infant may have resulted from transmission of the organism from the family cat to the mother and then to the infant.[704] The epidemiologic link between cats and dogs and infection in young infants suggests that parents should limit contact between pets and infants.

Fever in the First Month of Life

Reviews of fever in the first weeks of life indicate that elevation of temperature (>38.8° C [101.8° F])[705-712] is relatively uncommon. However, when fever occurs in the young infant, the incidence of severe disease, including sepsis, meningitis, and pneumonia, is sufficiently high to warrant careful evaluation and conservative management. A careful history of the pregnancy, delivery, nursery experience, interval since discharge from the nursery, and infections in the household should be obtained. Physical examination should establish the presence or absence of signs associated with congenital infection and late-onset diseases. Culture of blood and urine should be performed if no other focus is apparent, and culture of the CSF and a chest radiograph should be considered if the infant is believed to have systemic infection.

Practice guidelines prepared by Baraff and colleagues[705] for the management of infants and children with fever without source state that all febrile infants younger than 28 days should be hospitalized for parenteral antibiotic therapy. The group designated that a rectal temperature of 38.0° C (100.4° F) or higher should be used as the definition of fever. The sepsis evaluation includes a culture of blood, urine, and CSF; a complete blood cell and differential count; examination of CSF for cells, glucose, and protein; and a urinalysis.

Acknowledgment

Dr. S. Michael Marcy was a co-author of this chapter in the first four editions. The authors are indebted to Dr. Marcy for his continued interest in the preparation of this chapter.

REFERENCES

1. Gaynes RP, Edwards JR, Jarvis WR, et al. Nosocomial infections among neonates in high-risk nurseries in the United States. Pediatrics 93:357, 1996.
2. Dunham EC. Septicemia in the newborn. Am J Dis Child 45:229, 1933.

3. Nyhan WL, Fousek MD. Septicemia of the newborn. Pediatrics 22:268, 1958.
4. Gluck L, Wood HF, Fousek MD. Septicemia of the newborn. Pediatr Clin North Am 13:1131, 1966.
5. Freedman RM, Ingram DL, Cross I, et al. A half century of neonatal sepsis at Yale. Am J Dis Child 35:140, 1981.
6. Gladstone IM, Ehrenkranz RA, Edberg SC, Baltimore RS. A ten-year review of neonatal sepsis and comparison with the previous fifty-year experience. Pediatr Infect Dis J 9:819, 1990.
7. Baltimore RS, Huie SM, Meek JI, et al. Early-onset neonatal sepsis in the era of group B streptococcal prevention. Pediatrics 108:1094, 2001.
8. Silverman WA, Homan WE. Sepsis of obscure origin in the newborn. Pediatrics 3:157, 1949.
9. Smith RT, Platou ES, Good RA. Septicemia of the newborn: current status of the problem. Pediatrics 17:549, 1956.
10. Moorman RS Jr, Sell SH. Neonatal septicemia. South Med J 54:137, 1961.
11. Buetow KC, Klein SW, Lane RB. Septicemia in premature infants. Am J Dis Child 110:29, 1965.
12. Hodgman JE. Sepsis in the neonate. Perinatol Neonatol 5:45, 1981.
13. Kumar SP, Delivoria-Papadopoulos M. Infections in newborn infants in a special care unit. Ann Clin Lab Sci 15:351, 1985.
14. Stevens DC, Kleiman MB, Schreiner RL. Early-onset *Pseudomonas* sepsis of the neonate. Perinatol Neonatol 6:75, 1982.
15. Hall RT, Kurth CG, Hall SL. Ten-year survey of positive blood cultures among admissions to a neonatal intensive care unit. J Perinatol 7:122, 1987.
16. Fanaroff AA, Korones SB, Wright LL, et al. Incidence, presenting features, risk factors and significance of late onset septicemia in very low birth weight infants. Pediatr Infect Dis 17:593, 1998.
17. Karlowicz, MG, Buescher ES, Surka AE. Fulminant late-onset sepsis in a neonatal intensive care unit, 1988-1997, and the impact of avoiding empiric vancomycin therapy. Pediatrics 106:1387, 2000.
18. Stoll BJ, Hansen N, Fanaroff AA, et al. Late-onset sepsis in very low birth weight neonates: the experience of the NICHD neonatal research network. Pediatrics 110:285, 2002.
19. Spigelblatt L, Saintonge J, Chicoine R, et al. Changing pattern of neonatal streptococcal septicemia. Pediatr Infect Dis J 4:56, 1985.
20. Vesikari R, Janas M, Gronroos P, et al. Neonatal septicemia. Arch Dis Child 60:542, 1985.
21. Vesikari T, Isolauri E, Tuppurainen N, et al. Neonatal septicaemia in Finland 1981-85. Acta Paediatr Scand 78:44, 1989.
22. Hensey OJ, Hart CA, Cooke RWI. Serious infection in a neonatal intensive care unit: a two-year survey. J Hyg (Camb) 95:289, 1985.
23. Speer C, Hauptmann D, Stubbe P, et al. Neonatal septicemia and meningitis in Gottingen, West Germany. Pediatr Infect Dis J 4:36, 1985.
24. Tessin I, Trollfors B, Thiringer K. Incidence and etiology of neonatal septicaemia and meningitis in western Sweden 1975-1986. Acta Paediatr Scand 79:1023, 1990.
25. Battisi O, Mitchison R, Davies PA. Changing blood culture isolates in a referral neonatal intensive care unit. Arch Dis Child 56:775, 1981.
26. de Louvois J, Blackbourn J, Hurley R, et al. Infantile meningitis in England and Wales: a two year study. Arch Dis Child 66:603, 1991.
27. Hervás JA, Alomar A, Salva F, et al. Neonatal sepsis and meningitis in Mallorca, Spain, 1977-1991. Clin Infect Dis 16:719, 1993.
28. Bruun B, Paerregaard A. Septicemia in a Danish neonatal intensive care unit, 1984 to 1988. Pediatr Infect Dis J 10:159, 1991.
29. Ronnestad A, Abrahamsen TG, Gaustad P, Finne PH. Blood culture isolates during 6 years in a tertiary neonatal intensive care unit. Scand J Infect Dis 30:245, 1998.
30. Karpuch J, Goldberg M, Kohelet D. Neonatal bacteremia: a 4-year prospective study. Isr J Med Sci 19:963, 1983.
31. Greenberg D, Shinwell ES, Yagupsky P, et al. A prospective study of neonatal sepsis and meningitis in Southern Israel. Pediatr Infect Dis J 16:768, 1997.
32. Winfred I. The incidence of neonatal infections in the nursery unit at the Ahmadu Bello University Teaching Hospital, Zaria, Nigeria. East Afr Med J 61:197, 1984.
33. Ghiorghis B. Neonatal sepsis in Addis Ababa, Ethiopia: a review of 151 bacteremic neonates. Ethiop Med J 35:169, 1997.
34. Saloojee H, Liddle B, Gous H, Pooe M. Changing antibiotic resistance patterns in a neonatal unit and its implications for antibiotic usage. International Congress of Paediatric Surgery and Paediatrics. Cape Town, South Africa. February 1-6, 1998 (abstract).
35. Karan S. Purulent meningitis in the newborn. Childs Nerv Syst 2:26, 1986.
36. Sanghvi KP, Tudehope DI. Neonatal bacterial sepsis in a neonatal intensive care unit: a 5-year analysis. J Paediatr Child Health 32:333, 1996.
37. Makhoul IR, Sujov P, Smolkin T, et al. Epidemiology, clinical, and microbiological characteristics of late-onset sepsis among very low birth weight infants in Israel: a national survey. Pediatrics 109:34, 2002.
38. Ziai M, Haggerty RJ. Neonatal meningitis. N Engl J Med 259:314, 1958.
39. Mathies AW Jr, Wehrle PF. Management of bacterial meningitis. *In* Kagan BM (ed). Antimicrobial Therapy. Philadelphia, WB Saunders, 1974, pp 234-243.
40. Yow MD, Baker CJ, Barrett FF, et al. Initial antibiotic management of bacterial meningitis. Medicine (Baltimore) 52:305, 1973.
41. McCracken GH Jr. Personal communication, 1976.
42. Mulder CJJ, van Alphen L, Zanen HC. Neonatal meningitis caused by *Escherichia coli* in the Netherlands. J Infect Dis 150:935, 1984.
43. de Louvois J, Blackbourn J, Hurley R, et al. Infantile meningitis in England and Wales: a two year study. Arch Dis Child 66:603, 1991.
44. Unhanand M, Mustafa MM, McCracken GH Jr, Nelson JD. Gram-negative enteric bacillary meningitis: a twenty-one-year experience. J Pediatr 122:15, 1993.
45. Holt DE, Halket S, de Louvois J, Harvey D. Neonatal meningitis in England and Wales: 10 years on. Br Med J 84:F85, 2001.
46. Moreno MT, Vargas S, Poveda R, Sáez-Llorens X. Neonatal sepsis and meningitis in a developing Latin American country. Pediatr Infect Dis J 13:516, 1994.
47. Bennhagen R, Svenningsen NW, Bekassy AN. Changing pattern of neonatal meningitis in Sweden: a comparative study 1976 vs. 1983. Scand J Infect Dis 19:587, 1987.
48. Lancefield RC. Serologic differentiation of human and other groups of hemolytic streptococci. J Exp Med 57:571, 1933.
49. Hood M, Janney A, Dameron G. Beta hemolytic *Streptococcus* group B associated with problems of the perinatal period. Am J Obstet Gynecol 82:809, 1961.
50. Baker CJ, Barrett FF, Gordon RC, Yow MD. Suppurative meningitis due to streptococci of Lancefield group B: a study of 33 infants. J Pediatr 82:724, 1973.
51. Schlievert PM, Gocke JE, Deringer JR. Group B streptococcal toxic shock-like syndrome: report of a case and purification of an associated pyrogenic toxin. Clin Infect Dis 17:26, 1993.
52. Charles D, Larsen B. Streptococcal puerperal sepsis and obstetric infections: a historical perspective. Rev Infect Dis 8:411, 1986.
53. Loudon I. Puerperal fever, the streptococcus, and the sulphonamides, 1911-1945. BMJ 295:485, 1987.
54. Watson BP. An outbreak of puerperal sepsis in New York City. Am J Obstet Gynecol 16:159, 1928.
55. Jewett JF, Reid DE, Safon LE, Easterday CL. Childbed fever: a continuing entity. JAMA 206:344, 1968.
56. McCabe WR, Abrams AA. An outbreak of streptococcal puerperal sepsis. N Engl J Med 272:615, 1965.
57. Geil CC, Castle WK, Mortimer EA. Group A streptococcal infections in newborn nurseries. Pediatrics 46:849, 1970.
58. Gezon HM, Schaberg MJ, Klein JO. Concurrent epidemics of *Staphylococcus aureus* and group A *Streptococcus* disease in a newborn nursery-control with penicillin G and hexachlorophene bathing. Pediatrics 51:383, 1973.
59. Peter G, Hazard J. Neonatal group A streptococcal disease. J Pediatr 87:454, 1975.
60. Nelson JD, Dillon HC Jr, Howard JB. A prolonged nursery epidemic associated with a newly recognized type of group A *Streptococcus.* J Pediatr 89:792, 1976.
61. Campbell JR, Arango CA, Garcia-Prats JA, Baker CJ. An outbreak of M serotype 1 group A *Streptococcus* in neonatal intensive care unit. J Pediatr 129:396, 1996.
62. Cartwright RY. Neonatal septicaemia due to group A beta-haemolytic *Streptococcus.* BMJ 1:146, 1977.
63. Wong VK, Wright HT Jr. Group A β-hemolytic streptococci as a cause of bacteremia in children. Am J Dis Child 142:831, 1988.
64. Murphy DJ Jr. Group A streptococcal meningitis. Pediatrics 71:1, 1983.
65. Rathore MH, Barton LL, Kaplan EL. Suppurative group A β-hemolytic streptococcal infections in children. Pediatrics 89:743, 1992.
66. Wilschanski M, Faber J, Abramov A, et al. Neonatal septicemia caused by group A beta-hemolytic *Streptococcus.* Pediatr Infect Dis J 8:536, 1989.
67. Panaro NR, Lutwick LI, Chapnick EK. Intrapartum transmission of group A *Streptococcus.* Clin Infect Dis 17:79, 1993.

68. Mahieu LM, Holm SE, Goossens HJ, Van Acker KJ. Congenital streptococcal toxic shock syndrome with absence of antibodies against streptococcal pyrogenic exotoxins. J Pediatr 127:987, 1995.
69. Acharya U, Lamont CAR, Cooper K. Group A beta-hemolytic *Streptococcus* causing disseminated intravascular coagulation and maternal death. Lancet 1:595, 1988.
70. Kavi J, Wise R. Group A beta-hemolytic *Streptococcus* causing disseminated intravascular coagulation and maternal death. Lancet 1:993, 1988.
71. Swingler GR, Bigrigg MA, Hewitt BG, McNulty CAM. Disseminated intravascular coagulation associated with group A streptococcal infection in pregnancy. Lancet 1:1456, 1988.
72. Stevens DL, Tanner MH, Winship J, et al. Severe group A streptococcal infections associated with a toxic shock-like syndrome and scarlet fever toxin A. N Engl J Med 321:1, 1989.
73. Stevens DL. Invasive group A streptococcal infections. Clin Infect Dis 14:2, 1992.
74. Cleary PP, Kaplan EL, Handley JP, et al. Clonal basis for resurgence of serious *Streptococcus pyogenes* disease in the 1980s. Lancet 339:518, 1992.
75. Stevens DL, Bryant AS, Hackett SP, et al. Group A streptococcal bacteremia: the role of tumor necrosis factor in shock and organ failure. J Infect Dis 173:619, 1996.
76. Greenberg D, Leibovitz E, Shinnwell ES, et al. Neonatal sepsis caused by *Streptococcus pyogenes*—resurgence of an old etiology? Pediatr Infect Dis J 18:479, 1999.
77. Patamasucon P, Siegel JD, McCracken GH Jr. Streptococcal submandibular cellulitis in young infants. Pediatrics 67:378, 1981.
78. Stewardson-Krieger P, Gotoff SP. Neonatal meningitis due to group C beta hemolytic *Streptococcus.* J Pediatr 90:103, 1977.
79. Hervas JA, Labay MV, Rullan G, et al. Neonatal sepsis and meningitis due to *Streptococcus equisimilis.* Pediatr Infect Dis J 4:694, 1985.
80. Arditi M, Shulman ST, Davis AT, Yogev R. Group C β-hemolytic streptococcal infections in children: nine pediatric cases and review. Rev Infect Dis 11:34, 1989.
81. Baker CJ. Unusual occurrence of neonatal septicemia due to group G *Streptococcus.* Pediatrics 53:568, 1974.
82. Appelbaum PC, Friedman Z, Fairbrother PF, et al. Neonatal sepsis due to group G streptococci. Acta Paediatr Scand 69:599, 1980.
83. Dyson AE, Read SE. Group G streptococcal colonization and sepsis in neonates. J Pediatr 99:944, 1981.
84. Carstensen H, Pers C, Pryds O. Group G streptococcal neonatal septicemia: two case reports and a brief review of the literature. Scand. J Infect Dis 20:407, 1988.
85. Auckenthaler R, Hermans PE, Washington JA II. Group G streptococcal bacteremia: clinical study and review of the literature. Rev Infect Dis 5:196, 1983.
86. McNeeley DF, Brown AE, Noel GJ, et al. An investigation of vancomycin-resistant *Enterococcus faecium* within the pediatric service of a large urban medical center. Pediatr Infect Dis J 17:184, 1998.
87. Deville, JG, Adler S, Azimi PH, et al. Linezolid versus vancomycin in the treatment of known or suspected resistant Gram-positive infections in neonates. Pediatr Infect Dis J 22:S158, 2003.
88. Siegel JD, McCracken GH Jr. Group D streptococcal infections. J Pediatr 93:542, 1978.
89. McNeeley DF, Saint-Louis F, Noel GJ. Neonatal enterococcal bacteremia: an increasingly frequent event with potentially untreatable pathogens. Pediatr Infect Dis J 15:800, 1996.
90. Alexander JB, Giacoia GP. Early onset nonenterococcal group D streptococcal infection in the newborn infant. J Pediatr 93:489, 1978.
91. Headings DL, Herrera A, Mazzi E, et al. Fulminant neonatal septicemia caused by *Streptococcus bovis.* J Pediatr 92:282, 1978.
92. Fikar CR, Levy J. *Streptococcus bovis* meningitis in a neonate. Am J Dis Child 133:1149, 1979.
93. Bavikatte K, Schreiner RL, Lemons JA, et al. Group D streptococcal septicemia in the neonate. Am J Dis Child 133:493, 1979.
94. Hellwege HH, Ram W, Scherf H, et al. Neonatal meningitis caused by *Streptococcus mitis.* Lancet 1:743, 1984.
95. Bignardi GE, Isaacs D. Neonatal meningitis due to *Streptococcus mitis.* Rev Infect Dis 11:86, 1989.
96. Dobson SRM, Baker CJ. Enterococcal sepsis in neonates: features by age at onset and occurrence of focal infection. Pediatrics 85:165, 1990.
97. Buchino JJ, Ciambarella E, Light I. Systemic group D streptococcal infection in newborn infants. Am J Dis Child 133:270, 1979.
98. Boulanger JM, Ford-Jones EL, Matlow AG. Enterococcal bacteremia in a pediatric institution: a four-year review. Rev Infect Dis 13:847, 1991.
99. Coudron PE, Mayhall CG, Facklam RR, et al. *Streptococcus faecium* outbreak in a neonatal intensive care unit. J Clin Microbiol 20:1044, 1984.
100. Lugenbuhl LM, Rotbart HA, Facklan RR, et al. Neonatal enterococcal sepsis: case-control study and description of an outbreak. Pediatr Infect Dis J 6:1022, 1987.
101. Broughton RA, Krafka R, Baker CJ. Non-group D alpha-hemolytic streptococci: new neonatal pathogens. J Pediatr 99:450, 1981.
102. Espersen F, Frimodt-MÀller N, Rosdahl VT, Jessen O. *Staphylococcus aureus* bacteremia in children below the age of one year. Acta Paediatr Scand 78:56, 1989.
103. Baumgart S, Hall SE, Campos JM, et al. Sepsis with coagulase-negative staphylococci in critically ill newborns. Am J Dis Child 137:461, 1983.
104. Hall RT, Hall SL, Barnes WG, et al. Characteristics of coagulase negative staphylococci from infants with bacteremia. Pediatr Infect Dis J 6:377, 1987.
105. Freeman J, Goldmann DA, Smith NE, et al. Association of intravenous lipid emulsion and coagulase-negative staphylococcal bacteremia in neonatal intensive care units. N Engl J Med 323:301, 1990.
106. Kumar ML, Jenson HB, Dahms BD. Experience and reason—briefly recorded. Pediatrics 76:110, 1985.
107. Centers for Disease Control and Prevention. Public health dispatch: outbreak of listeriosis—Northeastern United States 2002. MMWR Morb Mortal Wkly Rep 51:950, 2002.
108. Bingen E, Picard B, Brahimi N, et al. Phylogenetic analysis of *Escherichia coli* strains causing neonatal meningitis suggests horizontal gene transfer from a predominant pool of highly virulent B2 group strains. J Infect Dis 177:642, 1998.
109. Robbins JB, McCracken GH Jr, Gotschuch EC, et al. *Escherichia coli* K_1 capsular polysaccharide associated with neonatal meningitis. N Engl J Med 290:1216, 1974.
110. McCracken GH Jr, Sarff LD, Glode MP, et al. Relation between *Escherichia coli* K_1 capsular polysaccharide antigen and clinical outcome in neonatal meningitis. Lancet 2:246, 1974.
111. McCracken GH Jr, Sarff LD. Current status and therapy of neonatal *E. coli* meningitis. Hosp Pract 9:57, 1974.
112. Sarff LD, McCracken GH Jr, Schiffer MS, et al. Epidemiology of *Escherichia coli* K_1 in healthy and diseased newborns. Lancet 1:1099, 1975.
113. Peter G, Nelson JS. Factors affecting neonatal *E. coli* K_1 rectal colonization. J Pediatr 93:866, 1978.
114. Guerina NG, Kessler TW, Guerina VJ, et al. The role of pili and capsule in the pathogenesis of neonatal infection with *Escherichia coli* K_1. J Infect Dis 148:395, 1983.
115. Tullus K. Epidemiological aspects of P-fimbriated *Escherichia coli* fecal colonization of newborn children and relation to development of extraintestinal *E. coli* infections. Stockholm, Kongl Karolinska Medico Chirurgiska Institutetet, Danderyl, 1986.
116. Hervás JA, Ballesteros F, Alomar A, et al. Increase of *Enterobacter* in neonatal sepsis: a twenty-two-year study. Pediatr Infect Dis J 20:1134, 2001.
117. Gupta A. Hospital-acquired infections in the neonatal intensive care unit—*Klebsiella pneumoniae.* Semin Perinatol 26:340, 2002.
118. Sood SK, Mulvihill D, Daum RS. Intrarenal abscess caused by *Klebsiella pneumoniae* in a neonate: modern management and diagnosis. Am J Perinatol 6:367, 1989.
119. Basu S, Mukherjee KK, Poddar B, et al. An unusual case of neonatal brain abscess following *Klebsiella pneumoniae* septicemia. Infection 29:283, 2001
120. Ozkan H, Kumtepe S. Turan A, et al. Perianal necrotizing fasciitis in a neonate. Indian J Pediatr 64:116, 1997.
121. Podschun R, Acktun H, Okpara J. Isolation of *Klebsiella planticola* from newborns in a neonatal ward. J Clin Microbiol 36:2331, 1998.
122. Westbrook GL, O'Hara CM, Roman SB, et al. Incidence and identification of *Klebsiella planticola* in clinical isolates with emphasis on newborns. J Clin Microbiol 38:1495, 2000.
123. Leibovitz E, Flidel-Rimon O, Juster-Reicher A, et al. Sepsis at a neonatal intensive care unit: a four-year retrospective study (1989-1992). Israel J Med Sci 33:734, 1997.
124. Pessoa-Silva CL, Meurer Moreira B, Camara Almeida V, et al. Extended-spectrum beta-lactamase-producing *Klebsiella pneumoniae* in a neonatal intensive care unit: risk factors for infection and colonization. J Hosp Infect 53:198, 2003.
125. Roilides E, Kyriakides G, Kadiltsoglou I, et al. Septicemia due to multiresistant *Klebsiella pneumoniae* in a neonatal unit: a case-control study. Am J Perinatol 17:35, 2000.

126. Stone PW, Gupta A, Loughrey M, et al. Attributable costs and length of stay of an extended-spectrum beta-lactamase-producing *Klebsiella pneumoniae* outbreak in a neonatal intensive care unit. Infect Control Hosp Epidemiol 24:601, 2003.
127. Kleiman MB, Allen SD, Neal P, et al. Meningoencephalitis and compartmentalization of the cerebral ventricles caused by *Enterobacter sakazakii*. J Clin Microbiol 14:352, 1981.
128. Willis J, Robinson JE. *Enterobacter sakazakii* meningitis in neonates. Pediatr Infect Dis J 7:196, 1988.
129. Bonadio WA, Margolis D, Tovar M. *Enterobacter cloacae* bacteremia in children: a review of 30 cases in 12 years. Clin Pediatr 30:310, 1991.
130. Harbarth S, Sudre P, Dharan S, et al. Outbreak of *Enterobacter cloacae* related to understaffing, overcrowding, and poor hygiene practices. Infect Control Hosp Epidemiol 20:598, 1999.
131. Wenger PJ, Tokars JI, Brennan P, et al. An outbreak of *Enterobacter hormaechei* infection and colonization in an intensive care nursery. Clin Infect Dis 24:1243, 1997.
132. da Silva CL, Miranda LE, Moreira BM, et al. *Enterobacter hormaechei* bloodstream infection at three neonatal intensive care units in Brazil. Pediatr Infect Dis J 21:175, 2002.
133. Gurses N. *Enterobacter* septicemia in neonates. Pediatr Infect Dis J 14:638, 1995.
134. Jain A, Roy I, Gupta MK, et al. Prevalence of extended-spectrum beta-lactamase-producing Gram-negative bacteria in septicaemic neonates in a tertiary care hospital. J Med Microbiol 52:421, 2003.
135. Muytjens HL, Kollee LAA. *Enterobacter sakazakii* meningitis in neonates: causative role of formula? Pediatr Infect Dis J 9:372, 1990.
136. Noriega FR, Kotloff KL, Martin MA, Schwalbe RS. Nosocomial bacteremia caused by *Enterobacter sakazakii* and *Leuconostoc mesenteroides* resulting from extrinsic contamination of infant formula. Pediatr Infect Dis J 9:447, 1990.
137. Fok TF, Lee CH, Wong EMC, et al. Risk factors for *Enterobacter* septicemia in a neonatal unit: case-control study. Clin Infect Dis 27:1204, 1998.
138. Tresoldi AT, Padoveze MC, Trabasso P, et al. *Enterobacter cloacae* sepsis outbreak in a newborn unit caused by contaminated total parenteral nutrition solution. Am J Infect Control 28:258, 2000.
139. Cheng HS, Lin HC, Peng CT, Tsai CH. Outbreak investigation of nosocomial *Enterobacter cloacae* bacteraemia in a neonatal intensive care unit. Scand J Infect Dis 32:293, 2000.
140. Doran TI. The role of *Citrobacter* in clinical disease of children: review. Clin Infect Dis 28:384, 1999.
141. Graham DR, Band JD. *Citrobacter diversus* brain abscess and meningitis in neonates. JAMA 245:1923, 1981.
142. Graham DR, Anderson RL, Ariel FE, et al. Epidemic nosocomial meningitis due to *Citrobacter diversus* in neonates. J Infect Dis 144:203, 1981.
143. Kaplan AM, Itabashi HH, Yoshimori R, et al. Cerebral abscesses complicating neonatal *Citrobacter freundii* meningitis. West J Med 127:418, 1977.
144. Lin FYC, Devol WF, Morrison C, et al. Outbreak of neonatal *Citrobacter diversus* meningitis in a suburban hospital. Pediatr Infect Dis J 6:50, 1987.
145. Eppes SC, Woods CR, Mayer AS, Klein JD. Recurring ventriculitis due to *Citrobacter diversus*: clinical and bacteriologic analysis. Clin Infect Dis 17:437, 1993.
146. Foreman SD, Smith EE, Ryan NJ, et al. Neonatal *Citrobacter* meningitis; pathogenesis of cerebral abscess formation. Ann Neurol 16:655, 1984.
147. Morris JG, Lin F-YC, Morrison CB, et al. Molecular epidemiology of neonatal meningitis due to *Citrobacter diversus*: a study of isolates from hospitals in Maryland. J Infect Dis 154:409, 1986.
148. Kline MW, Mason EO Jr, Kaplan SL. Characterization of *Citrobacter diversus* strains causing neonatal meningitis. J Infect Dis 157:101, 1988.
149. Assadian O, Berger A, Aspock C, et al. Nosocomial outbreak of *Serratia marcescens* in a neonatal intensive care unit. Infect Control Hosp Epidemiol 23:457, 2002.
150. Fleisch F, Zimmermann-Baer U, Zbinden R, et al. Three consecutive outbreaks of *Serratia marcescens* in a neonatal intensive care unit. Clin Infect Dis 34:767, 2002.
151. Jang TN, Fung CP, Yang TL, et al. Use of pulsed-field gel electrophoresis to investigate an outbreak of *Serratia marcescens* infection in a neonatal intensive care unit. J Hosp Infect 48:13, 2001.
152. Newport MT, John JF, Michel YM, Levkoff AH. Endemic *Serratia marcescens* infection in a neonatal intensive care nursery associated with gastrointestinal colonization. Pediatr Infect Dis 4:160, 1985.
153. Berthelot P, Grattard F, Amerger C, et al. Investigation of a nosocomial outbreak due to *Serratia marcescens* in a maternity hospital. Infect Control Hosp Epidemiol 20:233, 1999.
154. Zaidi M, Sifuentes J, Bobadilla M, et al. Epidemic of *Serratia marcescens* bacteremia and meningitis in a neonatal unit in Mexico City. Infect Control Hosp Epidemiol 10:14, 1989.
155. Campbell JR, Diacovo T, Baker CJ. *Serratia marcescens* meningitis in neonates. Pediatr Infect Dis J 11:881, 1992.
156. Ries M, Deeg KH, Heininger U, Stehr K. Brain abscesses in neonates—report of three cases. Eur J Pediatr 152:745, 1993.
157. Ghosal SP, SenGupta PC, Mukherjee AK. Noma neonatorum: its aetiopathogenesis. Lancet 2:289, 1978.
158. Shah SS, Gallagher PG. Complications of conjunctivitis caused by *Pseudomonas aeruginosa* in a newborn intensive care unit. Pediatr Infect Dis J 17:97, 1998.
159. Centers for Disease Control. Reported isolates of *Salmonella* from CSF in the United States, 1968-1979. J Infect Dis 143:504, 1981.
160. Totan M, Kucukoduk S, Dagdemir A, Dilber C. Meningitis due to *Salmonella* in preterm neonates. Turkish J Pediatr 44:45, 2002.
161. Reed RP, Klugman KP. Neonatal typhoid fever. Pediatr Infect Dis J 13:774, 1994.
162. Schuchat A, Robinson K, Wenger JD, et al. Bacterial meningitis in the United States in 1995. N Engl J Med 337:970, 1997.
163. Sunderland WA, Harris HH, Spence CA, et al. Meningococcemia in a newborn infant whose mother had meningococcal vaginitis. J Pediatr 81:856, 1972.
164. Jones RN, Stepack J, Eades A. Fatal neonatal meningococcal meningitis: association with maternal cervical-vaginal colonization. JAMA 236:2652, 1976.
165. Fiorito SM, Galarza PG, Sparo M, et al. An unusual transmission of *Neisseria meningitidis*: neonatal conjunctivitis acquired at delivery from the mother's endocervical infection. Sex Transm Dis 28:29, 2001.
166. Cher DJ, Maxwell WJ, Frusztajer N, et al. A case of pelvic inflammatory disease associated with *Neisseria meningitidis* bacteremia. Clin Infect Dis 17:134, 1993.
167. Bhutta ZA, Khan IA, Agha Z. Fatal intrauterine meningococcal infection. Pediatr Infect Dis J 10:868, 1991.
168. Chugh K, Bhalla CK, Joshi KK. Meningococcal abscess and meningitis in a neonate. Pediatr Infect Dis J 7:136, 1988.
169. Arango CA, Rathore MH. Neonatal meningococcal meningitis: case reports and review of literature. Pediatr Infect Dis J 15:1134, 1996.
170. Shepard CW, Rosenstein NE, Fischer M. Active Bacterial Core Surveillance Team. Neonatal meningococcal disease in the United States, 1990 to 1999. Pediatr Infect Dis J 22:418, 2003.
171. Manginello FP, Pascale JA, Wolfsdorf J, et al. Neonatal meningococcal meningitis and meningococcemia. Am J Dis child 133:651, 1979.
172. Clegg HW, Todres ID, Moylan FM, et al. Fulminant neonatal meningococcemia. Am J Dis Child 134:354, 1980.
173. Adams WG, Deaver KA, Cochi SL, et al. Decline of childhood *Haemophilus influenzae* type b (Hib) disease in the Hib vaccine era. JAMA 269:221, 1993.
174. Peltola H, Kilpi T, Anttila M. Rapid disappearance of *Haemophilus influenzae* type b meningitis after routine childhood immunization with conjugate vaccines. Lancet 340:592, 1992.
175. Bisgard KM, Kao A, Leake J, et al. *Haemophilus influenzae* invasive disease in the United States, 1994-1995: near disappearance of a vaccine-preventable childhood disease. Emerg Infect Dis 4:229, 1998.
176. Takala AK, Eskola J, Leinonen M, et al. Reduction of oropharyngeal carriage of *Haemophilus influenzae* type b (Hib) in children immunized with Hib conjugate vaccine. J Infect Dis 164:982, 1991.
177. Murphy TV, Pastor P, Medley R, et al. Decreased *Haemophilus* colonization in children vaccinated with *Haemophilus influenzae* type b conjugate vaccine. J Pediatr 122:517, 1993.
178. Mohle-Boetani JC, Ajello G, Breneman E, et al. Carriage of *Haemophilus influenzae* type b in children after widespread vaccination with *Haemophilus influenzae* type b vaccines. Pediatr Infect Dis J 12:589, 1993.
179. Urwin G, Krohn JA, Deaver-Robinson K, et al. Invasive disease due to *Haemophilus influenzae* serotype f: clinical and epidemiologic characteristics in the *H. influenzae* serotype b vaccine era. Clin Infect Dis 22:1069, 1996.
180. Heath PT, Booy R, Azzopardi HJ, et al. Non-type b *Haemophilus influenzae* disease: clinical and epidemiologic characteristics in the *Haemophilus influenzae* type b vaccine era. Pediatr Infect Dis J 20:300, 2001.

181. Perdue DG, Bulkow LR, Gellin GB. Invasive *Haemophilus influenzae* disease in Alaskan residents aged 10 years and older before and after infant vaccination programs JAMA 283:3089, 2000.
182. Barton LL, Cruz RD, Walentik C. Neonatal *Haemophilus influenzae* type C sepsis. Am J Dis Child 136:463, 1982.
183. Campognone P, Singer DB. Neonatal sepsis due to nontypeable *Haemophilus influenzae.* Am J Dis Child 140:117, 1986.
184. Wallace RJ Jr, Baker CJ, Quinones FJ, et al. Nontypable *Haemophilus influenzae* (biotype 4) as a neonatal, maternal and genital pathogen. Rev Infect Dis 5:123, 1983.
185. Falia TJ, Dobson SRM, Crook DWM, et al. Population-based study of non-typeable *Haemophilus influenzae* invasive disease in children and neonates. Lancet 341:851, 1993.
186. Friesen CA, Cho CT. Characteristic features of neonatal sepsis due to *Haemophilus influenzae.* Rev Infect Dis 8:777, 1986.
187. Lilien LD, Yeh TF, Novak GM, et al. Early-onset *Haemophilus* sepsis in newborn infants: clinical, roentgenographic, and pathologic features. Pediatrics 62:299, 1978.
188. Silverberg K, Boehm FH. *Haemophilus influenzae* amnionitis with intact membranes: a case report. Am J Perinatol 7:270, 1990.
189. Bradley JS. *Haemophilus parainfluenzae* sepsis in a very low birth weight premature infant: a case report and review of the literature. J Perinatol 19:315, 1999.
190. Holt RN, Taylor CD, Schneider HJ, et al. Three cases of *Hemophilus parainfluenzae* meningitis. Clin Pediatr (Phila) 13:666, 1974.
191. Zinner SH, McCormack WM, Lee Y-H, et al. Puerperal bacteremia and neonatal sepsis due to *Hemophilus parainfluenzae:* report of a case with antibody titers. Pediatrics 49:612, 1972.
192. Miano A, Cipolloni AP, Casadei GP, et al. Neonatal *Haemophilus aphrophilus* meningitis. Helv Paediatr Acta 31:499, 1977.
193. Bortolussi R, Thompson TR, Ferrieri P. Early-onset pneumococcal sepsis in newborn infants. Pediatrics 60:352, 1977.
194. Shaw PJ, Robinson DL, Watson JG. Pneumococcal infection in a mother and infant. Lancet 2:47, 1984.
195. Westh H, Skibsted L, Korner B. *Streptococcus pneumoniae* infections of the female genital tract and in the newborn child. Rev Infect Dis 12:416, 1990.
196. Robinson EN Jr. Pneumococcal endometritis and neonatal sepsis. Rev Infect Dis 12:799, 1990.
197. Hughes BR, Mercer JL, Gosbel LB. Neonatal pneumococcal sepsis in association with fatal maternal pneumococcal sepsis. Aust N Z J Obstet Gynaecol 41:457, 2001.
198. Hoffman JA, Mason EO, Schutze GE, at al. *Streptococcus pneumoniae* infections in the neonate. Pediatrics 112:1095, 2003.
199. Gorbach SL, Bartlett JG. Anaerobic infections. N Engl J Med 290:1177, 1974.
200. Gorbach SL, Menda KB, Thadepalli H, et al. Anaerobic microflora of the cervix in healthy women. Am J Obstet Gynecol 117:1053, 1973.
201. Chow AW, Guze LB. Bacteroidaceae bacteremia: clinical experience with 112 patients. Medicine (Baltimore) 53:93, 1974.
202. Finegold SM. Anaerobic infections. Surg Clin North Am 60:49, 1980.
203. Brook I. Bacteremia due to anaerobic bacteria in newborns. J Perinatol 10:351, 1990.
204. Chow AW, Leake RD, Yamauchi T, et al. The significance of anaerobes in neonatal bacteremia: analysis of 23 cases and review of the literature. Pediatrics 54:736, 1974.
205. Noel GJ, Laufer DA, Edelson PJ. Anaerobic bacteremia in a neonatal intensive care unit: an eighteen year experience. Pediatr Infect Dis J 7:858, 1988.
206. Mitra S. Panigrahi D. Narang A. Anaerobes in neonatal septicaemia: a cause for concern. J Trop Pediatr 43:153, 1997.
207. Ohta S, Shimizu S, Fujisawa S, et al. Neonatal adrenal abscess due to *Bacteroides.* J Pediatr 93:1063, 1978.
208. Lee Y-H, Berg RB. Cephalhematoma infected with *Bacteroides.* Am J Dis Child 121:72, 1971.
209. Siddiqi SF, Taylor PM. Necrotizing fasciitis of the scalp: a complication of fetal monitoring. Am J Dis Child 136:226, 1982.
210. Feder HM Jr. *Bacteroides fragilis* meningitis. Rev Infect Dis 9:783, 1987.
211. Harrod JR, Stevens DA. Anaerobic infections in the newborn infant. J Pediatr 85:399, 1974.
212. Dunkle LM, Brotherton TJ, Feigin RD. Anaerobic infections in children: a prospective survey. Pediatrics 57:311, 1976.
213. Airede AI. Pathogens in neonatal omphalitis. J Trop Pediatr 38:129, 1992.
214. Kosloske A, Cushing AH, Borden TA, et al. Cellulitis and necrotizing fasciitis of the abdominal wall in pediatric patients. J Pediatr Surg 16:246, 1981.
215. Chaney NE. *Clostridium* infection in mother and infant. Am J Dis Child 134:1175, 1980.
216. Spark RP, Wike DA. Nontetanus clostridial neonatal fatality after home delivery. Arizona Med 40:697, 1983.
217. Motz RA, James AG, Dove B. *Clostridium perfringens* meningitis in a newborn infant. Pediatr Infect Dis J 15:708, 1996.
218. Pascual FB, McGinley EL, Zanardi LR, et al. Tetanus surveillance—United States, 1998-2000. MMWR Surveill Summ 52:1, 2003.
219. Craig AS, Reed GW, Mohon RT, et al. Neonatal tetanus in the United States: a sentinel event in the foreign-born. Pediatr Infect Dis J 16:955, 1997.
220. Kumar S, Malecki LM. A case of neonatal tetanus. South Med J 84:396, 1991.
221. Centers for Disease Control. Neonatal tetanus—Montana, 1998. MMWR Morb Mortal Wkly Rep 47:928, 1998.
222. Vandelaer J, Birmingham M, Gasse F, et al. Tetanus in developing countries: an update on the Maternal and Neonatal Tetanus Elimination Initiative. Vaccine 21:3442, 2003.
223. Quddus A, Luby S, Rahbar M, Pervaiz Y. Neonatal tetanus: mortality rate and risk factors in Loralai District, Pakistan. Int J Epidemiol 31:648, 2002.
224. Idema CD, Harris BN, Ogunbanjo GA, Durrheim DN. Neonatal tetanus elimination in Mpumalanga Province, South Africa. Trop Med Int Health 7:622, 2002.
225. Mustafa BE, Omer MI, Aziz MI, Karrar ZE. Neonatal tetanus in rural and displaced communities in the East Nile Province. J Trop Pediatr 42:110, 1996.
226. Arnold RB, Soewarso TI, Karyadi A. Mortality from neonatal tetanus in Indonesia: results of two surveys. Bull World Health Organ 64:259, 1986.
227. Herrero JIH, Beltran RR, Sanchanz AMM. Failure of intrathecal tetanus antitoxin in the treatment of tetanus neonatorum. J Infect Dis 164:619, 1991.
228. Abrutyn E, Berlin JA. Intrathecal therapy in tetanus. JAMA 266:2262, 1991.
229. Traverso HP, Kahn AJ, Rahim H, et al. Ghee application to the umbilical cord: a risk factor for neonatal tetanus. Lancet 1:486, 1989.
230. Oudesluys-Murphy AM. Umbilical cord care and neonatal tetanus. Lancet 1:843, 1989.
231. Centers for Disease Control and Prevention. Progress toward the global elimination of neonatal tetanus, 1989-1993. JAMA 273:196, 1995.
232. Black RE, Huber DH, Curlin GT. Reduction of neonatal tetanus by mass immunization of nonpregnant women: duration of protection provided by one or two doses of aluminum-adsorbed tetanus toxoid. Bull World Health Organ 58:927, 1980.
233. Schofield F. Selective primary health care: strategies for control of disease in the developing world. XXII. Tetanus: a preventable problem. Rev Infect Dis 8:144, 1986.
234. Gromisch DS, Gordon SG, Bedrosian L, et al. Simultaneous mixed bacterial meningitis in an infant. Am J Dis Child 119:284, 1970.
235. Pacifico L, Chiesa C, Mirabella S, et al. Early-onset *Pseudomonas aeruginosa* sepsis and *Yersinia enterocolitica* neonatal infection: a unique combination in a preterm infant. Eur J Pediatr 146:192, 1987.
236. Faix RG, Kovarik SM. Polymicrobial sepsis among intensive care nursery infants. J Perinatol 9:131, 1989.
237. Jarvis WR, Hybsmith AK, Allen JR, et al. Polymicrobial bacteremia associated with lipid emulsion in a neonatal intensive care unit. Pediatr Infect Dis J 2:203, 1983.
238. Sferra TJ, Pacini DL. Simultaneous recovery of bacterial and viral pathogens from CSF. Pediatr Infect Dis J 7:552, 1988.
239. Giacoia GP. Uncommon pathogens in newborn infants. J Perinatol 14:134, 1994.
240. Boukadida J, Monastiri K, Snoussi N, et al. Nosocomial neonatal meningitis by *Alcaligenes xylosoxidans* transmitted by aqueous eosin. Pediatr Infect Dis J 12:696, 1993.
241. Hearn YR, Gander RM. *Achromobacter xylosoxidans.* An unusual neonatal pathogen. Am J Clin Path 96:211, 1991.
242. Manjra AI, Moosa A, Bhamjee A. Fatal neonatal meningitis and ventriculitis caused by multiresistant *Achromobacter xylosoxidans.* A case report. S Afr Med J 76:571, 1989.
243. Huang YC, Su LH, Wu TL, et al. Outbreak of *Acinetobacter baumannii* bacteremia in a neonatal intensive care unit: clinical implications and genotyping analysis. Pediatr Infect Dis J 21:1105, 2002.
244. Melamed R, Greenberg D, Porat N, et al. Successful control of an *Acinetobacter baumannii* outbreak in a neonatal intensive care unit. J Hosp Infect 53:31, 2003.

245. Mittal N, Nair D, Gupta N, et al. Outbreak of *Acinetobacter* spp septicemia in a neonatal ICU. Southeast Asian J Trop Med Pub Health 34:365, 2003.
246. Park JW, Grossman O. *Aerococcus viridans* infection: case report and review. Clin Pediatr 29:525, 1990.
247. Tokieda K, Morikawa Y, Maeyama K, et al. Clinical manifestations of *Bacillus cereus* meningitis in newborn infants. J Paediatr Child Health 35:582, 1999.
248. van der Zwet WC, Parlevliet GA, Savelkoul PH, et al. Outbreak of *Bacillus cereus* infections in a neonatal intensive care unit traced to balloons used in manual ventilation. J Clin Microbiol 38:4131, 2000.
249. Hilliard NJ, Schelonka RL, Waites KB. *Bacillus cereus* bacteremia in a preterm neonate. J Clin Microbiol 41:3441, 2003.
250. van Holten J, Tiems J, Jongen VH. Neonatal *Borrelia duttoni* infection: a report of three cases. Trop Doctor 27:115, 1997.
251. Melkert PW, Stel HV. Neonatal *Borrelia* infections (relapsing fever): report of 5 cases and review of the literature. East Afr Med J 68:999, 1991.
252. Chheda S, Lopez SM, Sanderson EP. Congenital brucellosis in a premature infant. Pediatr Infect Dis J 16:81, 1997.
253. Shamo'on H, Izzat M. Congenital brucellosis. Pediatr Infect Dis J 18:1110, 1999.
254. Giannacopoulos I, Eliopoulou MI, Ziambaras T, Papanastasiou DA. Transplacentally transmitted congenital brucellosis due to *Brucella abortus*. J Infect 45:209, 2002.
255. Kahyaoglu O, Nolan B, Kumar A. *Burkholderia cepacia* sepsis in neonates. Pediatr Infect Dis J 14:815, 1995.
256. Morooka T, Umeda A, Fujita M, et al. Epidemiologic application of pulsed-field gel electrophoresis to an outbreak of *Campylobacter fetus* meningitis in a neonatal intensive care unit. Scand J Infect Dis 28:269, 1996.
257. Wolfs TF, Duim B, Geelen SP, et al. Neonatal sepsis by *Campylobacter jejuni*: genetically proven transmission from a household puppy. Clin Infect Dis 32:E97, 2001.
258. Viejo G, Gomez B, De Miguel D, et al. *Campylobacter fetus* subspecies fetus bacteremia associated with chorioamnionitis and intact fetal membranes. Scand J Infect Dis 33:126, 2001.
259. Feldman JD, Kontaxis EN, Sherman MP. Congenital bacteremia due to *Capnocytophaga*. Pediatr Infect Dis J 4:415, 1985.
260. Edwards C, Yi CH, Currie JL. Chorioamnionitis caused by *Capnocytophaga*: case report. Am J Obstet Gynecol 173:244, 1995.
261. Rosenman JR, Reynolds JK, Kleiman MB. *Capnocytophaga canimorsus* meningitis in a newborn: an avoidable infection. Pediatr Infect Dis J 22:204, 2003.
262. Beckwith DG, Jahre JA, Haggerty S. Isolation of *Corynebacterium aquaticum* from spinal fluid of an infant with meningitis. J Clin Microbiol 23:375, 1986.
263. Berner R, Pelz K, Wilhelm C, et al. Fatal sepsis caused by *Corynebacterium amycolatum* in a premature infant. J Clin Microbiol 35:1011, 1997.
264. Vohra K, Torrijos E, Jhaveri R, et al. Neonatal sepsis and meningitis caused by *Edwardsiella tarda*. Pediatr Infect Dis J 7:814, 1988.
265. Mowbray EE, Buck G, Humbaugh KE, Marshall GS. Maternal colonization and neonatal sepsis caused by *Edwardsiella tarda*. Pediatrics 111:e296, 2003.
266. Ginsberg HG, Daum RS. *Escherichia hermanii* sepsis with duodenal perforation in a neonate. Pediatr Infect Dis J 6:300, 1987.
267. Tizer KB, Cervia JS, Dunn A, et al. Successful combination vancomycin and rifampin therapy in a newborn with community-acquired *Flavobacterium meningosepticum* neonatal meningitis. Pediatr Infect Dis J 14:916, 1995.
268. Chiu CH, Waddingdon M, Greenberg D, et al. Atypical *Chryseobacterium meningosepticum* and meningitis and sepsis in newborns and the immunocompromised, Taiwan. Emerg Infect Dis 6:481, 2000.
269. Hoque SN, Graham J, Kaufmann ME, Tabaqchali S. *Chryseobacterium (Flavobacterium) meningosepticum* outbreak associated with colonization of water taps in a neonatal intensive care unit. J Hosp Infect 47:188, 2001.
270. Tekerekoglu MS, Durmaz R, Ayan M, et al. Analysis of an outbreak due to *Chryseobacterium meningosepticum* in a neonatal intensive care unit. New Microbiol 26:57, 2003.
271. Berardi-Grassias L, Roy O, Berardi JC, et al. Neonatal meningitis due to *Gardnerella vaginalis*. Eur J Clin Microbiol Infect Dis 7:406, 1988.
272. Moran DJ, Payne A. Subclinical intra-amniotic infection with *Gardnerella vaginalis* associated with preterm delivery. Case report. Br J Obstet Gynaecol 96:489, 1989.
273. Catlin BW. *Gardnerella vaginalis*: characteristics, clinical considerations, and controversies. Clin Microbiol Rev 5:213, 1992.
274. Amaya RA, Al-Dossary F, Demmler GJ. *Gardnerella vaginalis* bacteremia in a premature neonate. J Perinatol 22:585, 2002.
275. Orlicek SI, Welch DF, Kuhls TL. Septicemia and meningitis caused by *Helicobacter cinaedi* in a neonate. J Clin Microbiol 31:569, 1993.
276. Broughton RA, Gruter WC, Haffar AAM, et al. Neonatal meningitis due to *Lactobacillus*. Pediatr Infect Dis J 2:382, 1983.
277. Thompson C, McCarter YS, Krause PJ, Herson VC. *Lactobacillus acidophilus* sepsis in a neonate. J Perinatol 21:258, 2001.
278. Gsell HO Jr, Olafsson A, Sonnabend W, et al. Intrauterine *Leptospirosis pomona*. Dtsch Med Wochenschr 31:1263, 1971.
279. Lindsay S, Luke IW. Fatal leptospirosis in a newborn infant. J Pediatr 7:90, 1947.
280. Shaked Y, Shpilberg O, Samra D, Samra Y. Leptospirosis in pregnancy and its effect on the fetus: case report and review. Clin Infect Dis 17:241, 1993.
281. Hardy S, Ruoff KL, Catlin E, et al. Catheter-associated infection with a vancomycin-resistant gram-positive coccus of the *Leuconostoc* species. Pediatr Infect Dis J 7:519, 1988.
282. Handwerger S, Horowitz H, Coburn K, et al. Infection due to *Leuconostoc* species: six cases and review. Rev Infect Dis 12:602, 1990.
283. Friedland IR, Snipelisky M, Khoosal M. Meningitis in a neonate caused by *Leuconostoc* sp. J Clin Microbiol 28:2125, 1990.
284. Carapetis J, Bishop S, Davis J, et al. *Leuconostoc* sepsis in association with continuous enteral feeding: two case reports and a review. Pediatr Infect Dis J 13:816, 1994.
285. Rowen JL, Lopez SM. *Morganella morganii* early onset sepsis. Pediatr Infect Dis J 17:1176, 1998.
286. Valencia GB, Piecuch S. Fatal early onset infection in an extremely low birth weight infant due to *Morganella morganii*. J Perinatol 19:533, 1999.
287. Casanova-Roman M, Sanchez-Porto A, Casanova-Bellido M. Early-onset neonatal sepsis caused by vertical transmission of *Morganella morganii*. Scand J Infect Dis 34:534, 2002.
288. Clapp DW, Kleiman MB, Reynolds JK, et al. *Pasteurella multocida* meningitis in infancy: an avoidable infection. Am J Dis Child 140:444, 1986.
289. Escande F, Borde M, Pateyron F. Maternal and neonatal *Pasteurella multocida* infection. Arch Pediatr 4:1116, 1997.
290. Zaramella P, Zamorani E, Freato F, et al. Neonatal meningitis due to a vertical transmission of *Pasteurella multocida*. Pediatr Int 41:307, 1999.
291. Ahmed K, Sein PP, Shahnawaz M, Hoosen AA. *Pasteurella gallinarum* neonatal meningitis. Clin Microbiol Infect 8:55, 2002.
292. Terpeluk C, Goldmann A, Bartmann P, Pohlandt F. *Plesiomonas shigelloides* sepsis and meningoencephalitis in a neonate. Eur J Pediatr 151:499, 1992.
293. Fujita K, Shirai M, Ishioka T, Kakuya F. Neonatal *Plesiomonas shigelloides* septicemia and meningitis: a case and review. Acta Paediatr Japonica 36:450, 1994.
294. Gupta P, Ramachandran VG, Seth A. Early onset neonatal septicemia caused by *Aeromonas hydrophilia*. Indian Pediatr 33:703, 1996.
295. Velvis H, Carrasco N, Hetherington S. Trimethoprim-sulfamethoxazole therapy of neonatal *Proteus mirabilis* meningitis unresponsive to cefotaxime. Pediatr Infect Dis 5:591, 1986.
296. Hervás JA, Ciria L, Henales V, et al. Nonsurgical management of neonatal multiple brain abscesses due to *Proteus mirabilis*. Helv Paediatr Acta 42:451, 1987.
297. Kassim Z, Aziz AA, Haque QM, Cheung HA. Isolation of *Proteus mirabilis* from severe neonatal sepsis and central nervous system infection with extensive pneumocephalus. Eur J Pediatr 162:644, 2003.
298. Lumbiganon P, Pengsaa K, Puapermpoonsiri S, Puapairoj A. Neonatal melioidosis: a report of 5 cases. Pediatr Infect Dis J 7:634, 1988.
299. Halder D, Zainal N, Wah CM, Haq JA. Neonatal meningitis and septicaemia caused by *Burkholderia pseudomallei*. Ann Trop Paediatr 18:161, 1998.
300. Barbaro DJ, Mackowiak PA, Barth SS, Southern PM. *Pseudomonas testosteroni* infections: eighteen recent cases and a review of the literature. Rev Infect Dis 9:124, 1987.
301. Lloyd-Puryear M, Wallace D, Baldwin T, Hollis DG. Meningitis caused by *Psychrobacter immobilis* in an infant. J Clin Microbiol 29:2041, 1991.
302. Ruderman JW, Stoller KP, Pomerance JJ. Bloodstream invasion with *Shigella sonnei* in an asymptomatic newborn infant. Pediatr Infect Dis J 5:379, 1986.
303. Rebarber A, Star Hampton B, Lewis V, Bender S. Shigellosis complicating preterm premature rupture of membranes resulting in congenital infection and preterm delivery. Obstet Gynecol 100:1063, 2002.

304. Langbaum M, Eyal FG. *Stomatococcus mucilaginosus* septicemia and meningitis in a premature infant. Pediatr Infect Dis J 11:334, 1992.
305. Bose A, Philip JK, Jesudason M. Neonatal septicemia caused by *Vibrio cholerae* O:139. Pediatr Infect Dis J 19:166, 2000.
306. Kerketta JA, Paul AC, Kirubakaran VB, et al. Non-01 *Vibrio cholerae* septicemia and meningitis in a neonate. Indian J Pediatr 69:909, 2002.
307. Challapalli M, Cunningham DG. *Yersinia enterocolitica* septicemia in infants younger than three months of age. Pediatr Infect Dis J 12:168, 1993.
308. White ME, Rosenbaum RJ, Canfield TM, et al. Plague in a neonate. Am J Dis Child 135:418, 1981.
309. Public Health Laboratory Service Report. Neonatal meningitis: a review of routine national data 1975-83. BMJ 290:778, 1985.
310. Schuchat A, Oxtoby M, Cochi S, et al. Population-based risk factors for neonatal group B streptococcal disease: results of a cohort study in metropolitan Atlanta. J Infect Dis 162:672, 1990.
311. Cordero L, Sananes M, Ayers LW. Bloodstream infections in a neonatal intensive-care unit: 12 years' experience with an antibiotic control program. Infect Control Hosp Epidemiol 20:242, 1999.
312. Persson E, Trollfors B, Brandberg LL, Tessin I. Septicaemia and meningitis in neonates and during early infancy in the Goteborg area of Sweden. Acta Paediatr 91:1087, 2002.
313. Simon C, Schroder H, Beyer C, Zerbst T. Neonatal sepsis in an intensive care unit and results of treatment. Infection 19:146, 1991.
314. Stoll BJ, Hansen N. Infections in VLBW infants: studies from the NICHD Neonatal Research Network. Semin Perinatol 27:293, 2003.
315. Barton L, Hodgman JE, Pavlova Z. Causes of death in the extremely low birth weight infant. Pediatrics 103:446, 1999.
316. Bhutta ZA, Yusuf K. Early-onset neonatal sepsis in Pakistan: a case control study of risk factors in a birth cohort. Am J Perinatol 14:577, 1997.
317. Boyer KM, Gadzala CA, Burd LI, et al. Selective intrapartum chemoprophylaxis of neonatal group B streptococcal early-onset disease. I. Epidemiologic rationale. J Infect Dis 148:795, 1983.
318. Lieberman E, Lang JM, Frigoletto F Jr, et al. Epidural analgesia, intrapartum fever, and neonatal sepsis evaluation. Pediatrics 99:415, 1997.
319. Niswander KR, Gordon M. The women and their pregnancies. The Collaborative Perinatal Study of the National Institute of Neurological Diseases and Stroke. U.S. Department of Health, Education and Welfare Publication No. (NIH) 73-379. Washington, DC, U.S. Government Printing Office, 1972.
320. National Center for Health Statistics. Healthy People 2000. Maternal and infant health progress review. Live broadcast from Washington, DC, May 5, 1999.
321. Fiscella K. Race, perinatal outcome, and amniotic infection. Obstet Gynecol Surv 51:60, 1996.
322. Centers for Disease Control and Prevention. Group B streptococcal disease in the United States, 1990: report from a multistate active surveillance system. *In* CDC Surveillance Summaries, November 20, 1992. MMWR Morb Mortal Wkly Rep 41(No. SS-6):25, 1992.
323. Benirschke K, Driscoll S. The Pathology of the Human Placenta. New York, Springer-Verlag, 1967.
324. Washburn TC, Medearis DN Jr, Childs B. Sex differences in susceptibility to infections. Pediatrics 35:57, 1965.
325. Torday JS, Nielsen HC, Fencl MD, et al. Sex differences in fetal lung maturation. Am Rev Respir Dis 123:205, 1981.
326. Sinha A, Yokoe D, Platt R. Epidemiology of neonatal infections: experience during and after hospitalization. Pediatr Infect Dis J 22:244, 2003.
327. Schuchat A, Zywicki SS, Dinsmoor MJ, et al. Risk factors and opportunities for prevention of early-onset neonatal sepsis: a multicenter case-control study. Pediatrics 105, 21, 2000.
328. Sohn AH, Garret DO, Sinkowitz-Cochran RL, et al. Prevalence of nosocomial infections in neonatal intensive care unit patients: results from the first national point-prevalence study. J Pediatr 139, 821, 2001.
329. MacFarlane DE. Neonatal group B streptococcal septicaemia in a developing country. Acta Paediatr Scand 76:470, 1987.
330. Ako-Nai AK, Adejuyigbe EA, Ajayi FM, Onipede AO. The bacteriology of neonatal septicaemiae in Ile-Ife, Nigeria. J Trop Pediatr 45:146, 1999.
331. Kuruvilla KA, Pillai S, Jesudason M, Jana AK. Bacterial profile of sepsis in a neonatal unit in South India. Indian Pediatr 35:851, 1998.
332. Ohlsson A, Bailey T, Takieddine F. Changing etiology and outcome of neonatal septicemia in Riyadh, Saudi Arabia. Acta Paediatr Scand 75:540, 1986.
333. Kilani RA, Basamad M. Pattern of proven bacterial sepsis in a neonatal intensive care unit in Riyadh-Saudi Arabia: a 2-year analysis. J Med Liban 48:77, 2000.
334. Amin A, Abdulrazzaq YM, Uduman S. Group B streptococcal serotype distribution of isolates from colonized pregnant women at the time of delivery in United Arab Emirates. J Infect 45:42, 2002.
335. Tsolia M, Psoma M, Gavrili S, et al. Group B streptococcus colonization of Greek pregnant women and neonates: prevalence, risk factors and serotypes. Clin Microbiol Infect 9:832, 2003.
336. Stoll BJ and Schuchat A. Maternal carriage of group B streptococci in developing countries. Pediatr Infect Dis J 17:499, 1998.
337. Cogwill K, Taylor TH Jr, Schuchat A, Schrag S. Report from the CDC. Awareness of perinatal group B streptococcal infection among women of childbearing age in the United States, 1999 and 2002. J Womens Health 12:527, 2003.
338. Beck-Sague CM, Azimi P, Fonseca SN, Baltimore RS. Blood stream infections in neonatal intensive care unit patients: results of a multicenter study. Pediatr Infect Dis J 13:1110, 1994.
339. Adams WG, Kinney JS, Schuchat A, et al. Outbreak of early onset group B streptococcal sepsis. Pediatr Infect Dis J 12:565, 1993.
340. Cheasty T, Robertson R, Chart H, et al. The use of serodiagnosis in the retrospective investigation of a nursery outbreak associated with *Escherichia coli* O157:H7. J Clin Pathol 51:498, 1998.
341. Hoyen C, Rice L, Conte S, et al. Use of real time pulsed field gel electrophoresis to guide interventions during a nursery outbreak of *Serratia marcescens* infection. Pediatr Infect Dis J 18:357, 1999.
342. Olive DM, Bean P. Principles and applications of methods for DNA-based typing of microbial organisms. J Clin Microbiol 37:1661, 1999.
343. Dent A, Toltzis P. Descriptive and molecular epidemiology of Gram-negative bacilli infections in the neonatal intensive care unit. Curr Opin Infect Dis 16:279, 2003.
344. van der Zwet WC, Parlevliet GA, Savelkoul PH, et al. Nosocomial outbreak of gentamicin-resistant *Klebsiella pneumoniae* in a neonatal intensive care unit controlled by a change in antibiotic policy. J Hosp Infect 42:295, 1999.
345. Raz R, Sharir R, Shmilowitz L, et al. The elimination of gentamicin-resistant gram-negative bacteria in newborn intensive care unit. Infection 15:32, 1987.
346. Gibbs RS, Duff P. Progress in pathogenesis and management of clinical intraamniotic infection. Am J Obstet Gynecol 164:1317, 1991.
347. Charles D, Edwards WR. Infectious complications of cervical cerclage. Am J Obstet Gynecol 141:1065, 1981.
348. Aarts JM. Brons JT. Bruinse HW. Emergency cerclage: a review. Obstet Gynecol Surv 50:459, 1995.
349. Fejgin M, Amiel A, Kaneti H, et al. Fulminant sepsis due to group B beta-hemolytic streptococci following transcervical chorionic villi sampling. Clin Infect Dis 17:142, 1993.
350. Wilkins I, Mezrow G, Lynch L, et al. Amnionitis and life-threatening respiratory distress after percutaneous umbilical blood sampling. Am J Obstet Gynecol 160:427, 1989.
351. Morison JE. Foetal and Neonatal Pathology, 3rd ed. Washington, DC, Butterworth, 1970.
352. St. Geme JW Jr, Murray DL, Carter J, et al. Perinatal bacterial infection after prolonged rupture of amniotic membranes: an analysis of risk and management. J Pediatr 104:608, 1984.
353. Blanc WA. Pathways of fetal and early neonatal infection: viral placentitis, bacterial and fungal chorioamnionitis. J Pediatr 59:473, 1961.
354. Hillier SL, Krohn MA, Kiviat NB, et al. Microbiologic causes and neonatal outcomes associated with chorioamnion infection. Am J Obstet Gynecol 165:955, 1991.
355. Yoder PR, Gibbs RS, Blanco JD, et al. A prospective, controlled study of maternal and perinatal outcome after intra-amniotic infection at term. Am J Obstet Gynecol 145:695, 1983.
356. Larsen B, Snyder IS, Galask RP. Bacterial growth inhibition by amniotic fluid. I. In vitro evidence for bacterial growth-inhibiting activity. Am J Obstet Gynecol 119:492, 1974.
357. Kitzmiller JL, Highby S, Lucas WE. Retarded growth of *E. coli* in amniotic fluid. Obstet Gynecol 41:38, 1973.
358. Axemo P, Rwamushaija E, Pettersson M, et al. Amniotic fluid antibacterial activity and nutritional parameters in term Mozambican and Swedish pregnant women. Gynecol Obstet Invest 42:24, 1996.
359. Scane TM, Hawkins DF. Antibacterial activity in human amniotic fluid: relationship to zinc and phosphate. Br J Obstet Gynaecol 91:342, 1984.
360. Nazir MA, Pankuch GA, Botti JJ, Appelbaum PC. Antibacterial activity of amniotic fluid in the early third trimester: its association with preterm labor and delivery. Am J Perinatol 4:59, 1987.
361. Baker SM, Balo NN, Abdel Aziz FT. Is vernix a protective material to the newborn? A biochemical approach. Indian J Pediatr 62:237, 1995.

362. Florman AL, Teubner D. Enhancement of bacterial growth in amniotic fluid by meconium. J Pediatr 74:111, 1969.
363. Hoskins IA, Hemming VG, Johnson TRB, et al. Effects of alterations of zinc-to-phosphate ratios and meconium content on group B *Streptococcus* growth in human amniotic fluid *in vitro*. Am J Obstet Gynecol 157:770, 1988.
364. Altieri C, Maruotti G, Natale C, Massa S. In vitro survival of *Listeria monocytogenes* in human amniotic fluid. Zentralbl Hyg Umweltmed 202:377, 1999.
365. Evaldson G, Nord CE. Amniotic fluid activity against *Bacteroides fragilis* and group B streptococci. Med Microbiol Immunol 170:11, 1981.
366. Eidelman AI, Nevet A, Rudensky B, et al. The effect of meconium staining of amniotic fluid on the growth of *Escherichia coli* and group B streptococcus. J Perinatol 22:467, 2002.
367. Marston G, Wald ER. *Hemophilus influenzae* type b sepsis in infant and mother. Pediatrics 58:863, 1976.
368. Tarpay MM, Turbeville DV, Krous HF. Fatal *Streptococcus pneumoniae* type III sepsis in mother and infant. Am J Obstet Gynecol 136:257, 1980.
369. Hughes BR, Mercer JL, Gosbel LB. Neonatal pneumococcal sepsis in association with fatal maternal pneumococcal sepsis. Aust N Z J Obstet Gynaecol 41:457, 2001.
370. Panaro NR, Lutwick LI, Chapnick EK. Intrapartum transmission of group A Streptococcus. Clin Infect Dis 17:79, 1993.
371. Bhutta ZA, Khan IA, Agha A. Fatal intrauterine meningococcal infection. Pediatr Infect Dis J 11:868, 1991.
372. Mastrobattista JM, Parisi VM. Vertical transmission of a *Citrobacter* infection. Am J Perinatol 14:465, 1997.
373. Boussemart T, Piet-Duroux S, Manouana M, et al. *Morganella morganii* and early-onset neonatal infection. Arch Pediatr 11:37, 2004.
374. Tempest B. Pneumococcal meningitis in mother and neonate. Pediatrics 53:759, 1974.
375. Grossman J, Tompkins RL. Group B beta-hemolytic streptococcal meningitis in mother and infant. N Engl J Med 290:387, 1974.
376. Pyati SP, Pildes RS, Jacobs NM, et al. Penicillin in infants weighing two kilograms or less with early-onset group B streptococcal disease. N Engl J Med 308:1383, 1983.
377. Maberry MC, Gilstrap LC. Intrapartum antibiotic therapy for suspected intraamniotic infection: impact on the fetus and neonate. Clin Obstet Gynecol 34:345, 1991.
378. Sacks LM, McKitrick JC, MacGregor RR. Surface cultures and isolation procedures in infants born under unsterile conditions. Am J Dis Child 137:351, 1983.
379. Brook I, Frazier EH. Microbiology of scalp abscess in newborn. Pediatr Infect Dis J 11:766, 1992.
380. Dobson SR, Baker CJ. Enterococcal sepsis in neonates: features by age at onset and occurrence of focal infection. Pediatrics 85:165, 1990.
381. Freedman RM, Baltimore R. Fatal *Streptococcus viridans* septicemia and meningitis: a relationship to fetal scalp electrode monitoring. J Perinatol 10:272, 1990.
382. Cordero L, Anderson CW, Zuspan FP. Scalp abscess: a benign and infrequent complication of fetal monitoring. Am J Obstet Gynecol 146:126, 1983.
383. Storm W. Transient bacteremia following endotracheal suctioning in ventilated newborns. Pediatrics 65:487, 1980.
384. Singer DB. Infections of fetuses and neonates. *In* Wigglesworth JS, Singer DB (eds). Textbook of Fetal and Perinatal Pathology. Boston, Blackwell Scientific Publications, 1991, pp 525-591.
385. Sorokin Y, Weintraub Z, Rothschild A, et al. Cerebrospinal fluid leak in the neonate—complication of fetal scalp electrode monitoring. Case report and review of the literature. Isr J Med Sci 26:633, 1990.
386. Nieburg P, Gross SJ. Cerebrospinal fluid leak in a neonate with fetal scalp electrode monitoring. Am J Obstet Gynecol 147:839, 1983.
387. Nagle RC, Taekman MS, Shallat RF, et al. Brain abscess aspiration in nursery with ultrasound guidance. J Neurosurg 65:557, 1986.
388. Renier D, Flandin C, Hirsch E, et al. Brain abscesses in neonates: a study of 30 cases. J Neurosurg 69:877, 1988.
389. Jadavji T, Humphreys RP, Prober CG. Brain abscesses in infants and children. Pediatr Infect Dis 4:394, 1985.
390. Volpe JJ. Neurology of the Newborn, 2nd ed. Philadelphia, WB Saunders, 1987, p 625.
391. Dillon HC, Khare S, Gray BM. Group B streptococcal carriage and disease: a 6-year prospective study. J Pediatr 110:31, 1987.
392. Maisels MJ, Kring E. Risk of sepsis in newborns with severe hyperbilirubinemia. Pediatrics 90:741, 1992.
393. Haber BA, Lake AM. Cholestatic jaundice in the newborn. Clin Perinatol 17:483, 1990.
394. Rooney JC, Hills DJ, Danks DM. Jaundice associated with bacterial infection in the newborn. Am J Dis Child 122:39, 1971.
395. Dagan R, Gorodischer R. Infections in hypothermic infants younger than 3 months old. Am J Dis Child 138:483, 1984.
396. Johanson RB, Spencer SA, Rolfe P, et al. Effect of post-delivery care on neonatal body temperature. Acta Paediatr 81:859, 1992.
397. Michael M, Barrett DJ, Mehta P. Infants with meningitis without CSF pleocytosis. Am J Dis Child 140:851, 1986.
398. El-Radhy AS, Jawad M, Mansor N, et al. Sepsis and hypothermia in the newborn infant: value of gastric aspirate examination. J Pediatr 104:300, 1983.
399. Barr PH. Association of *Escherichia coli* sepsis and galactosemia in neonates. J Am Board Fam Pract 5:89, 1992.
400. Levy HL, Sepe SJ, Shih VE, et al. Sepsis due to *Escherichia coli* in neonates with galactosemia. N Engl J Med 297:823, 1977.
401. Kelly S. Septicemia in galactosemia. JAMA 216:330, 1971.
402. Shurin SB. *Escherichia coli* septicemia in neonates with galactosemia. Letter to the editor. N Engl J Med 297:1403, 1977.
403. Kobayashi RH, Kettelhut BV, Kobayashi AL. Galactose inhibition of neonatal neutrophil function. Pediatr Infect Dis J 2:442, 1983.
404. Odievre M, Gentil C, Gautier M, et al. Hereditary fructose intolerance. Diagnosis management and course in 55 patients. Am J Dis Child 132:605, 1978.
405. Guerra-Moreno J, Barrios N, Santiago-Borrero PJ. Severe neutropenia in an infant with methylmalonic acidemia. Bol Assoc Med P R 95:17, 2003.
406. Hutchinson RJ, Bunnell K, Thoene JG. Suppression of granulopoietic progenitor cell proliferation by metabolites of the branched-chain amino acids. J Pediatr 106:62, 1985.
407. Weinberg ED. Iron and susceptibility to infectious disease. Science 184:952, 1974.
408. Barry DMJ, Reeve AW. Increased incidence of gram-negative neonatal sepsis with intramuscular iron administration. Pediatrics 60:908, 1977.
409. Farmer K. The disadvantages of routine administration of intramuscular iron to neonates. N Z Med J 84:286, 1976.
410. Usta IM, Nassar AH, Awwad JT, et al. Comparison of the perinatal morbidity and mortality of the presenting twin and its co-twin. J Perinatol 22:391, 2002.
411. Benirschke K. Routes and types of infection in the fetus and newborn. Am J Dis Child 99:714, 1960.
412. Pass MA, Khare S, Dillon HC Jr. Twin pregnancies: incidence of group B streptococcal colonization and disease. J Pediatr 97:635, 1980.
413. Edwards MS, Jackson CV, Baker CJ. Increased risk of group B streptococcal disease in twins. JAMA 245:2044, 1981.
414. Nieburg PI, William ML. Group A beta-hemolytic streptococcal sepsis in a mother and infant twins. J Pediatr 87:453, 1975.
415. Larsen JG, Harra BA, Bottone EJ, et al. Multiple antibiotic resistant *Salmonella agora* infection in malnourished neonatal twins. Mt Sinai J Med 46:542, 1979.
416. Devlin HR, Bannatyne RM. Neonatal malaria. Can Med Assoc J 116:20, 1977.
417. Romand S, Bouree P, Gelez J, et al. Congenital malaria. A case observed in twins born to an asymptomatic mother. Presse Med 23:797, 1994.
418. Shafai T. Neonatal coccidioidomycosis in premature twins. Am J Dis Child 132:634, 1978.
419. Saigal S, Eisele WA, Chernesky MA. Congenital cytomegalovirus infection in a pair of dizygotic twins. Am J Dis Child 136:1094, 1982.
420. Duvekot JJ, Theewes BA, Wesdorp JM, et al. Congenital cytomegalovirus infection in a twin pregnancy: a case report. Eur J Pediatr 149:261, 1990.
421. Lazzarotto T, Gabrielli L, Foschini MP, et al. Congenital cytomegalovirus infection in twin pregnancies: viral load in the amniotic fluid and pregnancy outcome. Pediatrics 112:e153, 2003.
422. Montgomery RC, Stockdell K. Congenital rubella in twins. J Pediatr 76:772, 1970.
423. Forshall I. Septic umbilical arteritis. Arch Dis Child 32:25, 1957.
424. Cruickshank JN. Child Life Investigations: The Causes of Neo-natal Death. Medical Research Council Special Report Series No. 145. London, His Majesty's Stationery Office, 1930, p 26.
425. Cushing AH. Omphalitis: a review. Pediatr Infect Dis J 4:282, 1985.
426. Rotimi VO, Duerden BI. The development of the bacterial flora in normal neonates. J Med Microbiol 14:51, 1981.
427. Mason WH, Andrews R, Ross LA, et al. Omphalitis in the newborn infant. Pediatr Infect Dis J 8:521, 1989.

428. Ameh EA, Nmadu PT. Major complications of omphalitis in neonates and infants. Pediatr Surg Int 18:413, 2002.
429. Meyer WW, Lind J. The ductus venosus and the mechanism of its closure. Arch Dis Child 41:597, 1966.
430. Morison JE. Umbilical sepsis and acute interstitial hepatitis. J Pathol Bacteriol 56:531, 1944.
431. Elliott RIK. The ductus venosus in neonatal infection. Proc R Soc Med 62:321, 1969.
432. Bedtke K, Richarz H. Nabelsepsis mit Pylephlebitis, multiplen Leberabscessen, Lungenabscessen und Osteomyelitis. Ausgang in Heilung. Monatsschr Kinderheilkd 105:70, 1957.
434. Beaven DW. Staphylococcal peritonitis in the newborn. Lancet 1:869, 1958.
435. Thompson EN, Sherlock S. The aetiology of portal vein thrombosis with particular reference to the role of infection and exchange transfusion. Q J Med 33:465, 1964.
436. Navarro C, Blanc WA. Subacute necrotizing funisitis: a variant of cord inflammation with a high rate of perinatal infection. J Pediatr 85:689, 1974.
437. Ohlsson A. Treatment of preterm premature rupture of the membranes: a meta-analysis. Am J Obstet Gynecol 160:890, 1989.
438. Crowley P, Chalmers I, Keirse MJ. The effects of corticosteroid administration before preterm delivery: an overview of the evidence from controlled trials. Br J Obstet Gynaecol 97:11, 1990.
439. Vermillion ST, Soper DE, Bland ML, Newman RB. Effectiveness of antenatal corticosteroid administration after preterm premature rupture of the membranes. Am J Obstet Gynecol 183:925, 2000.
440. Gottesfeld Z, Ullrich SE. Prenatal alcohol exposure selectively suppresses cell-mediated but not humoral immune responsiveness. Int J Immunopharmacol 17:247, 1995.
441. Johnson S, Knight R, Marmer DJ, et al. Immune deficiency in fetal alcohol syndrome. Pediatr Res 15:908, 1981.
442. Culver KW, Ammann AJ, Partridge JC, et al. Lymphocyte abnormalities in infants born to drug-abusing mothers. J Pediatr 111:230, 1987.
443. Chasnoff IJ (ed). Chemical dependency and pregnancy. Clin Perinatol 18:1, 1991.
444. Woods JR Jr (ed). Drug abuse in pregnancy. Clin Obstet Gynecol 36:221, 1993.
445. Chasnoff IJ (ed). Drug Use in Pregnancy: Mother and Child. Boston, MTP Press, 1986.
446. Ojala R, Ikonen S, Tammela O. Perinatal indomethacin treatment and neonatal complications in preterm infants. Eur J Pediatr 159:153, 2000.
447. Major CA, Lewis DF, Harding JA, et al. Tocolysis with indomethacin increases the incidence of necrotizing enterocolitis in the low-birth-weight neonate. Am J Obstet Gynecol 170:102, 1994.
448. Herson VC, Krause PJ, Einsenfeld LI, et al. Indomethacin-associated sepsis in very-low-birth-weight infants. Am J Dis Child 142:555, 1988.
449. O'Shea TM, Kothadia JM, Klinepeter KL, et al. Follow-up of preterm infants treated with dexamethasone for chronic lung disease. Am J Dis Child 147:658, 1993.
450. Heymann MA. Prostaglandins and leukotrienes in the perinatal period. Clin Perinatol 14:857, 1987.
451. Barson AJ. A postmortem study of infection in the newborn from 1976 to 1988. *In* de Louvois J, Harvey D (eds). Infection in the Newborn. New York, John Wiley & Sons, 1990, pp 13-34.
452. Berman PH, Banker BQ. Neonatal meningitis: a clinical and pathological study of 29 cases. Pediatrics 38:6, 1966.
453. Stocker JT, Dehner LP. Pediatric Pathology. Philadelphia, JB Lippincott, 1992.
454. Hoffman HJ, Hendrick EB, Hiscox JL. Cerebral abscesses in early infancy. J Neurosurg 33:172, 1970.
455. Watson DG. Purulent neonatal meningitis: a study of forty-five cases. J Pediatr 50:352, 1957.
456. Volpe JJ. Neurology of the Newborn, 3rd ed. Philadelphia, WB Saunders, 1995, pp 734-742.
457. Perlman JM, Rollins N, Sanchez PJ. Late-onset meningitis in sick, very-low-birth-weight infants: clinical and sonographic observations. Am J Dis Child 146:1297, 1992.
458. Gilles FH, Jammes JL, Berenberg W. Neonatal meningitis: the ventricle as a bacterial reservoir. Arch Neurol 34:560, 1977.
459. Schiano MA, Hauth JC, Gilstrap LC. Second-stage fetal tachycardia and neonatal infection. Am J Obstet Gynecol 148:779, 1984.
460. Soman M, Green B, Daling J. Risk factors for early neonatal sepsis. Am J Epidemiol 121:712, 1985.
461. Hegyi T, Carbone T, Anwar M, et al. The Apgar Score and its components in the preterm infant. Pediatrics 101:77, 1998.
462. Powell KR. Evaluation and management of febrile infants younger than 60 days of age. Pediatr Infect Dis J 9:153, 1990.
463. Bonadio WA, Hennes H, Smith D, et al. Reliability of observation variables in distinguishing infectious outcome of febrile young infants. Pediatr Infect Dis J 12:111, 1993.
464. Fielkow S, Reuter S, Gotoff SP. Cerebrospinal fluid examination in symptom-free infants with risk factors for infection. J Pediatr 119:971, 1991.
465. Albers WH, Tyler CW, Boxerbaum B. Asymptomatic bacteremia in the newborn infant. J Pediatr 69:193, 1966.
466. Petanovic M, Zagar Z. The significance of asymptomatic bacteremia for the newborn. Acta Obstet Gynecol Scand 80:813, 2001.
467. Howard JB, McCracken GH. The spectrum of group B streptococcal infections in infancy. Am J Dis Child 128:815, 1974.
468. Weisman LE, Stoll BJ, Cruess DF, et al. Early-onset group B streptococcal sepsis: a current assessment. J Pediatr 121:428, 1992.
469. Yagupsky P, Menegus MA, Powell KR. The changing spectrum of group B streptococcal disease in infants: an eleven-year experience in a tertiary care hospital. Pediatr Infect Dis J 10:801, 1991.
470. Ramsey PG, Zwerdling R. Asymptomatic neonatal bacteremia. Letter to the editor. N Engl J Med 295:225, 1976.
471. Yu JS, Grauang A. Purulent meningitis in the neonatal period. Arch Dis Child 38:391, 1963.
472. Solomon SL, Wallace EM, Ford-Jones EL, et al. Medication errors with inhalant epinephrine mimicking an epidemic of neonatal sepsis. N Engl J Med 310:166, 1984.
473. Bonadio WA, Hegenbarth M, Zachariason M. Correlating reported fever in young infants with subsequent temperature patterns and rate of serious bacterial infections. Pediatr Infect Dis J 9:158, 1990.
474. Messaritakis J, Anagnostakis D, Laskari H, et al. Rectal-skin temperature difference in septicaemic newborn infants. Arch Dis Child 65:380, 1990.
475. Dinarello CA, Shparber M, Kent EF Jr, et al. Production of leukocytic pyrogen from phagocytes of neonates. J Infect Dis 144:337, 1981.
476. Mayfield SR, Bhatia J, Nakamura K, et al. Temperature measurement in term and preterm neonates. J Pediatr 104:271, 1984.
477. Johnson KJ, Bhatia P, Bell EF. Infrared themometry of newborn infants. Pediatrics 87:34, 1991.
478. Schuman AJ. The accuracy of infrared auditory canal thermometry in infants and children. Clin Pediatr 32:347, 1993.
479. Anagnostakis D, Matsaniotis N, Grafakos S, et al. Rectal-axillary difference in febrile and afebrile infants and children. Clin Pediatr 32:268, 1993.
480. Weisse ME, Reagen MS, Boule L, et al. Axillary vs. rectal temperatures in ambulatory and hospitalized children. Pediatr Infect Dis J 10:541, 1991.
481. Freed GL, Fraley JK. Lack of agreement of tympanic membrane temperature assessments with conventional methods in a private practice setting. Pediatrics 89:384, 1992.
482. Voora S, Srinivasan G, Lilien LD, et al. Fever in full-term newborns in the first four days of life. Pediatrics 69:40, 1982.
483. Osborn LM, Bolus R. Temperature and fever in the full-term newborn. J Fam Pract 20:261, 1985.
484. Garcia FJ, Nager AL. Jaundice as an early diagnostic sign of urinary tract infection in infancy. Pediatrics 109:846, 2002.
485. Zamora-Castorena S, Murguia-de-Sierra MT. Five year experience with neonatal sepsis in a pediatric center. Rev Invest Clin 50:463, 1998.
486. Airede AI. Urinary-tract infections in African neonates. J Infect 25:55, 1992.
487. Seeler RA. Urosepsis with jaundice due to hemolytic *Escherichia coli.* Am J Dis Child 126:414, 1973.
488. Ashkenazi S, Mimouni F, Merlob P, et al. Size of liver edge in full-term, healthy infants. Am J Dis Child 138:377, 1984.
489. Reiff MI, Osborn LM. Clinical estimation of liver size in newborn infants. Pediatrics 71:46, 1983.
490. Sfeir J, Bloomfield J, Aspillaga C, Ferreiro M. Early onset neonatal septicemia caused by *Listeria monocytogenes*. Rev Chil Pediatr 61:330, 1990.
491. Bamji M, Stone RK, Kaul A, et al. Palpable lymph nodes in healthy newborns and infants. Pediatrics 78:573, 1986.
492. Embree J, Muriithi J. Palpable lymph nodes. Letter to the editor. Pediatrics 81:598, 1988.
493. Monfort Gil R, Castells Vilella L, Pagone Tangorra F, et al. Group B Streptococcus late-onset disease presenting as cellulitis-adenitis syndrome. Ann Pediatr 60:75, 2004.

494. Artigas Rodriguez S, Diaz Gonzalez P, et al. Group B streptococcus cellulitis-adenitis syndrome in neonates. Is it a marker of bacteremia? An Esp Pediatr 56:251, 2002.
495. Albanyan EA, Baker CJ. Is lumbar puncture necessary to exclude meningitis in neonates and young infants: lessons from the group B streptococcus cellulitis-adenitis syndrome. Pediatrics 102:985, 1998.
496. Volpe JJ. Neurology of the Newborn, 2nd ed. Philadelphia, WB Saunders, 1987, p 608.
497. Bell AH, Brown D, Halliday HL, et al. Meningitis in the newborn: a 14 year review. Arch Dis Child 64:873, 1989.
498. Weintraub MI, Otto RN. Pneumococcal meningitis and endophthalmitis in a newborn. JAMA 219:1763, 1972.
499. Matasova K, Hudecova J, Zibolen M. Bilateral endogenous endophthalmitis as a complication of late-onset sepsis in a premature infant. Eur J Pediatr 162:346, 2003.
500. Nejat F, Ardakani SB, Khotaei GT, Roodsari NN. Spinal epidural abscess in a neonate. Pediatr Infect Dis J 21:797, 2002.
501. Walter RS, King JC, Manley J, et al. Spinal epidural abscess in infancy: successful percutaneous drainage in a nine-month-old and review of the literature. Pediatr Infect Dis J 19:860, 1991.
502. Tang K, Xenos C, Sgouros S. Spontaneous spinal epidural abscess in a neonate. With a review of the literature. Childs Nerv Syst 17:629, 2001.
503. Steele RW. A revised strategy for the prevention of group B streptococcal infection in pregnant women and their newborns. Medscape Womens Health 1:2, 1996.
504. American College of Obstetricians and Gynecologists. ACOG Committee Opinion: number 279, December 2002. Prevention of early-onset group B streptococcal disease in newborns. Obstet Gynecol 100:1405, 2002.
505. Evans ME, Schaffner W, Federspiel CF, et al. Sensitivity, specificity, and predictive value of body surface cultures in a neonatal intensive care unit. JAMA 259:248, 1988.
507. Hertz D, Fuller D, Davis T, et al. Comparison of DNA probe technology and automated continuous-monitoring blood culture systems in the detection of neonatal bacteremia. J Perinatol 19:290, 1999.
508. Nolte FS, Williams JM, Jerris RC, et al. Multicenter clinical evaluation of a continuous monitoring blood culture system using fluorescent-sensor technology (BACTEC 9240). J Clin Microbiol 31:552, 1993.
509. Anderson JD, Trombley C, Cimolai N. Assessment of the BACTEC NR660 blood culture system for the detection of bacteremia in young children. J Clin Microbiol 27:721, 1989.
510. Campos JM, Spainhour JR. Rapid detection of bacteremia in children with modified lysis direct plating method. J Clin Microbiol 22:674, 1985.
511. St. Geme JW III, Bell LM, Baumgart S, et al. Distinguishing sepsis from blood culture contamination in young infants with blood cultures growing coagulase-negative staphylococci. Pediatrics 86:157, 1990.
512. Kurlat I, Stoll BJ, McGowan JE Jr. Time to positivity for detection of bacteremia in neonates. J Clin Microbiol 27:1068, 1989.
513. Pichichero MD, Todd JK. Detection of neonatal bacteremia. J Pediatr 94:958, 1979.
514. Rowley AH, Wald ER. Incubation period necessary to detect bacteremia in neonates. Pediatr Infect Dis J 5:590, 1986.
515. Sprunt K. Commentary. *In* Gellis SS (ed). The Year Book of Pediatrics 1973. Chicago, Year Book Medical Publishers, 1973, p 15.
516. Wiswell TE, Hachey WE. Multiple site blood cultures in the initial evaluation for neonatal sepsis during the first week of life. Pediatr. Infect Dis J 10:365, 1991.
517. Neal PR, Kleiman MB, Reynolds JK, et al. Volume of blood submitted for culture from neonates. J Clin Microbiol 24:353, 1986.
518. Dietzman DE, Fischer GW, Schoenknecht FD. Neonatal *Escherichia coli* septicemia—bacterial counts in blood. J Pediatr 85:128, 1974.
519. Kennaugh JK, Gregory WW, Powell KR, Hendley JO. The effect of dilution during culture on detection of low concentrations of bacteria in blood. Pediatr Infect Dis J 3:317, 1984.
520. Jawaheer G, Neal TJ, Shaw NJ. Blood culture volume and detection of coagulase negative staphylococcal septicaemia in neonates. Arch Dis Child 76:57F, 1997
521. Kellogg JA, Manzella JP, Bankert DA. Frequency of low-level bacteremia in children from birth to fifteen years of age. J Clin Microbiol 28:2181, 2000.
522. Kellogg JA, Ferrentino FL, Goodstein MH, et al. Frequency of low-level bacteremia in infants from birth to two months of age. Pediatr Infect Dis J 16:381, 1997.
523. Schelonka RL, Chai MK, Yoder BA, et al. Volume of blood required to detect common neonatal pathogens. J Pediatr 129:275, 1996.
524. Pourcyrous M, Korones SB, Bada HS, et al. Indwelling umbilical arterial catheter: a preferred sampling site for blood cultures. Pediatrics 81:621, 1988.
525. Bhandari V, Eisenfeld L, Lerer T, et al. Nosocomial sepsis in neonates with single lumen vascular catheters. Indian J Pediatr 64:529, 1997.
526. Benjamin DK Jr, Miller W, Garges H, et al. Bacteremia, central catheters, and neonates: when to pull the line. Pediatrics 107:1272, 2001.
527. Hammerberg O, Bialkowska-Hobrzanska H, Gregson D, et al. Comparison of blood cultures with corresponding venipuncture site cultures of specimens from hospitalized premature neonates. J Pediatr 120:120, 1992.
528. Healy CM, Palazzi DL, Edwards MS, et al. Distinctive features of neonatal invasive staphylococcal disease. Pediatrics 114:953, 2004.
529. Humphrey AA. Use of the buffy layer in the rapid diagnosis of septicemia. Am J Clin Pathol 14:358, 1944.
530. Boyle RJ, Chandler BD, Stonestreet BS, et al. Early identification of sepsis in infants with respiratory distress. Pediatrics 62:744, 1978.
531. Faden HS. Early diagnosis of neonatal bacteremia by buffy-coat examination. J Pediatr 88:1032, 1976.
532. Storm W. Early detection of bacteremia by peripheral smears in critically ill newborns. Acta Paediatr Scand 70:415, 1981.
533. Kleiman MB, Reynolds JK, Schreiner RL, et al. Rapid diagnosis of neonatal bacteremia with acridine orange-stained buffy coat smears. J Pediatr 105:419, 1984.
534. Kite P, Millar MR, Gorham P, et al. Comparison of five tests used in diagnosis of neonatal bacteremia. Arch Dis Child 63:639, 1988.
535. Tak SK, Bhandari PC, Bhandari B. Value of buffy coat examination in early diagnosis of neonatal septicemia. Indian Pediatr 17:339, 1980.
536. Powers DL, Mandell GL. Intraleukocytic bacteria in endocarditis patients. JAMA 227:312, 1974.
537. Cattermole HEJ, Rivers RPA. Neonatal *Candida* septicaemia: diagnosis on buffy smear. Arch Dis Child 62:302, 1987.
538. Ascuitto RJ, Gerber MA, Cates KL, et al. Buffy coat smears of blood drawn through central venous catheters as an aid to rapid diagnosis of systemic fungal infections. J Pediatr 106:445, 1985.
539. Selby DM, Gautier G, Luban NLC, Campos JM. Overwhelming neonatal septicemia diagnosed upon examination of peripheral blood smears. Clin Pediatr 29:706, 1990.
540. Strom W. Early detection of bacteremia by peripheral blood smears in critically ill newborns. Acta Paediatr Scand 70:415, 1981.
541. Rodwell RL, Leslie AL, Tudehope DI. Evaluation of direct and buffy coat films of peripheral blood for the early detection of bacteraemia. Aust Paediatr J 25:83, 1989.
542. Visser VE, Hall RT. Urine culture in the evaluation of suspected neonatal sepsis. J Pediatr 94:635, 1979.
543. DiGeronimo RJ. Lack of efficacy of the urine culture as part of the initial workup of suspected neonatal sepsis. Pediatr Infect Dis J 9:764, 1992.
544. Tobiansky R, Evans N. A randomized controlled trial of two methods for collection of sterile urine in neonates. J Paediatr Child Health 34:460, 1998.
545. Garcia Munoz MT, Cerezo Pancorbo JM, et al. Suprapubic bladder aspiration. Utility and complication. An Esp Pediatr 45:377, 1996.
546. Nelson JD, Peters PC. Suprapubic aspiration of urine in premature and term infants. Pediatrics 36:132, 1965.
547. Lau YL, Hey E. Sensitivity and specificity of daily tracheal aspirate cultures in predicting organisms causing bacteremia in ventilated neonates. Pediatr Infect Dis J 10:290, 1991.
548. Finelli L, Livengood JR, Saiman L. Surveillance of pharyngeal colonization: detection and control of serious bacterial illness in low birth weight infants. Pediatr Infect Dis J 13:854, 1994.
549. Klein JO, Gellis SS. Diagnostic needle aspiration in pediatric practice: with special reference to lungs, middle ear, urinary bladder, and amniotic cavity. Pediatr Clin North Am 18:219, 1971.
550. Eisenfeld L, Ermocilla R, Wirtschaffer D, et al. Systemic bacterial infections in neonatal deaths. Am J Dis Child 137:645, 1983.
551. Minckler TM, Newell GR, O'Toole WF, et al. Microbiology experience in human tissue collection. Am J Clin Pathol 45:85, 1966.
552. Pierce JR, Merenstein GB, Stocker JT. Immediate postmortem cultures in an intensive care nursery. Pediatr Infect Dis J 3:510, 1984.
553. Levin J, Poore TE, Zauber NP, et al. Detection of endotoxin in the blood of patients with sepsis due to gram-negative bacteria. N Engl J Med 283:1313, 1970.
554. Levin I, Poore TE, Young NS. Gram-negative sepsis. Detection of endotoxemia with the limulus test. Ann Intern Med 76:1, 1972.

555. Stumacher RI, Kovnat MJ, McCabe WR. Limitations of the usefulness of the limulus assay for endotoxin. N Engl J Med 288:1261, 1973.
556. Elin RJ, Robinson RA, Levine AS, et al. Lack of clinical usefulness of the limulus test in the diagnosis of endotoxemia. N Engl J Med 293:521, 1975.
557. McCracken GH Jr, Sarff LD. Endotoxin in CSF detection in neonates with bacterial meningitis. JAMA 235:617, 1976.
558. McGowan KL. Diagnostic value of latex agglutination tests for bacterial infections. Rep Pediatr Infect Dis 8:31, 1992.
559. Sanchez PJ, Siegel JD, Cushion NB, Threlkeld N. Significance of a positive urine group B streptococcal latex agglutination test in neonates. J Pediatr 116:601, 1990.
560. Weiss MG, Ionides SP, Anderson CL. Meningitis in premature infants with respiratory distress: role of admission lumbar puncture. J Pediatr 119:973, 1991.
561. Hendricks-Munoz KD, Shapiro DL. The role of the lumbar puncture in the admission sepsis evaluation of the premature infant. J Perinatol 10:60, 1990.
562. Eldadah M, Frenkel LD, Hiatt IM, Hegyi T. Evaluation of routine lumbar punctures in newborn infants with respiratory distress syndrome. Pediatr Infect Dis J 6:243, 1987.
563. Schwersenski J, McIntyre L, Bauer CR. Lumbar puncture frequency and CSF analysis in the neonate. Am J Dis Child 145:54, 1991.
564. Fielkow S, Reuter S, Gotoff SP. Clinical and laboratory observations: cerebrospinal fluid examination in symptom-free infants with risk factors for infection. J Pediatr 119:971, 1991.
565. Wiswell TE, Baumgart S, Gannon CM, Spitzer AR. No lumbar puncture in the evaluation for early neonatal sepsis: will meningitis be missed? Pediatrics 95:803, 1995.
566. Gleason CA, Martin FJ, Anderson JV, et al. Optimal position for a spinal tap in preterm infants. Pediatrics 71:31, 1983.
567. Pinheiro JMB, Furdon S, Ochoa LF. Role of local anesthesia during lumbar puncture in neonates. Pediatrics 91:379, 1993.
568. Porter FL, Miller JP, Cole S, Marshall RE. A controlled clinical trial of local anesthesia for lumbar punctures in newborns. Pediatrics 88:663, 1991.
569. Fiser DH, Gober GA, Smith CE, et al. Prevention of hypoxemia during lumbar puncture in infancy with preoxygenation. Pediatr Emerg Care 9:81, 1993.
570. Weisman LE, Merenstein GB, Steenbarger JR. The effect of lumbar puncture position in sick neonates. Am J Dis Child 137:1077, 1983.
571. Visser VE, Hall RT. Lumbar puncture in the evaluation of suspected neonatal sepsis. J Pediatr 96:1063, 1980.
572. Franco SM, Cornelius VE, Andrews BF. Should we perform lumbar punctures on the first day of life? Am J Dis Child 147:133, 1993.
573. Naidoo BT. The CSF in the healthy newborn infant. S Afr Med J 42:933, 1968.
574. Sarff LD, Platt LH, McCracken GH Jr. Cerebrospinal fluid evaluation in neonates: comparison of high-risk infants with and without meningitis. J Pediatr 88:473, 1976.
575. Bonadio WA, Stanco L, Bruce R, et al. Reference values of normal CSF composition in infants ages 0 to 8 weeks. Pediatr Infect Dis J 11:589, 1992.
576. Ahmed A, Hickey SM, Ehrett S, et al. Cerebrospinal fluid values in the term neonate. Pediatr Infect Dis J 15:298, 1996.
577. Wolf H, Hoepffner L. The CSF in the newborn and premature infant. World Neurol 2:871, 1961.
578. Otila E. Studies on the CSF in premature infants. Acta Paediatr Scand 35(Suppl 8):9, 1948.
579. Gyllensward A, Malmstrom S. The CSF in immature infants. Acta Paediatr Scand 135(Suppl):54, 1962.
580. Widell S. On the CSF in normal children and in patients with acute abacterial meningoencephalitis. Acta Pediatr 47:711, 1958.
581. McCracken GH Jr. The rate of bacteriologic response to antimicrobial therapy in neonatal meningitis. Am J Dis Child 123:547, 1972.
582. Rodriguez AF, Kaplan SL, Mason EO Jr. Cerebrospinal fluid values in the very low birth weight infant. J Pediatr 116:971, 1990.
583. Yeager AS, Bruhn FW, Clark J. Cerebrospinal fluid: presence of virus unaccompanied by pleocytosis. J Pediatr 85:578, 1974.
584. Moore CM, Ross M. Acute bacterial meningitis with absent or minimal CSF abnormalities: a report of three cases. Clin Pediatr (Phila) 12:117, 1973.
585. Sarman G, Moise AA, Edwards MS. Meningeal inflammation in neonatal gram-negative bacteremia. Pediatr Infect Dis J 14:701, 1995.
586. Hedner T, Iversen K, Lundborg P. Aminobutyric acid concentrations in the CSF of newborn infants. Early Hum Dev 7:53, 1982.
587. Engelke S, Bridgers S, Saldanha RL, et al. Cerebrospinal fluid lactate dehydrogenase in neonatal intracranial hemorrhage. Am J Med Sci 29:391, 1986.
588. Worley G, Lipman B, Gewolb IH, et al. Creatine kinase brain isoenzyme: relationship of CSF concentration to the neurologic condition of newborns and cellular localization in the human brain. Pediatrics 76:15, 1985.
589. Lin C-Y, Ishida M. Elevation of cAMP levels in CSF of patients with neonatal meningitis. Pediatrics 71:932, 1983.
590. Corrall CJ, Pepple JM, Moxon ER, Hughes WT. C-reactive protein in spinal fluid of children with meningitis. J Pediatr 99:365, 1981.
591. BenGershom E, Briggeman-Mol GJJ, de Zegher F. Cerebrospinal fluid C-reactive protein in meningitis: diagnostic value and pathophysiology. Eur J Pediatr 145:246, 1986.
592. Philip AGS, Baker CJ. Cerebrospinal fluid C-reactive protein in neonatal meningitis. J Pediatr 102:715, 1983.
593. Martin-Ancel A, Garcia-Alix A, Pascual-Salcedo D, et al. Interleukin-6 in the cerebrospinal fluid after perinatal asphyxia is related to early and late neurological manifestations. Pediatrics 100:789, 1997.
594. Sayman K, Blennow M, Gustafson K, et al. Cytokine response in cerebrospinal fluid after birth asphyxia. Pediatr Res 43:746, 1998.
595. Chow G, Schmidley JW. Lysis of erythrocytes and leukocytes in traumatic lumbar punctures. Arch Neurol 41:1084, 1984.
596. Steele RW, Marmer DJ, O'Brien MD, et al. Leukocyte survival in CSF. J Clin Microbiol 23:965, 1986.
597. Osborne JP, Pizer B. Effect on the white cell count of contaminating CSF with blood. Arch Dis Child 56:400, 1981.
598. Novak RW. Lack of validity of standard corrections for white blood cell counts of blood-contaminated CSF in infants. Am J Clin Pathol 82:95, 1984.
599. Mayefsky JH, Roghmann KJ. Determination of leukocytosis in traumatic spinal tap specimens. Am J Med 82:1175, 1987.
600. Mehl AL. Interpretation of traumatic lumbar puncture: a prospective experimental model. Clin Pediatr 25:523, 1986.
601. Mehl AL. Interpretation of traumatic lumbar puncture: predictive value in the presence of meningitis. Clin Pediatr 25:575, 1986.
602. Bonadio WA, Smith DS, Goddard S, et al. Distinguishing CSF abnormalities in children with bacterial meningitis and traumatic lumbar puncture. J Infect Dis 162:251, 1990.
603. Naqvi SH, Dunkle LM, Naseer S, Barth C. Significance of neutrophils in CSF samples processed by cytocentrifugation. Clin Pediatr 22:608, 1983.
604. Bonadio WA. Bacterial meningitis in children whose CSF contains polymorphonuclear leukocytes without pleocytosis. Clin Pediatr 27:198, 1988.
605. Weirich E, Rabin RL, Maldonado Y, et al. Neutrophil CD11b expression as a diagnostic marker for early-onset neonatal infection. J Pediatr 132:445, 1998.
606. Kennon C, Overturf G, Bessman S, et al. Granulocyte colony-stimulating factor as a marker for bacterial infection in neonates. J Pediatr 128:765, 1996.
607. Kuster H, Weiss M, Willeitner AE, et al. Interleukin-1 receptor antagonist and interleukin-6 for early diagnosis of neonatal sepsis 2 days before clinical manifestation. Lancet 352:1271, 1998.
608. Doellner H, Arntzen KJ, Haereid PE, et al. Interleukin-6 concentrations in neonates evaluated for sepsis. J Pediatr 132:295, 1998.
609. Panero A, Pacifico L, Rossi N, et al. Interleukin 6 in neonates with early and late onset infection. Pediatr Infect Dis J 16:370, 1997.
610. Harding D, Dhamrait S, Millar, et al. Is interleukin-6-174 genotype associated with the development of septicemia in preterm infants? Pediatr 112:800, 2003.
611. Resch B, Gusenleitner W, Muller WD. Procalcitonin and interleukin-6 in the diagnosis of early-onset sepsis of the neonate. Acta Paediatr 92:243, 2003.
612. Kordek A, Giedrys-Kalemba S, Pawlus B, et al. Umbilical cord blood serum procalcitonin concentration in the diagnosis of early neonatal infection. J Perinatol 23:148, 2003.
613. Chiesa C, Panero A, Rossi N, et al. Reliability of procalcitonin concentrations for the diagnosis of sepsis in critically ill neonates. Clin Infect Dis 26:664, 1998.
614. Yoon BH, Romero R, Yang SH, et al. Interleukin-6 concentrations in umbilical cord plasma are elevated in neonates with white matter lesions associated with periventricular leukomalacia. Am J Obstet Gynecol 174:1433, 1996.
615. Dammann O, Leviton A. Maternal intrauterine infection, cytokines, and brain damage in the preterm newborn. Pediatr Res 42:1, 1997.

616. Mehr S, Doyle LW. Cytokines as markers of bacterial sepsis in newborn infants: a review. Pediatr Infect Dis J 19:879, 2000.
617. Fernandez M, Hickman ME, Baker CJ. Antimicrobial susceptibilities of group B streptococci isolated between 1992 and 1996 from patients with bacteremia or meningitis. Antimicrob Agents Chemother 42:1517, 1998.
618. Swingle HM, Bucciarelli RL, Ayoub EM. Synergy between penicillins and low concentrations of gentamicin in the killing of group B streptococci. J Infect Dis 152:515, 1985.
619. Baker CN, Thornsberry C, Facklam RR. Synergism, killing kinetics, and antimicrobial susceptibility of group A and B streptococci. Antimicrob Agents Chemother 19:716, 1981.
620. Schauf V, Deveikis A, Riff L, et al. Antibiotic-killing kinetics of group B streptococci. J Pediatr 89:194, 1976.
621. Deveikis A, Schauf V, Mizen M, et al. Antimicrobial therapy of experimental group B streptococcal infection in mice. Antimicrob Agents Chemother 11:817, 1977.
622. Backes RJ, Rouse MS, Henry NK, et al. Activity of penicillin combined with an aminoglycoside against group B streptococci in vitro and in experimental endocarditis. J Antimicrob Chemother 18:491, 1986.
623. Odio CM, Umana MA, Saenz A, et al. Comparative efficacy of ceftazidime vs. carbenicillin and amikacin for treatment of neonatal septicemia. Pediatr Infect Dis J 6:371, 1987.
624. Begue P, Floret D, Mallet E, et al. Pharmacokinetics and clinical evaluation of cefotaxime in children suffering from purulent meningitis. J Antimicrob Chemother 14(Suppl):161, 1984.
625. Odio CM, Faingezicht I, Salas JL, et al. Cefotaxime vs. conventional therapy for treatment of bacterial meningitis of infants and children. Pediatr Infect Dis J 5:402, 1986.
626. Odio CM. Cefotaxime for treatment of neonatal sepsis and meningitis. Diagn Microbiol Infect Dis 22:111, 1995.
627. Bryan CS, John JF Jr, Pai MS, et al. Gentamicin vs. cefotaxime for therapy of neonatal sepsis. Am J Dis Child 139:1086, 1985.
628. Man P, Verhoeven BA, Verbrugh HA, et al. An antibiotic policy to prevent emergence of resistant bacilli. Lancet 355:973, 2000.
629. Feigin RD, McCracken GH, Klein JO. Diagnosis and management of meningitis. Pediatr Infect Dis J 11:785, 1992.
630. Bradley JS, Ching DLK, Wilson TA, Compogiannis LS. Once-daily ceftriaxone to complete therapy of uncomplicated group B streptococcal infection in neonates: a preliminary report. Clin Pediatr 31:274, 1992.
631. Kaplan SL, Patrick CC. Cefotaxime and aminoglycoside treatment of meningitis caused by gram-negative enteric organisms. Pediatr Infect Dis J 9:810, 1990.
632. Jackson MA, Abdel-Rahman SM, Kearns GL. Pharmacology of antibiotics in the neonate. Semin Pediatr Infect Dis 10:91, 1999.
633. Group B Streptococcal Infections in Pregnancy. ACOG Technical Bulletin, vol 170. Washington, DC, American College of Gynecology, 1996.
634. American Academy of Pediatrics Committee on Infectious Diseases and Committee on Fetus and Newborn. Guidelines for prevention of group B streptococcal (GBS) infection by chemoprophylaxis. Pediatrics 90:775, 1992.
635. Centers for Disease Control and Prevention. Prevention of perinatal group B streptococcal: a public health perspective. MMWR Morb Mortal Wkly Rep 45:1, 1996.
636. American Academy of Pediatrics, Committee on Infectious Diseases/ Committee on Fetus and Newborn. Revised guidelines for prevention of early-onset group B streptococcal infection. Pediatrics 99:489, 1997.
637. Schrag S, Gorwitz R, Fultz-Butts K, Schuchat A. Prevention of perinatal group B streptococcal disease. Revised guidelines from CDC. MMWR Morb Mortal Wkly Rep 51(RR-11):1, 2002.
638. Uy IP, D'Angio CT, Menegus M, Guillet R. Changes in early-onset group B beta hemolytic streptococcus disease with changing recommendations for prophylaxis. J Perinatol 22:516, 2002.
639. MacAulay MA, Abou-Sabe M, Charles D. Placental transfer of ampicillin. Am J Obstet Gynecol 96:943, 1966.
640. Nau H. Clinical pharmacokinetics in pregnancy and perinatology. II. Penicillins. Dev Pharmacol Ther 10:174, 1987.
641. Adamkin DH, Marshall E, Weiner LB. The placental transfer of ampicillin. Am J Perinatol 1:310, 1984.
642. Brozanski BS, Jones JG, Krohn MA, Sweet RL. Effect of a screening-based prevention policy on prevalence of early-onset group B streptococcal sepsis. Obstet Gynecol 95:496, 2000.
643. Moore MR, Schrag SJ, Schuchat A. Effects of intrapartum antimicrobial prophylaxis for prevention of group-B-streptococcal disease on the incidence and ecology of early-onset neonatal sepsis. Lancet Infect Dis 3:201, 2003.
644. Schrag SJ, Zywicki S, Farley MM, et al. Group B streptococcal disease in the era of intrapartum antibiotic prophylaxis. N Engl J Med 342:15, 2000.
645. Gotoff SP, Boyer KM. Prevention of early-onset neonatal group B streptococcal disease. Pediatr 99:866, 1997.
646. Squire E, Favara B, Todd J. Diagnosis of neonatal bacterial infection: hematologic and pathologic findings in fatal and nonfatal cases. Pediatrics 64:60, 1979.
647. McCracken GH Jr, Mize SG. A controlled study of intrathecal antibiotic therapy in gram-negative enteric meningitis of infancy. Report of the Neonatal Meningitis Cooperative Study Group. J Pediatr 89:66, 1976.
648. McCracken GH Jr, Mize SG, Threlkeld N. Intraventricular gentamicin therapy in gram-negative bacillary meningitis of infancy. Lancet 1:787, 1980.
649. Koksal N, Hacimustafaoglu M, Bagci S, Celebi S. Meropenem in neonatal severe infections due to multiresistant gram-negative bacteria. Ind J Pediatr 68:15, 2001.
650. Khaneja M, Naprawa J, Kumar A, Piecuch S. Successful treatment of late-onset infection due to resistant *Klebsiella pneumoniae* in an extremely low birth weight infant using ciprofloxacin. J Perinatol 19:311, 1999.
651. van den Oever HL, Versteegh FG, Thewessen EA, et al. Ciprofloxacin in preterm neonates: case report and review of the literature. Eur J Pediatr 157:843, 1998.
652. Wessalowski R, Thomas L, Kivit J, Voit T. Multiple brain abscesses caused by *Salmonella enteritidis* in a neonate: successful treatment with ciprofloxacin. Pediatr Infect Dis J 12:683, 1993.
653. Levitz RE, Quintiliani R. Trimethoprim-sulfamethoxazole for bacterial meningitis. Ann Intern Med 100:881, 1984.
654. Spirer Z, Jurgenson U, Lazewnick R, et al. Complete recovery from an apparent brain abscess treated without neurosurgery: the importance of early CT scanning. Clin Pediatr (Phila) 21:106, 1982.
655. Lauterbach R, Zembala M. Pentoxifylline reduces plasma tumour necrosis factor-alpha concentration in premature infants with sepsis. Eur J Pediatr 155:404, 1996.
656. Schibler KR, Osborn RA, Leung LY, et al. A randomized, placebo-controlled trial of granulocyte colony-stimulating factor administration to newborn infants with neutropenia and clinical signs of early-onset sepsis. Pediatrics 102:6, 1998.
657. Kocherlakota P, LaGamma EF. Preliminary Report: rhG-CSF may reduce the incidence of neonatal sepsis in prolonged preeclampsia-associated neutropenia. Pediatrics 102:1107, 1998.
658. Bilgin K, Yaramis A, Haspolat K, Tas MA, et al. A randomized trial of granulocyte-macrophage colony-stimulating factor in neonates with sepsis and neutropenia. Pediatrics 107:36, 2001.
659. Ahmad A, Laborada G, Bussel J, Nesin M. Comparison of recombinant granulocyte colony-stimulating factor, recombinant human granulocyte-macrophage colony-stimulating factor and placebo for treatment of septic preterm infants. Pediatr Infect Dis J 21:1061, 2002.
660. Hill HR. Intravenous immunoglobulin use in the neonate: role in prophylaxis and therapy of infection. Pediatr Infect Dis J 12:549, 1993.
661. Jenson HB, Pollock BH. The role of intravenous immunoglobulin for the prevention and treatment of neonatal sepsis. Semin Perinatol 22:50, 1998.
662. Noya FDN. Use of intravenous immunoglobulin in neonates. Rep Pediatr Infect Dis 3:30, 1993.
663. Shenoi A, Nagesh NK, Maiya PP, et al. Multicenter randomized placebo controlled trial of therapy with intravenous immunoglobulin in decreasing mortality due to neonatal sepsis. Indian Pediatr 36:1113, 1999.
664. Gladstone IM, Ehrenkranz RA, Edberg SC, et al. A ten-year review of neonatal sepsis and comparison with the previous fifty-year experience. Pediatr Infect Dis J 9:819, 1990.
665. Speer CP, Hauptmann D, Stubbe P, et al. Neonatal septicemia and meningitis in Gottingen, West Germany. Pediatr Infect Dis J 4:36, 1985.
666. Bennet R, Bergdahl S, Eriksson M, et al. The outcome of neonatal septicemia during fifteen years. Acta Paediatr Scand 78:40, 1989.
667. Placzek MM, Whitelaw A. Early and late neonatal septicaemia. Arch Dis Child 58:728, 1983.
668. de Louvois J. Septicaemia and meningitis in the newborn. *In* de Louvois J, Harvey D (eds). Infection in the Newborn. New York, John Wiley & Sons, 1990, pp 107-115.

669. Harvey DC, Holt DE, Bedford H. Bacterial meningitis in the newborn: a prospective study of mortality and morbidity. Semin Perinatol 23:218, 1999.
670. Klinger G, Chin C-N, Beyene J, Perlman M. Predicting the outcome of neonatal bacterial meningitis. Pediatr 106:477, 2000.
671. Wald E, Bergman I, Chiponis D, et al. Long-term outcome of group B streptococcal meningitis. Pediatrics 77:217, 1986.
672. Franco SM, Cornelius VE, Andrews BF. Long-term outcome of neonatal meningitis. Am J Dis Child 146:567, 1992.
673. Horn KA, Zimmerman RA, Knostman JD, et al. Neurological sequelae of group B streptococcal neonatal infection. Pediatrics 53:501, 1974.
674. Edwards MS, Rench MA, Haffar AAM, et al. Long-term sequelae of group B streptococcal meningitis in infants. J Pediatr 106:717, 1985.
675. Yang YJ, Liu CC, Wang SM. Group B streptococcal infections in children: the changing spectrum of infections in infants. J Microbiol Immunol Infect 3:107, 1998.
676. McCracken GH Jr, Mustafa M, Ramilo O, et al. Cerebrospinal fluid interleukin-1B and tumor necrosis factor concentrations and outcome from neonatal gram-negative enteric bacillary meningitis. Pediatr Infect Dis J 8:155, 1989.
677. McCracken GH Jr, Threlkeld N, Mize S, et al. Moxalactam therapy for neonatal meningitis due to gram-negative enteric bacilli: a prospective controlled evaluation. JAMA 252:1427, 1984.
678. Baier J, Bocchini JA Jr, Brown EG. Selective use of vancomycin to prevent coagulase-negative staphylococcal nosocomial bacteremia in high risk very low birth weight infants. Pediatr Infect Dis J 17:179, 1998.
679. Van de Perre P. Transfer of antibody via mother's milk. Vaccine 21:3374, 2003.
680. Hanson LA, Karlsson B, Jalil F, et al. Antiviral and antibacterial factors in human milk. *In* Hanson LA (ed). Biology of Human Milk. New York, Raven Press, 1988, pp 141-157.
681. Mathus NB, Dwarkadas AM, Sharma VK, et al. Anti-infective factors in preterm human colostrum. Acta Paediatr Scand 79:1039, 1990.
682. Isaacs CF, Kashyap S, Heird WC, et al. Antiviral and antibacterial lipids in human milk and infant formula feeds. Arch Dis Child 65:861, 1990.
683. Winberg J, Wessner G. Does breast milk protect against septicaemia in the newborn? Lancet 1:1091, 1971.
684. Ashraf RN, Jalil F, Zaman S, et al. Breast feeding and protection against neonatal sepsis in a high risk population. Arch Dis Child 66:488, 1991.
685. Coppa GV, Gabrielli OR, Giorgi P, et al. Preliminary study of breast-feeding and bacterial adhesion to uroepithelial cells. Lancet 1:569, 1990.
686. Pabst HF, Godel J, Grace M, et al. Effect of breast-feeding on immune response to BCG vaccination. Lancet 1:295, 1989.
687. Englund JA, Glezen WP. Maternal immunization for the prevention of infection in early infancy. Semin Pediatr Infect Dis 2:225, 1991.
688. Vicari M, Dodet B, Englund J. Protection of newborns through maternal immunization. Vaccine 21:3351, 2003.
689. Baker CJ, Rench MA, McInnes P. Immunization of pregnant women with group B streptococcal type III capsular polysaccharide-tetanus toxoid conjugate vaccine. Vaccine 21:3468, 2003.
690. Sandberg K, Fasth A, Berger A, et al. Preterm infants with low immunoglobulin G levels have increased risk of neonatal sepsis but do not benefit from prophylactic immunoglobulin G. J Pediatr 137:623, 2000.
691. Sidiropoulos D, Herrman U Jr, Morell A, et al. Transplacental passage of intravenous immunoglobulin in the last trimester of pregnancy. J Pediatr 109:505, 1986.
692. Cairo MS, Dana R, Park L, et al. Reduced cytokine production (IL-3, G-CSF, GM-CSF) from stimulated cord mononuclear cells compared to adult but normal cytokine receptor expression on newborn effector cells: possible mechanism in the dysregulation of neonatal granulopoiesis. Pediatr Res 29:273A, 1991.
693. Cairo MS. Cytokines: a new immunotherapy. Clin Perinatol 18:343, 1991.
694. Roilides E, Pizzo PA. Modulation of host defenses by cytokines: evolving adjuncts in prevention and treatment of serious infections in immunocompromised patients. Clin Infect Dis 15:508, 1992.
695. Roberts RL, Szelc CM, Scates SM, et al. Neutropenia in an extremely premature infant treated with recombinant human granulocyte colony-stimulating factor. Am J Dis Child 145:808, 1991.
696. Cairo MS, Agosti J, Ellis R, et al. A randomized, double-blind, placebo-controlled trial of prophylactic recombinant human granulocyte-macrophage colony-stimulating factor to reduce nosocomial infections in very low birth weight neonates. J Pediatr 134:64, 1999.
697. Yang KD, Bohnsack FJ, Hill HR. Fibronectin in host defense: implications in the diagnosis, prophylaxis and therapy of infectious diseases. Pediatr Infect Dis J 12:234, 1993.
698. Yoder MC. Therapeutic administration of fibronectin: current uses and potential applications. Clin Perinatol 18:325, 1991.
699. Dyke MP, Forsyth KD. Decreased plasma fibronectin concentrations in preterm infants with septicemia. Arch Dis Child 68:557, 1993.
700. Goldmann DA, Pier GB. Pathogenesis of infections related to intravascular catheterization. Clin Microbiol Rev 6:176, 1993.
701. Klein JO. Family spread of staphylococcal disease following a nursery outbreak. N Y State J Med 60:861, 1960.
702. Damato JJ, Eitzman DV, Baer H. Persistence and dissemination in the community of R-factors of nosocomial origin. J Infect Dis 129:205, 1974.
703. Thompson CM, Pappu L, Leukoff AH, et al. Neonatal septicemia and meningitis due to *Pasteurella multocida*. Pediatr Infect Dis J 3:559, 1984.
704. Bhave SA, Guy LM. *Pasteurella multocida* meningitis in an infant with recovery. BMJ 2:741, 1977.
705. Baraff LJ, Bass JW, Fleisher GR, et al. Practice guideline for the management of infants and children 0 to 36 months of age with fever without source. Agency for Health Care Policy and Research. Ann Emerg Med 22:1198, 1993.
706. Baker MD. Evaluation and management of infants with fever. Pediatr Clin North Am 46:1061, 1999.
707. Ferrera PC, Bartfield JM, Snyder HS. Neonatal fever: utility of the Rochester criteria in determining low risk for serious bacterial infections. Am J Emerg Med 15:299, 1997.
708. Dagan R, Sofer S, Phillip M, et al. Ambulatory care of febrile infants younger than 2 months of age classified as being at low risk for having serious bacterial infections. J Pediatr 112:355, 1988.
709. King JC Jr, Berman ED, Wright PF. Evaluation of fever in infants less than 8 weeks old. South Med J 80:948, 1987.
710. Klein JO, Schlessinger PC, Karasic RB. Management of the febrile infant under three months of age. Pediatr Infect Dis J 3:75, 1984.
711. Crain EF, Shelov SP. Febrile infants: predictors of bacteremia. J Pediatr 101:686, 1982.
712. Pantell RH, Naber M, Lamar R, et al. Fever in the first six months of life. Clin Pediatr (Phila) 19:77, 1980.

Chapter 7

BACTERIAL INFECTIONS OF THE RESPIRATORY TRACT

Elizabeth D. Barnett • Jerome O. Klein

INFECTIONS OF THE ORAL CAVITY AND NASOPHARYNX

Pharyngitis, Retropharyngeal Cellulitis, and Retropharyngeal Abscess

Neonates with bacterial infection of the oropharynx may present with pharyngeal inflammation with or without exudate or with retropharyngeal cellulitis or abscess. Extension of infection to the surrounding structures may occur, leading to deep neck abscess formation. Microorganisms identified as the etiologic agents of these infections and their manifestations of disease include the following:

Staphylococcus aureus. Although many children are colonized in the throat and nasopharynx with *S. aureus*, this organism is rarely a primary agent in the etiology of pharyngitis in infants (or adults). There have, however, been reports of localized abscesses in the oral cavity related to *S. aureus*. Clark and Barysh, in 1936, reported a case of retropharyngeal abscess in a 6-week-old infant.[1] The child was critically ill but recovered after incision and drainage of the abscess. Steinhauer reported a case of cellulitis of the floor of the mouth (Ludwig's angina) in a 12-day-old infant.[2] The child was febrile and toxic; examination of the mouth revealed swelling under the tongue. Purulent material was subsequently drained from this lesion, and *S. aureus* was isolated from the pus. A laceration was noted in the floor of the mouth, and the author considered this wound to be the portal of entry of the infection.

Streptococcus pyogenes. Fever and pharyngeal inflammation may result from infection with this organism in the neonate.[3]

Streptococcus agalactiae. Retropharyngeal cellulitis has been associated with bacteremia caused by group B streptococci.[4,5] The affected neonates presented with poor feeding, noisy breathing, and widening of the retropharyngeal space on radiographs of the lateral neck. Stridor also may be associated with retropharyngeal abscess, as reported in a 13-day-old infant in Hong Kong.[6] A retropharyngeal abscess caused by group B streptococci occurred in one of three neonates reported in a series of 31 cases of retropharyngeal abscess seen in children in Camperdown, Australia, between 1954 and 1990.[7,8] This infant was found to have a third branchial arch pouch that was subject to recurrent infection until age 5 years.

Listeria monocytogenes. Small focal granulomas on the mucous membrane of the posterior pharynx have been observed in neonates with *L. monocytogenes* infection. Necrosis of some of the granulomas results in ulcers on the pharynx and tonsils.

Treponema pallidum. Mucous patches occur on the lips, tongue, and palate of congenitally infected infants. Rhinitis may appear after the first week of life.

Neisseria gonorrhoeae. A yellow mucoid exudate of the pharynx may be present simultaneously with ophthalmia (A Yu, personal communication, 1981). A case report of in utero gonococcal infection with involvement of multiple tissues included pharyngeal abscess.[9]

Enterococcus faecalis. A case of retropharyngeal abscess in which culture of aspirated pus grew *E. faecalis* as well as two strains of coagulase-negative staphylococci occurred in a 2-week-old full-term infant from Australia.[8] The infant was severely ill and had atlanto-axial dislocation resulting in paraplegia. At autopsy the findings included bacterial endocarditis, diffuse bilateral pneumonia, and renal infarcts.

Escherichia coli. This organism can be a rare cause of infection of the pharyngeal cavity. Pus from a retropharyngeal abscess in a 1-week-old infant grew two strains of *E. coli.*[8] The infant was afebrile on presentation and had a large midline pharyngeal swelling.

Infants may have coryza and other signs of upper respiratory tract disease due to infection with respiratory viruses. Infections with respiratory viruses may damage the respiratory mucosa, thereby increasing susceptibility to bacterial infection of the respiratory tract. Eichenwald[10] described an apparent synergy of respiratory viruses and staphylococci that produced an upper respiratory tract infection called the "stuffy nose syndrome." The syndrome occurred only when both organisms were present. He and his group also documented increased dissemination of bacteria by newborns carrying staphylococci and echovirus 20 or adenovirus type 2 in the nasopharynx and coined the term *cloud babies* for these infants.[11] These studies have not been repeated by other investigators, and the significance of synergy of two or more microorganisms in neonatal respiratory infections remains uncertain.

Noma

Noma (cancrum oris) is a destructive gangrenous process that may affect the nose, lips, and mouth. It occurs almost exclusively in malnourished children in developing countries; nutrient deficiencies have been postulated to play a role in its pathogenesis.[12] Although it is usually a chronic, destructive process in older children, in neonates it may be rapidly fatal. Affected neonates are usually premature and of low birth weight. In older children and adults, noma is caused by fusospirochetes such as *Fusobacterium necrophorum.*[13] The disease in neonates is usually due to *Pseudomonas aeruginosa.* Ghosal and co-workers, from Calcutta, reported bacteriologic and histologic findings in 35 cases of noma in neonates.[14] *P. aeruginosa* was isolated from blood or the gangrenous area in more than 90% of the cases. An Israeli full-term infant with bilateral choanal atresia who required an airway developed gangrenous lesions of the cheek on day 11 and palatal lesions that progressed to ulceration and development of an oronasal fistula. Cultures of material from the lesions grew *P. aeruginosa.*[15] Freeman and associates reported the development of noma neonatorum in the third week of life in a 26-week-gestation premature infant; they suggest that this entity represents a neonatal form of ecthyma gangrenosum.[16]

Epiglottitis

Epiglottitis caused by *S. aureus* in an 8-day-old infant was reported by Baxter in a survey of experience with the disease at Montreal Children's Hospital between 1951 and 1965.[17] A second case of epiglottitis due to *S. aureus* in a 5-day-old infant was reported by Rosenfeld and associates.[18] The infant presented with bradycardia, hoarseness, and inspiratory stridor and had diffuse inflammation of the arytenoids and epiglottis. *S. aureus* was cultured from pus on the epiglottic surface; blood culture was negative. Epiglottitis due to group B streptococci was reported in an 11-week-old infant in 1996.[19]

Laryngitis

Laryngitis in the newborn is rare. The child with congenital syphilis may have laryngitis and an aphonic cry. Hazard and co-workers described a case of laryngitis caused by *Streptococcus pneumoniae.*[20] A term infant was noted at 12 hours to have a hoarse cry, which progressed to aphonia during the next 3 days. Direct examination of the larynx revealed swelling and redness of the vocal cords. The child was febrile (38.5° C), but the physical examination was unremarkable. *S. pneumoniae* was isolated from the amniotic fluid, the maternal cervix, and the larynx of the infant. The child responded rapidly to treatment with parenteral penicillin G.

Infection of the Paranasal Sinuses

The paranasal sinuses of the fetus begin to differentiate at about the fourth month of gestation. The sinuses develop by local evagination of nasal mucosa and concurrent resorption of overlying bone. The maxillary and ethmoid sinuses are developed at birth and may be sites for suppurative infection. The sphenoid and frontal sinuses are rudimentary at birth and are not well defined until about 6 years of age.[21,22]

Inflammatory reaction may occur simultaneously in the paranasal sinuses, the middle ears, and the lungs. Autopsy may reveal that purulent exudate and leukocytic infiltration of the mucosa are present at one or more of these sites. Infection of the ethmoid and maxillary sinuses may be severe and life-threatening in the newborn. Clinical manifestations include general signs of infection such as fever, lethargy, irritability, and poor feeding as well as focal signs indicative of sinus involvement (i.e., nasal congestion, purulent drainage from the nostrils, and periorbital redness and swelling). Proptosis may occur in severely affected children. Although any of the organisms responsible for neonatal sepsis may cause sinusitis, *S. aureus* and group A and group B streptococci are responsible for most infections.[23-25] Suppurative infection of the maxillary sinus may progress to osteomyelitis of the superior maxilla (see Chapter 8).[24]

Blood specimens, nasopharyngeal secretions, and purulent drainage material (if present) should be obtained for culture before treatment. Antibacterial therapy must include a penicillinase-resistant penicillin or cephalosporin for activity against *Staphylococcus* and group A and group B streptococci. If no material is available for examination of Gram-stained pus or if results of the preparation are ambiguous, initial therapy should include an aminoglycoside or a third-generation cephalosporin to ensure activity against gram-negative enteric bacilli (see discussion of management in Chapter 6). Surgical drainage of the infected site should be considered. Drainage of the suppurative maxillary sinus should be performed through the nose to avoid scars on the face and damage to the developing teeth.[24]

Diphtheria

Neonatal diphtheria, although now extremely rare in the United States, was common before the development and extensive use of immunization with diphtheria toxoid.

Outbreaks occurred in hospital nurseries. One of the most striking reports describes three separate epidemics in a "foundling hospital" in Tipperary, Ireland, between 1937 and 1941; 36 infants younger than 1 month of age were afflicted, and 26 died.[26] Goebel and Stroder described 109 infants younger than 1 year of age with diphtheria in Germany during the period extending from the fall of 1945 to the summer of 1947: 59 infants were younger than 1 month of age, and 26 died.[27] In a report from the Communicable Disease Unit of the Los Angeles County Hospital covering the 10-year period ending June 1950, 1433 patients were admitted to the hospital with diphtheria; 19 patients were younger than 1 year of age, but just 2 patients were younger than 1 month of age.[28] Elsewhere, the disease also appears to be on the wane; only three cases of neonatal diphtheria were identified in India between 1974 and 1984 by Mathur and associates.[29]

Respiratory diphtheria has been well controlled in the United States since the introduction of diphtheria toxoid in the 1920s, although it remained endemic in some states through the 1970s.[30] The results of a survey of cases of diphtheria reported to the Centers for Disease Control [and Prevention] (CDC) of the U.S. Public Health Service, Atlanta, Georgia, for the period 1971 to October 1975 showed that no cases involved children younger than 1 month of age and that only six cases occurred in children younger than 1 year of age (the youngest was 5 months old) (G Filice, personal communication, 1981). During the period 1980 through 1995, 41 cases of respiratory diphtheria were reported to the CDC; 4 (10%) were fatal, all of which occurred in unvaccinated children.[31] Importation of diphtheria from countries where diphtheria remains endemic, including areas of the world experiencing a resurgence of disease such as in the former Soviet Union, account for a majority of the cases in industrialized nations.[32] Reemergence of diphtheria in these newly independent states of the former Soviet Union underscores the need to maintain control measures in the United States, including universal childhood immunization, adult boosters, and maintenance of surveillance activities.[33] Maternal immunization may provide some protection to infants in the neonatal period before diphtheria vaccine is given.[34]

The newborn receives antibodies to *Corynebacterium diphtheriae* from the mother if she is immune, and the titers of mother and child at birth are approximately equivalent.[35] Protection of some degree results in the neonate from this passively transferred antibody. Serologic surveys performed in the United States in the 1970s and 1980s suggested that 20% to 60% of adults older than 20 years of age may be susceptible to diphtheria.[36,37] Additional data from Europe confirmed that many adults remain susceptible to diphtheria.[38,39] As is the case in general with passively transferred immunity, protection depends on the level of maternal antibody at the time of the infant's birth, and protection decreases during the months after birth unless the infant is immunized.[40,41]

Neonatal diphtheria usually is localized to the nares. Diphtheria of the fauces is less common. The skin and mucous membranes may be affected; the two infants in Los Angeles included an 8-day-old neonate with diphtheritic conjunctivitis.[28] Because isolation of *C. diphtheriae* requires inoculation of special culture media, notification of the laboratory about the possibility of diphtheria is important. Specimens of both nasal and pharyngeal secretions may improve yield of positive cultures.[42] Infants with suspected diphtheria should be isolated and receive penicillin or erythromycin to eradicate the organism from the respiratory tract or other foci of infection to terminate toxin production and decrease likelihood of transmission. The mainstay of therapy, however, is diphtheria antitoxin, which should be administered as soon as the diagnosis of diphtheria is considered. This product is available in the United States from the CDC.[43]

Pertussis

Infants and young children in the United States are at the highest risk for pertussis and its complications.[44] Although the incidence of pertussis has declined markedly since 1934, when more than 250,000 cases were recorded, resurgence of disease since the early 1980s underscores the need for continued awareness of this disease.[45] There were 29,134 cases of pertussis in the US in the years 1997 to 2000; 29% occurred in infants younger than 1 year of age, representing an 11% increase from surveillance data for 1994 to 1996.[46] The number of deaths in infants younger than 4 months of age increased from 49 (64% of deaths from pertussis) in 1980 to 1989 to 84 (82% of deaths) in 1990 to 1999.[47] There were 17 deaths due to pertussis in the United States in 2000; in all cases, onset of symptoms was before 4 months of age.[48]

Pertussis occurs in exposed and unprotected newborns.[49] Between 1959 and 1977, pertussis was diagnosed in 400 children in Dallas hospitals; 69 patients (17%) were younger than 12 weeks of age. An adult in the household with undiagnosed mild disease was the usual source of infection for these neonates and young infants.[50] A report of a nursery outbreak in Cincinnati highlights the persistent threat of pertussis in the young infant and in hospital personnel.[51] Between February and May 1974, pertussis developed in six newborns, eight physicians, and five nurses (documented by isolation of *Bordetella pertussis* from the nasopharynx). Four additional infants had clinical illness, but the organism was not isolated from the upper respiratory tract. Two mothers of uninfected infants became ill. The initial case was that of a 1-month-old infant managed in a ward whose infection spread to the nursery when house officers became infected and transmitted the organism to other newborns.

In the United States in the early 1990s, cases of pertussis were reported from every state, and large outbreaks occurred in Cincinnati and Chicago.[52] In the Chicago outbreak, the highest attack rate was in infants younger than 6 months of age; factors associated with transmission of pertussis in this age group included young maternal age and cough lasting 7 days or longer in their mothers.[53] Another risk factor for pertussis may be low birth weight. A study of cases of pertussis in Wisconsin infants and young children concluded that children of low birth weight were more likely than their normal-birth-weight counterparts to contract pertussis and to be hospitalized with the disease.[54] Fatal pertussis was identified through a pediatric hospital–based active surveillance system in 16 infants in Canada from 1991 to 2001; 15 of 16 infants were 2 months of age or younger. When fatal cases were matched with 32 nonfatal cases by age, date, and geography, pneumonia and leukocytosis were identified as independent predictors of a fatal outcome in hospitalized infants.[55]

Antibody to *B. pertussis* crosses the placenta, and titers in immune mothers and their newborns are approximately equal.[35,56] If high titers of the passively transferred antibody are present, the antibody is protective for the newborn. This was demonstrated by Cohen and Scadron, who observed protection of 6 months' duration in the offspring of recently immunized women.[56] Three cases of clinical pertussis occurred among six infants who were exposed to infection and whose mothers had not been immunized, whereas no cases occurred among eight similarly exposed infants of immunized mothers. In the group of infants aged 7 to 12 months, there were two cases of clinical pertussis in offspring of immunized and unimmunized mothers, which suggests that passively transferred immunity was no longer present in the infants whose mothers had been immunized during pregnancy. Many women who were vaccinated during infancy have low levels of antibody when they reach childbearing age, and this concentration of antibody may be insufficient to protect offspring if the infants are exposed to pertussis during the first few months of life (before they are immunized). Older children and adults are important sources of infection for infants.[57] These findings suggest that maternal immunization would provide sufficient antibody to protect infants before durable immunity could be provided by infant immunization. In addition, adolescent and adult immunization could reduce the number of individuals able to contract pertussis and infect infants.[58]

Clinical presentation of pertussis in newborns is similar to that in older children but may lack some features typical of disease in older children. The incubation period may vary, ranging from 5 to 10 days. The initial sign usually is mild coughing, which may progress over a period of several days to severe paroxysms with regurgitation and vomiting of food. The characteristic "whoop" may be absent in infants. The clinical picture of the most severely affected infants may be dominated by marked respiratory distress, cyanosis, and apnea, rather than significant cough. Fever is usually absent. Lymphocyte counts are frequently in excess of $30,000/mm^3$. Cockayne described a case of clinical pertussis in a neonate whose mother and brother were infectious at the time of birth.[59] The infant began to cough on the fifth day of life and had a high white blood cell count ($36,000/mm^3$), with a majority of lymphocytes. Phillips reported two cases of pertussis in newborns who were infected by an obstetric nurse.[60] The infants began to cough on the eighth and tenth days of life, respectively. Clinical signs of respiratory infection caused by *Chlamydia trachomatis* are similar to those of pertussis (see Chapter 11).

Complications of pertussis in young infants include convulsions, bronchopneumonia, and hemorrhage. Bacterial and viral superinfection may occur. In a study of 182 infants and children younger than age 2 hospitalized with pertussis from 1967 to 1986 in Dallas, apnea and convulsions occurred significantly more frequently in infants younger than 3 months of age; the three deaths all were in 1-month-old infants with secondary bacterial infection.[61] Mortality among infants younger than 3 months is high; in the earlier Dallas series, 5 of 69 infants (7%) with onset of signs at between 2 and 6 weeks died.[50] *B. pertussis* pneumonia may progress rapidly; pulmonary hypertension resulting from difficulty perfusing the congested lung may result in right-sided heart failure or fatal cardiac arrhythmias.[62] Long-term sequelae of whooping cough in infancy and early childhood were studied by Johnston and co-workers; there was a significant reduction in forced vital capacity in adulthood in persons who had pertussis before age 7 compared with those who did not have pertussis.[63] A case of hemolytic uremic syndrome in a neonate has been reported following pertussis.[64]

Diagnostic methods for pertussis depend on the age of the patient and the duration of cough. In children younger than 11 years of age and older patients with cough lasting less than 14 days, nasopharyngeal specimens should be obtained for bacterial culture using Dacron or calcium alginate swabs. Best results will be obtained if specimens are inoculated at the bedside or taken immediately to the laboratory in appropriate transport media. It is helpful to inform the laboratory of suspicion of pertussis because specialized agar (Regan-Lowe or Bordet-Gengou) is required. The organism is isolated most easily during the catarrhal or early paroxysmal stage of illness and rarely is found after the fourth week of illness. Direct fluorescent antibody testing of nasopharyngeal secretions has low sensitivity and variable specificity and cannot be relied on to diagnose pertussis. Polymerase chain reaction (PCR) assay shows promise as a diagnostic tool,[65,65a] but it is not yet widely available or standardized between laboratories.

Serologic testing is the diagnostic method of choice for patients 11 years of age or older and has excellent sensitivity and specificity when done in an experienced laboratory on paired specimens, the first having been collected as early as possible during the course of illness. No single serologic marker has been identified as diagnostic for pertussis; efforts to standardize serologic studies are under way.

Antimicrobial therapy may lessen severity of the disease if it is given in the catarrhal stage, but it has no clinical effect once paroxysms occur. Antibiotic therapy does eliminate carriage of the organisms from the upper respiratory tract and is of value in limiting communicability of infection, even if given late in the clinical course. The antibiotic of choice for treatment of pertussis is erythromycin estolate, 40 to 50 mg/kg per day orally in four divided doses, with a maximum daily dose of 2 g. Resistance of *B. pertussis* to erythromycin has been reported[66] but does not appear to be widespread. The newer macrolide antibiotics—azithromycin (10 to 12 mg/kg per day orally, in one dose for 5 days; maximum daily dose of 600 mg) and clarithromycin (15 to 20 mg/kg per day orally, in two divided doses, for 7 days; maximum daily dose of 1 g)—may be as effective as erythromycin and have the advantage of fewer side effects and better adherence but are not approved for use in neonates.[66a] Penicillins and first- and second-generation cephalosporins are ineffective against *B. pertussis*. One study demonstrated clinical efficacy in treating pertussis with high-dose specific pertussis globulin from donors immunized with acellular pertussis vaccine,[67] although efficacy of this regimen on a larger scale has not been proved. One investigator has proposed a role for inhaled corticosteroids in the treatment of pertussis.[68] There are no data available to evaluate the role of albuterol or other beta-adrenergic agents in the treatment of pertussis.

Erythromycin also is of value in prevention of pertussis in exposed infants. Granstrom and colleagues described its use in 28 newborns of mothers with pertussis.[69] The women had serologic or culture-confirmed pertussis at the time of labor. Mothers and their newborns received a 10-day course of erythromycin. The infected and treated mothers were allowed to nurse their infants. None of the infants developed signs or serologic evidence of pertussis. Erythromycin has also been shown to be effective in preventing secondary spread within households in which infants resided.[70]

Erythromycin (40 to 50 mg/kg per day, orally in four doses, maximum 2 g per day) for 14 days is recommended for household[70] and other close contacts, such as those in the hospital, including medical and surgical personnel.[71] Although their efficacies have not been established, clarithromycin, azithromycin, and trimethoprim-sulfamethoxazole may be alternatives for patients who cannot tolerate erythromycin.[71a] Azithromycin (10-12 mg/kg per day orally in one dose for 5 days) or clarithromycin (15-20 mg/kg per day orally in two divided doses for 7 days) may have fewer adverse effects and better compliance than erythromycin for treatment of the infected infant.[71]

Reports of clusters of cases of pyloric stenosis among infants given erythromycin for prophylaxis after exposure to pertussis have raised concern about using erythromycin in this setting.[72,73] A study of 469 infants given erythromycin during the first 3 months of life confirmed an association between systemic (but not ophthalmic) erythromycin and pyloric stenosis and identified that risk was highest in the first 2 weeks of life.[74] Because erythromycin remains the only medication proven effective for this purpose, and pertussis can be life-threatening in the neonate, the drug remains the recommended agent until alternative regimens can be shown to be safe and effective. Health care professionals who prescribe erythromycin to newborns should inform parents of the risk of pyloric stenosis and counsel them about signs and symptoms of pyloric stenosis.

OTITIS MEDIA

Otitis media in the newborn may be an isolated infection, or it may be associated with sepsis, pneumonia, or meningitis. Acute otitis media is defined as the presence of fluid in the middle ear (middle ear effusion) accompanied by an acute sign of illness. Middle ear effusion may be present without other signs of acute illness. Diagnostic criteria for otitis media in the newborn are the same as in the older child, but the vulnerability of the newborn infant and potential differences in the microbiology of otitis media in the neonate, especially in the first 2 weeks of life, make it necessary to exercise special considerations in choosing antimicrobial therapy.

Pathogenesis and Pathology

During fetal life, amniotic fluid bathes the entire respiratory tree, including the lungs, paranasal sinuses, and middle ear cleft. Amniotic fluid and cellular debris usually are cleared from the middle ear in most infants within a few days after birth.[75] In term infants, the middle ear usually is well aerated, with normal middle ear pressure and normal tympanic membrane compliance, within the first 24 hours.[76] A study of 68 full-term infants examined by otoscopy, tympanometry, and acoustic reflectometry within the first 3 hours of life revealed the presence of middle ear effusion in all neonates; fluid was absent at 72 hours of life in almost all infants.[77]

Studies of the middle ear at autopsy provide important information about the development of otitis media in the neonate. Inflammation in the lungs or paranasal sinuses usually was accompanied by inflammation in the middle ear.[75-80] DeSa examined 130 infants, including 36 stillborn infants, 74 neonates who died within 7 days of life, and 20 infants who died between 8 and 28 days. In 56 cases, the middle ear was aerated or contained a small amount of clear fluid. In 55 cases, amniotic debris was present; in 2 additional cases, cellular material was mixed with mucus. A purulent exudate was present in the middle ear of 17 infants; these exudates were cultured, and a bacterial pathogen was isolated from 13. Amniotic material was present in specimens obtained from most of the stillborn infants. Purulent exudate was not seen in the stillborns; the frequency of its presence increased with postnatal age at time of death. Of the 20 infants who lived for 7 or more days, 11 had purulent exudate in the middle ear. Each of the 17 infants with otitis media had one or more significant infections elsewhere; 12 had pneumonia, and 6 had meningitis.[75] The author subsequently identified mucosal metaplasia and chronic inflammation in the middle ears of newborns receiving ventilatory support.[81]

Factors that may affect the development of otitis media in the neonate include the nature of the amniotic fluid, the presence of other infectious processes, the need for resuscitative efforts (especially positive-pressure ventilation), the presence of anatomic defects such as cleft palate, the immunologic status of the infant, and the general state of health of the infant. Aspiration of infected amniotic fluid through the eustachian tube may be one factor in the development of otitis media in the neonate; dysfunction of the eustachian tube, which is shorter, wider, and more horizontal than in the older child,[82] and failure to clear aspirated material from the middle ear probably have etiologic roles as well. Piza and associates[83] speculate that infants born through thick meconium fluid may be at greater risk for otitis media because of the inflammatory nature of this fluid. DeSa noted that many infants in whom otitis media developed had required assistance in respiration and speculated that the pressure of ventilation efforts was responsible for propelling infected material into the middle ear.[75] In infants, as in older children, middle ear effusion appears to be frequent in patients with nasotracheal tubes, and the effusion occurs first on the side of intubation.[84] Berman and colleagues[85] described an association between nasotracheal intubation for more than 7 days and the presence of middle ear effusion.

Infants with cleft palate are at high risk for recurrent otitis media and conductive hearing loss due to the persistence of middle ear effusion. Attempts to reduce the incidence of permanent hearing impairment have included intensive monitoring of children with cleft palate for middle ear effusion and repair of these defects earlier in infancy. One study, however, found that early cleft palate repair did not reduce significantly the subsequent need for ventilating tubes in these children.[86]

Breast-fed infants are at lower risk than bottle-fed infants for acute otitis media. Results of studies of Canadian Eskimo infants[87] and of infants in India,[88] Finland,[89] Denmark,[90] and the United States[91] indicate a significant decrease in the incidence of infection of the middle ear in breast-fed compared with bottle-fed infants. A study from Cooperstown, New York, identified a significantly lower incidence of acute lower respiratory tract infection in infants who were breast-fed compared with infants who were bottle-fed; the incidence of otitis media was lower in the breast-fed infants, but this difference was not statistically significant.[92] Boston infants who were breast-fed had a lower risk for either having had one or more episodes of acute otitis media or having had recurrent acute otitis media (three or more episodes) during the first year of life. Of interest was the fact that the protective association of breast-feeding did not increase with increased duration of breast-feeding; infants who were breast-fed for 3 months had an incidence of otitis media in the first year of life that was as low as infants who were breast-fed for 12 months.[93]

The beneficial effects of breast-feeding may be due to immunologic factors in breast milk or to development of musculature in the breast-fed infant that may affect eustachian tube function and assist in promoting drainage of middle ear fluid. Alternatively, the findings could indicate harmful effects of bottle-feeding, including the reclining or horizontal position of the bottle-fed infant that allows fluid to move readily into the middle ear,[94,95] allergy to one or more components in cow's milk or formula, or aspiration of fluids into the middle ear during feeding. The hypothesis that breast milk is protective is substantiated by the results of studies of a special feeding bottle for infants with cleft palate. Among infants who were fed by this bottle containing breast milk, the number of days with middle ear effusion was less than in infants fed by this device containing formula, which suggests that protection was more likely to be a quality of the milk rather than of the mode of feeding.[96] Adherence of *S. pneumoniae* and *Haemophilus influenzae* to buccal epithelial cells was inhibited by human breast milk.[97]

Early onset of pneumococcal otitis media has been associated with low levels of cord blood pneumococcal immunoglobulin G (IgG) antibodies. Among a group of infants who had siblings with middle ear disease, low concentrations of cord blood antibody to pneumococcal serotype 14 or 19F were associated with earlier onset of otitis media.[98] Low cord blood antibody concentrations to serotype 19F predicted more episodes of otitis media over the first year of life in a cohort of 415 infants whose mothers enrolled in the study during pregnancy.[99] In these infants, early otitis media was associated significantly with type 14 IgG1 in the lowest quartile, but not with type 19F IgG1 antibody or with either IgG2 antibody.[100] These findings prompted study of maternal immunization to prevent pneumococcal disease in neonates. Immunization of pregnant chinchillas with heptavalent pneumococcal vaccine resulted in reduced incidence and severity of experimental otitis in their infants.[101] Immunization of pregnant women in Bangladesh, the Gambia, and the United States with pneumococcal polysaccharide vaccine resulted in pneumococcal antibody concentrations that were higher at birth in infants of immunized mothers than in controls.[102-104] In addition, pneumococcal IgG antibody acquired by infants of immunized mothers had greater opsonophagocytic activity than that in control infants.[104] A trial is under way to assess the role of maternal pneumococcal immunization in prevention of early infant otitis media.[105]

Antibody to pneumococci in breast milk has been proposed to have a role in prevention of early otitis media. Early colonization with pneumococci or other bacteria is associated with early otitis media.[106] The role of antibodies to pneumococci in human milk in prevention of nasopharyngeal colonization of infants with pneumococci remains controversial. A study in Sweden involving 448 mother-infant pairs failed to demonstrate reduction in carriage of pneumococci in neonates fed milk with anticapsular and antiphosphorylcholine activity and showed an increase in colonization when infants were fed milk with anti–cell wall polysaccharide antibody activity.[107] Maternal immunization with pneumococcal polysaccharide vaccine resulted in higher breast milk IgA antibodies to serotype 19F, but not type 6B.[102]

Epidemiology

The incidence of acute otitis media or middle ear effusion in the newborn is uncertain because of the paucity of definitive studies. Warren and Stool examined 127 consecutive infants whose birth weights were less than 2300 g and found 3 with middle ear effusions (at 2, 7, and 26 days of life).[108] Jaffe and co-workers examined 101 Navajo infants within 48 hours of birth and identified 18 with impaired mobility of the tympanic membrane.[109] Berman and co-workers identified effusion in the middle ear of 30% of 125 consecutively examined infants who were admitted to a neonatal intensive care unit (NICU).[85] The clinical diagnosis was corroborated by aspiration of middle ear fluid. The basis for the differences in incidence in the various studies is uncertain, but there may be an association with procedures used in the nurseries.

Acute otitis media is common in early infancy. In the prospective study of Boston children, 9% of children had an episode of middle ear infection by 3 months of age.[93] Age at the time of first episode of acute otitis media appears to be an important predictor for recurrent otitis media.[93,109,110] Children who experience a first episode during the first months of life are more likely to experience repeated infection than children whose first episode occurs after the first birthday. Additional risk factors include parental smoking and low socioeconomic status.[111,112]

Some host factors that also are present in infants with neonatal sepsis have been identified in infants with middle ear infection. The incidence of infection is higher in premature infants than in those delivered at term in some studies,[113,114] but not in the prospective study of Boston children.[93] Male infants are more frequently infected than female infants.[113] Otitis media also is associated with a prolonged interval after rupture of maternal membranes and with other obstetric difficulties.[75,115] Middle ear infection is more severe in Native Americans and Canadian Eskimos than in the general population, and it is likely that this is true in neonates and older infants as well.[87,109] Children with cleft palate have a high incidence of otitis media, which may begin soon after birth.[116] Prenatal, innate, and early environmental exposures were assessed in relation to early otitis media in a cohort of 596 infants followed prospectively from birth. In multivariable analysis, prenatal factors were not associated with early onset of otitis media, but environmental (day care, upper respiratory infection, birth in the fall) and innate factors (parental and sibling history of otitis media) were associated with early and/or recurrent otitis media.[117]

Microbiology

The bacteriology of otitis media in infants has been studied by investigators in Honolulu,[113] Dallas,[114] Huntsville,[118] Boston,[118] Denver,[85,85a] Milwaukee,[119] Tampere Hospital in Finland,[120] and Beer-Sheva, Israel (see Table 7-1).[121] *S. pneumoniae* and *H. influenzae* are isolated frequently from fluid aspirated from the middle ear in the very young, as is the case in older infants and children. Although it has been suggested that otitis media in the youngest neonates (younger than 2 weeks of age) is caused more frequently by organisms associated with neonatal sepsis, such as group B streptococci, *S. aureus*, and gram-negative enteric bacilli, this pattern does not emerge consistently when multiple studies are examined. Pneumococci were isolated from middle ear fluid in the first 2 weeks of life, and otitis associated with gram-negative enteric organisms and group B streptococci occurred in older infants. Microbiology of middle ear disease in infants who are in neonatal intensive care nurseries may be an exception to the pattern associated with otitis media in previously healthy infants and may reflect pathogens present in the NICU setting. In a small series of 13 such infants, only gram-negative enteric organisms and staphylococcal species were identified in the 10 samples of middle ear fluid from which bacteria were identified.[85] Table 7-1 shows the microbiology of middle ear isolates from 8 studies of otitis media in infants; when possible, data from the youngest neonates have been separated from data from older infants.

Susceptibility patterns of organisms causing otitis media in newborns reflect local patterns. In general, trends toward increasing resistance of pneumococci to antibacterial agents, and colonization and disease due to pneumococcal serotypes not present in the pneumococcal conjugate vaccine used routinely in the United States and other countries, have been observed.

Gram-negative enteric bacilli have been the predominant organisms isolated at autopsy from purulent effusions of the middle ear. Of 17 infants studied by deSa, 7 were found to have *E. coli* and 6 had *P. aeruginosa*.[75] Beta-hemolytic streptococci (not further identified) were isolated from one infant, and no organism was recovered from the remaining three. Because pneumonia and meningitis accompanied the otitis in all of these cases, the predominance of gram-negative pathogens in this series is not unexpected.

Congenital tuberculosis of the ear[122] and of the ear and parotid gland[123] has been reported in preterm infants from Hong Kong and Turkey. Both cases were notable for significant regional lymphadenopathy, lack of response to antibacterial therapy, and presence of active pulmonary tuberculosis in the mother. Authors of both reports suggest that there is continued need for a high index of suspicion for this disease in appropriate circumstances. Otitis media and bacteremia due to *P. aeruginosa* occurring at 19 days of life was thought to occur following inoculation of the organism during a water birth.[124] *B. pertussis* was isolated from middle ear fluid in a 1-month-old infant hospitalized with pertussis; intubation of the child's airway may have facilitated spread of the organism from the nasopharynx to the middle ear.[125]

Diagnosis

During the first few weeks of life, examination of the ear requires patience and careful appraisal of all of the structures of the external canal and the middle ear.[126] The diagnostic criteria for acute otitis media in the neonate are the same as those in the older child: presence of fluid in the middle ear accompanied by signs of acute illness. Middle ear effusion and its effect on tympanic membrane mobility are best measured with a pneumatic otoscope. The normal tympanic membrane moves inward with positive pressure and outward with negative pressure. The presence of fluid in the middle ear dampens tympanic membrane mobility.

In the first few days of life, the ear canal is filled with vernix caseosa; this material is readily removed with a small curette or suction tube. The canal walls of the young infant are pliable and tend to expand and collapse with insufflation during pneumatic otoscopy. Continuing pneumatic insufflation as the speculum is advanced is helpful because the positive pressure expands the pliable canal walls. The tympanic membrane often appears thickened and opaque, and mobility may be limited during the first few days of life.[127] In many infants, the membrane is in an extreme oblique position, with the superior aspect proximal to the observer (Fig. 7-1). The tympanic membrane and the superior canal wall may appear to lie almost in the same plane, so it is often difficult to distinguish the point where the canal ends and the pars flaccida of the membrane begins. The inferior canal wall may bulge loosely over the inferior position of the tympanic membrane and move with positive pressure, simulating movement of the tympanic membrane. The examiner must distinguish between the movement of the canal walls and the movement of the membrane. The following considerations are helpful in recognition of these structures: Vessels are seen within the tympanic membrane but are less apparent in the skin of the ear canal; and the tympanic membrane moves during crying or respiration when the middle ear is aerated. The ear canals of most neonates permit entry of only a 2-mm-diameter speculum. Because the entire eardrum cannot be examined at one time, owing to the small diameter of the speculum, quadrants must be examined sequentially. By 1 month of age, the infant's tympanic membrane has assumed an oblique position that is less marked than in the first few weeks of life and is similar to the position in the older child.

Tympanometry is of limited value in diagnosis of middle ear effusion in the neonate. The flat tympanogram indicative of effusion in children 6 months of age or older often is not present in the younger infant, even when fluid is documented by aspiration.[128] Acoustic reflectometry may be advantageous compared with tympanometry in the neonate because it does not require insertion into the ear canal or the achievement of a seal within the canal, but there are insufficient data to identify sensitivity and specificity.[129]

Culture of the throat or nasopharynx is an imperfect method of identifying the bacterial pathogens responsible for otitis media. Many studies have demonstrated the diagnostic value of needle aspiration of middle ear effusions (tympanocentesis) in acute otitis media. The specific microbiologic diagnosis defines the appropriate antimicrobial therapy and is sufficiently important in the sick neonate to warrant consideration of aspiration of the middle ear fluid. Aspiration of middle ear fluid is more difficult in the neonate than in the older child, and usually the assistance of an otolaryngologist (using an otoscope with a surgical head or an otomicroscope) is required.

Table 7–1 Microbiology of Otitis Media in Newborn Infants

Author(s)	Site (year[s])	Patients: Age Range	Patients: No. in Series	Causative Organism: No. of Cases (%): *S. pneumoniae*	*H. influenzae*	Staphylococcal Species	Enteric Gram-Negative Species	Other	Comment
Bland[113]	Honolulu (1970-1971)	10-14 days	2	1 (50)			1 (50)		Outpatients
		15-42 days	19[a]	0 (0)	3 (12)	5 (20)	13 (52)	1 (4)	
Tetzlaff et al[114]	Dallas (1974-1976)	0-5 wk	42[a]	13 (30)	11 (26)	NA[b]	8 (19)	12 (28)[c]	Outpatients
Balkany et al[85a]	Denver (1975-1976)	0-4 mo	21	9 (43)	5 (24)	5 (24)	1 (4)	1 (4)	Outpatients
Berman et al[85]	Denver (1975-1976)	0-4 mo	13[a]	0 (0)	0 (0)	6 (60)	4 (40)	—	NICU patients
Shurin et al[118]	Huntsville, Boston (1976)	0-6 wk	17	4 (24)	2 (12)		1 (6)	3 (18)	3 nursery patients ages 4, 4, and 26 days
Karma et al[120]	Finland (1980-1985)	0-1 mo	14	1 (7)	2 (14)	5 (35)	0	2 (14)	
		1-2 mo	93	19 (20)	8 (9)	55 (60)	5 (5)	11 (11)	
Nozicka et al[119]	Milwaukee (1994-1995)	0-2 wk	Unknown[a]	1 (14)	1 (14)	0	2 (28)	3 (43)	"Nontoxic" outpatients
		2-8 wk	Unknown[a]	5 (19)	0	9 (35)	3 (12)	9 (35)	
Turner et al[121]	Israel (1995-1999)	0-2 wk	5	2 (40)			3 (60)	0	Outpatients
		2-8 wk	109[a]	54 (44)	41 (34)	0	7 (6)	15 (12)	

[a]In some infants, more than one organism was identified, or cultures of middle ear fluid yielded no growth.
[b]Nonpathogen in this study.
[c]Includes group A and group B streptococci, *Staphylococcus* species, *Neisseria* species, diphtheroids, and hemolytic streptococci.
H. influenzae, Haemophilus influenzae; NA, not applicable; NICU, neonatal intensive care unit; *S. pneumoniae, Streptococcus pneumoniae*.

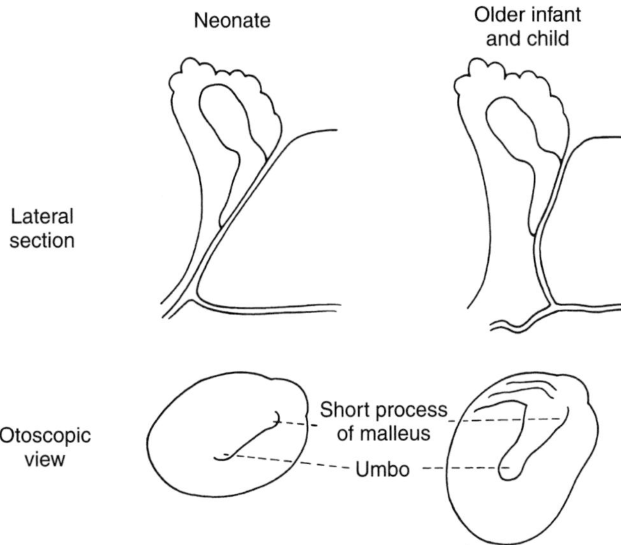

Figure 7–1 Lateral section of the middle ear and otoscopic view of the tympanic membrane in the neonate and older infant and child. (Courtesy of Charles D. Bluestone, MD.)

When spontaneous perforation has occurred, the fluid exuding into the external canal from the middle ear is contaminated by the microflora from the canal. Appropriate cultures may be obtained by carefully cleaning the canal with 70% alcohol and obtaining cultures from the area of perforation as the fluid emerges or by needle aspiration through the intact membrane.

Treatment

Initial therapy for febrile or ill-appearing infants with otitis media during the first 2 weeks of life is similar to that for children with neonatal sepsis. Both a penicillin and an aminoglycoside or third-generation cephalosporin should be used. Specific therapy can be provided if needle aspiration is performed and the pathogen is identified. Infants who remain in the nursery because of prematurity, low birth weight, or illness require similar management during the first 4 to 6 weeks of life. If the infant was born at term, had a normal delivery and course in the nursery, has been in good health since discharge from the nursery, is not ill-appearing, and is 2 weeks of age or older, the middle ear infection probably is due to *S. pneumoniae* or *H. influenzae* and may be treated with an appropriate oral antimicrobial agent such as amoxicillin or amoxicillin-clavulanate.[130] The infant may be managed outside the hospital if he or she does not appear to have a toxic condition. For infants born at term who have acute otitis media and are in a toxic condition, the physician must consider hospitalization, cultures of blood and cerebrospinal fluid, and use of parenterally administered antimicrobial agents because of possible systemic infection, a focus of infection elsewhere, or presence of a resistant organism.

Prognosis

Infants who have infections of the middle ear in the neonatal period appear to be susceptible to recurrent episodes of otitis media.[93,109,110] The earlier in life the child has an episode of otitis media, the more likely the child is to have recurrent infections. It is uncertain whether this means that an early episode of otitis media damages the mucosa of the middle ear and makes the child more prone to subsequent infection, or whether early infection merely identifies children with dysfunction of the eustachian tube or subtle or undefined immune system abnormalities who have a propensity to infection of the middle ear because of these abnormalities.

MASTOIDITIS

The mastoid air cells are not developed at birth and usually consist of only a single space each. Therefore, mastoiditis rarely occurs in the neonate. One report, however, cited a case of meningitis and mastoiditis caused by *H. influenzae* in a newborn.[131] Roentgenograms of the mastoid area demonstrated a cloudy right antrum. At operation, the middle ear was normal but the antrum was filled with infected mesenchymal tissue.

PNEUMONIA

Pneumonia, inflammation of the lungs, in the fetus and newborn can be classified into four categories according to the time and mode of acquisition of inflammation:

1. *Congenital pneumonia acquired by the transplacental route:* The pneumonia is one component of generalized congenital disease.
2. *Intrauterine pneumonia:* This is an inflammatory disease of the lungs found at autopsy in stillborn or live-born infants who die within the first few days of life, usually associated with fetal asphyxia or intrauterine infection and thus includes infectious and noninfectious causes.
3. *Pneumonia acquired during birth:* The signs of pneumonia occur within the first few days of life, and infection is due to microorganisms that colonize the maternal birth canal.
4. *Pneumonia acquired after birth:* The illness manifests itself during the first month of life, either in the nursery or at home; sources of infection include human contacts and contaminated equipment.

Although helpful as a general framework for understanding neonatal pneumonia, these four categories have clinical features and pathologic characteristics that overlap. Thus, management of pneumonia is essentially the same for all four categories, requiring aggressive supportive measures for the respiratory and circulatory systems along with treatment for the specific underlying infectious disorder.

Pneumonia in the neonate may be caused by viruses, bacteria, or parasitic organisms. Detailed information about causative organisms mentioned in this chapter other than bacteria is found in the appropriate chapters in this book; bacterial disease is covered in detail here.

Pneumonia acquired by the transplacental route may be caused by rubella, cytomegalovirus, herpes simplex virus, adenoviruses,[132] mumps virus,[133] *Toxoplasma gondii*, *L. monocytogenes*, or *T. pallidum*. Some of these organisms and the enteroviruses, genital mycoplasmas, *C. trachomatis*, and *Mycobacterium tuberculosis* are also responsible for intrauterine pneumonia resulting from aspiration of infected amniotic fluid. Fatal pneumonitis due to echovirus has also been reported in newborns (see Chapter 24).[134] Isolation of *Trichomonas vaginalis* from the tracheal aspirates of infants with pneumonia suggests a possible association of this organism with respiratory tract disease in the neonate.[135,136]

Group B streptococci constitute the most frequent cause of bacterial pneumonia acquired at delivery. Pneumonia due to group B streptococci and to other bacteria such as *E. coli* or *L. monocytogenes* may resemble hyaline membrane disease.

Pneumonias acquired after birth, either in the nursery or at home, include those caused by respiratory viruses such as respiratory syncytial virus, influenzavirus, or adenoviruses; gram-positive bacteria such as pneumococci and *S. aureus*; gram-negative enteric bacilli; *C. trachomatis*; *Mycoplasma*; and *Pneumocystis carinii*.[137] Pneumonia caused by non-bacterial microorganisms is discussed in the appropriate chapters. Bacterial pneumonia and neonatal sepsis acquired during or soon after birth share many features of pathogenesis, epidemiology, and management, and these aspects are discussed in Chapter 6. This section consists of a discussion of pneumonia in the fetus and newborn not presented elsewhere in the text.

Pathogenesis and Pathology

Congenital or Intrauterine Pneumonia

Histologic features of congenital or intrauterine pneumonia have been described from autopsy findings in infants who are stillborn or who die shortly after birth (usually within 24 hours). An inflammatory reaction is found in histologic sections of lung. Polymorphonuclear leukocytes are present in the alveoli and often are mixed with vernix and squamous cells. Infiltrates of round cells may be present in interstitial tissue of small bronchioles and interalveolar septa.[138-143] Alveolar macrophages may be present and have been associated with both duration of postnatal life and inflammatory pulmonary lesions.[144] The inflammation is diffuse and usually is uniform throughout the lung. Bacteria are seen infrequently, and cultures for bacteria are often negative. Davies and Aherne[141] noted that the usual characteristics of bacterial pneumonia are missing in congenital pneumonia; among these characteristics are pleural reaction, infiltration or destruction of bronchopulmonary tissue, and fibrinous exudate in the alveoli.

The pathogenesis of congenital pneumonia is not well understood.[145] Asphyxia and intrauterine infection, acting alone or together, appear to be the most important factors.[141] It is thought that microorganisms of the birth canal contaminate the amniotic fluid by ascending infection after early rupture of maternal membranes or through minimal and often unrecognized defects in the membranes. Evidence of aspiration of amniotic fluid is frequent.[141] Naeye and colleagues proposed that microbial invasion of the fetal membranes and aspiration of infected amniotic fluid constitute a frequent cause of chorioamnionitis and congenital pneumonia.[146-148] Bacteriologic studies, however, have given equivocal results. Many infants with congenital pneumonia do not have bacteria in their lungs, yet cultures of the lung of some infants without pneumonia do yield bacteria.[149] Fetal asphyxia or hypoxia appears to be a factor in most cases of congenital pneumonia. The asphyxia may cause death directly or by eliciting a pulmonary response consisting of hemorrhage, edema, and inflammatory cells. From his studies of congenital pneumonia, Barter concluded that hypoxia or infection may produce similar inflammation in the lungs.[150] In addition, Bernstein and Wang found that evidence of fetal asphyxia was frequently present at autopsy in infants with congenital pneumonia who also had generalized petechial hemorrhage, subarachnoid and intracerebral hemorrhage, liver cell necrosis, or ulceration of the gastrointestinal mucosa.[151]

Although it is likely that asphyxia and infection can produce similar inflammatory patterns in lungs of the fetus, available information is insufficient to determine which is more important or more frequent. In a review of fetal and perinatal pneumonia, Finland concluded that "pulmonary lesions certainly play a major role in the deaths of the stillborn and of infants in the early neonatal period. Infection, on the other hand, appears to play only a minor role in what has been called 'congenital pneumonia,' that is, the inflammatory lesion seen in the stillborn or in those dying within the first few hours, or possibly the first day or two; it assumes greater importance in pneumonias that cause death later in the neonatal period."[152] Davies noted that the histologic presentation of congenital pneumonia appears to represent aspiration of materials in amniotic fluid, including maternal leukocytes and amniotic debris, rather than infection originating in the pulmonary airspaces. Evidence of infiltration of alveoli or destruction of bronchopulmonary tissue is rarely present.[153]

Pneumonia Acquired during the Birth Process and in the First Month of Life

The pathology of pneumonia acquired during or after birth is similar to that in older children or adults. The lung contains areas of densely cellular exudate with vascular congestion, hemorrhage, and pulmonary necrosis.[141,151,154] Bacteria often are seen in sections of the lung. *S. aureus* (see Chapter 17) and *Klebsiella pneumoniae*[155,156] may produce extensive tissue damage, microabscesses, and empyema. Pneumatoceles are a common manifestation of staphylococcal pneumonia but also may occur in infections with *K. pneumoniae*[155,156] and *E. coli*.[157] Hyaline membranes similar to those seen in respiratory distress syndrome have been observed in the lungs of infants who died with pneumonia caused by group B streptococci. Cocci were present within the membranes, and in some cases, exuberant growth that included masses of organisms was apparent. Although most thoroughly documented in cases of pneumonia caused by group B streptococci, similar membranes have been seen in histologic sections of the lungs of infants who died with pneumonia caused by *H. influenzae* and gram-negative enteric bacilli.[158]

The pathogenesis of pneumonia acquired at or immediately after birth is similar to that of neonatal sepsis and is discussed in Chapter 6. Presumably, aspiration of infected amniotic fluid or secretions of the birth canal are responsible for most cases of pneumonia acquired during delivery. After birth, the infant may become infected through human contact or contaminated equipment. Infants who receive assisted ventilation are at risk because of the disruption of the normal barriers to infection due to the presence of the endotracheal tube and possible irritation of tissues near the tube. Bacteria or other organisms may invade the damaged tissue, which may result in tracheitis or tracheobronchitis.[159] Ventilator-associated pneumonia may be prevented by reducing bacterial colonization of the aerodigestive tract and decreasing the incidence of aspiration. A recent review highlighted strategies for prevention of pneumonia in patients receiving mechanical ventilation, including nonpharmacologic strategies such as attention to hand washing and standard precautions, positioning of patients, avoiding abdominal distention, avoiding nasal intubation, and maintaining ventilator circuits and suction catheters and tubing, as well as pharmacologic strategies such as appropriate use of antimicrobial agents.[160] Newborns with congenital anomalies such as tracheoesophageal fistula, choanal atresia, and diaphragmatic hernia have an increased risk of developing pneumonia.

Lung abscess and empyema are uncommon in neonates and usually occur as complications of severe pneumonia. Abscesses also may occur as a result of infection of congenital cysts of the lung.

Microbiology

Most information about the bacteriology of fetal and neonatal pneumonia has been derived from studies done at autopsy of stillborn infants and of infants who die during the first month of life. A study reviewing causes of death of very low birth weight infants concluded, on the basis of histologic studies done at autopsy, that pneumonia was an underrecognized cause of death in these infants.[161] Bacteriologic studies at autopsy of infants with and without pneumonia were reported by Barter and Hudson.[149] The incidence of bacteria in the lungs increased with age in infants dying with and without pneumonia; among those infants with pneumonia, bacteria were cultured from the lungs of 55% of stillborn infants and infants who died during the first day of life, 70% of infants who died between 24 hours and 7 days of age, and 100% of infants who died between 7 and 28 days of age. Among those infants without pneumonia, bacteria were cultured from the lungs of 36% of stillborn infants and infants who died within the first 24 hours, 53% of infants who died between 24 hours and 7 days of age, and 75% of infants who died between 7 and 28 days of age. The bacterial species were similar in the infants with and without pneumonia, with the exception of group B streptococci, which was found only in infants with pneumonia.

These results were corroborated by Penner and McInnis: Bacteria were cultured from 92% of the lungs of fetuses and neonates with pneumonia and from 40% of the lungs of fetuses and neonates without pneumonia.[143] Davies did lung punctures in stillborn and live-born infants immediately after death, and bacteria were cultured from the lungs of 74% of 93 infants, although pneumonia was diagnosed in only 9 cases.[162] Barson identified bacteria in lung cultures at autopsy of 252 infants dying with bronchopneumonia; positive cultures were obtained in 60% of infants dying on the first day of life and in 78% of infants dying between 8 and 28 days of age.[163] Thus, bacteria were cultured at autopsy from the lungs of many infants with and without pneumonia.

Information about bacterial etiology of pneumonia also can be obtained by culturing blood, tracheal aspirates and pleural fluid and by needle aspiration of the lungs of living children with pneumonia.

The bacterial species responsible for fetal and neonatal pneumonia are those present in the maternal birth canal; included in this flora are gram-positive cocci such as group A, group B, and group F[164] streptococci and gram-negative enteric bacilli, predominantly *E. coli* and, to a lesser extent, *Proteus*, *Klebsiella*, and *Enterobacter* species. Microorganisms acquired postnatally may, for those infants who remain hospitalized, reflect the microbial environment of the inpatient setting. For those infants who develop pneumonia in the community, typical organisms causing community-acquired pneumonia predominate. In the 1950s and 1960s, *S. aureus* was a common cause of neonatal pneumonia; this is uncommon now. Few data exist about relative frequency of specific etiologic agents of neonatal pneumonia or incidence of pneumonia due to specific organisms. One review of invasive pneumococcal disease monitored prospectively by the U.S. Pediatric Multicenter Pneumococcal Surveillance Group identified 29 cases of pneumococcal infection in infants younger than 30 days of age among 4428 cases in children; 4 of these were bacteremic pneumonia.[165] In addition to *S. pneumoniae*,[166-168] *H. influenzae*[158,169] and *Moraxella catarrhalis*[170] also are infrequent causes of pneumonia in the newborn. Pneumonia caused by these organisms is frequently associated with bacteremia, and sometimes with meningitis.[141,166,168,169] Many other organisms have been reported in association with pneumonia in neonates, including a fatal case of congenital pneumonia caused by *Pasteurella multocida* in a full-term neonate associated with maternal infection and colonization of the family cat with the same organism.[171] A case of pneumonia and sepsis due to ampicillin-resistant *Morganella morganii* was reported from Texas[172]; the authors speculate about the role of increased use of intrapartum antibiotics in predisposing to colonization and infection with ampicillin-resistant organisms.

Certain bacteria are associated with a predilection for developing lung abscess or empyema. During the 1950s and 1960s, outbreaks of staphylococcal pneumonia occurred; many times these infections were accompanied by empyemas and pneumatoceles. This is now seen infrequently. Although rare in newborns, *H. influenzae* was associated with pneumonia and empyema[173] until its virtual disappearance after initiation of universal immunization in the early 1990s. Single or multiple abscesses may also be caused by group B streptococci, *E. coli*, and *K. pneumoniae*.[174,175] Cavitary lesions may develop in pneumonia due to *Legionella pneumophila*.[176] Lung abscess and meningitis caused by *Citrobacter koseri* was reported recently in a previously health 1-month-old infant.[177] Nosocomial infection due to *L. pneumophila* has been reported, including cases of fatal necrotizing pneumonia and cavitary pneumonia.[178] Reports have identified *Citrobacter diversus* as a cause of lung abscess[179] and *Bacillus cereus* as a cause of a necrotizing pneumonia in premature infants.[180]

Empyema can also be associated with extensive pneumonia. Empyema due to *E. coli* and *Klebsiella* has been reported in 6- and 8-day-old infants,[181] and *Serratia marcescens* was isolated from blood, tracheal aspirate, and empyema fluid in

Table 7–2 Incidence of Congenital and Neonatal Pneumonia Based on Findings at Autopsy

Place (Reference No.), Year(s) of Study	No. with Pneumonia/Total No. of Infants (%)						Age or Weight of Infants at Death
	Stillbirths			*Live-Born Infants*			
	Premature	*Term*	*Total*	*Premature*	*Term*	*Total*	
Helsinki (138), 1951	5/13 (38)	9/32 (28)	14/45 (31)				
Helsinki (154), 1946-1952				218/361 (60)	210/315 (67)	428/676 (63)	<29 days
Newcastle (139), 1955-1956			13/70 (19)			10/31 (32)	<7 days
Adelaide (140), 1950-1951	5/44 (11)	10/53 (19)	15/97 (15)	9/32 (28)	3/8 (38)	12/40 (30)	Lived <6 hr after birth
Detroit (151), 1956-1959						55/231 (24)	<7 days
Winnipeg (186), 1954-1960	15/46 (33)						<750 g
Winnipeg (187), 1954-1957						27/110 (25)	<7 days
Edinburgh (188), 1922						22/80 (26)	8 hr to 5 wk
NIH Collaborative Study (189), 1959-1964				67/387 (17)	33/125 (26)	100/512 (20)	<48 hr
Manchester (142), 1950-1954			28/275 (10)			59/219 (27)	<7 days
Los Angeles (185), 1990-1993				25/111 (23)			<1000 g, <48 hr

a premature neonate.[182] The past decade was characterized by emergence of increased incidence of invasive disease due to group A streptococci. Cases of pleural empyema due to group A streptococci have been reported from the United Kingdom and Sweden[183,184]; it remains to be seen whether these reports represent isolated cases or are part of a generalized increase in this disease.

Epidemiology

INCIDENCE

The incidence of pneumonia at autopsy of stillborn and live-born infants is given in Table 7-2. Pneumonia remains a significant cause of death in the neonatal period,[185] and infection of amniotic fluid leading to pneumonia may be the most common cause of death in extremely premature infants.[186] The definition of pneumonia in the autopsy studies usually was based on the presence of polymorphonuclear leukocytes in the pulmonary alveoli or interstitium or both. The presence or absence of bacteria was not important in the definition of pneumonia. The incidence rates for congenital and neonatal pneumonia at autopsy are similar despite the different times of study (1922 to 1999) and different locations[138-140,142,151,184-189] (with the single exception of a report from Helsinki[154]): 15% to 38% of stillborn infants and 20% to 32% of live-born infants had evidence of pneumonia. The incidence rates for pneumonia were similar in premature and in term infants. Rates of pneumonia derived from epidemiologic studies are scarce. Sinha and colleagues report an attack rate of 0.4 per 100 infants diagnosed during a nursery stay, and 0.03 and 0.01 per 100 infants diagnosed at pediatric office visits and in hospital or emergency department visits, respectively. They acknowledged a paucity of data with which to compare their rates, which they derived from retrospective review of data from a large health maintenance organization.[190]

RACE AND SOCIOECONOMIC STATUS

In two studies, black infants had pneumonia at autopsy significantly more often than did white infants. The Collaborative Study of the National Institutes of Health[189] considered the incidence of pneumonia in live-born infants who died within the first 48 hours of life: 27.7% of black infants had evidence of pneumonia, whereas only 11.3% of white infants showed signs of this disease, and this difference was present in every weight group. In New York City, Naeye and co-workers studied 1044 consecutive autopsies of newborn and stillborn infants; black infants had significantly more pneumonia (38%) than did Puerto Rican infants (22%) or white infants (20%).[146] The same study showed that the incidence of pneumonia in the infant was inversely related to the level of household income. Infants from the families with the lowest income had significantly more pneumonia than infants from the families with the highest income. At comparable levels of household income, black infants had a higher incidence of neonatal pneumonia than that seen in Puerto Rican or white infants. These racial and economic differences were not readily explained by the authors or by other investigators.

EPIDEMIC DISEASE

Pneumonia may be epidemic in a nursery because of a single source of infection, such as a suppurative lesion caused by *S. aureus* in a nursery employee or contamination of a common solution or piece of equipment, usually caused by *Pseudomonas*, *Flavobacterium*, or *S. marcescens*. Infection may also spread by droplet nuclei among infants or between personnel and infants. Epidemics of respiratory infection related to viruses also have been reported (see Chapters 34 and 35).

DEVELOPING COUNTRIES

Pneumonia is a particular threat to neonates in developing countries. A survey of a rural area in central India revealed that the mortality rate for pneumonia in the first 29 days of life was 29 per 1000 live-born children (the rate during the first year was 49.6 per 1000 live-born children).[191] The aerobic bacteria grown from the vagina of rural women were used as a surrogate for likely pathogens of pneumonia in neonates.[192] Vaginal flora included *E. coli* and other gram-negative enteric bacilli and staphylococcal species in expected proportions but a relatively low rate of β-hemolytic streptococci (3.2%). Management of pneumonia cases (those that did not necessitate immediate referral to a hospital) included continued breast-feeding and trimethoprim-sulfamethoxazole. Because of the lack of microbiologic information, syndrome-based management of infectious diseases is encouraged in the developing world. A meta-analysis of this approach found a reduction of pneumonia mortality of 42% in neonates managed in this fashion.[193]

Singhi and Singhi studied the clinical signs of illness in Chandigarh infants younger than 1 month of age with radiologically confirmed pneumonia to determine how to increase accuracy of diagnosis of pneumonia by health care workers.[194] Rural health care workers (most were illiterate) used revised World Health Organization (WHO) criteria for pneumonia in infants, including respiratory rate greater than 60 breaths per minute, presence of severe chest indrawing (retraction), or both.[195] Cough and respiratory rate greater than 50 breaths per minute missed 25% of cases; decreasing the threshold respiratory rate to 40 breaths per minute increased the sensitivity. In the absence of cough, chest retraction and/or respiratory rate greater than 50 breaths per minute had maximum accuracy.

Clinical Manifestations

Onset of respiratory distress at or soon after birth is characteristic of intrauterine or congenital pneumonia. Before delivery, fetal distress may be evident: The infant may be tachycardic, and the fetal tracing may demonstrate poor beat-to-beat variability or evidence of deep decelerations. Meconium aspiration may have occurred before delivery, suggesting fetal asphyxia and gasping. The infant may have episodes of apnea or may have difficulty establishing regular respiration. In some cases, severe respiratory distress is delayed, but it may be preceded by increasing tachypnea, apneic episodes, and requirement for increasing amounts of oxygen. The infant may have difficulty feeding, temperature instability, and other signs of generalized sepsis, including poor peripheral perfusion, disseminated intravascular coagulation, and lethargy.

Infants who acquire pneumonia during the birth process or postnatally may have signs of systemic illness such as lethargy, anorexia, and fever. Signs of respiratory distress may be present at the onset of the illness or may develop later; these signs include tachypnea, dyspnea, grunting, coughing, flaring of the alae nasi, irregular respirations, cyanosis, intercostal and supraclavicular retractions, rales, and decreased breath sounds. Severe disease may progress to apnea, shock, and respiratory failure. Signs of pleural effusion or empyema may be present in suppurative pneumonias associated with staphylococcal infections, group A[196] and group B streptococcal infections, and *E. coli* infections.[197]

An outpatient study demonstrated the rarity of pneumonia in infants younger than 60 days of age. Infants with the following characteristics did not have pneumonia: illness in the summer; absence of cough, dyspnea, and respiratory distress (grunting, flaring, retracting); respiratory rate lower than 60 breaths per minute; absence of rales and decreased breath sounds; presence of normal color; and white blood cell count lower than 19,000/mm^3.[198]

Diagnosis

CLINICAL DIAGNOSIS

A history of premature delivery, prolonged interval between rupture of maternal membranes and delivery, prolonged labor, excessive obstetric manipulation, and presence of foul-smelling amniotic fluid frequently are associated with neonatal infection, including sepsis and pneumonia. The clinical manifestations of pneumonia may be subtle and nonspecific at the onset, and specific signs of respiratory infection may not be evident until late in the course of illness. Most commonly, pneumonia is associated with evidence of respiratory distress, including tachypnea, retractions, flaring of nasal alae, and increasing requirement for oxygen.

RADIOLOGIC DIAGNOSIS

A chest roentgenogram is the most helpful tool for making the diagnosis of pneumonia. The roentgenogram of the infant with intrauterine pneumonia, however, may contribute no information or show only the coarse mottling of aspiration. If the radiologic examination is done early in the course of meconium or other aspiration pneumonias, typical radiologic features may not yet have developed. The roentgenogram of the child with pneumonia acquired during or after birth may show streaky densities or confluent opacities. Peribronchial thickening, indicating bronchopneumonia, may be present. Pleural effusion, abscess cavities, and pneumatoceles are frequent in infants with staphylococcal infections but also may occur in pneumonia caused by group A streptococci, *E. coli*,[157] or *K. pneumoniae*.[156] Diffuse pulmonary granularity or air bronchograms similar to that seen in respiratory distress syndrome have been observed in infants with pneumonia related to group B streptococci.[199] Computed tomography with contrast medium enhancement is of benefit in localizing pulmonary lesions such as lung abscess and distinguishing abscess from empyema, pneumatoceles, or bronchopleural fistulas.[175] Ultrasound examination was used to diagnose hydrothorax in utero at 32 weeks of gestation.[200]

Although it is not possible to distinguish bacterial from viral pneumonia on the basis of a chest radiograph alone, several features may help distinguish between the two. Findings that are more characteristic of viral pneumonias include hyperexpansion, atelectasis, parahilar peribronchial infiltrates, and hilar adenopathy, which is associated almost exclusively with adenovirus infection. Alveolar disease, consolidation, air bronchograms, pleural effusions, pneumatoceles, and necrotizing pneumonias are more characteristic of bacterial processes.[201]

MICROBIOLOGIC DIAGNOSIS

Because of the difficulty in accessing material from a suppurative focus in the lower respiratory tree, microbiologic diagnosis of pneumonia is problematic. Although cultures of material obtained from lung aspiration have been shown to yield bacterial pathogens in about one third of a group of seriously ill infants with lung lesions accessible to needle aspiration,[202] this rate of positive results is unlikely to be obtained in an unselected group of infants with pneumonia. Diagnosis may be based on isolating pathogens from other sites. When generalized systemic infection is present, cultures of blood, urine, or cerebrospinal fluid may yield a pathogen. Bacteremia may be identified in about 10% of febrile children with pneumonia.[203] If a pleural effusion is present and the bacterial diagnosis is not yet evident, pleural fluid biopsy and/or culture may be helpful. Bacterial cultures of the throat and nasopharynx are unrevealing or misleading because of the high numbers of respiratory pathogens present.

Tracheal aspiration through a catheter is frequently valuable when performed by direct laryngoscopy, but the aspirate may be contaminated when the catheter is passed through the nose or mouth. Sherman and colleagues performed a careful study of the use of tracheal aspiration in diagnosis of pneumonia in the first 8 hours of life.[204] Tracheal aspirates were obtained from 320 infants with signs of cardiorespiratory disease and abnormalities on the chest radiograph; 25 infants had bacteria present in the smear of the aspirate, and the same organisms were isolated from cultures of 14 of 25 aspirates. Thureen and colleagues found that tracheal aspirate cultures failed to define an infectious cause of deterioration in ventilated infants. Positive tracheal aspirates were found with equal frequency among infants with clinically suspected lower respiratory tract infection and in "well" controls.[205] Tracheal aspirate cultures may provide useful information about potential pathogens in pneumonia or bacteremia but rarely indicate the risk or timing of such complications.[206] Often, surveillance cultures of tracheal aspirate material are used to guide empirical therapy when a new illness develops in an infant with a prolonged course on a ventilator.

Bronchoscopy can provide visual, cytologic, and microbiologic evidence of bacterial pneumonia.[207] Aspiration of pulmonary exudate (lung puncture or "lung tap") can be used to provide direct, immediate, and unequivocal information about the causative agent of pneumonia.[208] This procedure is now performed rarely; most reports of its use in infants and young children precede the introduction of antimicrobial agents.[209,210]

Open lung biopsy has been used to identify the etiology of lung disease in critically ill infants and appears to have been most helpful at a time when corticosteroids for bronchopulmonary dysplasia were withheld if there was concern about pulmonary infection. Cheu and colleagues identified three infections in 17 infants who had open lung biopsies: respiratory syncytial virus in 1 infant and *Ureaplasma urealyticum* in 2 infants.[211] Although the optimal indications for use of corticosteroids in bronchopulmonary dysplasia remain a topic of controversy,[212,212a] generally corticosteroids are not withheld if indicated because of low likelihood of an infectious process.[212b]

HISTOLOGIC AND CYTOLOGIC DIAGNOSIS

The data of Naeye and co-workers indicate that congenital pneumonia or pneumonia acquired during birth is almost always accompanied by chorioamnionitis, although chorioamnionitis may be present in the absence of pneumonia or other neonatal infections.[146] These and other studies[213] suggest that the presence of leukocytes in sections of placental membranes and of umbilical vessels or in Wharton's jelly is valuable in diagnosing fetal and neonatal infections, including pneumonia and sepsis. Other investigators are less certain and believe that the presence of inflammation in the placenta or umbilical cord does not distinguish changes caused by hypoxia from those caused by infection.[150,151]

Culture of material obtained by aspiration of stomach contents usually is not helpful in diagnosing pneumonia because this material is contaminated by the flora of the upper respiratory tract. In addition, infants with pneumonia may have no evidence of the organism in the gastric aspirate.[199,214] There is some evidence, however, that microscopic examination of gastric contents may be useful in defining the presence of an inflammatory process in the lung after the first day of life. Because infants so afflicted are unable to expectorate, they swallow bronchial secretions. During the first few hours of life, inflammatory cells present in the gastric aspirate are of maternal origin; however, after the first day, any polymorphonuclear leukocytes present are those of the infant. Tam and Yeung demonstrated that if more than 75% of the cells in the gastric aspirate obtained from infants after the first day of life were polymorphonuclear leukocytes, pneumonia was usually present.[214] However, a study by Pole and McAllister did not confirm the value of gastric aspirate cytology in the diagnosis of pneumonia.[215]

Primary ciliary dyskinesia is congenital and may manifest in the newborn period as respiratory distress. Infants with situs inversus are at risk for this condition. Consultation with a geneticist may be warranted; a biopsy of nasal epithelium may be needed to identify the characteristic abnormal morphology of cilia of the immotile cilia syndrome.[216-218]

IMMUNOLOGIC DIAGNOSIS

Immunologic response to various microorganisms responsible for pneumonia is used extensively as an aid to diagnosis, including infections related to group B streptococci, *S. aureus* (see Chapters 13 and 17) and organisms that cause congenital infection (rubella virus, *T. gondii*, herpes simplex virus, cytomegalovirus, and *T. pallidum*). Giacoia and colleagues prepared antigens from microorganisms isolated from bronchial aspirates and correlated specific antibodies and nonspecific IgM antibody with clinical and radiologic evidence of pneumonia.[219] A significant immune response was identified in approximately one fourth of the patients studied. These data are of interest but remain of uncertain significance because of the difficulty of distinguishing immune response to organisms responsible for lower respiratory tract disease from the response to organisms colonizing the respiratory tree.[220]

Though controversial, testing of blood, urine, and cerebrospinal fluid for antigens to group B streptococci, pneumococci, *H. influenzae*, and *Neisseria meningitidis* may provide helpful information for selected infants with generalized sepsis and pneumonia.[220a] Interpretation of results must take into account possible contamination by organisms colonizing the area around the urethra (in the case of a bag specimen of urine) and possible interference with the test result caused by recent immunization against *H. influenzae* type b or pneumococci or recent infection due to these organisms. Bedside cold agglutination testing may be helpful in the case of *Mycoplasma* infection, but the test has low sensitivity, so a negative result remains undiagnostic. Although PCR testing has provided diagnostic information for many conditions, it does not at present offer any specific advantages in the diagnosis of pneumonia.

Differential Diagnosis

A variety of noninfectious diseases and conditions may simulate infectious pneumonia. Respiratory distress syndrome (hyaline membrane disease), atelectasis, aspiration pneumonia, pneumothorax or pneumomediastinum, pulmonary edema and hemorrhage, pleural effusions of the lung (e.g., chylothorax), cystic lung disease, hypoplasia or agenesis, pulmonary infarct, and cystic fibrosis all have some signs and symptoms similar to those of pneumonia. Meconium aspirated into the distal air passages may produce chemical pneumonitis or segmental atelectasis.[221] Multifocal pulmonary infiltrates have been associated with feeding supplements containing medium-chain triglycerides.[222] Infants with immotile cilia syndrome may present within the first 24 hours of life with tachypnea, chest retraction, and rales. Results of prospective epidemiologic studies of neonatal respiratory diseases from Sweden[223] for the period 1976 to 1977 and from Lebanon[224] for the period 1976 to 1984 indicate that infection was second in frequency to hyaline membrane disease in both surveys. Clues to the diagnosis of diseases and conditions producing respiratory distress based on information from the maternal history and signs in the infant were presented in a convenient table by Avery and coworkers (Table 7-3).[225]

Pneumonia may be superimposed on hyaline membrane disease. One survey showed that histologic evidence of pneumonia was present at autopsy in 16% of 1535 infants with hyaline membrane disease.[226] Foote and Stewart

Table 7–3 Clues to Diagnosis of Types of Respiratory Distress

Information from Maternal History	Most Probable Condition in Infant
Peripartum fever	Pneumonia
Foul-smelling amniotic fluid	Pneumonia
Excessive obstetric manipulation at delivery	Penumonia
Infection	Pneumonia
Premature rupture of membranes	Pneumonia
Prolonged labor	Pneumonia
Prematurity	Hyaline membrane disease
Diabetes	Hyaline membrane disease
Hemorrhage in days before premature delivery	Hyaline membrane disease
Meconium-stained amniotic fluid	Meconium aspiration
Hydramnios	Tracheoesophageal fistula
Excessive medications	Central nervous system depression
Reserpine	Stuffy nose
Traumatic or breech delivery	Central nervous system hemorrhage; phrenic nerve paralysis
Fetal tachycardia or bradycardia	Asphyxia
Prolapsed cord or cord entanglements	Asphyxia
Postmaturity	Aspiration
Amnion fluid loss	Hypoplastic lungs
Signs in the Infant	**Most Probable Associated Condition**
Single umbilical artery	Congenital anomalies
Other congenital anomalies	Associated cardiopulmonary anomalies
Situs inversus	Kartagener's syndrome
Scaphoid abdomen	Diaphragmatic hernia
Erb's palsy	Phrenic nerve palsy
Inability to breathe with mouth closed	Choanal atresia; stuffy nose
Gasping with little air exchange	Upper airway obstruction
Overdistention of lungs	Aspiration; lobar emphysema or pneumothorax
Shift of apical pulse	Pneumothorax, chylothorax, hypoplastic lung
Fever or rise in body temperature in a constant-temperature environment	Pneumonia
Shrill cry, hypertonia or flaccidity	Central nervous system disorder
Atonia	Trauma, myasthenia, poliomyelitis, amyotonia
Frothy blood from larynx	Pulmonary hemorrhage
Head extended in the absence of neurologic findings	Laryngeal obstruction or vascular rings
Choking after feedings	Tracheoesophageal fistula or pharyngeal incoordination
Plethora	Transient tachypnea

From Avery ME, Fletcher BD, Williams RG. The Lung and Its Disorders in the Newborn Infant. Philadelphia, WB Saunders, 1981.

demonstrated, by chest roentgenography, that pneumonia modifies the reticulogranular pattern of hyaline membrane disease by replacing the air in the alveoli with inflammatory exudate.[227] Therefore, any modification of the radiographic pattern typical of hyaline membrane disease should lead the physician to consider superinfection.

Ablow and colleagues reported that infants with pneumonia caused by group B streptococci who also demonstrated clinical and radiologic signs of respiratory distress syndrome were easier to ventilate than were infants who had hyaline membrane disease with a clinical picture suggestive of respiratory distress syndrome unassociated with infection.[228] These findings are of limited value in identifying infection in individual infants and were not confirmed in a subsequent study by Menke and colleagues.[229]

Pleural fluid, usually limited to the lung fissures, occurs in many infants and may be related to slow resorption of fetal lung fluid, to transient tachypnea of the newborn, or to respiratory distress syndrome of noninfectious etiology. Large collections of fluid in the pleural space may represent bacterial empyema; noninfectious causes include chylothorax, hydrothorax (associated with hydrops fetalis, congestive heart failure, or transient tachypnea), meconium aspiration pneumonitis, or hemothorax related to hemorrhagic disease of the newborn.

The symptoms of cystic fibrosis may begin in early infancy. Thirty percent of patients with newly diagnosed cases seen in a 5-year period at Children's Hospital Medical Center in Boston were younger than 1 year of age.[230] The authors described the histories of four children whose respiratory symptoms began before the infants were 1 month of age. The clinical course of the disease in young infants is characterized by a bronchiolitis-like syndrome with secondary chronic obstructive pulmonary disease and respiratory distress, coughing, wheezing, poor exchange of gases, cyanosis, hypoxia, and failure to thrive.

Management

Infants with bacterial pneumonia must receive prompt treatment with appropriate antimicrobial agents. Culture of blood and urine may identify a bacterial pathogen, especially in patients with generalized sepsis. Cerebrospinal fluid culture may be helpful if the infant is not too unstable for lumbar puncture. In intubated infants, tracheal aspirate smears may indicate presence of inflammatory cells and cultures may provide information about organisms colonizing the trachea.

Because the microbiology of pneumonia in the newborn is the same as that of sepsis, the guidelines for management discussed in Chapter 6 are applicable. Initial antimicrobial therapy should include a penicillin (penicillin G or ampicillin) or a penicillinase-resistant penicillin (if staphylococcal infection is a possibility) and an aminoglycoside or a third-generation cephalosporin. In situations in which resistant pneumococci or methicillin-resistant *Staphylococcus aureus* may be the cause of the pneumonia, vancomycin may be used for initial therapy until microbiologic data are available. The oxazolidinone antibiotic linezolid, an agent with a unique mechanism of action with activity against gram-positive organisms, has been studied in neonates. Sixty-three neonates with known or suspected resistant gram-positive infections were randomized to receive linezolid or vancomycin. No difference in efficacy of the two agents was noted, and the authors concluded that linezolid is a safe and effective alternative to vancomycin in treatment of resistant gram-positive infections.[231] Other agents available for treatment of resistant gram-positive pathogens include linezolid, quinupristin-dalfopristin (Synercid), and daptomycin (Cubicin), although data on use of these agents in neonates are unavailable.

Duration of therapy depends on the causative agent: pneumonia caused by gram-negative enteric bacilli or group B streptococci is treated for 10 days; disease caused by *S. aureus* may require 3 to 6 weeks of antimicrobial therapy according to the severity of the pneumonia and the initial response to therapy. Empyema or lung abscesses may also require longer courses of therapy.

When clinical and radiologic signs of hyaline membrane disease are present, infection caused by group B streptococci or gram-negative organisms, including *H. influenzae*, is not readily distinguished from the respiratory distress syndrome of noninfectious etiology. Until techniques are developed that can distinguish infectious from noninfectious causes of respiratory distress syndrome, it is reasonable to treat all infants who present with clinical and radiologic signs of the syndrome. Therapy is instituted for sepsis, as outlined earlier, after appropriate cultures have been taken. If the results of cultures are negative and the clinical course subsequently indicates that the illness was not infectious, the antimicrobial regimen is stopped. Because of concern over respiratory signs as a part of the initial presentation of sepsis and the rapid progression of bacterial pneumonia in the neonate with associated high mortality rate, particularly that due to group B streptococci, early and aggressive therapy is warranted in infants with respiratory distress syndrome.

Antibiotics are only part of the management of the newborn with pneumonia; supportive measures such as maintaining fluid and electrolyte balance, providing oxygen or support of respiration with continuous positive airway pressure, or intubation and ventilation are equally important. Drainage of pleural effusions may be necessary when the accumulation of fluid results in respiratory embarrassment. Single or multiple thoracocenteses may be adequate when the volumes of fluid are small. If larger amounts are present, a closed drainage system with a chest tube may be needed. The tube should be removed as soon as its drainage function is completed because delay may result in injury to local tissues, secondary infection, and sinus formation. Empyema and abscess formation are uncommon but serious complications of pneumonia. They may occur in association with pneumonia due to *S. aureus* and are discussed in detail in Chapter 17.

Prognosis

Available data on the significance of pneumonia during early life have been obtained in large measure from autopsy studies. There is information about the natural course of pneumonia caused by *S. aureus* in infants (see Chapter 17), but few studies of the sequelae of pneumonia caused by other agents exist. Even autopsy studies are equivocal in determining the importance of pneumonia because respiratory disease may have been the cause of death, a contributing factor in death, or incidental to and apart from the main cause of death.[232,233] Pneumonia was said to be the sole cause of death in about 15% of neonatal deaths studied by Ahvenainen.[154] In the British Perinatal Mortality Study,[234] pulmonary infections were considered to be the cause of death in 5.5% of stillborn infants and those dying in the neonatal period.

Ahvenainen[154] noted that pneumonia often is a fatal complicating factor in infants with certain underlying conditions; these children include those with central nervous system malformations or disease, congenital heart disease, and anomalies of the gastrointestinal tract such as intestinal atresia. Ventilator-associated pneumonia is a known complication of critical illness. A prospective study of premature newborns found ventilator-associated pneumonia to occur frequently and to be significantly associated with death in extremely premature infants who remained in an NICU for more than 30 days.[235]

Presence of pneumonia in the neonatal period has been implicated as a cause of chronic pulmonary disease in infancy and childhood. Pacifico and associates found that isolation of *U. urealyticum* from the respiratory tract of premature low-birth-weight infants in the first 7 days of life was associated with early development of bronchopulmonary dysplasia and severe pulmonary outcome.[236] Brasfield and colleagues studied a group of 205 infants hospitalized with pneumonitis during the first 3 months of life and identified radiographic and pulmonary function abnormalities that persisted for more than a year.[237]

REFERENCES

1. Clark RH, Barysh N. Retropharyngeal abscess in an infant of six weeks, complicated by pneumonia and osteomyelitis, with recovery: report of case. Arch Pediatr 53:417, 1936.
2. Steinhauer PF. Ludwig's angina: report of a case in a 12-day-old boy. J Oral Surg 25:251, 1967.
3. Langewisch WH. An epidemic of group A, type 1 streptococcal infections in newborn infants. Pediatrics 18:438, 1956.
4. Asmar BI. Neonatal retropharyngeal cellulitis due to group B streptococcus. Clin Pediatr (Phila) 26:183, 1987.
5. Smith WL, Yousefzadeh DK, Yiu-Chi VS, et al. Percutaneous aspiration of retropharyngeal space in neonates. AJR Am J Roentgenol 139:1005, 1982.
6. Abdullah V, Ng SK, Chow SN, Yau FT, van Hasselt CA. A case of neonatal stridor. Arch Dis Child Fetal Neonatal Ed 87:224, 2002.
7. Coulthard M, Isaacs D. Retropharyngeal abscess. Arch Dis Child 66:1227, 1991.
8. Coulthard M, Isaacs D. Neonatal retropharyngeal abscess. Pediatr Infect Dis J 10:547, 1991.
9. Oppenheimer EH, Winn KJ. Fetal gonorrhea with deep tissue infection occurring in utero. Pediatrics 69:74, 1982.
10. Eichenwald HF. "Stuffy nose syndrome" of premature infants: an example of bacterial-viral synergism. Am J Dis Child 96:438, 1958.
11. Eichenwald HF, Kotsevalov O, Fasso LA. The "cloud baby": an example of bacterial-viral interaction. Am J Dis Child 100:161, 1960.
12. Enwonwu CO, Galkler WA, Idigbe EO, et al. Pathogenesis of cancrum oris (noma): confounding interactions of malnutrition with infection. Am J Trop Med Hyg 60:223, 1999.
13. Falkler WA, Enwonwu JCO, Idigbe EO. Isolation of *Fusobacterium necrophorum* from cancrum oris (noma). Am J Trop Med Hyg 60:150, 1999.
14. Ghosal SP, SenGupta PC, Mukherjee AK, et al. Noma neonatorum: its aetiopathogenesis. Lancet 2:289, 1978.
15. Alkalay A, Mogilner BM, Nissim F, et al. Noma in a full-term neonate. Clin Pediatr (Phila) 24:528, 1985.
16. Freeman AF, Mancini AJ, Yogev R. Is noma neonatorum a presentation of ecthyma gangrenosum in the newborn? Pediatr Infect Dis J 21:83, 2002.
17. Baxter JD. Acute epiglottitis in children. Laryngoscope 77:1358, 1967.
18. Rosenfeld RM, Fletcher MA, Marban SL. Acute epiglottitis in a newborn infant. Pediatr Infect Dis J 11:594, 1992.
19. Young N, Finn A, Powell C. Group B streptococcal epiglottitis. Pediatr Infect Dis J 15:95, 1996.
20. Hazard, GW, Porter PJ, Ingall D. Pneumococcal laryngitis in the newborn infant: report of a case. N Engl J Med 271:361, 1964.
21. Davis WB. Anatomy of the nasal accessory sinuses in infancy and childhood. Ann Otol Rhinol Laryngol 27:940, 1918.
22. Wasson WW. Changes in the nasal accessory sinuses after birth. Arch Otolaryngol 17:197, 1933.
23. Benner MC. Congenital infection of the lungs, middle ears and nasal accessory sinuses. Arch Pathol 29:455, 1940.
24. Cavanagh F. Osteomyelitis of the superior maxilla in infants: a report on 24 personally treated cases. BMJ 1:468, 1960.
25. Howard JB, McCracken GH Jr. The spectrum of group B streptococcal infections in infancy. Am J Dis Child 128:815, 1974.
26. O'Regan JB, Heenan M, Murray J. Diphtheria in infants. Ir J Med Sci 6:116, 1943.
27. Goebel F, Stroder J. Diphtheria in infants. Dtsch Med Wochenschr 73:389, 1948.
28. Naiditch MJ, Bower AG. Diphtheria: a study of 1433 cases observed during a ten-year period at the Los Angeles County Hospital. Am J Med 17:229, 1954.
29. Mathur NB, Narang P, Bhatia BD. Neonatal diphtheria. Indian J Pediatr 21:174, 1984.
30. Centers for Disease Control and Prevention. Toxigenic *Corynebacterium diphtheriae*—Northern Plains Indian Community, August-October 1996. MMWR Morb Mortal Wkly Rep 46:506, 1997.
31. Bisgard KM, Hardy IRB, Popovic T, et al. Virtual elimination of respiratory diphtheria in the United States (abstract no. G12). In Abstracts of the 36th Interscience Conference on Antimicrobial Agents and Chemotherapy. Washington, DC, American Society for Microbiology, 1995, p 160.
32. Centers for Disease Control and Prevention. Diphtheria acquired by US citizens in the Russian Federation and Ukraine—1994. MMWR Morb Mortal Wkly Rep 44:237, 1995.
33. Golaz A, Hardy IR, Strebel P, et al. Epidemic diphtheria in the newly independent states of the former Soviet Union: implications for diphtheria control in the United States. J Infect Dis 2000;18 (Suppl 1):S237.
34. Durbaca S. Antitetanus and antidiphtheria immunity in newborns. Rom Arch Microbiol Immunol 58:267, 1999.
35. Vahlquist B. The transfer of antibodies from mother to offspring. Adv Pediatr 10:305, 1958.
36. Crossley K, Irvine P, Warren JB, et al. Tetanus and diphtheria immunity in urban Minnesota adults. JAMA 242:2298, 1979.
37. Koblin BA, Townsend TR. Immunity to diphtheria and tetanus in inner-city women of child-bearing age. Am J Public Health 79:1297, 1989.
38. Maple PA, Efstratiou A, George RC, et al. Diphtheria immunity in UK blood donors. Lancet 345:963, 1995.
39. Galazka A. The changing epidemiology of diphtheria in the vaccine era. J Infect Dis 181(Suppl 1):S2, 2000.
40. Barr M, Glenny AT, Randall KJ. Concentration of diphtheria antitoxin in cord blood and rate of loss in babies. Lancet 2:324, 1949.
41. Cohen P, Scadron SJ. The effects of active immunization of the mother upon the offspring. J Pediatr 29:609, 1946.
42. Farizo KM, Strebel PM, Chen RT, et al. Fatal respiratory disease due to *Corynebacterium diphtheriae*: case report and review of guidelines for management, investigation, and control. Clin Infect Dis 16:59, 1993.
43. Centers for Disease Control and Prevention. Availability of diphtheria antitoxin through an investigational new drug protocol. MMWR Morb Mortal Wkly Rep 46:380, 1997.
44. Centers for Disease Control and Prevention. Pertussis vaccination: use of acellular pertussis vaccines among infants and young children-recommendations of the Advisory Committee on Immunization Practices (ACIP). MMWR Morb Mortal Wkly Rep 46(RR-7):2, 1997.
45. Centers for Disease Control and Prevention. Pertussis-United States, January 1992–June 1995. MMWR Morb Mortal Wkly Rep 44:525, 1995.
46. Centers for Disease Control and Prevention. Pertussis—United States, 1997-2000. MMWR 51:73, 2002.
47. Vitek CR, Pascual FB, Baughman AL, Murphy TV. Increase in deaths from pertussis among young infants in the United States in the 1990s. Pediatr Infect Dis J 22:628, 2003.

48. Centers for Disease Control and Prevention. Pertussis deaths—United States, 2000. MMWR Morb Mortal Wkly Rep 51:616, 2002.
49. Sutter RW, Cochi SL. Pertussis hospitalizations and mortality in the United States. JAMA 267:386, 1992.
50. Nelson JD. The changing epidemiology of pertussis in young infants. Am J Dis Child 132:371, 1978.
51. Linnemann CC Jr, Ramundo N, Perlstein PH, et al. Use of pertussis vaccine in an epidemic involving hospital staff. Lancet 2:540, 1975.
52. Centers for Disease Control and Prevention. Resurgence of pertussis—United States, 1993. MMWR Morb Mortal Wkly Rep 42:952, 1993.
53. Izurieta HS, Kenyon TA, Strebel PM, et al. Risk factors for pertussis in young infants during an outbreak in Chicago in 1993. Clin Infect Dis 22:503, 1996.
54. Langkamp DL, Davis JP. Increased risk of reported pertussis and hospitalization associated with pertussis in low birth weight children. J Pediatr 128:654, 1996.
55. Mikelova LK, Halperin SA, Scheifele D, et al. Predictors of death in infants hospitalized with pertussis: a case-control study of 16 pertussis deaths in Canada. J Pediatr 143:576, 2003.
56. Cohen P, Scadron SJ. The placental transmission of protective antibodies against whooping cough by inoculation of the pregnant mother. JAMA 121:656, 1943.
57. Deen JL, Mink CM, Cherry JD, et al. Household contact study of *Bordetella pertussis* infections. Clin Infect Dis 21:1211-1219, 1995.
58. Hoppe JE. Neonatal pertussis. Pediatr Infect Dis J 19:244, 2000.
59. Cockayne EA. Whooping-cough in the first days of life. Br J Child Dis 10:534, 1913.
60. Phillips J. Whooping-cough contracted at the time of birth, with report of two cases. Am J Med Sci 161:163, 1921.
61. Gan VN, Murphy TV. Pertussis in hospitalized children. Am J Dis Child 144:1130, 1990.
62. Lovell MA, Miller AM, Hendley O. Pathologic case of the month: pertussis pneumonia. Arch Pediatr Adolesc Med 152:925, 1998.
63. Johnston IDA, Strachan DP, Anderson HR. Effect of pneumonia and whooping cough in childhood on adult lung function. N Engl J Med 338:581, 1998.
64. Berner R, Krause MF, Gordjani N, et al. Hemolytic uremic syndrome due to an altered factor H triggered by neonatal pertussis. Pediatr Nephrol 17:190, 2002.
65. Edelman K, Nikkari S, Ruuskanen O, et al. Detection of *Bordetella pertussis* by polymerase chain reaction and culture in the nasopharynx of erythromycin-treated infants with pertussis. Pediatr Infect Dis J 15:54, 1996.
65a. Dragsted DM, Dohn B, Madsen J, Jensen JS. Comparison of culture and PCR for detection of *Bordetella pertussis* and *Bordetella pertussis* under routine laboratory conditions. J Med Microbiol 53:749-754, 2004.
66. Centers for Disease Control and Prevention. Erythromycin-resistant *Bordetella pertussis*—Yuma County, Arizona, May-October 1994. MMWR Morb Mortal Wkly Rep 43:807, 1994.
66a. Pichichero ME, Hoeger WJ, Casey JR. Azithromycin for the treatment of pertussis. Pediatr Infect Dis J 22:847-849, 2003.
67. Granstrom M, Olinder-Nielsen AM, Holmblad P, et al. Specific immunoglobulin for treatment of whooping cough. Lancet 33:1230, 1991.
68. Winrow AP. Inhaled steroids in the treatment of pertussis. Pediatr Infect Dis J 14:922, 1995.
69. Granstrom G, Sterner G, Nord CE, et al. Use of erythromycin to prevent pertussis in newborns of mothers with pertussis. J Infect Dis 155:1210, 1987.
70. Sprauer MA, Cochi JSL, Zell ER, et al. Prevention of secondary transmission of pertussis in households with early use of erythromycin. Am J Dis Child 146:177, 1992.
71. American Academy of Pediatrics. Pertussis. *In* Pickering LK (ed). Red Book: 2003 Report of the Committee on Infectious Diseases, 26th ed. Elk Grove Village, Ill, American Academy of Pediatrics, 2003, p 472.
71a. Friedman DS, Curtis CR, Schaver SL, et al. Surveillance for transmission and antibiotic adverse events among neonates and adults exposed to a healthcare worker with pertussis. Infect Control Hosp Epidemiol 25:967-973, 2004.
72. Hoey J. Hypertrophic pyloric stenosis caused by erythromycin. Can Med Assoc J 162:1198, 2000.
73. Centers for Disease Control and Prevention. Hypertrophic pyloric stenosis in infants following pertussis prophylaxis with erythromycin—Knoxville, Tennessee, 1999. MMWR Morb Mortal Wkly Rep 48:1117, 1999.
74. Mahon BE, Rosenman MB, Kleiman MB. Maternal and infant use of erythromycin and other macrolide antibiotics as risk factors for infantile hypertrophic pyloric stenosis. J Pediatr 139:380, 2001.
75. deSa DJ. Infection and amniotic aspiration of middle ear in stillbirth and neonatal deaths. Arch Dis Child 48:872, 1973.
76. Keith RW. Middle ear function in neonates. Arch Otolaryngol 101:376, 1975.
77. Roberts DG, Johnson CE, Carlin SA, et al. Resolution of middle ear effusion in newborns. Arch Pediatr Adolesc Med 149:873, 1995.
78. McLellan MS, Strong JP, Johnson QR, et al. Otitis media in premature infants: a histopathologic study. J Pediatr 61:53, 1962.
79. Johnson WW. A survey of middle ears: 101 autopsies of infants. Ann Otol Rhinol Laryngol 70:377, 1961.
80. Benner MC. Congenital infection of the lungs, middle ears and nasal accessory sinuses. Arch Pathol 29:455, 1940.
81. deSa DJ. Mucosal metaplasia and chronic inflammation in the middle ear of infants receiving intensive care in the neonatal period. Arch Dis Child 158:24, 1983.
82. Bluestone CD. Pathogenesis of otitis media: role of eustachian tube. Pediatr Infect Dis J 15:281-291, 1996.
83. Piza J, Gonzalez M, Northrop CC, Eavey RD. Meconium contamination of the neonatal middle ear. J Pediatr 115:910, 1989.
84. Persico M, Barker GA, Mitchell DP. Purulent otitis media—a "silent" source of sepsis in the pediatric intensive care unit. Otolaryngol Head Neck Surg 93:330, 1985.
85. Berman SA, Balkany TJ, Simmons MA. Otitis media in neonatal intensive care unit. Pediatrics 62:198, 1978.
85a. Balkany TJ, Berman SA, Simmons MA, Jafek BW. Middle ear effusions in neonates. Laryngoscope 88:398-405, 1978.
86. Nunn DR, Derkay CS, Darrow DH, et al. The effect of very early cleft palate closure on the need for ventilation tubes in the first years of life. Laryngoscope 105:905, 1995.
87. Schaefer O. Otitis media and bottle feeding: an epidemiological study of infant feeding habits and incidence of recurrent and chronic middle ear disease in Canadian Eskimos. Can J Public Health 62:478, 1971.
88. Chandra RK. Prospective studies of the effect of breast feeding on incidence of infection and allergy. Acta Paediatr Scand 68:691, 1979.
89. Pukander J. Acute otitis media among rural children in Finland. Int J Pediatr Otorhinolaryngol 4:325, 1982.
90. Saarinen UM. Prolonged breast feeding as prophylaxis for recurrent otitis media. Acta Paediatr Scand 71:567, 1982.
91. Dewey KG, Heinig J, Nommsen-Rivers LA. Differences in morbidity between breast-fed and formula-fed infants. J Pediatr 126:696, 1995.
92. Cunningham AS. Morbidity in breast fed and artificially fed infants. J Pediatr 90:726, 1977.
93. Teele DW, Klein JO, Rosner B, and the Greater Boston Otitis Media Study Group. Epidemiology of otitis media during the first seven years of life in children in Greater Boston: a prospective cohort study. J Infect Dis 160:83, 1989.
94. Duncan RB. Positional otitis media. Arch Otolaryngol 72:454, 1960.
95. Beauregard WG. Positional otitis media. J Pediatr 79:294, 1971.
96. Paradise JL, Elster BA. Breast milk protects against otitis media with effusion. Pediatr Res 18:283a, 1984.
97. Andersson B, Porras O, Hanson LA, et al. Inhibition of attachment of *Streptococcus pneumoniae* and *Haemophilus influenzae* by human milk and receptor oligosaccharides. J Infect Dis 153:232, 1986.
98. Salazar JC, Kaly KA, Giebink GS, et al. Low cord blood pneumococcal immunoglobulin G (IgG antibodies predict early onset acute otitis media in infancy). Am J Epidemiol 145:1048, 1997.
99. Becken ET, Daly K, Lindgren BR, Meland MH, Giebink GS. Low cord blood pneumococcal antibody concentrations predict more episodes of otitis media. Arch Otolaryngol Head Neck Surg 127:517, 2001.
100. Lockhart NJ, Daly KA, Lindgren BR, et al. Low cord blood type 14 pneumococcal IgG1 but not IgG2 antibody predicts early infant otitis media. J Infect Dis 181:1979, 2000.
101. Hajek DM, Quartey M, Giebink GS. Maternal pneumococcal conjugate immunization protects infant chinchillas in the pneumococcal otitis media model. Acta Otolaryngol 122:262, 2002.
102. Shahid NS, Steinhoff MC, Hoque SS, et al. Serum, breast milk, and infant antibody after maternal immunization with pneumococcal vaccine. Lancet 346:1252, 1995.
103. O'Dempsey TJD, McArdle T, Ceesay SJ, et al. Immunization with a pneumococcal capsular polysaccharide vaccine during pregnancy. Vaccine 14:963, 1996.

104. Munoz FM, Englund JA, Cheesman CC, et al. Maternal immunization with pneumococcal polysaccharide vaccine in the third trimester of gestation. Vaccine 20:826, 2001.
105. Daly KA, Toth JA, Giebink GS. Pneumococcal conjugate vaccines as maternal and infant immunogens: challenges of maternal recruitment. Vaccine 21:3473, 2003.
106. Faden H, Duffy L, Wasielewski R, et al. Relationship between nasopharyngeal colonization and the development of otitis media in children. J Infect Dis 175:1440, 1997.
107. Rosen IAV, Hakansson A, Aniansson G, et al. Antibodies to pneumococcal polysaccharides in human milk: lack of relationship to colonization and acute otitis media. Pediatr Infect Dis J 15:498, 1996.
108. Warren WS, Stool SJE. Otitis media in low-birth-weight infants. J Pediatr 79:740, 1971.
109. Jaffe BF, Hurtado F, Hurtado E. Tympanic membrane mobility in the newborn (with seven months' followup). Laryngoscope 80:36, 1970.
110. Howie VM, Ploussard JH, Sloyer J. The "otitis-prone" condition. Am J Dis Child 129:676, 1975.
111. Ey JL, Holberg CG, Aldous MB, et al. Passive smoke exposure and otitis media in the first year of life. Pediatrics 95:670, 1995.
112. Stahlberg M-R, Ruuskanen O, Virolainen E. Risk factors for recurrent otitis media. Pediatr Infect Dis J 5:30, 1986.
113. Bland, RD. Otitis media in the first six weeks of life: diagnosis, bacteriology and management. Pediatrics 49:187, 1972.
114. Tetzlaff TR, Ashworth C, Nelson JD. Otitis media in children less than 12 weeks of age. Pediatrics 59:827, 1977.
115. McLellan MS, Strong JP, Vautier T, et al. Otitis media in the newborn: relationship to duration of rupture of amniotic membrane. Arch Otolaryngol 85:380, 1967.
116. Paradise JL, Bluestone CD. Early treatment of universal otitis media of infants with cleft palate. Pediatrics 53:48, 1974.
117. Daly KA, Brown JE, Lindgren BR, et al. Epidemiology of otitis media onset by six months of age. Pediatrics 103:1158, 1999.
118. Shurin PA, Howie VM, Pelton SI, et al. Bacterial etiology of otitis media during the first six weeks of life. J Pediatr 92:893, 1978.
119. Nozicka CA, Hanly JG, Beste DJ, et al. Otitis media in infants aged 0-8 weeks: frequency of associated serious bacterial disease. Pediatr Emerg Care 15:252, 1999.
120. Karma PH, Pukander JS, Sipila MM, et al. Middle ear fluid bacteriology of acute otitis media in neonates and very young infants. Int J Pediatr Otorhinolaryngol 14:141, 1987.
121. Turner D, Leibovitz E, Aran A, et al. Acute otitis media in infants younger than two months of age: microbiology, clinical presentation and therapeutic approach. Pediatr Infect Dis J 21:669, 2002.
122. Ng PC, Hiu J, Fok TF, et al. Isolated congenital tuberculosis otitis in a pre-term infant. Acta Paediatr 84:955, 1995.
123. Senbil N, Sahin F, Caglar, et al. Congenital tuberculosis of the ear and parotid gland. Pediatr Infect Dis J 16:1090, 1997.
124. Parker PC, Boles RG. *Pseudomonas* otitis media and bacteremia following a water birth. Pediatrics 99:653, 1997.
125. Decherd ME, Deskin RW, Rowen JL, Brindley MB. *Bordetella pertussis* causing otitis media: a case report. Laryngoscope 113:226, 2003.
126. Eavey RD, Stool SE, Peckham GJ, et al. How to examine the ear of the neonate. Clin Pediatr 15:338, 1976.
127. Cavanaugh RM Jr. Pneumatic otoscopy in healthy full-term infants. Pediatrics 79:520, 1987.
128. Pestalozza G, Cusmano G. Evaluation of tympanometry in diagnosis and treatment of otitis media of the newborn and of the infant. Int J Pediatr Otorhinolaryngol 2:73, 1980.
129. Barnett ED, Klein JO, Hawkins KA, et al. Comparison of spectral gradient acoustic reflectometry and other diagnostic techniques for detection of middle ear effusion in children with middle ear disease. Pediatr Infect Dis J 17:556, 1998.
130. Dowell SF, Butler JC, Giebink S, et al. Acute otitis media: management and surveillance in an era of pneumococcal resistance—a report from the Drug-Resistant *Streptococcus pneumoniae* Therapeutic Working Group. Pediatr Infect Dis J 18:1, 1999.
131. Lee BT, Stingle WH, Ombres P, et al. Neonatal meningitis and mastoiditis caused by *Haemophilus influenzae.* JAMA 235:407, 1976.
132. Meyer K, Girgis N, McGravey V. Adenovirus associated with congenital pleural effusion. J Pediatr 107:433, 1985.
133. Reman O, Freymuth F, Laloum D, et al. Neonatal respiratory distress due to mumps. Arch Dis Child 61:80, 1986.
134. Boyd MT, Jordan SW, Davis LE. Fatal pneumonitis from congenital echovirus type 6 infection. Pediatr Infect Dis J 6:1138, 1987.
135. McLaren LC, Davis LE, Healy GR, et al. Isolation of *Trichomonas vaginalis* from the respiratory tract of infants with respiratory disease. Pediatrics 71:888, 1983.
136. Hiemstra I, Van Bel F, Berger HM. Can *Trichomonas vaginalis* cause pneumonia in newborn babies? BMJ 289:355, 1984.
137. Hostoffer RW, Litman A, Smith PG, et al. *Pneumocystis carinii* pneumonia in a term newborn infant with a transiently depressed T lymphocyte count, primarily of cells carrying the CD4 antigen. J Pediatr 122:792, 1993.
138. Ahvenainen EK. On congenital pneumonia. Acta Paediatr 40:1, 1951.
139. Anderson GS, Green CA, Neligan GA, et al. Congenital bacterial pneumonia. Lancet 2:585, 1962.
140. Barter R. The histopathology of congenital pneumonia: a clinical and experimental study. J Pathol Bacteriol 66:407, 1953.
141. Davies PA, Aherne W. Congenital pneumonia. Arch Dis Child 37:598, 1962.
142. Langley FA, McCredie Smith JA. Perinatal pneumonia: a retrospective study. J Obstet Gynaecol Br Commonw 66:12, 1959.
143. Penner DW, McInnis AC. Intrauterine and neonatal pneumonia. Am J Obstet Gynecol 69:147, 1955.
144. Alenghat E, Esterly JR. Alveolar macrophages in perinatal infants. Pediatrics 74:221, 1984.
145. Schaffer AJ. The pathogenesis of intrauterine pneumonia: I. A critical review of the evidence concerning intrauterine respiratory-like movements. Pediatrics 17:747, 1956.
146. Naeye RL, Dellinger WS, Blanc WA. Fetal and maternal features of antenatal bacterial infection. J Pediatr 79:733, 1971.
147. Naeye RL, Tafari N, Judge D, et al. Amniotic fluid infections in an African city. J Pediatr 90:965, 1977.
148. Naeye RL, Peters EC. Amniotic fluid infections with intact membranes leading to perinatal death: a prospective study. Pediatrics 61:171, 1978.
149. Barter RA, Hudson JA. Bacteriological findings in perinatal pneumonia. Pathology 6:223, 1974.
150. Barter RA. Congenital pneumonia. Lancet 1:165, 1962.
151. Bernstein J, Wang J. The pathology of neonatal pneumonia. Am J Dis Child 101:350, 1961.
152. Finland M. Fetal and perinatal pneumonia. *In* Charles D, Finland M (eds). Obstetric and Perinatal Infections. Philadelphia, Lea & Febiger, 1973, p 122.
153. Davies PA. Pathogen or commensal? Arch Dis Child 55:169, 1980.
154. Ahvenainen EK. Neonatal pneumonia: I. Incidence of pneumonia during first month of life. Ann Med Intern Fenn 42(Suppl 17):1, 1953.
155. Thaler MM. *Klebsiella-Aerobacter* pneumonia in infants: a review of the literature and report of a case. Pediatrics 30:206, 1962.
156. Papageovgiou A, Bauer CR, Fletcher BD, et al. *Klebsiella* pneumonia with pneumatocele formation in a newborn infant. Can Med Assoc J 109:1217, 1973.
157. Kunh JP, Lee SB. Pneumatoceles associated with *Escherichia coli* pneumonias in the newborn. Pediatrics 51:1008, 1973.
158. Jeffery H, Mitchison R, Wigglesworth JS, et al. Early neonatal bacteraemia: comparison of group B streptococcal, other gram-positive and gram-negative infections. Arch Dis Child 52:683, 1977.
159. Rojas J, Flanigan TH. Postintubation tracheitis in the newborn. Pediatr Infect Dis J 5:714, 1986.
160. Kollef MH. The prevention of ventilator-associated pneumonia. N Engl J Med 340:627, 1999.
161. Barton L, Hodgman JE, Pavlova Z. Causes of death in the extremely low birth weight infant. Pediatrics 103:446, 1999.
162. Davies PA. Pneumonia in the fetus and newborn. Pediatr Digest 1996, p 93.
163. Barson AF. A postmortem study of infection in the newborn from 1976 to 1988. *In* de Louvois J, Harvey D (eds). Infection in the Newborn. New York, John Wiley, 1990, p 13.
164. Wells DW, Keeney GT. Group F *Streptococcus* associated with intrauterine pneumonia. Letter to the editor. Pediatrics 66:820, 1980.
165. Hoffman JA, Mason EO, Schutze GE, et al. *Streptococcus pneumoniae* infections in the neonate. Pediatrics 112:1095-2000, 2003.
166. Rhodes PG, Burry VF, Hall RT, et al. Pneumococcal septicemia and meningitis in the neonate. J Pediatr 86:593-595, 1975.
167. Moriartey RR, Finer NN. Pneumococcal sepsis and pneumonia in the neonate. Am J Dis Child 133:601, 1979.
168. Naylor JC, Wagner KR. Neonatal sepsis due to *Streptococcus pneumoniae.* Can Med Assoc J 133:1019, 1985.

169. Collier AM, Connor JD, Nyhan WL. Systemic infection with *Haemophilus influenzae* in very young infants. J Pediatr 70:539, 1967.
170. Ohlsson A, Bailey T. Neonatal pneumonia caused by *Branhamella catarrhalis*. Scand J Infect Dis 17:225, 1985.
171. Andersson S, Larinkari U, Vartia T. Fatal congenital pneumonia caused by cat-derived *Pasteurella multocida*. Pediatr Infect Dis J 13:74, 1994.
172. Rowen JL, Lopez SM. *Morganella morganii* early onset sepsis. Pediatr Infect Dis J 17:1176, 1998.
173. Brook I. Microbiology of empyema in children and adolescents. Pediatrics 85:722, 1990.
174. Siegel JD, McCracken GH Jr. Neonatal lung abscess. Am J Dis Child 133:947, 1979.
175. Mayer T, Matlak ME, Condon V, et al. Computed tomographic findings of neonatal lung abscess. Am J Dis Child 139:39, 1982.
176. Famiglietti RF, Bakerman PR, Saubolle MA, Rudinsky M. Cavitary legionellosis in two immunocompetent infants. Pediatrics 99:899, 1997.
177. Adler SC, Chusid MJ. *Citrobacter koseri* pneumonia and meningitis in an infant. J Infect 45:65, 2002.
178. Holmberg RE, Pavia AT, Montgomery D, et al. Nosocomial *Legionella* pneumonia in the neonate. Pediatrics 92:450, 1993.
179. Shamir R, Horev G, Merlob P, et al. *Citrobacter diversus* lung abscess in a preterm infant. Pediatr Infect Dis J 9:221, 1990.
180. Vevon GP, Dunne WM, Hicks MJ, et al. *Bacillus cereus* pneumonia in premature neonates: a report of two cases. Pediatr Infect Dis J 12:251, 1993.
181. Gupta R, Faridi MM, Gupta P. Neonatal empyema thoracis. Indian Jour Pediatr 63:704, 1996.
182. Khan EA, Wafelman LS, Garcia-Prats, Taber LH. *Serratia marcescens* pneumonia, empyema and pneumatocele in a preterm neonate. Pediatr Infect Dis J 16:1003, 1997.
183. Thaarup J, Ellermann-Eriksen S, Sternholm J. Neonatal pleural empyema with group A *Streptococcus*. Acta Paediatr 86:769, 1997.
184. Nathavitharana KA, Watkinson M. Neonatal pleural empyema caused by Group A *Streptococcus*. Pediatr Infect Dis J 13:671, 1994.
185. Barton L, Hodgman JE, Pavlova Z. Causes of death in the extremely low birth weight infant. Pediatrics 103:446, 1999.
186. Briggs EJN, Hogg G. Pneumonia found at autopsy in infants weighing less than 750 grams. Can Med Assoc J 85:6, 1961.
187. Briggs EJN, Hogg G. Perinatal pulmonary pathology. Pediatrics 22:41, 1958.
188. Browne FJ. Pneumonia neonatorum. BMJ 1:469, 1922.
189. Fujikura T, Froehlich LA. Intrauterine pneumonia in relation to birth weight and race. Am J Obstet Gynecol 97:81, 1967.
190. Sinha A, Yokoe D, Platt R. Epidemiology of neonatal infections: experience during and after hospitalization. Pediatr Infect Dis J 22:244, 2003.
191. Bang AT, Bang RA, Morankar VJP, et al. Pneumonia in neonates: can it be managed in the community? Arch Dis Child 68:550, 1993.
192. Kishore K, Decorarai AK, Meharban S, et al. Early onset neonatal sepsis-vertical transmission from maternal genital tract. Indian Pediatr J 24:45, 1987.
193. Sazawal S, Black RE. Effect of pneumonia case management on mortality in neonates, infants, and preschool children: a meta-analysis of community-based trials. Lancet Infect Dis 3:547, 2003.
194. Singhi S, Singhi PD. Clinical signs in neonatal pneumonia. Lancet 336:1072, 1990.
195. World Health Organization. Acute respiratory infections in children: case management in small hospitals in developing countries. Geneva, World Health Organization, 1990 (WHO/ARI/90.5).
196. Petersen S, Astvad K. Pleural empyema in a newborn infant. Acta Paediatr Scand 65:527, 1976.
197. Gustavson EE. *Escherichia coli* empyema in the newborn. Am J Dis Child 140:408, 1986.
198. Losek JD, Kishaba RG, Berens RF, et al. Indications for chest roentgenogram in the febrile young infant. Pediatr Emerg Care 5:149, 1989.
199. Ablow RC, Gross I, Effmann EL, et al. The radiographic features of early onset group B streptococcal neonatal sepsis. Radiology 124:771, 1977.
200. Thomas DB, Anderson JC. Antenatal detection of fetal pleural effusion and neonatal management. Med J Aust 2:435, 1979.
201. Steele RW, Thomas MP, Kolls JK. Current management of community-acquired pneumonia in children: an algorithmic guideline recommendation. Infect Med Jan 1999, p 46.
202. Klein JO. Diagnostic lung puncture in the pneumonias of infants and children. Pediatrics 44:486, 1969.
203. Teele DW, Pelton SI, Grant MJA, et al. Bacteremia in febrile children under 2 years of age: results of cultures of blood of 600 consecutive febrile children seen in a "walk-in" clinic. J Pediatr 87:227, 1975.
204. Sherman MP, Goetzman BW, Ahlfor CE, et al. Tracheal aspiration and its clinical correlates in the diagnosis of congenital pneumonia. Pediatrics 65:258, 1980.
205. Thureen PJ, Moreland S, Rodden DJ, et al. Failure of tracheal aspirate cultures to define that cause of respiratory deteriorations in neonates. Pediatr Infect Dis J 12:560, 1993.
206. Lau YL, Hey E. Sensitivity and specificity of daily tracheal aspirate cultures in predicting organisms causing bacteremia in ventilated neonates. Pediatr Infect Dis J 10:290, 1991.
207. Fan LL, Sparks LM, Dulinski JP. Applications of an ultrathin flexible bronchoscope for neonatal and pediatric airway problems. Chest 89:673, 1986.
208. Klein JO. Diagnostic lung puncture in the pneumonias of infants and children. Pediatrics 44:486, 1969.
209. Alexander HE, Craig HR, Shirley RG, et al. Validity of etiology diagnosis of pneumonia in children by rapid typing from nasopharyngeal mucus. J Pediatr 18:31, 1941.
210. Bollowa JGM. Primary pneumonias of infants and children. Public Health Rep 51:1076, 1903.
211. Cheu MHW, Lally MKP, Clark MR, et al. Open lung biopsy in the critically ill newborn. Pediatrics 86:561, 1990.
212. Greenough A. Gains and losses from dexamethasone for neonatal chronic lung disease. Lancet 352:835, 1998.
212a. Yeh TF, Lin YJ, Lin HC, et al. Outcomes at school age after postnatal dexamethasone therapy for lung disease of prematurity. N Engl J Med 350:1304-1313, 2004.
212b. Lister P, Isles R, Shaw B, Ducharme F. Inhaled steroids for neonatal chronic lung disease. The Cochrane Database of Systematic Reviews 4, 2004.
213. Aherne W, Davies PA. Congenital pneumonia. Lancet 1:234, 1962.
214. Tam ASY, Yeung CY. Gastric aspirate findings in neonatal pneumonia. Arch Dis Child 47:735, 1972.
215. Pole VRG, McAllister TA. Gastric aspirate analysis in the newborn. Acta Paediatr Scand 64:109, 1975.
216. Whitelaw A, Evans A, Corrin B. Immotile cilia syndrome: a new cause of neonatal respiratory distress. Arch Dis Child 56:432, 1981.
217. Ramet J, Byloos J, Delree M, et al. Neonatal diagnosis of the immotile cilia syndrome. Chest 89:138, 1986.
218. Ciliary dyskinesia and ultrastructural abnormalitiesin respiratory disease. Annotation. Lancet 1:1370,1988.
219. Giacoia GP, Neter E, Ogra P. Respiratory infections in infants on mechanical ventilation: the immune response as a diagnostic aid. J Pediatr 98:691, 1981.
220. Marks MI, Law B. Respiratory infections vs. colonization. J Pediatr 100:508, 1982.
220a. Nigrovic LE, Kuppermann N, McAdam AJ, Malley R. Cerebrospinal latex agglutination fails to contribute to the microbiologic diagnosis of pre-treated children with meningitis. Pediatr Infect Dis J 23:786-788, 2004.
221. Lung function in children after neonatal meconium aspiration. Annotation. Lancet 2:317, 1988.
222. Smith RM, Brumley GW, Stannard MW. Neonatal pneumonia associated with medium-chain triglyceride feeding supplement. J Pediatr 92:801, 1978.
223. Hjalmarson O. Epidemiology of classification of acute, neonatal respiratory disorders: a prospective study. Acta Paediatr Scand 70:773, 1981.
224. Mounla NA. Neonatal respiratory disorders. Acta Paediatr Scand 76:159, 1987.
225. Avery ME, Fletcher BD, Williams RE. The Lung and Its Disorders in the Newborn Infant. Philadelphia, WB Saunders, 1981.
226. Butler NR, Alberman ED. Clinicopathological associations of hyaline membranes, intraventricular haemorrhage, massive pulmonary haemorrhage and pulmonaryinfection. *In* British Perinatal Mortality Survey, Second Report: Perinatal Problems. Edinburgh, E & S Livingstone, 1969, p 184.
227. Foote GA, Stewart JH. The coexistence of pneumonia and the idiopathic respiratory distress syndrome in neonates. Br J Radiol 46:504, 1973.
228. Ablow RC, Driscoll SG, Effman EL, et al. A comparison of early-onset group B streptococcal infection and the respiratory distress syndrome of the newborn. N Engl J Med 294:65, 1976.

229. Menke JA, Giacoia GP, Jockin H. Group B beta hemolytic streptococcal sepsis and the idiopathic respiratory distress syndrome: a comparison. J Pediatr 94:467,1979.
230. Lloyd-Still JD, Khaw K-T, Schwachman H. Severe respiratory disease in infants with cystic fibrosis. Pediatrics 53:678, 1974.
231. Delville JG, Adler S, Azimi PH, et al. Linezolid versus vancomycin in the treatment of known or suspected resistant gram-positive infections in neonates. Pediatr Infect Dis J 22:S158, 2003.
232. Ahvenainen EK. A study of causes of neonatal deaths. J Pediatr 55:691, 1959.
233. Osborn GT. Discussion on neonatal deaths. Proc R Soc Med 51:840, 1958.
234. Butler NR, Bonham DG. Perinatal Mortality. London, E & S Livingstone, 1963.
235. Apisarnthanarak A, Holzmann-Pazgal G, Hamvas A, et al. Ventilator-associated pneumonia in extremely preterm neonates in a neonatal intensive care unit: characteristics, risk factors, and outcomes. Pediatrics 12:1283, 2003.
236. Pacifico L, Panero A, Roggini M, et al. *Ureaplasma urealyticum* and pulmonary outcome in a neonatal intensive care population. Pediatr Infect Dis J 16:579, 1997.
237. Brasfield DM, Stagno S, Whitley RJ, et al. Infant pneumonitis associated with cytomegalovirus, *Chlamydia*, *Pneumocystis* and *Ureaplasma*: follow-up. Pediatrics 79:76, 1987.

Chapter 8

BACTERIAL INFECTIONS OF THE BONES AND JOINTS

Gary D. Overturf

OSTEOMYELITIS

Introduction

Osteomyelitis occurring in the first 2 months of life is uncommon. During the worldwide pandemic of staphylococcal disease from the early 1950s to the early 1960s, pediatric centers in Europe,[1-5] Australia,[6] and North America[7-11] reported the infrequent occurrence of neonatal osteomyelitis, accounting for only one or two admissions per year at each institution.

With the introduction of invasive neonatal supportive care and the increased use of diagnostic and therapeutic procedures, there was concern that osteomyelitis and septic arthritis secondary to bacteremia might occur more frequently in the newborn.[12] Yet subsequent experience in Europe,[13-15] Canada,[16,17] and the United States[11,18,19] (JD Nelson, personal communication, 1987) during the decade 1970 to 1979 indicated little or no change in the incidence of this condition. Even in intensive care nurseries, despite an increasing problem with fungal (*Candida*) osteoarthritis,[20-24] the overall rate of occurrence of nosocomial bone and joint infections remained low at 2.6 or fewer per 1000 admissions.[22,25,26] However, infections associated with invasive procedures, such as placement of intravascular catheters, may not appear or be recognized until days or weeks after the perinatal period.[12,22]

Little has been published on the relative incidence of neonatal osteomyelitis during the 1980s and 1990s. An ongoing review of nursery infections at a Kaiser Permanente hospital in southern California revealed only three cases of osteomyelitis among 67,000 consecutive live births between 1963 and 1993, and none occurred in the final years (A Miller, personal communication, 1993). A similar survey performed at two pediatric referral centers in Texas showed no significant variation in the number of annual admissions for this condition from 1964 to 1986[27] (JD Nelson, personal communication, 1987). Physicians working in intensive care nurseries in Great Britain,[28] France,[29] Spain,[30] and various parts of the United States[31] (J Pomerance [Los Angeles, Calif], JS Bradley [Portland, Or], RT Hall [Kansas City, Mo], WJ Cashore [Providence, RI], personal communications, 1987) observe, on the average, one to three cases of bone or joint infection per 1000 admissions, an incidence almost identical to that noted 15 years ago.[22,25,26]

In a review of more than 300 cases of neonatal osteomyelitis, male infants predominated over females (1.6:1). Premature infants acquire osteomyelitis with relatively greater frequency than has been noted for term infants.[11,13,16,32-41] In a series of patients with osteomyelitis, 17 of 30 proven cases were in premature infants, 4 occurred in term infants receiving intensive care, and *Staphylococcus aureus* was responsible for 23 of the proven cases of osteomyelitis (methicillin-sensitive strains in 16 cases and methicillin-resistant in 7).[42] *Escherichia coli* and group B streptococci caused three and two cases, respectively. Risk factors for osteomyelitis and septic arthritis in premature infants have been mostly iatrogenic and include use of intravenous or intra-arterial catheters, ventilatory support, and bacteremia with nosocomial pathogens.

Although osteomyelitis was rare in the past, some recent series have suggested that its frequency may be increasing in the neonate. The spectrum of bacterial and fungal infections in Finland from 1985 to 1989 was studied in 2836 infections in children.[43] The incidence of osteomyelitis and septic arthritis in children 28 days of age or younger was 67.7 per 100,000 person years, compared with rates of 262.2 and 2013.1 per 100,000 for meningitis and bacteremia, respectively; both pneumonia (80.4 per 100,000) and pyelonephritis (143.8 per 100,000), however, also were more frequent than bone or joint infections. Studies from other countries have also suggested an increase in osteomyelitis; among 241 bone infections in Panamanian children, 9 occurred in neonates (3 cases were due to gram-negative bacilli, 3 cases to *S. aureus*, 1 case to group B streptococci, and 2 to other organisms).[44]

Microbiology

Because most cases of neonatal osteomyelitis arise as a consequence of bacteremia, it is not surprising that the organisms responsible for causing osteomyelitis reflect the changing trends in the etiology of neonatal sepsis. Before 1940, hemolytic streptococci were the predominant organisms responsible for sepsis in the newborn[45] and also frequently caused osteomyelitis.[46,47] Streptococci were implicated in a majority of the cases of osteomyelitis in neonates and infants younger than 6 months of age.[48]

After 1950, the incidence of *S. aureus* osteomyelitis rose. A review of reports between 1952 and 1972 showed that 85% of the infections were caused by *S. aureus*, 6% were caused by hemolytic streptococci (no groups specified), and 2% were due to *Streptococcus pneumoniae*; either no organisms or miscellaneous organisms (particularly gram-negative bacilli) were isolated in 7% of the cases.[2-6,11,35,38,49-56]

Recognition of group B streptococcal sepsis in the 1970s was associated with a concomitant rise in reported frequency of bone infections caused by this organism.[20,57] This change in spectrum was reflected in U.S. reviews of osteomyelitis in infants hospitalized between 1965 and 1978 showing that group B streptococci had become the single most frequent agent.[11,19,58] However, this experience was not universal: newborn centers in Canada,[16] Sweden,[13] Spain,[30] Switzerland,[14] Nigeria,[59] and even sections of the United States[27] continued to find *S. aureus* as the predominant cause of osteomyelitis, with group B streptococci accounting for only a small number of cases. Although their relative importance may vary by region or institution, these two organisms have remained the most common cause of neonatal osteomyelitis.[31-33,40] A review of cases of occult bacteremia due to group B streptococci identified 147 children.[60] Eleven of these children had nonmeningeal foci, including two with septic arthritis and two with osteomyelitis. More recent cases of unusual sites of group B streptococcal osteomyelitis in the iliac wing[61] and the vertebrae[62] emphasize the renewed importance and frequency of this infection.

Osteomyelitis caused by gram-negative enteric bacilli is relatively uncommon despite the frequency of neonatal bacteremia.[32,45,63,64] In Stockholm during 1969 to 1979, *E. coli* and *Klebsiella-Enterobacter* were responsible for about 30% of cases of neonatal septicemia[15] but only 5% of bone infections.[13] *S. aureus*, on the other hand, although also causing about 30% of neonatal bacteremia cases, was responsible for 75% of cases of osteomyelitis. Several other surveys performed within the past 20 years show about 10% of cases of neonatal osteomyelitis to be due to gram-negative enteric bacilli,[11,14,16,27,31,38] although rates as high as 19%[59] and 45%[30,39,40] have been observed. A review of the literature has revealed isolated instances of hematogenous osteomyelitis in newborns caused by *E. coli*,* *Proteus* species,[13,19,28,53,71-75] *Klebsiella pneumoniae*,[13,30,40,41,70,76-78] *Enterobacter*,[30,72,79,80] *Serratia marcescens*,[19,30] *Pseudomonas* species,[19,30,35,38,40,47,69,82] and *Salmonella*.[16,27,39,81-85]

Presumptively, bacteremia from infected invasive devices is the usual cause of enteric osteomyelitis, infection, but infection may occur directly by translocation from the gut or from urinary tract infection. Studies of neonatal rats have suggested that formula feeding enhances translocation of enteric organisms with subsequent infection of the bone,[86] although other organs were infected as well. Although translocation of bacteria occurred in 23% of breast-fed rats, compared with 100% of formula-fed rats, positive bone cultures developed in 77% of the formula-fed rats, whereas none of the breast-fed rats had positive cultures. A single case of a 4-week-old boy with urinary tract infection with *K. pneumoniae* and vesicoureteral reflux suggests that this site also may be a source of gram-negative enteric bone and joint infections.[87]

*See references 2, 8, 11, 13, 14, 19, 30, 34, 38-40, 47, 53, 65-70.

Although suppurative arthritis is the most common manifestation of gonococcal sepsis involving the skeletal system,[88] osteomyelitis rarely is associated with sepsis as well and probably represents the site of primary infection in many cases.[38,89,90] Syphilitic osteitis and osteochondritis, although frequent in former years,[91] have been largely eliminated through serologic detection of disease during routine antenatal testing and institution of appropriate therapy for infected mothers. Unfortunately, an increase in the incidence of syphilis among women of childbearing age has been reflected in a parallel increase in the frequency of neonatal syphilis and attendant problems of treponemal bone infection.[92,93]

Mycoplasma and *Ureaplasma* have been reported as rare causes of osteomyelitis in infants. In one infant, bone infection due to *Mycoplasma hominis* developed in a sternotomy wound after cardiac surgery[65]; in another, 900-g infant with osteomyelitis of the hip and femur, the infection was caused by *Ureaplasma urealyticum*.[66]

Tuberculous osteomyelitis is extremely rare in the neonate, even in the presence of disseminated congenital tuberculosis.[94,95] Among a group of infants with widespread disease acquired in the perinatal or neonatal period, the youngest with skeletal involvement was 3 months of age.[90]

Pathogenesis

Complications of pregnancy, labor, or delivery precede the occurrence of neonatal osteomyelitis in one third to one half of patients.[11,13,16,19,30,38-40] In the modern era of the neonatal intensive care unit, it is likely that the great majority of bone and joint infections occur in the small or premature infant as a result of prolonged nosocomial exposures and multiple invasive procedures. Although anoxia (as from placenta previa, breech extraction, or fetal distress) or exposure to microorganisms (from premature rupture of membranes) can explain this association in some cases, the means whereby maternal or obstetric problems influence the likelihood of acquiring bone infection is generally unknown.

Microorganisms may reach the skeletal tissues of the fetus and newborn in one of four ways: (1) by direct inoculation, (2) by extension from infection in surrounding soft tissues, (3) as a consequence of maternal bacteremia with transplacental infection and fetal sepsis, and (4) by blood-borne dissemination in the course of neonatal septicemia. Although hematogenous dissemination is responsible for most cases, examples of other routes of infection have appeared occasionally in the literature. As noted previously (see under "Microbiology"), other factors, such as preceding urinary tract infection or direct translocation of bacteria across the bowel wall, may explain bone or joint infection in some neonates.

Direct inoculation of bacteria resulting in osteomyelitis has followed femoral venipuncture,[36,59,75,96-98] radial artery puncture,[30] use of a fetal scalp monitor,[14,99-102] great toe[88] or heel[14,30,31,104-108] capillary blood sampling,[103] and serial lumbar punctures.[109] Infection after surgical invasion of bony structures (e.g., median sternotomy for cardiac surgery) is uncommon.[110] Nevertheless, trauma has been associated with osteomyelitis of the neonate (an association that has been noted for osteomyelitis in older children); *S. aureus* osteomyelitis has occurred in a neonate at 3 weeks of age at the site of a perinatal fracture of the clavicle.[111]

Osteomyelitis caused by extension of infection from surrounding soft tissues usually is associated with organisms from an infected cephalhematoma involving the adjacent parietal bone.[112-115] A series of patients with *S. aureus* osteomyelitis of the skull associated with overlying scalp abscesses was reported nearly 50 years ago.[116] Predisposing factors in these patients were thought to be prolonged, excessive pressure on the fetal head when it lay against the sacral promontory or symphysis pubis, secondary ischemic necrosis, and localization of infection. Paronychia during the newborn period, although most frequently a source of sepsis and hematogenous dissemination of organisms, may extend into bony structures and cause phalangeal infection.[47]

Transplacental bacterial bone infection is most characteristic of syphilis (see Chapter 18). A rare exception, published as a case report in 1933, described a premature infant who died at 19 hours of age with evidence of subacute parietal bone osteomyelitis, meningitis, and cerebritis. Rupture of the amniotic sac immediately before delivery, histopathologic evidence of the prolonged course (at least 2 weeks) of the infection, and the lack of involvement of the overlying scalp epidermis indicate that despite apparent absence of maternal illness, this child was infected transplacentally. The authors postulated that a primary infection occurred in the parietal bone, with secondary extension to the meninges and brain. Although organisms were not isolated, gram-positive diplococci were identified in infected tissues.[117]

Blood-borne dissemination of organisms, with metastatic seeding of the skeletal system through nutrient arteries, represents the major cause of neonatal osteomyelitis.[48,118] Before the advent of antibiotics, the long bones reportedly became infected in as many as 10% of infants with bacteremia.[47,119] Since that time, early recognition and effective empirical therapy for bacterial sepsis led to a marked decrease in the incidence of this complication. Candidal invasion of the bloodstream has become a more frequent cause of bone and joint infections in small infants (see Chapter 33).[20,22,23,33,120,121]

The use of intravascular catheters, mostly central and occasionally peripheral, frequently has been associated with bacterial and fungal osteomyelitis in neonates.* It is probable that septic embolization occurs from infected catheter-tip thrombi, producing relatively high-grade bacteremias; local hypoxia from partial occlusion of vessels by the catheter may also contribute to bone infections.[123,124] The most common etiologic agent has been *S. aureus*, but other microorganisms, such as *Klebsiella*,[78] *Proteus*,[64] *Enterobacter*,[79,80] and *Candida*,[20,22,72,120] have also been implicated. Because the iliac arteries are the most likely pathway for an arterial embolus originating in an aortic catheter tip, the hips or knees or both are involved in more than three fourths of patients.[11,78,80,123-125] There is a very close correlation between the site of the catheter and localization of osteomyelitis in the ipsilateral leg.[124] The distribution of infection originating in umbilical vein catheters is less predictable.[22,79,120,126-128] Although the incidence of osteoarthritis varies greatly, ranging from 1 in 30[123] to less than 1 in 600[124] infants with umbilical artery catheters, it can be reduced significantly by proper attention to aseptic technique and careful monitoring of catheter placement, combined with prompt catheter removal whenever possible.[124]

*See references 11, 13, 16, 20, 22, 23, 40, 78-80, 120, 122-129.

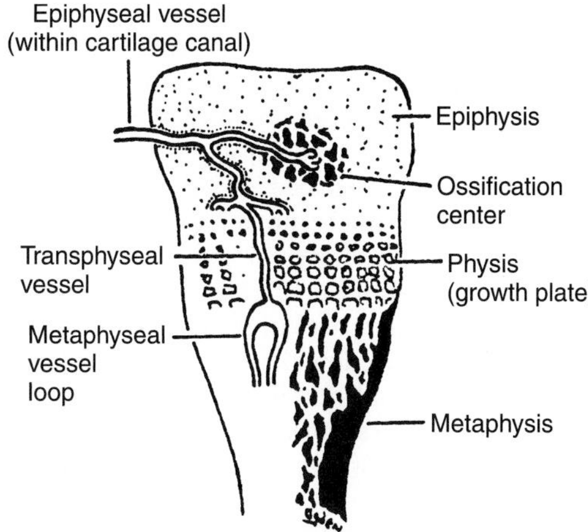

Figure 8–1 Schematic depiction of blood supply in the neonatal epiphysis. Normally in children there are two separate circulatory systems: (1) the metaphyseal loops, derived from the diaphyseal nutrient artery, and (2) the epiphyseal vessels, which course through the epiphyseal cartilage within structures termed *cartilage canals*. In the neonatal period, sinusoidal vessels termed the *transphyseal vessels* connect these two systems. With ensuing skeletal maturation, these vessels disappear, and the epiphyseal and metaphyseal systems become totally separated. (From Ogden JA, Lister G. The pathology of neonatal osteomyelitis. Pediatrics 55:474, 1975.)

The disseminating focus of a bacteremia-producing metastatic abscess in bones is often unknown. Common primary sources include an omphalitis,* pustular dermatitis,[4,11,19,30,33,39,49,53,75] purulent rhinitis,[5,55,132] paronychia,[4,5,37,52,55,75,132] and mastitis.[4,49] In a few infants, sepsis with subsequent osteomyelitis has arisen from infected circumcisions,[8,36] operative sites,[8,31,75] intramuscular injections,[49,75] or varicella lesions.[11] Although gonococcal osteoarthritis originates most commonly from a purulent conjunctivitis, virtually any orifice may provide a portal of entry.[88]

Hematogenous infection of long bones is initiated in dilated capillary loops of the metaphysis, adjacent to the cartilaginous growth plate (physis), where blood flow slows, providing pathogenic bacteria with an ideal environment to multiply, resulting in abscess formation (Fig. 8-1).[118,133,134] Once the infectious process localizes at this site, the following sequence may occur: (1) direct invasion and lysis of the cartilaginous growth plate; (2) spread from metaphyseal vessel loops into transphyseal vessels coursing through the growth plate and into epiphyseal vessels; or (3) rupture occurring laterally, through the cortex into the joint, subperiosteal space, or surrounding soft tissues.[133,134] Green and Shannon,[48] Blanche,[56] and others have pointed out that the large vascular spaces and thin spongy structure of metaphyseal cortex in infants permit early decompression of this primary abscess into the subperiosteal space. For this reason, the bone marrow compartment is seldom involved in neonates, and the term *osteitis* is probably more accurate than *osteomyelitis*.

After rupture into the subperiosteal space, the abscess dissects rapidly beneath loosely attached periosteum, often involving the entire length and circumference of the bone. As pressure increases from accumulating pus, there may be

*See references 4, 5, 11, 32, 39, 40, 49, 71, 75, 119, 130-132.

decompression through the thin, periosteal tissue into surrounding soft tissues, and a subcutaneous abscess may form. In the absence of surgical intervention, collected pus will "point" and drain spontaneously through the skin, forming a sinus tract. Once adequate decompression and drainage have been established, general supportive care often is sufficient to permit complete healing and resolution of osseous and soft tissue foci of infection.[46,48,135,136] Free communication between the original site of osteomyelitis and the subperiosteal space prevents the necrosis and extensive spread of infection through the bone shaft that occurs frequently in older children and adults. Cortical sequestra are therefore less common in infants, and because of the extreme richness of the newborn bone blood supply, sequestra often are completely absorbed if they do form.[48] In addition, the efficient vasculature and fertility of the inner layer of the periosteum encourage early development of profuse new bone formation (involucrum), permitting remodeling of bone within a very short period of time after the infectious process has been controlled.[48,118]

The same characteristics of neonatal bone that serve to prevent many of the features of chronic osteomyelitis seen in older children are also responsible for complications occurring in neonates and young infants, namely, epiphysitis and pyarthrosis. A consequence of the excellent bone blood supply in newborns is persistent fetal vessels that penetrate the cartilaginous epiphyseal plate and end in large venous lakes within the epiphysis.[118,133,134] Thus, localization of organisms at these sites early in the course of osteomyelitis leads to an epiphysitis, with resultant severe damage of the cartilage cells on the epiphyseal side of the growth plate. Once such damage occurs, it is generally irreparable[70,118] and ultimately results in arrest or disorganization of growth at the ends of the bone. By the age of 8 to 18 months, the vascular connections between metaphysis and epiphysis are obliterated, and the cartilaginous growth plate provides a barrier against the spread of infection that persists throughout childhood and adult life.[118,133,134]

Rapid decompression of the primary metaphyseal abscess through the adjacent cortex also permits ready entrance of pus into the articular space of those bones whose metaphyses lie within the articular capsule of the joint. Therefore, suppurative arthritis of the hips, shoulders, elbows, and knees is frequently associated with osteomyelitis of the humerus or femur in infants.* When the infection originates in the epiphysis, pyarthrosis also may occur by direct extension of the primary abscess through the articular cartilage and into the joint space. Once pus enters the joint, it causes distention of the joint capsule, and the increasing pressure may eventually produce a pathologic dislocation, particularly of the shoulder or hip joint. The lytic action of pyogenic exudate within the joint[140,141] and ischemia produced by the high intra-articular tension often are sufficient to cause dissolution or separation of the entire head of the femur or humerus, both of which are composed almost completely of cartilage during the neonatal period.[3,34,35,142-144] Although serious growth disturbances and deformities may result from septic arthritis at other sites, complete destruction of the joint is rare.

*See references 3, 4, 6, 11, 13, 16, 19, 20, 35, 58, 134, 137-141.

Clinical Manifestations

Greengard,[145] Thomson and Lewis,[37] and Dennison[3] have described two distinct clinical syndromes that may be associated with suppurative bone involvement in the newborn period: (1) a "benign form," with little or no evidence of infection (other than local swelling) or disability, related to an osteomyelitis involving one or more skeletal sites, and (2) a "severe form," with systemic manifestations of sepsis predominating until multiple sites of bone and visceral involvement are noted as manifestations of the infant's underlying condition. The most likely cause of the benign form of neonatal osteomyelitis is a mild, transient bacteremia that arises at a peripheral site and causes only minimal inflammation and suppuration. The experience of most investigators indicates that this form of illness represents a majority of the cases.* The few series in which high fever and evidence of sepsis were noted as common presenting signs probably represent instances in which diagnosis was delayed, resulting in more advanced disease at presentation.[2,3,39,49]

Infants with mild illness generally feed well, gain weight, and develop normally. Systemic manifestations are minimal, and the temperature is usually normal or only slightly elevated.[4,14,31,32,56,137,142] Thus, the diagnosis may be missed until 2 to 4 weeks have elapsed, by which time bone destruction may be severe and widespread.[47,54,56,146] Even in intensive care nurseries, where infants are under continuous professional observation, osteomyelitis may be missed for days or weeks. Bone involvement may be discovered during a skeletal survey or a generalized computed tomography (CT) or magnetic resonance imaging (MRI) scan as an unsuspected site or sites of infection in an infant without known bone involvement; osteomyelitis also has been diagnosed as an incidental finding on chest or abdominal radiographs.[16,22,147]

The first signs that may be noted by parents or physicians are diffuse edema and swelling of an extremity or joint, usually without discoloration, accompanied by excessive irritability of the infant. Handling the infant causes increased discomfort, and prolonged episodes of crying may be noted during after a diaper change or other physical manipulations of routine care. Examination reveals diminished spontaneous and reflex movement of the affected extremity, either as a result of pain (pseudoparalysis)[19,31,32,40,74,77,134] or because of weakness caused by an associated neuropathy.[148-151] Pyarthrosis of the hip joint is characterized by maintenznce of the hip in a flexed, abducted, and externally rotated ("frog-leg") position.[148] Because the slightest degree of passive motion of an extremity may cause severe pain and prolonged crying, attempts to elicit a point of maximal bone tenderness are often unsuccessful.

As the suppurative process extends through the metaphyseal cortex into the surrounding subperiosteal and subcutaneous tissues, external signs of inflammation become more intense, and points of maximal swelling, redness, and heat are more readily discernible. In most cases, an inflammatory mass is directly adjacent to the involved metaphysis or joint, although when deeper skeletal structures (e.g., vertebrae or pelvis) are involved, the abscess may point in

*See references 4, 6, 11, 13, 14, 16, 19, 31, 32, 38, 40, 51, 56, 135, 136.

distant sites. Thus, three infants have been described in whom vertebral osteomyelitis was not discovered, or even suspected, until after a large retroperitoneal abscess had developed.[6] An abscess arising from the proximal femur, ilium, or hip joint appears usually in the upper thigh, on the buttocks, or in the groin, but occasionally also in the iliac fossa, where it can be palpated through the abdominal wall or rectum.[51] Even when infection is localized in the distal extremities, it is difficult to determine solely on clinical grounds whether the bone or adjacent joint, or both, are involved. Radiologic examinations and diagnostic aspiration of suspected joints are generally necessary to establish a diagnosis.

The striking feature of the benign form of neonatal osteomyelitis is the satisfactory general condition of the infant, despite the intensity of the local process; feeding and weight gain are undisturbed, and there is no evidence of involvement of visceral structures. Although deformity and disability may follow such infections, the fatality rate is exceedingly low, and healing is prompt.

By contrast, signs and symptoms of the severe form of neonatal osteomyelitis are predominantly those of a septic process with prolonged and intense bacteremia. Infants with this condition usually demonstrate failure to thrive, with associated lethargy, refusal or vomiting of feedings, abdominal distention, jaundice, and other signs characteristic of sepsis in the newborn. Infection of the bones and joints may be noted almost simultaneously with onset of septicemia, or it may appear later, despite administration of antibiotics. The clinical evolution of the osteomyelitic process is identical to that in patients with the benign form of the disease. Early localizing signs and symptoms are frequently overshadowed by the systemic manifestations occurring in the infant. Evidence of a suppurative process in the bone may be discovered accidentally in the course of routine radiographic examinations, or it may not be apparent until formation of a local subcutaneous abscess directs attention to the underlying bone. The prognosis for these infants is guarded; death is generally caused by sepsis, with widespread and multiple foci of infection in the nervous system or viscera. The prognosis for the skeletal lesions among survivors is, however, not different from that described for the benign form.

As group B streptococcal infections have become increasingly prevalent, a distinctive clinical picture associated with osteomyelitis has emerged for this agent.[19,31,58,152-156] Most cases are caused by the type III serotype of streptococci and present as a late-onset illness during the third and fourth weeks of life (mean age at diagnosis, 25 days). Predisposing factors commonly seen with osteomyelitis caused by other agents, such as maternal obstetric complications, difficulties in the early neonatal period, use of vascular catheters, or other manipulative procedures, are unusual with group B streptococcal disease. The male preponderance usually identified with neonatal osteomyelitis is reversed, with a 1.5:1 excess of females. In almost 90% of the infants described with this condition, only a single bone has been involved, most commonly the humerus (50%) or femur (33%), affecting the shoulder or knee. In most cases, infants manifest the benign form of osteomyelitis without signs of systemic toxicity or involvement of other organ systems. Nevertheless, most are ill no more than 3 or 4 days before the diagnosis is established. Although affected joints are typically neither warm nor erythematous, local swelling, tenderness, and diminished movement of the affected extremity are usually severe enough for parents to seek early medical attention.

Table 8–1 Distribution of Bone Involvement in 485 Newborns with Osteomyelitis

Bone	No. of Sites[a]	% of Sites
Femur	287	39
62 Proximal		
91 Distal		
81 Unspecified		
Humerus	133	18
66 Proximal		
16 Distal		
51 Unspecified		
Tibia	102	14
47 Proximal		
11 Distal		
44 Unspecified		
Radius	34	5
5 Proximal		
17 Distal		
12 Unspecified		
Maxilla	30	4
Ulna	22	3
Clavicle	18	2
Tarsal bones	15	2
2 "Tarsus"		
3 Talus		
10 Calcaneus		
Metacarpals	14	2
Phalanges	12	2
Ribs	12	2
Skull	9	1
Fibula	9	1
Ilium	8	1
Metatarsals	7	1
Mandible	7	1
Scapula	7	1
Sternum	6	1
Vertebrae	5	1
Ischium	3	0.4
Patella	1	0.1

[a]Thirty-three percent of infants had disease in more than one bone.

The distribution of bone involvement reported in the literature is represented in Table 8-1, with 734 infected sites among 485 patients. A single bone was involved in 324 patients and multiple foci in 161 patients (33%).[157,158] Because radiographic or radionuclide skeletal surveys, which often identify unsuspected foci of osteomyelitis,[13,16,22,32,129,147] were generally not performed, the number of infants reported to have infection in multiple sites is probably falsely low. The high incidence of infections of the femur, humerus, and tibia in the neonate has also been noted in adults[159] and older infants and children.[8,10,137,160] The relatively large number of cases of maxillary osteomyelitis is, however, unique to the newborn period; therefore, this entity is discussed separately later on.

The exuberant new bone formation associated with osteomyelitis in the newborn period makes it difficult to determine the original foci of infection when radiographs are obtained late in the clinical course. For this reason, either the site of primary metaphyseal abscess was unspecified, or the infection was referred to as a "panosteitis" in many instances. In the femur, there are an equal distribution of proximal, distal, and uncertain sites of early infection, whereas localization in the tibia and humerus occurs most often at proximal ends of bones; in the radius, distal osteomyelitis predominates. The major consequence of these patterns of infection is the high incidence of secondary purulent arthritis of the hips, shoulders, knees, and wrists; this secondary arthritis has been noted in virtually every large series of newborns with bone infection.

Prognosis

From 1920 to 1940, reports of with neonatal osteomyelitis cited mortality rates of up to 40% in neonates and young infants[48] but stressed an overall benign nature of the disease and the good prognosis for life and function if sepsis was not present.[46,48,135,136] The introduction of antimicrobial agents effective against the common infecting organisms was associated with a considerable reduction in mortality rates. For example, only 24 deaths (mortality rate, 4.2%) were reported among approximately 575 newborns with osteomyelitis acquired between 1945 and 1990.*

The improved survival rate directed greater attention to a high incidence of residual joint deformities following neonatal osteomyelitis, particularly with hip and knee involvement or delayed diagnosis for more than 3 or 4 days.[34-36,38,39,56,70,75,161-163] Destruction or separation of the capital femoral epiphysis may result in serious disturbances of growth, usually combined with a marked coxa vara, valga, or magna; an unstable hip joint; flexion contractures; and abnormalities of gait.† Damage to the cartilaginous growth plate in the knees also is often followed by disturbances in longitudinal growth and angulation at the site of infection, leading to genu varum or valgum, restricted motion, and instability of the joint.[11,33,56,70,132,139] Although the consequences of shortening of bone and angular deformities are more serious in lower extremities, analogous growth disturbances may follow osteomyelitis of the humerus, radius, or ulna.[3,14,37,56,70,164] Most of these data have been collected from infants with staphylococcal bone or joint infection, whereas, in contrast, the prognosis for full recovery is excellent after group B streptococcal infection[19,58] (J Pomerance [Los Angeles, Calif], JS Bradley [Portland, Or], RT Hall [Kansas City, Mo], WJ Cashore [Providence, RI], personal communications, 1987).

Although vertebral osteomyelitis in the newborn is unusual, the consequences can be grave. Collapse or complete destruction of one or more vertebral bodies may occur,[13,22,164-168] with severe kyphosis or paralysis caused by spinal cord compression appearing as late complications.[13,164,165] In most cases, vertebral involvement is not recognized until after paraspinal abscesses appear.[6,169-171]

The full clinical consequences of osteomyelitis in the newborn period may not be apparent for months to years. Thus, despite a seemingly favorable outcome, even infants with minor bone or joint involvement should be followed to skeletal maturity to observe for the appearance of late deformity, dysfunction, or growth arrest.[70,75] Early evidence of skeletal destruction frequently requires multiple orthopedic procedures to stabilize a joint or to straighten a limb or equalize its length with that of the contralateral arm or leg. However, descriptions of late regeneration of femoral epiphyses despite severe injury emphasize the remarkable healing potential and unpredictability of this illness.[172-178]

Chronic osteomyelitis and sequestration of necrotic bone have been thought to be uncommon complications both before and after the availability of antibiotic therapy.[6,37,39,48,56,135,136] The apparent rarity of these complications in former years should be questioned, however, because approximately in 10% of infants with osteomyelitis who were studied by several groups of investigators, formation of sequestra occurred, and in many cases, sequestrectomy was required for complete cure.* A rare complication of neonatal osteomyelitis is osteochondroma (or exostosis) at the distal ulna, following *S. aureus* osteomyelitis.[178]

Diagnosis

Plain film radiographs remain the most useful means of establishing the diagnosis of neonatal osteomyelitis. Experience with CT and MRI in the evaluation of neonatal disease bone infection is limited. Often, transport of a small or sick neonate to MRI or CT diagnostic centers, and the need for monitoring of an anesthetized infant, preclude their use. Thus, these techniques are diagnostic methods that may be used if plain radiographs, ultrasonography (of joints), and bone scans have not yielded a diagnosis.[179]

The earliest radiographic sign is swelling of soft tissue around the site of primary infection. Although this finding reflects spreading edema and inflammation that occur as pus breaks through metaphyseal cortex, it is nonspecific and serves only to define an area of inflammation. The first distinct evidence of bone involvement appears as small foci of necrosis and rarefaction, most commonly located in the metaphysis adjoining the epiphyseal growth plate. This may be accompanied by capsular distention or widening of the joint space if inflammatory exudate or pus has entered the articular capsule. Unlike older children, in whom radiographic changes are commonly delayed for up to 3 weeks,[10,160] neonates almost always show definite signs of bone destruction after only 7 to 10 days.[5,11,19,38,53,55,124,129,177]

Extension of the suppurative process often produces widespread areas of cortical rarefaction, which, despite their appearance, infrequently result in significant bone sequestration. The presence of pus in the hip and shoulder joints may cause progressive lateral and upward displacement of the head of the femur[32,143,144,180] or humerus through stages of subluxation to pathologic dislocation. The absence in the newborn period of ossification centers, with the exception of those at the distal femur and proximal tibia, makes it very difficult to diagnose neonatal epiphysitis in any area but the knees.[139] For similar reasons, epiphyseal separation or destruction of the head of the femur or humerus is difficult to distinguish radiologically from simple dislocation.[143,144]

In most infants, the reparative phase begins within 2 weeks after onset of infection. The first sign of healing is the formation of a thin layer of subperiosteal bone, which rapidly

*See references 2, 4-6, 11, 13, 14, 16, 19, 30, 31, 38-40, 54, 56, 74, 129, 132.
†See references 35, 56, 75, 90, 97, 132, 143, 144, 164, 165.

*See references 2, 5, 16, 50, 51, 74, 116, 139, 176, 177.

enlarges to form a thick involucrum between the raised periosteum and the cortex. Although bone destruction may continue at the same time, necrotic foci are rapidly absorbed and filled in as new bone is deposited. The entire process from the first signs of rarefaction to restoration of the cortical structure may last no longer than 2 months; however, several months usually elapse before minimal deformities disappear and remodeling of the shaft is complete. In some cases, well-circumscribed defects involving the metaphysis and epiphysis may persist for years.[139]

The frequent benefit of utilizing radiologic skeletal surveys in newborns with osteomyelitis should be emphasized, particularly because the occurrence of multiple sites of osteomyelitis is much more common in the neonatal period. Thus, clinically unsuspected sites of infection can be discovered in a significant proportion of infants.[13,16,22,33,129,181] Demonstration of such lesions may be provide therapeutic benefits: In one series,[16] four of seven areas of occult infection required aspiration or drainage, whereas in another study,[13] 3 of 17 hip joint infections were discovered on routine radiographs taken because the infant had osteomyelitis elsewhere. Therefore, plain film skeletal surveys for occult bone and joint infection are recommended in any infant with osteomyelitis.

As mentioned, experience with CT and MRI in the diagnosis of neonatal musculoskeletal infection is limited.[182,183] Although both procedures can be helpful adjuncts to clinical diagnosis and conventional radiography, they are slow and require heavy sedation—usually undesirable in a febrile septic infant—to prevent movement artifact and loss of resolution. CT provides good definition of cortical bone and is sensitive for early detection of bone destruction, periosteal reaction, and formation of sequestra. It has been used to particular advantage in diagnosis of osteomyelitis of the skull associated with infected cephalhematoma.[112,113] Plain radiographs of uninfected cephalhematomas can show soft tissue swelling, periosteal elevation, calcification, and even underlying radiolucency caused by bone resorption[184]—findings also consistent with bone infection. In such cases, CT has been able to define foci of bone destruction more accurately, helping confirm the presence of osteomyelitis.

MRI, on the other hand, is of limited value in defining structural changes in cortical bone but provides excellent anatomic detail of muscle and soft tissue, superior to that of any other imaging technique.[183] It is therefore particularly useful in disclosing the early soft tissue edema seen adjacent to areas of bone involvement before the appearance of any osseous changes. It is also helpful in determining the presence of a periosteal abscess and assessing the need for surgical drainage. The major advantage of MRI over CT is the ability to detect inflammatory or destructive intramedullary disease. However, it is of greater advantage in older children and adults than in neonates, because involvement of the marrow compartment is uncommon in neonates.

Both modalities provide excellent spatial resolution and anatomic detail; however, CT is best suited to cross-sectional views, whereas MRI can display anatomy with equal clarity in coronal and sagittal planes, permitting visualization in the plane most advantageous for accurate diagnosis. Absence of ionizing radiation is another distinct advantage of MRI over CT.

In recent years, there has been increasing interest in the use of ultrasonography for the detection of bone infection and joint effusions.[185-189] Diagnosis of osteomyelitis is based on demonstration of periosteal thickening or the presence of abscess formation as indicated by periosteal elevation and separation from bone. The exact role of ultrasonography in diagnosis of neonatal osteoarthritis has continued to be defined. It currently appears most useful as a tool for defining the presence of fluid collections in joints or adjacent to bone and as a guide for needle aspiration or surgical drainage of these collections. The occurrence of false-positive or false-negative examinations, although infrequent, requires that infants with conflicting clinical findings be evaluated further by other techniques. Reports of successful diagnosis of osteomyelitis in neonates with ultrasonography include the diagnosis of rib infection in a 650-g infant with staphylococcal osteomyelitis.[190] Other series have included 2- to 6-week-old infants with osteomyelitis of the costochondral junction and ribs as well.[191,192]

Despite reports emphasizing the reliability of technetium-99m bone imaging in older infants and children,[193] experience with the use of this technique in neonates has been far less favorable.[16,33,40,129,194-198] In one study, among 10 newborns subsequently proved to have osteomyelitis involving 20 sites in all, only 8 of these sites were found to be abnormal or equivocal by technetium scan.[194] Of the 12 sites that were normal by scan at 1 to 33 days (mean, 8 days) after onset of symptoms, 9 showed destructive changes in the corresponding radiograph. The increased radioactivity in areas of inflammatory hyperemia surrounding an osteomyelitic lesion, usually present in the early "blood-pool" images in children,[195] also was not seen, even in those infants with ultimately positive delayed bone scans. Although false-negative bone scans also have been described in older infants,[199,200] the reason for the excessively high incidence among neonates is not known. It has been suggested that the discrepancy is due either to differences in the pathophysiology of neonatal disease or to the inability of earlier gamma cameras to separate the increased activity of the growth plate in the first weeks of life from that of infection.[147,193]

As indicated by clinical studies, use of newer high-resolution cameras combined with electronic magnification may provide greater diagnostic accuracy.[147] However, in these studies, the investigators also used significantly (four- to sixfold) larger doses of technetium, and almost all sites of involvement had radiographically detectable lesions at the time of diagnosis. At present, it appears reasonable to limit the use of technetium radionuclide scans to evaluation of infants with normal or equivocal radiographs in whom there is a strong clinical suspicion of osteomyelitis.

Among older patients, gallium-67 bone imaging has been shown to be of value when results of the technetium scan and appearance on plain films are normal and osteomyelitis is strongly suspected.[200] Studies performed in small infants and neonates have shown similar results.[199,201] Unfortunately, the radiation burden of this isotope is high, and the probability that the results of a scan will, by themselves, influence therapy is low. Thus, the role of gallium bone imaging in the diagnosis of neonatal bone and joint infections is very limited.

Needle aspiration of an inflammatory area may provide a rapid diagnosis.[19,31,38,40] Differentiation of subcutaneous from subperiosteal infection often is difficult; however, significant accumulations of pus aspirated from a periarticular abscess almost invariably are found to originate in bone rather than in the soft tissues.[2,134] Clinical or radiologic evidence of joint space infection, particularly in the hip and shoulder, requires immediate confirmation by needle aspiration. If no effusion is found and clinical signs persist, aspiration should be repeated within 8 to 12 hours. If there is doubt about whether the joint was actually entered, limited arthrography with small amounts of dye can readily be performed with an aspirating needle.[143,144] Most iodinated contrast materials will not interfere with bacterial growth from aspirated specimens.[202] Inserting a needle into the metaphyseal region or joint up to 24 hours before scanning does not interfere with the scintigraphic detection of osteomyelitis.[196-198]

The total peripheral white blood cell count is of little value in diagnosing neonatal osteomyelitis. In more than 150 cases in which these values were recorded, the median peripheral leukocyte count was approximately 17,000 cells per mm^3 (mean, 20,000; range, 4000 to 75,100). Polymorphonuclear leukocytes usually represented about 60% of the white blood cells counted; frequently, the number of immature forms was higher than normal. Neonates with osteomyelitis usually have a sedimentation rate higher than 20 mm per hour.[11,31,32,58,123,154] Like the leukocyte count, the sedimentation rate is helpful for diagnosis and follow-up evaluation when elevated but cannot be used to rule out osteomyelitis when normal.[11,13,14,203] Alternatively, the C-reactive protein is more useful than the erythrocyte sedimentation rate as an acute-phase reactant in neonate, and most methods for C-reactive protein determination require only 0.1 mL of blood, as opposed to the erythrocyte sedimentation rate, which may require 1 to 2 mL of blood.

Differential Diagnosis

The early descriptions of pyogenic neonatal osteomyelitis emphasized difficulties in distinguishing the pseudoparalysis and irritability that are characteristic of this condition from the symptoms of congenital syphilis and from true paralysis of congenital poliomyelitis.[204-206] The clinical course and radiologic examinations are generally sufficient to rule out polio; however, the periostitis and metaphyseal bone destruction that accompany congenital syphilis are frequently indistinguishable from bone alterations observed in infants with multicentric pyogenic osteomyelitis (see Chapter 18).[163,164] Similar osseous changes have been noted at birth in infants with congenital tumors or leukemia.[204,207]

Serial radiologic examinations may be necessary to distinguish a superficial cellulitis, subcutaneous abscess, or bursitis[208,209] from a primary bone infection, particularly when these conditions arise in a periarticular location. Similarly, a suppurative arthritis arising in the joint space rather than in the adjacent metaphysis can be defined as such only by determining that no destruction has occurred in bones contiguous to that joint.

The relative lack of any inflammatory sign other than edema is the only clinical feature that helps to differentiate between candidal and bacterial osteomyelitis.[20,22] The former condition has been observed more frequently in recent years, particularly in premature infants, in whom antibiotic therapy, placement of umbilical catheters, and use of parenteral hyperalimentation, together with immature host defense mechanisms, predispose to candidal infection and dissemination.[20,22-24,34-37,80,120,210,211] The lesions of *Candida albicans* infection typically are seen as well-defined ("punched-out") metaphyseal lucencies on radiographs but are less aggressive in appearance than those of staphylococcal osteitis, and often are surrounded by a slightly sclerotic margin.[20,22,34,37,38,80,211,212] Even when characteristic clinical circumstances and radiographic features are present, the diagnosis in almost all cases rests on identification of the organism by Gram stain or culture.

Several congenital viral lesions have also been associated with bone changes. Lesions caused by congenital rubella, although generally seen in the metaphyseal ends of the long bones, are distinct from those of bacterial osteomyelitis during the early stages of pathogenesis and show no evidence of periosteal reaction during the reparative phase.[213] There is little likelihood of confusion of the radiographic features of bone pathology resulting from congenital cytomegalic inclusion disease,[214,215] or from herpes simplex virus type 2 infections,[216] with those of hematogenous osteomyelitis, particularly when roentgenographic findings are considered in context with the characteristic clinical signs and symptoms of these infections.

A number of noninfectious conditions causing bone destruction or periosteal reaction may be confused with osteomyelitis on clinical and radiographic grounds as well as on the basis of radionuclide scan findings. These conditions include skeletal trauma caused by the birth process or caregiver abuse[147,217-219] or associated with osteogenesis imperfecta; congenital infantile cortical hyperostosis (Caffey's disease)[147,218,220]; congenital bone tumors, metastases, and leukemia[145,205]; extravasation of calcium gluconate at an infusion site[221]; and prostaglandin E_1 infusion.[222] The periosteal bone growth sometimes seen in normal infants, particularly the premature infant, may produce a "double-contour" effect in long bones that appears to be similar to the early involucrum of healing osteomyelitis but is unassociated with evidence of bone destruction and metaphyseal changes and is never progressive.[223]

Therapy

Successful treatment of osteomyelitis or septic arthritis depends on prompt clinical diagnosis and identification of the infectious agent. Every effort should be made to isolate responsible organism(s) before therapy is initiated. Pus localized in skin, soft tissues, joint, or bone should be aspirated under strict aseptic conditions and sent to the laboratory for Gram stain, culture, and antibiotic susceptibility testing. Blood specimens for culture should be obtained; such cultures may be the only source of the pathogen[16,27,35,38,52,55,224] (JD Nelson, personal communication, 1987). Because osteomyelitis generally is the consequence of a systemic bacteremia, a lumbar puncture should be considered. Any potential source of infection should be examined, including the tip of intravascular catheters.[225] Bacterial antigen testing of urine, blood, or cerebrospinal fluid can occasionally be helpful when direct examination of suppurative material fails to provide an etiologic diagnosis (see Chapter 6). Choice of therapy should be guided by results of Gram stain, culture, and antibiotic susceptibilities which in most cases should be available within 24 to 48 hours.

When the cause of infection cannot be immediately determined, the initial choice of antimicrobial agents must be based on the presumptive bacteriologic diagnosis. The penicillinase-resistant penicillins (e.g., nafcillin, oxacillin) and vancomycin are active against *S. aureus*, group A and group B streptococci, and *S. pneumoniae*, which together account for more than 90% of cases of osteoarthritis in neonates. Osteomyelitis caused by enteric organisms is sufficiently common to justify additional therapy with an aminoglycoside such as gentamicin, tobramycin, or amikacin or an extended-spectrum agent (cefotaxime). Both methicillin-resistant *S. aureus* (MRSA) and most strains of coagulase-negative staphylococci are increasingly frequent causes of sepsis and other focal infections in neonates. Numerous outbreaks of both nosocomial and community-acquired MRSA infections have been reported. Thus, infants who acquire infection in nurseries where MRSA is prevalent, or where community-acquired MRSA infections have occurred, should be started on vancomycin, rather than a penicillin antibiotic.[129] Alternative antibiotics recently approved and licensed for treatment of MRSA infections in older children and adults, including daptomycin, linezolid, and quinupristin-dalfopristin, have not been fully evaluated or approved for use in neonates in the first 2 months of life.

Once bacterial culture and sensitivity data are available, treatment should be changed to the single safest and most effective drug. If group B streptococcal infection is confirmed, combination therapy with penicillin G (or ampicillin) and gentamicin should be given for 2 to 5 days, after which time penicillin G (or ampicillin) alone is adequate.[226] Standard disk susceptibility tests may falsely indicate sensitivity of MRSA to cephalosporins.[227] Use of β-lactam antibiotics is inappropriate for MRSA infections and vancomycin should be continued for the full course of therapy. It is controversial whether the synergistic addition of an active aminoglycoside (e.g., gentamicin) to a penicillin antibiotic or vancomycin for a limited period of time (e.g., 5 days) enhances the clinical outcomes of infants with neonatal osteomyelitis caused by *S. aureus*.

All antibiotics should be given by the parenteral route, usually intravenously. There is no significant clinical advantage to intravenous over intramuscular administration, but the limited number of injection sites available in the newborn makes the intramuscular route impractical for use during prolonged periods. Intra-articular administration of antibiotics is unnecessary in the treatment of suppurative arthritis because adequate levels of activity have been demonstrated in joint fluid after parenteral doses of most drugs that would be used for therapy.[224] Antibiotic therapy for either osteomyelitis or suppurative arthritis should be continued for at least 4 or 6 weeks after defervescence. Monitoring serum acute-phase proteins (particularly C-reactive protein) has been proposed as a useful way to determine resolution of infection and duration of therapy.[112,228,229]

There are insufficient data on the absorption and efficacy of orally administered antibiotics in the neonate to routinely recommend their use in this age group for treatment of osteoarthritis. Nevertheless, after an initial course of intravenous therapy, newborns have been treated successfully with oral dicloxacillin,[203,230,231] flucloxacillin,[32] fusidic acid,[32,33] and penicillin V[32,181] for additional periods varying from 14 to 42 days. If sequential parenteral-oral therapy is used, adequacy of antibiotic absorption and efficacy must be closely monitored with regular clinical evaluation and and, possibly, serum bactericidal titers against the infecting organism.[181,231,232] It is likely, but unproved in the neonate, that the traditional antibiotics used for hematogenous osteomyelitis in older children (e.g., amoxicillin or cephalexin, in divided doses totally 100 to 150 mg/kg per day) would be tolerated and effective, but these agents should be used only after successful parenteral therapy has been established and only under the supervision of physicians with adequate training.

To overcome the uncertainties of oral absorption while still allowing discharge of the patient from the hospital, home intravenous antibiotic therapy has been advocated as an alternative form of treatment.[235] Although home management for older children and adults is now widely accepted, experience with newborns is still limited; however, with proper family and medical support, it can be a successful alternative to inpatient treatment.

Incision and drainage are indicated whenever there is a significant collection of pus in soft tissues. The need for drilling or "windowing" the cortex to drain intramedullary collections of pus is controversial.[11,13,14,32] There is no evidence, based on controlled studies, that these procedures are of any value in either limiting systemic manifestations or decreasing the extent of bone destruction. Open surgical drainage for relief of intra-articular pressure is, however, a critical measure for preserving the viability of the head of the femur or humerus in infants with suppurative arthritis of hip or shoulder joints.[6,35,35,161] Intermittent needle aspiration with saline irrigation usually is adequate for drainage of other, more readily accessible joints. Lack of improvement after 3 days, rapid reaccumulation of fluid, or loculation of pus and necrotic debris in the joint may indicate the need for open drainage of these joints as well.[234]

The affected extremity should be immobilized until inflammation has subsided and there is radiologic evidence of healing. Prolonged splinting in a brace or cast is necessary when pathologic dislocation of the head of the femur accompanies pyarthrosis of the hip joint. Maintenance of adequate nutrition and fluid requirements is critical in determining the ultimate course of the illness. Before the advent of antibiotics, attention to these factors alone often was adequate to ensure prompt healing of osseous lesions in those infants who survived the initial septic process.[48]

PRIMARY SEPTIC ARTHRITIS

Although septic arthritis often is a complication of neonatal osteomyelitis, it also can occur in the absence of demonstrable radiologic changes in adjacent bone. Infection usually is the result of synovial implantation of organisms in the course of a septicemia. Infrequently, traumatic inoculation of organisms into the articular capsule may occur as a consequence of femoral venipuncture.[36,59,96-98] As in osteomyelitis, there is a strong association between septic arthritis and placement of an umbilical catheter.[235] Whatever the source of infection, the presence of a concurrent osteomyelitis

Table 8–2 Organisms Isolated from Blood or Joints of Neonates with Primary Bacterial Arthritis (1972-1986)

Bacteria	No. of Infants
Staphylococcus aureus	9
Group B streptococci	4
Streptococci, unspecified	2
Staphylococcus epidermidis	1
Haemophilus influenzae type b	
Escherichia coli	
Klebsiella pneumoniae	1
Pseudomonas aeruginosa	1
Neisseria gonorrhoeae	1

Data from JD Nelson, personal communication, 1987; Pittard WB III, Thullen JD, Fanaroff AA. Neonatal septic arthritis. J Pediatr 88:621, 1976; and Jackson MA, Nelson JD. Etiology and medical management of acute suppurative bone and joint infections in pediatric patients. J Pediatr Orthop 2:313, 1982.

can never be ruled out completely because of the possibility that the original suppurative focus lay in the radiolucent cartilaginous portion of the bone, permitting entry of organisms to the joint by direct extension.

The spectrum of agents responsible for primary septic arthritis is similar to that of organisms causing arthritis secondary to a contiguous osteomyelitis. Bacteria that have been isolated from blood or joints of newborns in two series are listed in Table 8-2.

Signs and symptoms of purulent arthritis are virtually identical to those seen in newborns with osteomyelitis.[236,237] Limitation in use of an extremity progressing to pseudoparalysis is characteristic of both conditions, and although external signs of inflammation tend to be somewhat more localized to the periarticular area, recognition of this feature is of little diagnostic value in individual cases. Data are insufficient to provide any meaningful comparison between the skeletal distribution of septic arthritis and that of osteomyelitis. However, multiple joint involvement is common to both conditions. In one series of 16 consecutive newborns with pyarthrosis, 22 joints were involved; 4 (25%) infants had multifocal infections[27] (JD Nelson, personal communication, 1987). A migratory polyarthritis, which may precede localization in a single joint by several days, is particularly characteristic of gonococcal arthritis, as is an extremely high frequency of knee and ankle involvement.[88] A series from Malaysia emphasizes the frequency with which septic arthritis occurs within medical settings of newborn intensive care.[238] In this series, the knee, hip, and ankle were involved in 10 cases of septic arthritis, and 9 of the 10 cases were caused by MRSA, demonstrating the frequent occurrence of septic arthritis caused by nosocomial pathogens in premature infants in neonatal intensive care units.

The radiologic features, differential diagnosis, and therapy for septic arthritis are discussed under "Osteomyelitis." Studies of long-term evaluations are rare, precluding an accurate assessment of the prognosis for this condition.

OSTEOMYELITIS OF THE MAXILLA

Although most series of neonatal osteomyelitis have emphasized clinical features of infections of tubular bones, substantial literature is available concerning neonatal osteomyelitis of the maxilla as a distinct clinical entity. Early reports of neonatal osteomyelitis frequently focused exclusively on this entity, and the specific aspects of infection in the extremities have received serious attention only within the past 50 years. In terms of total numbers, maxillary osteomyelitis is a rare condition (there are fewer than 200 reported cases); yet in several surveys of neonatal bone infections, maxillary involvement was noted in approximately 25% of infants.[3,6,11,48,55,239] The far lower incidence in children[8,10] and adults[159] is probably explained by earlier recognition and treatment of sinusitis in these age groups and by the lack of predisposing factors unique to the newborn.

The causative organism is most frequently *S. aureus*,[240-242] although hemolytic streptococci have been isolated on rare occasions from drainage sites.[242] More than 85% of all maxillary infections in infants occur in the first 3 months of life; the incidence is highest during the second to fourth weeks.[241-244.]

In most cases, the predisposing cause remains obscure. Infants with sources of infection, such as skin abscesses or omphalitis, constitute a small minority.[242,243] It has been postulated that there is a relationship between breast abscess in the nursing mother and maxillary osteomyelitis[242,243,245]; however, it is unclear whether the maternal infection is a source or a result of the infant's condition.[246] The pathogenesis of bone infection after colonization of the infant by staphylococci is equally uncertain. In some cases, osteomyelitis is believed to result from extension from a contiguous focus of infection in the maxillary antrum. Alternatively, organisms may be blood-borne, establishing infection in the rich vascular plexus surrounding tooth buds.[244] Although the hematogenous route may be important in certain cases, particularly those involving the premaxilla,[240] this explanation is not compatible with the fact that mandibular osteomyelitis or associated metastatic involvement of other structures is uncommon.[242] Yet another theory is that trauma or abrasion of the gum overlying the first molar is the primary route of introduction of organisms.[243]

The clinical course of maxillary osteomyelitis begins with acute onset of fever and nonspecific systemic symptoms. Shortly thereafter, redness and swelling of the eyelid appear and are frequently accompanied by conjunctivitis with a purulent discharge. Thrombosis of nutrient vessels and increasing edema may cause a proptosis or chemosis of the affected eye. In most infants, an early and diffuse swelling and inflammation of the cheek may localize to form an abscess or draining fistula below the inner or outer canthus of the eye. This is nearly always followed or accompanied by a purulent unilateral nasal discharge that is increased by pressure on the abscess. The alveolar border of the superior maxilla on the affected side is swollen and soft, as is the adjacent hard palate. Within a few days, abscesses and draining fistulas may form in these areas.[247] Sepsis and death are frequent in untreated cases. In most infants, the illness pursues a relatively chronic course characterized by discharge of premature teeth or numerous small sequestra of necrotic bone through multiple palatal and alveolar sinuses that have formed. The entire course may evolve over several days in severe cases, or it may extend for several weeks in mild or partially treated cases.

Neonatal maxillary osteomyelitis is frequently confused with either orbital cellulitis or dacryocystitis.[13,243,248] The early edema and redness of the cheeks that accompany acute osteomyelitis constitute an important differentiating feature, which is not observed in orbital cellulitis and occurs only as a late sign in infection of the lacrimal sac. Neither of the latter conditions is associated with a unilateral purulent nasal discharge. The early onset, limited area of involvement, and Gram stain characteristic of ophthalmia neonatorum should be sufficient, in most cases, to permit diagnosis of this condition. CT can be helpful in assessing the extent of infection, as well as evaluating for possible complications such as cerebral abscess.[247]

Therapy for maxillary osteomyelitis should be directed toward early adequate drainage of the maxillary empyema and contiguous abscess and should include appropriate parenterally administered antibiotics. Because most infections are due to *S. aureus* and group A streptococci, systemic use of a penicillinase-resistant penicillin (or vancomycin) alone should be sufficient as initial therapy pending the results of bacterial cultures and sensitivity tests. The need for or desirability of instillation of antibiotics into the maxillary antrum is uncertain.

Before the advent of penicillin therapy, the mortality rate for maxillary osteomyelitis was high, ranging from 15% to 75% in various series.[242,243,245,249] Children who survived often had severe facial and dental deformities. Later studies[242,243,249] showed a mortality rate of closer to 5%, although sequelae such as stenosis of the lacrimal duct, ectropion, permanent loss of teeth, malocclusion, and facial hemiatrophy are still seen.[11,241-243] In many instances, these complications could have been prevented through early recognition of the nature of the illness and prompt institution of appropriate therapy.

REFERENCES

1. Craig WS. Care of the Newly Born Infant. Baltimore, Williams & Wilkins, 1962.
2. Boyes J, Bremner AD, Neligan GA. Haematogenous osteitis in the newborn. Lancet 1:544, 1957.
3. Dennison WM. Haematogenous osteitis in the newborn. Lancet 2:474, 1955.
4. Masse P. L'ostéomyelité du nouveau-né. Semaine Hôp Paris 34:2812, 1958.
5. Contzen H. Die sogennante Osteomyelitis des Neugeborenen. Dtsch Med Wochenschr 86:1221, 1961.
6. Clarke AM. Neonatal osteomyelitis: a disease different from osteomyelitis of older children. Med J Aust 1:237, 1958.
7. Hall JE, Silverstein EA. Acute hematogenous osteomyelitis. Pediatrics 31:1033, 1963.
8. Green M, Nyhan WL Jr, Fousek MD. Acute hematogenous osteomyelitis. Pediatrics 17:368, 1956.
9. Hung W, McGavisk DF. Acute hematogenous osteomyelitis: a report of 36 cases seen at Children's Hospital 1950 to 1958. Clin Proc Child Hosp 16:163, 1960.
10. Morse TS, Pryles CV. Infections of the bones and joints in children. N Engl J Med 262:846, 1960.
11. Fox L, Sprunt K. Neonatal osteomyelitis. Pediatrics 62:535, 1978.
12. Lim MO, Gresham EL, Franken EA Jr, et al. Osteomyelitis as a complication of umbilical artery catheterization. Am J Dis Child 131:142, 1977.
13. Bergdahl S, Ekengren K, Eriksson M. Neonatal hematogenous osteomyelitis: risk factors for long-term sequelae. J Pediatr Orthop 5:564, 1985.
14. Bamberger T, Gugler E. Die akute Osteomyelitis im Kindesalter. Schweiz Med Wochenschr 113:1219, 1983.
15. Bennet R, Eriksson M, Zetterström R. Increasing incidence of neonatal septicemia: causative organism and predisposing risk factors. Acta Paediatr Scand 70:207, 1981.
16. Mok PM, Reilly BJ, Ash JM. Osteomyelitis in the neonate with cerebral abscess. Radiology 145:677, 1982.
17. Dan M. Septic arthritis in young infants: Clinical and microbiologic correlations and therapeutic implications. Rev Infect Dis 6:147, 1984.
18. Barton LL, Dunkle LM, Habib FH. Septic arthritis in childhood: a 13-year review. Am J Dis Child 141:898, 1987.
19. Edwards MS, Baker CJ, Wagner ML, et al. An etiologic shift in infantile osteomyelitis: the emergence of the group B *Streptococcus*. J Pediatr 93:578, 1978.
20. Yousefzadeh DK, Jackson JH. Neonatal and infantile candidal arthritis with or without osteomyelitis: a clinical and radiographical review of 21 cases. Skeletal Radiol 5:77, 1980.
21. Pittard WB III, Thullen JD, Fanaroff AA. Neonatal septic arthritis. J Pediatr 88:621, 1976.
22. Brill PW, Winchester P, Krauss AN, et al. Osteomyelitis in a neonatal intensive care unit. Radiology 13:83, 1979.
23. Johnson DE, Thompson TR, Green TP, et al. Systemic candidiasis in very low-birth-weight infants (<1,500 grams). Pediatrics 73:138, 1984.
24. Turner RB, Donowitz LG, Hendley JO. Consequences of candidemia for pediatric patients. Am J Dis Child 139:178, 1985.
25. Goldmann DA, Durbin WA Jr, Freeman J. Nosocomial infections in a neonatal intensive care unit. J Infect Dis 144:449, 1981.
26. Townsend TR, Wenzel RP. Nosocomial bloodstream infections in a newborn intensive care unit. Am J Epidemiol 114:73, 1981.
27. Jackson MA, Nelson JD. Etiology and medical management of acute suppurative bone and joint infections in pediatric patients. J Pediatr Orthop 2:313, 1982.
28. Hensey JO, Hart CA, Cooke RWI. Serious infections in a neonatal intensive care unit: a two year survey. J Hyg 95:289, 1985.
29. Lejeune C, Maudiev P, Robin M, et al. Fréquence des infections bactériennes néonatales dans les unites de réanimation et/ou néonatologie. Pediatrie 41:95, 1986.
30. Coto-Cotallo GD, Solis-Sanchez G, Crespo-Hernandez M, et al. Osteomielitis neonatal: estudio de una serie de 35 casos. Ann Esp Pediatr 33:429, 1990.
31. Asmar BI. Osteomyelitis in the neonate. Infect Dis Clin North Am 6:117, 1992.
32. Knudsen CJ, Hoffman EB. Neonatal osteomyelitis. J Bone Joint Surg Br 72:846, 1990.
33. Williamson JB, Galasko CSB, Robinson MJ. Outcome after acute osteomyelitis in preterm infants. Arch Dis Child 65:1060, 1990.
34. Baitch A. Recent observations of acute suppurative arthritis. Clin Orthop 22:157, 1962.
35. Obletz BE. Suppurative arthritis of the hip joint in premature infants. Clin Orthop 22:27, 1962.
36. Ross DW. Acute suppurative arthritis of the hip in premature infants. JAMA 156:303, 1954.
37. Thomson J, Lewis IC. Osteomyelitis in the newborn. Arch Dis Child 25:273, 1950.
38. Weissberg ED, Smith AL, Smith DH. Clinical features of neonatal osteomyelitis. Pediatrics 53:505, 1974.
39. Kumari S, Bhargava SK, Baijal VN, et al. Neonatal osteomyelitis: a clinical and follow-up study. Indian J Pediatr 15:393, 1978.
40. Deshpande PG, Wagle SU, Mehta SD, et al. Neonatal osteomyelitis and septic arthritis. Indian J Pediatr 27:453, 1990.
41. Brill PW, Winchester P, Krauss AN, et al. Osteomyelitis in a neonatal intensive care unit. Radiology 131:83, 1979.
42. Wong M, Isaacs D, Howman-Giles R, Uren R. Clinical and diagnostic features of osteomyelitis in the first three months of life. Pediatr Infect Dis 14:1047, 1995.
43. Saarinen M, Takala AK, Koskenniemi E, et al. Spectrum of 2,836 cases of invasive bacterial or fungal infections in children: results of prospective nationwide five-year surveillance in Finland. Clin Infect Dis 21:1134, 1995.
44. Saez-Llorens X, Velarde J, Canton C. Pediatric osteomyelitis in Panama. Clin Infect Dis 19:323, 1994.
45. Freedman RM, Ingram DL, Gross I, et al. A half century of neonatal sepsis at Yale: 1928 to 1978. Am J Dis Child 135:140, 1981.
46. Dillehunt RB. Osteomyelitis in infants. Surg Gynecol Obstet 61:96, 1935.
47. Dunham EC. Septicemia in the newborn. Am J Dis Child 45:230, 1933.

48. Green WT, Shannon JG. Osteomyelitis of infants: a disease different from osteomyelitis of older children. Arch Surg 32:462, 1936.
49 Aractingi T-R. Étude de 32 cas d'ostéomyélité du nouveauné. Rev Chir Orthop 47:50, 1961.
50. Dennison WM, MacPherson DA. Haematogenous osteitis of infancy. Arch Dis Child 27:375, 1952.
51. DeWet IS. Acute osteomyelitis and suppurative arthritis of infants. S Afr Med J 28:81, 1954.
52. Hutter CG. New concepts of osteomyelitis in the newborn infant. J Pediatr 32:522, 1948.
53. Lindell L, Parkkulainen KV. Osteitis in infancy and early childhood: with special reference to neonatal osteitis. Ann Paediatr Fenn 6:34, 1960.
54. Kienitz M, Schulte M. Problematik bakterieller Infectionen des Frühund Neuegeborenen. Munch Med Wochenschr 109:70, 1967.
55. Wolman G. Acute osteomyelitis in infancy. Acta Paediatr Scand 45:595, 1956.
56. Blanche DW. Osteomyelitis in infants. J Bone Joint Surg Am 34:71, 1952.
57. Howard JB, McCracken GH Jr. The spectrum of group B streptococcal infections in infancy. Am J Dis Child 128:815, 1974.
58. Memon IA, Jacobs NM, Yeh TF, et al. Group B streptococcal osteomyelitis and septic arthritis: its occurrence in infants less than 2 months old. Am J Dis Child 133:921, 1979.
59. Omene JA, Odita JC. Clinical and radiological features of neonatal septic arthritis. Trop Geogr Med 31:207, 1979.
60. Garcia Pena BM, Harper MB, Fleisher GR. Occult bacteremia with group B streptococci in an outpatient setting. Pediatrics 102:67, 1998.
61. Choma TJ, Davlin LB, Wagner JS. Iliac osteomyelitis in the newborn presenting as nonspecific musculoskeletal sepsis. Orthopedics 17:632, 1994.
62. Barton LL, Villar RG, Rice SA. Neonatal group B streptococcal vertebral osteomyelitis. Pediatrics 98:459, 1996.
63. Speer CP, Hauptmann D, Stubbe P, et al. Neonatal septicemia and meningitis in Göttingen, West Germany. Pediatr Infect Dis 4:36, 1985.
64. Karpuch J, Goldberg M, Kohelet D. Neonatal bacteremia: a 4-year prospective study. Isr J Med Sci 19:963, 1983.
65. Lequier L, Robinson J, Vaudry W. Sternotomy infection with *Mycoplasma hominis* in a neonate. Pediatr Infect Dis J 14:1010, 1995.
66. Gjuric G, Prislin-Muskic M, Nikolic E, Zurga B. *Ureaplasma urealyticum* osteomyelitis in a very low birth weight infant. Perinat Med 22:79, 1994.
67. Scott JES. Intestinal obstruction in the newborn associated with peritonitis. Arch Dis Child 38:120, 1963.
68. Seeler RA, Hahn K. Jaundice in urinary tract infections in infancy. Am J Dis Child 118:553, 1969.
69. Bayer AS, Chow AW, Louie JS, et al. Gram-negative bacillary septic arthritis: clinical, radiographic, therapeutic, and prognostic features. Semin Arthritis Rheum 7:123, 1977.
70. Peters W, Irving J, Letts M. Long-term effects of neonatal bone and joint infection on adjacent growth plates. J Pediatr Orthop 12:806, 1992.
71. Levy HL, O'Connor JF, Ingall D. Neonatal osteomyelitis due to *Proteus mirabilis.* JAMA 202:582, 1967.
72. Müller WD, Urban C, Haidvogel M, et al. Septische Arthritis und Osteomyelitis als Komplikation neonataler Intensivpflege. Paediatr Paedol 14:469, 1979.
73. Bogdanovich A. Neonatal arthritis due to *Proteus vulgaris.* Arch Dis Child 23:65, 1948.
74. Omene JA, Odita JC, Okolo AA. Neonatal osteomyelitis in Nigerian infants. Pediatr Radiol 14:318, 1984.
75. Choi IH, Pizzutillo PD, Bowen JR, et al. Sequelae and reconstruction after septic arthritis of the hip in infants. J Bone Joint Surg Am 72:1150, 1990.
76. Berant M, Kahana D. *Klebsiella* osteomyelitis in a newborn. Am J Dis Child 118:634, 1969.
77. White AA, Crelin ES, McIntosh S. Septic arthritis of the hip joint secondary to umbilical artery catheterization associated with transient femoral and sciatic neuropathy. Clin Orthop 100:190, 1974.
78. Nathanson I, Giacoia GP. *Klebsiella* osteoarthritis in prematurity: complication of umbilical artery catheterization. N Y State J Med 79:2077, 1979.
79. Voss HV, Göbel U, Kemperdick H, et al. *Enterobacter*-Osteomyelitis bei zwei Säuglingen. Klin Paediatr 187:465, 1975.
80. Gordon SL, Maisels MJ, Robbins WJ. Multiple joint infections with *Enterobacter cloacae.* Clin Orthop 125:136, 1977.
81. Levinsky RJ. Two children with *Pseudomonas* osteomyelitis: the paucity of systemic symptoms may lead to delay in diagnosis. Clin Pediatr 14:288, 1975.
82. Gajzago D, Gottche O. *Salmonella suipestifer* infections in childhood. Am J Dis Child 63:15, 1942.
83. Konzert W. Über ein Salmonella-Osteomyelitis im Rahmen einer *Salmonella-typhimurium* Epidemia auf einer Neugeborenen Station. Wien Klin Wochenschr 81:713, 1969.
84. Tur AJ, Gartoch OO. Ein Fall von Erkrankung eines frühgeborenen Kindes im ersten Lebensmonate an multiplier Arthritis durch den Bacillus suipestifer. Z Kinderheilkd 56:696, 1934.
85. Adeyokunnu AA, Hendrickse RG. *Salmonella* osteomyelitis in childhood: a report of 63 cases seen in Nigerian children of whom 57 had sickle cell anemia. Arch Dis Child 55:175, 1980.
86. Steinwender G, Schimpl G, Sixl B, Wenzl HH. Gut-derived bone infection in the neonatal rat. Pediatr Res 50:767, 2001.
87. Nair S, Schoeneman MJ. Septic arthritis in an infant with vesicoureteral reflux and urinary tract infection. Pediatrics 111:e195, 2003.
88. Kohen DP. Neonatal gonococcal arthritis: three cases and review of the literature. Pediatrics 53:436, 1974.
89. Gregory JE, Chison JL, Meadows AT. Short case report: gonococcal arthritis in an infant. Br J Vener Dis 48:306, 1972.
90. Cooperman MB. End results of gonorrheal arthritis: a review of seventy cases. Am J Surg 5:241, 1928.
91. Nabarro D. Congenital Syphilis. London, Edward Arnold, 1954.
92. Zenker PN, Berman SM. Congenital syphilis: trends and recommendations for evaluation and management. Pediatr Infect Dis J 10:516, 1991.
93. Brion LP, Manuli M, Rai B, et al. Long-bone radiographic abnormalities as a sign of active congenital syphilis in asymptomatic newborns. Pediatrics 88:1037, 1991.
94. Hughesdon MR. Congenital tuberculosis. Arch Dis Child 21:121, 1946.
95. Mallet R, Ribierre M, Labrune B, et al. Diffuse bony tuberculosis in the newborn (spina ventosa generalisata). Sem Hôp Paris 44:36, 1968.
96. Nelson DL, Hable KA, Matsen JM. *Proteus mirabilis* osteomyelitis in two neonates following needle puncture. Am J Dis Child 125:109, 1973.
97. Asnes RS, Arendar GM. Septic arthritis of the hip: a complication of femoral venipuncture. Pediatrics 38:837, 1966.
98. Chacha PB. Suppurative arthritis of the hip joint in infancy: a persistent diagnostic problem and possible complication of femoral venipuncture. J Bone Joint Surg Am 53:538, 1971.
99. Overturf GD, Balfour G. Osteomyelitis and sepsis: severe complications of fetal monitoring. Pediatrics 55:244, 1975.
100. Plavidal FJ, Werch A. Fetal scalp abscess secondary to intrauterine monitoring. Am J Obstet Gynecol 125:65, 1976.
101. Brook I. Osteomyelitis and bacteremia caused by *Bacteroides fragilis*: a complication of fetal monitoring. Clin Pediatr 19:639, 1980.
102. McGregor JA, McFarren T. Neonatal cranial osteomyelitis: a complication of fetal monitoring. Obstet Gynecol 73:490, 1989.
103. Puczynski MS, Dvonch VM, Menendez CE, et al. Osteomyelitis of the great toe secondary to phlebotomy. Clin Orthop 190:239, 1984.
104. Lilien LD, Harris VJ, Ramamurthy RS, et al. Neonatal osteomyelitis of the calcaneus: complication of heel puncture. J Pediatr 88:478, 1976.
105. Myers MG, McMahon BJ, Koontz FP. Neonatal calcaneous osteomyelitis related to contaminated mineral oil. Clin Microbiol 6:543, 1977.
106. Blumenfeld TA, Turi GK, Blanc WA. Recommended site and depth of newborn heel skin punctures based on anatomical measurements and histopathology. Lancet 1:230, 1979.
107. Borris LC, Helleland H. Growth disturbance of the hind part of the foot following osteomyelitis of the calcaneus in the newborn: a report of two cases. J Bone Joint Surg Am 68:302, 1986.
108. Fernandez-Fanjul JL, Lopez-Sastre J, Coto-Cotallo D, et al. Osteomyelitis des Calcaneus beim Neugeborenen als Folge diagnostischer Fersenpunktionen. Monatsschr Kinderheilkd 127:515, 1979.
109. Bergman I, Wald ER, Meyer JD, et al. Epidural abscess and vertebral osteomyelitis following serial lumbar punctures. Pediatrics 72:476, 1983.
110. Edwards MS, Baker CJ. Median sternotomy wound infections in children. Pediatr Infect Dis 2:105, 1983.
111. Valerio PH. Osteomyelitis as a complication of perinatal fracture of the clavicle. Eur J Pediatr 154:497, 1995.
112. Mohon RT, Mehalic TF, Grimes CK, et al. Infected cephalohematoma and neonatal osteomyelitis of the skull. Pediatr Infect Dis 5:253, 1986.
113. Nightingale LM, Eaton CB, Fruehan AE, et al. Cephalohematoma complicated by osteomyelitis presumed due to *Gardnerella vaginalis.* JAMA 256:1936, 1986.

114. Plavidal FJ, Werch A. Fetal scalp abscess secondary to intrauterine monitoring. Am J Obstet Gynecol 125:65, 1976.
115. Lee PYC. Case report: infected cephalohematoma and neonatal osteomyelitis. J Infect 21:191, 1990.
116. McCarthy D, Walker AHC, Matthews S. Scalp abscesses in the newborn: a discussion of their causation. J Obstet Gynacol Br Emp 59:37, 1952.
117. Ladewig W. Über eine intrauterin entstandene umschriebene Osteomyelitis des Schädeldaches. Virchows Arch Pathol Anat 289:395, 1933.
118. Trueta J. Three types of acute haematogenous osteomyelitis. J Bone Joint Surg Br 41:671, 1959.
119. Todd RM. Septicaemia of the newborn: a clinical study of fifteen cases. Arch Dis Child 23:102, 1948.
120. Svirsky-Fein S, Langer L, Milbauer B, et al. Neonatal osteomyelitis caused by *Candida tropicalis:* report of two cases and review of the literature. J Bone Joint Surg Am 61:455, 1979.
121. Baley JE, Kliegman RM, Fanaroff AA. Disseminated fungal infections in very low-birth-weight infants: clinical manifestations and epidemiology. Pediatrics 73:144, 1984.
122. Randel SN, Tsang BHL, Wung J-T, et al. Experience with percutaneous indwelling peripheral arterial catheterization in neonates. Am J Dis Child 141:848, 1987.
123. Knudsen FU, Petersen S. Neonatal septic osteoarthritis due to umbilical artery catheterisation. Acta Paediatr Scand 66:225, 1977.
124. Lim MO, Gresham EL, Franken EA Jr, et al. Osteomyelitis as a complication of umbilical artery catheterization. Am J Dis Child 131:142, 1977.
125. Rhodes PG, Hall RT, Burry VF, et al. Sepsis and osteomyelitis due to *Staphylococcus aureus* phage type 94 in a neonatal intensive care unit. J Pediatr 88:1063, 1976.
126. deLorimier AA, Haskin D, Massie FS. Mediastinal mass caused by vertebral osteomyelitis. Am J Dis Child 111:639, 1966.
127. Qureshi ME. Osteomyelitis after exchange transfusion. BMJ 1:28, 1971.
128. Simmons PB, Harris LE, Bianco AJ. Complications of exchange transfusion: report of two cases of septic arthritis and osteomyelitis. Mayo Clin Proc 48:190, 1973.
129. Ish-Horowicz MR, McIntyre P, Nade S. Bone and joint infections caused by multiply resistant *Staphylococcus aureus* in a neonatal intensive care unit. Pediatr Infect Dis J 11:82, 1992.
130. Betke K, Richarz H. Nabelsepsis mit Pyelphlebitis, multiple Leberabscessen, Lungenabscessen, und Osteomyelitis. Ausgang in Heilung. Monatschr Kinderheilkd 105:70, 1957.
131. Fraser J. Discussion on acute osteomyelitis. BMJ 2:605, 1924.
132. Lindblad B, Ekingren K, Aurelius G. The prognosis of acute hematogenous osteomyelitis and its complications during early infancy after the advent of antibiotics. Acta Paediatr Scand 54:24, 1965.
133. Chung SMK. The arterial supply of the developing proximal end of the human femur. J Bone Joint Surg Am 58:961, 1976.
134. Ogden JA. Pediatric osteomyelitis and septic arthritis: the pathology of neonatal disease. Yale J Biol Med 52:423, 1979.
135. Cass JM. *Staphylococcus aureus* infection of the long bones in the newly born. Arch Dis Child 15:55, 1940.
136. Stone S. Osteomyelitis of the long bones in the newborn. Am J Dis Child 64:680, 1942.
137. Ingelrans P, Fontaine G, Lacheretz M, et al. Les ostéoarthrites du nouveau-né et du nourrison: particulariteés étiologiques, diagnostiques et thérapeutiques: à propos de 35 observations. Lille Med 13:390, 1968.
138. Nicholson JT. Pyogenic arthritis with pathologic dislocation of the hip in infants. JAMA 141:862, 1949.
139. Roberts PH. Disturbed epiphyseal growth at the knee after osteomyelitis in infancy. J Bone Joint Surg Br 52:692, 1970.
140. Curtis PH, Klein L. Destruction of articular cartilage in septic arthritis: I. In vitro studies. J Bone Joint Surg Am 45:797, 1963.
141. Curtis PH, Klein L. Destruction of articular cartilage in septic arthritis: II. In vivo studies. J Bone Joint Surg Am 47:1595, 1965.
142. Obletz BE. Acute suppurative arthritis of the hip in the neonatal period. J Bone Joint Surg Am 42:23, 1960.
143. Glassberg GB, Ozonoff MB. Arthrographic findings in septic arthritis of the hip in infants. Radiology 128:151, 1978.
144. Kaye JJ, Winchester PH, Freiberger RH. Neonatal septic "dislocation" of the hip: true dislocation or pathological epiphyseal separation? Radiology 114:671, 1975.
145. Greengard J. Acute hematogenous osteomyelitis in infancy. Med Clin North Am 30:135, 1946.
146. Chung SMK, Pollis RE. Diagnostic pitfalls in septic arthritis of the hip in infants and children. Clin Pediatr 14:758, 1975.
147. Bressler EL, Conway JJ, Weiss SC. Neonatal osteomyelitis examined by bone scintigraphy. Radiology 152:685, 1984.
148. Clay SA. Osteomyelitis as a cause of brachial plexus neuropathy. Am J Dis Child 136:1054, 1982.
149. Young RSK, Hawkes DL. Pseudopseudoparalysis. Letter to the editor. Am J Dis Child 137:504, 1983.
150. Isaacs D, Bower BD, Moxon ER. Neonatal osteomyelitis presenting as nerve palsy. BMJ 1:1071, 1986.
151. Obando I, Martin E, Alvarez-Aldeau J, et al. Group B *Streptococcus* pelvic osteomyelitis presenting as footdrop in a newborn infant. Pediatr Infect Dis J 10:703, 1991.
152. Lai TK, Hingston J, Scheifele D. Streptococcal neonatal osteomyelitis. Am J Dis Child 134:711, 1980.
153. Ancona RJ, McAuliffe J, Thompson TR, et al. Group B streptococcal sepsis with osteomyelitis and arthritis: its occurrence with acute heart failure. Am J Dis Child 133:919, 1979.
154. McCook TA, Felman AH, Ayoub E. Streptococcal skeletal infections: observations in four infants. AJR Am J Roentgenol 130:465, 1978.
155. Chilton SJ, Aftimos SF, White PW. Diffuse skeletal involvement of streptococcal osteomyelitis in a neonate. Radiology 134:390, 1980.
156. Broughton RA, Edwards MS, Haffar A, et al. Unusual manifestations of neonatal group B streptococcal osteomyelitis. Pediatr Infect Dis 1:410, 1982.
157. Einstein RAJ, Thomas CG Jr. Osteomyelitis in infants. AJR Am J Roentgenol 55:299, 1946.
158. Stack JK, Newman W. Neonatal osteomyelitis. Q Bull Northwestern Univ Med Sch 27:69, 1953.
159. Waldvogel FA, Medoff G, Swartz MN. Osteomyelitis. Clinical Features, Therapeutic Considerations, and Unusual Aspects. Springfield, Ill, Charles C Thomas, 1971.
160. Dich VQ, Nelson JD, Haltalin KC. Osteomyelitis in infants and children: a review of 163 cases. Am J Dis Child 129:1273, 1975.
161. Samilson RL, Bersani FA, Watkins MB. Acute suppurative arthritis in infants and children. Pediatrics 21:798, 1958.
162. Hallel T, Salvati EA. Septic arthritis of the hip in infancy: end result study. Clin Orthop 132:115, 1978.
163. Bennett OM, Namyak SS. Acute septic arthritis of the hip joint in infancy and childhood. Clin Orthop 281:123, 1992.
164. Ekengren K, Bergdahl S, Eriksson M. Neonatal osteomyelitis: radiographic findings and prognosis in relation to site of involvement. Acta Radiol Diagn 23:305, 1982.
165. Mallet JF, Rigault P, Padovani JP, et al. Les cyphoses par spondylodiscite grave du nourrisson et du jeune enfant. Rev Chir Orthop 70:63, 1984.
166. Ammari LK, Offit PA, Campbell AB. Unusual presentation of group B *Streptococcus* osteomyelitis. Pediatr Infect Dis J 11:1066, 1992.
167. Altman N, Harwood-Nash DC, Fitz CR, et al. Evaluation of the infant spine by direct sagittal computed tomography. AJNR Am J Neuroradiol 6:65, 1985.
168. Bolivar R, Kohl S, Pickering LK. Vertebral osteomyelitis in children: report of 4 cases. Pediatrics 62:549, 1978.
169. Bode H, Kunzer W. Dornfortsatzosteomyelitis der Brustwirbel 10 und 11 bei einem Neugeborenen. Klin Paediatr 197:65, 1985.
170. McCook TA, Felman AH, Ayoub E. Streptococcal skeletal infections: observations in four infections. AJR Am J Roentgenol 130:465, 1978.
171. Ein SH, Shandling B, Humphreys R, et al. Osteomyelitis of the cervical spine presenting as a neurenteric cyst. J Pediatr Surg 23:779, 1988.
172. Halbstein BM. Bone regeneration in infantile osteomyelitis: report of a case with 14-year follow-up. J Bone Joint Surg Am 49:149, 1967.
173. Miller B. Regeneration of the lateral femoral condyle after osteomyelitis in infancy. Clin Orthop 65:163, 1969.
174. Lloyd-Roberts GC. Suppurative arthritis of infancy: some observations upon prognosis and management. J Bone Joint Surg Br 42:706, 1960.
175. Singson RD, Berdon WE, Feldman F, et al. "Missing" femoral condyle: an unusual sequela to neonatal osteomyelitis and septic arthritis. Radiology 161:359, 1986.
176. Potter CMC. Osteomyelitis in the newborn. J Bone Joint Surg Br 36:578, 1954.
177. Troger J, Eissner D, Otte G, et al. Diagnose und Differentialdiagnose der akuten hämatogenen Osteomyelitis des Säuglings. Radiologe 19:99, 1979.
178. Vallcanera A, Moreno-Flores A, Gomez J, Cortina H. Osteochondroma post osteomyelitis. Pediatr Radiol 26:680, 1996.

179. Jaramillo D, Treves ST, Kasser JR, et al. Osteomyelitis and septic arthritis in children. Appropriate use of imaging to guide treatement. Am J Radiol 165:399, 1995.
180. Volberg FM, Sumner TE, Abramson JS, et al. Unreliability of radiographic diagnosis of septic hip in children. Pediatrics 74:118, 1984.
181. Perkins MD, Edwards KM, Heller RM, et al. Neonatal group B streptococcal osteomyelitis and suppurative arthritis: outpatient therapy. Clin Pediatr 28:229, 1989.
182. Schauwecker DS, Braunstein EM, Wheat LJ. Diagnostic imaging of osteomyelitis. Infect Dis Clin North Am 4:441, 1990.
183. Moore SG, Bisset GS III, Siegel MJ, et al. Pediatric musculoskeletal MR imaging. Radiology 179:345, 1991.
184. Harris VJ, Meeks W. The frequency of radiolucencies underlying cephalohematomas. Pediatr Radiol 129:391, 1978.
185. Einhorn M, Howard DB, Dagan R. The use of ultrasound in the diagnosis and management of childhood acute hematogenous osteomyelitis. Thirty-First Interscience Conference on Antimicrobial Agents and Chemotherapy, Anaheim, Calif, October 1992 (abstract Pub 77).
186. Williamson SL, Seibert JJ, Glasier CM, et al. Ultrasound in advanced pediatric osteomyelitis: a report of 5 cases. Pediatr Radiol 21:288, 1991.
187. Abiri MM, Kirpekar M, Ablow RC. Osteomyelitis: detection with US. Radiology 172:509, 1989.
188. Zeiger MM, Dorr U, Schulz RD. Ultrasonography of hip joint effusions. Skeletal Radiol 16:607, 1987.
189. Velkes S, Ganel A, Chechick A. Letter to the editor. Clin Orthop 260:309, 1990.
190. Rubin LP, Wallach MT, Wood BP. Radiological case of the month. Arch Pediatr Adolesc Med 150:217, 1996.
191. Riebel TW, Nasir R, Nazarenko O. The value of sonography in the detection of osteomyelitis. Pediatr Radiol 26:291, 1996.
192. Wright NB, Abbott GT, Carty HML. Ultrasound in children with osteomyelitis. Clin Radiol 50:623, 1995.
193. Harcke HT Jr. Bone imaging in infants and children: a review. J Nucl Med 19:324, 1978.
194. Ash JM, Gilday DL. The futility of bone scanning neonatal osteomyelitis: concise communication. J Nucl Med 21:417, 1980.
195. Gilday DL, Paul DJ. Diagnosis of osteomyelitis in children by combined blood pool and bone imaging. Radiology 117:331, 1975.
196. Canale ST, Harkness RM, Thomas PA, et al. Does aspiration of bones and joints affect results of later bone scanning? J Pediatr Orthop 5:23, 1985.
197. Traughber PD, Manaster BJ, Murphy K, et al. Negative bone scans of joints after aspiration or arthrography: experimental studies. AJR Am J Roentgenol 146:87, 1986.
198. Herndon WA, Alexieva BT, Schwindt ML, et al. Nuclear imaging for musculoskeletal infections in children. J Pediatr Orthop 5:343, 1985.
199. Lewin JS, Rosenfield NS, Hoffer PB, et al. Acute osteomyelitis in children: combined Tc-99m and Ga-67 imaging. Radiology 158:795, 1986.
200. Berkowitz ID, Wenzel W. "Normal" technetium bone scans in patients with acute osteomyelitis. Am J Dis Child 134:828, 1980.
201. Handmaker H, Giammona ST. Improved early diagnosis of acute inflammatory skeletal-articular diseases in children: a two-radiopharmaceutical approach. Pediatrics 73:661, 1984.
202. Melson GL, McDaniel RC, Southern PM, et al. In vitro effects of iodinated arthrographic contrast media on bacterial growth. Radiology 112:593, 1974.
203. Cole WG, Dalziel RE, Leitl S. Treatment of acute osteomyelitis in childhood. J Bone Joint Surg Br 64:218, 1982.
204. Rasool MN, Govender S. The skeletal manifestations of congenital syphilis: a review of 197 cases. J Bone Joint Surg Br 71:752, 1989.
205. Hiva SK, Ganapati JB, Patel JB. Early congenital syphilis: clinico-radiologic features in 202 patients. Sex Transm Dis 12:177, 1985.
206. McLean S. The roentgenographic and pathologic aspects of congenital osseous syphilis. Am J Dis Child 41:130, 363, 607, 887, 1128, 1411, 1931.
207. Ewerbeck V, Bolkenius M, Braun A, et al. Knochentumoren und tumorähnliche Veränderungen im Neugeborenen-und Säuglingsalter. Z Orthop 123:918, 1985.
208. Meyers S, Lonon W, Shannon, K. Suppurative bursitis in early childhood. Pediatr Infect Dis 3:156, 1984.
209. Brian MJ, O'Ryan M, Waagner D. Prepatellar bursitis in an infant caused by group B *Streptococcus*. Pediatr Infect Dis J 11:502, 1992.
210. Keller MA, Sellers BB Jr, Melish ME, et al. Systemic candidiasis in infants: a case presentation and literature review. Am J Dis Child 131:1260, 1977.
211. Reiser VM, Rupp N, Färber D. Röntgenologische Befunde bei der septischen Candida-Arthritis. Rofo 129:335, 1978.
212. Businco L, Iannaccone G, Del Principe D, et al. Disseminated arthritis and osteitis by *Candida albicans* in a two month old infant receiving parenteral nutrition. Acta Paediatr Scand 66:393, 1977.
213. Rudolph AJ, Singleton EB, Rosenberg HS, et al. Osseous manifestations of the congenital rubella syndrome. Am J Dis Child 110:428, 1965.
214. Merten DF, Gooding CA. Skeletal manifestations of congenital cytomegalic inclusion disease. Radiology 95:333, 1970.
215. Jenson HB, Robert MF. Congenital cytomegalovirus infection with osteolytic lesions: use of DNA hybridization in diagnosis. Clin Pediatr 26:448, 1987.
216. Chalhub EG, Baenziger J, Feigen RD, et al. Congenital herpes simplex type II infection with extensive hepatic calcification, bone lesions and cataracts: complete postmortem examination. Dev Med Child Neurol 19:527, 1977.
217. Madsen ET. Fractures of the extremities in the newborn. Acta Obstet Gynecol Scand 34:41, 1955.
218. Caffey J. Pediatric X-ray Diagnosis, 6th ed. Chicago, Year Book Medical Publishers, 1972.
219. Park H-M, Kernek CB, Robb JA. Early scintigraphic findings of occult femoral and tibial fractures in infants. Clin Nucl Med 13:271, 1988.
220. Marshall GS, Edwards KM, Wadlington WB. Sporadic congenital Caffey's disease. Clin Pediatr 26:177, 1987.
221. Ravenel SD. Cellulitis from extravasation of calcium gluconate simulating osteomyelitis. Am J Dis Child 137:402, 1983.
222. Ringel RE, Haney PJ, Brenner JI, et al. Periosteal changes secondary to prostaglandin administration. J Pediatr 103:251, 1983.
223. Ditkowsky SP, Goldman A, Barnett H, et al. Normal periosteal reactions and associated soft-tissue findings. Clin Pediatr 9:515, 1970.
224. Nelson JD. Follow up: the bacterial etiology and antibiotic management of septic arthritis in infants and children. Pediatrics 50:437, 1972.
225. Cooper GI, Hopkins CC. Rapid diagnosis of intravascular catheter-associated infection by direct Gram staining of catheter segments. N Engl J Med 312:1142, 1985.
226. Schauf V, Deveikis A, Riff L, et al. Antibiotic-killing kinetics of group B streptococci. J Pediatr 89:194, 1976.
227. Chambers HF, Hackbarth CJ, Drake TA, et al. Endocarditis due to methicillin-resistant *Staphylococcus aureus* in rabbits: expression of resistance to β-lactam antibiotics in vivo and in vitro. J Infect Dis 149:894, 1984.
228. Sann L, Bienvenu F, Bienvenu J, et al. Evolution of serum prealbumin, C-reactive protein, and orosomucoid in neonates with bacterial infection. J Pediatr 105:977, 1984.
229. Philip AGS. Acute-phase proteins in neonatal infection. J Pediatr 105:940, 1984.
230. Fajardo JE, Bass JW, Lugo EJ, et al. Oral dicloxacillin for the treatment of neonatal osteomyelitis. Letter to the editor. Am J Dis Child 138:991, 1984.
231. Schwartz GJ, Hegyi T, Spitzer A. Subtherapeutic dicloxacillin levels in a neonate: possible mechanisms. J Pediatr 89:310, 1976.
232. Nelson JD. Options for outpatient management of serious infections. Pediatr Infect Dis J 11:175, 1992.
233. Sudela KD. Nursing aspects of pediatric home infusion therapy for the treatment of serious infections. Semin Pediatr Infect Dis 1:306, 1990.
234. Dunkle LM. Towards optimum management of serious focal infections: the model of suppurative arthritis. Pediatr Infect Dis J 8:195, 1989.
235. Pittard WB III, Thullen JD, Fanaroff AA. Neonatal septic arthritis. J Pediatr 88:621, 1976.
236. Howard PJ. Sepsis in normal and premature infants with localization in the hip joint. Pediatrics 20:279, 1957.
237. Borella L, Goobar JE, Summitt RL, et al. Septic arthritis in childhood. J Pediatr 62:742, 1963.
238. Halder D, Seng QB, Malik AS, Choo KE. Neonatal septic arthritis. Southeast Asian J Trop Med Public Health 27:600, 1996.
239. Gilmour WN. Acute hematogenous osteomyelitis. J Bone Joint Surg Br 44:841, 1962.
240. Allibone EC, Mills CP. Osteomyelitis of the premaxilla. Arch Dis Child 36:562, 1961.
241. Boete G. Zur Frage der Spätschäden nach Kieferosteomyelitis von Säuglingen und Kleinkindern. Arch Klin Exp Ohren Nasen Kehlkopfheilkd 187:674, 1966.
242. Cavanagh F. Osteomyelitis of the superior maxilla in infants: a report on 24 personally treated cases. BMJ 1:468, 1960.
243. McCash CR, Rowe NL. Acute osteomyelitis of the maxilla in infancy. J Bone Joint Surg Br 35:22, 1953.

244. Wilensky AO. The pathogenesis and treatment of acute osteomyelitis of the jaws in nurslings and infants. Am J Dis Child 43:431, 1932.
245. Bass MH. Acute osteomyelitis of the superior maxilla in young infants. Am J Dis Child 35:65, 1928.
246. Webb JF. Newborn infants and breast abscesses of staphylococcal origin. Can Med Assoc J 70:382, 1954.
247. Wong SK, Wilhelmus KR. Infantile maxillary osteomyelitis. J Pediatr Ophthalmol Strabismus 23:153, 1986.
248. Burnard ED. Proptosis as the first sign of orbital sepsis in the newborn. Br J Ophthalmol 43:9, 1959.
249. Hahlbrock KH. Über die Oberkieferosteomyelitis des Säuglings. Klin Monatsbl Augenheilkd 145:744, 1964.

Chapter 9

BACTERIAL INFECTIONS OF THE URINARY TRACT

Sarah S. Long • Jerome O. Klein

In 1918, Helmholz recognized the cryptogenic nature and underdiagnosis of urinary tract infection (UTI) in the newborn.[1] His observations still hold true today. There are no specific signs of UTI in the newborn; the clinical presentation can vary, ranging from fever and other signs of septicemia to minimal changes such as alteration in feeding habits or poor gain in weight, or the infant may be without signs. The diagnosis of UTI in the neonate is made only by the examination and culture of a properly obtained specimen of urine.

The reported incidence, clinical manifestations, and prognosis of UTI in neonates have varied significantly. There are at least two reasons for discrepant results obtained in studies of UTI: different criteria have been used to define UTI, and infants with different characteristics have been studied. Before 1960, clean-voided specimens were used almost exclusively for examination and culture of urine. It is now clear that contamination is frequent when this method is used; Schlager and co-workers observed that 16 cultures of urine obtained by bag collection from 98 healthy newborns yielded greater than 10^4 colonies per mL of urine, with organisms that were found also on periurethral skin.[2] The only reliable methods for obtaining urine for bacteriologic study are percutaneous aspiration and urethral catheterization of bladder urine.

In the neonate, bacterial infections of the kidney and urinary tract usually are acquired at or after delivery. Fungal infections develop as opportunistic infections complicating a prolonged nursery stay in infants with risk factors such as prematurity and use of intravascular catheters, parenteral alimentation, and broad-spectrum antibiotics, or after prolonged or intermittent catheterization of the urinary tract.[3] Viral infections, including rubella, herpes simplex, and cytomegalovirus infections, are responsible for in utero infection, although the organisms can be excreted in the urine for months after birth. Bacterial infections of the urinary tract (other than those related to *Neisseria gonorrhoeae*, *Staphylococcus aureus*, and group B streptococci) are reviewed here. For information about infection and disease of the kidney and urinary tract caused by other microorganisms, the reader is referred to the respective chapters on toxoplasmosis, rubella, cytomegalovirus, herpes simplex, syphilis, the mycoplasmas, *Candida*, group B streptococci, gonorrhea, staphylococcal infection, and neonatal diarrhea (*Salmonella*).

EPIDEMIOLOGY

The incidence of UTI in infants in the first month of life varies, ranging from 0.1% to 1% in all infants,[4-10] and may be as high as 10% in low-birth-weight infants[11] and 12% to 25% in infants of very low birth weight evaluated for sepsis (Table 9-1).[12,13] In contrast with the increased incidence of bacteriuria among females in other age groups, infection of the urinary tract in the first 3 months of life is more frequent in males.[2,4-9,14-16]

Infection of the urinary tract is usually sporadic, but clusters of cases, closely related in time, have been reported from nurseries in Cleveland[17] and Baltimore.[18] A nursery epidemic caused by *Serratia marcescens* was responsible for UTI and balanitis. The outbreak was caused by contamination of a solution applied to the umbilical cord.[19]

Surveys of infants born in U.S. Army medical centers and subsequently hospitalized for UTI indicate that uncircumcised males have more UTIs than those reported in circumcised males in the first month and in months 2 to 12 of life (Table 9-2).[10,20,21] In 1982, Ginsburg and McCracken observed that 95% of 62 infant boys with UTI were uncircumcised.[22] A case-control study performed in 112 infant boys in whom suprapubic aspiration or bladder catheterization had been performed for investigation of acute illness showed that all infants with UTI were uncircumcised, compared with 32% of controls.[23] Infection was associated with anatomic abnormalities in 26% of cases. The records of more than 136,000 boys born in U.S. Army hospitals from 1980 to 1985 were reviewed through the first month of life to compare clinical courses in uncircumcised and circumcised boys.[24] Eighty-eight of 35,929 uncircumcised boys (0.24%) had UTI, 33 had concomitant bacteremia, 3 had meningitis,

Table 9–1 Incidence of Urinary Tract Infections in Newborn Infants: Results of Eight Studies

			Gender				Birth Weight			
			Male		*Female*		*<2500 g*		*>2500 g*	
Study[a]	Methods Used to Obtain Urine	No. Infected/ No. Studied (%)	*No. Surveyed*	*No. Infected*	*No. Surveyed*	*No. Infected*	*No. Surveyed*	*No. Infected*	*No. Surveyed*	*No. Infected*
Christchurch, N.Z. (4), 1968-1969	CVS, SPA	14/1460 (0.95)	757	11	703	3	N.S.	—	N.S.	—
Göteborg (5), 1960-1966	CVS	75[b]/57,000 (0.14)	N.S.	54	N.S.	21	N.S.	11	N.S.	64
New York (6), 1973[c]	CVS, SPA	12/1042 (1.2)	493	7	549	5	206	6	836	6
Leeds (7), 1967	CVS, SPA	8/600 (1.3)	309	7	291	1	N.S.	0	N.S.	8
Oklahoma City (11), 1974	SPA	10/102 (10)	N.S.	N.S.	N.S.	N.S.	102	10	—	—
Lausanne (8), 1978[c]	CVS, SPA	43/1762[d] (2.4)	1006	26	756	7	634[e]	10	1028[f]	33
Göteborg (9), 1977-1980[g]	CVS, SPA	26/198 (0.81)	1502	23	1696	3	—	—	—	—
U.S. Army (10), 1975-1984[h]	SPA, Ca	320/422,328 (0.08)	217,116	162	205,212	158	—	—	—	—

[a]Location (reference number), year(s) of study.
[b]Five male infants with infection and suspected or proven obstruction malformation of urinary tract not included.
[c]Date of published report; years of study not provided.
[d]Includes only infants younger than 28 days of age who were admitted to neonatal intensive care unit.
[e]Results reported for premature infants (<259 days' gestation)
[f]Results reported for term infants (≥259 days' gestation).
[g]Results reported for infants 1 wk to 2 mo of age.
[h]Results reported for infants 1 wk to 2 mo of age who were hospitalized.
Ca = catheter; CVS = clean-voided specimen; N.S. = not stated; SPA = suprapubic aspiration [of bladder urine].

Table 9–2 Incidence of Urinary Tract Infections during First Year of Life in Infants Born at U.S. Army Hospitals

Study Location and Parameters	Female Infants	Male Infants	
		Circumcised	*Not Circumcised*
Tripler Army Hosital[a] (January 1982–June 1983)			
No. infants	2759	1919	583
No. infants with UTI	13 (0.47%)	4 (0.21%)	24 (4.12%)
Mean age at diagnosis (mo)	2.5	1.4	1.7
Brooke Army Hospital[b] (January 1980–December 1983)			
No. infants	1905	1575	444
No. infants with UTI	8 (0.42%)	0	8 (1.8%)
Mean age at diagnosis (mo)	4.4	—	1.7
U.S. Army Hospital[b] (January 1975–December 1984)			
No. infants	205,212	175,317	41,799
No. infants with UTI	1164 (0.57%)	193 (0.11%)	468 (1.12%)
Mean age at diagnosis (mo)	3.9	2.7	2.5

[a]Data from Wiswell TE, Smith FR, Bass JW. Decreased incidence of urinary tract infection in circumcised males. Pediatrics 75:901, 1985.
[b]Data from Wiswell TE, Roscelli JD. Corroborative evidence for the decreased incidence of urinary tract infections in circumcised male infants. Pediatrics 78:96, 1986.

2 had renal failure, and 2 died. Complications followed 0.19% of 100,157 circumcisions (including 20 UTIs), and all were minor except for three episodes of hemorrhage leading to transfusion. Meta-analysis of nine published studies through 1992 yielded an overall 12-fold increased risk of infection in uncircumcised boys.[25]

In 1989, the American Academy of Pediatrics (AAP) rescinded a 1971 position against circumcision, recognizing the relative safety of the procedure and protection against UTI in the first year of life.[26] More recent studies using case-control and cohort design also support an association, although magnitude of risk for uncircumcised males is reduced to three- to sevenfold.[27,28] In 1999, the AAP revised the recommendation, citing that although existing scientific evidence demonstrates potential medical benefits of newborn male circumcision, data are not sufficient to recommend its routine performance.[29] Ritual Jewish circumcision performed on the eighth day of life, when periurethral bacterial colonization has been established, appears to have attendant risk for UTI. An epidemiologic study in Israel revealed excessive UTIs in males only from days 9 to 20 of life (the postcircumcision period).[30] A case-control study identified performance by a nonphysician (mohel) versus a physician as a risk factor for UTI (odds ratio 4.34); the authors postulate technique of hemostasis and duration of the shaft wrapping as responsible factors.[31]

Table 9–3 Pathogens Responsible for Urinary Tract Infections in Neonatal Intensive Care Units

Organism	Frequency (%) of Isolations of Each Pathogen		
	1969-1978[a]	*1989-1992*[b]	*1991-2001*[c]
Escherichia coli	75.3	10.5	13.6
Klebsiella spp.	13.4	10.5	30.0
Enterobacter spp.	1.4	12.3	16.4
Enterococcus spp.	2.1	14.0	5.5
Coagulase-negative staphylococci	1.4	31.6	6.4
Candida spp.	—	12.3	18.2
Other	6.4	8.8	7.2

[a]Data from 139 patients in nurseries and intensive care nurseries from references 4, 5, 7, and 8.
[b]Data from 50 patients in neonatal intensive care units from references 39 and 40.
[c]Data from 110 patients in neonatal intensive care units from references 12, 13, and 42.

MICROBIOLOGY

Escherichia coli continues to be responsible for the vast majority of community-acquired infections of the urinary tract in infants younger than 3 months of age, accounting for 90% to 93% of approximately 400 cases in reports from 1990 to 1998.[32-34] Many O serotypes of *E. coli* have been associated with these infections. UTI in neonates was associated with a limited number of O:K:H serotypes with P fimbriae, adhesive capacity, hemolysin production, and serum resistance.[35-37] The serotypes of *E. coli* associated with diarrhea, however, rarely cause UTI. Cultures of urine can be positive in infants with septicemia caused by group B streptococci, but primary infection of the urinary tract without septicemia is rare (see Chapter 13).[16,38] The incidence of neonatal UTI as a complication of intensive care has risen sharply in recent years; intensive care–associated UTI occurs in patients with and without urinary catheters.[3]

Microbiology of today's nosocomial UTI is dramatically different from that observed in the 1970s (Table 9-3), with *E. coli* supplanted by other Enterobacteriaceae genera, *Pseudomonas*, *Enterococcus*, *Candida*, and coagulase-negative staphylococci.[3,12,13,39-42] Multiple pathogens may be present;

Maherzi and colleagues identified more than one bacterial pathogen in 4 of 43 infants with UTI documented by aspiration of bladder urine.[8]

S. aureus and *E. coli* have been responsible for localized suppurative disease of the urinary tract in the neonate, including prostatitis, orchitis, and epididymitis.[43-48] Other examples of focal disease in the urinary tract include orchitis caused by *Pseudomonas aeruginosa*[49] and testicular abscess caused by *Salmonella enteritidis*.[50] Blood cultures frequently are positive in affected infants.

Bacteria responsible for infections of the circumcision site are discussed under "Infections of the Skin and Subcutaneous Tissue" in Chapter 10.

PATHOGENESIS

In older children and adults, most UTIs are thought to occur by the ascending route after introduction of bacteria through the urethral meatus. Less frequently, blood-borne infection of the kidney occurs. In the neonate, it is frequently difficult to know whether UTI was the cause or the result of bacteremia. The predominance of males among infants younger than 3 months of age with UTI contrasts with the predominance of females in all other age groups. This difference may reflect increased risk of UTI in young uncircumcised males, increased prevalence of urinary and renal anomalies in males, transient urodynamic dysfunction, and vesicoureteral reflux (VUR), which predominantly affects male infants,[51] and the occasional UTI that complicates circumcision. Additionally, bacteremia is more frequent in male infants, and it is likely that hematogenous invasion of the kidney can cause UTI in neonates.

Anatomic or physiologic abnormalities of the urinary tract play a role in the development and consequences of infection in some infants. Obstructive uropathy and VUR are the most important. Infection often is the first indication of an abnormality. Infection was the presenting sign in half of 40 infants younger than 2 months of age with anomalies of the kidneys or ureters reported in 1980.[52] Congenital obstruction of the urinary tract was diagnosed in 5 of 80 children with UTI studied in Göteborg[5] and in 2 of 60 children studied in Leeds[53]; important radiologic abnormalities of the urinary tract were identified in 10 of 46 male infants and 3 of 13 female infants younger than 3 months of age from 1972 to 1982 in Christchurch, New Zealand.[54] Increasingly, antenatal ultrasonography identifies fetuses with significant anatomic abnormalities, and early neonatal intervention (with prophylactic use of antibiotics with or without surgery) decreases likelihood of infection.

VUR is identified in many infants with UTI who are examined by radiologic techniques. It is frequently the result of infection but also can be a primary defect predisposing to UTI. VUR is not a prerequisite for upper tract infection (i.e., pyelonephritis); fewer than half of children with pyelonephritis by scintigraphy had VUR in two studies.[55,56] Majd and co-workers found that 23 of 29 (79%) children hospitalized for UTI who were found to have reflux had pyelonephritis by scintigraphy; so did 39 of 65 (60%) of children without reflux.[57] VUR can be a congenital abnormality. Fetal ultrasonography demonstrated that 30 of 107 infants with prenatally diagnosed urinary tract abnormalities had reflux, which was the only abnormality found postnatally in 10.[58] Gordon and colleagues observed that 16 of 25 infants with dilatation of the fetal urinary tract had reflux, which was of grade 3 to 5 severity in 79%.[59] Thirty-nine urinary tract abnormalities detected prenatally were compared with 46 urinary tract abnormalities found after first UTI in Austrian infants.[60] Obstructive lesions and multicystic dysplastic malformations of the kidneys accounted for 90% of all prenatally diagnosed malformations, and reflux accounted for only 10%. By contrast, reflux accounted for 59% of abnormalities detected after the first UTI. VUR detected prenatally has a male-to-female distribution of 6:1 (unlike VUR detected after UTI, when females predominate[61]), may be determined developmentally by the site of the origin of the ureteral bud from the wolffian duct, and in severe cases can be associated with congenital renal damage consisting of global parenchymal loss (so-called reflux nephropathy).[62] Gunn and colleagues performed ultrasound examinations of 3228 fetuses: No renal tract abnormalities were detected before 28 weeks of gestation.[63] Subsequently, 3856 fetuses were examined by ultrasonography after 28 weeks of gestation. Urinary tract anomalies were identified in 313 fetuses: 15 had major structural abnormalities, all of which were confirmed postnatally. In 298 (7.7%) of the fetuses, dilated renal pelvis with normal bladder was found; a majority of the cases resolved spontaneously, but 40 of the cases were confirmed postnatally to be due to serious abnormalities (usually obstruction or VUR).[64] Preterm infants in whom nosocomial UTI develops have a lower incidence of VUR than that noted in term infants with nosocomial UTI.[65] Isolated mild renal pyelectasis (i.e., less than 10 mm diameter of the collecting duct and without VUR) in fetuses is likely to be transient, unassociated with pathology or risk for UTI.[66,67] Fifty-four percent of such cases had resolved in the first postnatal month in one study, and 85% of the cases of moderate or severe pelviectasis had resolved or improved over the first 2 years of life.[68] In a long-term study performed in the United Kingdom of 425 infants with antenatally detected hydronephrosis, 284 had normal findings on neonatal ultrasound examination; negative predictive value of normal ultrasound findings for subsequent UTI in the first year of life was 99%.[69]

The relative contributions of reflux and infection in causing renal damage are debated, but there is growing consensus that postnatal damage correlates with episodes of infection. Follow-up of 108 cases of VUR diagnosed prenatally showed that when infections were prevented, 42% of cases with VUR grade 4 or greater followed medically resolved, and 16% of the patients improved within 18 months; renal damage did not progress in any case.[62] In another study, patients identified with VUR in early childhood were followed prospectively for an average of 9.5 years.[70] Either elimination of recurring UTIs or surgical correction of reflux prevented development of new renal scars. Four patients with unobstructed high-grade sterile reflux were followed for 6 to 10 years; none developed cortical scars. In a long-term study in Toronto of 260 infants with a diagnosis of prenatal hydronephrosis, 25 also had VUR (grade 3 or higher in 73%), received antibiotic prophylaxis, and did not have surgical correction during 4 years of follow-up. Breakthrough infection occurred in only 4 patients. Improvement was seen in a majority of the children with VUR, and there was no difference in renal growth in children who had resolved versus unresolved VUR or high-grade versus low-grade VUR.[71]

Bacterial virulence factors are likely to play an important role in the pathogenesis of UTIs. Strains of *E. coli* causing UTI are a selected sample of the fecal flora. Pyelonephritic isolates belong to a restricted number of serotypes, are resistant to the bactericidal effect of serum, attach to uroepithelial cells, and produce hemolysins.[72] Pili on the bacterial cell surface that adhere to specific receptors on epithelial cells may play a role in development of UTI.[35] Data from Stockholm,[35] Dallas,[36] and Copenhagen[37] suggest that some of these features of pyelonephritic strains of *E. coli* can be demonstrated in UTIs in newborns.

The increased rate of UTIs in the uncircumcised male is likely to be associated with periurethral bacterial flora. During the first 6 months of life, uncircumcised males have significantly higher total urethral bacterial colony counts and more frequent isolation and higher colony counts of uropathogenic organisms such as *E. coli*, *Klebsiella-Enterobacter* species, *Proteus*, and *Pseudomonas*.[73] With increasing age, the foreskin is more easily retracted and penile hygiene improves; by 12 months of age, both the excessive periurethral flora and UTIs in uncircumcised males almost disappear.[21,73]

Natural defenses in the urinary tract include antibacterial properties of urine, antiadherence mechanisms, mechanical effects of urinary flow and micturition, presence of phagocytic cells, antibacterial properties of the urinary tract mucosa, and immune mechanisms.[74] There is scant knowledge about these mechanisms in the newborn.

PATHOLOGY

The histologic appearance of acute pyelonephritis in newborns is similar to that in the adult.[75] Polymorphonuclear leukocytes are present in the glomeruli, the tubules, and the interstitial tissues. The renal pelvis can show signs of acute inflammation, with loss of the lining epithelium and necrosis. Focal suppuration can be present in the kidney, prostate, or testis. In disease of longer duration, the interstitial tissue is infiltrated with lymphocytes, plasma cells, and eosinophils. The number of glomeruli may be decreased, and some may be hyalinized. The epithelium of tubules is atrophic, and the lumen is filled with colloid casts. Pericapsular fibrosis is present in some infants. If the child dies within 6 months, there is little scarring or contraction of the kidney. Reversible hydronephrosis and hydroureter are observed manifestations of acute pyelonephritis in the neonate who has no anatomic abnormality or VUR. It is postulated that bacteria and endotoxins inhibit ureteral peristalsis.

Pathologic processes indicative of additional suppurative infections, such as otitis media, pneumonia, and meningitis, also can be seen in infants dying of acute infection of the urinary tract. Hepatocellular damage and bile stasis may be noted in liver sections from jaundiced infants.[76]

CLINICAL MANIFESTATIONS

The signs of UTI in neonates are varied and nonspecific. In general, five patterns are observed: (1) septicemia associated with early-onset (within the first 5 days of life) or late-onset (after 5 days of age) disease (see Chapter 21); (2) acute onset of fever without apparent source; (3) insidious illness marked by low-grade fever or failure to gain weight; (4) no apparent signs; and (5) localized signs of infection, including balanitis, prostatitis, urethritis, and orchitis.

Table 9–4 Clinical Manifestations of Urinary Tract Infections in Newborn Infants as Described in Selected Reports[a]

Clinical Manifestation	% of Infants with Manifestations[b]
Failure to thrive	50
Fever	39
Vomiting	37
Diarrhea	25
Cyanosis	23
Jaundice	18
Irritability or lethargy	17

[a]Data from references 4, 5, 7, and 8.
[b]When sign was not mentioned in report, the number of infants in the report was removed from the denominator used to determine percentage of infants with manifestations.

The most frequent signs of acute UTI are those associated with septicemia or fever, or both (see Chapter 21) (Table 9-4).[4,5,7,8] In infants with less acute infection, the presenting signs include poor weight gain or anorexia. Diarrhea and vomiting are common in these infants but do not appear to be the only factors responsible for failure to thrive. Fever is present in about half of such infants, although it may not be a presenting sign. Lethargy, irritability, seizures, and meningismus (in the absence of purulent meningitis) occur in some infants.[5] Enlargement of the liver and spleen and distention of the abdomen can be present. The kidneys may be enlarged or abnormal in shape or position, and anomalies of the urethra and penis also can occur. Signs associated with renal anomalies (e.g., a single umbilical artery, supernumerary nipples, spina bifida, low-set ears and anorectal abnormalities) are seen in some infants. Jaundice is an important feature of UTI and may be the presenting sign[76-78]; it is frequently sudden in onset and clears rapidly after adequate antimicrobial therapy. Many infants with UTI and jaundice have positive blood cultures.[18,78] Of 306 infants in one study admitted to hospital within 21 days of birth solely because of indirect hyperbilirubinemia (mean peak serum bilirubin level 18.5 mg/dL), 90% were breast-fed and none had a positive culture of urine or blood.[79] In another study, 12 of 160 (7.5%) infants younger than 8 weeks of age evaluated solely for jaundice had UTI confirmed by bladder catheterization. Renal ultrasound was abnormal in 6 of 11 infants. Infection was especially associated with elevated conjugated bilirubin and age of over 8 days.[80] A reported case of severe methemoglobinemia observed in a 3-week-old infant with *E. coli* UTI was postulated to be caused by nitrite-forming bacteria, but concurrent diarrhea, dehydration, and acidosis may have been precipitating factors.[81] Hyperammonemic encephalopathy due to *Proteus* infection in children with urinary tract obstruction or atony also has been described.[82]

UTI without apparent signs of illness also can occur. In some studies, infection detected during screening surveys was more frequent than infection identified after signs of illness[4,6,9,83]; infection was detected in 9 of 14 infants in a screening program in Christchurch[4] and in 8 of 10 premature infants whose UTI was diagnosed in a program in Oklahoma City.[11]

Abscesses of the prostate, testis, or epididymis usually present as signs of septicemia, including fever, vomiting, and diarrhea.[43-50] Local signs of inflammation, including tenderness and swelling over the surface of the infected organ, may be present. Urinary retention occurs in infants with prostatitis.[45,46] Renal abscess is rare in the neonate; at least case report in a neonate (with congenital nephrosis) has been published.[84]

UTI should be considered in the differential diagnosis for unexplained fever in early infancy. UTI was frequent in infants younger than 3 months of age with nonspecific signs of illness brought to the walk-in clinic at the Boston City Hospital; 3 of 9 febrile children (temperatures greater than 38.9° C) and 2 of 20 children with little or no temperature elevation (less than 38.9° C) had UTI.[85] Of 182 infants younger than 3 months of age presenting with fever at the Tripler Army Hospital in Hawaii, UTI was the most frequent bacterial infection; 20 of the infants (including 14 males) had UTI.[86] A 1-year study of children presenting to the emergency department of the Beilenson Hospital in Tel Aviv included 47 infants younger than 1 month of age; 8 of the infants had UTI, and 3 of these 8 also had bacteremia.[87] In Crain and Gershel's prospective study of 442 New York infants younger than 8 weeks of age with temperatures of 38.1° C (100.6° F) or more, 7.5% had UTI.[32] Of similarly aged infants studied by Hoberman and colleagues in Pittsburgh with temperatures of 38.3° C (101° F) or more, 14 of 306 (4.6%) infants had UTI.[88] Of 1298 febrile infants less than 90 days of age evaluated in Salt Lake City because of fever, 8% had serious bacterial infection and UTI accounted for 67% of infections identified.[89] In a study of 3066 infants under 3 months with fever who were evaluated by office-based pediatricians, 75% had laboratory testing performed; UTI was confirmed in 5.4%.[90] Rate of circumcision in the population can effect the rate of UTI. In the New York study, prevalence of UTI in boys (82% of whom were not circumcised) was 12.4%. In the Pittsburgh study, prevalence of UTI in boys (2% of whom were not circumcised) was only 2.9%. In a study of 162 febrile Japanese infants under 8 weeks of age, 22 (13.8%) has UTI; 18 were male, none of whom were circumcised.[91] In a study of 2411 febrile children younger than 24 months of age evaluated in an emergency department in Philadelphia, history of malodorous urine, prior history of UTI, and presence of abdominal tenderness were significantly associated with the diagnosis of UTI; findings, however, were present in less than 10% of infected infants, and only 8% to 13% of infants with findings had UTI confirmed.[34] In a retrospective study of 354 Boston infants younger than 24 months of age with UTI confirmed, irritability and decreased appetite were each reported in half of children; diarrhea, vomiting, lethargy, and congestion in one fourth; and malodorous urine, apparent dysuria, frequency of urination, and abdominal pain in less than 10%.[16]

DIAGNOSIS

Infection of the urinary tract is defined as the presence of bacteria in urine that was obtained without contamination from the urethra or external genitalia. UTI should be considered in all infants older than 3 days of age who have fever or other signs of septicemia or who have subtle and nonspecific signs of failure to thrive during the first months of life. At present, no clinical finding or simple laboratory test adequately defines the location of infection in the urinary tract of the infant. It is assumed that bacteriuria in the neonate indicates infection throughout the urinary tract (including the kidney).

Culture of Urine

Suprapubic needle aspiration of bladder urine is the most reliable technique for identifying bacteriuria. Although a negative result from culture of bag-collected urine indicates that the urine is sterile, 12% to 21% of bag-collected specimens yield results that are indeterminate or positive (colony count of 10^4/mL or greater),[2,32] and positive results must be verified by aspiration of bladder urine or by catheterization. There is infrequently insufficient time for this stepwise approach before institution of therapy. The technique of needle aspiration of the bladder has been used extensively, and the cumulative experience indicates that it is technically simple and safe and that it causes minimal discomfort to the infant.[92,93] Although most infected urine specimens will have bacterial colony counts of 10^5/mL or greater, any bacterial growth in urine obtained by suprapubic aspiration is believed to be significant.

Morbidity associated with suprapubic aspiration is minimal. Transient gross hematuria has been reported in 0.6% of 654 infants.[93] Gross bleeding that ceased only after cauterization was reported in one case.[94] Perforation of the bowel occurred in two cases, but this complication is avoided if the bladder is defined by palpation or percussion.[95] Hematoma of the anterior wall of the bladder,[96,97] peritonitis,[98] and anaerobic bacteremia[99] also have been reported after suprapubic aspiration. These reports warranted publication because the cases are very uncommon. The possibility of these complications should not deter the physician from using this technique for infants with suggested septicemia. However, suprapubic aspiration should not be performed if the infant has recently voided, has abdominal distention, has poorly defined anomalies of the urinary tract, or has a hematologic abnormality that might result in hemorrhage.

Suprapubic aspiration of bladder urine should be performed at least 1 hour after the patient has voided. The infant should lie supine, with the lower extremities held in a frog-leg position. The suprapubic area is cleansed with iodine and alcohol. A 20-gauge, 1½-inch needle attached to a syringe is used to pierce the abdominal wall and bladder approximately 1 inch above the symphysis pubis. The needle is directed caudally toward the fundus of the bladder, and urine is aspirated gently. Vigorous aspiration should be avoided because the mucosa can be drawn in to block the needle opening. The aspirated urine is sent to the laboratory immediately in a sterile tube. If the child urinates during the procedure, or if it cannot be done properly for other reasons, aspiration should be repeated after 1 to 2 hours. Ultrasound examination may be useful in detecting the presence of urine in the bladder before suprapubic aspiration[100,101]; with ultrasound-guided aspiration, the success rate for acquisition of an adequate sample of urine improved from 60% to 96.4%.[101]

When it is important to obtain an immediate sample of urine and suprapubic aspiration cannot be performed for technical reasons (lack of experience of the physician, dehydration, or recent voiding), catheterization of the bladder is appropriate. The incidence of infection related to catheterization in infants is unknown. Urine for culture should be transported to the laboratory as soon as possible, but if a delay is unavoidable, the specimen must be refrigerated. Colony counts of 10^3/mL of urine obtained by catheter may represent significant bacteriuria in this age group.[102] In multiple studies of young children evaluated because of fever (relatively few of whom were neonates), approximately 80% of those with bacteriuria had colony counts of 10^5/mL or greater. Significant pyuria, elevated serum level of C-reactive protein (CRP), isolation of a single enteric organism, and abnormality on renal scintigraphy were each decreasingly associated with lower colony counts, with only rare positive tests in those children with colony counts of less than10^4/mL.[15,16,33,103]

Culture of Blood and Cerebrospinal Fluid

Because bacteremia and meningitis frequently accompany UTI, cultures of the blood and cerebrospinal fluid should be obtained before therapy for UTI is begun if the neonate has fever or any signs of illness. Blood (but not necessarily cerebrospinal fluid) for culture also should be obtained from the neonate with UTI but without specific or nonspecific signs of infection. In the Göteborg studies,[5] lumbar puncture was performed before therapy in 31 neonates with UTI: 6 infants had purulent meningitis, and in 9 infants the cerebrospinal fluid was sterile but pleocytosis (22 to 200 white blood cells [WBCs] per mm^3) was also present. Blood was obtained for culture in 32 infants and was positive in 12.

Bacteremia was present in 11 of 35 (31%) Dallas infants younger than 30 days of age with UTI. The infants had been considered healthy when discharged from the nursery and were evaluated because of fever. Older infants with UTI were less likely to be bacteremic; positive cultures of blood occurred in 5 of 24 infants (21%) with UTI aged 1 to 2 months, 2 of 14 infants (14%) aged 2 to 3 months, and 1 of 18 infants (5.5%) aged 3 months or older.[22] Similarly, in Boston, bacteremia was present in 17 of 80 (21%) of febrile infants with UTI younger than 1 month, 8 of 59 (13%) 1 to 2 months of age, and 8 of 116 (7%) 2 to 6 months of age; 4 neonates had meningitis. No clinical finding or laboratory test discriminated between bacteremic and nonbacteremic infants.[16] In surveillance for UTI among 203,399 infants born in U.S. Army hospitals from 1985 to 1990, 23% of non-circumcised infant boys with UTI younger than 3 months of age had concomitant bacteremia; incidence of bacteremia associated with UTI was not different from that in circumcised boys or girls with UTI.[25] Incidence of bacteremia in neonatal nosocomial UTI is higher than in community-associated infection, up to 38% in one study.[12] Incidence of bacteremia in community-associated UTI is higher in infants younger than 2 months of age (22%) than in older infants (3%).[104]

Examination of Urine Sediment

Many studies and a meta-analysis assessing presence of WBCs in the urine of newborn infants have been performed.[5,22,71,105-111] Healthy infants can have up to 10 WBCs per mm^3 of clean-voided urine.[109] Lincoln and Winberg obtained uninfected and clean-voided specimens of urine from infants younger than 1 week of age: male infants had up to 25 WBCs per mm^3 and female infants up to 50 WBCs per mm^3.[110]

Neither presence nor absence of pyuria is completely reliable evidence for or against UTI. Many studies have assessed urine specimens for predictive values for UTI of WBCs, organisms, or detection by dipstick of leukocyte esterase or reduction of nitrate. The following results are limited to studies of acutely ill, usually febrile infants whose urine was obtained by catheterization (or suprapubic aspiration where stated). Methods of assessing pyuria and definitions of UTI vary. In 27% of unspun urine samples collected by suprapubic aspiration from Dallas infants with UTI (bacterial colony counts of 10^5/mL or greater), fewer than 10 WBCs per high-power field were present.[22] Landau and co-workers reported that among infants younger than 4 months of age with positive urine cultures (colony counts of 10^4/mL or greater), 4 of 49 (8.2%) with renal scintigraphy–diagnosed acute pyelonephritis had fewer than 5 WBCs per high-power field (400×) in fresh centrifuged urine, compared with 27 of 79 (34.2%) infants with UTI and negative results on scintigraphy.[15]

Quantifying WBCs in uncentrifuged urine using a counting chamber is the most reproducible test for pyuria. Hoberman and colleagues found pyuria (at least 10 WBCs per mm^3 of unspun urine) absent in 22 of 190 (20%) febrile infants younger than 24 months of age with positive urine cultures (colony counts of 5.0×10^4/mL or greater) and present in 6.7% with negative cultures; a single patient of 15 without pyuria in whom renal scintigraphy was performed under protocol had a positive result.[112] In Hansson and co-workers' study of 366 infants younger than 1 year of age with symptomatic UTI (colony counts of 10^3/mL or greater from suprapubic aspirate of urine), 80% had colony counts of 10^5/mL or greater, 13% had counts of 1×10^4 to 9×10^4 per mL, and 7% had counts of 1×10^3 to 9×10^3 per mL. Pyuria was significantly associated with colony count. In children with UTI with colony counts of less than 10^5/mL, sensitivity of pyuria (greater than 10 WBCs per mm^3) was 69%, compared with 88% for children with at least 10^5 colonies per mL. Nitrate reduction test was highly insensitive; 44% of the patients had a positive result when the colony count was at least 10^5/mL and 11% had a positive result with lower counts.[33] Renal scintigraphy was not performed in Hansson and co-workers' study to estimate significance of UTI, but VUR was present equally in infants with high (30%) and low (38%) colony counts.

Dipstick test for leukocyte esterase and nitrite is inadequate to exclude the diagnosis of UTI in infants. In Hoberman and colleagues' study, the test had sensitivity of 53% and positive predictive value of 82% for detecting 10 or more WBCs per mm^3; nitrite determination had sensitivity of 31% in identifying urine cultures with growth of at least 50,000 colonies per mL.[103] Shaw and co-workers reported dipstick results in 3873 febrile children younger than 2 years of age evaluated for UTI; sensitivity of a positive result (trace or greater for leukocyte esterase or positive nitrite) was 79% and positive predictive value was 46% for isolation of at least 10,000 colonies per mL from urine culture.[113]

Microscopic hematuria is present in some infants with UTI,[3,44] but gross hematuria usually is associated with other diseases (e.g., renal vein thrombosis, polycystic disease of the kidney, obstructive uropathy, Wilms' tumor).[114]

Usefulness of Gram stain of urine specimen in predicting bacteriuria has been studied prospectively in febrile infants younger than 24 months of age. Smears were prepared using 2 drops of uncentrifuged urine on a slide within a standardized marked area 1.5 cm in diameter, which was then air dried, fixed, and stained. Presence of at least one organism per 10 high-power fields examined using oil immersion lens was considered a positive result. Sensitivity and positive predictive value were 81% and 43%, respectively, for isolation of at least 1×10^4 colonies per mL of urine in Shaw and colleagues' study[113] and 93% and 57%, respectively, for isolation of at least 5.0×10^4 colonies per mL in Hoberman and co-workers' study.[103] Presence of both pyuria and bacteriuria increased positive predictive value for positive cultures in both studies to 85% and 88%, respectively.

Studies of neonates with early-onset septicemia indicate that the yield for culture of urine is low.[12,13,115,116] Thus, culture may be eliminated in evaluation of infants for presumed sepsis younger than 3 days of age. Examination of urine may occasionally assist in microbiologic diagnosis of early-onset septicemia, but initiation of antimicrobial therapy should not be delayed when there is difficulty in obtaining the specimen.

Examination of Blood

The peripheral blood leukocyte count varies among infants with UTI. Although significantly higher neutrophil and band counts and band-to-neutrophil ratios are documented in young children with UTI, these do not reliably discriminate among presence, absence, or level of infection in the urinary tract or presence of bacteremia.[15,16,112] In studies from New Zealand,[4] half of the neonates had a peripheral blood leukocyte count of greater than 16,000/mm^3, but no information was given about this measure in uninfected infants. Hemolytic anemia frequently accompanies jaundice when the latter is present in infants with UTI.[78] Results of the direct Coombs test are usually negative. The reticulocyte count can be normal or elevated.[78]

Signs of inflammatory response such as elevated erythrocyte sedimentation rate (ESR) or serum CRP or procalcitonin (PCT) have been shown to correlate significantly with abnormal renal scintigraphy findings suggestive of acute pyelonephritis in children with UTI. In 64 children studied, Majd and colleagues found abnormal scans in 78% of those with ESR of at least 25 mm/hour, compared with 33% of those with lower ESR.[57] Benador and co-workers found that ESR greater than 20 mm/hour or CRP level greater than 10 mg/L had sensitivity of 89% and specificity of 25% for identifying renal lesions among 73 children with UTI.[56] Stokland and colleagues correlated CRP level greater than 20 mg/L at the time of acute infection with resultant renal scar in 157 children reevaluated 1 year later; sensitivity of elevated CRP was 92%, and positive and negative predictive values were 41% and 80%, respectively.[117] In 153 children with fever and positive urine culture (colony count 5.0×10^4/mL or greater), Hoberman and co-workers reported significant correlations between evidence of pyelonephritis versus cystitis versus asymptomatic bacteriuria with mean peripheral WBC count (22.4/μL versus 14.6/μL versus 11.7×10^3/μL, respectively); ESR (44.0 versus 26.8 versus 15.3 mm/hour, respectively); and CRP (10.1 versus 2.7 versus 1.3 mg/L, respectively).[112] When cutoff values of 1 ng/mL for PCT and 20 mg/L for CRP were used, rates of sensitivity for detection of pyelonephritis in infants with UTI were similar (92%), but specificity of PCT (62%) exceeded that of CRP (34%).[118]

Chemical Determinations

Hyperbilirubinemia is present in many infants with UTI; the percentage of conjugated bilirubin often is determined by the age of the infant at the onset of jaundice.[76] During the first week of life, almost all of the bilirubin is unconjugated, but in the second week and thereafter, the fractionation is approximately equivalent. In 80 Boston infants younger than 1 month of age with UTI, 11 (14%) had jaundice and hyperbilirubinemia; only 4 had bacteremia.[16] With the exception of changes in serum bilirubin, the results of serum hepatic enzyme tests generally are normal or only slightly abnormal,[76,78] although toxic hepatitis and cholestasis unassociated with hemolysis were documented by liver biopsy in an older child with jaundice associated with UTI.[119] Azotemia and hyperchloremic acidosis are not unusual; serum bicarbonate measured less than 20 mEq/L in 34.1% of 354 young children with UTI in one study.[16]

Radiologic Examination of the Urinary Tract

The major goal of investigation of the urinary tract in infants with UTI (and those with abnormalities noted prenatally) is to identify important and correctable lesions (including urethral strictures, renal anomalies, severe VUR, obstructive uropathy, and urethral valves in males) and to provide the opportunity to begin antibiotic prophylaxis against recurring UTIs in those with reflux or hydronephrosis in whom surgery is not indicated. Multiple new imaging modalities are available and are safer than intravenous pyelography.[120] Each provides unique evaluations.[55,61,117,121-125] Ultrasound examination is capable of showing the size, shape, and location of kidneys and contributes to the diagnosis with hydronephrosis, hydroureter, ureterocele, bladder distention, and stones, but less so with VUR. It is the most noninvasive study, the accuracy of which is dependent on the experience of the interpreter. It is an insensitive test for pyelonephritis but sometimes shows kidney enlargement with abnormal echogenicity. Renal ultrasonography performed to follow up on fetal studies should be postponed for at least 48 hours after birth to avoid a false-negative result from dehydration or low glomerular filtration rate characteristic of newborns.[121]

Renal cortical scintigraphy using technetium-99m–labeled dimercaptosuccinic acid or gluceptate is the most sensitive test for identifying acute pyelonephritis (i.e., focally or diffusely decreased cortical uptake of tracer without evidence of cortical loss, sometimes in an enlarged kidney) or chronic scarring (i.e., decreased uptake with corresponding cortical volume loss); it also provides an estimate of renal function.

This modality is the "gold standard" for diagnosis of acute pyelonephritis; 66% of 66 infants younger than 1 year of age with febrile UTI had a positive result on the renal scan in one study,[56] as did 75% of 153 children younger than 2 years of age in another study[112] and 66% of 94 children in another study.[57]

Voiding cystourethrography using radiographic or radionuclide methodology is the best study to visualize the bladder and urethra and to detect VUR; radionuclide scan is superior to the dye study for detection of intermittent reflux but is inferior for detection of urethral and bladder wall abnormalities and cannot be used to grade VUR. Both are invasive and pose discomfort attendant with catheterization. A 24-day-old male infant with ureterovesical junction obstruction was found to have *E. coli* septicemia and UTI 6 days after elective vesicourethrography, which did not show VUR.[126] Toxic reaction to the cystourethrography dye can occur in infants but is very uncommon.

Ultrasonography and cystourethrography have been recommended for all neonates with UTI judged to be other than that secondary to septicemia. Male infants with community-associated first UTI diagnosed before 8 weeks of age have a higher incidence of VUR or anatomic abnormalities (22% of 45 male infants in one Israeli study) than that noted in older children.[127] Ultrasonography is performed at the time of infection to identify major renal and ureteral abnormalities. Cystourethrography sometimes can be delayed to permit resolution of inflammatory VUR; however, in clinical studies, less than 50% of children with acute pyelonephritis proved to have VUR.[33,57,122] Renal scintigraphy is useful in diagnosis and management of selective cases of UTI.[128,129] Computed tomography (CT) is performed infrequently—for example, when a mass lesion or abscess is suspected. For infants who have undergone prenatal ultrasonography in an experienced center after 30 to 32 weeks of gestation and whose study findings were normal, repeat ultrasonography at the time of first UTI is not recommended by some experts.[110,111]

MANAGEMENT

Management of UTI is aimed at halting infection rapidly, reconstituting normal fluid and acid-base status, and assessing medical or surgical interventions required to prevent subsequent episodes of UTI and kidney damage.

Antimicrobial Therapy

Antimicrobial agents should be administered as soon as culture specimens of the blood, cerebrospinal fluid (if indicated), and urine have been obtained. Because the physician must assume that bacteremia is present in the neonate who has UTI and signs of septicemia, the choice of antimicrobial agents for initial therapy and the dosage schedule is the same as that outlined in Chapter 6 for septicemia (a penicillin and an aminoglycoside). A penicillinase-resistant penicillin (methicillin or oxacillin) should be used if an abscess of the kidney, prostate, or testis is present, which suggests infection with *S. aureus*. Vancomycin may be appropriate when methicillin-resistant *S. aureus* organisms are prevalent in the community or nursery. Patients who have suspected hospital-acquired infection are frequently given vancomycin and an aminoglycoside as initial therapy because of the significant role of coagulase-negative staphylococci and *Enterococcus* species. The decision to use a third-generation cephalosporin is based on the patient's prior receipt of antibiotics, the patient's clinical state, and the knowledge of bacterial species indigenous in each neonatal intensive care unit (NICU). Extended-spectrum β-lactamase (ESBL)-producing organisms of the family Enterobacteriaceae are increasingly problematic in neonatal nosocomial infections, including UTI. Identification of such organisms may not be possible with routine susceptibility testing and may require special investigation. Infectious disease experts should be consulted to manage infections due to ESBL-producing pathogens and to aid in prospective surveillance for antibiotic-resistant microorganisms indigenous to a particular NICU. Gram stain of urine sediment is helpful in initiating empirical therapy for UTI, especially when use of amphotericin for potential *Candida* infection is considered. Therapeutic regimens should be reconsidered when the results of cultures and antimicrobial susceptibility tests are available.

Effective antimicrobial agents sterilize the urine within 24 to 48 hours. A second specimen of urine often is obtained for examination and culture at about 48 hours. Persistence of bacteriuria implies that treatment is ineffective or that a foreign body or obstruction is present.

The duration of antimicrobial therapy for UTI in neonates usually is 14 days. Longer therapy (up to 3 weeks) is necessary if there is a poor response or if an anatomic or physiologic abnormality suggests that relapse may occur if administration of the drug is not continued. Timing of change from parenterally to orally administered agents depends on rapidity of clinical and microbiologic response and the presence of bacteremia or anatomic, functional, or physiologic abnormalities and availability of a highly active oral agent. Parenteral therapy is usually given for at least 3 to 4 days in uncomplicated cases.[130] The urine should be examined and cultured frequently after conclusion of therapy so that relapse or recurrence of infection can be detected as soon as possible. Children with certain urinary tract anomalies, functional abnormalities, and higher grades of VUR are given prophylactic antibiotics continuously for extended periods until surgery is performed or the condition improves[63,121]; amoxicillin, 20 mg/kg per day divided in doses administered every 12 hours, is the agent most frequently used in the neonate. Systematic review of randomized controlled trials of prophylaxis reveals limited evidence for its efficacy.[131]

Ancillary Therapy

Severe dehydration, electrolyte imbalance, azotemia, and shock can accompany UTI in the newborn. Fluid replacement must be calculated carefully for correction of these abnormalities. Transfusion of blood may be necessary in infants with hemolytic anemia. Incision and drainage of abscesses of the prostate and testis should be considered.

PROGNOSIS

For patients with UTI and underlying genitourinary abnormalities, long-term control of infection is important. After that, prognosis is dependent on severity of the lesion. The natural history of UTI in the newborn without underlying abnormality is incompletely described. Some infants with asymptomatic bacteriuria have infection that clears without use of antimicrobial agents.[4,5,83,132] Some infants with symptomatic infection respond readily to therapy and have no subsequent infections, whereas others have recurrences, although the number appears to be smaller than that for older children and adults. In the series from Göteborg[5] and Leeds,[7] recurrences occurred in 26% and 19% of the infants, respectively; the second episode usually occurred during the first few months after the initial infection.

It is possible that inflammatory changes in the kidney early in life may lead to subsequent impairment of growth and development of the kidney and to epithelial damage, fibrosis, and vascular changes, but it is uncertain how frequently these events take place. In a study of 25 children with UTI in whom renal scintigraphy demonstrated evidence of acute pyelonephritis and who underwent repeat scanning an average of 10.5 months later, 16 (64%) had corresponding scars.[56] In another study, 38% of 157 children (with median age 0.4 year at the time of asymptomatic UTI) had renal scars documented 1 year later.[117] Infants do not appear to be at increased risk for scarring; in 50 infants younger than 1 year of age with UTI and acute renal lesions, repeat scintigraphy after an average of 3 months showed scars in 40%.[133]

Obstructive lesions associated with reflux during the neonatal period may be associated with progressive renal damage, whereas children with unobstructive reflux regardless of severity appear not to have progressive renal damage if infection is assiduously prevented.[51,58-60,63,121] Repeat ultrasonography for follow-up evaluation after UTI in children in whom findings on a postnatal ultrasound examination were normal is not indicated.[134] In a study of 102 children with end-stage renal disease in Missouri from 1986 to 1995, damage from VUR and UTIs accounted for less than 1% of cases.[135] A prospective population-based study in Italy suggests that primary vesiculoureteral reflux in males leads to congenital renal hypoplasia, which is the predominant cause of chronic renal failure.[136]

REFERENCES

1. Helmholz HF. Pyelitis in the newborn. Med Clin North Am 1:1451, 1918.
2. Schlager TA, Hendley JO, Dudley SM, et al. Explanation for false-positive urine cultures obtained by bay technique. Arch Pediatr Adolesc Med 149:170, 1995.
3. Lohr JA, Downs SM, Dudley S, et al. Hospital-acquired urinary tract infections in the pediatric patient: a prospective study. Pediatr Infect Dis J 13:8, 1994.
4. Abbott GD. Neonatal bacteriuria: a prospective study of 1460 infants. BMJ 1:267, 1972.
5. Bergström T, Larson H, Lincoln K, et al. Neonatal urinary tract infections. J Pediatr 80:859, 1972.
6. Edelman CM Jr, Ogwo JE, Fine BP, et al. The prevalence of bacteriuria in full-term and premature newborn infants. J Pediatr 82:125, 1973.
7. Littlewood JM, Kite P, Kite BA. Incidence of neonatal urinary tract infection. Arch Dis Child 44:617, 1969.
8. Maherzi M, Guignard JP, Torrado A. Urinary tract infection in high-risk newborn infants. Pediatrics 62:521, 1978.
9. Wettergren B, Jodal U, Jonasson G. Epidemiology of bacteriuria during the first year of life. Acta Paediatr Scand 74:925, 1985.
10. Wiswell TE, Roscelli JD. Corroborative evidence for the decreased incidence of urinary tract infections in circumcised male infants. Pediatrics 78:96, 1986.
11. Pendarvis BC Jr, Chitwood LA, Wenzl JE. Bacteriuria in the premature infant. Abstracts of papers presented at the Ninth Interscience Conference on Antimicrobial Agents and Chemotherapy, Washington, D.C., October 27-29, 1969. Washington, DC, American Society for Microbiology, 1969 (abstract).
12. Tamim MM, Alesseh H, Aziz H. Analysis of the efficacy of urine culture as part of sepsis evaluation in the premature infant. Pediatr Infect Dis J 22:805, 2003.
13. Bauer S, Eliakim A, Pomeranz A, et al. Urinary tract infection in very low birth weight preterm infants. Pediatr Infect Dis J 22:426, 2003.
14. Kunin CM. Detection, Prevention and Management of Urinary Tract Infections, 3rd ed. Philadelphia, Lea & Febiger, 1979.
15. Landau D, Turner M, Brennan J, et al. The value of urinalysis in differentiating acute pyelonephritis from lower urinary tract infection in febrile infants. Pediatr Infect Dis J 13:777, 1994.
16. Bachur R, Caputo GL. Bacteremia and meningitis among infants with urinary tract infections. Pediatr Emerg Care 11:280, 1995.
17. Sweet AY, Wolinsky E. An outbreak of urinary tract and other infections due to *E. coli*. Pediatrics 33:865, 1964.
18. Kenny JF, Medearis DN, Klein SW, et al. An outbreak of urinary tract infections and septicemia due to *Escherichia coli* in male infants. J Pediatr 68:530, 1966.
19. McCormack RC, Kunin CM. Control of a single source nursery epidemic due to *Serratia marcescens*. Pediatrics 37:750, 1966.
20. Wiswell TE, Smith FR, Bass JW. Decreased incidence of urinary tract infections in circumcised male infants. Pediatrics 75:901, 1985.
21. Wiswell TE, Enzenauer RW, Holton ME, et al. Declining frequency of circumcision: implications for changes in the absolute incidence and male to female sex ratio of urinary tract infections in early infancy. Pediatrics 79:338, 1987.
22. Ginsburg CM, McCracken GH Jr. Urinary tract infections in young infants. Pediatrics 69:409, 1982.
23. Herzog LW. Urinary tract infections and circumcision: a case-control study. Am J Dis Child 143:348, 1989.
24. Wiswell TE, Geschke DW. Risks from circumcision during the first month of life compared with those for uncircumcised boys. Pediatrics 83:1011, 1989.
25. Wiswell TE, Hachey WE. Urinary tract infections and the uncircumcised state: an update. Clin Pediatr 130, 1993.
26. Schoen EJ (chairman). American Academy of Pediatrics Task Force Report on Circumcision. Pediatrics 84:388, 1989.
27. To T, Agha M, Dick PT, et al. Cohort study on circumcision of newborn boys and subsequent risk of urinary-tract infection. Lancet 352:1813, 1998.
28. Craig JC, Knight JF, Sureshkumar P, et al. Effect of circumcision on incidence of urinary tract infection in preschool boys. J Pediatr 128:23, 1996.
29. Lannon CM. American Academy of Pediatrics Task Force Report on Circumcision. Pediatrics 103:686, 1999.
30. Cohen HA, Drucker MM, Vainer S, et al. Post-circumcision urinary tract infection. Clin Pediatr 31:322, 1992.
31. Harel L, Straussberg R, Jackson S, et al. Influence of circumcision technique on frequency of urinary tract infections in neonates. Pediatr Infect Dis J 21:879, 2002.
32. Crain EF, Gershel JC. Urinary tract infections in febrile infants younger than 8 weeks of age. Pediatrics 86:363, 1990.
33. Hansson S, Brandström P, Jodal U, et al. Low bacterial counts in infants with urinary tract infection. J Pediatr 132:179, 1998.
34. Shaw KN, Gorelick M, McGowan KL, et al. Prevalence of urinary tract infection in febrile young children in the emergency department. Pediatrics 102:390, 1998.
35. Tullus K, Sjoberg P. Epidemiological aspects of Pfimbriated *E. coli*. Acta Paediatr Scand 75:205, 1986.
36. Israele V, Darabi A, McCracken GH Jr. The role of bacterial virulence factors and Tamm-Horsfall protein in the pathogenesis of *Escherichia coli* urinary tract infection in infants. Am J Dis Child 141:1230, 1987.
37. Marild S, Wettergren B, Hellstrom M, et al. Bacterial virulence and inflammatory response in infants with febrile urinary tract infection screening bacteriuria. J Pediatr 112:348, 1988.
38. Pena BM, Harper MB, Fleisher GR. Occult bacteremia with group B streptococci in an outpatient setting. Pediatrics 102:67, 1998.
39. Lohr JA, Donowitz LG, Sadler JE III. Hospital-acquired urinary tract infection. Pediatrics 83:193, 1989.
40. Davies HD, Jones ELF, Sheng RY, et al. Nosocomial urinary tract infections at a pediatric hospital. Pediatr Infect Dis J 11:349, 1992.

41. Levy I, Leibovici L, Drucker M, et al. A prospective study of gram-negative bacteremia in children. Pediatr Infect Dis J 15:117, 1996.
42. Sohn AH, Garrett DO, Sinkowitz-Cochran RL, et al. Prevalence of nosocomial infections in neonatal intensive care unit patients: results from the first national point-prevalence survey. J Pediatr 139:821, 2001.
43. Giannattasio RC. Acute suppurative prostatitis in the neonatal period. N Y State J Med 60:3471, 1960.
44. Williams DI, Martins AG. Periprostatic haematoma and prostatic abscess in the neonatal period. Arch Dis Child 35:177, 1960.
45. Mann S. Prostatic abscess in the newborn. Arch Dis Child 35:396, 1960.
46. Heyman A, Lombardo LJ Jr. Metastatic prostatic abscess with report of a case in a newborn infant. J Urol 87:174, 1962.
47. Hendricks WM, Kellett GN. Scrotal mass in a neonate: testicular abscess. Am J Dis Child 129:1361, 1975.
48. Hemming VG. Bilateral neonatal group A streptococcal hydrocele infection associated with maternal puerperal sepsis. Pediatr Infect Dis 5:107, 1986.
49. McCartney ET, Stewart I. Suppurative orchitis due to *Pseudomonas aeruginosa*. J Pediatr 52:451, 1958.
50. Foster R, Weber TR, Kleiman M, et al. *Salmonella enteritidis*: testicular abscess in a newborn. J Urol 130:790, 1983.
51. Chandra M, Maddix H, McVicar M. Transient urodynamic dysfuncton of infancy: relationship to urinary tract infections and vesicoureteral reflux. J Urol 155:673, 1996.
52. Bensman A, Baudon JJ, Jablonski JP, et al. Uropathies diagnosed in the neonatal period: symptomatology and course. Acta Paediatr Scand 69:499, 1980.
53. Littlewood JM. 66 infants with urinary tract infection in first month of life. Arch Dis Child 57:218, 1972.
54. Bourcher D, Abbott ED, Maling TMJ. Radiological abnormalities in infants with urinary tract infection. Arch Dis Child 59:620, 1984.
55. Andrich MP, Majd M. Diagnostic imaging in the evaluation of the first urinary tract infection in infants and young children. Pediatrics 90:436, 1992.
56. Benador D, Benador N, Slosman DO, et al. Cortical scintigraphy in the evaluation of renal parenchymal changes in children with pyelonephritis. J Pediatr 124:17, 1994.
57. Majd M, Rushton HG, Jantausch B, et al. Relationships among vesico-ureteral reflux, P-fimbriated *Escherichia coli*, and acute pyelonephritis in children with febrile urinary tract infection. J Pediatr 119:578, 1991.
58. Najmaldin A, Burge DM, Atwell JD. Pediatric urology: fetal vesico-ureteric reflux. Br J Urol 65:403, 1990.
59. Gordon AC, Thomas DFM, Arthur RJ, et al. Prenatally diagnosed reflux: a follow-up study. Br J Urol 65:407, 1990.
60. Ring E, Zobel G. Urinary infection and malformations of urinary tract in infancy. Arch Dis Child 63:818, 1988.
61. Steele BT, De Maria J. A new perspective on the natural history of vesicoureteric reflux. Pediatrics 90:30, 1992.
62. Assael BM, Guez S, Marra G, et al. Congenital reflux nephropathy: a follow-up of 108 cases diagnosed perinatally. Br J Urol 82:252, 1998.
63. Gunn TR, Mora JD, Pease P. Outcome after antenatal diagnosis of upper urinary tract dilatation by ultrasonography. Arch Dis Child 63:1240, 1988.
64. Gunn TR, Mora JD, Pease P. Antenatal diagnosis of urinary tract abnormalities by ultrasonography after 28 weeks' gestation: incidence and outcome. Am J Obstet Gynecol 172:479, 1995.
65. Bauer S, Eliakim A, Pomeranz A, et al. Urinary tract infection in very low birth weight preterm infants. Pediatr Infect Dis J 22:426, 2003.
66. Dremsek PA, Gindl K, Void P, et al. Renal pyelectasis in fetuses and neonates: diagnostic value of renal pelvis diameter in pre- and postnatal sonographic screening. AJR Am J Roentgenol 168:1017, 1997.
67. Thomas DFM, Madden NP, Irving HC, et al. Mild dilatation of the fetal kidney: a follow-up study. Br J Urol 74:236, 1993.
68. Cheng AM, Phan V, Geary DF, et al. Outcome of isolated antenatal hydronephrosis. Arch Pediatr Adolesc Med 158:38, 2004.
69. Moorthy I, Joshi N, Cook JV, et al. Antenatal hydronephrosis: negative predictive value of normal postnatal ultrasound—a 5 year study. Clin Radiol 58:964, 2003.
70. Holland NH, Jackson EC, Kazee M, et al. Relation of urinary tract infection and vesicoureteral reflux to scars: follow-up of thirty-eight patients. J Pediatr 116:S65, 1990.
71. Upadhyay J, McLorie GA, Bolduc S, et al. Natural history of neonatal reflux associated with prenatal hydronephrosis: long-term results of a prospective study. J Urol 169:1837, 2003.
72. Svanborg C, Hausson S, Jodal U, et al. Host-parasite interaction in the urinary tract. J Infect Dis 157:421, 1988.
73. Wiswell TE, Miller GM, Gelston HM Jr, et al. Effect of circumcision status on periurethral bacterial flora during the first year of life. J Pediatr 113:442, 1988.
74. Sobel JD. Pathogenesis of urinary tract infections. Infect Dis Clin North Am 1:751, 1987.
75. Porter KA, Giles HM. A pathological study of live cases of pyelonephritis in the newborn. Arch Dis Child 31:303, 1956.
76. Bernstein J, Brown AK. Sepsis and jaundice in early infancy. Pediatrics 29:873, 1962.
77. Ng SH, Rawstron JR. Urinary tract infections presenting with jaundice. Arch Dis Child 46:173, 1971.
78. Seeler RA, Hahn K. Jaundice in urinary tract infection in infancy. Am J Dis Child 118:553, 1969.
79. Maisels MJ, Kring E. Risk of sepsis in newborns with severe hyperbilirubinemia. Pediatrics 90:741, 1992.
80. Garcia FJ, Nager AL. Jaundice as an early diagnostic sign of urinary tract infection in infancy. Pediatrics 112:1213, 2003.
81. Luk G, Riggs D, Luque M. Severe methemoglobinemia in a 3-week-old infant with a urinary tract infection. Crit Care Med 19:1325, 1992.
82. Das A, Henderson D. Your diagnosis, please. Pediatr Infect Dis J 15:922, 1996.
83. Abbott GD. Transient asymptomatic bacteriuria in infancy. BMJ 1:207, 1970.
84. Crawford DB, Rasoulpour M, Dhawan VM, et al. Renal carbuncle in a neonate with congenital nephrotic syndrome. J Pediatr 93:78, 1978.
85. Bauchner H, Philipp B, Dashefsky B, et al. Prevalence of bacteriuria in febrile children. Pediatr Infect Dis J 6:239, 1987.
86. Krober MS, Bass JW, Powell JM, et al. Bacterial and viral pathogens causing fever in infants less than 3 months old. Am J Dis Child 139:889, 1985.
87. Amir J, Alpert G, Reisner SH, et al. Fever in the first months of life. Isr J Med Sci 20:447, 1984.
88. Hoberman A, Chao H, Keller DM, et al. Prevalence of urinary tract infecton in febrile infants. J Pediatr 123:17, 1993.
89. Byington CL, Rittichier KK, Bassett KE, et al. Serious bacterial infections in febrile infants younger than 90 days of age: the importance of ampicillin-resistant pathogens. Pediatrics 111:964, 2003.
90. Pantell RH, Newman TB, Bernzweig J, et al. Management and outcomes of care of fever in early infancy. JAMA 10:1261, 2004.
91. Lin DS, Huang SH, Lin CC, et al. Urinary tract infection in febrile infants younger than eight weeks of age. Pediatrics 105:414, 2000.
92. Nelson JD, Peters PC. Suprapubic aspiration of urine in premature and term infants. Pediatrics 36:132, 1965.
93. Pryles CV, Saccharow L. Further experience with the use of percu-taneous suprapubic aspiration of the urinary bladder: bacteriologic studies in 654 infants and children. Pediatrics 43:1018, 1969.
94. Lanier B, Daeschner CW. Serious complication of suprabubic aspiration of the urinary bladder. J Pediatr 79:711, 1971.
95. Weathers WT, Wenzl JE. Suprapubic aspiration: perforation of a viscus other than the bladder. Am J Dis Child 117:590, 1969.
96. Morell RE, Duritz G, Oltorf C. Suprapubic aspiration associated with hematoma. Pediatrics 69:455, 1982.
97. Mandell J, Stevens PS. Supravesical hematoma following suprapubic urine aspiration. J Urol 119:286, 1978.
98. Schreiver RL, Skafish P. Complications of suprapubic bladder aspiration. Am J Dis Child 132:98, 1978.
99. Pass RF, Waldo FB. Anaerobic bacteremia following suprapubic bladder aspiration. J Pediatr 94:748, 1979.
100. Goldberg BB, Meyer H. Ultrasonically guided suprapubic urinary bladder aspiration. Pediatrics 51:70, 1973.
101. Kiernan SC, Pinckert TL, Kesler M. Ultrasound guidance of supra-pubic bladder aspiration in neonates. J Pediatr 123:789, 1993.
102. Pryles CV, Lüders D, Alkan MK. A comparative study of bacterial cultures and colony counts in paired specimens of urine obtained by catheter versus voiding from normal infants and infants with urinary tract infection. Pediatrics 27:17, 1961.
103. Hoberman A, Wald ER, Reynolds EA, et al. Pyuria and bacteriuria in urine specimens obtained by catheter from young children with fever. J Pediatr 124:513, 1994.
104. Pitetti RD, Choi S. Utility of blood cultures in febrile children with UTI. Am J Emerg Med 20:271, 2002.
105. Braude H, Forfar JO, Gould JC, et al. Cell and bacterial counts in the urine of normal infants and children. BMJ 4:697, 1967.

106. Houston IB. Urinary white cell excretion in childhood. Arch Dis Child 40:313, 1965.
107. Lam CN, Bremner AD, Maxwell JD, et al. Pyuria and bacteriuria. Arch Dis Child 42:275, 1967.
108. Hewstone AS, Lawson JS. Microscopic appearance of urine in the neonatal period. Arch Dis Child 39:287, 1964.
109. Littlewood JM. White cells and bacteria in voided urine of healthy newborns. Arch Dis Child 46:167, 1971.
110. Lincoln K, Winberg J. Studies of urinary tract infection in infancy and childhood: III. Quantitative estimation of cellular excretion in unselected neonates. Acta Paediatr Scand 53:447, 1964.
111. Huicho L, Campos-Sanchez M, Alamo C. Metaanalysis of urine screening tests for determining the risk of urinary tract infection in children. Pediatr Infect Dis J 21:1, 2002.
112. Hoberman A, Wald ER, Reynolds EA, et al. Is urine culture necessary to rule out urinary tract infection in young febrile children? Pediatr Infect Dis J 15:304, 1996.
113. Shaw KN, McGowan KL, Gorelick MH, et al. Screening for urinary tract infection in infants in the emergency department: which test is best? Pediatrics 101:1, 1998.
114. Emanuel B, Aronson N. Neonatal hematuria. Am J Dis Child 128:204, 1974.
115. Visser VE, Hall RT. Urine culture in the evaluation of suspected neonatal sepsis. J Pediatr 94:635, 1979.
116. DiGeronimo RJ. Lack of efficacy of the urine culture as part of the initial work up of suspected neonatal sepsis. Pediatr Infect Dis J 11:764, 1992.
117. Stokland E, Hellström M, Jacobsson B, et al. Renal damage one year after first urinary tract infection: role of dimercaptosuccinic acid scintigraphy. J Pediatr 129:815, 1996.
118. Prat C, Dominguez J, Rodrigo C, et al. Elevated serum procalcitonin values correlate with renal scarring in children with urinary tract infection. Pediatr Infect Dis J 22:438, 2003.
119. Hamdan JM, Rizk F. Jaundice complicating urinary tract infection in childhood. Pediatr Infect Dis 4:418, 1985.
120. Kassner EG, Elguezabal A, Pochaczevsky R. Death during intravenous urography: overdosage in young infants. N Y State J Med 73:1958, 1973.
121. Fine RN. Diagnosis and treatment of fetal urinary tract abnormalities. J Pediatr 121:333, 1992.
122. Strife CF, Gelfand MJ. Renal cortical scintigraphy: effect on medical decision making in childhood urinary tract infection. J Pediatr 129:785, 1996.
123. Hellerstein S. Evolving concepts in the evaluation of the child with a urinary tract infection. J Pediatr 124:589, 1994.
124. Conway JJ, Cohn RA. Evolving role of nuclear medicine for the diagnosis and management of urinary tract infection. J Pediatr 124:87, 1994.
125. Dick PT, Feldman W. Routine diagnostic imaging for childhood urinary tract infections: a systematic overview. J Pediatr 128:15, 1996.
126. Slyper AH, Olson JC, Nair RB. Overwhelming *Escherichia coli* sepsis in ureterovesical junction obstruction without reflux. Arch Pediatr Adolesc Med 148:1102, 1994.
127. Goldman M, Lahat E, Strauss S, et al. Imaging after urinary tract infection in male neonates. Pediatrics 105:1232, 2000.
128. Hoberman A, Charron M, Hickey RW, et al. Imaging studies after a first febrile urinary tract infection in young children. N Engl J Med 348:195, 2003.
129. Stapleton FB. Imaging studies for childhood urinary infections. N Engl J Med 348:251, 2003.
130. Hellerstein S. Antibiotic treatment for urinary tract infections in pediatric patients. Pediatrics 112:1213, 2003.
131. Williams G, Lee A, Craig J. Antibiotics for the prevention of urinary tract infection in children: a systematic review of randomized controlled trials. J Pediatr 138:868, 2001.
132. Hoffpauir CW, Guidry DJ. Asymptomatic urinary tract infection in premature infants. Pediatrics 45:128, 1970.
133. Benador D, Benador N, Slosman D, et al. Are younger children at highest risk of renal sequelae after pyelonephritis? Lancet 349:17, 1997.
134. Lowe LH, Patel MN, Gatti JM, et al. Utility of follow-up renal sonography in children with vesicoureteral reflux and normal initial sonogram. Pediatrics 113:548, 2004.
135. Sreenarasimhaiah S, Hellerstein S. Urinary tract infections per se do not cause end-stage kidney disease. Pediatr Nephrol 12:210, 1998.
136. Marra G, Oppezzo C, Ardissino G, et al. Severe vesiculoureteral reflux and chronic renal failure: a condition peculiar to male gender? Data from the ItalKid project. J Pediatr 144:677, 2004.

Chapter 10

FOCAL BACTERIAL INFECTIONS

Gary D. Overturf

INFECTIONS OF THE LIVER

Bacterial infection of the hepatic parenchyma frequently is recognized as multiple, small inflammatory foci (microabscesses) observed as an incidental finding in infants dying with sepsis. Diffuse hepatocellular damage, often in conjunction with infection of several organ systems, may be present after transplacental passage of microorganisms to the fetal circulation. On rare occasions, liver involvement may take the form of a solitary purulent abscess. Metastatic focal infections of the liver associated with bacteremia resolve with antimicrobial therapy, are not recognized, or are found only at postmortem examination. Rarely are they clinically apparent as solitary[1] or multiple[2] large abscesses diagnosed during life.

Although metastatic infections are rare, it is difficult to ascertain their true incidence. In a survey of more than 7500 autopsies of children performed between 1917 and 1967, Dehner and Kissane[3] found only three neonates with multiple, small, pyogenic hepatic abscesses, whereas a review of approximately 4900 autopsies[4] performed at Los Angeles Children's Hospital between 1958 and 1978 revealed 9 such infants.[5] Among 175,000 neonates admitted between 1957 and 1977 to Milwaukee Children's Hospital, 2 died with hepatic microabscesses[6]; 3 such patients were seen among 83,000 pediatric patients admitted to New York Hospital between 1945 and 1983,[7] and 1 was reported at the University of Texas Medical Branch in Galveston between 1963 and 1984.[8] Most reviewers who have discussed postmortem observations of infants dying with neonatal sepsis have not described the occurrence of such secondary sites of infection[9-16] or have presented them as an occasional ancillary finding.[17,18]

Similarly, solitary hepatic abscesses in the newborn have also been reported rarely. About 30 such cases have been described.[1,3,4,19-41] These infections frequently are associated with prematurity and umbilical vein catheterization,[5,6,21,22,25,28,32,34-41] whereas solitary abscesses may occur because of bacteremia. For example, Murphy and Baker[42] describe a solitary abscess after sepsis caused by *Staphylococcus aureus.*

Microbiology

Any bacteria that invade the bloodstream can cause multiple microabscesses in the liver. The etiologic agents in the infants described by Dehner and Kissane,[3] Moss and Pysher,[5] Chusid,[6] and Miedema and co-workers[7] included *Escherichia coli, S. aureus, Pseudomonas aeruginosa, Klebsiella* sp., *Enterobacter* sp., and *Listeria monocytogenes.* However, the causative bacteria of solitary abscesses are generally those colonizing the umbilical stump,[43] including *S. aureus* (11 cases); *E. coli* alone (3 cases); *E. coli* with *S. aureus* (2 cases) or enterococcus

(1 case); *Enterobacter* sp. (3 cases); *Klebsiella pneumoniae* alone (2 cases); *K. pneumoniae* with *Proteus* sp. (1 case); *P. aeruginosa* (1 case); *Staphylococcus epidermidis* with group F *Streptococcus* (1 case); and *Streptococcus pyogenes* (1 case). In three infants, the abscesses were described as "sterile."[19,28,31] Although one of these infants had received penicillin for 9 days before surgical drainage, it is possible that in all three cases the abscesses were caused by anaerobic bacteria that failed to grow under standard conditions of transport and culture. The presence of gas in seven abscesses[25,28,34,35,39] may indicate infection with anaerobes, a frequent cause of liver abscess in adults.[44]

The most common cause of intrauterine bacterial hepatitis, congenital listeriosis, characteristically involves the liver and adrenals (see Chapter 14). Typical lesions are histologically sharply demarcated areas of necrosis (miliary granulomatosis) or microabscesses containing numerous pleomorphic gram-positive bacilli.[15] Descriptions in the early 1900s of miliary necrosis of the liver related to "gram-positive argentophilic rodlike organisms" probably also represented infections with *L. monocytogenes,* which was not isolated and identified until 1926.[26]

Intrauterine tuberculosis results from maternal bacillemia with transplacental dissemination to the fetal bloodstream (see Chapter 19). Because the liver is perfused by blood with a high oxygen content[45] and is the first organ that encounters tubercle bacilli, it is often severely involved.[15,44,46] The presence of primary liver foci is considered prima facie evidence for the congenital nature of tuberculous lesions as a result of hematogenous spread through the umbilical vein.[47] However, closed-needle biopsy may be less accurate in the diagnosis of hepatic granulomas, and open biopsy may be required to confirm liver and regional node involvement.[48] Although generalized fetal infection may also arise through aspiration of contaminated amniotic fluid, the lesions acquired in this manner are usually most prominent in the lungs. In addition to hepatomegaly, a clinical picture of fever with elevated serum IgM and chorioretinitis (e.g., choroid tubercles) may be similar to that caused by other congenital infectious agents.[49] In a review by Abughal and co-workers,[49] positive sites of culture for tuberculosis included liver (8 of 9), gastric aspirate (18 of 23), tracheal aspirate (7 of 7), ear (5 of 6), and cerebrospinal fluid (3 of 10). Noncaseating granulomatous hepatitis, thought to be caused by a hypersensitivity reaction related to bacille Calmette-Guérin (BCG) vaccination, has also been described in a neonate,[50] but histologic and bacteriologic studies performed on liver biopsy specimens failed to identify the presence of acid-fast bacilli or BCG organisms.

On rare occasions, bacterial infection of the fetal liver has been reported in association with maternal tularemia,[51] anthrax,[52] typhoid fever,[53] and brucellosis.[54] It is uncertain whether the isolation of bacteria from the livers of stillborn fetuses is significantly associated with their clinical course.[55,56]

Treponema pallidum is the spirochete most commonly associated with transplacental hepatic infection (see Chapter 18). Pathologic changes in liver, found in up to 95% of infants dying with congenital syphilis,[57] may include those of diffuse hepatitis or focal areas of inflammation, both frequently accompanied by increased connective tissue and enlargement of the liver.[15,57-59] Involvement of liver has also been documented, on the basis of isolation of organisms or their identification in histologic sections, in newborns with intrauterine infection caused by various *Leptospira* species (*Leptospira icterohaemorrhagiae,*[60,61] *Leptospira pomona,*[62] *Leptospira canicola,*[63] *Leptospira kasman*[64]). Transplacental infection of the fetus with *Borrelia recurrentis* causes little or no inflammation of liver parenchyma or biliary epithelium despite the presence of large numbers of spirochetes in the sinusoids.[65-68] Congenital infection has been suggested with *Borrelia burgdorferi*[69] (cause of Lyme disease); hepatic, central nervous system, and cardiac lesions may be observed, and widely disseminated lesions were reported to occur in other tissues.

Pathogenesis

Infectious agents may reach the liver of the fetus or newborn by one of several pathways: transplacental or transorificial intrauterine infection; extension of thrombophlebitis of the umbilical vein; through the hepatic artery during the course of a systemic bacteremia; pylephlebitis due to a focus of infection in the drainage of the portal vein (mesenteric or splenic veins); direct invasion from contiguous structures or because of trauma or surgical inoculation; and extension up the biliary passages in cases of suppurative cholangitis. Abscesses with no apparent focus of infection seem to be relatively common in the newborn compared with older children.[30] Three such cases, all in infants with solitary hepatic abscesses, have been described.[23,24,31] Descriptions of the surgical findings, together with the nature of the lesions, suggest that an umbilical vein infection, obscured by the large collection of purulent material in the abscess, was the probable pathogenesis in all infants.

The mode of infection usually determines the pattern of hepatic involvement. Intense and prolonged seeding of the liver parenchyma, such as that which occurs in conjunction with intrauterine infection or neonatal sepsis, almost invariably results in diffuse hepatocellular damage or multiple small inflammatory lesions.[3,5,6] Umbilical vein thrombophlebitis, may cause an abscess of the falciform ligament[70] or extend into a single branch of the portal vein to produce a solitary pyogenic abscess,[6,21,22,26,29,32,33] or it can lead to disseminated foci of infection through dislodgment of septic emboli.[6,71-74]

The frequent use of umbilical catheters has been associated with an increase in the numbers of infants with solitary[5,6,20-22,32,34-40] or multiple[5,75,76] hepatic abscesses. In three large series, including almost 500 infants who died after placement of umbilical vein catheters, 29 infants were found to have purulent infections of hepatic vessels or parenchyma.[37,75,77] Use of venous catheters for infusion of hypertonic or acidic solutions may provide a necrotic focus for abscess formation,[21,32,34-36,76,77] and prolonged[5,22,32,77] or repeated[63] catheterization of a necrotic umbilical stump provides an ideal pathway for introduction of pathogenic organisms. It has been postulated that some hepatic abscesses have been caused by infusion of contaminated plasma[28] or by the use of nonsterile umbilical catheters.[75]

Although neonatal liver abscesses usually are caused by hematogenous dissemination of bacteria through the hepatic artery or umbilical vein, examples of infection arising from various other sources have been described. Solitary abscesses have followed a presumed portal vein bacteremia caused by amebic colitis.[19,20] Direct invasion of adjacent liver parenchyma from purulent cholecystitis[24] or postoperative perihepatic abscesses[5] also has been observed. Ascending cholangitis, the most frequent cause of hepatic purulent infections in adults,[30] has not been implicated in the causes of newborn infections.

Disease due to embryonic anatomic errors is unique to newborns. Shaw and Pierog[78] described a newborn with umbilical herniation of a pedunculated supernumerary lobe of the liver; histologic examination showed numerous small foci of early abscess formation. Although signs and symptoms of sepsis appeared at 18 days of age, possibly the result of bacterial spread from the liver to the umbilical vein, the infant improved and ultimately recovered after removal of the polypoid mass on the 19th day of life.

Descriptions of "umbilical sepsis" and "acute interstitial hepatitis" recorded by Morison seem to indicate that his patients had acquired bacterial infections of umbilical vessels with widespread extension into portal tracts.[79] Although mild periportal parenchymal necrosis was observed in a few infants, hepatocellular damage was minimal or absent in most. Similar lesions have been found in infants dying with sepsis[80] and infantile diarrhea.[81]

Clinical Manifestations

Multiple hepatic abscesses and diffuse hepatitis related to neonatal sepsis or transplacental fetal infection are usually recognized only at autopsy. Very few clinical manifestations referable to hepatocellular damage are evident before death. The signs and symptoms associated with these conditions are those of the underlying sepsis or of secondary metastatic complications such as meningitis, pneumonitis, or peritonitis.[2,3,29,33,72,75]

Solitary abscesses are indolent in terms of their development and clinical presentation. Although the suppurative umbilical focus or umbilical catheterization responsible for the introduction of microorganisms can usually be traced to the first week of life, evidence of hepatic involvement is usually not apparent before the second or third week. The abscess frequently becomes a source for the hematogenous dissemination of microorganisms, so that most infants have signs and symptoms of a bacteremia. Despite intense infection of the underlying vessels, inspection of the umbilical stump usually shows no evidence of inflammation or purulent discharge. The presence of hepatomegaly, a finding commonly associated with neonatal sepsis, also offers little aid in establishing a definitive diagnosis. In one half of infants for whom physical findings are clearly described, a well-delineated, often fluctuant or tender mass could be palpated in the epigastrium or right upper quadrant. On a few occasions, this mass was noticed by the infant's mother several days before the onset of systemic symptoms. Abscesses occur in the right or left lobe of the liver with almost equal frequency and are generally 3 cm or more in diameter at the time of surgical exploration.

Diagnosis

Hematologic studies are of little value in establishing a diagnosis; leukocyte counts and sedimentation rates may be normal or elevated. The serum levels of liver enzymes may also be normal[25,38] or elevated.[5,23,36]

Abdominal radiographs are usually normal or show nonspecific displacement of the lower edge of the liver. In five infants, diagnosis was suspected from plain x-ray films by the presence of gas within the hepatic shadow.[28,32,34,39] Radiologic findings that commonly accompany hepatic abscess in older children, such as an altered contour of the diaphragm, right pleural effusion, and platelike atelectasis,[82] are rarely present in the neonate.

Ultrasonography should be the initial imaging study in newborns with clinical evidence of a hepatic abscess.[83-86] If negative, and the diagnosis is still strongly suspected, more sensitive techniques such as computed tomography (CT) or magnetic resonance imaging (MRI) should be performed.[83-88] Enhancement with contrast agents may increase the definition of smaller abscesses. Because congenital cysts, arteriovenous malformations, and tumors with central necrosis or hemorrhage can mimic hepatic abscess, the diagnosis should always be confirmed by aspiration of purulent material at laparotomy or by means of percutaneous drainage with ultrasound or CT guidance.[84,89,90]

Prognosis

The prognosis for infants with diffuse liver involvement related to fetal or neonatal sepsis is that of the underlying condition because hepatic function is rarely compromised sufficiently to determine the outcome. In most cases, pathologic changes in the liver are unsuspected before postmortem examination.

Of 24 infants with solitary hepatic abscesses whose course was described, 8 died. Two infants died before antibiotics were available,[26] and the death of another was ascribed to cecal perforation.[20] Four newborns died with sepsis caused by organisms that were identical to those isolated from the abscess.[21,25,33,34] Prematurity was undoubtedly a major contributing factor in two of these deaths.[21,25]

Treatment

Newborns with a solitary hepatic abscess have traditionally been treated with open surgical drainage in conjunction with antibiotic therapy. Developments in the therapy for pyogenic liver abscess during the past few years suggest that a reassessment of this approach may be in order.

Several investigators have described the use of percutaneous drainage of intrahepatic abscesses and cysts, guided by CT or ultrasonography, in neonates[41,75,90] and children.[7,84,89] When combined with antibiotic therapy and monitored by ultrasonography to ensure resolution, this treatment has been highly effective. It is questionable whether drainage contributed to recovery other than by aiding the selection of antibiotic coverage. Subsequently, patients have been successfully treated with empirical antibiotic therapy alone.[91,92] Conservative medical management in infants has been described in only two neonates and a 5-month-old infant.[33,37,78]

The risk of bacteremia and disseminated infection is high in neonates, and the need to identify infecting organisms to guide antibiotic coverage is of greater urgency in the first weeks of life. It is appropriate to ascertain a microbiologic diagnosis with radiographically guided aspiration or drainage of any definable hepatic abscess in a newborn. When proper equipment (e.g., CT, ultrasonography) and experienced personnel are available, this can be attempted percutaneously.[89,90] When they are not available, open surgical drainage should be performed. Empirical antibiotic therapy should be reserved only for infants for whom it is believed that the risk of open or closed drainage would exceed the potential benefits.

If purulent material is obtained, initial antibiotic therapy can be selected on the basis of Gram staining results. In addition to *S. aureus* and the aerobic enteric organisms commonly associated with hepatic abscesses, anaerobic bacteria have been suspected as the cause of infection in a substantial number of patients.[25,28,32,33,35,39] If foul-smelling pus is aspirated or if Gram-stained smears show organisms with the characteristic morphology of anaerobes,[33] metronidazole, β-lactam and β-lactamase inhibitor combinations (e.g., piperacillin and tazobactam), clindamycin, or imipenem should be included in the initial regimen. Cultures of blood, cerebrospinal fluid, and urine should also be obtained before initiation of therapy.

If empirical antibiotic therapy is required, it must be adequate for infections caused by *S. aureus*, enteric organisms, and anaerobic bacteria. Oxacillin, gentamicin, and clindamycin is an appropriate combination. In nurseries where methicillin-resistant *S. aureus* or *S. epidermidis* infections have been a problem, substitution of vancomycin for oxacillin can provide coverage for these organisms. Gentamicin (and other aminoglycosides) and vancomycin levels must be monitored and dosages adjusted as necessary. Extended-spectrum cephalosporins (e.g., cefotaxime, cefepime, ceftazidime) may be used for enteric organisms and *Pseudomonas* sp., often obviating the need for aminoglycosides.

Definitive therapy is based on results of bacteriologic cultures that identify the bacteria and its antibiotic susceptibility. Adequate anaerobic transport and culture techniques must therefore be available if meaningful information is to be obtained. Duration of treatment is based on clinical response, cessation of drainage, and resolution of the abscess cavity as determined by serial ultrasonographic examinations. Parenteral therapy should be maintained for at least 2 weeks and may be individualized to longer therapy when necessary. In older children treated with multiple abscesses or in those for whom surgery is not feasible, therapy for up to 6 weeks or more has been recommended.

SPLENIC ABSCESS

Similar to hepatic abscesses, splenic abscesses have been rarely described in infants.[93] Only 1 of 55 splenic abscesses occurred in an infant younger than 6 months. *S. aureus*, *Candida* sp., and streptococci were the most frequent causes. In 20 of 48 cases, hepatic abscesses coexisted with splenic abscess. In the single infant case, torsion of the splenic vessels was present, whereas in older children, other distant infections of hematologic conditions (e.g., hemoglobinopathy, hematogenous malignancy) were the associated comorbid conditions.

INFECTIONS OF THE BILIARY TRACT

The development of ultrasonography has provided a safe and rapid means for evaluating the neonatal gallbladder. Consequently, an increasing number of reports have appeared within the past 10 years describing ultrasonographic changes seen in the first month of life, with hydrops,[94,95] cholelithiasis,[95-100] and transient distention of the gallbladder associated[94,95,99,101-104] or unassociated[99,102,103,105-108] with sepsis. Ultrasonographic criteria for separating normal from pathologically enlarged gallbladders and biliary tracts in neonates have also been described.[109,110]

Despite advanced technology and increased surveillance, cholecystitis in the neonate is observed infrequently. The literature has documented about 25 cases, of which 9 were seen in association with an epidemic of neonatal enteritis caused by *Salmonella enteritidis*.[111] Of the remaining infants, 16 were the subjects of isolated case reports[24,103,112-123] and 3 died of other causes with inflammatory changes in the gallbladder described as an incidental finding at autopsy.[81,95,124] A tissue diagnosis of "chronic cholecystitis" was established in an infant whose biliary disease apparently began at 6 days of age.[125]

The pathogenesis of this condition is uncertain; all but three cases[99,118,122] of cholecystitis in the newborn period have been acalculous. It is postulated that sepsis, dehydration, prolonged fasting (e.g., total parenteral nutrition), congenital obstruction, or a stone impacted in the cystic duct leads to biliary stasis and acute distention of the gallbladder. In most cases, resolution of the primary process permits restoration of the flow of bile and relief of distention. In some cases, prolonged obstruction leads to hydrops.[94] Cholecystitis rarely follows, perhaps because of a direct toxic effect of retained bile or because of ischemia related to elevated intraluminal pressure. Bacterial invasion by fecal flora is probably a secondary phenomenon.[114,115,126] Organisms that have been isolated from gallbladder contents or tissue include *E. coli*,[114-116,123] *Serratia marcescens*,[103,117] *Pseudomonas* sp.,[115] *Streptococcus faecalis*,[123] "*Streptococcus viridans*,"[121] *S. aureus*,[123] and *Clostridium welchii*.[123] "Gram-positive cocci" were identified by Gram stain in one patient.[113]

Infants with cholecystitis may become ill at any time during the first weeks of life; most cases are diagnosed in the third or fourth week. The typical clinical picture is one of sepsis together with signs of peritoneal inflammation and a palpable tender right upper quadrant or epigastric mass. Diarrhea frequently accompanies these findings. Although ultrasonography and radionuclide scintigraphy are helpful in suggesting the presence of gallbladder enlargement or inflammation, diagnosis can be confirmed only by surgical exploration.[94,102,103,106,108] Treatment consists of cholecystectomy or tube cholecystotomy, together with systemic antimicrobial therapy based on Gram stain, culture, and susceptibility studies. If a T tube is placed in the gallbladder, a cholangiogram should be done to confirm patency of the biliary system before the tube is removed.

Changes compatible with a diagnosis of ascending cholangitis have been described in histologic sections of liver specimens from infants who died with diarrhea accompanied by hepatocellular injury with cholestasis.[91] Bacteria were also identified in the biliary tree of 2 of 178 premature infants who died after placement of an umbilical venous catheter for an exchange transfusion or for delivery of parenteral fluids.[75] The reasons for this association, if any, are unclear. An infant with spontaneous cholangitis caused by *Enterobacter agglomerans,* presenting as a fever of unknown origin at 3 weeks of age, has also been reported.[127]

Severe inflammation and fibrosis of extrahepatic bile ducts and diffuse changes in the portal tracts, resembling those found in biliary atresia, were found in a premature infant who died when 3 hours old of listeriosis.[128] The investigator postulated that occult prenatal infections with *L. monocytogenes* might be a rare cause of ascending cholangitis presenting as idiopathic biliary atresia at birth.

INFECTIONS OF THE ADRENAL GLANDS

Multiple adrenal microabscesses are occasionally found as metastatic lesions associated with neonatal sepsis. Such abscesses are particularly characteristic of neonatal listeriosis (see Chapter 14). Solitary adrenal abscesses, however, are rare, and only about 25 such cases have been described.[17,129-150]

The spectrum of organisms responsible for adrenal abscesses is the same as that seen in neonatal sepsis, including *E. coli* (seven cases),[17,129,130,135-138] streptococcus group B (four cases),[138-141] *Proteus mirabilis* (three cases),[131,132,144] *S. aureus,*[142,143] *Bacteroides* sp.,[133,145] and two cases each of *Streptococcus pneumoniae* with *Bacteroides* sp.[134]; *Peptostreptococcus* sp.[146] was recovered from one case. Drainage of foul-smelling pus at surgery suggests that anaerobic bacteria may have been present in two infants from whom *E. coli* and *S. aureus* were isolated.[136,142] Cultures were not obtained from four patients.[147-150]

Fourteen abscesses were located on the right side, seven were located on the left, and three[138,139,147] were bilateral. Three fourths of the infants were male. The same laterality and sex predominance are seen with adrenal hemorrhage in the newborn,[147,150-152] and it has been postulated that formation of an adrenal abscess requires a preexisting hematoma as a nidus for bacterial seeding.[137,138] This theory of pathogenesis is further supported by clinical observations,[134,135,139,146,147] and by objective evidence (e.g., curvilinear calcifications[130,132]) documenting the presence of hemorrhage before development of an abscess.[134,138,142,145,150]

Most infants with adrenal abscess have presented in the third or fourth week of life with signs of sepsis and an abdominal or flank mass. A history of difficult delivery or intrapartum asphyxia has been observed in about one half of these infants and significant maternal fever or infection during labor in about one fourth.[138,140,141,150] Although a few infants are afebrile when first evaluated, a palpable mass is almost always present. Abscesses are usually 6 to 8 cm in diameter, with some containing as much as 200 mL of pus[133] and measuring up to 12 cm in diameter[134] or crossing the midline.[146]

Laboratory studies are helpful in the evaluation of a possible adrenal abscess. Most infants demonstrate a leukocytosis; about one third are anemic with a history of prolonged neonatal jaundice, both of which are features associated with adrenal hemorrhage. Urinary excretion of catecholamines and their metabolites (particularly vanillylmandelic acid and homovanillic acid), which is usually increased with neuroblastoma, is normal. Because most infants with adrenal abscess are seen for evaluation of possible sepsis, a blood culture, lumbar puncture, urine culture, and chest radiograph should be obtained.

Ultrasonography has become a widely accepted modality for initial evaluation of all neonatal abdominal masses. With the presence of an adrenal abscess, ultrasound examination can help to define the extent and cystic nature of the lesion and often can demonstrate movable necrotic debris in the abscess cavity.[132,137,138,141,142,144-148] With serial examinations, abscesses can be distinguished from those masses associated with liquefying hematoma, adrenal cyst, hydronephrosis of an obstructed upper pole duplication, or necrotic neuroblastoma.[138,140,150,153-154] Intravenous pyelography demonstrates downward displacement of the kidney and compression of the upper calyces, which confirms the presence of a suprarenal mass.[130-132,134,136,138,141,142,144-146,149] A round, suprarenal, radiopaque halo or rim with central lucency, which is characteristic of adrenal abscess, may also be seen on early films[137,139,143] but is not pathognomonic.[138] Intravenous pyelography adds little diagnostic information to that provided by ultrasound studies. Experience with radionuclide scanning,[140,142,143] CT,[138,144] and MRI[126] in this condition is limited, but these modalities are likely to be as useful as ultrasonography.

Whatever diagnostic methods are used, concern about persisting signs of sepsis and the more than possible presence of an adrenal neoplasm usually encourage early efforts to establish a diagnosis. In the past, recommended management has been incision and drainage or resection of the abscess.[134,138,141,144,150] Needle aspiration under ultrasonographic guidance, combined with placement of a catheter for drainage and irrigation, has proved to be a useful alternative method[88,130,131,143] and probably will supplant open drainage as the preferred method. Antibiotic therapy should be based on Gram stain, culture, and susceptibility studies of abscess fluid and should be continued for 10 to 14 days provided drainage can be established.

The adrenals are infected in about 15% of infants with congenital syphilis.[57,58] In addition to the presence of spirochetes, the most frequent and characteristic change is an extraordinary amount of cellular connective tissue in the capsule.

APPENDICITIS

Acute appendicitis is extremely rare in infants younger than 4 weeks of age. Reviews of more than 25,000 cases of appendicitis in infants and children in Great Britain,[156] Ireland,[157] Norway,[158] Germany,[159] and the United States[160-165] revealed only eight infants who presented during the neonatal period. Pediatric surgery centers in Germany,[166] Boston,[167] Cleveland,[168] Chicago,[169] and Detroit[170] found only four cases of neonatal appendicitis during the past 15 to 20 years. Since the condition was first described by Albrecht in 1905[171,172] and Diess in 1908,[173] approximately 65 cases of neonatal suppurative appendicitis have been reported in the literature with sufficient details to permit characterization of the clinical features,[156,161,162,165,174-211] and the following discussion is based on a review of those cases. Only infants with acute intra-abdominal appendicitis were considered. Those with appendicitis caused by other conditions, such as

Hirschsprung's disease,[212,213] necrotizing enterocolitis (NEC),[214] or incarceration in an inguinal hernia,[215,216] have not been included. An additional 25 to 30 cases that have been reported with incomplete clinical observations, listed in series of patients with neonatal peritonitis (see "Peritonitis") or mentioned in other review articles but not available for analysis, are also not included.

Inflammation of the appendix is more common in male newborns than in female newborns. In those reports in which the sex was stated, 40 cases occurred in males and 17 in females. Prematurity also appears to be a predisposing factor: 23 of the 49 infants whose birth weights were recorded weighed less than 2500 g at birth. The incidence of appendicitis in infants of multiple births (six twins and one triplet) appears to be higher than would be expected on the basis of low birth weight alone.

Microbiology

Because obstruction of the appendiceal lumen is responsible for almost all cases of appendicitis,[167] it is intuitive that gram-negative enteric organisms resident in the bowel are usually isolated from the peritoneal fluid or periappendiceal pus of about 75% of infants. Specific etiologic agents have included *E. coli, Klebsiella, Enterobacter* sp., *Pseudomonas, Proteus* sp., untyped *Streptococcus, S. aureus,* and *Bacteroides* sp. These bacterial species have also been isolated from the peritoneal fluid of older children with appendicitis.[164,167,217] Attempts at isolation of anaerobic bacteria have been rarely described.

A single case of perforated amebic appendicitis with secondary bacterial peritonitis and multiple hepatic abscesses in a premature infant born in Great Britain has been reported. The *Entamoeba histolytica* observed in the wall of the necrotic appendix was presumably acquired from the infant's father, who was a carrier.[20]

A patient with gangrenous appendicitis associated with *Rhizopus oryzae* has also been reported.[218] It was postulated that the fungus colonized the infant's gut by transfer from an adhesive bandage used to secure an endotracheal tube.

Pathogenesis

Obstruction of the appendiceal lumen has been generally accepted as the primary cause of appendicitis in all age groups. The relative rarity of this condition in the first month of life is therefore probably related to factors that serve to decrease the likelihood of obstruction. Such factors include a wide-based, funnel-shaped appendix; the predominantly liquid and soft-solid diet given to infants; the absence of prolonged periods in the upright position; and the infrequency of infections that cause hyperplasia of the appendiceal lymphoid tissue.[164,219,220]

The causes of luminal obstruction in the newborn period, when recognized, are often extrinsic to the appendix itself. Reports of appendicitis caused by the presence of ectopic pancreatic tissue,[161] a fecalith,[175] or meconium plug[168] are unusual exceptions. In 1911, it was suggested that sharp angulation of the appendix, bent on itself in the narrow retrocolic space, may be an important cause of obstruction,[221] however, this anatomy, found in 11 neonates with inflammatory changes in the appendix and noted among 200 consecutive autopsies in infants younger than 3 months at death, has not been repeated in the past 80 years.

Inflammation of the appendix with perforation has been described as the presenting illness in several infants with neonatal Hirschsprung's disease.[212,214] The association of these two conditions has been attributed to functional obstruction, increased intraluminal pressure, and fecal trapping that occur proximal to aganglionic segments. Suppurative appendicitis related to incarceration and strangulation of the cecum within an inguinal or scrotal hernia has been found in a significant number of infants.[215,216]

Clinical Manifestations

The onset of neonatal appendicitis generally occurs during the first 2 weeks of life. Only 3 of 54 infants with this condition presented between the 21st and 20th days. The reasons for this phenomenon are unclear, particularly in view of the relatively even distribution of cases during the remainder of the first year of life.[165] Five cases of "prenatal" appendicitis have been described.[222-226] Of the four available for analysis, only one showed definite evidence of a suppurative process in the appendix and signs of bowel obstruction clearly present at birth[222]; however, cultures and Gram stain of the pus found at surgery were free of bacteria. Poisoning by mercuric chloride was suspected in one[224] of the remaining three cases, and the other two, who were said to have prenatal rupture of the appendix, were asymptomatic until the second[222] and twelfth[226] days of life.

The signs of neonatal appendicitis correspond to those of any of the various forms of intestinal obstruction that occur during the newborn period (Table 10-1).[226] Prominent early findings include abdominal distention, progressive and frequently bilious vomiting, and evidence of pain, as manifested by persistent crying, irritability, or "colic." Clinical features such as diarrhea, constipation, lethargy, or refusal to feed may also be evident but are too nonspecific to be helpful in establishing a diagnosis. The presence or absence of fever is an unreliable sign in appendicitis as in other forms of neonatal infection; temperature has been recorded as normal or subnormal in more than 50% of newborns with this condition. Abdominal tenderness and guarding are inconstant findings and, when present, are rarely localized to the appendiceal area. Physical signs of

Table 10–1 Signs of Intra-abdominal Neonatal Appendicitis in 55 Infants

Sign	Incidence (%)
Abdominal distention	90
Vomiting	60
Refusal of feedings	40
Temperature ≥ 38° C	40
Temperature 37° C to 38° C	30
Temperature ≤ 37° C	30
Pain (crying, restlessness)	30
Lethargy	30
Erythema/edema of right lower quadrant	25
Mass in right lower quadrant	20
Diarrhea	20
Passage of bloody stools	20

sufficient specificity to indicate acute inflammation of the appendix are generally absent until late in the course of the illness, when gangrene and rupture may result in the formation of a localized intra-abdominal abscess or cellulitis of the anterior abdominal wall. Erythema or edema, or both, of the right lower quadrant has been observed in several patients. The presence of this finding, particularly when accompanied by a palpable mass in the right iliac fossa, indicates bowel perforation with peritonitis and should suggest a preoperative diagnosis of NEC or appendicitis (see "Necrotizing Enterocolitis").

Diagnosis

The diagnosis of appendicitis in the neonate is usually determined at surgery performed for evaluation of abdominal distention and suspected peritonitis. With the high incidence of prematurity associated with early appendicitis, bowel perforation from NEC has been a common preoperative consideration.[207] The two conditions can coexist, and in some cases, the appendix may participate in the process of ischemic necrosis and perforation.[206,214]

Laboratory studies are of little value in establishing a diagnosis of appendicitis in the newborn. White blood cell counts of less than 10,000/mm^3 were found in 10 of 30 infants for whom this determination was performed. Urinalyses are usually normal, although ketonuria, which reflects diminished caloric intake, hematuria, and proteinuria may be seen. Because bacteremia may accompany appendiceal perforation and peritonitis, a blood culture and evaluation for metastatic infection with lumbar puncture and chest radiography should be performed. The value of paracentesis for diagnosis of bowel perforation and peritoneal infection is discussed later (see "Necrotizing Enterocolitis").

Radiologic examinations are occasionally helpful, but in most cases serve only to confirm a clinical impression of small bowel obstruction. The presence of an increased soft tissue density displacing loops of intestine from the right iliac fossa generally indicates appendiceal perforation with abscess formation and is perhaps the most reliable sign of acute appendicitis in the neonate. Extraluminal gas may be localized briefly to the right lower quadrant after rupture of the appendix.[212] The rapid development of an extensive pneumoperitoneum, however, obscures the site of origin of the escaping gas in most infants within a short time.[227] Ultrasonography may aid in detection of a periappendiceal abscess[83] but lacks sensitivity and specificity to be of assistance in establishing an early diagnosis of appendicitis.

Prognosis

The overall mortality rate from appendicitis in the newborn is high but is improving. Eight of the newborns in the last 12 reported cases have survived, whereas of 60 infants with this condition for whom the outcome was recorded, 38 (64%) died. Survival was unrelated to birth weight. Among factors responsible for mortalities, three appear to be of primary importance: delay in diagnosis, a high incidence of perforation, and the rapid onset of diffuse peritonitis after appendiceal rupture.

Perforation has been identified at surgery or autopsy in 70% of newborns with acute appendicitis. The relative frequency of this complication has been attributed to delays in establishing a diagnosis and to certain anatomic features of the appendix in young infants that predispose it to early necrosis and rupture. These features include a meager blood supply that renders the organ more vulnerable to ischemia; a cecum that is relatively smaller and less distensible than that of adults, thereby forcing a greater intraluminal pressure on the appendix; and the presence of a thin muscularis and serosa that readily lose their structural integrity under the combined effects of ischemia and increased internal pressure.[164,182,183,192]

After the appendix ruptures, infants are unable to contain infection efficiently at the site of origin. Rapid dissemination of spilled intestinal contents produces a diffuse peritonitis within hours because of the small size of the infant's omentum, which fails to provide an efficient envelope for escaping material; the relatively longer and more mobile mesenteries, which favor widespread contamination; and the small size of the peritoneal cavity, which also permits access of infected material to areas distant from the site of perforation.[161,167,182,183]

Peritonitis, accompanied by sepsis and by the massive outpouring of fluids, electrolytes, and proteins from inflamed serosal surfaces, is generally the terminal event in neonatal appendicitis. Deterioration of the infant's condition is often extremely rapid; failure to recognize the underlying illness and to institute appropriate therapy promptly is inevitably followed by a fatal outcome.

Treatment

Surgical intervention is essential for survival of young infants with appendicitis. Because vomiting, diarrhea, and anorexia frequently accompany this condition, restoration of fluid and electrolyte balance is a major factor in ensuring a favorable outcome. Loss of plasma into the bowel wall and lumen of the dilated intestine may require additional replacement with whole blood, plasma, or an albumin equivalent. Optimal preparation often necessitates a delay of several hours but remains a major determining factor in the success of any surgical procedure done during the neonatal period.

The preoperative use of antibiotics has been recommended in infants with intestinal obstruction to achieve therapeutic blood levels of drug before the time of incision and possible contamination.[168,228,229] Although there are few data to support such a recommendation in neonates, any controversy regarding the need for prophylactic antibiotics is generally moot. Perforation, fecal spillage, and peritonitis occur so early in the course of neonatal appendicitis that almost all infants with this condition require treatment before the time of surgery. After the diagnosis of gangrenous or perforated appendicitis has been established and surgery performed, parenteral antibiotic therapy should be continued for 10 days. The combination of clindamycin (or metronidazole), gentamicin (or extended-spectrum cephalosporins), and ampicillin provides adequate coverage against most enteric pathogens and can be used for initial empirical therapy. Alternatively, β-lactam and β-lactamase inhibitor combinations such as ticarcillin plus clavulanate or piperacillin plus tazobactam or carbapenem antibiotics (e.g., imipenem) can be used alone to broadly cover enteric bacteria, *Pseudomonas* sp., and anaerobic bacteria. Until the infant is able to tolerate alimentation, careful attention to postoperative maintenance of body fluids, electrolyte balance, nutrition, and correction of blood and plasma losses is vital to survival (see "Peritonitis" and "Necrotizing Enterocolitis").

PERITONITIS

Peritonitis in the newborn is most commonly associated with perforation of the gastrointestinal tract, ruptured omphaloceles, or wound infections that follow abdominal surgery.[230,231] For this reason, diagnosis and treatment of neonatal peritonitis are less frequently the responsibility of the pediatrician or neonatologist than of the surgeon. It has been estimated that as many as 20% to 40% of gastrointestinal surgical problems in the neonatal period are complicated by bacterial peritonitis (see "Necrotizing Enterocolitis").[186,232] Between 1 and 10 cases per year have been reported in retrospective analyses of peritonitis diagnosed during the first month of life at pediatric surgical centers in the United States,[232-234] Great Britain,[231,235] Hungary,[236] Germany,[237,238] France,[239] and Zimbabwe.[240] Among almost 3000 infants admitted to a neonatal intensive care unit in Liverpool in 1981 to 1982, there were six cases of peritonitis, all from NEC perforation of the gastrointestinal tract.[241] Peritonitis was present in 4 (all of low birth weight) of 501 infants on whom consecutive autopsies were performed from 1960 through 1966 at St. Christopher's Hospital for Children in Philadelphia. These cases represented approximately 3% of all patients with inflammatory lesions associated with death in this age group.[242] Potter considered the peritoneum "one of the most frequent points of localization" in infants dying with sepsis.[15] Among 121 such infants autopsied from 1976 to 1988 at St. Mary's Hospital in Manchester, England, generalized peritonitis was found in 9 (7.4%).[231]

A preponderance of males (2.5:1)[191,240,241] and a high incidence of prematurity (33%)[232,235-237] have been found in unselected series of infants with this condition. These features are probably less a characteristic of bacterial peritonitis in the newborn than of the primary surgical and septic conditions that are responsible for its occurrence (particularly NEC). Among newborns with primary peritonitis, there appears to be a female preponderance.[236,244] A high incidence of congenital anomalies not involving the intestinal tract has also been observed among neonates with peritonitis.[232,237,243,245]

Microbiology

The condition that permits bacteria to colonize the peritoneal surface determines the nature of the infecting organisms. Most infants in whom rupture of a viscus and fecal spillage have caused peritonitis are infected by bacteria considered to be part of the normal enteric microflora; however, prior use of antimicrobial agents and colonization patterns within a nursery are important factors in determining which organisms predominate. Although a mixed flora of two to five species can often be recovered,[243] single isolates have been reported in as many as a third of infants with peritonitis.[246,247] The predominant aerobic organisms usually include *E. coli*, *Klebsiella* sp., *Enterobacter* sp., *Pseudomonas* sp., *Proteus* sp., coagulase-negative and coagulase-positive staphylococci, ungrouped streptococci, *Enterococcus*, and *Candida*.[231,232,238,240,247-249]

Techniques adequate for the isolation of anaerobic organisms have been used infrequently. In a series of 43 consecutive infants with gastrointestinal perforation and bacterial growth from peritoneal fluid, a mixed aerobic-anaerobic flora was isolated with *Bacteroides* sp. as the predominant anaerobes[243]; remaining specimens grew aerobic or facultative organisms alone and no culture yielded only anaerobes. In that series and others, the same organisms were frequently isolated from the peritoneal cavity and blood.[233,243,245,249]

In contrast to fecal flora isolated from infants with gastrointestinal perforation, gram-positive organisms predominated among neonates with "idiopathic primary peritonitis." This condition is caused by sepsis in most cases, but it also has often been associated with omphalitis. Specific organisms in one representative series included *S. pneumoniae* (three cases), ungrouped β-hemolytic *Streptococcus* (three cases), and *S. aureus*, *Pseudomonas* sp., and *E. coli* (one case each).[232] Gram-positive cocci were also the major isolates in other series of peritonitis associated with hematogenous dissemination of organisms or extension from a peripheral suppurative focus.[10,26,33,71,244-254] Many of the cases caused by *S. aureus* occurred before the advent of antibiotics or during the worldwide pandemic of staphylococcal disease in the late 1950s, whereas streptococci, particularly group B, have been a prominent cause in recent years.[244,250-254]

Rarely, peritonitis may be caused by *Candida albicans* in pure culture or mixed with gram-negative enteric organisms.[231,255] Because clinical findings in this condition are not different from those of bacterial peritonitis, the diagnosis is usually established by blood or peritoneal fluid culture. Severe hypothermia has been described as a possible predisposing cause of bowel perforation and peritonitis due to *Candida*.[256] In addition to well-recognized risk factors, such as prematurity, antibiotic therapy, and parenteral nutrition with deep venous catheters, NEC may also be a significant risk factor for systemic candidiasis, in which it was observed in 37% of 30 infants.[257] However, only a single infant in this series had a positive culture for *Candida* species from the peritoneum. Peritoneal catheters or peritoneal dialysis may also be a risk for direct inoculation of *Candida* organisms into the peritoneal space, which occurred in 1 of 26 children[258] (see Chapter 34).

Pathogenesis

Acute bacterial peritonitis may occur whenever bacteria gain access to the peritoneal cavity, through intestinal perforation, by extension from a suppurative focus, or by the hematogenous route. Intrauterine peritonitis due to *L. monocytogenes* has been reported[231]; however, cases of "fetal peritonitis" described in earlier reports were actually examples of meconium peritonitis caused by intrauterine intestinal perforation.[259,260] Although bacterial colonization of the gastrointestinal tract in the first days of life may lead to infection in this condition, it is an aseptic peritonitis in its initial stages. A similar condition with focal perforation of the ileum or colon occurring postnatally has been described in very low birth weight infants. Blue-black discoloration of the abdomen, caused by meconium staining of the tissues of

Table 10–2 Etiology of Bacterial Peritonitis in the Neonatal Period

Gastrointestinal perforation[191,231,232,235–240,243,245,249,262,263]
Necrotizing enterocolitis
Ischemic necrosis
Spontaneous focal gastrointestinal perforation[233,246,249,261,262,264]
Volvulus
Hirschsprung's disease
Meconium ileus (cystic fibrosis)[231,266]
Postoperative complications
Congenital anomalies
Internal hernia
Catheter-associated vascular thrombosis[231]
Indomethacin therapy (enteral or parenteral)[267,268]
Trauma
Feeding tubes[269]
Rectal thermometers, catheters, enema[279–275]
Intrauterine exchange transfusion[231,273]
Paracentesis of ascites fluid
Meconium peritonitis with postnatal bacterial contamination[243,259,260]
Peptic ulcer: stomach, duodenum, ectopic gastric mucosa
Acute suppurative appendicitis
Infection
Shigella or salmonella enterocolitis[274–276]
Congenital luetic enteritis with necrosis[58]
Ruptured omphalocele or gastroschisis
Postoperative: anastomotic leaks, wound dehiscence, wound contamination
Primary peritonitis
Prenatal sepsis: listeriosis, syphilis,[58] tuberculosis[46–49]
Neonatal sepsis[10,33,231,232,240,252–254,263,278]
Suppurative omphalitis[26,72,240,244,250,251,263,277]
Transmural migration (theory)[265,279]

the underlying skin, may be the first striking physical finding in these infants. Clinical, radiographic, and histopathologic evidence of infection or inflammation was notably absent in most cases.[229]

The various conditions that predispose to neonatal peritonitis are outlined in Table 10-2. The relative importance of each in the cause of this condition can be estimated from data collected in several large series. Among almost 400 newborns with peritonitis studied between 1959 and 1978, perforation of the intestinal tract was responsible for 72% of cases, with ruptured omphaloceles or gastroschisis responsible for 12%, hematogenous dissemination or "primary" peritonitis for 12%, and omphalitis and postoperative complications for 2% each.[191,230,231,237,262,263] A comprehensive review of neonatal peritonitis by Bell describes common sites and causes of gastrointestinal perforation and their relative frequencies (Figs. 10-1 and 10-2).[230,243]

No recent cases of neonatal peritonitis have been attributed to microorganisms entering the peritoneal cavity by traversing the bowel wall through the lymphatics or within macrophages (i.e., transmural migration). Evidence for the existence of this pathway is theoretical and is based primarily on retrospective analyses of pathologic data in humans, together with supporting observations made on laboratory animals.[265,279] Further confirmation is necessary before the transmural pathway can be accepted as an established source of peritoneal colonization by bacteria.

Clinical Manifestations

Neonatal peritonitis is a disease primarily of the first 10 days of life; a significant number of infants have evidence of

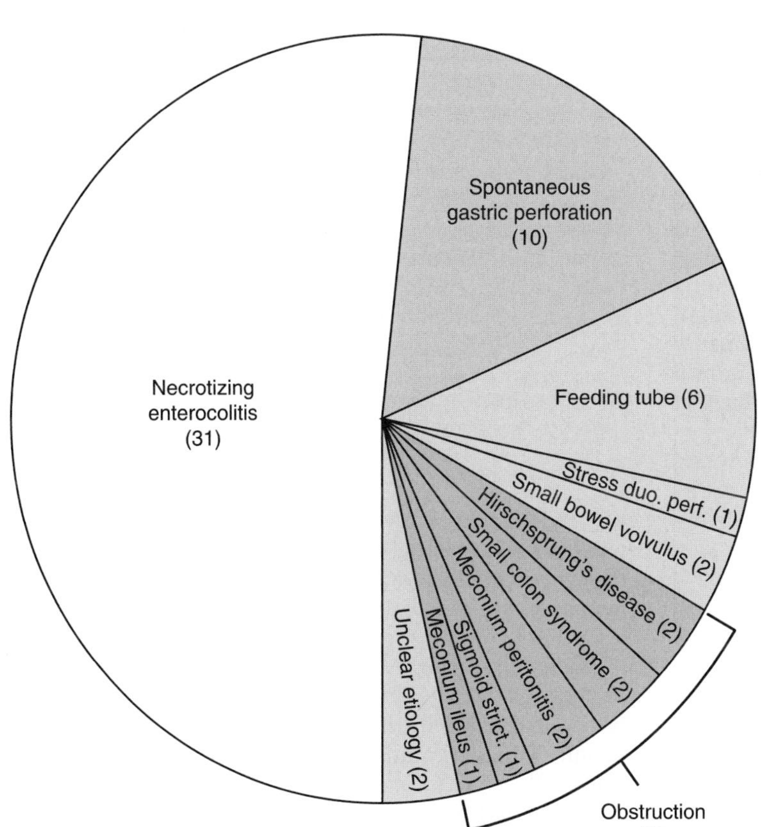

Figure 10–1 Causes of perforation in 60 neonates. (From Bell MJ. Peritonitis in the newborn—current concepts. duo. perf., duodenal perforation; strict., stricture. Pediatr Clin North Am 32:1181, 1985.)

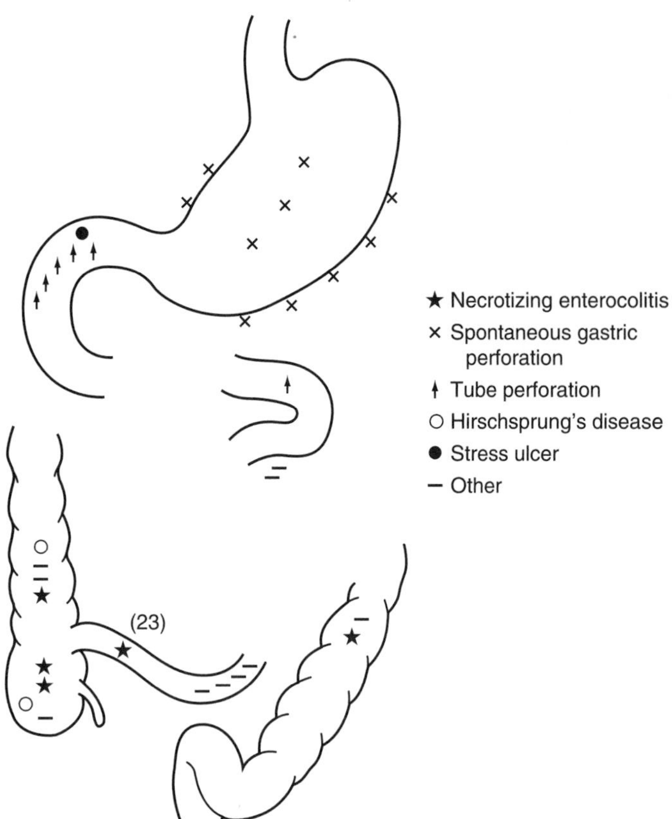

Figure 10–2 Sites of perforation in 60 neonates. (From Bell MJ. Peritonitis in the newborn—current concepts. Pediatr Clin North Am 32:1181, 1985.)

peritoneal infection within the first 24 hours.[232,233,240,245] An analysis of etiologic factors responsible for peritonitis in the newborn provides a ready explanation for this observation (see Table 10-2). Most cases of NEC[243,280] and spontaneous gastric perforation[233,243,249,262] occur within the first week. Ruptured omphaloceles and gastroschisis often develop early infections, and in infants with congenital obstruction, the onset of alimentation during the first 12 to 24 hours accentuates distention and ischemic necrosis of the bowel wall, which leads to early intestinal perforation. Exchange transfusions are performed most frequently within the first 1 or 2 days of life and may be followed by enterocolitis within 4 to 24 hours in infants in whom perforation ultimately occurs.[281,282] Neonatal sepsis, with potential peritoneal seeding of microorganisms, is more frequent during the first 48 hours of life than during any subsequent period.[283]

The variety of signs and symptoms present in a young infant with peritonitis were summarized most succinctly by Thelander[249] in 1939:

The little patient looks sick. He is cyanotic; the respirations are rapid and grunting; the abdomen is distended, and the abdominal wall, the flanks and the scrotum or vulva are usually edematous. Frequently brawny induration of the edematous area, which may resemble erysipelas, is also present. Food is taken poorly or not at all. Vomiting is frequent and persistent. The vomitus contains bile and may contain blood. The stools are either absent or scant; some mucus or blood may be passed. The temperature may be subnormal, but varying degrees of fever have been reported. The blood count is of little or no value. The hemoglobin content may be very high, which probably indicates only dehydration. The leukocytes may or may not respond with a rise.

Although this review was limited to neonates with perforation of the intestinal tract, subsequent reports have corroborated the presence of these findings in infants with peritonitis resulting from a wide variety of causes.[191,232,234-236,240,243,249] Not all of the symptoms described may be encountered in any one patient; however, some are always present (Table 10-3).

Table 10–3 Signs of Bacterial Peritonitis in the Neonate[a]

Sign	Incidence (%)
Abdominal distention	85
Shock	80
Vomiting	70
Constipation	60
Hypothermia	60
Respiratory distress	55
Fever	15
Diarrhea	15

[a]Data are based on patients described in references 232, 240, and 243. Redness, edema, and induration of the anterior abdominal wall, noted in only one series,[243] are also recognized as characteristic signs.

The large overlap between signs of neonatal peritonitis and sepsis can make it difficult to differentiate the two on the basis of clinical findings. Signs of intestinal obstruction such as abdominal distention and vomiting, which are seen in 10%to 20% of newborns with sepsis,[9,17,245] may reflect a coexistent unrecognized peritonitis. Because the early use of antibiotics often cures hematogenous peritonitis in infants with septicemia, the diagnosis may be missed in infants who survive. It is noteworthy that peritonitis unassociated with perforation was found at postmortem examination in 4 of 20 infants with sepsis in 1933,[10] 9 of 73 premature infants dying with septicemia between 1959 and 1964,[9] and 9 of 121 such infants dying between 1976 and 1988.[230]

Diagnosis

Demonstration of free intraperitoneal fluid by ultrasonography[284] or abdominal radiographs taken in the erect and recumbent positions can be helpful in the diagnosis of peritonitis, and is sometimes the only evidence of perforation. Absence of definition of the right inferior hepatic margin, increased density of soft tissue, and the presence of "floating" loops of bowel have been recorded as positive signs of ascites.[227,285] Diagnostic paracentesis can be useful in determining whether the fluid is caused by bacterial peritonitis,[244,252,286,287] hemoperitoneum, chylous ascites,[288] or bile peritonitis.[289]

The left lateral ("left-side down") decubitus film is of great value in showing small amounts of intraperitoneal gas.[243] Although pneumoperitoneum can be caused by mediastinal air dissecting from the chest into the abdomen,[290,291] free gas in the peritoneal cavity usually indicates intestinal perforation. An associated pneumatosis intestinalis should strongly suggest the diagnosis of NEC, but is not necessarily specific for this condition. Several patterns of intraperitoneal gas distribution have been described[281-293]: the air-dome sign, falciform ligament sign, football sign, lucent-liver sign, saddlebag sign, and gas in the scrotum. Absence of a gastric air-fluid level on an erect abdominal radiograph, together with a normal or decreased amount of gas in the small and large bowel, strongly favors a diagnosis of gastric perforation.[293] This finding is almost always accompanied by pneumoperitoneum.

In equivocal cases, metrizamide contrast studies of the bowel can be helpful in establishing a diagnosis of intestinal perforation.[246,290] Serial abdominal transillumination with a bright fiberoptic light is a useful bedside method for the early detection of ascites or pneumoperitoneum in the newborn.[294]

Failure to demonstrate free air in the peritoneal cavity does not, however, rule out a diagnosis of perforation, particularly if air swallowing has been reduced or prevented through orotracheal intubation, nasogastric suction, or use of neuromuscular blocking agents.[286,290,295] In some cases, the amount of gas in the bowel lumen is so small that even if perforation occurs the gas could escape detection. Alternatively, small leaks may become walled off and the free air reabsorbed.[290,296,297] In three large series of infants with peritonitis in whom a patent site of perforation was found at surgery, pneumoperitoneum was absent in 35% to 75%.[232,243,245]

Radiographic evidence of intestinal obstruction, although a common cause or consequence of peritonitis, lacks sufficient specificity to be a consistent aid to diagnosis. A diffuse granular appearance of the abdomen, with one or more irregular calcific densities lying within the bowel lumen or in the peritoneal cavity, should suggest a diagnosis of meconium peritonitis with possible bacterial superinfection.[260]

Prognosis

Prematurity, pulmonary infections, shock, and hemorrhage related to perforation of the intestinal tract, sepsis, and disseminated intravascular coagulopathy are often the factors responsible for the death of neonates, who may concurrently have peritonitis diagnosed at surgery or at postmortem examination. For this reason, case-fatality rates often represent the mortality rate among newborns dying with, rather than because of, infection of the peritoneal cavity.[231,237,243]

Before 1970, the incidence of fatalities was exceedingly high when peritonitis was associated with gastrointestinal perforation; mortality rates of 70% were observed in large series.[191,232,235,236,238-240,245,297] Heightened awareness of conditions associated with perforation, more rapid diagnosis, and improved surgical management have led to a doubling of survivors in recent years.[237,238] The cause of perforation appears to influence the likelihood of survival, with spontaneous gastric perforation having the lowest mortality rate (10%) and perforation of the duodenum caused by a feeding tube the highest (50%); NEC (40%) and all other causes (25%) occupy intermediate positions.[243]

As survival rates have improved, the number of nonlethal complications after perforation has risen proportionally. In one review, two thirds of surviving infants had significant postoperative complications pertaining to infection (e.g., bacteremia, wound infection, intra-abdominal abscess) or gastrointestinal tract dysfunction (e.g., esophageal reflux, obstruction, stomal stenosis).[243] Secondary surgical procedures to correct these problems were required in more than one half of the infants. Sixty percent required parenteral hyperalimentation for nutritional support during their recovery period.

The mortality rate among neonates with peritonitis from causes other than perforation of the bowel, such as sepsis,[191,232,236,240] omphalitis,[240,277] or a ruptured omphalocele,[232,237,240] although high in the past, has not been reassessed in the past few years.[243]

Early diagnosis and institution of appropriate surgical therapy are major factors in reducing the mortality rate.[243] It has been shown that infants operated on within 24 hours after the onset of symptoms have survival rates almost double those operated on between 24 and 48 hours and two and one half times higher than the rate for those whose surgery was delayed more than 48 hours.[245] Factors with an apparent adverse influence on prognosis include low birth weight,[232,237,240,243,263] low birth weight for gestational age,[230] congenital malformations,[237] male sex,[231] and initial serum pH of less than 7.30.[231]

Treatment

The treatment of bacterial peritonitis is directed primarily toward correction of the causative condition.[231] Careful attention to preoperative preparation of the infant is essential to survival. As soon as bowel obstruction or perforation is diagnosed, continuous nasogastric suction should be instituted for decompression and prevention of aspiration pneumonitis. Diagnostic needle paracentesis is also useful for relief of pneumoperitoneum and may facilitate exchange of gas by reducing the intra-abdominal pressure. Shock, dehydration, and electrolyte disturbances should be corrected through parenteral administration of appropriate electrolyte solutions, plasma, or plasma substitutes. If blood is discovered in fluid recovered by gastric suction or abdominal paracentesis, use of whole blood, packed red blood cells, or other fluids may be necessary to correct hypovolemia. Persistent bleeding must be evaluated for disseminated intravascular coagulation or thrombocytopenia, or both, and treated accordingly. Hypothermia, which frequently accompanies neonatal peritonitis, should be corrected before induction of anesthesia. Infants who are unable to tolerate oral or tube feedings within 2 or 3 postoperative days should be started on parenteral hyperalimentation.

If a diagnosis of peritonitis is established at the time of paracentesis or surgery, aerobic and anaerobic cultures of peritoneal contents should be taken before initiation of antibiotic therapy. Parenteral administration of a combination of gentamicin or an extended-spectrum cephalosporin with clindamycin and ampicillin should be continued for 7 to 10 days.[216,229] Other antibiotics that provide a broad spectrum against the enteric organisms, *Pseudomonas* sp., enterococci, and anaerobic organisms include the β-lactam and β-lactamase inhibitor compounds and the carbapenems. In the event of a poor clinical response, culture and susceptibility studies of the infecting organisms should be used as guides for modifying therapy.

Leakage of intestinal contents sometimes results in formation of a localized abscess rather than contamination of the entire peritoneal cavity. Management of infants with such an abscess should include antimicrobial therapy and surgical drainage of the abscess by the most convenient route.

NECROTIZING ENTEROCOLITIS

NEC with necrosis of the bowel wall is a severe, often fatal, disease occurring with increasing frequency in recent years. The average annual NEC mortality rate is 13.1 per 100,000 livebirths; black infants, particularly males, are three times more likely to die of NEC than are white infants, and mortality rates are highest in the southern United States.[298-308] NEC occurs in about 5% of infants admitted to neonatal intensive care units; however, the incidence varies widely among centers and even from year to year at the same institution.[309-322] NEC predominantly affects infants with birth weights below 2000 g[298,300,315,323-330]; in several series, the frequency in infants younger than 1500 g was as high as 10% to 15%.[298-301,316,317,321,329,331-335] Only 5% to 10% of all cases of classic NEC occur in term infants.[308,336-338] It has been stated that occasional cases of NEC may be the price to be paid for the benefits of modern neonatal intensive care.[339] Although most reports of NEC emanate from the United States, Canada, and Great Britain, the condition occurs worldwide in countries maintaining neonatal intensive care units. In a review of NEC in two neonatal intensive care units of academic centers, NEC increased the risk for death (OR = 24.5), infections (OR = 5.7), and the need for central line placement (OR = 14.0).[340] Infants with surgical and medical NEC had lengths of stay of 60 and 22 days greater, respectively, than infants without NEC with additional costs of $186,200 and $73,700, respectively, resulting in additional hospital charges of $216,666 per surviving infant.

Pathology and Pathogenesis

Bowel wall necrosis of variable length and depth is the characteristic feature of NEC, with perforation in up to one third of affected infants generally in the terminal ileum or cecum, where microcirculation is poor.[243,303,307,327,336,341-343] The pathogenesis of NEC is not established, but most investigators agree that the initiating event is some form of stress to the immature gastrointestinal tract, which leads to disruption of the mucosal barrier, bacterial invasion and proliferation, and gas formation within the bowel wall (Fig. 10-3).[315,323,324,345] Surgical specimens from early stages of the disease show mucosal edema, hemorrhage, and superficial ulceration with very little inflammation or cellular response. By the second or third day, after progression to pneumatosis and transmural necrosis of the bowel wall, bacterial proliferation and the acute inflammatory reaction become more prominent.[303,327]

There has been much investigation and little agreement on the importance of various perinatal events in the causation of NEC.[315,323,324,344] Except for immaturity and possibly polycythemia, other factors originally thought to predispose to NEC have, on further study, occurred with equal frequency in control populations of infants.[316,321,324,328,329,338,346,347] Maternal complications of pregnancy, labor, and delivery and neonatal respiratory distress syndrome are thought to be unrelated to the development of NEC, whereas evidence linking NEC to birth asphyxia, hypotension, hypothermia, use of vascular catheters, exchange transfusion, feeding history, abnormalities of gut motility, neonatal achlorhydria, and the presence of patent ductus arteriosus is often contradictory. Each of these conditions, singly or together, may act as a stress leading to mucosal injury, but none has been consistently associated with NEC.[348,349] NEC has occurred among apparently healthy infants with no known predisposing risk factors.[298,307,336,345] Several studies (discussed later) suggest that early feeding of premature neonates may play a causal role in NEC. Dvorak and coinvestigators[344] have shown that maternal milk may be protective compared with artificial formulas in a neonatal rat model of NEC; similar to human NEC, artificial feeding of maternal milk reduced the incidence and severity of NEC injury and IL-10 expression was significantly increased when neonates were fed maternal milk.

Some epidemiologic observations suggest that NEC is an infectious contagious disease of nosocomial origin. The temporal clustering of cases at institutions, the association of some outbreaks with single infectious agents or alterations in bowel flora, and the possible beneficial effects of breastfeeding, oral nonabsorbable antibiotics, or infection control measures in reducing the incidence of disease suggest a possible nosocomial cause. Unfortunately, the evidence linking NEC to a specific infectious agent is often circumstantial or open to alternative interpretation. Evidence suggests that

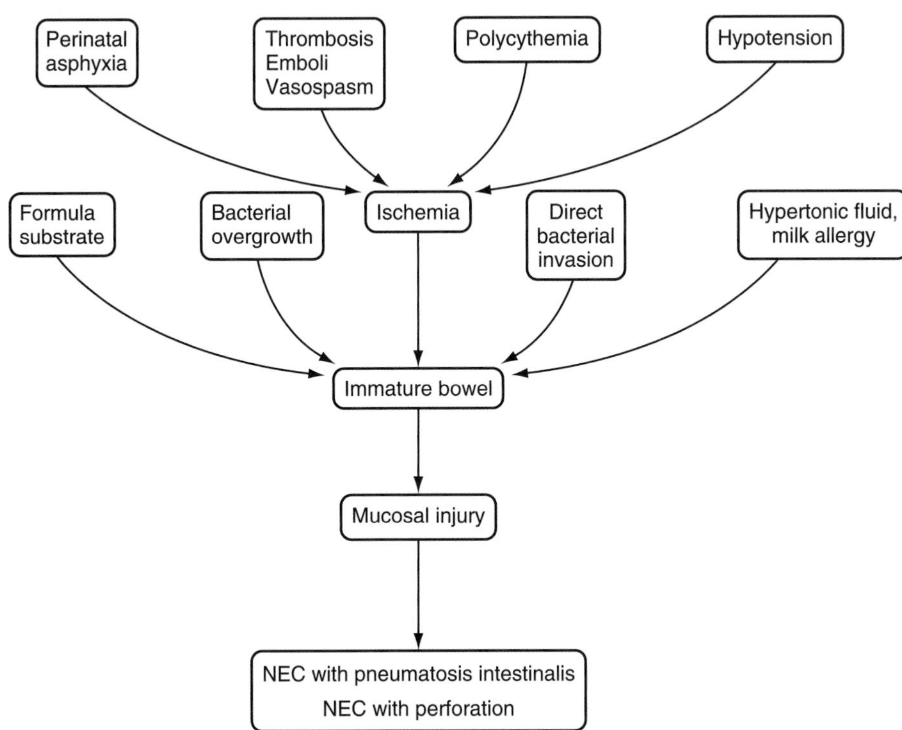

Figure 10–3 Pathogenesis of mucosal injury leading to necrotizing enterocolitis (NEC). (Adapted from Walsh MC, Kliegman RM. Necrotizing enterocolitis. Pediatric Basics 40:5, 1985.)

NEC is the end response of the immature gastrointestinal tract to multiple factors acting alone or in concert to produce mucosal injury, with colonization or invasion by the microorganisms representing only one part of the continuum of that disease process.[282,289,290,307]

Microbiology

Descriptions of sporadic outbreaks of NEC in neonatal intensive care units have led to a search for transmissible agents, including bacterial, viral, and fungal pathogens.[304,315,323,324,345,350-355] Predominance of a single organism in stool, blood, bowel wall, or peritoneal cavity of infants during epidemics of NEC has implicated a number of agents including *Klebsiella* sp.,[301,312,330,343,356-358] *Enterobacter* sp.,[359] *E. coli,*[360,361] *Pseudomonas* sp.,[362,363] *Salmonella* sp.,[364] *S. epidermidis* and other coagulase-negative staphylococci,[365] *S. aureus,*[366] rotavirus,[367,368] coronavirus,[369] coxsackievirus B2,[370] and *Torulopsis glabrata.*[371]

The analogous pathology of necrotizing enteritis caused by *Clostridium septicum*[3672]and *Clostridium perfringens* in domestic animals,[314,358,373] older children, and adults[374] favored suggestions that *Clostridium* species might act as a primary pathogen in NEC.[315,323,324,345,355,375] Several reports provided evidence that *C. perfringens,*[314,376-379] *Clostridium difficile,*[347,380] or *Clostridium butyricum,* acting alone[381,382] or synergistically with *Klebsiella,*[383] was able to evoke NEC. Subsequent studies, however, indicated that these species were often acquired from the nursery environment[385,386] and could frequently be recovered from healthy neonates.[374,386-392] Clostridial cytotoxin, which had been recovered from the stool of infants involved in an outbreak of NEC,[347,380] has also been found in the stool of up to 90% of normal infants.[347,379,385,391-393] The role of *Clostridium* sp. in NEC remains unclear.[355,375]

The δ-toxins, hemolysins of coagulase-negative staphylococci[394] and *S. aureus,* have also been proposed as possible primary toxins capable of producing NEC in infants. Frequent colonization by δ-toxin staphylococci and higher levels of toxin production by associated strains causing NEC have been reported,[395] as well as one outbreak with δ-toxin–producing *S. aureus* strains.[366] Prospective studies have documented significant shifts in aerobic bacterial bowel flora within 72 hours before onset of clinical NEC[396]; the observed shift results from preclinical changes in the intestinal environment. This suggests that bacteria isolated at the time of onset were present because of possible intraluminal changes and are not directly involved in NEC.

Pending further experimental or epidemiologic observations, the weight of evidence indicates that although bacteria or bacterial toxins may play a primary or secondary role in the pathogenesis of NEC, the occasional association of this condition with a single organism probably reflects patterns of intestinal colonization prevalent in the nursery at the time of an outbreak.[315,323,324,345] Despite intensive efforts to identify a specific infectious agent or toxin in the cause of NEC, there have yet to be convincing reports implicating the same pathogen in more than one outbreak.[355]

Clinical Manifestations

Signs of NEC usually develop in the first 7 days of life,[308,336,397] and 50% or more cases are recognized within 5 days of birth.[298,327,330,398,399] Small, immature newborns often develop illness later, during the second to the eighth week,[332,334] whereas low-risk, term infants may become ill shortly after delivery, as early as the first 24 hours.[337]

NEC is a disease with a wide spectrum of manifestations, ranging from a mild gastrointestinal disturbance to a fulminant course characterized by early bowel perforation,

Table 10–4 Modified Bell's Staging Criteria and Recommendations for Therapy for Necrotizing Enterocolitis

	Signs			
Stage	***Systemic***	***Intestinal***	***Radiologic***	**Treatment**
IA (suspected)	Temperature instability apnea, bradycardia, lethargy	Elevated residuals, mild abdominal distention emesis guaiac-positive stools	Normal, mild ileus	NPO, antibiotics for 3 days
IB (suspected)	Same as IA	Frank rectal blood	Same as IA	Same as IA
IIA (definite), mild	Same as IB	Same as IB plus absent bowel sounds ± abdominal tenderness	Dilatation, ileus, pneumatosis intestinalis	NPO, antibiotics for 7-14 days if examination is normal in 24-48 hr
IIB (definite), moderate	Same as IIA with mild metabolic acidosis, mild thrombocytopenia	Same as IIA with definite abdominal tenderness ± abdominal cellulitis or right lower quadrant mass	Same as IIA plus portal gas ± ascites	NPO, antibiotics for 14 days
IIIA (advanced), bowel intact	Same as IIB plus hypotension, bradycardia, severe apnea, respiratory/ metabolic acidosis, disseminated intravascular coagulation, neutropenia	Same as IIB plus peritonitis, marked tenderness, abdominal distention	Same as IIB with ascites	Same as IIB plus 200 mL/kg fluid, inotropic agents, assisted ventilation, paracentesis
IIIB (advanced), bowel perforated	Same as IIIA	Same as IIIA	Same as IIIA plus pneumoperitoneum	Same as IIIA plus surgery

NPO, nothing by mouth.
Adapted from Walsh MC, Kliegman RM. Necrotizing enterocolitis: treatment based on staging criteria. Pediatr Clin North Am 33:179, 1986.

peritonitis, sepsis, and shock.[323,400,402] A staging system (Table 10-4) taking these clinical variations into account may be useful in guiding patient evaluation and therapy.[323,403] The apparent stage of disease for an individual infant disease usually can be defined on the second day of illness. An infant who exhibits only mild systemic and intestinal signs 24 to 48 hours after onset is unlikely to develop a more serious illness.[323]

The classic presentation of NEC includes a triad of abdominal distention, retention of gastric contents, and gastrointestinal bleeding.* These findings are often preceded or accompanied by signs consistent with sepsis, such as lethargy, poor feeding, temperature instability, apnea, and bradycardia. Diarrhea is variable, rarely observed in some series[323] but common in others.[334,361] Progression of bowel wall necrosis leading to perforation, peritonitis, and sepsis is reflected in deteriorating vital signs accompanied by persistent acidosis,[404] clotting disorders, and circulatory collapse. Redness, induration, and edema of the anterior abdominal wall are commonly described in the advanced stages of NEC. In the absence of aggressive medical and surgical intervention, the course is rapidly downhill once late signs appear.

*See references 292, 303, 316, 318, 320, 325, 333, 338, 387, 392.

Diagnosis

Radiographic signs of NEC are largely nonspecific,[402] and interobserver variability in the interpretation of films is substantial.[404] However, roentgenographic examination of the abdomen remains the most reliable aid in establishing a diagnosis of NEC.[298,319,327,404,405] Ileus with generalized bowel dilatation and abdominal distention are the earliest radiologic findings. Increasing distention, separation of loops by peritoneal fluid or edema of the bowel wall, a gasless abdomen, pneumatosis intestinalis, and hepatic or portal air occur as NEC worsens. A persistent single dilated loop of bowel remaining relatively unchanged in shape and position in serial films is strongly suggestive[406-408] but not diagnostic[407,409] of localized bowel ischemia with impending perforation.

If free air or ascites is absent on initial abdominal examination, supine and left lateral decubitus films should be obtained every 6 to 8 hours until improvement or definitive surgery or invasive diagnostic measures have ruled out the presence of perforation. When perforation occurs, it is usually within the first day after diagnosis[341] but may be delayed for as long as 5 or 6 days.[410] Although the presence of pneumoperitoneum[245,281,292] or intraperitoneal fluid generally indicates perforation, its absence does not exclude perforation.[222,243,245] In one study,[341] only 63% of infants with NEC and proven perforation had free air, 21% had ascites, and 16% had neither.

When plain films are normal or equivocal, other studies may be diagnostic. A metrizamide gastrointestinal series may demonstrate intestinal perforation or abnormalities of the bowel wall, mucosa, or lumen.[246,290,411] Real-time ultrasonography may reveal portal venous and hepatic parenchymal gas in standard radiographs.[341,412,413] Serial abdominal transillumination with a fiberoptic light has been described as a bedside method for early detection of ascites or pneumoperitoneum, although its sensitivity when compared with standard radiographic methods has not been determined.[294]

A rapid and direct means of establishing the presence of intestinal necrosis or perforation is by abdominal paracentesis.[414-416] Use of the procedure is unnecessary in infants to rule out NEC or in those improving on medical therapy. It is generally reserved for infants suspected, on the basis of clinical, radiographic, and laboratory findings, of having intestinal gangrene. When performed properly, paracentesis is safe and accurate, as described by Kosloske[416]: The abdomen is palpated to locate any masses or enlarged viscera. After an antiseptic skin preparation, a small needle (22 or 25 gauge) is inserted carefully in the flank, at a 45-degree angle. It is advanced slowly and aspirated gently until free flow of 0.5 mL or more of peritoneal fluid is obtained. Any volume less than 0.5 mL is considered a dry tap and cannot be accurately interpreted. The color and appearance of the fluid are noted, and the fluid is transported immediately to the laboratory—preferably in the syringe with air expelled and the needle covered with a cork or rubber stopper—for Gram staining and for aerobic and anaerobic cultures. A positive paracentesis consists of brown fluid or bacteria on the unspun fluid.

The accuracy of paracentesis in determining the need for an operation is between 90% and 95%.[415,416] False-positive results are rare; false-negative results are quite common. Patients with a dry tap should be closely observed under medical therapy with continuing serial paracenteses until indications for or against surgical intervention are clearly defined. Infants with a positive result should undergo exploratory surgery immediately.

Thrombocytopenia and disseminated intravascular coagulation are the most common hematologic complications,[298,330,354,414,417-419] particularly in the presence of bowel gangrene or perforation.[303,419,420] Platelet-activating factor (PAF) has been used to assist in the staging of NEC[421]; a cut-off level of 10.2 ng/mL had a positive predictive value of 100% in identifying infants with stage II or III NEC. Leukopenia and absolute granulocytopenia, apparently caused by margination of white blood cells rather than bone marrow depletion,[422] also have occurred during early stages of the illness.[417,418] A low absolute granulocyte count persisting for 2 to 3 days is associated with a poor prognosis. Hemolytic anemia has been reported in association with NEC related to *C. perfringens*.[378] No consistent urinary abnormalities have been described for NEC, although increased D-lactate excretion, reflecting heightened enteric bacterial activity, may occur.[423] Increased amounts of fecal-reducing substances have been found in almost three fourths of formula-fed premature infants during early stages of NEC, before the onset of abdominal distention, poor feeding, or emesis.[424] Although not readily available, levels of growth factors in urine have been found to be much higher in children with stage II and III NEC[425]; such an analysis might identify children at higher risk of complications and the need for surgical intervention.

The evaluation of patients with NEC should include culture of blood, cerebrospinal fluid, urine, and stool. The likelihood of bacteremia accompanying NEC depends on the severity of bowel involvement; the reported incidence has varied from 10% to 67% among symptomatic infants. Combined data from several large studies showed positive blood cultures in about one third of newborns with NEC.[303,304,353,410] The usual organisms have been *E. coli*, *Klebsiella* sp., *S. aureus*, and *Pseudomonas* sp., whereas enterococci and anaerobic bacteria were isolated occasionally. A spectrum of organisms similar to those causing sepsis have been isolated from the peritoneal fluid.[303,312,334,354,410] Meningitis may accompany bacteremia, occurring in approximately 1% of NEC cases.[337,426]

Treatment

Early and aggressive treatment must be initiated for any infant suspected of having NEC.[315,323] The modified Bell staging system of NEC may guide diagnostic studies, management, antibiotics, and surgical consultation and intervention (see Table 10-4). Umbilical catheters should be removed whenever possible, oral feedings should be stopped, and nasogastric tube drainage should be instituted. Fluid and electrolyte deficits and maintenance require rigorous attention; blood, plasma, or colloid infusions are often necessary for volume expansion and maintenance of tissue perfusion.

After appropriate cultures (i.e., blood, cerebrospinal fluid, urine, and stool) are obtained, parenteral antibiotic therapy should be started with clindamycin and gentamicin or an extended-spectrum cephalosporin and ampicillin. In nurseries where coagulase-negative staphylococcal colonization or infection is prevalent, initial therapy with vancomycin may replace ampicillin.[427] The β-lactamase and β-lactamase inhibitor combinations (e.g., piperacillin plus tazobactam), can replace gentamicin, ampicillin, and clindamycin, covering anaerobic, gram-negative enteric aerobic, and many gram-positive pathogens. Gentamicin and vancomycin dosages should be modified as necessary on the basis of serum levels. Despite anecdotal evidence that oral nonabsorbable aminoglycosides prevent gastrointestinal perforation in infants with NEC,[428] later controlled studies did not corroborate this finding[429]; their use is not routinely recommended. The need for inclusion of clindamycin to provide activity against anaerobic bacteria in the management of NEC has been questioned.[430]

After immediate treatment has been started, follow-up studies should be instituted. These include serial examinations with measurement of abdominal girth; testing of stools for blood; levels of serum electrolytes, blood glucose, and arterial blood gases; complete blood cell count and platelet count; urine-specific gravity; and supine and left lateral decubitus abdominal radiographs. These tests should be considered as often as every 6 to 8 hours until the infant's clinical condition stabilizes. Attention to vital functions should be provided as necessary on the basis of clinical, laboratory, or radiographic studies. Parenteral nutritional support through a central or peripheral vein must be started as soon as possible.

Early recognition and prompt initiation of medical therapy may reduce the need for surgery. Generally accepted criteria for surgical exploration are a deteriorating clinical condition despite appropriate medical therapy, signs of peritonitis, presence of free air within the abdomen, or a positive paracentesis result. The principles of surgical preparation and management have been discussed by several investigators.[305,416,431,432] In addition to laparotomy with removal of necrotic bowel, closed peritoneal drainage has been proposed as an alternative in very small infants, with a resultant survival of more than 50%.[433]

Prevention

The first observations implicating bacterial proliferation as a factor in pathogenesis of NEC prompted efforts at suppression of gut flora with topical antibiotics in the hope of preventing NEC. Attempts to prevent NEC by giving oral kanamycin or gentamicin prophylactically in the first hours of life, before any signs of bowel involvement are recognized, have generated contradictory data. In controlled clinical trials, a significant reduction in the incidence of NEC in treated premature infants was shown in some,[331,434-437] whereas in others, investigators were unable to demonstrate any protective effect.[437,438] Studies of vancomycin[439] have shown a significant reduction in NEC in high-risk infants. Previous studies revealed selective growth of resistant organisms in bowel flora[331,438,440] and evidence of significant systemic absorption of aminoglycoside antibiotics,[429,441,442] suggesting that oral aminoglycoside prophylaxis is not free of potential risks. Potential risk factors, however, have not been examined in vancomycin trials. Until additional evidence is presented indicating clear-cut benefits from the use of oral aminoglycosides or vancomycin, it does not appear that either should be used routinely for prevention of NEC in premature infants. Epidemiologic evidence that early use of parenteral ampicillin and aminoglycoside therapy may delay or decrease the risk of NEC has not been confirmed in controlled studies.[343] Oral probiotics have been suggested to alter the bowel flora of the infant to reduce the incidence and severity of NEC. Infants fed breast milk and a product including *Lactobacillus acidophilus* and *Bifidobacterium infantis* had a reduced incidence and severity of NEC compared with those of infants fed breast milk alone.[343a]

Excessive or accelerated feedings have been associated with increased frequency of endemic NEC,[443] and some have recommended a schedule of slow advancement of daily feeding volumes limited to about 20 mL/kg/day. NEC infants are more likely to have been fed earlier, to have received full-strength formulas sooner, and to have received larger feeding volumes and increments, and stress and associated respiratory problems may make such infants more vulnerable to NEC.[245,309-314,444] Prior studies of the use of a feeding regimen employing prolonged periods of bowel rest in high-risk infants has been successful in preventing NEC in some nurseries[315] but totally without value in others.[317,324] Later studies have added additional support for standardized feeding schedules in low-birth-weight infants (500 to 2500 g); all have used maximum volumes no greater than 20 mL/kg/day, with feeding beginning at 24 to 72 hours after birth, depending on birth weight and gestational age.[325,326] Both synthetic formulas and breast milk have been successful. Carrion and Egan[445] have suggested that relative hypochlorhydria of the neonate may contribute to NEC and found that hydrochloric acid supplements (0.01 to 0.02 1.0 N HCl/mL of formula) significantly reduced NEC rates and lowered gastric pH. Additional studies have shown that standardized feedings begun at a median of 4 days after onset of NEC can be associated with an abbreviated time until institution of full enteral feedings, a reduced incidence of the use of central catheters and catheter infections, and ultimately, a shorter hospital stay.[446]

Many NEC "epidemics" in neonatal intensive care units, lasting 2 weeks to 7 months, have been reported from centers worldwide.[343,354,355,447,448] Although the microbiologic agents associated with these outbreaks have varied, institution of strict infection control measures was often useful in bringing about a significant decrease in the incidence of NEC; the reasons for success are less clear. However, results have been sufficiently impressive to recommend that enforcement of bedside enteric precautions, together with cohorting of infants and staff, be instituted when two or more cases of NEC occur in a nursery.[323,355,449]

The use of human breast milk has been claimed, largely on the basis of experimental evidence, to exert a protective effect against the development of NEC. Unfortunately, there are no prospective, controlled studies demonstrating any benefit from the feeding of colostrum or breast milk to human neonates. A study demonstrating the protective effect of an orally administered IgA-IgG preparation suggests a possible way to provide benefits of high levels of functionally active antibodies in the gastrointestinal tract.[450]

Prognosis

The mortality rate of NEC is difficult to determine because mild cases of suspected NEC are probably more common than is recognized.[323,400,401] In studies in which analysis has been limited to infants with "definite NEC," mortality figures vary from 20% to 40%.[308,315,324,334-338,397,402,404,415] Several longitudinal studies have shown a significant improvement in outcome.[308,319,404,451] A poor prognosis has been linked with very low birth weight, associated congenital defects, bacterial sepsis, disseminated intravascular coagulation, intestinal perforation, and persistent hemodynamic or respiratory instability.[329,350,397,410] Surgical intervention, generally reserved for the sickest infants with more extensive bowel involvement, is also associated with higher mortality rates.[329,397,401,404,416]

Infants who survive the acute phase of illness generally do well, although NEC may recur in 5% to 10%.[308,334,451,452] In addition to surgical complications (e.g., short-bowel syndrome, anastomotic leaks, fistula formation), enteric strictures are probably the most common delayed complication in surviving infants, occurring in 4% to 20%. Usually found at sites of ischemia and necrosis in terminal ileum or colon,[298,327,453] these strictures often become apparent within a few weeks but may be delayed as long as 18 months. When multiple strictures occur, the intervening normal bowel may form an enterocyst.[405,454] Clinically, strictures present as frequent episodes of abdominal distention, often with vomiting, obstipation, or hematochezia. Diagnosis is confirmed by gastrointestinal contrast studies. Surgery with removal of the stenotic site is necessary to effect a cure.

Long-term follow-up of low-birth-weight infants with severe NEC (i.e., Bell's stages II and III) has documented higher rates of subnormal body weight (15% to 39%) and head circumference (30%) in addition to significant neurodevelopmental impairment (83%).[455] Clinical observations suggest that infants with bowel resection for NEC are at increased risk of sepsis, occurring from 1 week to 3 years (mean, 4 months) later. Almost all had had a central venous catheter in place for parenteral nutrition at the time of infection. Enteric bacilli were responsible for more than 40% of the bacteremias, whereas only 20% were caused by staphylococcal species, which are the usual causes of catheter sepsis. Several infants had two or more episodes of sepsis, and 2 of 19 died as a direct consequence of infection.[445]

ENDOCARDITIS

Neonatal bacterial endocarditis, previously uncommon, has been recognized more frequently in recent years. About 60 cases that meet clinical and bacteriologic criteria sufficient to establish this diagnosis have been reported in the literature[457-485]; 35 have been reported in the past 2 decades. The prolonged survival of critically ill infants and the increased use of intravascular catheters, together with advances in the diagnostic sensitivity and availability of echocardiography, may be responsible for rising recognition of endocarditis. In a 35-year review of 76 cases of endocarditis in children, 10% of patients were younger than 1 year; the youngest patient was 1 month old.[486] Sixty-two (83%) had congenital heart disease, and 77% had had prior surgery. Central venous catheters were additional significant risk factors. For example, at the University of New Mexico in a level III nursery with 3200 to 3500 admissions annually, 12 cases of endocarditis occurred in children younger than 3 months.[487] Organisms isolated from these 10 cases included *S. aureus* (6 cases), *Klebsiella pneumoniae* (1 case), *Enterobacter cloacae* (2 cases), *Candida* sp. (1 case), alpha-streptococci (1 case), and coagulase-negative staphylococci (1 case). Three patients had congenital heart disease with early surgical intervention; all had surgically implanted catheters or intravenous access devices, one had NEC, and one had an associated osteomyelitis.

Etiologic agents of bacterial endocarditis in the newborn have been identified by isolation from blood cultures or morphologic characteristics of organisms entrapped within valvular vegetations examined at autopsy. On this basis, the causative organisms have included *S. aureus* in 36 infants*; streptococci in 6 infants[443,460,489]; *S. epidermidis*[468,469,488] and streptococcus group B[462,472,476] each in 5 infants; *S. pneumoniae,*[460,489] *P. aeruginosa,*[461,467] and *S. marcescens*[465,477] in 2 each; and *Neisseria gonorrhoeae,*[460] *S. faecalis,*[490] *Streptococcus salivarius,*[71] and mixed alpha-hemolytic *Streptococcus, K. pneumoniae,* and *P. mirabilis*[468] in 1 each. Despite widespread cardiovascular involvement associated with congenital syphilis, there is no conclusive evidence that this disease produces valvular heart lesions in infected infants.[58] *Candida* endocarditis has become increasingly prevalent, particularly associated with the use of central venous catheters.

*See references 445-447, 450, 453-455, 457, 458, 465-477, 479-500.

Factors that predispose a newborn to endocarditis are not well understood, although intravascular catheters are certainly associated with endocarditis. Unlike older children, in whom congenital heart disease is often associated with endocarditis,[492] cardiac anomalies were found in only nine of the reported cases in neonates in series before 1994.[458,463,465,468,472,473,478,494] Bacteremia arising from an infected umbilical stump,[459-461] conjunctivitis,[460] and skin lesions[460,482] were the presumed sources of valvular involvement in six infants; the invasive organisms associated with these conditions and with neonatal endocarditis in general can infect normal heart valves.[495] Nevertheless, the greater frequency of bacterial and fungal[481,493,496-502] endocarditis in newborns in recent years, particularly in association with prematurity or placement of central vessel catheters or both, indicates that other, more complex mechanisms may also be operative in some cases.[467-470,484,488,493,503]

Observations in laboratory animals and autopsy studies of adults have shown that damage to the intracardiac endothelium with formation of a sterile platelet-fibrin thrombus at the site of the injury is often the initiating event in a patient with endocarditis.[504] Endocardial trauma caused by placement of cardiac catheters, disseminated intravascular coagulation, and various nonspecific stresses associated with prematurity such as hypotension and hypoxia has been implicated in the genesis of thrombi.[468,484,488,495,505,506] Nonbacterial thrombotic endocarditis or verrucous endocarditis usually remains uninfected and is described as an incidental finding at autopsy.[467,484,506,507] With bacteremia, however, implantation of organisms may lead to valvular infection. Whether this mechanism or that of direct bacterial invasion is primarily responsible for valvulitis is not known. A similar pathogenesis has been postulated for formation of mycotic aortic aneurysms in newborns.[480,510,511]

Endocarditis should be suspected in any neonate, particularly a premature infant, with an indwelling vascular catheter, evidence of sepsis, and new or changing heart murmurs. When these findings are accompanied by persistent bacteremia or signs of congestive heart failure in the absence of underlying heart disease, the diagnosis must be considered seriously. Although Janeway's lesions,[484] a generalized petechial rash,[479,490,493] and splinter hemorrhages[490] have been seen, murmurs characteristic of semilunar valve insufficiency, Osler's nodes, Roth's spots, arthritis, and other findings typical of valvular infection in adults and older children have not been observed in neonates. However, multiple septic emboli with involvement of the skin, bones, viscera, and central nervous system are relatively common findings.*

Two-dimensional echocardiography has proved to be an invaluable rapid, noninvasive method for diagnosing endocarditis.[469-472,478,504,515] Although it cannot differentiate between infected and sterile vegetations and other valvular lesions (discussed later), imaging is quite specific, and false-positive readings are uncommon. Unfortunately, less certainty can be placed on a negative report. Despite detection of vegetations with echocardiography as small as 2 mm, the number of false-negative examinations is significant[478,484,516]; in one series, two of three infants with thrombotic valvular lesions 3 to 7 mm in diameter had normal two-dimensional

*See references 445, 447, 449, 450, 454-456, 458-464, 468, 469, 471, 475, 477, 479, 498-500.

echocardiograms.[484] A diagnosis of bacterial endocarditis should be considered in any infant with a compatible history and physical findings regardless of the results obtained by echocardiography. Widespread use of new techniques such as transesophageal echocardiography, which provides detailed views of the mitral and tricuspid valves, and color flow Doppler imaging, which can identify areas of turbulence as blood passes over vegetations or through narrowed valve leaflets, may greatly improve diagnostic accuracy in the future.[515]

When endocarditis is suspected, specimens of blood, cerebrospinal fluid, and urine obtained by catheterization or suprapubic aspiration should be sent for bacterial and fungal culture. Because blood drawn from a central catheter often contains organisms colonizing the line but not necessarily present in the systemic circulation, at least two *peripheral* venous blood cultures should be obtained before antimicrobial therapy is initiated. Volumes of 1 to 5 mL, depending on the infant's size, should be adequate.[504]

Routine laboratory studies are helpful in supporting a diagnosis of endocarditis in the newborn. The leukocyte count, differential count, and platelet count are usually indicative of sepsis rather than cardiac valve infection in particular. Microhematuria has been reported, although rarely.[484,490] A chest radiograph should be obtained to determine signs of cardiac failure or pulmonary or pleural space infection. CT or MRI of the brain can be helpful in an infant with neurologic signs, particularly if left-sided endocarditis or a right-to-left shunt exists. Baseline determinations of inflammatory markers are useful and can be used for assessing the efficacy of the therapy; both the erythrocyte sedimentation rate (ESR) and C-reactive protein (CRP) level have been used.

Intravenous therapy with a penicillinase-resistant penicillin and an aminoglycoside should be started after appropriate cultures have been obtained. In nurseries where methicillin-resistant *S. aureus* or *S. epidermidis* infections have been a problem, vancomycin should be substituted initially for the penicillin antibiotic.[504,515,516] If endocarditis caused by *Enterococcus* sp. is suspected, ampicillin should be added or substituted for the penicillinase-resistant penicillin. After the infecting organism is isolated and antibiotic susceptibilities have been determined, specific antimicrobial therapy can be instituted. Between 4 and 8 weeks of parenteral treatment is usually adequate, depending on the susceptibility of the organism, response to therapy assessed clinically by reduction or elimination of the observed vegetations, and laboratory response. The CRP level often normalizes 2 to 3 weeks before the ESR, and blood cultures are usually sterile after 3 to 5 days of effective therapy. However, *Candida* sp. may persist for weeks despite the use of active antifungal drugs. Dosage and efficacy should be monitored weekly with clinical and bacteriologic response with or without serum antibiotic and bactericidal levels.[515,517] Determination of serum bactericidal titers (Schlichter's assay) is of uncertain value and has never been validated in neonatal endocarditis.[504,515,518] Efficacy of treatment may also be monitored with serial echocardiograms taken until vegetations remain stable in size or disappear.[478,479,481,488,493]

Intravascular catheters must be removed whenever possible and the tip of the removed catheter should be cultured.[504,519] Extremely large or mobile vegetations occluding an outflow tract or posing a high risk of embolism may have to be removed surgically.[476,478,481] In infants with right-sided endocarditis, demonstration of decreased pulmonary blood flow through the use of ventilation-perfusion scan can be of value in confirming the presence of emboli, particularly if there is clinical evidence of increasing respiratory effort and diminished peripheral oxygen saturation.[476]

With the availability of echocardiography, improved clinical awareness, and early diagnosis, prognosis has improved. Although there were infrequent survivors before 1973,[495] the first survivors with proven endocarditis were reported in 1983.[478,479,484] Approximately two thirds of subsequent cases have been cured. Death is usually the result of overwhelming sepsis, often in conjunction with cardiac failure. Early reconstructive surgery for infants who fail medical management may be helpful but has been reported in only a limited number of cases.[520,521]

Inspection of the heart at autopsy has shown the mitral valve to be infected, alone or in combination with other valves, in about one half the patients. The tricuspid valve was involved in 12 infants, pulmonary valve in 7, aortic valve in 6, infected mural thrombi in 12, and an unspecified site in 3. Microscopic examination of valve cusps has revealed the characteristic lesions of endocarditis, with multiple small, confluent, friable vegetations composed principally of bacteria and thrombi surrounded by inflammatory exudate.[458,482,484] On gross inspection, these vegetations are easily confused with noninflammatory lesions such as those of nonbacterial thrombotic endocarditis, blood cysts,[522] developmental valvular defects,[523] or hemangiomas or other vascular anomalies.[524] Cases described as fetal endocarditis in the literature are almost certainly examples of these types of lesions.[508,523,525]

PERICARDITIS

Purulent pericarditis is a very unusual complication of neonatal sepsis. Approximately 20 cases of proven bacterial origin have been reported within the past 50 years.[512,527-538] No single causative agent has predominated. *S. aureus* was responsible for seven cases,[512,527-529] *E. coli* was isolated from three patients,[529,534,535] *Haemophilus influenzae* was found in two,[530,537] and *Salmonella wichita*,[531] *Klebsiella*,[538] and *P. aeruginosa*[536] were isolated from single cases. One early review of *Pseudomonas* sepsis described suppurative pericarditis in four neonates.[532] Another report on the recovery of *Pseudomonas* from the pericardium of premature infants dying of septicemia and meningitis during a nursery outbreak is difficult to evaluate because details of clinical and autopsy findings were not given.[539] Cases caused by *Candida* sp. and *Mycoplasma hominis* have also been described.[493,499,540] The causes of a pericardial effusion in three fetuses with multiple congenital anomalies, myocardial hypertrophy, and pericarditis are uncertain. Although the inflammatory exudate found at autopsy contained polymorphonuclear leukocytes in addition to lymphocytes, no evidence of bacterial infection was found.[541]

Virtually every infant with pericarditis has associated septic foci; pneumonia and multiple pulmonary abscesses are the most common sites. Involvement of pericardium may occur by direct extension from adjoining lung abscesses or by hematogenous spread of bacteria.[527] The presence of infectious processes elsewhere is sufficiently frequent to warrant the suggestion that pericarditis should be suspected in all infants who develop clinical signs of "heart failure" or a sudden increase in the size of the cardiac silhouette during the course of a purulent infection such as meningitis, pneumonia, or omphalitis.[530,542]

Neonates with bacterial pericarditis generally present with signs and symptoms suggesting sepsis and respiratory distress. Poor feeding, listlessness, emesis, or abdominal distention may be seen in the presence of tachypnea, tachycardia, and cyanosis of various degrees. More specific signs of cardiac involvement became apparent with the accumulation of increasing amounts of pericardial effusion. Unfortunately, the clinical findings of cardiac tamponade are extremely subtle and difficult to differentiate from those of myocardial disease with right-sided heart failure. A rapid pulse, quiet precordium, muffled heart sounds, neck vein distention, and hepatomegaly are findings common to both entities. More specific signs of tamponade, such as narrow pulse pressure or respiratory variations in pulse volume of more than 20 mm Hg (i.e., pulsus paradoxus), are technically difficult to obtain in neonates without an arterial catheter in place. A pericardial friction rub is absent in more than 50% of older infants and children and in most neonates with purulent pericarditis.

Rapid enlargement of the cardiac silhouette, a globular heart shape with widening of the base on tilting, and diminished cardiac pulsation on fluoroscopic examination are of little value in differentiating pericardial effusion from cardiac dilation.[543] The early ST segment elevation and subsequent T wave inversion seen on the electrocardiogram reflect subepicardial damage or inflammation and are similar to changes seen with primary myocarditis. Diminution in the amplitude of the QRS complex by fluid surrounding the heart is not a constant finding. Confirmation of the presence of a pericardial effusion is usually obtained by two-dimensional echocardiography.[512,543] In some cases, CT scan can also be helpful in delineating the extent of a pericardial effusion.[544]

The causes of neonatal pericardial effusion include viral pericarditis,[545] intrapericardial teratoma,[546] maternal lupus,[547] immune and nonimmune[548] fetal hydrops, congenital diaphragmatic defects,[549] chylopericardium,[550] and central venous catheter perforation of the right atrium.[551]

A definitive diagnosis of purulent pericarditis can be made only by obtaining fluid at surgery or through needle aspiration. Care and experience are necessary to facilitate aspiration while avoiding the risks of cardiac puncture or laceration.[541] Accurate monitoring of needle position can usually be obtained through CT guidance, with echocardiographic or fluoroscopic imaging, or by attaching the exploring electrode (V lead) of an electrocardiograph to the needle and by looking for injury current if contact is made with the epicardial surface of the heart.

When fluid is obtained, it should be sent for analysis to the laboratory in the aspirating syringe with the air expelled and the needle covered with a cork or rubber stopper. In addition to cell count and protein and glucose levels, Gram and acid-fast stains should be performed together with cultures for bacteria, viruses, mycobacteria, and fungi. Rapid identification of bacterial antigens by latex agglutination or by counterimmunoelectrophoresis of pericardial fluid, urine, or serum may also help to establish an etiologic diagnosis.[552]

Purulent pericarditis is a medical and surgical emergency. Therapy must be directed toward relief of the cardiac tamponade through adequate pericardial drainage and toward resolution of the infection. Both modes of treatment are essential for successful therapy for bacterial pericarditis in the newborn. Not a single infant with suppurative pericarditis has recovered when treated by antibiotics alone.[527] Although repeated needle aspirations or catheter drainage[553] may be sufficient, the frequent occurrence of loculations of pus, particularly with staphylococcal infection, suggests that open surgical pericardiostomy is the method of choice to achieve adequate drainage.

Cultures of blood, cerebrospinal fluid, and urine should be obtained before instituting antimicrobial therapy. Initial therapy should be based on results of Gram stain or antigen detection tests of the pericardial fluid. If no organisms can be identified, treatment can be started with penicillinase-resistant penicillin and an aminoglycoside (or extended-spectrum cephalosporin) until definitive culture and susceptibility data are available. In nurseries where methicillin-resistant *S. aureus* infection has been a problem, vancomycin should be substituted for penicillin.[517]

The prognosis of neonatal purulent pericarditis is very poor; only three survivors have been reported[512,529,538] before the last decade of the 20th century. Treatment of these patients consisted of needle aspirations, drainage, and systemic antibiotic therapy, and in one case, treatment was combined with local instillation.

MEDIASTINITIS

Purulent mediastinitis has been reported in 11 infants younger than 6 weeks, although it is likely that a great many more cases occur than have been reported in the literature and that it is a frequent complication of cardiothoracic surgery performed in the neonatal period. Six of the reported patients acquired their mediastinal abscess through blood-borne dissemination of organisms[554-556] or by extension from a focus of infection in an adjacent retropharyngeal abscess,[557] pleural or pulmonary abscess,[527,555] or vertebral osteomyelitis.[558] One infant developed infection as a complication of surgery for esophageal atresia.[555] *S. aureus* was the causative organism in four infants, and *S. pneumoniae*, *Clostridium* sp., and mixed *S. aureus* and *E. coli* were causative in one infant each. Organisms were not identified in four cases.

Traumatic perforation of the posterior pharynx or esophagus, often the result of resuscitative efforts in infants involving endotracheal or gastric intubation, produces a potential site for entry of microorganisms.[559-566] Although retropharyngeal abscess,[567] an infected pseudodiverticulum, or pyopneumothorax may occur as a consequence, purulent mediastinitis has been reported only three times as a complication,[556,560,561] but it is probably more common than is reported. At least one case of mediastinitis has occurred as the result of overly vigorous passage of a nasogastric tube through an atretic esophageal pouch.[560] Low (intrathoracic) perforations are said to have a higher risk of mediastinitis and abscess formation than those in the cervical region.[562]

Early symptoms are nonspecific and are similar to those of any septic process in a neonate. As purulent fluid accumulates in the mediastinum, it places increasing pressure on the esophagus, trachea, and tributaries of the superior vena cava and thoracic duct, bringing about rapid development of dysphagia, dyspnea, neck vein distention, and facial cyanosis or edema. To maintain a patent tracheal airway, an afflicted infant will lie in an arched position with head extended in a manner very similar to that seen in neonates with congenital vascular ring. A halting, inspiratory, staccato type of breathing, probably because of pain, is also characteristic. Ultimately, the abscess may point on the anterior chest wall or in the suprasternal notch.

Usually, mediastinitis is first suspected when widening of the mediastinum is observed on a chest radiograph obtained for evaluation of respiratory distress. Forward displacement of the trachea and larynx may accompany these findings when retropharyngeal abscess is associated with mediastinitis. Infection after traumatic perforation of the esophagus or pharynx is often accompanied by pneumomediastinum with or without a pneumothorax.[560,562]

Contrast studies performed to define the cause of respiratory or feeding difficulties in infants with mediastinitis may result in flow of radiopaque fluid into an esophageal laceration, mimicking the findings of an atresia, duplication, or diverticulum of the esophagus.[562,563] In such cases, endoscopy often demonstrates a mucosal tear confirming the diagnosis.[563,564]

Treatment should be directed toward establishment of drainage and relief of pressure on vital structures through a mediastinotomy and placement of drainage tubes. The use of a tracheostomy or endotracheal tube may be necessary for maintenance of an adequate airway.

Initial empirical antimicrobial therapy with clindamycin (or metronidazole), ampicillin, and an aminoglycoside (or extended-spectrum cephalosporin) should be started after cultures of the blood and cerebrospinal fluid have been obtained. More limited empirical antibiotic therapy could be provided with a β-lactam and β-lactamase inhibitor combination alone, such as piperacillin plus tazobactam, ampicillin plus sulbactam, or ticarcillin plus clavulanate. Specific therapy can subsequently be determined by the results of bacteriologic studies of these sources or purulent fluid obtained at surgery.

ESOPHAGITIS

The esophagus is infrequently a focus for infection of the fetus or newborn.[568] Esophageal atresia is associated with congenital rubella (see Chapter 28). Severe esophagitis has also been reported in neonates with congenital cytomegaloviral infection.[569] The esophagus may be involved in infants with congenital Chagas' disease identified by signs of dysphagia, regurgitation, and megaesophagus.[570] Esophageal disease may follow mediastinitis in the neonate (discussed earlier). Only occasional cases of bacterial esophagitis in a neonate have been reported; for example, a 940-g male infant developed signs of sepsis on the fifth day of life and died 5 hours later.[569] Premortem blood cultures were positive for *Bacillus* sp. Examination at autopsy revealed histologic evidence of esophagitis with pseudomembranous necrosis of squamous epithelium and many gram-positive bacilli. No other focus of infection was evident.

INFECTIONS OF ENDOCRINE ORGANS

Endocrine glands other than the adrenal are rarely involved in fetal or neonatal infection. Neonatal suppurative thyroiditis in a term Laotian infant was reported by Nelson.[571] The infant presented with a left anterior neck mass at 3 days of age. At surgery, a cystic mass within the left lobe of the thyroid was identified. Purulent material within the mass grew *S. viridans* and nonhemolytic streptococci.

Orchitis has been described in a 10-week-old neonate caused by *S. enteridis.*[572] This infant presented with symptoms of sepsis and diarrhea, subsequently developing unilateral scrotal swelling and erythema on the fifth day after onset of illness. Ultrasound examination of the testis showed a patchy increased echo intensity; the diagnosis was confirmed at exploratory surgery to rule out testicular torsion. Three other cases of infection of the testes caused by *Salmonella* sp. in infants younger than 3 months have been described.[572]

INFECTIONS OF THE SALIVARY GLANDS

Neonatal infections of salivary glands are uncommon, but when such infections occur, involvement of the parotid is the most frequent,[573-578] and submandibular gland infection is infrequent.[574-579] Most infections are caused by *S. aureus,*[573-576] but *E. coli,*[576] *P. aeruginosa,*[576] and group B streptococci (see Chapter 13) have also been implicated in suppurative parotitis. Not surprisingly, oral anaerobic bacteria, including *Bacteroides* sp. and *Peptostreptococcus* sp., may be found in mixed or isolated infections in more than one half of the cases.[577] Infections of the salivary glands occur more frequently in premature and male infants[576,579] and most commonly present during the second week of life. The oral cavity is the probable portal of entry for the infecting organism. However, blood-borne bacteria may invade the salivary glands. Dehydration with resultant decreased salivary flow may be a predisposing cause in some infants.

The clinical manifestations of salivary gland infection include fever, anorexia, irritability, and failure to gain weight. There may be swelling, tenderness, or erythema over the involved gland. Purulent material may be expressed from the ductal opening with or without gentle pressure over the gland.

The diagnosis is made by culture, Gram stain, or both, of the pus exuding from the duct or by percutaneous aspiration of a fluctuant area. If microscopic examination of the Gram stain does not suggest a responsible pathogen, initial antibiotic therapy should be directed against *S. aureus, E. coli,* and *P. aeruginosa* (i.e., penicillinase-resistant penicillin or vancomycin plus an aminoglycoside or extended-spectrum cephalosporin with activity against *Pseudomonas* organisms). If there is a strong suspicion of involvement with anaerobic bacteria (i.e., negative aerobic cultures or failure to respond to therapy directed at aerobic pathogens), consideration should be given to adding or substituting antibiotics appropriate for anaerobic bacteria (e.g., clindamycin, metronidazole in combination with other antibiotics or a β-lactam and β-lactamase antibiotic alone). The duration of therapy should extend throughout the period of inflammation, continuing 3 to 5 days after signs of local inflammation have disappeared. Incision and drainage often may be required; surgical drainage should be considered if there is not a prompt response to therapy within 72 hours or if fluctuance of the gland becomes apparent. Careful attention to preservation of the function of the seventh cranial nerve is important when considering incision and drainage.

INFECTIONS OF THE SKIN AND SUBCUTANEOUS TISSUE

Bacterial infections of the skin of the newborn may manifest as maculopapular rash, vesicles, pustules, bullae, abscesses, cellulitis, impetigo, erythema multiforme, and petechiae or purpura. In a review of 2836 neonatal infections in Finland, only 6 were characterized as cellulitis.[579a] Most infections of skin are caused by *S. aureus;* such staphylococcal diseases include bullous impetigo, chronic furunculosis, scalded skin syndrome, and breast abscesses (see Chapter 17). Cellulitis frequently accompanied by adenitis and bacteremia may be caused by group B streptococci (see Chapter 13). Cutaneous infections caused by many other bacteria are discussed in this section; however, most microorganisms that cause disease in the neonate may produce cutaneous infections, and when relevant, those infections are discussed in other chapters. For additional information on bacterial infections of the skin, the reader is referred to the text by Solomon and Esterly[580] and the reviews by Swartz and Weinberg[581] and Frieden.[582] Excellent color photographs are included in the *Color Atlas of Pediatric Dermatology* by Weinberg and co-workers.[583]

Pathogenesis

The skin of the newborn has unique characteristics, including absent microflora at birth; the presence of vernix caseosa; a less acid pH than that of older children; and often the presence of surgical wounds, including the severed umbilical cord, a circumcision site, and catheter wounds. The infant is immediately exposed to other infants, personnel, and the nosocomial environment. After the staphylococcal pandemic of the 1950s, information on the colonization of the skin, predisposing factors responsible for neonatal skin infection, bacterial transmission in the nursery, the inflammatory response of the skin to bacterial invasion, virulence factors of staphylococci, and methods of prevention of cross-infection became available. These studies are described in part in Chapters 17 and 35 and have been reviewed elsewhere.[584]

Cutaneous bacterial infection may be a primary event or the result of systemic infection. Septicemic embolic infection may occur at widely separated sites, whereas local infections often occur at a site with an identifiable predisposing cause. Procedures resulting in breaks in the cutaneous continuity, such as forceps abrasions or wounds at fetal electrodes or at venipuncture sites, may be readily identified. The necrotic umbilical cord is a site for proliferation of microorganisms that may invade local tissues.

Infection of the circumcision site remains a concern, because it is the most common surgical procedure in children in the United States. Speert[585] found that cleanliness was frequently disregarded by professional circumcisers as late as the 19th century. Operators were frequently uneducated, were dirty, and often spat on their instruments. Erysipelas, tetanus, and diphtheria have long been recognized as complications of unsterile surgical technique performed on newborns. In a now obsolete and prohibited part of the Orthodox Jewish circumcision ritual, the operator applied his lips to the fresh circumcision wound and sucked a few drops of blood. Such practices were responsible for transmission of syphilis and tuberculosis in neonates in the past. In one report,[586] a 4-month-old infant presented with a penile ulcer, bilateral inguinal adenopathy, and a draining inguinal sinus caused by *Mycobacterium tuberculosis* after the "barber" spat on his razor before circumcision. Reports of 43 cases of tuberculosis associated with circumcision had been published by 1916.[585] Subsequent case reports of severe infection after circumcision include bacteremia related to group B streptococci,[587] local infection and fatal staphylococcal pneumonia,[588] staphylococcal scalded skin syndrome,[589,590] necrotizing fasciitis,[591] and bullous impetigo.[592] Two reports of necrotizing fasciitis after Plastibell circumcision emphasize severe infection as a potential risk of this procedure.[593] One infection caused by *S. aureus* and *Klebsiella* sp. was associated with prolonged convalescent and multiple surgical repairs, whereas a second infant survived staphylococcal necrotizing fasciitis after 14 days of intravenous antibiotic treatment.

The incidence of infection after elective circumcision was investigated at the University of Washington Hospital[594] during the period 1963 to 1972. Infection, defined as the presence of pus or erythema, occurred in 0.41% of 5521 infants and was more frequently associated with the use of a disposable plastic bell (Plastibell, 0.72%) than with the use of a metal clamp (Gomco, 0.14%). Wound cultures were infrequently available, and the microbiologic diagnosis was uncertain for most infants. It is clear that circumcision infection is uncommon, but local spread of infection may be devastating and lead to systemic infection.

Intrapartum fetal monitoring with scalp electrodes and intrauterine pressure catheters and measurements of fetal blood gases through scalp punctures have been associated with infections related to herpesvirus (see Chapter 26), *Mycoplasma* (see Chapter 16), and a variety of aerobic and anaerobic bacteria. Bacterial infections have varied from pustules to abscesses or fasciitis.[578-581] Infection rates are relatively low, varying from 0.1% to 4.5%[597,598]; however, severe infections, including fasciitis, meningitis, and osteomyelitis have occurred as severe complications. A review[599] of causative organisms in fetal scalp monitor infections found that 61% of infections were polymicrobial, involving anaerobic bacteria, aerobic gram-positive cocci, and gram-negative bacilli.

A multitude of specific virulence factors may be important determinants of disease. Some phage types of *S. aureus* are responsible for local tissue damage and systemic disease; other staphylococci elaborate toxins that result in bullae and other cutaneous pathology. Groups A and B streptococci are responsible for cellulitis and impetigo in the infant. *P. aeruginosa* may invade and proliferate in small blood vessels, thereby causing local necrosis and eschar formation (i.e., ecthyma gangrenosum). Infections with *Clostridium* sp. cause disease in devitalized tissues such as the umbilical stump.[600] Similarly, organisms usually considered commensals, such as diphtheroids, might be responsible for infection of the cord and fetal membranes.[601]

Microbiology

The skin of the infant is colonized initially by microorganisms present in the maternal birth canal. The skin of infants delivered by cesarean section is usually sterile at birth. After birth, microorganisms may be transferred to the skin during handling by the parents and nursery personnel. The prevalent organisms on the skin during the first few days of life include coagulase-negative staphylococci, diphtheroids, and gram-negative enteric bacilli (including *E. coli*).[602,603] The umbilicus, genitalia, and adjacent skin areas (groin and abdomen) are colonized first; and organisms then spread to the nose, throat, conjunctivae, and other body sites. Organisms present in the nursery environment colonize neonatal skin after a few days in the nursery. *S. aureus*, group B streptococci, and various species of gram-negative bacilli may be present, but the microbiologic flora differs among nurseries and from time to time in the same nursery. Use of soaps and antiseptic solutions modifies the flora on the skin of the newborn. Hexachlorophene decreases colonization with staphylococci and diphtheroids, but gram-negative organisms are unaffected or may increase after use of this agent.[604]

Epidemiology

Male infants are more susceptible to skin infections caused by *S. aureus* than are female infants. Thompson and co-workers[605] demonstrated that males were colonized more frequently in every body site cultured, including the nose, groin, rectum, and umbilicus. Their review of studies indicated that in England, the United States, and Australia, approximately 50% more males had skin lesions than did females. Although the incidence of breast abscesses is equal in males and females during the first 2 weeks of life, such abscesses are more frequent thereafter in females.[606] The reason for this pattern is unclear, but Rudoy and Nelson[606] hypothesized that physiologic breast enlargement may play a role. Hormone production in the female infant after the second week might account for the increase in abscesses of the breast.

Infections caused by methicillin-resistant *S. aureus* (MRSA) involving the skin of children and neonates have markedly increased. The *mecA* gene responsible for resistance to oxacillin and nafcillin is often closely linked to a gene responsible for skin invasion. Before 1997, epidemic MRSA infections occurred in neonatal units involving infections of the respiratory tract, nasopharynx, gastrointestinal tract, eye, blood, wounds or umbilicus[607]; these infections were usually restricted to single nurseries and involved a single genetic variant of MRSA. Since 1990, MRSA infections acquired in the community have been reported with increased frequency,[608] including in infants as young as 2 weeks old. Up to 91% of these infections have involved the skin and soft tissues and, unlike typical nosocomial MRSA, community-acquired MRSA organisms have frequently remained susceptible to trimethoprim-sulfamethoxazole and clindamycin. At the University of New Mexico, continued surveillance of MRSA-colonized and -infected infants in the neonatal intensive care units has shown that by 2003, more than one half of all isolates are now community acquired.

Seasonal variation in the frequency of neonatal skin infections has been reported by Evans and co-workers, who conducted a series of studies at Harlem Hospital (New York).[609] The prevalence of *S. aureus*, *E. coli*, and streptococci in the nares and umbilicus of infants was lowest in the autumn and usually highest in the summer or spring. No seasonal variation was observed for *S. epidermidis* or *Enterobacter* sp. The investigators concluded that seasonal differences must be considered in investigations of bacterial colonization of the newborn skin and that high humidity may favor gram-negative colonization.

The time of onset of skin lesions associated with sepsis may be early (during the first week of life) or late (up to several weeks or months after birth). Disease acquired in the nursery usually becomes apparent after 5 days of age. Many skin lesions do not appear until after the infant has left the nursery; the observed incidence of skin disease caused by bacteria should include surveillance of infants in the home during the first month of life. Physicians responsible for neonatal care must be alert to the unusual occurrence of skin lesions. The introduction of a new and virulent bacterium, an alteration in technique, or the use of contaminated materials must be considered as possible causes of an increased incidence of such infections.

Clinical Manifestations

Infants who have skin infections that remain localized that are not invasive or part of a systemic infection have few general signs of disease, such as fever, alteration in feeding habits, vomiting, or diarrhea. These signs may be present when significant tissue invasion occurs, as in abscesses or extensive cellulitis. The various cutaneous manifestations that result from infectious diseases are listed in Table 10-5.

Among the common and least specific lesions are maculopapular rashes; these rashes may be caused by viruses (measles, rubella, or enteroviruses), fungi (*Candida* sp.), or bacteria (streptococci or staphylococci), or they may be unassociated with any infectious process. Erythema multiforme lesions have been observed in cases of sepsis related to *S. aureus*,[610] streptococci,[580] and *P. aeruginosa*.[611] Virtually any rash may be associated with bacterial infection. In an outbreak of sepsis caused by *Achromobacter* in premature infants,[612] illness was marked by respiratory distress, including apnea and cyanosis, but was characterized by a rash consisting of indurated, erythematous lesions with sharply defined borders that began on the cheeks or chest and spread rapidly to adjacent areas.

Cellulitis, erysipelas, and impetigo are usually associated with streptococcal infection (group A or B),[613] although impetigo caused by *S. aureus* or *E. coli* has also been reported in infants.

Vesicles, commonly associated with infections by herpesviruses, also are seen on occasion during early stages of skin lesions caused by *S. aureus*, *H. influenzae*,[614] *L. monocytogenes*,[615] and *P. aeruginosa*. *Streptococcus* group B,[616] *S. aureus*, *P. aeruginosa*, herpes simplex virus, and *T. pallidum* may also be responsible for bullous lesions. Pustules commonly occur in staphylococcal diseases but also occur in infections caused by *L. monocytogenes* and, rarely, in skin infections with *H. influenzae*.[617]

Ecthyma gangrenosum is a local manifestation of infection with *P. aeruginosa*.[618,619] Lesions begin as a vesicular eruption on a wide erythematous base. Vesicles

Table 10–5 Manifestations and Etiologies of Some Infections of the Skin in Newborns

Clinical Manifestation	Etiologic Agent[a]: Bacterial	Etiologic Agent[a]: Nonbacterial
Maculopapular rash	*Treponema pallidum*[b,c] *Listeria monocytogenes* *Streptococcus*[b] *Staphylococcus*[b]	Measles virus[b] Rubella virus[b] Enteroviruses[b] Molluscum contagiosum (639) *Candida* sp.[b]
Cellulitis (erysipelas)	Groups A and B streptococci *Achromobacter* sp. (612)	
Impetigo	Groups A and B streptococci (613)[b] *Staphylococcus aureus*[b] *Escherichia coli*	
Erythema multiforme	Beta-hemolytic *Streptococcus* (610) *Staphylococcus aureus*[b] *Pseudomonas aeruginosa* (611)	
Vesicular or bullous lesions	*Staphylococcus aureus* *Pseudomonas aeruginosa* *Treponema pallidum* *Haemophilus influenzae* type b (614) *Listeria monocytogenes* (615)	Herpes simplex virus[b,c] Cytomegalovirus[b] Varicella virus[b,c] Variola virus[c] Coxsackieviruses[b] *Candida* sp[b] *Aspergillus* sp.[b] *Drosophila* larvae (640) *Sarcoptes scabei* (641)
Pustular rashes	*Staphylococcus aureus*[b] *Listeria monocytogenes*[b] *Haemophilus influenzae* (617)	
Ecthyma gangrenosa	*Pseudomonas aeruginosa* (618-620)	
Abscesses and wound infections	*Staphylococcus aureus*[b] *Staphylococcus epidermidis*[b] Beta-hemolytic streptococci (623) Group B streptococci (624) *Escherichia coli* (625-627) *Klebsiella* sp. (628) *Proteus mirabilis* (629) *Pseudomonas aeruginosa* (630) *Salmonella* sp. (631) *Serratia marcescens* (633) *Haemophilus influenzae* (634) *Haemophilus parainfluenzae* (635) *Corynebacterium vaginalis* (636) *Neisseria gonorrhoeae* (644) *Gardnerella vaginalis* (637) *Bacteroides* sp. (638)	*Mycoplasma hominis*[b] *Candida albicans* (642)
Petechiae, purpura, and ecchymoses	Gram-positive cocci[b] and gram-negative bacilli[b] associated with sepsis *Listeria monocytogenes* (615) *Streptococcus pneumoniae* (615) *Treponema pallidum*[b,c]	Rubella virus[b,c] Cytomegalovirus[b,c] Herpes simplex virus[b,c] Coxsackievirus B[b,c] *Toxoplasma gondii*[b,c]

[a]Numbers in parentheses refer to references.
[b]See appropriate chapter for further discussion.
[c]Including infections acquired in utero.

rupture and form an indurated black eschar followed by larger sharply demarcated, painless necrotic areas, resulting from a small vessel vasculitis with necrosis of the adjacent tissue. The organisms are present in purulent material underlying the necrotic membrane. These lesions are particularly more common adjacent to nose, lip, ear, mouth, and perineum, resulting in avascular necrosis and loss of tissue. *P. aeruginosa* may be grown in pure culture from blood and lesions. Among 48 infants described in one outbreak, lesions appeared within the first 2 weeks of life; most infants died within 3 days of onset.[620] Ecthyma is relatively specific for *Pseudomonas* infections, but similar or identical lesions have rarely been described in infections due to *S. aureus, Aeromonas hydrophila, S. marcescens, Aspergillus* sp., or *Mucor* sp.[621]

Many infants with *Candida* infections have cutaneous manifestations. In a report by Baley and Silverman,[622] 18 infants with systemic candidiasis were described; 8 had a burnlike truncal erythema, and 9 other infants had typical candidal diaper rashes or maculopapular rashes of the axillae or neck.

Abscesses of the skin and subcutaneous tissue are usually caused by *S. aureus* and, less frequently, by streptococci of groups A or B[623,624] or by gram-negative enteric bacilli.[625-633] Community-acquired MRSA organisms are even more likely to produce skin infections with abscess formation. Organisms that colonize the skin over an area that has been disrupted by an abrasion or other wound may invade the subcutaneous tissue and produce an abscess. *Haemophilus* sp.,[634-636] *Gardnerella vaginalis,*[637] *Bacteroides* sp.,[638] molluscum contagiosum,[639] *Drosophila myiasis,*[640] scabies,[641] and *Candida*[642] are examples of diverse causes of cutaneous abscesses; virtually any bacterial, fungal, or parasitic agent that is normally or transiently on skin may become a pathogen. *E. coli, Klebsiella* sp., *P. aeruginosa,*[623,628,643] *N. gonorrhoeae,*[644] and *Bacteroides fragilis*[645] have caused wound infections in infants whose scalps were lacerated by forceps, fetal electrodes, or instruments used for obtaining blood from the scalp in utero. An extensive outbreak of systemic disease caused by *S. marcescens* in a neonatal intensive care nursery in Puerto Rico included wound infections at the site of intravenous infusions.

A cephalohematoma may become infected during sepsis or from manipulation of the cephalohematoma, such as through diagnostic or therapeutic needle puncture[646] or by puncture from a fetal monitor. Infections may be caused by *Bacteroides* sp.,[638] *E. coli,*[625,626] and *P. aeruginosa.*[647] The infection may be associated with meningitis[647] or with osteomyelitis of the underlying skull.[625,626]

S. aureus is the most frequent etiologic agent in breast abscess, but gram-negative enteric bacilli may becoming more common.[627,631,632] Of 36 cases with mastitis seen in Dallas during a 16-year period, 32 cases were caused by *S. aureus,* 1 was caused by *E. coli,* and 2 were caused by *Salmonella* sp.; and both *E. coli* and *S. aureus* were isolated from one abscess.[648] Forty-one cases of mastitis in neonates were managed at Children's Hospital (Boston) from 1947 to 1983.[649] *S. aureus* was responsible for 29 of 34 cases with an identifiable bacterial pathogen. All cases occurred in term infants during weeks 1 to 5 of life. Bilaterality and extramammary foci were rare. One third of infants were febrile, and most had elevated white blood cell counts (>15,000 cells/mm^3). Other reports have identified group B streptococci[624] and *P. mirabilis*[629] as causes of breast abscesses. Brook[632] found that 5 of 14 breast abscesses contained anaerobic bacteria (i.e., *Bacteroides* sp. and *Peptostreptococcus*), but *S. aureus,* group B streptococci, or enteric bacteria predominated; anaerobic bacteria occurred alone in only 2 of 14 cases.

Paronychia may occur in neonates after injury to the cuticle. The lesion is usually caused by *S. aureus* or β-hemolytic streptococci.[650] The authors of a report on an outbreak of paronychia in a Kuala Lumpur nursery suggest but do not prove that the lesions were caused by an anaerobic *Veillonella* sp.[651]

Omphalitis is defined by the presence of erythema or serous or purulent discharge from the umbilical stump or periumbilical tissues. A review by Cushing[652] provided a useful discussion of the pathophysiology, microbiology, diagnosis, and management of omphalitis. The incidence of infection is more frequent in low-birth-weight infants and in those with complications of delivery. A survey of infants born at the Royal Woman's Hospital in Brisbane[653] identified an incidence of approximately 2% among term infants. The mean age of presentation of omphalitis was 3.2 days. Perhaps because hexachlorophene bathing was used, gram-negative bacilli were more frequently associated with infection than were gram-positive cocci. However, microbiologic results are difficult to interpret because swabs of the site of infection do not exclude surface contaminants unless cultures are taken with extreme care and precision.

A series from the United States[654] found that periumbilical fasciitis was more frequent in males but did not find that umbilical catheterization, low birth weight, or septic delivery was associated with a high risk; overall, the incidence of omphalitis was equal in males and females. In this series, omphalitis presented as discharge, cellulitis, or fasciitis; gram-positive organisms were found in 94% of cultures, and gram-negative bacteria were found in 64%. *S. aureus* was the most frequent isolate, with *E. coli* and *Klebsiella* sp. the next most common. Group A streptococci have been responsible for nursery outbreaks that may include an indolent form of omphalitis characterized by erythema and oozing of the umbilical stump for days to weeks, accompanied by pustular lesions of the abdominal wall in some cases.[655] Neonatal tetanus usually occurs as a result of contamination of the umbilical wound by *Clostridium tetani* at delivery.

Acute necrotizing fasciitis is a bacterial infection of subcutaneous tissue and fascial sheath.[630,656,657] Infection can arise in an operative wound or in a focal infection such as a breast abscess, or there may be no apparent predisposing cause. Necrotizing fasciitis has been reported after circumcision[591] and as a complication of insertion of a fetal monitor.[595] The trunk and extremities are the areas most commonly involved; inflammation spreads rapidly along fascial planes, producing thrombosis and extensive necrosis, with infarcts developing in overlying skin. Vesicles and bullae appear, and the skin may become blue-gray or black. Myositis and bacteremia may accompany fasciitis. Staphylococci, group B streptococci,[658] *E. coli, P. aeruginosa,* anaerobic bacteria,[596] and mixtures of gram-positive and gram-negative bacteria have been associated with this disease. The bacteria are present in skin lesions, deep fascia, and in some cases, blood. The mortality is high despite the use of fasciotomy, wide debridement, and antibiotics.

Perirectal abscesses may occur in newborns. Unlike older children, most newborns with perirectal abscess do not have underlying immunodeficiency, although infants with acquired or congenital immunodeficiency often present with this condition. The most common cause of perirectal abscess is *S. aureus, E. coli,* or other enteric bacilli[659,660]; however, anaerobic bacteria can also be involved. *S. aureus* and enteric bacilli may be more common in infants and newborns.[660] Recent rectal surgery for conditions such as Hirschsprung's disease or imperforate anus (myotomy or rectal dilatation) may be predisposing causes in infants; as in older children, neutropenia may be associated with an increased risk for perirectal abscess.

Otitis externa is uncommon in the newborn. Victorin[661] described an outbreak of neonatal infections in which *P. aeruginosa* was cultured from seven infants with suppuration of the auditory canal. The author suggested that this outbreak was caused by contaminated bath water used in the nursery.

Diagnosis

The appearance of a skin lesion alone may be sufficiently typical to suspect certain etiologic agents (e.g., ecthyma gangrenosum), but more often, the appearance is nonspecific. A microbiologic diagnosis should be sought to provide specific therapy. The lesion and the surrounding tissue should be cleaned with 70% ethanol to prevent contamination from organisms that colonize the surface. If crusts are present, they should be lifted with a sterile swab to provide drainage, and cultures should be obtained from the base of the lesion. Vesicles and pustules can be aspirated with a needle (20 to 25 gauge) attached to a syringe, or they can be opened and exudate collected on a sterile swab. In general, swabs are not preferred for specimen collection because swab materials bind or inactivate bacterial organisms. Aspiration of abscesses is important; more than one aspiration may be required because the suppurative focus may not be easily distinguished from the surrounding inflammatory tissue. Aspiration of the leading edge or point of maximal inflammation of an area of cellulitis may be of value and should be performed if no other suppurative or purulent sites are available for culture. A small needle (25 or 26 gauge) should be attached to a tuberculin or other small-volume syringe filled with 0.25 to 0.50 mL of sterile non-bacteriostatic saline; the needle should be inserted into the area of soft tissue to be sampled, with continuous, gentle aspiration applied to the syringe. If no fluid is returned to the syringe, a small amount of fluid should be injected and immediately aspirated back into the syringe. Collected material may be sent to the laboratory in the syringe for Gram stain and culture, or, alternatively, the contents may be washed into a tube of bacteriologic broth medium for transport and subsequent culture.

If swabs are used, care must be taken that the material does not dry before it is plated on bacteriologic media. Swabs preferentially should be directly inoculated or rinsed in bacteriologic media and immediately transported to the microbiology laboratory. Alternatively, they may be refrigerated or placed in appropriate transport media if more than a few hours will elapse before inoculation of media in the laboratory. Whenever sufficient material is available (on swabs or in liquid), several slides should be prepared for Gram staining.

It is often difficult to distinguish petechiae from vascular dilatation. Pressure with a glass slide on the border of the lesion is a simple and reliable method for detecting extravasation of red blood cells. If the lesion disappears on pressure, it is probably caused by dilatation of small vessels, whereas persistence of the lesion after application of pressure indicates extravasation of red blood cells. Bacteria may be present in petechial lesions that occur in infants with bacterial sepsis. Blood obtained by aspiration or gentle scraping with a scalpel at the center of the petechiae may reveal the causative organism on Gram stain or culture.

Differential Diagnosis

Sclerema neonatorum, milia, and erythema toxicum are noninfectious lesions that are often confused with infections of the skin.[662] Bullous and purpuric lesions may be caused by noninfectious disorders, including mast cell diseases (e.g., urticaria pigmentosa), histiocytosis X, acrodermatitis enteropathica, dermatitis herpetiformis, epidermolysis bullosa, congenital porphyria,[580] and pemphigus vulgaris.[663] A syndrome of generalized erythroderma, failure to thrive, and diarrhea has been associated with various forms of immunodeficiency.[664]

Sclerema neonatorum is a diffuse, spreading, waxy hardness of the skin and subcutaneous tissue that occurs during the first weeks of life.[646,666] The subcutaneous tissue seems to be bound to underlying muscle and bone. This condition is usually seen on the thighs, buttocks, and trunk. Although associated with sepsis in some infants, sclerema also afflicts infants with dehydration, acidosis, and shock. Most evidence supports the hypothesis that sclerema is a manifestation of shock and insufficiency of the peripheral circulation. When it occurs in infants with generalized infection, sclerema is associated with a poor prognosis. In a review of cases of sepsis at The New York Hospital, sclerema was detected in 6 of 71 infants, 5 of whom died.[667]

Milia are yellow or pearly white papules that are 1 mm in diameter and usually found scattered over the cheeks, forehead, and nose.[662,668] The lesion is a small cyst formed from retention of sebum in sebaceous glands. Because the cyst is capped by a shiny surface of epidermis, it may be confused with a small pustule. Milia are common; Gordon[668] estimated that 40% of healthy newborns have milia. The lesions are common in the first few weeks of life. These cysts may be distinguished from staphylococcal pustules by aspiration and Gram stain of the material.

Erythema toxicum consists of several types of lesions, including 1- to 3-mm, yellow-white papules or pustules on an erythematous base, erythematous macules, or diffuse erythema. These lesions are usually present on the trunk but may involve the head and neck and extremities as well. Most lesions appear within the first hours of life and are uncommon after 2 days of age. Erythema toxicum is uncommon in low-birth-weight or premature infants.[669] The affected infants have no signs of systemic illness or local irritation. A smear of the contents of pustules reveals the presence of eosinophils and an absence of bacteria. Other noninfectious pustular lesions of newborns include neonatal pustular melanosis, which is marked by a mixed infiltrate that has a predominance of neutrophils,[670] and infantile acropustulosis, which is characterized by an eosinophilic infiltration of the skin.[671,672]

Bullae may occur on the skin of the wrist or forearm and usually are caused by trauma.[673] Sucking of the extremity by the infant is believed to cause the bullae, which contain sterile serous fluid.

Purpura may be caused by noninfectious causes, including trauma, erythroblastosis fetalis, or less frequently, coagulation disorders, maternal drug ingestion, congenital leukemia, and congenital Letterer-Siwe disease.

Diaper rash is primarily a contact dermatitis associated with soilage of the skin by urine and stool.[674-676] The rash may occur as a mild erythema or scaling, a sharply demarcated and confluent erythema, or discrete shallow ulcerations. A beefy red, confluent rash with raised margins, satellite (e.g., folliculitis) oval lesions, or discrete vesicular-pustular lesions indicates secondary invasion by *C. albicans* or *S. aureus.* Systemic infectious illnesses that manifest as disseminated rashes (e.g., herpes, varicella, syphilis) may be characterized by early typical lesions in the diaper area.

Treatment

The treatment of localized skin lesions consists of the use of local antiseptic materials, systemic antimicrobial agents, and appropriate incision and drainage or debridement.

Hexachlorophene (3% detergent emulsion) and chlorhexidine (4% solution) are of value in cleaning small, abraded areas and discrete pustular lesions. Because of the concern over its neurotoxicity and cutaneous absorption, hexachlorophene should not be used on large open areas of skin (see Chapter 17).

Systemic antibiotics should be considered for therapy whenever there is significant soft tissue infection with abscess or cellulitis. The specific antibiotic choice should be made on the basis of the microbiology of the lesion; streptococci may be treated effectively with penicillin G, ampicillin, or extended-spectrum cephalosporins (i.e., cefotaxime or ceftriaxone), whereas staphylococci generally must be treated with penicillinase-resistant penicillins or vancomycin. Infections due to gram-negative enteric bacilli may be treated with aminoglycosides or extended-spectrum cephalosporins based on the results of susceptibility testing. Infections due to *Pseudomonas* organisms can be effectively treated with aminoglycosides or ceftazidime.

Local heat and moist dressings over areas of abscess formation may facilitate localization or spontaneous drainage. Indications for incision and drainage of abscesses in infants are the same as for those in older children and adults.

Prevention

Prevention of local skin infections is best provided by appropriate routine hygiene, maintenance of the integrity of skin (i.e., avoidance of drying, trauma, or chemical contact), frequent diaper changes, and hygienic care of the umbilicus or other wounds or noninfectious skin inflammation. The following measures of skin care are recommended by the Committee of the Fetus and Newborn of the American Academy of Pediatrics[676] to prevent infection:

1. The first bath should be postponed until the infant is thermally stable.
2. Nonmedicated soap and water should be used; sterile sponges (not gauze) soaked in warm water may be used.
3. The buttocks and perianal should be cleaned with fresh water and cotton or with mild soap and water at diaper changes.
4. Ideally, agents used on the newborn skin should be dispensed in single-use containers.
5. No single method of cord care has proved to be superior, and none is endorsed.[676]

Cord care may include application of alcohol, triple dye (i.e., brilliant green, proflavine hemisulfate, and crystal violet) or antimicrobial agents such as bacitracin. Alcohol hastens drying of the cord but is probably not effective in preventing cord colonization and omphalitis. A randomized study of triple dye, povidone-iodine, silver sulfadiazine, and bacitracin ointment showed comparability in antimicrobial control.[677]

During nursery outbreaks, the Centers for Disease Control and Prevention recommend the judicious use of hexachlorophene bathing.[678] Daily hexachlorophene bathing of the diaper area[679] and umbilical cord care with 4% chlorhexidine solution[680] have demonstrated efficacy for prevention of staphylococcal disease (see Chapter 17).

CONJUNCTIVITIS AND OTHER EYE INFECTIONS

Conjunctivitis in the newborn usually results from one of four causes: infection with *N. gonorrhoeae,* infection with *S. aureus,* inclusion conjunctivitis caused by *Chlamydia trachomatis,* or chemical conjunctivitis induced by silver nitrate solution.[681,682] Less commonly, other microorganisms have been implicated as a cause of conjunctivitis, including group A and B streptococci, *S. pneumoniae, H. influenzae* (nontypeable[609] and group b[683]), *P. aeruginosa, Moraxella (Neisseria) catarrhalis,*[684] *Neisseria meningitidis,*[685] *Corynebacterium diphtheriae,*[686] *Pasteurella multocida,*[687] *Clostridium* sp.,[688] herpes simplex virus, echoviruses, *M. hominis,* and *Candida* sp. In addition to meningococcal infections, other neisserial species can be confused with gonococcal infections; *Neisseria cinerea* has been reported to cause conjunctivitis that was indistinguishable from gonococcal infection.[689] An epidemic of erythromycin-resistant *S. aureus* conjunctivitis affected 25 of 215 newborns during a 10-month period; control of the epidemic was achieved by identification of staff carriers and substitution of silver nitrate prophylaxis for erythromycin.[690] The major causes of conjunctivitis in the neonate are discussed in Chapter 12 and Chapter 17. Cultures of the conjunctivae of neonates with purulent conjunctivitis and from the comparable eyes of a similar number of infants chosen as controls revealed significant differences, suggesting causality for *S. viridans, S. aureus, E. coli,* and *Haemophilus* sp.[691,692]

Compared with chemical (e.g., silver nitrate) conjunctivitis, other noninfectious causes for conjunctivitis occur only rarely. Eosinophilic pustular folliculitis has been described since 1970[693]; although this disease usually occurs after 3 months of age, some infants younger than 4 to 6 weeks have been described. These infants present with recurrent crops of pruritic papules primarily affecting the scalp and brow. Biopsy specimens reveal folliculitis with a predominant eosinophilic infiltrate; most infants also have a leukocytosis and eosinophilia. Other acute or chronic cutaneous conditions may also manifest as conjunctival or periorbital inflammation, such as seborrhea, atopic dermatitis, acropustulosis of infancy, and erythema toxicum (see "Infections of the Skin and Subcutaneous Tissue").

In a review by Hammerschlag,[694] the incidence of the two major pathogens ranged from 17% to 32% for *C. trachomatis* and 0% to 14.2% for *N. gonorrhoeae* in four United States studies. In other developed countries such as England,[695] investigators found 8 cases of gonococcal infection and 44 cases of chlamydial infection among 86 newborns with ophthalmia neonatorum; in Denmark,[696] investigators found that 72% of infants with conjunctivitis at 4 to 6 days after birth had positive cultures, but 70% were caused by staphylococci (both *S. aureus* and *S. epidermidis*), and that chlamydiae were isolated from only 2 of 300 newborns. The incidence and microbiology of neonatal conjunctivitis is dependent on the incidence of transmissible infections in the maternal genital tract or the nursery and the use and efficacy of chemoprophylaxis. In Nairobi, Kenya, in a hospital where ocular prophylaxis had been discontinued, the incidence of gonococcal and chlamydial ophthalmitis was 3.6 and 8.1 cases per 100 livebirths, respectively[697]; whereas in Harare, Zimbabwe, in a hospital where prophylaxis also was not used, the most common cause of conjunctivitis was *S. aureus*.[698] The introduction of tetracycline ointment for prophylaxis at Bellevue Hospital (New York City) led to an overall increase in conjunctivitis associated with an increase in the incidence of gonococcal infection[699] because of the emergence of tetracycline resistance among gonococci.

Infections related to *P. aeruginosa* deserve special attention. Although uncommon, pseudomonal conjunctivitis may be a devastating disease if not recognized and treated appropriately.[699] The infection is usually acquired in the nursery, and the first signs of conjunctivitis appear between the 5th and 18th days of life. At first, the clinical manifestations are localized to the eye and include edema and erythema of the lid and purulent discharge. In some children, the conjunctivitis progresses rapidly, with denuding of the corneal epithelium and infiltration with neutrophils. With extension of the corneal infiltration, perforation of the cornea may occur. The anterior chamber may fill with fibrinous exudate, and the iris can adhere to the cornea. Subsequent invasion of the cornea by small blood vessels (pannus) is characteristic of pseudomonal conjunctivitis. The late ophthalmic complications may be followed by bacteremia and septic foci in other organs.[700]

Pseudomonal eye infections in neonates can occur in epidemic form, with subsequent high rates of mortality and ophthalmic morbidity. Burns and Rhodes[700] reported a series of eye infections caused by *P. aeruginosa* in premature infants with purulent conjunctivitis rapidly progressing to septicemia, shock, and death in four infants. Five other children with conjunctivitis alone survived, but one child required enucleation. Drewett and co-workers[701] described a nursery outbreak of pseudomonal conjunctivitis believed to be caused by contaminated resuscitation equipment; of 14 infected infants, 1 became blind, and another had severe corneal opacities. Rapidity of the course of this infection is indicated in a case report of a 10-day-old infant who developed a corneal ulcer with perforation within 2 days after first observation of a purulent discharge.[702] An outbreak of four cases of *Pseudomonas* conjunctivitis in premature infants occurred within a period of 2 weeks at the American University of Beirut Medical Center[703]; no cause for the outbreak was found.

A review by Lohrer and Belohradsky[704] of bacterial endophthalmitis in neonates underlines the importance of *P. aeruginosa* in invasive bacterial eye infections ranging from keratitis to panophthalmitis. The literature review included 16 cases of invasive eye infections in neonates; 13 were caused by *P. aeruginosa,* and the others were cases of endophthalmitis caused by group B streptococci and *S. pneumoniae*. Other opportunistic gram-negative pathogens associated with outbreaks of infections in nurseries may also include conjunctivitis as a part of the infection syndrome. In a report by Christensen and co-workers,[705] a multiply antibiotic-resistant *S. marcescens* was responsible for 15 cases of pneumonia, sepsis, and meningitis and for 20 cases of conjunctivitis, cystitis, and wound infection over a 9-month period in a neonatal intensive care unit.

Dacryocystitis may complicate a congenital lacrimal sac distention (i.e., dacryocystocele). Harris and DiClementi[706] described an infant who presented on day 4 of life with edema and erythema of the lower lid. Purulent material emerged from the puncta after moderate pressure over the lacrimal sac; *S. marcescens* was grown from the material.

The physician responsible for management of the child with purulent conjunctivitis must consider the major causes of the disease and must be alert to the rare pathogen. In hospitals that practice Credé's method (i.e., silver nitrate application), purulent conjunctivitis during the first 48 hours of life is almost always caused by chemical toxicity.[707] After the first 2 days, the pus of an exudative conjunctivitis must be carefully examined by Gram stain for the presence of gram-negative intracellular diplococci, gram-positive cocci in clusters, and gram-negative bacilli. Appropriate cultures should be used for isolation of the organisms concerned. If the smears are inconclusive and no pathogens are isolated on appropriate media and if the conjunctivitis persists, a diagnosis of inclusion or chlamydial infection is likely.[706,798,709]

The treatment of gonococcal and staphylococcal conjunctivitis is discussed in Chapters 12 and 17. Chlamydial conjunctivitis is reviewed in Chapter 11.

If infection with *Pseudomonas* species is suspected, treatment should be started at once with an effective parenteral antibiotic such as an aminoglycoside (e.g., tobramycin, amikacin, or gentamicin) with or without an antipseudomonal penicillin or ceftazidime (see Chapter 35) and with a locally applied ophthalmic ointment. The use of subconjunctival gentamicin or other antipseudomonal aminoglycoside is of uncertain value; however, if the cornea appears to be extensively involved, there is a risk of rapid development of endophthalmitis, and the subconjunctival injection of antibiotics should be considered in consultation with an ophthalmologist. If the diagnosis is confirmed, this regimen is continued until the local signs of *Pseudomonas* infection resolve.

Recommendations for ocular chemoprophylaxis are discussed in chapter 12 on gonococcal and Chapter 11 on chlamydial infections. Additional information is available in the 2000 edition of the Report of the Committee on Infectious Diseases published by the American Academy of Pediatrics.[710]

REFERENCES

Infections of the Liver

1. Murphy FM, Baker CJ. Solitary hepatic abscess: a delayed complication of neonatal bacteremia. Pediatr Infect Dis J 7:414, 1988.
2. Guillois B, Guillemin MG, Thoma M, et al. Staphylococcie pleuropulmonaire néonatale avec abcès hépatiques multiples. Ann Pediatr 36:681, 1989.
3. Dehner LP, Kissane JM. Pyogenic hepatic abscesses in infancy and childhood. J Pediatr 74:763, 1969.
4. Wright HT Jr. Personal communication, 1987.
5. Moss TJ, Pysher TJ. Hepatic abscess in neonates. Am J Dis Child 135:726, 1981.
6. Chusid MJ. Pyogenic hepatic abscess in infancy and childhood. Pediatrics 62:554, 1978.
7. Dineen P. Personal communication, Cornell University Medical College, New York, NY.
8. Bilfinger TV, Hayden CK, Oldham KT, et al. Pyogenic liver abscesses in nonimmunocompromised children. South Med J 79:37, 1986.
9. Beutow KC, Klein SW, Lane RB. Septicemia in premature infants: the characteristics, treatment, and prevention of septicemia in premature infants. Am J Dis Child 110:29, 1965.
10. Dunham EC. Septicemia in the newborn. Am J Dis Child 45:229, 1933.
11. Nyhan W, Fousek MD. Septicemia of the newborn. Pediatrics 22:268, 1958.
12. Gotoff SP, Behrman RE. Neonatal septicemia. J Pediatr 76:142, 1970.

13. Hamilton JR, Sass-Kortsak A. Jaundice associated with severe bacterial infection in young infants. J Pediatr 63:121, 1963.
14. Hänninen P, Terhe P, Toivanen A. Septicemia in a pediatric unit: a 20-year study. Scand J Infect Dis 3:201, 1971.
15. Potter E. Pathology of the Fetus and Infant, 3rd ed. Chicago, Year Book Medical Publishers, 1975.
16. Silverman WA, Homan WE. Sepsis of obscure origin in the newborn. Pediatrics 3:157, 1949.
17. Smith RT, Platau ES, Good RA. Septicemia of the newborn: current status of the problem. Pediatrics 17:549, 1956.
18. Gersony WM, McCracken GH Jr. Purulent pericarditis in infancy. Pediatrics 40:224, 1967.
19. Axton JHM. Amoebic proctocolitis and liver abscess in a neonate. S Afr Med J 46:258, 1972.
20. Botman T, Ruys PJ. Amoebic appendicitis in newborn infant. Trop Geogr Med 15:221, 1963.
21. Brans YW, Ceballos R, Cassady G. Umbilical catheters and hepatic abscesses. Pediatrics 53:264, 1974.
22. Cohen HJ, Dresner S. Liver abscess following exchange transfusion for erythroblastosis fetalis. Q Rev Pediatr 16:148, 1961.
23. deBeaujeu J, Bethenod M, Mollard P, et al. Abcès hépatique à forme tumorale chez un nourrisson. Pediatrie 23:363, 1968.
24. Heck W, Rehbein F, Reismann B. Pyogene Leberabszesse im Säuglingsalter. Z Kinderchir Suppl 1:49, 1966.
25. Kandall SR, Johnson AB, Gartner LM. Solitary neonatal hepatic abscess. J Pediatr 85:567, 1974.
26. Kutsunai T. Abscess of the liver of umbilical origin in infants: report of two cases. Am J Dis Child 51:1385, 1936.
27. Madsen CM, Secouris N. Solitary liver abscess in a newborn. Surgery 47:1005, 1960.
28. Martin C, Saint-Supery G, Babin JP, et al. Abcès gazeux du foie avec coagulopathie chez le nouveau-né: guérison (à propos de 2 observations). Bordeaux Med 5:1181, 1972.
29. Pouyanne, Martin D. Abcès du foie à staphylococques chez un nouveau-né, compliqué de suppuration sous-phrénique puis de péritonite à évolution subaiguë. Guerison J Med Bordeaux 130:929, 1953.
30. Pyrtek LJ, Bartus SA. Hepatic pyemia. N Engl J Med 272:551, 1965.
31. Sharma K, Kumar R. Solitary abscess of the liver in a newborn infant. Surgery 61:812, 1967.
32. Williams JW, Rittenberry A, Dillard R, et al. Liver abscess in newborn: complication of umbilical vein catheterization. Am J Dis Child 125:111, 1973.
33. Beaven DW. Staphylococcal peritonitis in the newborn. Lancet 1:869, 1958.
34. Fraga JR, Javate BA, Venkatessan S. Liver abscess and sepsis due to *Klebsiella pneumoniae* in a newborn. Clin Pediatr 13:1081, 1974.
35. Tariq AA, Rudolph NA, Levin EJ. Solitary hepatic abscess in a newborn infant: a sequel of umbilical vein catheterization and infusion of hypertonic glucose solutions. Clin Pediatr 16:577, 1977.
36. Cushman P, Ward OC. Solitary liver abscess in a neonate: complication of umbilical vein catheterization. Ir J Med Sci 147:374, 1978.
37. Wiedersberg H, Pawlowski P. Pyelophlebitis nach Nabelvenenkatheterismus. Monatsschr Kinderheilkd 128:128, 1980.
38. Gonzalez Rivera F, Montoro Burgos M, Cabrera Molina A. Absceso hepático en un recién nacido. An Esp Pediatr 23:59, 1985.
39. Nars PW, Klco L, Fliegel CP. Successful conservative management of a solitary liver abscess in a premature baby. Helv Paediatr Acta 38:489, 1983.
40. Larsen LR, Raffensperger J. Liver abscess. J Pediatr Surg 14:329, 1979.
41. Montoya F, Alam M-M, Couture A, et al. Abcès du foie chez un nouveau-né guerison après ponction percutanée sous controle échographique. Pediatrie 38:547, 1983.
42. Murphy SM, Baker CJ. Solitary hepatic abscess: a delayed complication of neonatal bacteremia. Pediatr Infect Dis J 7:414, 1988.
43. Anagnostakis D, Kamba A, Petrochilou V, et al. Risk of infection associated with umbilical vein catheterization: a prospective study in 75 newborn infants. J Pediatr 86:759, 1975.
44. Sabbaj J, Sutter V, Finegold SM. Anaerobic pyogenic liver abscess. Ann Intern Med 77:629, 1972.
45. Meyer WW, Lind J. Postnatal changes in the portal circulation. Arch Dis Child 41:606, 1966.
46. Hageman J, Shulman S, Schreiber M, et al. Congenital tuberculosis: critical reappraisal of clinical findings and diagnostic procedures. Pediatrics 66:980, 1980.
47. Hughesdon MR. Congenital tuberculosis. Arch Dis Child 21:121, 1946.
48. Cantwell MF, Shehab ZM, Costello AM, et al. Brief report: congenital tuberculosis. N Engl J Med 330:1051, 1994.
49. Abughal N, van der Kuyp F, Amable W, et al. Congenital tuberculosis. Pediatr Infect Dis J 13:738, 1994.
50. Simma B, Dietze O, Vogel W, et al. Bacille Calmette-Guérin–associated hepatitis. Eur J Pediatr 150:423, 1991.
51. Lide TN. Congenital tularemia. Arch Pathol 43:165, 1947.
52. Regan JC, Litvak A, Regan C. Intrauterine transmission of anthrax. JAMA 80:1769, 1923.
53. Hicks HT, French H. Typhoid fever and pregnancy with special reference to foetal infection. Lancet 1:1491, 1905.
54. Sarram M, Feiz J, Foruzandeh M, et al. Intrauterine fetal infection with *Brucella melitensis* as a possible cause of second-trimester abortion. Am J Obstet Gynecol 119:657, 1974.
55. Brim A. A bacteriologic study of 100 stillborn and dead newborn infants. J Pediatr 15:680, 1939.
56. Madan E, Meyer MP, Amortegui AJ. Isolation of genital mycoplasmas and *Chlamydia trachomatis* in stillborn and neonatal autopsy material. Arch Pathol Lab Med 112:749, 1988.
57. Oppenheimer EH, Hardy JB. Congenital syphilis in the newborn infant: clinical and pathological observations in recent cases. Johns Hopkins Med J 129:63, 1971.
58. Stokes JH, Beerman H, Ingraham NR Jr. Modern Clinical Syphilology: Diagnosis, Treatment, Case Study, 3rd ed. Philadelphia, WB Saunders, 1944.
59. Venter A, Pettifor JM, Duursma J, et al. Liver function in early congenital syphilis: does penicillin cause a deterioration? J Pediatr Gastroenterol Nutr 12:310, 1991.
60. Lindsay S, Luke JW. Fetal leptospirosis (Weil's disease) in a newborn infant: case of intrauterine fetal infection with report of an autopsy. J Pediatr 34:90, 1949.
61. Topciu V, Manu E, Strubert L, et al. Voie transplacentaire dans un cas de leptospirose humaine. Gynecol Obstet 65:617, 1966.
62. Gsell HO Jr, Olafsson A, Sonnabend W, et al. [Intrauterine leptospirosis pomona: 1st reported case of an intrauterine transmitted and cured leptospirosis.] Dtsch Med Wochenschr 96:1263, 1971. German.
63. Cramer HHW. Abortus bein Leptospirosis canicola. Arch Gynecol 177:167, 1950.
64. Chung H, Ts'ao W, Mo P, et al. Transplacental or congenital infection of leptospirosis: clinical and experimental observations. Chin Med J 82:777, 1963.
65. Fuchs PC, Oyama AA. Neonatal relapsing fever due to transplacental transmission of *Borrelia.* JAMA 208:690, 1969.
66. Yagupsky P, Moses S. Neonatal *Borrelia* species infection (relapsing fever). Am J Dis Child 139:74, 1985.
67. Fuchs PC. Personal communication, 1973.
68. Weber K, Bratzke H-J, Neubert U, et al. *Borrelia burgdorferi* in a newborn despite oral penicillin for Lyme borreliosis during pregnancy. Pediatr Infect Dis J 7:286, 1988.
69. Steere AC. Lyme disease. N Engl J Med 321:586, 1989.
70. Lipinski JK, Vega JM, Cywes S, et al. Falciform ligament abscess in the infant. J Pediatr Surg 20:556, 1985.
71. Betke K, Richarz H. Nabelsepsis mit Pyelphlebitis, multiplen Leberabscessen, Lungenabscessen, und Osteomyelitis. Ausgang in Heilung. Monatsschr Kinderheilkd 105:70, 1957.
72. Elliott RIK. The ductus venosus in neonatal infection. Proc R Soc Med 62:321, 1969.
73. McKenzie CG. Pyogenic infection of liver secondary to infection in the portal drainage area. BMJ 4:1558, 1964.
74. Menzel K, Buttenberg H. Pyelophlebitis mit multiplen Leberabszessen als Komplikation mehrfacher Sondierung der Nabelvene. Kinderaerztl Prax 40:14, 1972.
75. Sarrut S, Alain J, Alison F. Les complications précoces de la perfusion par la veine ombilicale chez le premature. Arch Fr Pediatr 26:651, 1969.
76. Santerne B, Morville P, Touche D, et al. Diagnostic et traitement d'une abcédation hépatique néo-natale multifocale par l'échographie. Presse Med 16:12, 1987.
77. Scott J. Iatrogenic lesions in babies following umbilical vein catheterization. Arch Dis Child 40:426, 1965.
78. Shaw A, Pierog S. "Ectopic" liver in the umbilicus: an unusual focus of infection in a newborn infant. Pediatrics 44:448, 1969.
79. Morison JE. Umbilical sepsis and acute interstitial hepatitis. J Pathol Bacteriol 56:531, 1944.
80. Bernstein J, Brown AK. Sepsis and jaundice in early infancy. Pediatrics 29:873, 1962.

81. Parker RGF. Jaundice and infantile diarrhea. Arch Dis Child 33:330, 1958.
82. Gwinn JL, Lee FA. Radiologic case of the month: pyogenic liver abscess. Am J Dis Child 123:50, 1972.
83. Martin DJ. Neonatal disorders diagnosed with ultrasound. Clin Perinatol 12:219, 1985.
84. Pineiro-Carrero VM, Andres JM. Morbidity and mortality in children with pyogenic liver abscess. Am J Dis Child 143:1424, 1989.
85. Caron KH. Magnetic resonance imaging of the pediatric abdomen. Semin Ultrasound CT MR 12:448, 1991.
86. Halvorsen RA Jr, Foster WL Jr, Wilkinson RH Jr, et al. Hepatic abscess: sensitivity of imaging tests and clinical findings. Gastrointest Radiol 13:135, 1988.
87. Weinreb JC, Cohen JM, Armstrong E, et al. Imaging the pediatric liver: MRI and CT. AJR Am J Roentgenol 147:785, 1986.
88. Cohen MD. Clinical utility of magnetic resonance imaging in pediatrics. Am J Dis Child 140:947, 1986.
89. Diament MJ, Stanley P, Kangarloo H, et al. Percutaneous aspiration and catheter drainage of abscesses. J Pediatr 108:204, 1986.
90. Rubinstein Z, Heyman Z, Morag B, et al. Ultrasound and computed tomography in the diagnosis and drainage of abscesses and other fluid collections. Isr J Med Sci 19:1050, 1983.
91. Reynolds TB. Medical treatment of pyogenic liver abscess. Ann Intern Med 96:373, 1982.
92. Loh R, Wallace G, Thong YH. Successful non-surgical management of pyogenic liver abscess. Scand J Infect Dis 19:137, 1987.
93. Keidl CM, Chusid MJ. Splenic abscesses in childhood. Pediatr Infect Dis J 8:368, 1989.

Infections of the Biliary Tract

94. Bowen A. Acute gallbladder dilatation in a neonate: emphasis on ultrasonography. J Pediatr Gastroenterol Nutr 3:304, 1984.
95. Goldthorn JF, Thomas DW, Ramos AD. Hydrops of the gallbladder in stressed premature infants. Clin Res 28:122A, 1980.
96. Brill PW, Winchester P, Rosen MS. Neonatal cholelithiasis. Pediatr Radiol 12:285, 1982.
97. Callahan J, Haller JO, Cacciarelli AA, et al. Cholelithiasis in infants: association with total parenteral nutrition and furosemide. Radiology 143:437, 1982.
98. Keller MS, Markle BM, Laffey PA, et al. Spontaneous resolution of cholelithiasis in infants. Radiology 157:345, 1985.
99. Schirmer WJ, Grisoni ER, Gauderer MWL. The spectrum of cholelithiasis in the first year of life. J Pediatr Surg 24:1064, 1989.
100. Debray D, Pariente D, Gauthrer F, et al. Cholelithiasis in infancy: a study of 40 cases. J Pediatr 122:38, 1993.
101. Neu J, Arvin A, Ariagno RL. Hydrops of the gallbladder. Am J Dis Child 134:891, 1980.
102. Leichty EA, Cohen MD, Lemons JA, et al. Normal gallbladder appearing as abdominal mass in neonates. Am J Dis Child 136:468, 1982.
103. Peevy KJ, Wiseman HJ. Gallbladder distension in septic neonates. Arch Dis Child 57:75, 1982.
104. Dutta T, George V, Sharma GD, et al. Gallbladder disease in infancy and childhood. Prog Pediatr Surg 8:109, 1975.
105. Saldanha RL, Stein CA, Kopelman AE. Gallbladder distention in ill preterm infants. Am J Dis Child 137:1179, 1983.
106. El-Shafie M, Mah CL. Transient gallbladder distention in sick premature infants: the value of ultrasonography and radionuclide scintigraphy. Pediatr Radiol 16:468, 1986.
107. Modi N, Keay AJ. Neonatal gallbladder distention. Arch Dis Child 57:562, 1982.
108. Amodio JB, Fontanetta E, Cohen M, et al. Neonatal hydrops of the gallbladder: evaluation by cholescintigraphy and ultrasonography. N Y State J Med 85:565, 1985.
109. McGahan JP, Phillips HE, Cox KL. Sonography of the normal pediatric gallbladder and biliary tract. Radiology 144:873, 1982.
110. Haller JO. Sonography of the biliary tract in infants and children. AJR Am J Roentgenol 157:1051, 1991.
111. Guthrie KJ, Montgomery GL. Infections with *Bacterium enteritidis* in infancy with the triad of enteritis, cholecystitis, and meningitis. J Pathol Bacteriol 49:393, 1939.
112. Faller W, Berkelhamor JE, Esterly JR. Neonatal biliary tract infection coincident with maternal methadone therapy. Pediatrics 48:997, 1971.
113. Jamieson PN, Shaw DG. Empyema of gallbladder in an infant. Arch Dis Child 50:482, 1975.
114. Arnspiger LA, Martin JG, Krempin HO. Acute noncalculous cholecystitis in children: report of a case in a 17-day-old infant. Am J Surg 100:103, 1960.
115. Ternberg JL, Keating JP. Acute acalculous cholecystitis: complication of other illnesses in childhood. Arch Surg 110:543, 1975.
116. Crystal RF, Fink RL. Acute acalculous cholecystitis in childhood: a report of two cases. Clin Pediatr 10:423, 1971.
117. Robinson AE, Erwin JH, Wiseman HJ, et al. Cholecystitis and hydrops of the gallbladder in the newborn. Radiology 122:749, 1977.
118. Snyder WH Jr, Chaffin L, Oettinger L. Cholelithiasis and perforation of the gallbladder in an infant, with recovery. JAMA 149:1645, 1952.
119. Washburn ME, Barcia PJ. Uncommon cause of a right upper quadrant abdominal mass in a newborn: acute cholecystitis. Am J Surg 140:704, 1980.
120. Thurston WA, Kelly EN, Silver MM. Acute acalculous cholecystitis in a premature infant treated with parenteral nutrition. Can Med Assoc J 135:332, 1986.
121. Pieretti R, Auldist AW, Stephens CA. Acute cholecystitis in children. Surg Obstet Gynecol 140:16, 1975.
122. Hanson BA, Mahour GH, Woolley MM. Diseases of the gallbladder in infancy and childhood. J Pediatr Surg 6:277, 1971.
123. Dewan PA, Stokes KB, Solomon JR. Paediatric acalculous cholecystitis. Pediatr Surg Int 2:120, 1987.
124. Denes J, Gergely K, Mohacsi A, et al. Die Frühgeborenen-Appendicitis. Z Kinderchir 5:400, 1968.
125. Traynelis VC, Hrabovsky EE. Acalculous cholecystitis in the neonate. Am J Dis Child 139:893, 1985.
126. Aach RD. Cholecystitis in childhood. *In* Feigin RD, Cherry JD (eds). Textbook of Pediatric Infectious Diseases, 2nd ed. Philadelphia, WB Saunders, 1987, pp 742-743.
127. Wyllie R, Fitzgerald JF. Bacterial cholangitis in a 10-week-old infant with fever of undetermined origin. Pediatrics 65:164, 1980.
128. Becroft DMO. Biliary atresia associated with prenatal infection by *Listeria monocytogenes*. Arch Dis Child 47:656, 1972.

Infections of the Adrenal Glands

129. Favara BE, Akers DR, Franciosi RA. Adrenal abscess in a neonate. J Pediatr 77:682, 1970.
130. Mondor C, Gauthier M, Garel L, et al. Nonsurgical management of neonatal adrenal abscess. J Pediatr Surg 23:1048, 1988.
131. François A, Berterottiere D, Aigrain Y, et al. Abcès surrénalien neonatal à *Proteus mirabilis*. Arch Fr Pediatr 48:559, 1991.
132. Lizardo-Barahona JR, Nieto-Zermño J, Bracho-Blanchet E. Absceso adrenal en el recien nacido: informe de un caso y revision de la literatura. Bol Med Hosp Infant Mex 47:401, 1990.
133. Torres-Simon JM, Figueras-Aloy J, Vilanova-Juanola JM, et al. Absceso suprarenal en el recien nacido. An Esp Pediatr 31:601, 1989.
134. Zamir O, Udassion R, Aviad I, et al. Adrenal abscess: a rare complication of neonatal adrenal hemorrhage. Pediatr Surg Int 2:117, 1987.
135. Van de Water JM, Fonkalsrud EW. Adrenal cysts in infancy. Surgery 60:1267, 1966.
136. Blankenship WJ, Borgen H, Stadalnik R, et al. Suprarenal abscess in the neonate: a case report and review of diagnosis and management. Pediatrics 55:239, 1975.
137. Gibbons DM, Duckett JW Jr, Cromie WJ, et al. Abdominal flank mass in the neonate. J Urol 119:671, 1978.
138. Atkinson GO Jr, Kodroff MB, Gay BB Jr, et al. Adrenal abscess in the neonate. Radiology 155:101, 1985.
139. Carty A, Stanley P. Bilateral adrenal abscesses in a neonate. Pediatr Radiol 1:63, 1973.
140. Walker KM, Coyer WF. Suprarenal abscess due to group B *Streptococcus*. J Pediatr 94:970, 1979.
141. Camilleri R, Thibaud D, Gruner M, et al. Abcédation d'un hématome surrénal avec hypertension artérielle. Arch Fr Pediatr 41:705, 1984.
142. Rajani K, Shapiro SR, Goetsman BW. Adrenal abscess: complication of supportive therapy of adrenal hemorrhage in the newborn. J Pediatr Surg 15:676, 1980.
143. Wells RG, Sty JR, Hodgson NB. Suprarenal abscess in the neonate: technetium-99m glucoheptonate imaging. Clin Nucl Med 11:32, 1986.
144. Cadarso BA, Mialdea AMR. Absceso adrenal en la epoca neonatal. An Esp Pediatr 21:706, 1984.
145. Ohta S, Shimizu S, Fujisawa S, et al. Neonatal adrenal abscess due to *Bacteroides*. J Pediatr 93:1063, 1978.
146. Bekdash BA, Slim MS. Adrenal abscess in a neonate due to gas-forming organisms: a diagnostic dilemma. Z Kinderchir 32:184, 1981.

147. Gross M, Kottmeier PK, Waterhouse K. Diagnosis and treatment of neonatal adrenal hemorrhage. J Pediatr Surg 2:308, 1967.
148. Vigi V, Tamisari L, Osti L, et al. Suprarenal abscess in a newborn. Helv Paediatr Acta 36:263, 1981.
149. Suri S, Agarwalla ML, Mitra S, et al. Adrenal abscess in a neonate presenting as a renal neoplasm. Br J Urol 54:565, 1982.
150. Mittelstaedt CA, Volberg FM, Merten DF, et al. The sonographic diagnosis of neonatal adrenal hemorrhage. Radiology 131:453, 1979.
151. Rey A, Arena J, Nogues A, et al. Hemorragia suprarenal encapsulada en el recien nacido: estudio de ocho casos. An Esp Pediatr 21:238, 1984.
152. Black J, Williams DI. Natural history of adrenal hemorrhage in the newborn. Arch Dis Child 48:173, 1973.
153. Iklof O, Mortensson W, Sandstedt B. Suprarenal haematoma versus neuroblastoma complicated by haemorrhage: a diagnostic dilemma in the newborn. Acta Radiol Diagn 27:3, 1986.
154. White SJ, Stuck KJ, Blane CE, et al. Sonography of neuroblastoma. Am J Radiol 141:465, 1983.
155. Shkolnik A. Applications of ultrasound in the neonatal abdomen. Radiol Clin North Am 23:141, 1985.

Appendicitis*

156. Etherington-Wilson WE. Appendicitis in newborn: report of a case 16 days old. Proc R Soc Med 38:186, 1945.
157. Puri P, O'Donnell B. Appendicitis in infancy. J Pediatr Surg 13:173, 1978.
158. Landaas B. Diagnosis of appendicitis in young children. Tidsskr Nor Laegeforen 68:335, 1948.
159. Reuter G, Krause I. Beitrag zur Problematik der Appendizitis des Neugeborenen. Kinderaerztl Prax 47:289, 1975.
160. Norris WJ. Appendicitis in children. West J Surg Obstet Gynecol 54:183, 1946.
161. Parsons JM, Miscall BG, McSherry CK. Appendicitis in the newborn infant. Surgery 67:841, 1970.
162. Schaupp W, Clausen EG, Ferrier PK. Appendicitis during the first month of life. Surgery 48:805, 1960.
163. Stanley-Brown EG. Acute appendicitis during the first five years of life. Am J Dis Child 108:134, 1964.
164. Snyder WH Jr, Chaffin L. Appendicitis during the first 2 years of life: report of 21 cases and review of 447 cases from the literature. Arch Surg 64:549, 1952.
165. Fields IA, Naiditch MJ, Rothman PE. Acute appendicitis in infants. Am J Dis Child 93:287, 1957.
166. Dick W, Hirt H-J, Vogel W. Die Appendizitis im Säglings- und Kleinkindesalter. Fortschr Med 94:125, 1976.
167. Gross RE. The Surgery of Infancy and Childhood: Its Principles and Techniques. Philadelphia, WB Saunders, 1953.
168. Grosfeld JL, Weinberger M, Clatworthy HW Jr. Acute appendicitis in the first two years of life. J Pediatr Surg 8:285, 1973.
169. Janik JS, Firor HV. Pediatric appendicitis: a 20-year study of 1,640 children at Cook County (Illinois) Hospital. Arch Surg 114:717, 1979.
170. Benson CD, Coury JJ Jr, Hagge DR. Acute appendicitis in infants: fifteen-year study. Arch Surg 64:561, 1952.
171. Massad M, Srouji M, Awdeh A, et al. Neonatal appendicitis: case report and a review of the English literature. Z Kinderchir 41:241, 1986.
172. Schorlemmer GR, Herbst CA Jr. Perforated neonatal appendicitis. South Med J 76:536, 1983.
173. Diess F. Die Appendizitis im Basler Kinderspital. Basle Dissertations, 1908, Case No. 36, p 63. Cited in reference 138 and in Abt. I A: Appendicitis in infants. Arch Pediatr 34:641, 1917.
174. Bartlett RH, Eraklis AJ, Wilkinson RH. Appendicitis in infancy. Surg Gynecol Obstet 130:99, 1970.
175. Broadbent NRG, Jardine JL. Acute appendicitis in a premature infant: a case report. Aust N Z J Surg 40:362, 1971.
176. Bryant LR, Trinkle JK, Noonan JA, et al. Appendicitis and appendiceal perforation in neonates. Am Surg 36:523, 1970.
177. Creery RDG. Acute appendicitis in the newborn. BMJ 1:871, 1953.
178. Hardman RP, Bowerman D. Appendicitis in the newborn. Am J Dis Child 105:99, 1963.
179. Klimt F, Hartmann G. Appendicitis perforata mit tiefsitzenden Dündarmverschluss beim Neugeborenen. Paediatr Prax 1:271, 1962.
180. Kolb G, Schaeffer EL. Über Appendizitis mit Perforation in den ersten Lebenwochen. Kinderaerztl Prax 1:1, 1955.
181. Liechti RE, Snyder WH Jr. Acute appendicitis under age 2. Am Surg 29:92, 1963.
182. Meigher SC, Lucas AW. Appendicitis in the newborn: case report. Ann Surg 136:1044, 1952.
183. Meyer JF. Acute gangrenous appendicitis in a premature infant. J Pediatr 41:343, 1952.
184. Neve R, Quenville NF. Appendicitis with perforation in a 12-day-old infant. Can Med Assoc J 94:447, 1966.
185. Nilforoushan MA. Fever and ascites in a newborn. Clin Pediatr 14:878, 1975.
186. Nuri M, Hecker WC, Duckert W. Beitrag zur Appendicitis im Neugeborenenalter. Z Kinderheilkd 91:1, 1964.
187. Parkhurst GF, Wagoner SC. Neonatal acute appendicitis. N Y State J Med 69:1929, 1969.
188. Phillips SJ, Cohen B. Acute perforated appendicitis in newborn children. N Y State J Med 71:985, 1971.
189. Smith AL, MacMahon RA. Perforated appendix complicating rhesus immunization in a newborn infant. Med J Aust 2:602, 1969.
190. Tabrisky J, Westerfeld R, Cavanaugh J. Appendicitis in the newborn. Am J Dis Child 111:557, 1966.
191. Vinz H, Erben U, Winkelvoss H. Neugeborenen peritonitis. Bruns Beitr Klin Chir 215:321, 1967.
192. Walker RH. Appendicitis in the newborn infant. J Pediatr 51:429, 1958.
193. Morehead CD, Houck PW. Epidemiology of *Pseudomonas* infections in a pediatric intensive care unit. Am J Dis Child 124:564, 1972.
194. Trojanowski JQ, Gang DL, Goldblatt A, et al. Fatal postoperative acute appendicitis in a neonate with congenital heart disease. J Pediatr Surg 16:85, 1981.
195. Ayalon A, Mogilner M, Cohen O, et al. Acute appendicitis in a premature baby. Acta Chir Scand 145:285, 1979.
196. Schellerer W, Schwemmle K, Decker R. Perforierte Appendizitis bei einem Frühgeborenen im Alter von 14 Tagen. Z Kinderchir 9:434, 1971.
197. Golladay ES, Roskes S, Donner L, et al. Intestinal obstruction from appendiceal abscess in a newborn infant. J Pediatr Surg 13:175, 1978.
198. Hemalatha V, Spitz L. Neonatal appendicitis. Clin Pediatr 18:621, 1979.
199. Tucci P, Holgersen L, Doctor D, et al. Congenital uretero-pelvic junction obstruction associated with unsuspected acute perforated appendicitis in a neonate. J Urol 120:247, 1978.
200. Fowkes GL. Neonatal appendicitis. BMJ 1:997, 1978.
201. Kwong MS, Dinner M. Neonatal appendicitis masquerading as necrotizing enterocolitis. J Pediatr 96:917, 1980.
202. Shaul WL. Clues to the early diagnosis of neonatal appendicitis. J Pediatr 98:473, 1981.
203. Grussner R, Pistor G, Engelskirchen R, et al. Appendicitis in childhood. Monatsschr Kinderheilkd 133:158, 1985.
204. Lassiter HA, Werner MH. Neonatal appendicitis. South Med J 76:1173, 1983.
205. Carol MJ, Creixell GS, Hernandez GJV, et al. Apendicitis neonatal: aportacion de un nuevo caso. An Esp Pediatr 20:807, 1984.
206. Bax NMA, Pearse RG, Dommering N, et al. Perforation of the appendix in the neonatal period. J Pediatr Surg 15:200, 1980.
207. Buntain WL. Neonatal appendicitis mistaken for necrotizing enterocolitis. South Med J 75:1155, 1982.
208. Heydenrych JJ, DuToit DF. Unusual presentations of acute appendicitis in the neonate: a report of 2 cases. S Afr Med J 62:1003, 1982.
209. Ruff ME, Southgate WM, Wood BP (eds). Radiological case of the month: neonatal appendicitis with perforation. Am J Dis Child 145:111, 1991.
210. Pathania OP, Jain SK, Kapila H, et al. Fatal neonatal perforation of appendix. Indian Pediatr J 26:1166, 1989.
211. Arora NK, Deorari AK, Bhatnagar V, et al. Neonatal appendicitis: a rare cause of surgical emergency in preterm babies. Indian Pediatr J 28:1330, 1991.
212. Srouji MN, Chatten J, David C. Pseudodiverticulitis of the appendix with neonatal Hirschsprung disease. J Pediatr 93:988, 1978.
213. Arliss J, Holgersen LO. Neonatal appendiceal perforation and Hirschsprung's disease. J Pediatr Surg 25:694, 1990.
214. Kliegman RM, Fanaroff AA. Necrotizing enterocolitis. N Engl J Med 310:1093, 1984.
215. Srouji MN, Buck BE. Neonatal appendicitis: ischemic infarction in incarcerated inguinal hernia. J Pediatr Surg 13:177, 1978.

*The list of references for intra-abdominal neonatal appendicitis is not exhaustive; additional cases can be found in the articles listed here.

216. Charif P. Perforated appendicitis in premature infants: a case report and review of the literature. Johns Hopkins Med J 125:92, 1969.
217. Stone HH, Sanders SL, Martin JD Jr. Perforated appendicitis in children. Surgery 69:673, 1971.
218. Dennis JE, Rhodes KH, Cooney DR, et al. Nosocomial *Rhizopus* infection (zygomycosis) in children. J Pediatr 96:824, 1980.
219. Buschard K, Kjaeldgaard A. Investigation and analysis of the position, fixation, length, embryology of the vermiform appendix. Acta Chir Scand 139:293, 1973.
220. Jones WR, Kaye MD, Ing RMY. The lymphoid development of the fetal and neonatal appendix. Biol Neonatal 20:334, 1972.
221. Smith GM. Inflammatory changes in the appendix during early infancy. Am J Dis Child 1:299, 1911.
222. Hill WB, Mason CC. Prenatal appendicitis with rupture and death. Am J Dis Child 29:86, 1925.
223. Corcoran WJ. Prenatal rupture of the appendix. Am J Dis Child 39:277, 1930.
224. Jackson WF. A case of prenatal appendicitis. Am J Med Sci 127:710, 1904.
225. Kümmell EW. Cited in Etherington-Wilson WE. Appendicitis in newborn: report of a case 16 days old. Proc R Soc Med 38:186, 1945.
226. Martin LW, Glen PM. Prenatal appendiceal perforation: a case report. J Pediatr Surg 21:73, 1986.
227. Wilkinson RH, Bartlett RH, Eraklis AJ. Diagnosis of appendicitis in infancy: the value of abdominal radiographs. Am J Dis Child 118:687, 1969.
228. Holder TM, Leape LL. The acute surgical abdomen in the neonate. N Engl J Med 278:605, 1968.
229. Chang JHT. The use of antibiotics in pediatric abdominal surgery. Pediatr Infect Dis 3:195, 1984.

Peritonitis

230. Bell MJ. Peritonitis in the newborn-current concepts. Pediatr Clin North Am 32:1181, 1985.
231. Barson AJ. A postmortem study of infection in the newborn from 1976 to 1988. *In* deLouvois J, Harvey D (eds): Infection in the Newborn. New York, John Wiley & Sons, 1990, pp 13-34.
232. Fonkalsrud EW, Ellis DG, Clatworthy HW Jr. Neonatal peritonitis. J Pediatr Surg 1:227, 1966.
233. Lloyd JR. The etiology of gastrointestinal perforations in the newborn. J Pediatr Surg 4:77, 1969.
234. McDougal WS, Izant RJ, Zollinger RM Jr. Primary peritonitis in infancy and childhood. Ann Surg 181:310, 1975.
235. Rickham PP. Peritonitis in the neonatal period. Arch Dis Child 30:23, 1955.
236. Denes J, Leb J. Neonatal peritonitis. Acta Paediatr Acad Sci Hung 10:297, 1969.
237. Daum R, Schütze U, Hoffman H. Mortality of preoperative peritonitis in newborn infants without intestinal obstruction. Prog Pediatr Surg 13:267, 1979.
238. Schütze U, Fey KH, Hess G. Die Peritonitis im Neugeborenen-, Säglings-, und Kindesalter. Munch Med Wochenschr 116:1201, 1974.
239. Prevot J, Grosdidier G, Schmitt M. Fatal peritonitis. Prog Pediatr Surg 13:257, 1979.
240. Singer B, Hammar B. Neonatal peritonitis. S Afr Med J 46:987, 1972.
241. Hensey OJ, Hart CA, Cooke RWI. Serious infection in a neonatal intensive care unit: a two-year survey. J Hyg (Camb) 95:289, 1985.
242. Valdes-Dapeña MA, Arey JB. The causes of neonatal mortality: an analysis of 501 autopsies on newborn infants. J Pediatr 77:366, 1970.
243. Bell MJ. Perforation of the gastrointestinal tract and peritonitis in the neonate. Surg Gynecol Obstet 160:20, 1985.
244. Duggan MB, Khwaja MS. Neonatal primary peritonitis in Nigeria. Arch Dis Child 50:130, 1975.
245. Birtch AG, Coran AG, Gross RE. Neonatal peritonitis. Surgery 61:305, 1967.
246. Lacheretz M, Debeugny P, Krivosic-Horner R, et al. Péritonite néonatale par pérforation gastrique: à propos de 21 observations. Chirurgie 109:887, 1983.
247. Mollitt DL, Tepas JJ, Talbert JL. The microbiology of neonatal peritonitis. Arch Surg 123:176, 1988.
248. Scott JES. Intestinal obstruction in the newborn associated with peritonitis. Arch Dis Child 38:120, 1963.
249. Thelander HE. Perforation of the gastrointestinal tract of the newborn infant. Am J Dis Child 58:371, 1939.
250. Dinari G, Haimov H, Geiffman M. Umbilical arteritis and phlebitis with scrotal abscess and peritonitis. J Pediatr Surg 6:176, 1971.
251. Forshall I. Septic umbilical arteritis. Arch Dis Child 32:25, 1957.
252. Chadwick EG, Shulman ST, Yogev R. Peritonitis as a late manifestation of group B streptococcal disease in newborns. Pediatr Infect Dis 2:142, 1983.
253. Reyna TM. Primary group B streptococcal peritonitis presenting as an incarcerated inguinal hernia in a neonate. Clin Pediatr 25:422, 1987.
254. Serlo W, Heikkinen E, Kouvalainen K. Group A streptococcal peritonitis in infancy. Ann Chir Gynaecol 74:183, 1985.
255. Johnson DE, Conroy MM, Foker JE, et al. *Candida* peritonitis in a newborn infant. J Pediatr 97:298, 1980.
256. Kaplan M, Eidelman AI, Dollberg L, et al. Necrotizing bowel disease with *Candida* peritonitis following severe neonatal hypothermia. Acta Paediatr Scand 79:876, 1990.
257. Butler KM, Bench MA, Baker CJ. Amphotericin B as a single agent in the treatment of systemic candidiasis in neonates. Pediatr Infect Dis J 9:51, 1990.
258. MacDonald L, Baker CJ, Chenoweth C. Risk factors for candidemia in a children's hospital. Clin Infect Dis 26:642, 1998.
259. Abt IA. Fetal peritonitis. Med Clin North Am 15:611, 1931.
260. Pan EY, Chen LY, Yang JZ, et al. Radiographic diagnosis of meconium peritonitis: a report of 200 cases including six fetal cases. Pediatr Radiol 13:199, 1983.
261. Aschner JL, Deluga KS, Metlay LA, et al. Spontaneous focal gastrointestinal perforation in very low birth weight infants. J Pediatr 113:364, 1988.
262. Holgersen LO. The etiology of spontaneous gastric perforation of the newborn: a reevaluation. J Pediatr Surg 16:608, 1981.
263. Rickham PP. Neugeborenen-peritonitis. Langenbecks Arch Klin Chir 292:427, 1959.
264. Kadowaki H, Takeuchi S, Nakahira M, et al. Neonatal gastric perforations; a diagnostic clue in pre-perforative phase. Jpn J Surg 13:446, 1983.
265. Fowler R. Primary peritonitis: changing aspects 1956-1970. Aust Paediatr J 7:73, 1971.
266. Donnison AB, Schwachman H, Gross RE. A review of 164 children with meconium ileus seen at the Children's Hospital Medical Center, Boston. Pediatrics 37:833, 1966.
267. Alpan G, Eyal F, Vinograd I, et al. Localized intestinal perforations after enteral administration of indomethacin in premature infants. J Pediatr 106:277, 1985.
268. Wolf WM, Snover DC, Leonard AS. Localized intestinal perforation following intravenous indomethacin in premature infants. J Pediatr Surg 24:409, 1989.
269. Hayhurst EG, Wyman M. Morbidity associated with prolonged use of polyvinyl feeding tubes. Am J Dis Child 129:72, 1975.
270. Fonkalsrud EW, Clatworthy HW Jr. Accidental perforation of the colon and rectum in newborn infants. N Engl J Med 272:1097, 1956.
271. Frank JD, Brown S. Thermometers and rectal perforations in the neonate. Arch Dis Child 53:824, 1978.
272. Horwitz MA, Bennett JV. Nursery outbreak of peritonitis with pneumoperitoneum probably caused by thermometer-induced rectal perforation. Am J Epidemiol 104:632, 1976.
273. deVeber LL, Marshall DG, Robinson ML. Peritonitis, peritoneal adhesions and intestinal obstruction as a complication of intrauterine transfusion. Can Med Assoc J 99:76, 1968.
274. Haltalin KC. Neonatal shigellosis: report of 16 cases and review of the literature. Am J Dis Child 114:603, 1967.
275. Abramson H, Frant S, Oldenbusch C. *Salmonella* infection of the newborn: its differentiation from epidemic diarrhea and other primary enteric disorders of the newborn. Med Clin North Am 23:591, 1939.
276. Starke JR, Baker CJ. Neonatal shigellosis with bowel perforation. Pediatr Infect Dis 4:405, 1985.
277. Opitz K. Beitrag zur Klinik und Pathologie der Nabelschnurinfektionen. Arch Kinderheilkd 150:174, 1955.
278. Gluck L, Wood HF, Fousek MD. Septicemia of the newborn. Pediatr Clin North Am 13:1131, 1966.
279. Wells CL, Maddaus MA, Simmons RL. Proposed mechanisms for the translocation of intestinal bacteria. Rev Infect Dis 10:958, 1988.
280. Wilson R, Kanto WP Jr, McCarthy BJ, et al. Short communication: age at onset of necrotizing enterocolitis: an epidemiologic analysis. Pediatr Res 16:82, 1982.
281. Caralaps-Riera JM, Cohn BD. Bowel perforation after exchange transfusion in the neonate: review of the literature and report of a case. Surgery 68:895, 1970.

282. Touloukian RJ, Kadar A, Spencer RP. The gastrointestinal complications of neonatal umbilical venous exchange transfusion: a clinical and experimental study. Pediatrics 51:36, 1973.
283. Freedman RM, Ingram DL, Gross I, et al. A half century of neonatal sepsis at Yale: 1928 to 1978. Am J Dis Child 135:140, 1981.
284. Martin DJ. Neonatal disorders diagnosed with ultrasound. Clin Perinatol 12:219, 1985.
285. Griscom NT, Colodny AH, Rosenberg HK, et al. Diagnostic aspects of neonatal ascites: report of 27 cases. AJR Am J Roentgenol 128:961, 1977.
286. Kosloske AM, Lilly JR. Paracentesis and lavage for diagnosis of intestinal gangrene in neonatal necrotizing enterocolitis. J Pediatr Surg 13:315, 1978.
287. Töllner U, Pohlandt F. Aszitespunktion zur Differentialdiagnose beim akuten Abdomen des Neugeborenen. Klin Paediatr 196:319, 1984.
288. McKendry JBJ, Lindsay WK, Gerstein MC. Congenital defects of the lymphatics in infancy. Pediatrics 19:21, 1959.
289. Lees W, Mitchell JE. Bile peritonitis in infancy. Arch Dis Child 41:188, 1966.
290. Cohen MD, Weber TR, Grosfeld JL. Bowel perforation in the newborn: diagnosis with metrizamide. Radiology 150:65, 1984.
291. Rosenfeld DL, Cordell CE, Jadeja N. Retrocardiac pneumomediastinum: radiographic finding and clinical implications. Pediatrics 85:92, 1989.
292. Wind ED, Pillari GP, Lee WJ. Lucent liver in the newborn: a roentgenographic sign of pneumoperitoneum. JAMA 237:2218, 1977.
293. Pochaczevsky R, Bryk D. New roentgenographic signs of neonatal gastric perforation. Radiology 102:145, 1972.
294. Gellis SS, Finegold M. Picture of the month: pneumoperitoneum demonstrated by transillumination. Am J Dis Child 130:1237, 1976.
295. Thomas S, Sainsbury C, Murphy JF. Pancuronium belly. Lancet 2:870, 1984.
296. Ein SH, Stephens CA, Reilly BJ. The disappearance of free air after pediatric laparotomy. J Pediatr Surg 20:422, 1985.
297. Emanuel B, Zlotnik P, Raffensperger JG. Perforation of the gastrointestinal tract in infancy and childhood. Surg Gynecol Obstet 146:926, 1978.

Necrotizing Enterocolitis

298. Yu VYH, Tudehope DI, Gill GJ. Neonatal necrotizing enterocolitis. 1. Clinical aspects and 2. Perinatal risk factors. Med J Aust 1:685, 688, 1977.
299. Holman RC, Stehr-Green JK, Zelasky MT. Necrotizing enterocolitis mortality in the United States, 1979-85. Am J Public Health 79:987, 1989.
300. Finer NN, Moriartey RR. Reply, letter to the editor. J Pediatr 96:170, 1980.
301. Book LS, Herbst JJ, Atherton SO, et al. Necrotizing enterocolitis in low-birth-weight infants fed an elemental formula. J Pediatr 87:602, 1975.
302. O'Neill JA Jr, Stahlman MT, Meng HC. Necrotizing enterocolitis in the newborn: operative indications. Ann Surg 182:274, 1975.
303. Moore TD (ed). Necrotizing Enterocolitis in the Newborn Infant: Report of the Sixty-Eighth Ross Conference on Pediatric Research. Columbus, Ohio, Ross Laboratories, 1975.
304. Virnig NL, Reynolds JW. Epidemiological aspects of neonatal necrotizing enterocolitis. Am J Dis Child 128:186, 1974.
305. Touloukian RJ. Neonatal necrotizing enterocolitis: an update on etiology, diagnosis, and treatment. Surg Clin North Am 56:281, 1976.
306. Bell MJ, Ternberg JL, Bower RJ. The microbial flora and antimicrobial therapy of neonatal peritonitis. J Pediatr Surg 15:569, 1980.
307. Emanuel B, Zlotnik P, Raffensperger JG. Perforation of the gastrointestinal tract in infancy and childhood. Surg Gynecol Obstet 146:926, 1978.
308. Kliegman RM, Fanaroff AA. Neonatal necrotizing enterocolitis: a nine-year experience: I. Epidemiology and uncommon observations. Am J Dis Child 135:603, 1981.
309. Goldman HI. Feeding and necrotizing enterocolitis. Am J Dis Child 134:553, 1980.
310. Brown EG, Sweet AY. Preventing necrotizing enterocolitis in neonates. JAMA 240:2452, 1978.
311. Book LS, Herbst JJ, Jung AL. Comparison of fast- and slow-feeding rate schedules to the development of necrotizing enterocolitis. J Pediatr 89:463, 1976.
312. Bell MJ, Shackelford P, Feigin RD, et al. Epidemiologic and bacteriologic evaluation of neonatal necrotizing enterocolitis. J Pediatr Surg 14:1, 1979.
313. Eidelman AI, Inwood RJ. Marginal comments: necrotizing enterocolitis and enteral feeding: is too much just too much? Am J Dis Child 134:545, 1980.
314. Kliegman RM, Fanaroff AA, Izant R, et al. Clostridia as pathogens in neonatal necrotizing enterocolitis. J Pediatr 95:287, 1979.
315. Brown EG, Sweet AY. Neonatal necrotizing enterocolitis. Pediatr Clin North Am 29:1149, 1982.
316. Kanto WP Jr, Wilson R, Breart GL, et al. Perinatal events and necrotizing enterocolitis in premature infants. Am J Dis Child 141:167, 1987.
317. Ostertag SG, LaGamma EF, Reisen CE, et al. Early enteral feeding does not affect the incidence of necrotizing enterocolitis. Pediatrics 77:275, 1986.
318. Merritt CRB, Goldsmith JP, Sharp MJ. Sonographic detection of portal venous gas in infants with necrotizing enterocolitis. AJR Am J Roentgenol 143:1059, 1984.
319. Cikrit D, Mastandrea J, Grosfeld JL, et al. Significance of portal venous air in necrotizing enterocolitis: analysis of 53 cases. J Pediatr Surg 20:425, 1985.
320. Maguire GC, Nordin J, Myers MG, et al. Infections acquired by young infants. Am J Dis Child 135:693, 1981.
321. Yu VYH, Joseph R, Bajuk B, et al. Perinatal risk factors for necrotizing enterocolitis. Arch Dis Child 59:430, 1984.
322. Uauy RD, Fanaroff AA, Korones SB, et al, for the National Institute of Child Health and Human Development Neonatal Research Network. Necrotizing enterocolitis in very low birth weight infants: biodemographic and clinical correlates. J Pediatr 119:630, 1991.
323. Walsh MC, Kliegman RM. Necrotizing enterocolitis: treatment based on staging criteria. Pediatr Clin North Am 33:179, 1986.
324. Kliegman RM, Fanaroff AA. Necrotizing enterocolitis. N Engl J Med 310:1093, 1984.
325. Kamitsuka MD, Horton MK, Williams MA. The incidence of necrotizing enterocolitis after introducing standardized feeding schedules for infants between 1250 and 2500 grams and less than 35 weeks of gestation. Pediatrics 105:379, 2000.
326. Rayyis SF, Ambalavanan N, Wright L, Carlo WA. Randomized trial of slow versus fast feed advancements on the incidence of necrotizing enterocolitis in very low birth weight infants. J Pediatr 134:293, 1999.
327. Santulli TV, Schullinger JN, Heird WC, et al. Acute necrotizing enterocolitis in infancy: a review of 64 cases. Pediatrics 55:376, 1975.
328. Kliegman RM, Hack M, Jones P, et al. Epidemiologic study of necrotizing enterocolitis among low-birth-weight infants: absence of identifiable risk factors. J Pediatr 100:440, 1982.
329. Stoll BJ, Kanto WP Jr, Glass RI, et al. Epidemiology of necrotizing enterocolitis: a case control study. J Pediatr 96:447, 1980.
330. Frantz ID III, L'Heureux P, Engel RR, et al. Necrotizing enterocolitis. J Pediatr 86:259, 1975.
331. Egan EA, Mantilla G, Nelson RM, et al. A prospective controlled trial of oral kanamycin in the prevention of neonatal necrotizing enterocolitis. J Pediatr 89:467, 1976.
332. Wilson R, Kanto WP Jr, McCarthy BJ, et al. Age at onset of necrotizing enterocolitis: an epidemiologic analysis. Pediatr Res 16:82, 1982.
333. Gerard P, Bachy A, Battisti O, et al. Mortality in 504 infants weighing less than 1501 g at birth and treated in four neonatal intensive care units of South-Belgium between 1976 and 1980. Eur J Pediatr 144:219, 1985.
334. Yu VYH, Joseph R, Bajuk B, et al. Necrotizing enterocolitis in very low birthweight infants: a four-year experience. Aust Paediatr J 20:29, 1984.
335. Palmer SR, Biffin A, Gamsu HR. Outcome of neonatal necrotising enterocolitis: results of the BAPM/CDSC surveillance study, 1989-84. Arch Dis Child 64:388, 1989.
336. de Gamarra E, Helardot P, Moriette G, et al. Necrotizing enterocolitis in full-term neonates. Biol Neonate 44:185, 1983.
337. Thilo EH, Lazarte RA, Hernandez JA. Necrotizing enterocolitis in the first 24 hours of life. Pediatrics 73:476, 1984.
338. Wilson R, del Portillo M, Schmidt E, et al. Risk factors for necrotizing enterocolitis in infants weighing more than 2,000 grams at birth: a case-control study. Pediatrics 71:19, 1983.
339. Necrotizing enterocolitis. Editorial. Lancet 1:459, 1977.
340. Bisquera JA, Cooper TR, Berseth CL. Impact of necrotizing enterocolitis on length of stay and hospital charges in very low birth weight infants. Pediatrics 109:423, 2002.
341. Frey EE, Smith W, Franken EA Jr, et al. Analysis of bowel perforation in necrotizing enterocolitis. Pediatr Radiol 17:380, 1987.
342. Kliegman RM, Pittard WB, Fanaroff AA. Necrotizing enterocolitis in neonates fed human milk. J Pediatr 95:450, 1979.

343. Guinan M, Schaberg D, Bruhn FW, et al. Epidemic occurrence of neonatal necrotizing enterocolitis. Am J Dis Child 133:594, 1979.
343a. Lin HC, Su BH, Chen AC, et al. Oral probiotics reduce the incidence and severity of necrotizing enterocolitis in very low birthweight infants. Pediatrics 115:1-4, 2005.
344. Dvorak B, Halpern MD, Holubec H, et al. Maternal milk reduces the severity of necrotizing enterocolitis and increases intestinal IL-10 in a neonatal rat model. Pediatr Res 55:426, 2003.
345. Kosloske AM. Pathogenesis and prevention of necrotizing enterocolitis: a hypothesis based on personal observation and a review of the literature. Pediatrics 74:1086, 1984.
346. Gaynes RP, Palmer S, Martone WJ, et al. The role of host factors in an outbreak of necrotizing enterocolitis. Am J Dis Child 138:1118, 1984.
347. Han VKM, Sayed H, Chance GW, et al. An outbreak of *Clostridium difficile* necrotizing enterocolitis: a case for oral vancomycin therapy? Pediatrics 71:935, 1983.
348. McClead RE Jr (ed). Neonatal necrotizing enterocolitis: current concepts and controversies. J Pediatr 17(Suppl):S1, 1990.
349. Jona JZ. Advances in neonatal surgery. Pediatr Clin North Am 45:605, 1998.
350. Milner ME, de la Monte SM, Moore GW, et al. Risk factors for developing and dying from necrotizing enterocolitis. J Pediatr Gastroenterol Nutr 5:359, 1986.
351. Wiswell TE, Hankins CT. Twins and triplets with necrotizing enterocolitis. Am J Dis Child 142:1004, 1988.
352. DeCurtis M, Paone C, Vetrano G, et al. A case control study of necrotizing enterocolitis occurring over 8 years in a neonatal intensive care unit. Eur J Pediatr 146:398, 1987.
353. Kliegman RM. Neonatal necrotizing enterocolitis: implications for an infectious disease. Pediatr Clin North Am 26:327, 1979.
354. Book LS, Overall JC Jr, Herbst JJ, et al. Clustering of necrotizing enterocolitis: interruption by infection-control measures. N Engl J Med 297:984, 1977.
355. Rotbart HA, Levin MJ. How contagious is necrotizing enterocolitis? Pediatr Infect Dis 2:406, 1983.
356. Roback SA, Foker J, Frantz IF, et al. Necrotizing enterocolitis. Arch Surg 109:314, 1974.
357. Stanley MD, Null DM Jr, deLemos RA. Relationship between intestinal colonization with specific bacteria and the development of necrotizing enterocolitis. Pediatr Res 11:543, 1977.
358. Hill HR, Hunt CE, Matsen JM. Nosocomial colonization with *Klebsiella*, type 26, in a neonatal intensive-care unit associated with an outbreak of sepsis, meningitis, and necrotizing enterocolitis. J Pediatr 85:415, 1974.
359. Powell J, Bureau MA, Paré C, et al. Necrotizing enterocolitis: epidemic following an outbreak of *Enterobacter cloacae* type 3305573 in a neonatal intensive care unit. Am J Dis Child 134:1152, 1980.
360. Speer ME, Taber LH, Yow MD, et al. Fulminant neonatal sepsis and necrotizing enterocolitis associated with a "nonenteropathogenic" strain of *Escherichia coli*. J Pediatr 89:91, 1976.
361. Cushing AH. Necrotizing enterocolitis with *Escherichia coli* heat-labile enterotoxin. Pediatrics 71:626, 1983.
362. Henderson A, Maclaurin J, Scott JM. *Pseudomonas* in a Glasgow baby unit. Lancet 2:316, 1969.
363. Waldhausen JA, Herendeen T, King H. Necrotizing colitis of the newborn: common cause of perforation of the colon. Surgery 54:365, 1963.
364. Stein H, Beck J, Solomon A, et al. Gastroenteritis with necrotizing enterocolitis in premature babies. BMJ 2:616, 1972.
365. Gruskay JA, Abbasi S, Anday E, et al. *Staphylococcus epidermidis*–associated enterocolitis. J Pediatr 109:520, 1986.
366. Overturf GD, Sherman MP, Wong L, et al. Neonatal necrotizing enterocolitis associated with delta toxin producing methicillin-resistant *S. aureus*. Pediatr Infect Dis J 9:88, 1990.
367. Rotbart HA, Nelson WL, Glode MP, et al. Neonatal rotavirus-associated necrotizing enterocolitis: case control study and prospective surveillance during an outbreak. J Pediatr 112:87, 1988.
368. Rotbart HA, Yolken RH, Nelson WL, et al. Confirmatory testing of Rotazyme results in neonates. J Pediatr 107:289, 1985.
369. Rousset S, Moscovici O, Lebon P, et al. Intestinal lesions containing coronavirus-like particles in neonatal necrotizing enterocolitis: an ultrastructural analysis. Pediatrics 73:218, 1984.
370. Johnson FE, Crnic DM, Simmons MA, et al. Association of fatal coxsackie B2 viral infection and necrotizing enterocolitis. Arch Dis Child 52:802, 1977.
371. Baley JE, Kliegman RM, Annable WL, et al. *Torulopsis glabrata* sepsis appearing as necrotizing enterocolitis and endophthalmitis. Am J Dis Child 138:965, 1984.
372. *Clostridium septicum* and neutropenic enterocolitis. Editorial. Lancet 2:608, 1987.
373. Finegold SM. Anaerobic Bacteria in Human Diseases. New York, Academic Press, 1977.
374. Lawrence G, Walker PD. Pathogenesis of enteritis necroticans in Papua, New Guinea. Lancet 1:125, 1976.
375. Kliegman RM. The role of clostridia in the pathogenesis of neonatal necrotizing enterocolitis. *In* Borriello SP (eds). Clostridia in Gastrointestinal Disease. Boca Raton, Fla, CRC Press, 1985, pp 68-92.
376. Volsted-Pedersen P, Hansen FH, Halveg AB, et al. Necrotising enterocolitis of the newborn—is it gas gangrene of the bowels? Lancet 2:715, 1976.
377. Kosloske AM, Ulrich JA, Hoffman H. Fulminant necrotising enterocolitis associated with clostridia. Lancet 2:1014, 1978.
378. Warren S, Schreiber JR, Epstein MF. Necrotizing enterocolitis and hemolysis associated with *Clostridium perfringens*. Am J Dis Child 138:686, 1984.
379. Blakey JL, Lubitz L, Campbell NT, et al. Enteric colonization in sporadic neonatal necrotizing enterocolitis. J Pediatr Gastroenterol Nutr 4:591, 1985.
380. Cashore WJ, Peter G, Lauermann M, et al. Clostridia colonization and clostridial toxin in neonatal necrotizing enterocolitis. J Pediatr 98:308, 1981.
381. Sturm R, Staneck JL, Stauffer LR, et al. Neonatal necrotizing enterocolitis associated with penicillin-resistant, toxigenic *Clostridium butyricum*. Pediatrics 66:928, 1980.
382. Howard FM, Flynn DM, Bradley JM, et al. Outbreak of necrotising enterocolitis caused by *Clostridium butyricum*. Lancet 2:1099, 1977.
383. Riser E, Bradley J, Flynn D, et al. Synergy in necrotizing enterocolitis. Am J Dis Child 135:291, 1981.
384. Zedd AJ, Sell TL, Schaberg DR, et al. Nosocomial *Clostridium difficile* reservoir in a neonatal intensive care unit. Pediatr Infect Dis 3:429, 1984.
385. Al-Jumaili IJ, Shibley M, Lishman AH, et al. Incidence and origin of *Clostridium difficile* in neonates. J Clin Microbiol 19:77, 1984.
386. Smith MF, Borriello SP, Clayden GS, et al. Clinical and bacteriological findings in necrotizing enterocolitis: a controlled study. J Infect 2:23, 1980.
387. Gothefors L, Blenkharn I. *Clostridium butyricum* and necrotising enterocolitis. Lancet 1:52, 1978. (Reply in Bradley JM, Szawatkowski M, Noone P, et al. Clostridia in necrotising enterocolitis. Lancet 1:389, 1978.)
388. Laverdière M, Robert A, Chicoine R, et al. Clostridia in necrotising enterocolitis. Lancet 2:377, 1978.
389. Kelsey MC, Vince AJ. Clostridia in neonatal feces. Lancet 2:100, 1979.
390. Kindley AD, Roberts PJ, Tulloch WH. Neonatal necrotising enterocolitis. Lancet 1:649, 1977.
391. Lishman AH, Al-Jumaili IJ, Elshibly E, et al. *Clostridium difficile* isolation in neonates in a special care unit: lack of correlation with necrotizing enterocolitis. Scand J Gastroenterol 19:441, 1984.
392. Westra-Meijer CM, Degener JE, Dzoljic-Danilovic G, et al. Quantitative study of the aerobic and anaerobic faecal flora in neonatal necrotizing enterocolitis. Arch Dis Child 58:523, 1983.
393. Thomas DFM, Fernie DS, Bayston R, et al. Clostridial toxins in neonatal necrotizing enterocolitis. Arch Dis Child 59:270, 1984.
394. Scheifele DW, Bjornson GL. Delta toxin activity in coagulase-negative staphylococci from the bowel of neonates. J Clin Microbiol 26:279, 1988.
395. Scheifele DW, Bjornson GL, Dyer RA, et al. Delta-like toxin produced by coagulase-negative staphylococci is associated with neonatal necrotizing enterocolitis. Infect Immun 55:2268, 1988.
396. Hoy C, Millar MR, MacKay P, et al. Quantitative changes in faecal microflora preceding necrotizing enterocolitis in premature neonates. Arch Dis Child 65:1057, 1990.
397. Dykes EH, Gilmour WH, Azmy AF. Prediction of outcome following necrotizing enterocolitis in a neonatal surgical unit. J Pediatr Surg 20:3, 1985.
398. Wayne ER, Burrington JD, Hutter J. Neonatal necrotizing enterocolitis: evolution of new principles in management. Arch Surg 110:476, 1975.
399. Wilson R, Kanto WP Jr, McCarthy BJ, et al. Age at onset of necrotizing enterocolitis. Am J Dis Child 136:814, 1982.
400. Leonidas JC, Hall RT. Neonatal pneumatosis coli: a mild form of neonatal necrotizing enterocolitis. J Pediatr 89:456, 1976.
401. Richmond JA, Mikity V. Benign form of necrotizing enterocolitis. AJR Am J Roentgenol 123:301, 1975.

402. Barnard JA, Cotton RB, Lutin W. Necrotizing enterocolitis. Variables associated with the severity of the disease. Am J Dis Child 139:375, 1985.
403. Bell MJ, Ternberg JL, Feigin RD, et al. Neonatal necrotizing enterocolitis: therapeutic decisions based upon clinical staging. Ann Surg 187:1, 1978.
404. Buras R, Guzzetta P, Avery G, et al. Acidosis and hepatic portal venous gas: indications for surgery in necrotizing enterocolitis. Pediatrics 78:273, 1986.
405. Daneman A, Woodward S, de Silva M. The radiology of neonatal necrotizing enterocolitis (NEC): a review of 47 cases and the literature. Pediatr Radiol 7:70, 1978.
406. Mata AG, Rosengart RM. Interobserver variability in the radiographic diagnosis of necrotizing enterocolitis. Pediatrics 66:68, 1980.
407. Johnson JF, Robinson LH. Localized bowel distension in the newborn: a review of the plain film analysis and differential diagnosis. Pediatrics 73:206, 1984.
408. Leonard T Jr, Johnson JF, Pettett PG. Critical evaluation of the persistent loop sign in necrotizing enterocolitis. Radiology 142:385, 1982.
409. Weinstein MM. The persistent loop sign in neonatal necrotizing enterocolitis: a new cause. Pediatr Radiol 16:71, 1986.
410. Kliegman RM, Fanaroff AA. Neonatal necrotizing enterocolitis: a nine-year experience: II. Outcome assessment. Am J Dis Child 135:608, 1981.
411. Keller MS, Chawla HS. Neonatal metrizamide gastrointestinal series in suspected necrotizing enterocolitis. Am J Dis Child 139:713, 1985.
412. Lindley S, Mollitt DL, Seiberty JJ, et al. Portal vein ultrasonography in the early diagnosis of necrotizing enterocolitis. J Pediatr Surg 21:530, 1986.
413. Malin SW, Bhutani VK, Ritchie WW, et al. Echogenic intravascular and hepatic microbubbles associated with necrotizing enterocolitis. J Pediatr 103:637, 1983.
414. Kosloske AM, Lilly JR. Paracentesis and lavage for diagnosis of intestinal gangrene in neonatal necrotizing enterocolitis. J Pediatr Surg 13:315, 1978.
415. Ricketts RR. The role of paracentesis in the management of infants with necrotizing enterocolitis. Am Surg 52:61, 1986.
416. Kosloske AM. Surgery of necrotizing enterocolitis. World J Surg 9:277, 1985.
417. Patel CC. Hematologic abnormalities in acute necrotizing enterocolitis. Pediatr Clin North Am 24:579, 1977.
418. Hutter JJ Jr, Hathaway WE, Wayne ER. Hematologic abnormalities in severe neonatal necrotizing enterocolitis. J Pediatr 88:1026, 1976.
419. Hyman PE, Abrams CE, Zipser RD. Enhanced urinary immunoreactive thromboxane in neonatal necrotizing enterocolitis: a diagnostic indicator of thrombotic activity. Am J Dis Child 141:688, 1987.
420. Scheifele DW, Olson EM, Pendray MR. Endotoxinemia and thrombocytopenia during neonatal necrotizing enterocolitis. Am J Clin Pathol 83:227, 1985.
421. Rabinowitz SS, Dzakpasu P, Piccuh S, et al. Platelet-activating factor in infants at risk for necrotizing enterocolitis. Journal of Pediatrics 138:81, 2001.
422. Christensen RD, Rothstein G, Anstall HB, et al. Granulocyte transfusion in neonates with bacterial infection, neutropenia, and depletion of mature marrow neutrophils. Pediatrics 70:1, 1982.
423. Garcia J, Smith FR, Cucinell SA. Urinary D-lactate excretion in infants with necrotizing enterocolitis. J Pediatr 104:268, 1984.
424. Book LS, Herbst JJ, Jung AL. Carbohydrate malabsorption in necrotizing enterocolitis. Pediatrics 57:201, 1976.
425. Scott S, Rogers C, Angelus P, et al. Effect of necrotizing enterocolitis on urinary epidermal growth factor levels. Am J Dis Child 145:804, 1991.
426. Kliegman RM, Walsh MC. The incidence of meningitis in neonates with necrotizing enterocolitis. Am J Perinatol 4:245, 1987.
427. Scheifele DW, Olsen E, Ginter G, et al. Comparison of two antibiotic regimens in neonates with necrotizing enterocolitis. Clin Invest Med 8:A183, 1985 (abstract).
428. Bell MJ, Kosloske AM, Benton C, et al. Neonatal necrotizing enterocolitis: prevention of perforation. J Pediatr Surg 8:601, 1973.
429. Hansen TN, Ritter DA, Speer ME, et al. A randomized controlled study of oral gentamicin in the treatment of neonatal necrotizing enterocolitis. J Pediatr 97:836, 1980.
430. Faix RB, Polley TZ, Grasela TH. A randomized, controlled trial of parenteral clindamycin in neonatal necrotizing enterocolitis. J Pediatr 112:271, 1988.
431. Burrington JD. Necrotizing enterocolitis in the newborn infant. Clin Perinatol 5:29, 1978.
432. Ghory MJ, Sheldon CA. Newborn surgical emergencies of the gastrointestinal tract. Surg Clin North Am 65:1083, 1985.
433. Ein SH, Shandling B, Wesson D, et al. A 13-year experience with peritoneal drainage under local anesthesia for necrotizing enterocolitis perforation. J Pediatr Surg 25:1034, 1990.
434. Grylack LJ, Scanlon JW. Oral gentamicin therapy in the prevention of neonatal necrotizing enterocolitis: a controlled double-blind trial. Am J Dis Child 132:1192, 1978.
435. Egan EA, Nelson RM, Mantilla G, et al. Additional experience with routine use of oral kanamycin prophylaxis for necrotizing enterocolitis in infants under 1500 grams. J Pediatr 90:331, 1977.
436. Brantley VE, Hiatt IM, Hegyi T. The effectiveness of oral gentamicin in reducing the incidence of necrotizing enterocolitis (NEC) in treated and control infants. Pediatr Res 14:592, 1980.
437. Rowley MP, Dahlenburg GW. Gentamicin in prophylaxis of neonatal necrotizing enterocolitis. Lancet 2:532, 1978.
438. Boyle R, Nelson JS, Stonestreet B, et al. Alterations in stool flora resulting from oral kanamycin prophylaxis of necrotizing enterocolitis. J Pediatr 93:857, 1978.
439. Dear PRF, Thomas DEM. Oral vancomycin in preventing necrotizing enterocolitis. Arch Dis Child 63:1390, 1988.
440. Conroy MM, Anderson R, Cates KL. Complications associated with prophylactic oral kanamycin in preterm infants. Lancet 1:613, 1978.
441. Bhat AM, Meny RG. Alimentary absorption of gentamicin in preterm infants. Clin Pediatr 23:683, 1984.
442. Grylack LJ, Boehnert J, Scanlan JW. Serum concentration of gentamicin following oral administration to preterm newborns. Dev Pharmacol Ther 5:47, 1982.
443. Anderson DM, Kleigman RM. Relationship of neonatal alimentation practices to the occurrence of endemic neonatal necrotizing enterocolitis. Am J Perinatol 8:62, 1991.
444. McKeown RE, Marsh D, Amarnath U, et al. Role of delayed feeding and of feeding increments in necrotizing enterocolitis. J Pediatr 121:764, 1992.
445. Carrion V, Egan EA. Prevention of neonatal necrotizing enterocolitis. J Pediatr Gastroenterol Nutr 11:317, 1990.
446. Bohnhorst B, Muller S, Dordelmann M, et al. Early feeding after necrotizing enterocolitis in preterm infants. J Pediatr 143:484, 2003.
447. Anderson CL, Collin MF, O'Keefe JP, et al. A widespread epidemic of mild necrotizing enterocolitis of unknown cause. Am J Dis Child 138:979, 1984.
448. Gerber AR, Hopkins SR, Lauer BA, et al. Increased risk of illness among nursery staff caring for neonates with necrotizing enterocolitis. Pediatr Infect Dis J 4:246, 1985.
449. Little GA (ed). American Academy of Pediatrics Committee on the Fetus and Newborn: Guidelines for Perinatal Care, 2nd ed. Elk Grove Village, Ill, American Academy of Pediatrics, 1988, pp 182-183.
450. Eibl MA, Wolf HM, Fürnkranz H, et al. Prevention of necrotizing enterocolitis in low-birth-weight infants by IgA-IgG feeding. N Engl J Med 319:1, 1988.
451. Schullinger JN, Mollitt DL, Vinocur CD, et al. Neonatal necrotizing enterocolitis: survival, management, and complications: a 25-year study. Am J Dis Child 136:612, 1981.
452. Abbasi S, Pereira GR, Johnson L, et al. Long-term assessment of growth, nutritional status and gastrointestinal function in survivors of necrotizing enterocolitis. J Pediatr 104:550, 1984.
453. Janik JS, Ein SH, Mancer K. Intestinal structure after necrotizing enterocolitis. J Pediatr Surg 16:438, 1981.
454. Ball TI, Wyly JB. Enterocyst formation: a late complication of neonatal necrotizing enterocolitis. AJR Am J Roentgenol 147:806, 1986.
455. Walsh MC, Simpser EF, Kliegman RM. Late onset of sepsis in infants with bowel resection in the neonatal period. J Pediatr 112:468, 1988.
456. Walsh MC, Kliegman RM, Hack M. Severity of necrotizing enterocolitis: influence on outcome at 2 years of age. Pediatrics 84:808, 1989.

Endocarditis

457. Scott J. Iatrogenic lesions in babies following umbilical vein catheterization. Arch Dis Child 40:426, 1965.
458. Blieden LC, Morehead RR, Burke B, et al. Bacterial endocarditis in the neonate. Am J Dis Child 124:747, 1972.
459. Lewis IC. Bacterial endocarditis complicating septicemia in an infant. Arch Dis Child 29:144, 1954.
460. Macaulay D. Acute endocarditis in infancy and early childhood. Am J Dis Child 88:715, 1954.

461. Shanklin DR. The pathology of prematurity. *In* Prematurity and the Obstetrician. New York, Appleton-Century-Crofts, 1969, p 471.
462. Steinitz H, Schuchmann L, Wegner G. Leberzirrhose, Meningitis, und Endocarditis ulceropolyposa bei einer Neugeborenensepsis durch B-Streptokokken (Streptokokkus agalactiae). Arch Kinderheilkd 183:382, 1971.
463. Johnson DH, Rosenthal A, Nadas AS. Bacterial endocarditis in children under 2 years of age. Am J Dis Child 129:183, 1975.
464. Mendelsohn G, Hutchins GM. Infective endocarditis during the first decade of life: an autopsy review of 33 cases. Am J Dis Child 133:619, 1979.
465. Liersch R, Nessler L, Bourgeois M, et al. Gegenwärtige Merkmale der bakteriellen Endokarditis im Kindersalter. Z Kardiol 66:501, 1977.
466. Colville J, Jeffries I. Bilateral acquired neonatal Erb's palsy. Ir Med J 68:399, 1975.
467. Symchych PS, Krauss AN, Winchester P. Endocarditis following intracardiac placement of umbilical venous catheters in neonates. J Pediatr 90:287, 1977.
468. Edwards K, Ingall D, Czapek E, et al. Bacterial endocarditis in 4 young infants: is this complication on the increase? Clin Pediatr 16:607, 1977.
469. McGuiness GA, Schieken RM, Maguire GF. Endocarditis in the newborn. Am J Dis Child 134:577, 1980.
470. Bender RL, Jaffe RB, McCarthy D, et al. Echocardiographic diagnosis of bacterial endocarditis of the mitral valve in a neonate. Am J Dis Child 131:746, 1977.
471. Lundström N-R, Björkhem G. Mitral and tricuspid valve vegetations in infancy diagnosed by echocardiography. Acta Paediatr Scand 68:345, 1979.
472. Weinberg AG, Laird WP. Group B streptococcal endocarditis detected by echocardiography. J Pediatr 92:335, 1978.
473. Barton CW, Crowley DC, Uzark K, et al. A neonatal survivor of group B beta-hemolytic streptococcal endocarditis. Am J Perinatol 1:214, 1984.
474. Agarwala BN. Group B streptococcal endocarditis in a neonate. Pediatr Cardiol 9:51, 1988.
475. Chattapadhyay B. Fatal neonatal meningitis due to group B streptococci. Postgrad Med J 51:240, 1975.
476. Cabacungan ET, Tetting G, Friedberg DZ. Tricuspid valve vegetation caused by group B streptococcal endocarditis: treatment by "vegetectomy." J Perinatol 13:398, 1993.
477. Kramer H-H, Bourgeois M, Liersch R, et al. Current clinical aspects of bacterial endocarditis in infancy, childhood, and adolescence. Eur J Pediatr 140:253, 1983.
478. Kavey R-EW, Frank DM, Byrum CJ, et al. Two-dimensional echocardiography assessment of infective endocarditis in children. Am J Dis Child 137:851, 1983.
479. Ward KE, Matson JR, Chartrand SR, et al. Successfully treated pulmonary valve endocarditis in a normal neonate. Am J Dis Child 137:913, 1983.
480. Nakayama DK, O'Neill JA Jr, Wagner H, et al. Management of vascular complications of bacterial endocarditis. J Pediatr Surg 21:636, 1986.
481. Morville P, Mauran P, Motte J, et al. Intérêt de l'échocardiographie dans le diagnostic des endocardités néonatales: à propos de trois observations. Ann Pediatr 32:389, 1985.
482. Eliaou J-F, Montoya F, Sibille G, et al. Endocardité infectieuse en période néo-natale. Pediatrie 38:561, 1983.
483. McCartney JE. A case of acute ulcerative endocarditis in a child aged three and a half weeks. J Pathol Bacteriol 25:277, 1922.
484. Oelberg DG, Fisher DJ, Gross DM, et al. Endocarditis in high-risk neonates. Pediatrics 71:392, 1983.
485. Gossius G, Gunnes P, Rasmussen K. Ten years of infective endocarditis: a clinicopathologic study. Acta Med Scand 217:171, 1985.
486. Noel GJ, O'Loughlin JE, Edelson PJ. Neonatal *Staphylococcus epidermidis* right-sided endocarditis: description of five catheterized infants. Pediatrics 82:234, 1988.
487. No reference provided.
488. Bannon MJ. Infective endocarditis in neonates. Letter to the editor. Arch Dis Child 63:112, 1998.
489. Giddings ES. Two cases of endocarditis in infants. Can Med Assoc J 35:71, 1936.
490. Berkowitz FE, Dansky R. Infective endocarditis in Black South African children: report of 10 cases with some unusual features. Pediatr Infect Dis J 8:787, 1989.
491. Soo SS, Boxman DL. *Streptococcus faecalis* in neonatal infective endocarditis. J Infect 23:209, 1991.
492. Zakrzewski T, Keith JD. Bacterial endocarditis in infants and children. J Pediatr 67:1179, 1965.
493. O'Callaghan C, McDougall P. Infective endocarditis in neonates. Arch Dis Child 63:53, 1988.
494. Prandstraller D, Marata AM, Picchio FM. *Staphylococcus aureus* endocarditis in a newborn with transposition of the great arteries: successful treatment. Int J Cardiol 14:355, 1987.
495. Weinstein L, Schlesinger JJ. Pathoanatomic, pathophysiologic and clinical correlations in endocarditis. N Engl J Med 291(Pt 1):832, 1974.
496. Morand P, Laugier J, Lain J-L, et al. Endocardité triscupidienne calcifée du nourisson. Arch Mal Coeur 66:901, 1973.
497. Luke JL, Bolande RP, Gross S. Generalized aspergillosis and *Aspergillus* endocarditis in infancy: report of a case. Pediatrics 31:115, 1963.
498. Wiley EL, Hutchins GM. Superior vena cava syndrome secondary to *Candida* thrombophlebitis complicating parenteral alimentation. J Pediatr 91:977, 1977.
499. Walsh TJ, Hutchins GM. Postoperative *Candida* infections of the heart in children: clinicopathologic study of a continuing problem of diagnosis and therapy. J Pediatr Surg 15:325, 1980.
500. Faix R, Feick HJ, Frommelt P, et al. Successful medical treatment of *Candida parapsilosis* endocarditis in a premature infant. Am J Perinatol 7:272, 1990.
501. Zenker PN, Rosenberg EM, Van Dyke RB, et al. Successful medical treatment of presumed *Candida* endocarditis in critically ill infants. J Pediatr 119:472, 1991.
502. Sanchez PJ, Siegel JD, Fishbein J. *Candida* endocarditis: successful medical management in three preterm infants and review of the literature. Pediatr Infect Dis J 10:239, 1991.
503. Walsh TJ, Hutchins GM. Postoperative *Candida* infections of the heart in children: clinicopathologic study of a continuing problem of diagnosis and therapy. J Pediatr Surg 15:325, 1980.
504. Millard DD, Shulman ST. The changing spectrum of neonatal endocarditis. Clin Perinatol 15:587, 1988.
505. Morrow WR, Haas JE, Benjamin DR. Nonbacterial endocardial thrombosis in neonates: relationship to persistent fetal circulation. J Pediatr 100:117, 1982.
506. Kronsbein H. Pathogenesis of endocarditis verrucosa simplex in the newborn. Beitr Pathol 161:82, 1977.
507. Favara BE, Franciosi RA, Butterfield LJ. Disseminated intravascular and cardiac thrombosis of the neonate. Am J Dis Child 127:197, 1974.
508. Kunstadter RH, Kaltenekker F. Acute verrucous endocarditis in the newborn. J Pediatr 61:58, 1962.
509. Krous HF. Neonatal nonbacterial thrombotic endocarditis. Arch Pathol Lab Med 103:76, 1979.
510. Bergsland J, Kawaguchi A, Roland JM, et al. Mycotic aortic aneurysms in children. Ann Thorac Surg 37:314, 1984.
511. Thompson TR, Tilleli J, Johnson DE, et al. Umbilical artery catheterization complicated by mycotic aortic aneurysm in neonates. Adv Pediatr 27:275, 1980.
512. Bannon MJ. Infective endocarditis in neonates. Letter to the editor. Arch Dis Child 63:1112, 1988.
513. Hernandez I, Arcil G, Garru O, et al. Endocardités infecteuses néonatales: à propos de cinq observations. Arch Mal Coeur 83:627, 1990.
514. Bullaboy CA, Coulson JD, Jennings RB Jr, et al. Neonatal mitral valve endocarditis: diagnosis and successful management. Clin Pediatr 29:398, 1990.
515. Baltimore RS. Infective endocarditis in children. Pediatr Infect Dis J. 11:907, 1992.
516. Popp RL. Echocardiography and infectious endocarditis. Curr Clin Topics Infect Dis 4:98, 1983.
517. Watanakunakorn C. Treatment of infections due to methicillin-resistant *Staphylococcus aureus*. Ann Intern Med 97:376, 1982.
518. Wolfson JS, Swartz MN. Serum bactericidal activity as a monitor of antibiotic therapy. N Engl J Med 312:968, 1985.
519. Cooper GI, Hopkins CC. Rapid diagnosis of intravascular catheter–associated infection by direct Gram staining of catheter segments. N Engl J Med 312:1142, 1985.
520. Perelman MJ, Sugimoto J, Arcilla RA, et al. Aortic root replacement for complicated bacterial endocarditis in an infant. J Pediatr Surg 24:1121, 1989.
521. Tulloh RMR, Silove ED, Abrams LD. Replacement of an aortic valve cusp after neonatal endocarditis. Br Heart J 64:204, 1990.

522. Levinson SA, Learner A. Blood cysts on the heart valves of newborn infants. Arch Pathol 14:810, 1932.
523. Gross P. Concept of fetal endocarditis: a general review with report of an illustrative case. Arch Pathol 31:163, 1941.
524. Begg JG. Blood-filled cysts in the cardiac valve cusps in foetal life and infancy. J Pathol Bacteriol 87:177, 1964.
525. Menahem S, Robbie MJ, Rajadurai VS. Valvular vegetations in the neonate due to fetal endocarditis. Int J Cardiol 32:103, 1991.
526. Charaf L, Lundell B, Abon P, et al. A case of neonatal endocarditis. Acta Pediatr Scand 79:704, 1990.

Pericarditis

527. Gersony WM, McCracken GH Jr. Purulent pericarditis in infancy. Pediatrics 40:224, 1967.
528. Schaffer AJ, Avery ME. Diseases of the Newborn, 3rd ed. Philadelphia, WB Saunders, 1971, p 252.
529. Neimann N, Pernot C, Gentin G, et al. Les péricardités purulentes néonatales: à propos du premier cas guéri. Arch Fr Pediatr 22:238, 1965.
530. Collier AM, Connor JD, Nyhan WL. Systemic infection with *Hemophilus influenzae* in very young infants. J Pediatr 70:539, 1967.
531. McKinlay B. Infectious diarrhea in the newborn caused by an unclassified species of *Salmonella.* Am J Dis Child 54:1252, 1937.
532. Chiari H. Zur Kenntnis der Pyozyaneus-infektion bei Säuglingen. Zentralb Allg Pathol 38:483, 1926.
533. Jaiyesimi F, Abioye AA, Anita AU. Infective pericarditis in Nigerian children. Arch Dis Child 54:384, 1979.
534. Wynn RJ. Neonatal *E. coli* pericarditis. J Perinatol Med 7:23, 1979.
535. Kachaner J, Nouaille J-M, Batisse A. Les cardiomegalies massives du nouveau-né. Arch Fr Pediatr 34:297, 1977.
536. Graham JPA, Martin A. *B. pyocyaneus* pericarditis occurring four days after birth. Cent Afr J Med 1:101, 1955.
537. Feldman WE. Bacterial etiology and mortality of purulent pericarditis in pediatric patients: review of 162 cases. Am J Dis Child 133:641, 1979.
538. Morgan RJ, Stephenson LW, Woolf PK, et al. Surgical treatment of purulent pericarditis in children. Thorac Cardiovasc Surg 85:527, 1983.
539. Jellard CH, Churcher GM. An outbreak of *Pseudomonas aeruginosa (pyocyanea)* infection in a premature baby unit, with observations on the intestinal carriage of *Pseudomonas aeruginosa* in the newborn. J Hyg 65:219, 1967.
540. Miller TC, Baman SI, Albers WW. Massive pericardial effusion due to *Mycoplasma hominis* in a newborn. Am J Dis Child 136:271, 1982.
541. Shenker L, Reed KL, Anderson CF, et al. Fetal pericardial effusion. Am J Obstet Gynecol 160:1505, 1989.
542. Cayler GG, Taybi H, Riley HD Jr. Pericarditis with effusion in infants and children. J Pediatr 63:264, 1963.
543. Noren GR, Kaplan EL, Staley NA. Nonrheumatic inflammatory diseases. *In* Adams FH, Emmanouilides GC (eds). Moss' Heart Disease in Infants, Children, and Adolescents, 3rd ed. Baltimore, Williams & Wilkins, 1983, pp 585-594.
544. Kanarek KS, Coleman J. Purulent pericarditis in a neonate. Pediatr Infect Dis J 10:549, 1991.
545. Cherry JD. Enteroviruses, polioviruses (poliomyelitis), coxsackieviruses, echoviruses, and enteroviruses. *In* Feigin RD, Cherry JD (eds). Textbook of Pediatric Infectious Diseases, 3rd ed. Philadelphia, WB Saunders, 1992, pp 1705-1752.
546. Zerella JT, Halpe DCE. Intrapericardial teratoma-neonatal cardiorespiratory distress amenable to surgery. J Pediatr Surg 15:961, 1980.
547. Doshi N, Smith B, Klionsky B. Congenital pericarditis due to maternal lupus erythematosus. J Pediatr 96:699, 1980.
548. Sasidharan P, Al-Mohsen I, Abdul-Karim A, et al. Nonimmune hydrops fetalis: case reports and brief review. J Perinatol 12:338, 1992.
549. deFonseca JMB, Davies MRQ, Bolton KD. Congenital hydropericardium associated with the herniation of part of the liver into the pericardial sac. J Pediatr Surg 22:851, 1987.
550. Jafa AJ, Barak S, Kaysar N, et al. Antenatal diagnosis of bilateral congenital chylothorax with pericardial effusion. Acta Obstet Gynaecol Scand 64:455, 1985.
551. Mupanemunda RH, Mackanjee HR. A life-threatening complication of percutaneous central venous catheters in neonates. Am J Dis Child 146:1414, 1992.
552. Dennehy PH. New tests for the rapid diagnosis of infection in children. *In* Aronoff S, Hughes W, Kohl S, et al (eds). Advances in Pediatric Infectious Disease, vol 8. St. Louis, Mosby–Year Book, 1993, pp 91-129.
553. Zeevi B, Perry S, Keane J, et al. Interventional cardiac procedures. Clin Perinatol 15:633, 1988.

Mediastinitis

554. Achenbach S. Mediastinalabszess bei einmen 3 Wochen alten Säugling. Arch Kinderheilkd 74:193, 1924.
555. Grewe HE, Martini Pape M. Die eitrige Mediastinitis im frühen Saüglingsalter. Kinderaerztl Prax 32:305, 1964.
556. Weichsel M. Mediastinitis in a newborn. Proc Rudolf Virchow Med Soc City N Y 22:67, 1963.
557. Weber G. Retropharyngeal und Mediastinalabszess bei einem 3 Wochen alten Säugling. Chirurg 21:308, 1950.
558. deLorimier AA, Haskin D, Massie FS. Mediastinal mass caused by vertebral osteomyelitis. Am J Dis Child 111:639, 1966.
559. Talbert JL, Rodgers BM, Felman AH, et al. Traumatic perforation of the hypopharynx in infants. J Thorac Cardiovasc Surg 74:152, 1977.
560. Grunebaum M, Horodniceanu C, Wilunsky E, et al. Iatrogenic transmural perforation of the oesophagus in the preterm infant. Clin Radiol 31:257, 1980.
561. Sands T, Glasson M, Berry A. Hazards of nasogastric tube insertion in the newborn infant. Lancet 2:680, 1989.
562. Krasna IH, Rosenfeld D, Benjamin BG, et al. Esophageal perforation in the neonate: an emerging problem in the newborn nursery. J Pediatr Surg 22:784, 1987.
563. Topsis J, Kinas HY, Kandall SR. Esophageal perforation—a complication of neonatal resuscitation. Anesth Analg 69:532, 1989.
564. Vandenplas Y, Delree M, Bougatef A, et al. Cervical esophageal perforation diagnosed by endoscopy in a premature infant. J Pediatr Gastroenterol Nutr 8:390, 1989.
565. Touloukian RJ, Beardsley GP, Ablow RC, et al. Traumatic perforation of the pharynx in the newborn. Pediatrics 59:1019, 1977.
566. Johnson DE, Foker J, Munson DP, et al. Management of esophageal and pharyngeal perforation in the newborn infant. Pediatrics 70:592, 1982.
567. Coulthard M, Isaacs D. Neonatal retropharyngeal abscess. Pediatr Infect Dis J 10:547, 1991.

Esophagitis

568. Bittencourt AL. Congenital Chagas disease. Am J Dis Child 130:97, 1976.
569. Azimi PH, Willert J, Petru A. Severe esophagitis in a newborn. Pediatr Infect Dis J 15:385, 1966.
570. Walsh TJ, Belitsos NJ, Hamilton SR. Bacterial esophagitis in immunocompromised patients. Arch Intern Med 146:1345, 1986.

Infections of the Endocrine Glands

571. Nelson AJ. Neonatal suppurative thyroiditis. Pediatr Infect Dis 2:243, 1983.
572. Berner R, Schumacher RF, Zimmerhackl LB, et al. *Salmonella enteritidis* orchitis in a 10-week old boy. Acta Pediatr 83:922, 1994.

Infections of the Salivary Glands

573. Sanford HN, Shmigelsky I. Purulent parotitis in the newborn. J Pediatr 26:149, 1945.
577. Shulman BH. Acute suppurative infections of the salivary glands in the newborn. Am J Dis Child 80:413, 1950.
575. Campbell WAB. Purulent parotitis in the newborn: report of a case. Lancet 2:386, 1951.
576. Leake D, Leake R. Neonatal suppurative parotitis. Pediatrics 46:203, 1970.
577. Brook I, Frazier EH, Thompson DH. Aerobic and anaerobic microbiology of acute suppurative parotitis. Laryngoscope 101:170, 1991.
578. David RB, O'Connell EJ. Suppurative parotitis in children. Am J Dis Child 119:332, 1970.
579. Banks WW, Handler SD, Glade GB, et al. Neonatal submandibular sialadenitis. Am J Otolaryngol 1:261, 1980.
579a. Saarinen M, Takala AK, Koskenniemi E, et al. Spectrum of 2,836 cases of invasive bacterial or fungal infections in children: results of prospective nationwide five-year surveillance in Finland. Finnish Pediatric Invasive Infection Study Group. Clin Infect Dis 21: 1134-1144, 1995.

Infections of the Skin and Subcutaneous Tissue

580. Solomon LM, Esterly NB. Neonatal Dermatology. Philadelphia, WB Saunders, 1973.

581. Swartz MN, Weinberg AN. Bacterial diseases with cutaneous involvement. *In* Fitzpatrick TB, Arndt KA, Clark WH Jr, et al (eds). Dermatology in General Medicine. New York, McGraw-Hill, 1971.
582. Frieden IJ. Blisters and pustules in the newborn. Curr Probl Pediatr 19:553, 1989.
583. Weinberg S, Leider M, Shapiro L. Color Atlas of Pediatric Dermatology. New York, McGraw-Hill, 1975.
584. Maibach HI, Hildick-Smith G (eds). Skin Bacteria and Their Role in Infection. New York, McGraw-Hill, 1965.
585. Speert H. Circumcision of the newborn: an appraisal of its present status. Obstet Gynecol 2:164, 1953.
586. Annabil SH, Al-Hifi A, Kazi T. Primary tuberculosis of the penis in an infant. Tubercle 71:229, 1990.
587. Cleary TG, Kohl S. Overwhelming infection with group B beta-hemolytic *Streptococcus* associated with circumcision. Pediatrics 64:301, 1979.
588. Sauer L. Fatal staphylococcal bronchopneumonia following ritual circumcision. Am J Obstet Gynecol 46:583, 1943.
589. Annunziato D, Goldblum LM. Staphylococcal scalded skin syndrome. Am J Dis Child 132:1187, 1978.
590. Breuer GS, Walfisch S. Circumcision complications and indications for ritual recircumcision—clinical experience and review of the literature. Isr J Med Sci 23:252, 1987.
591. Woodside JR. Necrotizing fasciitis after neonatal circumcision. Am J Dis Child 134:301, 1980.
592. Stranko J, Ryan ME, Bowman AM. Impetigo in newborn infants associated with a plastic bell clamp circumcision. Pediatr Infect Dis 5:597, 1986.
593. Bliss DP, Healey PJ, Waldbraussen JHT. Necrotizing fasciitis after Plastibell circumscision. J Pediatr 131:459, 1997.
594. Gee WF, Ansell JS. Neonatal circumcision: a 10-year overview: with comparison of the Gomco clamp and the Plastibell device. Pediatrics 58:824, 1976.
595. Siddiqi SF, Taylor PM. Necrotizing fasciitis of the scalp. Am J Dis Child 136:226, 1982.
596. Okada DM, Chow AW, Bruce VT. Neonatal scalp abscess and fetal monitoring: factors associated with infection. Am J Obstet Gynecol 129:185, 1977.
597. Cordero L, Anderson CW, Hon EH. Scalp abscess: a benign and infrequent complication of fetal monitoring. Am J Obstet Gynecol 146:126, 1983.
598. Wagener MM, Rycheck RR, Yee RB, et al. Septic dermatitis of the neonatal scalp and maternal endomyometritis with intrapartum internal fetal monitoring. Pediatrics 74:81, 1984.
599. Brook I. Microbiology of scalp abscesses in newborns. Pediatr Infect Dis J 11:766, 1992.
600. Bogdan JC, Rapkin RH. Clostridia infection in the newborn. Pediatrics 58:120, 1976.
601. Fitter WF, DeSa DJ, Richardson H. Chorioamnionitis and funisitis due to *Corynebacterium kutscheri.* Arch Dis Child 55:710, 1979.
602. Sarkany I, Gaylarde CC. Skin flora of the newborn. Lancet 1:589, 1967.
603. Evans HE, Akpata SO, Baki A. Factors influencing the establishment of neonatal bacterial flora. I. The role of host factors. Arch Environ Health 21:514, 1970.
604. Sarkany I, Arnold L. The effect of single and repeated applications of hexachlorophene on the bacterial flora of the skin of the newborn. Br J Dermatol 82:261, 1970.
605. Thompson DJ, Gezon HM, Rogers KD, et al. Excess risk of staphylococcal infection and disease in newborn males. Am J Epidemiol 84:314, 1966.
606. Rudoy RC, Nelson JD. Breast abscess during the neonatal period: a review. Am J Dis Child 129:1031, 1975.
607. Reboli AC, John JF, Levkoff AH. Epidemic methicillin-gentamicin–resistant *Staphylococcus aureus* in a neonatal intensive care unit. Am J Dis Child 143:34, 1989.
608. Fergie JE, Purcell K. Community-acquired methicillin-resistant *Staphylococcus aureus* infection in south Texas children. Pediatr Infect Dis J 20:860, 2001.
609. Evans HE, Akpata SO, Baki A, et al. Flora in newborn infants: annual variation in prevalence of *Staphylococcus aureus, Escherichia coli,* and streptococci. Arch Environ Health 26:275, 1973.
610. Starr HJ, Holliday PB Jr. Erythema multiforme as a manifestation of neonatal septicemia. J Pediatr 38:315, 1951.
611. Washington JL, Fowler REL, Guarino GJ. Erythema multiforme in a premature infant associated with sepsis due to *Pseudomonas.* Pediatrics 39:120, 1967.
612. Foley JF, Gravelle CR, Englehard WE, et al. *Achromobacter* septicemia-fatalities in prematures. I. Clinical and epidemiological study. Am J Dis Child 101:279, 1961.
613. Belgaumkar TK. Impetigo neonatorum congenita due to group B beta-hemolytic *Streptococcus* infection. Letter to the editor. J Pediatr 86:982, 1975.
614. Halal F, Delorme L, Brazeau M, et al. Congenital vesicular eruption caused by *Hemophilus influenzae* type b. Pediatrics 62:494, 1978.
615. Martin MO, Wallach D, Bordier C, et al. Les signes cutanés des infections bacteriennes néonatales. Arch Fr Pediatr 42:471, 1985.
616. Kline A, O'Connell E. Group B *Streptococcus* as a cause of neonatal bullous skin lesions. Pediatr Infect Dis J 12:165, 1993.
617. Khuri-Bulos N, McIntosh K. Neonatal *Haemophilus influenzae* infection: report of eight cases and review of the literature. Am J Dis Child 129:57, 1975.
618. Bray DA. Ecthyma gangrenosum: full thickness nasal slough. Arch Otolaryngol 98:210, 1973.
619. Heffner RW, Smith GF. Ecthyma gangrenosum in *Pseudomonas* septicemia. Am J Dis Child 99:524, 1960.
620. Ghosal SP, SenGupta PC, Mukherjee AK, et al. Noma neonatorum: its aetiopathogenesis. Lancet 1:289, 1978.
621. Bodey GP, Bolivar R, Fainstein V, et al. Infections caused by *Pseudomonas aeruginosa.* Rev Infect Dis 5:279, 1983.
622. Baley JE, Silverman RA. Systemic candidiasis: cutaneous manifestations in low birth weight infants. Pediatrics 82:211, 1988.
623. Cordero L Jr, Hon EH. Scalp abscess: a rare complication of fetal monitoring. J Pediatr 78:533, 1971.
624. Nelson JD. Bilateral breast abscess due to group B *Streptococcus.* Am J Dis Child 130:567, 1976.
625. Levy HL, O'Connor JF, Ingall D. Bacteremia, infected cephalhematoma, and osteomyelitis of the skull in a newborn. Am J Dis Child 114:649, 1967.
626. Ellis SS, Montgomery JR, Wagner M, et al. Osteomyelitis complicating neonatal cephalhematoma. Am J Dis Child 127:100, 1974.
627. Stetler H, Martin E, Plotkin S, et al. Neonatal mastitis due to *Echerichia coli.* J Pediatr 76:611, 1970.
628. Balfour HH Jr, Block SH, Bowe ET, et al. Complications of fetal blood sampling. Am J Obstet Gynecol 107:288, 1970.
629. McGuigan MA, Lipman RP. Neonatal mastitis due to *Proteus mirabilis.* Am J Dis Child 130:1296, 1976.
630. Wilson HD, Haltalin KC. Acute necrotizing fasciitis in childhood. Am J Dis Child 125:591, 1973.
631. Burry VF, Beezley M. Infant mastitis due to gram-negative organisms. Am J Dis Child 124:736, 1972.
632. Brook I. The aerobic and anaerobic microbiology of neonatal breast abscess. Pediatr Infect Dis J 10:785, 1991.
633. Centers for Disease Control. Nosocomial *Serratia marcescens* infections in neonates—Puerto Rico. MMWR Morbid Mortal Wkly Rep 23:183, 1974.
634. Todd JK, Bruhn FW. Severe *Haemophilus influenzae* infections: spectrum of disease. Am J Dis Child 129:607, 1975.
635. Zinner SH, McCormack WM, Lee Y-H, et al. Puerperal bacteremia and neonatal sepsis due to *Hemophilus parainfluenzae:* report of a case with antibody titers. Pediatrics 49:612, 1972.
636. Platt MS. Neonatal *Hemophilus vaginalis (Corynebacterium vaginalis)* infection. Clin Pediatr 10:513, 1971.
637. Leighton PM, Bulleid B, Taylor R. Neonatal cellulitis due to *Gardnerella vaginalis.* Pediatr Infect Dis 1:339, 1982.
638. Lee Y-H, Berg RB. Cephalhematoma infected with *Bacteroides.* Am J Dis Child 121:77, 1971.
639. Mandel MJ, Lewis RJ. Molluscum contagiosum of the newborn. Br J Dermatol 84:370, 1970.
640. Clark JM, Weeks WR, Tatton J. *Drosophila myiasis* mimicking sepsis in a newborn. West J Med 136:443, 1982.
641. Burns BR, Lampe RM, Hansen GH. Neonatal scabies. Am J Dis Child 133:1031, 1979.
642. Hensey OJ, Hart CA, Cooke RWI. *Candida albicans* skin abscesses. Arch Dis Child 59:479, 1984.
643. Turbeville DF, Heath RE Jr, Bowen FW Jr, et al. Complications of fetal scalp electrodes: a case report. Am J Obstet Gynecol 122:530, 1975.
644. Centers for Disease Control. Gonococcal scalp-wound infection—New Jersey. MMWR Morbid Mortal Wkly Rep 24:115, 1975.
645. Brook I. Osteomyelitis and bacteremia caused by *Bacteroides fragilis.* Clin Pediatr 19:639, 1980.
646. Mohon RT, Mehalic TF, Grimes CK, et al. Infected cephalhematoma and neonatal osteomyelitis of the skull. Pediatr Infect Dis 5:253, 1986.

647. Cohen SM, Miller BW, Orris HW. Meningitis complicating cephalhematoma. J Pediatr 30:327, 1947.
648. Rudoy RC, Nelson JD. Breast abscess during the neonatal period: a review. Am J Dis Child 129:1031, 1975.
649. Walsh M, McIntosh K. Neonatal mastitis. Clin Pediatr 25:395, 1986.
650. Langewisch WH. An epidemic of group A, type 1 streptococcal infections in newborn infants. Pediatrics 18:438, 1956.
651. Sinniah D, Sandiford BR, Dugdale AE. Subungual infection in the newborn: an institutional outbreak of unknown etiology, possibly due to *Veillonella.* Clin Pediatr 11:690, 1972.
652. Cushing AH. Omphalitis: a review. Pediatr Infect Dis 4:282, 1985.
653. McKenna H, Johnson D. Bacteria in neonatal omphalitis. Pathology 7:11, 1977.
654. Mason WH, Andrews R, Ross LA, et al. Omphalitis in the newborn infant. Pediatr Infect Dis J 8:521, 1989.
655. Geil CC, Castle WK, Mortimer EA Jr. Group A streptococcal infections in newborn nurseries. Pediatrics 46:849, 1970.
656. Kosloske AM, Cushing AH, Borden TA, et al. Cellulitis and necrotizing fasciitis of the abdominal wall in pediatric patients. J Pediatr Surg 16:246, 1981.
657. Goldberg GN, Hansen RC, Lynch PJ. Necrotizing fasciitis in infancy: report of three cases and review of the literature. Pediatr Dermatol 2:55, 1984.
658. Ramamurthy RS, Srinivasan G, Jacobs NM. Necrotizing fasciitis and necrotizing cellulitis due to group B *Streptococcus.* Am J Dis Child 131:1169, 1977.
659. Krieger RW, Chusid MJ. Perirectal abscess in childhood. Am J Dis Child 133:411, 1979.
660. Arditi M, Yogev R. Perirectal abscess in infants and children: report of 52 cases and review of the literature. Pediatr Infect Dis J 9:411, 1990.
661. Victorin L. An epidemic of otitis in newborns due to infection with *Pseudomonas aeruginosa.* Acta Paediatr Scand 56:344, 1967.
662. Laubo EJ, Paller AS. Common skin problems during the first year of life. Pediatr Clin North Am 41:1105, 1994.
663. Merlob P, Metzker A, Hazaz B, et al. Neonatal pemphigus vulgaris. Pediatrics 78:1102, 1986.
664. Glover MT, Atherton DJ, Levinsky RJ. Syndrome of erythroderma, failure to thrive, and diarrhea in infancy: a manifestation of immunodeficiency. Pediatrics 81:66, 1988.
665. Prod'hom LS, Choffat J-M, Frenck N, et al. Care of the seriously ill neonate with hyaline membrane disease and with sepsis (sclerema neonatorum). Pediatrics 53:170, 1974.
666. Hughes WE, Hammond ML. Sclerema neonatorum. J Pediatr 32:676, 1948.
667. McCracken GH Jr, Shinefield HR. Changes in the pattern of neonatal septicemia and meningitis. Am J Dis Child 112:33, 1966.
668. Gordon I. Miliary sebaceous cysts and blisters in the healthy newborn. Arch Dis Child 24:286, 1949.
669. Carr JA, Hodgman JE, Freedman RI, et al. Relationship between toxic erythema and infant maturity. Am J Dis Child 112:219, 1966.
670. Merlob P, Metzker A, Reisner SH. Transient neonatal pustular melanosis. Am J Dis Child 136:521, 1982.
671. Kahn G, Rywlin AM. Acropustulosis of infancy. Arch Dermatol 115:831, 1979.
672. Lucky AW, McGuire JS. Infantile acropustulosis with eosinophilic pustules. J Pediatr 100:428, 1982.
673. Murphy WF, Langley AL. Common bullous lesions—presumably self-inflicted—occurring in utero in the newborn infant. Pediatrics 32:1099, 1963.
674. Weston WL, Lane AT, Weston JA. Diaper dermatitis: current concepts. Pediatrics 66:532, 1980.
675. Nappy rashes. Editorial. BMJ 282:420, 1981.
676. Hauth JC, Merenstein GB (eds). Guidelines for Perinatal Care, 4th ed. Elks Grove, Ill, American Academy of Pediatrics and American College of Obstetricians and Gynecologists, 1997.
677. Gladstone IM, Clapper L, Thorp JW, et al. Randomized study of six umbilical cord care regimens. Clin Pediatr 27:127, 1988.
678. Centers for Disease Control. National nosocomial infections study report: nosocomial infections in nurseries and their relationship to hospital infant bathing practices—a preliminary report. Atlanta, Centers for Disease Control, 1974, pp 9-23.
679. Gezon HM, Schaberg MJ, Klein JO. Concurrent epidemics of *Staphylococcus aureus* and group A *Streptococcus* disease in a newborn nursery—control with penicillin G and hexachlorophene bathing. Pediatrics 51:383, 1973.
680. Seeberg S, Brinkhoff B, John E, et al. Prevention and control of neonatal pyoderma with chlorhexidine. Acta Paediatr Scand 73:498, 1984.

Conjunctivitis and Other Eye Infections

681. de Toledo AR, Chandler JW. Conjunctivitis of the newborn. Infect Dis Clin North Am 6:807, 1992.
682. Whitcher JP. Neonatal ophthalmia: have we advanced in the last 20 years? Int Ophthalmol Clin 30:39, 1990.
683. Millard DD, Yogev R. *Haemophilus influenzae* type b: a rare case of congenital conjunctivitis. Pediatr Infect Dis 7:363, 1988.
684. McLeod DT, Ahmad F, Calder MA. *Branhamella catarrhalis* (beta lactamase positive) ophthalmia neonatorum. Lancet 2:647, 1984.
685. Ellis M, Weindling DC, Ho N, et al. Neonatal conjunctivitis associated with meningococcal meningitis. Arch Dis Child 67:1219, 1992.
686. Naiditch MJ, Bower AG. Diphtheria: a study of 1433 cases observed during a ten year period at Los Angeles County Hospital. Am J Med 17:229, 1954.
687. Khan MS, Stead SE. Neonatal *Pasteurella multocida* conjunctivitis following zoonotic infection of mother. J Infect Dis 1:289, 1979.
688. Brook I, Martin WJ, Finegold SM. Effect of silver nitrate application on the conjunctival flora of the newborn, and the occurrence of clostridial conjunctivitis. J Pediatr Ophthalmol Strabismus 15:179, 1978.
689. Bourbeau P, Holla V, Piemontese S. Ophthalmia neonatorum caused by *Neisseria cinerea.* J Clin Microbiol 28:1640, 1990.
690. Hedberg K, Ristinen TL, Soler JT, et al. Outbreak of erythromycin-resistant staphylococcal conjunctivitis in a newborn nursery. Pediatr Infect Dis J 9:268, 1990.
691. Paentice MJ, Hutchinson GR, Taylor-Robinson D. A microbiological study of neonatal conjunctivitis. Br J Ophthalmol 61:9, 1977.
692. Sandstrom KI, Bell TA, Chandler JW, et al. Microbial causes of neonatal conjunctivitis. J Pediatr 105:706, 1984.
693. Duarte AM, Kramer J, Yusk W, et al. Eosinophilic pustular folliculitis in infancy and childhood. Am J Dis Child 147:197, 1993.
694. Hammerschlag MR. Conjunctivitis in infancy and childhood. Pediatr Rev 5:285, 1984.
695. Wincelaus J, Goh BT, Dunlop EM, et al. Diagnosis of ophthalmia neonatorum. BMJ 295:1377, 1987.
696. Molgaard I-L, Nielsen PB, Kaern J. A study of the incidence of neonatal conjunctivitis and of its bacterial causes including *Chlamydia trachomatis.* Acta Ophthalmol 62:461, 1984.
697. Laga M, Nzanze H, Brunham RC, et al. Epidemiology of ophthalmia neonatorum in Kenya. Lancet 2:1145, 1986.
698. Nathoo KJ, Latif AS, Trijssenaar JES. Aetiology of neonatal conjunctivitis in Harare. Cent Afr J Med 30:123, 1984.
699. Stenson S, Newman R, Fedukowicz H. Conjunctivitis in the newborn: observations on incidence, cause, and prophylaxis. Ann Ophthalmol 13:329, 1981.
700. Burns RP, Rhodes DH Jr. *Pseudomonas* eye infection as a cause of death in premature infants. Arch Ophthalmol 65:517, 1961.
701. Drewett SE, Payne DJH, Tuke W, et al. Eradication of *Pseudomonas aeruginosa* infection from a special-care nursery. Lancet 1:946, 1972.
702. Cole GA, Davies DP, Austin DJ. *Pseudomonas* ophthalmia neonatorum: a cause of blindness. BMJ 281:440, 1980.
703. Traboulsi EI, Shammas IV, Ratl HE, et al. *Pseudomonas aeruginosa* ophthalmia neonatorum. Am J Ophthalmol 98:801, 1984.
704. Lohrer R, Belohradsky BH. Bacterial endophthalmitis in neonates. Eur J Pediatr 146:354, 1987.
705. Christensen GD, Korones SB, Reed L, et al. Epidemic *Serratia marcescens* in a neonatal intensive care unit: importance of the gastrointestinal tract as a reservoir. Infect Control 3:127, 1982.
706. Harris GJ, DiClementi D. Congenital dacryocystocele. Arch Ophthalmol 100:1763, 1982.
707. Nishida H, Risemberg HM. Silver nitrate ophthalmic solution and chemical conjunctivitis. Pediatrics 56:3368, 1975.
708. Kripke SS, Golden B. Neonatal inclusion conjunctivitis: a report of three cases and a discussion of differential diagnosis and treatment. Clin Pediatr 11:261, 1972.
709. Naib ZM. Cytology of TRIC agent infection of the eye of newborn infants and their mothers' genital tracts. Acta Cytol 14:390, 1970.
710. Peter G (ed). Prevention of neonatal ophthalmia. *In* Report of the Committee on Infectious Diseases, 24th ed. Elk Grove Village, Ill, American Academy of Pediatrics, 1997, pp 601-603.

Chapter 11

CHLAMYDIA INFECTIONS

Toni Darville

In 1911, Lindner and colleagues identified typical intracytoplasmic inclusions in infants with a nongonococcal form of ophthalmia neonatorum called inclusion conjunctivitis of the newborn (ICN) or inclusion blennorrhea.[1] Mothers of affected infants were found to have inclusions in their cervical epithelial cells, and fathers of such infants had inclusions in their urethral cells. For 50 years, cytologic demonstration of chlamydial inclusions in epithelial cells was the only diagnostic procedure available. When methods to isolate *Chlamydia trachomatis* were developed, first in the yolk sac of the embryonated hen's egg and then in tissue culture, studies again demonstrated this organism as the etiologic agent for conjunctivitis in the newborn infant and then confirmed the maternal genital tract reservoir for transmission of this agent.[2] Although ICN was studied for 60 years, it was not until the late 1970s, with the impetus of the report by Beem and Saxon[3], that the importance of chlamydial infection of the respiratory tract in infants was recognized.

C. trachomatis now is appreciated as the most common sexually transmitted pathogen in Western industrialized society.[4] Although most *C. trachomatis* infections in men and women are asymptomatic, infection can lead to severe reproductive complications in women. The infection can be transmitted from an infected mother to her newborn during delivery, producing conjunctivitis or pneumonia. *C. trachomatis* is the most common cause of conjunctivitis in infants younger than 1 month of age worldwide and often is a cause of afebrile pneumonia in infants younger than 3 months of age.

EPIDEMIOLOGY AND TRANSMISSION

C. trachomatis is the most common bacterial cause of sexually transmitted infections in the United States.[5,6] Reported prevalence rates in the United States have ranged from 2% to 7% among female college students, from 4% to 12% among women attending a family planning clinic, and from 6% to 20% among men and women attending a clinic for sexually transmitted diseases or persons entering correctional facilities.[7,8] In the United Kingdom, recent data suggest that the rate of infection among young women exceeds 10%.[9] Prevalence rates have declined in areas where screening and treatment programs have been implemented.[10] Many men and most women infected with *C. trachomatis* are either asymptomatic or minimally symptomatic, and presentation for diagnosis is a result of a routine screening program, or of presence of symptoms in a contact. In gonococcal infections, by contrast, symptoms develop in most infected persons, who then present acutely for care. Regional estimates are hampered by underdiagnosis and underreporting of cases. Because symptoms are absent or minimal in most women and many men, a large reservoir of asymptomatic infection is present that can sustain the pathogen within a community.

Age younger than 20 years is the demographic factor in women most strongly associated with chlamydial infection (relative risk is 2 to 3.5 among women younger than 25 years compared with older women).[6] Although the prevalence of chlamydial infection is increased among black or economically disadvantaged persons, broad socioeconomic and geographic distribution of infection exists.[5,11,14,17] Other risk factors for cervical chlamydial infection in women are anatomic or hormonal (e.g., use of depot forms of medroxyprogesterone acetate[18] or ectopy following use of oral contraceptives),[13,19] behavioral (e.g., number of sexual partners),[11,12] and microbiologic (e.g., concurrent gonorrhea).[5,12]

For purposes relevant to this chapter, the major method of transmission of *C. trachomatis* is sexual. The child-to-child and intrafamilial infecting patterns that predominate in trachoma-endemic areas have not been proved to cause disease in newborns.[20] Chlamydiae cause between one third and one half of nongonococcal urethritis cases in men, and concomitant infections with gonococci are common in men and women.[6,21]

An infant born to a mother with a chlamydial infection of the cervix has a 60% to 70% risk of acquiring the infection during passage through the birth canal.[22-24] Conjunctivitis develops in 20% to 50% of exposed infants, and pneumonia in 10% to 20%. The rectum and vagina of infants exposed during delivery also may be infected, but a clear-cut relationship with disease in these sites has not yet been elucidated.[25,26] In utero transmission is not known to occur. Infection after cesarean section occurs rarely, usually in association with at-term or premature rupture of the membranes. No evidence exists to support postnatal transmission from the mother or other family members.

Studies in the 1980s identified *C. trachomatis* in 14% to 46% of infants younger than 1 month of age with conjunctivitis.[27-29] The prevalence of neonatal *Chlamydia* inclusion conjunctivitis has decreased in recent years in areas where screening and treatment of chlamydial infection in pregnant women constitute routine practice.[30]

No evidence exists to suggest that infants with chlamydial infections should be isolated. Transmission of the organism to other infants in nurseries or intensive care units has not been reported. Standard precautions consisting of hand hygiene between patient contacts is recommended. Use of protective gloves, masks or face shields, and nonsterile gowns are recommended for performing procedures likely to generate splashes of body fluids, secretions, or excretions.

MICROBIOLOGY

The Pathogen

Chlamydiae are obligate intracellular parasites that cause a variety of diseases in animal species at virtually all phylogenic levels. Traditionally, the order Chlamydiales has contained one genus with four recognized species: *Chlamydia trachomatis*, *Chlamydia psittaci*, *Chlamydia pneumoniae*, and *Chlamydia pecorum*. Recent taxonomic analysis involving the 16S and 23S rRNA genes have found that the order Chlamydiales contains at least four distinct groups at the family level and suggested splitting the genus *Chlamydia* into two genera, *Chlamydia* and *Chlamydophila*.[31] The genus *Chlamydophila* would contain *C. pneumoniae*, *C. pecorum*, and *C. psittaci*. This new classification continues to be controversial, and for the purposes of this chapter these organisms all are referred to as *Chlamydia*.

C. psittaci is responsible for psittacosis, a chlamydial infection contracted by human beings from infected birds that is characterized by interstitial pneumonitis. It should be suspected in any patient with atypical pneumonia who has had contact with birds. *C. pneumoniae* causes pneumonia, pharyngitis, and bronchitis in humans and may accelerate atherosclerosis. Epidemiologic studies have revealed that *C. pneumoniae* is a fairly common cause of infection in school-aged children and young adults; along with *Mycoplasma*, it probably is the most common cause of community-acquired pneumonia in these age groups. It is not known to cause disease in newborns and therefore is not discussed further.

The species *C. trachomatis* is associated with a spectrum of diseases and contains serologically distinct variants (up to 18) known as serovars. Serovars A, B, Ba, and C cause ocular trachoma, a major cause of blindness in many developing countries. Ocular trachoma is considered the most common cause of preventable blindness in the world. Three serovars, L_1, L_2, and L_3, are associated with lymphogranuloma venereum, a sexually transmitted disease that is rare in the United States but remains quite prevalent in many developing countries, and are particularly prevalent in tropical and subtropical areas. Perinatal transmission is rare with lymphogranuloma venereum. Serovars D to K produce infection of the genital tract—urethritis and epididymitis in the male, cervicitis and salpingitis in the female—the most prevalent chlamydial diseases. Major complications of female genital tract disease include acute pelvic inflammatory disease, ectopic pregnancy, infertility, and infant pneumonia and conjunctivitis.

Like gram-negative bacteria, chlamydiae have an outer membrane that contains lipopolysaccharide and membrane proteins, but their outer membrane contains no detectable peptidoglycan, despite the presence of genes encoding proteins for its synthesis.[32] This recent genomic finding is the basis for the so-called chlamydial peptidoglycan paradox, for it has been known for years that chlamydial development is inhibited by β-lactam antibiotics. Although chlamydiae contain DNA, RNA, and ribosomes, during growth and replication they obtain high-energy phosphate compounds from the host cell. Consequently, they are considered energy parasites. The chlamydial genome size is only 660 kDa, which is smaller than that of any other prokaryote except mycoplasmas. All chlamydiae encode an abundant protein, the major outer membrane protein (MOMP) that is surface exposed in *C. trachomatis* and *C. psittaci*, but not in *C. pneumoniae*.[33] MOMP is the major determinant of the serologic classification of *C. trachomatis* and *C. psittaci* isolates.

Chlamydial Developmental Cycle

The biphasic developmental cycle of chlamydiae is unique among microorganisms and involves two highly specialized morphologic forms shown in Figure 11-1. The extracellular form, or elementary body (EB), contains extensive disulfide cross-links both within and between outer membrane proteins, giving it an almost sporelike structure that is stable outside of the cell. The small (350 nm in diameter) infectious EB is inactive metabolically. The developmental cycle is initiated when an EB attaches to a susceptible epithelial cell. A number of candidate adhesions have been proposed, but their identity and that of associated epithelial cell receptors remain uncertain. One documented mechanism of entry into the epithelial cell is by receptor-mediated endocytosis through clathrin-coated pits,[34] but evidence suggests that chlamydiae may exploit multiple mechanisms of entry.[35] The process of EB internalization is very efficient, suggesting that EBs trigger their own internalization by cells that are not considered professional phagocytes.

Once the EB is inside the cell, surface antigens of the EB appear to prevent fusion of the endosome with lysosomes, protecting itself from enzymatic destruction. Evading host attack by antibody- or cell-mediated defenses, it reorganizes into the replicative form, the reticulate body (RB). RBs successfully parasitize the host cell and divide and multiply. As the RB divides by binary fission, it fills the endosome—now a cytoplasmic inclusion—with its progeny. After 48 to 72 hours, multiplication ceases, and nucleoid condensation occurs as the reticulate bodies transform to new infectious EBs. The EBs then are released from the cell by cytolysis,[36] or

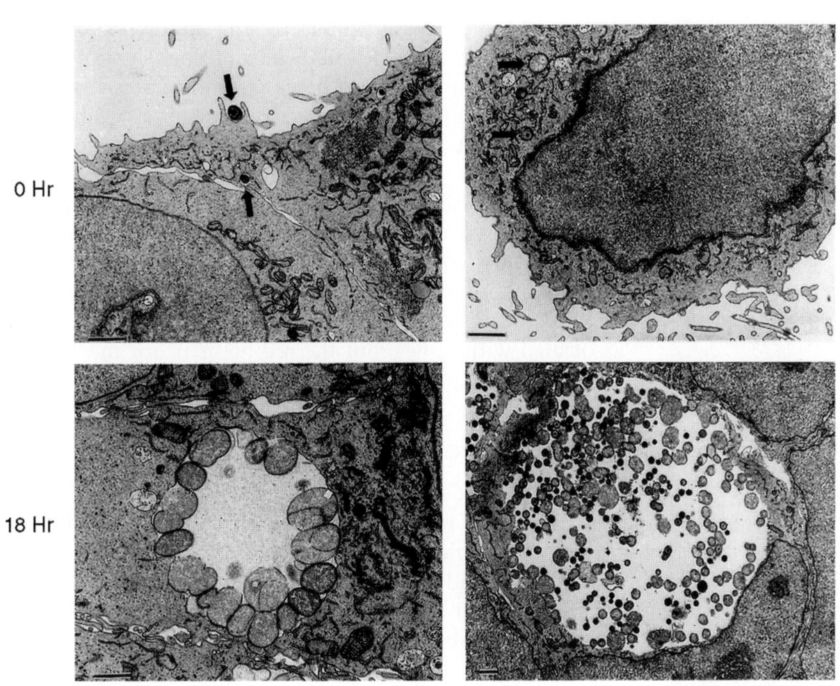

Figure 11–1 The *Chlamydia trachomatis* developmental cycle. Infection is initiated by elementary bodies (EBs). **0 Hr,** Immediately after endocytosis, EBs are found within tightly associated membrane vesicles. **2 Hr,** Within a few hours, EBs differentiate into the larger, metabolically active reticulate bodies (RBs). **18 Hr,** As the RBs multiply, the inclusion increases in size to accommodate the bacterial progeny. RBs are typically observed juxtaposed to the inclusion membrane. **36 Hr,** As the infection progresses, increasing numbers of chlamydiae are observed unattached in the interior of the inclusion. These unattached organisms are, for the most part, EBs and intermediate developmental forms. EBs accumulate within the inclusion even as RBs, still associated with the inclusion membrane, continue to multiply, until the cell undergoes lysis at 40 to 48 hours following infection. (*In* Stephens RS [ed]. Chlamydia, Intracellular Biology, Pathogenesis, and Immunity. Washington, D.C., ASM Press, p 102.)

by a process of exocytosis or by extrusion of the whole inclusion,[37] leaving the host cell intact. The last mechanism may explain the frequency of asymptomatic or subclinical chlamydial infections. The release of the infectious EBs allows infection of new host cells to occur.

PATHOGENESIS

Conjunctivitis

Chlamydiae replicate extensively in epithelial cells of the conjunctiva and cause considerable inflammation. The cells of the inflammatory reaction are mostly polymorphonuclear leukocytes. Conjunctivitis in a majority of untreated patients resolves spontaneously during the first few months of life. Occasionally, infants maintain persistent conjunctivitis, and the pannus formation (neovascularization of the cornea) and scarring typical of trachoma have been reported.[2,38] Loss of vision is rare. Micropannus and some scarring may occur in infants if they do not receive treatment within the first 2 weeks of the disease course.[39] If the infection is treated early, no ocular sequelae develop.

Pneumonia

The nasopharynx is the most frequent site of perinatally acquired chlamydial infection, with approximately 70% of infected infants demonstrating a positive result on cultures at that site.[40,41] Most of these infections are asymptomatic and may persist for up to 29 months.[42] Chlamydial pneumonia develops in only about 30% of infants with nasopharyngeal infection. Conjunctivitis is not a prerequisite for development of pneumonia.

PATHOLOGY

In inclusion conjunctivitis, the affected conjunctiva is highly vascularized and edematous. Inclusions are found in the conjunctival epithelial cells. A massive polymorphonuclear leukocyte infiltration occurs, and pseudomembrane formation may be seen. Lymphoid follicles such as are seen in adults or older children with chlamydial infection of the conjunctiva usually are not observed until the disease has been active for 1 to 2 months. Because in most infants the conjunctivitis spontaneously resolves by that time, lymphoid follicles are not commonly observed.

Because the pneumonia is rarely fatal and in most infants the course is relatively benign, there has been little occasion to obtain lung specimens. When such specimens have been obtained, no characteristic features have been described. Examination of biopsy material has shown pleural congestion and alveolar and bronchiolar mononuclear cell infiltrates with eosinophils, along with focal aggregations of neutrophils.[43,44]

CLINICAL MANIFESTATIONS

The principal clinical manifestations in infants are conjunctivitis, occurring in the first 3 weeks of life (usually 7 to 10 days), and pneumonia, which occurs within the first 3 months (typically about 6 to 8 weeks).

Conjunctivitis

Inclusion conjunctivitis (ICN) usually has an incubation period of 5 to 14 days after delivery, or onset may be earlier if amniotic membranes ruptured prematurely. Conjunctivitis develops in approximately one third of infants exposed to

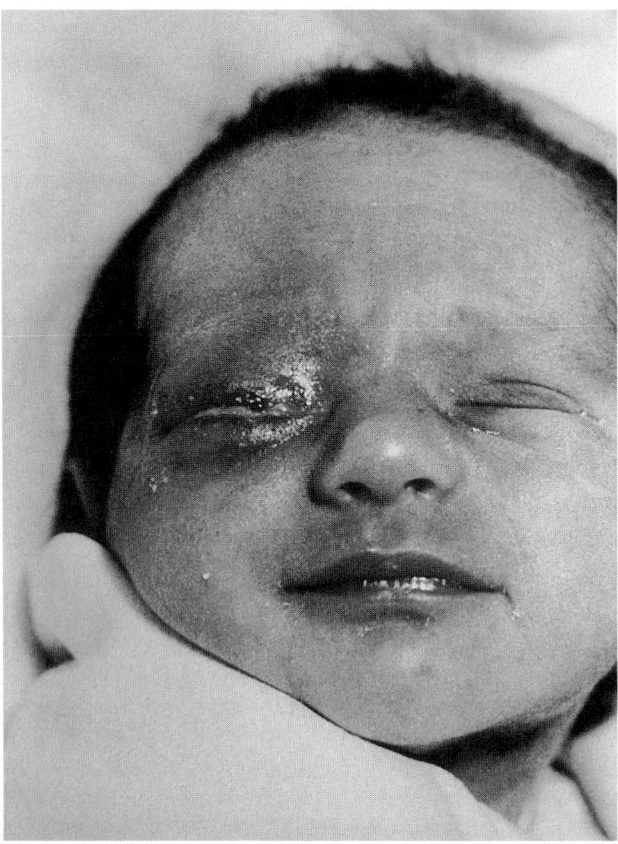

Figure 11–2 An infant with chlamydial conjunctivitis. (*In* Long S, Pickering LK, Prober CG [eds]. Principles and Practice of Pediatric Infectious Diseases. New York, Churchill Livingstone, 2003, p 904.)

chlamydiae during vaginal delivery.[22,33,45-47] Disease manifestations can vary widely and range from mild conjunctival injection with scant mucoid discharge to severe mucopurulent conjunctivitis with chemosis and pseudomembrane formation. The eyelids swell, and the conjunctivae become injected and swollen (Fig. 11-2). The"pseudomembrane" consists of inflammatory exudate that adheres to the inflamed surface of the conjunctiva. Except for micropannus formation, the cornea usually is spared. The duration of the illness typically is 1 to 2 weeks but ICN can last a few days to several weeks.

Pneumonia

Neonatal chlamydial pneumonia was first reported in 1975, and the characteristic clinical picture was described in 1977.[3,48] Most infants with chlamydial pneumonia are symptomatic before the eighth week of life. The illness is characterized by the insidious development of nasal obstruction or discharge, tachypnea, and a repetitive staccato cough. In some infants, these clinical features appear as early as the second week of life, initially involving the upper respiratory tract. Characteristically, infants have been symptomatic for 3 or more weeks before presentation. Most are only mildly or moderately ill and are afebrile. A history of conjunctivitis can be elicited, or the presence of conjunctivitis noted, in half of the cases.[49] Apnea may develop in some infants. Bilateral crepitant inspiratory rales are prominent and out of proportion to the degree of comfort indicated by the infant's breathing; expiratory wheezes are distinctly uncommon. Hyperinflation of the lungs usually accompanies the infiltrates found on chest radiographs, but in most infants this is quite mild. Infiltrates most commonly are bilateral and interstitial; reticulonodular patterns and atelectasis also have been described.[50] Possible laboratory findings include a distinctive peripheral eosinophilia (fewer than 400 cells per mm^3), mild arterial hypoxemia in some patients, and elevated serum immunoglobulins. Untreated disease can linger or recur. In very young infants, infection may be more severe and associated with apnea, but the requirement for mechanical ventilation for this illness is rare.

Perinatal Infections at Other Sites

Infants born to *Chlamydia*-positive mothers also can become infected in the rectum and urogenital tract.[24] Despite the presence of clinical abnormalities, these infections may go undiagnosed and persist for up to 3 years.[24] Consequently, differentiating infection acquired perinatally from infection due to sexual abuse can be particularly difficult in young children.

DIAGNOSIS

Conjunctivitis

Several nonculture methods are approved by the Food and Drug Administration (FDA) for the diagnosis of chlamydial conjunctivitis. These methods include enzyme immunoassays (EIAs)—specifically, Chlamydiazyme (Abbott Diagnostics, Chicago) and MicroTrak EIA (Genetic Systems, Seattle)—and direct fluorescent antibody assays (DFAs) using fluorescein-conjugated monoclonal antibodies to stain chlamydial EBs in a smear, including Syva MicroTrak (Genetic Systems) and Pathfinder (Sanofi-Pasteur, Chaska, Minn.). These tests perform well on conjunctival specimens, with sensitivities of greater than 90% and specificities of 95% or greater.[28,51,52]

In resource-poor settings, a useful diagnostic method is examination of Giemsa-stained conjunctival scrapings for the presence of blue-stained intracytoplasmic inclusions within epithelial cells. The sensitivity of this diagnostic method varies, ranging from 22% to 95%, depending on the technique of specimen collection and the examiner's expertise. This method also allows visualization of bacteria, such as gonococci, and of cytologic features suggestive of viral infection. Isolation of the chlamydiae from conjunctival scrapings inoculated into tissue cell culture is a more reliable, although more costly, method of diagnosis. Serologic diagnosis of chlamydial conjunctivitis (in contrast to pneumonia) is not reliable because of the presence of maternally transmitted IgG antibody and the unreliable appearance of IgM antibody in this infection.

Even if a firm diagnosis of chlamydial conjunctivitis is established, the possibility of a dual infection, particularly with *Neisseria gonorrhoeae*, should be kept in mind. For this reason, appropriate studies by stain and culture of the conjunctival exudate always should be performed.

Highly sensitive nucleic acid amplification tests (NAATs) are commercially available for the diagnosis of genital chlamydial infection in adolescents and adults.[53,54] NAATs have FDA approval for cervical swabs from women, urethral swabs from men, and urine from men and women. These tests have a high sensitivity, detecting perhaps 10% to 20% more cases of genital chlamydial infection than is possible with culture, while retaining high specificity.[55] Information on the use of NAATs in children is limited, but preliminary data suggest that polymerase chain reation (PCR) assay is equivalent to culture for the detection of *C. trachomatis* in the conjunctiva and nasopharynx of infants with conjunctivitis.[56]

Pneumonia

EIAs and DFAs for chlamydia do not perform well with nasopharyngeal specimens and are not approved for this purpose. The definitive diagnosis of pneumonia can be made by culture of the organism from the respiratory tract. *Chlamydia* culture has been defined by the Centers for Disease Control and Prevention (CDC) as isolation of the organism in tissue culture and confirmation by microscopic identification of the characteristic inclusions by fluorescent antibody staining.[5] The likelihood of obtaining a positive culture result is enhanced by obtaining a specimen by deep suction of the trachea or by collecting a nasopharyngeal aspirate rather than obtaining a specimen with a swab.[3,57] An acute microimmunofluorescence serum titer of *C. trachomatis*–specific immunoglobulin (Ig) M greater than 1:32 also is diagnostic. Detection of *C. trachomatis*–specific IgG is not diagnostic because passively transferred maternal antibodies may persist at high titers for months. The serologic test of choice is the microimmunofluorescence procedure of Wang and Grayston,[58] in which elementary bodies are used as antigen. Only a few clinical laboratories perform this test.

Indirect evidence of chlamydial pneumonia includes hyperinflation and bilateral diffuse infiltrates on chest radiographs, eosinophilia with peripheral blood counts of 0.3 to 0.4×10^9/L (300 to 400/μL) or more, and increased total serum IgG (less than 5 g/L [500 mg/dL]) and IgM (greater than 1.1 g/L [110 mg/dL]) concentrations. The absence of these findings, however, does not exclude the diagnosis of *C. trachomatis* infection.

DIFFERENTIAL DIAGNOSIS

Conjunctivitis

Inclusion conjunctivitis must be distinguished from that produced by pyogenic bacteria, particularly *N. gonorrhoeae.* Gonococcal ophthalmia usually occurs at an earlier age, typically 2 to 5 days after birth, although overlap in age at onset can occur. Gonococcal disease usually is more rapidly progressive than that due to *C. trachomatis.* Gonococcal infection can be diagnosed presumptively by examination of the Gram-stained smear of the exudate and confirmed by culture of the exudate. Staphylococcal conjunctivitis usually is acquired in the nursery or home environment. It is characterized more by purulent discharge than by redness. This and other forms of pyogenic conjunctivitis—which may be due to *Streptococcus pneumoniae*, *Haemophilus* species, or gram-negative bacteria such as *Pseudomonas aeruginosa*—can easily be diagnosed by Gram stain and culture of the exudate.

Of the viral infections, neonatal herpes simplex (see Chapter 26) is the most important. This infection is characterized by vesicle formation and lesions of the skin as well as the conjunctiva. Corneal involvement may occur. Adenovirus infection of the newborn is very rare but has been described.

Chemical conjunctivitis related to instillation of silver nitrate at birth also can produce marked redness and a purulent discharge. These signs begin on the first day of life and disappear after a few days, however, thereby distinguishing this entity from a chlamydial infection.

Pneumonia

The afebrile, tachypneic infant presenting with a staccato cough in the first 3 months of life is very likely to have chlamydial disease. Cytomegalovirus (CMV) can produce an interstitial pneumonia in preterm newborns who receive transfusions from CMV-positive donors; however, it often produces clinical signs in other organ systems. Congenital infection by the rubella virus and *Toxoplasma gondii* also produces multiorgan involvement, as does perinatal infection with the herpes simplex virus. Adenovirus or parainfluenza virus infection can cause an interstitial pneumonia, but without the characteristic staccato cough or eosinophilia. Respiratory syncytial virus (RSV), a common cause of pneumonia in early infancy, often produces fever in the early stages, and wheezing due to airway obstruction is typical. RSV infection is not associated with eosinophilia. RSV infection can be rapidly diagnosed by performing an EIA of a nasopharyngeal wash specimen. Many pyogenic bacteria may produce lower respiratory tract infections in infancy. Group B β-hemolytic streptococci, *S. pneumoniae*, *Staphylococcus aureus*, *Haemophilus influenzae*, and the coliform group of bacteria are the most common. Affected infants generally are much sicker, are more toxic and febrile, and have pulmonary consolidation rather than interstitial infiltrates. *Bordetella pertussis* classically causes a paroxysmal cough with or without accompanying fever, but lymphocytosis is a nonspecific diagnostic clue, and apnea occurs in infants younger than 6 months of age. In infants with *Pneumocystis jiroveci* pneumonia, a characteristic syndrome develops that includes subacute diffuse pneumonitis with dyspnea at rest, tachypnea, oxygen desaturation, nonproductive cough, and fever. Most have an underlying immune disorder.

PROGNOSIS

Conjunctivitis

If untreated, inclusion conjunctivitis can persist for many weeks, but it usually resolves spontaneously without complications. The scarring that occurs in trachoma that leads to lid deformities is not seen. Superficial corneal vascularization and conjunctival scar formation can occur, however.[38,39,59]

Pneumonia

Without treatment, affected infants usually are ill for several weeks, with frequent cough, poor feeding, and poor weight gain. A small number require oxygen, and fewer require ventilatory support. Beem and colleagues[60] found in a series of 11 infants that the duration of the clinical course was between 24 and 61 days, with a mean of 43 days, and that death was exceptionally rare. Follow-up evaluation of a small cohort of children who had *C. trachomatis* pneumonia in infancy demonstrated an increased prevalence of chronic cough and abnormal lung function when compared with that in age-matched controls.[61]

THERAPY

Topical treatment of inclusion conjunctivitis is not recommended, primarily because of failure to eliminate concurrent nasopharyngeal infection. Recommended therapy for conjunctivitis or pneumonia is oral erythromycin, 40 mg/kg/day in 4 divided doses for 14 days. The failure rate is around 20%, and a second course of therapy may be required.[62,63] Problems with compliance and tolerance are frequent. Oral sulfonamides can be used after the immediate neonatal period for infants who do not tolerate erythromycin. Convincing evidence suggests that this treatment shortens the clinical course of pneumonia and eliminates the organism from the respiratory tract. Beyond specific antimicrobial therapy, the infants require standard supportive care measures, with attention to nutrition and to fluid status. Oxygen and ventilatory therapy may be required in a minority of cases. A specific diagnosis of *C. trachomatis* infection in an infant should prompt treatment of the mother and her sexual partner(s).

An association between orally administered erythromycin and infantile hypertrophic pyloric stenosis (IHPS) has been reported in infants younger than 6 weeks of age who were given the drug for prophylaxis after nursery exposure to pertussis.[64,65] The risk of IHPS after treatment with other macrolides (e.g., azithromycin dihydrate, clarithromycin) is unknown. Because confirmation of erythromycin as a contributor to cases of IHPS requires additional investigation and because alternative therapies are not as well studied, the American Academy of Pediatrics continues to recommend use of erythromycin for treatment of *C. trachomatis* infection in infants. Parents of infants given erythromycin should be informed about the signs and potential risks of developing IHPS. Cases of pyloric stenosis developing after use of oral erythromycin should be reported to the Food and Drug Administration as an adverse drug reaction. One small study suggests that a short course of orally administered azithromycin, 20 mg/kg in a single daily dose for 3 days, may be effective.[30]

Prophylactic therapy of infants born to mothers known to have untreated chlamydial infection is not indicated, because the efficacy of such prophylaxis is unknown. Such infants should be monitored for signs of infection and to ensure appropriate treatment if infection develops. If adequate follow-up cannot be ensured, prophylaxis may be considered.

PREVENTION

Because *C. trachomatis* infections are transmitted vertically from mother to infant during delivery, an effective prevention measure is screening and treatment of pregnant women for *C. trachomatis* infection before delivery. The CDC currently recommends screening all pregnant women during their first prenatal visit, and during the third trimester if they are at high risk (age younger than 25 years or other risk factors such as new or multiple sexual partners).[5] Either erythromycin base (2 g/day in four divided doses) or amoxicillin (1.5 g/day in three divided doses) for 7 days is the recommended treatment regimen for pregnant women. Half-doses of erythromycin daily for 14 days may be given in pregnant women intolerant of the full-dose regimen. Because these regimens are not highly efficacious, a second course of therapy may be needed. Azithromycin (1 g orally in a single dose) is an alternative; preliminary data suggest that it is safe and effective.[66] Doxycycline and ofloxacin are contraindicated during pregnancy.

Ocular prophylaxis with topical erythromycin or tetracycline has reduced the incidence of gonococcal ophthalmia but does not appear to be effective against *C. trachomatis*.[67] Thus, the only means of preventing chlamydial infection of the newborn is treatment of maternal infection before delivery.

Ongoing efforts to develop a *C. trachomatis* vaccine to protect persons from genital tract infection have concentrated primarily on the use of peptides derived from the MOMP or recombinant synthetic MOMP polypeptides as immunogens. Future work may incorporate molecular technology and our increasing understanding of the host response to chlamydiae to develop one or more new vaccines. Stimulation of long-term mucosal immunity in the genital tract is a challenge; it is unclear whether all genital infections could be prevented or whether only more invasive disease, such as salpingitis, might be preventable using vaccine technology.

REFERENCES

1. Lindner L. Zur Aetiologie der gonokokkenfreien Urethritis. Wiem Klin Wochenschr 22:1555, 1910.
2. Jonesboro Al-Hussaini MK, Dunlop EMC. Genital infection in association with TRIC virus infection of the eye: I. Isolation of virus from urethra, cervix, and eye: preliminary report. Br J Vener Dis 40:19-24, 1964.
3. Beem MO, Saxon EM. Respiratory tract colonization and a distinctive pneumonia syndrome in infants infected with *Chlamydia trachomatis*. N Engl J Med 296:306-310, 1977.
4. Schachter J. Chlamydial infections (third of three parts). N Engl J Med 298:540-549, 1978.
5. Sexually transmitted diseases treatment guidelines 2002. Centers for Disease Control and Prevention. MMWR Recomm. Rep 51:30-36, 2002.
6. Sexually transmitted disease surveillance. 9-1-2002. Atlanta, Centers for Disease Control and Prevention, 2002.
7. Stamm WE. *Chlamydia trachomatis* infections of the adult. *In* Holmes KK, Mardh PA, Sparling PF (eds). Sexually Transmitted Diseases. New York, McGraw-Hill, 1999, pp 407-422.
8. Hardick J, Hsieh YH, Tulloch S, et al. Surveillance of *Chlamydia trachomatis* and *Neisseria gonorrhoeae* infections in women in detention in Baltimore, Maryland. Sex Transm Dis 30:64-70, 2003.
9. Tobin JM. *Chlamydia* screening in primary care: is it useful, affordable and universal? Curr Opin Infect Dis 15:31-36, 2002.
10. Herrmann B, Egger M. Genital *Chlamydia trachomatis* infections in Uppsala County, Sweden, 1985-1993: declining rates for how much longer? Sex Transm Dis 22:253-260, 1995.
11. Blythe MJ, Katz BP, Orr DP, et al. Historical and clinical factors associated with *Chlamydia trachomatis* genitourinary infection in female adolescents. J Pediatr 112:1000-1004, 1988.
12. Chacko MR, Lovchik JC. *Chlamydia trachomatis* infection in sexually active adolescents: prevalence and risk factors. Pediatrics 73:836-840, 1984.

13. Shafer MA, Beck A, Blain B, et al. *Chlamydia trachomatis*: important relationships to race, contraception, lower genital tract infection, and Papanicolaou smear. J Pediatr 104:141-146, 1984.
14. Burstein GR, Gaydos CA, Diener-West M, et al. Incident *Chlamydia trachomatis* infections among inner-city adolescent females. JAMA 280:521-526, 1998. (See comments.)
15. Gaydos CA, Howell MR, Pare B, et al. *Chlamydia trachomatis* infections in female military recruits. N Engl J Med 339:739-744, 1998. (See comments.)
16. Eagar RM, Beach RK, Davidson AJ, Judson FN. Epidemiologic and clinical factors of *Chlamydia trachomatis* in black, Hispanic and white female adolescents. West J Med 143:37-41, 1985.
17. Fraser JJ Jr, Rettig PJ, Kaplan DW. Prevalence of cervical *Chlamydia trachomatis* and *Neisseria gonorrhoeae* in female adolescents. Pediatrics 71:333-336, 1983.
18. Jacobson DL, Peralta L, Farmer M, et al. Relationship of hormonal contraception and cervical ectopy as measured by computerized planimetry to chlamydial infection in adolescents. Sex Transm Dis 27:313-319, 2000.
19. Louv WC, Austin H, Perlman J, Alexander WJ. Oral contraceptive use and the risk of chlamydial and gonococcal infections. Am J Obstet Gynecol 160:396-402, 1989.
20. Jones BR. The prevention of blindness from trachoma. Trans Ophthalmol Soc UK 95:16-33, 1975.
21. Holmes KK, Handsfield HH, Wang SP, et al. Etiology of nongonococcal urethritis. N Engl J Med 292:1199-1204, 1975.
22. Chandler JW, Alexander ER, Pheiffer TA, et al. Ophthalmia neonatorum associated with maternal chlamydial infections. Trans Am Acad Ophthalmol Otolaryngol 83:302-308, 1977.
23. Hammerschlag MR, Anderka M, Semine DZ, et al. Prospective study of maternal and infantile infection with *Chlamydia trachomatis*. Pediatrics 64:142-148, 1979.
24. Schachter J, Grossman M, Sweet RL, et al. Prospective study of perinatal transmission of *Chlamydia trachomatis*. JAMA 255:3374-3377, 1986.
25. Schachter J, Grossman M, Holt J, et al. Prospective study of chlamydial infection in neonates. Lancet 2:377-380, 1979.
26. Schachter J, Grossman M, Holt J, et al. Infection with *Chlamydia trachomatis*: involvement of multiple anatomic sites in neonates. J Infect Dis 139:232-234, 1979.
27. Hammerschlag MR, Roblin PM, Gelling M, Worku M. Comparison of two enzyme immunoassays to culture for the diagnosis of chlamydial conjunctivitis and respiratory infections in infants. J Clin Microbiol 28:1725-1727, 1990.
28. Rapoza PA, Quinn TC, Kiessling LA, et al. Assessment of neonatal conjunctivitis with a direct immunofluorescent monoclonal antibody stain for *Chlamydia*. JAMA 255:3369-3373, 1986.
29. Roblin PM, Hammerschlag MR, Cummings C, et al. Comparison of two rapid microscopic methods and culture for detection of *Chlamydia trachomatis* in ocular and nasopharyngeal specimens from infants. J Clin Microbiol 27:968-970, 1989.
30. Hammerschlag MR, Gelling M, Roblin PM, et al. Treatment of neonatal chlamydial conjunctivitis with azithromycin. Pediatr Infect Dis J 17:1049-1050, 1998.
31. Everett KD, Bush RM, Andersen A. Emended description of the order Chlamydiales, proposal of Parachlamydiaceae fam. nov. and Simkaniaceae fam. nov., each containing one monotypic genus, revised taxonomy of the family Chlamydiaceae, including a new genus and five new species, and standards for the identification of organisms. Int J Syst Bacteriol 49:2:415-440, 1999.
32. Kalman S, Mitchell W, Marathe R, et al. Comparative genomes of *Chlamydia pneumoniae* and *C. trachomatis*. Nat Genet 21:385-389, 1999.
33. Rockey DD, Lenart J, Stephens RS. Genome sequencing and our understanding of chlamydiae. Infect Immun 68:5473-5479, 2000.
34. Wyrick PB, Choong J, Davis CH, et al. Entry of genital *Chlamydia trachomatis* into polarized human epithelial cells. Infect Immun 57:2378-2389, 1989.
35. Wyrick PB. Cell biology of chlamydial infection. *In* Stephens RS, Byrne GI, Christiansen G (eds). Proceedings of the 9th International Symposium of Human Chlamydial Infection. San Francisco, International Chlamydia Symposium, 1998, p 69.
36. de la Maza LM, Peterson EM. Scanning electron microscopy of McCoy cells infected with *Chlamydia trachomatis*. Exp Mol Pathol 36:217-226, 1982.
37. Todd WJ, Caldwell HD. The interaction of *Chlamydia trachomatis* with host cells: ultrastructural studies of the mechanism of release of a biovar II strain from HeLa 229 cells. J Infect Dis 151:1037-1044, 1985.
38. Mordhorst CH, Wang SP, Grayston JT. Childhood trachoma in a nonendemic area in Danish trachoma patients and their close contacts, 1963 to 1973. JAMA 239:1765-1771, 1978.
39. Mordhorst CH, Dawson C. Sequelae of neonatal inclusion conjunctivitis and associated disease in parents. Am J Ophthalmol 71:861-867, 1971.
40. Hammerschlag MR. Chlamydial infections. J Pediatr 114:727-734, 1989.
41. Hammerschlag MR, Chandler JW, Alexander ER, et al. Longitudinal studies on chlamydial infections in the first year of life. Pediatr Infect Dis 1:395-401, 1982.
42. Bell TA, Stamm WE, Wang S, et al. Chronic *Chlamydia trachomatis* infections in infants. JAMA 267:400-402, 1992.
43. Frommell GT, Bruhn FW, Schwartzman JD. Isolation of *Chlamydia trachomatis* from infant lung tissue. N Engl J Med 296:1150-1152, 1977.
44. Arth C, Von Schmidt B, Grossman M, Schachter J. Chlamydial pneumonitis. J Pediatr 93:447-449, 1978.
45. Schachter J: Chlamydial infections (third of three parts). N Engl J Med 298:540-549, 1978. (Review.)
46. Frommell GT, Rothenberg R, Wang S, McIntosh K. Chlamydial infection of mothers and their infants. J Pediatr 95:28-32, 1979.
47. Hammerschlag MR, Anderka M, Semine DZ, et al. Prospective study of maternal and infantile infection with *Chlamydia trachomatis*. Pediatrics 64:142-148, 1979.
48. Schachter J, Lum L, Gooding CA, Ostler B. Pneumonitis following inclusion blennorrhea. J Pediatr 87:779-780, 1975.
49. Tipple MA, Beem MO, Saxon EM. Clinical characteristics of the afebrile pneumonia associated with *Chlamydia trachomatis* infection in infants less than 6 months of age. Pediatrics 63:192-197, 1979.
50. Radkowski MA, Kranzler JK, Beem MO, Tipple MA. *Chlamydia* pneumonia in infants: radiography in 125 cases. Am J Resp Dis 137:703-706, 1981.
51. Hammerschlag MR, Roblin PM, Gelling M, Worku M. Comparison of two enzyme immunoassays to culture for the diagnosis of chlamydial conjunctivitis and respiratory infections in infants. J Clin Microbiol 28:1725-1727, 1990.
52. Roblin PM, Hammerschlag MR, Cummings C, et al. Comparison of two rapid microscopic methods and culture for detection of *Chlamydia trachomatis* in ocular and nasopharyngeal specimens from infants. J Clin Microbiol 27:968-970, 1989.
53. Schachter J, Stamm WE, Quinn TC, et al. Ligase chain reaction to detect *Chlamydia trachomatis* infection of the cervix. J Clin Microbiol 32:2540-2543, 1994.
54. Jaschek G, Gaydos CA, Welsh LE, Quinn TC. Direct detection of *Chlamydia trachomatis* in urine specimens from symptomatic and asymptomatic men by using a rapid polymerase chain reaction assay. J Clin Microbiol 31:1209-1212, 1993.
55. Black CM. Current methods of laboratory diagnosis of *Chlamydia trachomatis* infections. Clin Microbiol Rev 10:160-184, 1997.
56. Hammerschlag MR, Roblin PM, Gelling M, et al. Use of polymerase chain reaction for the detection of *Chlamydia trachomatis* in ocular and nasopharyngeal specimens from infants with conjunctivitis. Pediatr Infect Dis J 16:293-297, 1997.
57. Harrison HR, English MG, Lee CK, Alexander ER. *Chlamydia trachomatis* infant pneumonitis: comparison with matched controls and other infant pneumonitis. N Engl J Med 298:702-708, 1978.
58. Wang SP, Grayston JT, Alexander ER, Holmes KK. Simplified microimmunofluorescence test with trachoma lymphogranuloma venereum (*Chlamydia trachomatis*) antigens for use as a screening test for antibody. Clin Microbiol 1:250-255, 1975.
59. Schachter J, Dawson CR. Human Chlamydial Infections. Littleton, Mass, PSG Publishing Company, 1978.
60. Beem MO, Saxon E, Tipple MA. Treatment of chlamydial pneumonia of infancy. Pediatrics 63:198-203, 1979.
61. Harrison HR, Taussig LM, Fulginiti VA. *Chlamydia trachomatis* and chronic respiratory disease in childhood. Pediatr Infect Dis J 1:29-33, 1982.
62. Hammerschlag MR, Chandler JW, Alexander ER, et al. Longitudinal studies on chlamydial infections in the first year of life. Pediatr Infect Dis J 1:395-401, 1982.
63. Patamasucon P, Rettig PJ, Faust KL, et al. Oral v topical erythromycin therapies for chlamydial conjunctivitis. Am J Dis Child 136:817-821, 1982.
64. Hypertrophic pyloric stenosis in infants following pertussis prophylaxis with erythromycin—Knoxville, Tennessee, 1999. MMWR Morb Mortal Wkly Rep 48:1117-1120, 1999.

65. Centers for Disease Control and Prevention. Hypertrophic pyloric stenosis in infants following pertussis prophylaxis with erythromycin—Knoxville, Tennessee, 1999. JAMA 283:471-472, 2000.
66. Miller JM, Martin DH. Treatment of *Chlamydia trachomatis* infections in pregnant women. Drugs 60:597-605, 2000.
67. Hammerschlag MR, Cummings C, Roblin PM, et al. Efficacy of neonatal ocular prophylaxis for the prevention of chlamydial and gonococcal conjunctivitis. N Engl J Med 320:769-772, 1989.

Chapter 12

GONOCOCCAL INFECTIONS

Joanne E. Embree

Infections of the fetus and newborn infant due to *Neisseria gonorrhoeae* are restricted primarily to mucosal surfaces of the newborn infant. The most common condition related to infection by this organism during the neonatal period is ophthalmia neonatorum, or neonatal conjunctivitis. *N. gonorrhoeae* produces purulent conjunctivitis in the newborn that, if untreated may lead to blindness. This is the primary disease entity discussed in this chapter.

Ophthalmia neonatorum had been a well-recognized entity, affecting between 1% and 15% of newborns, in Europe and North America when Hirschberg and Krause first described neonatal infection due to *N. gonorrhoeae* in an infant with purulent conjunctivitis in 1881.[1] Shortly thereafter, the topical instillation of silver nitrate into the newborn's eyes immediately after birth dramatically reduced the incidence of this disease due to *N. gonorrhoeae*, albeit with the complication in most infants of milder conjunctivitis, limited to the first 24 hours of life, due to the silver nitrate.[2,3] Use of erythromycin or tetracycline ointments for this purpose has proved to be efficacious for preventing gonococcal ophthalmia, with markedly reduced problems related to the chemical conjunctivitis seen with silver nitrate.[4-6] Systemic neonatal infection is unusual, but infants may present with a variety of clinical syndromes (in particular, arthritis), which implies that dissemination of the bacteria does occur.[7,8] Maternal systemic infection during pregnancy also is rare, and transplacental congenital infection of the fetus has not been described. Maternal genital mucosal infection, however, may result in an ascending infection, with chorioamnionitis leading to premature rupture of the placental membranes and preterm delivery.[9] In developed countries, screening and treatment of pregnant women for gonococcal infections with tracing of named contacts, along with the use of neonatal ophthalmic prophylaxis, have substantially reduced the incidence of gonococcal ophthalmia neonatorum. In medically developing areas, improvements in access to medical care, as well as aggressive pilot programs for prevention and treatment of sexually transmitted diseases (STDs) in conjunction with HIV infection/acquired immunodeficiency syndrome (AIDS) prevention strategies, have continued to decrease the incidence of gonococcal infection and its complications, such as ophthalmia neonatorum, in areas where these interventions have been introduced.[10] Despite the overall decreasing prevalence of *N. gonorrhoeae* infection worldwide, however, gonococcal ophthalmia neonatorum remains a significant illness.

EPIDEMIOLOGY AND TRANSMISSION

The incidence of neonatal gonococcal illnesss is related to the prevalence of *N. gonorrhoeae* colonization among women of childbearing age, and to the rates of acute infection during pregnancy. This is quite variable worldwide and now is heavily influenced by the human immunodeficiency virus type 1 infection (HIV-1) epidemic. In general, once antibiotic treatment for gonorrhea became available in the mid-20th century, rates of infection among women decreased worldwide, as these agents became more readily accessible and heath care programs improved. With the emergence of penicillin chromosomal resistance, the development of penicillinase production by some strains, and the expansion of the AIDS epidemic in the 1990s, however, rates began to rise again during that decade. In response, efforts to control this infection—which some authorities had hoped could ultimately be eliminated by the middle of this century—have been increased.

Estimates by the World Health Organization (WHO) of the burden of gonorrheal disease in various regions at the end of the twentieth century are presented in Table 12-1.[11] Although these estimates are useful in indicating areas of high burden of disease, considerable variation within regions exists. This variation is reflected in the differences seen in the number of reported cases of gonorrhea among women in North America. In the United States, during 2001, 361,705 cases of gonorrhea were tallied, resulting in a reported prevalence of 128 cases per 100,000 population, which was similar to that reported in 2000 (129 per 100,000), 1999 (132 per 100,000), and 1998 (131 per 100,000).[12] Overall, no changes have been noted in the prevalence rate among women in the United States during these years. The prevalence among women has equaled that among men since 1998. Infection rates have fallen since 1986, when the prevalence among women was approximately 310 cases per 100,000 population. Further significant differences are noted among populations in the United States, however, when rates are compared for groups of different races or ethnicity and for location. The prevalence among blacks in the United States is still considerably higher than in other ethnic groups but dropped

Table 12–1 WHO Estimated Numbers of Cases of Gonorrhea in Adults 1999

Geographical Location	Estimated No. of Cases
North America	1.5 million
Latin America	7.5 million
Western Europe	1 million
Eastern Europe and Central Asia	3.5 million
East Asia	3 million
South and Southeast Asia	27 million
North Africa and the Middle East	1.5 million
Sub-Saharan Africa	17 million
New Zealand and Australia	120,000

WHO, World Health Organization.
Data from World Health Organization. Global prevalence and incidence of selected curable sexually transmitted infections. Overview and estimates. WHO/CDS/CSR/EDC/2001. 10:1-50, 2001.

from approximately 2100 cases per 100,000 population in 1986 to around 800 per 100,000 in 2001. The background prevalence also differs significantly among the various states, with 6 states reporting rates greater than 200 per 100,000 in 2001, 17 states reporting between 100 and 200 cases per 100,000 and the rest reporting less than 100 per 100,000. The United States has set a goal of reducing the national prevalence of gonorrhea to less than 19 cases per 100,000 among adults. In 2001, 8 states reported a prevalence of disease below this target goal. In Canada, however, rates of gonorrhea are considerably lower than in the United States. Canada has placed an emphasis on STD control as well but has an exclusively publicly funded health care system. Gonorrhea prevalence rates have decreased steadily from 1980, when the prevalence among women was 166 per 100,000 population. The highest rates at that time were among women 15 to 19 and 20 to 24 years of age, which were extremely high at 510 and 598, respectively, per 100,000. In 2000, the prevalence among women was approximately 15 per 100,000, which actually represented an increase from 1997, when rates had dropped to a low of 11 per 100,000. The increase occurred primarily among women aged 15 to 19 and 20 to 24 years; in these age groups, rates increased from 69 and 60, respectively, per 100,000 in 1997 to 96 and 73 per 100,000. In 1997, Canada had set as its goal the elimination of endemic transmission of *N. gonorrhoeae* by the year 2010. This increase in prevalence has led to a call for an assessment of STD control and reporting procedures in Canada to determine why the previously observed declines in prevalence had stopped.[13]

Factors that increase a pregnant woman's risk of acquiring *N. gonorrhoeae* infection are similar to those that increase the risk of acquisition of any other sexually transmitted infection.[14] The prevalence of *N. gonorrhoeae* in the population or network in which she socializes and chooses her sexual partners will determine the likelihood of exposure to this pathogen. Women who have multiple sexual partners or whose partners have multiple sexual contacts increase their risk of exposure to *N. gonorrhoeae*. Women who do not use condoms or other barrier protection will increase their risk of acquisition of *N. gonorrhoeae* infection on exposure to the organism. It is unknown whether women who are HIV positive have an increased risk of infection by *N. gonorrhoeae* on exposure to it. Factors associated with an increased likelihood of at-risk behavior that results in an increased risk of gonococcal infection among pregnant women include younger age, unmarried status, homelessness, problems with drug or alcohol abuse, prostitution, low-income professions, and, in the United States, being black. Gonococcal infections are diagnosed more frequently in the summer months in the United States, probably reflecting transient changes in social behavior during vacations.[15] Varying gonococcal rates reported in various studies worldwide reflect the differences in risk among the populations studied. In a recent study in Brazil, involving a cross-sectional study of 200 women aged 14 to 29 years who attended an HIV testing site in central Rio de Janeiro, the prevalence of gonorrhea was high at 9.5%. Of the 200 women, 8% were HIV infected, confirming that the population studied had a high risk of STD exposure.[16] The prevalence of gonorrhea among 547 pregnant women attending a first-visit antenatal hospital clinic during 1999 and 2000 in Vila, Vanuatu, was 5.9%, but no women were found to be HIV infected at that time.[17] The occurrence rates of gonorrhea were quite high among this population, reflecting the prevalence in the general population. A study in Thailand in 1996 that investigated the prevalence of STDs among pregnant women, where case reporting suggested a marked decrease in STDs following a campaign promoting condom use during commercial sex, showed that the prevalence of gonorrhea was extremely low at 0.2%.[18] By contrast, in a population in Nairobi, where condom use was advocated for commercial sex workers but not promoted to the same extent as in Thailand and not routinely practiced by the at-risk general population, in a cross-sectional study of 520 women seeking treatment at an STD clinic, 4% were infected with gonorrhea and 29% were HIV positive.[19] In Nigeria, where the prevalence of HIV infection is low, the rate of gonorrhea also is lower among pregnant women. In a cross-sectional study, 230 pregnant women attending the antenatal clinic of a teaching hospital in Nigeria from January 2000 to December 2000 were screened randomly to determine the prevalence of common STDs; 1.3% were found to have gonorrhea.[20]

N. gonorrhoeae usually is transmitted from the infected maternal cervix during vaginal delivery. Ascending infection does occur, however, in the instance of prolonged ruptured membranes and has been observed after cesarean section delivery following ruptured membranes.[21-24] It has been estimated that colonization and infection of the neonate occur in only one third of instances in which the mother is infected.[25] The infant's mucous membranes become colonized when swallowing contaminated fluid during labor and delivery.

In instances of congenital infection, it is speculated that the chorioamnion is infected through an ascending infection.[26] Premature rupture of membranes then occurs, with early onset of labor and premature delivery or septic abortion.[9,27-29] This association was dramatically shown in one study in which premature rupture of membranes occurred in 6 (43%) of 14 women with untreated gonococcal infection during pregnancy, compared with 4 (3%) of 144 women whose infection had been treated.[29] Thus, screening and treatment programs for gonococcal infections during pregnancy are appropriate to reduce the risk of adverse pregnancy outcomes related to maternal infection.

MICROBIOLOGY

N. gonorrhoeae is a gram-negative diplococcus. It utilizes glucose for growth but not maltose, sucrose, or lactose. This is one of the characteristics used to distinguish *N. gonorrhoeae* isolates from *N. meningitidis* and other colonizing *Neisseria* species such as *N. cinerea*, *N. flava*, *N. subflava*, *N. lactamica*, *N. mucosa*, and *N. sicca*. *N. gonorrhoeae* produces acid only when grown in glucose. In addition, the organism is oxidase positive, hydroxyprolylaminopitidase positive, nitrate negative, DNase negative, catalase positive, strongly superoxol positive, and colistin resistant.[30] It is an obligate aerobe but lacks superoxide dismutase, which moderates the effects of oxygen radicals in most other aerobic bacteria. When grown in anaerobic conditions, virulent strains express a lipoprotein called Pan 1. Its function is unknown, but it elicits an immunoglobulin M (IgM) antibody response in acute infection.

When cultured in the laboratory, *N. gonorrhoeae* forms four different colony types. Pinpoint colonies, classified as type 1 and type 2, usually are only seen on primary isolation. What distinguishes these colony types from the large granular colonies classified as types 3 and 4 is the presence of pili, which are thin bacterial appendages on the cell surface that are involved in attachment to mammalian cells. *N. gonorrhoeae* has the genetic capacity to turn on and turn off the expression of pili.[31] With repeated subculturing at 37° C, the genes are no longer expressed and the pili disappear, resulting in colonial-type changes, with type 1 colonies shifting to type 4 and type 2 colonies to type 3. Associated with this change is a reduction in virulence.[32] *N. gonorrhoeae* also may form colonies that are either opaque or clear. This characteristic is related to the presence of a specific surface protein called outer membrane protein II. Transparent colonies lack outer membrane protein II and are more resistant to phagocytosis. Individual strains can also shift from forming opaque to forming clear colonies.[33]

Colonial morphology is of no use in differentiating gonococcal types or strains. Strains can be differentiated by auxotyping. Different strains have differing stable auxotrophic requirements for amino acids, purines, pyrimidines, or vitamins. Typing based on these requirements has been useful in some epidemiologic surveys. Additionally, enzyme-linked immunosorbent typing, based on differences in protein I, can be done. Nine distinct strains are detectable with this typing system. It is clinically relevant in that type 1 and type 2 strains are more likely to disseminate in adult patients. Use of serologic typing schemes can detect three serogroups: WI, WII, and WIII. Strains 1 to 3 are usually found in serogroup WI, strains 4 to 8 in serogroup WII, and strain 9 in serogroup WIII.[34] Finally, strains also are typed by coagulation testing following exposure to monoclonal antibodies made against the outer membrane protein I. Two major serogroups exist: 1A, which has 26 subgroups, and 1B, with 32 subgroups.[35] The combination of auxotyping and serologic typing is now used in most epidemiologic studies to determine the linkages among infected persons.[36]

PATHOGENESIS

To produce infection, *N. gonorrhoeae* first attaches to epithelial cells, penetrates into them, and then destroys the infected cells. Attachment to epithelial cells is related to the presence of pili, as well as the outer membrane protein II.[37] Penetration of the gonococcus into cells is through either phagocytosis or endocytosis.[38-40] Several bacteria usually are present in each infected cell, but whether this represents invasion of the cell by multiple organisms or growth and multiplication of organisms within the infected cell is unknown. Gonococci possess a cytotoxic lipopolysaccharide and produce proteases, phospholipases, and elastases that ultimately destroy the infected cells. Some strains of gonococci appear to be relatively less susceptible to phagocytosis and are thus thought to be more capable of causing disseminated infection. Gonococci are found in the subepithelial connective tissue very quickly after infection. This dissemination may be due to the disruption of the integrity of the epidermal surface with cell death, or the gonococci may migrate into this area by moving between cells. Epithelial cell death triggers a vigorous inflammatory response, initially with neutrophils and then macrophages and lymphocytes in untreated patients.

Human serum contains IgM antibody directed against lipopolysaccharide antigens on the gonococcus, which inhibits invasion. An IgG antibody against a surface protein antigen, however, also is normally present on some gonococci that are classified as serum-resistant gonococci; this antibody blocks the bactericidal action of the antilipopolysaccharide IgM antibody.[41,42] These serum-resistant strains are the most common ones involved in systemic infections in adults and probably in neonates as well.[43] Of note, infants' sera, in which maternal IgM antibody is absent, do not demonstrate serum bactericidal activity against *N. gonorrhoeae*[44]; thus, in theory, infants should be highly susceptible to invasive infection. Because such infection does not occur frequently, additional protective factors must function to prevent it.

N. gonorrhoeae produces IgA1 protease, which inactivates secretory IgA by cleaving it at the hinge region. This inactivation facilitates mucosal colonization and probably plays a role in the poor mucosal protection seen against subsequent gonococcal reinfection. It also is a proinflammatory protein and can trigger the release of proinflammatory cytokines from human monocytic subpopulations and a dose-dependent T_H1-type T-cell response.[45] Although symptomatic gonococcal infection triggers a brisk inflammatory response, it does not produce a significant immunologic response.[46] There is very little immunologic memory; as a result, recurrent infections occur easily on re-exposure. Epidemiologic evidence suggests that at least partial protection is obtained against subsequent infection with the same serotype.[47] In general, however, antibody responses are modest after initial infection, and no evidence of a boosting effect has been found when antibody levels are studied in response to subsequent infections. Also, adults with mucosal gonococcal infections have a discernible decreased $CD4^+$ count, which recovers with treatment or clearance of the infection. Thus, it has been speculated that the gonococci actually have a suppressive effect on the host immune response. In support of this theory, *N. gonorrhoeae* Opa proteins recently were shown to be able to bind CEACAM1 expressed by primary $CD4^+$ T lymphocytes and to suppress their activation and proliferation.[48] This immune suppressive effect may have significant consequences in populations with co-existing epidemics of gonorrhea and

HIV infection/AIDS. In a study of prostitutes in Nairobi, the presence of gonococcal cervicitis has been shown to reduce the interferon-g production by HIV-1 epitope-specific $CD8^+$ T-lymphocyte populations, demonstrating a deleterious effect of gonococcal cervicitis on HIV-1 immune control and susceptibility.[49]

Because only approximately one third of neonates exposed to *N. gonorrhoeae* during vaginal delivery become colonized and infected, additional protective innate factors obviously are in effect. Recently, significant antibacterial polypeptide activity has been demonstrated both in human amniotic fluid and within the vernix caseosa.[50,51] The presence of a number of antibacterial polypeptides in the vernix may be important for surface defense against gonococcal infection, but specific studies have yet to be done.

Antibiotic resistance to penicillin, tetracycline, the quinolones, and spectinomycin has become problematic in many regions.[52] Penicillin resistance can be a result of either alterations in the penicillin-binding protein or the production of penicillinase.[53-55] By 1991, 11% of all strains of *N. gonorrhoeae* in the United States were penicillinase producing, and 32% of all strains were resistant to at least one antimicrobial agent. As a result, penicillin is no longer recommended for primary therapy for gonococcal disease in the United States and in other regions where these strains are commonly found.

PATHOLOGY

In most affected infants, gonococcal disease manifests itself as infection of mucosal membranes. The eye is most frequently involved, but funisitis and infant vaginitis, rhinitis, and urethritis also have been observed.[56-59] Primary mucosal infection by *N. gonorrhoeae* involves the columnar and transitional epithelia. When pharyngeal colonization is looked for, it is found in 35% of ophthalmia neonatorum cases.[60] Systemic infection is rarely observed among neonates, but cases of meningitis and arthritis have been described.[61-70] Gonococcal scalp abscesses attributed to intrauterine fetal monitoring, omphalitis, and gingival abscess also have been reported.[71-77] One case of gonococcal ventriculitis has been reported in an infant who received a ventriculoamniotic shunt in utero.[78]

CLINICAL MANIFESTATIONS

Ophthalmia neonatorum due to *N. gonorrhoeae* is classically an acute purulent conjunctivitis that appears from 2 to 5 days after birth. Occasionally, however, the initial presentation is more subacute, or the onset may be delayed beyond 5 days of life.[79,80] Asymptomatic colonization has been documented.[81] Infants who become infected in utero may have symptoms at or shortly following birth.[21,22,79] Typically, early in the illness, tense edema of both lids develops, followed by profuse purulent conjunctival exudates (Fig. 12-1). If treatment is delayed, the infection progresses beyond the superficial epithelial layers of the eye to involve the subconjunctival connective tissue of the palpebral conjunctivae and the cornea. Infection of the cornea can lead to ulcerations, perforation, or rarely panophthalmitis. In some instances it may result in loss of the eye.[82] Neonatal sepsis, arthritis, and skin abscesses due to *N. gonorrhoeae* are not clinically distinguishable from conditions caused by other bacterial pathogens more commonly associated with these syndromes in this age group.

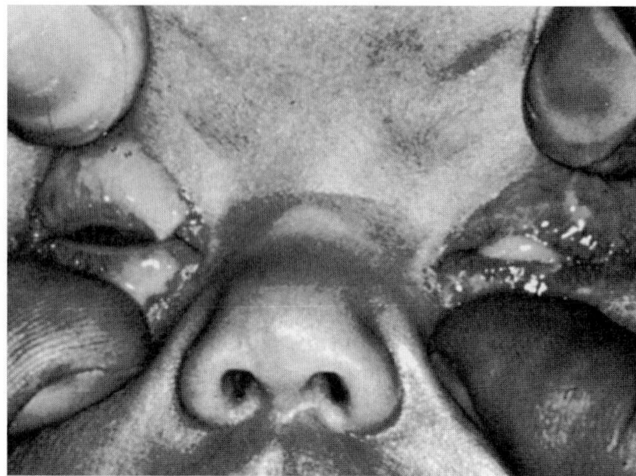

Figure 12–1 Bilateral acute gonococcal ophthalmia neonatorum. Appearance after inappropriate topical therapy for 2 weeks with neomycin–polymyxin B–bacitracin (Neosporin), sulfonamide, and chloramphenicol ophthalmic ointments.

DIAGNOSIS

Clinicians should suspect gonococcal ophthalmia neonatorum in an infant in whom purulent conjunctivitis develops during the first week of life, or if what was thought to be chemical conjunctivitis is prolonged beyond 24 to 48 hours.

Gram stain of the exudate usually reveals the gram-negative intracellular bean-shaped diplococci typical of *N. gonorrhoeae*, which will provide a presumptive diagnosis. Other *Neisseria* species—in particular, *N. meningitidis*—cannot be distinguished from the gonococcus by Gram stain appearance. *N. gonorrhoeae* must be isolated and tested for antibiotic susceptibility before a definitive diagnosis is made. A definitive diagnosis is important because of the public health and social consequences of the diagnosis of gonorrhea in an infant. If gonococcal ophthalmia neonatorum is suspected on the basis of the Gram stain appearance, cultures should be obtained from additional mucosal sites in the infant. The mother and her sexual partner(s) also should be tested for gonorrhea. Additional testing of the infant, the mother, and her sexual partner(s) for other sexually transmitted infections, including HIV infection, is strongly recommended.[83,84]

Isolation of *N. gonorrhoeae* from the exudate by culture is the diagnostic "gold standard." Samples of the exudate should be collected by swabbing and should be inoculated directly onto blood agar, MacConkey's agar, and chocolate agar or chocolate-inhibitory media. The inhibitory medium should be placed in a commercial carbon dioxide incubator or candle jar to provide an adequate concentration of carbon dioxide and should then be incubated at 36° C. Cultures are examined daily for the presence of typical colonies. Colonies resembling

N. gonorrhoeae are further identified by Gram stain, by a positive oxidase test, and by utilization of glucose but not maltose, sucrose, or lactose. Antibiotic sensitivity and penicillinase production should be tested. Further testing to confirm the identification of the isolate may be carried out in a reference laboratory if desired. Newer DNA- and polymerase chain reaction (PCR)–based technologies have replaced gonococcal cultures in many laboratories.[85-87] These assays have a high degree of sensitivity and actually detect more true cases of gonorrheal infection in adults than can be achieved by current culture methods. When correctly used, they also are very specific. Their suitability for diagnosis of gonorrheal infections in children without the additional use of culture methods, with the associated legal implications in older children, has not been extensively studied, however. Additionally, extensive use of these methods for primary diagnosis impairs the tracking of antimicrobial resistance patterns.

If gonococcal ophthalmia neonatorum is presumptively or definitively diagnosed, then testing also should be conducted for other sexually transmitted pathogens, in particular, *Chlamydia trachomatis*, because the two organisms frequently are found to co-infect pregnant women.[88] Also, the diagnosis of gonococccal infection in the neonate should trigger an investigation of the infant's mother and her sexual partner or partners for STDs.

DIFFERENTIAL DIAGNOSIS

At present, *N. gonorrhoeae* causes less than 1% of cases of ophthalmia neonatorum in North America, western Europe, Australia, and New Zealand and in areas and communities elsewhere where there is access to prenatal care and STD prevention programs. In other areas, the risk of gonococcal ophthalmia is higher depending on the prevalence of gonococcal infection among the pregnant women in the population. Even in areas with high prevalence rates, however, ophthalmia due to *N. gonorrhoeae* accounts for less than 5% of the cases of neonatal conjunctivitis. The other organisms that can produce conjunctivitis in the newborn period and the relative overall frequency of resultant infections, the usual time of presentation since birth, and relative severity are shown in Table 12-2. In general, conjunctivitis seen within 24 hours of birth usually is assumed to be a reaction to silver nitrate, if this has been used for prophylaxis. As described previously, however, in the instance of prolonged rupture of membranes and premature delivery, symptomatic gonococcal ophthalmia may be observed during this period as well. Also, some infants have a less acute course, with appearance of symptoms after 5 days of age. Therefore, reliance on the timing between 2 and 5 days after delivery of the onset of symptoms may be an unreliable clinically distinguishing feature. The possibility of gonococcal infection should be considered in every neonate with conjunctivitis present after 24 hours of birth, and the appropriate diagnostic testing to detect the organism should be done. In some instances, neonates with gonococcal ophthalmia neonatorum may be infected by additional pathogens, in particular, *C. trachomatis*.

The differential diagnosis of cutaneous or systemic gonococcal infection of the neonate includes the bacterial or fungal pathogens that are frequently involved in these types of infections during this time period and are discussed in more detail in Chapters 6 and 10.

TREATMENT (THERAPY/MANAGEMENT)

The principles of management of STDs in any age group apply when a neonate is determined to have a suspected or confirmed gonococcal infection. As stated previously, investigation and treatment of the mother and her sexual contacts for *N. gonorrhoeae* are essential, as is the investigation of the infant, the mother, and her sexual contacts for other sexually transmitted infections. STDs are like wolves—they travel in packs.

As discussed previously, because a significant proportion of gonococci worldwide is resistant to penicillin, either by decreased penicillin binding or by penicillinase production, this antibiotic is no longer recommended for therapy unless the infecting isolate has been tested and found to be sensitive. Most recommendations and guidelines for the treatment of gonococcal ophthalmia neonatorum identify

Table 12–2 Differential Diagnosis of Ophthalmia Neonatorum

Etiologic Condition/Agent	Percentage of Cases	Relative Severity	Usual Time of Onset after Delivery
Chemical conjunctivitis	Dependent on use	+	6-24 hours
Neisseria gonorrhoeae	<1	+++	2-5 days
Neisseria meningitidis	<1	++	2 days-2 weeks
Neisseria cinerea	<1	+	2 days-2 weeks
Herpes simplex virus	<1	++	2-14 days
Chlamydia trachomatis	2-40	+	5 days-2 weeks
Other bacteria	30-50	++	2 days-2 weeks
Group A and B streptococci			
Staphylococcus aureus			
Haemophilus species			
Klebsiella pneumoniae			
Escherichia coli			
Pseudomonas aeruginosa			
Enterococcus			
Pneumococcus			

Table 12–3 Recommended Treatment for Neonatal Gonococcal Infections

Condition	Recommended Therapy
Ophthalmia neonatorum	Ceftriaxone 25-50 mg/kg IV or IM in a single dose, not to exceed 125 mg; topical antibiotic therapy alone is inadequate and is unnecessary if systemic treatment is administered
Gonococcal meningitis, arthritis, or scalp lesions	Ceftriaxone 25-50 mg/kg/day IV or IM in a single daily dose for 7 days OR cefotaxime 25 mg/kg IV or IM every 12 hours for 7 days, with a duration of 10-14 days if meningitis is documented or 14 days if arthritis is documented
Known exposure at birth but asymptomatic	Ceftriaxone 25-50 mg/kg IV or IM in a single dose, not to exceed 125 mg

ceftriaxone as the agent of choice (Table 12-3).[83,84] Regimens using this drug have been studied and shown to be effective.[89-91] Kanamycin is an alternative but is not as effective, with a failure rate of approximately 5%.[92] Ceftriaxone should be administered cautiously to hyperbilirubinemic infants, especially those born prematurely. Infants who have gonococcal ophthalmia should be hospitalized and evaluated for signs of disseminated infection (e.g., sepsis, arthritis, meningitis). One dose of ceftriaxone is adequate therapy for gonococcal conjunctivitis. Treatment of disseminated infection in the neonate should be done in consultation with an expert in infectious diseases. Infants born to mothers who have documented untreated infection are at high risk of acquiring *N. gonorrhoeae*. If the membranes have been ruptured, if the infant is premature, or if close follow-up cannot be ensured, treatment for ophthalmia neonatorum rather than use of eye prophylaxis is recommended.

PROGNOSIS

With early recognition and appropriate treatment, cure rates for gonococcal ophthalmia and other neonatal manifestations of gonococcal infection in the newborn are close to 100%. By contrast, permanent corneal damage after gonococcal ophthalmia neonatorum was usual in the preantibiotic era.

PREVENTION

Prevention of gonococcal infection of the fetus and neonate is best done by preventing gonococcal infection of the mother. One way to accomplish this goal is by the reduction of the prevalence of *N. gonorrhoeae* in the core high-risk populations that serve as its reservoir for pregnant women. Targeted treatment and prevention campaigns among commercial sex workers, sexually active adolescents and young adults who have multiple partners, and groups with other risk factors that result in increased high-risk sexual activity, such as those with street drug and alcohol abuse problems and homosexual men who have multiple contacts, will reduce the prevalence in the general population. Education of youth before sexual maturity about the risks of STDs and about ways in which they can protect themselves from acquiring such diseases does not increase the rates of sexual activity among adolescents and should be encouraged as a joint responsibility of their parents or primary care providers and the schools. Provision of accessible health care with readily available antibiotics that are appropriate and effective against circulating strains of *N. gonorrhoeae* also is imperative for this purpose. Finally, to support optimal health behaviors, persons of all ages need to be able to feel confident that they will not be stigmatized for seeking health care for an STD.

Because infection with *N. gonorrhoeae* during pregnancy may result in adverse pregnancy outcomes, such as premature rupture of membranes and preterm delivery, screening of pregnant women for infection in early pregnancy is advisable. Women identified as having gonococcal infection should receive prompt treatment.[83,84] Recommended treatment includes the use of cefixime 400 mg orally, in a single dose if available, or ceftriaxone 125 mg intramuscularly in a single dose. Women for whom a third-generation cephalosporin is contraindicated should receive spectinomycin 2 g intramuscularly as a single dose. Either erythromycin or amoxicillin is recommended for treatment of presumptive or diagnosed co-infection with *C. trachomatis*. Follow-up cultures to ensure eradication of the infection are imperative. Testing for other STDs should be done, and the mother should be offered HIV testing. In addition, counseling related to avoidance of further infection is an important component of management. Tracing and treatment of sexual contacts are necessary to reduce the risk of subsequent infection. In one recent study in Louisiana, of 751 pregnant women whose charts were reviewed retrospectively, 5.1% were diagnosed with gonorrhea at the first prenatal visit and 2.5% acquired the infection during their pregnancy.[93] Therefore, women whose sexual behavior or social circumstances place them at risk of acquiring sexually transmitted infection during pregnancy should be retested for gonorrhea (and other STDs), in the third trimester. Retesting is most conveniently done at the time of screening for group B β-streptococci.

Since the late 1800s, eye prophylaxis has been the hallmark of prevention of gonococcal ophthalmia neonatorum. Currently, many jurisdictions mandate the use of ocular prophylaxis for newborns through legislation. Most others recommend and encourage its use. The issue is controversial in areas of low prevalence of *N. gonorrhoeae* infection and among populations with extremely low risk of the disease. In these situations, the concerns regarding the complications of the use of the prophylactic agents must be balanced against the actual risk of the disease and the ability, or the wish, to provide an alternate management approach involving close observation of the infant with early therapy if necessary.

At present, data from clinical trials support the use of 1% silver nitrate, 0.5% erythromycin, 1% tetracycline, or

2.5% povidone-iodine for prophylaxis against gonococcal ophthalmia neonatorum.[4-6,83,84,94-98] All of the agents are less effective against chlamydial conjunctivitis, however, and to date, there is no truly effective ocular agent to prevent this infection. Most agents are well tolerated, although a chemical conjunctivitis commonly is seen after instillation of silver nitrate. This reaction involves epithelial desquamation and a polymorphonuclear leukocytic exudate[99] and usually appears within 6 to 8 hours and disappears within 24 to 48 hours. A mild chemical conjunctivitis may be seen in from 10% to 20% of infants who received povidone-iodine prophylaxis as well. Use of antibiotic agents has the potential to lead to increased antibiotic resistance in other colonizing bacteria, which could lead to outbreaks of infection in the nursery.[100]

Failure of prophylaxis does occur. If the illness is established by the time of delivery, ocular prophylaxis is ineffective. Irrigation of the eyes with saline too soon after the application of silver nitrate has been suggested by some experts to be the cause of such failure. In extremely rare instances, infection may be acquired after prophylaxis had been provided. On occasion, the erythromycin eye ointment may not have penetrated to the eye itself as a result of difficulties in keeping the infant's eye exposed during application of the ointment.

At present, specific prophylaxis given immediately (minimum delay of 1 hour) after birth, using any of the following regimens, is recommended by most professional societies and government bodies: (1) 1% silver nitrate in single-dose ampules, (2) 0.5% erythromycin ophthalmic ointment in single-use tubes, or (3) 1% tetracycline ophthalmic ointment in single-use tubes. Povidone-iodine also is a safe and effective alternative in resource-poor countries.

REFERENCES

1. Hirschberg, J and Krause F. Zentralbl. Prakt Augen 5:39,1881.
2. Howe, L. Credé's method for prevention of purulent ophthalmia in infancy in public institutions. Trans Am Ophthalmol Soc 8:52-57, 1897.
3. Forbes, G. and Forbes, GM. Silver nitrate and the eyes of the newborn. Am J Dis Child 121:1-3, 1971.
4. Laga M, Plummer FA, Piot P, et al. Prophylaxis of gonococcal and chlamydial ophthlmia neonatorum. A comparison of silver nitrate and tetracycline. N Engl J Med 17:653-657, 1988.
5. Hammerschlag, MR, Cummings C, Roblin PM, et al. Efficacy of neonatal ocular prophylaxis for the prevention of chlamydial and gonococcal conjunctivitis. N Engl J Med 320:769-772, 1989.
6. Chen J-Y. Prophylaxis of ophthalmia neonatorum: comparison of silver nitrate, tetracycline, erythromycin and no prophylaxis. Pediatr Infect Dis J 11:1026-1030, 1992.
7. Kohen DP. Neonatal gonococcal arthritis: three cases and review of the literature. Pediatrics 53:436-440, 1974.
8. Babl FE, Ram S, Barnett ED, et al. Neonatal gonococcal arthritis after negative prenatal screening and despite conjunctival prophylaxis. Pediatr Infect Dis J 19:346-349, 2000.
9. Elliott B, Brunham RC, Laga M, et al. Maternal gonococal infection as a preventable risk factor for low birth weight. J Infect Dis 161:531-53, 1990.
10. Moses S, Ngugi EN, Costigan A et al. Response of a sexually transmitted infection epidemic to a treatment and prevention programme in Nairobi, Kenya. Sex Trans Infect 78(Suppl 1):114-120, 2002.
11. World Health Organization. Global prevalence and incidence of selected curable sexually transmitted infections. Overview and estimates. WHO/CDS/CSR/EDC/2001.10, 2001, pp 1-50.
12. CDC. Sexually transmitted disease surveillance 2001. Atlanta, U.S. Department of Health and Human Services publication, 2002.
13. Hansen L, Wong T, Perrin M. Gonorrhoea resurgence in Canada. Int J STD AIDS 14:727-731, 2003.
14. Klausner JD, Barrett DC, Dithmer D, et al. Risk factors for repeated gonococcal infections: San Francisco, 1990-1992. J Infect Dis 177:1766-1769, 1998.
15. Cornelius CE III. Seasonality of gonorrhea in the United States. HSMHA Health Rep 86:157-160, 1971.
16. Cook RL, May S, Harrison LH, et al. High prevalence of sexually transmitted diseases in young women seeking HIV testing in Rio de Janeiro, Brazil. Sex Transm Dis 31:67-72, 2004.
17. Sullivan EA, Abel M, Tabrizi S, et al. Prevalence of sexually transmitted infections among antenatal women in Vanuatu, 1999-2000. Sex Transm Dis 30:362-366, 2003.
18. Kilmarx PH, Black CM, Limpakarnjanarat K, et al. Rapid assessment of sexually transmitted diseases in a sentinel population in Thailand: prevalence of chlamydial infection, gonorrhoea, and syphilis among pregnant women—1996. Sex Transm Infect 74:189-193, 1998.
19. Fonck K, Kidula N, Kirui P, et al. Pattern of sexually transmitted diseases and risk factors among women attending an STD referral clinic in Nairobi, Kenya. Sex Transm Dis 27:417-423, 2000.
20. Aboyeji AP, Nwabuisi C. Prevalence of sexually transmitted diseases among pregnant women in Ilorin, Nigeria. J Obstet Gynecol 23:637-639, 2003.
21. Thompson TR, Swanson RE, Wiesner PJ. Gonococcal ophthalmia neonatorum: relationship of time of infection to relevant control measures. JAMA 228:186-188, 1974.
22. Diener B. Cesarean section complicated by gonococcal ophthalmia neonatorum. J Fam Pract 13:739-744, 1981.
23. Nickerson CW. Gonorrhea amnionitis. Obstet Gynecol 48:815-817, 1973.
24. Varady E, Nsanze H, Slattery T. Gonococcal scalp abscess in a neonate delivered by caesarean section. Sex transm Infect 74:451, 1998.
25. Rothenberg R. Ophthalmic neonatorum due to *Neisseria gonorrhoeae*: prevention and treatment. Sex Transm Dis 6(Suppl 2):187-191, 1979.
26. Rothbard MJ, Gregory T, Salerno LJ. Intrapartum gonococcal amnionitis. Am J Obstet Gynecol 121:565-566, 1975.
27. Sarrell PM, Pruett KA. Symptomatic gonorrhea during pregnancy. Obstet Gynecol 32:670-673, 1968.
28. Amstey MS, Steadman KT. Symptomatic gonorrhea and pregnancy. J Am Vener Dis Assoc 3:14-16, 1976.
29. Charles AG, Cohen S, Kass MB, et al. Asymptomatic gonorrhea in prenatal patients. Am J Obstet Gynecol 108:595-599, 1970.
30. Handsfield HH, Sparling PF. *Neisseria gonorrhoeae*. *In* Mandell GL, Bennett JE, Dolin R (eds). Principles and Practice of Infectious Diseases, 4th ed. New York, Churchill Livingstone, 1995, pp 1909-1926.
31. Juni E, Heym GA. Simple method for distinguishing gonococcal colony types. J Clin Microbiol 6: 511-517, 1977.
32. Swanson J. Studies on gonococcus infection. IV. Pili: their role in attachment of gonococci to tissue culture cells. J Exp Med 137:571-589, 1973.
33. Sparling PF, Cannon JG, and So, M. Phase and antigenic variation of pili and outer membrane protein II of *Neisseria gonorrhoeae*. J Infect Dis 153:196-2001, 1986.
34. Sandstrom EG, Bygdeman S. Serological classification of *Neisseria gonorrhoeae*. Clinical and epidemiological applications. *In* Poolman JT, Zanen HC, Meyer TF, et al (eds). Gonococci and Meningococci. Dordrecht, The Netherlands, Kluwer Academic Publishers, 1986, pp 45-50.
35. Knapp JS, Tam MR, Nowinski RC et al. Serological classification of *Neisseria gonorrhoeae* with use of monoclonal antibodies to gonococcal outer membrane protein I. J Infect Dis 150:44-48, 1984.
36. Handsfield HH, Sandstrom EG, Knapp JS et al. Epidemiology of penicillinase-producing *Neisseria gonorrhoeae* infections: analysis by auxotyping and serogrouping. N Engl J Med 306:950-954, 1982.
37. Bessen D, Gotschlich EC. Interactions of gonococci with HeLa cells: attachment, detachment, replication, penetration, and the role of protein II. Infect Immun 54:154-160, 1986.
38. Ward ME, Watt PJ. Adherence of *Neisseria gonorrhoeae* to urethral mucosal cells: an electron microscopic study of human gonorrhea. J Infect Dis 126:601-605, 1972.
39. McGee ZA, Jolinson AP, Taylor-Robinson D. Pathogenic mechanisms of *Neisseria gonorrhoeae*: observations on damage to human fallopian tubes in organ culture by gonococci of colony type 1 and type 4. J Infect Dis 143:413-422, 1981.
40. Ward ME, Glynn AA, Watt PJ. The fate of gonococci in polymorphonuclear leukocytes: an electron microscopic study of the natural disease. Br J Exp Pathol 53:289-294, 1972.
41. Rice PA, Kasper DL. Characterization of serum resistance of gonococci that disseminate. J Clin Invest 70:157-167, 1982.

42. Joiner KA, Scales R, Warren KA, et al. Mechanism of action of blocking immunoglobulin G for *Neisseria gonorrhoeae.* J Clin Invest 76:1765-1772, 1985.
43. Schoolnik GK, Buchanan TM, Holmes KK. Gonococci causing disseminated gonococcal infection are resistant to the bactericidal action of normal human sera. J Clin Invest 58:1163-1173, 1976.
44. Schoolnik GK, Ochs HD, Buchanan TM. Immunoglobulin class responsible for bactericidal activity of normal human sera. J Immunol 122:1771-1779, 1979.
45. Tsirpouchtsidis A, Hurwitz R, Brinkmann V, et al. Neisserial immunoglobulin A1 protease induces specific T-cell responses in humans. Infect Immunol 70:335-344, 2002.
46. Hedges SR, Mayo MS, Mestecky J, et al. Limited local and systemic antibody responses to *Neisseria gonorrhoeae* during uncomplicated genital infections. Infect Immun 67:3937-3946, 1999.
47. Buchanan TM, Eschenbach D, Knapp JS, et al. Gonococcal salpingitis is less likely to recur with *Neisseria gonorrhoeae* of the same principal outer membrane protein (POMP) antigenic type. Am J Obstet Gynecol 135:978-980, 1980.
48. Boulton IC, Gray-Owen SD. Neisserial binding to CEACAM1 arrests the activation and proliferation of CD4+ T lymphocytes. Nat Immunol 3:229-236, 2002.
49. Kaul R, Rowland-Jones SL, Gillespie G, et al. Gonococcal cervicitis is associated with reduced systemic CD8+ T cell responses in human immunodeficiency virus type-1–infected and exposed, uninfected sex workers. J Infec Dis 185:1525-1529, 2002.
50. Yoshio H, Tollin M, Gudmundsson GH, et al. Antimicrobial polypeptides of human vernix caseosa and amniotic fluid: implications for newborn innate defense. Pediatr Res 53:211-216, 2003.
51. Marchini G, Lindow S, Brismar H, et al. The newborn infant is protected by an innate antimicrobial barrier: peptide antibiotics are present in the skin and vernix caseosa. Br J Dermatol 147:127-134, 2002.
52. Dougherty TJ. Genetic analysis and penicillin-binding protein alterations in *Neisseria gonorrhoeae* with chromosomally mediated resistance. Antimicrob Agents Chemother 30:649-652, 1986.
53. Thirumoorthy T, Rajan VS, Goh CL. Penicillinase-producing *Neisseria gonorrhoeae* ophthalmia neonatorum in Singapore. Br J Vener Dis 58:308-310, 1982.
54. Pang R, Teh LB, Rajan VS, et al. Gonococcal ophthalmia neonatorum caused by beta-lactamase–producing *Neisseria gonorrhoeae.* BMJ 1:380, 1979.
55. Doraiswamy B, Hammerschlag MR, Pringle GF, et al. Ophthalmia neonatorum caused by β-lactamase–producing *Neisseria gonorrhoeae.* JAMA 250:790-791, 1983.
56. Hunter GW, Fargo ND. Specific urethritis (gonorrhea) in a male newborn. Am J Obstet Gynecol 38:520-521, 1939.
57. Stark AR, Glode MP. Gonococcal vaginitis in a neonate. J Pediatr 94:298-299, 1979.
58. Barton LL, Shuja M. Neonatal gonococcal vaginitis. J Pediatr 98:171-172, 1981.
59. Kirkland H, Storer RV. Gonococcal rhinitis in an infant. BMJ 1:263-267, 1931.
60. Fransen L, Nsanze H, Klaus V, et al. Ophthalmia neonatorum in Nairobi, Kenya: the roles of *Neisseria gonorrhoeae* and *Chlamydia trachomatis.* J Infect Dis 153:862-869, 1986.
61. Bradford WL, Kelley HW. Gonococcal meningitis in a newborn infant. Am J Dis Child 46:543-549, 1933.
62. Holt LE. Gonococcus infections in children with especial reference to their prevalence in institutions and means of prevention. N Y Med J 81:521-527, 1905.
63. Cooperman MB. Gonococcus arthritis in infancy. Am J Dis Child 33:932-948, 1927.
64. Babl FE, Ram S, Barnett ED, et al. Neonatal gonococcal arthritis after negative prenatal screening and despite conjunctival prophylaxis. Pediatr Infect Dis J 19:346-349, 2000.
65. Kohen DP. Neonatal gonococcal arthritis: three cases and review of the literature. Pediatrics 53:436-440, 1974.
66. Parrish PP, Console WA, Battaglia J. Gonococcic arthritis of a newborn treated with sulfonamide. JAMA 114:241-242, 1940.
67. Jones JB, Ramsey RC. Acute suppurative arthritis of hip in children. US Armed Forces Med J 7:1621-1628, 1956.
68. Soonzilli EE, Calabro JJ. Gonococcal arthritis in the newborn. JAMA 177:919-921, 1961.
69. Glaser S, Boxerbaum B, Kennell JH. Gonococcal arthritis in the newborn. Am J Dis Child 112:185-188, 1966.
70. Gregory JE, Chisom JL, Meadows AT. Gonococcal arthritis in an infant. Br J Vener Dis 48:306-307, 1972.
71. Kleiman MB, Lamb GA. Gonococcal arthritis in a newborn infant. Pediatrics 52:285-287, 1973.
72. D'Auria A, Tan L, Kreitzer M, et al. Gonococcal scalp wound infection. MMWR Morb Mortal Wkly Rep 24:115-116, 1975.
73. Thadepalli H, Rambhatla K, Maidman JE, et al. Gonococcal sepsis secondary to fetal monitoring. Am J Obstet Gynecol 126:510-512, 1976.
74. Plavidal FJ, Werch A. Gonococcal fetal scalp abscess: a case report. Am J Obstet Gynecol 127:437-438, 1977.
75. Reveri M, Krishnamurthy C. Gonococcal scalp abscess. J Pediatr 94:819-820, 1979.
76. Brook I, Rodriguez WJ, Controni G, et al. Gonococcal scalp abscess in a newborn. South Med J 73:396-397, 1980.
77. Urban MN, Heruada AR. Gonococcal gum abscess in a 10-week-old infant. Clin Pediatr 16:193-194, 1977.
78. Bland RS, Abramson JS, Nelson LH, et al. Gonococcal ventriculitis associated with ventriculoamniotic shunt placement. Pediatr Res 17:265A, 1983 (abstract).
79. Armstrong JH, Zacarias F, Rein MF. Ophthalmia neonatorum: a chart review. Pediatrics 57:884-892, 1976.
80. Brown WM, Cowper HH, Hodgman JE. Gonococcal ophthalmia among newborn infants at Los Angeles County General Hospital, 1957-1963. Public Health Rep 81:926-928, 1966.
81. Wald ER, Woodward CL, Marston A, et al. Gonorrheal disease among children in a university hospital. Sex Transm Dis 7:41-43, 1980.
82. Pearson HE. Failure of silver nitrate prophylaxis for gonococcal ophthalmia neonatorum. Am J Obstet Gynecol 73:805-807, 1957.
83. Centers for Disease Control and Prevention. Sexually transmitted diseases treatment guidelines—2002. MMWR 51(RR06):1-80, 2002.
84. LCDC Expert Working Group on Canadian Guidelines for Sexually Transmitted Diseases. Canadian STD Guidelines, 1998 edition. Ottawa, Health Canada (ISBN 0-662-27208-0), 1998, pp 1-230.
85. Van Der Pol B, Ferrero DV, Buck-Barrington L, et al. Multicenter evaluation of the BDProbeTec ET System for detection of *Chlamydia trachomatis* and *Neisseria gonorrhoeae* in urine specimens, female endocervical swabs, and male urethral swabs. J Clin Microbiol 39:1008-1016, 2001.
86. van Doornum GJ, Schouls LM, Pijl A, et al. Comparison between the LCx Probe system and the COBAS AMPLICOR system for detection of *Chlamydia trachomatis* and *Neisseria gonorrhoeae* infections in patients attending a clinic for treatment of sexually transmitted diseases in Amsterdam, The Netherlands. J Clin Microbiol 39:829-835, 2001.
87. Carroll KC, Aldeen WE, Morrison M, et al. Evaluation of the Abbott LCx ligase chain reaction assay for detection of *Chlamydia trachomatis* and *Neisseria gonorrhoeae* in urine and genital swab specimens from a sexually transmitted disease clinic population. J Clin Microbiol 36:1630-1633, 1998.
88. Fransen L, Nsanze H, D'Costa LJ, et al. Parents of infants with ophthalmia neonatorum: a high-risk group for sexually transmitted diseases. Sex Transm Dis 12:150-154, 1985.
89. Haase DA, Nash RA, Nsanze H, et al. Single-dose ceftriaxone therapy for gonococcal ophthalmia neonatorum. Sex Transm Dis 13:53-55, 1986.
90. Rawston SA, Hammerschlag MR, Gullans C, et al. Ceftriaxone treatment of penicillinase-producing *Neisseria gonorrhoeae* infections in children. Pediatr Infect Dis J 8:445-448, 1989.
91. Laga M, Naamara W, Brunham RC, et al. Single-dose therapy of gonococcal ophthalmia neonatorum with ceftriaxone. N Engl J Med 315:1382-1385, 1986.
92. Fransen L, Nsanze H, D'Costa L, et al. Single dose kanamycin therapy of gonococcal ophthalmia neonatorum. Lancet 2:1234-1236, 1984.
93. Miller JM Jr, Maupin RT, Mestad RE, et al. Initial and repeated screening for gonorrhea during pregnancy. Sex Trans Dis 30:728-730, 2003.
94. American Academy of Pediatrics. Prevention of neonatal ophthalmia. *In* Pickering LK (ed). Red Book: Report of the Committee on Infectious Diseases, 26th ed. Elk Grove Village, Ill., American Academy of Pediatrics, 2003, pp 778-781.
95. Isenberg SJ, Apt L, Del Signore M, et al. A double application approach to ophthalmia neonatorum prophylaxis. Br J Ophthalmol 87:1449-1452, 2003.
96. Isenberg SJ, Apt L, Wood M. A controlled trial of povidone-iodine as prophylaxis against ophthalmia neonatorum. N Engl J Med 332:562-566, 1995.

97. Benevento WJ, Murray P, Reed CA et al. The sensitivity of *Neisseria gonorrhoeae*, *Chlamydia trachomatis*, and herpes simplex type II to disinfection with povidone-iodine. Am J Ophthalmol 109:329-333, 1990.
98. Zanoni D, Isenberg SJ, Apt L. A comparison of silver nitrate with erythromycin for prophylaxis against ophthalmia neonatorum. Clin Pediatr 31:295-298, 1992.
99. Norn MS. Cytology of the conjunctival fluid in newborn with references to Credé's prophylaxis. Acta Ophthalmol 38:491-495, 1960.
100. Hedberg K, Ristinan TL, Soler JT, et al. Outbreak of erythromycin-resistant staphylococcal conjunctivitis in a newborn nursery. Pediatr Infect Dis J 9:268-273, 1990.

Chapter 13

GROUP B STREPTOCOCCAL INFECTIONS

Morven S. Edwards • Victor Nizet • Carol J. Baker

Lancefield group B β-hemolytic streptococci were first recorded as a cause of human infection in 1938, when Fry[1] described three patients with fatal puerperal sepsis. Sporadic cases were reported during the next 3 decades, but this microorganism remained unknown to most clinicians until the 1970s, when a dramatic increase in the incidence of septicemia and meningitis in neonates caused by group B streptococci was documented from geographically diverse regions.[2-4] The emergence of group B streptococcal infections in neonates was accompanied by an increasing number of these infections in pregnant women and nonpregnant adults. In pregnant women, these infections commonly were manifested as localized uterine infections or chorioamnionitis, often with bacteremia, and had an almost uniformly good outcome with therapy. In other affected adults, who typically had underlying medical conditions, however, group B streptococcal infection often resulted in a fatal outcome.[8]

The reason for the emergence of group B streptococci as a significant neonatal pathogen remains obscure. The severity and magnitude of infections attributed to these microorganisms stimulated intense investigational effort, in the hope that an understanding of the epidemiology and pathogenesis of these infections could result in the development of methods for their effective control and prevention. Even so, the incidence of perinatal infection associated with group B streptococci remained stable until the early 1990s.[9,10] Case-fatality rates had fallen but remained substantial in comparison with those reported for other invasive bacterial infections in infants.

Within the past decade, several notable events have occurred. A shift in the distribution of serotypes causing invasive infection has been noted. Serotype V group B streptococci now are responsible for a substantial proportion of infections in the newborn, as well as among pregnant women and nonpregnant adults.[11-15] Capsular serotypes VII and VIII have been described, bringing the number of serotypes causing invasive human disease to nine.[16] Infections caused by serotype Ia have increased, those due to type II have decreased, and type III remains a dominant cause of meningitis and of late-onset infection. The reason for this serotype shift is not known, but it has important implications for the development of vaccines to prevent group B streptococcal infections. The complete genomes of serotype III and serotype V group B streptococci have now been sequenced by two groups of investigators, opening new avenues for the identification of novel potential vaccine targets.[17,18]

The consensus guidelines developed in 1996 by the Centers for Disease Control and Prevention (CDC), the American College of Obstetricians and Gynecologists (ACOG), and the American Academy of Pediatrics (AAP) to prevent early-onset disease in neonates through intrapartum maternal chemoprophylaxis represent a notable achievement of the past decade.[19-21] The implementation of these guidelines effected a substantial decline in the incidence of neonatal infection for the first time in 2½ decades.[22] A population-based comparison of strategies concluded that routine culture-based screening for group B streptococci during pregnancy is more effective than the risk-based approach in prevention of early-onset disease.[23] In 2002, this finding led to the adoption of revised guidelines for prevention of perinatal group B streptococcal disease by universal screening for colonization of all pregnant women during the third trimester of gestation.[24] Finally, ongoing testing of group B streptococcal vaccines in healthy adults offers promise that immunoprophylaxis to prevent maternal and infant group B streptococcal disease may become a reality in the near future.

THE ORGANISM

Streptococcus agalactiae is the species designation for streptococci belonging to Lancefield group B. This bacterium is a facultative gram-positive diplococcus with an ultrastructure similar to that of other gram-positive cocci.[25] Before Lancefield's classification of hemolytic streptococci in 1933,[26] this microorganism was known to microbiologists by its characteristic colonial morphology, its narrow zone of β-hemolysis surrounding colonies on blood agar plates, and its double zone of hemolysis that appeared when plates were refrigerated an additional 18 hours beyond the initial incubation.[27] Occasional strains (approximately 1%) are designated α-hemolytic or nonhemolytic streptococci because they either produce a lesser zone of hemolysis or demonstrate none at all, respectively; these strains can cause human infection, although infrequently.[28,29] Group B streptococci are readily cultivated in a variety of bacteriologic media. Isolation from certain body sites (the respiratory, genital, and gastrointestinal tracts) can be enhanced by use of broth medium containing antimicrobial agents that inhibit growth of other bacterial species indigenous to these sites.[30,31]

Colonial Morphology and Identification

Colonies of group B streptococci grown on sheep blood agar medium are 3 to 4 mm in diameter, produce a narrow zone of β-hemolysis, are gray-white, and are flat and mucoid. β-Hemolysis for some strains is apparent only when colonies are removed from the agar.

Definitive identification of group B streptococci requires detection of the group B–specific antigen common to all strains through use of hyperimmune grouping antiserum. Laboratory tests that permit presumptive identification[28,32] include bacitracin and sulfamethoxazole-trimethoprim disk susceptibility testing (92% to 98% of strains are resistant),[28,32] hydrolysis of sodium hippurate broth (99% of strains are positive),[28,32] hydrolysis of bile esculin agar (99% to 100% of strains fail to react),[28,32] pigment production during anaerobic growth on certain media (96% to 98% of strains produce an orange pigment),[33,34] and CAMP (Christie–Atkins–Munch-Petersen) testing (98% to 100% of strains are CAMP positive).[32,35,36] This last test is based on the production of CAMP factor, a thermostable extracellular protein[37] that, in the presence of the beta toxin of *Staphylococcus aureus* (a sphingomyelinase), produces synergistic hemolysis when grown on sheep blood agar. A "spot" CAMP test, employing a crude beta toxin–containing filtrate derived from a broth culture of *S. aureus*, allows rapid (30-minute) identification of group B streptococci from a single colony of the primary isolation plate with an accuracy equal to that of the standard CAMP test.[38] Hippurate hydrolysis is an accurate method for presumptive identification of group B streptococci, but the requirement for 24 to 48 hours of incubation limits its usefulness. Group B strains can be differentiated from other streptococci by a combination of the CAMP test, the bile esculin reaction, and bacitracin sensitivity testing.[32] Biochemical micromethods identify group B streptococci with reasonable accuracy after a 4-hour incubation period.[39]

Definitive microbiologic identification of group B streptococci requires serologic methods to detect the group B carbohydrate antigen. Lancefield's original method required acid treatment of large volumes of broth-grown cells to extract or solubilize the group B antigen from the cell wall.[40] Supernatants were brought to neutral pH and mixed with hyperimmune rabbit antiserum prepared by immunization with the group B–variant strain (090R) (devoid of type-specific antigen), and precipitins in capillary tubes were recorded. Less time-consuming techniques subsequently were developed, but all employ hyperimmune group-specific antiserum to identify the group B antigen in intact cells, broth culture supernatants, or cell extracts. Commercial availability and simplicity make latex agglutination-based assays the most practical and frequently used methods by hospital laboratories.[41]

Strains of Human and Bovine Origin

Before the dramatic increase in the incidence of human group B streptococcal infections in the 1970s, these microorganisms were associated principally with bovine mastitis.[42] Modern veterinary practices have largely controlled epidemics of bovine mastitis due to *S. agalactiae*, but sporadic cases still occur. The relationship between strains of human and bovine origin has been questioned for years. To date, no studies have shown that cattle are a reservoir for transmission of group B streptococci to humans. Substantial evidence indicates several biochemical, biologic, and serologic differences between human and bovine isolates.[43,44] Pattison and associates[43] were unable to serotype 75% of their bovine strains employing antisera that had enabled them to classify all of their human isolates. This nontypeability of bovine strains has been confirmed by others.[42] Among typeable bovine strains, patterns of serotype distribution distinct from those of human isolates have been noted. Using the concept of "herd type" for serologic typing, Jensen[45] demonstrated that the distribution of group B streptococci from newly infected herds was not the same as that of human urogenital strains. Other distinguishing characteristics for bovine strains include their unique fermentation reactions, their decreased frequency of pigment production, and their usual susceptibility to bacitracin. Protein X, rarely found in human strains, is commonly present in pathogenic bovine isolates.[46]

Serologic Classification

Lancefield defined two cell wall carbohydrate antigens for group B streptococci employing hydrochloric acid (HCl)-extracted cell supernatants and hyperimmune rabbit antisera: (1) the group B–specific or "C" substance common to all strains of this species and (2) the type-specific or "S" substance that allowed classification into four serotypes: Ia, Ib, II, and III.[47-49] Group B streptococcal strains originally were classified as serotypes I, II, and III. Strains designated as type I were later shown by Lancefield[48] to have both cross-reactive and antigenically distinct polysaccharides. When antisera raised to two different type I strains were made type specific by reciprocal cross-absorption with streptococcal cells, the antigenically distinct type Ia and type Ib polysaccharides were defined.[48] The serotype of group B streptococci historically designated as type Ic was characterized by Wilkinson and her co-workers.[50] These strains possessed the type Ia capsular polysaccharide and a protein antigen common to type Ib, up to 60% of type II, and rare type III strains.[51,52] This protein antigen originally was called the "type Ibc antigen" and now has been renamed *C protein.*

The nomenclature of antigens was revised in the 1980s. Now, the polysaccharide antigens of group B streptococci are designated as type antigens and the protein antigens as additional markers for supplementary characterization of serotypes.[53,54] The formerly designated type Ic strains are now designated type Ia/c because they possess the Ia polysaccharide antigen and the C protein antigen. Type IV was identified as a new serotype in 1979, when 62 strains were described that possessed type IV polysaccharide alone or with one of the protein antigens.[51] More recently, new antigenically distinct serotypes, V through VIII, have been recognized and characterized.[55-61] Strains of group B streptococci from patients with serious infections that cannot be serologically classified continue to account for less than 3% of isolates.

The serotyping scheme of Lancefield is based on precipitin reactions of whole cell acid extracts with group B–specific and capsular type–specific rabbit antisera. The biologic relevance of these serologically defined type-specific antigens has been investigated employing mouse protection experiments. Rabbit antibodies directed against the capsular polysaccharides provide passive protection to mice challenged with lethal doses of mouse virulent strains containing homologous but not heterologous polysaccharide antigens.[48,58] Cross-protection also occurs when antibodies against the C protein and the type Ia and Ib strains that share this antigenic determinant are tested. Rabbit antibodies directed against the group B–specific antigen do not protect mice from lethal challenge.[62]

The C protein antigen consists of two components, one sensitive to trypsin and pepsin and the other sensitive only to pepsin.[50] Rabbit antibodies raised to these proteins are partially mouse protective.[63] The β C protein is present in about 10% of human group B streptococcal isolates. The α components of C proteins are present in approximately one half of isolates and in most of those strains bearing capsular polysaccharides other than III.[51] Strains expressing α C are less readily opsonized, ingested, and killed by leukocytes in the absence of specific antibody than are α -negative strains.[64] Strains bearing both the α and the β C protein components possess increased resistance to opsonization in vitro.

The α C protein consists of a series of tandem repeating units, and in naturally occurring strains, the repeat numbers may vary. The number of repeating units expressed alters antigenicity and influences the repertoires of antibodies elicited.[65] Two distinct protective epitopes are present within the α C protein. The use of one or two repeat units of α C proteins elicits antibodies that bind all α C proteins with equal affinity, suggesting their potential usefulness as vaccine candidates.[66,67] The β antigen appears as a single protein of molecular mass between 124 and 134 kDa. The β antigen, but not the α antigen, binds the Fc region of human IgA.[68-70]

In addition to the group B, capsular polysaccharide type–specific, and C protein antigens, some group B streptococci contain surface proteins designated X and R antigens. These were first described by Pattison and co-workers,[71] who introduced reagents for their detection in an attempt to further classify nontypeable strains. The X and R antigens are immunologically cross-reactive. R antigens are found in a majority of type II and type III strains but are rare in type Ia or Ib strains.[72] Four distinct immunologic species of R antigen have been described. Of these, R4 is the most prevalent in isolates recovered from humans, and it is expressed almost exclusively in type II and type III strains.[73] A distinct surface protein, designated Rib, is expressed by most invasive strains, including almost all serotype III strains. It is immunologically unrelated but, like alpha C protein, has an extremely repetitive structure.[74] A new R-like protein designated BPS (group B–protective surface protein) is expressed by a number of clinically relevant group B streptococcal serotypes and is a protective antigen in a mouse model.[75] It has a repetitive structure but shows no sequence similarity to Rib or alpha C protein. By contrast, a laddering protein from type V group B streptococci does share sequence homology with alpha C protein.[76] Thus, a family of surface proteins with a repetitive structure exists that may have a role in immunity to infection. The role of the R proteins in human immunity, if any, remains to be defined, however. A recently described protein named Sip (for *s*urface *i*mmunogenic *p*rotein) is distinct from other known surface proteins. It is produced by all serotypes of group B streptococci and confers protection against experimental infection.[77]

Ultrastructure

Early concepts regarding the cellular structure of β-hemolytic streptococci suggested a thick, rigid peptidoglycan layer external to the cytoplasmic membrane, which was surrounded by concentric layers of cell wall antigens. The group-specific carbohydrate was believed to be "covered" by the surface type-specific antigen, which for group A streptococci is M protein and for group B is capsular polysaccharide. Electron microscope definition indicated that the group B antigenic determinant was not accessible for binding to group B–specific antibody.[25] Evidence now supports a model of the group B streptococcal cell surface in which the group B carbohydrate and the capsular polysaccharide are independently linked to the cell wall peptidoglycan (Fig. 13-1).[78]

Standard techniques for demonstrating bacterial capsules (India ink or "quellung reaction") do not visualize capsules on group B streptococci, but these microorganisms are encapsulated. Immunoelectron techniques reveal abundant capsular polysaccharide on the surface of Lancefield prototype strains Ia, II, and III, whereas less dense capsules are found on type Ib/c and type Ia/c strains (Fig. 13-2).[25] Similarly, incubation of the reference strains of serotypes IV, V, and VI with homologous type-specific antisera led to visualization of a thick capsular layer.[58,79] The type-specific polysaccharides are surface structures on group B streptococcal cells. Ultrastructural studies also demonstrate that the C protein antigen also has a surface location on type Ia and type Ib cells.[25] The degree of encapsulation of group B streptococcal strains is a function of in vitro manipulation and of serotype. Expression of the capsular polysaccharide is not constitutive; rather, such

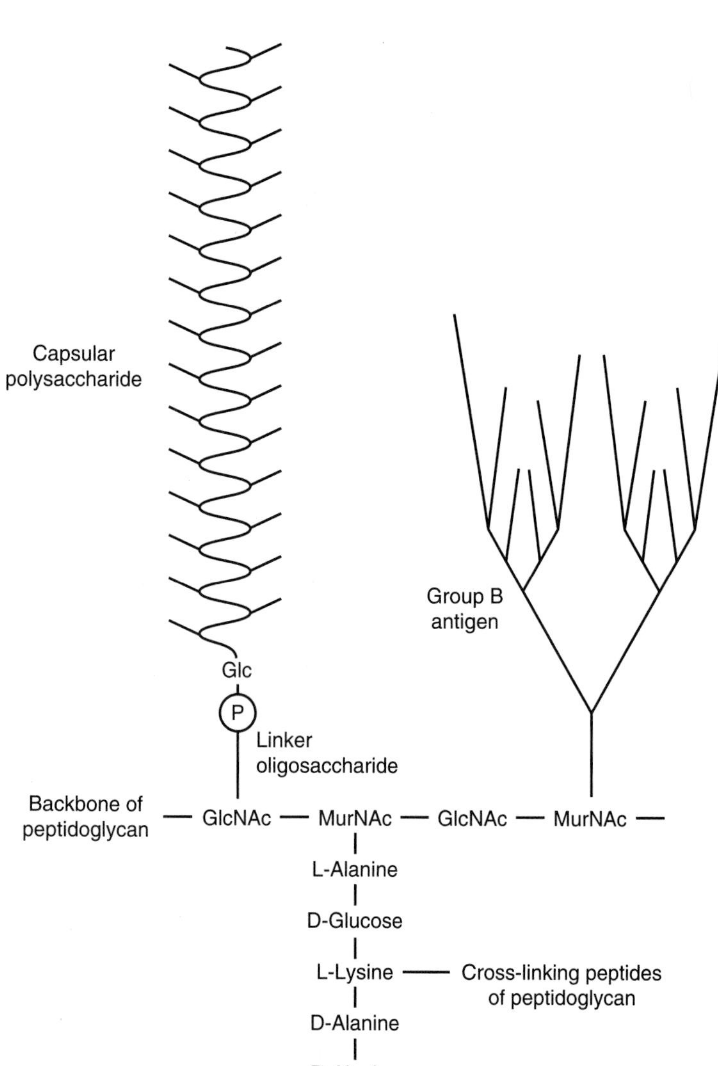

Figure 13–1 Schematic representation of a proposed model for the independent linkage of capsular polysaccharide and group B carbohydrate to peptidoglycan of the group B streptococcus. Group B carbohydrate is linked to *N*-acetylmuramic acid (MurNAc), and capsular polysaccharide is linked by a phosphodiester bond and oligosaccharide linker to *N*-acetylglucosamine (GlcNAc).[78] (From Deng L, Kasper DL, Krick TP, Wessels MR. Characterization of the linkage between the type III capsular polysaccharide and the bacterial cell wall of group B *Streptococcus*. J Biol Chem 275:7497, 2000.)

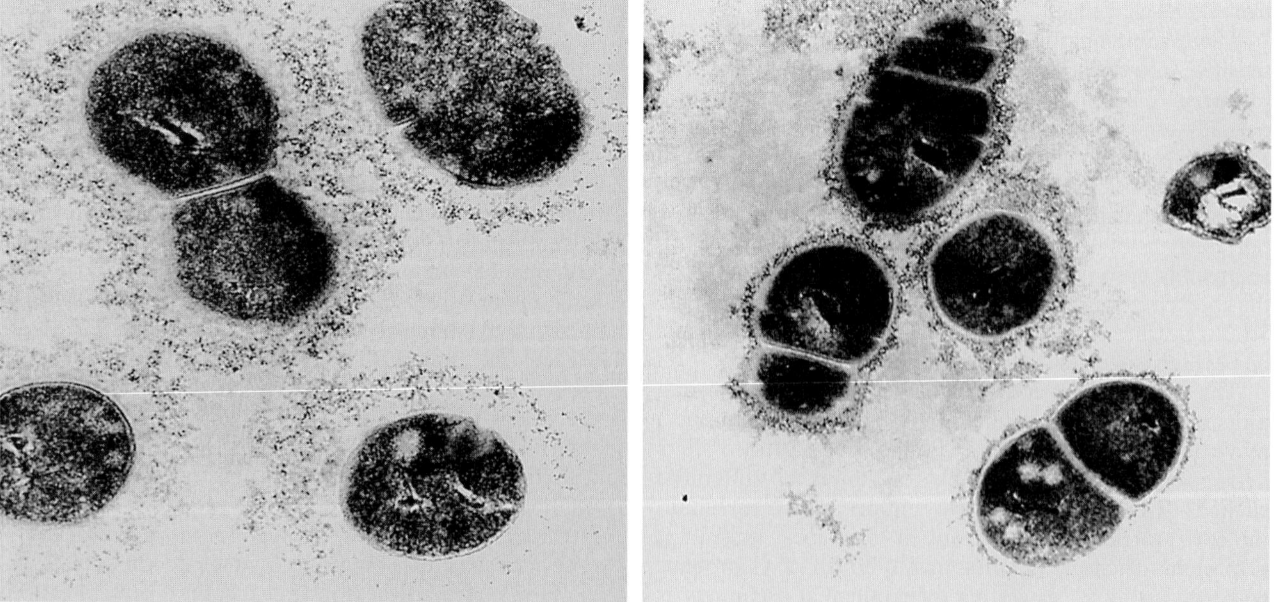

Figure 13–2 Electron micrographs of thin sections of group B streptococcal strains: **A,** type Ia (090); **B,** type Ia/c (A909). Both are stained with ferritin-conjugated type Ia–specific rabbit antibodies. The type Ia strain is representative of the large capsules found in Lancefield prototype II strain (18RS21) and type III isolates from infants with meningitis (M732), whereas the type Ia/c strain is representative of the much smaller capsules occurring in Lancefield prototype strains Ia/c (A909) and Ib/c (H36B). (Micrographs courtesy of Dennis L. Kasper, M.D.)

expression varies during growth in vitro and in primary cultures isolated from different sites of infection.[80,81]

Immunochemistry of Polysaccharide Antigens

Lancefield's serologic definition of the antigens of group B streptococci was achieved by their extraction from whole cells by dilute HCl and heat treatment.[48,49] Additional purification methods were necessary for isolation of the group B–specific from type-specific polysaccharide antigens. The chemical composition of the group B polysaccharide initially was determined for B antigen extracted from whole cells of the laboratory-adapted variant strain 090R, devoid of capsular polysaccharide.[82,83] In later studies, group B antigen was isolated from type III cells employing alcohol fractionation techniques with hot formamide extracts of whole cells.[84] With the use of rigorous biochemical methods for structural determination, the group B antigen was shown to contain L-rhamnose, D-galactose, 2-acetamido-2-deoxy-D-glucose, and D-glucitol. It is composed of four different oligosaccharides, designated I, II, III, and IV, that are linked by one type of phosphodiester bond to form a complex, highly branched multiantennary structure.[85] Inhibition studies have shown that antibodies to the group B polysaccharide are dominated by those specific for a trirhamnopyranoside epitope.

Extensive studies of the HCl-extracted type-specific polysaccharides have been reported in the past. The HCl antigens from type Ia, Ib, II, and III organisms are small-molecular-mass (1.5 to 5.0 × 10^4 daltons), neutral polysaccharides that contain identical constituents—galactose, glucose, and 2-acetamido-2-deoxyglucose—in repeating units of a core structure. When more gentle techniques are employed for the extraction of these type-specific capsular polysaccharides from whole cells, large-molecular-mass (5 × 10^5 to 1 × 10^6 daltons), acidic polysaccharides with an additional antigenic determinant are isolated. These "native" antigens form a partial identity with the HCl antigens from homologous strains by immunodiffusion with type-specific antisera. The additional antigenic determinant on the more complete type-specific polysaccharides is the acid-labile sugar sialic acid.[86] Acid hydrolysis of "native" polysaccharides results in degradation to core structures that are immunochemically identical to the homologous HCl-extracted antigens. Isolation of the immunologically more complete polysaccharides requires that growth of cells and extraction of antigens be performed under conditions that maintain neutral pH.[86]

The capsular polysaccharides of type Ia, type Ib, and type III group B streptococci have a five-sugar repeating unit containing galactose, glucose, *N*-acetylglucosamine, and sialic acid in a ratio of 2:1:1:1.[86-89] The type II and type V polysaccharides have a seven-sugar repeating unit, whereas those of types IV and VII consist of six-sugar repeating units, and that of type VIII consists of four.[57-59,90-92] The molar ratios vary, but the component monosaccharides are the same, with two exceptions. First, no *N*-acetylglucosamine is present in the type VI polysaccharide. In addition, the recently described type VIII capsular polysaccharide is the only structure that contains rhamnose in the backbone structure.[60] Each antigen has a backbone repeating unit of two (Ia, Ib), four (II), or three (II, IV, V, VII, VIII) monosaccharides to which one or two side chains are linked. Sialic acid as a terminal side chain residue is a consistent feature of the group B streptococcal capsular polysaccharides. With the exception of type II polysaccharide, which has a galactose terminal side chain sugar, sialic acid is the exclusive terminal sugar of the side chain(s).

The repeating unit structures of the group B streptococcal polysaccharides, determined by methylation analysis combined with gas-liquid chromatography/mass spectrometry, are schematically represented in Figure 13-3. The structures of the type Ia and type Ib polysaccharides differ only in a single monosaccharide side chain linkage, although there are differences in the tertiary configuration of the molecules.[93] These monosaccharide linkages are critical to their immunologic specificity and also explain their immunologic cross-reactivity.[48,94]

The type Ia, Ib, and III polysaccharides have a high degree of structural homology with two human serum glycoproteins. The terminal α-D sialic acid [2→3]-β-D-galactose of these polysaccharides is identical to the end group of human M and N blood group substances.[95] The type Ib polysaccharide has a repeating unit that is virtually identical to those of certain oligosaccharides present in human milk.[96] For the type III polysaccharide, a graded increase in relative affinity of antigen-antibody binding was observed as oligosaccharide size increased from 3 to 92 repeating units.[97] One implication of this difference in antibody-binding affinity, estimated to exceed 300-fold, is that binding interaction with an oligosaccharide on a host glycoprotein would be of very low affinity, and unlikely to result in activation of potentially damaging immune effector mechanisms. The type III polysaccharide also can form extended helices. The position of the conformational epitope along these helices is potentially important to binding site interactions.[98,99] Another structural homology is that between the HCl-extracted type III polysaccharide and the immunochemically identical type 14 pneumococcal polysaccharide.[100] This observation stimulated investigations concerning the immunodeterminant specificity of human immunity to type III group B streptococci and of antibody recognition of conformational epitopes as a facet of the host immune response.[101]

Because human immunity to type III strains correlates with antibody to the intact rather than to the desialylated capsular polysaccharide antigen, isolation of intact polysaccharides with sialic acid moieties has been necessary for the study of human immunity. Growth of cells in highly buffered media or by pH titration achieves the conditions of neutral pH necessary for isolation of immunologically complete antigens.[82] Yield of polysaccharides extracted from whole cells by these gentle neutral buffer techniques is low, however. Improvements in preparative methods through use of chemically defined, pH-controlled growth medium, treatment of bacterial cells with enzymes[102] to release capsule into the medium, and serial chromatographic procedures to ensure purity[89] now allow for isolation of large quantities of intact polysaccharides.

Growth Requirements and Bacterial Products

The nutritional requirements of several human and bovine strains of group B streptococci, examined in a chemically defined medium, reveal reasonable homogeneity in vitamin requirements. Group B streptococci also are quite homo-

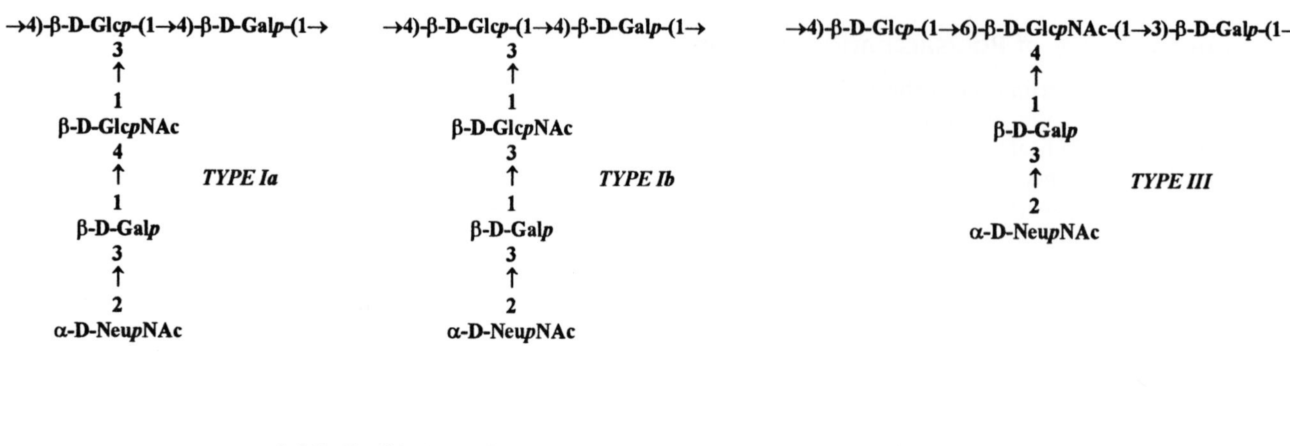

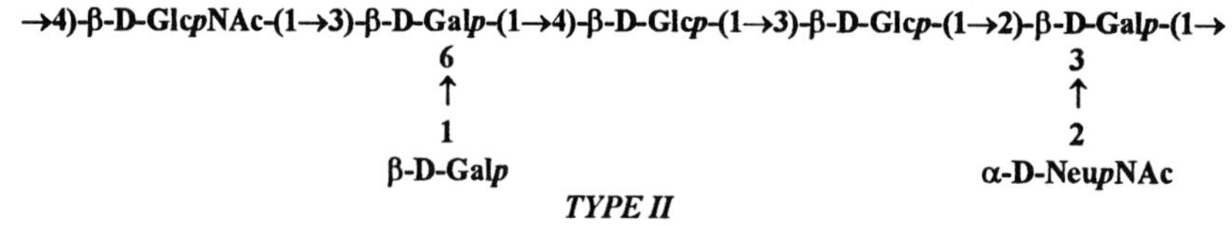

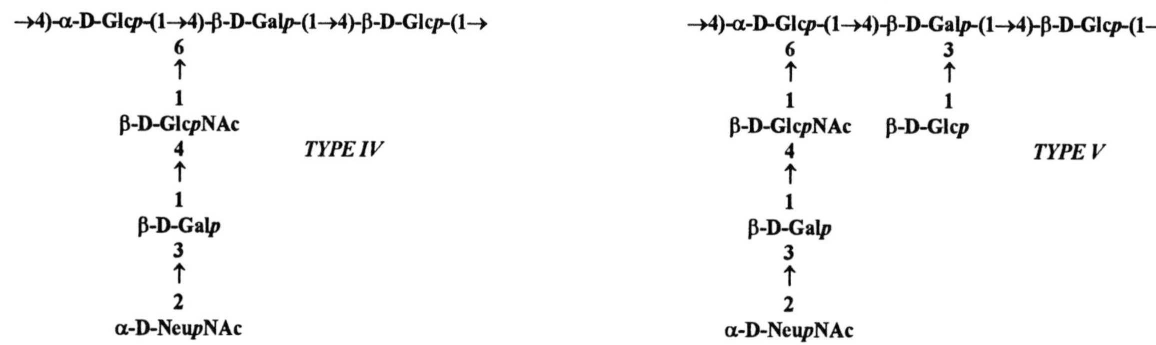

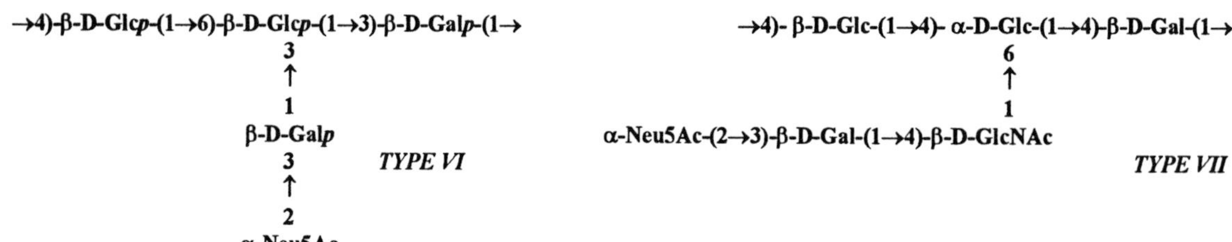

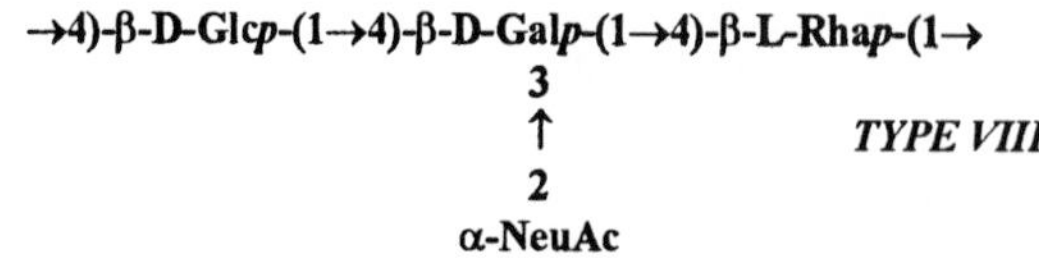

Figure 13–3 Repeating unit structures of group B streptococcal capsular polysaccharides type Ia,[93] type Ib,[93,94] type II,[90,92] type III,[88,89] type IV,[91] type V,[57] type VI,[61] type VII,[59] and type VIII.[60]

geneous in their amino acid requirements during aerobic or anaerobic growth.[103] Provision of a glucose-rich environment enhances the number of viable group B streptococci during stationary phase and the amount of capsular polysaccharide present on type III cells elaborated into the growth medium.[104] In a modified chemically defined medium, the expression of capsule during continuous growth is regulated by the growth rate.[80] Group B streptococcal invasiveness is enhanced by a fast growth rate and is optimal in the presence at least 5% oxygen.[105,106]

Group B streptococci elaborate a number of products, including the soluble type-specific capsular polysaccharides,[86] hemolysin,[107] pigment,[108] CAMP factor,[35] hippuricase,[28,109] nucleases,[110] superoxide dismutase,[111] protease,[112] an oligopeptidase, and lipoteichoic acid (LTA).[113] The hemolysin or hemolysins of group B streptococci are an extracellular product of almost all strains and are active against the erythrocytes from several mammalian species. The hemolysin that produces the β-hemolysis surrounding group B colonies on blood agar plates has been isolated and characterized.[106] When it was tested with known inhibitors of other streptococcal hemolysins (phospholipids, trypan blue, proteases, cholesterol), it was inhibited only by phospholipids. The hemolysin was not detected in supernatants of broth cultures, suggesting either that it exists in a cell-bound form or that it is released by cells and rapidly inactivated.

After growth to stationary phase, group B streptococci produce two types of pigment resembling a beta carotenoid.[108] Pigment, like hemolysin, is formed and released by an active metabolic process, retaining its properties only in the presence of a carrier molecule. A potential role for pigment as a virulence factor is proposed but unproved. No relationship between the group B streptococcal hemolysin and CAMP factor has been determined.[106]

The CAMP phenomenon—the elaboration of CAMP factor by group B streptococci—was described in 1944 by Christie, Atkins, and Munch-Petersen.[35] Skalka and Smola[114] reported that a partially purified CAMP factor was lethal in experimental infection. Subsequently, the finding of nonspecific binding of the CAMP factor to immunoglobulins in a protein A–like fashion led Jürgens and co-workers[115] to suggest the term *protein B* for CAMP factor. The cloning and expression of CAMP factor in *Escherichia coli* will aid investigations of its mode of action and role, if any, in the pathogenesis of human infections.

Group B streptococci can hydrolyze hippuric acid to benzoic acid and glycine, and this property has been useful historically to distinguish group B streptococci from other β-hemolytic groups.[28,104] Ferrieri and co-workers isolated and characterized the hippuricase of group B streptococci.[109] This enzyme is cell associated and is trypsin and heat labile. It is antigenic in rabbits, but its relationship to bacterial virulence, if any, has not been studied.

Most strains of group B streptococci have an enzyme that inactivates complement component C5a by cleaving a peptide at the carboxyl terminus.[116,117] Group B streptococcal C5a-ase appears to be a serine esterase; it is distinct from the C5a-cleaving enzyme (termed *streptococcal C5a peptidase*) produced by group A streptococci,[118] although the genes that encode these enzymes are similar.[119] C5a-ase contributes to the pathogenesis of group B streptococcal disease by rapidly inactivating the neutrophil agonist C5a, thereby preventing the accumulation of neutrophils at the site of infection.[116] Naturally occurring immunoglobulin G (IgG) antibodies can neutralize the enzyme in serum or plasma, but C5a-ase associated with the bacterial surface of encapsulated type III group B streptococci is not inactivated by IgG, suggesting that this capsule provides protection from neutralization of the enzyme.[120]

Another group of enzymes elaborated by nearly all group B streptococci are the extracellular nucleases.[110] Three distinct nucleases—designated I, II, and III by Ferrieri and colleagues[109]—have been physically and immunologically characterized. All are maximally activated by divalent cations of calcium plus manganese. These group B streptococcal nucleases are immunogenic in animals, and neutralizing antibodies to these antigens are detectable in sera from pregnant women known to be genital carriers of group B streptococci. The relationship between this latter observation and the pathogenesis of human infection, if any, is unknown.

An extracellular product that may relate to the virulence of group B streptococci in humans is neuraminidase (sialidase), considered by some investigators to be a hyaluronate lyase.[121,122] Maximal levels are detected during late exponential growth in a chemically defined medium. Subsequently, proteases may degrade neuraminidase. The neuraminidases from some of the serotypes of group B streptococci have been purified and partially characterized. These have a molecular size of approximately 1×10^5 daltons and a limited range of activity on sialic acid substrates when compared with other bacterial neuraminidases. Type III polysaccharide is resistant to type III group B streptococcal neuraminidase.[123,124]

Elaboration of large quantities of neuraminidase may be a virulence factor for type III group B streptococci. Almost all type Ia, Ib, and II strains are low producers, whereas type III strains are either high producers or nonproducers.[125] When type III strains isolated from infants with invasive infection were compared with those isolated from healthy colonized infants, the former were significantly more often high neuraminidase producers. Musser and co-workers[126] identified a high neuraminidase-producing subset of type III strains that were responsible for a majority of serious group B streptococcal infections.

The role of type-specific polysaccharides as virulence factors acting independently has been evaluated in a murine model.[127] The amount of extracellular capsular polysaccharide produced by type III strains correlated with virulence in chick embryos[128] and mice[129] and with invasiveness in susceptible infants. Mutants defective in capsular polysaccharide synthesis were cleared efficiently in a murine model.[130] The finding that group B streptococcal strains with low buoyant density produce higher amounts of type-specific capsular polysaccharide and are more resistant to phagocytic killing than are high-density variants, coupled with the identification of a group of genetically related organisms with increased capsule production that causes a majority of the cases of invasive type III disease, corroborates this concept.[131]

Group B streptococci synthesize acylated (lipoteichoic) and deacylated glycerol teichoic acids that are cell associated and can be readily extracted and purified.[113] Strains from infants with early- or late-onset disease have higher levels of cell-associated and native deacylated LTA,[113] and this product may contribute to attachment to human cells.[132,133]

EPIDEMIOLOGY AND TRANSMISSION

Historically, *S. agalactiae* was known to cause bovine mastitis rather than human perinatal infection. When the organism became recognized as a human pathogen, epidemiologic studies examined whether bovine and human strains were biologically related and whether transmission from bovine sources to humans might occur. Employing culture, physiologic, and serologic properties as strain markers, investigators concluded that transmission from cows was exceedingly rare.[42-44,71,134] In addition, during the past decades when it has been a dominant human pathogen in the United States, a majority of the population has lacked exposure to the two possible modes of transmission: (1) proximity to dairy cattle (direct contact) and (2) ingestion of unpasteurized milk.

Asymptomatic Infection (Colonization) in Adults

Group B streptococcal infection limited to mucous membrane sites has been designated as *asymptomatic infection*, *colonization*, or *carriage*. Direct comparisons of the prevalence of colonization reported in the literature are virtually impossible because of differences in the ascertainment techniques employed for study. Several factors influence the accuracy of detecting colonization in a given population: the choice of bacteriologic media, the body sites sampled, the number of cultures obtained, and the time interval chosen for study. Isolation rates are significantly higher with use of broth rather than solid agar media; with media containing substances inhibitory for normal flora (usually antibiotics); and with selective broth rather than selective solid agar media.[135] Among selective broth media chosen, Todd-Hewitt broth with gentamicin (4 to 8 μg/mL) or colistin (or polymyxin B) (10 μg/mL) *and* nalidixic acid (15 μg/mL), with or without sheep red blood cells, has been the most useful for accurate detection of group B streptococci from genital and rectal cultures.[135,136] These media inhibit the growth of most gram-negative enteric bacilli, as well as other normal flora, that make isolation of streptococci from these sites difficult. Use of broth media enables detection of low numbers of organisms that escape detection when inoculation of swabs is directly onto solid agar.[30,135-137]

Isolation rates also are influenced by body sites selected for culture. Female genital culture isolation rates double with progression from the cervical os to the vulva.[138,139] In addition, culture sampling of both lower genital tract *and* rectal sites increases group B streptococcal colonization rates 10% to 15% above that found if a single site is cultured.[9,140,141] The urinary tract also is an important site of group B streptococcal infection, especially during pregnancy, when infection usually is manifested as asymptomatic bacteriuria.[142,143] Therefore, to accurately predict the likelihood of neonatal exposure to group B streptococci at delivery, maternal culture specimens from the lower vagina, vulva, or periurethral area *and* rectum should be collected (see "Prevention" later on).

In neonates, selection of optimal body sites for detection of colonization also influences prevalence rates. In the first 24 hours of life, external auditory canal cultures are more likely to yield group B streptococci than those from anterior nares, throat, umbilicus, or rectum,[3,140] and isolation of organisms from the ear canal is a surrogate for the degree of contamination from amniotic fluid and vaginal secretions sequestered during the birth process. After the first 48 hours of life, throat and rectal sites are the most common sources of group B streptococci,[144,145] and positive cultures indicate true colonization (multiplication of organisms at mucous membrane sites), not just maternal exposure. Beyond the neonatal period, the throat and the rectum continue to be the most common sites for detection of group B streptococcal colonization, and this predominance persists until sexual debut, when the genitourinary tract becomes a common site of colonization in both sexes.[146-150]

The prevalence of group B streptococcal colonization also is influenced by the number of cultures obtained from a single site and the interval during which these are collected in an individual patient. An early longitudinal study in which women were evaluated throughout pregnancy with sequential lower vaginal cultures identified colonized women as having chronic, transient, intermittent, or indeterminant carriage of group B streptococci.[151] A more recent longitudinal cohort study of 1248 nonpregnant young women found that, among women who were culture negative at enrollment, almost one half acquired vaginal colonization during follow-up study at three 4-month intervals.[152] Other longitudinal studies found that nearly one half of women vaginally colonized at delivery had negative antenatal culture results.[153,154] In a longitudinal study of 5586 pregnant women by Boyer and associates,[154] initial cultures were performed during the second trimester in two thirds of the women; the overall predictive value of a positive prenatal vaginal *or* rectal culture result for colonization at delivery was 67%. The predictive value of a positive prenatal culture result was highest (73%) in women with vaginal *and* rectal colonization and lowest (60%) in those with rectal colonization only. Thus, if colonization is to be detected with maximal accuracy on a single occasion, lower vaginal and rectal cultures should be performed. Cultures performed from 1 to 5 weeks before delivery are accurate in predicting group B streptococcal colonization status at delivery in term parturients. Within this interval, the positive predictive value is 87% (95% confidence interval [CI] 83 to 92) and the negative predictive value is 96% (95% CI 95 to 98). Culture specimens collected within this interval perform significantly better than those collected 6 or more weeks before delivery.[155]

The primary reservoir for group B streptococci is the lower gastrointestinal tract.[3,156] The recovery of group B streptococci from the rectum alone is three to five times more common than from the vagina,[141] the rectal-to-vaginal isolation ratio exceeds 1,[154] and the rectal site more accurately predicts persistence[141] or chronicity of carriage.[143] These observations support the rationale for obtaining rectal as well as lower vaginal cultures to define maternal carriage during pregnancy. Fecal carriage or rectal colonization with group B streptococci has been documented in patients ranging in age from 1 day[157] to 70 to 80 years.[158] Additional compelling evidence supporting the intestine as the primary reservoir of colonization by group B streptococci includes their isolation from the small intestine of adults[159] and their association with infections resulting from surgery of the upper or lower intestinal tract.[160] Rectal colonization also may contribute to the importance of group B streptococci as a urinary tract pathogen and for the resistance of genital tract colonization to eradication by antibiotics.[161]

Table 13–1 **Group B Streptococcal Colonization Rates in Diverse Populations of Women and Men**

Population	Sites Cultured	Prevalence Rates (%)	Representative Reference Nos.
Pregnant women	Throat	2-5	2, 3, 15, 152, 171
	Vaginal and/or rectal	20-36	164, 165, 172
	Rectal	16-22	135, 156, 164
Nonpregnant women	Throat	3-12	3, 136
	Vaginal and/or rectal	29-34	155, 163
Venereal disease clinic enrollment	Vaginal and/or rectal	11-37	139, 148, 173, 174
	Rectal	24-40	173, 174
Heterosexual men	Throat	4-11	136, 175
	Urethra or urine	2-27	138, 163
Homosexual men	Throat	19	176
	Urethra	23	176

Outlining methods to prevent group B streptococcal infection have relied on data from prospective active surveillance studies.[162] Group B streptococci are common constituents of the genital microflora at delivery, and the prevalence rates of colonization in a given population are similar for each trimester of gestation.[2,151,153] Pregnancy does influence colonization rates, but few data are available for matched populations of pregnant and nonpregnant women.[9,148] Several factors have been assessed for their possible influence on genital carriage in women. Sexual activity is an important risk factor for vaginal colonization, but not for rectal-only colonization, in young nonpregnant women. In a longitudinal cohort study of 1248 nonpregnant young women, specific factors—African American race, having multiple sex partners during a preceding 4-month interval, having frequent sexual intercourse within the same interval, and having sexual intercourse within the 5 days before the follow-up visit—were independently associated with vaginal acquisition of group B streptococci.[152] These findings suggest either that the organism is sexually transmitted or that sexual activity alters the microenvironment to make it more permissive to colonization. In another study of 499 college women, group B streptococci were isolated significantly more often from sexually experienced women, women studied during the first half of the menstrual cycle, those with an intrauterine device, and women 20 years of age or younger.[148] Colonization with group B streptococci also occurs at a high rate in healthy college students and is associated with having engaged in sexual activity, tampon use, milk consumption, and hand washing done four times daily or less.[163]

Colonization with group B streptococci can elicit a systemic immune response. In a group of pregnant women evaluated at the time of admission for delivery, vaginal or rectal colonization with serotype Ia, II, III, or V was associated with significantly higher serum concentrations of IgG specific for the colonizing serotype compared with non-colonization.[164] Moderate concentrations of Ia, Ib, II, III, and V capsular polysaccharide–specific IgG also were found in association with colonization during pregnancy.[165] Maternal colonization with type III was least likely to be associated with these serotype-specific antibodies.

A higher prevalence of colonization with group B streptococci has been found among pregnant diabetic patients than among controls.[166] Prolonged carriage (over a 3-year interval) has been reported significantly more often in women who use tampons than in women who do not.[167] Colonization also appears to be more frequent among teenage women than among those 20 years of age or older,[148,151,153] and among women with three or fewer pregnancies than in those with more than three.[151,153,168] Ethnicity is related to colonization rates. In one large multicenter U.S. pregnancy study, colonization rates were highest in Hispanic women of Caribbean origin, followed by African Americans, whites, and other Hispanics (predominantly Mexicans).[168] In other recent assessments of geographically and ethnically diverse populations, the rate of colonization at delivery was significantly higher among African American women than in other racial or ethnic groups.[152,164,169] A large inoculum of vaginal group B streptococcal colonization also was more common among African American than among Hispanic or white women.[170]

Factors that do not influence the prevalence of genital colonization in nonpregnant women include use of oral contraceptives[148]; marital status; presence of vaginal discharge or other gynecologic signs or symptoms,[148] carriage of *Chlamydia trachomatis*, *Ureaplasma urealyticum*, *Trichomonas vaginalis*, or *Mycoplasma hominis*[168]; and infection with *Neisseria gonorrhoeae*.[138,139]

Asymptomatic infection of the genital or lower gastrointestinal tract with group B streptococci occurs in men as well as in women (Table 13-1). Of sexual partners of genitally colonized women, urethral isolation of group B streptococci can be found in at least one half.[2,9,138,149] Genital isolation rates are significantly greater in sexually active than in virgin women[148] and in patients attending venereal disease clinics than in those attending other outpatient facilities.[138,177] Molecular typing techniques have confirmed that sexual partners often carry identical strains. In contrast with agents such as *N. gonorrhoeae* or genital mycoplasmas, genital infection with group B streptococci is not related to genital symptoms.[148,174,177]

Group B streptococci have been isolated from vaginal or rectal sites or both in 15% to 30% of pregnant women (Table 13-2). These variations in colonization rates relate to intrinsic differences in populations (age, parity, socioeconomic status, geographic location) and to lack of standardization in culture methods employed for study. True population differences account for some of the disparity in these reported prevalence rates. When selective broth media are used and vaginal and rectal samples are cultured, the overall prev-

Table 13–2 Group B Streptococcal Colonization Rates in Geographically Diverse Populations of Pregnant Women

Country	Site(s) Cultured	Colonization Rates (%)[a]	Reference Nos.
Brazil	Vagina	18.6 [25.6]	178
Canada	Vagina, rectum	19.5	165
China	Endocervix, perineum, rectum[b]	19.0	179
Colombia	Vagina, rectum, throat	2	180
Denmark	Cervicovaginal	10	181
Fiji	Cervix, vagina	2	182
Greece	Vagina, rectum	6.6	183
India	Endocervix, vagina	5.8	184
Ireland	Vagina, perianal	25.6	185
Israel	Vagina or cervix	10.3-12.3	186, 187
Italy	Cervix, vagina	6.0, 7.3 [7.5]	188
Japan	Vagina	2.9	189
Jordan	Vagina, rectum, urine	30	190
Libya	Vagina	5	191
Mexico	Vagina, cervix	10	192, 193
Netherlands	Vagina, cervix	7.9, 6.3 [13.9]	194
Nigeria	Vagina	19.5	195
Peru	Cervix	6	196
Saudi Arabia	Vagina	5.1-9.2 [13.9]	197, 198
Scotland	Cervix, urethra	16	199
Spain	Vagina and/or rectum[b]	11.5	200
Thailand	Genital	6	201
The Gambia	Vagina, rectum	22	202
Trinidad	Vagina, rectum	31.4	203
United Arab Emirates	Vagina	10.1	204
United Kingdom	Vagina	10.5 [20]	205
United States	Vagina, rectum	25-28	164, 168, 169

[a]Overall carrier rate, multiple sites, given in brackets.
[b]Not specified by site positive.

alence of maternal colonization with group B streptococci by region is 12% in India and Pakistan, 19% in Asia and the Pacific Islands, 19% in sub-Saharan Africa, 22% in the Middle East and North Africa, 14% in Central and South America, and 26% in the United States.[164,205] The reported rates of colonization among pregnant women range from 1.5% to 22% in eastern Europe, from 7% to 30% in western Europe, from 10% to 25% in Scandinavia, and from 2.3% to 18.5% in the southern part of Europe.[206] The prevalence rates of pharyngeal colonization among pregnant and nonpregnant women and heterosexual men are similar[3,136,175]; however, the rate approaches nearly 20% in homosexual men.[176] No definite relationship between isolation of group B streptococci from throat cultures of adults or children and symptoms of pharyngitis has been proved,[207] but some investigators have suggested that these organisms can produce acute pharyngitis.[175]

Asymptomatic Infection in Infants and Children

The prevalence of group B streptococcal colonization in children appears to differ from that in adults. In a study of 100 girls between 2 months and 16 years of age, Hammerschlag and co-workers[146] isolated group B streptococci from cultures of samples from lower vaginal, rectal, or pharyngeal sites or all three in 20%. Although the prevalence of positive pharyngeal cultures in girls 11 years of age or older (5%) was similar to that reported for women, the prevalence in younger girls (15%) resembled that reported for neonates.[3,144,145] Rectal colonization was detected frequently in girls younger than 3 or older than 10 years of age (about 25%) but was uncommon in those between 3 and 10 years of age. In a similar study of prepubertal boys and girls, Mauer and colleagues[147] isolated group B streptococci from cultures of vaginal, anal, or pharyngeal specimens or all three in 11% of patients. Pharyngeal (5% each) and rectal (10% and 7%) isolation rates were similar for boys and for girls, respectively. Persson and co-workers[157] detected a lower (4%) rate of fecal carriage of group B streptococci among healthy boys and girls, and Cummings and Ross[208] found that only 2% of English schoolchildren had pharyngeal carriage of group B streptococci. Thus, the gastrointestinal tract is the most frequent site for carriage during infancy and childhood in both boys and girls, and genital colonization in girls is uncommon before puberty.[209] Whether the latter finding is related to environmental influences in the prepubertal vagina or to lack of sexual experience before puberty or both awaits further study.

Transmission of Group B Streptococci to Neonates

The presence of group B streptococci in the maternal genital tract at delivery is a significant determinant of colonization and infection in the neonate. Exposure of the neonate to the organism occurs either by the ascending route in utero through ruptured membranes or by contamination during passage through the birth canal. Prospective studies have

Table 13–3 Transmission of Group B Streptococci to Neonates from Maternal or Nosocomial Sources

Reference No.	Location	Maternal Colonization at Delivery (%)	Colonized Neonates Born to Mothers Colonized at Delivery[a] (%)	Colonized Neonates Born to Noncolonized Mothers (%)	Neonates Colonized from Nosocomial Source (%)
3	Houston	22.5	72	12	ND
140	Minneapolis	8.3	50	1	ND
144	Houston	27.7	65	ND	~43[b]
145	Los Angeles	28.8	63	9	ND
152	Houston	20.4	42	1.2	0
169	Houston	28.0	54	4.9	ND
210	Atlanta	23.2	58	ND	13
211	Dallas	26.6	50	ND	ND
178	Brazil	25.6	55	ND	ND
212	India	5.8	56	0	ND
188	Italy	7.1	45	2.1	ND
195	Nigeria	19.5	29	4.4	ND
212	Pakistan	24.0	85	9	ND
199	Scotland	2.9	33	1.3	ND
213	Spain	ND	69	5.6	ND
214	Turkey	8.2	67	0	ND
215	United Kingdom	15.0	35	4.7	22.2
216	United Kingdom	15.0	43	4.2	17.8

[a]Time of newborn culture collection varied from <30 minutes after birth to 48-72 hours of age in these studies; therefore, rates of colonization depended on maternal inoculum when assessment was performed shortly after birth.
[b]Exact data are not listed.
ND, not determined.

indicated vertical transmission rates of 29% to 85%, with a mean rate of approximately 50% (Table 13-3), among neonates born to women in whom group B streptococci were isolated from cultures of vagina or rectum, or both, at delivery. Conversely, only about 5% of infants delivered of culture-negative women become asymptomatically infected at one or more sites during the first 48 hours of life.

The risk of a neonate's acquiring colonization by the vertical route correlates directly with the intensity of colonization (inoculum size). Neonates born to heavily colonized women are more likely to acquire carriage at mucous membrane sites than those born to women with low colony counts of group B streptococci in vaginal cultures at delivery.[217] Boyer and associates[154] found that rates of vertical transmission were substantially higher in women with heavy than in those with light colonization (65% versus 17%) and that colonization at multiple sites and development of early-onset disease were more likely among infants born to heavily colonized mothers.

The likelihood of colonization in a neonate born to a woman who is culture positive at delivery is unrelated to maternal age, race, parity, or blood type or to duration of labor or method of delivery.[2,3,135,144,179,217] Whether preterm or low-birth-weight neonates are at higher risk for colonization from maternal sources than term infants remains unclear.

Most infected neonates have group B streptococci that are limited to surface or mucous membrane sites. This results from contamination of the oropharynx, gastric contents, or gastrointestinal tract by swallowing of infected amniotic fluid or maternal vaginal secretions. Healthy infants colonized from a maternal source demonstrate persistence of infection at mucous membrane sites for weeks.[9,144] The distribution of serotypes in group B streptococcal isolates from mothers is comparable to that in isolates from healthy neonates.

Besides exposure during birth, other sources for group B streptococcal colonization in the neonate have been established. Horizontal transmission from hospital or community sources to neonates is an important, albeit less frequent, mode for transmission of infection.[144,145,210,215,216,218] Cross-contamination from maternally infected to uninfected neonates can occur from hands of nursery personnel.[215] Unlike group A streptococci, which can produce epidemic disease in nurseries, group B streptococci rarely exhibit this potential, and isolation of neonates with a positive result on skin, umbilical, throat, or gastric cultures is not indicated. An epidemic cluster of five infants with late-onset bacteremic infection related to type Ib group B streptococci occurred among very low birth weight infants in a neonatal intensive care unit.[219] None of the index cases were colonized at birth, establishing that nosocomial acquisition had occurred. Phage typing identified two overlapping patterns of susceptibility believed to represent a single epidemic strain. Epidemiologic analysis suggested infant-to-infant spread by means of the hands of personnel, although acquisition from two nurses colonized with the same phage-type serotype Ib strain was not excluded. The control measures instituted prevented additional cases. This and other reports[210,215] indicate that cohorting of culture-positive infants during an outbreak coupled with implementation of strict hand hygiene for infant contact significantly diminishes nosocomial acquisition.

Community sources afford potential for transmission of group B streptococci to the neonate. Indirect evidence has suggested that this mode of infection is infrequent.[2,15,144,152,199] Only 2 of 46 neonates culture-negative for group B streptococci when discharged from the newborn nursery acquired

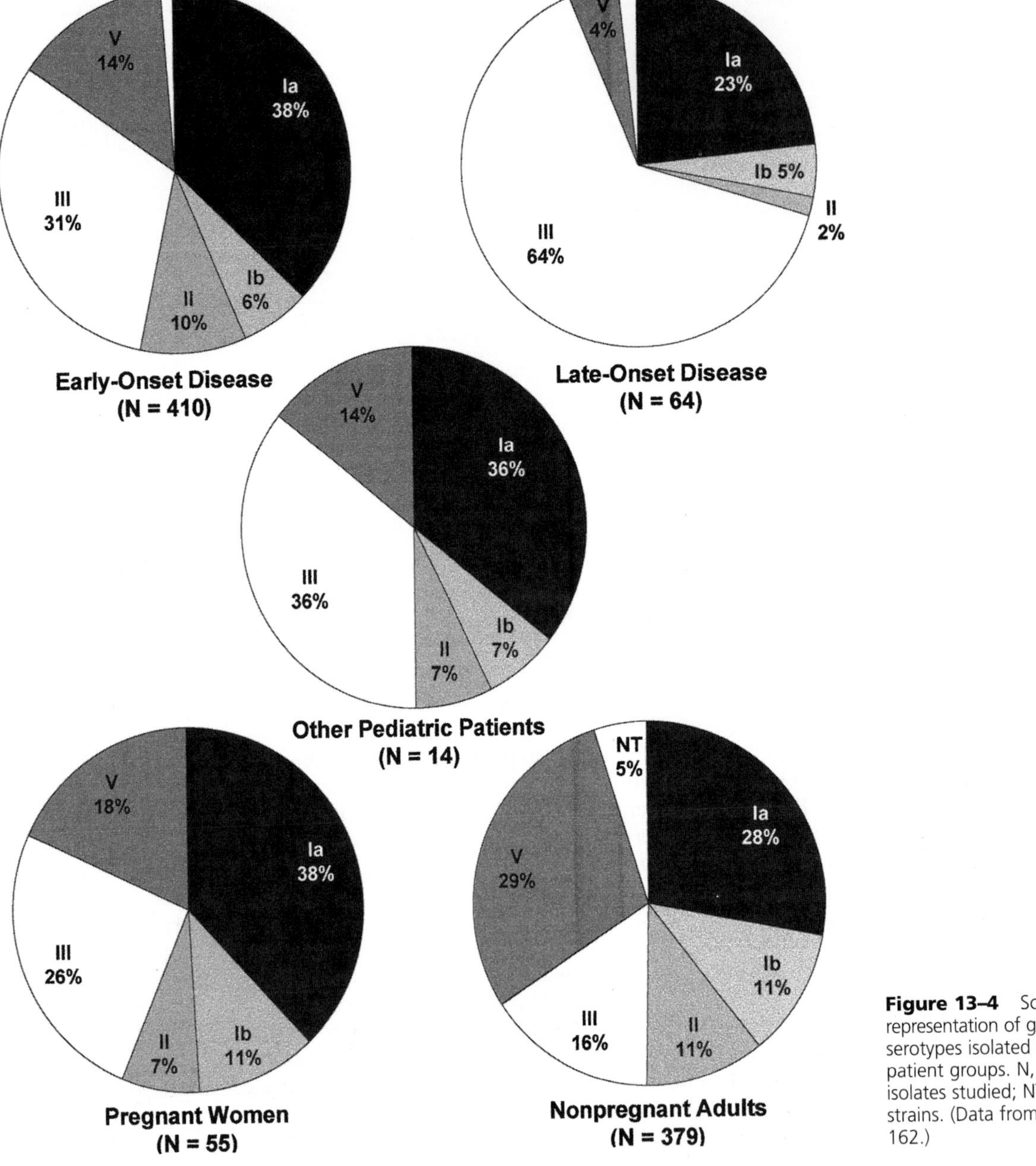

Figure 13–4 Schematic representation of group B streptococcal serotypes isolated from a variety of patient groups. N, number of patient isolates studied; NT, nontypeable strains. (Data from refs. 11, 12, 13, 162.)

mucous membrane infection at 2 months of age.[220] Presumably, the mode of transmission is fecal-oral. Whether acquired by vertical or horizontal mode, infection of mucous membrane sites in neonates usually persists for weeks or months.[144,172,210]

Serotype Distribution of Isolates

The differentiation of group B streptococcal strains into serotypes based on capsular polysaccharide or cell surface protein antigens has provided an invaluable tool in defining the epidemiology of human infection. In the 1970s and 1980s, virtually all studies in which a large number of group B streptococcal strains were isolated from asymptomatic neonates, children, or adults revealed an even distribution into serotypes I, II, and III. This distribution also was reported for isolates from neonates with early-onset infection without meningitis.[52,221,222] As late as 1990, serotypes other than I, II, or III accounted for less than 5% of isolates.

Since 1992, a number of reports from hospitals representing diverse regions throughout the United States and Canada have documented the emergence of serotype V as a frequent cause of colonization and invasive disease.[11-16,162,223,224] The serotype distribution of group B streptococcal strains isolated from different patient groups during the 1990s is shown in Figure 13-4. In two reports, type V has been the predominant serotype among invasive isolates from nonpregnant adults.[12,13] Type V causes a substantial proportion of cases of early-onset disease and of infection among pregnant women. During the 1990s, serotype Ia increased in prevalence and a corresponding decline occurred in serotype II strains as a cause of perinatal group B streptococcal disease.[162] Serotype III strains, which account for approximately 90% of isolates from infants with meningitis, continue to be isolated from two thirds to three quarters of infants with late-onset disease.[224] The emergence of type V is not due to a clone, but a majority of type V isolates do have one subtype pattern that has been present in the United States since 1975.[15] Serotypes VI, VII, and VIII rarely cause human disease in the United States, but recent reports indicate that types VI and VIII are the most common serotypes isolated from healthy Japanese women.[225,226]

Molecular Epidemiology

Epidemiologic investigation of group B streptococcal infections was hampered for many years by the lack of a discriminatory typing system.[227] Initial investigations employed phage typing in combination with serologic classification to differentiate between infant acquisition of group B streptococci from maternal or nosocomial sources.[228] This technique proved useful in determining the source of infection in the nursery environment.[219] Although plasmids have been described in a few group B streptococci,[229] their usefulness as epidemiologic markers is limited.

More recently, multilocus enzyme electrophoresis,[230-232] restriction enzyme fragment length polymorphism (RFLP) analysis, pulsed-field gel electrophoresis (PFGE),[233] and a random-amplified polymorphic DNA (RAPD) assay[234] have been employed for molecular characterization of group B streptococcal isolates associated with human disease. RFLP analysis has indicated that some geographically and epidemiologically distinct isolates have identical patterns, suggesting dissemination of a limited number of clones in the United States.[235] These techniques have shown the molecular relatedness of mother-infant and twin-twin strains[226,234] and have documented mother-to-infant transmission associated with ingestion of infected mother's milk.[235] Compared with conventional electrophoresis, PFGE generates more easily defined patterns with fewer and better-separated bands.[233] Although additional study will be required to define their role for subspecies strain differentiation, it is clear that PFGE and RAPD assay have distinct advantages over some of the previously employed typing schemes.

Molecular characterization has been employed to explore the role of virulence clones in contributing to invasive disease.[9] Type III group B streptococci have been classified into three major phylogenetic lineages on the basis of bacterial DNA restriction digest patterns (RDPs).[236] Most cases of type III neonatal invasive disease appear to be caused by strains with the RDP type III-3. The genetic variation that distinguishes RDP type III-3 strains appears to occur within localized areas of the genome that contain known or putative virulence genes.[237-239] Using genomic subtractive hybridization to identify regions of the genome unique to virulent RDP type III-3 strains, a surface protein was identified that mediates epithelial cell invasion.[240] Using multilocus sequence typing (MLST), 10 allelic profiles were identified among type III isolates recovered from neonates with invasive disease and from colonized pregnant women.[241] The allelic profiles converged into three groups on concatenation. There was an equal distribution of these groups among colonizing and invasive isolates. The finding that isolates with different capsular serotypes have the same sequence type suggests that capsular switching may occur.[241,242] One PFGE group bearing a gene from the capsular synthesis operon has been demonstrated in type III strains causing neonatal meningitis but not in type III colonizing strains.[243] Additional studies will be required to elucidate the difference in virulence between the clones identified by these techniques.[244]

Incidence of Infection in Neonates and Parturients

Two clinical syndromes occur among young infants with group B streptococcal disease that are epidemiologically distinct and relate to age at onset.[2,245] Historically, the attack rates for the first of these syndromes, designated *early-onset* because it appears within the first 6 days of life (mean onset, 12 to 18 hours), have ranged from 0.7 to 3.7 per 1000 live births (Table 13-4). The attack rates for *late-onset* infection (at 7 to 89 days of age) have ranged from 0.5 to 1.8 per 1000. A multistate active surveillance program that identified cases of invasive disease in a population of 10.1 million persons in 1990 reported an incidence of 1.4 and 0.3 per 1000 live births for early- and late-onset disease, respectively.[250] The incidence of disease was significantly higher among African Americans than among whites. The crude incidence was higher among Hispanic whites than among the non-Hispanic white population. The multistate surveillance findings are in accord with a cohort study conducted in Atlanta indicating a higher risk for early- or late-onset disease among African American infants than among those of other ethnic origins.[10] There was a statistically significant decline in the incidence of early-onset disease in some surveillance areas from 1993 to 1995.[253] The rates for late-onset and adult disease remained stable. This decline occurred in association with the implementation of measures to prevent early-onset infection through intrapartum chemoprophylaxis. Current data indicate that the incidence of early-onset disease decreased by 65% from 1993 to 1998, from 1.7 to 0.6 per 1000 live births. It is estimated that 3900 early-onset infections and 200 neonatal deaths were prevented in 1998 by the use of intrapartum antibiotics.[22]

The male-to-female ratio for early- and late-onset group B streptococcal infection is approximately 1:1. Before 1996, 20% to 25% of all infants with group B streptococcal disease had onset after the first 6 days of life. Although attack rates for early-onset group B streptococcal disease are stratified by birth weight, the highest rates occur in lower-birth-weight categories.[247,256] Nevertheless, full-term infants still account for a majority of the early-onset cases.

The importance of the group B streptococcus as a common pathogen for the perinatal period relates to the pregnant woman as well as her infant. Multistate surveillance data indicate that 5% to 10% of cases of invasive group B streptococcal disease occur in pregnant women.[22,250] Bacteremia is the most common manifestation, accounting for approximately two thirds of cases. Bacteremic chorioamnionitis and endometritis each account for approximately 10% of cases, and infection can manifest earlier in gestation as septic abortion.[22] Colonization with group B streptococci has been reported to increase the occurrence of post–cesarean section morbidity manifested as fever, endometritis, and

Table 13–4 **Attack Rates for Group B Streptococcal Disease in Infants**

Year(s) of Study	Location	Attack Rate per 1000 for Bacteremic Early-Onset Infection (Late-Onset Rate)	Ratio of Maternal Colonization at Delivery to Neonatal Invasive Disease	Reference No
1971	Denver	2.0	23:1[a]	2
1972	Houston	2.9	78:1	3
1976	Los Angeles	3.0 (1.6)[b]	100:1	245
1977	Birmingham	3.7 (1.7)	51:1	246
1978	Houston	2.3	102:1	9
1977-1981	Dallas	1.2 (0.5)	225:1	211
1978-1983	Birmingham	1.8 (1.8)	111:1	247
1982-1984	Madrid	0.7	164:1	200
1980-1989	Houston	2.1	175:1	248
1985-1994	Norway	0.4[b]	ND	249
1990	Multistate (USA)	1.4 (0.3)	ND	250
1991-1992	Multistate (USA)	1.8	ND	251
1992-1994	Australia	3.3 (0.1)	ND	252
1993-1995	Multistate (USA)	1.7 (0.5) (1993)	ND	253
1993-1996	Multistate (USA)	0.8	ND	169
		1.3 (0.5) (1995)	ND	253
1993-1998	Multistate (USA)	0.6-1.8	ND	22
1995-1999	Canada	0.6	ND	224
1995-2000	Finland	0.6-0.7	ND	254
2000-2001	Ireland	0.7 (0.5)	ND	255

[a]Calculated from literature review.
[b]Based on surveys carried out during the first 25 months of 41-month study.
ND, not done.

bacteremia,[257] as well as the overall frequency of pelvic infection in the puerperium.[258] Postpartum endometritis occurs with a frequency of 2.0% and clinically diagnosed intra-amniotic infection occurs in 2.9% of women vaginally colonized with group B streptococci at the time of delivery. The risk of intra-amniotic infection is greater in women with heavy colonization.[259] Implementation of intrapartum chemoprophylaxis has been associated with a significant decline in the incidence of invasive disease in pregnant women, from 0.29 per 1000 live births in 1993 to 0.23 per 1000 live births in 1998.[22]

IMMUNOLOGY AND PATHOGENESIS

Host-Bacterial Interactions Related to Pathogenesis

The prevalence and severity of group B streptococcal disease in neonates have stimulated intensive investigation to elucidate the pathogenesis of infection. The unique epidemiologic and clinical features of group B streptococcal disease pose several basic questions that provide a framework for hypothesis development and experimental testing: How does the organism colonize pregnant women and gain access to the infant prior to or during delivery? Why are newborn infants, especially those born prematurely, uniquely susceptible to infection? What allows group B streptococci to evade host immune defenses? How do these organisms gain entry to the bloodstream and cross the blood-brain barrier to produce meningitis? Do specific factors that injure host tissues induce the sepsis syndrome?

Advances in knowledge of pathogenesis have been achieved through development of in vitro systems and animal models. Refinement of molecular genetic techniques has yielded isogenic mutant strains varying solely in the production of a particular component (e.g., capsular polysaccharide). Such mutants are important in establishing the biological relevance of a given trait and its requirement for virulence in vivo. The recent sequencing of two complete group B streptococcus genomes has provided additional context for interpretation of experimental data and comparison to other well-studied pathogens.[17,18]

Although the group B streptococcus has adapted well to asymptomatic colonization of healthy adults, it remains a potentially devastating pathogen to susceptible infants. This section reviews the current understanding of virulence mechanisms, many of which are revealed or magnified by the unique circumstances of the birth process and the deficiencies of neonatal immune defense. The group B streptococcal virulence factors defined to date, with mode of action and proposed role in pathogenesis, are shown in Table 13-5. Key stages in the molecular, cellular, and immunologic pathogenesis of newborn infection are summarized schematically in Figure 13-5.

Maternal Colonization

The presence of group B streptococci in the genital tract of the mother at delivery determines whether or not a newborn infant is at risk for invasive disease. Among infants born to colonized women, the risk of early-onset disease is approximately 30-fold that for infants born to women with a negative result on prenatal cultures.[260] A direct relationship exists between the degree (inoculum size) of group B streptococcal vaginal colonization, the risk of vertical trans-

Table 13–5 **Group B Streptococcal Virulence Factors in Pathogenesis of Neonatal Infection**

Virulence Factor	Molecular or Cellular Action(s)	Proposed Role in Pathogenesis
Host Cell Attachment/Invasion		
C surface protein	Binds cervical epithelial cells	Epithelial cell adherence, invasion
Fibrinogen receptor, FbsA	Binds fibrinogen in extracellular matrix	Epithelial cell attachment
Lipoteichoic acid	Binds host cell surfaces	Epithelial cell attachment
C5a peptidase, ScpB	Binds fibronectin in extracellular matrix	Epithelial cell adherence, invasion
Surface protein Lmb	Binds laminin in extracellular matrix	Epithelial cell attachment
Spb1 surface protein	Promotes epithelial cell uptake	Invasion of epithelial barriers
iagA gene	?Alteration in bacterial cell surface	Promotes blood-brain barrier invasion
Injury to Host Tissues		
β-Hemolysin/cytolysin	Lyses epithelial and endothelial cells	Damage and spread through tissues
Hyaluronate lyase	Cleaves hyaluronan or chondroitin sulfate	Promotes spread through host tissues
CAMP factor	Lyses host cells (co-hemolysin)	Direct tissue injury
Resistance to Immune Clearance		
Exopolysaccharide capsule	Impairs complement C3 deposition/activation	Blocks opsonophagocytic clearance
C5a peptidase, ScpB	Cleaves and inactivates human C5a	Inhibits neutrophil recruitment
CAMP factor	Binds to Fc portion of IgG, IgM	Impairment of antibody function
Serine protease, CspA	Cleaves fibrinogen, coats GBS surface with fibrin	Blocks opsonophagocytosis
Fibrinogen receptor, FbsA	?Steric interference with complement function	Blocks opsonophagocytosis
C protein	Nonimmune binding of IgA	Blocks opsonophagocytosis
β-hemolysin/cytolysin	Lyses neutrophils macrophages, proapoptotic	Impairment of phagocyte killing
Superoxide dismutase	Inactivates superoxide	Impairment of oxidative burst killing
Carotenoid pigment	Antioxidant effect blocks H_2O_2, singlet oxygen	Impairment of oxidative burst killing
Dlt operon genes	Alanylation of lipoteichoic acid	Interferes with antimicrobial peptides
Penicillin-binding protein 1a	Alteration in cell wall composition	Interferes with antimicrobial peptides
Activation of Inflammatory Mediators		
Cell wall lipoteichoic acid	Binds host pattern recognition receptors (TLRs)	Cytokine activation
Cell wall peptidoglycan	Binds host pattern recognition receptors (TLRs)	Cytokine activation
β-Hemolysin/cytolysin	Activation of host cell stress response pathways	Triggers iNOS, cytokine release

mission, and the likelihood of serious disease in the newborn.[217,246] Consequently, a critical step in the pathogenesis of invasive disease in the newborn caused by group B streptococci is colonization of pregnant women.

To establish colonization of the female genital tract, group B streptococci must adhere successfully to the vaginal epithelium. Compared with other microorganisms, group B streptococci bind very efficiently to exfoliated human vaginal cells or vaginal tissue culture cells,[261,262] with maximal adherence at the acidic pH characteristic of vaginal mucosa.[263,264] A low-affinity interaction with epithelial cells is mediated by its amphiphilic cell wall–associated LTA, whereas higher-affinity interactions with host cells are mediated by hydrophobic surface proteins. Soluble LTA competitively inhibits epithelial cell adherence[265,266] and decreases vaginal colonization of pregnant mice.[267] Epithelial cell binding is inhibited by pretreatment of the organism with a variety of proteases,[264,268,269] by preincubating the cells with hydrophobic group B streptococcal surface proteins, or by preincubating the organism with antibodies to these proteins.[270]

Recent investigations reveal that high-affinity protein-mediated interactions with epithelium generally proceed through an intermediary. Group B streptococci effectively bind the extracellular matrix components fibronectin, fibrinogen, and laminin, which in turn interact with host cell–anchored proteins such as integrins. Binding occurs to immobilized fibronectin in the solid but not the liquid phase, suggesting that this interaction requires close proximity of multiple fibronectin molecules and group B streptococcal adhesins.[271] Recently, a genome-wide phage display technique revealed a fibronectin-binding property associated with the surface-anchored group B streptococcal C5a peptidase, ScpB.[272] The dual functionality of ScpB was confirmed by decreased fibronectin binding of isogenic ScpB mutants and the direct interaction of recombinant ScpB with solid-phase fibronectin.[272,273] Similar targeted mutagenesis studies demonstrate that adherence of group B streptococci to laminin involves a protein adhesin called Lmb,[274] whereas attachment to fibrinogen is mediated by repetitive motifs within the surface-anchored protein FbsA.[275]

Ascending Amniotic Infection

Group B streptococci can reach the fetus in utero through ascending infection of the placental membranes and amniotic fluid. Alternatively, the newborn may become contaminated with the organism on passage through the birth canal. Infection by the ascending route plays a pivotal

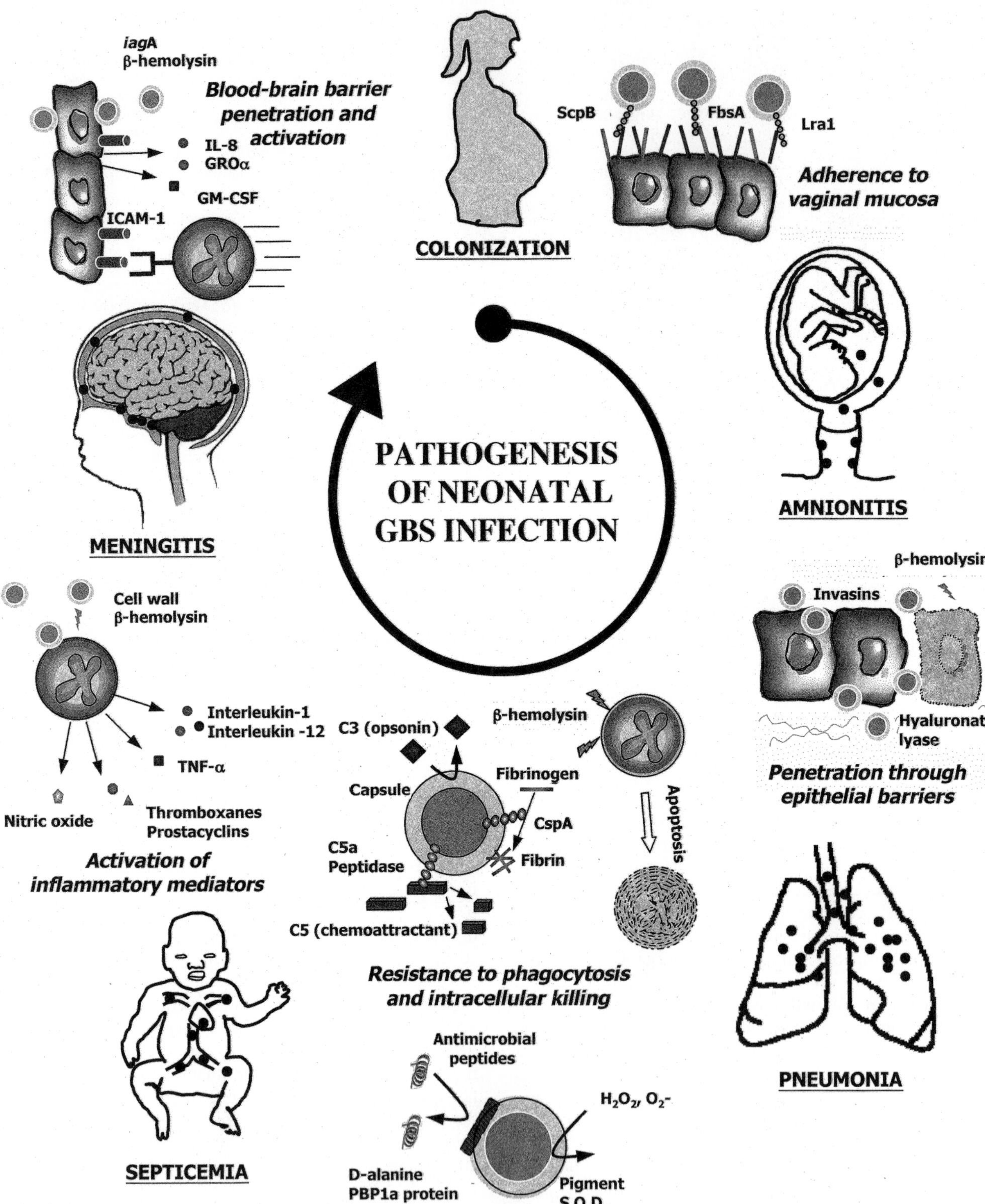

Figure 13–5 Pathomechanisms for different types of neonatal group B streptococcal infection. GM-CSF, granulocyte-macrophage colony-stimulating factor; ICAM, intercellular adhesion molecule; SOD, superoxide dismutase; TNF-α, tumor necrosis factor-α. (Adapted from Doran KS, Nizet V. Molecular pathogenesis of neonatal group B streptococcal infection: no longer in its infancy. Mol Microbiol 54:23-31, 2004.)

role in early-onset disease. A direct relationship exists between the duration of membrane rupture prior to delivery and attack rate for early-onset disease,[276] whereas an inverse relation exists between the duration of membrane rupture and the age at which clinical signs of early-onset pneumonia and sepsis first appear.[277] When the duration of membrane rupture was 18 hours or less, the attack rate was 0.7 per 1000 live births; when it was more than 30 hours, the attack rate increased to 18.3 per 1000.[276] Histologic examination of placentas from women with group B streptococcal chorioamnionitis shows bacterial infiltration along a choriodecidual course, implying that ascending infection may be a primary trigger in many instances of premature rupture.[278]

Group B streptococci may promote membrane rupture and premature delivery by several mechanisms. Isolated chorioamniotic membranes exposed to the organism have decreased tensile strength and elasticity and therefore are prone to rupture.[279] Peptide fragments released from these membranes indicate that proteases are produced that degrade placental tissue. The presence of group B streptococci at the cervix activates the maternal decidua cell peroxidase–hydrogen peroxide–halide system, promoting oxidative damage to adjacent fetal membranes.[280] Group B streptococci also can modify the arachidonic acid metabolism of cultured human amnion cells, favoring production of prostaglandin E_2,[281,282] which is known to stimulate the onset of labor. Stimulation of chorionic cell release of macrophage inflammatory protein-lα (MIP-lα) and interleukin-8 (IL-8) from human chorion cells recruits inflammatory cells that may contribute to infection-associated preterm labor.[283]

It appears that on occasion, group B streptococci can penetrate into the amniotic cavity through intact membranes. Clinically, this mechanism of entry is suggested by anecdotal reports of neonates with fulminant early-onset infection following delivery by cesarean section and no identifiable obstetric risk factors.[9,284,285] Migration of the organism through freshly isolated chorioamniotic membranes has been documented by scanning and transmission electron microscopy.[286] Group B streptococci invade primary chorion cells efficiently in vitro and are capable of transcytosing through intact chorion cell monolayers without disruption of intracellular junctions.[287] They also secrete an enzyme that degrades hyaluronic acid, an important component of the extracellular matrix that is abundant in placental tissues.[288] Theoretically, the action of the group B streptococcal hyaluronate lyase on the extracellular matrix could facilitate amniotic invasion by the organism.[289]

Amniotic fluid supports the proliferation of group B streptococci,[290] although some strains replicate more efficiently than others.[291] When group B streptococci gain access to the uterine cavity and proliferate in the amniotic fluid, a large inoculum can be delivered to the fetal lung. This results in a continuum of intrapartum (stillbirth) to early postpartum infant death.[246,291-295] In utero infection probably accounts for the 40% to 60% of newborns with early-onset disease who have poor Apgar scores and in whom pulmonary signs develop within a few hours of birth.[276,292] Such infants almost invariably display clinical or histologic evidence of congenital pneumonia. Conversely, when group B streptococci are encountered in the immediate peripartum period or on passage through the birth canal, a lesser inoculum is delivered to the neonate. Although a small but meaningful risk of subsequent invasive disease exists, the great majority of newborns who are contaminated with group B streptococci through swallowing of infected vaginal secretions will have asymptomatic colonization limited to mucosal surfaces and remain healthy.

Pulmonary and Bloodstream Entry

Early-onset group B streptococcal disease is heralded by respiratory symptoms including tachypnea, hypoxia, cyanosis, and pulmonary hypertension.[296] One third to more than one half of infants are symptomatic at birth or within 4 to 6 hours after delivery. Autopsies in fatal early-onset cases reveal that 80% have histologic evidence of lobar or multilobar pneumonia,[295,297] characterized by dense bacterial infiltration, epithelial cell damage, alveolar hemorrhage, interstitial inflammatory exudate, and hyaline membrane formation.[294,298] When pneumonia develops in newborn primates exposed by intra-amniotic injection of group B streptococci, bacterial density reaches 10^9 to 10^{11} organisms per gram of lung tissue.[299] Also, in experimental animals, an inverse relationship exists between age and ability to clear group B streptococci from the lung following aerosol challenge.[300,301] The poorer resolution of pneumonia in preterm than in term rabbits reflects quantitative deficiency of pulmonary alveolar macrophages, mandating the recruitment of neutrophils as a secondary phagocytic defense mechanism.[302]

Group B streptococcal disease rarely is limited to the initial pulmonary focus but spreads to the bloodstream and is circulated through other organs and tissues. The capacity of group B streptococci to cause disruption of the lung epithelial and endothelial barrier evidently involves the process of intracellular invasion, direct cytolytic injury, and damage induced by the inflammatory response of the newborn host. Intracellular invasion of both alveolar epithelial and pulmonary endothelial cells by group B streptococci was first noted in newborn macaques following intra-amniotic challenge[299] and later confirmed in human tissue culture lines derived from both cellular barriers.[303,304] Electron microscopy studies in vivo and in vitro demonstrate that host cytoskeletal changes are triggered that lead to endocytotic uptake of the bacterium within a membrane-bound vacuole. Uptake requires induction of protein kinase signal transduction pathways in the host cell that are mediated by calmodulin and phosphatidylinositol-3 (PI-3) kinase.[305,306]

Cellular invasion is correlated with virulence potential. Clinical isolates of group B streptococci from infants with bloodstream infections invade epithelial cells better than do strains from the vaginal mucosa of asymptomatic women.[307] Invasion is reduced by trypsin treatment or protein synthesis inhibition, suggesting the involvement of specific bacterial surface proteins in the process.[303,307] Genetic phenotyping of type III strains identified a particular restriction digest pattern (RDP III-3) characteristic of a majority of the isolates from invasive neonatal infection.[308] Subtractive hybridization studies identified a gene unique to these strains encoding the surface-anchored protein, Spb1, required for maximal epithelial cell invasion.[240] Similarly, elimination of the genes encoding the fibronectin-binding C5a peptidase, ScpB, or the antiphagocytic α C surface protein each significantly reduced epithelial cell invasion by group B streptococci.[273,309] By contrast, the capsular polysaccharide decreases intracellular invasion, presumably through steric interference of certain receptor-ligand interactions.[310]

Although cellular invasion may play a principal role in bloodstream penetration in late-onset group B streptococcal infection, damage to the lung barrier often is evident in severe early-onset infection. Alveolar exudate and hemorrhage in autopsy studies of infants with group B streptococcal pneumonia attest to significant pulmonary epithelial and endothelial cell injury.[294,311] The cellular damage appears to result largely from the actions of the β-hemolysin/cytolysin. This toxin is responsible for the characteristic β-hemolytic phenotype displayed by the organism when grown on sheep's blood agar. Mutagenesis and heterologous expression studies have identified a single open reading frame, cylE, as necessary for group B streptococcal β-hemolysin/cytolysin expression and sufficient to confer β-hemolysis when cloned in *E. coli*.[312,313] CylE is a predicted 79-kDa protein sharing no homology to the toxin, streptolysin S, that is responsible for β-hemolysis in group A, C, F, and G streptococci.[314] This pore-forming toxin lyses lung epithelial and endothelial cells and compromises their barrier function.[315,316] At subcytolytic doses, it promotes intracellular invasion and triggers the release of IL-8, the principal chemoattractant for human neutrophils.[317] Mutants lacking hemolysin expression are less virulent than the corresponding wild-type strains in mouse, rat, and rabbit models of group B streptococcal pneumonia.[318-320]

The cytolytic, pro-invasive, and pro-inflammatory effects of the group B streptococcal β-hemolysin/cytolysin all are neutralized by dipalmitoyl phosphatidylcholine (DPPC), the major phospholipid constituent of human lung surfactant.[315,317] This finding may explain in part the enhanced risk in premature, surfactant-deficient neonates for severe lung injury and invasive disease from group B streptococcal infection. Treatment with exogenous surfactant reduces histologic evidence of lung inflammation, improves lung compliance, and mitigates bacterial growth in preterm rabbits infected with group B streptococci.[321,322] Clinical studies exploring the effect of surfactant administration on human infants with group B streptococcal sepsis also suggest a beneficial effect.[323,324]

Capsular Polysaccharide and Immune Resistance

On penetration of group B streptococci into the lung tissue or bloodstream of the newborn infant, an immunologic response is recruited to clear the organism. Central to this response are host phagocytic cells including neutrophils and macrophages. Effective uptake and killing by these cells require opsonization of the bacterium by specific antibodies in the presence of complement.[325-327] Neonates are particularly prone to invasive disease because of their quantitative or qualitative deficiencies in phagocytic cell function, specific antibody, or the classic and alternate complement pathways. In addition to these newborn host susceptibilities, group B streptococci possess a number of virulence determinants that seek to thwart each of the key components of effective opsonophagocytic killing. Chief among these factors is the sialylated group B streptococcal polysaccharide capsule.

The serotype-specific epitopes of group B streptococcal capsular polysaccharides are created by different arrangements of four monosaccharides (glucose, galactose, *N*-acetylglucosamine, and sialic acid) into a unique repeating unit (see "Immunochemistry of Polysaccharide Antigens" under "The Organism" earlier), but unfailingly these structures contain a terminal sialic acid bound to galactose in an $\alpha2\rightarrow3$ linkage. The enzymatic machinery for capsule biosynthesis is encoded in the single long transcript of a 16-gene operon now fully sequenced in type Ia, type III, and type V strains. Recently, elegant experiments have shown that the heterologous expression of a single polymerase gene (*cps*H) from this operon can cause a group B streptococcal type Ia strain to express type III capsule epitopes, and vice versa.[328]

The conserved group B streptococcal terminal $\alpha2\rightarrow3$ sialic acid capsular component is identical to a sugar epitope widely displayed on the surface of all mammalian cells.[329] Furthermore, the terminal $\alpha2\rightarrow3$–linked sialic acid is overexpressed in humans, who in evolution have lost the genes to produce the alternative sialic acid, Neu5Gc. One can hypothesize that the group B *Streptococcus* is a particularly troublesome newborn pathogen because its sialylated capsule has undergone selection to resemble host "self" and avoid immune recognition. In fact, in comparison with wild-type strains, isogenic capsule-deficient mutants of group B streptococci elicit greater degrees of pro-inflammatory cytokine release from human cells.[330] These observations probably reflect a combination of decreased immune recognition as a result of capsule molecular mimicry of host epitopes, and increased access of host pattern recognition molecules (e.g., Toll-like receptors) to the cell wall components LTA and peptidoglycan hidden beneath the "cloak" of the polysaccharide capsule.

The properties of group B streptococcal capsular polysaccharide have been studied most thoroughly in serotype III organisms. Sialic acid is a critical element in the epitope of the type III capsule that confers protective immunity. After treatment with sialidase, the altered capsular polysaccharide fails to elicit protective antibodies against group B streptococcal infection. Moreover, protective antibodies derived from native type III capsule do not bind to the altered (asialo) capsule backbone structure.[331] Human infants who possess antibodies that react only to the desialylated capsule remain at high risk for invasive disease.

The correlation of capsular sialic acid and virulence was first noted in studies employing sialidase to remove the critical surface epitope. Sialidase-treated type III group B streptococci are opsonized more effectively by complement through the alternative pathway and are consequently more readily phagocytosed by human neutrophils in vitro.[332] Sialidase treatment also results in diminished lethality of the organism in neonatal rats.[333] Serial subculture of a wild-type strain in the presence of type III–specific antiserum allows identification of variants that do not express the terminal sialic acid component of the polysaccharide capsule. These strains possess a 1000-fold greater median lethal dose (LD_{50}) following tail-vein injection in mice.[334]

More definitive evidence for the role of type III capsule in virulence is provided by the construction of isogenic capsule-deficient mutants by transposon mutagenesis or targeted allelic replacement.[335-337] In comparison with the parent strains, isogenic capsule mutants are susceptible to opsonophagocytosis in the presence of complement and healthy adult neutrophils.[338] Situated at the convergence of the classic and alternative pathways, deposition of C3 on the bacterial surface, with subsequent cleavage and degradation to opsonically active fragments C3b and iC3b, is a pivotal element in host defense against invasive infections. C3 deposition and degradation occur on the surface of group B streptococci representing a variety of serotypes.[339] The extent of C3 deposition by the alternative pathway, however, is inversely related to the size and density of the polysaccharide capsule present on the surface of type Ib and type III strains.[338,340] C3 fragments bound to the acapsular mutant are predominantly in the active form, C3b, whereas the inactive form, C3bi, is predominantly bound to the surface of the parent strain. Less C3b is bound by the asialo capsule mutant than by the acapsular mutant, and less C3bi is bound by asialo capsule mutant than by the wild-type strain.[338] These studies prove that type III capsular polysaccharide—in particular, the sialic acid residues—inhibit the alternative complement pathway by blocking binding of C3 to the organism and promoting inactivation of C3b.

The type III group B streptococcal acapsular mutants also are significantly less virulent in animal models of infection. In a model of pneumonia and bacteremia, neonatal rats have been inoculated with either the parent strain or an acapsular mutant by intratracheal injection. In animals that receive the acapsular mutant, fewer group B streptococci are recovered per gram of lung, more bacteria are associated with resident alveolar macrophages, and the animals become significantly less bacteremic than animals that receive the parent strain.[341] Subcutaneous injection of the acapsular or asialo mutants in neonatal rats results in similar LD_{50} values that are at least 100-fold greater than those obtained with the parent strain.[336,342] Mouse passage of various serotypes of group B streptococci is followed by increases in sialylated capsule content that correlate with increased virulence.[343] Taken together, these data provide compelling evidence that the capsule protects the organism from phagocytic clearance during both the initial pulmonary phase and the later bacteremic phase of early-onset infection.

Noncapsular Factors That Interfere with Immune Clearance

The ability of group B streptococci to avoid opsonophagocytosis is enhanced by surface proteins that can act in concert with capsular polysaccharide. For example, serotype II strains displaying both components of the C protein antigen are more resistant to phagocytic killing than are serotype II strains lacking C protein.[344,345] A potential mechanism is that strains bearing the C protein antigen display increased nonimmune binding to serum IgA and decreased C3 deposition on their surface.[346] The β antigen of C protein binds human IgA,[347,348] and IgA deposited nonspecifically on the bacterial surface probably inhibits interactions with complement or IgG.[346] A cell surface protease, CspA, targets host fibrinogen, producing adherent fibrin-like cleavage products that coat the bacterial surface and interfere with opsonophagocytic clearance.[349] Mutational studies also have attributed an antiphagocytic property to a group B streptococcal surface fibrinogen-binding protein.[275]

Following phagocytic uptake of pathogens, neutrophils and macrophages seek to kill the engulfed bacteria by generation of reactive oxygen products and other antimicrobial substances. Streptococci are often thought of as "extracellular pathogens," but these organisms can survive for prolonged periods within the phagolysosome of macrophages.[350,351] Although group B streptococci lack the neutralizing enzyme catalase, they are more than 10 times resistant to killing by hydrogen peroxide than is catalase-positive *S. aureus.*[352] Several mechanisms for enhanced intracellular survival have been identified. The organism possesses a endogenous source of the oxygen metabolite scavenger glutathione.[352] Another defense against oxidative burst killing is the enzyme superoxide dismutase (SodA), as evidenced by the fact that a SodA mutant is highly susceptible to macrophage killing and survives poorly in vivo.[353] Finally, group B streptococci produce an orange carotenoid pigment, a property unique among hemolytic streptococci and genetically linked to the *cyl* operon encoding the β-hemolysin/cytolysin. The free-radical scavenging properties of the carotenoid neutralize hydrogen peroxide, superoxide, hypochlorite, and singlet oxygen, thereby providing a shield against several elements of phagocyte oxidative burst killing.[354] The antioxidant effects of glutathione, SodA, and carotenoid pigment appear to compensate for the lack of catalase and explain the unexpected persistence of group B streptococci within host phagolysomes.

Cationic antimicrobial peptides, such as defensins and cathelicidins produced by host phagocytes, also are an important component of immune defense.[355,356] The group B streptococcal *pon*A gene codes for an extracytoplasmic penicillin-binding protein (PBP1a) that promotes resistance to phagocytic killing independent of capsule.[357] Group B streptococcal mutants with deletion of the PBP1a gene are less virulent following both lung and systemic challenge, and this is correlated to an increased susceptibility to defensins and cathelicidins.[358] Another way in which the organism avoids antimicrobial peptide clearance is through the D-alanylation of LTA in the bacterial cell wall. This requires activity of gene products that are encoded by the *dlt* operon. A *dlt*A mutant exhibits decreased negative surface charge that impedes cationic host defense peptides from reaching their cell membrane target of action.[359]

Direct cytotoxicity to host phagocytes represents another important virulence mechanism for immune resistance. The *cyl*E-encoded β-hemolysin/cytolysin toxin produces direct cytolytic injury to macrophages and induces macrophage apoptosis over a longer interval. With highly hemolytic strains or with a large bacterial inoculum, killing of the phagocyte appears to outpace the phagocyte's microbicidal mechanisms, allowing bacterial proliferation in vitro in a murine bacteremia model.[354] Group B streptococci may trigger macrophage apoptosis by β-hemolysin/cytolysin–dependent[360] and β-hemolysin/cytolysin–independent mechanisms.[361] Addition of an inhibitor of β-hemolysin/cytolysin blocks cytolysis and reduces apoptosis of macrophages, thereby restoring phagocytic killing.[354]

Deficiencies in the neutrophil response to group B streptococci have been documented in newborn infants. Neutropenia and depletion of the marrow neutrophil storage pool are frequent findings in infants with septicemia[362] and are correlated with poor clinical outcome.[296] Whereas neutrophilia and an increase in granulocytic stem cells develop in adult rats infected with group B streptococci, severe neutropenia without a change in stem cell counts develops in neonatal rats.[363] Fatal infection in neonatal rats is associated with failure of recovery of depleted myeloid storage pools.[364] The explanation for this finding may be that the proliferative rate of neutrophils in noninfected neonatal animals already is maximal or near maximal and cannot further increase in response to bacterial challenge.[365]

Group B streptococci actively contribute to poor mobilization of neutrophils by production of an enzyme that cleaves and inactivates human C5a, a complement component that stimulates neutrophil chemotaxis.[366] Expression of C5a peptidase reduces the acute neutrophil response to sites of infection in C5a knockout mice reconstituted with human C5a.[367] The enzymatic activity of soluble C5a peptidase is neutralized by serum from normal human adults, in large part because of naturally occurring IgG antibodies.[366] IgG also neutralizes C5a peptidase on the surface of a capsule-deficient group B streptococcal mutant but fails to neutralize the enzyme on the surface of the intact encapsulated type III parent strain. Thus, the capsule serves to protect the cell-associated C5a peptidase from inactivation by naturally occurring antibodies.

Inflammatory Mediators and Sepsis

When failures in epithelial barrier function and immunologic clearance allow group B streptococci to establish bacteremia in the neonate, development of sepsis or septic shock is the consequence. Intravenous infusion of group B streptococci in animal models produces similar pathophysiologic changes to human newborn infection, including hypotension, persistent pulmonary hypertension, tissue hypoxemia and acidosis, temperature instability, disseminated intravascular coagulation, neutropenia, and ultimately, multiple organ system failure. These similarities have allowed in vivo experiments to elucidate the patterns in which the organism activates host inflammatory mediators to induce sepsis and circulatory shock.

Animal models in which group B streptococci are infused intravenously demonstrate a biphasic host inflammatory response.[368-370] The acute phase (up to 1 hour following infusion) is manifested by increased pulmonary artery pressure and decreased arterial oxygenation and is associated with a rise in serum levels of thromboxanes. Pulmonary hypertension and hypoxemia persist through the late phase (2 to 4 hours), in which a progressive pattern of systemic hypotension, decreased cardiac output, and metabolic acidosis develops together with hematologic abnormalities, organ system dysfunction, and increase in inflammatory markers, such as thromboxanes, tumor necrosis factor-α (TNF-α), and prostacyclins. If thromboxane and prostacyclin production is blocked by inhibition of the cyclooxygenase pathway in rabbits or lambs infused with group B streptococci, decreased myocardial dysfunction and a significant rise in systemic blood pressure are observed.[371-373]

Infusion of group B streptococci produces pulmonary hypertension in piglets and isolated piglet lung preparations, suggesting a direct interaction of the organism with target cells in lung microvasculature.[374,375] Live but not heat-killed organisms induce release of the vasoactive eicosanoids, prostacyclin and prostaglandin E_2, from cultured lung microvascular cells.[376] Experiments using specific antagonists have further implicated the host inflammatory mediators leukotriene D_4[377] and thromboxane A_2[378] as components of the pulmonary vascular response in pneumonia.

The cytokine interleukin-12 (IL-12) has an important role in the systemic response to group B streptococcal infection. IL-12 elevation occurs 12 to 72 hours after challenge in the neonatal rat. Pretreatment with a monoclonal antibody against IL-12 results in greater mortality and intensity of bacteremia, whereas therapeutic administration of IL-12 is associated with a lower mortality rate and bloodstream replication of the organism.[379] By contrast, interleukin-1 (IL-1), a known stimulator of cyclooxygenase and lipooxygenase pathways, appears to occupy a proximal position in the deleterious cytokine cascade of septic shock.[380] Treatment with an IL-1 receptor antagonist improves cardiac output and mean arterial pressure and increases duration of survival in piglets receiving a continuous infusion of group B streptococci.[381]

Controversy exists regarding the precise role of TNF-α in neonatal septicemia. TNF-α often is detected in the blood, urine, or cerebrospinal fluid (CSF) of infants with invasive disease.[382] Although infusion of group B streptococci in piglets is associated with TNF-α release during the late phase of hemodynamic response, the TNF-α inhibitor pentoxifylline has only modest effects on pulmonary hypertension, hypoxemia, and systemic hypotension.[383] Marked improvement in these hemodynamic parameters is seen only when pentoxifylline treatment is combined with indomethacin inhibition of thromboxane and prostacyclin synthesis.[384] Serum TNF-α levels in the mouse and rat also rise after challenge; however, administration of polyclonal or monoclonal anti-TNF-α antibody does not affect overall mortality rate in these animal models.[384,385]

Studies have sought to establish the components of group B streptococci cell wall that trigger the host cytokine cascade. Host release of IL-l and IL-6 is stimulated by soluble cell wall antigens.[386] Cell wall preparations also cause nuclear factor kappa-B (NF-κB) activation and TNF-α release from human monocytes in a manner requiring CD14 and complement receptor types 3 and 4.[387] The group B polysaccharide and peptidoglycan are more effective stimulators of TNF-α release from monocytes than is LTA or capsular polysaccharide.[388] Knockout mouse studies indicate that cell wall peptidoglycan-induced activation of p38 and NF-κB depends on the cytoplasmic toll-like receptor (TLR) adapter protein MyD88 but does not require the pattern recognition receptor TLR2 or TLR4.[389] An additional, undefined secreted factor appears to activate phagocytes through TLR2 and TLR6.[390]

Another pro-inflammatory molecule contributing to the pathogenesis of group B streptococcal septicemia is the β-hemolysin/cytolysin. The β-hemolysin/cytolysin acts to stimulate inducible nitric oxide synthase in macrophages, leading to release of nitric oxide, an important factor in the early sepsis cascade.[391] In a mouse model of bacteremia and arthritis, β-hemolysin/cytolysin expression is associated with higher mortality, increased bacterial loads, greater degrees of joint injury, and release of the pro-inflammatory cytokines IL-6 and IL-1α systemically and intra-articularly.[392] Challenge of rabbits with isogenic group B streptococcal mutants showed that β-hemolysin/cytolysin production was associated with significantly higher degrees of hypotension, increased mortality, and evidence of liver necrosis with hepatocyte apoptosis.[393] Partially purified β-hemolysin/cytolysin preparations produce significant hypotensive actions when infused in rats and rabbits, including death due to shock.[394]

Blood-Brain Barrier Penetration and Meningitis

The pathophysiology of group B streptococcal meningitis varies according to age at onset. In early-onset disease, autopsy studies demonstrate little or no evidence of leptomeningeal inflammation, despite the presence of abundant bacteria, vascular thrombosis, and parenchymal hemorrhage.[2,311] By contrast, infants with late-onset disease usually have diffuse purulent arachnoiditis with prominent involvement of the base of the brain.[395] Similar age-related differences in central nervous system pathology are evident in the infant rat model of invasive disease.[396] These histopathologic differences reflect underdevelopment of the host immunologic response in the immediate neonatal period, with a higher proportion of deaths resulting from overwhelming septicemia.

To produce meningitis, group B streptococci must penetrate human brain microvascular endothelial cells, the single-cell layer constituting the blood-brain barrier. Intracellular invasion and transcytosis of human brain microvascular endothelial cell tissue culture monolayers have been shown in vitro.[397] Serotype III strains, which account for a majority of the isolates causing meningitis, invade more efficiently than strains of other common serotypes. Recently, a transposon mutant library of type III group B streptococci was screened in tissue culture assays for alterations in invasiveness. Hypoinvasive mutants were identified with disruptions in *iag*A, sharing homology to genes encoding diglucosyldiacylglycerol synthase. Allelic replacement of *iag*A confirms the in vitro phenotype, and the *iag*A knockout mutant does not produce meningitis in mice.[397] At high bacterial densities, invasion by group B streptococci of brain microvascular endothelial cells is accompanied by evidence of β-hemolysin/cytolysin–induced cellular injury.[398] Correspondingly, β-hemolysin/cytolysin knockout mutants show decreased blood-brain barrier penetration and decreased lethality from meningitis in vivo.[330]

The host inflammatory response to group B streptococci contributes significantly to the pathogenesis of meningitis and central nervous system injury. The initiation of the inflammatory response is triggered through the sentinel function of the blood-brain barrier endothelium, which activates a specific pattern of gene transcription for neutrophil recruitment, including production of chemokines (e.g., IL-8, Groα), endothelial receptors (intercellular adhesion molecule-1 [ICAM-1]), and neutrophil activators (granulocyte-macrophage colony-stimulating factor [GM-CSF]).[330] A vascular distribution of cortical lesions in neonatal rats with group B streptococcal meningitis indicates that disturbances of cerebral blood flow contribute to neuronal damage.[399] Inflammation of individual brain vessels can lead to focal lesions, whereas diffuse alterations of cerebral blood flow could cause generalized hypoxic/ischemic injury and cerebral edema.[399,400] Arteriolar dysfunction is associated with the presence of oxygen free radicals thought to be a byproduct of the phagocytic killing by infiltrating neutrophils.[401]

In the neonatal rat, simultaneous intracisternal administration of dexamethasone with group B streptococci leads to a marked reduction in subarachnoid inflammation, vasculopathy, and neuronal injury.[399] In the neonatal rat model of meningitis, TNF-α production by astrocytes, microglial cells, and infiltrating leukocytes appears to contribute to apoptosis of hippocampal neurons,[402] further increasing blood-brain barrier permeability.[403] Intraventricular inoculation of newborn piglets with group B streptococci results in an early sharp rise in CSF TNF-α levels, followed shortly by prostaglandin release and neutrophil influx.[404] The magnitude of the observed TNF-α response and inflammatory cascade is markedly increased when an isogenic nonencapsulated mutant is tested in place of the type III parent strain,[404] suggesting that a component of the underlying cell wall and not capsule is responsible for inducing the central nervous system inflammatory response.

Table 13–6 Risk Factors for Early-Onset Group B Streptococcal Disease

Risk Factor	Representative Reference Nos.
Maternal colonization at delivery	3, 148, 247
High-density maternal colonization	153, 217, 246
Rupture of membranes before onset of labor	246, 251
Preterm delivery	251
Prolonged rupture of membranes	251, 405
Chorioamnionitis	406
Intrapartum fever	251
Intrauterine monitoring	251, 405
Maternal postpartum bacteremia	7
Twin pregnancy	407, 408
Group B streptococcal bacteriuria or urinary tract infection	251
Cesarean section	245, 246
Low level of antibody to infecting serotype	409
Young maternal age (<20 years)	251, 405
Previous infant with group B streptococcal infection	407, 408
Maternal race/ethnicity	10, 162, 164, 251

Host Factors Relating to Pathogenesis

Risk Factors for Early-Onset Infection

Infant and maternal factors that increase risk for early-onset group B streptococcal infection are summarized in Table 13-6. The most obvious risk determinant is exposure to the organism through maternal colonization at delivery. Maternal race or ethnicity is correlated significantly with early-onset group B streptococcal disease, with enhanced risk for infants born to African American and Hispanic mothers compared with that for infants born to white mothers.[162,164,251] Risk correlates directly with density of maternal genital inoculum.[217] Although symptomatic early-onset disease develops in only 1% to 2% of infants born to colonized women, this rate is considerably increased if there is premature onset of labor (before 37 weeks of gestation) (15%),[247] chorioamnionitis or interval between rupture of membranes and delivery longer than 18 hours (11%),[246,247] twin pregnancy (35%),[407,408] or maternal postpartum bacteremia (10%).[7]

Women who report a history of asymptomatic bacteriuria or urinary tract infection are more likely to deliver infants with group B streptococcal infection. Group B streptococcal bacteriuria is a predictor of high inoculum colonization, which is a known risk factor.[410] Heavy group B streptococcal colonization in the second trimester of pregnancy was associated in one study with increased risk of delivering a preterm, low-birth-weight infant.[411] Among infants born to mothers with premature rupture of membranes at term gestation, maternal chorioamnionitis and colonization with group B streptococci are strong predictors of neonatal infection.[412] Vaginal colonization with group B streptococci also is an independent risk factor for the development of chorioamnionitis.[413]

Although prolonged interval after rupture of membranes (more than 18 hours) before delivery and preterm delivery (before 37 weeks of gestation) often are concomitant risk factors in neonates with early-onset group B streptococcal infection, the latter is an independent contributor to neonatal risk, probably from immaturity of host defense mechanisms. It is estimated that the incidence of early-onset group B streptococcal infection is 10 to 15 times higher in premature than in term neonates.[246,276] Even when incidence is corrected for preterm gestation (less than 37 weeks) and low birth weight (less than 2500 g), Pass and co-workers[407] reported that twin pregnancy was an independent risk factor for invasive early-onset group B streptococcal septicemia. The explanation for this increased risk in twins[407,408] is undefined but may be related to genetic factors regulating host susceptibility or to virulence of disease-producing strains.

Antibody to Capsular Polysaccharide

Lancefield's studies demonstrated that antibodies directed against the type-specific surface antigens of group B streptococci protected mice from lethal challenge with strains containing these antigens.[62] Baker and Kasper[409] demonstrated in 1976 that neonates at risk for early- or late-onset group B streptococcal disease involving type III strains were those whose mothers had very low serum concentrations of antibodies to the type III capsular polysaccharide at delivery. A similar correlation was reported for neonates with type II and type III early-onset disease.[414] Absence of opsonic activity in response to the infecting strains was associated with a low concentration of these type-specific IgG antibodies in maternal serum or with failure to actively transport sufficient concentrations transplacentally before delivery of a premature infant.[415-419] Extremely premature infants have low total IgG concentrations in their sera, because approximately 60% of maternally derived IgG is transported to the fetus during the last 10 weeks of pregnancy.

Employing a radioactive antigen-binding assay, Baker and colleagues[420] detected low levels (less than 1.7 μg/mL) of type III capsular polysaccharide–specific antibodies in sera from each of 32 infants with invasive disease. Women with type III group B streptococcal genital colonization at delivery whose infants remained well had greater than 2.0 μg/mL of type III–specific antibodies significantly more often than did women in whose infants type III early-onset disease developed. Quantitative determination of antibodies to type III group B streptococcal polysaccharide by enzyme-linked immunosorbent assay (ELISA) indicates that these antibodies are predominantly of the IgG isotype.[421,422]

Capsular type–specific antibodies also are important in the pathogenesis of early-onset infection related to serotypes Ia, Ib, and II.[416,423] Using ELISA standardized by quantitative precipitation,[424] 1.0, 0.2, and 1.3 μg/mL of IgG to serotypes Ia, Ib, and III, respectively, were protective in experimental models of infection.[418,425-427] Among pregnant women at delivery, approximately 15% to 20% have capsular polysaccharide type–specific IgG in levels presumed to protect against invasive disease. These concentrations of IgG are significantly more likely to be found in the sera of women colonized with the homologous group B streptococcal serotype.[164,165,428] A recent prospective, multicenter hospital-based, case-control study of mothers delivering infants with type Ia, III, or V early-onset sepsis and matched colonized control mothers delivering healthy infants has quantified the maternal serum concentrations of type Ia, III, and V capsular polysaccharide–specific IgG at delivery that protects neonates from early-onset disease. For types Ia and III, maternal IgG concentrations of 0.5 μg/mL or higher corresponded to 90% risk reduction. For type V, the same antibody concentration corresponded to 70% risk reduction.[429] Gray and co-workers[430] noted a similar correlation between low concentrations of type II–specific antibodies in maternal delivery sera and susceptibility of infants to invasive infection. Human antibody to the group B polysaccharide is not protective against invasive infant disease.[431]

Antibodies to the capsular polysaccharides of group B streptococci correlate with in vitro opsonic activity (on chemiluminescence[414,432] and opsonophagocytic[344,345,346,433] assays) and with in vivo protection in experimental animal models of infection.[434-436] The factor or factors that explain the apparent relationship between asymptomatic mucosal infection and acquired specific humoral immunity in adults are unknown. A majority of adults and children have very low, presumably nonprotective levels of serotype-specific antibodies in their sera; nevertheless, the colonized pregnant woman who is likely to infect her neonate with group B streptococci at birth is also the one in whom passive protection of her infant is most likely. These antibodies appear to persist at a given concentration throughout gestation in the overwhelming majority of women.[417]

Although neonates with early-onset type III group B streptococcal sepsis are uniformly deficient in type III–specific IgG, most neonates born to women with type III genital colonization and low levels of type III IgG in their sera remain well.[415-417] Kim and co-workers[437] demonstrated opsonic and protective activity by cord sera that appeared to be independent of type-specific antibody or complement. Boyer and associates[438] reported that IgM-specific antibody, absent in serum from neonates, was detectable by 3 months of age and exceeded 0.5 μg/mL in sera from all infants after 7 months. They proposed that the development of IgM-specific antibody in infancy may account for the marked decline in type III group B streptococcal infection after early infancy, but this finding has not been confirmed, and is unlikely in view of the short half-life of IgM.

Low concentrations of IgG to type III capsular polysaccharide are uniformly found in the acute sera of infants with late-onset type III infection.[409,414-416] In a study of 28 infants with late-onset bacteremia and 51 with meningitis, Baker and co-workers[420] detected low levels of antibodies to type III capsular polysaccharide in acute sera from all infants. These low levels in term infants with late-onset type III group B streptococcal infection correlated with maternal levels at delivery.[415,420]

It is important to employ antigens with "native" or intact type III polysaccharide specificity in evaluating human immunity to type III group B streptococci.[439,440] Kasper and colleagues[331] used gently extracted (native) and HCl-treated (core) type III group B streptococcal and pneumococcal type 14 antigens to study sera from infants with invasive type

III infection and their mothers. Concentrations of type III–specific antibodies in sera of sick infants and their mothers had uniformly low binding to fully sialylated, type III polysaccharide. Opsonic immunity correlated with antibodies to fully sialylated but not to desialylated type III polysaccharide or to type 14 pneumococcal antigen. Among infants recovering from type III disease in whom a significant increase in antibodies to the fully sialylated polysaccharide developed, no detectable rise in the acid-degraded or core antigen was seen. Thus, human immunity to type III group B streptococci relates to antibodies to capsular type III polysaccharide with an intact protective epitope.

An extension of this concept comes from studies in which adults have been immunized with either type III polysaccharide or pneumococcal polysaccharide vaccine.[439,440] Adults with low concentrations of type III antibodies in their sera before immunization responded to type III polysaccharide vaccine with a significant increase in type III–specific antibodies. This response was not observed when the structurally related type 14 pneumococcal polysaccharide was used as an immunizing agent. Among adults with moderate to high levels of antibodies to type III polysaccharide, however, significant rises in level of this antibody developed after pneumococcal polysaccharide vaccine. This finding suggests that the structurally similar antigen could elicit secondary B cell proliferation in previously primed adults.

Mucosal Immune Response

Genital colonization with group B streptococci may elicit specific antibody responses in cervical secretions. Women with group B streptococcal type Ia, II, or III rectal or cervical colonization have markedly elevated levels of both IgA and IgG to the colonizing serotype in their cervical secretions when compared with those in cervical secretions from non-colonized women. Elevated amounts of IgA and IgG to the protein antigen, R4, also have been found in women colonized with type III strains (most type III strains contain R4 antigen) compared with those in noncolonized women.[441,442] These findings suggest that a mucosal immune response occurs in response to colonization with group B streptococci. Induction of mucosal antibodies to surface group B streptococcal polysaccharide or protein antigens may prevent genital colonization, thereby diminishing vertical transmission of infection from mothers to infants.

Serum Opsonins

The interactions between antibodies to group B streptococcal capsular polysaccharides and serum complement components have been explored in detail. Shigeoka and co-workers[325] demonstrated that type-specific antibody was required for opsonization of type Ia, type II, and type III group B streptococci by adult and neonatal sera and that classic complement pathway participation was necessary for maximal opsonization of type I, type II, and several type III strains.[443] Capsular type–specific antibodies also facilitate alternative complement pathway–mediated opsonization and phagocytosis of type III group B streptococci.[332] A linear relationship between concentration of type III polysaccharide–specific antibodies and the rate constant of killing of type III strains has been reported.[444] Furthermore, the efficacy of these specific antibodies is determined, at least in part, by the number of antibody molecules that bind to each bacterium.[445]

Opsonic activity against type III group B streptococci has been shown in vitro for IgG subclasses 1, 2, and 3, as well as for IgM antibodies.[446-449] An IgA monoclonal antibody to the type III capsular polysaccharide activated C3 and conferred protection against lethal infection.[450] Type III–specific antibodies also facilitate C3 fragment deposition in the early phases of opsonization, although both encapsulated and genetically derived acapsular mutants can deposit C3 and support its degradation.[451] An inverse correlation between extent of encapsulation and C3 deposition by the alternative pathway has been verified.[452]

In contrast with these findings for type III strains, clinical isolates of type Ia group B streptococci can be efficiently opsonized, phagocytosed, and killed by neutrophils from healthy adults by the classic complement pathway in the absence of antibodies.[453] Surface-bound capsular polysaccharide of type Ia strains mediates C1 binding and activation.[454,455] Thus, an intact classic complement pathway is necessary for opsonization of clinical isolates of type Ia group B streptococci. For type Ib group B streptococci, a role for capsule size and density in modulating C3 deposition has been reported using a whole-bacterial-cell ELISA.[340] Variability among these strains in their capacity for C3 deposition by the alternative pathway also has been shown.[456]

The strain-to-strain variability in opsonization of type II strains of group B streptococci, originally identified by Shigeoka and associates,[325] has been confirmed. Type II strains possessing α and β components of the C protein antigen are more resistant to opsonization than are strains lacking both components.[344] Strains lacking type II polysaccharide but having both components of protein antigen C are readily opsonized. However, neither the presence of the C antigen components nor the concentration of type II polysaccharide–specific antibodies in a serum fully explains all strain variation. Contribution by other opsonically active antigens (e.g., R proteins) or an IgA-mediated blocking effect may modulate phagocytosis of some type II strains. The IgA receptor for group B streptococci is antigenically unrelated to that of group A streptococci, but it binds to the same region in IgA.[457,458] Despite the complexity of type II opsonins, it is clear that complement is essential for effective opsonophagocytosis and that integrity of the classic complement pathway is critical.

Evaluation of neutrophil-mediated killing of type IV and type V group B streptococci also reveals that complement and capsular polysaccharide–specific antibodies are participants in opsonophagocytosis.[459,460] When complement is limited, type-specific antibodies have an important role in facilitating killing. In sufficient concentration, however, the complement in agammaglobulinemic serum promotes opsonization, phagocytosis, and killing of type IV and type V group B streptococci.

Quantitative deficiencies of complement components from both the classic and the alternative complement pathways have been defined in sera from normal newborns, when compared with those of their mothers or with levels in healthy adults. Maturation occurs in an age-related fashion by 6 months of age.[461] Efficient function of the alternative pathway has been demonstrated in neonatal sera for a variety of bacteria, including group B streptococci.[462] Deficient classic pathway activity in newborn sera correlated significantly with low C4 and C1q levels; this could be corrected by addition of fresh-frozen plasma.[463] The results of the study by Baker and co-workers,[464] in which pregnant women were immunized with purified type III group B streptococcal polysaccharide, suggest that deficient function of the alternative pathway may be overcome in neonatal as in adult sera if the concentration of type III–specific antibodies is sufficient. Among infants surviving type III group B streptococcal meningitis, transient development of type-specific antibodies, predominantly of the IgM isotype, has been noted, and efficient opsonophagocytosis occurs during convalescence.[465] Once specific IgM concentrations decline, however, and despite maturation of complement synthesis to adult capacity, opsonophagocytosis of type III organisms is poor to nil.

During the course of septic shock caused by group B streptococci, complement components are consumed. Cairo and co-workers[466] found a significant association between low levels of total hemolytic complement and fatal outcome from neonatal sepsis related to a variety of bacterial pathogens, including group B streptococci. Recently, a critical role for C3 activation through the alternative pathway has been shown for potent group B streptococcus–induced TNF-α release.[467] This finding and the observation that complement-dependent uptake of capsular polysaccharide by marginal zone B cells appears necessary for an effective immune response to the capsular polysaccharide[468] may in part explain this observation. The β component of C protein also may bind human factor F, a negative regulator of complement activation, thereby evading complement attack.[469]

Phagocyte Function

The role of neutrophil function in host defense against group B streptococci has been explored extensively.[326] Group B streptococcal antigens incubated in the absence of serum may enhance neutrophil adherence to endothelial cells and may impair the influx of neutrophils to sites of infection, such as the alveoli.[470] This enhanced adherence to endothelium could contribute to the pulmonary edema and hypertension observed in early-onset group B streptococcal infection.[471] With granulocyte depletion, there is significant attenuation of the pulmonary hypertension and hypoxemia characterizing the early phase of experimental infection. Chemiluminescence responses elicited by a type III group B streptococcal strain were significantly depressed for neutrophils from infants with group B streptococcal infection compared with values for neutrophils from healthy infants or adults.[472] "Stressed" infants with infections caused by organisms other than group B streptococci or those with noninfectious illnesses similarly had depressed chemiluminescence responses.

Smith and associates[473] examined the role of complement receptors CR1 and CR3 in the opsonic recognition of type Ia and type III group B streptococci by neutrophils from healthy neonates and adults. Selective blockade of CR3 or of both CR1 and CR3 inhibited killing for each serotype by neutrophils from neonates. These experiments indicated the importance of CR function to opsonization, phagocytosis, and killing of group B streptococci by neutrophils. Whether deficient CR function contributes to susceptibility of neonates to invasive infection is not known. Of interest, a role for CR3 also has been shown in nonopsonic recognition of group B streptococci by macrophages.[474]

Yang and co-workers[475] carried out selective blockade of neutrophil receptors in experiments with type III group B streptococci opsonized with immune globulin. Antibodies to neutrophil Fc receptor III (FcR III) inhibited phagocytosis of opsonized bacteria to an extent exceeding that of CR3. Noya and colleagues[476] demonstrated a substantial role for neutrophil FcR II in mediating ingestion of type III group B streptococci opsonized in complement-inactivated serum. When CR function was allowed, FcR II participation no longer was requisite for occurrence of phagocytosis. Participation by FcR and CR in phagocytosis of group B streptococci by peritoneal macrophages also has been reported.[477]

Christensen and co-workers[363,365] and others[362] have addressed the explanations for the profound neutropenia often observed in fulminant group B streptococcal infection in neonates. The nearly maximal proliferative rate of granulocytic stem cells in noninfected neonatal animals led to the suggestion that neutrophil transfusion might improve the survival of human neonates with group B streptococcal infection in whom neutrophil storage pool depletion was documented.[362,466] In experimental infection with type III group B streptococci, monoclonal IgM antibody to type III polysaccharide stimulated the release of neutrophils from storage pools into the bloodstream and improved neutrophil migration to the site of infection.[478] This facilitation of neutrophil function by type III–specific antibody improved survival in animals only if the antibody was administered when neutrophil reserves were intact (very early in infection).[479] Antibody recipients did not become neutropenic and did not experience depletion of their neutrophil reserves. These and similar in vitro and in vivo studies using commercial preparations of immune globulin for intravenous administration[480-482] emphasize the importance of IgG in facilitating the neutrophil inflammatory response.

Reticuloendothelial clearance of opsonized group B streptococci also is less efficient in experimental infection of young animals,[483,484] as are lung macrophage postphagocytic oxidative metabolic responses.[301] An age-related impairment in clearance of group B streptococci from the lungs has been reported for infant compared with adult rats and for preterm compared with term animals.[300,485] Animal age is a more important determinant of bacterial elimination from the lung than is amount of polysaccharide capsule, although encapsulated strains are ingested less efficiently and in fewer numbers in infant rats than in adult rats.[486]

Other Factors Relating to Pathogenesis

Fibronectin is a high-molecular-weight glycoprotein that participates in adherence and functions as a nonspecific opsonin. The observation that septic neonates have significantly lower fibronectin levels than those of healthy age-matched controls stimulated evaluation of its possible role in the pathogenesis of group B streptococcal infection.[487] Soluble fibronectin binds poorly to group B streptococci in the absence of other opsonins.[488] Group B streptococci do adhere to immobilized fibronectin, however. Fibronectin also enhances ingestion by neutrophils, monocytes, or macrophages of group B streptococci opsonized with type-specific antibody[489-491] and may promote TNF-α production by macrophages.[492] It also has been shown that interaction of type III capsular polysaccharide with the lectin site of CR3 effectively triggers phagocytosis of type III organisms by nonimmune serum. Use of this mechanism provides a potential explanation for the infrequency with which invasive infection develops in susceptible persons exposed to group B streptococci.[493]

It has been hypothesized that some persons may have a genetically based predisposition to infection with group B streptococci. Grubb and co-workers[494] identified a surplus of people possessing G3m(5) and a deficit of those with G1m(1) among 34 Swedish mothers of infants with group B streptococcal disease. Thom and colleagues[495] found deficits of G1m(1) and Km(1) and an increased incidence of G2m(23) among mothers of infected infants. The distribution of allotypic markers may influence responses to protein and polysaccharide antigens. For example, G2m(23) is a marker of IgG_2, the subclass most often associated with brisk immune responses to polysaccharide antigens. Thus, there could be genetically determined explanations for the deficiency of IgG subclasses,[496] high IgM concentration with divergent ratio of IgG to IgM,[497,498] and the chronic colonization state without immunologic response[499] described among Swedish mothers of infants with group B streptococcal disease. However, in a study of U.S. women who delivered infants with invasive type III group B streptococcal disease, postpartum immunization with type III group B streptococcal polysaccharide elicited immune responses similar to those in control women.[464]

PATHOLOGY

The morphologic features characteristic of early-onset neonatal infection are dependent on the type and duration of exposure to group B streptococci before or during birth. Intrauterine death has been attributed to group B streptococcal infection,[293,500,501] and it may be a relatively common cause of mid-gestational fetal loss in women who have experienced either vaginal hemorrhage or septic abortion.[501,502] Increasing evidence indicates that fetal membrane infection with group B streptococci may result in spontaneous abortion or premature rupture of membranes or both, as suggested by Hood and associates in 1961.[503-505] Becroft and colleagues[506] noted histologic changes consistent with congenital pneumonia in live-born neonates whose autopsy lung cultures yielded group B streptococci. Six of 10 placentas available for examination showed amnionitis; in each of the six cases, the infant had had pneumonia and died within 36 hours of birth. The evidence was sufficient in four of six stillborn infants to suggest that death was a direct result of group B streptococcal amnionitis and intrauterine pneumonia. deSa and Trevenen[502] documented pneumonitis with pulmonary interstitial and intra-alveolar inflammatory exudates in each of 15 infants weighing less than 1000 g with intrauterine group B streptococcal infection. Six infants were stillborn, and nine died within 6 hours of birth. Placental examination revealed chorioamnionitis. In a nonhuman primate model of infection, intra-amniotic inoculation of group B streptococci elicited fulminant early-onset neonatal infection.[299] Transmission electron microscopy of lung tissue revealed group B streptococci within membrane-bound vacuoles of alveolar epithelial cells and interstitial fibroblasts. The presence of organisms within tissue macrophages of the liver, spleen, and brain documents rapid dissemination to other viscera.

The finding of a high frequency of associated amnionitis and early death is not always so striking. However, it is clear that amnionitis in association with early-onset group B streptococcal sepsis (1) is more frequently detected when death occurs shortly after birth, (2) is a common finding when membranes have been ruptured 24 hours or more before delivery,[295,502,503] and (3) can be clinically silent in some women. It is obvious that group B streptococci can enter the amniotic cavity through ruptured or intact membranes,[507] thus allowing fetal aspiration of infected fluid and subsequent pulmonary lesions or bacteremia, *without* eliciting a local inflammatory response or maternal signs of amniotic fluid infection.

Among neonates with fatal early-onset group B streptococcal infection, pulmonary lesions represent the predominant pathologic feature. The association between pulmonary inflammation and hyaline membrane formation was first noted by Franciosi and co-workers.[2] Subsequently, autopsy findings in early-onset disease indicated "atypical" pulmonary hyaline membranes in a majority of the cases,[2,294,295] a finding that corresponds with radiographic features consistent with hyaline membrane disease in about 50% of neonates with early-onset sepsis.[9] Morphologically, the distribution of these membranes may be typical of those found in hyaline membrane disease, but in neonates who survive more than 20 hours, it may be less uniform. Group B streptococci frequently are found within these membranes, which in some patients are composed almost entirely of streptococci, rendering them basophilic in hematoxylin and eosin preparations.[298] Katzenstein and colleagues[298] postulated that invasion of alveolar pneumatocytes and capillary endothelial cells by group B streptococci resulted in exudation of plasma proteins into the alveoli, deposition of fibrin, and hyaline membrane formation. Immune complex–mediated injury to the lung was proposed by Pinnas and associates[508] as a mechanism for the hyaline membrane formation in early-onset group B streptococcal pneumonia. These investigators demonstrated C3, IgG, and fibrin deposition in the lungs of infants with fatal early-onset group B streptococcal sepsis.

Histologic evidence for pneumonia is found in approximately 80% of patients with fatal early-onset group B streptococcal pneumonia diagnosed by chest radiography.[294,508,509] The radiographic pattern can be focal or extensive or lobular or bronchial, involving one or more lobes. The typical histologic features of congenital pneumonia (i.e., alveolar exudates composed of neutrophils, erythrocytes, and aspirated squamous cells, with edema and congestion) can be observed either independently or in association with hyaline membrane formation. In neonates with fulminant, rapidly fatal infection, the cellular inflammatory response is less pronounced. A consistent feature is an interstitial inflammatory exudate. Also noted is progressive atelectasis, which is prominent in infants surviving more than 20 hours. Group B streptococci have been detected in hyaline membranes, within the alveoli, or in the alveolar septa beneath the membranes in most neonates for whom the location has been specified. Pulmonary hemorrhage, ranging from focal interstitial to extensive intra-alveolar, has been a common finding at autopsy.

In central nervous system infection, age at onset predicts distinctive morphologic findings in the brain and meninges. In early-onset meningitis, little or no evidence of lepto-

Table 13–7 Features of Group B Streptococcal Disease in Neonates and Infants

Feature	Early-Onset (<7 days)	Late-Onset (≥7 days)	Late, Late-Onset
Median age at onset[10]	1 hour	27 days	>3 months
Incidence of prematurity	Increased	Not increased	Common
Maternal obstetric complications	Frequent (70%)	Uncommon	Varies
Common manifestations[9, 10, 245, 516]	Septicemia (25-40%)	Meningitis (30-40%)	Bacteremia without a focus (common)
	Meningitis (5-10%)	Bacteremia without focus (40-50%)	Bacteremia with a focus (occasional)
	Pneumonia (35-55%)	Osteoarthritis (5-10%)	
Serotypes isolated[52, 222, 245]	Ia, Ib, Ia/c (30%) II (30%) III (40% nonmeningeal; 80% meningeal isolates)	III (~75-80%)	Several
Mortality rate[9, 10, 516, 517]	5-10%	2-6%	Low

meningeal inflammation is seen in up to three quarters of reported cases,[2,246,311] although purulent meningitis may be observed occasionally. This lack of inflammatory response may be the result of rapidly progressive infection, with an interval of only a few hours from onset of clinical illness until death, or may reflect deficient host response to infection, or both mechanisms may be involved. Bacteria generally are found in large numbers, and perivascular inflammation, thrombosis in small vessels, and parenchymal hemorrhage frequently are noted.[311] In some preterm infants surviving septic shock caused by early-onset group B streptococcal infection, periventricular leukomalacia, a condition characterized by infarction of the white matter surrounding the lateral ventricles, develops.[510] Those infants with fatal late-onset meningitis almost always have diffuse purulent leptomeningitis, especially at the base of the brain, with or without perivascular inflammation and hemorrhage.[2,511] In infants with severe meningitis who survive, multiple areas of necrosis and abscess formation may be found throughout the brain by neuroimaging or at later autopsy.

This age-related inflammatory response in infants with group B streptococcal infection has a parallel in the infant rat model of meningitis.[396] In infant rats 5 to 10 days of age, numerous bacteria distributed in a perivascular pattern are present, and in some animals, organisms extend transmurally into vessel lumina. These animals generally have no evidence of acute inflammation or edema in the leptomeninges. By contrast, 11- to 15-day-old animals have leptomeningitis and cerebritis characterized by a pronounced infiltration of neutrophils and macrophages around meningeal vessels and in perivascular spaces within the cerebral cortex. Because host response to infection becomes more efficient within a few weeks after birth, the absence of inflammation in the brain and meninges of infant rats as well as of human neonates with early-onset group B streptococcal infection may relate to chemotactic defects,[326] exhaustion of neutrophil stores,[365,512] immaturity of the reticuloendothelial system,[483] or other deficits in the host response to infection.

CLINICAL MANIFESTATIONS AND OUTCOME

Early-Onset Infection

When the incidence of neonatal infection caused by group B streptococci rose dramatically in the 1970s,[513] a bimodal distribution of cases according to age at onset of signs became apparent. Thus, two syndromes related to age were described in 1973 by Franciosi and associates[2] (acute and delayed) and by Baker and colleagues[245] (early and late). Early-onset infection almost always manifests itself within 24 hours of birth (an estimated 90% of cases; median age, 8 hours), but it may appear during the second 24 hours of life (an estimated 5% of cases) or at any time during the subsequent 5 days.[9,245,514] Premature infants often experience onset at or within 6 hours of birth; when onset is after the first 24 hours infants usually are term gestation.[292,407] Late-onset infections occur at 7 to 90 days of age (median age, 27 days).[9] Although this classification of syndromes by age at onset has been useful to enhance our understanding of the pathogenesis of infection, there is a continuum in age at onset. A few patients with early-onset disease may present at 5 or 6 days of age, and very late-onset infection occasionally affects 3- to 7-month-old infants, especially those with gestational age of less than 28 weeks.[9,245] Onset beyond 6 months of age may herald the presentation of human immunodeficiency virus (HIV) infection or other immune system abnormalities.[515]

Early-onset group B streptococcal infection often affects neonates whose mothers have obstetric complications associated with risk for neonatal sepsis (onset of labor before 37 weeks of gestation, prolonged interval at any gestation between rupture of membranes and delivery, rupture of membranes 18 or more hours before delivery, intrapartum fever, chorioamnionitis, early postpartum febrile morbidity, and twin births) (Table 13-7). A nearly threefold risk of early-onset group B streptococcal disease has occurred when six or more vaginal examnations are performed before delivery.[518] The incidence of infection correlates inversely with the degree of prematurity, and a contemporary report reveals that the group B streptococcus is the most frequent pathogen associated with early-onset sepsis in neonates of very low birth weight (less than 1500 g).[519] Early-onset group B streptococcal infection often develops in term neonates with no defined maternal risk factors other than colonization. In such cases, diagnosis and treatment often are delayed until the appearance of definite signs of sepsis (fever, tachypnea, apnea, hypotension), but more subtle signs usually precede these clinical manifestations. One recent report found that one third of healthy term neonates with early-onset group B streptococcal infection were identified solely on the basis of evaluation for maternal intrapartum temperature exceeding 100.4° F.[520]

The three most common manifestations of early-onset infection are septicemia (signs of sepsis in association with bacteremia *without* a defined focus of infection), pneumonia, and meningitis. Septicemia without a focus occurs in 25% to 40%, pneumonia in 35% to 55%, and meningitis in 5% to 10% of cases.[9,10,245,517,519] Bacteremia often is detected in neonates with the latter two presentations. Irrespective of site of involvement, respiratory signs (apnea, grunting respirations, tachypnea, or cyanosis) are the initial clinical findings in more than 80% of neonates. Hypotension is an initial finding in approximately 25%. Infants with fetal asphyxia related to group B streptococcal infection in utero may have shock and respiratory failure at delivery.[511,516] Other associated signs include lethargy, poor feeding, hypothermia or fever, abdominal distention, pallor, tachycardia, and jaundice. Five percent to 10% of neonates with early-onset infection have meningitis.[9,10,162,516,517] Neonates with meningitis often have a clinical presentation identical to those without meningeal involvement. In one study, respiratory distress was the most common initial sign, and among 27 infants with early-onset meningitis, seizures were never a presenting feature.[521] Examination of CSF is the only means to exclude meningitis, a finding that requires modification of supportive and specific chemotherapy (see "Treatment" later on). Seizures occur during the first 24 hours of therapy in nearly 50% of infants with meningitis. Persistent seizures, semicoma, or coma is associated with a poor prognosis.[245,522,523]

Pulmonary involvement occurs in 35% to 55% of patients with early-onset infection, and virtually all of these infants have acute respiratory signs (grunting, tachypnea, apnea). Of 175 neonates with pulmonary involvement, 84% had respiratory signs in the first few hours of life (many at birth), and in an additional 11%, these signs developed within the first 24 hours of life.[292,294,295,298,524] Among 19 infants with congenital pneumonia at autopsy, 89% had 1-minute Apgar scores of 4 or less, indicating in utero onset of infection.[292] Radiographically, features consistent with and indistinguishable from those of hyaline membrane disease are present in more than one half of neonates with group B streptococcal bacteremia and pulmonary infection (Fig. 13-6). Treatment with surfactant improves gas exchange in a majority of these infants, although the response is slower than in noninfected infants, and repeated surfactant doses often are needed.[525] Infiltrates suggesting congenital pneumonia (Fig. 13-7) are present in one third. Increased vascular markings suggesting the diagnosis of transient tachypnea of the newborn or pulmonary edema can occur. Occasionally, respiratory distress is present in the absence of radiographic abnormalities, appearing as persistent fetal circulation.[509,526] Small pleural effusions and cardiomegaly also have been described.[509,527]

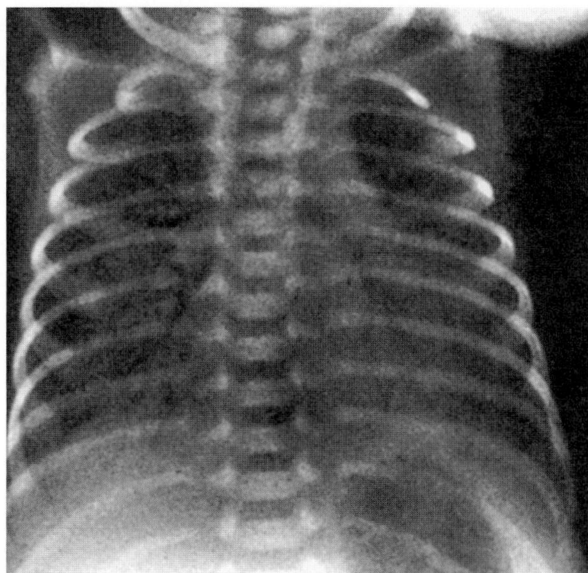

Figure 13–6 Chest radiograph from an infant with early-onset group B streptococcal septicemia showing features consistent with respiratory distress syndrome of the newborn.

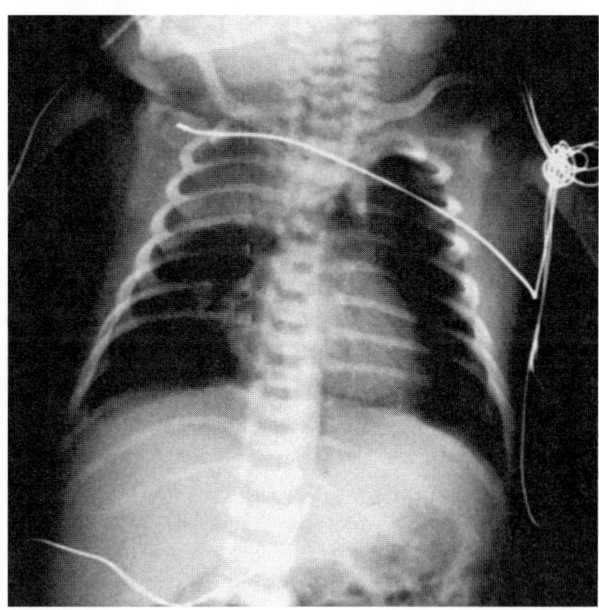

Figure 13–7 Chest radiograph demonstrating right upper and lower lobe infiltrates as manifestations of early-onset group B streptococcal pneumonia in an infant.

The case-fatality rate for the nearly 300 neonates with early-onset infection summarized by Anthony and Okada[513] in 1977 was 55%. More recent reports[9,516,517] suggest lower rates, ranging from 2% to 10%. Features associated with fatal outcome include a low 5-minute Apgar score, shock, neutropenia, pleural effusion, apnea, and delay in treatment after the onset of symptoms.[10,516,527] Fatal infection also occurs significantly more often among premature than among term neonates (Table 13-8). Pyati and colleagues[530] reported a fatality rate of 61% among 101 neonates who had early-onset group B streptococcal infection. However, infants with a birth weight in excess of 1500 g had a fatality rate of 14%. Recent data suggest a 15-fold increase when infants with a gestational age of 33 weeks or less are compared with term infants.[22] A contemporary case-fatality rate of 42% was reported for infants weighing less than 2500 g at birth. This was significantly higher than the case-fatality rate of 7% among infants who weighed 2500 grams or more at birth.[162]

Table 13–8 Fatality Rates in Early-Onset Group B Streptococcal Infection

	Fatality Rate (%) by Birth Weight (g) or Gestational Age				
Study	**500-1000**	**1001-1500**	**1501-2000**	**2001-2500**	**>2500**
Boyer et al[528] (1973-1981)	90	25	29	33	3
Baker[529] (1982-1989)	60	25	26	18	5
Weisman et al[516] (1987-1989)	75	40	20	15	6
Schrag et al[22] (1993-1998)		30 (≤33 wk)		10 (34-36 wk)	2 (≥37 wk)

Late-Onset Infection

Late-onset group B streptococcal infection typically affects the term infant from 7 days to 90 days of age. Such infants frequently have an unremarkable early neonatal history, although late-onset disease may occur in premature infants.[247,529] One report found that group B streptococci accounted for 2% of late-onset sepsis episodes in very low birth weight neonates.[531] Late-onset disease has a lower fatality rate (2% to 6%) than that of early-onset disease,[22,516,517,532] and meningitis is a frequent clinical manifestation (occurring in an estimated 35% to 40% of cases). Serotype III strains are isolated from two thirds to three quarters of patients, irrespective of focus of infection.[12] An exception to the usual pattern for late-onset infection is in the neonatal intensive care unit setting, where prematurity can dominate as a risk factor and where clusters of nosocomially acquired disease among low-birth-weight infants may occur.[219,517,531] In these infants, the spectrum of clinical expression is similar to that in early-onset disease, and serotypes other than type III have been implicated.

The initial signs in infants with late-onset meningitis almost always include fever, irritability or lethargy or both, poor feeding, and tachypnea. Upper respiratory tract infection precedes late-onset meningitis in 20% to 30% of infants, suggesting that alteration of mucosal barriers might facilitate entry of group B streptococci into the bloodsream.[2,3,245] In contrast with early-onset infection, grunting respirations and apnea are less frequent initial findings, and their presence suggests a more rapidly progressive, fulminant infection. Apnea or hypotension is observed in less than 15% of patients, but there is a spectrum in clinical severity of illness at presentation. Some neonates with late-onset meningitis are clinically well a few hours before their initial hospital evaluation, when they are noted to have seizures, poor perfusion, neutropenia, and large numbers of gram-positive cocci in the CSF. Such patients often have a rapidly fatal course, or if they survive, they are left with devastating neurologic sequelae. Leukopenia or neutropenia at the time of admission has been correlated with fatal outcome in such infants.[527] Other admission findings associated with increased risk for fatal outcome or permanent neurologic sequelae include hypotension, coma or semicoma, status epilepticus, an absolute neutrophil count of less than 1000/mm^3, a CSF protein level exceeding 300 mg/dL, and a high concentration of type III group B streptococcal antigen in CSF.[245,513,527] This last prognostic factor and the observation indicating prolonged antigenuria in meningitis survivors who are left with neurologic abnormalities probably reflect a larger bacterial inoculum in the CSF than is found in that of survivors with a normal outcome. Subdural effusions, which usually are small, unilateral, and asymptomatic, are found in up to 20% of patients with late-onset meningitis. These are not associated with any permanent sequelae.[9,516] Subdural empyema as a complication is rare.[533]

The outcomes with meningeal infection are based on reports of infants cared for nearly 20 years ago. Whether or not the prognosis has improved must await additional data. Of greater than 200 neonates with early- or late-onset meningitis, one quarter died in the hospital as the direct result of meningitis.[245,521-523] A substantial number of survivors (25% to 50%) had permanent neurologic sequelae of variable severity. In three series assessing a total of 112 survivors at mean intervals ranging from 2 to 8 years after diagnosis, major neurologic sequelae were observed in 21% of children. The most serious of these included profound mental retardation, spastic quadriplegia, cortical blindness, deafness, uncontrolled seizures, hydrocephalus, and hypothalamic dysfunction with poor thermal regulation and central diabetes insipidus.[521,523,534,535] Mild or moderate sequelae persisted in 21% of survivors evaluated at a mean of 6 years after diagnosis.[523] These problems included profound unilateral sensorineural hearing loss, borderline mental retardation, spastic or flaccid monoparesis, and expressive or receptive speech and language delay. In a sibling-controlled follow-up study, Wald and co-workers[535] found that the psychometric performance did not differ significantly for children who had had group B streptococcal meningitis and their siblings. More postmeningitis children than control children had seizure disorders and hydrocephalus that required shunting procedures, but they were functioning in a manner comparable with that of their siblings. More subtle deficits such as delayed language development and mild hearing loss may not be detected by routine examination,[523] and all patients should undergo auditory brain-stem evoked response testing during convalescence as well as careful long-term neurologic and developmental assessments.

Bacteremia without a detectable focus of infection now is the most common clinical expression of late-onset group B streptococcal disease.[536] Osteomyelitis, septic arthritis, cellulitis, and adenitis are less frequent manifestations of late-onset disease. The infant with bacteremia without a focus typically has an uncomplicated perinatal course and presents

Table 13–9 **Clinical Features of Group B Streptococcal Bone and Joint Infections**[a]

Feature	Septic Arthritis without Osteomyelitis (20 Patients)[4, 415, 544-549]	Osteomyelitis (45 Patients)[4, 541-544, 550-561]
Mean age at diagnosis (range)	20 days (5-37)	31 days (8-60)
Mean duration of symptoms (range)	1.5 days (<1-3)	9 days (1-28)
Male-to-female ratio	2:5	2:3
Site (%)	Hip (56) Knee (38) Ankle (6)	Humerus (56) Femur (24) Tibia, talus (4) Other[b] (16)
Group B streptococcal serotype (no. of patients)	III (12)	III (15), Ib/c (3), Ia/c (1)
Mean duration of parenteral therapy (range)	2 wk (2-3)	3 wk (1-6)

[a]Includes authors' unpublished data for seven patients.
[b]Ilium, acromion, clavicle, skull, digit, vertebrae; ribs—one patient each.

with nonspecific signs (fever, poor feeding, irritability, rhinorrhea) in either an inpatient or an outpatient setting. Diagnosis results from the practice of obtaining blood cultures in febrile infants in the first few weeks of life to exclude serious bacterial infection as an underlying cause. These infants are mildly ill, but failure to initiate antimicrobial therapy *before* the availability of blood culture findings can result in extension of infection to distant sites such as the central nervous system. Both transient and persistent bacteremia have been described in symptomatic and healthy patients.[4,537,538] Fatal outcome has not been reported among patients with late-onset bacteremia without a focus, and survivors recover without sequelae after treatment.

Late, Late-Onset Infection

One report suggests that infections in infants older than 3 months of age account for 20% of cases of late-onset disease.[517] The terms *very late onset*, *late late-onset*, and *beyond early infancy* have been applied to disease in these infants. Most of these infants have a gestational age of less than 35 weeks. The need for prolonged hospitalization and its attendant monitoring, as well as the immature host status of these infants, probably contributes to infection beyond the interval for term neonates. Bacteremia without a focus is a common presentation. Occasionally a focus for infection, such as the central nervous system, intravascular catheter, or soft tissues, is identified (see Table 13-7). In the outpatient setting, infants older than 3 months of age are likely to have a temperature higher than 39° C and a white blood cell count exceeding 15,000/mm^3.[536] When there are no other apparent risk factors, immune deficiency including HIV infection should be considered in the setting of a very late-onset infection.[539,540]

Septic Arthritis and Osteomyelitis

Group B streptococcal bone and joint infection has an indolent onset and a good prognosis. Less than 20% of affected infants demonstrate poor feeding,[541] respiratory distress,[542] meconium aspiration,[543] or mild elevation of serum bilirubin levels during the early neonatal period.[544] Manipulations known to predispose neonates to bone and joint infection caused by other pathogens (heel or needle puncture, umbilical vessel catheterization, exchange transfusion) have not been reported.

The clinical features of 20 infants with arthritis alone and 45 with osteomyelitis (with or without concomitant septic arthritis) related to group B streptococci are summarized in Table 13-9. The mean age at diagnosis of osteomyelitis (31 days) is greater than that for septic arthritis (20 days) or other manifestations of late-onset disease (27 days). In septic arthritis, the onset is acute (mean duration of clinical signs, 1.5 days), whereas in osteomyelitis, the course is often protracted (mean, 9 days). In some infants with osteomyelitis, failure to move the involved extremity since hospital discharge after birth, or shortly thereafter, may be noted; this lack of movement may persist for as long as 4 weeks before the diagnosis is made.[550]

Decreased motion of the involved extremity and evidence of pain with manipulation, such as lifting or diaper changing, are the most common signs of group B streptococcal bone or joint infection. Inflammatory signs (warmth or redness) occasionally are described[556,557]; a history of fever is reported in only 20% of infants. Lack of signs suggesting infection and the finding of pseudoparalysis has led to an initial diagnosis of Erb's palsy and to assessment for possible child abuse.[541,550,561] In several infants, findings on nerve conduction studies were consistent with brachial plexus neuropathy associated with group B streptococcal osteomyelitis of the proximal humerus,[558,562] and in one infant, sciatic nerve injury at the level of the pelvis caused footdrop as a result of iliac osteomyelitis.[563]

Signs frequently observed include fixed flexion of the involved extremity, mild swelling, evidence of pain with passive motion, decreased spontaneous movement, and, in a minority of infants, erythema and warmth. Lack of associated systemic involvement is the rule, although osteomyelitis in association with meningitis, peritonitis, and overwhelming sepsis with congestive heart failure has been reported.[541,544,557,559,564]

When infants with septic arthritis alone are compared with those with osteomyelitis, those with septic arthritis more often have lower extremity involvement, with the hip joint predominating.[544,548] By contrast, over one half of the reported infants with osteomyelitis have had exclusive involvement of the humerus, and in those for whom the location was specified, the proximal humerus was affected in greater than 90%.[541,544,550,554] Osteomyelitis involving both proximal humeri has been described.[559] The next most common site of involvement is the femur, and small, flat, and vertebral bone infections occur occasionally.[565,566] Single bone involvement predominates for group B streptococcal osteomyelitis, although infection involving two adjacent bones or multiple nonadjacent bones has been described.[542,551,559] The rarity of multiple bone involvement contrasts with its common occurrence (estimated at 70%) in neonatal osteomyelitis caused by *S. aureus* or gram-negative enteric bacilli. Although most infants with humeral osteomyelitis have had concomitant infection in the shoulder joint, isolated septic arthritis of the shoulder joint has not been reported.

Impaired function after neonatal osteomyelitis caused by bacteria other than group B streptococci occurs in one fourth to one third of patients. By contrast, in 17 (90%) of 19 infants with group B streptococcal osteomyelitis evaluated 6 months to 4 years after diagnosis, no functional impairment of the affected extremity was found.[4,543,544,546,550,556,558,559] Residual shortening and limitation of motion of the humerus were noted in a patient who had overwhelming sepsis of acute onset, with congestive heart failure and osteomyelitis involving noncontiguous sites.[544] Growth disturbance can result as a consequence of subluxation of the hip joint.

Although both septic arthritis and osteomyelitis are considered manifestations of late-onset disease, osteomyelitis may represent a clinically silent early-onset bacteremia with secondary spread to a metaphysis and then late-onset expression of infection. An episode of asymptomatic bacteremia with a birth trauma–induced nidus in the proximal humerus could allow localization of bacteria to the bone. Because lytic lesions take more than 10 days to become radiographically visible, the presence of such lesions on radiographs obtained at hospital admission is suggestive of long-standing disease (Fig. 13-8). Also, non–type III strains are overrepresented among infants with osteomyelitis. These findings are consistent with the hypothesis that, in at least some patients, early-onset acquisition may have occurred.

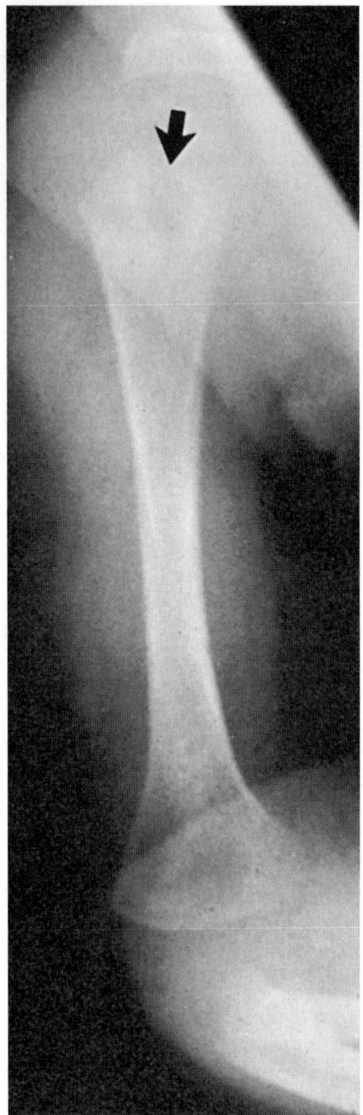

Figure 13–8 Radiograph showing a lytic lesion (*arrow*) of the proximal humerus in an infant whose bone biopsy demonstrated osteomyelitis caused by type III group B streptococci.

Cellulitis or Adenitis

The manifestation of late-onset group B streptococcal infection designated facial cellulitis,[567] submandibular cellulitis,[568] cellulitis/adenitis,[569] or lymphadenitis[570] has been reported in at least 25 infants.[571-574] Presenting signs include poor feeding, irritability, fever, and unilateral facial, preauricular, or submandibular swelling, usually but not always accompanied by erythema. The mean age at onset is 5 weeks (range, 2 to 11 weeks), and in contrast with all other patients with group B streptococcal infection, there is a striking male predominance (72%). The most common sites are the submandibular and parotid areas, and enlarged adjacent nodes become palpable within 2 days after onset of the soft tissue infection. Four of the five infants with facial or submandibular cellulitis described by Baker[569] had ipsilateral otitis media at the time of diagnosis. Less common sites of involvement with cellulitis are the face, preauricular or inguinal areas, scrotum, anterior neck region, and prepatellar spaces (Fig. 13-9).[569,573,574] In one patient, cellulitis of the neck occurred in association with an infected thyroglossal duct cyst.[569]

Bacteremia almost always is detected in these infants (92%), and cultures of soft tissue or lymph node aspirates have yielded group B streptococci in 83% of the children in whom aspiration was performed. These patients usually are not seriously ill, few have associated meningitis, and recovery within a few days of initiation of appropriate antimicrobial therapy is the rule. However, fulminant and fatal facial cellulitis has been described in a 7-hour-old neonate[4] and associated meningitis in two infants.[575]

Unusual Manifestations of Infection

A number of uncommon clinical manifestations of early- and late-onset group B streptococcal infection have been recorded (Table 13-10). Peritonitis[576] and adrenal abscess[577-579] have been described as abdominal manifestations of early-

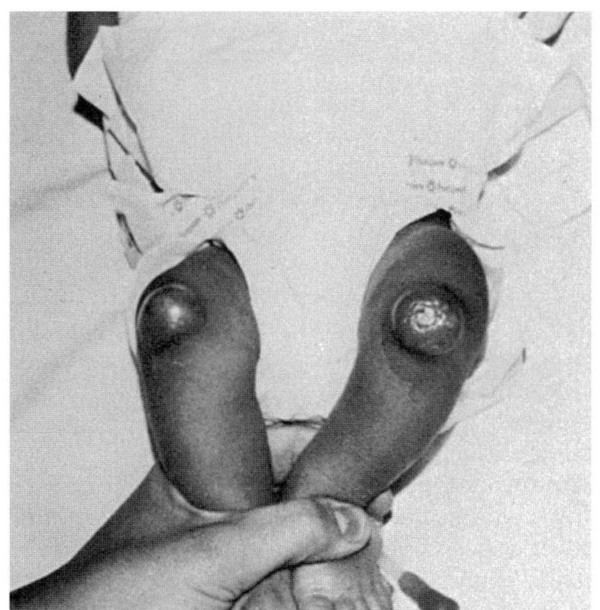

Figure 13–9 Prepatellar bursitis of both knees in an infant who had abraded his knees on the bedsheets. Aspiration of purulent material from the prepatellar space yielded type III group B streptococci. The knee joints were not affected.

and late-onset infection. Adrenal abscess is thought to be the result of bacteremic seeding associated with adrenal hemorrhage and subsequent abscess formation. One neonate thought to have neuroblastoma underwent en bloc resection of a large mass with nephrectomy before the diagnosis of adrenal abscess was established.[578] Gallbladder distention is a nonspecific manifestation of early-onset sepsis that usually resolves with medical management.[580] Late-onset bacteremia can occur in association with jaundice, elevated levels of liver enzymes, and increased direct-reacting bilirubin fraction. Possibly, hemolysis and "toxic" hepatocellular damage contribute to the development of jaundice. Underlying liver disease, a known predisposing factor for development of group B streptococcal bacteremia in adults, was suggested as an explanation for group B streptococcal bacteremia in a 22-month-old child.[628]

Brain abscess rarely occurs in association with recurrence of group B streptococcal meningitis. One infant recovered after craniotomy and excision of a well-encapsulated frontal mass but had neurologic sequelae.[581] Sokol and colleagues[583] described a 5-week-old infant with a cerebellar cyst believed to represent an astrocytoma. This infant proved to have obstructive hydrocephalus and chronic group B streptococcal ventriculitis. Rarely, anterior fontanelle herniation may complicate severe meningitis. The presence of a noncystic doughy mass over the fontanelle indicates that brain herniation may have occurred, and head ultrasonography or computed tomography may be used for confirmation. This finding is a poor prognostic sign.[582] One patient with cervical myelopathy initially had absence of extremity movement but made a good recovery and was able to walk at age 3 years.[585] Another unusual complication of group B streptococcal meningitis is subdural empyema, which has been described in patients with both early- and late-onset infections.[533,534] The diagnosis was established by needle aspiration of the subdural space at the time of hospital admission[534] or within the first 5 days of treatment. Irritability, vomiting, seizures, increasing head circumference, focal neurologic signs, a tense anterior fontanelle, or a combination of these prompted evaluation.[533,629] Sterilization of the subdural space was accomplished by drainage, open or closed, in conjunction with antimicrobial therapy. Basal ganglia and massive cerebral infarction also have been described.[584]

Cardiovascular manifestations of group B streptococcal infection are rare. However, endocarditis,[219,564,589,590] pericarditis,[591] myocarditis,[543] and mycotic aneurysm of the aorta[592] have been documented. Echocardiography has been useful in determining the nature of cardiac involvement, and this technique was employed successfully to delineate a 0.7-cm vegetation on the anterior leaflet of the mitral valve in a 4-week-old infant with endocarditis caused by a serotype III strain.[564] Paroxysmal atrial tachycardia may be a presenting feature of group B streptococcal bacteremia in the absence of focal infection of the heart.[9]

Group B streptococci are an uncommon cause of otitis media in the first few weeks of life (2% to 3% of cases).[594] However, otitis media is not infrequently associated with late-onset disease manifesting as meningitis or submandibular cellulitis.[593,595,596] The finding of acute mastoiditis at autopsy in one infant with otitis media and meningitis suggests that the middle ear may serve as a portal of entry in some patients.[596]

Conjunctivitis related to group B streptococci occurs with such rarity that no cases were identified among 302 neonates with ophthalmia neonatorum described by Armstrong and associates.[597] However, exudative conjunctivitis has been reported in association with early-onset bacteremia.[597] More severe ocular involvement is rare, but endophthalmitis has been noted in infants with bacteremia and meningitis.[599,600] As is the case for other agents producing endophthalmitis, high-grade bacteremia is a likely prelude to this unusual metastatic focus of group B streptococcal infection.

Supraglottitis was described in a 3-month-old infant with acute onset of stridor.[604] Swelling of the left aryepiglottic fold but not the epiglottis was noted at laryngoscopy. An infant with bacterial tracheitis had a similar presentation.[607] Although pulmonary infection caused by group B streptococci is common, pleural involvement is rare, but it has been reported as a complication of both early-onset[606] and late-onset[605] pneumonia. An interesting but as-yet inexplicable association is that of delayed development of right-sided diaphragmatic hernia and early-onset group B streptococcal sepsis.[602,603,630,631] In affected infants, the onset of respiratory distress invariably occurs at or within hours of birth, whereas the mean age at diagnosis of right-sided diaphragmatic hernia is 12 days (range, 3 to 35 days).[602] Ashcraft and associates[602] postulate that the insufficient diaphragmatic motion predisposes a neonate with peripartum exposure to group B streptococci to the development of pneumonia and that subsequent respiratory effort accounts for the ultimate herniation of viscera into the pleural space. This phenomenon should be remembered and considered in the infant with group B streptococcal infection whose condition continues to deteriorate despite appropriate management. Radiographic features include increased density in the right lower lung or

Table 13–10 Unusual Clinical Manifestations of Group B Streptococcal Infections

Site and Manifestation	Associated with Early- or Late-Onset Infection	Reference Nos.
Abdomen		
Peritonitis	Both	576
Adrenal abscess	Both	577-579
Gallbladder distention	Early	580
Brain		
Abscess	Late	581
Anterior fontanelle herniation	Both	582
Chronic meningitis	Late	583
Subdural empyema	Both	533, 534
Cerebritis	Late	584
Myelopathy/myelitis	Early	585, 586
Ventriculitis complicating myelomeningocele	Both	587
Cardiovascular		
Asymptomatic bacteremia	Both	4, 276, 537, 538
Endocarditis	Both	219, 564, 588-590
Pericarditis	Not listed	591
Myocarditis	Late	543
Mycotic aneurysm	Late	592
Ear and sinus		
Ethmoiditis	Late	4
Otitis media/mastoiditis	Both	569, 593-596
Eye		
Conjunctivitis/ophthalmia neonatorum	Early	2, 597, 598
Endophthalmitis	Late	599, 600
Retrobulbar abscess	Early	601
Respiratory Tract		
Diaphragmatic hernia	Both	602, 603
Supraglottitis	Late	604
Pleural empyema	Both	4, 605, 606
Tracheitis	Late	607
Skin and soft tissue		
Abscess of cystic hygroma	Late	608
Breast abscess	Late	609, 610
Bursitis	Late	611
Cellulitis/adenitis	Both	4, 529, 567-571, 612, 613
Dactylitis	Late	614
Fasciitis	Late	615-617
Impetigo neonatorum	Early	618, 619
Purpura fulminans	Both	620, 621
Omphalitis	Both	511, 622
Rhabdomyolysis	Late	623
Retropharyngeal cellulitis	Late	624, 625
Scalp abscess	Both	626
Urinary tract infection	Both	517, 627

irregular aeration or both, followed by progression to elevation of right bowel gas and liver shadow.

In addition to cellulitis and adenitis, group B streptococci uncommonly can produce a variety of unusual skin and soft tissue manifestations. These include violaceous cellulitis,[632] perineal cellulitis and septicemia after circumcision,[633] scrotal ecchymosis as a sign of intraperitoneal hemorrhage,[613] purpura fulminans,[620,621] necrotizing fasciitis,[615-617] impetigo neonatorum,[618,619] omphalitis,[511,622] scalp abscess secondary to fetal scalp electrode,[626] abscess complicating cystic hygroma,[608] retropharyngeal cellulitis[624,625] and breast abscess.[609] In patients with impetiginous lesions and abscess formation, bacteremia is unusual, but it is a frequent accompaniment to omphalitis and necrotizing fasciitis.

Among infants with early-onset bacteremia, isolation of group B streptococci from the urine is frequent when this body fluid is cultured, but primary urinary tract infection with these organisms is rare. An infant with severe bilateral ureterohydronephrosis and group B streptococci in his urine has been decribed.[627] The isolation of group B streptococci from a urine culture of a patient *without bacteremia* is an indication for evaluation for possible structural anomalies of the genitourinary tract.

Sudden death occurred in three infants ranging from 3 to 8 months of age. The deaths were attributed at the time of autopsy to group B streptococcal infection.[500]

Relapse or Recurrence of Infection

Recurrent infection has been reported in an estimated 0.5% to 3% of infants[572,581,612,633-640] in whom signs developed either during treatment or after an interval of 3 to 101 days after completion of antibiotic therapy. In one retrospective review, eight of nine infants were born at 25 to 36 weeks of gestation, and male infants predominated.[639] The first episode occurred at a mean age of 10 days (range, 1 to 27), and recurrence was noted at a mean age of 42 days (range, 23 to 68 days). In a recent report that included a set of fraternal twins, seven of eight infants were born before 37 weeks of gestation (mean 30 weeks), and each had a birth weight of less than 2500 g.[641] Each of the infections was late-onset. The mean age at initial presentation was 38 days (range, 13 to 112), and recurrence occurred at a mean age of 57 days (range, 34 to 130 days). Two separate episodes have been documented in several infants.[637,640,642,643] In some cases, circumstances that potentially predisposed the infant to relapse or reinfection were reported (maternal mastitis, protracted focal seizures in an infant with a brain abscess,[581,644] endocarditis with underlying congenital heart disease[634]). Identical isolates were recovered from the maternal genital and breast milk cultures, suggesting that breast-feeding might have been the source of repeated exposure both when signs of mastitis were noted and when the mother had no clinical features of mastitis.[640,645] Recurrent infection usually has a clinical expression similar to that of the initial episode, but some affected infants have had new sites of involvement with the relapse or recurrence (meninges, ventricular or subdural fluid, or both[634,636,637]; brain parenchyma[581]; and soft tissue[572,612]). In most patients, the second episode of group B streptococcal disease was treated in a similar manner with a β-lactam antibiotic, most often penicillin or ampicillin, but typically the duration was longer.[641]

One possible explanation for some early reports of relapse or recurrence was failure to administer penicillin G or ampicillin at an optimal dosage or for a sufficient duration. In two patients, penicillin-tolerant organisms were isolated at the time of the second infection[581,634]; isolates from the initial episode were not available for susceptibility testing. Because the finding of in vitro penicillin tolerance is not uncommon among group B streptococcal isolates (estimated at 4%[645]), the relationship between tolerance and relapse is unknown, and it is suggested that the phenomenon of penicillin tolerance may be one factor contributing to persistent mucosal carriage (see "Treatment" later on).[646]

Because infants who receive treatment for invasive infection frequently remain colonized with group B streptococci at mucous membrane sites, pharyngeal or gastrointestinal colonization may be the source for another episode of bacteremia. In addition, among infants recovering from invasive infection with type III strains, protective levels of antibody infrequently develop during convalescence. Moylett and colleagues[641] and others[643] used restriction endonuclease analysis to document that isolates from patients with recurrent episodes of group B streptococcal disease in an infant were identical and were derived from a single clone. Sets of isolates analyzed from first and second episodes and from maternal and infant colonizing and invasive strains were genotypically identical using pulsed-field gel electrophoresis.[639,641] Thus, recurrent infection in most infants results from reinvasion from persistently colonized mucous membrane sites or reexposure to a household carrier. However, a minority of infants encounter a new strain and have a second episode based on exposure other than maternal.

Maternal Infections Caused by Group B Streptococci

In 1938, Fry[1] described three fatal cases of endocarditis in postpartum women. This finding was the first indication that the group B streptococcus was a human pathogen and could cause puerperal infection. For the next several decades, additional postpartum infections including septic abortion, bacteremia, chorioamnionitis, endometritis, pneumonia, and septic arthritis were recorded sporadically.[503,647,648] However, before 1970, group B streptococcal infection in the postpartum woman, as in the neonate, was uncommon.[9] The increase in neonatal infections during the past 4 decades has been paralleled by an increasing number of infections in adults.[5,7,506] It is now obvious that group B streptococci constitute a significant common cause of febrile morbidity in pregnant women.

Before institution of intrapartum antibiotic prophylaxis, group B streptococci accounted for 10% to 20% of blood culture isolates from febrile women on obstetric services.[6,9] These women have a clinical picture generally characterized by fever, malaise, moderate uterine tenderness with normal lochia, and occasionally chills. A detailed study of group B streptococcal infection in postpartum patients was reported by Faro.[7] Forty women with endometritis and endoparametritis related to group B streptococci were observed among 3106 women giving birth over a 12-month interval, an incidence of 1.3 per 1000 deliveries. The diagnosis was established by isolation of group B streptococci from the endometrium either alone (in 35% of the cases) or in addition to other organisms; one third of the women had concomitant bacteremia. In many (94%) of these women, infection developed after cesarean section. Fever characteristically developed early in the postpartum course (mean time to onset, 11.7 hours; range, 1 to 24 hours). Additional clinical features included chills, tachycardia, abdominal distention, and exquisite uterine, parametrial, or adnexal tenderness. Temperature of 38.5° C or higher correlated with an increased risk of concomitant bacteremia. Recovery was uniform after administration of one of a number of antimicrobial agents to which group B streptococci were susceptible. However, group B streptococcal septicemia developed in 6 (13.3%) of 45 infants delivered to these women, and fatal infection occurred in 3. Febrile morbidity in a mother can be the single early clue of bacteremic infection in her neonate,[7,9] and the infants of such women should be carefully evaluated.

The contemporary incidence of invasive disease in pregnant women is 0.2 to 0.3 per 1000 live births.[22,162] This incidence has declined significantly in association with implementation of recommendations for maternal antibiotic prophylaxis to prevent early-onset neonatal disease. Bacteremia is the primary manifestation of infection, accounting for 64% of cases in one series.[22] Bacteremia in association with chorioamnionitis or endometritis each occurred in 10% of cases, and septic abortion in 7%. Maternal infection carries a toll for the infant, both for clinical illness with survival (17%) and for spontaneous abortion, stillbirth, or fatal infection (occurring in 29% of infants born to mothers with invasive infection).[22] Most obstetric patients with group B streptococcal infection, even in the presence of bacteremia, demonstrate a rapid response after initiation of appropriate therapy, but potentially fatal complications rarely occur, including meningitis,[649] ventriculoperitoneal shunt infection,[650] abdominal abscess,[651] endocarditis,[13,652-654] vertebral osteomyelitis,[655] epidural abscess,[656] and necrotizing fasciitis.[657]

Group B streptococcal bacteriuria during pregnancy is a risk factor for intrauterine or neonatal infection. Asymptomatic bacteriuria and cystitis or pyelonephritis occur in 6% to 8% of women during pregnancy. In those with asymptomatic bacteriuria, approximately 20% are caused by group B streptococci.[658] Pass and associates[659] observed three patterns of urinary tract infection among 20 patients: symptomatic lower urinary tract infection in the antenatal period; asymptomatic bacteriuria at delivery; and postpartum lower and upper tract infection. Eleven infants born to these women were colonized with group B streptococci, and early-onset sepsis developed in one. In the series reported by Moller and associates,[504] the 68 women with asymptomatic bacteriuria caused by group B streptococci had a significantly increased risk of delivery before 37 weeks of gestation compared with controls, but a causal relationship was not established. Among women with spontaneous abortion, the occurrence of group B streptococci in the urine has been significantly associated with fetal loss.[660] Women with group B streptococcal bacteriuria are those with heavy colonization, and both conditions are associated with enhanced risk for maternal and neonatal infection.[154]

DIAGNOSIS

Isolation and Identification of the Organism

The diagnosis of invasive group B streptococcal infection is established by isolation of the organism on culture of blood, CSF, or other specimen from the site of suppurative focus (e.g., bone, joint fluid, empyema fluid). Isolation of group B streptococci from surfaces such as the skin or umbilicus, or from mucous membranes, is of no clinical significance.

A selective approach to performing a lumbar puncture in the evaluation of neonates with possible sepsis has been advocated by some clinicians. Exclusion of meningeal infection by lumbar puncture always is indicated when either early- or late-onset group B streptococcal infection is suspected, however, because meningeal penetration occurs in 5% to 10% of cases[9,10,162,516,517] and early clinical features cannot distinguish between meningitis and bacteremia without meningitis. In many neonates with meningitis, group B streptococci are isolated from blood at initial evaluation, but the organism cannot be identified in a substantial minority (10% to 15%) of infants so affected. Wiswell and colleagues[661] found that if lumbar puncture was omitted as part of the early neonatal sepsis evaluation, the diagnosis of bacterial meningitis would have been missed or delayed in more than one third of infants. Infants with late-onset infection can have meningitis even when another site of infection, such as cellulitis, is apparent.[575] If lumbar puncture must be deferred initially because an infant is clinically unstable, penicillin G or ampicillin at the doses recommended for treatment of group B streptococcal meningitis (see "Treatment" later on) should be administered until meningeal involvement can be excluded.

Antigen Detection Methods

The difficulty of clinically differentiating neonates with group B streptococcal infection from those infected with other agents or with noninfectious disorders 3 decades ago prompted the development of tests to provide a presumptive diagnosis. These techniques included countercurrent immunoelectrophoresis (CIE),[662,663] latex particle agglutination (LPA),[664-666] staphylococcal coagglutination (SCA),[664,667,668] and enzyme immunoassay.[669] Each was based on the detection of group B– or type-specific polysaccharide antigens in body fluids using hyperimmune polyclonal antisera or monoclonal antibodies. The methods all have the attributes of simplicity, rapidity, and the ability to detect antigen after antimicrobial therapy has been initiated.

Antigen tests are not a substitute for appropriately performed bacterial cultures and now are rarely used for the diagnosis of group B streptococcal infection. A positive result indicates the presence of group B streptococcal antigen and not necessarily the presence of viable organisms. The only specimens recommended for antigen detection testing are serum and CSF.[670] In neonates with meningitis, the reported sensitivity of CSF assays is 72% to 89%. Serum is less likely to have detectable antigen (estimated sensitivity is 30% to 40%). LPA is more sensitive than CIE.[664,665] False-positive results have been encountered for antigen testing of serum and CSF, and the estimated specificity of assays varies, ranging from 95% to 98%. These assays should not be employed to monitor treatment efficacy.

Other Laboratory Tests

Elevation of levels of acute-phase reactants such as C-reactive protein may be observed acutely during group B streptococcal infection.[671,672] The usefulness of elevated serial C-reactive protein responses for detecting bacteremia was shown by Pourcyrous and colleagues.[672] Philip[671] suggests that C-reactive protein may not be a good indicator of neonatal infection during the first 12 hours after birth. However, the return to normal of the C-reactive protein level has been used to assist in minimizing antibiotic exposure in the nursery setting.[673] Levels of inflammatory cytokines such as interleukin-6 (IL-6) also are frequently elevated acutely during group B streptococcal sepsis. In one report, production of IL-6 was noted in all 16 neonates with bacteremic early- or late-onset group B streptococcal infection in samples collected within 48 hours of initiation of antimicrobial therapy.[674]

Abnormalities in the white blood cell count, including relative leukopenia, absolute neutropenia, leukocytosis, and a tendency for a decline in the total white blood cell count in the first 24 hours of life, are thought by some investigators to be useful in identifying neonates with group B streptococcal pneumonia.[295,298,675,676] In a study designed to determine the usefulness of the differential white blood cell count for distinguishing early-onset group B streptococcal infection from noninfectious causes of respiratory distress, Manroe and co-workers[675] found that each infected infant was identified by abnormalities in two or more of the following indices: (1) absolute neutrophil count indicating neutropenia or neutrophilia (87%), (2) elevation of the absolute immature neutrophil count (42%), and (3) abnormal ratio of immature neutrophils to the total number of neutrophils. The most useful index was the ratio of absolute immature neutrophils to absolute total neutrophils, which was elevated (greater than 0.20) in 91% of infants with infection and in only 1 of 23 noninfected infants with respiratory disease.[675] Greenberg and Yoder[677] caution that repeat testing at 12 to 24 hours of age may enhance sensitivity in comparison with testing between 1 and 7 hours of age. Fatal early-onset group B streptococcal sepsis can occur with a normal leukocyte count, however.[678] In general, measurements of peripheral blood leukocytes or inflammatory mediators are nonspecific and should be employed as adjuncts to blood and CSF cultures.

Differential Diagnosis

The clinical features in neonates with early-onset group B streptococcal infection mimic those in infants with sepsis caused by other etiologic agents and by some noninfectious illnesses. Radiographic findings characteristic of pneumonia are present in only one-third of neonates with early-onset group B streptococcal sepsis. At least one half of the neonates with proven bacteremia and pulmonary disease have radiographic abnormalities consistent with respiratory distress syndrome. Neonates with early-onset group B streptococcal pulmonary disease are more likely to have an interval after rupture of membranes of more than 12 hours before delivery, apnea and shock within the first 24 hours of life, a 1-minute Apgar score of 5 or less, and an unusually rapid progression of pulmonary disease than are neonates with noninfectious causes for respiratory distress.[292] Group B streptococcal infection also should be considered in a neonate with persistent fetal circulation associated with respiratory distress, neutropenia, and systemic hypotension.[527]

The differential diagnosis for late-onset group B streptococcal infection depends on the clinical presentation. For infants with meningitis, the characteristic CSF Gram stain findings can provide a presumptive diagnosis. When this is inconclusive or if partial treatment may have altered the CSF culture, other organisms, including viruses, *Neisseria meningitidis*, *Streptococcus pneumoniae*, and nontypeable *Haemophilus influenzae*, must be considered. Fever usually is a presenting feature, and empirical therapy with broad-spectrum antibiotics customarily is employed until results of cultures permitting a specific diagnosis of bacteremia are available. The paucity of signs characteristic of group B streptococcal osteomyelitis and the occasional history that signs have been present since birth have caused its confusion with Erb's palsy and neuromuscular disorders. Nevertheless, the characteristic bone lesion in the affected metaphysis, the common finding of tenderness of the extremity when a careful examination is performed, and the isolation of the organism from blood, bone, or joint fluid usually provide a definitive diagnosis.[550] Finally, the lengthy list of uncommon manifestations of group B streptococcal infection between 1 week and 3 months of age and beyond indicates that the group B streptococcus should be suspected as an etiologic agent, irrespective of site of infection, for infants in this age group.

TREATMENT

Group B streptococci have been a frequent cause of infection in neonates for more than 3 decades, resulting in increased awareness of associated risk factors and need for prompt and aggressive therapy. Despite striking declines, however, death and permanent sequelae from these infections remain all-too-frequent outcomes. In addition, relapses or reinfections, although uncommon, occur in the face of optimal therapy by conventional standards. These facts should prompt efforts to develop improved treatment modalities.

In Vitro Susceptibility

Uniform susceptibility of group B streptococci to penicillin G has continued for almost 50 years of usage.[679-683] In vitro susceptibility of these organisms to ampicillin, semisynthetic penicillins, vancomycin, teicoplanin, linezolid, quinopristin/dalfopristin, gatifloxacin, levofloxacin, and first-, second- (excluding cefoxitin), and third-generation cephalosporins also is the rule, although the degree of in vitro activity varies.[682-690] Ceftriaxone is the most active of the cephalosporins in vitro. Imipenem and meropenem are highly active.[680,684] Ciprofloxacin has moderate in vitro activity.[686] Resistance to erythromycin and clindamycin has increased dramatically. Contemporary data indicate that 20% to 30% of isolates are resistant to erythromycin and that 10% to 20% of isolates are resistant to clindamycin.[682,683,690-692] These rates of resistance have been reported from such geographically diverse areas as Turkey, France, Spain, and Taiwan, as well as North America.[693-696] The most frequently encountered macrolide resistance mechanisms in streptococci are ribosomal modification by a methylase encoded by an *erm* gene and drug efflux by a membrane-bound protein encoded by an *mef* gene.[691] The *erm*(A), *erm*(B), and *mef*(A) genes, either alone or in combination, are responsible for erythromycin resistance.[681] Erythromycin-resistant isolates that are constitutively resistant, inducibly resistant, or susceptible to clindamycin are described.[697] A higher proportion with resistance to erythromycin has been reported for serotype V strains than for other group B streptococcal serotypes.[683,698] Both tigecycline and telithromycin are very active in vitro against macrolide-resistant group B streptococci, but data are not yet available confirming their clinical effectiveness.[699,700] Tetracycline resistance has increased significantly; the percentage of resistant strains has increased from about 30% in 1957[701] to nearly 90%.[685] Resistance of group B streptococci to bacitracin, nalidixic acid, trimethoprim-sulfamethoxazole, metronidazole, and aminoglycosides is uniform.

Despite the in vitro resistance of most group B streptococcal strains to aminoglycosides, when one of these drugs (especially gentamicin) is combined with a penicillin, in vitro[702-705] and in vivo synergy[703,706-708] often is observed. The best combination to theoretically accelerate the killing of group B streptococci in vivo is penicillin, or ampicillin, plus gentamicin. By contrast, the rapid and predictable bactericidal effect of penicillin or ampicillin on group B streptococci in vitro is ablated by the addition of rifampin.[709,710] Although in vivo data are lacking, the in vitro antagonism of rifampin when combined with penicillins suggests that they should not be employed concurrently in the treatment of proven or suspected group B streptococcal disease.

Among the newer β-lactam antibiotics reputed to attain high concentrations of drug in the CSF, only cefotaxime,

Table 13–11 Antimicrobial Regimens Recommended for Treatment of Group B Streptococcal Infections in Infants[a]

Manifestation of Infection	Drug	Daily Dose (intravenous)	Duration
Bacteremia without meningitis	Ampicillin plus gentamicin	150-200 mg/kg plus 7.5 mg/kg	Initial treatment before culture results (48-72 hr)
	Penicillin G	200,000 units/kg	Complete a total treatment course of 10 days
Meningitis	Ampicillin plus gentamicin	300-400 mg/kg plus 7.5 mg/kg	Initial treatment (until cerebrospinal fluid is sterile)
	Penicillin G	500,000 units/kg	Complete a minimum total treatment course of 14 days[b]
Septic arthritis	Penicillin G	200,000 units/kg	2-3 wk
Osteomyelitis	Penicillin G	200,000 units/kg	3-4 wk
Endocarditis	Penicillin G	400,000 units/kg	4 wk[c]

[a]No modification of dose by postnatal age is recommended. Oral therapy is never indicated.
[b]Longer treatment (up to 4 wk) may be required for ventriculitis.
[c]In combination with gentamicin for the first 14 days.

ceftriaxone, meropenem, and imipenem achieve minimal bactericidal concentrations (MBCs) comparable with those of penicillin G and ampicillin (0.008 to 0.4 µg/mL, respectively).[680,684,691,708] Only a few infants have received treatment with these agents,[711-713] and limited data suggest that their efficacy is equivalent to that of penicillin G. Thus, no compelling reason exists to consider use of these alternative therapeutic agents.

Despite their uniform susceptibility to penicillin G, group B streptococci require higher concentrations for growth inhibition in vitro than are required for strains belonging to group A. The minimal inhibitory concentration (MIC) of penicillin G to group B streptococci is 4- to 10-fold greater (range, 0.003 to 0.4 µg/mL) than that for group A strains.[679,685,702] This observation, combined with that indicating the significant influence of inoculum size on in vitro susceptibility to penicillin G may have clinical relevance.[679,714] If the inoculum of group B streptococci is reduced from 10^5 to 10^4 colony-forming units (CFU)/mL, a twofold decrease in the concentration of penicillin G is sufficient to inhibit in vitro growth. Similarly, if the inoculum is increased from 10^4 to 10^7 CFU/mL, the MBC of ampicillin is increased from 0.06 to 3.9 µg/mL. Such in vitro findings may have in vivo correlates, because some infants with group B streptococcal meningitis have CSF bacterial concentrations of 10^7 to 10^8 CFU/mL.[714] At the initiation of therapy for meningitis, achievable CSF levels of penicillin G or ampicillin may be only $^1/_{10}$ of serum levels. This inoculum effect also has been noted with cefotaxime and imipenem.[685] Therefore, the dose chosen to treat group B streptococcal meningitis may be crucial to the prompt sterilization of CSF.

Although group B streptococci are susceptible to penicillin G, in vitro tolerance among 4% to 6% of strains has been noted.[581,634,645,715] Defined as an MBC in excess of 16 to 32 times the MIC, tolerance in vitro corresponds with delayed bacterial killing, additive rather than synergistic effects when gentamicin is used in combination with penicillin G, and possibly an autolytic enzyme defect in such strains.[716,717] Detection of tolerance among group B streptococcal isolates, however, is highly dependent on choice of growth medium, growth phase of bacterial inoculum, and quantitative definition of MBC employed for testing.[685] Although some infants with recurrence of group B streptococcal infection have had tolerant strains,[583,634] the clinical significance of this in vitro phenomenon is doubtful.

Antimicrobial Therapy

Although other penicillins are equally active in vitro, penicillin G remains the drug of choice for the treatment of group B streptococcal infections. This recommendation is undisputed, yet suggestions for dosage have varied considerably. The recommended dosage of penicillin for treatment of meningitis is relatively high because of (1) the relatively high MIC of penicillin G for group B streptococci (median, 0.04 µg/mL) with respect to attainable levels of this drug in the CSF,[718] (2) the large initial inoculum in the CSF of some infants,[9,714] (3) reports of relapse in infants with meningitis treated for 14 days with 200,000 units/kg per day of penicillin G, and (4) the safety of higher doses of penicillin G in the newborn. To ensure rapid bactericidal effects, particularly in the CSF, we recommend penicillin G (500,000 units/kg per day) or ampicillin (300 to 400 mg/kg per day) for the treatment of group B streptococcal meningitis (Table 13-11). There is no evidence to suggest increased risk for adverse reactions to these drugs at these higher doses even in premature infants.

In the usual clinical setting, antimicrobial therapy will be initiated before definitive identification of the organism. Initial therapy should include ampicillin and an aminoglycoside appropriate for the treatment of early-onset neonatal pathogens including group B streptococci. Such a combination has been shown more effective than penicillin G or ampicillin alone for in vitro and in vivo killing of group B streptococci.[702-704] It is our practice to continue combination therapy until the isolate has been identified as group B streptococci and, in patients with meningitis, until a CSF specimen obtained 24 to 48 hours into therapy is sterile. Kim[717] suggested that MIC and MBC determinations be considered in the following clinical circumstances: (1) a poor bacteriologic response to antimicrobial therapy, (2) relapse or recurrence of infection without a discernible cause, and (3) infections manifested as meningitis or endocarditis.

If tolerance is demonstrated in one of these circumstances, the clinician has the choice of empirically continuing the combination of penicillin G or ampicillin and gentamicin, or of using penicillin G or ampicillin alone, or of employing cefotaxime. No data are available to indicate the best choice.[719]

For the infant with late-onset disease in whom the CSF Gram stain reveals gram-positive cocci in pairs or short chains, initial therapy should include ampicillin and gentamicin or cefotaxime, rather than penicillin G alone. The rationale for this recommendation rests on several observations. First, group B streptococci are a frequent cause of meningitis in infants from 1 to 8 weeks of age. In this setting, combination therapy may provide for added efficacy early in the course of infection. Second, meningitis caused by *Listeria monocytogenes* can produce a CSF Gram stain indistinguishable from that with meningitis caused by group B streptococci, especially to an inexperienced observer. Ampicillin and gentamicin are synergistic in vitro against most strains of *Listeria*. If pneumococcal meningitis is a consideration, cefotaxime in combination with vancomycin should be included in the empirical regimen pending culture confirmation. Because group B streptococcal meningitis occurs uncommonly beyond 8 weeks of age, no change is suggested from the use of conventional agents as the initial treatment of meningitis in term infants older than 2 months of age. For the premature infant remaining in the hospital since birth, empirical therapy can include vancomycin and an aminoglycoside. However, if meningitis is suspected, an additional agent should be added (i.e., either ampicillin or cefotaxime), because vancomycin achieves low CSF concentration and has a substantially higher MBC against group B streptococci than that of ampicillin.

Once the bacteriologic diagnosis of group B streptococcal infection is known *and* the CSF of patients with meningeal infections 24 to 48 hours into therapy is shown to be sterile, treatment can be completed with penicillin G alone. Although the total duration of treatment is arbitrary, good outcomes have been noted when parenteral therapy is given for 10 days for bacteremia without a focus or with soft tissue infection, 2 to 3 weeks for meningitis or pyarthrosis,[544] and 3 to 4 weeks for osteomyelitis[550] or endocarditis[5,720] (see Table 13-11). Limited evidence suggests that a somewhat shorter course of therapy (6 to 7 days) may suffice for uncomplicated bacteremia, but additional data are needed to support a change in the current recommendations.[721] In the management of infants with meningitis, failure to achieve sterility suggests the presence of an unsuspected suppurative focus (subdural empyema, brain abscess, ventriculitis, septic thrombophlebitis) or failure to administer an appropriate drug in sufficient dosage. At the completion of therapy (minimum 14 days), another lumbar puncture should be considered to determine whether the CSF findings are compatible with adequacy of treatment or are of sufficient concern to warrant further treatment or further diagnostic evaluation. For example, polymorphonuclear cells in excess of 30% of the total or a protein concentration in excess of 200 mg/dL would merit additional investigation. These findings also can be observed in patients with a fulminant course manifested by severe cerebritis, extensive parenchymal destruction with focal suppuration, or severe vasculitis, or all three.

Infants with septic arthritis should receive at least 2 weeks of parenteral therapy; those with bone involvement require 3 to 4 weeks of therapy to optimize the chance for an uncomplicated outcome. Drainage of the suppurative focus is an adjunct to antibiotic therapy. In infants with septic arthritis excluding the hip or shoulder, needle aspiration of the involved joint on one occasion usually achieves adequate drainage.[4,544,545,550] With hip or shoulder involvement, immediate open drainage is warranted. For many infants with osteomyelitis, some type of drainage procedure, whether closed or open, is required for diagnosis because most patients have sterile blood cultures. Such procedures must be performed before or early in the course of antimicrobial therapy to ensure the successful isolation of the infecting organism.

With recurrent infection, three points should be considered. First, appropriate antimicrobial therapy fails to eliminate mucous membrane colonization with group B streptococci in up to 50% of infants.[722] Second, community exposure of the infant may result in colonization with a new strain that subsequently invades the bloodstream. Systemic infection in neonates does not result in protective levels of type-specific antibodies.[420] Therefore, even in the absence of an underlying immunologic abnormality or an unsuspected suppurative focus, recurrent systemic infections do occur. In this event, an evaluation to exclude underlying immune abnormality (e.g., HIV infection or hypogammaglobulinemia) should be considered. Most infants, however, will have no defined abnormalities. Therapy in those infants with recurrent infection need not be extended beyond that recommended by site of infection. Finally, although it is logical to suggest that colonization be eliminated, an efficacious regimen has not been identified. Rifampin has uniform in vitro activity against group B streptococci, but this agent is bacteriostatic. One small prospective study revealed that administration of oral rifampin (20 mg/kg per day for 4 days) to infants after completion of parenteral therapy eliminated mucous membrane colonization in some subjects.[723] Further study is needed to identify a means to eliminate colonization in infants who have invasive disease.

Supportive Management

Prompt, vigorous, and careful supportive therapy is important to the successful outcome of most group B streptococcal infections. In neonates with early-onset disease accompanied by respiratory distress, the need for ventilatory assistance should be anticipated before onset of apnea, because its appearance can herald a poor outcome.[245,277] The early treatment of shock, often not suspected during its initial phase, when systolic pressure is maintained by peripheral vasoconstriction, is crucial. Persistent metabolic acidosis and reasonably normal color are characteristic of this early phase. Any indication of poor peripheral perfusion after initial attempts to achieve adequate volume expansion merits placement of a central venous pressure monitoring device and treatment with appropriate inotropic agents. This concept applies also to patients with late-onset meningitis. Fluid management should include packed red blood cell transfusions if anemia is significant. In patients with meningitis, effective seizure control is required to achieve proper oxygenation, to decrease metabolic demands, to prevent additional cerebral edema, and to optimize cerebral blood flow. Attention to the details of urine output and electrolyte balance and osmolality is necessary to detect and manage the early complications of meningitis, such as inappropriate secretion of antidiuretic hormone and increased intracranial pressure. Such intense and careful supportive management requires treatment in an intensive care unit of a tertiary care facility.

Extracorporeal membrane oxygenation (ECMO) has been used as rescue therapy for neonates with overwhelming early-onset group B streptococcal sepsis. Hocker and associates[724] reported a retrospective study that compared conventional treatment and ECMO for neonates with early-onset disease. A fatal outcome occurred in three (11%) of 28 of infants in the conventional treatment group and in nine (17%) of 53 infants placed on ECMO. If only hypotensive neonates were considered, 13 of 15 ECMO patients survived, compared with 11 of 18 of those who received conventional treatment (P = .06). The authors concluded that neonates with suspected early-onset sepsis in whom acidosis or hypotension develops should be considered for early referral to an ECMO center. Commenting on these results, LeBlanc[725] emphasizes the difficulty of interpreting this study, citing the retrospective design and the fact that the most ill infants die before ECMO can be initiated. He also stressed that fatal complications of ECMO, such as brain hemorrhage, can occur. Until a prospective, controlled trial is performed, ECMO therapy should be considered controversial.

Adjunctive Therapies

Despite prompt initiation of antimicrobial therapy and aggressive supportive care, death and neurologic morbidity can result from group B streptococcal infection. Adjunctive therapy directed toward improvement of neonatal host defenses against group B streptococci has received considerable investigative effort. Reports indicating increases in mortality rate for neutropenic neonates prompted clinical evaluation of granulocyte transfusions as adjunctive therapy for early-onset group B streptococcal sepsis.[362,466,726,727] In three trials, 13 infants with neutrophil storage pool depletion (documented by bone marrow aspiration) were assessed.[362,466,726] The results seemed promising, but the logistics of providing timely transfusion and the concern for adverse effects (graft-versus-host reaction, transmission of viral agents, pulmonary leukocyte sequestration) make this mode of therapy impractical.

Recombinant human cytokine molecules stimulatory for granulocyte progenitor cells, namely, granulocyte colony-stimulating factor (G-CSF) and GM-CSF, are widely available. G-CSF promotes proliferation of granulocyte progenitors in bone marrow, enhances chemotactic activities and superoxide anion production, and increases expression of neutrophil C3bi receptors. Because many of these attributes might improve the limited bone marrow neutrophil reserve and the defective neutrophil functions in human neonates, several investigators have evaluated the use of these agents as adjunctive therapy in experimental infection. Taken together, these studies suggest that G-CSF or GM-CSF might be useful as adjunctive agents in the treatment of group B streptococcal neonatal sepsis, possibly when they are used in combination with intravenous immune globulin (IGIV).[728-731] Any clinical recommendations must await evaluation of their safety and efficacy in controlled clinical trials.

Another proposed therapy is human immune globulin modified for intravenous use to provide type-specific antibodies for more efficient opsonization and phagocytosis of group B streptococci.[732-738] IGIV has been shown in an animal model[739] and in septic neonates[740] to improve complement activation and chemotaxis by neonatal sera and to hasten resolution of neutropenia. Administration of sufficient human type-specific antibodies against capsular polysaccharides to animals before lethal challenge with group B streptococci of the homologous serotype is protective.[427,732-736]

Despite the sound theoretical basis on which use of IGIV as adjunctive therapy is based, several concerns remain. First, commercially available preparations contain relatively low concentrations of protective antibodies (directed at either protein or polysaccharide surface antigens),[735-738,740-745] suggesting that large doses would be required and raising concern for reticuloendothelial system blockade.[734,737] Second, the in vitro functional activity of the currently licensed globulins varies by method of preparation and by lot.[733,734,740-746] Third, the increase in type-specific antibodies after infusion may be only transient.[741,747]

Development of hyperimmune group B streptococcal globulin or of human-human monoclonal antibodies would theoretically circumvent many of these potential problems. Raff and co-workers[748] developed a human IgM monoclonal antibody specific for the group B cell wall polysaccharide. This antibody reacted with all group B streptococcal serotypes and was evaluated for safety and pharmacokinetics in two neonatal nonhuman primates.[749] Both it and a hyperimmune globulin[744] prepared by vaccination of healthy adults with polysaccharides from type Ia, Ib, II, and III group B streptococci were protective against experimental challenge with type I, II, and III strains in doses as low as 4 to 20 mg/kg.[750]

At present, any application of these intriguing experimental findings to the clinical setting is unclear. Clinical trials provide some insights. A prospective, multicenter, placebo-controlled trial included 753 neonates with birth weights from 500 to 2000 g receiving empirical treatment for possible sepsis; in 12, the causative agent was group B streptococci. Administration of IGIV at a dose of 500 mg/kg within 12 hours of birth was well tolerated and resulted in a survival rate for infants with group B streptococcal sepsis similar to that for placebo recipients. Christensen and colleagues[751] administered either IGIV (750 mg/kg) or albumin to 22 neonates with severe, early-onset sepsis. All infants survived. Eleven patients had neutropenia, but in IGIV recipients, this abnormality resolved within 24 hours of infusion, whereas it persisted in albumin (control) recipients. Each of the IGIV recipients had a significant elevation of immature to total neutrophil ratios 1 hour after infusion when compared with controls. The IGIV was considered to stimulate release of neutrophils into the circulation from bone marrow storage pools. It can be concluded that administration of IGIV in a single dose ranging from 500 to 750 mg/kg in neonates with clinical sepsis is safe and may provide some hematologic and immunologic benefit.

PROGNOSIS

Despite the extensive investigation of group B streptococcal disease, a relative paucity of information exists concerning the prognosis for infants surviving invasive neonatal infection. Several reports have assessed sequelae among survivors of meningitis, but these reports do not reflect outcome for infants who received intensive supportive care subsequent to improvements in such care since the late 1980s. In 1977, Haslam and associates[522] reported major neurologic sequelae in 2 of 15 survivors of meningitis. No differences were evident between survivors and sibling controls in tests of hearing, speech, or adaptive skills. In a prospective assessment of 20 survivors of early-onset meningitis treated between 1974 and 1982, 14 (70%) were considered to be normal.[521] Major handicaps were found in 15%, and three had mild cognitive impairments. Similarly, 50% of children assessed at a mean age of 6 years after surviving meningitis during the 1970s were functioning normally.[523] Another 29% had severe sequelae, including global mental retardation, cortical blindness, and spasticity. Among the 21% with mild or moderate sequelae, deficits such as borderline mental retardation, spastic or flaccid monoparesis, or language delay still permitted function at or near age-expected norms. In a study of 74 children who survived early- or late-onset group B streptococcal meningitis, 9 (12%) had major neurologic sequelae when evaluated at 3 to 18 years of age.[535] When these 9 children were excluded, there were no significant differences, as rated by parents, between the children with meningitis and their siblings for academic achievement, measures of intelligence quotient, fine motor dexterity, or behavior difficulties. These investigators concluded that "children not identified early, after appropriate examination, as having serious sequelae can be expected to perform intellectually, socially, and academically in a manner similar to other family members."[11,535]

Several clinical scoring systems exist for predicting a fatal outcome with neonatal group B streptococcal infection.[523,527,752] Payne and colleagues[527] described a score, derived from five variables, that, together with an initial blood pH less than 7.25, enabled prediction of outcome accurately in 93% of infants with early-onset group B streptococcal infection. These features were birth weight less than 2500 g, absolute neutrophil count less than 1500 cells per mm^3, hypotension, apnea, and a pleural effusion seen on the initial chest radiograph.

A fatal outcome can be predicted with reasonable accuracy, but little information is available concerning the long-term prognosis for survivors of neonatal group B streptococcal sepsis. One group at potential risk for sequelae consists of preterm infants with septic shock, who could develop periventricular leukomalacia. Among these survivors, substantial neurodevelopmental sequelae have been identified at evaluation during the second year of life. The correlates of severity and duration of shock with periventricular leukomalacia and with long-term morbidity from group B streptococcal disease have not been assessed, however.

PREVENTION

Theoretically, early- and late-onset group B streptococcal disease could be prevented if susceptible hosts were not exposed to the microorganism or if exposure occurred in the setting of protective immunity. Several approaches to prevention have been advocated; conceptually, these are directed at either eliminating exposure or enhancing host resistance—that is, chemoprophylaxis or immunoprophylaxis. Both strategies have limitations with respect to implementation, could be targeted for the prevention of maternal as well as neonatal infections, and are theoretically achievable.[19,24,406,753]

Chemoprophylaxis

Historical Precedents

Chemoprophylaxis as a method for preventing early-onset group B streptococcal infection was first suggested by Franciosi and colleagues in 1973.[2] Because vertical transmission was documented to be the prelude to early-onset disease, investigators proposed oral penicillin treatment for colonized women late in pregnancy to interrupt maternal exposure of the neonate at delivery. Group B streptococcal carriers were identified with third-trimester vaginal cultures; culture-positive women received oral antimicrobial agents for 1 to 2 weeks. Approximately 20% to 30% remained colonized at the end of therapy, and in nearly 70%, group B streptococci were isolated from vaginal cultures at delivery.[149,754,755] A suggested mechanism for treatment failure was reinfection of women by colonized sexual partners.[2] When colonized pregnant women and their spouses received concurrent treatment, 70% of women and 40% of their husbands remained infected after treatment.[149] Somewhat better results were reported by Lewin and Amstey,[756] who administered penicillin intramuscularly to colonized women in their third trimester of pregancy and their husbands: Only 18% of women remained colonized at delivery. One explanation for failure of antimicrobial therapy to eliminate group B streptococcal colonization is the inherent difficulty of eradicating a constituent of the bowel flora even when high doses of intravenous penicillin G or ampicillin are employed.[149]

The next method evaluated in the attempt to prevent early-onset group B streptococcal neonatal infection by interrupting perinatal exposure was use of intravenously administered antibiotic in women during labor. Yow and colleagues[757] gave intravenous ampicillin (500 mg) at hospital admission to 34 third-trimester women colonized with group B streptococci. Ampicillin uniformly interrupted vertical transmission to the neonates of women who received treatment, contrasting with an expected rate of approximately 50%. This observation was confirmed by others.[169,758-760]

The first documentation that intrapartum chemoprophylaxis was effective in preventing early-onset neonatal disease as well as group B streptococcal–associated maternal morbidity was reported by Boyer and Gotoff in 1986.[760] Women colonized with group B streptococci who had risk factors for early-onset infection (delivery at less than 37 weeks of gestation, membrane rupture at 12 hours before delivery or earlier, or intrapartum fever) were randomized to receive routine care or intrapartum intravenous ampicillin. Group B streptococcal sepsis developed in 5 of 79 neonates born to women in the routine care group (one death), whereas each of the 85 infants born to women in the ampicillin treatment group remained well ($P = .024$). Intrapartum ampicillin chemoprophylaxis for group B streptococcal carriers also resulted in reduced maternal morbidity.[761]

These and other data[758,762-764] established the efficacy of intrapartum chemoprophylaxis in group B streptococcal carriers identified antenatally in the prevention of early-onset neonatal disease and group B streptococcus–associated maternal morbidity. The cost effectiveness of this prevention method also has been validated.[765-769]

Rapid Assays for Antenatal Detection of Group B Streptococci

There are inherent difficulties in determining group B streptococcal colonization status at hospital admission even when assays can be processed 24 hours a day. Several methods using cervical or lower vaginal swab specimens have been evaluated to rapidly ascertain the colonization status at hospital admission. When secretions from vaginal swabs are immediately extracted and tested for group B streptococcal antigen by LPA, the sensitivity ranges from 15% to 28% for all culture-positive women and from 57% to 67% for heavily colonized women; the specificity ranges from 95% to 99%.[763,770-772] The sensitivity of enzyme immunoassays ranges from 12% to 44% for all colonized women and from 36% to 100% for heavily colonized women; the specificity is 95% to 99%.[771,773-776] Thus, these assays have limited sensitivity to detect group B streptococcal carriers, especially among women with a small inoculum of organisms. Although attack rates for early-onset disease are significantly higher in neonates born to heavily colonized women, risk does exist for those born to lightly colonized women (approximately 1.0%).[217,247,763,773] If commercially available latex assays are positive, the result is highly reliable. An optical immunoassay (Strep B OIA test, Biostar, Boulder, Colo.) is more sensitive for detecting light (13% to 67%) and heavy (42% to 100%) or overall (81%) colonization and outperforms enzyme immunoassays in direct comparisons.[776-780] Assays using a DNA hybridization methodology have shown variable sensitivity.[781,782] None of these rapid tests is sufficiently accurate for routine use in the intrapartum detection of maternal colonization with group B streptococci. A bulletin from the Food and Drug Administration (FDA) in 1996 provided guidelines stipulating that antigen tests "cannot be relied upon to exclude group B streptococcal colonization in a pregnant woman. Negative group B streptococcal antigen test results should be confirmed using selective broth culture which is more sensitive than antigen tests."

A recent study evaluated a new rapid polymerase chain reaction (PCR) assay as an alternative screening tool for rapid identification of colonized women at admission for delivery.[783] The sensitivity of both a rapid and a conventional PCR assay was 97%, and the negative predictive value was 99%. Both the specificity and the positive predictive value were 100%. The time required to obtain results by the rapid PCR assay was 30 to 45 minutes. The test has now been licensed by the FDA, and although its performance in nonresearch settings awaits further study, a cost-benefit analysis suggests that its widespread implementation would afford benefit over the current culture-based strategy.[784]

Intrapartum Antimicrobial Prophylaxis

The rationale for offering intrapartum antibiotic prophylaxis (IAP) to women who are antenatal culture positive for group B streptococci evolved from two concerns. First, selective intrapartum chemoprophylaxis based on clinically identifiable maternal risk factors fails to prevent 25% to 30% of cases and about 10% of deaths.[10,760,785] These cases represent term infants born to women with no risk factors for early-onset infant disease except vaginal or rectal colonization. The number of cases missed by selective chemoprophylaxis diminishes if maternal risk factors are expanded to include premature rupture of membranes at any gestational stage,[195] asymptomatic bacteriuria caused by group B streptococci,[251,504,786] nongestational diabetes mellitus,[10,786] maternal age younger than 20 years, and black race.[10,250,406] Second, the pregnant woman informed that she carries a potential pathogen for her newborn often desires prophylaxis in the absence of risk factors, especially when she is told that a culture-based prevention approach is more effective than a risk factor–based approach in preventing neonatal infection.[23] Thus, one approach to the prevention of early-onset group B streptococcal sepsis in neonates through intrapartum maternal chemoprophylaxis is to target all colonized women. Garland and Fliegner[762] identified Australian vaginal carriers of group B streptococci at 32 weeks of gestation and gave intravenous penicillin G during labor to all culture-positive women. From 1981 to 1988, no cases of early-onset disease occurred in neonates born to culture-positive women given IAP.

For the prevention of early-onset disease, intrapartum maternal chemoprophylaxis should be administered at least 4 hours before delivery. This interval allows sufficient time to achieve concentrations of penicillin, ampicillin, or cefazolin in the fetal blood (an estimated 30 minutes) and the amniotic fluid (approximately 2 to 4 hours)[787-789] that are bactericidal for group B streptococci. Also, when high doses of penicillin G (5 million units), ampicillin (2 g), or presumably cefazolin are given intravenously 4 or more hours before delivery, vertical transmission is interrupted[790] and infant disease prevented. Intrapartum chemoprophylaxis has no known efficacy in the prevention of late-onset infant infection.

In 1992, the ACOG[791] and the AAP[792] published separate documents regarding maternal intrapartum chemoprophylaxis for the prevention of early-onset group B streptococcal infection. Both documents concurred that selective IAP prevented early-onset group B streptococcal disease and reduced maternal puerperal morbidity. Both concurred that preterm labor at less than 37 weeks of gestation, preterm premature rupture of membranes at less than 37 weeks of gestation, rupture of membranes at any gestation beyond 18 hours, fever during labor, and previous delivery of a sibling with invasive group B streptococcal disease enhanced risk for early-onset neonatal disease.[793,794] Whereas the ACOG technical bulletin[791] was educational, the AAP guidelines[792] were more directive. The latter recommended that *if* culture screening was performed antenatally, culture specimens from both lower vaginal and anorectal sites should be obtained, and that culture-positive women with one or more risk factors and group B streptococcal colonization should be given intrapartum intravenous penicillin G or ampicillin. The ACOG proposed that culture screening could be avoided by providing treatment for all women with risk factors. Neither approach was adequately implemented, and invasive disease rates remained unacceptably high.

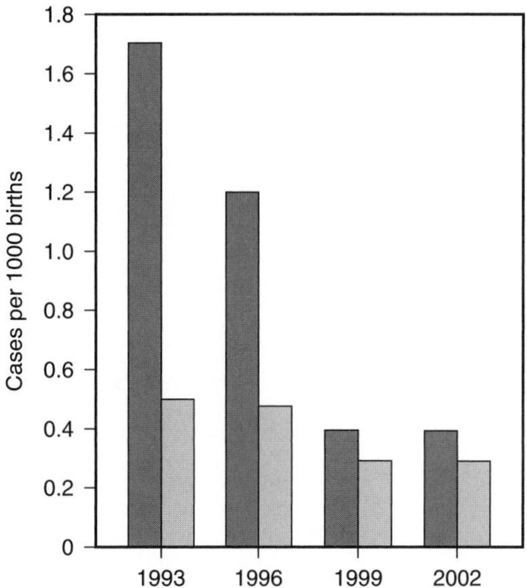

Figure 13–10 Incidence of early-onset (*dark bars*) and late-onset (*light bars*) group B streptococcal disease from 1993 to 2002. Data for 1993 and 1996 reflect aggregate disease rates from the state of Maryland, as well as from three counties in California, eight in Georgia, and five in Tennessee, which represent approximately 190,000 births annually. Data for 1999 and 2002 are from the Active Bacterial Core Surveillance (ABCS) Emerging Infections Program Network, which represents 425,404 children younger than 1 year of age. (Adapted from Schuchat A. Group B *Streptococcus*. Lancet 353:51-56, 1999; and data from the CDC National Center for Infectious Diseases website on group B streptococcal infection [http://www.cdc.gov/ncidod/dbmd/abcs/survreports/gbs02.pdf].)

In 1996, consensus guidelines for the prevention of early-onset group B streptococcal disease were published by the CDC, the ACOG, and the AAP.[19-21] These guidelines recommended that obstetric care providers and hospitals adopt a policy for group B streptococcal infection prevention based on one of two strategies, one culture-based and the other risk factor–based, to identify women who require IAP.[19-21] The culture-based approach employed the results of lower vaginal and rectal cultures obtained at 35 to 37 weeks of gestation to determine candidates for prophylaxis. Most women prefer self-obtaining of cultures, and there is a high correlation of patient-collected and of nurse-collected samples for accuracy.[795,796] Furthermore, pregnant women place a high priority on knowing their group B streptococcal colonization status.[797] The risk factor–based strategy favored by the ACOG identified IAP recipients by factors known to increase the likelihood of neonatal group B streptococcal disease: labor onset or membrane rupture before 37 weeks of gestation, intrapartum fever, and rupture of membranes 18 or more hours before delivery. In both strategies, women with previous delivery of an infant with group B streptococcal disease or with group B streptococcal bacteriuria during the current pregnancy always received IAP. These strategies each result in the administration of IAP to an estimated 25% of pregnant women.[19]

In association with active efforts to promote IAP in the 1990s, the incidence of early-onset disease declined by 70% from 1.7 per 1000 live births to 0.5 per 1000 live births by 1999 (Fig. 13-10) and remains stable.[24,798] For the years 1998 to 1999, an estimated 3900 to 4500 early-onset infections and 200 to 225 neonatal deaths were prevented annually by the use of IAP.[22,24] By contrast, the rate of late-onset disease has remained constant at 0.5 to 0.6 per 1000 live births throughout the 1990s and into the 21st century. The incidence of invasive group B streptococcal disease among pregnant girls and women declined significantly (21%) with implementation of IAP, from 0.29 per 1000 live births in 1993 to 0.23 in 1998.[22,24]

Surveys of physicians' practices have documented significant increases in the number of obstetric care providers who were screening at least 75% of pregnant women in their practices, and in the number of group B streptococcus–positive women who received IAP in the late 1990s.[799-801] Implementation of the consensus guidelines was associated with a reduction in the number and incidence of early-onset disease in a number of geographic regions in the United States and Canada.[799,801-803] By 1999, two thirds of U.S. hospitals in a multistate survey had a formal prevention policy, and a high number of individual practitioners had adopted policies.[24,804]

The proportion of disease theoretically prevented by the culture-based approach is higher (85% to 90%) than that using the risk factor–based approach (50% to 65%).[19] Group B streptococcal carriers without risk factors can be delivered of infants with early-onset disease, and approximately 45% of infants with early-onset disease are born to such women.[785] By 2002, it was evident that a further reduction in the incidence of early-onset disease could be accomplished only by adoption of universal culture screening. A direct comparison of the two methods in 5144 births demonstrated that culture screening was 50% more effective than a risk-based strategy in preventing early-onset disease in neonates.[23] Culture-based screening not only was more effective but was more often associated with administration of IAP more than 4 hours before delivery. The 2002 revised guidelines from the CDC for the prevention of perinatal group B streptococcal disease have been endorsed by the AAP and the Committee on Obstetric Practice of the ACOG.[24,805,806]

All pregnant women now should be screened in each pregnancy for group B streptococcal carriage at 35 to 37 weeks of gestation. The risk-based approach is not an acceptable alternative except in circumstances in which the culture results are not available before delivery. Culture specimens should be obtained from the lower vagina and the rectum using the same or two different swabs. These should be placed in a non-nutritive transport medium, incubated overnight in a selective broth medium, and subcultured onto 5% sheep blood agar medium for isolation of group B streptococci. At the time of labor or rupture of membranes, IAP should be given to all pregnant women identified as group B streptococcal carriers. The indications for IAP are shown in Figure 13-11. Delivery of a previous infant with invasive disease and group B streptococcal bacteriuria are always indications for IAP, and screening is not necessary for these women. If the results of culture are not known at the onset of labor, the risk factors listed in Figure 13-11 should be used to determine the need to institute IAP.

Planned cesarean section before rupture of membranes and onset of labor constitutes an exception to the need for IAP among women colonized with group B streptococci. These women are at low risk for having an infant with early-onset disease. Similarly, women documented to have negative

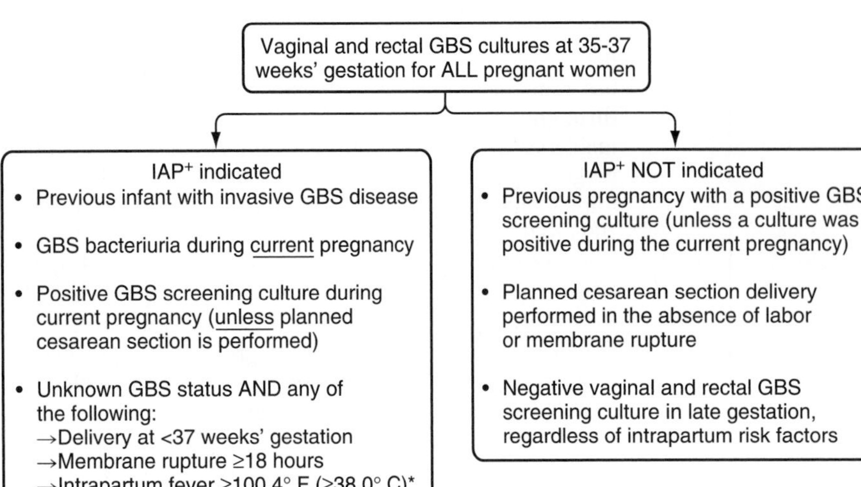

Figure 13–11 Revised recommendations for culture-based screening for maternal colonization with group B streptococci (GBS) and administration of intrapartum antibiotic prophylaxis (IAP). (Adapted from Centers for Disease Control and Prevention. Prevention of perinatal group B streptococcal disease: revised guidelines from CDC. MMWR Morb Mortal Wkly Rep 51[RR-11]:1-22, 2002.)

screening cultures for group B streptococci delivered at 37 weeks or later need not receive IAP routinely, even when a risk factor is present. Of course, therapeutic use of antibiotics in labor should be employed as is appropriate for maternal indications.

The current recommendations also include an algorithm for IAP for women with threatened preterm delivery.[24] If the results of screening cultures are not available and if onset of labor or rupture of membranes occurs before 37 weeks of gestation with a substantial risk for imminent preterm delivery, IAP should be provided pending culture results. For women who are culture positive, penicillin should be administered for a total of at least 48 hours, unless delivery occurs sooner. If tocolysis is successful, IAP should be reinitiated when labor that is likely to proceed to delivery occurs. If a negative culture result within the previous 4 weeks is on record, or if labor can be successfully arrested, IAP should not be initiated.

The recommended maternal intrapartum chemoprophylaxis regimen consists of penicillin G (5 million units initially and 2.5 million units every 4 hours thereafter until delivery).[24] Prophylaxis should be initiated as soon as possible, because penicillin given 4 or more hours before delivery prevents vertical transmission and early-onset disease more reliably than doses given at shorter intervals. Ampicillin administered as a 2-g intravenous loading dose and then 1 g every 4 hours until delivery is the alternative antimicrobial agent.[24]

Prophylaxis for penicillin-allergic women takes into account increasing resistance among group B streptococci to erythromycin and clindamycin. Women who are not at at high risk for anaphylaxis should receive cefazolin, 2 g intravenously as an initial dose and then 1 g every 8 hours until delivery. When anaphylaxis to β-lactams is considered a risk, IAP can be based on the results of susceptibility testing for erythromycin and clindamycin, if available. Women with erythromycin- and clindamycin-susceptible isolates can be given either clindamycin (900 mg intravenously every 8 hours) or erythromycin (500 mg intravenously every 6 hours until delivery). If susceptibility testing is not available or the results are not known, or when isolates are resistant to erythromycin and clindamycin, vancomycin 1 g intravenously every 12 hours until delivery is an alternative for women with immediate penicillin hypersensitivity.

The risk of anaphylaxis from administration of penicillin is low. Estimates range from 4 events per 10,000 to 4 per 100,000 recipients. There are reports of anaphylaxis associated with administration of a penicillin as IAP for the prevention of early-onset group B streptococcal infection.[23,807-809] No fatalities in association with IAP have been reported, and the risk of a fatal event is low, because the antimicrobials are administered in a hospital setting, in which intervention is readily available.

A number of residual problems, barriers to implementation, and missed opportunities remain that must be overcome to achieve the maximal benefit from IAP.[810-812] Procedural issues such as suboptimal culture techniques and collection of cultures earlier than 5 weeks before delivery constitute one set of barriers. Socioeconomic barriers also remain. Women who are not screened adequately are more likely to be in their teens. Blacks and Hispanics are more likely than whites to receive inadequate prenatal care and prenatal testing and are less likely to receive recommended prevention interventions. Increased awareness of perinatal group B streptococcal infection is needed. In one report, only 47% of women younger than 50 years of age reported ever having heard of group B streptococci.[813] Women with a high school education or less, low household income, or reporting black, Asian/Pacific Islander, or "other" race had lower awareness than that noted in other women. Efforts to raise awareness should target women from groups that traditionally are underserved in the health care system. Hospital infection control teams also can contribute to these efforts by spearheading educational efforts to effective implementation among hospital staff and laboratory personnel.[814]

Impact of Intrapartum Antibiotic Prophylaxis on Neonatal Sepsis

The efficacy of IAP in preventing early-onset group B streptococcal infection has been shown in a number of observational studies and in countries other than the United States when guidelines have been implemented.[23,518,815-817] The impact of increased use of IAP on the occurrence of sepsis caused by organisms other than group B streptococci is a subject of ongoing evaluation. Concern has been raised that neonatal sepsis caused by organisms other than group B streptococci may be increasing while group B streptococcal sepsis is decreasing and that the organisms causing non–group B streptococcal sepsis are more likely to be ampicillin resistant.[818] Reports that document such increases have found that they are restricted to preterm or low-birth-weight infants.[819] Among multicenter studies of the incidence of neonatal sepsis, a significant increase in the rate of early-onset sepsis caused by *E. coli* has been observed, but only infants of very low birth weight were evaluated.[820] In another multisite surveillance of trends in incidence and antimicrobial resistance of early-onset sepsis, stable rates of sepsis caused by other organisms were found, but an increase in ampicillin-resistant *E. coli* was observed among preterm but not term infants.[821]

A relationship between neonatal death caused by ampicillin-resistant *E. coli* and prolonged antepartum exposure to ampicillin was noted by Terrone and colleagues.[822] The frequency with which ampicillin-resistant Enterobacteriaceae were isolated, however, was similar after exposure to ampicillin to that after exposure to penicillin in another report.[823] Repeat cultures at 6 weeks post partum revealed no increase in antibiotic resistance in either group B streptococci or *E. coli* from women who had received antibiotics in labor.[824] To date, no causal link has been demonstrated between IAP and increasing numbers of infections caused by *E. coli* or ampicillin-resistant gram-negative sepsis among low-birth-weight neonates.[825] Fluctuations in the incidence of non–group B streptococcal sepsis and in the annual incidence of ampicillin-resistant infections indicates that ongoing population-based surveillance will be needed to monitor these trends and to identify possible reasons for the increase in ampicillin-resistant *E. coli* infections in preterm neonates.[826,827]

Management of Neonates Born to Mothers Receiving Intrapartum Antimicrobial Prophylaxis

Management of the infant born to a mother given intrapartum chemoprophylaxis is based on the infant's clinical status and gestational age as well as the duration of maternal chemoprophylaxis before delivery (Fig. 13-12).[24] If a woman receives IAP for suspected chorioamnionitis, her infant should have a full diagnostic evaluation and empirical therapy pending culture results regardless of the clinical condition at birth, gestational age, or duration of IAP before birth. This approach is based on the infant's exposure to suspected established infection. If the infant has signs of infection at or shortly following birth, full diagnostic evaluation including a complete blood cell count and differential, blood culture, and chest radiograph (if the neonate has respiratory signs) is indicated. A lumbar puncture, if feasible, also should be performed. A minimum of 10% to 15% of infants with meningitis will have a negative blood culture.[661] If lumbar puncture is deferred and therapy is continued for more than 48 hours because of suspected infection, CSF should be obtained for routine studies and culture. Empirical therapy for neonatal sepsis then is initiated. The duration of therapy is based on results of cultures and the infant's clinical course (see "Treatment" section). If the infant is healthy in appearance but has a gestational age of less than 35 weeks, a limited evaluation, including complete blood count and a blood culture, is performed without regard to the duration of maternal chemoprophylaxis. Empirical therapy need not be initiated unless signs of sepsis develop or the infant is very immature. Healthy-appearing infants with a gestational age of 35 weeks or more whose mothers received intravenous penicillin, ampicillin, or cefazolin less than 4 hours before delivery also should be evaluated and observed closely. If the infant is healthy, has a gestational age of 35 weeks or more, and has a mother given penicillin, ampicillin, or cefazolin 4 hours or more before delivery, then neither a diagnostic evaluation nor empirical antimicrobial therapy is recommended. The recommended observation interval for neonates undergoing a limited evaluation is 48 hours. The approach presented in Figure 13-12, however, is not an exclusive management pathway. Hospital discharge as early as 24 hours of age may be reasonable under certain circumstances, specifically when the infant is born after 4 or more hours of maternal β-lactam IAP, has a gestational age of 38 weeks or more, and is healthy-appearing. Other discharge criteria should be met, and the infant should be under the care of a person able to comply with instructions for home observation.[24,828] The risk of bacterial infection in healthy-appearing newborns is low. Outcomes among infants whose mothers receive IAP are better than among those whose mothers do not. Rehospitalization is uncommon among these infants.[829]

The influence of maternal IAP on the clinical spectrum of early-onset infection in term infants has been evaluated.[829-831] Exposure to antibiotics in labor does not change the clinical spectrum of disease or the onset of clinical signs of infection within 24 hours of birth for infants with early-onset group B streptococcal infection. Infants whose mothers have received IAP are less likely to be ill, to require assisted ventilation, or to have bacterial infection.[829] These infants are not more likely to undergo invasive procedures or to receive antibiotics.[830] The number of infants undergoing evaluation for sepsis has decreased in association with implementation of IAP guidelines, and among group B streptococcus–negative women, ordering of laboratory tests has diminished by almost 40%.[800]

Chemoprophylaxis for the Neonate

Chemoprophylaxis for neonates at birth continues to be advocated by some investigators. Three decades ago, Steigman and associates[832] found no cases of early-onset group B streptococcal infection among 130,000 newborns who received a single intramuscular injection of penicillin G (50,000 units) at birth as prophylaxis for gonococcal infection. Neonates with possible in utero acquisition of infection (those ill at birth) did not receive prophylaxis and were excluded from the analysis. Pyati and co-workers[833] evaluated over 1000 neonates with birth weights of less than 2000 g in whom a blood culture was obtained before penicillin was administered. In these high-risk infants, penicillin prophylaxis at

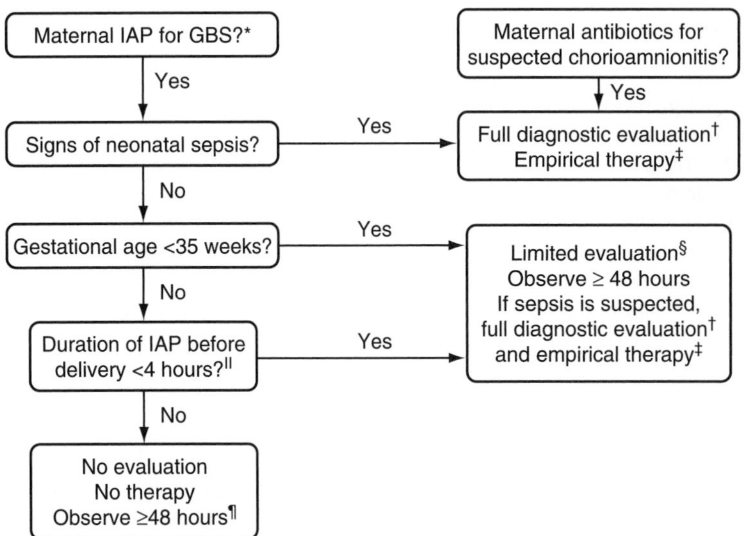

* If no maternal IAP for GBS was administered despite an indication of being present, data are insufficient on which to recommend a single management strategy.

† Includes complete blood cell (CBC) count and differential, blood culture, and chest radiograph if respiratory abnormalities are present. When signs of sepsis are present, a lumbar puncture, if feasible, should be performed.

‡ Duration of therapy varies depending on results of blood culture, cerebrospinal fluid findings, if obtained, and clinical course of the infant. If laboratory results and clinical course do not indicate bacterial infection, duration may be as short as 48 hours.

§ CBC with differential and blood culture.

|| Applies only to penicillin, ampicillin, or cefazolin and assumes recommended dosing regimens.

¶ A healthy-appearing infant who was ≥38 weeks' gestation at delivery and whose mother received ≥4 hours of IAP before delivery may be discharged home after 24 hours IF other discharge criteria have been met and a person able to comply fully with instructions for home observation will be present. If any one of these conditions is not met, the infant should be observed in the hospital for at least 48 hours and until criteria for discharge are achieved.

Figure 13–12 Recommended management of newborn infants exposed to maternal intrapartum antibiotic prophylaxis (IAP) for group B streptococcal (GBS) infection. (Adapted from Centers for Disease Control and Prevention. Prevention of perinatal group B streptococcal disease: revised guidelines from CDC. MMWR Morb Mortal Wkly Rep 51[RR-11]:1-22, 2002.)

birth was not effective in preventing group B streptococcal bacteremia or in altering the mortality rate associated with infection.

A few centers employ a combined maternal and neonatal protocol that consists of a risk-based maternal IAP approach combined with a single dose of intramuscular penicillin given to all infants within 1 hour of birth.[834,835] This policy is based on uncontrolled observational studies showing declines in early-onset group B streptococcal disease coincident with a policy of universal administration of penicillin to all infants.[836] A 76% reduction in early-onset infection has been noted, to 0.47 per 1000 live births, when the infection rate for the 5 years from 1986 to 1994 was compared with that from 1994 to 1999.

A special circumstance merits consideration for infant chemoprophylaxis: the non-affected sibling in a twin or multiple birth with early-onset[407,408] or late-onset[408] group B streptococcal disease. In this situation, the infant sibling of a neonate with invasive infection has a 25-fold increased risk of developing group B streptococcal disease. At the time of diagnosis of group B streptococcal disease in one infant of a multiple birth, the other infant or infants should be clinically evaluated.[408] If any sign of infection is noted, culture samples of blood *and* CSF are obtained, and empirical antimicrobial treatment is initiated and continued until cultures have been sterile for 48 hours. Obviously, if cultures are positive, a full course of treatment is recommended. If findings on the initial clinical evaluation are unremarkable, management should be individualized. The high incidence of infection in both twins and the poor outcome noted when the second twin was not evaluated until the onset of clinical signs of infection merit caution in this circumstance. Even when empirical therapy is given and invasive infection excluded, later onset is possible[837]

Immunoprophylaxis

The most promising and potentially lasting method for prevention of early- *and* late-onset infant infections as well as maternal infectious morbidity is immunoprophylaxis.[406,753] The underlying principle is that serum IgG directed against the type-specific capsular polysaccharide of group B streptococci, critical for protection against invasive group B streptococcal disease, is provided by passive or active immunization. Human sera containing sufficient amounts of type III–specific antibody has been demonstrated to be protective against lethal challenge in animal models of infection.[838] Studies of the other serotypes also indicate the importance of type-specific antibody in protection.[425-429,839,840] Provision of protective levels of type-specific immunity to the newborn theoretically may be achieved through passive or active immunization of the mother. Passive immune therapy for the mother would require development of hyperimmune preparations of human immune globulin for intravenous use, but animal studies indicate the potential usefulness of such an approach.[727,841]

The first candidate group B streptococcal vaccine, a purified type III capsular polysaccharide, underwent initial testing in healthy adults in 1978.[440] Subsequently, type Ia and type II capsular polysaccharides were studied.[842] Although these vaccines were well tolerated and elicited primarily IgG class response within 2 weeks, the immunogenicity was variable. It was discovered that nearly 90% of adults had very low preimmunization serum concentrations of capsular polysaccharide–specific antibodies in association with presumed immunologic naïvete. These low levels predicted a poor immune response in many, so that only 40% and 60% developed significant type-specific antibody responses after immunization with type Ia and type III polysaccharides, respectively. By contrast, 88% of those immunized with type II polysaccharide responded.

These early trials verified the feasibility of immunization as an approach to prevent group B streptococcal disease and revealed the need to develop candidate vaccines with enhanced immunogenicity. The first study conducted in pregnant women was an encouragement to the ultimate potential success of a group B streptococcal vaccine program.[464] Among 25 pregnant responders to a type III group B streptococcal polysaccharide vaccine, 90% delivered infants with substantial levels of specific antibody to the type III capsular polysaccharide in cord sera that promoted functional activity in vitro throughout the first 3 months of life in most.

Development of the first group B streptococcal conjugate vaccine, type III polysaccharide–tetanus toxoid, was driven by the prominence of type III among infant early- and late-onset disease–causing isolates, and by its dominance as a cause of meningitis. The type III polysaccharide was linked covalently to monomeric tetanus toxoid by reductive amination coupling chemistry.[843] Group B streptococcal capsular polysaccharide–protein conjugate vaccines of all clinically important serotypes subsequently were produced and found to be immunogenic and protective in experimental animals.[843-849] In the first clinical evaluation of the type III conjugate, greater than fourfold rises were achieved in 90% of healthy nonpregnant women who received the conjugate vaccine.[850] The vaccine was well tolerated, and the antibodies, predominantly of the IgG class, were functional in vitro and protective in a murine model of infection.

Since 1996, conjugate vaccines to each of the clinically relevant group B streptococcal serotypes causing invasive disease have been developed and tested in nearly 500 healthy adults 18 to 50 years of age.[850-853] Systemic responses, such as low-grade fever, chills, headache, or myalgias, which were short-lived, have been observed in less than 2% of these volunteers. Immune responses to each of the conjugate vaccines, with the exception of type V, are dose dependent. Doses of 4 to 15 μg of the capsular polysaccharide component have elicited greater than fourfold increases in capsular polysaccharide–specific IgG in 80% to 93% of recipients of type Ia, Ib, II, III and V conjugates at 8 weeks after immunization. Preliminary evaluation of a vaccine combining type II and type III capsular polysaccharide, each conjugated to tetanus toxoid, have shown no immune interference when compared with response following administration of the monovalent vaccine.[854]

As with the uncoupled purified polysaccharide, a phase 1 randomized placebo-controlled, double-blinded trial of type III capsular polysaccharide–tetanus toxoid conjugate vaccine has been conducted in 30 women at 30 to 32 weeks of gestation.[855] Immunization was well tolerated. Geometric mean concentrations of IgG antibody to type III capsular polysaccharide from immunized women were significantly increased from preimmunization values and correlated well with infant cord values. Sera from the infants of vaccinated women collected at 1 and 2 months of age promoted in vitro opsonization and killing of type III group B streptococci by neutrophils.

One alternate strategy for the preparation of group B streptococcal conjugate vaccines is to construct "designer" glycoconjugate vaccines with size-specific antigens and site-controlled coupling that optimizes the magnitude and specificity of the antipolysaccharide response.[856] An oligosaccharide-based tetanus toxoid conjugate vaccine against type III group B streptococci was synthesized to retain the antigenic specificity of the native polysaccharide and has been shown to be immunogenic in mice.[857] Conjugate size, polysaccharide size, and the degree of polysaccharide-protein cross-linking all are important considerations in optimizing immunogenicity of candidate vaccines.[858]

Use of proteins that are conserved across most group B streptococcal serotypes offers another vaccine development strategy. The C protein may be a promising alternative to tetanus toxoid as the protein component of a conjugate vaccine.[840,847,859] A type III polysaccharide–C protein conjugate vaccine theoretically could prevent a majority of systemic infections.[12] The group B streptococcal surface proteins Rib, Sip, and C5a peptidase each have been shown to elicit antibodies that are protective in experimental models of group B streptococcal infection.[860-862]

Because a majority of women have low concentrations of type-specific antibody in their sera, the most practical approach for future immunoprophylaxis is active immunization of all women of childbearing age, either before or later in pregnancy (i.e., early third trimester) or perhaps at the time of adolescent vaccinations.[753] Furthermore, in view of the substantial disease burden in nonpregnant adults, especially those with diabetes mellitus or age 65 or more years, targeted adult immunization is an attractive prevention strategy. Taken together, type Ia, type III, and type V group B streptococci now account for 75% to 85%, and five serotypes (Ia, Ib, II, III, and V), for nearly 100% of disease in infants and adults.[12,162,863,864] The production of a trivalent or a pentavalent conjugate is technically achievable. Physicians and their patients *and* pharmaceutical industry leaders must perceive this mode of prevention to be of high benefit and negligible risk, especially if pregnant women are to be the target population. The cost of developing suitable vaccines, although substantial, is considerably less than that of loss of life and of treating these infections and, for some infants, their lifelong sequelae.[766,769] If the prevention of group B streptococcal disease is to become a reality, however, obstetricians, pediatricians, public health officials, parents, and legislators must join together as advocates for the pregnant woman, her neonate, and high-risk adults.

REFERENCES

1. Fry RM. Fatal infections by haemolytic streptococcus group B. Lancet 1:199-201, 1938.
2. Franciosi RA, Knostman JD, Zimmerman RA. Group B streptococcal neonatal and infant infections. J Pediatr 82:707-718, 1973.
3. Baker CJ, Barrett FF. Transmission of group B streptococci among parturient women and their neonates. J Pediatr 83:919-925, 1973.
4. Howard JB, McCracken GH Jr. The spectrum of group B streptococcal infections in infancy. Am J Dis Child 128:815-818, 1974.
5. Bayer AS, Chow AW, Anthony BF, et al. Serious infections in adults due to group B streptococci. Am J Med 61:498-503, 1976.
6. Ledger WJ, Norman M, Gee C, et al. Bacteremia on an obstetric-gynecologic service. Am J Obstet Gynecol 121:205-212, 1975.
7. Faro S. Group B beta-hemolytic streptococci and puerperal infections. Am J Obstet Gynecol 139:686-689, 1981.
8. Farley MM, Harvey RC, Stull T, et al. A population-based assessment of invasive disease due to group B *Streptococcus* in nonpregnant adults. N Engl J Med 328:1807-1811, 1993.
9. Baker CJ, Edwards MS. Group B streptococcal infections: perinatal impact and prevention methods. Ann N Y Acad Sci 549:193-202, 1988.
10. Schuchat A, Oxtoby M, Cochi S, et al. Population-based risk factors for neonatal group B streptococcal disease: results of a cohort study in metropolitan Atlanta. J Infect Dis 162:672-677, 1990.
11. Lin F-YC, Clemens JD, Azimi PH, et al. Capsular polysaccharide types of group B streptococcal isolates from neonates with early-onset systemic infection. J Infect Dis 177:790-792, 1998.
12. Harrison LH, Elliott JA, Dwyer DM, et al. Serotype distribution of invasive group B streptococcal isolates in Maryland: implications for vaccine formulation. J Infect Dis 177:998-1002, 1998.
13. Blumberg HM, Stephens DS, Modansky M, et al. Invasive group B streptococcal disease: the emergence of serotype V. J Infect Dis 173:365-373, 1996.
14. Kvam AI, Efstratiou A, Bevanger L, et al. Distribution of serovariants of group B streptococci in isolates from England and Norway. J Med Microbiol 42:246-250, 1995.
15. Elliott JA, Farmer KD, Facklam RR. Sudden increase in isolation of group B streptococci, serotype V, is not due to emergence of a new pulsed-field gel electrophoresis type. J Clin Microbiol 36:2115-2116, 1998.
16. Lachenauer CS, Kasper DL, Shimada J, et al. Serotypes VI and VIII predominate among group B streptococci isolated from pregnant Japanese women. J Infect Dis 179:1030-1033, 1999.
17. Tettelin H, Masignani V, Cieslewicz MJ, et al. Complete genome sequence and comparative genomic analysis of an emerging human pathogen, serotype V *Streptococcus agalactiae*. Proc Natl Acad Sci U S A 99:12391-12396, 2002.
18. Glaser P, Rusniok C, Buchrieser C, et al. Genome sequence of *Streptococcus agalactiae*, a pathogen causing invasive neonatal disease. Mol Microbiol 45:1499-1513, 2002.
19. Centers for Disease Control and Prevention. Prevention of perinatal group B streptococcal disease: a public health perspective. MMWR Morb Mortal Wkly Rep 45:1-24, 1996.
20. American Academy of Pediatrics Committee on Infectious Diseases and Committee on Fetus and Newborn. Revised guidelines for prevention of early-onset group B streptococcal (GBS) infection. Pediatrics 99:489-496, 1997.
21. American College of Obstetricians and Gynecologists Committee on Obstetric Practice. Prevention of early-onset group B streptococcal disease in newborns. ACOG Committee Opinion. Washington, DC, American College of Obstetricians and Gynecologists, 1996 (Bulletin No. 173).
22. Schrag SJ, Zywicki S, Farley MM, et al. Group B streptococcal disease in the era of intrapartum antibiotic prophylaxis. N Engl J Med 342:15-20, 2000.
23. Schrag SJ, Zell ER, Stat M, et al. A population-based comparison of strategies to prevent early-onset group B streptococcal disease in neonates. N Engl J Med 347:233-239, 2002.
24. Centers for Disease Control and Prevention. Prevention of perinatal group B streptococcal disease: revised guidelines from CDC. MMWR Morb Mortal Wkly Rep 51(RR-11):1-22, 2002.
25. Kasper DL, Baker CJ. Electron microscopic definition of surface antigens of group B *Streptococcus*. J Infect Dis 139:147-151, 1979.
26. Lancefield RC. A serological differentiation of human and other groups of hemolytic streptococci. J Exp Med 57:571-595, 1933.
27. Brown JH. Appearance of double-zone beta-hemolytic streptococci in blood agar. J Bacteriol 34:35-48, 1937.
28. Facklam RR, Padula JF, Thacker LG, et al. Presumptive identification of groups A, B and D streptococci. Appl Microbiol 27:107-113, 1974.
29. Roe MH, Todd JK, Favara BE. Non-hemolytic group B streptococcal infections. J Pediatr 89:75-77, 1976.
30. Baker CJ, Clark DJ, Barrett FF. Selective broth medium for isolation of group B streptococci. Appl Microbiol 26:884-885, 1973.
31. Lim DV, Morales WJ, Walsh AF. Lim group B strep broth and coagglutination for rapid identification of group B streptococci in preterm pregnant women. J Clin Microbiol 25:452-453, 1987.
32. Facklam RR, Padula JF, Wortham EC, et al. Presumptive identification of group A, B and D streptococci on agar plate medium. J Clin Microbiol 9:665-672, 1979.
33. Merritt K, Jacobs NJ. Characterization and incidence of pigment production by human clinical group B streptococci. J Clin Microbiol 8:105-107, 1978.
34. de la Rosa M, Perez M, Carazo C, et al. New Granada medium for detection and identification of group B streptococci. J Clin Microbiol 30:1019-1021, 1992.
35. Christie R, Atkins NE, Munch-Petersen E. A note on a lytic phenomenon shown by group B streptococci. Aust J Exp Biol Med Sci 22:197-200, 1944.
36. Tapsall JW, Phillips EA. Presumptive identification of group B streptococci by rapid detection of CAMP factor and pigment production. Diagn Microbiol Infect Dis 7:225-228, 1987.
37. Bernheimer AW, Linder R, Avigad LS. Nature and mechanism of action of the CAMP protein of group B streptococci. Infect Immun 23:838-844, 1979.
38. Ratner HB, Weeks LS, Stratton CW. Evaluation of Spot-CAMP test for identification of group B streptococci. J Clin Microbiol 24:296-297, 1986.
39. Facklam R, Bosley GS, Rhoden D, et al. Comparative evaluation of the API 20S and automicrobic gram-positive identification systems for non-beta-hemolytic streptococci and aerococci. J Clin Microbiol 21:535-541, 1985.
40. Lancefield RC. A microprecipitin technic for classifying hemolytic streptococci, and improved methods for producing antisera. Proc Soc Exp Biol Med 38:473-478, 1938.
41. Daly JA, Seskin KC. Evaluation of rapid, commercial latex techniques for serogrouping beta-hemolytic streptococci. J Clin Microbiol 26:2429-2431, 1988.
42. Stableforth AW. Incidence of various serological types of *Streptococcus agalactiae* in herds of cows in Great Britain. J Pathol Bacteriol 46:21-29, 1938.
43. Pattison IH, Matthews PRJ, Maxted WR. Type classification by Lancefield's precipitin method of human and bovine group B streptococci isolated in Britain. J Pathol Bacteriol 69:51-60, 1955.
44. Finch LA, Martin DR. Human and bovine group B streptococci: two distinct populations. J Appl Bacteriol 57:273-278, 1984.
45. Jensen NE. Epidemiological aspects of human/animal interrelationships in GBS. Antibiot Chemother 35:40-48, 1985.
46. Wibawan IWT, Lämmler C. Properties of group B streptococci with protein surface antigens X and R. J Clin Microbiol 28:2834-2836, 1990.
47. Lancefield RC, Hare R. The serological differentiation of pathogenic and non-pathogenic strains of hemolytic streptococci from parturient women. J Exp Med 61:335-349, 1935.
48. Lancefield RC. Two serological types of group B hemolytic streptococci with related, but not identical, type-specific substances. J Exp Med 67:25-40, 1938.
49. Freimer EH. Type-specific polysaccharide antigens of group B streptococci: II. The chemical basis for serological specificity of the type II HCI antigen. J Exp Med 125:381-392, 1967.
50. Wilkinson HW, Eagon RG. Type-specific antigens of group B type Ic streptococci. Infect Immun 4:596-604, 1971.
51. Johnson DR, Ferrieri P. Group B streptococcal Ibc protein antigen: distribution of two determinants in wild-type strains of common serotypes. J Clin Microbiol 19:506-510, 1984.

52. Wilkinson HW. Analysis of group B streptococcal types associated with disease in human infants and adults. J Clin Microbiol 7:176-179, 1978.
53. Jelínková J, Motlová J. The nomenclature of GBS. Antibiot Chemother 35:49-52, 1985.
54. Henrichsen J, Ferrieri P, Jelínková J, et al. Nomenclature of antigens of group B streptococci. Int J Syst Bacteriol 34:500, 1984.
55. Perch B, Kjems E, Henrichsen J. New serotypes of group B streptococci isolated from human sources. J Clin Microbiol 10:109-110, 1979.
56. Jelínková J, Motlová J. Worldwide distribution of two new serotypes of group B streptococci: type IV and provisional type V. J Clin Microbiol 21:361-362, 1985.
57. Wessels MR, DiFabio JL, Benedí V-J, et al. Structural determination and immunochemical characterization of the type V group B *Streptococcus* capsular polysaccharide. J Biol Chem 266:6714-6719, 1991.
58. von Hunolstein C, D'Ascenzi S, Wagner B, et al. Immunochemistry of capsular type polysaccharide and virulence properties of type VI *Streptococcus agalactiae* (group B streptococci). Infect Immun 61:1272-1280, 1993.
59. Kogan G, Brisson J-R, Kasper DL, et al. Structural elucidation of the novel type VII group B *Streptococcus* capsular polysaccharide by high resolution NMR spectroscopy. Carbohydr Res 277:1-9, 1995.
60. Kogan G, Uhrín D, Brisson J-R, et al. Structural and immunochemical characterization of the type VIII group B *Streptococcus* capsular polysaccharide. J Biol Chem 271:8786-8790, 1996.
61. Kogan G, Uhrín D, Brisson J-R, et al. Structure of the type VI group B *Streptococcus* capsular polysaccharide determined by high resolution NMR spectroscopy. J Carbohydr Chem 13:1071-1078, 1994.
62. Lancefield RC, McCarty M, Everly WN. Multiple mouse-protective antibodies directed against group B streptococci. J Exp Med 142:165-179, 1975.
63. Bevanger L, Naess AI. Mouse-protective antibodies against the Ibc proteins of group B streptococci. Acta Pathol Microbiol Immunol Scand 93:121-124, 1985.
64. Madoff LC, Hori S, Michel JL, et al. Phenotypic diversity in the alpha C protein of group B streptococci. Infect Immun 59:2638-2644, 1991.
65. Madoff LC, Michel JL, Gong EW, et al. Group B streptococci escape host immunity by deletion of tandem repeat elements of the alpha C protein. Proc Natl Acad Sci U S A 93:4131-4136, 1996.
66. Kling DE, Gravekamp C, Madoff LC, et al. Characterization of two distinct opsonic and protective epitopes within the alpha c protein of the group B *Streptococcus*. Infect Immun 65:1462-1467, 1997.
67. Gravekamp C, Horensky DS, Michel JL, et al. Variation in repeat number within the alpha c protein of group B streptococci alters antigenicity and protective epitopes. Infect Immun 64:3576-3583, 1996.
68. Jerlström PG, Chhatwal GS, Timmis KN. The IgA-binding β antigen of the c protein complex of group B streptococci: sequence determination of its gene and detection of two binding regions. Mol Microbiol 54:843-849, 1991.
69. Brady LJ, Boyle MDP. Identification of non-immunoglobulin A-Fc-binding forms and low-molecular-weight secreted forms of the group B streptococcal β antigen. Infect Immun 57:1573-1581, 1989.
70. Jerlström PG, Talay SR, Valentin-Weigand P, et al. Identification of an immunoglobulin A binding motif located in the β-antigen of the c protein complex of group B streptococci. Infect Immun 64:2787-2793, 1996.
71. Pattison IH, Matthews PRJ, Howell DG. The type classification of group B streptococci with special reference to bovine strains apparently lacking in type polysaccharide. J Pathol Bacteriol 69:41-50, 1955.
72. Flores AE, Ferrieri P. Molecular species of R-protein antigens produced by clinical isolates of group B streptococci. J Clin Microbiol 27:1050-1054, 1989.
73. Fasola EL, Flores AE, Ferrieri P. Immune responses to the R4 protein antigen of group B streptococci and its relationship to other streptococcal R4 proteins. Clin Diagn Lab Immunol 3:321-325, 1996.
74. Stålhammar-Carlemalm M, Stenberg L, Lindahl G. Protein rib: a novel group B streptococcal cell surface protein that confers passive immunity and is expressed by most strains causing invasive infection. J Exp Med 177:1593-1603, 1993.
75. Erdogan S, Fagan PK, Talay SR, et al. Molecular analysis of group B protective surface protein, a new cell surface protective antigen of group B streptococci. Infect Immun 70:803-811, 2002.
76. Lachenauer CS, Madoff LC. A protective surface protein from type V group B streptococci shares N-terminal sequence homology with the alpha c protein. Infect Immun 64:4255-4260, 1996.
77. Rioux S, Martin D, Ackermann H-W, et al. Localization of surface immunogenic protein on group B *Streptococcus*. Infect Immun 69:5162-5265, 2001.
78. Deng L, Kasper DL, Krick TP, Wessels MR. Characterization of the linkage between the type III capsular polysaccharide and the bacterial cell wall of group B *Streptococcus*. J Biol Chem 275:7497-7504, 2000.
79. Rýc M, Jelínková J, Motlová J, et al. Immuno-electronmicroscopic demonstration of capsules on group-B streptococci of new serotypes and type candidates. J Med Microbiol 25:147-149, 1988.
80. Paoletti LC, Ross RA, Johnson KD. Cell growth rate regulates expression of group B *Streptococcus* type III capsular polysaccharide. Infect Immun 64:1220-1226, 1996.
81. Sellin M, Håkansson S, Norgren M. Phase-shift of polysaccharide capsule expression in group B streptococci, type III. Microb Pathog 18:401-415, 1995.
82. Kasper DL, Goroff DK, Baker CJ. Immunochemical characterization of native polysaccharides from group B *Streptococcus*: the relationship of the type III and group B determinants. J Immunol 121:1096-1105, 1978.
83. Russell H, Norcross NL. The isolation of some physiochemical and biologic properties of the type III antigen of group B *Streptococcus*. J Immunol 109:90-96, 1972.
84. Michon F, Katzenellenbogen E, Kasper DL, et al. Structure of the complex group-specific polysaccharide of group B *Streptococcus*. Biochemistry 26:476-486, 1987.
85. Michon F, Brisson J-R, Dell A, et al. Multiantennary group-specific polysaccharide of group B *Streptococcus*. Biochemistry 27:5341-5351, 1988.
86. Baker CJ, Kasper DL, Davis CE. Immunochemical characterization of the native type III polysaccharide of group B *Streptococcus*. J Exp Med 143:258-270, 1976.
87. Tai JY, Gotschlich EC, Lancefield RC. Isolation of type-specific polysaccharide antigen from group B type Ib streptococci. J Exp Med 149:58-66, 1979.
88. Jennings HJ, Rosell K-G, Kasper DL. Structural determination and serology of the native polysaccharide antigen of the type III group B *Streptococcus*. Can J Biochem 58:112-120, 1980.
89. Wessels MR, Pozsgay V, Kasper DL, et al. Structure and immunochemistry of an oligosaccharide repeating unit of the capsular polysaccharide of type III group B *Streptococcus*. J Biol Chem 262:8262-8267, 1987.
90. Kasper DL, Baker CJ, Galdes B, et al. Immunochemical analysis and immunogenicity of the type II group B streptococcal capsular polysaccharide. J Clin Invest 72:260-269, 1983.
91. Wessels MR, Benedí V-J, Jennings HJ, et al. Isolation and characterization of type IV group B *Streptococcus* capsular polysaccharide. Infect Immun 57:1089-1094, 1989.
92. Jennings HJ, Rosell K-G, Katzenellenbogen E, et al. Structural determination of the capsular polysaccharide antigen of type II group B *Streptococcus*. J Biol Chem 258:1793-1798, 1983.
93. Jennings HJ, Katzenellenbogen E, Lugowski C, et al. Structure of native polysaccharide antigens of type Ia and type Ib group B *Streptococcus*. Biochemistry 22:1258-1264, 1983.
94. Schifferle RE, Jennings HJ, Wessels MR, et al. Immunochemical analysis of the types Ia and Ib group B streptococcal polysaccharides. J Immunol 135:4164-4170, 1985.
95. Sadler JE, Paulson JC, Hill RL. The role of sialic acid in the expression of human MN blood group antigens. J Biol Chem 254:2112-2119, 1979.
96. Pritchard DG, Gray BM, Egan ML. Murine monoclonal antibodies to type Ib polysaccharide of group B streptococci bind to human milk oligosaccharides. Infect Immun 60:1598-1602, 1992.
97. Wessels MR, Muñoz A, Kasper DL. A model of high-affinity antibody binding to type III group B *Streptococcus* capsular polysaccharide. Proc Natl Acad Sci U S A 84:9170-9174, 1987.
98. Brisson J-R, Uhrinova S, Woods RJ, et al. NMR and molecular dynamics studies of the conformational epitope of the type III group B *Streptococcus* capsular polysaccharide and derivatives. Biochemistry 36:3278-3292, 1997.
99. Zou W, Jennings HJ. The conformational epitope of type III group B *Streptococcus* capsular polysaccharide. Adv Exp Med Biol 491:473-484, 2001.
100. Lindberg B, Lönngren J, Powell DA. Structural studies of the specific type 14 pneumococcal polysaccharide. Carbohydr Res 58:117-186, 1977.
101. Wessels MR, Kasper DL. Antibody recognition of the type 14 pneumococcal capsule. Evidence for a conformational epitope in a neutral polysaccharide. J Exp Med 169:2121-2131, 1989.

102. Yeung MK, Mattingly SJ. Biosynthesis of cell wall peptidoglycan and polysaccharide antigens by protoplasts of type III group B *Streptococcus*. J Bacteriol 154:211-220, 1983.
103. Milligan TW, Doran TI, Straus DC, et al. Growth and amino acid requirements of various strains of group B streptococci. J Clin Microbiol 7:28-33, 1978.
104. Baker CJ, Kasper DL. Microcapsule of type III strains of group B *Streptococcus*: production and morphology. Infect Immun 13:189-194, 1976.
105. Malin G, Paoletti LC. Use of a dynamic in vitro attachment and invasion system (DIVAS) to determine influence of growth rate on invasion of respiratory epithelium by group B *Streptococcus*. Proc Natl Acad Sci U S A 98:13335-13340, 2001.
106. Johri AK, Padilla J, Malin G, Paoletti LC. Oxygen regulates invasiveness and virulence of group B *Streptococcus*. Infect Immun 71:6707-6711, 2003.
107. Weiser JN, Rubens CE. Transposon mutagenesis of group B *Streptococcus* beta-hemolysin biosynthesis. Infect Immun 55:2314-2316, 1987.
108. Tapsall JW. Pigment production by Lancefield-group B streptococci (*Streptococcus agalactiae*). J Med Microbiol 21:75-81, 1986.
109. Ferrieri P, Wannamaker LW, Nelson J. Localization and characterization of the hippuricase activity of group B streptococci. Infect Immun 7:747-752, 1973.
110. Ferrieri P, Gray ED, Wannamaker LW. Biochemical and immunological characterization of the extracellular nucleases of group B streptococci. J Exp Med 151:56-68, 1980.
111. Poyart C, Pellegrini E, Gaillot O, et al. Contribution of Mn-cofactored superoxide dismutase (SodA) to the virulence of *Streptococcus agalactiae*. Infect Immun 69:5098-5106, 2001.
112. Milligan TW, Straus DC, Mattingly SJ. Extracellular neuraminidase production by group B streptococci. Infect Immun 18:189-195, 1977.
113. Nealon TJ, Mattingly SJ. Association of elevated levels of cellular lipoteichoic acids of group B streptococci with human neonatal disease. Infect Immun 39:1243-1251, 1983.
114. Skalka B, Smola J. Lethal effect of CAMP-factor and UBERIS-factor—a new finding about diffusible exosubstances of *Streptococcus agalactiae* and *Streptococcus uberis*. Zentralbl Bakteriol Mikrobiol Hyg 249:190-194, 1981.
115. Jürgens D, Sterzik B, Fehrenbach FJ. Unspecific binding of group B streptococcal cocytolysin (CAMP factor) to immunoglobulins and its possible role in pathogenicity. J Exp Med 165:720-732, 1987.
116. Hill HR, Bohnsack JF, Morris EZ, et al. Group B streptococci inhibit the chemotactic activity of the fifth component of complement. J Immunol 141:3551-3556, 1988.
117. Bohnsack JF, Mollison KW, Buko AM, et al. Group B streptococci inactivate complement component C5a by enzymic cleavage at the C-terminus. Biochem J 273:635-640, 1991.
118. Bohnsack JF, Zhou XN, Williams PA, et al. Purification of a protease from group B streptococci that inactivates human C5a. Biochim Biophys Acta 1079:222-228, 1991.
119. Cleary PP, Handley J, Suvorov AN, et al. Similarity between the group B and A streptococcal C5a peptidase genes. Infect Immun 60:4239-4244, 1992.
120. Bohnsack JF, Zhou X, Gustin JN, et al. Bacterial evasion of the antibody response: human IgG antibodies neutralize soluble but not bacteria-associated group B streptococcal C5a-ase. J Infect Dis 165:315-321, 1992.
121. Pritchard DG, Lin B, Willingham TR, et al. Characterization of the group B streptococcal hyaluronate lyase. Arch Biochem Biophys 315:431-437, 1994.
122. Hayano S, Tanaka A. Sialidase-like enzymes produced by group A, B, C, G, and L streptococci and by *Streptococcus sanguis*. J Bacteriol 97:1328-1333, 1969.
123. Milligan TW, Mattingly SJ, Straus DC. Purification and partial characterization of neuraminidase from type III group B streptococci. J Bacteriol 144:164-172, 1980.
124. Brown JG, Straus DC. Characterization of neuraminidases produced by various serotypes of group B streptococci. Infect Immun 55:1-6, 1987.
125. Milligan TW, Baker CJ, Straus DC, et al. Association of elevated levels of extracellular neuraminidase with clinical isolates of type III group B streptococci. Infect Immun 21:738-746, 1978.
126. Musser JM, Mattingly SJ, Quentin R, et al. Identification of a high-virulence clone of type III *Streptococcus agalactiae* (group B *Streptococcus*) causing invasive neonatal disease. Proc Natl Acad Sci U S A 86:4731-4735, 1989.
127. Durham DL, Straus DC. Extracellular products of type III *Streptococcus agalactiae* and their relationship to virulence. Curr Microbiol 8:89-94, 1983.
128. Klegerman ME, Boyer KM, Papierniak CK, et al. Type-specific capsular antigen is associated with virulence in late-onset group B streptococcal type III disease. Infect Immun 44:124-129, 1984.
129. Yeung MK, Mattingly SJ. Biosynthetic capacity for type-specific antigen synthesis determines the virulence of serotype III strains of group B streptococci. Infect Immun 44:217-221, 1984.
130. Yeung MK, Mattingly SJ. Isolation and characterization of type III group streptococcal mutants defective in biosynthesis of the type-specific antigen. Infect Immun 42:141-151, 1983.
131. Håkansson S, Granlund-Edstedt M, Sellin M, et al. Demonstration and characterization of buoyant-density subpopulations of group B *Streptococcus* type III. J Infect Dis 161:741-746, 1990.
132. Nealon TJ, Mattingly SJ. Role of cellular lipoteichoic acids in mediating adherence of serotype III strains of group B streptococci to human embryonic, fetal, and adult epithelial cells. Infect Immun 43:523-530, 1984.
133. Goldschmidt JC Jr, Panos C. Teichoic acids of *Streptococcus agalactiae*: chemistry, cytotoxicity, and effect on bacterial adherence to human cells in tissue culture. Infect Immun 43:670-677, 1984.
134. Wanger AR, Dunny GM. Identification of a *Streptococcus agalactiae* protein antigen associated with bovine mastitis isolates. Infect Immun 55:1170-1175, 1987.
135. Anthony BF, Eisenstadt R, Carter J, et al. Genital and intestinal carriage of group B streptococci during pregnancy. J Infect Dis 143:761-766, 1981.
136. Ferrieri P, Blair LL. Pharyngeal carriage of group B streptococci: detection by three methods. J Clin Microbiol 6:136-139, 1977.
137. Baker CJ, Goroff DK, Alpert SL, et al. Comparison of bacteriological methods for the isolation of group B streptococcus from vaginal cultures. J Clin Microbiol 4:46-48, 1976.
138. Christensen KK, Ripa T, Agrup G, et al. Group B streptococci in human urethral and cervical specimens. Scand J Infect Dis 8:74-78, 1976.
139. MacDonald SW, Manuel FR, Embil JA. Localization of group B beta-hemolytic streptococci in the female urogenital tract. Am J Obstet Gynecol 133:57-59, 1979.
140. Ferrieri P, Cleary PP, Seeds AE. Epidemiology of group B streptococcal carriage in pregnant women and newborn infants. J Med Microbiol 10:103-114, 1976.
141. Dillon HC, Gray E, Pass MA, et al. Anorectal and vaginal carriage of group B streptococci during pregnancy. J Infect Dis 145:794-799, 1982.
142. Wood EG, Dillon HC Jr. A prospective study of group B streptococcal bacteriuria in pregnancy. Am J Obstet Gynecol 140:515-520, 1981.
143. Persson K, Bjerre B, Elfström L, et al. Longitudinal study of group B streptococcal carriage during late pregnancy. Scand J Infect Dis 19:325-329, 1987.
144. Paredes A, Wong P, Mason EO Jr, et al. Nosocomial transmission of group B streptococci in a newborn nursery. Pediatrics 59:679-682, 1976.
145. Anthony BF, Okada DM, Hobel CJ. Epidemiology of the group B *Streptococcus*: maternal and nosocomial sources for infant acquisitions. J Pediatr 95:431-436, 1979.
146. Hammerschlag MR, Baker CJ, Alpert S, et al. Colonization with group B streptococci in girls under 16 years of age. Pediatrics 60:473-477, 1977.
147. Mauer M, Thirumoorthi MC, Dajani AS. Group B streptococcal colonization in prepubertal children. Pediatrics 64:65-67, 1979.
148. Baker CJ, Goroff DK, Alpert S, et al. Vaginal colonization with group B *Streptococcus*: a study in college women. J Infect Dis 135:392-397, 1977.
149. Gardner SE, Yow MD, Leeds LJ, et al. Failure of penicillin to eradicate group B streptococcal colonization in the pregnant woman. Am J Obstet Gynecol 135:1062-1065, 1979.
150. Lewis RFM. Beta-haemolytic streptococci from the female genital tract: clinical correlates and outcome of treatment. Epidemiol Infect 102:391-400, 1989.
151. Anthony BF, Okada DM, Hobel CJ. Epidemiology of group B *Streptococcus*: longitudinal observations during pregnancy. J Infect Dis 137:524-530, 1978.
152. Meyn L, Moore DM, Hillier SL, Krohn MA. Association of sexual activity with colonization and vaginal acquisition of group B *Streptococcus* in nonpregnant women. Am J Epidemiol 155:949-957, 2002.

153. Yow MD, Leeds LJ, Thompson PK, et al. The natural history of group B streptococcal colonization in the pregnant woman and her offspring: I. Colonization studies. Am J Obstet Gynecol 137:34-38, 1980.
154. Boyer KM, Gadzala CA, Kelly PD, et al. Selective intrapartum chemoprophylaxis of neonatal group B streptococcal early-onset disease: II. Predictive value of prenatal cultures. J Infect Dis 148:802-809, 1983.
155. Yancey MK, Schuchat A, Brown LK, et al. The accuracy of late antenatal screening cultures in predicting genital group B streptococcal colonization at delivery. Obstet Gynecol 88:811-815, 1996.
156. Badri MS, Zawaneh S, Cruz AC, et al. Rectal colonization with group B *Streptococcus*: relation to vaginal colonization of pregnant women. J Infect Dis 135:308-312, 1977.
157. Persson KM-S, Bjerre B, Elfström L, et al. Faecal carriage of group B streptococci. Eur J Clin Microbiol 5:156-159, 1986.
158. Kaplan EL, Johnson DR, Kuritsky JN. Rectal colonization by group B β-hemolytic streptococci in a geriatric population. J Infect Dis 148:1120, 1983.
159. Anthony BF, Carter JA, Eisenstadt R, et al. Isolation of group B streptococci from the proximal small intestine of adults. J Infect Dis 147:776, 1983.
160. Barnham M. The gut as a source of the haemolytic streptococci causing infection in surgery of the intestinal and biliary tracts. J Infect 6:129-139, 1983.
161. Easmon CSF. The carrier state: group B *Streptococcus*. J Antimicrob Chemother 18(Suppl A):59-65, 1986.
162. Zaleznik DF, Rench MA, Hillier S, et al. Invasive disease due to group B *Streptococcus* in pregnant women and neonates from diverse population groups. Clin Infect Dis 30:276-281, 2000.
163. Bliss SJ, Manning SD, Tallman P, et al. Group B *Streptococcus* colonization in male and nonpregnant female university students: a cross-sectional prevalence study. Clin Infect Dis 34:184-190, 2002.
164. Campbell JR, Hillier SL, Krohn MA, et al. Group B streptococcal colonization and serotype-specific immunity in pregnant women at delivery. Obstet Gynecol 96:498-503, 2000.
165. Davies HD, Adair C, McGeer A, et al. Antibodies to capsular polysaccharides of group B *Streptococcus* in pregnant Canadian women: relationship to colonization status and infection in the neonate. J Infect Dis 184:285-291, 2001.
166. Ramos E, Gaudier FL, Hearing LR, et al. Group B *Streptococcus* colonization in pregnant diabetic women. Obstet Gynecol 89:257-260, 1997.
167. Christensen KK, Dykes A-K, Christensen, P. Relation between use of tampons and urogenital carriage of group B streptococci. BMJ 289:731-732, 1984.
168. Regan JA, Klebanoff MA, Nugent RP, et al. The epidemiology of group B streptococcal colonization in pregnancy. Obstet Gynecol 77:604-610, 1991.
169. Hickman ME, Rench MA, Ferrieri P, et al. Changing epidemiology of group B streptococcal (GBS) colonization. Pediatrics 104:203-209, 1999.
170. Newton ER, Butler MC, Shain RN. Sexual behavior and vaginal colonization by group B *Streptococcus* among minority women. Obstet Gynecol 88:577-582, 1996.
171. Beachler CW, Baker CJ, Kasper DL, et al. Group B streptococcal colonization and antibody status in lower socioeconomic parturient women. Am J Obstet Gynecol 133:171-173, 1979.
172. Hansen SM, Uldbjerg N, Kilian M, Sørensen UBS. Dynamics of *Streptococcus agalactiae* colonization in women during and after pregnancy and in their infants. J Clin Microbiol 42:83-89, 2004.
173. Jackson DH, Hinder SM, Stringer J, et al. Carriage and transmission of group B streptococci among STD clinic patients. Br J Vener Dis 58:334-337, 1982.
174. Ross PW, Cumming CG. Group B streptococci in women attending a sexually transmitted diseases clinic. J Infect 4:161-166, 1982.
175. Chretien JH, McGinniss CG, Thompson, J, et al. Group B beta-hemolytic streptococci causing pharyngitis. J Clin Microbiol 10:263-266, 1979.
176. Sackel SG, Baker CJ, Kasper DL, et al. Isolation of group B *Streptococcus* from men. 18th Interscience Conference on Antimicrobial Agents and Chemotherapy, 1978 [Abstract 467].
177. Wallin J, Forsgren A. Group B streptococci in venereal disease clinic patients. Br J Vener Dis 51:401-404, 1975.
178. Benchetrit LC, Fracalanzza SEL, Peregrino H, et al. Carriage of *Streptococcus agalactiae* in women and neonates and distribution of serological types: a study in Brazil. J Clin Microbiol 15:787-790, 1982.
179. Liang ST, Lau SP, Chan SH, et al. Perinatal colonization of group B *Streptococcus*: an epidemiological study in a Chinese population. Aust N Z J Obstet Gynaecol 26:138-141, 1986.
180. Trujillo H. Group B streptococcal colonization in Medellín, Columbia. Pediatr Infect Dis J 9:224-225, 1990.
181. Feikin DR, Thorsen P, Zywicki S, et al. Association between colonization with group B streptococci during pregnancy and preterm delivery among Danish women. Am J Obstet Gynecol 184:427-433, 2001.
182. Gyaneshwar R, Nsanze H, Singh KP, et al. The prevalence of sexually transmitted disease agents in pregnant women in Suva. Aust N Z J Obstet Gynaecol 27:213-215, 1987.
183. Tsolia M, Psoma M, Gavrili S, et al. Group B *Streptococcus* colonization of Greek pregnant women and neonates: prevalence, risk factors and serotypes. Clin Microbiol Infect 9:832-838, 2003.
184. Mani V, Jadhav M, Sivadasan K, et al. Maternal and neonatal colonization with group B *Streptococcus* and neonatal outcome. Indian Pediatr 21:357-363, 1984.
185. Kieran E, Matheson M, Mann AG, et al. Group B *Streptococcus* (GBS) colonisation among expectant Irish mothers. Ir Med J 91:21-22, 1998.
186. Schimmel MS, Eidelman AI, Rudensky B, et al. Epidemiology of group B streptococcal colonization and infection in Jerusalem, 1989-91. Isr J Med Sci 30:349-351, 1994.
187. Marchaim D, Hallak M, Gortzak-Uzan L, et al. Risk factors for carriage of group B *Streptococcus* in southern Israel. Isr Med Assoc J 5:646-648, 2003.
188. Visconti A, Orefici G, Notarnicola AM. Colonization and infection of mothers and neonates with group B streptococci in three Italian hospitals. J Hosp Infect 6:265-276, 1985.
189. Yamane N, Yuki M, Kyono K. Isolation and characterization of group B streptococci from genitourinary tracts in Japan. Tohoku J Exp Med 141:327-335, 1983.
190. Sunna E, El-Daher N, Bustami K, et al. A study of group B streptococcal carrier state during late pregnancy. Trop Geogr Med 43:161-164, 1991.
191. Elzouki AY, Vesikari T. First international conference on infections in children in Arab countries. Pediatr Infect Dis J 4:527-531, 1985.
192. Solórzano-Santos F, Diáz-Ramos RD, Arredondo-Garciá JL. Diseases caused by group B *Streptococcus* in Mexico. Pediatr Infect Dis J 9:66, 1990.
193. Solórzano-Santos F, Echaniz-Aviles G, Conde-Glez CJ, et al. Cervicovaginal infection with group B streptococci among pregnant Mexican women. J Infect Dis 159:1003-1004, 1989.
194. Hoogkamp-Korstanje JAA, Gerards LJ, Cats BP. Maternal carriage and neonatal acquisition of group B streptococci. J Infect Dis 145:800-803, 1982.
195. Dawodu AH, Damole IO, Onile BA. Epidemiology of group B streptococcal carriage among pregnant women and their neonates: an African experience. Trop Geogr Med 35:145-150, 1983.
196. Collins TS, Calderon M, Gilman RH, et al. Group B streptococcal colonization in a developing country: its association with sexually transmitted disease and socioeconomic factors. Am J Trop Med Hyg 59:633-636, 1998.
197. Gosling PJ, Morgos FW. Group B streptococci: colonization of women in labour and neonatal acquisition in the western region of Saudi Arabia. J Hosp Infect 4:324, 1983.
198. Uduman SA, Chatterjee TK, Al-Mouzan MI, et al. Group B streptococci colonization among Saudi women in labor and neonatal acquisition. Int J Gynaecol Obstet 23:21-24, 1985.
199. Ross PW, Neilson JR. Group B streptococci in mothers and infants: Edinburgh studies. Health Bull 40:234-239, 1982.
200. Teres FO, Matorras R, Perea AG, et al. Prevention of neonatal group B streptococcal sepsis. Pediatr Infect Dis J 6:874, 1987.
201. Pengsa K, Puapermpoonsiri S, Taksaphan S, et al. Group B streptococcal colonization in mothers and their neonates. Ramathibodi Med J 7:83-90, 1984.
202. Suara RO, Adegbola RA, Baker CJ, et al. Carriage of group B streptococci in pregnant Gambian mothers and their infants. J Infect Dis 170:1316-1319, 1994.
203. Orrett FA, Olagundoye V. Prevalence of group B streptococcal colonization in pregnant third trimester women in Trinidad. J Hosp Infect 27:43-48, 1994.
204. Amin A, Abdulrazzaq YM, Uduman S. Group B streptococcal serotype distribution of isolates from colonized pregnant women at the time of delivery in United Arab Emirates. J Infect 45:42-46, 2002.

205. Stoll BJ, Schuchat A. Maternal carriage of group B streptococci in developing countries. Pediatr Infect Dis J 17:499-503, 1998.
206. Trijbels-Smeulders MAJM, Kollée LAA, Adriaanse AH, et al. Neonatal group B streptococcal infection: incidence and strategies for prevention in Europe. Pediatr Infect Dis J 23:172-173, 2004.
207. Hayden GF, Murphy TF, Hendley JO. Non-group A streptococci in the pharynx. Pathogens or innocent bystanders? Am J Dis Child 143:794-797, 1989.
208. Cummings CG, Ross PW. Group B streptococci (GBS) in the upper respiratory tract of schoolchildren. Health Bull 40:81-86, 1982.
209. Shafer MA, Sweet RL, Ohm-Smith MJ, et al. Microbiology of the lower genital tract in postmenarchal adolescent girls: differences by sexual activity, contraception, and presence of nonspecific vaginitis. J Pediatr 107:974-981, 1985.
210. Band JD, Clegg HW, Hayes PS, et al. Transmission of group B streptococci. Am J Dis Child 135:355-358, 1981.
211. Siegel JD, McCracken GH Jr, Threlkeld N, et al. Single-dose penicillin prophylaxis against neonatal group B streptococcal infections: a controlled trial in 18,738 newborn infants. N Engl J Med 303:769-775, 1980.
212. Akhtar T, Zai S, Khatoon J, et al. A study of group B streptococcal colonization and infection in newborns in Pakistan. J Trop Pediatr 33:302-304, 1987.
213. Matorras R, Garcia-Perea A, Usandizaga JA, et al. Natural transmission of group B *Streptococcus* during delivery. Int J Gynecol Obstet 30:99-103, 1989.
214. Gökalp A, Oguz A, Bakici Z, et al. Neonatal group B streptococcal colonization and maternal urogenital or anorectal carriage. Turk J Pediatr 30:17-23, 1988.
215. Easmon CSF, Hastings MJG, Clare AJ, et al. Nosocomial transmission of group B streptococci. BMJ 283:459-461, 1981.
216. Easmon CSF, Hastings MJG, Blowers A, et al. Epidemiology of group B streptococci: one year's experience in an obstetric and special care baby unit. Br J Obstet Gynaecol 90:241-246, 1983.
217. Ancona RJ, Ferrieri P, Williams PP. Maternal factors that enhance the acquisition of group B streptococci by newborn infants. J Med Microbiol 13:273-280, 1980.
218. Gerards LJ, Cats BP, Hoogkamp-Korstanje JAA. Early neonatal group B streptococcal disease: degree of colonization as an important determinant. J Infect 11:119-124, 1985.
219. Noya FJD, Rench MA, Metzger TG, et al. Unusual occurrence of an epidemic of type Ib/c group B streptococcal sepsis in a neonatal intensive care unit. J Infect Dis 155:1135-1144, 1987.
220. Gardner SE, Mason EO Jr, Yow MD. Community acquisition of group B *Streptococcus* by infants of colonized mothers. Pediatrics 66:873-875, 1980.
221. Wilkinson HW, Facklam RR, Wortham EC. Distribution by serological type of group B streptococci isolated from a variety of clinical material over a five-year period (with special reference to neonatal sepsis and meningitis). Infect Immun 8:228-235, 1973.
222. Baker CJ, Barrett FF. Group B streptococcal infection in infants: the importance of the various serotypes. JAMA 230:1158-1160, 1974.
223. Rench MA, Baker CJ. Neonatal sepsis caused by a new group B streptococcal serotype. J Pediatr 122:638-640, 1993.
224. Davies HD, Raj S, Adair C, et al. Population-based active surveillance for neonatal group B streptococcal infections in Alberta, Canada: implications for vaccine formulation. Pediatr Infect Dis J 20:879-884, 2001.
225. Lachenauer CS, Kasper DL, Shimada J, et al. Serotypes VI and VIII predominate among group B streptococci isolated from pregnant Japanese women. J Infect Dis 179:1030-1033, 1999.
226. Matsubara K, Katayama K, Baba K, et al. Seroepidemiologic studies of serotype VIII Group B *Streptococcus* in Japan. J Infect Dis 186:855-858, 2002.
227. Blumberg HM, Stephens DS, Licitra C, et al. Molecular epidemiology of group B streptococcal infections: use of restriction endonuclease analysis of chromosomal DNA and DNA restriction fragment length polymorphisms of ribosomal RNA genes (ribotyping). J Infect Dis 166:574-579, 1992.
228. Stringer J. The development of a phage typing system for group-B streptococci. J Med Microbiol 13:133-144, 1980.
229. Horodniceanu T, Bougueleret L, El-Solh N, et al. Conjugative R plasmids in *Streptococcus agalactiae* (group B). Plasmid 2:197-206, 1979.
230. Mattingly SJ, Maurer JJ, Eskew EK, et al. Identification of a high-virulence clone of serotype III *Streptococcus agalactiae* by growth characteristics at 40°C. J Clin Microbiol 28:1676-1677, 1990.
231. Musser JM, Mattingly SJ, Quentin R, et al. Identification of a high-virulence clone of type III *Streptococcus agalactiae* (group B *Streptococcus*) causing invasive neonatal disease. Proc Natl Acad Sci U S A 86:4731-4735, 1989.
232. Quentin R, Huet H, Wang F-S, et al. Characterization of *Streptococcus agalactiae* strains by multilocus enzyme genotype and serotype: identification of multiple virulent clone families that cause invasive neonatal disease. J Clin Microbiol 33:2576-2581, 1995.
233. Gordillo ME, Singh KV, Baker CJ, et al. Comparison of group B streptococci by pulsed field gel electrophoresis and by conventional electrophoresis. J Clin Microbiol 31:1430-1434, 1993.
234. Limansky AS, Sutich EG, Guardati MC, et al. Genomic diversity among *Streptococcus agalactiae* isolates detected by a degenerate oligonucleotide-primed amplification assay. J Infect Dis 177:1308-1313, 1998.
235. Bingen E, Denamur E, Lambert-Zechovsky N, et al. Analysis of DNA restriction fragment length polymorphism extends the evidence for breast milk transmission in *Streptococcus agalactiae* late-onset neonatal infection. J Infect Dis 165:569-573, 1992.
236. Adderson EE, Takahashi S, Bohnsack JF. Bacterial genetics and human immunity to group B streptococci. Mol Genet Metab 71:451-454, 2000.
237. Bohnsack JF, Whiting AA, Bradford RD, et al. Long-range mapping of the *Streptococcus agalactiae* phylogenetic lineage restriction digest pattern type III-3 reveals clustering of virulence genes. Infect Immun 70:134-139, 2002.
238. Bohnsack JF, Takahashi S, Detrick SR, et al. Phylogenetic classification of serotype III group B streptococci on the basis of *hyl*B gene analysis and DNA sequences specific to restriction digest pattern type III-3. J Infect Dis 183:1694-1697, 2001.
239. Takahashi S, Detrick S, Whiting AA, et al. Correlation of phylogenetic lineages of group B streptococci, identified by analysis of restriction-digestion patterns of genomic DNA, with *inf*B alleles and mobile genetic elements. J Infect Dis 186:1034-1038, 2002.
240. Adderson EE, Takahashi S, Wang Y, et al. Subtractive hybridization identifies a novel predicted protein mediating epithelial cell invasion by virulent serotype III group B *Streptococcus agalactiae*. Infect Immun 71:6857-6863, 2003.
241. Davies HD, Jones N, Whittam TS, et al. Multilocus sequence typing of serotype III group B *Streptococcus* and correlation with pathogenic potential. J Infect Dis 189:1097-1102, 2004.
242. Jones N, Bohnsack JF, Takahashi S, et al. Multilocus sequence typing system for group B *Streptococcus*. J Clin Microbiol 41:2530-2536, 2003.
243. Bidet P, Brahimi N, Chalas C, et al. Molecular characterization of serotype III group B-*Streptococcus* isolates causing neonatal meningitis. J Infect Dis 188:1132-1137, 2003.
244. Dore N, Bennett D, Kaliszer M, et al. Molecular epidemiology of group B streptococci in Ireland: associations between serotype, invasive status and presence of genes encoding putative virulence factors. Epidemiol Infect 131:823-833, 2003.
245. Baker CJ, Barrett FF, Gordon RC, et al. Suppurative meningitis due to streptococci of Lancefield group B: a study of 33 infants. J Pediatr 82:724-729, 1973.
246. Pass MA, Gray BM, Khare S, et al. Prospective studies of group B streptococcal infections in infants. J Pediatr 95:437-443, 1979.
247. Dillon HC Jr, Khare S, Gray BM. Group B streptococcal carriage and disease: a 6-year prospective study. J Pediatr 110:31-36, 1987.
248. Baker CJ. Unpublished observations, 1993.
249. Aavitsland P, Høiby EA, Lystad A. Systemic group B streptococcal disease in neonates and young infants in Norway 1985-94. Acta Paediatr 85:104-105, 1996.
250. Zangwill KM, Schuchat A, Wenger JD. Group B streptococcal disease in the United States, 1990: report from a multistate active surveillance system. MMWR Morb Mortal Wkly Rep 41:25-32, 1992.
251. Schuchat A, Deaver-Robinson K, Plikaytis BD, et al. Multistate case-control study of maternal risk factors for neonatal group B streptococcal disease. Pediatr Infect Dis J 13:623-629, 1994.
252. Collignon PJ, Dreimanis DE, Vaughan TM, et al. Group B streptococcal infections in neonates. Med J Aust 164:125-126, 1996.
253. Centers for Disease Control and Prevention. Decreasing incidence of perinatal group B streptococcal disease-United States, 1993-1995. MMWR Morb Mortal Wkly Rep 46:473-477, 1997.
254. Lyytikäinen O, Nuorti JP, Halmesmäki E, et al. Invasive group B streptococcal infections in Finland: a population-based study. Emerg Infect Dis 9:469-473, 2003.

255. Heath PT, Balfour G, Weisner AM, et al. Group B streptococcal disease in UK and Irish infants younger than 90 days. Lancet 363:292-294, 2004.
256. Pyati SP, Pildes RS, Jacobs NM, et al. Penicillin in infants weighing two kilograms or less with early-onset group B streptococcal disease. N Engl J Med 308:1383-1389, 1983.
257. Minkoff HL, Sierra MF, Pringle GF, et al. Vaginal colonization with group B beta-hemolytic *Streptococcus* as a risk factor for post-cesarean section febrile morbidity. Am J Obstet Gynecol 142:992-995, 1982.
258. Bobitt JR, Damato JD, Sakakini J. Perinatal complications in group B streptococcal carriers: a longitudinal study of prenatal patients. Am J Obstet Gynecol 151:711-717, 1985.
259. Krohn MA, Hillier SL, Baker CJ. Maternal peripartum complications associated with vaginal group B streptococcal colonization. J Infect Dis 179:1410-1415, 1999.
260. Boyer KM, Gotoff SP. Strategies for chemoprophylaxis of GBS early-onset infections. Antibiot Chemother 35:267-280, 1985.
261. Sobel JD, Myers P, Levison ME, Kaye D. Comparison of bacterial and fungal adherence to vaginal exfoliated epithelial cells and human vaginal epithelial tissue culture cells. Infect Immun 35:697-701, 1982.
262. Jelínková J, Grabovskaya KB, Ryc M, et al. Adherence of vaginal and pharyngeal strains of group B streptococci to human vaginal and pharyngeal epithelial cells. Zentralbl Bakteriol Mikrobiol Hyg [A] 262:492-499, 1986.
263. Zawaneh SM, Ayoub EM, Baer H, et al. Factors influencing adherence of group B streptococci to human vaginal epithelial cells. Infect Immun 26:441-447, 1979.
264. Tamura GS, Kuypers JM, Smith S, et al. Adherence of group B streptococci to cultured epithelial cells: roles of environmental factors and bacterial surface components. Infect Immun 62:2450-2458, 1994.
265. Nealon TJ, Mattingly SJ. Role of cellular lipoteichoic acids in mediating adherence of serotype III strains of group B streptococci to human embryonic, fetal, and adult epithelial cells. Infect Immun 43:523-530, 1984.
266. Teti G, Tomasello F, Chiofalo MS, et al. Adherence of group B streptococci to adult and neonatal epithelial cells mediated by lipoteichoic acid. Infect Immun 55:3057-3064, 1987.
267. Cox F. Prevention of group B streptococcal colonization with topically applied lipoteichoic acid in a maternal-newborn mouse model. Pediatr Res 16:816-819, 1982.
268. Bulgakova TN, Grabovskaya KB, Ryc M, et al. The adhesin structures involved in the adherence of group B streptococci to human vaginal cells. Folia Microbiol 31:394-401, 1986.
269. Miyazaki S, Leon O, Panos C. Adherence of *Streptococcus agalactiae* to synchronously growing human cell monolayers without lipoteichoic acid involvement. Infect Immun 56:505-512, 1988.
270. Wibawan IT, Lammler C, Pasaribu FH. Role of hydrophobic surface proteins in mediating adherence of group B streptococci to epithelial cells. J Gen Microbiol 138:1237-1242, 1992.
271. Tamura GS, Rubens CE. Group B streptococci adhere to a variant of fibronectin attached to a solid phase. Mol Microbiol 15:581-589, 1995.
272. Beckmann C, Waggoner JD, Harris TO, et al. Identification of novel adhesins from Group B streptococci by use of phage display reveals that C5a peptidase mediates fibronectin binding. Infect Immun 70:2869-2876, 2002.
273. Cheng Q, Stafslien D, Purushothaman SS, et al. The group B streptococcal C5a peptidase is both a specific protease and an invasin. Infect Immun 70:2408-2413, 2002.
274. Spellerberg B, Rozdzinski E, Martin S, et al. Lmb, a protein with similarities to the LraI adhesin family, mediates attachment of *Streptococcus agalactiae* to human laminin. Infect Immun 67:871-878, 1999.
275. Schubert A, Zakikhany K, Schreiner M, et al. A fibrinogen receptor from group B *Streptococcus* interacts with fibrinogen by repetitive units with novel ligand binding sites. Mol Microbiol 46:557-569, 2002.
276. Stewardson-Krieger PB, Gotoff SP. Risk factors in early-onset neonatal group B streptococcal infections. Infection 6:50-53, 1978.
277. Tseng PI, Kandall SR. Group B streptococcal disease in neonates and infants. N Y State J Med 74:2169-2173, 1974.
278. Evaldson GR, Malmborg AS, Nord CE. Premature rupture of the membranes and ascending infection. Br J Obstet Gynaecol 89:793-801, 1982.
279. Schoonmaker JN, Lawellin DW, Lunt B, et al. Bacteria and inflammatory cells reduce chorioamniotic membrane integrity and tensile strength. Obstet Gynecol 74:590-596, 1989.
280. Sbarra AJ, Thomas GB, Cetrulo CL, et al. Effect of bacterial growth on the bursting pressure of fetal membranes in vitro. Obstet Gynecol 70:107-110, 1987.
281. Lamont RF, Rose M, Elder MG. Effect of bacterial products on prostaglandin E production by amnion cells. Lancet 2:1331-1333, 1985.
282. Bennett PR, Rose MP, Myatt L, et al. Preterm labor: stimulation of arachidonic acid metabolism in human amnion cells by bacterial products. Am J Obstet Gynecol 156:649-655, 1987.
283. Dudley DJ, Edwin SS, Van Wagoner J, et al. Regulation of decidual cell chemokine production by group B streptococci and purified bacterial cell wall components. Am J Obstet Gynecol 177:666-672, 1997.
284. Ferrieri P, Cleary PP, Seeds AE. Epidemiology of group-B streptococcal carriage in pregnant women and newborn infants. J Med Microbiol 10:103-114, 1977.
285. Eickhoff TC, Klein JO, Daly AK, et al. Neonatal sepsis and other infections due to group B beta-hemolytic streptococci. N Engl J Med 271:1221-1228, 1964.
286. Galask RP, Varner MW, Petzold CR, et al. Bacterial attachment to the chorioamniotic membranes. Am J Obstet Gynecol 148:915-928, 1984.
287. Winram SB, Jonas M, Chi E, et al. Characterization of group B streptococcal invasion of human chorion and amnion epithelial cells In vitro. Infect Immun 66:4932-4941, 1998.
288. Lin B, Hollingshead SK, Coligan JE, et al. Cloning and expression of the gene for group B streptococcal hyaluronate lyase. J Biol Chem 269:30113-30116, 1994.
289. Pritchard DG, Lin B, Willingham TR, et al. Characterization of the group B streptococcal hyaluronate lyase. Arch Biochem Biophys 315:431-437, 1994.
290. Hemming VG, Nagarajan K, Hess LW, et al. Rapid in vitro replication of group B *Streptococcus* in term human amniotic fluid. Gynecol Obstet Invest 19:124-129, 1985.
291. Abbasi IA, Hemming VG, Eglinton GS, et al. Proliferation of group B streptococci in human amniotic fluid in vitro. Am J Obstet Gynecol 156:95-99, 1987.
292. Baker CJ. Early onset group B streptococcal disease. J Pediatr 93:124-125, 1978.
293. Bergqvist G, Holmberg G, Rydner T, et al. Intrauterine death due to infection with group B streptococci. Acta Obstet Gynecol Scand 57:127-128, 1978.
294. Ablow RC, Driscoll SG, Effmann EL, et al. A comparison of early-onset group B streptococcal neonatal infection and the respiratory-distress syndrome of the newborn. N Engl J Med 294:65-70, 1976.
295. Vollman JH, Smith WL, Ballard ET, et al. Early onset group B streptococcal disease: clinical, roentgenographic, and pathologic features. J Pediatr 89:199-203, 1976.
296. Payne NR, Burke BA, Day DL, et al. Correlation of clinical and pathologic findings in early onset neonatal group B streptococcal infection with disease severity and prediction of outcome. Pediatr Infect Dis J 7:836-847, 1988.
297. Hemming VG, McCloskey DW, Hill HR. Pneumonia in the neonate associated with group B streptococcal septicemia. Am J Dis Child 130:1231-1233, 1976.
298. Katzenstein A, Davis C, Braude A. Pulmonary changes in neonatal sepsis due to group B β-hemolytic streptococcus: relation to hyaline membrane disease. J Infect Dis 133:430-435, 1976.
299. Rubens CE, Raff HV, Jackson JC, et al. Pathophysiology and histopathology of group B streptococcal sepsis in *Macaca nemestrina* primates induced after intraamniotic inoculation: evidence for bacterial cellular invasion. J Infect Dis 164:320-330, 1991.
300. Martin TR, Rubens CE, Wilson CB. Lung antibacterial defense mechanisms in infant and adult rats: implications for the pathogenesis of group B streptococcal infections in the neonatal lung. J Infect Dis 157:91-100, 1988.
301. Sherman MP, Lehrer RI. Oxidative metabolism of neonatal and adult rabbit lung macrophages stimulated with opsonized group B streptococci. Infect Immun 47:26-30, 1985.
302. Sherman MP, Johnson JT, Rothlein R, et al. Role of pulmonary phagocytes in host defense against group B streptococci in preterm versus term rabbit lung. J Infect Dis 166:818-826, 1992.
303. Rubens CE, Smith S, Hulse M, et al. Respiratory epithelial cell invasion by group B streptococci. Infect Immun 60:5157-5163, 1992.
304. Gibson RL, Lee MK, Soderland C, et al. Group B streptococci invade endothelial cells: type III capsular polysaccharide attenuates invasion. Infect Immun 61:478-485, 1993.

305. Valentin-Weigand P, Jungnitz H, Zock A, et al. Characterization of group B streptococcal invasion in HEp-2 epithelial cells. FEMS Microbiol Lett 147:69-74, 1997.
306. Tyrrell GJ, Kennedy A, Shokoples SE, et al. Binding and invasion of HeLa and MRC-5 cells by *Streptococcus agalactiae*. Microbiology 148:3921-3931, 2002.
307. Valentin-Weigand P, Chhatwal GS. Correlation of epithelial cell invasiveness of group B streptococci with clinical source of isolation. Microb Pathog 19:83-91, 1995.
308. Takahashi S, Adderson EE, Nagano Y, et al. Identification of a highly encapsulated, genetically related group of invasive type III group B streptococci. J Infect Dis 177:1116-1119, 1998.
309. Bolduc GR, Baron MJ, Gravekamp C, et al. The alpha C protein mediates internalization of group B Streptococcus within human cervical epithelial cells. Cell Microbiol 4:751-758, 2002.
310. Hulse ML, Smith S, Chi EY, et al. Effect of type III group B streptococcal capsular polysaccharide on invasion of respiratory epithelial cells. Infect Immun 61:4835-4841, 1993.
311. Quirante J, Ceballos R, Cassady G. Group B beta-hemolytic streptococcal infection in the newborn. I. Early onset infection. Am J Dis Child 128:659-665, 1974.
312. Spellerberg B, Pohl B, Haase G, et al. Identification of genetic determinants for the hemolytic activity of *Streptococcus agalactiae* by ISS1 transposition. J Bacteriol 181:3212-3219, 1999.
313. Pritzlaff CA, Chang JC, Kuo SP, et al. Genetic basis for the beta-haemolytic/cytolytic activity of group B *Streptococcus*. Mol Microbiol 39:236-247, 2001.
314. Nizet V, Beall B, Bast DJ, et al. Genetic locus for streptolysin S production by group A *Streptococcus*. Infect Immun 68:4254-4254, 2000.
315. Nizet V, Gibson RL, Chi EY, et al. Group B streptococcal beta-hemolysin expression is associated with injury of lung epithelial cells. Infect Immun 64:3818-3826, 1996.
316. Gibson RL, Nizet V, Rubens CE. Group B streptococcal beta-hemolysin promotes injury of lung microvascular endothelial cells. Pediatr Res 45:626-634, 1999.
317. Doran KS, Chang JC, Benoit VM, et al. Group B streptococcal beta-hemolysin/cytolysin promotes invasion of human lung epithelial cells and the release of interleukin-8. J Infect Dis 185:196-203, 2002.
318. Wennerstrom DE, Tsaihong JC, Crawford JT. Evaluation of the role of hemolysin and pigment in the pathogenesis of early onset group B streptococcal infection. *In* Kimura Y, Kotami S, Shiokowa Y (eds). Recent Advances in Streptococci and Streptococcal Diseases. Bracknell, UK, Reedbooks, 1985, pp 155-156.
319. Nizet V, Gibson RL, Rubens CE. The role of group B streptococci beta-hemolysin expression in newborn lung injury. Adv Exp Med Biol 418:627-630, 1997.
320. Hensler ME, Sobczak SM, Liu GY, et al. The role of the beta-hemolysin/cytolysin in group B streptococcal infection in a neonatal rabbit model. Pediatric Academic Societies' Annual Meeting, San Francisco, 2004.
321. Herting E, Jarstrand C, Rasool O, et al. Experimental neonatal group B streptococcal pneumonia: effect of a modified porcine surfactant on bacterial proliferation in ventilated near-term rabbits. Pediatr Res 36:784-791, 1994.
322. Herting E, Sun B, Jarstrand C, et al. Surfactant improves lung function and mitigates bacterial growth in immature ventilated rabbits with experimentally induced neonatal group B streptococcal pneumonia. Arch Dis Child Fetal Neonatal Ed 76:F3-8, 1997.
323. Auten RL, Notter RH, Kendig JW, et al. Surfactant treatment of full-term newborns with respiratory failure. Pediatrics 87:101-107, 1991.
324. Hertig E, Gefeller O, Land M, et al. Surfactant treatment of neonates with respiratory failure and group B streptococcal infection. Members of the Collaborative European Multicenter Study Group. Pediatrics 106:957-964, 2000.
325. Shigeoka AO, Hall RT, Hemming VG, et al. Role of antibody and complement in opsonization of group B streptococci. Infect Immun 21:34-40, 1978.
326. Anderson DC, Hughes BJ, Edwards MS, et al. Impaired chemotaxigenesis by type III group B streptococci in neonatal sera: relationship to diminished concentration of specific anticapsular antibody and abnormalities of serum complement. Pediatr Res 17:496-502, 1983.
327. Edwards MS, Nicholson-Weller A, Baker CJ, et al. The role of specific antibody in alternative complement pathway–mediated opsonophagocytosis of type III, group B Streptococcus. J Exp Med 151:1275-1287, 1980.
328. Chaffin DO, Beres SB, Yim HH, et al. The serotype of type Ia and III group B streptococci is determined by the polymerase gene within the polycistronic capsule operon. J Bacteriol 182:4466-4477, 2000.
329. Angata T, Varki A. Chemical diversity in the sialic acids and related alpha-keto acids: an evolutionary perspective. Chem Rev 102:439-469, 2002.
330. Doran KS, Liu GY, Nizet V. Group B streptococcal beta-hemolysin/cytolysin activates neutrophil signaling pathways in brain endothelium and contributes to development of meningitis. J Clin Invest 112:736-744, 2003.
331. Kasper DL, Baker CJ, Baltimore RS, et al. Immunodeterminant specificity of human immunity to type III group B streptococcus. J Exp Med 149:327-339, 1979.
332. Edwards MS, Kasper DL, Jennings HJ, et al. Capsular sialic acid prevents activation of the alternative complement pathway by type III, group B streptococci. J Immunol 128:1278-1283, 1982.
333. Shigeoka AO, Rote NS, Santos JI, et al. Assessment of the virulence factors of group B streptococci: correlation with sialic acid content. J Infect Dis 147:857-863, 1983.
334. Yeung MK, Mattingly SJ. Isolation and characterization of type III group B streptococcal mutants defective in biosynthesis of the type-specific antigen. Infect Immun 42:141-151, 1983.
335. Rubens CE, Wessels MR, Kuypers JM, et al. Molecular analysis of two group B streptococcal virulence factors. Semin Perinatol 14:22-29, 1990.
336. Rubens CE, Wessels MR, Heggen LM, et al. Transposon mutagenesis of type III group B *Streptococcus*: correlation of capsule expression with virulence. Proc Natl Acad Sci U S A 84:7208-7212, 1987.
337. Yim HH, Nittayarin A, Rubens CE. Analysis of the capsule synthesis locus, a virulence factor in group B streptococci. Adv Exp Med Biol 418:995-997, 1997.
338. Marques MB, Kasper DL, Pangburn MK, et al. Prevention of C3 deposition by capsular polysaccharide is a virulence mechanism of type III group B streptococci. Infect Immun 60:3986-3993, 1992.
339. Campbell JR, Baker CJ, Edwards MS. Influence of serotype of group B streptococci on C3 degradation. Infect Immun 60:4558-4562, 1992.
340. Smith CL, Pritchard DG, Gray BM. Role of polysaccharide capsule in C3 deposition by type Ib group B streptococci (GBS). Thirty-first Interscience Conference on Antimicrobial Agents and Chemotherapy, Washington, DC, 1991.
341. Martin TR, Ruzinski JT, Rubens CE, et al. The effect of type-specific polysaccharide capsule on the clearance of group B streptococci from the lungs of infant and adult rats. J Infect Dis 165:306-314, 1992.
342. Wessels MR, Rubens CE, Benedi VJ, et al. Definition of a bacterial virulence factor: sialylation of the group B streptococcal capsule. Proc Natl Acad Sci U S A 86:8983-7898, 1989.
343. Orefici G, Recchia S, Galante L. Possible virulence marker for *Streptococcus agalactiae* (Lancefield Group B). Eur J Clin Microbiol Infect Dis 7:302-305, 1988.
344. Payne NR, Ferrieri P. The relation of the Ibc protein antigen to the opsonization differences between strains of type II group B streptococci. J Infect Dis 151:672-681, 1985.
345. Baker CJ, Webb BJ, Kasper DL, et al. The role of complement and antibody in opsonophagocytosis of type II group B streptococci. J Infect Dis 154:47-54, 1986.
346. Payne NR, Kim YK, Ferrieri P. Effect of differences in antibody and complement requirements on phagocytic uptake and intracellular killing of "c" protein-positive and -negative strains of type II group B streptococci. Infect Immun 55:1243-1251, 1987.
347. Russell-Jones GJ, Gotschlich EC, Blake MS. A surface receptor specific for human IgA on group B streptococci possessing the Ibc protein antigen. J Exp Med 160:1467-1475, 1984.
348. Jerlström PG, Chhatwal GS, Timmis KN. The IgA-binding beta antigen of the c protein complex of Group B streptococci: sequence determination of its gene and detection of two binding regions. Mol Microbiol 5:843-849, 1991.
349. Harris TO, Shelver DW, Bohnsack JF, et al. A novel streptococcal surface protease promotes virulence, resistance to opsonophagocytosis, and cleavage of human fibrinogen. J Clin Invest 111:61-70, 2003.
350. Cornacchione P, Scaringi L, Fettucciari K, et al. Group B streptococci persist inside macrophages. Immunology 93:86-95, 1998.
351. Teixeira CF, Azevedo NL, Carvalho TM, et al. Cytochemical study of *Streptococcus agalactiae* and macrophage interaction. Microsc Res Tech 54:254-259, 2001.
352. Wilson CB, Weaver WM. Comparative susceptibility of group B streptococci and *Staphylococcus aureus* to killing by oxygen metabolites. J Infect Dis 152:323-329, 1985.

353. Poyart C, Pellegrini E, Gaillot O, et al. Contribution of Mn-cofactored superoxide dismutase (SodA) to the virulence of *Streptococcus agalactiae*. Infect Immun 69:5098-5106, 2001.
354. Liu GY, Doran KS, Lawrence T, et al. Sword and shield: linked group B streptococcal β-hemolysin/cytolysin and carotenoid pigment act synergistically to subvert host phagocyte defenses. Proc Natl Acad Sci U S A 101:14491-14496, 2004.
355. Nizet V, Ohtake T, Lauth X, et al. Innate antimicrobial peptide protects the skin from invasive bacterial infection. Nature 414:454-457, 2001.
356. Dorschner RA, Lin KH, Murakami M, et al. Neonatal skin in mice and humans expresses increased levels of antimicrobial peptides: innate immunity during development of the adaptive response. Pediatr Res 53:566-572, 2003.
357. Jones AL, Needham RH, Clancy A, et al. Penicillin-binding proteins in *Streptococcus agalactiae*: a novel mechanism for evasion of immune clearance. Mol Microbiol 47:247-256, 2003.
358. Hamilton A, Mertz RH, Needham RH, et al. Evasion of innate immunity: a novel function for GBS penicillin-binding protein 1a. American Society for Microbiology General Meeting. New Orleans, 2004.
359. Poyart C, Pellegrini E, Marceau M, et al. Attenuated virulence of *Streptococcus agalactiae* deficient in D-alanyl-lipoteichoic acid is due to an increased susceptibility to defensins and phagocytic cells. Mol Microbiol 49:1615-1625, 2003.
360. Fettucciari K, Rosati E, Scaringi L, et al. Group B *Streptococcus* induces apoptosis in macrophages. J Immunol 165:3923-3933, 2000.
361. Ulett GC, Bohnsack JF, Armstrong J, et al. Beta-hemolysin-independent induction of apoptosis of macrophages infected with serotype III group B streptococcus. J Infect Dis 188:1049-1053, 2003.
362. Wheeler JG, Chauvenet AR, Johnson CA, et al. Neutrophil storage pool depletion in septic, neutropenic neonates. Pediatr Infect Dis 3:407-409, 1984.
363. Christensen RD, MacFarlane JL, Taylor NL, et al. Blood and marrow neutrophils during experimental group B streptococcal infection: quantification of the stem cell, proliferative, storage and circulating pools. Pediatr Res 16:549-553, 1982.
364. Zeligs BJ, Armstrong CD, Walser JB, et al. Age-dependent susceptibility of neonatal rats to group B streptococcal type III infection: correlation of severity of infection and response of myeloid pools. Infect Immun 37:255-263, 1982.
365. Christensen RD, Hill HR, Rothstein G. Granulocytic stem cell (CFUc) proliferation in experimental group B streptococcal sepsis. Pediatr Res 17:278-280, 1983.
366. Hill HR, Bohnsack JF, Morris EZ, et al. Group B streptococci inhibit the chemotactic activity of the fifth component of complement. J Immunol 141:3551-3556, 1988.
367. Bohnsack JF, Widjaja K, Ghazizadeh S, et al. A role for C5 and C5a-ase in the acute neutrophil response to group B streptococcal infections. J Infect Dis 175:847-855, 1997.
368. Rojas J, Larsson LE, Hellerqvist CG, et al. Pulmonary hemodynamic and ultrastructural changes associated with Group B streptococcal toxemia in adult sheep and newborn lambs. Pediatr Res 17:1002-1008, 1983.
369. Hemming VG, O'Brien WF, Fischer GW, et al. Studies of short-term pulmonary and peripheral vascular responses induced in oophorectomized sheep by the infusion of a group B streptococcal extract. Pediatr Res 18:266-269, 1984.
370. Gibson RL, Truog WE, Henderson WR, Jr, et al. Group B streptococcal sepsis in piglets: effect of combined pentoxifylline and indomethacin pretreatment. Pediatr Res 31:222-227, 1992.
371. Peevy KJ, Chartrand SA, Wiseman HJ, et al. Myocardial dysfunction in group B streptococcal shock. Pediatr Res 19:511-513, 1985.
372. Peevy KJ, Panus P, Longenecker GL, et al. Prostaglandin synthetase inhibition in group B streptococcal shock: hematologic and hemodynamic effects. Pediatr Res 20:864-866, 1986.
373. O'Brien WF, Golden SM, Bibro MC, et al. Short-term responses in neonatal lambs after infusion of group B streptococcal extract. Obstet Gynecol 65:802-806, 1985.
374. Gibson RL, Redding GJ, Truog WE, et al. Isogenic group B streptococci devoid of capsular polysaccharide or beta-hemolysin: pulmonary hemodynamic and gas exchange effects during bacteremia in piglets. Pediatr Res 26:241-245, 1989.
375. Bowdy BD, Aziz SM, Marple SL, et al. Organ-specific disposition of group B streptococci in piglets: evidence for a direct interaction with target cells in the pulmonary circulation. Pediatr Res 27:344-348, 1990.
376. Gibson RL, Soderland C, Henderson WR Jr, et al. Group B streptococci (GBS) injure lung endothelium in vitro: GBS invasion and GBS-induced eicosanoid production is greater with microvascular than with pulmonary artery cells. Infect Immun 63:271-279, 1995.
377. Schreiber MD, Covert RF, Torgerson LJ. Hemodynamic effects of heat-killed group B beta-hemolytic streptococcus in newborn lambs: role of leukotriene D4. Pediatr Res 31:121-126, 1992.
378. Pinheiro JM, Pitt BR, Gillis CN. Roles of platelet-activating factor and thromboxane in group B Streptococcus-induced pulmonary hypertension in piglets. Pediatr Res 26:420-424, 1989.
379. Mancuso G, Cusumano V, Genovese F, et al. Role of interleukin 12 in experimental neonatal sepsis caused by group B streptococci. Infect Immun 65:3731-3735, 1997.
380. Dinarello CA. The role of interleukin-1 in host responses to infectious diseases. Infect Agents Dis 1:227-236, 1992.
381. Vallette JD, Jr., Goldberg RN, Suguihara C, et al. Effect of an interleukin-1 receptor antagonist on the hemodynamic manifestations of group B streptococcal sepsis. Pediatr Res 38:704-708, 1995.
382. Williams PA, Bohnsack JF, Augustine NH, et al. Production of tumor necrosis factor by human cells in vitro and in vivo, induced by group B streptococci. J Pediatr 123:292-300, 1993.
383. Gibson RL, Redding GJ, Henderson WR, et al. Group B streptococcus induces tumor necrosis factor in neonatal piglets. Effect of the tumor necrosis factor inhibitor pentoxifylline on hemodynamics and gas exchange. Am Rev Respir Dis 143:598-604, 1991.
384. Teti G, Mancuso G, Tomasello F, et al. Production of tumor necrosis factor-alpha and interleukin-6 in mice infected with group B streptococci. Circ Shock 38:138-144, 1992.
385. Teti G, Mancuso G, Tomasello F. Cytokine appearance and effects of anti-tumor necrosis factor alpha antibodies in a neonatal rat model of group B streptococcal infection. Infect Immun 61:227-235, 1993.
386. von Hunolstein C, Totolian A, Alfarone G, et al. Soluble antigens from group B streptococci induce cytokine production in human blood cultures. Infect Immun 65:4017-4021, 1997.
387. Medvedev AE, Flo T, Ingalls RR, et al. Involvement of CD14 and complement receptors CR3 and CR4 in nuclear factor-kappa B activation and TNF production induced by lipopolysaccharide and group B streptococcal cell walls. J Immunol 160:4535-4542, 1998.
388. Vallejo JG, Baker CJ, Edwards MS. Roles of the bacterial cell wall and capsule in induction of tumor necrosis factor alpha by type III group B streptococci. Infect Immun 64:5042-5046, 1996.
389. Henneke P, Takeuchi O, Malley R, et al. Cellular activation, phagocytosis, and bactericidal activity against group B streptococcus involve parallel myeloid differentiation factor 88-dependent and independent signaling pathways. J Immunol 169:3970-3977, 2002.
390. Henneke P, Takeuchi O, van Strijp JA, et al. Novel engagement of CD14 and multiple Toll-like receptors by group B streptococci. J Immunol 167:7069-7076, 2001.
391. Ring A, Braun JS, Nizet V, et al. Group B streptococcal beta-hemolysin induces nitric oxide production in murine macrophages. J Infect Dis 182:150-157, 2000.
392. Puliti M, Nizet V, von Hunolstein C, et al. Severity of group B streptococcal arthritis is correlated with beta-hemolysin expression. J Infect Dis 182:824-832, 2000.
393. Ring A, Depnering C, Pohl J, et al. Synergistic action of nitric oxide release from murine macrophages caused by group B streptococcal cell wall and beta-hemolysin/cytolysin. J Infect Dis 186:1518-1521, 2002.
394. Griffiths BB, Rhee H. Effects of haemolysins of groups A and B streptococci on cardiovascular system. Microbios 69:17-27, 1992.
395. Berman PH, Banker BQ. Neonatal meningitis. A clinical and pathological study of 29 cases. Pediatrics 38:6-24, 1966.
396. Ferrieri P, Burke B, Nelson J. Production of bacteremia and meningitis in infant rats with group B streptococcal serotypes. Infect Immun 27:1023-1032, 1980.
397. Nizet V, Kim KS, Stins M, et al. Invasion of brain microvascular endothelial cells by group B streptococci. Infect Immun 65:5074-5081, 1997.
398. Engelson E, Nizet V, Doran KS. A newly identified gene, *iag*A, from group B streptococcus mediates invasion of the blood-brain barrier. American Society for Microbiology General Meeting, New Orleans, 2004.
399. Kim YS, Sheldon RA, Elliott BR, et al. Brain injury in experimental neonatal meningitis due to group B streptococci. J Neuropathol Exp Neurol 54:531-539, 1995.

400. Wahl M, Unterberg A, Baethmann A, et al. Mediators of blood-brain barrier dysfunction and formation of vasogenic brain edema. J Cereb Blood Flow Metab 8:621-634, 1988.
401. McKnight AA, Keyes WG, Hudak ML, et al. Oxygen free radicals and the cerebral arteriolar response to group B streptococci. Pediatr Res 31:640-644, 1992.
402. Bogdan I, Leib SL, Bergeron M, et al. Tumor necrosis factor-alpha contributes to apoptosis in hippocampal neurons during experimental group B streptococcal meningitis. J Infect Dis 176:693-697, 1997.
403. Kim KS, Wass CA, Cross AS. Blood-brain barrier permeability during the development of experimental bacterial meningitis in the rat. Exp Neurol 145:253-257, 1997.
404. Ling EW, Noya FJ, Ricard G, et al. Biochemical mediators of meningeal inflammatory response to group B streptococcus in the newborn piglet model. Pediatr Res 38:981-987, 1995.
405. Adair CE, Kowalsky L, Quon H, et al. Risk factors for early-onset group B streptococcal disease in neonates: a population based case-control study. Can Med Assoc J 169:198-203, 2003.
406. Schuchat A. Epidemiology of group B streptococcal disease in the United States: shifting paradigms. Clin Microbiol Rev 11:497-513, 1998.
407. Pass MA, Khare S, Dillon HC. Twin pregnancies: incidence of group B streptococcal colonization and disease. J Pediatr 97:635-637, 1980.
408. Edwards MS, Jackson CV, Baker CJ. Increased risk of group B streptococcal disease in twins. JAMA 245:2044-2046, 1981.
409. Baker CJ, Kasper DL. Correlation of maternal antibody deficiency with susceptibility to neonatal group B streptococcal infection. N Engl J Med 294:753-756, 1976.
410. Schuchat A. Group B *Streptococcus*. Lancet 353:51-56, 1999.
411. Regan JA, Klebanoff MA, Nugent RP, et al. Colonization with group B streptococci in pregnancy and adverse outcome. Am J Obstet Gynecol 174:1354-1360, 1996.
412. Seaward PG, Hannah ME, Myhr TL, et al. International multicenter term PROM study: evaluation of predictors of neonatal infection in infants born to patients with premature rupture of membranes at term. Am J Obstet Gynecol 179:635-639, 1998.
413. Yancey MK, Duff P, Clark P, et al. Peripartum infection associated with vaginal group B streptococcal colonization. Obstet Gynecol 84:816-819, 1994.
414. Hemming VG, Hall RT, Rhodes PG, et al. Assessment of group B streptococcal opsonins in human and rabbit serum by neutrophil chemiluminescence. J Clin Invest 58:1379-1387, 1976.
415. Baker CJ, Kasper DL, Tager IB, et al. Quantitative determination of antibody to capsular polysaccharide in infection with type III strains of group B *Streptococcus*. J Clin Invest 59:810-818, 1977.
416. Vogel LC, Kretschmer RR, Boyer KM, et al. Human immunity to group B streptococci measured by indirect immunofluorescence: correlation with protection in chick embryos. J Infect Dis 140:682-689, 1979.
417. Baker CJ, Webb BJ, Kasper DL, et al. The natural history of group B streptococcal colonization in the pregnant woman and her offspring: II. Determination of serum antibody to capsular polysaccharide from type III group B *Streptococcus*. Am J Obstet Gynecol 137:39-42, 1980.
418. Boyer KM, Papierniak CK, Gadzala CA, et al. Transplacental passage of IgG antibody to group B *Streptococcus* serotype Ia. J Pediatr 104:618-620, 1984.
419. Christensen KK, Christensen P, Duc G, et al. Correlation between serum antibody-levels against group B streptococci and gestational age in newborns. Eur J Pediatr 142:86-88, 1984.
420. Baker CJ, Edwards MS, Kasper DL. Role of antibody to native type III polysaccharide of group B *Streptococcus* in infant infection. Pediatrics 68:544-549, 1981.
421. Guttormsen H-K, Baker CJ, Edwards MS, et al. Quantitative determination of antibodies to type III group B streptococcal polysaccharide. J Infect Dis 173:142-150, 1996.
422. Berg S, Kasvi S, Trollfors B, et al. Antibodies to group B streptococci in neonates and infants. Eur J Pediatr 157:221-224, 1998.
423. Stewardson-Krieger PB, Albrandt K, Nevin T, et al. Perinatal immunity to group B β-hemolytic *Streptococcus* type Ia. J Infect Dis 136:649-654, 1977.
424. Papierniak CK, Klegerman ME, Boyer KM, et al. An enzyme-linked immunosorbent assay (ELISA) for human IgG antibody to the type Ia polysaccharide of group B *Streptococcus*. J Lab Clin Med 100:385-398, 1982.
425. Klegerman ME, Boyer KM, Papierniak CK, et al. Estimation of the protective level of human IgG antibody to the type-specific polysaccharide of group B *Streptococcus* type Ia. J Infect Dis 148:648-655, 1983.
426. Boyer KM, Kendall LS, Papierniak CK, et al. Protective levels of human immunoglobulin G antibody to group B streptococcus type Ib. Infect Immun 45:618-624, 1984.
427. Gotoff SP, Odell C, Papierniak CK, et al. Human IgG antibody to group B *Streptococcus* type III: comparison of protective levels in a murine model with levels in infected human neonates. J Infect Dis 153:511-519, 1986.
428. Gotoff SP, Papierniak CK, Klegerman ME, et al. Quantitation of IgG antibody to the type-specific polysaccharide of group B *Streptococcus* type 1b in pregnant women and infected infants. J Pediatr 105:628-630, 1984.
429. Baker CJ, Carey VJ, Rench MA, et al. Quantity of maternal antibody at delivery that protects neonates from group B streptococcal disease. Unpublished paper, 2004.
430. Gray BM, Pritchard DG, Dillon HC Jr. Seroepidemiological studies of group B *Streptococcus* type II. J Infect Dis 151:1073-1080, 1985.
431. Anthony BF, Concepcion NF, Concepcion KF. Human antibody to the group-specific polysaccharide of group B *Streptococcus*. J Infect Dis 151:221-226, 1985.
432. Anderson DC, Edwards MS, Baker CJ. Luminolenhanced chemiluminescence for evaluation of type III group B streptococcal opsonins in human sera. J Infect Dis 141:370-381, 1980.
433. Edwards MS, Baker CJ, Kasper DL. Opsonic specificity of human antibody to the type III polysaccharide of group B *Streptococcus*. J Infect Dis 140:1004-1007, 1979.
434. Baltimore RS, Baker CJ, Kasper DL. Antibody to group B *Streptococcus* type III in human sera measured by a mouse protection test. Infect Immun 32:56-61, 1981.
435. Larsen JW Jr, Harper JS III, London WT, et al. Antibody to type III group B *Streptococcus* in the rhesus monkey. Am J Obstet Gynecol 146:958-962, 1983.
436. Itoh T, Yan X-J, Nakano H, et al. Protective efficacy against group B streptococcal infection in neonatal mice delivered from preimmunized pregnants. Microbiol Immunol 30:297-305, 1986.
437. Kim KS, Wass CA, Hong JK, et al. Demonstration of opsonic and protective activity of human cord sera against type III group B *Streptococcus* that are independent of type-specific antibody. Pediatr Res 24:628-632, 1988.
438. Boyer KM, Klegerman ME, Gotoff SP. Development of IgM antibody to group B *Streptococcus* type III in human infants. J Infect Dis 165:1049-1055, 1992.
439. Baker CJ, Kasper DL, Edwards MS, et al. Influence of preimmunization antibody level on the specificity of the immune response to related polysaccharide antigens. N Engl J Med 303:173-178, 1980.
440. Baker CJ, Edwards MS, Kasper DL. Immunogenicity of polysaccharides from type III group B *Streptococcus*. J Clin Invest 61:1107-1110, 1978.
441. Hordnes K, Tynning T, Kvam AI, et al. Cervical secretions in pregnant women colonized rectally with group B streptococci have high levels of antibodies to serotype III polysaccharide capsular antigen and protein R. Scand J Immunol 47:179-188, 1998.
442. Hordnes K, Tynning T, Kvam AI, et al. Colonization in the rectum and uterine cervix with group B streptococci may induce specific antibody responses in cervical secretions of pregnant women. Infect Immun 64:1643-1652, 1996.
443. Hill HR, Shigeoka AO, Hall RT, et al. Neonatal cellular and humoral immunity to group B streptococci. Pediatrics S64:787-794, 1979.
444. De Cueninck BJ, Eisenstein TK, McIntosh TS, et al. Quantitation of in vitro opsonic activity of human antibody induced by a vaccine consisting of the type III–specific polysaccharide of group B streptococcus. Infect Immun 39:1155-1160, 1983.
445. Pincus SH, Shigeoka AO, Moe AA, et al. Protective efficacy of IgM monoclonal antibodies in experimental group B streptococcal infection is a function of antibody avidity. J Immunol 140:2779-2785, 1988.
446. Givner LB, Baker CJ, Edwards MS. Type III group B *Streptococcus*: functional interaction with IgG subclass antibodies. J Infect Dis 155:532-539, 1987.
447. Kim JS, Kim KW, Wass CA, et al. A human IgG 3 is opsonic in vitro against type III group B streptococci. J Clin Immunol 10:154-159, 1990.
448. Anthony BF, Concepcion NF. Opsonic activity of human IgG and IgM antibody for type III group B streptococci. Pediatr Res 26:383-387, 1989.
449. Campbell JR, Baker CJ, Metzger TG, et al. Functional activity of class-specific antibodies to type III, group B *Streptococcus*. Pediatr Res 23:31-34, 1988.

450. Bohnsack JF, Hawley MM, Pritchard DG, et al. An IgA monoclonal antibody directed against type III antigen on group B streptococci acts as an opsonin. J Immunol 143:3338-3342, 1989.
451. Campbell JR, Baker CJ, Edwards MS. Deposition and degradation of C3 on type III group B streptococci. Infect Immun 59:1978-1983, 1991.
452. Marques MB, Kasper DL, Pangburn MK, et al. Prevention of C3 deposition by capsular polysaccharide is a virulence mechanism of type III group B streptococci. Infect Immun 60:3986-3993, 1992.
453. Baker CJ, Edwards MS, Webb BJ, et al. Antibody-independent classical pathway–mediated opsonophagocytosis of type Ia, group B *Streptococcus*. J Clin Invest 69:394-404, 1982.
454. Levy NJ, Kasper DL. Surface-bound capsular polysaccharide of type Ia group B *Streptococcus* mediates C1 binding and activation of the classic complement pathway. J Immunol 136:4157-4162, 1986.
455. Levy NJ, Kasper DL. Antibody-independent and -dependent opsonization of group B *Streptococcus* requires the first component of complement C1. Infect Immun 49:19-24, 1985.
456. Smith CL, Smith AH. Strain variability of type Ib group B streptococci: unique strains are resistant to C3 deposition by the alternate complement pathway. Clin Res 40:823A, 1992.
457. Lindahl G, Åkerström B, Vaerman J-P, et al. Characterization of an IgA receptor from group B streptococci: specificity for serum IgA. Eur J Immunol 20:2241-2247, 1990.
458. Hedén L-O, Frithz E, Lindahl G. Molecular characterization of an IgA receptor from group B streptococci: sequence of the gene, identification of a proline-rich region with unique structure and isolation of N-terminal fragments with IgA-binding capacity. Eur J Immunol 21:1481-1490, 1991.
459. Hall MA, Edwards MS, Baker CJ. Complement and antibody participation in opsonophagocytosis of type IV and V group B streptococci. Infect Immun 60:5030-5035, 1992.
460. Hall MA, Hickman ME, Baker CJ, et al. Complement and antibody in neutrophil-mediated killing of type V group B *Streptococcus*. J Infect Dis 170:88-93, 1994.
461. Davis CA, Vallota EH, Forristal J. Serum complement levels in infancy: age-related changes. Pediatr Res 13:1043-1046, 1979.
462. Máródi L, Leijh PCJ, Braat A, et al. Opsonic activity of cord blood sera against various species of microorganism. Pediatr Res 19:433-436, 1985.
463. Edwards MS, Buffone GJ, Fuselier PA, et al. Deficient classical complement pathway activity in newborn sera. Pediatr Res 17:685–688, 1983.
464. Baker CJ, Rench MA, Edwards MS, et al. Immunization of pregnant women with a polysaccharide vaccine of group B *Streptococcus*. N Engl J Med 319:1180-1185, 1988.
465. Edwards MS, Hall MA, Rench MA, et al. Patterns of immune response among survivors of group B streptococcal meningitis. J Infect Dis 161:65-70, 1990.
466. Cairo MS, Worcester C, Rucker R, et al. Role of circulating complement and polymorphonuclear leukocyte transfusion in treatment and outcome in critically ill neonates with sepsis. J Pediatr 110:935-941, 1987.
467. Levy O, Jean-Jacques RM, Cywes C, et al. Critical role of the complement system in group B *Streptococcus*–induced tumor necrosis factor alpha release. Infect Immun 71:6344-6353, 2003.
468. Pozdnyakova O, Guttormsen H-K, Lalani FN, et al. Impaired antibody response to group B streptococcal type III capsular polysaccharide in C3- and complement receptor 2–deficient mice. J Immunol 170:84-90, 2003.
469. Areschoug T, Stalhammar-Carlemalm M, Karlsson I, et al. Streptococcal beta protein has separate binding sites for human factor H and IgA-Fc. J Biol Chem 277:12642-12648, 2002.
470. McFall TL, Zimmerman GA, Augustine NH, et al. Effect of group B streptococcal type-specific antigen on polymorphonuclear leukocyte function and polymorphonuclear leukocyte-endothelial cell interaction. Pediatr Res 21:517-523, 1987.
471. Olson TA, Fischer GW, Hemming VG, et al. A group B streptococcal extract reduces neutrophil counts and induces neutrophil aggregation. Pediatr Res 21:326-330, 1987.
472. Shigeoka AO, Chavette RP, Wyman ML, et al. Defective oxidative metabolic responses of neutrophils from stressed neonates. J Pediatr 98:392-398, 1981.
473. Smith CL, Baker CJ, Anderson DC, et al. Role of complement receptors in opsonophagocytosis of group B streptococci by adult and neonatal neutrophils. J Infect Dis 162:489-495, 1990.
474. Antal JM, Cunningham JV, Goodrum KJ. Opsonin-independent phagocytosis of group B streptococci: role of complement receptor type three. Infect Immun 60:1114-1121, 1992.
475. Yang KD, Bathras JM, Shigeoka AO, et al. Mechanisms of bacterial opsonization by immune globulin intravenous: correlation of complement consumption with opsonic activity and protective efficacy. J Infect Dis 159:701-707, 1989.
476. Noya FJD, Baker CJ, Edwards MS. Neutrophil Fc receptor participation in phagocytosis of type III group B streptococci. Infect Immun 61:1415-1420, 1993.
477. Noel GJ, Katz SL, Edelson PJ. The role of C3 in mediating binding and ingestion of group B *Streptococcus* serotype III by murine macrophages. Pediatr Res 30:118-123, 1991.
478. Christensen RD, Rothstein G, Hill HR, et al. The effect of hybridoma antibody administration upon neutrophil kinetics during experimental type III group B streptococcal sepsis. Pediatr Res 17:795-799, 1983.
479. Christensen RD, Rothstein G, Hill HR, et al. Treatment of experimental group B streptococcal infection with hybridoma antibody. Pediatr Res 18:1093-1096, 1984.
480. Harper TE, Christensen RD, Rothstein G, et al. Effect of intravenous immunoglobulin G on neutrophil kinetics during experimental group B streptococcal infection in neonatal rats. Rev Infect Dis 8:S401-S408, 1986.
481. Fischer GW, Hunter KW, Hemming VG, et al. Functional antibacterial activity of a human intravenous immunoglobulin preparation: in vitro and in vivo studies. Vox Sang 44:296-299, 1983.
482. Givner LB, Edwards MS, Anderson DC, et al. Immune globulin for intravenous use: enhancement of in vitro opsonophagocytic activity of neonatal serum. J Infect Dis 151:217-220, 1985.
483. Shigeoka AO, Bathras JM, Pincus SH, et al. Reticuloendothelial clearance of type III group B streptococci opsonized with type III specific monoclonal antibodies of IgM or IgG2a isotypes in an experimental rat model. Pediatr Res 21:334A, 1987.
484. Poutrel B, Dore J. Virulence of human and bovine isolates of group B streptococci (types Ia and III) in experimental pregnant mouse models. Infect Immunol 47:94-97, 1985.
485. Hall SL, Sherman MP. Intrapulmonary bacterial clearance of type III group B *Streptococcus* is reduced in preterm compared with term rabbits and occurs independent of antibody. Am Rev Respir Dis 145:1172-1177, 1992.
486. Martin TR, Ruzinski JT, Rubens CE, et al. The effect of type-specific polysaccharide capsule on the clearance of group B streptococci from the lungs of infant and adult rats. J Infect Dis 165:306-314, 1992.
487. Domula M, Bykowska K, Wegrzynowicz Z, et al. Plasma fibronectin concentrations in healthy and septic infants. Eur J Pediatr 144:49-52, 1985.
488. Butler KM, Baker CJ, Edwards MS. Interaction of soluble fibronectin with group B streptococci. Infect Immunol 55:2404-2408, 1987.
489. Hill HR, Shigeoka AO, Augustine NH, et al. Fibronectin enhances the opsonic and protective activity of monoclonal and polyclonal antibody against group B streptococci. J Exp Med 159:1618-1628, 1984.
490. Jacobs RF, Kiel DP, Sanders ML, et al. Phagocytosis of type III group B streptococci by neonatal monocytes: enhancement by fibronectin and gammaglobulin. J Infect Dis 152:695-700, 1985.
491. Yang KD, Bohnsack JF, Hawley MM, et al. Effect of fibronectin on IgA-mediated uptake of type III group B streptococci by phagocytes. J Infect Dis 161:236-241, 1990.
492. Peat EB, Augustine NH, Drummond WK, et al. Effects of fibronectin and group B streptococci on tumour necrosis factor-α production by human culture–derived macrophages. Immunology 84:440-445, 1995.
493. Albanyan, EA, Edwards MS. Lectin site interaction with capsular polysaccharide mediates nonimmune phagocytosis of type III group B streptococci. Infect Immun 68:5794-5802, 2000.
494. Grubb R, Christensen KK, Christensen P, et al. Association between maternal Gm allotype and neonatal septicaemia with group B streptococci. J Immunogenet 9:143-147, 1982.
495. Thom H, Lloyd DL, Reid TMS. Maternal immunoglobulin allotype (Gm and Km) and neonatal group B streptococcal infection. J Immunogenet 13:309-314, 1986.
496. Oxelius VA, Linden V, Christensen KK, et al. Deficiency of IgG subclasses in mothers of infants with group B streptococcal septicemia. Int Arch Allergy Appl Immunol 72:249-252, 1983.
497. Rundgren ÅK, Christensen KK, Christensen P. Increased frequency of high serum IgM among mothers of infants with neonatal group-B streptococcal septicemia. Int Arch Allergy Appl Immunol 77:372-373, 1985.
498. Christensen KK, Christensen P, Faxelius G, et al. Immune response to pneumococcal vaccine in mothers to infants with group B streptococcal septicemia: evidence for a divergent IgG/IgM ratio. Int Arch Allergy Appl Immunol 76:369-372, 1985.

499. Christensen KK, Christensen P, Hagerstrand I, et al. The clinical significance of group B streptococci. J Perinatol Med 10:133-146, 1982.
500. Christensen KK. Infection as a predominant cause of perinatal mortality. Obstet Gynecol 59:499-508, 1982.
501. Singer DB, Campognone P. Perinatal group B streptococcal infection in midgestation. Pediatr Pathol 5:271-276, 1986.
502. deSa DJ, Trevenen CL. Intrauterine infections with group B beta-haemolytic streptococci. Br J Obstet Gynaecol 91:237-239, 1984.
503. Hood M, Janney A, Dameron G. Beta-hemolytic *Streptococcus* group B associated with problems of perinatal period. Am J Obstet Gynecol 82:809-818, 1961.
504. Moller M, Thomsen AC, Borch K, et al. Rupture of fetal membranes and premature delivery associated with group B streptococci in urine of pregnant women. Lancet 2:69-70, 1984.
505. Novak RW, Platt MS. Significance of placental findings in early-onset group B streptococcal neonatal sepsis. Clin Pediatr 24:256-258, 1985.
506. Becroft DMO, Farmer K, Mason GH, et al. Perinatal infections by group B β-hemolytic streptococci. Br J Obstet Gynaecol 83:960-965, 1976.
507. Varner MW, Turner JW, Petzold CR, et al. Ultrastructural alterations of term human amnionic epithelium following incubation with group B beta-hemolytic streptococci. Am J Reprod Immunol Microbiol 9:27-32, 1985.
508. Pinnas JL, Strunk RC, Fenton LJ. Immunofluorescence in group B streptococcal infection and idiopathic respiratory distress syndrome. Pediatrics 63:557-561, 1979.
509. Leonidas JC, Hall RT, Beatty EC, et al. Radiographic findings of early onset neonatal group B streptococcal septicemia. Pediatrics 59:S1006-S1011, 1977.
510. Faix RG, Donn SM. Association of septic shock caused by early-onset group B streptococcal sepsis and periventricular leukomalacia in the preterm infant. Pediatrics 76:415-419, 1985.
511. Van Peenen PF, Cannon RE, Seibert DJ. Group B beta-hemolytic streptococci causing fatal meningitis. Mil Med 130:65-67, 1965.
512. Zeligs BJ, Armstrong CD, Walser JB, et al. Age-dependent susceptibility of neonatal rats to group B streptococcal type III infection: correlation of severity of infection and response of myeloid pools. Infect Immunol 37:255-263, 1982.
513. Anthony BF, Okada DM. The emergence of group B streptococci in infections of the newborn infant. Ann Rev Med 28:355-369, 1977.
514. Oddie S, Embleton ND, for the Northern Neonatal Network. Risk factors for early onset neonatal group B streptococcal sepsis: case-control study. BMJ 325:308-312, 2002.
515. DiJohn D, Krasinski K, Lawrence R, et al. Very late onset of group B streptococcal disease in infants infected with the human immunodeficiency virus. Pediatr Infect Dis J 9:925-928, 1990.
516. Weisman LE, Stoll BJ, Cruess DF, et al. Early-onset group B streptococcal sepsis: a current assessment. J Pediatr 121:428-433, 1992.
517. Yagupsky P, Menegus MA, Powell KR. The changing spectrum of group B streptococcal disease in infants: an eleven-year experience in a tertiary care hospital. Pediatr Infect Dis J 10:801-808, 1991.
518. Schuchat A, Zywicki SS, Dinsmoor MJ, et al. Risk factors and opportunities for prevention of early-onset neonatal sepsis: a multicenter case-control study. Pediatrics 105:21-26, 2000.
519. Stoll BJ, Gordon T, Korones SB, et al. Early-onset sepsis in very low birth weight neonates: a report from the National Institute of Child Health and Human Development Neonatal Research Network. J Pediatr 129:72-80, 1996.
520. Chen KT, Ringer S, Cohen AP, et al. The role of intrapartum fever in identifying asymptomatic term neonates with early-onset neonatal sepsis. J Perinatol 22:653-657, 2002.
521. Chin KC, Fitzhardinge PM. Sequelae of early-onset group B streptococcal neonatal meningitis. J Pediatr 106:819-822, 1985.
522. Haslam RHA, Allen JR, Dorsen MM, et al. The sequelae of group B β-hemolytic streptococcal meningitis in early infancy. Am J Dis Child 131:845-849, 1977.
523. Edwards MS, Rench MA, Haffar AAM, et al. Long-term sequelae of group B streptococcal meningitis in infants. J Pediatr 106:717-722, 1985.
524. Lilien LD, Harris VJ, Pildes RS. Significance of radiographic findings in early-onset group B streptococcal infection. Pediatrics 60:360-365, 1977.
525. Herting E, Gefeller O, Land M, et al. Surfactant treatment of neonates with respiratory failure and group B streptococcal infection. Pediatrics 106:957-964, 2000.
526. Hammerman C, Lass N, Strates E, et al. Prostanoids in neonates with persistent pulmonary hypertension. J Pediatr 110:470-472, 1987.
527. Payne NR, Burke BA, Day DL, et al. Correlation of clinical and pathologic findings in early onset neonatal group B streptococcal infection with disease severity and prediction of outcome. Pediatr Infect Dis J 7:836-847, 1988.
528. Boyer KM, Gadzala CA, Burd LI, et al. Selective intrapartum chemoprophylaxis of neonatal group B streptococcal early-onset disease: I. Epidemiologic rationale. J Infect Dis 148:795-801, 1983.
529. Baker CJ. Unpublished observations, 1990.
530. Pyati SP, Pildes RS, Ramamurthy RS, et al. Decreasing mortality in neonates with early-onset group B streptococcal infection: reality or artifact? J Pediatr 98:625-628, 1981.
531. Stoll BJ, Hansen N, Fanaroff AA, et al. Late-onset sepsis in very low birth weight neonates: the experience of the NICHD Neonatal Research Network. Pediatrics 110:285-291, 2002.
532. Lin F-YC, Weisman LE, Troendle J, et al. Prematurity is the major risk factor for late-onset group B *Streptococcus* disease. J Infect Dis 188:267-271, 2003.
533. erguson L, Gotoff SP. Subdural empyema in an infant due to group B β-hemolytic *Streptococcus.* Am J Dis Child 131:97, 1977.
534. McReynolds EW, Shane R. Diabetes insipidus secondary to group B beta streptococcal meningitis. J Tenn Med Assoc 67:117-120, 1974.
535. Wald ER, Bergman I, Taylor HG, et al. Long-term outcome of group B streptococcal meningitis. Pediatrics 77:217-221, 1986.
536. Garcia Peña BM, Harper MB, Fleisher GR. Occult bacteremia with group B streptococci in an outpatient setting. Pediatrics 102:67-72, 1998.
537. Ramsey PG, Zwerdling R. Asymptomatic neonatal bacteremia. N Engl J Med 295:225, 1977.
538. Roberts KB. Persistent group B *Streptococcus* bacteremia without clinical "sepsis" in infants. J Pediatr 88:1059-1060, 1976.
539. Hussain SM, Luedtke GS, Baker CJ, et al. Invasive group B streptococcal disease in children beyond early infancy. Pediatr Infect Dis J 14:278-281, 1995.
540. De Witt CC, Ascher DP, Winkelstein J. Group B streptococcal disease in a child beyond early infancy with a deficiency of the second component of complement (C2). Pediatr Infect Dis J 18:77-78, 1999.
541. Ashdown LR, Hewson PH, Suleman SK. Neonatal osteomyelitis and meningitis caused by group B streptococci. Med J Aust 2:500-501, 1977.
542. McCook TA, Felman AH, Ayoub EM. Streptococcal skeletal infections: observations in four infants. Roentgenology 130:465-467, 1978.
543. Ancona RJ, McAuliffe J, Thompson TR, et al. Group B streptococcal sepsis with osteomyelitis and arthritis. Am J Dis Child 133:919-920, 1979.
544. Memon IA, Jacobs NM, Yeh TF, et al. Group B streptococcal osteomyelitis and septic arthritis. Am J Dis Child 133:921-923, 1979.
545. Pittard WB, Thullen JD, Fanaroff AA. Neonatal septic arthritis. J Pediatr 88:621-624, 1976.
546. McCracken GH Jr. Septic arthritis in a neonate. Hosp Pract 14:158-164, 1979.
547. Nelson JD. The bacterial etiology and antibiotic management of septic arthritis in infants and children. Pediatrics 50:437-440, 1972.
548. Anthony BF, Concepcion NF. Group B *Streptococcus* in a general hospital. J Infect Dis 132:561-567, 1975.
549. Dan M. Neonatal septic arthritis. Isr J Med Sci 19:967-971, 1983.
550. Edwards MS, Baker CJ, Wagner ML, et al. An etiologic shift in infantile osteomyelitis: the emergence of the group B *Streptococcus.* J Pediatr 93:578-583, 1978.
551. Siskind B, Galliguez P, Wald ER. Group B beta hemolytic streptococcal osteomyelitis/purulent arthritis in neonates: report of three cases. J Pediatr 87:659, 1975.
552. Fox L, Sprunt K. Neonatal osteomyelitis. Pediatrics 62:535-542, 1978.
553. Lai TK, Hingston J, Scheifele D. Streptococcal neonatal osteomyelitis. Am J Dis Child 134:711, 1980.
554. Hutto JH, Ayoub EM. Streptococcal osteomyelitis and arthritis in a neonate. Am J Dis Child 129:1449-1451, 1975.
555. Henderson KC, Roberts RS, Dorsey SB. Group B β-hemolytic streptococcal osteomyelitis in a neonate. Pediatrics 59:1053-1054, 1977.
556. Ragnhildstreit E, Ose L. Neonatal osteomyelitis caused by group B streptococci. Scand J Infect Dis 8:219-221, 1976.
557. Kexel G. Occurrence of B streptococci in humans. Z Hyg Infektionskr 151:336-348, 1965.
558. Clay SA. Osteomyelitis as a cause of brachial plexus neuropathy. Am J Dis Child 136:1054-1056, 1982.

559. Broughton RA, Edwards MS, Haffar A, et al. Unusual manifestations of neonatal group B streptococcal osteomyelitis. Pediatr Infect Dis J 1:410-412, 1982.
560. Mohon RT, Mehalic TF, Grimes CK, et al. Infected cephalhematoma and neonatal osteomyelitis of the skull. Pediatr Infect Dis J 5:253-256, 1986.
561. Baevsky RH. Neonatal group B beta-hemolytic *Streptococcus* osteomyelitis. Am J Emerg Med 17:619-622. 1999.
562. Sadleir LG, Connolly MB. Acquired brachial-plexus neuropathy in the neonate: a rare presentation of late-onset group-B streptococcal osteomyelitis. Dev Med Child Neurol 40:496-499, 1998.
563. Ammari LK, Offit PA, Campbell AB, et al. Unusual presentation of group B *Streptococcus* osteomyelitis. Pediatr Infect Dis J 11:1066-1067, 1992.
564. Weinberg AG, Laird WP. Group B streptococcal endocarditis detected by echocardiography. J Pediatr 92:335-336, 1978.
565. Obando I, Martin E, Alvarez-Aldean J, et al. Group B *Streptococcus* pelvic osteomyelitis presenting as footdrop in a newborn infant. Pediatr Infect Dis J 10:703-705, 1991.
566. Barton LL, Villar RG, Rice SA. Neonatal group B streptococcal vertebral osteomyelitis. Pediatrics 98:459-461, 1996.
567. Hauger SB. Facial cellulitis: an early indicator of group B streptococcal bacteremia. Pediatrics 67:376-377, 1981.
568. Patamasucon P, Siegel JD, McCracken GH Jr. Streptococcal submandibular cellulitis in young infants. Pediatrics 67:378-380, 1981.
569. Baker CJ. Group B streptococcal cellulitis/adenitis in infants. Am J Dis Child 136:631-633, 1982.
570. Fluegge K, Greiner P, Berner R. Late onset group B streptococcal disease manifested by isolated cervical lymphadenitis. Arch Dis Child 88:1019-1020, 2003.
571. Pathak A, Hwu H-H. Group B streptococcal cellulitis. South Med J 78:67-68, 1985.
572. Haque KN, Bashir O, Kambal AMM. Delayed recurrence of group B streptococcal infection in a newborn infant: a case report. Ann Trop Paediatr 6:219-220, 1986.
573. Rand TH. Group B streptococcal cellulitis in infants: a disease modified by prior antibiotic therapy or hospitalization? Pediatrics 81:63-65, 1988.
574. Brady MT. Cellulitis of the penis and scrotum due to group B *Streptococcus.* J Urol 137:736-737, 1987.
575. Albanyan EA, Baker CJ. Is lumbar puncture necessary to exclude meningitis in neonates and young infants: lessons from group B *Streptococcus* cellulitis-adenitis syndrome. Pediatrics 102:985-986, 1998.
576. Chadwick EG, Shulman ST, Yogev R. Peritonitis as a late manifestation of group B streptococcal disease in newborns. Pediatr Infect Dis J 2:142-143, 1983.
577. Walker KM, Coyer WF. Suprarenal abscess due to group B streptococcus. J Pediatr 94:970-971, 1979.
578. Atkinson GO Jr, Kodroff MB, Gay BB, et al. Adrenal abscess in the neonate. Radiology 155:101-104, 1985.
579. Carty A, Stanley P. Bilateral adrenal abscesses in a neonate. Pediatr Radiol 1:63-64, 1973.
580. Peevy KJ, Wiseman HJ. Gallbladder distension in septic neonates. Arch Dis Child 57:75-76, 1982.
581. Siegel JD, Shannon KM, De Passe BM. Recurrent infection associated with penicillin-tolerant group B streptococci: a report of two cases. J Pediatr 99:920-924, 1981.
582. Cueva JP, Egel RT. Anterior fontanel herniation in group B *Streptococcus* meningitis in newborns. Pediatr Neurol 10:332-334, 1994.
583. Sokol DM, Demmler GJ, Baker CJ. Unusual presentation of group B streptococcal ventriculitis. Pediatr Infect Dis J 9:525-527, 1990.
584. Kim KS, Kaye KL, Itabashi HH, et al. Cerebritis due to group B *Streptococcus.* Scand J Infect Dis 14:305-308, 1982.
585. Coker SB, Muraskas JK, Thomas C. Myelopathy secondary to neonatal bacterial meningitis. Pediatr Neurol 10:259-261, 1994.
586. Schimmel MS, Schlesinger Y, Berger I, et al. Transverse myelitis: unusual sequelae of neonatal group B *Streptococcus* disease. J Perinatol 22:580-581, 2002.
587. Ellenbogen RG, Goldmann DA, Winston KR. Group B streptococcal infections of the central nervous system in infants with myelomeningocele. Surg Neurol 29:237-242, 1988.
588. Chattopadhyay B. Fatal neonatal meningitis due to group B streptococci. Postgrad Med J 51:240-243, 1975.
589. Barton CW, Crowley DC, Uzark K, et al. A neonatal survivor of group B beta-hemolytic streptococcal endocarditis. Am J Perinatol 1:214-215, 1984.
590. Horigome H, Okada Y, Hirano T, et al. Group B streptococcal endocarditis in infancy with a giant vegetation on the pulmonary valve. Eur J Pediatr 153:140-142, 1994.
591. Harper IA. The importance of group B streptococci as human pathogens in the British Isles. J Clin Pathol 24:438-441, 1971.
592. Agarwala BN. Group B streptococcal endocarditis in a neonate. Pediatr Cardiol 9:51-53, 1988.
593. Sapir-Ellis S, Johnson A, Austin TL. Group B streptococcal meningitis associated with otitis media. Am J Dis Child 130:1003-1004, 1976.
594. Shurin PA, Howie VM, Pelton SI, et al. Bacterial etiology of otitis media during the first six weeks of life. J Pediatr 92:893-896, 1978.
595. Tetzlaff TR, Ashworth C, Nelson JD. Otitis media in children less than 12 weeks of age. Pediatrics 59:827-832, 1977.
596. Ermocilla R, Cassady G, Ceballos R. Otitis media in the pathogenesis of neonatal meningitis with group B beta-hemolytic *Streptococcus.* Pediatrics 54:643-644, 1974.
597. Armstrong JH, Zacarias F, Rein MF. Ophthalmia neonatorum: a chart review. Pediatrics 57:884-892, 1976.
598. Poschl JM, Hellstern G, Ruef P, et al. Ophthalmia neonatorum caused by group B *Streptococcus.* Scand J Infect Dis 34:921-922, 2002.
599. Greene GR, Carroll WL, Morozumi PA, et al. Endophthalmitis associated with group B streptococcal meningitis in an infant. Am J Dis Child 133:752, 1979.
600. Berger BB. Endophthalmitis complicating group B streptococcal septicemia. Am J Ophthalmol 92:681-684, 1981.
601. Klusmann A, Engelbrecht V, Unsöld R, et al. Retrobulbar abscess in a neonate. Neuropediatrics 32:219-220, 2001.
602. Ashcraft KW, Holder TM, Amoury RA, et al. Diagnosis and treatment of right Bochdalek hernia associated with group B streptococcal pneumonia and sepsis in the neonate. J Pediatr Surg 18:480-485, 1983.
603. Vachharajani AJ, Shah JK, Paes BA. Late-onset left diaphragmatic hernia after group B streptococcal sepsis: an unusual presentation. 37:932-933, 2002.
604. Lipson A, Kronick JB, Tewfik L, et al. Group B streptococcal supraglottitis in a 3-month-old infant. Am J Dis Child 140:411-412, 1986.
605. LeBovar Y, Trung PH, Mozziconacci P. Neonatal meningitis due to group B streptococci. Ann Pediatr 17:207-213, 1970.
606. Sokal MM, Nagaraj A, Fisher BJ, et al. Neonatal empyema caused by group B beta-hemolytic *Streptococcus.* Chest 81:390-391, 1982.
607. Park JW. Bacterial tracheitis caused by *Streptococcus agalactiae.* Pediatr Infect Dis J 9:450-451, 1990.
608. Wiswell TE, Miller JA. Infections of congenital cervical neck masses associated with bacteremia. J Pediatr Surg 21:173-174, 1986.
609. Nelson JD. Bilateral breast abscess due to group B *Streptococcus.* Am J Dis Child 130:567, 1976.
610. Rench MA, Baker CJ. Group B streptococcal breast abscess in a mother and mastitis in her infant. Obstet Gynecol 73:875-877, 1989.
611. Brian MJ, O'Ryan M, Waagner D. Prepatellar bursitis in an infant caused by group B *Streptococcus.* Pediatr Infect Dis J 11:502-503, 1992.
612. Ruiz-Gomez D, Tarpay MM, Riley HD. Recurrent group B streptococcal infections: report of three cases. Scand J Infect Dis 11:35-38, 1979.
613. Amoury RA, Barth GW, Hall RT, et al. Scrotal ecchymosis: sign of intraperitoneal hemorrhage in the newborn. South Med J 75:1471-1478, 1982.
614. Frieden IJ. Blistering dactylitis caused by group B streptococci. Pediatr Dermatol 6:300-302, 1989.
615. Ramamurthy RS, Srinivasan G, Jacobs NM. Necrotizing fasciitis and necrotizing cellulitis due to group B *Streptococcus.* Am J Dis Child 131:1169-1170, 1977.
616. Goldberg GN, Hansen RC, Lynch PJ. Necrotizing fasciitis in infancy: report of three cases and review of the literature. Pediatr Dermatol 2:55-63, 1984.
617. Lang ME, Vaudry W, Robinson JL. Case report and literature review of late-onset group B streptococcal disease manifesting as necrotizing fasciitis in preterm infants: Is this a new syndrome? Clin Infect Dis 37:e132-e135, 2003.
618. Lopez JB, Gross P, Boggs TR. Skin lesions in association with β-hemolytic *Streptococcus* group B. Pediatrics 58:859-860, 1976.
619. Belgaumkar TK. Impetigo neonatorum congenita due to group B beta-hemolytic *Streptococcus* infection. J Pediatr 86:982-983, 1975.
620. Isaacman SH, Heroman WM, Lightsey AL. Purpura fulminans following late-onset group B beta-hemolytic streptococcal sepsis. Am J Dis Child 138:915-916, 1984.
621. Lynn NJ, Pauly TH, Desai NS. Purpura fulminans in three cases of early-onset neonatal group B streptococcal meningitis. J Perinatol 11:144-146, 1991.

622. Jacobs MR, Koornhof HJ, Stein H. Group B streptococcal infections in neonates and infants. S Afr Med J 54:154-158, 1978.
623. Turner MC, Naumburg EG. Acute renal failure in the neonate: two fatal cases due to group B streptococci with rhabdomyolysis. Clin Pediatr 26:189-190, 1987.
624. Bourgeois FT, Shannon MW. Retropharyngeal cellulitis in a 5-week-old infant. Pediatrics 109:e51-e53, 2002.
625. Kelly CP, Isaacman DJ. Group B streptococcal retropharyngeal cellulitis in a young infant: a case report and review of the literature. J Emerg Med 23:179-182, 2002.
626. Feder AM Jr, MacLean WC, Moxon R. Scalp abscess secondary to fetal scalp electrode. J Pediatr 89:808-809, 1976.
627. St. Laurent-Gagnon T, Weber ML. Urinary tract *Streptococcus* group B infection in a 6-week-old infant. JAMA 240:1269, 1978.
628. Callanan DL, Harris GG. Group B streptococcal infection in children with liver disease. Clin Pediatr 21:99-100, 1982.
629. Dorand RD, Adams G. Relapse during penicillin treatment of group B streptococcal meningitis. J Pediatr 89:188-190, 1976.
630. Kenny JD. Right-sided diaphragmatic hernia of delayed onset in the newborn infant. South Med J 70:373-375, 1977.
631. Suresh BR, Rios A, Brion LP, et al. Delayed onset right-sided diaphragmatic hernia secondary to group B streptococcal infection. Pediatr Infect Dis J 10:166-168, 1991.
632. Nudelman R, Bral M, Sakhai Y, et al. Violaceous cellulitis. Pediatrics 70:157-158, 1982.
633. Barton LL, Kapoor NK. Recurrent group B streptococcal infection. Clin Pediatr 21:100-101, 1982.
634. Broughton DD, Mitchell WG, Grossman M, et al. Recurrence of group B streptococcal infection. J Pediatr 89:183-185, 1976.
635. Walker SH, Santos AQ, Quintero BA. Recurrence of group B III streptococcal meningitis. J Pediatr 89:187-188, 1976.
636. Kenny JF, Zedd AJ. Recurrent group B streptococcal disease in an infant associated with the ingestion of infected mother's milk. J Pediatr 91:158-159, 1977.
637. McCrory JH, Au-Yeung YB, Sugg VM, et al. Recurrent group B streptococcal infection in an infant: ventriculitis complicating type Ib meningitis. J Pediatr 92:231-233, 1978.
638. Truog WE, Davis RF, Ray CG. Recurrence of group B streptococcal infection. J Pediatr 89:185-186, 1976.
639. Green PA, Singh KV, Murray BE, et al. Recurrent group B streptococcal infections in infants: clinical and microbiologic aspects. J Pediatr 125:931-938, 1994.
640. Atkins JT, Heresi GP, Coque TM, et al. Recurrent group B streptococcal disease in infants: who should receive rifampin? J Pediatr 132:537-539, 1998.
641. Moylett EH, Fernandez M, Rench MA, et al. A 5-year review of recurrent group B streptococcal disease: lessons from twin infants. Clin Infect Dis 30:282-287, 2000.
642. Simón JL, Bosch J, Puig A, et al. Two relapses of group B streptococcal sepsis and transient hypogammaglobulinemia. Pediatr Infect Dis J 8:729-730, 1989.
643. Denning DW, Bressack M, Troup NJ, et al. Infant with two relapses of group B streptococcal sepsis documented by DNA restriction enzyme analysis. Pediatr Infect Dis J 7:729-732, 1988.
644. Kotiw M, Zhang GW, Daggard G, et al. Late-onset and recurrent neonatal group B streptococcal disease associated with breast-milk transmission. Pediatr Dev Pathol 6:251-256, 2003.
645. Kim KS, Anthony BF. Penicillin tolerance in group B streptococci isolated from infected neonates. J Infect Dis 144:411-419, 1981.
646. Cunningham R. Recurrent group B streptococcal disease in infants: a possible explanation. Clin Infect Dis 31:627, 2000.
647. Ramsay AM, Gillespie M. Puerperal infection associated with haemolytic streptococci other than Lancefield's group A. J Obstet Gynaecol Br Emp 48:569-585, 1941.
648. Butter MNW, de Moor CE. *Streptococcus agalactiae* as a cause of meningitis in the newborn, and of bacteremia in adults. Antonie van Leeuwenhoek 33:439-450, 1967.
649. Aharoni A, Potasman I, Levitan Z, et al. Postpartum maternal group B streptococcal meningitis. Rev Infect Dis 12:273-276, 1990.
650. Kane JM, Jackson K, Conway JH. Maternal postpartum group B beta-hemolytic streptococcus ventriculoperitoneal shunt infection. Arch Gynecol Obstet 269:139-141, 2004.
651. Sexton DJ, Rockson SG, Hempling RE, et al. Pregnancy-associated group B streptococcal endocarditis: a report of two fatal cases. Obstet Gynecol 66:44S-47S, 1985.
652. Backes RJ, Wilson WR, Geraci JE. Group B streptococcal infective endocarditis. Arch Intern Med 145:693-696, 1985.
653. Seaworth BJ, Durack DT. Infective endocarditis in obstetric and gynecologic practice. Am J Obstet Gynecol 154:180-188, 1986.
654. Vartian CV, Septimus EJ. Tricuspid valve group B streptococcal endocarditis following elective abortion. Rev Infect Dis 13:997-998, 1991.
655. Lischke JH, McCreight PHB. Maternal group B streptococcal vertebral osteomyelitis: an unusual complication of vaginal delivery. Obstet Gynecol 76:489-491, 1990.
656. Jenkin G, Woolley IJ, Brown GV, et al. Postpartum epidural abscess due to group B *Streptococcus*. Clin Infect Dis 25:1249, 1997.
657. Sutton GP, Smirz LR, Clark DH, et al. Group B streptococcal necrotizing fasciitis arising from an episiotomy. Obstet Gynecol 66:733-736, 1985.
658. Wood EG, Dillon HC. A prospective study of group B streptococcal bacteriuria in pregnancy. Am J Obstet Gynecol 140:515-520, 1981.
659. Pass MA, Gray BM, Dillon HC Jr. Puerperal and perinatal infections with group B streptococci. Am J Obstet Gynecol 143:147-152, 1982.
660. Daugaard HO, Thomsen AC, Henriques U, et al. Group B streptococci in the lower urogenital tract and late abortions. Am J Obstet Gynecol 158:28-31, 1988.
661. Wiswell TE, Baumgart S, Gannon CM, et al. No lumbar puncture in the evaluation for early neonatal sepsis: will meningitis be missed? Pediatrics 95:803-806, 1995.
662. Edwards MS, Baker CJ. Prospective diagnosis of early onset group B streptococcal infection by countercurrent immunoelectrophoresis. J Pediatr 94:286-288, 1979.
663. Typlin BL, Koranyi K, Azimi P, et al. Counterimmunoelectrophoresis for the rapid diagnosis of group B streptococcal infections. Clin Pediatr 18:366-369, 1979.
664. Hamoudi AC, Marcon MJ, Cannon HJ, et al. Comparison of three major antigen detection methods for the diagnosis of group B streptococcal sepsis in neonates. Pediatr Infect Dis J 2:432-435, 1983.
665. Rench MA, Metzger TG, Baker CJ. Detection of group B streptococcal antigen in body fluids by a latex-coupled monoclonal antibody assay. J Clin Microbiol 20:852-854, 1984.
666. Baker CJ, Rench MA. Commercial latex agglutination for detection of group B streptococcal antigen in body fluids. J Pediatr 102:393-395, 1983.
667. Webb BJ, Edwards MS, Baker CJ. Comparison of slide coagglutination test and countercurrent immunoelectrophoresis for detection of group B streptococcal antigen in cerebrospinal fluid from infants with meningitis. J Clin Microbiol 11:263-265, 1980.
668. Drow DL, Welch DF, Hensel D, et al. Evaluation of the Phadebact CSF Test for detection of the four most common causes of bacterial meningitis. J Clin Microbiol 18:1358-1361, 1983.
669. Morrow DL, Kline JB, Douglas SD, et al. Rapid detection of group B streptococcal antigen by monoclonal antibody sandwich enzyme assay. J Clin Microbiol 19:457-459, 1984.
670. FDA Alert. Safety alert re risk of misdiagnosis of group B streptococcal infection. JAMA 277:1343, 1997.
671. Philip AGS. Response of C-reactive protein in neonatal group B streptococcal infection. Pediatr Infect Dis J 4:145-148, 1985.
672. Pourcyrous M, Bada HS, Korones SB, et al. Significance of serial C-reactive protein responses in neonatal infection and other disorders. Pediatrics 92:431-435, 1993.
673. Philip AG, Mills PC. Ue of C-reactive protein in minimizing antibiotic exposure: experience with infants initially admitted to a well-baby nursery. Pediatrics 106:e4, 2000.
674. Vallejo JG, Baker CJ, Edwards MS. Interleukin-6 production by human neonatal monocytes stimulated by type III group B streptococci. J Infect Dis 174:332-337, 1996.
675. Manroe BL, Rosenfeld CR, Weinberg AG, et al. The differential leukocyte count in the assessment and outcome of early-onset neonatal group B streptococcal disease. J Pediatr 91:632-637, 1977.
676. Manroe BL, Weinberg AG, Rosenfeld CR, et al. The neonatal blood count in health and disease: I. Reference values for neutrophilic cells. J Pediatr 95:89-98, 1979.
677. Greenberg DN, Yoder BA. Changes in the differential white blood cell count in screening for group B streptococcal sepsis. Pediatr Infect Dis J 9:886-889, 1990.
678. Christensen RD, Rothstein G, Hill HR, et al. Fatal early onset group B streptococcal sepsis with normal leukocyte counts. Pediatr Infect Dis J 4:242-245, 1985.

679. Baker CJ, Webb BJ, Barrett FF. Antimicrobial susceptibility of group B streptococci isolated from a variety of clinical sources. Antimicrob Agents Chemother 10:128-131, 1976.
680. Fernandez M, Hickman ME, Baker CJ. Antimicrobial susceptibilities of group B streptococci isolated between 1992 and 1996 from patients with bacteremia or meningitis. Antimicrob Agents Chemother 42:1517-1519, 1998.
681. Meyn LA, Hillier SL. Ampicillin susceptibilities of vaginal and placental isolates of group B *Streptococcus* and *Escherichia coli* obtained between 1992 and 1994. Antimicrob Agents Chemother 41:1173-1174, 1997.
682. Biedenbach DJ, Stephen JM, Jones RN. Antimicrobial susceptibility profile among β-haemolytic *Streptococcus* spp. collected in the SENTRY Antimicrobial Surveillance Program-North America, 2001. Diag Microbiol Infect Dis 46:291-294, 2003.
683. Manning SD, Foxman B, Pierson CL, et al. Correlates of antibiotic-resistant group B Streptococcus isolated from pregnant women. Obstet Gynecol 101:74-79, 2003.
684. Kim KS. Efficacy of imipenem in experimental group B streptococcal bacteremia and meningitis. Chemotherapy 31:304-309, 1985.
685. Kim KS. Antimicrobial susceptibility of GBS. Antibiot Chemother 35:83-89, 1985.
686. Persson KM-S, Forsgren A. Antimicrobial susceptibility of group B streptococci. Eur J Clin Microbiol 5:165-167, 1986.
687. Liberto MC, Carbone M, Fera MT, et al. Cefixime shows good effects on group A and group B β-hemolytic streptococci. Drugs Exp Clin Res 17:305-308, 1991.
688. Sheppard M, King A, Phillips I. In vitro activity of cefpodoxime, a new oral cephalosporin, compared with that of nine other antimicrobial agents. Eur J Clin Microbiol Infect Dis 10:573-581, 1991.
689. Kim KS, Kang JH, Bayer AS. Efficacy of teicoplanin in experimental group B streptococcal bacteremia and meningitis. Chemotherapy 33:177-182, 1987.
690. Manning SD, Pearlman MD, Tallman P, et al. Frequency of antibiotic resistance among group B *Streptococcus* isolated from healthy college students. Clin Infect Dis 33:e137-e139, 2001.
691. de Azavedo JCS, McGavin M, Duncan C, et al. Prevalence and mechanisms of macrolide resistance in invasive and noninvasive group B Streptococcus isolates from Ontario, Canada. Antimicrob Agents Chemother 45:3504-3508, 2001.
692. Pearlman MD, Pierson CL, Faix RG. Frequent resistance of clinical group B streptococci isolates to clindamycin and erythromycin. Obstet Gynecol 92:258-261, 1998.
693. Fitoussi F, Loukil C, Gros I, et al. Mechanisms of macrolide resistance in clinical group B streptococci isolated in France. Antimicrob Agents Chemother 45:1889-1891, 2001.
694. Betriu C, Culebras E, Gómez M, et al. Erythromycin and clindamycin resistance and telithromycin susceptibility in *Streptococcus agalactiae*. Antimicrob Agents Chemother 47:1112-1114, 2003.
695. Acikgoz ZC, Almayanlar E, Gamberzade S, et al. Macrolide resistance determinants of invasive and noninvasive group B streptococci in a Turkish hospital. Antimicrob Agents Chemother 48:1410-1412, 2004.
696. Hsueh P-R, Teng L-J, Lee L-N, et al. High incidence of erythromycin resistance among clinical isolates of *Streptococcus agalactiae* in Taiwan. Antimicrob Agents Chemother 45:3205-3208, 2001.
697. Heelan JS, Hasenbein ME, McAdam AJ. Resistance of group B *Streptococcus* to selected antibiotics, including erythromycin and clindamycin. J Clin Microbiol 42:1263-1264, 2004.
698. Lin F-YC, Azimi PH, Weisman LE, et al. Antibiotic susceptibility profiles for group B streptococci isolated from neonates, 1995-1998. Clin Infect Dis 31:76-79, 2000.
699. Betriu C, Culebras E, Rodríguez-Avial I, et al. In vitro activities of tigecycline against erythromycin-resistant *Streptococcus pyogenes* and *Streptococcus agalactiae*: mechanisms of macrolide and tetracycline resistance. Antimicrob Agent Chemother 48:323-325, 2004.
700. Bingen E, Doit C, Bidet P, et al. Telithromycin susceptibility and genomic diversity of macrolide-resistant serotype III group B streptococci isolated in perinatal infections. Antimicrob Agent Chemother 48:677-680, 2004.
701. Jones WF, Feldman HA, Finland M. Susceptibility of hemolytic streptococci, other than those of group D, to eleven antibiotics in vitro. Am J Clin Pathol 27:159-169, 1957.
702. Schauf V, Deveikis A, Riff L, et al. Antibiotic-killing kinetics of group B streptococci. J Pediatr 89:194-198, 1976.
703. Deveikis A, Schauf V, Mizen M, et al. Antimicrobial therapy of experimental group B streptococcal infection in mice. Antimicrob Agents Chemother 11:817-820, 1977.
704. Cooper MD, Keeney RE, Lyons SF, et al. Synergistic effects of ampicillin-aminoglycoside combinations on group B streptococci. Antimicrob Agents Chemother 15:484-486, 1979.
705. Swingle HM, Bucciarelli RL, Ayoub EM. Synergy between penicillins and low concentrations of gentamicin in the killing of group B streptococci. J Infect Dis 152:515-520, 1985.
706. Scheld WM, Alliegro GM, Field MR, et al. Synergy between ampicillin and gentamicin in experimental meningitis due to group B streptococci. J Infect Dis 146:100, 1982.
707. Backes RJ, Rouse MS, Henry NK, et al. Activity of penicillin combined with an aminoglycoside against group B streptococci in vitro and in experimental endocarditis. J Antimicrob Chemother 18:491-498, 1986.
708. Kim KS. Effect of antimicrobial therapy for experimental infections due to group B *Streptococcus* on mortality and clearance of bacteria. J Infect Dis 155:1233-1241, 1987.
709. Smith SM, Eng RHK, Landesman S. Effect of rifampin on ampicillin killing of group B streptococci. Antimicrob Agents Chemother 22:522-524, 1982.
710. Maduri-Traczewski M, Szymczak EG, Goldmann DA. In vitro activity of penicillin and rifampin against group B streptococci. Rev Infect Dis 5:S586-S592, 1983.
711. Hall MA, Ducker DA, Lowes JA, et al. A randomized prospective comparison of cefotaxime versus netilmicin/penicillin for treatment of suspected neonatal sepsis. Drugs 35(Suppl 2):169-188, 1988.
712. Bradley JS, Ching DLK, Wilson TA, et al. Once-daily ceftriaxone to complete therapy of uncomplicated group B streptococcal infection in neonates. Clin Pediatr 31:274-278, 1992.
713. Kim KS. Effect of antimicrobial therapy for experimental infections due to group B *Streptococcus* on mortality and clearance of bacteria. J Infect Dis 155:1233-1241, 1987.
714. Feldman WE. Concentrations of bacteria in cerebrospinal fluid of patients with bacterial meningitis. J Pediatr 88:549-552, 1976.
715. Kim KS, Anthony BF. Penicillin tolerance in group B streptococci isolated from infected neonates. J Infect Dis 144:411-419, 1981.
716. Kim KS, Yoshimori RN, Imagawa DT, et al. Importance of medium in demonstrating penicillin tolerance by group B streptococci. Antimicrob Agents Chemother 16:214-216, 1979.
717. Kim KS. Clinical perspectives on penicillin tolerance. J Pediatr 112:509-514, 1988.
718. McCracken GH Jr, Feldman WE. Editorial comment. J Pediatr 89:203-204, 1976.
719. Baker CJ. Antibiotic susceptibility testing in the management of an infant with group B streptococcal meningitis. Pediatr Infect Dis J 6:1073-1074, 1987.
720. Wilson WR. Antimicrobial therapy of streptococcal endocarditis. J Antimicrob Chemother 20(Suppl A):147-159, 1987.
721. Poschl JM, Hellstern G, Dertlioglou N, et al. Six day antimicrobial therapy for early-onset group B streptococcal infection in near-term and term neonates. Scand J Infect Dis 35:302-305, 2003.
722. Paredes A, Wong P, Yow MD. Failure of penicillin to eradicate the carrier state of group B *Streptococcus* in infants. J Pediatr 89:191-193, 1976.
723. Fernandez M, Rench MA, Albanyan EA, et al. Failure of rifampin to eradicate group B streptococcal colonization in infants. Pediatr Infect Dis J 20:371-376, 2001.
724. Hocker JR, Simpson PM, Rabalais GP, et al. Extracorporeal membrane oxygenation and early-onset group B streptococcal sepsis. Pediatrics 89:1-4, 1992.
725. LeBlanc MH. ECMO and sepsis. Pediatrics 90:127, 1992.
726. Christensen RD, Rothstein G, Anstall HB, et al. Granulocyte transfusions in neonates with bacterial infection, neutropenia, and depletion of mature marrow neutrophils. Pediatrics 70:1-6, 1982.
727. Givner LB, Baker CJ. The prevention and treatment of neonatal group B streptococcal infections. Adv Pediatr Infect Dis 3:65-90, 1988.
728. Cairo MS, Mauss D, Kommareddy S, et al. Prophylactic or simultaneous administration of recombinant human granulocyte colony stimulating factor in the treatment of group B streptococcal sepsis in neonatal rats. Pediatr Res 27:612-616, 1990.
729. Cairo MS, Plunkett JM, Nguyen A, et al. Effect of stem cell factor with and without granulocyte colony-stimulating factor on neonatal hematopoiesis: in vivo induction of newborn myelopoiesis and reduction of mortality during experimental group B streptococcal sepsis. Blood 80:96-101, 1992.
730. Iguchi K, Inoue S, Kumar A. Effect of recombinant human granulocyte colony-stimulating factor administration in normal and experimentally infected newborn rats. Exp Hematol 19:352-358, 1991.

731. Wheeler JG, Givner LB. Therapeutic use of recombinant human granulocyte-macrophage colony-stimulating factor in neonatal rats with type III group B streptococcal sepsis. J Infect Dis 165:938-941, 1992.
732. Hill HR, Shigeoka AO, Pincus S, et al. Intravenous IgG in combination with other modalities in the treatment of neonatal infection. Pediatr Infect Dis J 5(Suppl):S180-S184, 1986.
733 Givner LB. Human immunoglobulins for intravenous use: comparison of available preparations for group B streptococcal antibody levels, opsonic activity, and efficacy in animal models. Pediatrics 86:955-962, 1990.
734. Kim KS. Efficacy of human immunoglobulin and penicillin G in treatment of experimental group B streptococcal infection. Pediatr Res 21:289-292, 1987.
735. Givner LB, Baker CJ. Pooled human IgG hyperimmune for type III group B streptococci: evaluation against multiple strains in vitro and in experimental disease. J Infect Dis 163:1141-1145, 1991.
736. Fischer GW, Hemming VG, Gloser HP, et al. Polyvalent group B streptococcal immune globulin for intravenous administration: overview. Rev Infect Dis 12(Suppl 4):S483-S491, 1990.
737. Kim KS. High-dose intravenous immune globulin impairs antibacterial activity of antibiotics. J Allergy Clin Immunol 84:579-588, 1989.
738. Baker CJ, Noya FJD. Potential use of intravenous immune globulin for group B streptococcal infection. Rev Infect Dis 12(Suppl 4):S476-S482, 1990.
739. Redd H, Christensen RD, Fischer GW. Circulating and storage neutrophils in septic neonatal rats treated with immune globulin. J Infect Dis 157:705-712, 1988.
740. Christensen KK, Christensen P. Intravenous gamma-globulin in the treatment of neonatal sepsis with special reference to group B streptococci and pharmacokinetics. Pediatr Infect Dis J 5(Suppl):S189-S192, 1986.
741. Christensen KK, Christensen P, Bucher HU, et al. Intravenous administration of human IgG to newborn infants: changes in serum antibody levels to group B streptococci. Eur J Pediatr 143:123-127, 1984.
742. van Furth R, Leijh PCJ, Klein F. Correlation between opsonic activity for various microorganisms and composition of gammaglobulin preparations for intravenous use. J Infect Dis 149:511-517, 1984.
743. Kim KS, Wass CA, Kang JH, et al. Functional activities of various preparations of human intravenous immunoglobulin against type III group B *Streptococcus*. J Infect Dis 153:1092-1097, 1986.
744. Gloser H, Bachmayer H, Helm A. Intravenous immunoglobulin with high activity against group B streptococci. Pediatr Infect Dis J 5(Suppl):S176-S179, 1986.
745. Linden V, Christensen KK, Christensen P. Low levels of antibodies to surface antigens of group B streptococci in commercial IgG preparation. Int Arch Allergy Appl Immunol 68:193-195, 1982.
746. Fischer GW, Hemming VG, Hunter KW, et al. Intravenous immunoglobulin in the treatment of neonatal sepsis: therapeutic strategies and laboratory studies. Pediatr Infect Dis J 5(Suppl):S171-S175, 1986.
747. Noya FJD, Rench MA, Garcia-Prats JA, et al. Disposition of an immunoglobulin intravenous preparation in very low birth weight neonates. J Pediatr 112:278-283, 1988.
748. Raff HV, Siscoe PJ, Wolff EA, et al. Human monoclonal antibodies to group B *Streptococcus*: reactivity and in vivo protection against multiple serotypes. J Exp Med 168:905-917, 1988.
749. Raff HV, Shuford W, Wolff E, et al. Pharmacokinetic and pharmacodynamic analysis of a human immunoglobulin M monoclonal antibody in neonatal *Macaca fascicularis*. Pediatr Res 29:310-314, 1991.
750. Hill HR, Gonzales LA, Knappe WA, et al. Comparative protective activity of human monoclonal and hyperimmune polyclonal antibody against group B streptococci. J Infect Dis 163:792-798, 1991.
751. Christensen RD, Brown MS, Hall DC, et al. Effect on neutrophil kinetics and serum opsonic capacity of intravenous administration of immune globulin to neonates with clinical signs of early-onset sepsis. J Pediatr 118:606-614, 1991.
752. Lannering B, Larsson LE, Rojas J, et al. Early onset group B streptococcal disease. Seven year experience and clinical scoring system. Acta Paediatr Scand 72:597-602, 1983.
753. Baker CJ. Immunization to prevent group B streptococcal disease: victories and vexations. J Infect Dis 161:917-921, 1990.
754. Gordon JS, Sbara AJ. Incidence, technique of isolation, and treatment of group B streptococci in obstetric patients. Am J Obstet Gynecol 126:1023-1026, 1976.
755. Hall RT, Barnes W, Krishnan L, et al. Antibiotic treatment of parturient women colonized with group B streptococci. Am J Obstet Gynecol 124:630-634, 1976.
756. Lewin EB, Amstey MS. Natural history of group B *Streptococcus* colonization and its therapy during pregnancy. Am J Obstet Gynecol 139:512-515, 1981.
757. Yow MD, Mason EO, Leeds LJ, et al. Ampicillin prevents intrapartum transmission of group B *Streptococcus*. JAMA 241:1245-1247, 1979.
758. Morales WJ, Lim DV, Walsh AF. Prevention of neonatal group B streptococcal sepsis by the use of a rapid screening test and selective intrapartum chemoprophylaxis. Am J Obstet Gynecol 155:979-983, 1986.
759. Boyer KM, Gadzala CA, Kelly PD, et al. Selective intrapartum chemoprophylaxis of neonatal group B streptococcal early-onset disease: III. Interruption of mother-to-infant transmission. J Infect Dis 148:810-816, 1983.
760. Boyer KM, Gotoff SP. Prevention of early-onset neonatal group B streptococcal disease with selective intrapartum chemoprophylaxis. N Engl J Med 314:1665-1669, 1986.
761. Matorras R, García Perea A, Madero R, et al. Maternal colonization by group B streptococci and puerperal infection; analysis of intrapartum chemoprophylaxis. Eur J Obstet Gynecol Reprod Biol 38:203-207, 1990.
762. Garland SM, Fliegner JR. Group B *Streptococcus* (GBS) and neonatal infections: the case for intrapartum chemoprophylaxis. Aust NZ J Obstet Gynaecol 31:119-122, 1991.
763. Tuppurainen N, Hallman M. Prevention of neonatal group B streptococcal disease: intrapartum detection and chemoprophylaxis of heavily colonized parturients. Obstet Gynecol 73:583-587, 1989.
764. Morales WJ, Lim D. Reduction of group B streptococcal maternal and neonatal infections in preterm pregnancies with premature rupture of membranes through a rapid identification test. Am J Obstet Gynecol 157:13-16, 1987.
765. Strickland DM, Yeomans ER, Hankins GDV. Cost-effectiveness of intrapartum screening and treatment for maternal group B streptococci colonization. Am J Obstet Gynecol 163:4-8, 1990.
766. Mohle-Boetani JC, Schuchat A, Plikaytis BD, et al. Comparison of prevention strategies for neonatal group B streptococcal infection: an economic analysis. JAMA 270:1442-1448, 1993.
767. Rouse DJ, Goldenberg RL, Cliver SP, et al. Strategies for the prevention of early-onset neonatal group B streptococcal sepsis: a decision analysis. Obstet Gynecol 83:483-494, 1994.
768. Yancey MK, Duff P. An analysis of the cost-effectiveness of selected protocols for the prevention of neonatal group B streptococcal infection. Obstet Gynecol 83:367-371, 1994.
769. Committee to Study Priorities for Vaccine Development, Division of Health Promotion and Disease Prevention, Institute of Medicine: Stratton KR, Durch JS, Lawrence RS (eds). Vaccines for the 21st Century: A Tool for Decision Making. Washington, DC, National Academy of Sciences, 1999.
770. Kontnick CM, Edberg SC. Direct detection of group B streptococci from vaginal specimens compared with quantitative culture. J Clin Microbiol 28:336-339, 1990.
771. Skoll MA, Mercer BM, Baselski V, et al. Evaluation of two rapid group B streptococcal antigen tests in labor and delivery patients. Obstet Gynecol 77:322-326, 1991.
772. Green M, Dashefsky B, Wald ER, et al. Comparison of two antigen assays for rapid intrapartum detection of vaginal group B streptococcal colonization. J Clin Microbiol 31:78-82, 1993.
773. Towers CV, Garite TJ, Friedman WW, et al. Comparison of a rapid enzyme-linked immunosorbent assay test and the Gram stain for detection of group B *Streptococcus* in high-risk antepartum patients. Am J Obstet Gynecol 163:965-967, 1990.
774. Granato PA, Petosa MT. Evaluation of a rapid screening test for detecting group B streptococci in pregnant women. J Clin Microbiol 29:1536-1538, 1991.
775. Gentry YM, Hillier SL, Eschenbach DA. Evaluation of a rapid enzyme immunoassay test for detection of group B *Streptococcus*. Obstet Gynecol 78:397-401, 1991.
776. Baker CJ. Inadequacy of rapid immunoassays for intrapartum detection of group B streptococcal carriers. Obstet Gynecol 88:51-55, 1996.
777. Carroll KC, Ballou D, Varner M, et al. Rapid detection of group B streptococcal colonization of the genital tract by a commercial optical immunoassay. Eur J Clin Microbiol Infect Dis 15:206-210, 1996.

778. Park CH, Ruprai D, Vandel NM, et al. Rapid detection of group B streptococcal antigen from vaginal specimens using a new optical immunoassay technique. Diagn Microbiol Infect Dis 24:125-128, 1996.
779. Reisner DP, Haas MJ, Zingheim RW, et al. Performance of a group B streptococcal prophylaxis protocol combining high-risk treatment and low-risk screening. Am J Obstet Gynecol 182:1335-1343, 2000.
780. Thinkhamrop J, Limpongsanurak S, Festin MR, et al. Infections in international pregnancy study: performance of the optical immunoassay test for detection of group B *Streptococcus*. J Clin Microbiol 41:5288-5290, 2003.
781. Rosa C, Clark P, Duff P. Performance of a new DNA probe for the detection of group B streptococcal colonization of the genital tract. Obstet Gynecol 86:509-511, 1995.
782. Kircher SM, Meyer MP, Jordan JA. Comparison of a modified DNA hybridization assay with standard culture enrichment for detecting group B streptococci in obstetric patients. J Clin Microbiol 34:342-344, 1996.
783. Bergeron MG, Ke D, Ménard C, et al. Rapid detection of group B streptococci in pregnant women at delivery. N Engl J Med 343:175-179, 2000.
784. Haberland CA, Benitz WE, Sanders GD, et al. Perinatal screening for group B streptococci: cost-benefit analysis of rapid polymerase chain reaction. Pediatrics 110:471-480, 2002.
785. Rosenstein NE, Schuchat AE. Opportunities for prevention of perinatal group B streptococcal disease: a multistate surveillance analysis. Obstet Gynecol 90:901-906, 1997.
786. Thomsen AC, Mårup L, Hansen KB. Antibiotic elimination of group-B streptococci in urine in prevention of preterm labour. Lancet 1:591-593, 1987.
787. Mitchell TF, Pearlman MD, Chapman RL, et al. Maternal and transplacental pharmacokinetics of cefazolin. Obstet Gynecol 98:1075-1079, 2001.
788. Bray RE, Boe RW, Johnson WL. Transfer of ampicillin into fetus and amniotic fluid from maternal plasma in late pregnancy. Am J Obstet Gynecol 96:938-942, 1966.
789. Hirsch HA, Dreher E, Perrochet A, et al. Transfer of ampicillin to the fetus and amniotic fluid during continuous infusion (steady state) and by repeated single intravenous injections to the mother. Infection 2:207-212, 1974.
790. de Cueto M, Sanchez MJ, Sampedro A, et al. Timing of intrapartum ampicillin and prevention of vertical transmission of group B *Streptococcus*. Obstet Gynecol 91:112-114, 1998.
791. Group B streptococcal infections in pregnancy. ACOG Tech Bull 170:1-5, 1992.
792. Committee on Infectious Diseases and Committee on Fetus and Newborn. Guidelines for prevention of group B streptococcal (GBS) infection by chemoprophylaxis. Pediatrics 90:775-778, 1992.
793. Christensen KK, Dahlander K, Linden V, et al. Obstetrical care in future pregnancies after fetal loss in group B streptococcal septicemia: a prevention program based on bacteriological and immunological follow up. Eur J Obstet Gynecol Reprod Biol 12:143-147, 1981.
794. Dykes AK, Christensen KK, Christensen P. Chronic carrier state in mothers of infants with group B streptococcal infections. Obstet Gynecol 66:84-88, 1985.
795. Mercer BM, Taylor MC, Fricke JL, et al. The accuracy and patient preference for self-collected group B *Streptococcus* cultures. Am J Obstet Gynecol 173:1325-1328, 1995.
796. Taylor MC, Mercer BM, Engelhardt KF, et al. Patient preference for self-collected cultures for group B *Streptococcus* in pregnancy. J Nurse Midwifery 42:410-413, 1997.
797. Peralta-Carcelen M, Fargason CA Jr, Coston D, et al. Preferences of pregnant women and physicians for two strategies for prevention of early-onset group B streptococcal sepsis in neonates. Arch Pediatr Adolesc Med 151:712-718, 1997.
798. Schuchat A. Group B streptococcal disease: from trials and tribulations to triumph and trepidation. Clin Infect Dis 33:751-756, 2001.
799. Davies HD, Adair CE, Schuchat A, et al. Physicians' prevention practices and incidence of neonatal group B streptococcal disease in 2 Canadian regions. Can Med Assoc J 164:479-485, 2001.
800. Davis RL, Hasselquist MB, Cardenas V, et al. Introduction of the new Centers for Disease Control and Prevention group B streptococcal prevention guideline at a large West Coast health maintenance organization. Am J Obstet Gynecol 184:603-610, 2001.
801. Brozanski BS, Jones JG, Krohn MA, et al. Effect of a screening-based prevention policy on prevalence of early-onset group B streptococcal sepsis. Obstet Gynecol 95:496-501, 2000.
802. Factor SH, Whitney CG, Zywicki SS, et al. Effects of hospital policies based on 1996 group B streptococcal disease consensus guidelines. Obstet Gynecol 95:377-382, 2000.
803. Gilson GJ, Christensen F, Romero H, et al. Prevention of group B *Streptococcus* early-onset neonatal sepsis: comparison of the Center for Disease Control and Prevention screening-based protocol to a risk-based protocol in infants at greater than 37 weeks' gestation. J Perinatol 20:491-495, 2000.
804. Centers for Disease Control and Prevention. Hospital-based policies for prevention of perinatal group B streptococcal disease—United States, 1999. MMWR Morb Mortal Wkly Rep 49:936-940, 2000.
805. American Academy of Pediatrics. Group B streptococcal infections. *In* Pickering LK (ed). Red Book: 2003 Report of the Committee on Infectious Diseases, 26th ed. Elk Grove Village, Ill, American Academy of Pediatrics, 2003, pp 584-591.
806. ACOG Committee Opinion No. 279, December 2002. Prevention of early-onset group B streptococcal disease in newborns. Obstet Gynecol 100:1405-1412, 2002.
807. Pylipow M, Gaddis M, Kinney JS. Selective intrapartum prophylaxis for group B streptococcus colonization: management and outcome of newborns. Pediatrics 93:631-635, 1994.
808. Dunn AB, Blomquist J, Khousami V. Anaphylaxis in labor secondary to prophylaxis against group B streptococcus: a case report. J Reprod Med 44:381-384, 1999.
809. Heim K, Alge A, Marth C. Anaphylactic reaction to ampicillin and severe complication in the fetus. Lancet 337:859-860, 1991.
810. Pinto NM, Soskolne EI, Pearlman MD, et al. Neonatal early-onset group B streptococcal disease in the era of intrapartum chemoprophylaxis: residual problems. J Perinatol 23:265-271, 2003.
811. Cárdenas V, Davis RL, Hasselquist MB, et al. Barriers to implementing the group B streptococcal prevention guidelines. Birth 29:285-290, 2002.
812. Schrag SJ, Arnold KE, Mohle-Boetani JC, et al. Prenatal screening for infectious diseases and opportunities for prevention. Obstet Gynecol 102:753-760, 2003.
813. Cowgill K, Taylor TH Jr, Schuchat A, et al. Report from the CDC: awareness of perinatal group B streptococcal infection among women of childbearing age in the United States, 1999 and 2002. J Womens Health 12:527-532, 2003.
814. Schrag SJ, Whitney CG, Schuchat A. Neonatal group B streptococcal disease: how infection control teams can contribute to prevention efforts. Infect Control Hosp Epidemiol 21:473-483, 2000.
815. Schuchat A. Impact of intrapartum chemoprophylaxis on neonatal sepsis. Pediatr Infect Dis J 22:1087-1088, 2003.
816. Isaacs D, Royle JA, for the Australasian Study Group for Neonatal Infections. Intrapartum antibiotics and early onset neonatal sepsis caused by group B *Streptococcus* and by other organisms in Australia. Pediatr Infect Dis J 18:524-528, 1999.
817. Lin FYC, Brenner RA, Johnson YR, et al. The effectiveness of risk-based intrapartum chemoprophylaxis for the prevention of early-onset neonatal group B streptococcal disease. Am J Obstet Gynecol 184:1204-1210, 2001.
818. Joseph TA, Pyati SP, Jacobs N. Neonatal early-onset *Escherichia coli* disease: the effect of intrapartum ampicillin. Arch Pediatr Adolesc Med 152:35-40, 1998.
819. Levine EM, Ghai V, Barton JJ, et al. Intrapartum antibiotic prophylaxis increases the incidence of gram-negative neonatal sepsis. Infect Dis Obstet Gynecol 7:210-213, 1999.
820. Stoll BJ, Hansen N, Fanaroff AA, et al. Changes in pathogens causing early-onset sepsis in very-low-birth-weight infants. N Engl J Med 347:240-247, 2002.
821. Hyde TB, Hilger TM, Reingold A, et al. Trends in incidence and antimicrobial resistance of early-onset sepsis: population-based surveillance in San Francisco and Atlanta. Pediatrics 110:690-695, 2002.
822. Terrone DA, Rinehart BK, Einstein MH, et al. Neonatal sepsis and death caused by resistant *Escherichia coli*: possible consequences of extended maternal ampicillin administration. Am J Obstet Gynecol 180:1345-1348, 1999.
823. Edwards RK, Clark P, Sistrom CL, et al. Intrapartum antibiotic prophylaxis 1: relative effects of recommended antibiotics on gram-negative pathogens. Obstet Gynecol 100:534-539, 2002.
824. Spaetgens R, DeBella K, Ma D, et al. Perinatal antibiotic usage and changes in colonization and resistance rates of group B Streptococcus and other pathogens. Obstet Gynecol 100:525-533, 2002.
825. Schrag SJ, Schuchat A, Mohle-Boetani J. Prevention of early-onset group B streptococcal disease in neonates. Letter to the editor. N Engl J Med 347:1798-1799, 2002.

826. Baltimore RS, Huie SM, Meek JI, et al. Early-onset neonatal sepsis in the era of group B streptococcal prevention. Pediatrics 108:1094-1098, 2001.
827. Byington CL, Rittichier KK, Bassett KE, et al. Serious bacterial infections in febrile infants younger than 90 days of age: the importance of ampicillin-resistant pathogens. Pediatrics 111:964-968, 2003.
828. Mohle-Boetani JC, Lieu TA, Ray GT, et al. Preventing neonatal group B streptococcal disease: cost-effectiveness in a health maintenance organization and the impact of delayed hospital discharge for newborns who received intrapartum antibiotics. Pediatrics 103:703-710, 1999.
829. Escobar GJ, Li D-K, Armstrong MA, et al. Neonatal sepsis workups in infants ≥2000 grams at birth: a population-based study. Pediatrics 106:256-263, 2000.
830. Balter S, Zell ER, O'Brien KL, et al. Impact of intrapartum antibiotics on the care and evaluation of the neonate. Pediatr Infect Dis J 22:853-857, 2003.
831. Bromberger P, Lawrence JM, Braun D, et al. The influence of intrapartum antibiotics on the clinical spectrum of early-onset group B streptococcal infection in term infants. Pediatrics 106:244-250, 2000.
832. Steigman AJ, Bottone EJ, Hanna BA. Control of perinatal group B streptococcal sepsis: efficacy of single injection of aqueous penicillin at birth. Mt Sinai J Med 45:685-693, 1978.
833. Pyati SP, Pildes RS, Jacobs NM, et al. Early penicillin in infants ≤2,000 grams with early onset GBS: is it effective? Pediatr Res 16:1019, 1982.
834. Velaphi S, Siegel JD, Wendel GD Jr, et al. Early-onset group B streptococcal infection after a combined maternal and neonatal group B streptococcal chemoprophylaxis strategy. Pediatrics 111:541-547, 2003.
835. Wendel GD Jr, Leveno KJ, Sanchez PJ, et al. Prevention of neonatal group B streptococcal disease: a combined intrapartum and neonatal protocol. Am J Obstet Gynecol 186:618-626, 2002.
836. Siegel JD, Cushion NB. Prevention of early-onset group B streptococcal disease: another look at single-dose penicillin at birth. Obstet Gynecol 87:692-698, 1996.
837. Rubin EE, McDonald JC. Group B streptococcal disease in twins: failure of empiric therapy to prevent late onset disease in the second twin. Pediatr Infect Dis J 10:921-923, 1991.
838. Rodewald AK, Onderdonk AB, Warren HB, et al. Neonatal mouse model of group B streptococcal infection. J Infect Dis 166:635-639, 1992.
839. Paoletti LC, Wessels MR, Michon F, et al. Group B *Streptococcus* type II polysaccharide-tetanus toxoid conjugate vaccine. Infect Immunol 60:4009-4014, 1992.
840. Madoff LC, Michel JL, Gong EW, et al. Protection of neonatal mice from group B streptococcal infection by maternal immunization with beta C protein. Infect Immun 60:4989-4994, 1992.
841. Paoletti LC, Pinel J, Rodewald AK, et al. Therapeutic potential of human antisera to group B streptococcal glycoconjugate vaccines in neonatal mice. J Infect Dis 175:1237-1239, 1997.
842. Baker CJ, Kasper DL. Group B streptococcal vaccines. Rev Infect Dis 7:458-467, 1985.
843. Wessels MR, Paoletti LC, Kasper DL, et al. Immunogenicity in animals of a polysaccharide-protein conjugate vaccine against type III group B *Streptococcus*. J Clin Invest 86:1428-1433, 1990.
844. Paoletti LC, Kennedy RC, Chanh TC, et al. Immunogenicity of group B *Streptococcus* type III polysaccharide–tetanus toxoid vaccine in baboons. Infect Immun 64:677-679, 1996.
845. Wessels MR, Paoletti LC, Pinel J, et al. Immunogenicity and protective activity in animals of a type V group B streptococcal polysaccharide–tetanus toxoid conjugate vaccine. J Infect Dis 171:879-884, 1995.
846. Paoletti LC, Wessels MR, Rodewald AK, et al. Neonatal mouse protection against infection with multiple group B streptococcal (GBS) serotypes by maternal immunization with a tetravalent GBS polysaccharide–tetanus toxoid conjugate vaccine. Infect Immun 62:3236-3243,1994.
847. Madoff LC, Paoletti LC, Tai JY, et al. Maternal immunization of mice with group B streptococcal type III polysaccharide–beta C protein conjugate elicits protective antibody to multiple serotypes. J Clin Invest 94:286-292, 1994.
848. Paoletti LC, Pinel J, Johnson KD, et al. Synthesis and preclinical evaluation of glycoconjugate vaccines against group B *Streptococcus* types VI and VIII. J Infect Dis 180:892-895, 1999.
849. Paoletti LC, Madoff LC. Vaccines to prevent neonatal GBS infection. Semin Neonatol 7:315-323, 2002.
850. Kasper DL, Paoletti LC, Wessels MR, et al. Immune response to type III group B streptococcal polysaccharide–tetanus toxoid conjugate vaccine. J Clin Invest 98:2308-2314, 1996.
851. Baker CJ, Paoletti LC, Wessels MR, et al. Safety and immunogenicity of capsular polysaccharide–tetanus toxoid conjugate vaccines for group B streptococcal types Ia and Ib. J Infect Dis 179:142-150, 1999.
852. Baker CJ, Paoletti LC, Rench MA, et al. Use of capsular polysaccharide–tetanus toxoid conjugate vaccine for type II group B *Streptococcus* in healthy women. J Infect Dis 182:1129-1138, 2000.
853. Baker CJ, Paoletti LC, Rench MA, et al. Immune response of healthy women to 2 different group B streptococcal type V capsular polysaccharide–protein conjugate vaccines. J Infect Dis 189:1103-1112, 2004.
854. Baker CJ, Rench MA, Fernandez M, et al. Safety and immunogenicity of a bivalent group B streptococcal conjugate vaccine for serotypes II and III. J Infect Dis 188:66-73, 2003.
855. Baker CJ, Rench MA, McInnes P. Immunization of pregnant women with group B streptococcal type III capsular polysaccharide–tetanus toxoid conjugate vaccine. Vaccine 21:3468-3472, 2003.
856. Paoletti LC, Kasper DL, Michon F, et al. An oligosaccharide–tetanus toxoid conjugate vaccine against type III group B *Streptococcus*. J Biol Chem 265:18278-18283, 1990.
857. Wang JY, Chang AHC, Guttormsen H-K, et al. Construction of designer glycoconjugate vaccines with size-specific oligosaccharide antigens and site-controlled coupling. Vaccine 21:1112-1117, 2003.
858. Wessels MR, Paoletti LC, Guttormsen H-K, et al. Structural properties of group B streptococcal type III polysaccharide conjugate vaccines that influence immunogenicity and efficacy. Infect Immun 66:2186-2192, 1998.
859. Michel JL, Madoff LC, Kling DE, et al. Cloned alpha and beta C-protein antigens of group B streptococci elicit protective immunity. Infect Immun 59:2023-2028, 1991.
860. Larsson C, Holmgren J, Lindahl G, et al. Intranasal immunization of mice with group B streptococcal protein Rib and cholera toxin B subunit confers protection against lethal infection. Infect Immun 72:1184-1187, 2004.
861. Martin D, Rioux S, Gagnon E, et al. Protection from group B streptococcal infection in neonatal mice by maternal immunization with recombinant Sip protein. Infect Immun 70:4897-4901, 2002.
862. Cheng Q, Debol S, Lam H, et al. Immunization with C5a peptidase or peptidase-type III polysaccharide conjugate vaccines enhances clearance of group B streptococci from lungs of infected mice. Infect Immun 70:6409-6415, 2002.
863. Weisner AM, Johnson AP, Lamagni TL, et al. Characterization of group B streptococci recovered from infants with invasive disease in England and Wales. Clin Infect Dis 38:1203-1208, 2004.
864. Baker CJ, Edwards MS. Group B streptococcal conjugate vaccines. Arch Dis Child 88:375-378, 2003.

Chapter 14

LISTERIOSIS

Robert Bortolussi • Timothy L. Mailman

Listeria monocytogenes is a gram-positive, motile bacterium and a frequent veterinary pathogen that causes abortion and meningoencephalitis in sheep and cattle. Infection in a wide variety of other mammals is recognized. Uncommon in humans, listeriosis has potential for significant morbidity and mortality and occurs most frequently in the neonatal period, during pregnancy, and in elderly or immunosuppressed patients. Nyfeldt described "*Listerella hominis*" as the cause of human infectious mononucleosis in 1929,[1] but later descriptions indicate that human disease parallels that found in animals, with sepsis and meningoencephalitis occurring most commonly.

Murray and co-workers provided the first adequate description of the organism in 1926.[2] An epizootic among laboratory rabbits and guinea pigs provided an isolate, subsequently named *Bacterium monocytogenes*. The clinical characteristics were of dramatic wasting, lack of appetite, and lethargy leading to death. The greatest incidence and mortality rates were for newborn animals that had recently been weaned. Later, Pirie isolated the organism from South African gerbils and called it *Listerella hepatolytica*, in honor of Lord Lister.[3] Pirie subsequently revised the name to *Listeria monocytogenes*, the currently accepted species name.[4]

THE ORGANISM

Morphology

The morphology of *L. monocytogenes* varies with the age of the culture. In clinical specimens, Gram stains typically demonstrate short intracellular and extracellular gram-positive rods. Over-decolorized direct examinations may lead to a misdiagnosis of *Haemophilus influenzae* meningitis.[5] On primary culture, early bacterial growth may have a slightly pointed coccoid morphology with short chains occasionally seen. Older cultures may be gram variable.

Motility

All strains of *L. monocytogenes* are motile, distinguishing the organism from *Erysipelothrix* and most species of *Corynebacterium*. A characteristic tumbling motility is seen in hanging drop preparations of primary cultures grown at room temperature.[6] Tubes of semi-solid motility medium produce a distinctive umbrella pattern at room temperature when inoculated with the stab technique. Electron microscopic studies and protein electrophoresis have demonstrated that *L. monocytogenes* fails to express flagellar protein at 37° C.[7]

Culture and Identification

L. monocytogenes grows well on common media, including brain-heart infusion, trypticase soy, and thioglycollate broths. Primary isolation from normally sterile sites can be made on blood agar. Growth occurs between 4° C and 37° C, with fastest growth rates occurring between 30° C and 37° C. Selective media, such as Oxford, modified Oxford, or PALCAM agar, should be used for isolation from contaminated specimens, and they have largely replaced cold-enrichment techniques.[8,9]

After 48 hours at 37° C on 5% sheep blood agar, colonies are 0.2 to 1.5 mm in diameter. Narrow zones of β-hemolysis may often be visualized only by moving the colony. *Listeria seeligeri* and *Listeria ivanovii* are also β-hemolytic but nonpathogenic in humans. Speciation is aided by performance of the CAMP test using *Staphylococcus aureus* for *L. monocytogenes* and *L. seeligeri* and *Rhodococcus equi* for *L. ivanovii*.[10]

Discrimination between *Listeria* species is aided by sugar fermentation patterns. *L. monocytogenes* produces acid from L-rhamnose and α-methyl-D-mannoside but not from xylose. *L. ivanovii* and *L. seeligeri* produce acid from D-xylose only. Automated systems, commercial biochemical strips, and DNA probes are available to aid in the identification for clinical microbiology laboratories.

Antigenic Structure and Typing Systems

Thirteen serotypes of *Listeria* have been described and are distinguished on the basis of somatic (O) and flagellar (H) antigens.[11,12] Serotypes 1/2a, 1/2b, and 4b are responsible for most animal and human disease. Determining serotypes has no impact on clinical management but has a public health role in epidemiologic investigations. A commercial kit for serotyping *Listeria* has become available (Denka Seiken, Tokyo, Japan).

Before the advent of molecular methods, phage typing with an international bacteriophage set was used for epidemiologic investigations.[13,14] It proved useful in tracing sources of foodborne outbreaks of *Listeria* when serotyping failed to discriminate between epidemic and nonepidemic strains.[14,15] Some strains remained nontypeable, however, and phage typing has largely been replaced by molecular methods.

Molecular typing methods have provided investigators with new levels of discriminatory power. Multilocus enzyme electrophoresis (MLEE), although not directly DNA based, has proved reliable in distinguishing strains based on electrophoretic mobility of enzymes.[16] MLEE is limited, however, by the failure of many nucleotide and amino acid changes to alter net enzyme charge and hence electrophoretic mobility.[17,18]

Analysis of *Listeria* DNA and RNA is now the gold standard for strain typing.[19,20] One approach is generating restriction endonuclease and the creation of microrestriction patterns by using high-frequency-cutting enzymes. The technique has been used successfully in epidemiologic investigations, but its complex results can make strain comparison difficult. Ribotyping simplifies this by examining only DNA fragments from the ribosomal genes.[17] The automation of ribotyping into commercially available systems (RiboPrinter, Qualicon, Wilmington, Del) has enabled rapid identification of disease clusters and immediate typing of *Listeria* detected in food processing centers.

DNA macrorestriction pattern analysis using pulsed-field gel electrophoresis (PFGE) has become the method adopted by the World Health Organization (WHO) for standardizing international typing.[12] It is a highly discriminating and reproducible method—even for serotype 4b, which is poorly typed by most other methods. The Centers for Disease Control and Prevention (CDC) in the United States have created PulseNet, a network of laboratories using standardized PFGE protocols to subtype foodborne bacterial pathogens. Using the Internet for reporting and comparing PFGE patterns, laboratories are able to identify regional or national clusters that could be missed with localized reporting.

DNA amplification-based typing methods such as random amplification of polymorphic DNA (RAPD) have been shown to have a high degree of discriminatory power. The primary drawback is the lack of standardization. The combination of DNA amplification with automated sequencing provides ultimate discrimination—to the nucleotide level—but is not available on a widespread basis.

Virulence Factors

Foodborne outbreaks of *L. monocytogenes* infections have precipitated an intense interest in organism-specific virulence factors to determine the pathogenesis of infection. As the steps are characterized, *L. monocytogenes* has become a paradigm for intracellular parasitism. A review of virulence factors summarizes the progress made.[21,22]

Entry into host cells occurs by engulfment within a phagosome and involves several key bacterial proteins. The internalin (Inl) family of bacterial surface proteins mediate attachment to mammalian cells.[23,24] InlA, an 80-kDa protein, promotes internalization of bacteria by normally nonphagocytic intestinal epithelial cells. Its glycoprotein receptor, E-cadherin, is present on the surface of host cells known to be potential targets for *Listeria*: intestinal epithelial cells, brain microvascular endothelial cells, hepatocytes, and epithelial cells lining the choroid plexus and placental chorionic villi. Lecuit and colleagues[25] identified a proline residue in E-cadherin that mediates species specificity—the first potential molecular explanation of bacterial-host species specificity. InlB, a 67-kDa protein, has two receptors, Met and gC1q-R (a cellular ligand for the C1q complement fraction) that confer a tropism for hepatocytes and brain microvascular epithelial cells. A third protein, invasion-associated protein (iap or p60), with a molecular mass of 60 kDa, is secreted by invasive *Listeria* strains and is a major antigen in the protective response against *L. monocytogenes*.[26,27]

Invasive strains of *L. monocytogenes* produce listeriolysin O (LLO), a sulfhydryl-activated hemolysin similar to streptolysin O. Nonhemolytic mutants display a loss of virulence in animal models.[28] Listeriolysin O (*hly* gene) lyses phagosomes, releasing *Listeria* into the cytosol, where it begins intracellular growth.[29,30] Once in the cytosol, the bacterial surface protein ActA—product of the *actA* gene—triggers polymerization of host cell actin, enabling intracellular movement and cell-to-cell spread.[30-32]

L. monocytogenes also produces phospholipase C (*plcA* gene) and a lecithinase (*plcB* gene), which contribute to lysis of the primary phagosome and secondary phagosomes formed during cell-to-cell spread. Mutations of the *plcA* and *plcB* genes reduce virulence.[24,34] A metalloprotease encoded by the gene *mpl* converts lecithinase into its active form.[35]

The regulatory gene, *prfA* (positive regulatory factor A), controls expression of *hly* and *plcB* through PrfA, its protein product.[36] PrfA is the main switch of a regulon containing most of the virulence genes in *Listeria*. It promotes expression of certain genes (*hly, plcB*) and downregulates others (the motility-associated genes *motA* and *flaA*),[37] implying a global regulatory role.[38] PrfA/*prfA*-induced regulation is influenced by the bacteria's physicochemical environment. Thermoregulation is one example. PrfA-dependent transcription is minimal below 30° C (environmental temperature) but is induced at 37° C (body temperature of mammals).[39,40]

Other putative virulence factors include stress response mediators; a set of conserved proteins that upregulate after exposure to thermal stress, acidic pH, toxic molecules, and various stimuli that threaten survival.[41,42] They may play a role in repair and removal of damaged bacterial proteins, enabling adaptation to hostile conditions. In animal models, acid-adapted *Listeria* have enhanced survival in low gastric pH, resulting in higher bacterial loads in the intestine and mesenteric lymph nodes after oral infection.[43,44] The monocytosis initially observed in animals infected with *L. monocytogenes* has been partially explained. A phospholipid, monocytosis-producing agent (MPA) that produces monocytosis in rabbits, has been isolated.[45] Monocyte production is stimulated by an endogenous mediator induced by MPA.[46]

EPIDEMIOLOGY AND TRANSMISSION

Natural Reservoir and Human Transmission

Listeria species are ubiquitous in nature and can be isolated from diverse environmental sources including a variety of foods, soil, water, and feces of humans and animals. The natural habitat of the organism is in decaying plant matter.[47] Spoiled silage appears to be a source of infection for ruminant animals.[48] Fecal carriage of *L. monocytogenes* in animals probably plays a key role in the organism's persistence by providing an enrichment cycle through ingestion of contaminated silage.

Although direct transmission of *L. monocytogenes* to humans and veterinarians from infected animals has been described,[49-50] almost all human cases of infection are acquired through ingestion of contaminated food.[51,52] In the early and mid-1980s, large outbreaks of *L. monocytogenes* infection occurred in pregnant women and immunocompromised hosts. The first outbreak, reported from Canada,[15] suggested indirect transmission from an animal reservoir. In this outbreak, *Listeria*-contaminated sheep manure was used to fertilize cabbage, which was placed in cold storage over the winter; clinical disease developed in pregnant women and immunocompromised patients who subsequently consumed the cabbage. Large outbreaks caused by contaminated dairy products were first reported in the 1950s and continue to occur in North America and Europe.[53-55] The relative resistance of *Listeria* to high temperatures and its ability to multiply at low temperatures provide opportunities for heavy contamination of dairy products if pasteurization has been done improperly.[54,56] In recent years, outbreaks have been more commonly associated with prepared meat products, including deli meats, pâté, and hot dogs,[57-61] and occasionally seafood.[62]

Whether outbreaks are related to a high inoculum of *L. monocytogenes* in food or enhanced virulence of the epidemic strain is unknown. Host susceptibility appears to be constant in the population, although Schwartz and associates[63] have proposed that other gastrointestinal pathogens might be a predisposing factor in translocation of *L. monocytogenes* from the intestine and development of disseminated disease.

The improved ability to culture *L. monocytogenes* with selective media has offered the opportunity to examine food eaten by patients who have developed sporadic cases of listeriosis.[64] However, proof that most cases of sporadic listeriosis are caused by ingestion of contaminated foodstuffs was not confirmed until studies in the United States by the Listeriosis Study Group at the CDC clearly demonstrated this relationship.[65,66] These studies implicated undercooked chicken and soft cheeses as significant sources of sporadic disease. The conclusion is supported by sampling surveys carried out by regulatory agencies. A review of foodborne listeriosis has been published.[54,67]

Occurrence

L. monocytogenes causes an estimated 2500 serious illnesses and 500 deaths annually in the United States. Active surveillance programs in several countries have suggested an annual incidence of 0.4 to 0.7 cases per 100,000 people.[68,69] Slightly lower figures have been reported from Australia,[70] England,[71] and Denmark.[72] However, these studies relied on passive reporting programs. *L. monocytogenes* may cause symptomatic gastroenteritis, a nonreportable condition. Fecal carriage of listeriosis is uncommon but may be as high as 26% in household contacts of patients with listeriosis.[73] In the Canadian outbreak, fecal surveys demonstrated carriage rate in approximately 5% of family contacts.[15] During another outbreak carriage rates in the community were approximately 8%.[74]

The distribution of serovars causing disease may not be uniform. In the United States, serovars 4b and 1/2 account for 95% of strains, with serotype 4b being the most common overall. In Canada, serovar 1/2b occurred in 42% of clinical isolates.[75] In Spain and Germany, serovar 4b was predominant.[76,77] The significance of these geographic differences is unknown.

The incidence in the United States for neonatal listeriosis is estimated at 13 per 100,000 livebirths. This represents approximately one third of the total caseload in humans.[68] Two forms of neonatal listeriosis can occur: perinatal and nonperinatal listeriosis. The incidence of perinatal disease reported from other countries is similar.[76-78] However, the true incidence is probably much higher because abortion and stillbirth due to *Listeria* are largely unrecognized unless bacterial cultures are obtained from tissue. Epidemics of foodborne listeriosis have disproportionately involved perinatal cases. It is possible that lower inocula are needed to infect pregnant women compared with the general population. No differences in carriage rates between pregnant women and nonpregnant individuals have been found in fecal and vaginal specimens.[79] Fecal carriage may lead to vaginal colonization and be responsible for the development of late-onset infection in infants born of healthy mothers.

Two thirds of cases of listeriosis occur in immunocompromised adults, in whom sepsis and meningitis are the most frequent presenting illnesses.[69] Louria and co-workers[80] initially described this infection in patients with malignancies, but many other conditions have been reported in association with invasive listeriosis.[81,82] Susceptibility in laboratory animals is increased by the administration of corticosteroids,[83] cyclosporine,[84] and prostaglandins,[85] and the human experience parallels these studies. Renal transplantation appears to be a particularly significant risk factor, and a nosocomial outbreak has been reported in this population.[86] Hemochromatosis with increased iron stores may also predispose to infection. Patients with HIV infection have a 400- to 1000-fold increased risk of acquiring invasive listeriosis.[87] Alcoholism, diabetes, and cirrhosis also contribute to infection, although community-acquired listeriosis may occur spontaneously in patients with no underlying predisposing conditions.[88] Animal studies[89] and one outbreak of human listeriosis[90] suggest that decreased gastric acidity may also predispose to invasive infection in patients with immunosuppressive conditions.

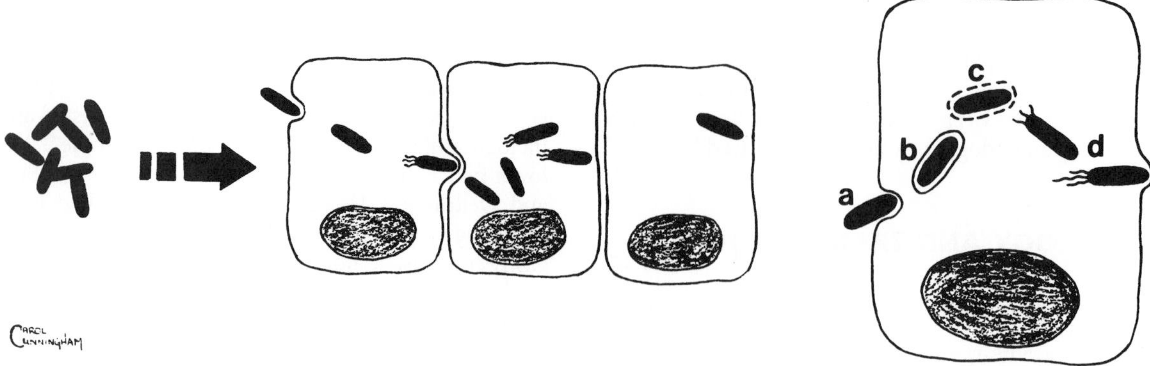

Figure 14–1 Cellular invasion by *Listeria monocytogenes.* Attachment of *L. monocytogenes* to the surface of cell membrane **(a)** is determined by a family of bacterial surface proteins, including internalins (IntA and IntB). Once internalized **(b)** within a vacuole **(c)**, listeriolysin O (LLO) can lyse the vacuole membrane, liberating the bacteria into the cytoplasm. Bacterial surface protein ActA induces polymerization of cellular actin, which concentrates at one end of the bacterium. This "rocket tail" **(d)** provides propulsion for the organism to move through the cytoplasm and into adjacent cells, where the intracellular process will begin again.

Nosocomial Transmission

Although most large outbreaks of listeriosis have occurred in the community, case clusters of nosocomial listeriosis in neonates and adults have been described.[91-97] Person-to-person transmission caused by poor infection-control techniques is likely responsible for most of these small clusters. Often, the patient with the index case presents with early-onset infection, and subsequent cases have typical late-onset listeriosis. Multiple cases of early-onset disease may suggest the possibility of foodborne disease in the community. Nosocomial infection among adults in the Boston outbreak[90] was probably related to ingestion of contaminated food in the hospital environment or within 2 weeks of hospitalization. Clear-cut nosocomial infection has been demonstrated in a neonatal outbreak in Costa Rica.[98] In that outbreak, the index case had early-onset disease and was bathed with mineral oil that became contaminated with the epidemic isolate. Subsequent bathing of other infants with the same oil led to late-onset disease in those infants.

PATHOGENESIS

Host Response in Normal Adults

Innate Immune Response

The pathogenesis of listeriosis in humans remains poorly understood. Most of the hypothetical evidence is derived from observations made on animal models of infection. Given that food is the most common source of outbreak and sporadic cases, the gastrointestinal tract is thought to be the usual portal of entry into the host. Although *L. monocytogenes* is probably ingested frequently through contaminated food sources, the incidence of clinical disease in humans is relatively low.[69] This suggests the organism has relatively low virulence, a concept supported by the high concentration of organisms required to cause infection in animal models.

Translocation of *Listeria* across the intestinal mucosa occurs very rapidly and without histologic evidence of inflammation in the bowel wall. The organism is transported to the liver within minutes of ingestion. This rapid process appears to be independent of the known listerial virulence factors, because mutant strains lacking these factors arrive at the liver at roughly the same time as their parent wild strains.[22]

In the liver, the first stage of the battle between bacteria and host occurs.[99] Within hours of ingestion, macrophages of the liver (Kupffer cells) and spleen capture and destroy most of the inoculum. Over the next 3 days, a nonspecific, T cell–independent phase of host resistance, called innate resistance is operative. Since the 1960s, it was known that *L. monocytogenes* could survive within Kupffer cells that line the hepatic sinusoids. In the late 1980s, it was also appreciated that *Listeria* could infect nonphagocytic cells (i.e., epithelial, hepatocellular, and fibroblast cell lines), providing the organism with an intracellular environment temporarily sheltered from more hostile host defense.[100-102]

Although proteins on the surface of *Listeria,* such as InlA, InlB, and p60, may identify important factors associated with entrance into the cell in vitro,[24,26,103] they do not fully explain intracellular spread and multiplication of the organism in vivo.[104] During the early course of infection, *L. monocytogenes* resides within a vacuole (for nonphagocytic cells) or a phagosome (in monocyte/macrophage-derived cells) (Fig. 14-1). Lysis of the phagosome or vacuole is mediated by LLO and non–LLO-derived proteins.[30,105-108] Bacteria-derived phospholipase C, a metalloprotease-mediated lysin and other virulence factors may also contribute to escape of *L. monocytogenes* from vacuoles and phagosomes.[22,109,110] Release of *L. monocytogenes* from intracellular vacuoles precipitates intracellular growth and actin polymerization.[31,111] Actin polymerization is important in the cell-to-cell transfer of *L. monocytogenes* and is mediated by ActA product of the *actA* gene.[33] A surface protein, ActA causes host-cell actin to assemble into filaments around the bacterium. After 2 or 3 hours, the actin filaments polarize at one end of the organism. This "rocket tail" provides propulsive force for the organism to move through the cytoplasm. When the bacterium reaches the cell membrane, it forms a filipod that is ingested by adjacent cells. In the process, the organism avoids exposure to the extracellular environment. In addition to hepatocytes, enterocytes, and phagocytic cells, *Listeria* can grow and spread in fibroblasts, epithelial cells, vascular endothelial cells, and renal tubular epithelial cells.[111] The

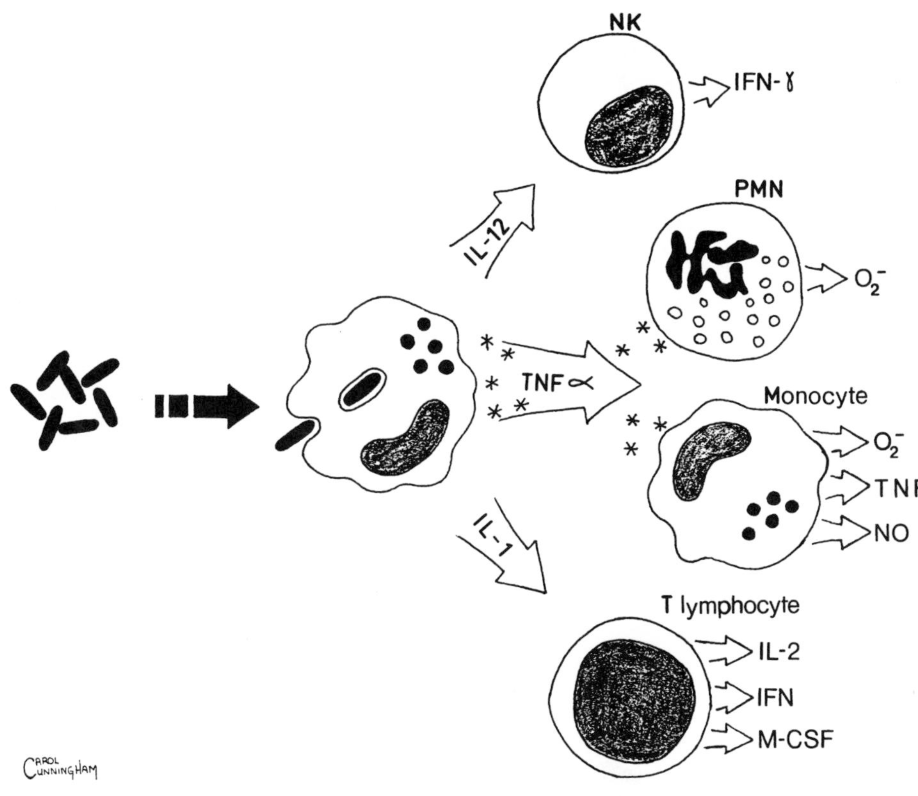

Figure 14–2 Interferon and cytokine production. Blood monocytes and tissue macrophages produce a variety of cytokines after ingestion of live *Listeria*. Interleukin (IL)-12 causes activation of natural killer (NK) cells, which release high concentrations of interferon-γ (IFN-γ). Tumor necrosis factor-α (TNF-α) is produced in high concentrations by monocytes and macrophages after ingestion of *Listeria*. TNF-α leads to priming of polymorphonuclear leukocytes (PMNs) and activation of other macrophage cells, with increased production of superoxide (O_2^-), nitric oxide (NO), and TNF-α. Macrophage-produced IL-1 leads to proliferation of T cells that produce immunomodulating proteins such as IL-2, macrophage colony-stimulating factor (M-CSF), and IFN-γ.

intracytoplasmic environment provides abundant growth conditions and a protected environment for this organism to survive.[100,112]

Between 3 and 4 days after infection begins, there is normally a decrease in viable bacteria in the monocyte-macrophage phagocytic system. This heralds the onset of the T cell–dependent stage of anti-*Listeria* defense, called acquired resistance.[113] Development of acquired anti-*Listeria* activity is seen by day 5 of infection and can be demonstrated by adoptive transfer of resistance using immune T cells. At this stage, the number of activated macrophages in infected tissue rapidly increases (Fig. 14-2).

Cellular Response

For adult animals, the process leading to acquired immunity to *Listeria* has been partially elucidated, and the sequence of cell-to-cell interaction resulting in cytolytic activity is becoming clear. In adult immunocompetent animals, *Listeria* are phagocytosed by "professional" phagocytes (i.e., macrophages and monocytes) and by "nonprofessional" phagocytic cells (e.g., fibroblasts, hepatocytes) (see Fig. 14-1). Once ingested, partial degradation of *Listeria* occurs and transfer of the *Listeria* protein antigen fragments to the macrophage cell surface takes place.[114]

Peptides resulting from digestion of *Listeria* in the cytoplasm are actively processed by the endoplasmic reticulum, where the peptides bind to major histocompatibility complex (MHC) class I molecules (Fig. 14-3).[11] The *Listeria*-peptide-MHC complex is transported to the cell surface, where it can be recognized by cytolytic T lymphocytes (i.e., CD8 phenotype).

Bacterial peptides that are digested within phagosomes are transported to the plasma membrane, where they attach to MHC class II molecules. CD4 T lymphocytes recognize specific antigens that are presented by MHC class II membrane receptors.[115] Development of T helper (T_H) subset during an immune response is pivotal because *L. monocytogenes* infection is most effectively controlled through this immune response.[115] *L. monocytogenes* induction of T_H1 development in vitro is mediated by macrophage-produced interleukin-12 (IL-12). Cells with T_H1 phenotype secrete IL-2 and interferon-γ (IFN-γ) during primary infection.[116,117] Although a small number of T_H2 cells may develop during *Listeria* infection, they play little role in the clearance of *Listeria*.[118]

In the presence of *Listeria* antigens and IL-2, T cells divide, producing *Listeria*-specific clones. In vitro evidence demonstrates that *L. monocytogenes*–immune CD8 T cells are cytolytic for *Listeria*-infected macrophages and hepatocytes (see Fig. 14-3).[119,120] A robust CD8 T cell response is induced during *L. monocytogenes* infection. *Listeria*-specific CD8 T cells confer protective immunity to naïve animals. However, such T cells lose antibacterial activity within days.[121] Neutrophils and monocytes that migrate to the site of primary infection may participate in the lysis of infected cells and, more importantly, play a role in the elimination of bacteria that are released to the surrounding tissue. By this stage of infection, phagocytic cells have been primed or activated by IFN-γ or cytokines, making them more effective killers.[121-127]

Roles of Toll-like Proteins, Interferon, and Cytokines

Toll-like receptors (TLRs) are conserved primitive membrane proteins found in cells that have been identified as key to initiation of innate immunity.[128] Ten TLRs have been identified. TLR-2 and TLR-6 are heterodimers for gram-positive peptidoglycan. Surface TLRs stimulate an innate immune

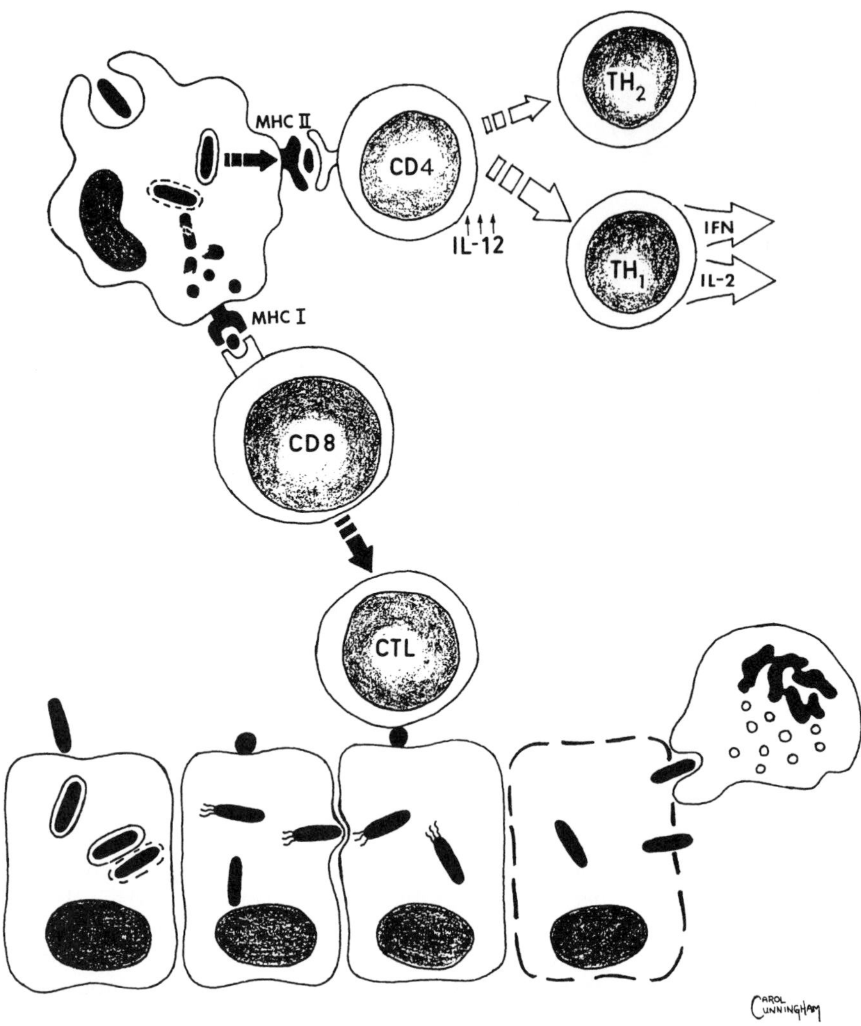

Figure 14–3 Activation of cytolytic cell mechanisms. Within an antigen-presenting cell, organisms killed and digested within a phagosome release bacterial peptides that are transported to the plasma membrane, where they attach to major histocompatibility complex (MHC) class II molecules. CD4 T lymphocytes recognize specific antigens that are presented by MHC class II receptors. CD4 T lymphocytes differentiate predominantly into T_H1 cells through stimulation by interleukin-12 (IL-12). Such cells secrete high concentrations of IL-2 and interferon-γ (IFN-γ) during primary infection. Bacterial peptides may also come from proteolytic digestion of intracytoplasmic organisms. Such peptides are processed by the endoplasmic reticulum, where they bind to MHC class I receptors. The bacterial-peptide-MHC I complex is transported to the cell membrane, where it is recognized by cytolytic T lymphocytes (CTLs, CD8 phenotype). Such cells cause lysis of *Listeria*-infected cells, which are recognized by the presence of listerial peptides on their surface. Lysis of *Listeria*-infected cells leaves the organism exposed to phagocytosis and killing by activated phagocytic cells, polymorphonuclear leukocytes, and monocytes.

response through a signal pathway involving intracellular kinases and transcription factors. The first intracellular adapter molecule in this cascade is myeloid differentiation antigen 88 (MyD88), which functions as a critical first adapter protein of several TLRs, including TLR-2 and TLR-6.[129] The role of the TLR and the TLR pathway in innate immunity to *Listeria* has become clear over the past 5 years. TLR-2–deficient mice show partial impairment in their resistance to *Listeria.*[130] However, MyD88 has an even more critical role in early clearance of *Listeria* and cytokine signaling.[130,131]

In mature immunocompetent animals, *Listeria* infection induces circulating IFN-γ and IFN-α/β on the second or third day in the acquired phase of immunity. Cytokines such as macrophage colony-stimulating factor (M-CSF)[118] and tumor necrosis factor-α (TNF-α) also appear during the first 5 days and have been implicated as mediators of listerial clearance.[126,132-137] However, peak immunity to *Listeria* is expressed about the sixth day of infection, which coincides with maximal T_H1 cell synthesis of IFN-γ.[138-139] A role for endogenous IFN-γ in resolution of *L. monocytogenes* infection has been shown.[140,141] Adult animals treated with monoclonal antibody directed against IFN-γ do not develop activated macrophages, and clearance of *Listeria* from liver and spleen is decreased.[140]

There is clear evidence that the cytokine cascade involving various interleukins, interferon, and TNF-α is essential for host response to listerial infection. MyD88-initiated signaling pathways are required for IL-1, IL-12, and IL-18 and for TNF induction in monocytes and other early responsive cells.[130,142-145] All of these interleukins and cytokines are involved in an early response to *Listeria* infection through activation of resident macrophage cells, circulating monocytes, and polymorphonuclear leukocytes (PMNs). Early activation through the innate immune system leads to removal of 90% of the bacterial burden in the liver within 6 hours of infection in animal models.[145]

TNF is a key cytokine to enhance antibacterial or antiparasitic resistance mechanisms (see Fig. 14-2).[147-150] Many cell types produce TNF, including natural killer (NK) cells[151]; however, monocytes and macrophages are probably the most abundant source. Endotoxins (lipopolysaccharides) and other agents, including mitogens, viruses, protozoa, and cytokines such as M-CSF, IL-1, IL-2, and IFN-γ have been identified as inducers of TNF.[152-155] When administered before infection, TNF-inducing agents enhanced resistance of the host to bacterial infection.[157]

Endogenously produced TNF during sublethal *Listeria* infection in adult animals appears to function as an inducer of resistance.[132-135] Injection of mice with anti-TNF immunoglobulin results in a striking proliferation of bacteria during the first 2 or 3 days of infection; however, administration of anti-TNF immunoglobulin on day 5 of infection has virtually no effect on *Listeria* replication in the spleen and liver.[126,127,134] These results suggest that TNF-dependent mechanisms limit intracellular infection early in the course of infection. Localized production of TNF is demonstrated in supernatants of organ homogenates from the liver or spleen.[158]

IL-12 participates in the differentiation of T_H1 cells, IFN-γ production, and NK cell activation.[115,137,159] In the absence of T_H1 activation, animals are more susceptible to *L. monocytogenes* infection.[115,159] IL-1, IL-12, and IL-18, molecules whose receptor signaling require MyD88, are all required for normal host defense against *Listeria*.[131,160]

Host Response in the Neonate

Cell Activation

In newborn animals, susceptibility to *Listeria* appears to be associated with delayed activation of macrophages.[161,162] Studies on the afferent and efferent arms of the immune system in fetal and newborn mice have shown that macrophage–T lymphocyte interaction and macrophage activation are impaired.[101,158,163-167] A perinatal rhesus monkey model of human listeriosis has also been established.[168] In the model, animals exposed to *L. monocytogenes* at the beginning of the third trimester had increased risk of stillbirth delivery and showed pathology similar to humans. Antibody and *Listeria*-induced cell proliferation was increased in mothers after delivery of stillborn rhesus monkey infants. The relevance of animal studies to human infection remains to be determined; however, Issekutz and co-workers[169] reported similar immunologic findings among mothers and infants surviving natural *Listeria* infection.

Functional capacity of monocytic and macrophage cells is decreased in newborn animals. Chemotaxis, phagocytosis, and killing of *Candida albicans*, for example, is markedly impaired in neonatal rhesus monkey alveolar macrophages compared with those in juveniles and adults.[170]

NK cells also appear to be important in early response to *L. monocytogenes* infection. The proportion of mononuclear cells expressing NK cell phenotype and NK cell activity is decreased at birth, particularly in premature infants.[171,172] NK cell phenotype and function increase rapidly in the weeks after birth.

Toll-like Proteins, Interferon, and Cytokines in Newborns

In adult animals and adult derived cells, *Listeria* infection induces production of IL-12 and IL-18, which mediates T_H1 differentiation, NK cell activation, and IFN-γ production.[103] The major cellular source of IL-12 and IL-18 are monocytes, macrophages, and dendritic cells. After lipopolysaccharide stimulation, IL-12 messenger RNA (mRNA) expression and protein production in cord blood mononuclear cells is also greatly decreased compared with adult cells.[173] The half-life of IL-12 p40 mRNA is shortened in activated cord blood cells compared with adult cells.[174] However, cord blood mononuclear cells from humans are capable of responding in vitro to exogenous IL-12 in high concentrations.

In adult animals, interferon and agents that induce or augment interferon production confer protection against lethal listeriosis.[175,176] Synthesis of interferon, IL-2 and IL-4, all of which modulate the immune response and macrophage activation, is deficient in newborns.[167,177-179] Although production of these factors may be defective, newborn animals do respond to exogenous interferon; pretreatment with interferon or its inducers[180] protects against subsequent infection.

The ontogeny of cytokine-related host defense mechanisms has not been studied in depth. TNF is decreased among newborn rats infected with *L. monocytogenes*.[158] In one study on *L. monocytogenes*–infected newborn rats, TNF was detected only among animals older than 8 days. The age at which TNF is measurable corresponds to the approximate age at which increased resistance to *L. monocytogenes* is seen. The study showed that IFN-γ might enhance resistance to *L. monocytogenes* in newborn animals by permitting them to respond to exogenous TNF-γ.

The pattern of delayed or diminished cytokine response in human newborns is similar to the response in animals deficient in TLR protein. This possibility has been explored in human newborns. However, TLR-2 and TLR-4 expressions are normal on mononuclear and PMN cells of newborns.[143] TLRs require membrane-associated proteins to initiate intracellular messenger activation and cytokine secretion. Chief among these proteins is MyD88, an intracellular myeloid differentiating antigen needed for intracellular signaling of all TLR proteins. Yan and colleagues[143] reported diminished TNF secretion in newborn monocytes associated with significantly diminished intracellular MyD88 protein.

Serum Factors

Opsonic activity of newborn serum for *Listeria* is minimal.[181,182] *Listeria* is opsonized primarily by IgM together with the classic complement pathway. Because newborn serum has negligible amounts of IgM and low concentrations of the classic complement pathway, its poor opsonic activity may contribute to the severity of infection in newborns. Adult serum may also contain specific antibodies to inhibit *L. monocytogenes* invasion of brain microvascular endothelial cells.[183] The inhibitory antibody, which is absent in newborn cord serum, reacts with the *Listeria* surface protein InlB, described earlier as a key virulence factor.

PATHOLOGY

In tissues, human listeriosis is characterized by miliary granulomas and focal necroses or by suppuration. The term *listerioma* has been coined for *Listeria*-associated granulomas. In the newborn, *Listeria* infection of organs produces multiple, tiny nodules that can be visualized on gross examination.[184] Massive involvement of the liver is typical, reflecting the abundance of internalin receptors on hepatocytes. Often, as in miliary tuberculosis, the liver is seeded with grayish yellow nodules. Analogous findings are observed in the spleen, adrenal glands, lungs, esophagus, posterior pharyngeal wall, and tonsils. Subepithelial granulomas often undergo necrosis. Focal granulomas may also be detected in the lymph nodes, thymus, bone marrow, myocardium, testes, and skeletal muscles. The intestinal tract is affected to a variable degree, with a preference for the lymphatic structures of the small

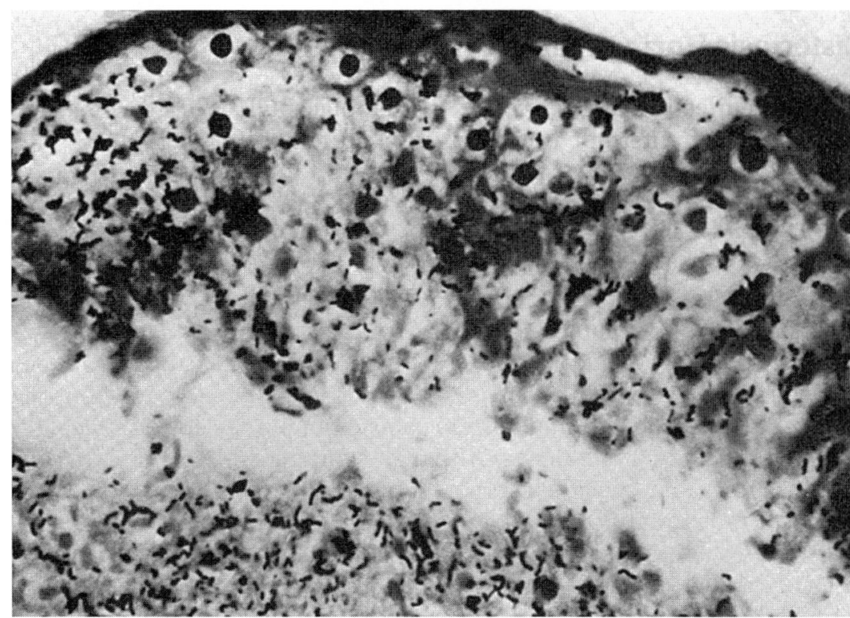

Figure 14–4 Cutaneous listeriosis. Notice the numerous gram-positive rods that extend from the dermis into the epidermis above.

intestine and appendix. Cutaneous lesions of neonatal listeriosis were first described by Reiss, [185] and occur most commonly on the back and lumbar region (Fig. 14-4).

In listeriosis of the central nervous system (CNS), granuloma formation is typical.[186] A characteristic histologic picture is seen in *Listeria* encephalitis, consisting of cerebral tissue necrosis with a loosening of the reticulum and an infiltration of leukocytes and lymphocytes leading to abscess formation.

Suppurative inflammation is the second form of tissue reaction to listeriosis. It is predominantly found in the meninges, the conjunctiva, and the epithelial linings of the middle ear and nasal sinuses. In meningitis, the subarachnoid space becomes filled with thick purulent exudate.

The histologic changes in human listeriosis are the same as those observed in animals. The organisms cause necrosis, followed by a proliferation of reticuloendothelial cells, resulting in the development of granulomas. The granuloma's center is necrotic, and the periphery contains an abundance of chronic inflammatory cells. *Listeria* are present in variable numbers within these necrotic foci and can be demonstrated with a Gram stain or Levaditi silver impregnation. Similar changes are found in all affected organs, independent of the age of the infected individual.

The gross and microscopic appearance of the placenta in listeriosis, although not pathognomonic, is sufficiently distinct to enable a presumptive diagnosis by the experienced pathologist (Fig. 14-5). *Listeria* placentitis is characterized grossly by multiple, minute, white or gray necrotic areas within the villous parenchyma and decidua; the largest tend to occur in basal villi and the decidua basalis.[187-189] These necrotic foci are macroabscesses identical to those described in other fetal organs.[184] Typically, localized collections of PMNs are found between the villous trophoblast and stroma, and inflamed or necrotic chorionic villi are enmeshed in intervillous inflammatory material and fibrin. Chorioamnionitis, deciduitis, villitis, and funisitis (in order of frequency) are seen. Cord lesions may be confined to superficial foci. Gram-positive rods are usually demonstrable within the necrotic centers of villous and decidual microabscesses, the membranes, and the umbilical cord. An immunohistochemical stain using polyclonal antibody directed at LLO has also been used.[190]

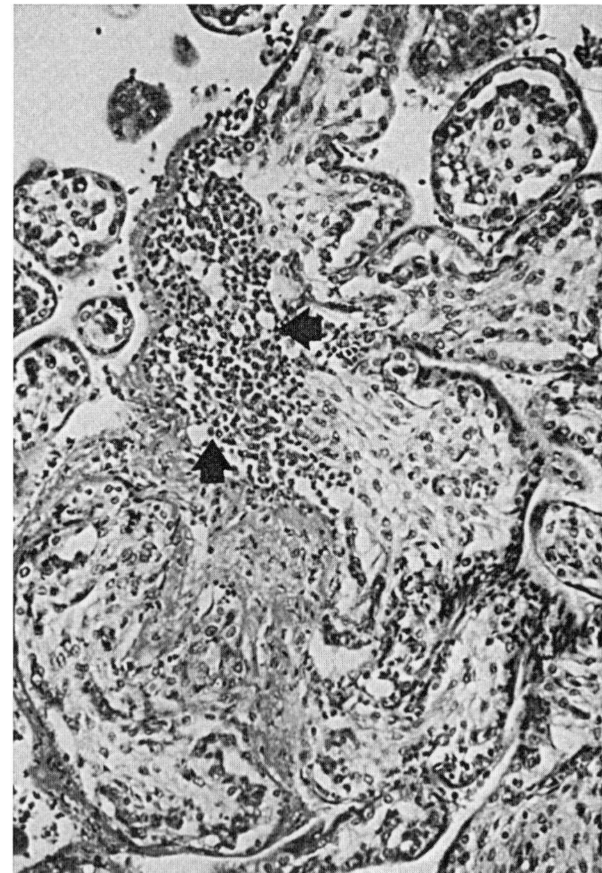

Figure 14–5 *Listeria* placentitis. Notice the microabscess between the necrotic villous trophoblast and the stroma *(arrows)*. Chorionic villi are enmeshed by intervillous and inflammatory material.

CLINICAL MANIFESTATIONS

The clinical features of listeriosis have considerable variability and may mimic other infections or other disease states. Based on the most common clinical manifestations, four or more clinical groups may be distinguished.

Listeriosis during Pregnancy

The predilection of *Listeria* for the fetoplacental unit and intrauterine infection is well documented.[191-195] Maternal listeriosis can be transmitted to the fetus by an ascending or transplacental route. Although early gestational listeriosis is associated with septic abortion, most clinically identified cases of perinatal listeriosis occur after the fifth month of pregnancy, with stillbirth or premature delivery of a septic infant the result.

Maternal influenza-like illness with fever and chills, fatigue, headache, and muscle pains often precedes delivery by 2 to 14 days. Although symptoms in the mother may subside before delivery, infection and fever precipitating delivery are common. Blood cultured from such women can yield *Listeria* at the same time or after these initial symptoms appear. Premature labor in mothers with listeriosis is common; length of gestation is less than 35 weeks in approximately 70%. The mortality rate, including stillbirth and abortion, is 40% to 50%. Early treatment of *Listeria* sepsis in pregnancy can prevent infection and sequelae in the fetus and newborn.[196,197] At the time of delivery, maternal symptoms of infection may be pronounced; however, symptoms in the mother usually subside with or without antibiotic treatment soon after delivery.

The pathogenesis of fetal listeriosis is not clear. Because the heaviest foci for neonatal infection are lung and gut, the fetus is probably infected by swallowing contaminated amniotic fluid and by the transplacental hematogenous route. Although ascending pathway from the lower genital tract may occur, infection through the transplacental route is favored by most experts. *L. monocytogenes* chorioamnionitis diagnosed by transabdominal amniocentesis before membrane rupture has been reported and supports a blood-borne route of infection.[184,193,197-199] Placental chorionic vascular thrombi can be associated with maternal coagulopathy. Emboli originating from *Listeria*-infected placental vessels have been described as a cause of congenital stroke in an infant.[190]

Susceptibility to *L. monocytogenes* is markedly increased in pregnant animals.[167,200,201] Immunoregulation during pregnancy is poorly understood. The fetoplacental unit must survive in the potentially hostile maternal immunologic environment throughout gestation. Evidence supports the hypothesis that the placenta and the immediately adjacent tissue constitute an immunologically privileged site, with local uterine immune response being suppressed.[195,202,203] Such regulation may be necessary to protect the fetus from immunologic rejection by the mother. However, if infection in this area occurs, bacterial proliferation may be overwhelming because of slow cell-mediated immune response.

Early-Onset Neonatal Listeriosis

The first descriptions of neonatal listeriosis were published in the 1930s by Burn.[204-206] Since then, it has become recognized that neonatal infection is the most common clinical form of human listeriosis. Infection in the neonatal period is usually divided into two clinical groups defined by age: early-onset and late-onset listeriosis.

Table 14–1 Clinical and Laboratory Findings of Early-Onset and Late-Onset Neonatal Listeriosis

Feature	Early Onset[a]	Late Onset[b]
Mortality (%)	25	15
Median age in days (range)	1 (0-6)	14 (7-35)
Male (%)	60	67
Preterm (%)	65	20
Respiratory involvement (%)	50	10
Meningitis (%)	25	95
Blood isolate (%)	75	20
Maternal perinatal illness (%)	50	0

[a]Data from references 77, 82, 191, 199, 207-211.
[b]Data from references 69, 207, 211-213, 287.

Some clinical and laboratory manifestations of early-onset neonatal listeriosis are outlined in Table 14-1, which is compiled from clinical cases published since 1970 in which early and late forms of the disease could be differentiated.[69,77,82,191,199,207-213] Classically, early-onset neonatal listeriosis develops within 1 or 2 days of life. However, in one outbreak involving 10 infants with nosocomially acquired listeriosis, an atypical clinical picture was described.[98] Nine of these infants were bathed with *L. monocytogenes*–contaminated mineral oil shortly after birth. Clinical features of infection developed 4 to 8 days later and were similar to those seen in late-onset infection (insidious onset of illness with fever and meningitis was common).

Evidence of preceding maternal illness is often described in infants with early-onset disease. Although some maternal symptoms are vague and nonspecific (e.g., malaise, myalgia), others are sufficiently distinctive (e.g., fever, chills) to alert physicians to the risk of prenatally acquired listeriosis. Blood cultures may be positive for *Listeria* from such mothers.

Although early-onset disease may occur in infants up to 7 days old, most cases are clinically apparent at delivery and demonstrate meconium staining, cyanosis, apnea, respiratory distress, and pneumonia. Meconium-stained amniotic fluid is a common feature in such infants and may occur at any gestational age. Pneumonia is also common, but radiographic features are nonspecific (i.e., peribronchial to widespread infiltration). In long-standing infection, a coarse, mottled, or nodular pattern has been described. Assisted ventilation is frequently necessary in such infants. Persistent hypoxia despite ventilator assistance is seen in severely affected infants.

In severe infection, a granulomatous rash—granulomatosis infantisepticum—has been described (Fig. 14-6). Slightly elevated pale patches (1 to 2 mm in diameter) with a bright erythematous base are seen. Biopsy of these areas demonstrates leukocytic infiltrates with multiple bacteria present (see Fig. 14-4).

Laboratory features are nonspecific; a leukocytosis with presence of immature cells may be seen, or if infection is severe, neutropenia may occur. Thrombocytopenia may also occur.[191,208] Many of the infants are anemic, perhaps attributable to hemolysin produced by the organism. These

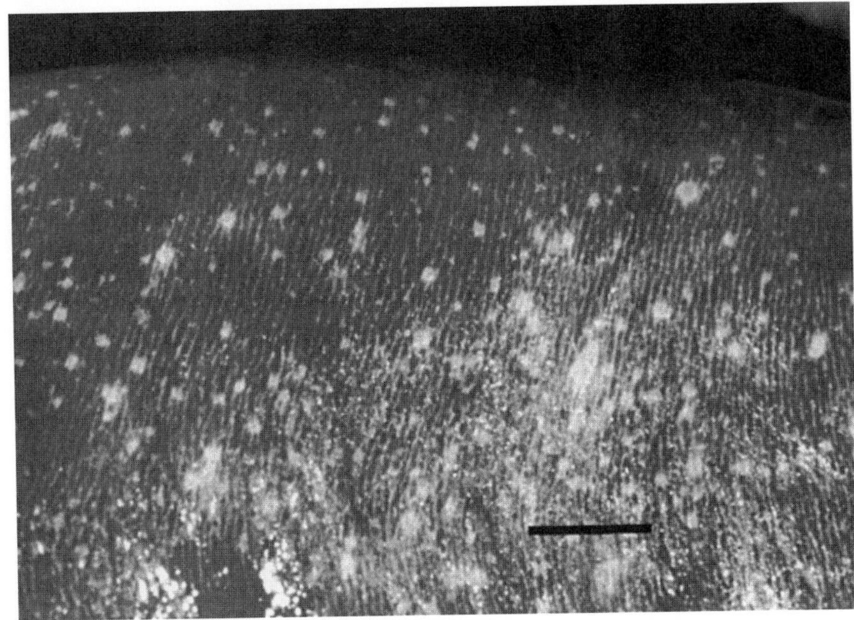

Figure 14–6 Rash of neonatal *Listeria monocytogenes* infection. Areas of small, elevated, pale pustules are surrounded by a deep red erythematous base on the abdomen of a premature neonate (horizontal bar ≈1 cm long).

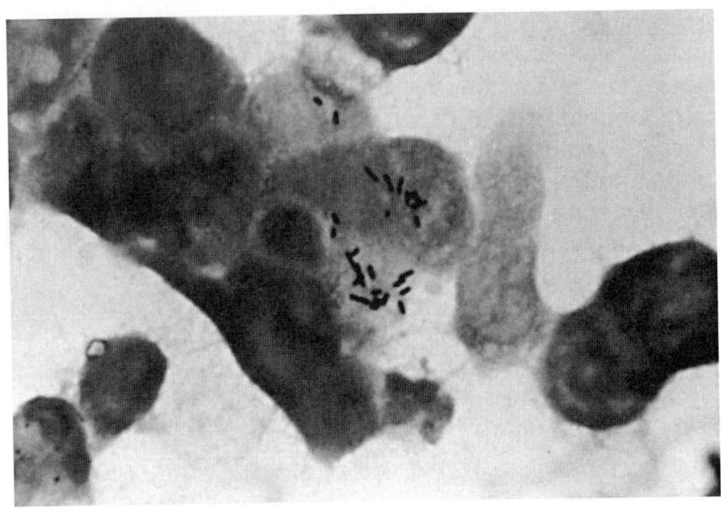

Figure 14–7 Short, gram-positive intracellular organisms with variable lengths and rounded ends are arranged irregularly.

laboratory and clinical features fail to distinguish listeriosis from early-onset group B streptococcal or other bacterial infection. The association of early-onset listeriosis with prematurity and maternal infection suggests the presence of intrauterine infection. The frequent presence of chorioamnionitis in the absence of ruptured membranes[77,211] supports the hypothesis of *Listeria* infection occurring by a transplacental route, which differs from the pathogenesis of group B streptococcal infection.

Late-Onset Neonatal Listeriosis

Neonatal listerial infection that occurs after 7 days of life is called *late-onset infection*. Although there is some overlap between early- and late-onset forms of listeriosis, the clinical patterns are usually distinct. Common clinical and laboratory features of late-onset neonatal listeriosis are shown in Table 14-1. By far the most common form of *Listeria* infection over this period is meningitis, which is present in 94% of late-onset cases. In many centers, *Listeria* ranks second only to streptococcus group B as a cause of bacterial meningitis in this age group, causing approximately 20% of such infections.[207]

Clinical features do not distinguish listerial meningitis in this age group from other causes. A striking predominance of male infants has been observed in most series. Fever and irritability are predominant clinical features. Often, infants do not appear excessively ill and may therefore elude diagnosis for several days. Other clinical forms of disease at this age are less common but include *Listeria*-induced colitis with associated diarrhea, and sepsis without meningitis.[214,215]

Laboratory features of late-onset infection are nonspecific as well. Cell counts in cerebrospinal fluid are usually high, with a predominance of neutrophils and band forms. Occasionally, in long-standing disease, a high number of monocytes may be seen. Gram stain of cerebrospinal fluid may not always suggest a diagnosis, because the organism may be rare or the morphology is atypical. Variable decolorization during staining may result in organisms appearing as gram-negative rods or gram-positive cocci. The appearance of organisms as illustrated in Figure 14-7 is characteristic of listeriosis in the early phase of severe meningitis.

Mortality of late-onset newborn infection is generally low unless diagnosis is delayed by more than 3 or 4 days after onset. Long-term sequelae and morbidity are uncommon.

Central Nervous System Infection

Acute or subacute bacterial meningitis accounts for two thirds of adult cases of listeriosis. Rhombencephalitis with ataxia, cranial nerve palsies, and multiple microabscesses on magnetic resonance imaging or computed tomography appears to be a distinct *Listeria* syndrome in humans, as it is in ruminants ("circling disease").[186] Survival of *Listeria* in the CNS is probably helped through cell-to-cell spread of the organism.[216] Morbidity and mortality rates are high for patients with CNS infection.[82]

Bacteremia

In immunocompromised patients, bacteremia is the most common manifestation of *Listeria* infection, with meningitis second in frequency.[68] Clinical signs are indistinguishable from bacteremia due to other organisms and typically include fever and myalgias after a prodromal illness of nausea and diarrhea. The risk of invasive listeriosis in patients with a malignancy, HIV infection, or after organ transplantation, may be 1000 times the risk in otherwise healthy persons.[77,217] During the bacteremic phase, an accompanying conjunctivitis is sometimes observed. Anton's eye test[218] resulted from a laboratory accident in which a technician accidentally contaminated his face.

Other Clinical Forms of Infection

Increasingly, a febrile gastroenteritis syndrome similar to salmonellosis has been described in adults and children. Processed meats have been repeatedly implicated,[219] but other outbreaks have involved contaminated shrimp salad,[220] rice salad,[221] and chocolate milk.[215] Only a few patients developed invasive disease (i.e., sepsis) in these outbreaks, and the level of *Listeria* contamination appeared to be very high.[222]

Papular cutaneous lesions are often observed in newborns when listeriosis is disseminated. These are to be distinguished from the primary skin lesions caused by *Listeria* as observed in adults,[223,224] which are the result of direct contact, such as the handling of a cow's placenta after abortion by a veterinarian or farmer.[50] Other unusual forms of listeriosis, such as endocarditis,[225] endophthalmitis,[226,227] liver abscesses,[228] peritonitis,[229,230] osteomyelitis, and septic arthritis,[231] have been described in adults but are rare in infants.

DIAGNOSIS

The clinical signs and symptoms of listeriosis overlap considerably with other illnesses, making a specific diagnosis difficult, if not impossible, when patients are first seen.

Serology

The agglutination reaction (Widal's test) demonstrates antibodies against O and H antigens of the various *Listeria* serovars. Unfortunately, because of the antigenic complexity of *L. monocytogenes*, no agreement has been reached on the interpretation of agglutination reactions for diagnostic purposes.

Attempts to demonstrate complement-fixing *Listeria* antibodies date back to the 1930s.[232] In one study, serum samples collected from 32 mothers with perinatal *Listeria* infection were compared with 128 samples from matched controls.[233] The sensitivity and specificity of the complement fixation test were found to be 78% and 91%, respectively; however, the positive predictive value was only 75%. A titer of 1:8 or more is accepted as significant.[233,234]

Detection of antibodies to LLO has also been used to diagnose human listeriosis.[235] Purified LLO incorporated into nitrocellulose filters is tested with serial dilutions of sera. Absorbed anti-LLO is identified using enzyme-labeled anti-human IgG. Sensitivity and specificity of the test is over 90%, and during a febrile gastroenteritis outbreak, it correlated well with clinical illness.[215] Although these results are impressive, the technique is not available commercially. A precipitin test,[236] indirect hemagglutination reaction,[237] and antigen fixation test[238] have also been described, showing apparent success but remaining unavailable on a widespread basis.

Isolation of the Organism

Cultivation of *L. monocytogenes* is the gold standard of diagnosis. Culture of venous blood, ascitic and other fluids, cervical material, urine, placenta, amniotic fluid, lochia and meconium, and tissues at biopsy or autopsy offers the best chances for identifying *Listeria* in persons with disease. Culture of the stool is not done routinely, because feces are positive for *Listeria* in 1% to 5% of healthy women.[73,239] In an outbreak setting, stool culture with selective media may recover organisms for comparative typing.

Microscopic diagnosis may be attempted by use of Gram stain only in specimens that normally do not contain bacteria: cerebrospinal fluid, meconium, and tissue smears. The finding of short, sometimes coccoid, gram-positive rods, strongly supports a suspicion of listeriosis and is indicative of this infection in meconium smears. Occasionally, *L. monocytogenes* may appear gram-variable or even predominantly coccoid. With long-standing disease or when the patient has received antibiotics, *Listeria* may appear gram-negative and be confused with *H. influenzae* when observed in the cerebrospinal fluid. In other instances, *Listeria* has been mistaken for pneumococci and corynebacteria.

Molecular Detection

Polymerase chain reaction (PCR)–based methods are used to detect *Listeria* in clinical samples such as cerebrospinal fluid[240] and endophthalmitis.[241] Spurred by the food industry's demand for rapid *Listeria* detection, techniques such as real-time PCR[242] and amplification with sequencing of *Listeria* 16S ribosomal RNA genes[243] are being reported in the literature. Although few clinical laboratories use these methods, the increasing availability of PCR technology is already changing this pattern.

PROGNOSIS

Neonatal listeriosis accounts for the largest recognizable group of infections caused by *L. monocytogenes*. Fetal loss with early gestational infection is a recognized complication of maternal infection. In late-gestational maternal infection, sparing of the fetus has been reported,[244] but it is probably uncommon unless antepartum antibiotic treatment has been given to the mother.[245,246]

Although fetal or neonatal infection with *L. monocytogenes* is known to have a high fatality rate, the long-term morbidity is unclear. Rotheberg and associates[247] found an increased incidence of developmental delay assessed at a mean age of 29.5 months among small (<1250 g at birth), *Listeria*-infected infants who required assisted ventilation. Naege,[248] studying children 4 to 7 years after they recovered from early-onset listeriosis, found increased neurodevelopmental handicaps. Others have reported hydrocephalus.[249]

In contrast, Evans and co-workers[250] found no evidence of neurodevelopmental sequelae in six of eight survivors studied at a mean age of 15 months and again at 32 months. The two infants with neurodevelopmental sequelae had severe acute perinatal sepsis with meningitis. Both had spastic diplegia. The investigators concluded that long-term sequelae after neonatal early-onset listeriosis was uncommon. If meningitis does not occur, the outcome may be generally good. The prognosis for infants with late-onset neonatal sepsis and meningitis has not been studied extensively.

THERAPY

Listeria remains susceptible to antibiotics commonly used in its treatment.[251,252] However, the high mortality rate and risk of relapse[253,254] have prompted a search for newer therapeutic regimens, including quinolones,[255] trimethoprim-sulfamethoxazole,[256,257] and rifampin.[258] Transferable plasmid-mediated antibiotic resistance has been reported[259] conferring resistance to chloramphenicol, tetracycline, and erythromycin.

In Vitro Studies

Conflicting reports of in vitro activity of antibiotics against clinical isolates of *L. monocytogenes* probably reflect a variable pattern of susceptibility for strains and differences in laboratory technique. Several large in vitro studies of antibiotic susceptibility of clinical isolates of *L. monocytogenes* have been reported using broth dilution susceptibility methods.[260-262] Most studies found that the strains represented a homogeneous population susceptible to ampicillin, penicillin, erythromycin, and tetracycline. In vitro results, however, are greatly influenced by methodology: inoculum size, media, and definition of end points. Since 1988, several strains have been isolated showing various degrees of relative resistance to non–β-lactam antibiotics such as tetracycline and gentamicin.[261,262] The minimal bactericidal concentration of antibiotics is often much higher than levels attainable clinically. Most antibiotics tested are bacteriostatic but not bactericidal. Although bacteriostatic antibiotics have been used in the past, bactericidal antibiotics have a potential advantage for patients with impaired host defense mechanisms.[263]

Studies with cephalosporin antibiotics using in vitro and in vivo models have been consistently disappointing.[264] The organism is uniformly resistant to cephalosporin antibiotics.[265] Cephalosporins may be incorporated into media to inhibit other bacteria while permitting growth of *Listeria*.[201] Activity of newer fluoroquinolones against *L. monocytogenes* is promising.[266,267] For example, moxifloxacin was found to have bactericidal activity for *Listeria* and was the most effective antibiotic tested for eradication of the organism from the intracellular compartment.[266]

In Vivo Studies

Several combinations of antibiotics[249,267-269] or altered methods of preparation such as liposome-entrapment[270] have been compared for their bactericidal activity against *L. monocytogenes* in vivo. Animal models appear to provide the only practical way to assess therapeutic regimens, because large clinical studies in humans are not available. Murine models employing normal adults,[257,270,271] cortisone-treated adults,[272] immunodeficient adults,[273-275] or animals infected by inhalation of aerosolized *Listeria*[257] have been reported. A rabbit model using animals injected intracisternally with *Listeria* has also been described.[276] The model most analogous to neonatal disease was described by Hawkins and colleagues.[277] In their study, neonatal rats were injected intraperitoneally with bacteria and then randomized to begin antibiotic regimens 2 days later.

Interpretation of in vivo models is difficult because conflicting results have been reported. In addition to variability accounted for by technique (e.g., route of injection, bacterial strain, inoculum size), consideration should also be given to the pharmacokinetics for each antibiotic in the various animal species. For example, animal species differ widely in their metabolism of rifampin,[276-278] and the half-life of ampicillin is much longer in human neonates than in most of the adult animal models in which it has been assessed. In one study involving adult mice infected with a virulent strain of *L. monocytogenes*, no synergy was demonstrated using a combination of ampicillin and gentamicin.[279] However, in the in vivo model of neonatal listeriosis described by Hawkins and associates, the combination of ampicillin with gentamicin gave significantly better eradication of organisms in spleen compared with ampicillin alone.[277] Similarly, the combination trimethoprim-sulfamethoxazole was found to be superior to either drug alone.[277] Reports of efficacy of other antibiotics in vivo are conflicting. Rifampin has been found by some authors to be highly effective in eradicating organisms,[257,278] whereas others have found it to be ineffective.[280] Sensitivity of individual strains to rifampin may account for the widely discrepant results. Rifampin resistance may develop in vivo when it is used as monotherapy. The use of ciprofloxacin in animal models has not suggested any therapeutic advantage over ampicillin.[272,281]

Clinical Reports

There have been no prospective clinical trials reported for human infection with *L. monocytogenes*. Anecdotal reports of single cases or reviews of outbreaks support the conclusions drawn from in vivo models. In one review of clinical management of 119 cases of listeriosis from three centers in the United States, excellent therapeutic results were seen for patients treated empirically with penicillin or ampicillin; all had a reduction of fever and clinical improvement. However, patients treated initially with cephalosporins had persistent fever and infection.[281] In the largest assessment of treatment regimens during a single outbreak,[282] a lower mortality was reported for children given ampicillin (16% of 57 children) compared with those treated with chloramphenicol, tetracycline, or streptomycin (33% of 82 children). As summarized by McLauchlin,[253] there have been several reports of treatment failure and recurrent human listeriosis. In some cases, weeks or months elapse between episodes. Patients have been treated with bacteriostatic (e.g., erythromycin) or β-lactam antibiotics during initial treatment. Nevertheless, in the absence of controlled clinical trials, a definitive recommendation for treatment cannot be made.

Suggested Management

Listeriosis during Pregnancy

If amnionitis is present, initial treatment should be given by the intravenous route to ensure adequate tissue levels (ampicillin, 4 to 6 g/day divided into four equal doses plus an aminoglycoside). If amnionitis is not present or if acute symptoms of amnionitis have subsided, oral antibiotics are probably adequate (amoxicillin, 1 to 2 g/day divided into three equal doses). In both situations, treatment should continue for 14 days. If the patient has a significant allergy to ampicillin, therapeutic options are limited. Erythromycin may be given. The estolate form of this drug should be avoided because there is increased liver toxicity during pregnancy. Trimethoprim-sulfamethoxazole should not be used because premature delivery of the infant may occur as a consequence of infection, in which case the drug may be toxic to the infant.

Early-Onset Neonatal Listeriosis

Ampicillin in combination with an aminoglycoside is the preferred management for early-onset infection. For infants with body weight less than 2000 g, 100 mg/kg/day (divided into two equal doses) should be administered for the first week of life. For infants with body weight of more than 2000 g, 150 mg/kg/day (divided into three equal doses) should be administered for the first week of life. For the second week of life, the appropriate dosages are 150 mg/kg/day and 200 mg/kg/day for infants weighing less than and more than 2000 g, respectively. Aminoglycoside doses vary with the agent chosen. For gentamicin, the suggested dosages are for full-term infants 5 mg/kg/day (divided into two equal doses) for the first week of life and 7.5 mg/kg/day (divided into three equal doses) for the second week of life. Fourteen days of treatment is recommended for early-onset neonatal sepsis due to *L. monocytogenes*; however, a longer course of treatment should be given in the uncommon event of early-onset neonatal listeriosis with meningitis.

Late-Onset Neonatal Listeriosis

Meningitis commonly coexists with late-onset listeriosis. Delayed eradication of the organism may be seen in such cases. Ampicillin (200 to 400 mg/kg/day divided into four to six equal doses) in combination with an aminoglycoside is recommended. Lumbar punctures should be repeated daily until the organism has been cleared. In the event of delayed clearance (>2 days), further investigations are indicated and should include computed tomography or cranial ultrasound evaluation to assess for the presence of cerebritis or intracranial hemorrhage. If the organism remains present in the cerebrospinal fluid after several days, the addition of moxifloxacin, rifampin, or use of trimethoprim-sulfamethoxazole may be considered if the organism is sensitive in vitro. Experience with these antibiotics and with this organism in neonates is limited.[283] Cephalosporin antibiotics have no role in treatment because *Listeria* organisms are uniformly resistant. Length of treatment is variable. If prompt clinical improvement and sterilization of cerebrospinal fluid occur, 10 to 14 days of treatment is probably adequate. However, if response is slow, treatment for as long as 21 days may be considered.

PREVENTION AND OUTBREAK MANAGEMENT

Foodborne outbreaks of listeriosis are unpredictable and may occur in a wide geographic area. Reporting of sporadic cases of listeriosis to public health authorities may be the only method of distinguishing sporadic from epidemic disease. The epidemic threshold is unknown and may be determined only in retrospect. Studies suggesting that sporadic listeriosis is also a foodborne pathogen have important public health implications.[284]

Sampling of foodstuffs associated with sporadic cases of listeriosis is not warranted. Case-control studies to determine potential vehicles of transmission in outbreaks may help define the source, and environmental sampling may be an important part of such outbreak investigations. Strains of *Listeria* from clinical and environmental isolates should be forwarded to a reference laboratory for appropriate epidemiologic typing. At a minimum, serotyping, phage typing, and multifocus enzyme electrophoresis typing should be performed to characterize the epidemic strain.

During an outbreak of listeriosis, pregnant women presenting with sepsis syndrome or a flulike illness should be empirically treated with ampicillin and an aminoglycoside after appropriate cultures of blood, rectum, and vagina have been obtained. Amniocentesis for diagnosis of chorioamnionitis may be appropriate.[198] If membranes have ruptured and contamination is suspected, use of selective media may enhance the isolation of *Listeria* from these patients.

Identification of early- or late-onset listeriosis in a newborn nursery should prompt appropriate epidemiologic and clinical history taking from the mother and postpartum cultures of the rectum and vagina. Infection-control precautions with gowning, gloves, and careful hand washing can prevent nosocomial transmission between infected infants and is consistent with current procedures for all forms of neonatal sepsis.

The recognition that sporadic cases of listeriosis are primarily foodborne has also prompted publication of preventive guidelines by the CDC (Table 14-2).[285] Guidelines for preventing listeriosis are similar to those for preventing other foodborne illnesses and include thorough cooking of

Table 14–2 Dietary Recommendations for Preventing Foodborne Listeriosis

For All Persons

1. Thoroughly cook raw food from animal sources (e.g., beef, pork, poultry).
2. Thoroughly wash raw vegetables before eating.
3. Keep uncooked meats separate from vegetables, cooked foods, and ready-to-eat foods.
4. Avoid consumption of raw (unpasteurized) milk or foods made from raw milk.
5. Wash hands, knives, and cutting boards after handling uncooked foods.

Additional Recommendations for Persons at High Risk[a]

1. Avoid soft cheeses (e.g., Mexican-style feta, Brie, Camembert, blue-veined cheeses). There is no need to avoid hard cheeses, cream cheese, cottage cheese, or yogurt.
2. Leftover foods or ready-to-eat foods (e.g., hot dogs) should be reheated until steaming hot before eating.
3. Although the risk for listeriosis associated with foods from delicatessen counters is relatively low, pregnant women and immunosuppressed persons may choose to avoid these foods or to thoroughly reheat cold cuts before eating them.

[a]Persons immunocompromised by illness or medications, pregnant women, and the elderly.

From Centers for Disease Control. Update: foodborne listeriosis—United States, 1988-1990. MMWR Morb Mortal Wkly Rep 41:251, 1992.

raw food from animals and thorough washing of vegetables and utensils. Persons at high risk, such as pregnant women, should also avoid soft cheeses and prepared salads, meats, and cheeses from deli counters. Thoroughly heating leftover foods until steaming hot has also been recommended.[61] Following these guidelines may be difficult for all pregnant women, and their effectiveness in reducing sporadic cases of perinatal listeriosis will be difficult to ascertain. However, a decrease in the rates of listeriosis in some geographic areas in the United States has been temporally associated with the publication of these guidelines and industry efforts directed at removing foodborne pathogens from the food chain.[285,286,287]

REFERENCES

1. Nyfeldt A. Étiologie de la mononucléose infectieuse. Compt Rend Biol 101:590, 1929.
2. Murray EGD, Webb RA, Swann MBR. A disease of rabbits characterized by a large mononuclear leucocytosis, caused by a hitherto undescribed bacillus: *Bacterium monocytogenes* (n. sp.). J Pathol Bacteriol 29:407, 1926.
3. Pirie JHH. A new disease of veld rodents, "Tiger River disease." S Afr Inst Med Res 3:163, 1927.
4. Pirie JHH. Change of name for a genus of bacteria. Nature 145:264, 1940.
5. Bille J, Doyle MP. *Listeria* and *Erysipelothrix*. *In* Balows A, Hausler WJ Jr, Hermann, KL, et al (eds). Manual of Clinical Microbiology, 5th ed. Washington, DC, American Society of Microbiology, 1991, pp 287-295.
6. Seeliger HPR. Listeriosis. Basel, S Karger, 1961.
7. Peel M, Donachie W, Shaw A. Temperature-dependent expression of flagella of *Listeria monocytogenes* studied by electron microscopy, SDS-PAGE, and Western blotting. J Gen Microbiol 134:2171, 1988.
8. van Netten P, Perales I, van de Moosdijk A, et al. Liquid and solid selected differential media for the detection and enumeration of *L. monocytogenes* on the *Listeria* species. Int J Food Microbiol 8:299, 1989.
9. Gray ML, Stafseth HJ, Thorp F Jr, et al. A new technique for isolating listerellae from the bovine brain. J Bacteriol 55:471, 1948.
10. Seeliger HPR, Jones D. Genus *Listeria*. *In* Sneath PHA, Mair HS, Sharp ME, et al (eds). Berge's Manual of Systematic Bacteriology, vol 2. Baltimore, Williams & Wilkins, 1986.
11. Seeliger HPR, Finger H. Analytical serology of *Listeria*. *In* Kwapinski JBG (ed). Analytical Serology of Microorganisms. New York, John Wiley, 1969, p 549.
12. Bille RJ, Swaminathan B. Listeria and erysipelothrix. *In* Murray PR, Baron EJ, Jorgensen JH, et al (eds). Manual of Clinical Microbiology, 8th ed. Washington, DC, ASM Press, 2003, pp 461-471.
13. Sword CP, Pickett MJ. Isolation and distribution of bacteriophages from *Listeria monocytogenes*. J Gen Microbiol 25:241, 1961.
14. McLauchlin J, Andurier A, Taylor AG. The evaluation of a phage typing system for *Listeria monocytogenes* for use in epidemiologic studies. J Med Microbiol 22:357, 1986.
15. Schlech WF 3d, Lavigne PM, Bortolussi R, et al. Epidemic listeriosis—evidence for transmission by food. N Engl J Med 308:203, 1983.
16. Piffaretti JC, Kressebuch H, Aeschbacher M, et al. Genetic characterization of clones of bacterium *Listeria monocytogenes* causing epidemic disease. Proc Natl Acad Sci U S A 86:3818, 1989.
17. Graves LM, Swaminathan B, Reeves MW, et al. Ribosomal DNA fingerprinting of *Listeria monocytogenes* using digoxin genum DNA probe. Eur J Epidemiol 7:77, 1991.
18. Richardson BP, Adams M. Allozyme Electrophoresis: A Handbook for Animal Systematics and Population Studies. Orlando, Fla, Academic Press, 1986.
19. Carriere C, Allardet-Servent A, Bourg G, et al. DNA polymorphism in strains of *Listeria monocytogenes*. J Clin Microbiol 29:1351, 1991.
20. Slade PJ, Collins-Thompson DL. Differentiation of the genus *Listeria* from other gram-positive species based on low molecular weight (LMW) RNA profiles. J Appl Bacteriol 70:355, 1991.
21. Portnoy DA, Chakraborty T, Goebel W, et al. Molecular determinants of *Listeria monocytogenes* pathogenesis. Infect Immun 60:1263, 1992.
22. Vazquez-Boland JA, Kuhn M, Berche P, et al. *Listeria* pathogenesis and molecular virulence determinants. Clin Microbiol Rev 14:584, 2001.
23. Gaillard JL, Berche P, Frehel C, et al. Entry of *L. monocytogenes* into cells is mediated by internalin, a repeat protein reminiscent of surface antigens from gram-positive cocci. Cell 65:1127, 1991.
24. Ireton K, Cossart P. Host-pathogen interactions during entry and actin-based movement of *Listeria monocytogenes*. Ann Rev Genet 31:113, 1997.
25. Lecuit M, Dramsi S, Gottardi C, et al. A single amino acid in E-cadherin responsible for host specificity towards the human pathogen *Listeria monocytogenes*. EMBO J 18:3956, 1999.
26. Hess J, Gentschev I, Szalay G, et al. *Listeria monocytogenes* p60 supports host cell invasion by and in vivo survival of attenuated *Salmonella typhimurium*. Infect Immun 63:2047, 1995.
27. Harty JT, Pamer EG. CD8 T lymphocytes specific for the secreted p60 antigen protect against *Listeria monocytogenes* infection. J Immunol 154:4642, 1995.
28. Cossart P, Vincente MF, Mengaud J, et al. Listeriolysin O is essential for virulence of *Listeria monocytogenes*: direct evidence by gene complementation. Infect Immun 57:3629, 1989.
29. Portnoy DA, Jacks PS, Hinrichs DJ. Role of hemolysin for the intracellular growth of *Listeria monocytogenes*. J Exp Med 167:1459, 1988.
30. Moors MM, Levitt B, Youngman P, Portnoy DA. Expression of listeriolysin O and ActA by intracellular and extracellular *Listeria monocytogenes*. Infect Immun 67:131, 1999.
31. Shetron-Rama LM, Marquis H, Bouwer HG, Freitag NE. Intracellular Induction of *Listeria monocytogenes* actA expression. Infect Immun 70:1087, 2002.
32. Kocks C, Hellio R, Gounon P, et al. Polarized distribution of *Listeria monocytogenes* surface protein ActA at the site of directional actin assembly. J Cell Sci 105(Pt 3):699, 1993.
33. Kocks C, Gouin E, Tabouret M, et al. *Listeria monocytogenes* induced actin assembly requires the *actA* gene product, a surface protein. Cell 68:521, 1992.
34. Vazquez-Boland J, Kocks C, Dramsi S, et al. Nucleotide sequence of lethicinase operon of *Listeria monocytogenes* and possible role of lethicinase in cell-to-cell spread. Infect Immun 60:219, 1992.
35. Raveneau J, Jeoffroy C, Beretti JL, et al. Reduced virulence of a *Listeria monocytogenes* phospholipase-deficient mutant obtained by transposon insertion into the zinc metalloproteinase gene. Infect Immun 60:916, 1992.
36. Mengaud J, Dramsi S, Gouin E, et al. Pleotrophic control of *Listeria monocytogenes* virulence factors by a gene that is auto regulated. Mol Microbiol 5:2273, 1991.

37. Domann E, Zechel S, Lingnau A, et al. Identification and characterization of a novel PrfA-regulated gene in *Listeria monocytogenes* whose product, IrpA, is highly homologous to internalin proteins, which contain leucine-rich repeats. Infect Immun 65:101, 1997.
38. Michel E, Mengaud J, Galsworthy S, Cossart P. Characterization of a large motility gene cluster containing the cheR, motAB genes of *Listeria monocytogenes* and evidence that PrfA downregulates motility genes. FEMS Microbiol Lett 169:341, 1998.
39. Liu PV, Bates JL. An extracellular haemorrhagic toxin produced by *Listeria monocytogenes*. Can J Microbiol 7:107, 1961.
40. Leimeister-Wachter M, Domann E, Chakraborty T. The expression of virulence genes in *Listeria monocytogenes* is thermoregulated. J Bacteriol 174:947, 1992.
41. Zipplies G. Über bakterielle Reizstoffe aus *Listeria monocytogenes* und ihre Wirkung am Kaninchen (Intrakutantest). Arch Exp Vet Med 11:816, 1964.
42. Gottesman S, Wickner S, Maurizi MR. Protein quality control: triage by chaperones and proteases. Genes Dev 11:815, 1997.
43. McIlwain P, Eveleth DF, Doubly JA. Pharmacologic studies of a toxic cellular component of *Listeria monocytogenes*. Am J Vet Res 25:774, 1964.
44. Saklani-Jusforgues H, Fontan E, Goossens PL. Effect of acid-adaptation on *Listeria monocytogenes* survival and translocation in a murine intragastric infection model. FEMS Microbiol Lett 193:155, 2000.
45. Stanley NF. Studies on *Listeria monocytogenes*: I. Isolation of a monocytosis-producing agent (MPA). Aust J Exp Biol 27:123, 1949.
46. Shum DT, Galsworthy SB. Stimulation of monocyte production by an endogenous mediator induced by a component of *Listeria monocytogenes*. Immunology 46:343, 1982.
47. Welshimer HJ. Isolation of *Listeria monocytogenes* from vegetation. J Bacteriol 95:300, 1968.
48. Low JC, Renton CP. Septicemia, encephalitis, and abortions in a housed flock of sheep caused by *Listeria monocytogenes* type 1/2. Vet Rec 114:147, 1985.
49. Owen CR, Meis A, Jackson JW, et al. A case of primary cutaneous listeriosis. N Engl J Med 262:1026, 1960.
50. McLauchlin J, Low JC. Primary cutaneous listeriosis in adults: an occupational disease in veterinarians and farmers. Vet Rec 135:615, 1994.
51. Elischerova K, Stupalova S. Listeriosis in professionally exposed persons. Acta Microbiol Acad Sci Hung 19:379, 1972.
52. Bojsen-Moller J. Human listeriosis: diagnostic, epidemiologic and clinical studies. Acta Pathol Microbiol Scand 229(Suppl):1, 1992.
53. Linnan JM, Mascola L, Lou XD, et al. Epidemic listeriosis associated with Mexican-style cheese. N Engl J Med 319:823, 1988.
54. Schlech WF 3d. Foodborne listeriosis. Clin Infect Dis 31:770, 2000.
55. Fleming DW, Cochi SL, MacDonald KL, et al. Pasteurized milk as a vehicle of infection in an outbreak of listeriosis. N Engl J Med 312:404, 1985.
56. Tienungoon S, Ratkowsky DA, McMeekin TA, Ross T. Growth limits of *Listeria monocytogenes* as a function of temperature, pH, NaCl, and lactic acid. Appl Environ Microbiol 66:4979, 2000.
57. McLauchlin J, Hall SM, Velani SK, Gilbert RJ. Human listeriosis and pâté: a possible association. Br Med J 303:773, 1991.
58. Multistate outbreak of listeriosis—United States, 1998. MMWR Morb Mortal Wkly Rep 47:1985, 1998.
59. Lepoutre A, Moyse C, Roure C, et al. Epidemie de listerioses en France. Bull Epidemiol Hebdonv 25:115, 1992.
60. Centers for Disease Control and Prevention. Multistate outbreak of listeriosis—United States, 2000. MMWR Morb Mortal Wkly Rep 49:1129, 2000.
61. Centers for Disease Control and Prevention. Outbreak of listeriosis—northeastern United States, 2002. MMWR Morb Mortal Wkly Rep 51:950, 2002.
62. Rorvik LM, Aase B, Alvestad T, Caugant DA. Molecular epidemiological survey of *Listeria monocytogenes* in seafoods and seafood-processing plants. Appl Environ Microbiol 66:4779, 2000.
63. Schwartz B, Hexter D, Broome CV, et al. Investigation of an outbreak of listeriosis: new hypothesis for the etiology of epidemic *Listeria monocytogenes* infections. J Infect Dis 159:680, 1989.
64. McLaughlin J, Greenwood MH, Pini PM. The occurrence of *Listeria monocytogenes* in cheese from a manufacturer associated with a case of listeriosis. Int J Food Microbiol 10:255, 1990.
65. Schuchat A, Deaver K, Wenger JD, et al. Role of foods in sporadic listeriosis. I. Case-control study of dietary risk factors. JAMA 267:2041, 1992.
66. Pinner RW, Schuchat A, Swaminathan B, et al. Role of foods in sporadic listeriosis. II. Microbiologic and epidemiologic investigations. JAMA 267:2046, 1992.
67. Schlech WF III. Listeriosis: epidemiology, virulence and the significance of contaminated foodstuffs. J Hosp Infect 19:211, 1991.
68. Gellin BG, Broome CV, Bibb WF, et al. The epidemiology of listeriosis in the United States—1986. Am J Epidemiol 133:392, 1991.
69. Siegman-Igra Y, Levin R, Weinberger M, et al. *Listeria monocytogenes* infection in Israel and review of cases worldwide. Emerg Infect Dis 8:305, 2002.
70. Paul ML, Dwyer DE, Chow C, et al. Listeriosis—a review of eighty-four cases. Med J Aust 160:489, 1994.
71. Newton L, Hall SM, PeLerin M, et al. Listeriosis surveillance: 1990. CDR (Lond Eng Rev) 1:R110-113, 1991.
72. Fredericksen B, Samuelsson S. Vito-maternalistic listeriosis in Denmark 1981-1988. J Infect 24:277, 1992.
73. Bojsen-Miller J. Human listeriosis: diagnostic, epidemiologic and clinical studies. Acta Pathol Microbiol Scand 229(Suppl):72, 1972.
74. Mascola L, Sorvillo F, Goulet V, et al. Fecal carriage of *Listeria monocytogenes*: observations during a community-wide, common-source outbreak. Clin Infect Dis 15:557, 1992.
75. Varughese PV, Carter AO. Human listeriosis in Canada—1988. Can Dis Wkly Rep 15:213, 1989.
76. Schmidt-Wolf G, Seeliger HPR, Schrettenbrunner A. Menschliche listeriosise-erkrankungen in der Bundesrepublik Deutschland, 1969-1985. Zentralbl Bakteriol Hyg 472, 1985.
77. Nolla-Salas J, Bosch J, Gasser I, et al. Perinatal listeriosis: a population-based multicenter study in Barcelona, Spain (1990-1996). Am J Perinatol 15:461, 1998.
78. McLaughlin J. Human listeriosis in Britain, 1967-1985: a summary of 722 cases: 1. Listeriosis during pregnancy and the newborn. Epidemiol Infect 104:181, 1990.
79. Lamont RJ, Postlethwaite R. Carriage of *Listeria monocytogenes* and related species in pregnant and non-pregnant women in Aberdeen, Scotland. J Infect 13:187, 1986.
80. Louria DB, Hentle T, Armstrong D, et al. Listeriosis complicating malignant disease: a new association. Ann Intern Med 67:261, 1967.
81. Schuchat A, Broome CV, Swaminathan B. Epidemiology of human listeriosis. Clin Microbiol Rev 4:169, 1991.
82. Lorber B. Listeriosis. Clin Infect Dis 24:1, 1997.
83. Miller JK, Hedberg M. Effects of cortisone on susceptibility of mice to *Listeria monocytogenes*. Am J Clin Pathol 43:248, 1965.
84. Hugin AW, Cerny A, Wrann M, et al. Effect of cyclosporin A on immunity to *Listeria monocytogenes*. Infect Immun 52:12, 1986.
85. Petit JC, Richard G, Burghoffer B, et al. Suppression of cellular immunity to *Listeria monocytogenes* by activated macrophages: mediation by prostaglandins. Infect Immun 49:383, 1985.
86. Stamm AM, Dismukes WE, Simmons BP, et al. Listeriosis in renal transplant recipients: report of an outbreak and review of 102 cases. Rev Infect Dis 4:665, 1982.
87. Gellin BG, Broome CV. Listeriosis. JAMA 261:1313, 1989.
88. Nieman RE, Lorber B. Listeriosis in adults: a changing pattern. Report of eight cases and review of the literature, 1968-1978. Rev Infect Dis 2:207, 1980.
89. Schlech WF 3d, Chase DP, Badley A. A model of foodborne *Listeria monocytogenes* infection in the Sprague-Dawley rats using gastric inoculation: development and effect of gastric acidity on infective dose. Int J Food Microbiol 18:15, 1993.
90. Ho JL, Shands KN, Friedland G, et al. An outbreak of type 4b *Listeria monocytogenes* infection involving patients from eight Boston hospitals. Arch Intern Med 145:520, 1986.
91. Florman AL, Sundararajan V. Listeriosis among nursery mates. Pediatrics 41:784, 1968.
92. Larson S. *Listeria monocytogenes* causing hospital-acquired enterocolitis and meningitis in newborn infants. Br Med J 2:473, 1978.
93. Filice GA, Cantrell HF, Smith AB, et al. *Listeria monocytogenes* infection in neonates: investigation of an epidemic. J Infect Dis 138:17, 1978.
94. Campbell AN, Sill PR, Wardle JK. *Listeria* meningitis acquired by cross-infection in a delivery suite. Lancet 2:752, 1981.
95. Nelson KE, Warren D, Tomasi AM, et al. Transmission of neonatal listeriosis in a delivery room. Am J Dis Child 139:903, 1985.
96. Simmons MD, Cockcroft PM, Okubadejo OA. Neonatal listeriosis due to cross-infection in an obstetric theatre. J Infect 13:235, 1986.
97. Graham JC, Lanser S, Bignardi G, et al. Hospital-acquired listeriosis. J Hosp Infect 51:136, 2002.

98. Schuchat A, Lizano C, Broome CV, et al. Outbreak of neonatal listeriosis associated with mineral oil. Pediatr Infect Dis J 10:183, 1991.
99. Mitsuyama M, Takeya K, Nomoto K, et al. Three phases of phagocyte contribution to resistance against *Listeria monocytogenes.* J Gen Microbiol 106:165, 1978.
100. Cossart P, Mengaud J. *Listeria monocytogenes*: a model system for the molecular study of intracellular parasitism. Mol Biol Med 6:463, 1989.
101. Lu CY. The delayed ontogenesis of Ia-positive macrophages: implications for host defense and self-tolerance in the neonate. Clin Invest Med 7:263, 1984.
102. Denis M. Growth of *Listeria monocytogenes* in murine macrophages and its modulation by cytokines; activation of bactericidal activity by interleukin-4 and interleukin-6. Can J Microbiol 37:253, 1991.
103. Kolb-Maurer A, Gentschev I, Fries HW, et al. *Listeria monocytogenes*–infected human dendritic cells: uptake and host cell response. Infect Immun 68: 3680, 2000.
104. Gregory SH, Sagnimeni AJ, Wing EJ. Expression of the *inlAB* operon by *Listeria monocytogenes* is not required for entry into hepatic cells in vivo. Infect Immun 64:3983, 1996.
105. Marquis H, Doshi V, Portnoy DA. The broad-range phospholipase C and a metalloprotease mediate listeriolysin O–independent escape of *Listeria monocytogenes* from a primary vacuole in human epithelial cells. Infect Immun 63:4531, 1995.
106. Jones S, Portnoy DA. Characterization of *Listeria monocytogenes* pathogenesis in a strain expressing perfringolysin O in place of listeriolysin O. Infect Immun 62:5608, 1994.
107. Bouwer HGA, Gibbins BL, Jones S, Hinrichs DJ. Antilisterial immunity includes specificity to listeriolysin O (LLO) and non-LLO–derived determinants. Infect Immun 62:1039, 1994.
108. Gedde MM, Higgins DE, Tilney LG, Portnoy DA. Role of listeriolysin O in cell-to-cell spread of *Listeria monocytogenes.* Infect Immun 68:999, 2000.
109. Dubail I, Autret N, Beretti JL, et al. Functional assembly of two membrane-binding domains in listeriolysin O, the cytolysin of *Listeria monocytogenes.* Microbiology 147:2679, 2001.
110. Bonnemain C, Raynaud C, Reglier-Poupet H, et al. Differential roles of multiple signal peptidases in the virulence of *Listeria monocytogenes.* Mol Microbiol 51:1251, 2004.
111. Southwick FS, Purich DL. Intracellular pathogenesis of listeriosis. N Engl J Med 334:770, 1996.
112. De Chastellier C, Berche P. Fate of *Listeria monocytogenes* in murine macrophages: evidence for simultaneous killing and survival of intracellular bacteria. Infect Immun 62:543, 1994.
113. McGregor DD, Chen-Woan M. The cell response to *Listeria monocytogenes* is mediated by a heterogeneous population of immunospecific T cells. Invest Med 7:243, 1984.
114. Shen H, Miller JF, Fan X, et al. Compartmentalization of bacterial antigens: differential effects on priming of CD8 T cells and protective immunity. Cell 92:535, 1998.
115. Kaufmann SHE, Ladel CH. Application of knockout mice to the experimental analysis of infections with bacteria and protozoa. Trends Microbiol 2:235, 1994.
116. Havell EA, Spitalny GL, Patel PJ. Enhanced production of murine interferon gamma by T-cells generated in response to bacterial infection. J Exp Med 156:112, 1982.
117. Hsieh C-S, Macatonia SE, Tripp CS, et al. Development of T_H1 $CD4^+$ T cells through IL-12 producted by *Listeria*-induced macrophages. Science 206:547, 1993.
118. Serody JS, Poston RM, Weinstock D, et al. $CD4^+$ cytolytic effectors are inefficient in the clearance of *Listeria monocytogenes.* Immunology 88:544, 1996.
119. Harty JT, Bevan MJ. CD8 T-cell recognition of macrophages and hepatocytes results in immunity to *Listeria monocytogenes.* Infect Immun 64:3632, 1996.
120. Conlan JW, North RJ. Early pathogenesis of infection in the liver with the facultative intracellular bacteria *Listeria monocytogenes, Francisella tularensis,* and *Salmonella typhimurium* involves lysis of infected hepatocytes by leukocytes. Infect Immun 60:5164, 1992.
121. Tuma RA, Giannino R, Guirnalda P, et al. Rescue of CD8 T cell–mediated antimicrobial immunity with a nonspecific inflammatory stimulus. J Clin Invest 110:1493, 2002.
122. Chen-Woan M, McGregor DD, Goldschneider I. Activation of *Listeria monocytogenes*–induced prekiller T cells by interleukin-2. Clin Invest Med 7:287, 1984.
123. Kaufmann SHE, Hug E, de Libero G. *Listeria monocytogenes*–reactive T lymphocyte clones with cytolytic activity against infected target cells. J Exp Med 164:363, 1986.
124. Guo Y, Neisel DW, Ziegler HK, et al. *Listeria monocytogenes* activation of human peripheral blood lymphocytes: induction of non-major histocompatibility complex-restricted cytotoxic activity and cytokine production. Infect Immun 60:1813, 1992.
125. Conlan W, North R. Neutrophil-mediated lysis of infected hepatocytes: selective lysis of permissive host cells is a strategy for controlling intracellular infection in the liver parenchyma. Am Soc Microbiol News 59:563, 1993.
126. Boockvar KS, Granger DL, Poston RM, et al. Nitric oxide produced during murine listeriosis is protective. Infect Immun 62:1089, 1994.
127. Beckerman KP, Rogers HW, Corbett JA, et al. Release of nitric oxide during the T cell–independent pathway of macrophage activation: its role in resistance to *Listeria monocytogenes.* J Immunol 150:888, 199
128. Lien E, Ingalls RR. Toll-like receptors. Crit Care Med 30:S1, 2002.
129. Marr KA, Balajee SA, Hawn TR, et al. Differential role of MyD88 in macrophage-mediated responses to opportunistic fungal pathogens. Infect Immun 71:5280, 2003.
130. Seki E, Tsutsui H, Tsuji NM, et al. Critical roles of myeloid differentiation factor 88-dependent proinflammatory cytokine release in early phase clearance of *Listeria monocytogenes* in mice. J Immunol 169:3863, 2002.
131. Edelson BT, Unanue ER. MyD88-dependent but toll-like receptor 2-independent innate immunity to *Listeria*: no role for either in macrophage listericidal activity. J Immunol 169:3869, 2002.
132. Nakane A, Minagawa T, Kohanawa M, et al. Interactions between endogenous gamma interferon and tumor necrosis factor in host resistance against primary and secondary *Listeria monocytogenes* infections. Infect Immun 57:3331, 1989.
133. Havell EA. Production of tumor necrosis factor during murine listeriosis. J Immunol 139:4225, 1987.
134. Havell EA. Evidence that tumor necrosis factor has an important role in antibacterial resistance. J Immunol 143:2894, 1989.
135. Nakane A, Minagawa T, Kato K. Endogenous tumor necrosis factor (cachectin) is essential to host resistance against *Listeria monocytogenes* infection. Infect Immun 56:2563, 1988.
136. van Furth R, van Zwet TL, Buisman AM, van Dissel JT. Anti-tumor necrosis factor antibodies inhibit the influx of granulocytes and monocytes into an inflammatory exudate and enhance the growth of *Listeria monocytogenes* in various organs. J Infect Dis 170:234, 1994.
137. Wagner RD, Czuprynski CJ. Cytokine mRNA expression in livers of mice infected with *Listeria monocytogenes.* J Biol 53:525, 1993.
138. Buchmeier NA, Schreiber RD. Requirement of endogenous interferon-gamma production for resolution of *Listeria monocytogenes* infection. Proc Natl Acad Sci U S A 82:7404, 1985.
139. Tsukada H, Kawamura I, Arakawa M, et al. Dissociated development of T cells mediating delayed-type hypersensitivity and protective T cells against *Listeria monocytogenes* and their functional difference in lymphokine production. Infect lmmun 59:3589, 1991.
140. Havell E. Augmented induction of interferons during *Listeria monocytogenes* infection. J Infect Dis 153:960, 1986.
141. Suzue K, Asai T, Takeuchi T, Koyasu S. In vivo role of IFN-gamma produced by antigen-presenting cells in early host defense against intracellular pathogens. Eur J Immunol 33:2666, 2003.
142. Wang Q, Dziarski R, Kirschning CJ, et al. Micrococci and peptidoglycan activate TLR2→MyD88→IRAK→TRAF→NIK→IKK→NF-kappaB signal transduction pathway that induces transcription of interleukin-8. Infect Immun 69:2270, 2001.
143. Yan SR, Qing B, Byers DM, et al. Role of myD88 in diminished tumor necrosis factor alpha production by newborn mononuclear cells in response to lipopolysaccharide. Infect Immun 72:1223, 2004.
144. Miller MA, Skeen MJ, Lavine CL, Ziegler KH. IL-12-assisted immunization generates CD4+ T cell-mediated immunity to *Listeria monocytogenes.* Cell Immunol 222:1, 2003.
145. Neighbors M, Xu X, Barrat FJ, et al. A critical role for interleukin 18 in primary and memory effector responses to *Listeria monocytogenes* that extends beyond its effects on interferon gamma production. J Exp Med 194:343, 2001.
146. LaCourse R, Ryan L, North RJ. Expression of NADPH oxidase-dependent resistance to listeriosis in mice occurs during the first 6 to 12 hours of liver infection. Infect Immun 70:7179, 2002.
147. Grau GE, Taylor TE, Molyneux ME, et al. Tumor necrosis factor and disease severity in children with falciparum malaria. N Engl J Med 320:1586, 1989.

148. Bermudez LEM, Young LS. Tumor necrosis factor, alone or in combination with IL-2, but not IFN-γ, is associated with macrophage killing of *Mycobacterium avium* complex. J Immunol 140:3006, 1988.
149. Flesch IEA, Kaufmann SHE. Activation of tuberculostatic macrophage functions by gamma interferon, interleukin-4, and tumor necrosis factor. Infect Immun 58:2675, 1990.
150. Bazzoni F, Beutler B. The tumor necrosis factor ligand and receptor families. N Engl J Med 334:1717, 1996.
151. Sung SS, Jung LK, Walters JA, et al. Production of tumor necrosis factor cachectin by human B cell lines and tonsillar B cells. J Exp Med 168:1539, 1988.
152. Cui W, Lei MG, Silverstein R, Morrison DC. Differential modulation of the induction of inflammatory mediators by antibiotics in mouse macrophages in response to viable gram-positive and gram-negative bacteria. J Endotoxin Res 9:225, 2003.
153. Nishimura H, Emoto M, Hiromatsu K, et al. The role of gamma delta T cells in priming macrophages to produce tumor necrosis factor-alpha. Eur J Immunol 25:1465, 1995.
154. Mira JP, Cariou A, Grall F, et al. Association of TNF2, a TNF-alpha promoter polymorphism, with septic shock susceptibility and mortality: a multicenter study. JAMA 282:561, 1999.
155. Ferrante A, Staugas REM, Rowan-Kelly B, et al. Production of tumor necrosis factors alpha and beta by human mononuclear leukocytes stimulated with mitogens, bacteria, and malarial parasites. Infect Immun 58:3996, 1990.
156. Michie HR, Manogue KR, Spriggs DR, et al. Detection of circulating tumor necrosis factor after endotoxin administration. N Engl J Med 318:1481, 1988.
157. Galleli A, LeGarreo Y, Chadid L. Increased resistance and depressed delayed-type hypersensitivity to *Listeria monocytogenes* induced by pretreatment with lipopolysaccharide. Infect Immun 31:88, 1981.
158. Bortolussi R, Rajaraman K, Serushago B. Role of tumor necrosis factor-alpha and interferon gamma in newborn host defense against *Listeria monocytogenes* infection. Pediatr Res 32:460, 1992.
159. Brunda MJ. Interleukin-12. J Leukoc Biol 55:280, 1994.
160. Serbina NV, Kuziel W, Flavell R, et al. Sequential MyD88-independent and -dependent activation of innate immune responses to intracellular bacterial infection. Immunity 19:891, 2003.
161. McKay D, Lu C. Listeriolysin as a virulence factor in *Listeria monocytogenes* infection of neonatal mice and murine decidual tissue. Infect Immun 59:4286, 1991.
162. Bortolussi R. Neonatal listeriosis. Semin Perinatol 14:44, 1990.
163. Lu CY, Unanue ER. Ontogeny of murine macrophages: functions related to antigen presentation. Infect Immun 36:169, 1982.
164. Lu CY, Calamai EG, Unanue ER. A defect in the antigen-presenting function of macrophages from neonatal mice. Nature 282:327, 1979.
165. Darmochwal-Kolarz D, Rolinski J, Buczkowski J, et al. CD1c(+) immature myeloid dendritic cells are predominant in cord blood of healthy neonates. Immunol Lett 91:71, 2004.
166. Hamrick TS, Horton JR, Spears PA, et al. Influence of pregnancy on the pathogenesis of listeriosis in mice inoculated intragastrically. Infect Immun 71:5202, 2003.
167. Wilson CB. The ontogeny of T lymphocyte maturation and function. J Pediatr 118:S4, 1991.
168. Smith MA, Takeuchi K, Brackett RE, et al. Nonhuman primate model for *Listeria monocytogenes*–induced stillbirths. Infect Immun 71:1574, 2003.
169. Issekutz TB, Evans J, Bortolussi R. The immune response of human neonates to *Listeria monocytogenes* infection. Clin Invest Med 7:281, 1984.
170. Kurland G, Cheung ATW, Miller ME, et al. The ontogeny of pulmonary defenses: alveolar macrophage function in neonatal and juvenile rhesus monkeys. Pediatr Res 23:293, 1988.
171. McDonald T, Sneed J, Valenski WR, et al. Natural killer cell activity in very low birth weight infants. Pediatr Res 31:376, 1992.
172. Dominguez E, Madrigal JA, Layriss Z, Cohen SB. Fetal natural killer cell function is suppressed. Immunology 94:109, 1998.
173. Lee SM, Suen Y, Chang L, et al. Decreased interleukin-12 (IL-12) from activated cord versus adult peripheral blood mononuclear cells and upregulation of interferon-gamma, natural killer and lymphokine-activated killer activity by IL-12 in cord blood mononuclear cells. Blood 88:945, 1996.
174. Lau AS, Sigaroudinia M, Yeung MC, Kohl S. Interleukin-12 induces interferon-γ expression and natural killer cytotoxicity in cord blood mononuclear cells. Pediatr Res 39:150, 1996.
175. Bortolussi R, Issekutz T, Burbridge S, et al. Neonatal host defense mechanisms against *Listeria monocytogenes* infection: the role of lipopolysaccharides and interferons. Pediatr Res 25:311, 1989.
176. Murray HW. Gamma interferon, cytokine-induced macrophage activation, and antimicrobial host defense: in vitro, in animal models, and in humans. Diagn Microbiol Infect Dis 13:411, 1990.
177. Cederblad B, Riesenfeld T, Alm GV. Deficient herpes simplex virus-induced interferon-γ production by blood leukocytes of preterm and term newborn infants. Pediatr Res 27:7, 1990.
178. Lewis DB, Larsen A, Wilson CB. Reduced interferon-gamma mRNA levels in human neonates: evidence for an intrinsic T cell deficiency independent of other genes involved in T cell activation. J Exp Med 163:1018, 1986.
179. Lewis DB, Yu CC, Meyer J, et al. Cellular and molecular mechanisms for reduced interleukin-4 and interferon-γ production by neonatal T cells. J Clin Invest 87:194, 1991.
180. Bortolussi R, Burbridge S, Durnford P, et al. Neonatal *Listeria monocytogenes* infection is refractory to interferon. Pediatr Res 29:400, 1991.
181. Bortolussi R. *Escherichia coli* infection in neonates: humoral defense mechanisms. Semin Perinatol 14:40, 1990.
182. Bortolussi R, Issekutz A, Faulkner A. Opsonization of *Listeria monocytogenes* type 4b by human adult and newborn sera. Infect Immun 52:493, 1986.
183. Hertzig T, Weber M, Greiffenberg L, et al. Antibodies present in normal human serum inhibit invasion of human brain microvascular endothelial cells *by Listeria monocytogenes.* Infect Immun 71:95, 2003.
184. Klatt EC, Pavlova Z, Teberg AJ, et al. Epidemic perinatal listeriosis at autopsy. Hum Pathol 17:1278, 1986.
185. Reiss HJ, Potel J, Krebbs A. Granulomatosis infantiseptica eine durch einen spezifischen Erreger hervorgerufene fatale sepsis. Klin Wochenschr 29:29, 1951.
186. Armstrong RW, Fung PC. Brainstem encephalitis (rhombencephalitis) due to *Listeria monocytogenes*: case report and review. Clin Infect Dis 16:689, 1993.
187. Steele PE, Jacobs DS. *Listeria monocytogenes*: macroabscesses of placenta. Obstet Gynecol 53:124, 1979.
188. Topalovski M, Yang S, Boonpasat Y. Listeriosis of the placenta: clinicopathologic study of seven cases. Am J Obstet Gynecol 169:616, 1993.
189. Infections and inflammatory lesions of the placenta. *In* Fox H (ed). Pathology of the Placenta, 2nd ed. Toronto, WB Saunders, 1997, pp 309-311.
190. Presentation of case 15—1997. N Engl J Med 336:1439, 1997.
191. Ahlfors CE, Goetzman BW, Halstad CC, et al. Neonatal listeriosis. Am J Dis Child 131:405, 1977.
192. Krause VW, Embree JE, MacDonald SW, et al. Congenital listeriosis causing early neonatal death. Can Med Assoc J 127:36, 1982.
193. Hood M. Listeriosis as an infection of pregnancy manifested in the newborn. Pediatrics 27:390, 1961.
194. Kelly CS, Gibson JL. Listeriosis as a cause of fetal wastage. Obstet Gynecol 40:91, 1972.
195. Redline RW, Lu CY. Specific defects in the anti-listerial immune response in discrete regions of the murine uterus and placenta account for susceptibility to infection. J Immunol 140:3947, 1988.
196. Kalstone C. Successful antepartum treatment of listeriosis. Am J Obstet Gynecol 164:57, 1991.
197. Liner RI. Intrauterine *Listeria* infection: prenatal diagnosis by biophysical assessment and amniocentesis. Am J Obstet Gynecol 163:1596, 1990.
198. Petrilli ES, d'Ablaing G, Ledger WJ. *Listeria monocytogenes* chorioamnionitis: diagnosis by transabdominal amniocentesis. Obstet Gynecol 55:5S, 1964.
199. Loeb MB, Ford-Jones EL, Styliadis S, et al. Perinatal listeriosis. J Soc Obstet Gynecol Can 18:164, 1996.
200. Luft BJ, Remington JS. Effect of pregnancy on resistance to *Listeria monocytogenes* and *Toxoplasma gondii* infections in mice. Infect Immun 38:1164, 1982.
201. Bortolussi R, Campbell N, Krause V. Dynamics of *Listeria monocytogenes* type 4b infection in pregnant and infant rats. Clin Invest Med 7:273, 1984.
202. Menu E, Kinsky R, Hoffman M, et al. Immunoactive products of human placenta. IV. Immunoregulatory factors obtained from cultures of human placenta inhibit in vivo local and systemic allogeneic and graft-versus-host reactions in mice. J Reprod Immunol 20:195, 1991.
203. Guleria I, Pollard JW. The trophoblast is a component of the innate immune system during pregnancy. Nat Med 6:589, 2000.

204. Burn CG. Unidentified gram-positive bacillus associated with meningo-encephalitis. Proc Soc Exp Biol Med 31:1095, 1934.
205. Burn CG. Characteristics of a new species of the genus *Listerella* obtained from human sources. J Bacteriol 30:573, 1935.
206. Burn CG. Clinical and pathological features of an infection caused by a new pathogen of the genus *Listerella*. Am J Pathol 12:341, 1936.
207. Albritton WL, Wiggins GL, Feeley JC. Neonatal listeriosis: distribution of serotypes in relation to age at onset of disease. J Pediatr Infect Dis 4:237, 1976.
208. Evans JR, Allen AC, Stinson DA, et al. Perinatal listeriosis: report of an outbreak. Pediatr Infect Dis J 4:237, 1985.
209. Lennon D, Lewis B, Mantell C, et al. Epidemic perinatal listeriosis. Pediatr Infect Dis J 3:30, 1984.
210. Becroft DMO, Farmer K, Seddon RJ, et al. Epidemic listeriosis in the newborn. Br Med J 3:747, 1971.
211. McLachlin J. Human listeriosis in Britain, 1967-85: a summary of 722 cases. I. Listeriosis during pregnancy and the newborn. Epidemiol Infect 104:181, 1990.
212. Filice GA, Cantrell HF, Smith AB, et al. *Listeria monocytogenes* infection in neonates: investigation of an epidemic. J Infect Dis 138:17, 1978.
213. Visintine AM, Oleske JM, Nahmias AJ. *Listeria monocytogenes* infection in infants and children. Am J Dis Child 131:339, 1977.
214. Pron B, Boumaila C, Jaubert F, et al. Comprehensive study of the intestinal stage of listeriosis in a rat ligated ileal loop system. Infect Immun 66:747, 1998.
215. Dalton CB, Austin CC, Sobel J, et al. An outbreak of febrile gastroenteritis and fever due to *Listeria monocytogenes* in milk. N Engl J Med 336:100, 1997.
216. Dramsi S, Levi S, Triller A, Cossart P. Entry of *Listeria monocytogenes* into neurons occurs by cell-to-cell spread: an in vitro study. Infect Immun 66:4461, 1998.
217. Jurado RL, Farley MM, Pereira E, et al. Increased risk of meningitis and bacteremia due to *Listeria monocytogenes* in patients with human immunodeficiency virus infection. Clin Infect Dis 17:224, 1993.
218. Anton W. Kritisch-experimenteller Beitrag zur Biologie des Bacterium-monocytogenes mit besenderer Berücksichtigung seiner Beziehung zur infektiösen Mononukleose des Menschen. Zentralbl Bakteriol Hyg 131:89, 1934.
219. Frye DM, Zweig R, Sturgeon J, et al. An outbreak of febrile gastro-enteritis associated with delicatessen meat contaminated with *Listeria monocytogenes*. Clin Infect Dis 35:943, 2002.
220. Riedo FX, Pinner RW, Tosca ML, et al. A point-source foodborne listeriosis outbreak: documented incubation period and possible mild illness. J Infect Dis 170:693, 1994.
221. Salamina G, Niccolini A, Dalle Donne E, et al. A foodborne outbreak of gastroenteritis due to *Listeria monocytogenes*. Epidemiol Infect 117:429, 1996.
222. Schlech WF. *Listeria* gastroenteritis—old syndrome, new pathogen. N Engl J Med 336:130, 1997.
223. Felsenfeld O. Diseases of poultry transmissible to man. Iowa State Coll Vet 13:89, 1951.
224. Owen RC, Meis A, Jackson JW, et al. A case of primary cutaneous listeriosis. N Engl J Med 262:1026, 1960.
225. Spyrou N, Anderson M, Foale R. Listeria endocarditis: current management and patient outcome—world literature review. Heart 77:380, 1997.
226. Jackson TL, Eykyn SJ, Graham EM, Stanford MR. Endogenous bacterial endophthalmitis: a 17-year prospective series and review of 267 reported cases. Surv Ophthalmol 48:403, 2003.
227. Betriu C, Fuentemilla S, Mendez R, et al. Endophthalmitis caused by *Listeria monocytogenes*. J Clin Microbiol 39:2742, 2001.
228. Braun TI, Travis D, Dee RR, Nieman RE. Liver abscess due to *Listeria monocytogenes*: case report and review. Clin Infect Dis 17:267, 1993.
229. Sivalingam JJ, Martin P, Fraimow HS, et al. *Listeria monocytogenes* peritonitis: case report and literature review. Am J Gastroenterol 87:1839, 1992.
230. Dylewski JS. Bacterial peritonitis caused by *Listeria monocytogenes*: case report and review of the literature. Can J Infect Dis 7:59, 1996.
231. Louthrenoo W, Schumacher HR. *Listeria monocytogenes* osteomyelitis complicating leukemia: report and literature review of *Listeria* osteoarticular infections. J Rheumatol 17:107, 1990.
232. Kolmer JA. *Listerella monocytogenes* in relation to the Wasserman and flocculation reactions in normal rabbits. Proc Soc Exp Biol Med 42:183, 1939.
233. Hudak AP, Lee SH, Issekutz AC, et al. Comparison of three serological methods—enzyme-linked immunoabsorbent assay, complement fixation, and microagglutination—in the diagnosis of human perinatal *Listeria monocytogenes* infection. Clin Invest Med 7:349, 1984.
234. Winblad S. Studies of antibodies in human listeriosis. Acta Pathol Microbiol Scand 58:123, 1963.
235. Berche P, Reiche KA, Bonnichon M, et al. Detection of anti-listeriolysin O for serodiagnosis of human listeriosis. Lancet 335:624, 1990.
236. Drew RM. Occurrence of two immunological groups within the genus *Listeria*: studies based upon precipitation reactions. Proc Soc Exp Biol Med 61:30, 1946.
237. Schierz G, Bürger A. The Detection of *Listeria* Antibodies by Passive Hemagglutination. Proceedings of the Third International Symposium on Listeriosis, Bilthoven, 1966, p 77.
238. Njoku-Obi AN. An antigen-fixation test for the serodiagnosis of *Listeria monocytogenes* infections. Cornell Vet 52:415, 1962.
239. Kampelmacher EH, Huysinga MT, van Noorle-Jansen ML. Het voorkomen van *Listeria monocytogenes* in faecesvan gravidae en pasgeborenen. Ned Tijdschr Geneeskd 116:1685, 1972.
240. Backman A, Lantz P, Radstrom P, Olcen P. Evaluation of an extended diagnostic PCR assay for detection and verification of the common causes of bacterial meningitis in CSF and other biological samples. Mol Cell Probes 13:49, 1999.
241. Lohmann CP, Gabel VP, Heep M, et al. *Listeria monocytogenes*–induced endogenous endophthalmitis in an otherwise healthy individual: rapid PCR—diagnosis as the basis for effective treatment. Eur J Ophthalmol 9:53, 1999.
242. Huijsdens XW, Linskens RK, Taspinar H, et al. *Listeria monocytogenes* and inflammatory bowel disease: detection of *Listeria* species in intestinal mucosal biopsies by real-time PCR. Scand J Gastroenterol 38:332, 2003.
243. Chiba M, Kono M, Hoshina S, et al. Presence of bacterial 16S ribosomal RNA gene segments in human intestinal lymph follicles. Scand J Gastroenterol 35:824, 2000.
244. Hune OS. Maternal *Listeria monocytogenes* septicemia with sparing of the fetus. Obstet Gynecol 48:335, 1976.
245. Katz VL, Weinstein L. Antepartum treatment of *Listeria monocytogenes* septicemia. South Med J 75:1353, 1982.
246. Fuchs S, Hochner-Celnikier D, Shalev O. First trimester listeriosis with normal fetal outcome. Eur J Clin Microbiol Infect Dis 13:656, 1994.
247. Rotheberg AD, Maisels MJ, Bagnato S, et al. Outcome for survivors of mechanical ventilation weighing less than 1200 gm at birth. J Pediatr 98:106, 1981.
248. Naege RL. Amnionic fluid infections, neonatal hyperbilirubinemia and psychomotor impairment. Pediatrics 62:497, 1978.
249. Line FG, Appleton FG. *Listeria* meningitis in a premature infant. J Pediatr 41:97, 1952.
250. Evans JR, Allen AC, Bortolussi R, et al. Follow-up study of survivors of fetal and early onset neonatal listeriosis. Clin Invest Med 7:329, 1984.
251. Espaze EP, Roubeix YG, LeBerre JY, et al. In vitro susceptibility of *Listeria monocytogenes* to some antibiotics and their combinations. Zentralbl Bakteriol Hyg 240:76, 1988.
252. Hof H. Therapeutic activities of antibiotics in listeriosis. Infection 19:S229, 1991.
253. McLauchlin J, Audurier A, Taylor AG. Treatment failure and recurrent human listeriosis. J Antimicrob Chemother 27:851, 1991.
254. Watson GW, Fuller TJ, Elms J, et al. *Listeria* cerebritis: relapse of infection in renal transplant patients. Arch Intern Med 138:83, 1978.
255. Hof H. Treatment of experimental listeriosis by CI 934, a new quinolone. J Antimicrob Chemother 25:121, 1990.
256. Spitzer PG, Hammer SM, Karchmer AW. Treatment of *Listeria monocytogenes* infection with trimethoprim-sulfamethoxazole: case report and review of the literature. Rev Infect Dis 8:427, 1986.
257. Armstrong RW, Slater B. *Listeria monocytogenes* meningitis treated with trimethoprim-sulfamethoxazole. Pediatr Infect Dis J 5:712, 1986.
258. Vischer WA, Rominger C. Rifampicin against experimental listeriosis in the mouse. Chemotherapy 24:104, 1978.
259. Poyart-Salmeran C, Carlier C, Trieu-Cuot P, et al. Transferable plasmid-mediated antibiotic resistance in *Listeria monocytogenes*. Lancet 355:1422, 1990.
260. MacGowan AP, Holt HA, Bywater MJ, et al. In vitro antimicrobial isolated in the UK and other *Listeria* species. Eur J Clin Microbiol Infect Dis 9:767, 1990.
261. Soriano F, Zapardiel J, Nieto E. Antimicrobial susceptibilities of *Corynebacterium* species and other non-spore-forming gram-positive bacilli to 18 antimicrobial agents. Antimicrob Agents Chemother 39:208, 1995.
262. Charpentier E, Gerbaud G, Jacquet C, et al. Incidence of antibiotic resistance in *Listeria* species. J Infect Dis 172:277, 1995.

263. Hof H, Nichterlein L, Kretschmar M. Management of listeriosis. Clin Microbiol Rev 10:345, 1997.
264. Traub WH. Perinatal listeriosis: tolerance of a clinical isolate of *Listeria monocytogenes* for ampicillin and resistance against cefotaxime. Chemotherapy 27:423, 1981.
265. Gordon RC, Barrett FF, Clark DJ. Influence of several antibiotics, singly and in combination, on the growth of *Listeria monocytogenes*. J Pediatr 80:667, 1972.
266. Carryn S, Van Bambeke F, Mingeot-Leclercq MP, Tulkens PM. Comparative intracellular (THP-1 macrophage) and extracellular activities of beta-lactams, azithromycin, gentamicin, and fluoroquinolones against *Listeria monocytogenes* at clinically relevant concentrations. Antimicrob Agents Chemother 46:2095, 2002.
267. Martinez-Martinez L, Joyanes P, Suarez AI, Perea EJ. Activities of gemifloxacin and five other antimicrobial agents against *Listeria monocytogenes* and coryneform bacteria isolated from clinical samples. Antimicrob Agents Chemother 45:2390, 2001.
268. Lavetter A, Leedom JM, Mathies AW Jr, et al. Meningitis due to *Listeria monocytogenes*: a review of 25 cases. N Engl J Med 285:598, 1971.
269. Eliopoulos GM, Moellering RC. Susceptibility of enterococci and *Listeria monocytogenes* to *n*-formimidoyl thienamycin alone and in combination with an aminoglycoside. Antimicrob Agents Chemother 19:789, 1981.
270. Fattal E, Rojas J, Youssef M, et al. Liposome-entrapped ampicillin in the treatment of experimental murine listeriosis and salmonellosis. Antimicrob Agents Chemother 35:770, 1991.
271. Edminsten CE, Gordon RC. Evaluation of gentamicin and penicillin as a synergistic combination in experimental murine listeriosis. Antimicrob Agents Chemother 16:862, 1979.
272. VanOgtrop ML, Mattie H, Razab SB, et al. Comparison of the antibacterial efficacies of ampicillin and ciprofloxacin against experimental infections with *Listeria monocytogenes* in hydrocortisone-treated mice. Antimicrob Agents Chemother 36:2375, 1992.
273. Hof P, Emmerling P, Seeliger HPR. Murine model for therapy of listeriosis in the compromised host. Chemotherapy 27:214, 1981.
274. Bakker-Woudenberg IAJM, de Bos P, van Leeuwen WB, et al. Efficacy of ampicillin therapy in experimental listeriosis in mice with impaired T-cell-mediated immune response. Antimicrob Agents Chemother 19:76, 1981.
275. Bakker-Woudenberg IAJM, Lokerse AF, Roerdink FH, et al. Free versus liposome-entrapped ampicillin in treatment of infection due to *Listeria monocytogenes* in normal and athymic (nude) mice. J Infect Dis 151:917, 1985.
276. Scheld WM, Fletcher DD, Fink FN, et al. Response to therapy in an experimental rabbit model of meningitis due to *Listeria monocytogenes*. J Infect Dis 140:287, 1979.
277. Hawkins AE, Bortolussi R, Issekutz AC. In vitro and in vivo activity of various antibiotics against *Listeria monocytogenes* type 4b. Clin Invest Med 7:335, 1984.
278. Dans PE, McGehee RF, Wilcox C, et al. Rifampin: antibacterial activity in vitro and absorption and excretion in normal young men. Am J Med Sci 259:120, 1970.
279. Hof H, Gukel H. Lack of synergism of ampicillin and gentamicin in experimental listeriosis. Infection 15:40, 1987.
280. Scheld WM. Evaluation of rifampin and other antibiotics against *Listeria monocytogenes* in vitro and in vivo. Rev Infect Dis 5:S593, 1983.
281. Cherubin CE, Appleman MD, Heseltine PNR, et al. Epidemiologic spectrum and current treatment of listeriosis. Rev Infect Dis 13:1108, 1991.
282. Weingartner L, Ortel S. Zur Behandlung der Listeriose mit Ampicillin. Dtsch Med Wochenschr 92:1098, 1967.
283. Fanos V, Dall'Agnola A. Antibiotics in neonatal infections: a review. Drugs 58:405, 1999.
284. Schlech WF. Expanding the horizons of foodborne listeriosis. JAMA 267:2081, 1992.
285. Centers for Disease Control and Prevention. Update: foodborne listeriosis—United States, 1988-1990. MMWR Morbid Mortal Wkly Rep 41:251, 1992.
286. Tappero JW, Schuchat A, Deaver KA, et al. Reduction in the incidence of human listeriosis in the United States. JAMA 273:1118, 1995.
287. Kessler SL, Dajani AS. Listeria meningitis in infants and children. Pediatr Infect Dis J 9:61, 1990.

Chapter 15

LYME DISEASE

Eugene D. Shapiro • Michael A. Gerber

Lyme disease, caused by the spirochete *Borrelia burgdorferi*, is the most common vector-borne illness in the United States. Although, in retrospect, a form of the illness had been recognized in Scandinavia in the early 1900s, modern awareness of Lyme disease began after a cluster of cases of "juvenile rheumatoid arthritis" in children living on one small street was reported by their parents in the mid-1970s. Investigation of this unexplained "epidemic" of arthritis led to the description of "Lyme arthritis" in 1976 and, ultimately, to the discovery of its bacterial etiology.[1-3] Both the reported incidence of Lyme disease and its geographic range have increased dramatically in recent years.[4]

Several spirochetes are known to cause transplacental infections in a variety of animals and in humans.[5-11] *Treponema pallidum* is the spirochete that has been the most thoroughly investigated with respect to transplacental transmission in humans.[5] Infection of the mother with *T. pallidum* during pregnancy frequently is associated with transplacental infection, resulting in congenital syphilis in the offspring. Congenital syphilis often is associated with clinically significant neurologic disease such as hydrocephalus, cerebral palsy, deafness, blindness, convulsive disorders, and mental retardation.[5] Adverse fetal outcomes also have been documented in gestational infections with *Leptospira canicola*, the etiologic agent of leptospirosis, and with other *Borrelia* species including *Borrelia recurrentis*, the etiologic agent of relapsing fever.[6-10] Because *B. burgdorferi* is a spirochete, whether it too can cause congenital infection naturally is of considerable interest.

*See references 75, 76, 80, 83, 85, 87, 88, 93, 96, 98, 101, 115, 121-124, 134, 140, 143.

EPIDEMIOLOGY AND TRANSMISSION

B. burgdorferi is transmitted by ticks of the ixodid species. In the United States, in both the Northeast and the upper Midwest, the usual vector is *Ixodes scapularis* (the black-legged tick), commonly called the deer tick, whereas *Ixodes pacificus* (the Western black-legged tick) is the usual vector on the Pacific Coast.[12] In Europe, the most important vector for the spirochete is *Ixodes ricinus*, which commonly feeds on sheep and cattle.

The life cycle of *I. scapularis* consists of three stages—larva, nymph, and adult—that develop during a 2-year period.[12] Ticks feed once during each stage of the life cycle. The larvae emerge in the early summer from eggs laid in the spring by the adult female tick. More than 95% of the larvae are born uninfected with *B. burgdorferi*, because transovarial transmission rarely occurs. The larvae feed on a wide variety of small mammals, such as the white-footed mouse, which are natural reservoirs for *B. burgdorferi*. Larvae become infected by feeding on animals that are infected with the spirochete. The tick emerges the following spring in the nymphal stage. It is this stage of the tick that is most likely to transmit infections to humans,[13] presumably because it is active at times during which humans are most likely to be in tick-infested areas and because it is very small and difficult to see. Consequently, it is more likely to be able to feed for a relatively long time, which increases the likelihood of transmission. If the nymphal tick is not infected with *B. burgdorferi*, it may subsequently become infected if it feeds on an infected animal in this stage of its development. The nymphs molt in the late summer or early fall and re-emerge as adults. If the adult is infected, it also may transmit *B. burgdorferi* to humans. The adult deer tick may spend the winter on an animal host, a favorite being white-tailed deer (hence its name, the deer tick). In the spring the females lay their eggs and die, thereby completing the 2-year life cycle.

A number of factors are associated with the risk of transmission of *B. burgdorferi* from infected ticks to humans. The proportion of infected ticks varies greatly, both by geographic area and by the stage of the tick in its life cycle. *I. pacificus* often feeds on lizards, which are not a competent reservoir for *B. burgdorferi*. Consequently, less than 5% of these ticks are infected with *B. burgdorferi*, so Lyme disease is rare in the Pacific states. By contrast, *I. scapularis* feeds on small mammals that are competent reservoirs for *B. burgdorferi*. As a result, in highly endemic areas the rates of infection for different stages of deer ticks are, approximately, 2% for larvae, 15% to 30% for nymphs, and 30% to 50% for adults.

B. burgdorferi is transmitted when an infected tick inoculates saliva into the blood vessels of the skin of its host. The risk of transmission of *B. burgdorferi* from infected deer ticks has been shown to be related to the duration of feeding.

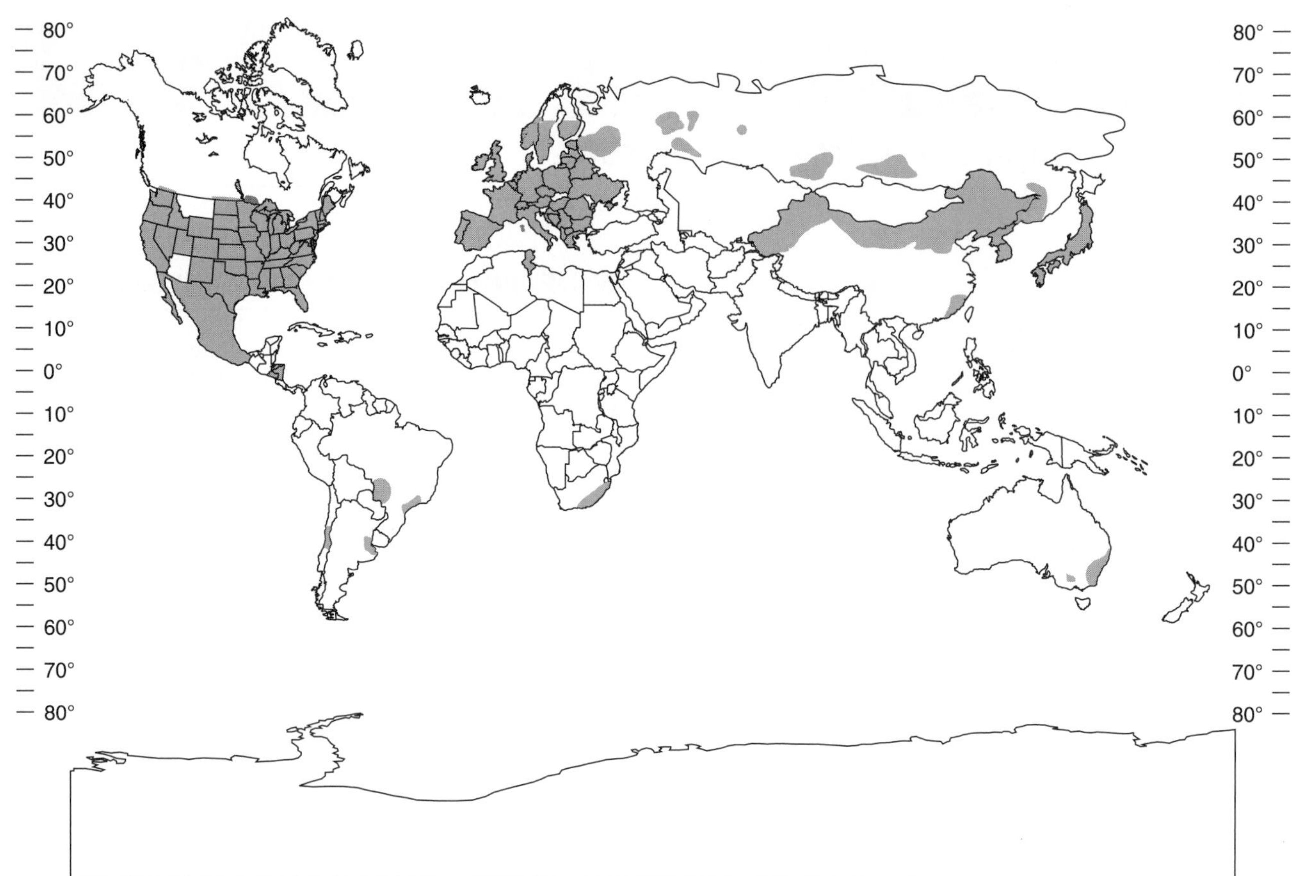

Figure 15–1 Worldwide geographic distribution of reported Lyme disease.

It takes hours for the mouth parts of ticks to implant in the host, and much longer (days) for the tick to become fully engorged from feeding. *B. burgdorferi* is found primarily in the midgut of the tick, but as the tick feeds and becomes engorged, the bacteria migrate to the salivary glands, from which they can be transmitted. Experiments with animals have shown that infected nymph-stage ticks must feed for 48 hours or longer and infected adult ticks must feed for 72 hours or longer before the risk of transmission of *B. burgdorferi* becomes substantial.[14-16] Results of a study of transmission of Lyme disease to humans are consistent with these experimental results.[13] Among persons bitten by nymphal stage ticks for which the duration of feeding could be estimated, the risk of Lyme disease was zero among persons bitten by nymphs that had fed for less than 72 hours but was 25% among persons bitten by nymphs that had fed for 72 hours or more. Approximately 75% of persons who recognize that they have been bitten by a deer tick remove the tick within 48 hours after it has begun to feed.[17] This may explain why only a small proportion of persons who recognize that they have been bitten by deer ticks subsequently develop Lyme disease. Indeed, the risk of Lyme disease probably is greater from *unrecognized* bites, because in such instances the tick is able to feed for a longer time.

Substantial evidence indicates that the risk of Lyme disease after a recognized deer tick bite, even in hyperendemic areas, is only 1% to 3%.[13,18,19] Unfortunately, the expertise to identify the species, stage, and degree of engorgement of a tick, and thereby to assess the degree of risk, is rarely available to persons who are bitten. Many "ticks" submitted for identification by physicians turned out actually to be spiders, lice, scabs, or dirt, none of which can transmit Lyme disease. In addition, estimates by patients of the duration for which the tick fed are unreliable.[20]

Lyme disease occurs throughout the world (Fig. 15-1). In the United States, most cases occur in a few highly endemic areas—southern New England, New York, New Jersey, Pennsylvania, Minnesota, and Wisconsin (Fig. 15-2).[21] In Europe, most cases occur in the Scandinavian countries and in central Europe (especially in Germany, Austria, and Switzerland), although cases have been reported from throughout the region.

Although an increase in frequency and an expansion of the geographic distribution of Lyme disease in the United States have occurred in recent years, the incidence of Lyme disease even in endemic areas varies substantially, both from region to region and within local areas. Information about the incidence of the disease is complicated by reliance, in most instances, on passive reporting of cases as well as by the high frequency of misdiagnosis of the disease. Furthermore, studies have indicated that some patients in whom serologic evidence of recent infection with *B. burgdorferi* develops are asymptomatic.[22,23]

A total of 17,730 cases of Lyme disease were reported to the Centers for Disease Control and Prevention (CDC) by 44 states and the District of Columbia in 2000 (a 9% increase

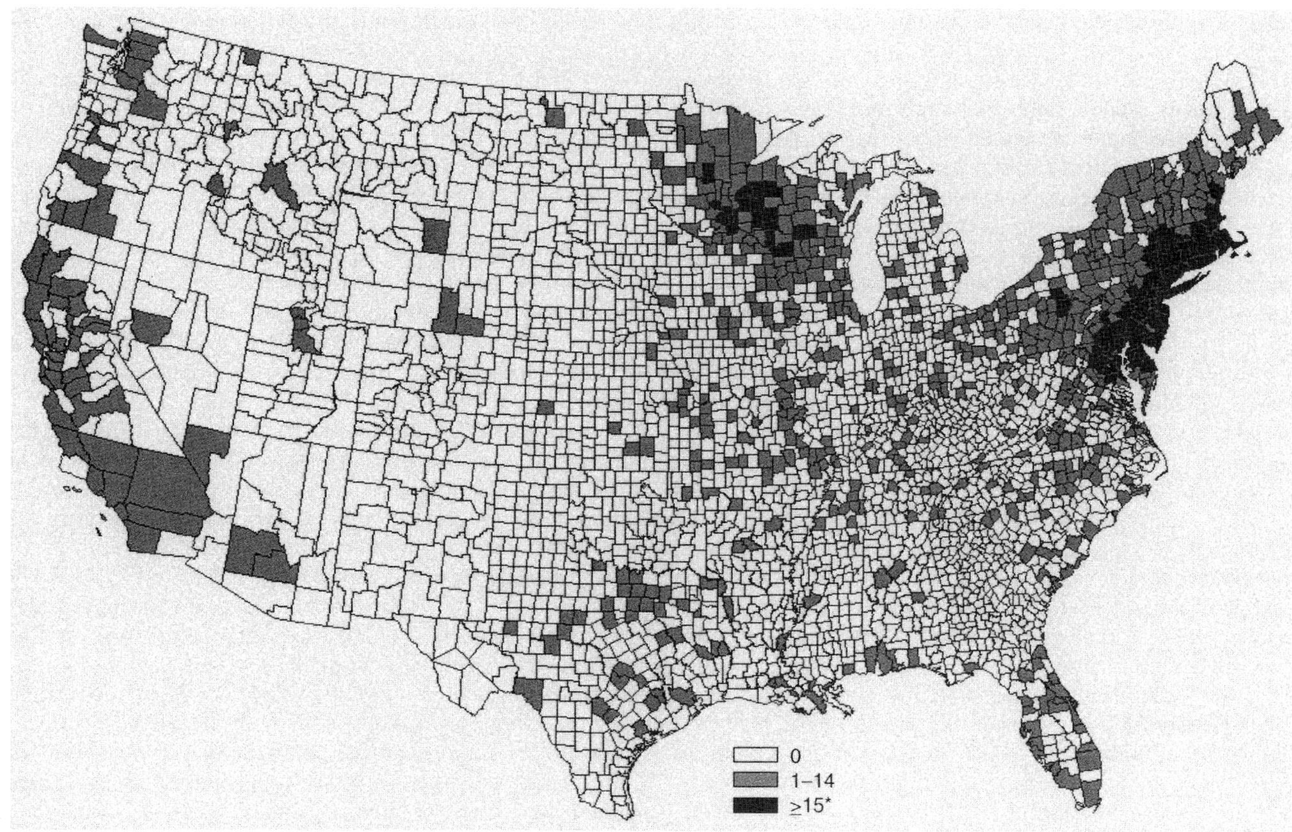

Figure 15–2 Number of cases of Lyme disease, by county: United States, 2000. (From MMWR Morb Mortal Wkly Rep 5:31, 2002 [available at http://www.cdc.gov/mmwr/PDF/wk/mm5102.pdf].)

from 1999).[21] Approximately 90% of the reported cases occurred in just 124 counties (see Fig. 15-2).

MICROBIOLOGY

The spirochetal bacterium *B. burgdorferi* is a fastidious, microaerophilic organism that in vitro must be grown on special media. It is a slow-growing bacterium with a cell membrane that is covered by flagella and a loosely associated outer membrane. Major antigens of the bacteria include the outer-surface lipoproteins OspA, OspB, and OspC (highly charged basic proteins of molecular masses of about 31, 34, and 23 kDa, respectively), as well as the 41-kDa flagellar protein. The organism is more properly classified as the *Borrelia burgdorferi* sensu lato ["in the broad sense"] species complex, which has been subclassified into several genospecies, among which the major ones that cause human diseases are *Borrelia burgdorferi* sensu stricto ["in the strict sense"], *Borrelia garinii*, and *Borrelia afzelii*. In the United States only *B. burgdorferi* sensu stricto has been isolated from humans. By contrast, substantial variability exists in the species of *B. burgdorferi* isolated from humans in Europe, most of which are either *B. garinii* or *B. afzelii*. The complete genome of the organism has been sequenced.[24] The biology of *B. burgdorferi* is complex, as might be expected in view of the complicated life cycle of this vector-borne bacterium, part of which is spent in ticks (with a primitive immune system) and part of which is spent in mammals, which have a highly evolved immune system. The reader is referred to other sources for detailed discussion of the biology of this organism.[25]

PATHOGENESIS AND PATHOLOGY

In approximately 90% of patients in the United States, Lyme disease begins with the characteristic expanding skin lesion, erythema migrans, at the site of the tick bite.[26,27] The spirochete subsequently disseminates by means of the bloodstream, producing the malaise, fatigue, headache, arthralgia, myalgia, fever, and regional lymphadenopathy that may be associated with early Lyme disease, as well as the clinical manifestations of early disseminated and, ultimately, of late Lyme disease. The spirochete's ability to spread through skin and other tissues may be facilitated by the binding of human plasminogen and its activators to the surface of the organism.[28] During dissemination, *B. burgdorferi* attaches to certain host integrins,[29,30] matrix glycosaminoglycans,[31] and extracellular matrix proteins,[32] which may explain the organism's particular tissue tropisms (e.g., collagen fibrils in the extracelluar matrix in the heart, nervous system, and joints).[31] In addition, the sequences of OspC vary considerably among strains, and only a few groups of sequences are associated with disseminated disease.[33]

Studies in mice have clearly demonstrated the importance of inflammatory innate immune responses in controlling early disseminated Lyme disease.[34,35] In humans with erythema migrans, infiltrates of macrophages and T cells produce both inflammatory and anti-inflammatory cytokines.[36] In addition, evidence suggests that in disseminated infections, adaptive T cell and B cell responses in lymph nodes produce antibodies against many components of the spirochete.[37,38]

A nonhuman primate animal model of neuroborreliosis has been developed to help elucidate the spread of *B. burgdorferi* within the nervous system.[39] In immunosuppressed monkeys with an exceptionally large spirochetal burden, *B. burgdorferi* infiltrated the leptomeninges, motor and sensory nerve roots, and dorsal root ganglia, but not the brain parenchyma.[40] *B. burgdorferi* also infiltrated the perineurium (the connective tissue sheath surrounding each bundle of peripheral nerve fibers) in the peripheral nervous system of these monkeys.

A C3H mouse model of Lyme carditis has been developed in which cardiac infiltrates of macrophages and T cells produce inflammatory cytokines.[41] In these mice, the killing of spirochetes through cellular immune mechanisms appears to be the dominant factor in the resolution of cardiac disease.[42]

Synovial tissue from patients with Lyme arthritis typically shows synovial hypertrophy, vascular proliferation, and a marked mononuclear cell infiltrate. Sometimes pseudolymphoid follicles are present that are reminiscent of peripheral lymph nodes.[43] During the attack of Lyme arthritis, innate immune responses to *B. burgdorferi* lipoprotein, as well as marked adaptive immune responses to many spirochetal proteins, are found.[38,44,45] A *Borrelia*-specific, inflammatory T_H1 response can be seen in the joint fluid; however, anti-inflammatory (T_H2) cytokines also may be present.[46,47] In addition, patients with Lyme arthritis typically have higher *Borrelia*-specific antibody titers than those in patients with other manifestation of Lyme disease.[38,48]

Investigations of Lyme arthritis in inbred strains of mice have demonstrated that severe, acute arthritis develops in certain strains of mice that are infected with *B. burgdorferi* but not in other strains.[49] The components of the immune response that account for these differences have yet to be identified. Effective innate immune responses, however, appear to be important in resistance to arthritis produced by infection with *B. burgdorferi*.[34,35] About 10% of adult patients with Lyme arthritis, particularly those with HLA-DRB1* 0401 or related alleles, will develop a chronic, antibiotic treatment–resistant, autoimmune arthritis.[50-52]

Several spirochetes have demonstrated the ability to cause transplacental infections in a variety of animals and in humans.[5-11] Transplacental transmission of *B. burgdorferi* has been documented in several animal studies, including case reports, case series, and transmission studies. *B. burgdorferi* has been cultured from fetal tissues of a coyote and a white-footed mouse, as well as from the blood of a newborn calf.[53-55] The presence of *B. burgdorferi* in fetal tissues of a white-footed mouse and a house mouse also has been demonstrated by polymerase chain reaction (PCR) assay.[56] Serologic evaluations also have been used to document in utero fetal infection with *B. burgdorferi* in an aborted calf, a newborn foal, and four beagle pups.[54,55,57] Several animal studies have linked infection with *B. burgdorferi* during pregnancy with fetal wastage and reproductive failure in cows and beagles.[55,57] Infection with *B. burgdorferi* during pregnancy also has been associated with reproductive failure and severe fetal infection in horses,[58] as well as with increased fetal loss in mice.[59]

In animal experiments, transplacental transmission of *B. burgdorferi* was documented by PCR assay in 19 of 40 pups born to female beagles that had been intradermally inoculated with this spirochete multiple times during pregnancy.[57] Only 4 of the 19 pups had culture-positive tissues, and none of the pups had any evidence of inflammation. In other studies, however, female rats inoculated with *B. burgdorferi* intraperitoneally at 4 days of gestation and pregnant hamsters infected by tick bite just before gestation showed no evidence by culture of transplacental transmission of *B. burgdorferi* to their offspring.[60,61] In another study, offspring of naturally infected white-footed mice were unable to transmit *B. burgdorferi* to spirochete-free deer ticks allowed to feed on them.[62]

Transplacental transmission of *B. burgdorferi* in humans has been demonstrated in association with adverse fetal outcome in several case reports. The first was a report by Schlesinger and co-workers in 1985[63] that described a 28-year-old woman with untreated Lyme disease during the first trimester of pregnancy, who gave birth, at 35 weeks of gestation, to an infant with widespread cardiovascular abnormalities. This infant died during the first week of life, and postmortem examination showed spirochetes morphologically compatible with *B. burgdorferi* in the infant's spleen, kidneys, and bone marrow, but not in the heart. In contrast with the mononuclear cell infiltrate and proliferation of fibroblasts usually seen with congenital syphilis,[64] there was no evidence of inflammation, necrosis, or granuloma formation in the infant's heart or other organs. In 1987, MacDonald and co-workers[65] described a 24-year-old woman with untreated Lyme disease in the first trimester of pregnancy who gave birth at term to a 2500-g stillborn infant. *B. burgdorferi* was cultured from the liver, and spirochetes were seen in the heart, adrenal glands, liver, brain, and placenta with both immunofluorescence and silver staining techniques. No evidence of inflammation was seen, however, and no abnormalities were noted except for a small ventricular septal defect. Weber and co-workers in 1988[66] described a 37-year-old woman who received penicillin orally for 1 week for erythema migrans during the first trimester of pregnancy. She subsequently gave birth to a 3400-g infant at term who died at 23 hours of age, of what was believed to be "perinatal brain damage." *B. burgdorferi* was identified in the newborn's brain using immunochromogenic staining with monoclonal antibodies. No significant inflammation or other abnormalities, however, were found in any organ, including the brain, on postmortem examination. In 1997, Trevisan and co-workers[67] described an otherwise healthy child who presented with multiple annular, erythematous lesions, fever, and generalized lymphadenopathy at 3 weeks of age. These clinical abnormalities recurred throughout the first 3 years of life despite oral therapy with amoxicillin and josamycin. A skin biopsy revealed spirochetes by silver stain and was positive for *B. burgdorferi* by PCR assay. In addition, serologic studies were positive for infection with *B. burgdorferi*. The patient's mother had no history of either a tick bite or Lyme disease, but she had been involved in outdoor activities in an endemic area and had a weakly positive serologic test for Lyme disease.

Several case reports have described pregnant women with either erythema migrans or neuroborreliosis who received appropriate antimicrobial therapy at different stages of their pregnancies.[68-72] In none of these reports was there an association between Lyme disease in the mother and an adverse outcome of the pregnancy.

Transplacental transmission of *B. burgdorferi* also has been investigated in a study of 60 placentas from asymptomatic women who lived in an area endemic for Lyme disease and whose results on serologic testing by enzyme-linked immunosorbent assay (ELISA) were either positive or equivocal for antibodies to *B. burgdorferi*.[73] All 60 placentas were examined with a Warthin-Starry silver stain for evidence of infection with *B. burgdorferi*; 3 (5%) were positive for spirochetes. PCR assays for *B. burgdorferi* nucleotide sequences were performed on 2 of these 3 placentas and were positive in both. The women from whom these 3 placentas were obtained all had equivocal results on ELISAs and negative results on Western blot analysis for Lyme disease as well as negative results on serologic tests for syphilis. In addition, none of these women had a history of either a tick bite or a clinical course consistent with Lyme disease. All of these pregnancies had entirely normal outcomes.

In addition to the individual case reports, several published case series have assessed the relationship between Lyme disease in pregnant women and fetal outcomes. Two of these case studies were conducted by the CDC. The first was a retrospective investigation conducted in 19 women with Lyme disease during pregnancy who were identified by the investigators without knowing the fetal outcomes.[74] The adverse outcomes included prematurity, cortical blindness, intrauterine fetal death, syndactyly, and a generalized neonatal rash. Infection with *B. burgdorferi* could not be directly implicated as the cause of any of these outcomes, however. The second case series included 17 women who acquired Lyme disease during pregnancy and were evaluated prospectively.[75] One woman had a spontaneous abortion with no evidence of an infection with *B. burgdorferi* on either stains or cultures of the fetal tissue, one woman had an infant with isolated syndactyly, and 15 women were delivered of normal infants with no clinical or serologic evidence of infection with *B. burgdorferi*.

In 1999, Maraspin and co-workers[76] reported a series of 105 women with erythema migrans during pregnancy. Ninety-three (88.6%) of the 105 women had healthy infants delivered at term, 2 (1.9%) pregnancies ended with a miscarriage, and 6 (5.7%) ended with a preterm birth. One of the preterm infants had cardiac abnormalities, and 2 died shortly after birth. Four (3.8%) babies born at term had congenital anomalies (1 with syndactyly and 3 with urologic abnormalities). As with a previous study, infection with *B. burgdorferi* could not be directly implicated as the cause of any of these adverse outcomes.

Several epidemiologic studies of Lyme disease during pregnancy also have been conducted. In the first, Williams and co-workers[77] examined 421 serum specimens obtained from cord blood and found no association between the presence of IgG antibodies to *B. burgdorferi* and congenital malformations. In another study, Nadal and co-workers[78] investigated outcomes in 1434 infants of 1416 women for the presence of antibodies to *B. burgdorferi* at the time of delivery. Twelve (0.85%) of the women were found to be seropositive, but only 1 woman had a history consistent with Lyme disease during pregnancy. Of the infants born to the 12 seropositive women, 2 had transient hyperbilirubinemia; 1 had transient hypotonia; 1 was post term and small for gestational age, with evidence of chronic placental insufficiency; 1 had transient macrocephaly; and 1 had transient supraventricular extra beats. The infant born to the woman with a clinical history of Lyme disease during pregnancy had a ventricular septal defect. At follow-up evaluations approximately 9 to 17 months later, all of the children except for the child with the cardiac defect were entirely well, and none had serologic evidence of infection with *B. burgdorferi*.

In 1994, Gerber and Zalneraitis[79] surveyed neurologists in areas of the United States in which Lyme disease was endemic at that time to determine how many had seen a child with clinically significant neurologic disease whose mother had been diagnosed as having Lyme disease during pregnancy. None of the 162 pediatric and 37 adult neurologists who responded to the survey had ever seen a child whose mother had been diagnosed with Lyme disease during pregnancy. The investigators concluded that congenital neuroborreliosis was either not occurring or occurring at an extremely low frequency in areas endemic for Lyme disease. In a retrospective case-control study carried out in an area endemic for Lyme disease, 796 "case" children with congenital cardiac anomalies were compared with 704 "control" children without cardiac defects with respect to Lyme disease in their mothers either during or before the pregnancy.[80] No association was found between congenital heart defects and either a tick bite or Lyme disease in the mothers either within 3 months of conception or during pregnancy.

Investigators in New York performed two studies of the relationship between Lyme disease in pregnant women and adverse outcomes of the pregnancies. The first was an unselected, prospective, population-based investigation in an area endemic for Lyme disease in which approximately 2000 women in Westchester County, New York, were evaluated for clinical and serologic evidence of Lyme disease at the first prenatal visit and again at delivery.[81] Of these women, 11 (0.7%) were seropositive and 79 (4%) reported at the first prenatal visit that they had had Lyme disease sometime in the past. One woman with an untreated influenza-like illness in the second trimester had a negative result on serologic testing for Lyme disease at the prenatal visit but a positive result at delivery. In addition, during the study period, clinical Lyme disease was diagnosed in 15 pregnant women. No association was found between exposure of the mother to *B. burgdorferi* either before conception or during pregnancy and fetal death, prematurity, or congenital malformations. In the second study, the researchers compared 5000 infants, half from an area in which Lyme disease was endemic and half from an area without Lyme disease, who served as controls. The researchers found no significant difference in the overall incidence of congenital malformations between the two groups.[82] Although there was a statistically significant higher rate of cardiac malformations in the endemic area compared with that in the control area, no relationship was noted between a cardiac malformation and either a clinical history or serologic evidence of Lyme disease. The researchers concluded from the findings of these two studies that a pregnant woman with a past infection with *B. burgdorferi*, either treated or untreated, did not have an increased risk of early fetal loss or of having a low-birth-weight infant or an infant with congenital malformations.[82]

Two reports have documented the presence of *B. burgdorferi* in cow's milk. In 1988, Burgess[55] cultured *B. burgdorferi* from

1 of 3 samples of colostrum from cows but from none of 44 samples of cow's milk. Lischer and co-workers[83] used a PCR assay to identify nucleotide sequences of *B. burgdorferi* in the milk of a cow with clinical Lyme disease. In a similar investigation of human milk, Schmidt and co-workers[84] examined breast milk from two lactating women with erythema migrans and from three lactating women with no clinical evidence of Lyme disease. The breast milk samples from both women with erythema migrans tested positive for *B. burgdorferi* by PCR assay, whereas the breast milk samples from all three healthy women tested negative. No other reports have corroborated these findings in human milk, however, and transmission of Lyme disease through breast-feeding has never been documented.

CLINICAL MANIFESTATIONS

The clinical manifestations of Lyme disease depend on the stage of the illness—early localized disease, early disseminated disease, or late disease.[4,85] Erythema migrans, the manifestation of *early localized Lyme disease*, appears at the site of the tick bite, 3 to 30 days (typically 7 to 10 days) after the bite. Erythema migrans is found in about 90% of patients with objective evidence of infection with *B. burgdorferi*.[26,27,86] Erythema migrans begins as a red macule or papule and expands for days to weeks to form a large, annular, erythematous lesion that is at least 5 cm and as much as 70 cm in diameter (median, 15 cm). This rash may be uniformly erythematous, or it may appear as a target lesion with a variable degree of central clearing. It can vary greatly in shape and, occasionally, may have vesicular or necrotic areas in the center. Erythema migrans is usually asymptomatic but may be pruritic or painful, and it may be accompanied by systemic findings such as fever, malaise, headache, regional lymphadenopathy, stiff neck, myalgia, or arthralgia.

The most common manifestation of *early disseminated Lyme disease* in the United States is multiple erythema migrans. The secondary skin lesions, which usually appear from 3 to 5 weeks after the tick bite, consist of multiple annular erythematous lesions similar to, but usually smaller than, the primary lesion. Other common manifestations of early disseminated Lyme disease are cranial nerve palsies, especially facial nerve palsy, and meningitis. Systemic symptoms such as fever, myalgia, arthralgia, headache, and fatigue also are common in this stage of Lyme disease. Carditis, which usually is manifested by various degrees of heart block, is a rare manifestation of early disseminated disease.[27]

The most common manifestation of *late Lyme disease*, which occurs weeks to months after the initial infection, is arthritis. The arthritis is usually monoarticular or oligoarticular and affects the large joints, particularly the knee. Although the affected joint often is swollen and tender, the intense pain associated with a septic arthritis usually is not present; not infrequently, the swollen joint is only mildly symptomatic. Encephalitis, encephalopathy, and polyneuropathy also are manifestations of late Lyme disease, but they are rare.

The clinical manifestations of Lyme disease also may depend on which subspecies of *B. burgdorferi* is causing the infection.[26] The differences in subspecies found in Europe and in North America may account for differences in the frequencies of certain clinical manifestations of Lyme disease in these areas. For example, neurologic manifestations of Lyme disease are more common in Europe, whereas rheumatologic manifestations are more common in North America. In addition, certain skin and soft tissue manifestations of Lyme disease, such as acrodermatitis chronica atrophicans and lymphocytomas, occur in Europe but are extremely rare in the United States.

Ixodes ticks may transmit other pathogens in addition to *B. burgdorferi*, including *Babesia*, *Ehrlichia*, other *Borrelia* species, and viruses. These agents may be transmitted either separately from or simultaneously with *B. burgdorferi*. The frequency with which co-infection occurs is unknown, however, and its impact on both the clinical presentation and the response to treatment of Lyme disease is not well established.

DIAGNOSIS

The CDC clinical case definition for Lyme disease initially was intended for epidemiologic surveillance purposes.[87] When used in conjunction with CDC and Food and Drug Administration (FDA) guidelines for diagnostic tests,[87-89] however, this case definition has been widely accepted as a means to standardize the clinical diagnosis of Lyme disease (Table 15-1).

Table 15–1 CDC Lyme Disease Case Definition for Public Health Surveillance Purposes

Erythema migrans

Single primary red macule or papule, expanding over days to weeks to large round lesion ≥5-cm diameter (physician-confirmed), ± central clearing, ± secondary lesions, ± systemic symptoms (fever, fatigue, headache, mild neck stiffness, arthralgia, myalgia)

PLUS

Known exposure ≤30 days before onset to an endemic area (in which ≥2 confirmed cases have been acquired, or in which *B. burgdorferi*–infected tick vectors are established)

OR

One or more late manifestations without other etiology:

1. Musculoskeletal
   –Recurrent brief episodes of monarticular or pauciarticular arthritis with objective joint swelling, ± chronic arthritis
2. Neurologic
   –Lymphocytic meningitis, facial palsy, other cranial neuritis, radiculoneuropathy, encephalomyelitis (confirmed by CSF *B. burgdorferi* antibody > serum *B. burgdorferi* antibody)
3. Cardiovascular
   –Acute second- or third-degree atrioventricular conduction defects, lasting days to weeks, ± myocarditis

PLUS

Laboratory confirmation by either:

1. Isolation of *B. burgdorferi* from patient specimen
2. Diagnostic levels of *B. burgdorferi* IgM or IgG antibodies in serum or CSF (initial ELISA or IFA screen followed by Western blot of positive or equivocal results)

CDC, Centers for Disease Control and Prevention; CSF, cerebrospinal fluid; ELISA, enzyme-linked immunosorbent assay; IFA, immunofluorescence assay.

Adapted from Centers for Disease Control and Prevention. MMWR Morb Mortal Wkly Rep 46(RR):20–21, 1997.

For patients in locations endemic for Lyme disease who present with the characteristic lesion of erythema migrans, the diagnosis of Lyme disease should be based on the clinical presentation alone. In such situations, laboratory testing is neither necessary nor recommended. With the exception of erythema migrans, however, the clinical manifestations of Lyme disease are nonspecific. Therefore, for patients who do not have erythema migrans, the diagnosis of Lyme disease should be based on clinical findings supported by results of laboratory tests. These laboratory tests may consist of either direct identification of *B. burgdorferi* in the patient or demonstration of a serologic response to the organism.

Methods for identifying the presence of *B. burgdorferi* in a patient (e.g., culture, histopathologic examination, antigen detection) generally have poor sensitivity and/or specificity and may require invasive procedures (such as a biopsy of the skin) to obtain an appropriate specimen for testing. Isolation of *B. burgdorferi* from a symptomatic patient should be considered diagnostic of Lyme disease. *B. burgdorferi* has been isolated from blood, skin biopsies, cerebrospinal fluid (CSF), myocardial biopsies, and the synovium of patients with Lyme disease. The medium in which *B. burgdorferi* is cultured is expensive, however, and it can take as long as 6 weeks for the spirochete to grow in culture. The best chance of culturing *B. burgdorferi* from a patient is when erythema migrans is present,[90] although at this stage of the disease, the diagnosis should be largely clinical. During the later stages of Lyme disease, culture is much less sensitive. In addition, it is necessary for patients to undergo an invasive procedure, such as a biopsy, to obtain appropriate tissue or fluid for culture. Therefore, culture is indicated only in rare circumstances.

B. burgdorferi has been identified with silver stains (Warthin-Starry or modified Dieterle) and with immunohistochemical stains (with monoclonal or polyclonal antibodies) in skin, synovial, and myocardial biopsies. *B. burgdorferi* can be confused with normal tissue structures, however, or it may be missed, because it often is present in low concentrations. Considerable training and experience are needed for skill in identifying spirochetes in tissues. Therefore, direct detection of *B. burgdorferi* in tissue is of limited practical value.

Attempts have been made to develop antigen-based diagnostic tests for Lyme disease, but no convincing data indicating the accuracy of any of these tests are available. All of these tests should be considered experimental until additional studies confirm their validity and reproducibility. Assays to detect *B. burgdorferi* antigens in CSF or urine, including the Lyme urine antigen test (LUAT) based on the procedure of Hyde and colleagues,[91,92] have both poor specificity and poor sensitivity and therefore are not recommended.[93]

Tests that use PCR techniques to identify *B. burgdorferi* may be helpful. However, results of such tests may be positive for some time after the spirochetes are no longer viable. In addition, the risk of false-positive results on PCR assays is great, especially when they are performed in commercial laboratories. If a PCR test is done, it should be performed in a reference laboratory that meets the highest standards of quality control for diagnostic PCR assays.[92] Because of its limited availability, expense, and insufficient evidence of its value in the management of most patients, PCR is at present reserved for special situations.[94] Use of PCR assay may be appropriate in testing of specimens such as synovial tissue or fluid from patients with persistent arthritis after a course of appropriate antibiotic therapy for late Lyme disease; samples of abnormal CSF from patients who are seropositive for antibodies to *B. burgdorferi* and have a neurologic illness that is compatible with, but not typical of, Lyme disease; and skin biopsy specimens from patients who have a localized rash that is consistent with erythema migrans but have no history of possible exposure or either residence in, or travel to, areas where Lyme disease is endemic.[94] Currently there is insufficient evidence of the accuracy, predictive value, or clinical significance of a PCR test of urine for *B. burgdorferi*, and its use for decisions regarding the management of patients has been strongly discouraged.[94]

Because of the limitations of laboratory tests designed to identify directly the presence of *B. burgdorferi* in a patient, the confirmation of Lyme disease in patients without erythema migrans usually is based on the demonstration of antibodies to *B. burgdorferi* in the serum. The normal antibody response to acute infection with *B. burgdorferi* is well described.[95] Specific immunoglobulin M (IgM) antibodies appear first, usually 3 to 4 weeks after the infection begins. These antibodies peak after 6 to 8 weeks and subsequently decline. However, a prolonged elevation of IgM antibodies sometimes is seen even after effective antimicrobial treatment.[96] Consequently, the results of serologic tests for specific IgM antibodies should not be used as the sole indicator of the timing of an infection. Specific IgG antibodies usually appear 6 to 8 weeks after the onset of the infection. These antibodies peak in 4 to 6 months. The IgG antibody titer may decline after treatment, but even after the patient is clinically cured, these antibodies usually remain detectable for many years.[97,98]

The immunofluorescent antibody test was the initial serologic test for diagnosing Lyme disease. It requires subjective interpretation and is time-consuming to perform, however, and has largely been replaced by ELISA. The ELISA method may give false-positive results because of cross-reactive antibodies in patients with other spirochetal infections (e.g., syphilis, leptospirosis, relapsing fever), certain viral infections (e.g., varicella), and certain autoimmune diseases (e.g., systemic lupus erythematosus). Unlike patients with syphilis, those with Lyme disease do not have positive results on nontreponemal tests for syphilis such as the Venereal Disease Research Laboratory (VDRL) test or rapid plasma reagin (RPR) determination. In addition, antibodies directed against bacteria in the normal oral flora may cross-react with antigens of *B. burgdorferi* to produce a false-positive ELISA result.

The first-generation ELISA method uses either whole cells of *B. burgdorferi* or the supernatant of sonicated spirochetes as the antigen. To improve the specificity of the ELISA, new assays have been developed that use less complex fractions of the spirochetes, such as the bacterial membrane, or purified native or recombinant proteins, alone or in combination.[94]

Immunoblot (Western blot) analysis for serum antibodies to *B. burgdorferi* also is used as a serologic test for Lyme disease. Although some investigators have suggested that the immunoblot is both more sensitive and more specific than the ELISA, there is still some debate about its interpretation. The immunoblot is most useful for validating a positive or equivocal ELISA result, especially in patients with a low clinical likelihood of having Lyme disease. For serologic testing for Lyme disease, it is recommended that a sensitive ELISA be performed, and, if results are either positive or equivocal, that a Western blot analysis be done to confirm the specificity of the result.[88] Specimens that give a negative result on a sensitive ELISA do not require immunoblot testing.

One reason for the poor sensitivity of serologic tests for Lyme disease is that erythema migrans, which is the clinical finding that usually brings patients to medical attention, usually appears within 2 to 3 weeks of onset of infection with *B. burgdorferi.* Antibodies to *B. burgdorferi* often are not detected at this early stage of the disease. The antibody response to *B. burgdorferi* also may be abrogated in patients with early Lyme disease who receive prompt treatment with effective antimicrobial agent; in these patients, antibodies against *B. burgdorferi* may never develop, at least as a result of that exposure. Most patients with early, disseminated Lyme disease and virtually all patients with late Lyme disease, however, have serum antibodies to *B. burgdorferi.* Seropositivity may persist for years even after successful antimicrobial therapy. Ongoing seropositivity, even persistence of IgM, is not necessarily a marker of active infection. Likewise, serologic tests should not be used to assess the adequacy of antimicrobial therapy.

Unfortunately, serologic tests for Lyme disease have not been adequately standardized. Both the accuracy and the reproducibility of currently available serologic tests, especially widely used, commercially produced kits, are poor.[99-103] Use of these commercial diagnostic test kits for Lyme disease will result in a high rate of misdiagnosis. Moreover, as with any diagnostic test, the predictive value of serologic tests for Lyme disease depends primarily on the probability that the patient has Lyme disease based on the clinical and epidemiologic history and the physical examination (the "pretest probability" of Lyme disease). Use of serologic tests to "rule out" Lyme disease in patients with a low probability of the illness will result in a very high proportion of test results that are falsely positive.[104] Therefore, antibody tests for Lyme disease should *not* be used as screening tests.[89,104,105] With few exceptions, the probability that a patient has Lyme disease will be very low in areas in which Lyme disease is rare. Even in areas with a high prevalence of Lyme disease, patients with *only* nonspecific signs and symptoms, such as fatigue, headache, and arthralgia, are not likely to have Lyme disease.[104,105] Although such nonspecific symptoms are common in patients with Lyme disease, they are almost always accompanied by more specific objective findings such as erythema migrans, facial nerve palsy, or arthritis. Even when more accurate tests performed by reference laboratories are available, clinicians should order serologic tests for Lyme disease selectively, reserving them for patients from populations with a relatively high prevalence of Lyme disease who have specific objective clinical findings that are suggestive of Lyme disease, so that the predictive value of a positive result is high.[104-106]

Clinicians should realize that even though a symptomatic patient has a positive result on serologic testing for antibodies to *B. burgdorferi,* Lyme disease may not be the cause of that patient's symptoms. In addition to the possibility that it is a falsely positive result (a common occurrence), the patient may have been infected with *B. burgdorferi* previously, and the patient's symptoms may be unrelated to that previous infection. As noted earlier, once serum antibodies to *B. burgdorferi* do develop, they may persist for many years despite adequate treatment and clinical cure of the illness.[97,98] In addition, because symptoms never develop in some people who become infected with *B. burgdorferi,* in endemic areas there will be a background rate of seropositivity among patients who have never had clinically apparent Lyme disease.

The diagnosis of an infection of the central nervous system with *B. burgdorferi* is made by demonstrating the presence of inflammation in the CSF as well as *Borrelia*-specific intrathecal antibodies.[92,107] Most patients with typical cases of Lyme neuroborreliosis have antibodies to *B. burgdorferi* in serum, and testing for the presence of antibodies in the CSF usually is not necessary.[94] In some instances, however, examination of the CSF for antibodies to *B. burgdorferi* may be indicated. Because antibodies to *B. burgdorferi* may be present in the CSF as the result of passive transit through a leaky blood-brain barrier, detection of antibodies in the CSF is not proof of infection of the CNS by the organism. Better evidence of CNS disease is the demonstration of intrathecal production of antibodies. This is accomplished by simultaneously measuring the antibodies in the serum and CSF by ELISA and calculating the "CSF index."[94] As noted previously, a PCR test of the CSF may be helpful in confirming the diagnosis of CNS Lyme disease.[92,94]

A lymphoproliferative assay that assesses the cell-mediated immune response to *B. burgdorferi* has been developed and used as a diagnostic test for Lyme disease. This assay has not been standardized, however, and is not approved by the FDA. The indications for this lymphoproliferative assay are few, if any.[94]

The diagnosis of Lyme disease in a pregnant woman should be made in accordance with the currently accepted CDC case definition (see Table 15-1). There is no indication for routine prenatal serologic screening of asymptomatic healthy women. Serosurveys have demonstrated that the seroprevalence rates among pregnant women were comparable with those in the general population[81,82,108] and that asymptomatic seroconversion during pregnancy was unusual.[81]

MANAGEMENT AND TREATMENT

Pediatricians are sometimes confronted with the challenge of how to manage a baby born to a woman who was diagnosed with Lyme disease during her pregnancy. The difficulty arises because of the paucity of evidence that congenital Lyme disease is a clinical problem. In addition, for reasons cited earlier, the diagnosis in the mother often is not accurate. First, parents should be reassured that there is no evidence that the child is at increased risk of any problem from maternal Lyme disease. Next, an attempt should be made to ascertain the accuracy of the diagnosis in the mother; if the mother did not have objective signs of Lyme disease (e.g., erythema migrans) or if the diagnosis was based on nonspecific symptoms (e.g., fatigue, myalgia) and a positive serology, it is likely that the diagnosis is not accurate. There is no reason to order serologic tests for Lyme disease in infants who are asymptomatic (even if diagnosis of Lyme disease in the mother is accurate). If such tests are ordered, it is important to remember that if the mother did have Lyme disease and is seropositive, the infant may have passively acquired antibodies from the mother and so may remain seropositive for many months even in the absence of infection.

Table 15–2 Antimicrobial Treatment of Lyme Disease

Early Disease

Localized Erythema Migrans

Doxycycline, 2-4 mg/kg/day divided bid (maximum: 100 mg/dose) for 10-21 days (do not use in children < 8 years of age), or amoxicillin, 50 mg/kg/day divided tid (maximum: 500 mg/dose) for 14-21 days. The preferred alternative agent for those who cannot take either amoxicillin or doxycycline is cefuroxime axetil, 30 mg/kg/day divided bid (maximum: 500 mg/dose) for 14-21 days. Erythromycin or azithromycin are less effective alternatives for patients who cannot take the other recommended agents.

Early Disseminated Disease

Multiple Erythema Migrans

Treat as for localized erythema migrans but for 21 days

Neurologic Disease

1. Isolated seventh nerve or other cranial nerve palsy

Treat as for localized erythema migrans but for 21-28 days

2. Meningitis (with or without encephalitis or radiculoneuritis)

Ceftriaxone: 75-100 mg/kg once daily (maximum: 2 g/dose) for 14-28 days

Alternatives include penicillin G, 200,000-400,000 units/kg/day (maximum: 18-24 million units/day) divided q4h or cefotaxime 150 mg/kg/day (maximum: 2 g/dose) divided q8h for 14-28 days

Carditis

1. First- or second-degree heart block

Treat as for localized erythema migrans

2. Third-degree heart block or other evidence of severe carditis

Treat as for meningitis

Late Disease

Arthritis

Doxycycline, 2-4 mg/kg/day divided bid (maximum: 100 mg/dose) for 28 days (do not use in children <8 years of age), or amoxicillin, 50 mg/kg/day divided tid (maximum: 500 mg/dose) for 28 days. The preferred alternative agent for those who cannot take either amoxicillin or doxycycline is cefuroxime axetil, 30 mg/kg/day divided bid (maximum: 500 mg /dose) for 28 days. For recurrent or persistent arthritis for which oral treatment has failed, either a second course of one of the orally administered agents for 28 days or a course of parenteral treatment for 14-28 days (as for meningitis) is indicated.

Neurologic Disease

As for meningitis above for 14-28 days

Because of the high frequency of false-positive test results, a positive test for IgM antibodies against *B. burgdorferi* in an asymptomatic child should be interpreted with a high degree of skepticism.

The choice of antibiotic and the duration of treatment for Lyme disease depend on the stage of the disease that is being treated (Table 15-2). In general, pregnant women should receive the same treatment as for other patients, except that use of doxycycline is not recommended during pregnancy.

Early Localized Disease

Doxycycline is the drug of choice for children 8 years of age and older with early localized Lyme disease.[109] Exposure to the sun should be avoided by persons who are taking doxycycline, because a rash develops in sun-exposed areas 20% to 30% of the time. Use of sunscreen may decrease this risk. Amoxicillin is recommended for children younger than 8 years of age, for pregnant women, and for patients who cannot tolerate doxycycline. For patients allergic to penicillin, alternative drugs are cefuroxime axetil, erythromycin, and azithromycin. Erythromycin and azithromycin may be less effective than other agents. Most experts recommend a 14- to 21-day course of therapy for early localized Lyme disease, although evidence indicates that 10 days of doxycycline constitutes adequate treatment in adults with uncomplicated infection.[110] A prompt clinical response to treatment is usual, with resolution of the erythema migrans within several days of initiating therapy. Occasionally, a Jarisch-Herxheimer reaction, which usually consists of an elevated temperature and worsening myalgia, develops shortly after antimicrobial treatment is initiated. These reactions typically last 1 to 2 days and do not constitute an indication to discontinue antimicrobial therapy, and symptoms respond to nonsteroidal anti-inflammatory agents. Appropriate treatment of erythema migrans almost always prevents development of the later stages of Lyme disease.

Early Disseminated and Late Disease

Multiple erythema migrans and initial episodes of arthritis should be treated with orally administered antimicrobial agents. If peripheral facial nerve palsy is the only neurologic manifestation of Lyme disease, the patient can be given an oral regimen of antimicrobials. If the facial nerve palsy is accompanied by clinical evidence of central nervous system involvement (e.g., severe headache, nuchal rigidity), a lumbar puncture should be performed. If there is pleocytosis, parenterally administered antimicrobials should be prescribed. Meningitis and recurrent or persistent arthritis also should be treated with parenterally administered antimicrobial agents. Some experts, however, will prescribe a second course of an orally administered antimicrobial agent for recurrent or persistent arthritis before using a parenterally administered agent. Nonsteroidal anti-inflammatory agents are a useful adjunct to antimicrobial therapy for patients with arthritis. Although mild carditis is usually treated orally with either doxycycline or amoxicillin, most experts recommend parenterally administered therapy for severe carditis. Other neurologic manifestations of late Lyme disease (e.g., encephalitis, encephalopathy, polyneuropathy) should be treated with antimicrobials administered parenterally.

The optimal duration of antimicrobial therapy for the various stages of Lyme disease is not well established, but there is no evidence that children with any manifestation of Lyme disease benefit from prolonged (longer than 4 weeks) courses of either orally or parenterally administered antimicrobial agents. Lyme disease, like other infections, may trigger a fibromyalgia syndrome that does not respond to additional courses of antimicrobials but may be managed with symptomatic therapy.

PROGNOSIS

Attempts to determine the potential impact of gestational Lyme disease on the outcome of the pregnancy have been limited for several reasons.[111] First, the prevalence of Lyme disease among pregnant women, even in highly endemic areas, is low, making it difficult to perform studies with sufficient statistical power. Second, diagnoses of gestational Lyme disease that are based on seropositivity, a history of a tick bite, or even a retrospective clinical history are often unreliable. Finally, because of increased awareness and concern about Lyme disease, it is difficult to find women with suspected gestational Lyme disease who did not receive antimicrobial treatment.

Despite these limitations, it is clear that *B. burgdorferi* can cross the placenta, presumably during a period of spirochetemia. The frequency and clinical significance of transplacental transmission of *B. burgdorferi* are unclear, however. Although a temporal relationship between Lyme disease during pregnancy and adverse outcomes has been documented, a causal relationship has not been established. The claims for the existence of a congenital Lyme disease syndrome are undermined by the absence of an inflammatory response in fetal tissue, absence of a fetal immunologic response, and lack of a consistent clinical outcome in affected pregnancies. An analysis of the current data indicates that there is no evidence of increased risk of abnormal outcomes with Lyme disease during pregnancy.

It is difficult to conduct high-quality studies of clinical outcome in persons with Lyme disease. On the basis of the available data, the long-term prognosis for adults or children who receive appropriate antimicrobial therapy for Lyme disease, regardless of the stage of the disease, appears to be excellent.[112] The most common reason for a lack of response to appropriate antimicrobial therapy for Lyme disease is misdiagnosis (i.e., the patient actually does not have Lyme disease). In approximately 10% of adults and less than 5% of children with Lyme arthritis, inflammatory joint disease develops that typically affects one knee for months to years and does not respond to antimicrobial therapy. An increased frequency of certain HLA-DR4 alleles has been noted among these patients, and recent findings suggest that an autoimmune process is involved.[52]

Nonspecific symptoms (such as fatigue, arthralgia, or myalgia) may persist for several weeks, even in patients with successfully treated early Lyme disease; their presence should not be regarded as an indication for additional treatment with antimicrobials. These symptoms usually respond to nonsteroidal anti-inflammatory agents. Within 6 months of completion of the initial course of antimicrobial therapy, these vague, nonspecific symptoms usually resolve without additional antimicrobial therapy. For those unusual patients who have symptoms persisting longer than 6 months after the completion of antimicrobial therapy, an attempt should be made to determine whether these symptoms are the result of a postinfectious phenomenon or have another etiology.

Klempner and co-workers recently reported the results of two controlled trials of antibiotic treatment for adult patients with chronic musculoskeletal pain, neurocognitive symptoms, or both that persisted after antibiotic treatment for Lyme disease.[113] One study included patients who were seropositive for IgG antibodies to *B. burgdorferi* at the time of enrollment; the other study included patients who were seronegative. In both studies, patients were randomly assigned to receive either ceftriaxone administered intravenously for 30 days, followed by doxycycline orally for 60 days, or matching regimens with placebos administered intravenously and orally in a double-blind manner. No significant differences were noted in the outcomes of patients in the antibiotic treatment group compared with those in the placebo group among either the seropositive or the seronegative patients. These findings support earlier recommendations that such patients are best managed with symptomatic treatment, rather than with prolonged courses of antibiotic therapy, which have been associated with serious adverse side effects.

PREVENTION

Reducing the risk of tick bites is one obvious strategy to prevent Lyme disease. In endemic areas, clearing brush and trees, removing leaf litter and woodpiles, and keeping grass mowed may reduce exposure to ticks. Application of pesticides to residential properties is effective in suppressing populations of ticks but may be harmful both to other wildlife and to people. Erecting fences to exclude deer from residential yards and maintaining tick-free pets also may reduce exposure to ticks.

Tick and insect repellents that contain *n,n*-diethylmeta-toluamide (DEET) applied to the skin provide additional protection, but most preparations require reapplication every 1 to 2 hours for maximum effectiveness. Serious neurologic complications in children from either frequent or excessive application of DEET-containing repellents have been reported, but they are rare and the risk is low when these products are used according to instructions on the label. Use of products with concentrations of DEET greater than 30% is not necessary and increases the risk of adverse effects. DEET should be applied sparingly only to exposed skin, but not to a child's face, hands, or skin that is either irritated or abraded. After the child returns indoors, skin that was treated should be washed with soap and water. Permethrin (a synthetic pyrethroid) is available in a spray for application to clothing only and is particularly effective because it kills ticks on contact.

Because most persons (approximately 75%) who recognize that they were bitten by a tick remove the tick within 48 hours,[17] the risk of Lyme disease from recognized deer tick bites is low—approximately 1% to 3% in areas with a high incidence of Lyme disease. Indeed, the risk of Lyme disease probably is higher from unrecognized bites (because in those cases the tick will feed for a longer time). A recent study of antimicrobial prophylaxis following tick bites among adults found that a single, 200-mg dose of doxycycline was 87% effective in preventing Lyme disease, although the 95% confidence interval around this estimate of efficacy was wide (the lower bound was 25% or less, depending on the method used).[13] In that study, the only persons in whom Lyme disease developed had been bitten by nymph-stage ticks that were at least partially engorged; the risk of Lyme disease in this group was 9.9% (among recipients of placebo), whereas it was zero for bites by all larval and adult deer ticks. Unfortunately, the expertise to identify the species, stage and degree of engorgement of a tick, and thereby to assess the degree of risk, is rarely available to persons who are bitten. Consequently, routine use of antimicrobial agents to prevent Lyme disease in persons who are bitten by a deer tick, even in highly endemic areas, generally is not recommended because the overall risk of Lyme disease is low. Only doxycycline (which is not recommended for children younger than 8 years of age) has been shown to be effective in prophylaxis of Lyme disease.[19] In the unusual instance in which doxycycline prophylaxis is used (e.g., in a nonpregnant patient older than 8 years of age who removes a fully engorged nymph-stage deer tick in an endemic area), only a single dose of doxycycline (200 mg) should be prescribed, and it should be taken with food to minimize nausea.

There is no evidence that pregnant women are at increased risk of Lyme disease after a deer tick bite. Moreover, the only drug that has been shown to be effective in preventing Lyme disease after a tick bite—doxycycline—is not recommended for use during pregnancy because of its possible effect on the developing fetus. Consequently, antimicrobial prophylaxis is not recommended for pregnant women.

Serologic testing for Lyme disease after a recognized tick bite also is not recommended. Antibodies to *B. burgdorferi* that are present at the time that the tick is removed likely would be due either to a false-positive test result or to an earlier infection with *B. burgdorferi*, rather than to a new infection from the recent bite. Likewise, in this setting the predictive value of a positive result is very low.

Ascertainment of whether the tick is infected, using tests such as the PCR assay, is also not recommended. Although testing ticks with a PCR assay may provide important epidemiologic information, the predictive values for infection of humans of either a positive or a negative PCR test result is unknown. The result may be positive even if only very few organisms are present, and it provides no information about the duration of feeding, a key determinant of the risk of transmission. In addition, the problems of both false-positive results due to contamination with amplification products and false-negative results due to inhibition of PCR by substances in the sample (such as blood) limit the test's validity.

People should be taught to inspect themselves and their children's bodies and clothing daily after possible exposure to ixodid ticks. An attached tick should be grasped with medium-tipped tweezers as close to the skin as possible and removed by gently pulling the tick straight out. If some of the mouth parts remain embedded in the skin, they should be left alone, because they usually are extruded eventually; additional attempts to remove them often result in unnecessary damage to tissue and may increase the risk of local bacterial infection.

REFERENCES

1. Steere AC, Malawista SE, Snydman DR, et al. Lyme arthritis: an epidemic of oligoarticular arthritis in children and adults in three Connecticut communities. Arth Rheum 20:7-17, 1977.
2. Burgdorfer W, Barbour AG, Hayes SF, et al. Lyme disease: a tick-borne spirochetosis? Science 216:1317-1319, 1982.
3. Steere AC, Grodzicki RL, Kornblatt AN, et al. The spirochetal etiology of Lyme disease. N Engl J Med 308:733-740, 1983.
4. Steere AC. Lyme disease. N Engl J Med 345:115-125, 2001.
5. Ingall D, Dobson SRM, Musher D. Syphilis. *In* Remington JS, Klein JD (eds). Infectious Diseases of the Fetus and Newborn Infant, 3rd ed. Philadelphia, WB Saunders, 1990, pp 367-394.
6. Fuchs PC, Oyama AA. Neonatal relapsing fever due to transplacental transmission of *Borrelia*. JAMA 208:690-692, 1969.
7. Coghlan JD, Bain AD. Leptospirosis in human pregnancy followed by death of the foetus. BMJ 1:228-230, 1969.
8. Lindsay S, Luke IW. Fatal leptospirosis (Weil's disease) in a newborn infant. J Pediatr 34:90-94, 1949.
9. Steenbarger JR. Congenital tick-borne relapsing fever: report of a case with first documentation of transplacental transmission. Birth Defects 18:39-45, 1982.
10. Yagupsky P, Moses S. Neonatal *Borrelia* species infection (relapsing fever). Am J Dis Child 139:74-76, 1985.
11. Lane RS, Burgdorfer W, Hayes SF, Barbour AG. Isolation of a spirochete from the soft tick, *Ornithodoros coriaceus*: a possible agent of epizootic bovine abortion. Science 230:85-87, 1985.
12. Lane RS, Piesman J, Burgdorfer W. Lyme borreliosis: relation of its causative agent to its vectors and hosts in North America and Europe. Annu Rev Entomol 36:587-609, 1991.
13. Nadelman RB, Nowakowski J, Fish D, et al. Prophylaxis with single-dose doxycycline for the prevention of Lyme disease after an *Ixodes scapularis* tick bite. N Engl J Med 345:79-84, 2001.
14. Piesman J, Mather TN, Sinsky R. Duration of tick attachment and *Borrelia burgdorferi* transmission. J Clin Microbiol 25:557-558, 1987.
15. Piesman J, Maupin GO, Campos EG, et al. Duration of adult female *Ixodes dammini* attachment and transmission of *Borrelia burgdorferi*, description of a needle aspiration isolation method. J Infect Dis 163:895-897, 1991.
16. Piesman J. Dynamics of *Borrelia burgdorferi* transmission by nymphal *Ixodes dammini* ticks. J Infect Dis 167:1082-1085, 1993.
17. Falco RC, Fish D, Piesman J. Duration of tick bites in a Lyme disease–endemic area. Am J Epidemiol 143:187-192, 1996.
18. Shapiro ED, Gerber MA, Holabird NB, et al. A controlled trial of antimicrobial prophylaxis for Lyme disease after deer-tick bites. N Engl J Med 327:1769-1773, 1992.
19. Shapiro ED. Doxycycline for tick bites—not for everyone. N Engl J Med 345:133-134, 2001.
20. Schwartz B, Nadelman RB, Fish D, et al. Entomologic and demographic correlates of anti-tick saliva antibody in a prospective study of tick bite subjects in Westchester County, New York. Am J Trop Med Hyg 48:50-57, 1993.
21. CDC. Lyme disease: United States, 2000. MMWR Morb Mortal Wkly Rep 51:29-31, 2002.
22. Hanrahan JP, Benach JL, Coleman JL, et al. Incidence and cumulative frequency of endemic Lyme disease in a community. J Infect Dis 150:489-496, 1984.
23. Steere AC, Taylor E, Wilson ML, et al. Longitudinal assessment of the clinical and epidemiological features of Lyme disease in a defined population. J Infect Dis 154:94-300, 1986.
24. Fraser CM, Casjens S, Huang WM, et al. Genomic sequence of a Lyme disease spirochaete, *Borrelia burgdorferi*. Nature 390:580-586, 1997.
25. Bergstrom S, Noppa L, Gylfe A, Ostberg Y. Molecular and cellular biology of *Borrelia burgdorferi* sensu lato. *In* Gray JS, Kahl O, Lane RS, Stanek G (eds). Lyme Borreliosis: Biology, Epidemiology and Control. Wallingford, UK, CABI Publishing, 2002, pp 47-90.
26. Nadelman RB, Wormser GP. Lyme borreliosis. Lancet 352:557-565, 1998.
27. Gerber MA, Shapiro ED, Burke GS, et al. Lyme disease in children in southeastern Connecticut. Pediatric Lyme Disease Study Group. N Engl J Med 335:1270-1274, 1996.
28. Coleman JL, Gebbia JA, Piesman J, et al. Plasminogen is required for efficient dissemination of *B. burgdorferi* in ticks and for enhancement of spirochetemia in mice. Cell 89:1111-1119, 1997
29. Coburn J, Leong JM, Erban JK. Integrin alpha IIb beta 3 mediates binding of the Lyme disease agent *Borrelia burgdorferi* to human platelets. Proc Natl Acad Sci U S A 90:7059-7063, 1993.
30. Coburn J, Magoun L, Bodary, Leong KM. Integrins alpha(v)beta3 and alpha5beta1 mediate attachment of Lyme disease spirochetes to human cells. Infect Immun 66:1946-1952, 1998.
31. Guo BP, Brown EL, Dorward DW. Decorin-binding adhesins from *Borrelia burgdorferi*. Mol Microbiol 30:711-723, 1998.
32. Probert WS, Johnson BJ. Identification of a 47 kDa fibronectin-binding protein expressed by *Borrelia burgdorferi* isolate B31. Mol Microbiol 30:1003-1015, 1998.
33. Seinost G, Dykhuizen DE, Dattwyler RJ, et al. Four clones of *Borrelia burgdorferi* sensu stricto cause invasive infection in humans. Infect Immun 67:3518-24, 1999.
34. Weiss JJ, McCracken BA, Ma Y, et al. Identification of quantitative trait loci governing arthritis severity and humoral responses in the murine model of Lyme disease. J Immunol 162:948-956, 1999.
35. Barthold SW, de Souza M. Exacerbation of Lyme arthritis in beige mice. J Infect Dis 172:778-784, 1995.
36. Mullegger RR, McHugh G, Ruthazer R, et al. Differential expression of cytokine mRNA in skin specimens from patients with erythema

migrans or acrodermatitis chronica atrophicans. J Invest Dermatol 115:1115-1123, 2000.

37. Krause A, Brade V, Schoerner C, et al. T cell proliferation induced by *Borrelia burgdorferi* in patients with Lyme borreliosis. Autologous serum required for optimum stimulation. Arthritis Rheum 34:393-402, 1991.
38. Akin E, McHugh GL, Flavell RA, et al. The immunoglobulin (IgG) antibody response to OspA and OspB correlates with severe and prolonged Lyme arthritis and the IgG response to P35 correlates with mild and brief arthritis. Infect Immun 67:173-181, 1999.
39. Roberts ED, Bohm RP Jr, Lowrie RC Jr, et al. Pathogenesis of Lyme neuroborreliosis in the rhesus monkey: the early disseminated and chronic phases of disease in the peripheral nervous system. J Infect Dis 178:722-732, 1998.
40. Cadavid D, O'Neill T, Schaefer H, Pachner AR. Localization of *Borrelia burgdorferi* in the nervous system and other organs in a nonhuman primate model of Lyme disease. Lab Invest 80:1043-1054, 2000.
41. Kelleher Doyle M, Telford SR III, Criscione L, et al. Cytokines in murine Lyme carditis: T_H1 cytokine expression follows expression of proinflammatory cytokines in a susceptible mouse strain. J Infect Dis 177:242-246, 1998.
42. Barthold SW, Feng S, Bockenstedt LK, et al. Protective and arthritis-resolving activity in sera of mice infected with *Borrelia burgdorferi*. Clin Infect Dis 25(Suppl 1):S9-S17, 1997.
43. Steere AC, Duray PH, Butcher EC. Spirochetal antigens and lymphoid cell surface markers in Lyme synovitis. Comparison with rheumatoid synovium and tonsillar lymphoid tissue. Arthritis Rheum 31:487-495, 1988.
44. Vincent MS, Roessner K, Sellati T, et al. Lyme arthritis synovial gamma delta T cells respond to *Borrelia burgdorferi* lipoproteins and lipidated hexapeptides. J Immunol 161:5762-5771, 1998.
45. Chen J, Field JA, Glickstein L, et al. Association of antibiotic treatment-resistant Lyme arthritis with T cell responses to dominant epitopes of outer surface protein A of *Borrelia burgdorferi*. Arthritis Rheum 42: 1813-1822, 1999.
46. Gross DM, Steere AC, Huber BT. T helper 1 response is dominant and localized to the synovial fluid in patients with Lyme arthritis. J Immunol 160:1022-1028, 1998.
47. Yin Z, Braun J, Neure L, et al. T cell cytokine pattern in the joints of patients with Lyme arthritis and its regulation by cytokines and anticytokines. Arthritis Rheum 40:69-79, 1997.
48. Dressler F, Whalen JA, Reinhardt BN, Steere AC. Western blotting in the serodiagnosis of Lyme disease. J Infect Dis 167:392-400, 1993.
49. Barthold SW, Beck DS, Hansen GM, et al. Lyme borreliosis in selected strains and ages of laboratory mice. J Infect Dis 162:133-138, 1990.
50. Steere AC, Baxter-Lowe LA. Association of chronic, treatment-resistant Lyme arthritis with rheumatoid arthritis (RA) alleles. Arthritis Rheum 41(Suppl):S81, 1998.
51. Steere AC, Levin RE, Molloy PJ, et al. Treatment of Lyme arthritis. Arthritis Rheum 37:878-888, 1994.
52. Gross DM, Forsthuber T, Tary-Lehmann M, et al. Identification of LFA-1 as a candidate autoantigen in treatment-resistant Lyme arthritis. Science 281:703-706, 1998.
53. Anderson JF, Johnson RC, Margnarelli LA. Seasonal prevalence of *Borrelia burgdorferi* in natural populations of white-footed mice, *Peromyscus leucopus*. J Clin Microbiol 25:1564-1566, 1987.
54. Burgess EC, Windberg LA. *Borrelia* sp. infection in coyotes, black-tailed jack rabbits and desert cottontails in southern Texas. J Wildl Dis 25:47-51, 1989.
55. Burgess EC. *Borrelia burgdorferi* infection in Wisconsin horses and cows. Ann N Y Acad Sci 539:235-243, 1988.
56. Burgess EC, Wachal MD, Cleven TD. *Borrelia burgdorferi* infection in dairy cows, rodents, and birds from four Wisconsin dairy farms. Vet Microbiol 35:61-77, 1993.
57. Gustafson JM, Burgess EC, Wachal MD, Steinberg H. Intrauterine transmission of *Borrelia burgdorferi* in dogs. Am J Vet Res 54:882-890, 1993.
58. Burgess EC, Gendron-Fitzpatrick A, Mattison M. Foal mortality associated with natural infection of pregnant mares with *Borrelia burgdorferi*. *In* Powell DG (ed). Proceedings of the 5th International Conference on Equine Infectious Diseases. Lexington, Ky, University Press of Kentucky, 1989, pp 217-220.
59. Silver RM, Yang L, Daynes RA, et al. Fetal outcome in murine Lyme disease. Infect Immun 63: 66-72, 1995.
60. Moody KD, Barthold SW. Relative infectivity of *Borrelia burgdorferi* in Lewis rats by various routes of inoculation. Am J Trop Med Hyg 44:135-139, 1991.
61. Woodrum JE, Oliver JH Jr. Investigation of venereal, transplacental, and contact transmission of the Lyme disease spirochete, *Borrelia burgdorferi*, in Syrian hamsters. J Parasitol 85:426-430, 1999.
62. Mather TN, Telford SR III, Adler GH. Absence of transplacental transmission of Lyme disease spirochetes from reservoir mice (*Peromyscus leucopus*) to their offspring. J Infect Dis 164:564-567, 1991.
63. Schlesinger PA, Duray PH, Burke BA, et al. Maternal-fetal transmission of the Lyme disease spirochete, *Borrelia burgdorferi*. Ann Intern Med 103:67-68, 1985.
64. Oppenheimer EH, Hardy JB. Congenital syphilis in the newborn infant: clinical and pathological observations in recent cases. Johns Hopkins Med J 129:63-82, 1971.
65. MacDonald AB, Benach JL, Burgdorfer W. Stillbirth following maternal Lyme disease. N Y State J Med 87:615-616, 1987.
66. Weber K, Bratzke HJ, Neubert U, et al. *Borrelia burgdorferi* in a newborn despite oral penicillin for Lyme borreliosis during pregnancy. Pediatr Infect Dis J 7:286-289, 1988.
67. Trevisan G, Stinco G, Cinco M. Neonatal skin lesions due to a spirochetal infection: a case of congenital Lyme borreliosis? Int J Dermatol 36:677-680, 1997.
68. Grandsaerd MJ. Lyme borreliosis as a cause of facial palsy during pregnancy. Eur J Obstet Gynecol Reprod Biol 91:99-101, 2000.
69. Mikkelson AL, Palle C. Lyme disease during pregnancy. Acta Obstet Gynecol Scand 6:477-478, 1987.
70. Schaumann R. Facial palsy caused by *Borrelia* infection in a twin pregnancy in an area of nonendemicity. Clin Infect Dis 29:955-956, 1999.
71. Schutzer SE, Janniger CK, Schwartz RA. Lyme disease during pregnancy. Cutis 47:267-268, 1991.
72. Stiernstedt G. Lyme borreliosis during pregnancy. Scand J Infect Dis 71(Suppl):99-100, 1990.
73. Figueroa R, Bracero LA, Aguero-Rosenfeld M, et al. Confirmation of *Borrelia burgdorferi* spirochetes by polymerase chain reaction in placentas of women with reactive serology for Lyme antibodies. Gynecol Obstet Invest 41:240-243, 1996.
74. Markowitz LE, Steere AC, Benach JL, et al. Lyme disease during pregnancy. JAMA 255:3394-3396, 1986.
75. Ciesielski CA, Russell H, Johnson S, et al. Prospective study of pregnancy outcome in women with Lyme disease. Twenty-seventh International Conference of Antimicrobial Agents and Chemotherapy, New York, 1987. Abstract 39.
76. Maraspin V, Cimperman J, Lotric-Furlan S, et al. Erythema migrans in pregnancy. Wien Klin Wochenschr 111:933-940, 1999.
77. Williams CL, Benach JL, Curran AS, et al. Lyme disease during pregnancy: a cord blood serosurvey. Ann N Y Acad Sci 539:504-506, 1988.
78. Nadal D, Hunziker UA, Bucher HU, et al. Infants born to mothers with antibodies against *Borrelia burgdorferi* at delivery. Eur J Pediatr 148:426-427, 1989.
79. Gerber MA, Zalneraitis EL. Childhood neurologic disorders and Lyme disease during pregnancy. Pediatr Neurol 11:41-43, 1994.
80. Strobino B, Abid S, Gewitz M. Maternal Lyme disease and congenital heart disease: a case-control study in an endemic area. Am J Obstet Gynecol 180:711-716, 1999.
81. Strobino BA, Williams CL, Abid S, et al. Lyme disease and pregnancy outcome: a prospective study of two thousand prenatal patients. Am J Obstet Gynecol 169:367-374, 1993
82. Williams CL, Strobino B, Weinstein A, et al. Maternal Lyme disease and congenital malformations: a cord blood serosurvey in endemic and control areas. Paediatr Perinat Epidemiol 9:320-330, 1995.
83. Lischer CJ, Leutenegger CM, Lutz BH. Diagnosis of Lyme disease in two cows by the detection of *Borrelia burgdorferi* DNA. Vet Rec 146:497-499, 2000.
84. Schmidt BL, Aberer E, Stockenhiber C, et al. Detection of *Borrelia burgdorferi* DNA by polymerase chain reaction in the urine and breast milk of patients with Lyme borreliosis. Diagn Microbiol Infect Dis 21:121-128, 1995.
85. Shapiro ED, Gerber MA. Lyme disease. Clin Infect Dis 31:533-542, 2000.
86. Steere AC, Sikand VK, Meurice F, et al. Vaccination against Lyme disease with recombinant *Borrelia burgdorferi* outer-surface lipoprotein A with adjuvant. N Engl J Med. 339:209-216, 1998.

87. Case definitions for public health surveillance. MMWR Morb Mortal Wkly Rep 39(RR-13):1-43, 1990.
88. Centers for Disease Control and Prevention. Recommendations for test performance and interpretation from the Second National Conference on Serologic Diagnosis of Lyme Disease. MMWR Morb Mortal Wkly Rep 44:590-591, 1995.
89. Food and Drug Administration. FDA Public Health Advisory: Assays for Antibodies to *Borrelia burgdorferi*: Limitations, Use, and Interpretation for Supporting a Clinical Diagnosis of Lyme Disease. July 7, 1997.
90. Wormser GP, Forseter G, Cooper D, et al. Use of a novel technique of cutaneous lavage for diagnosis of Lyme disease associated with erythema migrans. JAMA 268:1311-1313, 1992.
91. Hyde FW, Johnson RC, White TJ, et al. Detection of antigens in urine of mice and humans infected with *Borrelia burgdorferi*, etiologic agent of Lyme disease. J Clin Microbiol 27:58-61, 1989.
92. Hengge UR, Tannapfel A, Tyring SK, et al. Lyme borreliosis. Lancet Infect Dis 3:489-500, 2003.
93. Klempner MS, Schmid CH, Hu L, et al. Intralaboratory reliability of serologic and urine testing for Lyme disease. Am J Med 110:217-219, 2001.
94. Bunikis J, Barbour AG. Laboratory testing for suspected Lyme disease. Med Clin North Am 86:311-340, 2002.
95. Craft JE, Grodzicki RL, Steere AC. Antibody response in Lyme disease: evaluation of diagnostic tests. J Infect Dis 149:789-795, 1984.
96. Hilton E, Tramontano A, DeVoti J, Sood SK. Temporal study of immunoglobin M seroreactivity to *Borrelia burgdorferi* in patients treated for Lyme borreliosis. J Clin Microbiol 35: 774-776, 1997.
97. Feder HM Jr, Gerber MA, Luger SW, Ryan RW. Persistence of serum antibodies to *Borrelia burgdorferi* in patients treated for Lyme disease. Clin Infect Dis 15:788-793, 1992.
98. Kalish RA, Kaplan RF, Taylor E, et al. Evaluation of study patients with Lyme disease, 10-20-year follow-up. J Infect Dis 183:453-460, 2001.
99. Bacterial Zoonoses Branch, Centers for Disease Control and Prevention. Evaluation of serologic tests for Lyme disease: report of a national evaluation. Lyme Dis Surveill Summ 1:1-8, 1991.
100. Bakken LL, Callister SM, Wand PJ, Schell RF. Interlaboratory comparison of test results for detection of Lyme disease by 516 participants in the Wisconsin State Laboratory of Hygiene/College of American Pathologists Proficiency Testing Program. J Clin Microbiol 35:537-543, 1997.
101. Schwartz BS, Goldstein MD, Ribeiro JMC, et al. Antibody testing in Lyme disease. A comparison of results in four laboratories. JAMA 262:3431-3434, 1989.
102. Bakken LL, Case KL, Callister SM, et al. Performance of 45 laboratories participating in a proficiency testing program for Lyme disease serology. JAMA 268:891-895, 1992.
103. Luger SW, Krauss E. Serologic tests for Lyme disease. Interlaboratory variability. Arch Intern Med 150:761-761990.
104. Seltzer EG, Shapiro ED. Misdiagnosis of Lyme disease: when not to order serologic tests. Pediatr Infect Dis J 15:762-763, 1996.
105. Tugwell P, Dennis DT, Weinstein A, et al. Laboratory evaluation in the diagnosis of Lyme disease. Ann Intern Med 127:1109-1123, 1997.
106. Nichol G, Dennis DT, Steere AC, et al. Test-treatment strategies for patients suspected of having Lyme disease: a cost-effectiveness analysis. Ann Intern Med 128:37-48, 1998.
107. Steere AC, Berardi VP, Weeks KE, et al. Evaluation of the intrathecal antibody response to *Borrelia burgdorferi* as a diagnostic test for Lyme neuroborreliosis. J Infect Dis 161:1203-1209, 1990.
108. Bracero LA, Wormser GP, Leikin E, Tejani N. Prevalence of seropositivity to the Lyme disease spirochete during pregnancy in an epidemic area. A preliminary report. J Matern Fetal Invest 2:265-268, 1992.
109. Wormser GP, Nadelman RB, Dattwyler RJ, et al. Practice guidelines for the treatment of Lyme disease. Clin Infect Dis 31(Suppl 1):S1-S14, 2000.
110. Wormser GP, Ramanathan R, Nowakowski J, et al. Duration of antibiotic therapy for early Lyme disease. A randomized, double-blind, placebo-controlled trial. Ann Intern Med 138:697-704, 2003.
111. Elliott DJ, Eppes SC, Klein JD. Teratogen update: Lyme disease. Teratology 64:276-281, 2001.
112. Shapiro ED. Long-term outcomes of persons with Lyme disease. Vector Borne Zoonotic Dis 2:279-281, 2002.
113. Klempner MS, Hu LT, Evans J, et al. Two controlled trials of antibiotic treatment in patients with persistent symptoms and a history of Lyme disease. N Engl J Med 345:85-92, 2001.

Chapter 16

MYCOPLASMAL INFECTIONS

R. Doug Hardy • Octavio Ramilo

Mycoplasmas are prokaryotes of the class Mollicutes and represent the smallest known free-living organisms. Notably, they lack a cell wall and are bound by a cell membrane. Many of the biologic properties of mycoplasmas are due to the absence of a rigid cell wall, including resistance to β-lactam antibiotics and marked pleomorphism among individual cells. The mycoplasmal cell membrane contains phospholipids, glycolipids, sterols, and various proteins. Their small size of 150 to 350 nm is more on the order of viruses than of bacteria. Mycoplasmas are able to grow in cell-free media and possess both RNA and DNA. The entire genomes of many of the *Mycoplasma* species have been sequenced and have been found to be among the smallest of prokaryotic genomes, with the *Mycoplasma genitalium* genome consisting of only 580,070 DNA base pairs. The elimination of genes related to synthesis of amino acids, fatty acid metabolism, and cholesterol necessitates a parasitic dependence on their host for exogenous nutrients, such as nucleic acid precursors, amino acids, fatty acids, and sterols. In mammals, *Mycoplasma* species most commonly colonize mucosal surfaces, such as those of the respiratory and genital tracts. At least 16 different species of Mollicutes colonize the mucosa of humans.

Ureaplasma urealyticum and *Mycoplasma hominis* are the mycoplasmas most commonly isolated from the genital tract of females and are associated with maternal and fetal infection. Therefore, this chapter focuses on these two species in the maternal-fetal/neonatal and very young infant populations. Mycoplasmal illnesses in other populations, such as immunocompromised older children and nonpregnant adults, are not discussed. *Mycoplasma pneumoniae*, *M. genitalium*, and *Mycoplasma fermentans* are mentioned briefly.

UREAPLASMA UREALYTICUM AND *MYCOPLASMA HOMINIS*: COLONIZATION AND DISEASES OF THE URINARY AND REPRODUCTIVE TRACTS IN ADULTS

Colonization

U. urealyticum and *M. hominis* are commensal organisms in the lower female genital tract. Colonization of the female lower urogenital tract by *U. urealyticum* and *M. hominis* generally occurs as a result of sexual activity. In fact, sexual contact is the major mode of transmission of these organisms, and colonization increases dramatically with increasing numbers of sexual partners.[1,2,28]

In the asymptomatic female, these mycoplasmas may be found throughout the lower urogenital tract, including the external cervical os, vagina, labia, and urethra.[30,31] The vagina yields the largest number of organisms, followed by the periurethral area and the cervix.[31] *U. urealyticum* is isolated less often from urine than from the cervix, but *M. hominis* is present both in the urine and the cervix with approximately the same frequency. In the asymptomatic adult male, mycoplasmas also have been isolated from urine, semen, and the distal urethra.[33]

U. urealyticum can be isolated from the vagina of 40% to 80% of sexually active, asymptomatic women; *M. hominis* is found in 21% to 70%. Both microorganisms can be found concurrently in 31% to 60% of women.[6,7] In males, colonization with each is less prevalent. In women, colonization has been linked to younger age, lower socioeconomic status, multiple sexual partners, black ethnicity, oral contraceptive use, and recent antimicrobial therapy.[28,35] Additionally, mycoplasmas are prevalent in the lower genital tract of pregnant women.[6,36,37] When genital mycoplasmas are present at the first prenatal visit, usually they persist throughout the pregnancy. Studies of postmenopausal women suggest that this population is infrequently colonized with genital mycoplasmas.[38]

Urinary Tract

Three disease associations have been established for *U. urealyticum* and *M. hominis* in the urinary tract. These are urethritis in men caused by *U. urealyticum*, urinary calculi from *U. urealyticum*, and pyelonephritis due to *M. hominis*.[53]

Intraurethral inoculation of human volunteers and nonhuman primates with *U. urealyticum* produces urethritis.[53] Serologic studies and antimicrobial treatment trials also support a causative role of this organism in urethritis.[53] The common presence of ureaplasmas in the urethra of asymptomatic men suggests either that only certain serovars of ureaplasmas are pathogenic or that predisposing factors, such as lack of mucosal immunity, must exist in those persons in whom symptomatic infection develops. Alternatively, disease may develop only on initial exposure to ureaplasmas. *U. urealyticum* also has been implicated in urethroprostatitis and epididymitis.[9]

U. urealyticum has been shown to have a limited role in the production of urinary calculi. *U. urealyticum* produces urease, which splits urea into ammonia and carbon dioxide, and has been demonstrated to induce crystallization of struvite and calcium phosphates in artificial urine in vitro, demonstrating the capacity of *U. urealyticum* to induce stone formation.[39,40] Renal calculi have been induced experimentally by inoculation of pure cultures of *U. urealyticum* directly into the bladder and renal pelvis of rats. *U. urealyticum* has been isolated from stones recovered by surgery in 6 of 15 patients. In 4 of these 6, no other urease-producing organisms were isolated either in the stone or in urine sampled from the renal pelvis. *Proteus mirabilis* is the most common cause of similar stones in humans. The frequency with which *U. urealyticum* reaches the kidney, the predisposing factors that allow this to occur, and the relative frequency of renal calculi induced by this organism compared with that of calculi induced by other organisms are not known.

Even with the high incidence of *M. hominis* in the lower urogenital tract, this organism has been isolated from the upper urinary tract only in patients with symptoms of acute infection.[41] In one study, *M. hominis* was recovered from samples of ureteral urine collected during surgery from 7 of 80 patients (4 in pure culture) with acute pyelonephritis, and in a second study from 3 of 18 patients with acute exacerbation of chronic pyelonephritis. *M. hominis* was not found in the upper urinary tract of 22 patients with chronic pyelonephritis without acute exacerbation, or from 60 patients with noninfectious urinary tract disease.

Reproductive Tract

M. hominis is considered an etiologic agent of pelvic inflammatory disease.[42,43,49,50] Inoculation of *M. hominis* into fallopian tubes of primates induces parametritis and salpingitis within 3 days,[51] whereas inoculation of human fallopian tube explants produces ciliostasis.[52] The organism has been isolated in pure cultures from the fallopian tubes of approximately 8% of women with salpingitis diagnosed by laparoscopy, but not in any women without salpingitis.[42] The organism also can be isolated from the endometrium. A role for this organism in cases of pelvic inflammatory disease not associated with either *Neisseria gonorrhoeae* or *Chlamydia trachomatis* is supported by significant increases in specific antibodies to *M. hominis*.[49] *U. urealyticum* is not considered to be a cause of pelvic inflammatory disease.[9]

CHORIOAMNIONITIS, CLINICAL AMNIONITIS, AND MATERNAL SEPTICEMIA

Histologic Chorioamnionitis

Isolation of *U. urealyticum*, but not *M. hominis*, from the chorioamnion uniformly has shown a significant association with histologic chorioamnionitis.[3,5,10-14] Studies in which extensive culture for other agents was performed reported that women whose amniotic membranes contained *U. urealyticum* were more likely to have histologic evidence of chorioamnionitis than were women without *U. urealyticum*, even after adjusting for duration of labor, premature rupture of membranes, duration of membrane rupture, and the presence of other bacteria.[11] *U. urealyticum* in the chorioamnion was found to be significantly associated with histologic chorioamnionitis in the presence of intact membranes when delivery was by cesarean section.[15] In some cases, *U. urealyticum* was the only organism isolated. Case reports[5,17,18] indicate that *U. urealyticum* can persist in the amniotic fluid for as long as 7 weeks in the presence of an intense inflammatory response and in the absence of ruptured membranes or labor and can be isolated as a single microorganism when cultures for multiple agents are performed. These findings demonstrate that ureaplasmas can produce histologic evidence of chorioamnionitis.

Infection of the Amniotic Fluid and Clinical Amnionitis

Although *U. urealyticum* and *M. hominis* can invade the amniotic fluid as early as 16 to 20 weeks of gestation in the presence of intact membranes and in the absence of other microorganisms, these infections tend to be clinically silent and chronic (Fig. 16-1).[5,17] *U. urealyticum* and *M. hominis* have been isolated more frequently from the chorioamnion than from the amniotic fluid. Isolation of organisms from the chorioamnion or amniotic fluid has been significantly associated with histologic evidence of chorioamnionitis but not with clinical amnionitis.[15] Ureaplasmas can be detected in the amniotic fluid in up to 50% of both asymptomatic and symptomatic persons.[8] These reports indicate that the role of *U. urealyticum* in clinical amnionitis is not clear.

In an investigation by Yoon and colleagues,[57] amniocentesis was performed in 154 patients with preterm premature rupture of membranes. Amniotic fluid was cultured for aerobic and anaerobic bacteria and for mycoplasmas. Polymerase chain reaction (PCR) assay for *U. urealyticum* also was performed on the fluid. These investigators found that amniotic fluid culture for mycoplasmas missed 42% of cases identified as positive by *U. urealyticum* PCR assay. Patients with a negative result on amniotic fluid culture for *U. urealyticum* but a positive result on PCR assay had a significantly shorter interval from amniocentesis to delivery, higher amniotic fluid interleukin-6 (IL-6) concentrations, and higher white blood cell counts compared with patients with no detection of *U. urealyticum* by culture or PCR assay. Subsequently, in a similar investigation by Yoon and colleagues[58] in 257 patients with preterm labor and intact membranes, significant findings were similar, except that the prevalence of *U. urealyticum* was lower.

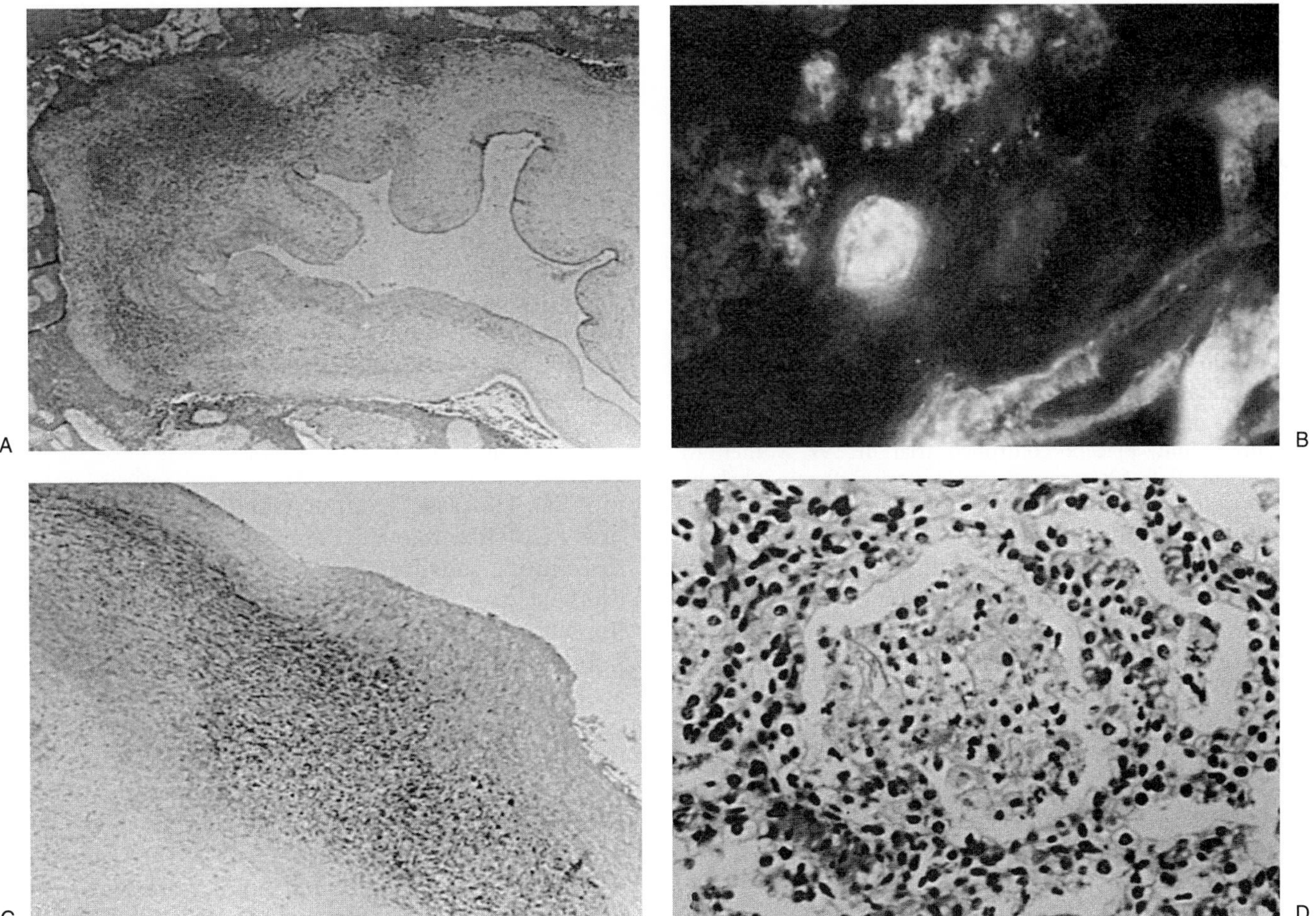

Figure 16–1 **A,** Section of placenta at 24 weeks of gestation showing extensive inflammation in the amnion and chorion (25×). *Ureaplasma urealyticum* was isolated from the amniotic fluid 7 weeks before delivery and from multiple fetal organs at postmortem examination. **B,** Adjacent section of placenta stained with rabbit anti–*U. urealyticum* serovar 1 serum and reacted with fluorescein-labeled goat anti-rabbit immunoglobulin G (IgG) (750×). **C,** Photomicrograph of the umbilical cord from the same case as in A and B demonstrates extensive inflammation (25×). **D,** Photomicrograph of lung tissue shows histologic evidence of pneumonia (50×).

The detection of *M. hominis* does not correlate with clinical symptoms. *M. hominis* commonly invades the chorioamnion and amniotic fluid, but such invasion rarely occurs in the absence of other organisms, particularly ureaplasmas. Thus, it is unclear whether this organism alone is a cause of histologic chorioamnionitis or clinical amnionitis.[15]

Postpartum and Postabortal Fever

M. hominis[64-67] and *U. urealyticum*[68,69] have been isolated from blood cultures from women with postpartum fever and septic abortion. Serologic investigations indicate that *M. hominis* is a common cause of postpartum fever, as demonstrated by a fourfold or greater rise in mycoplasmacidal antibody titer.[70] In a study at Boston City Hospital,[71] blood was obtained from 327 women shortly after vaginal delivery. Ten of these 327 women had blood cultures that grew *M. hominis*; 15 grew *U. urealyticum*; and in 1 woman, both *M. hominis* and *U. urealyticum* were isolated. The frequency of mycoplasma isolation was inversely related to the interval between delivery and the time at which the blood was obtained for culture. Twenty women whose blood culture grew mycoplasmas at the time of delivery were re-evaluated with a second culture 1 or more days later; in only 1 of these women was a positive result obtained on the second blood culture. Pathogenic bacteria were cultured from the blood of 16 of these 327 women, including 4 of the 11 women with *M. hominis*, but none from the women with *U. urealyticum*.

In a prospective study of 620 blood cultures from febrile obstetric patients,[73] *U. urealyticum* was the second and *M. hominis* the third most common microorganism isolated. All specimens were obtained during febrile postpartum or postabortum episodes. Mycoplasmas were isolated on a number of occasions from blood drawn more than 2 days after the procedure. Endometritis or histologically documented chorioamnionitis was present in one half of the patients, and fever persisted after delivery or abortion in many of the cases despite administration of antimicrobial agents directed at organisms other than mycoplasmas. Fever resolved after tetracycline therapy.

It has been shown that colonization of the chorioamnion with ureaplasmas in women with intact membranes undergoing cesarean delivery is a significant and independent predictor of ensuing endometritis.[74] Endometritis occurred in 28% of women with ureaplasmas isolated from the chorioamnion at cesarean delivery, compared with only 8.4%

if the culture result was negative, and 8.8% if only bacteria but no ureaplasmas were isolated.

Roberts and associates[75] found ureaplasmas to be the most common microorganism isolated from postcesarean wound infections. Of 47 cultures with a positive result from 939 wounds, ureaplasmas were recovered from 29. Additionally, one third of the cultures positive for ureaplasmas yielded no other microorganisms. Additionally, *M. hominis* has been recovered from the joint fluid of women post partum. These women had been febrile during the immediate postpartum period, and signs of arthritis developed 7 days to 3 weeks after delivery.[76] Cases of postpartum pneumonia with isolation of *M. hominis* from pleural fluid and cases of *M. hominis* wound infections after cesarean section also have been reported.[77-80]

Andrews and co-workers[61] performed a randomized, double-blind, placebo-controlled trial in 597 women to compare rates of postcesarean endometritis after prophylaxis with cefotetan versus cefotetan plus doxycycline and azithromycin. The frequency of postcesarean endometritis and wound infection was significantly lower in the group that received cefotetan plus doxycycline and azithromycin. The investigators concluded that this extended-spectrum antibiotic prophylaxis regimen, with activity against mycoplasmas, reduced the frequency of postcesarean endometritis and wound infection. *Mycoplasma* cultures were not obtained in this investigation, however, so it is not clear that the improved outcome was due to the addition of doxycycline and azithromycin prophylaxis aimed specifically at *Mycoplasma* infections.

ADVERSE PREGNANCY OUTCOME

Fetal Loss

Although studies have found the presence of *U. urealyticum* and *M. hominis* in the genital tract to be significantly associated with spontaneous abortion and early pregnancy loss,[62] their actual role in these events remains uncertain. Both organisms have been isolated from the lungs, brain, heart, and viscera of aborted fetuses and stillborn infants, in some cases in the presence of an inflammatory response and in the absence of other organisms.[5,13,81,82] In these cases, however, it was not clear whether death of the fetus occurred before these organisms "invaded." *U. urealyticum* has been found more frequently in the products of early abortions and midtrimester fetal losses than in products of induced abortions.[83,84] Furthermore, *U. urealyticum* has been isolated more frequently from the placentas of aborted fetuses than from controls.[10,13]

Although rates of isolation of ureaplasmas from the lower genital tract of habitual aborters are not different from those of normal controls, ureaplasmas are isolated more frequently from the endometrium of habitual aborters.[83,84] When only those patients with a positive result on cervical culture are considered, no higher endometrial colonization rates are found, however.[85] Antibody titers to *U. urealyticum* are higher in mothers with a history of fetal loss.[86] Those epidemiologic studies are difficult to interpret, however, because the comparability of the various groups of women is uncertain and the role of other potential infectious agents was not always taken into account.

Isolation of *U. urealyticum* from amniotic fluid in pure culture from women with intact membranes and subsequent fetal loss in the presence of histologic chorioamnionitis has been reported.[5,18,87] Berg and associates[60] performed a retrospective analysis of 2718 amniocentesis specimens obtained for genetic indications and cultured for *U. urealyticum* and *M. hominis*. Of the 2718 patients, 49 (1.8%) patients were found to be positive for one or both organisms. Of 43 evaluable patients, 35 were given oral erythromycin at the discretion of the physician caring for the patient. Rates of midtrimester loss were 11.4% and 44.4% ($P = .04$) in the treated and untreated groups, respectively. This study demonstrated that treatment of amniotic mycoplasmal colonization with erythromycin may decrease midtrimester losses. Prospective controlled trials are necessary to validate this hypothesis, however.

Preterm Birth

Multiple studies involving almost 12,000 patients have been conducted to evaluate the association of cervical ureaplasmal infection with prematurity.[4,88] The evidence suggests no consistent relationship between the presence of *U. urealyticum* in the lower genital tract of the mother and prematurity or low birth weight in the infant.

At least six prospective studies have evaluated the role of ureaplasmal infection of the amniotic fluid in etiology of prematurity. Three of these studies investigated the outcome of pregnancy when ureaplasmas were detected at the time of genetic amniocentesis between 12 and 20 weeks of gestation, when membranes were intact and when labor had not begun.[5,87,89] In an investigation by Cassell and colleagues,[5] two infants with *U. urealyticum* isolated from amniotic fluid were born preterm; both infants died, and both had evidence of pneumonia. *U. urealyticum* was isolated in pure culture at postmortem examination in both cases. In a study by Gray and associates,[87] 7 of 10 patients from whom ureaplasmas were isolated by culture of the amniotic fluid subsequently aborted within 4 to 7 weeks after amniocentesis and at less than 25 weeks of gestation. The 3 remaining infants were born at less than 37 weeks of gestation; 2 of these died. Histologic evidence of chorioamnionitis was present in all 10 placentas, and histologic evidence of pneumonia was present in all 8 fetuses. Placentas grew *U. urealyticum*, but results were negative for cultures of all other microorganisms in 6 of 7 evaluated at delivery and from 4 of the 6 fetal lungs that were evaluated. The third and largest investigation by Gerber and co-workers[89] utilized PCR assay and detected *U. urealyticum* in 29 of 254 (11.4%) amniotic fluid specimens. As might be expected, a higher percentage of *U. urealyticum*–positive amniotic fluid samples were found in this study that used PCR than in previous investigations that relied solely on culture. Subsequent preterm labor occurred in 17 (58.6%) *U. urealyticum*–positive women, compared with 10 (4.4%)of those whose cultures were *U. urealyticum* negative ($P < .0001$). Preterm birth occurred in 7 (24.1%) *U. urealyticum*–positive women compared with 1 (0.4%) *U. urealyticum*–negative woman ($P < .0001$). Of note, *U. urealyticum*–positive women did have a higher prevalence of preterm labor in a prior pregnancy (20.7%) than that in the *U. urealyticum*–negative women (2.7%; $P < .0008$).

In contrast with the foregoing studies, in the remaining three studies culture of amniotic fluid was performed on women hospitalized with preterm labor and intact membranes. *U. urealyticum* in the amniotic fluid was not consistently associated with preterm birth in these studies.[90-92] It must be noted that in these later studies of women with preterm labor, the mean gestation was 31.5 weeks, compared with 12 to 20 weeks of gestation in the previous studies of women with no labor.

A significant relationship between isolation of *U. urealyticum* from the chorioamnion and preterm birth has been documented in three of six prospective studies.[10-12,16,93,94] In most patients in these investigations, however, membrane rupture had occurred, which could have led to intrapartum microbial invasion of the chorioamnion, potentially confounding the results even if the duration of membrane rupture is taken into account.

As noted previously, Berg and associates[60] performed a retrospective analysis of 2718 genetic amniocentesis specimens cultured for *U. urealyticum* and *M. hominis*. Of the 2718 specimens, 49 (1.8%) were found to be positive for either organism. Of 43 evaluable patients in this study, 35 received treatment with oral erythromycin. Preterm delivery rates were similar in the treated and untreated groups at 19.4% and 20%, respectively. The investigators speculated that the lack of a treatment effect may have been due to recolonization with mycoplasmas.

The sum of the evidence suggests that the risk of preterm labor and delivery is increased when ureaplasmas are detected at amniocentesis between 12 to 20 weeks of gestation in women with intact membranes before onset of labor. Otherwise, the association between preterm birth and ureaplasmas is uncertain.

TRANSMISSION OF *UREAPLASMA UREALYTICUM* AND *MYCOPLASMA HOMINIS* TO THE FETUS AND NEWBORN

U. urealyticum and *M. hominis* can be transmitted to a fetus from an infected female either in utero or at the time of delivery by passage through a colonized birth canal. The isolation of *U. urealyticum* in pure culture from the chorioamnion, amniotic fluid, and internal fetal organs in the presence of funisitis and pneumonia[5] and a specific immunoglobulin M (IgM) response[95] can be taken as evidence that fetal infection can occur in utero. Investigators[21,26] also have found that *U. urealyticum* and *M. hominis* can be isolated from endotracheal specimens collected within 30 minutes to 24 hours after birth from infants who were delivered by cesarean section with intact membranes. It is thought that the acquisition of *U. urealyticum* and *M. hominis* can occur in utero either by an ascending route secondary to colonization of the mother's genital tract or transplacentally from the mother's blood. Each of these organisms has been isolated from maternal and umbilical cord blood at the time of delivery.[72,73]

The rate of vertical transmission of *U. urealyticum* and *M. hominis* ranges from 18% to 88%.[47,96-99] Chua and colleagues[99] prospectively investigated the transmission and colonization of *U. urealyticum* and *M. hominis* from mothers to term and preterm newborns delivered by the vaginal route. The rates of maternal cervical colonization with *U. urealyticum* and *M. hominis* were 57.5% and 15.8%, respectively, whereas the rates for isolation of *U. urealyticum* and *M. hominis* from nasopharyngeal secretions of the newborns were 50.8% and 6.6%, respectively. The vertical transmission rates were 88.4% for *U. urealyticum* and 42.1% for *M. hominis*. Maternal transmission was not associated with gestational age. In preterm neonates, the isolation of mycoplasmas was not associated with gestational age or birth weight. There was a tendency for *U. urealyticum* to persist in preterm newborns, especially in those with birth weight less than 2 kg. Colonization of full-term infants appears to be relatively transient, with a sharp drop in isolation rates after 3 months of age.[100] In premature infants with ureaplasmal infection, persistence of the organism in the lower respiratory tract and cerebrospinal fluid (CSF) has been documented for weeks to months.[19,21]

PERINATAL *UREAPLASMA UREALYTICUM* AND *MYCOPLASMA HOMINIS* INFECTION

A number of prospective studies based on direct culture of the affected site indicate that both *U. urealyticum* and *M. hominis* can cause invasive disease in infants, particularly in infants born prematurely. It must be noted, however, that the presence of mycoplasmas in the chorioamnion or amniotic fluid does not necessarily result in infection of the fetus. Similarly, the isolation of mycoplasmas from surface cultures (e.g., eyes, ears, nose, throat, gastric aspirates, vagina) is not necessarily indicative of invasive disease.

Pneumonia

Case reports,[17,27,29,87] retrospective studies,[103] and prospective studies[5,13,17] indicate an association of *U. urealyticum* with congenital and neonatal pneumonia. The organism has been isolated from affected lungs in the absence of other pathogens, such as chlamydiae, viruses, fungi, and bacteria, in the presence of chorioamnionitis and funisitis[5] and has been demonstrated within fetal membranes by immunofluorescence[5] and in lung lesions by electron and immunofluorescent microscopy.[95] A specific IgM response has been demonstrated in some cases of neonatal pneumonia.[95]

In a study of 98 infants,[21] respiratory distress syndrome, the need for assisted ventilation, severe respiratory insufficiency, and death were significantly more common among those born at less than 34 weeks of gestation from whom *U. urealyticum* was recovered from endotracheal aspirates at delivery than among those with a negative culture result. In another series of 292 infants with birth weights of less than 2500 g who were studied by follow-up evaluation for 4 weeks after birth, isolation of *U. urealyticum* from the endotracheal aspirate within a week of birth (mean age, 1.3 days) was significantly associated with radiographic pneumonia, whereas no such association was found for uninfected infants.[34] *U. urealyticum* was the most common organism isolated (15% of infants) among these 292 patients, and it was isolated in pure culture in 71%.

Conversely, other investigators have found a possibly protective effect associated with the isolation of *U. urealyticum* from preterm infants. Hannaford and co-workers,[105] in a prospective consecutive investigation of 143 ventilated newborns born at than 28 weeks of gestation, isolated *U. urealyticum* from endotracheal aspirates of 39 (27%) infants. Respiratory distress syndrome occurred significantly less often in infants from whom *U. urealyticum* was isolated than in infants from whom it was not isolated ($P = .002$). In addition, a trend for lower mortality rates in the first 28 days of life was identified among *U. urealyticum*–positive infants. Berger and associates[106] also found an apparently protective effect of *U. urealyticum* isolated from the amniotic cavity at the time of delivery against hyaline membrane disease in infants with a mean gestational age of 29 to 30 weeks, although nonsignificant. Again, no increase in acute morbidity or mortality was found to be associated with *U. urealyticum* isolation.

The baboon model of prematurity has been employed to investigate the pathogenicity of *U. urealyticum*. At age 140 days, baboons demonstrate physiologic and pathologic characteristics similar to those of human neonates of 30 to 32 weeks of gestation (e.g., they have hyaline membrane disease).[108] Endotracheal inoculation of premature baboons with *U. urealyticum* isolated from human infants results in histologic pulmonary lesions, including acute bronchiolitis with epithelial ulceration and polymorphonuclear infiltration, that are indistinguishable from those of hyaline membrane disease.[32]

Yoder and colleagues[181] performed an investigation in premature baboons that offers explanation for the divergent findings in human studies of *U. urealyticum* and respiratory status in preterm infants. Premature baboon infants were delivered 48 to 72 hours after maternal intra-amniotic inoculation with *U. urealyticum*. Two distinct patterns of disease were observed in the baboon infants. Baboons with persistent *U. urealyticum* tracheal colonization manifested worse lung function and prolonged elevated tracheal cytokines. Conversely, colonized baboons that subsequently cleared *U. urealyticum* from tracheal cultures demonstrated improved lung function compared with unexposed control animals.

In addition, pneumonia with persistent pulmonary hypertension has been described in newborn infants with *U. urealyticum* isolated from the lower respiratory tract.[27,29] Although cases of ureaplasmal pneumonia have been documented in full-term infants, pneumonia due to this agent is thought to occur much less frequently than in premature neonates. Case reports indicate that *M. hominis* can be a cause of pneumonia in newborns, but it has not been implicated as a common etiologic agent in prospective studies. These mycoplasmas are not thought to be a significant cause of acute respiratory disease in otherwise healthy infants after the first month of life.[59]

Chronic Lung Disease

U. urealyticum frequently colonizes the neonatal respiratory tract. Although a majority of the investigations support a significant association between ureaplasmas and chronic lung disease (CLD) in preterm infants, its role in causation of CLD remains uncertain. CLD is most often defined as a requirement for supplemental oxygen at 28 days of age or at 36 weeks of postconceptional age. Presence of concurrent chest radiographic changes compatible with CLD sometimes is included in this definition.

Wang and co-workers,[109] in a meta-analysis of 17 investigations published before 1995, explored the association between *U. urealyticum* and CLD. The studies in this analysis included preterm and term neonates. CLD was defined as a requirement for oxygen at 28 to 30 days of age, and diagnosis of *Ureaplasma* colonization required the recovery of *U. urealyticum* from a respiratory or surface specimen. The estimates of relative risk exceeded 1 in all of the investigations; however, the lower confidence interval included 1 in 7 (41%). The meta-analysis concluded that the relative risk for the development of CLD in colonized infants was 1.72 (95% confidence interval 1.5 to 1.96) times that for noncolonized infants. In the analysis, investigations that focused on extremely premature, very low birth weight (VLBW) neonates did not identify a significantly different relative risk from that for investigations that included all neonates. Also, the relative risk did not differ significantly between those studies in which only endotracheal aspirates were used to define colonization and other studies.

Subsequent to this meta-analysis, the association of *U. urealyticum* with chronic pulmonary disease, including bronchopulmonary dysplasia (or CLD), has been confirmed in multiple studies[101,102,104-106,110-115] but not in others.[116-122] Perzigian and colleagues[102] prospectively investigated a cohort of 105 VLBW (less than 1500 g) infants; in 22 (21%), results of tracheal aspirate cultures were positive for *U. urealyticum* at birth. At 28 days, *U. urealyticum*–positive patients were significantly more likely to have CLD than were *U. urealyticum*–negative patients, despite routine use of exogenous surfactant. The *U. urealyticum*–positive infants also required significantly longer duration of oxygen therapy and of mechanical ventilation. No significant differences were found for CLD at 36 weeks or for duration of hospitalization, however.

Because the relationship of neither *Ureaplasma* species nor the concentration of ureaplasmas with the development of CLD had yet been investigated, a prospective study was designed to look for such an association. In 175 VLBW infants, endotracheal aspirates were obtained at birth for quantitative culture; the results were analyzed for correlation with the development of CLD.[120] Ureaplasmas were isolated from 66 (38%) of the 175 infants. No statistically significant associations were identified between the development of CLD and the *Ureaplasma* species isolated (*U. urealyticum* or *Ureaplasma parvum*) or the concentration of ureaplasmas in the lower respiratory tract secretions.

Because the observed disparities in these studies might be explained in part by the variable persistence of *Ureaplasma* colonization of the infant respiratory tract, a prospective longitudinal study was performed to investigate this possibility. In 125 VLBW infants, culture and PCR assay were used to frequently sample for *U. urealyticum* in the respiratory tract over the course of their neonatal intensive care unit stay. It was found that the pattern of colonization was predictive for the development of CLD.[104] In this study, 40 (32%) of 125 infants had at least one specimen positive for *U. urealyticum*; however, only 18 (45%) of the 40 had persistent colonization throughout their hospitalization. Only persistent *U. urealyticum* colonization was associated with a significantly increased risk of development of CLD, both at 28 days of age and at 36 weeks after conception. Neither early transient colonization nor late acquisition of *U. urealyticum* was associated with CLD. The study by Yoder and colleagues[181] in premature baboons similarly found that the pattern of tracheal colonization was important in the manifestations of respiratory disease.

Inadequate detection of *U. urealyticum* in neonates can be another confounding factor in CLD research. False-negative results for isolation of *U. urealyticum* from respiratory specimens could weaken the association with CLD. Utilizing in situ hybridization (ISH) for *U. urealyticum* on lung autopsy tissue from 7 infants with positive cultures and 7 infants with negative cultures for *U. urealyticum* from the lower respiratory tract, Benstein and co-workers[101] found all 7 culture-positive infants were positive for *U. urealyticum* by ISH; 2 of the culture negative were positive by ISH. The ISH results had a 100% correlation with the presence of histopathologic evidence of bronchopulmonary dysplasia at autopsy of these 14 infants.

Although properly conducted antimicrobial agent trials showing reduction in CLD incidence and severity in neonates with *U. urealyticum* would support a causal role for this microorganism, failure of amelioration with effective therapy does not necessarily indicate that *U. urealyticum* does not have some role in the development of CLD. Small trials of therapy with erythromycin or clarithromycin have failed to provide evidence that therapy, predicted by in vitro testing to be effective, decreases CLD severity or produces clinical improvement in neonates with *U. urealyticum*.[106,121,123-127] Only two randomized, controlled trials have been conducted, together involving a total of 37 VLBW infants with *U. urealyticum* isolated from their respiratory tract; each failed to demonstrate a reduction in the incidence of CLD after 7 to 10 days of erythromycin therapy.[123] In one of these trials, erythromycin treatment significantly reduced the isolation of *U. urealyticum* from the respiratory tract, but it did not significantly alter required length of time with supplemental oxygen.[121] A large, definitive, well-controlled trial is needed, perhaps with more prolonged antimicrobial therapy.

Debate over the concept that initiating therapy after birth may be too late to influence the outcome of an inflammatory process with possible onset in utero was partially addressed in the Overview of Role of Antibiotics in the Curtailment of Labour and Early Delivery (ORACLE) I and ORACLE II prenatal trials (erythromycin or amoxicillin–clavulanic acid, or both, in a randomized double-blind, placebo-controlled design) involving a combined total of 11,121 women with preterm, prelabor rupture of fetal membranes or spontaneous preterm labor.[128,129] One of the primary outcomes of these trials was CLD, defined as the need for daily supplementary oxygen at age 36 weeks after conception; the other primary outcomes were neonatal death and major cerebral abnormality. ORACLE I and ORACLE II revealed no statistically significant reduction in any primary outcome. *U. urealyticum* colonization was not specifically addressed in these trials, however, so the results should not be generalized to directly address *U. urealyticum* and CLD.

To investigate for the presence of a long-term detrimental effect of perinatal *U. urealyticum* infection, a cohort of 40 preterm infants was prospectively followed for 12 months.[130] In 22 (55%), *U. urealyticum* was present in samples obtained from the trachea and/or blood at birth. The infants with perinatal *U. urealyticum* required significantly more days of hospitalization than the number of days for infants without *U. urealyticum*. The difference was attributed to an increase in respiratory tract disease among the infants with perinatal *U. urealyticum*. In addition, CLD was associated with significantly more admissions in the infants with perinatal *U. urealyticum* than in those without it. Syrogiannopoulos and associates[47] monitored 108 full-term infants during the first 3 months of life. These researchers were unable to demonstrate an increased risk of lower respiratory illness during this period of observation in the 51 of 108 infants with persistent pharyngeal *Ureaplasma* colonization over that in the infants who were not pharyngeally colonized at 3 months of life.

Although *U. urealyticum* has not been definitively shown to cause CLD, investigations have identified possible pathogenic mechanisms through which it may contribute to CLD. *U. urealyticum* has been hypothesized to induce lung injury through immunopathogenic mechanisms involving the release of pulmonary cytokines and chemokines after exposure to this microorganism either in utero or postnatally. It also has been proposed that *U. urealyticum* infection potentiates oxygen-induced lung injury.[101,104]

Although much effort has been expended to define the role of *U. urealyticum* in CLD, no clear conclusions can be made at present, although a majority of the investigations seem to indicate a significant association. Novel strategies need to be instituted to further explore the link between these entities.

Bloodstream Infections

Ureaplasmas have been isolated from blood cultures from neonates.[19,23,26,72,73,107,131,132] Case reports also have described the isolation of ureaplasmas from the bloodstream of neonates with pneumonia.[21,29] Cassell and associates[26] found that 26% of preterm infants with endotracheal aspirates that grew *U. urealyticum* also had a positive result on blood cultures for this organism, suggesting that bacteremia with ureaplasmas can be common in preterm infants. Cases of *M. hominis* bacteremia with systemic symptoms accompanied by an antibody response also have been reported.[56,133]

Not all investigations have been successful in recovering mycoplasmas from the blood of infants.[22-24] Mycoplasmas were not isolated from blood cultures obtained within 30 minutes of birth from 146 preterm infants in Israel.[23] In addition, investigators did not isolate mycoplasmas from the 191 blood cultures in a prospective study of older infants hospitalized for possible sepsis.[24] The frequency of clinical signs of infection in infants with *U. urealyticum* or *M. hominis* bacteremia is not clear.

Central Nervous System Infections

In general, the clinical significance of recovering *U. urealyticum* or *M. hominis* from a central nervous system (CNS) specimen from a neonate remains uncertain. In some situations, an association with a disease process appears plausible, whereas in others, no corresponding disease state is apparent. Multiple cases of *M. hominis* CNS infection (meningitis, brain abscess) have been described in full-term and preterm infants.[25,54,134-142] *U. urealyticum* also has been isolated from the CSF of infants with suspected sepsis and meningitis.[19-22,28,48,143]

In a prospective trial in 100 mostly premature infants, *U. urealyticum* was isolated from the CSF of 8 and *M. hominis* from the CSF of 5 who were undergoing investigation for

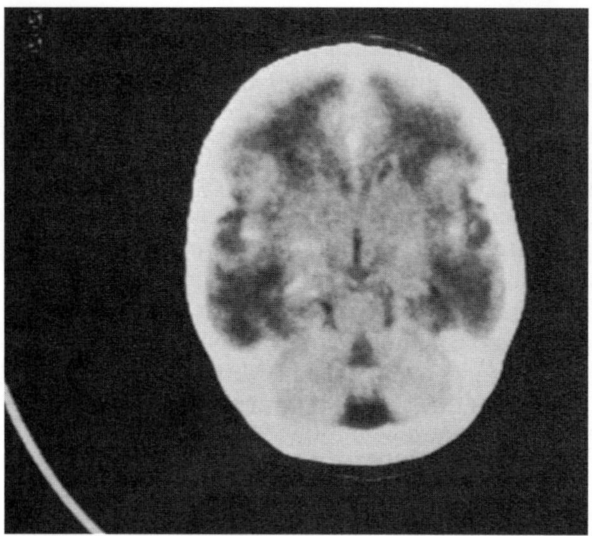

Figure 16–2 A 37-week-gestation newborn who had hypothermia, hypotonia, and lethargy noted at age 3 days. Computed tomography showed decreased attenuation predominantly of the supratentorial white matter symmetrically with punctate early-calcified lesions. Examination of the cerebrospinal fluid (CSF) demonstrated mononuclear pleocytosis, and *Mycoplasma hominis* was isolated. CSF culture was sterile after 5 days of doxycycline treatment, but the infant had spastic quadriplegia at 6 months of age.

suspected sepsis or treatment of hydrocephalus.[19] Of the 8 neonates with *U. urealyticum*, 6 had severe intraventricular hemorrhage, 3 had hydrocephalus, and 4 had ureaplasmas isolated several times in the CSF. *Ureaplasma* infection was significantly associated with severe intraventricular hemorrhage ($P < .001$). *U. urealyticum* was isolated from the respiratory tract of 4 of the 8 infants with CSF infections. Five infants received treatment with erythromycin or doxycycline. Three *Ureaplasma*-infected infants died. All 5 of the neonates from whom *M. hominis* was isolated from the CSF were being investigated for suspected sepsis; prominent neurologic signs and CSF pleocytosis were noted in only 1. This infant received doxycycline treatment and improved but had substantial neurologic sequelae (Fig. 16-2).[19] No *M. hominis*–infected infants died. A subsequent study by the same group of investigators in 318 infants isolated *U. urealyticum* from the CSF of 5 and *M. hominis* from 9. Spontaneous clearance of the organisms was documented in 5 of the infants, and 12 infants had a good outcome.[145]

Shaw and colleagues[144] performed a prospective study of 135 preterm infants undergoing lumbar puncture and found *U. urealyticum* in the CSF of 1 neonate and *M. hominis* in none. Ureaplasmas continued to be isolated from this 1 infant over the course of 16 weeks, despite treatment with erythromycin. The organism maintained in vitro susceptibility to erythromycin. Doxycycline treatment was associated with the disappearance of the organism.

In a prospective study by Ollikainen and co-workers,[21] *U. urealyticum* was isolated from the CSF of four of six infants born at less than 34 weeks of gestation. None had pleocytosis or hypoglycorrhachia in the CSF. Three had the organism also isolated from blood, and one from a tracheal sample. One died and had a postmortem brain culture positive for *U. urealyticum*. None had intracranial hemorrhage.

Valencia and associates[22] isolated *M. hominis* from 9 and *U. urealyticum* from 1 of 69 consecutive infants in whom CSF was cultured within the first 3 months of life for suspected sepsis. The CSF indices, except for bloody specimens, were considered to be within normal limits for newborns. Only 1 of the infants whose CSF culture grew *M. hominis* had clinical signs compatible with systemic infection. The other infants were healthy but were evaluated secondary to maternal fever and prolonged rupture of membranes. All 10 infants received ampicillin and gentamicin, antimicrobial agents without good activity against these organisms, and had a good clinical outcome.

In cultures of CSF from 920 infants in a neonatal intensive care unit, *U. urealyticum* was isolated from 2 (0.2%) and *M. hominis* from none.[124] Likitnukul and colleagues[24] and Mardh[25] failed to recover mycoplasmas from CSF of infants in prospective investigations. The study by Likitnukul's group involved infants who had been previously discharged from the hospital and had returned because of suspected sepsis. No mycoplasmas were recovered from the CSF of 47 preterm infants cultured within the first week of life by Izraeli and co-workers.[23] The reason for the frequent isolation of mycoplasmas in some studies but not in others remains uncertain. Possible technical reasons are discussed by Waites[148] and Heggie[149] and their colleagues.

The question of whether mycoplasmas are linked to abnormalities on CNS imaging also has been investigated, although in an indirect manner. Perzigian and associates[102] prospectively investigated a cohort of 105 VLBW infants in whom 22 (21%) results of tracheal aspirate culture were positive for *U. urealyticum* at birth. No differences were found between the groups for intraventricular hemorrhage or cystic periventricular leukomalacia. Similarly, in a study of 464 VLBW infants, Dammann and co-workers[150] addressed the question of whether *U. urealyticum* or *M. hominis* cultured from the placenta was associated with an increased risk of ultrasonographic cerebral white matter echolucency as a measure of white matter damage. The cranial ultrasound studies were performed up to a median of 22 days of life. Culture results were as follows: 139 of 464 (30%) were positive for *U. urealyticum*, 27 (6%) were positive for *M. hominis*, and 21 (5%) were positive for both. It was found that with a positive result on culture for *U. urealyticum*, the infants were not at increased risk of cerebral white matter damage. The presence of *M. hominis* was associated with a trend toward an increased risk of echolucency ($P = .08$).

The clinical findings in newborns with *U. urealyticum* and *M. hominis* isolated from the CSF are variable. *U. urealyticum* and *M. hominis* may produce abnormal CSF indices with pleocytosis, or an inflammatory reaction in CSF may be absent.[19,21,22,25] In some infants, mycoplasmas are cleared spontaneously from the CSF, whereas in others, the organisms have been shown to persist for weeks to months even after appropriate treatment.[44,59,139,146,147]

Other Sites of Infection in the Neonate

M. hominis also has been isolated from the pericardial fluid,[55] subcutaneous abscesses,[151,152,154] and the submandibular lymph node of neonates.[153] *U. urealyticum* and *M. hominis* have been isolated from the urine, but the clinical significance was uncertain.[24]

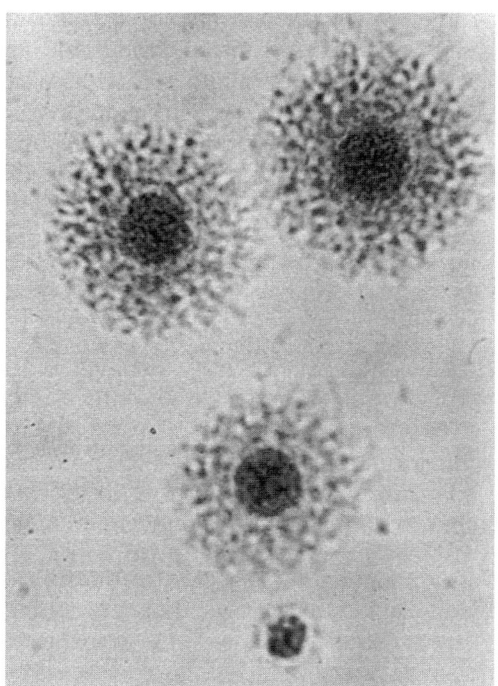

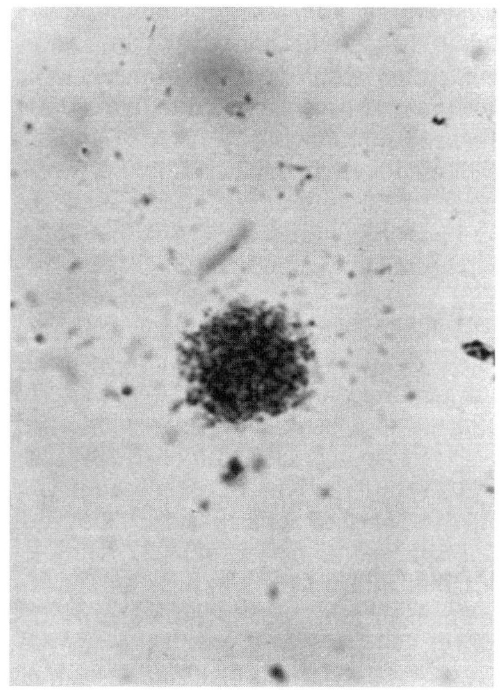

Figure 16–3 **A,** *Mycoplasma hominis* (original magnification 100×). **B,** *Ureaplasma urealyticum* (original magnification 1000×). (From Klein JO. Mycoplasmas, genitourinary tract infection, and reproductive failure. Hosp Pract 6:127-133, 1971, with permission.)

OTHER MYCOPLASMAS

The role of other mycoplasmas, such as *M. genitalium*, *M. fermentans*, and *M. pneumoniae*, in maternal/fetal and neonatal infections is not thought to be prominent, although investigations are limited. *M. genitalium* was not isolated by culture of the chorioamnion of 609 women or by culture or PCR assay of 232 amniotic fluid samples tested.[155] To evaluate the impact of *M. genitalium* on the outcome of pregnancy, cervical samples from 1014 women were assayed by PCR techniques for the presence of *M. genitalium*.[156] Among those women, *M. genitalium* was isolated in 6.2%, but its isolation was not significantly associated with adverse outcomes of pregnancy (preterm delivery, small for gestational age, spontaneous abortion, stillbirth). Taylor-Robinson[157] recently reviewed disease associations with *M. genitalium*.

M. fermentans was detected in amniotic fluid collected at the time of cesarean section from 4 of 232 women with intact membranes.[155] Placental tissue also was PCR assay positive for *M. fermentans* in 3 women. Villitis and chorioamnionitis were present in two of the four positive specimens, and no other organisms were detected.

DIAGNOSIS

Culture and PCR assay both are appropriate methods for the diagnosis of *Mycoplasma* and *Ureaplasma* infections. Culture of *U. urealyticum* and *M. hominis*, however, requires special handling with techniques and media generally not available outside major medical centers or reference laboratories. Detailed laboratory techniques for culture and identification of mycoplasmas and ureaplasmas have been reviewed by others.[59,160]

Ureaplasmas and mycoplasmas are extremely susceptible to adverse environmental conditions. Accordingly, correct methods of collecting, processing, and transporting specimens are important for reliable and interpretable culture results. A specific ureaplasmal transport medium, such as Shepard's 10B broth,[161,162] for *U. urealyticum* and *M. hominis* should be available for direct inoculation of clinical specimens and swabs at the time of collection. If specimens are allowed to sit at room temperature and are not inoculated into appropriate media, the recovery of these organisms is unlikely. Only calcium alginate– or Dacron-tipped swabs with plastic or wire shafts should be utilized for sampling of mucosal surfaces. Blood should be collected free of anticoagulants and immediately inoculated into the transport medium in a 1:5 to 1:10 ratio.[59] Specimens should be refrigerated at 4° C and protected from drying in a sealed container until transported to the laboratory. If transport to a suitable laboratory is not possible within 6 to 12 hours after collection, the specimen in appropriate transport medium should be stored at −70° C and shipped frozen on dry ice. Ureaplasmas and mycoplasmas are stable for long periods when kept frozen at −70° C in a protein-containing support medium such as Shepard's 10B. Storage at −20° C is less reliable and will result in a significant loss in number of organisms in a relatively short time.[59] Before collecting a clinical sample for culture, it is appropriate to arrange processing of samples with the microbiology laboratory.

U. urealyticum and *M. hominis* grow within 2 to 5 days. Broth cultures are incubated at 37° C under atmospheric conditions; agar plates are incubated under 95% nitrogen and 5% carbon dioxide. Colonies of *U. urealyticum* can be identified on A8 agar by urease production. The colonies often are amorphous. Colonies of other mycoplasmas are urease negative and have a typical "fried egg" appearance (Fig. 16-3).

PCR assays for the detection of *U. urealyticum* and *M. hominis*[63,118,163,164] have been developed. These assays appear to have greater sensitivity than culture in most studies.[57,58,104,165,166] A combination of PCR assay and culture should give the most reliable results.

Although enzyme-linked immunosorbent assays (ELISAs) have been developed to detect *U. urealyticum*– and *M. hominis*–specific antibodies in sera, serologic testing is not recommended for the routine diagnosis of *U. urealyticum* and *M. hominis* infections. The use of these assays is limited to the research setting.

Owing to the fastidiousness and slow growth of *M. genitalium* and *M. fermentans*, PCR assay, in situ hybridization, and/or immunohistochemistry are recommended for detection of these mycoplasmas.[155,158,159]

TREATMENT OF NEONATAL INFECTIONS

A positive result on culture or PCR assay for *U. urealyticum* or *M. hominis* from a normally sterile site, particularly in the absence of other microorganisms, is justification to consider treatment for infants with evidence of infectious inflammation. On the basis of the current understanding of these organisms, however, the isolation of *U. urealyticum* or *M. hominis* in the absence of disease generally does not warrant treatment.

Formulation of guidelines for treatment when these organisms are isolated from a maternal/fetal or neonatal specimen is difficult, in view of the following considerations as reviewed in this chapter:

- Causation has not been clearly established for many of the conditions associated with *U. urealyticum* and *M. hominis* (all maternal/fetal and neonatal associations, except postpartum and postabortal fever).
- Organisms often are present (in CSF, bloodstream, respiratory tract, amniotic fluid, or lower genital tract, for example) with little or no adverse clinical outcome.
- Organisms often are spontaneously cleared (from CSF, bloodstream, or respiratory tract, for example) without treatment.
- No definitive controlled trials have been performed for many sites of infection (e.g., CSF, bloodstream, amniotic fluid, lung in acute pneumonia).
- Small randomized, controlled trials have not shown benefit of treatment for CLD.
- Evidence that treatment can be useful comes from uncontrolled case reports for which the outcome without treatment is not known.
- Comparative clinical trials among antimicrobials have not been performed to assess their relative efficacy.
- Often the clinical indication for culture or PCR assay has resolved before the positive result is reported.

Treatment may be warranted in some situations, so decisions must be made on a case-by-case basis, to ensure full consideration of the risk-benefit ratio related to disease and treatment. The relative contribution of *U. urealyticum* and *M. hominis* infection to morbidity and mortality is difficult to establish, because most cases have been reported in VLBW preterm infants with multiple complications or in infants with clinical problems that probably contribute to the poor outcome. An authoritative reference states that antimicrobial therapy for *U. urealyticum* cannot be recommended for pregnant women to prevent preterm delivery or in preterm infants to prevent pulmonary disease, because trials of antimicrobial therapy for these indications generally have not demonstrated efficacy.[167] It also suggests that definitive efficacy of antimicrobial agents in the treatment of CNS *U. urealyticum* infections in infants is lacking.[167]

The treatment of some non-neonatal *U. urealyticum* and *M. hominis* infections is better established. For instance, *U. urealyticum* urethritis and *M. hominis* pyelonephritis, pelvic inflammatory disease, postabortal fever, and postpartum fever, as well as infections with either organism in immunocompromised patients (especially those with hypogammaglobulinemia), generally are considered to warrant treatment.

Erythromycin generally has been considered the antimicrobial agent of choice for neonatal ureaplasmal infections (not involving the CNS), although clinical superiority over other agents has not been investigated.[175] Erythromycin has been employed in most clinical trials in infants with *U. urealyticum*.[121,123-127] Other agents with in vitro activity against *U. urealyticum* and variable clinical experience include clarithromycin, azithromycin, doxycycline, and chloramphenicol.[106,171,172,174,176] Resistance to macrolides, doxycycline, and chloramphenicol has been reported.[168,173,175] The in vitro activities of newer agents, such as quinolones and ketolides, against *Ureaplasma* have been reported; clinical experience is lacking.[175,177-180]

M. hominis is resistant to erythromycin, as well as to other macrolides and azolides.[171,172,174,175] Doxycycline is the drug of choice for treatment of *M. hominis* infections, although resistance has been reported.[46,53,139,169,170] Clindamycin and chloramphenicol also are generally active in vitro against *M. hominis*.[175] The in vitro activity of newer antimicrobials against *M. hominis* has been reported; clinical experience is lacking, however.[175,177-180]

Antimicrobial susceptibility testing should be considered when it is deemed necessary to treat a *U. urealyticum* or *M. hominis* infection in a neonate, especially for the persistent isolation of either organism from a normally sterile site, because resistance to commonly used antibiotics is not rare. Some tetracycline-resistant strains of *U. urealyticum* can be erythromycin resistant, but high-level erythromycin resistance in *U. urealyticum* is uncommon.[175] Penetration of the blood-brain barrier by antimicrobials should be considered in treating a CNS infection, as should the safety and pharmacokinetics of antimicrobials in newborns in making treatment decisions.

REFERENCES

1. McCormack WM, Lee YH, Zinner SH. Sexual experience and urethral colonization with genital mycoplasmas. Ann Intern Med 78:696-698, 1973.
2. McCormack WM, Almeida PC, Bailey PE, et al. Sexual activity and vaginal colonization with genital mycoplasmas. JAMA 221:1375-1377, 1972.
3. Cassell GH (ed). Proceedings of the International Symposium: Ureaplasmas of humans with emphasis on maternal and neonatal infections. Pediatr Infect Dis 5(Suppl 6), 1986.
4. Cassell GH, Waites KB, Watson HL, et al. *Ureaplasma urealyticum* intrauterine infection: role in prematurity and disease in newborns. Clin Microbiol Rev 6:69-87, 1993.

5. Cassell GH, Davis RO, Waites KB, et al. Isolation of *Mycoplasma hominis* and *Ureaplasma urealyticum* from amniotic fluid at 16-20 weeks gestation: potential effect on pregnancy outcome. Sex Transm Dis 10:294-302, 1983.
6. Faye-Kette H, La Ruche G, Ali-Napo L, et al. Genital mycoplasmas among pregnant women in Cote d'Ivoire, West Africa: prevalence and risk factors. Int J STD AIDS 11:599-602, 2000.
7. Clegg A, Passey M, Yoannes M, et al. High rates of genital *Mycoplasma* infection in the highlands of Papua New Guinea determined both by culture and by a commercial detection kit. J Clin Microbiol 35:197-200, 1997.
8. Cassell GH, Waites KB, Gibbs RS, et al. The role of *Ureaplasma urealyticum* in amnionitis. Pediatr Infect Dis J 5(Suppl):247-252, 1986.
9. Taylor-Robinson, D. *Ureaplasma urealyticum, Mycoplasma hominis,* and *Mycoplasma genitalium*. *In* Mandell GL, Bennett JE, Dolin R (eds). Principles and Practice of Infectious Diseases, 5th ed. Philadelphia, Churchill Livingstone, 2000, pp 2027-2032.
10. Embree JE, Krause VW, Embil JA, et al. Placental infection with *Mycoplasma hominis* and *Ureaplasma urealyticum*: clinical correlation. Obstet Gynecol 56:475-481, 1980.
11. Hillier SL, Martius J, Krohn M, et al. A case-control study of chorioamnionic infection and histologic chorioamnionitis in prematurity. N Engl J Med 319:972-978, 1988.
12. Kundsin RB, Driscoll SG, Monson RR, et al. Association of *Ureaplasma urealyticum* in the placenta with perinatal morbidity and mortality. N Engl J Med 310:941-945, 1984.
13. Quinn PA, Butany J, Chipman M, et al. A prospective study of microbial infection in stillbirths and early neonatal death. Am J Obstet Gynecol 151:238-249, 1985.
14. Quinn PA, Butany J, Taylor J, et al. Chorioamnionitis: its association with pregnancy outcome and microbial infection. Am J Obstet Gynecol 156:379-387, 1987.
15. Cassell GH, Waites KB, Crouse DT. Mycoplasmal infections. *In* Remington JS, Klein JO (eds). Infectious Diseases of the Fetus and Newborn Infant, 5th ed. Philadelphia, WB Saunders Company, 2001, pp 733-767.
16. Hillier SL, Krohn MA, Kiviat NB, et al. Microbiologic causes and neonatal outcomes associated with chorioamnion infection. Am J Obstet Gynecol 165:955-961, 1991.
17. Gray DJ, Robinson HB, Malone J, et al. Adverse outcome in pregnancy following amniotic fluid isolation of *Ureaplasma urealyticum*. Prenat Diagn 12:111-117, 1992.
18. Foulon W, Naessens A, Dewaele M, et al. Chronic *Ureaplasma urealyticum* amnionitis associated with abruptio placentae. Obstet Gynecol 68:280, 1986.
19. Waites KB, Rudd PT, Crouse DT, et al. Chronic *Ureaplasma urealyticum* and *Mycoplasma hominis* infections of central nervous systems in preterm infants. Lancet 2:17-21, 1988.
20. Waites KB, Cox NR, Crouse DT, et al. *Mycoplasma* infection of the central nervous system in humans and animals. Int J Med Microbiol 20(Suppl):379-386, 1990.
21. Ollikainen J, Heikkaniemi H, Korppi M, et al. *Ureaplasma urealyticum* infection associated with acute respiratory insufficiency and death in premature infants. J Pediatr 122:756-760, 1993.
22. Valencia GB, Banzon F, Cummings M, et al. *Mycoplasma hominis* and *Ureaplasma urealyticum* in neonates with suspected infection. Pediatr Infect Dis J 12:571-573, 1993.
23. Izraeli S, Samra Z, Sirota L, et al. Genital mycoplasmas in preterm infants: prevalence and clinical significance. Eur J Pediatr 150:804-807, 1991.
24. Likitnukul S, Kusmiesz H, Nelson JD, et al. Role of genital mycoplasmas in young infants with suspected sepsis. J Pediatr 109:971-974, 1986.
25. Mardh PA. *Mycoplasma hominis* infections of the central nervous system in newborn infants. Sex Transm Dis 10:331-334, 1983.
26. Cassell GH, Waites KB, Crouse DT, et al. Association of *Ureaplasma urealyticum* infection of the lower respiratory tract with chronic lung disease and death in very low birthweight infants. Lancet 2:240-245, 1988.
27. Waites KB, Crouse DT, Phillips JB, et al. *Ureaplasma* pneumonia and sepsis .associated with persistent pulmonary hypertension of the newborn. Pediatrics 83:84-89, 1991.
28. McCormack WM. *Ureaplasma urealyticum*: ecologic niche and epidemiologic considerations. Pediatr Infect Dis J 5:S232-S233, 1986.
29. Brus F, van Waarde WM, Schoots C, et al. Fatal ureaplasmal pneumonia and sepsis in a newborn infant. Eur J Pediatr 150:782-783, 1991.
30. McCormack WM, Rankin JS, Lee YH. Localization of genital mycoplasmas in women. Am J Obstet Gynecol 112:920-923, 1972.
31. Braun P, Klein JO, Lee YH, et al. Methodologic investigations and prevalence of genital mycoplasmas in pregnancy. J Infect Dis 121:391-400, 1970.
32. Walsh WF, Butler J, Coalson J, et al. A primate model of *Ureaplasma urealyticum* infection in the premature infant with hyaline membrane disease. Clin Infect Dis 17(Suppl 1):S158-162, 1993.
33. Taylor-Robinson D, McCormack WM. The genital mycoplasmas. N Engl J Med 302:1003-1010, 1980.
34. Crouse DT, Odrezin GT, Cutter GR, et al. Radiographic changes associated with tracheal isolation of *Ureaplasma urealyticum* from neonates. Clin Infect Dis 17(Suppl 1):S122-S130, 1993.
35. McCormack WM, Rosner B, Alpert S, et al. Vaginal colonization with *Mycoplasma hominis* and *Ureaplasma urealyticum*. Sex Transm Dis 134:67-70, 1986.
36. McCormack WM, Rosner B, Lee YH. Colonization with genital mycoplasmas in women. Am J Epidemiol 97:240-245, 1973.
37. Braun P, Lee Y-H, Klein JO, et al. Birth weight and genital mycoplasmas in pregnancy. N Engl J Med 284:167-171, 1971.
38. Mardh PA, Westrom L. T-mycoplasmas in the genitourinary tract of the female. Acta Pathol Microbiol Scand 78B:367-374, 1970.
39. Becopoulos T, Tsagatakis E, Constantinides C, et al. *Ureaplasma urealyticum* and infected renal calculi. J Chemother 3:39-41, 1991.
40. Grenabo L, Hedelin H, Pettersson S. Urinary stones caused by *Ureaplasma urealyticum*: a review. Scand J Infect Dis Suppl 53:46-49, 1988.
41. Thomsen AC, Taylor-Robinson D, Hanson KB, et al. The infrequent occurrence of mycoplasmas in amniotic fluid from women with intact fetal membranes. Acta Obstet Gynecol Scand 3:425-429, 1983.
42. Mardh PA, Westrom L. Tubal and cervical cultures in acute salpingitis with special reference to *Mycoplasma hominis* and T-strain mycoplasmas. Br J Vener Dis 46:179-186, 1970.
43. Mardh PA. Mycoplasmal PID: a review of natural and experimental infections. Yale J Biol Med 56:529, 1983.
44. Shaw NJ, Pratt BC, Weindling AM. *Ureaplasma* and *Mycoplasma* infections of the central nervous system in preterm infants. Lancet 23:1530-1531, 1989.
45. Likitnukul S, Nelson JD, McCracken GH, et al. Role of genital *Mycoplasma* infection in young infants with aseptic meningitis. J Pediatr 110:998, 1987.
46. Mardh PA. *Mycoplasma hominis* infection of the central nervous system in newborn infants. Sex Transm Dis 10:332-334, 1983.
47. Syrogiannopoulos GA, Kapatais-Zoumbos K, Decavalas GO, et al. *Ureaplasma urealyticum* colonization of full term infants: perinatal acquisition and persistence during early infancy. Pediatr Infect Dis J 9:236-240, 1990.
48. Waites KB, Duffy LB, Crouse DT, et al. Mycoplasmal infection of cerebrospinal fluid in newborn infants from a community hospital population. Pediatr Infect Dis J 9:241-245, 1990.
49. Miettinen A, Paavonen J, Jansson E, et al. Enzyme immunoassay for serum antibody to *Mycoplasma hominis* in women with acute pelvic inflammatory disease. Sex Transm Dis 10(Suppl):289, 1983.
50. Henry-Suchet J, Catalan F, Loffredo V, et al. Microbiology of specimens obtained by laparoscopy from controls and from patients with pelvic inflammatory disease or infertility with tubal obstruction. *Chlamydia trachomatis* and *Ureaplasma urealyticum*. Am J Obstet Gynecol 138:1022, 1980.
51. Moller BR, Freundt EA, Black FT, et al. Experimental infection of the genital tract of female grivet monkeys by *Mycoplasma hominis*. Infect Immun 20:248, 1978.
52. Mardh PA, Westrom L, Mecklenburg C. Studies on ciliated epithelia of the human genital tract: I. Swelling of the cilia of fallopian tube epithelium in organ cultures infected with *Mycoplasma hominis*. Br J Vener Dis 52:52, 1976.
53. Cassell GH, Davis JK, Waites KB, et al. Pathogenesis and significance of urogenital mycoplasmal infections. *In* Bondi A, Stieritz D, Campos J, et al (eds). Urogenital Infections. New Developments in Laboratory Diagnosis and Treatment. New York, Plenum Publishing, 1987, pp 93-115.
54. McDonald JC. *Mycoplasma hominis* meningitis in a premature infant. Pediatr Infect Dis J 7:795-798, 1988.
55. Miller TC, Baman SI, Albers WH. Massive pericardial effusion due to *Mycoplasma hominis* in a newborn. Am J Dis Child 136:271-272, 1982.
56. Dan M, Tyrrel DL, Stemke GW, et al. *Mycoplasma hominis* septicemia in a burned infant. J Pediatr 99:743-744, 1981.

57. Yoon BH, Romero R, Kim M, et al. Clinical implications of detection of *Ureaplasma urealyticum* in the amniotic cavity with the polymerase chain reaction. Am J Obstet Gynecol 183:1130-7, 2000.
58. Yoon BH, Romero R, Lim JH, et al. The clinical significance of detecting *Ureaplasma urealyticum* by the polymerase chain reaction in the amniotic fluid of patients with preterm labor. Am J Obstet Gynecol 189:919-24, 2003.
59. Cassell GH, Waites KB, Crouse DT. Mycoplasmal infections. *In* Remington JS, Klein JO (eds). Infectious Diseases of the Fetus and Newborn Infant, 5th ed. Philadelphia, WB Saunders Company, 2001, pp 733-767.
60. Berg TG, Philpot KL, Welsh MS, et al. *Ureaplasma/Mycoplasma*-infected amniotic fluid: pregnancy outcome in treated and nontreated patients. J Perinatol 19:275-7, 1999.
61. Andrews WW, Hauth JC, Cliver SP, et al. Randomized clinical trial of extended spectrum antibiotic prophylaxis with coverage for *Ureaplasma urealyticum* to reduce post-cesarean delivery endometritis. Obstet Gynecol 101:1183-9, 2003.
62. Donders GG, Van Bulck B, Caudron J, et al. Relationship of bacterial vaginosis and mycoplasmas to the risk of spontaneous abortion. Am J Obstet Gynecol 183:431-7, 2000.
63. Blanchard A, Hentschel J, Duffy L, et al. Detection of *Ureaplasma urealyticum* by polymerase chain reaction in the urogenital tract of adults, in amniotic fluid, and in the respiratory tract of newborns. Clin Infect Dis 17(Suppl 1):S148-S153, 1993.
64. Stokes EJ. Human infection with pleuropneumonia-like organisms. Lancet 1:276-279, 1955.
65. Harwick HJ, Purcell RH, Iuppa JB, et al. *Mycoplasma hominis* and abortion. J Infect Dis 121:260-268, 1970.
66. Harwick HJ, Iuppa JB, Purcell RH, et al. *Mycoplasma hominis* septicemia associated with abortion. Am J Obstet Gynecol 99:725-727, 1967.
67. Tully JG, Brown MS, Sheagren JN, et al. Septicemia due to *Mycoplasma hominis* type 1. N Engl J Med 273:648-650, 1965.
68. Caspi E, Herczeg E, Solomon F, et al. Amnionitis and T strain mycoplasmemia. Am J Obstet Gynecol 111:1102-1106, 1971.
69. Sompolinsky D, Solomon F, Leiba H, et al. Puerperal sepsis due to T-strain *Mycoplasma*. Isr J Med Sci 7:745-748, 1971.
70. Edelin KC, McCormack WM. Infection with *Mycoplasma hominis* in postpartum fever. Lancet 2:1217-1221, 1980.
71. McCormack WM, Rosner B, Lee YH, et al. Isolation of genital mycoplasmas from blood obtained shortly after vaginal delivery. Lancet 1:596-599, 1975.
72. Kelly VN, Garland SM, Gilbert GL. Isolation of genital mycoplasmas from the blood of neonates and women with pelvic infection using conventional SPS-free blood culture media. Pathology 19:277-280, 1987.
73. Neman-Simha V, Renaudin H, de Barbeyrac B, et al. Isolation of genital mycoplasmas from blood of febrile obstetrical-gynecologic patients and neonates. Scand J Infect Dis 24:317-321, 1992.
74. Andrews W, Shah S, Goldenberg R, et al. Post-cesarean endometritis: role of asymptomatic antenatal colonization of the chorioamnion with *Ureaplasma urealyticum*. Am J Obstet Gynecol 170:416, 1994.
75. Roberts S, Maccato M, Faro S, et al. The microbiology of post-cesarean wound morbidity. Obstet Gynecol 81:383-386, 1993.
76. *Mycoplasma hominis*. Newsnotes. BMJ 2:816, 1974.
77. Word BM, Baldridge A. *Mycoplasma hominis* pneumonia and pleural effusion in a postpartum adolescent. Pediatr Infect Dis J 9:295-296, 1990.
78. Young MJ, Cox RA. Near fatal puerperal fever due to *Mycoplasma hominis*. Postgrad Med J 66:147-149, 1990.
79. Phillips LE, Faro S, Pokorny S, et al. Postcesarean wound infection by *Mycoplasma hominis* in a patient with persistent postpartum fever. Diagn Microbiol Infect Dis 7:193-197, 1987.
80. Maccato M, Faro S, Summers KL. Wound infections after cesarean section with *Mycoplasma hominis* and *Ureaplasma urealyticum*: a report of three cases. Diagn Microbiol Infect Dis 13:363-365, 1990.
81. Cassell GH, Cole BC. Mycoplasmas as agents of human disease. N Engl J Med 304:80-89, 1981.
82. McCormack WM, Taylor-Robinson D. The genital mycoplasmas. *In* Holmes KK, Mardh PA, Sparling PF, et al (eds). Sexually Transmitted Diseases. New York, McGraw-Hill, 1984, pp 408-419.
83. Sompolinsky D, Solomon F, Elkina L, et al. Infections with *Mycoplasma* and bacteria in induced midtrimester abortion and fetal loss. Am J Obstet Gynecol 121:610-616, 1975.
84. Stray-Pederson B, Engard J, Reikvam TM. Uterine T-*Mycoplasma* colonization in reproductive failure. Am J Obstet Gynecol 130:307, 1978.
85. Naessens A, Foulon W, Cammu H, et al. Epidemiology and pathogenesis of *Ureaplasma urealyticum* in spontaneous abortion and early preterm labor. Acta Obstet Gynecol Scand 66:513-516, 1987.
86. Quinn PA, Shewchuk AB, Shuber J, et al. Serologic evidence of *Ureaplasma urealyticum* infection in women with spontaneous pregnancy loss. Am J Obstet Gynecol 145:245-250, 1983.
87. Gray DJ, Robinson HB, Malone J, et al. Adverse outcome in pregnancy following amniotic fluid isolation of *Ureaplasma urealyticum*. Prenat Diagn 12:111-117, 1992.
88. Romero R, Mazor M, Oyarzun E, et al. Is genital colonization with *Mycoplasma hominis* or *Ureaplasma urealyticum* associated with prematurity/low birth weight? Obstet Gynecol 73:532-536, 1989.
89. Gerber S, Vial Y, Hohlfeld P, et al. Detection of *Ureaplasma urealyticum* in second-trimester amniotic fluid by polymerase chain reaction correlates with subsequent preterm labor and delivery. J Infect Dis 187:518-521, 2003.
90. Gravett MG, Hummel D, Eschenbach D, et al. Preterm labor associated with subclinical amniotic fluid infection and with bacterial vaginosis. Obstet Gynecol 67:229-237, 1986.
91. Romero R, Sirtori M, Oyarzun E, et al. Infection and labor: V. Prevalence, microbiology, and clinical significance of intraamniotic infection in women with preterm labor and intact membranes. Am J Obstet Gynecol 161:817-824, 1989.
92. Watts DH, Krohn MA, Hillier SL, et al. The association of occult amniotic fluid infection with gestational age and neonatal outcome among women in preterm labor. Obstet Gynecol 79:351-357, 1992.
93. Naessens A, Foulon W, Breynaert J, et al. Postpartum bacteremia and placental colonization with genital mycoplasmas and pregnancy outcome. Am J Obstet Gynecol 160:647-650, 1989.
94. Zlatnik FJ, Gellhaus TM, Benda JA, et al. Histologic chorioamnionitis, microbial infection, and prematurity. J Obstet Gynaecol 76:355-359, 1990.
95. Quinn PA, Gillian JE, Markestad T, et al. Intrauterine infection with *Ureaplasma urealyticum* as a cause of fatal neonatal pneumonia. Pediatr Infect Dis J 4:538-543, 1985.
96. Sanchez P, Regan JA. Vertical transmission of *Ureaplasma urealyticum* in full term infants. Pediatr Infect Dis J 6:825-828, 1988.
97. Sanchez PJ, Regan JA. Vertical transmission of *Ureaplasma urealyticum* from mothers to preterm infants. Pediatr Infect Dis J 9:398-401, 1990.
98. Dinsmoor MJ, Ramamurthy RS, Gibbs RS. Transmission of genital mycoplasmas from mother to neonate in women with prolonged membrane rupture. Pediatr Infect Dis J 8:483-487, 1989.
99. Chua KB, Ngeow YF, Lim CT, et al. Colonization and transmission of *Ureaplasma urealyticum* and *Mycoplasma hominis* from mothers to full and preterm babies by normal vaginal delivery. Med J Malaysia 54:242-6, 1999.
100. Foy HM, Kenny GE, Levinsohn EM, et al. Acquisition of mycoplasmata and T-strains during infancy. J Infect Dis 121:579-587, 1970.
101. Benstein BD, Crouse DT, Shanklin DR, et al. *Ureaplasma* in lung. 2. Association with bronchopulmonary dysplasia in premature newborns. Exp Mol Pathol 75:171-7, 2003.
102. Perzigian RW, Adams JT, Weiner GM, et al. *Ureaplasma urealyticum* and chronic lung disease in very low birth weight infants during the exogenous surfactant era. Pediatr Infect Dis J 17:620-625, 1998.
103. Tafari N, Ross S, Naeye RL, et al. Mycoplasma "T" strains and perinatal death. Lancet 1:108-109, 1976.
104. Castro-Alcaraz S, Greenberg EM, Bateman DA, et al. Patterns of colonization with *Ureaplasma urealyticum* during neonatal intensive care unit hospitalizations of very low birth weight infants and the development of chronic lung disease. Pediatrics 110:e45, 2002.
105. Hannaford K, Todd DA, Jeffery H, et al. Role of *Ureaplasma urealyticum* in lung disease of prematurity. Arch Dis Child Fetal Neonatal Ed 81:F162-7, 1999.
106. Berger A, Witt A, Haiden N, et al. Microbial invasion of the amniotic cavity at birth is associated with adverse short-term outcome of preterm infants. J Perinat Med 31:115-21, 2003.
107. Taylor-Robinson D, Furr PM, Liberman MM. The occurrence of genital mycoplasmas in babies with and without respiratory diseases. Acta Paediatr Scand 73:383-386, 1984.
108. Escobedo MB, Hilliard JL, Smith F, et al. A baboon model of bronchopulmonary dysplasia. Exp Mol Pathol 37:323-324, 1982.
109. Wang EEL, Ohlsson A, Kellner JD. Association of *Ureaplasma urealyticum* colonization with chronic lung disease of prematurity: results of a metaanalysis. J Pediatr 127:640-644, 1995.

110. Garland SM, Bowman ED. Role of *Ureaplasma urealyticum* and *Chlamydia trachomatis* in lung disease in low birth weight infants. Pathology 28:266-269, 1996.
111. Iles R, Lyon A, Ross P, McIntosh N. Infection with *Ureaplasma urealyticum* and *Mycoplasma hominis* and the development of chronic lung disease in pre-term infants. Acta Paediatr 85:482-484, 1996.
112. Pacifico L, Panero A, Roggini M, et al. *Ureaplasma urealyticum* and pulmonary outcome in a neonatal intensive care population. Pediatr Infect Dis J 16:579-586, 1997.
113. Kafetzis DA, Skevaki CL, Skouteri V, et al. Maternal genital colonization with *Ureaplasma urealyticum* promotes preterm delivery: association of the respiratory colonization of premature infants with chronic lung disease and increased mortality. Clin Infect Dis 39:1113-1122, 2004.
114. Abele-Horn M, Genzel-Boroviczeny O, Uhlig T, et al. *Ureaplasma urealyticum* colonization and bronchopulmonary dysplasia: a comparative prospective multicentre study. Eur J Pediatr 157:1004-1011, 1998.
115. Agarwal P, Rajadurai VS, Pradeepkumar VK, et al. *Ureaplasma urealyticum* and its association with chronic lung disease in Asian neonates. J Paediatr Child Health 36:487-490, 2000.
116. Da Silva O, Gregson D, Hammerberg O. Role of *Ureaplasma urealyticum* and *Chlamydia trachomatis* in development of bronchopulmonary dysplasia in very low birth weight infants. Pediatr Infect Dis J 16:364-369, 1997.
117. Van Waarde WM, Brus F, Okken A, Kimpen JLL. *Ureaplasma urealyticum* colonization, prematurity and bronchopulmonary dysplasia. Eur Respir J 10:886-890, 1997.
118. Couroucli XI, Welty SE, Ramsay PL, et al. Detection of microorganisms in the tracheal aspirates of preterm infants by polymerase chain reaction: association of adenovirus infection with bronchopulmonary dysplasia. Pedatr Res 47:225-232, 2000.
119. Cordero L, Coley BD, Miller RL, Mueller CF. Bacterial and *Ureaplasma* colonization of the airway: radiologic findings in infants with bronchopulmonary dysplasia. J Perinatol 17:428-433, 1997.
120. Heggie AD, Bar-Shain D, Boxerbaum B, et al. Identification and quantification of ureaplasmas colonizing the respiratory tract and assessment of their role in the development of chronic lung disease in preterm infants. Pediatr Infect Dis J 20:854-859, 2001.
121. Jonsson B, Rylander M, Faxelius G. *Ureaplasma urealyticum*, erythromycin and respiratory morbidity in high-risk preterm neonates. Acta Paediatr 87:1079-1084, 1998.
122. Ollikainen J, Korppi M, Heiskanen-Kosma T, et al. Chronic lung disease of the newborn is not associated with *Ureaplasma urealyticum*. Pediatr Pulmonol 32:303-307, 2001.
123. Buhrer C, Hoehn T, Hentschel J. Role of erythromycin for treatment of incipient chronic lung disease in preterm infants colonised with *Ureaplasma urealyticum*. Drugs 61:1893-1899, 2001.
124. Heggie AD, Jacobs MR, Butler VT, et al. Frequency and significance of isolation of *Ureaplasma urealyticum* and *Mycoplasma hominis* from cerebrospinal fluid and tracheal aspirate specimens from low birth weight infants. J Pediatr 124:956-961, 1994.
125. Lyon AJ, McColm J, Middlemist L, et al. Randomised trial of erythromycin on the development of chronic lung disease in preterm infants. Arch Dis Child Fetal Neonatal Ed 78:F10-F14, 1998.
126. Bowman ED, Dharmalingam A, Fan WQ, et al. Impact of erythromycin on respiratory colonization of *Ureaplasma urealyticum* and the development of chronic lung disease in extremely low birth weight infants. Pediatr Infect Dis J 17:615-620, 1998.
127. Pacifico L, Panero A, Roggini M, et al. *Ureaplasma urealyticum* and pulmonary outcome in a neonatal intensive care population. Pediatr Infect Dis J 16:579-586, 1997.
128. Kenyon SL, Taylor DJ, Tarnow-Mordi W. Broad-spectrum antibiotics for preterm, prelabour rupture of fetal membranes: the ORACLE I randomised trial. ORACLE Collaborative Group. Lancet 357:979-988, 2001.
129. Kenyon SL, Taylor DJ, Tarnow-Mordi W. Broad-spectrum antibiotics for spontaneous preterm labour: the ORACLE II randomised trial. ORACLE Collaborative Group. Lancet 357:989-994, 2001.
130. Ollikainen J. Perinatal *Ureaplasma urealyticum* infection increases the need for hospital treatment during the first year of life in preterm infants. Pediatr Pulmonol 30:402-405, 2000.
131. Steytler JG. Statistical studies on mycoplasma-positive human umbilical cord blood cultures. S Afr J Obstet Gynecol 8:10-13, 1970.
132. Ollikainen J, Hiekkaniemi H, Korppi M, et al. *Ureaplasma urealyticum* cultured from brain tissue of preterm twins who died of intraventricular hemorrhage. Scand J Infect Dis 25:529-531, 1993.
133. Unsworth PF, Taylor-Robinson D, Shoo EE, et al. Neonatal mycoplasmemia: *Mycoplasma hominis* as a significant cause of disease? J Infect 10:163-168, 1985.
134. Wealthall SR. *Mycoplasma* meningitis in infants with spina bifida. Dev Med Child Neurol 17(Suppl 35):117-122, 1975.
135. Siber GR, Alpert S, Smith DL, et al. Neonatal central nervous system infection due to *Mycoplasma hominis*. J Pediatr 90:625-627, 1977.
136. Kirk N, Kovar I. *Mycoplasma hominis* meningitis in a preterm infant. J Infect 15:109-110, 1987.
137. Hjelm E, Jousell E, Linglof T, et al. Meningitis in a newborn infant caused by *Mycoplasma hominis*. Acta Paediatr Scand 69:415-418, 1980.
138. Gewitz M, Dinwiddle R, Rees L, et al. *Mycoplasma hominis*: a cause of neonatal meningitis. Arch Dis Child 54:231-233, 1979.
139. Gilbert GL, Law F, Macinnes SJ. Chronic *Mycoplasma hominis* infection complicating severe intraventricular hemorrhage, in a premature neonate. Pediatr Infect Dis J 7:817-818, 1988.
140. Boe O, Diderichsen J, Matre R. Isolation of *Mycoplasma hominis* from cerebrospinal fluid. Scand J Infect Dis 5:285-288, 1973.
141. Rao RP, Ghanayem NS, Kaufman BA, et al. *Mycoplasma hominis* and *Ureaplasma* species brain abscess in a neonate. Pediatr Infect Dis J 21:1083-1085, 2002.
142. Knausz M, Niederland T, Dosa E, et al. Meningo-encephalitis in a neonate caused by maternal *Mycoplasma hominis* treated successfully with chloramphenicol. J Med Microbiol 51:187-188, 2002.
143. Waites KB, Crouse DT, Cassell GH. Systemic neonatal infection due to *Ureaplasma urealyticum*. Clin Infect Dis 17(Suppl 1):S131-S135, 1993.
144. Shaw NJ, Pratt BC, Weindling AM. *Ureaplasma* and *Mycoplasma* infections of central nervous systems in preterm infants. Lancet 2:1530-1531, 1989.
145. Waites KB, Duffy LB, Crouse DT, et al. Mycoplasmal infections of cerebrospinal fluid in newborn infants from a community hospital population. Pediatr Infect Dis J 9:241-245, 1990.
146. Waites KB, Brown M, Greenberg S, et al. Association of genital mycoplasmas with exudative vaginitis in a 10 year old: a case of misdiagnosis. Pediatrics 71:250-252, 1983.
147. Garland SM, Murton LJ. Neonatal meningitis caused by *Ureaplasma urealyticum*. Pediatr Infect Dis J 6:868-870, 1987.
148. Waites KB, Cassell GH, Duffey LB, Searcey KB. Isolation of *Ureaplasma urealyticum* from low birth weight infants. J Pediatr 126:502, 1995.
149. Heggie AD, Jacobs MR, Butler VT, et al. Isolation of *Ureaplasma urealyticum* from low birth weight infants. J Pediatr 126:503-504, 1995.
150. Dammann O, Allred EN, Genest DR, et al. Antenatal *Mycoplasma* infection, the fetal inflammatory response and cerebral white matter damage in very-low-birthweight infants. Paediatr Perinat Epidemiol 17:49-57, 2003.
151. Glaser JB, Engelbert M, Hamerschlag M. Scalp abscess associated with *Mycoplasma hominis* infection complicating intrapartum monitoring. Pediatr Infect Dis J 2:468-470, 1983.
152. Sacker I, Brunell PA. Abscess in newborn infants caused by *Mycoplasma*. Pediatrics 46:303-304, 1970.
153. Powell DA, Miller K, Clyde WA Jr. Submandibular adenitis in a newborn caused by *Mycoplasma hominis*. Pediatrics 63:789-799, 1979.
154. Abdel-Haq N, Asmar B, Brown W. *Mycoplasma hominis* scalp abscess in the newborn. Pediatr Infect Dis J 21:1171-1173, 2002.
155. Blanchard A, Hamrick W, Duffy L, et al. Use of the polymerase chain reaction for detection of *Mycoplasma fermentans* and *Mycoplasma genitalium* in the urogenital tract and amniotic fluid. Clin Infect Dis 17(Suppl 1):S272-S279, 1993.
156. Labbe AC, Frost E, Deslandes S, et al. *Mycoplasma genitalium* is not associated with adverse outcomes of pregnancy in Guinea-Bissau. Sex Transm Infect 78:289-291, 2002.
157. Taylor-Robinson D. *Mycoplasma genitalium*—an up-date. Int J STD AIDS 13:145-151, 2002.
158. de Barbeyrac B, Bernet-Poggi C, Febrer F, et al. Detection of *Mycoplasma pneumoniae* and *Mycoplasma genitalium* in clinical samples by polymerase chain reaction. Clin Infect Dis 17(Suppl 1):S83-S89, 1993.
159. Lo S-C, Dawson MS, Wong DM, et al. Identification of *Mycoplasma incognitus* infection in patients with AIDS: an immunohistochemistry, in situ hybridization and ultrastructural study. Am J Trop Med Hyg 41:601-616, 1989.
160. Cassell GH, Blanchard A, Duffy L, et al. Mycoplasmas. *In* Howard BJ, Klaas J III, Rubin SJ, et al (eds). Clinical and Pathogenic Microbiology. St. Louis, Mosby–Year Book, 1994, pp 491-502.
161. Shepard MC, Masover GK. Special features of ureaplasmas. *In* Barile MF, Razin S (eds). The Mycoplasmas I. Cell Biology. New York, Academic Press, 1979, pp 452-494.

162. Shepard MC. Culture media for ureaplasmas. *In* Razin S, Tully JG (eds). Methods in Mycoplasmology. New York, Academic Press, 1983.
163. Blanchard A, Yanez A, Dybvig K, et al. Evaluation of intraspecies genetic variation within the 16S rRNA gene of *Mycoplasma hominis* and detection by polymerase chain reaction. J Clin Microbiol 31:1358-1361, 1993.
164. Luki N, Lebel P, Boucher M, et al. Comparison of polymerase chain reaction assay with culture for detection of genital mycoplasmas in perinatal infections. Eur J Clin Microbiol Infect Dis 17:255-263, 1998.
165. Abele-Horn M, Wolff C, Dressel P, et al. Polymerase chain reaction versus culture for detection of *Ureaplasma urealyticum* and *Mycoplasma hominis* in the urogenital tract of adults and the respiratory tract of newborns. Eur J Clin Microbiol Infect Dis 15:595-598, 1996.
166. Cunliffe NA, Fergusson S, Davidson F, et al. Comparison of culture with the polymerase chain reaction for detection of *Ureaplasma urealyticum* in endotracheal aspirates of preterm infants. J Med Microbiol 45:27-30, 1996.
167. American Academy of Pediatrics. *Ureaplasma urealyticum* infections. *In* Pickering LK (ed). Red Book: 2003 Report of the Committee on Infectious Diseases, 26th ed. Elk Grove Village, Ill, American Academy of Pediatrics, 2003, pp 671-672.
168. Braun P, Klein JO, Kass EH. Susceptibility of *Mycoplasma hominis* and T-strains to 14 antimicrobial agents. Appl Microbiol 19:62-70, 1970.
169. Koutsky LA, Stamm WE, Brunham RC, et al. Persistence of *Mycoplasma hominis* after therapy: importance of tetracycline resistance and of co-existing vaginal flora. Sex Transm Dis 10(Suppl):374-381, 1983.
170. Cummings MC, McCormack WM. Increase in resistance of *Mycoplasma hominis* to tetracyclines. Antimicrob Agents Chemother 34:2297-2299, 1990.
171. Waites KB, Crouse DT, Cassell GH. Antibiotic susceptibilities and therapeutic options for *Ureaplasma urealyticum* infections in neonates. Pediatr Infect Dis J 11:23-29, 1992.
172. Waites KB, Crouse DT, Cassell GH. Therapeutic consideration for *Ureaplasma urealyticum* infections in neonates. Clin Infect Dis 17(Suppl 1):S208-S214, 1993.
173. Thornsberry C, Barry AJ. Methods for dilution-anti-microbial susceptibility tests for bacteria that grow aerobically. *In* Tentative Standards, 2nd ed. NCCLS document M7-T2. Villanova, Pa, National Committee for Clinical Laboratory Standards, 1988.
174. Waites KB, Cassell GH, Canupp KC, et al. In vitro susceptibilities of mycoplasmas and ureaplasmas to new macrolides and aryl-fluoroquinolones. Antimicrob Agents Chemother 32:1500-1502, 1988.
175. Taylor-Robinson D, Bebear C. Antibiotic susceptibilities of mycoplasmas and treatment of *Mycoplasma* infections. J Antimicrob Chemother 40:622-630, 1997.
176. Kober MB, Mason BA. Colonization of the female genital tract by resistant *Ureaplasma urealyticum* treated successfully with azithromycin. Clin Infect Dis 278:401-402, 1998.
177. Waites KB, Crabb DM, Bing X, et al. In vitro susceptibilities to and bactericidal activities of garenoxacin (BMS-284756) and other anti-microbial agents against human mycoplasmas and ureaplasmas. Antimicrob Agents Chemother 47:161-165, 2003.
178. Kenny GE, Cartwright FD. Susceptibilities of *Mycoplasma hominis, M. pneumoniae*, and *Ureaplasma urealyticum* to GAR-936, dalfopristin, dirithromycin, evernimicin, gatifloxacin, linezolid, moxifloxacin, quinupristin-dalfopristin, and telithromycin compared to their susceptibilities to reference macrolides, tetracyclines, and quinolones. Antimicrob Agents Chemother 45:2604-2608, 2001.
179. Waites KB, Crabb DM, Duffy LB. In vitro activities of ABT-773 and other antimicrobials against human mycoplasmas. Antimicrob Agents Chemother 47:39-42, 2003.
180. Bebear CM, Renaudin H, Charron A, et al. In vitro activity of trova-floxacin compared to those of five antimicrobials against mycoplasmas including *Mycoplasma hominis* and *Ureaplasma urealyticum* fluoro-quinolone-resistant isolates that have been genetically characterized. Antimicrob Agents Chemother 44:2557-2560, 2000.
181. Yoder BA, Coalson JJ, Winter VT, et al. Effects of antenatal colonization with ureaplasma urealyticum on pulmonary disease in the immature baboon. Pediatr Res 54:797-807, 2003.

Chapter 17

STAPHYLOCOCCAL INFECTIONS

Rachel C. Orscheln • Henry R. Shinefield • Joseph W. St. Geme III

Staphylococcal disease has been recognized in neonates for hundreds of years, identified at least as early as 1773, when pemphigus neonatorum was described.[1] Outbreaks of staphylococcal disease in nurseries were first noted in the late 1920s[2] and continue to occur sporadically today, although fortunately with less frequency than in the past.[3]

Up through the 1970s, staphylococcal disease in newborn infants was caused most often by *Staphylococcus aureus*.[4] In the past 3 decades, however, coagulase-negative staphylococci (CoNS) have assumed an equally important role, especially in premature infants in neonatal intensive care units (NICUs).[5-14] Indeed, in some NICUs, CoNS are responsible for almost half of all cases of serious bacterial disease.[12-21]

In recent years, management of staphylococcal disease in infants has become more complicated, reflecting the increasing incidence of methicillin resistance and the threat of vancomycin resistance among isolates of *S. aureus* and CoNS. Antibiotic-resistant isolates are particularly troublesome when they are responsible for epidemics in NICUs.[22-31]

This chapter summarizes current information about the medical aspects of *S. aureus* and CoNS, with a focus on the diseases these organisms produce in young infants.

EPIDEMIOLOGY AND TRANSMISSION

Staphylococcus aureus

Many factors are involved in the transmission of staphylococci among newborns, including nursery design, density of infant population, and obstetric and nursery practices. Other factors important in transmission include biologic properties of the organism and undefined host factors. The difficulty of isolating and investigating each variable in the epidemiologic equation accounts for the disagreement among various workers about which factors predominate in transmission and prevention of staphylococcal disease. Of note, a particular factor that is critical in one epidemic may not operate under different circumstances.

Quantitative studies demonstrate that very small numbers of *S. aureus* are capable of initiating colonization in the newborn. Fewer than 10 bacteria can initiate umbilical colonization in 50% of newborns, and approximately 250 organisms achieve a similar effect on the nasal mucosa.[32] These findings provide a plausible explanation for the challenge of defining any factor in the environment (e.g., fomites, hands, clothes) as a potential source of infection.

Most evidence indicates that the initial and perhaps major source of infection is medical and nursing personnel.[32,33] The *S. aureus* strain common among medical attendants is far more likely than a maternal strain to colonize a given infant.[3] Data collected by Wolinsky and colleagues suggest that in 85% of cases, infant colonization with *S. aureus* results from an attendant's touch.[34] In one group of 37 infants handled by a study nurse for 10 minutes through the window of an isolette, 20 infants (54%) acquired the nurse's strain of *S. aureus*.[35] Of note, the disseminating capacity of attendants varies.[36] Persons with overt lesions or disease often are highly infectious, but asymptomatic carriers can be infectious as well,[37] and carriage on the skin, in the anterior nares, and in the perineal area is relevant.[36,38]

Colonization of the newborn umbilicus, nares, and skin takes place early in life. By the fifth day in the nursery, the colonization rate among nursery inhabitants may be as high as 90%.[39-41] The incidence of colonization is higher in males than in females,[42] suggesting that genetic factors may be important, although studies of twins argue against this hypothesis.[43] The umbilicus or rectum usually is colonized before the nares are.[44,45] During the next 4 to 8 weeks in the infant's life, the likelihood of colonization of the umbilicus falls off rapidly and approaches zero and then stabilizes at approximately 20% for the balance of the first year of life.[40,41]

Despite the high rate of colonization during the newborn period, the incidence of disease in neonates is generally low, except when epidemic strains are involved. In one epidemic, the disease rate in infants and family members who were colonized with a virulent hospital strain of *S. aureus* approached 70%, whereas colonization with nonepidemic strains was associated with a disease rate of 3%.[46] Epidemics of staphylococcal disease resulting from colonization that occurs in well-infant nurseries usually are not revealed by infections in the nursery. Skin disease typically appears 1 to 3 weeks after hospital discharge, and breast abscesses and pneumonia may not develop until 2 weeks to 2 months of age. In NICUs, disease becomes apparent in the unit because of prolonged hospital stays.

Shortly after the introduction of methicillin in 1960, methicillin-resistant *S. aureus* (MRSA) emerged as an important nosocomial pathogen.[47] For MRSA, resistance is mediated through the *mecA* gene, which codes for an altered penicillin-binding protein (called PBP2a or PBP2′) that has a dramatically reduced affinity for β-lactam antibiotics.[48] Beyond possessing *mecA*, MRSA isolates frequently harbor other antibiotic resistance determinants as well, further limiting treatment options. Risk factors for infection with MRSA include treatment with antimicrobials, prolonged hospitalization, and stay within an intensive care unit.[49] Fortunately, although MRSA has become endemic in many adult hospitals, most infant nurseries have been unaffected by these organisms.[22-31,50-54] In a recent survey of neonatologists practicing in NICUs, 70% reported no cases of MRSA infection.[55] The incidence of MRSA infection in neonates is likely to increase over time, however.

Since the mid-1990s, infection with community-acquired MRSA (CA-MRSA) isolates has been reported increasingly in patients without hospital contact or traditional risk factors for MRSA.[56] Several features of CA-MRSA isolates differentiate them from health care–associated MRSA.[57] CA-MRSA strains typically have a distinct antibiotic susceptibility profile, with retained susceptibility to multiple classes of antimicrobials. CA-MRSA strains frequently cause skin and soft tissue infections, as with methicillin-sensitive *S. aureus* (MSSA). Several cases of invasive disease, bacteremia, and death caused by CA-MRSA have been reported, however.[58] These isolates appear to be readily transmitted between family members and close contacts,[57] but transmission in a health care setting has been limited to date. Health care transmission of CA-MRSA has been reported as the cause of infection among a cohort of postpartum women, although no infants were affected in this instance.[59] Unfortunately, unlike health care–associated MRSA, isolates of CA-MRSA are particularly well adapted to survive in the community, and introduction into and transmission within hospitals are likely to increase in the near future.

When clusters of staphylococcal disease associated with hospital exposure occur, temporal clustering of cases suggests the possibility of an outbreak caused by a single strain.[60] It is clear that strain identity as determined by phenotypic methods (i.e., phage types, antibiograms, and even plasmid profiles) may not be precise enough to identify *S. aureus* strains for epidemiologic investigatory purposes. In these situations, strain identity requires characterization based on a molecular technique, such as pulsed-field gel electrophoresis (PFGE).

PFGE generally is considered the most discriminating molecular typing approach for evaluating strains present during local outbreaks.[61] The performance of PFGE requires time and specialized equipment, however, and this technique is not universally available for routine clinical applications. Additionally, PFGE relies on examination of banding patterns on a gel and may not be useful for comparisons of strains between laboratories[62] or of strains reponsible for outbreaks that are separated in time. Multilocus sequence typing (MLST) is a sequence-based typing system that utilizes the sequence of seven housekeeping genes to evaluate the genetic relatedness of strains of staphylococci.[63] The discriminatory power of this approach is less than that of PFGE, so the usefulness for the evaluation of local outbreaks is less.[64] Nevertheless, MLST allows the user to compare sequences from isolates of various locations through a central database (http://www.mlst.net). Additional molecular approaches that have been applied to strain evaluation for epidemiologic purposes include staphylococcal protein A typing (*spa* typing),[65] random amplification of polymorphic DNA (RAPD),[66] repetitive element–based polymerase chain reaction (PCR) (rep-PCR) assay,[67] and multilocus restriction fragment typing (MLRFT).[64]

Coagulase-Negative Staphylococci

CoNS are common inhabitants of human skin and mucous membrane sites.[68] *S. epidermidis* is the species found most commonly as a member of the normal flora of the nasal mucosa and the umbilicus of the newborn.[69] Colonization occurs early and at many sites. With sensitive culture techniques, the nose, umbilicus, and chest skin are colonized with CoNS in up to 83% of neonates by 4 days of age.[70] In one study, rates of colonization with *S. epidermidis* among 63 infants in a NICU were as follows: nose, 89%; throat, 84%; umbilicus, 90%; and stool, 86%. Comparable percentages for *S. aureus* were 17%, 17%, 21%, and 10%, respectively.[69]

In other studies in which isolates were characterized by species, biotype, antibiotic susceptibility pattern, and the capacity to form biofims (using an assay for slime), colonization rates were 50% to 80% by 4 to 7 days after admission to the NICU.[71-73] After 2 weeks in the unit, 75% to 100% of infants were colonized with CoNS at some mucosal site. In one study, biofilm-forming strains selectively colonized infants over a 4-week period, with nearly 90% of infants eventually harboring a single predominant *S. epidermidis* biotype.[72] Although most infants acquire CoNS from environmental sources, including hospital personnel, a small percentage are colonized by vertical transmission.[74,75] The ubiquity of these organisms and their tolerance to both drying and temperature changes offer an explanation for the high prevalence of colonization among infants.

Ecologic relationships between the microbial flora of various body sites have been well studied, and factors that reduce colonization at one site with one organism tend to increase colonization at that site with others.[71] Current nursery practices that decrease colonization with *S. aureus* contribute to the increased presence of CoNS in neonates. These practices include the extensive use of antimicrobial agents and the use of skin and umbilical cleansing techniques. Furthermore, isolates of *S. epidermidis* and other CoNS resistant to multiple antibiotic agents are becoming increasingly common.[71] In a study involving premature neonates, D'Angio and associates demonstrated that the incidence of strains resistant to multiple antibiotics rose from 32% to 82% by the end of the first week of life.[72]

The observation that CoNS are important nosocomial pathogens among newborns, especially low-birth-weight infants in NICUs, is explained by the prevalence of colonization with these organisms at multiple sites and the widespread use of invasive therapeutic modalities. Examples of invasive treatments include endotracheal intubation; mechanical ventilation; placement of umbilical catheters, central venous catheters, chest tubes, and ventriculoperitoneal shunts; and the use of feeding tubes.[10,11,16,17,20,21] In this setting, CoNS account for greater than 50% of bloodstream isolates obtained from neonates with late-onset sepsis.[12,13]

An inverse relationship exists between the rate of infection with CoNS and both birth weight and gestational age. Additional factors that appear to be associated with CoNS bacteremia among very low birth weight (VLBW) neonates include respiratory distress syndrome, bronchopulmonary dysplasia, patent ductus arteriosus, severe intraventricular hemorrhage, and necrotizing enterocolitis.[14]

Certain nutritional factors are associated with the development of late-onset sepsis, including delayed initiation of enteral feeding, prolonged period to reach full enteral feeding status, delayed reattainment of birth weight, and prolonged parenteral hyperalimentation.[13] Administration of intralipids through a Teflon catheter has been shown in a case-control study to be associated with an increased risk of bacteremia due to CoNS.[76] The significant pathogenic factors include capacity of the organism to form biofilms, lipid infusion, and presence of the Teflon catheter, all of which interfere with neutrophil and macrophage function. Whether lipids infused through catheters made of other materials are associated with a similar risk remains to be determined.

Considered together, the clinical and experimental data suggest that CoNS have not become more virulent over time. Rather, these ubiquitous organisms have become more common pathogens because therapeutic approaches have become increasingly invasive and because premature infants, with compromised immunity, are surviving for longer periods of time.

MICROBIOLOGY

Staphylococci are members of the family Micrococcaceae and are nonmotile, non–spore-forming bacteria that are catalase negative. Species of staphylococci are defined by DNA-DNA hybridization studies and are separated into two large groups on the basis of ability to produce the extracellular enzyme coagulase. Organisms that produce coagulase are known as coagulase-positive staphylococci, or *S. aureus*,[77] and organisms that produce no coagulase are referred to as CoNS. The presence of coagulase can be evaluated either by assessing broth medium for secreted enzyme, which reacts with coagulase-reacting factor in plasma and results in formation of a fibrin clot, or by testing for cell-bound enzyme, which results in clumping when a suspension of organisms is incubated with plasma.

Staphylococci grow best in an aerobic environment but are capable of growing under anaerobic conditions as well. They grow readily on most routine laboratory media and usually are isolated from clinical specimens using sheep blood agar. Gram staining reveals gram-positive cocci that range from 0.7 to 1.2 μM in diameter and are usually visible in irregular grapelike clusters (Fig. 17-1A). Growth in liquid culture often results in a predominance of single cocci, pairs, tetrads, and chains of three or four cells. Of note, dying organisms and bacteria in stationary phase or ingested by phagocytes may appear to be gram-negative. Growth on blood agar results in round, convex, shiny opaque colonies that are 1 to 2 mm in diameter after 24 hours of incubation. Colonies of *S. aureus* often are deep yellow or golden and typically are surrounded by a zone of β-hemolysis (see Fig. 17-1B). By contrast, colonies of CoNS usually are chalk-white, often lacking surrounding hemolysis.

Staphylococcus aureus

For clinical purposes, many of the key characteristics of *S. aureus* can be determined by simple procedures performed with commercial rapid identification kits and automated systems.[77] *S. aureus* strains can be subdivided by their capacity to be lysed by certain bacteriophages.[78] Historically, phage typing and serologic typing were the most common systems for differentiating strains of *S. aureus* for epidemiologic purposes.[79] However, in recent years molecular approaches have become the standard for defining strain identity in a patient with multiple isolates or in a possible outbreak involving multiple patients.[80-82]

Studies of the subcellular structure of *S. aureus* have generated an increasing body of information. Of particular interest is knowledge about the chemical composition, biosynthesis, and antigenicity of the staphylococcal cell wall, which is made up of two major components, peptidoglycan and teichoic acid.[83] *S. aureus* peptidoglycan is composed of chains of acetylglucosamine, acetylmuramic acid, alanine, glutamic acid, and lysine or diaminopimelic acid, with pentaglycine bridges that cross-link these chains.[84] Studies on the inhibition of peptidoglycan biosynthesis have led to a recognition of the mode of action of several antibiotics and staphylolytic enzymes.[85] Four penicillin-binding proteins called PBP1, PBP2, PBP3, and PBP4 play an important role in peptidoglycan biosynthesis and are inactivated by β-lactams.[86] (PBP2a is present in isolates of MRSA and is resistant to β-lactams.) Teichoic acid is a polymer of ribitol phosphate that is held in the cell wall by covalent attachment to the insoluble peptidoglycan. Staphylococcal teichoic acid is antigenic, and antibodies to this substance cause agglutination of isolated staphylococcal cell walls.[87] Antibodies to teichoic acid enhance opsonophagocytic killing of nonencapsulated strains of *S. aureus* but have little effect on encapsulated isolates.[88,89] By way of contrast, antibodies to peptidoglycan play a key role in the opsonization of *S. aureus*.[90-93] Of note, antibodies to both teichoic acid and peptidoglycan are widespread in the population.[93]

In addition to peptidoglycan and teichoic acid, other components of the *S. aureus* cell wall include group antigen known as protein A and a number of other surface-exposed proteins. Similar to the situation with other gram-positive bacteria, many *S. aureus* proteins anchored in the cell wall possess a carboxy-terminal LPXTG motif, which serves as a sorting signal for a membrane enzyme called sortase (SrtA).[94,95]

A

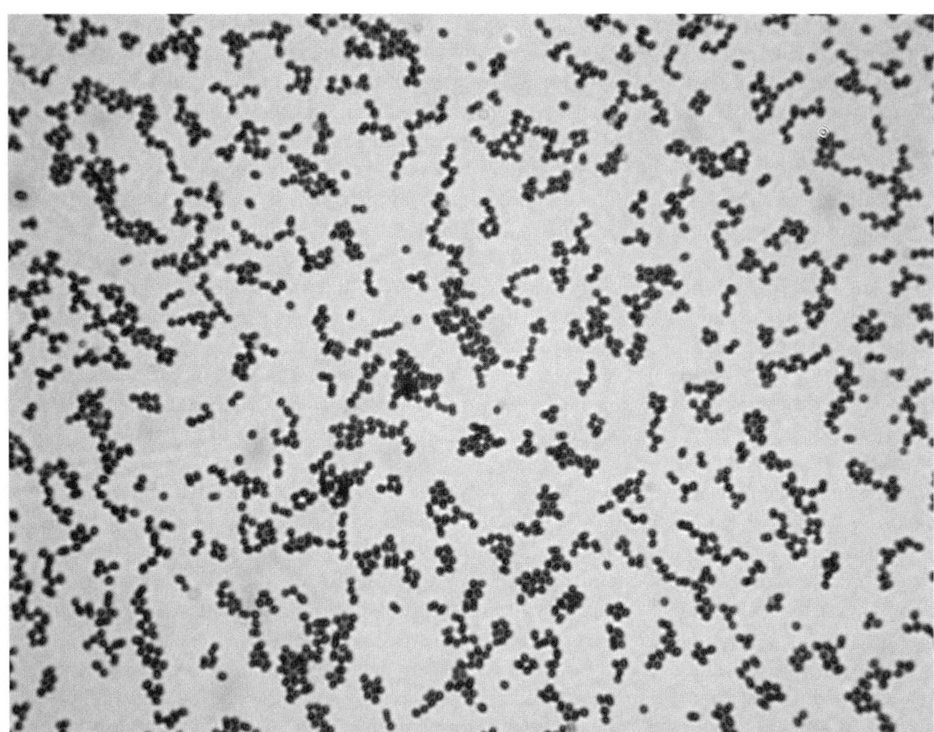

B

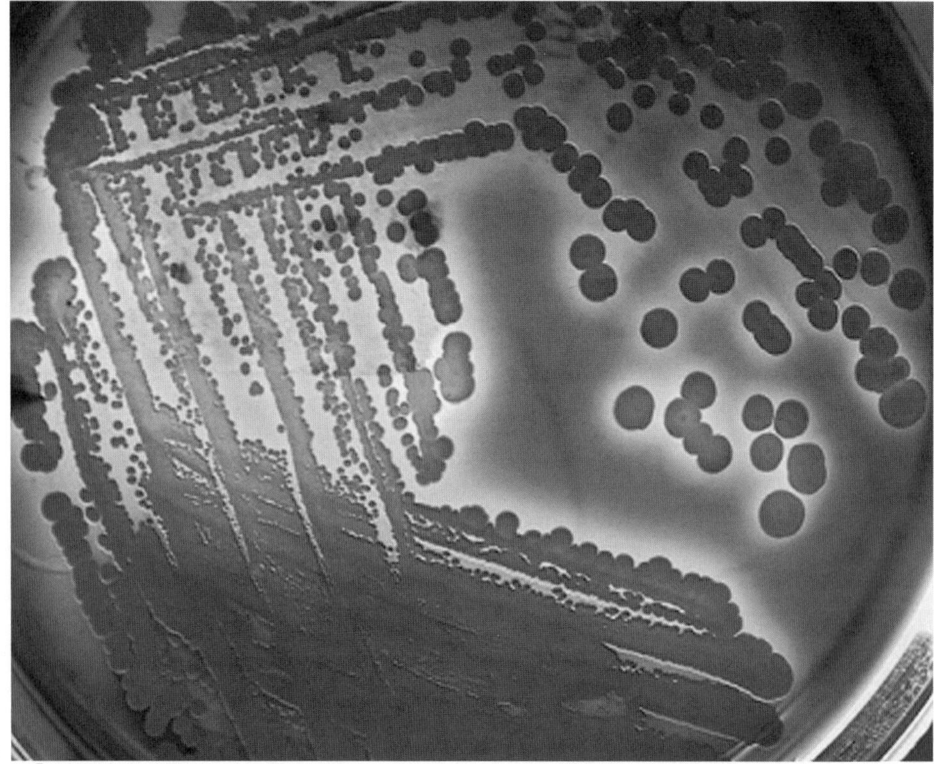

Figure 17–1 **A,** Gram stain of *Staphylococcus aureus* showing characteristic clusters. **B,** Blood agar plate showing growth of *S. aureus* with zone of β-hemolysis surrounding colonies.

This enzyme cleaves polypeptides between the threonine and the glycine of the LPXTG motif and catalyzes formation of an amide bond between the carboxy group of threonine and the amino group of peptidoglycan cross-bridges.[96] Sortase is encoded by *srtA* and is a 206-amino-acid protein with a putative amino-terminal membrane-spanning domain and a carboxy-terminal catalytic domain that is presumably translocated across the cytoplasmic membrane.[96] Of interest, BLAST searches using the *srtA* gene as a query have identified a second sortase gene called *srtB*.[97] Existing evidence indicates that the *srtA* and *srtB* gene products do not have redundant functions, raising the possibility that they catalyze similar reactions using different protein substrates.

S. aureus produces a capsular layer external to the cell wall. The staphylococcal capsule has aroused interest both because of its role in pathogenesis[98,99] and because of its ability to stimulate antibody production. Although the thick mucoid capsule produced by the prototype Smith strain is uncommon, most *S. aureus* stains produce a microcapsule.[100,101]

Nucleotide sequencing of the whole genome for several isolates of *S. aureus* established that the genome is 2.8 to 2.9 megabases in size, with approximately 2600 to 2700 open reading frames and an overall guanine:cytosine content of approximately 33%.[102,103] Much of the *S. aureus* genome appears to have been acquired by lateral gene transfer. Most antibiotic resistance genes are carried on mobile genetic elements, including a unique resistance island. Pathogenicity islands belonging to at least three different classes have been identified, including toxic shock syndrome toxin islands, exotoxin islands, and enterotoxin islands. Of interest, the exotoxin and enterotoxin islands are closely linked to other gene clusters encoding putative virulence factors.

Coagulase-Negative Staphylococci

CoNS are a heterogeneous group of organisms that have been divided into 32 species.[77] The following 15 species of CoNS are found as members of the normal human flora: *S. epidermidis*, *Staphylococcus haemolyticus*, *Staphylococcus saprophyticus*, *Staphylococcus capitis*, *Staphylococcus warnerii*, *Staphylococcus hominis*, *Staphylococcus xylosus*, *Staphylococcus cohnii*, *Staphylococcus simulans*, *Staphylococcus auricularis*, *Staphylococcus saccharolyticus*, *Staphylococcus caprae*, *Staphylococcus pasteuri*, *Staphylococcus lugdunensis*, and *Staphylococcus schleiferi*.[77,104] Among these species, several occupy very specific niches on the skin. For example, *S. capitis* is most abundant on the head, where sebaceous glands are plentiful. *S. auricularis* has a striking predilection for the external auditory canal. *S. hominis* and *S. haemolyticus* are most common in the axillae and the pubic area, where apocrine glands are numerous.

Speciation of CoNS is accomplished on the basis of a series of biochemical characteristics. In recent years, species identification has been simplified by the introduction of commercially available miniaturized kits.[77] Differentiation of two strains belonging to the same species (subspeciation) represents a more difficult problem, however. Biotyping and antibiotic susceptibility patterns together have been used for this purpose with some success.[105] Phage typing is another method that has been useful at times.[105-107] Analogous to the situation with *S. aureus*, more powerful techniques for distinguishing strains of a given species include PFGE, random amplification of a polymorphic DNA, rep-PCR assay, and MLRFT.[108]

The composition of CoNS is similar to the makeup of *S. aureus*, except that the teichoic acid contains glycerol in place of ribose and the cell wall lacks protein A. Determination of the genome of *S. epidermidis* strain ATCC 12228 (a commensal isolate not associated with disease) revealed a genome approximately 2.5 megabases in size with 2419 open reading frames, greater than 10% smaller than the published genomes of *S. aureus* isolates.[109] In comparison with the available *S. aureus* genomes, ATCC 12228 contains fewer antibiotic resistance genes and lacks pathogenicity islands and a capsule locus. A homologue of the *S. aureus srtA* gene is present, along with nine proteins predicted to contain an LPXTG motif.

PATHOGENESIS OF DISEASE

Role of the Organisms

Staphylococcus aureus

S. aureus has a diverse array of cellular and extracellular virulence proteins.[110] With the possible exception of toxic shock syndrome, staphylococcal scalded skin syndrome, and staphylococcal toxin–mediated enteritis, the pathogenesis of staphylococcal disease is dependent on the coordinated activity of multiple virulence factors (rather than a single predominant factor). The pathogenic process begins with colonization of host skin or mucosal surfaces and involves bacterial attachment to host cells or extracellular matrix. To persist, the organism produces molecules that resist phagocytosis and interfere with the function of specific antistaphylococcal antibodies. Ultimately, the organism expresses specific factors that attack host cells and others that degrade components of the extracellular matrix, contributing to persistence and facilitating spread.

S. aureus produces a number of adhesive factors referred to as MSCRAMMs (*m*icrobial *s*urface *c*omponents *r*ecognizing *a*dhesive *m*atrix *m*olecules), including clumping factor (ClfA), fibrinogen-binding protein (Fbp), fibronectin-binding protein A (FnbpA), fibronectin-binding protein B (FnbpB), collagen-binding protein (Cna), elastin-binding protein (EbpS), laminin receptor, bone sialoprotein-binding protein (Bbp), IsdA (which binds fibronectin and fibrinogen), and SdrC-D-E (which bind fibronectin), among others.[111-116] In addition, *S. aureus* is capable of binding to vitronectin[117] and thrombospondins,[118] although the specific genes and proteins responsible for these activities have not yet been identified. Studies suggest that the *S. aureus* MSCRAMMs and these additional adhesive activities play an important role in colonizing host tissues and binding to foreign objects such as catheters and prosthetic devices.[119-121] In the case of *S. aureus* Fnbp-mediated binding to fibronectin, the major binding sites on fibronectin reside in the amino-terminal type 1 module and toward the carboxy terminus. Proteins encoded by the *icaA-D* genes mediate interbacterial interactions and promote biofilm formation.

Bacterial survival during infection is dependent on the ability of the organism to circumvent host defenses. Staphylococci have developed several strategies for this purpose. Protein A is a surface-associated protein that binds to the Fc portion of IgG antibodies, presumably blocking opsonization and providing the organism with a protective cover.[122,123] *S. aureus* V8 protease is a serine protease that is capable of cleaving and inactivating IgG antibodies in vitro, leading to speculation that this protein functions to block the action of antibodies during natural infection. It is possible that V8 and other proteases also function to degrade antimicrobial peptides such as the neutrophil defensins and the platelet microbicidal proteins.[124,125] Catalase counteracts the toxic effects of oxygen free radicals produced by phagocytes and promotes survival inside and around neutrophils. The staphylococcal enterotoxins (SEA, SEB, SEC, SED, SEE, and SEH), toxic shock syndrome toxin 1 (TSST-1), and exfoliative (epidermolytic) toxins (ETA, ETB, ETC, and ETD) all have superantigen properties, binding to major histocompatibility complex class II proteins and activating specific subsets of T cells through the variable regions of T cell receptor β chains (Vβ chains).[126,127] This relatively nonspecific stimulation of lymphocyte populations results in activation of nearly 30% of circulating lymphocytes, possibly serving to prevent the host from elaborating antibodies to other staphylococcal antigens. The mature pyrogenic toxin superantigens are small, nonglycosylated proteins with molecular masses ranging from 20,000 to 30,000 daltons. Leukocidin, β-hemolysin, and γ-hemolysin are *S. aureus* extracellular proteins that have leukocytolytic activity[128-132] and may enable the organism to circumvent neutrophil infiltration and phagocytosis. Panton-Valentine leukocidin (PV leukocidin) causes lysis of rabbit and human phagocytes and is associated with an often lethal necrotizing pneumonia in patients. In addition, more than 90% of clinical isolates of *S. aureus* express a polysaccharide microcapsule, with 11 different known capsular types.[133] Although the role of the capsule in pathogenesis is unclear, more than 75% of human isolates express either the type 5 or the type 8 polysaccharide.[134] One hypothesis is that the capsule prevents the interaction of antibodies with the bacterial surface. In response to an infection, the host can produce a variety of fatty acids and other lipid molecules that act as surfactants to disrupt the bacterial membrane, especially when an abscess is formed. Virtually all strains of *S. aureus* express lipases and are lipolytic,[50] potentially counteracting the effects of host lipids.

A number of *S. aureus* factors have been postulated to promote tissue invasion. Perhaps the best-studied is α-toxin (also referred to as α-hemolysin), which forms heptamers in the membranes of a variety of cell types, creating pores.[135,136] Pore formation is associated with release of nitric oxide from endothelial cells and appears to stimulate apoptosis in lymphocytes.[137,138] On the basis of comparison of wild-type and mutant strains, α-toxin has been implicated in virulence in animal models of keratitis and mastitis.[139,140] β-Hemolysin is an enzyme with sphingomyelinase activity and acts on the membrane of red blood cells in vitro and potentially other cells during natural infection.[141] δ-Hemolysin is a 26-amino-acid peptide that potentiates the activity of β-hemolysin in vitro, causing membrane damage by a detergent-like action and enhancing hemolysis.[142] Additional proteins that may facilitate tissue invasion include hyaluronidase and hyaluronate lyase,[143] enzymes that digest hyaluronic acid, which is a straight-chain polymer found in skin, bone, synovial fluid, umbilical cord, and vitreous humor.[144] Of note, individual isolates of *S. aureus* have been shown to produce multiple electrophoretic forms of these enzymes, suggesting that families exist.

Of interest, many of the *S. aureus* cell wall–associated adhesive factors that facilitate the initial stages of infection are selectively produced during the exponential phase of in vitro growth.[145] It is noteworthy that these proteins can be anchored to the cell only while the cell wall is being assembled. By contrast, almost all *S. aureus* extracellular proteins presumed to participate in evasion of the immune system and to spread to adjacent tissues are synthesized predominantly in the postexponential phase of growth.[145,146] A notable exception is enterotoxin A, which is produced constitutively.[147] This differential expression of specific sets of virulence determinants probably is fundamental to the pathogenic process and is under control of the accessory gene regulator (*agr*) locus, the staphylococcal accessory gene regulator (*sar*) locus, and a catabolite repression system, with influence from the *sae*, the *srr* (also referred to as *srh*), and the *arl* two-component systems.[148-150] The *agr* locus responds to cell density (mediating quorum sensing) and is activated in midexponential phase. The *sae* system appears to respond to both cell density and environmental conditions.[151,152] The *arl* system serves to downregulate overall exoprotein synthesis, presumably by downregulating *agr*.[153] The *srr* system inhibits *agr* activation and in turn is downregulated by *agr*.[154] Of note, this system is especially important under microaerobic conditions and is a prerequisite for normal growth in the absence of oxygen.

S. aureus is capable of existing harmlessly as a commensal on the skin or a mucous membrane and also is able to produce disease in the blood and a variety of tissue sites. This versatility probably is a reflection of the capacity to regulate gene expression in response to environmental signals, in large part through the *agr*, the *sar*, the *sae*, the *srr*, and the *arl* loci.[148]

Coagulase-Negative Staphylococci

Until recently, the pathogenic potential of CoNS received little attention. With the emergence of these organisms as prominent pathogens, investigation has intensified in an effort to identify important virulence factors and develop new approaches to treatment and prevention. Attention has centered primarily on *S. epidermidis*, the species most commonly associated with clinical disease, usually in association with central intravascular catheters. Other species that have been examined, although to a lesser extent, include *S. lugdunensis*, *S. schleiferi*, and *S. saprophyticus*.

In CoNS infections involving indwelling catheters and other prosthetic devices, bacterial adherence to the foreign body is an important step in the pathogenic process (Fig. 17-2). Early evidence suggested that nonspecific factors, including long-range electromagnetic forces and surface hydrophobicity, promote initial attachment.[155] More recent studies have demonstrated that a polysaccharide capsular adhesin composed of *N*-acetylglucosamine also is involved in adherence.[156,157] This material is referred to as PIA or PS/A and is encoded by the *ica* locus. It promotes adherence to plastic polymers and functions as an antiphagocytic capsule, preventing C3 deposition and phagocytosis. A second factor suggested to promote attachment to plastic surfaces is AtlE, which shows significant homology with the major autolysin of *S. aureus*.[158] AtlE contains two bacteriologically active domains, including a 60-kDa amidase and a 52-kDa glucosaminidase domain, generated by proteolytic processing.[158] The 60-kDa domain is located on the bacterial surface and is a prerequisite for AtlE-related adhesion. Of note, AtlE also has vitronectin-binding activity,[158] suggesting that this protein plays a role in bacterial attachment both to a naked plastic surface early in infection and to plasma protein–coated surfaces later in infection. SSP-1 and SSP-2 are antigenically

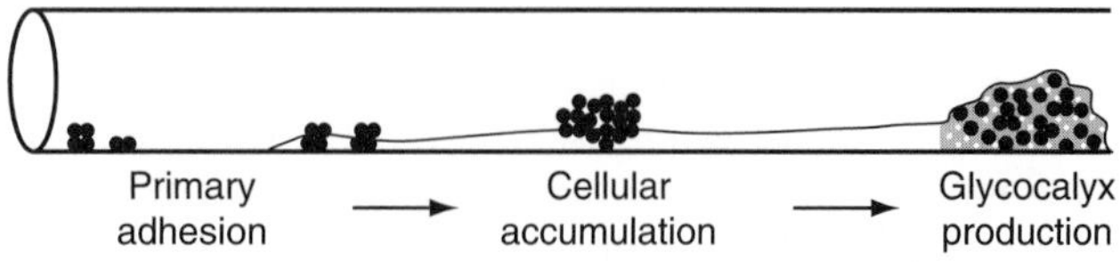

Figure 17–2 Schematic model of the phases involved in *Streptococcus epidermidis* biofilm formation.

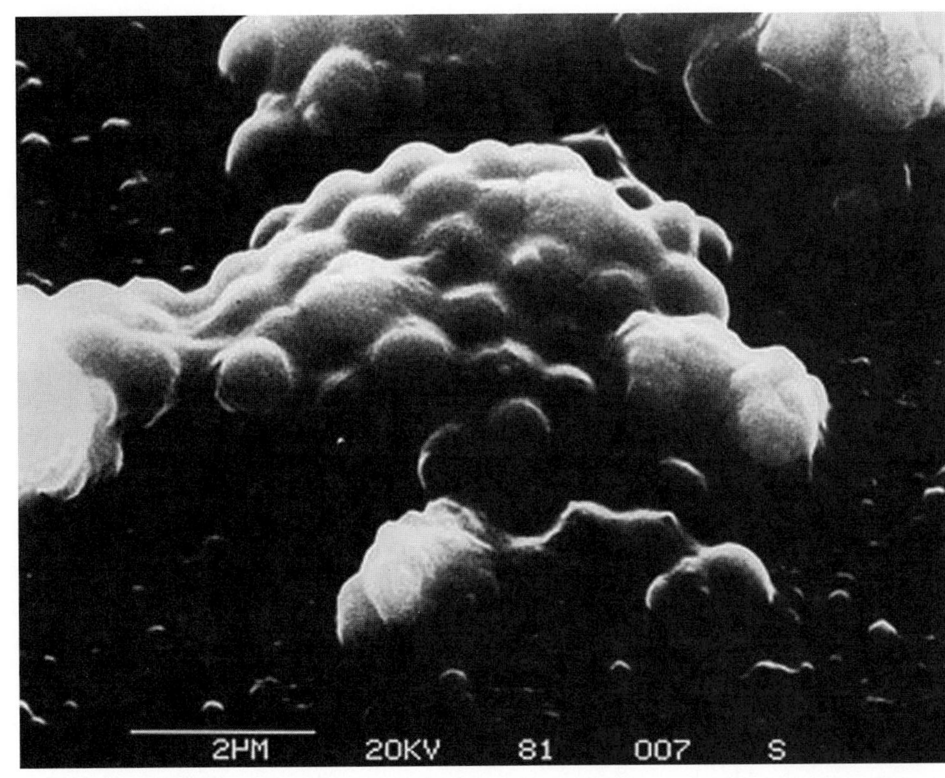

Figure 17–3 Scanning electron micrograph showing the presence of a *Streptococcus epidermidis* biofilm on an explanted intravascular catheter. The biofilm is characterized by multilayered cell clusters embedded in an extracellular polysaccharide. (From von Eiff C, Peters G, Heilmann C. Pathogenesis of infections due to coagulase-negative staphylococci. Lancet Infect Dis 2:677-685, 2002.)

related proteins that also contribute to binding to plastic. These proteins were identified in *S. epidermidis* strain 354 and form fiber-like structures on the surface of the organism.[159,160]

A variety of *S. epidermidis* factors promote attachment to host extracellular matrix proteins that may coat catheters and other foreign bodies (see Fig. 17-2). For example, AtlE mediates binding to vitronectin and is essential for full virulence in an intravascular catheter–associated infection model in rats.[158,161] Similarly, the Fbe protein mediates bacterial binding to fibrinogen, promoting interaction with the fibrinogen β chain.[162,163] Fbe is a member of the serine–aspartic acid–repeat–containing (Sdr) family of cell wall–anchored surface proteins. Other members of the family include SdrG, SdrF, and SdrH.[164] SdrG is 95% identical to Fbe and shares the capacity to bind to the fibrinogen β-chain. Recent evidence indicates that *S. epidermidis* cell wall teichoic acid facilitates adherence to fibronectin, perhaps serving as a bridging molecule between bacteria and fibronectin-coated surfaces.[165]

After initial attachment to a biomaterial, organisms multiply and form complex multilayered aggregates that involve intercellular adhesion and are referred to as biofilms (Fig. 17-3; see also Fig. 17-2). In recent work, Mack and colleagues found that a *S. epidermidis* mutant with a transposon in the *ica* locus was unable to form multilayered cell clusters.[166] Expression of the poly-*N*-acetylglucosamine adhesin is subject to reversible on and off switching, referred to as *phase variation* and resulting, at least in some cases, from reversible insertion and excision of an insertion sequence element in the *ica* operon.[167] Phase variation may be important in allowing for release of planktonic (free-floating) cells from mature biofilms. Of note, an *ica* mutant was less virulent than the wild-type strain in both a mouse model of subcutaneous foreign body infection and a rat model of central venous catheter–associated infection.[168,169] A second factor important for *S. epidermidis* intercellular adhesion and biofilm formation is a 140-kDa extracellular protein referred to as accumulation-associated protein (AAP).[170] Elimination of expression of AAP has no effect on initial adhesion to glass and polystyrene surfaces but disrupts bacterial accumulation. Consistent with this result, antibody against AAP almost completely blocks accumulation.[171] Of interest, expression of this protein is found only in bacteria grown under sessile conditions (attached to a surface).[171]

Historically, isolates of CoNS were often described as elaborating "slime" and "slime-associated antigen," terms that we now realize refer to biofilms and the presence of abundant quantities of poly-*N*-acetylglucosamine. In a hospital-wide survey, Ishak and colleagues noted slime production in 13 of 14 clinically significant bloodstream isolates of *S. epidermidis*, compared with only 3 of 13 blood culture contaminants and 4 of 27 skin isolates.[172] Studies in infants have revealed similar results. For example, in independent studies, Hall and co-workers and Gruskay and associates detected slime production by 82% of isolates from infants with invasive disease.[173,174] CoNS biofilm formation presumably provides a nonspecific physical barrier to cellular and humoral defense mechanisms. In addition, biofilm-associated polysaccharide inhibits neutrophil chemotaxis and phagocytosis and suppresses lymphocyte blastogenesis.[175,176] CoNS biofilm-associated polysaccharide also is capable of inhibiting the antimicrobial action of both vancomycin and teichoplanin.[177] Relevant to the issue of treatment, formation of biofilms makes eradication of CoNS infection more difficult.[178,179] With regard to regulation of CoNS biofilm formation, it is interesting that homologues of the *S. aureus agr* and *sar* loci have been identified in

S. epidermidis and that a *S. epidermidis agr* knockout mutant is deficient in biofilm formation.[180-182]

Recent work indicates that CoNS produce a variety of exoproteins, including urease, lipase/esterase, fibrinolysin, DNase, and a number of proteases.[183] In addition, selected isolates produce delta-like toxin, an extracellular hemolysin that is similar in size, biologic properties, and antigenicity to the enteropathic δ-toxin of *S. aureus*. Studies by Scheifele and colleagues suggest that delta-like toxin may play a role in the pathogenesis of necrotizing enterocolitis.[184,185]

Selected strains of CoNS produce a polysaccharide capsule. By analogy with other encapsulated pathogens, it is possible that capsule plays a role in the pathogenesis of disease. Among fresh clinical isolates, however, capsular material is present in fewer than 10%.[186,187] Further studies are needed to establish the precise relationship between capsule production and disease.

Role of the Host

Even under the most ideal conditions, infants in the hospital are surrounded by staphylococci. Physical barriers such as the skin and mucous membranes represent a major defense against staphylococcal disease. Bacteremic disease most often develops when organisms colonizing the skin gain access to the bloodstream through the portal created by an intravascular catheter. Other routes for entry into the bloodstream include the intestinal tract after injury to the epithelial barrier, the respiratory tract in patients receiving mechanical ventilation, the umbilicus when the umbilical cord is still in place, and occasionally the circumcision site. Localized disease occurs when colonizing organisms are implanted into deeper tissues, often related to a break in skin or mucous membrane integrity and sometimes during placement of a foreign body. On occasion, a foreign body becomes contaminated after placement, with organisms from the hands of medical personnel, from contaminated disinfectants, or from the patient.

As with other pathogenic bacteria, the presence of intact neutrophil phagocytic function is probably the single most important factor involved in controlling replication and spread of staphylococci.[188] Effective phagocytosis requires sufficient numbers of cells along with the ability to sense and migrate toward a site of infection and then ingest and kill microorganisms. In term infants, the peripheral neutrophil count is higher than in adults, but there is little capacity to respond to infection with an outpouring of additional cells. As a result, the number of neutrophils at a site of infection is relatively low in infants compared with that in adults.[189] In addition, neutrophils from newborns exhibit relatively diminished motility toward chemoattractants compared with that in cells from older children and adults.[190] Potential mechanisms for this diminished chemotaxis include decreased circulating levels of fibronectin,[191] abnormal polymerization of actin,[192] and decreased production of chemotactic factors such as C5a and interleukin-8 (IL-8).[193,194] Neutrophils from young infants also exhibit decreased migration across endothelium, possibly because of impaired capacity to upregulate endothelial cell expression of the CR3 receptor.[195,196] Beyond decreases in neutrophil number, chemotaxis, and transepithelial migration, the capacity for neutrophil adherence and phagocytosis is reduced in neonates, largely owing to deficiencies in opsonins, including complement, specific antibody, and fibronectin. Phagocytic killing appears to be intact in normal newborns but may be compromised in stressed infants, at least in part because of reduced production of hydroxyl radicals.[188,197,198]

Specific antibody is less important than complement in opsonization of *S. aureus* and plays a limited role in defense against neonatal staphylococcal disease, the possible exception being antibody directed against leukocidin and other toxins.[199-201] For example, in general, there is no correlation between antibody titers against *S. aureus* and the likelihood of asymptomatic carriage versus clinical disease.[202,203] Consistent with this information, an attempt many years ago to protect the newborn from staphylococcal disease by immunizing the mother near term was unsuccessful.[204]

In most cases of neonatal staphylococcal disease, the role of T cells is unclear. T cells are centrally involved, however, in the immune response to several *S. aureus* toxins, including TSST-1, the staphylococcal enterotoxins, and the staphylococcal exfoliative toxins (ETA, ETB, ETC, and ETD). All of these toxins appear to function as superantigens, interacting with major histocompatibility complex class II proteins on the surface of T cells and activating specific subsets of cells through the variable regions of T cell receptor β-chains. The consequence of this T cell activation is proliferation of a large proportion of T cells and release of a number of cytokines, including tumor necrosis factors TNF-α and TNF-β, interleukins IL-1 and IL-2, and interferon-γ.[205] These molecules are major contributors to the systemic manifestations of staphylococcal scalded skin syndrome, toxic shock syndrome, and food poisoning.

PATHOLOGY

The most characteristic pathologic lesion associated with *S. aureus* infection is a local abscess, consisting of necrotic tissue, fibrin, and a large number of live and dead neutrophils. Similarly, CoNS infection is characterized by infiltration of neutrophils, usually with moderate necrosis. Other pathologic findings are described next in the sections on clinical manifestations.

CLINICAL MANIFESTATIONS

Bullous Impetigo and Staphylococcal Scalded Skin Syndrome

S. aureus produces a spectrum of clinical skin diseases as a result of the elaboration of exfoliative (epidermolytic) toxins (ETs). The most serious of these is staphylococcal scalded skin syndrome (SSSS), also known as *Ritter's disease* after the physician who first described the condition among orphans in 1878. When the disease is localized, it is referred to most frequently as *bullous impetigo*.[206]

Large epidemiologic surveys have found that between 4% and 6.2% of *S. aureus* isolates produce ETs.[207-210] Neonates, children younger than 5 years of age, and adults with renal insufficiency or immunocompromise are the most susceptible to SSSS, the generalized form of staphylococcal ET-related disease.[211] When occurring in neonates, the illness usually

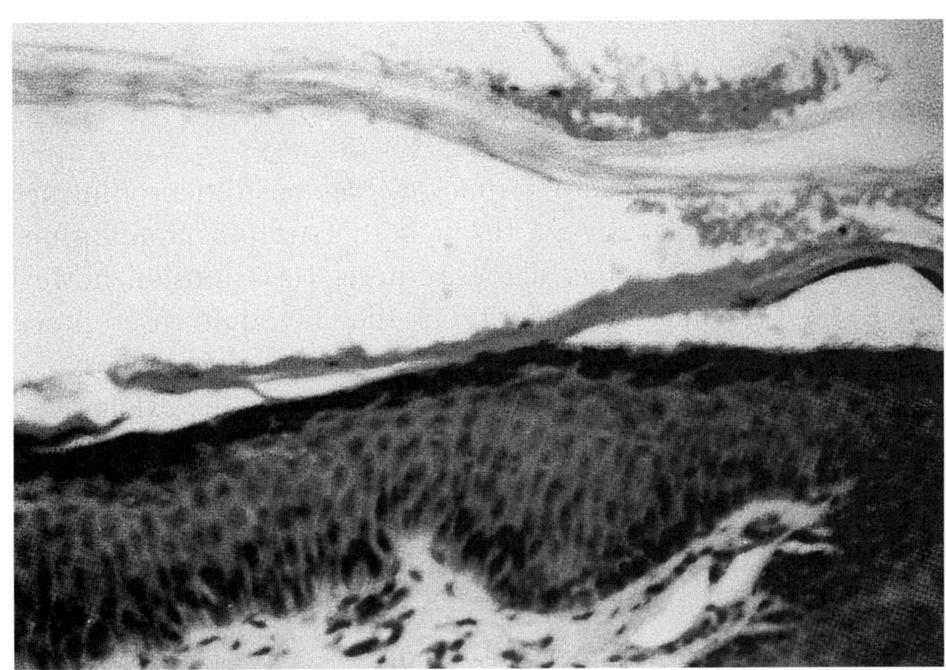

Figure 17–4 Photomicrograph of a skin biopsy from a patient with staphylococcal scalded skin syndrome, stained with hematoxylin and eosin. The histologic appearance is characterized by epidermal splitting at the granular layer of the epidermis. Magnification is approximately 200×. (From Hardwick N, Parry CM, Sharpe GR. Staphylococcal scalded skin syndrome in an adult. Influence of immune and renal factors. Br J Dermatol 132:468-471, 1995.)

develops between days 3 and 16 of life, but both intrauterine and congenital infections have been reported.[211-213] Outbreaks of SSSS have been reported to occur both in the normal newborn nursery[208,214] and among premature infants in NICUs.[60] Rates of both bullous impetigo and SSSS appear to be increasing, and some authors have postulated that this increase may be due to a reduction in the application of triple dye to the umbilical cord, a procedure traditionally used to reduce early colonization with *S. aureus*.[215]

Localized infection of the upper respiratory tract, inner ear, conjunctiva, or umbilical stump,[216] or, rarely, a more invasive site, is the initial step in both bullous impetigo and SSSS. Blister formation results from the elaboration of ETs by *S. aureus*. Four ETs, designated ETA, ETB, ETC, and ETD, have now been described.[127] These toxins are secreted extracellularly by staphylococci and are subsequently absorbed into the systemic circulation, where they ultimately reach the epidermis without significant binding to other organs.[217] Recently, the molecular mechanism of action of these toxins has been elucidated, revealing that they act as glutamic acid–specific serine proteases that target desmoglein-1, a transmembrane glycoprotein of desmosomes.[211,218,219]

The characteristic histologic feature of SSSS is intraepidermal cleavage through the granular layer, without evidence of epidermal necrosis or inflammatory cell infiltrate (Fig. 17-4).[220] This appearance is distinct from that in toxic epidermal necrolysis, characterized by a subepidermal split-and full-thickness necrosis of the epidermis.

The clinical spectrum of staphylococcal ET-related disease varies from a few localized blisters to diffuse exfoliation covering greater than 90% of the body surface area (Fig. 17-5). When localized blisters are present, as in bullous impetigo, they occur primarily in the perineal and periumbilical regions. The bullae are fragile and thin-roofed and rupture easily to release fluid that may be thin and amber-colored or purulent. For SSSS, the illness may begin with fever, lethargy, poor feeding, and an erythematous rash that rapidly becomes bullous and may involve the entire skin surface and spare the mucous membranes.[206]

The diagnoses of bullous impetigo and SSSS are made primarily on the basis of clinical presentation. A biopsy of the lesion showing the characteristic histologic features is the most useful test, but biopsies are rarely performed.[221,222] Attempts to isolate *S. aureus* from patient specimens may not be clinically useful, because the confirmatory tests to determine toxin production by a specific strain are available only at specialized centers. Isolating *S. aureus* from a patient specimen without confirmation of ET production is neither sensitive nor specific for SSSS.[222] Currently, rapid serologic tests are under development to provide more rapid confirmation of the diagnosis of SSSS.[223] Considerations in the differential diagnosis in infants with blistering skin disease include drug-induced toxic epidermal necrolysis, epidermolysis bullosa, bullous mastocytosis, herpetic lesions, and neonatal pemphigus.[224]

Treatment of bullous impetigo and SSSS generally involves systemic antibiotics targeted at *S. aureus*, together with appropriate local management of skin lesions. Oral antibiotics may be appropriate for bullous impetigo, but topical antibiotics are often ineffective owing to unpredictable absorption through the damaged skin.[206,221]

The prognosis for infants with bullous impetigo or SSSS is good, with a mortality rate from the latter of less than 5%.[210] Prevention of SSSS generally involves strict isolation of affected patients and relatively simple measures such as appropriate hand hygiene and cleansing of equipment that comes in contact with the patient to prevent cross-contamination.

Mastitis and Breast Abscess

Mastitis and breast abscesses are common problems among nursing mothers. The usual time to occurrence is between 2 weeks and 2 months post partum. The causative organism

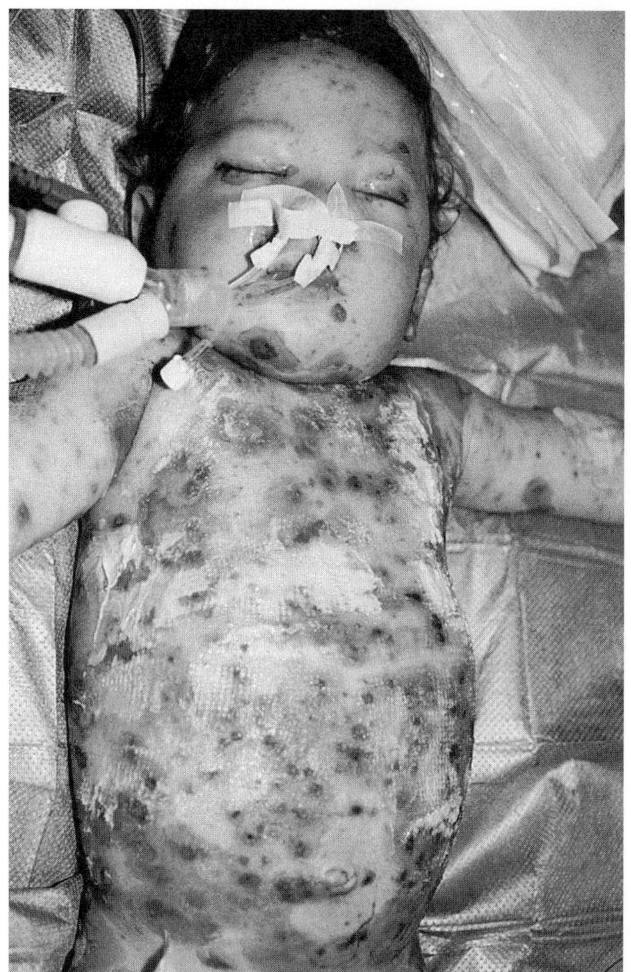

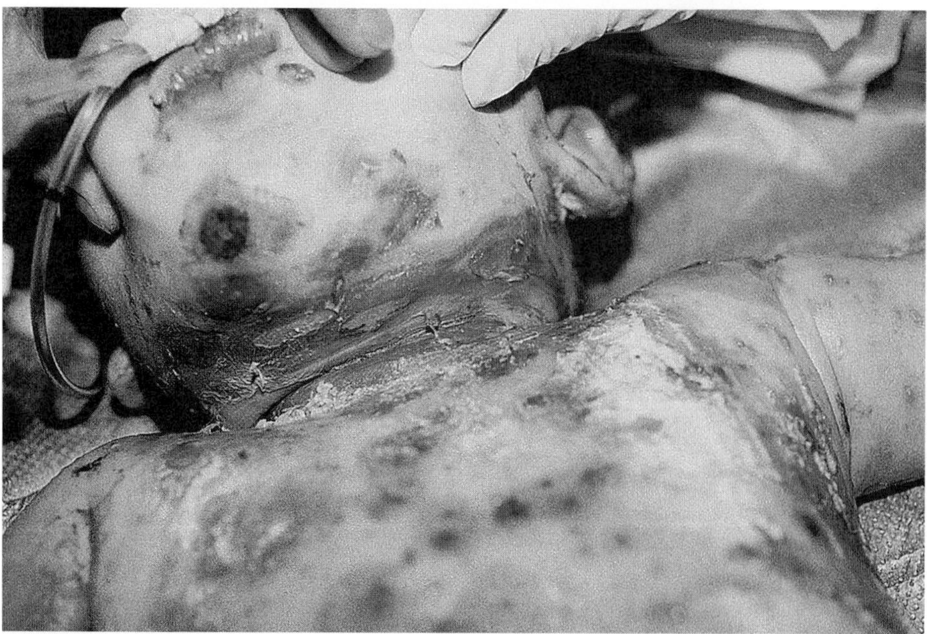

Figure 17–5 Generalized staphylococcal scalded skin syndrome in a previously well newborn infant. **A** and **B,** The characteristic well-demarcated erythematous superficial exfoliation, with areas of skin sparing, can be seen. (From Ladhani S, Joannou CL, Lochrie DP, et al. Clinical, microbial, and biochemical aspects of the exfoliative toxins causing staphylococcal scalded-skin syndrome. Clin Microbiol Rev 12:224-242, 1999.)

most frequently is *S. aureus* and originates from the mother's skin or the infant's nasopharynx,[225-228] generally gaining access to the interstitial tissues of the breast through a crack in the skin or nipple.[226,227] In addition to nipple breakdown, milk stasis secondary to incomplete emptying of the breasts has been proposed as a risk factor for breast infection among nursing mothers.[226,229-231]

Clinically, mastitis manifests as focal redness, warmth, tenderness, and induration of the breast. A breast abscess is diagnosed when the inflammatory findings are complemented by a fluctuant mass. Ultrasound examination is useful in confirming the diagnosis of breast abscess.[226,232,233] In addition to the focal findings, systemic signs of infection such as fever may be present. Culture of the milk or abscess fluid most frequently yields *S. aureus* as the causative organism.[226,227,234,235] Of note, however, staphylococci can be recovered from the milk of 25% to 50% of normal lactating women.[236-239]

The recommended therapy for mastitis involves systemic antibiotics and emptying the breast of milk.[225,226,240,241] Breast-feeding may be continued during the course of maternal therapy, with no adverse effects on the mother or the infant.[227] In the case of abscess formation, antibiotic treatment should be accompanied by needle aspiration or incision and drainage. Progression from mastitis to abscess formation may result from a delay in antibiotic therapy. Despite appropriate treatment, both mastitis and breast abscesses have relatively high rates of recurrence in the same or subsequent lactation periods.[242]

In neonates, breast disease usually occurs between the 10th and the 14th days of life. The disease can progress rapidly and involve the breast plus the surrounding subcutaneous tissue down to the abdomen and up to the shoulder and the back (Fig. 17-6). The extensive involvement is associated with systemic signs and symptoms of infection and a considerable amount of pus. Diagnosis can be made by Gram stain and culture of milk expressed from the infant's breast. Collections of pus should be incised, drained, and examined by Gram stain and culture.

Neonatal breast abscess can affect subsequent breast development and result in a decrease in breast size in adult life.[243] In one series of cases in which follow-up histories were obtained, a decrease in breast size was noted in two of six individuals who were examined at the ages of 8 and 15 years, respectively.[244]

Omphalitis

Omphalitis in the newborn is uncommon in resource-rich areas of the world but continues to be a significant cause of death and morbidity in resource-limited settings.[245] Risk factors for the development of this infection include home delivery, low birth weight, and factors associated with neonatal sepsis, such as chorioamnionitis, preterm labor, and rupture of membranes for greater than 8 hours.[246]

Neonatal omphalitis occurs along a spectrum of severity ranging from an unhealthy-appearing umbilical stump with purulent discharge to severe abdominal wall inflammation associated with necrotizing fasciitis. In a recent study by Sawardekar,[246] neonatal omphalitis was separated into four grades according to the level of severity: (1) funisitis/umbilical discharge: an unhealthy-appearing umbilical cord with purulent malodorous discharge; (2) omphalitis with abdominal wall cellulitis: periumbilical erythema and tenderness in addition to an unhealthy-appearing cord with discharge; (3) omphalitis with systemic sepsis: the findings of grade 2 with the addition of systemic signs of infection; and (4) omphalitis with necrotizing fasciitis: umbilical necrosis with periumbilical ecchymosis, crepitus bullae, and evidence of involvement of superficial and deep fascia, in addition to the signs and symptoms of overwhelming sepsis and shock.

The laboratory findings in neonatal omphalitis vary with the extent of the illness. When signs of systemic sepsis are present, a causative organism is isolated from the blood in approximately 60% of cases.[246] In addition, cultures of the umbilicus often yield a pathogen, most commonly *S. aureus*.[246,247] Infection is polymicrobial in approximately 10% of cases.[246]

A

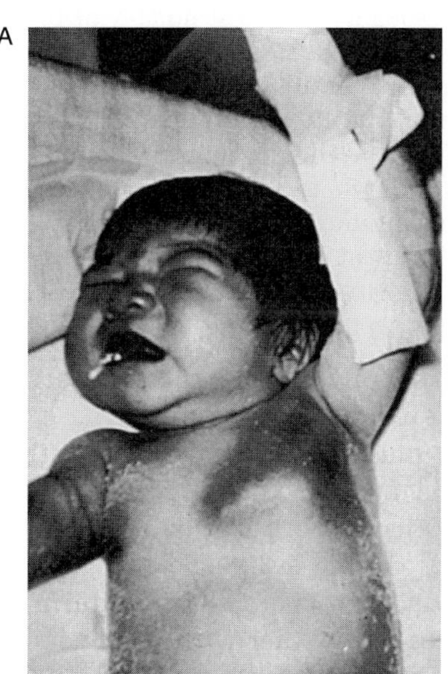

B

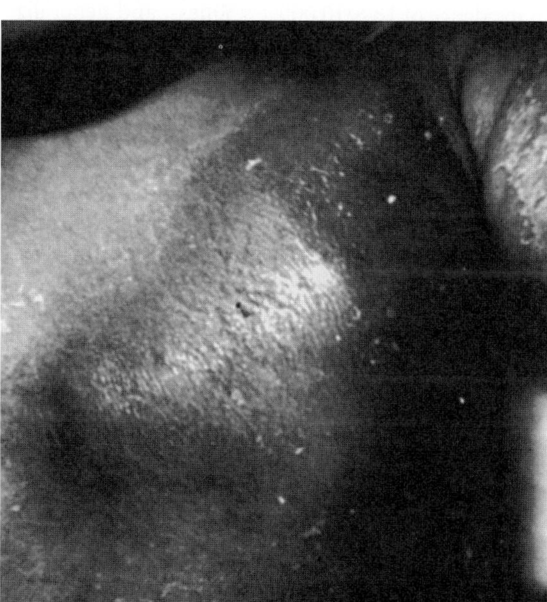

Figure 17–6 **A** and **B,** Left breast abscess in a 12-day-old infant. The abscess extends toward the right side of chest and up over the arm. The infant responded well to incision and drainage and antibiotic treatment.

Treatment of omphalitis is directed by the extent of the infection. When an infant presents with an unhealthy-appearing cord but evidence of cellulitis or systemic infection is lacking, local cord care may be sufficient. If cellulitis is present, the addition of systemic antibiotics is advisable. Constitutional symptoms should trigger an evaluation for sepsis and administration of parenteral antimicrobial therapy.[248] Signs of necrotizing fasciitis represent a critical situation and warrant prompt surgical consultation and intensive medical support. Empirical therapy in this circumstance should be directed at a polymicrobial infection with coverage for gram-positive, gram-negative, and anaerobic organisms.[247,248] Despite aggressive support, the mortality rate for neonatal omphalitis with necrotizing fasciitis remains high.[246,247]

Eye, Ear, Nose, and Throat Infections

One of the common sites of staphylococcal infection is the conjunctiva. Purulent staphylococcal conjunctivitis cannot be distinguished clinically from conjunctivitis caused by other organisms. The disease responds to local, nonspecific treatment and results in no residual damage, unlike gonococcal ophthalmitis.

Ethmoiditis with concomitant periorbital cellulitis is a serious infection that can evolve from *S. aureus* colonization of the nasopharynx. The periorbital tissues become red, edematous, and swollen. Disease progresses rapidly and leads to proptosis and limitation of eye movement. A variety of organisms other than staphylococci can cause this infection, which is dangerous because it is sometimes complicated by retrobulbar abscess and cavernous sinus infection and thrombosis. Intense parenteral treatment with antibiotics is required early.

Careful studies have suggested that staphylococci are occasionally true middle ear pathogens, *S. epidermidis* being the species most frequently encountered. Staphylococci are recovered from middle ear fluid in roughly 3% of premature infants with otitis media and can result in recurrent purulent or serous otitis.[249]

Neonatal suppurative parotitis is an uncommon infection among newborns, occurring with an incidence of 13.8/10,000 admissions.[250] Premature neonates and males appear to be at highest risk for suppurative parotitis,[251,252] which most frequently is caused by *S. aureus*.[251-253] Diagnosis of suppurative parotitis relies on the clinical findings of parotid swelling and purulent exudate from Stensen's duct on compression of the parotid gland, as well as growth of a pathogenic bacterium from culture of the pus.[254] Laboratory findings are most frequently nonspecific.[252] Antibiotic therapy without drainage is sufficient treatment in most cases of neonatal suppurative parotitis.[250,252] The lack of clinical improvement within 24 to 48 hours should prompt further evaluation for an intraparotid abscess that may require surgical drainage.

Cervical Adenitis

In the newborn, *S. aureus* cervical adenitis can be another manifestation of nursery colonization. At least two outbreaks of cervical adenitis resulting from nursery infection have been described in England. One outbreak involving 25 infants had an attack rate of 1.9%, and another involving 9 infants had an attack rate of 5.6%.[255,256] As with other manifestations of nursery-associated *S. aureus* disease, illness usually appears after discharge from the hospital. The mean incubation periods in the two epidemics in England were 86 and 72 days, respectively. Because of the delay in onset of disease, confirmation of a nursery as the source of the infection may be difficult and necessitates careful epidemiologic investigation.

Although the disease may be mild, serious complications occasionally have been reported. Dissection of the infection along the fascial sheaths of the neck into the thorax can result in secondary pneumonia and pyothorax.[257]

To guide treatment of *S. aureus* cervical adenitis, it is wise to obtain material for smear and culture by performing needle aspiration of the infected lymph node.[258,259]

Toxic Shock Syndrome

Toxic shock syndrome (TSS) is caused by pyrogenic toxin superantigens produced by *S. aureus*. These superantigens include TSST-1 and several enterotoxins, most commonly staphylococcal enterotoxin serotype B or C.[260,261] Before the 1980s, TSS occurred most commonly in menstruating women, particularly in those who used tampons.[262] More recently, disease has been recognized in persons with focal infection or surgical wound infection due to *S. aureus*, including MRSA. The disease is characterized by sudden onset of fever, diarrhea, shock, hyperemia of the mucous membranes, and a diffuse macular erythematous rash, followed by desquamation of the hands and feet.

Although this condition was first described in children,[263] it is uncommon in pediatric patients and occurs only rarely in young infants.[264] Several probable cases of TSS have been reported in newborns,[265,266] and recently an even more convincing case was described, with the infant fulfilling the Centers for Disease Control and Prevention (CDC) diagnostic criteria for TSS.[267] That infant presented with respiratory distress, hypotension, and fever and had laboratory evidence of renal insufficiency, hepatitis, coagulopathy, and muscular dysfunction. A diffuse macular erythroderma with mucous membrane involvement developed by day 4 of his illness, and generalized desquamation, most notably of the hands and feet, occurred subsequently. Other laboratory features included leukopenia, thrombocytopenia, and an elevated C-reactive protein level. Results of blood cultures were negative. The infant recovered with intensive support and administration of vancomycin and netilmicin.

Fluid loss and shock constitute a common cause of death in TSS; accordingly, replacement of fluid and electrolytes should be a management priority. Antibiotic therapy should be aimed at eliminating the toxin-producing organism. Intravenous immunoglobulin (IGIV) has been shown to be effective in reducing the mortality rate in adults with streptococcal TSS,[268] but efficacy of this intervention in staphylococcal TSS remains unknown.

Neonatal Toxic Shock Syndrome–like Exanthematous Disease

In 1997, researchers in Japan described a new neonatal exanthematous disease[269] that was later termed neonatal toxic shock syndrome–like exanthematous disease (NTED).[270]

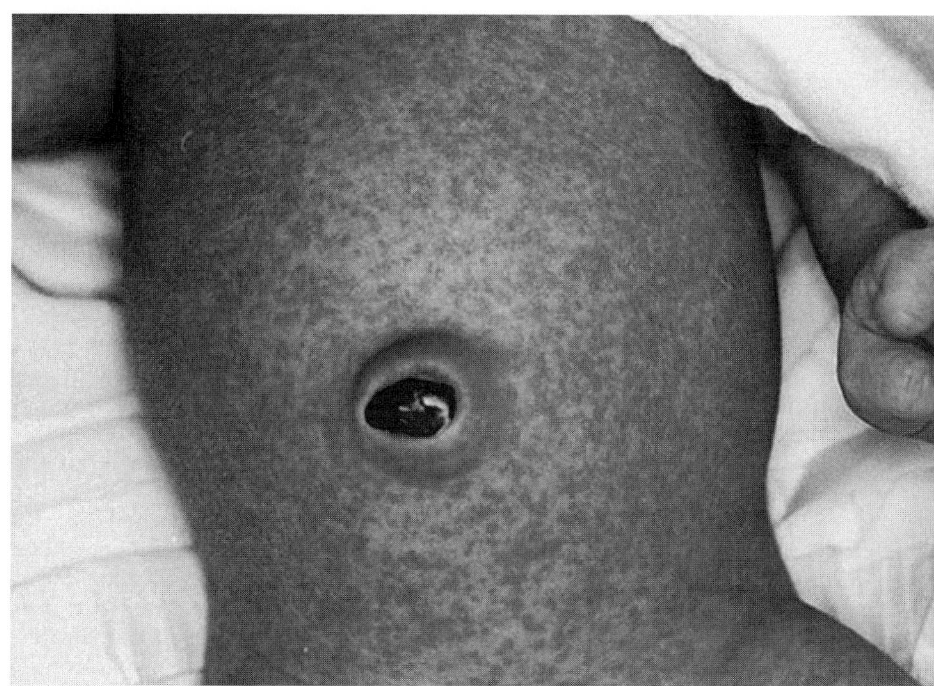

Figure 17–7 Typical exanthem in a full-term infant with neonatal toxic shock syndrome–like exanthematous disease (NTED). (From Takahashi N, Nishida H, Kato H, et al. Exanthematous disease induced by toxic shock syndrome toxin 1 in the early neonatal period. Lancet 351:1614-1619, 1998.)

Since the time of the first description, surveys in Japan have shown that up to 70% of Japanese hospitals have reported a similar illness in neonates.[271] Of interest, to date only three cases of probable NTED had been reported from countries other than Japan.[265,266]

The pathophysiology of NTED begins with colonization with MRSA, a common occurrence among Japanese newborns.[272] Typically, the colonizing strain of MRSA produces TSST-1,[272] and the symptoms of the disease are related to the overactivation of TSST-1–reactive T cells.[270] NTED does not develop in all infants who are colonized with TSST-1–producing MRSA, suggesting that protection from this illness may be mediated by the transplacental transfer of maternal antibody directed against TSST-1.[271]

The clinical criteria proposed for the diagnosis of NTED include erythema plus at least one of the following: thrombocytopenia, a low-positive serum C-reactive protein value, and fever.[269,270] In the initial description of the illness, fever occurred very early in the neonatal period, on the second or third day of life. Fever was absent from most preterm infants who were affected. With the resolution of fever came the development of a diffuse exanthem (Fig. 17-7), appearing on postnatal days 2 to 5 in full-term infants. The macular rash spread from the trunk to involve the face and extremities, including the palms and soles, often becoming confluent. Occasionally, petechiae were seen, but desquamation was absent. Abnormal laboratory studies in this condition include an elevated white blood cell count, low platelet count, and a C-reactive protein measurement that is above the upper limit of normal but usually below 50 mg/L. Hyperbilirubinemia requiring intervention is seen in both term and preterm infants with NTED. The most common site of colonization with MRSA is the umbilicus.[271]

Despite the apparently similar pathogenesis of NTED and TSS, these two entities can be easily differentiated by the absence of shock, desquamating rash, or multiple organ involvement in infants with NTED.[270] In most full-term infants, NTED resolves spontaneously without any specific treatment. By contrast, in preterm infants, NTED has been associated with serious illness, including symptomatic patent ductus arteriosus, mucosal damage, apnea, and death.[269,270]

Pneumonia

The incidence of *S. aureus* pneumonia in infants younger than 6 months of age is directly related to outbreaks of severe *S. aureus* disease in nurseries. In the late 1950s and early 1960s, many nurseries throughout the United States harbored virulent staphylococci (phage type 80/81). A sharp rise in the incidence of *S. aureus* pneumonia was noted during that period.[273-275] Over the years, *S. aureus* pneumonia has diminished in frequency, but the isolated cases that occur are still serious and should be cause for grave concern.[276] Recently, neonatal *S. aureus* pneumonia resulting from intrafamilial spread of virulent strains has been reported.[277,278]

S. aureus pneumonia can be secondary to a primary distant site of staphylococcal infection that results in bacteremia and seeding of the lung.[279] Most cases of *S. aureus* pneumonia in infants, however, occur in the setting of viral upper respiratory tract infection, with contiguous spread of bacteria from the upper respiratory tract to the alveoli, often resulting in microabscesses that rupture and produce empyema. The occlusion of terminal bronchioles leads to formation of pneumatoceles. The course of *S. aureus* pneumonia in infants typically is fulminant. In older series, mortality rates as high as 12% to 15% have been reported.[273,274] Because *S. aureus* pneumonia can be associated with either primary or secondary bacteremia, the possibility of distant metastatic staphylococcal lesions must be considered.

The clinical course of *S. aureus* pneumonia in infants is usually characterized by viral upper respiratory symptoms followed by rapid onset of tachypnea, dyspnea, and tachycardia. Patients typically appear restless and acutely ill. Most but not all patients have fever. Ileus and abdominal distention are common. Early radiologic examination reveals extensive pulmonary infiltrates, pneumothorax, and pleural effusion.

S. aureus pneumonia in infants almost always is associated with empyema, and needle aspiration of the pleural cavity is the most reliable way to establish a microbiologic diagnosis.[276] Ultimately, the empyema must be drained by continuous closed underwater suction, which should be continued until the pleural space is evacuated and the lung is re-expanded. In general, a bactericidal drug such as oxacillin or another semisynthetic penicillinase-resistant penicillin is indicated in this disease. The duration of therapy usually is 3 weeks but depends on the clinical condition of the infant and the ancillary laboratory data. Supportive therapy includes blood transfusion if significant anemia is present, supplemental oxygen, and appropriate fluids.

After the patient recovers from the acute infection, residual pulmonary abnormalities such as pneumatoceles are relatively common. Pneumatoceles are most common with staphylococcal pneumonia, but they also are occasionally seen with acute pyogenic lung infections caused by *Streptococcus pneumoniae*, *Streptococcus pyogenes*, or *Haemophilus influenzae*. They may persist for many months and usually require no therapy. The long-term prognosis for complete recovery is excellent, even after extensive bilateral lung disease.[280-282]

Pneumonia due to CoNS has also been described. In general, this diagnosis is assigned when CoNS are isolated from the blood of an infant with respiratory distress and a pulmonary infiltrate. The largest series was reported by Hall and colleagues, who identified 12 infants with hospital-acquired pneumonia among a total of 27 infants with CoNS bacteremia.[18] These authors noted an association between the presence of an endotracheal tube and development of pneumonia. Nine of their 12 patients were intubated at the time of the positive blood culture and pulmonary infiltrate, and the remaining 3 had been intubated previously.

Osteomyelitis

In interepidemic periods, *S. aureus* osteomyelitis is uncommon in neonates.[18] During nursery epidemics of *S. aureus* disease, however, osteomyelitis can occur secondary to skin infections and bacteremia.[283] Other factors that influence the pathogenesis of neonatal osteomyelitis include fetal monitoring[284] and manipulations related to the routine care of sick neonates, such as repeated heel punctures[285-287] and insertion of umbilical[288,289] and peripheral[290] intravascular catheters. Neonatal osteomyelitis is a different disease from the bone infection that is seen in older children.[290-295] For example, although the long, tubular bones are the most frequent sites of infection, membranous bones such as the scapula and maxilla also are frequently involved,[292,293,296] often with a relatively subtle clinical presentation.[297] Multifocal disease also is more common in neonates,[297-299] and an aggressive search for clinically silent sites may be necessary to identify all involved areas.[297] As in older infants and children, newborn infants develop bone infections at the metaphysis; however, because the cortex is thin and the periosteum strips easily in the bones of neonates, the sequestra that develop in older children usually are not seen.[300,301] Greater contiguous spread of the infection is possible because the bones of neonates have larger intraosseous vascular spaces. Secondary joint involvement occurs relatively often,[297-299] and the hip and shoulder are particularly vulnerable because in these joints the synovial capsule reaches beyond the metaphysis.

The signs and symptoms of neonatal osteomyelitis include redness, swelling, and reduced movement of the involved extremity, but these findings are not always present. In some cases, the infant is afebrile, and the white blood cell count is normal.[298] In an infant who is inexplicably irritable, the loss of function as manifested by pseudoparalysis is sometimes the only manifestation of disease. Osteomyelitis of the vertebrae can be particularly difficult to diagnose and should be suspected in an irritable infant who is uncomfortable lying supine or has pain on palpation. The diagnostic problem is exaggerated with vertebral osteomyelitis, because roentgenographic evidence of disease may not become visible until 2 or 3 weeks after infection. Radioisotope studies may be helpful in these cases.[302] Rupture through the cortex of a vertebra can result in epidural abscess with attendant cord compression.[303] Typical signs of sepsis such as lethargy, poor perfusion, apnea and bradycardia, feeding intolerance, and temperature instability can be present, especially in premature infants.[299] In infants, roentgenographic evidence of bone destruction and new bone formation can be evident as early as 7 days after infection,[293] earlier than in older children. Roentgenograms sometimes reveal soft tissue changes around the site of a bone infection before changes are visible in the bone itself. The earliest changes usually are seen with radionuclide imaging. In some cases, evidence of bone infection is present as early as 16 hours after the appearance of clinical signs.[304,305]

Organisms can be obtained from the blood early in the course of disease in about 50% of cases.[293] Because optimal antibiotic therapy depends on isolation of the etiologic agent, a vigorous attempt should be made to recover the organism from the blood and from the lesion itself by needle aspiration or bone biopsy. This approach is especially important in the era of MRSA, which has been reported as a cause of bone and joint infections in NICUs, primarily among preterm neonates.[289,299] Because sequestra seldom occur in neonates and the bone infection is not localized, early operative intervention is not indicated. If signs of localized collections of pus are present, these must be evacuated.

In cases of osteomyelitis, antibiotic therapy should be parenteral and continued for 4 to 6 weeks. Regimens combining parenteral and oral antibiotics that are common for the management of osteomyelitis in older infants and children are not suitable for treatment for neonates.[306,307] In the newborn, serum levels are unpredictable when antistaphylococcal antimicrobial agents are administered orally.[308] Following the sedimentation rate is a reasonable method for assessing the course of disease. If there is concomitant joint involvement, however, values may remain abnormal for a prolonged time.[309] Measurement of serum C-reactive protein is an alternative approach to monitoring response to therapy.

Despite early intensive therapy, neonatal osteomyelitis can result in severe long-term sequelae. In a study of 40 neonates followed for 7 months to 11 years after infection, the prognosis of neonatal osteomyelitis was correlated with both appropriate surgical measures and perinatal risk factors.[310]

Thirteen of 21 infants with sequelae had one or more of the following risk factors: low birth weight, low gestational age, catheterization of a large vessel, and respiratory distress syndrome. In neonates without such risk factors, however, the prognosis for acute osteomyelitis after adequate therapy is excellent unless the epiphysis of the bone is completely destroyed. Of interest, partially destroyed epiphyses of neonates show a remarkable ability to regenerate.[311] Chronic disease that results in draining sinuses is rarely observed, although permanent sequelae are possible if a joint is involved.

Neonatal osteomyelitis due to CoNS is unusual but has been reported at the site of a scalp clip.[284] In addition, osteomyelitis involving the sternum has been reported on occasion in neonates who have undergone sternotomy for intrathoracic surgery.[312]

Septic Arthritis

Septic arthritis in the neonate can be secondary either to osteomyelitis or to a distant focus of infection. Some cases have been associated with femoral venipuncture.[313] *S. aureus* is the most common cause of this disease throughout infancy, including during the neonatal period. The disease typically is difficult to diagnose, because the only indication in an infant may be irritability and crying with movement. Some edema or discoloration surrounding the affected joint is sometimes evident. Occasionally, localized abnormalities are not detected when the infant is examined initially but are noted several days later. Roentgenograms can be normal or show soft tissue swelling or capsular distention.[314]

To facilitate appropriate treatment, it is important to establish an etiologic diagnosis. Joint fluid should be aspirated for Gram stain and culture. Blood specimens for culture also should be collected, because they will sometimes yield an organism even when the joint fluid culture is sterile. Analysis of joint fluid usually reveals a white blood cell count greater than 50,000/mm^3, with a predominance of polymorphonuclear leukocytes, and a depressed glucose concentration.

Although satisfactory treatment in many cases consists only of repeated needle aspirations of purulent material in combination with antibiotic therapy, open drainage is advisable in infants to prevent destructive debilitating disease, particularly if the hip joint is involved. The femoral head may disappear within 4 days after onset of symptoms because of the extreme susceptibility of the articular cartilage to the ravages of *S. aureus*.[314]

In most cases, patients should receive treatment with a parenteral antibiotic for 3 to 4 weeks, provided that there is no evidence of osteomyelitis. If concomitant osteomyelitis is present, treatment should be continued for 4 to 6 weeks. In infants with delayed response to treatment, the possibility of a collection of pus should be explored, because even high concentrations of antibiotic may lack activity in the presence of pus. There is no evidence that instillation of antibiotics into the joint space itself hastens recovery.

Septicemia

CoNS and *S. aureus* are well-recognized causes of septicemia in the newborn period.[315,316] Among patients in the NICU, CoNS cause between 40% and 60% of all bacteremic episodes.[14,317-319] Septicemia is the most common manifestation of neonatal infection with CoNS and usually occurs in the setting of a central intravascular catheter. With *S. aureus*, septicemia often is associated with a focal site of infection and is more common when a virulent strain is present in the nursery.

The signs and symptoms associated with staphylococcal septicemia usually are nonspecific and include disturbances of temperature regulation, respiration, circulation, gastrointestinal function, and central nervous system activity. Hypothermia is more common than fever and often is observed as the initial sign. Respiratory distress frequently manifests as episodes of apnea and bradycardia, particularly in infants who weigh less than 1500 g. Other abnormalities related to respiration include tachypnea, retractions, and cyanosis. In 20% to 30% of infants, gastrointestinal abnormalities develop, including poor feeding, regurgitation, abdominal distention, diarrhea, and bloody stools. Evidence of poor perfusion can include mottling, poor capillary refill, and metabolic acidosis. In some infants, lethargy, irritability, or poor suck may be noted.

In infants who have septicemia with a focal site of infection, persistent bacteremia often is observed. Thus, when blood culture results remain positive after more than 72 hours of appropriate antibiotic therapy, a search for focal infection is advisable. The most common examples of such infection include skin or soft tissue infection, osteomyelitis, septic arthritis, endocarditis, and meningitis.

Of interest, Patrick and co-workers recently described a group of 13 low-birth-weight infants with persistent CoNS bacteremia who had no indwelling central intravascular catheter and lacked evidence of focal infection.[320] These infants had positive blood culture results for 6 to 25 days despite appropriate antibiotic therapy. Abdominal distention and thrombocytopenia were especially common findings. Although the bacteremia eventually cleared and no infants died, the explanation for the delayed response to therapy was elusive.

The diagnosis of staphylococcal septicemia is established by isolating organisms from the blood. To facilitate interpretation of positive results of cultures, especially those growing CoNS, multiple culture specimens should be obtained if at all possible. Recovery of the same strain (as defined by speciation, antibiotic susceptibility profile, and possibly molecular analysis) from two or more cultures provides strong evidence for true infection. On the other hand, when a single culture specimen is collected and CoNS is recovered, assessment of the likelihood of true infection is often difficult. At least one study suggests that quantitative blood cultures may be useful in this situation.[321] In that study, peripheral blood cultures yielding more than 50 colony-forming units per milliliter (CFU/mL) occurred exclusively in infants with proven septicemia. By contrast, low colony counts were observed with both septicemia and culture contamination. Infants with septicemia were significantly more likely to have a central catheter or an abnormal hematologic value (white blood cell count more than 20,000/mm^3 or less than 5000/mm^3, immature-to-total neutrophil ratio more than 0.12, or platelet count less than 150,000/mm^3), regardless of the magnitude of bacteremia. Infants who lacked these clinical features were more likely to have culture contamination. Several other studies have corroborated the usefulness of an elevated immature-to-total neutrophil ratio in identifying infants with CoNS septicemia.[7,20,320]

In an era of increasing methicillin resistance among staphylococci, the use of vancomycin is increasingly necessary for the treatment of both *S. aureus* and CoNS bacteremia. In a study by Krediet and co-workers, the *mecA* gene was identified in 78% of bloodstream isolates of CoNS from infants in the NICU.[322] Combination antibiotic therapy is sometimes necessary in infants who have persistent bacteremia. The addition of rifampin has been shown in selected patients to facilitate sterilization of the bloodstream.[323,324]

The decision to remove an indwelling catheter from a neonate with bacteremia often is difficult, especially when securing further intravascular access may be challenging but necessary for the delivery of life-sustaining therapies. Delayed removal of a central catheter in the setting of bacteremia may be associated with an increased risk of infection-related complications, including prolonged bacteremia and end-organ damage, however.[325] For infants with CoNS bacteremia, successful treatment of bacteremia may be possible with the central venous catheter in situ.[325] However, if bacteremia persists for longer than 4 days, the chance for subsequent clearance is reduced[326] and the risk of end-organ damage may be increased.[325,327] The presence of a ventricular reservoir or ventriculoperitoneal shunt increases the chance of the development of meningitis in the setting of prolonged catheter-related bacteremia. Thus, prompt removal of an indwelling central venous catheter should be considered in infants with central nervous system hardware.[326]

Endocarditis

Historically, infective endocarditis (IE) in the neonatal period has been a rare clinical diagnosis. Autopsy studies from the 1970s, however, revealed unsuspected IE in 0.2% to 3% of neonates who came to autopsy.[328,329] Nonbacterial thrombotic endocarditis is a condition that may predispose the patient to IE and was found in up to 10% of neonatal autopsies.[328,330] In the 1990s several authors described series of neonates with IE,[331-334] with incidence ranging from 0.07% of admissions to the NICU[334] to 4.3% of patients of the same gestational age.[333] The increased reporting of IE may be due to either improved diagnostic capabilities or to a true increase in incidence reflecting the increasing use of invasive techniques in the care of sick neonates.[335]

In older children with IE, α-hemolytic streptococci are the organisms recovered most frequently. By contrast, in neonates staphylococcal species appear to account for a majority of the cases of IE.[335] Historically, *S. aureus* has been the predominant bacterial pathogen among neonates with IE,[335] but more recent reports indicate that CoNS may be most common now.[331-334]

Most case reports of IE in the neonatal period involve infants with normal hearts who are receiving intensive medical care related to prematurity or serious congenital anomalies. These infants often have indwelling catheters and are at risk for bacteremia complicating invasive procedures. The initial step in the development of IE may be the formation of nonbacterial thrombotic endocarditis. In animal models, injury to the endocardium and subsequent thrombus formation can be induced by brief insertion of an intravascular catheter into the right atrium.[336-338] The finding of a catheter that has migrated to the right atrium is frequently reported as a preceding event in infants with IE.[328,331] Other factors that may lead to thrombus formation include hypoxia, respiratory distress syndrome of prematurity, and disseminated intravascular coagulation.[335] Bacterial colonization of the thrombus may occur as a consequence of transient bacteremia that develops during procedures that traumatize the skin or mucous membranes.

The signs and symptoms of IE in neonates often are nonspecific and similar to those of other conditions such as sepsis or congenital heart disease, including poor feeding, tachycardia, and respiratory distress.[335] While a new or changing cardiac murmur may raise the suspicion of IE, this finding may be absent.[331] Traditional manifestations of IE in older children and adults, such as hepatosplenomegaly, petechiae, skin abscesses, arthritis, and central nervous system abnormalities, are less common in neonates. Classic findings in IE in adults, such as Osler nodes and Roth spots, have not been described in neonates,[335] and only one case in the literature describes Janeway lesions in this age group.[339] Fever frequently is absent in neonates with IE, although temperature instability may be observed.[334]

The diagnosis of IE should be considered in any neonate with bacteremia that persists despite catheter removal and appropriate antimicrobial therapy. In the presence of IE, the yield of a single blood culture has been reported to be between 77% and 97%. When three blood cultures are obtained, the yield approaches 100%.[340-342] Additional laboratory abnormalities that are frequently reported in neonates with IE include thrombocytopenia,[331-334] neutropenia or neutrophilia,[332,334] and an elevated C-reactive protein.[331,332,334] The thin chest wall and often normal cardiac anatomy of neonates with IE make echocardiography a highly sensitive tool for diagnosis of IE in this age group. The limitations of this technique include the inability to detect lesions less than 2 mm in diameter and to differentiate between vegetations and other masses such as thrombi.[332] Additional studies that should be included in the evaluation of a neonate with suspected IE are listed in Table 17-1.

Table 17–1 Appropriate Laboratory Evaluation and Diagnostic Tests for Neonates with Suspected Endocarditis

1. Cultures:
   - Blood (at least two)
   - Urine
   - Cerebrospinal fluid
   - Other usually sterile body fluids, if available
2. Complete blood count including white blood cell differential
3. Erythrocyte sedimentation rate (micromethod may be used)[a]
4. Coagulation profile:
   - Prothrombin time
   - Partial thromboplastin time
   - Fibrinogen
   - Fibrin split products
5. Rheumatoid factor (of uncertain value in neonate)
6. Urinalysis
7. Chest radiograph
8. Echocardiogram
9. Ultrasound examination of great vessels and abdomen, including renal vessels
10. Computed tomography of head (if indicated)

[a]Data from Adler SM, Denton RL. The erythrocyte sedimentation rate in the newborn period. Pediatrics 86:942, 1986.

Traditional classification systems for the diagnosis of IE in adults, such as the von Reyn classification[343] and the Duke criteria,[344] may have reduced sensitivity when applied to children and have not been studied in neonates.[345] A suggested set of criteria for the diagnosis of IE in neonates has been proposed but has not been studied prospectively.[332]

The choice of antimicrobial therapy for the treatment of neonatal IE should be based on the susceptibility of the infecting organism. A bactericidal agent should be used when possible. The addition of a second agent, such as an aminoglycoside or rifampin, should be considered if the patient fails to improve on monotherapy. A course of parenteral therapy that continues for at least 4 to 6 weeks from the first negative blood culture result is indicated in neonates with IE.[335]

Historically, the prognosis for neonates with IE has been grave. A number of series published in recent years report disease-specific survival rates ranging from 40% to greater than 85%.[331-334,342,346,347] Survival of neonates with IE is likely to be improved with early diagnosis and aggressive management.[335]

Central Nervous System Infections

S. aureus and CoNS have long been recognized as causes of meningitis and ventriculitis, particularly in patients with intraventricular shunts or ventriculostomy catheters.[348-350] Before the extensive use of shunts and catheters to divert the flow of cerebrospinal fluid in patients with congenital or acquired obstructions, most staphylococcal infections of the central nervous system involved the dura and venous sinuses and were sequelae of infections near the face. In recent years, several authors have reported the development of neonatal staphylococcal meningitis in the absence of an intraventricular foreign body or a contiguous site of infection. In affected patients, meningitis appers to develop as a sequela of bacteremia.[320,351] In a recent series examining neonatal meningitis in VLBW infants, CoNS were the most frequently isolated organisms.[352] This change may be a consequence of the increased survival of VLBW infants and the resultant increased incidence of nosocomial infections including bacteremia with CoNS.

Neonatal staphylococcal meningitis typically is associated with nonspecific signs and symptoms, including lethargy, hypotonia, temperature instability, increased oxygen requirement, apnea and bradycardia, and feeding intolerance.[352] Among patients with a shunt or catheter, examination of the cerebrospinal fluid most often reveals a mild pleocytosis, typically with an elevated protein and sometimes with a slightly depressed glucose; however, occasionally, the cerebrospinal fluid is completely normal. Gruskay and associates described 10 infants with *S. epidermidis* bacteremia and meningitis who had unremarkable cerebrospinal fluid cell counts and normal glucose and protein levels; the mean cerebrospinal fluid white blood cell count was 6/mm^3, with a range of 0 to 14/mm^3, and the mean glucose and protein values were 2.8 mmol/L and 1.15 g/L, respectively.[351] The lack of cerebrospinal fluid pleocytosis during episodes of CoNS meningitis has been demonstrated by other investigators as well, especially among infants before 33 weeks of postconceptional age.[352] Although the pathogenesis of neonatal meningitis appears to involve preceding bacteremia, a concurrent positive blood culture may be found in only about half of infants with meningitis.[353,354]

Traditionally, management of staphylococcal meningitis in an infant with a shunt or catheter involves removal of the contaminated foreign body and administration of appropriate antibiotic therapy. Recently, however, several investigators have advocated simply externalizing the distal end of the shunt, administering both intravenous and intraventricular antibiotics (usually for 7 to 10 days after sterilization of the cerebrospinal fluid), and then replacing the distal catheter.[355,356] This approach can be effective in some patients but is less likely to succeed if the infecting organism elaborates polysaccharide and forms biofilms.[179,357] For *S. aureus*, oxacillin or nafcillin generally is recommended, unless the organism is methicillin resistant. For CoNS, vancomycin usually is the antibiotic of choice. In cases refractory to initial treatment, combination therapy with rifampin or gentamicin may be useful, especially if the intraventricular shunt or catheter cannot be removed.[358]

Diffuse glomerulonephritis can develop in patients with a ventriculoatrial shunt and CoNS bacteremia.[359] The renal disease results from immune-complex deposition in the renal parenchyma, rather than from direct bacterial embolization to the kidney. Improvement in renal function occurs after removal of the shunt.

Despite the frequent absence of significant neurologic and cerebrospinal fluid abnormalities, staphylococcal meningitis can have a significant detrimental effect on neurodevelopemental outcome, especially among VLBW infants. In a study by Doctor and associates, the presence of meningitis in VLBW infants was associated with higher rates of major neurologic abnormalities and cognitive impairment at 20 months of corrected age, compared with control infants admitted to the same NICU without meningitis.[352]

Abscesses in the central nervous system are infrequent in neonates and most often are secondary to infection with gram-negative bacilli.[360] Staphylococcal brain abscesses can occur in neonates and young infants, however, especially in the setting of prolonged bacteremia.[361] Additional risk factors for the development of brain abscesses in infants and children include the presence of congenital heart disease; head trauma; ventriculoperitoneal shunting; preceding ear, nose, or throat infection; sepsis; and meningitis.[362,363] A polymicrobial brain abscess including *S. aureus* has been reported as a complication of fetal scalp electrode monitoring.[364]

The signs and symptoms of abscesses of the central nervous system may be variable, depending on the location of the lesion and the identity of the infecting organism. In published studies of infants with brain abscesses, the most frequent presenting complaints include lethargy, irritability, poor feeding, respiratory symptoms, vomiting, a bulging fontanelle or splayed sutures, focal neurologic deficits, and seizures.[360,365-367] Fever is present in some infants[366] but is not a consistent finding.

Imaging of the brain with computed tomography (CT) or magnetic resonance imaging (MRI) is critical to establishing the diagnosis of a brain abscess.[361] Cerebrospinal fluid studies typically are unrevealing, and culture of the cerebrospinal fluid often is negative. In patients with a suspected brain abscess, lumbar puncture generally should be avoided until a CT or MRI study is performed and reveals no midline shift or mass.[361]

The treatment of brain abscesses in infancy and childhood typically involves both surgical and medical management, although in some cases, medical management alone is sufficient.[363,365] Despite appropriate treatment, the outcome for infants with brain abscesses often is poor, with death and disability occurring in a majority of the cases.[363,368]

Enteric Infections

S. aureus is a common colonizer of the gastrointestinal tract of newborns, present in up to 93% of asymptomatic infants.[369] The prevalence of colonization is not surprising, considering that large numbers of *S. aureus* can be recovered from samples of breast milk expressed from normal breasts of lactating and nonlactating women.[238]

On rare occasions, *S. aureus* may be associated with enterocolitis in the newborn infant. The first case was reported in 1947 and involved an infant whose mother suffered from staphylococcal mastitis.[370] Since that time, additional reports have emerged describing *S. aureus* enterocolitis in neonates. A number of etiologic factors have been implicated in the development of staphylococcal enterocolitis, including prior broad-spectrum antibiotic usage, gastrointestinal foreign bodies (feeding tubes), gastrointestinal surgery, influenzavirus A infection, and possibly starvation.[371] The pathophysiology of *S. aureus* enterocolitis may be secondary to the elaboration of toxins and the capacity of some isolates to invade intestinal epithelium, resembling invasion by *Shigella* spp.[371]

Infants with staphylococcal enterocolitis often present with systemic signs of infection, including lethargy, cyanosis, and bradycardia, associated with frequent watery, sometimes green-hued diarrhea that may contain blood or mucus. Typical laboratory features include leukocytosis, thrombocytopenia, acidosis, disseminated intravascular coagulation, and an elevated C-reactive protein level. Stool cultures have yielded growth of *S. aureus* in all reported cases, and blood cultures are positive in a subset of patients. Treatment of staphylococcal enterocolitis with oral vancomycin has been successful in resolving symptoms in affected neonates, although colonic stenosis after severe MRSA enterocolitis has been reported.[372]

The role of CoNS in neonatal enteric disease has been the subject of much debate. An association between necrotizing enterocolitis and CoNS was first suggested by Fabia and associates in 1983.[373] In 1986, Gruskay and colleagues described a series of 19 newborns with *S. epidermidis* bacteremia and associated acute enterocolitis.[374] In this series, the diagnosis of enterocolitis was assigned in infants who had blood and mucus in their stools, signs and symptoms of gastrointestinal distress, and abnormalities on the abdominal radiograph. Pneumatosis intestinalis developed in only one infant, and none had portal venous or free intraperitoneal air. Furthermore, none of these patients experienced prolonged feeding intolerance, and none required surgery. An association between necrotizing enterocolitis and delta-like toxin produced by CoNS was proposed by Scheifele and co-workers, who found toxin production in the stools of CoNS-colonized infants with NEC more frequently than in control infants who were similarly colonized.[184] Several authors have reported cases of necrotizing enterocolitis associated with CoNS bacteremia, but a causal function for CoNS remains to be established.[10,20,375-377]

ANTIBIOTIC TREATMENT

Staphylococcus aureus

The therapeutic approach to *S. aureus* infection is influenced by the special biologic properties of this organism, including the ability to persist under adverse conditions, the tendency to form deep-seated abscesses, and the capacity for resistance to a variety of antibiotics. In general, therapy consists of a sound antimicrobial regimen, in some cases coupled with surgery. Aside from superficial skin lesions, staphylococcal infection in the newborn is a serious disease. Accordingly, in general, infants should be hospitalized and receive parenteral antibiotic therapy.

Approximately 95% of *S. aureus* isolates produce β-lactamase, a serine protease that hydrolyzes the β-lactam ring and confers resistance to penicillin. In addition, an increasing percentage of isolates contain the *mecA* gene, which encodes PBP2a (also referred to as PBP2′) and confers resistance to methicillin and all other penicillinase-resistant penicillins (oxacillin, nafcillin, dicloxacillin, and cloxacillin) and cephalosporins.[48] Methicillin resistance is defined as a methicillin minimum inhibitory concentration (MIC) greater than 8 μg/mL or an oxacillin MIC greater than 4 μg/mL, and as noted earlier, isolates are referred to as methicillin-resistant *S. aureus* (MRSA) or sometimes oxacillin-resistant *S. aureus* (ORSA). The presence of the *mecA* gene can be detected by DNA probes or PCR assays directed at *mecA* or by a latex agglutination reaction specific for the PBP2a protein. The *mecA* gene is contained on a 21- to 67-kilobase genetic element that harbors a variety of other antibiotic resistance genes, accounting for the fact that MRSA isolates are typically resistant to multiple antibiotics.[48] This genetic element is integrated into the *S. aureus* chromosome and is called the staphylococcal cassette chromosome *mec* (SCC*mec*). At least four different variations of SCC*mec* exist, designated type I to type IV SCC*mec*.[48] Type IV SCC*mec* is being recognized with increasing frequency and is a smaller element that usually lacks resistance genes for aminoglycosides, tetracyclines, trimethoprim-sulfamethoxazole, and clindamycin. Occasional isolates of *S. aureus* display borderline resistance to methicillin, with a methicillin MIC less than 8 μg/mL and no *mecA* gene. In these isolates, resistance is a consequence of hyperproduction of β-lactamase and can be overcome by use of high doses of penicillinase-resistant penicillins.[378]

In recent years, isolates with intermediate susceptibility to vancomycin have been identified with increasing frequency (MIC of 8 to 16 μg/mL), in almost all cases having evolved from strains that are methicillin resistant.[379] These isolates are referred to as VISA, for vancomycin-intermediate *S. aureus*, or GISA, for glycopeptide-intermediate *S. aureus* (reflecting intermediate resistance to other antibiotics in the same class as that of vancomycin). They lack the *vanA*, *vanB*, *vanC*, *vanD*, *vanE*, and *vanG* genes associated with vancomycin resistance in enterococci. Biochemical studies have revealed increased rates of cell wall synthesis, increased quantities of cell wall precursors, and a disorganized, thickened cell wall with an increased number of vancomycin-binding sites.[380,381] The precise mechanism of reduced susceptibility is unclear, but it appears that "affinity trapping" may prevent vancomycin from reaching the cytoplasmic membrane, where nascent peptidoglycan synthesis occurs and where vancomycin exerts its antibiotic effect. In 2002, the first documented infections due to high-level vancomycin-resistant *S. aureus* were reported.[382,383] The original isolate was recovered from a catheter exit site in an adult diabetic patient undergoing chronic dialysis and had a vancomycin MIC of 1024 μg/mL.[382,384] Additional susceptibility testing revealed resistance to teichoplanin (a glycopeptide antibiotic, in the same class as that of vancomycin), oxacillin (MIC greater than 128 μg/mL), aminoglycosides, fluoroquinolones, macrolides, rifampin, and tetracycline, but susceptibility to chloramphenicol, linezolid, quinupristin-dalfopristin, and trimethoprim-sulfamethoxazole. Using a PCR assay, vancomycin resistance was identified as *vanA* mediated.[385] Further analyses suggested that *vanA* was acquired from a co-isolate of *Enterococcus faecalis* through interspecies transfer of Tn*1546*, a 10.8-kb transposon that contains *vanA* and the associated resistance gene cluster (*vanR*, *vanS*, *vanH*, *vanX*, *vanY*, and *vanZ*).[385] Analysis of another isolate, recovered from a foot ulcer in an adult male, demonstrated a vancomycin MIC of 32 μg/mL and the presence of *vanA*. This isolate was susceptible to chloramphenicol, linezolid, minocycline, quinupristin-dalfopristin, and trimethoprim-sulfamethoxazole. Of interest, additional testing revealed susceptibility to teichoplanin, an atypical finding for strains of *Enterococcus* with the *vanA* gene.[386]

For isolates susceptible to penicillin, the drug of choice is penicillin. For isolates that produce β-lactamase, oxacillin or nafcillin is preferred; alternatives include first-generation cephalosporins such as cephalothin and cefazolin, although these agents are sometimes less stable to β-lactamase, resulting in occasional reports of treatment failure. Vancomycin also is an alternative for β-lactamase–producing isolates but is less rapidly bactericidal than the β-lactam antibiotics and should be reserved for patients with hypersensitivity to β-lactams.[387] Isolates of *S. aureus* that test resistant to methicillin also are resistant to oxacillin and nafcillin and should be considered resistant to penicillin and all cephalosporins as well, even if in vitro susceptibility testing suggests otherwise. With these isolates, vancomycin usually is the antibiotic of choice, occasionally in conjunction with gentamicin or rifampin. Some methicillin-resistant isolates are susceptible to clindamycin, which therefore can be used for treatment of infection in such cases, especially if testing reveals no evidence of inducible resistance to clindamycin and infection is outside the central nervous system. Linezolid may be another option for treatment of infection in which methicillin-resistant isolates have been identified. Other antibiotics that often have activity against MRSA include trimethoprim-sulfamethoxazole and fluoroquinolones, although these agents generally are avoided in neonates. Treatment of infection involving isolates with reduced susceptibility to vancomycin should be guided by results of in vitro susceptibility testing, but potential agents generally include gentamicin, rifampin, and linezolid. In patients with endocarditis, other serious infections, or infections refractory to monotherapy, synergistic treatment with a β-lactam or vancomycin and either gentamicin or rifampin may be considered.

The pharmacokinetics of aqueous penicillin G, the semisynthetic penicillins (oxacillin, nafcillin, and methicillin), and the first-generation cephalosporins (cephalothin and cefazolin) have been well characterized in newborns.[104,388-400] In general, clearance of these antibiotics increases as postnatal age advances from birth to 4 weeks, and dosing intervals should be adjusted accordingly. Recommended doses and dosing intervals are summarized in Table 17-2.[401] Doses for both vancomycin and gentamicin are best calculated on the basis of postconceptional age (gestational age at birth plus postnatal age). Dosages of these agents used at St. Louis Children's Hospital are outlined in Tables 17-3 and 17-4. Even with careful dosing, serum concentrations of these antibiotics

Table 17–2 Drugs Useful in Treatment of Staphylococcal Disease in Term Neonates

Agent	Dosage: Age Birth–1 Wk	Dosage: Age 1-4 Wk
Penicillin G	25,000-50,000 units/kg q12h	Same dose q8h
Oxacillin	25-50 mg/kg q12h	25-40 mg/kg q6-8h
Nafcillin	25-50 mg/kg q12h	
Cefazolin	25 mg/kg q12h	Same dose q8h
Rifampin	5-10 mg/kg q12h	Same dose
Clindamycin	2.5-3.75 mg/kg q12h	Same dose q8h
Linezolid	10 mg/kg q12h	Same dose q8h
Synercid	7.5 mg/kg q12h	Same dose
Vancomycin	See Table 17-3	
Gentamicin	See Table 17-4	

Table 17–3 Dosing of Vancomycin in Term and Preterm Neonates

Postconceptional Age[a]	Postnatal Age	Dosage
<28 wk	0-14 d	15 mg/kg q8h
	>14 d	15 mg/kg q12h
28-34 wk	0-14 d	15 mg/kg q12h
	>14 d	15 mg/kg q8h
34-42 wk	0-7 d	15 mg/kg q12h
	>7 d	15 mg/kg q8h
>42 wk	All	15 mg/kg q8h

[a]Postconceptional age = gestational age at birth + postnatal age.

Table 17–4 Dosing of Gentamicin in Term and Preterm Neonates

Postconceptional Age[a]	Postnatal Age	Dosage
<26 wk	0-30 d	3 mg/kg q24h
	>30 d	5 mg/kg q24h
26-30 wk	0-21 d	3 mg/kg q24h
	21-45 d	5 mg/kg q24h
	45-60 d	2.5 mg/kg q12h
	>60 d	2.5 mg/kg q8h[b]
30-32 wk	0-14 d	3 mg/kg q24h
	14-45 d	5 mg/kg q24h
	>45 d	2.5 mg/kg q8h[b]
>32 wk	0-30 d	5 mg/kg q24h
	>30 d	2.5 mg/kg q8h[b]

[a]Postconceptional age = gestational age at birth + postnatal age.
[b]In patients with renal or cardiac dysfunction, use 2.5 mg/kg/dose q12-24h.

exhibit significant patient-to-patient variability, potentially compounded by medications, such as indomethacin, that impair glomerular filtration and delay excretion.[392] Accordingly, to maximize therapeutic effect and minimize renal toxicity and ototoxicity, serum levels of gentamicin and probably vancomycin should be monitored, allowing modification of dosing as necessary. With gentamicin, peak levels of 4 to 15 μg/mL and trough levels less than 2 μg/mL are desirable. With vancomycin, the ideal levels are unclear, although some experts recommend peak levels between 20 and 40 μg/mL and predose trough levels of 5 to 12 μg/mL.

Coagulase-Negative Staphylococci

As with infections due to *S. aureus*, antibiotic treatment is critical in the management of disease due to CoNS. Resistance to penicillin, the semisynthetic penicillins, and gentamicin is common among hospital-acquired isolates.[18,20,393] Resistance to vancomycin is rare but has been reported among isolates of *S. haemolyticus*.[394,395] With this information in mind, most experts recommend use of vancomycin as empirical therapy when CoNS infection is suspected or proved. The treatment regimen is then modified based on antibiotic susceptibility testing.

In considering antibiotic susceptibility results, several caveats are in order. First, as with *S. aureus*, penicillin resistance in CoNS frequently is mediated by production of β-lactamase.[396] Because this resistance often is not detected by routine microdilution methods, all isolates that appear susceptible to penicillin or ampicillin should be tested for β-lactamase production. Such testing involves first exposing organisms to oxacillin, which induces expression of β-lactamase. Second, although each organism in a population may have the genetic information necessary for resistance to semisynthetic penicillins, only a small minority express resistance under in vitro testing conditions.[104] To avoid overlooking these organisms, the clinical microbiology laboratory should attempt to optimize expression of resistance by culturing on salt-containing media at 30° C to 35° C.[397] Third, routine susceptibility testing sometimes indicates that an isolate resistant to methicillin is susceptible to cephalosporins. As described with *S. aureus*, however, cross-resistance is extensive; therefore, all isolates of CoNS found to be resistant to semisynthetic penicillins also should be considered resistant to cephalosporins for clinical purposes.[398-400]

For infection due to the few isolates that are rigorously established to be penicillin susceptible and β-lactamase negative, penicillin is a suitable antibiotic. With isolates that are resistant to penicillin but truly susceptible to the semisynthetic penicillins, therapy with oxacillin or nafcillin is appropriate. Vancomycin is the preferred antibiotic for infection due to CoNS that are resistant to semisynthetic penicillins and also for the rare neonate allergic to penicillin. One report indicates that the combination of rifampin and clindamycin is an alternative regimen for patients allergic to penicillin.[402] For multiresistant isolates, considerations include other glycopeptide antibiotics (for example, teicoplanin) or quinolone derivatives. Resistance to these agents has also been reported, however.

In patients with endocarditis or cerebrospinal fluid shunt infection, synergistic therapy may be indicated.[403,404] In vitro synergy studies have been performed with vancomycin in combination with rifampin, gentamicin, or β-lactams (with isolates susceptible to each), and synergy has been demonstrated with all of these combinations.[350,405] In view of the high frequency of resistance to gentamicin and the β-lactams, vancomycin plus rifampin probably is the best regimen in most cases. Although rifampin alone also has good antistaphylococcal activity, resistance emerges rapidly unless this antibiotic is used together with other antimicrobial agents.[405]

PREVENTION

Staphylococcus aureus

Control of nursery infection has been directed toward the three important links in the chain of events that leads to colonization of infants: the environment, nursery attendants, and the infants themselves.[406-408]

Staphylococci may be spread through the air; thus, overcrowding of infants in an NICU increases the risk of colonization and the potential for disease. In an outbreak situation, attempts to control the spread of staphylococci through remediation of overcrowding and isolation of infected or colonized patients have been shown to be effective in helping to curtail the outbreak.[409]

In the well-infant nursery, "rooming in," a practice of placing the neonate in a room with the mother, is utilized as a method of environmental control of staphylococcal transmission.[410,411] Because newborns may be colonized within the first few hours of life, however, and the usual rooming-in practice involves at least a short time in a common nursery, this approach has often failed. A variation of rooming in is "cohort isolation," which involves clustering a small number of infants born within 1 or 2 days of each other in the same nursery so that they can be discharged as a "cohort." The intent is to prevent contact between newly born, uncolonized neonates and older, contaminated infants. Several reports describe the successful interruption of epidemics using this technique.[410,412,413]

The primary determinant of infant colonization is nursing care. Maintaining an appropriate nurse-to-infant ratio is an important factor in reducing disease once a disease-associated *S. aureus* strain gains entrance to a nursery, especially in an NICU.[23,30] In addition, there are a variety of preventive maneuvers directed at nurses, including frequent mask, gown, and glove changes before handling of infants[414,415]; nasal application of antimicrobial or antiseptic ointment or spray[415-418]; and elimination of carriers from the nursery area.[419,420] In some situations, control of an epidemic requires removal of the nurse carrier from the nursery.[421] Fortunately, such situations are uncommon.

Proper hand hygiene among nursery health care providers is a fundamental factor in reducing colonization rates. Mortimer and associates achieved a reduction in infant colonization from 92% to 53% by insisting that attendants wash their hands.[422] Proper education and monitoring of hand hygiene practices are critical to the effectiveness of this intervention.[423,424] Hands must be cleansed before and after patient contact or contact with equipment that is used for patient care. Hands also should be cleansed after glove removal. Proper hand hygiene involves applying alcohol-based waterless rubs if hands are not soiled,[425] or washing the hands for at least 10 to 15 seconds with either chlorhexidine gluconate or triclosan hand-washing agents.[426]

Because of the limited success in controlling transmission of staphylococci to infants, efforts have been made to protect the sites on the infant that are easily colonized and to eliminate colonization that has occurred. Protection from colonization has been attempted through anointing or otherwise covering the skin or umbilicus of the newborn with some protective material. Application of antimicrobial ointments[24,29,427,428] or antiseptic dyes[27,429-431] to the umbilicus or repeated washing of infants with hexachlorophene-containing powders or washes[44,430,432-438] has been attempted both to protect the infant from colonization and to reduce colonization that has occurred. All of these approaches have achieved varying degrees of success. Because very few organisms are necessary for colonization,[429] success or failure in particular instances probably is related to the strain involved and a variety of host and environmental factors.

Before the appearance of MRSA, some nursery epidemics were controlled with the use of systemic antibiotics.[439] Because health care–acquired MRSA isolates generally exhibit resistance to multiple antibiotics, it is doubtful that this approach will be successful if the epidemic strain is MRSA. Currently, the CDC recommends contact isolation for patients colonized or infected with MRSA.[440] This practice was shown to reduce nosocomial transmission of MRSA by 16-fold during an outbreak of MRSA in an NICU.[441]

In the early 1960s, attempts were made to stop virulent *S. aureus* epidemics in 10 NICUs throughout the United States using the technique of bacterial interference.[442-446] This technique involved deliberate implantation of an *S. aureus* strain of low virulence (502A) on the nasal mucosa and umbilicus of newborns to prevent colonization with the virulent *S. aureus* strain. Although this procedure was successful in curtailing all 10 epidemics,[447] it is not widely used or recommended currently.

It also was found in the early 1960s that meticulous hexachlorophene newborn infant body washes and cord care resulted in reduced colonization with *S. aureus*.[433] This approach was used as an interepidemic technique in many nurseries in an attempt to prevent *S. aureus* epidemics.[432,435,436,438] Although epidemics of *S. aureus* infection have been associated with high colonization rates, they also have occurred on occasion in NICUs with low colonization rates.[448,449] Furthermore, high colonization rates do not necessarily lead to the development of epidemic disease.[449-451]

If hexachlorophene is to be effective in reducing colonization rates, the application must be carried out in an almost ritualistic fashion and continued at home after hospital discharge.[428,432,435,452] Hexachlorophene washes have been shown to be neurotoxic, particularly in premature infants, however.[375,453-460] For these reasons, application of hexachlorophene is not recommended as a routine interepidemic newborn body cleansing preventive measure.

Several additional routine approaches to minimize interepidemic colonization of newborns have been investigated, including umbilical application of triple dye (brilliant green, proflavine hemisulfate, and crystal violet),[461] bacitracin,[462] silver sulfadiazine,[463,464] or mupirocin.[24,29] All have shown some effect in reducing *S. aureus* colonization. It remains to be seen whether the long-term application of these materials results in the development of resistant organisms.

A novel approach to the prevention of staphylococcal disease among hospitalized patients involves vaccination. Several vaccines that show some protective effect in animal models have been developed.[465-468] A recently conducted trial involving adult hemodialysis patients demonstrated a significant reduction in *S. aureus* bacteremia in patients who were vaccinated with *S. aureus* capsular polysaccharide vaccine compared with controls.[469] The efficacy and immunogenicity of staphylococcal vaccines in the neonatal population remain unknown.

Coagulase-Negative Staphylococci

With the rise in prominence of CoNS as nosocomial pathogens, strategies for disease prevention have become increasingly important. Strict hand hygiene is of primary importance in minimizing staff-to-patient and patient-to-patient spread of CoNS. In addition, meticulous surgical technique to limit intraoperative bacterial contamination is critical in minimizing infection related to foreign bodies. Strict attention to protocols for the insertion and management of intravenous and intra-arterial catheters may decrease the risk of catheter-related infections. In patients who require intravenous access for prolonged periods of time, percutaneous placement of a small-diameter Silastic catheter is preferred when possible. In one study, these catheters were maintained for as long as 80 days, with an infection rate of less than 10% in infants weighing less than 1500 g.[338]

Studies of CoNS using scanning and transmission electron microscopy suggest that bacterial attachment to catheters is a dynamic process, dependent on properties intrinsic to the catheter surface.[470-472] Peters and co-workers have suggested that catheter components may even serve as a nutrient source for these organisms.[470] With this information in mind, a number of investigators have explored the possibility of developing catheters that are inert and resistant to bacterial colonization. Thus far, these attempts have been disappointing, however.

Over the years, clinicians have employed prophylactic antibiotic therapy during implantation of a foreign body, intending to prevent infection due to CoNS and other nosocomial pathogens. Although this practice is now routine during neurosurgical, cardiac, and orthopedic surgery, efficacy remains unproved, and selection for antibiotic resistance is a significant concern. More recent efforts have focused on the possibility of preventing infection by using catheters and other prosthetic materials that have been impregnated with antibiotics. Thus far, central catheters impregnated with cefazolin, minocycline-rifampin, or chlorhexidine–silver sulfadiazine have been studied in adults,[473-476] and these studies have generally shown a significant reduction in both catheter colonization and catheter-related bloodstream infection.[477,478] In one study comparing catheters impregnated with either minocycline-rifampin or chlorhexidine–silver sulfadiazine, impregnation with minocycline-rifampin was found to be superior.[479] Unfortunately, antibiotic-impregnated catheters are both unstudied and unavailable for use in the neonatal population.

In recent years, a number of investigators have examined the use of low-dose intravenous vancomycin to prevent nosocomial bacteremia due to CoNS in low-birth-weight infants. Spafford and associates performed a randomized, double-blind, controlled study involving 70 neonates weighing less than 1000 g who had central venous catheters in place.[480] Among these infants, 35 received the standard total parenteral nutrition (TPN) solution, and the remaining 35 received a constant infusion of vancomycin (25 μg/mL) mixed with their total TPN solution. In infants receiving vancomycin, the rate of colonization of catheters by CoNS was reduced from 40% to 18%, and the rate of catheter-related sepsis was reduced from 15% to zero. Kacica and colleagues conducted a similar study in infants weighing less than 1500 g and found that gram-positive bacteremia developed in 1 of 71 infants receiving vancomycin, compared with 24 of 70 control infants.[481] Cooke and co-workers, employing a slightly different protocol, administered vancomycin in a dose of 5 mg/kg twice daily.[482] Among 72 neonates weighing less than 1500 g, 11 of 37 who received vancomycin, compared with 17 of 35 who received standard TPN, had one or more episodes of CoNS bacteremia. The results of these studies certainly are encouraging. On the other hand, the potential risks associated with prophylactic vancomycin, including ototoxicity, nephrotoxicity, and selection for resistant bacteria, remain poorly defined. At present, the routine use of prophylactic vancomycin is not recommended.

A collaborative approach to the reduction of nosocomial infections in the NICU has been shown to be effective in reducing rates of CoNS bacteremia in the NICU.[483] The development of this process involved collaboration among six neonatal intensive care units (members of the Vermont Oxford National Evidence-Based Quality Improvement Collaborative for Neonatology) to reduce rates of nosocomial infection. Through a critical review of the literature, review of internal practices, benchmark studies, and analysis of the experience with implemented changes, strategies were developed to decrease rates of nosocomial infections in the NICU.[484] Each participating institution made clinical changes related to three areas of consensus: hand hygiene, intravascular catheter care, and accuracy of diagnosis of CoNS bacteremia. With the intervention related to these three areas, the incidence of CoNS bacteremia decreased from 24.6% to 16.4%.[483]

Recently, an antistaphylococcal monoclonal antibody called BSYX-A110 has been developed for the prevention of CoNS sepsis. This antibody targets staphylococcal lipoteichoic acid and has been shown to be safe and tolerable when administered by intravenous infusion to high-risk neonates.[485] The efficacy of the antibody in preventing CoNS infections and related morbidity and deaths remains to be seen.

CONCLUSION

Staphylococci continue to be common pathogens in both term and preterm infants. In recent years, our understanding of important staphylococcal virulence factors has expanded considerably. With the availability of the *S. aureus* and *S. epidermidis* genomes and advances in knowledge of neonatal immunity, it is likely that novel approaches to the treatment and prevention of staphylococcal disease will be forthcoming in the near future.

REFERENCES

1. Fox T. Epidemic pemphigus of newly born (impetigo contagiosa et bullosa neonatorum). Lancet 1:1323, 1935.
2. Rulison ET. Control of impetigo neonatorum: advisability of a radical departure in obstetrical care. JAMA 93:903, 1929.
3. Schaffer TE, Sylvester RF, Baldwin JN, et al. Staphylococcal infections in newborn infants: II. Report of 19 epidemics caused by an identical strain of *Staphylococcus pyogenes*. Am J Public Health 47:990, 1957.
4. Dixon RE, Kaslow RA, Mallinson GF, et al. Staphylococcal disease outbreaks in hospital nurseries in the United States—December 1971 through March 1972. Pediatrics 51:413, 1973.
5. Patrick CC. Coagulase-negative staphylococci: pathogens with increasing clinical significance. J Pediatr 116:497, 1990.
6. Hall SL. Coagulase-negative staphylococcal infections in neonates. Pediatr Infect Dis J 10:57, 1991.
7. Schmidt BK, Kirpalani HM, Corey M, et al. Coagulase-negative staphylococci as true pathogens in newborn infants: a cohort study. Pediatr Infect Dis J 6:1026, 1987.
8. Ponce de Leon S, Wenzel EP. Hospital-acquired bloodstream infections with *Staphylococcus epidermidis*. Am J Med 77:639, 1984.
9. Kumar ML, Jenson HB, Dahms BB. Fatal staphylococcal epidermidis infections in very low-birth-weight infants with cytomegalovirus infection. Pediatrics 76:110, 1985.
10. Noel GJ, Edelson DJ. *Staphylococcus epidermidis* bacteremia in neonates: further observations and the occurrence of focal infection. Pediatrics 74:832, 1984.
11. Fleer A, Senders RC, Visser MR, et al. Septicemia due to coagulase-negative staphylococci in a neonatal intensive care unit: clinical and bacteriologic features and contaminated parenteral fluids as a source of sepsis. Pediatr Infect Dis J 2:426, 1983.
12. Gaynes RP, Edwards JR, Jarvis WR, et al. Nosocomial infections among neonates in high-risk nurseries in the United States. National Nosocomial Infections Surveillance System. Pediatrics 98:357, 1996.
13. Stoll BJ, Hansen N, Fanaroff AA, et al. Late-onset sepsis in very low birth weight neonates: the experience of the NICHD Neonatal Research Network. Pediatrics 110:285, 2002.
14. Stoll BJ, Gordon T, Korones SB, et al. Late-onset sepsis in very low birth weight neonates: a report from the National Institute of Child Health and Human Development Neonatal Research Network. J Pediatr 129:63, 1996.
15. LaGamma EF, Drusin LM, Mackles AW, et al. Neonatal infections: an important determinant of late NICU mortality in infants less than 1,000 g at birth. Am J Dis Child 137:838, 1983.
16. Battisti O, Mitchison R, Davies DA. Changing blood culture isolates in a referral neonatal intensive care unit. Arch Dis Child 56:775, 1981.
17. Placzek MM, Whitelaw A. Early and late septicemia. Arch Dis Child 58:728, 1983.
18. Hall R, Kurth CG, Hall SL. Ten year survey of positive blood cultures among admissions to a neonatal intensive care unit. J Perinatol 7:122, 1987.
19. Donowitz LG, Haley CE, Gregory WW, et al. Neonatal intensive care unit bacteremia: emergence of gram-positive bacteria as major pathogens. Am J Infect Control 15:141, 1987.
20. Baumgart S, Hall SE, Campos JM, et al. Sepsis with coagulase-negative staphylococci in critically ill newborns. Am J Dis Child 137:461, 1983.
21. Munson DP, Thompson TR, Johnson DE, et al. Coagulase-negative staphylococcal septicemia: experience in a newborn intensive care unit. J Pediatr 101:602, 1982.
22. Dunkle LM, Naqvi SH, McCallum R, et al. Eradication of epidemic methicillin-gentamicin–resistant *Staphylococcus aureus* in an intensive care nursery. Am J Med 70:455, 1981.
23. Haley RW, Bregman DA. The role of understaffing and overcrowding in recurrent outbreaks of staphylococcal infection in a neonatal special-care unit. J Infect Dis 145:875, 1982.
24. Davies EA, Emmerson AM, Hogg GM, et al. An outbreak of infection with a methicillin-resistant *Staphylococcus aureus* in a special care baby unit: value of topical mupirocin and of traditional methods of infection control. J Hosp Infect 10:120, 1987.
25. Millar MR, Keyworth N, Lincoln C, et al. Methicillin-resistant *Staphylococcus aureus* in regional neonatal unit. J Hosp Infect 7:187, 1987.
26. Reboli AC, John JF, Leukoff AH. Epidemic methicillin-gentamicin resistant *Staphylococcus aureus* in a neonatal intensive care unit. Am J Dis Child 143:34, 1989.

27. Rosenfeld CR, Laptook AR, Jeffery J. Limited effectiveness of triple dye in preventing colonization with methicillin-resistant *Staphylococcus aureus* in a special care nursery. Pediatr Infect Dis J 9:291, 1990.
28. Noel GJ, Kreiswirth BN, Edelson PJ, et al. Multiple methicillin-resistant *Staphylococcus aureus* strains as a cause for a single outbreak of severe disease in hospital neonates. Pediatr Infect Dis J 11:184, 1992.
29. Haddad Q, Sobayo EI, Basit OBA, et al. Outbreak of methicillin-resistant *Staphylococcus aureus* in a neonatal-intensive care unit. J Hosp Infect 23:211, 1993.
30. Haley RW, Cushion NB, Tenover FC, et al. Eradication of endemic methicillin-resistant *Staphylococcus aureus* infections from a neonatal intensive care unit. J Infect Dis 171:614, 1995.
31. Back NA, Linnemann CC, Staneck JL, et al. Control of methicillin-resistant *Staphylococcus aureus* in a neonatal-intensive care unit: use of intensive microbiological surveillance and mupirocin. Infect Control Hosp Epidemiol 17:227, 1996.
32. Shinefield HR, Ribble JC, Boris M, et al. Bacterial interference: its effect on nursery-acquired infection with *Staphylococcus aureus*: I. Preliminary observations. Am J Dis Child 105:646, 1963.
33. Allison VD, Hobbs BC. Inquiry into epidemiology of pemphigus neonatorum. BMJ 2:1, 1947.
34. Wolinsky E, Lipsitz PJ, Mortimer EA, Jr. Acquisition of staphylococci by newborns: direct versus indirect transmission. Lancet 2:620, 1960.
35. Rammelkamp CH, Jr., Mortimer EA, Jr., Wolinsky E. Transmission of streptococcal and staphylococcal infections. Ann Intern Med 60:753, 1964.
36. Hare R, Thomas CGA. The transmission of *Staphylococcus aureus*. BMJ 2:840, 1956.
37. Shinefield HR, Ribble JC, Sutherland JM, et al. Bacterial interference: its effect on nursery-acquired infection with *Staphylococcus aureus*: II. The Ohio epidemic. Am J Dis Child 105:655, 1963.
38. Ridely M. Perineal carriage of *Staphylococcus aureus*. BMJ 1:270, 1959.
39. Fairchild JP, Graber CD, Vogel EH, et al. Flora of the umbilical stump: 2479 cultures. J Pediatr 53:538, 1958.
40. Hurst V. *Staphylococcus aureus* in the infant upper respiratory tract: I. Observations on hospital-born babies. J Hyg (Lond) 55:299, 1957.
41. Torrey JC, Reese MK. Initial anaerobic flora of newborn infants; selective tolerance of upper respiratory tract bacteria. Am J Dis Child 69:208, 1945.
42. Thompson DJ, Gezon HM, Hatch TF, et al. Sex distributions of *Staphylococcus aureus* colonization and disease in newborn infants. N Engl J Med 269:337, 1963.
43. Aly R, Shinefield HR. Staphylococcal colonization in identical and non-identical twins. Am J Dis Child 127:486, 1974.
44. Gillespie WA, Simpson K, Tozer RC. Staphylococcal infection in a maternity hospital: epidemiology and control. Lancet 2:1075, 1958.
45. Hurst V. Transmission of hospital staphylococci among newborn infants: II. Colonization of the skin and mucous membranes of the infants. Pediatrics 25:204, 1960.
46. Boris M, Shinefield HR, Ribble JC, et al. Bacterial interference: its effect on nursery-acquired infection with *Staphylococcus aureus*: IV. The Louisiana epidemic. Am J Dis Child 105:674, 1963.
47. Thompson RL, Cabezudo I, Wenzel RP. Epidemiology of nosocomial infections caused by methicillin-resistant *Staphylococcus aureus*. Ann Intern Med 97:309, 1982.
48. Hiramatsu K, Cui L, Kuroda M, et al. The emergence and evolution of methicillin-resistant *Staphylococcus aureus*. Trends Microbiol 9:486, 2001.
49. Boyce JM. Methicillin-resistant *Staphylococcus aureus*. Detection, epidemiology, and control measures. Infect Dis Clin North Am 3:901, 1989.
50. Elek SD. *Staphylococcus pyogenes*. London, E & S Livingstone, 1959.
51. Graham DR, Correa-Villasinor A, Anderson RJ, et al. Epidemic neonatal gentamicin-methicillin resistant *Staphylococcus aureus* infection associated with nonspecific topical use of gentamicin. J Pediatr 97:972, 1980.
52. Holzman RS, Florman AL, Lyman M. Gentamicin resistant and sensitive strains of *Staphylococcus aureus*: factors affecting colonization and virulence for infants in a special care nursery. Am J Epidemiol 112:352, 1980.
53. Parks YA, Nuy MF, Aukett MA. Methicillin-resistant *Staphylococcus aureus* in milk. Arch Dis Child 62:82, 1987.
54. Ribner BS. Endemic, multiply resistant *Staphylococcus aureus* in a pediatric population. Am J Dis Child 141:1183, 1987.
55. Rubin LG, Sanchez PJ, Siegel J, et al. Evaluation and treatment of neonates with suspected late-onset sepsis: a survey of neonatologists' practices. Pediatrics 110:e42, 2002.
56. Salgado CD, Farr BM, Calfee DP. Community-acquired methicillin-resistant *Staphylococcus aureus*: a meta-analysis of prevalence and risk factors. Clin Infect Dis 36:131, 2003. [See comment.]
57. Eady EA, Cove JH. Staphylococcal resistance revisited: community-acquired methicillin resistant *Staphylococcus aureus*—an emerging problem for the management of skin and soft tissue infections. Curr Opin Infect Dis 16:103, 2003.
58. Centers for Disease Control and Prevention. Four pediatric deaths from community-acquired methicillin-resistant *Staphylococcus aureus*—Minnesota and North Dakota, 1997-1999. JAMA 282:1123, 1999.
59. O'Keefe M, Graham PL, Wu F, et al. Healthcare-associated transmission of community-acquired methicillin-resistant *Staphylococcus aureus* (CA-MRSA) infections in postpartum women. 13th Annual Scientific Meeting of the Society for Healthcare Epidemiology of America, Arlington, Va., 2003.
60. Saiman L, Jakob K, Holmes KW, et al. Molecular epidemiology of staphylococcal scalded skin syndrome in premature infants. Pediatr Infect Dis J 17:329, 1998.
61. Tenover FC, Arbeit RD, Goering RV, et al. Interpreting chromosomal DNA restriction patterns produced by pulsed-field gel electrophoresis: criteria for bacterial strain typing. J Clin Microbiol 33:2233, 1995.
62. van Belkum A, van Leeuwen W, Kaufmann ME, et al. Assessment of resolution and intercenter reproducibility of results of genotyping *Staphylococcus aureus* by pulsed-field gel electrophoresis of *SmaI* macrorestriction fragments: a multicenter study. J Clin Microbiol 36:1653, 1998.
63. Enright MC, Day NP, Davies CE, et al. Multilocus sequence typing for characterization of methicillin-resistant and methicillin-susceptible clones of *Staphylococcus aureus*. J Clin Microbiol 38:1008, 2000.
64. Diep BA, Perdreau-Remington F, Sensabaugh GF. Clonal characterization of *Staphylococcus aureus* by multilocus restriction fragment typing, a rapid screening approach for molecular epidemiology. J Clin Microbiol 41:4559, 2003.
65. Shopsin B, Gomez M, Montgomery SO, et al. Evaluation of protein A gene polymorphic region DNA sequencing for typing of *Staphylococcus aureus* strains. J Clin Microbiol 37:3556, 1999.
66. Welsh J, McClelland M. Fingerprinting genomes using PCR with arbitrary primers. Nucleic Acids Res 18:7213, 1990.
67. van der Zee A, Verbakel H, van Zon JC, et al. Molecular genotyping of *Staphylococcus aureus* strains: comparison of repetitive element sequence-based PCR with various typing methods and isolation of a novel epidemicity marker. J Clin Microbiol 37:342, 1999.
68. Noble WC, Somerville DA. Microbiology of Human Skin. London, WB Saunders, 1974.
69. Goldmann DA. Bacterial colonization and infection in the neonate. Am J Med 70:417, 1981.
70. Simpson RA, Spencer AF, Speller DCE, et al. Colonization by gentamicin-resistant *Staphylococcus epidermidis* in a special care baby unit. J Hosp Infect 7:108, 1986.
71. Speck WT, Driscoll JM, Polin RA, et al. Effect of bacterial flora on staphylococcal colonization of the newborn. J Clin Pathol 31:153, 1978.
72. D'Angio CT, McGowan KL, Baumgart S, et al. Surface colonization with coagulase-negative staphylococci in premature neonates. J Pediatr 114:1029, 1989.
73. Hall SL, Riddell SW, Barnes WG, et al. Evaluation of coagulase-negative staphylococcal isolates from serial nasopharyngeal cultures of premature infants. Diagn Microbiol Infect Dis 13:17, 1990.
74. Hall SL, Hall RT, Barnes WG, et al. Relationship of maternal to neonatal colonization with coagulase-negative staphylococci. Am J Perinatol 7:384, 1990.
75. Patrick CH, John JF, Levkoff A, et al. Relatedness of strains of methicillin-resistant coagulase-negative *Staphylococcus* colonizing hospital personnel and producing bacteremias in a neonatal intensive care unit. Pediatr Infect Dis J 11:935, 1992.
76. Freeman J, Goldmann DA, Smith NE, et al. Association of intravenous lipid emulsion and coagulase negative staphylococcal bacteremia in neonatal intensive care units. N Engl J Med 323:301, 1990.
77. Kloos W. Taxonomy and systemics of staphylococci indigenous to humans. *In* Crossley KB, Archer GL (eds). The Staphylococci in Human Disease. New York, Churchill Livingstone, 1997, p 127.
78. Blair JE, Williams REO. Phage typing of staphylococci. Bull World Health Organ 24:771, 1961.

79. Parker MT, Roundtree PM. Report (1966B1970) of the Subcommittee on Phage Typing of Staphylococci to the International Committee on Nomenclature of Bacteria. Int J Syst Bacteriol 21:167, 1971.
80. Mulligan ME, Arbeit RD. Epidemiologic and clinical utility of typing systems for differentiating among strains of methicillin-resistant *Staphylococcus aureus*. Infect Control Hosp Epidemiol 12:20, 1991.
81. Prevost G, Jaulhoc B, Piedmont Y. DNA fingerprinting of pulsed-field gel electrophoresis is more effective than ribotyping in distinguishing among methicillin-resistant *Staphylococcus aureus* isolates. J Clin Microbiol 30:967, 1992.
82. Tenover FC, Arbeit R, Archer G, et al. Comparison of traditional and molecular methods of typing isolates of *Staphylococcus aureus*. J Clin Microbiol 32:407, 1994.
83. Braddiley J, Brock JH, Davidson AL, et al. The wall composition of micrococci. J Gen Microbiol 54:393, 1968.
84. Strominger JL. The Bacteria. New York, Academic Press, 1962.
85. Strominger JL, Ghuysen JM. Mechanisms of enzymatic bacteriolysis: cell walls of bacteria are solubilised by action of either specific carbohydrases or specific peptidases. Science 156:213, 1967.
86. Labischinski H. Consequences of interaction of β-lactam antibiotics with penicillin binding proteins from sensitive and resistant *Staphylococcus aureus* strains. Med Microbiol Immunol (Berl) 181:241, 1992.
87. Juergens WG, Sanderson AR, Strominger JL. Chemical basis for the immunological specificity of a strain of *Staphylococcus aureus*. Bull Soc Chim Biol (Paris) 42:110, 1960.
88. Mudd A, Yoshida A, Lenhart NA. Identification of a somatic antigen of *Staphylococcus aureus* critical for phagocytosis by human blood leucocytes. Nature 199:1200, 1963.
89. Lee JC, Pier GB. Vaccine-based strategies for prevention of staphylococcal diseases. *In* Crossley KB, Archer GL (eds). The Staphylococci in Human Disease. New York, Churchill Livingstone, 1997, p 640.
90. Shayegani M. Failure of immune sera to enhance significantly phagocytosis-promoting factors. Infect Immun 2:742, 1970.
91. Shayegani M, Hisatsune K, Mudd S. Cell wall component which affects the ability of serum to promote phagocytosis and killing of *Staphylococcus aureus*. Infect Immun 2:750, 1970.
92. Peterson PK, Wilkinson BJ, Kim Y, et al. The key role of peptidoglycan in the opsonization of *Staphylococcus aureus*. J Clin Invest 61:597, 1978.
93. Verburgh HA, Peters R, Rozenberg-Arska M, et al. Antibodies to cell wall peptidoglycan of *Staphylococcus aureus* in patients with serious staphylococcal infections. J Infect Dis 144:1, 1981.
94. Fischetti VA, Pancholi V, Schneewind O. Conservation of a hexapeptide sequence in the anchor region of surface proteins from gram-positive cocci. Mol Microbiol 4:1603, 1990.
95. Mazmanian SK, Liu G, Ton-That H, et al. *Staphylococcus aureus* sortase, an enzyme that anchors surface proteins to the cell wall. Science 285:760, 1999.
96. Mazmanian SK, Ton-That H, Schneewind O. Sortase-catalysed anchoring of surface proteins to the cell wall of *Staphylococcus aureus*. Mol Microbiol 40:1049, 2001.
97. Pallen MJ, Lam AC, Antonio M, et al. An embarrassment of sortases—a richness of substrates. Trends Microbiol 9:97, 2001.
98. Wiley BB, Maverakis NH. Capsule production and virulence among strains of *Staphylococcus aureus*. Ann N Y Acad Sci 236:221, 1974.
99. Morse SI. Isolation and properties of a surface antigen of *Staphylococcus aureus*. J Exp Med 115:295, 1962.
100. Wilkinson BJ. Staphylococcal capsules and slime. *In* Easmon CFS, Adlam C (eds). Staphylococci and Staphylococcal Infections. London, Academic Press, 1983, p 481.
101. Christensson B, Boutonnier A, Ryding U, et al. Diagnosing *Staphylococcus aureus* endocarditis by detecting antibodies against *S. aureus* capsular polysaccharide types 5 and 8. J Infect Dis 163:530, 1991.
102. Kuroda M, Ohta T, Uchiyama I, et al. Whole genome sequencing of meticillin-resistant *Staphylococcus aureus*. Lancet 357:1225, 2001.
103. Baba T, Takeuchi F, Kuroda M, et al. Genome and virulence determinants of high virulence community-acquired MRSA. Lancet 359:1819, 2002.
104. Pfaller MA, Herwaldt LA. Laboratory, clinical and epidemiological aspects of coagulase-negative staphylococci. Clin Microbiol Rev 1:281, 1988.
105. Christensen GD, Parisi JT, Bisno AL, et al. Characterization of clinically significant strains of coagulase-negative staphylococci. J Clin Microbiol 18:258, 1983.
106. Pulverer G, Pillich J, Klein A. New bacteriophages of *Staphylococcus epidermidis*. J Infect Dis 132:524, 1975.
107. Jefferson SH, Parisi JT. Bacteriophage typing of coagulase-negative staphylococci in critically ill newborns. Am J Dis Child 137:461, 1983.
108. Wu F, Della-Latta P. Molecular typing strategies. Semin Perinatol 26:357, 2002.
109. Zhang Y-Q, Ren S-X, Li H-L, et al. Genome-based analysis of virulence genes in a non-biofilm-forming *Staphylococcus epidermidis* strain (ATCC 12228). Mol Microbiol 49:1577, 2003.
110. Foster TJ, Höök M. Surface protein adhesions of *Staphylococcus aureus*. Trends Microbiol 12:484, 1998.
111. Projan SJ, Novik RP. The medical basis for pathogenicity. *In* Crossley KB, Archer GL (eds). The Staphylococci in Human Disease. New York, Churchill Livingstone, 1997, p 61.
112. Vercellotti GM, McCarthy JB, Lindholm P, et al. Extracellular matrix proteins (fibronectin, laminin, and type IV collagen) bind and aggregate bacteria. Am J Pathol 120:13, 1985.
113. Park PW, Roberts DD, Grosso LE, et al. Binding of elastin to *Staphylococcus aureus*. J Biol Chem 266:23399, 1991.
114. Tung H, Guss B, Hellman U, et al. A bone sialoprotein-binding protein from *Staphylococcus aureus*: a member of the staphylococcal Sdr family. Biochem J 345:611, 2000.
115. Josefsson E, McCrea KW, Ni-Eidhin D, et al. Three new members of the serine-aspartate repeat protein multigene family of *Staphylococcus aureus*. Microbiology 144:3387, 1998.
116. Clarke SR, Wittshire MD, Foster SJ. IsdA of *Staphylococcus aureus* is a broad spectrum, iron-regulated adhesin. Mol Microbiol 51:1509, 2004.
117. Chhatwal GS, Preissner KT, Muller-Berghaus G, et al. Specific binding of the human S protein (vitronectin) to streptococci, *Staphylococcus aureus*, and *Escherichia coli*. Infect Immun 55:1878, 1987.
118. Hermann M, Suchard SJ, Boxer LA, et al. Thrombospondin binds to *Staphylococcus aureus* and promotes staphylococcal adherence to surfaces. Infect Immun 59:279, 1991.
119. Cheung AL, Eberhardt KJ, Chung E, et al. Diminished virulence of a *sar-/agr*-mutant of *Staphylococcus aureus* in the rabbit model of endocarditis. J Clin Invest 94:1815, 1994.
120. Vaudaux P, Pittet D, Haeberli A, et al. Host factors selectively increase staphylococcal adherence on catheters: a role for fibronectin and fibrinogen or fibrin. J Infect Dis 160:865, 1989.
121. Pati JM, Allen BL, McGavin MJ, et al. MSCRAMM-mediated adherence of microorganisms to host tissues. Annu Rev Microbiol 48:585, 1994.
122. Forsgren A, Sjoquist J. "Protein A" from *S. aureus* pseudo-immune reaction with human gamma-globulin. J Immunol 97:822, 1966.
123. Verhoef J, Peterson PK, Verburgh HA. Host-parasite relationship in staphylococcal infections: the role of the staphylococcal cell wall during the process of phagocytosis. Antonie Van Leeuwenhoek 45:49, 1979.
124. Selsted ME, Tang YQ, Morris WL, et al. Purification, primary structures, and antibacterial activities of beta-defensins, a new family of antimicrobial peptides from bovine neutrophils. J Biol Chem 268: 6641, 1993.
125. Yeaman MR, Sullam PM, Dazin PF, et al. Platelet microbicidal protein alone and in combination with antibiotics reduces *Staphylococcus aureus* adherence to platelets in vitro. Infect Immun 62:3416, 1994.
126. Bohach GA, Dinges MH, Mitchell DT, et al. Exotoxins. *In* Crossley KB, Archer GL (eds). The Staphylococci in Human Disease. New York, Churchill Livingstone, 1997, p 83.
127. Prevost G, Couppie P, Monteil H. Staphylococcal epidermolysins. Curr Opin Infect Dis 16:71, 2003.
128. Supersac G, Prevost G, Piemont Y. Sequencing of leucocidin R from *Staphylococcus aureus* P83 suggests that staphylococcal leucocidins and gamma-hemolysin are members of a single, two-component family of toxins. Infect Immun 61:580, 1993.
129. Rahman A, Izaki K, Kato I, et al. Nucleotide sequence of leukocidin S-component gene (*lukS*) from methicillin resistant *Staphylococcus aureus*. Biochem Biophys Res Commun 181:138, 1991.
130. Rahman A, Nariya H, Izaki K, et al. Molecular cloning and nucleotide sequence of leukocidin F-component gene (*lukF*) from methicillin-resistant *Staphylococcus aureus*. Biochem Biophys Res Commun 184: 640, 1992.
131. Choorit W, Kaneko J, Muramoto K, et al. Existence of a new protein component with the same function as the LukF component of leukocidin or gamma-hemolysin and its gene in *Staphylococcus aureus* P83. FEBS Lett 357:260, 1995.
132. Cooney J, Kienle Z, Foster TJ, et al. The gamma-hemolysin locus of *Staphylococcus aureus* comprises three linked genes, two of which are identical to genes for the F and S components of leukocidin. Infect Immun 61:768, 1993.

133. Sau S, Lee CY. Cloning of type 8 capsule genes and analysis of gene clusters for the production of different capsular polysaccharides in *Staphylococcus aureus*. J Bacteriol 178:2118, 1996.
134. Arbeit R, Karakawa WW, Van WF, et al. Predominance of two newly described capsular polysaccharide types among clinical isolates of *Staphylococcus aureus*. Diagn Microbiol Infect Dis 2:85, 1984.
135. Gouaux JE, Braha O, Hobaugh MR, et al. Subunit stoichiometry of staphylococcal alpha-hemolysin in crystals and on membranes: a heptameric transmembrane pore. Proc Natl Acad Sci U S A 91:12828, 1994.
136. Bhakdi S, Tranum-Jensen J. Alpha-toxin of *Staphylococcus aureus*. Microbiol Rev 55:733, 1991.
137. Suttorp N, Fuhrmann M, Tannert-Otto S, et al. Pore-forming bacterial toxins potently induce release of nitric oxide in porcine endothelial cells. J Exp Med 178:337, 1993.
138. Jonas D, Waley I, Berger T, et al. Novel path to apoptosis: small transmembrane pores created by staphylococcal alpha-toxin in T lymphocytes evoke internucleosomal DNA degradation. Infect Immun 62:1304, 1994.
139. Callegan MC, Engels LS, Hill JM, et al. Corneal virulence of *Staphylococcus aureus*: roles of alpha-toxin and protein A in pathogenesis. Infect Immun 62:2478, 1994.
140. Bramley AJ, Patel AH, O'Reilly M, et al. Roles of alpha-toxin and beta-toxin in virulence of *Staphylococcus aureus* for the mouse mammary gland. Infect Immun 57:2489, 1989.
141. Wadstrom T, Mollby R. Studies on extracellular proteins from *Staphylococcus aureus*: VII. Studies on beta-hemolysin. Biochim Biophys Acta 242:308, 1972.
142. Ruzickova V. A rapid method for the differentiation of *Staphylococcus aureus* hemolysins. Folia Microbiol (Praha) 39:112, 1994.
143. Farrell AM, Taylor D, Holland KT. Cloning, nucleotide sequence determination and expression of the *Staphylococcus aureus* hyaluronate lyase gene. FEMS Microbiol Lett 130:81, 1995.
144. Meyer K, Palmer JW. The polysaccharide of the vitreous humor. J Biol Chem 107:629, 1934.
145. Bjorklind A, Arvidson S. Mutants of *Staphylococcus aureus* affected in the regulation of exoprotein synthesis. FEMS Microbiol Lett 7:203, 1980.
146. Coleman G, Jakeman C, Martin N. Patterns of extracellular protein secretion by a number of clinically isolated strains of *Staphylococcus aureus*. J Gen Microbiol 107:189, 1978.
147. Tremaine M, Brockman DK, Betley MJ. Staphylococcal enterotoxin A gene (*sea*) expression is not affected by the accessory gene regulator (*agr*). Infect Immun 61:356, 1993.
148. Novick RP. Autoinduction and signal transduction in the regulation of staphylococcal virulence. Mol Microbiol 48:1429, 2003.
149. Peng HL, Novick RP, Kreiswirth B, et al. Cloning, characterization, and sequencing of an accessory gene regulator (*agr*) in *Staphylococcus aureus*. J Bacteriol 170:4365, 1988.
150. Cheung AL, Koomey JM, Butler CA, et al. Regulation of exoprotein expression in *Staphylococcus aureus* by a locus (*sar*) distinct from *agr*. Proc Natl Acad Sci U S A 89:6462, 1992.
151. Giraudo A, Raspanti C, Calzolari A, et al. Characterization of a Tn551-mutant of *Staphylococcus aureus* defective in the production of several exoproteins. Can J Microbiol 8:677, 1994.
152. Giraudo AT, Calzolari A, Cataldi AA, et al. The sea locus of *Staphylococcus aureus* encodes a two-component regulatory system. FEMS Microbiol Lett 177:15, 1999.
153. Fournier B, Klier A, Rapoport G. The two-component system ArlS-ArlR is a reulator of virulence gene expression in *Staphylococcus aureus*. Mol Microbiol 41:247, 2001.
154. Yarwood JM, McCormick JK, Schlievert PM. Identification of a novel two-component regulatory system that acts in global regulation of virulence factors of *Staphylococcus aureus*. J Bacteriol 183:1113, 2001.
155. Hogt AH, Dankert J, Hulstaert CE, et al. Cell surface characteristics of coagulase-negative staphylococci and their adherence to fluorinated poly(ethylenepropylene). Infect Immun 51:294, 1986.
156. Tojo M, Yamashita N, Goldmann DA, et al. Isolation and characterization of a capsular polysaccharide adhesin from *Staphylococcus epidermidis*. J Infect Dis 157:713, 1988.
157. McKenney D, Hubner J, Muller E, et al. The *ica* locus of *Staphylococcus epidermidis* encodes production of the capsular polysaccharide/adhesin. Infect Immun 66:4711, 1998.
158. Heilman C, Hussain M, Peters G, et al. Evidence for autolysin-mediated primary attachment of *Staphylococcus epidermidis* to a polystrene surface. Mol Microbiol 24:1013, 1997.
159. Timmerman CP, Fleer A, Besnier JM, et al. Characterization of a proteinaceous adhesion of *Staphylococcus epidermidis* which mediates attachment to polystrene. Infect Immun 59:4187, 1991.
160. Veenstra GJC, Cremers FFM, Van Dijk H, et al. Ultrastructural organization and regulation of a biomaterial adhesin of *Staphylococcus epidermidis*. J Bacteriol 178:537, 1996.
161. Rupp ME, Fey PD, Heilman C, et al. Characterization of the importance of *Staphylococcus epidermidis* autolysin and polysaccharide intercellular adhesin in the pathogenesis of intravascular catheter–associated infection in a rat model. J Infect Dis 183:1038, 2001.
162. Nilsson M, Frykberg L, Flock JI, et al. A fibrinogen-binding protein of *Staphylococcus epidermidis*. Infect Immun 66:2666, 1998.
163. Pei L, Flock JI. Lack of *fbe*, the gene for a fibrinogen-binding protein from *Staphylococcus epidermidis*, reduces its adherence to fibrinogen coated surfaces. Microb Pathog 31:185, 2001.
164. McCrea KW, Hartford O, Davis S, et al. The serine-aspartate repeat (Sdr) protein family in *Staphylococcus epidermidis*. Microbiology 146:1535, 2000.
165. Hussain M, Heilman C, Peters G, et al. Teichoic acid enhances adhesion of *Staphylococcus epidermidis* to immobilized fibronectin. Microb Pathog 31:261, 2001.
166. Mack D, Nedelmann M, Krokotsch A, et al. Characterization of transposon mutants of biofilm-producing *Staphylococcus epidermidis* impaired in the accumulative phase of biofilm production: genetic identification of a hexosamine-containing polysaccharide intercellular adhesion. Infect Immun 62:3244, 1994.
167. Ziebuhr W, Krimmer V, Rachid S, et al. A novel mechanism of phase variation of virulence in *Staphylococcus epidermidis*: evidence for control of the polysaccharide intercellular adhesin synthesis by alternating insertion and excision of the insertion sequence element IS256. Mol Microbiol 32:345, 1999.
168. Rupp ME, Ulphani JS, Fey PD, et al. Characterization of the importance of polysaccharide intercellular adhesion/hemagglutinin of *Staphylococcus epidermidis* in the pathogenesis of biomaterial-based infection in a mouse foreign body infection model. Infect Immun 67:2627, 1999.
169. Rupp ME, Ulphani JS, Fey PD, et al. Characterization of *Staphylococcus epidermidis* polysaccharide intercellular adhesion/hemagglutinin in the pathogeneisis of intravascular catheter-associated infection in a rat model. Infect Immun 67:2656, 1999.
170. Schumacher-Perdreau F, Heilmann C, Peters G, et al. Comparative analysis of a biofilm forming *Staphylococcus epidermidis* strain and its adhesion-positive accumulation-negative isogenic mutant. FEMS Microbiol Lett 117:71, 1994.
171. Hussain M, Herrmann M, von Eiff C, et al. A 140-kilodalton extracellular protein is essential for the accumulation of *Staphylococcus epidermidis* strains on surfaces. Infect Immun 65:519, 1997.
172. Ishak MA, Groschel DHM, Mandell GL, et al. Association of slime with pathogenicity of coagulase-negative staphylococci causing nosocomial septicemia. J Clin Microbiol 22:1025, 1985.
173. Hall RT, Hall SL, Barnes WG, et al. Characteristics of coagulase-negative staphylococci from infants with bacteremia. Pediatr Infect Dis J 6:377, 1987.
174. Gruskay JA, Nachamkin I, Baumgart S, et al. Predicting the pathogenicity of coagulase-negative *Staphylococcus* in the neonate: slime production, antibiotic resistance, and predominance of *Staphylococcus epidermidis* species. Pediatrics 20:397A, 1986.
175. Gray ED, Peters G, Verstegen M, et al. Effect of extracellular slime substance from *Staphylococcus epidermidis* on the human cellular immune response. Lancet 1:365, 1984.
176. Johnson GM, Lee DA, Regelmann WE, et al. Interference with granulocyte function by *Staphylococcus epidermidis* slime. Infect Immun 54:13, 1986.
177. Farber BF, Kaplan MH, Clogston AG. *Staphylococcus epidermidis* extracted slime inhibits the antimicrobial action of glycopeptide antibodies. J Infect Dis 161:37, 1990.
178. Kristinson KG, Spencer RC. Slime production as a marker for clinically significant infection with coagulase-negative staphylococci. J Infect Dis 154:728, 1986.
179. Younger JJ, Christensen GD, Bartley DL, et al. Coagulase-negative staphylococci isolated from cerebrospinal fluid shunts: importance of slime production, species identification, and shunt removal to clinical outcome. J Infect Dis 156:548, 1987.
180. Van Wamel WJB, Van Rossum G, Verhoef J, et al. Cloning and characterization of an accessory gene regulator (agr)–like locus from *Staphylococcus epidermidis*. FEMS Microbiol Lett 163:1, 1998.

181. Fluckiger U, Wolz C, Cheung AL. Characterization of a sar homolog of *Staphylococcus epidermidis*. Infect Immun 66:2871, 1998.
182. Vuong C, Götz F, Otto M. Construction and characterization of an *agr* deletion mutant of *Staphylococcus epidermidis*. Infect Immun 68:1048, 2000.
183. Gemmel CG, Schumacher-Perdreau F. Extracellular toxins and enzymes elaborated by coagulase-negative staphylococci. *In* Easmon CFS, Adlam C (eds). Staphylococci and Staphylococcal Infections. New York, Academic Press, 1983, p 809.
184. Scheifele DW, Bjornson GL, Dyer RA, et al. Delta-like toxin produced by coagulase-negative staphylococci is associated with neonatal necrotizing enterocolitis. Infect Immun 55:2268, 1987.
185. Scheifele DW, Bjornson GL. Delta toxin activity in coagulase-negative staphylococci from the bowels of neonates. J Clin Microbiol 26:279, 1988.
186. Breckenridge JC, Bergdoll MS. Food borne gastroenteritis due to coagulase-negative *Staphylococcus*. N Engl J Med 284:541, 1971.
187. Males BM, Rogers WA, Parisi JT. Virulence factors of biotypes of *Staphylococcus epidermidis* from clinical sources. J Clin Microbiol 1:256, 1975.
188. Shigeoka AO, Santos JI, Hill HR. Functional analysis of neutrophil granulocytes from healthy, infected, and stressed neonates. J Pediatr 95:454, 1979.
189. Mease AD. Tissue neutropenia: the newborn neutrophil in perspective. J Perinatol 10:55, 1990.
190. Anderson DC, Hughes B, Smith CW. Abnormality motility of neonatal polymorphonuclear leukocytes. J Clin Invest 68:863, 1981.
191. Polin RA. Role of fibronectin in diseases of newborn infants and children. Rev Infect Dis 12:S428, 1990.
192. Hilmo A, Howard TH. F-actin content of neonate and adult neutrophils. Blood 69:945, 1987.
193. Schibler KR, Trautman MS, Liechty KW, et al. Diminished transcription of interleukin-8 by monocytes from preterm neonates. J Leukoc Biol 53:399, 1993.
194. Yoshimura TK, Matsuskima K, Tanaka S, et al. Purification of a human monocyte derived neutrophil chemotactic factor that shares sequence homology with other host defense cytokinese. Proc Natl Acad Sci U S A 84:9233, 1987.
195. Anderson DC, Rothlein R, Marlin SD, et al. Impaired transendothelial migration by neonatal neutrophils: abnormalities of Mac-1 (CD11b/CD18)-dependent adherence reactions. Blood 76:2613, 1990.
196. Zimmerman GA, Prescott SM, McIntyre TM. Endothelial cell, interactions with granulocytes: tethering and signaling molecules. Immunol Today 13:93, 1992.
197. Shigeoka AO, Charette RP, Wyman ML, et al. Defective oxidative metabolic responses of neutrophils from stressed infants. J Pediatr 98:392, 1981.
198. Strauss RG, Snyder EL. Activation and activity of the superoxide-generating system of neutrophils from human infants. Pediatr Res 17:662, 1983.
199. Banffer JR. Anti-leucocidin and mastitis puerperalis. BMJ 2:1224, 1962.
200. Johanovsky J. Importance of antileucocidin and antitoxin in immunity against staphylococcal infections. Z Immunitatsforsch Allerg Klin Immunol 116:318, 1959.
201. Banffer JRJ, Franken JF. Immunization with leucocidin toxoid against staphylococcal infection. Pathol Microbiol (Basel) 30:166, 1967.
202. Lack CH, Towers AG. Serological tests for staphylococcal infection. BMJ 2:1227, 1962.
203. Florman AL, Lamberston GH, Zepp H, et al. Relation of 7S and 19S staphylococcal hemagglutinating antibody to age of individual. Pediatrics 32:501, 1963.
204. Lavoipierre GJ, Newell KW, Smith MHD, et al. A vaccine trial for neonatal staphylococcal disease. Am J Dis Child 122:377, 1971.
205. Marrach P, Kappler J. The staphylococcal enterotoxin and their relatives. Science 248:705, 1990.
206. Ladhani S, Joannou CL, Lochrie DP, et al. Clinical, microbial, and biochemical aspects of the exfoliative toxins causing staphylococcal scalded-skin syndrome. Clin Microbiol Rev 12:224, 1999.
207. Adesiyun AA, Lenz W, Schaal KP. Exfoliative toxin production by *Staphylococcus aureus* strains isolated from animals and human beings in Nigeria. Microbiologica 14:357, 1991.
208. Dancer SJ, Simmons NA, Poston SM, et al. Outbreak of staphylococcal scalded skin syndrome among neonates. J Infect 16:87, 1988.
209. Piemont Y, Rasoamananjara D, Fouace JM, et al. Epidemiological investigation of exfoliative toxin-producing *Staphylococcus aureus* strains in hospitalized patients. J Clin Microbiol 19:417, 1984.
210. Gemmell CG. Staphylococcal scalded skin syndrome. J Med Microbiol 43:318, 1995.
211. Hanakawa Y, Schechter NM, Lin C, et al. Molecular mechanisms of blister formation in bullous impetigo and staphylococcal scalded skin syndrome. J Clin Invest 110:53, 2002.
212. Hargiss C, Larson E. The epidemiology of *Staphylococcus aureus* in a newborn nursery from 1970 through 1976. Pediatrics 61:348, 1978.
213. Loughead JL. Congenital staphylococcal scalded skin syndrome: report of a case. Pediatr Infect Dis J 11:413, 1992.
214. Dancer SJ, Poston SM, East J, et al. An outbreak of pemphigus neonatorum. J Infect 20:73, 1990.
215. Faden H. Neonatal staphylococcal skin infections. Pediatr Infect Dis J 22:389, 2003.
216. Bailey CJ, Lockhart BP, Redpath MB, et al. The epidermolytic (exfoliative) toxins of *Staphylococcus aureus*. Med Microbiol Immunol (Berl) 184:53, 1995.
217. Fritsch P, Elias P, Varga J. The fate of staphylococcal exfoliation in newborn and adult mice. Br J Dermatol 95:275, 1976.
218. Amagai M, Yamaguchi T, Hanakawa Y, et al. Staphylococcal exfoliative toxin B specifically cleaves desmoglein 1. J Invest Dermatol 118:845, 2002.
219. Amagai M, Matsuyoshi N, Wang ZH, et al. Toxin in bullous impetigo and staphylococcal scalded-skin syndrome targets desmoglein 1. [comment]. Nat Med 6:1275, 2000.
220. Farrell AM. Staphylococcal scalded-skin syndrome. Lancet 354:880, 1999.
221. Ladhani S, Joannou CL. Difficulties in diagnosis and management of the staphylococcal scalded skin syndrome. Pediatr Infect Dis J 19:819, 2000.
222. Ladhani S, Robbie S, Chapple DS, et al. Isolating *Staphylococcus aureus* from children with suspected staphylococcal scalded skin syndrome is not clinically useful. Pediatr Infect Dis J 22:284, 2003.
223. Ladhani S, Robbie S, Garratt RC, et al. Development and evaluation of detection systems for staphylococcal exfoliative toxin A responsible for scalded-skin syndrome. J Clin Microbiol 39:2050, 2001.
224. Makhoul IR, Kassis I, Hashman N, et al. Staphylococcal scalded-skin syndrome in a very low birth weight premature infant. Pediatrics 108:e16, 2001.
225. Jonsson S, Pulkkinen MO. Mastitis today: incidence, prevention and treatment. Ann Chir Gynaecol Suppl 208:84, 1994.
226. Benson EA. Management of breast abscesses. World J Surg 13:753, 1989.
227. Marshall BR, Hepper JK, Zirbel CC. Sporadic puerperal mastitis: an infection that need not interrupt lactation. JAMA 233:1377, 1975.
228. Schwartz GF. Benign neoplasms and "inflammations" of the breast. Clin Obstet Gynecol 25:373, 1982.
229. Scott-Conner CE, Schorr SJ. The diagnosis and management of breast problems during pregnancy and lactation. Am J Surg 170:401, 1995.
230. Kaufmann R, Foxman B. Mastitis among lactating women: occurrence and risk factors. Soc Sci Med 33:701, 1991.
231. Inch S, Fisher C. Mastitis: infection or inflammation? Practitioner 239:472, 1995.
232. O'Hara RJ, Dexter SP, Fox JN. Conservative management of infective mastitis and breast abscesses after ultrasonographic assessment. Br J Surg 83:1413, 1996.
233. Hayes R, Michell M, Nunnerley HB. Acute inflammation of the breast—the role of breast ultrasound in diagnosis and management. Clin Radiol 44:253, 1991.
234. Bedinghaus JM. Care of the breast and support of breast-feeding. Prim Care 24:147, 1997.
235. Matheson I, Aursnes I, Horgen M, et al. Bacteriological findings and clinical symptoms in relation to clinical outcome in puerperal mastitis. Acta Obstet Gynecol Scand 67:723, 1988.
236. Foster D, Harris RE. The incidence of *Staphylococcus pyogenes* in normal human breast milk. J Obstet Gynaecol Br Emp 67:463, 1960.
237. Montgomery TL, Wise MDI, Land WR, et al. A study of staphylococci colonization of postpartum mothers and newborn infants. Am J Obstet Gynecol 66:1227, 1959.
238. Ottenheimer EJ, Minchew IBH, Cohen LS, et al. Studies of the epidemiology of staphylococcal infection. Bull Johns Hopkins Hosp 109:114, 1961.
239. Burbianka M, Dluzniewska A, Windyga B. Enterogenic staphylococci and enterotoxin in human milk. *In* Jeljaszewicz J, Hryniewicz W (eds). Staphylococci and Staphylococcal Infections: Recent Progress. Warsaw, Polish Medical Publishers, 1973, p 444.

240. Ogle KS, Davis S. Mastitis in lactating women. J Fam Pract 26:139, 1988.
241. Thomsen AC, Espersen T, Maigaard S. Course and treatment of milk stasis, noninfectious inflammation of the breast, and infectious mastitis in nursing women. Am J Obstet Gynecol 149:492, 1984.
242. Dener C, Inan A. Breast abscesses in lactating women. World J Surg 27:130, 2003.
243. Kalwbow H. Über Mastitis neonatorum und ihre Folgen. Zentralbl Gynakol 60:1821, 1936.
244. Rudoy RC, Nelson JD. Breast abscess during the neonatal period. Am J Dis Child 129:1031, 1975.
245. Faridi MM, Rattan A, Ahmad SH. Omphalitis neonatorum. J Indian Med Assoc 91:283, 1993.
246. Sawardekar KP. Changing spectrum of neonatal omphalitis. Pediatr Infect Dis J 23:22, 2004.
247. Mason WH, Andrews R, Ross LA, et al. Omphalitis in the newborn infant. Pediatr Infect Dis J 8:521, 1989.
248. Cushing AH. Omphalitis: a review. Pediatr Infect Dis 4:282, 1985.
249. Warren WS, Stool SE. Otitis in low birth-weight infants. J Pediatr 79:740, 1971.
250. Sabatino G, Verrotti A, de Martino M, et al. Neonatal suppurative parotitis: a study of five cases. Eur J Pediatr 158:312, 1999.
251. Raad II, Sabbagh MF, Caranasos GJ. Acute bacterial sialadenitis: a study of 29 cases and review. Rev Infect Dis 12:591, 1990.
252. Spiegel R, Miron D, Sakran W, et al. Acute neonatal suppurative parotitis: case reports and review. Pediatr Infect Dis J 23:76, 2004.
253. Chiu CH, Lin TY. Clinical and microbiological analysis of six children with acute suppurative parotitis. Acta Paediatr 85:106, 1996.
254. David RB, O'Connel EJ. Suppurative parotitis in children. Am J Dis Child 119:332, 1970.
255. Ayliffe GA, Brightwell KM, Ball PM, et al. Staphylococcal infection in cervical glands of infants. Lancet 2:479, 1972.
256. Dewar J, Porter IA, Smylie GH. Staphylococcal infection in cervical glands of infants. Lancet 2:712, 1972.
257. Hieber HP, Davis AT. Staphylococcal cervical adenitis in young infants. Pediatrics 57:424, 1976.
258. Scobie WG. Acute suppurative adenitis in children. Scott Med J 14:352, 1969.
259. Barton LL, Feigin RD. Childhood cervical lymphadenitis: a reappraisal. J Pediatr 84:846, 1974.
260. Schlievert PM. Alteration of immune function by staphylococcal pyrogenic exotoxin type C: possible role in toxic-shock syndrome. J Infect Dis 147:391, 1983.
261. Schlievert PM. Staphylococcal enterotoxin B and toxic-shock syndrome toxin-1 are significantly associated with non-menstrual TSS. Lancet 1:1149, 1986.
262. Shands KN, Schmid GP, Dan BB, et al. Toxic shock syndrome in menstruating women: association with tampon use and *Staphylococcus aureus* and clinical features in 52 cases. N Engl J Med 303:1436, 1980.
263. Todd J, Fishaut M, Kapral F, et al. Toxic shock syndrome associated with phage group I staphylococci. Lancet 2:1116, 1978.
264. Rizkallah MF, Tolaymat A, Martinez JS, et al. Toxic shock syndrome caused by a strain of *Staphylococcus aureus* that produces enterotoxin C but not toxic shock syndrome toxin-1. Am J Dis Child 143:848, 1989.
265. Chow AW, Wittmann BK, Bartlett KH, et al. Variant postpartum toxic shock syndrome with probable intrapartum transmission to the neonate. Am J Obstet Gynecol 148:1074, 1984.
266. Green SL, LaPeter KS. Evidence for postpartum toxic-shock syndrome in a mother-infant pair. Am J Med 72:169, 1982.
267. Carvalho L, Neves JF. Toxic shock syndrome in a neonate? Acta Paediatr 87:699, 1998.
268. Kaul R, McGeer A, Norrby-Teglund A, et al. Intravenous immunoglobulin therapy for streptococcal toxic shock syndrome—a comparative observational study. The Canadian Streptococcal Study Group. Clin Infect Dis 28:800, 1999.
269. Takahashi N, Nishida H. New exanthematous disease with thrombocytopenia in neonates. Arch Dis Child Fetal Neonatal Ed 77:F79, 1997.
270. Takahashi N, Nishida H, Kato H, et al. Exanthematous disease induced by toxic shock syndrome toxin 1 in the early neonatal period. Lancet 351:1614, 1998.
271. Takahashi N, Kato H, Imanishi K, et al. Immunopathophysiological aspects of an emerging neonatal infectious disease induced by a bacterial superantigen. J Clin Invest 106:1409, 2000.
272. Kikuchi K, Takahashi N, Piao C, et al. Molecular epidemiology of methicillin-resistant *Staphylococcus aureus* strains causing neonatal toxic shock syndrome-like exanthematous disease in neonatal and perinatal wards. J Clin Microbiol 41:3001, 2003.
273. Koch R, Carson MJ, Donnell G. Staphylococcal pneumonia in children: a review of 83 cases. J Pediatr 55:473, 1959.
274. Hendren WH, III. Staphylococcal pneumonia in infancy and childhood: analysis of 75 cases. JAMA 168:6, 1958.
275. Bevaen DW, Burry AF. Staphylococcal pneumonia in the newborn: an epidemic with eight fatal cases. Lancet 2:211, 1956.
276. Turner JAP. Staphylococcal pneumonia: a contemporary rarity. Clin Pediatr (Phila) 2:69, 1972.
277. Hollis RJ, Barr JL, Doebbeling BN, et al. Familial carriage of methicillin-resistant *Staphylococcus aureus* and subsequent infection in a premature neonate. Clin Infect Dis 21:328, 1995.
278. Le Thomas I, Mariani-Kurkdjian P, Collignon A, et al. Breast milk transmission of a Panton-Valentine leukocidin-producing *Staphylococcus aureus* strain causing infantile pneumonia. J Clin Microbiol 39:728, 2001.
279. Kanof A, Kramer B, Carnes M. *Staphylococcus* pneumonia: a clinical, pathologic, and bacteriologic study. J Pediatr 14:712, 1939.
280. Huxtable KA, Tucker AS, Wedgwood RJ. Staphylococcal pneumonia in childhood. Am J Dis Child 108:262, 1964.
281. Wise MB, Beaudry PH, Bates DV. Long-term follow-up of staphylococcal pneumonia. Pediatrics 38:398, 1966.
282. Ceruti E, Contreras J, Neira M. Staphylococcal pneumonia in childhood: long-term follow-up including pulmonary function studies. Am J Dis Child 122:386, 1971.
283. Rhodes PG, Hall RT, Burry VE, et al. Sepsis and osteomyelitis due to *Staphylococcus aureus* phage type 94 in a neonatal intensive care unit. Letter to the editor. J Pediatr 88:1063, 1976.
284. Overturf GD, Balfour G. Osteomyelitis and sepsis: severe complications of fetal monitoring. Pediatrics 55:244, 1975.
285. Lilien LD, Harris VJ, Ramamurthy RS, et al. Neonatal osteomyelitis of the calcaneus: complication of heel puncture. J Pediatr 88:478, 1976.
286. Lauer BA, Altenburger KM. Outbreak of *Staphylococcus* infections following heel puncture for blood sampling. Am J Dis Child 135:277, 1981.
287. Myers MG, McMahon BJ, Koontz FP. Neonatal calcaneous osteomyelitis related to contaminated mineral oil. J Clin Microbiol 6:543, 1977.
288. Lim MO, Gresham EL, Franken EA Jr, et al. Osteomyelitis as a complication of umbilical artery catheterization. Am J Dis Child 131:142, 1977.
289. Weeks JL, Garcia-Prat JA, Baker C. Methicillin-resistant *Staphylococcus aureus* osteomyelitis in a neonate. JAMA 245:1662, 1981.
290. Blanche DW. Osteomyelitis in infants. J Bone Joint Surg Am 34A:578, 1954.
291. Potter CMC. Osteomyelitis in the newborn. J Bone Joint Surg 36B:578, 1954.
292. Clarke AM. Neonatal osteomyelitis: a disease different from osteomyelitis of older children. Med J Aust 45:237, 1958.
293. Gilmour WN. Acute hematogenous osteomyelitis. J Bone Joint Surg Am 44B:841, 1962.
294. Ogden JA, Lister G. The pathology of neonatal osteomyelitis. Pediatrics 55:474, 1975.
295. Ogden JA. Pediatric osteomyelitis and septic arthritis: pathology of neonatal disease. Yale J Biol Med 52:423, 1979.
296. Fardon DF. Osteomyelitis of the scapula in an infant: case report. Mo Med 67:299, 1970.
297. Wong M, Isaacs D, Howman-Giles R, et al. Clinical and diagnostic features of osteomyelitis occurring in the first three months of life. Pediatr Infect Dis J 14:1047, 1995.
298. Weissberg ED, Smith AL, Smith DH. Clinical features of neonatal osteomyelitis. Pediatrics 53:505, 1974.
299. Ish-Horowicz MR, McIntyre P, Nade S. Bone and joint infections caused by multiply resistant *Staphylococcus aureus* in a neonatal intensive care unit. Pediatr Infect Dis J 11:82, 1992.
300. Einstein RAJ, Thomas CG. Osteomyelitis in infants. AJR Am J Roentgenol 55:299, 1946.
301. Green WT. Osteomyelitis in infancy. JAMA 105:1835, 1935.
302. Ambrose GB, Alpert M, Neer CS. Vertebral osteomyelitis: a diagnostic problem. JAMA 197:101, 1966.
303. Miller WH, Hesch JA. Nontuberculous spinal epidural abscess: report of a case in a 5-week old infant. Am J Dis Child 104:269, 1962.
304. Magd M. Radionuclide imaging in early detection of childhood osteomyelitis and its differentiation from cellulitis and bone infarction. Ann Radiol (Paris) 20:9, 1977.

305. Treves S, Khettry J, Broher FH, et al. Osteomyelitis: early scintigraphic detection in children. Pediatrics 57:173, 1976.
306. Prober CG, Yeager AS. Use of the serum bactericidal titer to assess the adequacy of oral antibiotic therapy in the treatment of acute hematogenous osteomyelitis. J Pediatr 95:131, 1979.
307. Tetzloff TR, McCracken GH, Nelson JD. Oral antibiotic therapy for skeletal infections of children: II. Therapy of osteomyelitis and suppurative arthritis. J Pediatr 92:485, 1978.
308. Schwartz GJ, Hegyi T, Spitzer A. Subtherapeutic dicloxacillin levels in a neonate: possible mechanisms. J Pediatr 89:310, 1976.
309. Dich VC, Nelson JD, Haltalin KC. Osteomyelitis in infants and children. Am J Dis Child 129:1273, 1975.
310. Bergdahl S, Ekengren K, Eriksson M. Neonatal hematogenous osteomyelitis: risk factors for long-term sequelae. J Pediatr Orthop 5:564, 1985.
311. Halbstein BM. Bone regeneration in infantile osteomyelitis. J Bone Joint Surg Am 49A:149, 1967.
312. Edwards MS, Baker CJ. Median sternotomy wound infections in children. Pediatr Infect Dis 2:105, 1983.
313. Chacha PB. Suppurative arthritis of the hip in infancy: a persistent diagnostic problem and possible complication of femoral vein puncture. J Bone Joint Surg Am 53A:538, 1971.
314. Obletz BE. Acute suppurative arthritis of the hip in the neonatal period. J Bone Joint Surg Am 42A:23, 1960.
315. Buetow KC, Klein SW, Lane RB. Septicemia in premature infants. Am J Dis Child 110:29, 1965.
316. McCracken GH, Jr., Shinefield HR. Changes in the pattern of neonatal septicemia and meningitis. Am J Dis Child 112:33, 1966.
317. Isaacs D, Barfield C, Clothier T, et al. Late-onset infections of infants in neonatal units. J Paediatr Child Health 32:158, 1996.
318. Sanghvi KP, Tudehope DI. Neonatal bacterial sepsis in a neonatal intensive care unit: a 5 year analysis. J Paediatr Child Health 32:333, 1996.
319. Beck-Sague CM, Azimi P, Fonseca SN, et al. Bloodstream infections in neonatal intensive care unit patients: results of a multicenter study. Pediatr Infect Dis J 13:1110, 1994.
320. Patrick CC, Kaplan SL, Baker CJ, et al. Persistent bacteremia due to coagulase-negative staphylococci in low birthweight neonates. Pediatrics 84:977, 1989.
321. St Geme JW III, Bell LM, Baumgart S, et al. Distinguishing sepsis from blood culture contamination in young infants with blood cultures growing coagulase-negative staphylococci. Pediatrics 86:157, 1990.
322. Krediet TG, Jones ME, Janssen K, et al. Prevalence of molecular types and *mecA* gene carriage of coagulase-negative staphylococci in a neonatal intensive care unit: relation to nosocomial septicemia. J Clin Microbiol 39:3376, 2001.
323. Tan TQ, Mason EO Jr, Ou CN, et al. Use of intravenous rifampin in neonates with persistent staphylococcal bacteremia. Antimicrob Agents Chemother 37:2401, 1993.
324. Shama A, Patole SK, Whitehall JS. Intravenous rifampicin in neonates with persistent staphylococcal bacteraemia. Acta Paediatr 91:670, 2002.
325. Benjamin DK, Jr., Miller W, Garges H, et al. Bacteremia, central catheters, and neonates: when to pull the line. Pediatrics 107:1272, 2001.
326. Karlowicz MG, Furigay PJ, Croitoru DP, et al. Central venous catheter removal versus in situ treatment in neonates with coagulase-negative staphylococcal bacteremia. Pediatr Infect Dis J 21:22, 2002.
327. Chapman RL, Faix RG. Persistent bacteremia and outcome in late onset infection among infants in a neonatal intensive care unit. Pediatr Infect Dis J 22:17, 2003.
328. Symchych PS, Krauss AN, Winchester P. Endocarditis following intracardiac placement of umbilical venous catheters in neonates. J Pediatr 90:287, 1977.
329. Johnson DH, Rosenthal A, Nadas AS. Bacterial endocarditis in children under 2 years of age. Am J Dis Child 129:183, 1975.
330. Krous HF. Neonatal nonbacterial thrombotic endocarditis. Arch Pathol Lab Med 103:76, 1979.
331. Mecrow IK, Ladusans EJ. Infective endocarditis in newborn infants with structurally normal hearts. Acta Paediatr 83:35, 1994.
332. Daher AH, Berkowitz FE. Infective endocarditis in neonates. Clin Pediatr (Phila) 34:198, 1995.
333. Pearlman SA, Higgins S, Eppes S, et al. Infective endocarditis in the premature neonate. Clin Pediatr (Phila) 37:741, 1998.
334. Opie GF, Fraser SH, Drew JH, et al. Bacterial endocarditis in neonatal intensive care. J Paediatr Child Health 35:545, 1999.
335. Millard DD, Shulman ST. The changing spectrum of neonatal endocarditis. Clin Perinatol 15:587, 1988.
336. Garrison PK, Freedman LR. Experimental endocarditis: I. Staphylococcal endocarditis in rabbits resulting from placement of polyethylene catheter in the right side of the heart. Yale J Biol Med 42:394, 1970.
337. Durack DT, Beeson PG, Petersdorf RG. Experimental bacterial endocarditis: II. Production and progress of the disease in rabbits. Br J Exp Pathol 54:142, 1973.
338. Durand M, Ramanathan R, Martinelli B, et al. Prospective evaluation of percutaneous central venous Silastic catheters in newborn infants with birth weights of 510 to 3,920 grams. Pediatrics 78:245, 1986.
339. Oelberg DG, Fisher DJ, Gross DM, et al. Endocarditis in high-risk neonates. Pediatrics 71:392, 1983.
340. Washington JA. The microbiological diagnosis of infective endocarditis. J Antimicrob Chemother 20(Suppl A):29, 1987.
341. Johnson DH, Rosenthal A, Nadas AS. A forty-year review of bacterial endocarditis in infancy and childhood. Circulation 51:581, 1975.
342. O'Callaghan C, McDougall P. Infective endocarditis in neonates. Arch Dis Child 63:53, 1988.
343. Von Reyn CF, Levy BS, Arbeit RD, et al. Infective endocarditis: an analysis based on strict case definitions. Ann Intern Med 94:505, 1981.
344. Durack DT, Lukes AS, Bright DK. New criteria for diagnosis of infective endocarditis: utilization of specific echocardiographic findings. Duke Endocarditis Service. Am J Med 96:200, 1994. [See comment.]
345. Tissieres P, Gervaix A, Beghetti M, et al. Value and limitations of the von Reyn, Duke, and modified Duke criteria for the diagnosis of infective endocarditis in children. Pediatrics 112:e467, 2003.
346. Durack DT, Lukes AS, Bright DK. New criteria for diagnosis of infective endocarditis: utilization of specific echocardiographic findings. Duke Endocarditis Service. Am J Med 96:200, 1994.
347. Noel JG, O'Loughlin JE, Edelson PJ. Neonatal *Staphylococcus epidermidis* right side endocarditis: description of five catheterized infants. Pediatrics 82:234, 1988.
348. Wellman WE, Senft RA. Bacterial meningitis: III. Infections caused by *Staphylococcus aureus*. Proc Staff Meet Mayo Clin 39:263, 1964.
349. Mulcare RJ, Harter DH. Changing patterns of staphylococcal meningitis. Arch Neurol 7:114, 1962.
350. Shurtleff DB, Foltz EL, Weeks RD, et al. Therapy of *Staphylococcus epidermidis*: infection associated with cerebrospinal fluid shunts. Pediatrics 53:55, 1974.
351. Gruskay J, Harris MC, Costarino AT, et al. Neonatal *Staphylococcus epidermidis* meningitis with unremarkable CSF examination results. Am J Dis Child 143:580, 1989.
352. Doctor BA, Newman N, Minich NM, et al. Clinical outcomes of neonatal meningitis in very-low birth-weight infants. Clin Pediatr (Phila) 40:473, 2001.
353. Franco SM, Cornelius VE, Andrews BF. Long-term outcome of neonatal meningitis. Am J Dis Child 146:567, 1992. [See comment.]
354. Hack M, Horbar JD, Malloy MH, et al. Very low birth weight outcomes of the National Institute of Child Health and Human Development Neonatal Network. Pediatrics 87:587, 1991. [See comment.]
355. McLaurin RL, Frame PT. Treatment of infections of cerebrospinal fluid shunts. Rev Infect Dis 9:595, 1987.
356. Wald SL, McLaurin RL. Cerebrospinal fluid antibiotic levels during treatment of shunt infections. J Neurosurg 52:41, 1980.
357. Diaz-Mitoma F, Harding GKM, Hoban DJ, et al. Clinical significance of a test for slime production in ventriculoperitoneal shunt infections caused by coagulase-negative staphylococci. J Infect Dis 156:555, 1987.
358. Conners JM. Cure of Ommaya reservoir–associated *Staphylococcus epidermidis* ventriculitis with a simple regimen of vancomycin and rifampin without reservoir removal. Med Pediatr Oncol 10:549, 1982.
359. Stickler GB, Shin MH, Burke EC, et al. Diffuse glomerulonephritis associated with infected ventriculo-atrial shunt. N Engl J Med 279:1077, 1968.
360. Renier D, Flandin C, Hirsch E, et al. Brain abscesses in neonates. A study of 30 cases. J Neurosurg 69:877, 1988.
361. Yogev R, Bar-Meir M. Management of brain abscesses in children. Pediatr Infect Dis J 23:157, 2004.
362. Idriss ZH, Gutman LT, Kronfol NM. Brain abscesses in infants and children: current status of clinical findings, management and prognosis. Clin Pediatr (Phila) 17:738, 1978.
363. Wong TT, Lee LS, Wang HS, et al. Brain abscesses in children—a cooperative study of 83 cases. Childs Nerv Syst 5:19, 1989.
364. Koot RW, Reedijk B, Tan WF, et al. Neonatal brain abscess: complication of fetal monitoring. Obstet Gynecol 93:857, 1999.
365. Daniels SR, Price JK, Towbin RB, et al. Nonsurgical cure of brain abscess in a neonate. Childs Nerv Syst 1:346, 1985.

366. Hoffman HJ, Hendrick EB, Hiscox JL. Cerebral abscesses in early infancy. J Neurosurg 33:172, 1970.
367. Regev RH, Dolfin TZ, Zamir C. Multiple brain abscesses in a premature infant: complication of *Staphylococcus aureus* sepsis. Acta Paediatr 84:585, 1995.
368. Fischer EG, McLennan JE, Suzuki Y. Cerebral abscess in children. Am J Dis Child 135:746, 1981.
369. Barrie D. Staphylococcal colonization of the rectum in the newborn. BMJ 1:1574, 1966.
370. Selberg L. Fatal staphylococcal poisoning of breast fed infant whose mother suffered from staphylococcal mastitis. Acta Obstet Gynecol Scand 27:275, 1947.
371. Christie CDC, Lynch-Ballard E, Andiman WA. Staphylococcal enterocolitis revisited: cytotoxic properties of *Staphylococcus aureus* from a neonate with enterocolitis. Pediatr Infect Dis J 7:791, 1988.
372. Masunaga K, Mazaki R, Endo A, et al. Colonic stenosis after severe methicillin-resistant *Staphylococcus aureus* enterocolitis in a newborn. Pediatr Infect Dis J 18:169, 1999.
373. Fabia C, Pearlman MA, Leon EF, et al. *Staphylococcus epidermidis*: a new pathogen in necrotizing enterocolitis (NEC). Pediatr Res 17:312A, 1983.
374. Gruskay JA, Abbasi S, Anday E, et al. *Staphylococcus epidermidis*-associated enterocolitis. J Pediatr 109:520, 1986.
375. Shuman RM, Leech RW, Alvord EC, Jr. Neurotoxicity of hexachlorophene in humans: II. A clinical-pathologic study of 46 premature infants. Arch Neurol 32:320, 1975.
376. Curtis J, Stobie PE. Necrotizing enterocolitis and staphylococcal sepsis. J Pediatr 111:953, 1987.
377. Mollit DL, Tepas JJ, Talbert JL. The role of coagulase-negative staphylococci in neonatal necrotizing enterocolitis. J Pediatr Surg 23: 60, 1988.
378. Jorgensen J. Mechanisms of methicillin resistance in *Staphylococcus aureus* and methods for laboratory detection. Infect Control Hosp Epidemiol 12:14, 1991.
379. Srinivasan A, Dick JD, Perl TM. Vancomycin resistance in staphylococci. Clin Microbiol Rev 15:430, 2002.
380. Hanaki H, Kuwahara-Arai K, Boyle-Vavra S, et al. Activated cell-wall synthesis is associated with vancomycin resistance in methicillin-resistant *Staphylococcus aureus* clinical strains Mu3 and Mu50. J Antimicrob Chemother 42:199, 1998.
381. Cui L, Murakami H, Kuwahara-Arai K, et al. Contribution of a thickened cell wall and its gluatmine nonamidated component to the vancomycin resistance expressed by *Staphylococcus aureus* Mu50. Antimicrob Agents Chemother 44:2276, 2000.
382. Centers for Disease Control and Prevention. *Staphylococcus aureus* resistant ot vancomycin—United States, 2002. MMWR Morb Mortal Wkly Rep 51:565, 2002.
383. Centers for Disease Control and Prevention. Vancomycin-resistant *Staphylococcus aureus*—Pennsylvania, 2002. MMWR Morb Mortal Wkly Rep 51:902, 2002.
384. Chang S, Sievert DM, Hageman JC, et al. Infection with vancomycin-resistant *Staphylococcus aureus* containing the *vanA* resistance gene. N Engl J Med 348:1342, 2003.
385. Weigel LM, Clewell DB, Gill SR, et al. Genetic analysis of a high-level vancomycin-resistant isolate of *Staphylococcus aureus*. Science 302:1569, 2003.
386. Bozdogan B, Esel D, Whitener C, et al. Antibacterial susceptibility of a vancomycin-resistant *Staphylococcus aureus* strain isolated at the Hershey Medical Center. J Antimicrob Chemother 52:864, 2003.
387. Levine DP, Fromm BS, Reddy BR. Slow response to vancomycin or vancomycin plus rifampin in mthicillin-resistant *Staphylococcus aureus* endocarditis. Ann Intern Med 115:674, 1991.
388. Nu HC. Structure-activity relations of new beta-lactam compounds and in vitro activity against common bacteria. Rev Infect Dis 5:S319, 1983.
389. Nelson SJ, Boies EG, Shackelford PG. Ceftriaxone in the treatment of infections caused by *Staphylococcus aureus* in children. Pediatr Infect Dis J 4:27, 1985.
390. Odio CM, Umana MA, Saenz A, et al. Comparative efficacy of ceftazidime vs. carbenicillin and amikacin for treatment of neonatal septicemia. Pediatr Infect Dis J 6:371, 1987.
391. Beldhradsky BH, Bruch K, Geiss D, et al. Intravenous cefotaxime in children with bacterial meningitis. Lancet 1:61, 1980.
392. Spivey JM, Gal P. Vancomycin pharmacokinetics in neonates. Letter to the editor. Am J Dis Child 140:859, 1986.
393. Dunne WM, Nelson DB, Chusid MJ. Epidemiologic markers of pediatric infections caused by coagulase-negative staphylococci. Pediatr Infect Dis J 6:1031, 1987.
394. Schwalbe RW, Stapleton JT, Gilligan PH. Emergence of vancomycin resistance in coagulase-negative staphylococci. N Engl J Med 16:927, 1987.
395. Froggatt JW, Johnston JL, Galetto DW, et al. Antimicrobial resistance in nosocomial isolates of *Staphylococcus haemolyticus*. Antimicrob Agents Chemother 33:460, 1989.
396. Gill VJ, Manning CB, Ingalls CM. Correlation of penicillin minimum inhibitory concentrations and penicillin zone edge appearance with staphylococcal beta-lactamase production. J Clin Microbiol 14:437, 1981.
397. Sabath LD. Chemical and physical factors influencing methicillin-resistance of *Staphylococcus aureus* and *Staphylococcus epidermidis*. J Antimicrob Chemother 3:47, 1977.
398. Archer GL. Antimicrobial susceptibility and selection of resistance among *Staphylococcus epidermidis* isolates recovered from patients with infections of indwelling foreign devices. Antimicrob Agents Chemother 14:353, 1978.
399. John JF, Jr., McNeill WF. Activity of cephalosporins against methicillin-susceptible and methicillin-resistant coagulase-negative staphylococci: minimal effect of beta-lactamase. Antimicrob Agents Chemother 17:179, 1980.
400. Lowy FD, Hammer SM. *Staphylococcus epidermidis* infections. Ann Intern Med 99:834, 1983.
401. Young TE, Mangum B. Neofax: A Manual of Drugs Used in Neonatal Care, 16th ed. Raleigh, NC, Acorn Publishing, 2003.
402. Arditi M, Yogev R. In vitro interactions between rifampin and clindamycin against pathogenic coagulase-negative staphylococci. Antimicrob Agents Chemother 33:245, 1989.
403. Massanari RM, Donta ST. The efficacy of rifampin as adjunctive therapy in selected cases of staphylococcal endocarditis. Chest 73:371, 1978.
404. Karchmer AW, Archer GL, Dismukes WE. *Staphylococcus* endocarditis prosthetic value endocarditis: microbiological and clinical observations as guide to therapy. Ann Intern Med 98:447, 1983.
405. Lowy FD, Chang DS, Lash PR. Synergy of combinations of vancomycin, gentamicin, and rifampin against methicillin-resistant, coagulase-negative staphylococci. Antimicrob Agents Chemother 23: 932, 1983.
406. Gezon HM, Roger KD, Thompson DJ, et al. Environmental aspects of staphylococcal infections acquired in hospitals: II. Some controversial aspects in the epidemiology of hospital nursery staphylococcal infections. Am J Public Health 50:473, 1960.
407. Shinefield HR, Ribble JC. Current aspects of infections and diseases related to *Staphylococcus aureus*. Annu Rev Med 16:263, 1965.
408. Daschner FD. Nosocomial infections in maternity wards and newborn nurseries: rooming-in or not. J Hosp Infect 7:1, 1986.
409. Andersen BM, Lindemann R, Bergh K, et al. Spread of methicillin-resistant *Staphylococcus aureus* in a neonatal intensive unit associated with understaffing, overcrowding and mixing of patients. J Hosp Infect 50:18, 2002.
410. Call EL. An epidemic of pemphigus neonatorum. Am J Obstet Gynecol 50:473, 1904.
411. Seidemann I, Andeisenoff H. Rooming-in service in a medium-sized community hospital. Report on four and one-half years observation. N Y State J Med 56:2533, 1956.
412. Frazer MJL. A study of neonatal infections in the nurseries of a maternity hospital. Arch Dis Child 23:107, 1948.
413. Anthong BF, Guiliano DM, Oh W. Nursery outbreak of staphylococcal scalded-skin syndrome: rapid identification of the epidemic bacterial strain. Am J Dis Child 124:41, 1972.
414. Gillespie WA, Adler VG. Control of an outbreak of staphylococcal infection in a hospital. Lancet 1:632, 1957.
415. Rountree PM, Heseltine M, Rheuben J, et al. Control of staphylococcal infection of newborn by treatment of nasal carriers in staff. Med J Aust 1:528, 1956.
416. Monroe JA, Markham NP. Staphylococcal infection in mothers and infants: maternal breast abscesses and antecedent neonatal sepsis. Lancet 2:186, 1958.
417. Martin WJ, Nichols DR, Henderson ED. The problem of management of nasal carriers of staphylococci. Proceedings of the staff Meetings of the Mayo Clinic 35:282, 1960.
418. Williams JD, Waltho CA, Ayliffe GAJ, et al. Trials of five antibacterial creams in the control of nasal carriage of *Staphylococcus aureus*. Lancet 2:390, 1967.
419. Smith RT. The role of the chronic carrier in an epidemic of staphylococcal disease in a newborn nursery. Am J Dis Child 95:461, 1958.

420. Wysham DN, Mulhern ME, Navarre GC, et al. Staphylococcal infections in an obstetric unit: I. Epidemiologic studies of pyoderma neonatorum. N Engl J Med 257:295, 1957.
421. Belani A, Sherertz RJ, Sullivan ML, et al. Outbreak of staphylococcal infection in two hospital nurseries traced to a single nasal carrier. Infect Control 7:487, 1986.
422. Mortimer EA, Jr., Lipsitz PJ, Wolinsky E, et al. Transmission of staphylococci between newborns: importance of the hands of personnel. Am J Dis Child 104:289, 1962.
423. Kretzer EK, Larson EL. Behavioral interventions to improve infection control practices. Am J Infect Control 26:245, 1998.
424. Tibballs J. Teaching hospital medical staff to handwash. Med J Aust 164:395, 1996. [See comment.]
425. Pittet D. Improving compliance with hand hygiene in hospitals. Infect Control Hosp Epidemiol 21:381, 2000.
426. Ehrenkranz NJ, Alfonso BC. Failure of bland soap handwash to prevent hand transfer of patient bacteria to urethral catheters. Infect Control Hosp Epidemiol 12:654, 1991.
427. Klainer LM, Agrawal HS, Mortimer EA, Jr., et al. Bacitracin ointment and neonatal staphylococci. Am J Dis Child 103:72, 1962.
428. Gezon HM, Thompson DJ, Roger KD, et al. Control of staphylococcal infections and disease in the newborn through the use of hexachlorophene bathing. Pediatrics 51:331, 1973.
429. Jellard J. Umbilical cord as reservoir of infection in a maternity hospital. BMJ 1:925, 1957.
430. Pildes RS. Effect of triple dye on staphylococcal colonization in the newborn infant. J Pediatr 82:987, 1973.
431. Ramamurthy RS, Pildes RS, Gorbach SL. Nursery epidemic caused by a nontypable gray colony variant of *Staphylococcus aureus*. Pediatrics 51:608, 1973.
432. Gluck L, Wood HF. Effect of an antiseptic skin-care regimen in reducing staphylococcal colonization in newborn infants. N Engl J Med 265:1177, 1961.
433. Simon HJ, Yaffe SJ, Gluck L. Effective control of staphylococci in a nursery. N Engl J Med 265:1171, 1961.
434. Plueckhahn VD, Banks J. Antisepsis and staphylococcal disease in the newborn child. Med J Aust 2:519, 1963.
435. Gezon HM, Thompson DJ, Roger KD, et al. Hexachlorophene bathing in early infancy: effect on staphylococcal disease and infection. N Engl J Med 270:379, 1964.
436. Pleuckhaln VD. Hexachlorophene and the control of staphylococcal sepsis in a maternity unit in Geelong, Australia. Pediatrics 51:368, 1973.
437. Gezon HM, Schaberg MJ, Klein JO. Concurrent epidemics of *Staphylococcus aureus* and group A *Streptococcus* disease in a newborn nursery-control with penicillin G and hexachlorophene bathing. Pediatrics 51:383, 1973.
438. Hyams PJ, Counts WG, Monkus E, et al. Staphylococcal bacteremia and hexachlorophene bathing: epidemic in a newborn nursery. Am J Dis Child 129:595, 1975.
439. Shaffer TE, Baldwin JN, Rheins M, et al. Staphylococcal infections in newborn infants: study of epidemics among infants and nursing mothers. Pediatrics 18:750, 1956.
440. Garner JS. Guideline for isolation precautions in hospitals. The Hospital Infection Control Practices Advisory Committee. Infect Control Hosp Epidemiol 17:53, 1996 [erratum appears in Infect Control Hosp Epidemiol 17:214, 1996].
441. Jernigan JA, Titus MG, Groschel DH, et al. Effectiveness of contact isolation during a hospital outbreak of methicillin-resistant *Staphylococcus aureus*. Am J Epidemiol 143:496, 1996 [erratum appears in Am J Epidemiol 143:107, 1996].
442. Shinefield HR, Ribble JC, Boris M, et al. Bacterial interference: its effect on nursery-acquired infection with *Staphylococcus aureus*: V. An analysis and interpretation. Am J Dis Child 105:683, 1963.
443. Shinefield HR, Ribble JC, Boris M. Bacterial interference between strains of *Staphylococcus aureus*, 1960 to 1970. Am J Dis Child 121:148, 1971.
444. Eichenwald HF, Shinefield HR, Boris M, et al. Bacterial interference and staphylococcal colonization in infants and adults. Ann N Y Acad Sci 128:365, 1965.
445. Light IJ, Walton RL, Sutherland JM, et al. Use of bacterial interference to control a staphylococcal nursery outbreak. Am J Dis Child 113:291, 1967.
446. Light IJ, Sutherland JM, Schott JE. Control of a staphylococcal outbreak in a nursery—use of bacterial interference. JAMA 193:699, 1965.
447. Shinefield HR. Bacterial interference. Ann N Y Acad Sci 236:444, 1974.
448. Kwong MS, Loew AD, Anthony BF, et al. The effect of hexachlorophene on staphylococcal colonization rates in the newborn infant: a controlled study using a single-bath method. J Pediatr 82:982, 1973.
449. Light IJ, Sutherland JM. What is the evidence that hexachlorophene is not effective? Pediatrics 51:345, 1973.
450. Najem GR, Riley HD Jr, Ordway NK, et al. Clinical and microbiologic surveillance of neonatal staphylococcal disease: relationship to hexachlorophene whole-body bathing. Am J Dis Child 129:297, 1975.
451. Gooch JJ, Britt EM. *Staphylococcus aureus* colonization and infection in newborn nursery patients. Am J Dis Child 132:893, 1978.
452. Neumann LL, Rager R, Brickman A, et al. Gram-Positive Umbilical Flora in a Nursery Using Alcohol Cord Care. Atlantic City, NJ, Society for Pediatric Research, 1971, p 258.
453. Kimbrough RD. Review of recent evidence of toxic effects of hexachlorophene. Pediatrics 51:391, 1973.
454. Mullick FG. Hexachlorophene toxicity. Pediatrics 51:395, 1973.
455. Kopelman AE. Cutaneous absorption of hexachlorophene in low birth-weight infants. J Pediatr 82:972, 1973.
456. Committee on the Fetus and Newborn, American Academy of Pediatrics. Skin care of newborns. Pediatrics 54:682, 1974.
457. Powell H, Swarner O, Gluck L, et al. Hexachlorophene myelinopathy in premature infants. J Pediatr 82:976, 1973.
458. Shuman RM, Leech RW, Alvord EC, Jr. Neurotoxicity of hexachlorophene in the human: I. A clinical-pathologic study of 248 children. Pediatrics 54:90, 1974.
459. Shuman RM, Leech RW, Alvord EC, Jr. Neurotoxicity of topically applied hexachlorophene in the young rat. Arch Neurol 32:315, 1975.
460. Tyrala EE, Hillman CS, Hillman RE, et al. Clinical pharmacology of hexachlorophene in newborn infants. Pediatrics 91:481, 1977.
461. Pyati S, Ramamurthy RS, Krauss T, et al. Povidone-iodine (PI), ethyl alcohol (AL) and triple dye (TD): control of neonatal staphylococcal (*Staphylococcus aureus*) colonization. Pediatr Res 10:431, 1976.
462. Johnson JD, Malachowski NC, Vosti KL, et al. A sequential study of various modes of skin and umbilical care and the incidence of staphylococcal colonization and infection in the neonate. Pediatrics 58:354, 1976.
463. Speck WT, Driscoll JM, Polin RA, et al. Staphylococcal and streptococcal colonization of the newborn infant: effect of antiseptic cord care. Am J Dis Child 131:1005, 1977.
464. Barrett FF, Mason EO, Fleming D. The effect of three cord care regimens on bacterial colonization of normal neonates. Pediatr Res 11:497, 1977.
465. Balaban N, Goldkorn T, Nhan RT, et al. Autoinducer of virulence as a target for vaccine and therapy against *Staphylococcus aureus*. Science 280:438, 1998. [See comment.]
466. McKenney D, Pouliot K, Wang Y, et al. Vaccine potential of poly-1-6 beta-D-*N*-succinylglucosamine, an immunoprotective surface polysaccharide of *Staphylococcus aureus* and *Staphylococcus epidermidis*. J Biotechnol 83:37, 2000.
467. McKenney D, Pouliot KL, Wang Y, et al. Broadly protective vaccine for *Staphylococcus aureus* based on an in vivo–expressed antigen. Science 284:1523, 1999.
468. Senna JP, Roth DM, Oliveira JS, et al. Protective immune response against methicillin resistant *Staphylococcus aureus* in a murine model using a DNA vaccine approach. Vaccine 21:2661, 2003.
469. Shinefield H, Black S, Fattom A, et al. Use of *Staphylococcus aureus* conjugate vaccine in patients receiving hemodialysis. N Engl J Med 346:491, 2002.
470. Peters G, Locci R, Pulverer G. Adherence and growth of coagulase-negative staphylococci on surface of intravenous catheters. J Infect Dis 146:479, 1982.
471. Franson TR, Sheth NK, Rose HD, et al. Scanning electron microscopy of bacteria adherent to intavascular catheters. J Clin Microbiol 20:500, 1984.
472. Marrie TJ, Costerton JW. Scanning and transmission electron microscopy of in situ bacterial colonization of intravenous and intraarterial catheters. J Clin Microbiol 19:687, 1984.
473. Kamal GD, Pfaller MA, Rempe LE, et al. Reduced intravascular catheter infection by antibiotic bonding: a prospective, randomized, controlled trial. JAMA 265:2364, 1991.
474. Bach A. Clinical studies on the use antibiotic- and antiseptic-bonded catheters to prevent catheter-related infection. Int J Med Microbiol Virol Parasitol 283:208, 1995.
475. Radd I, Darouiche R, Dupuis J, et al. Central venous catheters coated with minocycline and rifampin for the prevention of catheter-related

colonization and bloodstream infections: a randomized, double-blind trial. Ann Intern Med 127:267, 1997.
476. Darouiche R, Raad I, Heard S, et al. A prospective randomized, multicenter clinical trial comparing central venous catheters impregnated with minocycline and rifampin vs. chlorhexidine gluconate and silver sulfadiazine. Crit Care Med 26:A128, 1998.
477. Veenstra DL, Saint S, Saha S, et al. Efficacy of antiseptic-impregnated central venous catheters in preventing catheter-related bloodstream infection. JAMA 281:261, 1999.
478. Hanna HA, Raad II, Hackett B, et al. Antibiotic-impregnated catheters associated with significant decrease in nosocomial and multidrug-resistant bacteremias in critically ill patients. Chest 124:1030, 2003.
479. Darouiche R, Raad I, Heard S, et al. A comparison of two antimicrobial-impregnated central venous catheters. N Engl J Med 340:1, 1999.
480. Spafford PS, Sinkin RA, Cox C, et al. Prevention of central venous catheter–related coagulase-negative staphylococcal sepsis in neonates. J Pediatr 125:259, 1994.
481. Kacica MA, Horgan MJ, Ochoa L, et al. Prevention of Gram-positive sepsis in neonates weighing less than 1500 grams. J Pediatr 125:253, 1994.
482. Cooke RWI, Nycyk JA, Okuonghuae H, et al. Low-dose vancomycin prophylaxis reduces coagulase-negative *Staphylococcus* bacteraemia in very low birthweight infants. J Hosp Infect 37:297, 1997.
483. Kilbride HW, Wirtschafter DD, Powers RJ, et al. Implementation of evidence-based potentially better practices to decrease nosocomial infections. Pediatrics 111:e519, 2003.
484. Kilbride HW, Powers R, Wirtschafter DD, et al. Evaluation and development of potentially better practices to prevent neonatal nosocomial bacteremia. Pediatrics 111:e504, 2003.
485. Weisman LE, Thackray HM, Cracia-Prats JA. Phase I/II double blind, placebo controlled, dose escalation, safety and pharmacokinetics study in very low birth weight neonates of BSYX-a110, an anti-staphylococcal monoclonal antibody for the prevention of staphylococcal bloodstream infections. San Francisco, PAS Late-Breaker Abstract Presentations, 2004.

Chapter 18

SYPHILIS

David Ingall • Pablo J. Sanchez • Carol J. Baker

Foetal syphilis is the malady that most medical men think of when reference is made to foetal disease. It has been studied in all its aspects and at very considerable length by a multitude of careful observers. It has been taken as the type of antenatal maladies, as the typical disease of the foetus; it may almost be said that, to some investigators, foetal pathology and foetal syphilis have been synonymous terms.[1]

Many decades have passed since Ballantyne wrote his congenital syphilis treatise in 1902,[1] but despite a complete understanding of the disease and the transmission of the organism and the availability of effective therapy and prevention strategies, congenital syphilis remains a disease of the 21st century.

The first major work on syphilis, written by Francisco Lopez de Villalobos, appeared in 1498,[2,3] and in 1530, Hieronymus Fracastorius[3,4] wrote an epic poem that featured a shepherd named Syphilus, and described the disease. A generation later, Gale[5] introduced the word *syphilis* into the English language. Lopez and Fracastorius mentioned syphilis of the newborn, but they and others[2,5,6] thought that infants became infected through contact at delivery or post partum by ingestion of infected breast milk. Because many mothers of infants with congenital syphilis had no obvious signs of infection, some investigators believed that congenital disease was transmitted by the father. Nevertheless, by 1850, it was believed that an infant could not have syphilis unless the mother was infected.

A lengthy account of the signs of syphilis in infants was published in 1854 by Diday,[5] but he failed to recognize that children who were without symptoms by 6 months of age could still be infected. In 1858, Sir Jonathan Hutchinson[7] described the famous triad of late congenital syphilis: notched incisor teeth, interstitial keratitis, and eighth cranial nerve deafness. Rosebury[8] has provided an eminently readable account of the history of syphilis and other venereal diseases.

THE ORGANISM

Although given various names following its discovery, the causative organism of syphilis was ultimately named *Treponema* because of its resemblance to a twisted thread and *pallidum* because of its pale color. This species is a member of the order Spirochaetales, family Spirochaetaceae, and genus *Treponema*. The other five genera of the order are *Borrelia*, *Spirochaeta*, *Leptospira*, and *Cristispira*. Originally, the pathogenic treponemes that cause syphilis and yaws were designated as subspecies of *Treponema pallidum* because no differences were detected by electron microscopy, DNA analysis (greater than 95% homology), or polyacrylamide gel electrophoresis of outer membrane proteins. These subspecies designations are *T. pallidum* subsp. *pallidum* and *T. pallidum* subsp. *pertenue*.[9-14] Moreover, because the etiologic agent of endemic (nonvenereal) syphilis is a variant of *T. pallidum*, it has been designated *T. pallidum* subsp. *endemicum*. The designation for the causative agent of pinta remains *Treponema carateum*. Recently, a genetic signature was defined in the 5′ flanking region of the 15-kilodalton (kDa) lipoprotein gene (*tpp*15) that distinguished *T. pallidum* subsp. *pallidum* from *T. pallidum* subsp. *pertenue*.[13] The genome of *T. pallidum* subsp. *pallidum* has been sequenced.[14]

Only *T. pallidum* and possibly *T. pertenue*[15] can cause congenital infection.[16-18] Neither of these organisms has been cultivated successfully in vitro, although the viability and virulence of *T. pallidum* can be maintained for days to weeks in artificial media. A limited degree of replication has been documented, especially in the presence of mammalian cells.[19-21]

The fact that these virulent treponemes cannot be readily cultivated in vitro is, to a great extent, responsible for our incomplete understanding of their properties. The problem of elucidating the biology of *T. pallidum* is further compounded by the relative unavailability of good animal models for the study of syphilitic infection. Atypical lesions develop in guinea pigs after challenge with *T. pallidum*.[16] Vigorously immunosuppressed mice may be susceptible to infection.[22] Aside from primates, however, only the rabbit is readily infected with *T. pallidum*, with development of lesions that resemble those seen in humans, even progressing to secondary infection.

No animal model for tertiary syphilis exists. A nonhuman primate model of central nervous system (CNS) invasion by *T. pallidum* was developed for elucidation of the immune mechanisms responsible for clearance of the organism from the CNS.[23] Initial results demonstrated the participation of locally produced interferon-γ in this process. Rabbit,[24] guinea pig,[25] and hamster[26] models for congenital infection have been described, but the relevance to human congenital syphilis is not yet defined. Vertical transmission of *T. pallidum* to various litters and generations of guinea pigs has been reported,[27] supporting the observation that a woman congenitally infected with syphilis that was never treated is able to transmit the disease to her fetus (third-generation syphilis).

Morphology

T. pallidum varies in size, ranging from 0.10 to 0.18 μm in diameter and from 6 to 20 μm in length, making it below the resolution of the light microscope. These spirochetes can be detected by darkfield microscopy, revealing the characteristic pattern of motion. The organism has pointed ends and lacks the hook shape found in some commensal human spirochetes. Electron microscopy shows wavelike organisms with tapered ends. They have tight, regular spirals with a wavelength of 1.1 μm and amplitude of 0.2 to 0.3 μm.[9,10]

Morphologically, *T. pallidum* consists of an outer membrane that surrounds the endoflagella, cytoplasmic membrane, and protoplasmic cylinder of the organism.[28,29] Three sheathed flagella or axial fibrils emerge from each end of the organism. Although it might seem reasonable to assume that, by analogy to bacterial flagella, the axial fibrils are responsible for motility, their location within the outer membrane and the failure of antiflagellar antibody to immobilize certain spirochetes make this less certain. A glycosaminoglycan layer that has been demonstrated in vitro[19,30,31] may function as an antiphagocytic capsule. Intracytoplasmic tubules are present, but their characteristics and function are as yet undefined.

Composition

The development of polyacrylamide gel electrophoresis techniques allowed characterization of some of the major constituent proteins of *T. pallidum*; 16 major proteins have been described.[30-32] By phase partitioning analysis utilizing the nonionic detergent Triton X-114, integral membrane proteins with apparent molecular masses of 47, 38, 36, 34, 32, 17, and 15 kDa have been identified.[33-40] These proteins, particularly the 47-, 34- and 17-kDa antigens, are proteolipids containing covalently linked fatty acids.[35-37] Cell fractionation studies of *T. pallidum* have demonstrated that the outer membrane consists of a lipid bilayer with a paucity of proteins.[28] Freeze-fracture and freeze-etch electron microscopy studies have provided more direct support for these findings.[38,39] Genomic analysis indicates 22 putative lipoproteins. Potential virulence factors are suggested by the presence of a large number of duplicated genes (tprA through tprL) that encode putative membrane proteins that may function as porins and adhesions.

The complete genome of *T. pallidum* subsp. *pallidum* (Nichols strain) has been sequenced by the whole-genome random sequencing method.[14,41-44] The *T. pallidum* genome is a circular chromosome containing 1,138,006 base pairs with 1041 predicted coding sequences (open reading frames). Systems for DNA replication, transcription, translation, and repair are intact, but catabolic and biosynthetic activities are minimized. Potential virulence factors include a family of 12 potential membrane proteins and several putative hemolysins. Motility-associated genes are highly conserved, consistent with the importance of this activity; 36 genes encode proteins in the flagellar structure.

Metabolism

Most information on of the physiology and metabolism of *T. pallidum* is derived from the Nichols strain, which has been maintained in rabbits since 1912. In the past, *T. pallidum* was regarded as an anaerobe; however, this organism takes up oxygen[45] and degrades glucose aerobically to carbon dioxide and acetate, as well as anaerobically to pyruvate and lactate.[46] Of 22 carbon sources studied, only glucose and pyruvate were metabolized aerobically.[47] *T. pallidum* is better able to incorporate amino acids into proteins in the presence of 10% oxygen under anaerobic conditions.[47] The aerobic capabilities of *T. pallidum* have been substantiated by finding a functional flavoprotein-cytochrome electron transport system[48] and by demonstrating oxygen consumption with oxidative phosphorylation.[49] Studies of in vitro growth of *T. pallidum* generally have found best survival or slight replication, or both, at oxygen atmospheres of 3% to 6%.[50,51] Thus, *T. pallidum* should be considered microaerophilic.

Immunity

Humoral immunity has been a subject of study in syphilis since the serendipitous discovery of antibody to cardiolipin by Wassermann early in this century. By the time patients seek medical attention for primary syphilis, antibodies to *T. pallidum* can be detected by immunofluorescence and hemagglutination techniques in 90% of cases and antibody to cardiolipin in 75% of cases.[58] Western blot techniques show both immunoglobulin M (IgM) and IgG class antibody responses to a wide repertoire of *T. pallidum* proteins,[37] the 47-kDa antigen being the most immunogenic.[45] A small percentage of patients have antibodies that, together with complement, inhibit motility and eliminate infectivity of the organism (*T. pallidum*–immobilizing antibodies).[59,60] Despite this ample evidence for an immune response, syphilis progresses and secondary lesions develop in nearly all patients unless specific therapy is given. *T. pallidum*–immobilizing antibody is present in a majority of patients who have active secondary syphilis,[59] and one could argue either that this antibody is protective, on the verge of controlling the disease, or that it is not protective because active disease is still present. After 1 to 3 months of secondary lesions, spontaneous remission occurs; this condition is called *latency* because the organism persists in lymph and other tissues, and tertiary syphilis may appear at a later date. Moreover, in the preantibiotic era, relapse to active infection occurred in up to 25% of persons who received no treatment after their infection had become latent.[61] Most recurrences occur toward the end of the first year after infection; recurrence is rare after 2 years and presumably does not occur after 4 years. Accordingly, *early latent* syphilis has been designated as being 1 year or less in duration, and *late latent* syphilis as being greater than 1 year in duration. Passive immunization with large amounts of serum from rabbits (that have recovered from experimental infection and are immune to rechallenge with *T. pallidum*) delays and attenuates infection but does not prevent the ultimate development of syphilitic lesions.[62-65] Immune serum facilitates uptake of *T. pallidum* by human polymorphonuclear leukocytes.[66] What remains unclear is why the disease progresses despite abundant evidence for antibody responses; these observations all suggest that humoral immunity is insufficient and that cellular mechanisms play a significant role.

Although an overwhelming majority of treponemes in syphilitic lesions are found in extracellular spaces, treponemes occasionally have been found within macrophages and other cells.[67] Radolf and associates[68] have shown that *T. pallidum* lipoproteins induce macrophages to secrete tumor necrosis factor by a mechanism distinct from that of lipopolysaccharide. The direct interaction of *T. pallidum* with vascular endothelium may be an important early event in the initiation of the host immune response to syphilitic infection[69]; purified 47-kDa lipoprotein can activate human vascular endothelial cells to upregulate the expression of intercellular adhesion molecule-1 and procoagulant activity on its surface.[70] The enhanced adhesiveness and coagulability may result in the fibrin deposition and perivasculitis that are characteristic histopathologic findings in syphilis.

Delayed-type hypersensitivity to treponemal antigens appears late in secondary syphilis and may be related to the onset of latency. Although infection with *T. pallidum* stimulates acquired cellular resistance,[71] infection with unrelated organisms such as *Mycobacterium bovis* (bacille Calmette-Guérin) or *Propionibacterium acnes* does not protect animals against challenge with *T. pallidum*.[72-74] Schell and associates, however, have transferred resistance to infection with *T. pallidum* strain Bosnia by transfusing T cells from immune hamsters.[75] T lymphocytes responsive to *T. pallidum* appear in syphilitic lesions as the number of treponemes decreases,[76] which gives further evidence, albeit circumstantial, for a role of cellular immunity in controlling infection.

Some findings suggest that immune responses may be impaired early in syphilis. In early syphilis, (1) in vitro blastogenic transformation of lymphocytes after stimulation with a variety of antigens is depressed[67]; (2) paracortical (thymus-dependent) areas of lymph nodes are depleted[77,78]; (3) delayed hypersensitivity to several antigens may be depressed[79,80]; and (4) ability to produce IgG in response to sensitization with sheep red blood cells (a T cell–dependent antigen) is markedly inhibited.[81,82] On the other hand, some authorities believe that the evolution of immunity is slow, albeit for unknown reasons, but that suppression of immunity is not responsible.[36]

It is even possible that true immunity to *T. pallidum* does not exist. Active lesions may be brought under control and animals may become resistant to rechallenge with *T. pallidum*, but the host is unable to rid itself completely of the infecting organism, which persists in lymph nodes. Premunition, resistance to rechallenge, or, in the case of syphilis, a "chancre-fast" state without biologic cure may best describe this situation. It is known that persons with untreated secondary syphilis or true latent infection are resistant to rechallenge with *T. pallidum*, as are those with untreated congenital syphilis.[83]

Some observations from studies of congenital syphilis helped to contribute to the understanding of immunity. Nineteenth-century physicians knew that a degree of maternal immunity is acquired during infection. Nabarro[84] observed that an infected infant did not infect the mother's breast. Paré speculated that an infant who acquired the infection from a syphilitic wet nurse could pass infection to the mother through contact with contagious lesions.[3] In 1846, Kassowitz observed that the longer syphilis exists untreated in a woman before pregnancy occurs, the more likely it is that when she does become pregnant, her treponemes will be held in check, and the less likely it is that her fetus will die in utero or be born with congenital syphilis; this observation is called *Kassowitz's law*.[8,84]

It remains unclear what factors determine which mothers, particularly those in the latent stage of infection, will pass disease to their fetuses. It also is not clear why some infants who are infected in utero are born without any clinical manifestations, with the subsequent development of overt disease in the first weeks or months of life or even later at puberty.

Modern immunology has only recently started to pay attention to the problem of congenital syphilis. As would be suspected by transplacental transfer of immunoglobulin, the IgG levels of infected infants largely match those of the mother. Moreover, by immunoblotting, the IgG reactivity of infant sera is indistinguishable from that of the mother, again indicating the transplacental nature of the IgG antibodies.[85-88] The range of IgM antibody responses to the proteins of *T. pallidum* in the sera of overtly infected newborns is comparable to that for disseminated (secondary) infection in adults.[85] The IgM response of the infant, however, is distinct from that of the mother and is uniformly directed against the 47-kDa membrane lipoprotein antigen.[85,86,88]

TRANSMISSION

Humans are the natural host of *T. pallidum*. Sexual contact is almost exclusively the mode of transmission. Rarely is the disease passed to health care workers or others who accidentally come into contact with infectious lesions or to laboratory personnel who handle infected animals. The newborn infant typically is infected in utero by transplacental passage of *T. pallidum* from an infected, untreated or inadequately treated mother, but the newborn also can be infected following contact with an active genital lesion at delivery. In utero transmission has been supported by isolation of the organism from umbilical cord blood and amniotic fluid,[88-90] detection of spirochetes in the placenta and umbilical cord with associated typical histopathologic changes,[91,92] and detection of IgM to *T. pallidum* in neonatal serum obtained at birth.[85-88] Lucas and associates[90] reported that *T. pallidum* can be isolated from approximately 74% of amniotic fluid samples from women with early syphilis; it is possible that *T. pallidum* can infect the fetus by traversing the fetal membranes to reach the amniotic fluid, resulting in fetal infection. Alternatively, infection may occur from contact with an infectious lesion during passage through the birth canal.[1,84] Centuries ago, when it was common for infants to be fed by a wet nurse, small epidemics of syphilis sometimes were caused by an infectious lesion on the nipple of the wet nurse. No recent data indicate that breast milk is associated with transmission of *T. pallidum*.

The risk of syphilis to the fetus or infant appears to vary considerably by interval when the mother acquired syphilis.[93,94] In 1951, Ingraham[94] described 220 women who had untreated early syphilis (up to 4 years duration); 41% of their infants were born alive and had congenital syphilis, 25% were stillborn, 14% died in the neonatal period, 21% weighed less than 2.3 kg at birth but had no evidence of congenital syphilis, and only 18% were healthy infants born at term gestation. By contrast, only 2% of infants born to 82 mothers with untreated late syphilis (longer than 4 years' duration) had congenital syphilis. Fiumara and colleagues[93] stated that when primary or secondary maternal syphilis went untreated, half of the infants were premature, stillborn, or died as neonates, and congenital syphilis developed in the other half; the chance of the mother's giving birth to a healthy full-term infant was very small. In the case of early latent syphilis, 20% to 60% of the infants were healthy, 20% were premature, and 16% were stillborn; 4% died as neonates, and 40% had congenital syphilis. In the case of untreated late syphilis, about 70% of the infants were healthy, 10% were stillborn, and approximately 9% were premature; about 1% died as neonates, and 10% had congenital syphilis.[93]

Recent data indicate that among women with untreated early syphilis, 40% of pregnancies result in spontaneous abortion, stillbirth, or perinatal death.[95] Infection can be transmitted to the fetus at any stage of disease, but the rate ranges from 60% to 100% during primary or secondary syphilis and slowly decreases with time. In a prospective cohort analysis of 428 women with untreated syphilis from 1988 to 1998, untreated primary syphilis at delivery resulted in a transmission rate of 29% (3% stillbirths and 26% live births with congenital syphilis). Untreated secondary syphilis at delivery resulted in congenital infection in 59% of the infants (20% stillborn, 39% live-born), whereas with early latent disease, the transmission rate was 50% (17% stillborn, 33% live-born). On the other hand, maternal late latent infection resulted in 5% stillbirths and only 8% live births with congenital syphilis.[96]

These statistical estimates put Kassowitz's law into epidemiologic terms. An interesting family study illustrating this law described a syphilitic mother who had five pregnancies resulting in eight children.[97] The first pregnancy produced a stillborn child; the second a full-term infant with congenital syphilis; the third, triplets, two of whom had congenital syphilis; the fourth, twins, one of whom had congenital syphilis; and the fifth, a healthy full-term infant. Although in keeping with Kassowitz's law, the effect of syphilis on the fetus was less severe with each succeeding pregnancy, the sobering point is that the mother, whose syphilis had escaped detection and treatment during the time she was delivering the syphilitic infants, was able to transmit congenital syphilis over the span of a decade. Two unusual aspects of this report are the unavailability of data to identify during which pregnancy the mother became infected and the fact that the diagnosis of infection in the parents occurred 4 years after the fifth pregnancy.

A majority of infants born to mothers with untreated or inadequately treated syphilis have no clinical or laboratory evidence of infection at birth. Nevertheless, manifestations of disease can develop a few weeks, months, or years later if these infants go untreated. The exact pathogenesis of this "late-onset" type of infection is unknown.

The effect of concurrent maternal infection with *T. pallidum* and human immunodeficiency virus (HIV) on the risk of fetal infection with *T. pallidum* and HIV is not fully understood.[98-100] Cellular immune dysfunction associated with HIV infection may permit a greater degree of treponemal proliferation and lead to a higher rate of fetal infection. HIV-infected women who acquire syphilis during pregnancy may not respond adequately to currently recommended benzathine penicillin therapy, thereby increasing the risk of fetal infection with *T. pallidum*.[101] Preliminary studies by Sanchez[98] indicate that infants born to co-infected mothers with early syphilis are significantly more likely to have clinical or laboratory evidence of congenital syphilis at delivery than infants born to women with early syphilis without HIV infection. Alternatively, untreated syphilis during a pregnancy complicated by maternal HIV may result in an increased risk of fetal HIV infection by producing a placentitis, allowing transmission of the virus from the maternal to fetal circulation.[99] The finding by Theus and colleagues[102] that virulent *T. pallidum* can directly promote the induction of HIV gene expression in macrophages, possibly resulting in increased systemic HIV levels with more rapid progression of the HIV infection, supports the notion of possible increased vertical transmission of HIV from a co-infected mother to the fetus.

T. pallidum is present in open, moist mucocutaneous lesions of primary or secondary syphilis, as well as in body fluids such as blood and cerebrospinal fluid (CSF), of infected infants. Health care workers should observe standard precautions when caring for infected infants, and infants and adults with infectious lesions should be placed in contact isolation for the first 24 hours of therapy. Once antimicrobial therapy has been initiated, the risk of transmission is virtually nonexistent because penicillin in sufficient dosage causes a complete disappearance of viable treponemes from syphilitic lesions within a few hours.[103] *T. pallidum* does not survive well outside the host and is easily killed by heat, drying, and soap and water.[104,105]

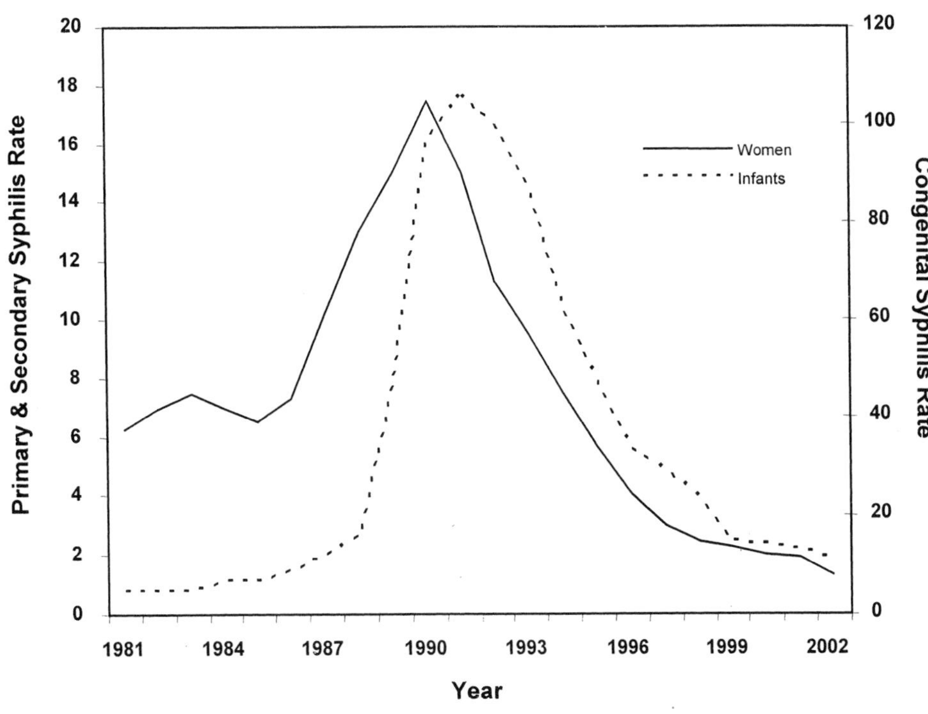

Figure 18–1 Rates of congenital syphilis among infants (per 100,000 live-born infants) and primary and secondary syphilis among women (per 100,000 population) by year in the United States, 1981 to 2002. (From Centers for Disease Control and Prevention. Congenital syphilis—United States, 2002. MMWR Morb Mortal Wkly Rep 53:717, 2004.)

EPIDEMIOLOGY

Early treatments for syphilis included mercury, first used in 1497; arsphenamine; other heavy metals; and malaria inoculation for paretic cases.[106] The breakthrough in treatment came in 1943 when Mahoney and colleagues[107] successfully used penicillin to treat primary syphilis in four patients. Because of the exquisite susceptibility of *T. pallidum* to penicillin, it was believed that use of this antimicrobial agent would lead to the virtual disappearance of syphilis. Indeed, a dramatic decline in the number of cases did occur, the incidence reaching a low point in the mid-1950s. Unfortunately, often when a disease approaches eradication, the control program rather than the disease is eradicated. As the incidence of syphilis decreased remarkably, the funding allocated for syphilis control was drastically reduced. By the early 1960s, the disease was resurgent, and more resources were again committed to control efforts. The incidence of syphilis subsequently declined in the 1970s, only to increase dramatically in the 1980s.[108,109] From 1986 to 1991, a steady increase was observed in the incidence of primary and secondary syphilis among women in the United States (Fig. 18-1).[98] This increase was greatest among blacks and Hispanic Americans in large urban centers such as New York City, Detroit, Miami, and Los Angeles.[108,110-112] The exchange of illegal drugs, particularly "crack cocaine," for sex with multiple partners appears to play a major role in the transmission of syphilis.[108,110,113-115] Because the identities of sexual partners often are unknown among persons trading sex for drugs, partner notification, a traditional syphilis control strategy, is virtually impossible. Other factors implicated in the dramatic increase of syphilis included a reduction in resources for syphilis control programs that are coordinated in sexually transmitted disease clinics of local public health departments,[116,117] as well as the use of spectinomycin for treatment of infections due to penicillinase-producing *Neisseria gonorrhoeae*, because spectinomycin is not effective against incubating syphilis.[118,119]

Between 1991 and 1996, the incidence of primary and secondary syphilis in the United States decreased by 86% (see Fig. 18-1). Several factors contributed to this significant decrease.[120-126] Awareness of the syphilis epidemic of the late 1980s has led to wider screening practices and identification of infected persons. Increased state and federal resources were invested in syphilis control programs for traditional (e.g., partner notification, clinical services) and nontraditional (e.g., community-based screening, outreach and risk-reduction counseling) activities.[121,122] These programs helped identify particular locations with a high prevalence of syphilis and with core populations at high risk for infection.[121,122] The recognition of these demographics allowed presumptive treatment of syphilis based on epidemiologic indications. Other reasons for the decline included a decrease in crack cocaine use and exchange of sex for drugs, major contributors to the epidemic, as well as the introduction of HIV prevention programs that target prevention of other sexually transmitted diseases. The development of acquired immunity to syphilis that occurred among high-risk populations when syphilis was more prevalent also may have played a role. In addition, changing the treatment recommendation for other STDs to ceftriaxone could have treated incubating syphilis.[124] By 1997, the incidence of reported cases of syphilis had fallen to the lowest ever reported, a rate of 3.2 cases per 100,000 persons.

Despite this decline, syphilis remains endemic in the United States.[123,124] Syphilis is a reportable disease; the number of reported cases of primary and secondary syphilis has varied, ranging between 6999 and greater than 45,000 cases per year,[125,126] although it is estimated that only about 1 of every 3 cases is reported.[127] Differences across race and gender have been reported. African American and Hispanic races are strong markers for syphilis seroreactivity.[128] In 1998, the rate (number of cases per 100,000 population) of primary and secondary syphilis was substantially higher among blacks (17.1) than among Native American Indians or Alaskan Natives (2.8), Hispanic Americans (1.5), non-Hispanic whites (0.5), and Asians/Pacific Islanders (0.4).[126] People who live in "inner cities" on the East Coast and in the rural South[129] bear a disproportionate burden. In 1998, the rate of primary and secondary syphilis was higher in the South (5.1) than in the Midwest (1.9), West (1.0), and Northeast (0.8).[126,130] In fact, a majority of the total reported cases of primary and secondary syphilis occurred in the southeastern United States, which contains only 19% of the total U.S. population.[120]

Moreover, focal outbreaks of primary and secondary syphilis continue to occur, and these have been associated with illicit drug use, exchange of sex for drugs or money, and in certain groups of homosexual men with multiple partners.[126,129] Attention also has focused on the induced migration that results when public housing projects are dismantled and infected persons move to less impoverished areas that surround the inner city; this results in infection of new sexual partners, who often lack a history of drug use. These continuing outbreaks are disconcerting because cyclic national epidemics have occurred every 7 to 10 years; they underscore the need for syphilis elimination rather than enhanced control.[128]

Worldwide, syphilis remains a considerable public health problem, particularly in Eastern Europe and in the developing countries of Africa and Latin America.[131] In countries such as those of the former Soviet Union, the increase in syphilis has been related to changes in sexual behavior and in the patterns of provisions, use, and effectiveness of diagnostic treatment and contact tracing services.[132] In South America, the problem of syphilis and congenital syphilis only now is being unraveled. In a study in Buenos Aires, 10% of women with reactive serologic tests for syphilis had a history of stillbirth that was believed to be caused by syphilis.[133] In Bolivia, 26% of women in 1996 who were delivered of stillborn infants had syphilis, compared with only 4% of mothers of live-born infants.[134]

Nonetheless, in the United States, expectations currently are heightened for the possibility of the eventual control and elimination of endemic syphilis.[128] In 1998, the rate of primary and secondary syphilis declined to 2.6 cases per 100,000 population, the lowest rate ever reported in the United States.[126] No cases were reported in 78% of U.S. counties, and 90% of the counties had 4 or fewer cases per 100,000 population, reaching the Healthy People 2000 national objective. Moreover, syphilis today is occurring in fewer geographic areas, with 50% of new syphilis cases reported from less than 1% of U.S. counties. Because of these findings, the Centers for Disease Control and Prevention (CDC) has developed a National Plan for Elimination of Syphilis from the United States.[126,128] The CDC has defined syphilis elimination as the absence of sustained transmission. The national goal for syphilis elimination is to reduce primary and secondary syphilis cases to 1000 or less (rate: 0.4 per 100,000 population) and to increase the number of syphilis-free counties to 90% by 2005. The plan focuses on five key strategies: (1) enhanced community involvement and partnerships at local, state, and national levels; (2) intensified surveillance; (3) rapid outbreak response; (4) expanded access to health care for persons infected with or exposed to syphilis; and (5) improved health promotion.

Gestational syphilis primarily affects women who are young, unmarried, and of low socioeconomic status and who receive inadequate prenatal care.[112,135] The incidence of congenital syphilis closely correlates with that of primary and secondary disease in women; it is not surprising that the incidence of congenital syphilis increased dramatically in the late 1980s, coincident with the rise in early syphilis among women of childbearing age.

The dramatic increase in the number of cases of congenital syphilis in 1990 to 1991 was due both to an increase in actual cases and to the use of revised reporting guidelines beginning in 1989, which broadened the surveillance definition for congenital syphilis.[108,136,137] Previous criteria for reporting cases of congenital syphilis were based on a clinical case definition.[138] A "confirmed case" was that of an infant or stillborn infant in whom *T. pallidum* was identified with darkfield microscopy or specific stains in specimens from lesions. A "presumptive case" was that of an infant or a stillborn infant who had a reactive test for syphilis and abnormalities on physical examination and on long bone radiographs, a reactive CSF Venereal Disease Research Laboratory (VDRL) test, an elevated CSF cell count or protein concentration without another cause, a nontreponemal serologic titer that was four times higher than that of the mother's, or, in the live-born infant, persistence of a reactive treponemal test beyond the age of 1 year. In 1989, a new surveillance case definition for reporting congenital syphilis was approved by the CDC (Table 18-1).[108] *Congenital syphilis* then included all cases in infants with clinical evidence of active syphilis, as well as infants without clinical manifestations and stillborn infants born to women with untreated or inadequately treated syphilis. Use of these guidelines increased the number of reported cases of congenital syphilis almost fourfold,[98,139,140] although clearly some cases were reported that actually were not infections. This current definition acknowledges the public health burden of the disease, because these infants require medical and public health interventions.

The persistence of congenital syphilis despite the wide availability of effective penicillin therapy has prompted close scrutiny of those cases still occurring. Mascola and associates[141] reviewed 50 Texas cases of congenital syphilis reported during 1 year for epidemiologic characteristics that might have led to their prevention. Their findings, including unpublished observations of 659 cases (C Beck-Sague, A Hadgu, L Frau, et al, unpublished data), are summarized in Table 18-2. Similar data have been reported from Miami,[110] Detroit,[111] and New York.[142,143] Lack of prenatal care was, by far, the single most important cause. Congenital syphilis is preventable, but only if prenatal care is available to, as well as sought by, those often hard-to-reach groups that are most at risk, such as teenage and/or unwed mothers, drug users, women who are sexually promiscuous, and members of disadvantaged minority groups (Table 18-3). Syphilis needs to be considered and ruled out with serologic tests in the first trimester of all pregnancies and with additional screenings at the beginning of the third trimester (28 weeks) and at delivery for mothers who live in areas with high incidences of infection.[108,112,135,139,144,145]

Table 18–1 Surveillance Case Definitions for Congenital Syphilis

A *confirmed case* of congenital syphilis is that in an infant in whom *Treponema pallidum* is identified by darkfield microscopy, fluorescent antibody testing, or use of other specific stains in specimens from lesions, placenta, umbilical cord, amniotic fluid, or autopsy material.

A *presumptive case* of congenital syphilis is that in either of the following:

A. Any infant whose mother had untreated or inadequately treated[a] syphilis at delivery, regardless of findings in the infant; OR

B. Any infant or child who has a reactive treponemal test for syphilis AND any one of the following:

1. Any evidence of congenital syphilis on physical examination; OR
2. Any evidence of congenital syphilis on long bone radiographs; OR
3. Reactive CSF VDRL test; OR
4. Elevated CSF cell count or protein content (without other defined cause); OR
5. Quantitative nontreponemal serologic titers that are four times higher than the mother's (both specimens drawn at time of birth)

A *syphilitic stillbirth* is defined as a death of a fetus weighing greater than 500 g or having reached a gestational age of greater than 20 weeks when the mother had untreated or inadequately treated syphilis.

[a]Inadequate treatment consists of any nonpenicillin therapy or penicillin therapy given less than 30 days before delivery.

CSF, cerebrospinal fluid; VDRL, Venereal Disease Research Laboratory.

Adapted from Centers for Disease Control and Prevention. Congenital syphilis, New York City, 1986-1988. MMWR Morb Mortal Wkly Rep 38:825, 1989.

Table 18–2 Factors Contributing to Occurrence of Congenital Syphilis

Factor	No. of Cases	% of Total
No prenatal care, STS result positive at delivery	301	46
Prenatal care received, STS result negative at first trimester, not repeated	96	15
No STS performed during prenatal care	27	4
Negative result on maternal STS at delivery	44	7
Laboratory error in testing	2	0.3
Delay in treatment	50	8
Prenatal treatment failures	95	14
Insufficient data	36	6
Other	8	1
TOTAL	659	

STS, serologic test for syphilis.

Data from Mascola L, Pelosi R, Blout JH, et al. Congenital syphilis. Why is it still occurring? JAMA 252:1719-1722, 1984 and C Beck-Sagne et al, unpublished data.

Table 18–3 Epidemiologic Factors Associated with High Risk for Syphilis Exposure

- Being an unmarried or teenage mother
- Inadequate or no prenatal care
- Illicit drug use in the mother or sexual partner
- Multiple sexual partners
- History of sexually transmitted disease[a]
- Sexual contact with anyone known to have a sexually transmitted disease[a]
- Racial/ethnic minority mothers of low socioeconomic status

[a]Including human immunodeficiency virus infection.

The CDC has identified factors contributing to the occurrence of congenital syphilis in 2002.[146] From 2000 to 2002 the rate of congenital syphilis decreased 21%, from 14.2 to 11.2 cases per 100,000 population. Primary and secondary syphilis rates among women during this same interval declined 35.3%, from 1.7 to 1.1 cases per 100,000. Thus, every year since 1991, congenital syphilis rates and primary and secondary syphilis rates in women have declined (see Fig. 18-1). Furthermore, congenital syphilis rates declined in all ethnic minority populations; rates declined 50.6% among Native American Indian/Alaskan Natives, 22.4% among Hispanic Americans, 21.4% among Asians/Pacific Islanders and 19.8% among non-Hispanic black infants. Rates also decreased in every region of the United States except the Northeast, where the rate increased by 0.9%. In 2002, only 4.4% of U.S. countries reported cases of congenital syphilis, compared with 5.4% in 2000.

Among the 451 cases of congenital syphilis reported during 2002, 333 (73.8%) occurred because the mother received either no penicillin or inadequate treatment before or during pregnancy (Fig. 18-2).[146] In 130 cases (28.8%), the mother received no prenatal care. Of the 288 mothers who received prenatal care, 86 initiated care during the first trimester, 93 during the second trimester, and 59 during the third trimester; 30.5% of the those initiating care in the third trimester did so less than 30 days before delivery. Of the 451 infants with congenital syphilis, 18 (4%) were stillborn, and 8 (1.8%) died within 30 days of delivery (overall case-fatality ratio, 5.8%). These mortality data represent a modest improvement from those reported from 1982 to 1998 by Gust and colleagues.[147] In that study, the case-fatality ratio was 6.4% (stillborns and neonatal deaths) for 14,627 infants with congenital syphilis. More than half of the deaths occurred when the infant was born before 30 weeks of gestation. Also, an inverse relationship was noted between number of prenatal visits and risk of fatal outcome.[147]

Several investigators have called attention to problems with antenatal management and communication crucial to the prevention of congenital syphilis.[148,149] These problems include failure to (1) obtain an appropriate and complete maternal history, (2) perform routine screening at appropriate times during the pregnancy, (3) correctly interpret

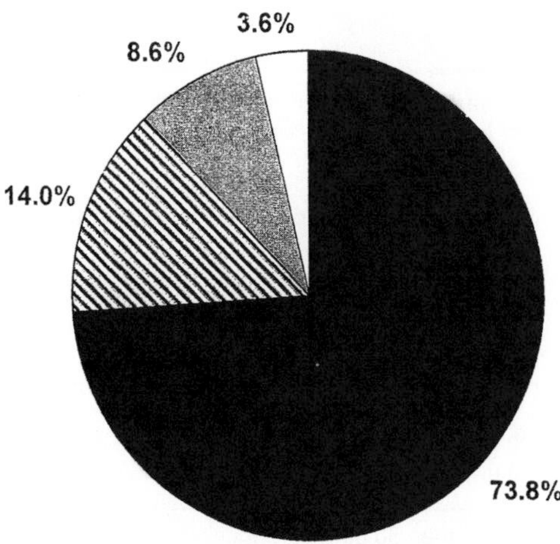

Figure 18–2 Diagnosis of congenital syphilis (CS) in the United States, 2002. (From Centers for Disease Control and Prevention. Congenital syphilis—United States, 2002. MMWR Morb Mortal Wkly Rep 53:717, 2004.)

serologic results, (4) recognize signs of maternal syphilis, (5) provide treatment for the pregnant sexual partner of an acutely infected man, and (6) communicate pertinent maternal history and results of screening tests to the infant's health care practitioner. Local health departments and clinicians must improve the exchange of information between obstetric and pediatric services. These issues further underscore the need for education of health care providers on the management of sexually transmitted diseases.

Sexually transmitted infections potentially threaten everyone regardless of demographic probabilities. As shown in Table 18-2, 44 cases occurred in women who were incubating syphilis at the time of delivery, which highlights the limitation of the screening serologic tests to detect early cases. Serologic tests are poor diagnostic tools during the incubation or early primary stage of syphilis. During those times, results of the nontreponemal (rapid plasma reagin [RPR] or VDRL) tests may not show reactivity because reactivity occurs 4 to 8 weeks after the infection is acquired and several days to 1 week after the development of a chancre.[150,151] In primary syphilis, nonreactivity on nontreponemal testing is reported to occur in one fourth to one third of cases.[152,153] Nonreactivity on the microhemagglutination–*T. pallidum* (MHA-TP) assay and the fluorescent treponemal antibody (FTA) test occurs in as many as 36% and 18% of cases of primary syphilis, respectively.[155] A prenatal prevention strategy that uses only currently available serologic tests, therefore, cannot eliminate all congenital syphilis,[155] and contact tracing of sexual partners, careful physical examination of women in labor for evidence of primary syphilis, and additional testing of postpartum women at 4 weeks after delivery will be necessary.[98,120,156,157] Moreover, if a woman with an infant younger than 1 year is diagnosed with early syphilis, that infant should be evaluated serologically and receive appropriate treatment.[156]

PATHOLOGY AND PATHOGENESIS

Controversy about the pathogenesis of congenital syphilis is ongoing. Historically, it was taught that infection of the fetus by a syphilitic mother could not occur before the fifth month of pregnancy, because pathologic changes in fetal tissue could not be demonstrated before this point in gestation. It was thought that the Langhans' cell layer of the cytotrophoblast formed a placental barrier against *T. pallidum* invasion of the fetus.[158,159] This theory was disproved by the electron microscopic demonstration of persistence of the Langhans' cell layer throughout pregnancy.[160] Moreover, using silver stains and immunofluorescence techniques, Harter and Benirschke[161] demonstrated spirochetes in fetal tissue from spontaneous abortions at 9 and 10 weeks of gestation. Infectivity testing that would have proved the presence of *T. pallidum* conclusively was not performed by these investigators, however. The lack of pathologic changes in fetal tissues earlier than the fifth month of pregnancy could be a result of fetal immunoincompetence during early gestation.[162] Moreover, viable spirochetes in amniotic fluid obtained by amniocentesis from a woman with early syphilis have been reported as early as 14 weeks of gestation, proving that the fetus can be exposed to *T. pallidum* early in pregnancy.[163]

Pathologic changes in congenital syphilis are similar to those that occur in acquired syphilis, except for the absence of a primary or chancre stage. Because infection involves the placenta[164] and spreads hematogenously to the fetus, widespread involvement is characteristic. No matter which organ is involved, the essential microscopic appearance of lesions is that of perivascular infiltration of lymphocytes, plasma cells, and histiocytes, with obliterative endarteritis and extensive fibrosis.[165-167] These typical histopathologic features of the inflammatory response to invasion by *T. pallidum* in tissues and blood vessels suggest an important role for cytokines as mediators of immunopathogenesis during syphilis.[68] Radolf and associates[68] have shown that *T. pallidum* lipoproteins induce macrophages to secrete tumor necrosis factor, as well as to activate vascular endothelium.

In addition, Brightbill and colleagues[168] have shown that the 47-kDa lipoprotein of *T. pallidum* induced production of interleukin-12 (IL-12) messenger RNA from human macrophages, a key signal of the innate immune system. The spirochete also has been shown to activate human promyelomonocytic cell line THP-1 cells in a CD14-dependent manner.[169] These findings lend further support to the concept that lipoproteins are the principal components of intact spirochetes and that they are responsible for monocyte activation, indicating that surface exposure of lipoproteins is an important determinant of a spirochetal pathogen's proinflammatory capacity.

Placenta

The infected placenta is larger, thicker, and paler than normal.[170] Histopathologic examination of the placenta, especially if unexpectedly large, and of the umbilical cord is a useful adjunct for the diagnosis of congenital syphilis.[112,170-175] The histologic features consist of focal villositis with endovascular and perivascular proliferation and relative immaturity of the villi, which become enlarged and hypercellular and have bullous projections[171,172]; these larger villi, with respect to the amount of blood in the capillaries, are the cause of the pallor. Sheffield and colleagues[175] have correlated villous enlargement as well as placental erythroblastosis with stillbirth due to congenital syphilis. In addition, an increased amount of connective tissue surrounds the capillaries and also makes up the stroma.

Treponemes are demonstrable with silver stains,[164,171,172] although tissue membrane artifacts may in fact be difficult to distinguish from these organisms. Necrotizing funisitis, a deeply seated inflammatory process within the matrix of the umbilical cord, has been associated with congenital syphilis and can provide a diagnostic clue to its presence at birth.[173-175] Spirochetes have been identified within the umbilical cord lesions by silver stain. Bromberg and co-workers[176] have detected *T. pallidum* in umbilical specimens by an immunofluorescent antigen detection assay (IFA). Using polymerase chain reaction (PCR) assay to detect *T. pallidum* DNA, Genest and colleagues[91] confirmed the strong association between the placental histopathologic features (enlarged hypercellular villi, proliferative fetal vascular changes, and acute or chronic villitis) and congenital syphilis and suggested that PCR assay may identify additional cases of histologically unidentified congenital syphilis.

The Fetus and Newborn

A stillborn syphilitic infant often has a macerated appearance, with a collapsed skull and protuberant abdomen. The skin shows vesicular or bullous lesions, which have a fluid rich in treponemes. Guarner and associates[177] reported that a constant feature throughout the tissues was concentric macrophage (CD68-positive) infiltrate around vessels, giving an onionskin appearance. Immunohistochemical analyses have identified macrophages as the prime immune response to congenital syphilis. The liver and spleen are enlarged and show fibrosis and extramedullary hematopoiesis.[178] Roentgenographs of long bones show evidence of osteochondritis and periostitis.[179]

A divergence of opinion exists as to the nature and extent of hepatic involvement in congenital syphilis. The traditional view has been that diffuse interstitial inflammation is present and can progress to disrupt the normal hepatic architecture by extensive scarring.[180,181] Oppenheimer and Hardy[178] found that 15 of 16 livers from infants who died before 9 weeks of age were abnormal; lesions varied considerably in severity but included inflammation in the interstitial stroma and perivascular network, especially in the area of the portal triads, with diffuse hepatitis and excessive extramedullary hematopoiesis.[178] When Wright and Berry[182] reviewed liver sections from which Nabarro[84] had previously described intercellular fibrosis, they found that 50 of 59 sections stained with hematoxylin and eosin were histologically normal, although silver stains revealed heavy infiltration with treponemes. The discrepancies in the observations of these workers may be related to the different ages of the patients and the severity of the infections. The patients described by Wright and Berry were as old as 1 year of age. Rarely, gummas have been described in the liver in infants with congenital syphilis; cirrhosis appears to be an uncommon complication.[178] The spleen is enlarged because of an extensive nonspecific inflammatory reaction[183]; it also demonstrates extramedullary hematopoiesis.

The "pneumonia alba" of congenital syphilis is characterized grossly by yellowish white, heavy, firm, and grossly enlarged lungs.[167,183] A marked increase in the amount of connective tissue in the interalveolar septa and the interstitium associated with collapse and loss of alveolar spaces explains the increased weight and density of the lung. This obliterative fibrosis of the lung is now reported only rarely,[178] most probably owing to treatment of mothers earlier in gestation.

Attention has been called to the unique submucosal inflammation and fibrosis of the gastrointestinal tract in infants who died during the first 2 months of life.[178] An initial mucosal and submucosal infiltration with mononuclear cells is associated with a striking submucosal fibroblastic proliferation, resulting in a remarkable increase in the width of the submucosa. These changes are found more often in the small intestine than in the colon and stomach.[177,184] An intense pancreatitis[178] is present, with a perivascular inflammatory infiltrate, obliteration of ductules and acini, reduction in the number of islets, and extensive fibrosis.

Renal involvement appears to be the consequence of injury to the glomeruli by immune complex deposition,[185] just as has been described for the glomerulitis of secondary syphilis in adults.[186] An epimembranous glomerulopathy[187] is common and is associated with two different forms of immune complex injury, one involving complement deposition in addition to IgA, IgM, and IgG and the other involving immune complexes without complement deposition along the basement membrane.[185] A perivascular inflammatory infiltrate, consisting of plasma cells and lymphocytes involving the interstitial tissues, is prominent. The visceral and parietal epithelial cells of the glomeruli are swollen and increased in number. Increased matrix, collagen, and cells broaden axial regions in each tuft. Numerous electron-dense nodular deposits are noted on the epithelial aspect of the thickened glomerular basement membrane.[185,187] Elution studies have demonstrated the presence of antitreponemal antibodies in the eluate and of treponemal antigen in the eluted sections.[188] A seemingly more rare proliferative glomerulonephritis also has been described, with mesangioendothelial proliferation and crescent formation.[189]

The neuropathologic features of congenital syphilis are comparable with those of acquired syphilis, except that the parenchymatous processes (general paresis, tabes dorsalis) that were infrequently described in the older literature now are extremely rare.[190] Meningeal involvement is apparent as a discoloration and thickening of the basilar meninges,[167,190] especially around the brain stem and the optic chiasm. Microscopically, endarteritis typically is present; depending on the severity and chronicity of the infection as well as on the blood vessels involved, various degrees of neuronal injury can ensue. As the infection resolves, fibrosis can occur, with formation of adhesions that obliterate the subarachnoid space, leading to an obstructive hydrocephalus or to a variety of cranial nerve palsies.[190] Interstitial inflammation and fibrosis of the anterior lobe of the pituitary gland, at times accompanied by focal necrosis, also have been reported among infants with congenital syphilis.[191] The posterior lobe remains unaffected. An evolving anterior pituitary gumma was noted at autopsy in a 3-day-old infant with congenital syphilis that did not respond to treatment.[192]

Widespread involvement of bones is characteristic of congenital syphilis. Osteochondritis, periostitis, and osteomyelitis are present, especially in the long bones and ribs. The osteochondritis is recognized grossly by the presence of a moderate and irregular yellow line in the zone of provisional calcification.[193] The trabeculae are irregular, discontinuous, and variable in size and shape. The excessive fibrosis occurring at the osseous-cartilaginous junction is referred to as syphilitic granulation tissue and contains numerous blood vessels surrounded by the inflammatory infiltrate.[167,194,195] The characteristic saw-toothed appearance described historically is now uncommonly found in radiographs[196]; however, xeroradiography of long bones of stillborn infants with congenital syphilis often demonstrates this classic pattern,[179] which is produced by irregularity in the provisional zone of calcification, corresponding to an irregularity in growth of capillaries. Small islands of cartilage may persist in the ossified bone.[178]

A subperiosteal deposit of osteoid, which can completely encircle the shaft of the long bone, is a feature of the periostitis.[84,197] An associated osteomyelitis (osteitis) usually is present and, when it involves the long bones, is called *diaphysitis*.[196] Microscopically, an inflammatory infiltrate with erosion of the trabeculae and prominent fibrosis is seen.[196] In the skull, the periosteal reaction eventually can lead to the radiographic feature of frontal bossing. The basic process of the osseous disturbance seems to involve a failure to convert cartilage in the normal sequence to mature bone. Controversy about the pathogenesis of these bone changes has been ongoing for years.[186,198] One view is that they are specific results of local infection by the spirochete; the other is that they represent nonspecific trophic changes on endochondral bone formation caused by severe generalized disease. The fact that they heal without specific antibiotic therapy tends to favor the latter view.

Pathologic observations do not provide a basis for hematologic manifestations of congenital syphilis, which are thought to reflect physiologic changes of unknown pathogenesis (discussed later in the chapter). Adequate numbers of megakaryocytes are present.[199] Severe anemia initially represents an acute hemolytic process, compounded by splenomegaly and excessive cellular destruction. This is followed by a chronic progressive anemia, accentuated by physiologic marrow hypoplasia.[200]

CLINICAL MANIFESTATIONS

General Considerations

The spectrum of perinatal syphilis is similar in many ways to that of other infections in which the infecting organism spreads hematogenously from the pregnant woman to involve the placenta and infect the fetus. The extent of damage to the fetus presumably depends on the stage of development when infection occurs and elapsed time before treatment. With early infection and in the absence of therapy, miscarriage, stillbirth, premature delivery, or neonatal death can occur.[84,94,95,147,164,170,201-203] Infection can be clinically recognizable or silent at birth; if the infection goes untreated, its expression is delayed for several months to years.[159,204,205]

Congenital syphilis has been divided somewhat arbitrarily into early and late stages.[166] Clinical manifestations appearing within the first 2 years of life are designated *early*, and those occurring after this time are called *late*. The clinical manifestations of early congenital syphilis are a direct result of active infection and inflammation. The clinical manifestations of late congenital syphilis represent the scars induced by initial lesions of early congenital syphilis or reactions to persistent and ongoing inflammation. These so-called stigmata of late congenital syphilis reflect the delayed expression of a prenatal insult in a fashion comparable with the occurrence of deafness beyond infancy that is related to congenital rubella.[206]

Syphilis in the Pregnant Woman

Clinical manifestations of acquired syphilis[131,135] are not altered by pregnancy. Genital chancres, the principal manifestation of primary infection, occur about 3 weeks after contact. They often are unrecognized in women because they cause no symptoms, and their location within the vagina or on the cervix, labia, or the perineum makes detection difficult. Extragenital chancres can occur (e.g., lips, tongue, tonsil, nipple, finger, anus). Syphilitic chancres are painless, clearly demarcated ulcers 0.5 to 2 cm in diameter and generally associated with enlargement of the regional lymph nodes. Multiple lesions are not uncommon.[207] Because these lesions are painless and may be hidden, the diagnosis of primary syphilis in women often is not made until the secondary or latent stage. Accordingly, ulcerating lesions always warrant evaluation by darkfield microscopy and serologic tests. If untreated, syphilitic chancres heal spontaneously 3 to 8 weeks after their appearance. The mechanism for healing is obscure; it is believed that local immunity is partly responsible, because secondary lesions appear during or after the regression of the primary one.

Lesions of secondary syphilis result from the dissemination of *T. pallidum* from syphilitic chancres, and the term *disseminated syphilis* probably is more appropriate.[19,208] More than 3 weeks elapse between the deposition of *T. pallidum* in the dermis and emergence of these lesions; this delay in development and failure of affected sites to evolve into lesions that resemble primary chancres probably reflect a degree of humoral or cellular immunity, or both. Thus, secondary syphilis manifests 4 to 10 weeks after the initial primary lesion; however, in some patients who present with disseminated lesions, a careful search leads to discovery of the primary chancre. The rash of secondary syphilis is macular, papular, follicular, papulosquamous, or pustular[166,209]; the vesiculobullous eruption that is common in congenital syphilis rarely occurs in adults. Lesions are symmetrical and generally involve the trunk, where they tend to follow skin lines, and the palms and soles. The rash has been misidentified as an allergic reaction, even though it seldom is pruritic. Mucous patches that appear as white plaques on erythematous bases represent superficial mucosal erosions and can involve the oral cavity, vulva, vagina, or cervix.[166] In warm, moist areas of the body such as the anogenital region and intertriginous surfaces, the papules enlarge and become exuberant, raised, wartlike lesions that are the highly infectious condylomata lata.[209]

Secondary syphilis is a systemic disease, and interest in the dermatologic manifestations should not prevent the physician from recognizing the presence of constitutional symptoms such as fever, weight loss, anorexia, headache, fatigue, and arthralgia that can precede or accompany the dermatologic manifestations. Generalized nontender lymphadenopathy usually is present. A variety of other complications occur, including hepatitis,[210,211] glomerulonephritis or nephrotic syndrome,[212-215] osteitis,[216-218] iritis, and meningitis (Table 18-4).[208] *T. pallidum* has been isolated from the CSF of 30% of adults with untreated primary and secondary syphilis.[101] With or without treatment, the lesions of secondary syphilis heal and infection enters a subclinical or latent phase that lasts for years and can be diagnosed only by serologic testing.[219,220] Too often its protean clinical manifestations are overlooked and misdiagnosed.[221-223]

Latent syphilis is subdivided into early (1 year or less from onset of infection) and late (later than 1 year from onset) latent stages based on the time when mucocutaneous lesions can recur and infection can still be transmitted.[156,166] Patients are diagnosed with early latent syphilis if, within the year preceding the evaluation, they had a documented seroconversion, symptoms or signs of primary or secondary syphilis, or a sexual partner who had primary, secondary, or early latent syphilis. If the time of infection cannot be ascertained, a diagnosis of syphilis of unknown duration is made and the patient is managed as if she had late latent syphilis.

A high index of suspicion (see Table 18-3) is needed by the obstetrician or perinatologist to consider the diagnosis of syphilis in pregnancy and to prevent adverse outcomes. Two caveats should be heeded: Any ulcer, regardless of location, that is painless, indurated, and indolent and fails to heal within 2 weeks warrants exclusion of syphilis as a diagnosis. Similarly, any generalized eruption, regardless of its morphology, should be viewed as secondary (disseminated) syphilis until proved otherwise. One of the most common sequelae of untreated syphilis during pregnancy that is recognized worldwide is spontaneous abortion during the second and early third trimesters.[92] Furthermore, untreated maternal syphilis can result in preterm delivery, perinatal death, and congenital infection. Antenatal ultrasonography can be helpful in the diagnosis of fetal syphilis; hydramnios, fetal hydrops, enlarged placenta, hepatosplenomegaly, and bowel dilatation have been described.[224,225] Ultrasonography performed in pregnant women with early syphilis has suggested that fetal hepatosplenomegaly can be an important early indicator of congenital infection.[225]

Table 18–4 Clinical Manifestations of Early Syphilis in the Pregnant Woman

- Asymptomatic
- Symptomatic
  - Chancre(s), genital and extragenital
  - Mucocutaneous lesions
  - Macular, papular, follicular, papulosquamous, pustular
  - Condylomata lata
  - Mucous patches
  - Lymphadenopathy
  - Constitutional symptoms
  - Less common manifestations (alopecia, hepatitis, glomerulonephritis or nephrotic syndrome, osteitis, iritis, meningitis)
  - Preterm labor (spontaneous abortion, stillbirth, preterm delivery)

Early Congenital Syphilis

The diagnosis of early congenital syphilis should be entertained in any infant who is born at less than 37 weeks of gestation with no other apparent explanation, or if unexplained hydrops fetalis or an enlarged placenta is present. In infancy, failure to move an extremity (pseudoparalysis of Parrot), persistent rhinitis (snuffles), a maculopapular or papulosquamous rash (especially in the diaper area), unexplained jaundice, hepatosplenomegaly or generalized lymphadenopathy, or an anemia or thrombocytopenia of uncertain cause should raise consideration of congenital syphilis (Table 18-5).

Hepatosplenomegaly. Hepatomegaly is present in nearly all infants with congenital syphilis and may occur in the absence of splenomegaly, although the reverse is not true.[226] Jaundice, which has been recorded in 33% of patients,[226] can be caused by syphilitic hepatitis (with elevated direct and indirect bilirubin levels) or by the hemolytic component of the disease. It may be the only manifestation of the disease. Hepatic dysfunction in the form of elevated serum aminotransferases, alkaline phosphatase,[227] and direct bilirubin[227-229] initially can worsen with initiation of penicillin therapy and can persist for several weeks.[228,229]

Table 18–5 Clues That Suggest a Diagnosis of Congenital Syphilis[a]

Epidemiologic Background	Clinical Findings
Untreated early syphilis in the mother	Osteochondritis, periostitis
Untreated latent syphilis in the mother	Snuffles, hemorrhagic rhinitis
An untreated mother who has contact with a known syphilitic during pregnancy	Condylomata lata Bullous lesions, palmar/plantar rash
Mother treated for syphilis during pregnancy with a drug other than penicillin	Mucous patches Hepatomegaly, splenomegaly
Mother treated for syphilis during pregnancy without follow-up to delivery	Jaundice Nonimmune hydrops fetalis
Any high-risk factor given in Table 18-3	Generalized lymphadenopathy Central nervous system signs; elevated cell count or protein in cerebrospinal fluid Hemolytic anemia, diffuse intravascular coagulation, thrombocytopenia Pneumonitis Nephrotic syndrome Placental villitis or vasculitis (unexplained enlarged placenta) Intrauterine growth restriction

[a]Arranged in decreasing order of confidence of diagnosis.
Data from Rathbun KC. Congenital syphilis: a proposal for improved surveillance, diagnosis and treatment. Sex Transm Dis 10:102, 1983.

Generalized Lymphadenopathy. Generalized lymphadenopathy usually occurs in association with hepatosplenomegaly and has been described in up to 50% of patients.[226] The lymph nodes themselves can be as large as 1 cm in diameter and typically are nontender and firm. Generalized enlargement of the lymph nodes can occur in other systemic illnesses but is quite uncommon in neonates and young infants. If an infant has palpable epitrochlear nodes, the diagnosis of syphilis is highly probable.

Hematologic Manifestations. Major hematologic findings include anemia, jaundice, leukopenia or leukocytosis, and thrombocytopenia. A characteristic feature in the immediate newborn period is that of a Coombs'-negative hemolytic anemia. After the neonatal period, chronic nonhemolytic anemia can develop, accentuated by the usual physiologic anemia of infancy.[199,200] The pathogenesis of this anemia is not known. Other findings include polychromasia and erythroblastemia with up to 500 nucleated red blood cells per 100 leukocytes. This pattern of anemia and erythropoietic response historically led to confusion with erythroblastosis fetalis.[84] Although the leukocyte count usually falls within the normal range,[199] leukopenia, leukocytosis, or a leukemoid reaction[226] can occur. Lymphocytosis and monocytosis may be features. Thrombocytopenia, related to decreased platelet survival rather than to insufficient production of platelets, often is present and can be the only manifestation of congenital infection. Hemophagocytosis has been described and may play an important role in the pathogenesis of anemia and thrombocytopenia.[230]

Hydrops fetalis also is a manifestation of congenital syphilis in newborns.[231] A negative Coombs' test result in a hydropic infant with hemolytic anemia should suggest this diagnosis. Paroxysmal cold hemoglobinuria, a disease mediated by an antibody to erythrocytes that meets even the most rigorous definition of an autoantibody, may develop in a few patients with congenital syphilis.[232,233]

Mucocutaneous Manifestations. Mucocutaneous manifestations occur in 15% to 60% of infants with syphilis.[226,234] Rhinitis (snuffles) can be an early feature, developing after the first week of life and usually before the end of the third month. It was reported in two thirds of patients in the early literature[234] but now is less common.[226] A mucous discharge develops, with character similar to that of discharge in upper respiratory tract infections. The discharge, which is teeming with spirochetes and is highly infectious, can become progressively more profuse and occasionally is blood-tinged. Secondary bacterial infection can occur, causing the discharge to become purulent. If ulceration of the nasal mucosa is sufficiently deep and involves the nasal cartilage, a "saddle nose" deformity, one of the later stigmata of congenital syphilis, can result. Snuffles also has been associated with laryngitis and an aphonic cry.[234] Mucous patches can appear in the mouth and are more prevalent in infants with severe systemic disease.

The most common cutaneous lesion is a maculopapular eruption that is oval and pink or red, subsequently becoming coppery brown.[235] As the rash changes color, very fine superficial desquamation or scaling can occur, particularly on the palms and soles. The lesions are more common on the posterior portion of the body (especially the buttocks, back, thighs, and soles) than on the anterior surface but also can involve the perioral area and palms. Other maculopapular types of eruptions uncommonly are found in early congenital syphilis. The lesions can be annular or circinate or can have the appearance of any other kind of lesion seen in acquired secondary syphilis.[209]

Pemphigus syphiliticus occurs most often in the neonatal period and is characterized by a widely disseminated vesiculobullous eruption that involves the palms and soles.[235] The lesions vary in size and can contain a cloudy hemorrhagic fluid that teems with treponemes. When these bullae rupture, they leave a denuded area that can undergo extensive maceration and crusting.

After the first 2 or 3 months of life, the perioral area, especially the nares and the angles of the mouth, and the perianal area can be affected by condylomata lata.[202,235] These highly infective areas are flat or wartlike and moist. The condylomata can be single or multiple and frequently accompany no other signs of infection. They can lead to deep fissures radial to the affected orifices and can result in fine scars designated *rhagades*. Comparable eruptions also can be found in other body folds or intertriginous areas but are considered to be more characteristic of the later stage of early congenital syphilis.

Other dermatologic manifestations of congenital syphilis have been described. Petechial lesions can result from thrombocytopenia. Generalized edema can be present[199,226] as a result of hypoproteinemia related to renal or hepatic disease.

Bone Lesions. Bone lesions are perhaps the most frequently encountered abnormalities in untreated early congenital syphilis. Most bone lesions are not clinically discernible (see "Radiographic Diagnosis" section) except in pseudoparalysis of Parrot.[236,237] Pseudoparalysis of Parrot, a syndrome in which pain is associated with a bone lesion or a superimposed fracture, or both, occurs infrequently in infants with congenital syphilis.[238] Clinically, it can manifest as irritability in an infant a few weeks of age who does not move one of the limbs.[239] The upper extremities are affected more frequently than lower extremities, and unilateral involvement predominates. This clinical picture can mimic Erb's palsy but rarely is present at birth. The correlation between the clinical and the radiologic findings is poor, inasmuch as other areas of bone involvement can look more severely affected on radiographs even though no clinical signs suggest their presence.

Renal Manifestations. The clinical picture of nephrotic syndrome usually appears at 2 or 3 months of age, the predominant manifestation being generalized edema, including pretibial, scrotal, and periorbital areas, together with ascites.[240-244] Rarely, the infant can have hematuria with less severe proteinuria but more profound azotemia, which suggests that a glomerulitis predominates.

Central Nervous System Manifestations. According to Platou, clinically inapparent involvement of the brain and spinal cord revealed by CSF abnormalities occurred in 60% of infants with congenital syphilis in 1949.[234] Of note, however, he empirically defined an abnormal CSF as having greater than 5 white blood cells per mm^3 and a protein content greater than 45 mg/dL. The overall incidence of neurosyphilis by these criteria could be challenged, because the CSF of neonates contains up to 25 white blood cells per mm^3, and a protein content as high as 150 mg/dL in full-term infants and 170 mg/dL in preterm infants can be considered normal.[245] Furthermore, the significance of a reactive CSF VDRL test in the absence of other diagnostic evidence of congenital syphilis is suspect, inasmuch as nontreponemal IgG can pass from the serum to the CSF.[246] Experiments using rabbit inoculation of CSF from infants born to mothers with untreated early syphilis documented a prevalence of spirochetal invasion of the CSF in 6 of 7 (86%) infants with clinical and laboratory evidence of congenital syphilis, but only 1 of 12 (8%) infants born to mothers with untreated early syphilis and whose findings on physical examination and laboratory evaluation were normal.[88] Neurologic manifestations, although well documented in the earlier literature,[190] are now infrequently reported. The clinical types of CNS involvement have been separated arbitrarily into supposedly well-defined groups, but frequently overlap exists.

Acute syphilitic leptomeningitis appears during the first year of life, usually between the ages of 3 and 6 months. Signs can suggest acute bacterial meningitis, including a stiff neck, progressive vomiting, Kernig's sign, bulging fontanelles, separation of the suture, and hydrocephalus.[247] In contrast with this clinical picture, CSF reveals abnormalities consistent with an aseptic meningitis, with up to 200 mononuclear cells per mm^3, a modest increase in protein (50 to 200 mg/dL), and a normal glucose value. The CSF VDRL test is positive. This is the one form of CNS involvement that always responds to specific therapy.[234]

Chronic meningovascular syphilis can have a protracted course, resulting in progressive hydrocephalus, cranial nerve palsies or vascular lesions of the brain, and gradual intellectual deterioration.[247] These complications develop toward the end of the first year. The hydrocephalus is of low grade, progressive, and communicating as a result of obstruction in the basilar cisterns. Cranial nerve palsies can complicate the picture.[190] The seventh nerve most often is involved, but the third, fourth, and sixth cranial nerves also can be affected. Optic atrophy can be preceded by papilledema.

A variety of cerebrovascular syndromes have been described, but they are rare.[190] Cerebral infarction results from syphilitic endarteritis and can occur between the first and second years of life, commonly manifesting as acute hemiplegia. Convulsions frequently complicate this clinical picture.

Ocular Manifestations. The occurrence of syphilitic involvement of the eye in early congenital syphilis is rare. Chorioretinitis, salt-and-pepper fundus, glaucoma, uveitis, cataract,[248] and chancres of the eyelid have been described.[84] Involvement by syphilis leads to a granular appearance of the fundus; pigmentary patches of various shapes and colors[84] are seen in the periphery of the retina. The young infant rarely manifests the signs of photophobia and diminution in vision that occur in older patients. Congenital glaucoma can occur[84] and should be a diagnostic consideration in the presence of blepharospasm, cloudy cornea, enlarged cornea (diameter exceeding 12 mm), and excessive tearing.

Inflammation of the uveal tract (including the iris and ciliary body anteriorly and the choroid posteriorly) affects the retina because of the close anatomic relationship of the cornea to the structures of the uveal tract. Consequently, chorioretinitis rather than uveitis is the more commonly diagnosed ocular problem in infancy. In a recent report, however, pathologic examination of an eye from a 3-day-old infant who died of congenital syphilis revealed a focal granulomatous reaction involving the anterior uvea and lens.[248] Rarely, a chancre of the eyelid appears 4 weeks after birth, presumably resulting from recently developed syphilitic lesions of the maternal genitalia.[84]

Intrauterine Growth Restriction. The effect of syphilis on the growth of the fetus in utero is likely to be related to the timing and severity of the fetal infection. In a carefully performed quantitative morphologic study, Naeye[249] demonstrated that syphilitic infection in utero did not seem to have a significant effect on the growth of the fetus, as manifested by a study of 36 perinatal deaths. Naeye's findings were similar to his previous results that showed a relative lack of effect on fetal growth from toxoplasmosis, contrasting with the intrauterine growth restriction associated with rubella and cytomegalovirus infections.[250] Case reports have indicated that infected newborns were small for their gestational age.[239] Whether this growth retardation is the result of syphilitic infection or other co-factors (e.g., use of illicit intravenous drugs by the mother[251]) that affect fetal growth is not known.

Other Findings. The classic historical description of the infant with congenital syphilis is a severely infected premature infant with marasmus, a pot belly, "old man" facies, and withered skin.[84,235] The degree of failure to thrive can be correlated with the frequently encountered pathologic finding of intense pancreatitis[178] and inflammation of the gastrointestinal tract.[178] Rectal bleeding due to syphilitic ileitis with ulcer formation and associated with intestinal obstruction has been reported.[185] Involvement of the anterior pituitary gland in congenital syphilis is manifested by persistent hypoglycemia beyond the early neonatal period.[191] Evaluation of pituitary function, including tests for thyroid function, and determination of growth hormone and cortisol levels, combined with magnetic resonance imaging of the pituitary, confirms the diagnosis of hypopituitarism.[191]

Other uncommon manifestations of congenital syphilis include pneumonia alba, or syphilitic pneumonitis, which is an obliterative fibrosis of the lung tissue. Myocarditis[178] has been found at autopsy in approximately 10% of infants who die, although the clinical significance of this finding is not clear. Fever has been reported to accompany other signs of congenital syphilis in infants beyond the immediate newborn period.[111,227]

Late Congenital Syphilis

As noted earlier, the clinical manifestations of late congenital syphilis are stigmata that represent scars induced by the initial lesions of early congenital syphilis or reactions to persistent and ongoing inflammation. In patients older than 2 years of age, late congenital syphilis can be manifested by (1) the stigmata of the disorder that represent the scars of initial lesions or developmental changes induced by the early infection; (2) ongoing inflammation that causes interstitial keratitis, nerve deafness, and Clutton's joints (although *T. pallidum* is not demonstrable); or (3) a persistently positive result on treponemal serologic tests for syphilis in the absence of apparent disease.[166] In reviewing the manifestations of late congenital syphilis (Table 18-6), Fiumara and Lessell[252] concluded that only Hutchinson's triad (Hutchinson's teeth, interstitial keratitis, and eighth nerve deafness), mulberry molars, or Clutton's joints are specific enough to confirm the diagnosis.

Table 18–6 Clinical Manifestations of Late Congenital Syphilis

Dentition:	Hutchinson's teeth, mulberry molars (Moon's, Fournier's)
Eye:	interstitial keratitis, healed chorioretinitis, secondary glaucoma (uveitis), corneal scarring
Ear:	eighth nerve deafness
Nose and face:	"saddle nose," protuberant mandible
Skin:	rhagades
Central nervous system:	mental retardation, arrested hydrocephalus, convulsive disorders, optic nerve atrophy, juvenile general paresis, cranial nerve palsies
Bones and joints:	"saber shins," Higouménakis' sign, Clutton's joints

Dentition. Vasculitis that occurs around the time of birth damages the developing tooth bud, which then leads to a number of dental abnormalities that appear in late congenital syphilis. The deciduous teeth do not seem to be affected, except for a possible increase in the incidence of dental caries.[84] Hutchinson's teeth are abnormalities of the permanent upper central incisors; these teeth are peg shaped and notched, usually with obvious thinning and discoloration of enamel in the area of the notching. The teeth are widely spaced and shorter than the lateral incisors. The width of the biting surface is less than that of the gingival margin.[252]

A diagnostic lesion, the mulberry molar (also known as Moon's or Fournier's molar) is always the first lower molar.[252] Characteristically, the tooth's grinding surface, which is narrower than that at the gingival margin, has many small cusps instead of the usual four well-formed cusps. The enamel itself tends to be poorly developed. Putkonen[253] examined 30 children whose infected mothers had received penicillin during the latter half of pregnancy and an additional 36 children whose initial therapy for congenital syphilis was initiated during the first few months of life. He noted distinct syphilitic dental changes in 7 of 15 children whose treatment began at age 4 months or later, but in none of the children whose mothers had received treatment during the last half of pregnancy or before age 3 months. He concluded that early treatment prevented the dental changes of syphilis.

Eye. Interstitial keratitis is the second manifestation of Hutchinson's triad. This lesion can be detected in patients between 5 and 20 years of age. A severe inflammatory reaction begins in one eye, generally becoming bilateral during the ensuing weeks or months. Spirochetes have not been found to be present.[201] Symptoms include photophobia, pain, excessive lacrimation, and blurred vision. Patients can have conjunctival injection, miosis, keratitis, or anterior uveitis, or a combination of these findings. Interstitial keratitis is considered preventable if treatment is given before age 3 months.[253] Interstitial keratitis usually appears at puberty and is not affected by penicillin therapy but responds transiently to corticosteroid treatment.[254] Keratitis often has a relapsing course that can result in secondary glaucoma or corneal clouding.

Ear. Eighth nerve deafness is the least common component of Hutchinson's triad, occurring in only 3% of patients with late congenital syphilis.[252,255,256] The histopathologic features of luetic involvement of the temporal bone include mononuclear leukocytic infiltration and obliterative endarteritis, with involvement of the periosteal, endochondral, and endosteal layers of bone. Osteochondritis affecting the otic capsule can lead to cochlear degeneration and fibrous adhesions, resulting in eighth nerve deafness as well as vertigo. Although the deafness usually occurs in the first decade, it may not appear until the third or fourth decade of life. The initial involvement can be unilateral or bilateral; deafness initially involves the higher frequencies, and normal conversational tones are affected later. It may respond to long-term corticosteroid therapy.

Nose and Face. The sequelae of syphilitic rhinitis include failure of the maxilla to grow fully, resulting in a concave configuration in the middle section of the face with relative protuberance of the mandible and an associated high palatal arch. Inflammation of the nasal mucosa can affect the cartilage, leading to destruction of the underlying bone and perforation of the nasal septum. The resulting depression of the roof of the septum gives the appearance of a "saddle nose."

Skin. An infrequent sign of late congenital syphilis is linear scars that become fissured or ulcerated, resulting in deeper scars called rhagades. These scars are located around body orifices, including the mouth, nostrils, and anus.[84]

Central Nervous System. The reported incidence of neurologic involvement in late congenital syphilis varies considerably, according to different authors. Some report that as many as one third of patients more than 2 years of age have CSF abnormalities that would justify a diagnosis of late asymptomatic neurosyphilis.[234] The neurologic manifestations can include mental retardation, arrested hydrocephalus, convulsive disorders, juvenile general paresis, and cranial nerve abnormalities, including deafness and blindness, which is due to optic nerve atrophy.[190,247] These findings are uncommon in cases described during the last 50 years.[252] Use of single photon emission computed tomography (SPECT) in a 5-year-old patient with late neurosyphilis clinically manifested as seizures demonstrated areas of hypoperfusion that closely agreed with abnormalities seen in the electroencephalogram.[257] Findings on cranial computed tomography, magnetic resonance imaging, and cerebral angiography, however, were normal.

Bones and Joints. Bone involvement in late congenital syphilis is relatively infrequent in comparison with the frequent occurrence of abnormalities in early congenital syphilis.[84] The sequelae of periosteal reactions can involve the skull, resulting in frontal bossing; the tibia, resulting in "saber shin"; or the sternoclavicular portion of the clavicle, resulting in a deformity called Higouménakis' sign.[252] For unknown reasons, the last-named finding tends to occur only on the side of dominant handedness.

Joint involvement is rare. Clutton's joints were found in only 1 of 271 patients described by Fiumara and Lessell.[252] In this condition, synovitis occurs with hydrarthrosis, local tenderness, and limitation of motion[258]; the knee is the most commonly affected joint. Roentgenograms do not show involvement of the bones, and examination of the joint fluid reveals a few mononuclear cells.

DIAGNOSIS

The ideal for the diagnosis of congenital syphilis would be to easily and accurately delineate the following groups: (1) infected mothers giving birth to infected infants with clinical manifestations of infection, (2) infected mothers giving birth to infected infants with no clinical signs of infection, (3) infected mothers giving birth to uninfected infants who appear healthy, (4) infected but seronegative mothers giving birth to infected infants who appear healthy, and (5) uninfected mothers. The problem of distinguishing among the latter four groups is a recurring problem in discussing identification of the infected infant and underscores the need for an "evaluate and treat when uncertain" approach to congenital syphilis.

A definitive diagnosis of congenital syphilis can be made in the unusual situation in which the organism can be identified by darkfield microscopy, histologic examination, or rabbit infectivity test (RIT) of specimens from suspicious lesions or amniotic fluid.[89,92,156,163,225,259] Seroconversion or a fourfold rise in titer on a syphilis serologic test, either the RPR or the VDRL test, with a positive result on a treponemal test (fluorescent treponemal antibody absorption [FTA-ABS] test or hemagglutination tests) also is sufficient for a definitive diagnosis to be made (Table 18-7).[88]

In most infants, the presence of one or more clinical features of congenital syphilis plus positive results on syphilis serologic testing usually is sufficient for a diagnosis of probable congenital syphilis (see Table 18-7).[260] The early manifestations of congenital syphilis (e.g., hepatosplenomegaly with or without jaundice or generalized lymphadenopathy), hematologic manifestations (e.g., hemolytic anemia or thrombocytopenia), nonimmune hydrops fetalis, mucocutaneous manifestations (vesiculobullous rash, snuffles, condylomata lata), bone involvement (osteochondritis), renal manifestations, or CNS or CSF abnormalities prompts serologic testing that will establish or refute probable infection. The diagnosis of possible congenital syphilis is made when a serologic test result is positive but clinical manifestations of infection are absent. The diagnosis of congenital syphilis can be excluded if both the RPR and FTA-ABS tests become nonreactive before the age of 6 months in an infant who has not received treatment, or if these serologic tests are nonreactive in the mother and the infant, barring the situation in which the mother is

Table 18–7 Suggested Diagnostic Categories of Congenital Syphilis Relative to Confidence of Diagnosis

Definite Diagnosis

1. Confirmation of presence of *T. pallidum* by darkfield microscopic or histologic examination or rabbit infectivity test (RIT)
2. STS (RPR, VDRL) titer increased fourfold or greater than maternal STS titer (both specimens drawn at time of evaluation)

Probable Diagnosis

1. STS (RPR or VDRL) reactive in presence of snuffles, condylomata lata, pemphigus syphiliticus, hepatosplenomegaly, or osseous lesions
2. STS (RPR or VDRL) reactive in presence of other clinical manifestations given in Table 18-5
3. STS (VDRL) reactive in cerebrospinal fluid
4. Reactive treponemal antibody test after the age of 15 months

Possible Diagnosis

STS (RPR or VDRL, FTA-ABS) reactive in absence of clinical disease

Unlikely Diagnosis

STS nonreactive before the age of 6 months

FTA-ABS, fluorescent treponemal antibody absorption (test); RPR, rapid plasma reagin (test); STS, serologic test for syphilis; VDRL, Venereal Disease Research Laboratory (test).

seronegative because she is in the incubation period of early syphilis.[157,227]

Because of the infrequent occurrence of congenital syphilis in most newborn infants and its protean clinical manifestations, the physician must be alert to the possibility of this diagnosis. Adding to the challenge is that the diagnosis of syphilis in the mother also can be difficult. Routine use of a serologic test for syphilis is recommended in the first trimester of pregnancy,[144,145] again at the beginning of the third trimester, and at delivery in women with demographic or behavioral factors placing then at risk for acquiring syphilis (see Table 18-3).[108,135,156] The diagnosis of syphilis in the first few weeks of life depends on epidemiologic evidence, careful physical examination, documentation of radiologic abnormalities consistent with the diagnosis, and confirmation of infection by appropriate serologic testing or, if possible, demonstration of spirochetes in suspicious lesions or amniotic fluid (such demonstration is rare, however).[89,156,163,225,259,261,262]

Radiographic Diagnosis

Bone involvement, the most common pathologic manifestation of congenital syphilitic infection,[234,263] involves multiple bones and is symmetrical. The metaphyses and diaphyses most often are involved, especially the long bones. The radiographic abnormalities include osteochondritis (metaphyseal dystrophy), osteomyelitis (osteitis-like dystrophy), and periostitis (periosteal dystrophy).

Characteristically, bone involvement is widespread; besides the long bones, the cranium, spine, and ribs also are affected. The earliest and most characteristic changes are found in the metaphysis, with sparing of the epiphysis.[198] The changes are nonspecific and variable, ranging from radiopaque bands to actual fragmentation and apparent destruction with mottled areas of radiolucency. Frequently, an enhanced zone of provisional calcification (radiopaque band) is associated with osteoporosis immediately beneath the dense zone. Variations of these paretic changes are seen, including peripheral (lateral) paresis only and alternating bands of density sandwiching a paretic zone (Fig. 18-3).[196] The classic saw-toothed appearance of the bone now is uncommon, although it can be seen on xeroradiographs of stillborn infants with congenital syphilis.[179] Metaphysitis or metaphyseal dystrophy (the choice of term depends on the concept of pathogenesis) of the long bones manifests at birth or can first appear after the first month of life.

In many of the long bones, the lesions are located on the lateral aspects of the metaphyses.[198] The tibia often exhibits metaphyseal defects on its upper medial aspect; bilateral presence of such defects is called Wimberger's sign (Fig. 18-4). Rarely, similar changes may occur at the upper ends of the humeri. Although Wimberger's sign formerly was thought to be pathognomonic of congenital syphilis,[264] it has been described[265] in other disease states, including osteomyelitis, hyperparathyroidism, and infantile generalized fibromatosis.

Focal areas of patchy cortical radiolucency with spreading of the medullary canal and irregularity of the endosteal and periosteal aspects of the cortex can be seen on radiographs. In severe cases, the radiolucent areas can appear as columns, giving a "celery stick" appearance of alternating bands of longitudinal translucency and relative density, a finding also seen in rubella and cytomegalovirus infection that probably represents a growth arrest abnormality.[196]

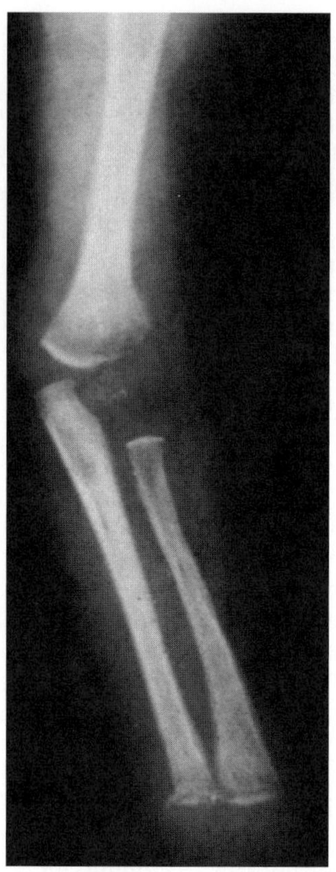

Figure 18–3 The patient was a 1-month-old male infant who presented with a respiratory illness and a positive result on VDRL testing. The radiograph of the forearm and distal humerus shows evidence of irregular metaphyseal demineralization associated with periosteal new bone formation. The changes are most marked in the distal radius and ulna, but the radial aspect of the distal humerus also is involved. The dense bands in the distal metaphysis of the radius and ulna as well as the distal humerus are nonspecific findings. Although these metaphyseal bands of density are seen in a significant number of infants with congenital syphilis, they are not diagnostic. The presence of symmetrical metaphyseal lesions is more typical and helps to differentiate the long bone lesions of congenital syphilis from other causes of osteomyelitis or osseous dysplasia associated with disseminated infection.

The inflammatory reaction in the diaphysis stimulates the periosteum to lay down new bone. The single or multiple layers of periosteal new bone extend along the cortex of the entire diaphysis. Unlike the other two forms of osseous involvement (metaphyseal dystrophy and osteitis-like dystrophy), diaphyseal abnormalities are less often present at birth. Osteochondritis is evident radiographically 5 weeks after fetal infection has occurred; periostitis requires 16 weeks for radiographic diagnosis.[266] Obstetric radiography[267] allows for the in utero diagnosis of fetal syphilis by demonstrating periosteal cloaking. Although maternal treatment has been associated with radiologic resolution of these lesions, the radiographic signs of congenital syphilis also resolve without therapy. Periostitis usually occurs during the early months of life and must be distinguished from that seen in healing rickets, battered child syndrome, infantile cortical hyperostosis, a variety of poorly understood disorders presumed

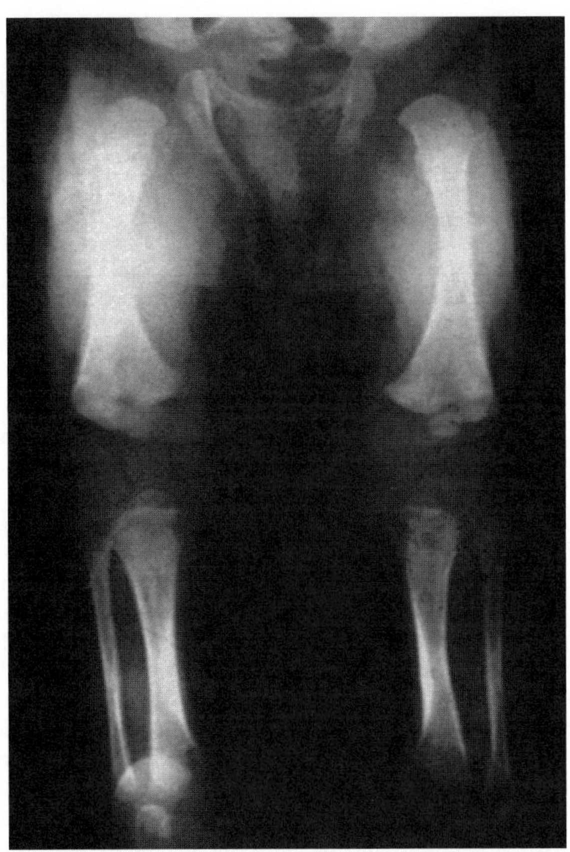

Figure 18–4 An anteroposterior film of both lower extremities of the same patient as in Figure 18-3 demonstrates demineralization and osseous destruction of the proximal medial tibial metaphysis bilaterally. These lesions are features of Wimberger's sign. Note the diffuse symmetrical periostitis and irregular demineralization of the metaphyses of the distal tibias and femurs.

to be related to nutritional deficiencies, occasionally pyogenic osteomyelitis,[198] and prostaglandin-induced periostitis.[268]

Involvement of the metacarpals, metatarsals, or proximal phalanges of the hand is rare. Dactylitis appears radiologically as a spindle-shaped enlargement of the bone and can occur from the ages of 3 to 24 months.[198] Unusual osseous manifestations also have been reported. A case of syphilitic arthritis of the hip and elbow in association with osteomyelitis of the femur and humerus has been described in the immediate newborn period.[269,270] Single bone involvement is unique, but solitary involvement of the radius has been described.[271] Solomon and Rosen[272,273] reported that in more than one third of 112 infants with congenital syphilis, radiographic findings were consistent with trauma of bone made more fragile by syphilitic infection. Bone scans have been performed in very few patients; they reveal diffuse abnormalities when performed,[274-276] but such scans are neither helpful nor recommended.

Demonstration of the Organism

The "gold standard" for the identification of *T. pallidum* in clinical specimens is inoculation into rabbits—the RIT.[88,89,101,277,278] RIT has excellent sensitivity, permitting detection of as few as 5 to 10 organisms. Within 30 to 60 minutes of collection, the clinical sample (serum, blood, CSF, or amniotic fluid) is injected into the testicle of a seronegative adult male rabbit. While housed at 10° C to 20° C, each animal is regularly examined over 3 months for evidence of infection by *T. pallidum* (orchitis) and also by serologic testing (RPR and treponemal tests). If after 3 months evidence of orchitis is lacking and the serologic test is nonreactive, the rabbit is considered to be noninfected and the specimen negative for viable *T. pallidum*. When treponemal infection in the rabbit is suspected because of seroconversion or development of orchitis, the rabbit is sacrificed, popliteal lymph nodes and testicular tissue are removed and minced in sterile saline, and the tissue extract is examined by darkfield microscopy. Positive findings on darkfield examination (i.e., visualization of spirochetes) of testicular extract are confirmatory. If the darkfield examination findings again are negative, 2 mL of the testicular homogenate is then injected into a second seronegative rabbit, and the previous procedure is repeated.

The RIT is performed only in research laboratories; in clinical situations, the definitive diagnosis of syphilis is made by detecting characteristic treponemes by darkfield microscopy.[279] Bullae can be aspirated with a sterile syringe and needle. Papules or condylomata can be abraded with a gauze square until oozing occurs. A sterile glass slide is applied to the exudate, which then is covered by a drop of normal saline and a coverslip and promptly examined. Negative findings on examination do not exclude the diagnosis of syphilis, and examinations should be repeated if the clinical findings are suggestive. The scaly eruption of syphilis is not a good source of material for darkfield microscopy.

Another definitive diagnostic test for the diagnosis of syphilis is darkfield microscopy of body fluid specimens. This procedure requires a darkfield microscope and specially trained personnel but usually is available in clinics for patients who have sexually transmitted infections. Although not evaluated for use in specimens from newborns, a modification called the "dark ground" microscopy method has been used in adults with primary and secondary syphilis, with sensitivities of 97% and 84%, respectively, and with good specificity.[280] This is a rapid and sensitive test but also requires a darkfield microscope and trained personnel.

Hematology

Blood should be obtained for determination of hematocrit and hemoglobin, red blood cell count, reticulocyte count, platelet count, and white blood cell count, as well as for a differential smear, direct Coombs' test, and serologic testing (RPR or VDRL). Performance of a serum treponemal test such as the FTA-ABS test is not necessary in the newborn period if the mother is known to have a reactive result (see later).

Serology

General Considerations

Serologic tests[155] have played a prominent role in the clinical diagnosis of syphilis since the early 1900s, when antibody to the mammalian membrane lipid cardiolipin (diphosphatidylglycerol) was serendipitously detected by Wassermann

Table 18–8 Serologic Tests for Syphilis

Tests to Detect Antibodies to Cardiolipin

1. VDRL (Venereal Disease Research Laboratory): usually done by reference laboratories
2. RPR (rapid plasma reagin): now used in offices and small laboratories

Tests to Detect Antibody to *T. pallidum*

1. TPI (*T. pallidum*–immobilizing): no longer available for diagnostic purposes
2. FTA-ABS (fluorescent treponemal antibody, absorbed with non-pallidum treponemes [*T. phagedenis*])
3. TP-PA (*T. pallidum* particle agglutination): hemagglutination test that detects antibody to *T. pallidum* components; hemagglutination assays have largely replaced FTA-ABS testing
4. ELISA (enzyme-linked immunosorbent assay): IgG and IgM antibody tests
5. FTA-ABS-IgM (fluorescent *T. pallidum* antibody-absorbed IgM): not recommended (see text)
6. Immunoblotting (IgG, IgM, IgA): not yet adapted for clinical use in diagnosing syphilis

IgA, IgG, IgM, immunoglobulins A, G, M.

Table 18–9 Seroreactivity of More Common Tests for Untreated Syphilis

	% Positive			
Test[a]	*Primary Stage*	*Secondary Stage*	*Latent Stage*	*Tertiary Stage*
VDRL or RPR	75	100	75	75
FTA-ABS, TP-PA	90	100	100	100

[a]See Table 18-8 for full test names.

in the serum of patients with active syphilis (Table 18-8). The test used to detect this antibody went through a number of modifications (by Kolmer, Kahn, and Mazzini), culminating in that of the Venereal Disease Research Laboratory (i.e., VDRL) of the Communicable Disease Center (as the CDC then was designated). Antibody to cardiolipin also was called reagin, a term that should be replaced because of potential confusion with IgE. The serologic test that has remained in use, however, is one that rapidly and easily detects antibody to cardiolipin, the RPR test, which has replaced the VDRL test in many laboratories. RPR results are reported as dilutions or titers so that the degree of reactivity can be determined; a high titer in the absence of treatment and especially a rising titer (a fourfold increase or greater) indicate the presence of active infection. The RPR titer often is one to two dilutions higher than results obtained from the VDRL test; therefore, caution must be exercised when making clinical decisions on the basis of results of these two different tests for the same patient. For similar reasons, so that appropriate comparisons can be made, the same nontreponemal test should be performed in the mother and her infant.[156] Because the RPR test generally is more sensitive than the VDRL test, it is the preferred test for screening pregnant women. The VDRL test is recommended for use with CSF.

Infection with *T. pallidum* causes the host to produce antitreponemal antibodies, which are detected by FTA testing. The more recently developed *T. pallidum* hemagglutination test—the *T. pallidum* particle agglutination (TP-PA) test—is easy to perform and can be done with small volumes of serum in an automated system. The microhemagglutination assay for *T. pallidum* antibody (MHA-TP) has similar performance characteristics but no longer is available commercially. The TP-PA provides results that are comparable with those of the FTA, although the FTA is slightly more sensitive and specific.[279] When syphilis is suspected in a patient who has a reactive RPR test but a negative TP-PA test result, an FTA test should be performed to exclude early syphilis as a diagnosis.

Nontreponemal Antibody Tests: Rapid Plasma Reagin and Venereal Disease Research Laboratory Tests. The VDRL and RPR tests often are called "nontreponemal antibody tests." Actually, the antigenic stimulus is uncertain. Diphosphatidylglycerol constitutes a small proportion of the lipids of *T. pallidum*,[281] but these organisms may be unable to synthesize this substance, and it is possible that they incorporate it from damaged host tissues. Thus, production of RPR antibody could reflect an autoimmune host response to a slightly altered or a differently presented cardiolipin. In this context, it is interesting that anticardiolipin antibody reflects ongoing tissue damage, its detection correlating closely with the amount of activity in the early stages of syphilis infection. These observations may explain why patients with autoimmune diseases, such as systemic lupus erythematosus, characteristically have positive RPR test results. The RPR test result also can be positive, generally not exceeding a titer of 1:8, in nonsyphilitic patients who have infections caused by viruses (especially Epstein-Barr and hepatitis viruses), *Mycoplasma*, or protozoa.[67,150,282] A reactive RPR test also is found in the absence of syphilis in heroin addicts, in elderly persons, and in patients with cirrhosis, malignancy (especially if associated with production of excess IgM), and autoimmune disease or, rarely, in pregnancy itself.[67,150,283-287] VDRL reactivity in these conditions has acquired the unfortunate designation "biologic false positive," to indicate an etiologic process other than *T. pallidum* infection.

The VDRL test is reactive in about 75% of adults at the time they seek medical attention for primary syphilis (Table 18-9). Secondary syphilis always is associated with a reactive VDRL, usually at a dilution greater than 1:16.[58,279] Persistence of a positive VDRL result after appropriate antibiotic therapy, sometimes called the serofast state, apparently is uncommon. The VDRL result usually becomes negative within 2 years of treatment.[155,288,289] Even without treatment, the VDRL titer slowly declines and is, in fact, negative in one third of patients with late syphilis.[58]

From 1% to 2% of sera from patients with secondary syphilis will exhibit a prozone phenomenon.[150-153] This phenomenon is due to presence of an excess amount of reagin antibody in the patient's undiluted serum. The excess in antibody prevents flocculation, resulting in a falsely negative test result. The prozone effect can be overcome by diluting the serum before testing, after which the serum usually will exhibit titers of 1:16 or greater. Failure to recognize a prozone effect in maternal serum tested during pregnancy has resulted in failure to diagnose congenital syphilis.[153]

Treponemal Antibody Tests. Other serologic tests detect an interaction between serum immunoglobulins and surface antigens of *T. pallidum*; these tests are distinguished from those for cardiolipin antibody and from all so-called treponemal antibody tests. The *T. pallidum*–immobilizing test was, for many years, foremost among these, being used as the "gold standard" to determine whether the patient had been infected with *T. pallidum*. This test was difficult to perform, required a source of viable organisms (usually obtained from an infected rabbit), a darkfield microscope, and a substantial investment of time; it no longer is available.

Antibody to treponemal antigens from lyophilized *T. pallidum* also can be detected by the FTA test. Because all of the antigens of *T. pallidum* are not unique and antibody reactivity with some of them may exist in normal serum, an absorption step was needed that used a nonpathogenic treponeme (*Treponema reiteri*, now called *Treponema phagedenis*). This gave rise to the more specific FTA-ABS test. Except for the rare instance in which antibody to DNA causes a positive FTA-ABS reaction in serum from a patient with lupus erythematosus or rheumatoid arthritis, this test is regarded as specific, and it essentially has replaced the *T. pallidum*–immobilizing test as the standard for determining whether prior infection with *T. pallidum* had ever occurred.[287] The FTA-ABS test, however, requires a fluorescence microscope and a highly trained technician.

The development of hemagglutination tests—for example, the TP-PA and MHA-TP—has provided specific assays that can be performed easily in most laboratories and require less specialized equipment. These tests use a lysate of pathogenic *T. pallidum* and yield results that are very similar to those obtained by the FTA-ABS. They largely have replaced the FTA-ABS as the most efficient and specific test to detect antibody to *T. pallidum*.[60,154,286,290-293] The MHA-TP, however, no longer is commercially available. The TP-PA test uses the same treponemal antigen as was required in the MHA-TP but utilizes gelatin particles rather than sheep red blood cells, which eliminates nonspecific reactions with serum or plasma samples. The TP-PA test was developed in Japan; its performance has been comparable with that of FTA-ABS tests.[294] Physicians out of habit continue to request an FTA-ABS test, although at present most laboratories perform a hemagglutination test; these terms—FTA-ABS assay and hemagglutination reaction—are used interchangeably throughout this chapter.

Immunoblotting has been studied by several investigators for detection of IgG and IgM antibodies to specific *T. pallidum* proteins in sera of adults with syphilis.[35,37,45] The sensitivity and specificity of immunoblotting are excellent; however, it has not been feasible to transfer this diagnostic method into the clinical laboratory.[295] Enzyme-linked immunosorbent assays (ELISAs)[295-300] are under study; some of them use *T. pallidum* outer membrane proteins that have been generated by recombinant techniques. For example, Van Voorhis and colleagues[300] studied six recombinant *T. pallidum* antigens in ELISA for their sensitivities and specificities in sera from patients with syphilis, Lyme disease, or leptospirosis as well as from uninfected patients. Two antigens (Tp0453 and Tp92) had sensitivities and specificities of 98% to 100% and 97% to 100%, respectively.

Another method recently evaluated is the immunochromatographic strip test.[301] This test detects antibodies specific for *T. pallidum* without reacting with the reagin in sera from patients with biologically false-positive tests. These newer tests ultimately should be helpful: Their sensitivity is sufficient to detect early syphilis cases, in which the currently used tests can be nonreactive, and they are now available commercially.

In approximately 90% of patients with a primary syphilitic chancre, the hemagglutination test result is positive by the time they seek medical attention.[60,279,285,286,288] All patients with secondary syphilis or late infection demonstrate a positive reaction. These tests are highly specific, as well as being extremely sensitive. A few disease states, such as systemic lupus erythematosus, polyarteritis or related conditions, and, in one report, even pregnancy, are said to cause a false-positive FTA-ABS result, but these diagnoses should be apparent, and the sophisticated observer often can detect a distinctive beaded pattern of fluorescence in these reactions.[67] Historically it was believed that, once positive results have been obtained on these tests, such results will remain so for life, even if the infection has been cured. Romanowski and co-workers,[302] however, found that 24% of first-episode primary syphilis patients exhibited a nonreactive result on FTA-ABS testing and 13% had a nonreactive result on MHA-TP testing at 36 months after treatment. Nevertheless, positive reactions are not helpful in determining whether active infection is present. Despite the exquisite sensitivity and specificity of these tests, therefore, a positive result may not be helpful diagnostically in an individual patient; a negative result excludes a diagnosis of all but early primary infection.

Serologic Diagnosis in the Infant

Rapid Plasma Reagin and Fluorescent Treponemal Antibody Absorption Tests. Maternal RPR and FTA-ABS test reactivity can be found in both IgG and IgM antibody isotypes.[37,303,304] If the placenta is intact, IgG is passively transferred to the newborn. Thus, a reactive serologic test in the neonate can be due to maternally derived IgG and does not necessarily indicate that the infant is infected. Furthermore, maternal antibody could have arisen from untreated, inadequately treated, or adequately treated disease. If the antibody titer is higher in the infant than in the mother by the same nontreponemal test (a fourfold or greater difference is required to exclude laboratory variation), this finding would signify congenital infection.[88] If the infant's reactive RPR test is caused by passively transferred antibody, the reactivity progressively declines as time passes and should disappear by 6 months of age. A persistently reactive RPR test in the infant beyond 12 to 15 months of age suggests an active infection, and a rising titer makes this diagnosis certain.

The CDC has recommended that serum from blood specimens drawn from the infant, rather than from umbilical cord blood obtained at birth, be used for serologic testing because the rates of false-positive and false-negative results are lower.[156] Owing to its ease of collection, however, umbilical cord blood continues to be a readily available specimen. Appropriate care in collection of umbilical cord blood should be taken to avoid contamination with maternal blood. Serologic testing of umbilical cord blood can be performed with either the RPR assay or the VDRL test. The RPR assay is more sensitive,[305] although false-positive reactions due to contamination of the sample with Wharton's jelly can occur. Both tests, however, may be nonreactive when the maternal serologic titer is low. It is best to screen the mother, rather than the newborn[306]; routine screening of umbilical cord blood is discouraged.[307]

If the mother has a false-positive RPR test result, the relevant antibody can be passively transferred to the infant. Naturally, in such a case, neither the mother nor the infant will have a reactive treponemal test. If the mother has a reactive treponemal test because of untreated or previously treated syphilis, the antibody also appears in the newborn by passive transfer. Thus, detection of such reactivity in the newborn indicates that the mother had at some point encountered *T. pallidum*, but it does not indicate whether her infection was treated, and it certainly does not diagnose active infection of the infant. Because the FTA-ABS test is performed without dilutions in the United States, sequential use of this test is not useful in infants suspected of having syphilis. Eventually, of course, any passively transferred maternal IgG antibody causing reactivity in a normal infant is catabolized until it is no longer detectable. Persistence of antibody beyond 12 to 18 months of age can be considered a reliable, but often retrospective, diagnostic finding, which is seen in 50% to 70% of infants with congenital syphilis.[308,309]

Fluorescent Treponemal Antibody Immunoglobulin M Test. Detection of IgM by FTA-ABS theoretically should be helpful in diagnosing congenital infection because IgM is not transferred across the placenta. In clinical studies, however, false-negative results have been obtained in 20% to 39% of cases, and false-positive results, perhaps related to rheumatoid factor,[310] in up to 10%. Prospective clinical investigations using rigorous case definitions and standardized methods have not been performed, and the place of the FTA IgM test in the clinical practice of pediatrics remains in question.[311] Stoll and associates[312] modified the original FTA-ABS IgM test by using the IgM fraction of neonatal serum. This FTA-ABS 19S IgM test had a sensitivity of 73% and a specificity of 100% among at-risk infants.

Enzyme-Linked Immunosorbent Assay. IgM ELISAs have been developed to detect both nontreponemal[87,313] and treponemal antibodies.[174,312,313] As currently marketed, these assays are of limited usefulness in diagnosis of congenital syphilis, owing to less than optimal sensitivity and specificity. Stoll and associates[312] used an IgM capture ELISA for *T. pallidum* and found a sensitivity of only 88% among infants with clinical and laboratory manifestations of congenital syphilis. Further refinement and evaluation of these assays will be important because the ELISA has the potential for rapid diagnosis of congenitally infected infants. Moreover, many clinical laboratories already are experienced with this technique.

Immunoglobulin M and Immunoglobulin A Immunoblotting. Immunoblotting has been used to detect and characterize the specific neonatal IgM and IgA[314] antibody responses to *T. pallidum*. Specific IgM antibody directed against *T. pallidum* membrane lipoprotein antigens with apparent molecular masses of 72, 47, 45, 42, 37, 17, and 15 kDa has been detected among sera of infants with clinical manifestations of congenital syphilis; reactivity against the 47-kDa antigen was uniformly present in all of the neonatal serum IgM immunoblots with a positive result.[85-88,315,316] Fractionation of sera into IgG and IgM components by high-performance liquid chromatography confirmed that serum reactivity to these treponemal antigens was not due to rheumatoid factors.[86] Similar IgA reactivity to a variety of *T. pallidum* antigens has been detected by immunoblotting in infants with possible congenital syphilis.[314]

IgM reactivity to the 47-kDa antigen also has been found in sera of 20% to 42% of subclinically infected infants born to mothers with untreated syphilis.[88,316] It has been detected in fetal blood obtained by cordocentesis at 24 weeks of gestation; the positive serum IgM immunoblot result was validated by the simultaneous detection of viable spirochetes in the blood of this hydropic fetus by RIT.[89] Moreover, 14 weeks later at delivery, after appropriate maternal therapy, the neonatal serum lacked IgM reactivity, suggesting that the fetal infection also had been successfully treated in utero. Dobson and colleagues[85] reported disappearance of neonatal IgM reactivity to *T. pallidum* 1 to 3 months after appropriate treatment.

The ability to detect IgM reactivity in neonatal sera has been enhanced when the antigen source for immunoblotting comprised the subset of membrane proteins selectively extracted by Triton X-114 phase partitioning (detergent-phase proteins), rather than whole-cell lysates of *T. pallidum*.[88] This improvement was particularly evident in evaluation of IgM reactivities to the 15- and 17-kDa immunogens, which are known to be present in *T. pallidum* in relatively low abundance. Recently, Sanchez and co-workers showed that immunoblot analysis with a recombinant form of the highly immunogenic 47-kDa lipoprotein of *T. pallidum* appeared to be even more sensitive than immunoblotting with native *T. pallidum* antigens.[317] In some infants with congenital syphilis, IgM reactivity was apparent only when the recombinant 47-kDa lipoprotein was used as the antigen source.

Similarly, IgM reactivity to the 47-kDa antigen also has been found in CSF of infants with congenital syphilis.[88,316,318] Lewis and associates[316] found 82% reactive CSF IgM immunoblots in infants with clinical and laboratory evidence of congenital syphilis, but 4% reactivity among infants at risk of having congenital infection with *T. pallidum* but with normal findings on clinical and laboratory evaluations. Sanchez and co-workers[88] detected IgM reactivity to the 47-kDa antigen in CSF of two of seven infants in whom findings on physical and laboratory examinations were consistent with a diagnosis of congenital syphilis; the significance of the reactive IgM immunoblot was confirmed by the finding of viable treponemes in the CSF by RIT.

Polymerase Chain Reaction Techniques. PCR tests for detection of specific *T. pallidum* DNA in tissues and body fluids have been developed.[319-324] PCR assay is said to be capable of detecting an amount of purified treponemal DNA equivalent to that of only a few organisms (about 0.01 pg).[319] Sanchez and co-workers[88] have reported on the use of PCR assay for congenital syphilis diagnosis; they compared results of PCR assay on neonatal serum and CSF with those obtained by RIT, the current reference standard.[88,324,325] Results for 5 CSF samples from 19 infants born to mothers with untreated early syphilis were positive by both PCR assay and RIT, were negative for 12 by both tests, and were positive for 2 by RIT but negative by PCR assay; none were positive by PCR assay and negative by RIT. Thus, the sensitivity of PCR assay relative to RIT was 71% for CSF, and the specificity was 100%. When the results of PCR assay and RIT on 29 serum and CSF samples were combined, 9 were positive by both tests, 17 were negative by both tests, and 3 were positive by RIT but negative by PCR assay; none that was negative by RIT was positive by PCR assay. Similarly, for amniotic fluid obtained from 12 pregnant women with early syphilis, 7 of 7 samples were positive by both tests, and all 5 that were negative by RIT were negative by PCR assay. The excellent agreement between results of RIT and of PCR assay substantiates the future use of PCR assay as a surrogate for RIT.

Cerebrospinal Fluid Examination

Using RIT of neonatal CSF, Sanchez and co-workers[88] studied the prevalence of CNS invasion by *T. pallidum* among 19 infants born to mothers with early syphilis. Seven of the infants had clinical and laboratory evidence of congenital syphilis, and 12 had no clinical or laboratory findings suggestive of congenital infection. These investigators found the prevalence of spirochetal invasion of the CSF to be 86% (6 of 7) among infants with clinically recognizable congenital syphilis, but only 8% (1 of 12) among infants who lacked clinical and laboratory evidence. The sensitivity and specificity of a reactive CSF VDRL test, presence of pleocytosis, and elevated CSF protein content were 71% and 92%, 43% and 92%, and 43% and 92%, respectively. All infants with a positive CSF RIT had a reactive serum IgM immunoblot (100% sensitivity) and a positive serum PCR assay result (100% sensitivity). No infant with a negative serum IgM immunoblot and a negative serum PCR assay result had a positive result on CSF RIT, leading the investigators to conclude that the diagnosis of congenital syphilis, particularly in the infant without clinical and laboratory evidence of infection, will ultimately require a comprehensive approach using assays for both specific neonatal IgM and *T. pallidum* DNA in serum and CSF. In a more recent study, Michelow and colleagues[326] evaluated 76 infants with untreated congenital syphilis using RIT. These investigators found spirochetes in the CSF of 17 of these 76 infants; all but one had clinical or laboratory findings suggestive of neurosyphilis. IgM immunoblotting of serum identified all infants who had *T. pallidum* infection of the CNS.

With use of currently available methodologies, leukocytosis (25 white blood cells per mm^3 or less) and elevated protein content (greater than 150 mg/dL in full-term and greater than 170 mg/dL in preterm infants) in the CSF in an infant who exhibits any features suggestive of congenital syphilis should be regarded as supportive of the diagnosis. Also, an infant with reactive CSF on VDRL testing should receive presumptive treatment for neurosyphilis, although such a result in the absence of other evidence of congenital syphilis is suspect, inasmuch as nontreponemal IgG can pass from serum to the CSF in neonates.[246]

An unsettling element has been introduced by the use of various modifications of the serum FTA technique to study CSF from syphilitic patients. Conflicting results have been obtained in adults,[327-329] and systematic studies have yet to be done for congenital syphilis. Thus, at present, the FTA-ABS and hemagglutination tests should not be done using CSF in infants suspected of having congenital syphilis; the results cannot be interpreted properly, and other means must be used to establish or exclude the diagnosis.

DIFFERENTIAL DIAGNOSIS

A diagnosis of syphilitic infection is highly likely in the presence of snuffles, a vesiculobullous eruption, hepatosplenomegaly, generalized lymphadenopathy, condylomata lata, symmetrical metaphyseal lesions, and a positive result on an RPR or VDRL test. Many of these findings, however, are features of multiple other disorders or closely resemble such features.

Dermatologic Manifestations

The vesiculobullous manifestations of congenital syphilis may be confused with other infections or with congenital disorders of the skin that can present as vesiculobullous eruptions.[330] Infection caused by *Staphylococcus aureus* can produce vesicles or bullae on any part of the body. Severe infection may result in confluent bullae with erythema and desquamation (Ritter's disease). Examination of aspirated fluid reveals many polymorphonuclear leukocytes and, on occasion, gram-positive cocci in clusters, and culture will yield the organism.

Pseudomonas aeruginosa septicemia can be accompanied by a cutaneous eruption consisting of clustered pearly vesicles on an erythematous background, which rapidly becomes purulent green or hemorrhagic.[331] When the lesion ruptures, a circumscribed ulcer with a necrotic base appears and may persist, surrounded by a purplish cellulitis. Culture of the lesion and the blood confirms the diagnosis.

In the septicemic early-onset form of listeriosis, a cutaneous eruption consisting of miliary lesions resembling papules, pustules, or papulopustules can occur over the entire body, with a predilection for the back.[332] Culture of these lesions and blood usually reveals *Listeria monocytogenes* as the etiologic agent. Additional infectious causes of vesicular or bullous lesions of the skin of the newborn include group B streptococci,[333] *Haemophilus influenzae* type b,[334] *Mycobacterium tuberculosis*,[335] and cytomegalovirus.[336]

In virus-induced eruptions, the vesicles are located in the mid-epidermis. In herpesvirus infection, vesicles are the most common dermatologic manifestation. They tend to be sparsely disseminated throughout the body, or they may occur in crops or clusters. Involvement of the palms and soles has been recorded, as has the formation of bullae. Recurrence of these skin lesions is not unusual. Scrapings from the base of these lesions, when fixed in alcohol and stained with Papanicolaou stain, may show intranuclear inclusions or multinucleated giant cells compatible with the diagnosis of herpes simplex or varicella-zoster infection, and cultures may yield the offending virus. The latter infection rarely occurs in the newborn period, and the diagnosis may be discarded on epidemiologic or clinical grounds. Variola and vaccinia can affect the fetus or newborn and cause vesicular eruptions. Appropriate epidemiologic evidence should be sought to exclude these diagnoses.

Mucocutaneous candidiasis may manifest as a vesicular dermatitis at the end of the first week of life. The vesicles usually become confluent and rupture, leaving a denuded area surrounded by satellite vesicles or pustules. Congenital candidiasis with skin manifestations also has been described, and severe systemic involvement may accompany this intrauterine infection.[337]

A variety of hereditary disorders of the skin appear at birth or in early infancy as vesiculobullous eruptions.[330] Epidermolysis bullosa is a group of specific genetic disorders. Erythema toxicum, miliaria rubra, incontinentia pigmenti, urticaria pigmentosa, epidermolytic hyperkeratosis, acrodermatitis enteropathica, Langerhans' cell histiocytosis (histiocytosis X), transient neonatal pustular melanosis, infantile acropustulosis, and aplasia cutis congenita should be included in the differential diagnosis.[338]

Hepatosplenomegaly

When the clinical presentation is that of hepatosplenomegaly with or without jaundice, the list of possiblities in the differential diagnosis is extensive and includes all causes of elevated direct and indirect bilirubin. The physician should consider isoimmunization (e.g., Rh incompatibility, ABO incompatibility), other infectious diseases (early-onset sepsis, cytomegalovirus infection, congenital rubella, herpes simplex infection, coxsackievirus B or other enteroviral infections, toxoplasmosis), neonatal hepatitis, diseases of the biliary tract (e.g., extrahepatic biliary atresia or choledochal cyst), and genetic and metabolic disorders (e.g., cystic fibrosis, galactosemia, and α_1-antitrypsin deficiency).[339]

Hydrops Fetalis

Hydrops fetalis can be caused by chronic anemia (isoimmunization disorder, homozygous α-thalassemia, fetomaternal or fetofetal transfusions), cardiac or pulmonary failure due to causes other than anemia (large arteriovenous malformations, premature closure of the foramen ovale, cystic adenomatoid malformation, pulmonary lymphangiectasia), perinatal tumors (neuroblastoma, chorioangioma), achondroplasia, renal disorders (congenital nephrosis, renal vein thrombosis), and infections, such as congenital cytomegalovirus infection, toxoplasmosis, parvovirus B19 infection,[340] and congenital hepatitis.[339]

Most cases of hydrops are caused by isoimmunization disorders, which can be excluded as a cause by a negative direct Coombs' test result. A normal hemoglobin electrophoresis pattern excludes the diagnosis of α-thalassemia. The Kleihauer-Betke technique of acid elution for identifying fetal cells in the maternal circulation can aid in ruling out the diagnosis of fetomaternal transfusion. Other diagnostic considerations can be discarded on the basis of appropriate radiographic studies, placental examination, urinalysis with microscopy, biopsy, and immunologic studies.

Renal Disease

In the neonate and young infant, the nephrotic syndrome and acute nephritis occur infrequently. The former more often is associated with infantile microcystic disease, minimal-lesion nephrotic syndrome, or renal vein thrombosis than with congenital syphilis. Neonatal nephritis can occur as a manifestation of congenital syphilis, hereditary nephritis, hemolytic-uremic syndrome, and, rarely, pyelonephritis. The clinical signs that distinguish syphilitic renal involvement from the other conditions mentioned include the presence of other manifestations of early congenital syphilis, a positive result on serologic tests for syphilis, elevated levels of IgG (in infantile microcystic disease, the levels of IgG are low), and the response to specific therapy for syphilis.

Ophthalmologic Involvement

Neonatal buphthalmos, an uncommon finding in syphilis, occurs as an isolated genetic disorder and may be associated with a variety of syndromes (e.g., aniridia, Hallermann-Streiff syndrome, Reiger's anomaly, Lowe's syndrome, Sturge-Weber syndrome, oculodentodigital syndrome, Pierre Robin syndrome); it also is associated with rubella.[341] Nasolacrimal duct obstruction is a more frequent cause of excessive lacrimation in the newborn period and early infancy.

THERAPY

The Pregnant Woman

A pregnant woman who has a suspicious lesion and a negative RPR test result may be in an early stage of infection. Detection of treponemes by darkfield microscopy should lead to therapy without regard to results of serologic tests; an RPR test should be repeated in 3 to 6 weeks (Table 18-10). A patient who has neither lesions nor positive results of serologic studies but who has been exposed sexually to a person who has syphilis should receive treatment for syphilis on the 25% to 50% likelihood that she has acquired syphilis and is in the early phase of the infection and able to infect the fetus.[157,227]

The finding of a positive RPR reaction should lead to a careful and complete evaluation of the pregnant patient for evidence of primary or secondary syphilis. If signs of active disease are not found and the treponemal test result also is reactive, then a diagnosis of latent syphilis is made, with the diagnosis being early latent disease if she was known to have a negative RPR result within the previous 1 to 2 years.

Failure of nontreponemal serologic titers to decrease appropriately is reason for CSF examination and retreatment unless reinfection can be established as the cause.[116] Moreover, persons with no decrease in titer should be reevaluated for HIV infection. In late latent syphilis or syphilis of unknown duration, a lumbar puncture is recommended in patients who are seropositive for antibody to HIV to exclude neurosyphilis.[156]

If the pregnant woman had positive results on RPR and treponemal tests before this pregnancy and it is certain that she received appropriate treatment, observation during the

Table 18–10 Therapeutic Decisions Involving the Pregnant Woman in Relation to Rapid Plasma Reagin (RPR) Status[a,b,c]

RPR Status	Decision
Negative RPR Result	
Signs of clinical disease	Treat[d,e]
No signs of clinical disease	*High risk*
	Repeat RPR at 28 wk and at term
	Low risk
	Repeat RPR at term
Positive RPR Result	
Signs of clinical disease[e]	Treat
No signs of clinical disease	
Known positive syphilis tests in past	
Adequate treatment	Observe[f]
Untreated	Treat
New positive TP-PA test	
If positive[e]	Evaluate and treat
If negative	Perform FTA-ABS
	If positive: Evaluate and treat[e]
	If negative: Observe[g] and repeat TP-PA in 3 wk
	If positive: Evaluate and treat[e]
	If negative: Observe[g]

[a]Positive result on RPR is the most common reason for medical evaluation.
[b]See text.
[c]See Table 18-8 for full test names.
[d]Test for possible prozone effect.
[e]Test for HIV antibody.
[f]Treat if RPR titer is greater than 1:4 (VDRL titer greater than 1:2) in a woman with a history of pre-pregnancy therapy—possible reinfection.
[g]Assume a biologically false-positive result (see text).
HIV, human immunodeficiency virus.

pregnancy, with clinical evaluation and RPR testing repeated in the third trimester and at delivery, constitutes adequate management. Serologic titers may be checked monthly in women at high risk for reinfection or in geographic areas in which the prevalence of syphilis is high.[156,342] Although it is expected that the nontreponemal test will eventually become nonreactive after appropriate treatment, some patients may have persistence of nontreponemal antibodies at a low titer for an extended period of time. This response is referred to as the *serofast reaction*, and the patient is not infectious.

If the pregnant woman has a positive RPR result but a nonreactive treponemal test, the result is referred to as a "biologically false-positive" result. Caution must be exercised to rule out the presence of early syphilis, because the RPR test becomes reactive earlier than do the treponemal tests. In cases of early syphilis, a second treponemal test performed 3 to 6 weeks later will be reactive, and the patient should be given treatment as noted earlier.

Penicillin

Parenteral penicillin G remains the drug of choice for the treatment of syphilis (Table 18-11).[156,343-345] A regimen of benzathine penicillin G (2.4 million units given as 1.2 million units in each buttock) appropriate for the stage of syphilis cures maternal infection and prevents or cures fetal infection.[156,343] For women with early syphilis, a second dose of benzathine penicillin (2.4 million units intramuscularly) can be administered 1 week after the initial dose, to minimize the occurrence of a fetal treatment failure.[156]

Failure rates for prevention of fetal infection ranging from 2%[270] to as high as 14% (see Table 18-2) have been reported. A majority of fetal treatment failures seem to occur after maternal treatment for secondary syphilis.[346] Treatment failure in such cases may be explained in part by the marked spirochetemia that occurs during secondary syphilitic infection. Other reasons for the presumptive treatment

Table 18–11 Recommended Treatment of Syphilis in Pregnant Patient[a]

Stage of Syphilis	Drug (Penicillin)	Route	Dose (units)
Early (duration less than 1 yr)	*Recommended*		
Primary, secondary, or early latent			
HIV antibody–negative	Benzathine	IM	2.4 million single dose; possibly repeat in 1 wk
HIV antibody–positive[b]	Benzathine	IM	2.4 million single dose; possibly repeat weekly × 3
	Alternative		
	Penicillin desensitization[c]		
Latent (duration longer than 1 yr)[d]	*Recommended*		
	Benzathine	IM	2.4 million weekly × 3 wk
	Alternative		
	Penicillin desensitization		
Neurosyphilis	*Recommended*		
	Aqueous	IV	3-4 million every 4 hr × 10-14 days
	Alternative		
	Procaine[e]	IM	2.4 million daily × 10-14 days

[a]See text.
[b]With normal cerebrospinal fluid findings, if performed.
[c]For details, see MMWR Morb Mortal Wkly Rep 51(RR-6):1, 2002.
[d]Lumbar puncture to exclude neurosyphilis is recommended for HIV antibody–positive patients.
[e]Probenecid, 500 mg orally qid × 10-14 days, also should be prescribed.
HIV, human immunodeficiency virus; IM, intramuscular; IV, intravenous.

failures have been related to possibly altered penicillin pharmacokinetics in pregnancy[347] or to advanced fetal disease.[348] Problems exist in the interpretation of these data because, by currently available methodologies, the accurate identification of an infected newborn is problematic at best. The clinical and laboratory manifestations of congenital syphilis may require several weeks to months for resolution despite adequate penicillin therapy. Likewise, the fetus may be adequately treated in utero by maternal penicillin therapy yet have persistent abnormalities that are detected at birth because insufficient time has elapsed for complete disappearance of the physical and laboratory abnormalities. Such a case would be erroneously classified as a treatment failure. Moreover, the improper use of the CDC surveillance case definitions as diagnostic criteria for congenital syphilis has led to the misclassification of infants as infected when the diagnosis is not certain.

Invasion of the CNS by *T. pallidum* can occur during any stage of syphilis.[101] Currently recommended therapy for neurosyphilis is aqueous crystalline penicillin G, 18 to 24 million units daily, administered as 3 to 4 million units intravenously every 4 hours for 10 to 14 days. If compliance can be ensured, an alternative regimen consists of procaine penicillin G, 2.4 million units intramuscularly daily, plus probenecid, 500 mg orally four times a day, both given for 10 to 14 days.[208,293] Benzathine penicillin G, 2.4 million units intramuscularly weekly for up to 3 weeks, often is provided after completion of either of these two neurosyphilis treatment regimens.[156]

Syphilis can be more difficult to eradicate in the presence of concurrent HIV infection.[101,344,349] Nevertheless, current recommendations include a regimen similar to that for patients who lack HIV antibody (see Table 18-11), along with careful and frequent clinical and serologic follow-up.[156] For HIV-infected patients with primary or secondary syphilis, some authorities recommend up to three once-weekly doses of 2.4 million units of benzathine penicillin G or other supplemental antibiotics,[156] in addition to a single intramuscular dose of benzathine penicillin G. HIV-infected patients who have either late latent syphilis or syphilis of unknown duration require a CSF examination before treatment. If nontreponemal antibody titers have not declined fourfold by 6 months with primary or secondary syphilis, or by 6 to 12 months in early latent syphilis, or if the titer has increased fourfold at any time, a CSF examination should be performed and the patient re-treated with 7.2 million units of benzathine penicillin G (administered as three once-weekly doses of 2.4 million units each) if CSF examination findings are normal. Patients who have CSF abnormalities consistent with neurosyphilis should receive treatment for neurosyphilis as described earlier (see Table 18-11).

Alternative Drugs

The pregnant syphilitic patient who has a history of penicillin allergy should be skin tested and, if necessary, desensitized according to the protocol of Wendel and co-workers.[350] Desensitization can be accomplished by providing the patient with gradually increasing doses of oral or intravenous penicillin during several hours until the objective of full tolerance is achieved. Such an approach must be attempted only under expert guidance and under circumstances in which emergency treatment is available.[156]

Multiple-dose regimens of ceftriaxone for treatment of primary and secondary syphilis, as well as for neurosyphilis, have been efficacious in limited studies.[351-357] A 10-day course of ceftriaxone is an alternative regimen for the nonpregnant, penicillin-allergic patient with early syphilis. Data are insufficient to recommend ceftriaxone treatment during pregnancy. In rabbits, a 7- to 10-day course of ceftriaxone failed to clear CNS infection with *T. pallidum* in a consistent fashion.[358] An occasional patient who is allergic to penicillin also is allergic to the cephalosporins, and cephalosporins should not be used if the penicillin allergy is potentially life-threatening.[156,352-357]

Erythromycin, which is effective in syphilis,[343,359] crosses the placenta in an unpredictable fashion, often poorly.[345] Erythromycin does not reliably cure the infected fetus, and it should not be used.[360]

Tetracycline given in a dosage of 28 g orally over a 14-day period (2 g per day in four doses) compares favorably in effectiveness with penicillin.[156,361] Because of its potential for damage to the liver of the pregnant woman[362,363] and its adverse effects on the teeth and long bones of the fetus,[364] tetracycline should not be used in pregnancy.

Preliminary data on use of azithromycin for treatment of syphilis in nonpregnant adults have shown efficacy.[365,366] Azithromycin treatment failures have occurred, however.[365,367] A mutation in ribosomal RNA recently has been described that confers azithromycin resistance to *T. pallidum*.[368] Caution is advised with use of azithromycin for therapy of syphilis; no data regarding its use in pregnancy are available to ensure its effectiveness in the prevention of fetal syphilis.

During a shortage of intravenous aqueous penicillin G in the United States,[369] the CDC recommended that for treatment of neurosyphilis, procaine penicillin G plus probenecid (see Table 18-11) be administered when intravenous penicillin is not available.[370] For persons with neurosyphilis who do not tolerate intramuscular procaine penicillin G, intravenous ampicillin (12 to 16 g per day in four divided doses for 10 to 14 days) or, alternatively, intravenous ceftriaxone (2 g daily, given as a single dose, for 10 to 14 days) could be considered for use only if careful clinical and serologic follow-up evaluation was ensured. For persons with neurosyphilis who are allergic to penicillin, desensitization to penicillin followed by treatment with either aqueous penicillin or procaine penicillin is preferred. These regimens for neurosyphilis can be followed by a single dose of benzathine penicillin G (see Table 18-11).

The Infant

Treatment for newborns with a reactive serologic test for syphilis is required in the following situations (Table 18-12)[156,371,372]:

- If the infant has clinical, laboratory, or radiographic abnormalities, or a combination of these, compatible with congenital syphilis
- If no maternal treatment before delivery was documented
- If maternal treatment was inadequate or unknown
- If maternal treatment was with drugs other than penicillin

Table 18–12 Therapeutic Decisions Involving the Infant in Relation to Rapid Plasma Reagin (RPR) Status

RPR Status	Decision
Negative RPR Result	
Possible early syphilis	
Without clinical findings	Treat
With clinical findings	Evaluate for other congenital infection; if none apparent, treat
Positive RPR Result	
With clinical manifestations	Treat
Without clinical manifestations, perform the following:	
1. Quantitative RPR in mother and infant—if infant titer fourfold higher	Treat
2. Hematologic studies—if abnormal	Treat
3. Bone radiography—if abnormal	Treat
4. Lumbar puncture—if abnormal	Treat
5. If mother	
a. Has no, inadequate, or undocumented treatment	Treat
b. Was treated with nonpenicillin	Treat
c. Was treated within 4 wk of delivery	Treat
d. Or if adequate follow-up of newborn in doubt	Treat

- If the mother received treatment within 4 weeks of delivery
- If the mother received treatment for early syphilis during the pregnancy with the appropriate penicillin regimen, but nontreponemal antibody titers did not decrease at least fourfold
- If the mother had serologic evidence of relapse or reinfection after treatment (a fourfold or greater increase in nontreponemal antibody titer)
- If adequate follow-up of the infant is uncertain

A practical approach is to provide treatment for congenital syphilis for all newborns who have a positive RPR test result even if the mother is not thought to have an active infection. This recommendation is based on a number of pragmatic considerations: (1) it may be difficult to document that the mother received adequate therapy and has a falling RPR titer; (2) a low-titer RPR test result may be compatible with untreated latent maternal syphilis; (3) the newborn, if infected, may not have any clinical manifestations at birth; and (4) compliance with follow-up visits is a monumental problem. Clearly, if the infant has a positive RPR test result and any signs consistent with congenital syphilis, treatment should be administered. If no clinical findings are present, however, a quantitative RPR test should be performed on blood from the mother and her newborn. Treatment is indicated if the infant has a titer four or more times higher than that of the mother.

In infants in whom findings on physical examination are normal and the quantitative RPR titer is not significantly higher than in the mother, the maternal history of infection with *T. pallidum* and treatment for syphilis must be considered in evaluation and treatment for the infant. If the infant may be infected, then hematologic investigation, skeletal radiographic survey, and lumbar puncture should be performed. If any of these reveal abnormalities that are consistent with the diagnosis of congenital syphilis, the infant must receive appropriate treatment.[156,372]

In the previous 2 decades, the need for examination of CSF obtained at lumbar puncture and for long bone radiographic evaluation has been questioned.[373,374] Beeram and colleagues[373] have reported that among infants who had normal findings on physical examination but were born to mothers with untreated or inadequately treated syphilis, a reactive CSF VDRL test was found in only 0.6% of evaluated infants. Mean CSF white blood cell count and protein content did not differ significantly from those in a control population of healthy infants who had negative evaluations for bacterial infection, including sterile cultures of blood and CSF. Using the stricter criteria of Platou (white blood cell count greater than 5 cells/mm^3; protein content greater than 40 mg/dL) in determination of abnormal CSF indices, 44% and 95% of control infants had CSF pleocytosis and elevated protein content, respectively. This study supports the recent recommendation by the CDC (see later) that if treatment for possible neurosyphilis is provided to infants at risk of being infected with *T. pallidum*, performance of a lumbar puncture is not necessary.[156] This study also highlights the need to use appropriate reference values in the evaluation of neonatal CSF.

Similarly, long bone radiographic findings frequently are abnormal among infants with clinical signs of congenital syphilis.[374] These infants require prolonged penicillin therapy irrespective of the results of the skeletal survey, and both the CDC and American Academy of Pediatrics no longer require that such surveys be routinely performed in these circumstances.[156,372] Nevertheless, because as many as 6% of normal infants born to mothers with untreated syphilis may have bone abnormalities as the sole manifestation of possible congenital syphilis,[374] radiographic examination should be performed before the decision to manage at-risk infants with only a single dose of benzathine penicillin therapy.[156]

If the meaning of a positive RPR test result in an otherwise normal infant is in doubt and the results of all other tests are negative, repeated quantitative RPR testing should be done. When antibody is passively acquired from the mother, serial quantitative tests show a declining titer. A falling titer suggests that the infant is free of infection; on the other hand, a stable or rising titer implies the presence of infection. The decision concerning treatment or observation of such a newborn depends on the clinical setting; whether the mother has received antibiotic therapy; the results of other tests such as skeletal radiography, liver function tests, and hematologic studies; and the opportunity for adequate follow-up. Antisyphilitic therapy is indicated in any circumstance in which the mother is unreliable and compliance with the therapeutic regimen and adequate follow-up care cannot be ensured.

It should not be forgotten that in the newborn, a negative RPR test result may not exclude incubating syphilis if maternal infection was in the earliest clinical stage and antibodies had not reached detectable levels.[157,227] Thus,

Table 18–13 Recommended Treatment of the Newborn[a, b]

Maternal Rx[c]	Clinical Findings in Newborn	Drug (Penicillin G)	Route	Dose (50,000 units/kg)
None or inadequate[d]	Present	Aqueous	IM or IV	Daily × 10-14 days in two (<7 days), three (8-30 days), or four (>1 mo) doses
		or		
		Procaine	IM	Daily dose × 10-14 days
None or inadequate[d]	Absent	Aqueous	IM or IV	Daily × 10-14 days in two (<7 days), three (8-30 days), or four (>1 mo) doses
		or		
		Procaine	IM	Daily dose × 10-14 days
		or		
		Benzathine	IM	Single dose
Adequate (during pregnancy)	Absent	Benzathine (CDC)	IM	Single dose
		or		
		Follow-up only (AAP)		
Adequate (before pregnancy)	Absent	Follow-up only	IM	Single dose
		or		
		Benzathine (only if follow-up cannot be ensured)		

[a]Close and frequent follow-up, including serologic test for syphilis, is essential.
[b]Test mother for HIV antibody.
[c]Inadequate maternal treatment: not documented, within 4 weeks of delivery, or with erythromycin or nonpenicillin drug; or serologic antibody titers do not fall appropriately (see text).
[d]Some experts would not treat if follow-up is ensured.
HIV, human immunodeficiency virus; IM, intramuscular; IV, intravenous.

such an infant without clinical abnormalities should undergo a second RPR test within 3 to 4 weeks. If the risk of exposure to the infant is considerable (e.g., if the child was born to a known syphilitic with no documented treatment history), a reasonable case can be made for immediate penicillin therapy. If the newborn has clinical manifestations that are thought to be consistent with the diagnosis of congenital syphilis, a negative RPR test result makes this clinical diagnosis highly questionable; reevaluation is indicated. Finally, the appearance of secondary or tertiary syphilis in the mother within the year after delivery should prompt a thorough reevaluation of the infant for the possibility of congenital syphilis.

Penicillin

Penicillin remains the drug of choice for treatment of congenital syphilis (Table 18-13).[88,98,136,156,359,371,372,375] Infants who are 4 weeks of age or younger and who have proven or highly probable disease are likely to have CNS invasion by *T. pallidum*.[88] These include (1) infants with physical findings compatible with congenital syphilis; (2) infants who lack such physical findings but have abnormalities on CSF examination, on bone radiographs, or on laboratory evaluation; (3) infants who have a serum quantitative nontreponemal serologic titer that is four times greater than the mother's titer; and (4) infants who have a positive result on darkfield or fluorescent antibody test of body fluids. The evaluation[156,372] of these infants should begin with CSF analysis to detect evidence of possible neurosyphilis and to establish a baseline for follow-up evaluation. A complete blood cell count and platelet count also should be performed, because anemia and thrombocytopenia may not be readily detected by physical examination only. Other tests such as chest radiography, cranial ultrasound study, ophthalmologic examination, and auditory-evoked brainstem response evaluation should be performed as clinically indicated.

Infants with proven or highly probable disease should receive treatment for 10 days with either (1) aqueous crystalline penicillin G, 50,000 units/kg intravenously every 12 hours for the first week of life and every 8 hours beyond 1 week of age or (2) aqueous procaine penicillin G, 50,000 units/kg administered intramuscularly once daily for 10 days.[156,372] If more than 1 day of therapy is missed, the entire course of penicillin be restarted.[156] Although the CSF levels of penicillin are higher in infants who receive intravenous aqueous penicillin G than in those given intramuscular procaine penicillin, the significance of this finding remains unclear, because both therapies have resulted in clinical and laboratory cure.[376] Similarly, infants and children who are identified as having congenital syphilis after the neonatal period (beyond 4 weeks of age) should receive aqueous penicillin G, 50,000 units/kg intravenously every 6 hours for 10 days.[156] For older children, the amount of penicillin should not exceed that recommended for adults (see Table 18-11). The efficacy of a 10-day course of penicillin for eradication of spirochetes from neonatal CSF has been documented.[88,326]

For infants who have normal findings on physical examination and a serum quantitative nontreponemal serologic titer that is the same as or less than four times the maternal titer, the evaluation is dependent on the maternal treatment history, maternal stage of infection, and planned infant treatment (see Table 18-13).[156] If maternal treatment for syphilis was not given, was undocumented, was a nonpenicillin regimen, or was administered 4 weeks or less before delivery, or if the adequacy of maternal treatment for early syphilis cannot be evaluated because the nontreponemal serologic titer has not decreased fourfold, or relapse or reinfection is suspected because of a fourfold increase in the maternal nontreponemal serologic titer, then the infant should receive the following treatment: (1) aqueous penicillin G or procaine penicillin G for 10 days or (2) benzathine penicillin G, 50,000 units/kg (single dose intramuscularly) with close serologic follow-up studies.[156,372] If the infant receives a 10-day course of parenteral penicillin, then a complete evaluation consisting of a lumbar puncture, complete blood cell count and platelet count, and bone radiographs may not be necessary, because the infant will receive adequate therapy for proven or highly probable disease (see earlier), including possible neurosyphilis.[116] Nevertheless, abnormalities found on these tests may further support a diagnosis of congenital syphilis, and performance of a lumbar puncture may document CSF abnormalities that would prompt close follow-up. On the other hand, if the infant is to receive a single intramuscular injection of benzathine penicillin G, then a complete evaluation (lumbar puncture, complete blood cell count with platelet count, and bone radiographs) is mandatory.[156,372] Using RIT as the diagnostic standard, Michelow and colleagues[326] have shown that most infants with *T. pallidum* infection of the CNS can be identified by this combination of tests. If any test has an abnormal result, or if any part of the evaluation is not done, then a 10-day course of penicillin is recommended.

The decision by both the CDC[116] and the American Academy of Pediatrics[372] to allow the expanded use of a single intramuscular dose of benzathine penicillin G is based on the finding that, in contrast with the infant with clinical manifestations of congenital syphilis, the prevalence of CNS invasion by *T. pallidum* as documented by RIT is very low in infants who lack physical, radiographic, or laboratory evidence of congenital infection.[88] Single-dose benzathine penicillin therapy has been widely used in the past, and its use allows for earlier hospital discharge of the infant with subsequent improved maternal-infant interaction and decrease in hospitalization costs.[377] This regimen has been supported by two small clinical studies.[378,379]

Nonetheless, failure of a single injection of benzathine penicillin G administered to three infants has been reported.[380,381] These infants were born to mothers with early syphilis and were not fully evaluated for evidence of congenital syphilis at delivery. These treatment failures have been attributed to the inability of benzathine penicillin G to adequately penetrate and achieve treponemicidal concentration in certain sites, such as the aqueous humor and CNS.[382,383] Michelow and colleagues[325] have documented the presence of spirochetes in the CSF of three infants without clinical manifestations who received a single injection of benzathine penicillin; at follow-up evaluation, findings on CSF examination were normal and the results of RIT for spirochetes were negative. These investigators recommend that if the evaluation for congenital syphilis is not complete or not performed, the infant should receive empirical therapy that will eradicate *T. pallidum* from the CNS.

For infants who appear healthy on physical examination and have a serum quantitative nontreponemal serologic titer that is the same as or less than four times the maternal titer, evaluation is unnecessary if during pregnancy the maternal treatment was appropriate for the stage of infection, and (1) it was given more than 4 weeks before delivery, (2) it was for early syphilis and the nontreponemal serologic titers decreased fourfold after appropriate therapy, or (3) it was for late latent syphilis, the nontreponemal titers remained stable and low, and evidence of maternal reinfection or relapse is lacking.[156] The CDC recommends that in these situations, a single intramuscular dose of benzathine penicillin G 50,000 units/kg be administered to the infant.[156] Some experts, however, would not treat these infants but would provide close serologic follow-up only.[156,372]

For infants who have normal findings on physical examination and a serum quantitative nontreponemal serologic titer that is the same as or less than four times the maternal titer, evaluation and treatment are unnecessary if the maternal treatment was before pregnancy and the nontreponemal serologic titers remained low and stable before and during the pregnancy and at delivery.[156] If compliance with follow-up is uncertain, a single intramuscular dose of benzathine penicillin G, 50,000 units/kg, may be given.

Infants born to mothers co-infected with syphilis and HIV do not require different evaluation or therapy for syphilis from that recommended for all infants.[156] These infants born to co-infected women may be at higher risk of infection with *T. pallidum*[98,100]; however, it is not known whether co-infected infants respond to treatment for congenital syphilis differently from infants uninfected with HIV. Close serologic follow-up evaluation of these infants is mandatory.

Alternative Drugs

Very few alternative regimens are available for infants with congenital syphilis. Clinical studies of the treatment of congenital syphilis with ampicillin or ceftriaxone, or other new cephalosporins that readily penetrate the blood-brain barrier, have not been reported, although theoretically these drugs should be effective.[384]

Infants with congenital syphilis should receive procaine penicillin or benzathine penicillin G for treatment (see Table 18-13).

The lack of adequate CNS penetration by erythromycin or oral tetracycline makes these drugs inappropriate for the treatment of congenital syphilis. In addition, tetracycline and doxycycline are not advised for children younger than 8 years of age because they may stain the teeth and possibly cause bone toxicity.

Jarisch-Herxheimer Reaction

The Jarisch-Herxheimer reaction, a common occurrence in the treatment of acquired early syphilis in adults,[385] consists of chills, fever, generalized malaise, hypotension, tachycardia, tachypnea, accentuation of the cutaneous lesions, leukocytosis, and, exceedingly rarely, death. It begins within 2 hours of treatment, peaks at approximately 8 hours, and disappears in 24 to 36 hours. The cause of the reaction is not known,[386] although release of *T. pallidum* membrane lipoproteins that stimulate pro-inflammatory cytokines likely explains this clinical phenomenon.[387]

Table 18–14 Follow-up after Treatment or Prophylaxis for Congenital Syphilis

Patient Category	Follow-up Procedures
Infants diagnosed as having congenital syphilis	1. RPR testing every 2-3 mo until negative or decreased fourfold. If RPR titer is stable or increasing after 6-12 mo after treatment, reevaluate and re-treat. 2. Perform treponemal antibody test after age of 15 mo. 3. If initial CSF was abnormal or infant showed signs of CNS disease, repeat CSF evaluation every 6 mo until normal. With abnormal CSF not due to intercurrent illness on re-testing, re-treat. 4. Careful developmental evaluation, vision testing, and hearing testing are indicated.
Infants who received treatment in utero or at birth because of maternal syphilis	1. RPR testing at birth and then every 3 mo until result is negative. 2. Treponemal antibody test after age of 15 mo.
Women who received treatment for syphilis during pregnancy	1. RPR testing as often as monthly until delivery, then every 6 mo until negative result obtained or titer decreased fourfold. 2. Re-treatment any time there is a fourfold rise in RPR titer.

CNS, central nervous system; CSF, cerebrospinal fluid; RPR, rapid plasma reagin.
Modified from Rathbun KC. Congenital syphilis: a proposal for improved surveillance, diagnosis and treatment. Sex Transm Dis 10:102, 1983, with permission; and MMWR Morb Mortal Wkly Rep 51(RR-6):1, 2002.

Approximately 40% of pregnant women who receive treatment for syphilis demonstrate a Jarisch-Herxheimer reaction.[388,389] In addition, these women may experience the onset of uterine contractions and preterm labor, with decreased fetal activity and fetal heart rate changes, including late decelerations, which last up to 24 to 48 hours and may lead to fetal death. These manifestations of the Jarisch-Herxheimer reaction in pregnancy possibly are mediated by the prostaglandin pathway. No prophylactic measure or treatment currently is available. Abnormal ultrasonographic findings in the fetus, as well as fetal monitoring for 24 hours, may identify pregnancies at highest risk.

In congenital syphilis, the incidence of the Jarisch-Herxheimer reaction is low, although it may be more common when treatment occurs later in infancy[227]; when it does occur, it varies in severity, ranging from fever to cardiovascular collapse and seizures.[88] In Platou's series,[234] almost half of the infants sustained a febrile reaction during the first 36 hours after initiation of penicillin therapy. No relationship was observed between the severity or the outcome of the infection and this temperature elevation.

Post-treatment Follow-up

Recommendations for follow-up evaluation are summarized in Table 18-14. It is advisable to monitor the outcome of therapy by repeated RPR testing. Patients responding to therapy should have falling titers (fourfold or better decrease), and as many as 70% to 93% should become seronegative within 1 year.[234,309] Re-treatment should be considered if signs persist or recur, if any increase in the titer of a non-treponemal test is noted, if an initially high-titer non-treponemal test fails to decrease fourfold in the first year, or if the repeated lumbar puncture plus CSF analysis at 6 months shows persistent abnormalities, including a positive VDRL test result.[156] The recommendation of a second treponemal test beyond 15 months as a way of retrospectively diagnosing congenital syphilis[308] is not merely for epidemiologic use—an established diagnosis can help in medical and developmental follow-up evaluation of the child.

PROGNOSIS

Although treatment can cure the infection, the prognosis in treated congenital syphilis depends on the degree of damage before the initiation of therapy. In general, the earlier treatment is initiated, the more likely it is that a satisfactory response can be obtained.[390] If marked damage to the fetus has occurred, treatment in utero may not prevent abortion, stillbirth, or neonatal death, and even if treatment keeps the newborn infant alive, stigmata can remain. If the treatment is provided prenatally or within the first 3 months of life, and such stigmata have not yet become apparent, they generally can be prevented.[253] Interstitial keratitis is an exception; this complication does not seem to be responsive to specific antibiotic therapy. On occasion, dramatic relief has been afforded by the use of corticosteroids and mydriatics, although relapses have occurred with cessation of corticosteroid therapy. The osseous lesions seem to heal independently of specific therapy. Treatment of congenital syphilis in the late stage does not reverse the stigmata.[194]

A number of reports describe the persistence of treponemes after therapy for syphilis in both humans and animals.[391-394] *T. pallidum* has been shown to survive in the lymph nodes, eye, and CSF after doses of penicillin that are presumed adequate. Silverstein[162,395] observed that monkeys inoculated in utero with *T. pallidum* had a significant number of viable treponemes in the aqueous humor of their clinically normal eyes 6 months after birth. Hardy and associates[396] described a newborn with congenital syphilis treated with penicillin in whom the aqueous humor contained virulent treponemes, and a number of cases of recrudescence of neurosyphilis in adults have been described after treatment with recommended doses of penicillin.[397-399] Survival of the organism in the eye or CSF is ascribed to inadequate penetration of penicillin, but this explanation does not account for persistence of treponemes in lymph nodes after treatment.

PREVENTION

Congenital syphilis is a preventable disease. To minimize the likelihood of its occurrence, every woman who becomes pregnant should undergo at least one serologic test for syphilis during the first trimester.[112,144,307,400] For communities and populations in which the prevalence of syphilis is high or for women in high-risk groups (see Table 18-3), repeated testing at the beginning of the third trimester (at 28 weeks of gestation)[135,139]and at delivery is recommended.[156,342] Sanchez and associates[139] have documented the importance of maternal serologic screening for syphilis at delivery in a high-risk inner-city population. During the years 1987 to 1990, approximately 3% of 58,387 pregnant women had reactive serologic tests for syphilis; in 5% of these women, an antepartum RPR test was nonreactive, but an RPR test at delivery was reactive.

Screening tests at delivery should be performed in mothers and not in infants.[112,156,306] An infant's serologic titer often is one to two dilutions less than that of the mother's; thus, an infant may have a nonreactive umbilical cord VDRL test but have a mother with a reactive serologic test for syphilis at delivery. From 1987 to 1990, Sanchez and co-workers[139] compared results of maternal serologic studies at delivery with those obtained from VDRL testing of umbilical cord blood. These investigators documented 534 cases with reactive maternal serologic tests at delivery but negative umbilical cord blood VDRL test results. Eighty-seven, or 16%, of these infants were born to mothers with untreated syphilis at delivery and were therefore at risk for infection if treatment was not given. It is clear that these infants would not have been identified if only the umbilical cord blood had been screened. No infant should be discharged from the nursery before results of maternal serologic screening have been documented. With the practice of early discharge at 48 hours or less, it becomes the responsibility of the health care provider to arrange for adequate follow-up in infants who are discharged before the result of the maternal serologic test is known.

In most clinical facilities, prenatal testing is required by law or as a matter of institutional procedure. Some states also mandate serologic screening at delivery for all women. The alternative of targeted testing is impractical to implement and would save little money, even as rates of syphilis decline in women and infants.[401] Printed requirements do not eliminate human error, and prenatal testing requirements are not applicable to a woman who does not enter the medical care system until the moment before delivery.

In an infant born to a woman who is incubating syphilis at delivery and whose serologic tests are nonreactive, congenital syphilis is, by current methods, impossible to prevent.[157,227] In areas with a high incidence of congenital syphilis, a postpartum serologic test for syphilis at 6 weeks can be helpful in detecting infants in this high-risk group.

Reporting of cases to the local health department will allow rapid-contact investigation of named sexual partners and appropriate follow-up for infected persons. Patients who have had sexual contact with an untreated person should have clinical evaluation, serologic testing, and treatment. The time periods before treatment used for identifying at-risk sexual partners are (1) 3 months plus duration of symptoms for primary syphilis; (2) 6 months plus duration of symptoms for secondary syphilis; and (3) 1 year for early latent syphilis.[156] Persons who were exposed within 90 days preceding the diagnosis of primary, secondary, or early latent syphilis in a sexual partner might be infected even if seronegative and should receive presumptive treatment.

As partner notification has become more challenging because of anonymous sex and the inability to locate sexual partners, attention has focused on identifying core environments and populations in which syphilis transmission is occurring.[402] Such knowledge has resulted in provision of prophylactic syphilis treatment to groups of people in high-risk populations. Recently, the CDC has designed a strategy to assist public health providers at both state and local levels to design interventions for targeted at-risk populations that are locally identified.[403] Called the rapid ethnographic community assessment process (RECAP), the assessment is a package of activities and tools designed to use ethnographic methods for improving community involvement, as well as developing interventions that fit a population's social and behavioral context. It has been used in North Carolina with success.[403] Ultimately, prevention of congenital syphilis will be accomplished only if elimination of syphilis becomes a reality.

REFERENCES

1. Ballantyne JW. Manual of Antenatal Pathology and Hygiene. Edinburgh, William Green & Son Publishers, 1902.
2. Goodman H. Notable Contributions to the Knowledge of Syphilis. New York, Froben Press, 1943.
3. Dennis CC. A History of Syphilis. Springfield, Ill, Charles C Thomas, 1962.
4. Truffi M. Hieronymous Fracastor's Syphilis: A Translation in Prose, 2nd ed. St Louis, Urologic and Cutaneous Press, 1931.
5. Pusey WA. The History and Epidemiology of Syphilis. Springfield, Ill, Charles C Thomas, 1933.
6. Brown WJ, Donohue JF, Axnick NW, et al. Syphilis and Other Venereal Diseases. Cambridge, Mass, Harvard University Press, 1970.
7. Hutchinson J. On the different forms of the inflammation of the eye consequent on inherited syphilis. Ophthalmol Hosp Rev 1:191, 1858.
8. Rosebury T. Microbes and Morals: The Strange Story of Venereal Disease. New York, Viking Press, 1971.
9. Hovind-Hougen K. Determination by means of electron microscopy of morphological criteria of value for classification of some spirochetes in particular treponemes. Acta Pathol Microbiol Scand B Suppl 225, 1976.
10. Canale-Parola E. Physiology and evolution of spirochetes. Bacteriol Rev 41:181, 1977. Treponemal Infection. New York, Marcel Dekker, 1982, p 3.
11. Fohn MJ, Wisnall S, Baker-Zander SA, et al. Specificity of antibodies from patients with pinta for antigens of *Treponema pallidum* subspecies *pallidum*. J Infect Dis 157:32, 1988.
12. Krieg NR, Holt JG (eds). Bergey's Manual of Systematic Bacteriology, vol 1. Baltimore/London, Williams & Wilkins, 1984, p 50.
13. Centurion-Lara A, Castro C, Castillo R, et al. The flanking region sequences of the 15-kD lipoprotein gene differentiate pathogenic treponemes. J Infect Dis 177:1036, 1997.
14. Fraser CM, Norris SJ, Weinstock GM, et al. Complete genome sequence of *Treponema pallidum*, the syphilis spirochete. Science 281:375, 1998.
15. Roman GC, Roman LN. Occurrence of congenital, cardiovascular, visceral, neurologic, and neuro-ophthalmologic complications in late yaws: a theme for future research. Rev Infect Dis 8:760, 1986.
16. Turner TB, Hollander DH. Biology of the treponematoses. WHO Monogr Ser 35:1, 1957.
17. Wilcox RR, Guthe T. *Treponema pallidum*: a bibliographical review of the morphology, culture and survival of *T. pallidum* and associated organisms. Bull World Health Organ 35:1, 1966.
18. Turner TB. Syphilis and the treponematoses. *In* Mudd S (ed). Infectious Agents and Host Reactions. Philadelphia, WB Saunders, 1970, p 346.

19. Jenkin HM, Banook PC. In vitro cultivation of treponemal infections. *In* Schell RF, Musher DM (eds). Pathogenesis and Immunology of Treponemal Infections. New York, Marcel Dekker, 1982, p 71.
20. Fieldsteel AH, Becker FA, Stout JG. Prolonged survival of virulent *Treponema pallidum* (Nichols strain) in cell-free and tissue culture systems. Infect Immun 18:173, 1977.
21. Fieldsteel AH, Cox DL, Moeckli RA. Cultivation of virulent *Treponema pallidum* in tissue culture. Infect Immun 32:908, 1981.
22. Klein JR, Monjan AA, Hardy PH Jr, et al. Abrogation of genetically controlled resistance of mice to *Treponema pallidum* by irradiation. Nature 283:572, 1980.
23. Marra CM, Castro CD, Kuller L, et al. Mechanisms of clearance of *Treponema pallidum* from the CSF in a nonhuman primate model. Neurol 51:957, 1998.
24. Fitzgerald TJ. Experimental congenital syphilis in rabbits. Can J Microbiol 31:757, 1985.
25. Wicher K, Baughn RE, Wicher V, et al. Experimental congenital syphilis: guinea pig model. Infect Immun 60:271, 1992.
26. Kajdacsy-Balla A, Howeedy A, Bagasra O. Experimental model of congenital syphilis. Infect Immun 61:3559, 1993.
27. Wicher K, Baughn RE, Abbruscato F, Wicher V. Vertical transmission of *Treponema pallidum* to various litters and generations of guinea pigs. J Infect Dis 179:1206, 1999.
28. Holt SC. Anatomy and chemistry of spirochetes. Microbiol Rev 42:114, 1978.
29. Johnson RC, Wachter MS, Ritzi DM. Treponeme outer cell envelope: solubilization and reaggregation. Infect Immun 7:249, 1973.
30. Norris SJ, Alderete JF, Axelson NH, et al. Identity of *Treponema pallidum* subsp. *pallidum* polypeptides: correlation of sodium dodecyl sulfate-polyacrylamide gel electrophoresis results from different laboratories. Electrophoresis 8:77, 1987.
31. Hanff PF, Fehniger TE, Miller JN, et al. Humoral immune response in human syphilis to polypeptides of *Treponema pallidum*. J Immunol 129:1287, 1982.
32. Baker-Zander SA, Hook EW III, Bonin P, et al. Antigens of *Treponema pallidum* recognized by IgG and IgM antibodies during syphilis in humans. J Infect Dis 151:264, 1985.
33. Radolf JD, Chamberlain NR, Clausell A, et al. Identification and localization of integral membrane proteins of virulent *Treponema pallidum* subsp. *pallidum* by phase partitioning with the nonionic detergent Triton X-114. Infect Immun 56:490, 1988.
34. Radolf JD, Norgard MV. Pathogen specificity of *Treponema pallidum* integral membrane proteins identified by phase partitioning with Triton X-114. Infect Immun 56:1825, 1988.
35. Cunningham TM, Walker EM, Miller JN, et al. Selective release of the *Treponema pallidum* outer membrane and associated polypeptides with Triton X-114. J Bacteriol 170:5789, 1988.
36. Chamberlain NR, Brandt ME, Erwin AL, et al. Major integral membrane protein immunogens of *Treponema pallidum* are proteolipids. Infect Immun 57:2872, 1989.
37. Swancutt MA, Radolf JD, Norgard MV. The 34-kilodalton membrane immunogen of *Treponema pallidum* is a lipoprotein. Infect Immun 58:384, 1990.
38. Walker EM, Zampighi GA, Blanco DR, et al. Demonstration of rare protein in the outer membrane of *Treponema pallidum* subsp. *pallidum* by freeze-fracture analysis. J Bacteriol 171:5005, 1989.
39. Radolf JD, Norgard MV, Schulz WW. Outer membrane ultrastructure explains the limited antigenicity of virulent *Treponema pallidum*. Proc Natl Acad Sci U S A 86:2051, 1989.
40. Jones SA, Marchitto KS, Miller JN, et al. Monoclonal antibody with hemagglutination, immobilization, and neutralization activities defines an immunodominant, 47,000 mol wt, surface-exposed immunogen of *Treponema pallidum* (Nichols). J Exp Med 160:1404, 1984.
41. Pennisi E. Genome reveals wiles and weak points of syphilis. Science 281:324, 1998.
42. Weinstock GM, Hardham JM, McLeod MP, et al. The genome of *Treponema pallidum*: new light on the agent of syphilis. FEMS Microbiol Rev 22:323, 1998.
43. Norris SJ, Fraser CM, Weinstock GM. Illuminating the agent of syphilis: the *Treponema pallidum* genome project. Electrophoresis 19:551, 1998.
44. Radolf JD, Steiner B, Shevchenko D. *Treponema pallidum*: doing a remarkable job with what it's got. Trends Microbiol 7:7, 1999.
45. Cox CD, Barber MK. Oxygen uptake by *Treponema pallidum*. Infect Immun 10:123, 1974.
46. Baseman JB, Nichols JC, Hayes NS. Virulent *Treponema pallidum*: aerobe or anaerobe. Infect Immun 13:704, 1976.
47. Nichols JC, Baseman JB. Carbon sources utilized by virulent *Treponema pallidum*. Infect Immun 12:1044, 1975.
48. Lysko PG, Cox CD. Terminal electron transport in *Treponema pallidum*. Infect Immun 16:885, 1977.
49. Lysko PG, Cox CD. Respiration and oxidative phosphorylation in *Treponema pallidum*. Infect Immun 21:462, 1978.
50. Norris SJ, Miller JN, Sykes JA, et al. Influence of oxygen tension, sulfhydryl compounds, and serum on the motility and virulence of *Treponema pallidum* (Nichols strain) in a cell-free system. Infect Immun 22:689, 1978.
51. Graves S, Billington T. Optimum concentrations of dissolved oxygen for the survival of virulent *Treponema pallidum* under conditions of low oxidation-reduction potential. Br J Vener Dis 55:387, 1979.
58. Olansky S, Norins LC. Current serodiagnosis and treatment of syphilis. JAMA 198:165, 1966.
59. Turner TB, Kluth FC, McLeod C, et al. Protective antibodies in the serum of syphilitic patients. Am J Hyg 48:173, 1948.
60. Garner MF, Backhouse JL, Daskalopoulos G, et al. *Treponema pallidum* haemagglutination test for syphilis: comparison with the TPI and FTA-ABS tests. Br J Vener Dis 48:470, 1972.
61. Clark EG, Danbolt N. The Oslo study of the natural course of untreated syphilis: an epidemiologic investigation based on a re-study of the Boeck-Bruusgaard material. Med Clin North Am 48:613, 1964.
62. Turner TB, Hardy PH, Newman B, et al. Effects of passive immunization on experimental syphilis in the rabbit. Johns Hopkins Med J 133:241, 1973.
63. Weiser RS, Erickson D, Perine PL, et al. Immunity to syphilis: passive transfer in rabbits using serial doses of immune serum. Infect Immun 13:1402, 1976.
64. Bishop NH, Miller JN. Humoral immunity in experimental syphilis: I. The demonstration of resistance conferred by passive immunization. J Immunol 117:191, 1976.
65. Graves S, Alden J. Limited protection of rabbits against infection with *Treponema pallidum* by immune rabbit sera. Br J Vener Dis 55:399, 1979.
66. Musher DM, Hague-Park M, Gyorkey F, et al. The interaction between *Treponema pallidum* and human polymorphonuclear leukocytes. J Infect Dis 147:77, 1983.
67. Musher DM, Baughn RE. Syphilis. *In* Samter M (ed). Immunologic Diseases, 3rd ed. Boston, Little, Brown, 1978, p 639.
68. Radolf JD, Norgard MY, Brandt ME, et al. Lipoproteins of *Borrelia burgdorferi* and *Treponema pallidum* activate cachectin/tumor necrosis factor synthesis: analysis using a CAT reporter construct. J Immunol 147:1968, 1991.
69. Thomas DD, Navab M, Haake DA, et al. *Treponema pallidum* invades intercellular junctions of endothelial cell monolayers. Proc Natl Acad Sci U S A 85:3608, 1988.
70. Riley BS, Oppenheimer-Marks N, Hansen EJ, et al. Virulent *Treponema pallidum* activates human vascular endothelial cells. J Infect Dis 165:484, 1992.
71. Schell RF, Musher DM, Jacobson K, et al. Induction of acquired cellular resistance following transfer of thymus-dependent lymphocytes from syphilitic rabbits. J Immunol 114:550, 1975.
72. Schell R, Musher D, Jacobson K, et al. Effect of macrophage activation on infection with *Treponema pallidum*. Infect Immun 12:505, 1973.
73. Graves SR, Johnson RC. Effect of pretreatment with *Mycobacterium bovis* (strain BCG) and immune syphilitic serum on rabbit resistance to *Treponema pallidum*. Infect Immun 12:1029, 1975.
74. Baughn RE, Musher DM, Knox JM. Effect of sensitization with *Propionibacterium acnes* on the growth of *Listeria monocytogenes* and *Treponema pallidum* in rabbits. J Immunol 118:109, 1977.
75. Schell RF, Chan JK, LeFrock JL, et al. Endemic syphilis: transfer of resistance to *Treponema pallidum* strain Bosnia A in hamsters with a cell suspension enriched in thymus-derived cells. J Infect Dis 141:752, 1980.
76. Lukehart SA, Baker-Zander SA, Lloyd RMC, et al. Characterization of lymphocyte responsiveness in early experimental syphilis: II. Nature of cellular infiltration and *Treponema pallidum* distribution in testicular lesions. J Immunol 124:461, 1980.
77. Festenstein HC, Abrahams C, Bokkenheuser V. Runting syndrome in neonatal rabbits infected with *Treponema pallidum*. Clin Exp Immunol 2:311, 1967.
78. Turner DR, Wright DJM. Lymphadenopathy in early syphilis. J Pathol 110:304, 1973.

79. From E, Thestrup-Pedersen K, Thulin H. Reactivity of lymphocytes from patients with syphilis towards *T. pallidum* antigen in the lymphocyte migration and lymphocyte transformation tests. Br J Vener Dis 56:224, 1976.
80. Wicher V, Wicher K. In vitro cell response to *Treponema pallidum*–infected rabbits: III. Impairment in production of lymphocyte mitogenic factor. Clin Exp Immunol 24:496, 1977.
81. Baughn RE, Musher DM. Altered immune responsiveness associated with experimental syphilis in the rabbit: elevated IgM and depressed IgG responses to sheep erythrocytes. J Immunol 120:1691, 1978.
82. Baughn RE, Musher DM. Aberrant secondary antibody responses to sheep erythrocytes in rabbits with experimental syphilis. Infect Immun 25:133, 1979.
83. Magnuson HJ, Thomas EW, Olansky S, et al. Inoculation syphilis in human volunteers. Medicine 35:33, 1956.
84. Nabarro D. Congenital Syphilis. London, E Arnold, 1954.
85. Dobson SRM, Taber LH, Baughn RE. Recognition of *Treponema pallidum* antibodies in congenitally infected newborns and their mothers. J Infect Dis 157:903, 1988.
86. Sanchez PJ, McCracken GH, Wendel GD, et al. Molecular analysis of the fetal IgM response to *Treponema pallidum* antigens: implications for improved serodiagnosis of congenital syphilis. J Infect Dis 159:508, 1989.
87. Lewis LL. Congenital syphilis: serologic diagnosis in the young infant. Infect Dis Clin North Am 6:31, 1992.
88. Sanchez PJ, Wendel GD, Grimprel K, et al. Evaluation of molecular methodologies and rabbit infectivity testing for the diagnosis of congenital syphilis and neonatal central nervous system invasion by *Treponema pallidum*. J Infect Dis 167:148, 1993.
89. Wendel GD Jr, Sanchez PJ, Peters MT, et al. Identification of *Treponema pallidum* in amniotic fluid and fetal blood from pregnancies complicated by congenital syphilis. Obstet Gynecol 78:890, 1991.
90. Lucas MJ, Theriot SK, Wendel GD. Doppler systolic-diastolic ratios in pregnancies complicated by syphilis. Obstet Gynecol 77:217, 1991.
91. Genest DR, Choi-Hong SR, Tate JE, et al. Diagnosis of congenital syphilis from placental examination. Hum Pathol 27:366, 1996.
92. Rawstron SA, Vetrano J, Tannis G, Bromberg K. Congenital syphilis: detection of *Treponema pallidum* in stillborns. Clin Infect Dis 24:24, 1997.
93. Fiumara NJ, Fleming WL, Downing JG, et al. The incidence of prenatal syphilis at the Boston City Hospital. N Engl J Med 247:48, 1952.
94. Ingraham NR. The value of penicillin alone in the prevention and treatment of congenital syphilis. Acta Derm Venereol 31(Suppl 24):60, 1951.
95. American Academy of Pediatrics. Syphilis. *In* Report of the Committee on Infectious Diseases (Red Book), 27th ed. Elk Grove Village, Ill, American Academy of Pediatrics, 2006.
96. Sheffield JS, Wendel GD Jr, Zeray F, et al. Congenital syphilis: the influence of maternal stage of syphilis on vertical transmission. Am J Obstet Gynecol 180:S85, 1999 (abstract).
97. Fiumara NJ. A legacy of syphilis. Arch Dermatol 92:676, 1965.
98. Sanchez PJ. Congenital syphilis. *In* Aronoff SC (ed). Advances in Pediatric Infectious Diseases. St. Louis, Mosby–Year Book, 1992, p 161.
99. Pollack M, Borkowsky W, Krasinski K. Maternal syphilis is associated with enhanced perinatal HIV transmission. *In* Program and Abstracts, 30th Interscience Conference on Antimicrobial Agents and Chemotherapy, Atlanta. Washington, DC, American Society for Microbiology, 1990, p 1274.
100. Chadwick, EG, Millard DD, Rowley AH. Congenital syphilis in HIV-infected and uninfected children in Chicago 1989-1991. Pediatr Res 31:89A, 1992.
101. Lukehart SA, Hook EW III, Baker-Zander SA, et al. Invasion of the central nervous system by *Treponema pallidum*: implications for diagnosis and treatment. Ann Intern Med 1:855, 1988.
102. Theus SA, Harrich DA, Gaynor R, et al. *Treponema pallidum*, lipoproteins, and synthetic lipoprotein analogues induce human immunodeficiency virus type 1 gene expression in monocytes via NF-kB activation. J Infect Dis 177:941, 1998.
103. Tucker HA, Robinson RCV. Disappearance time of *T. pallidum* from lesions of early syphilis following administration of crystalline penicillin G. Bull Johns Hopkins Hosp 80:169, 1947.
104. Turner TB, Bauer JA, Kluth FC. The viability of the spirochetes of syphilis and yaws in desiccated blood serum. Am J Med Sci 202:416, 1941.
105. Keller R, Morton HE. The effect of a hand soap and a hexachlorophene soap on the cultivatable treponemata. Am J Syph 36:524, 1952.
106. Singh AE and Romanowski B. Syphilis: review with emphasis on clinical, epidemiologic, and some biologic features. Clin Microbiol Rev 12:187, 1999.
107. Mahoney JK, Arnold RC, Harris AD. Penicillin treatment of early syphilis. Am J Public Health 33:1397, 1943.
108. Centers for Disease Control and Prevention. Congenital syphilis, New York City, 1986-1988. MMWR Morb Mortal Wkly Rep 38:825, 1989.
109. Rolfs RT, Nakashima AK. Epidemiology of early syphilis in the United States, 1981-89. JAMA 264:1432, 1990.
110. Ricci JM, Fojaco RM, O'Sullivan MJ. Congenital syphilis: the University of Miami/Jackson: Memorial Medical Center experience, 1986-1988. Obstet Gynecol 74:687, 1989.
111. Berry MC, Dajani AS. Resurgence of congenital syphilis. Infect Dis Clin North Am 6:19, 1992.
112. Reyes MP, Hunt N, Ostrea EM Jr, George D. Maternal/congenital syphilis in a large tertiary-care urban hospital. Clin Infect Dis 17:1041, 1993.
113. Rolfs RT, Goldberg M, Sharrar RG. Risk factors for syphilis: cocaine use and prostitution. Am J Public Health 80:853, 1990.
114. Klass PE, Brown ER, Pelton SL. The incidence of prenatal syphilis at the Boston City Hospital: a comparison across four decades. Pediatrics 94:24, 1994.
115. Sison CG, Ostrea EM Jr, Reyes MP, Salari V. The resurgence of congenital syphilis: a cocaine-related problem. J Pediatr 130:289, 1997.
116. Rathbun KC. Congenital syphilis: a proposal for improved surveillance, diagnosis, and treatment. Sex Transm Dis 10:102, 1983.
117. Centers for Disease Control and Prevention. Impact of closure of a sexually transmitted disease clinic on public health surveillance of sexually transmitted diseases—Washington, D.C., 1995. MMWR Morb Mortal Wkly Rep 47:1067, 1998.
118. Petzoldt D. Effect of spectinomycin on *T. pallidum* in incubating syphilis. Br J Vener Dis 51:305, 1975.
119. Schroeter AL, Turner RH, Lucas JB, et al. Therapy for incubating syphilis: effectiveness of gonorrhea treatment. JAMA 218:711, 1971.
120. Nakashima AK, Rolfs RT, Flock ML, et al. Epidemiology of syphilis in the United States, 1941-1993. Sex Transm Dis 23:16, 1996.
121. Centers for Disease Control and Prevention. Alternative case-finding methods in a crack-related syphilis epidemic—Philadelphia. MMWR Morb Mortal Wkly Rep 40:77, 1991.
122. Centers for Disease Control and Prevention. Selective screening to augment syphilis case-finding—Dallas, 1991. MMWR Morb Mortal Wkly Rep 42:424, 1993.
123. Centers for Disease Control and Prevention. Primary and secondary syphilis. MMWR Morb Mortal Wkly Rep 47:493, 1998.
124. Risser JMH, Hwang L, Risser WL et al. The epidemiology of syphilis in the waning years of an epidemic: Houston, Texas 1991-1999. Sex Transm Dis 26:121, 1999.
125. U.S. Department of Health, Education and Welfare, Public Health Service. VD Fact Sheet. Washington, DC, U.S. Government Printing Office, 1974.
126. Centers for Disease Control and Prevention. Primary and secondary syphilis—United States, 1998. MMWR Morb Mortal Wkly Rep 48:873, 1999.
127. Centers for Disease Control and Prevention. Epidemic of congenital syphilis—Baltimore, 1996-1997. MMWR Morb Mortal Wkly Rep 47:904, 1998.
128. Hahn RA, Magder LS, Aral SO, et al. Race and the prevalence of syphilis seroreactivity in the United States. Am J Public Health 79:467, 1989.
129. St. Louis ME, Wasserheit JM. Elimination of syphilis in the United States. Science 281:353, 1998.
130. Mobley JA, McKeown RE, Jackson KL, et al. Risk factors for congenital syphilis in infants of women with syphilis in South Carolina. Am J Public Health 88:597, 1998.
131. Report of WHO Scientific Group. Treponemal infections. World Health Organ Tech Rep Ser G74, 1982.
132. Tichonova L, Borisenko K, Ward H, et al. Epidemics of syphilis in the Russian Federation: trends, origins, and priorities for control. Lancet 350:210, 1997.
133. Pereyra N, Parisi A, Baptista G. Situación de la sífilis congénita en un municipio del gran Buenos Aires tres an os de evaluación 1994-97, San Isidro. *In* Program and Abstracts of the XI Latin American Congress on Sexually Transmitted Diseases/Fifth Pan-American Congress on AIDS, 1997, p 187.

134. Southwick K, Blanco S, Santander A, et al. Rapid assessment of maternal and congenital syphilis in Bolivia, 1996. *In* Program and Abstracts of the International Congress of Sexually Transmitted Diseases, 1997, p 96.
135. Wendel GD. Gestational and congenital syphilis. Clin Perinatol 15:287, 1988.
136. Zenker PN, Berman SM. Congenital syphilis: trends and recommendations for evaluation and management. J Pediatr Infect Dis 10:516, 1991.
137. Ikeda MK, Jenson HB. Evaluation and treatment of congenital syphilis. J Pediatr 117:843, 1990.
138. Mascola L, Pelosi R, Blount JH, et al. Congenital syphilis revisited. Am J Dis Child 139:575, 1985.
139. Sanchez PJ, Wendel GD, Hall M, et al. Congenital syphilis: the Dallas experience. Pediatr Res 29:286A, 1991.
140. Cohen DA, Boyd D, Pabhudas I, et al. The effects of case definition, maternal screening, and reporting criteria on rates of congenital syphilis. Am J Public Health 80:316, 1990.
141. Mascola L, Pelosi R, Blount JH, et al. Congenital syphilis. Why is it still occurring? JAMA 252:1729, 1984.
142. Rawstron SA, Jenkins S, Blanchard S, et al. Maternal and congenital syphilis in Brooklyn, NY: epidemiology, transmission and diagnosis. Am J Dis Child 146:727, 1993.
143. Webber MP, Lambert G, Bateman DA, Hauser WA. Maternal risk factors for congenital syphilis: a case-control study. Am J Epidemiol 137:415, 1993.
144. Monif GRG, Williams BR Jr, Shulman ST, et al. The problem of maternal syphilis after serologic surveillance during pregnancy. Am J Obstet Gynecol 117:268, 1973.
145. Bellingham FR. Syphilis in pregnancy: transplacental infection. Med J Aust 2:647, 1973.
146. Centers for Disease Control and Prevention. Congenital syphilis—United States, 2002. MMWR Morb Mortal Wkly Rep 53:716, 2004.
147. Gust DA, Levine WC, St Louis ME, et al. Mortality associated with congenital syphilis in the United States, 1992-1998. Pediatrics 109:e79, 2002.
148. Knight J, Richardson S, Petric M, et al. Contributions of suboptimal antenatal care and poor communication to the diagnosis of congenital syphilis. Pediatr Infect Dis 14:238, 1995.
149. Finelli L, Crayne EM, Spitalny KC. Treatment of infants with reactive syphilis serology, New Jersey: 1992 to 1996. Pediatrics 102:394, 1998.
150. Felman Y. How useful are the serologic tests for syphilis? Int J Dermatol 21:79, 1982.
151. Spangler AS, Jackson JH, Fiumara NJ, et al. Syphilis with a negative blood test reaction. JAMA 189:113, 1964.
152. Sparling PF. Diagnosis and treatment of syphilis. N Engl J Med 284:642, 1971.
153. Levine Z, Sherer DM, Jacobs A, Rotenberg O. Nonimmune hydrops fetalis due to congenital syphilis associated with negative intrapartum maternal serology screening. Am J Perinatol 15:233, 1998.
154. Larsen SA, Hambie EA, Pettit DE, et al. Specificity, sensitivity, and reproducibility among the fluorescent treponemal antibody-absorption test, the microhemagglutination assay for *Treponema pallidum* antibodies, and the hemagglutination treponemal test for syphilis. J Clin Microbiol 14:441, 1981.
155. Larsen SA, Steiner BM, Rudolph AH. Laboratory diagnosis and interpretation of tests for syphilis. Clin Microbiol Rev 8:1, 1995.
156. Centers for Disease Control and Prevention. Sexually transmitted diseases treatment guidelines. MMWR Morb Mortal Wkly Rep 51(RR-6), 2002.
157. Sanchez PJ, Wendel GD, Norgard MV. Congenital syphilis associated with negative results of maternal serologic tests at delivery. Am J Dis Child 145:967, 1991.
158. Dippel AL. The relationship of congenital syphilis to abortion and miscarriage, and the mechanism of intrauterine protection. Am J Obstet Gynecol 47:369, 1944.
159. Fiumara NJ. Venereal disease. *In* Charles D, Finland M (eds). Obstetric and Perinatal Infections. Philadelphia, Lea & Febiger, 1973.
160. Benirschke K. Syphilis—the placenta and the fetus. Am J Dis Child 128:142, 1974.
161. Harter CA, Benirschke K. Fetal syphilis in the first trimester. Am J Obstet Gynecol 124:705, 1976.
162. Silverstein AM. Congenital syphilis and the timing of immunogenesis in the human fetus. Nature 194:196, 1962.
163. Nathan L, Bohman VR, Sanchez PJ, et al. In utero infection with *Treponema pallidum* in early pregnancy. Prenat Diag 17:119, 1997.
164. Dorman HG, Sahyun PF. Identification and significance of spirochetes in the placenta: a report of 105 cases with positive findings. Am J Obstet Gynecol 33:954, 1937.
165. Turner TB. The spirochaetes. *In* Dubos RJ, Hirsch JG (eds). Bacterial and Mycotic Infection of Man, 4th ed. Philadelphia, JB Lippincott, 1965.
166. Syphilis: a synopsis. Public Health Service Publication No. 1660. Washington, DC, U.S. Government Printing Office, 1968.
167. Robbins SL. Pathologic Basis of Disease. Philadelphia, WB Saunders, 1974.
168. Brightbill HO, Libraty DH, Krutzik SR. Host defense mechanisms triggered by microbial lipoproteins through toll-like receptors. Science 285:732, 1999.
169. Sellati TJ, Bouis DA, Caimano MJ, et al. Activation of human monocytic cells by *Borrelia burgdorferi* and *Treponema pallidum* is facilitated by CD14 and correlates with surface exposure of spirochetal lipoproteins. J Immunol 163:2049, 1999.
170. Whipple DV, Dunham EC. Congenital syphilis: I. Incidence, transmission and diagnosis. J Pediatr 12:386, 1938.
171. Russell P, Altschuler G. Placental abnormalities of congenital syphilis. Am J Dis Child 128:160, 1974.
172. Qureshi F, Jacques SM, Reyes MP. Placental histopathology in syphilis. Hum Pathol 24:779, 1993.
173. Fojaco RM, Hensley GT, Moskowitz L. Congenital syphilis and necrotizing funisitis. JAMA 261:1788, 1989.
174. Jacques SM, Qureshi F. Necrotizing funisitis: a study of 45 cases. Hum Pathol 23:1278, 1992.
175. Sheffield JS, Sanchez PJ, Wendel GD, et al. Placental histopathology of congenital syphilis. Obstet Gynecol 100;126, 2002.
176. Bromberg K, Rawstron S, Tannis G. Diagnosis of congenital syphilis by combining *Treponema pallidum*–specific IgM detection with immunofluorescent antigen detection for *T. pallidum*. J Infect Dis 168:238, 1993.
177. Guarner J, Greer PW, Bartlett J, et al. Congenital syphilis in a newborn: an immunopathologic study. Mod Pathol 12:82, 1999.
178. Oppenheimer EH, Hardy JB. Congenital syphilis in the newborn infant: clinical and pathological observations in recent cases. Johns Hopkins Med J 129:63, 1971.
179. Cox SM, Wendel GD. Xeroradiography and skeletal survey in the diagnosis of congenital syphilis following fetal death. Meeting of the Society of Perinatal Obstetricians, February 1987 (abstract).
180. Stowens D. Pediatric Pathology, 2nd ed. Baltimore, Williams & Wilkins, 1966.
181. Kissane JM, Smith MG. Pathology of Infancy and Childhood. St. Louis, CV Mosby, 1967.
182. Wright DJM, Berry CL. Liver involvement in congenital syphilis. Br J Vener Dis 50:241, 1974.
183. Morison JE. Foetal and Neonatal Pathology. New York, Appleton-Century-Crofts, 1970.
184. Ajayi NA, Marven S, Kaschula RO, et al. Intestinal ulceration, obstruction and hemorrhage in congenital syphilis. Pediatr Surg Int 15:391, 1999.
185. Kaplan BS, Wiglesworth FW, Marks MI, et al. The glomerulopathy of congenital syphilis-an immune deposit disease. J Pediatr 81:1154, 1972.
186. Gamble CN, Reardon JB. Immune pathogenesis of syphilitic glomerulonephritis. N Engl J Med 292:449, 1975.
187. Hill LL, Singer DB, Falletta J, et al. The nephrotic syndrome in congenital syphilis: an immunopathy. Pediatrics 49:260, 1972.
188. Losito A, Cucciarelli E, Massi-Benedetti F, et al. Membranous glomerulonephritis in congenital syphilis. Clin Nephrol 12:32, 1979.
189. Wiggelinkhuizen J, Kaschula ROC, Uys CJ, et al. Congenital syphilis and glomerulonephritis with evidence for immune pathogenesis. Arch Dis Child 48:375, 1973.
190. Ford FR. Diseases of the Nervous System in Infancy, Childhood, and Adolescence. Springfield, Ill, Charles C Thomas, 1973.
191. Daaboul JJ, Kartchner W, Jones KL. Neonatal hypoglycemia caused by hypopituitarism in infants with congenital syphilis. J Pediatr 123:983, 1993.
192. Benzick AE, Wirthwein DP, Weinberg A, et al. Pituitary gland gumma in congenital syphilis after failed maternal treatment: a case report. Pediatrics 104:102, 1999.
193. Turnbull HM. Recognition of congenital syphilitic inflammation of the long bones. Lancet 1:1239, 1922.
194. Pendergrass EP, Bromer RS. Congenital bone syphilis: preliminary report: roentgenologic study with notes on the histology and pathology of the condition. AJR Am J Roentgenol 22:1, 1929.

195. Park EA, Jackson DA. The irregular extensions of the end of the shaft in the X-ray photograph in congenital syphilis, with pertinent observations. J Pediatr 13:748, 1938.
196. Cremin BJ, Fisher RM. The lesions of congenital syphilis. Br J Radiol 43:333, 1970.
197. Caffey J. Syphilis of the skeleton in early infancy: the nonspecificity of many of the roentgenographic changes. AJR Am J Roentgenol 42:637, 1939.
198. Caffey J. Pediatric X-ray Diagnosis. Chicago, Year Book Medical Publishers, 1973.
199. Whitaker JA, Sartain P, Shaheedy MD. Hematological aspects of congenital syphilis. J Pediatr 66:629, 1965.
200. Sartain P. The anemia of congenital syphilis. South Med J 58:27, 1965.
201. Thomas E. Syphilis: Its Course and Management. New York, Macmillan, 1949.
202. Willcox RR. A Text-Book of Venereal Disease. New York, Grune & Stratton, 1950.
203. Fiumara NJ. Congenital syphilis in Massachusetts. N Engl J Med 245:634, 1951.
204. Brown WJ, Moore MB Jr. Congenital syphilis in the United States. Clin Pediatr (Phila) 2:220, 1963.
205. Sever JL. Effects of infection on pregnancy risk. Clin Obstet Gynecol 16:225, 1973.
206. Sheridan MD. Final report of a prospective study of children whose mothers had rubella in early pregnancy. BMJ 2:536, 1964.
207. Chapel TA. The variability of syphilitic chancres. Sex Transm Dis 5:68, 1978.
208. Musher DM. Syphilis. Infect Dis Clin North Am 1:83, 1987.
209. Olansky S, Norins LC. Syphilis and other treponematoses. *In* Fitzpatrick TB, Arndt K, Clark WH, et al (eds). Dermatology in General Medicine. New York, McGraw-Hill, 1971, p 1955.
210. Feher J, Somogyi T, Timmer M, et al. Early syphilitic hepatitis. Lancet 2:896, 1975.
211. Jozsa L, Timmer M, Somogyi T, et al. Hepatitis syphilitica: a clinicopathological study of 25 cases. Acta Hepatogastroenterol 24:344, 1977.
212. Brophy EM, Ashworth CT, Aries M, et al. Acute syphilitic nephrosis in pregnancy. Obstet Gynecol 24:930, 1964.
213. Falls WF Jr, Ford KL, Answorth CT. The nephrotic syndrome in secondary syphilis: report of a case with renal biopsy findings. Ann Intern Med 63:1047, 1965.
214. Braunstein GD, Lewis EJ, Galvanek EG, et al. The nephrotic syndrome associated with secondary syphilis. Am J Med 48:643, 1970.
215. Bhorade MS, Carag HB, Lee HJ, et al. Nephropathy of secondary syphilis: a clinical and pathological spectrum. JAMA 216:1159, 1971.
216. Dismukes WE, Delgado DG, Mallernee SV, et al. Destructive bone disease in early syphilis. JAMA 236:2646, 1976.
217. Tight RR, Warner JF. Skeletal involvement in secondary syphilis detected by bone scanning. JAMA 235:2326, 1976.
218. Shore RN, Kiesel HA, Bennett HD. Osteolytic lesions in secondary syphilis. Arch Intern Med 137:1465, 1977.
219. Sanchez PJ, Wendel GD. Syphilis in pregnancy. Clin Perinatol 24:71, 1997.
220. Holder NR, Knox JM. Syphilis in pregnancy. Med Clin North Am 56:1153, 1972.
221. Blair EK, Lawson JM. Unsuspected syphilitic hepatitis in a patient with low-grade proteinuria and abnormal liver function. Mayo Clin Proc 65:1365, 1990.
222. Drusin LM, Topf-Olstein B, Levy-Zombek E. Epidemiology of infectious syphilis at a tertiary hospital. Arch Intern Med 139:901, 1979.
223. Scully RE, Mark EJ, McNeely WF, et al. Case records of the Massachusetts General Hospital. N Engl J Med 325:414, 1991.
224. Hill LM, Maloney JB. An unusual constellation of sonographic findings associated with congenital syphilis. Obstet Gynecol 78:895, 1991.
225. Nathan L, Twickler DM, Peters MT, et al. Fetal syphilis: correlation of sonographic findings and rabbit infectivity testing of amniotic fluid. J Ultrasound Med 2:97, 1993.
226. Saxoni F, Lapatsanis P, Pantelakis SN. Congenital syphilis: a description of 18 cases and re-examination of an old but ever-present disease. Clin Pediatr (Phila) 6:687, 1967.
227. Dorfman DH, Glaser JH. Congenital syphilis presenting in infants after the newborn period. N Engl J Med 323:1299, 1990.
228. Shah MC, Barton LL. Congenital syphilis hepatitis. Pediatr Infect Dis J 8:891, 1989.
229. Long WA, Ulshen MA, Lawson EE. Clinical manifestations of congenital syphilitic hepatitis: implications for pathogenesis. J Pediatr Gastroenterol Nutr 3:551, 1984.
230. Pohl M, Niemeyer CM, Hentschel R, et al. Hemophagocytosis in early congenital syphilis. Eur J Pediatr 158:553, 1999.
231. Bulova SI, Schwartz E, Harrer WV. Hydrops fetalis and congenital syphilis. Pediatrics 49:285, 1972.
232. Levine P, Celano MJ, Falkowski F. The specificity of the antibody in paroxysmal cold hemoglobinuria (P.C.H.). Ann N Y Acad Sci 124:456, 1965.
233. Shah AA, Desai AB. Paroxysmal cold hemoglobinuria (case report). Indian Pediatr 14:219, 1977.
234. Platou RV. Treatment of congenital syphilis with penicillin. Adv Pediatr 4:35, 1949.
235. King A, Nicol C. Venereal Diseases. Philadelphia, FA Davis, 1964.
236. Wilkinson RH, Heller RM. Congenital syphilis: resurgence of an old problem. Pediatrics 47:27, 1971.
237. Brion LP, Manuli M, Rai B, et al. Long bone radiographic abnormalities as a sign of active congenital syphilis in asymptomatic newborns. Pediatrics 88:1037, 1991.
238. Seckler AB, Kliner MM, Tunnessen W Jr. Pediatric Puzzler: play it again Sam. Contemp Pediatr 12:135, 1995.
239. Teberg A, Hodgman JE. Congenital syphilis in newborn. Calif Med 118:5, 1973.
240. Papaioannou AC, Asrow GG, Schuckmell NH. Nephrotic syndrome in early infancy as a manifestation of congenital syphilis. Pediatrics 27:636, 1961.
241. Pollner P. Nephrotic syndrome associated with congenital syphilis. JAMA 198:263, 1966.
242. Rosen EU, Abrahams C, Rabinowitz L. Nephropathy of congenital syphilis. S Afr Med J 47:1606, 1973.
243. Yuceoglu AM, Sagel I, Tresser G, et al. The glomerulopathy of congenital syphilis: a curable immune-deposit disease. JAMA 229:1085, 1974.
244. McDonald R, Wiggelinkhuizen J, Kaschula RO. The nephrotic syndrome in very young infants. Am J Dis Child 122:507, 1971.
245. Ahmed A, Hickey SM, Ehrett S, et al. Cerebrospinal fluid values in the term neonate. Pediatr Infect Dis J 15:298, 1996.
246. Thorley JD, Holmes RK, Kaplan JM, et al. Passive transfer of antibodies of maternal origin from blood to cerebrospinal fluid in infants. Lancet 1:651, 1975.
247. Wolf B, Kalangu K. Congenital neurosyphilis revisited. Eur J Pediatr 152:493, 1993.
248. Contreras F, Pereda J. Congenital syphilis of the eye with lens involvement. Arch Ophthalmol 96:1052, 1978.
249. Naeye RL. Fetal growth with congenital syphilis. Am J Clin Pathol 55:228, 1971.
250. Naeye RL. Judgment of fetal age: III. The pathologist's evaluation. Pediatr Clin North Am 13:849, 1966.
251. Bateman DA, Ng SKC, Hansen CA, et al. The effects of intrauterine cocaine exposure in newborns. Am J Public Health 83:190, 1993.
252. Fiumara NJ, Lessell S. Manifestations of late congenital syphilis: an analysis of 271 patients. Arch Dermatol 102:78, 1970.
253. Putkonen T. Does early treatment prevent dental changes in congenital syphilis? Acta Derm Venereol 43:240, 1963.
254. Azimi PH. Interstitial keratitis in a five-year old. Pediatr Infect Dis 18:299, 1999.
255. Hendershot EL. Luetic deafness. Otolaryngol Clin North Am 11:43, 1978.
256. Rothenberg R. Syphilitic hearing loss. South Med J 72:118, 1979.
257. Lapunzina PD, Alteca JM, Fuchman JC, Freilij H. Neurosyphilis in an eight-year old child: usefulness of the SPECT study. Pediatr Neurol 18:81, 1998.
258. Borella L, Goobar JE, Clark GM. Synovitis of the knee joints in late congenital syphilis. JAMA 180:84, 1962.
259. Wendel GD, Maberry MC, Christmas JT, et al. Examination of amniotic fluid in diagnosing congenital syphilis with fetal death. Obstet Gynecol 74:967, 1989.
260. Rathbun KC. Congenital syphilis: a proposal for improved surveillance, diagnosis and treatment. Sex Transm Dis 10:102, 1983.
261. Jensen HB. Congenital syphilis. Semin Pediatr Infect Dis 10:183, 1999.
262. Sanchez PJ. Laboratory tests for congenital syphilis. Pediatr Infect Dis J 17:70, 1998.
263. Hira SK, Bhat GJ, Patel JB, et al. Early congenital syphilis: clinicoradiologic features in 202 patients. Sex Transm Dis 12:77, 1985.

264. Woody NC, Sistrunk WF, Platou RV. Congenital syphilis: a laid ghost walks. J Pediatr 64:63, 1964.
265. Swischuk LE. Radiology of the Newborn and Young Infant. Baltimore, Williams & Wilkins, 1973.
266. Ingraham NR. The lag phase in early congenital osseous syphilis: a roentgenographic study. Am J Med Sci 191:819, 1936.
267. Cremin BJ, Shaff MI. Congenital syphilis diagnosed in utero. Br J Radiol 48:939, 1975.
268. Ringel RE, Brenner JI, Haney PJ, et al. Prostaglandin-induced periostitis: a complication of long-term PGE_1 infusion in an infant with congenital heart disease. Radiology 142:657, 1982.
269. Harris VJ, Jiminez CA, Vidyasager D. Congenital syphilis with syphilitic arthritis. Radiology 123:416, 1977.
270. Harris VJ, Jiminez CA, Vidvasager D. Congenital syphilis with unusual clinical presentations. Ill Med J 151:371, 1977.
271. Chipps BE, Swischuk LE, Voelter WW. Single bone involvement in congenital syphilis. Pediatr Radiol 5:50, 1976.
272. Solomon A, Rosen E. The aspect of trauma in the bone change of congenital lues. Pediatr Radiol 3:176, 1975.
273. Solomon A, Rosen E. Focal osseous lesions in congenital lues. Pediatr Radiol 7:36, 1978.
274. Heyman S, Mandell GA. Skeletal scintigraphy in congenital syphilis. Clin Nucl Med 8:531, 1983.
275. Wolpowitz A. Osseous manifestations of congenital lues. S Afr Med J 50:675, 1976.
276. Siegel D, Hirschman SZ. Syphilitic osteomyelitis with diffusely abnormal bone scan. Mt Sinai J Med 46:320, 1979.
277. Magnuson HJ, Eagle H, Fleischman R. The minimal infectious inoculum of *Spirochaeta pallida* (Nichols strain), and a consideration of its rate of multiplication in vivo. Am J Syph Gon Vener Dis 32:1, 1948.
278. Turner TB, Hardy PH, Newman B. Infectivity tests in syphilis. Br J Vener Dis 45:183, 1969.
279. Moore MB Jr, Knox JM. Sensitivity and specificity in syphilis serology: clinical implications. South Med J 48:963, 1965.
280. Wheeler HL, Agarwal S, Goh BT. Dark ground microscopy and treponemal serological tests in the diagnosis of early syphilis. Sex Transm Infect 80:411, 2004.
281. Matthews HM, Yang TK, Jenkin HM. Unique lipid composition of *Treponema pallidum* (Nichols virulent strain). Infect Immun 24:713, 1979.
282. Catterall RD. Systemic disease and the biological false positive reaction. Br J Vener Dis 48:1, 1972.
283. Buchanan CS, Haserick JR. FTA-ABS test in pregnancy: a probable false-positive reaction. Arch Dermatol 102:322, 1970.
284. Kostant GH. Familial chronic biologic false-positive seroreactions for syphilis: report of two families, one with three generations affected. JAMA 219:45, 1972.
285. Duncan WC, Knox JM, Wende RD. The FTA-ABS test in darkfield-positive primary syphilis. JAMA 228:859, 1974.
286. Rudolph AH. The microhemagglutination assay for *Treponema pallidum* antibodies (MHA-TP), a new treponemal test for syphilis: where does it fit? J Am Vener Dis Assoc 3:3, 1976.
287. Goodhard GL, Brown ST, Zaidi AA, et al. Blinded proficiency testing of the FTA-ABS test. Arch Intern Med 141:1245, 1981.
288. Schroeter AL, Lucas JB, Price EV, et al. Treatment for early syphilis and reactivity of serologic tests. JAMA 221:471, 1972.
289. Fiumara NJ. Treatment of primary and secondary syphilis: serological response. JAMA 243:2500, 1980.
290. O'Neill P, Warner RW, Nicol CS. *Treponema pallidum* haemagglutination assay in the routine serodiagnosis of treponemal disease. Br J Vener Dis 49:427, 1973.
291. Lesinski J, Krauch J, Kadziewicz E. Specificity, sensitivity and diagnostic value of the TPHA test. Br J Vener Dis 50:334, 1974.
292. Larsen SA, McCrew BE, Hunter EF, et al. Syphilis serology and dark field microscopy. *In* Holmes KK, Mardh PA, Sparling PF, et al (eds). Sexually Transmitted Diseases. New York, McGraw-Hill, 1984, p 875.
293. Musher DM. A positive VDRL reaction in an asymptomatic patient. *In* Remington JS, Swartz MN (eds). Current Clinical Topics in Infectious Diseases, no. 9. New York, McGraw-Hill, 1988, p 147.
294. Deguchi M, Hosotsubo H, Yamashita N, et al. Evaluation of gelatin particle agglutination method for detection of *Treponema pallidum* antibody. J Jpn Assoc Infect Dis 68:1271, 1994.
295. Norgard MV. Clinical and diagnostic issues of acquired and congenital syphilis encompassed in the current syphilis epidemic. Curr Opin Infect Dis 6:9, 1993.
296. Lefevre JC, Bertrand MA, Bauriaud R. Evaluation of the Captia enzyme immunoassays for detection of immunoglobulins G and M to *Treponema pallidum* in syphilis. J Clin Microbiol 28:1704, 1990.
297. Young H, Moyes A, McMillan A, Patterson J. Enzyme immunoassay for antitreponemal IgG: screening or confirmatory test? J Clin Pathol 45:37, 1992.
298. Ross J, Moyes A, Young H, McMillan A. An analysis of false positive reactions occurring with the Captia Syph-G EIA. Genitourin Med 67:408, 1991.
299. Lefevre JC, Bertrand MA, Bauriaud R, Lareng MB. False positive reactions occurring with the Captia Syphilis-G EIA, in sera from patients with Lyme disease. Genitourin Med 68:142, 1992.
300. Van Voorhis WC, Barrett LK, Lukehart SA, et al. Serodiagnosis of syphilis to pallidum recombinant Tp043, Tp92 and Gpd proteins are sensitive and specific indicators of infection by *Treponema pallidum.* J Clin Microbiol 41:3668, 2003.
301. Zarakolu P, Buchanan I, Tam M, et al. Preliminary evaluation of an immunochromatographic strip test for specific *Treponema pallidum* antibodies. J Clin Microbiol 40:3064, 2002.
302. Romanowski B, Sutherland R, Fick GH, et al. Serologic response to treatment of infectious syphilis. Ann Intern Med 114:1005, 1991.
303. Moskophidis M, Muller F. Molecular analysis of immunoglobulins M and G immune response to protein antigens of *Treponema pallidum* in human syphilis. Infect Immun 43:127, 1984.
304. Muller F. Specific immunoglobulin M and G antibodies in the rapid diagnosis of human treponemal infections. Diagn Immunol 4:1, 1986.
305. Sanchez PJ, Leos NK, Osorio MA, et al. Umbilical cord blood VDRL or RPR: what's the difference? Pediatr Res 35:303A, 1994.
306. Rawstron SA, Bromberg K. Comparison of maternal and newborn serologic tests for syphilis. Am J Dis Child 145:1383, 1991.
307. Chhabra RS, Brion LP, Castro M, et al. Comparison of maternal sera, cord blood and neonatal sera for detecting presumptive congenital syphilis: relationship with maternal treatment. Pediatrics 91:88, 1993.
308. Taber L, Baughn B. Long term follow-up of infants born of mothers with past or active infection with *T. pallidum*. 31st Interscience Conference on Antimicrobial Reagents and Chemotherapy, September 29–October 2, 1991, Chicago, p 155 (abstract 337).
309. Sanchez PJ, Wendel GD, Zeray F, et al. Serologic follow-up in congenital syphilis: what's the point? Program and Abstracts of the 34th Interscience Conference on Antimicrobial Agents and Chemotherapy, Orlando, Fla, 1994.
310. Reimer CG, Black CM, Phillips DJ, et al. The specificity of fetal IgM: antibody or anti-antibody? Ann N Y Acad Sci 254:77, 1975.
311. Kaufman RE, Olansky DC, Wiesner PJ. The FTA-ABS (IgM) test for neonatal congenital syphilis: a critical review. J Am Vener Dis Assoc 1:79, 1974.
312. Stoll BJ, Lee FK, Larsen S, et al. Clinical and serologic evaluation of neonates for congenital syphilis: a continuing diagnostic dilemma. J Infect Dis 167:1093, 1993.
313. Pedersen NS, Sheller JP, Ratnam AV, et al. Enzyme-linked immunosorbent assays for detection of immunoglobulin M to nontreponemal and treponemal antigens for the diagnosis of congenital syphilis. J Clin Microbiol 27:1835, 1989.
314. Schmitz JL, Gertis KS, Mauney C, et al. Laboratory diagnosis of congenital syphilis by immunoglobulin M (IgM) and IgA immunoblotting. Clin Diag Lab Immunol 1:32, 1994.
315. Meyer MP, Eddy T, Baughn RE. Analysis of Western blotting (immunoblotting) technique in diagnosis of congenital syphilis. J Clin Microbiol 32:629, 1994.
316. Lewis LL, Taber LH, Baughn RE. Evaluation of immunoglobulin M Western blot analysis in the diagnosis of congenital syphilis. J Clin Microbiol 28:296, 1990.
317. Sanchez PJ, Wendel GD Jr, Leos NK, et al. IgM immunoblotting utilizing recombinant 47- and 17-kDa antigens for the diagnosis of congenital syphilis. Thirty-fifth Interscience Conference on Antimicrobial Agents and Chemotherapy, San Francisco, Calif, Sept. 17-20, 1995.
318. Sanchez PJ, Wendel GD, Norgard MV. IgM antibody to *Treponema pallidum* in cerebrospinal fluid of infants with congenital syphilis. Am J Dis Child 146:1171, 1992.
319. Burstain JM, Grimprel E, Lukehart SA, et al. Sensitive detection of *Treponema pallidum* by using the polymerase chain reaction. J Clin Microbiol 29:62, 1991.
320. Wicher K, Noordhoek GT, Abbruscato F, et al. Detection of *Treponema pallidum* in early syphilis by DNA amplification. J Clin Microbiol 30:497, 1992.

321. Hay PE, Clarke JR, Strugnell RA, et al. Use of the polymerase chain reaction to detect DNA sequences specific to pathogenic treponemes in cerebrospinal fluid. FEMS Microbiol Lett 68:233, 1990.
322. Use of PCR in the diagnosis of early syphilis in the United Kingdom. Sex Transm Infect 79;479, 2003.
323. Noordhoek GT, Wolters EC, DeJonge MEJ, et al. Detection by polymerase chain reaction of *Treponema pallidum* in cerebrospinal fluid from neurosyphilis patients before and after antibiotic treatment. J Clin Microbiol 29:1976, 1991.
324. Grimprel E, Sannchez PJ, Wendel GD, et al. Use of the polymerase chain reaction and rabbit infectivity testing to detect *Treponema pallidum* in amniotic fluid, fetal and neonatal sera, and cerebrospinal fluid. J Clin Microbiol 29:1711, 1991.
325. Marra CM. Neurosyphilis. Curr Neurol Neurosci Rep 4:435, 2004.
326. Michelow IC, Wendel GD Jr, Norgard MV, et al. Central nervous system infection in congenital syphilis. N Engl J Med 346;1792, 2002.
327. LeClerc G, Giroux M, Birry A, et al. Study of fluorescent treponemal antibody test on cerebrospinal fluid using nonspecific anti-immunoglobulin conjugates IgG, IgM and IgA. Br J Vener Dis 54:303, 1978.
328. Muller F, Moskophidis M, Pranse HW. Demonstration of locally synthesized immunoglobulin M antibodies to *Treponema pallidum* in the central nervous system of patients with untreated syphilis. J Neuroimmunol 7:43, 1984.
329. Lee JB, Farshy CE, Hunter EF, et al. Detection of immunoglobulin M in cerebrospinal fluid for syphilis patients by enzyme-linked immunosorbent assay. J Clin Microbiol 47:736, 1986.
330. Esterly NB, Solomon LM. Neonatal dermatology: II. Blistering and scaling dermatoses. J Pediatr 77:1075, 1970.
331. Geppert LJ, Baker HJ, Copple BI, et al. *Pseudomonas* infections in infants and children. J Pediatr 41:555, 1952.
332. Ray CG, Wedgewood RJ. Neonatal listeriosis. Pediatrics 34:378, 1964.
333. Lopez JB, Gross P, Boggs TR. Skin lesions in association with β hemolytic *Streptococcus* group B. Pediatrics 58:859, 1976.
334. Halal F, Delorme L, Brazeau M, et al. Congenital vesicular eruption caused by *H. influenzae* type B. Pediatrics 62:494, 1978.
335. Hageman J, Shulman S, Schreiber M, et al. Congenital tuberculosis: critical reappraisal of clinical findings and diagnostic procedures. Pediatrics 66:980, 1980.
336. Blatt J, Kastner D, Hodes DS. Cutaneous vesicles in congenital cytomegalovirus infection. J Pediatr 92:509, 1978.
337. Dvorak AM, Gavaller B. Congenital systemic candidiasis. N Engl J Med 274:540, 1966.
338. Esterly NB, Spraker MK. Neonatal skin problems. *In* Moschella SL, Hurley HJ (eds). Dermatology. Philadelphia, WB Saunders, 1985, p 1882.
339. Oski FA, Naiman JL. Hematologic Problems in the Newborn. Philadelphia, WB Saunders, 1972.
340. Anand A, Gray ES, Brown T, et al. Human parvovirus infection in pregnancy and hydrops fetalis. N Engl J Med 316:183, 1987.
341. Weiss DI, Cooper LZ, Green RH. Infantile glaucoma. JAMA 195:105, 1966.
342. Coles FB, Hipp SS, Silberstein GS, Chen J. Congenital syphilis surveillance in upstate New York, 1989-1992: implications for prevention and clinical management. J Infect Dis 171:732, 1995.
343. Idsoe O, Guthe T, Willcox RR. Penicillin in the treatment of syphilis: the experience of three decades. Bull World Health Organ 47(Suppl):5-68, 1972.
344. Augenbraun MH, Rolfs R. Treatment of syphilis, 1998: nonpregnant adults. Clin Infect Dis 28(Suppl):S21, 1999.
345. Musher DM. How much penicillin cures early syphilis? Ann Intern Med 109:849, 1988.
346. Alexander JM, Sheffield JS, Sánchez PJ, et al. Efficacy of treatment for syphilis in pregnancy. Obstet Gynecol 93:5, 1999.
347. Conover CS, Reno CA, Miller GB Jr, Schmid GP. Congenital syphilis after treatment of maternal syphilis with a penicillin regimen exceeding CDC guidelines. Infect Dis Obstet Gynecol 6:134-137, 1998.
348. Nathan L, Bawdon RE, Sidawi JE, et al. Penicillin levels following administration of benzathine penicillin G in pregnancy. Obstet Gynecol 82:338, 1993.
349. Rolfs RT, Joesoef JR, Hendershot EF, et al. A randomized trial of enhanced therapy for early syphilis in patients with and without human immunodeficiency virus infection. N Engl J Med 337:307, 1997.
350. Wendel GD Jr, Stark BJ, Jamison RB, et al. Penicillin allergy and desensitization in serious infections during pregnancy. N Engl J Med 312:1229, 1985.
351. Shann S, Wilson J. Treatment of neurosyphilis with ceftriaxone. Sex Transm Infect 79:415, 2003.
352. Hook EW III, Roddy RE, Handsfield HH. Ceftriaxone therapy for incubating and early syphilis. J Infect Dis 158:881, 1988.
353. Moorthy TT, Lee CT, Lim KB, et al. Ceftriaxone for treatment of primary syphilis in men: a preliminary study. Sex Transm Dis 14:116, 1987.
354. Schofer H, Vogt HJ, Milbradt R. Ceftriaxone for the treatment of primary and secondary syphilis. Chemotherapy 35:140, 1989.
355. Vignale R, Burno J, Gibert P. Ceftriaxone in the treatment of primary and secondary syphilis: a comparative study with benzathine penicillin. *In* Hall TC (ed). Prediction of Response to Cancer Therapy. Proceedings of the 15th International Chemotherapy Congress, Istanbul, Turkey, July 19-24, 1987. New York, Alan R Liss, 1988, p 75.
356. Hook EW III, Baker-Zander SA, Moskovitz BL, et al. Ceftriaxone therapy for asymptomatic neurosyphilis: case report and Western blot analysis of serum and cerebrospinal fluid IgG response to therapy. Sex Transm Dis 13:185, 1986.
357. Dowell ME, Ross PG, Musher DM, et al. Response of latent syphilis or neurosyphilis to ceftriaxone therapy in persons infected with human immunodeficiency virus. Am J Med 93:481, 1992.
358. Marra C, Slatter V, Tartaglione T, et al. Comparison of ceftriaxone and aqueous crystalline penicillin G for central nervous system syphilis in an experimental model. 30th Interscience Conference on Antimicrobial Agents and Chemotherapy, Atlanta, Georgia, October 21-24, 1990, p 101 (abstract 87).
359. Philipson A, Sabath LD, Charles D. Transplacental passage of erythromycin and clindamycin. N Engl J Med 288:1219, 1973.
360. South MA, Short DH, Knox JM. Failures of erythromycin estolate therapy in in utero syphilis. JAMA 199:70, 1964.
361. Montgomery CH, Knox JM. Antibiotics other than penicillin in the treatment of syphilis. N Engl J Med 261:277, 1959.
362. Schultz JC, Adamson JS Jr, Workman WW, et al. Fatal liver disease after intravenous administration of tetracycline in high doses. N Engl J Med 269:999, 1963.
363. Tetracycline in pregnancy. Editorial. BMJ 1:743, 1965.
364. Demers P, Fraser RB, Goldbloom J, et al. Effects of tetracycline on skeletal growth dentition: a report to the Nutrition Committee of the Canadian Pediatric Society. Can Med Assoc J 99:849, 1968.
365. Verdon MS, Handsfield HH, Johnson RB. Pilot study of azithromycin for the treatment of primary and secondary syphilis. Clin Infect Dis 19:486, 1994.
366. Mashkilleyson AL, Gomberg MA, Mashkilleyson N. Treatment of syphilis with azithromycin. Int J STD AIDS 7:13, 1996.
367. Centers for Disease Control and Prevention. Azithromycin treatment failures in syphilis infections–San Francisco, California, 2002-2003. MMWR Morb Mortal Wkly Rep 53:197, 2004.
368. Lukehart SA, Godornes C, Molini BJ, et al. Macrolide resistance in *Treponema pallidum* in the United States and Ireland. N Engl J Med 351:122, 2004.
369. Notice to readers: shortage of intravenous penicillin G—United States. MMWR Morb Mortal Wkly Rep 48:974, 1999.
370. Alternatives to intravenous penicillin G for specific infections. Available at http://www.cdc.gov/nchstp/dstd/penicilllinG.htm
371. Sanchez PJ. Syphilis. *In* Burg FD, Ingelfinger JR, Wald ER (eds). Gellis and Kagan's Current Pediatric Therapy 14. Philadelphia, WB Saunders, 1993, p 590.
372. American Academy of Pediatrics. Syphilis. *In* Report of the Committee on Infectious Diseases (Red Book), 26th ed. Elk Grove Village, Ill, American Academy of Pediatrics, 2003, p 595.
373. Beeram MR, Chopde N, Dawood Y, et al. Lumbar puncture in the evaluation of possible asymptomatic congenital syphilis in neonates. J Pediatr 128:125, 1996.
374. Moyer VA, Schneider V, Yetman R, et al. Contribution of long-bone radiographs to the management of congenital syphilis in the newborn infant. Arch Pediatr Adolesc Med 152:353, 1998.
375. Centers for Disease Control and Prevention. 1993 Sexually transmitted diseases treatment guidelines. MMWR Morb Mortal Wkly Rep 42(No. RR-14):40, 1993.
376. Azimi PH, Janner D, Berne P, et al. Concentrations of procaine and aqueous penicillin in the cerebrospinal fluid of infants treated for congenital syphilis. J Pediatr 124:649, 1994.
377. Bateman DA, Phibbs CS, Joyce T, Heagarty MC. The hospital cost of congenital syphilis. J Pediatr 130:752, 1997.
378. Paryani SG, Vaughn AJ, Crosby M, Lawrence S. Treatment of asymptomatic congenital syphilis: benzathine versus procaine penicillin G therapy. J Pediatr 125:471, 1994.

379. Radcliffe M, Meyer M, Roditi D, et al. Single-dose benzathine penicillin in infants at risk of congenital syphilis: results of a randomized study. S Afr Med J 87:62, 1997.
380. Beck-Sague C, Alexander ER. Failure of benzathine penicillin G treatment in early congenital syphilis. Pediatr Infect Dis J 6:1061, 1987.
381. Woolf A, Wilfert C, Kelsey D, et al. Childhood syphilis in North Carolina. N C Med J 41:443, 1980.
382. McCracken GH, Kaplan JM. Penicillin treatment for congenital syphilis: a critical reappraisal. JAMA 228:855, 1974.
383. Speer ME, Taber LH, Clark DB, et al. Cerebrospinal fluid levels of benzathine penicillin G in the neonate. J Pediatr 91:966, 1977.
384. Norris SJ, Edmondson DG. In vitro culture system to determine MICs and MBCs of antimicrobial agents against *Treponema pallidum* subsp. *pallidum* (Nichols strain). Antimicrob Agents Chemotherapy 32:68, 1988.
385. Gelfano JA, Elin RJ, Berry FW Jr, et al. Endotoxemia associated with the Jarisch-Herxheimer reaction. N Engl J Med 295:211, 1976.
386. Young EJ, Weingarten NM, Baughn RE, et al. Studies on the pathogenesis of the Jarisch-Herxheimer reaction: development of animal model and evidence against a role for classical endotoxin. J Infect Dis 146:606, 1982.
387. Radolf JD, Norgard MV, Brandt ME, et al. Lipoproteins of *Borrelia burgdorferi* and *Treponema pallidum* activate cachectin/tumor necrosis factor synthesis: analysis using a CAT reporter construct. J Immunol 147:1968, 1991.
388. Klein VR, Cox SM, Mitchell MD, Wendel GD Jr. The Jarisch-Herxheimer reaction complicating syphilotherapy in pregnancy. Obstet Gynecol 75:375-380, 1990.
389. Myles TD, Elan G, Parik-Hwang E, Nguyen T. The Jarisch-Herxheimer reaction and fetal monitoring changes in pregnant women treated for syphilis. Obstet Gynecol 92:859, 1998.
390. Tan KL. The re-emergence of early congenital syphilis. Acta Paediatr Scand 62:661, 1973.
391. Goldman JN, Girard KF. Intraocular treponemes in treated congenital syphilis. Arch Ophthalmol 78:47, 1967.
392. Dunlop EMC, King AJ, Wickinson AE. Study of late ocular syphilis: demonstration of treponemes in aqueous humour and cerebrospinal fluid. 3. General and serological findings. Trans Ophthalmol Soc UK 88:275, 1969.
393. Dunlop EMC. Persistence of treponemes after treatment. BMJ 2:577, 1972.
394. Ryan SJ, Hardy PH, Hardy JM, et al. Persistence of virulent *Treponema pallidum* despite penicillin therapy in congenital syphilis. Am J Ophthalmol 73:259, 1972.
395. Report of the World Health Organization Expert Committee on Venereal Infections and Treponematoses. World Health Organ Tech Rep Ser 674:27, 1982.
396. Hardy JB, Hardy PH, Oppenheimer EH. Failure of penicillin in a newborn with congenital syphilis. JAMA 212:1345, 1970.
397. Bayne LL, Schmidley JW, Goodwin DS. Acute syphilitic meningitis: its occurrence after clinical and serologic cure of secondary syphilis with penicillin G. Arch Neurol 43:137, 1986.
398. Jorgensen J, Tikjob G, Weisman K. Neurosyphilis after treatment of latent syphilis with benzathine penicillin. Genitourin Med 62:129, 1986.
399. Markovitz DM, Beutner KR, Maggio RR, et al. Failure of recommended treatment for secondary syphilis. JAMA 256:1767, 1986.
400. Hurtig AK, Nicoll A, Carne C, et al. Syphilis in pregnant women and their children in the United Kingdom: results from national clinician reporting surveys, 1994-97. BMJ 317:1617, 1998.
401. Wendel GD Jr, Sheffield JS, Hollier LM et al. Treatment of syphilis in pregnancy and prevention of congenital syphilis. Clin Infect Dis 35(suppl 2):S200, 2002.
402. Williams LA, Klausner JD, Whittington AB, et al. Elimination and reintroduction of primary and secondary syphilis. Am J Public Health 89:1093, 1999.
403. Centers for Disease Control and Prevention. Outbreak of primary and secondary syphilis—Guilford County, North Carolina, 1996-1997. MMWR Morb Mortal Wkly Rep 47:1070, 1998.

TUBERCULOSIS

Jeffrey R. Starke

Tuberculosis is a classic familial disease.[1] The household is the main setting throughout the world for the person-to-person spread of *Mycobacterium tuberculosis*. With the recent resurgence of tuberculosis in many industrialized nations, issues concerning pregnant women and their children have been reexamined by practitioners of tuberculosis control.

Before 1985, tuberculosis in the pregnant woman and newborn had become an infrequent event in the United States. Although specific statistics concerning tuberculosis in pregnancy are not reported, the increase in total tuberculosis cases in the late 1980s and 1990s and the shift in numbers to young adults and children suggested that tuberculosis in pregnancy may become a more prevalent problem.[2,3] This problem disproportionately affects minority urban populations because they have very high tuberculosis case rates, a greater relative shift in cases to adults of childbearing age, and, in general, less access to prenatal care and screening for disease and infection caused by *M. tuberculosis*.

The influence of pregnancy on the occurrence and prognosis of tuberculosis has been discussed and debated for centuries. At various times, pregnancy has been thought to improve, worsen, or have no effect on the prognosis of tuberculosis. This controversy has lost much of its importance since the advent of effective antituberculosis chemotherapy. The greatest areas of debate at present concern (1) the use of chemotherapy to prevent the progression of *M. tuberculosis* infection to tuberculosis during pregnancy and the postpartum period and (2) the treatment of exposed infants to prevent the development of serious tuberculosis.[4]

TERMINOLOGY

A practical approach to tuberculosis terminology is to follow the natural history of the disease, which can be divided into three stages: exposure, infection, and disease.[5] Exposure implies that the patient has had recent (less than 3 months) and significant contact with an adult with suspected or confirmed contagious pulmonary tuberculosis. For example, an infant born into a family in which an adult has active tuberculosis would be in the exposure stage. In this stage, the child's tuberculin skin test is negative, the chest radiograph result is normal, and the child is free of signs and symptoms of tuberculosis. Unfortunately, it is impossible to know whether a young child in the exposure stage is truly infected with *M. tuberculosis*, because the development of delayed-type hypersensitivity to a tuberculin skin test for tuberculin may take up to 3 months after the organisms have been inhaled.

M. tuberculosis infection is present if an individual has a positive tuberculin skin test result but lacks signs or symptoms of tuberculosis. In this stage, findings on the chest radiograph either are normal or reveal only granuloma or calcification in the lung parenchyma or regional lymph nodes. The purpose of treating *M. tuberculosis* infection is to prevent future disease. In newborns, the progression from infection to disease can occur very rapidly, within several weeks to months.

Tuberculosis disease occurs if signs or symptoms or radiographic manifestations caused by *M. tuberculosis* become apparent. Because 25% to 35% of children with tuberculosis have extrapulmonary involvement, a thorough physical examination, in addition to a high-quality chest radiograph, is essential to rule out disease.[5] Genitourinary tuberculosis in women often causes only subtle symptoms until it is far advanced. Ten to 20% of immunocompetent adults and children with the disease initially have a negative tuberculin skin test result, usually because of immunosuppression by tuberculosis itself. The rate of negative skin test results with disease due to *M. tuberculosis*, however, is much higher in newborns and small infants, especially if they have life-threatening forms of tuberculosis such as disseminated disease or meningitis.

MYCOBACTERIOLOGY

Mycobacteria are nonmotile, non–spore-forming, pleomorphic, weakly gram-positive rods that are 1 to 5 μm long, usually slender, and slightly curved. *M. tuberculosis* may appear beaded or clumped. The cell wall constituents of mycobacteria determine their most striking biologic properties. The cell wall is composed of 20 to 60% lipids bound to proteins and carbohydrates. These and other properties make mycobacteria more resistant than most other bacteria to light, alkali, acid, and the bactericidal activity of antibodies. Growth of *M. tuberculosis* is slow, with a generation time of 12 to 24 hours on solid media.

Acid-fastness, the capacity to form stable mycolate complexes with certain aryl methane dyes that are not removed even by rinsing with 95% ethanol plus hydrochloric acid, is the hallmark of mycobacteria. The cells appear red when stained with carbol fuchsin (Ziehl-Neelsen or Kinyoun stains) or purple with crystal violet, or they exhibit yellow-green fluorescence under ultraviolet light when stained with auramine and rhodamine (Truant stain). Truant stain is considered the most sensitive stain, especially when small numbers of organisms are present. Approximately 10,000 cells per mm^3 must be present in a sample for them to be seen in an acid-fast stained smear.

Identification of mycobacteria depends on their staining properties and their biochemical and metabolic characteristics. Mycobacteria are obligate aerobes with simple growth requirements. *M. tuberculosis* can grow in classic media, whose essential ingredients are egg yolk and glycerin (Löwenstein-Jensen or Dorset media), or in simple synthetic media (Middlebrook, Tween-albumin). Isolation on solid media takes 2 to 6 weeks, followed by another 2 to 4 weeks for drug-susceptibility testing. More rapid isolation (7 to 21 days) can be achieved using a synthetic liquid medium in an automated radiometric system, the most common one being BACTEC (Becton, Dickinson, and Co. [BD], Sparks, Md). A specimen is inoculated into a bottle of medium containing carbon-14–labeled palmitic acid as a substrate. As mycobacteria metabolize the palmitic acid, carbon dioxide-14 accumulates in the head space of the bottle, where radioactivity can be measured. Unfortunately, because bottles are often analyzed in series by repetitive needle aspiration in an automated, single-needle system, cross-contamination leading to a false-positive culture can occur. Drug susceptibility testing can be performed on the same system using bottles with antimicrobial agents added to the medium. In this radiometric system, identification and drug-susceptibility testing often can be completed in 2 to 3 weeks, depending on the concentration of organisms in the patient sample.

Unfortunately, it is often difficult to isolate *M. tuberculosis* from infants and toddlers with tuberculosis.[6,7] Infants and children with pulmonary tuberculosis rarely produce sputum, the usual culture material for adults. The preferred source of culture for children is the gastric aspirate, performed early in the morning before the stomach has been emptied of the respiratory secretions swallowed overnight. For older children, the culture yield from gastric aspirates obtained on three consecutive mornings is 20% to 40%.[8] The yield from infants is usually higher, up to 75%.[9] For many infants with congenital pulmonary tuberculosis, *M. tuberculosis* can be cultured from a tracheal aspirate owing to the large number of organisms in the lungs.

Several types of nucleic acid amplification have been developed to detect *M. tuberculosis* in patient samples. The main form of nucleic acid amplification studied in children with tuberculosis is the polymerase chain reaction (PCR), which uses specific DNA sequences as markers for microorganisms. Various PCR techniques, most using the mycobacterial insertion element IS6110 as the DNA marker for *M. tuberculosis* complex organisms, have a sensitivity and specificity of more than 90% compared with sputum culture for detecting pulmonary tuberculosis in adults. However, test performance varies even among reference laboratories. The test is relatively expensive and requires fairly sophisticated equipment and scrupulous technique to avoid cross-contamination of specimens.

Use of PCR in childhood tuberculosis has been limited. Compared with a clinical diagnosis of pulmonary tuberculosis in children, the sensitivity of PCR has varied from 25 to 83% and specificity has varied from 80% to 100%.[10] The PCR of gastric aspirates may be positive in a recently infected child even when the chest radiograph result is normal, demonstrating the occasional arbitrariness of the distinction between *M. tuberculosis* infection and disease in children. The PCR may have a useful but limited role in evaluating children for tuberculosis. A negative PCR result never eliminates tuberculosis as a diagnostic possibility, and a positive result does not confirm it. The major use of PCR will be in evaluating children with significant pulmonary disease when the diagnosis is not established readily on clinical or epidemiologic grounds. PCR particularly may be helpful in evaluating immunocompromised children with pulmonary disease, especially children with human immunodeficiency virus (HIV) infection, although published reports of its performance in such children are lacking. PCR also may aid in confirming the diagnosis of extrapulmonary tuberculosis, although only a few case reports have been published. No information has been published concerning the accuracy of PCR or other techniques of nucleic acid amplification in samples from pregnant women or neonates with congenital or postnatally acquired tuberculosis.

Relatedness of strains of *M. tuberculosis* was determined in the past by analysis of bacteriophages, a cumbersome and difficult task. A newer technique, restriction fragment length polymorphism analysis of mycobacterial DNA, has become an accurate and powerful tool for determining strain relatedness.[11] It is used frequently in some communities and may help determine whether an infant with tuberculosis has true congenital infection or was infected by another source.

EPIDEMIOLOGY

Tuberculosis remains the leading infectious disease in the world.[12] The World Health Organization (WHO) estimates that during the 1990s 90 million individuals developed tuberculosis and 30 million people died of the disease worldwide. The WHO also estimates that, in the developing world, there are 1.3 million cases of tuberculosis and 400,000 tuberculosis-related deaths annually among children younger than 15 years of age. In most developing countries, the highest rates of tuberculosis occur among young adult men and women. Although much attention has been given recently to the growing number of children orphaned in developing countries by their parents' deaths from HIV-related illnesses, many orphans also are being created by tuberculosis.

In the United States from 1953 through 1984, the incidence of tuberculosis disease declined an average of 5% per year. From 1985 through 1992, there was a 20% increase in total cases of tuberculosis in the United States and a 40% increase in tuberculosis cases among children.[13] Most experts cite four major factors contributing to this increase: (1) the co-epidemic of HIV infection,[14] which is the strongest risk factor known for development of tuberculosis disease in an adult infected with *M. tuberculosis*[15]; (2) the increase in immigration of people to the United States from countries with a high prevalence of tuberculosis, enlarging the pool of infected individuals[16,17]; (3) the increased transmission of *M. tuberculosis* in congregate settings, such as jails, prisons, hospitals, nursing homes, and homeless shelters; and (4) the general decline in tuberculosis-related public health services and access to medical care for the indigent in many communities.[18] Fortunately, in 2003, the approximately 15,500 cases of tuberculosis in the United States was a 40% decline from the peak number of cases in 1992.

In the early 20th century in the United States, when tuberculosis was more prevalent, the risk of becoming infected with *M. tuberculosis* was high across the entire population. Currently, tuberculosis has retreated into fairly well-defined pockets of high-risk individuals, such as foreign-born persons from or persons who travel to high-prevalence countries, inmates of correctional institutions, illicit drug users, unprotected health care workers who care for high-risk patients, migrant families, homeless persons, and anyone likely to encounter people with contagious tuberculosis. One must distinguish the risk factors for becoming infected with *M. tuberculosis* from those that increase the likelihood that an infected individual will develop disease. A compromised immune system and recent infection with *M. tuberculosis* are the major risk factors for progression of infection to disease. Although tuberculosis occurs throughout the United States, cases are disproportionately reported from large urban areas. Cities with populations exceeding 250,000 account for only 18% of the nation's population but almost 50% of its tuberculosis cases.

The number of tuberculosis cases in the United States is increasing among foreign-born persons from countries with a high prevalence of tuberculosis. The percentage of total cases of tuberculosis in the United States that occurs in foreign-born individuals had increased from 22% in 1986 to more than 50% in 2003.[17] In previous estimates, two thirds of foreign-born individuals with tuberculosis were younger than 35 years of age when entering the United States, and in many cases their disease could have been prevented if they had been identified as infected after immigration and given appropriate treatment for *M. tuberculosis* infection. Unfortunately, new immigrants to the United States older than 15 years of age are required to have a chest radiograph but no tuberculin skin test to detect asymptomatic infection; children younger than 15 years old receive no tuberculosis testing as part of immigration.[19] Studies have estimated that 30% to 50% of the almost 1 million annual new immigrants to the United States are infected with *M. tuberculosis*.[17] Clearly, foreign-born women and adolescents of childbearing age should be one group targeted for appropriate tuberculosis screening and prevention.[20]

Another factor that has had a great impact on tuberculosis case rates in the United States has been the epidemic of HIV infection.[15] The proportion of women with HIV infection is increasing, and because risk factors for HIV infection intersect with those for tuberculosis the number of co-infected women will increase.[21-23] In most locales experiencing recent increases in tuberculosis cases, the demographic groups with the greatest tuberculosis morbidity rates are the same as those with high morbidity rates from HIV infection. HIV-infected persons with a reactive tuberculin skin test develop tuberculosis at a rate of 5% to 10% per year compared with a historical average of 5% to 10% for the lifetime of an immunocompetent adult. There is controversy concerning the infectiousness of adults with HIV-associated pulmonary tuberculosis. Although some studies have indicated dually infected adults are as likely as non–HIV-infected adults with tuberculosis to infect others, some studies have shown less transmission from HIV-infected adults.[24]

The current epidemiology of tuberculosis in pregnancy is unknown. From 1966 to 1972, the incidence of tuberculosis during pregnancy at New York Lying-In Hospital ranged from 0.6% to 1.0%.[25] During this time, 3.2% of the patients with culture-proven pulmonary tuberculosis were first diagnosed during pregnancy, a rate equal to that of nonpregnant women of comparable age. There have been only two series of pregnant women with tuberculosis reported from the United States in the past 2 decades.[26,27] Increased risk of tuberculosis is most striking for foreign-born women, who have high rates of tuberculosis infection, and poor minority women. In the United States, almost 40% of tuberculosis cases in minority women occur before 35 years of age. Approximately 80% of tuberculosis cases among children in the United States occur in minority populations.[13] Most of these cases occur after exposure to an ill family member. In all populations, whether the disease incidence is high or low, tuberculosis infection and disease tend to occur in clusters, often centered on the close or extended family, meaning that minority newborns are at greatly increased risk of congenital and postnatally acquired tuberculosis infection and disease.

TUBERCULOSIS IN PREGNANCY

Pathogenesis

The pathogenesis of tuberculosis infection and disease during pregnancy is similar to that for nonpregnant individuals.[28,29] The usual portal of entry for *M. tuberculosis* is the lung through inhalation of infected droplet nuclei discharged by an infectious individual. The inoculum of organisms necessary to establish infection is unknown but is probably fewer than 10.[30] Once tubercle bacilli are deposited in the lung, they multiply in the nonimmune host for several weeks. Usually, this uninhibited replication produces no symptoms, but a patient may experience low-grade fever, cough, or mild pleuritic pain. Shortly after infection, some organisms are carried from the initial pulmonary focus within macrophages

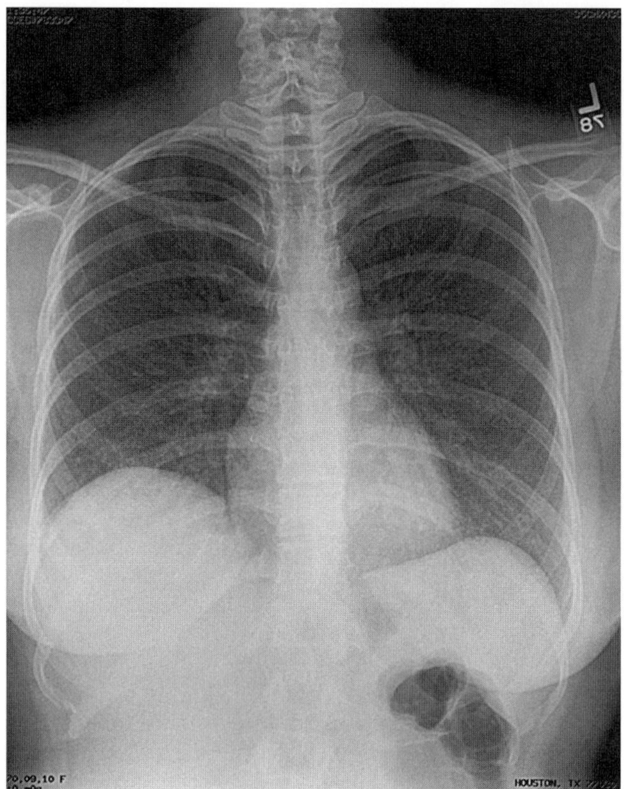

Figure 19–1 Chest radiograph of the mother of the child shown in Figure 19-2. This radiograph reveals early miliary tuberculosis.

to the regional lymph nodes.[31] From there, organisms enter lymphatic and blood vessels and disseminate throughout the body; the genitalia, endometrium, and, if the woman is pregnant, the placenta may be seeded.[32] By 1 to 3 months after infection, the host usually develops cell-mediated immunity and hypersensitivity to the tubercle bacillus, reflected by the development of a reactive tuberculin skin test.[33] As immunity develops, the primary infection in the lung and foci in other organs begin to heal through a combination of resolution, fibrosis, and/or calcification.[34] Although walling-off of these foci occurs, viable tubercle bacilli persist. If the host's immune system later becomes suppressed, these dormant bacilli may become active, leading to "reactivation" tuberculosis.[35]

There are two major ways that tuberculosis infection in the mother can lead to infection of the fetus in utero. If dissemination of organisms through the blood and lymphatic channels occurs during pregnancy, the placenta may be infected directly. This can occur either during the asymptomatic dissemination that is part of the mother's initial infection or during pulmonary, miliary, or disseminated tuberculosis disease in the mother.[36-50] Miliary tuberculosis in women can arise from a long-standing dormant infection but more often complicates a recent infection (Fig. 19-1). Therefore, infection with *M. tuberculosis* that occurs during pregnancy, as opposed to dormant infection that occurred before the pregnancy, probably poses a greater risk to the fetus. This is a major reason why pregnant women with new onset of *M. tuberculosis* infection usually should be treated carefully during the pregnancy; delay could result in disease in the mother, the infant, or both.

The second mechanism by which a fetus can become infected with *M. tuberculosis* is directly from established genitourinary tuberculosis in the mother. Genital tuberculosis is most likely to start around the time of menarche and can have a very long and relatively asymptomatic course. The fallopian tubes most often are involved (in 90%-100% of women), followed by the uterus (50%-60%), ovaries (20%-30%), and cervix (5%-15%).[25,32] Sterility often is the presenting complaint of tuberculosis endometritis, which diminishes the likelihood of congenital tuberculosis occurring.[51,52] If infection of the placenta occurs, it results more frequently from disseminated tuberculosis in the mother than from a local endometritis. Tuberculous endometritis, however, can lead to congenital infection of the newborn.[32,53-56] Tuberculosis in the mother as a complication of in vitro fertilization has been described.[57]

Effect of Pregnancy on Tuberculosis

Over the past 2 millennia, medical opinions regarding the interaction of pregnancy and tuberculosis have varied considerably. Hippocrates believed that pregnancy had a beneficial effect on tuberculosis, a view that persisted virtually unchallenged well into the 19th century.[58] In 1850, Grisolle reported 24 cases of tuberculosis that developed during pregnancy.[59] In all patients the progression of tuberculosis during pregnancy was more severe than that usually seen in nonpregnant women of the same age. Shortly thereafter, several other papers were published that implied that pregnancy had a deleterious effect on tuberculosis. This view gained so much support that by the early 20th century, the practice of induced abortion to deal with the consequences of tuberculosis during pregnancy became widely accepted.

The opinion that pregnancy had a deleterious effect on tuberculosis predominated until the late 1940s. In 1943, Cohen[60] detected no increased rate of progression of tuberculosis among 100 pregnant women with abnormal chest radiograph results. In 1953, Hedvall[59] presented a comprehensive review of published studies concerning tuberculosis in pregnancy. He cited studies totaling more than 1000 cases that reported deleterious effects of pregnancy on tuberculosis. He discovered a nearly equal number of reported cases, however, in which a neutral or favorable relationship between pregnancy and tuberculosis was observed. In his own study of 250 pregnant women with abnormal chest radiograph results thought to be due to tuberculosis, he noted that 9% improved, 7% worsened, and 84% remained unchanged during pregnancy. During the first postpartum year, 9% improved, 15% worsened, and 76% were stable. Cromie[61] noted that 31 of 101 pregnant women with quiescent tuberculosis experienced relapse after delivery. Twenty of the 31 relapses occurred in the first postpartum year. Several other investigators observed the higher risk of relapse during the puerperium. Several theories were proposed to explain this phenomenon, including postpartum descent of the diaphragm, nutritional stress of pregnancy and lactation, insufficient sleep for the new mother, rapid hormonal changes, and depression in immunity in late pregnancy and the postpartum period. A similar number of other studies, however, failed to support an increased risk of progression of tuberculosis in the postpartum period.[62-66] A study by Cohen and colleagues failed to demonstrate an increase in activity of tuberculosis during pregnancy or any postpartum interval.[62] Rosenbach and Gangemi[64] and Cohen and colleagues[62] showed that only 9% to 13% of women with long-standing tuberculosis had progression of disease during the pregnancy or first postpartum year, a rate thought to be comparable to that in nonpregnant women. Few of these studies had adequate control populations. From all the studies reported, it became clear that the anatomic extent of disease, the radiographic pattern, and the susceptibility of the individual patient to tuberculosis were more important than the pregnancy itself in determining the course and prognosis of the pregnant woman with tuberculosis.

The controversy concerning the effect of pregnancy or the postpartum period on tuberculosis has lost most of its importance with the advent of effective chemotherapy.[67,68] With adequate treatment, pregnant women with tuberculosis have the same excellent prognosis as nonpregnant women. Several studies document no adverse effects of pregnancy, birth, the postpartum period, or lactation on the course of tuberculosis in women receiving chemotherapy.[69,70]

Most studies have dealt with the risk of reactivation of tuberculosis among women with abnormal chest radiograph results but no evidence of active tuberculous lesions. It is not clear whether women with asymptomatic *M. tuberculosis* infection but no radiographic findings are at increased risk of developing tuberculosis during pregnancy or the postpartum period. In 1959, Pridie and Stradling[71] found that the incidence of pulmonary tuberculosis among pregnant women was the same as that in the nonpregnant female population of the area. From 1966 to 1972, Schaefer and associates[25] found that the annual pulmonary tuberculosis case rate among pregnant women in New York Lying-In Hospital was 18 to 29 per 100,000 population, comparable to the incidence of tuberculosis during the same period in women of childbearing age in of all New York City. Although no definitive study has been reported, it appears unlikely that progression from asymptomatic *M. tuberculosis* infection to tuberculosis disease is accelerated during pregnancy or the postpartum period.

Effect of Tuberculosis on Pregnancy

In the prechemotherapy era, active tuberculosis at an advanced stage carried a poor prognosis for both mother and child. Schaefer and associates[25] reported that the infant and maternal mortality rates from untreated tuberculosis were between 30% and 40%. In the chemotherapy era, the outcome of pregnancy rarely is altered by the presence of tuberculosis in the mother, except in the rare cases of congenital tuberculosis. One study from Norway revealed a higher incidence of toxemia, postpartum hemorrhage, and difficult labor in mothers with tuberculosis compared with that in control subjects.[72] The incidence of miscarriage was almost 10 times higher in the tuberculous mothers, but there was no significant difference in the rate of congenital malformations in children born to mothers with and without tuberculosis. Another study reported an incidence of prematurity for infants born to untreated mothers in a tuberculosis sanitarium ranging from 23% to 64%, depending on the severity of tuberculosis in the mother.[73] Most experts now believe, however, that with proper treatment of the pregnant woman with tuberculosis, the prognosis of the pregnancy should not be affected adversely by the presence of tuberculosis. Because of the excellent prognosis for the mother and child, the recommendation for therapeutic abortion has been abandoned.

Screening for Tuberculosis in Pregnancy

For all pregnant women, the history obtained in an early prenatal visit should include questions about a previously positive tuberculin skin test result, previous treatment for *M. tuberculosis* infection or disease, current symptoms compatible with tuberculosis, and known exposure to other adults with the disease.[74-76] Membership in a high-risk group is a sufficient reason for a tuberculin skin test. For many high-risk women, prenatal or peripartum care represents their only contact with the health care system, and the opportunity to test them for tuberculosis infection or disease should not be lost. Some experts believe that all pregnant women should receive a tuberculin skin test.[77] Most experts believe, however, that only women with specific risk factors for *M. tuberculosis* infection or disease should be tested. It must be emphasized that women co-infected with HIV and *M. tuberculosis* may show no reaction to a tuberculin skin test. Pregnant women with high risk for or with known HIV infection should have a thorough investigation for tuberculosis.

Changes in the interpretation of the Mantoux tuberculin skin test have been promoted by the Centers for Disease Control and Prevention, the American Thoracic Society, and the American Academy of Pediatrics.[76,78] The rationale for using different sizes of induration as representing a positive result in different populations has been discussed thoroughly in many publications. The current recommendation is that for individuals at the highest risk of having *M. tuberculosis* infection progress to tuberculosis—contacts of adults with infectious tuberculosis, patients with an abnormal chest radiograph result or clinical evidence of tuberculosis, or persons with HIV infection or other immunocompromise—a Mantoux tuberculin skin test reaction of at least 5 mm is classified as positive, indicating infection with *M. tuberculosis*. For other high-risk groups, a reaction of at least 10 mm is positive. For all other persons deemed at low risk for tuberculosis, a reaction of at least 15 mm is positive. Obviously, this classification scheme depends on the ability and willingness of the family and health care provider to develop a thorough epidemiologic history of tuberculosis exposures and risk. It also depends on accurate interpretation of the skin test result. One recent study implied that pediatricians tend to under-read induration in tuberculin skin tests.[79]

There have been no studies to verify whether the classification scheme for the Mantoux tuberculin skin test is valid in pregnant women, but there is no reason to suspect otherwise.[80,81] The effect of pregnancy on tuberculin hypersensitivity as measured by the tuberculin skin test is controversial.[82] Some studies have shown a decrease in in vitro lymphocyte reactivity to purified protein derivative during pregnancy.[83] In vivo studies using patients as their own controls, however, have demonstrated no effect of pregnancy on cutaneous delayed hypersensitivity to tuberculin.[84,85] Most experts believe the tuberculin skin test by the Mantoux technique is valid throughout pregnancy. There is no evidence that the tuberculin skin test has adverse effects on the pregnant mother or fetus or that skin testing reactivates quiescent foci of tuberculosis infection.[86]

One of the most difficult problems in the interaction of tuberculosis and pregnancy is deciding whether a pregnant woman with *M. tuberculosis* infection should receive immediate treatment or whether the treatment should be postponed until after the child is delivered.[87] Not all infected individuals have the same chance of developing tuberculosis during a short period of time. Individuals who were infected remotely (more than 2 years previously) have a low chance of developing tuberculosis during a given 9-month period. Individuals who have been infected more recently, however, particularly if their infection is discovered during a contact investigation of an adult with active tuberculosis, are at much higher risk; about half of the lifetime risk of progression of infection to disease occurs during the first 1 to 2 years after infection. Other vulnerable adults, particularly those co-infected with HIV, also are at greatly increased risk of having progression of infection to disease. In general, treatment for tuberculosis infection should be initiated during pregnancy if the woman likely has been infected recently (especially in the setting of a contact investigation of a recently diagnosed case) or if she is at increased risk of rapid development of tuberculosis. Although isoniazid (INH) is not thought to be teratogenic, some experts recommend waiting until the second trimester of pregnancy to begin treatment. Unfortunately, patient adherence to INH treatment for tuberculosis infection appears to be very low if the initiation of treatment is delayed until after the child is delivered. The reason for this low adherence is not clear, but several problems include the perception of nonimportance because a treatment delay of many months is allowed, transfer of care from one segment of the health care system to another, and, perhaps, the lack of reinforcement by health care professionals concerning the importance of the treatment. Although screening and treatment of high-risk pregnant women may seem to be an effective strategy to prevent future cases of tuberculosis, it has not yet been demonstrated that this strategy is successful in the U.S. health care system.[88]

Routine chest radiography is not advisable as a screening tool for pregnant women because the prevalence of tuberculosis remains fairly low.[89,90] With appropriate shielding, however, pregnant women with positive tuberculin skin test results should have chest radiographs to rule out tuberculosis.[91] In addition, a thorough review of systems and physical examination should be carried out to exclude extrapulmonary tuberculosis.

CONGENITAL TUBERCULOSIS

Tuberculosis in the Mother

In general, the clinical manifestations of tuberculosis in the pregnant woman are the same as those in nonpregnant individuals. The most important determinants of the clinical presentation are the extent and anatomic location of disease. In one series of 27 pregnant and postpartum women with pulmonary tuberculosis, the most common clinical findings were cough (74%), weight loss (41%), fever (30%), malaise and fatigue (30%), and hemoptysis (19%).[27] Almost 20% of patients had no significant symptoms; other studies also have found less significant symptoms in pregnant women with tuberculosis.[26] The tuberculin skin test result was positive in 26 of 27 patients. The diagnosis was established in all cases by culture of sputum for *M. tuberculosis*. Sixteen of the patients in this series had drug-resistant tuberculosis; their clinical course was marked by more extensive pulmonary involvement, a higher incidence of pulmonary complications, longer sputum conversion times, and a higher incidence of death. In other series, 5% to 10% of pregnant women with tuberculosis have had extrapulmonary disease, a rate comparable with nonpregnant women of the same age.[26]

Although the female genital tract may be the portal of entry for a primary tuberculosis infection, more often infection at this site originates by continuity from an adjacent focus of disease or by blood-borne seeding of the fallopian tubes.[51] Progression of disease usually is by descent in the genital tract. Mucosal ulceration within the fallopian tube develops, and pelvic adhesions occur frequently. Many patients are asymptomatic. The most common complaints are sterility and menstrual irregularity with menorrhagia or amenorrhea. These findings greatly diminish the likelihood of congenital tuberculosis. Other less frequent signs and symptoms include lower abdominal pain and tenderness, weight loss, fever, and night sweats. Diagnosis in the nonpregnant woman is usually established by culture and histologic examination of tissue recovered after uterine curettage. The highest recovery rates of *M. tuberculosis* are obtained from scrapings obtained just before or during menstruation.

Tuberculosis mastitis is very rare in the United States but occurs almost exclusively in childbearing-aged women.[92-94] The most common finding is a single breast mass, with or without a draining sinus. Nipple retraction and peau d'orange skin changes suggestive of carcinoma also may be present. The ipsilateral axillary lymph nodes usually are enlarged. Diagnosis is confirmed by biopsy of the mass or axillary node and culture of the tissue for *M. tuberculosis*. Transmission of *M. tuberculosis* to the infant through breast milk is exceedingly rare, if it occurs at all.

In Utero Routes of Transmission

Tuberculosis in the neonate can be either truly congenital (i.e., acquired in utero) or truly neonatal (i.e., acquired early in life from the mother, contagious members of the family, family friends, or caretakers). Each of these two kinds of perinatal tuberculosis may be subdivided. *Congenital tuberculosis* can be acquired in any one of three ways: (1) from the infected placenta via the umbilical vein, (2) by inhalation of infected amniotic fluid, and (3) by ingestion of infected amniotic fluid. *Neonatal tuberculosis* can be acquired in four different ways: (1) by inhalation of infected droplets, (2) by ingestion of infected droplets, (3) by ingestion of infected milk (theoretical), and (4) by contamination of traumatized skin or mucous membranes.

It is not always possible to be sure of the route of infection in a particular neonate, and, with effective chemotherapy at hand, it is not essential for the care of the infant. However, it is important to try to identify the source of infection so that the person infecting the infant can be treated and further transmission can be prevented.[95]

Table 19–1 Modes of Inoculation of the Fetus or Newborn with *Mycobacterium tuberculosis*

Maternal Focus	Mode of Spread
Placentitis	Hematogenous (umbilical vessel)
Amniotic fluid	Aspiration
Cervicitis	Direct contact
Pneumonitis	Airbone (postnatal)

The potential modes of inoculation of the fetus or newborn infant with *M. tuberculosis* from the mother are shown in Table 19-1.[96] Infection of the fetus through the umbilical cord has been rare, with fewer than 350 cases reported in the English-language literature.[97] These infants' mothers frequently suffer from tuberculous pleural effusion, meningitis, or disseminated disease during pregnancy or soon after.[39,42,44,47,98] In some series of congenital tuberculosis, however, fewer than 50% of the mothers were known to be suffering from tuberculosis at the time of delivery and beginning of symptoms in the newborn.[99,100] In most of these cases, diagnosis of the child led to the discovery of the mother's tuberculosis. The intensity of lymphohematogenous spread during pregnancy is one of the factors that determines whether congenital tuberculosis will occur. Hematogenous dissemination in the mother leads to infection of the placenta with subsequent transmission of organisms to the fetus. *M. tuberculosis* has been demonstrated in the decidua, amnion, and chorionic villi of the placenta. The organisms also have been shown to reach the placenta through direct extension from a tuberculous salpingeal tube. Even massive involvement of the placenta with tuberculosis, however, does not always give rise to congenital tuberculosis.[101] It is not clear whether the fetus can be infected directly from the mother's bloodstream without a caseous lesion forming first in the placenta, although this phenomenon has been demonstrated in experimental animal models.[102]

In hematogenous congenital tuberculosis, the organisms reach the fetus through the umbilical vein. If bacilli infect the liver, a primary focus develops with involvement of the periportal lymph nodes. The bacilli can pass through the liver, however, into the main circulation through the patent foramen ovale. Alternately, they can pass through the right ventricle into the pulmonary circulation, leading to a primary focus in the lung. The organisms in the lung often remain dormant until after birth when oxygenation and circulation increase significantly, leading to the growth of organisms and pulmonary tuberculosis in the young infant. In many children with congenital tuberculosis, multiple lesions occur throughout the body; it is not possible to determine whether they represent multiple primary foci or some occur secondary to primary lesions in the lung or liver. The only lesion of the neonate that is unquestionably associated with congenital infection is a primary complex in the liver.

Congenital infection of the infant also can occur through aspiration or ingestion of infected amniotic fluid.[103] If the caseous lesion in the placenta ruptures directly into the amniotic cavity, the fetus can inhale or ingest the bacilli. Inhalation or ingestion of infected amniotic fluid is the most likely cause of congenital tuberculosis if the infant has multiple primary foci in the lung, gut, or middle ear.[104] In congenital tuberculosis caused by aspiration, the primary complex can be in the liver, the lung, or both organs.

The pathology of congenital tuberculosis in the fetus and newborn usually demonstrates the predisposition to dissemination ensured by the modes of transmission, particularly through the umbilical vein. The liver and lungs are the primary affected organs, with bone marrow, bone, gastrointestinal tract, adrenal glands, spleen, kidneys, abdominal lymph nodes, and skin also frequently affected.[105,106] The histologic patterns of involvement are similar to those in adults; tubercles and granulomas are common. Central nervous system involvement occurs in fewer than 50% of cases.[99,106] In most recent series, the mortality rate of congenital tuberculosis has been close to 50%, primarily because of the failure to suspect the correct diagnosis. Most fatal cases are diagnosed at autopsy.[99,100]

Postnatal acquisition of *M. tuberculosis* through airborne inoculation is the most common route of infection of the neonate.[107-109] It may be impossible to differentiate postnatal infection from prenatal acquisition on clinical grounds alone.[110] Any adult in the neonate's environment can be a source of airborne tuberculosis, including health care workers.[111,112] Up to 40% of infants with untreated *M. tuberculosis* infection develop tuberculosis disease within 1 to 2 years. There are few data concerning the time of onset of tuberculosis when the infection is acquired at or shortly after birth. In one series of 48 infants exposed postnatally to mothers with pulmonary tuberculosis in the pretreatment era, 21 became infected; of those who became ill, signs such as fever, tachypnea, weight loss, and hepatosplenomegaly developed in 4 to 8 weeks.[113] Because newborns infected with the organism are at extremely high risk for developing severe forms of disease, investigation of an adult with tuberculosis whose household contacts include a pregnant woman or newborn should be considered a public health emergency. In addition, all adults in contact with an infant suspected of having *M. tuberculosis* infection or disease should undergo a thorough investigation for disease.

The skin and mucous membranes are rare portals of entry for *M. tuberculosis* in neonates. Infection through the skin has been mentioned several times in association with lesions of the head and face, very likely related to minor traumatic lesions being infected by kissing. Primary lesions of the mucous membranes of the mouth also have been recognized, although usually in infants beyond the newborn period. In both of these situations, the primary lesion was insignificant, but the enlarged regional lymph nodes called attention to the problem.

A previously well-known form of skin and mucous membrane infection was tuberculosis of the male genitalia after circumcision, in the years when it was customary for the individual performing the circumcision to suck the blood around the incision. This procedure was obviously dangerous if that individual happened to have bacilli in the sputum. The primary focus of inoculation on the penis was often inconspicuous, but within 1 to 4 weeks, ulceration, suppuration, and bilateral inguinal lymphadenopathy would develop. At first firm and nontender, the nodes might later break down with sinus formation to the exterior. Holt,[114] in his review of circumcision tuberculosis, described a case with extensive ulceration of the penis and scrotum, greatly swollen lymph nodes, a generalized rash resembling varicella, hepatosplenomegaly, fever, cough, rales, and a positive tuberculin test result, with recovery of tubercle bacilli from sputum and penile discharge. Of the 41 patients described by Holt, 16 died and 6 recovered, with the outcome of the others unknown.[114]

Criteria for Diagnosis of Congenital Tuberculosis

In 1935, Beitzke[115] suggested criteria for diagnosis of congenital tuberculosis in a thoughtful, detailed, and often-quoted review of the reported cases up to that time:

1. Tuberculosis in the child must be firmly established;
2. A primary complex in the liver is proof of congenital tuberculosis because this complex could arise only through perfusion of the liver with tubercle bacilli contained in umbilical cord blood;
3. If a primary complex is lacking in the liver, then tuberculosis can be considered to be congenital only if tuberculous lesions are present in a fetus or in a newborn only a few days old; *or* in an older infant, extrauterine infection can be excluded with certainty, that is, if the child was removed from the tuberculous mother at birth to a tuberculosis-free environment.

A study by Cantwell and co-workers,[97] based on a review of cases of congenital tuberculosis published before and after 1980, proposed the following modification of Beitzke's criteria: the infant must have proven tuberculous lesions and at least one of the following: (1) lesions in the first week of life; (2) a primary hepatic complex or caseating hepatic granulomas; (3) tuberculosis infection of the placenta or maternal genital tract, or both; or (4) exclusion of postnatal transmission by a thorough contact investigation. Although Beitzke's criteria are in fact fully met by many of the 350 or so reported cases of congenital tuberculosis, in other cases it is impossible to be certain whether infection was transmitted in utero or was acquired during the early days or weeks of life. In many cases of true congenital tuberculosis, the mother was not known to be suffering from active tuberculosis. Two articles contain tables with detailed information on 26 cases and 15 cases.[99,100] In only 10 of the 26 cases was tuberculosis diagnosed in the mother ante partum, although it became apparent in another 15 after diagnosis in the infant.[99] Five of the 26 mothers died of tuberculosis, an indirect confirmation of the fact that the diagnosis was made very late. In the series of 15 cases, 7 mothers were thought to be well at the time of delivery, but all 15 were subsequently found either to have had pleural effusion antepartum (four cases) or to have developed endometrial, miliary, or meningeal tuberculosis post partum.[100]

Clinical Features and Diagnosis of Congenital Tuberculosis

The clinical manifestations of tuberculosis in the fetus and newborn vary in relation to the site and size of the caseous lesions. Symptoms may be present at birth but more commonly begin by the second or third week of life. The most frequent signs or symptoms of true congenital tuberculosis are listed in Table 19-2.[97,99,116-147] Most infants have an abnormal chest radiograph result, with about half having a miliary pattern.[148] Some infants with a normal chest radiograph result early in the course develop profound radiographic abnormalities as the disease progresses (Fig. 19-2). The most common abnormalities are adenopathy and parenchymal infiltrates. Occasionally, the pulmonary involvement progresses very rapidly, leading to cavitation.[149,150] Tuberculosis of the middle ear in children with congenital tuberculosis has been described fairly often.[99,108,149,151-154] The eustachian tube in newborns permits ready access to infected pharyngeal fluids or vomitus. Multiple perforation or total destruction of the tympanic membrane, otorrhea, enlarged cervical lymph nodes, and facial paralysis are all possible sequelae.

Table 19–2 Most Frequent Signs and Symptoms of Congenital Tuberculosis

Symptom or Sign	Frequency (%)
Hepatosplenomegaly	76
Respiratory distress	72
Fever	48
Lymphadenopathy	38
Abdominal distention	24
Lethargy or irritability	21
Ear discharge	17
Papular skin lesions	14
Vomiting, apnea, cyanosis, jaundice, seizures, petechiae	<10 each

Adapted from Cantwell MF, Shebb ZM, Costello AM, et al. Brief report: congenital tuberculosis. N Engl J Med 330:1051–1054, 1994; with permission, copyright 1994, Massachusetts Medical Society. All rights reserved.

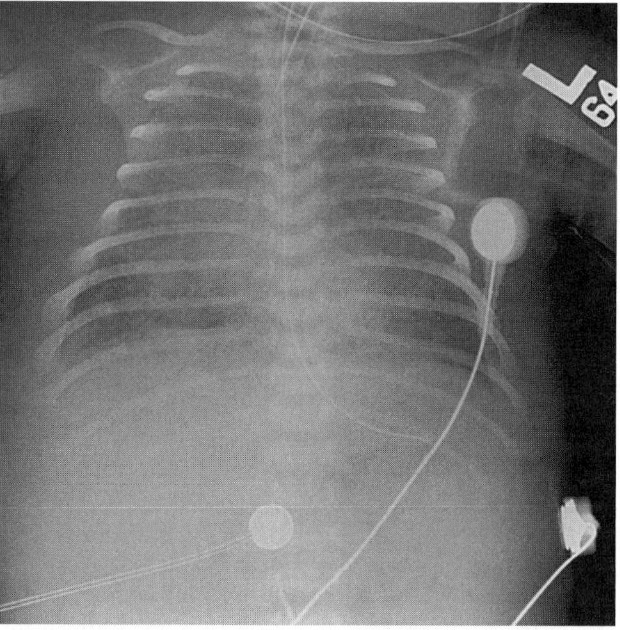

Figure 19–2 Chest radiograph of a 1-month-old infant with congenital tuberculosis.

Table 19–3 Antituberculosis Drugs in Children

Drugs	Dosage Forms	Daily Dose (mg/kg)	Twice-Weekly Dose (mg/kg/per dose)	Maximum Dose
Isoniazid	Scored tablets: 100 mg 300 mg Syrup: 10 mg/ml	10-15	20-40	Daily: 300 mg Twice weekly: 900 mg
Rifampin	Capsules: 150 mg 300 mg Syrup: formulated in syrup from capsules	10-20	10-20	600 mg
Pyrazinamide	Scored tablets: 500 mg	20-40	50-70	2 g
Streptomycin	Vials: 1 g, 4 g	20-40 (IM)	20-40 (IM)	1 g
Ethambutol	Scored tablets: 100 mg 400 mg	15-25	50	2.5 g

The clinical presentation of tuberculosis in the newborn is similar to that caused by bacterial sepsis[139-141] and congenital infections with syphilis and cytomegalovirus.[9] Abnormalities of liver function are common.[142,144] The diagnosis of congenital tuberculosis should be suspected in any infant with signs and symptoms of sepsis or viral infection who does not respond to vigorous antibiotic therapy and whose evaluation for other congenital infections is unrevealing. Of course, suspicion also should be high if the mother has or has had tuberculosis or if she is in a high-risk group for tuberculosis. The importance of obtaining an adequate history for the presence of risk factors for tuberculosis in the mother cannot be overemphasized. Suspicion should increase if the mother has suffered from unexplained pneumonia, bronchitis, pleural effusion, meningeal disease, or endometritis during, shortly before, or even after pregnancy. Evaluation of both parents and other family members can yield important clues about the presence of tuberculosis within the family.

The timely diagnosis of congenital or neonatal tuberculosis is often difficult.[95,155,156] Whenever possible, the placenta should be examined and cultured for *M. tuberculosis*. The tuberculin skin test result is always negative initially, although it may become positive after 1 to 3 months of treatment. The diagnosis must be established by finding acid-fast bacilli in body fluids or tissue or by culturing *M. tuberculosis*. A positive acid-fast bacilli smear of an early morning gastric aspirate obtained from a newborn should be considered indicative of tuberculosis, although false-positive results can occur.[8] Direct acid-fast bacilli smears from middle-ear fluid, bone marrow, tracheal aspirate, or biopsy tissue can be useful and should be obtained more often.[144,157] Hageman and colleagues[99] found positive cultures for *M. tuberculosis* in 10 of 12 gastric aspirates, three of three liver biopsies, three of three lymph node biopsies, and two of four bone marrow aspirations from children with congenital tuberculosis. Open-lung biopsy also has been used to establish the diagnosis.[158] The cerebrospinal fluid should be examined and cultured, although the yield for isolating *M. tuberculosis* is less than 20% and meningitis occurs in only one third of cases of congenital tuberculosis.

TREATMENT OF TUBERCULOSIS

The drugs used most commonly to treat *M. tuberculosis* infection and disease, their dosage forms, and doses are listed in Table 19-3.[159] Detailed discussion of the pharmacokinetics of each drug is beyond the scope of this chapter. No published study has examined in detail the pharmacokinetics of drugs used as antituberculosis agents in premature or term neonates.[160]

INH is the mainstay of treatment for tuberculosis infection and disease in infants, children, and adults. It is inexpensive, highly effective in preventing the multiplication of tubercle bacilli, of low molecular weight and therefore readily diffusible to all tissues in the body, and relatively nontoxic to children. It can be administered orally or intramuscularly. When it is taken orally, high plasma, sputum, and cerebrospinal fluid levels are reached within a few hours and persist for at least 6 to 8 hours. Because of the slow multiplication of *M. tuberculosis*, the total daily dose can be given at one time. The principal toxic effects of INH are peripheral neuritis and hepatitis. Peripheral neuritis, resulting from competitive inhibition of pyridoxine, is almost unknown in North American children because both cow's milk (or formula) and meat are the main dietary sources of pyridoxine. In some well-nourished children, serum pyridoxine concentrations are mildly depressed by INH, but clinical signs are not apparent. For most children, therefore, it is not necessary to use supplementary pyridoxine. However, in pregnancy, in teenagers whose diets may be inadequate, in children from ethnic groups with a low milk and meat intake, and in breast-fed babies, pyridoxine supplementation (25 to 50 mg/day) is important.

Hepatotoxicity from INH, rare in children, increases in frequency with age. Monitoring serum aspartate aminotransferase and serum alanine aminotransferase sometimes reveals transient increases during treatment with INH, but the levels usually return to normal spontaneously without interruption of treatment. Liver enzyme abnormalities in adolescents receiving INH likewise are rather common and usually disappear spontaneously, but severe hepatitis can occur. Although neonates usually tolerate INH well, some experts recommend routine biochemical monitoring in the first several months of therapy. The usual dosage of INH in children is 10 to 20 mg/kg per day, to a maximum of 300 mg per day. INH is available in tablets of 100 and 300 mg. A syrup of INH in sorbitol (10 mg/mL) appears to be satisfactory; however, it is unstable at room temperature and should be kept cool. Many children develop significant gastrointestinal intolerance (nausea, vomiting) while taking the INH suspension, but neonates and infants tolerate the lower required volume of suspension well. If tablets are used, they are easily crushed in a dessert spoon and given with some soft food such as applesauce, mashed banana, thawed undiluted frozen orange juice, or another palatable medium. The crushed tablets should not be added to the nursing bottle or offered in milk or water because they will be ingested only partially.

Rifampin (RIF) is a semisynthetic drug derived from *Streptomyces mediterranei.* The drug is absorbed readily from the gastrointestinal tract in the fasting state. Excretion mainly is through the biliary tract; however, effective levels are achieved in the kidneys and urine. In many patients receiving RIF treatment, the tears, saliva, urine, and stool turn orange as a result of a harmless metabolite, and the patient and parents always must be warned of this in advance. RIF can be made into a suspension easily for use in children. RIF is very well tolerated by neonates and infants. The incidences of hepatitis, leukopenia, and thrombocytopenia are extremely low. RIF should be used alone only when treating *M. tuberculosis* infection due to an INH-resistant organism. If one uses INH, 20 mg/kg, and RIF, 15 to 20 mg/kg, there is an appreciable incidence of hepatotoxicity. Therefore, when using the two together, one would be wise to approximate INH, 10 mg/kg, and RIF, 15 to 20 mg/kg.

Pyrazinamide (PZA) contributes to the killing of *M. tuberculosis*, particularly at a low pH such as that within macrophages. The exact mechanism of action of PZA is a subject of controversy. PZA has no effect on extracellular tubercle bacilli in vitro but clearly contributes to the killing of intracellular bacilli. Primary resistance is very rare, except that *Mycobacterium bovis* is resistant. The drug diffuses readily into all areas, including the cerebrospinal fluid. The usual adult daily dose is 20 to 40 mg/kg. The optimal dose for infants and children has not been established firmly because no formal pharmacokinetic studies have been reported. The adult dose is tolerated well by infants and children, results in high cerebrospinal fluid concentrations, and clearly is effective in therapy trials for active tuberculosis in children. PZA appears to exert its maximum effect during the first 2 months of therapy. Hepatotoxicity can occur at high doses but is rare at the usual dose. PZA routinely causes an increase in the serum uric acid concentration by inhibiting its excretion through the kidneys. Toxic reactions in adults include flushing, cutaneous hypersensitivity, arthralgia, and overt gout; however, the considerable experience with this drug in children in Latin American countries, Hong Kong, and the United States has revealed few problems.

Ethambutol (EMB) has been used for many years as a companion drug for INH in adults. The usual oral dose is 15 mg/kg per day. At this dose, the drug primarily is bacteriostatic, its major role being to prevent emergence of resistance to other drugs. However, at doses of 25 mg/kg per day or 50 mg/kg given twice a week, EMB has some bactericidal action. Unfortunately, at these higher doses, optic neuritis or red-green color blindness has occurred in some adults. Although the incidence of ophthalmologic toxicity in children is extremely low, if it occurs at all, EMB is not recommended for routine use in young children in whom visual field and color discrimination tests are difficult and inaccurate. However, it is used frequently and safely in children with life-threatening forms of tuberculosis or with drug-resistant tuberculosis.

Streptomycin (STM) is a valuable drug to be used in conjunction with INH and RIF in life-threatening forms of tuberculosis. It is bactericidal and tolerated well by children in the usual dose of 20 to 40 mg/kg per day intramuscularly up to 1 g. Usually, STM can be discontinued within 1 to 3 months if clinical improvement is definite.

General Principles

The tubercle bacillus can be killed only during replication, which occurs among organisms that are active metabolically. In one model, bacilli in a host exist in different populations.[5] They are active metabolically and replicate freely when oxygen tension is high and the pH is neutral or alkaline. Environmental conditions for growth are best within cavities, leading to a large bacterial population. Older children with pulmonary tuberculosis and patients of all ages with only extrapulmonary tuberculosis are infected with a much smaller number of tubercle bacilli because the cavitary population is not present. However, neonates with congenital tuberculosis tend to have a large burden of organisms at diagnosis.

Naturally occurring drug-resistant mutant organisms occur within large populations of tubercle bacilli even before chemotherapy is started. All known genetic loci for drug resistance in *M. tuberculosis* are located on the chromosome; no plasmid-mediated resistance is known. The rate of resistance within populations of organisms is related to the rate of mutations at these loci. Although a large population of bacilli as a whole may be considered drug susceptible, a subpopulation of drug-resistant organisms occurs at a fairly predictable rate. The mean frequency of these drug-resistant mutations is about 10^{-6} but varies among drugs: STM, 10^{-5}; INH, 10^{-6}; and RIF, 10^{-7}. A cavity containing 10^9 tubercle bacilli has thousands of single drug-resistant mutant organisms, whereas a closed caseous lesion contains few, if any, resistant mutants.

The population size of tubercle bacilli within a patient determines the appropriate therapy. For patients with a large bacterial population (adults with cavities or extensive infiltrates), many single drug-resistant mutants are present and at least two antituberculosis drugs must be used. Conversely, for patients with *M. tuberculosis* infection but no disease, the bacterial population is very small (about 10^3 to 10^4 organisms), drug-resistant mutants are rare, and a single drug can be used. Older children with pulmonary tuberculosis and patients of all ages with extrapulmonary tuberculosis have medium-sized populations in which drug-resistant mutants may or may not be present. In general, these patients should be treated with at least two drugs. Neonates and infants with tuberculosis disease have large mycobacterial populations, and several drugs are required to effect a cure.

Pregnant Women

The only drug with well-documented efficacy against *M. tuberculosis* infection in pregnant women is INH. Infants and children tolerate INH very well, and adverse reactions are rare. However, adverse reactions are more common in adults. Between 5% and 10% of young adults taking INH have an asymptomatic increase in serum liver transaminase levels; 1% to 2% suffer from symptomatic hepatitis, which is reversible if the medication is stopped immediately. For most young adults, monitoring for hepatitis is done clinically. Routine or periodic evaluation of serum liver enzyme tests is reserved for adults with underlying liver disease or those taking other potentially hepatotoxic drugs. However, some experts think that all pregnant women taking INH should have routine biochemical monitoring for hepatitis. Serum liver enzyme elevations of three to four times normal are common and do not necessitate discontinuation of the drug. There is no evidence that giving INH to a pregnant woman adversely affects the liver of the fetus. The other important adverse reaction of INH is peripheral neuritis caused by inhibition of pyridoxine metabolism. Pyridoxine should be given to pregnant adolescents or women and breast-feeding infants because breast milk has low concentrations of pyridoxine, even if the mother is receiving vitamin supplements.[161]

The current recommendation of the Centers for Disease Control and Prevention is to treat adults and children infected with *M. tuberculosis* with INH for 9 months.[76] Usually, the medication is taken daily under self-supervision. If poor patient adherence is likely and resources are available, INH can be given twice weekly using directly observed therapy.[162] Directly observed therapy requires that a health care worker, often from the local health department, observe the patient take antituberculosis medications. In general, directly observed therapy should be used for all patients with tuberculosis disease because of the difficulty in predicting patient adherence and the consequences of poor adherence (relapse and development of drug resistance). Directly observed therapy is often used for high-risk newborns with tuberculosis exposure or infants with *M. tuberculosis* infection.

For patients who cannot take INH for treatment of *M. tuberculosis* infection either because of side effects of the medication or because they are infected with an INH-resistant but RIF-susceptible strain of *M. tuberculosis*, the treatment of choice for *M. tuberculosis* infection is RIF, which also can be given daily or twice a week under directly observed therapy.[163] If the mother is known to be infected with a strain of tuberculosis that is resistant to both INH and RIF (multidrug-resistant tuberculosis), an expert should be consulted for the management of the mother and the child after delivery.[164]

Although treatment of a woman with active tuberculosis during pregnancy is unquestioned, treatment of a pregnant woman who has an asymptomatic *M. tuberculosis* infection is more controversial. Some clinicians prefer to delay therapy until after delivery, because pregnancy does not seem to increase the risk of developing active tuberculosis. Others believe that because recent infection can be accompanied by hematogenous spread to the placenta, it is preferable to treat without delay or to wait until the second trimester to start chemotherapy. A report by Franks and colleagues[165] suggests that the risk of INH-associated hepatitis and death is higher in women than in men and that women in the postpartum period are slightly more vulnerable to INH hepatotoxicity. These investigators suggest that it might be prudent to avoid INH during the postpartum period or at least to monitor postpartum women taking INH with frequent examinations and laboratory studies. The possible increased risk of INH hepatotoxicity must be weighed against the risk of developing active tuberculosis as well as the consequences to both mother and infant should active tuberculosis develop.

The indications for treatment and the basic principles of management for the pregnant woman with tuberculosis disease are no different from those for the nonpregnant patient. The recommendations for which drugs to use and how long to give them are slightly different, however, mostly because of possible effects of several of the drugs on the developing fetus.

The currently recommended treatment for drug-susceptible pulmonary tuberculosis in the United States in nonpregnant individuals is 6 months of INH and RIF, supplemented during the first 2 months with PZA and either EMB or STM.[159,166] With any of the regimens, the drugs usually are given every day for the first 2 weeks to 2 months; then they can be given daily or twice a week (under directly observed therapy) for the remainder of therapy with equal effectiveness and rates of adverse reactions.[167]

There is no doubt that untreated tuberculosis represents a far greater risk to a woman and her fetus than does appropriate treatment of the disease.[68,168-172] Extensive experience with the use of INH in pregnancy has been reported. Even though it crosses the placenta, it is not teratogenic even when given during the first 4 months of gestation.[173] EMB also appears to be safe during pregnancy. In 650 cases in which pregnant women were treated with EMB, no evidence of fetal malformations, including eye abnormalities, was found.[86,174-176] The action of RIF to inhibit DNA-dependent RNA polymerase combined with its ability to cross the placental barrier has created some concern about its use in pregnancy.[177] Only 3% of 446 fetuses exposed in utero to RIF had abnormalities, however, compared with 2% for EMB and 1% for INH.[86] The noted abnormalities included limb reductions, central nervous system abnormalities, and hypoprothrombinemia. Hemorrhagic disease of the newborn also has been described after the use of RIF in the mother. The incidence of abnormalities in fetuses not exposed to antituberculosis medications ranges from 1% to 6%. In general, the powerful antituberculosis effect of RIF outweighs concern about its effect on the fetus. Nonpregnant women receiving RIF should receive contraception counseling because receiving RIF can impair the efficacy of oral contraceptives, leading to unintended pregnancy in a tuberculous woman.[178]

Several antituberculosis drugs generally are not used in pregnant women because of possibly toxicity to the fetus.[179-182] STM has variable passage across the placental barrier. Its use in pregnancy is now limited by the availability of better drugs and its effect on the fetus.[181-184] In a review of 206 infants exposed in utero to STM, 34 (17%) had significant eighth nerve damage, the abnormalities ranging from mild vestibular damage to profound bilateral deafness.[86] The deleterious effects of STM are independent of the critical periods earlier in embryogenesis, and it is potentially hazardous throughout gestation. It is assumed that capreomycin, kanamycin, and amikacin, other aminoglycosides with antituberculosis activity, could have the same toxic potential as STM. Little is known about the specific effects of PZA on the fetus. Although there are no data, an increasing number of experts are using PZA during pregnancy with no reported adverse reactions. Nonspecific teratogenic effects have been attributed to ethionamide.[185] The central nervous system effects of cycloserine and the gastrointestinal effects of para-aminosalicylic acid in adults make their use in pregnancy undesirable.

The currently recommended initial treatment of drug-susceptible tuberculosis disease in pregnancy is INH and RIF daily, with the addition of EMB initially, under directly observed therapy.[186,187] Pyridoxine (50 mg daily) always should be given with INH during pregnancy because of the increased requirements for this vitamin in pregnant women. After drug susceptibility testing of the isolate of *M. tuberculosis* reveals it to be susceptible to both INH and RIF, the EMB can be discontinued. If PZA is not used in the initial regimen, INH and RIF must be given for 9 months instead of 6 months. After the first 2 weeks to 2 months of daily treatment, the drugs can be given twice a week under directly observed therapy, which is the preferred method of treatment by most experts. The treatment of any form of drug-resistant tuberculosis during pregnancy is extraordinarily difficult and should be handled by an expert with great experience with the disease.[188,189]

Because treatment of tuberculosis in pregnant women often continues after delivery, there is concern as to whether it is safe for the mother to breast-feed her infant. Snider and Powell[190] concluded that a breast-feeding infant would have serum levels of no more than 20% of the usual therapeutic levels of INH for infants and less than 11% of other antituberculosis drugs. Potential toxic effects of drugs delivered in breast milk have not been reported. Because pyridoxine deficiency in the neonate can cause seizures, however, and because breast milk has relatively low levels of pyridoxine, infants who are taking INH or whose breast-feeding mothers are taking INH should receive supplemental pyridoxine.[191]

Neonates and Infants

The optimal treatment of congenital tuberculosis has not been established, because the rarity of this condition precludes formal treatment trials. It would appear that the basic principles for treatment of other diseases in children and adults also apply to the treatment of congenital tuberculosis.[159,167,192] All children with suspected congenital tuberculosis should be started on four antituberculosis medications (INH, RIF, PZA, plus either EMB or STM) until the diagnostic evaluation and susceptibility testing of isolated organisms is concluded. Although the optimal duration of therapy has not been established, many experts treat infants with congenital or postnatally acquired tuberculosis for a total duration of 9 to 12 months because of the decreased immunologic capability of the young infant. INH given alone is known to be safe in neonates, including premature infants. There are no comparable data for INH given in combination with other drugs or for other drugs alone. Several studies have shown that RIF can be given safely to premature infants for indications other than tuberculosis. In addition, anecdotal information supports the notion that PZA, STM, and kanamycin are safe in neonates. Young infants taking these drugs should have biochemical monitoring of serum liver enzymes and uric acid (for PZA) performed on a regular basis. Although the pharmacokinetics of antituberculosis drugs in the neonate are essentially unknown, extensive clinical experience suggests that the doses listed in Table 19-3 are effective and safe. All neonates and infants with tuberculosis should be treated by directly observed therapy.

Following the Infant on Therapy

Follow-up of children treated with antituberculosis drugs has become somewhat more streamlined in recent years. While receiving chemotherapy, the patients should be seen monthly, both to encourage regular taking of the prescribed drugs and to check, by a few simple questions (concerning appetite, well-being) and a few observations (weight gain; appearance of skin and sclerae; palpation of liver, spleen, and lymph nodes), that the disease is not spreading and that toxic effects of the drugs are not appearing. Repeat chest radiographs probably should be obtained 1 to 2 months after the onset of chemotherapy to ascertain the maximal extent of disease before chemotherapy takes effect; thereafter, radiographs rarely are necessary. Chemotherapy has been so successful that follow-up beyond its termination is not usually necessary, except for children with serious disease, such as congential tuberculosis or meningitis, or those with extensive residual chest radiographic findings at the end of chemotherapy.

Every case of definite or suspected tuberculosis must, by law, be reported immediately by telephone to the health department to ensure (1) prompt contact investigation[193-199] and (2) free antituberculosis drugs, which are available for diagnosed cases and for intimate contacts in almost every state of the United States.

Prognosis

The prognosis for congenital tuberculosis was dismal in the prechemotherapy era.[200] In Hughesdon's report,[104] 3 infants died on the first day of life, 8 between 18 and 30 days, 15 between 31 and 60 days, and 3 between 65 and 112 days. Hageman and associates[99] reviewed 26 patients born since the introduction of INH in 1952: 12 died, and 9 of these were untreated, the diagnosis being established only at autopsy. The results in survivors were good, but the follow-up was usually short.[152,201] The child reported by Nemir and O'Hare,[100] who was treated intensively with INH, STM, and aminosalicylic acid in the 1950s, recovered, was followed for 27 years, and is herself the mother of two tuberculin-negative children.

There is little question that today's multidrug, short-course chemotherapeutic regimens should be extremely effective in bringing the disease under rapid and permanent control, if it is due to drug-susceptible organisms. Experience with treatment of disease due to drug-resistant organisms is so limited as to preclude prognosis.

VACCINATION AGAINST TUBERCULOSIS—BACILLE CALMETTE-GUÉRIN

Bacille Calmette-Guérin (BCG) vaccines are the oldest of the vaccines used throughout the world. They have been given to 4 billion people and have been used routinely since the 1960s in every country of the world except the United States and the Netherlands. However, despite their widespread use, tuberculosis remains among the most destructive infectious diseases in the world, indicating that the BCG vaccines alone will not be sufficient to eliminate or even control the disease.

History and Development of Bacille Calmette-Guérin Vaccines

The BCG vaccines are attenuated strains of *M. bovis*. Starting in 1908, the original strain was subcultured every 3 weeks for 13 years.[202] The genotype changes that resulted at various stages cannot be determined because the original cultures and subcultures were not preserved. This long process was marked by a loss of virulence first for calves, then for guinea pigs. In 1948, despite the complete lack of reported controlled trials or case-control studies, the First International BCG Congress stated that the BCG vaccines were effective and safe. After World War II, the WHO and UNICEF organized campaigns to promote vaccination with BCG in several countries. The seed lot system for BCG was established in 1956,[201] and the WHO developed requirements for freeze-dried BCG in 1966.[203] By the end of 1974, more than 1.5 billion individuals had received a BCG vaccination. Since 1977, BCG vaccination has been included in the WHO Expanded Programme on Immunization. Approximately 100 million children receive a BCG vaccination each year, expanding the total number of individuals who have received it to more than 4 billion.

The original strain of *M. bovis* used to make BCG was maintained by serial passage at the Pasteur Institute until it was lost or discarded. It previously was distributed to dozens of laboratories, each of which produced and maintained its own BCG stain. It soon became apparent that the conditions for culture used in the various laboratories resulted in the production of many "daughter" BCG strains that differed widely in growth characteristics, biochemical activity, ability to induce delayed hypersensitivity, and animal virulence.[204-207] The patterns of large restriction fragments created by the digestion of BCG DNA vary among strains.[208] In the 1960s, the WHO recommended stabilization of the biologic characteristics of the derivative strains by lyophilization and storage at low temperatures.[209]

Interlaboratory studies and genomic evaluation have shown that the BCG strains in use today vary widely in many characteristics.[210,211] However, the possible consequences on vaccine efficacy and adverse effects are not known. When comparing the various published clinical trials and case-control series, it is difficult to demonstrate that one strain of BCG is superior to another in the protection of humans against tuberculosis. Some laboratory and clinical observations have suggested that BCG strains can be separated into "strong" (Pasteur 1173 P2, Danish 1331) and "weak" (Glaxo 1077, Tokyo 172) groups. Although the relative efficacy of these two groups has been inconsistent, the strong strains have been associated with a higher rate of adverse reactions in neonates, including lymphadenitis and osteitis.[212-215] There is no consensus about which strain of BCG is optimal for general use. It has been postulated that investigators and public health authorities have selected BCG strains by their desire to maximize tuberculin reactivity and minimize adenitis, which may create strains that are the inverse of the ideal vaccine. It also appears that some BCG strains have lost efficacy over time.[216]

Vaccine Preparation and Administration

Seed lots are lyophilized bacilli that are part of the original harvest of the various BCG strains. The bacilli usually are grown in Sauton medium and are harvested early (day 6 to 9) to ensure good survival of organisms after lyophilization. The mass of mycobacterial cells is filtered, pressed, homogenized, diluted, then freeze dried. Reconstituted vaccines contain both live bacilli and dead bacteria. Regulating the ratio of live to dead organisms is an important aspect of quality control, and can affect both efficacy and rates of adverse reactions.

Most BCG vaccine programs favor the intradermal route of administration using a syringe and needle. Japan and most of South Africa use percutaneous administration with a multipuncture device. It is generally accepted that the intradermal method is more accurate and consistent because the dose is measured precisely and the administration is controlled. The deltoid region of the arm is the most common injection site, although many other body sites are used in individual patients. More than 90% of patients receiving their first BCG vaccination develop a local reaction (erythema, induration, tenderness) followed by healing and scar formation within 3 months.

Other methods of administration were developed to try to address problems of local reactions created by intradermal administration. Subcutaneous injection appears to be effective but often produces retracted scars. Other techniques, such as scarification, jet injection, and use of bifurcated needles, have yielded highly variable and, in some cases, inadequate results.[217] There have been no conclusive reported trials that compared the various techniques of BCG administration for protection against tuberculosis, but local complication rates generally are lowest with the multipuncture devices.

Adverse Reactions to Bacille Calmette-Guérin Vaccination

Local ulceration and regional lymphadenitis are the most common complications, occurring in less than 1% of immunocompetent recipients after intradermal administration of BCG.[218,219] These lesions usually occur within a few weeks to months after vaccination but can be delayed for months in immunocompetent persons and for years in immunocompromised hosts.[220] Axillary, cervical, or supraclavicular nodes may be involved on the ipsilateral side of vaccination. Outbreaks of lymphadenitis after BCG vaccination have followed the introduction of a new BCG strain into the vaccination program.[221,222] There is no evidence that children who experience local complications are more likely to have immune deficits or to have enhanced or diminished protection against tuberculosis.[221,222] Because the risk of lymphadenitis is significantly higher when newborns are given a full dose of BCG, the WHO recommends using a reduced dose in children younger than 30 days of age.

The treatment of local adenitis as a complication of BCG vaccination is controversial, ranging from observation to surgical drainage to administration of antituberculosis chemotherapy to a combination of surgery and chemotherapy.[223] Nonsuppurative lymph nodes usually resolve spontaneously, although resolution may take several months.[224,225] The WHO recommends drainage and direct instillation of an antituberculosis drug into the lesion for adherent or fistulated lymph nodes.[226] However, one study of 120 patients with BCG-induced lymphadenitis treated for 6 months with an oral antituberculosis drug showed that medical therapy was no better than observation and that the rate of spontaneous drainage of lymph nodes was higher among children who received isoniazid than among those who were only observed.[227] Most experts now agree that nonsuppurative adenitis associated with BCG vaccination should be managed by observation only.

Other complications of BCG vaccination are far less frequent. The mean risk of osteitis after BCG vaccination has varied from 0.01 per million in Japan to 300 per million in Finland.[228-230] As with lymphadenitis, osteitis rates occasionally have increased dramatically after introduction of a new vaccine strain into a vaccination program. Other very rare complications of BCG vaccination include lupus vulgaris, erythema nodosum, iritis, and osteomyelitis. In general, these complications should be treated with antituberculosis medications (except pyrazinamide, to which *M. bovis* is resistant).

Generalized BCG infection is extremely rare in immunocompetent hosts.[231-233] However, overall rates of fatal disseminated BCG disease in recently vaccinated persons have been reported at 0.19 to 1.56 cases per million vaccinated, most cases occurring in children with severe defects in cellular immunity, such as severe combined immunodeficiency, malnutrition, cancer, Di George syndrome, interferon-γ receptor deficiency, or symptomatic HIV infection.[218,234-240] It is likely that the real incidence of disseminated BCG infection is higher, as some cases undoubtedly are misdiagnosed as disseminated tuberculosis. The exact safety of BCG vaccination in children and adults with HIV infection is unknown. Disseminated BCG infection has been described in an HIV-infected adult 30 years after he received BCG.[241] One French study showed that 9 of 68 HIV-infected children given BCG vaccine developed complications: 7 had large satellite adenitis and 2 developed disseminated lesions.[242] The WHO recommends giving BCG vaccination to asymptomatic HIV-infected infants who live in high-risk areas for tuberculosis. BCG vaccine is not recommended for symptomatic HIV-infected children, even if local tuberculosis case rates are high.

Despite the presence of live BCG organisms in ulcerated vaccination sites, person-to-person transmission of BCG has never been documented.

Effect of Bacille Calmette-Guérin Vaccination on Tuberculin Skin Test Results

Although BCG vaccines have an effect on the result of the tuberculin skin test, the effect is variable, and no reliable method can distinguish tuberculin reactions caused by BCG vaccination from those caused by infection with *M. tuberculosis*. In various studies with different populations, the proportion of individuals who were vaccinated with BCG previously who have had significant skin test reactions has varied from 0% to 90%.[243-247] The size of the skin test reaction after BCG vaccination varies with the strain and dose of the vaccine, [245,248] the route of administration,[247,249] the age at vaccination,[244,250] the child's nutritional status, the time interval since vaccination,[244,250] and the frequency of skin testing.[251]

Several studies have demonstrated that when newborns are given a BCG vaccination, up to 50% have a negative tuberculin skin test reaction at 6 months of age and the vast majority have a negative reaction by 2 to 5 years of age.[244,252] However, interpretation of the skin test result in BCG-vaccinated children may be complicated by the booster phenomenon. The booster effect is the increase in reaction size caused by repetitive testing in a person sensitized to mycobacterial antigens.[253] Skin test reactions can be boosted in children who previously received a BCG vaccination, giving the false impression of "conversion" of a skin test from negative to positive, which usually indicates a new tuberculosis infection.[254]

Strong or severe reactions to a tuberculin skin test are rare in individuals who have been vaccinated with BCG previously who are *not* also infected with *M. tuberculosis*. Prior receipt of a BCG vaccine is never a contraindication for tuberculin skin testing. Most skin reactions due to BCG vaccination are less than 10 mm in size. In general, the tuberculin skin test should be interpreted in the same manner for an adult or child who has received a BCG vaccination as it is for a person with similar epidemiologic characteristics who has not received BCG.

Effectiveness of the Bacille Calmette-Guérin Vaccines

A detailed discussion of the effectiveness of the BCG vaccines and the variables that may have an impact on effectiveness is beyond the scope of this chapter. There have been eight major controlled trials conducted in a variety of populations and many published case-control and cohort studies of various BCG preparations.[255,256] Investigators at the Harvard School of Health found 15 prospective trials and 12 case-control studies that met their criteria for adequacy in study design and controls against potential bias. In the prospective trials, the protective effect of BCG vaccines against tuberculosis disease was 51%.[256] Analysis of eight studies involving only vaccination of newborns revealed a protective effort of 55%.[255] For trials that measured these outcomes, BCG vaccines showed 71% protection against death from tuberculosis, 64% protection against tuberculosis meningitis, and 72% protection against disseminated tuberculosis. Different BCG preparations and strains used in the same population gave similar levels of protection, whereas genetically identical BCG strains gave different levels of protection in different populations.[255,256] The duration of any protective effect is poorly studied and unknown but probably short-lived (less than 10 years at best).

It appears that BCG vaccines have worked well in some circumstances but poorly in others. Because only a small percentage of infectious cases of tuberculosis in adults are prevented by childhood BCG vaccination, BCG vaccination as currently practiced is not an effective instrument of disease control. The best use of BCG is the prevention of life-threatening forms of tuberculosis—meningitis and disseminated, severe pulmonary disease—in infants and young children.

MANAGEMENT OF A NEONATE BORN TO A MOTHER WITH A POSITIVE TUBERCULIN SKIN TEST RESULT

If the mother is well and her chest radiograph result is normal, no separation of the mother and infant is required. Although the mother is a candidate for treatment of *M. tuberculosis* infection, the infant does not need special evaluation or therapy. Other family members should have a tuberculin skin test and further evaluation, if indicated. The local health department, however, often does not have the resources to do this testing, which should be performed by the treating physicians. It is not necessary to delay discharge of the infant from the newborn nursery pending the results of this family investigation. The need for further skin testing of the infant depends on whether disease is found in the family or cannot be excluded within the family's environment.

If the radiograph result is abnormal, the mother and child should be separated until the mother has been evaluated thoroughly. If active tuberculosis is present in the mother, she should be started on effective antituberculosis medications right away. Examination of the mother's sputum for acid-fast organisms always is necessary even if obtaining a sample requires vigorous measures. All other household members and frequent visitors should be investigated for *M. tuberculosis* infection and disease.

If the mother's chest radiograph result is abnormal but the history, physical examination, sputum smear, and evaluation of the radiograph reveal no evidence of active tuberculosis, it is reasonable to assume that the infant is at low risk for infection and that the radiographic abnormality is due to another cause or a quiescent focus of previous infection with *M. tuberculosis*. If the mother remains untreated, however, she may develop reactivation tuberculosis and subsequently expose her infant. The mother, if not previously treated, should receive appropriate therapy, and she and her infant should receive frequent follow-up care. In this situation, the infant does not need chemotherapy. All household members should be evaluated for tuberculosis by a clinician.

If the mother has clinical and radiographic evidence of active, possibly contagious, tuberculosis, the local health department should be informed immediately about the mother so that a contact investigation can be performed. The infant should be evaluated for congenital tuberculosis with a physical examination and high-quality posteroanterior and lateral chest radiographs. If possible, serologic testing for HIV should be performed on the mother and her infant. The mother and infant should be separated until the infant is receiving chemotherapy or the mother is judged to be noncontagious.[257] Prophylactic INH (10 mg/kg per day) for newborns born to mothers with tuberculosis has been so efficacious that separation of the mother and infant is no longer considered mandatory once therapy is started.[258-260] Separation should occur only if the mother is ill enough to require hospitalization, if she has been or is expected to become nonadherent to her treatment, or if she is thought to be infected with a drug-resistant strain of *M. tuberculosis*. INH therapy should be continued in the infant at least until the mother has been shown to be culture negative for 3 months. At that time, a Mantoux tuberculin skin test is done on the child. If the result is positive, the infant should be investigated for the presence of tuberculosis with a physical examination and chest radiograph and further appropriate workup if disease is suggested. If disease is absent, the infant should continue INH for a total of 9 months. If the follow-up skin test result is negative and the mother or contact with tuberculosis has good adherence and response to treatment, INH many be discontinued in the infant. The infant needs close follow-up, and it is prudent to repeat a tuberculin skin test after 6 to 12 months.

If the mother or other family member with contagious tuberculosis has disease caused by a multidrug-resistant strain of *M. tuberculosis* or has poor adherence to treatment and better supervision of therapy for the adult and infant is not possible, the Centers for Disease Control and Prevention recommends that the infant be separated from the contagious adult and BCG vaccination be considered.[261,262] Vaccination with BCG appears to decrease the risk of tuberculosis in exposed infants, but the effect is variable.[263,264] Kendig[265] reported 117 infants born to mothers with active tuberculosis around the time of delivery; none of the 30 BCG-vaccinated infants developed tuberculosis, and 38 cases of tuberculosis and three deaths occurred among the 75 infants who received neither BCG vaccine nor INH therapy. However, 24 of the 30 infants who received BCG vaccine also were separated from their mother for at least 6 weeks; it is impossible to determine what degree of protection was conferred by this separation. Similar studies in England and Canada also describe the apparent efficacy of BCG given to neonates.[266] Usually, the child must be kept out of the household, away from the contagious case, until the skin test result becomes reactive (marking protection from infection). However, some infants who receive a BCG vaccination do not develop a reactive tuberculin skin test. It is unknown whether developing a reactive skin test correlates with protection. It is also unknown whether a second BCG vaccination given to a child who maintains a negative tuberculin skin test reaction after the first BCG vaccination will cause an enhanced level of protection. Although BCG vaccines have some protective effect for the exposed newborn, most experts in the United States feel that ensuring appropriate separation and taking whatever steps are necessary to provide adequate chemotherapy for the child and the contagious adult are a better approach than BCG vaccination. The use of directly observed therapy has made the need for BCG vaccination of infants in the United States almost nonexistent.

MANAGEMENT OF NEONATES AFTER POSTNATAL EXPOSURE

From time to time, workers in nurseries have been found to have infectious tuberculosis.[112,267] These experiments of nature provide useful data on the risk to the infants. In general, risk of infection of neonates in a modern hospital nursery appears to be low. Most nurseries have large air volumes, flows, and adequate air exchanges to decrease the risk of infection. Also, the minute volume of neonates is low, diminishing the risk of infection after a brief time of exposure. Light and co-workers[259] followed 437 infants exposed to a nurse with a cough and a sputum smear that was positive for tuberculosis. Of these infants, 160 were considered to be at greatest risk and received daily INH for 3 months; all infants remained tuberculin-negative. However, Steiner and colleagues[112] observed development of miliary tuberculosis in 2 of 1647 infants exposed in a nursery. Thus, infection is rare under nursery conditions, but it can and does occur. Strict control measures should prevent such episodes. Nursery personnel should undergo Mantoux testing before starting work and, if the result is negative, yearly thereafter. If the skin test is positive, a prospective employee should have a chest radiograph. If the radiograph result is normal, appropriate therapy for *M. tuberculosis* infection should be given, accompanied by careful medical follow-up. Prospective employees with positive skin tests and abnormal chest radiographs must be carefully and thoroughly evaluated. Many require antituberculosis therapy.

Theoretically, these same guidelines apply to workers in licensed and unlicensed daycare facilities, but in many cases they have not yet been implemented.

Children with primary tuberculosis are rarely contagious because of the nature of their pulmonary disease, absence of forceful cough, and small number of organisms in the diseased tissue.[268,269] Infants with congenital tuberculosis often have extensive pulmonary involvement with positive acid-fast stains of tracheal aspirates and large numbers of tubercle bacilli in the lungs and airways.[270,271] In several cases, there has been evidence of transmission of *M. tuberculosis* from congenitally infected infants to health care workers; transmission to other infants has not been reported.[272-276] Neonates with suspected congenital tuberculosis should be placed in appropriate isolation until it can be determined that they are not infectious, by acid-fast stain and culture of respiratory secretions.

If a member of the household other than the mother is found to have or to have had tuberculosis recently, the roles of chemotherapy and BCG vaccine for the infant remain controversial. If the tuberculous family member has completed treatment in the past, that individual should undergo a checkup before the infant enters the home. If the family member is still being treated, he or she should have been sputum culture negative for at least 3 months before contact with the infant. If the infant must return to a home in which one of the family members has only recently started treatment, he or she should receive daily INH for at least 3 to 4 months, which Dormer and associates[258] showed to be very effective in preventing the development of tuberculosis in infants born to mothers in a sanatorium. If the family cannot be relied on to administer daily medication, if directly observed therapy is impossible, or if there are a number of household members who may have tuberculosis, BCG vaccination of the neonate should be considered.

CONCLUSION

Perinatal tuberculosis, although rare, will continue to occur, particularly among high-risk groups such as blacks, Hispanics, Asian or Pacific Islanders, Native Americans Alaskan natives, and particularly among recent immigrants to the United States. Intrauterine transmission to the unborn child occurs particularly in pregnant women experiencing initial *M. tuberculosis* infection and disease such as pleural effusion or miliary tuberculosis; less often it is a complication of endometrial tuberculosis. Postnatal tuberculosis, on the other hand, is usually acquired from a mother, another close family member, or a caregiver with cavitary tuberculosis. Only by keeping the possibility of tuberculosis in mind and by carrying out appropriate history taking and tuberculin testing of pregnant patients, particularly those from high-risk groups, can tuberculosis be diagnosed and treated in time in the mother and newborn. If it does occur and is diagnosed in time, intensive treatment should result in an excellent outcome.

REFERENCES

1. Dubos R, Dubos J. The White Plague: Tuberculosis, Man and Society. Boston, Little, Brown, 1952.
2. Adhikari M, Pillay T, Pillay DG. Tuberculosis in the newborn: an emerging disease. Pediatr Infect Dis J 16:1108-1121, 1997.
3. Margono E, Mroueh J, Garely A, et al. Resurgence of active tuberculosis among pregnant women. Obstet Gynecol 83:911-914, 1994.
4. Starke JR. Pediatric tuberculosis: a time for a new approach. Tuberculosis 83:208-212, 2002.
5. Starke JR, Jacobs R, Jereb J. Resurgence of tuberculosis in children. J Pediatr 120:839-855, 1992.
6. Eamranond P, Jaramillo E. Tuberculosis in children: reassessing the need for improved diagnosis in global control strategies. Int J Tuberc Lung Dis 5:544-603, 2001.
7. Balaka B, N'dakena K, Bakonde B, et al. Tuberculosis in newborns in a tropical neonatology unit. Arch Pediatr 9:1156-1159, 2002.
8. Pomputius WF III, Rost J, Dennehy PH, et al. Standardization of gastric aspirate technique improves yield in the diagnosis of tuberculosis in children. Pediatr Infect Dis J 16:222-226, 1997.
9. Vallejo J, Ong L, Starke J. Clinical features, diagnosis and treatment of tuberculosis in infants. Pediatrics 94:1-7, 1994.
10. Smith KC, Starke JR, Eisenanch K, et al. Detection of *Mycobacterium tuberculosis* in clinical specimens from children using a polymerase chain reaction. Pediatrics 97:155-160, 1996.
11. Barnes PF, Cave MD. Molecular epidemiology of tuberculosis. N Engl J Med 349:1149-1156, 2003.
12. Raviglione MC, Snider D Jr, Kochi A. Global epidemiology of tuberculosis: morbidity and mortality of a worldwide epidemic. JAMA 273:220-226 1995.
13. Ussery XT, Valway SE, Mckenna M, et al. Epidemiology of tuberculosis among children in the United States: 1985 to 1994. Pediatr Infect Dis J 15:697-704, 1996.
14. Palme IB, Gudetta B, Bruchfeld J, et al. Impact of human immunodeficiency virus 1 infection on clinical presentation, treatment outcome and survival in a cohort of Ethiopian children with tuberculosis. Pediatr Infect Dis J 21:1053-1061, 2002.
15. Barnes PF, Bloch AB, Davidson PT, et al. Tuberculosis in persons with human immunodeficiency virus infection. N Engl J Med 324:1644-1650, 1991.
16. Cantwell MF, McKenna M, McCray E, et al. Tuberculosis and race/ethnicity in the United States: impact of socioeconomic status. Am J Respir Crit Care Med 157:1016-1020, 1997.
17. McKenna MT, McCray E, Onorato IM. The epidemiology of tuberculosis among foreign-born persons in the United States, 1986 to 1993. N Engl J Med 332:1071-1076, 1995.
18. Asch S, Leake B, Anderson R, et al. Why do symptomatic patients delay obtaining care for tuberculosis? Am J Respir Crit Care Med 157:1244-1248, 1998.
19. Chin DP, DeReimer K, Small PM, et al. Differences in contributing factors to tuberculosis incidence in U.S.-born and foreign-born persons. Am J Respir Crit Care Med 158:1797-1803, 1998.
20. Lobato MN, Hopewell PC. *Mycobacterium tuberculosis* infection after travel to or contact with visitors from countries with a high prevalence of tuberculosis. Am J Respir Crit Care Med 158:1871-1875, 1998.
21. Coovadia HM, Wilkinson D. Childhood human immunodeficiency virus and tuberculosis co-infections: reconciling conflicting data. Int J Tuberc Lung Dis 2:844-851, 1998.

22. Jeena PM, Mitha T, Samber S, et al. Effects of the human immunodeficiency virus on tuberculosis in children. Tubercle Lung Dis 77:437-443, 1996.
23. Mofenson LM, Rodriguez EM, Hershow R, et al. *Mycobacterium tuberculosis* infection in pregnant and nonpregnant women infected with HIV in the women and infants transmission study. Arch Intern Med 155:1066-1072, 1995.
24. Carvallo ACC, De Riemer K, Nunes ZB, et al. Transmission of *Mycobacterium tuberculosis* to contacts of HIV-infected tuberculosis patients. Am J Respir Crit Care Med 164:2166-2171, 2001.
25. Schaefer G, Zervondakis IA, Fuchs FF, et al. Pregnancy and pulmonary tuberculosis. Obstet Gynecol 46:706-715, 1975.
26. Carter EJ, Mates S. Tuberculosis during pregnancy: the Rhode Island experience, 1987 to 1991. Chest 106:1466-1470, 1994.
27. Good JT Jr, Iseman MD, Davidson PT, et al. Tuberculosis in association with pregnancy. Am J Obstet Gynecol 140:492-498, 1981.
28. Debré R, Lelong M, quoted by Rich AR. Pathogenesis of Tuberculosis, 2nd ed. Springfield, Ill, Charles C Thomas, 1951, p 72.
29. Weinberger SE, Weiss ST, Cohen WR, et al. Pregnancy and the lung. Am Rev Respir Dis 121:599-581, 1980.
30. Van Zwanenberg D. Influence of the number of bacilli on the development of tuberculous disease in children. Am Rev Respir Dis 83:31-44, 1960.
31. Rich AR. The Pathogenesis of Tuberculosis, 2nd ed. Springfield, Ill, Charles C Thomas, 1951.
32. Kini PG. Congenital tuberculosis associated with maternal asymptomatic endometrial tuberculosis. Ann Trop Paediatr 22:179-181, 2002.
33. Schluger NW, Rom WH. The host immune response to tuberculosis. Am J Respir Crit Care Med 157:679-691, 1998.
34. Wallgren A. The "time-table" of tuberculosis. Tubercle 29:245-251, 1948.
35. Smith S, Jacobs RF, Wilson CB. Immunobiology of childhood tuberculosis: a window on the ontogeny of cellular immunity. J Pediatr 131:16-26, 1997.
36. Abraham G, Teklu B. Miliary tuberculosis in pregnancy and puerperium: analysis of eight cases. Ethiop Med J 19:87-90, 1981.
37. Brar HS, Golde SH, Egan JE. Tuberculosis presenting as puerperal fever. Obstet Gynecol 70:488-491, 1987.
38. Brooks JH, Stirrat GM. Tuberculous peritonitis in pregnancy: case report. Br J Obstet Gynecol 93:1009-1010, 1986.
39. Centeno RS, Winter J, Bentson JR. Central nervous system tuberculosis related to pregnancy. J Comput Tomogr 6:141-145, 1982.
40. Freeman D. Abdominal tuberculosis in pregnancy. Tubercle 70:143-145, 1989.
41. Garrioch DB. Puerperal tuberculosis. Br J Clin Pract 29:280-281, 1975.
42. Golditch IM. Tuberculous meningitis and pregnancy. Am J Obstet Gynecol 110:1144-1146, 1971.
43. Govender S, Moodley SC, Grootboom MJ. Tuberculous paraplegia during pregnancy: a report of 4 cases. S Afr Med J 75:190-192, 1989.
44. Grenville-Mathers R, Harris WC, Trenchard HJ. Tuberculous primary infection in pregnancy and its relation to congenital tuberculosis. Tubercle 41:181-185, 1960.
45. Kingdom JCP, Kennedy DH. Tuberculous meningitis in pregnancy. Br J Obstet Gynecol 96:233-235, 1989.
46. Maheswaran C, Neuwirth RS. An unusual cause of postpartum fever: acute hematogenous tuberculosis. Obstet Gynecol 41:765-769, 1973.
47. Myers JP, Perlstein PH, Light IJ, et al. Tuberculosis in pregnancy with fatal congenital infection. Pediatrics 67:89-94, 1981.
48. Nsofor BI, Trivedi ON. Postpartum paraplegia due to spinal tuberculosis. Trop Doc 18:52-53, 1988.
49. Petrini B, Gente J, Winbladh B, et al. Perinatal transmission of tuberculosis: meningitis in mother, disseminated disease in child. Scand J Infect Dis 15:403-405, 1983.
50. Suvonnakote T, Obst D. Pulmonary tuberculosis with pregnancy. J Med Assoc Thor 64:26-30, 1981.
51. Bazaz-Malik G, Maheshwari B, Lal N. Tuberculosis endometritis: a clinicopathological study of 1000 cases. Br J Obstet Gynaecol 90:84-86, 1983.
52. Punnonen R, Kiilholma P, Meurman L. Female genital tuberculosis and consequent infertility. Int J Fertil 28:235-238, 1983.
53. Baumgartner W, Van Calker H, Eisenberger W. Congenital tuberculosis. Monatschr Kinderheilkd 128:563-566, 1980.
54. Cooper AR, Heneghan W, Mathew JD. Tuberculosis in a mother and her infant. Pediatr Infect Dis J 4:181-183, 1985.
55. Hallum JL, Thomas HE. Full term pregnancy after proved endometrial tuberculosis. J Obstet Gynaecol Br Emp 62:548-550, 1955.
56. Kaplan C, Benirschke K, Tarzy B. Placental tuberculosis in early and late pregnancy. Am J Obstet Gynecol 137:858-860, 1980.
57. Addis GM, Anthony GS, Semple P, et al. Miliary tuberculosis in an in-vitro fertilization pregnancy: a case report. Eur J Obstet Gynecol Reprod Biol 27:351-353, 1988.
58. Snider DE Jr. Pregnancy and tuberculosis. Chest 86(Suppl):10S-13S, 1984.
59. Hedvall E. Pregnancy and tuberculosis. Acta Med Scand 147(Suppl 286): 1-101, 1953.
60. Cohen RC. Effect of pregnancy and parturition on pulmonary tuberculosis. BMJ 2:775-776, 1943.
61. Cromie JB. Pregnancy and pulmonary tuberculosis. Br J Tuberc 48:97-101, 1954.
62. Cohen JD, Patton EA, Badger TL. The tuberculous mother. Am Rev Tuberc 65:1-23, 1952.
63. Edge JR. Pulmonary tuberculosis and pregnancy. Br J Med 2:845-846, 1952.
64. Rosenbach LM, Gangemi CR. Tuberculosis and pregnancy. JAMA 161:1035-1037, 1956.
65. Stewart CJ, Simmonds FAH. Child-bearing and pulmonary tuberculosis. BMJ 2:726-729, 1947.
66. Stewart CJ, Simmonds FAH. Prognosis of pulmonary tuberculosis in married women. Tubercle 35:28-30, 1954.
67. Wilson EA, Thelin TJ, Dilts PV Jr. Tuberculosis complicated by pregnancy. Am J Obstet Gynecol 115:526-529, 1973.
68. Cziezel AE, Rockenbauer M, Olsen J, et al. A population-based case control study of the safety of oral anti-tuberculosis drug treatment during pregnancy. Int J Tuberc Lung Dis 5:564-568, 2001.
69. de March AP. Tuberculosis and pregnancy: five to ten-year review of 215 patients in their fertile age. Chest 68:800-804, 1975.
70. Mehta BR. Pregnancy and tuberculosis. Dis Chest 39:505-511, 1961.
71. Pridie RB, Stradling P. Management of pulmonary tuberculosis during pregnancy. MBM 2:78-79, 1961.
72. Bjerkedal T, Bahna SL, Lehmann EH. Course and outcome of pregnancy in women with pulmonary tuberculosis. Scand J Respir Dis 56:245-250, 1975.
73. Ratner B, Rostler AE, Salgado PS. Care, feeding and fate of premature and full term infants born of tuberculous mothers. Am J Dis Child 81:471-482, 1951.
74. Bernsee Rush JJ. Protocol for tuberculosis screening in pregnancy. J Obstet Gynecol Neonat Nurs 14:225-230, 1986.
75. Hamadeh MA, Glassroth J. Tuberculosis and pregancy. Chest 101:1114-1120, 1992.
76. Pediatric Tuberculosis Collaborative Group. Targeted tuberculin skin testing and treatment of latent tuberculosis infection in children and adolescents. Pediatrics 114:1175-1201, 2004.
77. McIntyre PB, McCormack JG, Vacca A. Tuberculosis in pregnancy—implications for antenatal screening in Australia. Med J Aust 146:42-44, 1987.
78. Pediatric Tuberculosis Collaborative Group. Targeted tuberculin skin testing and treatment of latent tuberculosis infection in children and adolescents. Pediatrics 114:1175-1201, 2004.
79. Kendig EL Jr, Kirkpatrick BV, Carter WH, et al. Underreading of the tuberculin skin test reaction. Chest 113:1175-1177, 1998.
80. Covelli HD, Wilson RT. Immunologic and medical considerations in tuberculin-sensitized pregnant patients. Am J Obstet Gynecol 132:256-259, 1978.
81. Keller MA, Rodriguez AL, Alvarez S, et al. Transfer of tuberculin immunity from mother to infant. Pediatr Res 22:277-281, 1987.
82. Gillum MD, Maki DG. Brief report: tuberculin testing, BCG in pregnancy. Infect Cont Hosp Epidemiol 9:119-121, 1988.
83. Smith JK, Caspary EA, Field EJ. Lymphocyte reactivity to antigen pregnancy. Am J Obstet Gynecol 113:602-606, 1972.
84. Montgomery WP, Young RC Jr, Allen MP, et al. The tuberculin test in pregnancy. Am J Obstet Gynecol 100:829-831, 1968.
85. Present PA, Comstock GW. Tuberculin sensitivity in pregnancy. Am Rev Respir Dis 112:413-416, 1975.
86. Snider DE Jr, Layde PM, Johnson MW, et al. Treatment of tuberculosis during pregnancy. Am Rev Respir Dis 122:65-78, 1980.
87. Vallejo JG, Starke JR. Tuberculosis and pregnancy. Clin Chest Med 13:693-707, 1992.
88. Starke JR. Tuberculosis: an old disease but a new threat to the mother, fetus and neonate. Clin Perinatol 24:107-128, 1997.
89. Bonebrake CR, Noller KL, Loehnen PC, et al. Routine chest roentgenography in pregnancy. JAMA 240:2747-2748, 1978.

90. Maccato ML. Pneumonia and pulmonary tuberculosis in pregnancy. Obstet Gynecol Clin North Am 16:417-430, 1989.
91. Weinstein L, Murphy T. The management of tuberculosis during pregnancy. Clin Perinatol 1:395-405, 1974.
92. Hale JA, Peters GN, Cheek JH. Tuberculosis of the breast: rare but still extant. Am J Surg 150:620-624, 1985.
93. Jacobs RF, Abernathy RS. Management of tuberculosis in pregnancy and the newborn. Clin Perinatol 15:305-319, 1988.
94. Wapnir IL, Pallam TH, Gaudino J, et al. Latent mammary tuberculosis: a case report. Surgery 98:976-978, 1985.
95. Hageman JR. Congenital and perinatal tuberculosis: discussion of difficult issues in diagnosis and management. J Perinatol 18:389-394, 1998.
96. Smith KC. Congenital tuberculosis: a rare manifestation of a common infection. Curr Opin Infect Dis 15:269-274, 2002.
97. Cantwell MF, Shehab ZM, Costello AM, et al. Brief report: congenital tuberculosis. N Engl J Med 330:1051-1054, 1994.
98. Micozzi MS. Skeletal tuberculosis, pelvic contraction and parturition. Am J Phys Anthropol 58:441-445, 1982.
99. Hageman J, Shulman S, Schreiber M, et al. Congenital tuberculosis: critical reappraisal of clinical findings and diagnostic procedures. Pediatrics 66:980-984, 1980.
100. Nemir RL, O'Hare D. Congenital tuberculosis: review and guidelines. Am J Dis Child 139:284-287, 1985.
101. Rich AR, Follis RH Jr. Effect of low oxygen tension upon the development of experimental tuberculosis. Bull Johns Hopkins Hosp 71:345-357, 1942.
102. Vorwald AJ. Experimental tuberculous infection in the guinea-pig foetus compared with that in the adult. Am Rev Tuberc 35:260-295, 1937.
103. Hertzog AJ, Chapman S, Herring J. Congenital pulmonary aspiration tuberculosis. Am J Clin Pathol 19:1139-1142, 1949.
104. Hughesdon MR. Congenital tuberculosis. Arch Dis Child 21:121-139, 1946.
105. Corner BD, Brown NJ. Congenital tuberculosis: report of a case with necropsy findings in mother and child. Thorax 10:99-103, 1955.
106. Siegel M. Pathological findings and pathogenesis of congenital tuberculosis. Am Rev Tuberc 29:297-309, 1934.
107. Bate TWP, Sinclair RE, Robinson MJ. Neonatal tuberculosis. Arch Dis Child 61:512-514, 1986.
108. Devi PK, Mujumdar SS, Modadam NG, et al. Pregnancy and pulmonary tuberculosis: observations on the domiciliary management of 238 patients in India. Tubercle 45:211-216, 1964.
109. Kendig EL Jr. Tuberculosis in the very young: report of three cases in infants less than one month of age. Am Rev Respir Dis 70:161-165, 1954.
110. Watchi R, Lu K, Kahlstrom E, et al. Tuberculous meningitis in a five-week-old child. Int J Tuberc Lung Dis 2:255-257, 1998.
111. Burk JR, Bahar D, Wold FS, et al. Nursery exposure of 528 newborns to a nurse with pulmonary tuberculosis. South Med J 71:7-10, 1978.
112. Steiner P, Rao M, Victoria MS, et al. Miliary tuberculosis in two infants after nursery exposure: epidemiologic, clinical and laboratory findings. Am Rev Respir Dis 113:267-271, 1976.
113. Kendig EL Jr, Rodgers WL. Tuberculosis in the neonatal period. Am Rev Tuberc Pulm Dis 77:418-422, 1958.
114. Holt LE. Tuberculosis acquired through ritual circumcision. JAMA 61:99-102, 1913.
115. Beitzke H. Über de angeborene tuberkulöse Infektion. Ergeb Gesamte Tuerkuloseforsch 7:1-30, 1935.
116. Abughali N, Van der Kuyp F, Annable W, et al. Congenital tuberculosis. Pediatr Infect Dis J 13:738-741, 1994.
117. Arthur L. Congenital tuberculosis. Proc R Soc Med 60:19-20, 1967.
118. Asensi F, Otero MC, Perez-Tamarit D, et al. Congenital tuberculosis, still a problem. Pediatr Infect Dis J 9:223-224, 1990.
119. Blackall PB. Tuberculosis: maternal infection of the newborn. Med J Aust 42:1055-1058, 1969.
120. Foo AL, Tan KK, Chay DM. Congenital tuberculosis. Tubercle Lung Dis 74:59-61, 1993.
121. Hardy JB, Hartman JR. Tuberculous dactylitis in childhood. J Pediatr 30:146-156, 1947.
122. Hopkins R, Ermocilla R, Cassady G. Congenital tuberculosis. South Med J 69:1156, 1976.
123. Koutsoulieris K, Kaslaris E. Congenital tuberculosis. Arch Dis Child 45:584-586, 1970.
124. Krishnan L, Vernekar AV, Diwakar KK, et al. Neonatal tuberculosis: a case report. Ann Trop Paediatr 14:333-335, 1994.
125. McCray MK, Esterly NB. Cutaneous eruptions in congenital tuberculosis. Arch Dermatol 117:460-464, 1981.
126. Morens DH, Baublis JV, Heidelberger KP. Congenital tuberculosis and associated hypoadrenocorticism. South Med J 72:160-165, 1979.
127. Niles RA. Puerperal tuberculosis with death of infant. Am J Obstet Gynecol 144:131-132, 1982.
128. Pai PM, Parikh PR. Congenital miliary tuberculosis: case report. Clin Pediatr 15:376-378, 1976.
129. Polansky SM, Frank A, Ablow RC, et al. Congenital tuberculosis. AJR 130:994-996, 1978.
130. Ramos AD, Hibbard LT, Graig JR. Congenital tuberculosis. Obstet Gynecol 43:61-64, 1974.
131. Reisinger KS, Evans P, Yost G, et al. Congenital tuberculosis: report of case. Pediatrics 54:74-76, 1974.
132. Sauer P, Kuss JJ, Lutz P, et al. La tuberculose congénital. Pédiatrie 36:217-224, 1981.
133. Soeiro A. Congenital tuberculosis in a small premature baby. S Afr Med J 45:1025-1026, 1971.
134. Todd RM. Congenital tuberculosis: report of a case with unusual features. Tubercle 41:71-73, 1960.
135. Voyce MA, Hunt AC. Congenital tuberculosis. Arch Dis Child 41:299-300, 1966.
136. Vucicevic Z, Suskovic T, Ferencic Z. A female patient with tuberculous polyserositis and congenital tuberculosis in her new-born child. Tubercle Lung Dis 76:460-462, 1995.
137. Chen A, Shih SL. Congenital tuberculosis in two infants. Am J Roentgenol 182:253-256, 2004.
138. Grover SB, Taneja DK, Bhatia A, et al. Sonographic diagnosis of congenital tuberculosis: an experience with four cases. Abdom Imaging 25:622-626, 2000.
139. Weisoly DL, Khan AM, Elidemir O, et al. Congenital tuberculosis regarding extracorporeal membrane oxygenation. Pediatr Pulmonol 37:470-473, 2004.
140. Kobayashi K, Haruta T, Maeda H, et al. Cerebral hemorrhage associated with vitamin K deficiency in congenital tuberculosis treated with isoniazid and rifampin. Pediatr Infect Dis J 21:1088-1089, 2002.
141. Mazade MA, Evans EM, Starke JR, et al. Congenital tuberculosis presenting as sepsis syndrome: case report and review of the literature. Pediatr Infect Dis J 20:439-442, 2001.
142. Berk DR, Sylvester KG. Congenital tuberculosis presenting as progressive liver dysfunction. Pediatr Infect Dis J 23:78-80, 2004.
143. Sood M, Trehan A, Arora S, et al. Congenital tuberculosis manifesting as cutaneous disease. Pediatr Infect Dis J 19:1109-1111, 2000.
144. Chou YH. Congenital tuberculosis proven by percutaneous liver biopsy: report of a case. J Perinat Med 30:423-425, 2002.
145. Pejham S, Altman R, Li KI, et al. Congenital tuberculosis with facial nerve palsy. Pediatr Infect Dis J 21:1085-1086, 2002.
146. Hatzistamatiou Z, Kaleyias J, Ikonomidou U, et al. Congenital tuberculous lymphadenitis in a preterm infant in Greece. Acta Paediatr 92:392-394, 2003.
147. Grover SB, Pati NK, Mehta R, et al. Congenital spine tuberculosis: early diagnosis by imaging studies. Am J Perinatol 20:147-152, 2003.
148. Dische MR, Krishnan C, Andreychuk R, et al. Congenital tuberculosis in a twin of immigrant parentage. Can Med Assoc J 119:1068-1070, 1978.
149. Cunningham DG, McGraw TT, Griffin AJ, et al. Neonatal tuberculosis with pulmonary cavitation. Tubercle 63:217-219, 1982.
150. Teeratkulpisarn J, Lumbigagmon P, Pairojkul S, et al. Cavitary tuberculosis in a young infant. Pediatr Infect Dis J 13:545-546, 1994.
151. De Angelis P, Antonelli P, Esposito G, et al. Congenital tuberculosis in twins. Pediatrics 69:402-416, 1981.
152. Gordon-Nesbitt DC, Rajan G. Congenital tuberculosis successfully treated. Letter to the editor. BMJ 1:233-234, 1972.
153. Naranbai RC, Mathiassen W, Malan AF. Congenital tuberculosis localized to the ear. Arch Dis Child 63:738-740, 1989.
154. Senbil N, Sahin F, Coglar MK, et al. Congenital tuberculosis of the ear and parotid gland. Pediatr Infect Dis J 16:1090, 1997.
155. Schaaf HS, Smith J, Donald PR, et al. Tuberculosis presenting in the neonatal period. Clin Pediatr 28:474-475, 1989.
156. Schaaf HS, Gie RP, Beyers N, et al. Tuberculosis in infants less than 3 months of age. Arch Dis Child 69:371-374, 1993.
157. Khan EA, Starke JR. Diagnosis of tuberculosis in children: increased need for better methods. Emerg Infect Dis 1:115-123, 1995.
158. Stallworth JR, Brasfield DM, Tiller RE. Congenital miliary tuberculosis proved by open lung biopsy specimen and successfully treated. Am J Dis Child 14:320-321, 1980.

159. American Thoracic Society/Centers for Disease Control and Prevention/ Infectious Disease Society of America. Treatment of tuberculosis. Am J Respir Crit Care Med 167:603-662, 2003.
160. Mieeli JN, Olson WA, Cohen SN. Elimination kinetics of isoniazid in the newborn infant. Dev Pharmacol Ther 2:235-239, 1981.
161. Atkins JN. Maternal plasma concentration of pyridoxal phosphate during pregnancy: adequacy of vitamin B_6 supplementation during isoniazid therapy. Am Rev Respir Dis 126:714-717, 1982.
162. Sumartojo E. When tuberculosis treatment fails: a social behavior account of patient adherence. Am Rev Respir Dis 147:1311-1320, 1993.
163. Villarino ME, Ridzon R, Weismuller PC, et al. Rifampin preventive therapy for tuberculosis infection: experience with 157 adolescents. Am J Respir Crit Care Med 155:1735-1738, 1997.
164. Centers for Disease Control. Management of persons exposed to multidrug-resistant tuberculosis. MMWR Morb Mortal Wkly Rep 41(RR-11):1-8, 1992.
165. Franks AL, Binkin NJ, Snider DE Jr, et al. Isoniazid hepatitis among pregnancy and postpartum Hispanic patients. Public Health Rep 104:151-155, 1989.
166. Al-Dossary FS, Ong LT, Correa AG, et al. Treatment of childhood tuberculosis with a six month directly observed regimen of only two weeks of daily therapy. Pediatr Infect Dis J 21:91-97, 2002.
167. Shingadia D, Novelli V. Diagnosis and treatment of tuberculosis in children. Lancet 3:624-632, 2003.
168. Flanagan P, Hensler NM. The course of active tuberculosis complicated by pregnancy. JAMA 170:783-787, 1959.
169. Schaefer G, Douglas RG, Silverman F. A re-evaluation of the management of pregnancy and tuberculosis. J Obstet Gynecol Br Emp 66:990-997, 1959.
170. Schaeffer G, Birnbaum SJ. Present-day treatment of tuberculosis and pregnancy. JAMA 165:2163-2167, 1957.
171. Varpela E. On the effect exerted by first-line tuberculosis medicines on the foetus. Acta Tuberc Scand 35:53-69, 1964.
172. Wall MA. Treatment of tuberculosis during pregnancy. Am Rev Respir Dis 122:989-993, 1980.
173. Scheinhorn DJ, Angelillo VA. Antituberculous therapy in pregnancy: risks to the fetus. West J Med 127:195-198, 1977.
174. Bobrowitz ID. Ethambutol in pregnancy. Chest 66:20-24, 1974.
175. Lewit T, Nebel L, Terracina S, et al. Ethambutol in pregnancy: observations on embryogenesis. Chest 68:25-27, 1974.
176. Place VA Ethambutol administration during pregnancy: a case report. J New Drugs 4:206-208, 1964.
177. Steen JSM, Stainton-Ellis DM. Rifampin in pregnancy. Lancet 2:604-605, 1977.
178. Skolnick JL, Stoler BS, Katz DB, et al. Rifampin, oral contraceptives, and pregnancy. JAMA 236:1382, 1976.
179. Brock PG, Rooch M. Antituberculosis drugs in pregnancy. Lancet 1:43-44, 1981.
180. Byrd RB. Treating the pregnant tuberculous patient: curing the mother without harming the fetus. J Respir Dis 3:27-32, 1982.
181. Lowe CR. Congenital defects among children born to women under supervision or treatment for pulmonary tuberculosis. Br J Prev Soc Med 18:14-16, 1964.
182. Donald PR, Sellars SL. Streptomycin ototoxicity in the unborn child. S Afr Med J 60:316-318, 1981.
183. Robinson GC, Cambon KG. Hearing loss in infants of tuberculous mothers treated with streptomycin during pregnancy. N Engl J Med 271:949-951, 1964.
184. Varpela E, Hietalahti J, Aro MJT. Streptomycin and dihydrostreptomycin medication during pregnancy and their effect on the child's inner ear. Scand J Respir Dis 50:101-109, 1969.
185. Potworowska M, Sianozecka E, Szufladowicz R. Ethionamide treatment and pregnancy. Polish Med J 5:1152-1158, 1966.
186. Davidson PT. Managing tuberculosis during pregnancy. Lancet 346:199-200, 1995.
187. Medchill MT, Gillum M. Diagnosis and management of tuberculosis during pregnancy. Obstet Gynecol Rev 44:81-91, 1989.
188. Bloch A, Cauthen G, Onorato I, et al. Nationwide survey of drug-resistant tuberculosis in the United States. JAMA 271:665-671, 1994.
189. Pablos-Mendez A, Raviglione MC, Laszlo A. Global surveillance for anti-tuberculosis-drug resistance, 1994-1997. N Engl J Med 338:1641-1649, 1998.
190. Snider DE Jr, Powell KE. Should women taking antituberculosis drugs breast-feed? Arch Intern Med 144:589-590, 1984.
191. McKenzie SA, Macnab AJ, Katz G. Neonatal pyridoxine responsive convulsions due to isoniazid therapy. Arch Dis Child 51:567-569, 1976.
192. Steinhoff MC, Lionel J. Treatment of tuberculosis in newborn infants and their mothers. Indian J Pediatr 55:240-245, 1988.
193. Doerr CA, Starke JR, Ong LT. Clinical and public health aspects of tuberculous meningitis in children. J Pediatr 127:27-33, 1995.
194. Gessner BD, Weiss NS, Nolan CM. Risk factors for pediatric tuberculosis infection and disease after household exposure to adult index cases in Alaska. J Pediatr 132:509-513, 1998.
195. MacIntyre CR, Plant AJ. Preventability of incident cases of tuberculosis in recently exposed contacts. Int J Tuberc Lung Dis 2:56-61, 1998.
196. Mehta JB, Bentley S. Prevention of tuberculosis in children: missed opportunities. Am J Prev Med 8:283-286, 1992.
197. Nolan R Jr. Childhood tuberculosis in North Carolina: a study of the opportunities for intervention in the transmission of tuberculosis in children. Am J Public Health 76:26-30, 1986.
198. Rodrigo T, Cayla JA, de Olalla PG, et al. Characteristics of tuberculosis patients who generate secondary cases. Int J Tuberc Lung Dis 1:352-357, 1997.
199. Spark RP, Pock NA, Pedron SL, et al. Perinatal tuberculosis and its public health impact: a case report. Texas Med 92:50-53, 1996.
200. Kendig EL Jr. Prognosis of infants born of tuberculous mothers. Pediatrics 26:97-100, 1960.
201. Laurance BM. Congenital tuberculosis successfully treated. Letter to the editor. BMJ 2:55, 1973.
202. International Union against Tuberculosis. Phenotypes of BCG vaccine seed lot strains: results of an international cooperative study. Tubercle 59:139-142, 1978.
203. Milstein JB, Gibson JJ. Quality control of BCG vaccines by WHO: a review of factors that may influence vaccine effectiveness and safety. Bull World Health Org 68:93-108, 1990.
204. Osborn TW. Changes in BCG strains. Tubercule 64:1-13, 1983.
205. Jacox RF, Meade GM. Variation in the duration of tuberculin skin test sensitivity produced by two strains of BCG. Am Rev Tuberc 60:541-546, 1949.
206. Dubos RJ, Pierce CH. Differential characteristics in vitro and in vivo of several substrains of BCG. I. Multiplication and survival in vitro. Am Rev Tuber Pulm Dis 74:655-666, 1956.
207. Dubos RJ, Pierce CH. Differential characteristics in vitro and in vivo of several substrains of BCG. IV. Immunizing effectiveness. Am Rev Tuberc Pulm Dis 74:699-717, 1956.
208. Zhang Y, Wallace RJ Jr, Mazurek GH. Genetic differences between BCG substrains. Tuberc Lung Dis 76:43-50, 1995.
209. Gheorghiu M. The present and future role of BCG vaccine in tuberculosis control. Biologicals 18:135-141, 1990.
210. Gheorghiu M, Lagrange PH. Viability, heat stability and immunogenicity of four BCG vaccines prepared from four different BCG strains. Ann Immunol (Paris) 134C:125-147, 1983.
211. Behr MA. Correlation between BCG genomics and protective efficacy. Scan J Infect Dis 33:249-252, 2001.
212. Lehman HG, Englehardt H, Freudenstein H, et al. BCG vaccination of neonates, infants, school children and adolescents. II. Safety of vaccine with strain 1331 Copenhagen. Dev Biol Stand 43:133-135, 1979.
213. Expanded Programme on Immunization/Biologicals Unit. Lymphadenitis associated with BCG immunization. Wkly Epidemiol Rec 63:381-388, 1988.
214. Expanded Programme on Immunization/Biologicals Unit. BCG associated lymphadenitis in infants. Wkly Epidemiol Rec 30:231-323, 1989.
215. Kroger L, Brander E, Korppi M, et al. Osteitis after newborn vaccination with three different bacillus Calmette-Guérin vaccines: twenty-nine years of experience. Pediatr Infect Dis J 12:113-116, 1994.
216. Behr MA, Small PM. Declining efficacy of BCG strains over time? A new hypothesis for an old controversy [abstract]. Am J Respir Crit Care Med 155:A222, 1997.
217. Ten Dam HG. Research on BCG vaccination. Adv Tuberc Res 21: 79-106, 1984.
218. Lotte A, Wasz-Hockert O, Poisson N, et al. Second IUATLD study on complications induced by intradermal BCG-vaccination. Bull Int Union Tuberc 63:47-59, 1988.
219. Turnbull FM, McIntyre PB, Achat HM, et al. National study of adverse reactions after vaccination with bacille Calmette-Guérin. Clin Infect Dis 34:447-453, 2002.
220. Reynes J, Perez C, Lamaury I, et al. Bacille Calmette-Guérin adenitis 30 years after immunization in a patient with AIDS. Letter to the editor. J Infect Dis 160:727, 1989.

221. Helmick CG, D'Souza AJ, Goddard N. An outbreak of severe BCG axillary lymphadenitis in Saint Lucia, 1982-83. West Indies Med J 35:12-17, 1986.
222. Praveen KN, Smikle MF, Prabhakar P, et al. Outbreak of bacillus Calmette-Guérin–associated lymphadenitis and abscesses in Jamaican children. Pediatr Infect Dis J 9:890-893, 1990.
223. Goraya JS, Virdi VS. Treatment of Calmette-Guérin bacillus adenitis: a meta-analysis. Pediatr Infect Dis J 20:632-634, 2001.
224. Singla A, Singh S, Goraya JS, et al. The natural course of nonsuppurative Calmette-Guérin bacillus lymphadenitis. Pediatr Infect Dis J 21:446-448, 2002.
225. Oguz F, Mujgan S, Alper G, et al. Treatment of bacillus Calmette-Guérin associated lymphadenitis. Pediatr infect Dis J 11:887-888, 1992.
226. World Health Organization. BCG Vaccination of the Newborn: Rationale and Guidelines for Country Programs. Geneva, World Health Organization, 1986.
227. Micheli I, de Kantor IN, Colaicicovo D, et al. Evaluation of the effectiveness of BCG vaccination using the case control method in Buenos Aires, Argentina. Int J Epidemiol 17:629-634, 1988.
228. Lotte A, Wasz-Hockart O, Poisson N, et al. BCG complication: estimates of the risks among vaccinated subjects and statistical analysis of their main characteristics. Adv Tuberc Res 21:107-193, 1984.
229. Kroger L, Korppi M, Brander E, et al. Osteitis caused by bacillus Calmette-Guérin vaccination: a retrospective analysis of 222 cases. J Infect Dis 172:574-576, 1995.
230. Bottiger M. Osteitis and other complications caused by generalized BCGitis. Acta Paediatr Scand 71:471-478, 1982.
231. Pederson FK, Engbaek HC, Hertz H, Vergmann B. Fatal BCG infection in an immunocompetent girl. Acta Paediatr Scand 67:519-523, 1978.
232. Trevenen CL, Pagtakhan RD. Disseminated tuberculoid lesions in infants following BCG. Can Med J 15:502-504, 1982.
233. Tardieu M, Truffot-Pernot C, Carriere JP, et al. Tuberculosis meningitis due to BCG in two previously healthy children. Lancet 1:440-441, 1988.
234. Hesseling AC, Schaaf HS, Hanekom WA, et al. Danish bacilli Calmette-Guérin vaccine–induced disease in human immunodeficiency virus–infected children. Clin Infect Dis 37:1226-1233, 2003.
235. Casanova JL, Blanche S, Emile JF, et al. Idiopathic disseminated bacilli Calmette-Guérin infection: a French national retrospective study. Pediatrics 98:774-778, 1996.
236. Gonzalez B, Moreno S, Burdach R, et al. Clinical presentation of bacillus Calmette-Guérin infections in patients with immunodeficiency syndromes. Pediatr Infect Dis J 8:201-206, 1989.
237. Houde C, Dery P. *Mycobacterium bovis* sepsis in an infant with human immunodeficiency virus infection. Pediatr Infect Dis J 11:810-811, 1988.
238. Talbot EA, Perkins MD, Silva SFM, et al. Disseminated bacille Calmette-Guérin disease after vaccination: case report and review. Clin Infect Dis 24:1139-1146, 1997.
239. Jovanguy E, Altare F, Lamhamedi S, et al. Interferon-γ–receptor deficiency in an infant with fatal bacille Calmette-Guérin infection. N Engl J Med 335:1956-1961, 1996.
240. Elloumi-Zghal H, Barbouch MR, Chemli J, et al. Clinical and genetic heterogeneity of inherited autosomal recessive susceptibility to disseminated *Mycobacterium bovis* bacille Calmette-Guérin infection. J Infect Dis 185:1468-1475, 2002.
241. Armbruster C, Junker W, Vetter N, et al. Disseminated bacille Calmette-Guérin infection in AIDS patient 30 years after BCG vaccination. Letter to the editor. J Infect Dis 162:1216, 1990.
242. Besnard M, Sauvion S, Offredo C, et al. Bacillus Calmette-Guérin infection after vaccination of human immunodeficiency virus–infected children. Pediatr Infect Dis J 12:993-997, 1993.
243. Menzies R, Vissandjee B. Effect of bacille Calmette-Guérin vaccination on tuberculin reactivity. Am Rev Respir Dis 145:621-625, 1992.
244. Lifschitz M. The value of the tuberculin skin test as a screening test for tuberculosis among BCG vaccinated children. Pediatrics 36:624-627, 1965.
245. Horwitz O, Bunch-Christensen K. Correlation between tuberculin sensitivity after 2 months and 5 years among BCG-vaccinated subjects. Bull World Health Organ 47:49-58, 1972.
246. Comstock GW, Edwards LB, Nabangxang H. Tuberculin sensitivity eight to fifteen years after BCG vaccination. Am Rev Respir Dis 103:572-575, 1971.
247. Landi S, Ashley MJ, Grzybowski S. Tuberculin skin sensitivity following the intradermal and multiple puncture methods of BCG vaccination. Can Med Assoc J 97:222-225, 1967.
248. Ashley MJ, Seibenmann CO. Tuberculin skin sensitivity following BCG vaccination with vaccines of high and low viable counts. Can Med Assoc J 97:1335-1338, 1967.
249. Kemp EB, Belshe RB, Hoft DF. Immune responses stimulated by percutaneous and intradermal bacille Calmette-Guérin. J Infect Dis 174:113-119, 1996.
250. Joncas JH, Robitaille R, Gauthier T. Interpretation of the PPD skin test in BCG-vaccinated children. Can Med Assoc J 113:127-128, 1975.
251. Mangus K, Edwards LB. The effect of repeated tuberculin testing on post-vaccination allergy. Lancet 1:643-644, 1955.
252. Karalliede S, Katugha LP, Uragoda CG. The tuberculin response of Sri Lankan children after BCG vaccination at birth. Tubercle 68:33-38, 1987.
253. Thompson NJ, Glassroth JL, Snider DE, et al. The booster phenomenon in serial tuberculin testing. Am Rev Respir Dis 119:587-597, 1979.
254. Sepulveda RL, Burr C, Ferrer X, et al. Booster effect of tuberculin testing in healthy 6-year-old school children vaccinated with bacillus Calmette-Guérin at birth in Santiago, Chile. Pediatr Infect Dis J 7:578-581, 1988.
255. Colditz G, Berkey CS, Mosteller F, et al. The efficacy of bacillus Calmette-Guérin vaccination of newborns and infants in the prevention of tuberculosis: meta-analysis of the published literature. Pediatrics 96:29-35, 1995.
256. Colditz GA, Brewer TF, Berkey CS, et al. Efficacy of BCG vaccine in the prevention of tuberculosis: meta-analysis of the published literature. JAMA 271:698-702, 1994.
257. Avery ME, Wolfsdorf J. Diagnosis and treatment: approaches to newborn infants of tuberculous mothers. Pediatrics 42:519-521, 1968.
258. Dormer BA, Harrison I, Swart JA, et al. Prophylactic isoniazid protection of infants in a tuberculosis hospital. Lancet 2:902-903, 1959.
259. Light IJ, Saidleman M, Sutherland JM. Management of newborns after nursery exposure to tuberculosis. Am Rev Respir Dis 109:415-419, 1974.
260. Raucher HS, Grimbetz I. Care of the pregnant woman with tuberculosis and her newborn infant: a pediatrician's perspective. Mt Sinai J Med 53:70-75, 1986.
261. Centers for Disease Control and Prevention. The role of BCG vaccine in the prevention and control of tuberculosis in the United States: a joint statement by the Advisory Council for the Elimination of Tuberculosis and the Advisory Committee on Immunization Practices. MMWR Morb Mortal Wkly Rep 45(RR-4):1-18, 1996.
262. Sedaghatian MR, Hashem F, Hossain MM. Bacille Calmette Guérin vaccination in pre-term infants. Int J Tuberc Lung Dis 2:679-682, 1998.
263. Lorber J, Menneer PC. Long-term effectiveness of BCG vaccination of infants in close contact with infectious tuberculosis. BMJ 1:1430-1433, 1959.
264. Pabst HF, Godel J, Grace M, et al. Effect of breastfeeding on immune response to BCG vaccination. Lancet 1:295-297, 1989.
265. Kendig EL Jr. The place of BCG vaccine in the management of infants born to tuberculous mothers. N Engl J Med 281:520-523, 1969.
266. Curtis HM, Bamford FN, Leck I. Incidence of childhood tuberculosis after neonatal BCG vaccination. Lancet 1:145-148, 1984.
267. Nivin B, Nicholas P, Gayer M, et al. A continuing outbreak of multidrug-resistant tuberculosis with transmission in a hospital nursery. Clin Infect Dis 26:303-307, 1998.
268. Centers for Disease Control and Prevention. Guidelines for preventing the transmission of *Mycobacterium tuberculosis* in health-care facilities. MMWR Morb Mortal Wkly Rep 43(RR-13):1-133, 1994.
269. Starke JR. Transmission of *Mycobacterium tuberculosis* to and from children and adolescents. Sem Pediatr Infect Dis 12:115-123, 2001.
270. Lee HL, LeVea CM, Graman PS. Congenital tuberculosis in a neonatal intensive care unit: case report, epidemiological investigation, and management of exposures. Clin Infect Dis 27:474-477, 1998.
271. Manji KP, Msemo G, Tamian B, et al. Tuberculosis (presumed congenital) in a neonatal unit in Dar-es-Salaam, Tanzania. J Trop Pediatr 47:153-155, 2001.
272. Pillay T, Adhikari M. Congenital tuberculosis in a neonatal intensive care unit. Clin Infect Dis 29:467-268, 1999.
273. Machin GA, Honore LH, Fanning EA, et al. Perinatally acquired neonatal tuberculosis: report of two cases. Pediatr Pathol 12:707-716, 1992.
274. Rabalais G, Adams G, Stover B. PPD skin test conversion in healthcare workers after exposure to *Mycobacterium tuberculosis* infection in infants. Lancet 338:826, 1991.

275. Saitoh M, Ichiba H, Fujioka H, et al. Connatal tuberculosis in an extremely low birth weight infant: case report and management of exposure to tuberculosis in a neonatal intensive care nursery. Eur J Pediatr 160:88-90, 2001.

276. Laartz BW, Narvarte HJ, Hold D, et al. Congenital tuberculosis and management of exposures in a neonatal intensive care unit. Infect Control Hosp Epidemiol 23:573-579, 2002.

Chapter 20

MICROORGANISMS RESPONSIBLE FOR NEONATAL DIARRHEA

Miguel L. O'Ryan • James P. Nataro • Thomas G. Cleary

At the beginning of the 21st century, diarrheal disease continues to be a significant cause of morbidity and mortality worldwide. During the period of 1986 to 2000, an estimated 1.4 billion children younger than 5 years suffered an episode of acute diarrhea every year in developing countries; among these, 123.6 million required outpatient medical care, and 9 million required hospitalization. Approximately 2 million diarrhea-associated deaths occurred in this age group annually, primarily in the most impoverished areas of the world.[1] These estimates are somewhat lower than the more than 3 million annual deaths from diarrhea reported in the prior 10 years,[2] indicating progress in prevention and treatment of acute diarrhea. In the United States, approximately 400 childhood deaths per year were reported during the late 1980s,[3,4] although the actual number may be higher.[4]

Accurate incidence rates for acute diarrhea in neonates from different populations are not readily available. The relative sparing of the newborn probably results from low exposure to enteropathogens and protection associated with breast-feeding.[5-8] After the first few months of life, increasing interaction with other individuals and the environment, including introduction of artificial feeding, increases the risk of exposure to enteropathogens. For most pathogens, the incidence of acute diarrhea peaks in children between 6 months and 4 years old.[9] Neonatal diarrhea is more common in underdeveloped areas, where low educational levels, crowding, and poor standards of medical care, environmental sanitation, and personal hygiene favor early contact with enteropathogens. As the incidence of neonatal gastroenteritis rises, there is a proportional increase in neonatal deaths because medical care for the poor often is inadequate.[10,11] For very low birth weight infants (<1500 g), the death rate from diarrhea is 100-fold greater than for higher-birth-weight infants.[12]

This chapter discusses the pathogenesis, diagnosis, treatment, and prevention of gastroenteritis based on the available knowledge about pathogens that can cause neonatal diarrhea. Pathogens that rarely or never cause acute diarrhea in neonates are not discussed. After an overview of host defense mechanisms and protective factors in human milk, the remainder of the chapter is devoted to specific pathogens that cause inflammatory or noninflammatory diarrhea.

ENTERIC HOST DEFENSE MECHANISMS

The neonate is a host that is uniquely susceptible to enteric infections. Neonates have not had the opportunity to develop local or systemic immune responses, and in the first few days of life, they have not acquired the highly important enteric flora that protects the normal adult gastrointestinal tract.[13-18] Still less is known about the barrier effect of the neonate's gastric acidity,[19] intestinal mucus,[20] or motility,[21,22] each of which provides protection against gastrointestinal tract infections in older infants, children, and adults.

The gastric acid barrier appears to be least effective during the first months of life. The average gastric pH level of the newborn is high (pH 4 to 7; mean, 6).[23,24] Although the pH falls to low levels by the end of the first day of life (pH 2 to 3),[23] it subsequently rises again; by 7 to 10 days of life, the hydrochloric acid output of the neonatal stomach is far less than that of older infants and children.[24,25] The buffering action of frequent milk feedings and the short gastric emptying time[26-29] interpose additional factors in the neonate that would be expected to permit viable ingested organisms to reach the small intestine.

The intestinal epithelium serves as a nutrient absorptive machine, barrier to pathogen entry, and regulator of inflammation. Intestinal epithelial cells have receptors for bacterial products and produce chemokines (e.g., interleukin [IL]-8, monocyte chemotactic protein type 1 [MCP-1], granulocyte macrophage-cell stimulating factor [GM-CSF]) and proinflammatory cytokines (e.g., IL-6, tumor necrosis factor-α [TNF-α], IL-1) in response to invasion by enteropathogens.[30] The gut epithelium orchestrates the immune response. However, in the newborn, phagocytic, chemotactic, and complement functions are immature. B and T lymphocyte functions are impaired, resulting in a preferential IgM production in response to antigenic stimulation. IgG is actively transferred from mother to infant across the placenta at about 32 weeks' gestation and peaks by about 37 weeks; premature neonates, especially those born before 28 weeks' gestation, are deficient in these maternally derived serum antibodies.[31]

PROTECTIVE FACTORS IN HUMAN MILK

The importance of breast-feeding infants for the prevention of diarrheal disease has long been emphasized.[13,32-45] Published studies reporting the association between breast-feeding and diarrhea are extensive and suggest that infants who are breast-fed suffer fewer episodes of diarrhea than those who are not. This protection is greatest during a child's first 3 months of life and declines with increasing age. During the period of weaning, partial breast-feeding confers protection that is intermediate between that gained by infants who are exclusively breast-fed and that by those who are exclusively bottle-fed.

Table 20–1 Association between Antibodies in Human Milk and Protection against Enteropathogens

Organism	Antibody
Vibrio cholerae	Lipopolysaccharide, enterotoxin
Campylobacter jejuni	Surface proteins
Enteropathogenic *Escherichia coli*	Adherence proteins
Enterotoxigenic *E. coli*	Enterotoxin, adherence proteins
Shigatoxin producing *E. coli*	Adherence proteins
Shigella	Lipopolysaccharide, virulence plasmid–associated antigens
Giardia lamblia	Surface proteins

A striking demonstration of the protection afforded by breast-feeding of newborns has been provided by Mata and Urrutia[13] in their studies of a population of infants born in a rural Guatemalan village. Despite extremely poor sanitation and the demonstration of fecal organisms in the colostrum and milk of almost one third of mothers,[46] diarrheal disease did not occur in any newborns. The incidence of diarrhea rose significantly only after these infants reached 4 to 6 months old, at which time solids and other fluids were used to supplement the human milk feedings. At that time, *Escherichia coli* and gram-negative anaerobes (e.g., *Bacteroides*) were found to colonize the intestinal tract.[13] In contrast, urban infants of a similar ethnic background who were partly or totally artificially fed frequently acquired diarrheal disease caused by enteropathogenic *E. coli* (EPEC).

Multiple mechanisms by which breast-feeding protects against diarrhea have been postulated. Breast-feeding confers protection by active components in milk and by decreased exposure to organisms present on or in contaminated bottles, food, or water. Many protective components have been identified in human milk and generally are classified as belonging to the major categories of cells, antibody, anti-inflammatory factors, and glycoconjugates and other nonantibody factors.[47-50] Examples of milk antibodies are summarized in Table 20-1. For any given pathogen, multiple milk factors may help protect the infant. Human milk typically targets a major pathogenic mechanism using multiple, redundant strategies. Redundancy of milk protective factors and targeting of complex virulence machinery have created a formidable barrier to enteropathogens. Despite the fact that pathogens can rapidly divide and mutate, milk continues to protect infants. For example, human milk has secretory antibodies to *Shigella* virulence antigens and lipopolysaccharides,[51,52] neutral glycolipid Gb3 to bind Shiga toxin,[53,54] and lactoferrin to disrupt and degrade the surface-expressed virulence antigens.[55-57] In a similar way, milk contains antibodies directed toward the surface expressed virulence antigens of EPEC,[58] oligosaccharides that block cell attachment,[59] and lactoferrin that disrupts and degrades the surface expressed EPEC antigens.[60] Human milk can initiate and maintain the growth of *Bifidobacterium* and low pH in the feces of newborn infants, creating an environment antagonistic to the growth of *E. coli*.[13,17,18,61]

The protective effect of human milk antibodies against enteropathogen-specific disease has been described for *Vibrio cholerae*,[62] *Campylobacter jejuni*,[63] EPEC,[59] enterotoxigenic *E. coli* (ETEC),[64,65] *Shigella*,[66,67] and *Giardia lamblia*[68,69] and for bovine milk concentrate against ETEC,[70] rotavirus,[71] and *Shigella*.[72]

In 1933, the nonlactose carbohydrate fraction of human milk was found to consist mainly of oligosaccharides.[73] In 1960, Montreuil and Mullet[74] determined that up to 2.4% of colostrum and up to 1.3% of mature milk are oligosaccharides. Human milk contains a larger quantity of the oligosaccharides than does milk from other mammals, and its composition is singularly complex.[75] The metabolic fate of the oligosaccharides is of interest. Only water, lactose, and lipids are present in greater amounts than the oligosaccharides. Despite the fact that substantial energy must be expended by the mother to synthesize the many hundreds of different milk oligosaccharides, the infant does not use them as food. Most of the oligosaccharides pass through the gut undigested.[76,77] It is thought that they are present primarily to serve as receptor analogues that misdirect enteropathogen attachment factors away from gut epithelial carbohydrate receptors. Likewise, enteropathogens use the oligosaccharide portion of glycolipids and glycoproteins as targets for attachment of whole bacteria and toxins. Evidence is emerging that these glycoconjugates may have an important role in protection of the breast-fed infant from disease.[48]

Human milk protects suckling mice from the heat-stable enterotoxin (ST) of *E. coli*; on the basis of its chemical stability and physical properties, the protective factor has been deduced to be a neutral fucosyloligosaccharide.[79,80] Experiments have shown that EPEC attachment to HEp-2 cells can be inhibited by purified oligosaccharide fractions from human milk.[59] Oligosaccharides also may be relevant to protection from Norwalk virus and other caliciviruses, because these viruses attach to human ABO, Lewis, and secretor blood group antigens.[80,81] Human milk contains large amounts of these carbohydrates. The ganglioside fraction in human milk has been shown to inhibit the action of heat-labile toxin (LT) and cholera toxin on ileal loops more effectively than secretory IgA.[82,83] Lactadherin in human milk has been shown to bind rotavirus and to inhibit viral replication in vitro and in vivo.[84] A study of infants in Mexico showed that lactadherin in human milk protected infants from symptoms of rotavirus infection.[72]

ESCHERICHIA COLI

E. coli organisms promptly colonize the lower intestinal tracts of healthy infants in their first few days of life[85-88] and constitute the predominant aerobic coliform fecal flora throughout life in humans and in many animals. The concept that this species might cause enteric disease was first suggested in the late 19th and early 20th centuries, when several veterinary workers described the association of diarrhea (i.e., scours) in newborn calves with certain strains of *E. coli*.[89-94]

In 1905, Moro[95] observed that *Bacterium* (now *Escherichia*) *coli* was found more often in the small intestines of children with diarrhea than in children without diarrhea. Adam[96,97] confirmed these findings and noted the similarity with Asiatic cholera and calf scours. He further extended these observations by suggesting that *E. coli* strains from patients with diarrhea could be distinguished from normal coliform flora by certain sugar fermentation patterns. Although he called these disease-producing organisms *dyspepsicoli* and introduced the important concept that *E. coli* could cause enteric disease, biochemical reactions have not proved to be a reliable means of distinguishing nonpathogenic from pathogenic *E. coli* strains. There are now at least six recognized enteric pathotypes of *E. coli*.[98] The pathotypes can be distinguished clinically, epidemiologically, and pathogenetically (Table 20-2).[98-104]

ETEC organisms are defined by their ability to secrete the LT or the ST enterotoxin, or both. LT is closely related to cholera toxin and similarly acts by means of intestinal adenylate cyclase,[105,106] prostaglandin synthesis,[107,108] and possibly platelet activating factor.[109,110] ST (particularly the variant STa) causes secretion by specifically activating intestinal mucosal guanylate cyclase.[111-113] The STb toxin causes noncyclic, nucleotide-mediated bicarbonate secretion and appears to be important only in animals.[114-116] Enteroinvasive *E. coli* (EIEC) has the capacity to invade the intestinal mucosa, thereby causing an inflammatory enteritis much like shigellosis.[117,118] EPEC elicits diarrhea by a signal transduction mechanism,[98-102,119,120] which is accompanied by a characteristic attaching-and-effacing histopathologic lesion in the small intestine.[121] Enterohemorrhagic *E. coli* (EHEC) also induces an attaching-and-effacing lesion, but in the colon.[98] EHEC also secretes Shiga toxin, which gives rise to the sequela of hemolytic-uremic syndrome (HUS). Diffusely adherent *E. coli*[122] executes a signal transduction effect, which is accompanied by the induction of long cellular processes.[123] Enteroaggregative *E. coli* (EAEC) adheres to the intestinal mucosa and elaborates enterotoxins and cytotoxins.[98,103,125]

A major problem in the recognition of ETEC, EIEC, EPEC, and EHEC strains of *E. coli* is that they are indistinguishable from normal coliform flora of the intestinal tract by the usual bacteriologic methods. Serotyping is of value in recognizing EPEC serotypes[126] and EIEC, because these organisms tend to fall into a limited number of specific serogroups (see Table 20-2).[126,127] EIEC invasiveness is confirmed by inoculating fresh isolates into guinea pig conjunctivae, as described by Sereny.[128] The ability of organisms to produce enterotoxins (LT or ST) is encoded by a transmissible plasmid that can be lost by one strain of *E. coli* or transferred to a previously unrecognized strain.[129-131] Although the enterotoxin plasmids appear to prefer certain serogroups (different from EPEC or invasive serogroups),[132] ETEC is not expected to be strictly limited to a particular set of serogroups. Instead, these strains can be recognized only by examining for the enterotoxin. This is done in ligated animal loops,[133] in tissue culture,[134,135] or by enzyme-linked immunosorbent assay (ELISA)[136] for LT or in suckling mice for ST.[137,138] Specific DNA probes also are available for LT and ST.[98] Whether there are other mechanisms involved in the ability of the versatile *E. coli* species to cause enteric disease, such as by producing other types of enterotoxins[139] or by fimbriate adherence traits alone,[140,141] remains to be elucidated.

Table 20–2 Predominant Serogroups, Mechanisms, and Gene Codes Associated with Enterotoxigenic, Enteroinvasive, Enteropathogenic, Enterohemorrhagic, and Enteroaggregative *Escherichia coli*

ETEC	EIEC	EPEC	EHEC	EAEC
		Class I Serogroup		
LT O6:K15 O8:K40	O28ac O29, O112 O115, O124 O136, O144	 O55:K59 (B5) O111ab:K88 (B4) O119K6a (B14)	O157:H7 O26:H11/H- O128, O103:H2 O39	O3:H2 O44 O78:H33 O15:H11
LT and ST O11:H27 O15, O20:K79 O25:K7 O27, O63 O80, O85, O139	O147, O152 O164	O125ac:K70 (B15) O126:K71 (B16) O127a:K63 (B8) O128abc:K67 (B12) O142, O158	O111:K58:H8/H- O113:K75:H7/H21 O121:H-, O145:H- Rough And many others	O77:H18 O51:H11 And many others
		Class II Serogroup		
ST O groups 78, 115 128, 148, 149, 153 159, 166, 167		 O44:K74 O86a:K61 (B7) O114:H2		
Mechanisms				
Adenylate or guanylate cyclase activation	Colonic invasiveness (e.g., *Shigella*)	Localized attachment and effacement	Shiga toxins block protein synthesis; attachment and effacement	Aggregative adherence and toxins
Gene Codes				
Plasmid	Chromosomal and plasmid	Chromosomal and plasmid	Phage and chromosomal	Plasmid and chromosomal

ETEC, enterotoxigenic *Escherichia coli*; EIEC, enteroinvasive *E. coli*; EPEC, enteropathogenic *E. coli*; EHEC, enterohemorrhagic *E. coli*; EAEC, enteroaggregative *E. coli*; LT, heat-labile toxin; ST, heat-stable toxin.

Enterotoxigenic *Escherichia coli*

Although early work on the recognition of *E. coli* as a potential enteric pathogen focused on biochemical or serologic distinctions, there followed a shift in emphasis to the enterotoxins produced by previously recognized and entirely "new" strains of *E. coli*. Beginning in the mid-1950s with work by De and colleagues[142,143] in Calcutta, *E. coli* strains from patients with diarrhea were found to cause a fluid secretory response in ligated rabbit ileal loops analogous to that seen with *V. cholerae*. Work by Taylor and associates[144,145] showed that the viable *E. coli* strains were not required to produce this secretory response and that this enterotoxin production correlated poorly with classically recognized EPEC serotypes. In São Paulo, Trabulsi[146] made similar observations with *E. coli* isolated from children with diarrhea, and several veterinary workers demonstrated that ETEC was associated with diarrhea in piglets and calves.[147-150] A similar pattern was described in 1971 with acute undifferentiated diarrhea in adults in Bengal from whom *E. coli* could be isolated from the upper small bowel only during acute illness.[151,152] These strains of *E. coli* produced a nondialyzable, LT, ammonium sulfate–precipitable enterotoxin.[153] Analogous to the usually short-lived diarrheal illnesses of *E. coli* reported by several workers, a short-lived course of the secretory response to *E. coli* culture filtrates compared with the secretory response of cholera toxin was described.[154] However, like responses to cholera toxin, secretory responses to *E. coli* were associated with activation of intestinal mucosal adenylate cyclase that paralleled the fluid secretory response.[155,156]

The two types of enterotoxins produced by *E. coli*[157-159] have been found to be plasmid-encoded traits that are potentially separable from each other and from the equally important plasmid-encoded adherence traits for pathogenesis.[129-131,160] ST causes an immediate and reversible secretory response,[133] whereas the effects of LT (e.g., cholera toxin) follow a lag period necessitated by its intracellular site of action.[105,106,134] Only LT appears to cause fluid secretion by activating adenylate cyclase, which is accomplished by toxin-induced ADP-ribosylation of the $G_s\alpha$ signaling protein.[98,105] The activation of adenylate cyclase by LT and by cholera toxin is highly promiscuous, occurring in many cell types and resulting in development of nonintestinal tissue culture assay systems such as the Chinese hamster ovary (CHO) cell assay[134] and Y1 adrenal cell assay.[135] The antigenic similarity of LT and cholera toxin and their apparent binding to the monosialoganglioside GM_1 have enabled development of ELISAs for detection of LT and cholera toxin.[138,161-163]

ST is a much smaller molecule and is distinct antigenically from LT and cholera toxin.[134,137,138] Although it fails to alter cAMP levels, ST increases intracellular intestinal mucosal cyclic guanosine monophosphate (cGMP) concentrations and specifically activates plasma membrane–associated intestinal guanylate cyclase.[111-113] Like cAMP analogues, cGMP analogues cause intestinal secretion that mimics the response to ST.[111] The receptor for STa responds to an endogenous ligand called *guanylin*, of which STa is a structural homologue.[164] Because the capacity to produce an enterotoxin may be transmissible between different organisms by a plasmid or even a bacteriophage,[129-131] interstrain gene transfer may be expected to be responsible for occasional toxigenic non–*E. coli*. Enterotoxigenic *Klebsiella* and *Citrobacter* strains have been associated with diarrhea in a few reports, often in the same patients with ETEC.[165,166] Likewise, certain strains of *Salmonella* appear to produce an LT, CHO cell–positive toxin that may play a similar role in the pathogenesis of the watery, noninflammatory diarrhea sometimes seen with *Salmonella enteritidis* infection.[167,168] At least equally important as enterotoxigenicity for *E. coli* to cause disease is the ability of these organisms to colonize the upper small bowel, where the enterotoxin produced has its greatest effect. A separable, plasmid-encoded colonization trait was first recognized in porcine *E. coli*. Veterinary workers demonstrated that the fimbriate K-88 surface antigen was necessary for ETEC to cause disease in piglets.[160] An autosomal dominant allele appears to be responsible for the specific intestinal receptor in piglets. In elegant studies by Gibbons and co-workers,[169] the homozygous recessive piglets lacked the receptor for K-88 and were resistant to scours caused by ETEC. At least 15 analogous colonization factors have been described for human *E. coli* isolates[98,170,171] against which local IgA antibody may be produced. These antigens potentially may be useful in vaccine development.

Epidemiology and Transmission

Data on the epidemiology and transmission of ETEC remain scanty for the neonatal period. In the past 2 decades, these strains have been recognized among adults with endemic, cholera-like diarrhea in Calcutta, India, and in Dacca, Bangladesh,[105,151] and among travelers to areas such as Mexico and Central Africa.[173-175]

The isolation of ETEC is uncommon in sporadic diarrheal illnesses in temperate climates where sanitation facilities are good and where winter viral patterns of diarrhea predominate. ETEC is commonly isolated from infants and children with acute watery summer diarrhea in areas where sanitary facilities are less than optimal.[35,165,175-187] These include areas such as Africa,[165] Brazil,[35,175,181,186,187] Argentina,[177] Bengal,[178,179] Mexico,[180] and Native American reservations in the southwestern United States.[182,183] In a multicenter study of acute diarrhea in 3640 infants and children in China, India, Mexico, Myanmar, and Pakistan, 16% of cases (versus 5% of 3279 controls) had ETEC.[184] A case-control study from northwestern Spain showed a highly significant association of ETEC with 26.5% of neonatal diarrhea, often acquired in the hospital.[185] Although all types of ETEC (LT and/or ST producers) are associated with cholera-like, non inflammatory, watery diarrhea in adults in these areas, they probably constitute the major cause (along with rotaviruses) of dehydrating diarrhea in infants and young children in these areas. In this setting, peaks of illnesses tend to occur in the summer or rainy season, and dehydrating illnesses may be life threatening, especially in infants and young children.[35,181,186] Humans are probably the major reservoirs for the human strains of ETEC, and contaminated food and water probably constitute the principal vectors.[188,189] Although antitoxic immunity to LT and asymptomatic infection with LT-producing *E. coli* tends to increase with age, ST is poorly immunogenic, and ST-producing *E. coli* continues to be associated with symptomatic illnesses into adulthood in endemic areas.[183,187]

The association of ETEC with outbreaks of diarrhea in newborn nurseries is well documented. Ryder and colleagues[190] isolated an ST-producing *E. coli* from 72% of infants with diarrhea, from the environment, and in one instance, from an infant's formula during a 7-month period in a prolonged outbreak in a special care nursery in Texas. Another ST-producing *E. coli* outbreak was reported in 1976 by Gross and associates[191] from a maternity hospital in Scotland. ETEC and EPEC were significantly associated with diarrhea among infants younger than 1 year in Bangladesh.[192]

An outbreak of diarrhea in a newborn special care nursery that was associated with enterotoxigenic organisms that were not limited to the same serotype or even the same species has been reported.[193] The short-lived ETEC, *Klebsiella*, and *Citrobacter* species in this outbreak raised the possibility that each infant's indigenous bowel flora might become transiently toxigenic, possibly by receiving the LT genome from a plasmid or even a bacteriophage.

Clinical Manifestations

The clinical manifestations of ETEC diarrhea tend to be mild and self-limited, except in small or undernourished infants, in whom dehydration may constitute a major threat to life. In many parts of the developing world, acute diarrheal illnesses are the leading recognized causes of death. There is some suggestion that the diarrheal illnesses associated with ST-producing ETEC may be particularly severe.[179] Most probably the best definition of the clinical manifestations of ETEC infection comes from volunteer studies with adults. Ingestion of 10^8 to 10^{10} human ETEC isolates that produce LT and ST or ST alone resulted in a 30% to 80% attack rate of mild to moderate diarrheal illnesses within 12 to 56 hours that lasted 1 to 3 days.[117] These illnesses, typical for traveler's diarrhea, were manifested by malaise, anorexia, abdominal cramps, and sometimes explosive diarrhea. Nausea and vomiting occur relatively infrequently, and up to one third of patients may have a low-grade fever. Although illnesses usually resolve spontaneously within 1 to 5 days, they occasionally may persist for 1 week or longer. The diarrhea is noninflammatory, without fecal leukocytes or blood. In outbreaks in infants and neonates, the duration has been in the same range (1 to 11 days), with a mean of approximately 4 days.

Pathology

As in cholera, the pathologic changes associated with ETEC infection are minimal. From animal experiments in which Thiry-Vella loops were infected with these organisms and at a time when the secretory and adenylate cyclase responses were present, there was only a mild discharge of mucus from goblet cells and otherwise no significant pathologic change in the intestinal tract.[106] Unless terminal complications of severe hypotension ensue, ETEC organisms rarely disseminate beyond the intestinal tract. Like cholera, ETEC diarrhea is typically limited to being an intraluminal infection.

Diagnosis

The preliminary diagnosis of ETEC diarrhea can be suspected by the epidemiologic setting and the noninflammatory nature of stool specimens, which reveal few or no leukocytes. Although the ability of *E. coli* to produce enterotoxins may be lost or transmitted to other strains, there is a tendency for the enterotoxin plasmids to occur among certain predominant serotypes, as shown in Table 20-2.[132] These serotypes differ from EPEC or invasive serotypes, but their demonstration does not prove that they are enterotoxigenic. The only definitive way to identify ETEC is to demonstrate the enterotoxin itself by a specific gene probe for the toxin codon, by a bioassay such as tissue culture or ileal loop assays for LT or the suckling mouse assay for ST, or in the case of LT, by immunoassay such as ELISA. However, even these sensitive bioassays are limited by the unavailability of any selective media for detecting ETEC by culture. Even though substantial improvements have been made in enterotoxin assay (particularly for LT), the necessary random selection of *E. coli* from a relatively nonselective stool culture plate resulted in a sensitivity of only 43% of epidemiologically incriminated cases in an outbreak when 5 to 10 isolates were randomly picked and tested for enterotoxigenicity.[189] By also examining paired serum samples for antibody against LT, only 36% demonstrated significant serum antibody titer rises, for a total sensitivity of ETEC isolation or serum antibody titer rises of only 64%. Some have suggested that isolates may be pooled for LT or ST assay. The capacity to prove with radiolabeled or enzyme-tagged oligonucleotide gene sequences for the enterotoxins (LT or ST) further facilitates the identification of enterotoxigenic organisms.[194,195] A novel method of combining immunomagnetic separation (using antibody-coated magnetic beads) followed by DNA or polymerase chain reaction (PCR) probing may enhance the sensitivity of screening fecal or food specimens for ETEC or other pathogens.[196,197]

Therapy and Prevention

The mainstay of treatment of any diarrheal illness is rehydration.[198] This principle especially pertains to ETEC diarrhea, which is an intraluminal infection. The glucose absorptive mechanism remains intact in *E. coli* enterotoxin-induced secretion, much as it does in cholera, a concept that has resulted in the major advance of oral glucose-electrolyte therapy. This regimen can usually provide fully adequate rehydration in infants and children able to tolerate oral fluids, replacing the need for parenteral rehydration in most cases.[199,200] Its use is particularly critical in rural areas and developing nations, where early application before dehydration becomes severe may be lifesaving.

The standard World Health Organization solution contains 3.5 g NaCl, 2.5 g $NaHCO_3$, 1.5 g KCl, and 20 g glucose per liter of clean or boiled drinking water.[198] This corresponds to the following concentrations: 90 mmol/L of sodium, 20 mmol/L of potassium, 30 mmol/L of bicarbonate, 80 mmol/L of chloride, and 110 mmol/L of glucose. A variety of recipes for homemade preparations have been described,[201] but unless the cost is prohibitive, the premade standard solution is preferred. Each 4 ounces of this solution should be followed by 2 ounces of plain water. If there is concern about hypertonicity, especially in small infants in whom a high intake and constant direct supervision of feeding cannot be ensured, the concentration of salt can be reduced.[202] A reduced osmolality solution with 60 mmol/L of sodium and 84 mmol/L of glucose and a total osmolality of 224 (instead of 311) mOsm/kg has been found to reduce stool output by 28% and illness duration by 18% in a multicenter trial involving 447 children in four countries.[203] Commercially available rehydration solutions are increasingly available worldwide.[198]

The role of antimicrobial agents in the treatment or prevention of ETEC is controversial. This infection usually resolves within 3 to 5 days in the absence of antibacterial therapy.[198] Moreover, there is concern about the potential for coexistence of enterotoxigenicity and antibiotic resistance on the same plasmid, and co-transfer of multiple antibiotic resistance and enterotoxigenicity has been well documented.[204] Widespread use of prophylactic antibiotics in areas where antimicrobial resistance is common has the potential for selecting for rather than against enterotoxigenic organisms. The prevention and control of ETEC infections would be similar to those discussed under EPEC serotypes. The use of breast-feeding should be encouraged.

Enteroinvasive *Escherichia coli*

EIEC causes diarrhea by means of *Shigella*-like intestinal epithelial invasion (discussed later).[117,118] The somatic antigens of these invasive strains have been identified and seem to fall into 1 of 10 recognized O groups (see Table 20-2). Most, if not all, of these bacteria share cell wall antigens with one or another of the various *Shigella* serotypes and produce positive reactions with antisera against the cross-reacting antigen.[118] However, not all strains of *E. coli* belonging to the 10 serogroups associated with dysentery-like illness are pathogenic, because a large (140 MDa) invasive plasmid is also required.[205] Additional biologic tests, including the guinea pig conjunctivitis (Sereny) test or a gene probe for the plasmid, are used to confirm the property of invasiveness.[117]

Although an outbreak of foodborne EIEC diarrhea has been well documented among adults who ate an imported cheese,[118] little is known about the epidemiology and transmission of this organism, especially in newborns and infants. Whether the infectious dose may be as low as it is for *Shigella* is unknown; however, studies of adult volunteers suggest that attack rates may be somewhat lower after ingestion of even large numbers of EIEC than would be expected with *Shigella*. The outbreak of EIEC diarrhea resulted in a dysentery-like syndrome with an inflammatory exudate in stool and invasion and disruption of colonic mucosa.[118] Descriptions of extensive and severe ileocolitis in infants dying with *E. coli* diarrhea indicate that neonatal disease also can be caused by invasive strains capable of mimicking the pathologic features of shigellosis.[206] The immunofluorescent demonstration of *E. coli* together with an acute inflammatory infiltrate[207] in the intestinal tissue of infants tends to support this impression, although it has been suggested that the organisms may have invaded the bowel wall in the postmortem period.[117] There is still little direct evidence concerning the role of invasive strains of *E. coli* in the cause of neonatal diarrhea.[175] The infrequency with which newborns manifest a dysentery-like syndrome makes it unlikely that this pathogen is responsible for a very large proportion of the diarrheal disease that occurs during the first month of life.

The diagnosis should be suspected in infants who have an inflammatory diarrhea as evidenced by fecal polymorphonuclear neutrophils or even bloody dysenteric syndromes from whom no other invasive pathogens, such as *Campylobacter, Shigella, Salmonella, Vibrio,* or *Yersinia,* can be isolated. In this instance, it may be appropriate to have the fecal *E. coli* isolated and serotyped or tested for invasiveness in the Sereny test. Plasmid pattern analysis and chromosomal restriction endonuclease digestion pattern analysis by pulsed-field gel electrophoresis have been used to evaluate strains involved in outbreaks.[208] The management and prevention of EIEC diarrhea should be similar to those for acute *Shigella* or other *E. coli* enteric infections.

Enteropathogenic *Escherichia coli*: Classic Serotypes

The serologic distinction of *E. coli* strains associated with epidemic and sporadic infantile diarrhea was first suggested by Goldschmidt in 1933[209] and confirmed by Dulaney and Michelson in 1935.[205] These researchers found that certain strains of *E. coli* associated with institutional outbreaks of diarrhea would agglutinate with antisera on slides. In 1943, Bray[211] isolated a serologically homogeneous strain of *E. coli* (subsequently identified as serogroup O111) from 95% of infants with summer diarrhea in England. He subsequently summarized a larger experience with this organism isolated from only 4% of asymptomatic controls but from 88% of infants with diarrhea, one half of which was hospital acquired.[212] This strain (initially called *E. coli-gomez* by Varela in 1946) also was associated with infantile diarrhea in Mexico.[213] A second type of *E. coli* (called *beta* by Giles in 1948 and subsequently identified as O55) was associated with an outbreak of infantile diarrhea in Aberdeen, Scotland.[214,215]

From this early work primarily with epidemic diarrhea in infants has developed an elaborate serotyping system for certain *E. coli* strains that were clearly associated with infantile diarrhea.[216-218] These strains first were called enteropathogenic *E. coli* by Neter and colleagues[219] in 1955, and the association with particular serotypes can still be observed.[220] As shown in Table 20-1, these organisms are distinct from the enterotoxigenic or enteroinvasive organisms or those that inhabit the normal gastrointestinal tract. They exhibit localized adherence to HEp-2 cells, a phenotype that has been suggested to be useful for diagnosis and pathogenesis research.[119]

Epidemiology and Transmission

EPEC is an important cause of diarrhea in infants in developing or transitional countries.[98,221-223] Outbreaks have become rare in the United States and other industrialized countries, but they still occur.[224] Some have attributed the rarity of this recognition of illness in part to the declining severity of diarrheal disease caused by EPEC within the past 30 years, resulting in fewer cultures being obtained from infants with relatively mild symptoms.[98,225] However, several other variables influence the apparent incidence of this disease in the community. A problem arises with false-positive EPEC on the basis of the nonspecific cross-reactions seen with improper shortening of the serotyping procedure.[226,227] Because of their complexity and relatively low yield, neither slide agglutination nor HEp-2 cell adherence or DNA probe tests are provided as part of the routine identification of enteric pathogens by most clinical bacteriology laboratories. Failure to recognize the presence of EPEC in fecal specimens is the inevitable consequence.

The apparent incidence of EPEC gastroenteritis also varies with the epidemiologic circumstances under which stool cultures are obtained. The prevalence of enteropathogenic strains is higher among infants from whom cultures are obtained during a community epidemic compared with those obtained during sporadic diarrheal disease. Neither reflects the incidence of EPEC infection among infants involved in a nursery outbreak or hospital epidemic.

EPEC gastroenteritis is a worldwide problem, and socioeconomic conditions play a significant role in determining the incidence of this disease in different populations.[228] For instance, it is unusual for newborn infants born in a rural environment to manifest diarrheal disease caused by EPEC; most infections of the gastrointestinal tract in these infants occur after the first 6 months of life.[5,229] Conversely, among infants born in large cities, the attack rate of EPEC is high during the first 3 months of life. This age distribution reflects in large part the frequency with which EPEC causes cross-infection outbreaks among nursery populations[191,230-237]; however, a predominance of EPEC in infants in the first 3 months of life also has been described in community epidemics[238-240] and among sporadic cases of diarrhea acquired outside the hospital.[241-247] The disparity in the incidence of neonatal EPEC infection between rural and urban populations has been ascribed to two factors: the trend away from breast-feeding among mothers in industrialized societies and the crowding together of susceptible newborns in nurseries in countries in which hospital deliveries predominate over home deliveries.[5,229,248] Although the predominant serogroup can vary from year to year,[239,242,243,246,249,250] the same strains have been prevalent during the past 40 years in Great Britain,[251] Puerto Rico,[252] Guatemala,[5] Panama,[205] Israel,[247] Newfoundland,[240] Indonesia,[244] Thailand,[254] Uganda,[255] and South Africa.[256]

When living conditions are poor and overcrowding of susceptible infants exists, there is a rise in the incidence of neonatal diarrhea in general[257] and EPEC gastroenteritis in particular.[215,238,258] A higher incidence of asymptomatic family carriers is found in such situations.[238,239]

Newborn infants can acquire EPEC during the first days of life by one of several routes: (1) organisms from the mother ingested at the time of birth; (2) bacteria from other infants or toddlers with diarrheal disease or from asymptomatic adults colonized with the organism, commonly transmitted on the hands of nursery personnel or parents; (3) airborne or droplet infection; (4) fomites; or (5) organisms present in formulas or solid food supplements.[259] Only the first two routes have been shown conclusively to be of any real significance in the transmission of disease or the propagation of epidemics.

Most neonates acquire EPEC at the time of delivery through ingestion of organisms residing in the maternal birth canal or rectum. Stool cultures taken from women before, during, or shortly after delivery have shown that 10% to 15% carry EPEC at some time during this period.[85,86,88,260,261] Use of fluorescent antibody techniques[261] or cultures during a community outbreak of EPEC gastroenteritis[88] revealed twice this number of persons excreting the organism. Virtually none of the women carrying pathogenic strains of *E. coli* had symptoms referable to the gastrointestinal tract.

Many of the mothers whose stools contain EPEC transmit these organisms to their infants,[85,88] resulting in an asymptomatic infection rate of 2% to 5% among newborns cultured at random in nursery surveys.[85,86,191,262] These results must be considered conservative and are probably an artifact of the sampling technique. One study using 150 O antisera to identify as many *E. coli* as possible in fecal cultures showed a correlation between the coliform flora in 66% of mother-infant pairs.[263] Of particular interest was the observation that the O groups of *E. coli* isolated from the infants' mucus immediately after delivery correlated with those subsequently recovered from their stools, supporting the contention that these organisms were acquired orally at the time of birth. In mothers whose stools contained the same O group as their offspring, the mean time from rupture of membranes to delivery was about 2 hours longer than in those whose infants did not acquire the same serogroups, suggesting that ascending colonization before birth also can play a role in determining the newborn's fecal flora.

The contours of the epidemiologic curves in nursery[238,264-269] and community[238-240] outbreaks are in keeping with a contact mode of spread. Transmission of organisms from infant to infant takes place by way of the fecal-oral route in almost all cases, most likely on the hands of persons attending to their care.[86,267,269,270] Ill infants represent the greatest risk to those around them because of the large numbers of organisms found in their stools[271-274] and vomitus.[275-277] Cross-infection also has been initiated by infants who were healthy at the time of their admission to the nursery.[264,272,278-280]

A newborn exposed to EPEC is likely to acquire enteric infection if contact with a person excreting the organism is intimate and prolonged, as in a hospital or family setting. Stool culture surveys taken during outbreaks have shown that between 20% and 50% of term neonates residing in the nursery carry EPEC in their intestinal tracts.[102,230,231,234] Despite descriptions of nursery outbreaks in which virtually every neonate or low-birth-weight infant became infected,[262,264,281] there is ample evidence that exposure to pathogenic strains of *E. coli* does not necessarily result in greater likelihood of illness for premature infants than for term infants.[261,272,279,282] Any increased prevalence of cross-infections that may exist among premature infants can be explained more readily by the prolonged hospital stays, their increased handling, and the clustering of infants born in different institutions than by a particular susceptibility to EPEC based on immature defense mechanisms.

The most extensive studies on the epidemiology of gastroenteritis related to *E. coli* have dealt with events that took place during outbreaks in newborn nurseries. Unfortunately, investigations of this sort frequently regard the epidemic as an isolated phenomenon and ignore the strong interdependence that exists between community- and hospital-acquired illness.[280,283,284] Not surprisingly, the direction of spread is most often from the reservoir of disease within the community to the hospital. When the original source of a nursery outbreak can be established, frequently it is an infant born of a carrier mother who recently acquired her EPEC infection from a toddler living in the home. Cross-infection epidemics also can be initiated by infected newborns who have been admitted directly into a clean nursery unit from the surrounding district[270,272,285] or have been transferred from a nearby hospital.[278,280,286]

After a nursery epidemic has begun, it generally follows one of two major patterns. Some are explosive, with rapid involvement of all susceptible infants and a duration that seldom exceeds 2 or 3 months.[264,265,276,287] The case-fatality rate in these epidemics may be very high. Other nursery outbreaks have an insidious onset with a few mild, unrecognized cases; the patients may not even develop illness until after discharge from the hospital. During the next few days to weeks, neonates with an increased number of loose stools are reported by the nurses; shortly thereafter, the appearance of the first severely ill infants makes it apparent that an epidemic has begun. Unless oral antimicrobial therapy is instituted (see "Therapy"), nursery outbreaks like these may continue for months[266-269] or years,[270] with cycles of illness followed by periods of relative quiescence. This pattern can be caused by multiple strains (of different phage or antibiogram types) sequentially introduced into the nursery.[278,288,289]

The nursery can be a source of infection for the community. The release of infants who are in the incubation stages of their illness or are convalescent carriers about to relapse may lead to secondary cases of diarrheal disease among young siblings living in widely scattered areas.[238,239,243] These children further disseminate infection to neighboring households, involving playmates of their own age, young infants, and mothers.[238,239,242] As the sickest of these contact cases are admitted to different hospitals, they contaminate new susceptible persons, completing the cycle and compounding the outbreak. This feedback mechanism has proved to be a means of spreading infantile gastroenteritis through entire cities,[238,239,242] counties,[239,285,290] and even provinces.[240] One major epidemic of diarrhea related to EPEC O111:B4 that occurred in the metropolitan Chicago and northwestern Indiana region during the winter of 1961 involved more than 1300 children and 29 community hospitals during a period of 9 months.[240,291] Almost all of the patients were younger than 2 years old, and 10% were younger than 1 month, producing an age-specific attack rate of nearly 4% of neonates in the community. The importance of the hospital as a source of cross-infection in this epidemic was demonstrated through interviews with patients' families, indicating that a minimum of 40% of infants had direct or indirect contact with a hospital shortly before the onset of their illness.

It has been suggested, but not proved, that asymptomatic carriers of EPEC in close contact with a newborn infant, such as nursery personnel or family members, might play an important role in its transmission.[280,284,292] Stool culture surveys have shown that at any one time about 1% of adults[242,293] and 1% to 5% of young children[230,238,243] who are free of illness harbor EPEC strains. Higher percentages have been recorded during community epidemics.[238,239,243] Because this intestinal carriage is transitory,[238,280] the number of individuals who excrete EPEC at one time or another during the year is far higher than the 1% figure recorded for single specimens.[280,293]

Nursery personnel feed, bathe, and diaper a constantly changing population of newborns, about 2% to 5% of whom excrete EPEC.[238,280] Despite this constant exposure, intestinal carriage among nursery workers is surprisingly low. Even during outbreaks of diarrheal illness, when dissemination of organisms is most intense, less than 5% of the hospital personnel in direct contact with infected neonates are themselves excreting pathogenic strains of *E. coli*.[291,294,295]

Although adult asymptomatic carriers generally excrete fewer organisms than patients with acute illness do,[272] large numbers of pathogenic bacteria may nevertheless exist in their stools.[242,274] However, no nursery outbreak and few family cases[240] have been traced to a symptomless carrier. Instead, passive transfer of bacteria from infant to infant by the hands of personnel appears to be of primary importance in these outbreaks.

EPEC can be recovered from the throat or nose of 5% to 80% of infants with diarrheal illness[275,294,295] and from about 1% of asymptomatic infants.[232,243] The throat and nasal mucosa may represent a portal of entry or a source of transmission for EPEC. Environmental studies have shown that EPEC is distributed readily and widely in the vicinity of an infant with active diarrheal disease, often within 1 day of admission to the ward.[232,296] Massive numbers of organisms are shed in the diarrheal stool or vomitus of infected infants.[249,296] *E. coli* organisms may survive 2 to 4 weeks in dust[243,296] and can be found in the nursery air when the bedding or diapers of infected infants are disturbed during routine nursing procedures[243,296] or on floors, walls, cupboards, and nursery equipment such as scales, hand towels, bassinets, incubators, and oxygen tents of other infants.[88,243,267] Documentation of the presence of EPEC in nursery air and dust does not establish the importance of this route as a source of cross-infection. One study presented evidence of the respiratory transmission of EPEC; however, even in the cases described, the investigators pointed out that fecal-oral transmission could not be completely ruled out.[238] Additional clinical and experimental data are required to clarify the significance of droplet and environmental infection.

Coliform organisms have also been isolated in significant numbers from human milk,[46,297,298] prebottled infant formulas,[299] and formulas prepared in the home.[292] EPEC in particular has been found in stool cultures obtained from donors of human milk and workers in a nursery formula room.[260] In one instance, EPEC O111:B4 was isolated from a donor, and subsequently, the same serogroup was recovered in massive amounts in almost pure culture from her milk.[260] Pathogenic strains of *E. coli* have also been isolated from raw cow's milk[300] and from drinking water.[301] Likewise, EPEC has been isolated from flies during an epidemic, but this fact has not been shown to be of epidemiologic significance.[211,220]

Pathogenesis

Infection of the newborn infant with EPEC takes place exclusively by the oral route. Attempts to induce disease in adult volunteers by rectal instillation of infected material have been unsuccessful.[98] There are no reports of disease occurring after transplacental invasion of the fetal bloodstream by enteropathogenic or nonenteropathogenic strains of *E. coli.* Ascending intrauterine infection after prolonged rupture of the membranes has been reported only once; the neonate in this case suffered only from mild diarrhea.[86]

Bacterial cultures of the meconium and feces of newborns indicate that enteropathogenic strains of *E. coli* can colonize effectively the intestinal tract in the first days of life.[85-88] Although *E. coli* may disappear completely from stools of breast-fed children during the ensuing weeks, this disappearance is believed to be related to factors present in the human milk rather than the gastric secretions.[5,302,303] The use of breast-feeding or expressed human milk has even been effective in terminating nursery epidemics caused by EPEC O111:B4, probably by reducing the incidence of cross-infections among infants.[303,304] Although dose-effect studies have not been performed among newborns, severe diarrhea has occurred after ingestion of 10^8 EPEC organisms by very young infants.[305,306] The high incidence of cross-infection outbreaks in newborn nurseries suggests that a far lower inoculum can often effect spread in this setting.

The role of circulating immunity in the prevention of gastrointestinal tract disease related to EPEC has not been clearly established. Virtually 100% of maternal sera have been found to contain hemagglutinating,[219,307,308] bactericidal,[305,310] or bacteriostatic[280,312] antibodies against EPEC. The passive transfer of these antibodies across the placenta is extremely inefficient. Titers in blood of newborn infants are, on average, 4 to 100 times lower than those in the corresponding maternal sera. Group-specific hemagglutinating antibodies against the O antigen of EPEC are present in 10% to 20% of cord blood samples,[219,307,308] whereas bactericidal[307,311] or bacteriostatic[311] activity against these organisms can be found much more frequently. Tests for bacterial agglutination, which are relatively insensitive, are positive in only a small percentage of neonates.[219,311]

The importance of circulating antibodies in the susceptibility of infants to EPEC infection is unknown. Experiments with suckling mice have failed to demonstrate any effect of humoral immunity on the establishment or course of duration of intestinal colonization with *E. coli* O127 in mothers or their infants.[313] Similar observations have been made in epidemiologic studies among premature human infants using enteropathogenic (O127:B8)[310] and nonenteropathogenic (O4:H5)[269] strains of *E. coli* as the indicator organisms. In a cohort of 63 mothers and their infants followed from birth to 3 months old, Cooper and associates[85] were able to show a far higher incidence of clinical EPEC disease in infants of EPEC-negative mothers than in infants born of mothers with EPEC isolated from stool cultures. This finding suggested to the investigators the possibility that mothers harboring EPEC in their gastrointestinal tracts transfer specific antibodies to their infants that confer some protection during the first weeks of life.

Protection against enteric infections in humans often correlates more closely with levels of local secretory than serum antibodies. Although it is known that colonization of newborns with *E. coli* leads to the production of coproantibodies against the ingested organisms,[314,315] the clinical significance of this intestinal immunity is uncertain. The previously mentioned experiment with mice showed no effect of active intestinal immunity on enteric colonization.[313] In human infants, the frequency of bacteriologic and clinical relapse related to EPEC of the same serotype[264,265,279] and the capacity of one strain of EPEC to superinfect a patient already harboring a different strain[247,258,268] also cast some doubt on the ability of mucosal antibodies to inhibit or alter the course of intestinal infection. Studies of the protective effects of orally administered EPEC vaccines could help to resolve these questions.[248]

The mechanism by which EPEC causes diarrhea involves a complex array of plasmid and chromosomally encoded traits. EPEC serotypes usually do not make one of the recognized enterotoxins (LT or ST) as usually measured in tissue culture or animal models,[316-320] nor do these serotypes cause a typical invasive colitis or produce a positive Sereny test result.[315,316] Only uncommonly do EPEC strains invade the bloodstream or disseminate.[288] Nevertheless, EPEC strains that test negative in these tests are capable of causing diarrhea; inocula of 10^{10} *E. coli* O142 or O127 organisms caused diarrhea in 8 of 10 adult volunteers.[320]

Some EPEC strains may secrete weak enterotoxins,[321,322] but the consensus opinion is that the attaching and effacing lesion constitutes the critical secretory virulence phenotype.[98,121] Clinical pathologic reports reveal the characteristic attaching and effacing lesion in the small intestine of infected infants.[324] The lesion is manifested by intimate (about 10 nm) apposition of the EPEC to the enterocytes plasma membrane, with dissolution of the normal brush border and rearrangement of the cytoskeleton.[121,324] In some instances, the bacteria are observed to rise up on pedestal-like structures, which are diagnostic of the infection.[121] Villus blunting, crypt hypertrophy, histiocytic infiltration in the lamina propria, and a reduction in the brush border enzymes may also be observed.[324,325]

Two major EPEC virulence factors have been described; strains with both factors are designated as typical EPEC.[98,99,323] One such factor is the locus of enterocyte effacement (LEE), a type III secretion system encoded by the LEE chromosomal pathogenicity island.[326-328] The LEE secretion apparatus injects proteins directly from the cytoplasm of the infecting bacterium into the cytoplasm of the target enterocytes.[327] The injected proteins constitute cytoskeletal toxins, which together elicit the close apposition of the bacterium to the cell, cause the effacement of microvilli, and most likely give rise to the net secretory state.[98,99,121] One critical secreted protein, called Toll/interleukin-1 receptor (Tir),[120] inserts into the plasma membrane of the epithelial cell, where it serves as the receptor for a LEE-encoded EPEC outer membrane protein called intimin.[121] Animals infected with attaching and effacing pathogens mount antibody responses to intimin and Tir,[329] and both are considered potential immunogens. The lack of protection from EPEC reinfection suggests that natural antibody responses to Tir and intimin are not protective.

The second major virulence factor of typical EPEC is the bundle-forming pilus (BFP),[330] which is encoded on a partially conserved 60 MDa virulence plasmid called EPEC adherence factor (EAF).[331] BFP, a member of the type IV pilus family, mediates aggregation of the bacteria to each other and probably to enterocytes themselves, thereby facilitating mucosal colonization.[332] A BFP mutant was shown to be attenuated in adult volunteers.[333]

Pathology

The principal pathologic lesion with EPEC is the focal destructive adherence of the organism, effacing the microvillous brush border with villus blunting, crypt hypertrophy, histiocytic infiltration of the lamina propria, and reduced brush border enzymes. Rothbaum and colleagues[324] described similar findings with dissolution of the glycocalyx and flattened microvilli with the nontoxigenic EPEC strain O119:B14. There has been a wide range of pathologic findings reported in infants dying of EPEC gastroenteritis. Most newborns dying with diarrheal disease caused by EPEC show no morphologic changes of the gastrointestinal tract by gross or microscopic examination of tissues.[209,210] Bray[211] described such "meager" changes in the intestinal tract that "the impression received was that the term gastroenteritis is incorrect." At the other extreme, extensive and severe involvement of the intestinal tract, although distinctly unusual among neonates with EPEC diarrhea, has been discussed in several reviews of the pathologic anatomy of this disease.[247,319,334] Changes virtually identical to those found in infants dying with necrotizing enterocolitis have been reported.[334] Drucker and co-workers[319] found that among 17 infants who were dying of EPEC diarrhea, "intestinal gangrene, and/or perforation, and/or peritonitis were present in five, and intestinal pneumatosis in five."

The reasons for such wide discrepancies in EPEC disease pathology are not clear. The severity of intestinal lesions at the time of death does not correlate with the birth weight of the patient, the age of onset of illness, the serogroup of the infecting strain, or the prior administration of oral or systemic antimicrobial agents. The suggestion that the intensity of inflammatory changes may depend on the duration of the diarrhea[319] cannot be corroborated in autopsy studies[215,264,335] or small intestinal biopsies.[336,337] It is difficult to reconcile such a thesis with the observation that a wide range of intestinal findings can be seen at autopsy among newborns infected by a single serotype of EPEC during an epidemic. The nonspecific pathologic picture described by some researchers includes capillary congestion and edema of the bowel wall and an increase in the number of eosinophils, plasma cells, macrophages, and mononuclear cells in the mucosa and submucosa.[262,319,335] Villous patterns are generally well preserved, although some flattening and broadening of the villi are seen in the more severe cases. Almost complete absence of villi and failure of regeneration of small bowel mucosa have been reported in an extreme case.[338] Edema in and around the myenteric plexuses of Auerbach, a common associated finding, has been suggested as a cause of the gastrointestinal tract dilatation often seen at autopsy in infants with EPEC infections.[247,335,339] In general, the distal small intestine shows the most marked alterations; however, the reported pathologic findings may be found at all levels of the intestinal tract.

Several complications of EPEC infection have been reported. Candidal esophagitis accounted for significant morbidity in two series collected before[210] and during[247] the antibiotic era. Oral thrush has been seen in 50% of EPEC-infected infants treated with oral or systemic antibiotics.[245,264,335] Some degree of fatty metamorphosis of the liver has been reported by several investigators[210,215 335]; however, these changes are nonspecific and probably result from the poor caloric intake associated with persistent diarrhea or vomiting. Some degree of bronchopneumonia, probably a terminal event in most cases, exists in a large proportion of newborns dying of EPEC infection.[210,215,339] In one reported series of infant cases, EPEC was demonstrated by immunofluorescent staining in the bronchi, alveoli, and interalveolar septa.

Mesenteric lymph nodes are often swollen and congested with reactive germinal centers in the lymphoid follicles.[215,262,293] Severe lymphoid depletion, unrelated to the duration or severity of the antecedent illness, also has been described.[285] The kidneys frequently show tubular epithelial toxic changes. Various degrees of tubular degeneration and cloudy swelling of convoluted tubules are common findings.[215,285,335] Renal vein thrombosis or cortical necrosis may be observed in infants with disseminated intravascular coagulation in the terminal phases of the illness. The heart is grossly normal in most instances but may show minimal vacuolar changes of nonspecific toxic myocarditis on microscopic examination.[335,339] Candidal abscesses of the heart[339] and kidneys[285,335,339] have been described. With the exception of mild congestion of the pia arachnoid vessels and some edema of the meninges, examination of the central nervous system reveals few changes.[215,262] Despite the observation of Bray[211] that "inflammation of the middle ear [is] exceptional," strains of EPEC have been isolated from a significant number of specimens of the middle ear in case series in which dissection of the temporal bone has been performed.[209,215]

Clinical Manifestations

Exposure of newborns to EPEC may be followed by one of several possible consequences: no infection, infection without illness, illness with gastroenteritis of variable severity and duration, and rarely, septicemia with or without metastatic foci of infection accompanying gastroenteritis.

When infants are exposed to EPEC, a significant number become colonized as temporary stool[85,88,231] or pharyngeal[238] carriers with no signs of clinical disease. Although Laurell[340] showed that the percentage of asymptomatic infections rises steadily as age increases, this observation has not been confirmed by other investigators.[214,341] Similarly, the suggestion that prematurity per se is associated with a low incidence of inapparent EPEC infection has been documented in several clinical studies[262,264,265] but refuted in others.[252,279] Most neonates who acquire infection with EPEC eventually show some clinical evidence of gastroenteritis. The incubation period is quite variable. Its duration has been calculated mostly from evidence in outbreaks in newborn nurseries, where the time of first exposure can be clearly defined in terms of birth or admission dates. In these circumstances, almost all infants show signs of illness between 2 and 12 days after exposure, and most cases show signs within the first 7 days.[215,231,264] In some naturally acquired[85,86] and experimental[306] infections with heavy exposure, the incubation period may be as short as 24 hours; the stated upper limit is 20 days.[232,343] The first positive stool culture and the earliest recognizable clinical signs of disease occur simultaneously in most infants,[264,266] although colonization may precede symptoms by 7 to 14 days.[265,266,344] The gastroenteritis associated with EPEC infection in the newborn is notable for its marked variation in clinical pattern. Clinical manifestations vary from mild illness manifest only by transient anorexia and failure to gain weight to a sudden explosive fulminating diarrhea causing death within 12 hours of onset. Prematurity, underlying disease, and congenital anomalies often are associated with the more severe forms of illness.[214,233,345,346] Experienced clinicians have observed that the severity of EPEC gastroenteritis has declined markedly during the past 3 decades.[225] The onset of illness usually is insidious, with vague signs of reluctance to feed, lethargy, spitting up of formula, mild abdominal distention, or even weight loss that may occur for 1 or 2 days before the first loose stool is passed. Diarrhea usually begins abruptly. It may be continuous and violent, or in milder infections, it may run an intermittent course with 1 or more days of normal stools followed by 1 or more days of diarrhea. Emesis sometimes is a prominent and persistent early finding. Stools are loose and bright yellow initially, later becoming watery, mucoid, and green. Flecks or streaks of blood, which are commonly seen with enterocolitis caused by *Salmonella, Campylobacter,* or *Shigella,* are rarely a feature of EPEC diarrheal disease. A characteristic seminal smell may pervade the environment of infants infected with EPEC O111:B34,[232,262,347] and an odor variously described as "pungent," "musty," or "fetid" often surrounds patients excreting other strains in their stools.[231,256] Because the buttocks are repeatedly covered with liquid stools, excoriation of the perianal skin can be an early and persistent problem. Fever is an inconstant feature, and when it occurs, the patient's temperature rarely rises above 39° C. Convulsions occur infrequently; their occurrence should alert the clinician to the possible presence of electrolyte disturbances, particularly hypernatremia. Prolonged hematochezia, distention, edema, and jaundice are ominous signs and suggest an unfavorable prognosis.[215,240,285] Most infants receiving antimicrobial agents orally show a cessation of diarrhea, tolerate oral feedings, and resume weight gain within 3 to 7 days after therapy has been started.[242,245] Those with mild illness who receive no treatment can continue to have intermittent loose stools for 1 to 3 weeks. In one outbreak related to EPEC O142:K86, more than one third of the untreated or inappropriately treated infants had diarrhea for more than 14 days in the absence of a recognized enteric pathogen on repeated culturing.[267] Recurrence of diarrhea and vomiting after a period of initial improvement is characteristic of EPEC enteritis.[191,239,240] Although seen most often in newborns who have been treated inadequately or not treated at all, clinical relapses also occur after appropriate therapy. Occasionally, the signs of illness during a relapse can be more severe than those accompanying the initial attack of illness.[215,232,285] Not all clinical relapses result from persistent infection. A significant number of relapses, particularly those that consistently follow attempts at reinstitution of formula feedings,[262,265] are caused by disaccharide intolerance rather than bacterial proliferation. Intestinal superinfections, caused by another serotype of EPEC[283,347,348] or by completely different enteric pathogens, such as *Salmonella* or *Shigella,*[245] also can delay the resolution of symptoms. Rarely, infants suffer a "relapse" caused by an organism from the same O group as the original strain but differing in its H antigen. Unless complete serotyping is performed on all EPEC isolates, such an event easily could be dismissed as being a recurrence rather than a superinfection with a new organism.[258,268]

Antimicrobial agents to which the infecting organisms are susceptible often may not eradicate EPEC,[245,265,267] which may persist for weeks[264,283,344] or months[349] after the acute illness has subsided. Although reinfection cannot always be excluded, a significant number of infants are discharged from the hospital with positive rectal cultures.[231,233] Dehydration is the most common and serious complication of gastroenteritis caused by EPEC or a toxin-producing *E. coli.* Virtually all deaths directly attributable to the intestinal infection are caused by disturbances in fluids and electrolytes. When stools are frequent in number, large in volume, and violent in release, as they often are in severe infections with abrupt onset, a neonate can lose up to 15% of body weight in a few hours.[232,276] Rarely, fluid excretion into the lumen of the bowel proceeds so rapidly that reduction of circulating blood volume and shock may intervene before passage of even a single loose stool.[262] Before the discovery of the etiologic agent, epidemic diarrhea of the newborn was also known by the term *cholera infantum.*

Mild disease, particularly when aggravated by poor fluid intake, can lead to a subtle but serious deterioration of an infant's metabolic status. Sometimes, a week or more of illness elapses before it becomes apparent that an infant with borderline acidosis and dehydration who seemed to be responding to oral fluids alone requires parenteral therapy for improvement.[272] It is incumbent on the clinician caring for small infants with gastroenteritis to follow them closely, with particular attention to serial weights, until full recovery can be confirmed.

There are few other complications, with the possible exception of aspiration pneumonia, directly related to EPEC gastroenteritis. Protracted diarrhea and nutritional failure may occur as a consequence of functional damage to the small intestinal mucosa, with secondary intolerance to dietary sugars.[265,338] Necrotizing enterocolitis, which occasionally results in perforation of the bowel and peritonitis, has not been causally related to infection with EPEC.[247,264,266] A review of most of the large clinical series describing EPEC disease in infants who ranged in age from neonates to children aged 2 years revealed only three proven instances of bacteremia,[265,278] one possible urinary tract infection,[265] and one documented case of meningitis in an infant of unspecified age.[351] Focal infections among neonates were limited to several cases of otitis media[247,262] and a subcutaneous abscess[294] from which EPEC was isolated. Additional complications include interstitial pneumonia,[319] gastrointestinal bleeding with or without disseminated intravascular coagulation,[334,352] and methemoglobinemia caused by a mutant of EPEC O127:B8 that was capable of generating large quantities of nitrite from proteins present in the gastrointestinal tract.[353]

Diagnosis

The gold standard of EPEC diagnostics is identification in the stool of *E. coli* carrying genes for BFP and LEE. Identification of these genes can be accomplished by molecular methods (discussed later), but lack of access to these methods has led many labs to rely on surrogate markers, such as serotyping.[19] Classic EPEC has been recovered from the vomitus, stool, or bowel contents of infected newborns. Isolation from bile[233] and the upper respiratory tract[85,238,239] has been described in those instances in which a specific search has been made. Less commonly, EPEC is isolated from ascetic fluid[252] or purulent exudates[209,215,294]; occasionally, the organism has been recovered from blood cultures,[265,278] urine,[265] and cerebrospinal fluid. Stool cultures generally are more reliable than rectal swabs in detecting the presence of enteric pathogens, although a properly obtained swab should be adequate to demonstrate EPEC in most cases.[217,296,354] Specimens should be obtained as early in the course of the illness as possible because organisms are present in virtually pure culture during the acute phase of the enteritis but diminish in numbers during convalescence. Because of the preponderance of EPEC in diarrheal stools, two cultures are adequate for isolation of these pathogens in almost all cases of active disease. Studies using fluorescent antibody methods for identification of EPEC in stool specimens have demonstrated that during the incubation period of the illness, during convalescence, and among asymptomatic carriers of EPEC, organisms can be excreted in such small numbers that they escape detection by standard bacteriologic methods in a significant proportion of infants.[245,355,356] As many as 3 to 10 specimens may be required to detect EPEC using methods that identify individual EPEC isolates in the stool.[85,346] After a stool specimen is received, it should be plated as quickly as possible onto noninhibiting media or placed in a preservative medium if it is to be held for longer periods. Deep freezing of specimens preserves viable EPEC when a prolonged delay in isolation is necessary.[218] No selective media, biochemical reactions, or colonial variations permit differentiation of pathogenic and nonpathogenic strains. Certain features may aid in the recognition of two important serogroups. Cultures of serogroups O111:B4 and O55:B5, unlike many other coliforms, are sticky or stringy when picked with a wire loop and are rarely hemolytic on blood agar,[217,219] whereas O111:B4 colonies emit a distinctive evanescent odor commonly described as "seminal."[210,214] This unusual odor first led Bray[347] to suspect that specific strains of *E. coli* might be responsible for infantile gastroenteritis.

Because serotyping is simpler than molecular detection and because EPEC have long been known to belong to certain highly characteristic serotypes, serotyping can be used to identify likely EPEC strains, especially in outbreaks.[216] *E. coli*, like other Enterobacteriaceae members, possesses cell wall somatic antigens (O), envelope or capsular antigens (K), and if motile, flagellar antigens (H). Many of the O groups may be further divided into two or more subgroups (a, b, c), and the K antigens are divisible into at least three varieties (B, L, A) on the basis of their physical behavior. Organisms that do not possess flagellar antigens are nonmotile (designated NM). The EPEC B capsular surface antigen prevents agglutination by antibodies directed against the underlying O antigen. Heating at 100° C for 1 hour inactivates the agglutinability and antigenicity of the B antigen.

Slide agglutination tests with polyvalent O or OB antiserum may be performed on suspensions of colonies typical of *E. coli* that have been isolated from infants with diarrhea, especially in nursery outbreaks. However, because of numerous false-positive "cross-reactions," the O and K (or B) type must be confirmed by titration with the specific antisera.[227] The presence of EPEC does not prove that EPEC is the cause of diarrhea in an individual patient. Mixed cultures with two or three serotypes of EPEC have been demonstrated in 1% to 10% of patients.[244,245,352] This need not mean that two or three serotypes are causative agents. Secondary infection with hospital-acquired strains can occur during convalescence,[173,281,283,380] and some infants may have been asymptomatic carriers of one serotype at the time that another produced diarrheal disease. A similar explanation may pertain to mixed infections with EPEC and *Salmonella* or *Shigella*.[217,220,358] Nelson[245] reported the presence of these pathogens in combination with EPEC in 14% of infants who were cultured as part of an antibiotic therapy trial. *Salmonella* and *Shigella* that had not been identified on cultures obtained at admission were isolated only after institution of oral therapy with neomycin. The investigator postulated that the alteration in bowel flora brought about by the neomycin facilitated the growth of these organisms, which had previously been suppressed and obscured by coliform overgrowth.[245] The importance of seeking all enteric pathogens in primary and follow-up cultures of infantile diarrhea is apparent, particularly when the specimen originates from a patient in a newborn nursery or infants' ward.

Although EPEC gastroenteritis was once considered to be synonymous with "summer diarrhea," community outbreaks have occurred as frequently, if not more frequently, in the colder seasons.[133,160,172] It has been suggested that the increased incidence at that time of year might be related to the heightened chance of contact between infants and toddlers that is bound to occur when children remain indoors in close contact.[294] Nursery epidemics, which depend on the chance introduction and dissemination of EPEC within a relatively homogeneous population and stable environment, demonstrate no seasonal prevalence. Average relative humidity, temperature, and hours of daylight have no significant effect in determining whether an outbreak will follow the introduction of enteropathogenic strains of *E. coli* into a ward of infants.[243]

There are no clinical studies of the variations in peripheral leukocyte count, urine, or cerebrospinal fluid in neonatal enteritis caused by EPEC. Microscopic examination of stools of infants with acute diarrheal illness caused by these organisms usually has revealed an absence of fecal polymorphonuclear leukocytes,[214,256,320,359] although data on fecal lactoferrin in human volunteers suggest that an inflammatory process may be important in EPEC diarrhea.[360,361] Stool pH can be neutral, acid, or alkaline.[61,341] Serologic methods have not proved to be useful in attempting to establish a retrospective diagnosis of EPEC infection in neonates. Rising or significantly elevated agglutinin titers rarely could be demonstrated in early investigations[210,215,231]; hemagglutinating antibodies showed a significant response in no more than 10% to 20% of cases.[245,297] Fluorescent antibody techniques have shown promise for preliminary identification of EPEC in acute infantile diarrhea. This method is specific, with few false-positive results, and it is more sensitive than conventional plating and isolation techniques.[282,361,362] The rapidity with which determinations can be performed makes them ideally suited for screening ill infants and possible carriers in determining the extent and progression of a nursery[272,282] or community[238,291] outbreak. Because immunofluorescence does not depend on the viability of organisms and is not affected by antibiotics that suppress growth on culture plates, it can be used to advantage in following bacteriologic responses and relapses in patients receiving oral therapy.[210,363] The use of fluorescent antibody techniques offers many advantages in the surveillance and epidemiologic control of EPEC gastroenteritis. Immunofluorescent methods should supplement but not replace standard bacteriologic and serologic methods for identification of enteric pathogens.

Specific gene probes and PCR primers for the BFP adhesin, the intimin-encoding gene *(eae)* and for a cryptic plasmid locus (EAF) are available.[98] Detection of BFP or EAF are superior to detection of *eae*, because many non-EPEC, including nonpathogens, carry the *eae* gene.[98,364] PCR and gene probe analysis can be performed directly on the stools of suspect infants. However, confirmation of infection by the identification of the organism in pure culture should be pursued.

Before widespread use of molecular methods, the HEp-2 cell adherence assay was proposed for EPEC diagnosis.[119] The presence of a focal or localized adherence (LA)[119] pattern on the surface of HEp-2 or HeLa cells after 3-hour co-incubation is a highly sensitive and specific test for detection of EPEC.[365] The requirement for cell culture and expertise in reading this assay limits its utility to the research setting. An ELISA for the BFP has been described but is not readily available.[366] The capacity of LA + EPEC to polymerize F-actin can be detected in tissue culture cells stained with rhodamine-labeled phalloidin.[367] This fluorescence-actin staining (FAS) test is cumbersome and impractical for routine clinical use.

Prognosis

The mortality rate recorded previously in epidemics of EPEC gastroenteritis is impressive for its variability. During the 1930s and 1940s, when organisms later recognized as classic enteropathogenic serotypes were infecting infants, the case-fatality ratio among neonates was about 50%.[209,210] During the 1950s and 1960s, many nursery epidemics still claimed about one of every four infected infants, but several outbreaks involving the same serotypes under similar epidemiologic circumstances had fatality rates of less than 3%.[234,241,251] In the 1970s, reports appeared in the literature of a nursery epidemic with a 40% neonatal mortality rate[285] and of an extensive outbreak in a nursery for premature infants with 4% fatalities[265]; another report stated that among "243 consecutive infants admitted to the hospital for EPEC diarrheal disease, none died of diarrheal disease per se."[368]

A significant proportion of the infants who died during or shortly after an episode of gastroenteritis already were compromised by preexisting disease[233,283,330] or by congenital malformations[214,231,240] at the time they acquired their illness. These underlying pathologic conditions appear to exert a strongly unfavorable influence, probably by reducing the infant's ability to respond to the added stresses imposed by the gastrointestinal tract infection. Although prematurity is often mentioned as a factor predisposing to a fatal outcome, the overall mortality rate among premature infants with EPEC gastroenteritis has not differed significantly over the years from that recorded for term infants.[233,262,264]

Therapy

The management of EPEC gastroenteritis should be directed primarily toward prevention or correction of problems caused by loss of fluids and electrolytes.[198] Most neonates have a relatively mild illness that can be treated with oral rehydration. Infants who appear toxic, those with voluminous diarrhea and persistent vomiting, and those with increasing weight loss should be hospitalized for observation and treatment with parenteral fluids and careful maintenance of fluid and electrolyte balance and possibly with antimicrobial therapy. Clinical studies suggest that slow nasogastric infusion of an elemental diet can be valuable in treating infants who have intractable diarrhea that is unresponsive to standard modes of therapy.[369]

There is no evidence that the use of proprietary formulas containing kaolin or pectin is effective in reducing the number of diarrheal stools in neonates with gastroenteritis. Attempts to suppress the growth of enteric pathogens by feeding lactobacillus to the infant in the form of yogurt, powder, or granules have not been shown to be of value.[370] A trial of cholestyramine in 15 newborns with EPEC gastroenteritis had no effect on the duration or severity of the diarrhea.[265] The use of atropine-like drugs, paregoric, or loperamide to reduce intestinal motility or cramping should be avoided. Inhibition of peristalsis interferes with an efficient protective mechanism designed to rid the body of intestinal pathogens and may lead to fluid retention in the lumen of the bowel that may be sufficient to mask depletion of extracellular fluid and electrolytes.

The value of antimicrobial therapy in management of neonatal EPEC gastroenteritis, if any, is uncertain. There are no adequately controlled studies defining the benefits of any antibiotic in eliminating EPEC from the gastrointestinal tract, reducing the risk of cross-infection in community or nursery outbreaks, or modifying the severity of the illness. Proponents of the use of antimicrobial agents have based their claims for efficacy on anecdotal observations or comparative studies.[245] Nonetheless, several clinical investigations have provided sufficient information to guide the physician faced with the dilemma of deciding whether to treat an individual infant or an entire nursery population suffering from EPEC diarrheal disease. It should be emphasized, however, that these guidelines must be considered tentative until rigidly controlled, double-blind studies have established the efficacy of antibiotics on a more rational and scientific basis.

Oral therapy with neomycin,[234,251] colistin,[363] or chloramphenicol[344] appears to be effective in rapidly reducing the number of susceptible EPEC organisms in the stool of infected infants. Studies comparing the responses of infants treated orally with neomycin,[233] gentamicin,[265] polymyxin,[242] or kanamycin[371] with the responses of infants receiving supportive therapy alone have shown that complete eradication of EPEC occurs more rapidly in those receiving an antimicrobial agent. In most cases, stool cultures are free of EPEC 2 to 4 days after the start of therapy.[245,363] Bacteriologic failure, defined as continued isolation of organisms during or after a course of an antimicrobial agent, can be expected to occur in 15% to 30% of patients.[245,265] Such relapses generally are not associated with a recurrence of symptoms.[231,234,245] The effectiveness of oral antimicrobial therapy in reducing the duration of EPEC excretion serves to diminish environmental contamination and the spread of pathogenic organisms from one infant to another. Breaking the chain of fecal-oral transmission by administering antimicrobial agents simultaneously to all carriers of EPEC and their immediate contacts in the nursery has appeared to be valuable in terminating outbreaks that have failed to respond to more conservative measures.[234,264,372] The apparent reduction in morbidity and mortality associated with oral administration of neomycin,[230,233,234] colistin,[246,267,285] polymyxin,[242] or gentamicin[246] during nursery epidemics has led to the impression that these drugs also exert a beneficial clinical effect in severely or moderately ill infants. Reports describing clinical,[256] bacteriologic,[265] or histopathologic[319] evidence of tissue invasion by EPEC have persuaded some investigators to suggest the use of parenteral rather than oral drug therapy in debilitated or malnourished infants. On the basis of these data, there appears to be sufficient evidence to recommend oral administration of nonabsorbable antibiotics in the treatment of severely or moderately ill newborns with EPEC gastroenteritis. The drug most frequently used for initial therapy is neomycin sulfate in a dosage of 100 mg/kg/day administered orally every 8 hours in three divided doses.[245] In communities in which neomycin-resistant EPEC has been prevalent, treatment with colistin sulfate or polymyxin B in a dosage of 15 to 20 mg/kg/day orally and divided into three equal doses may be appropriate. However, it is rarely necessary to use this approach.

Treatment should be continued only until stool cultures become negative for EPEC.[245] Because of the unavoidable delay before cultures can be reported, most infants receive therapy for 3 to 5 days. If fluorescent antibody testing of rectal swab specimens is available, therapy can be discontinued as soon as EPEC no longer is identified in smears; this takes no more than 48 hours in more than 90% of cases.[245] After diarrhea and vomiting have stopped and the infant tolerates formula feedings, shows a steady weight gain, and appears clinically well, discharge with outpatient follow-up is indicated. Bacteriologic relapses do not require therapy unless they are associated with illness or high epidemiologic risks to other young infants in the household. Because the infecting organisms in these recurrences generally continue to show in vitro susceptibility to the original drug, it should be reinstituted pending bacteriologic results.[245]

When clinical judgment suggests that a neonate may be suffering from bacterial sepsis and EPEC diarrheal disease, parenteral antimicrobial therapy is indicated after appropriate cultures have been obtained. The routine use of systemic therapy in severe cases of EPEC enteritis is not appropriate on the basis of current clinical experience.

Antimicrobial susceptibility patterns of EPEC are an important determinant of the success of therapy in infections with these organisms.[233,246,247] These patterns are unpredictable, depending on the ecologic pressures exerted by local antibiotic usage[246,247] and on the incidence of transmissible resistance factors in the enteric flora of the particular population served by an institution.[373-378] For these reasons, variations in susceptibility patterns are apparent in different nurseries[246,376] and even from time to time within the same institution.[247,248,250] Sudden changes in clinical response may even occur during the course of a single epidemic as drug-susceptible strains of EPEC are replaced by strains with multidrug resistance.[233,291,375] Because differences can exist in the susceptibilities of different EPEC serogroups to various antimicrobial agents, regional susceptibility patterns should be reported on the basis of OB group or serotype rather than for EPEC as a whole.[250] Knowledge of the resistance pattern in one's area may help in the initial choice of antimicrobial therapy.

Prevention

The prevention of hospital outbreaks of EPEC gastroenteritis is best accomplished by careful attention to infection control policies for a nursery. All infants hospitalized with diarrhea should have a bacteriologic evaluation. If the laboratory is equipped and staffed to perform fluorescent antibody testing, infants transferred from another institution to a newborn, premature, or intensive care nursery and all infants with gastroenteritis on admission during an outbreak of EPEC diarrhea or in a highly endemic area can be held in an observation area for 1 or 2 hours until the results of the fluorescent antibody test or PCR are received. Because of the difficulty in diagnosing EPEC infection, reference laboratories, such as those at the Centers for Disease Control and Prevention (CDC), should be notified when an outbreak is suspected. Infants suspected to be excreting EPEC, even if healthy in appearance, then can be separated from others and given oral therapy until the test results are negative. Some experts have suggested that when the rapid results obtainable with fluorescent antibody procedures are not available, all infants admitted with diarrhea in a setting where EPEC is common may be treated as if they were excreting EPEC or some other enteric pathogen until contrary proof is obtained.[372] Stool cultures should be obtained at admission, and contact precautions should be enforced among all who come into contact with the infant. Additional epidemiologic studies are needed to establish the advantages of careful isolation and nursing techniques, particularly in smaller community hospitals in which the number of infants in a "gastroenteritis ward" may be small. The use of prophylactic antibiotics has been shown to be of no value and can select for increased resistance.[377-379]

Unfortunately, it can be difficult to keep a nursery continuously free of EPEC. Specific procedures have been suggested for handling a suspected outbreak of bacterial enteritis in a newborn nursery or infant care unit.[235,355,380] Evidence indicating that a significant proportion of *E. coli* enteritis may be caused by nontypeable strains has required some modification of these earlier recommendations. The following infection control measures may be appropriate:

1. The unit is closed, when possible, to all new admissions.
2. Cultures for enteric pathogens are obtained from nursing personnel assigned to the unit at the time of the outbreak.
3. Stool specimens obtained from all infants in the nursery can be screened by the fluorescent antibody or another technique and cultured. Identification of a classic enteropathogenic serotype provides a useful epidemiologic marker; however, failure to isolate one of these strains does not eliminate the possibility of illness caused by a nontypeable EPEC.
4. Antimicrobial therapy with oral neomycin or colistin can be considered for all infants with a positive fluorescent antibody test or culture result. The initial drug of choice depends on local patterns of susceptibility. Depending on the results of susceptibility tests, subsequent therapy may require modification.
5. If an identifiable EPEC strain is isolated, second and third stool specimens from all infants in the unit are reexamined by the fluorescent antibody technique or culture at 48-hour intervals. If this is not practical, exposed infants should be carefully followed.
6. Early discharge for healthy, mature, uninfected infants is advocated.
7. An epidemiologic investigation should be performed to seek the factor or factors responsible for the outbreak. A surveillance system may be established for all those in contact with the nursery, including physicians and other health care personnel, housekeeping personnel, and postpartum mothers with evidence of enteric disease. A telephone, mail, or home survey may be conducted on all infants who were residing in the involved unit during the 2 weeks before the outbreak.
8. When all patients and contacts are discharged and control of the outbreak is achieved, a thorough terminal disinfection of the involved nursery is mandatory.

Above all, personnel and parents should pay scrupulous attention to hand hygiene when handling infants.[381]

Enterohemorrhagic *Escherichia coli*

Since a multistate outbreak of enterohemorrhagic colitis was associated with *E. coli* O157:H7,[382] Shiga toxin–producing *E. coli* (STEC) have been recognized as emerging gastrointestinal pathogens in most of the industrialized world. A particularly virulent subset of STEC, EHEC, causes frequent and severe outbreaks of gastrointestinal disease[98,383]; the most virulent EHEC belong to serotype O157:H7. EHEC has a bovine reservoir and is transmitted by undercooked meat, unpasteurized milk, and contaminated vegetables such as lettuce, alfalfa sprouts, and radish sprouts (as occurred in more than 9000 schoolchildren in Japan).[384,387] It also spreads directly from person to person.[387,388] The clinical syndrome is that of bloody, noninflammatory (sometimes voluminous) diarrhea that is distinct from febrile dysentery with fecal leukocytes seen in shigellosis or EIEC infections.[98] Most cases of EHEC infections have been recognized in outbreaks of bloody diarrhea or HUS in daycare centers, schools, nursing homes, and communities.[388-390] Although EHEC infections often involve infants and young children, the frequency of this infection in neonates remains unclear; animal studies suggest that receptors for the Shiga toxin may be developmentally regulated and that susceptibility to disease may be age related.[391]

The capacity of EHEC to cause disease is related to the phage-encoded capacity of the organism to produce a Vero cell cytotoxin, subsequently shown to be one of the Shiga toxins.[392-394] Shiga toxin 1 is neutralized by antiserum against Shiga toxin, whereas Shiga toxin 2, although biologically similar, is not neutralized by anti-Shiga toxin.[395,396] Like Shiga toxin made by *Shigella dysenteriae*, both *E. coli* Shiga toxins act by inhibiting protein synthesis by cleaving an adenosine residue from position 4324 in the 28S ribosomal RNA (rRNA) to prevent elongation factor-1–dependent aminoacyl transfer RNA (tRNA) from binding to the 60S rRNA.[392,393] The virulence of EHEC also may be determined in part by a 60-MDa plasmid that encodes for a fimbrial adhesin in O157 and O26.[397,398] This phenotype is mediated by the LEE pathogenicity island, which is highly homologous to the island present in EPEC strains.[328]

EHEC and other STEC infections should be suspected in neonates who have bloody diarrhea or who may have been exposed in the course of an outbreak among older individuals. Because most cases are caused by ingestion of contaminated food, neonates have a degree of epidemiologic protection from the illness. Diagnosis of STEC diarrhea is made by isolation and identification of the pathogen in the feces. *E. coli* O157:H7 does not ferment sorbitol, and this biochemical trait is commonly used in the detection of this serotype.[98,399] Because some nonpathogenic *E. coli* share this characteristic, confirmation of the serotype by slide agglutination is required. These techniques can be performed in most clinical laboratories. However, detection of non-O157 serotypes is problematic and relies on detection of the Shiga toxin; available methods include Shiga toxin ELISA, latex agglutination, and molecular methods.[98,399] These should be performed by a reference laboratory.

HUS in infants is not necessarily caused by STEC infection. Even in older patients, however, the stool is typically negative for STEC at the time the that HUS develops.[400,401] Serum and fecal detection of cytotoxin has been performed in such patients, but no diagnostic modality is definitive once HUS has supervened.[400,401]

Antimicrobial therapy should not be administered to patients who may have STEC infection, although their role in inducing HUS remains controversial.[402,403] Management of the diarrhea and possible sequelae is supportive, with proper emphasis on fluid and electrolyte replacement. Aggressive rehydration is helpful in minimizing the frequency of serious sequelae.

Enteroaggregative *Escherichia coli*

The Hep-2 adherence assay is useful for the detection of EPEC, which exhibit a classic LA pattern.[119] Two other adherence patterns can be discerned in this assay: aggregative (AA) and diffuse (DA). These two patterns have been suggested to define additional pathotypes of diarrheogenic *E. coli.*[98] Strains exhibiting the AA pattern (i.e., EAEC) are common pathogens of infants.[125]

EAEC cause diarrhea by colonization of the intestinal mucosa and elaboration of enterotoxins and cytotoxins.[125,404] Many strains can be shown to elicit secretion of inflammatory cytokines in vitro, which may contribute to growth retardation associated with prolonged otherwise asymptomatic colonization.[103] Several virulence factors in EAEC are under the control of the virulence gene activator AggR.[404] Presence of the AggR regulator or its effector genes has been proposed as a means of detecting truly virulent EAEC strains (called typical EAEC),[404,405] and an empirical gene probe long used for EAEC detection has been shown to correspond to one gene under AggR control.[406,407]

Epidemiology and Transmission

The mode of transmission of EAEC has not been well established. In adult volunteer studies, the infectious dose is high (>10^8 colony-forming units [CFU]), suggesting that in adults at least, person-to-person transmission is unlikely.[408,409] Several outbreaks have been linked to consumption of contaminated food.[410,411] The largest of these outbreaks involved almost 2700 schoolchildren in Japan[410]; a contaminated school lunch was the implicated source of the outbreak. Some studies have demonstrated contamination of condiments or milk, which could represent vehicles of foodborne transmission.

Several nursery outbreaks of EAEC have been observed,[412,413] although in no case has the mechanism of transmission been established. The fist reported nursery outbreak involved 19 infants in Nis, Serbia, in 1995. Because these infants did not ingest milk from a common source, it is presumed that horizontal transmission by environmental contamination or hands of health care personnel was possible. Most of the infants were full term and previously well, and they were housed in two separate nursery rooms.

The earliest epidemiologic studies of EAEC implicated this organism as a cause of endemic diarrhea in developing countries.[414-416] In this setting, EAEC as defined by the AA pattern of adherence to Hep-2 cells can be found in upward of 30% of the population at any one time.[417] Newer molecular diagnostic modalities have revised this figure downward, although the organism remains highly prevalent in many areas. Several studies from the Indian subcontinent implicated EAEC among the most frequent enteric pathogens.[414,415,418] Other sites reproducibly reporting high incidence rates include Mexico[416] and Brazil.[417,419] There is evidence that EAEC may be emerging in incidence. A study from São Paulo, Brazil, implicated EAEC as the prevalent *E. coli* pathotypes in infants[419]; EPEC had previously been shown to be the most common pathogen in this community. Many other sites in developing countries of Africa,[421] Asia,[405,422] and South America[420] have described high endemic rates.

Several studies have suggested that EAEC is also a common cause of infant diarrhea in industrialized countries.[423-425] Using molecular diagnostic methods, a large prospective study in the United Kingdom implicated EAEC as the second most common enteric bacterial pathogen after *Campylobacter.*[426] A similar study from Switzerland found EAEC to be the most common bacterial enteropathogen.[423] Studies from the United States also have demonstrated a high rate of EAEC diarrhea in infants; using molecular diagnostic methods, EAEC was implicated in 11% and 8% of outpatient and inpatient diarrhea cohorts, respectively, compared with less than 2% of asymptomatic control infants ($P < .05$).[427] Although epidemiologic studies have shown that EAEC can cause diarrhea in all age groups, several studies suggest that the infection is particularly common in infants younger than 12 months old.[405,420]

Clinical Manifestations

Descriptions from outbreaks and volunteer studies suggest that EAEC diarrhea is watery in character with mucus but without blood or frank pus.[408,409,412] Patients typically are afebrile. Several epidemiologic studies have suggested that many infants may have bloody diarrhea,[416] but fecal leukocytes are uncommon.

The earliest reports of EAEC infection suggested that this pathogen may be particularly associated with persistent diarrhea (>14 days).[414-416] However, later studies suggest that persistent diarrhea may occur in only a subset of infected infants.[410] In the Serbian outbreak of 19 infected infants, the mean duration of diarrhea was 5.2 days[412]; diarrhea persisted more than 14 days in only three patients. Infants in this outbreak had frequent, green, odorless stools. In three cases, the stools had mucus, but none had visible blood. Eleven babies developed temperatures in excess of 38° C; only one had vomiting.

Despite a lack of clinical evidence suggesting inflammatory enteritis, several clinical studies have suggested that EAEC is associated with subclinical inflammation, including the shedding of fecal cytokines and lactoferrin.[103,428] Studies in Fortaleza, Brazil, suggest that children asymptomatically excreting EAEC may exhibit growth shortfalls compared with uninfected peers.[103] A study from Germany reported an association between EAEC isolation and infant colic in infants without diarrhea.[425] This observation has not been repeated. EAEC should be considered in the differential diagnosis of persistent diarrhea and failure to thrive in infants.

Diagnosis and Therapy

Diagnosis of EAEC requires identification of the organism in the patient's feces. The HEp-2 adherence assay can be used for this purpose[119]; some reports suggest that the adherence phenotype can be observed using formalin-fixed cells,[429,430] thereby obviating the need to cultivate eukaryotic cells for each assay. PCR and gene probe for typical EAEC are available.

Successful antibiotic therapy has been reported using fluoroquinolones in adult patients,[431] although preliminary studies suggest that azithromycin[432] or rifaximin[433] also may be effective. Therapy in infected infants should be guided by the results of susceptibility testing, as EAEC frequently is antibiotic resistant.[421]

Other *Escherichia coli* Pathotypes

Additional *E. coli* pathotypes have been described, including diffusely adherent *E. coli* (DAEC),[434] and cytodetaching *E. coli*.[435] DAEC has been specifically associated with diarrhea outside of infancy, as infants may have some degree of inherent resistance to infection.[436] Cytodetaching *E. coli* represent organisms that secrete the *E. coli* hemolysin.[437] It is not clear whether these latter organisms are true enteric pathogens.

SALMONELLA

Nature of the Organism

Salmonella classification tends to be confusing. Although taxonomists classify *Salmonella* narrowly as a single species, with *Salmonella typhi, Salmonella choleraesuis,* and *Salmonella enteritidis* technically being serovars or subspecies, for clinical purposes, these subspecies conventionally are referred to as *species*. For example, clinical laboratories tend to use the shorthand *S. typhimurium* rather than the more formal designation *Salmonella enterica* serovar *typhimurium.* Biochemical traits are used routinely by hospital laboratories to differentiate *S. typhi, S. choleraesuis,* and *S. enteritidis* from each other. *S. typhi* is unlike other salmonellae in that it does not produce gas from glucose.[438] Because there are several thousand serotypes included in the species *S. enteritidis,* serotyping of *S. enteritidis* is usually performed by state health departments rather than by hospital laboratories. The most common serogroups and representative serotypes are listed in Table 20-3. Infection of humans with the other serogroups (e.g., C_3, D_2, E_2, E_3, F, G, H, I) is uncommon.

Table 20–3 Common Serotypes and Serogroups of *Salmonella*

Serogroups	Serotypes
A	Paratyphi A
B	Agona
	Derby
	Heidelberg
	Paratyphi B *(schottmuelleri)*
	Saint-paul
	Typhimurium
C_1	Choleraesuis
	Eimsbuettel
	Infantis
	Montevideo
	Oranienburg
	Paratyphi C *(hirschfeldii)*
	Thompson
C_2	Blockley
	Hadar
	Muenchen
	Newport
C_3	Kentucky
D_1	Dublin
	Enteritidis
	Javiana
	Panama
	Typhi
D_2	Maarssen
E_1	Anatum
E_2	London Newington
E_3	Illinois
E_4	Krefeld
	Senftenberg

There are differences in invasiveness of *Salmonella* strains related to serotype. *S. typhi, S. choleraesuis, Salmonella heidelberg,*[439,440] and *Salmonella dublin*[441] are particularly invasive, with bacteremia and extraintestinal focal infections occurring frequently. *Salmonella* species possess genes closely related to those for the *Shigella* invasion plasmid antigens; these genes are probably essential to intestinal infection.[442,4436] Virulence plasmids, which increase invasiveness in some serotypes, have been recognized, although the precise mechanisms of virulence remain to be elucidated; resistance to complement-mediated bacteriolysis by inhibition of insertion of the terminal C5b-9 membrane attack complex into the outer membrane may be important.[444,445] Laboratory studies have demonstrated dramatic strain-related difference in the ability of *S. typhimurium* to evoke fluid secretion, to invade intestinal mucosa, and to disseminate beyond the gut.[446] Production of an enterotoxin immunologically related to cholera toxin by about two thirds of *Salmonella* strains may be related to the watery diarrhea often seen.[447] The significance of protein synthesis-inhibiting cytotoxins[448] remains to be proved, although such toxins can damage gut epithelium, which could facilitate invasion. The cytotoxins produced by *Salmonella* are not immunologically related to Shiga toxin made by *Shigella dysenteriae* type 1[449] or *E. coli* O157:H7.

Salmonellae have the ability to penetrate epithelial cells and reach the submucosa, where they are ingested by phagocytes.[450] In phagocytes, salmonellae are resistant to killing, in part because of the properties of their lipopolysaccharides.[451,452] Persistence of the organism within phagolysosomes of phagocytic cells may occur with any species of *Salmonella.* It is not completely clear how the organisms have adapted to survive in the harsh intracellular environment, but their survival has major clinical significance. It accounts for relapses after therapy. It explains the inadequacy of some antimicrobial agents that do not penetrate phagolysosomes. It perhaps is the reason for prolonged febrile courses that occur even in the face of appropriate therapy. Although humoral immunity and cell-mediated immunity are stimulated during *Salmonella* infections, it is believed that cell-mediated immunity plays a greater role in eradication of the bacteria.[453] T cell activation of macrophages appears to be important in killing intracellular *Salmonella.*[454] Defective interferon-γ production by monocytes of newborns in response to *S. typhimurium* lipopolysaccharide may explain in part the unusual susceptibility of infants to *Salmonella* infection.[455] Studies in mice suggest that helper T cell (T_H1) responses in Peyer's patches and mesenteric lymph nodes may be central to protection of the intestinal mucosa.[456] Humans who lack the IL-12 receptor and therefore have impaired T_H1 responses and interferon-γ production are at increased risk for *Salmonella* infection.[457]

In typhoid fever, presence of an envelope antigen, Vi, is known to enhance virulence. Patients who develop classic enteric fever have positive stool cultures in the first few days after ingestion of the organism and again late in the course after a period of bacteremia. This course reflects early colonization of the gut, penetration of gut epithelium with infection of mesenteric lymph nodes, and reseeding of the gut during a subsequent bacteremic phase.[458] Studies of *S. typhimurium* in monkeys suggest similar initial steps in pathogenesis (e.g., colonization of gut, penetration of gut epithelium, infection of mesenteric lymph nodes) but failure of the organism to cause a detectable level of bacteremia.[459]

Although both *Salmonella* and *Shigella* invade intestinal mucosa, the resultant pathologic changes are different. *Shigella* multiplies within and kills enterocytes with production of ulcerations and a brisk inflammatory response, whereas *Salmonella* passes through the mucosa and multiplies within the lamina propria, where the organisms are ingested by phagocytes; consequently, ulcer formation is less striking,[446] although villus tip cells are sometimes sloughed. Acute crypt abscesses can be seen in the stomach and small intestine, but the most dramatic changes occur in the colon, where acute diffuse inflammation with mucosal edema and crypt abscesses are the most consistent findings.[460,461] With *S. typhi* there also is hyperplasia of Peyer's patches in the ileum, with ulceration of overlying tissues.

Epidemiology and Transmission

Salmonella strains, with the exception of *S. typhi,* are well adapted to a variety of animal hosts; human infection often can be traced to infected meat, contaminated milk, or contact with a specific animal. Half of commercial poultry samples are contaminated with *Salmonella.*[462] Definition of the serotype causing infection can sometimes suggest the likely source. For example, *S. dublin* is closely associated with cattle; human cases occur with a higher-than-predicted frequency in people who drink raw milk.[441] For *S. typhimurium,* which is the most common serotype and accounts for more than one third of all reported human cases, a single source has not been established, although there is an association with cattle. Despite the 1975 ban by the U.S. Food and Drug Administration (FDA) on interstate commercial distribution of small turtles, these animals continue to be associated with infection, as illustrated by a series of cases in Puerto Rico.[463] Various pet reptiles are an important source of a variety of unusual *Salmonella* serotypes such as *Salmonella marina, Salmonella chameleon, Salmonella arizonae, Salmonella java, Salmonella stanley, Salmonella poona, Salmonella jangwain, Salmonella tilene, Salmonella pomona, Salmonella miami, Salmonella manhattan, Salmonella litchfield, Salmonella rubislaw,* and *Salmonella wassenaar.*[464-466] *Salmonella* organisms are hardy and capable of prolonged survival; organisms have been documented to survive in flour for nearly a year.[467] *Salmonella tennessee* has been shown to remain viable for many hours on non-nutritive surfaces (i.e., glass, 48 hours; stainless steel, 68 hours; enameled surface, 114 hours; rubber mattress, 119 hours; linen, 192 hours; and rubber tabletop, 192 hours).[468]

Infection with *Salmonella* is, like most enteric infections, more common in young children than in adults. The frequency of infection is far greater in the first 4 years of life; roughly equal numbers of cases are reported during each decade beyond 4 years of age. Although the peak incidence occurs in the second through sixth months of life, infection in the neonate is relatively common. Researchers at the CDC have estimated the incidence of *Salmonella* infection in the first month of life at nearly 75 cases per 100,000 infants.[469]

Adult volunteer studies suggest that large numbers of *Salmonella* (10^5 to 10^9) need to be ingested to cause disease.[470] However, it is likely that lower doses cause illness in infants. The occurrence of nursery outbreaks[468,471-496] and intrafamilial spread[497] suggests that organisms are easily spread from person to person; this pattern is typical of low-inoculum diseases transmitted by the fecal-oral route. The neonate with *Salmonella* infection infrequently acquires the organism from his or her mother during delivery. Although the index case in an outbreak can often be traced to a mother,[474-477,495] subsequent cases result from contaminated objects in the nursery environment[498,499] serving as a reservoir coming in contact with hands of attending personnel.[468,483] The mother of an index case may be symptomatic[479,480,500,501] or asymptomatic with preclinical infection,[484] convalescent infection,[477,481,502] or chronic carriage.[503] The risk of the newborn becoming infected once *Salmonella* is introduced into a nursery has been reported to be as high as 20% to 27%,[487,493] but the frequency of infection may be lower because isolated cases without a subsequent epidemic are unlikely to be reported.

Gastric acidity is an important barrier to *Salmonella* infection. Patients with anatomic or functional achlorhydria are at increased risk of developing salmonellosis.[504,505] The hypochlorhydria[25] and rapid gastric emptying typical of early life[28] may in part explain the susceptibility of infants to *Salmonella.* Premature and low-birth-weight infants appear to be at higher risk of acquiring *Salmonella* infection than term neonates.[483,485] Whether this reflects increased exposure because of prolonged hospital stays or increased susceptibility on the basis of intestinal or immune function is unclear. Contaminated food or water is often the source of *Salmonella* infection in older patients; the limited diet of the infant makes contaminated food a less likely source of infection. Although human milk,[506-508] raw milk,[509] powdered milk,[510-512] formula,[493] and cereal[513] have been implicated in transmission to infants, more often fomites, such as delivery room resuscitators,[471] rectal thermometers,[486,514] oropharyngeal suction devices,[515-517] water baths for heating formula,[517] soap dispensers,[518] scales,[468,472,519] "clean" medicine tables,[468] air-conditioning filters,[468] mattresses, radiant warmers,[498] and dust,[472] serve as reservoirs. One unusual outbreak involving 394 premature and 122 term infants was traced to faulty plumbing, which caused massive contamination of environment and personnel.[493] After *Salmonella* enters a nursery, it is difficult to eradicate. Epidemics lasting 6 to 7 weeks,[486,491] 17 weeks,[468] 6 months,[485,490] 1 year,[480] and 27 to 30 months[487,493] have been reported. Spread to nearby pediatric wards has occurred.[488,494]

The incubation period in nursery outbreaks has varied widely in several studies where careful attention has been paid to this variable. In one outbreak of *Salmonella oranienburg* involving 35 newborns, 97% of cases occurred within 4 days of birth.[487] In an outbreak of *S. typhimurium,* each of the ill infants presented within 6 days of birth.[477] These incubation periods are similar to those reported for *Salmonella newport* in older children and adults, 95% of whom have been reported to be ill within 8 days of exposure.[520,521] Conversely, one outbreak of *Salmonella nienstedten* involving newborns was characterized by incubation periods of 7 to 18 days.[488]

The usual incubation period associated with fecal-oral nursery transmission is not found with congenital typhoid. During pregnancy, typhoid fever is associated with bacteremic infection of the fetus. The congenitally infected infants are symptomatic at birth. They are usually born during the second to fourth week of untreated maternal illness.[522] Usually, the mother is a carrier; fecal-oral transmission of *S. typhi* can occur with delayed illness in the newborn.[523]

Clinical Manifestations

Several major clinical syndromes occur with nontyphoidal *Salmonella* infection in young infants. Colonization without illness may be the most common outcome of ingestion of *Salmonella* by the neonate. Such colonization usually is detected when an outbreak is under investigation. Most infected infants who become ill have abrupt onset of loose, green, mucus-containing stools, or they have bloody diarrhea; an elevated temperature is also a common finding in *Salmonella* gastroenteritis in the first months of life.[440] Grossly bloody stools are found in the minority of patients, although grossly bloody stools can occur in the first 24 hours of life. Hematochezia is more typically associated with non-infectious causes (e.g., swallowed maternal blood, intestinal ischemia, hemorrhagic diseases, anorectal fissures) at this early age.[524] There appear to be major differences in presentation related to the serotype of *S. enteritidis* causing infection. For example, in one epidemic of *S. oranienburg*[487] involving 46 newborns, 76% had grossly bloody stools, 11% were febrile, 26% had mucus in their stools, and only 11% were healthy. In a series of *S. newport* infections involving 11 premature infants,[474] 90% of infants with gastroenteritis had blood in their stools, 10% had fever, 10% had mucus in their stools, and 9% were asymptomatic. In an outbreak of *S. typhimurium*[477] involving 11 ill and 5 healthy infants, none had bloody stools; all of the symptomatic infants were febrile and usually had loose, green stools. Of 26 infants infected by *Salmonella virchow,* 42% were asymptomatic; the rest had mild diarrhea.[482] Seals and colleagues[488] described 12 infants with *S. nienstedten,* all of whom had watery diarrhea and low-grade fever; none had bloody stools. In a large outbreak in Zimbabwe of *S. heidelberg* infection reported by Bannerman,[485] 38% of 100 infants were asymptomatic, 42% had diarrhea, 16% had fever, 15% had pneumonia, and 2% developed meningitis. An outbreak of *Salmonella worthington* was characterized primarily by diarrhea, fever, and jaundice, although 3 of 18 infants developed meningitis and 17% died.[515] In dramatic contrast to these series, none of 27 infants with positive stool cultures for *S. tennessee* had an illness in a nursery found to be contaminated with that organism.[469] A few infants with *Salmonella* gastroenteritis have developed necrotizing enterocolitis,[492,525] but it is not clear whether *Salmonella* was the cause.

Although gastroenteritis is usually self-limited, chronic diarrhea has sometimes been attributed to *Salmonella.*[503,526] Whether chronic diarrhea is caused by *Salmonella* is uncertain. Although some infants develop carbohydrate intolerance after a bout of *Salmonella* enteritis[527,528] and *Salmonella* is typically listed as one of the causes of postinfectious protracted diarrhea,[529] it is difficult to be sure that the relationship is causal. The prolonged excretion of *Salmonella* after a bout of gastroenteritis may sometimes cause non-specific chronic diarrhea to be erroneously attributed to *Salmonella.*

Major extraintestinal complications of *Salmonella* infection may develop in the neonate who becomes bacteremic. Extraintestinal spread may develop in infants who initially present with diarrhea and in some who have no gastro-intestinal tract signs. Bacteremia appears to be more common in the neonate than in the older child.[530] A study of more than 800 children with *Salmonella* infection showed that extraintestinal infection occurred significantly more often (8.7% versus 3.6%) in the first 3 months of life.[531] Several retrospective studies suggest that infants in the first month of life may have a risk of bacteremia as high as 30% to 50%.[440] One retrospective study[439] suggests that the risk is not increased in infancy and estimates that the risk of bacteremia in childhood *Salmonella* gastroenteritis is between 8.5% and 15.6%. Prospective studies of infants in the first year of life suggest that the risk of bacteremia is 1.8% to 6.0%.[532,533] Although selection biases in these studies limit the reliability of these estimates, the risk is substantial. The *Salmonella* species isolated from infants include some serotypes that appear to be more invasive in the first 2 months of life than in older children or healthy adults *(S. newport, S. agona, S. blockley, S. derby, S. enteritidis, S. heidelberg, S. infantis, S. javiana, S. saint-paul,* and *S. typhimurium)* and serotypes that are aggressive in every age group *(S. choleraesuis* and *S. dublin).* Other serotypes appear more likely to cause bacteremia in adults (*S. typhi, S. paratyphi* A, and *S. paratyphi* B).[530]

Virtually any *Salmonella* serotype can cause bacteremic disease in neonates. A few infants with *Salmonella* gastro-enteritis have died with *E. coli* or *Pseudomonas aeruginosa* sepsis,[494] but the role of *Salmonella* in these cases is unclear. Unlike the situation in older children in whom bacteremic salmonellosis often is associated with underlying medical conditions, bacteremia may occur in infants who have no immunocompromising conditions.[534] *Salmonella* bacteremia is often not suspected clinically because the syndrome is not usually distinctive.[439,440] Even afebrile, well-appearing children with *Salmonella* gastroenteritis have been documented to have bacteremia that persists for several days.[535] Although infants with bacteremia may have spontaneous resolution without therapy,[536] a sufficient number develop complications to warrant empirical antimicrobial therapy when bacteremia is suspected. The frequency of complications is highest in the first month of life. Meningitis is the most feared complication of bacteremic *Salmonella* disease. Between 50% and 75% of all cases of nontyphoidal *Salmonella* meningitis occur in the first 4 months of life.[537] The serotypes associated with neonatal meningitis *(S. typhimurium, S. heidelberg, S. enteritidis, S. saint-paul, S. newport,* and *S. panama)*[497] are serotypes frequently associated with bacteremia. Meningitis has a high mortality rate, in part because of the high relapse rates. Relapse has been reported in up to 64% of cases.[538] In some studies, more than 90% of patients with meningitis have died,[539] although more typically, 30% to 60% of infants die.[540,541] The survivors suffer the expected complications of gram-negative neonatal meningitis, including hydrocephalus, seizures, ventriculitis, abscess formation, subdural empyema, and permanent neurologic impairment. Neurologic sequelae have included retardation, hemiparesis, epilepsy, visual impairment, and athetosis.[537]

In large nursery outbreaks, it is common to find infants whose course is complicated by pneumonia,[485] osteomyelitis,[542,543] or septic arthritis.[483,485] Other rare complications of salmonellosis include pericarditis,[544] pyelitis,[545] peritonitis,[477] otitis media,[477] mastitis,[546] cholecystitis,[547] endophthalmitis,[548] cutaneous abscesses,[492] and infected cephalohematoma.[542] Other focal infections seen in older children and adults, such as endocarditis and infected aortic aneurysms, rarely or never have been reported in neonates.[537,549] Although the mortality rate in two reviews of nursery outbreaks was 3.7% to 7.0%,[495,496] in some series, it reached 18%.[485]

Enteric fever, most often related to *S. typhi* but also occurring with *S. paratyphi* A, *S. paratyphi* B, *S. paratyphi* C, and other *Salmonella* species, is reported much less commonly in infants than in older patients. Infected infants develop typical findings of neonatal sepsis and meningitis. Current data suggest that mortality is about 30%.[550] In utero infection with *S. typhi* has been described. Typhoid fever[518,551] and nontyphoidal *Salmonella* infections[552] during pregnancy put women at risk of aborting the fetus. Premature labor usually occurs during the second to the fourth week of maternal typhoid if the woman is untreated.[522] In a survey of typhoid fever in pregnancy during the preantibiotic era, 24 of 60 women with well-documented cases delivered prematurely, with resultant fetal death; the rest delivered at term, although only 17 infants survived.[553] The outlook for carrying the pregnancy to term and delivering a healthy infant appears to have improved dramatically during the antibiotic era. However, one of seven women with typhoid in a series still delivered a dead fetus with extensive liver necrosis.[554] In the preantibiotic era, about 14% of pregnant women with typhoid fever died.[555] With appropriate antimicrobial therapy, pregnancy does not appear to put the woman at increased risk of death. Despite these well-described cases, typhoid fever is rare early in life.

Of 1500 cases of typhoid fever that Osler and McCrae[556] reported, only 2 were in the first year of life. In areas where typhoid fever is still endemic, systematic search for infants with enteric fever has failed to find many cases. The few infections with *S. typhi* documented in children in the first year of life often present as a brief nondescript "viral syndrome" or as pneumonitis.[557,558] Fever, diarrhea, cough, vomiting, rash, and splenomegaly may occur; the fever may be high, and the duration of illness may be many weeks.[522]

Diagnosis

The current practice of early discharge of newborn infants, although potentially decreasing the risk of exposure, can make recognition of a nursery outbreak difficult. Diagnosis of neonatal salmonellosis should trigger an investigation for other cases. Other than diarrhea, signs of neonatal *Salmonella* infection are similar to the nonspecific findings seen in most neonatal infections. Lethargy, poor feeding, pallor, jaundice, apnea, respiratory distress, weight loss, and fever are common. Enlarged liver and spleen are common in those neonates with positive blood cultures. Laboratory studies are required to establish the diagnosis because the clinical picture is not distinct. The fecal leukocyte examination reveals polymorphonuclear leukocytes in 36% to 82%[359,559] of persons with *Salmonella* infection, but it has not been evaluated in neonates. Obviously, the presence of fecal leukocytes is consistent with colitis of any cause and therefore is a nonspecific finding. Routine stool cultures usually detect *Salmonella* if two or three different enteric media (i.e., MacConkey's, eosin-methylene blue, *Salmonella-Shigella*, Tergitol 7, xylose-lysine-deoxycholate, brilliant green, or bismuth sulfite agar) are used. Stool, rather than rectal swab material, is preferable for culture, particularly if the aim of culture is to detect carriers.[560] On the infrequent occasions when proctoscopy is performed, mucosal edema, hyperemia, friability, and hemorrhages may be seen.[461] Infants who are bacteremic often do not appear sufficiently toxic to raise the suspicion of bacteremia.[561] Blood cultures should be obtained as a routine part of evaluation of neonates with suspected or documented *Salmonella* infection. Ill neonates with *Salmonella* infection should have a cerebrospinal fluid examination performed. Bone marrow cultures also may be indicated when enteric fever is suspected. There are no consistent abnormalities in the white blood cell count. Serologic studies are not helpful in establishing the diagnosis, although antibodies to somatic[562,563] and flagellar antigens[487] develop in many infected newborns.

If an outbreak of salmonellosis is suspected, further characterization of the organism is imperative.[464] Determination of somatic and flagellar antigens to characterize the specific serotype may be critical to investigation of an outbreak. When the serotype found during investigation of an outbreak is a common one (e.g., *S. typhimurium*), antimicrobial resistance testing[475,565] and use of molecular techniques such as plasmid characterization[565] can be helpful in determining whether a single-strain, common-source outbreak is in progress.

Therapy

As in all enteric infections, attention to fluid and electrolyte abnormalities is the first issue that must be addressed by the physician. Specific measures to eradicate *Salmonella* intestinal infection have met with little success. Multiple studies show that antibiotic treatment of *Salmonella* gastroenteritis prolongs the excretion of *Salmonella*.[566-573] Almost one half of the infected children in the first 5 years of life continue to excrete *Salmonella* 12 weeks after the onset of infection; more than 5% have positive cultures at 1 year.[574] No benefit of therapy has been shown in comparisons of ampicillin or neomycin versus placebo,[570] chloramphenicol versus no antibiotic treatment,[569] neomycin versus placebo,[571] ampicillin or trimethoprim-sulfamethoxazole versus no antibiotic,[568] and ampicillin or amoxicillin versus placebo.[572] In contrast to these studies, data suggest that there may be a role for quinolone antibiotics in adults and children,[573,575] but these drugs are not approved for use in neonates, and resistance has been encountered.[576] Because these studies have few data as to the risk-benefit ratio of therapy in the neonate, it is uncertain whether they should influence treatment decisions in neonates. Studies that have included a small number of neonates suggest little benefit from antimicrobial therapy.[477,487,568,577,578] However, because bacteremia is common in neonates, antimicrobial therapy for infants younger than 3 months who have *Salmonella* gastroenteritis often is recommended,[532,533,561] especially if the infant appears toxic. Premature infants and those who have other significant debilitating conditions also should probably be treated. The duration of therapy is debatable but should probably be no more than 3 to 5 days if the infant is not seriously ill and if blood cultures are sterile. If toxicity, clinical deterioration, or documented bacteremia complicates gastroenteritis, prolonged treatment is indicated. Even with antimicrobial therapy, some infants develop complications. The relatively low risk of extraintestinal dissemination must be balanced against the well-documented risk of prolonging the carrier state. For infants who develop chronic diarrhea and malnutrition, hyperalimentation may be required; the role of antimicrobial agents in this setting is unclear. The infant with typhoid fever should be treated with an antimicrobial agent; relapses sometimes occur after therapy.

Colonized healthy infants discovered by stool cultures during evaluation of an outbreak ought to be isolated but probably should not receive antimicrobial therapy. Such infants should be discharged from the nursery as early as possible and followed carefully as outpatients.

Antimicrobial treatment of neonates who have documented extraintestinal dissemination must be prolonged. Bacteremia without localization is generally treated with at least a 10-day course of therapy. Therapy for *Salmonella* meningitis must be given for at least 4 weeks to lessen the risk of relapse. About three fourths of patients who have relapses have been treated for three weeks or less.[537] Similar to meningitis, treatment for osteomyelitis must be prolonged to be adequate. Although cures have been reported with 3 weeks of therapy, 4 to 6 weeks of therapy is recommended.

In vitro susceptibility data for *Salmonella* isolates must be interpreted with caution. The aminoglycosides show good in vitro activity but poor clinical efficacy, perhaps because of the low pH of the phagolysosome. Aminoglycosides have poor activity in an acid environment. The stability of some drugs in this acid environment also may explain in vitro and in vivo disparities. The intracellular localization and survival of *Salmonella* within phagocytic cells also presumably explains the relapses encountered with virtually every regimen. Resistance to antibiotics has long been a problem with *Salmonella* infection.[566,579,580] There has been a steady increase in resistance to *Salmonella* in the United States over the last 20 years.[581] With the emergence of *typhimurium* type DT 104, resistance to ampicillin, chloramphenicol, streptomycin, sulfonamides, and tetracycline has increased from 0.6% in 1979 and 1980 to 34% in 1996.[582] Resistance plasmids have been selected and transmitted, partly because therapy has been given for mild illness that should not have been treated[566] and partly because of use of antibiotics in animal feeds. Resistance to chloramphenicol and ampicillin has made trimethoprim-sulfamethoxazole increasingly important for the treatment of *Salmonella* infection in those patients who require therapy. However, with increasing resistance to all three of these agents in Asia,[583] the Middle East,[584] Africa,[585] Europe,[586,587] Argentina,[580] and North America,[579,588,589] the third-generation cephalosporins and quinolones represent drugs of choice for invasive salmonellosis. The quinolones currently are not approved for persons younger than 18 years. Cefotaxime, ceftriaxone, and cefoperazone represent acceptable alternative drugs for typhoidal and nontyphoidal salmonellosis when resistance is encountered.[590,591] Because the second-generation cephalosporins, such as cefuroxime, are less active in vitro than the third-generation cephalosporins and are not consistently clinically effective, they should not be used.[590,592] Data suggest that cefoperazone may sterilize blood and cause patients with typhoid fever to become afebrile more rapidly than with chloramphenicol,[593] perhaps because cefoperazone is excreted into bile in high concentrations.[594] The third-generation cephalosporins may have higher cure and lower relapse rates than ampicillin or chloramphenicol in children with *Salmonella* meningitis.[595] The doses of ampicillin, chloramphenicol, or cefotaxime used in infants with gastroenteritis pending results of blood cultures are the same as those used in treatment of sepsis. Because of the risk of gray baby syndrome, chloramphenicol should not be used in neonates unless other effective agents are not available. Trimethoprim-sulfamethoxazole, although useful in older children and adults, is not used in neonates because of the risk of kernicterus. Nosocomial infection with strains of *Salmonella* resistant to multiple antibiotics, including third-generation cephalosporins, has emerged as a problem in South America.[580]

Nonantibiotic interventions are important in the control of *Salmonella* infections. Limited data suggest that intravenous immune globulin (IGIV) (500 mg/kg on days 1, 2, 3, and 8 of therapy) along with antibiotic therapy may decrease the risk of bacteremia and death in preterm infants with *Salmonella* gastroenteritis.[596]

Prevention

Early recognition and intervention in nursery outbreaks of *Salmonella* are crucial to control. When a neonate develops salmonellosis, a search for other infants who have been in the same nursery should be undertaken. When two or more cases are recognized, environmental cultures, cultures of all infants, cohorting and contact isolation of infected infants, rigorous enforcement of hand hygiene, early discharge of infected infants, and thorough cleaning of all possible fomites in the nursery and delivery rooms are important elements of control. If cases continue to occur, the nursery should be closed to further admissions. Cultures of nursery personnel are likely to be helpful in the unusual situation of an *S. typhi* outbreak in which a chronic carrier may be among the caretakers. Culture of health care personnel during outbreaks of salmonellosis caused by other *Salmonella* species is debatable, although often recommended. Data suggest that nurses infected with *Salmonella* rarely infect patients in the hospital setting.[597] The fact that nursing personnel are sometimes found to be colonized during nursery outbreaks[468,474,487,489,490] may be a result rather than a cause of those epidemics.

The potential role of vaccines in control of neonatal disease is minimal. For the vast number of non–*S. typhi* serotypes, there is no prospect for an immunization strategy. Multiple doses of the commercially available oral live attenuated vaccine (Ty21a; *Vivotif*, Berna), has been shown in Chilean schoolchildren to reduce typhoid fever cases by more than 70%.[598,599] However, the vaccine is not recommended for persons younger than 6 years, in part because immunogenicity of Ty21a is age dependent; children younger than 24 months fail to respond with development of immunity.[600] Vi capsular polysaccharide vaccine is available for children older than 2 years and is effective in a single dose. Whether some degree of protection of infants could

Table 20–4 *Shigella* Serogroups

Serogroups	Species	No. of Serotypes
A	*S. dysenteriae*	13
B	*S. flexneri*	15 (including subtypes)
C	*S. boydii*	18
D	*S. sonnei*	1

occur if stool carriage were reduced or could be transferred to infants by the milk of vaccinated mothers' remains to be studied. Data suggest that breast-feeding may decrease the risk of other *Salmonella* infections.[601]

SHIGELLA

Nature of the Organism

On the basis of DNA relatedness, shigellae and *E. coli* organisms belong to the same species.[602] However, for historical reasons and because of their medical significance, shigellae have been maintained as separate species. Shigellae are gram-negative bacilli that are unlike typical *E. coli* in that they do not metabolize lactose or do so slowly, are non-motile, and generally produce no gas during carbohydrate use. They are classically divided into four species (serogroups) on the basis of metabolic and antigenic characteristics (Table 20-4). The mannitol nonfermenters usually are classified as *S. dysenteriae.* Although the lipopolysaccharide antigens of the 13 recognized members of this group are not related to each other antigenically, these serotypes are grouped together as serogroup A. Serogroup D (*Shigella sonnei*) are ornithine decarboxylase positive and slow lactose fermenters. All *S. sonnei* share the same lipopolysaccharide (O antigen). Those shigellae that ferment mannitol (unlike *S. dysenteriae*) but do not decarboxylate ornithine or ferment lactose (*S. sonnei*) belong to serogroups B and C. Of these, the strains that have lipopolysaccharide antigens immunologically related to each other are grouped together as serogroup B (*Shigella flexneri*), whereas those whose O antigens are not related to each other or to other shigellae are included in serogroup C (*Shigella boydii*). There are six major serotypes of *S. flexneri* and 13 subserotypes (1a, 1b, 2a, 2b, 3a, 3b, 4a, 4b, 5a, 5b, 6, X and Y variant). There are 19 antigenically distinct serotypes of *S. boydii.* For *S. dysenteriae* and *S. boydii* serogroup confirmation, pools of polyvalent antisera are used.

The virulence of shigellae has been studied extensively since their recognition as major pathogens at the beginning of the 20th century. The major determinants of virulence are encoded by a 120- to 140-MDa plasmid.[603,604] This plasmid, which is found in all virulent shigellae, encodes the synthesis of proteins that are required for invasion of mammalian cells and for the vigorous inflammatory response that is characteristic of the disease.[605,606] Shigellae that have lost this plasmid, have deletions of genetic material from the region involved in synthesis of these proteins, or have the plasmid inserted into the chromosome lose the ability to invade eukaryotic cells and become avirulent[607]; maintenance of the plasmid can be detected in the clinical microbiology lab by ability to bind Congo red. The ability to invade cells is the basic pathogenic property shared by all shigellae[608,609] and by the *Shigella*-like invasive *E. coli,* which also possesses the *Shigella* virulence plasmid.[205,605,606,610-611] In the laboratory, *Shigella* invasiveness is studied in tissue culture (HeLa cell invasion), in animal intestine, or in rabbit or guinea pig eye, where instillation of the organism causes keratoconjunctivitis (Sereny test).[128] Animal model studies have shown that bacteria penetrate and kill colonic mucosal cells and then elicit a brisk inflammatory response.

In addition to the virulence plasmid, several chromosomal loci enhance virulence.[612,613] This has been best studied in *S. flexneri* in which multiple virulence-enhancing regions of the chromosome have been defined.[604,612-614] The specific gene products of some of the chromosomal loci are not known; one chromosomal virulence segment encodes for synthesis of the O repeat units of lipopolysaccharide. Intact lipopolysaccharide is necessary but not sufficient to cause virulence.[612,615] At least two cell-damaging cytotoxins that also are chromosomally encoded are produced by shigellae. One of these toxins (Shiga toxin) is made in large quantities by *S. dysenteriae* serotype 1 (the Shiga bacillus) and is made infrequently by other shigellae.[616] Shiga toxin is a major virulence factor in *S. dysenteriae*, enhancing virulence at the colonic mucosa and also giving rise to sequelae similar to those caused by STEC (discussed earlier). This toxin kills cells by interfering with peptide elongation during protein synthesis.[617-619] Additional toxins may also be secreted by shigellae, although their roles in virulence are not established.[620]

Epidemiology

Although much of the epidemiology of shigellosis is predictable based on its infectious dose, certain elements are unexplained. Shigellae, like other organisms transmitted by the fecal-oral route, are commonly spread by food and water, but the low infecting inoculum allows person-to-person spread. Because of this low inoculum, *Shigella* is one of the few enteric pathogens that can infect swimmers.[621] The dose required to cause illness in adult volunteers is as low as 10 organisms for *S. dysenteriae* serotype 1,[622] about 200 organisms for *S. flexneri,*[623] and 500 organisms for *S. sonnei.*[624] Person-to-person transmission of infection probably explains the continuing occurrence of *Shigella* in the developed world. Enteropathogens that require large inocula and hence are best spread by food or drinking water are less common in industrialized societies because of sewage disposal facilities, water treatment, and food-handling practices. In the United States, daycare centers currently serve as a major focus for acquisition of shigellosis.[625] Numerous outbreaks of shigellosis related to crowding, poor sanitation, and the low dose required for diseases have occurred in this setting.

Given the ease of transmission, it is not surprising that the peak incidence of disease is in the first 4 years of life. It is, however, paradoxical that symptomatic infection is uncommon in the first year of life.[626-629] The best data on the age-related incidence of shigellosis come from Mata's[625] prospective studies of Guatemalan infants. In these studies, stool cultures were performed weekly on a group of children followed from birth to 3 years old. The rate of infection was more than 60-fold lower in the first 6 months of life than

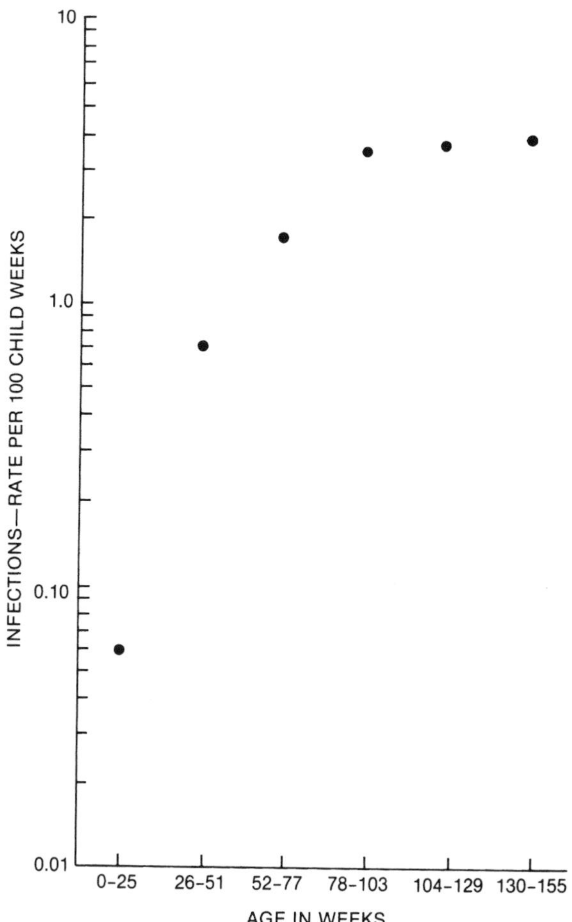

Figure 20–1 Age-related incidence of *Shigella* infection. (Data from Mata LG: The Children of Santa Maria Cauque: A Prospective Field Study of Health and Growth. Cambridge, Mass, MIT Press, 1978.)

between 2 and 3 years (Fig. 20-1).[626] The same age-related incidence has been described in the United States[629] and in a rural Egyptian village.[628] This anomaly has been explained by the salutary effects of breast-feeding.[630-632] However, it is likely that breast-feeding alone does not explain the resistance of infants to shigellosis.

A review of three large case series[633-635] suggests that about 1.6% (35 of 2225) of shigellosis cases occur in infants in the neonatal period. The largest series of neonatal shigellosis[632] suggests that the course, complications, and etiologic serogroups are different in neonates than in older children. Although newborns are routinely contaminated by maternal feces, neonatal shigellosis is rare.

Other aspects of the epidemiology of shigellosis elude simple explanation. The seasonality (summer-fall peak in the United States, rainy season peak in the tropics) is not well explained. The geographic variation in species causing infection likewise is not well understood. In the United States, most *Shigella* infections are caused by *S. sonnei* or, less commonly, *S. flexneri*. In most of the developing world, the relative importance of these two species is reversed, and other *Shigella* serotypes, especially *S. dysenteriae* serotype 1, are identified more frequently. As hygiene improves, the proportion of *S. sonnei* increases and that of *S. flexneri* decreases.[636] Data from Bangladesh suggest that *S. dysenteriae* is less common in neonates, but *S. sonnei* and *S. boydii* are more common.[632]

Clinical Manifestations

There appear to be some important differences in the relative frequencies of various complications of *Shigella* infection related to age. Some of these differences and estimates are based on data that are undoubtedly compromised by reporting biases. *S. dysenteriae* serotype 1 characteristically causes a more severe illness than other shigellae with more complications, including pseudomembranous colitis, hemolysis, and HUS. However, illnesses caused by various *Shigella* serotypes usually are indistinguishable from each other and conventionally are discussed together.

The incubation period of shigellosis is related to the number of organisms ingested, but in general, it is between 12 and 48 hours. Volunteer studies have shown that after ingestion, illness may be delayed for a week or more. Neonatal shigellosis seems to have a similar incubation period. More than one half of the neonatal cases occur within 3 days of birth, consistent with fecal-oral transmission during parturition. Mothers of infected neonates are sometimes carriers, although more typically they are symptomatic during the perinatal period. Intrauterine infection is rare. In the older child, the initial signs are usually high fever, abdominal pain, vomiting, toxicity, and large-volume watery stools; diarrhea may be bloody or may become bloody. Painful defecation and severe, crampy abdominal pain associated with frequent passage of small-volume stools with gross blood and mucus are characteristic findings in older children or adults who develop severe colitis. Many children, however, never develop bloody diarrhea. Adult volunteer studies have demonstrated that variations in presentation and course are not related to the dose ingested because some patients develop colitis with dysentery but others develop only watery diarrhea after ingestion of the same inoculum.[623] The neonate with shigellosis may have a mild diarrheal syndrome or a severe colitis.[633,637-645] Fever in neonates is usually low grade (<102° F) if the course is uncomplicated. The neonate has less bloody diarrhea, more dehydration, more bacteremia, and a greater likelihood of death than the older child.[632] Physical examination of the neonate may show signs of toxicity and dehydration, although fever, abdominal tenderness, and rectal findings are less striking than in the older child.[634]

Complications of shigellosis are common.[646] Although the illness is self-limited in the normal host, resolution may be delayed for a week or more. In neonates and malnourished children, chronic diarrhea may follow a bout of shigellosis.[637,645] Between 10% and 35% of hospitalized children with *Shigella* have convulsions before or during the course of diarrhea.[646-648] Usually, the seizures are brief, generalized, and associated with high fever. Seizures are uncommon in the first 6 months of life, although neonates have been described with seizures.[639,649] The cerebrospinal fluid generally reveals normal values in these children, but a few have mild cerebrospinal fluid pleocytosis. The neurologic outcome generally is good even with focal or prolonged seizures, but fatalities do occasionally occur, often associated with toxic encephalopathy.[650] Although the seizures had been postulated to result from the neurotoxicity of Shiga toxin, this explanation was proved to be incorrect because most shigellae make little or no Shiga toxin and the strains isolated from children with neurologic symptoms do not produce Shiga toxin.[616,651] Hemolysis with or without development of uremia is a complication primarily of *S. dysenteriae* serotype 1 infection.[652]

Sepsis during the course of shigellosis may be caused by the *Shigella* itself or by other gut flora that gain access to the bloodstream through damaged mucosa.[632,653,654] The risk of sepsis is higher in the first year of life, particularly in neonates,[632,637-639,649,656] in malnourished children, and in those with *S. dysenteriae* serotype 1 infection.[654] Sepsis occurs in up to 12% of neonates with shigellosis.[631,646,653,655] Given the infrequency of neonatal shigellosis, it is striking that 9% of reported cases of *Shigella* sepsis have involved infants in the first month of life.[657] One of the infants with bacteremia[658] reportedly had no discernible illness. Disseminated intravascular coagulation may develop in those patients whose course is complicated by sepsis. Meningitis has been described in a septic neonate. Colonic perforation has occurred in neonates,[630,659] older children,[660] and adults.[661] Although this complication of toxic megacolon is rare, it appears to be more common in neonates than in older individuals. Bronchopneumonia may complicate the course of shigellosis, but shigellae are rarely isolated from lungs or tracheal secretions.[662] The syndrome of sudden death in the setting of extreme toxicity with hyperpyrexia and convulsions but without dehydration or sepsis (i.e., Ekiri syndrome)[663-665] is rare in neonates. In the nonbacteremic child, other extraintestinal foci of infection, including vagina[666,667] and eye,[668] rarely occur. Reiter's syndrome, which rarely complicates the illness in children, has not been reported in neonates.

Although infection is less common in infants than in toddlers, case fatality rates are highest in infants.[669,670] The mortality rate in newborns appears to be about twice that of older children.[632] In industrialized societies, less than 1% of children with shigellosis die, whereas in developing countries, up to 30% die. These differences in mortality rates are related to nutrition,[633] availability of medical care, antibiotic resistance of many shigellae, the frequency of sepsis, and the higher frequency of *S. dysenteriae* serotype 1 infection in the less-developed world.[654]

Diagnosis

Although the diagnosis of shigellosis can be suspected on clinical grounds, other enteropathogens can cause illnesses that are impossible to distinguish clinically. Shigellosis in the neonate is rare. The neonate with watery diarrhea is more likely to be infected with *E. coli, Salmonella* or rotavirus than *Shigella.* Infants presenting with bloody diarrhea may have necrotizing enterocolitis or infection with *Salmonella,* EIEC, *Yersinia enterocolitica, C. jejuni,* or *Entamoeba histolytica.* Before cultures establish a diagnosis, clinical and laboratory data may aid in making a presumptive diagnosis. Abdominal radiographs demonstrating pneumatosis intestinalis suggest the diagnosis of necrotizing enterocolitis. A history of several weeks of illness not associated with fever and with few fecal leukocytes suggests *E. histolytica* rather than *Shigella* infection.[671]

The definitive diagnosis of shigellosis depends on isolation of the organism from stool. Unfortunately, culture may be insensitive.[672] In volunteer studies, daily stool cultures failed to detect shigellae in about 20% of symptomatic subjects.[623] Optimal recovery is achieved by immediate inoculation of stool (as opposed to rectal swabs) onto culture media. Use of transport media in general decreases the yield of cultures positive for *Shigella*[673] when compared with immediate inoculation.

Examination of stool for leukocytes as an indication of colitis is useful in support of the clinical suspicion of shigellosis. The white blood cell count and differential count also are used as supporting evidence for the diagnosis. Leukemoid reactions (white blood cells > 50,000/mm^3) occur in almost 15% of children with *S. dysenteriae* serotype 1 but in less than 2% of children with other shigellae.[651] Leukemoid reactions are more frequent in infants than in older children.[652] Even when the total white blood cell count is not dramatically elevated, there may be a striking left shift. Almost 30% of children with shigellosis have greater than 25% bands on the differential cell count.[674-676] Few reports address the white blood cell count in newborns, but those that do suggest that normal or low rather than elevated counts are more common. Although serum and fecal antibodies develop to lipopolysaccharides and the virulence plasmid-associated polypeptides,[677] serologic studies are not useful in the diagnosis of shigellosis. PCR can identify *Shigella* and EIEC in feces.[678] Colonoscopy typically shows inflammatory changes that are most severe in the distal segments of colon.[679]

Therapy

Because dehydration is particularly common in neonatal shigellosis, attention to correction of fluid and electrolyte disturbances is always the first concern when the illness is suspected. Although debate continues over the indications for antimicrobial therapy in the patient with shigellosis, the benefits of therapy generally appear to outweigh the risks. The chief disadvantages of antimicrobial therapy include cost, drug toxicity, and emergence of antibiotic-resistant shigellae. Because of the self-limited nature of shigellosis, it has been argued that less severe illness should not be treated. However, children can feel quite ill during the typical bout of shigellosis, and appropriate antimicrobial therapy shortens the duration of illness and eliminates shigellae from stool, decreasing secondary spread. Complications are probably decreased by antibiotics. Given the high mortality rates of neonatal shigellosis, therapy should not be withheld.

The empirical choice of an antimicrobial agent is dictated by susceptibility data for strains circulating in the community at the time the patient's infection occurs. Multiresistant shigellae complicate the choice of empirical therapy before availability of susceptibility data for the patient's isolate. Plasmid-encoded resistance (R factors) for multiple antibiotics has been observed frequently in *S. dysenteriae* serotype 1 outbreaks[682] and with other shigellae.[683-685] Antimicrobial resistance patterns fluctuate from year to year in a given locale.[686] However, despite the guesswork involved, early preemptive therapy is indicated when an illness is strongly suggestive of shigellosis. In vitro susceptibility does not always adequately predict therapeutic responses. Cefaclor,[687] furazolidone,[688] cephalexin,[689] amoxicillin,[690] kanamycin,[691] and cefamandole[692] all are relatively ineffective agents.

The optimal duration of therapy is debatable. Studies in children older than 2 years and in adults suggest that single-dose regimens may be as effective in relieving symptoms as courses given for 5 days. The single-dose regimens generally are not as effective in eliminating shigellae from the feces as are the longer courses. A third-generation cephalosporin, such as ceftriaxone, may be the best empirical choice. Optimal doses for newborns with shigellosis have not been established. Trimethoprim at a dose of 10 mg/kg/day (maximum, 160 mg/day) and sulfamethoxazole at a dose of 50 mg/kg/day (maximum, 800 mg/day) in two divided doses for a total of 5 days are recommended for the older child if the organism is susceptible.[693-695] If the condition of the infant does not permit orally administration, the drug usually is divided into three doses given intravenously over 1 hour.[696] Ampicillin at a dose of 100 mg/kg/day in four divided doses taken orally for 5 days may be used if the strain is susceptible.[676]

For the rare newborn who acquires shigellosis, appropriate therapy often is delayed until susceptibility data are available. This occurs because shigellosis is so rare in newborns that it is almost never the presumptive diagnosis of the child with watery or bloody diarrhea. Although a sulfonamide is as efficacious as ampicillin when the infecting strain is susceptible,[675] sulfonamides are avoided in neonates because of concern about the potential risk of kernicterus. The risk of empirical ampicillin therapy is that shigellae are frequently resistant to the drug; 50% of shigellae currently circulating in the United States are ampicillin resistant.[696,697] For the neonate infected with ampicillin-resistant *Shigella*, there are few data on which to base a recommendation. Ceftriaxone is generally active against shigellae, but in the neonate, this drug can displace bilirubin-binding sites and elicit clinically significant cholestasis. Data on children and adults suggest that clinical improvement occurs with ceftriaxone.[698,699] Quinolones, such as ciprofloxacin and ofloxacin, have been shown to be effective agents for treating shigellosis[700,701] in adults, but they are not approved for use in children younger than 18 years. Other drugs sometimes used to treat diarrhea pose special risks to the infant with shigellosis. The antimotility agents, in addition to their intoxication risk, may pose a special danger in dysentery. In adults, diphenoxylate hydrochloride with atropine has been shown to prolong fever and excretion of the organism.[702]

The response to appropriate antibiotic therapy is generally gratifying. Improvement is often obvious in less than 24 hours. Complete resolution of diarrhea may not occur until a week or more after the start of treatment. In those who have severe colitis or those infected by *S. dysenteriae* serotype 1, the response to treatment is somewhat delayed.

Prevention

For most of the developing world, the best strategy for prevention of shigellosis during infancy is prolonged breast-feeding. Specific antibodies in milk appear to prevent symptomatic shigellosis[66,68]; nonspecific modification of gut flora and the lack of bacterial contamination of human milk also may be important. Breast-feeding, even when other foods are consumed, decreases the risk of shigellosis; children who continue to consume human milk into the third year of life are still partially protected from illness.[703] In the United States, the best means of preventing infection in the infant is good hand hygiene when an older sibling or parent develops diarrhea. Even in unsanitary environments, secondary spread of shigellae can be dramatically decreased by hand hygiene after defecation and before meals.[704] Spread of shigellae in the hospital nursery can presumably be prevented by the use of contact isolation for infants with diarrhea and attention to thorough hand hygiene. Although nursery personnel have acquired shigellosis from infected newborns,[685] further transmission to other infants in the nursery, although described,[705] is rare. In contrast to *Salmonella*, large outbreaks of nosocomial shigellosis in neonates are rare.

Unfortunately, good hygiene is a particularly difficult problem in daycare centers. The gathering of susceptible children, breakdown in hand hygiene, failure to use different personnel for food preparation and diaper changing, and difficulty controlling the behavior of toddlers all contribute to daycare-focused outbreaks of shigellosis.

Immunization strategies have been studied since the turn of the 20th century, but no satisfactory immunization has been developed. Even if immunizations are improved, a role in managing neonates seems unlikely.

CAMPYLOBACTER

Nature of the Organism

Campylobacter was first recognized in an aborted sheep fetus in the early 1900s[706] and was named *Vibrio fetus* by Smith and Taylor in 1919.[707] This organism subsequently was identified as a major venereally transmitted cause of abortion and sterility and as a cause of scours in cattle, sheep, and goats.[708,709] It was not until 1947, when it was isolated from the blood culture of a pregnant woman who subsequently aborted at 6 months' gestation, that the significance of *Campylobacter* as a relatively rare cause of bacteremia and perinatal infections in humans was appreciated.[710-712] During the 1970s, *Campylobacter* was recognized to be an opportunistic pathogen in debilitated patients.[713,714] In 1963, *V. fetus* and related organisms were separated from the vibrios (such as *V. cholerae* and *V. parahaemolyticus*) and placed in a new genus, *Campylobacter* (Greek word for "curved rod").[715] Since 1973, several *Campylobacter* species have been recognized as a common cause of enteritis[716-732] and, in some cases, extraintestinal infections.

The genus *Campylobacter* contains 15 species, most of which are recognized as animal and human pathogens. The most commonly considered causes of human disease are *Campylobacter fetus, Campylobacter jejuni, Campylobacter coli, Campylobacter lari,* and *Campylobacter upsaliensis* (Table 20-5),[730-732] although *Campylobacter mucosalis* has been isolated from stool of children with diarrhea.[733] DNA hybridization studies have shown that these species are distinct, sharing less than 35% DNA homology under stringent hybridization conditions.[734,735] *Helicobacter pylori* was originally named *Campylobacter pylori,* but because of differences in DNA, it was reclassified and is no longer considered in the *Campylobacter* genus.

Strains of *C. fetus* are divided into two subspecies: *C. fetus* subsp. *fetus* and *C. fetus* subsp. *venerealis.* The first subspecies causes sporadic abortion in cattle and sheep[736,737]; in

Table 20–5 *Campylobacter* Species That Infect Humans

Current Nomenclature	Previous Nomenclature	Usual Disease Produced
C. fetus	*Vibrio fetus* *V. fetus* var. *intestinalis* *C. fetus* subsp. *intestinalis*	Bacteremia, meningitis, perinatal infection, intravascular infection
C. jejuni	*Vibrio jejuni*	Diarrhea
C. coli	*C. fetus* subsp. *jejuni*	Diarrhea
C. lari	Grouped with *C. jejuni,* nalidixic acid–resistant, thermophilic *Campylobacter,* *C. laridis I*	Diarrhea, bacteremia
C. upsaliensis	None	Diarrhea, bacteremia
C. hyointestinalis	None	Diarrhea, bacteremia
C. concisus	None	Diarrhea

the human fetus and newborn, it causes perinatal and neonatal infections that result in abortion, premature delivery, bacteremia, and meningitis.[710-712,736-748] Outside the newborn period, *Campylobacter* is a relatively infrequent cause of bacteremia, usually infecting those with impaired host defenses, including the elderly or the debilitated; less frequently, it causes intravascular infection.[713-715,749,750]

By far the most common syndrome caused by a *Campylobacter* species is enteritis. *C. jejuni* and *C. coli* cause gastroenteritis and generally are referred to collectively as *C. jejuni,* although DNA hybridization studies show them to be different. In the laboratory, *C. jejuni* can be differentiated from *C. coli* because it is capable of hydrolyzing hippurate, whereas *C. coli* is not. Most isolates that are associated with diarrhea (61% to 100%) are identified as *C. jejuni,*[751-754] and in some cases, individuals have been shown to be simultaneously infected with *C. jejuni* and *C. coli.*[752]

Because of the fastidious nature of *C. jejuni,* which is difficult to isolate from fecal flora, its widespread occurrence was not recognized until 1973.[716-732] Previously called *related vibrios* by King,[749] this organism had been associated with bloody diarrhea and colitis in infants and adults only when it had been associated with a recognized bacteremia.[755-757] In the late 1970s, development of selective fecal culture methods for *C. jejuni* enabled its recognition worldwide as one of the most common causes of enteritis in persons of all ages. It is an uncommon infection in neonates who generally develop gastroenteritis when infected.[718,758-881] Bacteremia with *C. jejuni* enteritis also is uncommon.[718,759,764,769,772-778] Maternal symptoms considered to be related to *C. jejuni* infection generally are mild and include fever (75%) and diarrhea (30%). In contrast to the serious disease in newborns that is caused by *C. fetus,* neonatal infections with *C. jejuni* usually result in a mild illness,[758,760,762,763,765-768,771,778] although meningitis occurs in rare instances.[761,769] Third trimester infection related to *C. fetus* or *C. jejuni* may results in abortion or stillbirth.

Pathogenesis

C. fetus does not produce recognized enterotoxins or cytotoxins and does not appear to be locally invasive by the Sereny test.[714,731] Instead, these infections may be associated with penetration of the organism through a relatively intact intestinal mucosa to the reticuloendothelial system and bloodstream.[714] Whether this reflects a capacity to resist serum factors or to multiply intracellularly remains to be determined.

C. jejuni is capable of producing illness by several mechanisms. These organisms have been shown to produce an LT enterotoxin and a cytotoxin.[779-782] This enterotoxin is known to be a heat-labile protein with a molecular mass of 60 to 70 MDa.[779,782] It shares functional and immunologic properties with cholera toxin and *E. coli* LT. *C. jejuni* and *C. coli* also elaborate a cytotoxin that is toxic for a number of mammalian cells.[783-785] The toxin is heat labile, trypsin sensitive, and not neutralized by immune sera to Shiga toxin or the cytotoxin of *Clostridium difficile.* The role of these toxins as virulence factors in diarrheal disease remains unproved.[779,784]

Several animal models have been tested for use in the study of this pathogen.[786] Potential models for the study of *C. jejuni* enteritis include dogs, which may acquire symptomatic infection[787]; 3- to 8-day old chicks[788-790]; chicken embryo cells, which are readily invaded by *C. jejuni*[725]; rhesus monkeys[791]; and rabbits by means of the removable intestinal tie adult rabbit technique. An established small mammal model that mimics human disease in the absence of previous treatment or surgical procedure has not been successful in adult mice.[792] An infant mouse model[793,794] and a hamster model[795] of diarrhea appear promising. *C. jejuni* is negative in the Sereny test for invasiveness,[796] and most investigators report no fluid accumulation in ligated rabbit ileal loops.

Pathology

The pathologic findings of *C. fetus* infection in the perinatal period include placental necrosis[711] and, in the neonate, widespread endothelial proliferation, intravascular fibrin deposition, perivascular inflammation, and hemorrhagic necrosis in the brain.[797] The tendency for intravascular location and hepatosplenomegaly in adults infected with *C. fetus* has been shown.[714]

The pathologic findings in infants and children infected with *C. fetus* can include an acute inflammatory process in the colon or rectum, as evidenced by the tendency for patients to have bloody diarrhea with numerous fecal leukocytes.[798] There also can be crypt abscess formation and an ulcerative colitis or pseudomembranous colitis–like appearance[799,800] or a hemorrhagic jejunitis or ileitis.[717,725,801,802] Mesenteric lymphadenitis, ileocolitis and acute appendicitis also have been described.

Epidemiology

Infection with *Campylobacter* species occurs after ingestion of contaminated food, including unpasteurized milk, poultry, and contaminated water.[726,803-812] Many farm animals and pets, such as chickens,[813] dogs,[814,815] and cats (especially young animals), are potential sources. The intrafamilial spread of infection in households,[717,816] the occurrence of outbreaks in nurseries,[769,770,817] and the apparent laboratory acquisition of *C. jejuni*[818] all suggest that *C. jejuni* infection may occur after person-to-person transmission of the organism. Outbreaks of *C. jejuni* in the child daycare setting are not common. Volunteer studies[819] have shown a variable range in the infecting dose, with many volunteers developing no illness. The report of illness after ingestion of 10^6 organisms in a glass of milk[728] and production of illness in a single volunteer by 500 organisms[819] substantiate the variation in individual susceptibility. The potential for low-inoculum disease has significant implications for the importance of strict enteric precautions when infected persons are hospitalized, particularly in maternity and nursery areas. When diarrhea in neonates caused by *C. jejuni* has been reported,[758-771] maternal-infant transmission during labor has generally been documented.[758-763,765-768,770,771] The Lior serotyping system, restriction length polymorphism, and pulse-field gel electrophoresis [820] have been used to confirm the identity of the infant and maternal isolates. Most mothers gave no history of diarrhea during pregnancy.[762,763,765,766] Outbreaks have occurred in neonatal intensive care units because of person-to-person spread.[820]

The frequency of asymptomatic carriage of *C. jejuni* ranges from 0% to 1.3%[716,717] to as high as 13% to 85%.[716,717,732,821-823] In a cohort study in Mexico, 66% of all infections related to *C. jejuni* were asymptomatic.[732] Infected children, if untreated, can be expected to excrete the organisms for 3 or 4 weeks; however, more than 80% are culture negative after 5 weeks.[721,722] Asymptomatic excreters pose a significant risk in the neonatal period, in which acquisition from an infected mother can be clinically important.[718,760,762,766] *C. jejuni* has increasingly been recognized as a cause of watery and inflammatory diarrhea in temperate and tropical climates throughout the world. It has been isolated from 2% to 11% of all fecal cultures from patients with diarrheal illnesses in various parts of the world.[716-724,728,824-829] There is a tendency for *C. jejuni* enteritis to occur in the summer in countries with temperate climates.[825]

The reservoir of *Campylobacter* is the gastrointestinal tract of domestic and wild birds and animals. It infects sheep, cattle, goats, antelope, swine, chickens, domestic turkeys, and pet dogs. *C. fetus* often is carried asymptomatically in the intestinal or biliary tracts of sheep and cattle. During the course of a bacteremic illness in pregnant animals, *C. fetus* organisms, which have a high affinity for placental tissue, invade the uterus and multiply in the immunologically immature fetus. The infected fetuses generally are aborted. Whether this organism is acquired by humans from animals or is carried asymptomatically for long periods in humans, who may then transmit the organism through sexual contact as appears to occur in animals, is unclear. It is believed that this subspecies rarely is found in the human intestine and that it is not a cause of human enteritis.[725] *C. fetus* infections predominantly occur in older men with a history of farm or animal exposure and in pregnant women in their third trimester.[710,711,716,717] Symptomatically or asymptomatically infected women may have recurrent abortions or premature deliveries and are the source of organisms associated with life-threatening perinatal infections of the fetus or newborn infant.[710,739-748,830] In several instances of neonatal sepsis and meningitis, *C. fetus* was isolated from culture of maternal cervix or vagina.[712,747,795] A nosocomial nursery outbreak has been associated with carriage in some healthy infants.[831] Other outbreaks have been associated with meningitis [832,833] Cervical cultures have remained positive in women who have had recurrent abortions and whose husbands have antibody titer elevations.[738]

The most commonly incriminated reservoir of *C. jejuni* is poultry.[808,812,834,835] Most chickens in several different geographic locations had a large number (mean, 4×10^6/g) of *C. jejuni* in the lower intestinal tract or feces. This occurred in some instances despite the use of tetracycline, to which the *Campylobacter* was susceptible in vitro, in the chicken feed.[828] The internal cavities of chickens remain positive for *Campylobacter* even after they have been cleaned, packaged, and frozen.[834] However, unlike *Salmonella, C. jejuni* organisms that survive usually do not multiply to high concentrations.[725] Domestic puppies or kittens with *C. jejuni* diarrhea also can provide a source for spread, especially to infants or small children.[717,755,812,836-838]

C. jejuni enteritis also has been associated in a number of outbreaks with consumption of unpasteurized milk.[725,809-811,839-841] In retrospect, the first reported human cases of *C. jejuni* enteritis were probably in a milk-borne outbreak reported in 1946.[842] Because *Campylobacter* infections of the udder are not seen, milk is probably contaminated from fecal shedding of the organism. These organisms are killed by adequate heating.

Fecally contaminated water is a potential vehicle for *C. jejuni* infections.[843] Several phenotypic and genotypic methods have been used for distinguishing *C. jejuni* strains from animals and humans involved in epidemics.[844] *C. jejuni* is associated with traveler's diarrhea among those traveling from England or the United States.[720]

Clinical Manifestations

Clinical manifestations of infection caused by *Campylobacter* depend on the species involved (see Table 20-5). Human infections with *C. fetus* are rare and generally are limited to bacteremia in patients with predisposing conditions[749,750] or to bacteremia or uterine infections with prolonged fever and pneumonitis that lasts for several weeks in women during the third trimester of pregnancy. Unless appropriately treated, symptoms usually resolve only after abortion or delivery of an infected infant.[710,712,739-748,750] These infected neonates, who are often premature, develop signs suggesting sepsis, including fever, cough, respiratory distress, vomiting, diarrhea, cyanosis, convulsions, and jaundice. The condition typically progresses to meningitis, which may be rapidly fatal or may result in serious neurologic sequelae.[712] Additional systemic manifestations include pericarditis, pneumonia, peritonitis, salpingitis, septic arthritis, and abscesses.[823]

C. jejuni infection typically involves the gastrointestinal tract, producing watery diarrhea or a dysentery-like illness with fever and abdominal pain and stools that contain blood and mucus.[715,732,800] Older infants and children generally are affected, but neonates with diarrhea have been reported. Infection in neonates generally is not clinically apparent or is mild. Stools can contain blood, mucus, and pus[712,721,762,763]; fever often is absent.[721,762] The illness usually responds to appropriate antimicrobial therapy,[760,762,816] which shortens the period of fecal shedding.[845] Extraintestinal infections related to *C. jejuni* other than bacteremia are rare but include cholecystitis,[846] urinary tract infection,[847] and meningitis.[761] Bacteremia is a complication of gastrointestinal infection,[848] especially in malnourished children.[849] Meningitis that appears to occur secondary to intestinal infection also has been reported in premature infants who have had intraventricular needle aspirations for neonatal hydrocephalus.[712] Complications in older children and adults that have been associated with *C. jejuni* enteritis include Reiter's syndrome,[850] Guillain-Barré syndrome,[851,852] and reactive arthritis.[853,854] Persistent *C. jejuni* infections have been described in patients infected with human immunodeficiency virus.[855] Extraintestinal manifestations generally occur in patients who are immunosuppressed or at the extremes of age.[714] *Campylobacter lari* has caused chronic diarrhea and bacteremia in a neonate.[856]

Diagnosis

Most important in the diagnosis of *Campylobacter* infection is a high index of suspicion based on clinical grounds. *C. fetus* and *C. jejuni* are fastidious and may be overlooked on routine fecal cultures. Isolation of *Campylobacter* from blood or other sterile body sites does not represent the same problem as isolation from stool. Growth occurs with standard blood culture media, but it may be slow. In the case of *C. fetus* infecting the bloodstream or central nervous system, blood culture flasks should be blindly subcultured and held for at least 7 days or the organism may not be detected because of slow or inapparent growth.[742] The diagnosis of *C. fetus* infection should be considered when there is an unexplained febrile illness in the third trimester of pregnancy or in the event of recurrent abortion, prematurity, or neonatal sepsis with or without meningitis. A high index of suspicion and prompt, appropriate antimicrobial therapy may prevent the potentially serious neonatal complications that may follow maternal *C. fetus* infection.

Campylobacter is distinguished from the *Vibrio* organisms by its characteristics of carbohydrate nonfermentation and by its different nucleotide base composition.[715,733-735,738] *Campylobacter* is 0.2 to 0.5 fm wide and 0.5 to 8.0 long. It is a fastidious, microaerophilic, curved, motile gram-negative bacillus that has a single polar flagellum and is oxidase and catalase positive, except for *C. upsaliensis,* which is generally catalase negative or weakly positive. *C. jejuni* and *C. fetus* are separated by growth temperature (*C. fetus* grows best at 25° C but can be cultured at 37° C; *C. jejuni* grows best at 42° C) and by nalidixic acid and cephalosporin susceptibilities, because *C. jejuni* is susceptible to nalidixic acid and resistant to cephalosporins. *C. jejuni* grows best in a microaerobic environment of 5% oxygen and 10% carbon dioxide at 42° C. It grows on a variety of media, including *Brucella* and Mueller-Hinton agars, but optimal isolation requires the addition of selective and nutritional supplements. Growth at 42° C in the presence of cephalosporins is used to culture selectively for *C. jejuni* from fecal specimens. In a study of six media, charcoal-based selective media and a modified charcoal cefoperazone deoxycholate agar were the most selective for identification of *Campylobacter* species. Extending the incubation time from 48 to 72 hours led to an increase in the isolation rate regardless of the medium used.[857] Its typical darting motility may provide a clue to identification, even in fresh fecal specimens, when viewed by phase-contrast microscopy.[721,858]

When the organism has been cultured, it is presumptively identified by motility and by its curved, sometimes sea gull–like appearance on carbolfuchsin stain. Polymorphonuclear leukocytes are usually found in stools when bloody diarrhea occurs and indicate the occurrence of colitis.[762,798] To avoid potentially serious *C. jejuni* infection in the newborn infant, careful histories of any diarrheal illnesses in the family should be obtained, and pregnant women with any enteric illness should have cultures for this and other enteric pathogens. Detection of *C. jejuni* and *C. coli* by PCR has been reported[859] and in the future may be useful for the rapid and reliable identification of this organism.

The differential diagnosis of *C. fetus* infections include the numerous agents that cause neonatal sepsis or meningitis, especially gram-negative bacilli. Diagnostic considerations for inflammatory or bloody enteritis include necrotizing enterocolitis, allergic proctitis, and *Salmonella;* rarely *Shigella,* and other infectious agents occur. Agglutination, complement fixation, bactericidal, immunofluorescence, and ELISA tests have been used for serologic diagnosis of *C. jejuni* infection and to study the immune response, but these assays are of limited value in establishing the diagnosis during an acute infection.[731]

Therapy

The prognosis is grave in newborn infants with sepsis or meningitis caused by *C. fetus.* In infants with *C. jejuni* gastroenteritis, limited data suggest that appropriate, early antimicrobial therapy results in improvement and rapid clearance of the organism from stool.[845] *Campylobacter* species are often resistant to β-lactams, including ampicillin and cephalosporins.[860,861] Most strains are susceptible to erythromycin, gentamicin, tetracycline, chloramphenicol, and the newer quinolones, although resistance to these agents has been reported.[862,863] It appears that a parenteral aminoglycoside is the drug of choice for *C. fetus* infections, pending in vitro susceptibility studies. In the case of central nervous system involvement, cefotaxime and chloramphenicol are potential alternative drugs. Depending on in vitro susceptibilities, which vary somewhat with locale, erythromycin is the drug of choice for treating *C. jejuni* enteritis.[717,721,722] If erythromycin therapy is initiated within the first 4 days of illness, a reduction in excretion of the organism and resolution of symptoms occur.[845] Although data regarding treatment of asymptomatic or convalescent carriers are not available, it seems appropriate to treat colonized pregnant women in the third trimester of pregnancy when there is a risk of perinatal or neonatal infection. The failure of prophylactic parenteral gentamicin in a premature infant has been documented, followed by successful resolution of symptoms and fecal shedding with erythromycin. Because there appears to be an increased risk of toxicity with erythromycin estolate during pregnancy and infancy,[864] other forms of erythromycin should probably be used in these settings. Azithromycin appears to be effective if the organism is susceptible.[865] Strains that are erythromycin resistant often are resistant to azithromycin.[866] *Campylobacter* tends to have higher minimal inhibitory concentrations for clarithromycin than for azithromycin.[867] Furazolidone has been used in children and ciprofloxacin in nonpregnant patients older than 17 years.

Prevention

Contact precautions should be employed during any acute diarrheal illness and until the diarrhea has subsided. Hand hygiene after handling raw poultry and washing cutting boards and utensils with soap and water after contact with raw poultry may decrease risk of infection. Pasteurization of milk and chlorination of water are critically important. Infected food handlers and hospital employees who are asymptomatic pose no known hazard for disease transmission if proper personal hygiene measures are maintained. Ingestion of human milk that contains anti–*C. jejuni* antibodies has been shown to protect infants from diarrhea due to *C. jejuni*.[63,868]

CLOSTRIDIUM DIFFICILE

Nature of the Organism and Pathophysiology

C. difficile is a spore-forming, gram-positive, anaerobic bacillus that produces two toxins. In the presence of antibiotic pressure, *C. difficile* colonic overgrowth and toxin production occur. The virulence properties of *C. difficile* are related to production of an enterotoxin that causes fluid secretion (toxin A) and a cytotoxin detectable by its cytopathic effects in tissue culture (toxin B).[869,870] Both toxin genes have been cloned and sequenced, revealing that they encode proteins with estimated molecular masses of 308 kDa for toxin A and 270 kDa for toxin B.[871]

A wide variety of antibacterial, antifungal, antituberculosis, and antineoplastic agents have been associated with *C. difficile* colitis, although penicillin, clindamycin, and cephalosporins are associated most frequently. Rarely, no precipitating drug has been given.[872-876] *C. difficile* and its toxins can be demonstrated in up to one third of patients with antibiotic-associated diarrhea and in about 98% of patients with pseudomembranous colitis.[877]

Epidemiology

C. difficile can be isolated from soil and frequently exists in the hospital environment. Spores of *C. difficile* are acquired from the environment or by fecal-oral transmission from colonized individuals or from items in the environment such as thermometers and feeding tubes.[878-883] *C. difficile* has been demonstrated to persist on a contaminated floor for 5 months.[879] Nosocomial spread is related to organisms on the hands of personnel[879,880,884] and to contaminated surfaces, which may serve as reservoirs.[885,886] Although all groups are susceptible to infection, newborn infants represent a special problem. Less than 5% of healthy children older than 2 years[887] and healthy adults carry *C. difficile*,[877] but more than 50% of neonates can be demonstrated to have *C. difficile* and its cytotoxin in their stools, usually in the absence of clinical findings.[880,886,888-890] Infants in neonatal intensive care units have high rates of colonization, in part because of frequent use of antimicrobial agents in these units.[889-890] Clustering of infected infants suggests that much of the colonization of newborn infants represents nosocomial spread[886] rather than acquisition of maternal flora. The number of *C. difficile* organisms present in stools of well infants is similar to that found in older patients with pseudomembranous colitis.[890] The high frequency of colonization has led to justified skepticism about the pathogenic potential of this organism in the very young.[891] Although some episodes of diarrhea in early infancy may be caused by *C. difficile*,[892] the diagnostic criteria used in older children and adults are inadequate to establish a definite diagnosis in this age group.

Clinical Manifestations

The usual manifestations of *C. difficile* disease in older children and adults include watery diarrhea, abdominal pain and tenderness, nausea, vomiting, and low-grade fever. Grossly bloody diarrhea is unusual, although occult fecal blood is common. Leukocytosis is present during severe illness. Diarrhea usually begins 4 to 9 days into a course of antimicrobial therapy but may be delayed until several weeks after completion of the therapeutic course. Usually, the illness is mild and self-limited if the offending drug is discontinued. Severe colitis with pseudomembranes is less common now than in previous years because the risk of diarrhea developing during antimicrobial therapy is recognized and the antimicrobial agent typically is stopped.

It is unclear whether this organism causes disease in newborns. One study from a newborn intensive care unit suggests that toxin A in stools is associated with an increased frequency of abnormal stools.[893]

Diagnosis

Endoscopic findings of pseudomembranes and hyperemic, friable rectal mucosa suggest the diagnosis of pseudomembranous colitis. Pseudomembranes are not always present in *C. difficile* colitis; mild cases are often described as nonspecific colitis. Several noninvasive techniques are used to establish the diagnosis, including enzyme immunoassay (EIA) for toxin detection and PCR.[893-896] Isolation of *C. difficile* from stool does not distinguish between toxigenic and nontoxigenic isolates. If *C. difficile* is isolated, testing for toxin by cell culture or EIA should be performed to confirm the presence of a toxigenic strain. There are multiple commercially available EIAs that detect either toxin A or both toxins A and B.[893-895] These assays are sensitive and easy to perform. Other assays are available for epidemiologic investigation of outbreaks of disease due to *C. difficile*.[896]

In older children and adults, the diagnosis is confirmed by culture of *C. difficile* and demonstration of toxin in feces. In neonates, these data are inadequate to prove that an illness is related to *C. difficile*. When the clinical picture is consistent, the stool studies are positive for *C. difficile* and no other cause for illness is found, a diagnosis of "possible" *C. difficile* is made. A favorable response to eradication of *C. difficile* is supportive evidence that the diagnosis is correct.[872]

Because of the uncertainty implicit in the ambiguity of neonatal diagnostic criteria, other diagnoses must be considered.

Therapy

When the decision is made that a neonate's illness might be related to *C. difficile,* the initial approach should include fluid and electrolyte therapy and discontinuation of the offending antimicrobial agent. If the illness persists or worsens or if the patient has severe diarrhea, specific therapy with metronidazole[886,897] should be instituted. Metronidazole is considered to be the treatment of choice for most patients with *C. difficile* colitis.[898] Rarely is there a need to consider orally administered vancomycin or bacitracin in neonates.[899,900]

After initiation of therapy, signs of illness generally resolve within several days, titers decrease, and fecal toxins disappear eventually. Recurrence of colitis after discontinuation of metronidazole or vancomycin has been documented in 10% to 20% of adults.[901] Relapses are treated with a second course of metronidazole or vancomycin. Drugs that decrease intestinal motility should not be administered.

Neutralizing antibody against *C. difficile* cytotoxin has been demonstrated in human colostrum.[902] Secretory component of sIgA binds to toxin A to inhibit its binding to receptors [903] Data show that there are nonantibody factors present in milk that interfere with the action of toxin B in addition to secretory IgA directed at toxin A.[904] Breast-feeding appears to decrease the frequency of colonization by *C. difficile.*[905]

Prevention

In addition to standard precautions, contact precautions are recommended for the duration of illness. Meticulous hand hygiene techniques, proper handling of contaminated waste and fomites, and limiting the use of antimicrobial agents are the best available methods for control of *C. difficile* infection.

VIBRIO CHOLERAE

Nature of the Organism

V. cholerae is a gram-negative, curved bacillus with a polar flagellum. Of the many serotypes, only enterotoxin-producing organisms of serotype O1 and O139 cause epidemics. *V. cholerae* O1 is divided into two serotypes, Inaba and Ogawa, and two biotypes, classic and El Tor; the latter is the predominant biotype. Nontoxigenic O1 strains and non-O1 strains of *V. cholerae* can cause diarrhea and sepsis but do not cause outbreaks.[906-908]

Pathogenesis

V. cholerae O group 1 is the classic example of an enteropathogen whose virulence is caused by enterotoxin production. Cholera toxin is an 84-MDa protein whose five B subunits cause toxin binding to the enterocyte membrane ganglioside GM_1 and whose A subunit causes adenosine diphosphate ribosylation of a guanosine triphosphate–binding regulatory subunit of adenylate cyclase.[105,908] The elevated cAMP levels that result from stimulation of enterocytes by cholera toxin cause secretion of salt and water with concomitant inhibition of absorption. Two other toxins are also encoded within the virulence cassette that encodes cholera toxin. These toxins, zona occludens toxin (zot) and accessory cholera toxin (ace), are consistently found in illness-causing strains of O1 and O139 but not usually in *V. cholerae* organisms that are less virulent.

Epidemiology

Since 1960, *V. cholerae* O1, biotype El Tor, has spread from India and Southeast Asia to Africa, the Middle East, southern Europe, and the southern, western, and central Pacific islands (Oceania). In late January of 1991, toxigenic *V. cholerae* O1, serotype Inaba, biotype El Tor, appeared in several coastal cities of Peru.[907,908] It rapidly spread to most countries in South and North America. In reported cases, travel from the United States to Latin America or Asia and ingestion of contaminated food transported from Latin America or Asia have been incriminated. *V. cholerae* O139 (Bengal) arose on the Indian subcontinent as a new cause of epidemic cholera in 1993.[910-915] It rapidly spread through Asia and continues to periodically reemerge as a cause of epidemic cholera. In the United States, an endemic focus of a unique strain of toxigenic *V. cholerae* O1 exists on the Gulf Coast of Louisiana and Texas.[906,916] This strain is different from the one associated with the epidemic in South America. Most cases of disease associated with the strain endemic to the U.S. Gulf Coast have resulted from the consumption of raw or undercooked shellfish. Humans are the only documented natural host, but free-living *V. cholerae* organisms can exist in the aquatic environment. The usual reported vehicles of transmission have included contaminated water or ice; contaminated food, particularly raw or undercooked shellfish; moist grains held at ambient temperature; and raw or partially dried fish. The usual mode of infection is ingestion of contaminated food or water. Boiling water or treating it with chlorine or iodine and adequate cooking of food kill the organism.[907] Asymptomatic infection of family contacts is common but direct person-to-person transmission of disease has not been documented. Persons with low gastric acidity are at increased risk for cholera infection.

Clinical Manifestations

Cholera acquired during pregnancy, particularly in the third trimester, is associated with a high incidence of fetal death.[917] Miscarriage can be attributed to a fetal acidosis and hypoxemia resulting from the marked metabolic and circulatory changes that this disease induces in the mother. It is not surprising that the likelihood of delivering a stillborn child is closely correlated with the severity of the maternal illness. The inability to culture *V. cholerae* from stillborn infants of infected mothers, together with the usual absence of bacteremia in cholera, suggests that transplacental fetal infection is not a cause of intrauterine death.

Neonatal cholera is a rare disease. This generalization also applies to the new O139 strains, although mild[918] and severe forms of illness have rarely been described in newborns.[919] Among 242 neonates admitted to a cholera research hospital in Dacca, Bangladesh, there were 25 infants ill with cholera.[920]

Even infants born to mothers with active diarrheal disease may escape infection, despite evidence that rice-water stools, almost certain to be ingested during the birth process, may contain as many as 10^9 organisms/mL.[920] The reason for this apparently low attack rate among newborns is not certain; however, it probably can be attributed in large part to the protection conferred by breast-feeding.[921] Human milk contains antibodies[62] and receptor-like glycoprotein that inhibit adherence of *V. cholerae*[64] and gangliosides that bind cholera toxin.[65] The role of transplacentally acquired vibriocidal maternal antibodies has not been determined.[922] Because *V. cholerae* causes neither bacteremia nor intestinal invasion, protection against illness is more likely to be a function of mucosal rather than serum antibodies.[923,924] Additional factors that may reduce the incidence of neonatal cholera include the large inoculum required for infection[925] and the limited exposure of the newborn to the contaminated food and water.[229]

Diagnosis

Clinicians should request that appropriate cultures be performed for stool specimens from persons suspected of having cholera. The specimen is plated on thiosulfate citrate bile salts sucrose agar directly or after enrichment in alkaline peptone water. Isolates of *V. cholerae* should be confirmed at a state health department and then sent to the CDC for testing for production of cholera toxin. A fourfold rise in vibriocidal antibody titers between acute and convalescent serum samples or a fourfold decline in titers between early and late (>2 months) convalescent serum specimens can confirm the diagnosis. Probes have been developed to test for cholera toxin.[926,927]

Therapy and Prevention

The most important modality of therapy is administration of oral or parenteral rehydration therapy to correct dehydration and electrolyte imbalance and maintain hydration.[907] Antimicrobial therapy can eradicate vibrios, reduce the duration of diarrhea, and reduce requirements for fluid replacement. One cholera vaccine, which is administered parenterally, is licensed in the United States but is of very limited value. Several experimental oral vaccines are being tested.[928-930]

YERSINIA ENTEROCOLITICA

Nature of the Organism, Epidemiology, and Pathogenesis

Y. enterocolitica is a major cause of enteritis in much of the industrialized world.[931,932] Enteritis due to this organism primarily occurs in infants and young children, and infections in the United States are reported to be more common in the North than in the South.[933-938] Animals, especially swine, have been shown to serve as the reservoir for *Y. enterocolitica*. A history of recent exposure to chitterlings (i.e., pig intestine) is common. Transmission has also occurred after ingestion of contaminated milk and infusion of contaminated blood products.[939,940]

Virulence of *Y. enterocolitica* is related primarily to a virulence plasmid, which is closely related to the virulence plasmids of *Yersinia pseudotuberculosis* and *Yersinia pestis*.[941,942] An ST enterotoxin, which is closely related to the ST of ETEC,[943] may also be important.

Clinical Manifestations

Infection with *Y. enterocolitica* is recognized as one of the causes of bacterial gastroenteritis in young children, but knowledge of neonatal infection with this organism is fragmentary. Even in large series, isolation of *Yersinia* from newborns is rare.[931,932,944]

The youngest infants whose clinical course has been described in detail were 11 days to several months old at the onset of their illness.[932,944-952] There were no features of the gastroenteritis to distinguish it from that caused by other invasive enteric pathogens such as *Shigella* or *Salmonella*. Infants presented with watery diarrhea or with stools containing mucus with streaks of blood. Sepsis was common in these infants particularly in the first 3 months of life when 28% of enteritis was complicated by sepsis.[948,949,953,954] Fever is not a consistent finding in children with bacteremia, and meningitis is rare. In older children, fever and right lower quadrant pain mimicking appendicitis are often found.[940]

Diagnosis

Y. enterocolitica can be recovered from throat swabs, mesenteric lymph nodes, peritoneal fluid, blood, and stool. Because laboratory identification of organisms from stool requires special techniques, laboratory personnel should be notified when *Yersinia* is suspected. Because avirulent environmental isolates occur, biotyping and serotyping are useful in assessing the clinical relevance of isolates. PCR has been used to detect pathogenic strains.[955,956]

Therapy

The effect of antimicrobial therapy on the outcome of gastrointestinal infection is uncertain. It has been recommended that antibiotics be reserved for sepsis or prolonged and severe gastroenteritis[931]; however, there are no prospective studies comparing the efficacy of various antimicrobial agents with each other or with supportive therapy alone. Most strains of *Y. enterocolitica* are susceptible to trimethoprim-sulfamethoxazole, the aminoglycosides, piperacillin, imipenem, third-generation cephalosporins, amoxicillin-clavulanate potassium, and chloramphenicol, and resistant to amoxicillin, ampicillin, carbenicillin, ticarcillin, and macrolides.[957-959] Therapy in individual cases should be guided by in vitro susceptibility testing, although cefotaxime has been successfully used in bacteremic infants.[954]

AEROMONAS HYDROPHILA

Nature of the Organism, Epidemiology, and Pathogenesis

Aeromonas hydrophila is widely distributed in animals and the environment. Although wound infection, pneumonia, and sepsis (especially in immunocompromised hosts) represent typical *Aeromonas* infections, gastroenteritis increasingly is being recognized. The organism is a gram-negative, oxidase-positive, facultatively anaerobic bacillus belonging to the family Vibrionaceae. Like other members of this family, it produces an enterotoxin[960] that causes fluid secretion in rabbit ileal loops.[961] Some strains cause fluid accumulation in the suckling mouse model,[962] whereas other strains are invasive[963] or cytotoxic.[964] The enterotoxin is not immunologically related to cholera toxin or the heat LT of *E. coli.*[965]

Although volunteer studies and studies with monkeys have failed to provide supportive evidence for enteropathogenicity,[966,967] there is good reason to believe that *A. hydrophila* does cause diarrhea in children. The earliest description of *Aeromonas* causing diarrhea was an outbreak that occurred in a neonatal unit.[968] Although several studies have failed to show an association with diarrhea,[969-974] most studies have found more *Aeromonas* isolates among children with gastroenteritis than among controls.[974-976] Part of the controversy may be caused by strain differences; some strains possess virulence traits related to production of gastroenteritis, whereas others do not.[970,977]

The diarrhea described in children is a disease of summer, primarily affecting children in the first 2 years of life. In one study, 7 (13%) of 55 cases of *Aeromonas* detected during a 20-month period occurred in infants younger than 1 month.

Clinical Manifestations

Typically, watery diarrhea with no fever has been described; although there are descriptions of watery diarrhea with fever.[978] However, in 22%, a dysentery-like illness occurred. Dysentery-like illness has been described in the neonate.[979] In one third of children, diarrhea has been reported to last for more than 2 weeks.[970] There may be species-related differences in clinical features of *Aeromonas*-associated gastroenteritis in children.[980] Organisms that were formerly classified as *A. hydrophila* are now sometimes labeled as *Aeromonas sobria* or *Aeromonas caviae.*[981,982] Fever and abdominal pain appear to be particularly common with *A. sobria.* One series of *A. hydrophila* isolates from newborns in Dallas showed more blood cultures than stool cultures positive for *Aeromonas.*[983]

Diagnosis and Therapy

Diagnosis of enteric infection associated with *Aeromonas* often is not made because this organism is not routinely sought in stool cultures. When the organism is suspected, the laboratory should be notified so that oxidase testing can be performed. The organism is usually susceptible to aztreonam, imipenem, meropenem, third-generation cephalosporins, trimethoprim-sulfamethoxazole, and chloramphenicol.[984-986]

PLESIOMONAS SHIGELLOIDES

Plesiomonas shigelloides is a gram-negative, facultative anaerobic bacillus that, like *Aeromonas,* is a member of the Vibrionaceae family. It is widely disseminated in the environment; outbreaks of disease are usually related to ingestion of contaminated water or seafood.[987] Although it has been associated with outbreaks of diarrheal disease[988] and has been found more commonly in ill than well controls, the role of *P. shigelloides* in diarrheal disease has remained controversial.[989] If it is a true enteropathogen, the mechanism by which it causes disease is unclear.[990,991] The role of this organism in neonatal diarrhea has not been extensively investigated. Infections of neonates have been reported,[992-995] but most cases of enteric disease currently reported in the United States are in adults.[987] Typical illness consists of watery diarrhea and cramps; sometimes, fever, bloody stools, and emesis occur and last for 3 to 42 days.

Diagnosis is not usually made by clinical microbiology laboratory testing because, as with *Aeromonas,* coliforms can be confused with *P. shigelloides* unless an oxidase test is performed.[996] The true frequency of infection is unknown. The organism has antibiotic susceptibilities similar to those of *Aeromonas.*[997,998]

OTHER BACTERIAL AGENTS AND FUNGI

Proving that an organism causes diarrhea is difficult, particularly when it may be present in large numbers in stools of healthy persons. Bacteria that have been associated with acute gastroenteritis may be considered causative when the following criteria are met:

1. A single specific strain of the organism should be found as the predominant organism in most affected infants by different investigators in outbreaks of enteric disease in different communities.
2. This strain should be isolated in a significantly lower percentage and in smaller numbers from stool specimens of healthy infants.
3. Available methods must be used to exclude other recognized enteropathogens, including viruses and parasites, enterotoxigenic agents, and fastidious organisms such as *Campylobacter.*
4. Demonstration of effective specific antimicrobial therapy and specific antibody responses and, ultimately, production of experimental disease in volunteers are helpful in establishing the identity of a microorganism as a pathogen.

Optimally, the putative pathogen should have virulence traits that can be demonstrated in model systems. Most bacteria that have been suggested as occasional causes of gastroenteritis in neonates fail to fulfill one or more of these criteria. Their role in the cause of diarrheal disease is questionable. This is particularly true of microorganisms described in early reports in which the possibility of infection with more recently recognized agents could not be excluded. Much of the clinical, bacteriologic, and epidemiologic data collected earlier linking unusual enteropathogens to infantile diarrhea must be reevaluated in light of current knowledge and methodology.

Several reports of acute gastroenteritis believed to have been caused by *Klebsiella* suggest that, rather than playing an etiologic role, these organisms had probably proliferated within an already inflamed bowel.[999-1001] The recovery of *Klebsiella-Enterobacter* in pure culture from diarrheal stools has led several investigators to suggest that these bacteria may occasionally play a causative role in infantile gastroenteritis and enterocolitis.[1002-1007] Ingestion of infant formula contaminated with *Enterobacter sakazakii* has been associated with development of bloody diarrhea and sepsis.[1008] However, *Klebsiella* species also may be isolated in pure culture from stools of newborns with no enteric symptoms.[1009-1011] In one study, certain capsular types of *Klebsiella* were more often isolated from infants with diarrheal disease than from normal infants.[1002] Later work has shown that *Klebsiella pneumoniae, Enterobacter cloacae,* and *Citrobacter* species are capable of producing enterotoxins.[139,166,167,175,193,1008,1012,1013] Reports of isolation of *Citrobacter* species, such as those of *Klebsiella* species, describe associations with enteric illnesses in up to 7% of cases.[1014-1016] There is inadequate evidence to define the roles of *Klebsiella, Enterobacter,* and *Citrobacter* species as etiologic agents of enteric illnesses.

Listeria monocytogenes, one of the classic causes of neonatal sepsis and meningitis (see Chapter 14), has been linked to outbreaks of febrile diarrheal disease in immunocompetent adults and children.[1017-1021] Seventy-two percent of ill individuals have had fever.[1022] Outbreaks have been related to ingestion of contaminated foods. *Listeria* has rarely been described as a cause of neonatal gastroenteritis.[1023-1026]

Infection with enterotoxin-producing *Bacteroides fragilis* has been associated with mild watery diarrhea.[1027] These infections have a peak incidence in 2- to 3-year-old infants.[1028] These toxin-producing organisms cannot be detected in routine hospital laboratories.

A variety of organisms has been isolated from infant stools during episodes of diarrhea. Most of these reports have failed to associate illness with specific organisms in a way that has stood the test of time. For example, *P. aeruginosa* [1029-1034] and *Proteus* [1017,1035-1041] have been associated with diarrhea, but there are few convincing data suggesting that either is a true enteropathogen. These organisms generally are recovered as frequently from healthy infants as from infants with diarrheal disease, suggesting that their presence in stool cultures is significant.[273,1042-1046] An association between *Providencia* and neonatal enteritis has been substantiated largely by anecdotal reports of nursery outbreaks.[215,271,1016,1047] These bacteria are rarely isolated from infants with sporadic or community-acquired diarrheal disease.[1042-1044,1048-1050]

Candida albicans usually is acquired during passage through the birth canal and is considered a normal, although minor, component of the fecal flora of the neonate (see Chapter 33).[1051] Intestinal overgrowth of these organisms frequently accompanies infantile gastroenteritis,[211,233,1051,1054] particularly after antimicrobial therapy.[233,247,1052-1055] The upper small gut may become colonized with *Candida* in malnourished children with diarrhea[1056]; whether the presence of the organism is cause or effect is unclear. Stool cultures obtained from infants with diarrheal disease are therefore inconclusive, and although *Candida* enteritis has been reported in adults,[1057] the importance of this organism as a primary cause of neonatal gastroenteritis has been difficult to prove. Clinical descriptions of nursery epidemics of candidal enteritis are poorly documented, generally preceding the recognition of EPEC and rotaviruses as a cause of neonatal diarrhea. Even well studied cases of intestinal involvement add little in the way of substantive proof because secondary invasion of *Candida* has been shown to be a complication of coliform enteritis.[211,233,247]

Although diarrhea has sometimes been described as a finding in neonatal disseminated candidiasis, more typically, gastrointestinal tract involvement with disseminated *Candida* is associated with abdominal distention and bloody stools mimicking necrotizing enterocolitis.[247,1056-1061] Typically, affected infants are premature and have courses complicated by antibiotic administration, intravascular catheter use, and surgical procedures during the first several weeks of life. A trial of oral anticandidal therapy may be helpful in neonates suffering from diarrhea in the presence of oral or cutaneous candidiasis. If the therapy is appropriate, a response should be forthcoming within 2 to 5 days.

Diarrhea sometimes occurs as a manifestation of systemic infection. Patients with staphylococcal toxic shock syndrome, for example, often have diarrhea. Loose stools sometimes occur in sepsis, but it is unclear whether the diarrhea is a cause or an effect. The organisms isolated from blood cultures in a group of Bangladeshi infants and children with diarrhea included *Staphylococcus aureus, Haemophilus influenzae, Streptococcus pneumoniae, P. aeruginosa,* and various gram-negative enteric bacilli.[1062] It is unknown whether the bacteriology of sepsis associated with diarrhea is similar in the well-nourished infants seen in industrialized countries.

PARASITES

Acute diarrhea associated with intestinal parasites is infrequent during the neonatal period. In areas with high endemicity, infection of the newborn is likely to be associated with inadequate maternal and delivery care, insufficient environmental sanitation, and poor personal hygiene standards. The occurrence of symptomatic intestinal parasitic infection during the first month of life requires acquisition of the parasite during the first days or weeks; the incubation period for *E. histolytica* and *G. lamblia* is 1 to 4 weeks, and for *Cryptosporidium parvum*, it is 7 to 14 days. The newborn can be infected during delivery by contact with maternal feces,[1063] in the hospital through contact with the mother or personnel, or in the household through contact with infected individuals in close contact with the child. Contaminated water can be an important source of infection for *G. lamblia* and *C. parvum.*

Entamoeba histolytica

Organisms formerly identified as *E. histolytica* have been reclassified into two species that are morphologically identical but genetically distinct: *E. histolytica* and *E. dispar*. The former can cause acute nonbloody and bloody diarrhea, necrotizing enterocolitis, ameboma, and liver abscess, and the latter is a noninvasive parasite that does not cause disease. Early acquisition of disease tends to be more severe in young infants; rarely, amebic liver abscess and rapidly fatal colitis have been reported in infants.[1064-1070] For example, a 19-day-old child from India who presented with 10 to 12 episodes of watery and mucous diarrhea, lethargy, jaundice, and mildly elevated liver enzymes has been described; the child recovered completely after 10 days of intravenous omidazole.[1064] However, asymptomatic colonization of neonates with various species of ameba is common in areas of high endemicity.[1071]

Diagnosis can be established by stool examination for cysts and trophozoites and by serologic studies.[1072] Through the use of PCR, isoenzyme analysis, and antigen detection assays, *E. histolytica* and *E. dispar* can be differentiated.[1073,1074] Serum antibody assays may be helpful in establishing the diagnosis of amebic dysentery and extraintestinal amebiasis with liver involvement. The efficacy of treatment with metronidazole for colitis or liver abscess has not been established for the newborn period, although this therapy has been used with success.[1065] Patients with colitis or liver abscess caused by *E. histolytica* are treated also with iodoquinol, as are asymptomatic carriers.

Giardia lamblia

G. lamblia is a binucleate, flagellated protozoan parasite with trophozoite and cyst stages. It is spread by the fecal-oral route through ingestion of cysts. Child-care center outbreaks reflecting person-to-person spread have demonstrated high infectivity.[1075-1078] Foodborne transmission and waterborne transmission also occur. Infection is often asymptomatic or mildly symptomatic; cases of severe symptomatic infection during the immediate newborn period have not been reported. Symptoms in giardiasis are related to the age of the patient, with diarrhea, vomiting, anorexia, and failure to thrive typical in the youngest children. Seroprevalence studies have demonstrated evidence of past or current infection in 40% of Peruvian children by the age of 6 months.[1081] In a study of lactating Bangladeshi mothers and their infants, 82% of women and 42% of infants excreted *Giardia* once during the study; in some infants, this occurred before they were 3 months old.[1082] Of these infected infants, 86% had diarrhea, suggesting that the early exposure to the parasite resulted in disease. In a prospective study of diarrhea conducted in Mexico, infants frequently were infected with *Giardia* from birth to 2 months, with a crude incidence rate of first *Giardia* infection of 1.4 infections per child-year in this age group.[6] The symptom status of these children was not reported but this study strongly suggests that *G. lamblia* may be more common than currently recognized among newborns living in developing areas.

The diagnosis of giardiasis can be made on the basis of demonstration of antigen by EIA or by microscopy of feces, duodenal fluid or, less frequently, duodenal biopsy.[1079,1080] Breast-feeding is believed to protect against symptomatic giardiasis.[6,69,1083] This protection may be mediated by cellular and humoral immunity[67,1084,1085] and nonspecifically by the antigiardial effects of unsaturated fatty acids.[1086] *Giardia* infections causing severe diarrhea may respond to metronidazole or furazolidone.[1080]

Cryptosporidium

C. parvum is a coccidian protozoon related to *Toxoplasma gondii, Isospora belli,* and *Plasmodium* species.[1087,1088] The life cycle involves ingestion of thick-walled oocysts; release of sporozoites, which penetrate intestinal epithelium; and development of merozoites. There is asexual and sexual reproduction, with the latter resulting in formation of new oocysts that can be passed in stools.

Cryptosporidium species are ubiquitous. Infection often occurs in persons traveling to endemic areas.[1089] Because *Cryptosporidium* infects a wide variety of animal species, there is often a history of animal contact among infected individuals.[1090] Person-to-person spread, particularly in household contacts[1091-1094] and daycare centers,[1095,1096] is well documented and suggests that the organism is highly infectious. Waterborne outbreaks of cryptosporidiosis occur and can be of massive proportions.[1097]

The clinical manifestations of illness in immunocompetent persons resemble those of *Giardia* infection but are somewhat shorter in duration[1098]; asymptomatic carriage is rare. Symptoms and signs include watery diarrhea, abdominal pain, myalgia, fever, and weight loss.[1089,1090,1095,1096,1098,1099] Infection in the first month of life has been described.[1100,1101] Because symptoms resolve before excretion of oocysts ceases, a newborn whose mother has been ill with cryptosporidiosis in the month before delivery might be at risk even if the mother is asymptomatic at the time of the child's birth.[1102] With the increasing frequency of human immunodeficiency virus infection, it is likely that women with symptomatic cryptosporidiosis occasionally will deliver an infant who will become infected. Infants infected early in life may develop chronic diarrhea and malnutrition.[1103]

The diagnosis of cryptosporidiosis is most typically made by examination of fecal smears using the Giemsa stain, Ziehl-Neelsen stain, auramine-rhodamine stain, Sheather's sugar flotation, an immunofluorescence procedure, a modified concentration-sugar flotation method, or an EIA.[1104,1105] Nitazoxanide is effective therapy of immunocompetent adults and children ill with cryptosporidiosis.[1106] Because illness is usually self-limited in the normal host, attention to fluid, electrolyte, and nutritional status usually suffices. Enteric isolation of hospitalized infants with this illness is appropriate because of the high infectivity. Several studies suggest that the risk of infection early in life may be decreased by breast-feeding.[1101,1107]

VIRUSES

Enteric Viruses

Viruses that infect the intestinal mucosa and cause primarily gastroenteritis are referred to as *enteric viruses*; they should not be confused with enteroviruses, members of Picornaviridae family that are associated primarily with systemic illnesses. Enteric viruses include rotaviruses, enteric adenoviruses, human caliciviruses, and astroviruses. Other viruses such as coronaviruses, Breda viruses, pestiviruses, parvoviruses, toroviruses, and picobirnaviruses have been sporadically associated with acute diarrhea but are currently considered of uncertain relevance. Extensive reviews on the role of enteric viruses in childhood diarrhea can be found elsewhere.[1108-1111]

All four enteric viruses could conceivably infect the newborn, but the extent of exposure and clinical manifestations are largely unknown for astrovirus, enteric adenovirus, and human caliciviruses. Rotavirus is the most extensively studied enteric virus. Neonatal rotavirus infections have similar virologic and clinical characteristics to infection in older children, although some differences exist.

Rotavirus

Rotavirus is a 75-nm, nonenveloped virus composed of three concentric protein shells: a segmented genome (11 segments), an RNA-dependent polymerase, and enzymes required for messenger RNA synthesis are located within the inner core. Each segment codes for at least one viral protein (VP). The VP can be part of the structure of the virus, or it may be a nonstructural protein (NSP) required for replication, viral assembly, budding, determination of host range, or viral pathogenesis.[1110]

Six distinct rotavirus groups (A through F) have been identified serologically based on common group antigens,[1112,1113] of which three (A, B, and C) have been identified in humans.[1108] Because group A rotaviruses represent more than 95% of isolated strains in humans worldwide, further discussion focuses on this group. Group A rotaviruses are subclassified into serotypes based on neutralization epitopes located on the outer capsid. Both rotavirus surface proteins, VP4 and VP7, can induce production of neutralizing antibodies.[1114,1115] At least 10 VP7 types (G serotypes: G1 to G6, G8 to G10, and G12) and nine VP4 types (P serotypes: P1A, P1B, P2A, P3, P3B, P4, P5, P8, and P12) have been detected among human rotaviruses.[1116-1123] By sequencing the VP4-coding gene, eight genomic P types (genotypes) have been identified that correspond to one or more of the described P antigenic types (genotype 8 to antigenic type P1A, 4 to P1B, 6 to P2A, 9 to P3, 13 to P3B, 10 to P4, 3 to P5, and 11 to P8).[1110] Combining G antigenic with P antigenic and genetic typing, a specific rotavirus strain can be identified: P antigenic type (P genetic type), G type. As an example, the human neonatal M37 strain is described as P2A[6], G1.

Four combined GP types: P1A[8], G1; P1B[4], G2; P1A[8], G3; and P1A[8], G4 account for more than 95% of the organisms isolated from children, and of these, P1A[8], G1 represents the single most common type.[1118-1123] Isolation of less common types appears to be more frequent among neonates with nosocomial rotavirus infections.[1123-1130] Some of these strains seem to be associated with occurrence of asymptomatic infections, although the existence of naturally acquired asymptomatic strains is controversial. Strains P2A[6], G9; P2A[6], G4; P2A[6], G2; and P2A[6], G8 have been reported[1128-1131] from newborn nurseries, some of which seem to be endemic to the newborn units with high rates of asymptomatic infection,[1129-1131] and less commonly, outbreaks of symptomatic infection.[1128] These findings suggest that specific conditions of the newborn environment (e.g., child, nursery, personnel) may increase the possibility of reassortments between human strains; such strains may persist in these settings possibly through constant transmission involving asymptomatic newborns, adults, and contaminated surfaces.

Pathogenesis

Rotavirus primarily infects mature enterocytes located in the mid and upper villous epithelium.[1132-1136] Lactase, which is present only on the brush border of the differentiated epithelial cells at these sites, may act as a combined receptor and uncoating enzyme for the virus, permitting transfer of the particles into the cell.[1137] Perhaps for this reason, infection is limited to the mature columnar enterocytes; crypt cells and crypt-derived cuboidal cells, which lack a brush border, appear to be resistant to rotaviral infection.[1137,1138] This concept also may explain why rotavirus infection is less common in infants younger than 32 weeks' gestational age than in more mature infants[1139]; between 26 and 34 weeks' gestational age, lactase activity is approximately 30% of that found in term infants.[1140]

The upper small intestine is most commonly involved, although lesions may extend to the distal ileum and rarely to the colon.[1141,1142] Interaction between intestinal cell and rotavirus structural and nonstructural proteins occurs, resulting in death of infected villous enterocytes.[1143] Once infected, the villous enterocyte is sloughed, resulting in an altered mucosal architecture that becomes stunted and flattened. The gross appearance of the bowel is usually normal; however, under the dissecting microscope, scattered focal lesions of the mucosal surface are apparent in most cases. Light microscopy also shows patchy changes in villous morphology, compatible with a process of infection, inflammation, and accelerated mucosal renewal. The villi take on a shortened and blunt appearance as tall columnar cells are shed and replaced by less mature cuboidal enterocytes.[1133,1135,1144] Ischemia may also play a role in the loss and stunting of villi[1145] and activation of the enteric nervous system; active secretion of fluid and electrolytes may be another pathogenic mechanism.[1146] During the recovery phase, the enteroblastic cells mature and reconstruct the villous structure. Because of the loss of mature enterocytes on the tips of the villi, the surface area of the intestine is reduced. Diarrhea that occurs may be a result of this decrease in surface area, disruption in epithelial integrity, transient disaccharidase deficiency, or altered countercurrent mechanisms and net secretion of water and electrolytes.[1133,1140,1142,1146,1147,1148] NSP4 has been found to induce age-dependent diarrhea in CD1 mice by triggering calcium-dependent chloride and water secretion.[1149] The potential role of this "viral enterotoxin" in human disease is not yet clear.[1150,1151]

Infection and Immunity

Infants with asymptomatic rotavirus infections in the nursery are less likely than uninfected nursery mates to experience severe rotavirus infection later in life[1152-1153]; this finding suggested protective immunity and supported vaccine development. Most studies have indicated that serum and intestinal antirotavirus antibody levels are correlated with protection against infection[1153-1161] although this correlation has not been universal.[1162-1163] Breast-feeding protects against rotavirus disease during the first year of life,[57] probably including newborns.[1146] The high prevalence of antirotaviral antibodies in colostrum and human milk has been demonstrated by numerous investigators in widely diverse geographic areas.[8] Maternal rotavirus infection or immunization is accompanied by the appearance of specific antibodies in milk, probably through stimulation of the enteromammary immune system.[1164-1169] Between 90% and 100% of women examined in London, Bangladesh, Guatemala, Costa Rica, and the United States had antirotaviral IgA antibodies in their milk for up to 2 years of lactation.[8,1164-1170] Rotavirus-specific IgG antibodies have been found during the first few postpartum days in about one third of human milk samples assayed,[1164,1167] whereas IgM antibodies were detectable in about one half.[1167]

Glycoproteins in human milk have been shown to prevent rotavirus infection in vitro and in an animal model.[1170] The concentration of one milk glycoprotein, lactadherin, was found to be significantly higher in human milk ingested by infants who developed asymptomatic rotavirus infection than in milk ingested by infants who developed symptomatic infection.[45]

Epidemiology

Rotaviruses probably infect neonates more commonly than previously recognized, although most infections seem to be asymptomatic or mildly symptomatic.[1128-1130,1131,1172-1187] In a prospective study, the prevalence of rotavirus infection among neonatal intensive care unit patients was 18.4%. Rotavirus has a mean incubation period of 2 days, with a range of 1 to 3 days in children and in experimentally infected adults. Fecal excretion of virus often begins a day or so before illness and maximal excretion usually occurs during the third and fourth days, and generally diminishes by the end of the first week, although low concentrations of virus have been detected in neonates for up to 8 weeks.[1140,1186-1189]

Rotavirus infections are markedly seasonal (autumn and winter) in many areas of the world, although in some countries seasonality is less striking; the reason for this is unclear.[1190-1195] In nurseries in which persisting endemic infection has permitted long-term surveillance of large numbers of neonates, rotavirus excretion can follow the seasonal pattern of the community but can also show no seasonal fluctuation.[1196-1198] It is not clear how units in which infection remains endemic for months or years differ from those with a low incidence of rotavirus. Some nurseries are free of rotavirus infection[1198-1200] or minimally affected[45,1201] whereas others have rotavirus diarrheal disease throughout the year or in outbreaks that involve 10% to 40% of neonates.[1128,1139,1179,1202-1203]

Low birth weight does not seem to be an important factor in determining the attack rate among infants at risk but may be important in mortality.[1204] Infants in premature or special-care nurseries, despite their prolonged stays and the increased handling necessary for their care, do not demonstrate a higher susceptibility to infection; data regarding shedding of the virus are inconsistent.[45,1200]

After infection is introduced into a nursery, rotavirus probably will spread steadily and remain endemic until the nursery is closed to new admissions or nursing practices permit interruption of the cycle.[1205] Exactly how the virus is introduced and transmitted is uncertain, although limited observations and experience with other types of enteric disease in maternity units suggest several possibilities. The early appearance of virus in stools of some neonates indicates that infection probably was acquired at delivery. Virus particles can be detected on the first[45,1186] or second[1198] day of life in a significant number of infected infants. By day 3 or 4, most infected infants who will shed virus, with or without signs of illness, are doing so.[1174,1186,1198] The large numbers of virus particles excreted[1174,1198] suggest a fairly large and early oral inoculum. It is unlikely that contamination from any source other than maternal feces could provide an inoculum large enough to cause infection by the second day.

Transfer of particles from infant to infant on the hands of nursing and medical staff is probably the most important means of viral spread. With 10^8 to 10^{11} viral particles usually present in 1 g of stool, the hands of personnel easily could become contaminated after infection is introduced into a nursery. There are numerous reports of nosocomial and daycare center rotavirus gastroenteritis outbreaks that attest to the ease with which this agent spreads through a hospital or institutional setting.[1108] Admission of a symptomatic child usually is the initiating event, although transfer of a neonate with inapparent infection from one ward to another also has been incriminated. The most important factors influencing the incidence of rotavirus diarrhea in a nursery are the proximity to other newborns and the frequency of handling.[1187] During a 4-month study, infants cared for by nursing staff and kept in communal nurseries experienced three epidemics of diarrhea with attack rates between 20% and 50%. During the same period, only 2% of infants rooming in with their mothers became ill, even though they had frequent contact with adult relatives and siblings.

There is no clear evidence of airborne or droplet infection originating in the upper respiratory tract or spread by aerosolization of diarrheal fluid while diapers are changed. Indirect evidence of airborne transmission includes the high infection rate in closed settings, the isolation of the virus from respiratory secretions,[1206] and the experimental observation of transmission by aerosol droplets in mice.[1207] However, the respiratory isolation achieved by placing an infant in a closed incubator is not fully protective.[1187] No evidence indicates that transplacental or ascending intrauterine infection occurs. Transmission of virus through contaminated fomites, formula, or food is possible but has not been documented in newborns. Rotavirus particles have not been found in human milk or colostrum.[1166,1170]

Clinical Manifestations

Exposure of a newborn to rotavirus can result in asymptomatic infection or cause mild or severe gastroenteritis.[1129,1130,1173,1179,1196,1197,1201,1208] Outbreaks with high attack rates as measured by rotavirus excretion have been described but the extent of symptomatic infection varies.[1175,1177,1186,1198,1203] Severe rotavirus infection is seldom reported during the newborn period[1203] but the extent of underreporting of severe disease, especially in the less developed areas of the world, has not been evaluated.

It has been hypothesized that asymptomatic infections during the newborn period are the result of naturally attenuated strains circulating in this environment. RNA electrophoretic patterns of rotaviruses found in certain nurseries have shown uniform patterns[1180,1182,1184,1208], and it has been suggested that these strains may be attenuated. The presence of unusual antigenic types such as the P2A[6] type within nurseries also suggests "less virulent strains." At least 10 rotavirus strains were documented to co-circulate in a tertiary care center during a 2-month period[1209] and in a different setting the same rotavirus strains by electropherotype produced asymptomatic infection in neonates and symptomatic infection in older infants.[1183] Newborns within a nursery exposed to a given rotavirus strain can develop symptomatic or asymptomatic infection.[1130,1210,1211] Because newborns routinely have frequent relatively loose stools, it is possible that mild diarrhea episodes caused by rotavirus are being wrongly labeled as asymptomatic episodes.

No clinical feature is pathognomonic of rotaviral gastroenteritis. Early signs of illness, such as lethargy, irritability, vomiting, and poor feeding, usually are followed in a few hours by the passage of watery yellow or green stools free of blood but sometimes containing mucus.[1187,1212-1214] Diarrhea usually decreases by the second day of illness and is much improved by the third or fourth day. Occasionally, intestinal fluid loss and poor weight gain may continue for 1 or 2 weeks, particularly in low-birth-weight infants.[1175] Although reducing substances frequently are present in early fecal samples[1139,175,1176,1187] this finding is not necessarily abnormal in neonates, particularly those who are breast-fed.[1215] Nevertheless, infants with prolonged diarrhea should be investigated for monosaccharide or disaccharide malabsorption or intolerance to cow's milk protein or both.[1216] In a prospective study,[1185] 49% of newborns with gastrointestinal symptoms in a neonatal intensive care unit had rotavirus detected in their stools. Frequent stooling (present in 60%), bloody mucoid stool (42%), and watery stools (24%) were risk factors for a rotavirus infection. Bloody mucoid stools, intestinal dilatation, and abdominal distention were significantly more common in preterm infants, but severe outcomes such as necrotizing enterocolitis and death did not differ among infected term and preterm infants.

Longitudinal studies in newborn nurseries and investigations of outbreaks among neonates rarely describe a severe adverse outcome or death.[1139,1168,1187] Because these infants are under constant observation, early detection of excessive fluid losses and the availability of immediate medical care are probably major factors in determining outcome. Rotavirus gastroenteritis causes almost 400,000 deaths of infants every year,[1217] concentrated largely in the poorest regions of the world. It is likely that in places where hospital-based care is uncommon, rotavirus causes neonatal deaths secondary to dehydration.

Group A rotavirus has been associated with a wide array of diseases in infants and children; Reye syndromes, encephalitis-aseptic meningitis, sudden infant death syndrome, inflammatory bowel disease, and Kawasaki syndrome have been described but not systematically studied.[1108] Case reports and small case series have associated neonatal rotavirus infection with necrotizing enterocolitis.[1218,1219] Rotavirus infection may play a role in a small proportion of cases of necrotizing enterocolitis, although it probably represents one of many potential triggering factors. A significant association between neonatal rotavirus infection and bradycardia-apnea episodes was detected in one prospective study.[1220] The possible association between natural rotavirus infection and intussusception[1221-1223] gained support after the association was made between the human-simian reassortant vaccine and intussusception in infants older than 2 months (attributable risk ≈ 1:10,000).[1224] Intussusception is extremely uncommon in the newborn; it is highly unlikely that rotavirus triggers this disease in neonates.

Diagnosis

There are many methods used for detection of rotavirus in stool specimens, including electron microscopy, immune electron microscopy, ELISA, latex agglutination, gel electrophoresis, culture of the virus, and reverse transcriptase–polymerase chain reaction. ELISA and latex agglutination currently are the most widely used diagnostic techniques for detection of rotavirus in clinical samples. Many commercial kits are available that differ in specificity and sensitivity.[1225-1229] In general, latex agglutination assays are more rapid than ELISAs but are less sensitive. The sensitivity and specificity of the commercially available ELISAs surpass 90%. Checking of the ELISA by another method such as gel electrophoresis or PCR amplification may be desirable if there is concern about false-positive results.

Fecal material for detection of rotavirus infection should be obtained during the acute phase of illness. Whole-stool samples are preferred, although suspensions of rectal swab specimens have been adequate for detection of rotavirus by ELISA.[1230,1231] Rotavirus are relatively resistant to environmental temperatures, even tropical temperatures,[1232] although 4°C is desirable for short-term storage and -70°C for prolonged storage.[1108] Excretion of viral particles may precede signs of illness by several days[1190]; maximal excretion by older infants and children usually occurs 3 to 4 days after onset of symptoms.[1233] Neonates can shed virus for 1 to 2 weeks after onset of symptoms.

Therapy and Prevention

The primary goal of therapy is restoration and maintenance of fluid and electrolyte balance. Despite the documented defect in carbohydrate digestion with rotavirus diarrhea, rehydration often can be accomplished with glucose-electrolyte or sucrose-electrolyte solutions given orally.[199,1234-1236] Intravenous fluids may be needed in neonates who are severely dehydrated, who have ileus, or who refuse to feed. Persistent or recurrent diarrhea after introduction of milk-based formulas or human milk warrants investigation for secondary carbohydrate or milk protein intolerance.[1139,1217] Disaccharidase levels and xylose absorption return to normal within a few days[1144] to weeks after infection.[1133]

Intractable diarrhea related to severe morphologic and enzymatic changes of the bowel mucosa is possible although rare in the newborn; it may require an elemental diet or parenteral nutrition. Efficacy of anti-rotavirus antibodies (e.g., hyperimmune colostrum, antibody-supplemented formula, human serum immunoglobulin) and of probiotics has been postulated,[1238-1241] although not convincingly shown[1242]; the widespread clinical use of these measures seems remote. One study suggests that use of lactobacillus during the diarrheal episode may decrease the duration of rotavirus-associated hospital stays, especially when used early in the course of the disease, although more studies are needed before recommending widespread use.[1241]

Hand hygiene before and after contact with each infant remains the single most important means of preventing the spread of infection. Because rotavirus is often excreted several days before illness is recognized, isolation of an infant with diarrhea may be too late to prevent cross-infection unless all nursing personnel and medical staff have adhered to this fundamental precaution. Infants who develop gastroenteritis should be moved out of the nursery area if adequate facilities are available and the infant's condition permits transfer. The use of an incubator is of value in reducing transmission of disease only by serving as a reminder that proper hand-hygiene and glove techniques are required, but is of little value as a physical barrier to the spread of virus.[1187] Encouraging rooming-in of infants with their mothers has been shown to be helpful in preventing or containing nursery epidemics.[1243] Temporary closure of the nursery may be required for clinically significant outbreaks that cannot be controlled with other measures.[1128]

Vaccines

Development of rotavirus vaccines began in the early 1980s. Candidate vaccines included bovine and rhesus monkey

Table 20–6 Differential Diagnosis of Neonatal Diarrhea

Diagnosis	Reference(s)
Anatomic Disorders	
Microvillous inclusion disease	1245
Hirschsprung's disease	1246
Massive intestinal resection (short-bowel syndrome)	1247
Intestinal lymphangiectasis	1248
Metabolic and Enzymatic Disorders	
Congenital disaccharidase deficiency (lactase, sucrase-isomaltase deficiency)	1249,1250
Congenital glucose-galactose malabsorption	1251,1252
Secondary disaccharide, monosaccharide malabsorption	337,528,1252-1258
After gastrointestinal surgery	
After infection	
With milk-soy protein sensitivity	
Cystic fibrosis	1259
Syndrome of pancreatic insufficiency and bone marrow dysfunction (Shwachman's syndrome)	1260
Physiologic deficiency of pancreatic amylase	1261
Intestinal enterokinase deficiency	1262
Congenital bile acid deficiency syndrome	1263
Alpha/beta-lipoproteinemia	1264
Acrodermatitis enteropathica	1265,1266
Congenital chloride diarrhea	1267,1268
Primary hypomagnesemia	1269
Congenital adrenal hyperplasia	1270
Intestinal hormone hypersecretion	1271,1272
Non–beta islet cell hyperplasia (Wolman's disease)	1273
Transcobalamin II deficiency	1274
Congenital iron storage	1275
Hartnup's disease	1276
Congenital Na^+ diarrhea	1277
Inflammatory Disorders	
Cow's milk protein intolerance	1278
Soy protein intolerance	1279,1280
Regional enteritis	1281
Ulcerative colitis	1282,1283
Primary Immunodeficiency Disorders	
Wiskott-Aldrich syndrome	1284
Thymic dysplasia	1284
Acquired immunodeficiency syndrome	1285
Miscellaneous	
Irritable colon of childhood (chronic nonspecific diarrhea)	1286
Phototherapy for hyperbilirubinemia	1287
Familial dysautonomia (Riley-Day syndrome)	1288
Familial enteropathy	1289,1290
High sulfates in water	1291
Phenolphthalein poisoning/child abuse	1292

attenuated strains, human attenuated strains, and bovine-human and rhesus-human reassortant strains.[1109] In August 1998, the first licensed rotavirus vaccine, Rotashield, an oral formulation of a simian-human quadrivalent reassortant vaccine, was recommended for use in children when they were 2, 4, and 6 months old. After approximately 500,000 children were vaccinated with more than 1 million doses, a significantly increased risk of intussusception was observed among vaccinated children, with an overall odds ratio of 1.8.[1244] Use of this vaccine was terminated. Two new vaccine candidates are undergoing phase III clinical trials: a "pentavalent" bovine-human reassortant vaccine including G types G1-G4 and P type P1A[8] and a monovalent human attenuated P1A[8]G1 vaccine. The epidemiology of rotavirus infection will change significantly if one or both candidates become widely available in the future. The impact on neonatal infection will depend on the effect of herd immunity in decreasing circulation of rotavirus strains.

DIFFERENTIAL DIAGNOSIS

Stools from breast-fed neonates are typically watery and yellow, green, or brown. The frequency of stooling can vary from one every other day to eight evacuations per day. In an active, healthy infant who is feeding well, has no vomiting, and has a soft abdomen, these varied patterns of stooling are not a cause for concern. Physicians need to consider the child's previous frequency and consistency of stools and establish a diagnosis of acute diarrhea on an individual basis. Close follow-up of weight increase in infants with nonformed stools can help confirm the clinical impression. A normal weight gain should direct medical action away from stool exams or treatment.

Diarrhea during the neonatal period is a clinical manifestation of a wide variety of disorders (Table 20-6). The most common initiating factor is a primary infection of the gastrointestinal tract that is mild to moderate in severity, self-limited, and responsive to supportive measures. Acute diarrhea can also be an initial manifestation of a systemic infection, including bacterial and viral neonatal sepsis. Infants with moderate to severe diarrhea require close monitoring until the etiologic diagnosis and the clinical evolution are clarified. There are noninfectious diseases leading to chronic intractable diarrhea that may result in severe nutritional disturbances or even death unless the specific underlying condition is identified and treated appropriately. The differential diagnosis of a diarrheal illness requires a careful clinical examination to determine whether the child has a localized or a systemic process. Lethargy, abnormalities in body temperature, hypothermia or hyperthermia, decreased feeding, abdominal distention, vomiting, pallor, respiratory distress, apnea, cyanosis, hemodynamic instability, hypotension, hepatomegaly or splenomegaly, coagulation or bleeding disorders, petechiae, and exanthemas should lead to an intense laboratory investigation directed at systemic viral or bacterial infection. If the process is deemed a localized intestinal infection, initial evaluation can be focused on differentiating an inflammatory-invasive pathogen from those that cause a noninflammatory process. For this, stool examination for fecal leukocytes, red blood cells, and lactoferrin can be a helpful indicator of the former.

Inflammatory diarrhea can be caused by *Shigella, Salmonella, Campylobacter, V. parahaemolyticus, Y. enterocolitica,* EIEC, EAEC, *C. difficile,* necrotizing enterocolitis, antibiotic-associated colitis, and allergic colitis (i.e., milk or soy intolerance). Noninflammatory causes of diarrhea include ETEC, EPEC, rotaviruses, enteric adenoviruses, calicivirus, astrovirus, *G. lamblia* and *Cryptosporidium.* Although supportive fluid therapy is mandatory for all types of diarrhea, the brief examination for fecal leukocytes and red blood cells can direct the diagnostic and therapeutic approach. Pathogens such as *Shigella, Salmonella,* and EHEC can cause watery or bloody diarrhea, depending on the specific host-pathogen interaction and the pathogenic mechanisms involved. Some of the noninfectious diseases responsible for neonatal diarrhea are listed in Table 20-6.[337,528,1245-1292] The evaluation and management of persistent infantile diarrhea has been reviewed.[1293]

REFERENCES

1. Prashar UD, Hummelman EG, Bresee JS, et al. Global illness and deaths caused by rotavirus disease in children. Emerg Infect Dis 9:565, 2003.
2. Guerrant RL. Lessons from diarrheal diseases: demography to molecular pharmacology. J Infect Dis 169:1206, 1994.
3. Ho MS, Glass RI, Pinsky PF, et al. Diarrheal deaths in American children: are they preventable? JAMA 260:3281, 1988.
4. Cohen ML. The epidemiology of diarrheal disease in the United States. Infect Dis Clin North Am 2:557, 1988.
5. Mata LJ, Urrutia JJ. Intestinal colonization of breastfed children in a rural area of low socioeconomic level. Ann N Y Acad Sci 176:93, 1971.
6. Morrow AL, Reves RR, West MS, et al. Protection against infection with *Giardia lamblia* by breast-feeding in a cohort of Mexican infants. J Pediatr 121:363, 1992.
7. Velásquez FR, Matson DO, Lourdes Guerrero M, et al. Serum antibody as a marker of protection against natural rotavirus infection and disease. J Infect Dis 182:1602, 2000.
8. Morrow AL, Pickering LK. Human milk protection against diarrheal disease. Semin Pediatr Infect Dis 5:236, 1994.
9. Prado V, O'Ryan M. Acute Gastroenteritis in Latin America. Infect Dis Clin North Am 8:77, 1994.
10. Guerrant RL, Hughes JM, Lima NL, et al. Diarrhea in developed and developing countries: magnitude, special settings, and etiologies. Rev Infect Dis 12:S41, 1990.
11. World Health Organization. Implementation of the Global Strategy for Health for All by the Year 2000, Second Evaluation, and Eighth Report of the World Health Situation. Forty-Fifth World Health Assembly. Geneva, World Health Organization, 1992, p A45/3.
12. Parashar UD, Kilgore PE, Holman RC, et al. Diarrheal mortality in US infants. Arch Pediatr Adolesc Med 152:47, 1998.
13. Mata LJ, Urrutia JJ. Intestinal colonization of breastfed children in a rural area of low socioeconomic level. Ann N Y Acad Sci 176:93, 1971.
14. Guerrant LR, Steiner TS, Lima AAM, Bobak DA. How intestinal bacteria cause disease. J Infect Dis 179:S331, 1999.
15. Pickering LK, Cleary TG. Approach to patients with gastrointestinal tract infections and food poisoning. *In* Feigin RD, Cherry JC (eds). Textbook of Pediatric Infectious Diseases, 4th ed. Philadelphia, WB Saunders, 1997, p 567.
16. Bettelheim KA, Lennox-King SMJ. The acquisition of *Escherichia coli* by newborn babies. Infection 4:174, 1976.
17. Gorden J, Small PLC. Acid resistance in enteric bacteria. Infect Immun 61:364, 1993.
18. Pickering LK. Biotherapeutic agents and disease in infants. Adv Exp Med Biol 501:365, 2001.
19. Giannella RA, Broitman SA, Zamcheck N. Influence of gastric acidity on bacterial and parasitic enteric infections: a perspective. Ann Intern Med 78:271, 1973.
20. Schrager J. The chemical composition and function of gastrointestinal mucus. Gut 11:450, 1970.
21. Challacombe DN, Richardson JM, Anderson CM. Bacterial microflora of the upper gastrointestinal tract in infants without diarrhea. Arch Dis Child 49:264, 1974.
22. Furuta GT, Walker WA. Nonimmune defense mechanisms of the gastrointestinal tract. *In* Blaser MJ, Smith PD, Ravdin JI, et al (eds). Infections of the Gastrointestinal Tract. New York, Raven Press, 1995, pp 89-97.
23. Avery G, Randolph JG, Weaver T. Gastric acidity in the first day of life. Pediatrics 37:1005, 1966.
24. Harries JT, Fraser AJ. The acidity of the gastric contents of premature babies during the first fourteen days of life. Biol Neonate 12:186, 1968.
25. Agunod M, Yamaguchi N, Lopez R, et al. Correlative study of hydrochloric acid, pepsin, and intrinsic factor secretion in newborns and infants. Am J Dig Dis 14:400, 1969.
26. Cavel B. Gastric emptying in infants. Acta Paediatr Scand 60:371, 1971.
27. Blumenthal I, Ebel A, Pildes RS. Effect of posture on the pattern of stomach emptying in the newborn. Pediatrics 66:482, 1980.
28. Silverio J. Gastric emptying time in the newborn and nursling. Am J Med Sci 247:732, 1964.
29. Cavell B. Gastric emptying in preterm infants. Acta Paediatr Scand 68:725, 1979.
30. Eckmann L, Kagnoff M, Fierer J. Intestinal epithelial cells as watchdogs for the natural immune system. Trends Microbiol 3:118, 1995.
31. Bernt K, Walker W. Human milk as a carrier of biochemical messages. Acta Paediatr Suppl 88:27, 1999.
32. Fallot ME, Boyd JL, Oski FA. Breast-feeding reduces incidence of hospital admissions for infection in infants. Pediatrics 65:1121, 1980.
33. Larsen SA, Homer DR. Relation of breast versus bottle feeding to hospitalization for gastroenteritis in a middle-class U.S. population. J Pediatr 92:417, 1978.
34. Cushing AH, Anderson L. Diarrhea in breast-fed and non–breast-fed infants. Pediatrics 70:921, 1982.
35. Guerrant RL, Kirchhoff LV, Shields DS, et al. Prospective study of diarrheal illnesses in northeastern Brazil: patterns of disease, nutritional impact, etiologies and risk factors. J Infect Dis 148:986, 1983.
36. Myers MG, Fomon SJ, Koontz FP, et al. Respiratory and gastrointestinal illnesses in breast- and formula-fed infants. Am J Dis Child 138:629, 1984.
37. Kovar MG, Serdula MK, Marks JS, et al. Review of the epidemiologic evidence for an association between infant feeding and infant health. Pediatrics 74:615, 1984.
38. Feachem RG, Koblinsky MA. Interventions for the control of diarrhoeal diseases among young children: promotion of breastfeeding. Bull World Health Organ 62:271, 1984.

39. Forman MR, Graubard BI, Hoffman HJ, et al. The Pima infant feeding study: breastfeeding and gastroenteritis in the first year of life. Am J Epidemiol 119:335, 1984.
40. Leventhal JM, Shapiro ED, Aten CB, et al. Does breastfeeding protect against infections in infants less than 3 months of age? Pediatrics 78:8896, 1986.
41. Rubin DH, Leventhal JM, Krsilnikoff PA, et al. Relationship between infant feeding and infectious illness: a prospective study of infants during the first year of life. Pediatrics 85:464, 1989.
42. Victora CG, Smith PG, Vaughan JP, et al. Infant feeding and deaths due to diarrhea. Am J Epidemiol 129:1032, 1989.
43. Popkin BM, Adair L, Akin JS, et al. Breast-feeding and diarrheal morbidity. Pediatrics 86:874, 1990.
44. Morrow AL, Pickering LK. Human milk and infectious diseases. *In* Long SS, Pickering LK, Prober CG (eds). Principles and Practice of Pediatric Infectious Diseases. New York, Churchill-Livingstone, 1997, pp 87-95.
45. Newburg DS, Peterson JA, Ruiz-Palacios GM, et al. High levels of lactadherin in human milk are associated with protection against symptomatic rotavirus infection amongst breast-fed infants. Lancet 351:1160, 1998.
46. Wyatt RG, Mata LJ. Bacteria in colostrum and milk in Guatemalan Indian women. J Trop Pediatr 15:159, 1969.
47. Grazioso CF, Werner AL, Alling DW, et al: Antiinflammatory effects of human milk on chemically induced colitis in rats. Pediatr Res 42:639, 1997.
48. Newburg DS. Oligosaccharides and glycoconjugates in human milk: their role in host defense. J Mammary Gland Biol Neoplasia 1:271, 1996.
49. Morrow AL, Pickering LK. Human milk protection against diarrheal disease. Semin Pediatr Infect Dis 5:236, 1994.
50. Pickering LK, Granoff DM, Erickson JE, et al. Modulation of the immune system by human milk and infant formula containing nucleotides. Pediatrics 101:242, 1998.
51. Hayani K, Guerrero M, Morrow A, et al. Concentration of milk secretory immunoglobulin A against *Shigella* virulence plasmid-associated antigens as a predictor of symptom status in *Shigella*-infected breast-fed infants. J Pediatr 121:852, 1992.
52. Hayani K, Guerrero M, Ruiz-Palacios G, et al. Evidence for long-term memory of the mucosal immune system: milk secretory immunoglobulin A against *Shigella* lipopolysaccharides. J Clin Microbiol 29:2599, 1991.
53. Newburg D, Ashkenazi S, Cleary T. Human milk contains the Shiga toxin and Shiga-like toxin receptor glycolipid Gb3. J Infect Dis 166:832, 1992.
54. Herrera-Insua I, Gomez H, Diaz-Gonzalez V, et al. Human milk lipids bind Shiga toxin. Adv Exp Med Biol 501:333, 2001.
55. Gomez H, Ochoa T, Carlin L, Cleary T. Human lactoferrin impairs virulence of *Shigella flexneri*. J Infect Dis 187:87, 2003.
56. Gomez H, Ochoa T, Herrera-Insua I, et al. Lactoferrin protects rabbits from *Shigella flexneri*–induced inflammatory enteritis. Infect Immun 70:7050, 2002.
57. Gomez H, Herrera-Insua I, Siddiqui M, et al. Protective role of human lactoferrin against invasion of *Shigella flexneri* M90T. Adv Exp Med Biol 501:457, 2001.
58. Noguera-Obenza M, Ochoa T, Gomez H, et al. Human milk secretory antibodies against attaching and effacing *Escherichia coli* antigens. Emerg Infect Dis 9:545, 2003.
59. Cravioto A, Tello A, Villafan H, et al. Inhibition of localized adhesion of enteropathogenic *Escherichia coli* to HEp-2 cells by immunoglobulin and oligosaccharide fractions of human colostrum and breast milk. J Infect Dis 163:1247, 1991.
60. Ochoa T, Noguera-Obenza M, Ebel F, et al. Lactoferrin impairs type III secretory system function in Enteropathogenic *Escherichia coli*. Infect Immun 71:5149, 2003.
61. Ross CA, Dawes EA. Resistance of the breast fed infant to gastro-enteritis. Lancet 1:994, 1954.
62. Glass RI, Svennerholm A, Stoll BJ, et al. Milk antibodies protect breastfed children against cholera. N Engl J Med 308:1389, 1983.
63. Ruiz-Palacios GM, Calva JJ, Pickering LK, et al. Protection of breastfed infants against *Campylobacter* diarrhea by antibodies in human milk. J Pediatr 116:707, 1990.
64. Holmgren J, Svennerholm AM, Lindblad M. Receptor-like glyco-compounds in human milk that inhibit classical and El Tor *Vibrio cholerae* cell adherence (hemagglutination). Infect Immun 39:147, 1983.
65. Laegreid A, Otnaess ABK, Fuglesang J. Human and bovine milk: comparison of ganglioside composition and enterotoxin-inhibitory activity. Pediatr Res 20:416, 1986.
66. Hayani KC, Guerrero ML, Morrow AL, et al. Concentration of milk secretory immunoglobulin A against *Shigella* virulence plasmid-associated antigens as a predictor of symptom status in *Shigella*-infected breast-fed infants. J Pediatr 121:852, 1992.
67. Miotti PG, Gilman RH, Pickering LK, et al. Prevalence of serum and milk antibodies to *Giardia lamblia* in different populations of lactating women. J Infect Dis 152:1025, 1985.
68. Hayani KC, Guerrero ML, Ruiz-Palacios GM, et al. Evidence for long-term memory of the mucosal immune system: milk secretory immuno-globulin A against *Shigella* lipopolysaccharides. J Clin Microbiol 29:2599, 1991.
69. Walterspiel JN, Morrow AL, Guerrero ML, et al. Protective effect of secretory anti-*Giardia lamblia* antibodies in human milk against diarrhea. Pediatrics 93:28, 1994.
70. Tacket CO, Losonsky G, Link H, et al. Protection by milk immuno-globulin concentrate against oral challenge with enterotoxigenic *E. coli*. N Engl J Med 318:1240, 1988.
71. Davidson GP, Whyte PBD, Daniels E, et al. Passive immunization of children with bovine colostrum containing antibodies to human rotavirus. Lancet 2:709, 1989.
72. Tacket CO, Binion SB, Bostwick E, et al. Efficacy of bovine milk immunoglobulin concentrate in preventing illness after *Shigella flexneri* challenge. Am J Trop Med Hyg 47:276, 1992.
73. Polonovsky M, Lespagnol A. Nouvelles acquisitions sur les composés glucidiques du lait de femme. Bull Soc Chem Biol 15:320, 1933.
74. Montreuil J, Mullet S. Etude des variations des constituants glucidiques du lait de femme au cours de la lactation. Bull Soc Chem Biol 42:365, 1960.
75. Kobata A. Milk glycoproteins and oligosaccharides. *In* Horowitz MI, Pigman W (eds). The Glycoconjugates. I. New York, Academic Press, 1978, p 423.
76. Gnoth M, Kunz C, Kinne-Saffran E, Rudloff S. Human milk oligo-saccharides are minimally digested in vitro. J Nutr 130:3014, 2000.
77. Chaturvedi P, Warren C, Buescher C, et al. Survival of human milk oligosaccharides in the intestine of infants. Adv Exp Med Biol 501:315, 2001.
78. Cleary TG, Chambers JP, Pickering LK. Protection of suckling mice from heat-stable enterotoxin of *Escherichia coli* by human milk. J Infect Dis 148:1114, 1983.
79. Newburg DS, Pickering LK, McCluer RH, et al. Fucosylated oligosaccharides of human milk protect suckling mice from heat-stable enterotoxin of *Escherichia coli*. J Infect Dis 162:1075, 1990.
80. Huang P, Farkas T, Marionneau S, et al. Noroviruses bind to human ABO, Lewis, and secretor histo-blood group antigens: identification of 4 distinct strain-specific patterns. J Infect Dis 188:19, 2003.
81. Lindesmith L, Moe C, Marionneau S, et al. Human susceptibility and resistance to Norwalk virus infection. Nat Med 9:548, 2003.
82. Otnaess AB, Svennerholm AM. Non-immunoglobulin fraction of human milk protects rabbits against enterotoxin-induced intestinal fluid secretion. Infect Immun 35:738, 1982.
83. Otnaess ABK, Laegreid A, Ertesvag K. Inhibition of enterotoxin from *Escherichia coli* and *Vibrio cholerae* by gangliosides from human milk. Infect Immun 40:563, 1983.
84. Yolken RH, Peterson JA, Vonderfecht SL, et al. Human milk mucin inhibits rotavirus replication and prevents experimental gastroenteritis. J Clin Invest 90:1984, 1992.
85. Cooper ML, Keller HM, Walters EW, et al. Isolation of enteropathogenic *Escherichia coli* from mothers and newborn infants. Am J Dis Child 97:255, 1959.
86. Ocklitz HW, Schmidt EF. Enteropathogenic *Escherichia coli* serotypes: infection of the newborn through mother. BMJ 2:1036, 1957.
87. Gareau FE, Mackel DC, Boring JR III, et al. The acquisition of fecal flora by infants from their mothers during birth. J Pediatr 54:313, 1959.
88. Rosner R. Antepartum culture findings of mothers in relation to infantile diarrhea. Am J Clin Pathol 45:732, 1966.
89. Nocard E, Leclainche E. Les Maladies Microbiennes des Animaux, 2nd ed. Paris, Masson, 1898, p 106.
90. Joest E. Untersuchungen über Kalberruhr. Z Tiermed 7:377, 1903.
91. Titze C, Weichel A. Die Ätiologie der Kalberruhr. Berl Tierarztl Wochenschr 26:457, 1908.
92. Jensen CO. Handbuch der pathogenen Microorganismen, vol 6. Jena, G Fischer, 1913, p 131.

93. Smith T, Orcutt ML. The bacteriology of the intestinal tract of young calves with special reference to the early diarrhea ("scours"). J Exp Med 41:89, 1925.
94. Tennant B (ed). Neonatal enteric infections caused by *Escherichia coli*. Ann N Y Acad Sci 176:1, 1971.
95. Moro E. Quoted in Adam A. Über die Biologie der Dyspepsiecoli und ihre Beziehungen zur Pathogenese der Dyspepsie und Intoxikation. Jahrb Kinderheilkd 101:295, 1923.
96. Adam, A. Über die Biologie der Dyspepsiecoli und ihre Beziehungen zur Pathogenese der Dyspepsie und Intoxikation. Jahrb Kinderheilkd 101:295, 1923.
97. Adam A. Zur Frage der bakteriellen Ätiologie der sogenannten alimentaren Intoxikation. Jahrb Kinderheilkd 116:8, 1927.
98. Nataro JP, Kaper JB. Diarrheagenic *Escherichia coli*. Clin Microbiol Rev 11:142, 1998.
99. Donnenberg MS, Kaper JB. Enteropathogenic *Escherichia coli*. Infect Immun 60:3953, 1992.
100. Levine MM. *Escherichia coli* that cause diarrhea: enterotoxigenic, enteropathogenic, enteroinvasive, enterohemorrhagic, and enteroadherent. J Infect Dis 155:377, 1987.
101. Guerrant RL, Thielman NM. Types of *Escherichia coli* enteropathogens. *In* Blaser MJ, Smith PD, Ravdin JL, et al (eds). Infections of the Gastrointestinal Tract. New York, Raven Press, 1995, p 687.
102. Schlager TA, Guerrant RL. Seven possible mechanisms for *Escherichia coli* diarrhea. Infect Dis Clin North Am 2:607, 1988.
103. Steiner TS, Lima AM, Nataro JP, Guerrant R. Enteroaggregative *Escherichia coli* produce intestinal inflammation and growth impairment and cause interleukin-8 release from intestinal epithelial cells. J Infect Dis 177:88, 1998.
104. Guerrant R, Steiner T. Principles and syndromes of enteric infections. *In* Mandell GL, Bennett J, Dolin R (eds). Mandell, Douglas, and Bennett's Principles and Practice of Infectious Diseases, 5th ed. Philadelphia, WB Saunders, 1999.
105. Spangler BD. Structure and function of cholera toxin and the related *Escherichia coli* heat-labile enterotoxin. Microbiol Rev 56:622, 1992.
106. Guerrant RL, Ganguly U, Casper AGT, et al. Effect of *Escherichia coli* on fluid transport across canine small bowel: mechanism and time-course with enterotoxin and whole bacterial cells. J Clin Invest 52:1707, 1973.
107. Peterson JW, Ochoa G. Role of prostaglandins and cAMP in the secretory effects of cholera toxin. Science 245:857, 1989.
108. Peterson JW, Reitmeyer JC, Jackson CA, et al. Protein synthesis is required for cholera toxin-induced stimulation or arachidonic acid metabolism. Biochim Biophys Acta 1092:79, 1991.
109. Thielman NM, Marcinkiewics M, Sarosiek J, et al. The role of platelet activating factor in Chinese hamster ovary cell responses to cholera toxin. J Clin Invest 99:1999, 1997.
110. Guerrant RL, Fang GD, Thielman NM, Fonteles MC. Role of platelet activating factor (PAF) in the intestinal epithelial secretory and Chinese hamster ovary (CHO) cell cytoskeletal responses to cholera toxin. Proc Natl Acad Sci U S A 91:9655, 1994.
111. Hughes JM, Murad F, Chang B, et al. Role of cyclic GMP in the action of heat-stable enterotoxin of *Escherichia coli*. Nature 271:755, 1978.
112. Field M, Graf LH Jr, Laird WJ, et al. Heat-stable enterotoxin of *Escherichia coli*: in vitro effects on guanylate cyclase activity, cyclic GMP concentration, and ion transport in small intestine. Proc Natl Acad Sci U S A 75:2800, 1978.
113. Guerrant RL, Hughes JM, Chang B, et al. Activation of intestinal guanylate cyclase by heat-stable enterotoxin of *Escherichia coli*: studies of tissue specificity, potential receptors and intermediates. J Infect Dis 142:220, 1980.
114. Kennedy DJ, Greenberg RN, Dunn JA, et al. Effects of *E. coli* heat stabile enterotoxin STb on intestines of mice, rats, rabbits, and piglets. Infect Immun 46:639, 1984.
115. Weikel CS, Nellans HN, Guerrant RL. *In vivo* and *in vitro* effects of a novel enterotoxin, STb, produced by *E. coli*. J Infect Dis 153:893, 1986.
116. Weikel CS, Tiemens KM, Moseley SL, et al. Species specificity and lack of production of STb enterotoxin by *E. coli* strains isolated from humans with diarrheal illness. Infect Immun 52:323, 1986.
117. DuPont HL, Formal SB, Hornick RB, et al. Pathogenesis of *Escherichia coli* diarrhea. N Engl J Med 285:1, 1971.
118. Tulloch EF, Ryan KJ, Formal SB, et al. Invasive enteropathic *Escherichia coli* dysentery. An outbreak in 28 adults. Ann Intern Med 79:13, 1973.
119. Nataro JP, Kaper JB, Robins-Browne R, et al. Patterns of adherence of diarrheagenic *E. coli* to HEp-2 cells. Pediatr Infect Dis J 6:829, 1987.
120. Kenny B, DeVinney R, Stein M, et al. Enteropathogenic *E. coli* (EPEC) transfers its receptor for intimate adherence into mammalian cells. Cell 91:511, 1997.
121. Nougayrede JP, Fernandes PJ, Donnenberg MS. Adhesion of enteropathogenic *Escherichia coli* to host cells. Cell Microbiol 5:359, 2003.
122. Giron JA, Fry J, Frankel G, et al. Diffuse-adhering *Escherichia coli* (DAEC) as a putative cause of diarrhea in Mayan children in Mexico. J Infect Dis 163:507, 1991.
123. Peiffer I, Bernet-Camard MF, Rousset M, Servin AL. Impairments in enzyme activity and biosynthesis of brush border-associated hydrolases in human intestinal Caco-2/TC7 cells infected by members of the Afa/Dr family of diffusely adhering *Escherichia coli*. Cell Microbiol 3:341, 2001.
124. Wanke CA, Schorling JB, Barrett LJ, et al. Adherence traits of *Escherichia coli*, alone and in association with other stool pathogens: potential role in pathogenesis of persistent diarrhea in an urban Brazilian slum. Pediatr J Infect Dis 10:746, 1991.
125. Okeke IN, Nataro JP. Enteroaggregative *Escherichia coli*. Lancet Infect Dis 1:304, 2001.
126. Rowe B, Scotland SM, Gross RJ. Enterotoxigenic *Escherichia coli* causing infantile enteritis in Britain. Lancet 1:90, 1977.
127. Trabulsi LR, Fernandes MFR, Zuliani ME. Novas bacterias patogenicas para o intestino do homen. Rev Inst Med Trop São Paulo 9:31, 1967.
128. Sereny B. Experimental *Shigella* keratoconjunctivitis: a preliminary report. Acta Microbiol Acad Sci Hung 2:293, 1955.
129. Skerman FJ, Formal SB, Falkow S. Plasmid-associated enterotoxin production in a strain of *Escherichia coli* isolated from humans. Infect Immun 56:22, 1972.
130. Takeda Y, Murphy J. Bacteriophage conversion of heat-labile enterotoxin in *Escherichia coli*. J Bacteriol 133:172, 1978.
131. Lathe R, Hirth P. Cell-free synthesis of enterotoxin of *E. coli* from a cloned gene. Nature 284:473, 1980.
132. Merson MH, Rowe B, Black RE, et al. Use of antisera for identification of enterotoxigenic *Escherichia coli*. Lancet 2:222, 1980.
133. Evans DG, Evans DJ Jr, Pierce NF. Differences in the response of rabbit small intestine to heat-labile and heat-stable enterotoxins of *Escherichia coli*. Infect Immun 7:873, 1973.
134. Sears CL, Kaper JB. Enteric bacterial toxins: mechanisms of action and linkage to intestinal secretion. Microbiol Rev 60:167, 1996.
135. Donta ST, Moon HW, Whipp SC. Detection of heat-labile *Escherichia coli* enterotoxin with the use of adrenal cells in tissue cultures. Science 183:334, 1974.
136. Yolken RH, Greenberg HB, Merson MH, et al. Enzyme-linked immunosorbent assay for detection of *Escherichia coli* heat-labile enterotoxin. J Clin Microbiol 6:439, 1977.
137. Dean AG, Ching YC, Williams RG, et al. Test for *Escherichia coli* enterotoxin using infant mice: application in a study of diarrhea in children in Honolulu. J Infect Dis 125:407, 1972.
138. Giannella RA. Suckling mouse model for detection of heat-stable *Escherichia coli* enterotoxin: characteristics of the model. Infect Immun 14:95, 1976.
139. Klipstein FA, Holdeman LV, Corcino JJ, et al. Enterotoxigenic intestinal bacteria in tropical sprue. Ann Intern Med 79:632, 1973.
140. Smith HW, Halls S. Observations by ligated intestinal segment and oral inoculation methods on *Escherichia coli* infections in pigs, calves, lambs and rabbits. J Pathol Bacteriol 93:499, 1967.
141. Evans DG, Silver RP, Evans DJ Jr, et al. Plasmid-controlled colonization factor associated with virulence in *Escherichia coli* enterotoxigenic for humans. Infect Immun 12:656, 1975.
142. De SN, Chatterjee DN. An experimental study of the mechanism of action of *Vibrio cholerae* on the intestinal mucous membrane. J Pathol Bacteriol 66:559, 1953.
143. De SN, Bhattachaya K, Sakar JK. A study of the pathogenicity of strains of *Bacterium coli* from acute and chronic enteritis. J Pathol Bacteriol 71:201, 1956.
144. Taylor J, Wilkins MP, Payne JM. Relation of rabbit gut reaction to enteropathogenic *Escherichia coli*. Br J Exp Pathol 42:43, 1961.
145. Taylor J, Bettelheim KA. The action of chloroform-killed suspensions of enteropathogenic *Escherichia coli* on ligated rabbit gut segments. J Gen Microbiol 42:309, 1966.
146. Trabulsi LR. Revelacao de colibacilos associados as diarreias infantis pelo metodo da infeccao experimental de alca ligade do intestino do coehlo. Rev Inst Med Trop São Paulo 6:197, 1964.
147. Moon HW, Sorensen DK, Sautter JH, et al. Association of *Escherichia coli* with diarrheal disease of the newborn pig. Am J Vet Res 27:1107, 1966.

148. Smith HW, Halls S. Studies on *Escherichia coli* enterotoxin. J Pathol Bacteriol 93:531, 1967.
149. Truszcynski M, Pilaszek J. Effects of injection of enterotoxin, endotoxin or live culture of *Escherichia coli* into the small intestine of pigs. Res Vet Sci 10:469, 1969.
150. Gyles CL, Barnum DA. A heat-labile enterotoxin from strains of *Escherichia coli* enteropathogenic for pigs. J Infect Dis 120:419, 1969.
151. Gorbach SL, Banwell JG, Chatterjee BD, et al. Acute undifferentiated human diarrhea in the tropics. I. Alterations in intestinal microflora. J Clin Invest 50:881, 1971.
152. Banwell JG, Gorbach SL, Pierce NF, et al. Acute undifferentiated human diarrhea in the tropics. II. Alterations in intestinal fluid and electrolyte movements. J Clin Invest 50:890, 1971.
153. Sack RB, Gorbach SL, Banwell JG, et al. Enterotoxigenic *Escherichia coli* isolated from patients with severe cholera-like disease. J Infect Dis 123:278, 1971.
154. Pierce NF, Wallace CK. Stimulation of jejunal secretion by a crude *Escherichia coli* enterotoxin. Gastroenterology 63:439, 1972.
155. Guerrant RL, Carpenter CCJ, Pierce NF. Experimental *E. coli* diarrhea: effects of viable bacteria and enterotoxin. Trans Assoc Am Physicians 86:111, 1973.
156. Kantor HS, Tao P, Gorbach SL. Stimulation of intestinal adenyl cyclase by *Escherichia coli* enterotoxin: comparison of strains from an infant and an adult with diarrhea. J Infect Dis 129:1, 1974.
157. Smith HW, Gyles CL. The relationship between two apparently different enterotoxins produced by enteropathogenic strains of *Escherichia coli* of porcine origin. J Med Microbiol 3:387, 1970.
158. Kohler EM. Observations on enterotoxins produced by enteropathogenic *Escherichia coli*. Ann N Y Acad Sci 176:212, 1971.
159. Moon HW, Whipp SC. Systems for testing the enteropathogenicity of *Escherichia coli*. Ann N Y Acad Sci 176:197, 1971.
160. Smith HW, Linggood MA. Observations on the pathogenic properties of the K88, HLY and ENT plasmids of *Escherichia coli* with particular reference to porcine diarrhea. J Med Microbiol 4:467, 1971.
161. Holmgren J, Svennerholm AM. Enzyme-linked immunosorbent assays for cholera serology. Infect Immun 7:759, 1973.
162. Svennerholm AM, Holmgren J. Identification of *Escherichia coli* heat-labile enterotoxin by means of a ganglioside immunosorbent assay (Gm1 ELISA) procedure. Curr Microbiol 1:19, 1978.
163. Sack DA, Huda S, Neogi PKB, et al. Microtiter ganglioside enzyme-linked immunosorbent assay for *Vibrio* and *Escherichia coli* heat-labile enterotoxins and antitoxin. J Clin Microbiol 11:35, 1980.
164. Currie MG, Fok KF, Kato J, et al. Guanylin: an endogenous activator of intestinal guanylate cyclase. Proc Natl Acad Sci U S A 89:947, 1992.
165. Wadstrom T, Aust-Kettis A, Habte D, et al. Enterotoxin-producing bacteria and parasites in stools of Ethiopian children with diarrhoeal disease. Arch Dis Child 51:865, 1976.
166. Wachsmuth K, Wells J, Shipley P, et al. Heat-labile enterotoxin production in isolates from a shipboard outbreak of human diarrheal illness. Infect Immun 24:793, 1979.
167. Sandefur PD, Peterson JW. Isolation of skin permeability factors from culture filtrates of *Salmonella typhimurium*. Infect Immun 14: 671, 1976.
168. Sandefur PD, Peterson JW. Neutralization of *Salmonella* toxin–induced elongation of Chinese hamster ovary cells by cholera antitoxin. Infect Immun 15:988, 1977.
169. Gibbons RA, Sellwood R, Burrows M, et al. Inheritance of resistance to neonatal *E. coli* diarrhoea in the pig: examination of the genetic system. Theor Appl Genet 51:65, 1977.
170. Wolf MK. Occurrence, distribution and associations of O and H serogroups, colonization factor antigens, and toxins of enterotoxigenic *Escherichia coli*. Clin Microbiol Rev 10:569, 1997.
171. Cassels FJ, Wolf MK. Colonization factors of diarrheagenic *E. coli* and their intestinal receptors. J Ind Microbiol 15:214, 1995.
172. Katz DE, DeLorimier AJ, Wolf MK, et al. Oral immunization of adult volunteers with microencapsulated enterotoxigenic *Escherichia coli* (ETEC) CS6 antigen. Vaccine 21:341, 2003.
173. Sack DA, Kaminsky DC, Sack RB, et al. Enterotoxigenic *Escherichia coli* diarrhea of travelers: a prospective study of American Peace Corps volunteers. Johns Hopkins Med J 141:63, 1977.
174. Guerrant RL, Rouse JD, Hughes JM, et al. Turista among members of the Yale Glee Club in Latin America. Am J Trop Med Hyg 29:895, 1980.
175. Guerrant RL, Moore RA, Kirschenfeld PM, et al. Role of toxigenic and invasive bacteria in acute diarrhea of childhood. N Engl J Med 293:567, 1975.
176. Echeverria P, Blacklow NR, Smith DH. Role of heat-labile toxigenic *Escherichia coli* and reovirus-like agent in diarrhoea in Boston children. Lancet 2:1113, 1975.
177. Viboud GI, Binsztein N, Svennerholm AM. Characterization of monoclonal antibodies against putative colonization factors of enterotoxigenic *Escherichia coli* and their use in an epidemiological study. J Clin Microbiol 31:558, 1993.
178. Ryder RW, Sack DA, Kapikian AZ, et al. Enterotoxigenic *Escherichia coli* and reovirus-like agent in rural Bangladesh. Lancet 1:659, 1976.
179. Nalin DR, McLaughlin JC, Rahaman M, et al. Enterotoxigenic *Escherichia coli* and idiopathic diarrhea in Bangladesh. Lancet 2:1116, 1975.
180. Lopez-Vidal Y, Calva JJ, Trujillo A, et al. Enterotoxins and adhesins of enterotoxigenic *Escherichia coli*: are they risk factors for acute diarrhea in the community? J Infect Dis 162:442, 1990.
181. McLean M, Brennan R, Hughes JM, et al. Etiology and oral rehydration therapy of childhood diarrhea in northeastern Brazil. Bull Pan Am Health Organ 15:318, 1981.
182. Sack RB, Hirschhorn N, Brownlee I, et al. Enterotoxigenic *Escherichia coli* associated diarrheal disease in Apache children. N Engl J Med 292:1041, 1975.
183. Hughes JM, Rouse JD, Barada AF, et al. Etiology of summer diarrhea among the Navajo. Am J Trop Med Hyg 29:613, 1980.
184. Huilan S, Zhen LG, Mathan MM, et al. Etiology of acute diarrhea among children in developing countries: a multicentre study in five countries. Bull World Health Organ 69:549, 1991.
185. Blanco J, Gonzalez EA, Blanco M, et al. Enterotoxigenic *Escherichia coli* associated with infant diarrhoea in Galicia, northwestern Spain. J Med Microbiol 35:162, 1991.
186. Nations MK, de Sousa MA, Correia LL, daSilva DM. Brazilian popular healers as effective promoters of oral rehydration therapy (ORT) and related child survival strategies. Bull Pan Am Health Organ 22:335, 1988.
187. Korzeniowski OM, Dantas W, Trabulsi CR, et al. A controlled study of endemic sporadic diarrhea among adult residents of southern Brazil. Trans R Soc Trop Med Hyg 78:363, 1984.
188. Kudoh Y, Hiroshi ZY, Matsushita S, et al. Outbreaks of acute enteritis due to heat-stable enterotoxin-producing strains of *Escherichia coli*. Microbiol Immunol 21:175, 1977.
189. Rosenberg ML, Koplan JP, Wachsmuth IK, et al. Epidemic diarrhea at Crater Lake from enterotoxigenic *Escherichia coli*: a large waterborne outbreak. Ann Intern Med 86:714, 1977.
190. Ryder RW, Wachsmuth IK, Buxton AE, et al. Infantile diarrhea produced by heat-stable enterotoxigenic *Escherichia coli*. N Engl J Med 295:849, 1976.
191. Gross RJ, Rowe B, Henderson A, et al. A new *Escherichia coli* O-group, O159, associated with outbreaks of enteritis in infants. Scand J Infect Dis 8:195, 1976.
192. Albert MJ, Faruque SM, Faruque AS, et al. Controlled study of *Escherichia coli* diarrheal infections in Bangladeshi children. J Clin Microbiol 33:973, 1995.
193. Guerrant RL, Dickens MD, Wenzel RP, et al. Toxigenic bacterial diarrhea: nursery outbreak involving multiple bacterial strains. J Pediatr 89:885, 1976.
194. Abe A, Komase K, Bangtrakulnonth A, et al. Trivalent heat-labile- and heat-stable-enterotoxin probe conjugated with horseradish peroxidase for detection of enterotoxigenic *Escherichia coli* by hybridization J Clin Microbiol 28:2616, 1990.
195. Sommerfelt H, Svennerholm AM, Kallard KH, et al. Comparative study of colony hybridization with synthetic oligonucleotide probes and enzyme-linked immunosorbent assay for identification of enterotoxigenic *E. coli*. J Clin Microbiol 26:530, 1988.
196. Lund A, Wasteson W, Olsvik O. Immunomagnetic separation and DNA hybridization for detection of enterotoxigenic *Escherichia coli* in a piglet model. J Clin Microbiol 29:2259, 1991.
197. Hornes E, Wasteson W, Olsvik O. Detection of *Escherichia coli* heat-stable enterotoxin genes in pig stool specimens by an immobilized, calorimetric, nested polymerase chain reaction. J Clin Microbiol 29:2375, 1991.
198. Guerrant RL, Van Gilder T, Steiner TS, et al. Practice guidelines for the management of infectious diarrhea. Clin Infect Dis 32:331, 2001.
199. Pizarro D, Posada G, Mata L, et al. Oral rehydration of neonates with dehydrating diarrheas. Lancet 2:1209, 1979.
200. Santosham M, Daum RS, Dillman L, et al. Oral rehydration therapy for infantile diarrhea. A controlled study of well nourished children

hospitalized in the United States and Panama. N Engl J Med 306:1070, 1982.
201. Molla AM, Molla A, Nath SK, et al. Food based oral rehydration salt solutions for acute childhood diarrhoea. Lancet 2:429, 1989.
202. Walker SH, Gahol VP, Quintero BA. Sodium and water content of feedings for use in infants with diarrhea. Clin Pediatr 20:199, 1981.
203. International Study Group on Reduced Osmolality ORS Solution. Multicentre evaluation of reduced-osmolality oral rehydration salts solution. Lancet 345:282, 1995.
204. Echeverria P, Ulyangco CV, Ho MT, et al. Antimicrobial resistance and enterotoxin production among isolates of *Escherichia coli* in the Far East. Lancet 2:589, 1978.
205. Harris JR, Wachsmuth IK, Davis BR, et al. High-molecular-weight plasmid correlates with *Escherichia coli* invasiveness. Infect Immun 37:1295, 1982.
206. De Assis A. *Shigella* guanabara, tipo serologico destacado do grupo B ceylonensis-dispar. O Hospital 33:508, 1948.
207. Lapatsanis PD, Irving IM. A study of specific *E. coli* infections occurring in a unit for surgical neonates. Acta Paediatr 52:436, 1963.
208. Gordillo ME, Reeve GR, Pappas J, et al. Molecular characterization of strains of enteroinvasive *Escherichia coli* O143, including isolates from a large outbreak in Houston, Texas. J Clin Microbiol 30:889, 1992.
209. Goldschmidt R. Untersuchungen zur Ätiologie der Durchfallserkrankungen des Säuglings. Jahrb Kinderheilkd 139:318, 1933.
210. Dulaney AD, Michelson ID. A study of *E. coli* mutable from an outbreak of diarrhea in the new-born. Am J Public Health 25:1241, 1935.
211. Bray J. Isolation of antigenically homogenous strains of *Bact. coli* neopolitanum from summer diarrhea of infants. J Pathol Bacteriol 57:239, 1945.
212. Bray J, Beaven TED. Slide agglutination of *Bacterium coli* var. neopolitanum in summer diarrhea. J Pathol Bacteriol 60:395, 1948.
213. Olarte J, Varela G. A complete somatic antigen common to *Salmonella adelaide*, *Escherichia coli-gomez* and *Escherichia coli* O111:B4. J Lab Clin Med (Lond) 40:252, 1952.
214. Giles C, Sangster, G. An outbreak of infantile gastroenteritis in Aberdeen. J Hyg 46:1, 1948.
215. Giles C, Sangster G, Smith J. Epidemic gastroenteritis of infants in Aberdeen during 1947. Arch Dis Child 24:45, 1949.
216. Kaufman F, Dupont A. *Escherichia* strains from infantile epidemic gastroenteritis. Acta Pathol Microbiol Scand 27:552, 1950.
217. Edwards PR, Ewing WH. Identification of Enterobacteriaceae, 3rd ed. Minneapolis, Minn, Burgess Publishing, 1972.
218. Neter E, Korns RF, Trussell RF. Association of *Escherichia coli* serogroup O111 with two hospital outbreaks of epidemic diarrhea of the newborn infant in New York State during 1947. Pediatrics 12:377, 1953.
219. Neter E, Westphal O, Luderitz O, et al. Demonstration of antibodies against enteropathogenic *Escherichia coli* in sera of children of various ages. Pediatrics 16:801, 1955.
220. Gronroos JA. Investigations on certain *Escherichia coli* serotypes, with special reference to infantile diarrhoea. Ann Med 32:9, 1954.
221. Donnenberg MS, Whittam TS. Pathogenesis and evolution of virulence in enteropathogenic and enterohemorrhagic *Escherichia coli*. J Clin Invest 107:539, 2001.
222. Trabulsi LR, Keller R, Tardelli Gomes TA. Typical and atypical enteropathogenic *Escherichia coli*. Emerg Infect Dis 8:508, 2002.
223. Moyenuddin M, Rahman KM. Enteropathogenic *Escherichia coli* diarrhea in hospitalized children in Bangladesh. J Clin Microbiol 22:838, 1985.
224. Bower JR, Congeni BL, Cleary TG, et al. *Escherichia coli* O114: nonmotile as a pathogen in an outbreak of severe diarrhea associated with a day care center. J Infect Dis 160:243, 1989.
225. Neter E. Discussion. Ann N Y Acad Sci 176:136, 1971.
226. Marker SC, Blazevic DJ. Enteropathogenic serotypes of *E. coli*. J Pediatr 90:1037, 1977.
227. Farmer JJ, Davis BR, Cherry WB, et al. "Enteropathogenic serotypes" of *Escherichia coli* which really are not. J Pediatr 90:1047, 1977.
228. Gordon JE. Diarrheal disease of early childhood—worldwide scope of the problem. Ann N Y Acad Sci 176:9, 1971.
229. Gordon JE, Chitkara ID, Wyon JB. Weanling diarrhea. Am J Med Sci 245:345, 1963.
230. Bernet CP, Graber CD, Anthony CW. Association of *Escherichia coli* O127:B8 with an outbreak of infantile gastroenteritis and its concurrent distribution in the pediatric population. J Pediatr 47:287, 1955.
231. Cooper ML, Walters EW, Keller HM, et al. Epidemic diarrhea among infants associated with the isolation of a new serotype of *Escherichia coli*: *E. coli* O127:B8. Pediatrics 16:215, 1955.
232. Laurell G, Magnusson JH, Frisell E, et al. Epidemic infantile diarrhea and vomiting. Acta Paediatr 40:302, 1951.
233. Martineau B, Raymond R, Jeliu G. Bacteriological and clinical study of gastroenteritis and enteropathogenic *Escherichia coli* O127:B8. Can Med Assoc J 79:351, 1958.
234. Wheeler WE, Wainerman B. The treatment and prevention of epidemic infantile diarrhea due to *E. coli* O111 by the use of chloramphenicol and neomycin. Pediatrics 14:357, 1954.
235. Kaslow RA, Taylor A Jr, Dweck HS, et al. Enteropathogenic *Escherichia coli* infection in a newborn nursery. Am J Dis Child 128:797, 1974.
236. Boyer KM, Peterson NJ, Farzaneh I, et al. An outbreak of gastroenteritis due to *E. coli* O142 in a neonatal nursery. J Pediatr 86:919, 1975.
237. Masembe RN. The pattern of bacterial diarrhea of the newborn in Mulago Hospital (Kampala). J Trop Pediatr 23:61, 1977.
238. Boris M, Thomason BM, Hines VD, et al. A community epidemic of enteropathogenic *Escherichia coli* O126:B16:NM gastroenteritis associated with asymptomatic respiratory infection. Pediatrics 33:18, 1964.
239. Kessner DM, Shaughnessy HJ, Googins J, et al. An extensive community outbreak of diarrhea due to enteropathogenic *Escherichia coli* O111:B4. I. Epidemiologic studies. Am J Hyg 76:27, 1962.
240. Severs D, Fardy P, Acres S, et al. Epidemic gastroenteritis in Newfoundland during 1963 associated with *E. coli* O111:B4. Can Med Assoc J 94:373, 1966.
241. Cooper ML, Keller HM, Walters EW. Comparative frequency of detection of enteropathogenic *E. coli*, *Salmonella* and *Shigella* in rectal swab cultures from infants and young children. Pediatrics 19:411, 1957.
242. Hinton NA, MacGregor RR. A study of infections due to pathogenic serogroups of *Escherichia coli*. Can Med Assoc J 79:359, 1958.
243. Hutchinson RI. *Escherichia coli* (O-types 111, 55, and 26) and their association with infantile diarrhea. A five-year study. J Hyg 55:27, 1957.
244. Joe LK, Sahab K, Yauw GS, et al. Diarrhea among infants and children in Djakarta, Indonesia, with special reference to pathogenic *Escherichia coli*. Am J Trop Med Hyg 9:626, 1960.
245. Nelson JD. Duration of neomycin therapy for enteropathogenic *Escherichia coli* diarrheal disease: a comparative study of 113 cases. Pediatrics 48:248, 1971.
246. Riley HD Jr. Antibiotic therapy in neonatal enteric disease. Ann N Y Acad Sci 176:360, 1971.
247. Rozansky R, Berant M, Rosenmann E, et al. Enteropathogenic *Escherichia coli* infections in infants during the period from 1957 to 1962. Pediatrics 64:521, 1964.
248. South MA. Enteropathogenic *Escherichia coli* disease: new developments and perspectives. J Pediatr 79:1, 1971.
249. Linzenmeier G. Wandel im Auftreten und Verhalten enteropathogene Colitypen. Z Bakteriol 184:74, 1962.
250. Nicolopoulos D, Arseni A. Susceptibility of enteropathogenic *E. coli* to various antibiotics. Letter to the editor. J Pediatr 81:426, 1972.
251. Ironside AG, Tuxford AF, Heyworth B. A survey of infantile gastroenteritis. BMJ 2:20, 1970.
252. Riley HD Jr. Clinical rounds. Enteropathogenic *E. coli* gastroenteritis. Clin Pediatr 3:93, 1964.
253. Kourany M, Vasquez MA. Enteropathogenic bacteria associated with diarrhea among infants in Panama. Am J Trop Med Hyg 18:930, 1969.
254. Gaines S, Achavasmith U, Thareesawat M, et al. Types and distribution of enteropathogenic *Escherichia coli* in Bangkok, Thailand. Am J Hyg 80:388, 1964.
255. Buttner DW, Lado-Kenyi A. Prevalence of *Salmonella*, *Shigella*, and enteropathogenic *Escherichia coli* in young children in Kampala, Uganda. Tropenmed Parasitol 24:259, 1973.
256. Coetzee M, Leary PM. Gentamicin in *Esch. coli* gastroenteritis. Arch Dis Child 46:646, 1971.
257. Kahn E. The aetiology of summer diarrhoea. S Afr Med J 31:47, 1957.
258. Taylor J. The diarrhoeal diseases in England and Wales. With special reference to those caused by *Salmonella*, *Escherichia*, and *Shigella*. Bull World Health Organ 23:763, 1960.
259. Epidemiological Research Laboratory of the Public Health Laboratory Service, United Kingdom and Republic of Ireland. *E. coli* gastroenteritis from food. BMJ 1:911, 1976.

260. Ocklitz HW, Schmidt E. F. Über das Vorkommen von Dispepsie-Coli bei Erwachsenen. Helv Paediatr Acta 10:450, 1955.
261. Schaffer J, Lewis V, Nelson J, et al. Antepartum survey for enteropathogenic *Escherichia coli*. Detection by cultural and fluorescent antibody methods. Am J Dis Child 106:170, 1963.
262. Kirby AC, Hall EG, Coackley W. Neonatal diarrhoea and vomiting. Outbreaks in the same maternity unit. Lancet 2:201, 1950.
263. Bettelheim KA, Breaden A, Faiers MC, et al. The origin of O-serotypes of *Escherichia coli* in babies after normal delivery. J Hyg 72:67, 1974.
264. Stulberg CS, Zuelzer WW, Nolke AC. An epidemic of diarrhea of the newborn caused by *Escherichia coli* O111:B4. Pediatrics 14:133, 1954.
265. Farmer K, Hassall IB. An epidemic of *E. coli* type O55:K59(B5) in a neonatal unit. N Z Med J 77:372, 1973.
266. Hugh-Jones K, Ross GIM. Epidemics of gastroenteritis associated with *E. coli* O119 infection. Arch Dis Child 33:543, 1958.
267. Senerwa D, Olsvik O, Mutanda LN, et al. Colonization of neonates in a nursery ward with enteropathogenic *Escherichia coli* and correlation to the clinical histories of the children. J Clin Microbiol 27:2539, 1989.
268. Wright J, Roden AT. *Escherichia coli* O55B5 infection in a gastroenteritis ward. Epidemiological applications of H antigen type determinations. Am J Hyg 58:133, 1953.
269. Balassanian N, Wolinsky E. Epidemiologic and serologic studies of *E. coli* O4:115 in a premature nursery. Pediatrics 41:463, 1968.
270. Jameson JE, Mann TP, Rothfield NJ. Hospital gastroenteritis. An epidemiological survey of infantile diarrhea and vomiting contracted in a children's hospital. Lancet 2:459, 1954.
271. Thomson S. The role of certain varieties of *Bacterium coli* in gastroenteritis in babies. J Hyg 53:357, 1955.
272. Page RH, Stulberg CS. Immunofluorescence in epidemiologic control of *E. coli* diarrhea. Incidence, cross-infections, and control in a children's hospital. Am J Dis Child 104:149, 1962.
273. Bertrams J, Pfortner M, Neusel H, et al. Colienteritis des Säuglings. Quantitative und fluoreszenzserologische Verlaufsuntersuchungen. Munch Med Wochenschr 112:38, 1970.
274. Thomson S. The numbers of pathogenic bacilli in faeces in intestinal diseases. J Hyg 53:217, 1955.
275. Herweg JC, Middlekamp JN, Thornton HK. *Escherichia coli* diarrhea. The relationship of certain serotypes of *Escherichia coli* to sporadic and epidemic cases of infantile diarrhea. J Pediatr 49:629, 1956.
276. Belnap WD, O'Donnell JJ. Epidemic gastroenteritis due to *Escherichia coli* 0-111. A review of the literature, with the epidemiology, bacteriology, and clinical findings of a large outbreak. J Pediatr 47:178, 1955.
277. Rogers KB, Koegler SJ. Inter-hospital cross-infection epidemic infantile gastroenteritis associated with type strains of *Bacterium coli*. J Hyg 49:152, 1951.
278. Stock AH, Shuman ME. Gastroenteritis in infants associated with specific serotypes of *Escherichia coli*. II. An epidemic of *Escherichia coli* O111:B4 gastroenteritis involving multiple institutions. Pediatrics 17:196, 1956.
279. Stulberg CS, Zuelzer WW, Nolke AC, et al. *Escherichia coli* O127:B8, a pathogenic strain causing infantile diarrhea. Epidemiology and bacteriology of a prolonged outbreak in a premature nursery. Am J Dis Child 90:125, 1955.
280. Thomson S, Watkins AG, Grapy PO. *Escherichia coli* gastroenteritis. Arch Dis Child 31:340, 1956.
281. Olarte J, Ramos-Alvarez M. Epidemic diarrhea in premature infants. Etiological significance of a newly recognized type of *Escherichia coli* (O142:K86:H6). Am J Dis Child 109:436, 1965.
282. Nelson JD, Whitaker JA, Hempstead B, et al. Epidemiological application of the fluorescent antibody technique. Study of a diarrhea outbreak in a premature nursery. JAMA 176:26, 1961.
283. Buttiaux R, Nicolle P, LeMinor S, et al. Etude épidémiologique des gastroentéritis à Escherichia coli dans un service hospitalier du nord de la France. Arch Mal Appar Dig Mal Nutr 45:225, 1956.
284. Harris AH, Yankauer A, Green DC, et al. Control of epidemic diarrhea of the newborn in hospital nurseries and pediatric wards. Ann N Y Acad Sci 66:118, 1956.
285. Jacobs SI, Holzel A, Wolman B, et al. Outbreak of infantile gastroenteritis caused by *Escherichia coli* O114. Arch Dis Child 46:656, 1970.
286. Curtin M, Clifford SH. Incidence of pathogenic serologic types of *Escherichia coli* among neonatal patients in the New England area. N Engl J Med 255:1090, 1956.
287. Greene DC, Albrecht RM. Recent developments in diarrhea of the newborn. N Y State J Med 55:2764, 1955.
288. Wheeler WE. Spread and control of *Escherichia coli* diarrheal disease. Ann N Y Acad Sci 66:112, 1956.
289. Buttiaux RR, Nicolle P, LeMinor L, et al. Etudes sur les *E. coli* de gastroentérite infantile. Ann Inst Pasteur 91:799, 1956.
290. Love WC, Gordon AM, Gross RJ, et al. Infantile gastroenteritis due to *Escherichia coli* O142. Lancet 2:355, 1972.
291. Shaughnessy HJ, Lesko M, Dorigan F, et al. An extensive community outbreak of diarrhea due to enteropathogenic *Escherichia coli* O111:B4. Am J Hyg 76:44, 1962.
292. Kendall N, Vaughan VC III, Kusakcioglu A. A study of preparation of infant formulas. A medical and sociocultural appraisal. Am J Dis Child 122:215, 1971.
293. Gamble DR, Rowson KEK. The incidence of pathogenic *Escherichia coli* in routine fecal specimens. Lancet 2:619, 1957.
294. Taylor J, Powell BW, Wright J. Infantile diarrhoea and vomiting. A clinical and bacteriological investigation. BMJ 2:117, 1949.
295. Modica RI, Ferguson WW, Ducey EF. Epidemic infantile diarrhea associated with *Escherichia coli* O111, B4. J Lab Clin Med 39:122, 1952.
296. Rogers KB. The spread of infantile gastroenteritis in a cubicled ward. J Hyg 49:140, 1951.
297. Mossel DAA, Weijers HA. Uitkomsten, verkregen bij bacteriologisch onderzoek van vrouwenmelk van diverse herkomst en de betekenis daarvan de pediatrische praktijk. Maandschr Kindergeneeskd 25:37, 1957.
298. Rantasalo I, Kauppinen MA. The occurrence of *Staphylococcus aureus* in mother's milk. Ann Chir Gynaecol 48:246, 1959.
299. Edwards LD, Tan-Gatue LG, Levin S, et al. The problem of bacteriologically contaminated infant formulas in a newborn nursery. Clin Pediatr 13:63, 1974.
300. Thomson S. Is infantile gastroenteritis fundamentally a milk-borne infection? J Hyg 54:311, 1956.
301. Danielssen D, Laurell G. Fluorescent antibody technique in the diagnosis of enteropathogenic *Escherichia coli*, with special reference to sensitivity and specificity. Acta Pathol Microbiol Scand 76:601, 1969.
302. Bullen CL, Willis AT. Resistance of the breast-fed infant to gastroenteritis. BMJ 2:338, 1971.
303. Svirsky-Gross S. Pathogenic strains of coli (0,111) among prematures and the use of human milk in controlling the outbreak of diarrhea. Ann Paediatr 190:109, 1958.
304. Tassovatz B, Kotsitch A. Le lait de femme et son action de protection contre les infections intestinales chez le nouveau-né. Ann Paediatr 8:285, 1961.
305. Adam A. Fortschritte in der Pathogenese und Therapie der Ernährungsstörungen. Arztl Forschung 6:59, 1952.
306. Neter E, Shumway CN. *E. coli* serotype D433; occurrence in intestinal and respiratory tracts, cultural characteristics, pathogenicity, sensitivity to antibiotics. Proc Soc Exp Biol Med 75:504, 1950.
307. Arnon H, Salzberger M, Olitzki AL. The appearance of antibacterial and antitoxic antibodies in maternal sera, umbilical cord blood and milk: observations on the specificity of antibacterial antibodies in human sera. Pediatrics 23:86, 1959.
308. Kenny JF, Boesman MI, Michaels RH. Bacterial and viral coproantibodies in breast-fed infants. Pediatrics 39:202, 1967.
309. Sussman S. The passive transfer of antibodies to *Escherichia coli* O111:B4 from mother to offspring. Pediatrics 27:308, 1961.
310. Stulberg CS, Zuelzer WW. Infantile diarrhea due to *Escherichia coli*. Ann N Y Acad Sci 66:90, 1956.
311. Yeivin R, Salzberger M, Olitzki AL. Development of antibodies to enteric pathogens: placental transfer of antibodies and development of immunity in childhood. Pediatrics 18:19, 1956.
312. Dancis J, Kunz HW. Studies of the immunology of the newborn infant. VI. Bacteriostatic and complement activity of the serum. Pediatrics 13:339, 1954.
313. Kenny JF, Weinert DW, Gray JA. Enteric infection with *Escherichia coli* O127 in the mouse. II. Failure of specific immunity to alter intestinal colonization of infants and adults. J Infect Dis 129:10, 1974.
314. Lodinova R, Jouja V, Wagner V. Serum immunoglobulins and coproantibody formation in infants after artificial intestinal colonization with *Escherichia coli* O83 and oral lysozyme administration. Pediatr Res 7:659, 1973.
315. McNeish AS, Gaze H. The intestinal antibody response in infants with enteropathic *E. coli* gastroenteritis. Acta Paediatr Scand 63:663, 1974.
316. Goldschmidt MC, DuPont HL. Enteropathogenic *Escherichia coli*: lack of correlation of serotype with pathogenicity. J Infect Dis 133:153, 1976.

317. Echeverria PD, Chang CP, Smith D. Enterotoxigenicity and invasive capacity of "enteropathogenic" serotypes of *Escherichia coli*. J Pediatr 89:8, 1976.
318. Gross RJ, Scotland SM, Rowe B. Enterotoxin testing of *Escherichia coli* causing epidemic infantile enteritis in the U.K. Lancet 1:629, 1976.
319. Drucker MM, Pollack A, Yeivin R, et al. Immunofluorescent demonstration of enteropathogenic *Escherichia coli* in tissues of infants dying with enteritis. Pediatrics 46:855, 1970.
320. Levine MM, Bergquist EJ, Nalin DR, et al. *Escherichia coli* strains that cause diarrhea but do not produce heat-labile or heat-stable enterotoxins and are non-invasive. Lancet 1:1119, 1978.
321. Wade WG, Thom BT, Evans N. Cytotoxic enteropathogenic *Escherichia coli*. Lancet 2:1235, 1979.
322. Mellies JL, Navarro-Garcia F, Okeke I, et al. EspC pathogenicity island of Enteropathogenic *Escherichia coli* encodes an enterotoxin. Infect Immun 69:315, 2001.
323. Vallance BA, Chan C, Robertson ML, Finlay BB. Enteropathogenic and enterohemorrhagic *Escherichia coli* infections: emerging themes in pathogenesis and prevention. Can J Gastroenterol 16:771, 2002.
324. Rothbaum RJ, Partin JC, McAdams AJ, et al. Enterocyte adherent *E. coli* O119:B14: a novel mechanism of infant diarrhea. Gastroenterology 80:1265, 1981.
325. Polotsky Y, Dragunskaya EM, Seliverstova VG, et al. Pathogenic effect of enterotoxigenic *Escherichia coli* and *Escherichia coli* causing infantile diarrhea. Acta Microbiol Acad Sci Hung 24:221, 1977.
326. McDaniel TK, Jarvis KG, Donnenberg MS, Kaper JB. A genetic locus of enterocyte effacement conserved among diverse enterobacterial pathogens. Proc Natl Acad Sci U S A 92:1664, 1995.
327. McDaniel TK, Kaper JB. A cloned pathogenicity island from enteropathogenic *Escherichia coli* confers the attaching and effacing phenotype on *E. coli* K-12. Mol Microbiol 23:399, 1997.
328. Elliott SJ, Wainwright LA, McDaniel TK, et al. The complete sequence of the locus of enterocyte effacement (LEE) from enteropathogenic *Escherichia coli* E2348/69. Mol Microbiol 28:1, 1998.
329. Ghaem-Maghami M, Simmons CP, Daniell S, et al. Intimin-specific immune responses prevent bacterial colonization by the attaching-effacing pathogen *Citrobacter rodentium*. Infect Immun 69:5597, 2001.
330. Giron JA, Ho ASY, Schoolnik GK. An inducible bundle-forming pilus of enteropathogenic *Escherichia coli*. Science 254:710, 1992.
331. Stone KD, Zhang HZ, Carlson LK, Donnenberg MS. A cluster of fourteen genes from enteropathogenic *Escherichia coli* is sufficient for the biogenesis of a type IV pilus. Mol Microbiol 20:325, 1996.
332. Knutton S, Shaw RK, Anantha RP, et al. The type IV bundle-forming pilus of enteropathogenic *Escherichia coli* undergoes dramatic alterations in structure associated with bacterial adherence, aggregation and dispersal. Mol Microbiol 33:499, 1999.
333. Bieber D, Ramer SW, Wu CY, et al. Type IV pili, transient bacterial aggregates, and virulence of enteropathogenic *Escherichia coli*. Science 280:2114, 1998.
334. Hopkins GB, Gould VE, Stevenson JK, et al. Necrotizing enterocolitis in premature infants. A clinical and pathologic evaluation of autopsy material. Am J Dis Child 120:229, 1970.
335. Rho Y, Josephson JE. Epidemic enteropathogenic *Escherichia coli*. Newfoundland, 1963: autopsy study of 16 cases. Can Med Assoc J 96:392, 1967.
335. Shwachman H, Lloyd-Still JD, Khaw KT, et al. Protracted diarrhea of infancy treated by intravenous alimentation. II. Studies of small intestinal biopsy results. Am J Dis Child 125:365, 1973.
337. Lucking T, Gruttner R. Chronic diarrhea and severe malabsorption in infancy following infections with pathogenic *E. coli*. Acta Paediatr Scand 63:167, 1974.
338. Handforth CP, Sorger K. Failure of regeneration of small bowel mucosa following epidemic infantile gastroenteritis. Can Med Assoc J 84:425, 1961.
339. McKay DG, Wahle GH Jr. Epidemic gastroenteritis due to *Escherichia coli* O111:B4. II. Pathologic anatomy (with special reference to the presence of the local and generalized Shwartzman phenomena). Arch Pathol 60:679, 1955.
340. Laurell G. Quoted in Ordway NK. Diarrhoeal disease and its control. Bull World Health Organ 23:93, 1960.
341. Braun OH, Henckel H. Über epidemische Säuglingsenteritis. Z Kinderheilkd 70:33, 1951.
342. Neter E. Enteritis due to enteropathogenic *Escherichia coli*. Present day status and unsolved problems. J Pediatr 55:223, 1959.
343. Rogers KB, Cracknell VM. Epidemic infantile gastroenteritis due to *Escherichia coli* type 0,114. J Pathol Bacteriol 72:27, 1956.
344. Todd RM, Hall EG. Chloramphenicol in prophylaxis of infantile gastroenteritis. BMJ 1:1359, 1953.
345. Gastroenteritis due to *Escherichia coli*. Editorial. Lancet 1:32, 1968.
346. Senerwa D, Olsvik O, Mutanda LN, et al. Enteropathogenic *Escherichia coli* serotype O111:HNT isolated from preterm neonates in Nairobi, Kenya. J Clin Microbiol 27:1307, 1989.
347. Bray J. Bray's discovery of pathogenic *Esch. coli* as a cause of infantile gastroenteritis. Arch Dis Child 48:923, 1973.
348. Ironside AG, Brennand J, Mandal BK, et al. Cross-infection in infantile gastroenteritis. Arch Dis Child 46:815, 1971.
349. Linetskaya-Novgorodskaya EM. Acute intestinal infections of non-dysenteric etiology. Bull World Health Organ 21:299, 1959.
350. Lloyd-Still JD, Shwachman H, Filler RM. Protracted diarrhea of infancy treated by intravenous alimentation. 1. Clinical studies of 16 infants. Am J Dis Child 125:358, 1973.
351. Drimmer-Hernheiser H, Olitzki AL. The association of *Escherichia coli* (serotypes O111:B4 and O55:B5) with cases of acute infantile gastroenteritis in Jerusalem. Acta Med Orient 10:219, 1951.
352. Linde K, Kodizt H, Funk G. Die Mehrfachinfektionen mit Dyspepsie-Coli, ihre Beurteilung in statistischer, bakteriologischer und klinischer Sicht. Z Hyg 147:94, 1960.
353. Fandre M, Coffin R, Dropsy G, et al. Epidemic of infantile gastroenteritis due to *Escherichia coli* O127:B8 with methemoglobinemic cyanosis. Arch Fr Pediatr 19:1129, 1962.
354. Garcia de Olarte D, Trujillo H, Agudelo ON, et al. Treatment of diarrhea in malnourished infants and children. A double-blind study comparing ampicillin and placebo. Am J Dis Child 127:379, 1974.
355. Yow MD. Prophylactic antimicrobial agents-panel. Statement of panelist. *In* Centers for Disease Control Proceedings of the International Conference on Nosocomial Infections, August 3-6, 1970. Chicago, American Hospital Association, 1971, pp 315-316.
356. Bettelheim KA, Faiers M, Sheeter RA. Serotypes of *Escherichia coli* in normal stools. Lancet 2:1227, 1972.
357. Stock AH, Shuman ME. Gastroenteritis in infants associated with specific serotypes of *Escherichia coli*. I. Incidence of specific *Escherichia coli* serotypes O111:B4 and O55:B5 in the Pittsburgh area. Pediatrics 17:192, 1956.
358. Mushin R. Multiple intestinal infection. Med J Aust 1:807, 1953.
359. Harris JC, DuPont HL, Hornick RB. Fecal leukocytes in diarrheal illness. Ann Intern Med 76:697, 1972.
360. Guerrant RL, Araujo V, Cooper WH, et al. Measurement of fecal lactoferrin as a marker of fecal leukocytes and inflammatory enteritis. J Clin Microbiol 30:1238, 1992.
361. Miller JR, Barrett LJ, Kotloff K, Guerrant RL. A rapid test for infectious and inflammatory enteritis. Arch Intern Med 154:2660, 1994.
362. Cherry WB, Thomason BM. Fluorescent antibody techniques for *Salmonella* and other enteric pathogens. Public Health Rep 84:887, 1969.
363. Murray WA, Kheder J, Wheeler WE. Colistin suppression of *Escherichia coli* in stools. I. Control of a nosocomial outbreak of diarrhea caused by neomycin-resistant *Escherichia coli* O111:B4. Am J Dis Child 108:274, 1964.
364. Bokete TN, Whittam TS, Wilson RA, et al. Genetic and phenotypic analysis of *Escherichia coli* with enteropathogenic characteristics isolated from Seattle children. J Infect Dis 175:1382, 1997.
365. Vial PA, Mathewson JJ, DuPont HL, Guers L, Levine MM. Comparison of two assay methods for patterns of adherence to HEp-2 cells of *Escherichia coli* from patients with diarrhea. J Clin Microbiol 28:882, 1990.
366. Albert MJ, Ansaruzzaman M, Faruque SM, et al. An ELISA for the detection of localized adherent classic enteropathogenic *Escherichia coli* serogroups. J Infect Dis 164:986, 1991.
367. Knutton S, Baldwin T, Williams PH, et al. Actin accumulation at sites of bacterial adhesion to tissue culture cells: basis of a new diagnostic test for enteropathogenic and enterohemorrhagic *Escherichia coli*. Infect Immun 57:1290, 1989.
368. Nelson JD. Comment. *In* Gellis S (ed). Yearbook of Pediatrics, 1973. St Louis, Mosby–Year Book, 1973.
369. Sherman JO, Hamly CA, Khachadurian AK. Use of an oral elemental diet in infants with severe intractable diarrhea. J Pediatr 86:518, 1975.
370. Pearce JL, Hamilton JR. Controlled trial of orally administered lactobacilli in acute infantile diarrhea. J Pediatr 84:261, 1974.
371. Marie J, Hennequet A, Roux C. La kanamycin "per os" dans le traitement des gastroentérites à colibacilles du nourrison. Ann Paediatr 9:97, 1962.
372. Valman HB, Wilmers MJ. Use of antibiotics in acute gastroenteritis among infants in hospital. Lancet 1:1122, 1969.

373. Dailey KM, Sturtevant AB, Feary TW. Incidence of antibiotic resistance and R-factors among gram-negative bacteria isolated from the neonatal intestine. J Pediatr 80:198, 1972.
374. Neu HC, Cherubin C, Vogt M, et al. Antibiotic resistance of fecal *Escherichia coli*. A comparison of samples from children of low and high socioeconomic groups. Am J Dis Child 126:174, 1973.
375. Watanabe T. Transferable antibiotic resistance in Enterobacteriaceae: relationship to the problems of treatment and control of coliform enteritis. Ann N Y Acad Sci 176:371, 1971.
376. McCracken GH. Changing pattern of the antimicrobial susceptibilities of *Escherichia coli* in neonatal infections. J Pediatr 78:942, 1971.
377. Kunin CM. Resistance to antimicrobial drugs—a worldwide calamity. Ann Intern Med 118:559, 1993.
378. Silver LL, Bostian KA. Discovery and development of new antibiotics: the problem of antibiotic resistance. Antimicrob Agents Chemother 37:377, 1993.
379. Nelson JD. Commentary. J Pediatr 89:471, 1976.
380. Committee on Fetus and Newborn. Guidelines for Perinatal Care, 3rd ed. American Academy of Pediatrics and American College of Obstetricians and Gynecologists, 1992.
381. Sprunt K, Redman W, Leidy G. Antibacterial effectiveness of routine handwashing. Pediatrics 52:264, 1973.
382. Multistate outbreak of *Escherichia coli* O157:H7 infections from hamburgers. MMWR Morb Mortal Wkly Rep 42:258, 1993.
383. MacDonald KL, Osterholm MT. The emergence of *Escherichia coli* O157:H7 infection in the United States. JAMA 269:2264, 1993.
384. Watanabe H, Wadam A, Inagaki Y, et al. Outbreaks of enterohemorrhagic *Escherichia coli* O157:H7 infection by two different genotype strains in Japan. Lancet 348:831, 1996.
385. Slutsker L, Ries AA, Maloney K, et al. A nationwide case-control study of *Escherichia coli* O157:H7 infection in the United States. J Infect Dis 177:962, 1998.
386. Rasmussen MA, Casey TA. Environmental and food safety aspects of *Escherichia coli* O157:H7 infections in cattle. Crit Rev Microbiol 27:57, 2001.
387. Ochoa TJ, Cleary TG. Epidemiology and spectrum of disease of *Escherichia coli* O157. Curr Opin Infect Dis 16:259, 2003.
388. Hemolytic-uremic syndrome associated with *Escherichia coli* O157:H7 enteric infections—United States. MMWR Morb Mortal Wkly Rep 34:20, 1985.
389. Belongia EA, Osterholm MT, Soler JT, et al. Transmission of *Escherichia coli* O157:H7 infection in Minnesota child day-care facilities. JAMA 269:883, 1993.
390. Besser RE, Lett SM, Weber JT, et al. An outbreak of diarrhea and hemolytic uremic syndrome from *Escherichia coli* O157:H7 in fresh-pressed apple cider. JAMA 269:2217, 1993.
391. Mobasellah M, Donohue-Rolfe A, Jacewicz M, et al. Pathogenesis of *Shigella* diarrhea: evidence for a developmentally regulated glycolipid receptor for Shigatoxin involved in the fluid secretory response of rabbit small intestine. J Infect Dis 157:1023, 1988.
392. Sandvig K. Shiga toxins. Toxicon 39:1629, 2001.
393. Ray PE, Liu XH. Pathogenesis of Shiga toxin–induced hemolytic uremic syndrome. Pediatr Nephrol 16:823, 2001.
394. Schmidt H. Shiga-toxin-converting bacteriophages. Res Microbiol 152:687, 2001.
395. Scotland SM, Smith HR, Rowe B. Two distinct toxins active on Vero cells from *Escherichia coli* O157. Lancet 2:885, 1985.
396. Karmali MA, Petric M, Louie S, et al. Antigenic heterogeneity of *Escherichia coli* verotoxins. Lancet 1:164, 1986.
397. Karch H, Heeseman J, Laufs R, et al. A plasmid of enterohemorrhagic *Escherichia coli* O157:H7 is required for expression of a new fimbrial antigen and for adhesion to epithelial cells. Infect Immun 55:455, 1987.
398. Levine MM, Jian-guo XU, Kaper JB. A DNA probe to identify enterohemorrhagic *Escherichia coli* of O157:H7 and other serotypes that cause hemorrhagic colitis and hemolytic uremic syndrome. J Infect Dis 156:175, 1987.
399. Paton JC, Paton AW. Methods for detection of STEC in humans. An overview. Methods Mol Med 73:9, 2003.
400. Klein EJ, Stapp JR, Clausen CR, et al. Shiga toxin–producing *Escherichia coli* in children with diarrhea: a prospective point-of-care study. J Pediatr 141:172, 2002.
401. Tarr PI. *Escherichia coli* O157:H7: clinical, diagnostic, and epidemiological aspects of human infection. Clin Infect Dis 20:1, 1995.
402. Wong CS, Jelacic S, Habeeb RL, et al. The risk of the hemolytic-uremic syndrome after antibiotic treatment of *Escherichia coli* O157:H7 infections. N Engl J Med 342:1930, 2000.
403. Safdar N, Said A, Gangnon RE, Maki DG. Risk of hemolytic uremic syndrome after antibiotic treatment of *Escherichia coli* O157:H7 enteritis: a meta-analysis. JAMA 288:996, 2002.
404. Nataro JP. Enteroaggregative *Escherichia coli*. *In* Hughes J, ed. Emerging Infections 6. Washington, DC, American Society for Microbiology Press, 2003.
405. Sarantuya J, Nishi J, Wakimoto K, et al. Typical enteroaggregative *Escherichia coli* are the most prevalent pathotypes causing diarrhea in Mongolian children. J Clin Microbiol. In press.
406. Baudry B, Savarino SJ, Vial P, et al. A sensitive and specific DNA probe to identify enteroaggregative *Escherichia coli*, a recently discovered diarrheal pathogen. J Infect Dis 161:1249, 1990.
407. Nishi J, Sheikh J, Mizuguchi K, et al. The export of coat protein from enteroaggregative *Escherichia coli* by a specific ATP-binding cassette transporter system. J Biol Chem 278:45680, 2003.
408. Mathewson JJ, Johnson PC, DuPont HL, et al. Pathogenicity of enteroadherent *Escherichia coli* in adult volunteers. J Infect Dis 154:524, 1986.
409. Nataro JP, Deng Y, Cookson S, et al. Heterogeneity of enteroaggregative *Escherichia coli* virulence demonstrated in volunteers. J Infect Dis 17:465, 1995.
410. Itoh Y, Nagano I, Kunishima M, Ezaki T. Laboratory investigation of enteroaggregative *Escherichia coli* O untypeable:H10 associated with a massive outbreak of gastrointestinal illness. J Clin Microbiol 35:2546, 1997.
411. Smith HR, Cheasty T, Rowe B. Enteroaggregative *Escherichia coli* and outbreaks of gastroenteritis in UK. Lancet 350:814, 1997.
412. Cobeljic M, Miljkovic-Selimovic B, Paunovic-Todosijevic D, et al. Enteroaggregative *E. coli* associated with an outbreak of diarrhea in a neonatal nursery ward. Epidemiol Infect 117:11, 1996.
413. Eslava CE, Villaseca J, Morales R, et al. Identification of a protein with toxigenic activity produced by enteroaggregative *Escherichia coli*. Abstracts of the General Meeting of the American Society for Microbiology, 1993 (abstract B-105).
414. Bhan MK, Raj P, Levine MM, et al. Enteroaggregative *Escherichia coli* associated with persistent diarrhea in a cohort of rural children in India. J Infect Dis 159:1061, 1989.
415. Bhan MK, Khoshoo V, Sommerfelt H, et al. Enteroaggregative *Escherichia coli* and Salmonella associated with non-dysenteric persistent diarrhea. Pediatr Infect Dis J 8:499, 1989.
416. Cravioto A, Tello A, Navarro A, et al. Association of *Escherichia coli* HEp-2 adherence patterns with type and duration of diarrhoea. Lancet 337:262, 1991.
417. Lima AAM, Fang G, Schorling JB, et al. Persistent diarrhea in Northeast Brazil: etiologies and interactions with malnutrition. Acta Paediatr Scand 381:39, 1992.
418. Dutta S, Pal S, Chakrabarti S, Dutta P, Manna B. Use of PCR to identify enteroaggregative *Escherichia coli* as an important cause of acute diarrhoea among children living in Calcutta, India. J Med Microbiol 48:1011, 1999.
419. Scaletsky IC, Fabbricotti SH, Silva SO, et al. HEp-2-adherent *Escherichia coli* strains associated with acute infantile diarrhea, São Paulo, Brazil. Emerg Infect Dis 8:855, 2002.
420. Gonzalez R, Diaz C, Marino M, et al. Age-specific prevalence of *Escherichia coli* with localized and aggregative adherence in Venezuelan infants with acute diarrhea. J Clin Microbiol 35:1103, 1997.
421. Okeke IN, Lamikanra A, Czeczulin J, et al. Heterogeneous virulence of enteroaggregative *Escherichia coli* strains isolated from children in Southwest Nigeria. J Infect Dis 181:252, 2000.
422. Bouzari S, Jafari A, Farhoudi-Moghaddam AA, Shokouhi F, Parsi M. Adherence of non-enteropathogenic *Escherichia coli* to HeLa cells. J Med Microbiol 40:95, 1994.
423. Pabst WL, Altwegg M, Kind C, et al. Prevalence of enteroaggregative *Escherichia coli* among children with and without diarrhea in Switzerland. J Clin Microbiol 41:2289, 2003.
424. Presterl E, Nadrchal R, Wolf D, et al. Enteroaggregative and enterotoxigenic *Escherichia coli* among isolates from patients with diarrhea in Austria. Eur J Clin Microbiol Infect Dis 18:209, 1999.
425. Huppertz HI, Rutkowski S, Aleksic S, Karch H. Acute and chronic diarrhoea and abdominal colic associated with enteroaggregative *Escherichia coli* in young children living in western Europe. Lancet 349:1660, 1997.
426. Tompkins DS, Hudson MJ, Smith HR, et al. A study of infectious intestinal disease in England: microbiological findings in cases and controls. Commun Dis Public Health 2:108, 1999.
427. Cohen M, Nataro JP. Unpublished observations, 2005.

428. Bouckenooghe AR, Dupont HL, Jiang ZD, et al. Markers of enteric inflammation in enteroaggregative *Escherichia coli* diarrhea in travelers. Am J Trop Med Hyg 62:711, 2000.
429. Miqdady MS, Jiang ZD, Nataro JP, DuPont HL. Detection of enteroaggregative *Escherichia coli* with formalin-preserved HEp-2 cells. J Clin Microbiol 40:3066, 2002.
430. Spencer J, Chart H, Smith HR, Rowe B. Improved detection of enteroaggregative *Escherichia coli* using formalin-fixed HEp-2 cells. Lett Appl Microbiol 25:325, 1997.
431. Wanke CA, Gerrior J, Blais V, et al. Successful treatment of diarrheal disease associated with enteroaggregative *Escherichia coli* in adults infected with human immunodeficiency virus. J Infect Dis 178:1369, 1998.
432. Adachi JA, Ericsson CD, Jiang ZD, et al. Azithromycin found to be comparable to levofloxacin for the treatment of US travelers with acute diarrhea acquired in Mexico. Clin Infect Dis 37:1165, 2003.
433. DuPont HL, Jiang ZD, Ericsson CD, et al. Rifaximin versus ciprofloxacin for the treatment of traveler's diarrhea: a randomized, double-blind clinical trial. Clin Infect Dis 33:1807, 2001.
434. Bilge SS, Clausen CR, Lau W, et al. Molecular characterization of a fimbrial adhesin, F1845, mediating diffuse adherences of diarrhea-associated *Escherichia coli* to HEp-2 cells. J Bacteriol 171:4281, 1989.
435. Gunzburg ST, Chang BJ, Elliott SJ, et al. Diffuse and enteroaggregative patterns of adherence of enteric *Escherichia coli* isolated from aboriginal children from the Kimberley region of western Australia. J Infect Dis 167:755, 1993.
436. Baqui AH, Sack RB, Black RE, et al. Enteropathogens associated with acute and persistent diarrhea in Bangladeshi children <5 years of age. J Infect Dis 166:792, 1992.
437. Elliott SJ, Srinivas S, Albert MJ, et al. Characterization of the roles of hemolysin and other toxins in enteropathy caused by alpha-hemolytic *Escherichia coli* linked to human diarrhea. Infect Immun 66:2040, 1998.
438. Ewing WH. Edwards and Ewing's Identification of Enterobacteriaceae, 4th ed. New York, Elsevier, 1986.
439. Meadow WL, Schneider H, Beem MO. *Salmonella enteritidis* bacteremia in childhood. J Infect Dis 152:185, 1985.
440. Hyams JS, Durbin WA, Grand RJ, et al. *Salmonella* bacteremia in the first year of life. J Pediatr 96:57, 1980.
441. Taylor DN, Bied JM, Munro JS, et al. *Salmonella dublin* infections in the United States, 1979-1980. J Infect Dis 146:322, 1982.
442. Zhou D, Galan J. *Salmonella* entry into host cells: the work in concert of type III secreted effector proteins. Microbes Infect 3:1293, 2001.
443. Zhang S, Kingsley RA, Santos RL, et al. Molecular pathogenesis of *Salmonella enterica* serotype typhimurium-induced diarrhea. Infect Immun 71:1, 2003.
444. Waterman SR, Holden DW. Functions and effectors of the *Salmonella* pathogenicity island 2 type III secretion system. Cell Microbiol 5:501, 2003
445. Fierer J, Krause M, Tauxe R, et al. *Salmonella typhimurium* bacteremia: association with the virulence plasmid. J Infect Dis 166:639, 1992.
446. Giannella RA, Formal SB, Dammin GJ, et al. Pathogenesis of salmonellosis: studies of fluid secretion, mucosal invasion, and morphologic reaction in the rabbit ileum. J Clin Invest 52:441, 1973.
447. Jiwa SF. Probing for enterotoxigenicity among the salmonellae: an evaluation of biological assays. J Clin Microbiol 14:463, 1981.
448. Koo FCW, Peterson JW, Houston CW, et al. Pathogenesis of experimental salmonellosis: inhibition of protein synthesis by cytotoxin. Infect Immun 43:93, 1984.
449. Ashkenazi S, Cleary T, Murray BE, et al. Cytotoxin production by *Salmonella* strains: quantitative analysis and partial characterization. Infect Immun 56:3089, 1988.
450. Takeuchi A. Electron microscope studies of experimental *Salmonella* infection. I. Penetration into the intestinal epithelium by *S. typhimurium*. Am J Pathol 50:109, 1967.
451. Modrazakowski MC, Spitznagel JK. Bactericidal activity of fractionated granule contents from human polymorphonuclear leukocytes: antagonism of granule cationic proteins by lipopolysaccharide. Infect Immun 25:597, 1979.
452. Weiss J, Victor M, Elsbach P. Role of charge and hydrophobic interaction in the action of the bactericidal/permeability increasing protein of neutrophils on gram-negative bacteria. J Clin Invest 71:540, 1983.
453. Mackaness GV. Resistance to intracellular infection. J Infect Dis 123:439, 1971.
454. Mackaness GV, Blander RV, Collins FM. Host parasite relations in mouse typhoid. J Exp Med 124:573, 1966.
455. McKenzie SE, Kline J, Douglas SD, Polin RA. Enhancement in vitro of the low interferon-gamma production of leukocytes from human newborn infants. J Leukoc Biol 53:691, 1993.
456. George A. Generation of gamma interferon responses in murine Peyer's patches following oral immunization. Infect Immun 64:4606, 1996.
457. de Jong R, Altare F, Haagen IA, et al. Severe mycobacterial and *Salmonella* infections in interleukin-12 receptor-deficient patients. Science 280:1435, 1998.
458. Hornick RB, Greisman SE, Woodward TE, et al. Typhoid fever: pathogenesis and immunologic control. N Engl J Med 283:686, 1970.
459. Kent TH, Formal SB, LaBrec EH. *Salmonella* gastroenteritis in rhesus monkeys. Arch Pathol 82:272, 1966.
460. Boyd JF. Pathology of the alimentary tract of *S. typhimurium* food poisoning. Gut 26:935, 1985.
461. Day DW, Mandel BK, Morson BC. The rectal biopsy appearances in *Salmonella colitis*. Histopathology 2:117, 1978.
462. Wilder AN, MacCready RA. Isolation of *Salmonella* from poultry, poultry products and poultry processing plants in Massachusetts. N Engl J Med 274:1453, 1966.
463. Pet turtle-associated salmonellosis—Puerto Rico. MMWR Morb Mortal Wkly Rep 33:141, 1984.
464. Sanyal D, Douglas T, Roberts R. *Salmonella* infection acquired from reptilian pets. Arch Dis Child 77:345, 1997.
465. Mermin J, Hoar B, Angulo FJ. Iguanas and *Salmonella* marina infection in children: a reflection of the increasing incidence of reptile-associated salmonellosis in the United States. Pediatrics 99:399, 1997.
466. Woodward DL, Khakhria R, Johnson WM. Human salmonellosis associated with exotic pets. J Clin Microbiol 35:2786, 1997.
467. Thomson S. Paratyphoid fever and Baker's confectionery: analysis of epidemic in South Wales 1952. Monthly Bull Ministry Health Public Health Serv 12:187, 1953.
468. Watt J, Wegman ME, Brown OW, et al. Salmonellosis in a premature nursery unaccompanied by diarrheal diseases. Pediatrics 22:689, 1958.
469. Hargrett-Bean NT, Pavia AT, Tauxe RV. *Salmonella* isolates from humans in the United States, 1984-1986. MMWR Morb Mortal Wkly Rep 37:25SS, 1988.
470. Blaser MJ, Newman LS. A review of human salmonellosis. I. Infective dose. Rev Infect Dis 4:1096, 1982.
471. Rubinstein AD, Fowler RN. Salmonellosis of the newborn with transmission by delivery room resuscitators. Am J Public Health 45:1109, 1955.
472. Bate JG, James U. *Salmonella typhimurium* infection dustborne in a children's ward. Lancet 2:713, 1958.
473. Rubbo SD. Cross-infection in hospital due to *Salmonella derby*. J Hyg 46:158, 1948.
474. Lamb VA, Mayhall CG, Spadora AC, et al. Outbreak of *S. typhimurium* gastroenteritis due to an imported strain resistant to ampicillin, chloramphenicol, and trimethoprim/sulfamethoxazole in a nursery. J Clin Microbiol 20:1076, 1984.
475. Abramas IF, Cochran WD, Holmes LB, et al. A *Salmonella newport* outbreak in a premature nursery with a one year follow up. Pediatrics 37:616, 1966.
476. Epstein HC, Hochwald A, Agha R. *Salmonella* infections of the newborn infant. J Pediatr 38:723, 1951.
477. Abramson H. Infections with *S. typhimurium* in the newborn. Am J Dis Child 74:576, 1947.
478. Leeder FS. An epidemic of *S. panama* infections in infants. Ann N Y Acad Sci 66:54, 1956.
479. Watt J, Carlton E. Studies of the acute diarrheal diseases. XVI. An outbreak of *S. typhimurium* infection among newborn premature infants. Public Health Rep 60(Pt 1):734, 1945.
480. Foley AR. An outbreak of paratyphoid B fever in a nursery of a small hospital. Can J Public Health 38:73, 1947.
481. Seligman E. Mass invasion of salmonellae in a babies' ward. Ann Paediatr 172:406, 1949.
482. Rowe B, Giles C, Brown GL. Outbreak of gastroenteritis due to *S. virchow* in a maternity hospital. BMJ 3:561, 1969.
483. Sasidharan CK, Rajagopal KC, Jayaram CK, et al. *S. typhimurium* epidemic in newborn nursery. Indian J Pediatr 50:599, 1983.
484. Borecka J, Hocmannova M, van Leeuwen WJ. Nosocomial infection of nurslings caused by multiple drug-resistant strain of *S. typhimurium*-utilization of a new typing method based on lysogeny of strains. Z Bakteriol 2336:262, 1976.
485. Bannerman CHS. Heidelberg enteritis—an outbreak in the neonatal unit of Harare Central Hospital. Cent Afr J Med 31:1, 1985.

486. McAllister TA, Roud JA, Marshall A, et al. Outbreak of *S. eimsbuettel* in newborn infants spread by rectal thermometers. Lancet 1:1262, 1986.
487. Szanton VL. Epidemic salmonellosis: a 30-month study of 80 cases of *S. oranienburg* infection. Pediatrics 20:794, 1957.
488. Seals JE, Parrott PL, McGowan JE, et al. Nursery salmonellosis: delayed recognition due to unusually long incubation period. Infect Control Hosp Epidemiol 4:205, 1983.
489. Hering E, Fuenzalida O, Lynch B, et al. Analises clinico-epidemiologica de un brote de infeccion por *S. bredeney* en recien nacidos. Rev Clin Pediatr 50:81, 1979.
490. Kumari S, Gupta R, Bhargava SK. A nursery outbreak with *S. newport*. Indian Pediatr 17:11, 1980.
491. Omland T, Gardborg O. *Salmonella* enteritidis infections in infancy with special reference to a small nosocomial epidemic. Acta Paediatr Belg 49:583, 1960.
492. Puri V, Thirupuram S, Khalil A, et al. Nosocomial *S. typhimurium* epidemic in a neonatal special care unit. Indian Pediatr 17:233, 1980.
493. Mendis NMP, de la Motte PU, Gunatillaka PDP, et al. Protracted infection with *S. bareilly* in a maternity hospital. J Trop Med Hyg 79:142, 1976.
494. Marzetti G, Laurenti F, deCaro M, et al. *Salmonella muenchen* infections in newborns and small infants. Clin Pediatr 12:93, 1973.
495. Baine WB, Gangarosa EJ, Bennett JV, et al. Institutional salmonellosis. J Infect Dis 128:357, 1973.
496. Schroeder SA, Aserkoff B, Brachman PS. Epidemic salmonellosis in hospitals and institutions. N Engl J Med 279:674, 1968.
497. Wilson R, Feldman RA, Davis J, et al. Salmonellosis in infants: the importance of intrafamilial transmission. Pediatrics 69:436, 1982.
498. Newman MJ. Multiple-resistant *Salmonella* group G outbreak in a neonatal intensive care unit. West Afr J Med 15:165, 1996.
499. Mahajan R, Mathur M, Kumar A, et al. Nosocomial outbreak of *Salmonella typhimurium* infection in a nursery intensive care unit (NICU) and paediatric ward. J Commun Dis 27:10, 1995.
500. Martyn-Jones DM, Pantin GC. Neonatal diarrhea due to *S. paratyphi* B. J Clin Pathol 9:128, 1956.
501. Rubinstein AD, Feemster RF, Smith HM. Salmonellosis as a public health problem in wartime. Am J Public Health 34:841, 1944.
502. Neter E. Observation on the transmission of salmonellosis in man. Am J Public Health 40:929, 1950.
503. Sanders DY, Sinal SH, Morrison L. Chronic salmonellosis in infancy. Clin Pediatr 13:640, 1974.
504. Waddell WR, Kunz LJ. Association of *Salmonella enteritis* with operations on the stomach. N Engl J Med 255:555, 1956.
505. Gray JA, Trueman AM. Severe *Salmonella* gastroenteritis associated with hypochlorhydria. Scott Med J 16:255, 1971.
506. Fleischhacker G, Vutue C, Werner H-P. Infektion eines Neugeborenen durch *S. typhimurium*-haltige Muttermilch. Wien Klin Wochenschr 24:394, 1972.
507. Ryder RW, Crosby-Ritchie A, McDonough B, et al. Human milk contaminated with *S. kottbus*. A cause of nosocomial illness in infants. JAMA 238:1533, 1977.
508. Revathi G, Mahajan R, Faridi MM, et al. Transmission of lethal *Salmonella senftenberg* from mother's breast-milk to her baby. Ann Trop Paediatr 15:159, 1995.
509. Small RG, Sharp JCM. A milkborne outbreak of *S. dublin*. J Hyg 82:95, 1979.
510. Weissman JB, Deen RMAD, Williams M, et al. An island-wide epidemic of salmonellosis in Trinidad traced to contaminated powdered milk. West Indian Med J 26:135, 1977.
511. *Salmonella anatum* infection in infants linked to dried milk. Commun Dis Rep CDR Wkly 7:33, 1997.
512. Usera MA, Echeita A, Aladuena A, et al. Interregional foodborne salmonellosis outbreak due to powdered infant formula contaminated with lactose-fermenting *Salmonella virchow*. Eur J Epidemiol 12:377, 1996.
513. Silverstope L, Plazikowski U, Kjellander J, et al. An epidemic among infants caused by *S. muenchen*. J Appl Bacteriol 24:134, 1961.
514. Im SWK, Chow K, Chau PY. Rectal thermometer-mediated cross-infection with *S. wadsworth* in a pediatric ward. J Hosp Infect 2:171, 1981.
515. Khan MA, Abdur-Rab M, Israr N, et al. Transmission of *S. worthington* by oropharyngeal suction in hospital neonatal unit. Pediatr Infect Dis J 10:668, 1991.
516. Umasankar S, Mridha EU, Hannan MM, et al. An outbreak of *Salmonella enteritidis* in a maternity and neonatal intensive care unit. J Hosp Infect 34:117, 1996.
517. Riley LW, Cohen ML. Plasmid profiles and *Salmonella* epidemiology. Lancet 1:573, 1982.
518. Michel J, Malpeach G, Godeneche P, et al. Etude clinique et bactériologique d'une épidémie de salmonellose en milieu hospitalier (*S. oranienburg*). Pediatrie 25:13, 1970.
519. Adler JL, Anderson RL, Boring JR, et al. A protracted hospital-associated outbreak of salmonellosis due to a multiple antibiotic-resistant strain of *S. indiana*. J Pediatr 77:970, 1970.
520. Bilie BO, Mellbin T, Nordbring F. An extensive outbreak of gastroenteritis caused by *S. newport*. Acta Med Scand 175:557, 1964.
521. Horwitz M, Pollard R, Merson M, et al. A large outbreak of foodborne salmonellosis on the Navajo Nation Indian Reservation: epidemiology and secondary transmission. Am J Public Health 67:1071, 1977.
522. Griffith JPC, Ostheimer M. Typhoid fever in children. Am J Med Sci 124:868, 1902.
523. Freedman ML, Christopher P, Boughton CR, et al. Typhoid carriage in pregnancy with infection of neonate. Lancet 1:310, 1970.
524. Chhabra RS, Glaser JH. *Salmonella* infection presenting as hematochezia on the first day of life. Pediatrics 94:739, 1994.
525. Stein H, Beck J, Solomon A, et al. Gastroenteritis with necrotizing enterocolitis in premature babies. BMJ 1:616, 1972.
526. Guarino A, Spagnuolo MI, Russo S, et al. Etiology and risk factors of severe and protracted diarrhea. J Pediatr Gastroenterol Nutr 20:173, 1995.
527. Lifshitz F, Coello-Ramirez P, Gutirrez-Topete G, et al. Monosaccharide intolerance and hypoglycemia in infants with diarrhea. I. Clinical course of 23 infants. J Pediatr 77:595, 1970.
528. Iyngkaran N, Abdin Z, Davis K, et al. Acquired carbohydrate intolerance and cow milk protein-sensitive enteropathy in young infants. J Pediatr 95:373, 1979.
529. Lo CW, Walker WA. Chronic protracted diarrhea of infancy: a nutritional disease. Pediatrics 72:786, 1983.
530. Blaser MJ, Feldman RA. *Salmonella* bacteremia: reports to the Centers for Disease Control, 1968-1979. J Infect Dis 143:743, 1981.
531. Schutze GE, Schutze SE, Kirby RS. Extraintestinal salmonellosis in a children's hospital. Pediatr Infect Dis J 16:482, 1997.
532. Davis RC. *Salmonella* sepsis in infancy. Am J Dis Child 135:1096, 1981.
533. Torrey S, Fleisher G, Jaffe D. Incidence of *Salmonella* bacteremia in infants with Salmonella gastroenteritis. J Pediatr 108:718, 1986.
534. Sirinavin S, Jayanetra P, Lolekha S, et al. Predictors for extraintestinal infection of *Salmonella enteritis* in Thailand. Pediatr Infect Dis J 7:44, 1988.
535. Katz BZ, Shapiro ED. Predictors of persistently positive blood cultures in children with "occult" *Salmonella* bacteremia. Pediatr Infect Dis J 5:713, 1986.
536. Yamamoto LG, Ashton MJ. *Salmonella* infections in infants in Hawaii. Pediatr Infect Dis J 7:48, 1988.
537. Cohen JI, Bartlett JA, Corey GR. Extraintestinal manifestations of *Salmonella* infections. Medicine (Baltimore) 66:349, 1987.
538. West SE, Goodkin R, Kaplan AM. Neonatal *Salmonella* meningitis complicated by cerebral abscesses. West J Med 127:142, 1977.
539. Applebaum PC, Scragg J. *Salmonella* meningitis in infants. Lancet 1:1052, 1977.
540. Cherubin CE, Marr JS, Sierra MF, et al. *Listeria* and gram-negative bacillary meningitis in New York City 1973-1979. Am J Med 71:199, 1981.
541. Low LC, Lam BC, Wong WT, et al. *Salmonella* meningitis in infancy. Aust Paediatr J 20:225, 1984.
542. Diwan N, Sharma KB. Isolation of *S. typhimurium* from cephalohematoma and osteomyelitis. Indian J Med Res 67:27, 1978.
543. Konzert W. Über eine *Salmonella*-Osteomyelitis in Rahmen einer *S. typhimurium* Epidemie auf einer Neugeborenen Station. Wien Klin Wochenschr 81:713, 1969.
544. McKinlay B. Infectious diarrhea of the newborn caused by an unclassified species of *Salmonella*. Am J Dis Child 54:1252, 1937.
545. Szumness W, Sikorska J, Szymanek E, et al. The microbiological and epidemiological properties of infections caused by *S. enteritidis*. J Hyg 64:9, 1966.
546. Nelson JD. Suppurative mastitis in infants. Am J Dis Child 125:458, 1973.
547. Guthrie KJ, Montgomery GI. Infections with *Bacterium enteritidis* in infancy with the triad of enteritis, cholecystitis and meningitis. J Pathol Bacteriol 49:393, 1939.
548. Corman LI, Poirier RH, Littlefield CA, et al. Endophthalmitis due to *S. enteritidis*. J Pediatr 95:1001, 1979.

549. Haggman DL, Rehm SJ, Moodie DS, et al. Nontyphoidal *Salmonella* pericarditis: a case report and review of the literature. Pediatr Infect Dis J 5:259, 1986.
550. Reed RP, Klugman KP. Neonatal typhoid fever. Pediatr Infect Dis J 13:774, 1994.
551. Stuart BM, Pullen RL. Typhoid: clinical analysis of 360 cases. Arch Intern Med 78:629, 1946.
552. Sengupta B, Ramachander N, Zamah N. *Salmonella* septic abortion. Int Surg 65:183, 1980.
553. Diddle AW, Stephens RL. Typhoid fever in pregnancy. Am J Obstet Gynecol 38:300, 1939.
554. Riggall F, Salkind G, Spellacy W. Typhoid fever complicating pregnancy. Obstet Gynecol 44:117, 1974.
555. Hicks HT, French H. Typhoid fever and pregnancy with special references to fetal infection. Lancet 1:1491, 1905.
556. Osler W, McCrae T. Typhoid fever. *In* Osler W. Principles and Practice of Medicine, 8th ed. New York, D Appleton, 1912, pp 1-46.
557. Ferreccio C, Levine MM, Manterola A, et al. Benign bacteremia caused by *S. typhi* and *S. paratyphi* in children younger than two years. J Pediatr 104:899, 1984.
558. Thisyakorn U, Mansuwan P, Taylor DN. Typhoid and paratyphoid fever in 192 hospitalized children in Thailand. Am J Dis Child 141:862, 1987.
559. Pickering LK, DuPont HL, Olarte J, et al. Fecal leukocytes in enteric infections. Am J Clin Pathol 68:562, 1977.
560. McCall CE, Martin WT Boring JR. Efficiency of cultures of rectal swabs and fecal specimens in detecting *Salmonella* carriers: correlation with numbers of *Salmonella* excreted. J Hyg 64:261, 1966.
561. Raucher HS, Eichenfield AH, Hodes HL. Treatment of *Salmonella* gastroenteritis in infants. The significance of bacteremia. Clin Pediatr 22:601, 1983.
562. Gotoff SP, Cochran WD. Antibody response to the somatic antigen of *S. newport* in premature infants. Pediatrics 37:610, 1966.
563. Hodes HL, Zepp HD, Ainbender E. Production of O and H agglutinins by a newborn infant infected with *S. saint-paul*. J Pediatr 68:780, 1966.
564. Taylor DN, Bopp C, Birkness K, et al. An outbreak of salmonellosis associated with a fatality in a healthy child: a large dose and severe illness. Am J Epidemiol 119:907, 1984.
565. Rivera MJ, Rivera N, Castillo J, et al. Molecular and epidemiological study of *Salmonella* clinical isolates. J Clin Microbiol 29:927, 1991.
566. Aserkoff B, Bennett JV. Effect of antibiotic therapy in acute salmonellosis on the fecal excretion of salmonellae. N Engl J Med 281:636, 1969.
567. Dixon JMS. Effect of antibiotic treatment on duration of excretion of *S. typhimurium* by children. BMW 2:1343, 1965.
568. Kazemi M, Bumpert TG, Marks MI. A controlled trial comparing trimethoprim/sulfamethoxazole, ampicillin, and no therapy in the treatment of *Salmonella* gastroenteritis in children. J Pediatr 83:646, 1973.
569. Neill MA, Opal SM, Heelan J, et al. Failure of ciprofloxacin to eradicate convalescent fecal excretion after acute salmonellosis: experience during an outbreak in health care workers. Ann Intern Med 114:195, 1991.
570. Pettersson T, Klemola E, Wager O. Treatment of acute cases of *Salmonella* infection and *Salmonella* carriers with ampicillin and neomycin. Acta Med Scand 175:185, 1964.
571. Association for Study of Infectious Diseases. Effect of neomycin in noninvasive *Salmonella* infections of the gastrointestinal tract. Lancet 2:1159, 1970.
572. Nelson JD, Kusmiesz H, Jackson LH, et al. Treatment of *Salmonella* gastroenteritis with ampicillin, amoxicillin, or placebo. Pediatrics 65:1125, 1980.
573. Asperilla MO, Smego RA, Scott LK. Quinolone antibiotics in the treatment of *Salmonella* infections. Rev Infect Dis 12:873, 1990.
574. Buchwald DS, Blaser MJ. A review of human salmonellosis. II. Duration of excretion following infection with nontyphi *Salmonella*. Rev Infect Dis 6:345, 1984.
575. Dutta P, Rasaily R, Saha MR, et al. Ciprofloxacin for treatment of severe typhoid fever in children. Antimicrob Agents Chemother 37:1197, 1993.
576. Piddock LJV, Griggs DJ, Hall MC, et al. Ciprofloxacin resistance in clinical isolates of *Salmonella typhimurium* obtained from two patients. Antimicrob Agents Chemother 37:662, 1993.
577. Edgar WM, Lacey BW. Infection with *S. heidelberg*. An outbreak presumably not foodborne. Lancet 1:161, 1963.
578. Rice PA, Craven PC, Wells JG. *S. heidelberg* enteritis and bacteremia. An epidemic on two pediatric wards. Am J Med 60:509, 1976.
579. MacDonald KL, Cohen ML, Hargrett-Bean NT, et al. Changes in antimicrobial resistance of *Salmonella* isolated from humans in the United States. JAMA 258:1496, 1987.
580. Maiorini E, Lopez EL, Morrow AL, et al. Multiply resistant nontyphoidal *Salmonella* gastroenteritis in children. Pediatr Infect Dis J 12:139, 1993.
581. Lee LA, Puhr ND, Maloney EK, et al. Increase in antimicrobial-resistant *Salmonella* infections in the United States, 1989-1990. J Infect Dis 170:128, 1994.
582. Glynn MK, Bopp C, Dewitt W, et al. Emergence of multidrug-resistant *Salmonella enterica* serotype typhimurium DT104 infections in the United States. N Engl J Med 338:1333, 1998.
583. Koshi G. Alarming increases in multi-drug resistant *S. typhimurium* in Southern India. Indian J Med Res 74:635, 1981.
584. Anderson ES, Threlfall EJ, Carr JM, et al. Clonal distribution of resistance plasmid carrying *S. typhimurium*, mainly in the Middle East. J Hyg 79:425, 1977.
585. Wamola IA, Mirza NB. Problems of *Salmonella* infections in a hospital in Kenya. East Afr Med J 58:677, 1981.
586. Falbo V, Capriola A, Moncello F, et al. Antimicrobial resistance among *Salmonella* isolates from hospitals in Rome. J Hyg 88:275, 1982.
587. Threlfall EJ, Ward LR, Ashley AS, et al. Plasmid encoded trimethoprim resistance in multi-resistant epidemic *S. typhimurium* phagotypes 204 and 193 in Britain. BMJ 280:1210, 1980.
588. French GI, Lowry MF. Trimethoprim-resistant *Salmonella*. Lancet 2:375, 1978.
589. Smith SM, Palumbo PE, Edelson PJ. *Salmonella* strains resistant to multiple antibiotics: therapeutic implications. Pediatr Infect Dis J 3:455, 1984.
590. Soe GB, Overturf GD. Treatment of typhoid fever and other systemic salmonellosis with cefotaxime, ceftriazone, cefoperazone, and other newer cephalosporins. Rev Infect Dis 9:719, 1987.
591. Moosa A, Rubidge CJ. Once daily ceftriaxone vs. chloramphenicol for treatment of typhoid fever in children. Pediatr Infect Dis J 8:696, 1989.
592. deCarvalho EM, Martinelli R, de Oliveira MMG, et al. Cefamandole treatment of *Salmonella* bacteremia. Antimicrob Agents Chemother 21:334, 1982.
593. Pape JW, Gerdes H, Oriol L, et al. Typhoid fever: successful therapy with cefoperazone. J Infect Dis 153:272, 1986.
594. Demmerich B, Lode H, Boner K, et al. Biliary excretion and pharmacokinetics of cefoperazone in humans. J Antimicrob Chemother 12:27, 1983.
595. Kinsella TR, Yogev R, Shulman ST, et al. Treatment of *Salmonella* meningitis and brain abscess with the new cephalosporins: two case reports and a review of the literature. Pediatr Infect Dis J 6:476, 1987.
596. Gokalp AS, Toksoy HB, Turkay S, et al. Intravenous immunoglobulin in the treatment of *Salmonella typhimurium* infections in preterm neonates. Clin Pediatr (Phila) 33:349, 1994.
597. Tauxe RV, Hassan LF, Findeisen KO, et al. Salmonellosis in nurses: lack of transmission to patients. J Infect Dis 157:370, 1988.
598. Levine MM, Ferraccio C, Cryz S, et al. Comparison of enteric coated capsules and liquid formulation of Ty21a typhoid vaccine in randomised controlled field trial. Lancet 336:4, 1990.
599. Cryz SJ Jr, Vanprapar N, Thisyakorn U, et al. Safety and immunogenicity of *Salmonella typhi* Ty21a vaccine in young Thai children. Infect Immun 61:1149, 1993.
600. Murphy JR, Grez L, Schlesinger L, et al. Immunogenicity of *S. typhi* Ty21a vaccine for young children. Infect Immun 59:4291, 1991.
601. France GL, Marmer DJ, Steele RW. Breast-feeding and *Salmonella* infection. Am J Dis Child 134:147, 1980.
602. Brenner DJ, Fannin GR, Skerman FJ, et al. Polynucleotide sequence divergence among strains of *E. coli* and closely related organisms. J Bacteriol 109:953, 1972.
603. Sansonetti PJ, Kopecko DJ, Formal SB. Involvement of a plasmid in the invasive ability of *Shigella flexneri*. Infect Immun 35:852, 1982.
604. Sansonetti P. Host-pathogen interactions: the seduction of molecular cross talk. Gut 50(Suppl 3):III2, 2002.
605. Fernandez MI, Sansonetti PJ. *Shigella* interaction with intestinal epithelial cells determines the innate immune response in shigellosis. Int J Med Microbiol 293:55, 2003.
606. Hale TL, Oaks EV, Formal SB. Identification and characterization of virulence associated, plasmid-coded proteins of *Shigella spp.* and enteroinvasive *E. coli*. Infect Immun 50:620, 1985.
607. Sasakawa C, Kamata K, Sakai T, et al. Molecular alteration of the 140-megadalton plasmid associated with the loss of virulence and

Congo red binding activity in *Shigella flexneri*. Infect Immun 51:470, 1986.
608. LaBrec EH, Schneider H, Magnani TJ, et al. Epithelial cell penetration as an essential step in the pathogenesis of bacillary dysentery. J Bacteriol 88:1503, 1964.
609. Ogawa H. Experimental approach in studies on pathogenesis of bacillary dysentery—with special reference to the invasion of bacilli into intestinal mucosa. Acta Pathol Jpn 20:261, 1970.
610. Sansonetti PJ, d'Hauteville H, Formal SB, et al. Plasmid-mediated invasiveness of "*Shigella*-like" *Escherichia coli*. Ann Microbiol 133A:351, 1982.
611. Sansonetti PJ, d'Hauteville H, Ecobiochon C, et al. Molecular comparison of virulence plasmids in *Shigella* and enteroinvasive *Escherichia coli*. Ann Microbiol 134A:295, 1983.
612. Sansonetti PJ, Hale TL, Dammin GI, et al. Alterations in the pathogenicity of *Escherichia coli* K-12 after transfer of plasmids and chromosomal genes from *Shigella flexneri*. Infect Immun 39:1392, 1983.
613. Wei J, Goldberg MB, Burland V, et al. Complete genome sequence and comparative genomics of *Shigella flexneri* serotype 2a strain 2457T. Infect Immun 71:2775, 2003.
614. Okada N, Sasakawa C, Tobe T, et al. Virulence associated chromosomal loci of *S. flexneri* identified by random Tn5 insertion mutagenesis. Mol Microbiol 5:187, 1991.
615. Okamura N, Nagai T, Nakaya R, et al. HeLa cell invasiveness and O antigen of *Shigella flexneri* as separate and prerequisite attributes of virulence to evoke keratoconjunctivitis in guinea pigs. Infect Immun 39:505, 1983.
616. Bartlett AV, Prado D, Cleary TG, et al. Production of Shiga toxin and other cytotoxins by serogroups of *Shigella*. J Infect Dis 154:996, 1986.
617. Olenick JG, Wolfe AD. *Shigella* toxin inhibition of binding and translation of polyuridylic acid by *Escherichia coli* ribosomes. J Bacteriol 141:1246, 1980.
618. Brown JE, Rothman SW, Doctor BP. Inhibition of protein synthesis in intact HeLa cells by *Shigella dysenteriae* 1 toxin. Infect Immun 29:98, 1980.
619. Al-Hasani K, Henderson IR, Sakellaris H, et al. The sigA Gene which is borne on the she pathogenicity island of *Shigella flexneri* 2a encodes an exported cytopathic protease involved in intestinal fluid accumulation. Infect Immun 68:2457, 2000.
620. Prado D, Cleary TG, Pickering LK, et al. The relation between production of cytotoxin and clinical features in shigellosis. J Infect Dis 154:149, 1986.
621. Makintubee S, Mallonee J, Istre GR. Shigellosis outbreak associated with swimming. Am J Public Health 77:166, 1987.
622. Levine MM, DuPont HL, Formal SB, et al. Pathogenesis of *Shigella dysenteriae* 1 (Shiga) dysentery. J Infect Dis 127:261, 1973.
623. DuPont HL, Hornick RB, Dawkins AT, et al. The response of man to virulent *Shigella flexneri* 2a. J Infect Dis 119:296, 1969.
624. Levine MM. Shigella infections and vaccines: experiences from volunteer and controlled field studies. *In* Rahaman MM, Greenough WB, Novak NR, et al (eds). Shigellosis: A Continuing Global Problem. Dacca, Bangladesh, International Centre for Diarrhoeal Disease Research, 1983, p 208.
625. Pickering LK, Hadler SC. Management and prevention of infectious diseases in day care. *In* Feigin RD, Cherry JC (eds). Textbook of Pediatric Infectious Diseases. Philadelphia, WB Saunders, 1992, p 2308.
626. Mata LG. The Children of Santa Maria Cauque: A Prospective Field Study of Health and Growth. Cambridge, Mass, MIT Press, 1978.
627. Stoll BJ, Glass RI, Huq MI, et al. Surveillance of patients attending a diarrhoeal disease hospital in Bangladesh. BMJ 285:1185, 1982.
628. Floyd T, Higgins AR, Kader M. A. Studies in shigellosis. V. The relationship of age to the incidence of *Shigella* infections in Egyptian children, with special reference to shigellosis in the newborn and infant in the first six months of life. Am J Trop Med Hyg 5:119, 1956.
629. Summary of notifiable diseases, United States, 1981. MMWR Morb Mortal Wkly Rep 40:10, 1992.
630. Clemens JS, Stanton B, Stoll B, et al. Breast-feeding as a determinant of severity in shigellosis. Am J Epidemiol 123:710, 1986.
631. Mata LJ, Urrutia JM, Garcia B, et al. *Shigella* infections in breast fed Guatemalan Indian neonates. Am J Dis Child 117:142, 1969.
632. Huskins WC, Griffiths JK, Faruque AS, Bennish ML. Shigellosis in neonates and young infants. J Pediatr 125:14, 1994.
633. Haltalin KC. Neonatal shigellosis. Am J Dis Child 114:603, 1967.
634. Scragg JN, Rubidge CJ, Appelbaum PC. *Shigella* infection in African and Indian children with special reference to *Shigella septicemia*. J Pediatr 93:796, 1978.
635. Burry VF, Thurn AN, Co TG. Shigellosis: an analysis of 239 cases in a pediatric population. Mo Med 65:671, 1968.
636. Enteric infection due to *Campylobacter, Yersinia, Salmonella* and *Shigella*. Bull World Health Organ 58:519, 1980.
637. Kraybill EN, Controni G. Septicemia and enterocolitis due to *S. sonnei* in a newborn infant. Pediatrics 42:529, 1968.
638. Moore EE. *Shigella sonnei* septicemia in a neonate. BMJ 1:22, 1974.
639. Aldrich JA, Flowers RP, Hall FK. *S. sonnei* septicemia in a neonate: a case report. J Am Osteopath Assoc 79:93, 1979.
640. Barton LL, Pickering LK. Shigellosis in the first week of life. Pediatrics 52:437, 1973.
641. Landsberger M. Bacillary dysentery in a newborn infant. Arch Pediatr 59:330, 1942.
642. Neter E. *S. sonnei* infection at term and its transfer to the newborn. Obstet Gynecol 17:517, 1961.
643. McIntire MS, Jahr HM. An isolated case of shigellosis in the newborn nursery. Nebr State Med J 39:425, 1954.
644. Greenberg M, Frant S, Shapiro R. Bacillary dysentery acquired at birth. J Pediatr 17:363, 1940.
645. Emanuel B, Sherman JO. Shigellosis in a neonate. Clin Pediatr 14:725, 1975.
646. Barret-Connor E, Connor JD. Extraintestinal manifestations of shigellosis. Am J Gastroenterol 53:234, 1970.
647. Fischler E. Convulsions as a complication of shigellosis in children. Helv Paediatr Acta 4:389, 1962.
648. Ashkenazi S, Dinari G, Zevalunov A, et al. Convulsions in childhood shigellosis. Am J Dis Child 141:208, 1987.
649. Whitfield C, Humphries JM. Meningitis and septicemia due to *Shigella* in a newborn infant. J Pediatr 70:805, 1967.
650. Goren A, Freier S, Passwell JH. Lethal toxic encephalopathy due to childhood shigellosis in a developed country. Pediatrics 89:1189, 1992.
651. Ashkenazi S, Cleary KR, Pickering LK, et al. The association of Shiga toxin and other cytotoxins with the neurologic manifestations of shigellosis. J Infect Dis 161:961, 1990.
652. Rahaman MM, Jamiul Alam AKM, Islam MR, et al. Shiga bacillus dysentery associated with marked leukocytosis and erythrocyte fragmentation. Johns Hopkins Med J 136:65, 1975.
653. Neglia TG, Marr TJ, Davis AT. *Shigella* dysentery with secondary *Klebsiella* sepsis. J Pediatr 63:253, 1976.
654. Struelens MJ, Patte D, Kabir I, et al. *Shigella* septicemia: prevalence, presentation, risk factors, and outcome. J Infect Dis 152:784, 1985.
655. Haltalin KC, Nelson JD. Coliform septicemia complicating shigellosis in children. JAMA 192:441, 1965.
656. Levin SE. *Shigella* septicemia in the newborn infant. J Pediatr 71:917, 1967.
657. Martin T, Habbick BF, Nyssen J. Shigellosis with bacteremia: a report of two cases and a review of the literature. Pediatr Infect Dis J 2:21, 1983.
658. Raderman JW, Stoller KP, Pomerance JJ. Blood-stream invasion with *S. sonnei* in an asymptomatic newborn infant. Pediatr Infect Dis J 5:379, 1986.
659. Starke JR, Baker CJ. Neonatal shigellosis with bowel perforation. Pediatr Infect Dis J 4:405, 1985.
660. Azad MAK, Islam M. Colonic perforation in *Shigella dysenteriae* 1 infection. Pediatr Infect Dis J 5:103, 1986.
661. O'Connor JH, O'Callaghan U. Fatal *S. sonnei* septicemia in an adult complemented by marrow aplasia and intestinal perforation. J Infect 3:277, 1981.
662. Alam AN, Chowdhurg AAKM, Kabir IAKM, et al. Association of pneumonia with under-nutrition and shigellosis. Indian Pediatr 21:609, 1984.
663. Hoefnagel D. Fulminating, rapidly fatal shigellosis in children. N Engl J Med 258:1256, 1958.
664. Sakamoto A, Kamo S. Clinical, statistical observations on Ekiri and bacillary dysentery. A study of 785 cases. Ann Paediatr 186:1, 1956.
665. Dodd K, Buddingh GJ, Rapoport S. The etiology of Ekiri, a highly fatal disease of Japanese children. Pediatrics 3:9, 1949.
666. Davis TC. Chronic vulvovaginitis in children due to *S. flexneri*. Pediatrics 56:41, 1975.
667. Murphy TV, Nelson JD. *Shigella* vaginitis: report on 38 patients and review of the literature. Pediatrics 63:511, 1979.
668. Tobias JD, Starke JR, Tosi MF. *Shigella* keratitis: a report of two cases and a review of the literature. Pediatr Infect Dis J 6:79, 1987.
669. Butler T, Dunn D, Dahms B, et al. Causes of death and the histopathologic findings in fatal shigellosis. Pediatr Infect Dis J 8:767, 1989.

670. Bennish ML, Harris JR, Wojtyniak BJ, et al. Death in shigellosis: incidence and risk factors in hospitalized patients. J Infect Dis 161:500, 1990.
671. Speelman P, McGlaughlin R, Kabir I, et al. Differential clinical features and stool findings in shigellosis and amoebic dysentery. Trans R Soc Trop Med Hyg 81:549, 1987.
672. Taylor WI, Harris B. Isolation of shigellae. II. Comparison of plating media and enrichment broths. Am J Clin Pathol 44:476, 1965.
673. Stypulkowska-Misiurewics H. Problems in bacteriological diagnosis of shigellosis. *In* Rahaman MM, Greenough WB, Novak NR, et al (eds). Shigellosis: A Continuing Global Problem. Dacca, Bangladesh, International Centre for Diarrhoeal Disease Research, 1983, p 87.
674. Haltalin KC, Nelson JD, Ring R III, et al. Double-blind treatment study of shigellosis comparing ampicillin, sulfadiazine, and placebo. J Pediatr 70:970, 1967.
675. Haltalin KC, Nelson JD, Kusmiesz HT, et al. Optimal dosage of ampicillin in shigellosis. J Pediatr 74:626, 1969.
676. Haltalin KC, Nelson JD, Kusmiesz HT. Comparative efficacy of nalidixic acid and ampicillin for severe shigellosis. Arch Dis Child 48:305, 1973.
677. Oaks EV, Hale TL, Formal SB. Serum immune response to *Shigella* protein antigens in rhesus monkeys and humans infected with *Shigella spp.* Infect Immun 53:57, 1986.
678. Frankel G, Riley L, Giron JA, et al. Detection of *Shigella* in feces using DNA amplification. J Infect Dis 161:1252, 1990.
679. Speelman P, Kabir I, Islam M. Distribution and spread of colonic lesions in shigellosis: a colonoscopic study. J Infect Dis 150:899, 1984.
680. Formal SB, Kent TH, Austin S, et al. Fluorescent antibody and histological studies of vaccinated control monkeys challenged with *Shigella flexneri*. J Bacteriol 91:2368, 1966.
681. LaBrec EH, Formal SB. Experimental *Shigella* infections. IV. Fluorescent antibody studies of an infection in guinea pigs. J Immunol 87:562, 1961.
682. Frost JA, Rowe B, Vandepitte J, et al. Plasmid characterization in the investigation of an epidemic caused by multiply resistant *S. dysenteriae* type 1 in Central Africa. Lancet 2:1074, 1981.
683. Haider K, Hug MI, Samadi AR, et al. Plasmid characterization of *Shigella spp.* isolated from children with shigellosis and asymptomatic excretors. J Antimicrob Chemother 16:691, 1985.
684. Tauxe RV, Puhr ND, Wells JG, et al. Antimicrobial resistance of *Shigella* isolates in the USA: the importance of international travelers. J Infect Dis 162:1107, 1990.
685. Salzman TC, Scher CD, Moss R. *Shigellae* with transferable drug resistance: outbreak in a nursery for premature infants. J Pediatr 71:21, 1967.
686. Bennish ML, Salam MA, Hossain MA, et al. Antimicrobial resistance of *Shigella* isolates in Bangladesh, 1983-1990: increasing frequency of strains multiply resistant to ampicillin, trimethoprim/sulfamethoxazole, and nalidixic acid. Clin Infect Dis 14:1055, 1992.
687. Ostrower VG. Comparison of cefaclor and ampicillin in the treatment of shigellosis. Postgrad Med J 55:82, 1979.
688. Haltalin KC, Nelson JD. Failure of furazolidone therapy on shigellosis. Am J Dis Child 123:40, 1972.
689. Nelson JD, Haltalin KC. Comparative efficacy of cephalexin and ampicillin for shigellosis and other types of acute diarrhea in infants and children. Antimicrob Agents Chemother 7:415, 1975.
690. Nelson JD, Haltalin KC. Amoxicillin less effective than ampicillin against *Shigella* in vitro and in vivo: relationship of efficacy to activity in serum. J Infect Dis 129:S222, 1974.
691. Tong MJ, Martin DG, Cunningham JJ, et al. Clinical and bacteriological evaluation of antibiotic treatment in shigellosis. JAMA 214:1841, 1970.
692. Orenstein WA, Ross L, Overturf GD, et al. Antibiotic treatment of acute shigellosis: failure of cefamandole compared to trimethoprim/sulfamethoxazole and ampicillin. Am J Med Sci 282:27, 1981.
693. Yunus MD, Rahaman MM, Faruque ASG, et al. Comparative treatment of shigellosis with trimethoprim/sulfamethoxazole and ampicillin. *In* Rahaman MM, Greenough WB, Novak NR, et al (eds). Shigellosis: A Continuing Global Problem. Dacca, Bangladesh, International Centre for Diarrhoeal Disease Research, 1983, p 166.
694. Nelson JD, Kusmiesz H, Jackson LH, et al. Trimethoprim/sulfamethoxazole therapy for shigellosis. JAMA 235:1239, 1976.
695. Nelson JD, Kusmiesz H, Jackson LH. Comparison of trimethoprim/sulfamethoxazole and ampicillin for shigellosis in ambulatory patients. J Pediatr 89:491, 1976.
696. Nelson JD, Kusmiesz H, Shelton S. Oral or intravenous trimethoprim/sulfamethoxazole therapy for shigellosis. Rev Infect Dis J 4:546, 1982.
697. Gilman RH, Spira W, Rabbani H, et al. Single dose ampicillin therapy for severe shigellosis in Bangladesh. J Infect Dis 143:164, 1981.
698. Varsano I, Elditz-Marcus T, Nussinovitch M, et al. Comparative efficacy of ceftriaxone and ampicillin for treatment of severe shigellosis in children. J Pediatr 118:627, 1991.
699. Kabir T, Butler T, Khanam A. Comparative efficacies of single intravenous doses of ceftriaxone and ampicillin for shigellosis in a placebo-controlled trial. Antimicrob Agents Chemother 29:645, 1986.
700. Bennish ML, Salam MA, Khan WA, et al. Treatment of shigellosis. III. Comparison of one- or two-dose ciprofloxacin with standard 5-day therapy. Ann Intern Med 117:727, 1992.
701. John JF Jr, Atkins LT, Maple PAH, et al. Activities of new fluoroquinolones against *Shigella sonnei*. Antimicrob Agents Chemother 36:2346, 1992.
702. DuPont HL, Hornick RB. Adverse effect of Lomotil therapy in shigellosis. JAMA 226:1525, 1973.
703. Ahmed F, Clemens JD, Rao MR, et al. Community based evaluation of the effect of breast feeding on the risk of microbiologically confirmed or clinically presumptive shigellosis in Bangladeshi children. Pediatrics 90:406, 1992.
704. Khan MU. Interruption of shigellosis by handwashing. Trans R Soc Trop Med Hyg 76:164, 1982.
705. Farrar WE, Edison M, Guerry P, et al. Interbacterial transfer of R-factor in the human intestine: in vitro acquisition of R-factor mediated kanamycin resistance by a multi-resistant strain of *S. sonnei.* J Infect Dis 126:27, 1972.
706. McFadyean F, Stockman S. Report of the Departmental Committee Appointed by the Board of Agriculture and Fisheries to Inquire into Epizootic Abortion, vol 3, London, His Majesty's Stationery Office, 1909.
707. Smith T, Taylor MS. Some morphological and biochemical characters of the spirilla (*Vibrio fetus*, n. *spp.*) associated with disease of the fetal membranes in cattle. J Exp Med 30:200, 1919.
708. Jones FS, Orcutt M, Little RB. Vibrios (*Vibrio jejuni*, n. *spp.*) associated with intestinal disorders of cows and calves. J Exp Med 53:853, 1931.
709. Bryner JH, Estes PC, Foley JW, et al. Infectivity of three *Vibrio fetus* biotypes for gallbladder and intestines of cattle, sheep, rabbits, guinea pigs, and mice. Am J Vet Res 32:465, 1971.
710. Vinzent R, Dumas J, Picard, N. Septicémie grave au cours de la grossesse due à un vibrion. Avortement consécutif. Bull Acad Natl Med 131:90, 1947.
711. Eden AN. Perinatal mortality caused by *Vibrio fetus*: review and analysis. J Pediatr 68:297, 1966.
712. Torphy DE, Bond WW. *Campylobacter fetus* infections in children. Pediatrics 64:898, 1979.
713. Bokkenheuser V. *Vibrio fetus* infection in man. I. Ten new cases and some epidemiologic observations. Am J Epidemiol 91:400, 1970.
714. Guerrant RL, Lahita RG, Winn WC, et al. Campylobacteriosis in man: pathogenic mechanisms and review of 91 bloodstream infections. Am J Med 65:584, 1978.
715. Sebald M, Veron M. Teneur en bases de l'ADN et classification des vibrions. Ann Inst Pasteur 105:897, 1963.
716. Butzler JP, Dekeyser P, Detrain M, et al. Related vibrio in stools. J Pediatr 82:493, 1973.
717. Skirrow MB. *Campylobacter* enteritis: a "new" disease. BMJ 2:9, 1977.
718. Communicable Disease Surveillance Centre and the Communicable Diseases (Scotland) Unit. *Campylobacter* infections in Britain 1977. BMJ 1:1357, 1978.
719. De Mol P, Bosmans E. *Campylobacter* enteritis in Central Africa. Lancet 1:604, 1978.
720. Lindquist B, Kjellander J, Kosunen T. *Campylobacter* enteritis in Sweden. BMJ 1:303, 1978.
721. Karmali MA, Fleming PC. *Campylobacter* enteritis in children. J Pediatr 94:527, 1979.
722. Pai CM, Sorger S, Lackman L, et al. *Campylobacter* gastroenteritis in children. J Pediatr 94:589, 1979.
723. Blaser MJ, Reller LB. *Campylobacter* enteritis. N Engl J Med 305:1444, 1981.
724. Dekeyser P, Gossuin-Detrain M, Butzler JP, et al. Acute enteritis due to related *Vibrio*: first positive stool cultures. J Infect Dis 125:390, 1972.

725. Butzler JP, Skirrow MB. *Campylobacter* enteritis. Clin Gastroenterol 8:737, 1979.
726. Blaser MJ, Berkowitz ID, LaForce FM, et al. *Campylobacter* enteritis: clinical and epidemiologic features. Ann Intern Med 91:179, 1979.
727. Karmali MA, Fleming PC. *Campylobacter* enteritis. Can Med Assoc J 120:1525, 1979.
728. Steele TW, McDermott S. *Campylobacter* enteritis in South Australia. Med J Aust 2:404, 1978.
729. Guandalini S, Cucchiara S, deRitis G, et al. *Campylobacter* colitis in infants. J Pediatr 102:72, 1983.
730. Walker RI, Caldwell MB, Lee EC, et al. Pathophysiology of *Campylobacter* enteritis. Microbiol Rev 50:81, 1986.
731. Penner JL. The genus *Campylobacter*: a decade of progress. Clin Microbiol Rev 1:157, 1988.
732. Calva JJ, Ruiz-Palacios GM, Lopez-Vidal AB, et al. Cohort study of intestinal infection with *Campylobacter* in Mexican children. Lancet 1:503, 1988.
733. Figura N, Guglielmetti P, Zanchi A, et al. Two cases of *Campylobacter mucosalis* enteritis in children. J Clin Microbiol 31:727, 1993.
734. Harvey SM, Greenwood JR. Relationships among catalase-positive campylobacters determined by deoxyribonucleic acid-deoxyribonucleic acid hybridization. Int J Syst Bacteriol 33:275, 1983.
735. Owen RJ. Nucleic acids in the classification of campylobacters. Eur J Clin Microbiol 2:367, 1983.
736. Hoffer MA. Bovine campylobacteriosis: a review. Can Vet J 22:327, 1981.
737. Grant CA. Bovine vibriosis: a brief review. Can J Comp Med 19:156, 1955.
738. Vinzent R. Une affection méconnue de la grossesse: l'infection placentaire à "*Vibrio* fetus." Presse Med 57:1230, 1949.
739. Wong S-N, Tam Y-CA, Yeun K-Y. *Campylobacter* infection in the neonate: case report and review of the literature. Pediatr Infect Dis J 9:665, 1990.
740. Hood M, Todd JM. *Vibrio fetus*—a cause of human abortion. Am J Obstet Gynecol 80:506, 1960.
741. van Wering RF, Esseveld H. *Vibrio fetus*. Ned Tijdschr Geneeskd 107:119, 1963.
742. Burgert W Jr, Hagstrom JWC. *Vibrio fetus* meningoencephalitis. Arch Neurol 10:196, 1964.
743. Willis MD, Austin WJ. Human *Vibrio fetus* infection: report of two dissimilar cases. Am J Dis Child 112:459, 1966.
744. Smith JP, Marymont JH Jr, Schweers J. Septicemia due to *Campylobacter fetus* in a newborn infant with gastroenteritis. Am J Med Technol 43:38, 1977.
745. West SE, Houghton DJ, Crock S, et al. *Campylobacter spp*. isolated from the cervix during septic abortion. Case report. Br J Obstet Gynaecol 89:771, 1982.
746. Lee MM, Welliver RC, LaScolea LJ. *Campylobacter* meningitis in childhood. Pediatr Infect Dis J 4:544, 1985.
747. Simor AE, Karmali MA, Jadavji T, et al. Abortion and perinatal sepsis associated with *Campylobacter* infection. Rev Infect Dis J 8:397, 1986.
748. Forbes JC, Scheifele DW. Early onset *Campylobacter* sepsis in a neonate. Pediatr Infect Dis J 6:494, 1987.
749. King EO. Human infections with *Vibrio fetus* and a closely related vibrio. J Infect Dis 101:119, 1957.
750. Francioli P, Herzstein J, Grobe JP, et al. *Campylobacter fetus* subspecies *fetus* bacteremia. Arch Intern Med 145:289, 1985.
751. Karmali MA, Penner JL, Fleming PC, et al. The biotype and biotype distribution of clinical isolates of *Campylobacter jejuni* and *Campylobacter coli* over a three-year period. J Infect Dis 147:243, 1983.
752. Albert MJ, Leach A, Asche V, et al. Serotype distribution of *Campylobacter jejuni* and *Campylobacter coli* isolated from hospitalized patients with diarrhea in Central Australia. J Clin Microbiol 30:207, 1992.
753. Riley LW, Finch MJ. Results of the first year of national surveillance of *Campylobacter* infections in the United States. J Infect Dis 151:956, 1985.
754. Georges-Courbot MC, Baya C, Beraud AM, et al. Distribution and serotypes of *Campylobacter jejuni* and *Campylobacter coli* in enteric *Campylobacter* strains isolated from children in the Central African Republic. J Clin Microbiol 23:592, 1986.
755. Wheeler WE, Borchers J. Vibrionic enteritis in infants. Am J Dis Child 101:60, 1961.
756. Middlekamp JN, Wolf HA. Infection due to a "related" *Vibrio*. J Pediatr 59:318, 1961.
757. Ruben FL, Wolinsky E. Human infection with *Vibrio fetus*. *In* Hobby GL (ed). Antimicrobial Agents and Chemotherapy. Bethesda, Md, American Society for Microbiology, 1967, p 143.
758. Mawer SL, Smith BAM. *Campylobacter* infection of premature baby. Lancet 1:1041, 1979.
759. *Campylobacter* in a mother and baby. Commun Dis Rep CDR 7917:4, 1979.
760. Karmali MA, Tan YC. Neonatal *Campylobacter* enteritis. Can Med Assoc J 122:192, 1980.
761. Thomas K, Chan KN, Riberiro CD. *Campylobacter jejuni/coli* meningitis in a neonate. BMJ 280:1301, 1980.
762. Anders BJ, Lauer BA, Paisley JW. *Campylobacter* gastroenteritis in neonates. Am J Dis Child 135:900, 1981.
763. Vesikari T, Huttunen L, Maki R. Perinatal *Campylobacter fetus ss. jejuni* enteritis. Acta Paediatr Scand 70:261, 1981.
764. Miller RC, Guard RW. A case of premature labour due to *Campylobacter jejuni* infection. Aust N Z Obstet Gynaecol 22:118, 1982.
765. Buck GE, Kelly MT, Pichanick AM, et al. *Campylobacter jejuni* in newborns: a cause of asymptomatic bloody diarrhea. Am J Dis Child 136:744, 1982.
766. Karmali MA, Norrish B, Lior H, et al. *Campylobacter* enterocolitis in a neonatal nursery. J Infect Dis 149:874, 1984.
767. Youngs ER, Roberts C, Davidson DC. *Campylobacter* enteritis and bloody stools in the neonate. Arch Dis Child 60:480, 1985.
768. Terrier A, Altwegg M, Bader P, et al. Hospital epidemic of neonatal *Campylobacter jejuni* infection. Lancet 2:1182, 1985.
769. Goossens H, Henocque G, Kremp L, et al. Nosocomial outbreak of *Campylobacter jejuni* meningitis in newborn infants. Lancet 2:146, 1986.
770. DiNicola AF. *Campylobacter jejuni* diarrhea in a 3-day old male neonate. Pediatr Forum 140:191, 1986.
771. Hershkowici S, Barak M, Cohen A, et al. An outbreak of *Campylobacter jejuni* infection in a neonatal intensive care unit. J Hosp Infect 9:54, 1987.
772. Gribble MJ, Salit IE, Isaac-Renton J, et al. *Campylobacter* infections in pregnancy: case report and literature review. Am J Obstet Gynecol 140:423, 1981.
773. Gilbert GL, Davoren RA, Cole ME, et al. Midtrimester abortion associated with septicaemia caused by *Campylobacter jejuni*. Med J Aust 1:585, 1981.
774. Jost PM, Galvin MC, Brewer JH, et al. *Campylobacter* septic abortion. South Med J 77:924, 1984.
775. Pearce CT. *Campylobacter jejuni* infection as a cause of septic abortion. Aust J Med Lab Sci 2:107, 1981.
776. Pines A, Goldhammer E, Bregman J, et al. *Campylobacter* enteritis associated with recurrent abortions in agammaglobulinemia. Acta Obstet Gynecol Scand 62:279, 1983.
777. Kist M, Keller KM, Niebling W, et al. *Campylobacter coli* septicaemia associated with septic abortion. Infection 12:88, 1984.
778. Reina J, Borrell N, Fiol M. Rectal bleeding caused by *Campylobacter jejuni* in a neonate. Pediatr Infect Dis J 6:500, 1992.
779. Ruiz-Palacios GM, Torres J, Escamilla NI. Cholera-like enterotoxin produced by *Campylobacter jejuni*: characterization and clinical significance. Lancet 2:250, 1983.
780. Johnson WM, Lior H. Toxins produced by *Campylobacter jejuni* and *Campylobacter coli*. Lancet 1:229, 1984.
781. Guerrant RL, Wanke CA, Pennie RA. Production of a unique cytotoxin by *Campylobacter jejuni*. Infect Immun 55:2526, 1987.
782. McCardell BA, Madden JM, Lee EC. *Campylobacter jejuni* and *Campylobacter coli* production of a cytotonic toxin immunologically similar to cholera toxin. J Food Prot 47:943, 1984.
783. Klipstein FA, Engert RF. Purification of *Campylobacter jejuni* enterotoxin. Lancet 1:1123, 1984.
784. Klipstein FA, Engert RF, Short H, et al. Pathogenic properties of *Campylobacter jejuni*: assay and correlation with clinical manifestations. Infect Immun 50:43, 1985.
785. Lee A, Smith SC, Coloe PJ. Detection of a novel *Campylobacter* cytotoxin. J Appl Microbiol 89:719, 2001.
786. Newell DG. Experimental studies of *Campylobacter* enteritis. *In* Butzler JP (ed). *Campylobacter* Infection in Man and Animals. Boca Raton, Fla, CRC Press, 1984, p 113.
787. Prescott JF, Barker IK, Manninen KI, et al. *Campylobacter jejuni* colitis in gnotobiotic dogs. Can J Comp Med 45:377, 1981.
788. Ruiz-Palacios GM, Escamilla E, Torres N. Experimental *Campylobacter* diarrhea in chickens. Infect Immun 34:250, 1981.
789. Sanyal SC, Islam KM, Neogy PKB, et al. *Campylobacter jejuni* diarrhea model in infant chickens. Infect Immun 43:931, 1984.

790. Welkos SL. Experimental gastroenteritis in newly hatched chicks infected with *Campylobacter jejuni*. J Med Microbiol 18:233, 1984.
791. Fitzgeorge RB, Baskerville A, Lander KP. Experimental infection of rhesus monkeys with a human strain of *Campylobacter jejuni*. J Hyg 86:343, 1981.
792. Field LH, Underwood JL, Berry LJ. The role of gut flora and animal passage in the colonization of adult mice with *Campylobacter jejuni*. J Med Microbiol 17:59, 1984.
793. Jesudason MV, Hentges DJ, Pongpeeh P. Colonization of mice by *Campylobacter jejuni*. Infect Immun 57:2279, 1989.
794. Kazmi SU, Roberson BS, Stern NJ. Animal-passed, virulence-enhanced *Campylobacter jejuni* causes enteritis in neonatal mice. Curr Microbiol 11:159, 1984.
795. Humphrey CD, Montag DM, Pittman FE. Experimental infection of hamsters with *Campylobacter jejuni*. J Infect Dis 151:485, 1985.
796. Manninen KI, Prescott JF, Dohoo IR. Pathogenicity of *C. jejuni* isolates from animals and humans. Infect Immun 38:46, 1982.
797. Eden AN. *Vibrio fetus* meningitis in a newborn infant. J Pediatr 61:33, 1962.
798. Maki M, Maki R, Vesikari T. Fecal leucocytes in *Campylobacter*-associated diarrhoea in infants. Acta Paediatr Scand 68:271, 1979.
799. Lambert ME, Schofield PF, Ironside AG, et al. *Campylobacter* colitis. BMJ 1:857, 1979.
800. Blaser MJ, Parsons RB, Wang WL. Acute colitis caused by *Campylobacter fetus spp. jejuni*. Gastroenterology 78:448, 1980.
801. King EO. The laboratory recognition of *Vibrio fetus* and a closely related *Vibrio* isolated from cases of human vibriosis. Ann N Y Acad Sci 78:700, 1962.
802. Evans RG, Dadswell JV. Human vibriosis. BMJ 3:240, 1967.
803. Butzler JP, Oosterom J. *Campylobacter*: pathogenicity and significance in foods. Int J Food Microbiol 12:1, 1991.
804. Gill CO, Harris LM. Contamination of red meat carcasses by *Campylobacter fetus* subsp. *jejuni*. Appl Environ Microbiol 43:977, 1982.
805. Palmer SR, Gulley PR, White JM, et al. Water-borne outbreak of *Campylobacter* gastroenteritis. Lancet 1:287, 1983.
806. Rogol M, Sechter I, Falk H, et al. Water-borne outbreaks of *Campylobacter* enteritis. Eur J Clin Microbiol 2:588, 1983.
807. Shankers S, Rosenfield JA, Davey GR, et al. *Campylobacter jejuni*: incidence in processed broilers and biotype distribution in human and broiler isolates. Appl Environ Microbiol 43:1219, 1982.
808. Hood AM, Pearson AD, Shahamat M. The extent of surface contamination of retailed chickens with *Campylobacter jejuni* serogroups. Epidemiol Infect 100:17, 1988.
809. Harris NV, Kimball TJ, Bennett P, et al. *Campylobacter jejuni* enteritis associated with raw goat's milk. Am J Epidemiol 126:179, 1987.
810. Korlath JA, Osterholm MT, Judy LA, et al. A point-source outbreak of campylobacteriosis associated with consumption of raw milk. J Infect Dis 152:592, 1985.
811. Klein BS, Vergeront JM, Blaser MJ, et al. *Campylobacter* infection associated with raw milk. JAMA 255:361, 1986.
812. Deming MS, Tauxe RV, Blake PA, et al. *Campylobacter* enteritis at a university: transmission from eating chicken and from cats. Am J Epidemiol 126:526, 1987.
813. Tenkate TD, Stafford RJ. Risk factors for *Campylobacter* infection in infants and young children: a matched case-controled study. Epidemiol Infect 127:399, 2001.
814. Hallett AF, Botha PL, Logan A. Isolation of *Campylobacter fetus* from recent cases of human vibriosis. J Hyp 79:381, 1977.
815. Wolfs TF, Duim B, Geelen Sp, et al. Neonatal sepsis by *Campylobacter jejuni*: genetically proven transmission from a household puppy. Clin Infect Dis 31:e97, 2001.
816. Blaser MJ, Waldman RJ, Barrett T, et al. Outbreaks of *Campylobacter* enteritis in two extended families: evidence for person-to-person transmission. J Pediatr 98:254, 1981.
817. Cadranel S, Rodesch P, Butzler JP, et al. Enteritis due to "related *Vibrio*" in children. Am J Dis Child 126:152, 1973.
818. Prescott JF, Karmali MA. Attempts to transmit *Campylobacter* enteritis to dogs and cats. Can Med Assoc J 119:1001, 1978.
819. Black RE, Levine MM, Clements ML, et al. Experimental *Campylobacter jejuni* infection in humans. J Infect Dis 157:472, 1988.
820. Llovo J, Mateo E, Munoz A, et al. Molecular typing of *Campylobacter jejuni* isolates involved in a neonatal outbreak indicates nosocomial transmission. J Clin Microbiol 41:3926, 2003.
821. Bokkenheuser VD, Richardson NJ, Bryner JH, et al. Detection of enteric campylobacteriosis in children. J Clin Microbiol 9:227, 1979.
822. Georges-Courbot MC, Beraud-Cassel AM, Gouandjika I, et al. Prospective study of enteric *Campylobacter* infections in children from birth to 6 months in the Central African Republic. J Clin Microbiol 25:836, 1987.
823. Rettig PJ. *Campylobacter* infections in human beings. J Pediatr 94:855, 1979.
824. Blaser MJ, Berkowitz ID, LaForce FM, et al. *Campylobacter* enteritis: clinical and epidemiological features. Ann Intern Med 91:179, 1979.
825. Butzler JP. Related vibrios in Africa. Lancet 2:858, 1973.
826. Lauwers S, DeBoeck M, Butzler JP. *Campylobacter* enteritis in Brussels. Lancet 1:604, 1978.
827. Severin WP. *Campylobacter* en enteritis. Ned Tijdschr Geneeskd 122:499, 1978.
828. Ribeiro CD. *Campylobacter* enteritis. Lancet 2:270, 1978.
829. Richardson NJ, Koornhof HJ. *Campylobacter* infections in Soweto. S Afr Med J 55:73, 1979.
830. Gribble MJ, Salit EI, Isaac-Renton J, et al. *Campylobacter* infections in pregnancy. Case report and literature review. Am J Obstet Gynecol 140:423, 1981.
831. Morooka T, Umeda A, Fujita M, et al. Epidemiologic application of pulsed-field gel electrophoresis to an outbreak of *Campylobacter fetus* meningitis in a neonatal intensive care unit. Scand J Infect Dis 28:269, 1996.
832. Morooka T, Takeo H, Yasumoto S, Mimatsu T, et al. Nosocomial meningitis due to *Campylobacter fetus* subspecies *fetus* in a neonatal intensive care unit. Acta Paediatr Jpn 34:350, 1992.
833. Norooka T, Takeo H, Yasumoto S, et al. Nosocomial meningitis due to *Campylobacter fetus* subspecies *fetus* in a neonatal intensive care unit. Acta Paediatr Jpn 34:530, 1992.
834. Smith MV, Muldoon AJ. *Campylobacter fetus* subspecies *jejuni* (*Vibrio fetus*) from commercially processed poultry. Appl Microbiol 27:995, 1974.
835. Grant IH, Richardson NJ, Bokkenheuser VD. Broiler chickens as potential source of *Campylobacter* infections in humans. J Clin Microbiol 2:508, 1980.
836. Blaser MJ, Weiss SH, Barrett TJ. *Campylobacter* enteritis associated with a healthy cat. JAMA 247:816, 1982.
837. Skirrow MB, Turnbull GL, Walker RE, et al. *Campylobacter jejuni* enteritis transmitted from cat to man. Lancet 1:1188, 1980.
838. Blaser MJ, Cravens J, Powers BW, et al. *Campylobacter* enteritis associated with canine infection. Lancet 2:979, 1978.
839. Taylor PR, Weinstein WM, Bryner JH. *Campylobacter fetus* infection in human subjects: association with raw milk. Am J Med 66:779, 1979.
840. *Campylobacter* enteritis in a household—Colorado. MMWR Morb Mortal Wkly Rep 27:273, 1979.
841. Robinson DA, Edgar WM, Gibson GL, et al. *Campylobacter* enteritis associated with the consumption of unpasteurized milk. BMJ 1:1171, 1979.
842. Levy AJ. A gastroenteritis outbreak probably due to bovine strain of *Vibrio*. Yale J Biol Med 18:243, 1946.
843. Vogt RL, Sours HE, Barrett T, et al. *Campylobacter* enteritis associated with contaminated water. Ann Intern Med 96:292, 1982.
844. Patton CM, Wachsmuth IK, Evins GM, et al. Evaluation of 10 methods to distinguish epidemic-associated *Campylobacter* strains. J Clin Microbiol 29:680, 1991.
845. Salazar-Lindo E, Sack B, Chea-Woo E, et al. Early treatment with erythromycin of *Campylobacter jejuni* associated dysentery in children. J Pediatr 109:355, 1986.
846. Darling WM, Peel RN, Skirrow MB. *Campylobacter* cholecystitis. Lancet 1:1302, 1979.
847. Davis JS, Penfold JB. *Campylobacter* urinary tract infection. Lancet 1:1091, 1979.
848. Hossain MA, Kabir I, Albert MJ, et al. *Campylobacter jejuni* bacteraemia in children with diarrhea in Bangladesh: report of six cases. J Diarrhoeal Dis Res 10:101, 1992.
849. Reed RP, Friedland IR, Wegerhoff FO, Khoosal M. *Campylobacter* bacteremia in children. Pediatr Infect Dis J 15:345, 1996.
850. Johonsen K, Ostensen M, Christine A, et al. HLA-B27-negative arthritis related to *Campylobacter jejuni* enteritis in three children and two adults. Acta Med Scand 214:165, 1983.
851. Kaldor J, Speed BR. Guillain-Barré syndrome and *Campylobacter jejuni*: a serological study. BMJ 288:1867, 1984.
852. Kuroki S, Haruta T, Yoshioka M, et al. Guillain-Barré syndrome associated with *Campylobacter* infection. Pediatr Infect Dis J 10:149, 1991.

853. Ebright JR, Ryay LM. Acute erosive reactive arthritis associated with *Campylobacter jejuni*–induced colitis. Am J Med 76:321, 1984.
854. Schaad UB. Reactive arthritis associated with *Campylobacter* enteritis. Pediatr Infect Dis J 1:328, 1982.
855. Perlman DM, Ampel NM, Schifman RB, et al. Persistent *Campylobacter jejuni* infections in patients infected with human immunodeficiency virus (HIV). Ann Intern Med 108:540, 1988.
856. Chiu CH, Kuo CY, Ou JT. Chronic diarrhea and bacteremia caused by *Campylobacter lari* in a neonate. Clin Infect Dis 21:700, 1995.
857. Endtz HP, Ruijs GJHM, Zwinderman AH, et al. Comparison of six media, including a semisolid agar for the isolation of various *Campylobacter* species from stool specimens. J Clin Microbiol 29:1007, 1991.
858. Paisley JW, Mirrett S, Lauer BA, et al. Darkfield microscopy of human feces for presumptive diagnosis of *Campylobacter fetus subsp. jejuni* enteritis. J Clin Microbiol 15:61, 1982.
859. Oyofo BA, Thornton SA, Burr DH, et al. Specific detection of *Campylobacter jejuni* and *Campylobacter coli* by using polymerase chain reaction. J Clin Microbiol 30:2613, 1992.
860. Kiehlbauch JA, Baker CN, Wachsmuth IK, et al. In vitro susceptibilities of aerotolerant *Campylobacter* isolates to 22 antimicrobial agents. Antimicrob Agents Chemother 36:717, 1992.
861. LaChance N, Gaudreau C, Lamothe F, et al. Susceptibilities of β-lactamase-positive and -negative strains of *Campylobacter coli* to β-lactam agents. Antimicrob Agents Chemother 37:1174, 1993.
862. Yan W, Taylor DE. Characterization of erythromycin resistance in *Campylobacter jejuni* and *Campylobacter coli*. Antimicrob Agents Chemother 35:1989, 1991.
863. Segretti J, Gootz TD, Goodman LJ, et al. High-level quinolone resistance in clinical isolates of *Campylobacter jejuni*. J Infect Dis 165:667, 1992.
864. Krowchuk D, Seashore JH. Complete biliary obstruction due to erythromycin estolate administration in an infant. Pediatrics 64:956, 1979.
865. Kuschner RA, Trofa AF, Thomas RJ, et al. Use of azithromycin for the treatment of *Campylobacter* enteritis in travelers to Thailand, an area where ciprofloxacin resistance is prevalent. Clin Infect Dis 21:536, 1995.
866. Rautelin H, Renkonen OV, Kosunen TU. Azithromycin resistance in *Campylobacter jejuni* and *Campylobacter coli*. Eur J Clin Microbiol Infect Dis 12:864, 1993.
867. Endtz HP, Broeren M, Mouton RP. In vitro susceptibility of quinolone-resistant *Campylobacter jejuni* to new macrolide antibiotics. Eur J Clin Microbiol Infect Dis 12:48, 1993.
868. Nachamkin I, Fischer SH, Yang XH, et al: Immunoglobulin A antibodies directed against *Campylobacter jejuni* flagellin present in breast-milk. Epidemiol Infect 112:359, 1994.
869. Borriello SP, Davies HA, Kamiya S, et al. Virulence factors of *Clostridium difficile*. Rev Infect Dis 12:S185, 1990.
870. Sears CL, Kaper JB. Enteric bacterial toxins: mechanisms of action and linkage to intestinal secretion. Microbiol Rev 60:167, 1996.
871. Wren BW. Molecular characterisation of *Clostridium difficile* toxins A and B. Rev Med Microbiol 3:21, 1992.
872. Hyams JS, Berman MM, Helgason H. Nonantibiotic-associated enterocolitis caused by *Clostridium difficile* in an infant. J Pediatr 99:750, 1981.
873. Larson HE, Price AB. Pseudomembranous colitis: presence of clostridial toxin. Lancet 1:1312, 1977.
874. Peikin SR, Galdibin J, Bartlett JG. Role of *Clostridium difficile* in a case of nonantibiotic-associated pseudomembranous colitis. Gastroenterology 79:948, 1980.
875. Wald A, Mendelow H, Bartlett JG. Nonantibiotic-associated pseudomembranous colitis due to toxin producing clostridia. Ann Intern Med 92:798, 1980.
876. Adler SP, Chandrika T, Berman WF. *Clostridium difficile* associated with pseudomembranous colitis. Am J Dis Child 135:820, 1981.
877. Willey S, Bartlett JG. Cultures for *C. difficile* in stools containing a cytotoxin neutralized by *C. sordellii* antitoxin. J Clin Microbiol 10:880, 1979.
878. Tabaqchali S. Epidemiologic markers of *Clostridium difficile*. Rev Infect Dis 12:S192, 1990.
879. Kim KH, Fekety R, Batts D, et al. Isolation of *C. difficile* from the environment and contacts of patients with antibiotic-associated colitis. J Infect Dis 143:42, 1981.
880. Sheretz RJ, Sarubb FA. The prevalence of *C. difficile* and toxin in a nursery population: a comparison between patients with necrotizing enterocolitis and an asymptomatic group. J Pediatr 100:435, 1982.
881. Clabots CR, Johnson S, Olson MM, et al. Acquisition of *Clostridium difficile* by hospitalized patients: evidence for colonized new admissions as a source of infection. J Infect Dis 166:561, 1992.
882. Bliss DZ, Johnson S, Savik K, et al. Acquisition of *Clostridium difficile* and *Clostridium difficile*-associated diarrhea in hospitalized patients receiving tube feeding. Ann Intern Med 129:1012, 1998.
883. Jernigan JA, Siegman-Igra Y, Guerrant RC, Farr BM. A randomized crossover study of disposable thermometers for prevention of *Clostridium difficile* and other nosocomial infections. Infect Control Hosp Epidemiol 19:494, 1998.
884. Johnson S, Gerding DN, Olson NM, et al. Prospective controlled study of vinyl glove use to interrupt *Clostridium difficile* transmission. Am J Med 88:137, 1990.
885. Zedd AJ, Sell TL, Schabert DR, et al. Nosocomial *C. difficile* reservoir in a neonatal intensive care unit. Pediatr Infect Dis J 3:429, 1984.
886. Johnson S, Gerding DN. *Clostridium difficile*–associated diarrhea. Clin Infect Dis 26:1027, 1998.
887. Fekety R, Shah AB. Diagnosis and treatment of *Clostridium difficile* colitis. JAMA 269:71, 1993.
888. Kelber M, Ament ME. *Shigella dysenteriae* 1. A forgotten cause of pseudomembranous colitis. J Pediatr 89:595, 1976.
889. Donta ST, Myers MG. *C. difficile* toxin in asymptomatic neonates. J Pediatr 100:431, 1982.
890. Al-Jumaili I, Shibley M, Lishman AH, et al. Incidence and origin of *C. difficile* in neonates. J Clin Microbiol 19:77, 1984.
891. Welch DF, Marks MT. Is *C. difficile* pathogenic in infants? J Pediatr 100:393, 1982.
892. Donta ST, Stuppy MS, Myers MG. Neonatal antibiotic-associated colitis. Am J Dis Child 135:181, 1981.
893. Enad D, Meislich D, Bodsky NL, Hurt H. Is *Clostridium difficile* a pathogen in the newborn intensive care unit? A prospective evaluation. J Perinatol 17:355, 1997.
894. Lyerly DM, Neville LM, Evans DT, et al. Multicenter evaluation of the *Clostridium difficile* TOX A/B TEST. J Clin Microbiol 36:184, 1998.
895. Kato H, Kato N, Watanabe K, et al. Identification of toxin A-negative, toxin B-positive *Clostridium difficile* by PCR. J Clin Microbiol 36:2178, 1998.
896. Rafferty ME, Baltch AL, Smith RP, et al. Comparison of restriction enzyme analysis, arbitrarily primed PCR, and protein profile analysis typing for epidemiologic investigation of an ongoing *Clostridium difficile* outbreak. J Clin Microbiol 36:2957, 1998.
897. Teasley DG, Gerding DN, Olson MM, et al. Prospective randomized trial of metronidazole vs. vancomycin for *C. difficile* associated diarrhoea and colitis. Lancet 2:1043, 1983.
898. Wenisch C, Parschalk B, Hasenhündl M, et al. Comparison of vancomycin, teicoplanin, metronidazole, and fusidic acid for the treatment of *Clostridum difficile*-associated diarrhea. Clin Infect Dis 22:813, 1996.
899. Young GP, Ward PB, Bayley N, et al. Antibiotic-associated colitis due to *C. difficile:* double-blind comparison of vancomycin with bacitracin. Gastroenterology 89:1039, 1985.
900. Dudley MN, McLaughlin JC, Carrington G, et al. Oral bacitracin vs. vancomycin therapy for *C. difficile*–induced diarrhea. Arch Intern Med 146:1101, 1986.
901. Bartlett JG, Tedesco FJ, Shull S, et al. Relapse following oral vancomycin therapy of antibiotic-associated pseudomembranous colitis. Gastroenterology 78:431, 1980.
902. Wada N, Nishida N, Iwak S, et al. Neutralizing activity against *C. difficile* toxin in the supernatants of cultures of colostral cells. Infect Immun 29:545, 1980.
903. Dallas S, Rolfe R. Binding of *Clostridium difficile* toxin A to human milk secretory component. J Med Microbiol 47:879, 1998.
904. Kim K, Pickering LK, DuPont HL, et al. *In vitro* and *in vivo* neutralizing activity of *C. difficile* purified toxins A and B by human colostrum and milk. J Infect Dis 150:57, 1984.
905. Cooperstock MS, Steffen E, Yolken R, et al. *C. difficile* in normal infants and sudden death syndrome: an association with infant formula feeding. Pediatrics 70:91, 1982.
906. Levine WC, Griffin PM, and the Gulf Coast Vibrio Working Group. *Vibrio* infections on the Gulf Coast: results of first year of regional surveillance. J Infect Dis 167:479, 1993.
907. Swerdlow DL, Ries AA. Cholera in the Americas: guidelines for the clinician. JAMA 267:1495, 1992.
908. Glass RI, Libel M, Brandling-Bennett AD. Epidemic cholera in the Americas. Science 256:1524, 1992.

909. Wachsmuth IK, Evins GM, Fields PI, et al. The molecular epidemiology of cholera in Latin America. J Infect Dis 167:621, 1993.
910. Siddique AK, Zaman K, Akram K, et al. Emergence of a new epidemic strain of *Vibrio cholerae* in Bangladesh. An epidemiological study. Trop Geogr Med 46:147, 1994.
911. Fisher-Hoch SP, Khan A, Inam-ul-Haq, et al. *Vibrio cholerae* O139 in Karachi, Pakistan. Lancet 342:1422, 1993.
912. Chongsa-Nguan M, Chaicumpa W, Moolasart P, et al. *Vibrio cholerae* O139 Bengal in Bangkok. Lancet 342:430, 1993.
913. Cholera Working Group, International Centre for Diarrhoeal Diseases Research, Bangladesh. Large epidemic of cholera-like disease in Bangladesh caused by *Vibrio cholerae* O139 synonym Bengal. Lancet 342:387, 1993.
914. Bhattacharya SK, Bhattacharya MK, Nair GB, et al. Clinical profile of acute diarrhoea cases infected with the new epidemic strain of *Vibrio cholerae* O139: designation of the disease as cholera. J Infect 27:11, 1993.
915. Garg S, Saha PK, Ramamurthy T, et al. Nationwide prevalence of the new epidemic strain of *Vibrio cholerae* O139 Bengal in India. J Infect 27:108, 1993.
916. Blake PA, Allegra DT, Snyder JD, et al. Cholera—a possible endemic focus in the United States. N Engl J Med 302:305, 1980.
917. Hirschhorn N, Chowdhury AAKM, Lindenbaum J. Cholera in pregnant women. Lancet 1:1230, 1969.
918. Khan AM, Bhattacharyl MK, Albert MJ. Neonatal diarrhea caused by *Vibrio cholerae* O139 Bengal. Diagn Microbiol Infect Dis 23:155, 1995.
919. Lumbiganon P, Kosalaraksa P, Kowsuwan P. *Vibrio cholerae* O139 diarrhea and acute renal failure in a three day old infant. Pediatr Infect Dis J 14:1105, 1995.
920. Haider R, Kabir I, Fuchs GJ, Habte D. Neonatal diarrhea in a diarrhea treatment center in Bangladesh: clinical presentation, breastfeeding management and outcome. Indian Pediatr 37:37, 2000.
921. Gunn RA, Kimball AM, Pollard RA, et al. Bottle feeding as a risk factor for cholera in infants. Lancet 2:730, 1979.
922. Ahmed A, Bhattacharjee AK, Mosley WH. Characteristics of the serum vibriocidal and agglutinating antibodies in cholera cases and in normal residents of the endemic and non-endemic cholera areas. J Immunol 105:431, 1970.
923. Merson MH, Black RE, Sack DA, et al. Maternal cholera immunisation and secretory IgA in breast milk. Lancet 1:931, 1980.
924. Cash RA, Music SI, Libonati JP, et al. Response of man to infection with *Vibrio cholerae*. I. Clinical, serologic and bacteriologic responses to a known inoculum. J Infect Dis 129:45, 1974.
925. Nalin DR, Levine RJ, Levine MM. Cholera, non–*Vibrio* cholera, and stomach acid. Lancet 2:856, 1978.
926. Wright AC, Guo Y, Johnson JA, et al. Development and testing of a nonradioactive DNA oligonucleotide probe that is specific for *Vibrio cholerae* cholera toxin. J Clin Microbiol 30:2302, 1992.
927. Yoh M, Miyagi K, Matsumoto Y, et al. Development of an enzyme-labeled oligonucleotide probe for the cholera toxin gene. J Clin Microbiol 31:1312, 1993.
928. Kotloff KL, Wasserman SS, O'Donnell S, et al. Safety and immunogenicity in North Americans of a single dose of live oral cholera vaccine CVD 103-HgR: results of a randomized, placebo-controlled, double-blind crossover trial. Infect Immun 60:4430, 1992.
929. Clemens JD, Sack DA, Rao MR, et al. Evidence that inactivated oral cholera vaccines both prevent and mitigate *Vibrio cholerae* O1 infections in a cholera-endemic area. J Infect Dis 166:1029, 1992.
930. Levine MM, Noriega F. A review of the current status of enteric vaccines. P N G Med J 38:325, 1995.
931. Kohl S. *Yersinia enterocolitica* infections in children. Pediatr Clin North Am 26:433, 1979.
932. Marks MI, Pai CH, Lafleur L, et al. *Yersinia enterocolitica* gastroenteritis: a prospective study of clinical, bacteriologic, and epidemiologic features. J Pediatr 96:26, 1980.
933. Lee LA, Gerber AR, Lonsway DR, et al. *Yersinia enterocolitica* 0:3 infections in infants and children, associated with the household preparation of chitterlings. N Engl J Med 322:984, 1990.
934. Krogstad P, Mendelman PM, Miller VL, et al. Clinical and microbiologic characteristics of cutaneous infection with *Yersinia enterocolitica*. J Infect Dis 165:740, 1992.
935. Lee LA, Taylor J, Carter GP, et al. *Yersinia enterocolitica* 0:3: an emerging cause of pediatric gastroenteritis in the United States. J Infect Dis 163:660, 1991.
936. Morris JG Jr, Prado V, Ferreccio C, et al. *Yersinia enterocolitica* isolated from two cohorts of young children in Santiago, Chile: incidence of and lack of correlation between illness and proposed virulence factors. J Clin Microbiol 29:2784, 1991.
937. Metchock B, Lonsway DR, Carter GP, et al. *Yersinia enterocolitica*: a frequent seasonal stool isolate from children at an urban hospital in the southeast United States. J Clin Microbiol 29:2868, 1991.
938. Kane DR, Reuman PD. *Yersinia enterocolitica* causing pneumonia and empyema in a child and a review of the literature. Pediatr Infect Dis J 11:591, 1992.
939. Black RE, Jackson RJ, Tsai T, et al. Epidemic *Yersinia enterocolitica* infection due to contaminated chocolate milk. N Engl J Med 298:76, 1978.
940. Pietersz RNI, Reesink HW, Pauw W, et al. Prevention of *Yersinia enterocolitica* growth in red blood cell concentrates. Lancet 340:755, 1992.
941. Kapperud G, Namork E, Skurnik M, et al. Plasmid-mediated surface fibrillae of *Y. pseudotuberculosis* and *Y. enterocolitica*. Relationship to the outer membrane protein YOP1 and possible importance for pathogenesis. Infect Immun 55:2247, 1987.
942. Brubaker RR. Factors promoting acute and chronic diseases caused by yersiniae. Clin Microbiol Rev 4:309, 1991.
943. Takao T, Tominaga N, Shimoniski Y, et al. Primary structure of heat-stable enterotoxin produced by *Y. enterocolitica*. Biochem Biophys Res Commun 125:845, 1984.
944. Paisley JW, Lauer BA. Neonatal *Yersinia enterocolitica* enteritis. Pediatr Infect Dis J 11:331, 1992.
945. Shapiro ED. *Yersinia enterocolitica* septicemia in normal infants. Am J Dis Child 135:477, 1981.
946. Chester B, Sanderson T, Zeller DJ, et al. Infections due to *Yersinia enterocolitica* serotypes 0:2, 3 and 0:4 acquired in South Florida. J Clin Microbiol 13:885, 1981.
947. Rodriguez WJ, Controni G, Cohen GJ, et al. *Y. enterocolitica* enteritis in children. JAMA 242:1978, 1979.
948. Challapalli M, Cunningham DG. *Yersinia enterocolitica* septicemia in infants younger than three months of age. Pediatr Infect Dis J 12:168, 1993.
949. Paisley JW, Lauer BA. Neonatal *Yersinia enterocolitica* enteritis. Pediatr Infect Dis J 11:332, 1992.
950. Antonio-Santiago MT, Kaul A, Lue Y, et al. *Yersinia enterocolitica* septicemia in an infant presenting as fever of unknown origin. Clin Pediatr 25:213, 1986.
951. Sutton JM, Pasquariell PS. *Yersinia enterocolitica* septicemia in a normal child. Am J Dis Child 137:305, 1983.
952. Kohl S, Jacobson JA, Nahmias A. *Yersinia enterocolitica* infections in children. J Pediatr 89:77, 1976.
953. Naqvi S, Swierkosz E, Gerard J, Mills J. Presentation of *Yersinia enterocolitica* enteritis in children. Pediatr Infect Dis J 12:386, 1993.
954. Abdel-Haq N, Asmar B, Abuhammour W, Brown W. *Yersinia enterocolitica* infection in children. Pediatr Infect Dis J 19:954, 2000.
955. Ibrahim A, Liesack W, Stackebrandt E. Polymerase chain reaction–gene probe detection system specific for pathogenic strains of *Yersinia enterocolitica*. J Clin Microbiol 30:1942, 1992.
956. Kwaga J, Iversen JO, Misra V. Detection of pathogenic *Yersinia enterocolitica* by polymerase chain reaction and digoxigenin-labeled polynucleotide probes. J Clin Microbiol 30:2668, 1992.
957. Stolk-Engelaar VM, Meis JF, Mulder JA, et al. *In-vitro* antimicrobial susceptibility of *Yersinia enterocolitica* isolates from stools of patients in the Netherlands from 1982-1991. J Antimicrob Chemother 36:839, 1995.
958. Alzugaray R, Gonzalez Hevia MA, Landeras E, Mendoza MC. *Yersinia enterocolitica* 0:3. Antimicrobial resistance patterns, virulence profiles and plasmids. New Microbiol 18:215, 1995.
959. Preston MA, Brown S, Borczyk AA, et al. Antimicrobial susceptibility of pathogenic *Yersinia enterocolitica* isolated in Canada from 1972 to 1990. Antimicrob Agents Chemother 38:2121, 1994.
960. James C, Dibley M, Burke V, et al. Immunological cross-reactivity of enterotoxins of *A. hydrophila* and cholera toxin. Clin Exp Immunol 47:34, 1982.
961. Sanyal SC, Singh SJ, Sen PC. Enteropathogenicity of *A. hydrophila* and *P. shigelloides*. J Med Microbiol 8:195, 1975.
962. Kirov SM, Rees B, Wellock RC, et al. Virulence characteristics of *Aeromonas spp*. in relation to source and biotype. J Clin Microbiol 24: 827, 1986.
963. Watson IM, Robinson JO, Burke V, et al. Invasiveness of *Aeromonas spp*. in relation to biotype, virulence factors, and clinical features. J Clin Microbiol 22:48, 1985.

964. Kindshuh M, Pickering LK, Cleary TG, et al. Clinical and biochemical significance of toxin production by *A. hydrophila*. J Clin Microbiol 25:916, 1987.
965. Ljungh A, Eneroth P, Wadstrom T. Cytotonic enterotoxin from *Aeromonas hydrophila*. Toxicon 20:787, 1982.
966. Morgan D, Johnson PC, DuPont HL, et al. Lack of correlation between known virulence properties of *A. hydrophila* and enteropathogenicity for humans. Infect Immun 50:62, 1985.
967. Pitarangsi C, Echeverria P, Whitemire R, et al. Enteropathogenicity of *A. hydrophila* and *P. shigelloides*: prevalence among individuals with and without diarrhea in Thailand. Infect Immun 35:666, 1982.
968. Martinez-Silva R, Guzmann-Urrego M, Caselitz FH. Zur Frage der Bedeutung von Aeromonasstammen bei Saüglingsenteritis. Z Tropenmed Parasitol 12:445, 1961.
969. Figura N, Marri L, Verdiani S, et al. Prevalence, species differentiation, and toxigenicity of *Aeromonas* strains in cases of childhood gastroenteritis and in controls. J Clin Microbiol 23:595, 1986.
970. Gracey M, Burke V, Robinson J. *Aeromonas*-associated gastroenteritis. Lancet 2:1304, 1982.
971. Shread P, Donovan TJ, Lee JV. A survey of the incidence of *Aeromonas* in human feces. Soc Gen Microbiol 8:184, 1981.
972. Escheverria P, Blacklow NR, Sanford LB, et al. Travelers' diarrhea among American Peace Corps volunteers in rural Thailand. J Infect Dis 143:767, 1981.
973. Bhat P, Shanthakumari S, Rajan D. The characterization and significance of *P. shigelloides* and *A. hydrophila* isolated from an epidemic of diarrhea. Indian J Med Res 62:1051, 1974.
974. Agger WA, McCormick JD, Gurwith MJ. Clinical and microbiological features of *A. hydrophila*–associated diarrhea. J Clin Microbiol 21:909, 1985.
975. Agger WA. Diarrhea associated with *A. hydrophila*. Pediatr Infect Dis J 5:S106, 1986.
976. Deodhar LP, Saraswathi K, Varudkar A. *Aeromonas spp.* and their association with human diarrheal disease. J Clin Microbiol 29:853, 1991.
977. Santoso H, Agung IGN, Robinson J, et al. Faecal *Aeromonas spp.* in Balinese children. J Gastroenterol Hepatol 1:115, 1986.
978. Gomez CJ, Munozz P, Lopez F, et al. Gastroenteritis due to *Aeromonas* in pediatrics. An Esp Pediatr 44:548, 1996.
979. Diaz A, Velasco AC, Hawkins F, et al. *A. hydrophila*–associated diarrhea in a neonate. Pediatr Infect Dis J 5:704, 1986.
980. San Joaquin VH, Pickett DA. *Aeromonas*-associated gastroenteritis in children. Pediatr Infect Dis J 7:53, 1988.
981. George WL, Jones MJ, Nakata MM. Phenotypic characteristics of *Aeromonas* species isolated from adult humans. J Clin Microbiol 23:1026, 1986.
982. Janda JM. Recent advances in the study of the taxonomy, pathogenicity, and infectious syndromes associated with the genus *Aeromonas*. Clin Microbiol Rev 4:397, 1991.
983. Freij BJ. *Aeromonas*: biology of the organism and diseases in children. Pediatr Infect Dis J 3:164, 1984.
984. Fainstein V, Weaver S, Bodey GP. *In vitro* susceptibilities of *A. hydrophila* against new antibiotics. Antimicrob Agents Chemother 22:513, 1982.
985. San Joaquin VH, Scribner RK, Pickett DA, et al. Antimicrobial susceptibility of *Aeromonas* species isolated from patients with diarrhea. Antimicrob Agents Chemother 30:794, 1986.
986. Jones BL, Wilcox MH. *Aeromonas* infections and their treatment. J Antimicrob Chemother 35:453, 1995.
987. Holmberg SD, Wachsmuth IK, Hickmann-Brenner FW, et al. *Plesiomonas* enteric infections in the United States. Ann Intern Med 105:690, 1986.
988. Tsukamoto T, Kinoshita Y, Shimada T, et al. Two epidemics of diarrhoeal disease possibly caused by *P. shigelloides*. J Hyg 80:275, 1978.
989. Holmberg SD, Farmer JJ. *A. hydrophila* and *P. shigelloides* as causes of intestinal infections. Rev Infect Dis 6:633, 1984.
990. Herrington DA, Tzipori S, Robins-Browne RM, et al. *In vitro* and *in vivo* pathogenicity of *P. shigelloides*. Infect Immun 55:979, 1987.
991. Brenden RA, Miller MA, Janda JM. Clinical disease spectrum and pathogenic factors associated with *P. shigelloides* infections in humans. Rev Infect Dis 10:303, 1988.
992. Pathak A, Custer JR, Levy J. Neonatal septicemia and meningitis due to *Plesiomonas shigelloides*. Pediatrics 71:389, 1983.
993. Fujita K, Shirai M, Ishioka T, Kakuya F. Neonatal *Plesiomonas shigelloides* septicemia and meningitis: a case review. Acta Paediatr Jpn 36:450, 1994.
994. Terpeluk C, Goldmann A, Bartmann P, Pohlandt F. *Plesiomonas shigelloides* sepsis and meningoencephalitis in a neonate. Eur J Pediatr 151:499, 1992.
995. Billiet J, Kuypers S, Van Lierde S, Verhaegen J. *Plesiomonas shigelloides* meningitis and septicaemia in a neonate: report of a case and review of the literature. J Infect 19:267, 1989.
996. Alabi SA, Odugbemi T. Biochemical characteristics and a simple scheme for the identification of *Aeromonas* species and *Plesiomonas shigelloides*. J Trop Med Hyg 93:166, 1990.
997. Reinhardt JF, George WL. Comparative in vitro activities of selected antimicrobial agents against *Aeromonas species* and *P. shigelloides*. Antimicrob Agents Chemother 27:643, 1985.
998. Visitsunthorn N, Komolpis P. Antimicrobial therapy in *Plesiomonas shigelloides*–associated diarrhea in Thai children. Southeast Asian J Trop Med Public Health 26:86, 1995.
999. Jampolis M, Howell KM, Calvin JK, et al. *Bacillus* mucosus infection of the newborn. Am J Dis Child 43:70, 1932.
1000. Olarte J, Ferguson WW, Henderson ND, et al. *Klebsiella* strains isolated from diarrheal infants. Human volunteer studies. Am J Dis Child 101:763, 1961.
1001. Murdoch MM, Janovski NA, Joseph S. *Klebsiella* pseudomembranous enterocolitis. Report of two cases. Med Ann Dist Columbia 38:137, 1969.
1002. Ujvary G, Angyal T, Voros S, et al. Beobachtungen Über die Ätiologie der Gastroenterocolitiden des Säuglings- und Kindesalters. II. Untersuchung der Rolle der Klebsiella-Stamme. Acta Microbiol Acad Sci Hung 10:241, 1964.
1003. Gergely K. Über eine Enteritis-Epidemie bei Frühgeborenen, verursacht durch den Bacillus Klebsiella. Kinderarztl Prax 9:385, 1964.
1004. Walcher DN. "*Bacillus mucosus capsulatus*" in infantile diarrhea. J Clin Invest 25:103, 1946.
1005. Cass JM. *Bacillus lactis aerogenes* infection in the newborn. Lancet 1:346, 1941.
1006. Sternberg SD, Hoffman C, Zweifler BM. Stomatitis and diarrhea in infants caused by *Bacillus mucosus capsulatus*. J Pediatr 38:509, 1951.
1007. Worfel MT, Ferguson WW. A new *Klebsiella* type (capsular type 15) isolated from feces and urine. Am J Clin Pathol 21:1097, 1951.
1008. Simmons BP, Gelfand MS, Haas M, et al. *Enterobacter sakazakii* infections in neonates associated with intrinsic contamination of a powdered infant formula. Infect Control Hosp Epidemiol 10:398, 1989.
1009. Ayliffe GAJ, Collins BJ, Pettit F. Contamination of infant feeds in a Milton milk kitchen. Lancet 1:559, 1970.
1010. Adler JL, Shulman JA, Terry PM, et al. Nosocomial colonization with kanamycin-resistant *Klebsiella* pneumoniae, types 2 and 11, in a premature nursery. J Pediatr 77:376, 1970.
1011. Hill HR, Hunt CE, Matsen JM. Nosocomial colonization with *Klebsiella*, type 16, in a neonatal intensive-care unit associated with an outbreak of sepsis, meningitis, and necrotizing enterocolitis. J Pediatr 85:415, 1974.
1012. Panigrahi D, Roy P, Chakrabarti A. Enterotoxigenic *Klebsiella pneumoniae* in acute childhood diarrhea. Indian J Med Res 93:293, 1991.
1013. Guarino A, Capano G, Malamisura B, et al. Production of *E. coli* STa-like heat stable enterotoxin by *Citrobacter freundii* isolated from humans. J Clin Microbiol 25:110, 1987.
1014. Lipsky BA, Hook EW, Smith AA, et al. *Citrobacter* infections in humans: experience at the Seattle Veterans Administration Medical Center and a review of the literature. Rev Infect Dis 2:746, 1980.
1015. Kahlich R, Webershinke J. A contribution to incidence and evaluation of *Citrobacter* findings in man. Cesk Epidemiol Mikrobiol Imunol 12:55, 1963.
1016. Parida SN, Verma IC, Deb M, et al. An outbreak of diarrhea due to *Citrobacter freundii* in a neonatal special care nursery. Indian J Pediatr 47:81, 1980.
1017. Heitmann M, Gerner-Smidt P, Heltberg O. Gastroenteritis caused by *Listeria monocytogenes* in a private day-care facility. Pediatr Infect Dis J 16:827, 1997.
1018. Sim J, Hood D, Finnie L, et al. Series of incidents of *Listeria monocytogenes* non-invasive febrile gastroenteritis involving ready-to-eat meats. Lett Appl Microbiol 35:409, 2002.
1019. Schlech W. *Listeria* gastroenteritis—old syndrome, new pathogen. N Engl J Med 336:130, 1997.
1020. Wing E, Gregory S. *Listeria monocytogenes*: clinical and experimental update. J Infect Dis 185:S18, 2002.

1021. Aureli P, Fiorucci G, Caroli D, et al. An outbreak of febrile gastroenteritis associated with corn contaminated by *Listeria monocytogenes*. N Engl J Med 342:1236, 2000.
1022. Dalton C, Austin C, Sobel J, et al. An outbreak of gastroenteritis and fever due to *Listeria monocytogenes* in milk. N Engl J Med 336:100, 1997.
1023. Hof H, Lampidis R, Bensch J. Noscomial *Listeria* gastroenteritis in a newborn, confirmed by random amplification of polymorphic DNA. Clin Microbiol Infect 6:683, 2000.
1024. Larsson S, Cederberg A, Ivarsson S, et al. *Listeria monocytogenes* causing hospital-acquired enterocolitis and meningitis in newborn infants. Br Med J 2:473, 1978.
1025. Edelbroek M, De Nef J, Rajnherc J. *Listeria* meningitis presenting as enteritis in a previously healthy infant: a case report. Eur J Pediatr 153:179, 1994.
1026. Norys H. Fetal chronic nonspecific enterocolitis with peritonitis in uniovular twins after *Listeria* infection in the mother. Monatsschr Kinderheilkd 108:59, 1960.
1027. Sack R, Albert M, Alam K, et al. Isolation of enterotoxigenic *Bacteroides fragilis* from Bangladeshi children with diarrhea: a controlled study. J Clin Microbiol 32:960, 1994.
1028. Sack R, Myers L, Almeido-Hill J, et al. Enterotoxigenic *Bacteroides fragilis*: epidemiologic studies of its role as a human diarrhoeal pathogen. J Diarrhoeal Dis Res 10:4, 1992.
1029. Kubota Y, Liu PV. An enterotoxin of *Pseudomonas aeruginosa*. J Infect Dis 123:97, 1971.
1030. Bassett DCJ, Thompson SAS, Page B. Neonatal infections with *Pseudomonas aeruginosa* associated with contaminated resuscitation equipment. Lancet 1:781, 1965.
1031. Ensign PR, Hunter CA. An epidemic of diarrhea in the newborn nursery caused by a milk-borne epidemic in the community. J Pediatr 29:620, 1946.
1032. Falcao DP, Mendonca CP, Scrassolo A, et al. Nursery outbreak of severe diarrhoea due to multiple strains of *Pseudomonas aeruginosa*. Lancet 2:38, 1972.
1033. Henderson A, Maclaurin J, Scott JM. *Pseudomonas* in a Glasgow baby unit. Lancet 2:316, 1969.
1034. Jellard CH, Churcher GM. An outbreak of *Pseudomonas aeruginosa* (pyocyanea) infection in a premature baby unit, with observations on the intestinal carriage of *Pseudomonas aeruginosa* in the newborn. J Hyg 65:219, 1967.
1035. Rowe B, Gross RJ, Allen HA. *Citrobacter koseri* II. Serological and biochemical examination of *Citrobacter koseri* strains from clinical specimens. J Hyg 75:129, 1975.
1036. Kalashnikova GK, Lokosova AK, Sorokina RS. Concerning the etiological role of bacteria belonging to *Citrobacter* and *Hafnia* genera in children suffering from diseases accompanied by diarrhea, and some of their epidemiological peculiarities. Zh Mikrobiol Epidemiol Immunobiol 6:78, 1974.
1037. Graber CD, Dodd MC. The role of *Paracolobactrum* and *Proteus* in infantile diarrhea. Ann N Y Acad Sci 66:136, 1956.
1038. Neter E, Goodale ML. Peritonitis due to the *Morgani bacillus*. With a brief review of literature on the pathogenicity of this organism. Am J Dis Child 56:1313, 1938.
1039. Neter ER, Farrar RH. *Proteus vulgaris* and *Proteus morgani* in diarrheal disease of infants. Am J Dig Dis 10:344, 1943.
1040. Neter E, Bender NC. *Bacillus morgani*, type I, in enterocolitis of infants. J Pediatr 19:53, 1941.
1041. Ujvary G, Lanyi B, Gregacs M, et al. Beobachtungen über die Ätiologie der Gastroenterocolitiden des Säuglings- und Kindesalters. III. Untersuchung der Rolle der Proteus vulgaris- und der Proteus mirabilis-Stamme. Acta Microbiol Acad Sci Hung 10:315, 1964.
1042. Moffet HL, Shulenberger HK, Burkholder ER. Epidemiology and etiology of severe infantile diarrhea. J Pediatr 72:1, 1968.
1043. Mohieldin MS, Gabr M, el-Hefny A, et al. Bacteriological and clinical studies in infantile diarrhoea. II. Doubtful pathogens: *Enterobacteriaceae, Pseudomonas, Alcaligenes* and *Aeromonas*. J Trop Pediatr 11:88, 1966.
1044. Singer JM, Bar-Hay J, Hoenigsberg R. The intestinal flora in the etiology of infantile infectious diarrhea. Am J Dis Child 89:531, 1955.
1045. Williams S. The bacteriological considerations of infantile enteritis in Sydney. Med J Aust 2:137, 1951.
1046. Ujvary G, Voros S, Angyal T, et al. Beobachtungen über die Ätiologie der Gastroenterocolitiden des Säuglings- und Kindesalters. IV. Untersuchung der Rolle der Proteus morgani-Stamme. Acta Microbiol Acad Sci Hung 10:327, 1964.
1047. Sharpe ME. Group D streptococci in the faeces of healthy infants and of infants with neonatal diarrhea. J Hyg 50:209, 1952.
1048. Kohler H, Kite P. Neonatal enteritis due to Providencia organisms. Arch Dis Child 45:709, 1970.
1049. Ridge LEL, Thomas MEM. Infection with the Providence type of *Paracolon bacillus* in a residential nursery. J Pathol Bacteriol 69:335, 1955.
1050. Bhat P, Myers RM, Feldman RA. Providence group of organisms in the aetiology of juvenile diarrhoea. Indian J Med Res 59:1010, 1971.
1051. Bishop RF, Barnes GL, Townley RRW. Microbial flora of stomach and small intestine in infantile gastroenteritis. Acta Paediatr Scand 63:418, 1974.
1052. Chaudhury A, Nath G, Shukla B, et al. Diarrhoea associated with *Candida spp.*: incidence and seasonal variation. J Diarrhoeal Dis Res 14:110, 1996.
1053. Enweani I, Obi C, Jokpeyibo M. Prevalence of *Candida species* in Nigerian children with diarrhea. J Diarrhoeal Dis Res 12:133, 1994.
1054. Klingspor L, Stitzing G, Johansen K, et al. Infantile diarrhea and malnutrition associated with *Candida* in a developing community. Mycoses 36:19, 1993.
1055. Ponnuvel K, Rajkumar R, Menon T, Sankaranarayanan V. Role of *Candida* in indirect pathogenesis of antibiotic associated diarrhea in infants. Mycopathologia 135:145, 1996.
1056. Omoike IU, Abiodun PO. Upper small intestine microflora in diarrhea and malnutrition in Nigerian children. J Pediatr Gastroenterol Nutr 9:314, 1989.
1057. Kane JG, Chretien JH, Garagusi VF. Diarrhea caused by *Candida*. Lancet 1:335, 1976.
1058. VonGerloczy F, Schmidt K, Scholz M. Beiträge zur Frage der Moniliasis in Säuglingsalter. Ann Pediatr (Paris) 187:119, 1956.
1059. Hill HR, Mitchell TG, Matsen JM, et al. Recovery from disseminated candidiasis in a premature neonate. Pediatrics 53:748, 1974.
1060. Faix RG. Systemic *Candida* infections in infants in intensive care nurseries: high incidence of central nervous system involvement. J Pediatr 105:616, 1984.
1061. Baley JE, Kliegman RM, Fanaroff AA. Disseminated fungal infections in very low birth weight infants: clinical manifestations and epidemiology. Pediatrics 73:144, 1984.
1062. Struelens MJ, Bennish ML, Mondal G, et al. Bacteremia during diarrhea: incidence, etiology, risk factors, and outcome. Am J Epidemiol 133:451, 1991.
1063. Rodriguez-García R, Rodriguez-Guzman LM, Sanchez-Maldonado MI, et al. Prevalence and risk factors associated with intestinal parasitoses in pregnant women and their relation to the infant's birth weight. Ginecol Obstet Mex 70:338, 2002.
1064. Guven A. Amebiasis in the newborn. Indian J Pediatr 70:437, 2003.
1065. Axton JHM. Amoebic proctocolitis and liver abscess in a neonate. S Afr Med J 46:258, 1972.
1066. Botman T, Rusy PJ. Amoebic appendicitis in a newborn infant. Trop Geogr Med 15:221, 1963.
1067. Hsiung CC. Amebiasis of the newborn: report of three cases. Chin J Pathol 4:14, 1958.
1068. Dykes AC, Ruebush TK, Gorelkin L, et al. Extraintestinal amebiasis in infancy: report of three patients and epidemiologic investigations of their families. Pediatrics 65:799, 1980.
1069. Gomez NA, Cozzarelli R, Alvarez LR, et al. Amebic liver abscess in newborn. Report of a case. Acta Gastroenterol Latinoam 29:115, 1999.
1070. Rennert W, Ray C. Fuliminant amebic colitis in a ten-day-old infant. Arch Pediatr 4:92, 1997.
1071. Kotcher E, Mata LJ, Esquivel R, et al. Acquisition of intestinal parasites in newborn human infants. Fed Proc 24:442, 1965 (abstract).
1072. Ravdin JI. Amebiasis. Clin Infect Dis 20:1453, 1995.
1073. Mirelman D, Nuchamowitz Y, Stolarsky T. Comparison of use of enzyme-linked immunosorbent assay–based kits and PCR amplification of rRNA genes for simultaneous detection of *Entamoeba histolytica* and *E. dispar*. J Clin Microbiol 35:2405, 1997.
1074. Haque R, Ali IKM, Petri WA Jr. Comparison of PCR, isoenzyme analysis, and antigen detection for diagnosis of *Entamoeba histolytica* infection. J Clin Microbiol 36:449, 1998.
1075. Black RE, Dykes AC, Sinclair SP, et al. Giardiasis in day care centers. Evidence of person-to-person transmission. Pediatrics 60:486, 1977.
1076. Keystone JS, Krajden S, Warren MR. Person-to-person transmission of *G. lamblia* in day care nurseries. Can Med Assoc J 119:241, 1978.

1077. Pickering LK, Evans DG, DuPont HL, et al. Diarrhea caused by *Shigella*, rotavirus, and *Giardia* in day care centers: prospective study. J Pediatr 99:51, 1981.
1078. Pickering LK, Woodward WE, DuPont HL, et al. Occurrence of *G. lamblia* in children in day care centers. J Pediatr 104:522, 1984.
1079. Adam RD. The biology of *Giardia spp*. Microbiol Rev 55:706, 1991.
1080. Pickering LK, Engelkirk PG. *Giardia lamblia*. Pediatr Clin North Am 35:565, 1988.
1081. Miotti PG, Gilman RH, Santosham M, et al. Age-related rate of seropositivity and antibody to *Giardia lamblia* in four diverse populations. J Clin Microbiol 24:972, 1986.
1082. Islam A, Stoll BJ, Ljungstrom I, et al. *Giardia lamblia* infections in a cohort of Bangladeshi mothers and infants followed for one year. J Pediatr 103:996, 1983.
1083. Gendrel D, Richard-Lenoble D, Kombila M, et al. Giardiasis and breastfeeding in urban Africa. Pediatr Infect Dis J 8:58, 1989.
1084. Stevens DP, Frank DM. Local immunity in murine giardiasis: is milk protective at the expense of maternal gut? Trans Assoc Am Physicians 91:268, 1978.
1085. Andrews JS Jr, Hewlett EL. Protection against infection with *Giardia muris* by milk containing antibody to *Giardia*. J Infect Dis 143:242, 1981.
1086. Rohrer L, Winterhalter KH, Eckert J, et al. Killing of *G. lamblia* by human milk mediated by unsaturated fatty acids. Antimicrob Agents Chemother 30:254, 1986.
1087. Current WL, Garcia LS. Cryptosporidiosis. Clin Microbiol Rev 4:325, 1991.
1088. Heyworth MF. Immunology of *Giardia* and *Cryptosporidium* infections. J Infect Dis 166:465, 1992.
1089. Wolfson IS, Richter JM, Waldron MA, et al. Cryptosporidiosis in immunocompetent patients. N Engl J Med 312:1278, 1985.
1090. Tzipori S. Cryptosporidiosis in animals and humans. Microbiol Rev 47:84, 1983.
1091. Stehr-Green JK, McCaig L, Remsen HM, et al. Shedding of oocysts in immunocompetent individuals infected with *Cryptosporidium*. Am J Trop Med Hyg 36:338, 1987.
1092. Soave R, Ma P. Cryptosporidiosis travelers' diarrhea in two families. Arch Intern Med 145:70, 1985.
1093. Collier AC, Miller RA, Meyers JD. Cryptosporidiosis after marrow transplantation, person-to-person transmission and treatment with spiramycin. Ann Intern Med 101:205, 1984.
1094. Navin TR. Cryptosporidiosis in humans: review of recent epidemiologic studies. Eur J Epidemiol 1:77, 1985.
1095. Alpert G, Bell LM, Kirkpatrick CE, et al. Outbreak of cryptosporidiosis in a day care center. Pediatrics 77:152, 1986.
1096. Taylor JP, Perdue JN, Dingley D, et al. Cryptosporidiosis outbreak in a day care center. Am J Dis Child 139:1023, 1986.
1097. Hoxie NJ, Davis JP, Vergeront JM, et al. Cryptosporidiosis-associated mortality following a massive waterborne outbreak in Milwaukee, Wisconsin. Am J Public Health 87:2032, 1997.
1098. Jokipii L, Pohiola S, Jokipii AM. *Cryptosporidium*: a frequent finding in patients with gastrointestinal symptoms. Lancet 2:358, 1983.
1099. Current WL, Reese NC, Ernst JV, et al. Human cryptosporidiosis in immunocompetent and immunodeficient persons: studies of an outbreak and experimental transmission. N Engl J Med 308:1252, 1983.
1100. Enriquez FJ, Avila CR, Santos JI, et al. *Cryptosporidium* infections in Mexican children: clinical, nutritional, enteropathogenic, and diagnostic evaluations. Am J Trop Med Hyg 56:254, 1997.
1101. Mata L, Bolanos H, Pizarro D, et al. Cryptosporidiosis in children from some highland Costa Rican rural and urban areas. Am J Trop Med Hyg 33:24, 1984.
1102. Jokipii L, Jokipii AMM. Timing of symptoms and oocyst excretion in human cryptosporidiosis. N Engl J Med 313:1643, 1986.
1103. Sallon S, Deckelbaum RI, Schmid II, et al. *Cryptosporidium*, malnutrition and chronic diarrhea in children. Am J Dis Child 142:312, 1988.
1104. Garcia LS, Shimizu RY. Evaluation of nine immunoassay kits (enzyme immunoassay and direct fluorescence) for detection of *Giardia lamblia* and *Cryptosporidium parvum* in human fecal specimens. J Clin Microbiol 35:1526, 1997.
1105. MacPherson DW, McQueen R. Cryptosporidiosis: multiattribute evaluation of six diagnostic methods. J Clin Microbiol 31:198, 1993.
1106. Rossignol FJ, Ayoub A, Ayers MS. Treatment of diarrhea caused by *Cryptosporidium parvum*: a prospective of randomized, double-blind, placebo-controlled study of nitazoxanide. J Infect Dis 184:103, 2001.
1107. Agnew DG, Lima AAM, Newman RD, et al. Cryptosporidiosis in northeastern Brazilian children: association with increased diarrhea morbidity. J Infect Dis 177:754, 1998.
1108. Matson DO, O'Ryan ML, Jiang X, Mitchell DK. Rotavirus, enteric adenoviruses, caliciviruses, astroviruses, and other viruses causing gastroenteritis. *In* Spector S, Hodinka RL, Young SA (eds). Clinical Virology Manual, 3rd ed. Washington, DC, ASM Press, 2000, p 270.
1109. Kapikian AZ, Chanock RM. Rotaviruses. *In* Fields BN, Knipe DM, Howley PM, et al (eds). Fields Virology, 3rd ed. Philadelphia, Lippincott-Raven Press, 1996, p 1657.
1110. Estes MK. Rotaviruses and their replication. *In* Fields BN, Knipe DM, Howley PM, et al (eds). Fields Virology, 3rd ed. Philadelphia, Lippincott-Raven Press, 1996, p 1625.
1111. Wilhelmi I, Roman E, Sanchez-Fauquier A. Viruses causing gastroenteritis. Clin Microbiol Infect 9:247, 2003.
1112. Bridger JC. Non-group A rotavirus. *In* Farthing M (ed). Viruses in the Gut. Welwyn Garden City, UK, Smith Kline & French, 1988, p 79.
1113. Desselberger U. Molecular epidemiology of rotavirus. *In* Farthing M (ed). Viruses in the Gut. Welwyn Garden City, UK, Smith Kline & French, 1988, p 55.
1114. Hoshino Y, Saif LJ, Sereno MM. Infection immunity of piglets to either VP3 or VP7 outer capsid protein confers resistance to challenge with a virulent rotavirus bearing the corresponding antigen. J Virol 62:74, 1988.
1115. Offit PA, Clark HF, Blavat G. Reassortant rotavirus containing structural proteins VP3 and VP7 from different parents are protective against each parental strain. J Virol 57:376, 1986
1116. Zhou Y, Li L, Okitsu S, et al. Distribution of human rotaviruses, especially G9 strains, in Japan from 1996 to 2000. Microbiol Immunol 47:591, 2003.
1117. O'Ryan ML, Matson DO, Estes MK, Pickering LK. Molecular epidemiology of rotavirus in children attending day care centers in Houston. J Infect Dis 162:810, 1990.
1118. Ramachandran M, Das B, Vij A, et al. Unusual diversity of human rotavirus G and P genotypes in India. J Clin Microbiol 34:436, 1996.
1119. Unicomb L, Podder G, Gentsch J, et al. Evidence of high-frequency genomic reassortment of group A rotavirus strains in Bangladesh: emergence of type G9 in 1995. J Clin Microbiol 37:1885, 1999.
1120. Santos N, Lima R, Pereira C, Gouvea V. Detection of rotavirus types G8 and G10 among Brazilian children with diarrhea. J Clin Microbiol 36:2727, 1998.
1121. Palombo E, Bishop R. Genetic an antigenetic characterization of a serotype G6 human rotavirus isolated in Melbourne, Australia. J Med Virol 47:348, 1995.
1122. Pongsuwanna Y, Guntapong R, Chiwakul M, et al. Detection of a human rotavirus with G12 and P[9] specificity in Thailand. J Clin Microbiol 40:1390, 2002.
1123. Gentsch JR, Woods PA, Ramachandran M, et al. Review of G and P typing results from a global collection of rotavirus strains: implications for vaccine development. J Infect Dis 174(Suppl 1):S30, 1996.
1124. Kilgore P, Unicomb L, Gentsch R, et al. Neonatal rotavirus infection in Bangladesh strain characterization and risk factors for nosocomial infection. Pediatr Infect Dis J 15:672, 1996.
1125. Tam JS, Zeng BJ, Lo SK, et al. Distinct population of rotaviruses circulating among neonates and older infants. J Clin Microbiol 28:1033, 1990.
1126. Jain V, Prashar UD, Glass RI, Bhan MK. Epidemiology of rotavirus in India. Indian J Pediatr 68:855, 2001.
1127. Mascarenhas JD, Linhares AC, Gabbay YB, Leite JP. Detection and characterization of rotavirus G and P types from children participating in a rotavirus vaccine trial in Belen, Brazil. Mem Inst Oswald Cruz 97:113, 2002.
1128. Widdowson MA, van Doornum GJ, van der Poel WH, et al. An outbreak of diarrhea in a neonatal medium care unit caused by a novel strain of rotavirus: investigation using both epidemiologival and microbiological methods. Infect Control Hosp Epidemiol 23:665, 2002.
1129. Steele D, Reynecke E, de Beer M, et al. Characterization of rotavirus infection in a hospital neonatal unit in Pretoria, South Africa. J Trop Pediatr 48:161, 2002.
1130. Linhares AC, Mascarenhas JD, Gusmao RH, et al. Neonatal rotavirus infection in Belem, northern Brazil: nosocomial transmission of a P[6] G2 strain. J Med Virol 67:418, 2002.
1131. Cunliffe NA, Rogerson S, Dove W, et al. Detection and characterization of rotaviruses in hospitalized neonates in Blantyre, Malawi. J Clin Microbiol 40:1534, 2002.

1132. Davidson GP, Bishop RF, Townley RR, Holmes IH. Importance of a new virus in acute sporadic enteritis in children. Lancet 1:242, 1975.
1133. Bishop RF, Davidson GP, Holmes IH, et al. Virus particles in epithelial cells of duodenal mucosa from children with acute nonbacterial gastroenteritis. Lancet 2:1281, 1973.
1134. Holmes IH, Ruck BJ, Bishop RF, et al. Infantile enteritis viruses: morphogenesis and morphology. J Virol 16:937, 1975.
1135. Suzuki H, Konno T. Reovirus-like particles in jejunal mucosa of a Japanese infant with acute infectious nonbacterial gastroenteritis. Tohoku J Exp Med 115:199, 1975.
1136. Graham DY, Estes MK. Comparison of methods for immunocytochemical detection of rotavirus infections. Infect Immun 26:686, 1979.
1137. Holmes IH, Rodger SM, Schnagl RD, et al. Is lactase the receptor and uncoating enzyme for infantile enteritis (rota) viruses? Lancet 1:1387, 1976.
1138. Shepherd RW, Butler DG, Cutz E, et al. The mucosal lesion in viral enteritis. Extent and dynamics of the epithelial response to virus invasion in transmissible gastroenteritis of piglets. Gastroenterology 76:770, 1979.
1139. Cameron DJS, Bishop RF, Veenstra A, et al. Noncultivable viruses and neonatal diarrhea. Fifteen-month survey in a newborn special care nursery. J Clin Microbiol 8:93, 1978.
1140. Lebenthal E. Lactose malabsorption and milk consumption in infants and children. Am J Dis Child 133:21, 1979.
1141. Philipps AD. Mechanisms of mucosal injury: human studies. *In* Farthing M (ed). Viruses in the Gut. Welwyn Garden City, UK, Smith Kline & French, 1988, p 30.
1142. Shepherd RW, Gall DG, Butler DG, et al. Determinants of diarrhea in viral enteritis. The role of ion transport and epithelial changes in the ileum in transmissible gastroenteritis in piglets. Gastroenterology 76:20, 1979.
1143. Hoshino Y, Saif LJ, Kang SY, et al. Identification of group A rotavirus genes associated with virulence of a porcine rotavirus and host range restriction of a human rotavirus in the gnotobiotic piglet model. Virology 209:274, 1995.
1144. Saulsbury FT, Winklestein JA, Yolken RH. Chronic rotavirus infection in immunodeficiency. J Pediatr 97:61, 1980.
1145. Stephen J. Functional abnormalities in the intestine. *In* Farthing M (ed). Viruses in the Gut. Welwyn Garden City, UK, Smith Kline & French, 1988, p 41.
1146. Lundgren O, Peregrin AT, Persson K, et al. Role of the enteric nervous system in the fluid and electrolyte secretion of rotavirus diarrhea. Science 287:491, 2000.
1147. Kerzner B, Kelly MH, Gall DG, et al. Transmissible gastroenteritis: sodium transport and the intestinal epithelium during the course of viral gastroenteritis. Gastroenterology 72:457, 1977.
1148. Gall DG, Chapman D, Kelly M, et al. Na^+ transport in jejunal crypt cells. Gastroenterology 72:452, 1977.
1149. Ball JM, Tian P, Zeng CQ, et al. Age-dependent diarrhea induced by a rotaviral nonstructural glycoprotein. Science 272:101, 1996.
1150. Ward RL, Mason B, Bernstein D, et al. Attenuation of a human rotavirus vaccine candidate did not correlate with mutations in the NSP4 protein gene. J Virol 71:6267, 1997.
1151. Zhang M, Zeng CQ, Dong Y, et al. Mutations in nonstructural glycoprotein NSP4 are associated with altered virus virulence. J Virol 72:3666, 1998.
1152. Bishop RF, Barnes GL, Cipriani E, et al. Clinical immunity after neonatal rotavirus infection. A prospective longitudinal study in young children. N Engl J Med 309:72, 1983.
1153. Bhan MK, Lew JF, Sazawal S, et al. Protection conferred by neonatal rotavirus infection against subsequent rotavirus diarrhea. J Infect Dis 168:282, 1993.
1154. Chiba S, Nakata S, Urasawa T, et al. Protective effect of naturally acquired homotypic and heterotypic rotavirus antibodies. Lancet 1:417, 1986.
1155. Greene KY, Kapikian AZ. Identification of VP7 epitopes associated with protection against human rotavirus illness or shedding in volunteers. J Virol 66:548, 1992.
1156. Hjelt K, Grauballe PC, Paerregaard A, et al. Protective effect of preexisting rotavirus-specific immunoglobulin A against naturally acquired rotavirus infection in children. J Med Virol 21:39, 1987.
1157. Matson DO, O'Ryan ML, Estes MK, et al. Characterization of serum antibody responses to natural rotavirus infections in children by VP7-specific epitope-blocking assays. J Clin Microbiol 30:1056, 1992.
1158. Ward RL, Knowlton DR, Schiff GM, et al. Relative concentrations of serum neutralizing antibody to VP3 and VP7 protein in adults infected with human rotavirus. J Virol 62:1543, 1988.
1159. Clemens JD, Ward RL, Rao MR, et al. Seroepidemiologic evaluation of antibodies to rotavirus as correlates of the risk of clinically significant rotavirus diarrhea in rural Bangladesh. J Infect Dis 165:161, 1992.
1160. Matson DO, O'Ryan M, Herrera I, et al. Fecal antibody responses to symptomatic and asymptomatic rotavirus infections. J Infect Dis 167:557, 1993.
1161. O'Ryan M, Matson DO, Estes MK, Pickering LK. Anti-rotavirus G type-specific and isotype-specific antibodies in children with natural rotavirus infections. J Infect Dis 169:504, 1994.
1162. Zheng BJ, Lo SK, Tam J Jr, et al. Prospective study of community-acquired rotavirus infection. J Clin Microbiol 27:2083, 1989.
1163. Ward RL, Clemens JD, Knowlton DR, et al. Evidence that protection against rotavirus diarrhea after natural infection is not dependent on serotype-specific neutralizing antibody. J Infect Dis 166:1251, 1992.
1164. Totterdell BM, Chrystie IL, Banatvala JE. Cord blood and breast milk antibodies in neonatal rotavirus infection. BMJ 1:828, 1980.
1165. Yolken RH, Wyatt RG, Zissis G, et al. Epidemiology of human rotavirus types 1 and 2 as studied by enzyme-linked immunosorbent assay. N Engl J Med 299:1156, 1978.
1166. McLean B, Holmes IH. Transfer of anti-rotaviral antibodies from mothers to their infants. J Clin Microbiol 12:320, 1980.
1167. McLean BS, Holmes IH. Effects of antibodies, trypsin, and trypsin inhibitors on susceptibility of neonates to rotavirus infection. J Clin Microbiol 13:22, 1981.
1168. Brhssow H, Sidoti J, Lerner L, et al. Antibodies to seven rotavirus serotypes in cord sera, maternal sera, and colostrum of German women. J Clin Microbiol 29:2856, 1991.
1169. Brhssow H, Benitez O, Uribe F, et al. Rotavirus-inhibitory activity in serial milk samples from Mexican women and rotavirus infections in their children during their first year of life. J Clin Microbiol 31:593, 1993.
1170. Yolken RH, Wyatt RG, Mata L, et al. Secretory antibody directed against rotavirus in human milk-measurement by means of enzyme-linked immunosorbent assay. J Pediatr 93:916, 1978.
1171. Yolken RH, Peterson JA, Vonderfecht SL, et al. Human milk mucin inhibits rotavirus replication and prevents experimental gastroenteritis. J Clin Invest 90:1984, 1992.
1172. Bishop RF, Barnes GL, Cipriani E, et al. Clinical immunity after neonatal rotavirus infection. A prospective longitudinal study in young children. N Engl J Med 309:72, 1983.
1173. Santosham M, et al. Neonatal rotavirus infection. Lancet 1:1070, 1982.
1174. Madeley CR, Cosgrove BP, Bell EJ. Stool viruses in babies in Glasgow. 2. Investigation of normal newborns in hospital. J Hyg 81:285, 1978.
1175. Glasgow JFT, McClure BG, Connolly J, et al. Nosocomial rotavirus gastroenteritis in a neonatal nursery. Ulster Med J 47:50, 1978.
1176. Cameron DJS, Bishop RF, Davidson G, et al. New virus associated with diarrhoea in neonates. Med J Aust 1:85, 1976.
1177. Bryden AS, Thouless ME, Hall CJ, et al. Rotavirus infections in a special-care baby unit. J Infect 4:43, 1982.
1178. Grillner L, Broberger U, Chrystie I, et al. Rotavirus infections in newborns: an epidemiological and clinical study. Scand J Infect Dis 17:349, 1985.
1179. Tufvesson B, Polberger L, Svanberg L, et al. A prospective study of rotavirus infections in neonatal and maternity wards. Acta Paediatr Scand 75:211, 1986.
1180. Hoshino Y, Wyatt RG, Flores J, et al. Serotypic characterization of rotaviruses derived from asymptomatic human neonatal infections. J Clin Microbiol 21:425, 1985.
1181. Crewe E, Murphy AM. Further studies on neonatal rotavirus infection. Med J Aust 1:61, 1980.
1182. Perez-Schael I, Daoud G, White L, et al. Rotavirus shedding by newborn children. J Med Virol 14:127, 1984.
1183. Vial PA, Kotloff KL, Losonsky GA. Molecular epidemiology of rotavirus infection in a room for convalescing newborns. J Infect Dis 157:668, 1988.
1184. Haffejee IE. Neonatal rotavirus infections. Rev Infect Dis 13:957, 1991.
1185. Rodriguez WJ, Kim HW, Brandt CD, et al. Rotavirus: a cause of nosocomial infection in a nursery. J Pediatr 101:274, 1982.
1186. Jesudoss ES, John TJ, Maiya PP, et al. Prevalence of rotavirus infection in neonates. Indian J Med Res 70:863, 1979.
1187. Bishop RF, Cameron DJS, Veenstra AA, et al. Diarrhea and rotavirus infection associated with differing regimens for postnatal care of newborn babies. J Clin Microbiol 9:525, 1979.

1188. Pickering LK, Bartlett AV, Reves RR, et al. Asymptomatic rotavirus before and after rotavirus diarrhea in children in day care centers. J Pediatr 112:361, 1988.
1189. Vesikari T, Sarkkinen HK, Maki M. Quantitative aspects of rotavirus excretion in childhood diarrhoea. Acta Paediatr Scand 70:717, 1981.
1190. Konno T, Suzuki H, Katsushima N, et al. Influence of temperature and relative humidity on human rotavirus infection in Japan. J Infect Dis 147:125, 1983.
1191. Bartlett AV III, Reeves RR, Pickering LK. Rotavirus in infant-toddler day care centers: epidemiology relevant to disease control strategies. J Pediatr 113:435, 1988.
1192. Matson DO, Estes MK, Burns JW, et al. Serotype variation of human group A rotaviruses in two regions of the United States. J Infect Dis 162:605, 1990.
1193. Ryan MJ, Ramsay M, Brown D, et al. Hospital admissions attributable to rotavirus infection in England. J Infect Dis 174(Suppl 1):S12, 1996.
1194. Glass R, Kilgore PE, Holmans RC, et al. The epidemiology of rotavirus diarrhea in the United States: surveillance and estimates of disease burden. J Infect Dis 74(Suppl 1):S5, 1996.
1195. O'Ryan M, Pérez-Schael I, Mamani N, et al. Rotavirus-associated medical visits and hospitalizations in South America: a prospective study at three large sentinel hospitals. Pediatr Infect Dis J 20:685, 2001.
1196. Duffy LC, Riepenhoff-Talty M, Byers TE, et al. Modulation of rotavirus enteritis during breast-feeding. Am J Dis Child 140:1164, 1986.
1197. van Renterghem L, Borre P, Tilleman J. Rotavirus and other viruses in the stool of premature babies. J Med Virol 5:137, 1980.
1198. Murphy AM, Albrey MB, Crewe EB. Rotavirus infections in neonates. Lancet 2:1149, 1977.
1199. Soenarto Y, Sebodo T, Ridho R, et al. Acute diarrhea and rotavirus infection in newborn babies and children in Yogyakarta, Indonesia from June 1978 to June 1979. J Clin Microbiol 14:123, 1981.
1200. Appleton H, Buckley M, Robertson MH, et al. A search for faecal viruses in newborn and other infants. J Hyg 81:279, 1978.
1201. Schnagl RD, Morey F, Holmes IH. Rotavirus and coronavirus-like particles in aboriginal and non-aboriginal neonates in Kalgoorlie and Alice Springs. Med J Aust 2:178, 1979.
1202. Grillner L, Broberger U, Chrystie I, et al. Rotavirus infections in newborns: an epidemiological and clinical study. Scand J Infect Dis 17:349, 1985.
1203. Dearlove J, Latham P, Dearlove B, et al. Clinical range of neonatal rotavirus gastroenteritis. BMJ 286:1473, 1983.
1204. Parashar UD, Holman RC, Bresee JS, et al. Epidemiology of diarrheal disease among children enrolled in four West Coast health maintenance organizations. Pediatr Infect Dis J 17:605, 1998.
1205. Leece JC, King MW, Dorsey WE. Rearing regimen producing piglet diarrhea (rotavirus) and its relevance to acute infantile diarrhea. Science 199:776, 1978.
1206. Santosham M, Yolken RH, Quiroz E, et al. Detection of rotavirus in respiratory secretions of children with pneumonia. J Pediatr 103:583, 1983.
1207. Prince DS, Astry C, Vonderfecht S, et al. Aerosol transmission of experimental rotavirus infection. Pediatr Infect Dis J 5:218, 1986.
1208. Steele AD, Alexander JJ. Molecular epidemiology of rotavirus in black infants in South Africa. J Clin Microbiol 25:2384, 1987.
1209. Rodriguez WJ, Kim HW, Brandt CD, et al. Use of electrophoresis of RNA from human rotavirus to establish the identity of stains involved in outbreaks in a tertiary care nursery. J Infect Dis 148:34, 1983.
1210. Srivinasan G, Azarcon E, Muldoon, et al. Rotavirus infection in a normal nursery: epidemic and surveillance. Infect Control 5:478, 1984.
1211. Gerna G, Forster J, Parea M, et al. Nosocomial outbreak of neonatal gastroenteritis caused by a new serotype 4, subtype 4B human rotavirus. J Med Virol 31:175, 1990.
1212. Tallet S, MacKenzie C, Middleton P, et al. Clinical, laboratory, and epidemiologic features of a viral gastroenteritis in infants and children. Pediatrics 60:217, 1977.
1213. Hieber JP, Shelton S, Nelson JD, et al. Comparison of human rotavirus disease in tropical and temperate settings. Am J Dis Child 132:853, 1978.
1214. Mutanda LN. Epidemiology of acute gastroenteritis in early childhood in Kenya. VI. Some clinical and laboratory characteristics relative to the aetiological agents. East Afr Med J 57:599, 1980.
1215. Whyte RK, Homes R, Pennock CA. Faecal excretion of oligosaccharides and other carbohydrates in normal neonates. Arch Dis Child 53:913, 1978.
1216. Hyams JS, Krause PJ, Gleason PA. Lactose malabsorption following rotavirus infection in young children. J Pediatr 99:916, 1981.
1217. Prashar UD, Hummelman EG, Breese J, et al. Global illness and deaths caused by rotavirus disease in children. Emerg Infect Dis 9:565, 2003.
1218. Dani C, Trevisanuto D, Cantarutti F, Zanardo V. A case of neonatal necrotizing enterocolitis due to rotavirus. Pediatr Med Chir 16:185, 1994.
1219. Goma Brufau AR, Vega Romero M, Martinez Ubieto P, et al. Epidemic outbreak of necrotizing enterocolitis coincident with an epidemic of neonatal rotavirus gastroenteritis. An Esp Pediatr 29:307, 1988.
1220. Riedel F, Kroener T, Stein K, et al. Rotavirus infection and bradycardia-apnoea-episodes in the neonate. Eur J Pediatr 155:36, 1996.
1221. Konno T, Suzuki H, Kutsuzawa T, et al. Human rotavirus infection in infants and young children with intussusception. J Med Virol 2:265, 1978.
1222. Mulcahy DL, Kamath KR, de Silva LM, et al. A two-part study of the aetiological role of rotavirus in intussusception. J Med Virol 9:51, 1982.
1223. Nicolas JC, Ingrand D, Fortier B, Bricout F. A one-year virological survey of acute intussusception in childhood. J Med Virol 9:267, 1982.
1224. Murphy TV, Gargiullo PM, Massoudi MS, et al. Intussusception among infants given an oral rotavirus vaccine. N Engl J Med 22:564, 2001.
1225. Dennehy P, Hartin M, Nelson S, Reising S. Evaluation of the inmunocardstat. Rotavirus assay for detection of group A rotavirus in fecal specimens. J Clin Microbiol 37:1977, 1999.
1226. Gilchrist MJR, Bretl TS, Moultney K, et al. Comparison of seven kits for detection of rotavirus in fecal specimens with a sensitive, specific enzyme immunoassay. Diagn Microbiol Infect Dis 8:221, 1987.
1227. Knisley CV, Bednarz-Prashad A, Pickering LK. Detection of rotavirus in stool specimens with monoclonal and polyclonal antibody-based assay systems. J Clin Microbiol 23:897, 1986.
1228. Thomas EE, Puterman ML, Kawano E, et al. Evaluation of seven immunoassays for detection of rotavirus in pediatric stool samples. J Clin Microbiol 26:1189, 1988.
1229. Miotti PG, Eiden J, Yolken RH. Comparative efficacy of commercial immunoassays for the diagnosis of rotavirus gastroenteritis during the course of infection. J Clin Microbiol 22:693, 1985.
1230. Brandt CD, Kim HW, Rodriguez WJ, et al. Comparison of direct electron microscopy, immune electron microscopy, and rotavirus enzyme-linked immunosorbent assay for detection of gastroenteritis viruses in children. J Clin Microbiol 13:976, 1981.
1231. Yolken RH, Kim HW, Clem T, et al. Enzyme-linked immunosorbent assay (ELISA) for detection of human reovirus-like agent of infantile gastroenteritis. Lancet 2:263, 1977.
1232. Fischer TK, Steinsland H, Valentiner-Branth P. Rotavirus particles can survive storage in ambient tropical temperatures for more than 2 months. J Clin Microbiol 40:4763, 2002.
1233. Viera de Torres B, Mazzali de Ilja R, Esparza J. Epidemiological aspects of rotavirus infection in hospitalized Venezuelan children with gastroenteritis. Am J Trop Med Hyg 27:567, 1978.
1234. Provisional Committee on Quality Improvement, Subcommittee on Acute Gastroenteritis. Practice parameter: the management of acute gastroenteritis in young children. Pediatrics 97:424, 1996.
1235. Sack DA, Eusof A, Merson MH, et al. Oral hydration in rotavirus diarrhoea: a double-blind comparison of sucrose with glucose electrolyte solution. Lancet 2:280, 1978.
1236. Black RE, Merson MH, Taylor PR, et al. Glucose vs. sucrose in oral rehydration solutions for infants and young children with rotavirus-associated diarrhea. Pediatrics 67:79, 1981.
1237. Saulsbury FT, Winklestein JA, Yolken RH. Chronic rotavirus infection in immunodeficiency. J Pediatr 97:61, 1980.
1238. Ebina T, Ohta M, Kanamura Y, et al. Passive immunizations of suckling mice and infants with bovine colostrum containing antibodies to human rotavirus. J Med Virol 38:117, 1992.
1239. Guarino A, Guandalini S, Albano F, et al. Enteral immunoglobulins for treatment of protracted rotaviral diarrhea. Pediatr Infect Dis J 10:612, 1991.
1240. Brunser O, Espinoza J, Figueroa G, et al. Field trial of an infant formula containing anti-rotavirus and anti-*Escherichia coli* milk antibodies from hyperimmunized cows. J Pediatr Gastroenterol Nutr 15:63, 1992.
1241. Rosenfeldt V, Fleischer K, Jakobsen M, et al. Effect of probiotic *Lactobacillus* strains in young children hospitalized with acute diarrhea. Pediatr Infect Dis J 21:411, 2002.
1242. Mohan P, Haque K. Oral immunoglobulin for the treatment of rotavirus infection in low birth weight infants. Cochrane Database Syst Rev 3:CD003742, 2003.

1243. Birch CJ, Lewis FA, Kennett ML, et al. A study of the prevalence of rotavirus infection in children with gastroenteritis admitted to an infectious disease hospital. J Med Virol 1:69, 1977.
1244. Kombo LA, Gerber MA, Pickering LK, et al. Intussusception, infection, and immunization: summary of a workshop on rotavirus. Pediatrics 108:E37, 2001.
1245. Wilson W, Scott RB, Pinto A, Robertson MA. Intractable diarrhea in a newborn infant: microvillous inclusion disease. Can J Gastroenterol 15:61, 2001.
1246. Stockdale EM, Miller CA. Persistent diarrhea as the predominant symptom of Hirschsprung's disease (congenital dilatation of colon). Pediatrics 19:91, 1957.
1247. Wilmore DW. Factors correlating with a successful outcome following extensive intestinal resection in newborn infants. J Pediatr 80:88, 1972.
1248. Fried D, Gotlieb A, Zaidel L. Intractable diarrhea of infancy due to lymphangiectasis. Am J Dis Child 127:416, 1974.
1249. Lebenthal E. Small intestinal disaccharidase deficiency. Pediatr Clin North Am 22:757, 1975.
1250. Ament ME, Perera DR, Esther LJ. Sucrase-isomaltose deficiency—a frequently misdiagnosed disease. J Pediatr 83:721, 1973.
1251. Marks JF, Norton JB, Fordtran JS. Glucose-galactose malabsorption. J Pediatr 69:225, 1969.
1252. Burke V, Anderson CM. Sugar intolerance as a cause of protracted diarrhea following surgery of the gastrointestinal tract in neonates. Aust Paediatr J 2:219, 1966.
1253. Bishop RF, Davidson GP, Holmes IH, et al. Virus particles in epithelial cells of duodenal mucosa from children with acute non-bacterial gastroenteritis. Lancet 2:1281, 1973.
1254. Coello-Ramirez P, Lifshitz F, Zuniga V. Enteric microflora and carbohydrate intolerance in infants with diarrhea. Pediatrics 49:233, 1972.
1255. Akesode F, Lifshitz F, Hoffman KM. Transient monosaccharide intolerance in a newborn infant. Pediatrics 51:891, 1973.
1256. Iyngkaran N, Davis K, Robinson MJ, et al. Cow's milk protein-sensitive enteropathy. An important contributing cause of secondary sugar intolerance in young infants with acute infective enteritis. Arch Dis Child 54:39, 1979.
1257. Ament ME. Malabsorption syndromes in infancy and childhood. I, II. J Pediatr 81:685, 867, 1972.
1258. Whyte RK, Homer R, Pennock CA. Faecal excretion of oligosaccharides and other carbohydrates in normal neonates. Arch Dis Child 53:913, 1978.
1259. Schwachman H, Redmond A, Khaw KT. Studies in cystic fibrosis. Report of 130 patients diagnosed under 3 months of age over a 20 year period. Pediatrics 46:335, 1970.
1260. Aggett PJ, Cavanagh NPC, Matthew DJ, et al. Schwachman's syndrome. A review of 21 cases. Arch Dis Child 55:331, 1980.
1261. Lilibridge CB, Townes PL. Physiologic deficiency of pancreatic amylase in infancy: a factor in iatrogenic diarrhea. J Pediatr 82:279, 1973.
1262. Lebenthal E, Antonowicz I, Schwachman H. Enterokinase and trypsin activities in pancreatic insufficiency and diseases of the small intestine. Gastroenterology 70:508, 1979.
1263. Powell GK, Jones LA, Richardson J. A new syndrome of bile acid deficiency—a possible synthetic defect. J Pediatr 83:758, 1973.
1264. Lloyd JK. Disorders of the serum lipoproteins. I. Lipoprotein deficiency states. Arch Dis Child 43:393, 1968.
1265. Cash R, Berger CK. Acrodermatitis enteropathica: defective metabolism of unsaturated fatty acids. J Pediatr 74:717, 1969.
1266. Garretts M, Molokhia M. Acrodermatitis enteropathica without hypozincemia. J Pediatr 91:492, 1977.
1267. McReynolds EW, Roy S III, Etteldorf JN. Congenital chloride diarrhea. Am J Dis Child 127:566, 1974.
1268. Minford AMB, Barr DGD. Prostaglandin synthetase inhibitor in an infant with congenital chloride diarrhea. Arch Dis Child 55:70, 1980.
1269. Woodard JC, Webster PD, Carr AA. Primary hypomagnesemia with secondary hypocalcemia, diarrhea and insensitivity to parathyroid hormone. Am J Dig Dis 17:612, 1972.
1270. Iversen T. Congenital adrenal hyperplasia with disturbed electrolyte regulation. Pediatrics 16:875, 1955.
1271. Iida Y, Nose O, Kai H, et al. Watery diarrhoea with a vasoactive intestinal peptide–producing ganglioneuroblastoma. Arch Dis Child 55:929, 1980.
1272. Ghishan FK, Soper RT, Nassif EG, et al. Chronic diarrhea of infancy: nonbeta islet cell hyperplasia. Pediatrics 64:46, 1979.
1273. Storm W, Wendel U, Sprenkamp M, Seidler A. Wolman's disease in an infant. Monatsschr Kinderheilkd 138:88, 1990.
1274. Hakami N, Neiman PE, Canellos GP, et al. Neonatal megaloblastic anemia due to inherited transcobalamin II deficiency in 2 siblings. N Engl J Med 285:1163, 1971.
1275. Verloes A, Lombert J, Lambert Y, et al. Tricho-hepato-enteric syndrome: further delineation of a distinct syndrome with neonatal hemochromatosis phenotype, intractable diarrhea, and hair anomalies. Am J Med Genet 68:391, 1997.
1276. Jonas AJ, Butler IJ. Circumvention of defective neutral amino acid transport in Hartnup disease using tryptophan ethyl ester. J Clin Invest 84:200, 1989.
1277. Holmberg C, Perheentipa J. Congenital Na+ diarrhea: a new type of secretory diarrhea. J Pediatr 106:56, 1985.
1278. Bayna SL, Heiner DC. Cow's milk allergy: manifestations, diagnosis and management. Adv Pediatr 25:1, 1978.
1279. Halpin TC, Byrne WJ, Ament ME. Colitis, persistent diarrhea, and soy protein intolerance. J Pediatr 91:404, 1977.
1280. Powell GK. Milk- and soy-induced enterocolitis of infancy. Clinical features and standardization of challenge. J Pediatr 93:553, 1978.
1281. Miller RC, Larsen E. Regional enteritis in early infancy. Am J Dis Child 122:301, 1971.
1282. Avery GB, Harkness M. Bloody diarrhea in the newborn infant of a mother with ulcerative colitis. Pediatrics 34:875, 1964.
1283. Ein SH, Lynch MJ, Stephens CA. Ulcerative colitis in children under one year: a twenty-year review. J Pediatr Surg 6:264, 1971.
1284. Sunshine P, Sinatra FR, Mitchell CH. Intractable diarrhoea of infancy. Clin Gastroenterol 6:445, 1977.
1285. Scott GB, Buck BE, Leterman JG, et al. Acquired immunodeficiency syndrome in infants. N Engl J Med 310:76, 1984.
1286. Davidson M, Wasserman R. The irritable colon of childhood (chronic nonspecific diarrhea syndrome). J Pediatr 69:1027, 1966.
1287. Ebbesen F, Edelsten D, Hertel J. Gut transit time and lactose malabsorption during phototherapy. I, II. Acta Paediatr Scand 69:65, 1980.
1288. Perlman M, Benady S, Saggi E. Neonatal diagnosis of familial dysautonomia. Pediatrics 63:238, 1979.
1289. Davidson GP, Cutz E, Hamilton JR, et al. Familial enteropathy: a syndrome of protracted diarrhea from birth, failure to thrive, and hypoplastic villous atrophy. Gastroenterology 75:783, 1978.
1290. Candy DCA, Larcher VF, Cameron DJS, et al. Lethal familial protracted diarrhea. Arch Dis Child 56:15, 1981.
1291. Chien L, Robertson H, Gerrard JW. Infantile gastroenteritis due to water with high sulfate content. Can Med Assoc J 99:102, 1968.
1292. Fleisher D, Ament ME. Diarrhea, red diapers, and child abuse. Clin Pediatr (Phila) 17:820, 1978.
1293. Ochoa TJ, Salazar-Lindo E, Cleary TG. Management of children with infection-associated persistent diarrhea. Semin Pediatr Infect Dis 15:229, 2004.

Section III

VIRAL INFECTIONS

Chapter 21

ACQUIRED IMMUNODEFICIENCY SYNDROME IN THE INFANT

Yvonne A. Maldonado

The first descriptions of the acquired immunodeficiency syndrome (AIDS) in infants and children were published in the early 1980s.[1-4] As of December 2002, 9300 AIDS cases in children younger than 13 years had been confirmed by the Centers for Disease Control and Prevention (CDC) in the United States.[5] However, this represents only a fraction of the 2.5 million children living with human immunodeficiency virus type 1 (HIV-1) infection worldwide.[6] Although HIV infection in children has been acquired in the past by the transfusion of contaminated blood or coagulation products, this route has been virtually eliminated in the United States. It is estimated that 1700 new perinatally acquired HIV infections occur every day in the world, with most occurring in developing countries. Sexual abuse has been associated with the acquisition of HIV infection by some children, and the use of contaminated needles and unprotected sexual intercourse account for most infections in teenagers.

In this chapter, the experience with HIV infection in children is reviewed, with the focus on the infection in neonates and infants. We have a sound knowledge of the clinical presentation of HIV infection in infants and children and have made major progress in preventing vertical transmission in industrialized countries. However, there is an urgent need for the development of simple and inexpensive interventions and a need to better understand the point at which transmission occurs and the role of potentially protective factors. Such knowledge will impact future recommendations for the treatment of pregnant women, the management of very young children, and the use of preventive measures, including immunization and other supportive care modalities before the onset of disease manifestations.

EPIDEMIOLOGY

HIV infection is a pandemic with cases reported to the World Health Organization (WHO) from virtually every country. Through December 2003, an estimated 40 million people were infected, including 2.5 million children younger than 15 years.[6] The epidemic continues unabated in Africa and is expanding rapidly in Southeast Asia, India, and Latin America.[7-10] It has been estimated that in 2003 alone, 4.2 million adults and 700,000 children were newly infected with HIV-1, and 2.5 million adults and 500,000 children younger than 15 years have died of HIV-related complications.

In contrast, in the United States, HIV-infected children younger than 13 years account for only 1% of all AIDS cases.[5] However, in developing nations, children constitute more than 5% of the people living with HIV/AIDS, and 17% of AIDS-related deaths have been children younger than 15 years. The Joint United Nations Programme on HIV/AIDS (UNAIDS) estimates that more than 13 million children have been orphaned by the AIDS epidemic.

As of December 2002, of the 9300 cases of AIDS in children younger than 13 years that have been reported to the CDC in the United States, more than one half have already died of their disease.[5] Minority groups are disproportionally affected, with 59% of cases occurring among black, non-Hispanic children (who account for only 14% of the U.S. pediatric population) and 23% in Hispanics (17% of the U.S. pediatric population), compared with 17% among white, non-Hispanic children (64% of the U.S. pediatric population).

Almost 80% of the children with AIDS are younger than 5 years, reflecting the predominant mode of transmission from mother to child, which accounts for 93% of HIV infections in children.[5] About 43% of the women in the United States have acquired HIV infection through intravenous drug use, but a growing number (53%) have been infected through sexual contact.[5] The increasing number of infected women of childbearing age will continue to greatly influence the number of infected children in the United States and worldwide.

TRANSMISSION

Data suggest that most children are infected during the immediate peripartum period. In the United States, the transmission rate without intervention is estimated to be 25% to 30%; in Europe, it is lower (13% to 20%); and a rate of 40% has been observed in Africa.[11,12] These differences in transmission rates are difficult to explain. However, it has been clear that maternal disease status, especially a high viral load or a CD4 count less than 200 cells/mm^3, is highly correlated with the risk for vertical transmission.[11,13-17]

In 1994, the results of the AIDS Clinical Trials Group protocol 076 (PACTG 076) employing zidovudine during pregnancy were published, resulting in guidelines issued by the CDC.[18-21] This trial, which resulted in a 67% reduction in perinatal transmission, has become the gold standard in the United States and western Europe to which future strategies for the prevention of perinatal transmission are being compared. In developing countries, other simpler and less expensive strategies have been used.[22-25]

Intrauterine Transmission

The female glandular epithelium can contain HIV between the columnar and squamous cells of the cervix, whereas swabs from the vagina yield fewer virus particles.[26,27] Sperm cells do not express CD4 receptors and are therefore unlikely to be directly infected with HIV, but the virus can be detected in seminal white cells and plasma.[27]

Virus has been detected in some aborted fetuses of 8 to 20 weeks' gestational age and in amniotic fluid.[28-31] Maternal decidual leukocytes, villous macrophages (Hofbauer cells), and endothelial cells stain positive for gp41 antigen and HIV nucleic acids.[32] The placenta can be infected through the CD4$^+$ trophoblasts or through the occasional occurrence of chorioamnionitis.[33,34] Notably, there is not a clear predictive value for the identification of HIV in the placenta and the infection of the fetus or newborn.[35] Moreover, there are important technical limitations to studies of fetal or placenta tissues, particularly because of the difficulty of excluding contamination with maternal blood.

Several factors that might correlate with a heightened risk for transmission have been assessed, including the maternal viral burden, specific viral phenotypes or genotypes, the disease stage of the mother, her immune response to HIV infection, placental disruption by coexistence of other infections, and fetal susceptibility (which may be influenced by genetic factors).[14-17,36-41] In the absence of prophylactic zidovudine treatment, HIV-positive mothers have a potentially higher risk for transmission if they have mastitis, positive p24 antigenemia, a high HIV RNA or DNA level, and a CD4 count of less than 400 cells/mm^3.[13,41,42] A high rate of transmission was reported with advanced clinical stage of disease, with 100% transmission among 10 patients with CDC class IV (symptomatic) disease, compared with 13% in 56 patients with CDC class II (asymptomatic) or CDC class III (lymphadenopathy as only symptom) disease.[43]

Intrapartum Infection

The bimodal course of disease in HIV-infected children and the fact that at the time of birth virus can only be recovered from less than 25% of the infants who are subsequently shown to be infected suggest that a large proportion of perinatal infections occur late during pregnancy or during delivery.[44] An infant is considered to have been infected in utero if the HIV-1 genome can be detected by polymerase chain reaction (PCR) or be cultured from blood within 48 hours of birth. In contrast, a child is considered to have intrapartum infection if diagnostic assays such as culture, PCR, and serum p24 antigen are negative in blood samples obtained during the first week of life but became positive during the period from day 7 to day 90 and the infant had not been breast-fed.[45]

In a study by the French Collaborative Study Group, timing of transmission was estimated with a mathematical model.[46] Data for the 95 infected infants (those seropositive at 18 months and those who died of HIV disease before this age and who were exclusively bottle-fed) were used in the model, which indicated that one third of the infants were infected in utero less than 2 months before delivery (95th percentile). In the remaining 65% of cases (95% confidence interval [CI], 22%-92%), the date of infection was estimated as the day of birth. Viral markers became positive after an estimated median time period of 10 days (95% CI, 6%-14%), and the 95th percentile was estimated at 56 days.[46]

Discordance of infection has been described among the progeny of different pregnancies and even more intriguingly among twins.[47-50] In a large multinational study, data were collected on 100 sets of twins and one set of triplets born to HIV-seropositive mothers.[49] HIV-1 infection was more common in first-born than in second-born twins ($P = .004$), with 50% of first-born twins delivered vaginally and 38% of first-born twins delivered by cesarean section being infected, compared with 19% of second-born twins delivered by either route. Because passage through or proximity to the birth canal appeared to be an important factor, prophylactic measures such as cleansing the birth canal before delivery were suggested to reduce the risk of intrapartum infection.[51] One study performed in Africa compared the HIV transmission rate of infants born to 3327 women whose infants were delivered in a conventional way with that of 3637 infants of women who were treated with manual cleansing of the birth canal with a cotton pad soaked in 0.25% chlorhexidine on admission for labor and every 4 hours until delivery.[52] Although the intervention had no significant impact on HIV transmission rates (27% in 505 intervention women compared with 28% in 477 control women), cleansing the birth canal with chlorhexidine reduced the hospitalization rates for early neonatal and maternal postpartum infectious problems.[53] In this and two other studies, the concentrations of chlorhexidine were relatively low (0.25% to 0.4%).[54-56] A study of the safety and tolerability of higher concentrations of chlorhexidine for use as peripartum maternal and infant washes demonstrated that a 1% solution was safe and well tolerated, whereas a 2% solution was associated with maternal vaginal and vulvar or perineal burning or itching.[56] Further studies of the efficacy of the 1% chlorhexidine solution in preventing perinatal HIV transmission are possible.

Cesarean section, although likely to reduce the risk of transmission to a certain degree (in one study from 32% to 18%, $P = .11$), does not prevent it altogether.[37,49] However, one meta-analysis of 15 prospective cohort studies demonstrated a 50% reduction of transmission with elective cesarean section compared with other modes of delivery and an 87% reduction of transmission with both elective cesarean section and receipt of antiretroviral therapy during the prenatal, intrapartum, and neonatal periods compared with other modes of delivery and the absence of therapy.[57] It has been demonstrated that prolonged rupture of membranes over 4 hours increases the risk of transmission considerably, regardless of the mode of delivery.[58,59]

Postpartum Infection

Breast-feeding has been implicated as a postnatal route of maternal-infant transmission of HIV disease.[60,61] HIV-1 has been demonstrated by culture or PCR in up to 73% of breast milk specimens from HIV-1–seropositive women.[62,63] The prevalence of cell-free HIV-1 appears to be higher in mature milk (47%) than in colostrum (27%; $P = .1$).[64] Guay and colleagues collected expressed breast milk specimens from 201 HIV-1–seropositive and 86 HIV-1–seronegative Ugandan women approximately 6 weeks after delivery. Forty-seven of the 201 HIV-1–infected women had HIV-1–infected children, 143 had children who seroconverted, and 11 had children of indeterminate status. Breast milk supernatants were available for p24 antigen testing from 188 of the HIV-1–infected women, and breast milk cell pellets were available and contained amplifiable DNA in 125 of them (20 transmitters, 104 nontransmitters, 1 indeterminate). HIV-1 DNA was detected by PCR in 72% (75 of 104) of nontransmitters and 80% (16 of 20) of the transmitters.[65] Other studies have also shown that most breast-fed infants appear to remain uninfected.[62,66] A study of breast-fed infants born to HIV-infected mothers was performed in Kinshasa, Democratic Republic of Congo (formerly Zaire).[68] Among 69 HIV-infected children (26% of the cohort), 23% (CI, 14%-35%) were estimated to have had intrauterine transmission, 65% (CI, 53%-76%) intrapartum or early postpartum transmission, and 12% (CI, 5%-22%) late postpartum transmission. The investigators estimated the risks for intrauterine, intrapartum or early postpartum, and late postpartum infection, respectively, to be 6% (16 of 261; CI, 4%-10%), 18% (45 of 245; CI, 14%-24%), and 4% (8 of 189, CI, 2%-8%).[67] Others have estimated that the maximum risk of breast-feeding transmission occurs in the first 6 months,[68] coinciding with a period of maximum benefits of breast-feeding. There is a 5% to 10% risk of transmission from breast-feeding through 6 months of age and an additional 5% to 10% risk from breast-feeding through 18 to 24 months of age.[69] Early weaning at 6 months of age has therefore been proposed as a way to maximize the benefits of breast-feeding while minimizing the risk of HIV infection.

The risk of transmission of HIV-1 by breast-feeding and subsequent associated mortality has been compared with the mortality resulting from bottle-feeding with potentially contaminated water, and it is yielding controversial results. One study demonstrated that the benefits of breast-feeding over bottle-feeding can substantially outweigh the risk of HIV transmission unless the prevalence of HIV infection is high or the difference in mortality of breast-fed and bottle-fed infants is very low[70]; however, another study did not support this conclusion.[71] The American Academy of Pediatrics (AAP) has issued the following policy statement (abbreviated form)[72]:

Transmission of human immunodeficiency virus type 1 (HIV-1) through breast-feeding has been conclusively demonstrated. The risk of such transmission has been quantified, the timing has been clarified, and certain risk factors for breast-feeding transmission have been identified. In areas where infant formula is accessible, affordable, safe, and sustainable, avoidance of breast-feeding has represented one of the main components of mother-to-child HIV-1 transmission prevention efforts for many years. In areas where affordable and safe alternatives to breast-feeding may not be available, interventions to prevent breast-feeding transmission are being investigated. Complete avoidance of breast-feeding by HIV-1–infected women has been recommended by the American Academy of Pediatrics and the Centers for Disease Control and Prevention and remains the only means by which prevention of breast-feeding transmission of HIV-1 can be absolutely ensured.

Several large studies have shown a lack of transmission of HIV infection to household contacts through casual interactions.[73-76] The AAP does not place any special restrictions on daycare or school attendance of HIV-infected children but recommends observance of universal precaution measures for all handling of blood and body fluids, regardless of the infection status of the child.[77,78] The same guidelines apply to the handling of *all* newborns during or after birth. Gloves should be worn when handling body fluids, including amniotic fluid, and only bulb or wall suction devices should be used to avoid exposure of medical personnel.[79]

MOLECULAR BIOLOGY

HIV-1 is an enveloped virus with a diameter of 80 to 120 nm and a cylindrical, electrodense core. HIV-1 and its close relative HIV-2 are members of the Lentiviridae family of retroviruses, which have a complex genomic structure.[80,81] Like all retroviruses, HIV-1 contains the genes for *gag*, which encodes the core nucleocapsid polypeptides (gp24, p17, p9), *env* for the surface-coat proteins of the virus (gp120 and gp41), and *pol*, which codes for the viral reverse transcriptase and other enzymatic activities (i.e., integrase and protease). There are at least six regulatory genes: *vif*, *vpr*, *vpx*, *tat*, *rev*, *vpu*, and *nef*.[82] The retroviral core also contains two copies of the viral single-stranded RNA associated with enzymes such as the reverse transcriptase, RNase H, integrase, and protease.[81]

The life cycle of HIV-1 is characterized by several distinct stages.[83] The first step in the entry process of HIV into a cell is the interaction of the virion envelope glycoproteins (gp120 and gp41) with the CD4 molecule and a chemokine receptor.[84-90] Human cord blood mononuclear cells are preferentially infected by macrophage-tropic (M-tropic) strains of HIV-1 using the CC chemokine receptor CCR5.[88,90,91] T cell–tropic strains replicate in $CD4^+$ T cells and macrophages. They use the chemokine receptor CXCR4, a member of the CXC chemokine family.[84,87,88,90]

The HIV virions enter the cell and are rapidly uncoated. The viral reverse transcriptase transforms the single-stranded viral RNA into linear double-stranded DNA, whereas the less specific ribonuclease H degrades and removes the RNA template.[92] This viral DNA is circularized and transferred to the nucleus, where it is inserted by the viral integrase at random sites as a provirus.[93,94] It is also a common feature of all retroviruses to accumulate large amounts of unintegrated viral DNA that are fully competent templates for HIV-1 core and envelope antigen production.[95] The inactive provirus in the form of HIV-1 DNA has been found in 0.1% to 13.5% of peripheral blood mononuclear cells, compared with viral mRNA, which is found in 0.002% to 0.25% of these cells.[96-98] The latent provirus is activated by host cell responses to antigens, mitogens, cytokines such as tumor necrosis factor, and different gene products of other viruses.[98-101]

HIV gene expression follows by using host cell RNA polymerase II (among other factors), forming a ribonucleoprotein core containing *gag* and *pol* gene products. The 53-kDa precursor of the *gag* protein is cleaved by the HIV-1–derived protease into the p24, p17, p9, and p7 proteins.[102-104] The assembly of new virions consists of the formation of the critical viral enzymes, including reverse transcriptase, integrase, ribonuclease, and a protease, and the aggregation into a ribonucleoprotein core.[80,81] This core then moves to the cell surface and buds as mature virions through the plasma membrane.

Perinatal HIV infection is characterized by plasma RNA levels that rapidly reach very high levels.[105-108] In a study of 106 HIV-infected infants, the median plasma HIV RNA value at 1 month old was 318,000 copies/mL, and it was not uncommon to see viral levels that exceeded 10^6 copies/mL. In the absence of antiretroviral therapy, the levels decrease only gradually over the first 24 to 36 months of life.[109] As in adults, higher viral loads correlate with a more rapid disease progression.[105,110-113] This provides a strong argument for early and aggressive intervention with antiretroviral therapy.

A controversial issue is the proposed clearance of HIV infection in some perinatally infected infants.[114-118] It was postulated that children rarely could have a positive culture of peripheral blood mononuclear cells for HIV-1 and positivity of plasma by PCR assay but later become negative as assessed by culture and PCR and remain seronegative without ever having received antiretroviral therapy. However, analysis of 42 cases of suspected "transient infection" among 1562 exposed seroreverting infants and one mother did not document a phylogenetic linkage between the infant's and the mother's virus in 17 cases, did not detect any HIV-1 *env* sequences in 20 cases, or demonstrated that the specimens were mistakenly attributed to the child (6 cases).[119]

IMMUNE PATHOGENESIS

Infection with HIV results in profound deficiencies in cell-mediated and humoral immunity caused by quantitative and qualitative defects, leading to a progressive dysfunction of the immune system with depletion of $CD4^+$ T cells. Flow cytometric analysis of lymphocyte subpopulations in healthy children has revealed age-related changes in the number of the different subgroups.[120-122] Comparison of lymphocytes subsets in HIV-infected versus noninfected children younger than 2 years demonstrated no difference for absolute CD8 counts but clearly decreased levels of CD4 cells.[123] In the absence of early antiretroviral therapy, an abnormal CD4 count (<10th percentile for uninfected children) was found in 83%, and an abnormally low absolute CD4 count was observed in 67% of the infected children. As in adults, the relative risks of death or disease progression are inversely related to the CD4 cell count, which is closely related to the viral load.[107,113,124] A rapid increase in HIV RNA levels correlates with early disease progression and loss of CD4 cells in vertically infected infants.[124]

Other immune abnormalities include decreased lymphocyte proliferation in response to an antigen, polyclonal B cell activation resulting in hypergammaglobulinemia, and altered function of monocytes and neutrophils.[125-128] In the European Collaborative Study, hypergammaglobulinemia (IgG, IgM, and IgA) identified 77% of infected children at the age of 6 months with 97% specificity.[129] In a group of 47 HIV-infected children (17 asymptomatic and 30 symptomatic), Roilides and co-workers[125] found an abnormality of at least one IgG subclass in 83%, including some patients who had IgG2, IgG4, or combined IgG2-IgG4 deficiencies. There was no clear correlation of the incidence of bacterial infections with specific subclass deficiencies. A virus-specific cytotoxic T lymphocyte response can be demonstrated at a very early age, even in the fetus, and becomes more pronounced with longer duration of infection.[130,131]

DIAGNOSIS

Diagnosis of HIV infection as part of routine prenatal care of pregnant women is very important, because preventive therapies are now widely available, even in developing countries. The CDC recommends voluntary HIV testing for all pregnant women and strongly encourages antiretroviral therapy for HIV-positive pregnant women.[20,21]

Prenatal diagnosis in the fetus is difficult because of the risk for bleeding and contamination of the sample with maternal blood or the possibility for accidental iatrogenic infection of the fetus. Amniotic fluid has been found to be positive for p24 antigen and HIV reverse transcriptase.[28,31] Chorionic villus sampling and percutaneous umbilical blood sampling are associated with a higher risk for the fetus, and noninvasive techniques such as fetal ultrasonography or the clinical assessment of the mother give unspecific and not very predictive information.

The diagnosis of HIV infection in an infant born to a seropositive mother used to pose a problem because of the passive transfer of maternal antibodies. However, measurement of viral RNA or DNA copy numbers and the culture technique have become standardized and are now widely available in industrialized countries.[132] The PCR assay should not be performed on cord blood, because there is a possibility of contamination with maternal blood. However, any positive test should be repeated for confirmation. It is assumed that children who have a positive HIV PCR result within the first 48 hours after birth were infected in utero, whereas those who are infected during the intrapartum period might become positive 2 to 6 weeks after birth. In a study using dried blood spot specimens, a technique yielding equivalent results to fresh blood specimens, only 19% (5 of 26) of infected children had detectable HIV DNA compared with a sensitivity of 96% (25 of 26) at 1 month old.[133]

In adults and in children older than 18 months, serologic tests for specific antibodies are still important tools to establish the diagnosis of HIV infection, especially if PCR assays or culture methods are not available. HIV-specific antibody is usually detectable within 4 to 24 weeks after initial infection.[134] These antibodies are directed against the envelope proteins gp160, gp120, and gp41; the core proteins p24, p55, and p18; and the enzyme bands p31 and p65/51. The response to the envelope proteins usually persists throughout life, but the antibodies to core (gag) proteins may become lost in more symptomatic patients, and severely hypogammaglobulinemic children do not produce detectable antibodies.[135] Most commercially available enzyme immunoassay tests measure IgG antibodies to HIV. Virtually all children born to seropositive mothers therefore are positive for HIV antibodies at birth, even though only a few are infected. Up to 75% of uninfected children lose these passively transferred antibodies between 6 and 12 months of age, but persistence of maternal antibodies has been documented in 2% up to 18 months of age.[129,136] Tests for IgM antibodies have been problematic, probably because of interaction with abundant IgG and the short duration of IgM production.[137] The 1994 revised CDC guidelines for the diagnosis of HIV infection in infants and children are shown in Table 21-1.

Clinical and nonspecific laboratory parameters may also suggest HIV infection. The newborn HIV-infected child is usually asymptomatic but can become seriously ill within the first weeks to months of life. Table 21-2 provides a diagram outlining the initial evaluation and the necessary follow-up tests for an asymptomatic child born to an HIV-positive mother, as recommended by the AAP.[79] Opportunistic infections, hepatosplenomegaly, and lymphadenopathy are indicators for infection in the antibody-positive child younger than 18 months. Hypergammaglobulinemia is a nonspecific but early finding of HIV infection, and CD4 counts must be interpreted within the bounds of the age-dependent normal range.[120-122,138] Diagnosis is established if an AIDS-defining disease occurs (Table 21-3). In developing countries with limited diagnostic resources, the diagnosis often has to be based on clinical symptoms, and a modified provisional definition for pediatric cases of AIDS has been issued by the WHO.[139]

Table 21–1 Centers for Disease Control and Prevention Definition of Human Immunodeficiency Virus Infection in Children Younger than 13 Years of Age

HIV Infected

A. A child <18 mo of age who is known to be HIV seropositive or born to an HIV-infected mother

and

Has positive results on two separate determinations (excluding cord blood) from one or more of the following HIV detection tests:

- HIV culture
- HIV polymerase chain reaction
- HIV antigen (p24)

or

Meets criteria for AIDS diagnosis based on the 1987 AIDS surveillance case definition

B. A child >18 mo of age born to an HIV-infected mother or any child infected by blood, blood products, or other known modes of infection who

- Is HIV antibody positive by repeatedly reactive EIA and confirmatory test (e.g., Western blot or immunofluorescence assay)

or

- Meets any of the criteria in A

Perinatally Exposed (Prefix E)

A child who does not meet the criteria above and who:

- Is HIV seropositive by EIA and confirmatory test and is <18 mo of age

or

- Has unknown antibody status but was born to a mother known to be HIV infected

Seroreverter (SR)

A child who is born to an HIV-infected mother and who:

- Has been documented as HIV-antibody negative (i.e., two or more negative EIA tests performed at 6-18 mo of age or one negative EIA test performed after 18 mo of age)

or

- Has had no laboratory evidence of infection

and

- Has not had an AIDS-defining condition

EIA, enzyme immunoassay.
Adapted from 1994 Revised classification system for human immunodeficiency virus infection in children less than 13 years of age. MMWR Morb Mortal Wkly Rep 431:1-10, 1994.

CLINICAL MANIFESTATIONS AND PATHOLOGY

HIV infection in infants and children has a different presentation from that in adults, and the CDC classifies HIV infection in children younger than the age of 13 years based on clinical and immunologic parameters (see Table 21-3). Children found to be HIV infected are reported to the CDC only at the time of diagnosis, and tables that list the incidence of certain marker diseases (Table 21-4) are necessarily incomplete because a child may show other symptoms after the initial registration. Growth delay is an early and frequent finding of untreated perinatal HIV infection, and the linear growth is most severely affected in children with high viral loads.[140] Children are more likely than adults to have serious bacterial infections, and lymphocytic interstitial pneumonitis is almost entirely restricted to the pediatric age group. However, toxoplasmosis, cryptococcal infection, and the occurrence of cancer, especially Kaposi's sarcoma, are less common in HIV-infected children.

The initial symptoms may be subtle and sometimes difficult to distinguish from manifestations caused by drug use during pregnancy, from problems associated with prematurity, or from congenital infections other than HIV. Premature birth has been reported in 19%, with no difference between children born to drug-using mothers and children of mothers who were infected through other routes.[129,141] However, children of drug-addicted mothers had significantly lower birth weights and smaller head circumferences.

Common clinical features seen during the course of HIV infection are lymphadenopathy, fevers, malaise, loss

Table 21–2 Evaluation Schedule for Asymptomatic Infants Born to Human Immunodeficiency Virus–Seropositive Mothers

	Age								
Test	*Birth*	*2 wk*	*4 wk*	*6 wk*	*2 mo*	*3 mo*	*4 mo*	*5 mo*	*6 mo*
History[a], physical examination (including weight, height, head circumference)	+	+	+	+[b]	+	+	+	+	+
Developmental testing	(+)		+		+	+	+	+	+
Complete blood cell test and platelets	+		+	+	+	+	+		+
Serum chemistry (blood urea nitrogen, creatinine, liver function tests)	+			+		+	+		+
Serum immunoglobulins							+		+
Lymphocyte subsets[c]			+			+			+
HIV peripheral blood culture and/or polymerase chain reaction[d]	+		+				+		+
Urine for cytomegalovirus	+				+				
Chest radiograph, computed tomography or magnetic resonance imaging of head[e]									(+)
Electrocardiogram or echocardiogram[e]									(+)

[a]The frequency of "common" pediatric problems, such as diaper rash, mucocutaneous *Candida* infection, diarrhea, otitis, and so on should be carefully monitored.
[b]Zidovudine to prevent perinatal transmission is discontinued at 6 wk of age; however, strongly consider initiation of other antiretroviral therapy in a child who is proved to be infected. Initiate prophylaxis for *Pneumocystis* pneumonia (PCP).
[c]T cell profile should be repeated at 6 mo if infection startus is unclear at 6 mo.
[d]Repeat PCR or viral culture immediately if positive to confirm infection. If the initial test is negative, repeat test at 4 wk to 2 mo (earlier if clinical or laboratory parameters suggest infection).
[e]Optional in the absence of clinical symptoms.

Table 21–3 1994 Centers for Disease Conrol and Prevention Revised Classification System for Human Immunodeficiency Virus (HIV) Infection in Children Younger than 13 Years of Age

Using this system children are classified according to three parameters: infection status, clinical status, and immunologic status. The categories are mutually exclusive. Once classified in a more severe category, a child is *not* reclassified in a less severe category even if the clinical or immunologic status improves.[a]

Pediatric HIV Virus Classification

	Clinical Categories			
Immune Categories	*(N) No Symptoms*	*(A) Mild Symptoms*	*(B)[b] Moderate Symptoms*	*(C)[b] Severe Symptoms*
(1) No suppression	N1	A1	B1	C1
(2) Moderate suppression	N2	A2	B2	C2
(3) Severe suppression	N3	A3	B3	C3

Immunologic Categories Based on Age-Specific $CD4^+$ T Lymphocyte Counts and Percent of Total Lymphocytes

The immunologic category classification is based on age-specific $CD4^+$ T lymphocyte count or percent of total lymphocytes and is designed to determine severity of immunosuppression attributable to HIV for age. If either CD4 count or percent results in classification into a different category, the child should be classified into the more severe category. A value should be confirmed before reclassified into a less severe category.

	Age Groups		
Immunologic Category	*0-11 mo*	*1-5 yr*	*>6 yr*
(1) No suppression	>1500 cells/μL (>25%)	>1000 cells/μL (>25%)	>500 cells/μL (>25%)
(2) Moderate suppression	750-1499 cells/μL (15-24%)	500-999 cells/μL (15-24%)	200-499 cells/μL (15-24%)
(3) Severe suppression	<750 cells/μL (<15%)	<500 cells/μL (<15%)	<200 cells/μL (<15%)

Clinical Categories for Children with HIV Infection

Category N: Not Symptomatic

Children who have no signs or symptoms considered to be the result of HIV infection or who have only one of the conditions listed in Category A

Category A: Mildly Symptomatic

Children with two or more of the conditions listed below but none of the conditions listed in Categories B and C

- Lymphadenopathy (>0.5 cm at more than two sites; bilateral = one site)
- Hepatomegaly
- Splenomegaly
- Dermatitis

continued

Table 21–3 1994 Centers for Disease Conrol and Prevention Revised Classification System for Human Immunodeficiency Virus (HIV) Infection in Children Younger than 13 Years of Age—*continued*

Clinical Categories for Children with HIV Infection *(continued)*

- Parotitis
- Recurrent or persistent respiratory infection, sinusitis, or otitis media

Category B: Moderately Symptomatic

Children who have symptomatic conditions other than those listed for Category A or C that are attributed to HIV infection. Examples of conditions in clinical Category B included but are not limited to:

- Anemia (<8 g/dL), neutropenia (<1000/mm^3), or thrombocytopenia (<100,000/mm^3) persisting >30 d
- Bacterial meningitis, pneumonia, or sepsis (single episode)
- Candidiasis, oropharyngeal thrush, persisting for >2 mo in children >6 mo of age
- Cardiomyopathy
- Cytomegalovirus infection, with onset before 1 mo of age
- Diarrhea, recurrent or chronic
- Hepatitis
- Herpes simplex virus stomatitis, recurrent (more than two episodes within 1 yr)
- Herpes simplex virus bronchitis, pneumonitis, or esophagitis with onset before 1 mo of age
- Herpes zoster (shingles) involving at least two distinct episodes or more than one dermatome
- Leiomyosarcoma
- Lymphoid interstitial pneumonia or pulmonary lymphoid hyperplasia complex
- Nephropathy
- Nocardiosis
- Persistent fever (lasting >1 mo)
- Toxoplasmosis, onset before 1 mo of age
- Varicella, disseminated (complicated chickenpox)

Category C: Severely Symptomatic

Children who have any condition listed in the 1987 surveillance case definition for AIDS, with the exception of lymphoid interstitial pneumonia

- Serious bacterial infections, multiple or recurrent (i.e., any combination of at least two culture-confirmed infections within a 2-yr period, of the following types: septicemia, pneumonia, meningitis, bone or joint infection, or abscess of an internal body organ or body cavity, excluding otitis media, superficial skin or mucosal abscesses, and indwelling catheter-related infections)
- Candidiasis, esophageal or pulmonary (bronchi, trachea, lungs)
- Coccidioidomycosis, disseminated (at site other than or in addition to lungs or cervical or hilar nodes)
- Cryptosporidiosis or isosporidiosis with diarrhea persisting >1 mo
- Cytomegalovirus disease with onset of symptoms at age >1 mo (other than liver, spleen, or lymph nodes)
- Encephalopathy (at least one of the following progressive findings present for at least 2 mo in the absence of a concurrent illness other than HIV infection that could explain the findings): (a) failure to attain or loss of development milestones or loss of inellectual ability verified by standard developmental scale or neuropsychological tests; (b) impaired brain growth or acquired microcephaly demonstrated by head circumference measurements or brain atrophy demonstrated by computed tomography or magnetic resonance imaging (serial imaging is required for children <2 yr of age); (c) acquired symmetrical motor deficit manifested by two or more of the following: paresis, pathologic, pathologic reflexes, ataxia, or gait disturbance
- Herpes simplex virus infection causing a mucocutaneous ulcer that persists for >1 mo or bronchitis, pneumonitis, or esophagitis for any duration affecting a child >1 mo of age
- Histoplasmosis, disseminated (other than or in addition to lungs or cervical lymph nodes)
- Kaposi's sarcoma
- Lymphoma, primary, in brain
- Lymphoma, small, noncleaved cell (Burkitt's), or immunoblastic or large cell lymphoma of B cell or unknown immunologic phenotype
- *Mycobacterium tuberculosis,* disseminated or extrapulmonary
- Mycobacterium, other species or unidentified species, disseminated (other than or in addition to lungs, skin, or cervical or hilar lymph nodes)
- *Mycobacterium avium-intracellulare* complex or *Mycobacterium kansasii,* disseminated (other than or in addition to lungs, skin, or cervical or hilar lymph nodes)
- *Pneumocystis carinii* pneumonia
- Progressive multifocal leukoencephalopathy
- *Salmonella* (nontyphgoid) septicemia, recurrent
- Toxoplasmosis of the brain with onset >1 mo of age
- Wasting syndrome in the absence of a concurrent illness other than HIV infection that could explain the following findings: (a) persistent weight loss >10% of baseline *or* (b) downward crossing of at least two of the following percentile on weight-for-height chart on two consecutive measurements >30 d apart *plus* (a) chronic diarrhea (i.e., at least two loose stools per day for >30 d) *or* (b) documented fever (for >30 d, intermitent or constant)

[a]Children whose HIV infection status is not confirmed are classified by using the grid with a letter E (for vertically exposed) placed before the appropriate classification code (e.g., EN2).

[b]Both category C and lymphoid interstitial pneumonitis in category B are reportable to state and local health departments as acquired immune deficiency syndrome.

From Centers for Disease Control and Prevention. Recommendations of the U.S. Public Health Service Task Force on the use of zidovudine to reduce perinatal transmission of human immunodeficiency virus. MMWR Morb Mortal Wkly Rep 43:1-20, 1994.

Table 21–4 Acquired Immunodeficiency Syndrome Indicator Diseases Diagnosed in 8086 Children Younger than Age 13 Years Reported to the Centers for Disease Control and Prevention Through 1997

Disease	No. of Children Diagnosed	Percent of Total[a]
Pneumocystis carinii pneumonia	2700	33
Lymphocytic interstitial pneumonitis	1942	24
Recurrent bacterial infections	1619	20
Wasting syndrome	1419	18
Encephalopathy	1322	16
Candida esophagitis	1266	16
Cytomegalovirus disease	658	8
Mycobacterium avium infection	639	8
Severe herpes simplex infection	370	5
Pulmonary candidiasis	307	4
Cryptosporidiosis	291	4
Cancer	162	2

[a]The sum of percentages is greater than 100 because some patients have more than one disease.
From Centers for Disease Control and Prevention (CDC). U.S. HIV and AIDS cases reported through December 1997. HIV/AIDS Surveillance report: year-end edition. MMWR Morb Mortal Wkly Rep 9:1-44, 1997.

of energy, hepatosplenomegaly, respiratory tract infections, and recurrent and chronic otitis and sinusitis. Other commonly encountered characteristics are failure to thrive, sometimes associated with chronic diarrhea; failure to grow; the presence and persistence of mucocutaneous candidiasis; and many nonspecific cutaneous manifestations.

Infectious Complications

Infections in the HIV-infected newborn or infant can be serious or life threatening. The difficulty in treating these infectious episodes, their chronicity, and their tendency to recur distinguish them from the normal infections of early infancy. It is therefore helpful to document each episode and to evaluate the course and frequency of their recurrences.

Bacterial Infections

Recurrent serious bacterial infections such as meningitis, sepsis, and pneumonia are so typical of HIV infection in children that they were included in the revised CDC definition of 1987.[142,143] In a study of 42 vertically infected children, a mean of 1.8 febrile visits per child-year of observation was reported.[144] Eleven of the 27 positive blood cultures grew *Streptococcus pneumoniae*, and 16 grew organisms that were considered central venous line related (coagulase-negative *Staphylococcus*, gram-negative enterics, *Staphylococcus aureus*, *Pseudomonas aeruginosa*, *Candida* species). This increased incidence of pneumococcal infections has been confirmed by other studies.[145,146]

Infections in the HIV-infected newborn have the same pattern as that seen commonly in the neonatal period. A syndrome of very-late-onset group B streptococcal disease (at the age of 3.5 to 5 months of life) has been described in HIV-infected children.[147] Other rare infections such as congenital syphilis or neonatal gonococcal disease may become more frequent in the future as the incidence rises among pregnant women.[148-150] Congenital syphilis may be missed if serologic tests are not performed on the mother and her child at the time of delivery and repeated later if indicated.

Mycobacterial infections have assumed an increasingly important role in the pathology of the HIV-infected infant and child. Although the number of HIV-infected children with *Mycobacterium tuberculosis* infection is still small, organisms resistant to multiple antituberculosis drugs cultured from adults and children pose a threat not only to other immunocompromised patients but also to health care providers.[151-155] An important issue for the neonatologist is whether the mother is infected with *M. tuberculosis* and may transmit the disease to her child. The diagnosis of *M. tuberculosis* infection is complicated in the HIV-infected patient because of the frequent anergy leading to a negative Mantoux test result even in the presence of infection. To diagnose anergy, a control (e.g., for mumps, *Candida*, or tetanus) should always be placed simultaneously with the Mantoux test.[154,156] Treatment of *M. tuberculosis* infection in children is complicated by the lack of pediatric formulations but usually includes isoniazid, rifampin, and during the first 2 months, pyrazinamide.[157]

Infection with *Mycobacterium avium-intracellulare* complex occurs in almost 20% of HIV-infected children with advanced disease and presents as nonspecific symptoms such as night sweats, weight loss, and low-grade fevers.[158,159] Treatment usually consists of three or more drugs (e.g., clarithromycin; ethambutol; rifampin or amikacin, or both; ciprofloxacin; clofazimine) but commonly provides only temporary symptomatic relief and not eradication of the infection. Prophylaxis with clarithromycin or azithromycin should be initiated in infants younger than 1 year with a CD4 count less than 750 cells/mm^3, in children 1 to 2 years old with a CD4 count less than 500 cells/mm^3, and in children 2 to 6 years old with a CD4 count less than 75 cells/mm^3. In children older than 6 years, the adult threshold of 50 cells/mm^3 can be used.[160]

Viral Infections

Viral infections are important causes for morbidity and mortality in HIV-infected children. Primary varicella can be unusually severe and can recur as zoster, often presenting with very few, atypical lesions. The virus may become resistant to standard treatment with acyclovir.[161-163] Cytomegalovirus infection can result in esophagitis, hepatitis, enterocolitis, or retinitis.[164-167] Cytomegalovirus can become resistant to the treatment with ganciclovir, necessitating the use of foscarnet or even combination regimens.[168,169]

Other commonly encountered viruses in the HIV-infected infant and child are hepatitis A, B, and C, often associated with a more fulminant or chronic aggressive course than in the non–HIV-infected patient.[170-172] Hepatitis C infection has been shown to be more common in children born to HIV-infected mothers in some studies,[172] but others have found no association between maternal HIV status and perinatal hepatitis C transmission.[173,174]

Infection with the measles virus is associated with a high mortality in HIV-infected children and often presents without the typical rash and can result in a fatal giant cell pneumonia.[175-178] Infection with respiratory syncytial virus or adenovirus, alone or in combination, can also result in rapid and sometimes fatal respiratory compromise and in chronic or persistent viral shedding or infection.[179-181]

An interesting observation is the occurrence of a polyclonal lymphoproliferative syndrome, often associated with evidence of primary or reactivated Epstein-Barr virus infection. These patients develop impressive lymphadenopathy and sometimes have concurrent lymphocytic interstitial pneumonitis or parotitis.[182] The distinction between a self-limited, benign hyperproliferation and the development of a monoclonal lymphoid malignancy is crucial for determining treatment and prognosis.

Fungal and Protozoal Infections

Oral candidiasis is common even in healthy, non–HIV-infected newborns and infants. However, infection beyond infancy, involvement of pharynx and esophagus, and persistence despite treatment with antifungal agents are more typical for the immunocompromised child. Disseminated candidiasis is, however, uncommon in the absence of predisposing factors such as central venous catheters or total parenteral nutrition.[183]

Infection with *Cryptococcus neoformans*, although common in adults with HIV infection, is less common in children.[184,185] Colonization with *Aspergillus* species and invasive disease has been described in adult patients with HIV infection, and we have observed at least one infant with perinatally acquired HIV infection and associated myelodysplastic syndrome who developed fatal pulmonary aspergillosis.[186-188] The incidence of other fungal infections varies with the prevalence of the organism in the specific geographic area. Disseminated histoplasmosis as the AIDS-defining illness has been described in a few infants.[189-191]

Early in the HIV epidemic, *Pneumocystis jiroveci* (formerly known as *Pneumocystis carinii)* pneumonia (PCP) was the AIDS indicator disease in almost 40% of the pediatric cases reported to the CDC.[192] However, this has changed dramatically since the introduction of guidelines for PCP prophylaxis in HIV-exposed infants and HIV-infected children and in 1997 accounted for only 25% of the AIDS cases.[193,194] The peak incidence of PCP in infancy occurs during the first 3 to 6 months of life, often as the first symptom of HIV infection. Presumably, this represents primary infection in these infants. At least one case of maternal-fetal transmission of PCP has also been documented.[195]

Most children with PCP present with an acute illness, hypoxemia, and without a typical radiographic picture.[196,197] The diagnosis is usually made by obtaining an induced sputum (which can be done by experienced therapists even in very young children) or by performing a bronchoalveolar lavage, and only rarely is an open lung biopsy necessary.[198,199] Treatment options are high-dose intravenous trimethoprim-sulfamethoxazole (TMP-SMX) or pentamidine as first-line drugs.[200] Early adjunctive treatment with corticosteroids has been beneficial in adults and children with moderate to severe PCP and is commonly recommended for patients with an initial arterial oxygen pressure of less than 70 mm Hg or an arterial-alveolar gradient of more than 35 mm Hg.[201-204]

Unfortunately, PCP has been associated with a mortality of 39% to 65% in infants despite improved diagnosis and treatment.[205,206] In 1991, the CDC issued guidelines for PCP prophylaxis in children, taking into account the age-dependent levels of normal CD4 cell numbers.[207] However, these recommendations were applicable only if a child was known to be HIV infected. A survey published in 1995 revealed basically no change between 1988 and 1992 in the incidence of PCP among infants born to HIV-infected mothers.[208] Two thirds of these infants had never received PCP prophylaxis, and 59% of those children were recognized as having been exposed to HIV infection within 30 days or less of PCP diagnosis. Among the infants known to be HIV infected who had a CD4 count performed within 1 month of PCP diagnosis, 18% had a CD4 count higher than 1500 cells/mm^3, the recommended threshold for initiation of PCP prophylaxis.[208] At the same time, it was shown that primary prophylaxis during the first year of life was highly effective in the prevention of PCP.[209] These pivotal studies led to revised guidelines in 1995.[193] The major new recommendation was that all infants born to HIV-infected women should be started on PCP prophylaxis at 4 to 6 weeks of age, regardless of their CD4 counts. More details are presented in Table 21-5.

The recommended prophylactic regimen is TMP-SMX with 150 mg/m^2/day of TMP and 750 mg/m^2/day of SMX given orally in divided doses twice each day during 3 consecutive days per week. If TMP-SMX is not tolerated, alternative regimens are dapsone taken orally (2 mg/kg/day, not to exceed 100 mg) once daily or aerosolized pentamidine. However, breakthrough infections can occur with every regimen and appear to be most frequent with intravenous pentamidine and least common with TMP-SMX.[210,211]

Encephalitis caused by *Toxoplasma gondii* is common in adults with HIV infection but only rarely seen in children.[109] However, several case reports of *T. gondii* encephalitis in infants between 5 weeks and 18 months old have been published. Some of these infants probably acquired toxoplasmosis infection in utero.[213,214] Toxoplasmosis remains an important differential diagnosis in the patient with an intracerebral mass.

Protozoal infections of the gastrointestinal tract often represent difficult diagnostic and therapeutic problems and can be associated with an intractable diarrhea. Infection with cryptosporidia has a prevalence of 3.0% to 3.6% among children with diarrhea.[215] HIV-infected children are at risk for prolonged diarrheal disease with often severe wasting.

Table 21–5 Recommendations for *Pneumocystis jiroveci* Pneumonia (PCP) Prophylaxis and CD4 Monitoring in HIV-Exposed Infants and HIV-Infected Children

Age/HIV-Infection Status	PCP Prophylaxis	CD4⁺ Monitoring
Birth to 4-6 wk, HIV exposed or infected	No prophylaxis (because PCP is rare and due to concerns regarding kernicterus with TMP/SMX)	1 mo
4-6 wk to 4 mo, HIV exposed	Prophylaxis	3 mo
4-12 mo		
• HIV infected or indeterminate	Prophylaxis	6, 9, 12 mo
• HIV infection reasonably excluded[a]	No prophylaxis	None
1-5 yr, HIV infected	Prophylaxis if • $CD4^+$ count is < 500 cells/mm^3 or • $CD4^+$ percentage is < 15%	Every 3-4 mo (more frequently if indicated)
Older than 6 yr, HIV infected	Prophylaxis if • $CD4^+$ count < 200 cells/mm^3 or • $CD4^+$ percentage is < 15%	Every 3-4 yr

[a]Two or more negative HIV diagnostic tests (i.e., HIV culture or polymerase chain reaction), both performed at ≥ 1 mo of age and one of which was performed at ≥ 4 mo of age, or ≥ 2 negative HIV IgG antibody tests performed at ≥ 6 mo of age among children without clinical evidence of HIV disease.

HIV, human immunodeficiency virus; TMP/SMX, trimethorprim-sulfamethoxazole.

From Centers from Disease control and Prevention. 1995 Revised guidelines for prophylaxis against *Pneumocystis carinii* pneumonia for children infected with or perinatally exposed to human immunodeficiency virus. MMWR Morb Mortal Wkly Rep 44:1-12, 1995.

Malignancies

Several case reports of malignancies associated with HIV infection in infants and children have been published; however, cancer is the AIDS-defining illness in only 2% of children, compared with 14% of the adults.[5,216] The most common cancer in HIV-infected children is non-Hodgkin's lymphoma as a systemic disease or as a primary central nervous system tumor.[217-219] Kaposi's sarcoma has been described in a few children, including a 6-day-old infant, but remains relatively uncommon.[220-222] Leiomyomas and leiomyosarcomas, soft tissue tumors associated with Epstein-Barr virus infection in immunocompromised patients, are increasingly common.[220,223,224]

Encephalopathy

Encephalopathy, often with early onset, was a frequent and typical manifestation of HIV infection in children before the introduction of antiretroviral therapy. Symptoms of encephalopathy in the newborn or young infant initially include delayed head control or delayed acquisition of a social smile and variable degrees of truncal hypotonia.[225-227] Subsequently, impairment of cognitive, behavioral, and motor functions becomes apparent. Typical findings included a loss of or failure to attain normal developmental milestones, weakness, intellectual deficits, or neurologic symptoms such as ataxia and pyramidal tract signs, including spasticity or rigidity.[228] Seizures are rare but have been described, and cerebrovascular disease resulting in strokes or the formation of giant aneurysms at the base of the brain has been reported.[229,230] The course can be static, wherein the child attains milestones, albeit at a slower rate than normal for age, or the development can reach a plateau and then the child ceases to acquire new milestones. The most severe form is manifested by a subacute-progressive course in which the child loses previously acquired capabilities.[231,232] The older child has impaired expressive language function, whereas receptive language appears to be slightly less affected.[233,234] Physical examination can reveal hypotonia or spasticity, and microencephaly may be present. Radiologic examination can suggest cerebral atrophy, calcifications in the basal ganglia and periventricular frontal white matter, and decreased attenuation in the white matter (Fig. 21-1).[235-239]

HIV-1 can be found in brain monocytes, macrophages, and microglia, and limited expression of the regulatory gene *nef*, but not of structural gene products, has been demonstrated in astrocytes.[240-243] Analysis of cerebrospinal fluid revealed HIV RNA in 90% of samples, and more than 10,000 copies/mL were associated with severe neurodevelopmental delay.[244,245] It is likely that immune-mediated mechanisms or the secretion of toxic cytokines by infected cells contributes to the pathogenesis of central nervous system disease in AIDS patients.[246] The level of quinolinic acid, a neurotoxin that has been implicated in the development of HIV-related encephalopathy, is elevated in children with symptomatic central nervous system disease and decreased during treatment with zidovudine.[247,248]

Postmortem examination shows variable degrees of white matter abnormalities, calcific deposits in the wall of blood vessels of the basal ganglia and the frontal white matter, and subacute encephalitis. At least one report described an HIV-related meningoencephalitis in a newborn, supporting the assumption of an intrauterine infection.[249] Spinal cord disease, manifested by vacuolar myelopathy, has been described in children but is less common than in adults.[250]

Dramatic improvements in the degree of encephalopathy have been achieved by treating the children with zidovudine, especially when given as a continuous intravenous infusion (see later).[251] Therapy with corticosteroids has also been shown to be beneficial in some patients.[252]

Ophthalmologic Pathology

The ophthalmologic complications associated with HIV infection can be particularly devastating. HIV-1 can infect

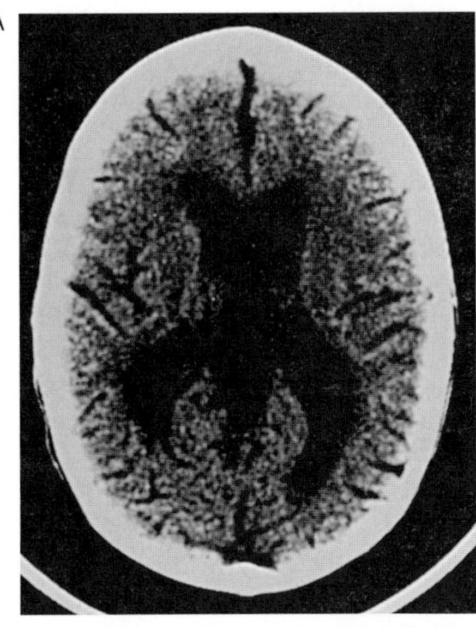

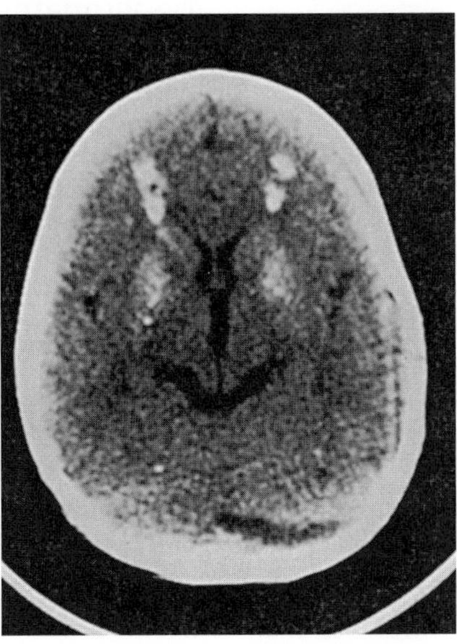

Figure 21–1 Computed tomographic scans of the brains of two infants with HIV-associated encephalopathy. **A,** Cerebral atrophy with enlarged ventricles and widened sulci. **B,** Calcifications in basal ganglia and frontal white matter.

the retina and manifest as cotton-wool spots on examination, but it rarely leads to impaired vision.[253,254] However, several other pathogens, some of them acquired in utero, can affect the eye and affect visual acuity. Fortunately, the incidence of blindness remains low in pediatric AIDS, but the infections caused by herpesviruses and especially by cytomegaloviral retinitis can be difficult to control and require intensive intravenous treatment.[164,166,167] A few children have been described with congenital toxoplasmosis and associated chorioretinitis, and one of the extrapulmonary manifestations of *P. juroveci* infection is involvement of the retina.[255-257] Early recognition and aggressive intervention are crucial to prevent progression of visual impairment, and routine ophthalmologic examinations should be part of the care of all HIV-infected children.

Interstitial Lung Disease

Lymphocytic interstitial pneumonitis, or pulmonary lymphoid hyperplasia, is seen almost exclusively in the pediatric patient with HIV infection and is still included into the CDC definition of AIDS-defining diseases for children younger than 13 years old (see Table 21-3). The incidence of lymphocytic interstitial pneumonitis is difficult to assess but may affect as many as 50% of the HIV-infected children.[258] Clinically, there is a wide spectrum in the severity of this disease; a child may be asymptomatic with only radiologic changes, or he or she can become severely compromised with exercise intolerance or even with oxygen dependency and the need for high-dose corticosteroid therapy. Children with lymphocytic interstitial pneumonitis are at higher risk to develop frequent bacterial and viral infections.[259]

A diffuse, interstitial, often reticulonodular infiltrative process is typically observed on radiologic examination and is sometimes associated with hilar or mediastinal lymphadenopathy (Fig. 21-2).[258] On biopsy, peribronchiolar lymphoid aggregates or a diffuse lymphoid infiltration of the alveolar septa and peribronchiolar areas is seen.[182] Treatment of lymphocytic interstitial pneumonitis is only indicated in the symptomatic child with hypoxia and consists of oral therapy with corticosteroids, to suppress the lymphocytic proliferation.[258] Lymphocytic interstitial pneumonitis has been associated in some studies with a better prognosis than other HIV-related manifestations such as encephalopathy or PCP, with a median survival of 72 months after diagnosis compared with 1 and 11 months, respectively.[260]

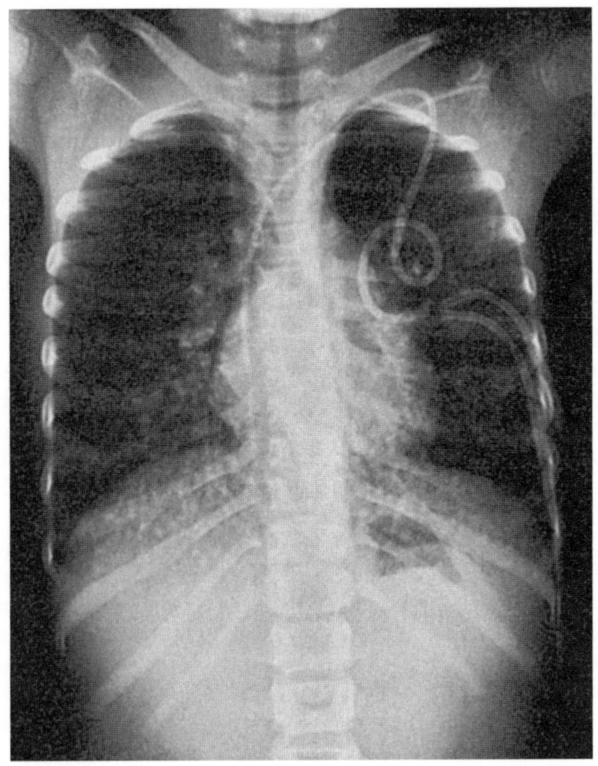

Figure 21–2 Chest radiograph of an 8-year-old girl with severe lymphocytic interstitial pneumonitis who is oxygen and steroid dependent.

Cardiovascular Complications

Cardiovascular abnormalities are seen in more than 50% of HIV-infected adults and have been described in children.[261,262] A progressive left ventricular dilatation and an increase in ventricular afterload were demonstrated in a group of 51 children with symptomatic HIV disease but with a normal initial echocardiogram.[262] Clinical manifestations include hepatosplenomegaly, tachypnea, and tachycardia, often with an S_3 gallop or another arrhythmia. Postmortem examination is remarkable for biventricular dilatation with grossly unremarkable valves and coronary arteries and, less frequently, a pericardial effusion. Cardiomyopathy is more commonly found in children with HIV-related encephalopathy (30%) than in those without this manifestation (2%).[227]

Microscopically, a hypertrophy of the myocardium with only rare foci of inflammatory lymphocytic infiltrates is usually present.[263,264] HIV RNA can be demonstrated in only a small number of cells, probably representing macrophages, monocytes, or endothelial cells, but the distribution does not correlate with the structural damage.[265,266]

Another poorly understood phenomenon is the formation of aneurysms of the cerebral and coronary arteries in association with HIV infection.[230,267,268] A child who developed large cerebral aneurysms, leading to hypothalamic dysfunction and neurologic impairment, has been described.[269]

Pathology of the Gastrointestinal Tract

Dysfunction of the digestive tract is a frequent problem in children with AIDS. In an Italian study of 200 HIV-infected children, Galli and colleagues[270] observed a higher incidence of hepatitis and diarrhea with onset during the first year of life (occurring in 20% to 50% of cases) than at any later time. Commonly encountered pathogens that may cause severe diarrhea are *Cryptosporidium*, *M. avium-intracellulare* complex, *Microsporidium*, *Salmonella*, and *Shigella*.[271] HIV nucleic acids have been found in the feces of children with persistent diarrheal disease.[272] However, many HIV-infected children have a gastrointestinal dysfunction due to disaccharide intolerance, and their clinical status can be improved with careful attention to dietary intake.[272]

Progressive weight loss, anorexia, and sometimes pathogen-negative diarrhea characterize the wasting syndrome often seen in association with HIV disease.[273-276] The cause is not clear but probably represents a combination of a metabolic imbalance with hypermetabolism, disturbed nitrogen balance, and increased cytokine levels. No specific treatment is available, but individual patients may benefit from appetite stimulants, dietary supplements, or parenteral nutrition.[277]

Liver dysfunction resulting from an infection, including that from cytomegalovirus, Epstein-Barr virus, the hepatitis viruses, *M. avium-intracellulare* complex, or HIV-1, is a common feature and can evolve into a chronic hepatitis or cholangitis.[278,279] *Candida albicans* and the herpesviruses are often the cause of infections of the oral cavity and of esophagitis. Esophagitis in the HIV-infected child does not necessarily manifest as the typical symptoms or dysphagia but may be the cause of poor appetite and weight loss. Pancreatitis is a rare complication of HIV infection in children and may occur as the result of opportunistic infections such as cytomegalovirus or as a side effect or therapeutic agents.[280,281]

Nephropathy

Renal disease in children with HIV infection presents most often as focal glomerulosclerosis or mesangial hyperplasia. In one study, 12 of 155 children between the ages of 7 months and 8 years were found to have proteinuria, and 5 of them developed severe renal failure within a year of diagnosis.[282,283] This nephrotic syndrome is often resistant to treatment with corticosteroids, but cyclosporins may induce a remission.[284] IgA nephritis has been observed in a few HIV-infected children and adults, clinically manifesting as recurrent gross hematuria.[285,286] However, an infection with cytomegalovirus or treatment with the protease inhibitor indinavir can also cause hematuria.[167,287,288]

Pathology of Endocrine Organs

Failure to thrive or grow is commonly seen in children with HIV infection. In a study of 35 HIV-positive hemophiliacs, a decrease of more than 15 percentile points in height or weight for age was a predictive marker for children who become symptomatic for AIDS.[289-291] Whereas a few patients may have some dysregulation of thyroid function or a lack of growth hormone, often there is no definable endocrine cause recognizable.[292,293] The exception is the child with adrenal insufficiency, which may be caused by cytomegalovirus infection of the adrenal gland.[294] One child with severe salt craving is described who required therapy with fluorocortisol. In a study of 167 HIV-infected children, Hirschfeld and associates[295] found low levels of free thyroxine in 18% and increased thyrotropin or thyroid binding globulin levels in 30% of children.

Involvement of Lymphoid Organs and Thymus

Thymic abnormalities have been found in 3 of 37 fetuses aborted between 20 and 27 weeks' gestation.[296] This may represent the initial injury to the lymphoid system. In children with AIDS, the thymus can show precocious involution, with marked depletion of lymphocytes and loss of corticomedullary differentiation, or a thymitis, characterized by the presence of lymphoid follicles with germinal centers or a diffuse lymphomononuclear infiltration.[297] An interesting phenomenon is the occurrence of multilocular thymic cysts, often detected as an incidental finding.[297] Lymphadenopathy is common among infected children and adults, and lymphoid organs function as reservoirs for HIV-1.[298-301]

Hematologic Problems

Anemia is the most common hematologic disorder observed in HIV-infected children, with the incidence depending on the severity of HIV disease, the age group, and the use of antiretroviral therapy.[302-304] In a retrospective study of 75 HIV-infected children, 19.7% had anemia at age 6 months, 32.9% at 9 months, and 37.3% at 12 months.[305] Bone marrow aspirate or biopsy specimens may show lymphoid aggregates, some degree of dysplasia, or an ineffective erythropoiesis.[306] Pure red cell aplasia from acute or persistent B19 parvovirus infection has been described in some HIV-infected children and adults and should be considered when the red blood cell production rate is less than expected for the degree of anemia.[307-309]

A white blood cell count of less than 3000 cells/mm^3 has been observed in 26% to 38% of untreated pediatric patients, and neutropenia, defined as an absolute neutrophil count of less than 1500 cells/mm^3, has been found in 43%.[302-304] This can result from HIV infection, infection with opportunistic pathogens such as *M. avium-intracellulare* complex or cytomegalovirus, or therapy with a myelotoxic drug, including zidovudine.

In the patient population at the National Cancer Institute, a platelet count of less than 50,000 cells/mm^3 was found in 19% of the children; thrombocytopenia has also been described in HIV-infected infants.[310-312] Treatment options are similar to those of noninfected children and include intravenous g-globulins, corticosteroids, and WinRho. However, improvement is often best achieved by optimizing the antiretroviral therapy and decreasing the circulating viral load.

Deficiency of the vitamin K–dependent factors II, VII, IX, and X is common in HIV-infected children and can result in a coagulopathy that is relatively easy to correct. Also commonly seen are autoimmune phenomena, such as lupus anticoagulants and antiphospholipid or anti-cardiolipid antibodies.[313-315] Disseminated intravascular coagulopathy has been described as a complication of fulminant infectious conditions, but there are no data to indicate that this complication occurs more frequently in HIV-infected individuals.

Skin

Mucocutaneous disease is very common in pediatric HIV infection but often manifests in an unusual or atypical form.[316,317] The most common lesions with an infectious cause are oral thrush and diaper rash *(C. albicans)*, chickenpox (acute or chronic), and recurrent shingles (varicella zoster virus), and molluscum contagiosum.[318] Bacterial infections and a highly contagious form of scabies have also been reported with some frequency. Severe seborrheic dermatitis or an unspecific intensely pruritic eczematous dermatitis can pose difficult and frustrating clinical problems, necessitating prolonged therapy. Because of the atypical presentations and wide variety of possible causes, it is often prudent to culture lesions for bacteria or for varicella zoster virus or even to perform a scraping or biopsy. Drug eruptions appear to be more common in HIV-infected patients and can develop into a toxic epidermal necrolysis.[316] However, most drug-related rashes resolve after stopping the causative agent.

MORBIDITY, MORTALITY, AND PROGNOSIS

Thanks to more effective treatment of HIV infection and associated complications and to improved guidelines for the prophylaxis of opportunistic infections, major decreases in the morbidity and mortality rates of HIV-infected children and adults have occurred. However, infants who are not known to be HIV infected or do not have access to early intervention are still at high risk for early and severe morbidity and continue to have a high mortality rate.[319-321]

Although the course of HIV infection in children is in general more accelerated than in adults, distinct subgroups are noticeable. Perinatally acquired HIV infection follows a bimodal course, with about one third of the children becoming symptomatic within the first 2 years of life and the remainder in the next several years. Only a minority of patients remains relatively asymptomatic until the age of 8 years or older. In a study of HIV-seropositive and HIV-seronegative women and their newborns in Nairobi, Kenya, no statistically significant difference was found between the groups regarding occurrence of congenital malformations, stillbirths, Apgar score, or gestational age. However, the mean birth weight of singleton neonates of HIV-positive mothers was significantly lower than that of controls.[322] Although not as pronounced, there was also a difference between the height and weight of birth of HIV-infected infants born in the United States compared with uninfected infants.[323] These studies of natural history of perinatal HIV infection were performed before the routine use of antiretroviral therapy in pregnant women and their infants.

In a European study of 392 HIV-infected children, Blanche and colleagues[319] found that 20% of children died or developed an AIDS-defining symptom (CDC category C; see Table 21-3) within the first year of life and 4.7% per year thereafter, reaching a cumulative incidence of 36% by 6 years of age. Two thirds of the children alive at 6 years of age had only minor symptoms, and one third had well preserved CD4 counts (<25%) despite prior clinical manifestations. Children with HIV infection acquired through a transfusion during the neonatal period tend to have a prolonged asymptomatic period.[324]

Both clinical and laboratory factors have been evaluated in regard to their prognostic value. Children born to mothers with low CD4 counts and high viral load tend to progress more rapidly to category C disease or death, emphasizing the importance of diagnosis and adequate treatment of HIV-infected pregnant women.[42,113,325] Early manifestation of clinical symptoms in the infant, especially opportunistic infections, encephalopathy, or hepatosplenomegaly, has repeatedly been associated with a poor prognosis.[305,326,327]

A high virus copy number in the blood has been shown to be a strong predictor for progression of HIV disease.[107,328-330] Infants with very high HIV RNA copy numbers shortly after birth are presumed to have been infected in utero and tend to have early onset of symptoms.[329] Dickover and associates,[329] when calculating HIV-infected infants followed for up to 8 years, found that a 1-log higher HIV-1 RNA copy number at birth increased the relative hazard of developing CDC class A or B symptoms by 40% ($P = .004$), to develop AIDS by 60% ($P = .01$), and the risk of death by 80% ($P = .023$). The peak HIV-1 RNA copy number during the period of primary viremia was also predictive of progression to AIDS (relative hazard 9.9; 95% CI, 1.8%-541%; $P = .008$) and death (relative hazard, 6.9; 95% CI, 1.1%-43.8%; $P = .04$).[329]

PREVENTION

An important goal in the care of HIV-infected people is the prevention of further infections and especially the transmission from mother to infant. Many countries have initiated large educational programs to halt the spread of the epidemic in the heterosexual community. However, the prevalence of HIV infection is so high in certain populations, especially in developing countries, that a change in behavior results in only a very slow decrease in the number of new infections. Identifying pregnant women who are HIV infected is essential for the potential initiation of therapy and for the coordination of optimal prenatal care.[330,331]

The birth order and delivery route appear to play a role in the infection rate. In the absence of zidovudine treatment, HIV infection occurred in 35% of first-born twins and 15% of second-born twins who were delivered vaginally, compared with 16% of first-born and 8% of second-born twins delivered by cesarean section.[50] The European Collaborative Study of 1254 HIV-infected mothers and their children estimated that cesarean section resulted in a 50% reduction of the transmission rate.[333] However, there is a potential bias in the indication for cesarean section. Obstetricians may be less likely to perform a surgical procedure in a mother with advanced HIV infection; emergency cesarean section is more common in the case of larger infants (who are less likely to be infected), and monitoring during vaginal deliveries may itself increase the risk for transmission, especially if fetal scalp electrodes are being used.[51] A European randomized clinical trial of 414 women demonstrated decreased perinatal HIV transmission among infants born by caesarean section versus vaginal delivery (1.7% versus 10.6%).[334,335] It has also been demonstrated that prolonged rupture of membranes (>4 hours before delivery) increases the risk for perinatal transmission and should therefore be avoided.[58,59]

The success of the AIDS Clinical Trials Group 076 (PACTG 076) protocol has had a major impact on the prevention of perinatal transmission of HIV-1 and has resulted in guidelines issued by the CDC.[18-21] In that landmark study, pregnant HIV-infected women received oral zidovudine starting at 14 to 34 weeks' gestation and intravenous zidovudine during labor and delivery, whereas the infants were treated with 6 weeks of oral zidovudine post partum (Table 21-6). This resulted in a 67% reduction in the perinatal transmission rate, from 25% to 8.3% ($P = .00006$).[19] It has also been demonstrated that a high maternal plasma concentration of HIV-1 is a risk factor for transmission to the infant.[13] The identification of HIV-infected pregnant women and their prompt treatment has already led to a marked decrease in the number of newly HIV-infected children in industrialized countries.[336,337]

Table 21–6 Pediatric AIDS Clinical Trials Group 076 Regimen

Time of Zidovudine Administration	Regimen
Anterpartum	100 mg zidovudine five times daily, initiated at 14-34 wk of gestation and continued throughout pregnancy
Intrapartum	During labor, intravenous administration of zidovudine in a 1-hr initial dose of 2 mg/kg, followed by continuous infusion of 1 mg/kg per hr until delivery
Postpartum	Oral zidovudine to the newborn (zidovudine syrup at 2 mg/kg per dose every 6 hr) for the first 6 wk of life, beginning at 8-12 hr after birth. If an infant cannot tolerate oral zidovudine, it can be given intravenously at a dosage of 1.5 mg/kg every 6 hr

From Centers for Disease Control and Prevention. Public Health Service task force recommendations for the use of antiretroviral drugs in pregnant women infected with HIV-1 for maternal health and for reducing perinatal HIV-1 transmission in the United States. MMWR Morb Mortal Wkly Rep 47:1-31, 1998.

This treatment regimen is not feasible for developing countries, where 1600 new perinatal infections occur per day. Discussions regarding the ethics of clinical trials in developing countries, especially trials involving a placebo group, occurred early in the course of developing strategies appropriate for developing countries.[338] Ultimately, a number of randomized clinical trials conducted in some of these countries led to a good understanding of the benefits and obstacles in developing effective and sustainable perinatal prevention programs. An attempt to decrease the transmission rate by cleansing the birth canal with dilute chlorhexidine solutions has unfortunately not been successful, although higher concentrations of chlorhexidine have been found to be safe and tolerable and may be studied as potential interventions.[52-56] Results from a study performed in Thailand as a collaboration between the Thailand Ministry of Health and the CDC demonstrated a 50% reduction in perinatal HIV transmission in a non–breast-feeding population.[22] This trial enrolled non–breast-feeding women who were treated with zidovudine (300 mg twice daily) beginning at week 36 of gestation. During labor and delivery, the oral dose of zidovudine was increased to 300 mg every 3 hours; the newborns were not treated. The estimated efficacy of this therapy was 51% (decrease from 18.6% transmission rate in placebo group to 9.2% in treated group). Although this transmission rate is somewhat higher than the one reported with the PACTG 076 regimen, it indicates that a two-part regimen without the intravenous and postnatal component (a more feasible alternative for developing countries) merits further investigation. Other studies, particularly in a variety of African countries, have demonstrated substantial reductions in perinatal transmission, especially with a simple and inexpensive two-dose nevirapine regimen studied in Uganda. This trial (HIVNET 012) demonstrated a 47% reduction in transmission at 14 to 16 weeks of age and a 41% reduction by 18 months of age when the mother was given a single 200-mg nevirapine tablet at the onset of labor and when a single 2-mg/kg oral dose of nevirapine suspension was given to the neonate at 72 hours after birth or at discharge from the hospital.[24,25]

A major challenge in the prevention of perinatal HIV transmission is the management of breast-feeding transmission in settings where replacement feeding is not feasible. The risks of acquiring HIV infection through breast-feeding may be lower than the risk of death from diarrheal diseases and malnutrition in areas where replacement feeding is not available or unsafe. Decision models to determine the optimal choice of interventions to reduce breast-feeding transmission have been proposed.[341] For developing areas of the world, the WHO recommends exclusive breast-feeding through the first 6 months of life with early weaning in countries where replacement feeding is "acceptable, feasible, affordable, sustainable, and safe."[342]

Immunoglobulins of the IgG class are readily transported through the placenta, and passive immunization of the mother may protect the fetus, a model that has been extensively used in the prevention of neonatal hepatitis B infection. Passive immunization of the fetus in combination with antiretroviral therapy has been studied in a U.S. study called ACTG 185. Pilot studies evaluating the safety and toxicity of highly purified human immune globulin prepared from asymptomatic HIV-seropositive persons were conducted and demonstrated that HIV immune globulin (HIVIG) appeared to be safe and well tolerated.[339,340] However, the results of ACTG 185 demonstrated no decrease in the perinatal transmission rate because of the widespread concurrent use of antiretroviral therapy among pregnant HIV-infected women in the United States.[343]

TREATMENT

Supportive Care and General Management

Optimizing prenatal care, including nutrition, avoidance of drugs and other harmful substances, and recognition and treatment of concurrent infections, is crucial to prevent the premature delivery of children with low birth weight. The general care of the newborn and infant is not different for children born to seropositive mothers, but special attention should be given to the documentation of developmental milestones, frequency and course of infections, and nutritional status.

The AAP recommends routine immunizations with some modifications for all seropositive children, whether they are infected or not.[79] Similar to other newborns, children born to HIV-infected mothers should receive hepatitis B vaccinations, but if the mother is HBsAg positive, the child should also receive HBIG within 12 hours after birth. The current recommendation is that live virus vaccine (oral poliovirus) or live bacterial vaccines (bacillus Calmette-Guérin) should not be given to patients with HIV infection. The exception is MMR, because the risk for measles in immunocompromised children is much higher than the risk associated with the vaccination, although only children with mild to moderate immunosuppression should have the MMR vaccine.[176] However, varicella-zoster immunization is contraindicated in HIV-infected children and adults. A recommended prophylaxis regimen in HIV-infected infants is the administration of intravenous immunoglobulin (IGIV) or specific hyperimmune globulin within 72 to 96 hours after the exposure to varicella-zoster virus or measles.[160,344] Immunization with the conjugated pneumoccocal vaccine series may be started at 2 months of age. Alternatively, children older than 2 years with HIV infection should be administered the 23-valent polysaccharide pneumococcal vaccine, and revaccination should be offered after 3 to 5 years in children younger than 10 years and after 5 years in older children.[160] However, prior immunization does not give complete protection from further infection, as has been described for pertussis occurring in previously immunized children.[345]

The monthly administration of IGIV has been studied in asymptomatic and symptomatic children with HIV infection. IGIV has been shown to prevent serious bacterial infections in patients with congenital immunodeficiencies. However, in a group of children who did not receive any antiretroviral treatment, only children with a CD4 count of 200 cells/mm^3 or more appeared to benefit from monthly IGIV administration.[346] A study evaluating children receiving antiretroviral therapy did not find a statistically significant difference between children who received IGIV and children treated with placebo (albumin), as long as they were also receiving PCP prophylaxis with TMP-SMX. The current recommendation is to use prophylactic IGIV (400 mg/kg per dose every 28 days) in HIV-infected children with hypogammaglobulinemia, poor functional antibody performance (i.e., lack of antibody response after immunizations), or significant recurrent infections despite therapy with appropriate antibiotics.[160]

Prophylactic measurements for the prevention of PCP have been discussed previously. Prophylaxis for *M. tuberculosis* exposure follows the guidelines used for immunocompetent children, but all children born to HIV-infected mothers should have a purified protein derivative test placed at or before 9 to 12 months of age and should be retested every 2 to 3 years.[160] Prophylaxis with clarithromycin or azithromycin for *M. avium-intracellulare* complex infection should be offered to children younger than 12 months if their CD4 count is less than 750 cells/µL, children 1 to 2 years old with CD4 counts less than 500 cells/µL, children 2 to 6 years old with CD4 counts less than 75 µL, and children older than 6 years if the CD4 count is less than 50 cells/µL.[160]

The evaluation and therapy for an infectious complication in the HIV-infected child mandates a high level of suspicion for unusual presentations, an aggressive approach for the establishment of the diagnosis, and the use of intravenous antibiotics, at least during the initial days. Chronic and recurrent infections can compromise the nutritional status of the child and influence the neurodevelopmental state. However, these symptoms are also typical for progressive HIV infection and should be monitored carefully.

Antiretroviral Therapy—General Guidelines

As our knowledge about the dynamics of viral replication and its implications for disease progression and prognosis has evolved, it has become clear that early and aggressive therapy offers the potential benefit of a prolonged asymptomatic time period. Panels of experts have developed guidelines for the use of antiretroviral agents in children, adolescents, and adults, including pregnant women, with HIV infection.[21,347,348] The indications for the initiation of antiretroviral therapy include clinical, immunologic, and virologic parameters (Table 21-7). Pediatric HIV experts agree that infected infants with clinical symptoms of HIV disease or with evidence of immune compromise should be treated, but there remains controversy regarding treatment of asymptomatic infants with normal immunologic status. Guidelines from The Working Group on Antiretroviral Therapy and Medical Management of HIV-Infected Children recommend initiation of therapy for infants younger than 12 months who have clinical or immunologic symptoms of HIV disease, regardless of HIV RNA level, and consideration of therapy for HIV-infected infants younger than 12 months who are asymptomatic and have normal immune parameters (see Table 21-7). Because of the high risk for rapid progression of HIV disease, many experts would treat all HIV-infected infants younger than 12 months, regardless of clinical, immunologic, or virologic parameters. Other experts would treat all infected infants younger than 6 months old and use clinical and immunologic parameters and assessment of adherence issues for decisions regarding initiation of therapy

Table 21–7 Indications for the Initiation of Antiretroviral Therapy

Initiation of Therapy

These recommendations are continuously updated by the Panel on Clinical Practices for Treatment of HIV Infection and reflect the opinions of the Panel. For information on a diversity of recommendations from other HIV experts and for the most up-to-date recommendations, the Panel summary statements can be viewed at http://aidsinfo.nih.gov/guidelines/.

Infants < 12 Months Old

- All HIV-infected infants < 12 months old, with clinical or immunologic symptoms of HIV disease, regardless of HIV RNA level, should be treated.
- Consideration of therapy should be made for those who are asymptomatic and have normal immune parameters

Children > 12 Months Old

- Therapy should be started for all children > 12 months old with AIDS (clinical category C [see Table 21-3]) or severe immune suppression (immune category 3)
- Therapy should be considered for children who have
  - Mild to moderate clinical symptoms (clinical categories A or B [see Table 21-3])
  - Moderate immunologic suppression (immune category 2)
  - And/or confirmed plasma HIV RNA levels ≥ 100,000 copies/mL

From Panel on Clinical Practices for Treatment of HIV Infection. Guidelines for the Use of Antiretroviral Agents in HIV-1 Infected Adolescents and Adults. http://aidsinfo.nih.gov/guidelines/, accessed January 2004.

in infants 6 to 12 months old. The Working Group recommends that treatment should be started for all children older than 12 months with AIDS (clinical category C) or severe immune suppression (immune category 3) and be considered for children who have mild to moderate clinical symptoms (clinical categories A or B), moderate immunologic suppression (immune category 2), or confirmed plasma HIV RNA levels higher than 100,000 copies/mL (see Table 21-7). Many experts would defer treatment in asymptomatic children older than 1 year with normal immune status in situations in which the risk for clinical disease progression is low (e.g., HIV RNA < 100,000 copies/mL) and when other factors (i.e., concern for adherence, safety, and persistence of antiretroviral response) favor postponing treatment. In such cases, the health care provider should closely monitor virologic, immunologic, and clinical status.

Monotherapy is no longer considered appropriate treatment for the HIV-infected child or adult. The only exception is the use of zidovudine monotherapy in infants of indeterminate HIV status during the first 6 weeks of life as part of the regimen to prevent perinatal transmission. As soon as a child is proved to be infected, therapy should be changed to a combination of agents.[348] Based on results from trials in adults, a recommended three-drug combination provides the best opportunity to preserve immune function and to prevent disease progression. This therapy should include a highly active protease inhibitor plus two dideoxynucleoside reverse transcriptase inhibitors (NRTIs) as the initial therapeutic regimen or two NRTIs and a non-nucleoside reverse transcriptase inhibitor (NNRTI).[348] As of January 2004, 20 antiretroviral drugs were approved for use in the United States in HIV-infected adolescents and adults; of those, 12 have approved pediatric indications. Therapeutic drugs fall into four major classes based on mechanism of action: nucleoside analogues or nucleotide reverse transcriptase inhibitors (NRTIs, NtRTIs), NNRTIs, protease inhibitors, and fusion inhibitors. More detailed information about these agents can be obtained at the U.S. federal AIDS information website (http://aidsinfo.nih.gov/guidelines). The most pediatric experience with NRTIs is with zidovudine (ZDV), lamivudine (3TC), didanosine (ddI), and stavudine (d4T). All are available in a liquid formulation. Dual NRTI combinations are the backbone of highly active antiretroviral therapy (HAART) in adults and children. The combinations of NRTIs with the most data available include zidovudine and didanosine (ZDV/ddI), zidovudine and lamivudine (ZDV/3TC), and stavudine and lamivudine (d4T/3TC). Added to this dual NRTI backbone is an NNRTI or a protease inhibitor The acceptable NNRTIs for pediatric use are nevirapine or efavirenz (approved for children > 3 years old); efavirenz is not available in a liquid formulation. Delavirdine is the other available NNRTI but is not approved for pediatric use. The one available NtNRTI, tenofovir, is approved only for adult use, and pediatric trials are underway. The protease inhibitors recommended for pediatric use are nelfinavir, ritonavir, and lopinavir plus ritonavir. These are available in powder or liquid formulations. Other protease inhibitors available for pediatric use are available in capsule formulation only and include indinavir, saquinavir, and amprenavir. However, no data are available for the long-term tolerance and efficacy of any of these combinations in children. Certain combinations are not recommended because of overlapping toxicities, including zalcitabine plus didanosine, zalcitabine plus stavudine, and zalcitabine plus lamivudine. The combination of stavudine and zidovudine is not recommended because of their antagonism.

The most commonly used antiretroviral agents in newborns and infants, the NRTIs zidovudine, didanosine, lamivudine, the NNRTI nevirapine, and the protease inhibitors nelfinavir and ritonavir, are briefly reviewed. More extensive reviews are available in specific textbooks or the current recommendations from the CDC and the federal guidelines website (http://aidsinfo.nih.gov).[348,349] Because the standards of care are still evolving, collaboration between the child's primary health care provider and an HIV treatment center is strongly suggested. Whenever possible, children should be enrolled in clinical trials; access and information can be obtained by calling 1-800-TRIALS-A (AIDS Clinical Trials Group [ACTG]), or 301-402-0696 (HIV & AIDS Malignancy Branch, National Cancer Institute).

Zidovudine

Only limited data are available regarding the appropriate dosing of antiretroviral drugs in the neonate. Zidovudine does cross the placenta and can be measured in amniotic fluid, cord blood, and fetal organs.[350,351] The total body clearance and terminal half-life of zidovudine is similar in nonpregnant women and in women during the third trimester of pregnancy, and the half-life in the neonate is about 10-fold longer than in the mother.[352,353] Elimination of the drug and its main metabolite is markedly prolonged during the first 24 to 36 hours of life, with a mean serum half-life after maternal ingestion of 14.4 ± 7.5 hours.[350,354-356] The total-body clearance of zidovudine increases rapidly within the first few weeks of life from 10.9 mL/min/kg in infants 14 days old or younger to 19.0 mL/min/kg in older infants ($P < .0001$).[357,358] Oral bioavailability decreases from 89% in the younger group to 61% in infants older than 14 days.

Some studies have demonstrated that zidovudine is incorporated into the DNA of newborn mice and monkeys and into the nuclear DNA of cord blood samples drawn from children whose mothers were being treated with zidovudine.[359,360] Studies of the offspring of mice who had been treated with zidovudine during the last trimester of pregnancy revealed an increased risk for developing tumors of the liver, lung, and reproductive organs. However, a similar study performed by Burroughs Wellcome, the manufacturer of zidovudine, was not able to support these findings. A panel convened by the National Institutes of Health, although acknowledging the validity of the findings, recognized that the benefit of preventing transmission of HIV disease in most children outweighs the potential concerns about carcinogenicity.

Common side effects of zidovudine include bone marrow suppression, myopathy, and liver toxicity.[357,361,362] Severe, unusual toxicity includes lactic acidosis and severe hepatomegaly with steatosis.

The recommended dosage of zidovudine (in combination with other antiretroviral agents as discussed earlier[348]) is as follows:

- Premature babies (under study): 1.5 mg/kg per dose given intravenously or 2 mg/kg given orally every 12 hours from birth to 2 weeks of age; then increase to 2 mg/kg per dose every 8 hours at 2 weeks (neonates ≥30 weeks gestational age) or at 4 weeks (neonates <30 weeks gestational age)
- Neonatal dosage: 2 mg/kg per dose every 6 hours given orally or 1.5 mg/kg every 6 hours administered intravenously
- Pediatric dosage: 160 mg/m^2 per dose every 8 hours given orally (range, 90 to 180 mg/m^2 every 6 to 8 hours); intermittent intravenous dosing at 120 mg/m^2 every 6 hours or continuous intravenous dosing at 20 mg/m^2/hour

Didanosine

Didanosine has a plasma half-life of about an hour but, in contrast to zidovudine, a lower oral absorption rate (19% ± 17%) that is further characterized by high interpatient variability and a low penetration rate into cerebrospinal fluid.[363] Some of the variation in bioavailability could be because didanosine is acid labile and has to be taken with an antacid. The amount of antacid necessary to neutralize gastric acidity may vary among patients. Pharmacokinetic data for neonates or young infants are limited because of these problems, but data from the macaque animal model indicate limited transplacental transport.[364-366]

Side effects of didanosine include dose-related peripheral neuropathy, diarrhea, abdominal pain, nausea, vomiting, pancreatitis, retinal depigmentation, and increased liver enzymes.[281,367-369] Cases of lactic acidosis and severe hepatomegaly with steatosis have been reported.

The recommended dosage of didanosine (in combination with other antiretroviral agents as discussed earlier[348]) is as follows:

- Premature babies: no data available
- Neonatal dosage (infants younger than 90 days old): 50 mg/m^2 per dose every 12 hours given orally
- Pediatric dosage: 120 mg/m^2 per dose every 12 hours orally (range, from 90 to 150 mg/m^2 per dose every 8 to 12 hours)

Lamivudine

Lamivudine has been approved for the use in combination with zidovudine. Lamivudine at doses between 0.5 to 20 mg/kg/day given to children in two daily doses was well tolerated.[370,371] Side effects include hyperactivity (2%), increase in liver function to more than 10 times normal (3%), neutropenia (3%), and reversible pancreatitis (8%). Other less common toxicities include peripheral neuropathy and lactic acidosis with severe hepatomegaly and steatosis. Lamivudine was rapidly absorbed after oral administration and 66% ± 25% of the oral dose was absorbed.

The recommended dosage of lamivudine (in combination with other antiretroviral agents as discussed earlier[348]) is as follows:

- Premature babies: no data available
- Neonatal dosage (infants < 30 days old): 2 mg/kg per dose given twice daily orally
- Pediatric dosage: 4 mg/kg per dose administered twice daily

Nevirapine

Nevirapine is also a reverse transcriptase inhibitor but, unlike zidovudine, didanosine, and lamivudine, does not belong to the dideoxynucleoside family of drugs.[372] Nevirapine therapy results in a rapid and marked decrease in HIV-1 RNA concentrations in plasma, which makes it a useful agent for the prevention of vertical transmission.[373] However, a drawback of nevirapine is that resistance develops rapidly during monotherapy because of several possible mutations.[346,374] Nevirapine was well tolerated in pediatric trials.[375,376] At doses of more than 240 mg/m^2/day, 5 of 10 children experienced a prolonged reduction in p24 antigenemia. Eight infants born to seven HIV-infected mothers were studied after the mothers received 200 mg of nevirapine during labor. The infants were treated with 2-mg/kg oral doses of nevirapine at a mean of 56.6 hours after birth.[377] No side effects were observed in mothers or children, and with a dose of nevirapine during labor and another 48 to 72 hours after birth, nevirapine levels of more than 100 ng/mL (10 times the IC_{50}) were achieved throughout the first week of life.

The recommended dosage of nevirapine (in combination with other antiretroviral agents as discussed earlier[348]) is as follows:

- Premature babies: no data available
- Neonatal dosage (under study in PACTG 356): 5 mg/kg per dose given once daily for 14 days, followed by 120 mg/m^2 every 12 hours for 14 days, followed by 200 mg/m^2 per dose every 12 hours
- Pediatric dosage: 120 to 200 mg/m^2 per dose every 12 hours. *Note*: Therapy should be initiated at 120 mg/m^2 per dose (maximum dose 200 mg every 12 hours) once

daily for 14 days to decrease the risk of cutaneous reactions.

Nelfinavir

Nelfinavir, a protease inhibitor approved for the use in children and adults with HIV infection, was studied in an open-label, uncontrolled clinical trial of 38 children 2 to 13 years old.[378] Nelfinavir should be taken with food to optimize absorption of the drug. The most common adverse event is diarrhea of mild to moderate intensity. Less common toxicities include asthenia, abdominal pain, rash, exacerbation of chronic liver disease, and fat redistribution and lipid abnormalities. Nelfinavir, as with all protease inhibitors, is metabolized by the hepatic cytochrome P-450 enzyme system, which can lead to drug interactions with a variety of commonly used medications.[379]

The recommended dosage of nelfinavir (in combination with other antiretroviral agents as discussed see earlier[348]) is as follows:

Premature babies: no data available
Neonatal dosage (under study in PACTG 353): 40 mg/kg every 12 hours
Pediatric dosage (limited data): 20 to 30 mg/kg per dose three times daily

Ritonavir

Ritonavir, another protease inhibitor approved for use in children, is extensively metabolized by the P-450 enzyme system, and drug interactions are very common.[379] In a phase I/II study performed by the National Cancer Institute, HIV-infected children between 6 months and 18 years old were eligible to enroll at four different dose levels of ritonavir oral solution (250, 300, 350, and 400 mg/m^2 given every 12 hours).[380] Ritonavir was administered alone for the first 12 weeks and then in combination with zidovudine or didanosine, or both. Dose-related nausea, diarrhea, and abdominal pain were the most common toxicities. Less common toxicities include circumoral paresthesias, increase in liver enzymes, fat redistribution, and lipid abnormalities. CD4 cell counts increased by a median of 79 cells/mm^3 after 4 weeks of monotherapy and were maintained throughout the study. Plasma HIV RNA levels decreased by 1 to 2 $\log_{10}$ copies/mL within 4 to 8 weeks of ritonavir monotherapy, and this level was sustained in patients enrolled at the highest dose level of 400 mg/m^2 for the 24-week period.

The recommended dosage of ritonavir (in combination with other antiretroviral agents as discussed earlier[348]) is as follows:

Premature babies: no data available
Neonatal dosage: no data available but being studied under PACTG 354
Pediatric dosage (limited data): 400 mg/m^2 (range, 350 to 400 mg/m^2) every 12 hours orally. To minimize nausea and vomiting, initiate therapy at 250 mg/m^2 every 12 hours and increase stepwise over 5 days to full dose.

FUTURE GOALS

The past decade has brought major advances in the understanding, prevention, and treatment of HIV disease. Application of the PACTG 076 protocol has led to a marked decrease in the perinatal transmission rate of HIV infection in industrialized countries. Better understanding of the interactions between viral load and immunologic status and their implications for prognosis has prompted earlier and more aggressive antiretroviral therapy. The advent of the protease inhibitors and the accelerated approval of antiretroviral drugs both children and adults have broadened the therapeutic armamentarium. However, many problems remain.

The most urgent need continues to be the prevention of further spread of HIV infection among adults and from a mother to her unborn child. Almost 2 decades after the description of the clinical syndrome of AIDS, we are still dealing with an ever-growing pandemic, affecting certain minorities, both sexes, and all age groups and social levels but targeting mainly the developing countries with already limited resources. The staggering demands put on public health systems and their financial resources could easily create tensions regarding the distribution of available funds. Before the widespread use of combination therapy and protease inhibitors, the estimated lifetime cost of hospital-based care for children with HIV infection was $408,307.[381] Assuming that hospital-based care represents 83% of the total charges, the mean overall lifetime cost would be about $500,000. The cost of current antiretroviral therapy is even higher and life expectancy longer, although this is partially offset by fewer hospitalizations. It has become very clear that major efforts are needed to make prevention and therapy for HIV infection feasible and affordable for developing nations, because they have the highest numbers of infected people with the fewest financial and organizational resources.

New and different antiretroviral agents are needed because of toxicities and emergence of resistance to provide more effective or even permanent inhibition of viral replication. We need to know the pharmacokinetic properties of drugs when given to the pregnant mother, the neonate, or the very young infant. Progress has been made in the early recognition and prophylaxis of opportunistic infections. However, as patients with HIV infection survive longer, problems with resistant organisms, multidrug allergies, altered organ function, and long-term side effects of medications emerge and complicate adequate therapy.

Advocacy for children and pregnant women, ensuring equal access to new drugs and providing sound data regarding dosing and potential toxicities, continues to be important. The U.S. Food and Drug Administration allows the approval of drugs for use in children based on efficacy data gathered in adults if the disease in children and adults is reasonably similar and if the pharmaceutical companies provide dosing (pharmacokinetic) and safety (toxicity) data from controlled trials performed in an adequate number of children. The treatment and care of HIV-infected children and adults has become increasingly complex, and close collaboration with physicians and centers specialized in their care is highly recommended.

REFERENCES

1. Centers for Disease Control. Unexplained immunodeficiency and opportunistic infections in infants—New York, New Jersey, California. MMWR Morb Mortal Wkly Rep 31:665-667, 1982.

2. Ammann AJ, Cowan MJ, Wara DW, et al. Acquired immunodeficiency in an infant: possible transmission by means of blood products. Lancet 1:956-958, 1983.
3. Oleske J, Minnefor A, Cooper R, et al. Immune deficiency syndrome in children. JAMA 249:2345-2349, 1983.
4. Rubinstein A, Sicklick M, Gupta A, et al. Acquired immunodeficiency with reversed T4/T8 ratios in infants born to promiscuous and drug-addicted mothers. JAMA 249:2350-2356, 1983.
5. Centers for Disease Control and Prevention. HIV/AIDS Surveillance report. 14:1-48, 2002.
6. Joint United Nations Programme on HIV/AIDS (UNAIDS), World Health Organization (WHO). AIDS Epidemic Update 2003. Geneva, World Health Organization, 2003.
7. Coleman RL, Wilkinson D. Increasing HIV prevalence in a rural district of South Africa from 1992 through 1995. J Acquir Immune Defic Syndr Hum Retrovirol 16:50-53, 1997.
8. Laga M, De Cock KM, Kaleeba N, et al. HIV/AIDS in Africa: the second decade and beyond. AIDS 11:S1-S53, 1997.
9. Foster G. Today's children—challenges to child health promotion in countries with severe AIDS epidemics. AIDS Care 10(Suppl 1):S17-S23, 1998.
10. Balter M. United Nations: global program struggles to stem the flood of new cases. Science 280:1863-1864, 1998.
11. The European Collaborative Study. Vertical transmission of HIV-1: maternal immune status and obstetric factors. AIDS 10:1675-1681, 1996.
12. The Working Group on Mother-To-Child Transmission of HIV. Rates of mother-to-child transmission of HIV-1 in Africa, America, and Europe: results from 13 perinatal studies. J Acquir Immune Defic Syndr Hum Retrovirol 8:506-510, 1995.
13. Sperling RS, Shapiro DE, Coombs RW, et al. Maternal viral load, zidovudine treatment, and the risk of transmission of human immunodeficiency virus type 1 from mother to infant. Pediatric AIDS Clinical Trials Group Protocol 076 Study Group. N Engl J Med 335:1621-1629, 1996.
14. Abrams EJ, Weedon J, Steketee RW, et al. Association of human immunodeficiency virus (HIV) load early in life with disease progression among HIV-infected infants. New York City Perinatal HIV Transmission Collaborative Study Group. J Infect Dis 178:101-8, 1998.
15. Garcia PM, Kalish LA, Pitt J, et al. Maternal levels of plasma human immunodeficiency virus type 1 RNA and the risk of perinatal transmission. Women and Infants Transmission Study Group. N Engl J Med 341:394-402, 1999.
16. John GC, Nduati RW, Mbori-Ngacha DA, et al. Correlates of mother-to-child human immunodeficiency virus type 1 (HIV-1) transmission: association with maternal plasma HIV-1 RNA load, genital HIV-1 DNA shedding, and breast infections. J Infect Dis 183:206-212, 2001. Epub Dec 15, 2000.
17. Montano M, Russell M, Gilbert P, et al. Comparative prediction of perinatal human immunodeficiency virus type 1 transmission, using multiple virus load markers. J Infect Dis 188:406-13, 2003. Epub Jul 14, 2003.
18. Connor EM, Sperling RS, Gelber R, et al. Reduction of maternal-infant transmission of immunodeficiency virus type 1 with zidovudine treatment. N Engl J Med 331:1173-1180, 1994.
19. Connor EM, Mofenson LK. Zidovudine for the reduction of perinatal human immunodeficiency virus transmission: Pediatric AIDS Clinical Trials Group protocol 076—results and treatment recommendations. Pediatr Infect Dis J 14:536-541, 1995.
20. Centers for Disease Control and Prevention. Recommendations of the U.S. Public Health Service Task Force on the use of zidovudine to reduce perinatal transmission of human immunodeficiency virus. MMWR Morb Mortal Wkly Rep 43:1-20, 1994.
21. Centers for Disease Control and Prevention. U.S. Public Health Service Task Force Recommendations for use of antiretroviral drugs in pregnant HIV-1–infected women for maternal health and interventions to reduce perinatal HIV-1 transmission in the United States. MMWR Morb Mortal Wkly Rep 51(RR18);1-38, 2002.
22. Shaffer N, Chuachoowong R, Mock PA, et al. Short-course zidovudine for perinatal HIV-1 transmission in Bangkok, Thailand: a randomised controlled trial. Bangkok Collaborative Perinatal HIV Transmission Study Group. Lancet 353:773-780, 1999.
23. Wiktor SZ, Ekpini E, Karon JM, et al. Short-course oral zidovudine for prevention of mother-to-child transmission of HIV-1 in Abidjan, Côte d'Ivoire: a randomised trial. Lancet. 6;353:781-785, 1999.
24. Guay L, Musoke P, Fleming T, et al. Intrapartum and neonatal single-dose nevirapine compared with zidovudine for prevention of mother-to-child transmission of HIV-1 in Kampala, Uganda: HIVNET 012 randomised trial. Lancet 354:795-802, 1999.
25. Jackson JB, Musoke P, Fleming T, et al. Intrapartum and neonatal single-dose nevirapine compared with zidovudine for prevention of mother-to-child transmission of HIV-1 in Kampala, Uganda: 18-month follow-up of the HIVNET 012 randomised trial. Lancet 1362:859-868, 2003.
26. Nuovo GJ, Forde A, MacConnell P, Fahrenwald R. In situ detection of PCR-amplified HIV-1 nucleic acids and tumor necrosis factor cDNA in cervical tissues. Am J Pathol 143:40-48, 1993.
27. Royce RA, Sena A, Cates W, Cohen MS. Sexual transmission of HIV. N Engl J Med 336:1072-1078, 1997.
28. Sprecher S, Soumenkoff G, Puissant F, Degueldre M. Vertical transmission of HIV in 15-week fetus. Lancet 2:288-289, 1986.
29. Jovaisas E, Koch MA, Schäfer A, et al. LAV/HTLV-III in 20-week fetus. Lancet 2:1129, 1985.
30. Mano H, Chermann JC. Fetal human immunodeficiency virus type 1 infection of different organs in the second trimester. AIDS Res Hum Retroviruses 7:83-88, 1991.
31. Mundy DC, Schinazi RF, Gerber AR, et al. Human immunodeficiency virus isolated from amniotic fluid. Lancet 2:459-460, 1987.
32. Lewis SH, Reynolds-Kohler C, Fox HE, Nelson JA. HIV-1 in trophoblastic and villous Hofbauer cells, and haematological precursors in eight-week fetuses. Lancet 335:565-568, 1990.
33. Amirhessami-Aghili N, Spector SA. Human immunodeficiency virus type 1 infection of human placenta: Potential route for fetal infection. J Virol 65:2231-2236, 1991.
34. Zachar V, Thomas RA, Jones T, Goustin AS. Vertical transmission of HIV: detection of proviral DNA in placental trophoblasts. AIDS 8:129-130, 1994.
35. Mattern CFT, Murray K, Jensen A, et al. Localization of human immunodeficiency virus core antigen in term human placentas. Pediatrics 89:207-209, 1992.
36. St. Louis ME, Kamenga M, Brown C, et al. Risk for perinatal HIV-1 transmission according to maternal immunologic, virologic, and placental factors. JAMA 269:2853-2859, 1993.
37. Thomas PA, Weedon J, Krasinski K, et al. Maternal predictors of perinatal human immunodeficiency virus transmission. Pediatr Infect Dis J 13:489-495, 1994.
38. Borkowsky W, Krasinski K, Cao Y, et al. Correlation of perinatal transmission of human immunodeficiency virus type 1 with maternal viremia and lymphocyte phenotypes. J Pediatr 125:345-351, 1994.
39. Fang G, Burger H, Grimson R, et al. Maternal plasma human immunodeficiency virus type 1 RNA level: A determinant and projected threshold for mother-to-child transmission. Proc Natl Acad Sci U S A 92:12100-12104, 1995.
40. Mayaux MJ, Blanche S, Rouzioux C, et al. Maternal factors associated with perinatal HIV-1 transmission: the French Cohort Study: 7 years of follow-up observation. J Acquir Immune Defic Syndr Hum Retrovirol 8:188-194, 1995.
41. Cao Y, Krogstad P, Korber BT, et al. Maternal HIV-1 viral load and vertical transmission of infection: the Ariel Project for the prevention of HIV transmission from mother to infant. Nature Med 3:549-552, 1997.
42. Lambert G, Thea DM, Pliner V, et al. Effect of maternal CD4+ cell count, acquired immunodeficiency syndrome, and viral load on disease progression in infants with perinatally acquired human immunodeficiency virus type 1 infection. J Pediatr 130:890-897, 1997.
43. D'Arminio Monforte A, Ravizza M, Muggiasca ML, et al. HIV-infected pregnant women: possible predictors of vertical transmission. Presented before the 7th International Conference on AIDS, Florence, Italy, 1991.
44. Peckham C, Gibb D. Mother-to-child transmission of the human immunodeficiency virus. N Engl J Med 333:298-302, 1995.
45. Bryson YJ, Luzuriaga K, Sullivan JL, Wara DW. Proposed definition for in utero versus intrapartum transmission of HIV-1. N Engl J Med 327:1246-1247, 1992.
46. Rouzioux C, Costagliola D, Burgard M, et al. Estimated timing of mother-to-child human immunodeficiency virus type 1 (HIV-1) transmission by use of a Markov model. The HIV Infection in Newborns French Collaborative Study Group. Am J Epidemiol 142:1330-1337, 1995.
47. Nesheim SR, Shaffer N, Vink P, et al. Lack of increased risk for perinatal human immunodeficiency virus transmission to subsequent

children born to infected women. Pediatr Infect Dis J 15:886-890, 1996.

48. Young KY, Nelson RP. Discordant human immunodeficiency virus infection in dizygotic twins detected by polymerase chain reaction. Pediatr Infect Dis J 9:454-456, 1990.
49. Goedert JJ, Duliege AM, Amos CI, et al. High risk of HIV-1 infection for first-born twins. Lancet 338:1471-1475, 1991.
50. Duliege A-M, Amos CI, Felton S, et al. Birth order, delivery route, and concordance in the transmission of human immunodeficiency virus type 1 from mothers to twins. J Pediatr 126:625-632, 1995.
51. Mofenson LM. A critical review of studies evaluating the relationship of mode of delivery to perinatal transmission of human immunodeficiency virus. Pediatr Infect Dis J 14:169-177, 1995.
52. Biggar RJ, Miotti PG, Taha TE, et al. Perinatal intervention trial in Africa: effect of a birth canal cleansing intervention to prevent HIV transmission. Lancet 347:1647-1650, 1996.
53. Taha TE, Biggar RJ, Broadhead RL, et al. Effect of cleansing the birth canal with antiseptic solution on maternal and newborn morbidity and mortality in Malawi: clinical trial. BMJ 315:216-219, 1997.
54. Biggar RJ, Miotti PG, Taha TE, et al. Perinatal intervention trial in Africa: effect of a birth canal cleansing intervention to prevent HIV transmission. Lancet 347:1647-1650, 1996.
55. Gaillard P, Mwanyumba F, Verhofstede C, et al. Vaginal lavage with chlorhexidine during labor to reduce mother-to-child HIV transmission: clinical trial in Mombassa, Kenya. AIDS 15:389-396, 2001.
56. Wilson CM, Gray G, Read JS, et al. Tolerance and safety of different concentrations of chlorhexidine for peripartum vaginal and infant washes: HIVNET 025. J Acquir Immune Defic Syndr 35:138-143, 2004.
57. The International Perinatal HIV Group. The mode of delivery and the risk of vertical transmission of human immunodeficiency virus type 1—a meta-analysis of 15 prospective cohort studies. N Engl J Med 340:977-987, 1999.
58. Landesman SH, Kalish LA, Burns DN, et al. Obstetrical factors and the transmission of human immunodeficiency virus type 1 from mother to child. N Engl J Med 334:1617-1623, 1996.
59. International Perinatal HIV Group. Duration of ruptured membranes and vertical transmission of HIV-1: a meta-analysis from 15 prospective cohort studies. AIDS 15:357-368, 2001.
60. Van De Perre P, Simonon A, Msellati P, et al. Postnatal transmission of human immunodeficiency virus type 1 from mother to infant. N Engl J Med 325:593-598, 1991.
61. Van de Perre P, Simonon A, Hitimana D-G, et al. Infective and anti-infective properties of breast milk from HIV-1 infected women. Lancet 341:914-918, 1993.
62. Ruff AJ, Halsey NA, Coberly J, Boulos R. Breast-feeding and maternal-infant transmission of human immunodeficiency virus type 1. J Pediatr 121:325-329, 1992.
63. Thiry L, Sprecher-Goldberger S, Jonckheer T, et al. Isolation of AIDS virus from cell-free breast milk of three healthy virus carriers. Lancet 2:891-892, 1985.
64. Lewis P, Nduati R, Kreiss JK, et al. Cell-free human immunodeficiency virus type 1 in breast milk. J Infect Dis 177:34-39, 1998.
65. Guay LA, Hom DL, Mmiro F, et al. Detection of human immunodeficiency virus type 1 (HIV-1) DNA and p24 antigen in breast milk of HIV-1–infected Ugandan women and vertical transmission. Pediatrics 98:438-444, 1996.
66. de Martino M, Tovo P-A, Tozzi AE, et al. HIV-1 transmission through breast milk: appraisal of risk according to duration of feeding. AIDS 6:991-997, 1992.
67. Bertolli J, St. Louis ME, Simonds RJ, et al. Estimating the timing of mother-to-child transmission of human immunodeficiency virus in a breast-feeding population in Kinshasa, Zaire. J Infect Dis 174:722-726, 1996.
68. Miotti PG, Taha TE, Kumwenda N, et al. HIV transmission through breastfeeding: a study in Malawi. JAMA 282:744-749, 1999.
69. De Cock KM, Fowler MG, Mercier E, et al. Prevention of mother-to-child HIV transmission in resource-poor countries: translating research into policy and practice. JAMA 283:1175-1182, 2000.
70. Lederman SA. Estimating infant mortality from human immunodeficiency virus and other causes in breast-feeding and bottle-feeding populations. Pediatrics 89:290-296, 1992.
71. Bobat R, Moodley D, Coutsoudis A, Coovadia H. Breastfeeding by HIV-1–infected women and outcome in their infants: a cohort study from Durban, South Africa. AIDS 11:1627-1633, 1997.
72. Read JS, for the American Academy of Pediatrics Committee on Pediatric AIDS. Human milk, breastfeeding, and transmission of human immunodeficiency virus type 1 in the United States. Pediatrics 112:1196-1205, 2003.
73. Friedland GH, Saltzman BR, Rogers MF, et al. Lack of transmission of HTLV-III/LAV infection to household contacts of patients with AIDS or AIDS-related complex with oral candidiasis. N Engl J Med 314:334-339, 1986.
74. Mann JM, Quinn TC, Francis H, et al. Prevalence of HTLV-III/LAV in household contacts of patients with confirmed AIDS and controls in Kinshasa, Zaire. JAMA 256:721-724, 1986.
75. Centers for Disease Control and Prevention. Human immunodeficiency virus transmission in household settings—United States. MMWR Morb Mortal Wkly Rep 43:347-356, 1994.
76. Lobato MN, Oxtoby MJ, Augustyniak L, et al. Infection control practices in the home: a survey of households of HIV-infected persons with hemophilia. Infect Control Hosp Epidemiol 17:721-725, 1996.
77. American Academy of Pediatrics Task Force of Pediatric AIDS. Education of children with human immunodeficiency virus infection. Pediatrics 88:645-648, 1991.
78. Committee on Infectious Diseases. Health guidelines for the attendance in day-care and foster care settings of children infected with human immunodeficiency virus. Pediatrics 79:466-470, 1987.
79. American Academy of Pediatrics. Evaluation and medical treatment of the HIV-exposed infant. Pediatrics 99:909-917, 1997.
80. Zeichner SL. The molecular biology of HIV: insights into pathogenesis and targets for therapy. Clin Perinatol 21:39-73, 1994.
81. Pavlakis GN. The molecular biology of human immunodeficiency virus type 1. *In* DeVita VT Jr, Hellman S, Rosenberg SA (eds): AIDS: Biology, Diagnosis, Treatment and Prevention. Philadelphia, Lippincott-Raven, 1997, pp 45-74.
82. Cullen BR. HIV-1 auxiliary proteins: making connections in a dying cell. Cell 93:685-692, 1998.
83. Fauci AS, Pantaleo G, Stanley S, Weissman D. Immunopathogenic mechanisms of HIV infection. Ann Intern Med 124:654-663, 1996.
84. Feng Y, Broder CC, Kennedy PE, Berger EA. HIV-1 entry cofactor: Functional cDNA cloning of a seven-transmembrane G protein–coupled receptor. Science 272:872-877, 1996.
85. Cocchi F, DeVico AL, Garzino-Demo A, et al. The V3 domain of the HIV-1 gp120 envelope glycoprotein is critical for chemokine-mediated blockade of infection. Nat Med 2:1244-1247, 1996.
86. Kinter AL, Ostrowski M, Goletti D, et al. HIV replication in CD4+ T cells of HIV-infected individuals is regulated by a balance between viral suppressive effects of endogenous β-chemokines and the viral inductive effects of other endogenous cytokines. Proc Natl Acad Sci U S A 93:14076-14081, 1996.
87. Lapham CK, Ouyang J, Chandrasekhar B, et al. Evidence for cell-surface association between fusin and the CD4-gp120 complex in human cell lines. Science 274:602-605, 1996.
88. Wu L, Gerard NP, Wyatt R, et al. CD4-induced interaction of primary HIV-1 gp120 glycoproteins with the chemokine receptor CCR-5. Nature 384:179-183, 1996.
89. Rollins BJ. Chemokines. Blood 90:909-928, 1997.
90. Cairns JS, D'Souza MP. Chemokines and HIV-1 second receptors: the therapeutic connection. Nat Med 4:563-568, 1998.
91. Reinhardt PP, Reinhardt B, Lathey JL, Spector SA. Human cord blood mononuclear cells are preferentially infected by non-syncytium-inducing, macrophage-tropic human immunodeficiency virus type 1 isolates. J Clin Microbiol 33:292-297, 1995.
92. Panganiban AT. Retroviral reverse transcription and DNA integration. Virology 1:187-194, 1990.
93. Bushman FD, Fujiwara T, Craigie R. Retroviral DNA integration directed by HIV integration protein in vitro. Science 249:1555-1558, 1990.
94. Brown PO, Bowerman B, Varmus HE, Bishop JM. Retroviral integration: structure of the initial covalent product and its precursor, and a role for the viral IN protein. Proc Natl Acad Sci U S A 86:2525-2529, 1989.
95. Stevenson M, Haggerty S, Lamonica CA, et al. Integration is not necessary for expression of human immunodeficiency virus type 1 protein products. J Virol 64:2421-2425, 1990.
96. Bagasra O, Hauptman SP, Lischner HW, et al. Detection of human immunodeficiency virus type 1 provirus in mononuclear cells by in situ polymerase chain reaction. N Engl J Med 326:1385-1391, 1992.
97. Chevret S, Kirstetter M, Mariotti M, et al. Provirus copy number to predict disease progression in asymptomatic human immunodeficiency virus type 1 infection. J Infect Dis 169:882-885, 1994.
98. Ho DD. Dynamics of HIV-1 replication in vivo. J Clin Invest 99:2565-2567, 1997.

99. Ho DD, Neumann AU, Perelson AS, et al. Rapid turnover of plasma virions and CD4 lymphocytes in HIV-1 infection. Nature 373:123-126, 1995.
100. Perelson AS, Neumann AU, Markowitz M, et al. HIV-1 dynamics in vivo: clearance rate, infected cell life-span, and viral generation time. Science 271:1582-1586, 1996.
101. Perelson AS, Essunger P, Cao Y, et al. Decay characteristics of HIV-1–infected compartments during combination therapy. Nature 387:188-191, 1997.
102. Kohl NE, Emini EA, Schleif WA, et al. Active human immunodeficiency virus protease is required for viral infectivity. Proc Natl Acad Sci U S A 85:4686-4690, 1988.
103. Swanstrom R, Kaplan AH, Manchester M. The aspartic proteinase of HIV-1. Semin Virol 1:175-186, 1990.
104. Perno C-F, Bergamini A, Pesce CD, et al. Inhibition of the protease of human immunodeficiency virus blocks replication and infectivity of the virus in chronically infected macrophages. J Infect Dis 168:1148-1156, 1993.
105. Shearer WT, Quinn TC, LaRussa P, et al. Viral load and disease progression in infants infected with human immunodeficiency virus type 1. N Engl J Med 336:1337-1342, 1997.
106. Palumbo PE, Kwok S, Wesley Y, et al. Viral measurement by polymerase chain reaction-based assays in human immunodeficiency virus–infected infants. J Pediatr 126:592-595, 1995.
107. Mofenson LM, Korelitz J, Meyer WA 3rd, et al. The relationship between serum human immunodeficiency virus type 1 (HIV-1) RNA level, CD4 lymphocyte percent, and long-term mortality risk in HIV-1–infected children. National Institute of Child Health and Human Development Intravenous Immunoglobulin Clinical Trial Study Group. J Infect Dis 175:1029-1038, 1997.
108. Abrams EJ, Weedon J, Steketee RW, et al. Association of human immunodeficiency virus (HIV) load early in life with disease progression among HIV-infected infants. New York City Perinatal HIV Transmission Collaborative Study Group. J Infect Dis 178:101-108, 1998.
109. McIntosh K, Shevitz A, Zaknun D, et al. Age- and time-related changes in extracellular viral load in children vertically infected by human immunodeficiency virus. Pediatr Infect Dis J 15:1087-1091, 1996.
110. Balotta C, Colombo MC, Colucci G, et al. Plasma viremia and virus phenotype are correlates of disease progression in vertically human immunodeficiency virus type 1–infected children. Pediatr Infect Dis J 16:205-211, 1997.
111. Mellors JW, Kingsley LA, Rinaldo CR, et al. Quantitation of HIV-1 RNA in plasma predicts outcome after seroconversion. Ann Intern Med 122:573-579, 1995.
112. Mellors JW, Rinaldo CR, Gupta P, et al. Prognosis of HIV-1 infection predicted by the quantity of virus in plasma. Science 272:1167-1170, 1996.
113. Rich KC, Fowler MG, Mofenson LM, et al. Maternal and infant factors predicting disease progression in human immunodeficiency virus type 1–infected infants. Women and Infants Transmission Study Group. Pediatrics 105:e8, 2000.
114. Bryson YJ, Pang S, Wei LS, et al. Clearance of HIV infection in a perinatally infected infant. N Engl J Med 332:833-838, 1995.
115. Bryson YJ. HIV clearance in infants—a continuing saga. AIDS 9:1373-1375, 1995.
116. Roques PA, Gras G, Parnet-Mathieu F, et al. Clearance of HIV infection in 12 perinatally infected children: clinical, virological and immunological data. AIDS 9:F19-F26, 1995.
117. Lepage P, Van de Perre P, Simonon A, et al. Transient seroreversion in children born to human immunodeficiency virus 1–infected mothers. Pediatr Infect Dis J 11:892-894, 1992.
118. Bakshi SS, Tetali S, Abrams EJ, et al. Repeatedly positive human immunodeficiency virus type 1 DNA polymerase chain reaction in human immunodeficiency virus–exposed seroreverting infants. Pediatr Infect Dis J 14:658-662, 1995.
119. Frenkel LM, Mullins JI, Learn GH, et al. Genetic evaluation of suspected cases of transient HIV-1 infection of infants. Science 280:1073-1077, 1998.
120. Erkeller-Yuksel FM, Deneys V, Hannet I, et al. Age-related changes in human blood lymphocyte subpopulations. J Pediatr 120:216-222, 1992.
121. The European Collaborative Study. Age-related standards for T lymphocyte subsets based on uninfected children born to human immunodeficiency virus 1–infected mothers. Pediatr Infect Dis J 11:1018-1026, 1992.
122. Comans-Bitter WM, de Groot R, van den Beemd R, et al. Immunophenotyping of blood lymphocytes in childhood. Reference values for lymphocyte subpopulations. J Pediatr 130:388-393, 1997.
123. McKinney RE, Wilfert CM. Lymphocyte subsets in children younger than 2 years old: normal values in a population at risk for human immunodeficiency virus infection and diagnostic and prognostic application to infected children. Pediatr Infect Dis J 11:639-644, 1992.
124. Dickover RE, Dillon M, Gillette SG, et al. Rapid increases in load of human immunodeficiency virus correlate with early disease progression and loss of CD4 cells in vertically infected infants. J Infect Dis 170:1279-1284, 1994.
125. Roilides E, Black C, Reimer C, et al. Serum immunoglobulin G subclasses in children infected with human immunodeficiency virus type 1. Pediatr Infect Dis J 10:134-139, 1991.
126. Luzuriaga K, Koup RA, Pikora CA, et al. Deficient human immunodeficiency virus type 1–specific cytotoxic T cell responses in vertically infected children. J Pediatr 119:230-236, 1991.
127. Monforte ADA, Novati R, Galli M, et al. T-cell subsets and serum immunoglobulin levels in infants born to HIV-seropositive mothers: a longitudinal evaluation. AIDS 4:1141-1144, 1990.
128. Borkowsky W, Rigaud M, Krasinski K, et al. Cell-mediated and humoral immune responses in children infected with human immunodeficiency virus during the first four years of life. J Pediatr 120:371-375, 1992.
129. European Collaborative Study. Children born to women with HIV-1 infection: natural history and risk of transmission. Lancet 337:253-260, 1991.
130. Luzuriaga K, Holmes D, Hereema A, et al. HIV-1–specific cytotoxic T lymphocyte responses in the first year of life. J Immunol 154:433-443, 1995.
131. Pikora CA, Sullivan JL, Panicali D, Luzuriaga K. Early HIV-1 envelope-specific cytotoxic T lymphocyte responses in vertically infected children. J Exp Med 185:1153-1161, 1997.
132. Kline MW, Lewis DE, Hollinger FB, et al. A comparative study of human immunodeficiency virus culture, polymerase chain reaction and anti–human immunodeficiency virus immunoglobulin A antibody detection in the diagnosis during early infancy of vertically acquired human immunodeficiency virus infection. Pediatr Infect Dis J 13:90-94, 1994.
133. Comeau AM, Pitt J, Hillyer GV, et al. Early detection of human immunodeficiency virus on dried blood spot specimens: sensitivity across serial specimens. J Pediatr 129:111-118, 1996.
134. Horsburgh CR, Ou CY, Jason J, et al. Duration of human immunodeficiency virus infection before detection of antibody. Lancet 2:637-640, 1989.
135. Rogers MF, Ou C-Y, Kilbourne B, Schochetman G. Advances and problems in the diagnosis of human immunodeficiency virus infection in infants. Pediatr Infect Dis J 10:523-531, 1991.
136. Chantry CJ, Cooper ER, Pelton SI, et al. Seroreversion in human immunodeficiency virus–exposed but uninfected infants. Pediatr Infect Dis J 14:382-387, 1995.
137. Tudor-Williams G. Early diagnosis of vertically acquired HIV-1 infection. AIDS 5:103-105, 1991.
138. Yanase Y, Tango T, Okumura K, et al. Lymphocyte subsets identified by monoclonal antibodies in healthy children. Pediatr Res 20:1147-1151, 1986.
139. Quinn TC, Ruff A, Halsey N. Pediatric acquired immunodeficiency syndrome: special considerations for developing nations. Pediatr Infect Dis J 11:558-568, 1992.
140. Pollack H, Glasberg H, Lee E, et al. Impaired early growth of infants perinatally infected with human immunodeficiency virus: correlation with viral load. J Pediatr 130:915-922, 1997.
141. Blanche S, Tardieu M, Duliege A-M, et al. Longitudinal study of 94 symptomatic infants with perinatally acquired human immunodeficiency virus infection. Am J Dis Child 144:1210-1215, 1990.
142. Centers for Disease Control. Revision of the CDC surveillance case definition for acquired immunodeficiency syndrome. MMWR Morb Mortal Wkly Rep 36(Suppl 1S):1S-15S, 1987.
143. Andiman WA, Mezger J, Shapiro E. Invasive bacterial infections in children born to women infected with human immunodeficiency virus type 1. J Pediatr 124:846-852, 1994.
144. Lichenstein R, King JC, Farley JJ, et al. Bacteremia in febrile human immunodeficiency virus–infected children presenting to ambulatory care settings. Pediatr Infect Dis J 17:381-385, 1998.
145. Janoff EN, Breiman RE, Daley CL, Hopewell PC. Pneumococcal disease during HIV infection: epidemiology, clinical, and immunologic perspectives. Ann Intern Med 117:314-324, 1992.

146. Farley JJ, King JC, Nair P, et al. Invasive pneumococcal disease among infected and uninfected children of mothers with human immunodeficiency virus infection. J Pediatr 124:853-858, 1994.
147. Di John D, Krasinski K, Lawrence R, et al. Very late onset of group B streptococcal disease in infants infected with the human immunodeficiency virus. Pediatr Infect Dis J 9:925-928, 1990.
148. Dorfman DH, Glaser JH. Congenital syphilis presenting in infants after the newborn period. N Engl J Med 323:1299-1302, 1990.
149. Dumois JA. Potential problems with the diagnosis and treatment of syphilis in HIV-infected pregnant women. Pediatr AIDS HIV Infect Fetus Adolesc 3:22-24, 1992.
150. McIntosh K. Congenital syphilis—breaking through the safety net. N Engl J Med 323:1339-1341, 1990.
151. Centers for Disease Control. Screening for tuberculosis and tuberculous infection in high-risk populations and the use of preventive therapy for tuberculous infections in the United States. MMWR Morb Mortal Wkly Rep 39:1-12, 1990.
152. Khoury YF, Mastrucci MT, Hutto C, et al. *Mycobacterium tuberculosis* in children with human immunodeficiency virus type 1 infection. Pediatr Infect Dis J 11:950-955, 1992.
153. Gutman LT, Moye J, Zimmer B, Tian C. Tuberculosis in human immunodeficiency virus–exposed or –infected United States children. Pediatr Infect Dis J 13:963-968, 1994.
154. Committee on Infectious Diseases. Screening for tuberculosis in infants and children. Pediatrics 93:131-134, 1994.
155. Adhikari M, Pillay T, Pillay DG. Tuberculosis in the newborn: an emerging disease. Pediatr Infect Dis J 16:1108-1112, 1997.
156. Committee on Infectious Diseases. Update on tuberculosis skin testing of children. Pediatrics 97:282-284, 1996.
157. Starke JR, Correa AG. Management of mycobacterial infection and disease in children. Pediatr Infect Dis J 14:455-470, 1995.
158. Lewis LL, Butler KM, Husson RN, et al. Defining the population of human immunodeficiency virus–infected children at risk for *Mycobacterium avium-intracellulare* infection. J Pediatr 121:677-683, 1992.
159. Rutstein RM, Cobb P, McGowan KL, et al. *Mycobacterium avium intracellulare* complex infection in HIV-infected children. AIDS 7:507-512, 1993.
160. USPHS/IDSA Prevention of Opportunistic Infections Working Group. USPHS/IDSA guidelines for the prevention of opportunistic infections in persons infected with human immunodeficiency virus. MMWR Morb Mortal Wkly Rep 46:1-46, 1997.
161. Jura E, Chadwick EG, Josephs SH, et al. Varicella-zoster virus infections in children infected with human immunodeficiency virus. Pediatr Infect Dis J 8:586-590, 1989.
162. Silliman CC, Tedder D, Ogle JW, et al. Unsuspected varicella-zoster virus encephalitis in a child with acquired immunodeficiency syndrome. J Pediatr 123:418-422, 1993.
163. Lyall EG, Ogilvie MM, Smith NM, Burns S. Acyclovir resistant varicella zoster and HIV infection. Arch Dis Child 70:133-135, 1994.
164. Chandwani S, Kaul A, Bebenroth D, et al. Cytomegalovirus infection in human immunodeficiency virus type 1–infected children. Pediatr Infect Dis J 15:310-314, 1996.
165. Nigro G, Krysztofiak A, Castelli Gattinara G, et al. Rapid progression of HIV disease in children with cytomegalovirus DNAemia. AIDS 10:1127-1133, 1996.
166. Doyle M, Atkins JT, Rivera-Matos IR. Congenital cytomegalovirus infection in infants infected with human immunodeficiency virus type 1. Pediatr Infect Dis J 15:1102-1106, 1996.
167. Kitchen BJ, Engler HD, Gill VJ, et al. Cytomegalovirus infection in children with human immunodeficiency virus infection. Pediatr Infect Dis J 16:358-363, 1997.
168. Zaknun D, Zangerle R, Kapelari K, et al. Concurrent ganciclovir and foscarnet treatment for cytomegalovirus encephalitis and retinitis in an infant with acquired immunodeficiency syndrome: case report and review. Pediatr Infect Dis J 16:807-811, 1997.
169. Walton RC, Whitcup SM, Mueller BU, et al. Combined intravenous ganciclovir and foscarnet for children with recurrent cytomegalovirus retinitis. Ophthalmology 102:1865-1870, 1995.
170. Bodsworth NJ, Cooper DA, Donovan B. The influence of human immunodeficiency virus type 1 infection on the development of the hepatitis B virus carrier state. J Infect Dis 163:1138-1140, 1991.
171. Eyster ME, Diamondstone LS, Lien J-M, et al. Natural history of hepatitis C virus infection in multitransfused hemophiliacs: effect of co-infection with human immunodeficiency virus. J Acquir Immune Defic 6:602-610, 1993.
172. Paccagnini S, Principi N, Massironi E, et al. Perinatal transmission and manifestation of hepatitis C virus infection in a high risk population. Pediatr Infect Dis J 14:195-199, 1995.
173. Conte D, Fraquelli M, Prati D, et al. Prevalence and clinical course of chronic hepatitis C virus (HCV) infection and rate of HCV vertical transmission in a cohort of 15,250 pregnant women. Hepatology 31:751-755, 2000.
174. Resti M, Azzari C, Galli L, et al. Maternal drug use is a preeminent risk factor for mother-to-child hepatitis C virus transmission: results from a multicenter study of 1372 mother-infant pairs. J Infect Dis 185: 567-72, 2002. Epub Feb 14, 2002.
175. Kaplan LJ, Daum RS, Smaron M, McCarthy CA. Severe measles in immunocompromised patients. JAMA 267:1237-1241, 1992.
176. Palumbo P, Hoyt L, Demasio K, et al. Population-based study of measles and measles immunization in human immunodeficiency virus–infected children. Pediatr Infect Dis J 11:1008-1014, 1992.
177. Nadel S, McGann K, Hodinka RL, et al. Measles giant cell pneumonia in a child with human immunodeficiency virus infection. Pediatr Infect Dis J 10:542-544, 1991.
178. Krasinski K, Borkowsky W. Measles and measles immunity in children infected with human immunodeficiency virus. JAMA 261:2512-2516, 1989.
179. Chandwani S, Borkowsky W, Krasinski K, et al. Respiratory syncytial virus infection in human immunodeficiency virus-infected children. J Pediatr 117:251-254, 1990.
180. Ellaurie M, Schutzbank TE, Rakusan TA, Lipson SM. Spectrum of adenovirus infection in pediatric HIV infection. Pediatr AIDS HIV Infect 4:211-214, 1993.
181. King JC, Burke AR, Clemens JD, et al. Respiratory syncytial virus illnesses in human immunodeficiency virus– and noninfected children. Pediatr Infect Dis J 12:733-739, 1993.
182. Joshi VV, Kauffman S, Oleske JM, et al. Polyclonal polymorphic B-cell lymphoproliferative disorder with prominent pulmonary involvement in children with acquired immune deficiency syndrome. Cancer 59:1455-1462, 1987.
183. Gonzales CE, Venson D, Lee S, et al. Risk factors for fungemia in children infected with human immunodeficiency virus: a case control study. Clin Infect Dis 23:515-521, 1996.
184. Leggiadro RJ, Kline MW, Hughes WT. Extrapulmonary cryptococcosis in children with acquired immunodeficiency syndrome. Pediatr Infect Dis J 10:658-662, 1991.
185. Gonzales GE, Shetty D, Lewis LL, et al. Cryptococcosis in human immunodeficiency virus–infected children. Pediatr Infect Dis J 15:796-800, 1996.
186. Minamoto GY, Barlam TF, Vander Els NJ. Invasive aspergillosis in patients with AIDS. Clin Infect Dis 14:66-74, 1992.
187. Denning DW, Follansbee SE, Scolaro M, et al. Pulmonary aspergillosis in the acquired immunodeficiency syndrome. N Engl J Med 324:654-662, 1991.
188. Shetty D, Giri N, Gonzales CE, et al. Invasive aspergillosis in human immunodeficiency virus–infected children. Pediatr Infect Dis 16:216-221, 1997.
189. Sarosi GA, Johnson PC. Disseminated histoplasmosis in patients infected with human immunodeficiency virus. Clin Infect Dis 14(Suppl 1):S60-S67, 1992.
190. Pappas PG, Pottage JC, Powderly WG, et al. Blastomycosis in patients with the acquired immunodeficiency syndrome. Ann Intern Med 116:847-853, 1992.
191. Byers M, Feldman S, Edwards J. Disseminated histoplasmosis as the acquired immunodeficiency syndrome–defining illness in an infant. Pediatr Infect Dis J 11:127-128, 1992.
192. Simonds RJ, Oxtoby MJ, Caldwell B, et al. *Pneumocystis carinii* pneumonia among US children with perinatally acquired HIV infection. JAMA 270:470-473, 1993.
193. Centers for Disease Control and Prevention. 1995 Revised guidelines for prophylaxis against *Pneumocystis carinii* pneumonia for children infected with or perinatally exposed to human immunodeficiency virus. MMWR Morb Mortal Wkly Rep 44:1-12, 1995.
194. Centers for Disease Control and Prevention. HIV AIDS Surveill Rep 9:1-43, 1997.
195. Mortier E, Pouchot J, Bossi P, Molinié V. Maternal-fetal transmission of *Pneumocystis carinii* in human immunodeficiency virus infection. N Engl J Med 332:825-826, 1995.
196. Bye MR, Bernstein LJ, Glaser J, Kleid D. *Pneumocystis carinii* pneumonia in young children with AIDS. Pediatr Pulmonol 9: 251-253, 1990.

197. Connor E, Bagarazzi M, McSherry G, et al. Clinical and laboratory correlates of *Pneumocystis carinii* pneumonia in children infected with HIV. JAMA 265:1693-1697, 1991.
198. Gosey LL, Howard RM, Witebsky FG, et al. Advantages of a modified toluidine blue O stain and bronchoalveolar lavage for the diagnosis of *Pneumocystis carinii* pneumonia. J Clin Microbiol 22:803-807, 1985.
199. Ognibene FP, Gill VJ, Pizzo PA, et al. Induced sputum to diagnose *Pneumocystis carinii* pneumonia in immunosuppressed pediatric patients. J Pediatr 115:430-433, 1989.
200. Sattler FR, Cowan R, Nielsen DM, Ruskin J. Trimethoprim-sulfamethoxazole compared with pentamidine for treatment of *Pneumocystis carinii* pneumonia in the acquired immunodeficiency syndrome: a prospective, noncrossover study. Ann Intern Med 109:280-287, 1988.
201. Gagnon S, Boota AM, Fischl MA, et al. Corticosteroids as adjunctive therapy for severe *Pneumocystis carinii* pneumonia in the acquired immunodeficiency syndrome. N Engl J Med 323:1444-1450, 1990.
202. Bozzette SA, Sattler FR, Chiu J, et al. A controlled trial of early adjunctive treatment with corticosteroids for *Pneumocystis carinii* pneumonia in the acquired immunodeficiency syndrome. N Engl J Med 1323:1451-1457, 1990.
203. The National Institutes of Health–University of California Expert Panel for Corticosteroids as Adjunctive Therapy for Pneumocystis Pneumonia. Consensus statement on the use of corticosteroids as adjunctive therapy for *Pneumocystis* pneumonia in the acquired immunodeficiency syndrome. N Engl J Med 323:1500-1504, 1990.
204. McLaughlin GE, Virdee SS, Schleien CL, et al. Effect of corticosteroids on survival of children with acquired immunodeficiency syndrome and *Pneumocystis carinii*–related respiratory failure. J Pediatr 126:821-824, 1995.
205. Bernstein LJ, Bye MR, Rubinstein A. Prognostic factors and life expectancy in children with acquired immunodeficiency syndrome and *Pneumocystis carinii* pneumonia. Am J Dis Child 143:775-778, 1989.
206. Kovacs A, Frederick T, Church J, et al. CD4 T-lymphocyte counts and *Pneumocystis carinii* pneumonia in pediatric HIV infection. JAMA 265:1698-1703, 1991.
207. Centers for Disease Control. Guidelines for prophylaxis against *Pneumocystis carinii* pneumonia for children infected with human immunodeficiency virus. MMWR Morb Mortal Wkly Rep 40:1-13, 1991.
208. Simonds RJ, Lindegren ML, Thomas P, et al. Prophylaxis against *Pneumocystis carinii* pneumonia among children with perinatally acquired human immunodeficiency virus infection in the United States. N Engl J Med 332:786-790, 1995.
209. Thea DM, Lambert G, Weedon J, et al. Benefit of primary prophylaxis before 18 months of age in reducing the incidence of *Pneumocystis carinii* pneumonia and early death in a cohort of 112 human immunodeficiency virus–infected infants. Pediatrics 97:59-64, 1996.
210. Mueller BU, Butler KM, Husson RN, Pizzo PA. *Pneumocystis carinii* pneumonia despite prophylaxis in children with human immunodeficiency virus infection. J Pediatr 119:992-994, 1991.
211. Nachman SA, Mueller BU, Mirochnik M, Pizzo PA. High failure rate of dapsone and pentamidine as *Pneumocystis carinii* pneumonia prophylaxis in human immunodeficiency virus–infected children. Pediatr Infect Dis J 13:1004-1006, 1994.
212. Mitchell CD. Toxoplasmosis. *In* Pizzo PA, Wilfert CM (eds): Pediatric AIDS: The Challenge of HIV Infection in Infants, Children, and Adolescents. Baltimore, Williams & Wilkins, 1994, pp 419-431.
213. Mitchell CD, Erlich SS, Mastrucci MT, et al. Congenital toxoplasmosis occurring in infants infected with human immunodeficiency virus 1. Pediatr Infect Dis J 9:512-518, 1990.
214. Medlock MD, Tilleli JT, Pearl GS. Congenital cardiac toxoplasmosis in a newborn with acquired immunodeficiency syndrome. Pediatr Infect Dis J 9:129-132, 1990.
215. Cordell RL, Addiss DG. Cryptosporidiosis in child care settings: a review of the literature and recommendations for prevention and control. Pediatr Infect Dis J 13:310-317, 1994.
216. Mueller BU. Cancers in human immunodeficiency virus–infected children. J Natl Cancer Inst Monogr 23:31-35, 1998.
217. Siskin GP, Haller JO, Miller S, Sundaram R. AIDS-related lymphoma: Radiologic features in pediatric patients. Radiology 196:63-66, 1995.
218. Nadal D, Caduff R, Frey E, et al. Non-Hodgkin's lymphoma in four children infected with the human immunodeficiency virus. Cancer 73:224-230, 1994.
219. Granovsky MO, Mueller BU, Nicholson HS, et al. HIV-associated tumors in children: a case series from the Children's Cancer Group and National Cancer Institute, Tenth Annual Meeting of the American Society of Pediatric Hematology/Oncology, San Francisco, CA, September 10-20, 1997.
220. Connor E, Boccon-Gibod L, Joshi V, et al. Cutaneous acquired immunodeficiency syndrome–associated Kaposi's sarcoma in pediatric patients. Arch Dermatol 126:791-793, 1990.
221. Buck BE, Scott GB, Valdes-Dapena M, Parks WP. Kaposi sarcoma in two infants with acquired immune deficiency syndrome. J Pediatr 103:911-913, 1983.
222. Gutierrez-Ortega P, Hierro-Orozco S, Sanchez-Cisneros R, Montana LF. Kaposi's sarcoma in a 6-day-old infant with human immunodeficiency virus. Arch Dermatol 125:432-433, 1989.
223. McClain KL, Leach CT, Jenson HB, et al. Association of Epstein-Barr virus with leiomyosarcomas in young people with AIDS. N Engl J Med 332:12-18, 1995.
224. Jenson HB, Leach CT, McClain KL, et al. Benign and malignant smooth muscle tumors containing Epstein-Barr virus in children with AIDS. J Acquir Immune Defic Syndr Hum Retrovirol 14:A49, 1997.
225. Lobato MN, Caldwell MB, Ng P, et al. Encephalopathy in children with perinatally acquired human immunodeficiency virus infection. J Pediatr 126:710-715, 1995.
226. Diaz C, Hanson C, Cooper ER, et al. Disease progression in a cohort of infants with vertically acquired HIV infection observed from birth: the Women and Infants Transmission Study (WITS). J Acquir Immune Defic Syndr Hum Retrovirol 18:221-228, 1998.
227. Cooper ER, Hanson C, Diaz C, et al. Encephalopathy and progression of human immunodeficiency virus disease in a cohort of children with perinatally acquired human immunodeficiency virus infection. Women and Infants Transmission Study Group. J Pediatr 132:808-812, 1998.
228. The European Collaborative Study. Neurologic signs in young children with human immunodeficiency virus infection. Pediatr Infect Dis J 9:402-406, 1990.
229. Park YD, Belman AL, Kim T-S, et al. Stroke in pediatric acquired immunodeficiency syndrome. Ann Neurol 28:303-311, 1990.
230. Lang C, Jacobi G, Kreuz W, et al. Rapid development of giant aneurysm at the base of the brain in an 8-year-old boy with perinatal HIV infection. Acta Histochem Suppl 42:S83-S90, 1992.
231. Belman AL, Diamond G, Dickson D, et al. Pediatric acquired immunodeficiency syndrome: neurologic symptoms. Am J Dis Child 142:29-35, 1988.
232. Epstein LG, Sharer LR, Goudsmit J. Neurological and neuropathological features of human immunodeficiency virus infection in children. Ann Neurol 23(Suppl):S19-S23, 1988.
233. Gay GL, Armstrong FD, Cohen D, et al. The effects of HIV on cognitive and motor development in children born to HIV-seropositive women with no reported drug use: birth to 24 months. Pediatrics 96:1078-1082, 1995.
234. Wolters PL, Brouwers P, Moss HA, Pizzo PA. Differential receptive and expressive language functioning of children with symptomatic HIV disease and relation to CT scan brain abnormalities. Pediatrics 95:112-119, 1995.
235. Brouwers P, Belman A, Epstein L. Central nervous system involvement: manifestations, evaluation, and pathogenesis. *In* Pizzo PA, Wilfert CA (eds): Pediatric AIDS. The Challenge of HIV Infection in Infants, Children, and Adolescents. Baltimore, Williams & Wilkins, 1994, pp 433-455.
236. Brouwers P, DeCarli C, Civitello L, et al. Correlation between computed tomographic brain scan abnormalities and neuropsychological function in children with symptomatic human immunodeficiency virus disease. Arch Neurol 52:39-44, 1995.
237. Brouwers P, DeCarli C, Tudor-Williams G, et al. Interrelations among patterns of change in neurocognitive, CT brain imaging and CD4 measures associated with anti-retroviral therapy in children with symptomatic HIV infection. Adv Neuroimmunol 4:223-231, 1994.
238. DeCarli C, Civitello LA, Brouwers P, Pizzo PA. The prevalence of computed tomographic abnormalities of the cerebrum in 100 consecutive children symptomatic with the human immunodeficiency virus. Ann Neurol 34:198-205, 1993.
239. DeCarli C, Fugate L, Falloon J, et al. Brain growth and cognitive improvement in children with human immunodeficiency virus–induced encephalopathy after 6 months of continuous infusion zidovudine therapy. J Acquir Immune Defic Syndr 4:585-592, 1991.
240. Sharer LR, Saito Y, Epstein LG, Blumberg BM. Detection of HIV-1 DNA in pediatric AIDS brain tissue by two-step ISPCR. Adv Neuroimmunol 4:283-285, 1994.

241. Sharer LR. Neuropathological aspects of HIV-1 infection in children. *In* Gendelman HE, Lipton SA, Epstein L, Swindells S (eds): The Neurology of AIDS. New York, Chapman & Hall, 1998, pp 408-418.
242. Saito Y, Sharer LR, Epstein LG, et al. Overexpression of nef as a marker for restricted HIV-1 infection of astrocytes in postmortem pediatric central nervous tissues. Neurology 44:474-481, 1994.
243. Baba TW, Liska V, Ruprecht RM. HIV-1/SIV infection of the fetal and neonatal nervous system. *In* Gendelman HE, Lipton SA, Epstein L, Swindells S (eds): The Neurology of AIDS. New York, Chapman & Hall, 1998, pp 443-456.
244. Pratt RD, Nichols S, McKinney N, et al. Virologic markers of human immunodeficiency virus type 1 in cerebrospinal fluid of infected children. J Infect Dis 174:288-293, 1996.
245. Sei S, Stewart SK, Farley M, et al. Evaluation of HIV-1 RNA levels in cerebrospinal fluid and viral resistance to zidovudine in children with HIV encephalopathy. J Infect Dis 174:1200-1206, 1996.
246. Gelbard HA. HIV-1–induced neurotoxicity in the developing central nervous system. In Gendelman HE, Lipton SA, Epstein L, Swindells S (eds): The Neurology of AIDS. New York, Chapman & Hall, 1998, pp 419-424.
247. Brouwers P, Heyes MP, Moss HA, et al. Quinolinic acid in the cerebrospinal fluid of children with symptomatic human immunodeficiency virus type 1 disease: relationships to clinical status and therapeutic response. J Infect Dis 168:1380-1386, 1993.
248. Sei S, Saito K, Stewart SK, et al. Increased human immunodeficiency virus (HIV) type 1 DNA content and quinolinic acid concentration in brain tissues from patients with HIV encephalopathy. J Infect Dis 172:638-647, 1995.
249. Srugo I, Wittek AE, Israele V, Brunell PA. Meningoencephalitis in a neonate congenitally infected with human immunodeficiency virus type 1. J Pediatr 120:93-95, 1992.
250. Sharer LR, Dowling PC, Michaels J, et al. Spinal cord disease in children with HIV-1 infection: a combined molecular biological and neuropathological study. Neuropathol Appl Neurobiol 16:317-331, 1990.
251. Brouwers P, Moss H, Wolters P, et al. Effect of continuous-infusion zidovudine therapy on neuropsychologic functioning in children with symptomatic human immunodeficiency virus infection. J Pediatr 117:980-985, 1990.
252. Stiehm ER, Bryson YJ, Frenkel LM, et al. Prednisone improves human immunodeficiency virus encephalopathy in children. Pediatr Infect Dis J 11:49-50, 1992.
253. Cunningham ET, Margolis TP. Ocular manifestations of HIV infection. N Engl J Med 339:236-244, 1998.
254. de Smet MD, Nussenblatt RB. Ocular manifestations of HIV in pediatric populations. *In* Pizzo PA, Wilfert CM (eds): Pediatric AIDS: The Challenge of HIV Infection in Infants, Children, and Adolescents. Baltimore, Williams & Wilkins, 1994, pp 457-466.
255. Bottoni F, Gonnella P, Autelitano A, Orzalesi N. Diffuse necrotizing retinochoroiditis in a child with AIDS and toxoplasmic encephalitis. Graefes Arch Clin Exp Ophthalmol 228:36-39, 1990.
256. Lopez JS, deSmet MD, Masur H, et al. Orally administered 566C80 for treatment of ocular toxoplasmosis in a patient with the acquired immunodeficiency syndrome. Am J Ophthalmol 113:331-333, 1992.
257. Telzak EE, Cote RJ, Gold JWM, et al. Extrapulmonary *Pneumocystis carinii* infections. Rev Infect Dis 12:380-386, 1990.
258. Connor EM, Andiman WA. Lymphoid interstitial pneumonitis. *In* Pizzo PA, Wilfert CM (eds): Pediatric AIDS: The Challenge of HIV Infection in Infants, Children, and Adolescents. Baltimore, Williams & Wilkins, 1994, pp 467-482.
259. Sharland M, Gibb DM, Holland F. Respiratory morbidity from lymphocytic interstitial pneumonitis (LIP) in vertically acquired HIV infection. Arch Dis Child 76:334-336, 1997.
260. Scott GB, Hutto C, Makuch RW, et al. Survival in children with perinatally acquired human immunodeficiency virus type 1 infection. N Engl J Med 321:1791-1796, 1989.
261. Luginbuhl LM, Orav EJ, McIntosh K, Lipshultz SE. Cardiac morbidity and related mortality in children with HIV infection. JAMA 269:2869-2875, 1993.
262. Lipshultz SE, Orav EJ, Sanders SP, et al. Cardiac structure and function in children with human immunodeficiency virus infection treated with zidovudine. N Engl J Med 327:1260-1265, 1992.
263. Lipshultz SE, Fox CH, Perez-Atayde AR, et al. Identification of human immunodeficiency virus-1 RNA and DNA in the heart of a child with cardiovascular abnormalities and congenital acquired immune deficiency syndrome. Am J Cardiol 66:246-250, 1990.
264. Joshi VV, Gadol C, Connor E, et al. Dilated cardiomyopathy in children with acquired immunodeficiency syndrome: a pathologic study of five cases. Hum Pathol 19:69-73, 1988.
265. Lewis W. AIDS: cardiac findings from 115 autopsies. Prog Cardiovasc Dis 32:207-215, 1989.
266. Grody WW, Cheng L, Lewis W. Infection of the heart by the human immunodeficiency virus. Am J Cardiol 66:203-206, 1990.
267. Joshi VV, Pawel B, Connor E, et al. Arteriopathy in children with acquired immune deficiency syndrome. Pediatr Pathol 7:261-275, 1987.
268. Kure K, Park YD, Kim T-S, et al. Immunohistochemical localization of an HIV epitope in cerebral aneurysmal arteriopathy in pediatric acquired immunodeficiency syndrome (AIDS). Pediatr Pathol 9:655-667, 1989.
269. Husson RN, Saini R, Lewis LL, et al. Cerebral artery aneurysms in children infected with human immunodeficiency virus. J Pediatr 121:927-930, 1992.
270. Galli L, de Martino M, Tovo P-A, et al. Onset of clinical signs in children with HIV-1 perinatal infection. AIDS 9:455-461, 1995.
271. Pickering LK. Infections of the gastrointestinal tract. *In* Pizzo PA, Wilfert CM (eds): Pediatric AIDS: The Challenge of HIV Infection in Infants, Children, and Adolescents. Baltimore, Williams & Wilkins, 1994, pp 377-404.
272. Yolken RH, Li S, Perman J, Viscidi R. Persistent diarrhea and fecal shedding of retroviral nucleic acids in children infected with human immunodeficiency virus. J Infect Dis 164:61-66, 1991.
273. Grunfeld C, Feingold KR. Metabolic disturbances and wasting in the acquired immunodeficiency syndrome. N Engl J Med 327:329-337, 1992.
274. Lewis JD, Winter HS. Intestinal and hepatobiliary diseases in HIV-infected children. Gastroenterol Clin North Am 24:119-132, 1995.
275. Kotloff KL, Johnson JP, Nair P, et al. Diarrheal morbidity during the first 2 years of life among HIV-infected infants. JAMA 271:448-452, 1994.
276. Thea DM, St. Louis ME, Atido U, et al. A prospective study of diarrhea and HIV-1 infection among 429 Zairian infants. N Engl J Med 329:1696-1702, 1993.
277. Miller TL. Nutritional assessment and its clinical application in children infected with the human immunodeficiency virus. J Pediatr 129:633-636, 1996.
278. Leggiadro RJ, Lewis D, Whitington GL, et al. Chronic hepatitis associated with perinatal HIV infection. AIDS Reader March/April:57-61, 1992.
279. Persaud D, Bangaru B, Greco A, et al. Cholestatic hepatitis in children infected with the human immunodeficiency virus. Pediatr Infect Dis J 12:492-498, 1993.
280. Miller TL, Winter HS, Luginbuhl LM, et al. Pancreatitis in pediatric human immunodeficiency virus infection. J Pediatr 120:223-227, 1992.
281. Butler KM, Venzon D, Henry N, et al. Pancreatitis in human immunodeficiency virus–infected children receiving dideoxyinosine. Pediatrics 91:747-751, 1993.
282. Strauss J, Abitol C, Zilleruelo G, et al. Renal disease in children with the acquired immunodeficiency syndrome. N Engl J Med 321:625-630, 1989.
283. Strauss J, Zilleruelo G, Abitbol C, et al. Human immunodeficiency virus nephropathy. Pediatr Nephrol 7:220-225, 1993.
284. Ingulli E, Tejani A, Fikrig S, et al. Nephrotic syndrome associated with acquired immunodeficiency syndrome in children. J Pediatr 119:710-716, 1991.
285. Schoeneman MJ, Ghali V, Lieberman K, Reisman L. IgA nephritis in a child with human immunodeficiency virus: a unique form of human immunodeficiency virus–associated nephropathy? Pediatr Nephrol 6:46-49, 1992.
286. Kimmel PL, Phillips TM, Ferreira-Centeno A, et al. Brief report: Idiotypic IgA nephropathy in patients with human immunodeficiency virus infection. N Engl J Med 327:702-706, 1992.
287. Mueller BU, Sleasman J, Nelson RP Jr, et al. A phase I/II study of the protease inhibitor indinavir in children with HIV infection. Pediatrics 102:101-109, 1998.
288. Bruce RG, Munch LC, Hoven AD, et al. Urolithiasis associated with the protease inhibitor indinavir. Urology 50:513-518, 1997.
289. Gertner JM, Kaufman FR, Donfield SM, et al. Delayed somatic growth and pubertal development in human immunodeficiency virus–infected hemophiliac boys: Hemophilia Growth and Development Study. J Pediatr 124:896-902, 1994.
290. Fisher GD, Rinaldo CR, Gbadero D, et al. Seroprevalence of HIV-1 and HIV-2 infection among children diagnosed with protein-calorie malnutrition in Nigeria. Epidemiol Infect 110:373-378, 1993.

291. Brettler DB, Forsberg A, Bolivar E, et al. Growth failure as a prognostic indicator for progression to acquired immunodeficiency syndrome in children with hemophilia. J Pediatr 117:584-588, 1990.
292. Laue L, Pizzo PA, Butler K, Cutler GB. Growth and neuroendocrine dysfunction in children with acquired immunodeficiency syndrome. J Pediatr 117:541-545, 1990.
293. Schwartz LJ, St. Louis Y, Wu R, et al. Endocrine function in children with human immunodeficiency virus infection. Am J Dis Child 145:330-333, 1991.
294. Grinspoon SK, Bilezikian JP. HIV disease and the endocrine system. N Engl J Med 327:1360-1365, 1992.
295. Hirschfeld S, Laue L, Cutler GB Jr, Pizzo PA. Thyroid abnormalities in children infected with human immunodeficiency virus. J Pediatr 128:70-74, 1996.
296. Papiernik M, Brossard Y, Mulliez N, et al. Thymic abnormalities in fetuses aborted from human immunodeficiency virus type 1 seropositive women. Pediatrics 89:297-301, 1992.
297. Joshi VV, Oleske JM, Saad S, et al. Thymus biopsy in children with acquired immunodeficiency syndrome. Arch Pathol Med 110:837-842, 1986.
298. Sei S, Kleiner DE, Kopp JB, et al. Quantitative analysis of viral burden in tissues from adults and children with symptomatic human immunodeficiency virus type 1 infection assessed by polymerase chain reaction. J Infect Dis 170:325-333, 1994.
299. Pantaleo G, Cohen OJ, Schacker T, et al. Evolutionary pattern of human immunodeficiency virus (HIV) replication and distribution in lymph nodes following primary infection: implications for antiviral therapy. Nat Med 4:341-345, 1998.
300. Pantaleo G, Fauci AS. HIV-1 infection in the lymphoid organs: a model of disease development. J NIH Res 5:68-72, 1993.
301. Mueller BU, Sei S, Anderson B, et al. Comparison of virus burden in blood and sequential lymph node biopsy specimens from children infected with human immunodeficiency virus. J Pediatr 129:410-418, 1996.
302. Scott GB, Buck BE, Leterman JG, et al. Acquired immunodeficiency syndrome in infants. N Engl J Med 310:76-81, 1984.
303. Ellaurie M, Burns ER, Rubinstein A. Hematologic manifestations in pediatric HIV infection: severe anemia as a prognostic factor. Am J Pediatr Hematol Oncol 12:449-453, 1990.
304. Mueller BU. Hematological problems and their management in children with HIV infection. *In* Pizzo PA, Wilfert CM (eds): Pediatric AIDS: The Challenge of HIV Infection in Infants, Children, and Adolescents. Baltimore, Williams & Wilkins, 1994, pp 591-602.
305. Forsyth BW, Andiman WA, O'Connor T. Development of a prognosis-based clinical staging system for infants infected with human immunodeficiency virus. J Pediatr 129:648-655, 1996.
306. Mueller BU, Tannenbaum S, Pizzo PA. Bone marrow aspirates and biopsies in children with human immunodeficiency virus infection. J Pediatr Hematol Oncol 18:266-271, 1996.
307. Parmentier L, Boucary D, Salmon D. Pure red cell aplasia in an HIV-infected patient. AIDS 6:234-235, 1992.
308. Nigro G, Castelli Gattinara G, et al. Parvovirus-B19–related pancytopenia in children with HIV infection. Lancet 340:115, 1992.
309. Abkowitz JL, Brown KE, Wood RW, et al. Clinical relevance of parvovirus B19 as a cause of anemia in patients with human immunodeficiency virus infection. J Infect Dis 176:269-273, 1997.
310. Holodniy M, Margolis D, Carroll R, et al. Quantitative relationship between platelet count and plasma virion HIV RNA. AIDS 10:232-233, 1996.
311. Ballem PJ, Belzberg A, Devine DV, et al. Kinetic studies of the mechanism of thrombocytopenia in patients with human immunodeficiency virus infection. N Engl J Med 327:1779-1789, 1992.
312. Rigaud M, Leibovitz E, Sin Quee C, et al. Thrombocytopenia in children infected with human immunodeficiency virus: long-term follow-up and therapeutic considerations. J Acquir Immune Defic Syndr 5:450-455, 1992.
313. Abuaf N, Laperche S, Rajoely B, et al. Autoantibodies to phospholipids and the coagulation proteins in AIDS. Thromb Haemost 77:856-861, 1997.
314. Sorice M, Griggi T, Arcieri P, et al. Protein S and HIV infection: the role of anticardiolipin and anti-protein S antibodies. Thromb Res 73:165-175, 1994.
315. Rodriguez-Mahou M, Lopez-Longo J, Lapointe N, et al. Autoimmune phenomena in children with human immunodeficiency virus infection and acquired immunodeficiency syndrome. Acta Paediatr Suppl 400:31-34, 1994.
316. Coopman SA, Johnson RA, Platt R, Stern RS. Cutaneous disease and drug reactions in HIV infection. N Engl J Med 328:1670-1674, 1993.
317. Prose NS. Skin problems. *In* Pizzo PA, Wilfert CM (eds): Pediatric AIDS: The Challenge of HIV Infection in Infants, Children, and Adolescents. Baltimore, Williams & Wilkins, 1994, pp 535-546.
318. von Seidlein L, Gillette SG, Bryson Y, et al. Frequent recurrence and persistence of varicella-zoster virus infections in children infected with human immunodeficiency virus type 1. J Pediatr 128:52-57, 1996.
319. Blanche S, Newell ML, Mayaux MJ, et al. Morbidity and mortality in European children vertically infected by HIV-1. The French Pediatric HIV Infection Study Group and European Collaborative Study. J Acquir Immune Defic Syndr Hum Retrovirol 14:442-450, 1997.
320. Palella FJ, Delaney KM, Moorman AC, et al. Declining morbidity and mortality among patients with advanced human immunodeficiency virus infection. N Engl J Med 338:853-860, 1998.
321. Jean SS, Reed GW, Verdier R-I, et al. Clinical manifestations of human immunodeficiency virus infection in Haitian children. Pediatr Infect Dis J 16:600-606, 1997.
322. Braddick MR, Kreiss JK, Embree JE, et al. Impact of maternal HIV infection on obstetrical and early neonatal outcome. AIDS 4:1001-1005, 1990.
323. Moye J Jr, Rich KC, Kalish LA, et al. Natural history of somatic growth in infants born to women infected by human immunodeficiency virus. Women and Infants Transmission Study Group. J Pediatr 128:58-69, 1996.
324. Frederick T, Mascola L, Eller A, et al. Progression of human immunodeficiency virus disease among infants and children infected perinatally with human immunodeficiency virus or through neonatal blood transfusion. Pediatr Infect Dis J 13:1091-1097, 1994.
325. Blanche S, Mayaux M-J, Rouzioux C, et al. Relation of the course of HIV infection in children to the severity of the disease in their mothers at delivery. N Engl J Med 330:308-312, 1994.
326. Blanche S, Rouzioux C, Guihard Moscato M-L, et al. A prospective study of infants born to women seropositive for human immunodeficiency virus type 1. N Engl J Med 320:1643-1648, 1989.
327. Mayaux M-J, Burgard M, Teglas J-P, et al. Neonatal characteristics in rapidly progressive perinatally acquired HIV-1 disease. JAMA 275:606-610, 1996.
328. Zaknun D, Orav J, Kornegay J, et al. Correlation of ribonucleic acid polymerase chain reaction, acid dissociated p24 antigen, and neopterin with progression of disease. J Pediatr 130:898-905, 1997.
329. Dickover RE, Dillon M, Leung KM, et al. Early prognostic indicators in primary perinatal human immunodeficiency virus type 1 infection: importance of viral RNA and the timing of transmission on long-term outcome. J Infect Dis 178:375-387, 1998.
330. Stoto MA, Almario DA, McCormik MC (eds). Reducing the Odds—Preventing Perinatal Transmission of HIV in the United States. Washington, DC, National Academy Press, 1999.
331. Peters V, Liu KL, Dominguez K, et al. Missed opportunities for perinatal HIV prevention among HIV-exposed infants born 1996-2000, pediatric spectrum of HIV disease cohort. Pediatrics 111:1186-1191, 2003.
332. Abrams EJ, Weedon J, Steketee RW, et al. Association of human immunodeficiency virus (HIV) load early in life with disease progression among HIV-infected infants. New York City Perinatal HIV Transmission Collaborative Study Group. J Infect Dis 178:101-108, 1998.
333. The European Collaborative Study. Caesarean section and risk of vertical transmission of HIV-1 infection. Lancet 343:1464-1467, 1994.
334. The European Mode of Delivery Collaboration. Elective caesarean-section versus vaginal delivery in prevention of vertical HIV-1 transmission: a randomized clinical trial. Lancet 353:1035-1039, 1999.
335. Ricci E, Parazzini F, Pardi G. Caesarean section and antiretroviral treatment. Italian trial on mode of delivery in HIV-positive women study group. Lancet 355:496, 2000.
336. Lindegren ML, Byers RH Jr, Thomas P, Davis SF, et al. Trends in perinatal transmission of HIV/AIDS in the United States. JAMA 282:531-318, 1999.
337. Italian Register for Human Immunodeficiency Virus Infection in Children. Determinants of mother-to-infant human immunodeficiency virus 1 transmission before and after the introduction of zidovudine prophylaxis. Arch Pediatr Adolesc Med 156:915-921, 2002.
338. Lurie P, Wolfe SM. Unethical trials of interventions to reduce perinatal transmission of the human immunodeficiency virus in developing countries. N Engl J Med 337:853-856, 1997.

339. Mofenson LM, Burns DN. Passive immunization to prevent mother-infant transmission of human immunodeficiency virus: current issues and future directions. Pediatr Infect Dis J 10:456-462, 1991.
340. Lambert JS, Mofenson LM, Fletcher CV, et al. Safety and pharmacokinetics of hyperimmune anti-human immunodeficiency virus (HIV) immunoglobulin administered to HIV-infected pregnant women and their newborns. Pediatric AIDS Clinical Trials Group Protocol 185 Pharmacokinetic Study Group. J Infect Dis 175:283-291, 1997.
341. Bertolli J, Hu DJ, Nieburg P, et al. Decision analysis to guide choice of interventions to reduce mother-to-child transmission of HIV. AIDS 17:2089-2098, 2003.
342. WHO. Breastfeeding and replacement feeding practices in the context of mother-to-child transmission of HIV—an assessment tool for research. RHR/01.12, 2001.
343. Stiehm ER, Lambert JS, Mofenson LM, et al. Efficacy of zidovudine and human immunodeficiency virus (HIV) hyperimmune immunoglobulin for reducing perinatal HIV transmission from HIV-infected women with advanced disease: results of Pediatric AIDS Clinical Trials Group Protocol 185. J Infect Dis 179:567-575, 1999.
344. American Academy of Pediatrics Committee on Infectious Diseases. Recommended timing of routine measles immunization for children who have recently received immune globulin preparations. Pediatrics 93:682-685, 1994.
345. Adamson PC, Wu TC, Meade BD, et al. Pertussis in a previously immunized child with human immunodeficiency virus infection. J Pediatr 115:598-592, 1989.
346. The National Institute of Child Health and Human Development Intravenous Immunoglobulin Study Group. Intravenous immune globulin for the prevention of bacterial infections in children with symptomatic human immunodeficiency virus infection. N Engl J Med 325:73-80, 1991.
347. Panel on Clinical Practices for Treatment of HIV Infection. Guidelines for the Use of Antiretroviral Agents in HIV-1 Infected Adolescents and Adults. http://aidsinfo.nih.gov/guidelines/, accessed January 2004.
348. The Working Group on Antiretroviral Therapy and Medical Management of HIV-Infected Children. Guidelines for the Use of Antiretroviral Agents in Pediatric HIV Infection. http://aidsinfo.nih.gov/guidelines/, accessed January 2004.
349. Working Group on Antiretroviral Therapy and Medical Management of Infants, Children, and Adolescents with HIV Infection. Antiretroviral therapy and medical management of pediatric HIV infection. Pediatrics 102:1005-1085, 1998.
350. Lyman WD, Tanaka KE, Kress Y, et al. Zidovudine concentrations in human fetal tissue: implications for perinatal AIDS. Lancet 335:1280-1281, 1990.
351. Garland M, Szeto HH, Daniel SS, et al. Placental transfer and fetal metabolism of zidovudine in the baboon. Pediatr Res 44:47-53, 1998.
352. Sperling RS, Roboz J, Dische R, et al. Zidovudine pharmacokinetics during pregnancy. Am J Perinatol 9:247-249, 1992.
353. O'Sullivan MJ, Boyer PJJ, Scott GB, et al. The pharmacokinetics and safety of zidovudine in the third trimester of pregnancy for women infected with human immunodeficiency virus and their infants: Phase I Acquired Immunodeficiency Syndrome Clinical Trials Group study (protocol 082). Am J Obstet Gynecol 168:1510-1516, 1993.
354. Watts DH, Brown ZA, Tartaglione T, et al. Pharmacokinetic disposition of zidovudine during pregnancy. J Infect Dis 163:226-232, 1991.
355. Lopez-Anaya A, Unadkat JD, Schumann LA, Smith AL. Pharmacokinetics of zidovudine (azidothymidine). I. Transplacental transfer. J Acquir Immune Defic Syndr 3:959-964, 1990.
356. Lopez-Anaya A, Unadkat JD, Schumann LA, Smith AL. Pharmacokinetics of zidovudine (azidothymidine): II. Development of metabolic and renal clearance pathways in the neonate. J Acquir Immune Defic Syndr 3:1052-1058, 1990.
357. Boucher FD, Au DS, Martin DM, et al. Pharmacokinetics and safety of azidothymidine (AZT) in infants less than three months old, exposed at birth to HIV. Clin Res 37:190A, 1989.
358. Boucher FD, Modlin JF, Weller S, et al. Phase I evaluation of zidovudine administered to infants exposed at birth to the human immunodeficiency virus. J Pediatr 122:137-144, 1993.
359. Olivero OA, Anderson LM, Diwan BA, et al. Transplacental effects of 3′-azido-2′,3′-dideoxythymidine (AZT): tumorigenicity in mice and genotoxicity in mice and monkeys. J Natl Cancer Inst 89:1602-1608, 1997.
360. Olivero OA, Anderson LM, Diwan BA, et al. AZT is a genotoxic transplacental carcinogen in animal models. J Acquir Immune Defic Syndr Hum Retrovirol 14:A29, 1997.
361. Dalakas MC, Illa I, Pezeshkpour GH, et al. Mitochondrial myopathy caused by long-term zidovudine therapy. N Engl J Med 322:1098-1105, 1990.
362. Brady MT, McGrath N, Brouwers P, et al. Randomized study of the tolerance and efficacy of high- versus low-dose zidovudine in human immunodeficiency virus–infected children with mild to moderate symptoms (AIDS Clinical Trial Group 128). J Infect Dis 173:1097-1106, 1996.
363. Balis FM, Pizzo PA, Butler KM, et al. Clinical pharmacology of 2′,3′-dideoxyinosine in human immunodeficiency virus–infected children. J Infect Dis 165:99-104, 1992.
364. Pons JC, Boubon MC, Taburet AM, et al. Fetoplacental passage of 2′,3′-dideoxyinosine. Lancet 337:732, 1991.
365. Pereira CM, Nosbisch C, Winter HR, et al. Transplacental pharmacokinetics of dideoxyinosine in pigtailed macaques. Antimicrob Agents Chemother 38:781-786, 1994.
366. Pereira CM, Nosbisch C, Unadkat JD. Pharmacokinetics of dideoxyinosine in neonatal pigtailed macaques. Antimicrob Agents Chemother 38:787-789, 1994.
367. Lai KR, Gang DL, Zawacki JK, Cooley TP. Fulminant hepatic failure associated with 2′,3′-dideoxyinosine (ddI). Ann Intern Med 115:283-284, 1991.
368. Whitcup SM, Butler KM, Caruso R, et al. Retinal toxicity in human immunodeficiency virus–infected children treated with 2′,3′-dideoxyinosine. Am J Ophthalmol 113:1-7, 1992.
369. Whitcup S, Butler K, Pizzo P, Nussenblatt R. Retinal lesions in children treated with dideoxyinosine. N Engl J Med 326:1226-1227, 1992.
370. Lewis LL, Venzon D, Church J, et al. Lamivudine in children with human immunodeficiency virus infection: a phase I/II study. J Infect Dis 174:16-25, 1996.
371. Mueller BU, Lewis LL, Yuen GJ, et al. Serum and cerebrospinal fluid pharmacokinetics of intravenous and oral lamivudine in human immunodeficiency virus–infected children. Antimicrob Agents Chemother 42:3187-3192, 1998.
372. Grob PM, Wu JC, Cohen KA, et al. Nonnucleoside inhibitors of HIV-1 reverse transcriptase: nevirapine as a prototype drug. AIDS Res Hum Retrovir 8:145-152, 1992.
373. Grob PM, Cao Y, Muchmore E, et al. Prophylaxis against HIV-1 infection in chimpanzees by nevirapine, a nonnucleoside inhibitor of reverse transcriptase. Nat Med 3:665-670, 1997.
374. Richman DD, Havlir D, Corbeil J, et al. Nevirapine resistance mutations of human immunodeficiency virus type 1 selected during therapy. J Virol 68:1660-1666, 1994.
375. Luzuriaga K, Bryson Y, McSherry G, et al. Pharmacokinetics, safety, and activity of nevirapine in human immunodeficiency virus type 1–infected children. J Infect Dis 174:713-721, 1996.
376. Shetty AK, Coovadia HM, Mirochnick MM, et al. Safety and trough concentrations of nevirapine prophylaxis given daily, twice weekly, or weekly in breast-feeding infants from birth to 6 months. J Acquir Immune Defic Syndr 34:482-490, 2003.
377. Mirochnik M, Sullivan J, Gagnier P, et al. Safety and pharmacokinetics (PK) of nevirapine in neonates born to HIV-1 infected women. Presented before the 4th Conference on Retroviruses and Opportunistic Infections, Washington, DC, 1997.
378. Krogstad P, Wiznia A, Luzuriaga K, et al. Treatment of human immunodeficiency virus 1–infected infants and children with the protease inhibitor nelfinavir mesylate. Clin Infect Dis 28:1109-1118, 1999.
379. Flexner C. HIV-protease inhibitors. N Engl J Med 338:1281-1292, 1998.
380. Mueller BU, Nelson RP Jr, Sleasman J, et al. A phase I/II study of the protease inhibitor ritonavir in children with human immunodeficiency virus infection. Pediatrics 101:335-343, 1998.
381. Havens PL, Cuene BE, Holtgrave DR. Lifetime cost of care for children with human immunodeficiency virus infection. Pediatr Infect Dis J 16:607-610, 1997.

Chapter 22

CHICKENPOX, MEASLES, AND MUMPS

Anne A. Gershon

The viruses that cause varicella, zoster, measles, and mumps may complicate the management of a mother, fetus, or newborn when maternal infection with one of these agents occurs during pregnancy or at term. In the United States, because most women of childbearing years are immune to measles and mumps and because there is little opportunity for exposure to these infections because the current population is highly immunized, these diseases posed more problems during pregnancy during the first half of the 20th century than they do now.

Because a licensed varicella vaccine is routinely used in the United States, the incidence of varicella among women of childbearing age can be predicted to decrease in the future. However, the varicella-zoster virus (VZV) still inflicts significant fetal damage as the cause of the congenital varicella syndrome, especially in locations where the vaccine is not being used routinely. Improved methods for control, including better diagnostic methods, antiviral therapy with acyclovir, passive immunization with varicella-zoster immune globulin (VZIG), and use of live-attenuated varicella vaccine, have decreased prenatal and postnatal morbidity from this virus. Understanding of this viral infection at the molecular level, including clarification of the cause of zoster by studies of viral DNA, RNA, and proteins in latency, and study of specific viral glycoproteins and their importance in the immune response have advanced our knowledge and can be expected to lead to improved therapeutic measures.

CHICKENPOX AND ZOSTER

Chickenpox (i.e., varicella) is an acute, contagious disease that most commonly occurs in childhood. It is characterized by a generalized exanthem consisting of vesicles that develop in successive crops and that rapidly evolve to pustules, crusts, and scabs. Zoster (i.e., herpes zoster, shingles) occurs in persons who have previously had chickenpox. It is typified by a painful vesicular eruption usually restricted to one or more segmental dermatomes. An abundance of virologic, epidemiologic, and immunologic evidence has been amassed, indicating that these two illnesses are caused by the same etiologic agent,[1] which therefore was designated *VZV*. Chickenpox is a manifestation of primary infection with VZV. After the acute infection subsides, VZV, like other herpesviruses, persists in a latent form. For VZV, the site of latent infection is in the dorsal root and cranial nerve ganglia, where certain early viral genes and proteins are expressed in latency.[2-4] VZV may subsequently be reactivated with expression of all of its genes as immunity wanes. The reactivated infection assumes the segmental distribution of the nerve cells in which latent virus resided, giving rise to zoster. A description of the historical recognition of disease caused by VZV follows.

Varicella is a modernized Latin word used since at least 1764 and intended to connote a diminutive of the more serious variola (i.e., smallpox).[5] The etymology of chicken in chickenpox is less clear. It may also be a diminutive derived from the French *pois chiche*, or "chick pea," a dwarf species of pea *(Cicer arietinum)*.[5] Other workers doubt this Latin origin and conjecture that the word originated from the farmyard fowl, in which case it has a Teutonic ancestry in the Old English *cicen* and the Middle High German *kuchen*.[6] Herpes has been used to designate a malady since 1398 ("this euyll callyd Herpes")[7] but derives from the Greek word meaning "to creep"; *zoster* is the Greek and Latin word meaning "girdle" or "belt." Shingles, from the Latin *cingulus* (meaning "girdle"), was also used in the 14th century as *schingles* to describe "icchynge and scabs wett and drye."[7]

The Organism

Classification and Morphology

The VZV (Herpesvirus varicellae) is a member of the herpesvirus family. In addition to a burgeoning number of animal herpesviruses, this group includes eight additional, closely related viruses that infect humans: herpes simplex viruses (HSV) types 1 and 2 (Herpesvirus hominis), cytomegalovirus

(CMV), Epstein-Barr virus (EBV), and human herpesviruses 6, 7, and 8. Only one antigenic type of VZV has been identified, but molecular studies have revealed some minor differences in VZV that have proved useful for epidemiologic studies.[8]

Common properties of the family include a DNA genome and enveloped virions exhibiting icosahedral symmetry with a diameter of 180 to 200 nm.[1] Nucleocapsids, which are assembled in the nucleus, have a diameter of about 100 nm and consist of a DNA core surrounded by 162 identical subunits, or capsomeres. Nucleocapsids acquire a temporary envelope at the nuclear membrane; they are further transported by means of the endoplasmic reticulum to the Golgi, where they receive a final envelope. In cell cultures, virions are packaged in vesicles identified as endosomes, which are acidic.[9,10] Virus particles are released from these structures at the cell surface by exocytosis. Extracellular virions are extremely pleomorphic compared with those of HSV. This pleomorphism, presumably reflecting injury to the envelope possibly caused by exposure to acid or enzymes in endosomes, is believed to account for the lability and lack of cell-free virus that characterizes VZV in tissue culture and in its spread through the body during varicella infection, and it distinguishes VZV from HSV.[9-11] In vivo, however, enveloped and well-formed VZV is released from skin cells, yielding highly infectious virions capable of airborne spread and with a great degree of communicability.

Molecular studies have elucidated some details concerning how latent VZV infection is established, maintained, and reactivated. Latent infection probably comes from virions present in skin during varicella. However, it is unlikely that complete viral replication occurs in the neuron during establishment of latency, because the neuron must survive, and replication would cause cell death. The replication process of VZV is begun during latent infection, but a block in the cascade of viral gene expression takes place. About six viral genes and their protein gene products are expressed in latently infected neurons. These proteins are confined to the cell cytoplasm. It appears that when these proteins are transduced into the nucleus by factors still to be determined, reactivation occurs, with production of all 70 VZV gene products and synthesis of infectious, enveloped virions in the nerve and skin.[12,13]

Propagation

VZV grows readily in diploid human fibroblasts such as WI 38 cells, the most commonly used cell type for virus isolation. VZV also can be propagated in certain epithelial cells, such as human embryonic kidney, primary human amnion cells, primary human thyroid cells, and Vero (African green monkey kidney) cells. Like CMV, the cytopathic effect of VZV is focal in cell culture because of its cell-associated character, and cytopathic effects develop more slowly (3 to 7 days) than with HSV. Animal models for varicella (guinea pigs)[14] and for zoster (rats)[15] have been described. An in vitro model of latency and reactivation in guinea pig enteric neurons has also been developed and provides a setting in which to study factors that influence latency and reactivation.[12]

Serologic Tests and Antigenic Properties of Varicella-Zoster Virus

Several serologic tests are available to measure antibodies to VZV. These tests include indirect immunofluorescence, often called *fluorescent antibody to membrane antigen* (FAMA)[16,17]; latex agglutination (LA)[18]; enzyme-linked immunosorbent assay (ELISA)[19-22]; radioimmunoassay[23]; immune adherence hemagglutination[24]; neutralization[19,25]; and complement-enhanced neutralization.[26] All of these methods are more sensitive than the complement fixation assay.[27] Data gathered from these assays show that antibody to VZV develops within a few days after the onset of varicella, persists for many years, and is present before the onset of zoster.

Serologic cross-reactions between HSV and VZV have been described.[28,29] HSV and VZV share common antigens, and similar polypeptides and glycoproteins have been identified for both viruses, but cross-protection has not been observed.[30-32] Rare simultaneous infections with one or more human herpesviruses have been reported.[33,34] Elevations in heterologous antibody titers in apparent HSV or VZV infections may result from cross-reactions of the viruses but also may indicate simultaneous infection by both viruses.

VZV produces at least eight major glycoprotein antigens—B, C, E, H, I, K, L, and M—all of which are on the envelope of the virus and on the surface of infected cells. The glycoproteins and internal antigens, such as the capsid and tegument, stimulate production of neutralizing and other types of antibodies, as well as cellular immunity.[35-37] Antibodies elaborated in varicella and zoster are of the immunoglobulin G (IgG), IgA, and IgM classes.[38,39]

Epidemiology and Transmission

Chickenpox ranks as one of the most communicable of human diseases. No extrahuman reservoir of VZV is known. Because the supply of susceptible persons, especially in the era before the urbanization of society, would be rapidly exhausted by so contagious a disease, virus latency may have adaptive evolutionary significance in perpetuating infection. In isolated communities, cases of zoster would be responsible for the reintroduction of VZV and its transmission as varicella to new generations of susceptible individuals.[1,40]

Communicability by Droplets and Contact

Historically, transfer of VZV was believed to occur by way of respiratory droplets, and epidemiologic evidence suggests that transmission can occur before the onset of rash.[41-43] It is rare, however, to isolate VZV from the pharynx of infected patients. A study using polymerase chain reaction (PCR) methods demonstrated that VZV DNA is present in the nasopharynx of a high percentage of children during the early stages of clinical varicella,[44] but PCR does not necessarily indicate the presence of infectious virus. In contrast, the vesicular lesions in varicella and zoster are full of infectious VZV that can readily be cultured. Moreover, in a study of leukemic recipients of live-attenuated varicella vaccine, only those with skin lesions as a side effect of varicella vaccination spread vaccine-type virus to varicella-susceptible close contacts.[45] Similarly, the rare instances of transmission of vaccine virus from healthy vaccines to other susceptibles occurred only when the vaccinee had a rash.[46] Cell-free VZV virions are known to be copiously produced in skin lesions and are the type of particle that could be aerosolized and involved in viral transmission. It appears that the major source of infectious VZV is the skin, although it is possible that transmission from the respiratory tract can occur.

Airborne spread of varicella has been documented,[47,48] but indirect transfer by fomites has not. VZV DNA has been detected in air samples for many hours in hospitals,[49] but the relation to infectivity of the virus is unclear. Varicella is most contagious at the time of onset of rash and for 1 to 2 days afterward,[50] but the period of infectivity probably encompasses 1 to 2 days before the rash is noticed until 5 days after onset of the rash.

Incubation Period

The usual incubation period for chickenpox is 13 to 17 days, with a mean of 15 days. The extremes are 10 and 21 days, unless passive immunization has been given, in which case the incubation period may be prolonged.[43,51]

Relationship between Varicella and Zoster

It is amply documented that exposure of susceptible persons to zoster may result in chickenpox. Vesicular fluid from patients with zoster produced chickenpox when inoculated into susceptible children.[52,53] Other studies have confirmed that a similar relationship exists under conditions of natural exposure.[54] Claims to the contrary notwithstanding,[55,56] it has not been documented that zoster is acquired from other patients with zoster or chickenpox. Instances that have been reported do not exclude the chance sporadic occurrence of zoster in persons who happen to have been exposed to chickenpox or zoster. It is difficult to reconcile this postulated mode of transmission with current concepts of the pathogenesis of zoster, particularly the strict segmental distribution of lesions and the demonstrated presence of VZV DNA, RNA, and certain viral proteins in ganglia during latency.[2,4,13,57] Studies have also determined that the VZV DNA from zoster isolates is identical to that which caused the primary infection, proving that zoster is caused by reactivation of latent VZV.[58-60]

Transplacental Transmission

In pregnancy, VZV may be transmitted across the placenta, resulting in congenital or neonatal chickenpox.[61] The consequences of transplacental infection are discussed in a later section.

Incidence and Distribution of Chickenpox

The distribution of chickenpox is worldwide. Because vaccination is routine for children in the United States, significant changes in the epidemiology of varicella have occurred, with evidence of personal and herd immunity.[62] Before the vaccine era in the United States, which began in 1995 with vaccine licensure, outbreaks of varicella occurred each year without major fluctuations between years.[63] Although the disease was seen in all months, more cases occurred in the winter and early spring. This seasonal variation was attributed primarily to the gathering of children in school but also may be related to changes in environmental temperature. With introduction of the vaccine, there is less varicella disease occurring in all age groups, and the seasonality of the disease is blurred.[62]

Chickenpox is more contagious than mumps but somewhat less so than measles.[57,64] After exposure within households, 61% of susceptible persons of all age groups (without a history of previous disease) developed chickenpox, compared with 76% for measles and 31% for mumps.[51] Compared with measles, chickenpox is about 80% as infectious in the household but only 35% to 65% as infectious in society. The reason probably is that chickenpox requires relatively intimate contact for transmission, such as that occurring in the household, whereas in society, there are more casual contacts. Measles may infect efficiently even through casual contacts.[64]

An estimated 4 million cases of chickenpox used to occur yearly in the United States. Varicella remains a nonreportable disease, but this is expected to change as more and more vaccine is used and there are fewer and fewer cases of varicella annually. The disease affects both sexes equally and is most commonly seen in children of early school age. Increasing urbanization was associated with acquisition of the disease at younger ages. In Massachusetts between 1952 and 1961, 29% of children reported with chickenpox were younger than 4 years old, 62% were 5 to 9 years old, 7% were 10 to 14 years old, and less than 3% were older than 15 years.[65] Later data also indicated that varicella is primarily a disease of young children.[66] Between 70% and 80% of young American adults report a history of varicella.[65,67] This compares with histories in the same age group in the prevaccine era of 92% for measles, 45% for mumps, and 31% for rubella. Subclinical varicella is uncommon. Data from family studies indicate that only 8% of adults without a history of varicella develop clinical disease when exposed to their own infected children.[68] The relative importance of faulty memory or past subclinical infection in this secondary attack rate is uncertain.

With the use of sensitive assays for the measurement of antibodies to VZV, it appears that less than 25% of adults with no history of chickenpox are susceptible.[69] Based on a population of adults in which 90% are immune, this suggests a subclinical attack rate of varicella of roughly 7%.

Incidence of Chickenpox, Mumps, and Measles in Pregnancy

Few studies have addressed the incidence of chickenpox, mumps, and measles during pregnancy. In these studies, two questions are posed. First, of all pregnancies, how many are complicated by measles, mumps, or chickenpox? Second, among all reported cases of those diseases, how many occur in pregnant women? In a prospective study of clinically recognized infections that occurred during 30,059 pregnancies between 1958 and 1964, the Collaborative Perinatal Research Study identified approximately 1600 women with presumed viral infections (excluding the common cold).[70] Serologic testing was used to confirm the diagnoses of measles, varicella, and mumps. Taking into account the many possible inaccuracies in such a study, the minimum frequency per 10,000 pregnancies of confirmed cases was 0.6 case for measles, 5 cases for varicella, and 10 cases for mumps.

In another study of maternal virus diseases in New York City between 1957 and 1964, Siegel and Fuerst[71] followed pregnant women for whom a clinical diagnosis of measles, mumps, chickenpox, or other viral infection had been made. Of the 826 virus-infected pregnant women who were identified, 417 were infected with rubella (50.5%), 150 with chickenpox (18.1%), 128 with mumps (15.5%), and 66 with measles (8.0%). Approximately 190,000 pregnancies per year were reported in this population. The calculated attack rates of varicella, mumps, and measles are shown in Table 22-1. The data in these studies are undoubtedly inaccurate because of incorrect clinical diagnoses, underreporting of mild or subclinical infections, and other factors. These figures reflect findings in the prevaccine era, and it seems likely that measles

Table 22–1 Attack Rates of Various Viral Infections during Pregnancy in the Prevaccine Era[a]

Study	Measles	Varicella-Zoster	Mumps
Cases per 10,000 pregnancies			
Collaborative[65]	0.6	5	10
New York[66]	0.4	0.8	1
Connecticut[67]	—	7	—
Predicted cases per year in the United States during pregnancy	120-180	240-2450	300-3000

[a]Based on 3.5 million U.S. births yearly.

occurred less frequently during pregnancy than mumps or chickenpox in the prevaccine era. The probable explanation is that in unvaccinated populations the greater communicability of measles resulted in fewer females reaching childbearing age without already having been infected.

Today, measles and mumps are rare in the United States, and varicella is becoming less common. In highly immunized populations such as exist in the United States, an even lower incidence of infection during pregnancy is predicted for measles, mumps, and varicella. It is possible that the incidence of varicella in pregnant women in the United States is affected by the influx of varicella-susceptible immigrants from countries with tropical climates. A calculation in 1992 projected an incidence of seven cases of varicella per 10,000 pregnancies.[72] Even these crude data, however, indicate that varicella, mumps, and measles are unusual during pregnancy.

The relative rarity of the association of each of these diseases with pregnancy, as indicated by these studies, highlights the difficulties involved in obtaining data on their effect on the outcome of pregnancy compared with a disease with a higher incidence during pregnancy, such as was once true for rubella. Answers can come only from uniform national reporting policies involving many collaborating agencies.

Incidence and Distribution of Zoster

In contrast to chickenpox, zoster is primarily a disease of adults, especially older adults or immunosuppressed patients. Hope-Simpson, describing patients of all ages in a general practice observed during a 16-year period, found an incidence of 3.4 cases per 1000 people per year.[40] Zoster occurs with approximately the same frequency each month, which is compatible with the concept that zoster results from reactivation of latent infection rather than exogenous reinfection with VZV. In the household or hospital, VZV-naïve persons exposed to zoster are not at increased risk of developing zoster but are likely to develop chickenpox in the absence of a previous history of varicella. Zoster "epidemics" have been claimed in special circumstances, such as in a hospitalized leukemic population,[55] but their documentation is not convincing.

Adults and children older than 2 years who have zoster usually give a history of a previous attack of varicella, whereas in younger infants a history of intrauterine exposure to VZV can often be elicited.[40] The latency period between primary infection and zoster is shorter if varicella occurs in prenatal rather than in postnatal life.[73] Chickenpox in the first year of life also increases the risk of childhood zoster, with a relative risk roughly between 3 and 21.[74,75] Possibly, this phenomenon is caused by immaturity of the immune response to chickenpox in young infants, permitting early viral reactivation.[76]

After infancy, the incidence of zoster rises progressively with age. The attack rate in octogenarians was 14 times that of children in Hope-Simpson's series.[40] Second attacks of zoster are unusual; 8 were observed among 192 cases in the previously cited series.[40] Four of those attacks involved the same dermatome as the first attack, suggesting a tendency for reactivation of VZV from the same ganglion cells in which the virus was dormant. Some of these cases, however, might have been caused by reactivation of HSV; in one study, HSV was isolated from 13% of a series of 47 immunocompetent patients with clinically diagnosed zoster.[77] Zoster in adults and children occurs with increased frequency in patients with malignant hematopoietic neoplasms (especially Hodgkin's disease), after organ transplantation, and in individuals infected with human immunodeficiency virus (HIV).[78-80] Spinal trauma, irradiation, and corticosteroid therapy may also be precipitating factors. The distribution of lesions in chickenpox, which primarily affects the trunk, head, and neck, is reflected in a proportionately greater representation of these regions in the segmental lesions of zoster.[40]

Incidence of Zoster in Pregnancy

Several reports describe the occurrence of zoster during pregnancy, but adequate statistics from which to calculate attack rates are not available. Brazin and associates[81] have projected an incidence of 6000 cases annually in pregnant women, which would mean that gestational zoster is more common than gestational chickenpox. Assuming that there are 3.5 million pregnant women yearly in the United States, this calculates to a rate of 20 cases per 10,000 pregnant women per year. Prospective studies of pregnant women in Sweden, however, have suggested that zoster is less common in pregnancy than varicella.[82] In any case, zoster, like varicella, appears to be a rarity in pregnancy. The severity or natural history of zoster does not appear to be worse in pregnant women than in the population at large. Implications of gestational zoster for the fetus are discussed in a subsequent section.

Nosocomial Chickenpox in the Nursery

The precise risk of horizontal transmission in maternity wards or the newborn nursery after VZV has been introduced is unclear, but based on experience, it is very low. This is in part because maternal immunity plays a role in protection of the infant. About 70% of persons give a history of chickenpox by age 20 years, and still others are immune in the absence of a positive history, so that most mothers and hospital personnel are not at risk. Many hospital workers require proof of immunity to varicella (or vaccination) for employment. It appears that only 5% to 10% of women born in the United States are susceptible to varicella and that more than 75% of those with no history of chickenpox are immune.[69,83-86] The percentage of susceptible persons among women raised in tropical climates is somewhat higher, probably because viral spread is impeded by high temperatures and the lack of urbanization.[83,87-90]

Because IgG antibodies to VZV cross the placenta,[83,91] the newborn infants of immune mothers should be at least partially protected. Using the sensitive FAMA assay to measure antibodies to VZV in a study of 67 infants, even among children 5 months old, 50% still had detectable VZV antibodies.[83] Even in premature and low-birth-weight infants, antibodies to VZV are likely to be detectable.[92-94] Nevertheless, perinatal chickenpox has been reported rarely in infants born to women with positive histories of chickenpox.[95-99] In Newman's study,[98] varicella developed in a mother and her baby after exposure to a student midwife with chickenpox. The mother had experienced varicella as a child and had a few remaining skin scars; apparently, she had developed a second attack as an adult. Readett and McGibbon[99] reported two cases of extrauterine infection in neonates whose mothers had histories of chickenpox. After delivery at home, each of these infants was exposed within 24 hours of birth to a sibling with chickenpox and subsequently developed skin lesions when 12 and 14 days old, respectively. Their mothers did not develop chickenpox in the perinatal period and were found to have serum-neutralizing antibodies to VZV. In the literature before 1975, VZV antibody titers were not often reported because sensitive tests for measuring these antibodies were not readily available. Since that time, infection of a few seropositive infants after postnatal exposure to VZV has been documented.[95,96] These infants had mothers with a history of varicella, and the VZV antibody in the infants' blood was transplacentally acquired. In one instance, mild varicella developed in a 2-week-old, 1040-g infant who was seropositive at exposure and was also passively immunized with VZIG 72 hours after the exposure.[96] In another study, five infants younger than 2 months old, all of whom were seropositive at exposure, developed varicella in a children's custodial institution.[95] Even when varicella develops in the presence of maternal antibodies, it appears to be modified. Although complete protection of every neonate against chickenpox is not guaranteed by immunity in the mother, protection is the exception rather than the rule.

Not unexpectedly, horizontal transmission of chickenpox in maternity wards and newborn nurseries is an uncommon event. In some reports, lack of transmission is difficult to explain. In 1965, Newman[98] reported two cases of varicella that occurred in mothers in the same prenatal ward 18 to 19 days after exposure to the index-infected infant and its mother. One mother developed chickenpox 7 days ante partum, and the other developed the disease 3 days post partum. Each mother was immediately isolated from the ward but not from her own infant; neither of the infants developed chickenpox. In all, 139 mothers, excluding the index case, were exposed, and 8 developed infection. Three of the 42 staff members also became infected. Remarkably, the index infant was the only neonate infected; all other infants, including those born to the eight infected mothers, remained free of disease. Gershon and co-workers[83] described an outbreak in which a woman developed varicella post partum and exposed 10 mothers, their infants, 1 antepartum woman, and approximately 25 staff members during a brief period while she was waiting in the hospital corridor. Her infant developed varicella 10 days afterward. About 2 weeks later, three cases of varicella developed in the exposed persons: a hospital employee and a postpartum woman and her infant. Gustafson and colleagues[96] described another mini-outbreak that took place during a 2-month period in a neonatal intensive care unit in which a total of 29 infants were exposed. Two of these infants, whose mothers gave a history of previous varicella, developed chickenpox after exposure to two hospital employees who had been infected nosocomially.[96]

Other reports largely confirm the low rate of transmissibility of chickenpox in neonates. Freud[100] described an infant who had transplacentally acquired disease and developed lesions on the second day of life. None of the other 17 neonates in the nursery became infected, but the index infant had been isolated immediately, so exposure had been very brief.[100] When transferred to another ward, this same infant transmitted the disease to two older children, who were 4 and 7 years old. Odessky[101] reported three instances of congenital varicella: two infants were immediately isolated, but the third was not recognized as having chickenpox and exposed other neonates for 4 days. The number at risk is not stated, but no instances of transmission were observed. In the report of Harris,[102] a total of 35 infants were exposed to two infants with congenital chickenpox for periods of 18 and 10 hours before isolation. None subsequently became infected, possibly because all the mothers had positive histories of chickenpox. In an additional case described by Matseoane and Abler,[103] an infant developed transplacentally acquired chickenpox at the age of 9 days and exposed 13 other neonates in the nursery for periods of 2 to 10 hours before isolation. Six mothers had a positive history of varicella, three did not, and four did not know. None of the exposed mothers or infants developed chickenpox. Lack of transmission despite hospital exposure to an adult with varicella in neonatal intensive care nurseries was also reported by Wang and associates (32 infants),[94] Lipton and Brunell (22 infants),[104] Patou and co-workers (15 infants),[105] Mendez and associates (16 infants),[92] and Gold and co-workers (29 infants).[106]

One experience in a neonatal intensive care unit in Mississippi is illustrative.[107] After the development of hemorrhagic varicella in a 25-week-gestation infant whose mother had varicella 2 weeks previously, 14 infants in the unit were exposed over a period of several days. None of the infants in isolettes became ill, but four who were in open warming units at exposure developed varicella 10 days later. All had received VZIG, and in each instance, the mother gave a history of varicella. The illnesses were mild with only a few papular skin lesions, but three of the four infants were positive for VZV on immunofluorescence testing of skin scrapings. Each child with varicella was treated with intravenous acyclovir. The incidence of disease was higher in infants with less than 29 weeks' gestation than in infants with longer gestational periods.

Of historical interest is an extensive epidemic lasting 5 months that was described by Apert in 1895.[108] Two infants in a newborn nursery developed chickenpox on January 7

Table 22–2 Nosocomial Chickenpox Infections in the Nursery

Reference No. (Year)	Case No.	Period Others Exposed after Onset of Rash	Prior History of Varicella in Mothers of Infants Exposed			No. of Persons Exposed	No. Subsequently Infected
			Yes	*No*	*Unknown*		
108 (1895)	1	Variable		No data		<40 young infants	19
101 (1954)	2	4 days		No data		Not stated	0
	3	0 (immed. isolation)		No data		Not stated	0
	4	0 (immed. isolation)		No data		Not stated	0
100 (1958)	5	0 (immed. isolation in nursery)	0	0	17	17 neonates	0
		3 days (other ward)		No data		Not stated	2[a]
102 (1963)	6	18 hr					
	7	10 hr	35	0	0	35 neonates	0
103 (1965)	8	2, 3, 8, 10 hr in susceptible neonates	6	3	4	13 neonates	0
98 (1965)	9	Variable	1	7	132	139 mothers	8
						?139 neonates	0[b]
83 (1976)	10	Brief	0	2	9	11 mothers	2
						10 infants	1 infant
						25 staff	1
94 (1983)	11	Brief		No data		32 infants	0
96 (1984)	12	Variable	8	0	21	29 infants	2 infants[c]
104 (1989)	13	Brief, intimate	22			22 infants	0
105 (1990)	14	Brief[c,d]	13	1	1	15 infants	0
92 (1992)	15	Brief[c,d]		No data		16 infants	0
106 (1993)	16	1 hr on each of 3 days		No data		29 infants	0
107 (1994)	17	Intimate	10		4	14 infants	4 infants
Total since 1990						218 infants	7 infants

[a]Infected infant transferred to another ward, where two older children (ages 4 and 7) later developed chickenpox.
[b]No cases of chickenpox in neonates, despite appearance of chickenpox in eight mothers from 34 days ante partum to 14 days post partum.
[c]In neonatal intensive care unit.
[d]Exposure 1-2 days before rash in index case.

and 8. They were immediately transferred with their mothers to another ward, where they were isolated, but a third infant (second generation of chickenpox) developed disease on January 24 and was likewise isolated with its mother. A fourth infant (third generation) developed varicella on February 7 but was not isolated until February 13 because the mother deliberately obscured the fact that the infant had lesions. Subsequently, a fifth infant (fourth generation) developed chickenpox on February 21. Because the number of infants exposed and the maternal histories of varicella are not stated, the attack rates are unclear. Although this was the last case of chickenpox in the newborn nursery, one of the infected neonates introduced the virus to another ward of 40 to 45 debilitated infants. Before the epidemic was over in May, nine generations of chickenpox separated with mathematical precision by 14 days had occurred. In all, 19 infants, 12 younger than 6 six months, were infected along with two mothers.

These experiences with nosocomial chickenpox in the newborn nursery are summarized in Table 22-2. In the 20th century, in reports in which the number of neonates exposed is explicitly stated, a total of 218 exposures resulted in only eight instances of transmission to infants. Most of the mothers had histories of varicella, although in many the history was unknown. Several factors undoubtedly contribute to the low rate of transmission of disease to neonates: passive immunity in most; relatively brief exposure compared with that in the household setting, where 80% to 90% of susceptibles become clinically infected[40,68]; and relative lack of intimacy of contact in the nursery, particularly for infants in isolettes.

Pathogenesis of Varicella and Zoster

In the usual case of chickenpox, the portal of entry and initial site of virus replication is probably the oropharynx, but attempts to demonstrate this directly have been surprisingly unrewarding. In five patients whose blood, throat secretions, and skin were cultured repeatedly during the prodromal period and after the appearance of cutaneous lesions, VZV was recovered from a throat swab in only one instance and from the blood in none. In contrast, vesicle fluid from these patients yielded VZV in all instances.[109] Attempts to isolate the virus from the blood of six additional patients were positive in only one instance: on the second day of rash in an immunosuppressed host. Other, more extensive searches for VZV in throat secretions of patients with varicella, even during the incubation period, proved essentially negative.[110,111] However, in one report, VZV was isolated from nasal swabs in 4 of 11 children on days 2 through 4 after onset of the rash. VZV could not be isolated during the incubation period or even during the first day of the rash. It was not clear whether the virus was multiplying in the nasal mucosa.[112]

VZV has been isolated from blood obtained from patients with varicella. Ozaki and colleagues[113] cultured blood from seven immunocompetent children; VZV was isolated a few days before the onset of rash or within 1 day after onset. Asano and co-workers[114] similarly isolated VZV from the blood of 7 of 12 otherwise healthy patients with early varicella. Those from whom virus could not be isolated had been studied after they had the rash for more than 4 days. Both investigators introduced an additional technical step into the blood culture process that might explain why they were successful in isolating VZV while many others before them had not been. The white blood cells were separated on Ficoll-Hypaque gradients and added to cell cultures. Although there was no evidence of viral growth in these cultures, they were blindly passaged onto new cell cultures. Evidence of growth of VZV was present in these second cultures after the blind passage within 2 to 5 days. Before these studies, VZV had been isolated only from blood obtained from immunocompromised patients with varicella or zoster.[110,115,116] The white blood cell infected with VZV is a mononuclear cell, but it is uncertain whether monocytes or lymphocytes, or both, are involved.[113,114] Experiments in the SCID-hu mouse model have shown that VZV is lymphotropic for human $CD4^+$ and $CD8^+$ T lymphocytes and that human T cells release some infectious virus.[117]

Data from PCR studies of patients with varicella are of interest, although they have yielded various results. In the study of Koropchak and colleagues,[118] performed 24 hours after rash onset in 12 patients, 3.3% of oropharyngeal samples, 67% of mononuclear cells, and 75% of skin vesicles were positive for VZV DNA. In the study by Ozaki and co-workers[119] of pharyngeal secretions of chickenpox patients, 26% and 90% were positive during the incubation period and after clinical onset, respectively.

Virus is readily recovered from cutaneous lesions soon after the onset of chickenpox. Isolation of VZV was successful in 23 of 25 cases in which vesicle fluid was cultured within 3 days after the onset of the rash but was successful in only 1 of 7 specimens collected between 4 and 8 days after onset.[109] In contrast, the virus apparently persists longer in vesicles of zoster patients, in whom 7 of 10 specimens collected later than 3 days after onset were positive.[104] PCR is more sensitive than virus culture. In the study of Koropchak and co-workers,[118] for example, VZV was recovered from only 21% of skin lesions, but 75% were positive by PCR. Unlike smallpox, chickenpox is no longer communicable by the time the lesions have crusted and scabbed.

The pathogenesis of chickenpox appears to be as follows. Transmission is probably effected by airborne spread of virus from cutaneous vesicles and by respiratory droplets from patients with varicella or zoster. After an initial period of virus replication in the oropharynx in the susceptible individual, there is invasion of the local lymph nodes and then a primary viremia of low magnitude, delivering virus to the viscera.[120] After several more days of virus multiplication, a secondary viremia of greater magnitude occurs, resulting in widespread cutaneous dissemination of virus and rash. Cropping of the vesicles is thought to represent several viremic phases. In the body, the virus spreads by cell-to-cell contact; viremia also is cell associated. Enveloped, cell-free infectious VZV is, however, present in the vesicular skin vesicles. Crusting and scabbing of the vesicles and pustules occur as host defense mechanisms, particularly as various forms of cell-mediated immunity become active. Latency is achieved from the cell-free VZV particles in the skin that are in proximity to sensory nerve endings.

The pathogenesis of zoster is different from that of varicella. Before development of zoster, latent VZV begins to reactivate and multiply in the sensory ganglion (or ganglia) because of unknown local factors.[2] The virus then travels down the axon to the skin supplied by that nerve. Development of a localized rash occurs if there is a deficiency in cell-mediated immunity to VZV.[121-124] This compromise in cell-mediated immunity may be obvious, as in patients who have had transplantation, therapy for malignant disease, or HIV infection,[125] or presumably, it may be transient, as in normal persons who develop zoster for no apparent reason. In immunosuppressed patients, a viremic phase with zoster has been documented occasionally,[126,127] and this probably happens after skin involvement has occurred, especially if there continues to be an inadequate immune response to VZV after the virus has reached the skin. The clinical manifestation of this viremia is disseminated zoster, in which vesicular lesions develop outside the original dermatome. A viremic phase in pregnant patients with disseminated zoster has not been documented, but it seems logical to assume that viremia would be a prerequisite for dissemination.

Pathology

Cutaneous Lesions

Histologic changes in the skin leading to the formation of vesicles are essentially identical for chickenpox, zoster, and HSV infection. The hallmark of each is the presence of multinucleated giant cells and intranuclear inclusions, changes that are not found in the vesicular lesions caused by vaccinia virus and coxsackieviruses. The lesion is primarily localized in the epidermis, where ballooning degeneration of cells in the deeper layers is accompanied by intercellular edema. As edema progresses, the cornified layers are separated from the more basal layers to form a delicate vesicle with a thin roof. An exudate consisting primarily of mononuclear cells is seen in the dermis, but the characteristic nuclear changes of epithelial cells are absent in this region.

The predominant cells in vesicular lesions are polymorphonuclear leukocytes. These cells may play a role in generating interferon in vesicular lesions, which may be important in recovery from the disease.[128] In vitro data also suggest that the polymorphonuclear leukocyte plays a role in host defense against VZV, possibly by mediating antibody-dependent cell-mediated cytotoxicity (ADCC).[129-131]

Visceral Lesions in the Fetus and Placenta

Few reports describe the appearance of the placenta in cases of congenital chickenpox with or without survival. Garcia[132] observed grossly visible necrotic lesions of the placenta in a case of chickenpox occurring in the fourth month of pregnancy that resulted in spontaneous abortion. Microscopically, central areas of necrosis were surrounded by epithelioid cells and rare giant cells of the foreign body type, giving a granulomatous appearance. Peripherally, these lesions in the villi were accompanied by an exudate of necrotic material, nuclear fragments, and leukocytes filling the intervillous spaces. Some decidual cells had typical intranuclear inclusions.

Table 22–3 Frequency of Gross and Microscopic Lesions in Seven Autopsied Cases of Fetal and Neonatal Chickenpox

Organ	No. of Cases/No. Examined	Percent	References
Skin	7/7	100	132-137
Lungs	7/7	100	132-137
Liver	7/7	100	132-137
Adrenals	6/7	86	132, 133, 135-137
Esophagus or intestines	5/6	83	127-132
	4/5	80	
Thymus	5/7	71	132, 133, 135, 137
Kidneys	4/7	56	132, 133, 135, 137
Spleen	3/7	43	132, 135-137
Pancreas	2/7	29	132, 133, 135
Heart	1/5	20	132, 136
Brain[a]			132
Miscellaneous			
Ovaries	1		133
Bone marrow	1		135
Placenta	1		132

[a]Not well documented; possibility of concomitant toxoplasmosis not definitely excluded.

Descriptions of the pathology of visceral lesions in fetal or neonatal chickenpox are necessarily restricted to autopsies in fatal cases.[132-137] Grossly, the lesions are small, punctate, white or yellow, and resemble miliary tuberculosis. Microscopically, their appearance resembles that of the lesions of the placenta: central necrotic areas, often resembling fibrinoid necrosis, surrounded by a few epithelioid cells and a scant infiltrate of mononuclear cells. Intranuclear inclusions are present. The skin, lungs, and liver are uniformly involved (Table 22-3). Slightly less frequently, the adrenals, gastrointestinal tract mucosa, and thymus are also involved. Less often, lesions appear in the kidneys, spleen, pancreas, and heart. Only one report describes necrotic foci in the brain.[132] In this case, the cortical, subependymal, and basilar structures of the cerebrum were totally destroyed and accompanied by extensive calcification. Although a search for *Toxoplasma* was negative, serologic data to rule out dual infection are lacking in the report. The gross and microscopic lesions of fatal perinatal chickenpox resemble those of disseminated HSV infection, including a preference for the liver and adrenal gland, but the provided data suggest that involvement of the brain is more common in neonatal HSV infection than it is in fatal neonatal chickenpox. A neonate with fatal hemorrhagic varicella with pneumonia and hepatitis is shown in Figure 22-1.

Visceral Lesions in the Mother

In fatal cases of chickenpox in pregnant women, maternal death is usually caused by pulmonary involvement. The pathologic course of chickenpox pneumonia in pregnant women is identical to that in nonpregnant women and in children.[138,139] The lungs are usually edematous and congested. Interstitial pneumonitis may follow a peribronchiolar distribution of disease. Edema, septal cell proliferation, and infiltration of the alveolar septa by mononuclear leukocytes occur. Intranuclear inclusions may be found in alveolar lining cells, macrophages, capillary endothelium, and tracheobronchial mucosa. Necrotic foci may be accompanied by hemorrhage, and hyaline membranes lining the alveoli are often prominent.

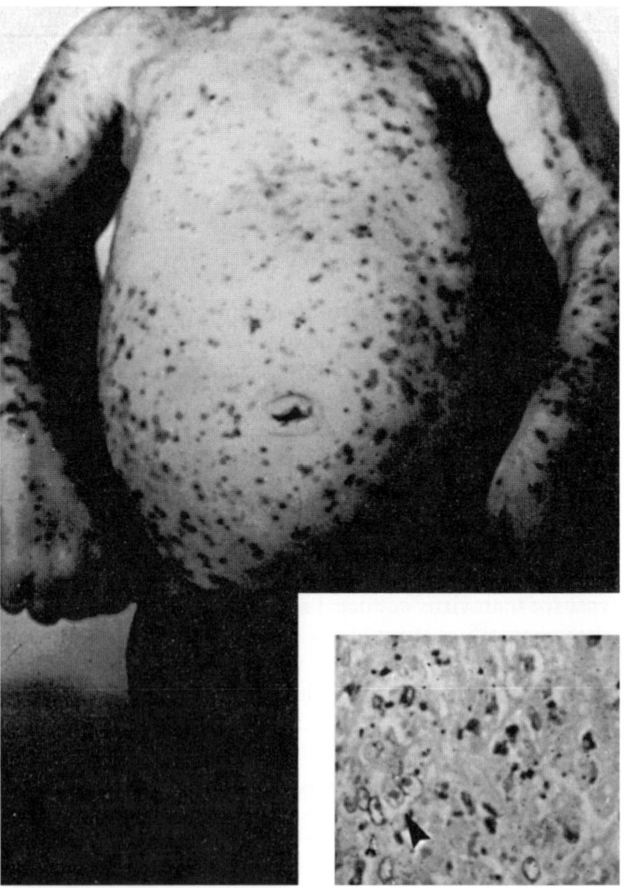

Figure 22–1 Congenital hemorrhagic varicella complicated by pneumonia and hepatitis. The mother of this infant developed varicella a few days before delivery. Zoster immune globulin was not available at that time. *Inset* shows a section of liver with intranuclear inclusion bodies obtained at autopsy.

Zoster

The pathologic picture of cutaneous lesions in zoster is indistinguishable from that of chickenpox lesions. The dorsal root ganglion of the affected dermatome exhibits a mononuclear inflammatory infiltrate. There may also be necrosis of ganglion cells and demyelination of the corresponding axon. There are no descriptions of these lesions in pregnant women or in neonates specifically.

Clinical Manifestations

Chickenpox Rash

After an incubation period of usually 13 to 17 days,[40,65] chickenpox is heralded by the approximately simultaneous occurrence of fever and rash. In adults, the exanthem is often preceded by a prodromal fever and constitutional symptoms lasting 2 or 3 days.[6] Occasionally, one or more isolated vesicles may precede a generalized exanthem by 1 or 2 days. The rash is characteristically centripetal, beginning on the face or scalp and spreading rapidly to the trunk, but with relative sparing of the extremities. The lesions begin as red macules but progress quickly to vesicles and crusts. Itching is the rule. There is a tendency for new lesions to occur in crops. Unlike smallpox, all stages of lesions—vesicles, pustules, and scabs—may occur simultaneously in the same anatomic region. New crops often continue to appear over a 2- to 5-day period. Lesions may be more numerous in skin folds or in the diaper area. The total number of vesicles varies from only two or three in very mild cases, especially in infants, to thousands of lesions that border on confluence, especially in adults.[6] In many cases, one or two mucosal lesions may occur in the mouth or, less commonly, on the vulva. Occasionally, the lesions may be bullous or hemorrhagic. Residual scarring is exceptional. Constitutional symptoms tend to be mild even in the presence of an extensive exanthem.

Complications of Chickenpox

The most common complication is secondary bacterial infection, usually caused by streptococci or staphylococci. Skin infections may lead to severe sequelae such as toxic shock syndrome and necrotizing fasciitis.[140-148] Septicemia was observed in 0.5% of 2534 cases seen at the Willard Parker Hospital from 1929 to 1934.[149] Central nervous system complications, which are uncommon, include encephalitis, cerebellar ataxia, aseptic meningitis, and myelitis.[150,151] Glomerulonephritis,[152,153] myocarditis,[154,155] and arthritis[156,157] have also been reported.

Chickenpox in Immunocompromised Children

It is widely appreciated that varicella may be severe and even fatal in children with an underlying malignancy, those with congenital deficits in cellular immunity, those receiving high doses of corticosteroids for any reason,[158] and children with underlying infection with HIV and the acquired immunodeficiency syndrome (AIDS).[80,159] Leukemic children have a mortality rate approaching 10% if untreated[160] and may develop what has been called *progressive varicella*. Instead of developing new vesicular lesions for several days, they continue to have fever and new lesions for as long as 2 weeks after the onset of illness. Frequently, their skin lesions become hemorrhagic, large, and umbilicated. Varicella pneumonia often ensues and is a major factor contributing to the death of a child. It is believed that this abnormal response to VZV represents a failure of the normal cell-mediated immunity response to eliminate the virus.[160] The cell-mediated immunity response to VZV includes ADCC, natural killer cells, and cytotoxic T cells, including CD4 and CD8 cells.[35,129-131,161-163]

Chickenpox Pneumonia

Primary varicella pneumonia is a dreaded complication of chickenpox and is responsible for most fatalities. It is most common in immunocompromised patients, in adults, and in most fatal cases of neonatal chickenpox,[132-134,164] but it is rarely seen in otherwise healthy children. It has been suggested that the incidence is about 15% in adults and that 90% of cases have occurred in persons older than 19 years.[164,165] The true incidence is difficult to determine because chest radiographs are not performed in most cases of chickenpox and extensive radiographic evidence of disease may be present when pulmonary symptoms are only minimal. In male military recruits with varicella, virtually all of whom had been hospitalized and had chest radiographs, radiographic evidence of pneumonia was found in 16.3% of 110 cases.[166]

Two reviews of chickenpox pneumonia in adults outline the major features.[139,167] The onset of pneumonia usually occurs in 2 to 4 days but sometimes occurs as long as 10 days after the appearance of the exanthem. Fever and cough are present in 87% to 100% of cases, and dyspnea occurs in 70% to 80%. Other symptoms and signs include cyanosis (42% to 55%), rales (55%), hemoptysis (35% to 38%), and chest pain (21%). Radiographic changes seem to correlate best with the severity of the rash rather than with the physical examination of the lungs. The radiograph typically reveals a diffuse nodular or miliary pattern, most pronounced in the perihilar regions. The radiographic appearance changes rapidly. The white blood cell count varies between 5000 and 20,000 cells/mm^3 and is of little help in differentiating viral from secondary bacterial pneumonia. Pneumonia is usually self-limiting, and recovery is temporally correlated with clearing of skin lesions. The fatality rate has been variously estimated at 10% to 30%, but it probably approximates the lower of these values if immunocompromised hosts are excluded.[139,167] Blood gas analyses and pulmonary function tests indicate a significant diffusion defect that may persist in some cases for months after clinical recovery.[168] The introduction of antiviral chemotherapy has greatly improved the outcome in this disease.

Maternal Effects of Chickenpox

Reports from the middle of the 20th century suggested that when chickenpox occurred during pregnancy, it was a highly lethal disease. Deaths usually resulted from varicella pneumonia, in some cases accompanied by glomerulitis and renal failure or myocarditis, occurring after the fourth month of gestation.[169,170] Harris and Rhoades[171] reviewed the literature to 1963 and found a reported mortality of 41% for 17 pregnant women with chickenpox pneumonia compared with 11% for 236 nonpregnant adults with chickenpox pneumonia. Other reports, however, question whether varicella, especially in the absence of pneumonia, is more serious in pregnant women than in the adult population at large.[136,172,173] Because most cases of gestational varicella with an uncomplicated course are undoubtedly not reported, the denominator of the case-fatality ratio is unknown. In a prospective study of 150 cases of chickenpox in pregnancy in 1966, only one maternal death related to chickenpox pneumonia was

Table 22–4 Maternal Mortality Associated with Gestational Varicella[a]

Reference	Year	No. of Cases	No. with Varicella Pneumonia	No. of Deaths	Onset of Rash[b] 0-3 Months	4-6 Months	7-9 Months	Immediately Post Partum
132	1963	2	0	0	0	1	1	0
177	1964	18	0	0	0	0	15	3
136	1964	16	1	1	0	0	16 (1)[c]	0
98	1965	9	0	0	0	0	5	4
178	1966	11[d]	0	0	0	4	7	0
171	1965[e]	17	17	7	2 (1)[c]	3 (2)	11 (4)	1 (0)
284	1968	1	1	1	0	1 (1)	0	0
180	1969	2	2	1	0	0	2 (1)	0
181	1971	1	1	0	0	0	1	1
182	1986	43	4	1	11	11 (1)	21	0
183	1989	3	3	1	0	1	2 (1)	0
185	1990	5	5	1	3	0	2 (1)	0
195	1991	1	1	0	0	2	0	0
186[f]	1991	21	21	3	0	7	14 (3)	0
173[g]	1996	28	1	0	7	7	11	0
184	1997	22	0	0	3	9	0	0
175, 176	2002[h]	347	18	0	140	122	100	0
Totals		545	75 (16) 21%	16 (3%)	166 (<1%)	168 (2%)	208 (5%)	

[a]The antiviral therapy era is considered to have begun after 1985.
[b]If specified.
[c]Numbers in parentheses give deaths at indicated gestational periods.
[d]Includes one patient with zoster whose gestational dates are not given.
[e]Includes review of the literature before 1963.
[f]Reports five new cases with a review of additional case reports in the literature.
[g]In a series of 28 pregnant women with varicella, 1 (3.6%) had pneumonia.
[h]In a series of 347 pregnant women with varicella, 18 (5.2%) had pneumonia.

recorded.[174] In a very large, collaborative, prospective study published in 2002, there were no fatalities in 347 consecutive pregnant women with varicella, although 18 (5.2%) had radiologic evidence of pneumonia.[175,176] Although the data did not reach statistical significance in this study, it seems striking that 16 (89%) of 18 of the reported cases of pneumonia occurred in women who developed varicella after the 16th week of pregnancy.

To a review of the literature on varicella pneumonia in pregnancy before 1964,[171] Table 22-4 adds data from subsequent case reports of gestational varicella, with and without pneumonia, and reports of perinatal varicella in which the outcome in the mother is described. Among 545 cases of chickenpox in pregnant women, there were 16 deaths (3%). All of the deaths occurred among the 75 women who had chickenpox pneumonia (21% fatality rate for pneumonia). One (<1%) of 166 women whose disease occurred during the first trimester died, as did 4 (2%) of 168 women with disease in the second trimester and 11 (5%) of 208 women who became ill in the third trimester. No deaths occurred among 8 women who were exposed to chickenpox in late pregnancy but did not develop an exanthem until the first few days post partum. In summary, it remains uncertain whether chickenpox pneumonia has a graver prognosis when it occurs during pregnancy. There is no definitive evidence that chickenpox in the absence of pneumonia is a more serious illness in pregnant women than in other adults; however, the risk of developing pneumonia may be increased after the 16th week of pregnancy. It seems likely that older mortality information on varicella in pregnancy reflected the pre-antiviral therapy era and was biased by selective reporting of fatal cases.

Some patients with varicella during pregnancy who were treated with acyclovir have been reported.[173,175,176,183,185-196] These reports suggest that acyclovir has improved the outcome of this complication of varicella, although controlled studies have not been performed. Although a wide variety of dosages has been used, the standard dosage of 30 mg/kg/day given intravenously would seem appropriate for treatment of pregnant women with varicella pneumonia. Congenital abnormalities from administration of acyclovir to women during pregnancy have not been observed.[197,198]

Controlled studies of the value of corticosteroids in pregnant women with varicella pneumonia have not been performed. Several reports indicate that 2 of 6 pregnant women treated with corticosteroids died, whereas 8 of 17 pregnant women given supportive therapy without corticosteroids died.[171,179-181,199] It seems that administration of an antiviral drug is of greater importance than administration of corticosteroids. VZIG may be administered to seronegative women after close exposure to VZV to attempt to modify the infection; although not certain, this approach may prevent fetal infection.[200,201] In a study from 1994, among 97 women who developed varicella after receiving VZIG, there were no observed cases of the congenital varicella syndrome.[201] About two abnormal infants could be expected in a series of this magnitude, but the number of women followed is too low to achieve statistical significance.

Table 22–5 Frequency of Low Birth Weight among Infants Born to Mothers with Selected Viral Infections during Pregnancy

	Virus-Infected Group			Control Group[a]		
Disease	*No. of Livebirths*	*No. with Low Birth Weight[b]*	%	*No. of Livebirths*	*No. with Low Birth Weight[b]*	%
Rubella	359	50	13.9	402	21	5.2
Chickenpox	135	5	3.7	146	13	8.9
Mumps	117	9	7.7	122	4	3.3
Measles	60	10	16.7	62	2	3.3

[a]Control group was matched for age, race, and parity of the mother and type of obstetric service.
[b]Low birth weight was defined as less than 2500 g.
Table modified from data of Siegel M, Fuerst HT. Low birth weight and maternal virus diseases: a prospective study of rubella, measles, mumps, chickenpox, and hepatitis. JAMA 197:88, 1966. Fetal deaths and multiple births were excluded from the analysis.

Effects of Gestational Varicella on the Fetus

CHROMOSOMAL ABERRATIONS

VZV can induce chromosomal abnormalities in vitro and in vivo. When human diploid fibroblasts are infected with the virus, a high proportion of cells is observed in metaphase arrest, as if they were under the influence of colchicine.[202] Twenty-four hours after infection, the incidence of chromatid and chromosomal breaks ranges from 26% to 45%, compared with 2% for control cultures. In the acute phase of chickenpox, up to the fifth day of rash, peripheral blood leukocytes show a 17% to 28% incidence of chromosomal breaks, compared with 6% in controls, but 1 month after infection, these abnormalities have disappeared.[203] A single case report suggests the possibility that chromosomal damage may be more lasting when chickenpox is acquired in utero. A boy with bird-headed dwarfism, born to a mother who contracted chickenpox in the sixth month of pregnancy, had a 26% incidence of chromosomal breakage in peripheral blood leukocytes when he was examined at 2 years of age.[204] However, chromosomal analyses in four infants with the congenital varicella syndrome, whose mothers had chickenpox at the 8th, 14th, 16th, and 20th week of gestation, respectively, were reported as normal.[205-208] Information on chromosomal aberrations in infants who have no congenital anomalies and are the offspring of mothers with gestational varicella is unfortunately lacking. Further concern about the possibility of persistent chromosomal abnormalities after intrauterine exposure to VZV is suggested by a prospective survey of deaths among children born in England and Wales between 1950 and 1952 whose mothers had chickenpox in pregnancy. Two deaths, both from acute leukemia, were reported among the offspring of 270 women; the two children developed acute leukemia at the ages of 3 and 4 years after intrauterine exposure at 25 and 23 weeks' gestation, respectively.[209] In the absence of confirmation, it remains questionable whether exposure to chickenpox in utero is a risk factor for leukemia or other malignancies.

ABORTION AND PREMATURITY

Several studies have addressed the question of whether gestational chickenpox and other viral diseases result in an increased incidence of spontaneous abortion or prematurity. In a retrospective study in 1948, only four cases of chickenpox were identified among 26,353 pregnant women.[210] No stillbirths occurred among these four. Prospective studies have tended to confirm that maternal chickenpox during pregnancy is not associated with a significant excess of prematurity[174] or fetal death.[178] Among 826 virus-infected pregnant subjects observed in New York City from 1957 to 1964, 150 women with chickenpox were followed to term. After exclusion of fetal deaths and multiple births, 5 of 135 live-born infants were found to have birth weights of less than 2500 g. This incidence of prematurity was lower than that in the control group of non–virus-infected pregnant women (Table 22-5). Similarly, in the study of Paryani and Arvin,[182] premature delivery occurred in 2 (5%) of 42 pregnancies, with delivery at 31 and 35 weeks' gestation. In a prospective study involving 194 women with gestational varicella and 194 control women, the rate of spontaneous abortion was 3% and 7%, respectively, in the first 20 weeks.[211] In the large prospective series of Enders and associates[201] of 1330 women in England and Germany who developed varicella, 36 (3%) experienced spontaneous abortions after varicella in the first 16 weeks. However, in the prospective study of Pastuszak and co-workers[212] involving 106 women with varicella in the first 20 weeks of pregnancy, there were more premature births (14.3%) among women with varicella than among controls (5.6%; $P = .05$). There is no question, however, that the congenital varicella syndrome is associated with low birth weight. Approximately one third of reported cases of the syndrome have been premature, had low birth weight, or were small for dates.

An accurate assessment of the incidence of fetal mortality after maternal chickenpox is difficult to obtain. Fetal wastage is probably unreported, in part because some spontaneous abortions occur before prenatal care is sought. In the prospective study of maternal viral diseases in New York City referred to earlier,[178] nine fetal deaths were observed among 144 instances of maternal chickenpox. Five fetal deaths occurred among 32 pregnancies in the first trimester, four among 60 second-trimester pregnancies, and none among 52 third-trimester pregnancies (Table 22-6). These do not represent significant increases in fetal wastage associated with chickenpox infection compared with control groups in which no maternal viral infection occurred. Only for mumps was there a significant excess of fetal deaths, and these occurred primarily in the first trimester. Only three of the nine fetal

Table 22–6 Fetal Deaths in Relation to Gestational Age after Selected Virus Infections during Pregnancy

Infection Groups	Weeks of Gestation		
	0-11	*12-27*	*>28*
Mumps			
No. of cases	33	51	43
No. of fetal deaths	9	1	0
%	27.3	2	—
Measles			
No. of cases	19	29	17
No. of fetal deaths	3	1	1.9
%	15.8	3.4	5.9
Chickenpox			
No. of cases	32	60	52
No. of fetal deaths	5	4	0
%	15.6	4.7	—
Controls			
No. of cases	1010[a]	392[b]	152[b]
No. of fetal deaths	131	15	1
%	13	3.8	0.7

[a]Subjects were attending prenatal clinic in first trimester without virus infections.
[b]Controls were matched for age, race, and parity of the mother and type of obstetric service.
Table modified from Siegel M, Fuerst HT, Peress NS. Comparative fetal mortality in maternal virus diseases: a prospective study on rubella, measles, mumps, chickenpox, and hepatitis. N Engl J Med 274:768, 1966.

deaths associated with maternal chickenpox occurred within 2 weeks of the onset of the mother's illness, and two of these were in the first trimester. Two additional deaths occurred 2 to 4 weeks after the onset of maternal chickenpox, two after 5 to 9 weeks, and two 10 or more weeks after the onset of maternal illness. The absence of a close temporal relationship between most fetal deaths and maternal disease provides further support for the concept that maternal chickenpox during pregnancy does not commonly result in fetal mortality.

Although the incidence of fetal death is not increased by maternal varicella, fetal deaths have been associated with maternal varicella. Deaths in utero may result from direct invasion of the fetus by VZV[132,201,213-215] or from the presumed toxic effects of high fever, anoxia, or metabolic changes caused by maternal disease.[178] The precise mechanisms of these toxic effects have not been elucidated. When maternal disease is unusually severe, particularly in cases of chickenpox pneumonia, fetal death may also result from premature onset of labor or death in utero caused by maternal death.[136,171,179,180,185,214]

CONGENITAL MALFORMATIONS

For many years, there was uncertainty about whether gestational varicella led to a symptomatic congenital infection. Intensive investigation during the past 30 years has led to the recognition that VZV can cause fetal malformations. Two types of investigations were carried out to determine whether chickenpox during pregnancy leads to a congenital syndrome. The first were retrospective analyses or case reports describing specific anomalies that occurred in the offspring of mothers who had gestational varicella. These reports were necessarily highly selective and did not define the incidence of such anomalies. However, they consistently described a syndrome of skin scarring, eye and brain damage, and limb hypoplasia that might follow intrauterine varicella.

The second type of analysis consisted of prospective studies of pregnant women followed throughout pregnancy and afterward. The problem was to delineate the coincidence of two events, each of which is itself uncommon—gestational chickenpox and congenital malformations—to determine the magnitude of risk to the fetus. Siegel,[71] despite an 8-year observation period encompassing approximately 190,000 pregnancies annually in New York City, was able to identify only four malformations among infants born to 135 mothers who had chickenpox during pregnancy, compared with five malformations among 146 matched controls. The follow-up period was 5 years and included psychomotor and audiometric tests. Only 27 of the pregnancies complicated by chickenpox occurred during the first trimester, and of these, 2 (7.4%) were associated with congenital anomalies, compared with three anomalies (3.4%) among 87 pregnancies in the control population. The largest single prospective series is that of Enders and associates.[201] In a joint prospective study in Germany and the United Kingdom between 1980 and 1993, Enders and associates[201] followed 1373 women with varicella and 366 with zoster during pregnancy. Of the women with varicella, 1285 continued to term, and 9 had defects attributed to the congenital varicella syndrome.[201] The incidence was 2 (0.4%) of 472 for infections between 0 and 12 weeks and 7 (2%) of 351 for infections between 13 and 20 weeks. In a collaborative prospective study in the United States, 347 women with gestational varicella were reported, and adequate follow-up of their infants was available in 231.[176] In this cohort, there was one case (0.4%) of the congenital syndrome and two cases of fetal demise, including one case of hydrops. If these cases are included, the rate of congenital varicella was 1.3%. The mother of the one child with the syndrome had varicella at 24 weeks; the child had skin, eye, and central nervous system involvement.

That the congenital varicella syndrome is a reality is now widely appreciated. Only recently has it become possible to make a tissue diagnosis of the congenital varicella syndrome, because affected infants do not chronically shed virus as is seen in congenital infections with rubella virus and CMV.[201,213,215-217] It may be prevented in the future by widespread use of varicella vaccine, analogous to the situation for congenital rubella.

The constellation of developmental abnormalities described in individual case reports of infants born to mothers who had varicella in early pregnancy and in prospective series is sufficiently distinctive to indicate that VZV is a teratogen. In 1947, LaForet and Lynch[218] described an infant with multiple congenital anomalies after maternal chickenpox in early pregnancy. The infant had hypoplasia of the entire right lower extremity, talipes equinovarus, and absent deep tendon reflexes on the right. There were cerebral cortical atrophy, cerebellar aplasia, chorioretinitis, right torticollis, insufficiency of the anal and vesical sphincters, and cicatricial cutaneous lesions of the left lower extremity. In 1974, Srabstein and coworkers[219] rekindled interest in the subject, reported another case, and reviewed the literature, concluding that although the virus could not be isolated from the infants, the congenital syndrome typically consisted of some combination of cicatricial skin lesions, ocular abnormalities, limb deformities,

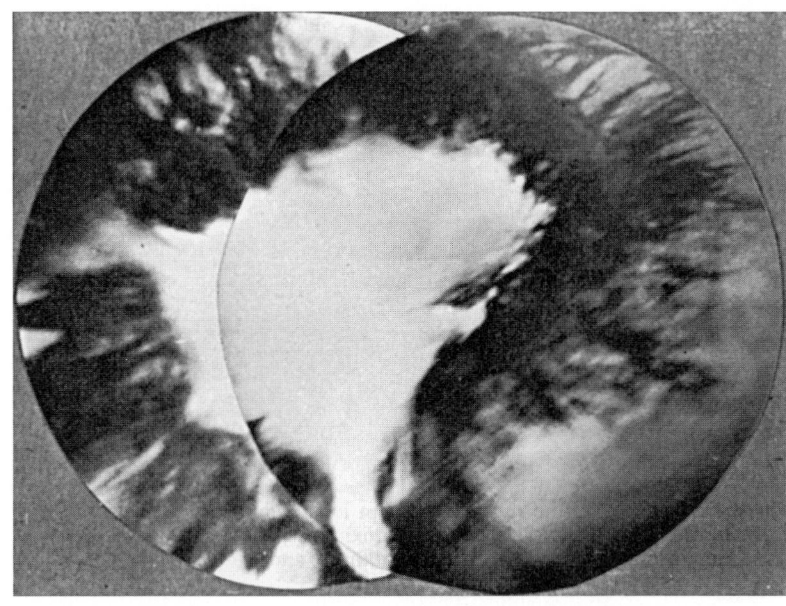

Figure 22–2 Fundus photograph of the right eye of a 13-month-old patient shows central gliosis with a surrounding ring of black pigment. The child's mother had varicella during the early fourth month of pregnancy. (Adapted from Charles N, Bennett TW, Margolis S. Ocular pathology of the congenital varicella syndrome. Arch Ophthalmol 95:2034, 1977.)

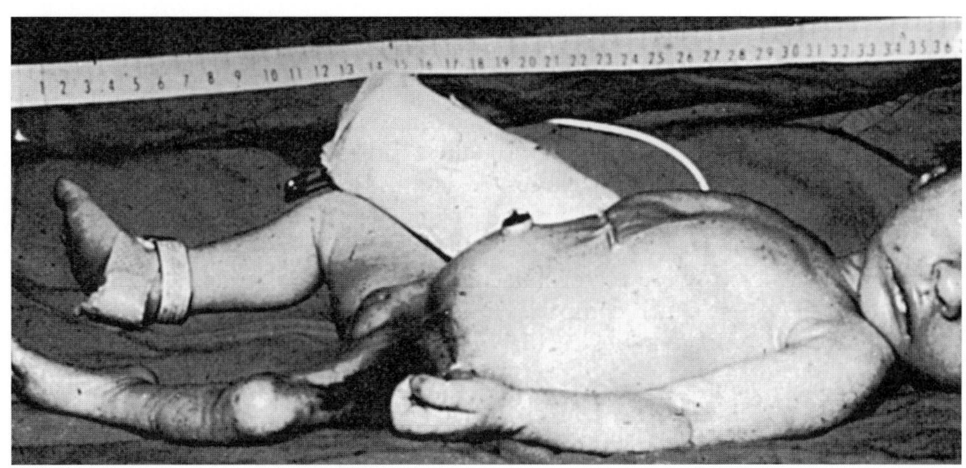

Figure 22–3 This infant, whose mother had varicella during the 13th to 15th weeks of pregnancy, had bilateral microphthalmia with cataracts and an atrophic left leg. The infant died of bronchopneumonia at age 6.5 months. (From Srabstein JC, Morris N, Larke RPB, et al. Is there a congenital varicella syndrome? J Pediatr 84:239, 1974.)

mental retardation, and early death after maternal varicella in early pregnancy (Figs. 22-2 to 22-4). There have been numerous additional reports in the literature of the syndrome, encompassing more than 100 cases, indicating that there is a wide spectrum of manifestations (Table 22-7).[71,73,182,201,205-286]

Whereas at one time it was thought that the syndrome occurred after maternal VZV infection in the first trimester of pregnancy, current evaluation of the data indicates that cases also occur in the second trimester. Of 82 cases for which data are available, 32 (39%) occurred after maternal varicella that developed before the 13th week, 47 (59%) occurred between weeks 13 and 26, and 1 (1%)[249] occurred during the 28th week. The average gestation when maternal varicella occurred was 15 weeks. Five cases occurring after maternal zoster have been reported[250,251,280,281]; four occurred after maternal zoster in the first trimester, and one followed zoster in the second trimester.[280] Of 108 reported affected infants, 103 (95%) cases followed maternal varicella, and 5 (5%) followed maternal zoster (disseminated in one instance).

Scars of the skin, usually cicatricial lesions, are the most prominent stigmata, although a few patients have had no rash whatsoever.[267,270,271,288] Eye abnormalities (i.e., chorioretinitis, microphthalmia, Horner's syndrome, cataract, and nystagmus) and neurologic damage are almost as common; other features include a hypoplastic limb, prematurity, and early death. The features of the syndrome are summarized in Table 22-7.

Cutaneous scars were usually observed overlying a hypoplastic limb but also have been seen in the contralateral limb.[218] Characteristically, the skin scars are cicatricial, depressed, and pigmented and often have a zigzag configuration. Such scars are thought to be the result of zoster that occurred before birth. In some patients, large areas of scarred skin have required skin grafting.[231,239] In other patients, the rash was bullous[238] or consisted of multiple, scattered, depressed, white scars.[242,246,259] In one infant, healing zoster was present at the T11 dermatome at birth; there was also spinal cord atrophy at the same level and aganglionosis of the intestine.[258]

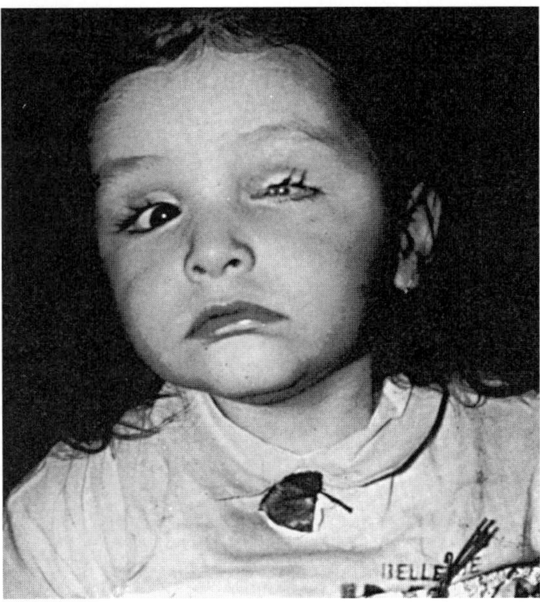

Figure 22–4 A child, whose mother had varicella during the 16th week of pregnancy, had atrophy of the left orbit, with blindness that required cosmetic enucleation. Severe chorioretinitis occurred in the right eye. Except for blindness, the child developed normally. She died of pneumonia when approximately 4 years old. (Adapted from Frey HM, Bialkin G, Gershon A: Congenital varicella: case report of a serologically proved long-term survivor. Pediatrics 59:110, 1977.)

Ocular abnormalities include chorioretinitis, Horner's syndrome or anisocoria, microphthalmia, cataract, and nystagmus.* Rarely, major abnormalities were confined to the eye. There was no apparent effect of timing of maternal varicella during gestation; the times of infection varied from 9 to 23 weeks in these infants. Figure 22-2 is a photograph showing retinal involvement in one of these patients.[242,253]

Neurologic involvement is about as common as skin and eye abnormalities in infants with this syndrome. Patients with cerebral cortical atrophy, diffuse brain involvement, or mental retardation (frequently accompanied by abnormal electroencephalograms and seizures or myoclonic jerks) have been described.[218,219,226-228,261] In a few patients, cerebrospinal fluid findings were normal[73,219,228,255]; in others, there were increased numbers of leukocytes or protein levels.[218,225,227] Bulbar palsy is suspected to result in dysphagia and bouts of aspiration pneumonia in some of these children.† Deep tendon reflexes were reported as normal in one infant[227] and diminished to absent in six,[207,208,218,219,223,224] and they were in some cases accompanied by sensory deficits.[73,219,224,228,255] Electromyography in some patients revealed a denervation pattern with loss of motor units.[219,228,229,251,255] Biopsy in one instance showed replacement of muscle bundles by fat.[219] At least five children with vocal cord paralysis have been reported.[261,269,272,273,274]

Abnormalities of the limbs can be extremely dramatic in presentation, and are seen in about half of affected infants. The most common limb abnormality, which first called attention to this congenital syndrome, is hypoplasia of a limb, most commonly unilateral involvement of a leg or arm (see Table 22-7). Hypoplasia or absence of digits has also been observed.[218,220,223,224,227-229] Talipes equinovarus or a calcaneovalgus deformity has also occurred.* This complex of abnormalities in the limbs, including the bony abnormalities, is probably attributable to a neuropathy caused by direct viral invasion of the ganglia and spinal cord.[270]

Table 22–7 Reported Symptoms in Infants with the Congenital Varicella Syndrome, 1947-2002

Symptom	Estimated Incidence (%)
Skin lesions (cicatricial scars, skin loss)	60-70
Ocular abnormalities (chorioretinitis, Horner's syndrome, anisocoria, microphthalmia, cataract, nystagmus)	60
Neurologic abnormalities (cortical atrophy, mental retardation, microcephaly, seizures, dysphagia, limb paresis)	60
Abnormal limbs (hypoplasia, equinovarus, abnormal or absent digits)	50
Prematurity, low birth weight	35
Death in early infancy	25
Abnormalities of gastrointestinal tract	10
Urinary tract abnormalities	10
Zoster in infancy	20

See references 71, 73, 182, 201, 205-286.

About one fourth of these infants died within the first 14 months of life. One child with the obvious syndrome was stillborn.[215] In one who died at 6 months, autopsy revealed a necrotizing encephalitis with various degrees of gliosis and inflammatory infiltrates. Focal calcification was observed in white and gray matter of the cerebrum, brain stem, and cerebellum. Atrophy of the anterior columns of the spinal cord and scarring in the ganglion corresponding to the distribution of the skin lesions and an atrophic limb were also present. No inclusion bodies were identified.[219] Among infants with a hypoplastic limb, 40% had evidence of mental retardation or died early. The presence of a hypoplastic limb on an ultrasound examination suggests a poor outcome.

About one third of affected infants were premature or had low birth weight for their gestational ages, and about 10% had various abnormalities of the gastrointestinal tract, including reflux, duodenal stenosis, jejunal dilatation, microcolon, atresia of the sigmoid colon, and sphincter malfunction.[70,217,218,225,239,254,257,253,258,260] A similar percentage had abnormalities of the urinary tract, often due to poor or absent bladder sphincter function.[73,182,218,219,222,237,250,255,258] Involvement of the cervical or lumbar spinal cord and the autonomic nervous system is thought to account for the observed hypoplasia or aplasia of limbs and digits, motor and

*See references 71,73,182,201,205,206,208,211-213,215-231,233-246, 248,249,252-255,258,259,280,281.

†See references 73,182,219,223,225,228,235,236,241,243,245,248,255, 261-263.

*See references 73,207,208,212,216,218,227,235,249,251,255,280.

sensory defects, decrease or absence of deep tendon reflexes, Horner's syndrome, and gastrointestinal and urinary tract abnormalities.[282]

Figures 22-3 and 22-4 depict two children with stigmata of the congenital varicella syndrome. One has severe[219] and one has relatively mild involvement.[242,253]

Zoster after the Congenital Varicella Syndrome. Fifteen percent of children with the congenital varicella syndrome develop clinical zoster in infancy or early childhood, almost all in the first year of life.* This is of particular interest because cell-mediated immunity to VZV in 2 of 10 of children with the syndrome has been reported to be absent as determined by lymphocyte transformation.[182,206] In Enders' series[201] of 1291 livebirths (without the congenital syndrome), of whom conservatively perhaps 25% were infected with VZV (the attack rate could be as high as 50%), the rate of zoster in childhood was 3%. It appears therefore that zoster is even more common in children with the congenital syndrome than in infants who were infected with VZV in utero but were asymptomatic at birth.

Diagnosis of the Congenital Varicella Syndrome. During the neonatal period or infancy, attempts to isolate VZV from the skin, cerebrospinal fluid, eye, and other tissues in infants with developmental defects were negative.[73,205,219,227,235,236,241,242] Although rubella virus and CMV are commonly isolated from young infants afflicted by these viruses, failure to isolate VZV in these cases is probably explained by the fact that the period of viral replication took place during early gestation and no replicating virus persisted by the time of birth. In children who developed zoster at an early age, it has been possible to isolate VZV from the rash.[210,229,254] In seven infants who died, autopsy results demonstrated apparent dissemination of VZV with varicella-like involvement of the lungs, liver, spleen, adrenals, or pancreas.[206-208,212,228-231]

Total IgM concentrations in the serum or cord blood of six infants were measured.[205,219,228,240-242] In three instances, the levels were clearly increased, with values of 48 to 100 mg/dL found when the infants were 1.5 to 6 weeks old. Specific VZV antibodies in the IgM fraction were not detected in seven cases in which they were sought,[182,228,242,248,282] but they were detectable in six other cases.[201,206,207,232,240] In one of these cases, VZV IgM was detected prenatally by obtaining blood by cordocentesis.[282] In most infants, a decline of antibodies in the serum was observed, a finding compatible with a fetal or a maternal origin. In 10 instances, however, persistence of or an increase in antibodies in the infant supported a presumption of intrauterine infection.[73,205,221,226,243,241,242,253,255]

It has been possible to document some reported cases of the congenital varicella syndrome but not all of them, because antibody titers may be inconclusive even in children with the apparent full-blown and rather distinctive constellation of abnormalities. Some children were diagnosed even before it was possible to measure antibody titers to VZV. The development of zoster at an early age can be interpreted as substantiating VZV infection in utero. Although many of the cases reported as the congenital varicella syndrome lack proof, it has been possible to show that some infants with characteristic stigmata were infected in utero with VZV, although an active, chronic infection does not exist. Modern molecular methods such as PCR and in situ hybridization have been useful for proving the congenital syndrome in a few reported infants and will undoubtedly be used to prove future cases.[201,213,215-217,261] In the future, it is expected that these will become the methods of choice rather than antibody testing. It is also predicted that with widespread use of varicella vaccine, the incidence of this unusual cause of congenital disease will become rare.

*See references 73,201,216,217,222,236,241,246,247,255,259,261,262,268.

MANAGEMENT OF PREGNANT WOMEN WITH VARICELLA-ZOSTER VIRUS INFECTION WITH REGARD TO FETAL MALFORMATIONS

In the decade of the 1990s, the incidence of fetal malformations after maternal VZV infection was clarified. Varicella is a significantly greater threat than zoster; 95% of reported cases of the congenital varicella syndrome have followed maternal chickenpox. In Enders' series[201] of 366 women with zoster in pregnancy, there were no cases of the congenital syndrome. This outcome is not unexpected, because zoster is probably less likely to be accompanied by a viremia than is varicella; many fetuses may escape VZV infection from maternal zoster. Because zoster is a secondary infection, residual maternal immunity to VZV may at least partially protect the fetus from damage, analogous to that seen when congenital CMV infection is caused by reactivation rather than to primary CMV infection.[288] As with CMV infection, however, it is possible, although rare, for fetal stigmata to follow secondary maternal infection.

The time at which maternal VZV infection occurs during gestation also influences whether the infant is likely to be severely damaged. Infection during the first and early second trimester appears to be the most critical. Most of the reported cases of the congenital syndrome have occurred when the onset of maternal infection was before the 20th week of pregnancy. Only six infants with some of the stigmata have been recorded as the result of maternal varicella after the 20th week.[213,176,247-249,257] When maternal varicella occurs after the 20th week, the infant may be infected, but usually the only evidence is a positive VZV antibody titer when the infant is older than 1 year and, in some cases, development of zoster at an early age.

Eleven prospective studies of the incidence of the congenital varicella syndrome have been published. Data from these studies are presented in Table 22-8. There are 14 cases of the congenital varicella syndrome in 858 (1.6%) women who developed varicella in the first 20 weeks of pregnancy. If the entire gestational period is considered, 2245 women who had varicella during pregnancy were delivered of live-born infants; the overall incidence of the congenital syndrome was 0.6%. These data indicate that the risk for development of the congenital varicella syndrome is mostly confined to the first 20 weeks of pregnancy, and even the risk after maternal varicella in the first 20 weeks of pregnancy is extremely low, on the order of 1% to 2%. Weeks 7 to 20 are the time of the greatest risk.[201] The tendency to develop overwhelming forms of VZV infection in the fetus indicates the increased ability of VZV to multiply in fetal tissues, which is similar to that of other viruses such as rubella virus and CMV.

Counseling of pregnant women who have acquired varicella during pregnancy can be very difficult. Because the congenital syndrome is rare, termination of pregnancy is not

Table 22–8 Incidence of the Congenital Varicella Syndrome: Results of Prospective Studies 1960-1997

		Incidence of Syndrome	
Reference	Year	*First Trimester/ First 20 Weeks*	*Total Gestation*
508	1960	0/70	0/288
71	1973	2/27	2/135
231	1984	0/23	
182	1986	1/11	1/38
72	1992	0/40	
212	1994	1/49	
201	1994	7/351	7/1291
211	1994	2/99	2/146
173	1996	0/26	
184	1997	0/22	
176	2002	0/140	1/347
Total reported		13/858 (1.6%)	14/2245 (0.6%)

routinely recommended, in contrast to recommendations for gestational rubella. When the syndrome does occur, however, it is likely to be severe. It would be helpful if prenatal diagnoses were available, but diagnostic attempts such as measurement of maternal antibody titers and amniocentesis have not proved useful. Although blood may be obtained by cordocentesis for antibody testing, even the presence of fetal VZV IgM does not mean that the infant has the congenital varicella syndrome but only that infection with VZV has taken place. Similarly, PCR may identify an infected fetus but not necessarily one with malformations.[286,287]

Ultrasound has been used successfully to identify the following fetal abnormalities after maternal varicella: hydrocephalus 12 weeks later[206]; clubfeet and hydrocephalus 13 weeks later[235]; a large, bullous skin lesion originally believed to be a meningocele 15 weeks later[238]; calcifications in the liver and other organs 9, 15, and 18 weeks later[216,236,263]; a hypoplastic limb and clubfoot 11 and 16 weeks later[201,216]; and a lacuna of the skull 25 weeks later.[232] Additional successes with ultrasound as a diagnostic tool to identify this syndrome prenatally have also been reported in cases with evidence of widespread infection.[275-278] Three published reports, however, indicate that ultrasound is not infallible. In two infants, ultrasound was normal 3 weeks after maternal varicella, but the fetus was later diagnosed as having the congenital varicella syndrome.[207,235] One infant was diagnosed with liver calcifications by ultrasonography at 27 weeks and a positive PCR for VZV; his mother had varicella at 12.5 weeks. At birth, no obvious anomalies were present, and the infant did well except for development of zoster at age 8 months.[286] Even defects detected by ultrasonography must be interpreted with some caution.

Because about 40% of reported patients with a hypoplastic limb also sustained brain damage or died in early infancy, the presence of a limb abnormality on ultrasound seems to suggest a poor overall prognosis for the fetus. Two women were reported to have terminated their pregnancies after the diagnosis of the congenital varicella syndrome was made based on abnormal limbs at ultrasound. At physical examination, the infants were found to be severely affected.[201,286]

Because abnormalities may not be detected by ultrasound immediately after maternal varicella, by the time any is noticed, it may be too late to consider interruption of pregnancy, depending on the time of onset of maternal varicella.

Although the congenital varicella syndrome varies in severity, most cases are severe. It would be helpful if maternal infection could be identified and appropriate management initiated as early as possible. It is not known whether administration of VZIG or acyclovir to a pregnant woman can prevent her fetus from developing the congenital varicella syndrome. In Enders' study,[201] there were no cases of the congenital syndrome in 97 women who were given VZIG on exposure; unfortunately, it is not known how many of these women were in the first 20 weeks of pregnancy.

Perinatal Chickenpox

Perinatal chickenpox includes disease that is acquired postnatally by droplet infection and that is transplacentally transmitted or congenital. Chickenpox is considered to be transplacentally transmitted when it occurs within 10 days of birth.

POSTNATALLY ACQUIRED CHICKENPOX

Postnatally acquired chickenpox, which begins between 10 and 28 days after birth, is generally mild.[289] The experiences with nosocomial chickenpox infections in the newborn nursery that were described in a previous section further corroborate the benign nature of the disease and the fact that transmission to neonates in this environment is inefficient and rarely reaches epidemic proportions.

Deaths among neonates caused by postnatally acquired disease are rare, but some data indicate an appreciably higher incidence of complications or deaths in neonates than in older children.[96,101-103,108,289,290] Preblud and associates[289] found that of 92 reported deaths caused by varicella from 1968 to 1978 in children younger than 1 year, only 5 occurred in newborns (8 hours to 19 days old). Although mortality was increased by a factor of four for infants younger than 1 year compared with older children, there was a low calculated death rate for varicella throughout childhood (8 in 100,000 patients if younger than 1 year and 2 in 100,000 patients 1 to 14 years old).[289] One 15-day-old infant with severe disseminated chickenpox born to a woman who developed varicella 7 days after delivery has been described.[290] The child survived; acyclovir was administered for 10 days. The only other report in the English literature of severe postnatally acquired varicella in an infant younger than 1 month is that of Gustafson and colleagues.[96] The term infant with Turner's syndrome was exposed to varicella when 7 days old, developed more than 200 vesicles, and died of pneumonia; however, the role of VZV in the child's death was unclear because no autopsy was performed.

CONGENITAL CHICKENPOX: MATERNAL INFECTION NEAR TERM

Congenital chickenpox is not inevitable when maternal chickenpox occurs in the 21 days preceding parturition. In only 8 (24%) of 34 reported cases of maternal disease with onset during this period did chickenpox develop in the neonate within the first 10 days of life.[98,136,172,174] An identical attack rate of 24% for congenital varicella after the occurrence of maternal varicella within 17 days preceding delivery was arrived at by Meyers,[291] who reviewed many cases in the literature and 14 examples reported to the Centers for Disease Control and Prevention in 1972 to 1973. However, attack rates on the order of 50% were reported in two studies on the efficacy of passive immunization to prevent severe neonatal varicella.[292,293] In Meyers' study,[291] there was no statistically significant relationship between day of onset of the rash in the mother and subsequent attack rates of congenital varicella. Seven of 22 neonates born to mothers whose rash appeared less than 5 days ante partum ultimately developed congenital chickenpox, whereas 4 of 24 infants born to mothers whose rash began 5 to 14 days ante partum had congenital disease.[291] These data indicate that the attack rate in congenital varicella (25% to 50%) is lower than that after household exposure to VZV (90%) and suggest that blood-borne transmission is less efficient than by the skin and respiratory routes.

The incubation period in congenital varicella, defined as the interval between the onset of rash in the mother and onset in the fetus or neonate, is usually 9 to 15 days.[294] This interval is slightly shorter than the normal postnatal incubation period, possibly because fetal tissues are more susceptible to VZV than more mature tissues. Rarely, presumably when fetal infection is caused by the primary maternal viremia, the exanthem appears in the mother and neonate within 3 days of each other[101] or even simultaneously.[294] The average incubation period in 36 cases reported in the literature was 11 days, with a maximum of 16 days. In only three instances was the incubation period less than 6 days.[291]

In contrast to postnatally acquired neonatal chickenpox, congenital chickenpox can be associated with significant mortality. Severe cases clinically resemble varicella in the immunocompromised host. A child who died of hemorrhagic varicella with pulmonary and liver involvement is shown in Figure 22-1. The spectrum of illness also includes extremely mild infections with only a handful of vesicles. Erlich and co-workers[133] first observed that infants born with the rash or who had an early onset of rash survived, whereas those who died had a relatively late onset of rash. It was hypothesized that for those neonates with early onset, maternal illness had occurred long enough before parturition to allow antibodies to be elaborated by the mother and to cross the placenta. Subsequent reports offer strong confirmation of these observations. There were no deaths among 22 infants with congenital chickenpox (reviewed by Meyers) whose onset of rash occurred between birth and 4 days of age. In contrast, 4 (21%) of 19 neonates in whom the rash began when they were 5 to 10 days old died (Table 22-9).[291] These four deaths occurred among 13 neonates (31%) whose mothers' exanthems developed within 4 days before birth, but no deaths were observed among 23 neonates with congenital chickenpox whose mothers developed a rash 5 or more days before birth.

Further support for the protective or modifying effect of maternal antibody has come from measurements of placental transfer of IgG to VZV.[91] When varicella occurred more than 1 week before delivery, complement-fixing antibody titers in maternal and cord blood were similar. In contrast, when infection occurred 3 to 5 days before delivery, maternal antibody was present at parturition, and antibodies to VZV in the neonate were absent or at least eightfold lower. These data suggest that a lag of several days occurs before IgG antibodies to VZV cross the placenta and equilibrate with the fetal circulation. The development of mild congenital varicella in the presence of placentally transferred maternal antibody has also been demonstrated using the more sensitive FAMA test.[61] The neonate may be at risk for developing severe varicella because the immune system is immature, as has been demonstrated by Kohl with regard to host defense against HSV.[295]

Zoster in Neonates and Older Children

The most characteristic feature of zoster is the localization of the rash. It is nearly always unilateral, does not cross the midline, and is typically limited to an area of skin served by one to three sensory ganglia. In children, prodromata of malaise, fever, headache, and nausea may be observed. Pain and paresthesias in the involved dermatome may precede the exanthem by 4 or 5 days. Involvement of the dermatomes of the head, neck, and trunk is more common than involvement of the extremities, a distribution that also reflects the density of lesions in chickenpox.[40] Erythematous papules give rise to grouped vesicles, which progress to pustules in 2 to 4 days. New crops of vesicles may keep appearing for a week. Pain may be associated with the exanthem and usually abates as the skin lesions scab; in elderly adults, severe and incapacitating neuralgia of the involved nerve may persist for months. Cutaneous dissemination of vesicles to sites distant from the involved dermatome is observed uncommonly and is more frequent in compromised hosts such as patients with lymphoma or immunologic deficiencies.

Zoster occurs as host defense mechanisms against VZV wane in a person who has previously experienced chickenpox. Because immunity is relatively durable, this hypothesis presumes that zoster will occur predominantly in the older population and will be rare in neonates. Among 192 patients with zoster in a general practice, the attack rate increased progressively with age.[40] Only six patients were younger than 10 years; the youngest was 2 years old. In two reported series describing zoster in a total of 22 children, only two cases occurred in children younger than 2 years old.[172,296] These reports confirm the rarity of zoster among infants. When zoster occurs in children who have not previously had chickenpox, there is often a history of intrauterine exposure to VZV. In these reports, the mothers contracted chickenpox

Table 22–9 Deaths from Congenital Varicella in Relation to Date of Onset of Rash in Mother or Neonate

Onset	Neonatal Deaths	Neonatal Cases	%
Day of onset of rash in neonate			
0-4	0	22	0
5-10	4	19	21
Onset of maternal rash, days ante partum			
≥5	0	23	0
0-4	4	13	31

Data from Meyers JD. Congenital varicella in term infants: risk reconsidered. J Infect Dis 129:215, 1974, with permission from the University of Chicago.

during gestation but gave birth to normal infants who, without ever developing chickenpox despite frequent childhood exposure, developed typical zoster at a young age, many in the first few months of life.[73,262,297-301] In most of these infants, the course of zoster was benign. One child developed a second attack of zoster when 10 months old; the first occurred when the child was 4 months old.[297]

Although there are six reports of zoster during the neonatal period,[302-307] it is doubtful whether any of these cases diagnosed on clinical grounds is an authentic example of zoster. HSV may produce a vesicular exanthem in the newborn that appears to have a dermatomal distribution. Virus isolation (or demonstration of VZV antigen from skin lesions) is required before a diagnosis of zoster can be accepted. Serologic studies are not useful in differentiating these diseases.

Diagnosis and Differential Diagnosis

Chickenpox

In a neonate with a widespread, generalized vesicular exanthem and a history of recent maternal varicella or postnatal exposure, a diagnosis of chickenpox can usually be made with confidence on clinical grounds alone. Greater difficulty is encountered when lesions are few or when there is no history of exposure.

DIAGNOSTIC TECHNIQUES

If laboratory diagnosis is required, it is best accomplished by demonstration of VZV antigen or DNA in skin lesions or isolation of virus from vesicular fluid. VZV antigen may be demonstrated by using immunofluorescence, employing a monoclonal antibody to VZV that is conjugated to fluorescein and is commercially available.[308-310] For virus isolation, fluid should be promptly inoculated onto tissue cultures because VZV is rather labile. PCR has proved extremely sensitive and accurate for diagnosis of VZV infections, although it remains a research test in most locations.[118,311-317] In situ hybridization is also a useful diagnostic technique.[217,318,319]

VZV infections may be documented by demonstration of a fourfold or greater rise in VZV antibody titer by using a sensitive test such as FAMA or ELISA. The presence of specific IgM in one serum specimen suggests recent VZV infection.[38,39,320] Persistence of VZV antibody beyond the age of 8 months is highly suggestive of intrauterine varicella, providing there is no history of clinical varicella after birth.[24] Persistence of VZV antibody with no fall in titer over several months in a young infant (as long as all sera are tested simultaneously) is highly suggestive of intrauterine infection. A FAMA or LA antibody titer of 1:4 or greater beyond 8 months of life is suggestive of immunity to varicella, provided that the patient has not received γ-globulin or other blood products in the previous 3 to 4 months. Physicians should be aware that no serologic test is 100% accurate for identifying individuals immune to varicella, although these antibody tests are generally reliable.[321]

DIFFERENTIAL DIAGNOSIS

Several diseases may be considered in the differential diagnosis of varicella in the newborn: neonatal HSV, smallpox, disseminated vaccinia, contact dermatitis, hand-foot-and-mouth syndrome, impetigo, and other conditions.

In *neonatal HSV*, cutaneous lesions may be relatively sparse and may be absent altogether despite widespread visceral dissemination. Vesicles tend to occur in clusters rather than in the more even distribution seen in chickenpox. Fever, marked toxicity, and encephalitis are more common in neonates with HSV. Stained smears of vesicle fluid (i.e., Tzanck preparation) are of no help in differentiating HSV from varicella because both are characterized by multinucleated giant cells and intranuclear inclusion bodies. In cell cultures, HSV typically produces a widespread cytopathic effect in 24 to 48 hours, whereas the cytopathic effect caused by VZV is cell associated and focal and develops more slowly. Indirect immunofluorescence using monoclonal antibodies conjugated to fluorescein can be performed on smears of skin scrapings; if positive, the assay can identify VZV, HSV-1, and HSV-2 within several hours. Paired serum samples can be examined for rising antibody titers to HSV and VZV antigens. It is exceedingly rare for varicella to develop in a newborn in the absence of any (i.e., infant or mother) exposure to varicella or zoster. In contrast, most infants with neonatal HSV have no recognized exposure to the virus.

Although 95% of cases of perinatal HSV are transmitted during delivery, a syndrome similar to the congenital varicella syndrome, with limb and eye abnormalities, skin scarring, and zosteriform rashes, has been observed after the unusual occurrence of intrauterine transmission of HSV.[322,323] In an infant with stigmata of the congenital varicella syndrome whose mother has no history of varicella during pregnancy, congenital HSV should be considered. It may not be possible to make a definitive diagnosis immediately unless the infant develops a vesicular rash from which the causative virus can be identified. Determination of antibody titers to HSV and VZV at presentation and when they are 8 to 12 months old may be useful to establish a diagnosis.

Smallpox is traditionally part of the differential diagnosis of vesicular lesions in neonates. Although smallpox was eradicated, there is concern that the disease may reemerge because of bioterrorism. Classically, the vesicles of smallpox appear to be at the same stage of development instead of showing the pattern of crops over a period of several days. Centrifugal distribution the skin rash distribution is prominent. The best approach in a suspicious situation is to rule out the possibility of VZV or HSV infection as described previously, preferably by immunofluorescence testing. If the test results are negative, a search for smallpox may then be indicated, especially if the history of the patient warrants it. Accurate diagnosis may be achieved in a matter of hours by electron microscopy of the vesicle fluid or crusts; such microscopic examination reveals virus particles whose morphology is very different from that of viruses of the herpes family. Smallpox modified by exposure to vaccinia in the distant past and alastrim (i.e., variola minor) may be particularly difficult to distinguish from chickenpox. In suspicious cases, the local health department should be promptly involved.

Disseminated vaccinia is rare today because smallpox vaccine (i.e., vaccinia virus) is not routinely used, although a bioterrorism attack could change the scenario. Vaccinia can be considered in a neonate exposed postnatally to a person who has been recently vaccinated. The lesions resemble those of smallpox. Impression smears of vesicle fluid do not show intranuclear inclusions or giant cells. Laboratory diagnosis may be achieved by electron microscopy and immunofluorescence.

In some cases of *contact dermatitis*, papules and vesicles may appear after exposure to specific chemical irritants. Typically, they appear on exposed body surfaces and do not have the characteristic distribution of chickenpox or smallpox.

In patients with *hand-foot-and-mouth syndrome,* a vesicular exanthem usually caused by coxsackievirus A16 or A5 may be observed during the enterovirus season (i.e., summer or early autumn). Vesicles rarely exceed a dozen and typically occur on the distal extremities, especially the palms and soles. Vesicular lesions that ulcerate quickly may also be seen in the oropharynx. The causative virus is readily isolated from vesicle fluid or from feces.

Impetigo may occur in neonates. In bullous impetigo (i.e., pemphigus neonatorum), large blebs are present instead of the smaller vesicles of chickenpox. This disease, which is caused by *Staphylococcus aureus,* may be associated with high fever, toxicity, septicemia, and death.

Alternative diagnoses include syphilis, group B streptococcal infection, and incontinentia pigmenti, which may cause vesiculobullous lesions in the neonate.

Zoster

Zoster usually is easily recognized by the typical dermatomal distribution of the vesicular lesions. In the differential diagnosis, the main entity to be distinguished in the neonatal period is HSV appearing in a linear pattern. Identification of VZV or HSV antigen by immunofluorescence or virus isolation is the only reliable means of differentiating these entities when the distribution of the exanthem is linear. Contact dermatitis should also be considered in the differential diagnosis of zosteriform lesions in the neonatal period.

Therapy

Treatment of the Mother

Acyclovir is the antiviral drug of choice for treatment of potentially severe or severe VZV infections.[324,325] Acyclovir itself has no antiviral action, but when it is phosphorylated by enzymes produced by cells infected with VZV, it is incorporated as a DNA chain terminator and it also inhibits viral DNA polymerase. Because these actions occur only in virus-infected cells, acyclovir is well tolerated and associated with little toxicity. The drug is available in topical, oral, and intravenous formulations.

The safety of acyclovir has been demonstrated in the past 30 years, and there is good reason to use this drug liberally in clinical situations for which it is indicated, even during pregnancy. Although most VZV infections in normal hosts are self-limited, there is a low but real fatality rate from varicella in adults. For this reason and because long-term toxicity of acyclovir in the fetus seems unlikely, acyclovir is recommended more often for use during pregnancy in women with varicella than previously. A registry of patients (and their offspring) who have received acyclovir during pregnancy has been established.[197,198] In general, pregnant women who develop varicella should be treated with orally administered acyclovir and observed carefully. Pregnant women who develop severe varicella while receiving oral therapy, especially those who develop pneumonia, should be promptly treated with intravenous acyclovir.[326] Supportive respiratory therapy (e.g., nasal oxygen, tracheostomy, ventilatory assistance) should be used as needed. Controlled studies of corticosteroids for varicella pneumonia are not available; therefore, steroids are not recommended. Antibiotics should be given if there is evidence of bacterial superinfection.

Anecdotal reports on the apparently successful use of acyclovir in pregnant women with varicella have been published, although controlled studies have not been performed. The data suggest that most women who develop varicella in pregnancy ultimately survive without sequelae.[175] This is undoubtedly the result of increasing awareness of the potential seriousness of the illness on the part of medical providers and also the more liberal use of acyclovir today.

There is little information on the use of acyclovir for pregnant women with zoster. Presumably, because zoster would be expected to be self-limited in most women of childbearing age, there would be little need for antiviral therapy in this situation. However, especially in the setting of an extensive rash or severe pain, use of acyclovir, particularly as oral therapy, should be strongly considered. Alternatively, one of the newer drugs, such as famciclovir or valacyclovir, can be used to treat pregnant women who develop severe zoster. The dose of famciclovir is 500 mg taken orally three times daily; the dose of valacyclovir is 1 g taken orally three times daily. Both medications are administered for 7 days. There is no information on the use of famciclovir or valacyclovir in pregnancy. Although famciclovir and valacyclovir are both converted to acyclovir, and acyclovir is the active drug in the blood, there is more safety information on use of acyclovir in pregnancy and for that reason it is probably preferable.

Acyclovir has been most effective when it is administered within 1 day after the onset of varicella and 3 days after onset of zoster. The usual adult dose for intravenous acyclovir is 10 mg/kg, given three times per day. Orally administered acyclovir has been found to have a modest effect on the fever and rash of varicella in otherwise healthy populations. A multicenter, double-blind, placebo-controlled, collaborative study involving 815 similarly treated children, who were given 20 mg/kg of acyclovir orally four times per day, shortened the course of illness by about 1 day.[327] The benefit to secondary household cases was not increased beyond that of primary cases. Similar results emerged from a study involving adolescents with varicella.[328] The modest benefit conferred by oral acyclovir therapy is not surprising in view of the self-limited nature of chickenpox in children and the poor oral absorption of acyclovir. There is a similar small benefit for adults with varicella who were given oral acyclovir (800 mg taken five times each day for 5 days) within 24 hours of onset of rash.[329,330] In the double-blind, placebo-controlled study of Wallace and associates,[330] involving 76 military recruits, the duration of illness was shortened by about 1 day and the personnel were able to return to work 1 day sooner on average, if they received acyclovir. There is no information regarding treatment of pregnant women, and physicians are reluctant to extrapolate to them from studies involving mainly healthy young men. However, given the possibility that acyclovir will help and is unlikely to harm, the drug should be strongly considered for most adults today with early varicella, pregnant or not.

Treatment of the Newborn Infant

Although there is little information on the use of acyclovir in newborns for varicella, it has been used to treat a great many infants with neonatal HSV infection. In a study in which 95 infants received acyclovir (30 mg/kg/day given intravenously), no short- or long-term toxicity was observed.[325-327] Neonates with HSV that is disseminated or involves the central nervous system should receive double this dose (60 mg/kg/day). Pharmacokinetic studies have indicated that dose adjustments for acyclovir may be necessary in premature infants and those with hepatic or renal dysfunction.[331-333] There are no data about the use of oral acyclovir for severe neonatal infections caused by VZV, and acyclovir is poorly absorbed when given by the gastrointestinal route. A dose of 1500 mg/m^2 of acyclovir, given intravenously in three divided daily doses, is recommended for infants with severe or rapidly progressing varicella. It is not recommended that infants with the congenital varicella syndrome receive treatment with acyclovir, except in the unusual setting of severe active zoster.

Prevention

Immunity to Varicella-Zoster Virus

Immunity to VZV may be incomplete in some persons. It was recognized years ago that waning of immunity to VZV might predispose a person to zoster.[40] That immunity to varicella might wane on occasion and result in a second case of chickenpox has been recognized only fairly recently. Immunologic evidence consistent with asymptomatic reinfection with VZV, manifested by an increase in VZV-specific IgG or IgA or the production of IgM, as well as an increase in the cell-mediated immune response to VZV, has been documented in adults with a household exposure to varicella.[334,335] Symptomatic reactivation with subsequent boosting of immunity is also possible but is difficult to substantiate. Clinical reinfection with VZV has been observed in some persons despite a positive antibody titer at exposure.[336-339] However, most clinical reinfections are mild, which suggests that partial immunity to the virus may be present. Cellular immunity as well as antibodies may play a role in protection. In a study by Bogger-Goren and coworkers,[340] children with positive cellular immune responses were likely to be protected against varicella after household exposure even if they were seronegative; in contrast, children with negative responses became infected. Secretory IgA against VZV has also been demonstrated after chickenpox.[341] Although it has not yet been demonstrated, it is hypothesized that cellular immunity at the mucosal level may play an important role in protection against clinical varicella.

In addition to predisposing to reinfection with the virus, incomplete immunity to VZV is associated with development of zoster. In addition to clinical zoster, silent reactivation of latent VZV in those who have had previous varicella probably occurs; this may be detected immunologically by an increase in antibody titer or the transient appearance of specific IgM, although it is difficult to rule out the possibility of an exogenous exposure.[39,342-344] Sometimes, clinical manifestations of zoster such as pain may occur in the absence of a rash, so-called zoster sine herpete. Silent reactivation of VZV in bone marrow transplant patients has been demonstrated by PCR.[345] Zoster results in patients who have latent VZV infection when specific cell-mediated immunity is depressed.[121,122,124,346] Defective antibody responses to VZV glycoproteins have not been associated with development of zoster in immunocompromised persons.[347] Similarly, the increased incidence of zoster in the elderly has been associated with loss of cell-mediated immunity to VZV,[348,349] whereas antibody to VZV does not wane with age but rather tends to increase.[350] Immunity to VZV may be seen as a complex interaction between humoral and cell-mediated immunity responses, with the possibility of partial as well as complete immunity to the virus.

It is possible to provide humoral immunity to persons at high risk for developing severe varicella by passive immunization with VZIG. Although used successfully to prevent severe varicella, passive immunization has not prevented zoster in those at high risk for it,[351] nor is it believed to be useful to treat patients with varicella or zoster.[352] Passive immunization should therefore not be employed to try to prevent development of varicella pneumonia in the pregnant woman with chickenpox or dissemination in an already infected infant. It is uncertain whether passive immunization of a woman with varicella can prevent infection of her fetus or development of the congenital varicella syndrome. It is possible to increase cell-mediated immunity to VZV by immunization, and whether this approach can prevent or modify zoster is being explored.[353-355] Results of a large, double-blind, controlled study in healthy vaccinees older than 60 years are expected to be available in 2005.

Passive Immunization: Zoster Immunoglobulin and Varicella-Zoster Immune Globulin

Controlled studies have indicated that pooled immunoglobulin attenuates but does not prevent chickenpox when administered to susceptible family contacts[63] and that zoster immune globulin (ZIG) prevents clinical chickenpox when given to susceptible healthy children within 72 hours of household exposure.[356] Additional uncontrolled studies of immunocompromised children, such as leukemics receiving maintenance chemotherapy, at high risk for developing severe or fatal varicella have indicated that ZIG administered within 3 to 5 days of a household exposure usually modifies varicella so that the infection is mild or subclinical.[357-359] ZIG that was prepared from plasma from donors with zoster has been supplanted by VZIG, which is prepared from normal donors with high antibody titers to VZV. The antibody content of the two preparations is similar,[360] as is the protective efficacy.[361] VZIG is licensed in the United States, and it is commercially available through the American Red Cross and local blood centers.[200] Passive immunization may prolong the incubation period of varicella.[358]

Passive immunization has also been studied for its possible efficacy in modifying severe congenital varicella that may occur in the infant of a woman who develops chickenpox close to term. Infants born to women with the onset of varicella more than 5 days before delivery can be expected to have mild infection,[61,133,291,362,363] and these infants do not require passive immunization. In contrast, infants born to women who develop varicella 5 days or less before delivery are at risk for developing disseminated or fatal varicella, and these infants can be expected to benefit from passive immunization. In an uncontrolled study by Hanngren and co-workers[292] of 41 neonates born to women who developed

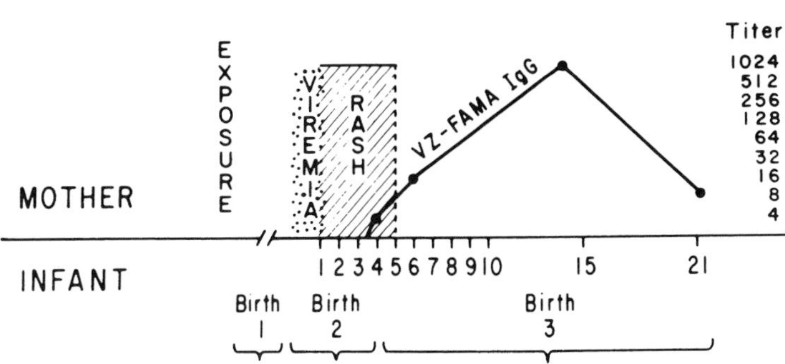

Figure 22–5 Diagrammatic representation of transmission of varicella-zoster virus (VZV) and VZV antibody to the fetus in maternal varicella near term. When the infant is born during the maternal incubation period (1), no varicella occurs unless the infant is exposed postnatally to the infection. When the infant is born 0 to 4 days after onset of maternal varicella (2), disseminated varicella may develop because the infection is not modified by maternal antibody. The onset of varicella occurs when the infant is 5 to 10 days old. Infants born 5 days or more after maternal varicella (3) receive maternal antibody, which leads to mild infection. This diagram is based on data for 50 newborn infants with varicella. (Adapted from Gershon A. Varicella in mother and infant: problems old and new. *In* Krugman S, Gershon A [eds]: Infection of the Fetus and Newborn Infant. New York, Alan R Liss, 1975, pp 79-95.)

varicella between 4 days before and 2 days after delivery, the illness appeared to be modified. These infants received 1 mL of ZIG. Although the attack rate was 51%, and the incubation period averaged 11 days, there were no fatalities instead of the expected mortality rate of about 30%, and 13 (62%) of 21 had fewer than 20 vesicles with no fever. Two (10%) had rather severe infections, and one was treated with interferon. In a similar study of VZIG by Preblud and colleagues,[293] a similar varicella attack rate of 45% was observed in 132 infants. In this study, a dose of 125 units (1.25 mL) of VZIG was administered. The illness also appeared to be modified, because of 53 infants with varicella, 74% had fewer than 50 vesicles, and only 10% had more than 100 vesicles. No antiviral therapy was given; there was one death in the group, but it was not clear that it was caused by varicella. The high attack rates of varicella in these studies in comparison with historical data have not been explained. In previous studies, infant attack rates of 24% in late[291] and overall[182] pregnancy have been reported. Successful passive immunization would, if anything, be expected to decrease the attack rate rather than increase it. Nevertheless, the mildness of the illness and absence of mortality in these two studies are suggestive if not proof positive of successful passive immunization of infants born to women with varicella at term. Since the introduction of ZIG and VZIG for use in appropriate neonates, fatalities from neonatal varicella have become rare.

It is recommended that VZIG be administered to infants whose mothers have the onset of varicella 5 days or less before delivery or in the first 48 hours after delivery.[200,364] A dose of 125 units (1.25 mL or one vial) should be administered intramuscularly as soon as possible after birth. Administration of VZIG to the mother before delivery of the infant is not recommended, because a larger dose would be required to passively immunize the infant, and no benefit to the mother will result. Early delivery of the infant of a mother with active varicella is also not recommended; the longer the infant remains in utero, the more likely there will be transplacental transfer of maternal antibody. A diagram of the relationship between maternal and infant varicella, development of maternal antibodies, and transplacental transfer of these antibodies is shown in Figure 22-5. Because women with zoster near term have high antibody titers to VZV, it is not necessary to administer VZIG to their infants.

A small number of infants have developed severe or fatal congenital varicella despite prompt administration of VZIG in adequate dosage.[365-370] The reason for the severity of these cases is not fully understood, but they appear to be unusual or rare. Presumably, they were immunologically normal infants. Many of these children were reported from the United Kingdom, and the VZIG used there might have been less potent than that produced in the United States. The antibody titers of the two preparations have not been compared. It seems obvious, however, that passively immunized infants should be observed carefully for the rare instance in which antiviral therapy may also be required. Rapid evolution of large numbers of vesicles, hemorrhagic manifestations, and respiratory involvement are indications for the use of intravenous acyclovir. Some investigators have recommended prophylactic use of intravenously administered acyclovir in any infant who develops varicella despite passive immunization,[366,367,371,372] but this strategy has not been formally studied. Based on the studies cited previously, most passively immunized infants who develop clinical illness will have mild or moderate infections. Administration of acyclovir to all such infants who develop clinical illness would result in needless hospitalization of many infants and potential iatrogenic problems and would not be cost effective. Unless additional data become available, acyclovir should be given only to infants who manifest early signs of potentially severe varicella.

Although it is recommended that VZIG be administered to infants born to women who develop varicella in the first 2 days after delivery, few reports indicate that this timing of birth at onset of maternal varicella is associated with increased risk to the infant. One of the reported infants with fatal varicella despite passive immunization was born to a woman who developed chickenpox on the second postpartum day.[368] A child with severe varicella whose mother developed chickenpox 3 days after delivery has also been reported.[373] This child was treated with a leukocyte transfusion from her mother and thymic hormone and survived. In view of the absence of data indicating efficacy and the potential danger of graft-versus-host reaction after leukocyte transfusion in immunocompromised patients,[374] this therapy cannot be recommended.

To minimize the possibility of infection of the infant, mother and infant should be separated until the mother's chickenpox vesicles have dried, even if the infant has been passively immunized. Normally, this will be 5 to 7 days after the onset of maternal rash. If the infant develops clinical varicella, the mother may care for the infant.

Pregnant women who are closely exposed to persons with varicella or zoster and who have no history of varicella and are seronegative may be passively immunized with VZIG.[200] Although precise information regarding dosage is not available, a dose of 5 mL (625 units) is usually recommended for adults. The rationale for passive immunization of the mother is to protect her from developing severe chickenpox.

Because some low-birth-weight infants may have low or absent levels of transplacentally acquired maternal VZV antibody, it is recommended that infants of less than 28 weeks' gestation or who weighed less than 1000 g at birth be passively immunized with VZIG after close exposure.[200,364] There is no recognized age at which passive immunization is no longer recommended for these infants, but presumably it would not be necessary in an infant more than several weeks old. Administration of VZIG to term infants who are 2 to 7 days old at the time of exposure is not recommended, but it may be done optionally to decrease morbidity from varicella in this age group.[375] VZIG should not be used to try to control nosocomial varicella because it does not necessarily prevent varicella but rather modifies it.

Guidelines for Preventive Measures and Isolation Procedures in the Nursery

In contrast to transplacentally transmitted chickenpox, there is little evidence that postnatally acquired chickenpox (defined as disease beginning after the infant is 10 days old) is significantly more serious in infants than in older children (discussed in the preceding section). Nevertheless, despite the evidence cited previously indicating that nosocomial chickenpox among infants in the nursery is relatively uncommon, it is desirable to institute preventive measures to minimize the possibility of transmission of infection to other neonates, mothers, and hospital personnel. Any hospital patient isolated because of chickenpox or zoster should be in a separate room with the door closed, preferably in a room with air pressure negative compared with that in the corridor. Visitors and staff should be limited to persons immune to varicella. They should wear a new gown for each entry and wash their hands when leaving. Bedding and tissues soiled with respiratory excreta of the patient should be bagged and autoclaved. Special precautions for feces, urine, and needles or blood products are not required. Terminal disinfection of the room is likewise unnecessary.

Guidelines for isolation procedures and other measures are summarized in Table 22-10. If there are siblings or others at home with active VZV infections at the time mother and infant are ready for discharge from the hospital, one of the following alternatives is recommended:

1. The mother and neonate may be sent home after boarding the older siblings with immune relatives until they are no longer infectious, generally when no new vesicles have appeared for 72 hours and all lesions have progressed to the stage of crusts.
2. The mother can return home while the neonate remains in the nursery.
3. The neonate can be boarded with a surrogate mother until the siblings are no longer infectious.
4. VZIG may be given to the newborn.

If siblings at home develop chickenpox at the time of delivery or shortly after birth and the mother lacks a definite history of previous chickenpox, the first or last alternative is recommended. Serologic determination of the mother's immune status to varicella is recommended. Women with detectable VZV antibodies may be discharged home. Those who are seronegative should be offered varicella vaccine. Theoretically, if a woman has a history of varicella, her newborn should be at least partially protected from varicella. It seems prudent, however, to use a conservative approach, such as outlined here, because the real risk of varicella to the newborn is unknown.

When a mother with a negative history is exposed to chickenpox or zoster 6 to 20 days ante partum, she may become infectious before the onset of exanthem, during hospitalization for labor and the puerperium, assuming an average stay of 72 hours. This calculation is based on a minimum incubation period (exposure until onset of rash) of 10 days and a period of communicability preceding the exanthem by 3 days. When maternal exposure occurs less than 6 days before the onset of labor, the mother is unlikely to become infectious until after she has returned home. In either case, if the mother is exposed to chickenpox during the 20-day period ante partum, it is advisable to send the mother and infant home at the earliest possible date.

No special management is necessary for other mothers and infants in the nursery or for physicians and nurses potentially exposed in the delivery room or the nursery if they have previously had chickenpox. In the absence of a positive history, immediate serologic testing to determine the immune status of exposed hospital personnel may be performed when diagnostic facilities are available. Exposed personnel with negative histories may continue to work in the nursery for a period of 8 days after exposure pending serologic results because they are not potentially infectious during this period. Personnel with positive VZV antibody titers in serum are probably immune. Nonimmune (seronegative) nursery and delivery personnel should be excluded from patient care activities between days 8 and 21 after exposure. Subsequently, they should be strongly encouraged to be immunized against varicella, and they may be given postexposure prophylaxis with varicella vaccine (discussed later).

The greatest risk of nosocomial chickenpox exists when a mother develops chickenpox lesions less than 5 days before delivery or in the immediate postpartum period. If the neonate is born with lesions (i.e., congenital chickenpox), the mother and her newborn should be isolated together and sent home as soon as they are clinically stable. Other exposed mothers and infants in the nursery may also be sent home at the earliest date possible. Restriction of patient care activities and serologic testing of exposed delivery and nursery personnel as described earlier should be instituted. Passive immunization of exposed infants is optional considering the usually benign course of postnatally acquired chickenpox.

When maternal chickenpox occurs within approximately 5 days of delivery or immediately post partum and no lesions are present in the neonate, the mother and the infant should be isolated separately. Transplacentally acquired chickenpox, beginning 7 to 15 days after disease appears in the mother, will ultimately develop in about one half of these neonates despite administration of VZIG. The remainder will be at risk for postnatally acquired chickenpox unless isolated from their mothers. If no lesions develop in the

Table 22–10 **Guidelines for Preventive Measures after Exposure to Chickenpox in the Nursery or Maternity Ward**

Type of Exposure or Disease	Chickenpox Lesions Present: *Mother*	Chickenpox Lesions Present: *Neonate*	Disposition
A. Siblings at home have active chickenpox when neonate and mother are ready for discharge from hospital	No	No	1. *Mother:* if she has a history of chickenpox, she may return home. Without a history, she should be tested for VZV antibody titer.[a] If test is positive, she may return home. If test is negative, VZIG[b] may be administered and she may be discharged home. If she is antibody negative, 3 months after VZIG she should be immunized. 2. *Neonate:* may be discharged home with mother if mother has history of varicella or is VZV antibody positive. If mother is susceptible, administer VZIG to infant and discharge home or place in protective isolation.
B. Mother with no history of chickenpox; exposed during period 6-20 days ante partum[d]	No	No	1. *Exposed mother and infant:* send home at earliest date unless siblings at home have communicable chickenpox.[c] If so, may administer VZIG and discharge home, as above. 2. *Other mothers and infants:* no special management indicated. 3. *Hospital personnel:* no precautions indicated if there is a history of previous chickenpox or zoster. In absence of history, immediate serologic testing is indicated to determine immune status.[a] Nonimmune personnel should be excluded from patient contact until 21 days after an intimate exposure. Vaccination of nonimmune personnel should be encouraged. Immunized personnel who develop a vaccine-associated rash should be excluded from work until rash has healed. 4. If mother develops varicella 1 to 2 days post partum, infant should be given VZIG.
C. Onset of maternal chickenpox ante partum[d] or post partum	Yes	No	1. *Infected mother:* isolate until no longer clinically infectious. If seriously ill, treat with acyclovir. 2. *Infected mother's infant:* administer VZIG[b] to neonates born to mothers with onset of chickenpox <5 days before delivery and isolate separately from mother. Send home with mother if no lesions develop by the time mother is noninfectious. 3. *Other mothers and infants:* send home at earliest date. VZIG may be given optionally to exposed neonates 4. *Hospital personnel:* same as B-3.
D. Onset of maternal chickenpox ante partum[c]			1. *Mother:* isolation unnecessary if no longer infectious. 2. *Infant:* isolate from other infants but not from mother. 3. *Other mothers and infants:* same as C-3 (if exposed). 4. *Hospital personnel:* same as B-3.
E. Congenital chickenpox	No	Yes	1. *Infected infant and mother:* same as D-1 and D-2. 2. *Other mothers and infants:* same as C-3. 3. *Hospital personnel:* same as B-3.

[a]Send serum to virus diagnostic laboratory for determination of antibodies to VZV by a sensitive technique such as FAMA, LA, or ELISA. Personnel may continue to work for 8 days after exposure pending serologic results because they are not potentially infectious during this period. Antibodies to VZV >1:4 probably are indicative of immunity.

[b]VZIG is available through the American Red Cross. The dose for a newborn is 1.25 mL (1 vial). The dose for a pregnant woman is conventionally 6.25 mL (5 vials).

[c]Considered noninfectious when no new vesicles have appeared for 72 hours and all lesions have crusted.

[d]If exposure occurred less than 6 days ante partum, mother would not be potentially infectious until at least 72 hours post partum.

ELISA, enzyme-linked immunosorbent assay; FAMA, fluorescent antibody to membrane antigen; LA, latex agglutination; VZIG, varicella-zoster immune globulin; VZV, varicella-zoster virus.

neonate by the time its mother is noninfectious, both may be sent home. Guidelines for exposed hospital personnel and patients are like those described previously.

In congenital chickenpox, lesions may be absent in the mother at the time of delivery but present in the neonate. This may occur after rare subclinical infection in the mother[98] or because the onset of the exanthem in the infant occurs after the lesions in the mother have already healed. In either circumstance, the mother is not at risk and may be isolated with her newborn infant.

Active Immunization against Chickenpox

A live-attenuated varicella vaccine was developed in Japan by Takahashi and colleagues.[376] This vaccine was licensed in 1995 by the U.S. Food and Drug Administration for varicella-susceptible healthy children older than 1 year, adolescents, and adults. The vaccine is also licensed for routine use in a number of countries in Europe and in Asia, including Japan. The vaccine has proved to be safe and highly effective,[46,377,378] and it is recommended for routine use by the American Academy of Pediatrics[364,379] and the Centers for Disease

Control and Prevention.[200] The vaccine protects against varicella in about 85% of those vaccinated and decreases the incidence of zoster in immunocompromised patients and presumably in healthy vaccinees.[122,377,378,380]

The major adverse effect of vaccination is development of a very mild transient rash about 1 month (range, few days to 6 weeks) after immunization. The main concern about the rash is the possibility of spread of the vaccine-type virus to varicella-susceptible persons intimately exposed to a vaccinee with a rash. Contagion has not been reported in the absence of rash, and contact cases have uniformly been mild. There is no evidence of clinical reversion to wild-type VZV.[45,158,377] The vaccine-type virus spreads less efficiently than the wild-type virus, by a factor of about four, in children with leukemia who were immunized.[45] There is a much greater tendency to develop rash and also to transmit vaccine-type VZV from immunocompromised vaccinees than from healthy vaccinated individuals. A quantitative comparison is difficult to make, but in household contacts of leukemic vaccinees with rash, transmission occurred in about 25%.[45] In contrast, since the licensure of vaccine in the United States, about 40 million doses of vaccine have been distributed by the manufacturer, with only three reported instances of spread.[46] (There is one additional recorded instance of spread of varicella vaccine from a healthy vaccinee involving an experimental varicella vaccine.[381]) Unfortunately, one instance of spread occurred when a healthy child was immunized and his pregnant mother developed mild varicella, from which the vaccine-type virus was identified by PCR.[382] The mother terminated the pregnancy; the products of conception were negative for VZV by PCR. It is important to immunize susceptible women of childbearing age before they become pregnant. The risk of immunizing healthy toddlers is calculated to be lower than not immunizing them and risking their development of natural varicella that would expose a pregnant varicella-susceptible pregnant mother to the fully virulent virus.[383] Widespread use of vaccine in the United States may decrease or even eliminate the problems of congenital malformations and severe varicella in the neonatal period, as has occurred with rubella. Although varicella vaccine-type virus has not been shown to cause the congenital varicella syndrome, immunization during pregnancy is contraindicated. It is also recommended that immunized women refrain from becoming pregnant for at least 3 months after receipt of vaccine.[200,364,379] Individuals older than 13 years are recommended to receive two doses of vaccine 4 to 8 weeks apart. The reported seroconversion rate after two doses of vaccine in healthy adults is about 90%.[158,377] Ideally, women should have serologic testing for immunity after immunization, but a negative antibody titer after immunization does not necessarily indicate vaccine failure because commercially available ELISA antibody tests may fail to identify some individuals who have responded to the vaccine.[384]

The vaccine program in the United States has been highly successful, with a decrease in varicella incidence in the vaccinated and unvaccinated in regions where there is active reporting of varicella.[46,385,386] There is evidence of herd immunity with this vaccine.

The vaccine is under scrutiny for two reasons. One concern is the possibility of rare primary (no take) and secondary (waning immunity) immune failure. Studies involving outbreaks of varicella in children in daycare have suggested that these phenomena can result in transmission and even lead to mini-epidemics. In one daycare study, protection against varicella was only 44% in vaccinees.[387] Considerable data have suggested that children younger than 15 months may respond slightly less effectively to vaccine than older children.[387-390] A two-dose schedule to obvert these unusual problems has been suggested, but the recommendations for vaccine use in the United States remain unchanged.[391]

The second issue surrounding varicella vaccine is whether its widespread use will lead to a significant increase in the incidence of zoster in the unvaccinated. It is thought that zoster is less common in those vaccinated than in those who have had natural infection.[392] This probably occurs because the vaccine virus is less likely to establish latent infection than the wild-type virus. After natural infection, however, reexposure to wild-type VZV can boost immunity to the virus, resulting in protection against zoster, presumably caused by control of reactivating virus before it results in illness.[392] The important question is how significant an increase in zoster is likely to occur in the vaccine era. Based mainly on epidemiologic evidence and computer modeling, some studies predict a serious increase in zoster with accompanying fatalities.[393,394] The incidence of zoster is roughly 2 cases per 1000 person-years of observation.[395] If this incidence doubles as a result of routine vaccination, it is unlikely to represent an epidemic of zoster. Moreover, zoster is rarely fatal even in immunocompromised patients, in contrast to varicella, which continues to cause fatalities and has a higher mortality rate than zoster.[396-399]

MEASLES

Measles (i.e., rubeola) is a highly communicable childhood disease whose hallmarks are fever, coryza, conjunctivitis, cough, and a generalized maculopapular rash that usually appears 1 to 2 days after a specific enanthem (i.e., Koplik's spots). The word *measles* means "little spots" and is derived from the Dutch word for the disease, *maeselen,* a diminutive of *maese,* meaning "spot" or "stain."[400] Although measles was described in medieval times, it was not until the 17th century that Sydenham differentiated the disease from smallpox and scarlet fever.

The Organism

Classification and Morphology

Measles virus is a paramyxovirus, but some of its properties, such as the lack of neuraminidase, are distinct from those of other members of this family. Like paramyxoviruses, measles virions have a diameter of 100 to 250 nm and consist of a helical ribonucleoprotein core surrounded by a lipid envelope.

In cell culture, virions replicate predominantly in the cytoplasm and are released from the cell surface by budding. The envelope of the virion is composed of at least two glycoproteins: E, which causes membrane fusion and is crucial for infectivity, and H, the hemagglutinin. A nonglycosylated matrix protein, M, also exists on the envelope. Antibodies to glycoprotein F inhibit viral infectivity.[401] Other internal structural proteins are the large protein (L), the phosphoprotein or polymerase (P), and the nucleocapsid protein (N). The cellular receptors for measles virus are the CD46 and

CD150 molecules expressed on human lymphocytes and many other human cell types.[402,403]

Measles virus has been fully sequenced. Genomic data indicate that the viruses that caused the resurgence of measles between 1989 and 1992 were not new strains, that most of the reported cases in 1994 and 1995 were the result of international importation of virus, and that aggressive control measures in 1992 resulted in control of the viruses circulating at that time.[404] The latest data support this contention and indicate that there is no endemic measles in the United States; the few circulating viruses identified are imported from other countries.[403,405]

Propagation of Measles Virus

Primary cultures of human embryonic kidney and rhesus monkey kidney cells have proved to be superior to all others for the isolation of measles virus, although the agent has been adapted after several passages to a number of continuous cell lines.[402] Cytopathic effect on primary isolation is not generally detected before 5 to 10 days. Rapid identification may be accomplished by use of immunofluorescent staining using monoclonal antibodies.[402]

Antigenic Properties and Serologic Tests

Measles virus isolates are antigenically homogeneous. Some cross-reactivity of soluble ribonucleoprotein antigens and hemagglutinins has been observed among measles and the related viruses of rinderpest and canine distemper but not with other paramyxoviruses. The hemagglutination inhibition (HI) test has essentially been replaced with more modern assays for antibodies.

ELISA is the most useful and sensitive method for measuring antibodies to measles virus.[402,406] A similar test that identifies specific IgM antibody and is useful diagnostically when only one serum specimen is available has also been developed.[402,407,408]

Transmission and Epidemiology

Transmission by Droplets and Fomites

Measles is the most communicable of the childhood exanthems.[51,64] The virus is spread chiefly by droplets expectorated by an infected subject in proximity to susceptible persons. Rarely, transmission may occur by means of articles soiled by respiratory secretions. There is some uncertainty concerning the precise portal of entry of the virus. Although the virus may gain access through the nose or the oropharynx, the work of Papp[409] suggests that the conjunctival mucosa is at least a possible portal of entry.

Measles occurs worldwide in temperate, tropical, and arctic climates. Before the introduction of live measles vaccines, urban areas of the United States typically experienced epidemics at intervals of 2 to 3 years. In interepidemic years, few cases of measles occur, probably because the supply of susceptible persons has been exhausted. Additional births add to this pool, permitting epidemic transmission when the pool is sufficiently large. In the United States, the disease had a peak incidence between March and May. Seasonal variation is attributed to the crowding of children indoors and in schools in the winter, resulting in increased transmission. Amplification of each cycle leads to a progressively larger number of cases of measles by the end of the winter. Attack rates are highest among the lowest socioeconomic populations.

Patterns of disease vary strikingly with respect to age, incidence, and severity in different geographic regions. In urban areas of industrialized countries, measles infects predominantly children between the ages of 2 and 6 years, and the disease is relatively mild. In rural areas of the same countries, children are characteristically older when they contract the disease and may reach adulthood without becoming infected. For this reason, measles in pregnant women may be observed more often among women from rural or otherwise geographically isolated localities (see later discussion). A different pattern of disease is seen in less developed areas, such as equatorial Africa, where measles occurs predominantly in children younger than 2 years and has a high fatality rate.[410] Protein deficiency is associated with an increased incidence of complications, such as bronchopneumonia and death. Still another pattern of infection has been observed in extremely isolated regions of the world, where whole populations may never have experienced measles before its exogenous introduction. In a classic description of such an epidemic in the Faroe Islands in 1846, measles was observed to spread rapidly through an entire population, irrespective of age, with an attack rate of virtually 100%.[411] Mortality rates tend to be higher in populations having little experience with measles. An extreme example is the Fiji Islands epidemic of 1875, in which 20,000 people, or about one fourth of the population, are said to have died.[411]

The use of live-attenuated measles vaccine in the United States since 1963 has decreased the incidence of measles to less than 1% of its former incidence. Before 1963, there were about 400,000 reported cases of measles annually; a record low of 1497 cases was reported in 1983, but in the late 1980s and early 1990s, there was an increase in the incidence of measles that has since come under control.[372] From 1989 to 1991, there were more than 55,000 reported cases with more than 120 measles-associated deaths reported to the Centers for Disease Control and Prevention, but after 1991, the number of reported cases dropped significantly.[412] Measles occurring despite vaccination may be the result of primary vaccine failure, a "no take" for the vaccine, or secondary vaccine failure due to loss of immunity to measles after vaccination.[413,414] There is little evidence, however, that secondary immune failure (i.e., that protective immunity induced by measles wanes with time) is significant.[413-416] Since the requirement for two doses of measles vaccine in childhood was instituted in 1993, the number of annual cases of measles has fallen to an all-time low. In 1995, 309 cases were reported, and in 1996, 508 cases were reported to the Centers for Disease Control and Prevention.[412] Measles has become a rare disease in the United States; in 2001, only 116 cases were reported.[403,405]

Incidence of Measles in Pregnant Women

Because measles is well controlled in the United States by immunization, it occurs even less frequently during pregnancy than chickenpox.

Pathogenesis

By analogy with other viral infections whose pathogenesis has been better delineated, the initial multiplication of measles virus is believed to occur in epithelial and lymphoid cells near the portal of entry. A transient viremia then delivers virus to the reticuloendothelial system, where further replication occurs. A second viremia, more severe and more sustained, disseminates virus to the skin, gut, respiratory tract, and other affected organs. In monkeys, this viremia may occur over a period as long as 1 week before the appearance of the prodrome or exanthem. Measles virus replicates in and probably destroys lymphocytes in the peripheral blood,[417] giving rise to a circulating lymphopenia. The symptoms of measles are probably attributable to inflammation accompanying necrosis of cells in which the virus is replicating. By the time the exanthem appears, 13 to 14 days after infection, measles virus is actively replicating in the skin, gut, and respiratory mucosa. Electron microscopy of biopsies of Koplik's spots and cutaneous lesions reveals syncytial giant cells whose nuclear and cytoplasmic inclusions contain aggregates of microtubules that are 15 to 20 nm in diameter and characteristic of paramyxovirus infection.[418] This finding and the observation that convalescent measles serum injected into the skin can prevent the local development of the exanthem[419] suggest that replication of virus per se is directly responsible for the lesions. Nevertheless, it is possible that an interaction between viral antigen and antibody is required. The latter hypothesis is supported by the observation that immunosuppressed children who develop giant cell pneumonia caused by measles virus do not develop a rash and do not elaborate antibodies.[420,421] Virus titers in the viscera have already diminished considerably by the time the exanthem appears, and serum antibodies are readily detectable within 24 hours. There is also experimental evidence that T lymphocytes are important in the development of some symptoms of measles such as the rash, as well as in recovery from the disease.[422]

Incubation Period for Measles Acquired by Droplet Infection

The usual interval between exposure to measles and onset of first symptoms (i.e., prodrome) is about 10 days; 12 to 14 days usually elapse before the onset of rash. However, considerable variation may be observed.[383] The incubation period in modified measles (see " Clinical Manifestations") may last as long as 17 to 21 days, because of the presence of low levels of measles antibodies.[423]

Incubation Period for Hematogenously Acquired Measles

It has been claimed that infantile measles may be acquired by transfusion of maternal blood presumably containing measles virus.[424] Two infants developed typical enanthems and exanthems 13 and 14 days after transfusion, and their mothers developed measles exanthems 4 and 2 days, respectively, after blood donation. The infants had not been visited by their mothers for 4 days and 1 day, respectively, before transfusion. Hematogenous transmission may not have occurred, however, because the mothers may well have been shedding virus from the respiratory tract at the time they last handled their infants.

Intrauterine hematogenous transmission is well documented (discussed later). In these cases, the onset of disease in the infant may occur almost simultaneously with that in the mother or after a variable interval that is less than the minimum time required for extrauterine infection by the respiratory route.

Period of Communicability

Measles is more communicable during the prodrome and catarrhal stage of infection than during the period of the exanthem. Dramatic corroboration of this observation was provided during an epidemic in Greenland in 1962.[425] Deliberate exposure of 400 susceptible persons to disease was achieved by having a patient on the first day of appearance of the exanthem cough twice in the face of each. Not a single transmission resulted. When the experiment was repeated with a patient during the pre-exanthematous period, measles was readily transmitted.

Patients with measles should be considered infectious from the onset of the prodrome (about 4 days before the appearance of the exanthem) until 3 days after the onset of the exanthem, although the risk of contagion abruptly diminishes 48 hours after the rash appears, concomitant with the appearance of circulating neutralizing antibodies. Measles virus is most readily recovered from respiratory secretions from 2 days before until 1 or 2 days after the onset of the rash.

Pathology

The replication of measles virus in epithelial cells of the mucous membranes and skin leads to the formation of intranuclear inclusions and syncytial giant cells with up to 100 nuclei per cell (i.e., Warthin-Finkeldey cells).[426] Focal hyaline necrosis of epithelial cells is accompanied by a subepithelial exudate containing predominantly mononuclear leukocytes. The pathology of cutaneous lesions and Koplik's spots is essentially similar.[418] It is likely that virus replicates simultaneously in the skin and mucous membranes, but Koplik's spots are detected earlier than the exanthem, probably because the epithelium that forms the roof of the lesions is thinner and more translucent in the mucous membranes.

Similar lesions containing the characteristic multinucleated giant cells may be widespread throughout the respiratory and gastrointestinal tracts. The pharynx, tonsils, bronchial epithelium, appendix, colon, and lymph nodes have been involved. Viral bronchitis occurs in most cases of measles. Necrotic columnar epithelial cells and giant cells are sloughed into the lumen of the bronchi and bronchioles. When this damage is extensive, the regenerating epithelium frequently undergoes squamous metaplasia and is accompanied by bronchial and peribronchial inflammation. Extension of the process into the alveolar septa results in interstitial pneumonitis. Secondary bacterial infection commonly supervenes, leading to a bronchopneumonia with purulent exudate.

Measles virus has been demonstrated, using immunofluorescence and immunoperoxidase methodology, in the placental syncytial trophoblastic cells and decidua, in a 25-week fetus of a woman who developed gestational measles. The fetus was spared. It is postulated that placental damage induced by the virus, leading to hypoxia, is responsible for fetal death during maternal measles.[427]

The pathologic signs of measles encephalitis are not readily distinguishable from those of other postinfectious encephalitides, such as those caused by vaccinia, chickenpox, and rubella. The characteristic lesion is perivenous demyelination, often accompanied by mild perivascular infiltrates of mononuclear leukocytes, petechial hemorrhages, and microglial proliferation. Neuronal damage and meningeal inflammation are not prominent. Nuclear or cytoplasmic inclusions and giant cells are inconstant. Measles virus has been isolated only infrequently from the brain or spinal cord, and it remains unclear whether the pathologic changes in the brain are a direct result of measles virus or an allergic response to a virus-induced product or antigen-antibody complexes.[428,429] Because of the spectrum of pathology, including acute demyelinating encephalitis and acute hemorrhagic leukoencephalitis, it has been postulated that measles encephalitis is an autoimmune process. Myelin basic protein has been demonstrated in the cerebrospinal fluid of patients with measles encephalitis, and the pathologic process has been likened to experimental allergic encephalitis as produced in animal models.[430] One theory regarding pathogenesis is that measles virus has an epitope similar to that of the encephalitogenic sequence in central nervous system myelin (i.e., an instance of molecular mimicry leading to disease).[431] A second form of encephalitis is caused by continued replication of measles virus in the brains of immunocompromised patients.[432]

Clinical Manifestations

Prodrome and Rash

The prodrome typically begins 10 to 11 days after exposure, with fever and malaise, followed within 24 hours by coryza, sneezing, conjunctivitis, and cough. During the next 2 to 3 days, this catarrhal phase is accentuated, with markedly infected conjunctivae and photophobia. Toward the end of the prodrome, Koplik's spots appear. They are tiny (no larger than a pinhead), granular, slightly raised white lesions surrounded by a halo of erythema. Beginning with fewer than a dozen specks on the lateral buccal mucosa, Koplik's spots may multiply during a 24-hour period to affect virtually all the mucous membranes of the cheeks and may extend to the lips and eyelids. Hundreds of spots may be present. At this stage, the lesions may be said to resemble grains of salt on a wet background. Koplik's spots appear 1 to 2 days before the exanthem.

The rash, which appears 12 to 14 days after exposure, begins on the head and neck, especially behind the ears and on the forehead. At first, the lesions are red macules 1 to 2 mm in diameter, but during a period of 2 or 3 days, they enlarge and coalesce. By the second day, the exanthem has spread to the trunk and upper extremities. The lower extremities are involved by the third day. The lesions are most prominent in those regions where the exanthem appears first, namely, the face and upper trunk. By the third or fourth day, the exanthem begins to fade in the order of its appearance. A brown staining of the lesions often persists for 7 to 10 days and is followed by fine desquamation.

The clinical course of measles may be greatly altered by administration of immunoglobulin during the incubation period. In modified measles, the catarrhal phase may be completely suppressed and the exanthem limited to a few macules on the trunk.

Complications and Mortality

The most frequent complications of measles involve the respiratory tract. Otitis media and mild croup are common in young children during the catarrhal phase, but bacterial pneumonia is the complication that results in death most frequently. If carefully sought, fine rales and radiologic evidence of bronchopneumonia can be found during the early exanthematous phase in most patients. Cough may persist beyond the peak of the exanthem in uncomplicated measles, but when the fever fails to decline or recurs as the rash is fading, a bacterial superinfection is usually present. The chest radiograph may show consolidation. A peripheral blood polymorphonuclear leukocytosis is present. When bacterial superinfection occurs, antimicrobial therapy is indicated and should be directed against the most likely etiologic agents: *Streptococcus pneumoniae, S. aureus,* and *Streptococcus pyogenes.* Smears and cultures of sputum should be obtained, but in young infants it may be necessary to treat bacterial superinfection without a specific etiologic diagnosis because of the difficulty in obtaining adequate sputum and the potential gravity of the illness (see "Therapy").

After otitis and pneumonia, encephalitis is the most frequent serious complication of measles. It is far less common than pneumonia. Encephalitis, including coma and gross cerebral dysfunction, is estimated to occur with a frequency of 1 per 1000 cases[428] but is probably more common if drowsiness, irritability, and transient electroencephalographic changes are accepted as evidence of encephalitis. This complication occurs in all age groups, including the neonatal period. A fatal outcome has been recorded in an infant, born in the hospital, who developed measles with encephalitis when 27 days old.[429] Measles encephalitis may occur at any stage of the illness but appears most commonly 3 to 7 days after the onset of the exanthem. The initial symptoms are drowsiness and irritability, followed by lethargy, convulsions, and coma. The cerebrospinal fluid changes are those of a mild aseptic meningitis. Mental obtundation may clear over a period of 1 to 4 days or may assume a more protracted course that is associated with a higher incidence of such sequelae as severe behavioral abnormalities and mental retardation. Death occurs in about 11% of cases.[428] Other complications of measles have been described. These include thrombocytopenic purpura, appendicitis, myocarditis, subacute sclerosing panencephalitis, and reactivation or exacerbation of previously acquired tuberculosis. In a study of 3220 U.S. Air Force recruits with measles, whose mean age was 19 years, between 1976 and 1979, bacterial superinfection and elevated serum transaminase levels were observed in 30%, otitis in 29%, sinusitis in 25%, bronchospasm in 17%, and pneumonia in 3%.[433]

The precise case-fatality ratio in measles is highly variable among different populations and at different periods in the history of the same population. Between 1920 and 1950 in Massachusetts, deaths caused by measles declined progressively during each successive 5-year period from 7.6 to 0.28 per 100,000 people, despite an approximately constant morbidity related to measles.[411] Because the decline preceded the widespread use of antibiotics, much of the change is attributed to improved social conditions, less crowding, improved nutrition, and medical care. In the United States since 1963 the case-fatality ratio has averaged about 0.1% based on reported cases, but it may be closer to 0.01% if estimated unreported cases of measles are included in the calculation.[434] However, the risk is considerably greater in children younger than 1 year old. The age-specific death rates for measles in the United States reported in 1949 (per 100,000 people) were 7.8 when younger than 1 year, 2.8 at 1 to 4 years old, 1.3 at 5 to 9 years old, and 0.4 at 10 to 14 years old. That death rates are higher for infants is confirmed by data obtained during an epidemic in Greenland in 1951, in which the age-specific death rates (per 1000 people) were 26 for infants younger than 1 year and 15 for infants 1 to 2 years old; no deaths were recorded in children between 2 and 14 years old.[435] In cases for which adequate information was available, all deaths of children younger than 1 year old apparently were caused by pneumonia, which appeared during the prodrome or shortly after the onset of the exanthem.

Children with underlying infection with HIV have been reported to be at risk for developing severe measles, and fatalities have been reported, especially in children who have developed AIDS.[436] In Africa, it has also been observed that infants born to HIV-infected women have lower titers of measles antibodies in cord sera than infants from women not infected with HIV. The outcome has been that these infants are at greater risk for developing measles early in infancy.[437] One adolescent with HIV infection who had previously received measles vaccine developed fatal measles pneumonia after the second dose.[438] Because the infection was proved to be from the vaccine virus, measles vaccine is no longer recommended for HIV-infected children who have developed AIDS or evidence of severe immunosuppression.[412]

Immunocompromised children with underlying malignant diseases who have not been immunized are also at risk for developing severe and even fatal measles.[439-441]

Maternal Effects of Measles

Is the pregnant woman with measles at greater risk of serious complications and death than other adults with this disease are? The answer is probably yes. Some of the published experiences leading to this conclusion are summarized in the following paragraphs.

In the early part of the 20th century, fatality rates for pregnant women with measles were reported to be approximately 15%, mostly caused by pneumonia in the puerperium.[442,443] In the 1951 Greenland epidemic, 4 deaths (4.9%) occurred among 83 women who had measles during pregnancy or the puerperium. In contrast, there were 19 deaths (1.7%) among 1099 nonpregnant women between the ages of 15 and 54.[435] This difference is probably significant ($\chi^2 = 3.9$, $P = .05$). There was no significant difference in the frequency of pneumonia as a complication of measles among pregnant and nonpregnant women in the same age group, but heart failure was observed far more often in pregnant women with measles. Heart failure was observed in seven patients with gestational measles. Of these, three were in the second half of pregnancy, and four were puerperal. Although in some patients heart failure occurred during the prodrome, in most women, it occurred within 2 weeks after onset of the exanthem.

Additional experience in the United States and Australia since 1940 supports the concept that measles during pregnancy is only rarely catastrophic. Among 24 women with gestational measles in an outbreak in rural Oklahoma, no deaths occurred and serious morbidity was likewise not increased.[444] In another epidemic, reported in 1950 from Australia, 18 cases of gestational measles were observed. In only one case—a woman in the third trimester with measles pneumonia—were complications reported.[445]

Between 1988 and 1992 in the United States, when there was a resurgence of measles, a number of pregnant women developed this infection. Thirteen such women who were hospitalized in Houston, Texas, were reported because 7 (54%) had respiratory complications that were the basis for their hospitalization. They required supplemental oxygen and monitoring in the intensive care unit, and 1 woman died.[446] These women appeared to have primary measles pneumonia rather than bacterial superinfection. Nine of these 13 women were treated with aerosolized ribavirin administered by facemask. Hepatitis, demonstrated by elevations of transaminases, also occurred frequently in these women, but this is a common finding in nonpregnant adults that seems to be of little clinical importance. During this same period, medical records from 58 pregnant women from Los Angeles with measles were reviewed. Thirty-five (60%) were hospitalized for measles, 15 (26%) developed pneumonia, and 2 (3%) died.[447] Although it is difficult to prove that measles is more severe in pregnant than nonpregnant women, it seems likely to be so.

Effects of Gestational Measles on the Fetus

CHROMOSOMAL ABERRATIONS

The possibility that measles occurring in pregnancy may potentially damage the fetus is suggested by the observation that there is a high frequency of chromosomal breaks in leukocyte metaphase preparations between the second and fifth day of the exanthem.[448] Other reports, however, have not fully confirmed the preceding observations. Miller[449] found no chromosomal breaks in leukocytes of patients with measles who were examined 1 to 12 days after onset of the rash, but he attributed this discrepancy to methodologic differences involving more gentle treatment of the leukocytes. A report from Japan[450] also failed to show an increased frequency of chromosomal breaks per cell in patients with measles compared with those in normal subjects. However, a significant increase in chromosomal breaks was observed in patients with Down syndrome who had measles and it was inferred that their chromosomes were more sensitive to measles infection.[450]

These chromosomal abnormalities are transient and disappear during convalescence. No studies have examined whether intrauterine exposure of the fetus to measles results in more lasting chromosomal aberrations.

ABORTION AND PREMATURITY

The consensus of several reports dealing with the frequency of premature births is that this untoward event occurs more often in association with measles during pregnancy than in the pregnant population at large. In contrast to rubella, in which there is retarded intrauterine development, prematurity caused by measles is associated with normal intrauterine development but premature expulsion of the fetus. Although there is no statistically valid proof that gestational measles also causes a higher rate of abortion, it seems probable that measles is responsible for some instances of abortion.

Among the retrospective studies is that of Dyer,[444] who reported 24 cases of gestational measles from rural Oklahoma in 1938 and 1939. Uterine contractions, which typically occurred during the illness, were identified in 11 of the 24 women and caused premature delivery of the fetus in 9 (38%). In one woman in whom measles occurred at 18 weeks' gestation, the exanthem was followed by spontaneous abortion 7 days later. Two additional pregnancies were associated with premature births at 33 weeks' gestation. No abortions were associated with eight cases of measles occurring in the first trimester.

Adverse outcomes of gestational measles on the fetus involving 18 pregnant women with measles were reported in the epidemic in South Australia in 1950.[445] There were three spontaneous abortions (17%), which occurred in one of seven women who had measles in the first trimester, one of eight in the second trimester, and one of three in the third trimester. Abortions followed the onset of the exanthem by 2 to 3 weeks in the patients who became ill in the first and second trimesters. The patient with measles in the third trimester had severe measles pneumonia and expelled a macerated fetus 7 weeks later. One live premature birth was recorded in the third trimester.

In the 1951 Greenland epidemic, birth or abortion occurred in 26 of the 76 pregnant women while they had measles.[435] Thirteen were term pregnancies. Of the remainder, spontaneous abortion at 3 to 5 months' gestation occurred in seven women (9%). There were six instances of premature delivery (8%), and perinatal death ensued in three. A retrospective analysis of 51 women in Greenland who developed measles during the first 3 months of pregnancy between 1951 and 1962 also suggested a high fetal death rate. One half with measles in the first 2 months and one fifth with measles in the third month had spontaneous abortions.[451] Five infants born to women with measles during an outbreak in 1981 and 1982 in Israel have been reported.[452] All were born prematurely (range, 28 to 34 weeks) with a mean duration between maternal onset of illness and delivery of 3.5 days and a mean birth weight of 1496 g. None had any signs of measles at birth or in the neonatal period.

Controlled, prospective studies carried out in New York City during the period from 1957 to 1964 demonstrated a significant association between maternal measles and prematurity but not between maternal measles and abortion. Low birth weight (<2500 g) was identified in 10 (16.7%) of 60 infants born to measles-infected mothers, compared with 2 (3.3%) of 62 matched controls ($\chi^2 = 6.2$, $P < .025$) (see Table 22-5).[178] When fetal mortality was examined in relation to gestational age (see Table 22-6), it was found that 3 deaths (15.8%) occurred in 19 cases of measles in the first trimester, 1 (3.4%) in 29 in the second trimester, and 1 (5.9%) in 17 in the third trimester.[178] These figures were not significantly different from those for fetal deaths in control pregnancies not involving measles. Of the five fetal deaths that occurred in pregnant women with measles, two of the deaths occurred within 2 weeks of maternal disease.

The resurgence of measles from 1989 to 1991 resulted in measles in a number of pregnant women. In the experience of Atmar and associates,[446] there was an adverse fetal outcome in 4 (31%) of 13 pregnancies complicated by maternal measles. Two women gave birth in the 34th and 35th weeks, and one spontaneously aborted at 16 weeks during measles. One additional woman and her fetus died at 20 weeks. In a report from Los Angeles of 58 women, the incidence of abortion was 5 (9%), and that of prematurity was 13 (22%).[447]

CONGENITAL DEFECTS

The teratogenic potential of gestational measles for the fetus has been neither proved nor refuted because of the rarity of the infection during pregnancy, particularly during the first trimester when the process of organogenesis is most active. It seems clear, however, that if measles causes congenital malformations, it does so far less frequently than does rubella. Unlike gestational chickenpox, no particular constellation of abnormalities has been found among the sporadic instances of congenital defects that have occurred because of measles in the mother during pregnancy.

Isolated instances of buphthalmos,[453] congenital heart disease,[454] cleft lip,[210] pyloric stenosis,[454] genu valgum,[453] cerebral leukodystrophy,[451] and cyclopia[451] have been reported in infants born to mothers with measles diagnosed during the organogenic period. In these and other cases, documentation that the maternal illness was measles and not rubella or other exanthems is often lacking.

No congenital malformations were observed among four infants born to mothers who had measles during the first 4 months of pregnancy in the Oklahoma outbreak.[444] Similarly, in the 1951 Greenland epidemic, there were no congenital malformations among the infants of 76 mothers with gestational measles, although the number of cases that occurred in the first trimester is unclear.[435] After the epidemic in South Australia,[445] two infants with congenital defects (one with Down syndrome and one with partial deafness) were recorded among those whose mothers had measles during the first trimester. No birth defects occurred in infants born to eight mothers with measles in the second trimester and three mothers who had been ill in the third trimester. Although one of the five infants born during the outbreak in 1981 and 1982 in Israel was severely malformed, this was not caused by maternal measles, which had begun only a few days before birth. Five additional reported Israeli infants had no congenital anomalies, but all their mothers had measles just before delivery.[452] In the Houston report of 13 pregnant women, the fetal gestational age at onset of maternal measles ranged from 16 to 35 weeks (mean, 27 weeks). Follow-up of eight of these infants, delivered a mean of 12 weeks later (range, 1 to 24 weeks), revealed that no infants had congenital malformations.[446] These analyses are incapable of establishing whether the incidence of congenital defects is increased as a result of gestational measles because they were uncontrolled. One controlled prospective study is inconclusive because only small numbers of pregnant women with measles could be studied. Among 60 children who were born to mothers who had gestational measles and were followed to the age of 5 years, only one congenital malformation was identified, compared with a virtually identical incidence of one defect among 62 controls.[174] The defect in the infected group was bilateral deafness in an infant weighing 1990 g born to a mother who had measles at 6 weeks' gestation. In summary, if there is any increased risk of malformations from gestational measles, this risk appears to be small if it exists at all.

Perinatal Measles

As in chickenpox, perinatal measles includes transplacental infection and disease acquired postnatally by the respiratory route. Because the usual incubation period from infection to the first appearance of the exanthem is 13 to 14 days, measles exanthems acquired in the first 10 days of life may be considered transplacental in origin, whereas disease appearing at 14 days or later is probably acquired outside the uterus.

POSTNATALLY ACQUIRED MEASLES

Several reports describe cases of measles in which the onset of the exanthem occurred in infants 14 to 30 days old. The course of the disease in these cases was generally mild.[444,455,456] In one infant with notably mild illness and little fever, the illness began at the age of 14 days. This neonate had been suckled by the mother, in whom the prodrome of measles developed on the first postpartum day. Because circulating and presumably also secretory antibodies appear within 48 hours of the onset of the exanthem, it is possible that the neonate's illness was modified by measles-specific IgA antibodies present in the mother's milk.[444,455,456] A report from Japan in 1997 described seven cases of measles in infants during the first month of life. No case was believed to be severe, although there were three infants with pneumonia, two of whom had received immunoglobulin at exposure.[457] Measles acquired postnatally may also cause more severe illness; when a mother developed the disease 20 days post partum, her infant was quite sick with measles 10 days later, but complications such as pneumonia or otitis apparently did not develop.[458]

Outbreaks of nosocomial measles in the newborn nursery apparently have not been recorded in the 20th century, probably because of the low incidence of measles in the United States and other developed countries, nearly universal immunity in mothers in urban areas, and corresponding protection of the newborn by passive antibodies.

CONGENITAL MEASLES

Congenital measles includes cases in which the exanthem is present at birth and infections acquired in utero in which the rash appears during the first 10 days of life. In congenital measles, the incubation period, defined as the interval between onset of exanthem in the mother and in the infant, varies between 2 days[444] and 10 days[459] (mean, 6 days). A nearly simultaneous onset in mother and neonate implies that measles virus in the maternal bloodstream may sometimes cross the placenta in sufficient quantity to cause disease in the fetus without the need for many additional cycles of replication. However, the placenta may act as a barrier of limited effectiveness, as suggested by those instances in which disease does not appear in the fetus until 10 days after its appearance in the mother. Even more cogent is the fact that maternal measles immediately preceding parturition by no means invariably involves the fetus. Of 44 pregnancies in which a maternal rash was present at delivery, only in 13 (30%) was exanthematous measles reported in the neonate.[443] Later reports include 13 instances in which maternal rashes with onsets ranging from 7 days ante partum to 3 days post partum were associated with clinically apparent measles in the infant in only 3 (23%).[444,452,458,460] However, eight of these children received immunoglobulin (0.25 mL/kg) at birth,

Table 22–11 Deaths in Neonates Whose Mothers Had Measles at Parturition

Exanthem in Neonate	Neonatal Deaths[a]	Neonatal Cases	%
Present at birth	4	12	33
Appeared after birth	3	10	30
Did not appear	7[b]	16	44

[a]Stillborns excluded.
[b]All of these were premature infants reported in a single series.[435]

Table 22–12 Deaths from Congenital Measles in Relation to Date of Onset of Rash in Mothers

Onset of Maternal Rash	Neonatal Deaths	Neonatal Cases	%
Ante partum	4	15	27
Post partum	3	11	27

including the three who developed measles.[452,460] During the Greenland epidemic of 1951, no examples of congenital measles were observed among infants born to 13 women who had measles at parturition.[435] It appears that most of these neonates do not experience subclinical measles without exanthem but simply are not infected. This conclusion is supported by the observation that infants whose mothers had measles late in the third trimester are fully susceptible to infection later in childhood.[443] During the Faroe Islands epidemic of 1846, many pregnant women had measles, but 36 years later, their infants were infected as adults in a new epidemic in 1882.[458]

As in congenital chickenpox, the spectrum of illness in congenital measles varies from a mild illness, in which the rash is transient and Koplik's spots may be absent, to rapidly fatal disease. The precise case-fatality ratio is uncertain because the course of measles in different populations has been so variable, even in older children and adults. Among 22 cases of congenital measles culled from the literature in which immunoglobulin prophylaxis was not given, there were seven deaths (Table 22-11).[443,444,458,459] Approximately the same case-fatality ratio (30% to 33%) was observed whether the rash was present at birth or appeared subsequently. Although the number of observations is small, it appears that for premature infants with congenital measles, the death rate is higher (5 of 9) than for infants with congenital measles delivered at term (2 of 10). The death rate has also been high among premature infants born to women who had measles at parturition even when the infant never developed clinically apparent measles (see Table 22-11).[435,443]

Insufficient data are available to evaluate whether transplacentally acquired antibodies to measles virus may diminish the case-fatality ratio in congenital measles when the mother's exanthem appears more than 48 hours ante partum. The death rate from congenital measles does not appear to differ appreciably whether the maternal rash appears ante partum or post partum (Table 22-12), but more precise information on the time of appearance of the maternal rash is needed to answer this question definitively. Although firm data are not available, administration of immunoglobulin at birth may also decrease mortality.[446,452,460]

Most reports of death related to congenital measles do not specify the immediate cause, but pneumonia is among the leading complications.[443,444,446,452,460,461] Because nearly all reports of deaths preceded the antibiotic era, the current case-fatality ratio may be significantly lower than it was previously because of improved supportive care and appropriate antimicrobial therapy of bacterial superinfections.

Diagnosis and Differential Diagnosis

The diagnosis of measles is easy when there is a history of recent exposure and the typical catarrhal phase is followed by Koplik's spots and a maculopapular exanthem in the characteristic distribution. Koplik's spots are pathognomonic. However, the diagnosis is more difficult during the prodrome (when the illness is maximally communicable) or when the illness and the exanthem are attenuated by passively acquired measles antibodies. Measles antibodies may be contained in transfused plasma or immunoglobulin, or they may cross the placenta to the neonate if the mother develops measles shortly before parturition. The atypical exanthem of measles in subjects who have been previously immunized with inactivated measles vaccine may potentially also cause diagnostic difficulties. When the diagnosis cannot be made confidently on clinical and epidemiologic grounds, laboratory confirmation is indicated so that appropriate measures can be taken to prevent the occurrence of nosocomial measles among susceptible persons. Aids to rapid diagnosis include examination of exfoliated cells from the pharynx, nasal and buccal mucosa, conjunctiva, or urinary tract by direct staining for epithelial giant cells[462,463] or identification of measles antigens by direct immunofluorescence.[464-466] PCR assays can diagnose acute measles.[402] These tests are positive in more than 90% of patients during the prodrome and the period of the early exanthem. At later stages of the illness, the diagnosis may be confirmed by detecting measles-specific IgM antibodies in serum or rising antibody titers in acute and convalescent sera.[406,407,467] Because serum antibodies appear within 48 hours of the exanthem, it is important that the acute-phase serum be collected at the onset of the rash or earlier.

Among the diseases and conditions to be considered in the differential diagnosis of measles are the following. None is likely to occur in the newborn.

1. *Drug eruptions and other allergies.* Maculopapular exanthems may be caused by a variety of drugs and chemicals in susceptible persons. A history of exposure is of paramount importance in distinguishing these causes from measles. An urticarial component may be seen in some instances of drug hypersensitivity but is not present in measles.
2. *Kawasaki disease.* This illness is often confused with measles and vice versa in children younger than 5 years. Classic signs include conjunctivitis, red cracked lips, strawberry tongue, morbilliform or scarlatiniform rash, induration of the hands and feet, and usually a solitary enlarged cervical lymph node. In confusing cases, viral diagnostic procedures may be necessary to rule measles in or out.
3. *Rubella.* The maculopapular exanthem of rubella is finer and more transient. It undergoes a more rapid evolution and does not assume the blotchy configuration often seen in measles. The posterior cervical and postauricular lymphadenopathies of rubella are not present in measles, and conversely the prominent catarrhal symptoms in the prodrome of measles are not a feature of rubella.
4. *Scarlet fever.* The rash of scarlet fever is punctate and extremely fine rather than papular. It blanches on pressure and is accentuated in skin folds. The onset is typically abrupt without a prodrome. There is an accompanying sore throat, and the cheeks are flushed. Peripheral blood leukocytosis is usual, in contrast to the leukopenia of measles.
5. *Meningococcemia.* When the early rash of meningococcemia is maculopapular rather than petechial, it may be confused with measles. Unlike measles, it has no characteristic distribution.
6. *Roseola.* The exanthem of roseola, which usually appears when the patient's temperature drops to normal, typically appears on the trunk before it is evident on the head. It lasts only 1 or 2 days. Roseola, which is caused by human herpesvirus type 6, is seen most often in children younger than 3 years and is almost never seen in adults.
7. *Atypical measles.* This hypersensitivity disease is related to infection with measles virus in persons who received killed measles vaccine years ago. Killed measles vaccine was removed from the U.S. market in 1968. Extremely high measles HI antibody titers (e.g., 1:1 million) have been observed in patients with this disease.
8. *Other infections.* Rocky Mountain spotted fever, toxoplasmosis, enterovirus infections, parvovirus infection, and infectious mononucleosis may cause maculopapular exanthems resembling measles.

Therapy

The treatment of uncomplicated measles is symptomatic. Immunoglobulin has no proven value in established disease. Antibiotics are not indicated for prophylaxis of bacterial superinfections (i.e., otitis and pneumonia). When these complications develop, antimicrobial therapy should be selected on the basis of Gram stain and culture of appropriate body fluids, such as sputum. If culture specimens cannot be obtained or if the illness is grave, broad-spectrum antibiotics may be selected on the basis of the most likely offending pathogens. The antibiotic regimen for pneumonia, most commonly caused by *S. pneumoniae* or *S. aureus*, should include a penicillinase-resistant penicillin; the drug of choice for otitis media, which is usually caused by *S. pneumoniae* or *Haemophilus influenzae*, is amoxicillin. Vitamin A (200,000 IU orally for 2 days) has been used to treat infants with measles and seems to decrease the severity of the infection.[468-470] The drug ribavirin has been used experimentally to treat severe measles in immunocompromised and other high-risk patients.[471,472]

Prevention

Passive Immunization

Passive immunization is recommended for the prevention of measles in exposed, susceptible pregnant women, neonates, and their contacts in the delivery room or newborn nursery (see "Nosocomial Measles in the Nursery"). Therapy with intramuscularly administered immunoglobulin should be given as soon as possible after exposure. A dose of 0.25 mL/kg given within 72 hours of exposure is a reliable means of prevention of clinical measles, although immunoglobulin given later (up to 7 days after exposure) or in smaller doses (0.04 mL/kg) may also prevent or at least modify the infection. It is recommended that passive prophylaxis be followed in 5 months or more by administration of live measles vaccine in those old enough to receive it.[364]

Active Immunization

The currently recommended live measles vaccines are derivatives of the Edmonston B strain that have been further attenuated. They produce a noncommunicable infection, which is mild or inapparent. Fever occurs in about 5% of susceptible recipients. A mild rash is observed in 10% to 20% of susceptible recipients 5 to 10 days after administration. The vaccines induce seroconversion in 95% and prevent clinical disease in more than 90% of exposed susceptible recipients. Live-attenuated measles vaccines are contraindicated in pregnant women.[364] In one small series, Edmonston B measles vaccine and γ-globulin were administered to seven pregnant women, 18 to 34 years old, who were in the second to eighth months of pregnancy. There were no serologic data. Three of the seven developed fever (>38.5° C) and rash. All were delivered of healthy infants at term.[473] Vaccination is likewise not usually recommended for infants younger than 12 months because the induction of immunity and the elaboration of antibodies may be suppressed by residual transplacentally acquired antibodies in the fetal circulation or other mechanisms. A single fatality in an HIV-infected young adult due to pneumonia after re-immunization has been reported.[438]

In exposed populations having little experience with measles or in populations in which the incidence of natural measles before the age of 1 year is high, live vaccines may be given when infants are 6 to 9 months old but should be followed by a second dose at 15 months to increase the seroconversion rate.[364] Data indicate that measles antibody titers are lower in women vaccinated as children than in women who have previously had natural measles and that the offspring of vaccinated women lose transplacentally acquired measles antibodies before they are 1 year old.[474,475] It is therefore predicted that routine vaccination against measles may be recommended at 12 rather than 15 months. Nevertheless, passive immunization should be given to protect young infants exposed during an epidemic.

Although the MMR vaccine had an excellent safety record in 2000, the question was raised about whether this vaccine might result in autism in previously healthy children.[476] After an extensive review by numerous experts, it was concluded that there was no relationship between MMR and development of autism.[476-479] Unfortunately, the public in the United Kingdom became so fearful of this possibility that use of measles vaccine has decreased significantly, leading to reported outbreaks.[480] Potentially this development could lead to an increase in measles in pregnant women in the United Kingdom and other countries where MMR coverage might fall off.

Nosocomial Measles in the Nursery: Guidelines for Prevention

Most women of childbearing age in urban areas are immune to measles because of previous natural infection or vaccination. Because it is amply documented that infants born to immune mothers are usually protected by transplacentally acquired antibodies, measles outbreaks in newborn nurseries are extraordinarily rare. Studies by Krugman and colleagues[481] indicated that before the introduction of live-attenuated measles vaccine, 94% of infants had passive HI antibodies when 1 month old, 47% had them at 4 months, and 26% had them at 6 months. The rarity of measles among mothers, newborns, and hospital staff in the newborn nursery makes it difficult to assess the precise risk once the virus has been introduced. Nonetheless, the fact that age-specific mortality rates related to measles are highest in the first year of life (see previous discussion) justifies instituting measures designed to prevent disease in those exposed and the spread of infection to neonates of uncertain immune status (Table 22-13).

Infants born to mothers with an unequivocal history of previous natural measles or vaccination with live-attenuated measles virus are assumed not to be at risk when exposed to measles in the neonatal period. If siblings at home have measles in a communicable stage, neonates born to immune mothers may be discharged from the hospital with no treatment. In the absence of a maternal history of measles or measles vaccine, the mother's serum should be tested for the presence of antibodies to measles. If the mother's serum contains detectable levels of measles antibodies by a reliable method, both mother and baby may be sent home. If specific antibodies are not detected in the mother's serum, the neonate and mother should not have contact with the older siblings until they are no longer infectious. The mother and neonate, as well as any nonimmune older siblings without disease, should receive immunoglobulin (0.25 mg/kg given intramuscularly) to prevent or modify subsequent measles infection that might have been incubating at the time of delivery.

If a mother without a history of previous measles or measles vaccination is exposed 6 to 15 days ante partum, she may be in the incubation period and capable of transmitting measles infection during the postpartum period before discharge from the hospital. In such a situation, it is optimal to test the mother for measles antibodies. If no antibodies are detected (or the test cannot be performed) and if she had been exposed less than 6 days ante partum, she could not transmit measles by the respiratory route until at least 72 hours post partum. By this time in most instances, the mother would have been discharged from the hospital and potential nosocomial transmission would not be a problem. In either event (exposure from 0 to 5 days or from 6 to 15 days ante partum), both the exposed susceptible mother and her neonate should receive immunoglobulin and be sent home as soon as possible unless siblings at home have measles in a communicable stage. If the mother's exposure occurred 6 to 15 days ante partum, prophylaxis with immunoglobulin should also be administered to the other mothers, neonates, and hospital personnel in the delivery room and nursery except those with a history of natural measles or vaccination with live-attenuated measles virus or who have detectable antibodies to measles virus. Globulin prophylaxis given within 72 hours of exposure prevents infection in nearly all instances, and in many cases it is effective for as long as 7 days.[411,482] Immunoglobulin given after this period but before the prodrome usually results in modified measles infection with diminished morbidity.[411,482] Those patients to

Table 22–13 Guidelines for Preventive Measures after Exposure to Measles in the Nursery or Maternity Ward

Type of Exposure or Disease	Measles Present (Prodrome or Rash)[a]		Disposition
	Mother	*Neonate*	
A. Siblings at home with measles[a] when neonate and mother are ready for discharge from hospital	No	No	1. *Neonate:* protective isolation and immune globulin (IG) indicated unless mother had unequivocal history of previous measles or measles vaccination.[b] 2. *Mother:* with history of previous measles or measles vaccination, she may remain with neonate or return to older children. Without previous history she may remain with neonate until older siblings are no longer infectious, or she may receive IG prophylactically and return to older children.
B. Mother without history of measles or measles vaccination exposed during period 6-15 days ante partum[c]	No	No	1. *Exposed mother and infant:* administer IG to each and send home at earliest date unless there are siblings at home with communicable measles. Test mothers for susceptibility if possible. If susceptible, administer live measles vaccine 5 months after IG. 2. *Other mothers and infants:* same unless clear history of previous measles or measles vaccination in the mother. 3. *Hospital personnel:* unless clear history of previous measles or measles vaccination administer IG within 72 hours of exposure. Vaccinate 5 months or more later.
C. Onset of maternal measles ante partum or post partum[d]	Yes	Yes	1. *Infected mother and infant:* isolate together until clinically stable, then send home. 2. *Other mothers and infants:* same as B-3 except infants should be vaccinated at 15 months of age. 3. *Hospital personnel:* same as B-3.
D. Onset of maternal measles ante partum or post partum[d]	Yes	No	1. *Infected mother:* isolate until no longer infectious.[d] 2. *Infected mother's infant:* isolate separately from mother. Administer IG immediately. Send home when mother is no longer infectious. Alternatively, observe in isolation for 18 days for modified measles,[e] expecially if IG administration was delayed more than 4 days. 3. *Other mothers and infants:* same as C-2. 4. *Hospital personnel:* same as B-3.

[a]Catarrhal stage or less than 72 hours after onset of exanthem.
[b]Vaccination with live attenuated measles virus (see text).
[c]With exposure less than 6 days ante partum, mother would not be potentially infectious until at least 72 hours post partum.
[d]Considered infectious from onset of prodrome until 72 hours after onset of exanthem.
[e]Incubation period for modified measles may be prolonged beyond the usual 10 to 14 days.

whom immunoglobulin had to be given should later be vaccinated, after allowing an interval of at least 5 months so that residual measles antibody does not interfere with the immune response to the vaccine.[411]

If a mother develops measles immediately ante partum or post partum and her infant is born with congenital measles, the mother and infant should be isolated together until 72 hours after the appearance of the exanthem. Close observation of the neonate for signs of bronchopneumonia and other complications is warranted. Other susceptible mothers, neonates, and hospital personnel should receive immediate prophylaxis with immunoglobulin as outlined previously, followed by vaccination at a later date.

If a mother develops perinatal measles but her infant is born without signs of infection, each should be isolated separately. The infant may be incubating transplacentally acquired measles or may be at risk for postnatally acquired droplet infection. In either case, the infant should receive immunoglobulin. The mother may be discharged with her infant after the third day of exanthem. The neonate should be followed closely and observed for signs of modified measles, which may require up to 18 days' observation because of the abnormally long incubation period of modified measles.[411]

The availability of virus diagnostic facilities varies, and the approach to potential nosocomial spread of measles therefore may differ from place to place. If serologic testing is expensive or unavailable, it may be simpler to administer immunoglobulin to all exposed persons who do not have an unequivocal history of previous measles or previous vaccination with live-attenuated measles virus vaccine. Serologic testing of those exposed who are thought to possibly be susceptible to measles, with administration of immunoglobulin to those exposed who are truly susceptible, would seem to be the ideal management for prevention of nosocomial measles.

Neonates or mothers isolated because of measles require a separate room with the door closed. Only immune visitors and staff should enter the room. Gown and hand-washing precautions must be observed, and containment of bedding and tissues soiled with respiratory excreta by double bagging and autoclaving is indicated. Because measles virus is excreted in the urine during the early exanthematous phase, it is also advisable to treat the urine as potentially infectious and to disinfect bedpans. Terminal disinfection of the room is recommended.

MUMPS

Mumps is an acute, generalized, communicable disease whose most distinctive feature is swelling of one or both parotid glands. Involvement of other salivary glands, the meninges, the pancreas, and the testes of postpubertal males is also common. The origin of the name is obscure but probably is related to the Old English verb *to mump*, meaning "to sulk," or to the Scottish verb meaning "to speak indistinctly."

The Organism

Properties and Propagation

Mumps virus is a member of the paramyxovirus family and therefore has most of the morphologic and physicochemical properties described for measles. Five antigens have been described: two envelope glycoproteins, a hemagglutinin-neuraminidase (H-N), a hemolysis cell fusion (F) glycoprotein antigen, and a matrix envelope protein. There are two internal antigens: a nucleocapsid protein (NP) and an RNA polymerase protein (P).[483]

Mumps virus is readily isolated after inoculation of appropriate clinical specimens into a variety of host systems. Rapid identification may be accomplished by use of cells grown in shell vials and use of fluorescein-labeled monoclonal antibodies.[484]

The virus may be recovered during the first few days of illness from saliva, throat washings, and urine and from the cerebrospinal fluid of patients with mumps meningitis. Shedding of virus in the urine may persist longer, sometimes up to 2 weeks. Less commonly, the virus is present in blood, milk, and testicular tissue.[483]

A highly sensitive ELISA useful for diagnosing and determining susceptibility to mumps has been described. This assay has also been used to diagnose acute mumps in one serum specimen by the presence of specific IgM.[483] The diagnosis may also be established by demonstrating a rising antibody titer in paired acute and convalescent sera.

Epidemiology and Transmission

Period of Communicability

Mumps occurs worldwide and is endemic in most urban areas where routine vaccination is not practiced. In the United States, before widespread vaccination against mumps, the incidence was highest in the winter, reaching a peak in March and April. Mumps was principally a disease of childhood, with most infections occurring between the ages of 5 and 15 years. Mumps in infancy is very uncommon (discussed later). In the prevaccine era, approximately one third of infections were subclinical. Epidemics tended to occur in confined populations such as those in boarding schools, the military, and other institutions. Since the introduction of mumps vaccine in 1967, the incidence of clinical mumps has declined dramatically in the United States and mumps remains an extremely uncommon disease.

Incubation Period

The usual incubation period, measured between exposure to infection and onset of parotitis, is 14 to 18 days, with extremes between 7 and 23 days. However, because the contact may be shedding virus before the onset of clinical disease or may have subclinical infection and therefore be unrecognizable, the incubation period in individual cases is often uncertain.

Incidence of Mumps in Pregnancy

The incidence of mumps in pregnancy is unknown. Because there is now little opportunity for exposure to mumps and many women are immune, the incidence is expected to be low. The incidence in prospective studies has been variously estimated as between 0.8 and 10 cases per 10,000 pregnancies.[70,174]

Pathogenesis

Mumps is transmitted by droplet nuclei, saliva, and fomites. The precise pathogenesis of infection has not been established because, although experimentally infected monkeys may develop parotitis, no animal model closely resembles human disease. After entry into the host, the virus initially replicates in the epithelium of the upper respiratory tract. A viremia ensues, after which there is localization in glandular or central nervous system tissues. Parotitis is believed to occur as a result of viremia rather than the reverse, because in many instances, generalized disease precedes involvement of the parotid gland, which may not be involved at all.

Pathology

Studies of the pathology of mumps are few because the disease is rarely fatal. The histologic changes that have been observed in the parotid gland and the testis are similar. The inflammatory exudate consists of perivascular and interstitial infiltrates of mononuclear cells accompanied by prominent edema. There is necrosis of acinar and duct epithelial cells in the salivary glands and of the germinal epithelium of the seminiferous tubules.

There are few reports of placental pathology in gestational mumps. Garcia and associates[485] described a 29-year-old Brazilian woman with a history of two bleeding episodes during pregnancy who developed mumps in her fifth month. A hysterotomy was subsequently performed, yielding a macerated 90-g fetus. Necrotizing villitis and accumulation of necrotic material, mononuclear cells, and nuclear fragments were found in the intervillous spaces of the placenta. Necrotizing granulomas and cytoplasmic inclusions consistent with mumps virus infection were also identified. Two additional women with mumps in the 10th week and second month of pregnancy underwent therapeutic abortions. Typical inclusion bodies were identified in both placentas and in the adrenal cortex of one fetus.[485] No serologic data were available on these three women, however, so that it is possible that their parotitis was caused by an agent other than mumps virus.

Clinical Manifestations

The prodrome of mumps consists of fever, malaise, myalgia, and anorexia. Parotitis, when present, usually appears within the next 24 hours but may be delayed for a week or even more. Swelling of the gland is accompanied by tenderness to palpation and obliteration of the space between the earlobe and the angle of the mandible. The swelling progresses for 2 to 3 days, then gradually subsides, and disappears in 1 week or less. The orifice of Stensen's duct is commonly red and swollen. In most cases, parotitis is bilateral, although the onset in each gland may be asynchronous by 1 or more days. The submaxillary glands are involved less often than the parotid and almost never by themselves. The sublingual glands are only rarely affected.

Orchitis is the most common manifestation other than parotitis in postpubertal males; it affects about 20% of this group of patients. Orchitis in infancy has been described but is not well documented.[486] Oophoritis is far less common. It is associated with lower abdominal pain, and the ovaries rarely may be palpable. Oophoritis does not lead to sterility.

Aseptic meningitis may occur in children and adults of either sex but is more common in males. Although pleocytosis of the cerebrospinal fluid may occur in up to 50% of cases of clinical mumps, signs of meningeal irritation occur in a smaller proportion of cases, variably estimated at 5% to 25%. The cerebrospinal fluid contains up to 1000 cells/mm^3. Within the first 24 hours, polymorphonuclear leukocytes may predominate, but by the second day, most cells are lymphocytes. In the absence of parotitis, the syndrome of aseptic meningitis in mumps is indistinguishable clinically from that caused by enteroviruses and other viruses. The course is almost invariably self-limited. Rarely, cranial nerve palsies have led to permanent sequelae, of which deafness is the most common.

Mumps pancreatitis may cause abdominal pain. The incidence of this manifestation is unclear because reliable diagnostic criteria are difficult to obtain. An elevated serum amylase level may be present in parotitis or pancreatitis. The character of the abdominal pain is rarely sufficiently distinctive to permit unequivocal diagnosis. Other complications of mumps include mastitis, thyroiditis, myocarditis, nephritis, and arthritis.

The peripheral blood cell count in mumps is not characteristic. The white blood cell count may be elevated, normal, or depressed, and the differential count may reveal a mild lymphocytosis or a polymorphonuclear leukocytosis.

Maternal Effects of Mumps

Unlike varicella and measles, when mumps occurs in pregnant women, the illness is generally benign and is not appreciably more severe than it is in other adult women.[486-495] In a 1957 "virgin soil" epidemic of mumps among the Inuit, 20 infections occurred in pregnant women. Of these, only 8 (40%) were clinically apparent, compared with an incidence of 57 clinically apparent cases (62%) among 92 nonpregnant women. Overt disease therefore does not appear to be more common during pregnancy.[492] Some complications such as mastitis and perhaps thyroiditis are more frequent in postpubertal women than in men but probably do not occur more commonly in pregnant women than in other adult women.[492] Mumps virus has been isolated on the third postpartum day from the milk of a woman who developed parotitis 2 days ante partum.[496] Her baby, who was not breastfed, did not develop clinically apparent mumps. Aseptic meningitis, apparently without unduly high incidence or severity, has also been reported in pregnant women.[497] In pregnant women, as well as in the population as a whole, deaths from mumps are exceedingly rare. One death has been reported in a woman who developed mumps complicated by glomerulonephritis at 8 months' gestation.[497]

Effects of Gestational Mumps on the Fetus

ABORTION

An excessive number of abortions is associated with gestational mumps when the disease occurs during the first trimester. In prospective studies of fetal mortality in virus diseases, Siegel and associates[178] observed 9 fetal deaths (27%) among 33 first-trimester pregnancies complicated by mumps, compared with 131 (13%) of 1010 matched uninfected controls (see Table 22-6). This difference is significant ($\chi^2 = 5.6$; $P < .02$). Mumps-associated fetal deaths occurred in only 1 of 51 second-trimester pregnancies and none of 43 third-trimester pregnancies. Unlike fetal deaths associated with measles, those associated with mumps were closely related temporally to maternal infection: 6 of the 10 deaths occurred within 2 weeks after the onset of maternal mumps.[178]

Many other reports describe isolated cases of abortion associated with gestational mumps. Most cases occurred in the first 4 months of pregnancy.[487,492,493,495,498-500] In one instance, mumps virus was isolated from a 10-week fetus spontaneously aborted 4 days after the mother developed clinical mumps.[500]

PREMATURITY

In the only prospective study of low birth weight in relation to maternal mumps infection, no significant association was found.[178] Nine (7.7%) of 117 pregnant women with mumps gave birth to infants with birth weights of less than 2500 g, compared with 4 (3.3%) of 122 uninfected pregnant women in a control group (see Table 22-5).

CONGENITAL MALFORMATIONS

In experimentally infected animals, mumps virus may induce congenital malformations.[501-503] Definitive evidence of a teratogenic potential for mumps virus in humans, however, has not been shown. Many reports describe the occurrence of congenital malformations after gestational mumps, but no data are available in most of these studies regarding the incidence of anomalies in uninfected matched control pregnancies. Swan[498] reviewed the literature in 1951 and found 18 anomalies in the offspring of 93 pregnancies complicated by mumps. These included four malformations originating in the first trimester (i.e., cutaneous nevus, imperforate anus, spina bifida, and Down syndrome) and nine originating in the second trimester (i.e., four had Down syndrome and miscellaneous other malformations). Other reports have described malformation of the external ear,[488] intestinal atresia,[495] chorioretinitis and optic atrophy in the absence of evidence of congenital toxoplasmosis,[504] corneal cataracts,[454] and urogenital abnormalities.[505] One case of hydrocephalus caused by obstruction of the foramen of Monro in an infant whose mother had serologically proven mumps during the fifth month of pregnancy has been described.[506] A similar phenomenon has been seen after extrauterine mumps with encephalitis[507] and in an animal model.[503] In the only controlled, prospective study, the rate of congenital malformations in children whose mothers had mumps during pregnancy (2 of 117) was essentially identical to the rate of those in infants born to uninfected mothers (2 of 123).[71] Neither of the two affected infants, both of whom were mentally retarded, was born to any of the 24 pregnant women who had mumps in the first trimester. Similarly, no association between gestational mumps and fetal malformations was reported by British investigators, who evaluated the outcomes of 501 pregnancies complicated by maternal mumps and found no significant differences compared with a control series.[508]

ENDOCARDIAL FIBROELASTOSIS

A postulated association between gestational mumps infection and endocardial fibroelastosis in the offspring was at one time the subject of much debate.[509] An extensive review of evidence for and against an etiologic role for mumps virus in this condition was made by Finland in the 1970s that was inconclusive, and there was little more information in the literature for the next 30 years.[510] The issue remains unresolved. The rarity of mumps during pregnancy and the rarity of endocardial fibroelastosis as a possible sequel in the fetus make it unlikely that conclusive data will ever be obtained.

Molecular approaches, however, seem to have shed new light on the issue. Using PCR, mumps virus genome was detected in two of two fatal cases of fibroelastosis.[511] In another study of 29 fatal cases of this disease, fragments of the mumps genome were identified in 20 cases.[512] Adenovirus was identified in the remainder. It was hypothesized that endocardial fibroelastosis is the end result of myocarditis. As mumps has become rare because of vaccination, endocardial fibroelastosis has also become rare.[512] The possible role of intrauterine mumps was not addressed in these two modern studies and may be impossible to evaluate further given the rarity of mumps in developed countries today.

Perinatal Mumps

In contrast to congenital chickenpox and measles, congenital mumps or even postnatally acquired perinatal mumps has rarely been documented virologically or serologically. Although several cases of parotitis have been reported in women near delivery and their neonates and infants,[492,513-516] the significance of these reports is often uncertain, especially when clinically apparent mumps only is present in the mother. Other viral, bacterial, and noninfectious causes are difficult to exclude without laboratory evidence of mumps infection.

Among the possible explanations for the rarity of transplacental and postnatally acquired mumps in neonates are the rarity of mumps today, protection of the neonate by passive maternal antibodies, exclusion of mumps virus from the fetus by a hypothetical placental barrier, relative insusceptibility of fetal and neonatal tissues to infection by mumps virus, and occurrence of infections that are predominantly subclinical.

Passage of mumps virus across the human placenta has occasionally been reported. Live-attenuated mumps virus has been recovered from the placenta of pregnant women (but not from fetal tissues) who were vaccinated 10 days before undergoing saline-induced abortion.[517] Mumps virus was isolated from two infants whose mothers had mumps at delivery. One infant had parotitis, and the other had pneumonia; presumably, transplacental transmission had occurred.[515] Mumps virus was also isolated from a fetus spontaneously aborted on the fourth day after the onset of maternal mumps.[485] However, transplacental passage of virus should not be assumed to occur invariably because in several instances passage could not be documented.[485,518,519]

A differentiation between lack of susceptibility and subclinical infection as explanations for failure of the neonate to develop parotitis or other manifestations of mumps can be made only by adequate serologic investigations and viral isolation attempts. Unfortunately, these data are not available. Several investigators have observed that clinically apparent mumps with parotitis[520,521] or orchitis[486] during the first year of life tends to be a very mild disease and that age-specific attack rates for manifest disease related to mumps increase progressively until the age of 5 years.[522] Antibodies to mumps virus are known to cross the placenta and to persist for several months.[523]

Diagnosis and Differential Diagnosis

The diagnosis of mumps is easy when there is acute, bilateral, painful parotitis with a history of recent exposure. More difficulty is encountered when the disease is unilateral or when the manifestations are confined to organs other than the parotid gland. In these cases, laboratory confirmation by virus isolation or demonstration of a rising antibody titer may be performed.

Among neonates, few conditions need be considered in the differential diagnosis. Clinical parotitis in this age group is rare. Suppurative parotitis of the newborn, usually caused by *S. aureus,* is most often unilateral.[524] Pus can be expressed from the parotid duct, and there is a polymorphonuclear leukocytosis of the peripheral blood. Other diagnostic considerations in the neonate include infection with parainfluenza viruses and coxsackieviruses, drug-induced parotitis, and facial cellulitis.

In addition to these conditions in the neonate, the differential diagnosis in pregnant women includes anterior cervical lymphadenitis, idiopathic recurrent parotitis, salivary gland calculus with obstruction, sarcoidosis with uveoparotid fever, and salivary gland tumors.

Other entities should be considered when the manifestations appear in organs other than the parotid. Testicular torsion in infancy may produce a painful scrotal mass resembling mumps orchitis.[486] Aseptic meningitis related to mumps typically occurs in the winter and early spring, and enterovirus aseptic meningitis is most common in the summer and early autumn. Other viruses may also cause aseptic meningitis that is clinically indistinguishable from mumps.

Therapy

Treatment of parotitis is symptomatic. Analgesics and application of heat or cold to the parotid area may be helpful. Mumps immune globulin has no proven value in the prevention or treatment of mumps. Mastitis may be managed by the application of ice packs and breast binders. Testicular pain may be minimized by the local application of cold and gentle support for the scrotum. In some instances, severe cases of orchitis have appeared to respond to the systemic administration of corticosteroids.

Prevention

Active Immunization

Live-attenuated mumps virus vaccine induces antibodies that protect against infection in more than 95% of recipients. The subcutaneously administered vaccine may be given to children older than 1 year, but its use in infants younger than this is not recommended because of possible interference by passive maternal antibodies. Usually, it is administered simultaneously with measles and rubella vaccines when children are 15 months old. The vaccine is recommended for older children and adolescents, particularly adolescent males who have not had mumps; it is not recommended for pregnant women, for patients receiving corticosteroids, or for other immunocompromised hosts.

Passive Immunization

Passive immunization for mumps is ineffective and unavailable.

Prevention of Nosocomial Mumps in the Newborn Nursery

In contrast to chickenpox and measles, mumps does not appear to be a potentially serious hazard in the newborn nursery. No outbreaks of nosocomial mumps have been described in this setting, and transmission of mumps in a hospital setting is highly unusual.[525] Most mothers are immune, and even neonates born to nonimmune mothers rarely develop clinically apparent mumps. Prudence dictates that mothers who develop parotitis or other manifestations of mumps in the period immediately ante partum or post partum should be isolated from other mothers and neonates. The case is less strong for isolating the puerperal mother with mumps from her own newborn. In the hospital setting, isolation of patients with mumps from the time of onset of parotitis has proved to be ineffective in preventing the spread of disease.[526] Infected subjects shed mumps virus in respiratory secretions for several days before the onset of parotitis or other manifestations recognizable as mumps.

At one time, exposed hospital personnel, particularly postpubertal males, and mothers with a negative history of mumps could be given mumps immunoglobulin, although the prophylactic effectiveness of this product was never established. This preparation is no longer available. Live-attenuated mumps virus vaccine has not been evaluated for protection after exposure but may theoretically modify or prevent disease by inducing neutralizing antibodies before the onset of illness because of the long incubation period of mumps. It should be considered for exposed susceptible hospital personnel and puerperal mothers. Some hospitals have the facilities to test for susceptibility to mumps by measurement of antibody titers, whereas others do not. Testing for susceptibility could eliminate some use of vaccine for the previously described situation.

Isolation procedures for mumps include the use of a single room for the patient with the door closed at all times except to enter. Immune personnel caring for the patient should exercise gown and hand-washing precautions. Isolation is continued until parotid swelling has subsided. Terminal disinfection of the room is desirable.

REFERENCES

1. Weller TH. Varicella and herpes zoster: changing concepts of the natural history, control, and importance of a not-so-benign virus. N Engl J Med 309:1362, 1983.
2. Lungu O, Annunziato P, Gershon A, et al. Reactivated and latent varicella-zoster virus in human dorsal root ganglia. Proc Natl Acad Sci U S A 92:10980, 1995.
3. Mahalingham R, Wellish M, Wolf W, et al. Latent varicella-zoster viral DNA in human trigeminal and thoracic ganglia. N Engl J Med 323:627, 1990.
4. Lungu O, Panagiotidis C, Annunziato P, et al. Aberrant intracellular localization of varicella-zoster virus regulatory proteins during latency. Proc Natl Acad Sci U S A 95:780, 1998.
5. Old English Dictionary. London, Oxford University Press, 1933.
6. Christie AB. Chickenpox. *In* Infectious Diseases: Epidemiology and Clinical Practice. Edinburgh, E & S Livingstone, 1969, p 238.
7. Angelicus B. De Propreitatibus Rerum. Liber septimus, vol xciii. London, Trevisa John, 1398.
8. Muir WB, Nichols R, Breuer J. Phylogenetic analysis of varicella-zoster virus: evidence of intercontinental spread of genotypes and recombination. J Virol 76:1971, 2002
9. Gabel C, Dubey L, Steinberg S, et al. Varicella-zoster virus glycoproteins are phosphorylated during posttranslational maturation. J Virol 63:4264, 1989.
10. Gershon A, Cosio L, Brunell PA. Observations on the growth of varicella-zoster virus in human diploid cells. J Gen Virol 18:21, 1973.
11. Cook ML, Stevens J. Labile coat: reason for noninfectious cell-free varicella zoster virus in culture. J Virol 2:1458, 1968.
12. Chen J, Gershon A, Silverstein S, et al. Latent and lytic infection of isolated guinea pig enteric and dorsal root ganglia by varicella zoster virus. J Med Virol 70:S71, 2003.
13. Chen J, Wan S, Bischoff S, et al. Latent, lytic, and reactivating infection of human and guinea pig enteric neurons by varicella zoster virus. Presented at the 28th Annual Herpesvirus Workshop, Madison, Wis, 2003.
14. Myers M, Connelly BL. Animal models of varicella. J Infect Dis 166:S48, 1992.
15. Sadzot-Delvaux C, Merville-Louis M-P, Delree P, et al. An in vivo model of varicella-zoster virus latent infection of dorsal root ganglia. J Neurosci Res 26:83, 1990.
16. Williams V, Gershon A, Brunell P. Serologic response to varicella-zoster membrane antigens measured by indirect immunofluorescence. J Infect Dis 130:669, 1974.
17. Zaia J, Oxman M. Antibody to varicella-zoster virus-induced membrane antigen: immunofluorescence assay using monodisperse glutaraldehyde-fixed target cells. J Infect Dis 136:519, 1977.
18. Gershon A, Steinberg S, LaRussa P. Measurement of Antibodies to VZV by Latex Agglutination. Anaheim, Calif, Society for Pediatric Research, 1992.
19. Forghani B, Schmidt N, Dennis J. Antibody assays for varicella-zoster virus: comparison of enzyme immunoassay with neutralization, immune adherence hemagglutination, and complement fixation. J Clin Microbiol 8:545, 1978.
20. Gershon A, Frey H, Steinberg S, et al. Enzyme-linked immunosorbent assay for measurement of antibody to varicella-zoster virus. Arch Virol 70:169, 1981.
21. LaRussa P, Steinberg S, Waithe E, et al. Comparison of five assays for antibody to varicella-zoster virus and the fluorescent-antibody-to-membrane-antigen test. J Clin Microbiol 25:2059, 1987.
22. Shehab Z, Brunell P. Enzyme-linked immunosorbent assay for susceptibility to varicella. J Infect Dis 148:472, 1983.
23. Friedman MG, Leventon-Kriss S, Sarov I. Sensitive solid-phase radioimmunoassay for detection of human immunoglobulin G antibodies to varicella-zoster virus. J Clin Microbiol 9:1, 1979.
24. Gershon A, Kalter Z, Steinberg S. Detection of antibody to varicella-zoster virus by immune adherence hemagglutination. Proc Soc Exp Biol Med 151:762, 1976.
25. Caunt AE, Shaw DG. Neutralization tests with varicella-zoster virus. J Hyg (Lond) 67:343, 1969.
26. Grose C, Edmond BJ, Brunell PA. Complement-enhanced neutralizing antibody response to varicella-zoster virus. J Infect Dis 139:432, 1979.
27. Gold E, Godek G. Complement fixation studies with a varicella-zoster antigen. J Immunol 95:692, 1965.
28. Schmidt NJ, Lennette EH, Magoffin RL. Immunological relationship between herpes simplex and varicella-zoster viruses demonstrated by

complement-fixation, neutralization and fluorescent antibody tests. J Gen Virol 4:321, 1969.
29. Schaap GJP, Huisman J. Simultaneous rise in complement-fixing antibodies against herpesvirus hominus and varicella-zoster virus in patients with chickenpox and shingles. Arch Gesamte Virusforsch 25:52, 1968.
30. Schmidt NJ. Further evidence for common antigens in herpes simplex and varicella-zoster virus. J Med Virol 9:27, 1982.
31. Shiraki K, Okuno T, Yamanishi K, Takahashi M. Polypeptides of varicella-zoster virus (VZV) and immunological relationship of VZV and herpes simplex virus (HSV). J Gen Virol 61:255, 1982.
32. Kitamura K, Namazue J, Campo-Vera H, et al. Induction of neutralizing antibody against varicella-zoster virus (VZV) by gp 2 and cross-reactivity between VZV gp 2 and herpes simplex viruses gB. Virology 149:74, 1986.
33. Lemon SM, Hutt LM, Huang Y-T, et al. Simultaneous infection with multiple herpesviruses. Am J Med 66:270, 1979.
34. Landry ML, Hsiung GD. Diagnosis of dual herpesvirus infection: varicella-zoster virus (VZV) and herpes simplex viruses. *In* Nahmias AJ, Dowdle WR, Schinazi RF (eds). The Human Herpesviruses. New York, Elsevier, 652, p 1981.
35. Arvin AM. Cell-mediated immunity to varicella-zoster virus. J Infect Dis 166:S35, 1992.
36. Davison A, Edson C, Ellis R, et al. New common nomenclature for glycoprotein genes of varicella-zoster virus and their products. J Virol 57:1195, 1986.
37. Arvin AM, Sharp M, Moir M, et al. Memory cytotoxic T cell responses to viral tegument and regulatory proteins encoded by open reading frames 4, 10, 29, and 62 of varicella-zoster virus. Viral Immunol 15:507, 2002.
38. Brunell P, Gershon AA, Uduman SA, Steinberg S. Varicella-zoster immunoglobulins during varicella, latency, and zoster. J Infect Dis 132:49, 1975.
39. Gershon A, Steinberg S, Borkowsky W, et al. IgM to varicella-zoster virus: demonstration in patients with and without clinical zoster. Pediatr Infect Dis 1:164, 1982.
40. Hope-Simpson RE. The nature of herpes zoster: a long-term study and a new hypothesis. Proc R Soc Med 58:9, 1965.
41. Brunell PA. Transmission of chickenpox in a school setting prior to the observed exanthem. Am J Dis Child 143:1451, 1989.
42. Evans P. An epidemic of chickenpox. Lancet 2:339, 1940.
43. Gordon JE, Meader FM. The period of infectivity and serum prevention of chickenpox. JAMA 93:2013, 1929.
44. Kido S, Ozaki T, Asada H, et al. Detection of varicella-zoster virus (VZV) DNA in clinical samples from patients with VZV by the polymerase chain reaction. J Clin Microbiol 29:76, 1991.
45. Tsolia M, Gershon A, Steinberg S, Gelb L. Live attenuated varicella vaccine: evidence that the virus is attenuated and the importance of skin lesions in transmission of varicella-zoster virus. J Pediatr 116:184, 1990.
46. Sharrar RG, LaRussa P, Galea, SA, et al. The postmarketing safety profile of varicella vaccine. Vaccine 19:916, 2000.
47. Gustafson TL, Lavely GB, Brauner ER, et al. An outbreak of nosocomial varicella. Pediatrics 70:550, 1982.
48. Leclair JM, Zaia J, Levin MJ, et al. Airborne transmission of chicken-pox in a hospital. N Engl J Med 302:450, 1980.
49. Sawyer M, Chamberlin C, Wu Y, et al. Detection of varicella-zoster virus DNA in air samples from hospital rooms. J Infect Dis 169:91, 1993.
50. Moore DA, Hopkins RS. Assessment of a school exclusion policy during a chickenpox outbreak. Am J Epidemiol 133:1161, 1991.
51. Hope-Simpson RE. Infectiousness of communicable diseases in the household (measles, mumps, and chickenpox). Lancet 2:549, 1952.
52. Kundratitz K. Experimentelle Übertragung von Herpes Zoster auf den Menschen und die Beziehungen von Herpes Zoster zu Varicellen. Monatsschr Kinderheilkd 29:516, 1925.
53. Bruusgaard E. The mutual relation between zoster and varicella. Br J Dermatol Syphilis 44:1, 1932.
54. Seiler HE. A study of herpes zoster particularly in its relationship to chickenpox. J Hyg (Lond) 47:253, 1949.
55. Schimpff S, Serpick A, Stoler B, et al. Varicella-zoster infection in patients with cancer. Ann Intern Med 76:241, 1972.
56. Berlin BS, Campbell T. Hospital-acquired herpes zoster following exposure to chickenpox. JAMA 211:1831, 1970.
57. Mahalingham R, Wellish M, Cohrs R, et al. Expression of protein encoded by varicella-zoster virus open reading frame 63 in latently infected human ganglionic neurons. Proc Natl Acad Sci U S A 93:2122, 1996.
58. Hayakawa Y, Torigoe S, Shiraki K, et al. Biologic and biophysical markers of a live varicella vaccine strain (Oka): identification of clinical isolates from vaccine recipients. J Infect Dis 149:956, 1984.
59. Straus SE, Reinhold W, Smith HA, et al. Endonuclease analysis of viral DNA from varicella and subsequent zoster infections in the same patient. N Engl J Med 311:1362, 1984.
60. Williams DL, Gershon A, Gelb LD, et al. Herpes zoster following varicella vaccine in a child with acute lymphocytic leukemia. J Pediatr 106:259, 1985.
61. Gershon A. Varicella in mother and infant: problems old and new. *In* Krugman S, Gershon A (eds). Infections of the Fetus and Newborn Infant. New York, Alan R Liss, 1975, p 79.
62. Seward JF, Watson BM, Peterson CL, et al. Varicella disease after introduction of varicella vaccine in the United States, 1995-2000. JAMA 287:606, 2002.
63. London WP, Yorke JA. Recurrent outbreaks of measles, chickenpox and mumps. I. Seasonal variation in contact rates. Am J Epidemiol 98:453, 1973.
64. Yorke JA, London WP. Recurrent outbreaks of measles, chickenpox and mumps: II. Systematic differences in contact rates and stochastic effects. Am J Epidemiol 98:469, 1973.
65. Gordon JE. Chickenpox: an epidemiologic review. Am J Med Sci 244:362, 1962.
66. Preblud S, Orenstein W, Bart K. Varicella: clinical manifestations, epidemiology, and health impact on children. Pediatr Infect Dis 3:505, 1984.
67. Preblud SR, D'Angelo LJ. Chickenpox in the United States, 1972-1977. J Infect Dis 140:257, 1979.
68. Ross AH, Lencher E, Reitman G. Modification of chickenpox in family contacts by administration of gamma globulin. N Engl J Med 267:369, 1962.
69. LaRussa P, Steinberg S, Seeman MD, Gershon AA. Determination of immunity to varicella by means of an intradermal skin test. J Infect Dis 152:869, 1985.
70. Sever J, White LR. Intrauterine viral infections. Annu Rev Med 19:471, 1968.
71. Siegel M. Congenital malformations following chickenpox, measles, mumps, and hepatitis: results of a cohort study. JAMA 226:1521, 1973.
72. Balducci J, Rodis JF, Rosengren S, et al. Pregnancy outcome following first-trimester varicella infection. Obstet Gynecol 79:5, 1992.
73. Brunell PA, Kotchmar GSJ. Zoster in infancy: failure to maintain virus latency following intrauterine infection. J Pediatr 98:71, 1981.
74. Baba K, Yabuuchi H, Takahashi M, Ogra P. Increased incidence of herpes zoster in normal children infected with varicella-zoster virus during infancy: community-based follow up study. J Pediatr 108:372, 1986.
75. Guess H, Broughton DD, Melton LJ, Kurland L. Epidemiology of herpes zoster in children and adolescents: a population-based study. Pediatrics 76:512, 1985.
76. Terada K, Kawano S, Yoshihiro K, Morita T. Varicella-zoster virus (VZV) reactivation is related to the low response of VZV-specific immunity after chickenpox in infancy. J Infect Dis 169:650, 1994.
77. Kalman CM, Laskin OL. Herpes zoster and zosteriform herpes simplex virus infections in immunocompetent adults. Am J Med 81:775, 1986.
78. Locksley RM, Flournoy N, Sullivan KM, Meyers J. Infection with varicella-zoster virus after marrow transplantation. J Infect Dis 152:1172, 1985.
79. Veenstra J, Krol A, van Praag R, et al. Herpes zoster, immunological deterioration and disease progression in HIV-1 infection. AIDS 9:1153, 1995.
80. Gershon A, Mervish N, LaRussa P, et al. Varicella-zoster virus infection in children with underlying HIV infection. J Infect Dis 175:1496, 1997.
81. Brazin SA, Simkovich JW, Johnson WT. Herpes zoster during pregnancy. Obstet Gynecol 53:175, 1979.
82. Sterner G, Forsgren M, Enocksson E, et al. Varicella-zoster infections in late pregnancy. Scand J Infect Dis 71:30, 1990.
83. Gershon A, Raker R, Steinberg S, et al. Antibody to varicella-zoster virus in parturient women and their offspring during the first year of life. Pediatrics 58:692, 1976.
84. Shehab Z, Brunell P, Cobb E. Epidemiological standardization of a test for susceptibility to mumps. J Infect Dis 149:810, 1984.
85. Sirpenski SP, Brennan T, Mayo D. Determination of infection and immunity to varicella-zoster virus with an enzyme-linked immuno-sorbent assay. J Infect Dis 152:1349, 1985.
86. Steele R, Coleman MA, Fiser M, Bradsher RW. Varicella-zoster in hospital personnel: skin test reactivity to monitor susceptibility. Pediatrics 70:604, 1982.

87. Kjersem H, Jepsen S. Varicella among immigrants from the tropics, a health problem. Scand J Soc Med 18:171, 1990.
88. Longfield JN, Winn RE, Gibson RL, et al. Varicella outbreaks in army recruits from Puerto Rico. Arch Intern Med 150:970, 1990.
89. Maretic Z, Cooray MPM. Comparisons between chickenpox in a tropical and a European country. J Trop Med Hyg 66:311, 1963.
90. Sinha DP. Chickenpox—a disease predominantly affecting adults in rural west Bengal, India. Int J Epidemiol 5:367, 1976.
91. Brunell P. Placental transfer of varicella-zoster antibody. Pediatrics 38:1034, 1966.
92. Mendez D, Sinclair MB, Garcia S, et al. Transplacental immunity to varicella-zoster virus in extremely low birthweight infants. Am J Perinatol 9:236, 1992.
93. Raker R, Steinberg S, Drusin L, Gershon A. Antibody to varicella-zoster virus in low birth weight infants. J Pediatr 93:505, 1978.
94. Wang E, Prober C, Arvin AM. Varicella-zoster virus antibody titers before and after administration of zoster immune globulin to neonates in an intensive care nursery. J Pediatr 103:113, 1983.
95. Baba K, Yabuuchi H, Takahashi M, Ogra P. Immunologic and epidemiologic aspects of varicella infection acquired during infancy and early childhood. J Pediatr 100:881, 1982.
96. Gustafson TL, Shehab Z, Brunell P. Outbreak of varicella in a newborn intensive care nursery. Am Dis Child 138:548, 1984.
97. Hyatt HW. Neonatal varicella. J Natl Med Assoc 59:32, 1967.
98. Newman CGH. Perinatal varicella. Lancet 2:1159, 1965.
99. Readett MD, McGibbon C. Neonatal varicella. Lancet 1:644, 1961.
100. Freud P. Congenital varicella. Am J Dis Child 96:730, 1958.
101. Odessky L, Newman B, Wein GB. Congenital varicella. N Y State J Med 54:2849, 1954.
102. Harris LE. Spread of varicella in nurseries. Am J Dis Child 105:315, 1963.
103. Matseoane SL, Abler C. Occurrence of neonatal varicella in a hospital nursery. Am J Obstet Gynecol 92:575, 1965.
104. Lipton S, Brunell PA. Management of varicella exposure in a neonatal intensive care unit. JAMA 261:1782, 1989.
105. Patou G, Midgley P, Meurisse EV, Feldman RG. Immunoglobulin prophylaxis for infants exposed to varicella in a neonatal unit. J Infect 20:207, 1990.
106. Gold WL, Boulton J, Goldman C, et al. Management of varicella exposures in the neonatal intensive care unit. Pediatr Infect Dis J 12:954, 1993.
107. Friedman CA, Temple DM, Robbins KK, et al. Outbreak and control of varicella in a neonatal intensive care unit. Pediatr Infect Dis J 13:152, 1994.
108. Apert ME. Une epidemic de varicelle dans une maternite. Bull Med (Paris) 9:827, 1985.
109. Gold E. Serologic and virus-isolation studies of patients with varicella or herpes zoster infection. N Engl J Med 274:181, 1966.
110. Myers MG. Viremia caused by varicella-zoster virus: association with malignant progressive varicella. J Infect Dis 140:229, 1979.
111. Nelson A, St. Geme J. On the respiratory spread of varicella-zoster virus. Pediatrics 37:1007, 1966.
112. Trlifajova J, Bryndova D, Ryc M. Isolation of varicella-zoster virus from pharyngeal and nasal swabs in varicella patients. J Hyg Epidemiol Microbiol Immunol 28:201, 1984.
113. Ozaki T, Ichikawa T, Matsui Y, et al. Lymphocyte-associated viremia in varicella. J Med Virol 19:249, 1986.
114. Asano Y, Itakura N, Hiroishi Y, et al. Viremia is present in incubation period in nonimmunocompromised children with varicella. J Pediatr 106:69, 1985.
115. Feldman S, Epp E. Isolation of varicella-zoster virus from blood. J Pediatr 88:265, 1976.
116. Feldman S, Epp E. Detection of viremia during incubation period of varicella. J Pediatr 94:746, 1979.
117. Moffat JF, Stein MD, Kaneshima H, Arvin AM. Tropism of varicella-zoster virus for human CD4+ and CD8+ T lymphocytes and epidermal cells in SCID-hu mice. J Virol 69:5236, 1995.
118. Koropchak C, Graham G, Palmer J, et al. Investigation of varicella-zoster virus infection by polymerase chain reaction in the immunocompetent host with acute varicella. J Infect Dis 163:1016, 1991.
119. Ozaki T, Miwata H, Asano Y, et al. Varicella-zoster virus DNA in throat swabs of vaccinees. Arch Dis Child 267:328, 1993.
120. Grose CH. Variation on a theme by Fenner. Pediatrics 68:735, 1981.
121. Arvin AM, Pollard RB, Rasmussen L, Merigan T. Selective impairment in lymphocyte reactivity to varicella-zoster antigen among untreated lymphoma patients. J Infect Dis 137:531, 1978.
122. Hardy IB, Gershon A, Steinberg S, et al. The incidence of zoster after immunization with live attenuated varicella vaccine: a study in children with leukemia. N Engl J Med 325:1545, 1991.
123. Rand KH, Rasmussen LE, Pollard RB, et al. Cellular immunity and herpesvirus infections in cardiac transplant patients. N Engl J Med 296:1372, 1977.
124. Ruckdeschel JC, Schimpff SC, Smyth AC, Mardiney MR. Herpes zoster and impaired cell-associated immunity to the varicella-zoster virus in patients with Hodgkin's disease. Am J Med 62:77, 1977.
125. Friedman-Kien A, Lafleur F, Gendler F, et al. Herpes zoster: a possible early clinical sign for development of acquired immunodeficiency syndrome in high-risk individuals. J Am Acad Dermatol 14:1023, 1988.
126. Feldman S, Chaudhary S, Ossi M, Epp E. A viremic phase for herpes zoster in children with cancer. J Pediatr 91:597, 1977.
127. Gershon A, Steinberg S, Silber R. Varicella-zoster viremia. J Pediatr 92:1033, 1978.
128. Stevens D, Ferrington R, Jordan G, Merigan T. Cellular events in zoster vesicles: relation to clinical course and immune parameters. J Infect Dis 131:509, 1975.
129. Szanton E, Sarov I. Interaction between polymorphonuclear leukocytes and varicella-zoster infected cells. Intervirology 24:119, 1985.
130. Ihara T, Starr S, Ito M, et al. Human polymorphonuclear leukocyte-mediated cytotoxicity against varicella-zoster virus-infected fibroblasts. J Virol 51:110, 1984.
131. Ihara T, Ito M, Starr SE. Human lymphocyte, monocyte and polymorphonuclear leucocyte mediated antibody-dependent cellular cytotoxicity against varicella-zoster virus–infected targets. Clin Exp Immunol 63:179, 1986.
132. Garcia AGP. Fetal infection in chickenpox and alastrim, with histopathologic study of the placenta. Pediatrics 32:895, 1963.
133. Erlich RM, Turner JAP, Clarke M. Neonatal varicella. J Pediatr 53:139, 1958.
134. Lucchesi PF, LaBoccetta AC, Peale AR. Varicella neonatorum. Am J Dis Child 73:44, 1947.
135. Oppenheimer EH. Congenital chickenpox with disseminated visceral lesions. Bull Johns Hopkins Hosp 74:240, 1944.
136. Pearson HE. Parturition varicella-zoster. Obstet Gynecol 23:21, 1964.
137. Steen J, Pederson RV. Varicella in a newborn girl. J Oslo City Hosp 9:36, 1959.
138. Ranney EK, Norman MG, Silver MD. Varicella pneumonitis. Can Med Assoc J 96:445, 1967.
139. Triebwasser JH, Harris RE, Bryant RE, Rhodes ER. Varicella pneumonia in adults: report of seven cases and a review of the literature. Medicine (Baltimore) 46:409, 1967.
140. Bradley JS, Schlievert PM, Sample TG. Streptococcal toxic shock-like syndrome as a complication of varicella. Pediatr Infect Dis J 10:77, 1991.
141. Brogan TV, Niozet V, Waldhausen JHT, et al. Group A streptococcal necrotizing fasciitis complicating primary varicella: a series of fourteen patients. Pediatr Infect Dis J 14:588, 1995.
142. Centers for Disease Control. Outbreak of invasive group A *Streptococcus* associated with varicella in a childcare center—Boston, MA, 1997. MMWR Morb Mortal Wkly Rep 46:944, 1997.
143. Davies HD, McGeer A, Schwarts B, et al. Invasive group A streptococcal infections in Ontario, Canada. N Engl J Med 335:547, 1996.
144. Doctor A, Harper MB, Fleischer GR. Group A beta-hemolytic streptococcal bacteremia: historical review, changing incidence, and recent association with varicella. Pediatrics 96:428, 1995.
145. Gonzalez-Ruiz A, Ridgway GL, Cohen SL, et al. Varicella gangrenosa with toxic shock-like syndrome due to group A *Streptococcus* infection in an adult. Clin Infect Dis 20:1058, 1995.
146. Mills WJ, Mosca VS, Nizet V, et al. Invasive group A streptococcal infections complicating primary varicella. J Pediatr Orthop 16:522, 1996.
147. Peterson CL, Vugia D, Meyers H, et al. Risk factors for invasive group A streptococcal infections in children with varicella: a case-control study. Pediatr Infect Dis J 15:151, 1996.
148. Wilson G, Talkington D, Gruber W, et al. Group A streptococcal necrotizing fasciitis following varicella in children: case reports and review. Clin Infect Dis 20:1333, 1995.
149. Bullowa JGM, Wishik SM. Complications of varicella. I. Their occurrence among 2,534 patients. Am J Dis Child 49:923, 1935.
150. Johnson R, Milbourn PE. Central nervous system manifestations of chickenpox. Can Med Assoc J 102:831, 1970.
151. Jenkins RB. Severe chickenpox encephalopathy. Am J Dis Child 110:137, 1965.

152. Minkowitz S, Wenk R, Friedman E, et al. Acute glomerulonephritis associated with varicella infection. Am J Med 44:489, 1968.
153. Yuceoglu AM, Berkovich S, Minkowitz S. Acute glomerular nephritis as a complication of varicella. JAMA 202:113, 1967.
154. Morales A, Adelman S, Fine G. Varicella myocarditis. Arch Pathol 91:29, 1971.
155. Moore CM, Henry J, Benzing G, et al. Varicella myocarditis. Am J Dis Child 118:899, 1969.
156. Priest JR, Groth KE, Balfour HH. Varicella arthritis documented by isolation of virus from joint fluid. J Pediatr 93:990, 1978.
157. Ward JR, Bishop B. Varicella arthritis. JAMA 212:1954, 1970.
158. Gershon A. Varicella-zoster virus: prospects for control. Adv Pediatr Infect Dis 10:93, 1995.
159. Jura E, Chadwick E, Josephs SH, et al. Varicella-zoster virus infections in children infected with human immunodeficiency virus. Pediatr Infect Dis J 8:586, 1989.
160. Feldman S, Hughes W, Daniel C. Varicella in children with cancer: 77 cases. Pediatrics 80:388, 1975.
161. Ihara T, Kamiya H, Starr SE, et al. Natural killing of varicella-zoster virus (VZV)–infected fibroblasts in normal children, children with VZV infections, and children with Hodgkin's disease. Acta Pediatr Jpn 31:523, 1989.
162. Arvin A, Sharp M, Smith S, et al. Equivalent recognition of a varicella-zoster virus immediate early protein (IE62) and glycoprotein I by cytotoxic T lymphocytes of either CD4+ or CD8+ phenotype. J Immunol 146:257, 1991.
163. Cooper E, Vujcic L, Quinnan G. Varicella-zoster virus-specific HLA-restricted cytotoxicity of normal immune adult lymphocytes after in vitro stimulation. J Infect Dis 158:780, 1988.
164. Krugman S, Goodrich C, Ward R. Primary varicella pneumonia. N Engl J Med 257:843, 1957.
165. Mermelstein RH, Freireich AW. Varicella pneumonia. Ann Intern Med 55:456, 1961.
166. Weber DM, Pellecchia JA. Varicella pneumonia: study of prevalence in adult men. JAMA 192:572, 1965.
167. Sargent EN, Carson MJ, Reilly ED. Varicella pneumonia: a report of 20 cases with postmortem examination in 6. Calif Med 107:141, 1967.
168. Bocles JS, Ehrenkranz NJ, Marks A. Abnormalities of respiratory function in varicella pneumonia. Ann Intern Med 60:183, 1964.
169. Fish SA. Maternal death due to disseminated varicella. JAMA 173:978, 1960.
170. Hackel DB. Myocarditis in association with varicella. Am J Pathol 29:369, 1953.
171. Harris RE, Rhoades ER. Varicella pneumonia complicating pregnancy: report of a case and review of the literature. Obstet Gynecol 25:734, 1965.
172. Brunell PA. Varicella-zoster infections in pregnancy. JAMA 199:315, 1967.
173. Baren J, Henneman P, Lewis R. Primary varicella in adults: pneumonia, pregnancy, and hospital admission. Ann Emerg Med 28:165, 1996.
174. Siegel M, Fuerst HT. Low birth weight and maternal virus diseases: a prospective study of rubella, measles, mumps, chickenpox, and hepatitis. JAMA 197:88, 1966.
175. Harger JH, Ernest JM, Thurnau GR, et al. Risk factors and outcome of varicella-zoster virus pneumonia in pregnant women. J Infect Dis 185:422, 2002.
176. Harger JH, Ernest JM, Thurnau GR, et al. Frequency of congenital varicella syndrome in a prospective cohort of 347 pregnant women. Obstet Gynecol 100:260, 2002.
177. Abler C. Neonatal varicella. Am J Dis Child 107:492, 1964.
178. Siegel M, Fuerst HT, Peress NS. Comparative fetal mortality in maternal virus diseases: a prospective study on rubella, measles, mumps, chickenpox, and hepatitis. N Engl J Med 274:768, 1966.
179. Pickard RE. Varicella pneumonia in pregnancy. Am J Obstet Gynecol 101:504, 1968.
180. Mendelow DA, Lewis GC. Varicella pneumonia during pregnancy. Obstet Gynecol 33:98, 1969.
181. Geeves RB, Lindsay DA, Robertson TI. Varicella pneumonia in pregnancy with varicella neonatorum: report of a case followed by severe digital clubbing. Aust N Z J Med 1:63, 1971.
182. Paryani SG, Arvin AM. Intrauterine infection with varicella-zoster virus after maternal varicella. N Engl J Med 314:1542, 1986.
183. Esmonde TF, Herdman G, Anderson G. Chickenpox pneumonia: an association with pregnancy. Thorax 44:812, 1989.
184. Figueroa-Damian R, Arrendondo-Garcia JL. Perinatal outcome of pregnancies complicated with varicella infection during the first 20 weeks of gestation. Am J Perinatol 14:411, 1997.
185. Cox SM, Cunningham FG, Luby J. Management of varicella pneumonia complicating pregnancy. Am J Perinatol 7:300, 1990.
186. Smego RA, Asperilla MO. Use of acyclovir for varicella pneumonia during pregnancy. Obstet Gynecol 78:1112, 1991.
187. Landsberger EJ, Hager WD, Grossman JH. Successful management of varicella pneumonia complicating pregnancy: a report of 3 cases. J Reprod Med 31:311, 1986.
188. Lotshaw RR, Keegan JM, Gordon HR. Parenteral and oral acyclovir for management of varicella pneumonia in pregnancy: a case report with review of literature. W V Med J 87:204, 1991.
189. Hockberger RS, Rothstein RJ. Varicella pneumonia in adults: a spectrum of disease. Ann Emerg Med 115:931, 1986.
190. Hollingsworth HM, Pratter MR, Irwin RS. Acute respiratory failure in pregnancy. J Intensive Care Med 4:11, 1089.
191. Hankins GDV, Gilstrap LC, Patterson AR. Acyclovir treatment of varicella pneumonia in pregnancy. Letter. Crit Care Med 15:336, 1987.
192. Glaser JB, Loftus J, Ferragamo V, et al. Varicella in pregnancy. Letter. N Engl J Med 315:1416, 1986.
193. Boyd K, Walker E. Use of acyclovir to treat chickenpox in pregnancy. BMJ 296:393, 1988.
194. White RG. Chickenpox in pregnancy. Letter. BMJ 196:864, 1988.
195. Broussard OF, Payne DK, George RB. Treatment with acyclovir of varicella pneumonia in pregnancy. Chest 99:1045, 1991.
196. Eder SE, Apuzzio JA, Weiss G. Varicella pneumonia during pregnancy: treatment of 2 cases with acyclovir. Am J Perinatol 5:16, 1988.
197. Andrews EB, Tilson HH, Hurn BAL, Cordero JF. Acyclovir in pregnancy registry. Am J Med 85:123, 1988.
198. Centers for Disease Control. Acyclovir registry. MMWR Morb Mortal Wkly Rep 42:806, 1993.
199. Pearse BM. Characterization of coated-vesicle adaptors: their reassembly with clathrin and with recycling receptors. Methods Cell Biol 31:229, 1989.
200. Centers for Disease Control. Prevention of varicella: recommendations of the Advisory Committee on Immunization Practices (ACIP). MMWR Morb Mortal Wkly Rep 45:1, 1996.
201. Enders G, Miller E, Cradock-Watson J, et al. Consequences of varicella and herpes zoster in pregnancy: prospective study of 1739 cases. Lancet 343:1548, 1994.
202. Benyesh-Melnick M, Stich HF, Rapp F, et al. Viruses and mammalian chromosomes. III. Effect of herpes zoster virus on human embryonal lung cultures. Proc Soc Exp Biol Med 117:546, 1964.
203. Aula P. Chromosomes and virus infections. Lancet 1:720, 1964.
204. Massimo I, Vianello MG, Dagna-Bricarelli F, et al. Chickenpox and chromosome aberrations. BMJ 2:172, 1965.
205. Collier E. Congenital varicella cataract. Am J Ophthalmol 86:627, 1978.
206. Cuthbertson G, Weiner CPW, Giller RH, Grose C. Prenatal diagnosis of second-trimester congenital varicella syndrome by virus-specific immunoglobulin M. J Pediatr 111:592, 1987.
207. Harding B, Bonner JA. Congenital varicella-zoster: a serologically proven case with necrotizing encephalitis and malformations. Acta Neuropathol 76:311, 1988.
208. Hammad E, Helin I, Pasca A. Early pregnancy varicella and associated congenital anomalies. Acta Paediatr Scand 78:963, 1989.
209. Adelstein AM, Donovan JW. Malignant disease in children whose mothers had chickenpox, mumps, or rubella in pregnancy. BMJ 2:629 1972.
210. Fox MJ, Krumpiegel ER, Teresi JL. Maternal measles, mumps, and chickenpox as a cause of congenital anomalies. Lancet 1:746, 1948.
211. Jones KL, Johnson KA, Chambers CD. Offspring of women infected with varicella during pregnancy: a prospective study. Teratology 49:29, 1994.
212. Pastuszak A, Levy M, Schick B, et al. Outcome after maternal varicella infection in the first 20 weeks of pregnancy. N Engl J Med 330:901 1994.
213. Michie CA, Acolet D, Charlton R, et al. Varicella-zoster contracted in the second trimester of pregnancy. Pediatr Infect Dis J 10:1050, 1992.
214. Connan L, Ayoubi J, Icart J, et al. Intra-uterine fetal death following maternal varicella infection. Eur J Obstet Gynecol 68:205, 1996.
215. Sauerbrai A, Muller D, Eichhorn U, Wutzler P. Detection of varicella-zoster virus in congenital varicella syndrome: a case report. Obstet Gynecol 88:687 1996.
216. Mouly F, Mirlesse V, Meritet JF, et al. Prenatal diagnosis of fetal varicella-zoster virus infection with polymerase chain reaction of amniotic fluid in 107 cases. Am J Obstet Gynecol 177:894, 1997.
217. Ussery XT, Annunziato P, Gershon A, et al. Congenital varicella-zoster infection and Barrett's esophagus. J Infect Dis 178:539, 1998.

218. LaForet EG, Lynch LL. Multiple congenital defects following maternal varicella. N Engl J Med 236:534, 1947.
219. Srabstein JC, Morris N, Larke B, et al. Is there a congenital varicella syndrome? J Pediatr 84:239, 1974.
220. Alfonso I, Palomino JA, DeQuesada G, et al. Picture of the month: congenital varicella syndrome. Am J Dis Child 138:603, 1984.
221. Alkalay AL, Pomerance JJ, Yamamura JM, et al. Congenital anomalies associated with maternal varicella infections during early pregnancy. J Perinatol 7:69, 1987.
222. Borzykowski M, Harris RF, Jones RWA. The congenital varicella syndrome. Eur J Pediatr 137:335, 1981.
223. Dietzsch H, Rabenalt P, Trlifajova J. Varizellen-Embryopathie: kliniche und serologische Verlaufsbeobachtungen. Kinderarztl Prax 3:139, 1980.
224. Fuccillo DA. Congenital varicella. Teratology 15:329, 1977.
225. Hajdi G, Meszner Z, Nyerges G, et al. Congenital varicella syndrome. Infection 14:177, 1986.
226. McKendry JBJ. Congenital varicella associated with multiple defects. Can Med Assoc J 108:66, 1973.
227. Rinvik R. Congenital varicella encephalomyelitis in surviving newborn. Am J Dis Child 117:231, 1969.
228. Savage MO, Moosa A, Gordon RR. Maternal varicella infection as a cause of fetal malformations. Lancet 1:352, 1973.
229. Schlotfeld-Schafer I, Schafer P, Llatz S, et al. Congenitales Varicellensyndrom. Monatsschr Kinderheilkd 131:106, 1983.
230. Broomhead. Cited in Dudgeon HA (ed). Viral Diseases of the Fetus and Newborn. Philadelphia, WB Saunders, 1982, p 161.
231. Enders G. Varicella-zoster virus infection in pregnancy. Prog Med Virol 29:166, 1984.
232. Essex-Cater A, Heggarty H. Fatal congenital varicella syndrome. J Infect 7:77, 1983.
233. Lamy M, Minkowski A, Choucroun J. Embryopathie d'origine infectieuse. Semaine Med 72, 1951.
234. Konig R, Gutjahr P, Kruel R, et al. Konnätale varizellen-embryo-fetopathy. Helv Paediatr Acta 40:391, 1985.
235. Scharf A, Scherr O, Enders G, Helftenbein E. Virus detection in the fetal tissue of a premature delivery with a congenital varicella syndrome. J Perinat Med 18:317, 1990.
236. DaSilva O, Hammerberg O, Chance GW. Fetal varicella syndrome. Pediatr Infect Dis J 9:854, 1990.
237. Magliocco AM, Demetrick DJ, Sarnat HB, Hwang WS. Varicella embryopathy. Arch Pathol Lab Med 116:181, 1992.
238. Alexander I. Congenital varicella. BMJ 2:1074, 1979.
239. Bailie FB. Aplasia cutis congenita of neck and shoulder requiring a skin graft: a case report. Br J Plastic Surg 36:72 1983.
240. Brice JEH. Congenital varicella resulting from infection during second trimester at pregnancy. Arch Dis Child 51:474, 1976.
241. Dodion-Fransen J, Dekegel D, Thiry L. Maternal varicella infection as a cause of fetal malformations. Scand J Infect Dis 5:149, 1973.
242. Frey H, Bialkin G, Gershon A. Congenital varicella: case report of a serologically proved long-term survivor. Pediatrics 59:110, 1977.
243. Pettay O. Intrauterine and perinatal viral infections. Ann Clin Res 11:258, 1979.
244. Taranger J, Blomberg J, Strannegard O. Intrauterine varicella: a report of two cases associated with hyper-A-immunoglobulinemia. Scand J Infect Dis 13:297, 1981.
245. Unger-Koppel J, Kilcher P, Tonz O. Varizellenfetopathie. Helv Paediatr Acta 40:399, 1985.
246. White MI, Daly BM, Moffat MA, Rankin R. Connective tissue naevi in a child with intra-uterine varicella infection. Clin Exp Dermatol 15:149, 1990.
247. Palmer CGS, Pauli RM. Intrauterine varicella infection. J Pediatr 112:506, 1988.
248. Lambert SR, Taylor D, Kriss A, et al. Ocular manifestations of the congenital varicella syndrome. Arch Ophthalmol 107:52, 1989.
249. Bai PVA, John TJ. Congenital skin ulcers following varicella in late pregnancy. J Pediatr 94:65, 1979.
250. Klauber GT, Flynn FJ, Altman BD. Congenital varicella syndrome with genitourinary anomalies. Urology 8:153, 1976.
251. Michon L, Aubertin D, Jager-Schmidt G. Deux observations de malformations congenitales paraissant relever d'embryopathies zosteriennes. Arch Fr Pediatr 16:695, 1959.
252. Enders G. Serodiagnosis of varicella-zoster virus infection in pregnancy and standardisation of the ELISA IgG and IgM antibody tests. Dev Biol Stand 52:221, 1982.
253. Charles N, Bennett TW, Margolis S. Ocular pathology of the congenital varicella syndrome. Arch Ophthalmol 95:2034, 1977.
254. Andreou A, Basiakos H, Hatsikoumi I, Lazarides A. Fetal varicella syndrome with manifestations limited to the eye. Am J Perinatol 12:347, 1995.
255. Kotchmar G, Grose C, Brunell P. Complete spectrum of the varicella congenital defects syndrome in 5-year-old child. Pediatr Infect Dis 3:142, 1984.
256. Grose C. Congenital varicella-zoster virus infection and the failure to establish virus-specific cell-mediated immunity. Mol Biol Med 6:453, 1989.
257. Salzman MB, Sood SK. Congenital anomalies resulting from maternal at 25 and a half weeks of gestation. Pediatr Infect Dis J 11:504, 1992.
258. Hitchcock R, Birthistle K, Carrington D, et al. Colonic atresia and spinal cord atrophy associated with a case of fetal varicella syndrome. J Pediatr Surg 30:1344, 1995.
259. Lloyd KM, Dunne JL. Skin lesions as the sole manifestation of the fetal varicella syndrome. Clin Exp Dermatol 15:149, 1990.
260. Scheffer IE, Baraitser M, Brett EM. Severe microcephaly associated with congenital varicella infection. Dev Med Child Neurol 33:916, 1991.
261. Randel R, Kearns DB, Sawyer MH. Vocal cord paralysis as a presentation of intrauterine infection with varicella-zoster virus. Pediatrics 97:127, 1996.
262. Bennet R, Forsgren M, Herin P. Herpes zoster in a 2-week-old premature infant with possible congenital varicella encephalitis. Acta Pediatr Scand 74:979, 1985.
263. Byrne JLB, Ward K, Kochenour NK, Dolcourt JL. Prenatal sonographic diagnosis of fetal varicella syndrome. Am J Hum Genet 47:A470, 1990.
264. Sauerbrai, A, Muller, D, Eichhorn, U, et al. Detection of varicella-zoster virus in congenital varicella syndrome: a case report. Obstet Gynecol 88:687, 1996.
265. Mazzella M, Arioni C, Bellini C, et al. Severe hydrocephalus associated with congenital varicella syndrome. CMAJ 168:561, 2003.
266. Huang CS, Lin SP, Chiu NC, et al. Congenital varicella syndrome as an unusual cause of congenital malformation: report of one case. Acta Paediatr Taiwan 42:239, 2001.
267. Dimova PS, Karparov AA. Congenital varicella syndrome: case with isolated brain damage. J Child Neurol 16:595, 2001.
268. Kent A, Paes B. Congenital varicella syndrome: a rare case of central nervous system involvement without dermatological features. Am J Perinatol 17:253, 2000.
269. Liang CD, Yu TJ, Ko SF. Ipsilateral renal dysplasia with hypertensive heart disease in an infant with cutaneous varicella lesions: an unusual presentation of congenital varicella syndrome. J Am Acad Dermatol 43:864, 2000.
270. Cooper C, Wojtulewicz J, Ratnamohan VM, et al. Congenital varicella syndrome diagnosed by polymerase chain reaction—scarring of the spinal cord, not the skin. J Paediatr Child Health 36:186, 2000.
271. Choong CS, Patole S, Whitehall J. Congenital varicella syndrome in the absence of cutaneous lesions. J Paediatr Child Health 36:184, 2000.
272. Forrest J, Mego S, Burgess M. Congenital and neonatal varicella in Australia. J Paediatr Child Health 36:108, 2000.
273. Gaynor EB. Congenital varicella and the newborn cry. Otolaryngol Head Neck Surg 104:541, 1991.
274. Taylor WG, Walkinshaw SA, Thompson MA. Antenatal assessment of neurological impairment. Arch Dis Child 68:604, 1993.
275. Kerkering KW. Abnormal cry and intracranial calcifications: clues to the diagnosis of fetal varicella-zoster syndrome. J Perinatol 21:131, 2001.
276. Hartung J, Enders G, Chaoui R, et al. Prenatal diagnosis of congenital varicella syndrome and detection of varicella-zoster virus in the fetus: a case report. Prenat Diagn 19:163, 1999.
277. Hofmeyr GJ, Moolla S, Lawrie T. Prenatal sonographic diagnosis of congenital varicella infection—a case report. Prenat Diagn 16:1148, 1996.
278. Petignat P, Vial Y, Laurini R, et al. Fetal varicella-herpes zoster syndrome in early pregnancy: ultrasonographic and morphological correlation. Prenat Diagn 21:121, 2001.
279. Verstraelen H, Vanzieleghem B, Defoort P, et al. Prenatal ultrasound and magnetic resonance imaging in fetal varicella syndrome: correlation with pathology findings. Prenat Diagn 23:705, 2003.
280. Duehr PA. Herpes zoster as a cause of congenital cataract. Am J Ophthalmol 39:157, 1955.
281. Webster MH, Smith CS. Congenital abnormalities and maternal herpes zoster. BMJ 4:1193, 1977.
282. Grose C, Itani O, Weiner C. Prenatal diagnosis of fetal infection: advances from amniocentesis to cordocentesis—congenital toxoplasmosis, rubella, cytomegalovirus, varicella virus, parvovirus and human immunodeficiency virus. Pediatr Infect Dis J 8:459, 1989.

283. Alkalay AL, Pomerance JJ, Rimoin D. Fetal varicella syndrome. J Pediatr 111:320, 1987
284. Pickard RE. Varicella pneumonia in pregnancy. Am J Obstet Gynecol 101:504, 1968.
285. Hofmeyer GJ, Moolla S, Lawrie T. Prenatal sonographic diagnosis of congenital varicella infection—a case report. Prenat Diagn 16:1148, 1996.
286. Lecuru F, Taurells R, Bernard JP, et al. Varicella-zoster virus infection during pregnancy: the limits of prenatal diagnosis. Eur J Obstet Gynecol Reprod Biol 56:67, 1994.
287. Isada NB, Paar DP, Johnson M, et al. In utero diagnosis of congenital varicella zoster infection by chorionic villus sampling and polymerase chain reaction. Am J Obstet Gynecol 165:1727, 1991.
288. Fowler KB, Stagno S, Pass RF, et al. The outcome of congenital cytomegalovirus infection in relation to maternal antibody status. N Engl J Med 326:663, 1992.
289. Preblud S, Bregman DJ, Vernon LL. Deaths from varicella in infants. Pediatr Infect Dis 4:503, 1985.
290. Rubin L, Leggiadro R, Elie MT, Lipsitz P. Disseminated varicella in a neonate: implications for immunoprophylaxis of neonates postnatally exposed to varicella. Pediatr Infect Dis 5:100, 1986.
291. Meyers J. Congenital varicella in term infants: risk reconsidered. J Infect Dis 129:215, 1974.
292. Hanngren K, Grandien M, Granstrom G. Effect of zoster immunoglobulin for varicella prophylaxis in the newborn. Scand J Infect Dis 17:343, 1985.
293. Preblud S, Nelson WL, Levin M, Zaia J. Modification of congenital varicella infection with VZIG. Interscience Conference on Antimicrobial Agents and Chemotherapy, New Orleans, 1986.
294. Nankervis GA, Gold E. Varicella-zoster viruses. *In* Kaplan AS (ed). The Herpesviruses. New York, Academic Press, 1973, p 327.
295. Kohl S. The neonatal human's immune response to herpes simplex virus infection: a critical review. Pediatr Infect Dis J 8:67, 1989.
296. Winkelman RK, Perry HO. Herpes zoster in children. JAMA 171:876, 1959.
297. David T, Williams M. Herpes zoster in infancy. Scand J Infect Dis 11:185, 1979.
298. Dworsky M, Whitely R, Alford C. Herpes zoster in early infancy. Am J Dis Child 134:618, 1980.
299. Helander I, Arstila P, Terho P. Herpes zoster in a 6 month old infant. Acta Dermatol 63:180, 1982.
300. Lewkonia IK, Jackson AA. Infantile herpes zoster after intrauterine exposure to varicella. BMJ 3:149, 1973.
301. Lyday JH. Report of severe herpes zoster in a 13 and one-half-year-old boy whose chickenpox infection may have been acquired in utero. Pediatrics 50:930, 1972.
302. Adkisson MA. Herpes zoster in a newborn premature infant. J Pediatr 66:956, 1965.
303. Bonar BE, Pearsall CJ. Herpes zoster in the newborn. Am J Dis Child 44:398, 1932.
304. Counter CE, Korn BJ. Herpes zoster in the newborn associated with congenital blindness: report of a case. Arch Pediatr 67:397, 1950.
305. Feldman GV. Herpes zoster neonatorum. Arch Dis Child 27:126, 1952.
306. Freud P, Rook GD, Gurian S. Herpes zoster in the newborn. Am J Dis Child 64:895, 1942.
307. Music SI, Fine EM, Togo Y. Zoster-like disease in the newborn due to herpes-simplex virus. N Engl J Med 284:24, 1971.
308. Gershon A, Steinberg S, LaRussa P. Varicella-zoster virus. *In* Lennette EH (ed). Laboratory Diagnosis of Viral Infections. New York, Marcel Dekker, 1992, p 749.
309. Rawlinson WD, Dwyer DE, Gibbons V, Cunningham A. Rapid diagnosis of varicella-zoster virus infection with a monoclonal antibody based direct immunofluorescence technique. J Virol Methods 23:13, 1989.
310. Vazquez M, LaRussa P, Gershon A, et al. The effectiveness of the varicella vaccine in clinical practice. N Engl J Med 344:955, 2001.
311. Hughes P, LaRussa PS, Pearce JM, et al. Transmission of varicella-zoster virus from a vaccinee with underlying leukemia, demonstrated by polymerase chain reaction. J Pediatr 124:932, 1994.
312. Ito M, Nishihara H, Mizutani K, et al. Detection of varicella zoster virus (VZV) DNA in throat swabs and peripheral blood mononuclear cells of immunocompromised patients with herpes zoster by polymerase chain reaction. Clin Diagn Virol 4:105, 1995.
313. LaRussa P, Lungu O, Hardy I, et al. Restriction fragment length polymorphism of polymerase chain reaction products from vaccine and wild-type varicella-zoster virus isolates. J Virol 66:1016, 1992.
314. LaRussa P, Steinberg S, Gershon A. Diagnosis and typing of varicella-zoster virus (VZV) in clinical specimens by polymerase chain reaction (PCR). Thirty-fourth International Conference on Antimicrobial Agents and Chemotherapy, Orlando, Fla, September 1994.
315. Mahalingham R, Cohrs R, Dueland AN, Gilden DH. Polymerase chain reaction diagnosis of varicella-zoster virus. *In* Becker Y, Darai G (eds). Diagnosis of Human Viruses by Polymerase Chain Reaction Technology, vol 1. New York, Springer-Verlag, 1992, p 134.
316. Puchhammer-Stockl E, Kunz C, Wagner G, Enders G. Detection of varicella zoster virus (VZV) in fetal tissue by polymerase chain reaction. J Perinat Med 22:65, 1994.
317. Sawyer M, Wu YN. Detection of varicella-zoster virus DNA by polymerase chain reaction in CSF of patients with VZV-related central nervous system complications. International Conference on Antimicrobial Agents and Chemotherapy, New Orleans, La, September 1993.
318. Annunziato P, Lungu O, Gershon A, et al. In situ hybridization detection of varicella zoster virus in paraffin-embedded skin biopsy specimens. Clin Diagn Virol 7:69, 1997.
319. Silliman CC, Tedder D, Ogle JW, et al. Unsuspected varicella-zoster virus encephalitis in a child with acquired immunodeficiency syndrome. J Pediatr 123:418, 1993.
320. Gershon AA, LaRussa P. Varicella-zoster virus. *In* Donowitz LG (ed). Hospital-Acquired Infection in the Pediatric Patient. Baltimore, Williams & Wilkins, 1988, p 139.
321. Le CT, Lipson M. Difficulty in determining varicella-zoster immune status in pregnant women. Pediatr Infect Dis J 8:650, 1989.
322. Vasileiadis GT, Roukema HW, Romano W, et al. Intrauterine herpes simplex infection. Am J Perinatol 20:55, 2003.
323. Grose C. Congenital infections caused by varicella zoster virus and herpes simplex virus. Semin Pediatr Neurol 1: 43. 1994.
324. Whitley RJ, Straus S. Therapy for varicella-zoster virus infections: where do we stand? Infect Dis Clin Pract 2:100, 1993.
325. Whitley RJ, Gnann JW. Acyclovir: a decade later. N Engl J Med 327:782, 1992.
326. Greffe BS, Dooley S, Deddish R, Krasny H. Transplacental passage of acyclovir. J Pediatr 108:1020, 1986.
327. Dunkel L, Arvin A, Whitley R, et al. A controlled trial of oral acyclovir for chickenpox in normal children. N Engl J Med 325:1539, 1991.
328. Balfour HH, Rotbart H, Feldman S, et al. Acyclovir treatment of varicella in otherwise healthy adolescents. J Pediatr 120:627, 1992.
329. Feder H. Treatment of adult chickenpox with oral acyclovir. Arch Intern Med 150:2061, 1990.
330. Wallace MR, Bowler WA, Murray NB, et al. Treatment of adult varicella with oral acyclovir: a randomized, placebo-controlled trial. Ann Intern Med 117:358, 1992.
331. Whitley RJ, Middlebrooks M, Gnann JW. Acyclovir: the past ten years. Adv Exp Med Biol 278:243, 1990.
332. Whitley R, Arvin A, Prober C, et al. A controlled trial comparing vidarabine with acyclovir in neonatal herpes simplex virus infection. N Engl J Med 324:444, 1991.
333. Englund J, Fletcher CV, Balfour HH. Acyclovir therapy in neonates. J Pediatr 119:129, 1991.
334. Gershon AA, Steinberg S, NIAID Collaborative Varicella Vaccine Study Group. Live attenuated varicella vaccine: protection in healthy adults in comparison to leukemic children. J Infect Dis 161:661, 1990.
335. Arvin A, Koropchak CM, Wittek AE. Immunologic evidence of reinfection with varicella-zoster virus. J Infect Dis 148:200, 1983.
336. Gershon AA, Steinberg S, Gelb L, NIAID Collaborative Varicella Vaccine Study Group. Clinical reinfection with varicella-zoster virus. J Infect Dis 149:137, 1984.
337. Junker AK, Angus E, Thomas E. Recurrent varicella-zoster virus infections in apparently immunocompetent children. Pediatr Infect Dis J 10:569, 1991.
338. Junker AK, Tilley P. Varicella-zoster virus antibody avidity and IgG-subclass patterns in children with recurrent chickenpox. J Med Virol 43:119, 1994.
339. Martin KA, Junker AK, Thomas EE, et al. Occurrence of chickenpox during pregnancy in women seropositive for varicella-zoster virus. J Infect Dis 170:991, 1994.
340. Bogger-Goren S, Bernstein JM, Gershon A, Ogra PL. Mucosal cell mediated immunity to varicella zoster virus: role in protection against disease. J Pediatr 105:195, 1984.
341. Bogger-Goren S, Baba K, Hurley P, et al. Antibody response to varicella-zoster virus after natural or vaccine-induced infection. J Infect Dis 146:260, 1982.

342. Ljungman P, Lonnqvist B, Gahrton G, et al. Clinical and subclinical reactivations of varicella-zoster virus in immunocompromised patients. J Infect Dis 153:840, 1986.
343. Weigle K, Grose C. Molecular dissection of the humoral immune response to individual varicella-zoster viral proteins during chickenpox, quiescence, reinfection, and reactivation. J Infect Dis 149:741, 1984.
344. Gilden DH, Wright R, Schneck S, et al. Zoster sine herpete, a clinical variant. Ann Neurol 35:530, 1994.
345. Wilson A, Sharp M, Koropchak C, et al. Subclinical varicella-zoster virus viremia, herpes zoster, and T lymphocyte immunity to varicella-zoster viral antigens after bone marrow transplantation. J Infect Dis 165:119, 1992.
346. Hardy IB, Gershon A, Steinberg S, et al. Incidence of zoster after live attenuated varicella vaccine. International Conference on Antimicrobial Agents and Chemotherapy, Chicago, Ill, September 1991.
347. LaRussa PL, Gershon AA, Steinberg S, Chartrand S. Antibodies to varicella-zoster virus glycoproteins I, II, and III in leukemic and healthy children. J Infect Dis 162:627, 1990.
348. Burke BL, Steele RW, Beard OW, et al. Immune responses to varicella-zoster in the aged. Arch Intern Med 142:291, 1982.
349. Miller AE. Selective decline in cellular immune response to varicella-zoster in the elderly. Neurology 30:582, 1980.
350. Gershon A, Steinberg S. Antibody responses to varicella-zoster virus and the role of antibody in host defense. Am J Med Sci 282:12, 1981.
351. Stevens D, Merigan T. Zoster immune globulin prophylaxis of disseminated zoster in compromised hosts. Arch Intern Med 140:52, 1980.
352. Gershon A. Immunoprophylaxis of varicella-zoster infections. Am J Med 76:672, 1984.
353. Levin M. Can herpes zoster be prevented? Eur J Clin Microbiol Infect Dis 15:1, 1996.
354. Levin M, Murray M, Rotbart H, et al. Immune response of elderly individuals to a live attenuated varicella vaccine. J Infect Dis 166:253, 1992.
355. Levin M, Murray M, Zerbe G, et al. Immune responses of elderly persons 4 years after receiving a live attenuated varicella vaccine. J Infect Dis 170:522, 1994.
356. Brunell P, Ross A, Miller L, Kuo B. Prevention of varicella by zoster immune globulin. N Engl J Med 280:1191, 1969.
357. Brunell P, Gershon A, Hughes W, et al. Prevention of varicella in high-risk children: a collaborative study. Pediatrics 50:718, 1972.
358. Gershon A, Steinberg S, Brunell P. Zoster immune globulin: a further assessment. N Engl J Med 290:243, 1974.
359. Orenstein W, Heymann D, Ellis R, et al. Prophylaxis of varicella in high risk children: response effect of zoster immune globulin. J Pediatr 98:368, 1981.
360. Zaia JA, Levin MJ, Wright GG, et al. A practical method for preparation of varicella-zoster immune globulin. J Infect Dis 137:601, 1978.
361. Zaia J, Levin M, Preblud S, et al. Evaluation of varicella-zoster immune globulin: protection of immunosuppressed children after household exposure to varicella. J Infect Dis 147:737, 1983.
362. Neustadt A. Congenital varicella. Am J Dis Child 106:96, 1963.
363. O'Neill RR. Congenital varicella. Am J Dis Child 104:391, 1962.
364. Committee on Infectious Diseases, American Academy of Pediatrics. Report of the Committee on Infectious Diseases. Elk Grove Village, Ill, American Academy of Pediatrics, 2003.
365. Bakshi S, Miller TC, Kaplan M, et al. Failure of VZIG in modification of severe congenital varicella. Pediatr Infect Dis 5:699, 1986.
366. Haddad J, Simeoni U, Willard D. Perinatal varicella. Lancet 1:494, 1986.
367. Holland P, Isaacs D, Moxon ER. Fatal neonatal varicella infection. Lancet 2:1156, 1986.
368. King S, Gorensek M, Ford-Jones EL, Read S. Fatal varicella-zoster infection in a newborn treated with varicella-zoster immunoglobulin. Pediatr Infect Dis 5:588, 1986.
369. Oglivie MM, Stephens JRD, Larkin M. Chickenpox in pregnancy. Lancet 1:915, 1986.
370. Williams H, Latif A, Morgan J, Ansari BM. Acyclovir in the treatment of neonatal varicella. J Infect 15:65, 1987.
371. Haddad J, Simeoni U, Messer J, Willard D. Acyclovir in prophylaxis and perinatal varicella. Lancet 1:161, 1987.
372. Sills J, Galloway A, Amegavie L, et al. Acyclovir in prophylaxis and perinatal varicella. Lancet 1:161, 1987.
363. Fried D, Hanukoglu A, Birk O. Leukocyte transfusion in severe neonatal varicella. Acta Pediatr Scand 71:147, 1982.
374. Betzhold J, Hong R. Fatal graft versus host reaction in a small leucocyte transfusion in a patient with lymphoma and varicella. Pediatrics 60:62, 1978.
375. Gershon A. Commentary on VZIG in infants. Pediatr Infect Dis J 6:469, 1987.
376. Takahashi M, Otsuka T, Okuno Y, et al. Live vaccine used to prevent the spread of varicella in children in hospital. Lancet 2:1288, 1974.
377. Arvin A, Gershon A. Live attenuated varicella vaccine. Annu Rev Microbiol 50:59, 1996.
378. White CJ. Varicella-zoster virus vaccine. Clin Infect Dis 24:753, 1997.
379. Committee on Infectious Diseases. Live attenuated varicella vaccine. Pediatrics 95:791, 1995.
380. Broyer M, Tete MT, Guest G, et al. Varicella and zoster in children after kidney transplantation: long term results of vaccination. Pediatrics 99:35, 1997.
381. LaRussa P, Steinberg S, Meurice F, Gershon A. Transmission of vaccine strain varicella-zoster virus from a healthy adult with vaccine-associated rash to susceptible household contacts. J Infect Dis 176:1072, 1997.
382. Salzman MB, Sharrar R, Steinberg S, LaRussa P. Transmission of varicella-vaccine virus from a healthy 12 month old child to his pregnant mother. J Pediatr 131:151, 1997.
383. Long S. Toddler-to-mother transmission of varicella-vaccine virus: how bad is that? J Pediatr 131:10, 1997.
384. Saiman L, Crowley K, Gershon A. Control of varicella-zoster infections in hospitals. *In* Abrutyn E, Goldmann DA, Scheckler WE (eds). Infection Control Reference Service. Philadelphia, WB Saunders, 1997, p 687.
385. Centers for Disease Control. Decline in annual incidence of varicella in selected states, 1990-2001. MMWR Morb Mortal Wkly Rep 52:884, 2003.
386. Clements DA, Zaref JI, Bland CL, et al. Partial uptake of varicella vaccine and the epidemiological effect on varicella disease in 11 day-care centers in North Carolina. Arch Pediatr Adolesc Med 155:455, 2001.
387. Galil K, Fair E, Strine T, et al. Younger age at vaccination may increase risk of varicella vaccine failure. J Infect Dis 186:102, 2002.
388. Dworkin MS, Jennings CE, Roth-Thomas J, et al. An outbreak of varicella among children attending preschool and elementary school in Illinois. Clin Infect Dis 35:102, 2002.
389. Vazquez M, LaRussa P, Steinberg S, et al. Effectiveness of varicella vaccine after 8 years. Presented at the 41st Annual Meeting of the Infectious Disease Society of America, San Diego, Calif, 2003.
390. Verstraeten T, Jumaan AO, Mullooly JP, et al. A retrospective cohort study of the association of varicella vaccine failure with asthma, steroid use, age at vaccination, and measles-mumps-rubella vaccination. Pediatrics 112:98, 2002.
391. Gershon A. Varicella vaccine: are two doses better than one? N Engl J Med 347:1962, 2002.
392. Gershon A, Takahashi M, Seward J. Varicella vaccine. *In* Plotkin S, Orenstein W (eds): Vaccines, 4th ed. Philadelphia, WB Saunders, 2003, pp 783-823.
393. Brisson M, Edmunds WJ, Gay NJ, et al. Varicella vaccine and shingles. JAMA 287:2211, 2002.
394. Brisson M, Gay N, Edmunds WJ, et al. Exposure to varicella boosts immunity to herpes-zoster: implications for mass vaccination against chickenpox. Vaccine 20:2500, 2002.
395. Donahue JG, Choo PW, Manson JE, et al. The incidence of herpes zoster. Arch Intern Med 155:1605, 1995.
396. Centers for Disease Control. Varicella-related deaths among children—United States, 1997. MMWR Morb Mortal Wkly Rep 279:1773, 1998.
397. Centers for Disease Control. Varicella-related deaths—Florida. MMWR Morb Mortal Wkly Rep 48:379, 1999.
398. Feldman S, Lott L. Varicella in children with cancer: impact of antiviral therapy and prophylaxis. Pediatrics 80:465, 1987.
399. Whitley, R, Soong, S, Dolin R, et al. Early vidarabine to control the complications of herpes zoster in immunosuppressed patients. N Engl J Med 307:971, 1982.
400. Wain H. The Story Behind the Word. Springfield, Ill, Charles C Thomas, 1958, p 199.
401. Choppin P, Richardson C, Merz D, et al. The functions and inhibition of the membrane glycoproteins of paramyxoviruses and myxoviruses and the role of the measles virus M protein in subacute sclerosing panencephalitis. J Infect Dis 143:352, 1981.
402. Bellini WJ, Icenogle J. Measles and rubella virus. *In* Murray PR, Baron EJ, Jorgenson JH, et al (eds). Manual of Clinical Microbiology. Washington, DC, ASM Press, 2003, pp 1389-1403.
403. Rota PA, Liffick SL, Rota JS, et al. Molecular epidemiology of measles viruses in the United States, 1997-2001. Emerg Infect Dis 8:902, 2002.

404. Rota PA, Rota JS, Bellini WJ. Molecular epidemiology of measles virus. Semin Virol 6:379, 1995.
405. Centers for Disease Control. Measles—United States, 2000. MMWR Morb Mortal Wkly Rep 51:120, 202.
406. Weigle K, Murphy D, Brunell P. Enzyme-linked immunosorbent assay for evaluation of immunity to measles virus. J Clin Microbiol 19:376, 1984.
407. Mayo DR, Brennan T, Cormier DP, et al. Evaluation of a commercial measles virus immunoglobulin M enzyme immunoassay. J Clin Microbiol 29:2865, 1991.
408. Lievens A, Brunell PA. Specific immunoglobulin M enzyme-linked immunosorbent assay for confirming the diagnosis of measles. J Clin Microbiol 24:391, 1986.
409. Papp K. Experiences prouvant que la voie d'infection de la rougeole est la contamination de la musqueuse conjunctivale. Rev Immunol 20:27, 1956.
410. Morley DC, Woodland M, Martin WJ. Measles in Nigerian children: a study of the disease in West Africa, and its manifestations in England and other countries during different epochs. J Hyg (Lond) 61:113, 1963.
411. Babbott FL Jr, Gordon JE. Modern measles. Am J Med Sci 225:334, 1954.
412. Centers for Disease Control. Measles, mumps, and rubella-vaccine use and strategies for elimination of measles, rubella, and congenital rubella syndrome and control of mumps. MMWR Morb Mortal Wkly Rep 47:1, 1998.
413. Frank J, Orenstein W, Bart K, et al. Major impediments to measles elimination. Am J Dis Child 139:881, 1985.
414. Markowitz LE, Preblud SR, Fine PE, et al. Duration of live measles vaccine-induced immunity. Pediatr Infect Dis J 9:101, 1990.
415. Krugman S. Further-attenuated measles vaccine: characteristics and use. Rev Infect Dis 5:477, 1983.
416. Mathias RG, Meekison WG, Arcand TA, et al. The role of secondary vaccine failures in measles outbreaks. Am J Public Health 79:475, 1989.
417. Berg RB, Rosenthal MS. Propagation of measles virus in suspensions of human and monkey leukocytes. Proc Soc Exp Biol Med 106:581, 1961.
418. Suringa DWR, Bank LJ, Ackerman AB. Role of measles virus in skin lesions and Koplik's spots. N Engl J Med 283:1139, 1970.
419. Debre R, Celers J. Measles: pathogenicity and epidemiology. *In* Debre R, Celers J (eds). Clinical Virology. Philadelphia, WB Saunders, 1970, p 336.
420. Enders J, McCarthy K, Mitus A, et al. Isolation of measles virus at autopsy in cases of giant cell pneumonia without rash. N Engl J Med 261:875, 1959.
421. Mitus A, Enders J, Crair JM, et al. Persistence of measles virus and depression of antibody formation in patients with giant cell pneumonia after measles. N Engl J Med 261:882, 1959.
422. Lachmann P. Immunopathology of measles. Proc R Soc Med 67:12, 1974.
423. Stillerman M, Thalhimer W. Attack rate and incubation period of measles. Am J Dis Child 67:15, 1944.
424. Baugess H. Measles transmitted by blood transfusion. Am J Dis Child 27:256, 1924.
425. Littauer J, Sorensen K. The measles epidemic at Umanak in Greenland in 1962. Dan Med Bull 12:43, 1965.
426. Warthin AS. Occurrence of numerous large giant cells in tonsils and pharyngeal mucosa in prodromal stage of measles: report of four cases. Arch Pathol 11:864, 1932.
427. Moroi K, Saito S, Kurata T, et al. Fetal death associated with measles virus infection of the placenta. Am J Obstet Gynecol 164:1107, 1991.
428. La Boccetta AC, Tornay AS. Measles encephalitis: report of 61 cases. Am J Dis Child 107:247, 1964.
429. Musser JH, Hauser GH. Encephalitis as a complication of measles. JAMA 90:1267, 1928.
430. Pearl PL, Abu-Farsakh H, Starke JR, et al. Neuropathology of two fatal cases of measles in the 1988-1989 Houston epidemic. Pediatr Neurol 6:126, 1990.
431. Jahnke U, Fischer EH, Alvord EC. Hypothesis-certain viral proteins contain encephalitogenic and/or neuritogenic sequences. J Neuropathol Exp Neurol 44:320, 1985.
432. Kipps A, Dick G, Moodie JW. Measles and the central nervous system. Lancet 2:1406, 1983.
433. Gremillion DH, Crawford GE. Measles pneumonia in young adults: an analysis of 106 cases. Am J Med 71:539, 1981.
434. Centers for Disease Control. Measles surveillance. MMWR Morb Mortal Wkly Rep 9:***, 1973.
435. Christensen PE, Schmidt H, Bang HO, et al. An epidemic of measles in southern Greenland, 1951. Acta Med Scand 144:430, 1953.
436. Krasinski K, Borkowsky W. Measles and measles immunity in children infected with human immunodeficiency virus. JAMA 261:2512, 1989.
437. Embree JE, Datta P, Stackiw W, et al. Increased risk of early measles in infants of human immunodeficiency type 1-seropositive mothers. J Infect Dis 165:262, 1992.
438. Angel JB, Walpita P, Lerch RA, et al. Vaccine-associated measles pneumonitis in an adult with AIDS. Ann Intern Med 129:104, 1998.
439. Kaplan LJ, Daum RS, Smaron M, McCarthy C. Severe measles in immunocompromised patients. JAMA 267:1237, 1992.
440. Kernahan J, McQuillin J, Craft A. Measles in children who have malignant disease. BMJ 295:15, 1987.
441. Breitfeld V, Hashida Y, Sherman FE, et al. Fatal measles infection in children with leukemia. Lab Invest 28:279, 1973.
442. Greenhill JP. Acute (extragenital) infections in pregnancy, labor, and the puerperium. Am J Obstet Gynecol 25:760, 1933.
443. Nouvat JR. Rougeole et Grossesse. Bordeaux, xxxx, 1904.
444. Dyer I. Measles complicating pregnancy: report of 24 cases with three instances of congenital measles. South Med J 33:601, 1940.
445. Packer AD. The influence of maternal measles (morbilli) on the newborn child. Med J Aust 1:835, 1950.
446. Atmar RL, Englund JA, Hammill H. Complications of measles during pregnancy. Clin Infect Dis 14:217, 1992.
447. Eberhart-Phillips JE, Fredrick PD, Baron RC, Mascola L. Measles in pregnancy: a descriptive study of 58 cases. Obstet Gynecol 82:797, 1993.
448. Nichols WW, Levan A, Hall B, et al. Measles-associated chromosome breakage. Preliminary communication. Hereditas 48:367, 1962.
449. Miller ZB. Chromosome abnormalities in measles. Lancet 2:1070, 1963.
450. Higurashi M, Tamura T, Nakatake T. Cytogenic observations in cultured lymphocytes from patients with Down's syndrome and measles. Pediatr Res 7:582, 1973.
451. Jespersen CS, Littauer J, Sigild U. Measles as a cause of fetal defects. Acta Pediatr Scand 66:367, 1977.
452. Gazala E, Karplus M, Sarov I. The effect of maternal measles on the fetus. Pediatr Infect Dis 4:202, 1985.
453. Rones B. The relationship of German measles during pregnancy to congenital ocular defects. Med Ann DC 13:285, 1944.
454. Swan C, Tostevin AL, Moore B, et al. Congenital defects in infants following infectious diseases during pregnancy, with special reference to relationship between German measles and cataract, deaf mutism, heart disease and microcephaly, and to period in pregnancy in which occurrence of rubella was followed by congenital abnormalities. Med J Aust 2:201, 1943.
455. Canelli AF. Sur le comportement normal et pathologique de l'immunity antimorbilleuse chez le nourison jeune. Rev Fr Pediatr 5:668, 1929.
456. Ronaldson GW. Measles at confinement with subsequent modified attack in the child. Br J Child Dis 23:192, 1926.
457. Narita M, Togashi T, Kikuta H. Neonatal measles in Hokkaido, Japan. Pediatr Infect Dis J 16:908, 1997.
458. Kohn JL. Measles in newborn infants (maternal infection). J Pediatr 23:192, 1933.
459. Richardson DL. Measles contracted in utero. R I Med J 3:13, 1920.
460. Muhlbauer B, Berns LM, Singer A. Congenital measles—1982. Isr J Med Sci 19:987, 1983.
461. Noren GR, Adams P Jr, Anderson RC. Positive skin reactivity to mumps virus antigen in endocardial fibroelastosis. J Pediatr 62:604, 1963.
462. Abreo F, Bagby J. Sputum cytology in measles infection: A case report. Acta Cytol 35:719, 1991.
463. Lightwood R, Nolan R. Epithelial giant cells in measles as an aid in diagnosis. J Pediatr 77:59, 1970.
464. Llanes-Rodas R, Liu C. Rapid diagnosis of measles from urinary sediments stained with fluorescent antibody. N Engl J Med 275:516, 1966.
465. Minnich LL, Goodenough F, Ray CG. Use of immunofluorescence to identify measles virus infections. J Clin Microbiol 29:1148, 1991.
466. Smaron MF, Saxon E, Wood L, et al. Diagnosis of measles by fluorescent antibody and culture of nasopharyngeal secretions. J Virol Methods 33:223, 1991.
467. Rossier E, Miller H, McCulloch B, et al. Comparison of immunofluorescence and enzyme immunoassay for detection of measles-specific immunoglobulin M antibody. J Clin Microbiol 29:1069, 1991.
468. Arrieta C, Zaleska M, Stutman H, Marks M. Vitamin A levels in children with measles in Long Beach, California. J Pediatr 121:75, 1992.

469. Frieden TR, Sowell AL, Henning K, et al. Vitamin A levels and severity of measles. Am J Dis Child 146:182, 1992.
470. Hussey GD, Klein M. A randomized, controlled trial of vitamin A in children with severe measles. N Engl J Med 323:160, 1990.
471. Forni AL, Schluger NW, Roberts RB. Severe measles pneumonitis in adults: evaluation of clinical characteristics and therapy with intravenous ribavirin. Clin Infect Dis 19:454, 1994.
472. Mustafa MM, Weitman SD, Winick NJ, et al. Subacute measles encephalitis in the young immunocompromised host: report of two cases diagnosed by polymerase chain reaction and treated with ribavirin and review of the literature. Clin Infect Dis 16:654, 1993.
473. Gudnadottir M, Black FL. Measles vaccination in adults with and without complicating conditions. Arch Gesamte Virusforsch 16:521, 1965.
474. Chui LW-L, Marusyk RG, Pabst HF. Measles virus specific antibody in infants in a highly vaccinated society. J Med Virol 33:199, 1991.
475. Lennon J, Black F. Maternally derived measles immunity in sera of vaccine-protected mothers. J Pediatr 108:671, 1986.
476. Wakefield AJ. Enterocolitis, autism and measles virus. Mol Psychiatry 7(Suppl 2):S44, 2002.
477. Fombone E, Chakrabarti S. No evidence for a new variant of MMR-induced autism. Pediatrics 108: E58, 2001
478. Taylor B, Lingam R, Simmons A, et al. Autism and MMR vaccination in North London; no causal relationship. Mol Psychiatry 7(Suppl 2): S7, 2002.
479. Taylor B, Miller E, Lingam R, et al. Measles, mumps, and rubella vaccination and bowel problems or developmental regression in children with autism: population study. BMJ 324:393, 2002.
480. Coughlan S, Connell J, Cohen B, et al. Suboptimal measles-mumps-rubella vaccination coverage facilitates an imported measles outbreak in Ireland. Clin Infect Dis 35:84, 2002.
481. Krugman S, Giles JP, Friedman H. Studies on immunity to measles. J Pediatr 66:471, 1965.
482. Stillerman M, Marks HH, Thalhimer W. Prophylaxis of measles with convalescent serum. Am J Dis Child 67:1, 1944.
483. Orvell C. The reactions of monoclonal antibodies with structural proteins of mumps virus. J Immunol 132:2622, 1984.
484. Lennette E. Laboratory Diagnosis of Viral Infections. New York, Marcel Dekker, 1992.
485. Garcia A, Periera J, Vidigal N, et al. Intrauterine infection with mumps virus. Obstet Gynecol 56:756, 1980.
486. Connolly NK. Mumps orchitis without parotitis in infants. Lancet 1:69, 1953.
487. Bowers D. Mumps during pregnancy. West J Surg Obstet Gynecol 61:72, 1953.
488. Greenberg MW, Beilly JS. Congenital defects in the infant following mumps during pregnancy. Am J Obstet Gynecol 57:805, 1949.
489. Hardy JB. Viral infection in pregnancy: a review. Am J Obstet Gynecol 93:1052, 1965.
490. Homans A. Mumps in a pregnant woman. Premature labor, followed by the appearance of the same disease in the infant, twenty-four hours after its birth. Am J Med Sci 29:56, 1855.
491. Moore JH. Epidemic parotitis complicating late pregnancy: report of a case. JAMA 97:1625, 1931.
492. Philip RN, Reinhard KR, Lackman DB. Observations on a mumps epidemic in a "virgin" population. Am J Epidemiol 69:91, 1959.
493. Schwartz HA. Mumps in pregnancy. Am J Obstet Gynecol 60:875, 1950.
494. Siddall RS. Epidemic parotitis in late pregnancy. Am J Obstet Gynecol 33:524, 1937.
495. Ylinen O, Jervinen PA. Parotitis during pregnancy. Acta Obstet Gynecol Scand 32:121, 1953.
496. Kilham L. Mumps virus in human milk and in milk of infected monkey. Am J Obstet Gynecol 33:524, 1951.
497. Dutta PC. A fatal case of pregnancy complicated with mumps. J Obstet Gynaecol Br Emp 42:869, 1935.
498. Swan C. Congenital malformations associated with rubella and other virus infections. *In* Banks HS (ed). Modern Practice in Infectious Fevers. New York, PB Hoeber, 1951, p 528.
499. Hyatt H. Relationship of maternal mumps to congenital defects and fetal deaths, and to maternal morbidity and mortality. Am Pract Dig Treat 12:359, 1961.
500. Kurtz J, Tomlinson A, Pearson J. Mumps virus isolated from a fetus. BMJ 284:471, 1982.
501. Robertson GG, Williamson AP, Blattner RJ. Origin and development of lens cataracts in mumps-infected chick embryos. Am J Anat 115:473, 1964.
502. St. Geme JW Jr, Davis CWC, Peralta HJ, et al. The biologic perturbations of persistent embryonic mumps virus infection. Pediatr Res 7:541, 1973.
503. Johnson RT, Johnson KP, Edmonds CJ. Virus-induced hydrocephalus: development of aqueductal stenosis in hamsters after mumps infection. Science 157:1066, 1967.
504. Holowach J, Thurston DL, Becker B. Congenital defects in infants following mumps during pregnancy: a review of the literature and a report of chorioretinitis due to fetal infection. J Pediatr 50:689, 1957.
505. Grenvall H, Selander P. Some virus diseases during pregnancy and their effect on the fetus. Nord Med 37:409, 1948.
506. Baumann B, Danon L, Weitz R, et al. Unilateral hydrocephalus due to obstruction of the foramen of Monro: another complication of intrauterine mumps infection? Eur J Pediatr 139:158, 1982.
507. Timmons G, Johnson K. Aqueductal stenosis and hydrocephalus after mumps encephalitis. N Engl J Med 283:1505, 1970.
508. Manson MM, Logan WPD, Loy RM. Rubella and Other Virus Infections During Pregnancy. London, Her Majesty's Stationery Office, 1960.
509. St. Geme JW Jr, Noren GR, Adams P. Proposed embryopathic relation between mumps virus and primary endocardial fibroelastosis. N Engl J Med 275:339, 1966.
510. Finland M. Mumps. *In* Charles D, Finland M (eds). Obstetric and Perinatal Infections. Philadelphia, Lea & Febiger, 1973, p 333.
511. Calabrese F, Rigo E, Milanese O, et al. Molecular diagnosis of myocarditis and dilated cardiomyopathy in children: clinicopathologic features and prognostic implications. Diagn Mol Pathol 11:212, 2002.
512. Ni J, Bowles NE, Kim YH, et al. Viral infection of the myocardium in endocardial fibroelastosis. Molecular evidence for the role of mumps virus as an etiologic agent. Circulation 95:133, 1997.
513. Zardini V. Eccezionale casso di parotite epidemica in neonato da madre convalescente della stessa malattia. Lattante 33:767, 1962.
514. Shouldice D, Mintz S. Mumps in utero. Can Nurse 51:454, 1955.
515. Jones JF, Ray G, Fulginiti VA. Perinatal mumps infection. J Pediatr 96:912, 1980.
516. Reman O, Freymuth F, Laloum D, et al. Neonatal respiratory distress due to mumps. Arch Dis Child 61:80, 1986.
517. Yamauchi T, Wilson C, St. Geme JW Jr. Transmission of live, attenuated mumps virus to the human placenta. N Engl J Med 290:710, 1974.
518. Chiba Y, Ogra PA, Nakao T. Transplacental mumps infection. Am J Obstet Gynecol 122:904, 1975.
519. Monif GR. Maternal mumps infection during gestation: observations on the progeny. Am J Obstet Gynecol 121:549, 1974.
520. Meyer MB. An epidemiologic study of mumps: its spread in schools and families. Am J Hyg 75:259, 1962.
521. Hoen E. Mumpsinfektion beim jungen Sugling. Kinderprtzl 36:27, 1968.
522. Harris RW, Turnball CD, Isacson P, et al. Mumps in a Northeast metropolitan community: epidemiology of clinical mumps. Am J Epidemiol 88:224, 1968.
523. Hodes D, Brunell P. Mumps antibody: placental transfer and disappearance during the first year of life. Pediatrics 45:99, 1970.
524. Sanford HN, Shmigelsky II. Purulent parotitis in the newborn. J Pediatr 26:149, 1945.
525. Wharton M, Cochi S, Hutcheson RH, Schaffner W. Mumps transmission in hospitals. Arch Intern Med 150:47, 1990.
526. Brunell PA, Brickman A, O'Hare D, et al. Ineffectiveness of isolation of patients as a method of preventing the spread of mumps. N Engl J Med 279:1357, 1968.

Chapter 23

CYTOMEGALOVIRUS INFECTIONS

Sergio Stagno • William Britt

Cytomegaloviruses (CMVs) comprise a group of agents in the herpesvirus family known for their ubiquitous distribution in humans and in numerous other mammals. In vivo and in vitro infections with CMVs are highly species specific and result in a characteristic cytopathology of greatly enlarged (cytomegalic) cells containing intranuclear and cytoplasmic inclusions.[1] The strikingly large, inclusion-bearing cells with a typical owl's-eye appearance were first reported by Ribbert[2] in 1904 from the kidneys of a stillborn infant with congenital syphilis. Subsequently, Jesionek and Kiolemenoglou[3] reported similar findings for another stillborn infant with congenital syphilis. In 1907, Lowenstein[4] described inclusions in 4 of 30 parotid glands obtained from children 2 months to 2 years old. Goodpasture and Talbot[5] observed the similarity of these cells to the inclusion-bearing cells (giant cells) found in cutaneous lesions caused by varicella virus, and they postulated that cytomegaly was the result of a similar agent. The observation of a similar cytopathic effect after infection with herpes simplex virus led Lipschutz[6] and then others to suggest that these characteristic cellular changes were a specific reaction of the host to infection with a virus. The observation by Cole and Kuttner[7] that inclusion-bearing salivary glands from older guinea pigs were infectious for younger animals after being passed through a Berkefeld N filter in a highly species-specific manner led to the denomination of these agents as *salivary gland viruses.* The cellular changes observed in tissue sections from patients with a fatal infection led to the use of the term *cytomegalic inclusion disease* (CID) years before the causative agent was identified.

In 1954, Smith[8] succeeded in propagating murine CMV in explant cultures of mouse embryonic fibroblasts. Use of similar techniques led to the independent isolation of human CMV (unless otherwise noted, CMV refers to human cytomegalovirus) shortly thereafter by Smith,[9] Rowe and coworkers,[10] and Weller and associates.[11] Smith[9] isolated the agent from two infants with CID. Rowe and associates[10] isolated three strains of CMV from adenoidal tissue of children undergoing adenoidectomy. The term *AD169*, used to designate a common laboratory-adapted strain of CMV, comes from these studies. Weller and associates[11] isolated the virus from the urine and liver of living infants with generalized CID. The term *cytomegalovirus* was proposed in 1960 by Weller and colleagues[12] to replace the names CID and salivary gland virus, which were misleading because the virus usually involved other organs and because the name *salivary gland virus* had been used to designate unrelated agents obtained from bats.

The propagation of CMV in vitro led to the rapid development of serologic methods such as neutralization and complement fixation. Using such antibody assays and viral isolation, several investigators quickly established that CMV was a significant pathogen in humans. This ancient virus, like other members of the herpesvirus family, infects almost all humans at some time during their lives.[13,14] Evidence of infection has been found in all populations tested. The age at acquisition of infection differs in various geographic groups and socioeconomic settings, which results in major differences in prevalence among groups. The natural history of human CMV infection is very complex. After a primary infection, viral excretion, occasionally from several sites, persists for weeks, months, or even years before the virus becomes latent. Episodes of recurrent infection with renewed viral shedding are common, even years after the primary infection. These episodes of recurrent infection are caused by reactivation of latent viruses or reinfections with an antigenically diverse strain of CMV. In immunocompetent hosts, CMV infections are generally subclinical. However, when infection occurs during pregnancy without consequences for the mother, it can have serious repercussions for the fetus. Even though most immunocompromised hosts tolerate CMV infections relatively well, in some instances, such as acquired immunodeficiency syndrome (AIDS) and bone marrow transplantation, CMV can cause disease of diverse severity, and the infection can be life threatening. Because of a long-standing and close host-parasite relationship, many—probably thousands—genetically different strains of CMV have evolved and circulate in the general population.[15]

THE VIRUS

CMV (human herpesvirus 5) is the largest and structurally most complex member of the family of human herpesviruses. It has been classified as a betaherpesvirus based on several biochemical criteria such as the genome size, guanosine and cytosine content, slow replicative cycle, and restricted in vivo and in vitro tropism. Other members of this subfamily of viruses include other mammalian CMVs and the agents associated with the exanthem roseola, human herpesviruses 6 and 7.[16-18] Early estimates of its size based on electron microscopic studies indicated that the CMV particle was approximately 200 nm in diameter, a finding consistent with its measurement by more contemporary techniques.[19,20] Intracellular and extracellular particles are heterogeneous in size, which is probably a reflection of the variability of envelope glycoprotein content. The virus genome consists of more than 250 kilobase pairs of linear double-stranded DNA, making CMV almost 50% larger than the alphaherpesviruses, herpes simplex virus and varicella-zoster virus.[21] In contrast to other betaherpesviruses, including other CMVs, CMV contains terminal and internal repeated nucleotide sequences that enable the genome to exist in four isomeric forms, similar to herpes simplex virus and other alphaherpesviruses.[22] The biologic advantages that favor four isomeric forms of the genome of this virus have not been determined but clearly depend on replication of the genome in a permissive cell.[23]

The nucleotide sequence of several clinical isolates of CMV has been determined, and from the analysis of these strains, it is estimated that CMVs could encode more than 250 open reading frames (ORFs). Individual viral genes and ORFs are designated by their location in the unique long (UL) region, unique short (US) region, or the internal or terminal repeat regions (IRS, IRL, TRS, TRL) of the prototypic genome of CMV.[22] In addition to the massive size of the genome, other post-transcriptional modifications can increase the complexity of the coding sequence of CMV. A limited number of CMV genes represent spliced transcripts, primarily those encoding immediate-early gene products. In some cases, multiple proteins can arise from a single gene by use of internal translational initiation sites. Although in most cases experimental verification of virus-specific proteins arising from predicted ORFs has not been accomplished, it is nevertheless obvious from this analysis that the proteomes of the virus and of the virus-infected cell are exceedingly complex. Consistent with this observation has been the complexity of the proteome of the virion revealed by mass spectrometry.[24] Organization of the CMV genome is similar to that of other herpesviruses in that conserved gene blocks that encode replicative and virion structural proteins can be found in similar locations. This organization of the genome has allowed assignment of positional homologues between members for different subfamilies of herpesviruses, an approach that has been instrumental in the identification of genomic coding sequences of CMV proteins. Outside of these conserved gene blocks are genes or gene families that are specific for individual betaherpesvirus. These genes are thought to impart specific in vivo tropism and the species-restricted growth of these viruses.

The CMV virion consists of three identifiable regions: the capsid containing the double-stranded DNA viral genome, the tegument, and the envelope. The CMV capsid consists of six proteins that have functional and structural homologues in other herpesviruses. These proteins and their counterparts found in herpes simplex virus are listed in Table 23-1.

The capsid of CMV has been studied by high-resolution cryoelectron microscopy, and its structure is almost identical to that of herpes simplex virus, with the exception that it has slightly different internal dimensions because it must incorporate a genome that is about 60% larger than herpes simplex virus. The capsid consists of 162 capsomere subunits consisting of 150 hexons and 12 pentons arranged in icosahedral symmetry.[19] The subunits of the capsid are thought to be partially assembled in the cytoplasm of the infected cell, followed by self-assembly using products of the UL80a

Table 23–1 Cytomegalovirus Proteins and Their Homologues in Herpes Simplex Virus

Protein	Herpes Simplex Virus	Cytomegalovirus
Major capsid protein	Vp5 (UL119)	MCP (UL86)[a]
Small capsid protein	Vp26 (UL35)	SCP (UL48-49)[a]
Minor capsid protein	Vp23(UL18)	MnCP (UL85)[a]
Minor capsid protein	Vp19c (UL38)	MnCP-bp (UL46)[a]
Assembly protein	Vp22a(UL26.5)	Assembly protein (UL80.5)
Assembly protein precursor	Vp21(UL26)	Assemblin $precursor_{COOH}$ (UL80a)
Assembly protein precursor	Vp24(UL26)	Assemblin (UL80a)[a]
Portal protein	UL6	UL104

[a]Indicates capsid proteins that have been demonstrated in infectious virions.

Data from Gibson W. Structure and assembly of the virion. Intervirology 39:389-400, 1996.

ORF.[25] Proteins encoded by this ORF serve as a scaffold for the assembly of the individual capsomeres.[25] After the shell is assembled, newly replicated concatemeric viral DNA enters the capsid shell through a portal generated by the portal protein and the action of a virus-encoded protein complex called the *terminase complex*, generating the intranuclear capsid.[26,27]

Several steps in the assembly of the viral DNA–containing capsid are unique to CMV, including the cleavage of unit length DNA and the formation of the capsid portal. At least one of these steps in virus replication have been demonstrated to be the target of antiviral drugs.[28] Capsids containing infectious DNA leave the nucleus by poorly understood pathways and are enveloped in the cytoplasm.

The tegument of CMV is the most complex and heterogeneous structure in the virion. An undetermined number of viral proteins and viral RNAs can be found in the tegument of infectious particles.[29] Although it is generally argued that the tegument has no identifiable structure and is usually described as an amorphous layer between the envelope and the capsid, some studies have argued that at least the innermost region of the tegument assumes the structure of the underlying icosahedral capsid.[19] Proteins within the tegument are characteristically phosphorylated and in many cases serve regulatory functions for virus replication. Some tegument proteins appear to have a primary role in maintenance of the structural integrity of the virion. Tegument proteins have a variety of functions in the infected cell, including direct stimulation of cell cycle progression from G_0 to G_1 by degradation of the retinoblastoma (Rb) protein and blocking progression at the G_1-S junction of the cell cycle.[30-33] Other tegument proteins enhance transcription from the immediate-early genes and accelerate the replication of viral DNA.[34] Some tegument proteins are thought to modify cellular structures such as the infected cell nucleus to facilitate nuclear egress of capsids containing viral DNA (Table 23-2).[35]

These examples illustrate the functional complexity of CMV tegument proteins and suggest that it will be difficult in some cases to assign a unique function to an individual protein in the replicative cycle of CMV. The tegument contains the most immunogenic proteins of the virions, including the immunodominant targets of T lymphocyte responses and antibody responses.[36-40] In the case of one of the most abundant tegument proteins, pp65 (UL83 ORF), studies have shown that approximately 2% to 5% of peripheral blood $CD8^+$ lymphocytes from CMV-infected hosts are specific for this single protein.[40] It remains unclear why the normal host has devoted such a large percentage of peripheral $CD8^+$ lymphocyte reactivity to a single CMV antigen.

The envelope of CMV rivals the tegument in terms of the number of unidentified proteins and the limited amount of information on the function of many envelope proteins. Sequence analysis of the CMV genome indicates that more than 50 ORFs exhibit predicted amino acid motifs found in glycoproteins.[21,41]

The number of glycoproteins in the envelope of CMV is unknown, but eight glycoproteins have been defined experimentally (Table 23-3). Results of studies have suggested that the gM/gN complex represents the most abundant proteins in the virion envelope, with gB and the gH/gL/gO complex being the second and third most abundant group of glycoproteins in the envelope, respectively. There appears to be a redundancy in function for several of these glycoproteins (see Table 23-3); however, it also is likely that these redundancies are a function of in vitro assays and that each of these proposed functions is essential for virus infectivity in vivo. The envelope glycoproteins induce a readily detectable

Table 23–2 Functions of Selected Cytomegalovirus Tegument Proteins

ORF	Protein	Proposed Function
UL25	ppUL25	Structural[a]
UL26	ppUL26	Regulatory[b]
UL32	pp150	Structural
UL47	ppUL47	Regulatory, structural
UL48	pp200	Structural
UL50	p35	Assembly[c]
UL53	ppUL53	Assembly, structural
UL76		Regulatory, structural
UL82	pp71	Regulatory, structural
UL83	pp65	Regulatory, structural
UL84		Regulatory
UL94	ppUL94	Structural
UL99	pp28	Structural

[a]Tegument proteins are considered structural if they are considered essential for assembly of an infectious particle.
[b]Tegument proteins with identified regulatory activities in the replicative cycle of the virus.
[c]The proteins are considered essential for assembly of an infectious particle, but in some cases, they have not been demonstrated to be in the particle.
ORF, open reading frame; UL, unique long region.

Table 23–3 Cytomegalovirus Envelope Glycoproteins

Glycoprotein	ORF	Complex Formation	Essential for Infectivity	Proposed Function
gB	UL55	Oligomer	Yes	Attachment/fusion
gH	UL75	gH/gL/gO	Yes	Fusion/penetration
gL	UL115	gH/gL/gO	Yes	Fusion/penetration
gO	UL74	gH/gL/gO	Yes	Fusion/penetration
gM	UL100	gM/gN	Yes	Unknown
gN	UL73	gM/gN	Yes	Unknown
gpTRL10	TRL10	Unknown	No	Unknown
gpUL132	UL132	Unknown	No	Unknown

ORF, open reading frame; TRL, terminal repeat location; UL, unique long region.

antibody response in the infected hosts and neutralizing antibodies directed against gB, gH, and the gM/gN complex can be demonstrated in human CMV immune serum.[42-49] Moreover, considerable amounts of data from human and animal studies have indicated that antiviral antibodies directed at proteins of the envelope are a major component of the host protective response to this virus. These and other findings further demonstrate that envelope glycoproteins play a key role in the early steps of viral infection.

Cytomegalovirus Replication

Virus replication begins when CMV attaches to the cell surface. The initial engagement of virion glycoproteins with cell surface proteoglycans is followed by more specific receptor interactions.[50-52] Suggested cellular receptors for CMV include the epidermal growth factor receptor and integrins.[53] Regardless of the specific receptor used by CMV, several studies have shown that CMV attachment and likely fusion with the host cell membrane result in a cascade of cellular responses mediated by signaling pathways.[54-57] Signaling pathways can be activated by the attachment of ultraviolet light–inactivated, noninfectious virus and by a single envelope glycoprotein, indicating that the process of binding and fusion with the cell membrane is sufficient to induce these cellular responses.[52,55-57] After infection with CMV, more than 1400 cellular genes are induced or repressed, suggesting that infection with this virus elicits myriad host cell responses.[56] Included in these early responses are activation of transcription factors such as nuclear factor-kappa B (NF-κB), increases in levels of second messengers such as phosphoinositide-3 (PI3) kinase, inhibition of cellular innate responses that block virus infection (e.g., RNA-activated protein kinase [PKR]), and progression to apoptosis of the infected cell.[22,55,56,58-60] CMV infection prepares the host cell for virus replication and inhibits host cell responses that can block virus infection.

After attachment and penetration, the DNA-containing viral capsid is rapidly transported to the nucleus, probably using the microtubular network of the cell. Once in the nucleus, the immediate-early genes of the virus are expressed in the absence of any de novo viral protein synthesis, suggesting that host or virion proteins are responsible for their induction. The replication cycle is divided into three classes according to time of synthesis after infection: immediate early, early, and late. The immediate-early genes are the first set of viral genes to become active within infected cells, usually within the first 4 hours after infection, and the most abundantly expressed products of these genes are the immediate-early 1 (IE1) and 2 (IE2) proteins. Both gene products arise from the same region of the genome and share some amino acid sequences. IE1 is a 72-kDa phosphoprotein (pp72) that is readily detectable throughout infection in permissive cells and is the target of antibody assays for detection of CMV-infected cells.[61-63] IE2 is a promiscuous *trans*-activating protein that probably is responsible for activating many of the early and late genes of CMV and some cellular genes.[22] IE1, IE2, and additional immediate-early genes encode inhibitors of cellular apoptotic responses.[64,65]

The remaining replication program of CMV is similar to that initially described for bacteriophages and for herpes simplex virus. It involves the coordinated and sequential temporal expression of viral genes and the coordinated inhibition of viral gene expression. This allows regulated expression of the viral genome. The next set of viral genes, the early or β genes, primarily encode viral proteins that are required for replication of viral DNA or alteration of cellular responses such as progression through the cell cycle or cellular apoptotic responses.[22] These include the viral DNA polymerase, alkaline exonuclease, ribonucleotide reductase, and other replicative enzymes. Some virion structural proteins are also made during this interval. The final set of viral genes, the late or γ genes, are expressed approximately 24 hours after infection. These genes encode virion structural proteins and are required for the assembly of an infectious particle. The entire replicative cycle is estimated to take between 36 and 48 hours in permissive cells. Abortive infections in nonpermissive cells have also been characterized, and viral gene expression usually is limited to the immediate-early genes and possibly to a limited number of early genes.

After viral DNA replication in the nucleus of infected cells, concatemeric DNA is cleaved during packaging into the procapsid by mechanisms that closely resemble the pathway of bacteriophage assembly. Studies[66,67] of the assembly of alphaherpesviruses have provided a better understanding of the mechanisms and pathways of viral capsid assembly and DNA packaging. The viral capsid leaves the nucleus by undetermined mechanisms and enters the cytoplasm as a partially tegumented, subviral particle. Assembly of the mature particle takes place in the cytoplasm of the infected cell in a specialized compartment that has been called the *assembly compartment*.[68] It is believed that this is a modified secretory compartment close to the *trans*-Golgi.[68,69] Virion structural proteins are transported to this compartment, and presumably through a series of protein interactions, the virus is assembled and enveloped. The latter step is of considerable complexity because of the large number of virion glycoproteins that constitute the envelope of infectious virion. Virus is presumably released by cell lysis in cells such as fibroblasts and by poorly defined exocytic pathways in certain other cell types.[69,70]

Latency is a common theme of herpesviruses, particularly of the betaherpesviruses. The concept of CMV latency is somewhat controversial in that viral persistence in the host is more likely associated with chronic, low-level productive infection and intermittent excretion. However, latent CMV infection has been demonstrated in macrophages obtained from infected nonimmunocompromised donors and in vitro models of infection with CMV.[71-74] The mechanisms that favor the establishment of latent infections are not known, but the viral genome is thought to be maintained as closed circular viral DNA that persists as an episome in latently infected cells, not by integration into the host DNA.[75] More definitive information is available on the signals that induce reactivation from latent infection. They include pro-inflammatory cytokines such as tumor necrosis factor-α (TNF-α) and possibly interferon-γ (IFN-γ).[73,74,76] It has been argued that latently infected cells of the monocytic lineage can become activated and replicate CMV after exposure to these cytokines in vivo, such as in the setting of rejection of an allograft. This mechanism may explain aspects of the pathogenesis of CMV infection in uninfected allograft recipients transplanted with an organ from a CMV-infected donor.[77,78]

Cytomegalovirus Cellular Tropism

CMV can be detected in a wide variety of cell types in vivo.[77,79-84] Studies using tissue from autopsies or biopsies have demonstrated virus in almost every cell type, including epithelial cells, endothelial cells, smooth muscle cells, neuronal cells and supporting cells in the central nervous system (CNS), retinal epithelium, dermal fibroblasts, and cells of the monocyte-macrophage lineage. There appears to be a very limited restriction of the host cellular tropism in vivo. Routine virus isolation and propagation in vitro requires that the host cell be permissive for CMV replication. Primary cells derived from a variety of organs such as primary astrocytes, primary endothelial cells, primary smooth muscle cells, primary macrophages, and primary fibroblasts are permissive for CMV replication in vitro. However, the yield of infectious virus from these various cell types is highly variable, ranging from very low (macrophages) to high (fibroblasts). Primary human fibroblasts are the most commonly employed cells for the recovery and propagation of CMV and if adequately maintained can yield up to 10^6 to 10^7 infectious particles per milliliter of supernatant from cultures infected with laboratory strains of CMV. In contrast, recent clinical isolates often yield a fraction of this amount of virus, and almost all of the progeny virions are cell associated. The explanation for the differences in replication phenotype is unknown. Clinical isolates often exhibit an extended tropism and infect primary endothelial cells, macrophages, and primary smooth muscle cells, whereas commonly used laboratory strains of CMV do not infect these cell types. Although not fully understood, studies have provided clues about possible mechanisms that lead to extended cellular tropisms of some recent clinical viral isolates. It has been argued that these clinical isolates contain a number of genes that facilitate their in vivo replication and spread. These genes are not required for in vitro replication in fibroblasts and perhaps even inhibit replication, particularly the production of extracellular virus.[85] They are selected against, and over time, viral mutants with deletions of genomic material can be isolated from these cultures. Loss of these viral genes restricts host cell tropism for cells such as endothelial cells and macrophages. The in vivo phenotype of these viral genes and their importance to in vivo replication and spread are not understood, but they are assumed to be essential because they are conserved in recent virus isolates.

EPIDEMIOLOGY

Overview

Human CMV is highly species specific, and humans are believed to be its only reservoir.[1] CMV infection is endemic and has no seasonal variation.[14] Seroepidemiologic surveys have found CMV infection in every human population that has been tested.[13,14] The prevalence of antibody to CMV increases with age, but according to geographic and ethnic and socioeconomic backgrounds, the patterns of acquisition of infection vary widely among populations (Fig. 23-1).[15]

In general, the prevalence of CMV infection is higher in developing countries and among the lower socioeconomic strata of the more developed nations. These differences are particularly striking during childhood. For instance, in sub-Saharan Africa, South America, and South Pacific, the rate of seropositivity was 95% to 100% among preschool children studied, whereas surveys in Great Britain and in certain populations in the United States have generally found that less than 20% of children of similar ages are seropositive.

The level of immunity among women of childbearing age, which is an important factor in determining the incidence and significance of congenital and perinatal CMV infections, varies widely among different populations. Several reports indicate that seropositivity rates in young women in the United States and Western Europe range from less than 50% to 85%.[13,14] In contrast, in sub-Saharan Africa, Central and South America, India, and the far East, the rate of seropositivity is greater than 90% by the end of the second decade of life. More important, from the point of view of congenital infection, prospective studies of pregnant women in the United States indicate that the rate of CMV acquisition for childbearing-aged women of middle to higher socioeconomic background is approximately 2% per year, whereas

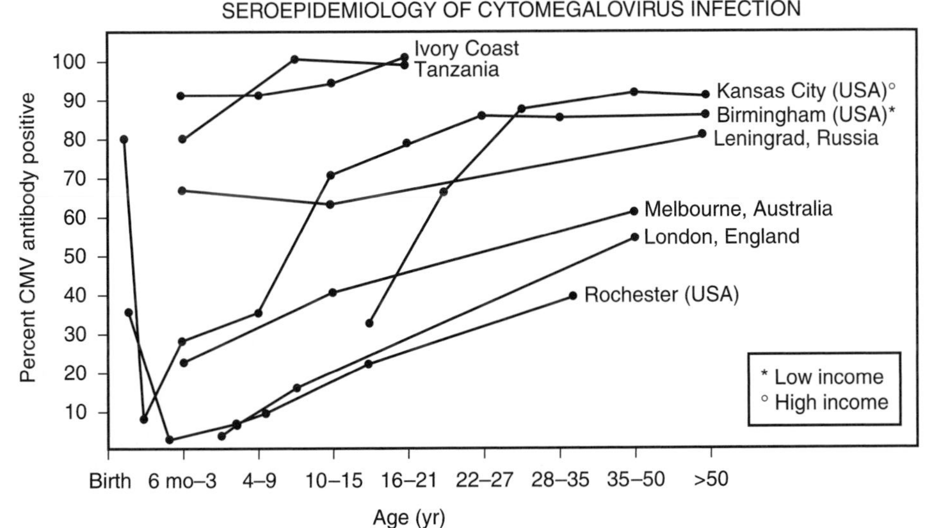

Figure 23–1 Age-related prevalence of antibody to cytomegalovirus (CMV) in various populations. (From Alford CA, Stagno S, Pass RF, et al. Epidemiology of cytomegalovirus. *In* Nahmias AJ, Dowdle WR, Schinazi RE [eds]. The Human Herpesviruses. New York, Elsevier/North-Holland, 1981, p 161.)

Table 23–4 Breast-feeding Patterns and Prevalence of Cytomegalovirus Infections in Young Children of Various Nations

Nation	Breast-feeding Rate		Percent Seropositive	
	Ever	*At 3 Months*	*Mothers*	*Children (Age)*
Solomon Islands	100	97	100	100 (5 mo-4 yr)
India				
Vellore	96	64	98	80 (1 yr)
Pondicherry			97	67 (1-5 yr)
Barbados	96	?	77	62 (1-5 yr)
Guatemala	95	?	98	47 (6 mo-1 yr)
Chile	89	?	92	42 (1-2 yr)
Japan				
Sapporo	?	56	67	42 (6 mo-2 yr)
Sendai			85	38 (1 yr)
Finland (Helsinki)	95	50	55	28 (1 yr)
United States				
Houston, Texas	46	?	48	15 (1 yr)
Birmingham, Alabama	8	?	85	8 (1 yr)
France (Paris)	85	?	56	10 (10 mo)
Canada (Nova Scotia)	49	26	34	12 (6 mo-1 yr)
U.K. (Manchester)	51	13	59	12 (3-11 mo)

Data from Pass RF. Transmission of viruses through human milk. *In* Howell RR, Morris FH Jr, Pickering K (eds). Role of Human Milk in Infant Nutrition and Health. Springfield, Ill, Charles C Thomas, 1986, pp 205-224.

it is 6% per year among women of lower socioeconomic background.[86]

The modes of transmission from person to person are incompletely understood. Several features of CMV infection make it difficult to study the modes of acquisition. In most individuals, CMV infections are subclinical, including those acquired in utero and during the perinatal period. Infected persons continue to expose other susceptible people to CMV. Virus excretion persists for years after congenital, perinatal, and early postnatal infections. Prolonged viral shedding, which lasts more than 6 months in most individuals, is also a feature of primary infection in older children and adults. Because recurrent infections are fairly common, intermittent excretion of virus can be anticipated in a significant proportion of seropositive adults. Regardless of whether CMV is maintained as a latent infection with periodic reactivation or as a chronic, persistent infection yielding low titers of infectivity, the virus readily spreads within a population.

A large reservoir of CMV exists in the population at all times. Transmission occurs by direct or indirect person-to-person contact. Sources of virus include urine, oropharyngeal secretions, cervical and vaginal secretions, semen, milk, tears, blood products, and organ allografts.[87-91]

CMV is not very contagious because the spread of infection appears to require close or intimate contact with infected secretions. The prevalence of CMV infection is higher for populations of low socioeconomic status, presumably reflecting factors that account for increased exposure to CMV, such as crowding, sexual practices, and increased exposure to infants and toddlers. Sexual contact contributes to the spread of CMV. Higher rates of seropositivity have been observed among males and females with multiple sex partners and histories of sexually transmitted diseases.[92-95]

Breast-feeding

CMV is commonly excreted in milk collected post partum from seropositive women.[87,96] The rates of excretion range from 13% to 32% by isolation of virus in tissue cultures to an excess of 70% when tested by polymerase chain reaction (PCR) methods. Peak excretion occurs between 2 weeks and 2 months post partum. The risk of transmission of CMV infection to the infants is 39% to 59%. The risk of transmission by lactating mothers correlates with viral loads of 7×10^3 genome equivalents/mL. CMV can be detected in different components of breast milk. There is consensus that milk whey is the material of choice to detect the virus during lactation. Fractions of milk containing milk cells are less likely to show the virus by culture or PCR methods. This may explain why rates of viral isolation are lower in colostrum than in mature milk. Most infected infants begin to excrete CMV between 22 days and 3 months after birth.

Conservatively, it is estimated that almost 40% of all infants nursed for at least 1 month by CMV-seropositive mothers become infected postnatally. Most of these infants become chronic excreters of CMV in urine and saliva, creating a large pool of infected infants. Because in most populations of the world the seroprevalence of CMV infection in women of childbearing age is high (80% to 100%) and most women breast-feed their infants for more than 1 month, the rate of transmission of CMV is quite high (Table 23-4).

Trends in infant feeding practices have undergone major changes in the industrialized world. In the United States, breast-feeding in the hospital setting declined progressively during the 20th century to reach a nadir in the early 1970s, when exclusive breast-feeding was reported by 19% of white and 9% of black mothers.

Table 23–5 **Prevalence of Cytomegalovirus Excretion among Children in Daycare Centers**

Investigator	Year	Location	Percent Infected (n/N)
Stangert	1976	Stockholm, Sweden	35 (7/20)
Strom	1979	Stockholm, Sweden	72 (13/18)
Pass	1982	Birmingham, Alabama, USA	51 (36/70)
Adler	1985	Richmond, Virginia, USA	24 (16/66)
Hutto	1985	Birmingham, Alabama, USA	41 (77/188)
MMWR	1985	Birmingham, Alabama, USA	29 (66/231)
Jones	1985	San Francisco, California, USA	22 (31/140)
Murph	1986	Iowa City, Iowa, USA	22 (9/41)
Adler	1987	Richmond, Virginia, USA	53 (55/104)

Data from Adler SP. Cytomegalovirus transmission among children in day care, their mothers and caretakers. Pediatr Infect Dis J 7:279-285, 1988.
MMWR, Morbidity and Mortality Weekly Report.

Young Children as a Source of Cytomegalovirus

Certain child-rearing practices influence the spread of CMV among children. In 1971, Weller[1] suggested that the high rate of seropositivity among Swedish children probably was caused by the frequent use of daycare centers. Swedish children had a rate of infection that was three to four times higher than that observed in London or in Rochester, New York. As shown in Table 23-5, high rates of CMV infection among children attending daycare centers were later confirmed in Sweden and have been reported in several studies in the United States.[97-101]

The studies, which included a control group of children, confirmed that the rate of CMV infection was substantially higher among those in daycare than in those who stayed at home.[97,98] In the study of Pass and co-workers[97] of a group of 70 children of middle- to upper-income background whose ages ranged from 3 to 65 months, the rate of CMV excretion in urine and saliva was 51%. The lowest rate of excretion (9%) occurred in infants younger than 1 year, and the highest rate (88%) was among toddlers in their second year of life. Twelve infants whose mothers were seronegative excreted CMV, which indicated that their infection was not congenitally or perinatally acquired. These findings have been corroborated by other investigators.

Similar results were reported by Adler and colleagues,[100] who found that more than 50% of initially seronegative children acquired daycare-associated strains of CMV as determined by restriction fragment length polymorphism analysis of viral DNA. The findings of Adler, which have been confirmed by others, demonstrate that CMV is very efficiently transmitted from child to child in the daycare setting and that it is not unusual to find excretion rates as high as 20% to 40% in young toddlers.[99,102] In many instances, these rates of infection are substantially higher than the seroprevalence rates for the parents of the children and young adults in the cities where the studies were done.[103] There is compelling evidence that the high rate of CMV infection among children in group daycare is caused by horizontal transmission from child to child. The route of transmission that appears most likely is the transfer of virus that occurs through saliva on hands and toys.[104,105] CMV can retain infectivity for hours on plastic surfaces and has been isolated from randomly selected toys and surfaces in a daycare center. No data have indicated CMV transmission through respiratory droplets.

These observations in daycare centers indicate that transmission of CMV between young children is very efficient. Once infected, these children excrete CMV in large quantities and for extended periods. With the changes in child-rearing practices occurring in the United States and the resurgence of breast-feeding, significant changes in the epidemiology of CMV can be expected within the next few decades.[103]

An important issue is whether children excreting CMV can become a source of infection for serosusceptible child-care personnel and parents, particularly women who may become pregnant. This type of transmission has been confirmed by restriction endonuclease mapping of CMV DNA.[106,107] Seroepidemiologic studies suggest that parents often acquire CMV from their children who became infected outside the family. For instance, Yeager[108] reported that 7 (47%) of 15 seronegative mothers of premature infants who acquired CMV in a nursery seroconverted within 1 year. Dworsky and colleagues[109] reported that the rate of seroconversion for women with at least one child living at home was 5.5%, significantly higher than the 2.3% rate for women from the same clinic who were pregnant for the first time or the rates for susceptible nursery nurses and for physicians in training. Taber and associates showed a significant association between seroconversion among children and seroconversion among susceptible parents and showed that, in most cases, the infection in a child preceded seroconversion in the parents.[466] There is also compelling evidence linking the acquisition of CMV by children in daycare with subsequent infection in their mothers and caregivers.[102,106,110-113] Several studies have demonstrated that CMV-seronegative parents have a significant risk of acquiring CMV infection if their infants and children attend daycare. The highest risk of seroconversion is approximately 20% to 45% for parents with a child shedding CMV at 18 months old. On average, parents acquire infection within 4.2 months (range, 3 to 7 months) after their children become infected. As determined by restriction fragment length polymorphism analysis of viral DNA, many of the strains isolated from the children, their parents, and their caretakers are epidemiologically related. For caretakers working with young children in daycare centers, the annual rate of seroconversion is approximately 10%, which is significantly higher than the 2% annual rate occurring in hospital employees matched for age, race, and marital status. These observations provide compelling evidence that serosusceptible parents and women who work with children in daycare centers have an occupational risk of

Table 23–6 Rate of Congenital Cytomegalovirus Infection in Relation to Rate of Maternal Immunity in Various Locations

Location and Date	No. of Infants	Rate of Congenital CMV Infection (%)	Rate of Maternal Seropositivity (%)
Manchester, England, 1978	6051	0.24	25
Aarhus-Viborg, Denmark, 1979	3060	0.4	52
Hamilton, Canada, 1980	15,212	0.42	44
Halifax, Canada, 1975	542	0.55	37
Birmingham, Alabama (upper SES), 1981	2698	0.6	60
Houston, Texas (upper SES), 1980	461	0.6	50
London, England, 1973	720	0.69	58
Houston, Texas (low SES), 1980	493	1.2	83
Abidjan, Ivory Coast, 1978	2032	1.38	100
Sendai, Japan, 1970	132	1.4	83
Santiago, Chile, 1978	118	1.7	98
Helsinki, Finland, 1977	200	2.0	85
Birmingham, Alabama (low SES), 1980	1412	2.2	85

CMV, cytomegalovirus; SES, socioeconomic status.
Data from Stagno S, Pass RF, Dworsky ME, et al. Maternal cytomegalovirus infection and perinatal transmission. Clin Obstet Gynecol 25:564, 1982.

acquiring CMV. It is reasonable to expect that as many as 50% of susceptible children between the ages of 1 and 3 years who attend daycare will acquire CMV from their playmates and become an important source of infection for susceptible parents and caregivers. Of particular concern is the risk to seronegative women who become pregnant.

Maternal Infection and Vertical Transmission

Because maternal CMV infection is the origin of congenital infections and of most perinatal infections, it is important to review the relevant issues that pertain to vertical transmission. As used here, *vertical transmission* implies transmission from mother to infant.

Congenital Infection

Congenital infection is assumed to be the result of transplacental transmission. In the United States, congenital CMV infection occurs in 0.2% to 2.2% (average, 1%) of all newborns. However, as shown in Table 23-6, the incidence of congenital infection is quite variable among different populations.

The natural history of CMV during pregnancy is particularly complex and has not been fully explained. Infections such as rubella and toxoplasmosis cannot serve as models. With these infections, in utero transmission occurs only as a result of a primary infection acquired during pregnancy, whereas the in utero transmission of CMV can occur as a consequence of primary and recurrent infections (i.e., reinfection or reactivation).[114,115] Congenital infection resulting from recurrent CMV infection is common, especially in highly immune populations. The initial clue was provided by three independent reports of congenital CMV infections that occurred in consecutive pregnancies.[116-118] In all three instances, the first infant was severely affected or died and the second born in each case was subclinically infected. More convincing evidence came from a prospective study of women known to be seroimmune before conception.[115] As shown in Table 23-7, the rate of congenital CMV infection was 1.9% among 541 infants born to these seropositive women. The 10 congenitally infected infants were not infected as a result of primary maternal CMV infection because all mothers were known to have been infected with CMV 1 year to several years before the onset of pregnancy. Shortly after our studies were published, Schopfer and associates[114] found that in an Ivory Coast population in which virtually all inhabitants are infected in childhood, the prevalence of congenital CMV infection was 1.4%.

Table 23–7 Incidence of Congenital Cytomegalovirus Infection in a Low-Income Population

Parameter	Total	No. Infected (%)
Incidence in general infant population	1412	31 (2.2)
Incidence with recurrent maternal infection		
Previously seropositive	457	8 (1.8)
Prior cytomegalovirus excretion	58	1 (1.7)
Prior intrauterine transmission	26	1 (3.8)
Total	541	10 (1.9)

Data from Stagno S, Pass RF, Dworsky ME, et al. Maternal cytomegalovirus infection and perinatal transmission. Clin Obstet Gynecol 25:567, 1982.

This remarkable phenomenon of intrauterine transmission that occurs in the presence of substantial immunity has been attributed to reactivation of endogenous virus in some cases and to reinfection with different strains of CMV in other instances. In support of reactivation is our observation that the viruses isolated from each of three pairs of congenitally infected siblings were identical when examined by restriction endonuclease analysis.[119] In two of these three pairs, the first-born infant was severely affected, whereas the second-born sibling was subclinically infected, which suggested that virulence of infection was not related to strain and that maternal immunity in some way attenuated the fetal infection.

Another study[120] indicates that women who are CMV seropositive can become reinfected with a different strain of CMV, leading to intrauterine transmission and symptomatic congenital infection. This study assessed maternal humoral immunity to strain-specific epitopes of CMV glycoprotein H. Serum specimens from women with preconceptional immunity were obtained during the previous and the current pregnancy. Of the 16 mothers with congenitally infected infants, 10 had acquired new antibody specificities against glycoprotein H, compared with only 4 of the 30 mothers of uninfected infants. The women participating in this study were from a group that is predominantly characterized by low socioeconomic rank, young age, unmarried status, high seroprevalence of CMV, and a strong background of sexually transmitted diseases, including high rates of CMV excretion. Whether the observations of this study can be extrapolated to other populations remains to be defined.

Intrauterine transmission in immune women accounts for the direct relationship between the incidence of congenital CMV infection and the rate of seropositivity shown in Table 23-6. It is extremely difficult to define by virologic or serologic markers which patient may undergo a reactivation of CMV, and it is almost impossible to define the time of intrauterine transmission with such reactivations or reinfections during pregnancy. The sites from which CMV reactivates to produce congenital infection are unknown and probably are inaccessible to sampling during pregnancy. Although CMV excretion is a relatively common event during and after pregnancy, the simple isolation of virus during pregnancy is a poor indicator of the risk of intrauterine infection.

Virus can be shed at variable rates from single or multiple sites after primary or recurrent infections in women whether pregnant or not. Sites of excretion include the genital tract, cervix, urinary tract, pharynx, and breast. In pregnant women, virus is excreted most commonly, in decreasing order, from the cervix, urinary tract, and the throat. In the immediate postpartum period, the frequency of viral shedding into breast milk can reach 40% of seropositive women. The rates of cervical and urinary tract shedding in nonpregnant women are comparable to those found in pregnant cohorts of similar demographic and socioeconomic characteristics. In general, rates of cervical shedding range from 5.2% for nonpregnant women drawn from private practice or family planning clinics to 24.5% among women attending a sexually transmitted disease clinic.[92-95]

Pregnancy per se has no discernible effect on the overall prevalence of viral shedding. However, the prevalence of excretion is lower (2.6%) in the first trimester than near term (7.6%).[119] This rate is comparable to the prevalence of genital excretion in nonpregnant women.

The rates of CMV excretion in the genital and urinary tracts of women are inversely related to age after puberty. In one study, the rate of genital CMV excretion fell from 15% in girls between 11 and 14 years old to undetectable levels in women 31 years old or older.[119] From a peak of 8% for the younger group, urinary excretion fell to zero among women 26 years old or older. No CMV excretion occurred from either site in postmenopausal women.

The transient depression of cellular immune responses to CMV antigens during the second and third trimesters is another peculiar aspect of the relationship between CMV and the pregnant human host.[121] In one study, there was no generalized depression of cellular immunity because numbers of T lymphocytes, T cell proliferative responses to other mitogens, and serum antibody titers remained unchanged. None of these mothers shed virus during the period of depressed cellular immune response, nor did they transmit the infection to their infants. It has been shown that antibody responses to glycoprotein B are significantly higher at the time of delivery in women with primary CMV infection who transmitted the infection in utero compared with those who did not, suggesting that the amount of antiviral antibody is not reflective of protection from transmission.[122] However, analysis of the qualitative antibody response revealed lower neutralizing antibody titers in transmitters, suggesting an association between neutralizing activity and intrauterine transmission. In this study, a significant correlation was found between neutralizing titers and antibody avidity, indicating that antibody avidity maturation is critical for production of high levels of neutralizing antibodies during primary CMV infection.[122] In a separate study, higher levels of transplacentally acquired maternal antibodies against glycoprotein B and neutralizing antibodies were observed in infants with symptomatic infection at birth and who went on to develop sequelae.[123]

Perinatal Infection

In contrast to the poor correlation that exists between CMV excretion during pregnancy and congenital infection, there is a good correlation between maternal shedding in the genital tract and milk and perinatal acquisition. As shown in Table 23-8, in one study,[90] the two most efficient sources of transmission in the perinatal period were infected breast milk, which resulted in a 63% rate of perinatal infection, and the infected genital tract, particularly in late gestation, which was associated with transmission in 26% and 57% of cases (i.e., natal infection). Viral shedding from the pharynx and urinary tract of the mother late in gestation and during the first months post partum has not been associated with perinatal transmission.

As shown in Table 23-4, there is considerable variability in perinatal transmission of CMV throughout the world.[124] The age of the mother and her prior experience with CMV,

Table 23–8 Association between Maternal Excretion of Cytomegalovirus from Various Sites and Subsequent Infection of the Infant

Only Site of Maternal Excretion	No. of Infants Infected/ No. Exposed (%)
Breast milk	
Breast-fed infant	19/30 (63)
Bottle-fed infant	0/9 (0)
Cervix	
Third trimester and post partum	8/14 (57)
Third trimester	18/68 (26)
First and second trimesters	1/8 (12)
Urine[a]	0/11 (0)
Saliva[b]	0/15 (0)
Nonexcreting women	
Bottle-fed infant	0/125 (0)
Breast-fed infant	0/11 (9)

[a]Late third trimester.
[b]Excretion 1 day post partum.
Data from Stagno S, Reynolds DW, Pass RF, et al. Breast milk and the risk of cytomegalovirus infection. N Engl J Med 302:1073, 1980.

which influence the frequency of viral excretion into the genital tract and breast milk, are important factors. Younger seropositive women who breast-feed are at a greater risk for transmitting virus in early infancy, especially in lower socioeconomic groups.[103] It is remarkable that in Japan, Guatemala, Finland, and India, where the rates of CMV excretion within the first year of life are extremely high (39% to 56%), the practice of breast-feeding is almost universal, and most women of childbearing age are seroimmune for CMV.

Sexual Transmission

Many epidemiologic studies support the classification of CMV as a sexually transmitted infection. This is consistent with excretion of this virus in cervical secretions, vaginal fluid, and semen. In general, in developing areas of the world, 90% to 100% of the population is infected during childhood, even before they are 5 years old. Sexual transmission in these populations plays a minor role as a source of primary CMV infection, but its importance in reinfection is unclear. In developed countries, the infection is acquired at a lower rate, and in some population groups, there is a burst in the prevalence of infection after puberty. Several lines of evidence indicate that sexual transmission of CMV is at least partly responsible for this increase in seroprevalence. Increased seroprevalence of CMV and excretion of virus have been found in women attending sexually transmitted disease clinics and in young male homosexuals.[92-95,125] Handsfield demonstrated that previously infected individuals could be reinfected by a different strain of CMV as assessed by restriction fragment length polymorphism.[125a] Evidence has also been provided for sexual transmission in less promiscuous populations.[94,95] Among the many variables investigated, a significant correlation was found among seropositivity to CMV, greater numbers of lifetime sexual partners, and past or present infection with other sexually transmitted diseases.

Nosocomial Transmission

Nosocomial CMV infection is an important hazard of blood transfusion and organ transplantation. In compromised hosts such as small premature newborns and bone marrow transplant recipients, transfusion-acquired CMV infection has been associated with serious morbidity and even fatal infection. The association between the acquisition of CMV infection and blood transfusion was first suggested in 1960 by Kreel and co-workers,[126] who described a syndrome characterized by fever and leukocytosis occurring 3 to 8 weeks after open heart surgery. The reports that followed soon after expanded the syndrome to include fever, atypical lymphocytosis, splenomegaly, rash, and lymphadenopathy.[127-131] The term *postperfusion mononucleosis* was then proposed. Prospective studies incriminated blood transfusion as the major risk factor and demonstrated that although the clinical syndrome occurred in approximately 3% of the patients undergoing transfusion, inapparent acquisition of CMV infection ranged from 9% to 58% as determined by seroconversion, a fourfold rise in complement-fixing antibody titers or viral excretion, or both, occurring between 3 and 12 weeks after surgery. It has been estimated that the percentage of blood donors capable of transmitting CMV ranges from 2.5% to 12%. In a study of seronegative children receiving blood for cardiac surgery, the risk of acquiring CMV was calculated to be 2.7% per unit of blood.[128] There is a significant correlation between the risk of acquisition of CMV by patients labeled seronegative and the number of units of blood (total volume) transfused. In one study, the incidence of primary infection increased from 7% among patients receiving 1 unit of blood to 21% among those receiving more than 15 units.[129] For seronegative marrow transplant recipients who receive standard blood products, the risk of CMV infection is between 28% and 57%.[132] Under conditions found in blood banks, CMV inoculated in whole blood persisted for 28 days and in fresh-frozen plasma for 97 days.

The observation that two newborns who received large volumes of fresh blood subsequently developed symptomatic CMV infections led McCracken and associates[133] to suggest an association between blood transfusion and clinically apparent postnatal CMV infection. A subsequent report indicated an association between postnatal CMV infection and exchange transfusions.[134] With exchange transfusions, the risk of infection can reach 50%, which is probably the result of the much larger volume (150 to 200 mL/kg) received by these infants.[134] Intrauterine transfusions have also been implicated in CMV infection of mothers and their infants.

CMV infections resulting from transfusion of blood products can cause significant disease in newborn infants, particularly in premature infants and infants born to women without immunity to CMV. Extremely premature infants born to seropositive mothers are also at increased risk because the transplacental transfer of specific antibodies does not occur until the later stages of gestation. Infected infants with passively acquired anti-CMV antibodies develop milder disease than infected infants without passively acquired antibodies. This observation is a compelling argument for the role of antiviral antibodies in protecting the host against severe disease.

Transmission of CMV by transplantation of an allograft from donors previously infected with CMV represents a major clinical problem in allograft transplantation. Transplantation of a kidney from a seropositive donor into a seronegative recipient results in primary CMV infection in 80% of the patients. The clinical manifestations of the infection vary widely, depending principally on immunosuppressive regimens. Most investigators have found that CMV infection has an adverse effect on the survival of the allograft. CMV is also a major cause of morbidity and mortality in bone marrow recipients.[135-137] Interstitial pneumonitis is the most significant manifestation of the infection; the mortality rate approaches 100% in some series. Between 70% and 100% of heart transplant recipients excrete CMV.[138,139] Primary CMV infection occurs in a high proportion (60%) of patients who are seronegative before surgery. Severe disease is more likely to be associated with primary than with reactivated infection, but primary infection is not associated with an increased risk of rejection of the transplant.[140,141] The demonstration of CMV nucleic acid in kidneys of infected donors and of latent CMV in cells of macrophage-monocyte lineage indicates that the transplanted organs and hematopoietic allografts can serve as the source of virus in transplant recipients.

Nosocomial transmission is possible in the nursery setting, which suggests that workers' hands or contaminated

Table 23–9 Rates of Primary Cytomegalovirus Infection among Health Care Workers and Others

Study	Group	No. in Group	Seroconversions (%/yr)
Yeager 1975[144]	Non-nurses	27	0
	Neonatal nurses	34	4.1
	Pediatric nurses	31	7.7
Dworsky et al, 1983[109]	Medical students	89	0.6
	Pediatric residents	25	2.7
	Neonatal nurses	61	3.3
Friedman et al,[a] 1984[145]	High risk: pediatric intensive care unit, blood/ intravenous fluids team	57	12.3
	Low risk: pediatric ward nurses, noncontact	151	3.3
Brady et al, 1985[145a]	Pediatric residents	122	3.8
Adler et al, 1986[148]	Pediatric nurses	31	4.4
	Neonatal nurses	40	1.8
Demmler et al, 1986[148a]	Pediatric nurses	43	0
	Pediatric "therapists"	76	0
Balfour and Balfour, 1986[148b]	Transplant/dialysis nurses	117	1.04
	Neonatal intensive care unit nurses	96	2.28
	Nursing students	139	2.25
	Blood donors	167	1.57
Stagno et al, 1986[86]	Middle-income pregnant women	4692	2.5
	Low-income pregnant women	507	6.8

[a]Only study in a children's hospital reporting a statistically significant difference in relation to occupational contact.
Data from Pass RF, Stagno S. Cytomegalovirus. *In* Donowitz LG (ed). Hospital Acquired Infection in the Pediatric Patient. Baltimore, Williams & Wilkins, 1988.

fomites might be involved.[104-107] CMV has been recovered from objects used in the care of an infected newborn and from surfaces in a daycare center, with recovery of virus for up to 8 hours.[104,105,142] However, the very low rate of CMV infection in newborn infants of seronegative mothers who are not exposed to other important sources such as banked human milk or seropositive blood products indicates that transmission of CMV by means of fomites or workers' hands is rare.

Transmission to Hospital Workers

Because hospital workers are often women of childbearing age, there has been concern about occupational risk through contact with patients shedding CMV. As illustrated in Table 23-9, most studies carried out during the past decade indicate that the risk is not significantly different from the general population.[143] The studies showing differences in the rate of seroconversion between health care workers and controls did not show that the risks were statistically significant.[144,145]

The risk for hospital personnel is a function of the prevalence of CMV excretion among patients, the prevalence of seronegativity in health care workers, and the degree of their exposure to infected patients. In general, among hospitalized infants and children, viruria occurs in approximately 1% of newborns and 5% to 10% of older infants and toddlers.

Working with hospitalized children inevitably leads to contact with a child shedding CMV; however, it is important that workers who develop a primary infection not assume that their occupational exposure or contact with a specific patient is the source of infection. Three reports illustrate this point well. Yow and co-workers,[146] Wilfert and associates,[147] and Adler and colleagues[148] described health care workers who acquired CMV while pregnant and after attending patients known to be excreting CMV. In each of these reports, assays of restriction fragment length polymorphisms from CMV isolates demonstrated that the source of CMV for the workers were not the patients under suspicion. With the implementation of universal precautions in the care of hospitalized patients, the risk of nosocomial transmission of CMV to health care workers is expected to be much lower than the risk of acquiring the infection in the community.

PATHOGENESIS

The disease manifestations that are associated with CMV infections can be conveniently divided into those associated with acute infection and those associated with chronic infections. Considerably more is known about acute infectious syndromes, because acute CMV infections can be temporally related to specific symptoms and associated with specific laboratory abnormalities. Infrequently, acute CMV syndromes can occur in presumably normal individuals and in these cases manifest as an infectious mononucleosis that is indistinguishable clinically from the infectious mononucleosis associated with Epstein-Barr virus infection.[149,150] Normal individuals with symptomatic infections often have increased viral burdens as measured by serologic responses compared with individuals with asymptomatic infections.[151] More commonly, acute CMV infections that result in symptomatic disease occur in immunocompromised hosts. In general, acute CMV syndromes that are associated with clinical disease often share several common characteristics, including occurrence in hosts with depressed cellular immunity, uncontrolled virus replication, multiorgan involvement, end-organ disease caused by direct viral cytopathic effects, and clinical manifestations of disease correlated with virus burden. In patients with invasive CMV infections, such as those in allograft recipients, organ dysfunction and often disease course can be correlated with increasing virus burden.[152-154] There is usually not an absolute level of viral replication as measured by viral genome copy number in the peripheral blood that is predictive of the onset of an invasive infection and end-organ disease. It appears that increasing levels of virus replication (i.e., genome copy number) is more useful in the identification of individuals at risk for invasive disease and presumably reflects ongoing viral replication with an increasing risk of dissemination.

Chronic disease syndromes associated with CMV include a variety of chronic inflammatory diseases of older populations such as atherosclerotic vascular disease and vascular processes associated with chronic allograft rejection.[155-164] The progressive and late-onset hearing loss associated with congenital CMV infection can be considered in this same category.[165-168] The characteristics of populations experiencing these manifestations of CMV infection are different from those described previously and do not include hosts with global immune dysfunction. Most individuals have normal immunity and allograft recipients undergoing chronic graft rejection may have increased immune responsiveness within the allograft. Viral replication appears to be a prerequisite for disease, but the level of virus replication has not been related to disease. The course of the disease in animal models of CMV-associated vascular disease is that of ongoing inflammation that is enhanced and prolonged by the presence of CMV.[169-172] Inhibition of virus replication early in the course of infection in animal models has been shown to dramatically alter the course of disease, suggesting that virus must seed these areas and establish a persistent infection.[169] The presence of the virus in areas of inflammation increases the expression of soluble mediators of inflammation such as cytokines and chemokines and in some cases, virus-infected cells actively recruit inflammatory cells, including monocytes, into the area of disease.[164,173] The bidirectional interactions between CMV and the host inflammatory response are unique and appear to favor virus persistence, viral gene expression, and likely virus dissemination.

Cytomegalovirus Infection and Cell-Associated Viremia

An important aspect of the pathogenesis of CMV infection is the route of infection and spread within the host. It is believed that virus is acquired at mucosal sites (i.e., community exposures) or by blood-borne transmission, such as after blood transfusion or transplantation of an infected allograft. Understanding the pathogenesis of these types of infections requires an understanding of the mode of virus transmission and virus dissemination. It is believed that cell-free virus is responsible for community-acquired CMV infection based on recovery of virus from saliva and from cell-free genital tract secretions, but only limited data directly support this claim. The most convincing evidence comes from studies in breast-feeding women that have demonstrated that infectious virus exists in the cell-free fraction of breast milk.[174] This finding suggests that cell-free virus can infect a mucosal surface. Animal models of CMV infection have most commonly used intraperitoneal or subcutaneous inoculations; however, oral infection with cell-free murine CMV has been accomplished (S. Jonjic, University of Rijeka, Rijeka, Croatia, personal communication, 2000).

After infection, local replication, and amplification of virus titer in regional sites, the spread of CMV within an infected host is likely to be cell associated based on findings from immunocompromised patients and experiments using animal models. In mucosal surface infection and blood-borne infections, the mode of spread and dissemination probably is the same, albeit with different kinetics and quantity of infected cells in the vasculature and infected organs. In all but the most severely immunocompromised patients, infectivity that can be demonstrated in the blood compartment is most frequently associated with endothelial cells and polymorphonuclear leukocytes (PMNs) from the buffy coat fraction of peripheral blood.[175-177] PMNs cannot support virus replication but have been shown to carry infectious virus and viral gene products.[178,179] It has been proposed that CMV-infected endothelial cells or fibroblasts can transfer infectious virus to PMNs, and these cells can transmit virus by a microfusion event between virus-containing vesicles and susceptible cells.[178] This mechanism has not been experimentally verified in animal models of CMV infection, but the role of PMNs in transmission of infectious CMV in vivo is accepted, and the correlation between CMV antigen-positive PMNs (antigenemia assay) and disseminated infection provides a diagnostic tool for the identification of patients at risk for invasive infection with CMV.[180-187] Antigen-positive PMNs can be detected in normal hosts infected with CMV, although with a drastically reduced frequency compared with immunocompromised patients, suggesting that even in normal hosts that PMNs may be a common mode of virus dissemination. Other cells within the leukocyte fraction of peripheral blood cells support CMV persistence and transmit infectious virus, including monocyte and macrophages derived by differentiation of blood monocytes.[188-197] Granulocyte-monocyte progenitor cells have been proposed as sites of latency based on in vitro infections and can be detected as antigen containing cells in immunocompromised patients with disseminated CMV infection.[72,73,189-190,192,198] Macrophages derived from peripheral blood monocytes have been shown to harbor infectious CMV on stimulation with specific cytokines, including TNF-α.[71,76,78] Viral replication and expression of a variety of early and late proteins can be demonstrated in macrophages after infection with recently derived CMV clinical isolates. Another cell lineage believed to be critical for the in vivo spread of CMV is endothelial cells in a variety of microvascular beds. Endothelial cells have been shown to support CMV replication in vitro and infection of these cells results in a variety of cellular responses, including the release of cytokines and chemokines.[70,79,80,191,199-206] Lytic and nonlytic productive infections have been described, suggesting that endothelial cells can respond very differently to infection.[70,200,207,208] Virus infection of endothelial cells is thought to be an initial step for infection of various tissues during CMV dissemination, and endothelial cell infection appears to be critical for the hematogenous spread from infected tissue.[178,191,205] Early studies in transplantation populations described viral antigen–containing endothelial cells circulating in the blood of viremic transplant recipients.[201,209,210] These cells are believed to be infected endothelium that slough into the circulation, presumably because of local infection or inflammation. A similar role for endothelial cells in spread of CMV in the murine model and guinea pig CMV model has been proposed.[204]

Virus-Encoded Pathogenic Functions

Specific CMV-encoded virulence factors have not been identified. Early studies attempted to correlate restriction fragment length polymorphism of viral isolates from congenitally infected infants with clinical outcome. This genetic analysis proved too crude to allow identification of subtle changes in the viral genome. Numerous studies have reported a possible linkage between polymorphisms in a gene encoding the major envelope glycoprotein gB and disease.[211-214] Most studies have failed to demonstrate any specific linkage between different gB genotypes and disease, and studies using other polymorphisms in several viral genes (UL73, UL74, UL144) have failed to establish any genetic linkage between a specific genotype and disease.[215-218] Although the explanation for the vast polymorphisms in CMVs is unclear, several characteristics of CMV infections, including frequent reinfections with new strains of virus in exposed populations and recombination between strains of virus, are likely reasons for the variability in the nucleotide sequences of different viral isolates.[120,213,219,220] However, there appear to be differences in the biologic behavior of CMVs, such that some strains exhibit extended tropism and can infect endothelial cells, macrophages, and epithelial cells in addition to permissive primary fibroblast cells. This extended tropism is found only in very recently derived isolates of CMV, and after these viruses are repeatedly passaged through fibroblast cells, their extended tropism is quickly lost. It is believed that one or more viral genes are responsible for their extended tropism in vivo and that without the selective pressure of replication in vivo, these genes are lost or mutated. Specific genes that permit extended tropism in vitro have not been identified, but the presence of large numbers of genes that modify the immune response to CMV point to the possibility that these genes can encode a function that inhibits an innate response from cells such as macrophages. Other viral genes encode functional chemokine receptors, viral cytokine-like molecules (vIL-10, vIL-8), and viral anti-apoptotic functions (vICA, UL37), all of which have been proposed to contribute to the in vivo replication and virulence of CMV infections.[65,221-223]

Although defining the function of viral genes in the in vivo replication and spread of CMV has been difficult because of the restricted tropism of CMV to cells of human origin, much information has been gathered from studies in animal models. Using the mouse model of murine CMV infection, several laboratories have identified specific viral genes that appeared to be required for efficient replication and spread in vivo.[195,224-229] Three viral genes encoded by m139, m140, and m141 ORFs of murine CMV (MCMV) have been shown to play a critical role in viral replication in monocytes and macrophages but have little or no effect on the replication of the virus in mouse fibroblasts.[230-233] The in vivo phenotype of viruses that lacked these genes indicated these genes were required for in vivo dissemination and spread of MCMV.[232,234] The mechanism that accounts for restricted replication in monocytes of MCMV with deletions in these specific genes is unknown. The CMV genes that permit replication in monocyte-macrophages has not been definitively identified, but the MCMV genes *M139*, *M140*, and *M141* are homologous to a family of CMV genes (US22 gene family). Another example of a viral gene that directly influences in vivo tropism and replication of CMV is the MCMV gene *M45*. Endothelial cell tropism of MCMV can be linked to this single viral gene (M45), and it is believed that expression of this gene limits resistance of endothelial cells to MCMV-induced apoptosis.[204] Deletion of the homologous reading frame in CMV (UL45) was not associated with the loss of endothelial tropism.[235]

Other genes in MCMV encode functional chemokines, such as the murine cytomegalovirus chemokine 1 (MCK-1) that exhibits activity similar to that of interleukin-8 (IL-8).[232,234] Studies in mice have suggested that the capacity of this gene product to recruit inflammatory cells into a site of virus replication is important for cell-associated virus spread within infected animals.[232] In the absence of this virus-encoded function, virus replication remains localized to the site of infection because of a failure to recruit and infect infiltrating inflammatory cells, limiting viral dissemination.[232] A functionally homologous viral gene in CMV (UL146) may influence the spread of CMV in vivo.[236] The protein encoded by UL146 is a secreted protein that appears to function as a CXCL chemokine (CXCL1) and can induce chemotaxis and degranulation of PMNs.[236] It has been postulated that this viral chemokine could recruit PMNs in vivo and promote CMV dissemination.[234] In severely immunocompromised hosts such as AIDS patients with gastrointestinal and retinal disease from disseminated CMV infection, neutrophil infiltration can be observed in the lamina propria and in the retina.[237-240] Infection of lamina propria macrophages with CMV in vitro results in the induction of IL-8 release from these cells, suggesting that CMV can induce IL-8 release and encode a viral IL-8–like molecule.[241] Such findings are consistent with the proposed mechanism of chemokine expression and CMV dissemination from sites of virus replication. This mechanism of dissemination is consistent with the histopathologic findings in severely immunocompromised patients. However, a neutrophil infiltrate is not an invariant feature of the histopathology of naturally acquired CMV infections, and interactions between other virus-encoded chemokines and chemokine receptors and peripheral blood leukocytes may contribute to virus dissemination. Research findings have demonstrated that CMV engages toll-like receptors with resultant induction of pro-inflammatory cytokines and chemokines cascades.[242] This observation raises the possibility that virus infection alone can recruit cells such as monocytes and PMNs to sites of infection without the requirement of a specific viral chemokine.[242] Other viral genes probably induce host cell genes that facilitate virus replication. Microarray and differential display experiments have demonstrated that CMV infection induces the expression of cyclooxygenase 2 (COX-2), an enzyme required for prostaglandin synthesis and initiation of early steps of inflammation.[55] Subsequent experiments have shown that when COX-2 activity is blocked, CMV replication was blocked.[243] Together, these experiments demonstrated that a CMV-encoded gene could induce a cellular enzyme that facilitated its replication possibly by increasing the inflammatory response to the infection. This host response presumably leads to the recruitment of inflammatory cells into the site of virus replication, thereby promoting infection of infiltrating cells and virus spread.

CMV encodes four G-coupled protein receptor (GPCR)–like molecules in ORFs UL33, UL78, US 27, and US28.[173,244-246]

The US28 gene encodes a GPCR that is constitutively activated and that can also signal after interaction with chemokines, including RANTES, MCP-1, and fractalkine.[173,247-248] Reports have detailed possible roles for this molecule in the spread of CMV in vivo, including as a chemokine sink to limit host cell chemotaxis to CMV-infected cells, providing an anti-apoptotic function, recruitment of infected mononuclear cells to the sites of inflammation leading to dissemination of virus, and perhaps even binding of virus or virus-infected cells to chemokine expressing endothelial cells.[246-251] Arterial smooth muscle cells expressing US28 have been shown to migrate down chemokine gradients, thereby providing a mechanism for the localization of CMV-infected cells to sites containing inflammatory cellular infiltrates.[173] Although the role of US28 in CMV-induced vascular disease has been well described and supported by in vitro models of smooth muscle cell migration, the importance of US28 in virus dissemination from local site of infection remains to be more completely defined. Together, these and other studies suggest that the large coding sequence of CMV encodes proteins that are essential for efficient replication and for spread within the infected animal but probably have little or no function in the in vitro replication of virus.

Host Immunity and the Pathogenesis of Cytomegalovirus Infections

In normal hosts, innate and adaptive cellular immune responses can limit but not prevent the spread of CMV from secondary sites such as the liver and spleen. The roles of innate and adaptive cellular immune responses in the control of virus replication and spread to other sites have been clearly shown in experimental animal models of CMV infection.[252-258] Increased levels of virus replication follow the loss of either class of cellular immune responses.[253,255] The loss of virus-specific $CD4^+$ or $CD8^+$ cytotoxic T lymphocyte (CTL) responses is associated with uncontrolled virus replication and lethal disease in these models.[255] The role of virus-specific antibodies has also been defined in these models and appears to contribute minimally to control of local virus replication but plays a key role in limiting blood-borne dissemination of the virus.[254] This finding is of some interest because in this model of CMV infection, virus spread is almost entirely by cell-associated virus and not cell-free virus, raising several interesting questions, including the mechanisms by which antiviral antibodies restrict virus dissemination.[226] Consistent with the findings in experimental animal models, studies in immunocompromised human hosts have repeatedly demonstrated that loss of normal T lymphocyte responses predisposes the host to CMV infection and, depending on the severity of the immune deficit, can lead to invasive disease resulting in considerable morbidity and mortality.[259-264] Several striking examples of the relationship between immunity and invasive CMV disease have been documented. These include the development of pneumonitis in bone marrow and cardiac allograft recipients, prolonged CMV viremia and end-organ disease such as retinitis in AIDS patients with high viral (i.e., human immunodeficiency virus [HIV]) burdens and low $CD4^+$ lymphocyte counts, and in fetuses infected in utero. Perhaps the most convincing evidence for the critical role of T lymphocyte responses in host resistance to invasive CMV infection were studies in bone marrow allograft recipients who received ex vivo expanded CMV-specific $CD8^+$ CTL and were protected from invasive CMV infection compared with historical control patients.[262] Another interesting finding from this study was that patients that failed to generate CMV-specific $CD4^+$ lymphocyte responses failed to generate long-term protection from CMV and developed invasive infections late in the course of transplantation.[262,264] This observation predated studies that showed that a $CD4^+$ response is required for maintenance of long-term immunity to an infectious agent.[265,266] Effector cells and mediators of the innate immune response have also been shown to be critical for control of CMV infections. Although most studies have used murine models of CMV infections, loss of natural killer (NK) cell activity and invasive CMV infection have been reported.[267,268] In murine models, NK cells and interferons have been shown to play a critical role in resistance to MCMV infection and appear to represent an initial host response that can limit virus replication and spread during the development of a more efficient effector function of the adaptive immune system.[255] In contrast to the role of antiviral antibodies in limiting dissemination of MCMV, the importance of antiviral antibodies in protective responses to CMV remains unclear. Several studies have demonstrated a correlation between antiviral antibody responses, particularly virus-neutralizing antibodies, and patient outcome.[269-273] Studies in solid organ transplant recipients given intravenous immunoglobulins containing anti-CMV antibodies have suggested that virus-specific antibodies can provide some degree of protection from invasive infections.[274-277] In other transplantation populations, such as bone marrow allograft recipients, the efficacy of anti-CMV immunoglobulins has not been proved, and its use varies among transplant centers.[275,276,278,279] Animal models other than mice have also indicated that antiviral antibodies could provide some degree of protection. This is most convincing in a guinea pig model of congenital CMV infection in which passive transfer of anti-guinea pig CMV (gpCMV) antibodies limited maternal disease and disease in infected offspring.[280,281] Available data argue for a role of antiviral antibodies in limiting disease caused by CMV, and in the case of intrauterine infections, antiviral antibodies could freely pass into the fetal circulation and, if protective, could alter the outcome of intrauterine infections.

Modulation of the Host Immune Response to Cytomegalovirus

Over the past 10 years, several laboratories have identified multiple viral genes whose products interfere with immune recognition and destruction of virus-infected cells. A description of these genes and their modes of action is provided in Table 23-10.

The importance of these genes in the biology of CMV in vivo is not completely understood; however, animal models of CMV infection have allowed investigators to determine the importance of homologous genes during virus replication. The results from these studies have indicated that these viral functions actively interfere with virus clearance during acute infection in experimental animals.[258,282,283] Although a complete discussion of these viral genes and their mechanisms of immune evasion is outside the scope of this chapter, several pertinent observations can be made about the

Table 23–10 Mechanisms of Cytomegalovirus Modulation of Host Immune Responses

Responses	Viral Gene ORFs[a]	Mechanism
Innate Immune responses		
↓ Interferon responses	UL83 (pp65)	↓ IRFs, ↓NF-κB
	TRS1	↓ PKR activity
↓ NK cell activity	UL18	MHC class I decoy
	UL40	↑HLA-E expression
Adaptive Immune Responses		
↓ CD8+, MHC restricted CTL	US2, US3, US11	↓ Class I expression
↓ CD4+ responses	US2	HLA-DR degradation
	US6	Blocks TAP transport
↓ Antibody activity	TRL11	Viral Fc receptor
Antigenic variation	UL73, UL55, UL75	Loss of antibody binding
Cytokines, Chemokine Responses		
Chemokine receptors (GPCRs)	US28, US27	GPCR acts as a sink for extracellular chemokines
Cytokine	UL111a	Viral IL-10

[a]Genes and ORFs are designated by their locations in the unique long region (UL), unique short region (US), or the internal or terminal repeat regions (IRS, IRL, TRS, TRL) of the prototypic genome of cytomegalovirus.
GPCRs, G-coupled protein receptors; HLA, human leukocyte antigen; IL, interleukin; IRFs, interferon regulatory factors; MHC, major histocompatibility complex; NF-κB, nuclear factor of kappa light polypeptide gene enhancer in B cells; ORFs, open reading frames, PKR, protein kinase activated by double-stranded RNA; TAP, transporter associated with antigen presentation.
Data from references 282, 475, 476, 477, 478, 479, 480, 481.

importance of these viral genes in the pathogenesis of CMV infections. These genes do not prevent recognition and control of CMV infections in normal hosts, as evidenced by the limited pathogenicity of this virus in normal individuals and in experimental animal models. Some investigators have argued that the phenotype of these viral genes can only be appreciated in the immunocompromised hosts. Moreover, vast amounts of literature describe the function of immune evasion genes in experimental animals and during acute infection. In most studies, the function of these viral genes has only been evaluated in a limited number of target organs, raising the question of whether some of these genes could be tissue specific. Other investigators have raised the question of whether these genes function to focus the immune response to a limited number of viral antigens, restricting the available antigens for immune recognition. However, these viruses have committed a large amount of their genome to immune evasion functions, the genes are conserved in animal and human CMVs, and experiments using animals have demonstrated that immune evasion functions facilitate a tissue-specific virus replication advantage in vivo.[283] These observations suggest that these genes likely play a critical role in the biology of these viruses.

Immune evasion functions encoded by CMVs interfere with innate immune responses and adaptive immune responses to virus-infected cells. Mutations that result in mutation in viral structural proteins and in viral proteins recognized by the immune system also appear to allow escape from immunologic control. Mutations in CMV viral genes encoding targets of dominant $CD8^+$ CTL responses have been reported.[284] One of the more interesting findings has been the observation that one MCMV gene, *M157*, previously shown to activate NK responses through NK receptor Ly49H in strains of mice that were genetically resistant to MCMV infection, can develop mutations within weeks of infection.[285] Viruses with mutations in *M157* were shown to replicate to higher titers in strains of resistant mice. This mutational event appears to be caused by immune selection because genetically susceptible strains of mice that do not use this NK cell activation pathway do not generate viruses with mutations in the m157 gene.[285] Antigenic variation in virion envelope glycoproteins that are targets of virus neutralizing antibodies have been well described. Strain-specific neutralizing antibody responses to the envelope glycoprotein B have been described.[48,286] One study[287] of the polymorphic envelope glycoprotein N suggested that immune selection was responsible for the variation in amino acid sequence of gN derived from different virus isolates. CMVs, including human CMV, can evade immune recognition by a variety of active mechanisms such as immune evasion genes and by more conventional strategies, such as loss of antigenic determinants or loss of key antigens required for activation and recognition by immune cells.

Pathogenesis of Acute Infections

Very early in the study of CMV infections, disease manifestations associated with congenital and perinatal CMV infections were related to the level of virus excretion, a marker for virus replication.[288] Subsequent studies in allograft recipients and in patients with AIDS have confirmed these findings and have consistently demonstrated that increased levels of CMV replication in these patients are a key predictor of invasive disease. Unchecked virus replication and dissemination leads to multiorgan disease as illustrated by autopsy studies of neonates with congenital CMV infections, allograft recipients, and AIDS patients. Studies using rhesus macaques infected with rhesus CMV (RhCMV) have yielded results consistent with the proposed pathogenesis of human infection and provided a more detailed view of infection with this virus.[289] In these studies, virus given intravenously or by a mucosal route resulted in blood-borne dissemination and widespread infection of a number of organs, including the liver and spleen.[289] The kinetics of the virus replication were different in the two groups, with a lag in peak virus titers and liver infection occurring in animals inoculated by a mucosal route. This result suggested that a local or regional amplification of virus was required after mucosal infection before blood-borne dissemination to the liver and spleen. This finding is consistent with experimental findings in guinea pigs and mice infected with their respective CMVs.[228,290-292] The rhesus macaques that were inoculated by mucosal exposure remained asymptomatic and failed to exhibit the clinical and laboratory abnormalities that were observed in animals given virus intravenously.[289] Together, these findings parallel clinical and laboratory findings in humans infected with CMV, and human infections that follow parenteral exposure to virus can exhibit clinical and laboratory abnormalities similar to those described in these experimental animal models.

The dissemination of CMV from the liver and spleen to distal sites probably occurs in the normal immunocompetent individual and in the immunocompromised host. However, it is also quite likely that the quantity and duration of the viral dissemination is quantitatively different in these two populations. In contrast to community-acquired CMV infections in normal adults, persistent viral DNAemia as detected by PCR is characteristic of populations with disseminated CMV infections, such as AIDS patients or infants with symptomatic congenital CMV infection.[153,293-299] It appears that the natural history of CMV infection includes local replication at mucosal sites followed by amplification of virus, locally and presumably in regional lymphoid tissue, and spread to the viscera such as liver and spleen. Virus replication in these organs further increases the quantity of viruses, and virus then spreads to distal organs and sites of persistence such as the salivary glands and renal tubules. From observations in humans and in experimental models of infection, symptomatic infection appears to be related to the level of virus replication in sites seeded by the primary viremia, such as the liver and spleen. It follows that parenteral exposure from sources such as contaminated blood are associated with symptomatic infections because a larger viral inoculum is delivered to the organs such as the liver, often in the absence of a developing immune response that would normally be present after infection of a mucosal surface.

Pathogenesis of Central Nervous System Infections in Congenitally Infected Infants

The disease manifestations of congenital CMV infections include manifestations seen in adult immunocompromised hosts with disseminated CMV infections and include visceral organ involvement, such as hepatitis and, infrequently, pneumonitis and adrenalitis.[300-303] Unique to congenital CMV infection is the presence of CNS disease, a manifestation rarely seen even in the most immunocompromised allograft recipients. CMV encephalitis has been reported in patients with AIDS, but this disease is distinctly different clinically and pathologically from CMV infection of the CNS associated with intrauterine infection. CNS involvement in infants with congenital CMV infections often is associated with ongoing disease, such as progressive hearing loss during the first few years of life, at a time when there is no apparent progression of structural damage in the CNS.[165-168,304] The pathogenesis of CMV CNS infection in the developing fetus is poorly understood for several reasons, including the lack of a sufficiently large number of autopsy studies. There are no well-developed animal models of CNS infection associated with congenital CMV infection. The MCMV model is useful for the study of many aspects of CMV infection, but congenital infection with MCMV does not occur in mice. The other widely employed small animal model, the guinea pig, can be used to study intrauterine infections, and early reports suggested that CNS infections developed in these animals.[305,306] However, the usefulness of this model for studying CNS infection has not been defined, and because only a limited number of observational studies have been reported, it has been difficult to assign its value as a model. The rhesus macaque offers perhaps the most relevant model for the study of CMV CNS infections for several reasons, including the similarities in brain development shared between macaques and humans. The rhesus CMV is more closely related to CMV than are the rodent and guinea pig CMVs. However, this model is expensive, and these experimental animals are in limited supply because of their use in studies of HIV. For these reasons, our understanding of CNS infection with CMV is limited.

Infection of the developing CNS is associated with a number of structural abnormalities, depending on the age of fetus at the time of CNS infection. Imaging studies of living infants and children with congenital CMV infections and clinical findings consistent with CNS disease have been informative. Commonly observed abnormalities include periventricular calcifications, ventriculomegaly, and loss of white-gray matter demarcation.[307-309] More refined imaging studies have detailed loss of normal brain architecture with loss of normal radial neuronal migration.[310] Limited autopsy studies have confirmed these imaging abnormalities and have demonstrated the presence of inflammatory infiltrates in the parenchyma of the brain.[308] The latter finding is consistent with the presence of increased protein and inflammatory cells in spinal fluid obtained from congenitally infected infants with CNS disease. Together these findings argue for a pathogenic spectrum that likely includes lytic infection of neuronal progenitor cells in the subventricular gray area, vasculitis with loss of supporting vessels in the developing brain, and meningoencephalitis with release of inflammatory mediators. It is unclear why the fetal and newborn brains are more susceptible to CMV infection compared with the adult brain; however, findings from experimental models suggest that the developing cells of the CNS are particularly susceptible to the lytic or possibly the apoptotic effects of CMVs. In animal models, including mice and rhesus macaques, infection of the developing CNS results in widespread lytic virus replication, including neuronal progenitor cells of the subventricular gray area and endothelium.[311-313] Lytic virus replication in this area would lead to loss of normal neuronal development, radial migration, and vascularity of the developing brain. Extravasation of blood from damaged microvasculature would lead to calcifications that are prominent findings in imaging studies of CMV-infected newborn infants. The more severe manifestations of CMV CNS infection can be explained by lytic virus infection of neuronal progenitor cells, glial cells in the CNS, and destruction of supporting vasculature. Intracerebral inoculation of fetal rhesus macaques with RhCMV results in findings similar to those described in severely affected human infants, suggesting that if CMV enters the CNS early in development, significant structural damage will ensue.

Other infants infected in utero with CMV exhibit clinical findings consistent with CNS involvement, including developmental delays and loss of perceptual functions, but do not have structural damage of the brain that can be detected by routine imaging techniques. At least one autopsy series has suggested that affected infants without calcifications can have neuronal migration deficits manifest as pachygyria and other abnormalities such as cerebellar hypoplasia.[308] The mechanisms leading to loss of normal architecture are unknown but could be related to ongoing inflammation in the CNS because of intrauterine meningoencephalitis. Various inflammatory mediators have been shown to cause loss of neuron and supporting cell function and can modify vascular permeability and endothelial function. Evidence from experimental animal models has suggested that cytokines and chemokines may directly influence neuronal radial migration.[314,315] Ongoing inflammation may result in loss of normal brain architecture from delayed or absent radial migration of neurons destined for the cerebral cortex.

Pathogenesis of Hearing Loss Associated with Congenital Cytomegalovirus Infection

Hearing loss represents one of the most common long-term sequelae of congenital CMV infection, and its pathogenesis is perhaps the least understood of any manifestation of CMV infection. As discussed in preceding sections, the hearing loss can vary between mild and profound and be unilateral or bilateral, and it can develop or progress after the perinatal period.[165-168,304,316] Hearing impairment may represent the common outcome of CMV infections in different parts of the auditory apparatus or result from infection at different stages in the development of the auditory system. Besides the potential complexity of the disease, several other reasons probably contribute to the lack of understanding of the pathogenesis of hearing loss that follows congenital CMV infection. One of the most apparent is the lack of adequate histopathologic examinations of affected tissue from infected infants. A literature review revealed that only 12 temporal bones from congenitally infected infants have been studied and described in the medical literature. Most of the studies were done without the aid of modern techniques of virus and viral antigen detection and relied almost entirely on conventional histologic examinations. These limitations, together with the lack of adequate information on the maternal and fetal infection, have resulted in the lack of solid clues to the possible mechanisms of virus-induced damage to the auditory system. Hearing loss in CNS infections in adults with AIDS or transplant-related infections is rare and not well described, presumably because these infections differ significantly from congenital CMV infection in the extent of CNS involvement, the underlying diseases, and type of treatment in these immunocompromised patients. Animal models of CMV-induced hearing loss have been developed and have provided some information regarding selected aspects of the hearing loss associated with CMV. In general, however, they have failed to recapitulate the disease, and in some cases, early findings have been difficult to reproduce. Investigators have attempted to combine the limited data from histopathologic studies with natural history studies of hearing loss from congenitally infected infants with findings from animal studies to develop a model of the pathogenesis of hearing loss associated with congenital CMV infections.

A comprehensive review of temporal bone pathology in infants with congenital CMV infection was published by Strauss.[317,318] The specimens in this series were from infants who died between the ages of 3 weeks and 5 months. A single case report of a 14-year-old patient with severe neuromuscular sequelae resulting from congenital CMV can be found.[319] Findings in the inner ear, cochlea, vestibular system, and auditory or vestibular neural structures were described in all patients. Five of the original nine specimens had evidence of endolabyrinthitis, and virus was isolated from the endolymph in three of the nine specimens.[318] Viral antigen was detected by immunofluorescence in two cases in which routine histology failed to demonstrate viral inclusions.[165] Cochlear and vestibular findings were variable and ranged from rare inclusion bearing cells in or adjacent to the sensory neuroepithelium of the cochlea or vestibular system to more extensive involvement of the nonsensory epithelium. Routine histologic analysis failed to detect viral inclusions in the auditory or vestibular neural structures, but viral antigens were detected in the spiral ganglion when specimens were examined by immunofluorescence.[165] Inflammatory infiltrates were minimal and reported in only three patients in this series.[318] Perhaps the most interesting results were those reported in the examination of tissue from the 14-year-old patient with extensive sequelae from congenital CMV infection. In this patient, extensive cellular degeneration, fibrosis, and calcifications were observed in the cochlea and vestibular systems.[319] Several generalizations can be made from these limited data. First, in all but two of these cases, virus, viral antigens, or histopathologic findings consistent with virus infection were detected in the cochlea or vestibular apparatus. These findings indicate that virus replication could have occurred in the sensory neuroepithelium and nonsensory epithelium and that cellular damage could have resulted from a direct viral cytopathic effect. Virus-induced damage can also result from bystander effects from immune-mediated cytopathology. CMV could induce loss of sensory neuroepithelium in the absence of direct infection of the sensory neuroepithelium but from infection of supporting epithelium followed by host immunopathologic responses. However, an inflammatory infiltrate was seen in only three of nine specimens, an unexpected finding based on the role that the inflammatory response is thought to play in CMV end-organ disease in other patient populations. However, it is well documented that infants with congenital CMV have a delay in the development of immunologic responses to CMV, and it can be argued that findings in the cochlea and vestibular apparatus are consistent with the ineffectual immune responses of congenitally infected infants. An alternative and not exclusive possibility is that infection of the inner ear structures is a late or, in some cases, a postnatal event. The relationship between susceptibility of cells of the sensory neuroepithelium and supporting epithelium to infection with CMV and their developmental status is unknown. These cells could be resistant to CMV infection until late in development. In this case, findings from specimens of the autopsy series described previously may reflect recent infection before host inflammatory responses. Such an explanation is, however, inconsistent with the course of fetal CMV infection in other parts of the CNS in most of the patients included in autopsy studies. The findings of extensive degenerative changes together with fibrosis and calcifications in the temporal bones from the oldest patient presumably reflect the natural history of CMV labyrinthitis and, depending on the rate at which these changes develop, may explain the progressive nature of hearing loss associated with congenital CMV infection. The loss of neuroepithelium from direct virus-mediated damage or from host-derived inflammation followed by fibrosis is consistent with the profound hearing impairment that develops in some children with congenital CMV infection. Findings in experimental animal models indicate that exaggerated deposition of extracellular matrix is part of the inflammatory response in the inner ear and that this host response possibly leads to the ossification that is observed in animals inoculated in the labyrinth with CMV.[320,321]

Studies in animal models have provided some limited insight into the pathogenesis of hearing loss after congenital CMV infection. Small animal models have provided some information and have mirrored findings in humans. Both virus and inflammation are required for the development of pathology in the inner ear. A study in guinea pigs demonstrated that virus infection in immunocompromised animals was not associated with the typical pathologic findings in virus-infected normal animals.[322] Similarly, blocking virus replication with antiviral compounds or pretreating the animals with virus-neutralizing antibodies limited the development of inner ear pathology.[323-325] From the available studies the pathogenesis of hearing loss associated with congenital CMV infection requires virus replication and a host immune response. Interrupting virus replication or the local host inflammatory response could offer some therapeutic benefit to these patients.

Nature of Maternal Infection

The nature of the maternal infection is a major pathogenetic factor for congenital CMV infection. Primary infections are more likely to be transmitted to the fetus and are likely to cause more fetal injury than recurrent infections.[326] With primary CMV infection, as in other infections during pregnancy, there appears to be some innate barrier against vertical transmission.[86,327-331] Intrauterine transmission after primary infection occurs in 30% to 40% of cases. How the placenta contains the infection is poorly defined. There have been a few reports of isolated placental involvement in the absence of fetal infection. Current information suggests that gestational age has no apparent influence on the risk of transmission of CMV in utero.[86,327,328,332] However, with regard to the role of gestational age on the expression of disease in the fetus and offspring, infection at an earlier gestational age produces the worst outcome.[86,327,333]

Congenital infection may also result from recurrences of infection.[114-118] The term *recurrence* is used here to represent reactivation of infection or reinfection with the same or a different strain of CMV during pregnancy. Evidence indicates that despite the inability of maternal immunity to prevent transmission of this virus to the fetus, congenital infections that result from recurrent infections are less likely to affect the offspring than those resulting from primary infections.[326] The risk of congenital CMV infection resulting from a recurrence of infection during pregnancy ranges from a high of 1.5% for a U.S. population of low socioeconomic background to 0.19% for women of middle or upper socioeconomic background from the United States,[86] Great Britain,[328] or Sweden.[334]

In recurrent infection, it is likely that preexisting immunity inhibits the occurrence of viremia, at least to some extent. Cellular immunity may be more important than humoral immunity; however, maternal IgG antibodies are transmitted to the fetus, although their precise role has not been elucidated. Several cases of symptomatic congenital infection have been reported after therapeutic immune suppression, in women with lupus or AIDS, and even in women with intact immune systems.[334-341]

Perinatal Infection

Naturally acquired perinatal CMV infections result from exposure to infected maternal genital secretions at birth or to breast milk during the first months of postnatal life.[89,90] The presence of CMV at these two sites may be the result of primary or recurrent maternal infection. Iatrogenic CMV infections are acquired predominantly from transfusions of blood or blood products and breast milk from CMV-infected donors. Exposure to CMV in the maternal genital tract has resulted in a 30% to 50% rate of perinatal infection. The transmission from mother to infant through breast milk occurs in 30% to 70% if nursing lasts for more than 1 month.[96,124,174,342-344] After ingestion of the virus, CMV infection is presumably established at a mucosal surface (i.e., buccal, pharyngeal, or esophageal mucosa) or in the salivary glands, for which CMV is known to have a special tropism. Occasionally, perinatal CMV infection and, rarely, congenital CMV infections are associated with pneumonitis. Although it is not proved, it is conceivable that CMV replicates in respiratory mucosa after aspiration of infected secretions or breast milk.

Transmission of CMV by blood transfusion is more likely to occur when large quantities of blood are transfused. The failure to isolate CMV from the blood or blood elements of healthy seropositive blood donors suggests that the virus exists in a latent state, presumably within leukocytes. It has been suggested that CMV becomes reactivated after transfusion, when infected cells encounter the allogeneic stimulus. CMV genomes are activated when transfused to a recipient, particularly if immunologically immature or deficient. Chou and colleagues[345] reported that if the recipient is human leukocyte antigen (HLA) matched with the donor, activation is more likely to occur, presumably because of better survival of infected cells.

Persistent Viral Excretion

Congenitally and perinatally acquired CMV infections are characterized by chronic viral excretion.[301] Virus is consistently shed into the urine for up to 6 years or longer and into saliva for 2 to 4 years. Not only does excretion persist much longer in these patients than in infected older children and adults, but the quantity of virus excreted is also much greater. Even asymptomatic congenitally or perinatally infected infants excrete quantities of virus that usually exceed those

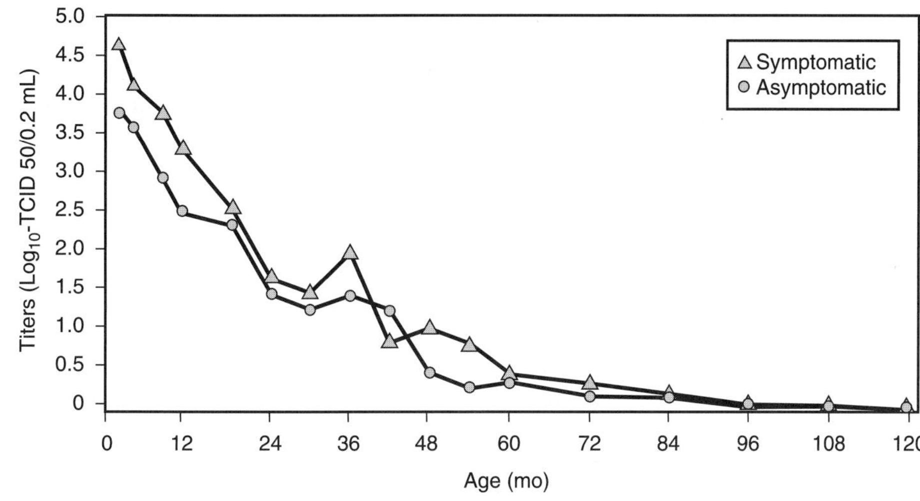

Figure 23–2 Quantitative assessment of cytomegalovirus excretion in subjects with congenital symptomatic *(triangles)* and congenital asymptomatic *(circles)* infections.

detectable in seriously ill immunocompromised older patients. As shown in Figure 23-2, the highest quantities of virus are excreted during the first 6 months of life. Infants with symptomatic congenital CMV infection excrete significantly larger amounts than those with asymptomatic congenitally or perinatally acquired infections.

PATHOLOGY

Overview

Early reports of histopathologic changes associated with CMV infections relied on a demonstration of classic changes characterized by cytomegaly and nuclear and cytoplasmic inclusions.[300,346] The distinctive features include large cells 20 to 35 mm in diameter with a large nucleus containing round, oval, or reniform inclusions. These large inclusions are separated from the nuclear membrane by a clear zone, which gives the inclusion the so-called owl's-eye appearance. The inclusions within the nucleus show DNA positivity by histochemical staining, whereas the cytoplasmic inclusions contain carbohydrates, as evidenced by periodic acid–Schiff positivity. The cytoplasmic inclusions vary from minute dots to distinct rounded bodies 3 to 4 mm in diameter. The cytoplasmic inclusions are usually aggregated opposite to the eccentrically placed inclusion-bearing nucleus. Unfortunately, the classic CMV inclusion-bearing cell may be only scattered throughout involved tissue and missed by routine sectioning. This finding has been confirmed when more refined techniques such as in situ DNA hybridization and immunofluorescence using CMV-specific monoclonal antibodies have been used to define the extent of infection with CMV in immunocompromised patients.

Disseminated disease can occur in the infected fetus and congenitally infected infant. CMV can cause a multisystem disease in which almost all major organ systems are involved.[300]

Commonly Involved Organ Systems

Central Nervous System

Involvement of the CNS is perhaps the most important consequence of fetal infection with CMV. Most descriptions of the pathology of CNS infection are relevant only to infants with severe CID, which is occasionally fatal.[347-349] The infection can be described grossly as focal encephalitis and periependymitis. The encephalitis can involve cells of the gray matter and white matter and cells within the choroid plexus. Inclusion-bearing cells have been identified in neurons, glia, ependyma, choroid plexus, meninges, and vascular endothelium, and in cells lying free in the ventricles. Rarely, inclusion-bearing cells have been identified in the cerebrospinal fluid.[350] Resolution of acute encephalitis leads to gliosis and calcification. Previous descriptions have emphasized the periventricular location of calcifications; however, these lesions can be located anywhere in the brain.[351,352] CMV has been isolated on a few occasions from cerebrospinal fluid.[353]

Viral inclusion-bearing cells and viral antigen-containing cells can also be found within structures of the inner ear, including the organ of Corti, and in epithelial cells of striae vascularis of the cochleae.[165,354-356] Involvement of the eye, including chorioretinitis, optic neuritis, cataract formation, colobomas, and microphthalmos, has been demonstrated.[165,349] The histopathologic changes associated with retinitis begin as an acute vasculitis that spreads into the choroid through the vascular basement membrane. CMV has been isolated from fluid of the anterior chamber of the eye.[357]

Liver

Involvement of the liver is common in congenital CMV infections. Clinical evidence of hepatitis as manifested by hepatomegaly, elevated levels of serum transaminases, and direct hyperbilirubinemia is frequently seen in infants with symptomatic congenital infections. Pathologic descriptions of hepatic involvement include mild cholangitis with CMV infections of bile duct cells, intralobular cholestasis, and obstructive cholestasis caused by extramedullary hematopoiesis.[348] Liver calcification has been detected radiologically in infants with congenital infections.[358,359] Clinical and laboratory evidence of liver disease eventually subsides in surviving infants.

Hematopoietic System

Hematologic abnormalities, including thrombocytopenia, anemia, and extramedullary hematopoieses, are common in symptomatically infected infants, but these abnormalities almost invariably resolve within the first year of life. The exact mechanism accounting for these disturbances is not certain, although congestive splenomegaly resulting in platelet and red blood cell trapping must play some part in the overall process. Major splenomegaly is common, and congestion, extramedullary hematopoiesis, and diminished size of lymphoid follicles can be seen histologically.

In congenital CMV infections, thrombocytopenia may persist for several months, even years, with or without petechiae. At least in animal models, direct infection of megakaryocytes has been found and postulated as a possible mechanism.[360] Anemia is another feature of symptomatic congenital CMV infection. The presence of indirect hyperbilirubinemia, extramedullary hematopoiesis, and erythroblastemia indicates active hemolysis, but mechanisms for these effects have not been elucidated.

Kidneys

Macroscopically, the kidneys show no alterations. Microscopically, inclusion-bearing cells are commonly seen, especially in the cells lining the distal convoluted tubules and collecting ducts.[361,362] Affected cells may desquamate into the lumina of the tubules and appear in the urine sediment. Inclusions can be found occasionally in Bowman's capsules and proximal tubules. Mononuclear cell infiltration may be present in the peritubular zones of the kidney.

Endocrine Glands

Secretory cells of endocrine glands commonly contain typical CMV inclusions. In the pancreas, the endocrine and exocrine cells are affected.[300] Some reports describe intralobular or periductal mononuclear infiltration, suggesting focal pancreatitis. There is no indication of an association between congenital CMV infection and diabetes mellitus. CMV inclusion-bearing cells have been documented in follicular cells of the thyroid, the adrenal cortex, and the anterior pituitary.

Gastrointestinal Tract

The salivary glands are commonly involved in congenital and perinatal CMV infections. However, there are no reliable figures on the frequency of involvement because the examination of the salivary glands is not always part of autopsies.[362] CMV inclusions have also been described in the mucosal surfaces of the esophagus, stomach, and intestine and in the vessels of ulcerative intestinal lesions.[363]

Lungs

Pulmonary CMV lesions are similar in the newborn and the adult. Microscopically, most inclusion-bearing cells are alveolar cells that lay free in terminal air spaces. In general, there is little inflammatory reaction; however, in the more severe cases, focal interstitial infiltration by lymphocytes and plasma cells can be found.

Placenta

Abnormalities occur in the placentas of most patients with symptomatic CMV infection and are uncommon with subclinical infections.[364] Placentas are not remarkable in size or macroscopic appearance. The most specific feature histologically is the presence of inclusion-bearing cells, which may be found in endothelial cells, in cells attached to the capillary walls, or in Hofbauer's or stromal cells.[364,365] Other lesions include focal necrosis, which in early gestation shows sparse infiltration by lymphocytes, macrophages, and a few plasma cells. The early lesions manifest as foci of necrosis of the stroma and occasionally of the vessels of the villi. The focus of necrosis is later invaded by inflammatory cells, histiocytes, and fibroblasts. At later gestational ages, these focal lesions become densely cellular, with plasma cells predominating over lymphocytes. Deposition of intracellular and extracellular hemosiderin can be found in stem and terminal villi and is presumably the result of fetal hemorrhage during the necrotizing phase or of maternal intervillous thrombosis. Calcification within villi or on basement membranes has been described as a late manifestation of placental CMV infection.

CLINICAL MANIFESTATIONS

Congenital Infection

Approximately 10% of the estimated 44,000 infants (1% of all livebirths) born annually with congenital CMV infection in the United States have signs and symptoms at birth that would lead the physician to suspect a congenital infection. Only one half of these symptomatic infants have typical generalized CID, characterized mainly by the clinical manifestations given in Table 23-9.[303,366] Another 5% of these infants present with milder or atypical involvement, and 90% are born with subclinical but chronic infection. Because early studies emphasized symptomatic infections, congenital CMV was considered a rare and often fatal disease. In the early reports, many patients were referred to the investigators because of developmental problems; this might have automatically highlighted a group of patients at a higher risk for persistent abnormalities and neurologic damage. The use of more sensitive and specific methods of diagnosis, particularly viral isolation, has allowed prospective longitudinal study of newborns with symptomatic and asymptomatic congenital CMV infections. This has resulted in a better understanding of the infection and its clinical spectrum.

Symptomatic Infection

ACUTE MANIFESTATIONS

Clinically apparent infections or CID is characterized by involvement of multiple organs, particularly the reticuloendothelial system and CNS, with or without ocular and auditory damage. Weller and Hanshaw[366] defined the abnormalities found most frequently in infants with symptomatic congenital infection as hepatomegaly, splenomegaly, microcephaly, jaundice, and petechiae. As shown in Table 23-11, petechiae, hepatosplenomegaly, and jaundice are the most common presenting signs.

The magnitude of the prenatal insult is demonstrated by the occurrence of microcephaly with or without cerebral calcification, intrauterine growth retardation, and prematurity.[86,303,307,309,327,367-370] Inguinal hernia in males and chorioretinitis with or without optic atrophy are less common. Clinical findings occasionally include hydrocephalus, hemolytic anemia, and pneumonitis. Among the most severely affected infants, the mortality rate may be as high as 30%.[301] Most

Table 23–11 Clinical and Laboratory Findings for 106 Infants with Symptomatic Congenital Cytomegalovirus Infection in the Newborn Period

Abnormality	Positive/Total Examined (%)
Prematurity (<38 wk)	36/106 (34)
Small for gestational age	53/106 (50)
Petechiae	80/106 (76)
Jaundice	69/103 (67)
Hepatosplenomegaly	63/105 (60)
Purpura	14/105 (13)
Neurologic findings	
One or more of the following	72/106 (68)
Microcephaly	54/102 (53)
Lethargy/hypotonia	28/104 (27)
Poor suck	20/103 (19)
Seizures	7/105 (7)
Elevated alanine aminotransferase (>80 U/L)	46/58 (83)
Thrombocytopenia	
$<100 \times 10^3/mm^3$	62/81 (77)
$<50 \times 10^3/mm^3$	43/81 (53)
Conjugated hyperbilirubinemia	
Direct serum bilirubin >4 mg/dL	47/68 (69)
Hemolysis	37/72 (51)
Increased cerebrospinal fluid protein (>120 mg/dL)[a]	24/52 (46)

[a]Determinations in the first week of life.

From Boppana S, Pass RF, Britt WS, et al. Symptomatic congenital cytomegalovirus infection: neonatal morbidity and mortality. Pediatr Infect Dis J 11:93-99, 1992.

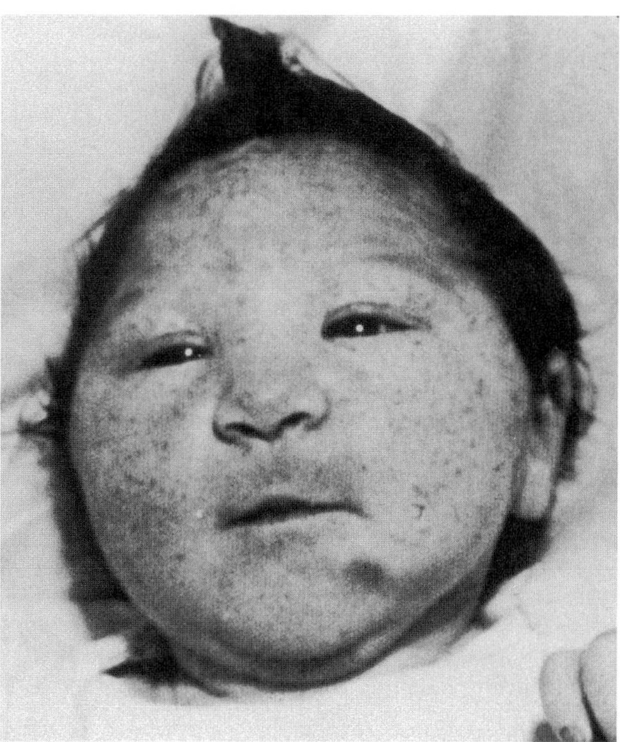

Figure 23–3 Symptomatic congenital cytomegalovirus infection is manifested by microcephaly and petechiae.

deaths occur in the neonatal period and usually are caused by multiorgan disease with severe hepatic dysfunction, bleeding, disseminated intravascular coagulation, and secondary bacterial infections. When death occurs after the first month but during the first year, it typically is caused by progressive liver disease with severe failure to thrive. Death after the first year usually is restricted to severely neurologically handicapped children and is caused by malnutrition, aspiration pneumonia, and overwhelming infections.

Hepatomegaly. This sign, along with splenomegaly, is probably the most common abnormality found in the newborn period in infants born with a symptomatic congenital CMV infection.[370] The liver edge is smooth and nontender and usually measures 4 to 7 cm below the right costal margin. Liver function tests are often abnormal but usually not markedly so. The persistence of hepatomegaly is variable. In some infants, liver enlargement disappears by the age of 2 months. In others, significant enlargement persists throughout the first year of life. However, massive hepatomegaly extending beyond the first 12 months of life is uncharacteristic of CID.

Splenomegaly. Enlargement of the spleen exists to a greater or lesser degree in all the common human congenital infections and is especially frequent in congenital CMV infections.[303,370] It may be the only abnormality present at birth. In some instances, splenomegaly and a petechial rash coexist as the only manifestations of the disease. Occasionally, the enlargement is such that the spleen may be felt 10 to 15 cm below the costal margin. Splenomegaly usually persists longer than hepatomegaly does.

Jaundice. Jaundice is a common manifestation of congenital CID. The pattern of hyperbilirubinemia may take several forms, ranging from high levels on the first day to undetectable jaundice on the first day with gradual elevation of the bilirubin level to clinically apparent jaundice. The level of jaundice in the early weeks of life may fluctuate considerably.[303,370] In some instances, jaundice is a transient phenomenon, beginning on the first day and disappearing by the end of the first week. More often, however, jaundice tends to persist beyond the time of physiologic jaundice. Transient jaundice may occasionally occur in early infancy with pronounced elevation of bilirubin levels during the third month. Bilirubin levels are high in the direct and the indirect components. Characteristically, the direct component increases after the first few days of life and may constitute as much as 50% of the total bilirubin level. It is rare for the indirect bilirubin component to rise high enough to require an exchange transfusion, but this has been reported.

Petechiae and Purpura. There is evidence that CMV has a direct effect on the megakaryocytes of the bone marrow that results in a depression of the platelets and a localized or generalized petechial rash.[360,370] In some patients, the rash is purpuric (Fig. 23-3), not unlike that observed in the expanded rubella syndrome. Unlike the latter infection, however, pinpoint petechiae are a more common manifestation. These petechiae are rarely present at birth but often appear within a few hours thereafter; they may be transient, disappearing within 48 hours. The petechiae may be the only clinical manifestation of CMV infection. More often, however, enlargement of the spleen and liver is associated. The petechiae may persist for weeks after birth. Crying, coughing, the application of a tourniquet, a lumbar puncture, or restraints of any kind may result in the appearance of petechiae even months after birth. Platelet counts in the first week of life range from less than 10,000 to 125,000, and most counts are in the 20,000 to 60,000 range. Some infants with petechial rashes do not have associated thrombocytopenia.

Microcephaly. Microcephaly, usually defined as a head circumference of less than the fifth percentile, affected 14 of 17 patients with CID in the early studies of Medearis in 1964.[371] As tissue culture methods became more widely used and clinical awareness of the infection increased, microcephaly became a less prominent symptom in subsequent series that included mainly infants born with less severe disease. In an examination of 106 surviving patients who were born with symptomatic CMV infection, 53% were microcephalic.[303] Not all infants with microcephaly continue to have head circumferences of less than the third percentile.[370] Microcephaly is the most specific predictor of mental retardation (this is especially true if the head measurement is close to the fifth percentile in an infant of low birth weight). Intracranial calcifications are an indication that the infant will have at least moderate and probably severe mental retardation.

Ocular Defects. The principal abnormality related to the eye in CMV infection is chorioretinitis, with strabismus and optic atrophy.[303,367,370] Microphthalmos, cataracts, retinal necrosis and calcification, blindness, anterior chamber and optic disk malformations, and pupillary membrane vestiges have also been described in association with generalized congenital CID. Despite these findings, the presence of abnormalities such as microphthalmos and cataracts is strong presumptive evidence that the disease process is not caused by CMV. Chorioretinitis occurs in approximately 14% of infants born with symptomatic congenital infection.[303,367] Although chorioretinitis occurs less frequently in symptomatic congenital CMV than in congenital toxoplasmosis, lesions caused by CMV and *Toxoplasma* cannot be differentiated on the basis of location or appearance.[165,367] *Toxoplasma gondii* and CMV can induce central retinal lesions. Occasionally, the appearance of strabismus with subsequent referral to an ophthalmologist is the means by which chorioretinitis is detected. Any infant with suspected CMV infection or strabismus in early life should be examined carefully for retinal lesions. Chorioretinitis caused by CMV differs from that caused by *Toxoplasma* in that postnatal progression is uncommon.[367]

Fetal Growth Retardation. Intrauterine growth retardation, occasionally severe, was reported in 50% of 106 patients with symptomatic congenital CMV infection, whereas prematurity occurred in 34% (see Table 23-11).[303] Infants with asymptomatic congenital infection in general show no intrauterine growth retardation or prematurity, and CMV cannot be considered an important cause of either condition.

Pneumonitis. Pneumonitis, a common clinical manifestation of CMV infection after bone marrow and renal transplantation in adults, is not usually a part of the clinical presentation of congenital CMV infection in newborns. Diffuse interstitial pneumonitis occurs in less than 1% of congenitally infected infants, even when the most severely affected cases are considered. As is discussed in greater detail later, CMV-associated pneumonitis is more likely to develop in infants with perinatally acquired CMV infections.[372]

Dental Defects. Congenital CMV infection is also associated with a distinct defect of enamel, which seems to affect mainly primary dentition.[373] This defect is more severe in children with the symptomatic form of the infection than in those born with asymptomatic infections (Fig. 23-4).

Clinically, this defect appears on all or most of the teeth and is characterized by generalized yellowish discoloration.

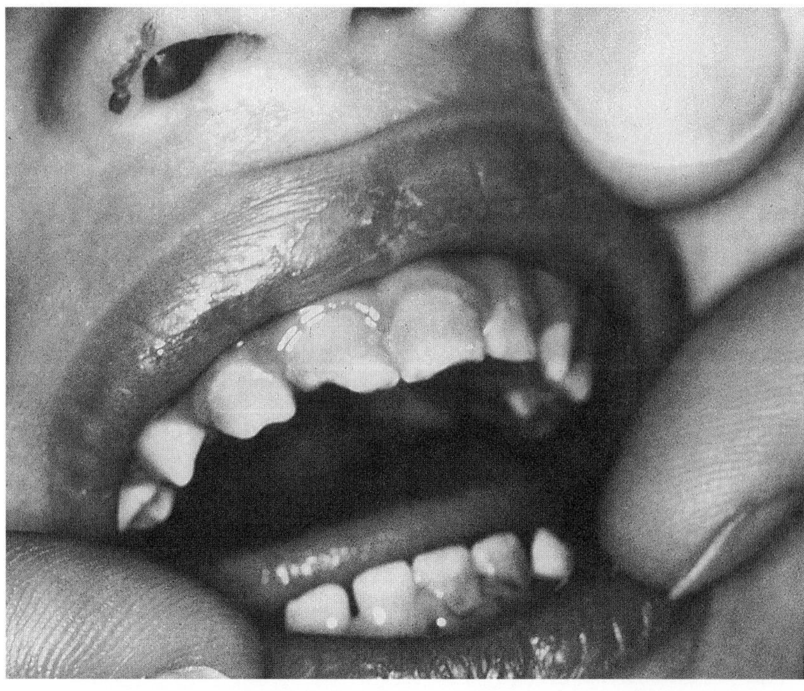

Figure 23–4 Cytomegalovirus (CMV)–affected teeth. This patient had a clinically severe congenital CMV infection. Notice the fractured borders and opaque and hypocalcified enamel.

The enamel is opaque and moderately soft and tends to chip away from dentin. Affected teeth tend to wear down rapidly, leading to dental caries frequently seen in these children. In our longitudinal studies, this defect of enamel was documented in 27% of 92 children born with symptomatic congenital CMV infection and in 4% of 267 who were born with the subclinical form and who were observed for at least 2 years.[373] These patients usually require extensive orthodontic therapy. It is evident that these defects do not involve permanent teeth to the same degree.

Deafness. Sensorineural deafness is the most common handicap caused by congenital CMV infection. Medearis[371] was the first investigator to call attention to the presence of deafness in symptomatic congenitally infected infants. Subsequent reports confirmed this association and provided evidence that CMV can also cause sensorineural hearing loss in children with subclinical congenital infection.[133,165-168,304,309,316,374-381] CMV is now one of the most important causes of deafness in childhood. CMV can replicate in many structures of the inner ear, as demonstrated by typical CMV-induced cytopathology in Reissner's membrane, stria vascularis, and semicircular canals or by CMV-specific immunofluorescence in the organ of Corti and neurons of the eighth nerve.[165,317,318,354-356] The distribution of viral antigens is far more extensive than viral cellular cytolysis. The presence of an inflammatory response suggests the possibility that immune damage in the inner ear may also be a contributing factor.

The frequency and severity of the hearing impairment are worse in patients with symptomatic infection (58%) compared with asymptomatic infection at birth (7.4%). In general, hearing loss is progressive in 50%, is bilateral in 50%, and has a late onset in 20% of cases. The predictors of hearing loss in children with symptomatic congenital CMV infection are intrauterine growth retardation, petechiae, hepatosplenomegaly, thrombocytopenia, and intracerebral calcifications. The presence of microcephaly and other neurologic abnormalities does not predict hearing loss. Using logistic regression analysis, only petechiae and intrauterine growth retardation are independent predictors of hearing loss.

LONG-TERM OUTCOME

The likelihood of survival with normal intellect and hearing after symptomatic congenital CMV infection is small.[133,303,316,367,368,371,375-377,382,383] As shown in Table 23-12, in our prospective studies, one or more handicaps have occurred in almost 90% of the patients with symptomatic congenital infection who survived.[303]

Psychomotor retardation, usually combined with neurologic complications and microcephaly, occurred in almost 70% of the patients. Sensorineural hearing loss was seen in 50%. The hearing loss is bilateral in 67% of patients with hearing loss and is progressive in 54%. Chorioretinitis or optic atrophy occurred in 20% of cases. Expressive language delays independent from hearing loss and mental impairment have also been described. Several studies have searched for clinical predictors of intelligence and developmental outcome and found that microcephaly at birth, development of neurologic problems during the first year of life, ocular lesions (e.g., chorioretinitis), and microcephaly that became apparent after birth were significantly associated with a low IQ and developmental quotient. The best predictor of adverse neurodevelopmental outcome is the presence of cranial computed tomographic (CT) abnormalities detected within the first month of life.[309] In infants with symptomatic congenital CMV infection, abnormal CT findings, particularly intracerebral calcifications, are common (70%). Almost 90% of children with abnormal newborn CT scans develop at least one sequela compared with 29% among those with a normal study.[309] In this particular study, which included 56 children with symptomatic congenital CMV, only 1 child with a normal CT scan had an IQ of less than 70, in contrast to 59% of those with imaging abnormalities. Newborn CT abnormalities were also associated with an abnormal hearing screen at birth and hearing loss on follow-up. None of the neonatal neurologic findings was predictive of an abnormal CT finding.[309] Overall, it can be anticipated that between 90% and 95% of infants with symptomatic

Table 23–12 Sequelae in Children after Congenital Cytomegalovirus Infection

Sequelae	Percent Symptomatic (n/N)	Percent Asymptomatic (n/N)
Sensorineural hearing loss	58 (58/100)	7.4 (22/299)
Bilateral hearing loss	37 (37/100)	2.7 (8/299)
Speech threshold moderate to profound (60-90 dB)[a]	27 (27/100)	1.7 (5/299)
Chorioretinitis	20.4 (19/93)	2.5 (7/281)
IQ <70	55 (33/60)	3.7 (6/159)
Microcephaly, seizures, or paresis/paralysis	51.9 (54/104)	2.7 (9/330)
Microcephaly	37.5 (39/104)	1.8 (6/330)
Seizures	23.1 (24/104)	0.9 (3/330)
Paresis/paralysis	12.5 (13/104)	0 (0/330)
Death[b]	5.8 (6/104)	0.3 (1/330)

[a]For the ear with better hearing.
[b]After the newborn period.
Data from Pass RF, Fowler KB, Boppana S. Progress in cytomegalovirus research. *In* Landini MP (ed). Proceedings of the Third International Cytomegalovirus Workshop, Bologna, Italy, June 1991. London, Excerpta Medica, 1991, pp 3-10.

congenital infections who survive will develop mild to severe handicaps.

Asymptomatic Infection

As indicated in the previous section, almost 90% of infants with congenital CMV infections have no early clinical manifestations, and their long-term outcome is much better. Nevertheless, there is solid evidence derived from controlled, prospective studies that at least 10% of these infants, and perhaps as many as 15%, are at risk of developing a multitude of developmental abnormalities, such as sensorineural hearing loss, microcephaly, motor defects (e.g., spastic diplegia or quadriplegia), mental retardation, chorioretinitis, dental defects, and others. These abnormalities usually become apparent within the first 2 years of life.[165,167,324,374,375,378,379,384-386] Table 23-12 shows results based on our prospective longitudinal study of 330 patients with asymptomatic congenital infection who were followed by using serial clinical, psychometric, audiometric, and visual assessments.[303] Follow-up studies of patients with inapparent congenital CMV infection have also been done by Kumar and colleagues,[378] Saigal and associates,[375] Melish and Hanshaw,[374] Pearl and co-workers,[380] Williamson and colleagues,[384] Preece and associates,[331] Harris and co-workers,[324] Conboy and colleagues,[381] Ivarsson and associates,[385] Fowler and colleagues,[167] Kashden and co-workers,[386] and Noyola and associates.[387] In general, their findings resemble the results of our study presented in Table 23-12. Most patients in these studies and their controls were from a low socioeconomic background.

The most significant abnormality in children born with subclinical congenital CMV infection is hearing loss. Fowler and associates[167] evaluated 307 children with documented asymptomatic congenital CMV infection and compared their audiometric assessments with 76 uninfected siblings of children with asymptomatic congenital CMV infection and 201 children whose neonatal screen for this infection showed negative results. Sensorineural hearing loss occurred only in children with congenital CMV infection. Among them, 22 (7.2%) had hearing loss. In 11 (50%) of the 22 children, the hearing loss was bilateral. Among the children with hearing loss, further deterioration of hearing occurred in 50% with a medial age at first progression of 18 months (range, 2 to 70 months). Delayed onset of sensorineural hearing loss occurred in 18% of the children with the medial age of detection at 27 months (range, 25 to 62 months). Fluctuating hearing loss was documented in 22.7% of the children with hearing loss. These results are very similar to those obtained by Williamson and co-workers in Houston.[384] A study in Sweden of more than 10,000 newborns screened for hearing loss and congenital CMV infection found that this congenital infection was the leading cause of sensorineural hearing loss accounting for 40% of the cases with hearing loss.[324] In our group, Hicks and co-workers[388] found 14 cases of congenital CMV infection with sensorineural hearing loss in 12,371 neonates screened for CMV, a rate of approximately 1.1 per 1000 livebirths. The rate was 0.6 per 1000 livebirths when only cases with bilateral loss of 50 dB or greater were considered. These results suggest that CMV infection accounts for at least one third of sensorineural hearing loss in young children.[388] Taken together, these studies indicate that the universal screening for hearing loss in vogue in the United States will detect less than one half of all the cases of sensorineural hearing loss caused by congenital CMV infection. Because most of these infants are asymptomatic at birth, they are not recognized as being at high risk for hearing loss and are not being further tested to detect late onset hearing loss. The universal screening of neonates for hearing loss needs to be combined with a screening for congenital CMV infections.

Prospective studies of children with subclinical congenital CMV infections have revealed a wide but significant spectrum of neurologic complications.[384] It has been estimated that within the first 2 years of life, 2% to 7% of the infants in this group develop microcephaly with various degrees of mental retardation and neuromuscular defects. How often milder forms of brain damage, such as learning or behavioral difficulties, will occur as these patients grow older is unknown. Studies of the intellectual development of children with asymptomatic congenital CMV infections have shown conflicting results. However, one study evaluated 204 prospectively followed children with asymptomatic congenital CMV infections and 177 uninfected siblings ranging in age from 6 to 203 months.[381] Parents were administered the Developmental Profile, and the children were administered an objective intelligence measure. Results showed that children with asymptomatic congenital CMV infection do not demonstrate intellectual impairment and that they perform similarly to uninfected siblings.

Children with asymptomatic congenital CMV infections are at low risk for developing chorioretinitis. The current estimate is that it occurs in 2% of these children, and like hearing loss, it may not exist at birth.

In summary, these observations underscore the need for longitudinal follow-up of patients with congenital CMV infection regardless of the initial clinical presentation. Careful assessments of perceptual functions (e.g., hearing, visual acuity), psychomotor development, and learning abilities must be made to recognize the full impact of CMV. With early identification of a problem, corrective measures can be instituted to reduce psychosocial and learning problems.

Effect of Type of Maternal Infection on Symptoms and Long-Term Outcome

Studies have clearly demonstrated that preexisting maternal immunity does not prevent CMV from reactivating during pregnancy and cannot reliably prevent transmission in utero nor symptomatic congenital infections.[114-118,120,326,334-341,389,390] A prospective study of young, predominantly African American women with one or more previous deliveries were evaluated to quantify the protection conferred by preconception maternal immunity.[391] For the almost 3500 multiparous women who had previously delivered newborns screened for congenital CMV infection and who subsequently became part of this study, the overall rate of congenital CMV infection was 1.3%. Congenital infection occurred in 18 (3.0%) of 604 newborns (95% CI, 1.8% to 4.7%) born to initially seronegative mothers compared with 29 (1.0%) among the 2857 births (95% CI, 0.7% to 1.4%) to immune mothers. Of the initially seronegative women, 23.5% seroconverted for an annualized seroconversion rate of 7.8% per year with 12.7% of these seroconversions resulting in congenital CMV infection. Only 1% of infants born to mothers immune to CMV before conception had congenital infection. These results show that young women who have immunity to CMV from naturally acquired infections are 69% less likely to have a baby with congenital CMV infections in the future than are those who are initially seronegative. This study also demonstrated a strong relationship between an increased rate of congenital CMV infection and short interval from initial CMV antibody test to subsequent birth among seropositive women. This observation indicates that some of the initially seropositive women had recently experienced primary infection and therefore had increased risk for congenital CMV infection.

It is generally recognized that primary infection has a higher risk of symptomatic infection; however, data that have emerged in recent years, including our own prospective studies, raise the possibility that recurrent maternal infection may result in adverse outcome more frequently than previously thought. In 1999, prospective studies carried out in Sweden[392] and the United States[393] reported the presence of symptomatology at birth and the development of long-term sequelae in children born with congenital CMV infection after a recurrence of maternal infection. Our study[393] included 246 children (1.18%) with congenital CMV infection from the screening of 20,885 neonates. Of the 246 infants, 47 were symptomatic at birth, and 8 (17%) of the 47 were born to mothers with recurrent CMV infection as defined by seropositive status at the time of a previous pregnancy. Demographically, the women in this study have been characterized as predominantly black (93%), single (96%), young (46% ≤20 years old), and without private insurance. A study of this population concluded that in women who are seropositive for CMV, reinfection with different strains of CMV rather than reactivation of the endogenous strain could lead to intrauterine transmission and symptomatic congenital infection. In contrast, the study of women who are predominantly white, married, of middle to high socioeconomic background, and somewhat older has not revealed the occurrence of symptomatic congenital CMV infection as a result of a recurrence of maternal infection.

Public Health Significance

The public health impact of congenital CMV infection in the United States is significant, as shown in Table 23-13. With an average incidence of 1% and a birth rate of 4 million per annum, approximately 40,000 infants are born each year with congenital CMV infections. Of these, as many as 2800 present with signs and symptoms of infection (e.g., CID). About 336 of them can be expected to die within the first year, and almost 2160 of the survivors develop handicaps. Another 5580 or so among the subclinically infected develop significant hearing and mental deficits. In addition to the personal and family suffering associated with these conditions, the cost to society for caring for all these children must amount to millions of dollars annually.

Table 23–13 Public Health Impact of Congenital Cytomegalovirus Infection in the United States

Parameter	Estimate
No. of live births per year	4,000,000
Rate of congenital CMV infection (average)	1%
No. of infected infants	40,000
No. of infants symptomatic at birth (5%-7%)	2800
No. with fatal disease (±12%)	336
No. with sequelae (90% of survivors)	2160
No. of infants asymptomatic at birth (93%-95%)	37,200
No. with late sequelae (15%)	5580
Total no. with sequelae or fatal outcome	8076

Perinatal Infection

Perinatal infections can be acquired from exposure to virus in the maternal genital tract at delivery, from breast milk, or through multiple blood transfusions.[89,90,96,342,344,394,395] To establish the diagnosis of perinatal CMV infection, the examiner must first exclude congenital infection by showing an absence of viral excretion during the first 2 weeks of life. The incubation period of perinatal CMV infection ranges between 4 and 12 weeks. Although the quantity of virus excreted by infants with perinatal infection is less than that seen with intrauterine acquisition, the infection is also chronic, with viral excretion persisting for years.[301]

Most infants with naturally acquired perinatal infections remain asymptomatic. Most of these infections result from reactivation of maternal virus, and infants therefore are born with variable levels of maternal antibody. Asymptomatic perinatal CMV infection in full-term and otherwise healthy infants does not appear to have an adverse effect on growth, perceptual functions, or motor or psychosocial development. CMV has been incriminated as a cause of pneumonitis in infants younger than 4 months.[90,344,372,396,397] In a study undertaken to define the possible association of CMV and other respiratory pathogens with pneumonitis in young infants, CMV was isolated in 21 (21%) of 104 patients enrolled.[372] Only 3% of 97 hospitalized controls were infected. CMV-associated pneumonitis occurs throughout the year in contrast to the common respiratory virus infections, which occur most often in winter and early spring.

CMV-associated pneumonitis is clinically and radiographically indistinguishable from other types of afebrile pneumonia caused by agents such as *Chlamydia trachomatis* and respiratory syncytial virus. Clinically, patients with CMV-associated pneumonitis have an afebrile course with tachypnea, cough (sometimes paroxysmal), occasional episodes of apnea, coryza, nasal congestion, intercostal retractions, and radiographic evidence of diffuse lower airway obstruction (e.g., air trapping, thickened bronchial walls with prominent pulmonary markings and various degrees of atelectasis). Expiratory wheezing is unusual. Laboratory findings include elevated levels of one or more serum immunoglobulins (especially IgM, in 66% of patients), leukocytosis of more than 12,000 white blood cells/mm^3 (59%), and absolute eosinophilia. The median time of hospitalization is 17 days. Some infants require oxygen therapy and ventilatory assistance. Long-term follow-up of patients with pneumonitis associated with CMV and other respiratory pathogens provides evidence that significant mortality and morbidity do occur irrespective of the etiologic agent.[397]

In premature and ill term infants, Yeager and colleagues[398] found that naturally acquired CMV infection may pose a greater risk. They found that premature infants weighing less than 1500 g at birth who acquired CMV from a maternal source often developed hepatosplenomegaly, neutropenia, lymphocytosis, and thrombocytopenia, coinciding with the onset of virus excretion. Frequently, infected patients required longer treatment with oxygen than uninfected patients. In a later study, Paryani and co-workers[399] from the same group reported a prospective study of 55 premature infants, including controls, and suggested that there might be a propensity for an increased incidence of neuromuscular impairments, particularly in premature infants with the onset of CMV excretion during the first 2 months of life. However, sensorineural hearing loss, chorioretinitis, and microcephaly occurred with similar frequency in both groups. Similar findings were reported by Vochem[342] and Maschmann.[344]

Transfusion-acquired perinatal CMV infection can cause significant morbidity and mortality, particularly in premature infants with a birth weight of less than 1500 g born to CMV-seronegative mothers.[134,394,395] The syndrome of post-transfusion CMV infection in premature newborns was characterized by Ballard and co-workers.[400] They isolated CMV from 16 of 51 preterm infants of a mean birth weight of 1000 g and found that 14 of the 16 virus-positive infants had a constellation of symptoms that resembled CID. This recognizable, self-limited syndrome consisted of deterioration of respiratory function, hepatosplenomegaly, unusual gray pallor with disturbing septic appearance, an atypical and an absolute lymphocytosis, thrombocytopenia, and hemolytic anemia. The syndrome was more severe in low-birth-weight infants and occurred 4 to 12 weeks after the transfusion, when the infants were progressing satisfactorily. Although the course of the disease was generally self-limited (lasting 2 to 3 weeks), death occurred in 20% of the ill infants. Subsequent work by Yeager and associates[269] and Adler[401] confirmed these observations. The risk of infection is greater with an increasing number of units of blood transfused. Yeager and associates[269] demonstrated that the risk of infection is related to the serologic status of the donor and that these infections could be prevented by transfusing seronegative newborns with blood from seronegative donors.

DIAGNOSIS

Detection of Virus

The diagnosis of congenital CMV infection should be entertained in any newborn with signs of congenital infection or if there is a history of maternal seroconversion or a mononucleosis-like illness during pregnancy. The best test is virus isolation in tissue culture, which is generally accomplished with urine or saliva or with demonstration of CMV genetic material by PCR (Table 23-14).[295,299,346,402-405]

CMV-IgM serology does not have adequate sensitivity or specificity for the diagnosis of congenital CMV infection. With diagnostic methods that detect the virus, viral antigens, and nucleic acids, it is possible to confirm the diagnosis from blood, cerebrospinal fluid, and biopsy material. Of particular interest is the possibility of diagnosis by PCR on blood stored on filter paper.[404] To confirm a congenital CMV infection, demonstration of virus must be attempted in the first 2 weeks of life because viral excretion after that time may represent an infection acquired at birth (natal) by exposure to an infected birth canal or one acquired in the neonatal period by exposure to breast milk or blood products. Although isolation of CMV during the first 2 weeks of life proves a congenital CMV infection, it does not necessarily confirm an etiologic relationship with an existing disease. Urine and saliva are the preferred specimens for culture because they contain larger amounts of virus. The viability of CMV is surprisingly good when specimens are properly stored. For instance, when positive urine specimens (without preservatives) are stored at 4° C for 7 days, the rate of isolation drops to 93%; it drops to only 50% after 1 month of storage.[404] However, storage and transport at ambient temperature or freezing should never be used because infectivity is rapidly and significantly reduced.

Table 23–14 Diagnostic Methods for Identification of Infants with Congenital Cytomegalovirus Infection

Method	Advantages	Disadvantages
Detection of Virus or Viral Antigens		
Standard tube culture method	Standard reference method	Takes 2-4 weeks, not suitable for screening
Shell vial assay[83]	Rapid, sensitive, commercially available	Expensive, not suitable for screening
Microtiter plate immunofluorescent antibody assay[84,85]	Rapid, sensitive, reliable, simple, inexpensive	Cell culture based, not commercially available
CMV antigenemia[86]	Rapid and simple	Unknown sensitivity and utility to screen newborns, expensive
Nucleic Acid Amplification Methods		
DNA hybridization assay[87]	Sensitive and reliable	Complicated, need for a radiolabeled probe
PCR amplification methods[88-90]	Simple and can be used to screen large numbers	Utility as a screening assay not proved
Serologic Methods		
Anti-CMV IgM antibody assay	Simple and widely available	Low sensitivity and not reliable for screening

CMV, cytomegalovirus; PCR, polymerase chain reaction.
Data from Boppana and Fowler, personal communication, 2004.

Tissue Culture

Standard tissue culture based viral isolation requires inoculation of specimen into monolayers of human fibroblasts. Typically, 2 to 4 weeks may be required for the appearance of the characteristic cytopathic effect. Since 1980, methods for rapid viral diagnosis have become available. Several modifications of the standard tissue culture method combined with immunologic detection of immediate-early CMV-induced antigens have maintained high specificity and sensitivity but allowed the confirmation of diagnosis within 24 hours of inoculation of the clinical specimen.[406-411]

Typically, tissue culture includes the use of monoclonal antibodies to CMV-specific early antigens with low-speed centrifugation of the clinical specimens onto the monolayer of fibroblasts growing on coverslips inside shell vials.[408-410] When this method was evaluated with clinical specimens (i.e., blood; urine; bronchoscopy lavage; lung, liver, and kidney biopsy samples; sputum; and others) obtained primarily from immunosuppressed patients, the sensitivity approached 80%, and the specificity ranged from 80% to 100%. Subsequently, another adaptation of this rapid immunofluorescent assay used 96-well microtiter plates and a monoclonal antibody that is reactive with the major immediate-early human CMV protein polypeptide 72.[411] This rapid assay detected all but 1 of 19 specimens identified by standard virus isolation method from 1676 newborn urine specimens, achieving a sensitivity of 94.5% and a specificity of 100%. This test retained high sensitivity and specificity when saliva instead of urine was tested.[403] This microtiter plate method using saliva or urine samples is the most rapid, simple to perform, and inexpensive alternative to the standard virus isolation method. It is perfectly suitable for mass screening, and there is no drop in sensitivity for specimens at 4° C for up to 3 days. This study also showed that the sensitivity of the microtiter plate method declined rapidly for specimens from older infants and children with congenital CMV infection and from virus-infected children attending daycare centers. It is not recommended for screening or diagnosing CMV infections in older infants and children.

DNA Hybridization

Rapid diagnosis of CMV can also be accomplished by DNA hybridization.[412-416] However, the methodology is cumbersome because of the need to concentrate virus at high speed centrifugation and the need to extract DNA and hybridize it with a DNA probe labeled with phosphorus 32. The sensitivity and specificity of this method is good when the specimens contain 10^3 or more tissue culture infective doses per milliliter.

Polymerase Chain Reaction Amplification

Detection of viral DNA by PCR amplification has proven extremely sensitive for the detection of CMV genetic material in a variety of clinical samples, including urine, cerebrospinal fluid, blood, plasma, saliva, and biopsy material.[293,295,299,402,404-405] Using primers directed at major immediate-early protein and late antigen genes, the initial report from Demmler and colleagues[402] found 41 urine specimens positive by PCR from a total of 44 specimens positive by tissue culture. No positive PCR results were found in 27 urine specimens that were negative by tissue culture.[402] Warren and co-workers[403] used the PCR technique to detect CMV in saliva from children who were between the ages of 1 month and 14 years and who had congenital or perinatal CMV infection and compared the results with a standard tissue culture method and microtiter plate detection of early antigen with tissue culture results as a reference. The sensitivity of PCR was 89.2%, and the specificity was 95.8%. Reproducibility was excellent. If primer selection and amplification conditions are carefully chosen, PCR can give results comparable to standard tissue culture test. Some advantages include the minute amount of specimen and the fact that infectious virus is not required, allowing for retrospective diagnosis of CMV infection if the appropriate specimens are available.[404] Nelson and colleagues[295] showed that PCR detection of CMV DNA in serum was a sensitive, specific, and rapid method for diagnosis of infants with symptomatic congenital CMV infection. The PCR detected CMV DNA in the serum of 18 infants with symptomatic infection, 1 of 2 with asymptomatic infection, and 0 of 32 controls. An exciting new development is the use of real-time PCR to detect and quantitate CMV DNA in dried blood spots obtained from a drop of neonatal blood applied to the IsoCode card (Schleicher and Schuell, Inc., Keene, NH) at the time of the newborn metabolic screen. IsoCode cards are preferred for this application because of ease of isolation of DNA from peripheral blood without the use of a lysis procedure.[404] Swedish investigators were able to detect CMV DNA in dried blood specimens of 13 (81%) of 16 infants with congenital CMV infection.[404] Italian investigators using a similar method obtained a sensitivity of 100% and a specificity of 98.5% in a study of 205 neonates, including 14 with congenital infections.[417] Both groups of investigators used a nested PCR method to detect CMV DNA in dried blood specimens, which adds to the complexity of the assay, reducing its potential use as a screening assay. Advantages of PCR-based methods to screen newborn infants include no need for tissue culture facilities and a minute amount of specimens. Once dried, the samples on filter paper are no longer infectious, reducing the biohazard risk. They are easy to ship and transport without occupational exposure to infectious material. They offer the possibility to quantitate CMV DNA in PCR-positive samples and the possibility for automation. They are available for retrospective diagnosis when appropriate specimens are available, and they can be stored at room temperature for many years.

Antigenemia

An assay to detect CMV antigenemia by means of monoclonal antibodies to pp65 in PMNs has shown good sensitivity compared with conventional methods (e.g., serology, culture) for the diagnosis of CMV disease in immunocompromised adult subjects.[183,299,418-420] Revello and colleagues[299,421] examined pp65 antigenemia, viremia, and DNAemia in peripheral blood leukocytes from 75 infants born to mothers who had primary CMV infection during pregnancy. The results of this study showed that compared with virus isolation from newborn urine, the sensitivity of PCR, antigenemia, and viremia were 100%, 42.5%, and 28%, respectively. The specificity of the three assays was 100%.

Detection of Immune Response

With congenital CMV infection, antibody production begins in utero and is continued probably during the life span of the host. Antibodies are also produced for prolonged periods after postnatally acquired infections.

Detection of IgG Antibodies

Serologic tests that measure IgG antibody are readily available and are easier to perform than are most virologic methods. However, their correct interpretation is complicated by the presence of antibodies (IgG class) that are normally transmitted from the mother to the fetus.[288] A negative antibody titer in cord and maternal sera is sufficient evidence to exclude the diagnosis of congenital CMV infection. In uninfected infants born to seropositive mothers, IgG antibodies serially decrease with a half-life of approximately 1 month and disappear when the children are between 4 and 9 months old. In contrast, in infected infants, IgG antibody levels persist for long periods at comparable or sometimes higher levels than in their mothers. CMV infections are commonly acquired during the neonatal period mostly from maternal sources (e.g., milk, genital secretions) and blood or blood products. When neonatal infections are transmitted from the mother, the distinction from congenital involvement is not possible by routine serologic means. In both situations, IgG antibody titers tend to remain stable for many months. A neonatal infection in the face of a negative maternal IgG antibody titer should point to transmission from other sources, such as a blood transfusion or nosocomial infection.

Many serologic assays have been described and evaluated for the detection of CMV IgG antibodies. Among these, complement fixation, enzyme-linked immunosorbent assay (ELISA), anticomplement immunofluorescence, radioimmunoassay, and indirect hemagglutination are adequate.

Detection of IgM Antibodies

Infected fetuses usually produce specific IgM antibodies. IgM antibodies are not transferred by the placenta, and their presence in cord or neonatal blood represents a fetal antibody response. There are a number of different means to test for IgM antibodies, but before deciding on the use of any particular test, it is important to know its specificity, sensitivity, and reproducibility. None has reached a level of specificity and sensitivity to match the virologic assays described in the previous section.

The solid-phase radioimmunoassay RIA described by Griffiths and Kangro[422] is among the best, with a reported sensitivity of 89% and a specificity of 100% for diagnosis of congenital CMV infections. With the IgM ELISA, the specificity was almost 95% with a sensitivity of approximately 70% when evaluating congenitally infected infants.[423] The IgM capture ELISA and radioimmunoassay have not fared much better when testing for congenital CMV infection. Modifications of the IgM tests yet to be appropriately tested in newborns include an ELISA test that uses purified recombinant CMV polypeptides shown to be highly immunogenic as the antigens for the assay.[424] Another version with proven greater sensitivity in blood donors, pregnant women, and transplant recipients with active CMV infection is a Western blot test for IgM antibodies against viral structural polypeptides pp150 and pp52.[425] Until IgM antibody tests are better perfected for general use, clinicians should not rely solely on one of these assays to diagnose congenital CMV infection. Continued research in this area may provide a simple and generally available method for rapid, definitive diagnosis of congenital infections in ill and asymptomatic neonates.

Diagnosis of Cytomegalovirus Infection during Pregnancy

Clinical Signs and Symptoms

Most primary CMV infections in immunocompetent hosts are subclinical and infections occurring in pregnant women are no exception. Less than 5% of pregnant women with proven primary CMV infections are symptomatic with an even smaller percentage manifesting mononucleosis-like syndrome. No clinical manifestations are expected with recurrent infections (i.e., reactivations or reinfections).

Laboratory Markers

The diagnosis of primary CMV infection can be easily confirmed by documenting seroconversion (i.e., the de novo appearance of virus-specific IgG antibodies in a pregnant woman who was seronegative). In the absence of serologic screening, this is seldom available in clinical practice. The presence of IgG antibodies denotes past infection from 2 weeks to many years in duration.

IgM Assays

Of the several tests that have undergone evaluation, the ELISA-IgM capture method seems to provide the best specificity (95%) and sensitivity (100%). The IgM antibody response varies widely from one patient to another. Seropositivity can be detected up to 16 weeks, but it is unusual to last more than 1 year. It is typical to see sharp drops in titers within the first 2 to 3 months of infection.

Recombinant IgM assays have been developed based on recombinant CMV proteins and peptides. Structural and nonstructural CMV-encoded proteins react with IgM antibodies. The detection of specific IgM antibodies can be accomplished by Western blot, immunoblot, or microparticle enzyme immunoassay.[426,427] With the immunoblot assay, the sensitivity was 100%, and the specificity was 98%.[426] The microparticle enzyme immunoassay had sensitivity and specificity of greater than 95%.[427]

IgG Avidity Assay

The IgG avidity assay is based on the observation that IgG antibodies of low avidity are present during the first months after the onset of infection. With time, IgG antibodies of increasingly higher avidity are produced and eventually only IgG of high avidity is detected in individuals with long-standing CMV infection. The results of the avidity test are reported as an index representing the percentage of IgG antibody bound to the antigen after denaturation treatment with 6M urea.[299,428,429] Similar approaches have been reported for other infectious agents. In one study, an avidity index value of approximately 20% was obtained in serum samples collected within 3 months after onset of primary infection, in contrast to an avidity index of 78% in sera from individuals with remote infection (Fig. 23-5).[430]

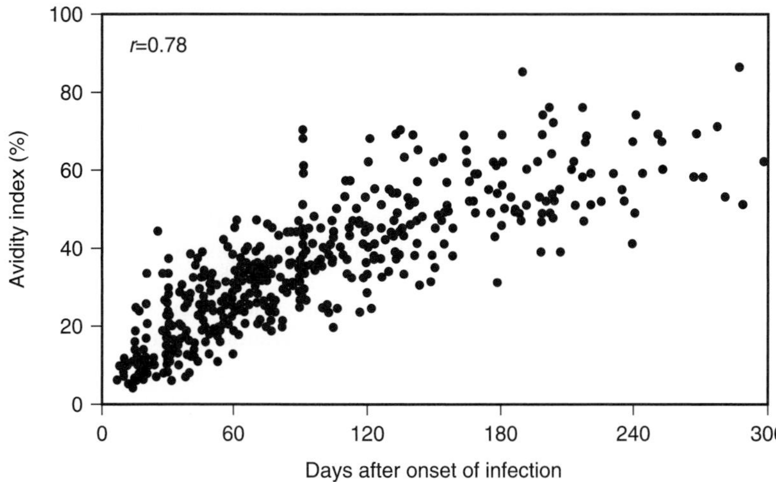

Figure 23–5 Kinetics of IgG avidity index. (From Revello MG, Gerna G. Diagnosis and management of human cytomegalovirus infection in the mother, fetus, and newborn infant. Clin Microbiol Rev 15:680-715, 2002.)

In determining the risk of congenital CMV, a moderate to high avidity index obtained before the 18th week of gestation[429,431] has a negative predictive value of 100%. When the avidity index is determined between 21 and 23 weeks' gestation, the negative predictive value dropped to 91%.[431] The explanation for this observation is that some of the women who transmitted the infection in utero had acquired the infection at a very early gestational age. One important limitation of the IgG avidity test is the lack of standardization. In one study, the ability of these IgG avidity assays to identify primary CMV infection almost reached 100%, whereas the ability to exclude a recent infection ranged from 20% to 96%.

Viral Cultures

CMV excretion from multiple sites such as urine, saliva, and genital secretions is common and can last weeks to several months after a primary infection. Unfortunately, the same occurs with reinfections and reactivations, making this diagnostic approach useless. Viremia, as determined by conventional tissue culture methods, is too insensitive to confirm the diagnosis of primary infection in immunocompetent hosts.

Other Viral Tests

Other diagnostic methods with greater sensitivity and specificity include the determination of antigenemia (number of pp65-positive peripheral blood leukocytes); quantification of CMV DNA in whole blood (DNAemia), leukocytes (leuko-DNAemia), or plasma; and determination of immediate-early and late mRNA (RNAemia) in blood.[299,432] Some of these assays are commercially available. The data supporting their diagnostic value are derived largely from studies in immunosuppressed patients with primary CMV infections, reactivations, and dissemination of infection and evaluation of antiviral treatments. One study of immunocompetent adults, including a large proportion of pregnant women with primary CMV infection, showed that pp65 antigenemia was detected in 57% of patients examined within the first month after the onset of primary infection.[433] The rate of positive results dropped to 25% a month later and to 0% 5 months later. Viremia was detected in 26% of patients during the first month only. Leuko-DNAemia (by PCR test) was detected in 100% of patients tested during the first month, in 89% of those tested on the second month, and in 47% of those tested 3 months after the onset of primary infection. DNAemia lasted 4 to 6 months in 26% of patients, and no patient remained positive beyond 6 months from the onset of infection. None of these three assays was positive for patients with old CMV infection, including nine subjects with proven recurrences. The results of this study[433] indicate that antigenemia and DNAemia when run on blood specimens can rapidly and specifically diagnose and provide an approximate date of onset for primary infection in pregnant women. The detection of immediate-early mRNA has been evaluated as a diagnostic tool for primary CMV infection in healthy individuals.[434,435] This test was consistently negative in all subjects with old or recurrent CMV infection. In contrast, all subjects within the first month of a primary infection tested positive. The proportion of positive results declined over time with all patients testing negative after 6 months of the onset of CMV infection. The kinetics of this test resemble that of DNA detection and, in at least one comparison, the immediate-early mRNA test was slightly more sensitive in the early phase of primary CMV infection.[435]

Maternal Laboratory Tests of Fetal Infection

In utero transmission of CMV infection occurs in approximately 40% of primary infections acquired during pregnancy. No reliable tests can define transmission of infection to the fetus. Moreover, there are no maternal prognostic markers of fetal infection with a recurrence of maternal infection. One study showed that reinfection with a different strain of CMV, as measured by new antibody specificity against epitopes of glycoprotein H, was capable of causing symptomatic congenital CMV infection. The methodology used in this study is far from becoming a standard laboratory assay.

Prenatal Diagnosis

The prenatal diagnosis of CMV is possible by testing fetal blood obtained by cordocentesis and amniotic fluid obtained by amniocentesis. Fetal blood can be used for determination of specific IgM antibodies and direct viral markers. IgM antibodies can be detected only after 20 weeks' gestation, but because of low sensitivity (approximately 50%), the test has very limited diagnostic value.[436-438] However, studies of viral load in fetal blood show that the sensitivity of antigenemia was approximately 58%; of viremia, 55%; and of leuko-DNAemia, 82%. The specificity is 100% for the three assays.[299] In one study, PCR in fetal blood had a sensitivity of 41%, but viral culture had a sensitivity of only 7%. With the use of fetal blood, even the most sensitive assays miss almost 15% to 20% of infected fetuses.

Results in amniotic fluid are far better, and this method is the standard for prenatal diagnosis. Viral isolation in tissue culture has a sensitivity of approximately 60%, whereas the sensitivity of PCR can reach 100%. The specificity of both assays is excellent.[436,439-442] A quantitative PCR method has shown that when the amniotic fluid contains 10^5 or more genome equivalents of CMV DNA, the risk of symptomatic congenital CMV infection is significantly higher than when the viral load is 10^3 genome equivalents or less.[443-445]

A confounding factor in prenatal diagnosis is the gestational age at the time of amniocentesis or cordocentesis. After a primary maternal infection, it may take weeks to months for transplacental transmission of CMV to occur. An interval of 7 weeks between maternal onset of infection and diagnostic tests for fetal infection has been suggested as a reasonable interval by some investigators.[439,440,446] Gestational age at the time of testing is important, because the sensitivity can be as low as 30% when amniotic fluid is obtained before the 21st week of gestation, and it can be 100% if the test is performed after 21 weeks' gestation.[437,438,442,447-452]

When counseling pregnant women, it is important to remember that 80% to 90% of children with congenital CMV infection escape CNS sequelae. In the absence of specific antiviral treatment, the only alternatives available after a prenatal diagnosis of congenital CMV infection are to terminate the pregnancy or do nothing. The presence or absence of ultrasonographic evidence of fetal abnormalities should be taken into consideration during counseling of women at risk.

Diagnosis of Perinatally Acquired Infections

For perinatally acquired infections, viral culture and CMV DNA detection by PCR using urine and saliva are the preferred diagnostic methods, but CMV excretion does not begin until 3 to 12 weeks after exposure.[89,288] For diagnostic specificity, it is imperative to have a negative result from urine or saliva specimens collected within the first 2 weeks of life. In early infancy, antibody assays have the same limitations described earlier for infants with congenital CMV infection. The desire to differentiate between congenital and perinatal CMV infections stems from the fact that their risks for acute morbidity and for long-term sequelae are very different.

DIFFERENTIAL DIAGNOSIS

During the newborn period, the constellation of hepatosplenomegaly, petechiae, and direct hyperbilirubinemia with or without pneumonitis, microcephaly, and ocular and neurologic abnormalities that characterize CID is common to several disease entities, including other congenital infections such as congenital rubella syndrome, toxoplasmosis, syphilis, neonatal herpes simplex virus infections, and less likely, hepatitis B and varicella virus infections.[370] The differential diagnosis of symptomatic congenital CMV infection also includes bacterial sepsis and noninfectious disorders such as hemolytic diseases related to Rh or ABO incompatibilities or red blood cell defects, metabolic disorders such as galactosemia and tyrosinemia, immune thrombocytopenia, histiocytosis X, congenital leukemia, and others. The list of diseases that must be considered in the differential diagnosis becomes broader as the clinical manifestations diminish in severity.

Infections may coexist in the same patient. Consequently, the laboratory workup for differential diagnosis must be thorough.

Congenital Rubella Syndrome

Congenital rubella has been virtually eliminated in the United States after the successful immunization program adopted years ago. Although symptomatic congenital rubella and CMV infections share many signs and symptoms, central cataracts, congenital heart defects, raised purpuric rather than petechial rash, salt-and-pepper lesions as opposed to chorioretinitis, and the absence of cerebral calcifications are more likely to occur with congenital rubella syndrome than with CID.[370]

Congenital Toxoplasmosis

Almost all of the manifestations observed in CID have been described for symptomatic congenital toxoplasmosis. Some differences merit discussion.[370] For instance, the calcifications of toxoplasmosis are generally scattered throughout the cerebral cortex, whereas the calcifications of CID tend to occur in the periventricular areas. The rash associated with toxoplasmosis is usually maculopapular but is not petechial or purpuric. Chorioretinitis in the two diseases cannot be differentiated on the basis of appearance or distribution. However, it is more likely that chorioretinitis related to CMV is associated with other major clinical manifestations, such as microcephaly. Not uncommonly, the chorioretinitis of toxoplasmosis is an isolated finding.

Congenital Syphilis

The most consistent signs of early congenital syphilis are osteochondritis and epiphysitis on the radiograph of the long bones.[370] These occur in approximately 90% of infected patients and are more likely to appear in patients who become symptomatic in the first week of life. Rhinitis, sometimes associated with laryngitis, is another common manifestation of congenital syphilis; it is often followed by a dark red maculopapular, spotted rash. Lesions of the skin and mucous membranes are also seen. Hepatosplenomegaly occurs but is less common in early syphilis than in CID. Calcifications of the brain are not characteristic of congenital syphilis. However, choroiditis may be seen.

Neonatal Herpes Simplex Virus Infections

Congenital herpes simplex virus infections are less common than neonatal herpes simplex virus infections, but they are more likely to pose a diagnostic dilemma because they may resemble CID. Microcephaly, intracranial calcifications, chorioretinitis with and without optic atrophy and hepatosplenomegaly are common clinical manifestations of intrauterine herpes simplex virus infections. The presence of skin vesicles or scarring present at birth is valuable for the differential diagnosis. The more common form of herpes simplex virus infection, neonatal infection, is acquired during parturition and does not usually manifest as an acute disease until the infants are 5 to 21 days old. Unlike the situation in typical CID, the infant is well during most of the first week of life. When illness does occur, it may be accompanied by seizures, encephalitis, respiratory distress, bleeding disorders, and vesicular lesions that tend to cluster. The presence of skin and mucous membranous lesions is valuable for the differential diagnosis of CID.

TREATMENT

Chemotherapy

A small number of systemically administered antiviral agents have been used in therapeutic trials of serious, life-threatening or sight-threatening CMV disease. Two antiviral agents, ganciclovir and foscarnet, are licensed for this purpose in immunocompromised patients. Foscarnet inhibits viral replication by inhibiting viral DNA polymerase, and ganciclovir acts as a chain terminator during elongation of the newly synthesized viral DNA.[453-457]

The Collaborative Antiviral Study Group (CASG) under the auspices of the National Institute of Allergy and Infectious Diseases first conducted a phase II pharmacokinetic-pharmacodynamic study that established the safe dose of ganciclovir to be used in young infants and demonstrated an antiviral effect with suppression of viruria.[453] A phase III, randomized, controlled study followed in newborn infants with symptomatic congenital infection involving the CNS.[456] A total of 100 patients were enrolled. Those in the ganciclovir treatment arm received doses of 6 mg/kg administered intravenously every 12 hours for 6 weeks of treatment. The primary end point was improved hearing (as assessed by brain-stem–evoked response) between baseline and 6 months of follow-up or, for those with normal hearing at enrollment, preservation of normal hearing at follow-up. Twenty-one (84%) of 25 ganciclovir-treated patients had hearing improvement or maintained normal hearing at 6 months, compared with 10 (59%) of 17 in the no-treatment group ($P = .06$). At 6 months of follow-up, none (0 of 25) of the ganciclovir-treated infants had hearing deterioration, compared with 7 (41%) of 17 in the no-treatment group ($P < .01$). Alternatively, 5 (21%) of 24 of ganciclovir recipients had worsening in hearing in their best ear between baseline and 1 year or longer, compared with 13 (68%) of 19 in the no-treatment group ($P < .01$).

As in the previous phase II study, the most significant toxicity in the treated group was neutropenia, with 29 (63%) of 46 patients developing moderate to severe neutropenia compared with 9 (21%) of 43 of the no-treatment group ($P < .01$). One half of the patients with neutropenia required dosage adjustment and 12% had discontinuation of therapy. This study demonstrates that 6 weeks of intravenous ganciclovir in symptomatic congenital CMV-infected infants prevents worsening of hearing loss at 6 months and 1 year of follow-up. Treated patients had a more rapid resolution of their liver function abnormalities and improvements in short-term growth and head circumference compared with controls. There are no reports on the therapeutic efficacy of combined therapy (i.e., foscarnet-ganciclovir). The CASG is conducting a phase I/II pharmacokinetic-pharmacodynamic study of valganciclovir, the orally bioavailable prodrug of ganciclovir, to determine the dose necessary to achieve a safe and effective concentration of ganciclovir in the bloodstream.

Intravenous ganciclovir treatment at a dose of 6 mg/kg that is administered every 12 hours for 42 days can be recommended for infants with proven symptomatic congenital CMV infection, particularly for those with no evidence of hearing loss. Although the phase III study sponsored by the CASG did not include infants without CNS involvement, the data suggest that treatment may speed the resolution of liver abnormalities. The decision to treat should be carefully discussed with parents and caregivers because treatment often requires a substantial commitment, including 42 days of intravenous therapy (preferably in the hospital), the use of secure intravenous access, and frequent blood sampling to check for ganciclovir toxicity. Anecdotal reports do not support the use of hyperimmune immunoglobulin or antiviral treatment with ganciclovir or foscarnet for treating the fetus in utero.

Passive Immunization

Hyperimmune plasma and immunoglobulin have been used with some success as prophylaxis for primary CMV infections in immunosuppressed transplant recipients. A meta-analysis of randomized, controlled trials of immunoglobulin as prophylaxis for CMV disease in adult transplant recipients found a significant beneficial effect.[458] Studies are being conducted to determine if a humanized monoclonal antibody, such as the one that binds to gH of CMV, is more efficacious for the prevention or treatment in patients at high risk for CMV infection.[459] It is unlikely that passive immunoprophylaxis will ever work for treatment of congenital infections because the cases are identified weeks and months after infection occurred in utero. However, it might be a means of preventing primary CMV infection and disease associated with transfusion-acquired infections in premature infants. No controlled studies are available.

Vaccines

In the United States, congenital CMV infection is a significant public health problem. It is the leading cause of sensorineural hearing loss and the leading infectious cause of brain damage in children.[460] Not surprisingly, the Institute of Medicine of the National Academy of Sciences concluded that a vaccine to prevent congenital CMV infection should be a top priority. Despite 30 years of research efforts, no such vaccine is available. The prevailing thought is that both neutralizing antibodies and cell-mediated immunity are necessary for prevention. Of the CMV proteins, gB, gH, pp65, and pp150 can induce neutralizing and CTL responses.[460-465]

The strategies for vaccine development include live-attenuated vaccine (i.e., Towne strain). This vaccine induces a significant antibody response and cell-mediated immunity, as determined by lymphoproliferative response. In CMV-seronegative recipients of kidneys from seropositive donors, this vaccine reduced disease severity but did not prevent infection.[461] It also protected against a low-dose virulent CMV challenge in normal volunteers. In a later trial, this vaccine failed to decrease the rate of acquisition of CMV in parents of children in daycare. The magnitude of the induced immune response was 10-fold lower than that generated by natural infection.[463] The Towne vaccine is not excreted by vaccinees.

Recombinant Virus Vaccine

The genome of the virulent Toledo strain of CMV, divided into four fragments, was inserted in the genetic background of the attenuated Towne strain, creating four chimeras. The ability of these four recombinant virus strains to generate antibody and cell-mediated immune responses in the absence of clinical side effects is being evaluated in a phase I study.[461]

Subunit Vaccines

A CMV vaccine based on the envelope glycoprotein gB combined with a novel adjuvant (MF59) was tested in a double-blind, placebo-controlled trial of seronegative adult volunteers.[464] Results showed that after three doses, the antibody responses to gB and neutralizing antibodies exceeded the levels in seropositive control subjects. Cell-mediated immunity was not evaluated. The major target of the cell-mediated immune response is pp65. In an effort to elicit this response, a study[465] made use of the nonreplicating canarypox expression vector in which CMV pp65 has been inserted. A phase I trial on seronegative volunteers found that pp65-specific CTLs were elicited after only two vaccinations. An antibody response to pp65 was also demonstrated. In this preliminary study, the canarypox CMV pp65 recombinant vaccine seems to generate an immune response similar to that provided by natural infection.[465] A canarypox CMV recombinant that contained gB did not induce neutralizing antibodies. It is possible to explore the immunogenicity of a vaccine combining canarypox CMV (pp65) with gB with an appropriate adjuvant such as MF59. This combination may generate sufficient CTLs and neutralizing antibodies to protect against CMV disease.

Other potential avenues for the development of CMV vaccine include peptide vaccines and DNA vaccines. All candidate vaccines must demonstrate that immunogenicity provides protection.

PREVENTION

CMV usually is not very contagious, and its horizontal transmission requires direct contact with infected material, such as secretions that contain the virus and, less likely, fomites.[97-113,466] With the exception of a few small studies that were designed to prevent infection through blood and blood products and grafted organs, no broad-based strategies for preventing the transmission of this virus have been tested.[269,395,467,468] Although there are still no effective means of preventing congenital CMV infections or most perinatally acquired CMV infections, a few common sense recommendations can be made.

Pregnant Women

An average of 2% of susceptible pregnant women acquire CMV infection during pregnancy in the United States; most of them have no symptoms, and only 40% of the episodes result in fetal infection (Fig. 23-6).[469] Because there is no effective drug therapy and the risk of fetal morbidity is low, several investigators have concluded that routine serologic screening of pregnant women for primary CMV infections during pregnancy is of limited value.[328,470] However, reliable and inexpensive serologic tests are available, and women of childbearing age can be informed of their immune status.[471] Those who are seronegative should be able to make informed decisions about the risks of CMV. Primary CMV infection should be suspected in pregnant women with symptoms compatible with a heterophil-negative, mononucleosis-like syndrome. To more precisely define a recent asymptomatic primary CMV infection, serologic tests such as IgM capture ELISA, IgG avidity index, and DNAemia (PCR) could be used. There are no reliable means to determine whether intrauterine transmission has occurred after symptomatic or subclinical primary infection in early gestation or to assess the relatively small number of fetuses at risk of disease. The sensitivity and specificity of prenatal diagnosis by testing fetal blood obtained by cordocentesis or amniotic fluid PCR and viral culture are good after 20 weeks' gestation. There is still limited information to serve as a basis for recommendations regarding termination of pregnancy after a primary CMV infection acquired in early gestation. Similarly, there is no conclusive information regarding how long conception should be delayed after documented primary infection is acquired in a woman of childbearing age. Viral excretion is not a good indicator because virus is shed into saliva for weeks or months after infection and into urine and the cervix for months or years.

The data on which to base recommendations for prevention of congenital CMV infection after recurrent maternal infection are even more inadequate. Preexisting immunity does not prevent the virus from reactivating or reinfection, nor does it effectively control the occasional spread to the fetus.[326] Preexisting maternal immunity affords significant protection to the fetus. However, evidence that in some high-risk populations reinfections with antigenically different virus can cause fetal disease and long-term sequelae may temper this statement. There are no techniques for identifying women with reactivation of CMV that result in intrauterine transmission. Because the risk of transmission is very low (see Fig. 23-6) and the risk of fetal disease even lower, women known to be seropositive before conception do not need to be virologically or serologically tested, nor do they need to be unduly worried about the very low risk of adverse effects on the fetus.

The principal sources of CMV infection among women of childbearing age are exposure to children excreting CMV and sexual contacts. Recommendations for prevention of sexual transmission of CMV are beyond the scope of this review. Suffice it to say that they are similar to those advocated for the prevention of other, more common sexually transmitted infections. As for the risk from exposure to children, at greater risk are susceptible pregnant mothers of CMV-infected children who attend daycare centers.[97,98,102,106-108,110-113] Hand washing and simple hygienic measures that are routine

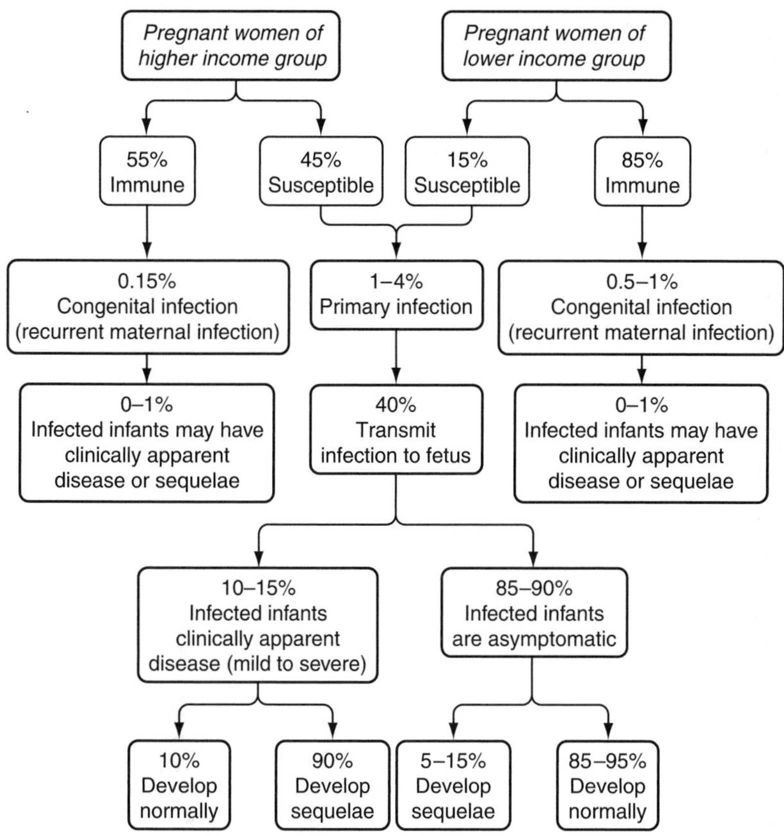

Figure 23–6 Characteristics of cytomegalovirus infection in pregnancy. (From Stagno S, Whitley RJ. Herpesvirus infection of pregnancy. N Engl J Med 313:1270-1274, 1985.)

for hospital care can be recommended, but it is unrealistic to expect all mothers to comply.

Because CMV has been found to be endemic in the daycare setting and is found everywhere in hospitals, questions often arise about the occupational risks to pregnant personnel in these facilities. Although hospital workers do not appear to be at increased risk for CMV infection,[109,143,145,148] personnel who work in daycare centers are.[97,98,102,104,105,110] In the hospital, routine procedures for hand washing and infection control should make nonparenteral acquisition of CMV infections less likely than in the community. Although most patients who shed CMV are asymptomatic and go unrecognized, when caring for known CMV-excreting patients, these routine measures should be combined with a special recommendation that pregnant caretakers be especially careful in handling such patients.[143] In the daycare setting, where hygiene is difficult at best, these preventive measures may be more difficult to implement. Although there is still debate about the need for routine serologic screening of female personnel and daycare workers, I believe that it should be recommended for potentially childbearing women whose occupation exposes them to CMV. Knowing their immune status can be helpful in counseling pregnant women at risk. Those found to be seropositive can be strongly reassured. Those found to be serosusceptible should be provided with information on prevention measures and reassured that common sense steps such as hand washing and avoiding contact with secretions should prevent acquisition of infection.[143] Attempts to identify all congenitally CMV-infected children and children excreting this virus in the workplace so that seronegative workers and parents can avoid contact with them pose serious logistic problems and would require frequent periodic testing.

Nosocomial Infection

Hospitalized patients who receive blood products and organ transplants are at risk for nosocomial CMV infection. Because the role of organ transplantation in transmission of CMV is insignificant in the newborn period, it is not discussed here. Transfusion of blood products can be an important source of perinatal CMV infections. The use of blood products from seronegative donors prevents the transmission of CMV and the subsequent risk of disease.[132,269,395,401] However, this method is not practical in areas where most of the donor population is seropositive. The availability of seronegative donors and the additional cost involved in serologic screening and processing the blood must be evaluated by regional blood banks.

The use of deglycerolized, frozen red blood cells and the use of filters to remove leukocytes are also effective means of eliminating post-transfusion CMV infection in adult dialysis patients and in newborns, even in low-birth-weight infants.[132,468,472] Both methods result in a significant disruption and depletion of leukocytes.

Many hospitals are using one of these three approaches to prevent transfusion-acquired perinatal CMV infections.[473] It is up to the local hospital and blood bank to determine whether transfusion-associated CMV disease is a problem and which method to choose. However, many nurseries have adopted the policy that all transfusions of blood or blood products should be with seronegative blood, irrespective of the infant's birth weight and maternal immune status.

The absence of CMV infection in premature infants born to seronegative mothers and who receive only seronegative blood products suggests that spread of CMV from hands of personnel or from fomites must be rare. Until more information is available, the only logical recommendation is hand washing and routine infection control measures.

Rarely is perinatal infection through breast milk a cause for concern, at least for full-term newborns who receive their mother's milk.[90,96] Premature infants, who generally do not receive sufficient quantities of specific transplacental antibodies, are at higher risk for morbidity.[342,344] We must also be cautious with expressed banked milk and wet nurses because CMV-infected milk might inadvertently be given to infants born to seronegative women. Storage of naturally infected breast milk at –20° C (freezer temperature) significantly reduces but does not eliminate infectivity.[474] Heat treatment of breast milk at 72° C for 10 seconds eliminates all infectious viruses without affecting the nutritional and immunologic properties of milk.[342]

REFERENCES

1. Weller TH. The cytomegaloviruses: ubiquitous agents with protean clinical manifestations. N Engl J Med 285:203-214, 1971.
2. Ribbert H. Uber protozoenartigen Zellen in der Nireeines syphilitischen Neugeboren und in der Parotis von Kindren. Zentralbl Allg Pathol 15:945-948, 1904.
3. Jesionek A, Kiolemenoglou B. Über einen Befund von protozoenartigen Gebilden in den Organen eines hereditarleustiochen Fotus. MMW Munch Med Wochenschr 51:1905-1907, 1904.
4. Lowenstein C. Über protozoenartigen Gebilden in den Organen von Dindern. Zentralbl Allg Pathol 18:513-518, 1907.
5. Goodpasture E, Talbot FB. Concerning the nature of "protozoan-like" cells in certain lesions of infancy. Am J Dis Child 21:415-425, 1921.
6. Lipschutz B. Untersuchungen uber die Aetiologic der Krankheiten d. herpes genitalis, usw. Arch Derm Syph 136:428-482, 1921.
7. Cole R, Kuttner AG. Filterable virus present in the salivary glands of guinea pigs. J Exp Med 44:855-873, 1926.
8. Smith MG. Propagation of salivary gland virus of the mouse in tissue culture. Proc Soc Exp Biol Med 86:435-440, 1954.
9. Smith MG. Propagation in tissue cultures of a cytopathogenic virus from human salivary gland virus (SGV) disease. Proc Soc Exp Biol Med 92:424-430, 1956.
10. Rowe WP, Hartley JW, Waterman S, et al. Cytopathogenic agent resembling salivary gland virus recovered from tissue cultures of human adenoids. Proc Soc Exp Biol Med 92:418-424, 1956.
11. Weller TH, Macauley JC, Craig JM, et al. Isolation of intranuclear inclusion-producing agents from infants with illnesses resembling cytomegalic inclusion disease. Proc Soc Exp Biol Med 94:4-12, 1957.
12. Weller TH, Hanshaw JB, Scott DE. Serologic differentiation of viruses responsible for cytomegalic inclusion disease. Virology 12:130-132, 1960.
13. Krech U, Jung M, Jung F. Cytomegalovirus Infections of Man. Basel, S Karger, 1971, p 28.
14. Gold E, Nankervis GA. Cytomegalovirus. *In* Evans AS (ed). Viral Infections of Humans: Epidemiology and Control. New York, Plenum, 1982, pp 167-186.
15. Alford CA, Stagno S, Pass RF, et al. Epidemiology of cytomegalovirus. *In* Nahmias A, Dowdle W, Schinazi R (eds). The Human Herpesviruses: An Interdisciplinary Perspective. New York, Elsevier, 1981, pp 159-171.
16. Black JB, Pellett PE. Human herpesvirus 7. Rev Med Virol 9:245-262, 1999.
17. Campadelli-Fiume G, Mirandola P, Menotti L. Human herpesvirus 6: an emerging pathogen. Emerg Infect Dis 5:353-366, 1999.
18. Clark DA. Human herpesvirus 6. Rev Med Virol 10:155-173, 2000.
19. Chen DH, Jiang H, Lee M, et al. Three-dimensional visualization of tegument/capsid interactions in the intact human cytomegalovirus. Virology 260:10-16, 1999.
20. Trus BL, Gibson W, Cheng N, Steven AC. Capsid structure of simian cytomegalovirus from cryoelectron microscopy: evidence for tegument attachment sites [erratum appears in J Virol 73:4530, 1999]. J Virol 73:2181-2192, 1999.
21. Murphy E, Yu D, Grimwood J, et al. Coding capacity of laboratory and clinical strains of human cytomegalovirus. Proc Natl Acad Sci U S A 100:14976-1981, 2003.
22. Mocarski ES, Tan Courcelle C. Cytomegaloviruses and their replication. *In* Fields BN, Howley PM, Griffin DE, et al (eds). Fields Virology. Philadelphia, Lippincott Williams & Wilkins, 2001, pp 2629-2673.
23. Borst EM, Hahn G, Koszinowski UH, Messerle M. Cloning of the human cytomegalovirus (HCMV) genome as an infectious bacterial artificial chromosome in *Escherichia coli*: a new approach for construction of HCMV mutants. J Virol 73:8320-8329, 1999.
24. Streblow DW, Varnum S, Hall L, et al. Relative viral and cellular protein composition of the AD169 HCMV proteome. The 28th International Herpes Workshop, Madison, Wis, 2003.
25. Gibson W. Structure and assembly of the virion. Intervirology 39:389-400, 1996.
26. Bogner E, Radsak K, Stinski MF, et al. The gene product of human cytomegalovirus open reading frame UL56 binds the pac motif and has specific nuclease activity. J Virol 72:2259-2264, 1998.
27. Scheffczik H, Savva CG, Holzenburg A, et al. The terminase subunits pUL56 and pUL89 of human cytomegalovirus are DNA-metabolizing proteins with toroidal structure. Nucleic Acids Res 30:1695-1703, 2002.
28. Krosky PM, Underwood MR, Turk SR, et al. Resistance of human cytomegalovirus to benzimidazole ribonucleosides maps to two open reading frames: UL89 and UL56. J Virol 72:4721-4728, 1998.
29. Bresnahan WA, Shenk T. A subset of viral transcripts packaged within human cytomegalovirus particles. Science 288:2373-2376, 2000.
30. Fortunato EA, Spector DH. P53 and RPA are sequestered in viral replication centers in the nuclei of cells infected with human cytomegalovirus. J Virol 72:2033-2039, 1998.
31. Salvant BS, Fortunato EA, Spector DH. Cell cycle dysregulation by human cytomegalovirus: influence of the cell cycle phase at the time of infection and effects on cyclin transcription. J Virol 72:3729-3741, 1998.
32. Hayashi ML, Blankenship C, Shenk T. Human cytomegalovirus UL69 protein is required for efficient accumulation of infected cells in the G1 phase of the cell cycle. Proc Natl Acad Sci U S A 97:2692-2696, 2000.
33. Kalejta RF, Bechtel JT, Shenk T, et al. Human cytomegalovirus pp71 stimulates cell cycle progression by inducing the proteasome-dependent degradation of the retinoblastoma family of tumor suppressors. Mol Cell Biol 23:1885-1895, 2003.
34. Baldick CJ, Marchini A, Patterson CE, Shenk T. Human cytomegalovirus tegument protein pp71 (ppUL82) enhances the infectivity of viral DNA and accelerates the infectious cycle. J Virol 71:4400-4408, 1997.
35. Muranyi W, Haas J, Wagner M, et al. Cytomegalovirus recruitment of cellular kinases to dissolve the nuclear lamina. Science 297:854-857, 2002.
36. Landini MP, LaPlaca M. Humoral immune response to human cytomegalovirus proteins: a brief review. Comp Immunol Microbiol Infect Dis 14:97-105, 1991.
37. McLaughlin-Taylor E, Pande H, Forman SJ, et al. Identification of the major late human cytomegalovirus matrix protein pp65 as a target antigen for CD8+ virus-specific cytotoxic T lymphocytes. J Med Virol 43:103-110, 1994.
38. Boppana SB, Britt WJ. Recognition of human cytomegalovirus gene products by HCMV-specific cytotoxic T cells. Virology 222:293-296, 1996.
39. Kern F, Faulhaber N, Frommel C, et al. Analysis of CD8 T cell reactivity to cytomegalovirus using protein-spanning pools of overlapping pentadecapeptides. Eur J Immunol 30:1676-1682, 2000.
40. Kern F, Bunde T, Faulhaber N, et al. Cytomegalovirus (CMV) phosphoprotein 65 makes a large contribution to shaping the T cell repertoire in CMV-exposed individuals. J Infect Dis 185:1709-1716, 2002.
41. Chee MS, Bankier AT, Beck S, et al. Analysis of the protein-coding content of the sequence of human cytomegalovirus strain AD169. Curr Top Microbiol Immunol 154:125-170, 1990.

42. Britt WJ, Vugler L, Butfiloski EJ, Stephens EB. Cell surface expression of human cytomegalovirus (HCMV) gp55-116 (gB): use of the HCMV-vaccinia recombinant virus infected cells in analysis of the human neutralizing antibody response. J Virol 64:1079-1085, 1990.
43. Meyer H, Masuho Y, Mach M. The gp116 of the gp58/116 complex of human cytomegalovirus represents the amino-terminal part of the precursor molecule and contains a neutralizing epitope. J Gen Virol 71:2443-2450, 1990.
44. Rasmussen L, Matkin C, Apaete R, et al. Antibody response to human cytomegalovirus glycoproteins gB and gH after natural infection in humans. J Infect Dis 164:835-842, 1991.
45. Marshall GS, Rabalais GP, Stout GG, Waldeyer SL. Antibodies to recombinant-derived glycoprotein B after natural human cytomegalovirus infection correlate with neutralizing activity. J Infect Dis 165:381-384, 1992.
46. Urban M, Klein M, Britt WJ, et al. Glycoprotein H of human cytomegalovirus is a major antigen for the neutralizing humoral immune response. J Gen Virol 77:1537-1547, 1996.
47. Navarro D, Lennette E, Tugizov S, Pereira L. Humoral immune response to functional regions of human cytomegalovirus glycoprotein B. J Med Virol 52:451-459, 1997.
48. Klein M, Schoppel K, Amvrossiadis N, Mach M. Strain-specific neutralization of human cytomegalovirus isolates by human sera. J Virol 73:878-886, 1999.
49. Mach M, Kropff B, Dal Monte P, Britt W. Complex formation by human cytomegalovirus glycoproteins M (gpUL100) and N (gpUL73). J Virol 74:11881-11892, 2000.
50. Compton T, Nowlin DM, Cooper NR. Initiation of human cytomegalovirus infection requires initial interaction with cell surface heparan sulfate. Virology 193:834-841, 1993.
51. Compton T. Towards a definition of the HCMV entry pathway. Scand J Infect Dis Suppl 99:30-32, 1995.
52. Boyle KA, Pietropaolo RL, Compton T. Engagement of the cellular receptor for glycoprotein B of human cytomegalovirus activates the interferon-responsive pathway. Mol Cell Biol 19:3607-3613, 1999.
53. Wang X, Huong SM, Chiu ML, et al. Epidermal growth factor receptor is a cellular receptor for human cytomegalovirus. Nature 424:456-461, 2003.
54. Zhu H, Cong JP, Shenk T. Use of differential display analysis to assess the effect of human cytomegalovirus infection on the accumulation of cellular RNAs: induction of interferon-responsive RNAs. Proc Natl Acad Sci U S A 94:13985-13990, 1997.
55. Zhu H, Cong JP. Cellular gene expression altered by human cytomegalovirus: global monitoring with oligonucleotide arrays. Proc Natl Acad Sci U S A 95:14470-14475, 1998.
56. Browne EP, Wing B, Coleman D, Shenk T. Altered cellular mRNA levels in human cytomegalovirus-infected fibroblasts: viral block to the accumulation of antiviral mRNAs. J Virol 75:12319-12330, 2001.
57. Simmen KA, Singh J, Luukkonen BG, et al. Global modulation of cellular transcription by human cytomegalovirus is initiated by viral glycoprotein B. Proc Natl Acad Sci U S A 98:7140-7145, 2001.
58. Sambucetti LC, Cherrington JM, Wilkinson GW, Mocarski ES. NF-kappa B activation of the cytomegalovirus enhancer is mediated by a viral transactivator and by T cell stimulation. EMBO J 8:4251-4258, 1989.
59. Child S, Jarrahian S, Harper V, Geballe A. Complementation of vaccinia virus lacking the double stranded RNA-binding protein gene E3L by human cytomegalovirus. J Virol 76:4912-4918, 2002.
60. Yu Y, Alwine JC. Human cytomegalovirus major immediate-early proteins and simian virus 40 large T antigen can inhibit apoptosis through activation of the phosphatidylinositide 3′-OH kinase pathway and the cellular kinase. Akt J Virol 76:3731-3738, 2002.
61. Gleaves CA, Smith TF, Shuster EA, Pearson GR. Comparison of standard tube and shell vial cell culture techniques for the detection of cytomegalovirus in clinical specimens. J Clin Microbiol 21:217-221, 1985.
62. Jespersen DJ, Drew WL, Gleaves CA, et al. Multisite evaluation of a monoclonal antibody reagent (Syva) for rapid diagnosis of cytomegalovirus in the shell vial assay. J Clin Microbiol 27:1502-1505, 1989.
63. Rabella N, Drew WL. Comparison of conventional and shell vial cultures for detecting cytomegalovirus infection. J Clin Microbiol 28:806-807, 1990.
64. Zhu H, Shen Y, Shenk T. Human cytomegalovirus IE1 and IE2 proteins block apoptosis. J Virol 69:7960-7970, 1995.
65. Goldmacher VS, Bartle LM, Skaletskaya A, et al. A cytomegalovirus-encoded mitochondria-localized inhibitor of apoptosis structurally unrelated to Bcl-2. Proc Natl Acad Sci U S A 96:12536-12541, 1999.
66. Newcomb WW, Homa FL, Thomsen DR, Brown JC. In vitro assembly of the herpes simplex virus procapsid: formation of small procapsids at reduced scaffolding protein concentration. J Struct Biol 133:23-31, 2001.
67. Heymann JB, Cheng N, Newcomb WW, et al. Dynamics of herpes simplex virus capsid maturation visualized by time-lapse cryo-electron microscopy. Nat Struct Biol 10:334-341, 2003.
68. Sanchez V, Greis KD, Sztul E, Britt WJ. Accumulation of virion tegument and envelope proteins in a stable cytoplasmic compartment during human cytomegalovirus replication. Characterization of a potential site of virus assembly. J Virol 74:975-986, 2000.
69. Homman-Loudiyi M, Hultenby K, Britt W, Soderberg-Naucler C. Envelopment of human cytomegalovirus occurs by budding into Golgi-derived vacuole compartments positive for gB, Rab 3, trans-Golgi network 46, and mannosidase II [erratum appears in J Virol Arch 77:8179, 2003]. J Virol 77:3191-3203, 2003.
70. Fish KN, Soderberg-Naucler C, Mills LK, et al. Human cytomegalovirus persistently infects aortic endothelial cells. J Virol 72: 5661-568, 1998.
71. Taylor-Wiedeman J, Sissons P, Sinclair J. Induction of endogenous human cytomegalovirus gene expression after differentiation of monocytes from healthy carriers. J Virol 68:1597-1604, 1994.
72. Kondo K, Xu J, Mocarski ES. Human cytomegalovirus latent gene expression in granulocyte-macrophage progenitors in culture and in seropositive individuals. Proc Natl Acad Sci USA 93:11137-11142, 1996.
73. Soderberg-Naucler C, Fish KN, Nelson JA. Interferon-gamma and tumor necrosis factor-alpha specifically induce formation of cytomegalovirus-permissive monocyte-derived macrophages that are refractory to the antiviral activity of these cytokines. J Clin Invest 100:3154-3163, 1997.
74. Soderberg-Naucler C, Fish KN, Nelson JA. Reactivation of latent human cytomegalovirus by allogeneic stimulation of blood cells from healthy donors. Cell 91:119-126, 1997.
75. Bolovan-Fritts CA, Mocarski ES, Wiedeman JA. Peripheral blood CD14(+) cells from healthy subjects carry a circular conformation of latent cytomegalovirus genome. Blood 93:394-398, 1999.
76. Soderberg-Naucler C, Streblow DN, Fish KN, et al. Reactivation of latent human cytomegalovirus in CD14(+) monocytes is differentiation dependent. J Virol 75:7543-7554, 2001.
77. Gnann JW, Ahlmen J, Svalander C, et al. Inflammatory cells in transplanted kidneys are infected by human cytomegalovirus. Am J Pathol 132:239-248, 1988.
78. Hummel M, Zhang Z, Yan S, et al. Allogeneic transplantation induces expression of cytomegalovirus immediate-early genes in vivo: a model for reactivation from latency. J Virol 75:4814-4822, 2001.
79. Sinzger C, Grefte A, Plachter B, et al. Fibroblasts, epithelial cells, endothelial cells and smooth muscle cells are major targets of human cytomegalovirus infection in lung and gastrointestinal tissues. J Gen Virol 76(Pt 4):741-750, 1995.
80. Plachter B, Sinzger C, Jahn G. Cell types involved in replication and distribution of human cytomegalovirus. Adv Virus Res 46:195-261, 1996.
81. Sinzger C, Jahn G. Human cytomegalovirus cell tropism and pathogenesis. Intervirology 39:302-319, 1996.
82. Halwachs-Baumann G, Wilders-Truschnig M, Desoye G, et al. Human trophoblast cells are permissive to the complete replicative cycle of human cytomegalovirus. J Virol 72:7598-7602, 1998.
83. Hemmings DG, Kilani R, Nykiforuk C, et al. Permissive cytomegalovirus infection of primary villous term and first trimester trophoblasts. J Virol 72:4970-4979, 1998.
84. Fisher S, Genbacev O, Maidji E, Pereira L. Human cytomegalovirus infection of placental cytotrophoblasts in vitro and in utero: implications for transmission and pathogenesis. J Virol 74:6808-6820, 2000.
85. Hahn G, Baldanti F, Gallina A, et al. Novel genes within the UL131-128 locus of human cytomegalovirus determine leukocyte and endothelial cell tropism. The 28th International Herpesvirus Workshop, 2003 (abstract 1.02).
86. Stagno S, Pass RF, Cloud G, et al. Primary cytomegalovirus infection in pregnancy: incidence, transmission to fetus and clinical outcome. JAMA 256:1904-1908, 1986.
87. Hayes K, Danks DM, Gibas H, et al. Cytomegalovirus in human milk. N Engl J Med 287:177-178, 1972.

88. Lang DJ, Krummer JF. Cytomegalovirus in semen: observations in selected populations. J Infect Dis 132:472-473, 1975.
89. Reynolds DW, Stagno S, Hosty TS, et al. Maternal cytomegalovirus excretion and perinatal infection. N Engl J Med 289:1-5, 1973.
90. Stagno S, Reynolds DW, Pass RF, et al. Breast milk and the risk of cytomegalovirus infection. N Engl J Med 302:1073-1076, 1980.
91. Bowden RA. Cytomegalovirus infection in transplant patients: methods of prevention of primary cytomegalovirus. Transplant Proc 23:136-138, 1991.
92. Jordan MC, Rousseau WE, Noble GR, et al. Association of cervical cytomegaloviruses with venereal disease. N Engl J Med 288:932-934, 1973.
93. Coonrod D, Collier AC, Ashley R, et al. Association between cytomegalovirus seroconversion and upper genital tract infection among women attending a sexually transmitted disease clinic: a prospective study. J Infect Dis 177:1188-1193, 1998.
94. Drew WL, Mintz L, Miner RC, et al. Prevalence of cytomegalovirus infection in homosexual men. J Infect Dis 143:188-192, 1981.
95. Chandler SJ, Holmes KK, Wentworth BB, et al. The epidemiology of cytomegaloviral infection in women attending a sexually transmitted disease clinic. J Infect Dis 152:597-605, 1985.
96. Stagno S. Breastfeeding and the transmission of cytomegalovirus infections. Ital J Pediatr 28:275-280, 2002.
97. Pass RF, August AM, Dworsky M, et al. Cytomegalovirus infection in a day care center. N Engl J Med 307:477-479, 1982.
98. Adler SP, Wilson MS, Lawrence LT. Cytomegalovirus transmission among children attending a day care center. Pediatr Res 19:285A, 1985 (abstract).
99. Murph JR, Bale JF, Perlman S, et al. The prevalence of cytomegalovirus infection in a Midwest day care center. Pediatr Res 19:205A, 1985 (abstract).
100. Adler SP. The molecular epidemiology of cytomegalovirus transmission among children attending a day care center. J Infect Dis 152:760-768, 1985.
101. Hutto C, Ricks R, Garvie M, et al. Epidemiology of cytomegalovirus infections in young children: day care vs. home care. Pediatr Infect Dis 4:149-152, 1985.
102. Pass RF, Little EA, Stagno S, et al. Young children as a probable source of maternal and congenital cytomegalovirus infection. N Engl J Med 316:1366-1370, 1987.
103. Stagno S, Cloud GA. Working parents: the impact of day care and breast feeding on cytomegalovirus infection in offspring. Proc Natl Acad Sci U S A 91:2384-2389, 1994.
104. Hutto C, Little A, Ricks R, et al. Isolation of cytomegalovirus from toys and hands in a day care center. J Infect Dis 154:527-530, 1986.
105. Faix RG. Survival of cytomegalovirus on environmental surfaces. J Pediatr 106:649-652, 1985.
106. Dworsky ME, Lakeman AD, Stagno S. Cytomegalovirus transmission within a family. Pediatr Infect Dis 3:236-238, 1984.
107. Spector SA, Spector DH. Molecular epidemiology of cytomegalovirus infection in premature twin infants and their mother. Pediatr Infect Dis 1:405-409, 1982.
108. Yeager AS. Transmission of cytomegalovirus to mothers by infected infants: another reason to prevent transfusion-acquired infections. Pediatr Infect Dis 2:295-297, 1983.
109. Dworsky ME, Welch K, Cassady G, et al. Occupational risk for primary cytomegalovirus infection. N Engl J Med 309:950-953, 1983.
110. Adler SP. Molecular epidemiology of cytomegalovirus: viral transmission among children attending a day care center, their parents, and caretakers. J Pediatr 112:366-372, 1988.
111. Pass RF, Hutto SC, Ricks R, et al. Increased rate of cytomegalovirus infection among parents of children attending day care centers. N Engl J Med 314:1414-1418, 1986.
112. Adler SP. Molecular epidemiology of cytomegalovirus: evidence for viral transmission to parents from children infected at a day care center. Pediatr Infect Dis 5:315-318, 1986.
113. Adler SP. Cytomegalovirus and child day care: evidence for an increased infection rate among day-care workers. N Engl J Med 321:1290-1300, 1989.
114. Schopfer K, Lauber E, Krech U. Congenital cytomegalovirus infection in newborn infants of mothers infected before pregnancy. Arch Dis Child 53:536, 1978.
115. Stagno S, Reynolds DW, Huang ES, et al. Congenital cytomegalovirus infection: occurrence in an immune population. N Engl J Med 296:1254-1258, 1977.
116. Embil JA, Ozere RJ, Haldane EV. Congenital cytomegalovirus infection in two siblings from consecutive pregnancies. J Pediatr 77:417-421, 1970.
117. Stagno S, Reynolds DW, Lakeman AD, et al. Congenital cytomegalovirus infection (C-CMV): consecutive occurrence with similar antigenic viruses. Pediatr Res 7:141, 1973 (abstract).
118. Krech U, Konjajev Z, Jung M. Congenital cytomegalovirus infection in siblings from consecutive pregnancies. Helv Paediatr Acta 26: 355-362, 1971.
119. Stagno S, Pass RF, Dworsky ME, et al. Maternal cytomegalovirus infection and perinatal transmission. Clin Obstet Gynecol 25:563-576, 1982.
120. Boppana SB, Rivera LB, Fowler KB, et al. Intrauterine transmission of cytomegalovirus to infants of women with preconceptional immunity. N Engl J Med 344:1366-1371, 2001.
121. Gehrz RC, Christianson WR, Linner KM, et al. Cytomegalovirus-specific humoral and cellular immune response in human pregnancy. J Infect Dis 143:391-395, 1981.
122. Boppana SB, Britt WJ. Antiviral antibody responses and intrauterine transmission after primary maternal cytomegalovirus infection. J Infect Dis 171:1115-1121, 1995.
123. Boppana SB, Miller J, Britt WJ. Transplacentally acquired antiviral antibodies and outcome in congenital human cytomegalovirus infection. Viral Immunol 9:211-218, 1996.
124. Pass RF. Transmission of viruses through human milk. *In* Howell RR, Morris FH Jr, Pickering K (eds). Role of Human Milk in Infant Nutrition and Health. Springfield, Ill, Charles C Thomas, 1986, pp 205-224.
125. Chretien JH, McGinnis CG, Muller A. Venereal causes of cytomegalovirus mononucleosis. JAMA 238:1644-1645, 1977.
125a. Handsfield HH, Chandler SH, Caine VA, et al. Cytomegalovirus in sex partners: evidence for sexual transmission. J Infect Dis 151:344–348, 1985.
126. Kreel I, Zaroff LI, Canter JW, et al. A syndrome following total body perfusion. Surg Gynecol Obstet 111:317-321, 1960.
127. Seaman AJ, Starr A. Febrile postcardiotomy lymphocytic splenomegaly: a new entity. Ann Surg 156:956-960, 1962.
128. Armstrong JA, Tarr GC, Youngblood LA, et al. Cytomegalovirus infection in children undergoing open-heart surgery. Yale J Biol Med 49:83-91, 1976.
129. Prince AM, Szmuness W, Millian SJ, et al. A serologic study of cytomegalovirus infections associated with blood transfusions. N Engl J Med 284:1125-1131, 1971.
130. Stevens DP, Barker LF, Ketcham AS, et al. Asymptomatic cytomegalovirus infection following blood transfusion in tumor surgery. JAMA 211:1341-1344, 1970.
131. Kaariainen L, Klemola E, Paloheimo J. Rise of cytomegalovirus antibodies in an infectious mononucleosis-like syndrome after transfusion. BMJ 1:1270-1272, 1966.
132. Bowden RA, Slichter SJ, Sayers M, et al. A comparison of filtered leukocyte-reduced and cytomegalovirus (CMV) seronegative blood products for the prevention of transfusion-associated CMV infection after bone marrow transplant. Blood 86:3598-3603, 1995.
133. McCracken GJ, Shinefield HR, Cobb K, et al. Congenital cytomegalic inclusion disease: a longitudinal study of 20 patients. Am J Dis Child 117:522-539, 1969.
134. Kumar A, Nankervis GA, Cooper AR, et al. Acquisition of cytomegalovirus infection in infants following exchange transfusion: a prospective study. Transfusion 20:327-331, 1980.
135. Neiman PE, Reeves W, Ray G, et al. A prospective analysis of interstitial pneumonia and opportunistic viral infection among recipients of allogeneic bone marrow grafts. J Infect Dis 136:754-767, 1977.
136. Winston DJ, Gale RP, Meyer DV, et al. Infectious complications of human bone marrow transplantation. Medicine (Baltimore) 58:1-31, 1979.
137. Meyers JD, Flournoy N, Thomas ED. Nonbacterial pneumonia after allogeneic marrow transplantation: a review of ten years' experience. Rev Infect Dis 4:1119-1132, 1982.
138. Preiksaitis JK, Rosno S, Grumet C, et al. Infections due to herpesviruses in cardiac transplant recipients: role of the donor heart and immunosuppressive therapy. J Infect Dis 147:974-981, 1983.
139. Dummer JS, Hardy A, Poorsattar A, et al. Early infections in the kidney, heart and liver transplant recipients on cyclosporine. Transplantation 36:259-267, 1983.
140. Pollard RB, Rand KH, Arvin AM, et al. Cell-mediated immunity to cytomegalovirus infection in normal subjects and cardiac transplant patients. J Infect Dis 137:541-549, 1978.

141. Pollard RB, Arvin AM, Gamberg P, et al. Specific cell-mediated immunity and infections with herpesviruses in cardiac transplant recipients. Am J Med 73:679-687, 1982.
142. Pass RF, Hutto SC, Reynolds DW, et al. Increased frequency of cytomegalovirus in children in group day care. Pediatrics 74:121-126, 1984.
143. Pass RF, Stagno S. Cytomegalovirus. *In* Donowitz LG (ed). Hospital Acquired Infection in the Pediatric Patient. Baltimore, Williams & Wilkins, 1988.
144. Yeager AS. Longitudinal, serological study of cytomegalovirus infections in nurses and in personnel without patient contact. J Clin Microbiol 2:448-452, 1975.
145. Friedman HM, Lewis MR, Nemerofsky DM, et al. Acquisition of cytomegalovirus infection among female employees at a pediatric hospital. Pediatr Infect Dis 3:233-235, 1984.
145a. Brady MT, Demmler GJ, Andersen DC. Cytomegalovirus infection in pediatric house officers. Susceptibility and risk of primary infection (abstract). Pediatr Res 19:179A, 1985.
146. Yow MD, Lakeman AD, Stagno S, et al. Use of restriction enzymes to investigate the source of a primary CMV infection in a pediatric nurse. Pediatrics 70:713-716, 1982.
147. Wilfert CV, Huang ES, Stagno S. Restriction endonuclease analysis of cytomegalovirus DNA as an epidemiological tool. Pediatrics 70:717-721, 1982.
148. Adler SP, Baggett J, Wilson M, et al. Molecular epidemiology of cytomegalovirus in a nursery: lack of evidence for nosocomial transmission. J Pediatr 108:117-123, 1986.
148a. Demmler GJ, Yow MD, Spector SA, et al. Nosocomial transmission of cytomegalovirus in a Children's Hospital (abstract). Pediatr Res 20:308A, 1986.
148b. Balfour CL, Balfour HH. Cytomegalovirus is not an occupational risk for nurses in renal transplant and neonatal units. JAMA 256:1909-1914, 1986.
149. Klemola E, Kaariainen L. Cytomegalovirus as a possible cause of a disease resembling infectious mononucleosis. BMJ 2:1099-1102, 1965.
150. Andersson J, Stern H. Cytomegalovirus as a possible cause of a disease resembling infectious mononucleosis. BMJ 1:672, 1966.
151. Hayes K, Alford CA, et al. Antibody response to infected cell proteins following primary symptomatic and subclinical cytomegalovirus infection. Program and abstracts of the 25th Interscience Conference on Antimicrobial Agents and Chemotherapy, Washington, DC, ASM Press, 1985, p 908.
152. Hassan-Walker AF, Kidd IM, Sabin C, et al. Quantity of human cytomegalovirus (CMV) DNAemia as a risk factor for CMV disease in renal allograft recipients: relationship with donor/recipient CMV serostatus, receipt of augmented methylprednisolone and anti-thymocyte globulin (ATG). J Med Virol 58:182-187, 1999.
153. Spector SA, Hsia K, Crager M, et al. Cytomegalovirus (CMV) DNA load is an independent predictor of CMV disease and survival in advanced AIDS. J Virol 73:7027-7030, 1999.
154. Emery VC, Sabin CA, Cope AV, et al. Application of viral-load kinetics to identify patients who develop cytomegalovirus disease after transplantation. Lancet 355:2032-2036, 2000.
155. Grattan MT, Moreno-Cabral CE, Starnes VA, et al. Cytomegalovirus infection is associated with cardiac allograft rejection and atherosclerosis. JAMA 261:3561-3566, 1989.
156. Melnick JL, Adam E, Debakey ME. Cytomegalovirus and atherosclerosis. Eur Heart J 14(Suppl K):30-38, 1993.
157. Nieto FJ, Adam E, Sorlie P, et al. Cohort study of cytomegalovirus infection as a risk factor for carotid intimal-medial thickening, a measure of subclinical atherosclerosis. Circulation 94:922-927, 1996.
158. Hosenpud JD. Coronary artery disease after heart transplantation and its relation to cytomegalovirus. Am Heart J 138(5 Pt 2):S469-S472, 1999.
159. Koskinen PK, Kallio EA, Tikkanen JM, et al. Cytomegalovirus infection and cardiac allograft vasculopathy. Transplant Infect Dis 1:115-126, 1999.
160. Valantine HA, Gao SZ, Menon SG, et al. Impact of prophylactic immediate posttransplant ganciclovir on development of transplant atherosclerosis: a post hoc analysis of a randomized, placebo-controlled study. Circulation 100:61-66, 1999.
161. Zhu J, Quyyumi AA, Norman JE, et al. Cytomegalovirus in the pathogenesis of atherosclerosis: the role of inflammation as reflected by elevated C-reactive protein levels. J Am Coll Cardiol 34:1738-1743, 1999.
162. Evans PC, Soin A, Wreghitt TG, et al. An association between cytomegalovirus infection and chronic rejection after liver transplantation. Transplantation 69:30-35, 2000.
163. Soderberg-Naucler C, Emery VC. Viral infections and their impact on chronic renal allograft dysfunction. Transplantation 71(Suppl):SS24-SS30, 2001.
164. Streblow DN, Orloff SL, Nelson JA. Do pathogens accelerate atherosclerosis? J Nutr 131:2798S-2804S, 2001.
165. Stagno S, Reynolds DW, et al. Auditory and visual defects resulting from symptomatic and subclinical congenital cytomegaloviral and toxoplasma infections. Pediatrics 59:669-678, 1977.
166. Dahle AJ, McCollister FP, Stagno S, et al. Progressive hearing impairment in children with congenital cytomegalovirus infection. J Speech Hear Disord 44:220-229, 1979.
167. Fowler KB, McCollister FP, Dahle AJ, et al. Progressive and fluctuating sensorineural hearing loss in children with asymptomatic congenital cytomegalovirus infection. J Pediatr 130:624-630, 1997.
168. Dahle AJ, Fowler KB, Wright JD, et al. Longitudinal investigation of hearing disorders in children with congenital cytomegalovirus. J Am Acad Audiol 11:283-290, 2000.
169. Lemstrom KB, Bruning JH, Bruggeman CA, et al. Triple drug immunosuppression significantly reduces immune activation and allograft arteriosclerosis in cytomegalovirus-infected rat aortic allografts and induces early latency of viral infection. Am J Pathol 144:1334-1347, 1994.
170. Lemstrom K, Koskinen P, Krogerus L, et al. Cytomegalovirus antigen expression, endothelial cell proliferation, and intimal thickening in rat cardiac allografts after cytomegalovirus infection. Circulation 92:2594-2604, 1995.
171. Li F, Yin M, Van Dam JG, et al. Cytomegalovirus infection enhances the neointima formation in rat aortic allografts: effect of major histocompatibility complex class I and class II antigen differences. Transplantation 65:1298-1304, 1998.
172. Zhou YF, Shou M, Guetta E, et al. Cytomegalovirus infection of rats increases the neointimal response to vascular injury without consistent evidence of direct infection of the vascular wall. Circulation 100:1569-1575, 1999.
173. Streblow DN, Soderberg-Naucler C, Vieira J, et al. The human cytomegalovirus chemokine receptor US28 mediates vascular smooth muscle cell migration. Cell 99:511-520, 1999.
174. Hamprecht K, Vochem M, Baumeister A, et al. Detection of cytomegaloviral DNA in human milk cells and cell free milk whey by nested PCR. J Virol Method 70:167-176, 1998.
175. Gerna G, Zipeto D, Percivalle E, et al. Human cytomegalovirus infection of the major leukocyte subpopulations and evidence for initial viral replication in polymorphonuclear leukocytes from viremic patients. J Infect Dis 166:1236-1244, 1992.
176. Schafer P, Tenschert W, Cremaschi L, et al. Cytomegalovirus cultured from different major leukocyte subpopulations: association with clinical features in CMV immunoglobulin G–positive renal allograft recipients. J Med Virol 61:488-496, 2000.
177. Liapis H, Storch GA, Hill DA, et al. CMV infection of the renal allograft is much more common than the pathology indicates: a retrospective analysis of qualitative and quantitative buffy coat CMV-PCR, renal biopsy pathology and tissue CMV-PCR. Nephrol Dial Transplant 18:397-402, 2003.
178. Gerna G, Percivalle E, Baldanti F, et al. Human cytomegalovirus replicates abortively in polymorphonuclear leukocytes after transfer from infected endothelial cells via transient microfusion events. J Virol 74:5629-5638, 2000.
179. Kas-Deelen AM, The TH, Blom N, et al. Uptake of pp65 in in vitro generated pp65-positive polymorphonuclear cells mediated by phagocytosis and cell fusion? Intervirology 44:8-13, 2001.
180. van der Bij W, Schirm J, Torensma R, et al. Comparison between viremia and antigenemia for detection of cytomegalovirus in blood. J Clin Microbiol 26:2531-2535, 1988.
181. The TH, van der Bij W, van den Berg AP, et al. Cytomegalovirus antigenemia. Rev Infect Dis 12:734-744, 1990.
182. Gerna G, Zipeto D, Parea M, et al. Monitoring of human cytomegalovirus infections and ganciclovir treatment in heart transplant recipients by determination of viremia, antigenemia, and DNAemia. J Infect Dis 164:488-498, 1991.
183. Erice A, Holm MA, Gill PC, et al. Cytomegalovirus (CMV) antigenemia assay is more sensitive than shell vial cultures for rapid detection of CMV in polymorphonuclear blood leukocytes. J Clin Microbiol 30:2822-2825, 1992.

184. Landry ML, Ferguson D. Comparison of quantitative cytomegalovirus antigenemia assay with culture methods and correlation with clinical disease. J Clin Microbiol 31:2851-2856, 1993.
185. Boeckh M, Gooley TA, Myerson D, et al. Cytomegalovirus pp65 antigenemia-guided early treatment with ganciclovir versus ganciclovir at engraftment after allogeneic marrow transplantation: a randomized double-blind study. Blood 88:4063-4071, 1996.
186. Nichols WG, Boeckh M. Recent advances in the therapy and prevention of CMV infections. J Clin Virol 16:25-40, 2000.
187. Singh N, Paterson DL, Gayowski T, et al. Cytomegalovirus antigenemia directed pre-emptive prophylaxis with oral versus I.V. ganciclovir for the prevention of cytomegalovirus disease in liver transplant recipients: a randomized, controlled trial. Transplantation 70:717-722, 2000.
188. Rice GPA, Schrier RD, Oldstone MBA, et al. Cytomegalovirus infects human lymphocytes and monocytes: virus expression is restricted to immediate-early gene products. Proc Natl Acad Sci U S A 81:6134-6139, 1984.
189. Taylor-Wiedeman J, Sissons JG, Borysiewicz LK, Sinclair JH. Monocytes are a major site of persistence of human cytomegalovirus in peripheral blood mononuclear cells. J Gen Virol 72(Pt 9):2059-2064, 1991.
190. Fish KN, Stenglein SG, Ibanez C, Nelson JA. Cytomegalovirus persistence in macrophages and endothelial cells. Scand J Infect Dis (Suppl 99):34-40, 1995.
191. Waldman WJ, Knight DA, Huang EH, Sedmak DD. Bidirectional transmission of infectious cytomegalovirus between monocytes and vascular endothelial cells: an in vitro model. J Infect Dis 171:263-272, 1995.
192. Sinclair J, Sissons P. Latent and persistent infections of monocytes and macrophages. Intervirology 39:293-301, 1996.
193. Guetta E, Guetta V, Shibutani T, Epstein SE. Monocytes harboring cytomegalovirus: interactions with endothelial cells, smooth muscle cells, and oxidized low-density lipoprotein. Possible mechanisms for activating virus delivered by monocytes to sites of vascular injury. Circulation Res 81:8-16, 1997.
194. Soderberg-Naucler C, Fish KN, Fish KN, Nelson JA. Growth of human cytomegalovirus in primary macrophages. Methods 16: 126-138, 1998.
195. Hanson LK, Slater JS, Karabekian Z, et al. Replication of murine cytomegalovirus in differentiated macrophages as a determinant of viral pathogenesis. J Virol 73:5970-5980, 1999.
196. Jahn G, Stenglein S, Riegler S, et al. Human cytomegalovirus infection of immature dendritic cells and macrophages. Intervirology 42:365-372, 1999.
197. Riegler S, Hebart H, Einsele H, et al. Monocyte-derived dendritic cells are permissive to the complete replicative cycle of human cytomegalovirus. J Gen Virol 81(Pt 2):393-399, 2000.
198. Hahn G, Jores R, Mocarski ES. Cytomegalovirus remains latent in a common precursor of dendritic and myeloid cells. Proc Natl Acad Sci U S A 95:3937-3942, 1998.
199. Waldman WJ, Roberts WH, Davis DH, et al. Preservation of natural endothelial cytopathogenicity of cytomegalovirus by propagation in endothelial cells. Arch Virol 117:143-164, 1991.
200. Sinzger C, Knapp J, Plachter B, et al. Quantification of replication of clinical cytomegalovirus isolates in culture endothelial cells and fibroblasts by a focus expansion assay. J Virol Methods 63:103-112, 1997.
201. Gerna G, Zavattoni M, Baldanti F, et al. Circulating cytomegalic endothelial cells are associated with high human cytomegalovirus (HCMV) load in AIDS patients with late-stage disseminated HCMV disease. J Med Virol 55:64-74, 1998.
202. Evans PC, Coleman N, Wreghitt TG, et al. Cytomegalovirus infection of bile duct epithelial cells, hepatic artery and portal venous endothelium in relation to chronic rejection of liver grafts. J Hepatol 31:913-920, 1999.
203. Kas-Deelen AM, de Maar EF, Harmsen MC, et al. Uninfected and cytomegalic endothelial cells in blood during cytomegalovirus infection: effect of acute rejection. J Infect Dis 181:721-724, 2000.
204. Brune W, Menard C, Heesemann J, Koszinowski UH. A ribonucleotide reductase homolog of cytomegalovirus and endothelial cell tropism. Science 291:303-305, 2001.
205. Maidji E, Percivalle E, Gerna G, et al. Transmission of human cytomegalovirus from infected uterine microvascular endothelial cells to differentiation/invasive placental cytotrophoblasts. Virology 304:53-69, 2002.
206. Odeberg J, Cerboni C, Browne H, et al. Human cytomegalovirus (HCMV)–infected endothelial cells and macrophages are less susceptible to natural killer lysis independent of the downregulation of classical HLA class I molecules or expression of the HCMV class I homologue, UL18. Scand J Immunol 55:149-161, 2002.
207. Kahl M, Siegel-Axel D, Stenglein S, et al. Efficient lytic infection of human arterial endothelial cells by human cytomegalovirus strains. J Virol 74:7628-7635, 2000.
208. Sinzger C, Kahl M, Laib K, et al. Tropism of human cytomegalovirus for endothelial cells is determined by a post-entry step dependent on efficient translocation to the nucleus. J Gen Virol 81(Pt 12): 3021-3035, 2000.
209. Grefte A, van der Giessen M, van Son W, The TH. Circulating cytomegalovirus (CMV)-infected endothelial cells in patients with an active CMV infection. J Infect Dis 167:270-277, 1993.
210. Percivalle E, Revello MG, Vago L, et al. Circulating endothelial giant cells permissive for human cytomegalovirus (HCMV) are detected in disseminated HCMV infections with organ involvement. J Clin Invest 92:663-670, 1993.
211. Fries BC, Chou S, Boeckh M, Torok-Storb B. Frequency distribution of cytomegalovirus envelope glycoprotein genotypes in bone marrow transplant recipients. J Infect Dis 169:769-774, 1994.
212. Rasmussen L, Hong C, Zipeto D, et al. Cytomegalovirus gB genotype distribution differs in human immunodeficiency virus–infected patients and immunocompromised allograft recipients. J Infect Dis 175:179-184, 1997.
213. Haberland M, Meyer-Konig U, Hufert FT. Variation within the glycoprotein B gene of human cytomegalovirus is due to homologous recombination. J Gen Virol 80(Pt 6):1495-1500, 1999.
214. Bale JF, Murph JR, Demmler GJ, et al. Intrauterine cytomegalovirus infection and glycoprotein B genotypes. J Infect Dis 182:933-936, 2000.
215. Lurain NS, Kapell KS, Huang DD, et al. Human cytomegalovirus UL144 open reading frame: sequence hypervariability in low-passage clinical isolates. J Virol 73:10040-10050, 1999.
216. Bale JF, Petheram SJ, Robertson M, et al. Human cytomegalovirus: a sequence and UL144 variability in strains from infected children. J Med Virol 65:90-96, 2001.
217. Rasmussen L, Geissler A, Cowan C, et al. The genes encoding the gCIII complex of human cytomegalovirus exist in highly diverse combinations in clinical isolates. J Virol 76:10841-10848, 2002.
218. Rasmussen L, Geissler A, Winters M. Inter- and intragenic variations complicate the molecular epidemiology of human cytomegalovirus. J Infect Dis 187:809-819, 2003.
219. Chou SW. Cytomegalovirus infection and reinfection transmitted by heart transplantation. J Infect Dis 155:1054-1056, 1987.
220. Chou SW. Reactivation and recombination of multiple cytomegalovirus strains from individual organ donors. J Infect Dis 160:11-15, 1989.
221. Hayajneh WA, Colberg-Poley AM, Skaletskaya A, et al. The sequence and antiapoptotic functional domains of the human cytomegalovirus UL37 exon 1 immediate early protein are conserved in multiple primary strains. Virology 279:233-240, 2001.
222. Skaletskaya A, Bartle LM, Chittenden T, et al. A cytomegalovirus-encoded inhibitor of apoptosis that suppresses caspase-8 activation. Proc Natl Acad Sci U S A 98:7829-7834, 2001.
223. Spencer JV, Lockridge KM, Barry PA, et al. Potent immunosuppressive activities of cytomegalovirus-encoded interleukin-10. J Virol 76:1285-1292, 2002.
224. Bale JF, O'Neil ME. Detection of murine cytomegalovirus DNA in circulating leukocytes harvested during acute infection of mice [erratum appears in J Virol 63:4120, 1989]. J Virol 63:2667-2673, 1989.
225. Collins TM, Quirk MR, Jordan MC. Biphasic viremia and viral gene expression in leukocytes during acute cytomegalovirus infection of mice. J Virol 68:6305-6311, 1994.
226. Stoddart CA, Cardin RD, Boname JM, et al. Peripheral blood mononuclear phagocytes mediate dissemination of murine cytomegalovirus. J Virol 68:6243-6253, 1994.
227. Mitchell BM, Leung A, Stevens JG. Murine cytomegalovirus DNA in peripheral blood of latently infected mice is detectable only in monocytes and polymorphonuclear leukocytes. Virology 223:198-207, 1996.
228. Kern ER. Animal models for cytomegalovirus infection: murine CMV. *In* Zak O, Sande M (eds). Handbook of Animal Models of Infection. London, Academic Press, 1999, pp 927-934.
229. Reddehase MJ, Podlech J, Grzimek NK. Mouse models of cytomegalovirus latency: overview. J Clin Virol 25(Suppl 2):S23-S36, 2002.

230. Saederup N, Lin YC, Dairaghi DJ, et al. Cytomegalovirus-encoded beta chemokine promotes monocyte-associated viremia in the host. Proc Natl Acad Sci U S A 96:10881-10886, 1999.
231. Hanson LK, Slater JS, Karabekian Z, et al. Products of US22 genes M140 and M141 confer efficient replication of murine cytomegalovirus in macrophages and spleen. J Virol 75:6292-6302, 2001.
232. Saederup N, Aguirre SA, Sparer TE, et al. Murine cytomegalovirus CC chemokine homolog MCK-2 (m131-129) is a determinant of dissemination that increases inflammation at initial sites of infection. J Virol 75:9966-9976, 2001.
233. Menard C, Wagner M, Ruzsics Z, et al. Role of murine cytomegalovirus US22 gene family members in replication in macrophages. J Virol 77:5557-5570, 2003.
234. Mocarski ES. Immunomodulation by cytomegaloviruses: manipulative strategies beyond evasion. Trends Microbiol 10:332-339, 2002.
235. Hahn G, Khan H, Baldanti F, et al. The human cytomegalovirus ribonucleotide reductase homolog UL45 is dispensable for growth in endothelial cells, as determined by a BAC-cloned clinical isolate of human cytomegalovirus with preserved wild-type characteristics. J Virol 76:9551-9555, 2002.
236. Penfold ME, Dairaghi DJ, Duke GM, et al. Cytomegalovirus encodes a potent alpha chemokine. Proc Natl Acad Sci U S A 96:9839-9844, 1999.
237. Pepose JS, Holland GN, Nestor MS, et al. Acquired immune deficiency syndrome. Pathogenic mechanisms of ocular disease. Ophthalmology 92:472-484, 1985.
238. Jacobson MA, O'Donnell JJ, Porteous D, et al. Retinal and gastrointestinal disease due to cytomegalovirus in patients with the acquired immune deficiency syndrome: prevalence, natural history and response to ganciclovir therapy. Q J Med 67:473-486, 1988.
239. Francis ND, Boylston AW, Roberts AH, et al. Cytomegalovirus infection in gastrointestinal tracts of patients infected with HIV-1 or AIDS. J Clin Pathol 42:1055-1064, 1989.
240. Wilcox CM, Chalasani N, Lazenby A, Schwartz DA. Cytomegalovirus colitis in acquired immunodeficiency syndrome: a clinical and endoscopic study. Gastrointest Endosc 48:39-43, 1998.
241. Redman TK, Britt WJ, Wilcox CM, et al. Human cytomegalovirus enhances chemokine production by lipopolysaccharide-stimulated lamina propria macrophages. J Infect Dis 185:584-590, 2002.
242. Compton T, Kurt-Jones EA, Boehme KW, et al. Human cytomegalovirus activates inflammatory cytokine responses via CD14 and Toll-like receptor 2. J Virol 77:4588-4596, 2003.
243. Zhu H, Cong JP, Bresnahan WA, Shenk TE. Inhibition of cyclooxygenase 2 blocks human cytomegalovirus replication. Proc Natl Acad Sci U S A 99:3932-3937, 2002.
244. Margulies BJ, Browne H, Gibson W. Identification of the human cytomegalovirus G protein-coupled receptor homologue encoded by UL33 in infected cells and enveloped virus particles. Virology 225:111-125, 1996.
245. Rosenkilde MM, Waldhoer M, Luttichau HR, Schwartz TW. Virally encoded 7TM receptors. Oncogene 20:1582-1593, 2001.
246. Beisser PS, Goh CS, Cohen FE, Michelson S. Viral chemokine receptors and chemokines in human cytomegalovirus trafficking and interaction with the immune system. CMV chemokine receptors. Curr Top Microbiol Immunol 269:203-234, 2002.
247. Bodaghi B, Jones TR, Zipeto D, et al. Chemokine sequestration by viral chemoreceptors as a novel viral escape strategy: withdrawal of chemokines from the environment of cytomegalovirus-infected cells. J Exp Med 188:855-866, 1998.
248. Billstrom Schroeder M, Worthen GS. Viral regulation of RANTES expression during human cytomegalovirus infection of endothelial cells. J Virol 75:3383-3390, 2001.
249. Kledal TN, Rosenkilde MM, Schwartz TW. Selective recognition of the membrane-bound CX3C chemokine, fractalkine, by the human cytomegalovirus-encoded broad-spectrum receptor US28. FEBS Lett 441:209-214, 1998.
250. Billstrom Schroeder M, Christensen R, Worther GS et al. Human cytomegalovirus protects endothelial cells from apoptosis induced by growth factor withdrawal. J Clin Virol 25(Suppl 2):S149-S157, 2002.
251. Randolph-Habecker JR, Rahill B, Rahill B, et al. The expression of the cytomegalovirus chemokine receptor homolog US28 sequesters biologically active CC chemokines and alters IL-1 production. Cytokine 19:37-46, 2002.
252. Jonjic S, del Val M, Keil GM, et al. A nonstructural viral protein expressed by a recombinant vaccinia virus protects against lethal cytomegalovirus infection. J Virol 62:1653-1658, 1988.
253. Jonjic S, Pavic I, Lucin P, et al. Efficacious control of cytomegalovirus infection after long-term depletion of CD8+ T lymphocytes. J Virol 64:5457-5464, 1990.
254. Jonjic S, Pavic I, Polic B, et al. Antibodies are not essential for the resolution of primary cytomegalovirus infection but limit dissemination of recurrent virus. J Exp Med 179:1713-1717, 1994.
255. Polic B, Hengel H, Krmpotic A, et al. Hierarchical and redundant lymphocyte subset control precludes cytomegalovirus replication during latent infection. J Exp Med 188:1047-1054, 1998.
256. Steffens HP, Kurz S, Holtappels R, Reddehase MJ. Preemptive CD8 T-cell immunotherapy of acute cytomegalovirus infection prevents lethal disease, limits the burden of latent viral genomes, and reduces the risk of virus recurrence. J Virol 72:1797-1804, 1998.
257. Krmpotic A, Messerle M, Crnkovic-Mertens I, et al. The immunoevasive function encoded by the mouse cytomegalovirus gene m152 protects the virus against T cell control in vivo. J Exp Med 190:1285-1296, 1999.
258. Krmpotic A, Busch DH, Bubic I, et al. MCMV glycoprotein gp40 confers virus resistance to CD8+ T cells and NK cells in vivo. Nat Immunol 3:529-535, 2002.
259. Reusser P, Riddell SR, Meyers JD, Greenberg PD. Cytotoxic T-lymphocyte response to cytomegalovirus after human allogeneic bone marrow transplantation: pattern of recovery and correlation with cytomegalovirus infection and disease. Blood 78:1373-1380, 1991.
260. Riddell SR, Gilbert MJ, Li CR, et al. Reconstitution of protective CD8+ cytotoxic T lymphocyte responses to human cytomegalovirus in immunodeficient humans by the adoptive transfer of T cell clones. *In* Michelson S, and Plotkin SA (eds). Multidisciplinary Approach to Understanding Cytomegalovirus Disease. Amsterdam, Elsevier Science, 1993, pp155-164.
261. Li CR, Greenberg PD, Gilbert MJ, et al. Recovery of HLA-restricted cytomegalovirus (CMV)-specific T-cell responses after allogeneic bone marrow transplant: correlation with CMV disease and effect of ganciclovir prophylaxis. Blood 83:1971-1979, 1994.
262. Walter EA, Greenberg PD, Gilbert MJ, et al. Reconstitution of cellular immunity against cytomegalovirus in recipients of allogeneic bone marrow by transfer of T-cell clones from the donor. N Engl J Med 333:1038-1044, 1995.
263. Lacey SF, Gallez-Hawkins G, Crooks M, et al. Characterization of cytotoxic function of CMV-pp65–specific CD8+ T-lymphocytes identified by HLA tetramers in recipients and donors of stem-cell transplants. Transplantation 74:722-732, 2002.
264. Boeckh M, Leisenring W, Riddell SR, et al. Late cytomegalovirus disease and mortality in recipients of allogeneic hematopoietic stem cell transplants: importance of viral load and T-cell immunity. Blood 101:407-414, 2003.
265. Matloubian M, Concepcion RJ, Ahmed R. CD4+ T cells are required to sustain CD8+ cytotoxic T-cell responses during chronic viral infection. J Virol 68:8056-8063, 1994.
266. Sun JC, Bevan MJ. Defective CD8 T cell memory following acute infection without CD4 T cell help. Science 300:339-342, 2003.
267. Biron CA, Byron KS, Sullivan JL. Severe herpesvirus infections in an adolescent without natural killer cells. N Engl J Med 320:1731-1735, 1989.
268. Biron CA, Brossay L. NK cells and NKT cells in innate defense against viral infections. Curr Opin Immunol 13:458-464, 2001.
269. Yeager AS, Grumet FC, Hafleigh EB, et al. Prevention of transfusion-acquired cytomegalovirus infections in newborn infants. J Pediatr 98:281-287, 1981.
270. Rasmussen L, Morris S, Wolitz R, et al. Deficiency in antibody response to human cytomegalovirus glycoprotein gH in human immunodeficiency virus-infected patients at risk for cytomegalovirus retinitis. J Infect Dis 170:673-767, 1994.
271. Boppana SB, Polis MA, Kramer AA, et al. Virus specific antibody responses to human cytomegalovirus (HCMV) in human immunodeficiency virus type 1–infected individuals with HCMV retinitis. J Infect Dis 171:182-185, 1995.
272. Schoppel K, Kropff B, Schmidt C, et al. The humoral immune response against human cytomegalovirus is characterized by a delayed synthesis of glycoprotein-specific antibodies. J Infect Dis 175:533-544, 1997.
273. Schoppel K, Schmidt C, Einsele H, et al. Kinetics of the antibody response against human cytomegalovirus-specific proteins in allogeneic bone marrow transplant recipients. J Infect Dis 178:1233-1243, 1998.
274. Snydman DR, Werner BG, Heinze-Lacey B, et al. Use of cytomegalovirus immune globulin to prevent cytomegalovirus disease in renal-transplant recipients. N Engl J Med 317:1049-1054, 1987.

275. Winston DJ, Ho WG, Lin CH, et al. Intravenous immune globulin for prevention of cytomegalovirus infection and interstitial pneumonia after bone marrow transplantation. Ann Intern Med 106:12-18, 1987.
276. Emanuel D, Cunningham I, Jules-Elysee K, et al. Cytomegalovirus pneumonia after bone marrow transplantation successfully treated with the combination of ganciclovir and high-dose intravenous immune globulin. Ann Intern Med 109:777-782, 1988.
277. Snydman DR, Werner BG, et al. Cytomegalovirus immune globulin prophylaxis in liver transplantation. A randomized, double-blind placebo-controlled trial. The Boston Center for Liver Transplantation CMVIG Study Group. Ann Intern Med 119:984-991, 1993.
278. Bowden RA, Sayers M, Flournoy N, et al. Cytomegalovirus immune globulin and seronegative blood products to prevent primary cytomegalovirus infection after marrow transplantation. N Engl J Med 314:1006-1010, 1986.
279. Bowden RA, Fisher LD, Rogers K, et al. Cytomegalovirus (CMV)–specific intravenous immunoglobulin for the prevention of primary CMV infection and disease after marrow transplantation. J Infect Dis 164:483-487, 1991.
280. Bratcher DF, Bourne N, Bravo FJ, et al. Effect of passive antibody on congenital cytomegalovirus infection in guinea pigs. J Infect Dis 172:944-950, 1995.
281. Chatterjee A, Harrison CJ, Britt WJ, Bewtra C. Modification of maternal and congenital cytomegalovirus infection by anti-glycoprotein b antibody transfer in guinea pigs. J Infect Dis 183:1547-1553, 2001.
282. Reddehase MJ. Antigens and immunoevasins: opponents in cytomegalovirus immune surveillance. Nat Rev Immunol 2:831-844, 2002.
283. Holtappels R, Podlech J, Pahl-Seibert MF, et al. Cytomegalovirus misleads its host by priming of CD8 T cells specific for an epitope not presented in infected tissues. J Exp Med 199:131-136, 2004.
284. Zaia JA, Gallez-Hawkins G, Li X, et al. Infrequent occurrence of natural mutations in the pp65 (495-503) epitope sequence presented by the HLA A*0201 allele among human cytomegalovirus isolates. J Virol 75:2472-2474, 2001.
285. Voigt V, Forbes CA, Tonkin JN, et al. Murine cytomegalovirus m157 mutation and variation leads to immune evasion of natural killer cells. Proc Natl Acad Sci U S A 100:13483-13488, 2003.
286. Britt WJ. Recent advances in the identification of significant human cytomegalovirus-encoded proteins. Transplant Proc 23:64-69, 1991.
287. Pignatelli S, Dal Monte P, Dal Monte P, et al. Human cytomegalovirus glycoprotein N (gpUL73-gN) genomic variants: identification of a novel subgroup, geographical distribution and evidence of positive selective pressure. J Gen Virol 84(Pt 3):647-655, 2003.
288. Stagno S, Reynolds DW, Tsiantos A, et al. Comparative serial virologic and serologic studies of symptomatic and subclinical congenitally and natally acquired cytomegalovirus infections. J Infect Dis 132: 568-577, 1975.
289. Lockridge KM, Sequar G, Zhou SS, et al. Pathogenesis of experimental rhesus cytomegalovirus infection. J Virol 73:9576-9583, 1999.
290. Griffith BP, Lucia HL, Bia FJ, Hsiung GD. Cytomegalovirus-induced mononucleosis in guinea pigs. Infect Immun 32:857-863, 1981.
291. Griffith BP, McCormick SR, Booss J, Hsiung GD. Inbred guinea pig model of intrauterine infection with cytomegalovirus. Am J Pathol 122:112-119, 1986.
292. Bernstein DI, Bourne N. Animal models for cytomegalovirus infection: guinea-pig CMV. *In* Zak O, Sande M (eds). Handbook of Animal Models of Infection. London, Academic Press, 1999, pp 935-941.
293. Spector SA, Merrill R, Wolf D, Dankner WM. Detection of human cytomegalovirus in plasma of AIDS patients during acute visceral disease by DNA amplification. J Clin Microbiol 30:2359-2365, 1992.
294. Bowen EF, Wilson P, Atkins M, et al. Natural history of untreated cytomegalovirus retinitis. Lancet 346:1671-1673, 1995.
295. Nelson CT, Istas AS, Wilkerson MK, Demmler GJ. PCR detection of cytomegalovirus DNA in serum as a diagnostic test for congenital cytomegalovirus infection. J Clin Microbiol 33:3317-3318, 1995.
296. Rasmussen L, Morris S, Zipeto D, et al. Quantitation of human cytomegalovirus DNA from peripheral blood cells of human immunodeficiency virus-infected patients could predict cytomegalovirus retinitis. J Infect Dis 171:177-182, 1995.
297. Bowen EF, Sabin CA, Wilson P, et al. Cytomegalovirus (CMV) viremia detected by polymerase chain reaction identifies a group of HIV-positive patients at high risk of CMV disease. AIDS 11:889-893, 1997.
298. Spector SA, Wong R, Hsia K, et al. Plasma cytomegalovirus (CMV) DNA load predicts CMV disease and survival in AIDS patients. J Clin Invest 101:497-502, 1998.
299. Revello MG, Gerna G. Diagnosis and management of human cytomegalovirus infection in the mother, fetus, and newborn infant. Clin Microbiol Rev 15:680-715, 2002.
300. Becroft DMO. Prenatal cytomegalovirus infection: epidemiology, pathology, and pathogenesis. *In* Rosenberg HS, Bernstein J (eds). Perspective in Pediatric Pathology. New York, Masson Press, 1981, pp 203-241.
301. Stagno S, Pass RF, Dworsky ME, Alford CA. Congenital and perinatal cytomegalovirus infections. Semin Perinatol 7:31-42, 1983.
302. Stagno S. Cytomegalovirus infection: a pediatrician's perspective. Curr Probl Pediatr 16:629-667, 1986.
303. Boppana SB, Pass RF, Britt WJ, et al. Symptomatic congenital cytomegalovirus infection: neonatal morbidity and mortality. Pediatr Infect Dis J 11:93-99, 1992.
304. Williamson WD, Demmler GJ, Percy AK, Catlin FI. Progressive hearing loss in infants with asymptomatic congenital cytomegalovirus infection. Pediatrics 90:862-866, 1992.
305. Griffith BP, Lucia HL, Hsiung GD. Brain and visceral involvement during congenital cytomegalovirus infection of guinea pigs. Pediatr Res 16:455-259, 1982.
306. Bia FJ, Griffith BP, Fong CK, Hsiung GD. Cytomegaloviral infections in the guinea pig: experimental models for human disease. Rev Infect Dis 5:177-195, 1983.
307. Bale JF, Bray PF, Bell WE. Neuroradiographic abnormalities in congenital cytomegalovirus infection. Pediatr Neurol 1:42-47, 1985.
308. Perlman JM, Argyle C. Lethal cytomegalovirus infection in preterm infants: clinical, radiological, and neuropathological findings. Ann Neurol 31:64-68, 1992.
309. Boppana SB, Fowler KB, Vaid Y, et al. Neuroradiographic findings in the newborn period and long-term outcome in children with symptomatic congenital cytomegalovirus infection. Pediatrics 99: 409-414, 1997.
310. Boesch C, Issakainen J, Kewitz G, et al. Magnetic resonance imaging of the brain in congenital cytomegalovirus infection. Pediatric Radiology 19:91-93, 1989.
311. Tarantal AF, Salamat MS, Britt WJ, et al. Neuropathogenesis induced by rhesus cytomegalovirus in fetal rhesus monkeys *(Macaca mulatta)*. J Infect Dis 177:446-450, 1998.
312. Chang WL, Tarantal AF, Zhou SS, et al. A recombinant rhesus cytomegalovirus expressing enhanced green fluorescent protein retains the wild-type phenotype and pathogenicity in fetal macaques. J Virol 76:9493-9504, 2002.
313. van den Pol AN, Reuter JD, Santarelli JG. Enhanced cytomegalovirus infection of developing brain independent of the adaptive immune system. J Virol 76:8842-8854, 2002.
314. Zou YR, Kottmann AH, Kuroda M, et al. Function of the chemokine receptor CXCR4 in haematopoiesis and in cerebellar development. Nature 393:595-599, 1998.
315. Zhu Y, Yu T, Nagasawa T, et al. Role of the chemokine SDF-1 as the meningeal attractant for embryonic cerebellar neurons. Nat Neurosci 5:719-720, 2002.
316. Williamson WD, Desmond MM, LaFevers N, et al. Symptomatic congenital cytomegalovirus: disorders of language, learning and hearing. Am J Dis Child 136:902-905, 1982.
317. Strauss M. A clinical pathologic study of hearing loss in congenital cytomegalovirus infection. Laryngoscope 95:951-962, 1985.
318. Strauss M. Human cytomegalovirus labyrinthitis. Am J Otolaryngol 11:292-298, 1990.
319. Rarey KE, Davis LE. Temporal bone histopathology 14 years after cytomegalic inclusion disease: a case study. Laryngoscope 103:904-909, 1993.
320. Harris JP, Heydt J, Keithley EM, Chen MC. Immunopathology of the inner ear: an update. Ann N Y Acad Sci 830:166-178, 1997.
321. Chen MC, Harris JP, Keithley EM. Immunohistochemical analysis of proliferating cells in a sterile labyrinthitis animal model. Laryngoscope. 108:651-656, 1998.
322. Harris JP, Fan JT, Keithley EM, et al. Immunologic responses in experimental cytomegalovirus labyrinthtis. Am J Otolaryngol 11:304-308, 1990.
323. Harris JP, Woolf NK, Ryan AF, et al. Immunologic and electrophysiological response to cytomegaloviral inner ear infection in the guinea pig. J Infect Dis 150:523-530, 1984.
324. Harris S, Ahlfors K, Ivarsson S, et al. Congenital cytomegalovirus infection and sensorineural hearing loss. Ear Hear 5:352-355, 1984.
325. Fukuda S, Keithley EM, Harris JP. Experimental cytomegalovirus infection: viremic spread to the inner ear. Am J Otolaryngol 9:135-141, 1988.

326. Fowler KB, Stagno S, Pass RF, et al. The outcome of congenital cytomegalovirus infection in relation to maternal antibody status. N Engl J Med 326:663-667, 1992.
327. Demmler GJ. Summary of a workshop on surveillance for congenital cytomegalovirus disease. Rev Infect Dis 13:315-319, 1991.
328. Griffiths PD, Baboonian C. A prospective study of primary cytomegalovirus infection during pregnancy: final report. Br J Obstet Gynaecol 91:307-315, 1984.
329. Granstrom ML. Perinatal cytomegalovirus in man. Thesis. Helsinki, Finland, University of Helsinki, 1979.
330. Monif GRG, Egan EA, Held B, et al. The correlation of maternal cytomegalovirus infection during varying stages in gestation with neonatal involvement. J Pediatr 80:17-20, 1972.
331. Preece PM, Pearl KN, Peckham CS. Congenital cytomegalovirus infection. Arch Dis Child 59:1120-1126, 1984.
332. Yow MD, Williamson DW, Leeds LJ, et al. Epidemiologic characteristics of cytomegalovirus infection in mothers and their infants. Am J Obstet Gynecol 158:1189-1195, 1988.
333. Pass RF, Fowler KB, Stagno S, et al. Gestational age at time of maternal infection and outcome of congenital cytomegalovirus infection. Pediatr Res 35:191A, 1994 (abstract).
334. Ahlfors K, Ivarsson SA, Harris S, et al. Congenital cytomegalovirus infection and disease in Sweden and the relative importance of primary and secondary maternal infections. Scand J Infect Dis 16:129-137, 1984.
335. Rutter D, Griffiths P, Trompeter RS. Cytomegalic inclusion disease after recurrent maternal infection. Lancet 2:1182, 1985.
336. Jones MM, Lidsky MD, Brewer EJ, et al. Congenital cytomegalovirus infection and maternal systemic lupus erythematosus: a case report. Arthritis Rheum 29:1402-1404, 1986.
337. Evans TJ, McCollum JPK, Valdimarssan H. Congenital cytomegalovirus infection after maternal renal transplantation. Lancet 1:1359-1360, 1975.
338. Portalini M, Cermelli S, Sabbatini AMT, et al. A fatal case of congenital cytomegalic inclusion disease following recurrent maternal infection. Microbiologica 18:427-428, 1995.
339. Morris DJ, Sims D, Chiswick M, et al. Symptomatic congenital cytomegalovirus infection after maternal recurrent infection. Pediatr Infect Dis J 13:61-64, 1994.
340. Laifer SA, Ehrlich GD, Haff DS, et al. Congenital cytomegalovirus infection in offspring of liver transplant recipient. Clin Infect Dis 20:52-55, 1995.
341. Muss-Pinhata MM, Yamamoto AY, Figueiredo LTM, et al. Congenital and perinatal cytomegalovirus infection in infants born to mothers infected with human immunodeficiency virus. J Pediatr 132:285-290, 1998.
342. Vochem M, Hamprecht K, Jahn G, et al. Transmission of cytomegalovirus to preterm infants through breast milk. Pediatr Infect Dis 17:53-58, 1998.
343. van der Strate BW, Harrisen MC, Schafer P, et al. Viral load in breast milk correlates with transmission of human cytomegalovirus to preterm neonates but lactoferrin concentrations do not. Clin Diagn Lab Immunol 8:812-818, 2001.
344. Maschmann J, Hamprecht K, Dietz K, et al. Cytomegalovirus infection of extremely low-birth weight infants via breast milk. Clin Infect Dis 33:1998-2003, 2001.
345. Chou S, Kim DY, Norman DJ. Transmission of cytomegalovirus by pretransplant leukocyte transfusions in renal transplant candidates. J Infect Dis 155:565-567, 1987.
346. Reynolds DW, Stagno S, Alford CA. Laboratory diagnosis of cytomegalovirus infections. *In* Lennette EH, Schmidt NJ (eds). Diagnostic Procedures for Viral, Rickettsial and Chlamydial Infections, 5th ed. Washington, DC, American Public Health Association, 1979, pp 399-439.
347. Wolf A, Cowen D. Perinatal infections of the central nervous system. J Neuropathol Exp Neurol 18:191-243, 1959.
348. Naeye RL. Cytomegalic inclusion disease, the fetal disorder. Am J Clin Pathol 47:738-744, 1967.
349. Hanshaw JB. Developmental abnormalities associated with congenital cytomegalovirus infection. Adv Teratol 4:64-93, 1970.
350. Arey JB. Cytomegalic inclusion disease in infancy. Am J Dis Child 88:525-526, 1954.
351. Mercer RD, Luse S, Guyton DH. Clinical diagnosis of generalized cytomegalic inclusion disease. Pediatrics 11:502-514, 1953.
352. Sackett GL, Ford MM. Cytomegalic inclusion disease with calcification outlining the cerebral ventricles. AJR Am J Roentgenol 76:512, 1956.
353. Jamison RM, Hathorn AW. Isolation of cytomegalovirus from cerebrospinal fluid of a congenitally infected infant. Am J Dis Child 132:63-64, 1978.
354. Keithley EM, Woolf NK, Harris JP. Development of morphological and physiological changes in the cochlea induced by cytomegalovirus. Laryngoscope 99:409-414, 1989.
355. Myers EN, Stool S. Cytomegalic inclusion disease of the inner ear. Laryngoscope 78:1904-1915, 1968.
356. Davis GL. Cytomegalovirus in the inner ear. Case report and electron microscopic study. Ann Otol Rhinol Laryngol 78:1179-1188, 1969.
357. Guyton TB, Ehrlich F, Blanc WA, et al. New observations in generalized cytomegalic inclusion disease of the newborn: reports of a case with chorioretinitis. N Engl J Med 257:803-807, 1957.
358. Ansari BM, Davis DB, Jones MR. Calcification in liver associated with congenital cytomegalic inclusion disease. J Pediatr 90:661-663, 1977.
359. Alix D, Castel Y, Gouedard H. Hepatic calcification in congenital cytomegalic inclusion disease. J Pediatr 92:856, 1978.
360. Osborn JE, Shahidi NT. Thrombocytopenia in murine cytomegalovirus infection. J Lab Clin Med 81:53-63, 1973.
361. Fetterman GH, Sherman FE, Fabrizio NS, et al. Generalized cytomegalic inclusion disease of the newborn: localization of inclusions in the kidney. Arch Pathol 86:86-94, 1968.
362. Donnellan WL, Chantra-Umporn S, Kidd JM. The cytomegalic inclusion cell: an electron microscopic study. Arch Pathol 82:336-348, 1966.
363. Reyes C, Pereira S, Warden MJ, Sills J. Cytomegalovirus enteritis in a premature infant. J Pediatr Surg 32:1545-1547, 1997.
364. Blanc WA. Pathology of the placenta and cord in some viral infections. *In* Hanshaw JB, Dudgeon JA (eds). Viral Diseases of the Fetus and Newborn. Philadelphia, WB Saunders, 1978, pp 237-258.
365. Benirschke K, Mendoza GR, Bazeley PL. Placental and fetal manifestations of cytomegalovirus infection. Virchows Arch B 16:121, 1974.
366. Weller TH, Hanshaw JB. Virologic and clinical observations on cytomegalic inclusion disease. N Engl J Med 266:1233-1244, 1962.
367. Anderson KS, Amos CS, Boppana S, Pass RF. Ocular abnormalities in congenital cytomegalovirus infection. J Am Optom Assoc 67:273-278, 1996.
368. Istes AS, Demmler GJ, Dobbins JG, et al. Surveillance for congenital cytomegalovirus disease: a report from the National Congenital Cytomegalovirus Disease Registry. Clin Infect Dis 20:665-670, 1995.
369. Demmler GJ. Congenital cytomegalovirus infection. Semin Pediatr Neurol 1:36-42, 1994.
370. Hanshaw JB, Dudgeon JA (eds). Viral Diseases of the Fetus and Newborn. Philadelphia, WB Saunders, 1978.
371. Medearis TN. Observations concerning human cytomegalovirus infection and disease. Bull Johns Hopkins Hosp 114:181-211, 1964.
372. Stagno S, Brasfield DM, Brown MC, et al. Infant pneumonitis associated with cytomegalovirus, *Chlamydia*, *Pneumocystis*, and *Ureaplasma*—a prospective study. Pediatrics 68:322-329, 1981.
373. Stagno S, Pass RF, Thomas JP, et al. Defects of tooth structure in congenital cytomegalovirus infection. Pediatrics 69:646-648, 1982.
374. Melish ME, Hanshaw JB. Congenital cytomegalovirus infection: developmental progress of infants detected by routine screening. Am J Dis Child 126:190-194, 1973.
375. Saigal S, Luynk O, Larke B, et al. The outcome in children with congenital cytomegalovirus infection: a longitudinal follow-up study. Am J Dis Child 136:896-901, 1982.
376. Berenberg W, Nankervis G. Long-term follow-up of cytomegalic inclusion disease of infancy. Pediatrics 37:403-410, 1970.
377. Conboy TJ, Pass RF, Stagno S, et al. Early clinical manifestations and intellectual outcome in children with symptomatic congenital cytomegalovirus infection. J Pediatr 111:343-348, 1987.
378. Kumar ML, Nankervis GA, Gold E. Inapparent congenital cytomegalovirus infection: a follow-up study. N Engl J Med 288:1370-1377, 1973.
379. Reynolds DW, Stagno S, Stubbs KG, et al. Inapparent congenital cytomegalovirus infection with elevated cord IgM levels: causal relationship with auditory and mental deficiency. N Engl J Med 290:291-296, 1974.
380. Pearl KN, Preece PM, Ades A, et al. Neurodevelopmental assessment after congenital cytomegalovirus infection. Arch Dis Child 61:232-236, 1986.
381. Conboy TJ, Pass RF, Stagno S, et al. Intellectual development in school aged children with asymptomatic congenital cytomegalovirus infection. Pediatrics 77:801-806, 1986.

382. Pass RF, Stagno S, Myers GJ, et al. Outcome of symptomatic congenital cytomegalovirus infection: results of long-term longitudinal follow-up. Pediatrics 66:758-762, 1980.
383. Ramsey MEB, Miller E, Peckham CS. Outcome of confirmed symptomatic congenital cytomegalovirus infection. Arch Dis Child 66:1068-1069, 1991.
384. Williamson WD, Percy AK, Yow MD, et al. Asymptomatic congenital cytomegalovirus infection. Audiologic, neuroradiologic and neurodevelopmental abnormalities during the first year. Am J Dis Child 144:1365-1368, 1990.
385. Ivarsson SA, Lernmark B, Svanberg L. Ten-year clinical, developmental and intellectual follow up of children with congenital cytomegalovirus infection without neurologic symptoms at one year of age. Pediatrics 99:800-803, 1997.
386. Kashden J, Frison S, Fowler K, et al. Intellectual assessment of children with asymptomatic congenital cytomegalovirus infection. J Dev Behav Pediatr 19:254-259, 1998.
387. Noyola DE, Demmler GJ, Williamson WD, et al. Cytomegalovirus urinary excretion and long term outcome in children with congenital cytomegalovirus infection. Congenital CMV Longitudinal Study Group. Pediatr Infect Dis J 19:505-510, 2000.
388. Hicks T, Fowler K, Richardson M, et al. Congenital cytomegalovirus infection and neonatal auditory screening. J Pediatr 123:779-782, 1993.
389. Hayes K, Symington G, Mackay IR. Maternal immunosuppression and cytomegalovirus infection of the fetus. Aust N Z J Med 9:430-433, 1979.
390. Stagno S, Pass RF, Dworsky ME, et al. Congenital cytomegalovirus infection: the relative importance of primary and recurrent maternal infection. N Engl J Med 306:945-949, 1982.
391. Fowler KB, Stagno S, Pass RF. Maternal immunity and prevention of congenital cytomegalovirus infection. JAMA 289:1008-1011, 2003.
392. Ahlfors K, Ivarsson SA, Harris S. Report on a long-term study of maternal and congenital cytomegalovirus infection in Sweden: review of prospective studies available in the literature. Scand J Infect Dis 31:443-57, 1999.
393. Boppana SB, Fowler KB, Britt WJ, et al. Symptomatic congenital cytomegalovirus infection in infants born to mothers with preexisting immunity to cytomegalovirus. Pediatrics 104:55-60, 1999.
394. Yeager AS. Transfusion-acquired cytomegalovirus infection in newborn infants. Am J Dis Child 128:478-483, 1974.
395. Adler SP, Chandrika T, Lawrence L, et al. Cytomegalovirus infections in neonates due to blood transfusions. Pediatr Infect Dis 2:114-118, 1983.
396. Whitley RJ, Brasfield D, Reynolds DW, et al. Protracted pneumonitis in young infants associated with perinatally acquired cytomegaloviral infection. J Pediatr 89:11-16, 1976.
397. Brasfield DM, Stagno S, Whitley RJ, et al. Infant pneumonitis associated with cytomegalovirus, *Chlamydia*, *Pneumocystis*, and *Ureaplasma*: follow-up. Pediatrics 79:76-83, 1987.
398. Yeager AS, Palumbo PE, Malachowski N, et al. Sequelae of maternally derived cytomegalovirus infections in premature infants. Pediatrics 102:918-922, 1983.
399. Paryani SG, Yeager AS, Hosford-Dunn H, et al. Sequelae of acquired cytomegalovirus infection in premature and sick term infants. J Pediatr 107:451-456, 1985.
400. Ballard RB, Drew WL, Hufnagle KG, et al. Acquired cytomegalovirus infection in preterm infants. Am J Dis Child 133:482-485, 1979.
401. Adler SP. Transfusion-associated cytomegalovirus infections. Rev Infect Dis 5:977-993, 1983.
402. Demmler GJ, Buffone GJ, Schimbor CM, et al. Detection of cytomegalovirus in urine from newborns by using polymerase chain reaction DNA amplification. J Infect Dis 158:1177-1184, 1988.
403. Warren WP, Balcarek K, Smith RJ, et al. Comparison of rapid methods of detection of cytomegalovirus in saliva with virus isolation in tissue culture. J Clin Microbiol 30:786-789, 1992.
404. Johansson PJH, Jonsson M, Ahlfors K, et al. Retrospective diagnosis of congenital cytomegalovirus infection performed by polymerase chain reaction in blood stored on filter paper. Scand J Infect Dis 29:465-468, 1997.
405. Dzierzahowska D, Augustynowicz E, Gzyl A, et al. Application of polymerase chain reaction (PCR) for the detection of DNA-HCMV in cerebrospinal fluid of neonates and infants with cytomegalovirus infection. Neurol Neurochir Pol 31:447-462, 1997.
406. Stagno S, Pass RF, Reynolds DW, et al. Comparative study of diagnostic procedures for congenital cytomegalovirus infection. Pediatrics 65:251-257, 1980.
407. Griffiths PD. Cytomegalovirus. *In* Zuckerman AJ, Banatvala JE, Pattison JR (eds). Principles and Practice of Clinical Virology. New York, John Wiley 1987, pp 75-109.
408. Shuster EA, Beneke JS, Tegtmeier GE, et al. Monoclonal antibody for rapid laboratory detection of cytomegalovirus infections: characterization and diagnostic application. Mayo Clin Proc 60:577-585, 1985.
409. Alpert G, Mazeron MC, Colimon R, et al. Rapid detection of human cytomegalovirus in the urine of humans. J Infect Dis 152:631-633, 1985.
410. Stirk PR, Griffiths PD. Use of monoclonal antibodies for the diagnosis of cytomegalovirus infection by the detection of early antigen fluorescent foci (DEAFF) in cell culture. J Med Virol 21:329-337, 1987.
411. Boppana SB, Smith RJ, Stagno S, et al. Evaluation of a microtiter plate fluorescent-antibody assay for rapid detection of human cytomegalovirus infection. J Clin Microbiol 30:721-723, 1992.
412. Chou S, Merigan TC. Rapid detection and quantitation of human cytomegalovirus in urine through DNA hybridization. N Engl J Med 308:921-925, 1983.
413. Spector SA, Rua JA, Spector DH, et al. Detection of human cytomegalovirus in clinical specimens by DNA-DNA hybridization. J Infect Dis 150:121-126, 1984.
414. Schuster V, Matz B, Wiegand H, et al. Detection of human cytomegalovirus in urine by DNA-DNA and RNA-DNA hybridization. J Infect Dis 154:309-314, 1986.
415. Virtanen M, Syvanen A, Oram J, et al. Cytomegalovirus in urine: detection of viral DNA by sandwich hybridization. J Clin Microbiol 20:1083-1088, 1984.
416. Lurain NS, Thompson SK, Farrand SK. Rapid detection of cytomegalovirus in clinical specimens by using biotinylated DNA probes and analysis of cross-reactivity with herpes simplex virus. J Clin Microbiol 24:724-730, 1986.
417. Barbi M, Binda S, Primache V, Clerici D. Congenital cytomegalovirus infection in a northern Italian region. NEOCMV Group. Eur J Epidemiol 14:791-796, 1998.
418. Mazzulli T, Rubin RH, Ferraro MJ, et al. Cytomegalovirus antigenemia: clinical correlations in transplant recipients and in persons with AIDS. J Clin Microbiol 31:2824-2827, 1993.
419. Dodt KK, Jacobsen PH, Hofmann B, et al. Development of cytomegalovirus (CMV) disease may be predicted in HIV-infected patients by CMV polymerase chain reaction and the antigenemia test. AIDS 11:F21-F28, 1997.
420. Wetherill PE, Landry ML, Alcabes P, Friedland G. Use of a quantitative cytomegalovirus (CMV) antigenemia test in evaluating HIV+ patients with and without CMV disease. J Acquir Immune Defic Syndr Hum Retrovirol 12:33-37, 1996.
421. Revello MG, Zavattoni M, Baldanti F, et al. Diagnostic and prognostic value of human cytomegalovirus load and IgM antibody in blood of congenitally infected newborns. J Clin Virol 14:57-66, 1999.
422. Griffiths PD, Kangro HO. A user's guide to the indirect solid-phase radioimmunoassay for the detection of cytomegalovirus specific IgM antibodies. J Virol Methods 8:271-282, 1984.
423. Stagno S, Tinker MK, Elrod C, et al. Immunoglobulin M antibodies detected by enzyme-linked immunosorbent assay and radioimmunoassay in the diagnosis of cytomegalovirus infections in pregnant women and newborn infants. J Clin Microbiol 21:930-935, 1985.
424. Vornhagen R, Hinderer W, Sonneborn HH, et al. IgM-specific serodiagnosis of acute human cytomegalovirus infection using recombinant autologous fusion proteins. J Virol Methods 60:73-80, 1996.
425. Lazzarotto T, Maine GT, DalMonte P, et al. A novel Western blot test containing both viral and recombinant proteins for anticytomegalovirus immunoglobulin M detection. J Clin Microbiol 35:393-397, 1997.
426. Lazzarotto T, Ripalti A, Bergamini G, et al. Development of a new cytomegalovirus (CMV) immunoglobulin M (IgM) immunoblot for detection of CMV-specific IgM. J Clin Microbiol 36:3337-3341, 1998.
427. Maine GT, Stricker R, Schuler M, et al. Development and clinical evaluation of a recombinant-antigen-based cytomegalovirus immunoglobulin M automated immunoassay using the Abbott AxSYM analyzer. J Clin Microbiol 38:1476-1481, 2000.
428. Lazzarotto T, Spezzacatena P, Pradelli P, et al. Avidity of immunoglobulin G directed against human cytomegalovirus during primary and secondary infections in immunocompetent and immunocompromised subjects. Clin Diagn Lab Immunol 4:469-473, 1997.
429. Lazzarotto T, Spezzacatena P, Varani S, et al. Anticytomegalovirus (anti-CMV) immunoglobulin G avidity in identification of pregnant

women at risk of transmitting congenital CMV infection. Clin Diagn Lab Immunol 6:127-129, 1999.

430. Revello MG, Gerna G. Diagnosis and implications of human cytomegalovirus infection in pregnancy. Fetal Matern Med Rev 11:117-134, 1999.
431. Maine GT, Lazzarotto T, Landini MP. New developments in the diagnosis of maternal and congenital CMV infection. Expert Rev Mol Diagn 1:19-29, 2001.
432. Boeckh M, Boivin G. Quantitation of cytomegalovirus: methodologic aspects and clinical applications. Clin Microbiol Rev 11:533-554, 1998.
433. Revello MG, Zavattoni M, Sarasini A, et al. Human cytomegalovirus in blood of immunocompetent persons during primary infection: prognostic implications for pregnancy. J Infect Dis 177:1170-1175, 1998.
434. Revello MG, Lilleri D, Zavattoni M, et al. Human cytomegalovirus immediate-early messenger RNA in blood of pregnant women with primary infection and of congenitally infected newborns. J Infect Dis 184:1078-1081, 2001.
435. Gerna G, Baldanti F, Lilleri D, et al. Human cytomegalovirus immediate-early mRNA detection by nucleic acid sequence-based amplification as a new parameter for preemptive therapy in bone marrow transplant recipients. J Clin Microbiol 38:1845-1853, 2000.
436. Donner C, Liesnard C, Content J, et al. Prenatal diagnosis of 52 pregnancies at risk for congenital cytomegalovirus infection. Obstet Gynecol 82:481-486, 1993.
437. Lamy ME, Mulongo KN, Gadisseux JF, et al. Prenatal diagnosis of fetal cytomegalovirus infection. Am J Obstet Gynecol 166:91-94, 1992.
438. Lynch L, Daffos F, Emanuel D, et al. Prenatal diagnosis of fetal cytomegalovirus infection. Am J Obstet Gynecol 165:714-718, 1991.
439. Liesnard C, Donner C, Brancart F, et al. Prenatal diagnosis of congenital cytomegalovirus infection: prospective study of 237 pregnancies at risk. Obstet Gynecol 95:881-888, 2000.
440. Lipitz S, Yagel S, Shalev E, et al. Prenatal diagnosis of fetal primary cytomegalovirus infection. Obstet Gynecol 89:763-767, 1997.
441. Revello MG, Baldanti F, Furione M, et al. Polymerase chain reaction for prenatal diagnosis of congenital human cytomegalovirus infection. J Med Virol 47:462-466, 1995.
442. Ruellan-Eugene G, Barjot P, Barjot P, et al. Evaluation of virological procedures to detect fetal human cytomegalovirus infection: avidity of IgG antibodies, virus detection in amniotic fluid and maternal serum. J Med Virol 50:9-15, 1996.
443. Ahlfors K, Ivarsson SA, Nilsson H. On the unpredictable development of congenital cytomegalovirus infection. A study in twins. Early Hum Dev 18:125-135, 1988.
444. Guerra B, Lazzarotto T, Quarta S, et al. Prenatal diagnosis of symptomatic congenital cytomegalovirus infection. Am J Obstet Gynecol 183:476-482, 2000.
445. Lazzarotto T, Varani S, Guerra B, et al. Prenatal indicators of congenital cytomegalovirus infection. J Pediatr 137:90-95, 2000.
446. Bodeus M, Hubinont C, Bernard P, et al. Prenatal diagnosis of human cytomegalovirus by culture and polymerase chain reaction: 98 pregnancies leading to congenital infection. Prenatal Diagn 19:314-17, 1999.
447. French MLV, Thompson JR, White A. Cytomegalovirus viremia with transmission from mother to fetus. Ann Intern Med 86:748-749, 1977.
448. Huikeshoven FJM, Wallenburg HCS, Jahoda MGJ. Diagnosis of severe fetal cytomegalovirus infection from amniotic fluid in the third trimester of pregnancy. Am J Obstet Gynecol 142:1053-1054, 1982.
449. Yambao TJ, Clark D, Weiner L, Aubry RH. Isolation of cytomegalovirus from the amniotic fluid during the third trimester. Am J Obstet Gynecol 141:937-938, 1981.
450. Grose C, Weiner CP. Prenatal diagnosis of congenital cytomegalovirus infection: two decades later. Am J Obstet Gynecol 163:447-450, 1990.
451. Grose C, Meehan T, Weiner CP. Prenatal diagnosis of congenital cytomegalovirus infection by virus isolation after amniocentesis. Pediatr Infect Dis J 11:605-608, 1992.
452. Pass RF. Commentary: is there a role for prenatal diagnosis of congenital cytomegalovirus infection? Pediatr Infect Dis J 11:608-609, 1992.
453. Collaborative DHPG Treatment Study Group. Treatment of serious cytomegalovirus infections with 9-(1,3-dihydroxy-2-propoxymethyl) guanine in patients with AIDS and other immunodeficiencies. N Engl J Med 314:801-805, 1986.
454. Chrisp P, Clissold SP. Foscarnet: a review of its antiviral activity, pharmacokinetic properties and therapeutic use in immunocompromised patients with cytomegalovirus retinitis. Drugs 41:104-129, 1991.
455. Faulds D, Heel RC. Ganciclovir: a review of its antiviral activity, pharmacokinetic properties and therapeutic efficacy in cytomegalovirus infections. Drugs 39:597-638, 1990.
456. Kimberlin DW, Lin CY, Sanchez PJ, et al. Effect of ganciclovir therapy on hearing in symptomatic congenital cytomegalovirus disease involving the central nervous system: a randomized, controlled trial. J Pediatr 16-25, 2003.
457. Michaels MG, Greenberg DP, Sabo DL, et al. Treatment of children with congenital cytomegalovirus infection with ganciclovir. Pediatr Infect Dis J 22:504-508, 2003.
458. Glowacki LS, Smaill FM. Meta-analysis of immune globulin prophylaxis in transplant recipients for the prevention of symptomatic cytomegalovirus disease. Transplant Proc 25:1408-1410, 1993.
459. Hamilton AA, Manuel DM, Grundy JE, et al. A humanized antibody against human cytomegalovirus (CMV) gp UL 75 (gH) for prophylaxis or treatment of CMV infections. J Infect Dis 176:59-68, 1997.
460. Pass RF, Burke RL. Development of cytomegalovirus vaccines: prospects for prevention of congenital CMV infection. Semin Pediatr Infect Dis 13:196-204, 2002.
461. Gonczol E, Plotkin S. Development of a cytomegalovirus vaccine: lessons from recent clinical trials. Exp Opin Biol Ther 1:401-412, 2001.
462. Britt WJ. Vaccines against human cytomegalovirus: time to test. Trends Microbiol 4:34-38, 1996.
463. Adler SP, Hempfling SH, Starr SE, et al. Safety and immunogenicity of the Towne strain cytomegalovirus vaccine. Pediatr Infect Dis J 17:200-206, 1998.
464. Pass RF, Duliege AM, Boppana S, et al. A subunit cytomegalovirus vaccine based on recombinant envelope glycoprotein B and a new adjuvant. J Infect Dis 180:970-975, 1999.
465. Berencsi K, Gyulai Z, Gonczol E, et al. A canarypox vector-expressing cytomegalovirus (CMV) phosphoprotein 65 induces long-lasting cytotoxic T cell responses in human CMV-seronegative subjects. J Infect Dis 183:1171-1179, 2001.
466. Taber LH, Frank AL, Yow MD, et al. Acquisition of cytomegaloviral infections in families with young children: a serological study. J Infect Dis 151:948-952, 1985.
467. Onorato IM, Morens DM, Martone WJ, et al. Epidemiology of cytomegalovirus infections: recommendations for prevention and control. Rev Infect Dis 7:479-497, 1985.
468. Brady MT, Milam JD, Anderson DC, et al. Use of deglycerolized red blood cells to prevent posttransfusion infection with cytomegalovirus in neonates. J Infect Dis 150:334-399, 1984.
469. Stagno S, Whitley RJ. Herpesvirus infection of pregnancy. N Engl J Med 313:1270-1274, 1327-1329, 1985.
470. Peckham CS, Chin KS, Coleman JC, et al. Cytomegalovirus infection in pregnancy: preliminary findings from a prospective study. Lancet 1:1352-1355, 1983.
471. Yow MD. Congenital cytomegalovirus disease: a NOW problem. J Infect Dis 159:163-167, 1989.
472. Gilbert GL, Hayes K, Hudson IL, et al. Prevention of transfusion-acquired cytomegalovirus infection in infants by blood filtration to remove leukocytes. Lancet 1:1228-1231, 1989.
473. Holland PV, Schmitt PJ. Standards for Blood Banks and Transfusion Services, 12th ed. Arlington, Va, Committee on Standards, American Association of Blood Banks, 1987, pp 30-31.
474. Dworsky ME, Stagno S, Pass RF, et al. Persistence of cytomegalovirus in human milk after storage. J Pediatr 101:440-443, 1982.
475. Ploegh HL. Viral strategies of immune evasion. Science 280:248-253, 1998.
476. Hengel H, Reusch U, Gutermann A, et al. Cytomegaloviral control of MHC class I function in the mouse. Immunol Rev 168:167-176, 1999.
477. Tomazin R, Boname J, Hegde NR, et al. Cytomegalovirus US2 destroys two components of the MHC class II pathway, preventing recognition by CD4+ T cells. Nat Med 5:1039-1043, 1999.
478. Alcami A, Koszinowski UH. Viral mechanisms of immune evasion. Immunol Today 21:447-455, 2000.
479. Tortorella D, Gewurz BE, Furman MH, et al. Viral subversion of the immune system. Annu Rev Immunol 18:861-926, 2000.
480. Gewurz BE, Gaudet R, Tortorella D, et al. Antigen presentation subverted: structure of the human cytomegalovirus protein US2 bound to the class I molecule HLA-A2. Proc Natl Acad Sci U S A 98:6794-6799, 2001.
481. Mocarski ES Jr. Immunomodulation by cytomegaloviruses: manipulative strategies beyond evasion. Trends Microbiol 10:332-339, 2002.

Chapter 24

ENTEROVIRUS AND PARECHOVIRUS INFECTIONS

James D. Cherry

Enteroviruses (i.e., coxsackieviruses, echoviruses, newer enteroviruses, and polioviruses) and parechoviruses are responsible for significant and frequent human illnesses, with protean clinical manifestations.[1-14] Enteroviruses and parechoviruses are two genera of the Picornaviridae.[13-16] Enteroviruses were first categorized together and named in 1957 by a committee sponsored by the National Foundation for Infantile Paralysis[17]; the human alimentary tract was believed to be the natural habitat of these agents. Enteroviruses and parechoviruses are grouped together because of similarities in physical, biochemical, and molecular properties, as well as shared features in their epidemiology and pathogenesis and the many disease syndromes that they cause.

Congenital and neonatal infections have been linked with many different enteroviruses and parechoviruses. Representatives of all four major enterovirus groups, as well as parechoviruses 1 and 2, have been associated with disease in the neonate.[1-14,18-32]

Poliomyelitis, the first enteroviral disease to be recognized and the most important one, has had a long history.[33] The earliest record is an Egyptian stele of the 18th dynasty (1580 to 1350 BC), which shows a young priest with a withered, shortened leg, the characteristic deformity of paralytic poliomyelitis.[34,35] Underwood,[36] a London pediatrician, published the first medical description in 1789 in his *Treatise on Diseases of Children.* During the 19th century, many reports appeared in Europe and the United States describing small clusters of cases of "infantile paralysis." The authors were greatly puzzled about the nature of the affliction; not until the 1860s and 1870s was the spinal cord firmly established as the seat of the pathologic process. The contagious nature of poliomyelitis was not appreciated until the latter part of the 19th century. Medin, a Swedish pediatrician, was the first to describe the epidemic nature of poliomyelitis (1890), and his pupil Wickman[37] worked out the basic principles of the epidemiology.

The virus was first isolated in monkeys by Landsteiner and Popper in 1908.[38] The availability of a laboratory animal assay system opened up many avenues of research that in the ensuing 40 years led to the demonstration that an unrecognized intestinal infection was common and that paralytic disease was a relatively uncommon event.

Coxsackieviruses and echoviruses have had a shorter history. Epidemic pleurodynia was first clinically described in northern Germany in 1735 by Hannaeus[3,39] more than 200 years before the coxsackieviral cause of this disease was discovered. In 1948, Dalldorf and Sickles[40] first reported the isolation of a coxsackievirus by using suckling mouse inoculation.

In 1949, Enders and associates[41] reported the growth of poliovirus type 2 in tissue culture, and their techniques paved the way for the recovery of a large number of other cytopathic viruses. Most of these "new" viruses failed to produce illness in laboratory animals. Because the relationships of many of these newly recovered agents to human disease were unknown, they were called orphan viruses.[4] Later, several agents were grouped together and called enteric cytopathogenic human orphan viruses, or echoviruses. Some studies[13-16] of the viral genome of echoviruses 22 and 23 found that they were distinctly different from other enteroviruses, and they have been placed in the new genus, parechovirus.

Live-attenuated oral poliovirus vaccines (OPV) became available 40 years ago, and the most notable advance during the past 20 years has been the dramatic reduction in worldwide poliomyelitis because of immunization with OPV and efforts of the global immunization initiative.[42-47] The last case of confirmed paralytic polio in the Western Hemisphere occurred in 1991.[42]

Aside from the polio immunization successes, there have been few major advances or new modes of treatment for enteroviral diseases. However, the use of nucleic acid detection systems for enteroviral diagnosis has progressed over the past 15 years, and rapid diagnosis of meningitis and other enteroviral illnesses has become possible.[31,48-64] There has been progress in the development of specific anti-enteroviral drugs.[65-67]

THE VIRUSES

Morphology and Classification

The enteroviruses are single-stranded RNA viruses belonging to the Picornaviridae (from *pico,* meaning "small"). They are grouped together because they share certain physical, biochemical, and molecular properties.[11,13,15 68-78] In electron micrographs, the virus is seen as a 30-nm particle consisting of a naked protein capsid that constitutes 70% to 75% of the mass; each particle has a dense central core (nucleoid) of RNA. Enterovirus capsids are composed of four structural proteins: VP1, VP2, VP3, and VP4. The capsid shell has icosahedral symmetry with 20 triangular faces and 12 vertices. The shell is formed by VP1, VP2, and VP3; VP4 lies on its inner surface.

The three surface proteins (VP1, VP2, VP3) have no sequence homology, but they have the same topology.[15] They form an eight-stranded, antiparallel β barrel that is wedge shaped and composed of two antiparallel β sheets. The amino acid sequences in the loops that connect the β strands and the N- and C-terminal sequences that extend from the β-barrel domain of VP1, VP2, and VP3 give each enterovirus its distinct antigenicity.

The coat proteins protect the RNA genome from nucleases and are important determinants of host range and tropism. They determine antigenicity, and they deliver the RNA genome into the cytoplasm of new host cells.

The genome of enteroviruses is a single-stranded, positive-strand RNA molecule.[71] It contains a 5′ noncoding region, which is followed by a single long open reading frame, a short 3′ noncoding region, and a poly(A) tail. The four capsid proteins (VP1 through VP4) and seven nonstructural proteins (2A, 2B, 2C, 3A, 3B, 3C, and 3D) result from a cleaved, long polyprotein that was translated from genomic RNA.

Viral components and complete virions are formed in the cytoplasm of infected cells. If the rate of virus assembly is rapid and many particles are formed in one area, crystallization may occur.

The original classification of human enteroviruses is shown in Table 24-1. The enteroviral subgroups were differentiated from each other by their different effects in tissue cultures and in animals. Although these differentiating factors are still useful, many strains have been isolated that do not conform to such rigid specificities. For example, several coxsackievirus A strains grow and have a cytopathic effect in monkey kidney tissue cultures, and some echovirus strains cause paralysis in mice. Since 1974, newly identified enteroviral types were assigned enterovirus type numbers instead of coxsackievirus or echovirus numbers. Prototype enteroviral strains Fermon, Toluca-1, J670/71, and BrCr were assigned enteroviral numbers 68 through 71, respectively. Sequencing studies of the VP1 protein of "untypeable" strains have identified at least six new enteroviral types.[78] Definitive identification of enteroviral types is made by neutralization with type-specific antiserum.

Because studies of the viral genomes of echoviruses 22 and 23 found that they were distinctly different from other enteroviruses, they were placed in the new genus, parechovirus; they are parechoviruses types 1 and 2.[14-16] The parechoviruses contain only three capsid polypeptides: VP1, VP2, and VP0, which is the uncleaved precursor to VP2 plus VP4.

Complete or partial genetic sequence data are available from all enteroviruses.[71-75] In general, sequence comparisons partially support the classic subgrouping of enteroviruses as provided in Table 24-1. However, in many instances, genetic relationships do not correlate with the original subdivisions.[13,64,71,77] All prototype human enterovirus strains fall into one of five genomically identified clusters.[13,64,71,76,77] Presented in Table 24-2 is the species designation by genetic analysis for the original enteroviral types.

The cellular receptors and co-receptors for attachment in the replication cycle for selected enteroviruses and parechoviruses are presented in Table 24-3. After attachment, the replication cycle takes 5 to 10 hours and occurs in the cytoplasm.

Table 24–1 Human Enteroviruses: Animal and Tissue Culture Spectrum

		Cytopathic Effect		Illness and Pathology	
Virus[a]	Antigenic Types[b]	*Monkey Kidney Culture*	*Human Tissue Culture*	*Suckling Mouse*	*Monkey*
Polioviruses	1-3	+	+	-	+
Coxsackieviruses A	1-24[c]	-	-	+	-
Coxsackieviruses B	1-6	+	+	+	-
Echoviruses	1-34[d]	+	±	-	-

[a]Many enteroviral strains have been isolated that do not conform to these categories.

[b]New types, beginning with type 68, were assigned enterovirus type numbers instead of coxsackievirus or echovirus numbers. Types 68 through 71 were identified.

[c]Type 23 was found to be the same as echovirus 9.

[d]Echovirus 10 was reclassified as a reovirus; echovirus 26 was reclassified as a rhinovirus; echoviruses 22 and 23 have been reclassified as parechoviruses.

Characteristics and Host Systems

Enteroviruses are relatively stable viruses in that they retain activity for several days at room temperature and can be stored indefinitely at ordinary freezer temperatures (−20° C).[11,13,35,69,70] They are rapidly inactivated by heat (>56° C), formaldehyde, chlorination, and ultraviolet light but are resistant to 70% alcohol, 5% Lysol, quaternary ammonium compounds, ether, deoxycholate, and detergents that are effective against lipid-containing viruses.

Enteroviral strains grow rapidly when adapted to susceptible host systems and cause cytopathology in 3 to 7 days. The typical tissue culture cytopathic effect is shown in Figure 24-1; characteristic pathologic findings in mice are shown in Figures 24-2 and 24-3. Final titers of virus recovered in the laboratory vary markedly among different viral strains and the host systems employed; usually, concentrations of 10^3 to 10^7 infectious doses per 0.1 mL of tissue culture fluid or tissue homogenate are obtained. Unadapted viral strains frequently require long periods of incubation in tissue cultures or suckling mice before visible evidence of growth is observed.

Table 24–2 Genomic Classification of Enteroviruses

Species Designation	Original Enteroviral Type
Poliovirus (PV)	Poliovirus types 1, 2, 3
Human enterovirus A (HEV A)	Enterovirus type 71, Coxsackievirus A types 2-8, 10, 12, 14, 16
Human enterovirus B (HEV-B)	Coxsackievirus type A9 Coxsackievirus types B1-6 Echovirus types 1-9, 11-21, 24-27, 29-33 Enterovirus type 69
Human enterovirus C (HEV-C)	Coxsackievirus A types 1, 11, 13, 15, 17-22, 24
Human enterovirus D (HEV-D)	Enterovirus types 68, 70

Data from Ishiko H, Shimada Y, Yonaha M, et al. Molecular diagnosis of human enteroviruses by phylogeny-based classification by use of the VP4 sequence. J Infect Dis 185:744-754, 2002, and from Pallansch MA, Roos RP. Enteroviruses: polioviruses, coxsackieviruses, and newer enteroviruses. *In* Knipe DM, Howley PM (eds). Fields Virology, vol. 1. Philadelphia, Lippincott Williams & Wilkins, 2001, pp 723-775.

Blind passage is occasionally necessary for cytopathic effects to become apparent.

Although many different primary and secondary tissue culture systems support the growth of various enteroviruses, it is generally accepted that primary rhesus monkey kidney cultures have the most inclusive spectrum. Other simian kidney tissue cultures, although less commonly used, also have the same broad spectrum.[79] Tissue cultures of human origin have a more limited spectrum, but several echovirus types have had more consistent primary isolation in human embryonic lung fibroblastic cell strains than in monkey kidney cultures.[80-82]

Most coxsackievirus A types do not grow and produce a cytopathic effect in simian kidney tissue cultures. However, most coxsackievirus A types (except A1, A19, and A22) replicate in the RD cell line derived from a human rhabdomyosarcoma.[83] A satisfactory system for the primary recovery of enteroviruses from clinical specimens would include primary rhesus, cynomolgus, or African green monkey kidney tissue cultures; a diploid, human embryonic lung fibroblast cell strain; the RD cell line; and the intraperitoneal and intracerebral inoculation of suckling mice younger than 24 hours old. Optimally, blind passage should be carried out in the tissue culture systems.

Antigenic Characteristics

Although some minor cross-reactions exist between several coxsackievirus and echovirus types, common group antigens of diagnostic importance are not well defined.[11,13,35,69] Heat treatment of virions and the use of synthetic peptides have produced antigens with broad enteroviral reactivity.[84,85] These antigens have been used in enzyme-linked immunosorbent assay (ELISA) and complement fixation tests to determine IgG and IgM enteroviral antibodies and for antigen detection. In one study, Terletskaia-Ladwig and colleagues[85] identified patients infected with enteroviruses with the use of an IgM enzyme immunoassay (EIA). This test employed heat-treated coxsackievirus B5 and echovirus 9 as antigens, and it identified patients infected with echoviruses 4, 11, and 30. The sensitivity of the test was 35%. In another study using heat-treated virus or synthetic peptides, the respective sensitivities were 67% and 62%.[84] However, both tests lacked specificity. Intratypic strain differences are common occurrences, and some strains (i.e., prime strains) are neutralized

Table 24–3 Cell Receptors and Co-receptors for Selected Enteroviruses and Parechoviruses

Virus Type	Receptor	Co-receptor
Polioviruses 1-3	Poliovirus receptor (PVR, CD155)	
Coxsackievirus A13, A18	Intercellular adhesion molecule-1 (ICAM-1)	
Coxsackievirus A21	Decay-accelerating factor (CD55)	ICAM-1
Coxsackievirus A9	$\alpha_V\beta_3$ (vitronectin receptor)	
Coxsackievirus B1-6	Coxsackievirus-adenovirus receptor (CAR) or decay-accelerating factor (CD55)	$\alpha_v\beta_6$ integrin
Echoviruses 1, 8	$\alpha_2\beta_1$ integrin (V1a-2)	β_2-microglobulin
Echoviruses 3, 6, 7, 11-13, 20, 21, 29, 33	Decay-accelerating factor (CD55)	β_2-microglobulin
Enteroviruses 70	Decay-accelerating factor (CD55)	
Parechovirus 1	$\alpha_v\beta_1$, $\alpha_v\beta_3$ (vitronectin receptor)	

Data from Racaniello VR. Picornaviridae: the viruses and their replication. *In* Knipe DM, Howeley PM (eds). Fields Virology, vol. 1. Philadelphia, Lippincott Williams & Wilkins, 2001, pp 685-722.

A 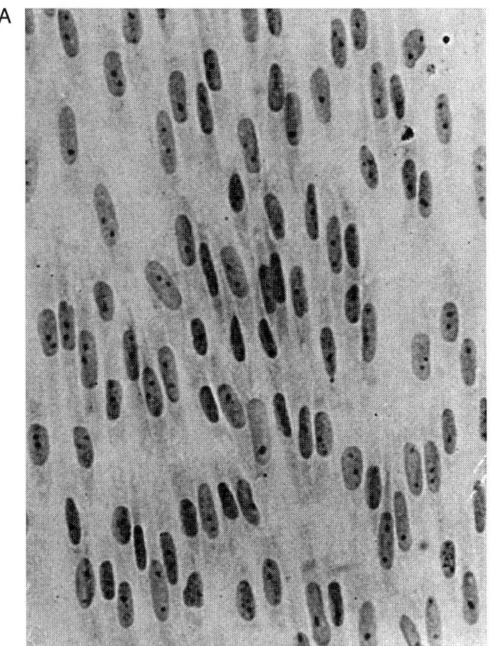 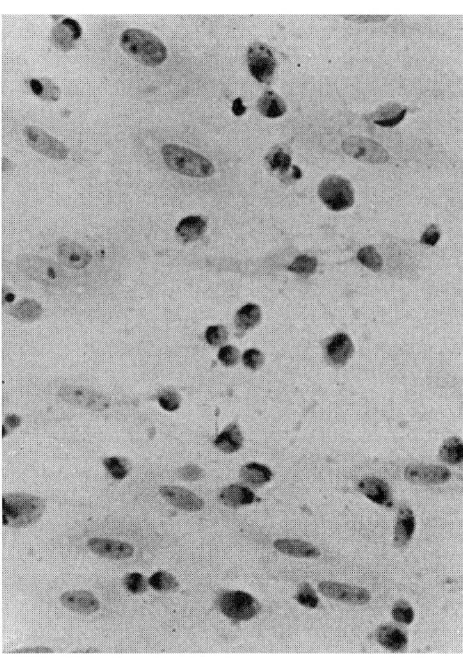 B

Figure 24–1 Fetal rhesus monkey kidney tissue culture (HL-8). **A**, Uninoculated tissue culture. **B**, Echovirus 11 cytopathic effect.

A 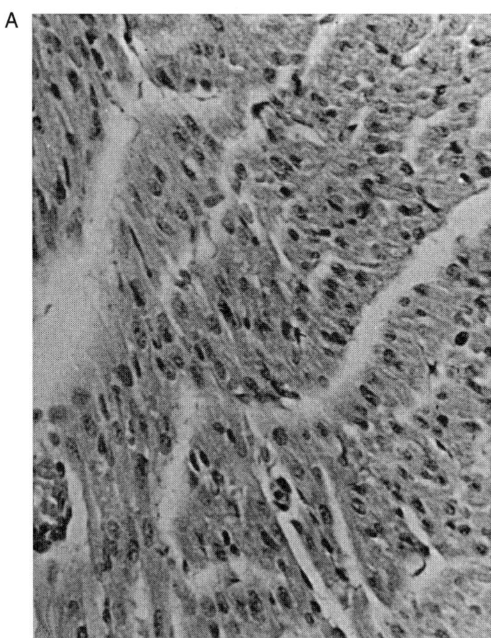 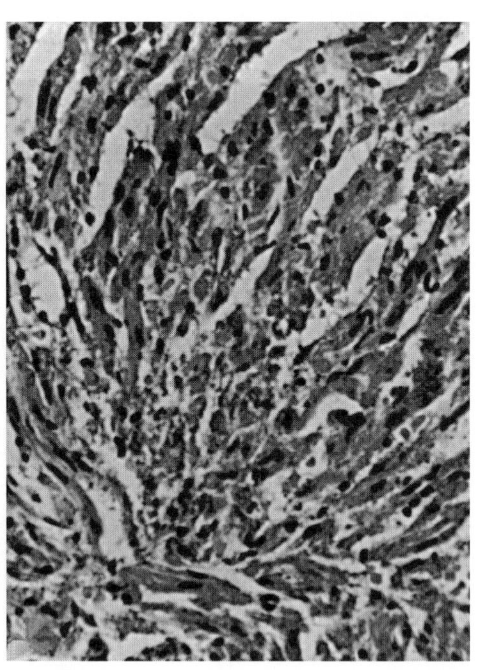 B

Figure 24–2 Suckling mouse myocardium. **A**, Normal suckling mouse myocardium. **B**, Myocardium of suckling mouse infected with coxsackievirus B1.

poorly by antiserums to prototype viruses. In animals, however, these prime strains induce antibodies that neutralize the specific prototype viruses.

Identification of polioviral, coxsackieviral, and echoviral types by neutralization in suckling mice or tissue cultures with antiserum pools is relatively well defined. Neutralization is induced by the epitopes on structural proteins VP1, VP2, and VP3; in particular, several epitopes are clustered on VP1. Prime strains do cause diagnostic difficulties because frequently they are not neutralized by the reference antiserums, which is a particular problem with echoviruses 4, 9, and 11 and with enterovirus 71. If these types or other possible prime strains are suspected, this problem sometimes can be overcome by employing antiserums in less-diluted concentrations or using antiserums prepared against several different strains of problem viruses. Kubo and associates[77] were able to type enteroviral isolates not identified by neutralization by nucleotide sequence analysis of the VP4 gene. They specifically identified prime strains of echovirus 18 and enterovirus 71. Sequence analysis of the VP1 gene also is useful for typing enteroviral prime strains not identified by neutralization.[86]

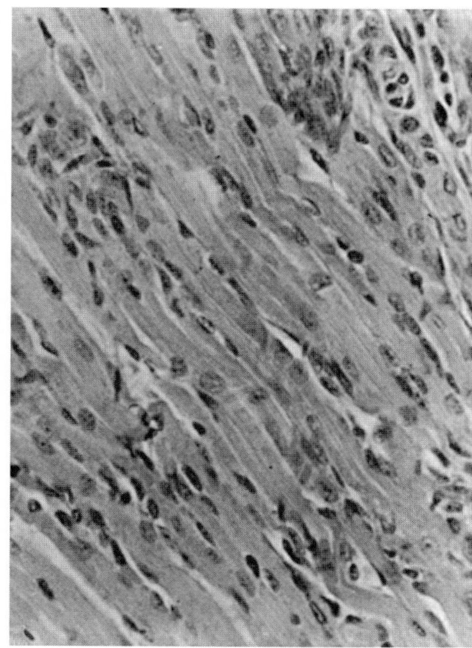

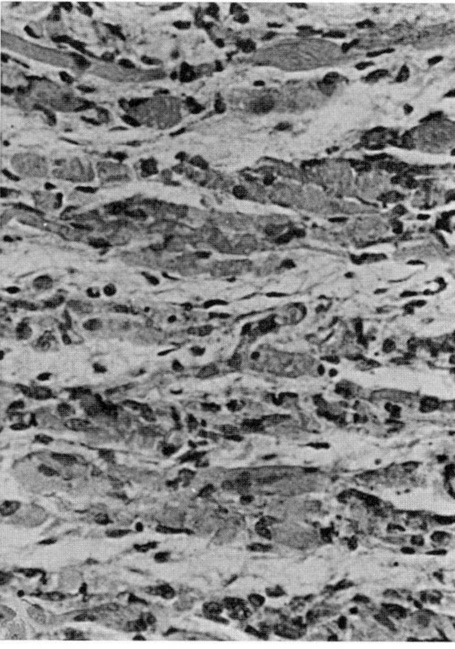

Figure 24–3 Suckling mouse skeletal muscle. **A**, Normal suckling mouse skeletal muscle. **B**, Skeletal muscle of a suckling mouse infected with coxsackievirus A16.

EPIDEMIOLOGY AND TRANSMISSION

General Considerations

Enteroviruses are spread from person to person by fecal-oral and possibly by oral-oral (respiratory) routes.[1-11,87] Swimming and wading pools may serve as a means of spread of enteroviruses during the summer.[88] Oral-oral transmission by way of the contaminated hands of health care personnel and transmission by fomites have been documented on a long-term care pediatric ward.[89] Enteroviruses have been recovered from trapped flies, and this carriage probably contributes to the spread of human infections, particularly in lower socioeconomic populations that have poor sanitary facilities.[90-92]

Children are the main susceptible cohort; they are immunologically susceptible, and their unhygienic habits facilitate spread. Spread is from child to child (by feces to skin to mouth) and then within family groups. Recovery of enteroviruses is inversely related to age; the prevalence of specific antibodies is directly related to age. The incidence of infections and the prevalence of antibodies do not differ between boys and girls.

Transplacental Transmission

Polioviruses

Poliovirus infections in pregnancy can result in abortion, stillbirth, neonatal disease, or no evidence of fetal involvement.[93] Gresser and associates[94] have shown that the human amniotic membrane in organ culture can be infected, resulting in a persistent low-grade infection. It has been observed on many occasions that maternal poliomyelitis occurring late in pregnancy has resulted in transplacental transmission of the virus to the fetus in utero.[95-116] The evidence that transplacental passage of virus occurs in early pregnancy is meager. Schaeffer and colleagues[98] were able to recover virus from the placenta and the fetus after a spontaneous abortion in a 24-year-old woman with poliomyelitis.

Although attenuated poliovirus vaccines have been given to pregnant women, there has never been a search for the transplacental passage of vaccine virus.[117-119] Viremia occurs after oral administration of polio vaccine, and occasionally, this virus probably is passed transplacentally to the fetus.[120-127]

Coxsackieviruses

Several investigators have studied coxsackievirus infections in pregnant animals and the transplacental passage of virus to the fetus. Dalldorf and Gifford[128] studied two strains of coxsackievirus B1 and one of coxsackievirus A8 in gravid mice. In only one instance (coxsackievirus B1) were they able to recover virus from a fetus. They thought that this result was inconclusive because they were unable to recover virus in five other instances. Berger and Roulet[129] observed muscle lesions in the young of gravid mice infected with coxsackieviruses A1 and B1. Selzer[130] studied several viruses in gravid mice; coxsackievirus A9 was found in the placentas of two mice but in no fetuses, and coxsackievirus A18 was not recovered from fetuses or placentas. Selzer[130] found that coxsackieviruses B3 and B4 passed the placental barrier. Soike[131] also observed that in the last week of pregnancy, coxsackievirus B3 reached fetal mice transplacentally. Modlin and Crumpacker[132] reported that infection in late gestational mice was more severe than that occurring in early pregnancy and that transplacental infection of the fetus occurred transiently during the maternal infection. Flamm[133] observed that coxsackievirus A9, when injected intravenously in rabbits, reached the blastocyst early in pregnancy and the amniotic fluid later in pregnancy. He also demonstrated congenital infection in mice with coxsackievirus A1.[134]

Palmer and co-workers[135] studied the gestational outcome in pregnant mice inoculated intravenously with Theiler's murine encephalomyelitis virus, a murine enterovirus. In early gestational infections they found a high rate of placental and fetal abnormalities. The rates of fetal abnormalities and placental infection were greater than the rate of fetal viral infection, suggesting that the adverse effects of the viral infections were direct and indirect. Gestational infection could result in virus passage to the fetus and fetal damage or in placental compromise with indirect fetal damage.

In another study using the same murine model with Theiler's murine encephalomyelitis virus, Abzug[136] found that maternal factors (i.e., compromised uteroplacental blood flow, concomitant infection, and advanced age) increased the risk of transplacental fetal infection.

In humans, the transplacental passage of coxsackieviruses at term has been documented on several occasions. Benirschke[137] studied the placentas in three cases of congenital coxsackievirus B disease and could find no histologic evidence of infection. In 1956, Kibrick and Benirschke[138] reported the first case of intrauterine infection with coxsackievirus B3. In this instance, the infant was delivered by cesarean section and had clinical evidence of infection several hours after birth. Brightman and colleagues[139] recovered coxsackievirus B5 from the placenta and rectum of a premature infant. No histologic abnormalities of the placenta were identified. Other evidence of intrauterine infection has been presented for coxsackieviruses A4 and B2 through B6.[140-148]

Evidence for intrauterine infection during the first and second trimesters of pregnancy with coxsackieviruses is less clear. Burch and co-workers[149] reported the results of immunofluorescent studies of two fetuses of 5 months' gestation and one fetus of 6 months' gestation; the 6-month-old fetus had evidence of coxsackievirus B4 myocarditis, one 5-month-old fetus showed signs of coxsackievirus B3 infection, and the other 5-month-old fetus showed evidence of coxsackievirus B2, B3, and B4 infections. Basso and associates[143] recovered coxsackievirus B2 from the placenta, liver, and brain of a fetus after a spontaneous abortion at 3 months' gestation. Plager and co-workers found no evidence of intrauterine viral transmission of coxsackievirus B5 infections during the first and second trimesters of pregnancy.[150]

Euscher and associates[151] detected coxsackievirus RNA in placental tissue from six of seven newborn infants with respiratory difficulties and other manifestations at birth. Of these infants, one died shortly after birth, and the other six suffered neurodevelopmental delays. The placentas of 10 normal infants were examined for coxsackievirus RNA, and results of these studies were negative. Three of the placentas from the affected infants showed focal chronic villitis, two showed focal hemorrhagic endovasculitis, and one showed focal calcifications. In addition to respiratory distress, two neonates had rashes, two had seizures, two had thrombocytopenia, and one had intraventricular hemorrhage.

Echoviruses, Enteroviruses, and Parechoviruses

Less is known about transplacental passage of echoviruses than about that of coxsackieviruses and polioviruses. Echovirus infections are regular occurrences in all populations. Women in all stages of pregnancy are frequently infected, and viremia is commonly seen in these infections.[152] In particular, epidemic disease related to echovirus 9 has been studied epidemiologically and serologically.[153-155] In these studies, a search for teratogenesis has been made, but no definitive virologic investigations have been carried out; asymptomatic transplacental infection might have occurred.

Cherry and colleagues[141] cultured samples from 590 newborns during a period of enteroviral prevalence without isolating an echovirus. Antepartum serologic study of a group of 55 mothers in this study showed that 5 (9%) were actively infected with echovirus 17 during the 6-week period before delivery. In two other large nursery studies, there was no suggestion of intrauterine echovirus infections.[156,157]

Berkovich and Smithwick[158] described a newborn without clinical illness who had specific IgM parechovirus 1 antibody in the cord blood, suggesting intrauterine infection with this virus. Hughes and colleagues[159] reported a newborn with echovirus 14 infection who had a markedly elevated level of IgM (190 mg/dL) on the sixth day of life. It seems likely that this infant was also infected in utero. Echoviruses 6, 7, 9, 11, 19, 27, and 33 have been identified in cases of transplacentally acquired infections.[143,160-168]

Chow and associates[169] described a 1300-g fetus, which was stillborn after 26 weeks' gestation, with unilateral hydrocephalus, hepatosplenomegaly, fibrotic peritonitis, and meconium staining. Enterovirus 71 was isolated from the amniotic fluid, and the same virus was identified by polymerase chain reaction (PCR) in the cord blood and by immunohistochemical staining in the fetal midbrain and liver. Otonkoski and coworkers[170] reported the occurrence of neonatal type 1 diabetes after a possible maternal echovirus 6 infection.

Ascending Infection and Contact Infection during Birth

Definitive evidence is lacking for ascending infection or contact infection with enteroviruses during birth. In prospective studies of genital herpes simplex and cytomegaloviral infections, there have been no enteroviral isolations.[171,172] These results suggest that ascending infections with enteroviruses, if they occur at all, are rare. However, Reyes and associates[173] recovered coxsackievirus B5 from the cervix of four third-trimester pregnant women. Three of the four positive cultures were obtained 3 weeks or more before delivery. In the fourth case, the cervical culture was obtained the day before delivery, and the child was delivered by cesarean section. All of the infants were healthy, but unfortunately, culture for virus was possible only from the infant delivered by cesarean section; the result was negative. In an earlier study, Reyes and colleagues[164] reported a child who died of a disseminated echovirus 11 infection. The illness had its onset on the third day of life, and the virus was recovered from the mother's cervix at that time.

Enteroviral infection during the birth process seems probable. The fecal carriage rate of enteroviruses in asymptomatic adult patients varies between 0% and 6% or higher in different population groups.[174-176] Cherry and associates[141] found that in 2 (4%) of 55 mothers, enteroviruses were present in the feces shortly after delivery. Katz,[177] in a discussion of a child with neonatal coxsackievirus B4 infection, suggested that the infant might have inhaled maternally excreted organisms during birth. The fact that this child had pneumonia tends to support the contention. Infections occurring 2 to 7 days after birth could have been acquired during passage through the birth canal.

Neonatal Infection

Neonatal infections and illnesses from enteroviruses are relatively common.[178] Transmission of enteroviruses to newborns is similar to that for populations of older people. The main factor in the spread of virus is human-to-human contact.

During the summer and fall of 1981 in Rochester, New York, 666 neonates were cultured for enteroviruses within 24 hours of birth and then weekly for 1 month.[164] The incidence of acquisition of nonpolio enteroviral infections during this period was 12.8%. Two risk factors were identified: lower socioeconomic status and lack of breast-feeding.

Polioviruses

Clinical poliomyelitis is rare in neonates, but the infection rate before the vaccine era was never determined. It is probable that the rarity of neonatal poliomyelitis was not related to lack of viral transmission but reflected the protection from disease offered by specific, transplacentally transmitted polioviral antibodies. From experience gained in vaccine studies, it is apparent that infants with passively acquired antibody can be regularly infected.[179-191]

In 1955, Bates[110] reviewed the literature on poliomyelitis in infants younger than 1 month. He described six infants who apparently were not infected by their mothers and who had had other likely contacts. A neighbor was the contact in one case, siblings in two cases, nursery nurses in two cases, and an uncle in the sixth case. In most other infants, the mother had had poliomyelitis shortly before the child was born and probably was the contact. The mode of transmission—intrauterine, during birth, or postnatal contact—is unknown.

Bergeisen and colleagues[192] reported a case of paralytic poliomyelitis from a type 3 vaccine viral strain. They suggested that the source of this virus might have been the child of the neonate's baby sitter, who was vaccinated about 2 weeks before the onset of the illness.

Coxsackieviruses

Several epidemics with coxsackieviruses B in newborn nurseries have been studied. Brightman and co-workers[139] observed an epidemic of coxsackievirus B5 in a premature nursery. Their data suggested that the virus was introduced into this nursery by an infant with a clinically inapparent infection who had been infected in utero. Secondary infections occurred in 12 infants and two nurses. The timing of the secondary cases suggested that three generations of infection had occurred and that the nurses had been infected during the second generation. The investigators suggested that the infection had spread from infant to infant and from infant to nurse.

Javett and colleagues[193] documented an acute epidemic of myocarditis associated with coxsackievirus B3 infection in a Johannesburg maternity home. Unfortunately, no epidemiologic investigation or search for asymptomatic infected infants was performed. However, analysis of the onset dates of the illnesses indicated that single infections occurred for five generations and then five children became ill within a 3-day period.

Kipps and colleagues[194] carried out epidemiologic investigations in two coxsackievirus B3 nursery epidemics. In the first epidemic, the initial infection was probably transmitted from a mother to her child; this infant was then the source of five secondary cases in newborns and one illness in a nurse. Infants with four of the five secondary cases were located on one side of the nursery, but only one cot was close to the cot of the index patient, and this cot did not adjoin the cots of the three other infants with contact cases. In the second outbreak, an infant who also was infected by his mother probably introduced the virus into the nursery. Infants with the three secondary cases were geographically far removed from the one with the primary case of infection.

There have been many other instances of isolated nursery infections and small outbreaks with coxsackieviruses, and it seems that the most consistent source of original nursery infection is transmission from a mother to her child,[193-233] but introduction of virus into the nursery by personnel also occurs.[233,234]

Echoviruses and Parechoviruses

Although many outbreaks of echovirus infections have been observed in newborn nurseries, information on viral transmission is incomplete.[30,235-265] Cramblett and co-workers[235] reported an outbreak of echovirus 11 disease in four infants in an intensive care nursery. All infants were in enclosed incubators, and three patients became ill within 24 hours; the fourth child became ill 4 days later. Echovirus 11 was recovered from two members of the nursery staff. These data suggest that transmission from personnel to infants occurred because of inadequate hand washing. In another outbreak in an intensive care unit, the initial patient was transferred to the nursery because of severe echovirus 11 disease.[250] After transfer, infection occurred in the senior house officer and a psychologist in the unit. It was inferred by the investigators that spread by respiratory droplets to nine other infants occurred from these infected personnel.

In a maternity unit outbreak of echovirus 11 involving six secondary cases,[257] infection spread through close contact between the infected newborns and the nurses. In another reported nosocomial echovirus 11 outbreak, infants in an intermediate care unit for more than 2 days were more likely to become infected than those who were there for less than 2 days. Illness was also associated with gavage feeding, mouth care, and being a twin.[258]

Modlin[260] reviewed reports of 16 nursery outbreaks involving 206 ill infants. In only 4 of the 16 outbreaks was the source identified, and in all 4, the primary case was an infant who acquired infection vertically from its mother. After introduction of an infected newborn into a nursery, spread to other infants by personnel is common.[262-265] Risk factors for nursery transmission as described by Rabkin and co-workers[262] were "lower gestational age or birth weight; antibiotic or transfusion therapy; nasogastric intubation or feeding; proximity in the nursery to the index patient; and care by the same nurse during the same shift as the index patient."

Wilson and associates[264] reported an intensive care nursery epidemic in which respiratory syncytial virus and echovirus 7 infections occurred concurrently. This epidemic persisted from January to June 1984 despite an aggressive isolation cohorting program. A major factor in persistence was asymptomatic infections with both viruses.

Sato and associates[266] reported a point-source outbreak of echovirus 33 infection in nine newborns related to one nursery over a 10-day period. The primary case was born to a mother who was febrile and who had a high echovirus 33 neutralizing antibody titer in a convalescent-phase serum specimen.

Jack and colleagues[236] observed the endemic occurrence of asymptomatic infection with parechovirus 1 in a nursery during an 8-month period. A total of 44 infants were infected during this time, and nursery infection occurred when there was no known activity of parechovirus 1 in the community at large. The investigators believed that the endemic viral infection was spread by fecal contamination of hands of nursery personnel.

Nakao and colleagues[246] and Berkovich and Pangan[237] also documented parechovirus 1 infections in nurseries. Like Jack and colleagues,[236] they observed that the infections seemed to be endemic to the nurseries rather than related to community epidemics.

Host Range

It is the general opinion that humans are the only natural hosts of enteroviruses.[87] However, enteroviruses have been recovered in nature from sewage,[91] flies,[90-92] swine,[267,268] dogs,[269,270] a calf,[271] a budgerigar (i.e., small Australian parakeet),[272] a fox,[273] mussels,[274] and oysters.[275] Serologic evidence of infection with enteroviruses similar to human strains has been found in chimpanzees,[276] cattle,[277] rabbits,[278] a fox,[279] a chipmunk,[280] and a marmot.[251] It is probable that infection of these animals was the result of their direct contact with an infected human or infected human excreta. Although enteroviruses do not multiply in flies, they appear to be a possible significant vector in situations of poor sanitation and heavy human infection. The contamination of shellfish is also intriguing[274,275,279-284] because in addition to their possible role in human infection, they offer a source of enteroviral storage during cold weather. Contaminated foods are another possible source of human infection.[284]

Geographic Distribution and Season

Enteroviruses have a worldwide distribution.[1,11,87,285,286] Neutralizing antibodies for specific viral types have been found in serologic surveys throughout the world, and most strains have been recovered in worldwide isolation studies. In any one area, there are frequent fluctuations in predominant types. Epidemics probably depend on new susceptible persons in the population rather than on reinfections; they may be localized and sporadic and may vary in cause from place to place in the same year. Pandemic waves of infection also occur.

In temperate climates, enteroviral infections occur primarily in the summer and fall, but in the tropics, they are prevalent all year.[11,87,287] A basic concept in understanding their epidemiology is the far greater frequency of unrecognized infection than that of clinical disease. This is illustrated by poliomyelitis, which remained an epidemiologic mystery until it was appreciated that unrecognized infections were the main source of contagion. Serologic surveys were instrumental in elucidating the problem. In populations living in conditions of poor sanitation and hygiene, epidemics do not occur; but wide dissemination of polioviruses has been confirmed by demonstrating the presence of specific antibodies to all three types in nearly 100% of children by the age of 5 years.

Epidemics of poliomyelitis first began to appear in Europe and the United States during the latter part of the 19th century; they continued with increasing frequency in the economically advanced countries until the introduction of effective vaccines in the 1950s and 1960s.[33,34,288,289] The evolution from endemic to epidemic follows a characteristic pattern, beginning with collections of a few cases, then endemic rates that are higher than usual, followed by severe epidemics with high attack rates.

The age group attacked in endemic areas and in early epidemics is the youngest one; more than 90% of paralytic cases begin in children younger than 5 years. After a pattern of epidemicity begins, it is irreversible unless preventive vaccination is carried out. Because epidemics recur over a period of years, there is a shift in age incidence such that relatively fewer cases are in the youngest children; the peak often occurs in the 5- to 14-year-old group, and an increasing proportion is in young adults. These changes are correlated with socioeconomic factors and improved standards of hygiene; when children are protected from immunizing infections in the first few years of life, the pool of susceptible persons builds up, and introduction of a virulent strain often is followed by an epidemic.[290] Extensive use of vaccines in the past 4 decades has resulted in elimination of paralytic poliomyelitis from large geographic areas, but the disease remains endemic in various parts of the world. Although seasonal periodicity is distinct in temperate climates, some viral activity does take place during the winter.[291] Infection and acquisition of postinfection immunity occur with greater intensity and at earlier ages among crowded, economically deprived populations with less efficient sanitation facilities.

Molecular techniques have allowed the study of genotypes of specific viral types in populations over time.[292-295] For example, Mulders and colleagues[295] studied the molecular epidemiology of wild poliovirus type 1 in Europe, the Middle East, and the Indian subcontinent. They found four major genotypes circulating. Two genotypes were found predominantly in Eastern Europe, a third genotype was circulating mainly in Egypt, and the fourth genotype was widely dispersed. All four genotypes were found in Pakistan.

The epidemiologic behavior of coxsackieviruses and echoviruses parallels that of polioviruses; unrecognized infections far outnumber those with distinctive symptoms. The agents are disseminated widely throughout the world, and outbreaks related to one or another type of virus occur regularly. These outbreaks tend to be localized, with different agents being prevalent in different years. In the late 1950s, however, echovirus 9 had a far wider circulation, sweeping through a large part of the world and infecting children and young adults. This behavior has been repeated occasionally with other enteroviruses; after a long absence, a particular agent returns and circulates among the susceptible persons of different ages who have been born since the previous epidemic occurred. Other agents remain endemic in a given area, surfacing as sporadic cases and occasionally as small outbreaks. Multiple types are frequently active at the same time, although one agent commonly predominates in a given locality.

There are no available data on the incidence of symptomatic congenital and neonatal enteroviral infections. From the frequency of reports in the literature, it appears that severe neonatal disease caused by enteroviruses decreased

Table 24–4 Predominant Types of Nonpolio Enteroviral Isolations in the United States, 1961-1999

	Five Most Common Viral Types per Year[a]				
Year	***First***	***Second***	***Third***	***Fourth***	***Fifth***
1961	Coxsackievirus B5	Coxsackievirus B2	Coxsackievirus B4	Echovirus 11	Echovirus 9
1962	Coxsackievirus B3	Echovirus 9	Coxsackievirus B2	Echovirus 4	Coxsackievirus B5
1963	Coxsackievirus B1	Coxsackievirus A9	Echovirus 9	Echovirus 4	Coxsackievirus B4
1964	Coxsackievirus B4	Coxsackievirus B2	Coxsackievirus A9	Echovirus 4	Echovirus 6, Coxsackievirus B1
1965	Echovirus 9	Echovirus 6	Coxsackievirus B2	Coxsackievirus B5	Coxsackievirus B4
1966	Echovirus 9	Coxsackievirus B2	Echovirus 6	Coxsackievirus B5	Coxsackievirus A9, A16
1967	Coxsackievirus B5	Echovirus 9	Coxsackievirus A9	Echovirus 6	Coxsackievirus B2
1968	Echovirus 9	Echovirus 30	Coxsackievirus A16	Coxsackievirus B3	Coxsackievirus B4
1969	Echovirus 30	Echovirus 9	Echovirus 18	Echovirus 6	Coxsackievirus B4
1970	Echovirus 3	Echovirus 9	Echovirus 6	Echovirus 4	Coxsackievirus B4
1971	Echovirus 4	Echovirus 9	Echovirus 6	Coxsackievirus B4	Coxsackievirus B2
1972	Coxsackievirus B5	Echovirus 4	Echovirus 6	Echovirus 9	Coxsackievirus B3
1973	Coxsackievirus A9	Echovirus 9	Echovirus 6	Coxsackievirus B2	Coxsackievirus B5, echovirus 5
1974	Echovirus 11	Echovirus 4	Echovirus 6	Echovirus 9	Echovirus 18
1975	Echovirus 9	Echovirus 4	Echovirus 6	Coxsackievirus A9	Coxsackievirus B4
1976	Coxsackievirus B2	Echovirus 4	Coxsackievirus B4	Coxsackievirus A9	Coxsackievirus B3, echovirus 6
1977	Echovirus 6	Coxsackievirus B1	Coxsackievirus B3	Echovirus 9	Coxsackievirus A9
1978	Echovirus 9	Echovirus 4	Coxsackievirus A9	Echovirus 30	Coxsackievirus B4
1979	Echovirus 11	Echovirus 7	Echovirus 30	Coxsackievirus B2	Coxsackievirus B4
1980	Echovirus 11	Coxsackievirus B3	Echovirus 30	Coxsackievirus B2	Coxsackievirus A9
1981	Echovirus 30	Echovirus 9	Echovirus 11	Echovirus 3	Coxsackievirus A9, echovirus 5
1982	Echovirus 11	Echovirus 30	Echovirus 5	Echovirus 9	Coxsackievirus B5
1983	Coxsackievirus B5	Echovirus 30	Echovirus 20	Echovirus 11	Echovirus 24
1984	Echovirus 9	Echovirus 11	Coxsackievirus B5	Echovirus 30	Coxsackievirus B2, A9
1985	Echovirus 11	Echovirus 21	Echovirus 6, 7[b]		Coxsackievirus B2
1986	Echovirus 11	Echovirus 4	Echovirus 7	Echovirus 18	Coxsackievirus B5
1987	Echovirus 6	Echovirus 18	Echovirus 11	Coxsackievirus A9	Coxsackievirus B2
1988	Echovirus 11	Echovirus 9	Coxsackievirus B4	Coxsackievirus B2	Echovirus 6
1989	Coxsackievirus B5	Echovirus 9	Echovirus 11	Coxsackievirus B2	Echovirus 6
1990	Echovirus 30	Echovirus 6	Coxsackievirus B2	Coxsackievirus A9	Echovirus 11
1991	Echovirus 30	Echovirus 11	Coxsackievirus B1	Coxsackievirus B2	Echovirus 7
1992	Echovirus 11	Echovirus 30	Echovirus 9	Coxsackievirus B1	Coxsackievirus A9
1993	Echovirus 30	Coxsackievirus B5	Coxsackievirus A9	Coxsackievirus B1	Echovirus 7
1994	Coxsackievirus B2	Coxsackievirus B3	Echovirus E6	Echovirus 30	Coxsackievirus A9
1995	Echovirus 9	Echovirus 11	Coxsackievirus A9	Coxsackievirus B2	Echovirus 30
1996	Coxsackievirus B5	Echovirus 17	Echovirus 6	Coxsackievirus A9	Coxsackievirus B4
1997	Echovirus 30	Echovirus 6	Echovirus 7	Echovirus 11	Echovirus 18
1998	Echovirus 30	Echovirus 9	Echovirus 11	Coxsackievirus B3	Echovirus 6
1999	Echovirus 11	Echovirus 16	Echovirus 9	Echovirus 14	Echovirus 25

[a]Most patients from whom viruses were isolated had neurologic illnesses.
[b]Third and fourth place tie.
Data from Cherry JD. Enteroviruses and parechoviruses. *In* Feigin RD, Cherry JD, Demmler GJ, Kaplan SL (eds). Textbook of Pediatric Infectious Diseases, 5th ed. Philadelphia, WB Saunders, 2004, p 1989.

slightly during the late 1960s and early 1970s and then became more common again. Shown in Table 24-4 are the five most prevalent nonpolio enterovirus isolations per year in the United States from 1961 through 1999. Most patients from whom viruses were isolated had neurologic illnesses. It is possible that other enteroviruses were also prevalent but did not produce clinical disease severe enough to cause physicians to submit specimens for study. Many coxsackievirus A infections, even in the epidemic situation, probably went undiagnosed because suckling mouse inoculation was not performed. Although 62 nonpolio enteroviral types and 2 parechovirus types have been identified, in the 39 years covered in Table 24-4, only 24 different virus types have been reported. In the earlier years, echovirus 9 was the most common type; echoviruses 6 and 11 and coxsackieviruses B2 and B4 were the next most common types. Since 1990, echoviruses 30 and 11 have been the most common circulating viral types. In 1999, three of the five most common viral types (echoviruses 14, 16, and 25) were new to the list.

Similar data are available for the most common enteroviral isolates in Spain from 1988 to 1997 and Belgium from 1980 to 1994.[296,297] The most common enterovirus isolated in both countries was echovirus 30. In 1997 and 1998, major epidemic disease caused by enterovirus 71 occurred in Taiwan, Malaysia, Australia, and Japan.[298-302]

An analysis of the Centers for Disease Control and Prevention nonpolio enterovirus data for 14 years found that early isolates in a particular year were predictive of isolates for the remainder of that year.[303] The six most common isolates during March, April, and May were predictive of 59% of the total isolates during July through December of the same year.

Although the use of live polioviral vaccine has eliminated epidemic poliomyelitis in the United States, it is hard to

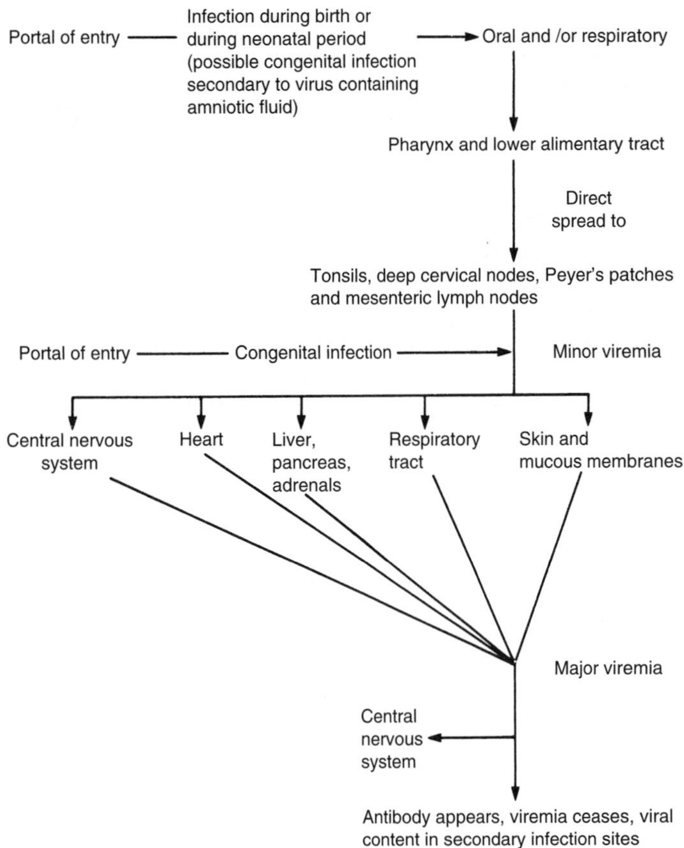

Figure 24–4 The pathogenesis of congenital and neonatal enteroviral infections.

determine what the effect of polio vaccine viruses has been on enteroviral ecology. In 1970, polioviruses accounted for only 6% of the total enteroviral isolations from patients with neurologic illnesses.[304] Although the figures are not directly comparable, more than one third of the enteroviral isolations in 1962 from similar patients were polioviruses.[305] However, Horstmann and associates[306] studied specimens from sewage and asymptomatic children during the vaccine era and found that the number of yearly polioviral isolations (presumably vaccine strains) was greater than the number of nonpolio enteroviruses. The prevalence of vaccine viruses did not seem to affect the seasonal epidemiology of other enteroviruses.

PATHOGENESIS

Events during Pathogenesis

Congenital infections with enteroviruses result from transplacental passage of virus to fetus. The method of transport from mother to fetus is poorly understood. Maternal viremia during enteroviral infections is common, and because virus has been recovered from the placenta on several occasions, it is probable that active infection of the placenta also occurs. Benirschke[137] found no histologic evidence of placental disease in three cases of established transplacentally acquired coxsackievirus B infections. Batcup and associates[307] found diffuse perivillous fibrin deposition with villous necrosis and inflammatory cell infiltration of the placenta in a woman who 2 weeks earlier, at 33 weeks' gestation, had coxsackievirus A9 meningitis. The woman was delivered of a macerated, stillborn infant. At birth, virus was recovered from the placenta but not from the stillborn infant.

It is assumed that infection in the fetus results from hematogenous dissemination initiated in the involved placenta. It is also possible that some in utero infection results from the ingestion of virus contained in amniotic fluid; in this situation, primary fetal infection involves the pharynx and lower alimentary tract. The portal of entry of infection during the birth process and the neonatal period is similar to that for older children and adults.

Figure 24-4 shows a schematic diagram of the events of pathogenesis. After initial acquisition of virus by the oral or respiratory route, implantation occurs in the pharynx and the lower alimentary tract. Within 1 day, the infection extends to the regional lymph nodes. On about the third day, minor viremia occurs, resulting in involvement of many secondary infection sites. In congenital infections, infection is initiated during the minor viremia phase. Multiplication of virus in secondary sites coincides with the onset of clinical symptoms. Illness can vary from minor to fatal infections. Major viremia occurs during the period of multiplication of virus in the secondary infection sites; this period usually lasts from the third to the seventh days of infection. In many echovirus and coxsackievirus infections, central nervous system involvement apparently occurs at the same time as other secondary organ involvement. This occasionally appears to happen with polioviral infections; however, more commonly, the central nervous system symptoms of poliomyelitis are delayed, suggesting that seeding occurred later in association with the major viremia.

Cessation of viremia correlates with the appearance of serum antibody. The viral concentration in secondary infection sites begins to diminish on about the seventh day. However, infection continues in the lower intestinal tract for prolonged periods.

Factors That Affect Pathogenesis

The pathogenesis and pathology of enterovirus infections depend on the virulence, tropism, and inoculum concentration of virus, as well as on many specific host factors. Enteroviruses have marked differences in tropism and virulence. Although some generalizations can be made in regard to tropism, there are marked differences even among strains of specific viral types. Differences in virulence of specific enteroviral types may be the result of recombination among enteroviruses or point mutations.[308-310]

Enterovirus infections of the fetus and neonate are thought to be more severe than similar infections in older individuals. This is undoubtedly true for coxsackievirus B infections and probably also true for coxsackievirus A, echovirus, and poliovirus infections. Although the reasons for this increased severity are largely unknown, several aspects of neonatal immune mechanisms offer clues. The similarity of coxsackievirus B infections in suckling mice to those in human neonates has provided a useful animal model. Heineberg and co-workers[311] compared coxsackievirus B1 infections in 24-hour-old suckling mice with similar infections in older mice. They observed that adult mice produced interferon in all infected tissues, whereas in suckling mice, only small amounts of interferon were identified in the liver. They thought that the difference in outcome of coxsackievirus B1 infections in suckling and older mice could be explained by the inability of the cells of the immature animal to elaborate interferon.

Others thought that the increased susceptibility of suckling mice to severe coxsackievirus infections was related to the transplacentally acquired, increased concentrations of adrenocortical hormones.[312,313] Kunin[314] suggested that the difference in age-specific susceptibility might be explained at the cellular level. He showed that a variety of tissues of newborn mice bound coxsackievirus B3, whereas tissues of adult mice were virtually inactive in this regard.[314,315] It has been suggested that the progressive loss of receptor-containing cells or of receptor sites on persisting cells with increasing age might be the mechanism that accounts for infections of lesser severity in older animals. Teisner and Haahr[316] suggested that the increased susceptibility of suckling mice to severe and fatal coxsackievirus infections might be from physiologic hypothermia and poikilothermia during the first week of life.

In the past, it was assumed that specific pathology in various organs and tissues in enteroviral infections was caused by the direct cytopathic effect and tropism of a particular virus. However, a large number of studies using murine myocarditis model systems have suggested that host immune responses contribute to the pathology.[13,308,317-332] These studies suggest that T cell–mediated processes and virus-induced autoimmunity cause acute and chronic tissue damage. Other studies suggest that the primary viral cytopathic effect is responsible for tissue damage and that various T cell responses are a response to the damage, not the cause.[333] From my review of various murine myocarditis model systems, it is apparent that the genetics of the hosts and of the viral strains determine the likelihood of autoimmune, cell-mediated cellular damage.[308,317-320,322-325,327,329,331] However, none of the model systems is appropriate for the evaluation of the pathogenesis of neonatal myocarditis. Although available studies suggest that enterovirus-induced myocarditis in older children and adults occasionally may have a delayed cell-mediated component, the short incubation period and fulminant nature of neonatal disease, as well as the similar infection in suckling mice, suggest that autoimmune factors are not major in the pathogenesis of myocarditis in neonates.

During the past 40 years, the clinical manifestations caused by several enteroviral serotypes have changed. For example, echovirus 11 infections initially were associated with exanthem and aseptic meningitis in children. They later were found to cause severe sepsis-like illnesses in neonates. These phenotypic changes in disease expression may be the result of recombination among enteroviruses.[310,334]

PATHOLOGY

General Considerations

Great variations in the clinical signs of congenital and neonatal enterovirus infections are paralleled by wide variations in pathology. Because pathologic material usually is available only from patients with fatal illnesses, the discussion in this section considers only the more severe enteroviral manifestations. It is worth emphasizing, however, that these fatal infections account for only a small portion of all congenital and neonatal enterovirus infections. The pathologic findings in infants with milder infections, such as nonspecific febrile illness, have not been described.

Polioviruses

The pathologic findings in fatal neonatal poliomyelitis are similar to those seen in disease of older children and adults.[19,102,108,109,111] The major findings have involved the central nervous system, specifically the anterior horns of the spinal cord and the motor nuclei of the cranial nerves. Involvement is usually irregularly distributed and asymmetric. Microscopically, the anterior horn cells show neuronal destruction, gliosis, and perivascular small round cell infiltration. Myocarditis has also been observed,[102] characterized by focal necrosis of muscle fibers and various degrees of cellular infiltration.

Coxsackieviruses A

Records of neonatal illnesses associated with coxsackieviruses A are rare.[335-337] Gold and co-workers,[336] in a study of sudden unexpected death in infants, recovered coxsackievirus A4 from the brains of three children. Histologic abnormalities were not identified in the brains or spinal cords of these patients. Baker and Phillips[337] reported the death of twins in association with coxsackievirus A3 intrauterine infections; the first twin was stillborn, and the second twin died when 2 days old of viral pneumonia.

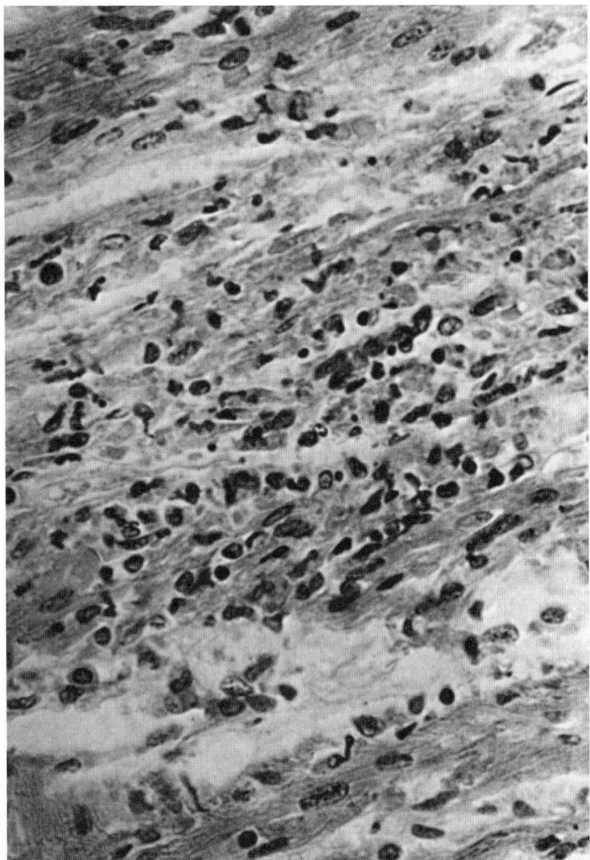

Figure 24–5 Coxsackievirus B4 myocarditis in a 9-day-old infant. Notice the myocardial necrosis and mononuclear cellular infiltration.

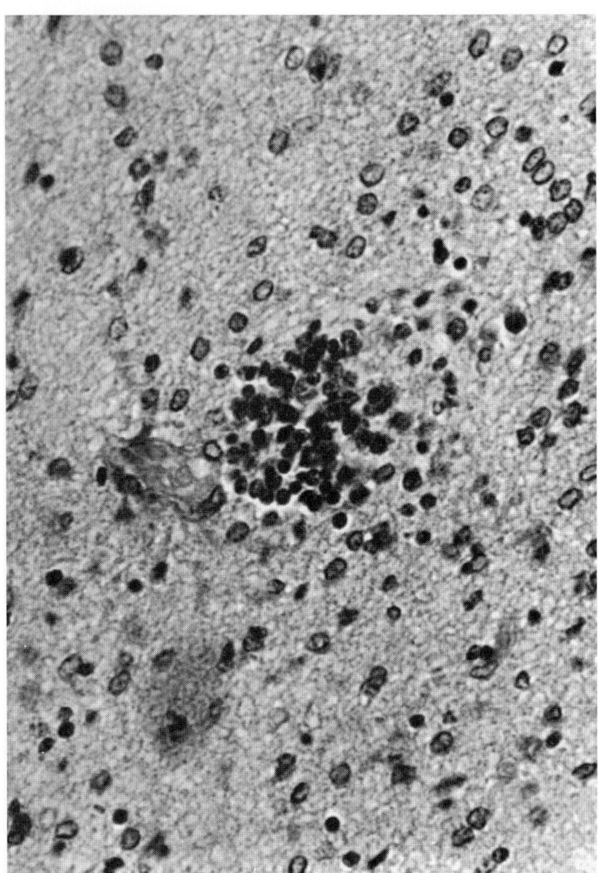

Figure 24–6 Coxsackievirus B4 encephalitis in a 9-day-old infant. Notice the focal infiltrate of mononuclear and glial cells.

Eisenhut and associates[338] described a full-term neonate with coxsackievirus A9 infection with meningitis, myocarditis, and disseminated intravascular coagulation who died on the seventh day of life.

Coxsackieviruses B

Of the enteroviruses, coxsackieviruses B have been most frequently associated with severe and catastrophic neonatal disease. The most common findings in these cases have been myocarditis or meningoencephalitis, or both. Involvement of the adrenals, pancreas, liver, and lungs has occurred.

Heart

Grossly, the heart is usually enlarged, with dilatation of the chambers and flabby musculature.[138,147,193,195,204] Microscopically, the pericardium frequently contains some inflammatory cells; and thickening, edema, and focal infiltrations of inflammatory cells may be found in the endocardium. The myocardium (Fig. 24-5) is congested and contains infiltrations of inflammatory cells (i.e., lymphocytes, mononuclear cells, reticulum cells, histiocytes, plasma cells, and polymorphonuclear and eosinophil leukocytes). Involvement of the myocardium is often patchy and focal but occasionally is diffuse. The muscle shows loss of striation, edema, and eosinophilic degeneration. Muscle necrosis without extensive cellular infiltration is common.

Brain and Spinal Cord

The meninges are congested, edematous, and occasionally mildly infiltrated with inflammatory cells.[138,147,177,195,201,204,339] Lesions in the brain and spinal cord are focal rather than diffuse but frequently involve many different areas. The lesions consist of areas of eosinophilic degeneration of cortical cells, clusters of mononuclear and glial cells (Fig. 24-6), and perivascular cuffing. Occasionally, areas of liquefaction necrosis unassociated with inflammation are seen.

Other Organs

The lungs commonly have areas of mild focal pneumonitis with peribronchiolar mononuclear cellular infiltrations.[138,177,195,201,340-342] Massive pulmonary hemorrhage has been observed. The liver is frequently engorged and occasionally contains isolated foci of liver cell necrosis and mononuclear cell infiltrations. A neonate with a coxsackievirus B1 infection developed a sepsis-like illness on the fourth day of life with severe hepatitis and subsequently developed progressive liver calcifications.[342] In the pancreas, infiltration of mononuclear cells, lymphocytes, and plasma cells has been observed, and occasional focal degeneration of the islet cells occurs. Congestion has been observed in the adrenal glands, with mild to severe cortical necrosis and infiltration of inflammatory cells.

Echoviruses

In an earlier period, although frequently responsible for neonatal illnesses, echoviruses were rarely associated with fatal infections. During the past 30 years, however, there have been many reports of fatal illnesses in newborns from echovirus type 11.[30,162,165,257,343-348] In virtually all cases, the major pathologic finding was massive hepatic necrosis; other findings included hemorrhagic necrosis of the adrenal glands, hemorrhage in other organs, myocardial necrosis, and acute tubular necrosis of the kidneys. Wang and colleagues[348] studied four neonates (three with echovirus 11 and one with echovirus 5 infections) with fulminant hepatic failure and observed two histopathologic patterns associated with minimal inflammation but extensive hemorrhagic necrosis. One pattern indicated ongoing endothelial injury with endotheliitis and fibrinoid necrosis. The second pattern, which was seen in the two neonates who initially survived, was that of veno-occlusive disease. Virus has not been identified in hepatocytes. Extensive myositis of the strap muscles of the neck occurred in one case.[347] Massive hepatic necrosis has also occurred in infections with echoviruses 3, 5, 6, 7, 9, 14, 19, 20, and 21.[159,160,254,343,349-353] Wreghitt and associates[354] described a neonate with a fatal echovirus 7 infection. This infant was found to have massive disseminated intravascular coagulation, with bleeding in the adrenal glands, renal medulla, liver, and cerebellum.

At autopsy, one infant with echovirus 6 infection was found to have cloudy and thickened leptomeninges, liver necrosis, adrenal and renal hemorrhage, and mild interstitial pneumonitis.[343] One infant with echovirus 9 infection had an enlarged and congested liver with marked central necrosis,[350] and another with this virus had interstitial pneumonitis without liver involvement.[161] Three infants with echovirus 11 infections had renal and adrenal hemorrhage and small-vessel thrombi in the renal medulla and in the medulla and the inner cortex of the adrenal glands.[250] In these patients, the livers were normal. Two infants, one with echovirus 6 and the other with echovirus 31 infection, had only extensive pneumonias.[256,355]

CLINICAL MANIFESTATIONS

Abortion

Polioviruses

Poliomyelitis is associated with an increased incidence of abortion. Horn[93] reported 43 abortions in 325 pregnancies complicated by maternal poliomyelitis. Abortion was directly related to the severity of the maternal illness, including the degree of fever during the acute phase of illness. However, abortion also was associated with mild, nonparalytic poliomyelitis. Schaeffer and colleagues[98] studied the placenta and abortus 12 days after the onset of illness in a mother. Poliovirus type 1 was isolated from the placenta and the fetal tissues.

Other investigators[356-360] have reported an increased incidence of abortions in cases of maternal poliomyelitis. Siegel and Greenberg[112] noticed that fetal death occurred in 14 (46.7%) of 30 instances of maternal poliomyelitis during the first trimester. Kaye and colleagues[360] reviewed the literature in 1953 and found 19 abortions in 101 cases of poliomyelitis in pregnancy. In a small study in Evanston Hospital in Illinois, the abortion rate associated with maternal poliomyelitis was little different from the expected rate.[357] In a study of 310 pregnant women who received trivalent oral poliovirus vaccine, there was no increase in abortions above the expected rate.[118] In a later study in Finland that involved about 9000 pregnant women immunized with oral poliovirus vaccine, there was no evidence of an increase in stillbirths.[361]

Coxsackieviruses

Although in the late 1950s and early 1960s there were extensive outbreaks of illness caused by coxsackievirus A16, there was no evidence of adverse outcomes of pregnancy related to this virus. Because infections with other coxsackieviruses rarely involve large segments of the population, rate studies have not been performed.

Frisk and Diderholm[362] found that 33% of women with abortions had IgM antibody to coxsackieviruses B, whereas only 8% of controls had similar antibody. In a second, larger study, the same research group confirmed their original findings.[363]

Echoviruses

There is no available evidence suggesting that echovirus infections during pregnancy are a cause of spontaneous abortion. Landsman and associates[155] studied 2631 pregnancies during an epidemic of echovirus 9 and could find no difference in antibody to echovirus 9 between mothers who aborted and those who delivered term infants. A similar study in Finland revealed no increase in the abortion rate among mothers infected in early pregnancy with echovirus 9.[153]

Congenital Malformations

Polioviruses

The congenital malformation rate associated with poliovirus infection as determined in the NIH-sponsored Collaborative Perinatal Research Project of 45,000 pregnancies was 4.1%.[364] Although isolated instances of congenital malformation and maternal poliomyelitis have been reported, there is little statistical evidence demonstrating that polioviruses are teratogens. In their review of the literature, Kaye and colleagues[360] identified six anomalies in 101 infants born to mothers with poliomyelitis during pregnancy. In the reviews of Horn,[93] Bates,[110] and Siegel and Greenberg,[112] there was no evidence of maternal poliovirus infection–induced anomalies.

The possibility of congenital anomalies associated with attenuated oral poliovirus vaccine has also been studied.[117,118,361,365-367] Pearson and co-workers[117] studied the fetal malformation rate in a community in which a large vaccine field trial had been carried out; although it is probable that pregnant women became infected with vaccine virus by secondary spread, there was no community increase in fetal malformations. Prem and associates[118] studied the infants of 69 women who received attenuated vaccine before 20 weeks' gestation and found that none had anomalies. In contrast, the rate of congenital defects in Blackburn, England, increased coincident with mass vaccination with trivalent poliomyelitis vaccine.[365] However, there is no evidence of cause and effect related to this observation. Connelly and colleagues[366] commented on a child with a unique renal disease acquired in utero. The child's mother had received oral polio vaccine during the second month of pregnancy.

In February 1985, a mass vaccination program with live oral poliovirus vaccine was carried out in Finland.[367] Although pregnant women received vaccine, there was no evidence that vaccine virus had a harmful effect on developing fetuses.

Coxsackieviruses

In a large prospective study, Brown[368-370] and colleagues (Evans[371,372] and Karunas[373]) made a serologic search for selected maternal enteroviral infections in association with congenital malformations. In one study,[373] serum samples from 22,935 women had been collected. From this group, serum samples from 630 mothers of infants with anomalies and from 1164 mothers of children without defects were carefully studied. Specifically, serologic evidence was sought for infection during the first trimester and last 6 months of pregnancy with coxsackieviruses B1 through B5 and A9 and with echoviruses 6 and 9. In this study, infants were examined for 113 specific abnormalities; these anomalies were grouped into 12 categories for analysis. The investigators demonstrated a positive correlation between maternal infection and infant anomaly with coxsackieviruses B2 through B4 and A9. The overall first-trimester infection rate with coxsackievirus B4 was significantly higher in patients with anomalies than that in controls. Maternal coxsackievirus B2 infection throughout pregnancy, coxsackievirus B4 infections during the first trimester of pregnancy, and infection with at least one of the five coxsackieviruses B during pregnancy were all associated with urogenital anomalies. Coxsackievirus A9 infection was associated with digestive anomalies, and coxsackieviruses B3 and B4 were associated with cardiovascular defects. When coxsackieviruses B were analyzed as a group (B1 to B5), there was an overall association with congenital heart disease; the likelihood of cardiovascular anomalies was increased when maternal infection with two or more coxsackieviruses B occurred. In this study, the mothers had been instructed to keep illness diary sheets. There was no correlation between reported maternal clinical illnesses and serologic evidence of infection with the selected enteroviruses. This suggests that many infections that may have been causally related to the anomalies were asymptomatic. A disturbing finding in this study was the lack of seasonal occurrence of the births of children with specific defects. Because enteroviral transmission is most common in the summer and fall, the birth rate of children with malformations should have been greatest in the spring and summer if coxsackieviruses were a major cause of malformation.

In the NIH-sponsored Collaborative Perinatal Research Project, Elizan and co-workers[374] were unable to find any relationships between maternal infections with coxsackieviruses B and congenital central nervous system malformations. Scattered case reports in the literature describe congenital anomalies associated with maternal coxsackievirus infections. Makower and colleagues[140] reported a child with congenital malformations who was born at 32 weeks' gestation and from whom a coxsackievirus A4 strain was recovered from the meconium. The child's mother had been well throughout pregnancy, except for a febrile illness during the first month. The relationship of the viral infection to the congenital malformations or to the prematurity is uncertain.

Gauntt and associates[375] studied the ventricular fluids from 28 newborn infants with severe congenital anatomic defects of the central nervous system. In four infants (two with hydranencephaly, one with an occipital meningocele, and one with aqueductal stenosis), neutralizing antibody to one or more coxsackievirus B types was found in the fluid. In one case, IgM-neutralizing antibody to coxsackievirus B6 was found. The investigators concluded that their data suggested the possibility of an association between congenital infections with coxsackieviruses B and severe central nervous system defects.

Echoviruses

In the large prospective study of Brown and Karunas,[373] the possible association of maternal infections with echoviruses 6 and 9 and congenital malformations was examined. Maternal infection with these selected echoviruses apparently was not associated with any anomaly. In three other studies,[153-155] no association was found between maternal echovirus 9 infection and congenital malformation.

Prematurity and Stillbirth

Polioviruses

In the study by Horn[93] of 325 pregnancies, nine infants died in utero. In each instance, the mother was critically ill with poliomyelitis. Horn[93] also observed that 45 infants weighed less than 6 pounds, and 17 of these had a birth weight of less than 5 pounds. These low-birth-weight infants were born predominantly to mothers who had had poliomyelitis early in pregnancy. A similar finding was reported by Aycock.[96,376] In New York City, Siegel and Greenberg[112] also documented an increase in prematurity after maternal poliomyelitis infection. This was specifically related to maternal paralytic poliomyelitis. There has been no observation of stillbirth or prematurity in relation to vaccine administration.[361]

Coxsackieviruses

Bates reported a fetus of 8 months' gestational age who was stillborn and had calcific pancarditis and hydrops fetalis at autopsy.[144] Fluorescent antibody study revealed coxsackievirus B3 antigen in the myocardium. Burch and colleagues[149] described three stillborn infants who had fluorescent antibody evidence of coxsackievirus B myocarditis, one each with coxsackieviruses B2, B3, or B4. They also reported a premature boy who had histologic and immunofluorescent evidence of cardiac infection with coxsackieviruses B2 through B4; he lived only 24 hours. A macerated stillborn girl was delivered 2 weeks after the occurrence of aseptic meningitis caused by coxsackievirus A9 in a 27-year-old woman.[307] Virus was recovered from the placenta but not from the infant. Coxsackievirus B6 has been recovered from the brain, liver, and placenta of a stillborn infant.[143]

Echoviruses and Enteroviruses

Freedman[377] reported the occurrence of a full-term, fresh stillbirth in a woman infected with echovirus 11. Because the infant had no pathologic or virologic evidence of infection, he attributed the event to a secondary consequence of maternal infection from fever and dehydration rather than

Table 24–5 **Major Manifestations of Neonatal Nonpolio Enteroviral and Parechoviral Infections**

Specific Involvement	Common	Rare
Inapparent infection	Par 1	Cox A9, B1, B2, B4, B5 Echo 3, 5, 9, 11, 13, 14, 20, 30, 31
Mild, nonspecific, febrile illness	Cox B5 Echo 5, 11, 33	Cox B1, B2, B3, B4, A9, A16 Echo 4, 7, 9, 17
Sepsis-like illness	Cox B2, B3, B4, B5 Echo 5, 11, 15	Cox B1, A9 Echo 2, 3, 4, 6, 9, 14, 19, 21 Par 1
Respiratory illness (general)	Echo 11 Par 1	Cox B1, B4, B5, A9 Echo 9, 17
Herpangina		Cox A5
Coryza		Cox A9 Echo 11, 17, 19 Par 1
Pharyngitis		Cox B4 Echo 11, 17, 18
Laryngotracheitis or bronchitis		Cox B1, B4 Echo 11
Pneumonia		Cox B4, A9 Echo 6, 9, 11, 17, 31 Par 1
Cloud baby		Echo 20
Gastrointestinal		
Vomiting or diarrhea	Echo 5, 17, 18	Cox B1, B2, B5 Echo 4, 6, 8, 9, 11, 16, 19, 21 Par 1 Entero 71
Hepatitis	Echo 11, 19	Cox B1, B3, B4, A9 Echo 5, 6, 7, 9, 14, 20, 21
Pancreatitis		Cox B3, B4, B5
Necrotizing enterocolitis		Cox B2, B3 Par 1
Cardiovascular		
Myocarditis and pericarditis	Cox B1, B2, B3, B4	Cox B5, A9 Echo 11, 19
Skin	Cox B5 Echo 5, 17 Par 1	Cox B1 Echo 4, 7, 9, 11, 18 Entero 71
Neurologic		
Aseptic meningitis	Cox B2, B3, B4, B5 Echo 3, 9, 11, 17	Cox B1, A9, A14 Echo 1, 5, 13, 14, 21, 30 Entero 71
Encephalitis	Cox B1, B2, B3, B4	Cox B5 Echo 6, 9, 23 Par 2 Entero 71
Paralysis		Cox B2
Sudden infant death		Cox B1, B3, B4, A4, A5, A8 Par 1

Cox, coxsackievirus; echo, echovirus; entero, enterovirus; par, parechovirus.
Data from Cherry JD. Enteroviruses and Parechoviruses. *In* Feigin RD, Cherry JD, Demmler GJ, Kaplan SL (eds). Textbook of Pediatric Infectious Diseases, 5th ed. Philadelphia, WB Saunders, 2004.

primary transplacental infection. Echovirus 27 has been associated with intrauterine death on two occasions.[143,166]

In an extensive study of neonatal enteroviral infections in Milwaukee in 1979, Piraino and associates[165] found that 12 of 19 stillbirths occurred from July through October coincident with a major outbreak of enterovirus disease. Echovirus 11 was the main agent isolated during this period. A 1300-g fetus, stillborn after 26 weeks' gestation, had hydrocephalus, fibrotic peritonitis, and hepatosplenomegaly and was found to have an enterovirus 71 infection by PCR and immunohistochemical study.[169]

Neonatal Infection

Nonpolio Enteroviruses and Parechoviruses

Illnesses caused by nonpolio enteroviruses and parechoviruses are discussed by clinical classification (Table 24-5) in the following sections.

INAPPARENT INFECTION

Although it is probable that inapparent infections in neonates occasionally occur with many different enteroviruses, there is little documentation of this assumption. Cherry and co-workers[141] studied 590 normal newborns during a 6-month period and found only one infection without clinical signs of illness. This was a child infected in utero or immediately thereafter with coxsackievirus B2. The mother had an upper respiratory illness 10 days before delivery. In a similar but more comprehensive study, Jenista and associates[178] failed to isolate any enteroviruses from cultures from 666 newborns on the first postpartum day. However, during weekly cultures during the month after birth, 75 enteroviruses were isolated. Symptomatic enteroviral disease occurred in 21% (16 of 75).

During a survey of perinatal virus infections, 44 infants were found to be infected with parechovirus 1 during the study period from May to December 1966.[236] The virus prevalence and the incidence of new infections during this period were fairly uniform. No illness was attributed to parechovirus 1 infection, and the virus disappeared from the nursery in mid-December 1966. Inapparent infections with parechovirus 1 have been reported on two other occasions.[237,246] Infections without evidence of illness have occurred with coxsackieviruses A9, B1, B4, and B5 and with echoviruses 3, 5, 9, 11, 13, 14, 20, 30, and 31.[9,156,157,178,210,250,256,340,378-381]

MILD, NONSPECIFIC FEBRILE ILLNESS

In a review of 338 enteroviral infections in early infancy, 9% were classified as nonspecific febrile illnesses.[378] Illness may be sporadic in nature or part of an outbreak with a specific viral type. In the latter situation, clinical manifestations vary depending on the viral type; some infants have aseptic meningitis and other signs and symptoms, and some have only nonspecific fever. Coxsackievirus B5 and echovirus types 5, 11, and 33 have been those found most commonly in nonspecific fevers; other agents identified have included coxsackieviruses A9, A16, and B1 through B4 and echoviruses 4, 7, 9, and 17.*

Mild, nonspecific febrile illness occurs most commonly in full-term infants after uneventful pregnancies and deliveries without complications. Illness can occur at any time during the first month of life. When the onset occurs after the infant is 7 days old, a careful history frequently reveals a trivial illness in a family member. The onset of illness is characterized by mild irritability and fever, which is usually in the range of 38° C to 39° C, but higher temperatures occasionally occur. Poor feeding is frequently observed. One or two episodes of vomiting or diarrhea, or both, may occur in some infants. The usual duration of illness is 2 to 4 days.

Routine laboratory study is not helpful, but cerebrospinal fluid (CSF) examination may reveal an increased protein concentration and leukocyte count indicative of aseptic meningitis. Although, by definition, illness in this category is mild, the degree of viral infection may be extensive. When looked for, virus may be isolated from the blood, urine, and spinal fluid of infants with mild illnesses.[211,379]

SEPSIS-LIKE ILLNESS

The major diagnostic problem in neonatal enteroviral infections is differentiation of bacterial from viral disease. Even in the infant with mild, nonspecific fever, bacterial disease must be strongly considered. The sepsis-like illness described here is always alarming. This illness is characterized by fever, poor feeding, abdominal distention, irritability, rash, lethargy, and hypotonia.[340,385-387] Other findings include diarrhea, vomiting, seizures, shock, disseminated intravascular coagulation, thrombocytopenia, hepatomegaly, jaundice, and apnea. The onset of illness is introduced by irritability, poor feeding, and fever and followed within 24 hours by other manifestations. In a group of 27 neonates, Lake and associates[286] observed that 54% had temperatures of 39° C or higher. The duration of fever varies from 1 to 8 days, most commonly 3 to 4 days. Barre and colleagues[388] reported a 3-day-old boy with an enterovirus-associated hemophagocytic syndrome. This neonate presented with a typical sepsis-like picture with fever, hepatosplenomegaly, coagulopathy, thrombocytopenia, and anemia. This child recovered and had no hemophagocytic relapses.

Sepsis-like illness is common. Morens[378] described its occurrence in one fifth of 338 enteroviral infections in infants. In an attempt to differentiate bacterial from viral disease, Lake and co-workers[340] studied 27 infants with enteroviral infections. White blood cell counts were not helpful because the total count, the number of neutrophils, and the number of band form neutrophils were elevated in most instances. Of most importance were historical data. Most mothers had evidence of a recent febrile, viral-like illness. Other factors often associated with bacterial sepsis, such as prolonged rupture of membranes, prematurity, and low Apgar scores, were unusual in the enteroviral infection group.

Sepsis-like illness has been identified most often with coxsackieviruses B2 through B5 and echovirus types 5, 11, and 16; other viruses detected include coxsackieviruses A9 and B1; echoviruses 2, 3, 4, 6, 9, 14, 19, and 21; and parechovirus 1.*

Since the early 1980s, echovirus 11 has been associated most frequently with fatal septic events, with hepatic necrosis, and disseminated intravascular coagulation.[30,163-165,257,344-348,354]

RESPIRATORY ILLNESS

Respiratory complaints are generally overshadowed by other manifestations of neonatal enteroviral disease. Only 7% of 338 enteroviral infections in early infancy were classified as respiratory illness.[378] Except for echoviruses 11 and parechovirus 1, respiratory illness associated with enteroviruses has been sporadic.[237,239]

Hercík and co-workers[239] reported an epidemic of respiratory illness in 22 newborns associated with echovirus 11 infection. All of these infants had rhinitis and pharyngitis, 50% had laryngitis, and 32% had interstitial pneumonitis. Berkovich and Pangan[237] studied respiratory illnesses in premature infants and reported 64 with illness, 18 of whom had virologic or serologic evidence of parechovirus 1 infection. Many had high but constant levels of serum antibody to parechovirus 1. Some of the 18 infants were probably also infected with parechovirus 1. The children with proven parechovirus 1 infections could not be clinically differentiated from those without evidence of parechovirus 1 infection. Ninety percent of the infants had coryza, and 39% had radiographic evidence of pneumonia.

*See references 29, 141, 165, 196, 207, 211, 229, 230, 238, 240-242, 249-251, 379, 382, 384.

*See references 28-30, 160, 161, 163-165, 168, 214, 234, 235, 243, 247, 250, 251, 257, 338, 340, 342, 344-346, 348, 350, 351, 354, 383, 385, 389-394.

Herpangina. Chawareewong and associates[396] described several infants with herpangina and coxsackievirus A5 infection. A vesicular lesion on an erythematous base on a tonsillar pillar in a 6-day-old infant with coxsackievirus B2 meningitis has also been reported.[397] Two 1-month-old infants were described in an outbreak of herpangina due to coxsackievirus B3 in a welfare home in Japan.[398]

Coryza. Several agents have been associated with coryza: coxsackievirus A9 and echoviruses 11, 17, 19, and 22.[158,239,243,246,399]

Pharyngitis. Pharyngitis is uncommon in neonatal enteroviral infections. In more than 50 infants with enteroviral infections studied by Linnemann and colleagues[383] and Lake and associates,[340] pharyngitis did not occur. Suzuki and coworkers[400] observed pharyngitis in 3 of 42 neonates with echovirus 11 infections. In contrast, in the same study, 67% of children 1 month to 4 years old had pharyngitis. Pharyngitis has been associated with coxsackievirus B4 and with echoviruses 11, 17, and 18.[207,239,253,400,401]

Laryngotracheobronchitis or Bronchitis. A few enteroviruses have been identified in cases of laryngotracheobronchitis or bronchitis: coxsackieviruses B1 and B4 and echovirus 11.[239,402] Specific clinical descriptions of laryngotracheobronchitis or bronchitis associated with enteroviral infections are scanty. Hercík and co-workers[239] observed laryngitis in 11 and croup in 4 of 22 neonates during an echovirus 11 outbreak. All of the affected infants had upper respiratory tract findings, vomiting, and lethargy. Many were also cyanotic and had hepatosplenomegaly.

Pneumonia. Pneumonia as the main manifestation of neonatal enteroviral infection is rare. Morens[378] documented only seven instances of pneumonia in 338 neonatal enteroviral infections. Outbreaks of pneumonia in neonates have been reported with echovirus 11 and parechovirus 1.[237,239] Pneumonia resulting from other enteroviruses is a sporadic event and has been reported for the following nonpolio enteroviruses: coxsackieviruses A9 and B4 and echoviruses 9, 17, and 31.

During a nursery echovirus 11 outbreak, 7 of 22 neonates had pneumonia.[239] All infants had signs of upper respiratory infection and general signs of sepsis-like illness. In infants with pneumonia associated with an echovirus 22 nursery epidemic, coryza, cough, and dyspnea were early signs.[237] The illnesses tended to be protracted, with radiographic changes persisting for 10 to 100 days.

Cloud Baby. Eichenwald and associates[248] recovered echovirus 20 from four full-term infants younger than 8 days. Although these infants apparently were well, it was found that they were extensively colonized with staphylococci and that they disseminated these organisms into the air around them. Because of this ability to disseminate staphylococci, they were called *cloud babies*. The investigators believed that these cloud babies contributed to the epidemic spread of staphylococci in the nursery. Because active staphylococcal dissemination occurred only during the time that echovirus 20 could be recovered from the nasopharynx, it was theorized that viral-bacterial synergism occurred.

GASTROINTESTINAL MANIFESTATIONS

Significant gastrointestinal illness occurs in about 7% of enteroviral infections during infancy.[378]

Vomiting or Diarrhea. Vomiting and diarrhea are common but usually just part of the overall illness complex and not the major manifestations. In 1958, Eichenwald and colleagues[244] described epidemic diarrhea associated with echovirus 18 infections.

In 22 infants with epidemic respiratory disease caused by echovirus 11, all had vomiting as a manifestation of the illness.[239] Linnemann and colleagues[383] reported vomiting in 36% and diarrhea in 7% of neonates with echoviral infections. In another study, Lake and associates[340] found diarrhea in 81% and vomiting in 33% of neonates with nonpolio enteroviral infections. Vomiting and diarrhea in neonates have been associated with coxsackieviruses B1, B2, and B5; echoviruses 4 through 6, 8, 9, 11, 16, 17, 18, 19, and 21; parechovirus 1; and enterovirus 71.*

Hepatitis. Morens[378] observed that 2% of neonates with clinically severe enteroviral disease had hepatitis. Lake and colleagues[340] found that 37% of neonates with enteroviral infections had hepatomegaly, and hepatosplenomegaly was observed by Hercík and associates[239] in 12 of 22 newborns with echovirus 11 respiratory illnesses.

Severe hepatitis, frequently with hepatic necrosis, has been associated with echoviruses 5, 6, 7, 9, 11, 14, 19, 20, and 21.[159,160,263,343,344,347-350,353,406,407] In 1980, Modlin[254] reported four fatal echovirus 11 illnesses in premature infants. All had hepatitis, disseminated intravascular coagulation, thrombocytopenia, lethargy, poor feeding, and jaundice. Since 1980, there have been many reports of sepsis-like illness with fatal hepatitis related to echovirus 11.[30,163,165,257,345,347,348,351]

Coxsackieviruses B1, B4, and other B types have been associated with neonatal hepatitis.[12,29,203,216,342,393-395] Abzug[408] reviewed medical records of 16 neonates with hepatitis and coagulopathy and found a case-fatality rate of 31%. All of the five patients who died had myocarditis, and three had encephalitis.

Pancreatitis. Pancreatitis was recognized in three of four newborns with coxsackievirus B5 meningitis[200] and in coxsackievirus B3 and B4 infections at autopsy.[197] In other fatal coxsackievirus B infections, pancreatic involvement has been identified, but clinical manifestations have rarely been observed.

Necrotizing Enterocolitis. Lake and associates[340] described three infants with necrotizing enterocolitis. Coxsackievirus B3 was recovered from two of these infants and coxsackievirus B2 from the third. Parechovirus 1 was associated with a necrotizing enterocolitis outbreak.[409]

CARDIOVASCULAR MANIFESTATIONS

In contrast with enteroviral cardiac disease in children and adults, in which pericarditis is common, neonatal disease virtually always involves the heart muscle.† Most cases of neonatal myocarditis are related to coxsackievirus B infections, and nursery outbreaks have occurred on several occasions. In 1961, Kibrick[20] reviewed the clinical findings in 45 cases of neonatal myocarditis; his findings are summarized in

---

*See references 157, 211, 214, 234, 238-240, 242-244, 247, 383, 385, 403-405.
†See references 6, 12, 28, 29, 138, 144, 147-149, 163, 165, 193-196, 201-206, 208-210, 213, 215, 218, 220, 221, 223, 225, 227-229, 341, 345, 346, 393-395, 410-414, 416.

Table 24–6 Findings in Neonatal Coxsackievirus B Myocarditis

Finding	Frequency (%)
Feeding difficulty	84
Listlessness	81
Cardiac signs	81
Respiratory distress	75
Cyanosis	72
Fever	70
Pharyngitis	64
Hepatosplenomegaly	53
Biphasic course	35
Central nervous system signs	27
Hemorrhage	13
Jaundice	13
Diarrhea	8

Modified from Kibrick S. Viral infections of the fetus and newborn. Perspect Virol 2:140, 1961.

Table 24-6. Many of the early experiences, particularly in South Africa, involved catastrophic nursery epidemics. Since the observation in 1972 of five newborns with echovirus 11 infections and myocarditis, there have been no further reports of nursery epidemics.[412]

The illness as described by Kibrick[20] most commonly had an abrupt onset and was characterized by listlessness, anorexia, and fever. A biphasic pattern was observed in about one third of the patients. Progression was rapid, and signs of circulatory failure appeared within 2 days. If death did not occur, recovery was occasionally rapid but usually occurred gradually during an extended period. Most patients had cardiac findings, such as tachycardia, cardiomegaly, electrocardiographic changes, and transitory systolic murmurs. Many patients showed signs of respiratory distress and cyanosis. About one third of the infants had signs suggesting neurologic involvement. Of the 45 patients analyzed by Kibrick, only 12 survived.

In the echovirus 11 nursery outbreak reported by Drew,[414] 5 of 10 infants had tachycardia out of proportion to their fevers. Three of these infants had electrocardiograms, supraventricular tachycardia occurred in all, and ST segment depression was observed in two of the records. Supraventricular tachycardia has also been seen in patients with coxsackievirus B infections.[210] Echovirus 19 has been associated with myocarditis.[399]

Neonatal myocarditis related to enteroviruses has been less common than it was 4 decades ago. In his review, Morens[378] reported only two instances among 248 severe neonatal enteroviral illnesses.

EXANTHEM

Exanthem as a manifestation of neonatal enteroviral infection has occurred with coxsackieviruses B1, B3, and B5; echoviruses 4, 5, 7, 9, 11, 16, 17, 18, and 21; and parechovirus 1.* In most instances, rash is just a minor manifestation of moderate to severe neonatal disease. Of 27 infants studied by Lake and colleagues, 41% had exanthem.[340] Similarly, Linnemann and co-workers[383] reported exanthem in 4 of 14 neonates with echoviral infections.

Cutaneous manifestations usually have their onset between the third and fifth day of illness. The rash is usually macular or maculopapular, and petechial lesions occasionally are seen. Surprisingly, vesicular lesions have been reported only once with coxsackievirus B3 infection and once with enterovirus 71 infection in neonates. Theodoridan and associates[417] described a full-term newborn boy with vesicular lesions at birth. PCR revealed coxsackievirus B3. A 1-month-old infant with enterovirus 71 infection and hand-foot-and-mouth syndrome has been reported.[418] Hall and associates[385] reported two neonates with echovirus 16 infections in which the illnesses were similar to roseola. The patients had fevers for 2 and 3 days, defervescence, and then the appearance of maculopapular rashes.

NEUROLOGIC MANIFESTATIONS

Meningitis and Meningoencephalitis. As shown in Table 24-5, meningitis and meningoencephalitis have been associated with coxsackieviruses B1 through B5 and with many echoviruses.* In most instances, the differentiation of meningitis from meningoencephalitis is difficult in neonates. Meningoencephalitis is common in infants with sepsis-like illness, and autopsy studies reveal many infants with disseminated viral disease (e.g., heart, liver, adrenals) in addition to central nervous system involvement. In the review of Morens,[378] 50% of the neonates with enteroviral infections had encephalitis or meningitis.

The initial clinical findings in neonatal meningitis or meningoencephalitis are similar to those in nonspecific febrile illness or sepsis-like illness. Most often, the child is quite normal and then becomes febrile, anorectic, and lethargic. Jaundice frequently affects newborns, and vomiting occurs in neonates of all ages. Less common findings include apnea, tremulousness, and general increased tonicity. Seizures occasionally occur.

CSF examination reveals considerable variation in protein, glucose, and cellular values. In seven newborns with meningitis related to coxsackievirus B5 studied by Swender and associates,[234] the mean CSF protein value was 244 mg/dL, and the highest value was 480 mg/dL. The mean CSF glucose value was 57 mg/dL, and one of the seven had pronounced hypoglycorrhachia (12 mg/dL). The mean CSF leukocyte count for the seven infants was 1069 cells/mm^3, with 67% polymorphonuclear cells. The highest cell count was 4526 cells/mm^3, with 85% polymorphonuclear cells. In another study involving 28 children younger than 2 months in whom coxsackievirus B5 was the implicated pathogen, 36% of the infants had CSF leukocyte counts of 500 cells/mm^3 or more.[391] In this same study, only 13% of the infants had CSF protein values of 120 mg/dL or more; 12% of the infants had glucose values of less than 40 mg/dL.

The CSF findings in cases of neonatal nonpolio enteroviral infections are frequently similar to those in bacterial disease. In particular, the most consistent finding in bacterial disease, hypoglycorrhachia, affects about 10% of newborns with enteroviral meningitis.[234,340,382,391,419]

*See references 28, 29, 147, 158, 161, 165, 198, 212, 224, 235, 238, 240, 243, 383, 385-387, 393, 399, 412, 415, 417.

*See references 28-30, 149, 157, 165, 212, 228, 234, 235, 238, 242, 247, 257, 259, 338, 339, 346, 380, 386, 387, 391, 395, 397, 403, 405, 409, 412, 415-437.

Paralysis. Johnson and associates[420] reported a 1-month-old boy with a right facial paralysis and loss of abdominal reflexes. The facial paralysis persisted through convalescence; the reflexes returned to normal within 2 weeks. The boy was infected with coxsackievirus B2. A 1-month-old boy with hand-foot-and-mouth syndrome and bilateral lower limb weakness due to enterovirus 71 infection has been described.[418]

SUDDEN INFANT DEATH

Balduzzi and Greendyke[335] recovered coxsackievirus A5 from the stool of a 1-month-old child after sudden infant death. In a similar investigation of sudden infant death, Gold and co-workers[336] recovered coxsackievirus A4 from the brains of three infants. Coxsackievirus A8 was recovered from the stool of a child in whom anorexia was diagnosed on the day before death. Coxsackievirus B3 was recovered at autopsy from an infant who died suddenly on the eighth day of life.[335] Morens and associates[6] reported eight cases of sudden infant death associated with enteroviral infection; parechovirus 1 was found on two occasions. In five instances of cot death in one study, echovirus 11 was isolated from the lungs in two children, from the myocardium in one, and from the nose or feces in the other two.[344]

Grangeot-Keros and co-workers[438] looked for evidence of enteroviral infections using PCR and an IgM immunoassay in cases of sudden and unexplained infant deaths. They divided their infant death population into two groups. One group had clinical, biologic, or histologic signs of viral infection, and the other group had no indicators of an antecedent infection. Fifty-four percent of infants with evidence of a preceding infection had PCR evidence of an enterovirus in samples from the respiratory tract or lung, or both, whereas none of those without evidence of a prior infection had similar positive PCR findings. Their IgM antibody studies supported their PCR findings.

Manifestations of Polioviruses

GENERAL CONSIDERATIONS

Polioviral infection in children classically results in a spectrum of clinical illness. As described by Paul[439] and accepted by others, 90% to 95% of infections in non-neonatal children are inapparent, 4% to 8% are abortive, and 1% to 2% are frank cases of poliomyelitis. Whether neonatal polioviral infection is acquired in utero, during birth, or after birth, it appears that the more severe manifestations of clinical illness are similar to those of older children. However, the available reports in the literature suggest that the frequencies of occurrence of inapparent, abortive, and frank cases are quite different from those in older children. Most reports describe severely affected infants.[95,98-106,108-116] Asymptomatic infection does occur, however.[96,97]

In the excellent review by Bates[110] in 1955, 58 cases of clinically overt poliomyelitis in infants younger than 1 month were described. Although complete data were not available on many of the cases, 51 had paralysis or died from their disease, or both. Of the total number of infants for whom there were clinical data, only one had nonparalytic disease. Because follow-up observation was recorded for only a short time in many infants, the evaluation of residual paralysis (presence or absence) may not be reliable. Pertinent clinical data from the study by Bates are presented in Table 24-7, and these data show that more than one half of the cases resulted from maternal disease. Because others have identified congenital infection without symptomatic maternal infection, it is probable that infection in the mothers was the source for an even greater percentage of the neonatal illnesses. Because the incubation period of neonatal poliomyelitis has not been determined, it is difficult to know how many infants were infected in utero. Most illnesses occurring within the first 5 days of life probably were congenital. Most neonates had symptoms of fever, anorexia or dysphagia, and listlessness. Almost one half the infants described in this review died, and of those surviving, 48% had residual paralysis.

INAPPARENT INFECTION

Shelokov and Habel[97] followed a virologically proven infected newborn without signs of illness. The infant was normal when 1 year old. Wingate and co-workers[107] studied an infant delivered by cesarean section from a woman with poliomyelitis who died 1 hour after delivery. Her infant was treated with gamma globulin intramuscularly at the postnatal age of 21 hours. He remained asymptomatic; poliovirus 1 was recovered from a stool specimen on the fifth day of life.

INFECTION ACQUIRED IN UTERO

Elliott and colleagues[111] described an infant girl in whom "complete flaccidity" was observed at birth. This child's mother had had mild paralytic poliomyelitis, with the onset of minor illness occurring 19 days before the infant's birth. Fetal movements had ceased 6 days before delivery, suggesting that paralysis had occurred at this time. On examination, the infant was severely atonic; when supported under the back, she was passively opisthotonic. Respiratory efforts were

Table 24–7 Clinical Findings in 58 Cases of Neonatal Poliomyelitis

Finding	No. of Cases with a Particular Finding/No. of Cases Evaluated (%)
Time of Onset after Birth	
≤5 days	13/55 (24)
6-14 days	25/55 (45)
≥15 days	17/55 (31)
Infection Source for Symptomatic Illness	
Mother	22/42 (52)
Other contact	6/42 (14)
Unknown	14/42 (34)
Acute Illness	
Fever	17/29 (59)
Anorexia or dysphagia	16/24 (67)
Listlessness	24/33 (73)
Irritability	3/33 (9)
Diarrhea	2/11 (18)
Paralysis	43/44 (98)
Outcome	
Death	21/44 (48)
Residual paralysis	12/44 (27)
Recovery without paralysis	11/44 (25)

Adapted from Bates T. Poliomyelitis in pregnancy, fetus, and newborn. Am J Dis Child 90:189, 1955.

abortive and confined to accessory muscles, and laryngoscopy revealed complete flaccidity in the larynx.

Johnson and Stimson[104] reported a case in which the mother's probable abortive infection occurred 6 weeks before the birth of the infant. The newborn was initially thought to be normal but apparently had no medical examination until the fourth day of life. At that time, the physician diagnosed a right hemiplegia. On the next day, a more complete examination revealed a lateral bulging of the right abdomen accompanied by crying and the maintenance of the lower extremities in a frog-leg position. Adduction and flexion at the hips were weak, and the knee and ankle jerks were absent. Laboratory studies were unremarkable except for the examination of the CSF, which revealed 20 lymphocytes/mm^3 and a protein concentration of 169 mg/dL. During a 6-month period, this child's paralysis gradually improved and resulted in only residual weakness of the left lower extremity.

Paresis of the left arm occurred in another child with apparent transplacentally acquired poliomyelitis shortly after birth.[114] The 2-day-old infant was quadriplegic, but patellar reflexes were present, and there were no respiratory or swallowing difficulties. This child had pneumonia when 3 weeks old, but general neurologic improvement occurred. Examination when the infant was 8 weeks old revealed bilateral atrophy of the shoulder girdle muscles. The CSF in this case revealed 63 leukocytes/mm^3, with 29% of them polymorphonuclear cells, and a protein value of 128 mg/dL.

All three of the infants previously discussed were apparently infected in utero several days before birth. Their symptoms were exclusively neurologic; fever, irritability, and vomiting did not occur.

POSTNATALLY ACQUIRED INFECTION

In contrast to infections acquired in utero, those acquired postnatally are more typical of classic poliomyelitis. Shelokov and Weinstein[99] described a child who was asymptomatic at birth. Onset of minor symptoms in the mother occurred 3 weeks before delivery, and major symptoms occurred 1 day before delivery. On the sixth day of life, the infant became suddenly ill with watery diarrhea. He looked grayish and pale. On the next day, he was irritable, lethargic, and limp and had a temperature of 38° C. Mild opisthotonos and weakness of both lower extremities developed. He was responsive to sound, light, and touch. The CSF had an elevated protein level and an increased number of leukocytes. His condition worsened during a total period of 3 days, and then gradual improvement began. At 1 year, he had severe residual paralysis of the right leg and moderate weakness in the left leg.

Baskin and associates[102] described two infants with neonatal poliomyelitis. The first child, whose mother had severe poliomyelitis at the time of delivery, was well for 3 days and then developed a temperature of 38.3° C. On the fifth day of life, the boy became listless and cyanotic. CSF examination revealed a protein level of 300 mg/dL and 108 leukocytes/mm^3. His condition worsened, and extreme flaccidity, irregular respiration, and progressive cyanosis developed; he died on the seventh day of life. The second infant was a boy who was well until he was 8 days old, but he then became listless and developed a temperature of 38.3° C. During the next 5 days, he developed flaccid quadriplegia; irregular, rapid, and shallow respirations; and an inability to swallow. The child died on the 14th day of life. His mother had developed acute poliomyelitis 6 days before the onset of his symptoms.

Abramson and colleagues[108] reported four children with neonatal poliomyelitis, two of whom died. In three of the children, the illnesses were typical of acute poliomyelitis seen in older children; they were similar to the cases of Baskin and associates[102] described previously. The fourth child died at 13 days of age with generalized paralysis. The onset of his illness was difficult to define, and he was never febrile. Swarts and Kercher[109] also described a child whose illness had an insidious onset. When 10 days old, the child gradually became lethargic and anorectic and regurgitated formula through his nose. On the next day, flaccid quadriplegia developed. Winsser and associates[115] and Bates[110] reported infants with acute poliomyelitis with clinical illnesses similar to those that occur in older individuals.

VACCINE VIRAL INFECTIONS

Administration of oral polio vaccines to newborns has been carried out in numerous studies.[118,179-191] Vaccine viral infection occurs in newborns with all three types of poliovirus, although the rate of infection is less than that for immunized older children. This rate is governed by the dose of virus, transplacentally acquired maternal antibody, and antibody acquired from colostrum and breast milk. Although clinical illness rarely has resulted from attenuated polioviral infections in older children and adults, there is only one specific report of paralytic poliomyelitis in a newborn associated with infection with a vaccine viral strain.[192] In that case, the possible source for the infection was the recently vaccinated child of the baby-sitter. In a review of 118 cases of vaccine-associated paralytic poliomyelitis in the United States between 1980 and 1992, the age of patients ranged from 1 month to 69 years, but details about neonates were not presented.[444]

Manifestations of Specific Nonpolio Enteroviruses

COXSACKIEVIRUSES

Coxsackievirus A. There have been few reports of neonatal coxsackievirus A infections. Baker and Phillips[337] reported a small-for-gestational-age infant with pneumonia and a sepsis-like illness with disseminated intravascular coagulation. This newborn died on the second day of life, and when cultured, the CSF grew coxsackievirus A3. Balduzzi and Greendyke[335] recovered a coxsackievirus A5 from the stool of a 1-month-old child with sudden infant death. In a similar investigation of sudden infant death, Gold and co-workers[336] recovered coxsackievirus A4 from the brains of three infants. Coxsackievirus A8 was also recovered from the stool of a child in whom anorexia was observed on the day before death. Berkovich and Kibrick[242] reported a 3-day-old neonate with nonspecific febrile illness (38.3° C) who was infected with coxsackievirus A9. Coxsackievirus A9 was also recovered from an 11-day-old infant with rhinitis, lethargy, anorexia, and fever.[243] This illness lasted 3 days. Jack and associates[236] described a 3-day-old newborn with fever, cyanosis, and respiratory distress who died on the seventh day of life; an autopsy revealed bronchopneumonia. Coxsackievirus A9 was isolated from the feces on the fourth and sixth days of life.

Lake and associates[340] reported two neonates with coxsackievirus A9 infections, but no clinical details were presented. Jenista and co-workers[178] recovered coxsackievirus A9 strains from seven nonhospitalized neonates who were thought to be well. In the Netherlands, a neonate with coxsackievirus A9 illness had pericarditis, meningitis, pneumonitis, and hepatitis; he recovered completely.[410] Krajden and Middleton[28] described a neonate with a sepsis-like illness who died. Coxsackievirus A9 was recovered from the liver and lung. Morens[378] also reported a death associated with this same virus type. Eisenhut and colleagues[338] reported an outbreak that included four neonates with coxsackievirus A9 infections. One infant who had meningitis, myocarditis, and disseminated intravascular coagulation died. A second neonate had vomiting, rhinitis, and abdominal distention, and two neonates had asymptomatic infections. Forty-eight of 598 neonates admitted to a regular nursery in Bangkok, Thailand, in the spring of 1977 had herpangina.[394] Coxsackievirus A5 was isolated from nine specimens from the afflicted infants, and a rise in the serum antibody titer was identified in 10 instances. Helin and colleagues[424] described 16 newborns with aseptic meningitis caused by coxsackievirus A14. During a 2.5-year follow-up period, they all developed normally, and no sequelae were identified. Coxsackievirus A16 was recovered from one newborn with nonspecific illness; his mother had had hand-foot-and-mouth syndrome 4 days previously.[230]

Coxsackievirus B1. Coxsackievirus B1 has only occasionally been recovered from newborns (Table 24-8). Eckert and co-workers[402] recovered a coxsackievirus B1 strain from the stool of a 1-month-old boy with bronchitis. Jahn and Cherry[211] described a 4-day-old infant who became febrile and lethargic. This illness persisted for 5 days without other signs or symptoms. An examination of the CSF showed a slight increase in the number of leukocytes, and most were mononuclear cells. Coxsackievirus B1 was recovered from the throat, stool, urine, and serum.

Wright and colleagues[216] reported an infant fatality associated with coxsackievirus B1 infection. This premature boy was well until he was 4 days old, when he had two episodes of cyanosis and apnea. After this, he became anorexic and listless and lost the Moro reflex. On the ninth day of life, he had shallow respirations, hepatomegaly, jaundice, petechiae, and thrombocytopenia. He was edematous and lethargic, and he had a temperature of 34.5° C, a pulse rate of 130 beats per minute, and a respiratory rate of 20 breaths per minute. He became weaker, unresponsive, and apneic and died. Positive laboratory findings included the following values: less than 10,000 platelets/mm^3, 283 mg of CSF protein/dL; 20.5 mg of serum bilirubin/dL; and 100 units of serum aspartate aminotransferase. Autopsy revealed hepatic necrosis, meningoencephalitis, and myocarditis. Coxsackievirus B1 was recovered from the throat, urine, liver, lung, kidney, and brain.

Twin boys with a sepsis-like illness with hepatitis and disseminated intravascular coagulation have been reported.[29] The first twin died on the 16th day of life, and the second twin survived. Another set of twins had coxsackievirus B1 infections shortly after birth; one twin had myocarditis, and the other had hepatitis with subsequent progressive liver calcifications.[342] A third set of twins had coxsackievirus B1 infections with illness that began when they were 5 days old.[395] One twin had disseminated intravascular coagulation, and the other had meningitis. Three other newborns with fatal sepsis-like illnesses with hepatitis have been described.[393,394]

Isacsohn[233] described four severe cases of neonatal illnesses due to coxsackievirus B1; three of the four neonates died. Of the three fatalities, one was caused by myocarditis, and the other two resulted from multiorgan dysfunction. The surviving

Table 24–8 Clinical and Pathologic Findings in Coxsackievirus B Infection of Newborns

	References for Coxsackievirus				
Finding	***B1***	***B2***	***B3***	***B4***	***B5***
Exanthem	224, 393		148		147, 198, 212, 415
Nonspecific febrile illness		142	229	196, 207	384
Sepsis-like illness	29, 215, 233, 393-395	29	28, 233	163, 337	29
Paralysis	394	420			
Diarrhea		404			
Sudden infant death	438		335, 438	438	
Pneumothorax					236
Aseptic meningitis, meningoencephalitis, encephalomyelitis	211, 214, 216, 395	149, 199, 209, 222, 337, 339, 382, 397, 434, 435	28, 29, 138, 145, 201, 212, 223	29, 198, 203, 204, 212, 227, 339	28, 139, 147, 149, 200, 202, 210, 231, 232, 234, 380, 391, 413, 423, 432
Myocarditis	214, 216-218, 233, 342, 393, 394	29, 149, 199, 209, 210, 219, 220, 337, 382, 431	28, 29, 138, 148, 207, 208, 215, 222, 243, 247, 376	28, 149, 165, 196, 198, 203, 204, 206, 213, 227, 337, 411, 416, 431	28, 147, 202, 380, 423
Hepatitis	216, 233, 342, 393, 396		233	203, 213	
Pancreatitis				197	200
Adrenocortical necrosis			201		
Bronchitis				402	

infant had hepatitis, congestive heart failure, thrombocytopenia, and residual neurologic damage.

McLean and colleagues[214] described a male newborn who had a temperature of 39° C, vomiting, and diarrhea on the fourth day of life. When 6 days old, he appeared gray and mottled and developed shallow respirations. He died on the seventh day of life after increased respiratory distress (90 breaths per minute), hepatomegaly, generalized edema, and cardiac enlargement. Coxsackievirus B1 was recovered from the heart and brain.

Gear[217] studied an extensive epidemic of Bornholm disease related to coxsackievirus B1 in Johannesburg in the summer of 1960 to 1961. After the first coxsackievirus B1 isolations, the medical officers of the area were on the alert for nursery infections and the prevention of nursery epidemics. Despite careful isolation procedures, Gear[217] reported that infection "was introduced into all the large maternity homes in Johannesburg." About 20 cases of neonatal myocarditis were documented, as were three deaths. The isolation procedures apparently prevented secondary nursery cases.

Volakova and Jandasek[218] reported epidemic myocarditis related to coxsackievirus B1. Cherry and Jahn[224] described a child with a mild febrile exanthematous illness, which had its onset within 10 minutes of birth.

Coxsackievirus B2. The reported instances of coxsackievirus B2 infections in neonates are provided Table 24-8. In most instances, the infants had myocarditis or neurologic manifestations. Eleven of 12 of the infants with myocarditis died. The one child with myocarditis who survived was reexamined when 2 years old and was found to be normal.[219] This child's mother became ill with sore throat, coryza, and malaise on the day after delivery. When 3 days old, the child became febrile (38.9° C) and had periods of apnea and cardiac irregularities. The cry was "pained." The electrocardiogram showed a left-sided heart pattern in the V leads and T wave abnormalities. The child's symptoms lasted less than 48 hours. Coxsackievirus B2 was isolated from the nose, urine, throat, and CSF of the child and from the mother's stool. The mother breast-fed the infant (while she wore a mask) during her illness. A later specimen of breast milk was cultured for virus without successful recovery of an agent.

Puschak[142] reported a child who became febrile (39.5° C) 8 hours after birth. During the next 9 days, the infant's temperature fluctuated between 36.7° C and 38.9° C. The patient had no other symptoms. Serologic evidence of coxsackievirus B2 infection was found.

Johnson and associates[420] described a 1-month-old infant with aseptic meningitis who developed a persistent right facial paralysis. In a study of undifferentiated diarrheal syndromes, Ramos-Alvarez[404] observed a child with coxsackievirus B2 infection. Eilard and associates[382] reported a nursery outbreak in which 12 infants were infected. All had aseptic meningitis, and 2 also had myocarditis. One of the two infants died on the 13th day of life. One child with thrombocytopenia and respiratory failure died.[340]

Coxsackievirus B3. Neonatal infections with coxsackievirus B3 are summarized in Table 24-8. Most reported cases have been severe illnesses with myocarditis or meningoencephalitis, or both. One case involved sudden infant death,[335] in which coxsackievirus B3 was recovered from a pool of organs from an infant who died on the eighth day of life.

Tuuteri and co-workers[229] studied a nursery outbreak of coxsackievirus B3 infection. Seven children had mild disease characterized by anorexia, listlessness, and fever, and two infants had fatal myocarditis. Of the 57 reported neonatal infections with coxsackievirus B3, 30 deaths occurred, and most were associated with myocarditis and sepsis-like illness. Three infants had febrile illnesses with meningitis and were reported to have suffered no residual effects; long-term follow-up is not available, however.[145,212]

Isacsohn and colleagues[233] reported two neonates with multiorgan dysfunction who survived. A full-term boy delivered by caesarean section had scattered vesicular lesions at birth.[417] New lesions appeared over a 5-day period, and the rash lasted for 10 days. The child had no other symptoms, and the mother had no febrile illness during pregnancy.

Chesney and associates[419] studied a 3-week-old girl with meningoencephalitis. This child had hypoglycorrhachia; the CSF glucose value on the sixth day of illness was 23 mg/dL, with a corresponding blood glucose level of 78 mg/dL. As described in another review,[340] two infants who died had thrombocytopenia and respiratory failure; a clinical picture suggestive of necrotizing enterocolitis also was observed.

During a 5-year period in Toronto, Krajden and Middleton[28] assessed 24 neonates with enteroviral infections who were admitted to the Hospital for Sick Children. Nine children were infected with coxsackievirus B3; of these, two infants had meningitis, three had myocarditis, and four had a sepsis-like illness. Of this group, one infant with meningitis, one with myocarditis, and all with sepsis-like illness died. All the neonates with sepsis-like illness had clinical evidence of multiorgan involvement; they had respiratory distress, hepatomegaly, hemorrhagic manifestations, and congestive heart failure. Two neonates with herpangina and coxsackievirus B3 infections were described in an outbreak involving 25 infants.[398]

Coxsackievirus B4. Table 24-8 summarizes coxsackievirus B4 neonatal infections. Most were severe and frequently were fatal illnesses with neurologic and cardiac involvement. An infant with less severe disease was described by Sieber and associates.[207] This child was well until 6 days after delivery, when he developed pharyngitis, diarrhea, and gradually increasing lethargy. This was followed by fever for 36 hours. No other signs or symptoms were observed, and the child was well when 11 days old. He had virologic and serologic evidence of coxsackievirus B4 infection.

Winsser and Altieri[197] studied an infant who suddenly became cyanotic and convulsed and died at 2 days of age. At autopsy, the only findings were bronchopneumonia, congestive splenomegaly, and chronic, interstitial pancreatitis. Coxsackievirus B4 was isolated from the spleen.

Barson and associates[411] reported the survival of an infant with myocarditis. Cardiac calcification was revealed on radiographs when the child was 4 weeks old, and the electrocardiogram revealed a left bundle branch block. When the child was 7 months old, the conduction defect remained, but the myocardial calcification had resolved.

Coxsackievirus B5. The spectrum of neonatal infection with coxsackievirus B5 is greater than that with the other coxsackieviruses B. Studies are summarized in Table 24-8. Meningitis and encephalitis are common neonatal manifestations of coxsackievirus B5 infection.* Nursery epidemics have been observed. Rantakallio and associates[231] studied 17 infants in one nursery with aseptic meningitis. None of the infants was severely ill. All had fever, with a temperature of 38° C to 40° C. Eleven of the 17 neonates were boys. Signs included irritability, nuchal rigidity, increased tone, anorexia, opisthotonos, whimpering, loose stools, and diminution of alertness. In another nursery outbreak, Farmer and Patten[380] found 28 infected infants. Of the group of 28, 15 had aseptic meningitis, 4 had diarrhea, and 9 had no signs of illness. Six years later, the 15 children who had had meningitis were studied. Thirteen were found to be physically normal and to have normal intelligence. Two children had intelligence levels below the mean for the group and had residual spasticity. At the time of the initial illness, these two infants and one additional child were twitching, irritable, or jittery.

Swender and associates[234] studied seven cases of aseptic meningitis in an intensive care nursery during a 6-week period during the summer of 1972. Two of the infants had apnea. One of the infants had a CSF glucose level of 12 mg/dL. During a community outbreak of coxsackievirus B5 infections, Marier and colleagues[391] studied 32 infants with aseptic meningitis. In this group, 36% had CSF leukocyte counts of 500 cells/mm^3 or higher, and in 19%, neutrophils accounted for 50% or more of the count. In 12% of patients, the CSF glucose level was less than 40 mg/dL. Thirty-eight percent of the infants had blood leukocyte counts of 15,000 cells/mm^3 or higher values.

Of particular interest is the observation of exanthem in four reports. Cherry and co-workers[415] described a 3-week-old boy with fever, a maculopapular rash, and enlarged cervical and postauricular lymph nodes. Examination of the CSF revealed 141 leukocytes/mm^3, of which 84% were lymphocytes, and a protein value of 100 mg/dL. An electrocardiogram was normal. In this child, the rash appeared before the fever. Coxsackievirus B5 was isolated from the pharynx and the CSF. Nogen and Lepow[212] reported an infant with a similar illness. This child had a nonspecific erythematous papular rash on the face and scalp. One week later, he became febrile and irritable. The CSF contained 440 white blood cells/mm^3, and 96% of them were mononuclear. Virus was isolated from the feces, throat, and CSF.

Artenstein and associates[198] reported a 23-day-old girl with a fever and an erythematous macular rash that spread from the scalp to the entire body, except the palms and soles, and lasted 4 days. Coxsackievirus B5 was recovered from the stool, but no evidence of serum antibody to this virus was found. McLean and co-workers[147] also described a child with a papular rash on the trunk and limbs that was present at birth. On the fourth day of life, the rash had disappeared, but the patient then developed a temperature of 39.4° C. Irritability, twitching, and fullness of the anterior fontanelle were observed, and CSF examination showed meningitis. During an 8-day period, the child had repeated episodes of vomiting and diarrhea. On the 11th day of life, the infant had hyperpnea, tachycardia, and an enlarging liver. The child died on the 13th day of life. Autopsy revealed extensive encephalitis and focal myocardial necrosis. Virus was recovered from the brain, heart, lungs, and liver.

*See references 28, 139, 147, 149, 200, 202, 231, 232, 234, 380, 391, and 423.

It appears that neonatal infection with coxsackievirus B5 is less likely to be fatal than infection with the other coxsackieviruses B. Only 6 of 36 infants described in Table 24-8 died. In contrast to coxsackieviruses B2, B3, and B4, coxsackievirus B5 appears to be more neurotropic than cardiotropic.

ECHOVIRUSES

Echovirus 1. Dömök and Molnár[228] described aseptic meningitis related to echovirus 1.

Echovirus 2. Krajden and Middleton[28] described three infants with echovirus 2 infections. Two of the neonates had meningitis and recovered. The third child, who died, had a sepsis-like illness. Virus was isolated from the CSF, lung, liver, and urine. One other neonate with echovirus 2 infection has been observed, but no details are available.[340]

Echovirus 3. In the summer of 1970, Haynes and co-workers[421] studied an epidemic of infection caused by echovirus 3. Three infected neonates were observed, all of whom had meningitis. One child, a full-term girl, developed tonic seizures and an inability to suck on the third day of life. The serum bilirubin level was 28 mg/dL. Shortly thereafter, the child became cyanotic, flaccid, and apneic and developed a bulging anterior fontanelle; she was in shock. She received assisted ventilation with a respirator for 3 days. When the child was 1 month old, severe neurologic damage with developing hydrocephalus was obvious. Echovirus 3 was recovered from the CSF, and the CSF protein level was 880 mg/dL on the sixth day of life.

The other two infants in this study apparently had uncomplicated aseptic meningitis. The CSF findings in one child revealed 1826 white blood cells/mm^3, and 91% of them were polymorphonuclear cells. The other child had 320 cells/mm^3, 98% of which were polymorphonuclear cells.

A 4-day-old infant from whom echovirus 3 was recovered from the CSF has been reported.[28] This child had fewer than 3 white blood cells/mm^3 in the CSF. Other neonates with echovirus 3 infection have been observed, but no details are available.[178,340]

Echovirus 4. Linnemann and associates[383] studied 11 infants with echovirus 4 infections. All infants had fevers, and most were irritable. Four infants had a fine maculopapular rash, which was located on the face or abdomen, or both. In two children, the extremities were also involved. Other neonates with echovirus 4 infections have been reported, but details of their illness are not available.[178,340]

Echovirus 5. There have been six reports of neonatal illnesses associated with echovirus 5 infections.[340,348,379,432] In one nursery epidemic, six infants were involved.[241] All infants had fever (38.3° C to 39.7° C) that lasted 4 to 8 days. Two neonates had tachycardia that was disproportionately rapid when compared with the degree of fever, but in neither was there evidence of myocarditis. Four infants had splenomegaly and enlarged lymph nodes; these findings persisted for several weeks.

In 1966 (July to October), an epidemic of echovirus 5 infection involved 23% of the infants in the maternity unit at the Royal Air Force Hospital in Chargi, Singapore.[240] Fifty-six infants were symptomatically infected, and 10 were asymptomatically infected. Those who were ill were 2 to 12 days old at the onset of disease. All 56 symptomatic infants had fever; 87% of them had a temperature of 38.3° C or greater. The mean duration of fever was 3.5 days, with a range of 2 to 7 days. Twenty infants had a faint erythematous macular rash that was most prominent on the limbs and buttocks but also occurred on the trunk and face. The rash, which began 24 to 36 hours after the beginning of fever, lasted 48 hours. Diarrhea occurred in 17 infants, 4 of whom passed blood and mucus. Vomiting was observed in about one half the neonates. All infants apparently recovered completely.

One newborn girl had a nonspecific, biphasic febrile illness.[327] Echovirus 5 was recovered from the CSF, but the cell count, protein level, and glucose value were normal.

Another study included a 9-day-old infant with aseptic meningitis.[432] During an epidemiologic investigation in Rochester, New York, 13 of 75 enteroviral isolates were echovirus 5.[178] Six of the infants were asymptomatic; no clinical details of the other seven patients were presented. A neonate with sepsis-like illness and hepatic failure died 9 days after birth.[348]

Echovirus 6. Sanders and Cramblett[243] reported a boy who was well until 9 days old, when he developed a fever (38° C), severe diarrhea, and dehydration. His white blood cell count was 27,900 cells/mm^3, and virologic and serologic evidence of echovirus 6 infection was found. Treatment consisted of intravenous hydration, to which there was a good response. Krous and colleagues[343] described an infant who died on the ninth day of life with a sepsis-like illness. The child had meningitis, disseminated intravascular coagulation, hepatic necrosis, and adrenal and renal hemorrhage. Ventura and associates[348] reported the death of a full-term neonate with sepsis-like syndrome who at postmortem examination had massive hepatic necrosis, adrenal hemorrhagic necrosis, renal medullary hemorrhage, hemorrhagic noninflammatory pneumonia, and severe encephalomalacia. Yen and co-workers[168] reported a premature boy who developed a sepsis-like illness on the fifth day of life. This infant had hepatic failure and was treated with intravenous immune globulin. He recovered gradually, but on the 62nd day of life, he died of a nosocomial *Enterobacter cloacae* infection. Echovirus type 6 has been associated with neonatal illness on two other occasions, but no clinical details are available.[340,383]

Echovirus 7. Piraino and colleagues[165] reported three infants with echovirus 7 infections. All three had fever, one had respiratory distress and exanthem, and one had irritability and loose stools. Two neonates with fatal sepsis-like illnesses with massive disseminated intravascular coagulation have been reported.[263,354] One neonate with severe hepatitis was treated with pleconaril and survived.[407]

Echovirus 8. In a search for etiologic associations in infantile diarrhea, Ramos-Alvarez[404] identified one neonate from whom echovirus 8 was recovered from the stool. The antibody titer to this virus rose fourfold.

Echovirus 9. Echovirus 9 is the most prevalent of all the enteroviruses (see Table 24-4). From 1955 to 1958, epidemic waves of infection spread throughout the world.[445] Since that time, echovirus 9 has been a common cause of human illness. Despite its prevalence and its frequent association with epidemic disease, descriptions of neonatal illness are uncommon. Unlike experiences with several other enteroviruses, newborn nursery epidemics caused by echovirus 9 have not often been described.

Table 24–9 Neonatal Infection with Echovirus 9

Study	Finding
Moscovici and Maisel[156]	Asymptomatic infection
Mirani et al.[403]	Meningitis (4 cases)
	Gastroenteritis (2 cases)
	Pneumonia (1 case)
Rawls et al.[350]	Hepatic necrosis
Cho et al.[389]	Severe, generalized disease
Jahn and Cherry[211]	Mild febrile illness
Eichenwald and Kostevalov[157]	Aseptic meningitis
	Gastroenteritis (2 cases)
Haynes et al.[422]	Meningoencephalitis
Cheeseman et al.[161]	Fatal interstitial pneumonia
Krajden and Middleton[28]	Meningitis

Neonatal echovirus 9 experiences are provided in Table 24-9. Moscovici and Maisel[156] described an asymptomatic infant with echovirus 9 infection. When echovirus 9 was prevalent in Erie County, New York, during the summer of 1971, seven neonatal cases were observed.[403] Four children had aseptic meningitis, but only moderate elevations of CSF protein values and white blood cells were observed. One child, a 15-day-old infant, had radiologic evidence of bronchopneumonia, and two infants had gastroenteritis. Rawls and co-workers[350] described an infant who was well until the seventh day of life, when progressive lethargy, anorexia, and irritability developed. The child became moribund, and jaundice, scattered petechiae, and hypothermia were observed. The pulse rate was 90 beats per minute, the respiratory rate was 40 breaths per minute, and the liver was enlarged. The infant died 3 days after the onset of symptoms. Echovirus 9 was recovered from the lung, brain, and CSF. Cho and colleagues[389] described a similar severe neonatal illness in a child from whom echovirus 9 was recovered from the CSF. This child was hypothermic and hypotonic on the third day of life. He had bilateral pneumonia and leukopenia. After a stormy course, which included an exchange transfusion for suspected sepsis and mechanical ventilation for apnea, he eventually recovered.

A child who became febrile (38.3° C), irritable, and anorectic on the sixth day of life was described by Jahn and Cherry.[211] This child became asymptomatic within 2 days; echovirus 9 was recovered from the throat, feces, serum, and CSF. Eichenwald and Kostevalov[157] reported two children with mild irritability, fever, and diarrhea and a third child with diarrhea and convulsions in whom laboratory findings showed aseptic meningitis. Haynes and colleagues[422] studied a large outbreak of meningoencephalitis caused by echovirus 9 and described nine children who were 2 weeks to 2 months old. Cheeseman and associates[161] studied a neonate with fatal interstitial pneumonia, and Krajden and Middleton[28] reported a 4-day-old infant from whom echovirus 9 was recovered from the CSF. This child had fewer than 3 white blood cells/mm^3 in the CSF.

Echovirus 11. Neonatal illness associated with echovirus 11 infection has been interesting and varied. Reported cases are

Table 24–10 Neonatal Infection with Echovirus 11

Study	Finding
Miller et al.[238]	Exanthem and pneumonia (1 case) Nonspecific febrile illness (1 case) Aseptic meningitis (1 case)
Sanders and Cramblett[243]	Gastroenteritis (2 cases)
Berkovich and Kibrick[242]	Gastroenteritis (1 case) Meningitis (1 case)
Cramblett et al.[235]	Meningitis (3 cases, 1 with rash) Severe, nonspecific febrile illness (1 case)
Hercík et al.[239]	Respiratory illness (22 cases)
Hasegawa[252]	Fever (31 cases) Stomatitis (4 cases) Fever and stomatitis (6 cases)
Davies et al.[251]	Encephalopathy (1 case) Nonspecific febrile illness (1 case) Sepsis-like illness with cardiac failure (1 death) Lower respiratory infection (1 case)
Jones et al.[162]	Sepsis-like illness with hepatitis and rash (1 case)
Lapinleimu and Hakulinen[253]	Aseptic meningitis (4 cases) Gastroenteritis and/or respiratory distress (3 cases)
Nagington et al.[250]	Sepsis-like illness with shock, diffuse bleeding, and renal hemorrhage (3 deaths)
Suzuki et al.[400]	Fever (100%); pharyngitis (7%) (42 cases)
Krous et al.[343]	Sepsis-like illness with disseminated intravascular coagulation, hepatic necrosis (1 death)
Modlin[254]	Sepsis-like illness with apnea, lethargy, poor feeding, jaundice, hepatitis, disseminated intravascular coagulation (4 deaths)
Drew[414]	Myocarditis (5 cases)
Piraino et al.[165]	Meningitis and rash (2 cases) Meningitis (4 cases) Fatal case with cardiac failure, interstitial pneumonia, and interventricular cerebral hemorrhage
Krajden and Middleton[28]	Meningitis
Mertens et al.[257]	Fever (2 cases) Meningitis (4 cases)
Reyes et al.[164]	Fatal sepsis-like illness
Berry and Nagington[344]	Sepsis-like illness (11 deaths) Sudden death
Gh et al.[345]	Sepsis-like illness (5 deaths)
Bose et al.[163]	Sepsis-like illness (1 death, 1 survived)
Bowen et al.[429]	Meningitis (34 infants ≤4 months old)
Halfon and Spector[346]	Sepsis-like illness (2 deaths)
Steinmann and Albrecht[259]	Sepsis-like illness with meningitis and apnea (5 cases) Meningitis (4 cases) Gastroenteritis (3 cases)
Gitlin et al.[347]	Sepsis-like illness with hepatic necrosis (4 deaths)
Kinney et al.[258]	Meningitis (8 cases with 1 death) Mild illness (4 cases) Inapparent infection (2 cases)
Rabkin et al.[262]	Sepsis-like illness (9 cases, 5 with meningitis) Inapparent infection (1 case)
Isaacs et al.[265]	Meningitis (2 cases, 1 with myocarditis) Pneumonia (1 case) Inapparent infection (7 cases) Apnea (1 case)
Wang et al.[348]	Sepsis-like illness with hepatic failure
Tarcan et al.[433]	Bone marrow failure

listed in Table 24-10. Eleven of the reports involved nursery outbreaks, and in five reports, the neonatal cases were part of a larger community epidemic. Miller and associates[238] studied an epidemic of aseptic meningitis and other acute febrile illnesses in New Haven, Connecticut, in the summer of 1965. This epidemic was unique in that one half of the patients with meningitis from whom virus was isolated were younger than 6 months. The echovirus 11 in this epidemic was a prime strain. Three neonatal illnesses were reported. One of the patients, a 1-month-old infant, was initially irritable and feverish and had diarrhea. Chest radiographs revealed bilateral pneumonitis. A generalized, discrete maculopapular rash, which lasted 24 hours, was seen on the third day of illness. Fever persisted for 6 days. A 12-day-old girl had fever (39.4° C) lasting 1 day but no other findings. Echovirus 11 was recovered from her throat. Another 1-month-old infant had aseptic meningitis.

Sanders and Cramblett[243] described two infants with diarrhea. Both infants were acutely ill; one was jaundiced and irritable and had feeding difficulty. In another study, two infants with echovirus 11 infections had diarrhea.[242] One infant had a temperature of 39.3° C and a "stuffy nose," and the other had a temperature of 39.8° C and aseptic meningitis. Cramblett and co-workers[235] observed an outbreak of nosocomial infections caused by echovirus 11 in a neonatal intensive care unit. In a 1-month-old, premature infant with frequent apneic episodes, the CSF contained 2200 white blood cells/mm^3, 89% of them polymorphonuclear cells, and the protein level was 280 mg/dL. The infant made a gradual recovery. Echovirus 11 was isolated from the CSF and stool. In another premature infant, apneic episodes and bradycardia suddenly began on the 20th day of life. Fever developed, the apneic spells continued, and digitalis therapy was necessary because of congestive heart failure. Examination of the CSF revealed aseptic meningitis, and echovirus 11 was recovered from the CSF, throat, and stool. A third child with aseptic meningitis had an exanthem. The disease began suddenly, and the child had shallow respirations and poor skin color. On the next day, generalized seizures occurred, and a maculopapular rash developed on the trunk, extremities, and face. The patient made a gradual recovery. A fourth child had a severe, nonspecific febrile illness.

A particularly noteworthy finding in neonatal echovirus 11 infection has been severe sepsis-like illness with hepatitis or hepatic necrosis, disseminated intravascular coagulation, and extensive hemorrhagic manifestations.[162-164,250,251,254,343-348,351] During the past 15 years, more than 40 such cases have been described, and most of the illnesses have been fatal.

Hercík and co-workers[239] reported an epidemic of respiratory illness in 22 newborns. Six of the infants were severely ill, and one subsequently died. The incubation period varied from 17 hours to 9 days, with an average of 3 days. Seven infants had an interstitial pneumonia, and all had rhinitis, pharyngitis, and vomiting. Toce and Keenan[167] reported two newborns with respiratory distress and pneumonia at birth. Both infants died of their echovirus 11 infections. Tarcan and colleagues[433] described a 5-day-old boy who developed fever and diarrhea. He developed a maculopapular rash on the face, generalized petechiae and hemorrhagic bullae, and pancytopenia due to bone marrow failure. This infant was treated with intravenous immune globulin and recovered.

Echovirus 13. Before 2000, infection with echovirus 13 was rare in neonates. The virus was isolated from one asymptomatic infant in a neonatal surveillance study.[178] In 2001 in the United States, echovirus 13 was the leading cause of aseptic meningitis, and during 2001 and 2002, aseptic meningitis outbreaks with this agent occurred in a number of countries.[440-443] A substantial number of cases were infants who were 3 months old or younger.[440] A 28-day-old boy in Tennessee had aseptic meningitis and hepatitis.[441] Neonatal cases were reported in Israel and Spain, but details were not presented.[442,443]

Echovirus 14. Hughes and colleagues[159] reported an infant boy who became febrile (38° C) and had cyanotic episodes on the third day of life. When 4 days old, his temperature was 38.9° C, and he experienced recurrent apneic spells. Liver enlargement, hypothermia, bradycardia, periodic breathing, and spontaneous ecchymoses developed, and the infant died on the seventh day of life. Laboratory studies revealed the presence of leukopenia and thrombocytopenia, and autopsy showed severe hepatic necrosis. Drouhet[446] described a child with aseptic meningitis and echovirus 14 infection, and Hinuma and associates[381] reported four newborns with apparent asymptomatic echovirus 14 infections.

Echovirus 16. In 1974, Hall and colleagues[385] studied five neonates with echovirus 16 infections. All five infants were admitted to the hospital because sepsis was suspected. Four of five were febrile, all were lethargic and irritable, and two had abdominal distention. Three of the neonates had erythematous maculopapular exanthems, and in two, the rash appeared after or with defervescence. Leukocyte counts in four infants revealed an increased percentage of band form neutrophils. Two neonates had aseptic meningitis. Lake and associates[340] observed three infants with echovirus 16 infections. In their study, clinical findings were not itemized by virus type, but it is inferred that sepsis-like illnesses occurred.

Echovirus 17. Neonatal infection with echovirus 17 has been observed by three investigators. Cherry and co-workers[141] reported two ill infants. A 19-day-old infant developed otitis media 5 days after his mother had a flulike illness. Echovirus 17 was isolated from his feces, and serologic evidence of echovirus 17 infection was found in the infant and the mother. The second child had a nonspecific febrile illness at the age of 4 weeks, which was severe enough to require hospitalization. Virus was isolated from the infant's throat, feces, and serum.

Sanders and Cramblett[243] described two neonates with exanthem associated with echovirus 17. The first child, a 3-week-old girl, became drowsy, anorectic, and febrile. She had a fine maculopapular rash on the trunk, a slightly injected pharynx, and a few petechiae on the soft palate. She remained febrile for 5 days. Echovirus 17 was recovered from the CSF and the feces. The second infant became ill when 3 weeks old. His symptoms were mild rhinitis and cough followed by lethargy and refusal to eat. Four days after the onset of symptoms, his temperature was 39° C, and his respiratory rate was 60 breaths per minute. A fine maculopapular rash appeared on the trunk, and radiographs revealed an infiltrate in the right lung. The patient's course was uneventful, and he was much improved 12 days after the onset of symptoms.

Faulkner and van Rooyen[247] described an outbreak of echovirus 17 infection with illness in a nursery in mid-August of 1971. Seven infants were involved, including one with aseptic meningitis who was 7 weeks old. All the infants had fever, four had central nervous system signs, three had abdominal distention, four had diarrhea, and three had a rash. One other infant from another community was also studied by the investigators. This child had a febrile pneumonitis when 3.5 weeks old. The findings abated in 5 days, but the child suddenly died 6 days later. Autopsy revealed interstitial pneumonitis with extensive edema and scattered petechial hemorrhages of the viscera. Echovirus 17 was isolated from the liver, lung, spleen, and kidney.

Echovirus 18. In 1958, Eichenwald and colleagues[244] described epidemic diarrhea associated with echovirus 18 infections. In a nursery unit of premature infants, 12 of 21 were mildly ill. Neither temperature elevation nor hypothermia occurred. Six infants were lethargic and listless, and two developed moderate abdominal distention. The diarrhea lasted 1 to 5 days; there were five or six watery, greenish stools per day, occasionally expelled explosively. In two infants, a small amount of blood was seen in the stools, but there was no mucus or pus cells. Five other infants in another nursery had similar diarrheal illness. Echovirus 18 was recovered from all ill infants.

Medearis and co-workers[401] reported a 3-week-old girl with fever, irritability, lethargy, pharyngitis, and postnasal drainage. Admitted to the hospital because of apneic spells, she developed a generalized erythematous blotchy macular rash and had frequent stools. The illness lasted about 7 days. Echovirus 18 was recovered from the blood, throat, and feces. Berkovich and Kibrick[242] found echovirus 18 in the stool of a 12-day-old twin infant with fever and a red throat. The relationship of echovirus 18 to the illness is uncertain because the patient's twin was infected with echovirus 11, and the patient also had serologic evidence of echovirus 11 infection. The fever and red throat may have been caused by echovirus 11 rather than echovirus 18 infection. Wilfert and associates[425] observed a 9-day-old infant with aseptic meningitis.

Echovirus 19. Cramblett and co-workers[399] described two neonates with echovirus 19 infections. One child had an upper respiratory infection, cough, and paroxysmal atrial tachycardia. The other child also had an upper respiratory infection, but in addition to echovirus 19 infection, coxsackievirus B4 was recovered from the throat of this infant. Butterfield and associates[245] isolated echovirus 19 post mortem from the brain, lung, heart, liver, spleen, lymph nodes, and intestine of a premature infant who had cystic emphysema. The relationship between the generalized viral infection and the pulmonary disease is not understood.

Philip and Larson[160] reported three catastrophic neonatal echovirus 19 infections, which resulted in hepatic necrosis and massive terminal hemorrhage. One infant, infected in utero, was symptomatic at birth. The Apgar score was 3, and multiple petechiae were observed. The infant had generalized ecchymoses and apneic episodes and died when 3.5 hours old. Thrombocytopenia was identified, and echovirus 19 was isolated from the brain, liver, spleen, and lymph nodes. The other two infants who died of echovirus 19 infection were twins. They were normal during the first 3 days of life but then became mildly cyanotic and lethargic. Shortly thereafter, apneic episodes occurred, and jaundice and petechiae developed. Both twins became oliguric, and they died on the eighth and ninth days of life, with severe gastrointestinal bleeding. Both twins were thrombocytopenic, and virus was recovered from systemic sites in both. Two similar catastrophic cases have been described.[406]

Purdham and associates[255] reported an outbreak of echovirus 19 in a neonatal unit in which 12 infants were affected. Eleven infants were febrile, 10 were irritable, 7 had marked abdominal distention with decreased bowel sounds, and 5 had apneic episodes. Bacon and Sims[392] described two neonates with sepsis-like illness. The infants were cyanotic with peripheral circulatory failure. In another study involving the same echovirus 19 epidemic, five infants younger than 3 months were reported.[390] All had sepsis-like illness with hypotonia and peripheral circulatory failure. Two infants had aseptic meningitis, and two others had diarrhea.

Echovirus 20. Eichenwald and Kostevalov[157] recovered echovirus 20 from four asymptomatic infants younger than 8 days (see "Cloud Baby"). Five neonates with severe illness due to echovirus 20 have also been described.[352,353] All had hepatitis, and two died.

Echovirus 21. Jack and co-workers[236] recovered echovirus 21 from the feces of a 7-day-old infant with jaundice and diarrhea. No other details of the child's illness are available. Chonmaitree and associates[412] studied a 19-day-old infant with aseptic meningitis and rash, and Georgieff and colleagues[351] reported a newborn with fulminant hepatitis. Lake and colleagues[340] also mentioned one infected infant but presented no specific details.

Echovirus 25. Linnemann and colleagues[383] reported one neonate with echovirus 25 infection. They gave no virus-specific details except that fever and irritability occurred.

Echovirus 30. Matsumoto and associates[428] described a nursery outbreak involving 11 infants during a 2-week period. All the neonates had aseptic meningitis, and all recovered. Two symptomatic and six asymptomatic neonates were reported in the Rochester, New York, surveillance study.[178]

Echovirus 31. McDonald and associates[256] described three neonates in an intensive care nursery with echovirus 31 infections. One infant had a fatal encephalitis-like illness, with hypertonicity, hyperreflexia, and apneic spells. The other two infants also experienced apneic spells, and in addition, one had pneumonia and meningitis.

Echovirus 33. In a study of epidemic illness related to echovirus 33 disease in the Netherlands, Kapsenberg[249] stated that 7- to 8-day-old neonates in a maternity ward had a febrile illness. No further data were presented.

ENTEROVIRUS 71

Schmidt and colleagues[426] mentioned one 3-week-old infant with meningitis and enterovirus 71 infection. Chonmaitree and colleagues[405] described one 9-day-old neonate with aseptic meningitis and one 14-day-old infant with gastroenteritis from enterovirus 71. Chen and associates[418] reported a child with bilateral lower limbs weakness in association with the hand-foot-and-mouth syndrome.

PARECHOVIRUSES

Parechovirus 1. Parechovirus 1 has been associated with three epidemics of nursery infections. During a survey of perinatal virus infections, 44 infants were found to be infected with parechovirus 1 during a study period from May to December 1966.[236] The virus prevalence and the incidence of new infections during this period were fairly uniform. No illness was attributed to parechovirus 1 infection, and the virus disappeared from the nursery in mid-December of 1966. Berkovich and Pangan[237] studied respiratory illnesses in premature infants and reported 64 infants with illness, 18 of whom had virologic or serologic evidence of parechovirus 1 infection. Many had high but constant levels of serum antibody to parechovirus 1. Some of these infants were probably also infected with parechovirus 1. The children with proven parechovirus 1 infections could not be clinically differentiated from those without evidence of parechovirus 1 infection. Of 18 infants with documented parechovirus 1 infections, 90% had coryza, 39% had pneumonia, and 11% had morbilliform rash or conjunctivitis, or both. In contrast to the studies of Jack and co-workers,[236] only 3 of 35 asymptomatic infants were found to be infected with parechovirus 1. Nakao and associates[246] recovered parechovirus 1 from 29 premature infants. Many of the infected infants were asymptomatic, and those who were ill had only mild symptoms of coryza, cough, and diarrhea. Jenista and colleagues[178] described 17 parechovirus 1 infections in nonhospitalized neonates. Clinical details were not presented, but it appears that all of these infants were asymptomatic. Parechovirus 1 infection was associated with a nosocomial necrotizing enterocolitis outbreak.[409]

Parechovirus 2. Ehrnst and Eriksson[437] reported a 1-month-old girl with encephalopathy resulting from a nosocomial parechovirus 2 infection. No further details of this case were provided.

DIAGNOSIS AND DIFFERENTIAL DIAGNOSIS

Clinical Diagnosis

The clinical differentiation of neonatal infectious diseases frequently seems to be an impossible task. Although it is true that treatable bacterial and viral illnesses should always be considered and treated first, it is also true that when all the circumstances of a particular neonatal illness are considered, enterovirus diseases can be suspected on clinical grounds. The most important factors in clinical diagnosis are season of the year, geographic location, exposure, incubation period, and clinical symptoms.

In temperate climates, enteroviral prevalence is distinctly seasonal, and disease is usually seen in the summer and fall. Neonatal enterovirus disease is unlikely in the winter. In the tropics, enteroviruses are prevalent throughout the year, and the season therefore is not helpful diagnostically.

As with all infectious illnesses, knowledge of exposure and incubation time is important. A careful history of maternal illness is vital, particularly the symptoms of maternal illness. For example, nonspecific mild febrile illness in the mother that occurs in the summer and fall should warn of the possibility of more severe neonatal illness. More specific findings in the mother (e.g., aseptic meningitis, pleurodynia, herpangina, pericarditis, myocarditis) should alert the clinician to look for more specific enteroviral illnesses. Minor illness in nursery personnel during enteroviral seasons and the short incubation period of enteroviral infections should be taken into consideration. Manifestations of neonatal nonpolio enteroviral infections are given in Table 24-5.

Laboratory Diagnosis

Virus Isolation

Most viral diagnostic laboratories have facilities for the recovery of most enteroviruses that cause congenital and neonatal illness. Three tissue culture systems—primary rhesus, cynomolgus, or African green monkey kidney tissue culture; a diploid, human embryonic lung fibroblast cell strain; and the RD cell line—allow the isolation of all polioviruses, coxsackieviruses B, echoviruses, newer enteroviruses, parechoviruses, and many coxsackieviruses A. In a 1988 study in which Buffalo green monkey kidney cells and subpassages of primary human embryonic kidney cells were used in addition to primary monkey kidney and human diploid fibroblast (MRC-5) cells, the enterovirus recovery rate was increased by 11%.[447] For a complete diagnostic isolation spectrum, suckling mouse inoculation should also be performed. Optimally, at least one blind passage should be carried out in each of the culture systems.

Proper selection and handling of specimens are most important in the isolation of viruses from ill neonates. Because infection in neonates tends to be generalized, collection of material from multiple sites is important. Specimens should be taken from any or all of the following: nasopharynx, throat, stool, blood, urine, CSF, and any other body fluids that are available. Swabs from the nose, throat, and rectum should be placed in a transport medium.

Transport medium provides a protective protein, neutral pH, and antibiotics for control of microbial contamination and, most importantly, prevents desiccation. Many viral transport and storage media are commercially available or are prepared readily in the laboratory; their utility has been reviewed elsewhere.[448] Convenient and practical collection devices, such as the Culturette (Becton-Dickinson, Cockeysville, Md) or Virocult (Medical Wire and Equipment Co., Victory Gardens, NY), consist of a swab, usually Dacron or rayon, on a plastic or aluminum shaft accompanied by a self-contained transport medium (Stuart or Amies) and are routinely available in most hospitals for bacteriologic culture. Calcium alginate swabs, which are toxic to herpes simplex virus, and wooden shafts, which may be toxic for viruses and the cell culture system itself, should not be used. Saline or holding media that contain serum also should be avoided. Useful liquid transport media (2-mL aliquots in screw-capped vials) consist of tryptose phosphate broth with 0.5% bovine albumin; Hanks' balanced salt solution with 5% gelatin or 10% bovine albumin; or buffered sucrose phosphate (0.2 M, 2-SP),[448,449] which has been used as a combined transport for viral, chlamydial, and mycoplasmal culture requests and is appropriate for long-term frozen storage of specimens and isolates.[450]

Fluid specimens should be collected in sterile vials. Specimens of autopsy material are best collected in vials that contain transport medium. In general, specimens should be refrigerated immediately after collection and during transportation to the laboratory. Specimens should not be exposed to sunlight during transportation. If an extended period is likely to elapse before a specimen can be processed in the laboratory, it is advisable to ship and store it frozen.

Contrary to popular belief, evidence of enteroviral growth from tissue cultures takes only a few days in many cases and less than a week in most.[451] The use of the spin amplification, shell vial technique, and monoclonal antibodies has significantly reduced the time for detection of enteroviral cultures.[59,452] After isolation of an enterovirus, identification of its type is conventionally done by neutralization, which is unfortunately an expensive and lengthy process.

Rapid Virus Identification

Because of the number of different serotypes of enteroviruses, the use of immunofluorescence, agglutination, counterimmunoelectrophoresis, and ELISA techniques for the direct detection of antigen in suspected enteroviral infections has not been useful. Nucleic acid techniques with cDNA and RNA probes have been useful for the direct identification of enteroviruses.[76,453-456] Of most importance has been the development of numerous PCR techniques. Since 1990, innumerable reports have described enteroviral PCR methods and their use in identifying enterovirus RNA in clinical specimens.[49-62,457-465] PCR has proved most useful for the direct identification of enteroviruses in the CSF of patients with meningitis. Compared with culture of CSF specimens, PCR is more rapid and sensitive, and the specificity is equal.

PCR also has proved useful in the identification of enteroviruses in blood, urine, and throat specimens.[31,51,56,58,459,460] Particularly impressive are the findings of Byington and associates.[31] Using PCR on specimens of blood and CSF, they found that more than 25% of infants admitted to the hospital for suspected sepsis in 1997 had nonpolio enterovirus infections. Based on this study and the work of Adréoletti and co-workers,[52] I believe the general workup for febrile neonates hospitalized for possible sepsis should include PCR for enteroviruses in blood and CSF. This is most important during enterovirus season (summer and fall in temperate climates), but because enteroviral circulation continues all year, it is reasonable to also perform PCR in the off seasons. Although PCR detects enterovirus RNA, the specific enteroviral type is not identified. Because of this shortcoming, I recommend that conventional culture should be performed along with PCR.

PCR has also identified enteroviruses in frozen and formalin-fixed biopsy and autopsy specimens of myocardium.[51,56,58,459,460] In one study, enteroviruses were identified in myocardial tissue from four neonates who died of myocarditis.[460] In one case, the specimen was obtained during life by a right ventricular endomyocardial biopsy, and in the other three, frozen or formalin-fixed autopsy samples were used. Most PCR methods can detect one tissue culture infective dose of enterovirus in CSF, stool, or throat specimen.[459] Polioviruses can be separated from other enteroviruses, and poliovirus vaccine strains can be rapidly identified by PCR.[461-466]

Enteroviral RNA has been identified in numerous tissue specimens from patients with chronic medical conditions, such as idiopathic dilated cardiomyopathy. However, the possibility of lack of specificity (false-positive results) is a concern.

Serology

Except in special circumstances, the use of serologic techniques in the primary diagnosis of suspected neonatal enterovirus infections is impractical. Standard serologic study depends on the demonstration of an antibody titer rise to a specific virus as an indication of infection with that agent. Although hemagglutination inhibition, ELISA, and complement fixation tests take only a short time to perform, these tests can be done only after the collection of a second, convalescent-phase blood specimen. These tests are also impractical in searching for the cause of a specific illness in a child because there are so many antigenically different enteroviruses. As discussed in "Antigenic Characteristics," group antigens can be produced that allow serologic diagnosis by IgM EIA and complement fixation, but these tests lack specificity.[84,85,467]

In the evaluation of an infant with a suspected enterovirus infection, serum should be collected as soon as possible after the onset of illness and then again 2 to 4 weeks later. This serum should be stored frozen. In most clinical situations, it is not necessary to carry out serologic tests on the collected serum because demonstration of an antibody titer rise in the serum of an infant from whom a specific virus has been isolated from a body fluid is obviously superfluous. However, collected serum can be useful diagnostically if the prevalence of specific enteroviruses in a community is known. In this situation, it is relatively easy to look for antibody titer changes to a selected number of viral types. More rapid diagnosis using a single serum sample is possible if a search for specific IgM enteroviral antibody is made.[207,468-476]

Unfortunately, enterovirus IgM antibody tests are not commercially available. Commercial laboratories do offer enteroviral complement fixation antibody panels. However, these tests are expensive, and their results in the clinical setting are almost always meaningless unless acute-phase and convalescent-phase sera are analyzed.

Histology

There are no specific histologic findings in enteroviral infections, such as those seen in cytomegalovirus or herpes simplex viral infections. However, tissues can be examined for specific enteroviral antigens by immunofluorescent study and by PCR.[149,457,477,478]

Differential Diagnosis

The differential diagnosis of congenital and neonatal enterovirus infections depends on the clinical manifestations. In general, the most important illness categories are generalized bacterial sepsis or meningitis, congenital heart disease, and congenital and neonatal infections with other viruses.

Hypothermia and hyperthermia associated with nonspecific signs such as lethargy and poor appetite are common in neonatal enteroviral infections; they are also the presenting manifestations in bacterial sepsis. Proper bacterial cultures are essential. Differentiation between congenital heart disease and neonatal myocarditis is frequently difficult. However, the occurrence of fever or hypothermia, generalized lethargy and weakness, and characteristic electrocardiographic changes should suggest a viral cause.

Congenital infections with rubella virus, cytomegalovirus, *Toxoplasma gondii*, or *Treponema pallidum* are frequently associated with intrauterine growth retardation; this is not usual with enterovirus infections. Generalized herpes simplex infections are clinically similar to severe infections with several enteroviruses; in herpes infections, skin lesions are common, and a scraping of a lesion and a culture should allow a rapid diagnosis. In infants with signs of central nervous system involvement, it is particularly important to consider herpes simplex virus infection as a possible cause because infection with this agent is treatable and early treatment is essential. In infants with meningitis, proper cultures and PCR testing are essential because the CSF findings in bacterial and viral illnesses are frequently similar.

PROGNOSIS

Polioviruses

As substantiated in the review by Bates[110] and the summary in Table 24-7, poliovirus infections in neonates are generally severe. Of the 44 cases with available follow-up data, there were 21 deaths; of the survivors, 12 had residual paralyses. Because infant survivors of poliomyelitis are susceptible to infection by the other two types of poliovirus, they should receive polio vaccine.

Nonpolio Enteroviruses

It is apparent that the immediate prognosis for patients with coxsackievirus and echovirus infections is related to the specific manifestations. Mortality rates are highest for infants with myocarditis, encephalitis, or sepsis-like illness with liver involvement. Differences in the severity of illness depend on viral type and strain variations. In general, infections with coxsackieviruses B1 to B4 and with echovirus 11 appear to carry the most ominous initial prognoses.

There is a surprising dearth of information related to long-term sequelae of neonatal coxsackievirus and echovirus infections. Gear,[195] in a 4-year follow-up study, found no evidence of permanent cardiac damage in several children who had coxsackievirus B myocarditis. For children with aseptic meningitis, there is little available evidence of neurologic damage. One of five infants studied by Nogen and Lepow,[212] from whom virus was recovered from the CSF, was suspected of having brain damage. Cho and colleagues[389] reported that a child who had had severe neonatal echovirus 9 disease was developing normally at 1 year of age. Tuuteri and associates[229] reported that two children who had had clinically mild neonatal coxsackievirus B3 infections were thriving when seen at 1 year of age. After an epidemic of mild febrile disease related to echovirus 5, 51 children were examined at 1 year of age and found to be normal.[240]

Farmer and colleagues[423] did a careful follow-up study of 15 children who had meningoencephalitis related to coxsackievirus B5 during the neonatal period. When 6 years old, two of the children were found to have developed spasticity, and their intelligence was below the mean for the study group as a whole and below the mean of a carefully selected control group. Three children who had myocarditis and meningoencephalitis had no cardiac sequelae at the age of 6 years. Sells and associates[427] described neurologic impairment at later follow-up study of some children who had central nervous system enteroviral infections during the first year of life.

In a study in which nine children with enteroviral meningitis during the first 3 months of life were compared with nine matched control children, Wilfert and associates[432] found that the receptive language functioning of patients was significantly less than that of the controls. Head circumference, hearing, and intellectual function were similar for patients and controls. Bergman and colleagues[431] reported an extensive study in which 33 survivors of enteroviral meningitis during infancy were compared with their siblings. In this comprehensive study, none of the survivors had major neurologic sequelae, and they performed as well as their siblings on a large number of cognitive, achievement, perceptual-motor skills, and language tests. Rantakallio and co-workers[413] found that 16 of 17 patients with neonatal meningitis related to coxsackievirus B5 had normal neurologic development on follow-up. The one exception was a child with suspected intrauterine myocarditis. In another study, 16 newborns with meningitis related to coxsackievirus A14 were normal 2.5 years later.

The most alarming report is that of Eichenwald,[479] who gave details of a 5-year follow-up study of infants who had had neonatal diarrhea associated with echovirus 18 infection.[244] Thirteen of 16 infants who had had an echovirus 18 infection during the neonatal period showed neurologic damage; these children had an IQ of less than 70, spasticity, deafness, blindness, or a combination of these effects.

In most instances, the antibody response of neonates after enterovirus infection is good. It is therefore to be expected that one attack of infection with a particular viral type provides immunity to the specific agent in the future. From the evidence derived from polio vaccine studies, it is probable that reinfection with all enteroviruses is common, but that after an initial antibody response, a secondary inapparent infection occurs and is confined to the gastrointestinal tract.

THERAPY

Specific Therapy

No specific therapy for any enterovirus infection is approved for use in the United States. In severe, catastrophic and generalized neonatal infection, it is likely that the infant received no specific antibody for the particular virus from the mother. In this situation, it is probably advisable to administer human immune serum globulin to the infant. Dagan and associates[480] examined three lots of human serum globulin and found the presence of neutralizing antibodies to several commonly circulating and infrequently circulating enteroviruses. Although there is no evidence that this therapy is beneficial in treating acute neonatal infections, there is evidence of some success in the treatment of chronic enteroviral infections in agammaglobulinemic patients.[481] Because it was found by Hammond and co-workers[482] that a single dose of intramuscular immunoglobulin resulted in little change in circulating neutralizing antibodies to coxsackievirus B4 and echovirus 11 in seven infants, it seems advisable when therapy is decided on to use high-dose intravenous immune globulin. One neonate with disseminated echovirus 11 infection with hepatitis, pneumonitis, meningitis, disseminated intravascular coagulation, decreased renal function, and anemia survived after receiving a large dose of intravenous immune globulin and supportive care.[483]

Abzug and colleagues[484] performed a small but controlled study in which nine enterovirus-infected neonates received intravenous immune globulin and seven similarly infected infants received supportive care. In this study, there was no significant difference in clinical scores, antibody values, or magnitude of viremia and viruria in those treated compared with the control infants. However, five infants received intravenous immune globulin with a high neutralizing antibody titer (≥1:800) to their individual viral isolates, and they had a more rapid cessation of viremia and viruria.

Jantausch and associates[485] reported an infant with a disseminated echovirus 11 infection who survived after maternal plasma transfusions. The role, if any, of these transfusions in the infant's recovery is unknown, and this form of therapy cannot be recommended. A neonate with an echovirus 11 infection–induced fulminant hepatitis survived after orthotopic liver transplantation.[486]

Many antipicornavirus drugs and biologicals have been studied during the past 30 years.[65,66] The antiviral drug pleconaril offers promise for the treatment of enteroviral infections.[65,395,407,487-489] This drug is a novel compound that integrates into the capsid of enteroviruses. It prevents the virus from attaching to cellular receptors and therefore prevents uncoating and subsequent release of viral RNA into the host cell. In a double-blinded, placebo-controlled study of 39 patients with enteroviral meningitis, a statistically significant shortening of the disease duration was noted from 9.5 days in controls to 4.0 days in drug recipients.[65] Pleconaril also has been used on a compassionate-release basis in the treatment of patients with life-threatening infection.[489] Several categories of enteroviral illnesses have been treated: chronic meningoencephalitis in patients with agammaglobulinemia or hypogammaglobulinemia, neonatal sepsis, myocarditis, poliomyelitis (wild-type or vaccine associated), encephalitis, and bone marrow transplant patients. Favorable clinical responses were observed in 22 of 36 treated patients, including 12 of 18 patients with chronic meningoencephalitis. However, in the absence of controls, the extent to which the favorable outcomes can be attributed to pleconaril is unknown.

In severe illnesses, such as neonatal myocarditis or encephalitis, it is frequently tempting to administer corticosteroids. Although some investigators thought this approach was beneficial in treating coxsackievirus myocarditis, I believe that corticosteroids should not be given during acute enterovirus infections. The deleterious effects of these agents in coxsackievirus infections of mice[490] are particularly persuasive. Immunosuppressive therapy for myocarditis of unknown origin with prednisone and cyclosporine or azathioprine was evaluated in a controlled trial of 111 adults, and no beneficial effect was observed.[491]

Because the possibility of bacterial sepsis cannot be ruled out in most instances of neonatal enteroviral infections, antibiotics should be administered for the most likely potential pathogens. Care in antibiotic selection and administration is urged so that drug toxicity is not added to the problems of the patient. In neonates with meningitis or meningoencephalitis and in some infants with sepsis-like illnesses, the possibility of herpes simplex virus infections should be strongly considered, and empirical treatment with intravenous acyclovir should be instituted after obtaining appropriate herpesvirus studies.

Nonspecific Therapy

Mild, Nonspecific Febrile Illness

In infants in whom fever is the only symptom, careful observation is most important. Many infants who eventually become severely ill have 2 to 3 days of fever initially without other localized findings. Care should be taken to administer adequate fluids to febrile infants, and excessive elevation of temperature should be prevented, if possible.

Sepsis-like Illness

In infants with severe sepsis-like illness, the major problems are shock, hepatitis and hepatic necrosis, and disseminated intravascular coagulation. For shock, attention should be directed toward treating hypotension and acidosis and ensuring adequate oxygenation.

For hepatitis, oral neomycin (25 mg/kg every 6 hours) or other nonabsorbable antibiotics to suppress intestinal bacterial flora may be helpful. The administration of blood (i.e., exchange transfusion) and vitamin K may be useful when bleeding occurs because of liver dysfunction. Heparin therapy should be considered when disseminated intravascular coagulation occurs.

Myocarditis

There is no specific therapy for myocarditis. However, congestive heart failure and arrhythmias should be treated by the usual methods. In administering digitalis preparations to infants with enteroviral myocarditis, careful attention to the initial dosage is most important because the heart is often extremely sensitive; frequently, only small amounts of digoxin are necessary.

Meningoencephalitis

In patients with meningoencephalitis, convulsions, cerebral edema, and disturbances of fluid and electrolyte balance occur frequently and respond to treatment. Seizures are best treated with phenobarbital, phenytoin (Dilantin), or lorazepam. Cerebral edema can be treated with urea, mannitol, or large doses of corticosteroids. However, it seems unwise to use corticosteroids in active enterovirus infections because the potential benefits may be outweighed by deleterious effects. Fluids should be monitored closely, and frequent determinations of serum electrolyte levels should be made because inappropriate antidiuretic hormone secretion is common.

Paralytic Poliomyelitis

Infants should be observed carefully for evidence of respiratory paralysis. If respiratory failure occurs, the early use of a positive-pressure ventilator is essential. In newborns, this is better performed without tracheotomy. Careful attention to pooling of secretions is important. Blood gas levels should be monitored frequently. Passive exercises of all involved extremities should be started if the infant has been afebrile for 3 days.

PREVENTION

Immunization

Congenital and neonatal poliomyelitis should be illnesses of historical interest only. However, because segments of populations in a few regions of the world have not been adequately immunized with polioviral vaccines, clinical poliomyelitis will continue to occur. In adequately immunized populations, congenital and neonatal poliomyelitis has been eliminated.

Attenuated viral vaccines for other enteroviruses are not available. However, if a virulent enteroviral type became prevalent, it is probable that a specific vaccine for active immunization could be developed.

Passive protection with intramuscular immune globulin (0.15 to 0.5 mL/kg) or perhaps intravenous immune globulin can be useful in preventing disease.[482,492-494] In practice, however, this approach seems to be worthwhile only in sudden and virulent nursery outbreaks. For example, if several cases of myocarditis occurred in a nursery, it would seem wise to administer immune globulin to all infants in the nursery. Pooled human immune globulin in most instances can be expected to contain antibodies against coxsackievirus types B1 through B5 and echovirus 11. This procedure could offer protection to infants without transplacentally acquired specific antibody who had not yet become infected.

Other Measures

Careful attention to routine nursery infection control procedures is important in preventing and controlling epidemics of enteroviral diseases. Nursery personnel should exercise strict care in washing their hands after handling each infant. It is also important to restrict the nursery area to personnel who are free of even minor illnesses.

Nursery infection, when it occurs, is best controlled in units that follow a cohort system. When illness occurs, the infant in question should be immediately isolated, and the nursery should be closed to all new admissions.

REFERENCES

1. Cherry JD, Nelson DB. Enterovirus infections: their epidemiology and pathogenesis. Clin Pediatr 5:659, 1966.
2. Bodian D, Horstmann DM. Polioviruses. *In* Horsfall FL Jr, Tamm I (eds). Viral and Rickettsial Infections of Man, 4th ed. Philadelphia, JB Lippincott, 1965, p 430.
3. Dalldorf G, Melnick JL. Coxsackie viruses. *In* Horsfall FL Jr, Tamm I (eds). Viral and Rickettsial Infections of Man, 4th ed. Philadelphia, JB Lippincott, 1965, p 474.
4. Melnick JL. Echoviruses. *In* Horsfall FL Jr, Tamm I (eds). Viral and Rickettsial Infections of Man, 4th ed. Philadelphia, JB Lippincott, 1965, p 513.
5. Kibrick S. Current status of coxsackie and ECHO viruses in human disease. Prog Med Virol 6:27, 1964.
6. Morens DM, Zweighaft RM, Bryan JM. Nonpolio enterovirus disease in the United States, 1971-1975. Int J Epidemiol 8:49, 1979.
7. Wenner HA, Behbehani AM. Echoviruses. *In* Gard S, Hallaner C, Meyer KF (eds). Virology Monographs, vol. 1. New York, Springer-Verlag, 1968, p 1.
8. Scott TFM. Clinical syndromes associated with entero virus and REO virus infections. Adv Virus Res 8:165, 1961.
9. Cherry JD. Enteroviruses and Parechoviruses. *In* Feigin RD, Cherry JD (eds). Textbook of Pediatric Infectious Diseases, 5th ed. Philadelphia, WB Saunders, 2003, p 1984.
10. Grist NR, Bell EJ, Assaad F. Enteroviruses in human disease. Prog Med Virol 24:114, 1978.
11. Melnick JL. Enteroviruses. *In* Evans AS (ed). Viral Infections of Humans: Epidemiology and Control, 3rd ed. New York, Plenum Publishing, 1989, p 191.
12. Gear JHS, Measroch V. Coxsackievirus infections of the newborn. Prog Med Virol 15:42, 1973.
13. Pallansch MA, Roos RP. Enteroviruses: polioviruses, coxsackieviruses, echoviruses, and newer enteroviruses. *In* Knipe DM, Howley PM (eds). Fields Virology, vol. 1. Philadelphia, Lippincott Williams & Wilkins, 2001, p 723.
14. Stanway G, Joki-Korpela P, Hyypiä T. Human parechoviruses—biology and clinical significance. Rev Med Virol 10:57, 2000.
15. Racaniello VR. *Picornaviridae*: the viruses and their replication. *In* Knipe DM and Howley PM (eds). Fields Virology, vol. 1, Philadelphia, Lippincott Williams & Wilkins, 2001, p 685.
16. Stanway G, Hyypiä T. Parechoviruses. J Virol 73:5249, 1999.
17. Melnick JL, Dalldorf G, Enders JF, et al. The enteroviruses. Am J Public Health 47:1556, 1957.
18. Overall JC Jr, Glasgow LA. Virus infections of the fetus and newborn infant. J Pediatr 77:315, 1970.
19. Monif GRG. Viral Infections of the Human Fetus. Toronto, Macmillan, 1969.
20. Kibrick S. Viral infections of the fetus and newborn. Perspect Virol 2:140, 1961.
21. Eichenwald HF, McCracken GH, Kindberg SJ. Virus infections of the newborn. Prog Med Virol 9:35, 1967.
22. Blattner RJ, Heys FM. Role of viruses in the etiology of congenital malformations. Prog Med Virol 3:311, 1961.
23. Hardy JB. Viral infection in pregnancy: a review. Am J Obstet Gynecol 93:1052, 1965.
24. Horstmann DM. Viral infections in pregnancy. Yale J Biol Med 42:99, 1969.
25. Hardy JB. Viruses and the fetus. Postgrad Med 43:156, 1968.
26. Plotz EJ. Virus disease in pregnancy. N Y J Med 65:1239, 1965.
27. Hanshaw JB, Dudgeon JA. Viral Diseases of the Fetus and Newborn. Philadelphia, WB Saunders, 1978.
28. Krajden S, Middleton PJ. Enterovirus infections in the neonate. Clin Pediatr 22:87, 1983.
29. Kaplan MH, Klein SW, McPhee J, et al. Group B coxsackievirus infections in infants younger than three months of age: a serious childhood illness. Rev Infect Dis 5:1019, 1983.
30. Modlin JF. Perinatal echovirus infection: insights from a literature review of 61 cases of serious infection and 16 outbreaks in nurseries. Rev Infect Dis 8:918, 1986.
31. Byington CL, Taggart W, Carroll KC, et al. A polymerase chain reaction-based epidemiologic investigation of the incidence of nonpolio enteroviral infections in febrile and afebrile infants 90 days and younger. Pediatrics 103:E27, 1999.
32. Wang S-M, Liu C-C, Yang Y-J, et al. Fatal coxsackievirus B infection in early infancy characterized by fulminant hepatitis. J Infect 37:270, 1998.
33. Paul JR. A History of Poliomyelitis. New Haven, Conn, Yale University Press, 1971.
34. Horstmann DM. The poliomyelitis story: a scientific hegira. Yale J Biol Med 58:79, 1985.
35. Melnick JL. Portraits of viruses: the picornaviruses. Intervirology 20:61, 1983.
36. Underwood M. A Treatise on the Diseases of Children, 2nd ed. London, J Mathews, 1789.
37. Wickman I. On the epidemiology of Heine-Medin's disease. Rev Infect Dis 2:319, 1980.
38. Landsteiner K, Popper E. Übertragung der Poliomyelitis acuta auf Affen. Z Immun Forsch 2:377, 1909.
39. Hannaeus G. Dissertation. Copenhagen, 1735.
40. Dalldorf G, Sickles GM. An unidentified, filtrable agent isolated from the feces of children with paralysis. Science 108:61, 1948.
41. Enders JF, Weller TH, Robbins FC. Cultivation of the Lansing strain of poliomyelitis virus in cultures of various human embryonic tissues. Science 109:85, 1949.
42. Robbins FC, de Quadros CA. Certification of the eradication of indigenous transmission of wild poliovirus in the Americas. J Infect Dis 175:S281, 1997.
43. Cochi SL, Hull HF, Sutter RW, et al. Commentary: the unfolding story of global poliomyelitis eradication. J Infect Dis 175:S1, 1997.
44. Centers for Disease Control and Prevention. Progress toward global poliomyelitis eradication, 1985-1994. MMWR Morb Mortal Wkly Rep 44:273, 1995.
45. Hull HF, Ward NA, Hull BP, et al. Paralytic poliomyelitis: seasoned strategies, disappearing disease. Lancet 343:1331, 1994.
46. World Health Organization. Poliomyelitis. Fact sheet no. 114, http://www.who.int/mediacentre/factsheets/fs114/en/ print.html, last revised 2003.
47. Centers for Disease Control and Prevention. Progress toward global eradication of poliomyelitis, 2002. MMWR Morb Mort Wkly Rep 52:366, 2003.
48. Romero JR, Rotbart HA. Sequence diversity among echoviruses with different neurovirulence phenotypes. Pediatr Res 33:181A, 1993.
49. Schlesinger Y, Sawyer MH, Storch GA. Enteroviral meningitis in infancy: potential role for polymerase chain reaction in patient management. Pediatrics 94:157, 1994.
50. Sawer MH, Holland D, Aintablian N, et al. Diagnosis of enteroviral central nervous system infection by polymerase chain reaction during a large community outbreak. Pediatr Infect Dis J 13:177, 1994.
51. Abzug MJ, Loeffelholz M, Rotbart HA. Clinical and laboratory observations. J Pediatr 126:447, 1995.
52. Andréoletti L, Blassel-Damman N, Dewilde A, et al. Comparison of use of cerebrospinal fluid, serum, and throat swab specimens in the diagnosis of enteroviral acute neurological infection by a rapid RNA detection PCR assay. J Clin Microbiol 36:589, 1998.
53. Rotbart HA. Reproducibility of AMPLICOR enterovirus PCR test results. J Clin Microbiol 35:3301, 1997.

54. Marshall GS, Hauck MA, Buck G, et al. Potential cost savings through rapid diagnosis of enteroviral meningitis. Pediatr Infect Dis J 16:1086, 1997.
55. Yerly S, Gervaix A, Simonet V, et al. Rapid and sensitive detection of enteroviruses in specimens from patients with aseptic meningitis. J Clin Microbiol 34:199, 1996.
56. Sharland M, Hodgson J, Davies EG, et al. Enteroviral pharyngitis diagnosed by reverse transcriptase-polymerase chain reaction. Arch Dis Child 74:462, 1996.
57. Tanel RE, Kao S, Niemiec TM, et al. Prospective comparison of culture vs genome detection for diagnosis of enteroviral meningitis in childhood. Arch Pediatr Adolesc Med 150:919, 1996.
58. Nielsen LP, Modlin JF, Rotbart HA. Detection of enteroviruses by polymerase chain reaction in urine samples of patients with aseptic meningitis. Pediatr Infect Dis J 15:125, 1996.
59. Klespies SL, Cebula DE, Kelley CL, et al. Detection of enterovirus from clinical specimens by spin amplification shell vial culture and monoclonal antibody assay. J Clin Microbiol 34:1465, 1996.
60. Uchio E, Yamazaki K, Aoki K, et al. Detection of enterovirus 70 by polymerase chain reaction in acute hemorrhagic conjunctivitis. Am J Ophthalmol 122:273, 1996.
61. Andréoletti L, Hober D, Belaich S, et al. Rapid detection of enterovirus in clinical specimens using PCR and microwell capture hybridization assay. J Virol Methods 62:1, 1996.
62. Lina B, Pozzetto B, Andréoletti L, et al. Multicenter evaluation of a commercially available PCR assay for diagnosing enterovirus infection in a panel of cerebrospinal fluid specimens. J Clin Microbiol 34:3002, 1996.
63. Oberste MS, Nix WA, Maher K, et al. Improved molecular identification of enteroviruses by RT-PCR and amplicon sequencing. J Clin Virol 26:375, 2003.
64. Ishiko H, Shimada Y, Yonaha M, et al. Molecular diagnosis of human enteroviruses by phylogeny-based classification by use of the VP4 sequence. J Infect Dis 185:744, 2002.
65. Rotbart HA, O'Connel JF, McKinlay MA. Treatment of human enterovirus infections. Antiviral Res 38:1, 1998.
66. Diana GD, Pevear DC. Antipicornavirus drugs: current status. Antivir Chem Chemother 8:401, 1997.
67. Rotbart HA, Webster AD. Treatment of potentially life-threatening enterovirus infections with pleconaril. Clin Infect Dis 32:228, 2001.
68. Fenner F. Classification and nomenclature of viruses: second report of the International Committee on Taxonomy of Viruses. Intervirology 7:1, 1976.
69. Melnick JL, Wenner HA. Enteroviruses. *In* Lennette EH, Schmidt NJ (eds). Diagnostic Procedures for Viral and Rickettsial Infections, 4th ed. New York, American Public Health Association, 1969.
70. Rueckert RR. Picornaviridae and their replication. *In* Fields BN, Knipe DM (eds). Virology, 2nd ed. New York, Raven Press, 1990, p 507.
71. Pöyry T, Kinnunen L, Hyypiä T, et al. Genetic and phylogenetic clustering of enteroviruses. J Gen Virol 77:1699, 1996.
72. Diedrich S, Driesel G, Schreier E. Sequence comparison of echovirus type 30 isolates to other enteroviruses in the 5′ noncoding region. J Med Virol 46:148, 1995.
73. Kew OM, Mulders MN, Lipskaya GY, et al. Molecular epidemiology of polioviruses. Virology 6:401, 1995.
74. Pöyry T, Hyypiä T, Horsnell C, et al. Molecular analysis of coxsackievirus A16 reveals a new genetic group of enteroviruses. Virology 202: 962, 1994.
75. Pulli T, Koskimies P, Hyypiä T. Molecular comparison of coxsackie A virus serotypes. Virology 212:30, 1995.
76. Hyypiä T, Hovi T, Knowles NJ, et al. Classification of enteroviruses based on molecular and biological properties. J Gen Virol 78:1, 1997.
77. Kubo H, Iritani N, Seto Y. Molecular classification of enteroviruses not identified by neutralization tests. Emerg Infect Dis 8:298, 2002.
78. Norder H, Bjerregaard L, Magnius L, et al. Sequencing of 'untypable' enteroviruses reveals two new types, EV-77 and EV-78, within human enterovirus type B and substitutions in the BC loop of the VP1 protein for known types. J Gen Virol 84:827, 2003.
79. Bryden AS. Isolation of enteroviruses and adenoviruses in continuous simian cell lines. Med Lab Sci 49:60, 1992.
80. Hatch MH, Marchetti GE. Isolation of echoviruses with human embryonic lung fibroblast cells. Appl Microbiol 22:736, 1971.
81. Kelen AE, Lesiak JM, Labzoffsky NA. An outbreak of aseptic meningitis due to ECHO 25 virus. Can Med Assoc J 90:1349, 1964.
82. Cherry JD, Bobinski JE, Horvath FL, et al. Acute hemangiomalike lesions associated with ECHO viral infections. Pediatrics 44:498, 1969.
83. Bell EJ, Cosgrove BP. Routine enterovirus diagnosis in a human rhabdomyosarcoma cell line. Bull World Health Organ 58:423, 1980.
84. Terletskaia-Ladwig E, Metzger C, Schalasta G, et al. Evaluation of enterovirus serological tests IgM-EIA and complement fixation in patients with meningitis, confirmed by detection of enteroviral RNA by RT-PCR in cerebrospinal fluid. J Med Virol 61:221, 2000.
85. Terletskaia-Ladwig E, Metzger C, Schalasta G, et al. A new enzyme immunoassay for the detection of enteroviruses in faecal specimens. J Med Virol 60:439, 2000.
86. Norder H, Bjerregaard L, Magnius LO. Homotypic echoviruses share aminoterminal VP1 sequence homology applicable for typing. J Med Virol 63:35, 2001.
87. Gelfand HM. The occurrence in nature of the coxsackie and ECHO viruses. Prog Med Virol 3:193, 1961.
88. Keswick BH, Gerba CP, Goyal SM. Occurrence of enteroviruses in community swimming pools. Am J Public Health 71:1026, 1981.
89. Johnson I, Hammond GW, Verma MR. Nosocomial coxsackie B4 virus infections in two chronic-care pediatric neurological wards. J Infect Dis 151:1153, 1985.
90. Downey TW. Polioviruses and flies: studies on the epidemiology of enteroviruses in an urban area. Yale J Biol Med 35:341, 1963.
91. Melnick JL, Emmons J, Coffey JH, et al. Seasonal distribution of coxsackie viruses in urban sewage and flies. Am J Hyg 59:164, 1954.
92. Melnick JL, Dow RP. Poliomyelitis in Hidalgo County, Texas 1948: poliomyelitis and coxsackie viruses from flies. Am J Hyg 58:288, 1953.
93. Horn P. Poliomyelitis in pregnancy: a twenty-year report from Los Angeles County, California. Obstet Gynecol 6:121, 1955.
94. Gresser I, Chany C, Enders JF. Persistent polioviral infection of intact human amniotic membrane without apparent cytopathic effect. J Bacteriol 89:470, 1965.
95. Blattner RJ. Intrauterine infection with poliovirus, type I. J Pediatr 62:625, 1963.
96. Aycock WL. The frequency of poliomyelitis in pregnancy. N Engl J Med 225:405, 1941.
97. Shelokov A, Habel K. Subclinical poliomyelitis in a newborn infant due to intrauterine infection. JAMA 160:465, 1956.
98. Schaeffer M, Fox MJ, Li CP. Intrauterine poliomyelitis infection. JAMA 155:248, 1954.
99. Shelokov A, Weinstein L. Poliomyelitis in the early neonatal period: report of a case of possible intrauterine infection. J Pediatr 38:80, 1951.
100. Lance M. Paralysis infantile (poliomyelité) constatée des la naissance. Bull Soc Pediatr (Paris) 31:2297, 1933.
101. Severin G. Case of poliomyelitis in newborn. Nord Med 1:55, 1939.
102. Baskin JL, Soule EH, Mills SD. Poliomyelitis of the newborn: pathologic changes in two cases. Am J Dis Child 80:10, 1950.
103. Kreibich H, Wold W. Ueber einen Fall von diaplazenter poliomyelitis Infektion des Feten in 9 Schwangerschaftsmonat. Zentralbl Gynaekol 72:694, 1950.
104. Johnson JF, Stimson PM. Clinical poliomyelitis in the early neonatal period. J Pediatr 40:733, 1956.
105. Carter HM. Congenital poliomyelitis. Obstet Gynecol 8:373, 1956.
106. Jackson AL, Louw JX. Poliomyelitis at birth due to transplacental infection. S Afr Med J 33:357, 1959.
107. Wingate MB, Meller HK, Ormiston G. Acute bulbar poliomyelitis in late pregnancy. Br Med J 1:407, 1961.
108. Abramson H, Greenberg M, Magee MC. Poliomyelitis in the newborn infant. J Pediatr 43:167, 1953.
109. Swarts CL, Kercher EF. A fatal case of poliomyelitis in a newborn infant delivered by cesarean section following maternal death due to poliomyelitis. Pediatrics 14:235, 1954.
110. Bates T. Poliomyelitis in pregnancy, fetus, and newborn. Am J Dis Child 90:189, 1955.
111. Elliott GB, McAllister JE, Alberta C. Fetal poliomyelitis. Am J Obstet Gynecol 72:896, 1956.
112. Siegel M, Greenberg M. Poliomyelitis in pregnancy: effect on fetus and newborn infant. J Pediatr 49:280, 1956.
113. Barsky P, Beale AJ. The transplacental transmission of poliomyelitis. J Pediatr 51:207, 1957.
114. Lycke E, Nilsson LR. Poliomyelitis in a newborn due to intrauterine infection. Acta Paediatr 51:661, 1962.
115. Winsser J, Pfaff ML, Seanor HE. Poliomyelitis viremia in a newborn infant. Pediatrics 20:458, 1957.
116. Wyatt HV. Poliomyelitis in the fetus and the newborn: a comment on the new understanding of the pathogenesis. Clin Pediatr 18:33, 1979.
117. Pearson RJC, Miller DG, Palmier ML. Reactions to the oral vaccine. Yale J Biol Med 34:498, 1962.

118. Prem KA, Fergus JW, Mathers JE, et al. Vaccination of pregnant women and young infants with trivalent oral attenuated live poliomyelitis vaccine. *In* Second International Conference on Live Poliovirus Vaccines, Washington, DC, June 6-10, 1960. Washington, DC, Pan American Sanitary Bureau, 1960.
119. Prem KA, McKelvey JL. Immunologic response of pregnant women to oral trivalent poliomyelitis vaccine. *In* First International Conference on Live Poliovirus Vaccines, Washington, DC, June 22-26, 1959. Washington, DC, Pan American Sanitary Bureau, 1959.
120. McKay HW, Fodor AR, Kokko UP. Viremia following the administration of live poliovirus vaccines. Am J Public Health 53:274, 1963.
121. Horstmann DM, Opton EM, Klemperer R, et al. Viremia in infants vaccinated with oral poliovirus vaccine (Sabin). Am J Hyg 79:47, 1964.
122. Melnick JL, Proctor RO, Ocampo AR, et al. Free and bound virus in serum after administration of oral poliovirus vaccine. Am J Epidemiol 84:329, 1966.
123. Cabasso VJ, Jungherr EL, Moyer AW, et al. Oral poliomyelitis vaccine, Lederle: thirteen years of laboratory and field investigation. N Engl J Med 263:1321, 1960.
124. Katz SL. Efficacy, potential and hazards of vaccines. N Engl J Med 270:884, 1964.
125. Payne AMM. Summary of the conference. *In* Second International Conference on Live Poliovirus Vaccines, Washington, DC, June 6-10, 1960. Washington, DC, Pan American Sanitary Bureau, 1960.
126. White LR. Comment. *In* Viral Etiology of Congenital Malformations, May 19-20, 1967. Washington, DC, U.S. Government Printing Office, 1968.
127. Horstmann DM. Epidemiology of poliomyelitis and allied diseases—1963. Yale J Biol Med 36:5, 1963.
128. Dalldorf G, Gifford R. Susceptibility of gravid mice to coxsackie virus infection. J Exp Med 99:21, 1954.
129. Berger E, Roulet F. Beitrage zur Ausscheidung und Tierpathogenitüt des Coxsackie-virus. Schweiz Z Allg Pathol 15:462, 1952.
130. Selzer G. Transplacental infection of the mouse fetus by Coxsackie viruses. Israel J Med Sci 5:125, 1969.
131. Soike K. Coxsackie B-3 virus infection in the pregnant mouse. J Infect Dis 117:203, 1967.
132. Modlin JF, Crumpacker CS. Coxsackievirus B infection in pregnant mice and transplacental infection of the fetus. Infect Immun 37:222, 1982.
133. Flamm H. Some considerations concerning the pathogenesis of prenatal infections. *In* Eichenwald HC (ed). The Prevention of Mental Retardation Through Control of Infectious Diseases. Washington, DC, U.S. Government Printing Office, 1966.
134. Flamm H. Untersuchungen über die diaplazentare Übertragung des Coxsackievirus. Schweiz Z Allg Pathol 18:16, 1955.
135. Palmer AL, Rotbart HA, Tyson RW, et al. Adverse effects of maternal enterovirus infection on the fetus and placenta. J Infect Dis 176:1437, 1997.
136. Abzug MJ. Maternal factors affecting the integrity of the late gestation placental barrier to murine enterovirus infection. J Infect Dis 176:41, 1997.
137. Benirschke K. Viral infection of the placenta. *In* Viral Etiology of Congenital Malformations, May 19-20, 1967. Washington, DC, U.S. Government Printing Office, 1968.
138. Kibrick S, Benirschke K. Acute aseptic myocarditis and meningo-encephalitis in the newborn child infected with Coxsackie virus group B, type 3. N Engl J Med 255:883, 1956.
139. Brightman VJ, Scott TFM, Westphal M, et al. An outbreak of coxsackie B-5 virus infection in a newborn nursery. J Pediatr 69:179, 1966.
140. Makower H, Skurska Z, Halazinska L. On transplacental infection with Coxsackie virus. Texas Rep Biol Med 16:346, 1958.
141. Cherry JD, Soriano F, Jahn CL. Search for perinatal viral infection: a prospective, clinical, virologic and serologic study. Am J Dis Child 116:245, 1968.
142. Puschak RB. Coxsackie virus infection in the newborn with case report. Harrisburg Polyclinic Hosp J, p 14, 1962.
143. Basso NGS, Fonseca MEF, Garcia AGP, et al. Enterovirus isolation from foetal and placental tissues. Acta Virol 34:49, 1990.
144. Bates HR. Coxsackie virus B3 calcific pancarditis and hydrops fetalis. Am J Obstet Gynecol 106:629, 1970.
145. Hanson L, Lundgren S, Lycke E, et al. Clinical and serological observations in cases of Coxsackie B3 infections in early infancy. Acta Paediatr Scand 55:577, 1966.
146. Benirschke K, Pendleton ME. Coxsackie virus infection: an important complication of pregnancy. Obstet Gynecol 12:305, 1958.
147. McLean DM, Donohue WL, Snelling CE, et al. Coxsackie B5 virus as a cause of neonatal encephalitis and myocarditis. Can Med Assoc J 85:1046, 1961.
148. Bendig J, Franklin O, Hebden A, et al. Coxsackievirus B3 sequences in the blood of a neonate with congenital myocarditis, plus serological evidence of maternal infection. J Med Virol 70:606, 2003.
149. Burch GE, Sun SC, Chu KC, et al. Interstitial and coxsackievirus B myocarditis in infants and children. JAMA 203:1, 1968.
150. Plager H, Beeve R, Miller JK. Coxsackie B-5 pericarditis in pregnancy. Arch Intern Med 110:735, 1962.
151. Euscher E, Davis J, Holzman I, et al. Coxsackievirus virus infection of the placenta associated with neurodevelopmental delays in the newborn. Obstet Gynecol 98:1019, 2001.
152. Yoshioka I, Horstmann DM. Viremia in infection due to ECHO virus type 9. N Engl J Med 262:224, 1960.
153. Rantasalo I, Penttinen K, Saxen L, et al. ECHO 9 virus antibody status after an epidemic period and the possible teratogenic effect of the infection. Ann Paediatr Fenn 6:175, 1960.
154. Kleinman H, Prince JT, Mathey WE, et al. ECHO 9 virus infection and congenital abnormalities: a negative report. Pediatrics 29:261, 1962.
155. Landsman JB, Grist NR, Ross CAC. Echo 9 virus infection and congenital malformations. Br J Prev Soc Med 18:152, 1964.
156. Moscovici C, Maisel J. Intestinal viruses of newborn and older prematures. Am J Dis Child 101:771, 1961.
157. Eichenwald HF, Kostevalov O. Immunologic responses of premature and full-term infants to infection with certain viruses. Pediatrics 25: 829, 1960.
158. Berkovich S, Smithwick EM. Transplacental infection due to ECHO virus type 22. J Pediatr 72:94, 1968.
159. Hughes JR, Wilfert CM, Moore M, et al. Echovirus 14 infection associated with fatal neonatal hepatic necrosis. Am J Dis Child 123:61, 1972.
160. Philip AGS, Larson EJ. Overwhelming neonatal infection with ECHO 19 virus. J Pediatr 82:391, 1973.
161. Cheeseman SH, Hirsch MS, Keller EW, et al. Fatal neonatal pneumonia caused by echovirus type 9. Am J Dis Child 131:1169, 1977.
162. Jones MJ, Kolb M, Votava HJ, et al. Intrauterine echovirus type 11 infection. Mayo Clin Proc 55:509, 1980.
163. Bose CL, Gooch WM III, Sanders GO, et al. Dissimilar manifestations of intrauterine infection with echovirus 11 in premature twins. Arch Pathol Lab Med 107:361, 1983.
164. Reyes MP, Ostrea EM Jr, Roskamp J, et al. Disseminated neonatal echovirus 11 disease following antenatal maternal infection with a virus-positive cervix and virus-negative gastrointestinal tract. J Med Virol 12:155, 1983.
165. Piraino FF, Sedmak G, Raab K. Echovirus 11 infections of newborns with mortality during the 1979 enterovirus season in Milwaukee, Wisc. Public Health Rep 97:346, 1982.
166. Nielsen JL, Berryman GK, Hankins GD. Intrauterine fetal death and the isolation of echovirus 27 from amniotic fluid. J Infect Dis 158:501, 1988.
167. Toce SS, Keenan WJ. Congenital echovirus 11 pneumonia in association with pulmonary hypertension. Pediatr Infect Dis J 7:360, 1988.
168. Yen H, Lien R, Fu R, et al. Hepatic failure in a newborn with maternal peripartum exposure to echovirus 6 and enterovirus 71. Eur J Pediatr 162:648, 2003.
169. Chow K, Lee C, Lin T, et al. Congenital enterovirus 71 infection: a case study with virology and immunochemistry. Clin Infect Dis 31:509, 2000.
170. Otonkoski T, Roivainen M, Vaarala O, et al. Neonatal type I diabetes associated with maternal echovirus 6 infection: a case report. Diabetologia 43:1235, 2000.
171. Kleger B, Prier JE, Rosato DJ, et al. Herpes simplex infection of the female genital tract. I. Incidence of infection. Am J Obstet Gynecol 102:745, 1968.
172. Montgomery R, Youngblood L, Medearis DN Jr. Recovery of cytomegalovirus from the cervix in pregnancy. Pediatrics 49:524, 1972.
173. Reyes MP, Zalenski D, Smith F, et al. Coxsackievirus-positive cervices in women with febrile illnesses during the third trimester in pregnancy. Am J Obstet Gynecol 155:159, 1986.
174. Cole RM, Bell JA, Beeman EA, et al. Studies of Coxsackie viruses: observations on epidemiologic aspects of group A viruses. Am J Public Health 41:1342, 1951.
175. Ramos-Alvarez M, Sabin AB. Intestinal viral flora of healthy children demonstrable by monkey kidney tissue culture. Am J Public Health 46:295, 1956.
176. Vandeputte M. L'endémicité des virus entériques à Léopoldville. Congo Bull WHO/OMS 22:313, 1960.

177. Katz SL. Case records of the Massachusetts General Hospital. Case 20-1965. N Engl J Med 272:907, 1965.
178. Jenista JA, Powell KR, Menegus MA. Epidemiology of neonatal enterovirus infection. J Pediatr 104:685, 1984.
179. Pagano JS, Plotkin SA, Cornely D. The response of premature infants to infection with type 3 attenuated poliovirus. J Pediatr 65:165, 1964.
180. Pagano JS, Plotkin SA, Koprowski H. Variations in the response of infants to living attenuated poliovirus vaccines. N Engl J Med 264:155, 1961.
181. Pagano JS, Plotkin SA, Cornely D, et al. The response of premature infants to infection with attenuated poliovirus. Pediatrics 29:794, 1962.
182. Murphy W. Response of infants to trivalent poliovirus vaccine (Sabin strains). Pediatrics 40:980, 1967.
183. Lepow ML, Warren RJ, Gray N, et al. Effect of Sabin type 1 poliomyelitis vaccine administered by mouth to newborn infants. N Engl J Med 264:1071, 1961.
184. Sabin AB, Michaels RH, Krugman S, et al. Effect of oral poliovirus vaccine in newborn children. I. Excretion of virus after ingestion of large doses of type 1 or of mixture of all three types, in relation to level of placentally transmitted antibody. Pediatrics 31:623, 1963.
185. Sabin AB, Michaels RH, Ziring P, et al. Effect of oral poliovirus vaccine in newborn children. II. Intestinal resistance and antibody response at 6 months in children fed type 1 vaccine at birth. Pediatrics 31:641, 1963.
186. Warren RJ, Lepow ML, Bartsch GE, et al. The relationship of maternal antibody, breast feeding, and age to the susceptibility of newborn infants to infection with attenuated polioviruses. Pediatrics 34:4, 1964.
187. Lepow ML, Warren RJ, Ingram VG, et al. Sabin type 1 (LSc2ab) oral poliomyelitis vaccine. Am J Dis Child 104:67, 1962.
188. Keller R, Dwyer JE, Oh W, et al. Intestinal IgA neutralizing antibodies in newborn infants following poliovirus immunization. Pediatrics 43:330, 1969.
189. Földes P, Bános A, Bános Z, et al. Vaccination of newborn children with live poliovirus vaccine. Acta Microbiol Acad Sci Hung 9:305, 1962.
190. Plotkin SA, Katz M, Brown RE, et al. Oral poliovirus vaccination in newborn African infants. Am J Dis Child 111:27, 1966.
191. Katz M, Plotkin SA. Oral polio immunization of the newborn infant: a possible method of overcoming interference by ingested antibodies. J Pediatr 73:267, 1968.
192. Bergeisen GH, Bauman RJ, Gilmore RL. Neonatal paralytic poliomyelitis: a case report. Arch Neurol 43:192, 1986.
193. Javett SN, Heymann S, Mundel B, et al. Myocarditis in the newborn infant. J Pediatr 48:1, 1956.
194. Kipps A, Naudé WDT, Don P, et al. Coxsackie virus myocarditis of the newborn. Med Proc 4:401, 1958.
195. Gear JHS. Coxsackie virus infection of the newborn. Prog Med Virol 1:106, 1958.
196. Montgomery J, Gear J, Prinsloo FR, et al. Myocarditis of the newborn: an outbreak in a maternity home in Southern Rhodesia associated with Coxsackie group-B virus infection. S Afr Med J 29:608, 1955.
197. Winsser J, Altieri RH. A three-year study of coxsackie virus, group B, infection in Nassau County. Am J Med Sci 247:269, 1964.
198. Artenstein MS, Cadigan FC, Buescher EL. Epidemic coxsackie virus infection with mixed clinical manifestations. Ann Intern Med 60:196, 1964.
199. Farber S, Vawter GF. Clinical pathological conference. J Pediatr 62:786, 1963.
200. Koch VF, Enders-Ruckle G, Wokittel E. Coxsackie B5-Infektionen mit signifikanter Antikörperentwicklung bei Neugeborenen. Arch Kinderheilkd 165:245, 1962.
201. Moossy J, Geer JC. Encephalomyelitis, myocarditis and adrenal cortical necrosis in coxsackie B3 virus infection. Arch Pathol 70:614, 1960.
202. Sussman ML, Strauss L, Hodes HL. Fatal Coxsackie group B infection in the newborn. Am J Dis Child 97:483, 1959.
203. Hosier DM, Newton WA. Serious Coxsackie infection in infants and children. Am J Dis Child 96:251, 1958.
204. Fechner RE, Smith MG, Middelkamp JN. Coxsackie B virus infection of the newborn. Am J Pathol 42:493, 1963.
205. Verlinde JD, Van Tongeren HAE, Kret A. Myocarditis in newborns due to group B Coxsackie virus: virus studies. Ann Pediatr 187:113, 1956.
206. Van Creveld S, De Jager H. Myocarditis in newborns, caused by Coxsackie virus: clinical and pathological data. Ann Pediatr 187:100, 1956.
207. Sieber OF, Kilgus AH, Fulginiti VA, et al. Immunological response of the newborn infant to Coxsackie B-4 infection. Pediatrics 40:444, 1967.
208. Butler N, Skelton MO, Hodges GM, et al. Fatal Coxsackie B3 myocarditis in a newborn infant. BMJ 1:1251, 1962.
209. Robino G, Perlman A, Togo Y, et al. Fatal neonatal infection due to Coxsackie B2 virus. J Pediatr 61:911, 1962.
210. Jack I, Townley RRW. Acute myocarditis of newborn infants, due to Coxsackie viruses. Med J Aust 2:265, 1961.
211. Jahn CL, Cherry JD. Mild neonatal illness associated with heavy enterovirus infection. N Engl J Med 274:394, 1966.
212. Nogen AG, Lepow ML. Enteroviral meningitis in very young infants. Pediatrics 40:617, 1967.
213. Kibrick S, Benirschke K. Severe generalized disease (encephalohepatomyocarditis) occurring in the newborn period and due to infection with Coxsackie virus, group B. Pediatrics 22:857, 1958.
214. McLean DM, Coleman MA, Larke RPB, et al. Viral infections of Toronto children during 1965. I. Enteroviral disease. Can Med Assoc J 94:839, 1966.
215. Rapmund G, Gauld JR, Rogers NG, et al. Neonatal myocarditis and meningoencephalitis due to Coxsackie virus group B, type 4: virologic study of a fatal case with simultaneous aseptic meningitis in the mother. N Engl J Med 260:819, 1959.
216. Wright HT Jr, Okuyama K, McAllister RM. An infant fatality associated with Coxsackie B1 virus. J Pediatr 63:428, 1963.
217. Gear J. Coxsackie virus infections in Southern Africa. Yale J Biol Med 34:289, 1961.
218. Volakova N, Jandasek L. Epidemic of myocarditis in newborn infants caused by Coxsackie B1 virus. Cesk Epidemiol 13:88, 1963.
219. Cherry JD, Lerner AM, Klein J, et al. Unpublished data, 1962.
220. Gear J, Measroch V, Prinsloo FR. The medical and public health importance of the coxsackie viruses. S Afr Med J 30:806, 1956.
221. Woodward TE, McCrumb FR Jr, Carey TN, et al. Viral and rickettsial causes of cardiac disease, including the Coxsackie virus etiology of pericarditis and myocarditis. Ann Intern Med 53:1130, 1960.
222. Hurley R, Norman AP, Pryse-Davies J. Massive pulmonary hemorrhage in the newborn associated with coxsackie B virus infection. BMJ 3:636, 1969.
223. Suckling PV, Vogelpoel L. Coxsackie myocarditis of the newborn. Med Proc 4:372, 1958.
224. Cherry JD, Jahn CL. Virologic studies of exanthems. J Pediatr 68:204, 1966.
225. Jennings RC. Coxsackie group B fatal neonatal myocarditis associated with cardiomegaly. J Clin Pathol 19:325, 1966.
226. Johnson WR. Manifestations of Coxsackie group B infections in children. Del Med J 32:72, 1960.
227. Delaney TB, Fakunaga FH. Myocarditis in a newborn with encephalomeningitis due to Coxsackie virus group B, type 5. N Engl J Med 259:234, 1958.
228. Dömök I, Molnár E. An outbreak of meningoencephalomyocarditis among newborn infants during the epidemic of Bornholm disease of 1958 in Hungary. II. Aetiological findings. Ann Pediatr 194:102, 1960.
229. Tuuteri L, Lapinleimu K, Meurman L. Fatal myocarditis associated with coxsackie B3 infection in the newborn. Ann Paediatr Fenn 9:56, 1963.
230. Archibald E, Purdham DR. Coxsackievirus type A16 infection in a neonate. Arch Dis Child 54:649, 1979.
231. Rantakallio P, Lapinleimu K, Mäntyjärvi R. Coxsackie B5 outbreak in a newborn nursery with 17 cases of serious meningitis. Scand J Infect Dis 2:17, 1970.
232. Lapinleimu K, Kaski U. An outbreak caused by coxsackievirus B5 among newborn infants. Scand J Infect Dis 4:27, 1972.
233. Isacsohn M, Eidelman AI, Kaplan M, et al. Neonatal coxsackievirus group B infections: experience of a single department of neonatology. Israel J Med Sci 30:371, 1994.
234. Swender PT, Shott RJ, Williams ML. A community and intensive care nursery outbreak of coxsackievirus B5 meningitis. Am J Dis Child 127:42, 1974.
235. Cramblett HG, Haynes RE, Azimi PH, et al. Nosocomial infection with echovirus type 11 in handicapped and premature infants. Pediatrics 51:603, 1973.
236. Jack I, Grutzner J, Gray N, et al. A survey of prenatal virus disease in Melbourne. Personal communication, July 21, 1967.
237. Berkovich S, Pangan J. Recoveries of virus from premature infants during outbreaks of respiratory disease: the relation of ECHO virus type 22 to disease of the upper and lower respiratory tract in the premature infant. Bull N Y Acad Med 44:377, 1968.
238. Miller DG, Gabrielson MO, Bart KJ, et al. An epidemic of aseptic meningitis, primarily among infants, caused by echovirus 11-prime. Pediatrics 41:77, 1968.

239. Hercík L, Huml M, Mimra J, et al. Epidemien der Respirationstrakterkrankunger bei Neugeborenen durch ECHO 11-Virus. Zentrabl Bakteriol 213:18, 1970.
240. German LJ, McCracken AW, Wilkie KM. Outbreak of febrile illness associated with ECHO virus type 5 in a maternity unit in Singapore. BMJ 1:742, 1968.
241. Hart EW, Brunton GB, Taylor CED, et al. Infection of newborn babies with ECHO virus type 5. Lancet 2:402, 1962.
242. Berkovich S, Kibrick S. ECHO 11 outbreak in newborn infants and mothers. Pediatrics 33:534, 1964.
243. Sanders DY, Cramblett HG. Viral infections in hospitalized neonates. Am J Dis Child 116:251, 1968.
244. Eichenwald HF, Ababio A, Arky AM, et al. Epidemic diarrhea in premature and older infants caused by ECHO virus type 18. JAMA 166:1563, 1958.
245. Butterfield J, Moscovici C, Berry C, et al. Cystic emphysema in premature infants: a report of an outbreak with the isolation of type 19 ECHO virus in one case. N Engl J Med 268:18, 1963.
246. Nakao T, Miura R, Sato M. ECHO virus type 22 in a premature infant. Tohoku J Exp Med 102:61, 1970.
247. Faulkner RS, van Rooyen CE. Echovirus type 17 in the neonate. Can Med Assoc J 108:878, 1973.
248. Eichenwald HF, Kostevalov O, Fasso LA. The "cloud baby": an example of bacterial-viral interaction. Am J Dis Child 100:161, 1960.
249. Kapsenberg JG. ECHO virus type 33 as a cause of meningitis. Arch Gesamte Virusforschl 23:144, 1968.
250. Nagington J, Wreghitt TG, Gandy G, et al. Fatal echovirus 11 infections in outbreak in special-care baby unit. Lancet 2:725, 1978.
251. Davies DP, Hughes CA, MacVicar J, et al. Echovirus-11 infection in a special-care baby unit. Lancet 1:96, 1979.
252. Hasegawa A. Virologic and serologic studies on an outbreak of echovirus type 11 infection in a hospital maternity unit. Jpn J Med Sci Biol 28:179, 1975.
253. Lapinleimu K, Hakulinen A. A hospital outbreak caused by ECHO virus type 11 among newborn infants. Ann Clin Res 4:183, 1972.
254. Modlin JF. Fatal echovirus 11 disease in premature neonates. Pediatrics 66:775, 1980.
255. Purdham DR, Purdham PA, Wood BSB, et al. Severe ECHO 19 virus infection in a neonatal unit. Arch Dis Child 51:634, 1976.
256. McDonald LL, St. Geme JW, Arnold BH. Nosocomial infection with ECHO virus type 31 in a neonatal intensive care unit. Pediatrics 47:995, 1971.
257. Mertens T, Hager H, Eggers HJ. Epidemiology of an outbreak in a maternity unit of infections with an antigenic variant of echovirus 11. J Med Virol 9:81, 1982.
258. Kinney JS, McCray E, Kaplan JE, et al. Risk factors associated with echovirus 11 infection in a hospital nursery. Pediatr Infect Dis 5:192, 1986.
259. Steinmann J, Albrecht K. Echovirus 11 epidemic among premature newborns in a neonatal intensive care unit. Zentralbl Bakteriol Mikrobiol Hyg 259:284, 1985.
260. Modlin JF. Perinatal echovirus infection: insights from a literature review of 61 cases of serious infection and 16 outbreaks in nurseries. Rev Infect Dis 8:918, 1986.
261. Modlin JF. Echovirus infections of newborn infants. Pediatr Infect Dis 7:311, 1988.
262. Rabkin CS, Telzak EE, Ho MS, et al. Outbreak of echovirus 11 infection in hospitalized neonates. Pediatr Infect Dis J 7:186, 1988.
263. Wreghitt TG, Sutehall GM, King A, et al. Fatal echovirus 7 infection during an outbreak in a special care baby unit. J Infect 19:229, 1989.
264. Wilson CW, Stevenson DK, Arvin AM. A concurrent epidemic of respiratory syncytial virus and echovirus 7 infections in an intensive care nursery. Pediatr Infect Dis J 8:24, 1989.
265. Isaacs D, Wilkinson AR, Eglin R, et al. Conservative management of an echovirus 11 outbreak in a neonatal unit. Lancet 1:543, 1989.
266. Sato K, Yamashita T, Sakae K, et al. A new-born baby outbreak of echovirus type 33 infection. J Infect 37:123, 1998.
267. Verlinde JD, Versteeg J, Beeuwkes H. Mogelijkheid van een besmetting van de mens door varkens lijdende aan een Coxsackievirus pneumonie. Ned Tijdschr Geneeskd 102:1445, 1958.
268. Moscovici C, Ginevri A, Felici A, et al. Virus 1956 R.C. Ann Ist Super Sanita 20:1137, 1957.
269. Lundgren DL, Clapper WE, Sanchez A. Isolation of human enteroviruses from beagle dogs. Proc Soc Exp Biol Med 128:463, 1968.
270. Lundgren DL, Sanchez A, Magnuson MG, et al. A survey for human enteroviruses in dogs and man. Arch Gesamte Virusforsch 32:229, 1970.
271. Koprowski H. Counterparts of human viral disease in animals. Ann N Y Acad Sci 70:369, 1958.
272. Sommerville RG. Type I poliovirus isolated from a budgerigar. Lancet 1:495, 1959.
273. Makower H, Skurska Z. Badania nad wirusami Coxsackie. Doniesienie III. Izolacja wirusa Coxsackie z mózgu lisa. Arch Immunol Ter Dosw 5:219, 1957.
274. Bendinelli M, Ruschi A. Isolation of human enterovirus from mussels. Appl Microbiol 18:531, 1969.
275. Metcalf TG, Stiles WC. Enterovirus within an estuarine environment. Am J Epidemiol 88:379, 1968.
276. Horstmann DM, Manuelidis EE. Russian Coxsackie A-7 virus ("AB IV" strain)—neuropathogenicity and comparison with poliovirus. J Immunol 81:32, 1958.
277. Bartell P, Klein M. Neutralizing antibody to viruses of poliomyelitis in sera of domestic animals. Proc Soc Exp Biol Med 90:597, 1955.
278. Morris JA, O'Connor JR. Neutralization of the viruses of the Coxsackie group by sera of wild rabbits. Cornell Vet 42:56, 1952.
279. Chang PW, Liu OC, Miller LT, et al. Multiplication of human enteroviruses in northern quahogs. Proc Soc Exp Biol Med 136:1380, 1971.
280. Metcalf TG, Stiles WC. Accumulation of enteric viruses by the oyster, *Crassostrea virginica.* J Infect Dis 115:68, 1965.
281. Liu OC, Seraichekas HR, Murphy BL. Viral depuration of the Northern quahaug. Appl Microbiol 15:307, 1967.
282. Duff MF. The uptake of enteroviruses by the New Zealand marine blue mussel *Mytilus edulis aoteanus.* Am J Epidemiol 85:486, 1967.
283. Atwood RP, Cherry JD, Klein JO. Clams and viruses. Hepat Surveill Rep 20:26, 1964.
284. Lynt RK. Survival and recovery of enterovirus from foods. Appl Microbiol 14:218, 1966.
285. Kalter SS. A serological survey of antibodies to selected enteroviruses. Bull World Health Organ 26:759, 1962.
286. Fox JP. Epidemiological aspects of coxsackie and ECHO virus infections in tropical areas. Am J Public Health 54:1134, 1964.
287. Centers for Disease Control. Enterovirus Surveillance, Summary 1970-1979. Issued November 1981.
288. Bodian D, Horstmann DM. Poliomyelitis. *In* Horsfall FL, Tamm I (eds). Viral and Rickettsial Infections of Man, 4th ed. Philadelphia, JB Lippincott, 1965, p 430.
289. Christie AB. Acute poliomyelitis. *In* Infectious Diseases: Epidemiology and Clinical Practice. Edinburgh, Churchill Livingstone, 1974, p 567.
290. Assaad F, Ljungars-Esteves K. World overview of poliomyelitis: regional patterns and trends. Rev Infect Dis 6:S302, 1984.
291. Phillips CA, Aronson MD, Tomkow J, et al. Enteroviruses in Vermont, 1969-1978: an important cause of illness throughout the year. J Infect Dis 141:162, 1980.
292. Drebit MA, Nguan CY, Campbell JJ, et al. Molecular epidemiology of enterovirus outbreaks in Canada during 1991-1992: identification of echovirus 30 and coxsackievirus B1 strains by amplicon sequencing. J Med Virol 44:340, 1994.
293. Ishiko H, Takeda N, Miyanura K, et al. Phylogenetic analysis of a coxsackievirus A24 variant: the most recent worldwide pandemic was caused by progenies of a virus prevalent around 1981. Virology 187: 748, 1992.
294. Lin KH, Wang HL, Sheu MM, et al. Molecular epidemiology of a variant of coxsackievirus A24 in Taiwan: two epidemics caused by phylogenetically distinct viruses from 1985 to 1989. J Clin Microbiol 31:1160, 1993.
295. Mulders MN, Lipskaya GY, van der Avoort HGAM, et al. Molecular epidemiology of wild poliovirus type 1 in Europe, the Middle East, and the Indian subcontinent. J Infect Dis 171:1399, 1995.
296. Druyts-Voets E. Epidemiological features of entero non-poliovirus isolations in Belgium 1980-94. Epidemiol Infect 119:71, 1997.
297. Trallero G, Casas I, Tenorio A, et al. Enteroviruses in Spain: virological and epidemiological studies over 10 years (1988-97). Epidemiol Infect 124:497, 2000.
298. Brown BA, Steven Oberste M, Alexander JP Jr, et al. Molecular epidemiology and evolution of enterovirus 71 strains isolated from 1970 to 1998. J Virol 73:9969, 1999.
299. Chan LG, Parashar UD, Lye MS, et al. Deaths of children during an outbreak of hand, foot, and mouth disease in Sarawak, Malaysia: clinical and pathological characteristics of the disease. Clin Infect Dis 31:678, 2000.
300. Ho M, Chen ER, Hsu KH, et al. An epidemic of enterovirus 71 infection in Taiwan. N Engl J Med 341:929, 1999.

301. Komatsu H, Shimizu Y, Takeuchi Y, et al. Outbreak of severe neurologic involvement associated with enterovirus 71 infection. Pediatr Neurol 20:17, 1999.
302. McMinn P, Stratov I, Nagarajan L, et al. Neurological manifestations of enterovirus 71 infection in children during an outbreak of hand, foot, and mouth disease in Western Australia. Clin Infect Dis 32:236, 2001.
303. Strikas RA, Anderson LJ, Parker RA. Temporal and geographic patterns of isolates of nonpolio enterovirus in the United States, 1970-1983. J Infect Dis 153:346, 1986.
304. Center for Disease Control. Neurotropic Diseases Surveillance, No. 3. Annual Summary. Washington, DC, U.S. Department of Health, Education, and Welfare, 1970.
305. Communicable Disease Center. Poliomyelitis Surveillance, No. 274. Washington, DC, U.S. Department of Health, Education, and Welfare, 1963.
306. Horstmann DB, Emmons J, Gimpel L, et al. Enterovirus surveillance following a community-wide oral poliovirus vaccination program: a seven-year study. Am J Epidemiol 97:173, 1973.
307. Batcup G, Holt P, Hambling MH, et al. Placental and fetal pathology in coxsackie virus A9 infection: a case report. Histopathology 9:1227, 1985.
308. Ramsingh AI, Collins DN. A point mutation in the VP4 coding sequence of coxsackievirus B4 influences virulence. J Virol 69:7278, 1995.
309. Rinehart JE, Gomez RM, Roos RP. Molecular determinants for virulence in coxsackievirus B1 infection. J Virol 71:3986, 1997.
310. Santti J, Hyypiä T, Kinnunen L, et al. Evidence of recombination among enteroviruses. J Virol 73:8741, 1999.
311. Heineberg H, Gold E, Robbins FC. Differences in interferon content in tissues of mice of various ages infected with coxsackie B1 virus. Proc Soc Exp Biol Med 115:947, 1964.
312. Behbehani AM, Sulkin SE, Wallis C. Factors influencing susceptibility of mice to coxsackie virus infection. J Infect Dis 110:147, 1962.
313. Boring WD, Angevine DM, Walker DL. Factors influencing host-virus interactions. I. A comparison of viral multiplication and histopathology in infant, adult, and cortisone-treated adult mice infected with the Conn-5 strain of coxsackie virus. J Exp Med 102:753, 1955.
314. Kunin CW. Cellular susceptibility to enteroviruses. Bacteriol Rev 28: 382, 1964.
315. Kunin CM. Virus-tissue union and the pathogenesis of enterovirus infections. J Immunol 88:556, 1962.
316. Teisner B, Haahr S. Poikilothermia and susceptibility of suckling mice to coxsackie B1 virus. Nature 247:568, 1974.
317. Arola A, Kalimo H, Ruuskanen O, et al. Experimental myocarditis induced by two different coxsackievirus B3 variants: aspects of pathogenesis and comparison of diagnostic methods. J Med Virol 47:251, 1995.
318. Gauntt CJ, Arizpe HM, Higdon AL, et al. Molecular mimicry, anti-coxsackievirus B3 neutralizing monoclonal antibodies, and myocarditis. J Immunol 154:2983, 1995.
319. Gauntt CJ, Higdon AL, Arizpe HM, et al. Epitopes shared between coxsackievirus B3 (CVB3) and normal heart tissue contribute to CVB3-induced murine myocarditis. Clin Immunol Immunopathol 68:129, 1993.
320. Henke A, Huber S, Stelzner A, et al. The role of CD8+ T lymphocytes in coxsackievirus B3-induced myocarditis. J Virol 69:6720, 1995.
321. Hosier DM, Newton WA Jr. Serious coxsackie infection in infants and children: myocarditis, meningoencephalitis, and hepatitis. Am J Dis Child 96:251, 1958.
322. Pague RE. Role of anti-idiotypic antibodies in induction, regulation, and expression of coxsackievirus-induced myocarditis. Prog Med Virol 39:204, 1992.
323. Rabausch-Starz I, Scwaiger A, Grünewald K, et al. Persistence of virus and viral genome in myocardium after coxsackievirus B3-induced murine myocarditis. Clin Exp Immunol 96:69, 1994.
324. Seko Y, Yoshifumi E, Yagita H, et al. Restricted usage of T-cell receptor Va genes in infiltrating cells in murine hearts with acute myocarditis caused by coxsackie virus B3. J Pathol 178:330, 1996.
325. Neu N, Beisel KW, Traystman MD, et al. Autoantibodies specific for the cardiac myosin isoform are found in mice susceptible to coxsackievirus B3-induced myocarditis. J Immunol 183:2488, 1987.
326. Herskowitz A, Beisel KW, Wolfgram LJ, et al. Coxsackievirus B3 murine myocarditis: wide pathologic spectrum in genetically defined inbred strains. Hum Pathol 16:671, 1985.
327. Wolfgram LJ, Rose NR. Coxsackievirus infection as a trigger of cardiac autoimmunity. Immunol Res 8:61, 1989.
328. Chehadeh W, Weill J, Vantyghem MC, et al. Increased level of interferon-alpha in blood of patients with insulin-dependent diabetes mellitus: relationship with coxsackievirus B infection. J Infect Dis 181:1929, 2000.
329. Hober D, Andréoletti L, Shen L, et al. Coxsackievirus B3-induced chronic myocarditis in mouse: use of whole blood culture to study the activation of TNF alpha-producing cells. Microbiol Immunol 40:837, 1996.
330. Juhela S, Hyöty H, Roivainen M, et al. T-cell responses to enterovirus antigens in children with type 1 diabetes. Diabetes 49:1308, 2000.
331. Lane JR, Neumann DA, Lafond-Walker A, et al. Role of IL-1 and tumor necrosis factor in coxsackie virus-induced autoimmune myocarditis. J Immunol 151:1682, 1993.
332. Roivainen M, Knip M, Hyöty H, et al. Several different enterovirus serotypes can be associated with prediabetic autoimmune episodes and onset of overt IDDM. Childhood Diabetes in Finland (DiMe) Study Group. J Med Virol 56:74, 1998.
333. McManus BM, Chow LH, Wilson JE, et al. Direct myocardial injury by enterovirus: a central role in the evolution of murine myocarditis. Clin Immunol Immunopathol 68:159, 1993.
334. Kew O, Morris-Glasgow V, Landaverde M, et al. Outbreak of poliomyelitis in Hispaniola associated with circulating type 1 vaccine-derived poliovirus. Science 296:356, 2002.
335. Balduzzi PC, Greendyke RM. Sudden unexpected death in infancy and viral infection. Pediatrics 38:201, 1966.
336. Gold E, Carver DH, Heineberg H, et al. Viral infection: a possible cause of sudden, unexpected death in infants. N Engl J Med 264:53, 1961.
337. Baker DA, Phillips CA. Maternal and neonatal infection with coxsackievirus. Obstet Gynecol 55:12S, 1980.
338. Eisenhut M, Algawi G, Wreghitt T, et al. Fatal coxsackie A9 virus infection during an outbreak in a neonatal unit. J Infect 40:297, 2000.
339. Estes ML, Rorke LB. Liquefactive necrosis in coxsackie B encephalitis. Arch Pathol Lab Med 110:1090, 1986.
340. Lake AM, Lauer BA, Clark JC, et al. Enterovirus infections in neonates. J Pediatr 89:787, 1976.
341. Iwasaki T, Monma N, Satodate R, et al. An immunofluorescent study of generalized coxsackie virus B3 infection in a newborn infant. Acta Pathol Jpn 35:741, 1985.
342. Konen O, Rathaus V, Bauer S, et al. Progressive liver calcifications in neonatal coxsackievirus infection. Pediatr Radiol 30:343, 2000.
343. Krous HF, Dietzman D, Ray CG. Fatal infections with echovirus types 6 and 11 in early infancy. Am J Dis Child 126:842, 1973.
344. Berry PJ, Nagington J. Fatal infection with echovirus 11. Arch Dis Child 57:22, 1982.
345. Gh MM, Lack EE, Gang DL, et al. Postmortem manifestations of echovirus 11 sepsis in five newborn infants. Hum Pathol 14:818, 1983.
346. Halfon N, Spector SA. Fatal echovirus type 11 infections. Am J Dis Child 135:1017, 1981.
347. Gitlin N, Visveshwara N, Kassel SH, et al. Fulminant neonatal hepatic necrosis associated with echovirus type 11 infection. West J Med 138:260, 1983.
348. Wang J, Atchinson R, Walpusk J, et al. Echovirus hepatic failure in infancy: report of four cases with speculation on the pathogenesis. Pediatr Dev Pathol 4:454, 2001.
349. Ventura K, Hawkins H, Smith M, et al. Fatal neonatal echovirus 6 infection: autopsy case report and review of the literature. Mod Pathol 14:85, 2001.
350. Rawls WE, Shorter RG, Herrmann EC Jr. Fatal neonatal illness associated with ECHO 9 (coxsackie A-23) virus. Pediatrics 33:278, 1964.
351. Georgieff MK, Johnson DE, Thompson TR, et al. Fulminant hepatic necrosis in an infant with perinatally acquired echovirus 21 infection. Pediatr Infect Dis 6:71, 1987.
352. Chambon M, Delage C, Bailly J, et al. Fatal hepatitis necrosis in a neonate with echovirus 20 infection: use of the polymerase chain reaction to detect enterovirus in the liver tissue. Clin Infect Dis 24:523, 1997.
353. Verboon-Maciolek MA, Swanink CM, Krediet TG, et al. Severe neonatal echovirus 20 infection characterized by hepatic failure. Pediatr Infect Dis J 16:524, 1997.
354. Wreghitt TG, Gandy GM, King A, et al. Fatal neonatal echo 7 virus infection. Lancet 2:465, 1984.
355. Boyd MT, Jordan SW, Davis LE. Fatal pneumonitis from congenital echovirus type 6 infection. Pediatr Infect Dis J 6:1138, 1987.
356. Aycock WL, Ingalls TH. Maternal disease as a principle in the epidemiology of congenital anomalies. Am J Med Sci 212:366, 1946.

357. Bowers VM Jr, Danforth DN. The significance of poliomyelitis during pregnancy—an analysis of the literature and presentation of twenty-four new cases. Am J Obstet Gynecol 65:34, 1953.
358. Schaefer J, Shaw EB. Poliomyelitis in pregnancy. Calif Med 70:16, 1949.
359. Anderson GW, Anderson G, Skaar A, et al. Poliomyelitis in pregnancy. Am J Hyg 55:127, 1952.
360. Kaye BM, Rosner DC, Stein I Sr. Viral diseases in pregnancy and their effect upon the embryo and fetus. Am J Obstet Gynecol 65:109, 1953.
361. Harjulehto-Mervaala T, Aro T, Hiilesmaa VK, et al. Oral polio vaccination during pregnancy: lack of impact on fetal development and perinatal outcome. Clin Infect Dis 18:414, 1994.
362. Frisk G, Diderholm H. Increased frequency of coxsackie B virus IgM in women with spontaneous abortion. J Infect 24:141, 1992.
363. Axelsson C, Bondestam K, Frisk G, et al. Coxsackie B virus infections in women with miscarriage. J Med Virol 39:282, 1993.
364. Berendes HW, Weiss W. The NIH collaborative study. A progress report. In Congenital Malformations. Proceedings of the Third International Conference on Congenital Malformations. The Hague, Netherlands, September 7-13, 1969. Fraser FC, McKusick VA, Eds. Excerpta Medica International Congress Series No. 204, 1969:293-298.
365. News and Notes. Polio vaccine and congenital defects. BMJ 1:510, 1967.
366. Connelly JP, Reynolds S, Crawford JD, et al. Viral and drug hazards in pregnancy. Clin Pediatr 3:587, 1964.
367. Harjulehto T, Hovi T, Aro T, et al. Congenital malformations and oral poliovirus vaccination during pregnancy. Lancet 1:771, 1989.
368. Brown GC. Maternal virus infection and congenital anomalies. Arch Environ Health 21:362, 1970.
369. Brown GC. Recent advances in the viral aetiology of congenital anomalies. Adv Teratol 1:55, 1966.
370. Brown GC. Coxsackie virus infections and heart disease. Am Heart J 75:145, 1968.
371. Evans TN, Brown GC. Congenital anomalies and virus infections. Am J Obstet Gynecol 87:749, 1963.
372. Brown GC, Evans TN. Serologic evidence of coxsackievirus etiology of congenital heart disease. JAMA 199:183, 1967.
373. Brown GC, Karunas RS. Relationship of congenital anomalies and maternal infection with selected enteroviruses. Am J Epidemiol 95: 207, 1972.
374. Elizan TS, Ajero-Froehlich L, Fabiyi A, et al. Viral infection in pregnancy and congenital CNS malformations in man. Arch Neurol 20:115, 1969.
375. Gauntt CJ, Gudvangen RJ, Brans YW, et al. Coxsackievirus group B antibodies in the ventricular fluid of infants with severe anatomic defects in the central nervous system. Pediatrics 76:64, 1985.
376. Aycock WL. Acute poliomyelitis in pregnancy: its occurrence according to month of pregnancy and sex of fetus. N Engl J Med 235:160, 1946.
377. Freedman PS. Echovirus 11 infection and intrauterine death. Lancet 1:96, 1979.
378. Morens DM. Enteroviral disease in early infancy. J Pediatr 92:374, 1978.
379. Barton LL. Febrile neonatal illness associated with echo virus type 5 in the cerebrospinal fluid. Clin Pediatr 16:383, 1977.
380. Farmer K, Patten PT. An outbreak of coxsackie B5 infection in a special care unit for newborn infants. N Z Med J 68:86, 1968.
381. Hinuma Y, Murai Y, Nakao T. Two outbreaks of echovirus 14 infection: a possible interference with oral poliovirus vaccine and a probable association with aseptic meningitis. J Hyg (Lond) 63:277, 1965.
382. Eilard T, Kyllerman M, Wennerblom I, et al. An outbreak of coxsackie virus type B2 among neonates in an obstetrical ward. Acta Paediatr Scand 63:103, 1974.
383. Linnemann CC Jr, Steichen J, Sherman WG, et al. Febrile illness in early infancy associated with ECHO virus infection. J Pediatr 84:49, 1974.
384. News and Notes. Coxsackie B virus infections in 1971. BMJ 1:453, 1972.
385. Hall CB, Cherry JD, Hatch MH, et al. The return of Boston exanthem. Am J Dis Child 131:323, 1977.
386. Abzug MJ, Levin MJ, Rotbart HA. Profile of enterovirus disease in the first two weeks of life. Pediatr Infect Dis J 12:820, 1993.
387. Haddad J, Gut JP, Wendling MJ, et al. Enterovirus infections in neonates: a retrospective study of 21 cases. Eur J Med 2:209, 1993.
388. Barre V, Marret S, Mendel I, et al. Enterovirus-associated haemophagocytic syndrome in a neonate. Acta Paediatr 87:467, 1998.
389. Cho CT, Janelle JG, Behbehani A. Severe neonatal illness associated with ECHO 9 virus infection. Clin Pediatr 12:304, 1973.
390. Codd AA, Hale JH, Bell TM, et al. Epidemic of echovirus 19 in the northeast of England. J Hyg (Lond) 76:307, 1976.
391. Marier R, Rodriguez W, Chloupek RJ, et al. Coxsackievirus B5 infection and aseptic meningitis in neonates and children. Am J Dis Child 129: 321, 1975.
392. Bacon CJ, Sims DG. Echovirus 19 infection in infants under six months. Arch Dis Child 51:631, 1976.
393. Grossman M, Azimi P. Fever, hepatitis and coagulopathy in a newborn infant. Pediatr Infect Dis J 11:1069, 1992.
394. Wong SN, Tam AYC, Ng THK, et al. Fatal coxsackie B1 virus infection in neonates. Pediatr Infect Dis J 8:638, 1989.
395. Bauer S, Gottesman G, Sirota L, et al. Severe coxsackie virus B infection in preterm newborns treated with pleconaril. Eur J Pediatr 161:491, 2002.
396. Chawareewong S, Kiangsiri S, Lokaphadhana K, et al. Neonatal herpangina caused by coxsackie A-5 virus. J Pediatr 93:492, 1978.
397. Murray D, Altschul M, Dyke J. Aseptic meningitis in a neonate with an oral vesicular lesion. Diagn Microbiol Infect Dis 3:77, 1985.
398. Nakayama T, Urano T, Osano M, et al. Outbreak of herpangina associated with coxsackievirus B3 infection. Pediatr Infect Dis J 8:495, 1989.
399. Cramblett HG, Moffet HL, Middleton GK Jr, et al. ECHO 19 virus infections. Arch Intern Med 110:574, 1962.
400. Suzuki N, Ishikawa K, Horiuchi T, et al. Age-related symptomatology of ECHO 11 virus infection in children. Pediatrics 65:284, 1980.
401. Medearis DN Jr, Kramer RA. Exanthem associated with ECHO virus type 18 viremia. J Pediatr 55:367, 1959.
402. Eckert HL, Portnoy B, Salvatore MA, et al. Group B Coxsackie virus infection in infants with acute lower respiratory disease. Pediatrics 39:526, 1967.
403. Mirani M, Ogra PL, Barron AL. Epidemic of echovirus type 9 infection: certain clinical and epidemiologic features. N Y J Med 73:403, 1973.
404. Ramos-Alvarez M. Cytopathogenic enteric viruses associated with undifferentiated diarrheal syndromes in early childhood. Ann N Y Acad Sci 67:326, 1957.
405. Chonmaitree T, Menegus MA, Schervish-Swierkosz EM, et al. Enterovirus 71 infection: report of an outbreak with two cases of paralysis and a review of the literature. Pediatrics 67:489, 1981.
406. Arnon R, Naor N, Davidson S, et al. Fatal outcome of neonatal echovirus 19 infection. Pediatr Infect Dis J 10:788, 1991.
407. Aradottir E, Alonso E, Shulman S. Severe neonatal enteroviral hepatitis treated with pleconaril. Pediatr Infect Dis J 20:e457, 2001.
408. Abzug MJ. Prognosis for neonates with enterovirus hepatitis and coagulopathy. Pediatr Infect Dis J 20:758, 2001.
409. Boccia D, Stolfi I, Lana S, et al. Nosocomial necrotising enterocolitis outbreaks: epidemiology and control measures. Eur J Pediatr 160:385, 2001.
410. Talsma M, Vegting M, Hess J. Generalised coxsackie A9 infection in a neonate presenting with pericarditis. Br Heart J 52:683, 1984.
411. Barson WJ, Craenen J, Hosier DM, et al. Survival following myocarditis and myocardial calcification associated with infection by coxsackie virus B4. Pediatrics 68:79, 1981.
412. Chonmaitree T, Menegus MA, Powell KR. The clinical relevance of "CSF viral culture." A two-year experience with aseptic meningitis in Rochester, N.Y. JAMA 247:1843, 1982.
413. Rantakallio P, Saukkonen AL, Krause U, et al. Follow-up study of 17 cases of neonatal coxsackie B5 meningitis and one with suspected myocarditis. Scand J Infect Dis 2:25, 1970.
414. Drew JH. ECHO 11 virus outbreak in a nursery associated with myocarditis. Aust Paediatr J 9:90, 1973.
415. Cherry JD, Lerner AM, Klein JO, et al. Coxsackie B5 infections with exanthems. Pediatrics 31:445, 1963.
416. Chan SH, Lun KS. Ventricular aneurysm complicating neonatal coxsackie B4 myocarditis. Pediatr Cardiol 22:247, 2001.
417. Theodoridou M, Kakourou T, Laina I, et al. Vesiculopapular rash as a single presentation in intrauterine coxsackie virus infection. Eur J Pediatr 161:412, 2002.
418. Chen CY, Chang YC, Huang CC, et al. Acute flaccid paralysis in infants and young children with enterovirus 71 infection: MR imaging findings and clinical correlates. Am J Neuroradiol 22:200, 2001.
419. Chesney PJ, Quennec P, Clark C. Hypoglycorrhachia and coxsackie B3 meningoencephalitis. Am J Clin Pathol 70:947, 1978.
420. Johnson RT, Shuey HE, Buescher EL. Epidemic central nervous system disease of mixed enterovirus etiology. I. Clinical and epidemiologic description. Am J Hyg 71:321, 1960.
421. Haynes RE, Cramblett HG, Hilty MD, et al. ECHO virus type 3 infections in children: clinical and laboratory studies. J Pediatr 80:589, 1972.
422. Haynes RE, Cramblett HG, Kronfol HJ. Echovirus 9 meningoencephalitis in infants and children. JAMA 208:1657, 1969.
423. Farmer K, MacArthur BA, Clay MM. A follow-up study of 15 cases of neonatal meningoencephalitis due to coxsackie virus B5. J Pediatr 87:568, 1975.

424. Helin I, Widell A, Borulf S, et al. Outbreak of coxsackievirus A-14 meningitis among newborns in a maternity hospital ward. Acta Paediatr Scand 76:234, 1987.
425. Wilfert CM, Lauer BA, Cohen M, et al. An epidemic of echovirus 18 meningitis. J Infect Dis 131:75, 1975.
426. Schmidt NJ, Lennette EH, Ho HH. An apparently new enterovirus isolated from patients with disease of the central nervous system. J Infect Dis 129:304, 1974.
427. Sells CJ, Carpenter RL, Ray CG. Sequelae of central-nervous-system enterovirus infections. N Engl J Med 293:1, 1975.
428. Matsumoto K, Yokochi T, Matsuda S, et al. Characterization of an echovirus type 30 variant isolated from patients with aseptic meningitis. Microbiol Immunol 30:333, 1986.
429. Bowen GS, Fisher MC, Deforest A, et al. Epidemic of meningitis and febrile illness in neonates caused by echo type 11 virus in Philadelphia. Pediatr Infect Dis 2:359, 1983.
430. Sumaya CV, Corman LI. Enteroviral meningitis in early infancy: significance in community outbreaks. Pediatr Infect Dis 1:151, 1982.
431. Bergman I, Painter MJ, Wald ER, et al. Outcome in children with enteroviral meningitis during the first year of life. J Pediatr 110:705, 1987.
432. Wilfert CM, Thompson RJ Jr, Sunder TR, et al. Longitudinal assessment of children with enteroviral meningitis during the first three months of life. Pediatrics 67:811, 1981.
433. Tarcan A, Özbek N, Gürakan B. Bone marrow failure with concurrent enteroviral infection in a newborn. Pediatr Infect Dis J 20:e719, 2001.
434. Schurmann W, Statz A, Mertens T, et al. Two cases of coxsackie B2 infection in neonates: clinical, virological, and epidemiological aspects. Eur J Pediatr 140:59, 1983.
435. Barson WJ, Reiner CB. Coxsackievirus B2 infection in a neonate with incontinentia pigmenti. Pediatrics 77:897, 1986.
436. Blokziji ML, Koskiniemi M. Echovirus 6 encephalitis in a preterm baby. Lancet 2:164, 1989.
437. Ehrnst A, Eriksson M. Echovirus type 23 observed as a nosocomial infection in infants. Scand J Dis 28:205, 1996.
438. Grangeot-Keros L, Broyer M, Briand E, et al. Enterovirus in sudden unexpected deaths in infants. Pediatr Infect Dis J 15:123, 1996.
439. Paul JR. Epidemiology of poliomyelitis. Monogr Ser World Health Organ 26:9, 1955.
440. Mullins JA, Khetsuriani N, Nix WA, et al. Emergence of echovirus type 13 as a prominent enterovirus. Clin Infect Dis 38:70, 2004.
441. Kirschke DL, Jones TF, Buckingham SC, et al. Outbreak of aseptic meningitis associated with echovirus 13. Pediatr Infect Dis J 21:1034, 2002.
442. Somekh E, Cesar K, Handsher R, et al. An outbreak of echovirus 13 meningitis in central Israel. Epidemiol Infect 130:257, 2003.
443. Trallero G, Casas I, Avellón CA, et al. First epidemic of aseptic meningitis due to echovirus type 13 among Spanish children. Epidemiol Infect 130:251, 2003.
444. Weibel RE, Benor DE. Reporting vaccine-associated paralytic poliomyelitis: concordance between the CDC and the National Vaccine Injury Compensation Program. Am J Public Health 86:734, 1996.
445. Sabin AB, Krumbiegel ER, Wigand R. ECHO type 9 virus disease. Am J Dis Child 96:197, 1958.
446. Drouhet V. Enterovirus infection and associated clinical symptoms in children. Ann Inst Pasteur 98:562, 1960.
447. Chonmaitree T, Ford C, Sanders C, et al. Comparison of cell cultures for rapid isolation of enteroviruses. J Clin Microbiol 26:2576, 1988.
448. Johnson FB. Transport of viral specimens. Clin Microbiol Rev 3:120, 1990.
449. Howell CL, Miller MJ. Effect of sucrose phosphate and sorbitol on infectivity of enveloped viruses during storage. J Clin Microbiol 18: 658, 1983.
450. August MJ, Warford AL. Evaluation of a commercial monoclonal antibody for detection of adenovirus antigen. J Clin Microbiol 25:2233, 1987.
451. Herrmann EC Jr. Experience in providing a viral diagnostic laboratory compatible with medical practice. Mayo Clin Proc 42:112, 1967.
452. Trabelsi A, Grattard F, Nejmeddine M, et al. Evaluation of an enterovirus group-specific anti-VPI monoclonal antibody, 5-D8/1, in comparison with neutralization and PCR for rapid identification of enteroviruses in cell culture. J Clin Microbiol 33:2454, 1995.
453. Carstens JM, Tracy S, Chapman NM, et al. Detection of enteroviruses in cell cultures by using in situ transcription. J Clin Microbiol 30:25, 1992.
454. De L, Nottay B, Yang CF, et al. Identification of vaccine-related polioviruses by hybridization with specific RNA probes. J Clin Microbiol 33:562, 1995.
455. Rotbart HA. Nucleic acid detection systems for enteroviruses. Clin Microbiol Rev 4:156, 1991.
456. Petitjean J, Freymuth F, Kopecka H, et al. Detection of enteroviruses in cerebrospinal fluids: enzymatic amplification and hybridization with a biotinylated riboprobe. Mol Cell Probes 8:15B22, 1994.
457. Redline RW, Genest DR, Tycko B. Detection of enteroviral infection in paraffin-embedded tissue by the RNA polymerase chain reaction technique. Am J Clin Pathol 96:568, 1991.
458. Muir P, Nicholson F, Jhetam M, et al. Rapid diagnosis of enterovirus infection by magnetic bead extraction and polymerase chain reaction detection of enterovirus RNA in clinical specimens. J Clin Microbiol 31:31, 1993.
459. Muir P, Ras A, Klapper PE, et al. Multicenter quality assessment of PCR methods for detection of enteroviruses. J Clin Microbiol 37:1409, 1999.
460. Martin AB, Webber S, Fricker FJ, et al. Acute myocarditis: rapid diagnosis by PCR in children. Circulation 90:330, 1994.
461. Abraham R, Chonmaitree T, McCombs J, et al. Rapid detection of poliovirus by reverse transcription and polymerase chain amplification: application for the differentiation between poliovirus and nonpoliovirus enteroviruses. J Clin Microbiol 31:295, 1993.
462. Chezzi C. Rapid diagnosis of poliovirus infection by PCR amplification. J Clin Microbiol 34:1722, 1996.
463. Egger D, Pasamontes L, Ostermayer M, et al. Reverse transcription multiplex PCR for differentiation between polio and enteroviruses from clinical and environmental samples. J Clin Microbiol 33:1442, 1995.
464. Gorgievski-Hrisoho M, Schumacher JD, Vilimomovic N, et al. Detection by PCR of enteroviruses in cerebrospinal fluid during a summer outbreak of aseptic meningitis in Switzerland. J Clin Microbiol 36:2408, 1998.
465. Ramers C, Billman G, Hartin M, et al. Impact of a diagnostic cerebrospinal fluid enterovirus polymerase chain reaction test on patient management. JAMA 283:2680, 2000.
466. Yang CF, De L, Holloway BP, et al. Detection and identification of vaccine-related polioviruses by the polymerase chain reaction. Viral Res 20:159B179, 1991.
467. Samuelson A, Glimåker M, Skoog E, et al. Diagnosis of enteroviral meningitis with IgG-EIA using heat-treated virions and synthetic peptides as antigens. J Med Virol 40:271, 1993.
468. Chan D, Hammond GW. Comparison of serodiagnosis of group B coxsackievirus infections by an immunoglobulin M capture enzyme immunoassay versus microneutralization. J Clin Microbiol 21:830, 1985.
469. Chomel JJ, Thouvenot D, Fayol V, et al. Rapid diagnosis of echovirus type 33 meningitis by specific IgM detection using an enzyme linked immunosorbent assay (ELISA). J Virol Methods 10:11, 1985.
470. Gong CM, Ho DWT, Field PR, et al. Immunoglobulin responses to echovirus type 11 by enzyme linked immunosorbent assay: single-serum diagnosis of acute infection by specific IgM antibody. J Virol Methods 9:209, 1984.
471. Pozzetto B, LeBihan JC, Gaudin OG. Rapid diagnosis of echovirus 33 infection by neutralizing specific IgM antibody. J Med Virol 18:361, 1986.
472. McCartney RA, Banatvala JE, Bell EJ. Routine use of mu-antibody-capture ELISA for the serological diagnosis of Coxsackie B virus infections. J Med Virol 19:205, 1986.
473. Dorries R, Ter Meulen V. Specificity of IgM antibodies in acute human coxsackievirus B infections, analysed by indirect solid phase enzyme immunoassay and immunoblot technique. J Gen Virol 64:159, 1983.
474. Bell EJ, McCartney RA, Basquill D, et al. Mu-antibody capture ELISA for the rapid diagnosis of enterovirus infections in patients with aseptic meningitis. J Med Virol 19:213, 1986.
475. Glimaker M, Ehrnst A, Magnius L, et al. Early diagnosis of enteroviral meningitis by a solid-phase reverse immunosorbent test and virus isolation. Scand J Infect Dis 22:519, 1990.
476. Gaudin O-G, Pozzetto B, Aouni M, et al. Detection of neutralizing IgM antibodies in the diagnosis of enterovirus infections. J Med Virol 28:200, 1989.
477. Martin AB, Webber S, Fricker FJ, et al. Acute myocarditis. Rapid diagnosis by PCR in children. Circulation 90:330, 1994.
478. Chambon M, Delage C, Bailly JL, et al. Fatal hepatic necrosis in a neonate with echovirus 20 infection: use of the polymerase chain reaction to detect enterovirus in liver tissue. Clin Infect Dis 24:523, 1997.

479. Eichenwald HC (ed). The Prevention of Mental Retardation Through Control of Infectious Diseases. Washington, DC, U.S. Government Printing Office, 1966, p 31.
480. Dagan R, Prather SL, Powell KR, et al. Neutralizing antibodies to nonpolio enteroviruses in human immune serum globulin. Pediatr Infect Dis 2:454, 1983.
481. McKinney RE Jr, Katz SL, Wilfert CM. Chronic enteroviral meningoencephalitis in agammaglobulinemic patients. Rev Infect Dis 9:334, 1987.
482. Hammond GW, Lukes H, Wells B, et al. Maternal and neonatal neutralizing antibody titers to selected enteroviruses. Pediatr Infect Dis 4:32, 1985.
483. Johnston JM, Overall JC Jr. Intravenous immunoglobulin in disseminated neonatal echovirus 11 infection. Pediatr Infect Dis J 8:254, 1989.
484. Abzug MJ, Keyerling HL, Lee ML, et al. Neonatal enterovirus infection: virology, serology, and effects of intravenous immune globulin. Clin Infect Dis 20:1201, 1995.
485. Jantausch BA, Luban NLC, Duffy L, et al. Maternal plasma transfusion in the treatment of disseminated neonatal echovirus 11 infection. Pediatr Infect Dis J 14:154, 1995.
486. Chuang E, Maller ES, Hoffman MA, et al. Successful treatment of fulminant echovirus 11 infection in a neonate by orthotopic liver transplantation. J Pediatr Gastroenterol Nutr 17:211, 1993.
487. Kearns GL, Bradley JS, Jacobs RF, et al. Single dose pharmacokinetics of pleconaril in neonates. Pediatric Pharmacology Research Unit Network. Pediatr Infect Dis J 19:833, 2000.
488. Pevear DC, Tull TM, Seipel ME, et al. Activity of pleconaril against enteroviruses. Antimicrob Agents Chemother 43:2109, 1999.
489. Rotbart HA, Abzug MJ, Levin MJ. Development and application of RNA probes for the study of picornaviruses. Mol Cell Probes 2:65, 1988.
490. Kilbourne ED, Wilson CB, Perrier D. The induction of gross myocardial lesions by a Coxsackie (pleurodynia) virus and cortisone. J Clin Invest 35:367, 1956.
491. Mason JW, O'Connell JB, Herskowitz A, et al. A clinical trial of immunosuppressive therapy for myocarditis. N Engl J Med 333:269, 1995.
492. Carolane DJ, Long AM, McKeever PA, et al. Prevention of spread of echovirus 6 in a special care baby unit. Arch Dis Child 60:674, 1985.
493. Nagington J, Walker J, Gandy G, et al. Use of normal immunoglobulin in an echovirus 11 outbreak in a special-care baby unit. Lancet 2:443, 1983.
494. Pasic S, Jankovic B, Abinun M, et al. Intravenous immunoglobulin prophylaxis in an echovirus 6 and echovirus 4 nursery outbreak. Pediatr Infect Dis J 16:718, 1997.

Chapter 25

HEPATITIS

John S. Bradley

Scientific and medical knowledge about the genetic composition, molecular structure, pathogenesis, and natural history of infection has dramatically increased over the past decade for the hepatotropic viruses (Table 25-1). Six viral agents have been documented or suspected to cause hepatitis as the primary clinical manifestation of infection in children and adults: hepatitis A virus (HAV); hepatitis B virus (HBV); hepatitis C virus (HCV); hepatitis D virus (HDV), an agent found to infect only patients simultaneously infected with HBV; hepatitis E virus (HEV); and hepatitis G virus (HGV), also known as GB virus type C (GB being the initials of the patient from whom the prototype virus in this group was first isolated). Fortunately, these viruses rarely cause transplacental in utero infection. As a result of the almost universal inoculation of the vaginally born infant with maternal blood, vaginal secretions, and stool, however, most of these agents may be transmitted perinatally (at the time of labor and delivery) when present in the mother.

This chapter reviews the characteristics of each of these viruses, pathogenesis and transmission of the disease, nature of the clinical illness, and diagnosis, therapy, and prevention of the infection.

HEPATITIS A

The Virus

HAV was first identified in the stool of a patient with the acute phase of hepatitis A (Fig. 25-1).[8] Although the size (27 nm in diameter), density, and structure (genetic organization, absence of lipid envelope) are similar to those of enteroviruses, HAV does not share any cross-reactive antigens, nucleic acid, or protein sequences with the enteroviruses.[2,19] It is classified as a picornavirus within the genus *Hepatovirus*.[4] The positive-sense, single-stranded RNA is 7.5 kilobases long and is composed of a single open reading frame, coding for at least four structural (VP1, VP2, VP3, and VP4) and seven nonstructural proteins (including an RNA polymerase and a protease).[3] The structural proteins are cleaved from a single precursor protein by the viral protease, with the capsid proteins VP1 and VP3 representing the antigenic structure against which neutralizing antibody is directed.[4] Although only one serotype is known to exist, genetic variability derives from isolates around the world, which have been categorized into four human genotypes.[3] HAV has been cultured in a variety of human and nonhuman primate cells in vitro.[32]

Pathogenesis

Virus is ingested, enters the gastrointestinal tract, and is transported from the gut to the liver where hepatocyte entry occurs.[4] The cellular receptor involved in viral uptake is a membrane glycoprotein of unknown function.[26] The pathogenesis of HAV-mediated liver injury is not well understood. HAV can be detected in the liver, bile, blood, and stool as early as 2 weeks after exposure following release of virions from hepatocytes into both bile and blood. HAV replication may occur within the hepatocyte without evidence of cell

Table 25–1 Hepatitis Viruses

Virus	Virus Structure	Primary Route of Neonatal Infection	Transmission in Children and Adults
HAV (picornavirus, genus *Hepatovirus*)	SS RNA, nonenveloped	Perinatal	Fecal-oral
HBV (*Hepadnavirus*)	DS circular DNA, enveloped	Perinatal	Blood-borne
HCV (flavivirus, genus *Hepacivirus*)	SS RNA, enveloped	Perinatal	Blood-borne
HDV (*Deltavirus*)	SS, circular RNA (HBV envelope)	Not reported	Blood-borne
HEV (provisionally togavirus)	SS RNA, nonenveloped	In utero; perinatal	Fecal-oral
HGV (flavivirus)	SS RNA, nonenveloped	In utero; perinatal	Blood-borne, sexual

DS, double-stranded; HAV, hepatitis A virus; HBV, hepatitis B virus; HCV, hepatitis C virus; HDV, hepatitis D virus; HEV, hepatitis E virus; HGV, hepatitis G virus (GB virus type C); SS, single-stranded.

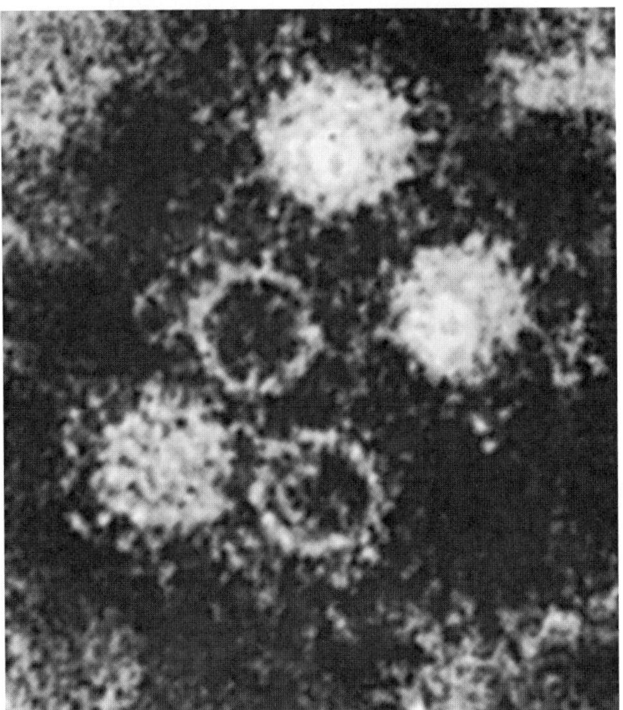

Figure 25–1 Hepatitis A virus (HAV) particles. Electron micrograph of the 27-nm HAV virions in a stool specimen. (Reprinted with permission from Feinstone SM, Kapikian AZ, Purcell RH. Hepatitis A: detection by immune electron microscopy of a viruslike antigen associated with acute illness. Science 182:1026. Copyright 1973 by the American Association for the Advancement of Science.)

injury; most tissue-cultured strains of HAV are not cytotoxic. Some clinical or environmental isolates are clearly cytopathic, however.[5] The role of the immune system in clearing the infection is poorly understood. The anti-HAV immune response in adults consists of specific cellular and humoral responses.[28,34] Hepatocyte injury is thought to be a result of of cytotoxic T cell responses.[34]

In one study of 11 acutely infected adults,[20] for the first 70 days after the appearance of jaundice, virus titers in serum were detectable in the range of 1×10^3 to 3×10^4 genome equivalents per mL. During the subsequent 4 months, the viral load generally decreased, although in 4 patients, the load increased after an apparent earlier decline, despite the presence of circulating antibody. In 3 patients, virus could be detected in blood for longer than 6 months. In these patients, anti-HAV immunoglobulin M (IgM) and total anti-HAV antibody also were measured, in addition to liver function testing. A correlation was found between peak serum virus and peak serum aminotransferase levels; however, peak anti-HAV IgM levels did not correlate with a decreasing viral load. Instead, viral loads decreased with increasing total anti-HAV antibody, suggesting a greater role for anti-HAV IgG, or specific antibody in the context of an ongoing cellular response, which was not assessed in these patients. Primate model evidence suggests that virus particles excreted into the bile and intestine may again be absorbed through the gut and transported back to the liver in an enterohepatic circulation, providing a mechanism for autoinoculation.[4]

The biochemical and histologic changes in hepatitis occur with the onset of the anti-HAV immune response. The histopathologic findings in HAV infection are nonspecific and include focal hepatocellular necrosis with balloon degeneration and hepatocyte regeneration, accompanied by a predominantly mononuclear inflammatory infiltrate. The areas of most marked inflammation are periportal.

Transmission

Hepatitis A is spread by the fecal-oral route. Transmission occurs by direct contact with a person with an acute HAV infection, such as an infected infant in a daycare center environment, or by ingestion of contaminated food and water.[4,18,24] The stool is highly contagious; in prospective evaluations of fecal excretion in symptomatic older children and adults, as well as in experimental animals, investigators found stool containing up to 10^8 HAV genome equivalents per mL.[16,31] Following infection, children may excrete virus for a more prolonged period than has been noted in adults; investigators unexpectedly also found HCV DNA in the stool during the second week of illness more often in children than in adults.[31] Excretion in the stool may be particularly prolonged in neonates. HAV RNA was detected in neonatal stool samples for 4 to 5 months in 23% of babies diagnosed with HAV infection.[22] In addition to prolonged excretion in clinically silent infection, transmission is facilitated by the fact that the quantity of virus in stool is highest before HAV-mediated illness becomes clinically detectable in children and adults, before the development of elevated serum concentrations of transaminases or bilirubin.[21,31] To further facilitate transmission, HAV is known to be stable in stool specimens for prolonged periods, as documented by animal infection following inoculation by

HAV-containing stool that had been dried and stored at 77°F for 30 days.[17]

In addition to fecal-oral transmission, parenteral transmission of HAV also is possible, both by blood transfusion and by injection drug use, because viremia has been well documented to occur with acute HAV infection.[4,16,22]

With respect to maternal-infant transmission of HAV, an early study of acute icteric hepatitis during pregnancy assessed six women with acute hepatitis A. All six women were symptomatic with jaundice at the time of hospitalization for delivery and had markedly increased serum alanine aminotransferase (ALT) levels. Clinical or laboratory signs of hepatitis did not develop in any of the infants born to mothers with acute hepatitis A during pregnancy, presumably owing to the fact that viral shedding had decreased substantially by the time clinical symptoms appeared.[33] Perinatal transmission, however, was documented in a neonate in the course of an investigation of a nursery outbreak of HAV, finding that the infant's mother had been diagnosed with an acute HAV infection 10 days before delivery.[35] Perinatal transmission also has been documented in infants born to mothers diagnosed with infection at 4 months before delivery[7] or at the time of delivery.[30] In both of these reports, the infants were asymptomatic for the first weeks of life, with documentation in one report[30] of the absence of HAV RNA in cord blood. Other reports have documented intrauterine transmission with fetal infection associated with polyhydramnios and ascites at 27 weeks of gestation, following maternal infection at 20 weeks of gestation.[15] Prospectively collected epidemiologic data on the true incidence of neonatal HAV infection following maternal infection, acquired either in utero or perinatally at the time of delivery, are not available.

Although a neonate may become infected from transfusion or from vertical transmission as outlined, spread within nurseries to other infants and health care workers also has been documented. Outbreaks of HAV infection once the virus was introduced into the nursery have been reported.[13,22,25]

No cases of transmission from breast milk as the sole means of exposure of the neonate to infectious virus have been reported.

Clinical Illness

Although biopsy-proven clinical HAV infection in a neonate has been reported,[7] the true incidence of clinical disease in HAV-infected neonates is unknown, because no prospective evaluation in exposed neonates has been possible. In infants and children, particularly those younger than 3 years of age, less than 20% are clinically symptomatic following infection[9,10,12] —far lower than in adults, of whom between 76% and 97% have clinical illness, with icterus in 40% to 70%.[4,14] The average incubation period from exposure to onset of symptoms is 30 days, with a range of 15 to 50 days. Nonspecific signs and symptoms associated with infection include fever, anorexia, nausea, myalgia, diarrhea, and abdominal discomfort. In adults, these symptoms may be present 5 to 7 days before the onset of jaundice. Duration of disease varies considerably, averaging 30 days in adults, but is shorter in children. Elevated values on liver function tests and abnormalities on liver biopsy, however, may persist in some cases for several months.[4] Approximately 100 cases of fulminant HAV infection with liver failure occur each year in the United States, representing less than 1% of cases of HAV infection. Acute liver failure occurs more often in older adults or in those with underlying liver disease but has been reported in children as well.[6,23,27]

Chronic, lifelong infection, as has been documented for HBV and HCV, has not been shown to occur with HAV infection.

Laboratory Diagnosis

Hepatitis A is diagnosed in the laboratory by demonstration of serum antibodies to HAV (anti-HAV) by a number of different enzyme immunoassays or radioimmunoassays. The most commonly used test to diagnose HAV infection is the determination of anti-HAV IgM, which is virtually always present at the first sign of clinical disease and persists for 4 to 6 months. The sensitivity and specificity of anti-HAV IgM assay were reported to be 100% and 99%, respectively, in one community outbreak,[29] but similar data are not available for the accuracy of the test in the neonate. Anti-HAV IgG remains detectable for years following infection. Research laboratories also can detect virus in blood or stool by means of reverse transcriptase–polymerase chain reaction (RT-PCR) tests or by in situ hybridization techniques on biopsy samples.

Therapy

No approved antiviral agents are available for treatment of hepatitis A infection. This state of affairs is likely to be a consequence of the widespread availability of effective vaccines and the self-limited nature of this infection.

Prevention of Infection

For infants born to mothers whose symptoms began between 2 weeks before to 1 week after delivery, current recommendations are to administer a single intramuscular injection of immune serum globulin (ISG), 0.02 mL/kg, to the infant, although the efficacy of ISG in this situation has not been documented.[1]

Prevention of infection in infants and health care workers in a nursery outbreak consists of strict infection control measures to prevent fecal-oral transmission of virus from infected infants to susceptible infants. For health care workers, previous immunization with one of the U.S. Food and Drug Administration (FDA)–approved HAV vaccines should be protective for those who are inadvertently exposed to an infected neonate, parent, or sibling and should prevent further nosocomial transmission within the nursery. If an outbreak of hepatitis A is documented in the nursery, postexposure prophylaxis with ISG (0.02 mL/kg) should provide sufficient anti-HAV antibody to prevent or modify illness in non–HAV-immunized, exposed health care workers, or in neonates who may have had close exposure to infectious secretions. No data are available to support the use of vaccine alone for postexposure prophylaxis.[1] Because HAV vaccines have not been tested in the neonate, immune prophylaxis is the only available preventive measure for this population following documented exposure.

HEPATITIS B

The Virus

HBV is a *hepadnavirus*, an enveloped virus that contains a partially double-stranded DNA molecule approximately 3200 nucleotides in length.[96] Although viruses with genetic organization and morphologic structure similar to those of HBV have been identified in birds and other mammals, the host range of HBV is limited to humans, gorillas, and chimpanzees.

The life cycle of HBV is largely understood because of extensive studies in animal models with species-specific hepadnaviruses. Early after infection, the virus infects primarily hepatocytes but also may infect cells of the kidney and pancreas and mononuclear cells. Although the hepatocyte cell surface receptor for HBV remains unknown, several possibilities are under investigation.[64] Following membrane fusion, the virus nucleocapsid ultimately arrives in the nucleus, where the partially double-stranded DNA molecule becomes covalently closed, circular DNA through the action of host cellular DNA repair enzymes, which not only complete the DNA strand but also release the attached viral polymerase.[52,64] This double-stranded DNA may then be associated with cellular histone proteins to form stable minichromosomes, which may represent a feature of intracellular stability of the virus, with implications for viral latency.[64] The double-stranded DNA also serves as the template for host RNA polymerase II, which provides the RNA required for translation to viral proteins and creates the pregenomic RNA destined for encapsidation in the process of forming new viral progeny.

The HBV DNA genome codes for four families of polypeptides (corresponding to overlapping open reading frames): the pre-S/S region proteins, the pre-C/C/e-antigen proteins, the P gene polymerase product, and the X gene product, HBx protein. The pre-S/S region codes for three envelope proteins that exist as both glycosylated and nonglycosylated forms: the large L (pre-S1) protein, the medium (middle) M (pre-S2) protein, and the small S (S, or major) protein.[51,54,64,91,96,103] The serum of patients with acute hepatitis B contains three morphologically distinct forms of virus or viral antigen (Fig. 25-2). These forms are distinct particles that can be readily aggregated by reaction with serum containing specific antibody against the hepatitis B surface antigen (HBsAg). The first particle to be described, and the most common form in the serum, is a spherical 22-nm particle composed of multiple subunits of the S envelope protein.[11] In addition, long microfilaments with the same 22-nm diameter as for the spherical particles can be seen scattered throughout an electron microscopic field. The third particle is a large spherical particle, 42 nm in diameter, with an outer shell and a dense inner core, which represents the complete infectious virus particle. The 22-nm particles are formed from HBsAg composed of 90% S (major) protein, with minor components of the medium and large proteins. About 70% of HBsAg protein on the filamentous and 42-nm particles consists of the S protein.[64]

The pre-C/C open reading frame provides the genetic material for the core protein (P21), which is serologically recognized by the host as HBcAg and is the major protein in the core, or nucleocapsid. The pre-C region also codes for a soluble antigen, detected in the blood as HBeAg.

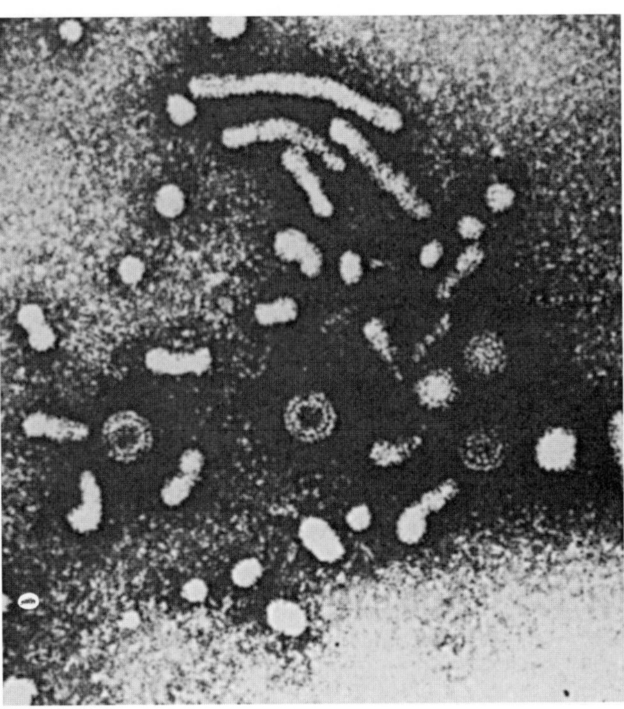

Figure 25–2 Hepatitis B virus (HBV) particles. Electron micrograph from a patient with acute HBV infection demonstrates three circulating particles: 20-nm structures and filamentous structures containing HBsAg envelope proteins (primarily the S, or major protein, but no HBV viral genome); and the 47-nm infectious virion structures containing both envelope proteins and nucleocapsid containing genomic HBV DNA. HBSAg, hepatitis B surface antigen. (Courtesy of Dr. June Almeida.)

The pol gene is the longest-segment open reading frame, coding for a multifunctional 90-kilodalton (kDa) polymerase protein, which has the ability to act as reverse transcriptase (creating double-stranded DNA, which is present in infectious virions), an RNase, and a DNA polymerase.

The X open reading frame leads to the formation of the 154-amino-acid-long nonstructural, regulatory HBx protein. The function of HBx is not well understood,[40] but it appears to be involved as a transactivator for a number of viral and cellular gene promoters, possibly in events that lead to dysregulation of cellular functions. These occurrences over time are believed to be factors leading to the development of hepatocellular carcinoma.

The core protein self-assembles into capsids in the cytoplasm, incorporating pregenomic single-stranded HBV RNA. Following assembly of the caspsid, however, the RNA is transcribed back into DNA by the multifunctional pol gene polymerase (also called the Pol protein, or P protein), exhibiting reverse transcriptase activity. Within the nucleocapsid, the pregenomic RNA is then degraded by this enzyme, and the viral polymerase subsequently completes the formation of the final double-stranded HBV DNA, and then attaches covalently to the 3′ end of the minus-strand DNA, to complete the formation of the nucleocapsid. These completed nucleocapsids are then capable of associating with cell membranes, binding to envelope proteins, and subsequent release.[64]

Possibly because of the extensive worldwide distribution of HBV, some diversity exists in its DNA sequences and the antigenicity of HBsAg.[112] Classically, three antigenic epitopes on HBsAg have been distinguished: a, d/y, and w/r.[48,110,111] The a antigen is common to HBsAg molecules derived from all strains of HBV and is a major neutralizing epitope. Because vaccination with HBsAg usually results in the development of antibodies to the a epitope, any form of HBsAg can be used to produce neutralizing antibodies. HBsAg usually is exclusively d or y and w or r, leading to serologic designations of ayw, ayr, adw, and adr. With the development of monoclonal antibodies to HBsAg and genetic sequencing data, more subtle differences in serotypes of HBsAg have become apparent; for example, four distinct subgroups have been identified within the ayw group.[112] The antigenic differences among viral isolates are of epidemiologic interest, although clinical outcomes of HBV infection as they relate to strain differences are currently under study.

Pathogenesis

HBV is noncytopathic to the hepatocyte. The pathogenesis of disease is closely associated with the appearance of the host immune response, most prominently that of circulating HBV-specific cytotoxic T cells.[52,81,85] The breadth and intensity of the response to the HBV antigenic epitopes have been correlated with the ability to clear the virus. In addition to direct cytotoxic mechanisms, HBV-specific T cells have the ability to decrease viral replication by noncytolytic mechanisms, primarily involving IFN-γ, which leads to an enhanced immune response both within the hepatocyte and with respect to recruitment of additional immune-competent ($CD4^+$ and natural killer [NK]) cells.[87,113] Accumulating evidence suggests that even in adults who recover clinically from the infection, persisting, perhaps lifelong HBV infection, is the rule, accompanied by a strong and continuing T cell response.[86] The actual immune parameters that are responsible for the persistent, chronic infection seen in neonates, however, have not been investigated in detail.

Acute infection in adults may be either asymptomatic or symptomatic, in the latter case accompanied by biochemical and histologic evidence of hepatitis. The pathogenesis of infection has been broadly separated into four categories: immune tolerance, immune/active clearance, nonreplicative, and reactivation.[108] Greater than 90% of neonatal infections result in chronic infection, whereas only 5% of infections in adults become persistent. Immune tolerance in the neonate may result either from cellular immune system immaturity or from suppression of immune responses. Immune suppression leading to chronic infection may either be specific to HBV, possibly linked to the transplacental passage of soluble HBeAg, or be a nonspecific function of the fetal immune suppression that normally occurs during gestation.

The serum concentration of HBV DNA varies markedly from patient to patient with different states of chronic HBV disease. Asymptomatic HBsAg-positive chronic carriers with little or no hepatocellular injury usually have very high concentrations of serum HBV DNA, validating the concept of immune tolerance, with poor host regulation of viral replication and minimal host-mediated injury to hepatocytes. On the other hand, persons who remain HBsAg positive but have ongoing evidence of hepatocellular injury, as assessed by serum aminotransferases and liver biopsy, will have a 20% chance of developing cirrhosis with their chronic HBV infection.

In general, circulating HBeAg in adults denotes a higher load of circulating virus, with less host control of the infection and less host-mediated damage to hepatocytes. Over time, a certain percentage of adults will revert from HBeAg seropositivity to anti-HBe seropositivity, usually accompanied acutely by increased liver inflammation.[106] One study showed that the vertical transmission rate of HBV infection was increased in women who were HBeAg positive, suggesting a correlation between viral load and transmission rates.[77] Of those with perinatal infection, the period of immune tolerance may last for the first 2 decades or longer.[108] Although HBeAg positivity may correlate with less inflammation, the risk of hepatocellular carcinoma is highest in those who are HBeAg positive, suggesting that altered molecular control of cellular function in HBV infected hepatocytes may correlate with the development of cancer.[40]

In addition to being present as extrachromosomal, covalently closed, double-stranded DNA, HBV DNA also may become integrated into host chromosomes and can be found within the chromosomes of most hepatocellular tumors. The viral DNA usually has been severely rearranged, with deletions, duplications, inversions, and insertions.[75] The role of HBV in carcinogenesis is not well defined and may be a function of random genetic integration events that facilitate the development of uncontrolled tumor growth through genetic expression of HBV enhancers or promoters within critical human genes, or may reflect a biologic effect of one of the HBV proteins, such as HBx, which may prevent mechanisms of cell homeostasis from operating normally. As the chronic infection progresses over many years, the lifetime risk of the development of hepatocellular carcinoma is estimated to be 40% to 50%.[38,61]

Following inoculation of a susceptible host with infectious virions, HBsAg appears in the bloodstream within 1 to 6 months during the acute phase of infection, correlating with high levels of circulating virus and contagiousness. A high risk of vertical transmission of HBV from mother to infant is present during the acute infection. In older children and adults, HBV-specific $CD8^+$ and $CD4^+$ lymphocytes clear the production of virus by both cytolytic and noncytolytic mechanisms.[88] In the neonate, the most common response following perinatal exposure is a chronic asymptomatic hepatitis with the histologic features of unresolved or persistent hepatitis.

Limited data exist on the hepatocellular characteristics of infection in the newborn or during the first year of life. Early studies by Schweitzer and colleagues demonstrated that in 13 of 17 HBsAg-positive infants, no signs of acute clinical hepatitis were present.[93] Physical findings for 12 infants with persistent antigenemia remained normal. In one child, hepatomegaly and splenomegaly were detected at 15 months of age. Liver biopsy specimens were obtained from 10 HBsAg-positive infants between 3 and 27 months of age; results from 8 of the 10 infants documented intact lobular architecture with no suggestion of nodular regeneration or fibrosis. Some liver cells were hydropic and polyhedral, giving a cobblestone appearance to the liver lobule. Liver cell nuclei were slightly enlarged, and small foci of liver cell necrosis were present. Only one liver biopsy specimen had increased amounts of fibrosis, but no bridging between portal areas was apparent.

Transmission

Transmission to the neonate most often occurs at the time of delivery, but some evidence suggests that some neonates may already be infected in utero, with virus present in cord blood at birth.[84] In Taiwan, where the prevalence of HBsAg positivity in the population is 5% to 20%, a high frequency of vertical transmission of HBsAg from asymptomatic carrier mothers was documented before the routine use of hepatitis B immune globulin (HBIG) and HBV vaccines. In natural history studies by Stevens and co-workers, HBsAg antigenemia was eventually documented in 63 infants born to 158 carrier mothers.[100] Fifty-one of these infants became HBsAg positive within the first 6 months of life. Furthermore, within this group, 21 of 103 infants born to carrier mothers had a positive cord blood sample for HBsAg, suggesting a high rate of in utero transmission. A relationship also was documented in this study between the level of the mother's viremia and the development of infection in the infant. This strikingly high frequency of transmission of the hepatitis virus noted in Taiwan also has been observed in other Asian and African populations.

A high incidence of maternal transmission of HBV from asymptomatic carrier mothers to infants also was reported in 1975 by investigators in Japan.[76] In a study of 5993 mothers in five municipal hospitals in Tokyo, 139 (2.3%) were positive for HBsAg. These women were judged to be asymptomatic carriers by three criteria: (1) HBsAg was present in a high titer (1:512 or greater) as determined by the immune adherence hemagglutination method; (2) the women were free of clinical liver disease; and (3) no laboratory-tested abnormalities of liver function were present. Of the infants born to the 139 HBsAg-positive mothers, none had congenital malformations. Of note, none of 59 cord blood specimens tested by the technique of immune adherence hemagglutination were positive for HBsAg. Outcomes in 11 infants of HBsAg-positive mothers were studied in follow-up evaluations. In 8 of these 11, HBsAg appeared in the serum within 6 months; 3 remained HBsAg negative for 7 to 14 months. In view of the lack of HBsAg in cord blood in this study, perinatal transmission, rather than in utero transmission appears to have been the major route of neonatal infection in this population studied in Japan.

Another early report from Japan[77] documented the presence of e antigen (a marker of higher viral load and less vigorous host response to HBV) in the blood of 10 asymptomatic carrier mothers, all 10 of whose infants became HBsAg positive. The infants born to mothers whose sera contained antibodies to e antigen (anti-e) did not become HBsAg positive. The importance of e antigen as a determinant in the transmission of HBV was confirmed in a prospective trial of pregnant women who were chronic carriers of HBsAg. Of the 70 pregnant women who delivered, 38 were HBeAg positive. Thirty-seven of the 38 HBeAg-positive mother-infant pairs were followed for 5 months or more. By 5 months, 26 of the 37 infants (70.3%) born to HBeAg-positive mothers were HBsAg positive.[63] Another study from Taiwan further supported the correlation between the presence of HBeAg in the serum of HBsAg carrier mothers and infection in their newborns: 85% of infants born to HBeAg-positive women became infected with HBV during the first year of life, and no vertical transmission was documented in HbeAg-negative mothers.[101] Circulating HBV DNA was measured during pregnancy in chronically infected pregnant women in Sweden, both HBeAg positive ($n = 9$) and HbeAg negative ($n = 46$).[99] Not unexpectedly, viral load was higher in HbeAg-positive women than in those who were HbeAg negative; the three infants who acquired the infection all were born to HbeAg-positive mothers.

In the United States, the rate of transmission of HBsAg from asymptomatic carrier mothers to their children appears to be lower. Schweitzer and colleagues found that only 1 of 21 infants born to HBsAg-positive mothers became positive for HBsAg.[94] In this study, HBsAg was found in the cord blood in 9 of 18 specimens, but none of these infants became HBsAg positive. The authors concluded that the presence of HBsAg in the cord blood bore no relationship to the development of antigenemia in the infant of an asymptomatic carrier mother. In Denmark, Skinhoj and co-workers[98] found no infections among 28 infants studied for 3 to 5 months after birth to asymptomatic carrier mothers.

In a recent study from China, a high rate of in utero transmission was again suggested in the population studied.[117] Among 59 infants born to HBV chronic carrier mothers, in utero transmission was documented in 40% by HBV DNA detected in peripherally drawn venous blood shortly after birth.

A fetal pulmonary or gastrointestinal route of infection in utero is theoretically possible in infants who may not be infected through a hematogenous route. Investigators in one study found HBsAg in 33% of amniotic fluid samples and in 95% of gastric aspirates from the newborn infants.[63] HBV DNA was found by PCR assay of amniotic fluid from 48% of chronic carrier mothers, although contamination of amniotic fluid from maternal blood may have been possible.[117]

Thus, in Taiwan, Japan, and China, the risk of infants acquiring hepatitis B from asymptomatic carrier mothers by perinatal as well as in utero routes appears to be high, whereas in the United States and other countries, the risk of acquiring neonatal hepatitis from HBsAg carrier mothers appears to be lower. It is not clear what role genetically determined immune responses, or socioeconomic or cultural conditions, may play in the epidemiology of transmission from mother to infant.

No evidence is available to suggest that the clinical course in the pregnant woman in whom acute hepatitis B develops during pregnancy is different from that in women who are not pregnant.[49] With acute infection during the first part of pregnancy, however, clearance of HBV virions usually occurs by the time of delivery. For those women with infection later in pregnancy who are HBsAg positive at the time of delivery, the rate of perinatal acquisition of infection in the infant is similar to the rate found in infants born to mothers with chronic infection. In the United States, Schweitzer and co-workers assessed the presence of HBsAg in 56 mother-infant pairs; the mothers had acute viral hepatitis during pregnancy or within 6 months after delivery.[92,94] This study indicated that HBsAg was transmitted from mother to infant by 10 of 26 mothers who had HBsAg-positive hepatitis. Of interest, infection was transmitted from 8 of 17 mothers whose hepatitis developed within 2 months after delivery. The investigators demonstrated that the frequency of HBV transmission from mother to infant is high (76%) when acute hepatitis B occurs in the third trimester or early in the postpartum period and low (10%) when hepatitis occurs in the first two trimesters of pregnancy.

Although infants may theoretically be infected through breast milk, which is known to contain virus,[41,67,104] this mode of transmission does not appear to add additional risk for the infant beyond other exposures from a chronically infected mother.[55,84] Infants who receive appropriate prophylaxis following delivery should be allowed to breast-feed.[1] For parents who refuse appropriate prophylaxis, or in situations in which prophylaxis is not available, the added risks of neonatal infection beyond those from exposures to HBV during the pregnancy and birth are minimal, particularly when balanced with the nutritional and immunologic benefits from breast milk.

Clinical Illness

A majority of infants who become positive for HBsAg after mother-to-infant transmission remain anicteric, show no signs of acute clinical hepatitis, and remain HBsAg positive for an extended period. The natural history of neonatal infection is best described by studies in which ongoing exposures to HBV from the community are minimal, giving the best insight into the evolution of virus-child interactions. A natural history study was recently published from England in which 73 infants diagnosed with perinatal infection were born to HBsAg-, HBeAg-positive mothers (comprising 53 women from the Indian subcontinent and 9 Asian, 6 African-Caribbean, and 5 white women).[42] These infants either were born before the era of routine perinatal prophylaxis (n = 51) or were prophylaxis failures (n = 22). The mean duration of follow-up was 10 years (range 2 to 20 years). All children were clinically well; none had evidence of liver enlargement by palpation or ultrasound examination. All were of normal height and weight. Of the 73 children, 3 had cleared HBsAg and had become seropositive for anti-HBs at follow-up testing. Sixty-five percent of children were seropositive for HBeAg, and 30% had seroconverted to become anti-HBe positive by an average of 10 years of age (range 4 to 19 years). Four of the five (80%) white children seroconverted, compared with 18 of the 50 (36%) children from the Indian subcontinent, with no seroconversions noted in the 9 Asian children. This finding of different rates of HBeAg seroreversion in different ethnic groups also has been reported by other investigators.[43]

Half of the Indian subcontinent children and two thirds of the Asian children had normal values for serum ALT. Elevated aminotransferase values tended to be stable over the period of follow-up evaluation. Liver biopsy samples were available in 48% of the children. In these children, 30% of biopsy specimens showed minimal or no inflammation, 63% showed mild hepatitis, and 6% demonstrated moderately severe hepatitis, as graded by Ishak scoring. Two children with moderately severe changes had "incomplete cirrhosis." No association was found between the severity of the histopathologic changes and age, gender, or ethnic origin. A weak association was found between elevation of liver function tests and the degree of inflammation present.Children who were HBeAg positive also were shown to have the highest levels of circulating HBV DNA.

Although none of the children in this series became clinically symptomatic, in earlier reports mild, self-limited hepatitis with variable elevations of ALT and abnormalities on liver biopsy were reported.[95] In the study carried out in Taiwan, however, in which 158 women who were carriers of HBsAg gave birth to 63 antigen-positive infants (40%), all of the infants remained healthy, without signs or symptoms of hepatitis.[100]

Although the vast majority of infants have benign clinical disease, fulminant hepatitis has been reported, particularly in infants born to HBeAg-negative mothers, although it may also occur in infants born to mothers who are HBeAg positive.[43,45,59,60]

Neonatal infection with HBV has been suggested to play a dominant role in the development of primary hepatocellular carcinoma in later life.[38] A progression of events from vertical HBV transmission leading to chronic infection, resulting in cirrhosis and hepatocellular carcinoma in adult life, has been implicated to explain findings in Senegal, West Africa, where primary hepatocellular carcinoma is a major cause of death among young adult men.[62] The finding that mothers of patients with hepatocellular carcinoma were positive for HBsAg four times more frequently than the fathers suggested that the virus was acquired from the mother by vertical transmission. The development of hepatocellular carcinoma also may relate to an associated high incidence of HBeAg positivity in HBsAg carriers in particular geographic regions. In the United States, only 3% to 5% of HBsAg carriers also are HBeAg positive, and hepatocellular carcinoma is uncommon, whereas 30% of HBsAg carriers also are HBeAg positive in Taiwan, Japan, and Uganda; these countries have a very high incidence of hepatocellular carcinoma. In several studies, between 37% and 90% of patients with hepatocellular carcinoma were HBsAg positive; these rates were 10 times higher than that in matched controls living in the same area.[105] Furthermore, preliminary data from Taiwan suggest that perinatal HBV prophylaxis programs, now in their third decade, have been associated with the decrease in hepatocellular carcinoma in the age groups immunized.[46]

In summary, it is evident that a majority of infants who become HBSAg positive by mother-to-infant transmission are clinically healthy, but they may have persistently elevated values on liver function tests, and approximately 5% will have moderately severe histopathologic changes on liver biopsy. These changes are not well predicted by the clinical or HBV serologic status, or by liver function testing. Late complications include cirrhosis and hepatocellular carcinoma.[52,61] Clinical illness in adults has recently been reviewed.[52,108]

Laboratory Diagnosis

The availability of reliable, reproducible methods for a variety of antigens and antibodies associated with HBV infection has played a major role in the accumulation of knowledge on the epidemiology and clinical relevance of HBV. These tests are widely available from both hospitals and regional reference laboratories. The patterns of HBV viral products and host responses in both acute, resolved infection and in chronic infection are summarized in Figure 25-3.[96]

HBsAg was one of the first detected virus-associated antigens. At present, most clinical laboratories use variations of the enzyme-linked immunoassay (EIA) methods or radioimmunoassay (RIA) and to detect HBsAg. HBsAg is

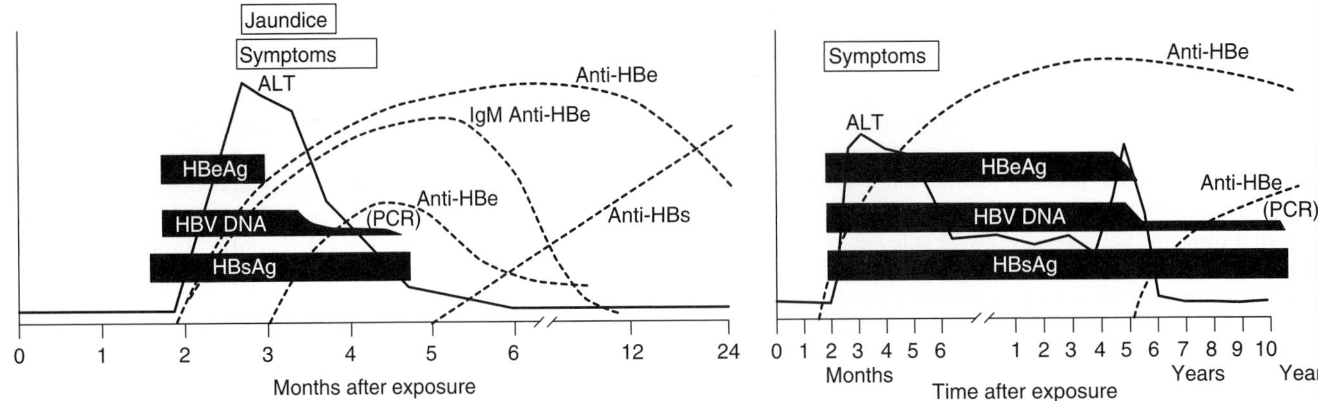

Figure 25–3 Viral and host serologic markers and clinical correlates of hepatitis B virus (HBV) infection. **A,** Acute infection with appropriate host response and resolution of infection. **B,** Chronic infection. (Data from Servoss JC, Friedman LS. Serologic and molecular diagnosis of hepatitis B virus.Clin Liver Dis 2004;8[2]:267-81.)

synthesized during viral replication and also may be synthesized from HBV DNA sequences integrated into the chromosomes of hepatocytes in the absence of viral production.[107] In general, the presence of HBsAg is an indication of active viral infection. Approximately 90% of adults will be HBsAg positive using a conventional enzyme-linked immunosorbent assay (ELISA) for HBsAg during the first 2 weeks of symptomatic acute viral hepatitis B. A single negative assay result early in the course of infection may represent a false-negative result, because the antigen concentration may be below the sensitivity of the immunoassays. Repeating the assay several weeks later may yield a positive result. In acute infection, the levels of HBsAg begins to fall 4 to 6 months after exposure.[96] In the neonate, HBsAg may be present at birth, as a consequence of in utero infection, or may not be detectable for several months following perinatal or postnatal inoculation. For infants born to chronically infected mothers who are provided immunoprophylaxis, HBsAg (and anti-HBs) should be checked at 9 to 15 months of age, or 1 to 3 months following completion of the primary immunization series.[1]

Anti-HBs antibody testing is widely available, usually performed by EIA or RIA techniques. This circulating antibody is directed against epitopes on the S protein of the pre-S/S ORF gene product. In self-limited HBV infections, it usually is assumed that the patient is no longer infectious after anti-HBs is detectable. With the development of more sensitive assays for HBsAg and anti-HBs, patients with self-limited infection may be transiently HBsAg and anti-HBs positive simultaneously.[97] Most patients with chronic HBV infections will never be anti-HBs positive. Conversely, less than 10% of chronic carriers have anti-HBs antibodies.[97] Anti-HBs positivity usually implies that an HBV infection has resolved or that the patient has mounted an antibody response to the hepatitis B vaccine. In persons with natural infection, anti-HBc also is positive. Evidence that an adult may both have anti-HBs and be intermittently positive for small amounts of HBV DNA suggests that anti-HBs is a marker for clinical cure, rather than for sterilizing immunity.[52,88]

Anti-HBc is formed against the nucleocapsid core protein during the course of infection. It is most commonly detected by EIA or RIA. Early in the infection, anti-HBc antibodies are predominantly of the IgM class and have been used to diagnose acute infection in adults. Symptomatic adults are anti-HBc positive 2 weeks after symptoms begin, and virtually all patients with asymptomatic HBV infections are anti-HBc positive at the time when other virus-associated antigens are detectable and the ALT rises. With time, the titer of anti-HBc IgM declines as the titer of anti-HBc IgG rises. At 6 months following infection, a majority of patients' anti-HBc antibodies are IgG, although a minority may have detectable anti-HBc IgM for up to 2 years. The anti-HBc antibody titer slowly declines but remains detectable for many years after self-limited infection. The anti-HBc titer usually remains high during the course of chronic infection. During recovery from an acute infection, the anti-HBc IgM may be detected in serum several weeks after infection at a time when the HBsAg is decreasing and no longer detectable in serum, and while anti-HBs is increasing but is not yet detectable in serum. The newborn infant's anti-HBc response following perinatal infection has not been prospectively studied. Of note is the fact that immunized infants born to mothers not infected by hepatitis B may be transiently positive for HBsAg from the vaccine but should not be positive for anti-HBc. In infants born to mothers with chronic infection, transplacental, maternal anti-HBc should be detectable for up to the first several months of life. In addition, in infants born to chronically infected mothers, passive immunization with hepatitis B immune globulin also may provide anti-HBc detectable in the infant's serum. Continued presence of anti-HBc at 12 to 18 months in these infants, however, should raise the suspicion of perinatal infection with HBV.

Both HBeAg and anti-HBe are detectable by both EIA and RIA. The HBeAg usually is detectable in adults when viral replication is occurring with little host response to limit the production of virions. Later in the course of infection, particularly in certain ethnic groups, a seroconversion from HBeAg to anti-HBe may be accompanied by decreasing viral titers, or even the eventual clearance of virus. The concentration of virus usually is higher in HBeAg-positive sera than in HBeAg-negative sera. The absence of HBeAg positivity, however, does not exclude the potential infectivity of HBsAg-positive sera in patients with HBV infections either caused by standard strains or caused by those with mutations in the precore region in which HBeAg is not produced.[65,66,83] At present, although the immunoassays for HBeAg and anti-HBe are readily available to the practitioner, the clinical use of these assays is limited to guiding antiviral therapy in helping to identify an HBeAg–to–anti-HBe seroconversion in the chronic HBV carrier. No other management decisions can be reliably based on these tests at this time. The decision of whether to perform immunoprophylaxis of a newborn of an HBsAg-positive mother with HBIG and HBV vaccine should not depend on her HBeAg/anti-HBe status, because vertical transmission may occur in either setting.

HBV DNA can be measured in commercial reference laboratories by a variety of techniques, either *qualitative* assays that detect the presence or absence of HBV DNA or *quantitative* HBV DNA assays. Techniques include signal amplification following molecular hybridization (including hybrid capture and branched-DNA methods) or nucleic acid target amplification (PCR and transcription-mediated amplification [TMA] techniques).[79,80] These tests most often are used to monitor response to antiviral therapy, rather than to diagnose an HBV infection.

HBV genotypes also can be determined in reference laboratories by using immunoassay and nucleic acid sequencing techniques. These assays most often are interpreted in conjunction with a pretreatment laboratory assessment, because different genotypes may respond differently to various antiviral and immune therapies.

Many other tests for hepatitis B virus and other techniques to measure HBV antigens, HBV antibody, and specific lymphocyte responses to various HBV epitopes have existed for several years. New molecular techniques are being used to provide more insight into the pathogenesis of infection, and to allow investigators to track response to antiviral therapy more closely.

Therapy

Therapy for HBV infection has not been studied systematically in the neonate. In older children, therapy is undertaken in those with biopsy evidence of liver disease.[43] Therapy for hepatitis B includes interferon-α (including pegylated formulations) and lamivudine and adefovir, the nucleoside analogues that act as polymerase inhibitors. In children, multiple studies have been conducted using interferon-α, with overall encouraging results. Response rates as high as 58% were noted in some studies.[39,43] In adults and children with chronic hepatitis B infection, lamivudine treatment has been associated with a rapid and profound decrease in serum HBV DNA levels, normalization of aminotransferase levels, and in adults, reversal of some histologic changes seen in liver biopsy specimens, with reduction in fibrosis and cirrhosis.[52,56,58,61] Unfortunately, emergence of lamivudine resistance may occur within 6 months of therapy, linked to nucleic acid mutations in the HBV genome.[79,96] Adefovir has been studied in both HbeAg-negative[53] and HbeAg-positive[70] adults. Limited data exist on adefovir therapy in children with chronic HBV infection, but no recommendations can yet be made. Other nucleotide analogues are currently investigational. The concept of multiple drug therapy to decrease the risk of the development of resistance also has been suggested.

In addition, pegylated interferon-α, used alone or in combination with lamivudine in adults, provided a better antiviral response than lamivudine alone, and the combination of lamivudine plus peginterferon-α did not significantly improve the outcome of infection beyond that achieved by peginterferon-α alone.[71] In two smaller studies involving 19 and 20 children, respectively, interferon-α plus lamivudine was used for treatment in (1) children who were noted to be interferon-α nonresponders, demonstrating a response rate of 37%,[89] and (2) those who were treatment naïve, resulting in a response rate of 55%.[90]

The decision of which child to treat is still evolving, and incorporates both the safety, side effects, tolerability, as well as efficacy in children who usually are asymptomatic with their HBV infections.[39,43]

Prevention of Infection

Prophylaxis for the HBV-exposed neonate may consist of passive immunization with hepatitis B immune globulin (HBIG), active immunization with HBV vaccines, or antiviral therapy with lamivudine, or a combination of these treatments. The role of HBIG in preventing vertical transmission of HBV to infants born to HBV carrier mothers has been well documented, but HBIG is currently being replaced by vaccine in some countries, particularly in infants born to mothers considered at low risk of transmitting the infection.[69,74,115] HBIG is used routinely with vaccine for all infants born to HbsAg-positive mothers in the United States.[1]

HBIG is derived from plasma collected from persons who have recovered from HBV infection and is processed to eliminate risk of infection from HIV or HCV.[44] The success of HBIG alone in preventing vertical transmission was documented in Taiwan by demonstrating a decrease in neonatal HBV infection from 92% in infants born to HBSAg- and HBEAg-positive mothers to 26% in infants given 0.5 mL of HBIG at birth, 3 months, and 6 months.[36] In an effort to further decrease transmission, subsequent studies employed both passive protection (HBIG) and active immunization with HBV vaccine. Immune serum globulin (ISG) is not considered to have sufficient antibody to HBV to be a reasonable substitute for HBIG for passive prophylaxis in the newborn.

The first hepatitis B vaccines were originally approved in the United States in 1981. They were composed of purified HBsAg from plasma of chronic carriers and were documented to be immunogenic and protective in infants born to chronic carrier mothers.[37,57,68,72,73,114,116] These vaccines were replaced a few years later by the currently available vaccines, all of which use recombinant DNA technology in *Saccharomyces cerevisiae* to produce HBsAg and are safer than but just as effective as previously available vaccines.[69,74,82,102] Currently available data on long-term protection suggest that booster doses of HBV vaccines may not be necessary for children who received either plasma-derived or recombinant vaccines, although the relevant studies were conducted largely in countries in which hepatitis B is endemic.

Current recommendations to achieve protection of the infant from vertically transmitted infection begin with universal screening of all pregnant women for the HBV carrier state. For infants born in the United States to women who are identified as chronic carriers (regardless of HBeAg serologic status), both HBIG (0.5 mL) and an initial dose of one of the FDA-approved hepatitis B vaccines (Recombivax

HB [Merck], 5 μg; or Engerix-B [GSK], 10 μg) should be administered at different sites, within 12 hours of birth.

For premature infants born at less than 2000 g whose mothers are HbsAg positive, the initial dose of vaccine at birth should not be considered as part of the immunizing series and should be regarded as just an additional dose. For infants born to women who are not HBV carriers, the first dose of vaccine should be provided in the neonatal period, not necessarily within 12 hours of birth. For women who have not been screened, vaccine should be administered within the first 12 hours of life while maternal testing is under way. If maternal testing indicates that the mother is a chronic HBV carrier, then HBIG should be administered as quickly as possible, preferably within 48 hours of birth, but may be given within 7 days of birth. For infants born at less than 2000 g whose mothers did not undergo screening or were screened too late for results to be available within 12 hours of birth, a dose of HBIG should be given in addition to vaccine, rather than waiting for the maternal HBV status to be determined. For infants born to HBSAg-positive mothers, follow-up testing should be performed for HBsAg and anti-HBs at 9 to 15 months of age, after completion of the series of immunizations for HBV. Testing of the infant shortly after vaccine administration may yield a positive result for HBsAg as a result of vaccination, rather than of infection. Detailed recommendations for immunization of neonates are available from the American Academy of Pediatrics[1] and the ACIP.[44]

In situations in which a chronic carrier mother has premature rupture of the membranes, the delivery management should not be altered in order to deliver the infant to provide prophylaxis, because no data are available to support an increased risk of HBV infection to the infant before delivery in this situation.[50]

Mutations in the viral genome responsible for the production of HBsAg with an altered antigenic structure are known to exist. These relatively rare mutations create HBV virions that are not neutralized by the immunity created with HBV immunization[47,78]; the clinical consequences in persons infected by these altered HBV virions are therefore not altered with available HBV vaccines.

The current recommendation to prevent HBV infection in infants born to mothers with chronic hepatitis also should apply to infants born to mothers who become infected by HBV in the last trimester of pregnancy and are HBsAg positive at the time of delivery, because risk of vertical transmission appears to be similar in both situations. Large-scale trials to document efficacy of HBIG and HBV vaccine in these infants do not exist, however.

In addition to providing immune prophylaxis with HBIG and vaccine to infants, lamivudine also has been used for treatment in mothers with high viral loads during the last month of pregnancy in an effort to reduce the risk of vertical transmission. Although the average viral load decreased in women who received lamivudine, one of eight infants who also received immune prophylaxis became infected with HBV.[109] At this time, antiviral therapy during the last month of pregnancy cannot be routinely recommended.

Intervention strategies with hepatitis vaccine and HBIG for the newborn infant, based on maternal screening for HBV infection and the gestational age of the infant, are summarized in Table 25-2.

HEPATITIS C

The Virus

After the development of definitive assays for both HAV and HBV in the mid-1970s, it became clear that other agents also were responsible for post-transfusion hepatitis, sporadic hepatitis, and occasional epidemics of maternally transmitted hepatitis.[119] Following the discovery of the virus by means of a "blind" recombinant immunoscreening approach, HCV was recognized as the agent most commonly responsible for parenterally transmitted non-A, non-B virus infection.[122] HCV is a single-stranded enveloped RNA virus approximately 9600 nucleotides long, belonging to the Flaviviridae family.[146,149] The single strand of positive-sense RNA codes for a single open reading frame, producing a single polyprotein of approximately 3000 amino acids that is cleaved into three *structural* proteins—core, E1, E2—and seven *nonstructural* proteins—p7, NS2, NS3, NS4A, NS4B, NS5A, and NS5B. Structural proteins E1 and E2 are involved in the viral envelope and are likely to be involved in cell receptor binding. Nonstructural proteins provide various intracellular functions, including a protease used to cleave a portion of the polyprotein into active components, a helicase, and an RNA-dependent RNA polymerase.

Entry into the cell follows attachment of the virus by means of the E2 envelope protein to CD81, a cell surface protein expressed on hepatocytes and other cells.[147] Following entry, events of viral replication and release are not well understood. Viral uncoating occurs, with release of viral RNA into the cytoplasm and subsequent translation into the polyprotein as well as the production of negative-sense RNA, from which further copies of RNA for virus production can be made. Core protein, formed from the first 191 amino acids of the polyprotein, polymerizes to form the icosahedral HCV nucleocapsid, which combines with positive-sense RNA to form virions, which then incorporate the envelope proteins E1 and E2 before release. The E2 protein genome contains a hypervariable region (HVR-1) that permits ongoing change in antigenic structure of the E2 protein, providing a mechanism by which HCV may continually elude targeted host defenses,[156] similar to that seen in HIV infections. The viral RNA polymerase lacks the "proofreading" capabilities normally found in mammalian polymerases, thereby facilitating ongoing base replacement and altered tertiary structure of the E2 protein.

Worldwide, six major genotypes exist, although each genotype comprises hundreds to thousands of subtypes resulting from the high mutation rates during virus replication. These subtypes are called *quasispecies* and provide some insight into the unique ability of this virus to continually alter its immunologically recognizable epitopes. In general, the genotypes of HCV are used as epidemiologic tools, but they also appear to respond differently to antiviral therapies.

Pathogenesis

Most of the information gathered on the pathogenesis of disease is based on primate models of infection, because cell culture systems and small animal models do not currently exist.[132] Following infection, the virus primarily enters

Table 25–2 Hepatitis B Neonatal Intervention Strategies Based on Maternal HBV Screening Status

Maternal HBV Status	Interpretation	Laboratory Evaluation at Birth and during Infancy	Infant Treatment
HBsAg negative	Mother is not considered infectious; no risk to the neonate	None required	*All newborn infants:* standard 3-dose immunization regimen with hepatitis B vaccine recommended: dose 1 given soon after birth, up to 2 months of age; dose 2 given at least 4 weeks after dose 1; dose 3 given at least 16 weeks after dose 1, and at least 8 weeks after dose 2, with last dose no earlier than 24 weeks of age
HBsAg positive	Mother is infectious; significant risk of neonatal infection	HBsAg on peripheral venous blood sampling to diagnose intrauterine infection (and less likely benefit from perinatal intervention); test infant for anti-HBs and HBsAg at 9-15 months of age for outcome of intervention	*All infants:* HBIG 0.5 mL within 12 hours of birth, in addition to the first dose of hepatitis B vaccine, also given within 12 hours of birth; second and third doses of vaccine for infants with birth weight 2000 g or greater, as above *Preterm infants less than 2000 g birth weight:* initial birth dose should not be counted as one of immunizing series because of an immature response to vaccine; subsequent 3 immunizations in primary immunizing series for these infants should start at age 1 month
HBsAg status unknown	Mother's infectious status unknown; do maternal HBsAg testing as soon as possible	None required at birth In infants whose mothers are subsequently found to be HBsAg positive, testing for anti-HBs and HBsAg at 9-15 months of age is recommended	*Full-term infants:* give first dose of hepatitis B vaccine within 12 hours of birth; if maternal HBsAg is positive, give HBIG 0.5 mL as soon as possible, within 7 days of age; if maternal HBsAg is negative, HBIG is not needed; subsequent doses as for HBsAg negative *Preterm infants less than 2000 g birth weight:* if maternal HBsAg status cannot be determined within 12 hours of birth, give HBIG in addition to hepatitis vaccine within 12 hours of birth; provide subsequent 3 hepatitis B immunizations for primary series, starting at 1 month of age, as above for preterm infants

HBIG, hepatitis B immune globulin; HBsAg, hepatitis B surface antigen; HBV, hepatitis B virus.

hepatocytes, although viral replication also may occur in other cell types, including dendritic cells and B cells. The virus is not cytopathic, similar to HBV. Within 10 to 14 weeks following inoculation, acute hepatitis develops, although virus can be detected in the liver many weeks before clinically evident disease. At the onset of illness, liver function test results become abnormal, and HCV-specific T cells appear in the liver.[121,124,138,140,149]

In a study of outcome in five persons following needle-stick exposure, viremia could first be detected within 1 to 2 weeks after exposure.[158] Clearance of virus occurred in only one subject in this study and was not seen until after the appearance of HCV-specific $CD8^+$ T cells accompanied by a strong HCV-specific $CD4^+$ response. Clinical hepatitis occurred at the time of appearance of $CD8^+$ T cells, although elevation of liver enzymes occurred as early as 2 weeks after exposure in persons who remained asymptomatic. In persons in whom persistent infection did not develop, no $CD8^+$-specific response was detected, although in some, strong $CD4^+$ T cell responses initially developed that subsequently faded during the 23 to 92 weeks of follow-up evaluation. Of note, the production of IFN-γ led to a

100,000-fold drop in circulating virus titer, suggesting that the noncytolytic mechanisms of T cell control of intracellular virus replication in HBV infections may be similar in HCV.

Other studies have documented strong $CD8^+$ T cell responses to multiple different epitopes of HCV among human subjects with resolution of infection.[137] The responses differed in the specific HCV epitopes recognized, suggesting that no single neutralizing epitope exists, and that a response to multiple epitopes simultaneously is more likely to lead to clearance of virus. Persons with persisting infection had responses that were weaker and more narrowly focused. Similar data exist in the chimpanzee model, suggesting that $CD8^+$ T cell responses, seen in cells resident within the liver, constitute an important component of the immune response.[121,149,155,159] Within the liver, complex interactions between virally infected cells and HCV-specific $CD8^+$ and $CD4^+$ T cells occur, leading to both cytolytic, destructive changes in hepatocytes and interferon production. With an extremely high replication rate of greater than 10^{10} virions per day, as well as rapid rates of mutation, the ever-changing antigenic structure provides a moving target for the immune system. The HCV-specific antibody, which is used to diagnose infection, recognizes epitopes on the various quasispecies of HCV virions, many of which may no longer exist in the circulation at the time antibody is detected. Likewise, epitopes that elicit a cellular immune response also are changing, providing a difficult challenge to the cellular immune system to find and neutralize virally infected cells. It is not difficult to understand that chronic infection develops in 80% of infected adults.

Transmission

HCV is primarily transmitted parenterally: by needlestick exposure (from reused needles in medical settings from the past decades, or in intravenous drug abuse) and by blood transfusion before screening of donated blood beginning in 1992. The infection may be transmitted vertically from chronically infected mother to infant, although the rate of infection in newborns is only about 3% to 7%.[152] Infection appears to be most often acquired perinatally, although some controversy exists as about what proportion of neonates might be infected in utero. The assessment of in utero infection usually is made by confirming the presence of HCV RNA by RT-PCR assay in cord blood. Inapparent contamination of the cord with maternal blood, however, may lead to false-positive results. In some of these situations, contamination is supported by follow-up studies in infants that failed to detect either HCV RNA by RT-PCR assay, or evidence of productive infection as assessed by the later appearance of anti-HCV antibody. In some studies, a rare infant who is negative for HCV by PCR assay at birth may become transiently positive during the first year of life without evidence of anti-HCV antibody at that time, or when tested later at follow-up evaluation. These observations of transient viremia may be explained either by false-positive test results or by inoculation and subsequent clearance of HCV in the infant without evidence of productive infection.

Many studies of vertical transmission have recently been published describing the rate of infection in the newborn and factors that may influence transmission.[123,126,150,152,157,160] The vast majority of infants who develop infection are born to viremic mothers; the viral load in the mother has been a significant factor in transmission in most studies in which viral load was determined, with the presence of greater than 10^6 genome equivalents per mL resulting in greater risk of transmission.[128,130] HIV co-infection has been associated with increased rates of HCV transmission four to five times higher than in women who are not also HIV infected.[126,129,142,154,160] Some investigators also have noted infantile hypoxia and intrapartum exposure to maternal blood as assessed by a history of perineal or vaginal laceration as additional risk factors.[157]

At present, universal screening during pregnancy for HCV is not recommended[118,145]; however, pregnant women at high risk for infection should be screened. Risk factors include HIV or HBV infection, parenteral drug abuse, transfusion or transplantation before 1992, presence of chronic infection with HCV/HBV/HIV in a sexual partner, attendance at a chronic dialysis unit or assocaition with staff of such units, elevated values on liver function tests, and history of body piercing.[133] Although most authorities do not advocate cesarean section for delivery in cases of maternal infection, some studies suggest a higher rate of transmission with vaginal delivery.[150] One analysis predicted the cost-effectiveness of cesarean section if the perinatal transmission rate in a group of HCV-positive pregnant women is at least 7.7%, estimating a reduction in transmission of more than 77%.[148]

Although breast milk may contain HCV DNA, breast-feeding does not appear to carry additional risk to the term infant born to a mother with HCV infection. Therefore, no restrictions should be placed on routine breast-feeding by the HCV-positive mother.[139,153]

Recommenations for testing the infant for evidence of vertical transmission, based on maternal laboratory screening tests for HCV infection, are summarized in Table 25-3.

Clinical Illness

HCV infection most often is asymptomatic in infants with perinatally acquired HCV.[134,151] Most infections in children are either found by screening those with exposure to HCV (receipt of blood products prior to 1992 or born to mothers with chronic HCV infection) or noted incidentally on examinations and laboratory testing unrelated to hepatitis. Long-term follow-up evaluation of 62 perinatally infected infants, defined by presence of HCV RNA in serum and presence of anti-HCV antibody beyond 18 months of age, suggests that chronic infection will develop in greater than 80%.[151] Elevated values on liver function tests were present in 93%, and liver biopsies performed in 11 asymptomatic children all demonstrated only mild abnormalities. Therefore, it is likely that a majority of infants will have not overt manifestations of infection, and that the first clinical symptoms attributable to HCV infection will appear in the third and fourth decades of life, when cirrhosis begins to produce clinical symptoms.[136] Unlike in HBV infections, in which the degree of abnormality of liver function tests correlates roughly with the degree of liver damage, the fluctuating host response in HCV infection suggests that liver function tests are not helpful in assessing the development of aggressive hepatitis and cirrhosis. Normal findings on these tests may simply reflect a period in which the child's immune surveillance has not yet recognized new quasi-

Table 25–3 Hepatitis C Management Strategy for Infants Born to Mothers Screened for HCV Due to Risk Factors

Maternal HCV Status	Interpretation	Laboratory Evaluation at Birth and during Infancy	Infant Treatment
Anti-HCV negative	Mother not considered infectious; no risk to neonate unless mother was infected within 6 months before testing and had not yet seroconverted at time of screening; for recent high-risk exposures for mother, request additional plasma HCV RT-PCR testing on mother at delivery	None required for infants born to mothers who are anti-HCV negative (or with negative result on HCV RT-PCR assay if obtained)	None
Anti-HCV positive	Mother has been previously infected and has an 80% chance of being chronically infected and persistently viremic with HCV Check maternal plasma HCV by RT-PCR assay; if result is positive, mother is infectious (5% risk of HCV vertical transmission), particularly if she also is HIV positive (30% risk of HCV vertical transmission)	No routine testing at birth; infant should be tested for anti-HCV antibody at 12 to 18 months of age Maternal, transplacental antibody should be reliably cleared by the infant at that time if no neonatal infection has occurred; if anti-HCV is present at age 12 to 18 months, do plasma HCV RT-PCR testing in infant; if result is positive, infant has been infected If anti-HCV test result is positive at age 18 months, and plasma HCV RT-PCR assay result is negative, repeat anti-HCV and HCV PCR testing every 6 months until both are negative (no infection) or both are positive (infection)	No HCV vaccine available; no effective immune globulin to prevent HCV transmission to neonate

anti-HCV, antibody to hepatitis C virus; HCV, hepatitis C virus; HIV, human immunodeficiency virus; RT-PCR, reverse transcriptase–polymerase chain reaction.

species within hepatocytes, and no acute inflammatory host response is present at that moment. Yet significant damage to the liver may have already occurred. Similarly, highly elevated liver function test values may reflect an ongoing immunologic response, with a liver that previously incurred minimal inflammatory changes.

Of perinatally infected children, about 20% have been documented to clear their infection during childhood—a higher proportion than in children who acquired infection through transfusion.[134] Of perinatally infected children who cleared their infection, liver inflammation as assessed by liver function tests was greater than in those who remained chronically infected. This finding suggests that greater host recognition of viral infection accompanied by liver damage may be a predictor of subsequent cure.[151] Routine liver biopsy in children with HCV is not currently recommended.[1,135]

In adults, jaundice will develop as part of the clinical presentation in only 20% of those with acute HCV infections.[141] Some patients will have a nonspecific prodrome of fatigue, lethargy, low-grade fever, nausea and vomiting, and abdominal discomfort beginning approximately 2 months following exposure (2 to 12 weeks), and lasting from 2 to 12 weeks. Of those adults who are clinically symptomatic, approximately 50% will clear the infection; of those who have clinically asymptomatic infection, the infection will become chronic in 80%.[140] The interval from acute infection to the development of cirrhosis may be 30 years or longer. Severe complications of cirrhosis will occur in 15% to 20% of chronically infected persons.[136] With HCV infection outbreaks associated with contaminated blood products, long-term follow-up evaluation suggests that the great majority of chronically infected adults have minimal cirrhosis as confirmed by biopsy performed 20 years after infection. Alcohol use and co-infection with other viruses causing hepatitis are associated with an acceleration of the inflammatory process. The genotype of HCV causing the infection does not appear to play a major role in the clinical course or progression of infection.[132]

Chronic HCV infection in adults also is a risk factor for the development of hepatocellular carcinoma. An HCV-attributable risk of 1% to 4% per year has been reported for persons in whom cirrhosis also developed.[136]

The status of HCV viral infection in pregnancy has been studied. Published reports suggest a decrease in the level of aminotransferases as the pregnancy progresses, as well as some variability in the viral load.[123,131]

Laboratory Diagnosis

The diagnosis of an HCV infection is based on the detection of anti-HCV antibodies, which reflect a host humoral response to a wide range of HCV viral antigens as measured by enzyme immunoassay (EIA). Unlike in HAV or HBV infection, however, the presence of antibody does not document recovery from infection, or lack of contagiousness. As in HIV infection, the EIAs are very sensitive, but serologic confirmation of infection also is available with the more specific recombinant immunoblot assay (RIBA), which detects the host response to specific viral products within infected cells. Current-generation EIA and RIBA tests are more sensitive and specific than previous tests, allowing more accuracy in diagnosis. The third-generation EIA tests detect antibodies to recombinant and synthetic peptides representing the core and NS3, NS4, and NS5 regions and are 99% specific.[127,143] RIBAs also are highly specific in measuring host antibody reactions to each of a number of specific HCV antigens, including two synthetic peptides, 5-1-1(p) and c100(p), from the NS4 region of the HCV genome; c33-c recombinant antigen derived from the NS3 region; c22(p) from the core portion of HCV; and the product of the NS5 region of the HCV genome.

Routine confirmation of positive third-generation EIA results with RIBA usually is not required to document infection.[143] Antibodies to HCV antigens develop as early as 2 to 4 weeks after infection; however, some HCV-infected persons, including neonates, may not seroconvert for up to 6 months or longer following the assumed time of exposure.

The diagnosis of active, chronic infection also relies on detection of HCV RNA, because the virus cannot be cultured. Both qualitative (nonquantitative) and quantitative assays are commercially available. Qualitative systems generally are more sensitive and include RT-PCR or TMA techniques, which can detect as few as 50 HCV genome copies per mL of blood. Quantitative assays, useful in following response to antiviral therapy, include PCR, TMA, and branched-DNA amplification techniques.[143] The quantity of HCV nucleic acid detected in serum in chronic infection appears to wax and wane, probably in response to the state of immunologic recognition by the host. When the host recognizes specific HCV epitopes and produces specific antibody and cellular immunity against that particular strain of circulating virus (quasispecies), it often will disappear from the circulation—only to be replaced by other quasispecies of HCV as the hypervariable genes continue to mutate to produce antigenically distinct epitopes, which then are no longer recognized by the host. At certain times during a chronic infection, the viral load of organisms detected in the serum may drop below the level of detection, producing a false-negative result. With time and further mutation during viral replication, however, new quasispecies will appear and will again be detected by assays for HCV RNA in chronically infected patients.

Additional tests that generally are not helpful in management of patients include RNA sequencing assays, to determine the genotype of infecting strain of HCV, and HCV core antigen levels (which correlate with HCV RNA levels).

Transplacentally acquired antibody in babies who are not documented to have chronic infection usually becomes undetectable during the first year of life. Antibody has not been detected in infants at 18 months of age but has been found in some infants up to 15 months of age.[120,126] Diagnosis of transplacental infection can be made by detecting persisting anti-HCV antibody at 18 months of age, with infection confirmed by qualitative PCR testing for HCV RNA. Although the presence of antibody before the age of 18 months may still represent maternal antibody, the presence of HCV RNA at any age suggests inoculation, if not infection. Clinicians may wish to test for HCV RNA (qualitative) in infants born to mothers with chronic HCV infection as early as 6 months of life, but if the result is positive, the test should be repeated at the age of 9 to 12 months to confirm vertical transmission.

Therapy

As with HBV infection in the newborn, the infection is clinically benign during the first years of life; therapy with either interferon-α or specific anti-HCV antivirals in the infant is more likely to cause unacceptable adverse reactions in these asymptomatic babies than it is to provide any long-term benefit in preventing cirrhosis or hepatocellular carcinoma. In general, therapy is not necessary during infancy. In view of the variability in clinical progression of disease during childhood, however, a liver biopsy in the school-aged child may help the clinician in assessing the risks versus benefits of anti-HCV therapy during childhood.

Interferon-α has been FDA approved for use in children with hepatitis C infection in children from 3 to 16 years of age. All children in pediatric clinical trials were biopsied before enrollment; all trials required some histologic evidence of hepatitis. Virologic response rates in children varied, ranging from 33% to 45%, with a consistently lower response rate for genotype 1.[135] Interferon-α in combination with ribavirin also has received FDA approval[125] for the same age group based on data from 118 children, with virologic response to genotype 1 ($n = 92$) of 36% and a response to non-1 genotypes of 81% ($n = 26$).

In adults, pegylated interferon-α in combination with ribavirin has produced the best overall virologic response among FDA-approved therapies, with response rates of about 55%.[144] Clinical trials of peginterferon are under way in children.

Prevention of Infection

No HCV vaccines have been approved for use in humans. No therapeutic trials in pregnancy have been undertaken during the last trimester to reduce the viral load at the time of delivery in an attempt to decrease the rate of vertical transmission. No immune globulins or antivirals have been used for the newborn infant to prevent the development of infection in those perinatally exposed to HCV.

HEPATITIS D

The Virus

Rizzetto and colleagues first noted that clinical deterioration of chronic HBV infection was associated with the appearance of a new (delta) antigen in the liver and antibody in the serum to this antigen.[170] This delta agent was subsequently isolated and analyzed and its nucleic acid cloned and sequenced.[162,165,171] HDV (delta agent) is a 37-nm negative-sense single-stranded RNA agent that requires co-infection with HBV. The unique circular RNA genome is only 1700 nucleotides long. HDV is unrelated to known animal RNA viruses but shares some similarities with plant viruses.[161,163,169] Reclassification of HDV as a new genus, *Deltavirus*, has been proposed.

Pathogenesis

Little is known about HDV infection. Cell entry is thought to be mediated by an HBsAg-associated cellular receptor. Once inside the cell, host cell RNA polymerase transcribes viral RNA by mechanisms that are poorly understood, because no RNA-dependent RNA polymerase activity usually exists for host enzymes.[161] HDV has multiple open reading frames, but only one, ORF5, leads to the production of a single, identifiable HDV protein. This protein can take two forms—HDAg-S (short) and HDAg-L (long), which contains an additional 19 amino acids and serves a different function. HDAg-S is involved in HDV RNA replication by stimulating transcription of viral nucleic acid by the host enzyme; HDAg-L is involved in virion assembly.[161,163] Genetic heterogeneity is well documented with HDV: Three genotypes, as well as numerous quasispecies within each genotype, have been described.[163] The RNA genome is capable of self-cleavage and self-ligation in the process of creating circular RNA; therefore, it is classified as a ribozyme. The virus uses the HBV S protein (HBsAg) as a coat protein, packaging the HDV RNA/HDAg within infectious virions. The virus may be directly cytotoxic to the hepatocyte.

Investigation of the immunologic response to HDV acute infection in patients chronically infected by HBV suggests clearance of HDV by $CD4^+$ helper T cells, which have been documented to respond to at least four specific viral epitopes.[168] Patients with HDV hepatitis in whom chronic HDV infections subsequently developed lacked these specific cellular responses. Recently, a set of HDV epitopes eliciting specific anti-HDV $CD8^+$ T cell responses were found in patients with evidence of past HDV infection, suggesting that cellular immune responses to HDV may be similar to these seen with HBV infection.[164]

The histopathology of hepatitis delta virus infection has been studied in carriers of HBsAg with serial biopsies in adults with acute HDV hepatitis associated with chronic infection. No feature distinguished HDV histopathology from other types of viral hepatitis. Portal and periportal inflammation with piecemeal necrosis was documented, often accompanied by cirrhosis. Biopsies also documented focal, confluent, and bridging necrosis. In patients with chronic HBV infection who are co-infected with HDV, more rapid progression to cirrhosis may occur, particularly in certain population groups.[169] HDV co-infection does not appear to confer additional risk of hepatocellular carcinoma, however.[169]

Overall, approximately 5% of persons infected chronically with HBV worldwide are co-infected with HDV, resulting in a public health burden of 15 million cases of HDV infection. As the epidemiology of hepatitis D is better understood, the worldwide distribution and clinical significance of HDV are becoming appreciated. HDV is present in 40% to 60% of all cases of fulminant HBV infection.

Transmission

HDV infection in adults in the developed world occurs primarily in association with parenteral drug abuse, although sexual transmission and intrafamilial transmission also may occur.[166] In underdeveloped areas within Africa and South America, the seroprevalence of HDV is much higher, although it may vary considerably even within regions of a single country. In these areas, identified risk factors include living in a household with an index case, sexual contact, and spread through open skin lesions in children.[169] In utero or vertical transmission of HDV from mother to neonate has not been reported.

Clinical Illness

HDV infections occur in three clinical settings: (1) acute HDV hepatitis with acute HBV hepatitis, (2) acute HDV hepatitis with chronic HBV hepatitis, and (3) chronic HDV hepatitis with chronic HBV hepatitis. The incidence, transmission, and clinical consequence of HDV infection in newborns and young children have not been defined.

Laboratory Diagnosis

Commercial anti-HDV EIA tests are widely available, including an anti-HDV IgM test. In acute self-limited HDV hepatitis, the IgM anti-HDV antibody is only transiently positive; therefore, serial samples may be necessary to confirm the diagnosis. In any HBsAg-positive, anti-HBc IgM antibody–negative patient who has acute hepatitis, a screening test for IgM anti-HDV antibody may help rule out concurrent HDV superinfection. In chronic HDV hepatitis, anti-HDV IgM or high-titer anti-HDV IgG antibodies are detectable. Serial samples that are positive for anti-HDV antibody confirm that the infection is chronic and not acute. In addition to detection of antibody, HDV antigen (HDAg) can be detected in serum by immunoblot technique in a majority of patients with chronic HDV infection. The most sensitive test for HDV infection is an assay for HDV RNA using RT-PCR, which also is commercially available.

Therapy

The only treatment that proved effective in HDV/HBV co-infection in adults is high-dose, prolonged therapy with interferon-α.[167] Courses of interferon longer than 1 year have been used in some patients.[163] No treatment has been used in children.

Prevention of Infection

The prevention of hepatitis D is accomplished through the prevention of hepatitis B, because available evidence does not suggest that HDV can infect a person who is HBsAg negative. Perinatal transmission has not yet been documented; accordingly, the need for intervention during pregnancy has not yet been defined.

HEPATITIS E

The Virus

HEV is a 7500-base, positive-sense, single-stranded RNA whose sequence is unique among those of other known viruses, most closely resembling that of togaviruses. The viral genome consists of three open reading frames, which code for at least five nonstructural and capsid proteins, including a protease, a helicase, and an RNA-dependent RNA polymerase. This virus is 27 to 32 nm in diameter and can be found in stool by immune electron microscopy during the acute phase of the infection. The virus does not have a lipid membrane and is labile to high salt concentrations and freezing but appears to be able to persist in sewage.[186,188]

Pathogenesis

HEV infection is found worldwide. Like HAV, this virus is a major cause of waterborne epidemics of acute hepatitis under conditions of poor sanitation. Infections occur predominantly in Asia, Africa, and Mexico. Recently developed EIAs for anti-HEV have detected antibodies to HEV-related antigens in 1% to 2% of U.S. volunteer blood donors, indicating that HEV also may be endemic in the United States. Most people infected with HEV are older than those infected with HAV, with seroepidemiologic investigations suggesting a peak incidence of infection between the ages of 15 and 40 years. Published data suggest negligible intrafamilial transmission from index cases identified during outbreaks of HEV infection, providing support for a more prominent role in exposure from contaminated water supplies.[172] Early childhood transmission, presumably through direct contact, also has been documented to occur.[180]

Very little is known about the pathophysiology of HEV infection in humans, although primate models have successfully been used to study productive infections. The virus first appears in the liver, followed by viremia, and subsequently by shedding of the virus in feces. Liver injury occurs with elevated serum aminotransferases and develops at the time of appearance of anti-HEV IgM antibody. Evidence of liver inflammation is accompanied by biopsy evidence of injury, but without the presence of significant clinical illness in the primate model. No chronic infection has been described in humans. In animal models and in humans, the severity of the disease may be genotype dependent. Passively administered neutralizing antibody to HEV capsid antigens is successful in preventing infection following challenge in the cynomolgus primate model.[187] Little is known about the human cellular immune response to HEV infection.

A number of studies of the natural history of hepatitis in pregnancy have documented HEV to play a dominant role in the progression to fulminant hepatic failure and death.[181,184,185] The pathogenesis of aggressive infection in pregnancy is not well understood.

Transmission

Hepatitis E virus (HEV) usually is transmitted to children and adults by the fecal-oral route.[173,174] With respect to the neonate, limited data point to in utero infection as suggested by the presence of specific HEV IgM in cord blood, as well as by the detection of virus by PCR assay.[182,185] In one report from India of a series of eight infants born to mothers with evidence of acute HEV infection in the third trimester, five infants had PCR evidence of in utero infection[182]; of these, four had elevated values of liver aminotransesterases, and three had anti-HEV IgM. Two of these five neonates died, with postmortem examination in one infant documenting hepatic necrosis.

In another report, also from India, three of six neonates born to mothers with acute HEV infection during the third trimester of pregnancy were PCR positive for HEV. Two of these three infants also were anti-HEV IgM positive in cord blood. One of these infants had intrauterine growth retardation and elevated values on liver function tests at the time of birth but recovered clinically from the illness.[185]

Prospectively collected, uncontrolled data on HEV transmission from mothers to infants in Saudi Arabia documented HEV RNA in colostrum of infected mothers. Of 57 pregnant women documented to be HEV seropositive for viral RNA during the last trimester, 6 experienced symptomatic liver disease in the perinatal period. Clinical hepatitis developed in 4 infants born to these 6 women by 6 to 8 weeks of age. None of these infants were breast-fed, because of maternal illness. All other infants born to HEV RNA-positive mothers were breast-fed for a mean of 3.6 months. Hepatitis did not develop in any of these infants. Therefore, available data suggest that breast-feeding does not increase the transmission of virus from mother to infant.[176]

Clinical Illness

The incubation period following exposure in children and adults is between 15 and 60 days. The clinical manifestations of illness usually are mild, with nausea, vomiting, and epigastric pain, followed by the onset of jaundice. Clinical symptoms and aminotransferase elevation usually resolve within 1 to 6 weeks.[183,188] In the animal model, clinical symptoms are dependent on the inoculum of virus.[177] Excretion generally continues for a few weeks following onset of illness.[175] Chronic HEV infection has not been documented.

Laboratory Diagnosis

Acute infection may be diagnosed by the presence of anti-HEV IgM, whereas past infection may be documented by the presence of anti-HEV IgG. Assays for both immunoglobulins are available commercially in reference laboratories.[175,179]

Therapy

Clinical studies of antiviral therapy in animal models or humans have not been reported. Nevertheless, antiviral therapy might provide benefit to specific populations, including pregnant women, in whom more serious disease may develop.

Prevention of Infection

Postexposure, passive administration of immune globulin does not appear to reduce the incidence of disease.[183] Based on the ability to passively neutralize virus and to prevent infection in animal models, vaccines have been developed for HEV infection. A vaccine that contains an epitope spanning all genotypes is now in clinical trials in Nepal.[178]

HEPATITIS G

The Virus

HGV, also known as GB virus type C (GBV-C), was identified in 1995 from the blood of hepatitis patients who had no other identifiable causes of viral hepatitis.[192] Since its discovery, however, no further association has been found with hepatitis as a clinical syndrome attributable to this virus—hence the preference of some experts for the name GBV-C.[197] The virus is classified as a flavivirus, containing a 9.4-kilobase single strand of positive-sense RNA. The single polyprotein encoded by the single open reading frame in the genome has approximately 30% homology with HCV. The polyprotein is cleaved into at least eight proteins, including two envelope proteins (E1, E2) and six nonstructural proteins (NS2, NS3, NS4A, NS4B, NS5A, NS5B), analogous to HCV. Unlike the genes that code for the HCV E2 protein, however, a hypervariable region does not appear to exist in HGV.[197]

Pathogenesis

In an attempt to define the HGV-attributable liver infection in patients known to be chronically infected with the virus because of persistent serum HGV RNA, investigators assayed HGV RNA in both liver and serum from patients undergoing liver transplantation (for a variety of underlying disorders) who were known to be infected either with HGV alone, infected with HCV alone, or coinfected with both viruses.[193] The investigators found a mean liver-to-serum ratio of HCV, known to be hepatotropic, of greater than 10^2, whereas the mean liver-to-serum ratio in HGV patients was only 0.3, leading to the conclusions that HGV was not hepatotropic and that HGV RNA found in the liver was related to blood circulation rather than to hepatocyte infection. Indeed, HGV has not been found to be pathogenic in any study in which patients were known to be infected.[196] Anti-HGV antibody was found in 13% of blood donors in the midwestern United States who passed the standard laboratory and questionnaire screening tests to permit donation. Furthermore, in 2% of these donors, HGV RNA was detected.

In epidemiologic studies worldwide, the prevalence of antibodies to HGV E2 protein varies, ranging from 20% in South Africa to 3% in the Philippines.[194] In studies in which both HGV RNA and anti-HGV antibody directed against the E2 protein are assayed, both are never found together in the same patient.[194,197]

Transmission

HGV has been shown to be transmitted by exposure to infected blood and blood products, by sexual exposure, and from mother to newborn infant.[196] In Sweden, three studies investigated vertical transmission, including one study of HIV-infected mothers. Of seven infants born to mothers not infected with HIV, one infant became HGV RNA positive in serum at 3 months, with persisting viremia during 42 months of follow-up and no evidence of liver disease.[191] In another investigation, 16 of 20 mothers (80%) with HGV viremia transmitted the infection, as documented by the presence of HGV RNA in their infants.[198] The time to acquisition of viremia in the infants was not well defined, but occurred in a majority of infants by 3 to 6 months of age. Symptomatic hepatitis did not develop in any of the infants. In mothers with HGV and HIV coinfection, the vertical transmission rate of HGV was assessed in the era prior to maternal antiretroviral antenatal prophylaxis. Of 17 mothers identified with HGV infection, 3 were viremic with HGV at the time of delivery, and 14 had anti-HGV antibody. None of the anti-HGV–antibody positive women had detectable serum HGV RNA. Only one of the infants born to the mothers with HGV viremia transmitted the infection to her infant; HIV was not co-transmitted to this infant.[190] HGV did not appear to influence the rate of transmission of HIV, noted to be 20% in this study.

The role of breast-feeding in transmission was investigated in one study, documenting the lack of detectable HGV RNA in the breast milk of 15 viremic women.[195] Nevertheless, the vertical transmission rate in this study was 20%, as assessed by HGV RNA in the infants. Because breast milk may not play a significant role in vertical transmission of HGV, and the consequences of neonatal chronic infection are not defined, breast-feeding should not be discouraged in women known to be HGV infected.

Laboratory Diagnosis

Most commercial laboratories do not offer routine testing for HGV. An EIA for antibody to the E2 protein has been developed to detect past infection, however, and is used in epidemiologic investigations.[196] HGV RNA can be detected by RT-PCR assay, which is available in some reference laboratories. Because the virus is not known to cause disease, recommendations for routine screening for HGV infection in any population, including blood donors, have not been made.

REFERENCES

Hepatitis A

1. American Academy of Pediatrics. The 2003 Report of the Committee on Infectious Diseases. Elk Grove, Ill, American Academy of Pediatrics, 2003.
2. Baroudy BM, Ticehurst JR, Miele TA, et al. Sequence analysis of hepatitis A virus cDNA coding for capsid proteins and RNA polymerase. Proc Natl Acad Sci U S A 82:2143-2147, 1985.

3. Costa-Mattioli M, Di Napoli A, Ferre V, et al. Genetic variability of hepatitis A virus. J Gen Virol 84:3191-3201, 2003.
4. Cuthbert JA. Hepatitis A: old and new. Clin Microbiol Rev 14:38-58, 2001.
5. Cromeans T, Fields HA, Sobsey MD. Replication kinetics and cytopathic effect of hepatitis A virus. J Gen Virol 70:2051-2062, 1989.
6. Debray D, Cullufi P, Devictor D, et al. Liver failure in children with hepatitis A. Hepatology 26:1018-1022, 1997.
7. Fagan EA, Hadzic N, Saxena R, Mieli-Vergani G. Symptomatic neonatal hepatitis A disease from a virus variant acquired in utero. Pediatr Infect Dis J 18:389-391, 1999.
8. Feinstone SM, Kapikian AZ, Purceli RH. Hepatitis A detection by immune electron microscopy of a virus-like antigen associated with acute illness. Science 182:1026-1028, 1973.
9. Gingrich GA, Hadler SC, Elder HA, Ash KO. Serologic investigation of an outbreak of hepatitis A in a rural day-care center. Am J Public Health 73:1190-1193, 1983.
10. Hadler SC, Webster HM, Erben JJ, et al. Hepatitis A in day-care centers. A community-wide assessment. N Engl J Med 302:1222-1227, 1980.
11. Krugman S. Viral hepatitis A identified by CF and immune adherence. N Engl J Med 292:1141-1143, 1975.
12. Krugman S.Viral hepatitis: A, B, C, D and E infection. Pediatr Rev 13:203-212, 1992.
13. Klein BS, Michaels JA, Rytel MW, et al. Nosocomial hepatitis A: a multinursery outbreak in Wisconsin. JAMA 252:2716-2721, 1984.
14. Lednar WM, Lemon SM, Kirkpatrick JW, et al. Frequency of illness associated with epidemic hepatitis A virus infections in adults. Am J Epidemiol 122:226-233, 1985.
15. Leikin E, Lysikiewicz A, Garry D, Tejani N. Intrauterine transmission of hepatitis A virus. Obstet Gynecol 88:690-691, 1996.
16. Lemon SM. The natural history of hepatitis A: the potential for transmission by transfusion of blood or blood products. Vox Sang 67(Suppl 4):19-23, 1994.
17. McCaustland KA, Bond WW, Bradley DW, et al. Survival of hepatitis A virus in feces after drying and storage for 1 month. J Clin Microbiol 16:957-958, 1982.
18. Muecke CJ, Beliveau C, Rahme E, et al. Hepatitis A seroprevalence and risk factors among day-care educators. Clin Invest Med 27:259-264, 2004.
19. Najarian R, Caput D, Gee W, et al. Primary structure and gene organization of human hepatitis A virus. Proc Natl Acad Sci U S A 82:2627-2631, 1985.
20. Normann A, Jung C, Vallbracht A, Flehmig B. Time course of hepatitis A viremia and viral load in the blood of human hepatitis A patients. J Med Virol 72:10-16, 2004.
21. Rakela J, Mosley JW. Fecal excretion of hepatitis A virus in humans. J Infect Dis 135:933-938, 1977.
22. Rosenblum LS, Villarino ME, Nainan OV, et al. Hepatitis A outbreak in a neonatal intensive care unit: risk factors for transmission and evidence of prolonged viral excretion among preterm infants. J Infect Dis 164:476-482, 1991.
23. Schiodt FV, Davern TJ, Shakil AO, et al. Viral hepatitis-related acute liver failure. Am J Gastroenterol 98:448-453, 2003.
24. Shapiro CN, Hadler SC. Hepatitis A and hepatitis B virus infections in day-care settings. Pediatr Ann 20:435-441, 1991.
25. Shaw FE Jr, Sudman JH, Smith SM, et al. A community-wide epidemic of hepatitis A in Ohio. Am J Epidemiol 123:1057-1065, 1986.
26. Silberstein E, Dveksler G, Kaplan GG. Neutralization of hepatitis A virus (HAV) by an immunoadhesin containing the cysteine-rich region of HAV cellular receptor-1. J Virol 75:717-725, 2001.
27. Sjogren M. Immunization and the decline of viral hepatitis as a cause of acute liver failure. Hepatology 38:554-556, 2003.
28. Stapleton JT. Host immune response to hepatitis A virus. J Infect Dis 171(Suppl 1):S9-S14, 1995.
29. Storch GA, Bodicky C, Parker M, et al. Use of conventional and IgM-specific radioimmunoassays for anti–hepatitis A antibody in an outbreak of hepatitis A. Am J Med 73:663-668, 1982.
30. Tanaka I, Shima M, Kubota Y, et al. Vertical transmission of hepatitis A. Lancet 345:397, 1995.
31. Tassopoulos NC, Papaevangelou GJ, Ticehurst JR, Purcell RH. Fecal excretion of Greek strains of hepatitis A virus in patients with hepatitis A and in experimentally infected chimpanzees. J Infect Dis 154:231-237, 1986.
32. Ticehurst JR. Hepatitis A virus: clones, cultures, and vaccines. Semin Liver Dis 6:46-55, 1986.
33. Tong MJ, Thursby M, Rakela J, et al. Studies on the maternal-infant transmission of the viruses which cause acute hepatitis. Gastroenterology 80:999-1004, 1981.
34. Vallbracht A, Maier K, Stierhof YD, et al. Liver-derived cytotoxic T cells in hepatitis A virus infection. J Infect Dis 160:209-217, 1989.
35. Watson JC, Fleming DW, Borella AJ, et al. Vertical transmission of hepatitis A resulting in an outbreak in a neonatal intensive care unit. J Infect Dis 167:567-571, 1993

Hepatitis B

36. Beasley RP, Hwang LY, Stevens CE, et al. Efficacy of hepatitis B immune globulin for prevention of perinatal transmission of the hepatitis B virus carrier state: final report of a randomized double-blind, placebo-controlled trial. Hepatology 3:135-141, 1983.
37. Beasley RP, Hwang LY, Lee GC, et al. Prevention of perinatally transmitted hepatitis B virus infections with hepatitis B virus infections with hepatitis B immune globulin and hepatitis B vaccine. Lancet 2:1099-1102, 1983.
38. Beasley RP. Hepatitis B virus. The major etiology of hepatocellular carcinoma. Cancer 61:1942-1956, 1988.
39. Bortolotti F. Treatment of chronic hepatitis B in children. J Hepatol 39(Suppl 1):S200-S205, 2003.
40. Bouchard MJ, Schneider RJ. The enigmatic X gene of hepatitis B virus. J Virol 78:12725-12734, 2004.
41. Boxall EH, Flewett TH, Dane DS, et al. Hepatitis B surface antigen in breast milk. Lancet 2:1007-1008, 1974.
42. Boxall EH, Sira J, Standish RA, et al. Natural history of hepatitis B in perinatally infected carriers. Arch Dis Child Fetal Neonatal Ed 89:F456-F460, 2004.
43. Broderick A, Jonas MM. Management of hepatitis B in children. Clin Liver Dis 8:387-401, 2004.
44. Centers for Disease Control and Prevention. Hepatitis B Virus: A Comprehensive Strategy for Eliminating Transmission in the United States Through Universal Childhood Vaccination: Recommendations of the Immunization Practices Advisory Committee (ACIP). MMWR 40(RR-130):1-19, 1991.
45. Chang MH, Lee CY, Chen DS, et al. Fulminant hepatitis in children in Taiwan: the important role of hepatitis B virus. J Pediatr 111:34-39, 1987.
46. Chang MH. Decreasing incidence of hepatocellular carcinoma among children following universal hepatitis B immunization. Liver Int 23:309-314, 2003.
47. Chen WN, Oon CJ. Human hepatitis B virus mutants: significance of molecular changes. FEBS Lett 453:237-242, 1999.
48. Dane DS, Cameron CH, Briggs M. Virus-like particles in serum of patients with Australia–antigen-associated hepatitis. Lancet 1:695, 1970.
49. Dinsmoor MJ. Hepatitis in the obstetric patient. Infect Dis Clin North Am 11:77-91, 1997.
50. Fiore AE. Chronic maternal hepatitis B infection and premature rupture of membranes. Pediatr Infect Dis J 21:357-358, 2002.
51. Ganem D. Assembly of hepadnaviral virions and subviral particles. Curr Top Microbiol Immunol 168:61-83, 1991.
52. Ganem D, Prince AM. Hepatitis B virus infection—natural history and clinical consequences. N Engl J Med 350:1118-1129, 2004.
53. Hadziyannis SJ, Tassopoulos NC, Heathcote EJ, et al. Adefovir dipivoxil for the treatment of hepatitis B e antigen-negative chronic hepatitis B. N Engl J Med 348:800-807, 2003.
54. Heerman KH, Goldmann U, Schwartz W, et al. Large surface proteins of hepatitis B virus containing the pre-S sequence. J Virol 52:396-402, 1984.
55. Hill JB, Sheffield JS, Kim MJ, et al. Risk of hepatitis B transmission in breast-fed infants of chronic hepatitis B carriers. Obstet Gynecol 99:1049-1052, 2002.
56. Hom X, Little NR, Gardner SD, Jonas MM. Predictors of virologic response to lamivudine treatment in children with chronic hepatitis B infection. Pediatr Infect Dis J 23:441-445, 2004.
57. Hwang LY, Beasley RP, Stevens CE, Szmuness W. Immunogenicity of HBV vaccine in healthy Chinese children. Vaccine 1:10-12, 1983.
58. Jonas MM, Mizerski J, Badia IB, et al. Clinical trial of lamivudine in children with chronic hepatitis B. N Engl J Med 346:1706-1713, 2002.
59. Kattamis CA, Demetrios D, Matsaurotis NS. Australia antigen and neonatal hepatitis syndrome. Pediatrics 54:157-164, 1974.
60. Komatsu H, Inui A, Morinishi Y, et al. Sequence analysis of hepatitis B virus genomes from an infant with acute severe hepatitis and a hepatitis B e antigen-positive carrier mother. J Med Virol 65:457-462, 2001.

61. Lai CL, Ratziu V, Yuen MF, Poynard T. Viral hepatitis B. Lancet 362:2089-2094, 2003.
62. Larouze B, et al. Host response to hepatitis-B infection in patients with primary hepatic carcinoma and families: a case/control study in Senegal, West Africa. Lancet 2:534-538, 1976.
63. Lee AKY, Ip HMH, Wong VCW. Mechanisms of maternal-fetal transmission of hepatitis B virus. J Infect Dis 138:668-671, 1978.
64. Lee JY, Locarnini S. Hepatitis B virus: pathogenesis, viral intermediates, and viral replication. Clin Liver Dis 8:301-320, 2004.
65. Lemon, SM. What is the role of testing for IgM antibody to core antigen of hepatitis B virus? Mayo Clin Proc 63:201-204, 1988.
66. Lindsay KL, Nizze JA, Koretz R, et al. Diagnostic usefulness of testing for anti-HBc IgM in acute hepatitis B. Hepatology 6:1325-1328, 1986.
67. Linnemann CC, Goldberg S. HBAg in breast milk. Lancet 2:155, 1974.
68. Lo KJ, Lee SD, Tsai YT, et al. Long-term immunogenicity and efficacy of hepatitis B vaccine in infants born to HBeAg-positive HBsAg-carrier mothers. Hepatology 8:1647-1650, 1988.
69. Lolekha S, Warachit B, Hirunyachote A, et al. Protective efficacy of hepatitis B vaccine without HBIG in infants of HBeAg-positive carrier mothers in Thailand. Vaccine 20:3739-3743, 2002.
70. Marcellin P, Chang TT, Lim SG, et al. Adefovir dipivoxil for the treatment of hepatitis B e antigen–positive chronic hepatitis B. N Engl J Med 348:808-816, 2003.
71. Marcellin P, Lau GK, Bonino F, et al. Peginterferon alfa-2a alone, lamivudine alone, and the two in combination in patients with HBeAg-negative chronic hepatitis B. N Engl J Med 351:1206-1217, 2004.
72. Maynard P, Barin F, Chiron JP, et al. Efficacy of hepatitis B vaccine in prevention of early HB_sAg carrier state in children. Lancet 1:289-292, 1981.
73. Mele A, Stroffolini T, Zanetti AR. Hepatitis B in Italy: where we are ten years after the introduction of mass vaccination. J Med Virol 67: 440-443, 2002.
74. Milne A, West DJ, Chinh DV, et al. Field evaluation of the efficacy and immunogenicity of recombinant hepatitis B vaccine without HBIG in newborn Vietnamese infants. J Med Virol 67:327-333, 2002.
75. Moroy T, Marchio A, Etiemble J, et al. Rearrangement and enhanced expression of c-myc in hepatocellular carcinoma of hepatitis virus infected woodchucks. Nature 324:276-279, 1986.
76. Okada K, Yarnada T, Mijakawa Y, et al. Hepatitis B surface antigen in the serum of infants after delivery from asymptomatic carrier mothers. J Pediatr 87:360-363, 1975
77. Okada K, Kamiyama I, Inomata M, et al. *e* antigen and anti-*e* in the serum of asymptomatic carrier mothers as indicators of positive and negative transmission of hepatitis B virus to their infants. N Engl J Med 294:746-749, 1976.
78. Oon CJ, Lim GK, Ye Z, et al. Molecular epidemiology of hepatitis B virus vaccine variants in Singapore. Vaccine 13:699-702, 1995.
79. Pawlotsky JM. Molecular diagnosis of viral hepatitis. Gastroenterology 122:1554-1568, 2002.
80. Pawlotsky JM. Hepatitis B virus (HBV) DNA assays (methods and practical use) and viral kinetics. J Hepatol 39(Suppl 1):S31-S35, 2003.
81. Penna A, Artini M, Cavalli A, et al. Long-lasting memory T cell responses following self-limited acute hepatitis B. J Clin Invest 98:1185-1194, 1996.
82. Poovorawan Y, Sanpavat S, Pongpunglert W, et al. Long term efficacy of hepatitis B vaccine in infants born to hepatitis B e antigen-positive mothers.Pediatr Infect Dis J 11:816-821, 1992.
83. Raimondo G, Schneider R, Stemler M, et al. A new hepatitis B virus variant in a chronic carrier with multiple episodes of viral reactivation and acute hepatitis. Virology 179:64-68, 1990.
84. Ranger-Rogez S, Denis F. Hepatitis B mother-to-child transmission. Expert Rev Anti Infect Ther 2:133-145, 2004.
85. Rehermann B, Chang KM, McHutchinson J, et al. Differential cytotoxic T-lymphocyte responsiveness to the hepatitis B and C viruses in chronically infected patients. J Virol 70:7092-7102, 1996.
86. Rehermann B, Ferrari C, Pasquinelli C, Chisari FV. The hepatitis B virus persists for decades after patients' recovery from acute viral hepatitis despite active maintenance of a cytotoxic T-lymphocyte response. Nat Med 2:1104-1108, 1996.
87. Rehermann B, Chisari FV. Cell mediated immune response to the hepatitis C virus. Curr Top Microbiol Immunol 242:299-325, 2000.
88. Rehermann B. Immune responses in hepatitis B virus infection. Semin Liver Dis 23:21-38, 2003.
89. Saltik-Temizel IN, Kocak N, Demir H. Interferon-alpha and lamivudine combination therapy of children with chronic hepatitis b infection who were interferon-alpha nonresponders. Pediatr Infect Dis J 23:466-468, 2004.
90. Saltik-Temizel IN, Kocak N, Demir H. Lamivudine and high-dose interferon-alpha combination therapy for naïve children with chronic hepatitis B infection. J Clin Gastroenterol 39:68-70, 2005.
91. Schmitt S, Glebe D, Tolle TK, et al. Structure of pre-S2 *N*- and *O*-linked glycans in surface proteins from different genotypes of hepatitis B virus.J Gen Virol 85:2045-2053, 2004.
92. Schweitzer IL, Wing A, McPeak C, et al. Hepatitis and hepatitis-associated antigen in 56 mother-infant pairs. JAMA 220:1092-1095, 1972.
93. Schweitzer IL, Dunn AE, Peters RL, et al. Viral hepatitis B in neonates and infants. Am J Med 55:762-771, 1973.
94. Schweitzer IL, Moseley JW, Ashcavai M, et al. Factors influencing neonatal infection by hepatitis B virus. Gastroenterology 65:227-283, 1973.
95. Schweitzer IL. Vertical transmission of the hepatitis B surface antigen. Am J Med Sci 270:287-291, 1975.
96. Servoss JC, Friedman LS. Serologic and molecular diagnosis of hepatitis B virus. Clin Liver Dis 8:267-281, 2004.
97. Shields MT, Taswell HF, Czaja AJ, et al. Frequency and significance of concurrent hepatitis B surface antigen and antibody in acute and chronic hepatitis B. Gastroenterology 93:675-680, 1987.
98. Skinhoj P, Sardemann H, Cohen J. Hepatitis associated antigen (HAA) in pregnant women and their newborn infants. Am J Dis Child 123:380-381, 1972.
99. Soderstrom A, Norkrans G, Lindh M. Hepatitis B virus DNA during pregnancy and post partum: aspects on vertical transmission. Scand J Infect Dis 35:814-819, 2003.
100. Stevens CE, Beasley RP, Tsui J, et al. Vertical transmission of hepatitis B antigen in Taiwan. N Engl J Med 292:771-774, 1975.
101. Stevens CE, Neurath RA, Beasley P, et al. HBeAg and anti HBe detection by radioimmunoassay correlation with vertical transmission of HBV in Taiwan. J Med Virol 3:237-241, 1979.
102. Stevens CE, Taylor PE, Tong MJ, et al. Yeast-recombinant hepatitis B vaccine. Efficacy with hepatitis B immune globulin in prevention of perinatal hepatitis B virus transmission. JAMA 257:2612-2616, 1987.
103. Stibbe W, Gerlich WH. Variable protein composition of hepatitis B surface antigen from different donors. Virology 123:436-442, 1982.
104. Stiehm ER, Keller MA. Breast milk transmission of viral disease. Adv Nutr Res 10:105-122, 2001.
105. Szmuness W. Hepatocellular carcinoma and the hepatitis B virus: evidence for a causal association. Prog Med Virol 24:40-69, 1978.
106. Tedder RS, Ijaz S, Gilbert N, et al. Evidence for a dynamic host – parasite relationship in e-negative hepatitis B carriers. J Med Virol 68:505-512, 2002.
107. Tiollais P, Dejean A, Brechot C, et al. Structure of hepatitis B virus DNA. *In* Vyas GN, Dienstag JL, Hoofnagle JH (eds). Viral Hepatitis and Liver Disease. New York, Grune & Stratton, 1984, pp 49-65.
108. Tran TT, Martin P. Hepatitis B: epidemiology and natural history. Clin Liver Dis 8:255-266, 2004.
109. van Zonneveld M, van Nunen AB, Niesters HG, et al. Lamivudine treatment during pregnancy to prevent perinatal transmission of hepatitis B virus infection. J Viral Hepat 10:294-297, 2003.
110. Vitvitski L, Trepo C, Prince AM, et al. Detection of virus-associated antigen in serum and liver of patients with non-A, non-B hepatitis. Lancet 32:1263-1267, 1979.
111. Wands JR, Fujita YK, Isselbacher KJ, et al. Identification and transmission of hepatitis B virus-related variants. Proc Natl Acad Sci U S A 83:6608-6612, 1986.
112. Wai CT, Fontana RJ. Clinical significance of hepatitis B virus genotypes, variants, and mutants. Clin Liver Dis 8:321-352, 2004.
113. Wieland S, Thimme R, Purcell RH, Chisari FV. Genomic analysis of the host response to hepatitis B virus infection. Proc Natl Acad Sci U S A 101:6669-6674, 2004.
114. Wu JS, Hwang LY, Goodman KJ, Beasley RP. Hepatitis B vaccination in high-risk infants: 10-year follow-up. J Infect Dis 179:1319-1325, 1999.
115. Yang YJ, Liu CC, Chen TJ, et al. Role of hepatitis B immunoglobulin in infants born to hepatitis B e antigen-negative carrier mothers in Taiwan. Pediatr Infect Dis J 22:584-588, 2003.
116. Young BW, Lee SS, Lim WL, Yeoh EK. The long-term efficacy of plasma-derived hepatitis B vaccine in babies born to carrier mothers. J Viral Hepat 10:23-30, 2003.
117. Zhang SL, Yue YF, Bai GQ, et al. Mechanism of intrauterine infection of hepatitis B virus. World J Gastroenterol 10:437-438, 2004.

Hepatitis C

118. ACOG educational bulletin. Viral hepatitis in pregnancy. No. 248, July 1998. American College of Obstetricians and Gynecologists. Int J Gynaecol Obstet 63:195-202, 1998.
119. Bradley DW, Maynard JE. Etiology and natural history of post-transfusion and enterically-transmitted non A, non-B hepatitis. Semin Liver Dis 6:56-66, 1986.
120. Caudai C, Battiata M, Riccardi MP, et al. Vertical transmission of the hepatitis C virus to infants of anti-human immunodeficiency virus-negative mothers: molecular evolution of hypervariable region 1 in prenatal and perinatal or postnatal infections. J Clin Microbiol 41:3955-3959, 2003.
121. Cerny A, Chisari FV. Pathogenesis of chronic hepatitis C: immunological features of hepatic injury and viral persistence. Hepatology 30: 595-601, 1999.
122. Choo QL, Weiner AJ, Overby LR, et al. Hepatitis C virus: the major causative agent of viral non-A, non-B hepatitis. Br Med Bull 46: 423-441, 1990.
123. Conte D, Colucci A, Minola E, et al. Clinical course of pregnant women with chronic hepatitis C virus infection and risk of mother-to-child hepatitis C virus transmission. Dig Liver Dis 33:366-371, 2001.
124. Darling JM, Wright TL. Immune responses in hepatitis C: is virus or host the problem? Curr Opin Infect Dis 17:193-198, 2004.
125. FDA, 2004 (http://www.fda.gov/cder/foi/label/2004/103132_5064lbl.pdf).
126. Ferrero S, Lungaro P, Bruzzone BM, et al. Prospective study of mother-to-infant transmission of hepatitis C virus: a 10-year survey (1990-2000). Acta Obstet Gynecol Scand 82:229-234, 2003.
127. Germer JJ, Zein NN. Advances in the molecular diagnosis of hepatitis C and their clinical implications. Mayo Clin Proc 76:911-920, 2001.
128. Giacchino R, Tasso L, Timitilli A, et al. Vertical transmission of hepatitis C virus infection: usefulness of viremia detection in HIV-seronegative hepatitis C virus–seropositive mothers. J Pediatr 132: 167-169, 1998.
129. Giles M, Hellard M, Sasadeusz J. Hepatitis C and pregnancy: an update. Aust N Z J Obstet Gynaecol 43:290-293, 2003.
130. Granovsky MO, Minkoff HL, Tess BH, et al. Hepatitis C virus infection in the mothers and infants cohort study. Pediatrics 102:355-359, 1998.
131. Hadzic N. Hepatitis C in pregnancy. Arch Dis Child Fetal Neonatal Ed 84:F201-F204, 2001.
132. Hoofnagle JH. Course and outcome of hepatitis C. Hepatology 36(5 Suppl 1):S21-S29, 2002.
133. Hupertz VF, Wyllie R. Perinatal hepatitis C infection. Pediatr Infect Dis J 22:369-372, 2003.
134. Jara P, Resti M, Hierro L, et al. Chronic hepatitis C virus infection in childhood: clinical patterns and evolution in 224 white children. Clin Infect Dis 36:275-280, 2003.
135. Jonas MM. Children with hepatitis C. Hepatology 36(5 Suppl 1): S173-S178, 2002.
136. Lauer GM, Walker BD. Hepatitis C virus infection. N Engl J Med 345:41-52, 2001.
137. Lauer GM, Barnes E, Lucas M, et al. High resolution analysis of cellular immune responses in resolved and persistent hepatitis C virus infection. Gastroenterology 127:924-936, 2004.
138. Li DY, Schwarz KB. Immunopathogenesis of chronic hepatitis C virus infection. J Pediatr Gastroenterol Nutr 35:260-267, 2002.
139. Mast EE. Mother-to-infant hepatitis C virus transmission and breastfeeding. Adv Exp Med Biol 554:211-216, 2004.
140. Neumann-Haefelin C, Blum HE, Chisari FV, Thimme R. T cell response in hepatitis C virus infection. J Clin Virol 32:75-85, 2005.
141. Orland JR, Wright TL, Cooper S. Acute hepatitis C. Hepatology 33:321-327, 2001.
142. Pappalardo BL. Influence of maternal human immunodeficiency virus (HIV) co-infection on vertical transmission of hepatitis C virus (HCV): a meta-analysis. Int J Epidemiol 32:727-734, 2003.
143. Pawlotsky JM. Use and interpretation of hepatitis C virus diagnostic assays. Clin Liver Dis 7:127-137, 2003.
144. Pearlman BL. Hepatitis C treatment update. Am J Med 117:344-352, 2004.
145. Pembrey L, Newell ML, Peckham C. Is there a case for hepatitis C infection screening in the antenatal period? J Med Screen 10:161-168, 2003.
146. Penin F, Dubuisson J, Rey FA, et al. Structural biology of hepatitis C virus. Hepatology 39:5-19, 2004.
147. Pileri P, Uematsu Y, Campagnoli S, et al. Binding of hepatitis C virus to CD81. Science 282:938-941, 1998.
148. Plunkett BA, Grobman WA. Elective cesarean delivery to prevent perinatal transmission of hepatitis C virus: a cost-effectiveness analysis. Am J Obstet Gynecol 191:998-1003, 2004.
149. Racanelli V, Rehermann B. Hepatitis C virus infection: when silence is deception. Trends Immunol 24:456-464, 2003.
150. Resti M, Azzari C, Mannelli F, et al. Mother to child transmission of hepatitis C virus: prospective study of risk factors and timing of infection in children born to women seronegative for HIV-1. Tuscany Study Group on Hepatitis C Virus Infection. BMJ 317:437-441, 1998.
151. Resti M, Jara P, Hierro L, et al. Clinical features and progression of perinatally acquired hepatitis C virus infection. J Med Virol 70: 373-377, 2003.
152. Roberts EA, Yeung L. Maternal-infant transmission of hepatitis C virus infection. Hepatology 36(5 Suppl 1):S106-S113, 2002.
153. Ruiz-Extremera A, Salmeron J, Torres C, et al. Follow-up of transmission of hepatitis C to babies of human immunodeficiency virus-negative women: the role of breast-feeding in transmission. Pediatr Infect Dis J 19:511-516, 2000.
154. Schuval S, Van Dyke RB, Lindsey JC, et al. Hepatitis C prevalence in children with perinatal human immunodeficiency virus infection enrolled in a long-term follow-up protocol. Arch Pediatr Adolesc Med 158:1007-1013, 2004.
155. Shoukry NH, Grakoui A, Houghton M, et al. Memory $CD8^+$ T cells are required for protection from persistent hepatitis C virus infection. J Exp Med 197:1645-1655, 2003.
156. Simmonds P. Genetic diversity and evolution of hepatitis C virus—15 years on. J Gen Virol 85:3173-3188, 2004.
157. Steininger C, Kundi M, Jatzko G, et al. Increased risk of mother-to-infant transmission of hepatitis C virus by intrapartum infantile exposure to maternal blood. J Infect Dis 187:345-351, 2003.
158. Thimme R, Oldach D, Chang KM, et al. Determinants of viral clearance and persistence during acute hepatitis C virus infection. J Exp Med 194:1395-1406, 2001.
159. Thimme R, Bukh J, Spangenberg HC, et al.Viral and immunological determinants of hepatitis C virus clearance, persistence, and disease. Proc Natl Acad Sci U S A 99:15661-15668, 2002.
160. Thomas SL, Newell ML, Peckham CS, et al. A review of hepatitis C virus (HCV) vertical transmission: risks of transmission to infants born to mothers with and without HCV viraemia or human immunodeficiency virus infection. Int J Epidemiol 27:108-117, 1998.

Hepatitis D

161. Casey JL. Hepatitis delta virus: molecular biology, pathogenesis and immunology. Antivir Ther 3(Suppl 3):37-42, 1998.
162. Denniston KJ, Hoyer BH, Smedile A, et al. Cloned fragment of the hepatitis delta virus RNA genome: sequence and diagnostic application. Science 232:873-875, 1986.
163. Farci P. Delta hepatitis: an update. J Hepatol 39(Suppl 1):S212-S219, 2003.
164. Huang YH, Tao MH, Hu CP, et al. Identification of novel HLA-A*0201-restricted $CD8^+$ T-cell epitopes on hepatitis delta virus. J Gen Virol 85:3089-3098, 2004.
165. Kos A, Dijkema R, Arnberg AC, et al. The hepatitis delta virus possesses a circular RNA. Nature 323:558-560, 1986.
166. Niro GA, Casey JL, Gravinese E, et al. Intrafamilial transmission of hepatitis delta virus: molecular evidence. J Hepatol 30:564-569, 1999.
167. Niro GA, Rosina F, Rizzetto M. Treatment of hepatitis D. J Viral Hepat 12:2-9, 2005.
168. Nisini R, Paroli M, Accapezzato D, et al. Human $CD4^+$ T-cell response to hepatitis delta virus: identification of multiple epitopes and characterization of T-helper cytokine profiles. J Virol 71:2241-2251, 1997.
169. Polish LB, Gallagher M, Fields HA, Hadler SC. Delta hepatitis: molecular biology and clinical and epidemiological features. Clin Microbiol Rev 6:211-229, 1993.
170. Rizzetto M, Canese MG, Gerin JL, et al. Transmission of the hepatitis B virus–associated delta antigen to chimpanzees J Infect Dis 141: 590-602, 1980.
171. Wang KS, Choo QL, Weiner AJ, et al. Structure, sequence and expression of the hepatitis delta viral genome. Nature 323:508-514, 1986.

Hepatitis E

172. Arankalle VA, Chadha MS, Mehendale SM, Tungatkar SP. Epidemic hepatitis E: serological evidence for lack of intrafamilial spread. Indian J Gastroenterol 19:24-28, 2000.
173. Balayan MS, Adnjaparidz AG, Savinskaya SS, et al. Evidence for a virus in non-A, non-B hepatitis transmitted via the fecal-oral route. Intervirology 20:23-31, 1983.

174. Balayan MS. HEV infection: historical perspectives, global epidemiology, and clinical features. *In* Hollinger FB, Lemon SM, Margolis HS (eds). Viral Hepatitis and Liver Disease. Baltimore, Williams & Wilkins, 1991, pp 498-501.
175. Bradley DW. Hepatitis E virus: a brief review of the biology, molecular virology, and immunology of a novel virus. J Hepatol 22(1 Suppl): 140-145, 1995.
176. Chibber RM, Usmani MA, Al-Sibai MH. Should HEV infected mothers breast feed? Arch Gynecol Obstet 270:15-20, 2004.
177. Emerson SU, Purcell RH. Hepatitis E virus. Rev Med Virol 13:145-154, 2003.
178. Emerson SU, Purcell RH. Running like water—the omnipresence of hepatitis E. N Engl J Med 351:2367-2368, 2004.
179. Favorov MO, Fields HA, Purdy MA, et al. Serologic identification of hepatitis E virus infections in epidemic and endemic settings. J Med Virol 36:246-250, 1992.
180. Fix AD, Abdel-Hamid M, Purcell RH, et al. Prevalence of antibodies to hepatitis E in two rural Egyptian communities. Am J Trop Med Hyg 62:519-523, 2000.
181. Jaiswal SP, Jain AK, Naik G, et al. Viral hepatitis during pregnancy. Int J Gynaecol Obstet 72:103-108, 2001.
182. Khuroo MS, Kamili S, Jameel S. Vertical transmission of hepatitis E virus. Lancet 22:1025-1026, 1995.
183. Krawczynski K, Aggarwal R, Kamili S. Hepatitis E. Infect Dis Clin North Am 14:669-687, 2000.
184. Kumar A, Beniwal B, Kar P, et al. Hepatitis E in pregnancy. Obstet Gynecol Surv 60:7-8, 2005.
185. Singh S, Mohanty A, Joshi YK, et al. Mother-to-child transmission of hepatitis E virus infection. Indian J Pediatr 70:37-39, 2003.
186. Ticehurst J. Identification and characterization of hepatitis E virus. *In* Hollinger FB, Lemon SM, Margolis HS (eds). Viral Hepatitis and Liver Disease. Baltimore, Williams & Wilkins, 1991, pp 501-513.
187. Tsarev SA, Tsareva TS, Emerson SU, et al. Successful passive and active immunization of cynomolgus monkeys against hepatitis E. Proc Natl Acad Sci U S A 91:10198-10202, 1994.
188. Worm HC, van der Poel WH, Brandstatter G. Hepatitis E: an overview. Microbes Infect 4:657-666, 2002.
189. Yarbough PO. Hepatitis E virus. Advances in HEV biology and HEV vaccine approaches. Intervirology 42:179-184, 1999.

Hepatitis G

190. Barqasho B, Naver L, Bohlin AB, et al. GB virus C coinfection and vertical transmission in HIV-infected mothers before the introduction of antiretroviral prophylaxis. HIV Med 5:427-430, 2004.
191. Fischler B, Lara C, Chen M, et al. Genetic evidence for mother-to-infant transmission of hepatitis G virus. J Infect Dis 176:281-285, 1997.
192. Linnen J, Wages J Jr, Zhang-Keck ZY, et al. Molecular cloning and disease association of hepatitis G virus: a transfusion-transmissible agent. Science 271:505-508, 1996.
193. Pessoa MG, Terrault NA, Detmer J, et al. Quantitation of hepatitis G and C viruses in the liver: evidence that hepatitis G virus is not hepatotropic. Hepatology 27:877-880, 1998.
194. Ross RS, Viazov S, Schmitt U, et al. Distinct prevalence of antibodies to the E2 protein of GB virus C/hepatitis G virus in different parts of the world. J Med Virol 54:103-106, 1998.
195. Schroter M, Polywka S, Zollner B, et al. Detection of TT virus DNA and GB virus type C/hepatitis G virus RNA in serum and breast milk: determination of mother-to-child transmission. J Clin Microbiol 38:745-747, 2000.
196. Stapleton JT. GB virus type C/hepatitis G virus. Semin Liver Dis 23:137-148, 2003.
197. Stapleton JT, Williams CF, Xiang J.GB virus type C: a beneficial infection? J Clin Microbiol 42:3915-3919, 2004.
198. Wejstal R, Manson AS, Widell A, Norkrans G. Perinatal transmission of hepatitis G virus (GB virus type C) and hepatitis C virus infections—a comparison. Clin Infect Dis 28:816-821, 1999.

Chapter 26

HERPES SIMPLEX VIRUS INFECTIONS

Ann M. Arvin • Richard J. Whitley • Kathleen M. Gutierrez

HISTORICAL BACKGROUND

Infections caused by herpes simplex viruses (HSVs) were recognized by the ancient Greeks. The word *herpes*, meaning "to creep or crawl," was used to describe skin lesions. Herodotus associated mouth ulcers and lip vesicles with fever[1] and called this event *herpes febrilis*. Genital herpetic infections were first described by Astruc, a physician to French royalty.[2] The transmissibility of these viruses was established unequivocally by passage of virus from lip and genital lesions of humans to the cornea or the scarified skin of the rabbit.[3] During the early 20th century, diseases associated with HSV infections became more clearly defined by numerous clinical and pathologic case reports.

Neonatal HSV infection was identified as a distinct disease 70 years ago. The first written descriptions of neonatal HSV infections were attributed to Hass, who described the histopathologic findings of a fatal case, and to Batignani, who described a newborn child with HSV keratitis.[4,5] During subsequent decades, our understanding of neonatal HSV infections was based on histopathologic descriptions of the disease, which indicated a broad spectrum of organ involvement in infants.

An important scientific breakthrough occurred in the mid-1960s, when Nahmias and Dowdle[6] demonstrated two antigenic types of HSV. The development of viral typing methods provided the tools required to clarify the epidemiology of these infections. HSV infections "above the belt," primarily of the lip and oropharynx, were found in most cases to be caused by HSV type 1 (HSV-1). Infections "below the belt," particularly genital infections, were usually caused by HSV type 2 (HSV-2). The finding that genital HSV infections and neonatal HSV infections were most often caused by HSV-2 suggested a cause-and-effect relationship between these two disease entities. This causal relationship was strengthened by detection of the virus in the maternal genital tract at the time of delivery, indicating that acquisition of the virus by the infant occurs by contact with infected genital secretions during birth.

During the past 25 years, our knowledge of the epidemiology, natural history, and pathogenesis of neonatal HSV infections has been enhanced greatly. The development of antiviral therapy represents a significant advance in the management of infected children, providing the opportunity to decrease mortality and reduce the morbidity associated with these infections. Neonatal HSV infection is more amenable to prevention and treatment than many other pathogens because it is acquired most often at birth rather than during gestation. As our understanding of the epidemiology of HSV infections has improved, postnatal acquisition of HSV-1 has been documented from nonmaternal sources, and more cases caused by HSV-1 infections of the maternal genital tract have been identified. New perspectives on the changing presentations of neonatal HSV infection, the obstacles to diagnosis, and the value of antiviral therapy are topics addressed in this chapter.

HERPES SIMPLEX VIRUS

Structure

The biologic, molecular, antigenic, and epidemiologic characteristics of HSV-1 and HSV-2 have been the subject of numerous publications. Reviews highlight the importance of these organisms as models for viral replication and as pathogens in human infection.[7,8]

The HSVs are members of a family of large DNA viruses that contain centrally located, linear, double-stranded DNA. Other members of the herpesvirus family include cytomegalovirus, varicella-zoster virus, Epstein-Barr virus, and human herpesviruses 6A, 6B, 7, and 8.[7,8] As a family, these viruses are virtually indistinguishable from each other by electron microscopy. The viral DNA is packaged inside a protein structure, the capsid, which confers icosahedral symmetry to the virus. The capsid consists of 162 capsomers and is surrounded by a tightly adherent membrane known as the tegument. An envelope consisting of glycoproteins, lipids, and polyamines loosely surrounds the capsid and tegument. The glycoproteins mediate attachment of the virus to cells.

The HSV genome consists of about 150,000 base pairs.[7] The DNA encodes for more than 80 polypeptides. The genome consists of two components, L and S, each of which contains unique sequences that can invert, which leads to four isomers. Viral DNA extracted from virions or infected cells consists of four equal populations differing solely with respect to the relative orientation of these two unique components.

The DNAs of HSV-1 and HSV-2 are colinear with respect to the order of genes encoding viral proteins. The percent homology of base pairs that constitute each gene varies from higher to lesser degrees of conservation. There is considerable overlap in the cross-reactivity between HSV-1 and HSV-2 glycoproteins, although unique regions of these gene products exist for each virus.[9,10] The two viral types can be distinguished by using restriction enzyme analysis of viral DNA, which allows precise epidemiologic investigations of virus transmission.

Replication

Replication of HSV is characterized by the expression of three gene classes: alpha, beta, and gamma. These genes are expressed temporally and in a cascade sequence.[7] Although herpesvirus genes carry transcriptional and translational signals similar to those of other DNA viruses that infect higher eukaryotic cells, the messenger RNAs arising from most genes are not spliced. The information density is lower than that encoded in the genes of smaller viruses. This relatively low density of genetic information is important in that it permits insertion and deletion of genes in the HSV genome without significant alteration of the genomic architecture. This point is relevant because it provides an opportunity for the use of genetically engineered herpesviruses as vaccines or vectors for antigen delivery.[11]

Alpha genes are expressed at immediate-early times after infection and are responsible for the initiation of replication. These genes are transcribed in infected cells in the absence of viral protein synthesis. Products of the beta genes, or early genes, include the enzymes necessary for viral replication, such as HSV thymidine kinase, and the regulatory proteins. These genes require functional alpha gene products for expression. The onset of expression of beta genes coincides with a decline in the rate of expression of alpha genes and an irreversible shutoff of host cellular macromolecular protein synthesis. Structural proteins are usually of the gamma, or late, gene class. The gamma genes are heterogeneous and are differentiated from beta genes solely by their requirement for viral DNA synthesis for maximal expression. Most glycoproteins are expressed as late genes. In addition to its regulatory and structural genes, the virus encodes genes that allow initial evasion of the host response, including gene products that block interferon-α and interferon-β responses. HSV-1 and HSV-2 also express an immediate-early protein, ICP47, that mediates the downregulation of major histocompatibility complex class I molecules.[12]

Replication of viral DNA occurs in the nucleus of the cell. Assembly of the virus begins with formation of nucleocapsids in the nucleus, followed by acquisition of the envelope at cytoplasmic locations. Virus is transported through the cytoskeleton to the plasma membrane, where progeny virions are released.

HSV specifies at least 11, and probably several more, glycoproteins. The glycoproteins have been designated as B, C, D, E, G, H, I, J, K, L, and M.[9] Glycoprotein D (gD) is required for infectivity and is the most potent inducer of neutralizing antibodies; glycoprotein B (gB) is required for infectivity and also induces neutralizing antibodies; glycoprotein C (gC) binds to the C3b component of complement; and glycoprotein E (gE) binds to the Fc portion of IgG. The amino acid sequences of the glycoprotein G (gG) produced by HSV-1 and HSV-2 are sufficiently different to elicit antibody responses that are specific for each virus type. The fact that the antibody response to the two G molecules exhibits minimal cross-reactivity has provided the basis for serologic methods that can be used to detect recent or past HSV-2 infection in individuals who have also been infected with HSV-1.[13-16]

The close antigenic relatedness between HSV-1 and HSV-2 interferes with the serologic diagnosis of these infections using standard serologic assays. These methods do not distinguish between individuals who have had past infection with HSV-1 only, past infection with HSV-2 only, or dual infection. Although laboratory reports often indicate antibody titers to each virus, the methods used by some commercial laboratories are based on use of crude antigen and do not eliminate the detection of cross-reactive antibodies. Commercial type-specific tests based on glycoprotein G are available in some laboratories and must be used for diagnosis of HSV-2 infection.[15] Clinicians must be knowledgeable regarding the type of testing performed by their referral laboratory to correctly interpret results.

Latency and Reactivation

All of the herpesviruses have a characteristic ability to establish latency, by mechanisms that remain unidentified, to persist in this latent state for various intervals of time and to reactivate, causing virus excretion at mucosal or other sites. After infection, the viral DNA persists in the host for the entire lifetime of the individual.

The biologic phenomenon of latency has been recognized and described since the beginning of the 20th century, particularly the association of HSV latency with neurons. In 1905, Cushing[17] observed that patients treated for trigeminal neuralgia by sectioning a branch of the trigeminal nerve developed herpetic lesions along the innervated areas of the sectioned branch. This specific association of HSV with the trigeminal ganglion was suggested by Goodpasture.[18] Past observations have demonstrated that microvascular surgery of the trigeminal nerve tract to alleviate pain associated with tic douloureux resulted in recurrent lesions in more than 90% of seropositive individuals.[19,20]

Accumulated experience in animal models and from clinical observations suggests that inoculation of virus at the portal of entry, usually oral or genital mucosal tissue, results in infection of sensory nerve endings, and the virus is transported to the dorsal root ganglia. Replication at the site of inoculation enhances access of the virus to ganglia but is usually not associated with signs of mucocutaneous disease. Only a fraction of new infections with HSV-1 and HSV-2 are associated with clinically recognizable disease. When reactivation is triggered at oral or genital sites, the virus is transported back down axons to mucocutaneous sites. Replication and shedding of infectious virus occur at these sites. Recognizing that excretion of infectious virus during reactivation is not usually associated with clinical signs of recurrent herpes lesions is essential for understanding the transmission of HSV to newborns. Clinically silent reactivations are much more common than recurrent lesions. Reactivation, with or without symptoms, appears in the presence of humoral and cell-mediated immunity. Reactivation is spontaneous, although symptomatic recurrences have been associated with physical or emotional stress, exposure to ultraviolet light, tissue damage, and suppression of the immune system. Persistence of viral DNA has been documented in neuronal tissue of animal models and humans.[7,8,21-23]

Animal model studies indicate that the transport of virus to the ganglia is by retrograde axonal flow.[24] After transport, virus replicates for several days in sensory ganglia that innervate the sites of inoculation. After latency is established in sensory ganglia, virus cannot be eradicated from the infected cells. Because the latent virus does not multiply, it is not susceptible to drugs, such as acyclovir, that affect viral DNA synthesis. Our understanding of the mechanisms by which HSV establishes a latent state and persists in this form remains limited, and this is a subject of intense research interest.

EPIDEMIOLOGY

Nature of Infection

Although many routes of infection have been suggested, transmission of HSV most often occurs as a consequence of intimate, person-to-person contact. Virus must come in contact with mucosal surfaces or abraded skin for infection to be initiated. Infection with HSV-1, generally limited to the oropharynx, can be transmitted by respiratory droplets or through direct contact of a susceptible individual with infected secretions. Acquisition often occurs during childhood.

Primary HSV-1 infection in the young child is usually asymptomatic, but clinical illness is associated with HSV gingivostomatitis. Primary infection in young adults has been associated with only pharyngitis or with a mononucleosis-like syndrome. Seroprevalence studies have demonstrated that acquisition of HSV-1 infection, like that of other herpesvirus infections, is related to socioeconomic factors. Antibodies, indicative of past infection, are found early in life among individuals of lower socioeconomic groups, presumably reflecting the crowded living conditions that provide a greater opportunity for direct contact with infected individuals. As many as 75% to 90% of individuals from lower socioeconomic populations develop antibodies to HSV-1 by the end of the first decade of life.[8,25-27] In middle and upper middle socioeconomic groups, only 30% to 40% of individuals are seropositive by the middle of the second decade of life.[8] A change in seroprevalence rates of HSV-1 has been recognized in the past few decades, which reflects a delay in acquisition of infection until later in life. The increase in the reported number of cases of genital herpes caused by HSV-2 may be related to a lower prevalence of prior HSV-1 infection in young adults. These individuals would not have the partial protection against HSV-2 infection that is probably conferred by cross-reactive HSV-1 immunity. Investigators have found that a substantial percentage of cases of genital HSV infection are caused by HSV-1 in certain populations.[28]

Because infections with HSV-2 are usually acquired through sexual contact, antibodies to this virus are rarely found until the age of onset of sexual activity.[26] A progressive increase in infection rates with HSV-2 in all populations begins in adolescence. Until recently, the precise seroprevalence of antibodies to HSV-2 had been difficult to determine because of cross-reactivity with HSV-1 antigens. During the late 1980s, seroepidemiologic studies performed using type-specific antigen for HSV-2 (glycoprotein G-2) identified antibodies to this virus in approximately 25% to 35% of middle-class women in several geographic areas of the United States.[14,29-31] Based on national health surveys, the seroprevalence of HSV-2 in the United States from 1988 to 1994 was 21.9% for individuals 12 years old or older.[31] Among those with serologic evidence of infection, fewer than 10% had a history of genital herpes symptoms. This seroprevalence represented a 30% increase compared with data collected from 1976 to 1980. HSV seroprevalence is highly variable and depends on geographic region, sex, age, race, and high-risk behaviors.[32] The increasing prevalence of genital HSV-1 infection in some countries suggests that use of type-specific tests for HSV-1 and HSV-2 may be helpful in determining the true incidence of genital HSV infections.[28]

The molecular epidemiology of HSV infections can be determined by restriction enzyme analysis of viral DNA obtained from infected individuals. Viruses have identical profiles when they are from the same host or are epidemiologically related.[33] In a few circumstances, however, it has been demonstrated that superinfection or exogenous reinfection with a new strain of HSV is possible. Such occurrences are uncommon in the nonimmunocompromised host with recurrent genital HSV infection.[33-35] Differences in the restriction endonuclease patterns of viral DNAs, indicating exogenous infections, are more common in immunocompromised individuals who are exposed to different HSVs, such as patients with acquired immunodeficiency syndrome (AIDS).

Maternal Infection

Infection with HSV-2, which reactivates and is shed at genital sites, is common in the pregnant woman. Using assays to detect type-specific antibodies to HSV-2, seroepidemiologic investigations have demonstrated that approximately one in five pregnant women has had HSV-2 infection.[30,36-40] Given the capacity of HSV to establish latency, the presence of antibodies is a marker of persistent infection of the host with the virus. The incidence of infection in women of upper socioeconomic class was 30% or higher in three large studies.[38,40,41] These investigations have demonstrated that most women with serologic evidence of HSV-2 infection have no history of symptomatic primary or recurrent disease. New HSV-2 infections also appear to be acquired during pregnancy with a frequency that is comparable to seroconversion rates among nonpregnant women, and these infections usually occur without clinical signs or symptoms.[37-41]

Evaluation of pregnant women and their partners has demonstrated that women can remain susceptible to HSV-2 despite prolonged sexual contact with a partner who has known genital herpes.[39] One in 10 women in this study were found to be at unsuspected risk for acquiring HSV-2 infection during pregnancy as a result of contact with a partner whose HSV-2 infection was asymptomatic.

Most maternal infections are clinically silent during gestation. However, infection during gestation may manifest in several clinical syndromes. An uncommon problem encountered with HSV infections during pregnancy is that of widely disseminated disease. As first reported by Flewett and co-workers[42] in 1969 and by others[43,44] subsequently, infection has been documented to involve multiple visceral sites in addition to cutaneous ones. In a limited number of cases, dissemination after primary oropharyngeal or genital infection has led to severe manifestations of disease, including necrotizing hepatitis with or without thrombocytopenia, leukopenia, disseminated intravascular coagulopathy, and encephalitis. Although only a few patients have suffered from disseminated infection, the mortality rate for these pregnant women is more than 50%. Fetal deaths were described in more than 50% of cases, although mortality did not necessarily correlate with the death of the mother. Surviving fetuses were delivered by cesarean section during the acute illness or at term, and none had evidence of neonatal HSV infection.

Earlier studies described an association of maternal primary infection before 20 weeks' gestation with spontaneous abortion in some women.[45] Although the original incidence of spontaneous abortion after a symptomatic primary infection during gestation was thought to be as high as 25%, this estimate was not substantiated by prospective studies and was erroneous because of the small number of women followed. More precise data obtained from a prospective analysis of susceptible women demonstrated that 2% or more acquired infection but that acquisition of infection was not associated with a risk of spontaneous abortion.[46] With the exception of rare case reports,[47] primary infection that develops later in gestation is not generally associated with premature rupture of membranes or premature termination of pregnancy.[47]

Localized genital infection, whether it is associated with lesions or remains asymptomatic, is the most common form of HSV infection during pregnancy. Overall, prospective investigations using cytologic and virologic screening indicate that genital herpes occurs with a frequency of about 1% in women tested at any time during gestation.[38,46] Most of these infections were classified as recurrent when HSV-2–specific serologic evaluation was done concurrently. Transmission of infection to the infant is most frequently related to the actual shedding of virus at the time of delivery. Because HSV infection of the infant is usually the consequence of contact with infected maternal genital secretions at the time of delivery, the incidence of viral excretion at this point has been of particular interest. The reported incidence of viral excretion at delivery is 0.01% to 0.39% for all women, regardless of their history of genital herpes.[38,41]

Several prospective studies have evaluated the frequency and nature of viral shedding in pregnant women with a known history of genital herpes. These women represent a subset of the population of women with HSV-2 infection because they had characteristic genital lesions from which virus was isolated. In a predominantly white, middle-class population, symptomatic recurrent infection occurred during pregnancy in 84% of pregnant women with a history of symptomatic disease.[48] Viral shedding from the cervix occurred in only 0.56% of symptomatic infections and 0.66% of asymptomatic infections. These data are similar to those obtained for other populations.[29] The incidence of cervical shedding in asymptomatic pregnant women has been reported to vary from 0.2% to 7.4%, depending on the numbers of cultures that were obtained between symptomatic episodes. Overall, these data indicate that the frequency of cervical shedding is low, which may reduce the risk of transmission of virus to the infant when the infection is recurrent. The frequency of shedding does not appear to vary by trimester during gestation. No increased incidence of premature onset of labor was apparent in these prospective studies of women with reactivation of HSV-2 infection.

The most important fact about maternal transmission is that most infants who develop neonatal disease are born to women who are completely asymptomatic for genital HSV infections during the pregnancy and at the time of delivery. These women usually have neither a past history of genital herpes nor a sexual partner reporting a genital vesicular rash and account for 60% to 80% of all women whose infants become infected.[49-51] Among women delivering children who developed neonatal HSV infection, only 27% had a history of or evidence of recurrent lesions indicative of HSV infection during the current pregnancy.[50] One half of these women reported genital HSV infection in their sexual partners.

Factors Influencing Transmission of Infection to the Fetus

The development of serologic assays that distinguish antibodies to HSV-1 from those elicited by HSV-2 infection has allowed an accurate analysis of risks related to perinatal transmission of HSV.[13-16] The category of maternal genital infection at the time of delivery influences the frequency of neonatal acquisition of infection. Maternal infections are classified as caused by HSV-1 or HSV-2 and as newly acquired or recurrent. These categories of maternal infection status are based on laboratory criteria and are independent of clinical signs. Women with recurrent infections are those who have preexisting antibodies to the virus type that is isolated from the genital tract, which is usually HSV-2. Most women classified as having recurrent infection have no history of symptomatic genital herpes. Infections that are newly acquired, which have been referred to as *first-episode* infections, are further categorized as *primary* or *first episode, nonprimary* based on type-specific serologic testing. This differentiation is made whether clinical signs are present or not. *Primary infections* are those in which the mother is experiencing a new infection with HSV-1 or HSV-2 and has not already been infected with the other virus type. These mothers are seronegative for any HSV antibodies (i.e., HSV-1 or HSV-2 negative) at the onset of infection. *Nonprimary infections* are those in which the mother has a new infection with one virus type, usually HSV-2, but has antibodies to the other virus type, usually HSV-1, because of an infection that was acquired previously. As transmission has been studied using type-specific serologic methods, it has become obvious that attempts to distinguish primary and recurrent disease by clinical criteria are not reliable. Serologic classification is an important advance because many "new" genital herpes infections in pregnancy represent the first symptomatic episode of infection acquired at some time in the past. In one study designed to evaluate acyclovir therapy, pregnant women who were thought to have recent acquisition of HSV-2 based on symptoms had all been infected previously. These women were experiencing genital symptoms, caused by the reactivation of latent virus, for the first time.[52]

A hierarchy of risk of transmission has emerged using laboratory tools to classify maternal infection. Infants born to mothers who have true primary infections at the time of delivery are at highest risk, with transmission rates of 50% or higher.[46,51] Those born to mothers with new infections that are first episode but nonprimary appear to be at lower risk; transmission rates are estimated to be about 30%. The lowest risk of neonatal acquisition occurs when the mother has active infection caused by shedding of virus acquired before the pregnancy or at stages of gestation before the onset of labor. The estimated attack rate for neonatal herpes among these infants is less than 2%. This estimate is reliable because it is based on the cumulative experience from large, prospective studies of pregnant women in which viral shedding was evaluated at delivery, regardless of the mother's history of genital herpes or contact with a partner with suspected or documented genital herpes.

The reasons for the higher risk of transmission to the infant when the mother has a new infection can be attributed to differences in the quantity and duration of viral shedding in the mother and in the transfer of passive antibodies from the mother to the infant before delivery. Primary infection is associated with larger quantities of virus replicating in the genital tract (>10^6 viral particles per 0.2 mL of inoculum) and a period of viral excretion that may persist for an average of 3 weeks.[53] Many women with new infections have no symptoms but shed virus in high titers. In some mothers, these infections cause signs of systemic illness, including fever, malaise, and myalgias. In a small percentage of cases, significant complications, such as urinary retention and aseptic meningitis, occur. In contrast, virus is shed for an average of only 2 to 5 days and at lower concentrations (approximately 10^2 to 10^3 viral particles per 0.2 mL of inoculum) in women with symptomatic recurrent genital infections. Asymptomatic reactivation is also associated with short periods of viral replication, often less than 24 to 48 hours. One of the most important observations about HSV infections that has emerged from the evaluation of pregnant women is that new HSV-1 and HSV-2 infections often occur without any of the manifestations that were originally described as the classic findings in primary and recurrent genital herpes.

In parallel with the classification of maternal infection, the mother's antibody status to HSV at delivery appears to be an additional factor that influences the likelihood of transmission and probably affects the clinical course of neonatal herpes. Transplacental maternal neutralizing antibodies appear to have a protective, or at least an ameliorative, effect on acquisition of infection for infants inadvertently exposed to virus.[54] Maternal primary infection late in gestation may not result in significant passage of maternal antibodies across the placenta to the fetus. Based on available evidence, the highest risk of transmission from mothers with newly acquired genital herpes is observed when the infant is born before the transfer of passive antibodies to HSV-1 or HSV-2, when the infant is exposed at delivery or within the first few days of life.[46,50,55]

The duration of ruptured membranes has also been described as an indicator of risk for acquisition of neonatal infection. Observations of a small cohort of women with symptomatic genital herpes indicated that prolonged rupture of membranes (>6 hours) increased the risk of acquisition of virus, perhaps as a consequence of ascending infection from the cervix.[45] It is recommended that women with active genital lesions at the time of onset of labor be delivered by cesarean section.[56]

Isolation of HSV from the genital tract at the time of delivery is a major risk factor for neonatal herpes infection. One study found that cesarean section significantly reduced the rate of HSV infection in infants born to women from whom HSV was isolated at the time of delivery (1.2% versus 7.7%, $P = .047$).[57] However, this effect of cesarean delivery was established by postdelivery analysis of data on viral shedding at delivery for a large cohort of pregnant women. In the absence of a reliable rapid test for HSV in the birth canal, it is difficult at this time to apply this information in clinical practice.

The benefit of cesarean section beyond 6 hours of ruptured membranes has not been evaluated. Although some protection may be expected, infection of the newborn has occurred despite delivery by cesarean section.[49,58]

Certain forms of medical intervention during labor and delivery may increase the risk of neonatal herpes if the mother has active shedding of the virus, although in most instances, viral shedding is not suspected clinically. For example, fetal scalp monitors can be a site of viral entry through skin.[57,59,60] The benefits and risks of these devices should be considered for women with a history of recurrent genital HSV infections. Because most women with genital infections caused by HSV are asymptomatic during labor and have no history of genital herpes, it is usually not possible to make this assessment.

Incidence of Newborn Infection

A progressive increase in the number of cases of neonatal HSV infection to a rate of approximately 1 in 1500 deliveries was reported in King County, Washington, during the period from 1966 to 1983, when adult infection rates were also increasing.[61] Overall, the United States, with approximately 4 million deliveries each year, has an estimated 11 to 33 cases of neonatal infection per 100,000 livebirths. This estimate has been confirmed by a review of comprehensive hospital discharge data recorded in California for the years 1985, 1990, and 1995. The diagnosis of HSV infection in infants 6 weeks old or younger was made in 11.7, 11.3, and 11.4 infants, respectively, per 100,000 livebirths in each of these years.[62]

In studies where maternal serologic status during pregnancy and virologic status at the time of delivery are evaluated prospectively, the rate of transmission leading to neonatal HSV infection varies from 12 to 54 newborn infections per

100,000 livebirths. Higher rates of transmission are seen in babies born to seronegative mothers and those infected with HSV-1.[57]

Neonatal HSV infection occurs far less frequently than might be expected given the high prevalence of genital HSV infections in women of childbearing age in the United States. Some countries do not report a significant number of cases of neonatal HSV infection despite a similar high prevalence of antibodies to HSV-2 in women. In the United Kingdom, genital herpes infection is relatively common, but very few cases of neonatal HSV infection are recognized. Although serologic studies in central Africa indicate that women have a high frequency of antibodies to HSV-2, the first case of neonatal herpes was reported less than 25 years ago. Neonatal HSV infection in the Netherlands occurs in only 2.4 of 100,000 newborns.[63]

Although underreporting of cases may explain some differences between countries, there may be unidentified factors that account for these differences. The interpretation of incidence data must also include the potential for postnatal acquisition of HSV infection. Not all cases of neonatal herpes are the consequence of intrapartum contact with infected maternal genital secretions, which alters the overall estimate of delivery-associated infections.

Times of Transmission of Infection

HSV infection of the newborn can be acquired in utero, intrapartum, or postnatally. The mother is the most common source of infection for the first two of these routes of transmission of infection. With regard to postnatal acquisition of HSV infection, the mother can be a source of infection from a genital or nongenital site, or other contacts or environmental sources of virus can lead to infection of the child. A maternal source is suspected when maternal herpetic lesions are discovered shortly after the birth of the child or when the infant's illness is caused by HSV-2. Although intrapartum transmission accounts for 85% to 90% of cases, in utero and postnatal infection must be recognized for public health and prognostic purposes.

Some infants acquire infection in utero, but this mode of transmission is rare.[64-69] Although it was originally presumed that in utero acquisition of infection resulted in a totally normal infant or premature termination of gestation,[45] it has become apparent that intrauterine acquisition of infection can lead to the clinical signs of congenital infection. By using stringent diagnostic criteria, more than 30 infants with symptomatic congenital disease have been described in the literature. These criteria include identification of infected infants with lesions present at birth, virologic confirmation of infection, and the exclusion of other infectious agents whose pathogenesis mimics the clinical findings of HSV infections, such as congenital cytomegalovirus infection, rubella, syphilis, or toxoplasmosis. Virologic diagnosis is a necessary criterion because no standard method for detection of IgM antibodies is available and infected infants often fail to produce IgM antibodies detectable by research methods.[55,70] The manifestations of disease in this group of children range from the presence of skin vesicles at the time of delivery to the most severe neurologic abnormalities.[49,64]

In utero infection can result from transplacental or ascending infection. The placenta can show evidence of necrosis and inclusions in the trophoblasts, which suggests a transplacental route of infection.[71] This situation can result in an infant who has hydranencephaly at the time of birth, or it may be associated with spontaneous abortion and intrauterine HSV viremia. Virus has been isolated from the products of conception under such circumstances. Histopathologic evidence of chorioamnionitis suggests ascending infection as an alternative route for in utero infection.[68] Risk factors associated with intrauterine transmission are not known. Primary and recurrent maternal infections can result in infection of the fetus in utero.

HSV DNA has been detected in the amniotic fluid of two women experiencing a first-episode nonprimary infection and in one woman during a symptomatic recurrent infection. All three infants were healthy at birth and demonstrated no clinical or serologic evidence of HSV infection during follow-up.[72]

The second and most common route of infection is intrapartum contact of the fetus with infected maternal genital secretions. Intrapartum transmission is favored by delivery of the infant to a mother with newly acquired infection.

Postnatal acquisition is the third route of transmission. Postnatal transmission of HSV-1 has been suggested as an increasing risk. Data from the National Institute of Allergy and Infectious Diseases (NIAID) Collaborative Antiviral Study Group indicate that the frequency of infants with neonatal HSV-1 infection ranges from approximately 25% to 30%.[49,73] HSV-1 infections appear to account for only about 5% to 17% of all genital HSV infections in the United States,[28] creating greater concern about postnatal acquisition of HSV-1 infection from nonmaternal sources.

Relatives and hospital personnel with orolabial herpes may be a reservoir of virus for infection of the newborn. The documentation of postnatal transmission of HSV-1 has focused attention on such sources of virus.[74-78] Postpartum transmission from mother to child has been reported as a consequence of nursing on an infected breast.[79] Transmission from fathers and grandparents has also been documented.[77] When the infant's mother has not had HSV infection, the infant may be inoculated with the virus from a nonmaternal contact in the absence of any possible protection from maternally derived passive antibodies.

Because of the prevalence of HSV-1 infections in the general population, many individuals have intermittent episodes of asymptomatic excretion of the virus from the oropharynx and therefore can provide a source of infection for the newborn. The occurrence of herpes labialis, commonly referred to as fever blisters or cold sores, has ranged from 16% to 46% in various groups of adults.[80] Population studies conducted in two hospitals indicated that 15% to 34% of hospital personnel had a history of nongenital herpetic lesions.[80,81] In both hospitals surveyed, at least 1 in 100 individuals documented a recurrent cold sore each week. As is true of genital herpes, many individuals have HSV-1 infection with no clinical symptoms at the time of acquisition or during episodes of reactivation and shedding of infectious virus in oropharyngeal secretions. Prospective virologic monitoring of hospital staff increased the frequency with which infection was detected by twofold; however, no case of neonatal HSV infection was documented in these nurseries.

The risk of nosocomial infection in the hospital environment is a concern. The demonstration of identity by restriction endonuclease analysis of virus recovered from an index case and a nursery contact leaves little doubt about the possibility of spread of virus in a high-risk nursery population.[75,76] The possible vectors for nosocomial transmission have not been defined. Whether personnel with herpes labialis should avoid working in the nursery while lesions are active remains a matter of debate. No cases of transmission of HSV from personnel to infants have been documented. Vigorous handwashing procedures and continuing education of personnel in newborn nurseries can be expected to contribute to the low frequency of HSV transmission in this environment. Herpetic whitlow in a health care provider should preclude direct patient contact, regardless of the nursing unit. Because more infants are born to seronegative women now, our nursery practice is to exclude personnel with active herpes labialis from direct patient care activities until the lesion is crusted.

Because most mothers have antibodies to HSV and these antibodies are transferred to their infants, exposures to the virus in the newborn period may not often result in neonatal disease. However, if the mother was seronegative, nosocomial exposure may pose a more significant risk to the infant.

IMMUNOLOGIC RESPONSE

The host response of the newborn to HSV is impaired compared with older children and adults.[55,70,82-86] There is no evidence for differences in virulence of particular HSV strains. The severity of the manifestations of HSV-1 and HSV-2 infections in the newborn, as described in "Neonatal Infection," can be attributed to immunologic factors. The relevant issues are protection of the fetus by transplacental antibodies, the innate immune response of the exposed infant and the acquisition of adaptive immunity by the infected newborn.

Passive antibodies to HSV influence the acquisition of infection and its severity and clinical signs.[40,51,55,70] Transplacentally acquired antibodies from the mother are not totally protective against newborn infection, but transplacentally acquired neutralizing antibodies correlate with a lower attack rate in exposed newborns.[51,54,55] Although the absence of any detectable antibodies has been associated with dissemination, the presence of antibodies at the time that clinical signs appear does not predict the subsequent outcome.[49,70] The most important example of the failure of passive antibodies to alter progression is the occurrence of encephalitis in untreated infants whose initial symptoms were limited to cutaneous lesions. Most infected newborns eventually produce IgM antibodies, but the interval to detection is prolonged, requiring at least 2 to 4 weeks.[55] This method cannot be used for diagnostic purposes to determine the need for antiviral therapy. These antibodies increase rapidly during the first 2 to 3 months, and they may be detectable for as long as 1 year after infection. The quantity of neutralizing antibodies and antibodies that mediate antibody-dependent cellular cytotoxicity in infants with disseminated infection is lower than that in those with more limited disease.[55,82] Humoral antibody responses to specific viral proteins, especially glycoproteins, have been evaluated by assays for antibodies to gG and by immunoblot.[13,70] Immunoblot studies indicate that the severity of infection correlates directly with the number of antibody bands to defined polypeptides. Children with a more limited infection, such as infection of the skin, eye, or mouth, have fewer antibody bands compared with those children with disseminated disease. A vigorous antibody response to the ICP4 alpha gene product, which is responsible for initiating viral replication, has been correlated with poor long-term neurologic outcome, suggesting that these antibodies reflect the extent of viral replication. A regression analysis that compared neurologic impairment with the quantity of antibodies to ICP4 identified the child at risk for severe neurologic impairment.[70]

Adaptive cellular immunity is a critical component of the host response to primary herpetic infections. Newborns with HSV infections have a delayed T lymphocyte proliferative response compared with older individuals.[55,84,85] Most infants have no detectable T lymphocyte responses to HSV when evaluated 2 to 4 weeks after the onset of clinical symptoms.[55] The delayed T lymphocyte response to viral antigens in infants whose initial disease is localized to the skin, eye, or mouth may be an important determinant of the frequent progression to more severe disease in infants.[55,85] Lack of cell-mediated immunity is likely to permit viremia and dissemination in infants, which is otherwise controlled by the host response in older children and adults with new HSV infections.

Infected newborns have decreased interferon-α and interferon-γ production in response to HSV antigen when compared with adults with primary HSV infection.[55,85] The importance of interferon-α may be related to its effect on the induction of innate immune mechanisms, such as natural killer cell responses.[86] Other mechanisms of the innate immune system of the newborn that may be deficient in controlling HSV include other nonspecific cytokine responses and complement-mediated effects. T lymphocytes from infected infants have decreased interferon-γ production during the first month of life. This defect can be predicted to limit the clonal expansion of helper and cytotoxic T lymphocytes specific for herpes viral antigens, allowing more extensive and prolonged viral replication and failure to establish latency.

Antibody-dependent cell-mediated cytotoxicity has been demonstrated to be an important component of adaptive immunity to viral infection.[82] Antibodies and lymphocytes, monocytes, macrophages or polymorphonuclear leukocytes, as well as antibodies and complement, lyse HSV-infected cells in vitro.[87] However, newborns appear to have fewer effector lymphocytes than older individuals do. The immaturity of neonatal monocytes and macrophage function against HSV infection has been demonstrated in vitro and in animal models.[88,89] Adhesion defects may be responsible for suboptimal antibody-mediated target-cell binding of neonatal natural killer cells.[90] Additional information regarding the immune response to HSV is provided in Chapter 4.

NEONATAL INFECTION

Background

After direct exposure, replication of HSV is presumed to occur at the portal of entry, which is probably the mucous membranes of the mouth or eye, or at sites where the skin has been damaged. Factors that determine whether the infection causes symptoms at the site of inoculation or disseminates to other organs are poorly understood. Sites of replication during the incubation period have not been defined, but the virus evades the host response during this early stage, probably by mechanisms such as blocking cell-mediated immune recognition of viral peptides by preventing major histocompatibility complex class I molecules from reaching the surface of infected cells. Intraneuronal transmission of viral particles may provide a privileged site that is inaccessible to circulating humoral and cell-mediated defense mechanisms, facilitating the pathogenesis of encephalitis. Transplacental maternal antibodies may be less effective under such circumstances. Disseminated infection appears to be the consequence of viremia. HSV DNA has been detected in peripheral blood mononuclear cells, even in infants who appear to have localized infection.[91] Extensive cell-to-cell spread could explain primary HSV pneumonia after aspiration of infected secretions.

After the virus has adsorbed to cell membranes and penetration has occurred, viral replication proceeds, leading to release of progeny virus and cell death. The synthesis of cellular DNA and protein ceases as large quantities of HSV are produced. Cell death in critical organs of the newborn, such as the brain, results in devastating consequences, as reflected by the long-term morbidity of herpes encephalitis. Cellular swelling, hemorrhagic necrosis, development of intranuclear inclusions, and cytolysis all result from the replicative process. Small, punctate, yellow-to-gray areas of focal necrosis are the most prominent gross lesions in infected organs. When infected tissue is examined by microscopy, there is extensive evidence of hemorrhagic necrosis, clumping of nuclear chromatin, dissolution of the nucleolus, cell fusion with formation of multinucleate giant cells, and ultimately, a lymphocytic inflammatory response.[92] Lymphocytic perivascular cuffing is particularly prominent in organs that exhibit extensive hemorrhagic necrosis, especially in the central nervous system.[93] Irreversible organ damage results from ischemia and direct viral destruction of cells.

Clinical Presentations

Pediatricians must be prepared to consider the diagnosis of neonatal herpes in infants who have clinical signs consistent with the disease regardless of the maternal history of genital herpes. Only about 30% of mothers whose infants develop neonatal herpes have had symptomatic genital herpes or sexual contact with a partner who has recognized HSV infection during or before the pregnancy.

The clinical presentation of infants with neonatal HSV infection depends on the initial site and extent of viral replication. In contrast to human cytomegalovirus, neonatal infections caused by HSV-1 and HSV-2 are almost invariably symptomatic. Case reports of asymptomatic infection in the newborn exist, but they are uncommon, and long-term follow-up of these children to document absence of subtle disease or sequelae was not described.

Classification of newborns with HSV infection is used for prognostic and therapeutic considerations.[94] Historically, infants with neonatal HSV infection were classified as having localized or disseminated disease, with the former group being subdivided into those with skin, eye, or mouth disease versus those with central nervous system infection. However, this classification system understates the significant differences in outcome within each category.[95] In a revised classification scheme, infants who are infected intrapartum or postnatally are divided into three groups, including those with disease localized to the skin, eye, or mouth; encephalitis, with or without skin, eye, or mouth involvement; and disseminated infection that involves multiple organs, including the central nervous system, lung, liver, adrenals, skin, eye, or mouth. A few infants with intrauterine infection constitute a fourth category.

Knowledge of the patterns of clinical disease caused by HSV-1 and HSV-2 in the newborn is based on prospectively acquired data obtained through the NIAID Collaborative Antiviral Study Group. These analyses have employed uniform case record forms from one study interval to the next. Of 186 infants enrolled in the NIAID Collaborative Antiviral Study Group studies of neonatal herpes virus infections between 1981 and 1997, 34% were classified with skin, eye, or mouth disease; 34% with central nervous system disease; and 32% with disseminated infection.[73] This analysis of the natural history of neonatal herpes infections likely underestimates the proportion of infants who present with skin, eye, or mouth disease. Patients with central nervous system or disseminated HSV infection were disproportionately enrolled in a high-dose acyclovir study conducted from 1989 to 1997.

The presentation and outcome of infection, including the effect of antiviral therapy on prognosis, varies significantly according to the clinical categories.[96] Table 26-1 summarizes disease classification and outcome of 291 infants with neonatal herpes simplex virus infections enrolled in NIAID Collaborative Antiviral Study Group protocols.

Intrauterine Infection

Intrauterine infection is rare. The manifestations are seen in approximately 3 of every 100 infected infants.[67] When infection occurs in utero, severe disease follows acquisition of infection at virtually any time during gestation. In the most severely afflicted group of infants, evidence of infection is apparent at birth and is characterized by a triad of findings, including skin vesicles or scarring, eye damage, and the severe manifestations of microcephaly or hydranencephaly. Central nervous system damage is caused by intrauterine encephalitis. Infants do not have evidence of embryopathy. Often, chorioretinitis in combination with other eye findings, such as keratoconjunctivitis, is a component of the clinical presentation. Serial ultrasound examination of the mothers of infants infected in utero has demonstrated the presence of hydranencephaly, but cases are seldom diagnosed before delivery. Chorioretinitis alone should alert the pediatrician to the possibility of this diagnosis, although it is a common sign for other congenital infections. A few infants have been described who have signs of HSV infection at birth after prolonged rupture of membranes. The infants may have no other findings of invasive multiorgan involvement—no chorioretinitis, encephalitis, or evidence of other diseased organs—and can be expected to respond to antiviral therapy. Antiviral therapy is not effective for infants who are born with hydranencephaly. Intrauterine HSV infection has been reported as a cause of hydrops fetalis.[97]

Table 26–1 Demographic and Clinical Characteristics of Infants Enrolled in the National Institute of Allergy and Infectious Diseases Collaborative Antiviral Study

	Disease Classification		
Demographic Characteristics	**Disseminated**	**Central Nervous System**	**Skin, Eye, or Mouth**
No. of infants (%)	93 (32)	95 (33)	102 (35)
No. male/no. female	54/39	50/46	51/51
Race			
No. white/no. other	60/33	73/23	76/26
No. premature, <36 wk (%)	33 (35)	20 (21)	24 (24)
Gestational age (wk)	36.5 ± 0.4	37.9 ± 0.4	37.8 ± 0.3
Enrollment age (wk)	11.6 ± 0.7	17.4 ± 0.8	12.1 ± 1.1
Maternal age (yr)	21.7 ± 0.5	23.1 ± 0.5	22.8 ± 0.5
No. of clinical findings (%)			
Skin lesions	72 (77)	60 (63)	86 (84)
Brain involvement	69 (74)	96 (100)	0 (0)
Pneumonia	46 (49)	4 (4)	3 (3)
Deaths at 1 yr[b] (%)	56 (60)	13 (14)	0 (0)
No. of survivors with neurologic impairment/total no. (%)			
Total	15/34 (44)	45/81[b] (56)	10/93[b] (11)
Adenine arabinoside	13/26[b] (50)	25/51[b] (49)	3/34[b] (9)
Acyclovir	1/6[b] (17)	18/27[b] (67)	4/51[b] (8)
Placebo	1/2[b] (50)	2/3[b] (67)	3/8[b] (38)

[a]Regardless of therapy.
[b]Denominators vary according to number with follow-up available.

Disseminated Infection

Infants whose initial diagnosis is disseminated herpes have the worst prognosis for mortality. Many of these infants are born to mothers who are experiencing a new HSV-1 or HSV-2 infection and may lack any passively acquired antibodies against the infecting virus type.[13,51,98] Infants with disseminated infection have signs of illness within the first week of life, although the diagnosis may be delayed until the second week. The onset of symptoms may occur less than 24 hours after birth, but most infants appear well at delivery. The short incubation period of disseminated herpes reflects an acute viremia, which allows transport of the virus to all organs; the principal organs involved are the adrenals and the liver, causing fulminant hepatitis in some cases.[94,99-101] Viremia is associated with infection of circulating mononuclear cells in these infants.[91,100-103] Infection can affect multiple organs, including the central nervous system, larynx, trachea, lungs, esophagus, stomach, lower gastrointestinal tract, spleen, kidneys, pancreas, and heart. Initial signs and symptoms are irritability, seizures, respiratory distress, jaundice, coagulopathy, and shock. The characteristic vesicular exanthem is usually not present when the symptoms begin. Untreated infants may develop cutaneous lesions resulting from viremia. More than one third of children with disseminated infection do not develop skin vesicles during the course of their illness.[49,73,100] Disseminated infections caused by HSV-1 and HSV-2 are indistinguishable by clinical criteria.

The diagnosis of disseminated neonatal herpes is exceedingly difficult because the clinical signs are often vague and nonspecific, mimicking those of neonatal enteroviral disease or bacterial sepsis. The diagnosis of disseminated herpes should be pursued by obtaining specimens of oropharyngeal and respiratory secretions and a rectal swab to be tested by viral culture and by polymerase chain reaction (PCR) testing if a qualified reference laboratory is available. Direct immunofluorescence methods are useful for rapid diagnosis of herpesvirus-infected cells in skin lesion specimens but must not be used to test oropharyngeal or other secretions. When discrete lesions are not available for obtaining infected cells, the virus can also be detected in the peripheral blood of some infants by viral culture or PCR, but confirmation of viremia is not necessary for clinical management.

Evaluation of the extent of dissemination is imperative to provide appropriate supportive interventions early in the clinical course. Infants should be assessed for hypoxemia, acidosis, hyponatremia, abnormal hepatic enzyme levels, direct hyperbilirubinemia, neutropenia, thrombocytopenia, and bleeding diathesis. Chest radiographs should be obtained, and depending on signs and whether the infant is stable enough, abdominal radiography, electroencephalography, and computed tomography or magnetic resonance imaging of the head should be used be to further determine the extent of disease. The radiographic picture of HSV lung disease is characterized by a diffuse, interstitial pattern, which progresses to a hemorrhagic pneumonitis and on rare occasions, a significant pleural effusion.[104] Not infrequently, necrotizing enterocolitis with pneumatosis intestinalis can be detected when gastrointestinal disease is present. Meningoencephalitis appears to be a common component of disseminated infection, occurring in about 60% to 75% of children. Usual examinations of cerebrospinal fluid, including viral culture and PCR, should be performed along with noninvasive neurodiagnostic tests to assess the extent of brain disease.

The mortality rate for disseminated HSV in the absence of therapy exceeds 80%, and many survivors are impaired. The most common causes of death of infants with disseminated disease are intravascular coagulopathy or HSV pneumonitis. There is evidence that the long-term neurologic outcome is better for infants who survive disseminated HSV-1 involving the central nervous system than for those who are infected with HSV-2.[96,105]

Encephalitis

Almost one third of all infants with neonatal HSV infection have encephalitis only as the initial manifestation of disease.[96,106] These infants have clinical manifestations distinct from those who have central nervous system infection associated with disseminated HSV. The pathogenesis of these two forms of brain infection is probably different. The virus is likely to reach brain parenchyma by a hematogenous route in infants with disseminated infection, resulting in multiple areas of cortical hemorrhagic necrosis. In contrast, neonates who present with only encephalitis are likely to develop brain disease because of retrograde axonal transport of the virus to the central nervous system. The evidence for this hypothesis is twofold. First, newborns with disseminated disease have documented viremia. Second, infants with encephalitis are more likely to have received transplacental neutralizing antibodies from their mothers, which may allow only intraneuronal transmission of virus to the brain.

Infants with localized HSV encephalitis as their initial manifestation of infection usually develop signs more than a week after birth, typically presenting in the second or third week but sometimes as late as 4 to 6 weeks. Clinical manifestations of encephalitis include seizures (focal and generalized), fever, lethargy, irritability, tremors, poor feeding, temperature instability, bulging fontanelle, and pyramidal tract signs. Similar signs are observed when disseminated herpesvirus is associated with encephalitis. As in cases of disseminated herpesvirus, many infants with encephalitis do not have skin vesicles when signs of illness begin. Some infants have a history or residual signs of lesions of the skin or eye that were not recognized as herpetic. If untreated, infants with encephalitis may develop skin vesicles later in the disease course. Anticipated findings on cerebrospinal fluid examination include a mononuclear cell pleocytosis, moderately low glucose concentrations, and elevated protein. A few infants with central nervous system infection, proven by brain biopsy done immediately after the onset of seizures, have no abnormalities of their cerebrospinal fluid, but most infants have some pleocytosis and mild reduction of the glucose level. The hemorrhagic nature of the encephalitis may result in an apparent "bloody tap." Although initial protein concentrations may be normal or only slightly elevated, infants with localized brain disease usually demonstrate progressive increases in protein (≥1000 mg/dL). The importance of cerebrospinal fluid examinations in all infants is underscored by the finding that even subtle abnormalities have been associated with significant developmental sequelae.[94]

Electroencephalography and computed tomography or magnetic resonance imaging can be very useful in defining the presence and extent of central nervous system abnormalities and should be done before discharge of all infants with this diagnosis.[107,108] These abnormalities may also be detected by ultrasound examination.[108] Typical abnormalities seen by neuroimaging include localized or multifocal areas of abnormal parenchymal attenuation, atrophy, edema, and hemorrhage involving the temporal, frontal, parietal, and subcortical regions of the brain[109] (Fig. 26-1).

Localized central nervous system disease is fatal in approximately 50% of infants who are not treated and is usually related to involvement of the brain stem. With rare exceptions, survivors are left with neurologic impairment.[94] The long-term prognosis is poor. As many as 50% of surviving children have some degree of psychomotor retardation, often in association with microcephaly, hydranencephaly, porencephalic cysts, spasticity, blindness, chorioretinitis, or learning disabilities.

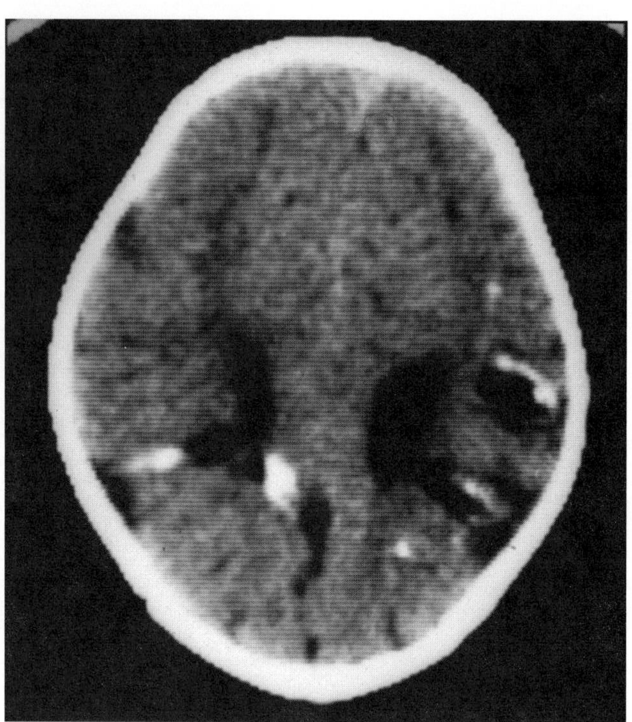

Figure 26–1 Herpes simplex encephalitis. Computed tomographic scan of an infant with herpes simplex virus type 2 infection and severe sequelae.

Quantitative PCR methods show a greater amount of HSV-2 DNA in cerebrospinal fluid from patients with more extensive neurologic impairment.[110] There is evidence that progressive neurologic damage occurs after neonatal HSV encephalitis, although many infants have obvious severe sequelae within a few weeks after onset of HSV encephalitis.[111,112]

Despite the presumed differences in pathogenesis, clinical manifestations of disease in children with encephalitis alone are virtually identical to the findings for brain infection in disseminated cases. For infants with encephalitis, approximately 60% develop evidence of a vesicular rash characteristic of HSV infection. A newborn with pleocytosis and proteinosis of the cerebrospinal fluid but without a rash can easily be misdiagnosed as having another viral or bacterial infection unless HSV infection is considered.

Skin, Eye, and Mouth Infections

Infection localized to the skin, eye, or mouth or some combination of these sites appears benign at the onset, but it is associated with a high risk of progression to serious disease. When infection is localized to the skin, the presence of discrete vesicles remains the hallmark of disease (Fig. 26-2). Vesicles occur in 90% of children with skin, eye, or mouth infection. The skin vesicles usually erupt from an erythematous base and are usually 1 to 2 mm in diameter. The formation of new lesions adjacent to the original vesicles is typical, creating a cluster that may coalesce into larger, irregular vesicles. In some cases, the lesions progress to large bullae larger than 1 cm in diameter. Clusters of vesicles may appear initially on the presenting part of the body, presumably because of prolonged contact with infected secretions during birth, or at sites of trauma (e.g., scalp monitor sites). Nevertheless, first herpetic lesions in infants with localized cutaneous disease have been described on the trunk, extremities, and other sites. Children with disease localized to the skin, eye, or mouth or some combination of these sites typically have symptoms within the first 7 to 10 days of life.

Although discrete vesicles are usually encountered, crops and clusters of vesicles are described, particularly before antiviral treatment was available or when the cause of the first lesions is not recognized. In these cases, the rash can progress to involve other cutaneous sites, presumably by viremia and hematogenous spread. The scattered vesicles resemble varicella. Although progression is expected without treatment, a few infants have had infection of the skin limited to one or two vesicles, with no further evidence of cutaneous disease. These infants may be identified after the newborn period and should have a careful evaluation because many are likely to have had neurologic disease that was not detected. A zosteriform eruption is another manifestation of herpetic skin disease reported in infants.[113]

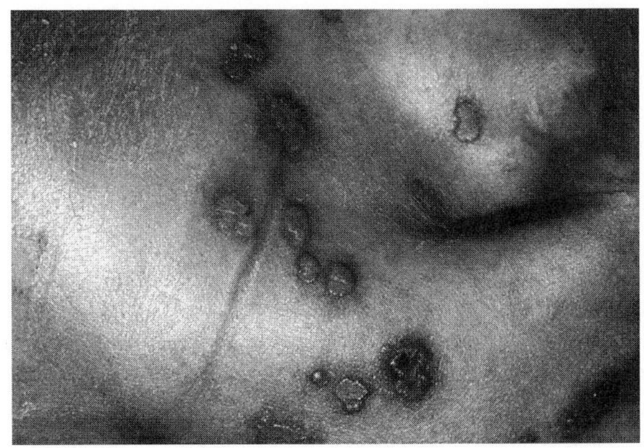

Figure 26–2 Cutaneous herpes simplex virus infection. Initial vesicular lesion in a premature infant with herpes simplex type 2 infection.

Infections involving the eye may manifest as keratoconjunctivitis. Ocular infection may be the only site of involvement in the newborn. When localized eye infection is observed in infants who also have microphthalmos and retinal dysplasia, intrauterine acquisition should be suspected, and a thorough neurologic evaluation should be done. Before antiviral therapy was available, persistent ocular disease resulted in chorioretinitis caused by HSV-1 or HSV-2.[114] Keratoconjunctivitis can progress to chorioretinitis, cataracts, and retinal detachment despite therapy. Cataracts have been detected as a long-term consequence in infants with perinatally acquired HSV infections.

Localized infection of the oropharynx involving the mouth or tongue occurs, but newborns do not develop the classic herpetic gingivostomatitis caused by primary HSV-1 infection in older children. Overall, approximately 10% of patients have evidence of HSV infection of the oropharynx by viral culture. Unfortunately, many of these children did not undergo a thorough oral examination to determine whether the detection of infectious virus in oropharyngeal secretions was associated with lesions.

Long-term neurologic impairment has been encountered in children whose disease appeared to be localized to the skin, eye, or mouth during the newborn period.[49,94,112] The significant findings include spastic quadriplegia, microcephaly, and blindness. Important questions regarding the pathogenesis of delayed-onset neurologic debility are raised by these clinical observations. Despite normal clinical examinations in these children, neurologic impairment became apparent between 6 months and 1 year of life. At this stage of the disease, the clinical presentation may be similar to that associated with congenitally acquired toxoplasmosis or syphilis.

Newborns who have skin lesions invariably suffer from recurrences for months or years. Continued recurrences are common, particularly when the infecting virus is HSV-2, whether or not antiviral therapy was administered.

Historically, although death was not associated with disease localized to the skin, eye, or mouth, approximately 30% of these children eventually developed some evidence of neurologic impairment.[49] Table 26-2 shows morbidity and mortality 12 months after infection by HSV viral type and disease classification in patients enrolled in two studies

Table 26–2 Morbidity and Mortality among Patients after 12 Months by Viral Type, 1981-1997

	Number of Patients by Disease Classification (%)[a]					
	Skin, Eye, or Mouth		CNS		Disseminated	
Outcome	*HSV-1*	*HSV-2*	*HSV-1*	*HSV-2*	*HSV-1*	*HSV-2*
Normal	24 (100)	19 (95)	4 (75)	7 (17.5)	3 (23)	14 (41)
Mild impairment	0 (0)	0 (0)	0 (0)	7 (17.5)	0 (0)	1 (3)
Moderate impairment	0 (0)	1 (5)	1 (14)	7 (17.5)	0 (0)	0 (0)
Severe impairment	0 (0)	0 (0)	2 (29)	13 (32.5)	1 (8)	3 (9)
Death	0 (0)	0 (0)	0 (0)	6 (15)	9 (69)	16 (47)
Unknown	Total of 20		Total of 16		Total of 16	

[a]Survival rate (by Cox regression analysis) of patients infected with HSV-2 was higher compared with that of patients infected with HSV-1; however, the difference was not statistically significant. Patients infected with HSV-2 were more likely to have neurologic abnormalities compared with those infected with HSV-1 (borderline significance, $P = .10$).

CNS, central nervous system; HSV, herpes simplex virus.

Data from Kimberlin DW, Lin CY, Jacobs RF, et al. Natural history of neonatal herpes simplex virus infections in the acyclovir era. Pediatrics 108:223-229, 2001.

conducted by the NIAID Collaborative Antiviral Study Group between 1981 and 1997. With parenteral acyclovir therapy, virtually all children with HSV-1 and most children with HSV-2 disease of the skin, eye, or mouth who enrolled and who were available for follow-up at 12 months had normal development.[73]

Subclinical Infection

A few cases of apparent subclinical infection with HSV proven by culture isolation of virus in the absence of symptoms have been described.[115] It has been difficult to document such cases in the course of prospective evaluations of several thousand infants from many centers around the United States. Conversely, infants who were exposed to active maternal infection at the time of delivery and who did not develop symptoms have been followed for the first year of life and did not have immunologic evidence of subclinical infection.[51] HSV-1 or HSV-2 may be recovered from the infant's oropharyngeal secretions transiently, without representing true infection. Because of the propensity of the newborn to develop severe or life-threatening disease, laboratory evidence of neonatal HSV infection requires careful follow-up for clinical signs and the administration of antiviral therapy.

DIAGNOSIS

Clinical Evaluation

The clinical diagnosis of neonatal HSV infection is difficult because the appearance of skin vesicles cannot be relied on as an initial component of disease presentation. Enteroviral sepsis is a major differential diagnostic possibility in infants with signs suggesting neonatal HSV. Bacterial infections of newborns can mimic neonatal HSV infection. Skin lesions may resemble those seen with bullous or crusted impetigo. Some infants infected by HSV have been described who had concomitant bacterial infections, including group B *Streptococcus, Staphylococcus aureus, Listeria monocytogenes,* and gram-negative bacteria. A positive culture for one of these pathogens does not rule out HSV infection if the clinical suspicion for neonatal herpes infection is present. Many other disorders of the newborn can be indistinguishable from neonatal HSV infections, including acute respiratory distress syndrome, intraventricular hemorrhage, necrotizing enterocolitis, and various ocular or cutaneous diseases.

When vesicles are present, alternative causes of exanthems should be excluded. Other diagnoses include enteroviral infection, varicella-zoster virus infection, and syphilis. Laboratory methods are available to differentiate these causes of cutaneous lesions in the newborn. Cutaneous disorders such as erythema toxicum, neonatal melanosis, acrodermatitis enteropathica, and incontinentia pigmenti often confuse physicians who suspect neonatal HSV infections. HSV lesions can be distinguished rapidly from those caused by these diseases using direct immunofluorescence stain of lesion scrapings or other methods for rapid detection of viral proteins and confirmed by viral culture.

HSV encephalitis is a difficult clinical diagnosis to make, particularly because many children with central nervous system infection do not have a vesicular rash at the time of clinical presentation. Infection of the central nervous system is suspected in the child who has evidence of acute neurologic deterioration, often associated with the onset of seizures, and in the absence of intraventricular hemorrhage and metabolic causes. PCR to detect the viral DNA in cerebrospinal fluid has become an important diagnostic method, largely replacing the need for diagnosis by brain biopsy.[116] Infants with localized encephalitis usually have serial increases in cerebrospinal fluid cell counts and protein concentrations and negative bacterial cultures of the cerebrospinal fluid. Noninvasive neurodiagnostic studies can be used to define the sites of involvement.

Laboratory Assessment

The appropriate use of laboratory methods is essential if a timely diagnosis of HSV infection is to be achieved.[117] Virus isolation remains the definitive diagnostic method. If skin lesions are present, a swab of skin vesicles, done vigorously enough to obtain cells from the base of the lesion, should be made and transferred in appropriate virus transport media to a diagnostic virology laboratory. Rapid diagnosis should be attempted by preparing material from skin lesion scrapings for direct immunofluorescence testing to detect the presence of virus-infected cells or for testing by enzyme immunoassays for viral proteins. Because of the possibility of false-positive results using immunofluorescence or other antigen detection methods, specimens should also be obtained for confirmation by viral isolation. Direct immunofluorescence staining for virus-infected cells is not reliable unless the specimen is obtained from a skin lesion. Cells from oropharyngeal swabs or from cerebrospinal fluid should not be tested using this method.

Clinical specimens should be transported to the diagnostic virology laboratory without being frozen and their processing expedited to permit the rapid confirmation of the clinical diagnosis. In addition to skin vesicles, other materials or sites from which virus may be isolated include the cerebrospinal fluid, stool, urine, throat, nasopharynx, and conjunctivae. The isolation of virus from swabs of superficial sites, such as the nasopharynx, may represent transient presence of the virus in secretions, when the culture is obtained within the first 24 hours after birth, and particularly when the specimen is taken immediately after birth. Typing of an HSV isolate may be done by one of several techniques. Because the outcome of antiviral treatment and risk of late sequelae may be related to the virus type, typing is of prognostic and epidemiologic importance.[94] Results of viral cultures of the cerebrospinal fluid may be positive for infants with disseminated HSV infections but are usually negative for those who have localized encephalitis.

Detection of HSV DNA in cerebrospinal fluid by PCR can allow a rapid presumptive diagnosis of HSV encephalitis in the newborn.[116-120] PCR was used in the retrospective analysis of materials collected from 34 infants enrolled in the NIAID Collaborative Antiviral Study Group antiviral studies.[118] HSV was detected by PCR assay of cerebrospinal fluid in 71% of infants before antiviral therapy was initiated. At least one specimen was positive in 76% of infants, and all samples that were positive by viral culture were positive by PCR. Similar findings were reported by Swedish investigators when stored cerebrospinal fluid specimens obtained from infants with neonatal HSV infection were tested for HSV by

PCR. HSV DNA was detected from cerebrospinal fluid in the acute phase of illness from 78% of patients with central nervous system disease.[121]

Use of HSV PCR methods on cerebrospinal fluid can potentially decrease the duration of time to diagnosis of some cases of HSV encephalitis; however, there are reports in older patients of initial negative HSV PCR results early in the course of illness. Cerebrospinal fluid obtained 4 to 7 days after the initial cerebrospinal fluid samples were obtained was subsequently positive for HSV DNA in a small number of patients.[122]

PCR tests of cerebrospinal fluid were positive in 7 (24%) of 29 infants enrolled in the NIAID Collaborative Antiviral Study Group antiviral studies whose clinical disease was limited to mucocutaneous lesions. Five of the six infants who were evaluated when 1 year old were developmentally normal.[118] The significance of this observation for disease classification and prognosis remains to be determined in prospective studies.

Most studies of PCR for the diagnosis of HSV central nervous system infections indicate the test is sensitive in approximately 75% to 100% of cases in small cohorts of infants.[118-121] Specificity of the test ranges from 71% to 100%. The broad range of values for sensitivity and specificity of HSV PCR probably results from different study methods and disease classifications.[123]

Some studies have shown that HSV PCR may be used to detect HSV DNA in peripheral blood mononuclear cells and plasma of infants with proven neonatal HSV infection. Using a sensitive and well-standardized PCR method, investigators found HSV DNA in peripheral blood mononuclear cells of 6 of 10 infants tested and in plasma of 4 of 6 infants tested.[91] Other investigators have reported the presence of HSV DNA in serum of 67% (20 of 30) infants with neonatal HSV infection.[121] Whether HSV PCR testing of peripheral blood mononuclear cells or plasma can be used to accurately diagnose neonatal HSV infection in the absence of positive cultures is unknown.

In clinical practice, there is considerable interlaboratory variability in HSV PCR test performance. Many clinical laboratories employ user-developed ("home-brew") protocols, further complicating interpretation of PCR results. Diagnostic laboratories that perform HSV PCR testing must be able to validate their test and participate in national and in-house proficiency testing programs.[124]

Until more information regarding the reliability of HSV PCR results obtained in clinical diagnostic laboratories has been determined, interpretation of negative or positive HSV PCR results must depend on clinical findings. A negative PCR result for HSV in cerebrospinal fluid in the setting of clinical, laboratory, or radiologic findings consistent with central nervous system infection does not rule out HSV infection. It is important to continue to use standard clinical and laboratory diagnostic methods for the evaluation of infants with possible neonatal HSV (Table 26-3).

Every effort should be made to confirm HSV infection by viral isolation. Cytologic examination of cells from the infant's lesions should not be used to diagnose HSV infection because reliable specific methods are available. Cytologic methods, such as Papanicolaou, Giemsa, or Tzanck staining, have a sensitivity of only approximately 60% to 70%. A negative result therefore must not be interpreted as excluding the diagnosis of HSV, and a positive result should not be the sole diagnostic determinant for HSV infection in the newborn. Intranuclear inclusions and multinucleated giant cells may be consistent with, but not diagnostic of, HSV infection.

In contrast to some other neonatal infections, serologic diagnosis of HSV infection has little clinical value. The interpretation of serologic assays is complicated by the fact that transplacentally acquired maternal IgG cannot be differentiated from endogenously produced antibodies, making it difficult to assess the neonate's antibody status during acute infection. Serial type-specific antibody testing may be useful for retrospective diagnosis if a mother without a prior history of HSV infection has a primary infection late in gestation and transfers little or no antibody to the fetus. Therapeutic decisions cannot await a diagnostic approach based on comparing acute-phase and convalescent-phase antibody titers. IgM production is delayed or does not occur in infected infants because of inherent immunodeficiencies in the response to systemic viral infections in the newborn, and commercially available assays for IgM antibodies to HSV have limited reliability.

The results of specific laboratory tests for HSV should be used in conjunction with clinical findings and general laboratory tests, such as platelet counts, cerebrospinal fluid analysis, and liver function tests, to establish a disease classification.

TREATMENT

Background

The cumulative experience of the past 2 decades demonstrates that perinatally acquired HSV infections are amenable to

Table 26–3 Initial Diagnostic Evaluation for Suspected Neonatal Herpes Simplex Virus Infection

A. Microbiologic studies
   1. Skin lesion: viral culture and direct viral examination
   2. Cerebrospinal fluid: viral culture and HSV PCR[a]
   3. Conjunctivae: viral culture
   4. Nasopharynx: viral culture
   5. Rectum: viral culture
   6. Urine: viral culture
B. Ancillary studies
   1. Cerebrospinal fluid cell count, glucose and protein levels
   2. Complete blood cell count with differential and platelet counts
   3. Liver function studies
   4. Coagulation studies
   5. Electroencephalogram
   6. Computed tomography or magnetic resonance imaging of head
   7. Chest radiograph
C. Not recommended
   1. Direct viral examination of samples from conjunctivae, nasopharynx, rectum, urine, or cerebrospinal fluid
   2. Herpes antibody from serum
   3. Tzanck smear

[a]The diagnostic reliability of herpes simplex virus polymerase chain reaction (HSV PCR) results from blood or skin lesions performed outside of the research setting is unknown.

treatment with antiviral agents. Acyclovir is the drug of choice.[96] Because most infants acquire infection at the time of delivery or shortly thereafter, antiviral therapy has the potential to decrease mortality and improve long-term outcome. The benefits that antiviral therapy can provide are influenced substantially by early diagnosis. The likelihood of disease progression in infants who acquire HSV infections is an established fact. Without treatment, approximately 70% of those presenting with disease localized to the skin, eye, or mouth develop involvement of the central nervous system or disseminated infection. Treatment initiated after disease progression is not optimal because many of these children die or are left with significant neurologic impairment. Regardless of the apparently minor clinical findings in some cases, the possibility of HSV infection in the newborn requires aggressive diagnostic evaluation and likely or proved infection mandates the immediate initiation of acyclovir therapy, which must be given intravenously.

Antiviral Drugs

Historically, four nucleoside analogues have been used to treat neonatal herpes: idoxuridine, cytosine arabinoside, vidarabine, and acyclovir. Of these compounds, the first three are nonspecific inhibitors of cellular and viral replication, and the fourth, acyclovir, is selectively activated by HSV thymidine kinase. Acyclovir acts as a competitive inhibitor of HSV DNA polymerase and terminates DNA chain elongation.[125] Idoxuridine and cytosine arabinoside have no value as systemic therapy for any viral infection because of toxicity and equivocal efficacy. Vidarabine was the first drug demonstrated to be efficacious; it decreased mortality and improved morbidity in cases of neonatal HSV infections.[126] A comparison of vidarabine with acyclovir suggests that these compounds have a similar level of activity for this disease; however, vidarabine is no longer available for clinical use.[112] Acyclovir is safe for use in newborns and is familiar to pediatricians from its other clinical uses.

Acyclovir has been established as efficacious for the treatment of primary genital HSV infection when administered by intravenous, oral, and topical routes.[127,128] Oral and intravenous administration of acyclovir to the immunocompromised host decreases the frequency of reactivation after immunosuppression and the duration of disease.[129] Acyclovir has been established to be superior to vidarabine for the treatment of HSV encephalitis in older children and adults.[130] Because this compound is a selective inhibitor of viral replication, it has a low frequency of side effects.

After pharmacokinetic and tolerance evaluations of acyclovir were done in infants,[131,132] the NIAID Collaborative Antiviral Study Group compared vidarabine and acyclovir for the treatment of neonatal HSV infection in a randomized trial.[112] The dose of vidarabine used was 30 mg/kg/day, and acyclovir was given at a dose of 10 mg/kg every 8 hours. The duration of therapy was 10 days. There were no significant differences in survival between the two treatment groups (Fig. 26-3). There were no differences in adverse effects or laboratory evidence of toxicity.

Survival with antiviral therapy depended on classification of the extent of disease at diagnosis (Fig. 26-4). Mortality and morbidity were also influenced by clinical status at the time of diagnosis and the virus type. Among infants with

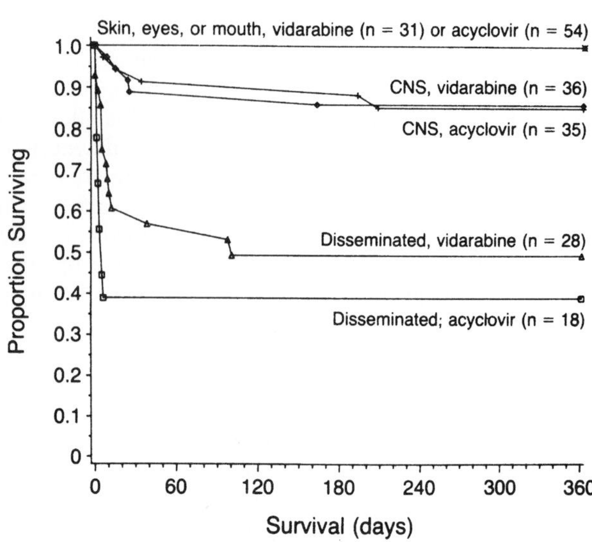

Figure 26–3 Survival of babies with neonatal herpes simplex virus infection according to treatment and the extent of disease. The infection was classified as confined to the skin, eyes, or mouth; affecting the central nervous system (CNS); or producing disseminated disease. After adjustment for the extent of disease with the use of a stratified analysis, the overall comparison of vidarabine with acyclovir was not statistically significant ($P = .27$) by a log-rank test. No comparison of treatments within disease categories was statistically significant. (From Whitley R, Arvin A, Prober C, et al. A controlled trial comparing vidarabine with acyclovir in neonatal herpes simplex virus infection. N Engl J Med 324:444, 1991.)

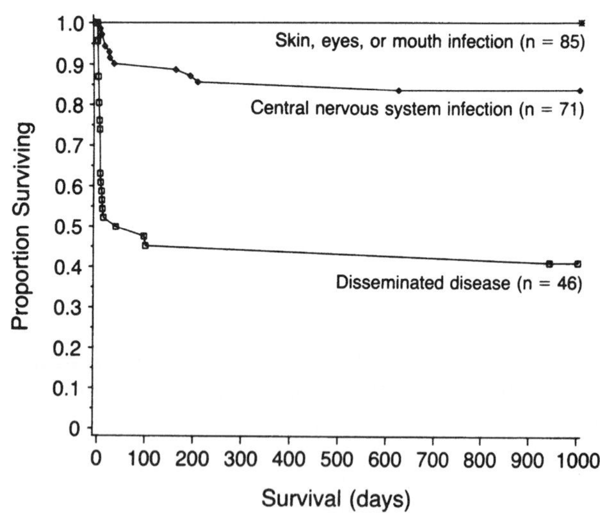

Figure 26–4 Survival of babies with neonatal herpes simplex virus infection according to the extent of disease ($P < .001$ for all comparisons). (From Whitley R, Arvin A, Prober C, et al. Predictors of morbidity and mortality in neonates with herpes simplex infections. N Engl J Med 324:450, 1991.)

skin, eye, or mouth disease, those with HSV-1 infections were all normal developmentally at 1 year compared with 86% of those with HSV-2 infections. Infants who were alert or lethargic when treatment was initiated had a survival rate of 91%, compared with 54% for those who were semi-comatose or comatose; similar differences in survival rates related to neurologic status were observed in infants with

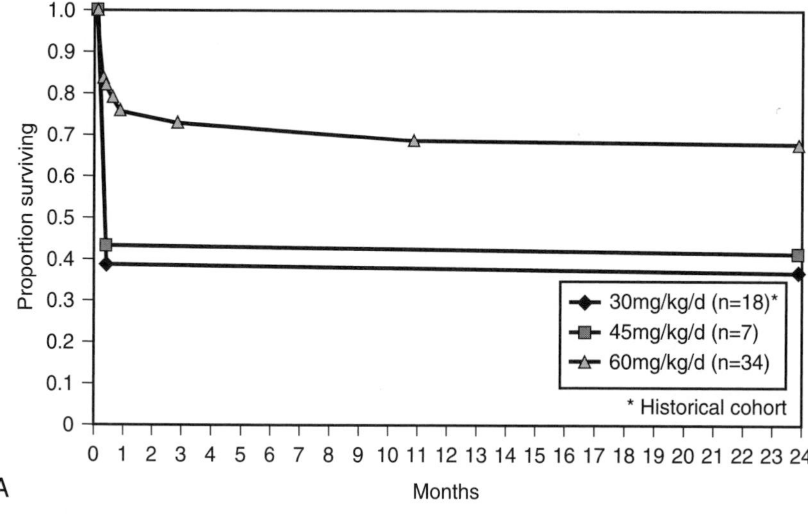

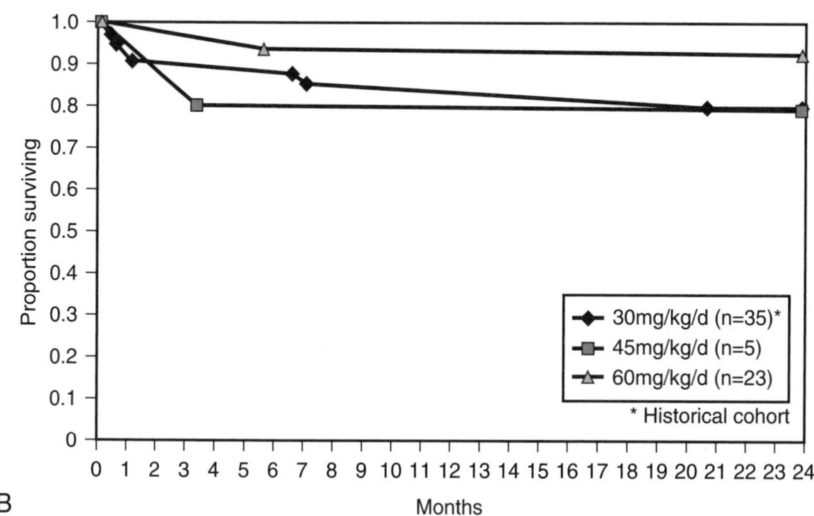

Figure 26–5 Mortality rates for patients with disseminated disease **(A)** and central nervous system disease **(B)** depending on the dose of acyclovir. (Data from Kimberlin DW, Chin-Yu L, Jacobs RF, et al. Safety and efficacy of high-dose intravenous acyclovir in the management of neonatal herpes simplex virus infections. Pediatrics 108:230-238, 2001.)

disseminated infection. Prematurity, pneumonitis, and disseminated intravascular coagulopathy were poor prognostic signs.[94]

The improved outcome compared with historical data probably reflects earlier diagnosis and institution of antiviral therapy, thereby preventing progression of disease from skin, eye, or mouth to more severe disease. The mean duration of symptoms before treatment for all participants, regardless of disease classification, was 4 to 5 days, indicating that therapy might have been instituted even sooner. These observations suggested that further advances in therapeutic outcome might be achieved by earlier intervention. Unfortunately, despite advances in laboratory diagnosis and treatment of neonatal HSV infection, the mean time between onset of disease symptoms and initiation of antiviral therapy has not changed.[73]

Despite the proven efficacy of antiviral therapy for neonatal HSV infection, the mortality rate remains high, and many infants who survive disseminated or central nervous system disease have serious sequelae. This circumstance dictated the need to evaluate high doses of acyclovir and longer treatment regimens. Infants were enrolled in an NIAID Collaborative Antiviral Study Group assessment of acyclovir given at an intermediate dose (45 mg/kg/day) or high dose (60 mg/kg/day). Mortality rates for infants with disseminated or central nervous system disease were lower for infants given high-dose acyclovir than observed in the earlier studies (Fig. 26-5).[133] There was no significant difference in morbidity status at 12 months of follow-up between high-dose and standard-dose acyclovir recipients for each of the three disease categories. Transient and reversible neutropenia occurred more frequently during high-dose therapy but resolved during or after cessation of treatment. The dose of acyclovir used had no impact on the duration of viral shedding.[133]

The current recommendation for treatment of neonatal HSV infection is acyclovir, 60 mg/kg/day in three doses (20 mg/kg/dose) given intravenously. Disseminated and central nervous system infections are treated at least 21 days. Duration of treatment for skin, eye, and mucous membrane infection, after disseminated and central nervous system infection have been ruled out, is a minimum of 14 days.[134]

The use of oral acyclovir is contraindicated for the treatment of acute HSV infections in newborns. Its limited oral bioavailability results in plasma and cerebrospinal fluid concentrations of drug that are inadequate for therapeutic effects on viral replication. The high risk of progression from localized mucocutaneous infections requires the administration of intravenous acyclovir to these infants, regardless of how well they appear at the time of diagnosis. In addition to intravenous therapy, infants with ocular involvement caused by HSV should receive one of the topical ophthalmic agents approved for this indication. Topical acyclovir is not necessary for treatment of mucocutaneous lesions caused by HSV because parenteral drug reaches these sites.

Acyclovir treatment is based on a laboratory diagnosis of neonatal HSV infection. Rapid methods, including direct antigen detection and PCR, should be used to facilitate early laboratory confirmation of suspected cases. Acyclovir prophylaxis is not recommended. Presumptive treatment may be a reasonable option when circumstances prevent rapid laboratory diagnosis and the clinical manifestations are those described for mucocutaneous infections, disseminated disease, or HSV encephalitis. In all cases, specimens should be obtained for laboratory testing to guide the decision to continue treatment. During the course of therapy, careful monitoring is important to assess the therapeutic response. Even in the absence of clinical evidence of encephalitis, evaluation of the central nervous system should be done for prognostic purposes. Serial evaluations of hepatic and hematologic parameters may indicate changes caused by the viral infection or by drug toxicity.

Intravenous acyclovir is tolerated well by infants. Adequate hydration is necessary to minimize the risk of nephrotoxicity, and dosage adjustments are necessary if renal clearance is impaired. As for all drugs, the possibility of acute toxicity should be considered in any child receiving parenteral antiviral therapy and should be assessed by serially evaluating bone marrow, renal, and hepatic functions. The potential for long-term harm from these drugs remains to be defined.

Acyclovir resistance has been reported in an infant with acute HSV infection of the larynx in the newborn period; in this case, the initial isolate was not inhibited by acyclovir, although the source of this infection could not be explained.[135] Acyclovir resistance has also been reported in a premature infant with cutaneous and central nervous system disease caused by an initially acyclovir-susceptible HSV. The infant developed recurrent disseminated HSV infection 8 days after a 21-day course of acyclovir. The virus isolated at the onset of recurrent symptoms was found to lack thymidine kinase activity on the basis of a frame-shift mutation in the thymidine kinase gene.[136] Another infant born to a mother with severe systemic primary HSV-2 infection developed an acyclovir resistant mutant during acyclovir therapy for disseminated HSV infection and eventually died. The use of steroids to treat blood pressure instability may further have hampered this baby's immune response to infection.[137]

Isolates of HSV recovered from infants who received intravenous acyclovir for cutaneous disease in the newborn period and had subsequent recurrent cutaneous lesions typically remain sensitive to acyclovir.[138] Emergence of viral resistance to acyclovir has been described in patients requiring prolonged or repeated treatment with this drug. One infant who was given long-term oral acyclovir for suppression of recurrences during the first 6 months of life had a resistant HSV isolated from a lesion after therapy was discontinued, but subsequent isolates were susceptible.[139]

Antiviral resistance does not generally explain the failure of infants with the disseminated or encephalitic form of the disease to respond well to antiviral therapy. Clinical deterioration, despite appropriate therapy and supportive care, can be attributed to virus-induced destruction of cells comprising infected organs, such as liver or brain, or irreversible changes, such as disseminated intravascular coagulopathy.

The observation of an association between late sequelae and frequent recurrences of skin lesions in infants who were treated for localized HSV-2 infections during the newborn period has raised questions about the potential efficacy of suppressive therapy with oral acyclovir. The NIAID Collaborative Antiviral Study Group has undertaken an assessment of the safety and efficacy of suppression as an adjunct after the recommended treatment of mucocutaneous disease with intravenous acyclovir.[139] Infants were given 300 mg/m^2 twice or three times per day for 6 months. Of 16 infants given the three daily doses, 13 (81%) had no recurrences of lesions while receiving therapy, compared with 54% of infants from earlier studies who received intravenous acyclovir only. Forty-six percent of the 26 infants developed neutropenia. In one infant, suppressive therapy was associated with a transient recurrence of infection due to an acyclovir-resistant isolate of HSV-2; subsequent recurrences were caused by susceptible isolates. Whether this effect on cutaneous recurrences, which was limited to periods of active oral suppressive therapy, has any effect on late neurologic sequelae is unknown. Oral acyclovir prophylaxis is not recommended for routine use, pending results from a larger NIAID Collaborative Antiviral Study Group trial of efficacy against this end point.

Other Issues in Acute Management

Isolation of the newborn with HSV infection is important to decrease the potential for nosocomial transmission. Many infants with this infection have life-threatening problems, including disseminated intravascular coagulation, shock, and respiratory failure, and they require supportive care that is available only at tertiary medical centers.

There is no indication that administration of immune globulin or hyperimmune globulin is of value for the treatment of neonatal HSV infection. Although a series of studies have suggested that the quantity of transplacental neutralizing antibodies affects the attack rate among exposed infants and may influence the initial disease manifestations, the presence of antibodies may or may not influence the subsequent course of infection.[49,51,54,55,82] The administration of standard preparations of intravenous immune globulin does not enhance the titers of functional antibodies against HSV in low-birth-weight infants.[140] The evaluation of virus-specific monoclonal antibodies in combination with antiviral therapy may become feasible as new technologies for deriving human or humanized antibody preparations are developed.[141]

No other forms of adjunctive therapy are useful for treating neonatal HSV infections. Various experimental modalities, including bacille Calmette-Guérin, interferon, immune modulators, and immunization, have been attempted, but none has produced demonstrable effects.

Long-Term Management of Infected Infants

With the advent of antiviral therapy, an increasing number of newborns who suffered from HSV infection are surviving and require careful long-term follow-up. The most common complications of neonatal HSV infection include neurologic and ocular sequelae that may be detected only on long-term follow-up. It is therefore necessary that these children receive serial long-term evaluation from qualified pediatric specialists in these areas, which should include neurodevelopmental, ophthalmologic, and hearing assessments.

Recurrent skin vesicles are present in many children, including those who did not have obvious mucocutaneous disease during the acute phase of the clinical illness. Skin vesicles provide a potential source for transmission of infection to other children or adults who have direct contact with these infants. The increasing use of daycare for children, including those surviving neonatal HSV infections, stimulates many questions from daycare providers about these children. There is some risk that children with recurrent HSV skin lesions will transmit the virus to other children in this environment. The most reasonable recommendation in this situation is to cover the lesions to prevent direct contact. It is much more likely that HSV-1 will be present in the daycare environment in the form of asymptomatic infection or gingivostomatitis. In both cases, virus is present in the mouth and pharynx, and the frequent exchange of saliva and other respiratory droplets that occurs among children in this setting makes this route of transmission more likely. Education of daycare workers and the general public about herpesvirus infections, their implications, and the frequency with which they occur in the population as a whole can calm fears and correct common misconceptions.

Parents of children with neonatal HSV infection often have significant guilt feelings. Parents often require support from psychologists, psychiatrists, or counselors. The family physician or pediatrician can provide a supportive role of great value to the family in this situation. Most parents and many physicians are unaware of the high prevalence of HSV-2 infection in the United States and of the lifelong persistence and subclinical nature of these infections. Concern about the risk of fetal and neonatal infection during subsequent pregnancies is often a major issue that can be addressed effectively based on the low risks as proved from large, prospective studies.

PREVENTION

Background

Despite the progress that has been made in antiviral treatment of neonatal HSV infection, the ideal approach is to prevent the exposure of infants to active maternal infection at the time of delivery. Unfortunately, genital infections caused by HSV are often clinically silent when they are acquired as new infections and when the virus reactivates. The high prevalence of HSV-2 infections in the U.S. population means that women are at risk for acquiring new genital infections during pregnancy and that at least one in five will become infected before pregnancy. The problem of asymptomatic genital HSV infection means that the transmission of HSV from mothers to infants cannot be eliminated even with the best obstetric management. It is futile to obtain sequential genital cultures during the last weeks of gestation in women with a history of genital herpes in an effort to identify those who will have asymptomatic infection at the onset of labor.[48] These cultures do not predict the infant's risk of exposure at delivery because of the usually brief duration of asymptomatic shedding and the time required for the culture to become positive. Because of the attention of the lay press to the devastating outcome of neonatal HSV infection, many women who know that they have genital herpes experience severe anxiety about the potential risks to the fetus and newborn. As a consequence, these women may have an unnecessarily high frequency of cesarean deliveries. The risk of neonatal HSV infection in the newborn is approximately equivalent for women who have no prior history of genital herpes or a partner with known infection (Table 26-4).

Table 26–4 Projected Risk of Transmission of HSV-2 from Mothers to Infants at Delivery in a Cohort of 100,000 Pregnant Women

25% with Past HSV-2 Infection	75% Susceptible to HSV-2 Infection
25,000 women	75,000 women
1.5% reactivation at delivery	0.02% seroconversion/wk
375 women with reactivation	30 women with infection <2 wk before delivery
<5% risk of transmission to infant	≈50% risk of transmission
19 infected infants	15 infected infants

Data from Arvin AM. The epidemiology of perinatal herpes simplex infections. *In* Stanberry L (ed). Genital and Neonatal Herpes. New York, John Wiley & Sons, 1996, pp 179-192.

Management of Pregnant Women with Known Genital Herpes

Women who have a history of recurrent genital herpes should be reassured that the risk of fetal or neonatal infection is very low. Intrauterine HSV infections are rare, with an estimated overall risk of 1 in 200,000 pregnancies.[64] Information about the risk of exposure to asymptomatic reactivation at delivery derived from six large-scale prospective studies is sufficient to conclude that the incidence of asymptomatic reactivation in these women is about 2% and that the attack rate for their exposed infants is approximately 3% or less; the risk of neonatal infection under these circumstances is less than 1 in 2000 deliveries.

Because laboratory methods cannot be used to detect asymptomatic infection in a timely manner, the current approach to management is to perform a careful vaginal examination at presentation and to elect cesarean delivery if the mother has signs or symptoms of recurrent genital herpes at the onset of labor. Given the low probability of neonatal infection, it is appropriate to deliver infants of women who have a history of recurrent genital herpes but who have no active clinical disease at delivery by the vaginal route.[56] An analysis of the occurrence of HSV infections in infants in California showed no change from 1985 to 1995, despite a documented decrease in deliveries by cesarean section and an increase in the proportion of women with a previous diagnosis of genital herpes whose infants were delivered vaginally.[62]

A culture for HSV obtained at the time of delivery may be useful in establishing whether the virus was present at delivery to facilitate recognition of neonatal infection if it occurs. However, the value of this approach has not been established. Alternative diagnostic approaches, such as those based on PCR to detect virus, are being developed to expedite identification of women at risk for delivering infected infants.[142,143] Evidence indicates that detection of viral presence in genital samples by PCR is more sensitive than culture methods. However, the significance of a positive PCR result in predicting risk of transmission of HSV to the infant is unknown.[144] Viral DNA can persist for a longer interval than infectious virus.

The utility of suppressive therapy of genital herpes in women with a known history of recurrent infection remains a question for clinical investigation because of risk-benefit considerations. It has already been established from the trials of suppressive therapy with acyclovir in individuals with frequently recurrent genital herpes that reactivation of virus can occur despite the administration of 200 mg of acyclovir three times daily.[145,146] Results of one study evaluating the efficacy of 400 mg of oral acyclovir three times daily indicate that prophylactic acyclovir significantly reduces the number of genital lesions. Despite prophylaxis, a few women continue to have virus detectable by PCR.[144]

The pharmacokinetics and metabolism of acyclovir in the human fetus are unknown. The possibility of fetal nephrotoxicity related to acyclovir is a potential risk that must be considered. Whether acyclovir treatment of mothers with primary genital herpes late in gestation can reduce the neonatal risk of these infections is also a research issue. However, signs of disseminated herpes in the mother warrant the administration of intravenous acyclovir.

Management of Infants of Mothers with Genital Herpes

Infants of mothers with histories of genital herpes delivered vaginally or by cesarean section and whose mothers have no evidence of active genital herpetic infection are at low risk for acquiring neonatal HSV infection. These children need no special evaluation during the newborn period.

Infants delivered vaginally to mothers with an active genital HSV infection or who have genital cultures done at delivery that are positive for HSV should be isolated from other infants for the duration of their hospitalization up to age 4 weeks. Parents and primary care physicians should be notified about the exposure of the infant so that the infant can be observed for the occurrence of nonspecific signs consistent with possible neonatal herpes. The parents and responsible family members should be educated about the low risk of transmission to relieve anxiety and to ensure prompt return for care in the unlikely event that signs of infection appear. Information regarding infection should include a description of the risks associated with transmission of infection to the newborn, the common signs and symptoms of neonatal herpes, the necessity for careful monitoring for the onset of illness as long as 4 weeks after birth, and the planned approach to treatment if symptoms occur.

It may be useful to obtain cultures from the exposed infant between 24 and 48 hours after delivery and at intervals during the first 4 weeks of life. Sites from which virus may be recovered include the eye, oropharynx, nasopharynx, and skin lesions that are suspected to be herpetic. Weekly viral cultures have been suggested for the surveillance of exposed infants; the utility of this approach has not been proved by prospective studies, and it should be considered an optional addition to clinical observation.

If cultures from any site in the infant are positive, a thorough diagnostic evaluation should be done, including obtaining additional specimens for viral culture from the site that was reported to be positive, the oropharynx, and the cerebrospinal fluid, and treatment with acyclovir should be initiated. Viral cultures of urine and viral culture and HSV PCR of peripheral blood mononuclear cells may also be considered to identify additional sites of viral infection. PCR testing must be performed by a laboratory with a validated HSV PCR assay and expertise in proper performance of PCR on specimens from various sources. A positive HSV PCR result in addition to the initial positive culture can provide additional evidence to support the diagnosis of HSV infection. A negative HSV PCR result does not in itself rule out infection.

No data are available to support the administration of acyclovir to exposed infants who have no clinical signs or laboratory evidence of infection. Parameters for duration of such prophylaxis cannot be defined. The experience from other clinical settings is that the virus is suppressed only for the period the drug is given and is not eradicated. Careful clinical follow-up of these infants, with immediate institution of antiviral therapy if symptoms occur, is an appropriate approach.

An issue of frequent concern is whether the mother with an active genital HSV infection at delivery should be isolated from her child after delivery. Women with recurrent orolabial HSV infection, as well as cutaneous HSV infections at other sites (e.g., breast lesions), are at similar risk for transmission of virus to their newborn. Because transmission occurs by direct contact with the virus, appropriate precautions by the mother, including careful hand washing before touching the infant, should prevent any need to separate mother and child. In some cases, it is possible to have the exposed infant room-in with the mother as a means of isolating the child from other newborns. Breast-feeding is contraindicated if the mother has vesicular lesions involving the breast.

CONCLUSIONS

Neonatal HSV infection remains a life-threatening disease in the newborn. With an increasing prevalence of genital herpes and the recognition that many infections are completely asymptomatic in the mother, pediatricians, neonatologists, obstetricians, and family practitioners must continue to remain alert to infants whose symptoms may be compatible with HSV infections. Early identification leads to prompt treatment. It is hoped that during this decade, the development of safe and efficacious vaccines and a better understanding of factors associated with transmission of virus from mother to infant will enable prevention of neonatal HSV infection.[147-149]

Acknowledgments

The databases on clinical presentations, diagnosis, and antiviral treatment of neonatal HSV infections have been generated through the efforts of the NIAID Collaborative Antiviral Study Group for more than 20 years, with support from the National Institute of Allergy and Infectious Diseases. The institute has also supported prognostic studies of HSV infection in pregnancy and the newborn in the United States.

REFERENCES

1. Mettler C. History of Medicine. Philadelphia, Blakiston, 1947, p 356.
2. Astruc J. De Morbis Venereis Libri Sex. Paris, G Cavelier, 1736, p 361.
3. Gruter W. Das Herpesvirus, seine atiologische und klinische Bedeutung. Munch Med Wochenschr 71:1058, 1924.
4. Hass M. Hepatoadrenal necrosis with intranuclear inclusion bodies: report of a case. Am J Pathol 11:127, 1935.
5. Batignani A. Conjunctivite da virus erpetico in neonato. Boll Ocul 13:1217, 1934.
6. Nahmias A, Dowdle WR. Antigenic and biological differences in herpesvirus hominis. Prog Med Virol 10:110-159, 1968.
7. Roizman B, Knipe D. Herpes simplex viruses and their replication. *In* Knipe D, Howley P (eds). Fields Virology. Philadelphia, Lippincott Williams & Wilkins, 2001, p 2399.
8. Whitley RJ. Herpes simplex viruses. *In* Knipe D, Howley P (eds). Fields Virology. Lippincott Williams & Wilkins, 2001, p 2461.
9. Spear PG. Glycoproteins of herpes simplex virus. *In* Bentz J (ed). Viral Fusion Mechanisms. Boca Raton, Fla, CRC Press, 1993, p 201.
10. Roizman B, Norrild B, Chan C, et al. Identification and preliminary mapping with monoclonal antibodies of a herpes simplex virus 2 glycoprotein lacking a known type 1 counterpart. Virology 133:242-247, 1984.
11. Roizman B, Jenkins FJ. Genetic engineering of novel genomes of large DNA viruses. Science 229:1208-1214, 1985.
12. Jugovic P, Hill AM, Tomazin R, et al. Inhibition of major histocompatibility complex type 1 antigen presentation in pig and primate cells by herpes simplex virus type 1 and 2 ICP47. J Virol 72:5076-5084, 1998.
13. Sullender WM, Yasukawa LL, Schwartz M, et al. Type-specific antibodies to herpes simplex virus type 2 (HSV-2) glycoprotein G in pregnant women, infants exposed to maternal HSV-2 infections at delivery, and infants with neonatal herpes. J Infect Dis 157:164-171, 1988.
14. Coleman RM, Pereira L, Bailey PD, et al. Determination of herpes simplex virus type-specific antibodies by enzyme-linked immunosorbent assay. J Clin Microbiol 18:287-291, 1983.
15. Wald A, Ashley-Morrow R. Serological testing for herpes simplex virus HSV-1 and HSV-2 infection. Clin Infect Dis 35(Suppl 2):S173-S182, 2002.
16. Ashley RL, Wu L, Pickering JW, et al. Pre-market evaluation of a commercial glycoprotein-G–based enzyme immunoassay for herpes simplex virus type-specific antibodies. J Clin Microbiol 36:294-295, 1998.
17. Cushing H. Surgical aspects of major neuralgia of trigeminal nerve: report of 20 cases of operation upon the gasserian ganglion with anatomic and physiologic notes on the consequence of its removal. JAMA 44:1002, 1905.
18. Goodpasture EW. Herpetic infections with special reference to involvement of the nervous system. Medicine (Baltimore) 8:223, 1929.
19. Carton CA, Kilbourne ED. Activation of latent herpes simplex by trigeminal sensory-root section. N Engl J Med 246:172, 1952.
20. Pazin GJ, Armstrong JA, Lam MT, et al. Prevention of reactivation of herpes simplex virus infection by human leukocyte interferon after operation on the trigeminal root. N Engl J Med 301:225-230, 1979.
21. Stevens JG, Cook ML. Latent herpes simplex virus in spinal ganglia of mice. Science 173:843-845, 1971.
22. Rock DL, Fraser NW. Detection of HSV-1 genome in central nervous system of latently infected mice. Nature 302:523-525, 1983.
23. Baringer JR. Recovery of herpes simplex virus from human trigeminal ganglions. N Engl J Med 291:828-830, 1974.
24. Hill TJ. Herpes simplex virus latency. *In* Roizman B (ed). The Herpesviruses, vol. 3. New York, Plenum Publishing, 1985, p 175.
25. Wentworth BB, Alexander ER. Seroepidemiology of infections due to members of the herpesvirus group. Am J Epidemiol 94:496-507, 1971.
26. Arvin AM. The epidemiology of perinatal herpes simplex infections. *In* Stanberry L (ed). Genital and Neonatal Herpes. New York, John Wiley & Sons, 1996, pp 179-192.
27. Nahmias AJ, Josey WE, Naib ZM, et al. Antibodies to Herpesvirus hominis types 1 and 2 in humans. Am J Epidemiol 91:539-546, 1970.
28. Lafferty WE, Downey L, Celum C, Wald A. Herpes simplex virus type 1 as a cause of genital herpes. Impact on surveillance and protection. J Infect Dis 18:1454-1457, 2000.
29. Wald A, Zeh J, Selke S, et al. Virologic characteristics of subclinical and symptomatic genital herpes infections. N Engl J Med 326:770-775, 1995.
30. Frenkel LM, Garratty E, Shen JP, et al. Clinical reactivation of herpes simplex virus type 2 in seropositive pregnant women with no history of genital herpes. Ann Intern Med 118:414-418, 1993.
31. Fleming DT, McQuillan GM, Johnson RE, et al. Herpes simplex virus type 2 in the United States, 1976 to 1994. N Engl J Med 337:1105-1111, 1997.
32. Smith JS, Robinson NJ. Age-specific prevalence of infection with herpes simplex virus types 2 and 1: a global review. J Infect Dis 186 (Suppl 1):S3-S28, 2002.
33. Buchman T, Roizman B, Nahmias AJ. Demonstration of exogenous genital reinfection with herpes simplex virus type 2 by restriction endonuclease fingerprinting of viral DNA. J Infect Dis 140:295-304, 1979.
34. Schmidt OW, Fife KH, Corey L. Reinfection is an uncommon occurrence in patients with symptomatic recurrent genital herpes. J Infect Dis 149:645-646, 1984.
35. Lakeman AD, Nahmias AJ, Whitley RJ. Analysis of DNA from recurrent genital herpes simplex virus isolates by restriction endonuclease digestion. Sex Transm Dis 13:61-66, 1986.
36. Boucher FD, Yasukawa LL, Bronzan RN, et al. A prospective evaluation of primary genital herpes simplex virus type 2 infections acquired during pregnancy. Pediatr Infect Dis J 9:499-504, 1990.
37. Brown ZA, Vontver LA, Benedetti J, et al. Genital herpes in pregnancy: risk factors associated with recurrences and asymptomatic viral shedding. Am J Obstet Gynecol 153:24-30, 1985.
38. Prober CG, Hensleigh PA, Boucher FD, et al. Use of routine viral cultures at delivery to identify neonates exposed to herpes simplex virus. N Engl J Med 318:887-891, 1988.
39. Kulhanjian JA, Soroush V, Au DS, et al. Identification of women at unsuspected risk of primary infection with herpes simplex virus type 2 during pregnancy. N Engl J Med 326:916-920, 1992.
40. Brown ZA, Vontver L, Bendetti J, et al. Effects on infants of first episode of genital herpes during pregnancy. N Engl J Med 317:1246-1251, 1987.
41. Brown ZA, Benedetti J, Ashley R, et al. Neonatal herpes simplex virus infection in relation to asymptomatic maternal infection at the time of labor. N Engl J Med 324:1247-1252, 1991.
42. Flewett TH, Parker RGF, Philip WM. Acute hepatitis due to herpes simplex virus in an adult. J Clin Pathol 22:60-66, 1969.
43. Young EJ, Killam AP, Greene JF Jr. Disseminated herpesvirus infection. Association with primary genital herpes in pregnancy. JAMA 235: 2731-2733, 1976.
44. Hensleigh PA, Glover DB, Cannon M. Systemic herpesvirus hominis in pregnancy. J Reprod Med 22:171-176, 1979.
45. Nahmias AJ, Josey WE, Naib ZM, et al. Perinatal risk associated with maternal genital herpes simplex virus infection. Am J Obstet Gynecol 110:825-837, 1971.
46. Brown ZA, Selke S, Zeh J, et al. The acquisition of herpes simplex virus during pregnancy. N Engl J Med 337:509-515, 1997.
47. Dietrich YM, Napolitano PG. Acyclovir treatment of primary herpes in pregnancy complicated by second trimester preterm premature rupture of membranes with term delivery: a case report. Am J Perinatol 19:235-238, 2002.
48. Arvin AM, Hensleigh PA, Prober CG, et al. Failure of antepartum maternal cultures to predict the infant's risk of exposure to herpes simplex virus at delivery. N Engl J Med 315:796-800, 1986.
49. Whitley RJ, Corey L, Arvin A, et al. Changing presentation of neonatal herpes simplex virus infection. J Infect Dis 158:109-116, 1988.
50. Prober CG, Arvin AM. Genital herpes and the pregnant woman. *In* Remington JS, Swartz M (eds). Current Clinical Topics in Infectious Diseases, vol. 10. Boston, Blackwell Scientific, 1989, p 1.
51. Prober CG, Sullender WM, Yasukawa LL, et al. Low risk of herpes simplex virus infections in neonates exposed to the virus at the time of vaginal delivery to mothers with recurrent genital herpes simplex virus infections. N Engl J Med 316:240-244, 1987.

52. Hensleigh PA, Andrews WW, Brown Z, et al. Genital herpes during pregnancy: inability to distinguish primary and recurrent infections clinically. Obstet Gynecol 89:891-895, 1997.
53. Corey L, Adams HG, Brown ZA, et al. Genital herpes simplex virus infections: clinical manifestations, course and complications. Ann Intern Med 98:958-972, 1983.
54. Yeager AS, Arvin AM, Urbani LJ, et al. Relationship of antibody to outcome in neonatal herpes simplex virus infections. Infect Immun 29:532-538, 1980.
55. Sullender WM, Miller JL, Yasukowa LL, et al. Humoral and cell-mediated immunity in neonates with herpes simplex virus infection. J Infect Dis 155:28-37, 1987.
56. ACOG Practice Bulletin. Management of herpes in pregnancy, no. 8, October 1999. Clinical management guidelines for obstetrician-gynecologists. Int J Gynaecol Obstet 68:165-173, 2000.
57. Brown ZA, Wald A, Ashley-Morrow RA, et al. Effect of serologic status and cesarean delivery on transmission rates of herpes simplex virus from mother to infant. JAMA 289:203-209, 2003.
58. Stone KM, Brooks CA, Guinan ME, et al. National surveillance for neonatal herpes simplex virus infection. Sex Transm Dis 16:152-156, 1989.
59. Parvey LS, Chien LT. Neonatal herpes simplex virus infection introduced by fetal monitor scalp electrode. Pediatrics 65:1150-1153, 1980.
60. Kaye EM, Dooling EC. Neonatal herpes simplex meningoencephalitis associated with fetal monitor scalp electrodes. Neurology 31:1045-1047, 1981.
61. Sullivan-Bolyai J, Hull HF, Wilson C, et al. Neonatal herpes simplex virus infection in King County, Washington: increasing incidence and epidemiologic correlates. JAMA 250:3059-3062, 1983.
62. Gutierrez KM, Halpern MF, Maldonado Y, Arvin AM. The epidemiology of neonatal herpes simplex virus (HSV) infections in California from 1985 to 1995. J Infect Dis 180:199-202, 1999.
63. Gaytant MA, Steegers EA, von Cromvoirt PL, et al. Incidence of herpes neonatorum in Netherlands. Ned Tijdschr Geneeskd 144:1832-1836, 2000.
64. Hutto C, Arvin A, Jacobs R, et al. Intrauterine herpes simplex virus infections. J Pediatr 110:97-101, 1987.
65. Florman AL, Gershon AA, Blackett PR, et al. Intrauterine infection with herpes simplex virus: resultant congenital malformations. JAMA 225:129-132, 1973.
66. South MA, Tompkins WA, Morris CR, et al. Congenital malformation of the central nervous system associated with genital type (type 2) herpesvirus. J Pediatr 75:13-18, 1969.
67. Baldwin S, Whitley RJ. Intrauterine HSV infection. Teratology 39:1-10, 1989.
68. Arvin AM. Fetal and neonatal infections. *In* Nathanson N, Murphy F (eds). Viral Pathogenesis. New York, Lippincott-Raven, 1996, pp 801-814.
69. Vasileiadis GT, Roukema HW, Romano W, et al. Intrauterine herpes simplex infection. Am J Perinatol 20:55-58, 2003
70. Kahlon J, Whitley RJ. Antibody response of the newborn after herpes simplex virus infection. J Infect Dis 158:925-933, 1988.
71. Garcia AG. Maternal herpes-simplex infection causing abortion. Histopathologic study of the placenta. Hospital (Rio J) 78:1267-1274, 1970.
72. Alanen A, Hukkanen V. Herpes simplex virus DNA in amniotic fluid with neonatal infection. Clin Infect Dis 30:363-367, 2000.
73. Kimberlin DW, Lin CY, Jacobs RF, et al. Natural history of neonatal herpes simplex virus infections in the acyclovir era. Pediatrics 108:223-229, 2001.
74. Light IJ. Postnatal acquisition of herpes simplex virus by the newborn infant: a review of the literature. Pediatrics 63:480-482, 1979.
75. Linnemann CC, Light IJ, Buchman TG, et al. Transmission of herpes simplex virus type 1 in a nursery for the newborn: identification of viral isolates by DNA finger-printing. Lancet 1:964-966, 1978.
76. Hammerberg O, Watts J, Chernesky M, et al. An outbreak of herpes simplex virus type 1 in an intensive care nursery. Pediatr Infect Dis 2:290-294, 1983.
77. Yeager AS, Ashley RL, Corey L. Transmission of herpes simplex virus from the father to neonate. J Pediatr 103:905-907, 1983.
78. Douglas JM, Schmidt O, Corey L. Acquisition of neonatal HSV-1 infection from a paternal source contact. J Pediatr 103:908-910, 1983.
79. Sullivan-Bolyai JZ, Fife KH, Jacobs RF, et al. Disseminated neonatal herpes simplex virus type 1 from a maternal breast lesion. Pediatrics 71:455-457, 1983.
80. Hatherley LI, Hayes K, Jack I. Herpesvirus in an obstetric hospital. Asymptomatic virus excretion in staff members. Med J Aust 2:273-275, 1980.
81. Hatherley LI, Hayes K, Jack I. Herpes virus in an obstetric hospital. III. Prevalence of antibodies in patients and staff. Med J Aust 2:325-329, 1980.
82. Kohl S, West MS, Prober CG, et al. Neonatal antibody-dependent cellular cytotoxic antibody levels are associated with the clinical presentation of neonatal herpes simplex virus infection. J Infect Dis 160:770-776, 1989.
83. Pass RF, Dworsky ME, Whitley RJ, et al. Specific lymphocyte blastogenic responses in children with cytomegalovirus and herpes simplex virus infections acquired early in infancy. Infect Immun 34:166-170, 1981.
84. Chilmonczyk BA, Levin MJ, McDuffy R, et al. Characterization of the human newborn response to herpesvirus antigen. J Immunol 134: 4184-4188, 1985.
85. Burchett SK, Corey L, Mohan K, et al. Diminished interferon-gamma and lymphocyte proliferation in neonatal and postpartum primary herpes simplex virus infection. J Infect Dis 165:813-818, 1992.
86. Kohl S, Harmon MW. Human neonatal leukocyte interferon production and natural killer cytotoxicity in response to herpes simplex virus. J Interferon Res 3:461-463, 1983.
87. Kohl S. Neonatal herpes simplex virus infection. Clin Perinatol 24: 129-150, 1997.
88. Mintz H, Drew WL, Hoo R, et al. Age dependent resistance of human alveolar macrophages to herpes simplex virus. Infect Immun 28: 417-420, 1980.
89. Hirsch MS, Zisman B, Allison AC. Macrophages and age-dependent resistance to herpes simplex virus in mice. J Immunol 104:1160-1165, 1970.
90. Kohl S, Sigouroudinia M, Engleman EG. Adhesion defects of antibody-mediated target cell binding of neonatal natural killer cells. Pediatr Res 46:755-759, 1999.
91. Diamond C, Mohan K, Hobson A, et al. Viremia in neonatal herpes simplex virus infections. Pediatr Infect Dis J 18:487-489, 1999
92. Singer DB. Pathology of neonatal herpes simplex virus infection. Perspect Pediatr Pathol 6:243-278, 1981.
93. Smith MC, Lennette EH, Reames HR. Isolation of the virus of herpes simplex and the demonstration of intranuclear inclusions in a case of acute encephalitis. Am J Pathol 17:538, 1971.
94. Whitley R, Arvin A, Prober C, et al. Predictors of morbidity and mortality in neonates with herpes simplex infections. N Engl J Med 324:450-454, 1991.
95. Nahmias A, Alford C, Korones S. Infection of the newborn with herpesvirus hominis. Adv Pediatr 17:185-226, 1970.
96. Whitley RJ, Kimberlin D. Infections in perinatology: antiviral therapy of neonatal herpes simplex virus infections. Clin Perinatol 24:267-283, 1997.
97. Anderson MS, Abzug MJ. Hydrops fetalis: an unusual presentation of intrauterine herpes simplex virus infection. Pediatr Infect Dis J 18:837-839, 1999.
98. Malm G, Berg U, Forsgren M. Neonatal herpes simplex: clinical findings and outcome in relation to type of maternal infection. Acta Paediatr 84:256-260, 1995.
99. Greenes DS, Rowitch D, Thorne G, et al. Neonatal herpes simplex virus infection presenting as fulminant liver failure. Pediatr Infect Dis J 14:242-244, 1995.
100. Arvin AM, Yeager AS, Bruhn FW, et al. Neonatal herpes simplex infection in the absence of mucocutaneous lesions. J Pediatr 100: 715-721, 1982.
101. Lee WS, Kelly DA, Tanner MS, et al. Neonatal liver transplantation for fulminant hepatitis caused by herpes simplex virus type 2. J Pediatr Gastroenterol Nutr 35:220-223, 2002.
102. Gressens P, Langston C, Martin JR. In situ PCR localization of herpes simplex virus DNA sequences in disseminated neonatal herpes encephalitis. J Neuropathol Exp Neurol 53:469-482, 1994.
103. Golden SE. Neonatal herpes simplex viremia. Pediatr Infect Dis J 7:425-427, 1987.
104. Langlet C, Gaugler C, Castaing M, et al. An uncommon case of disseminated neonatal herpes simplex infection presenting with pneumonia and pleural effusions. Eur J Pediatr 162:532-533, 2003.
105. Corey L, Stone EF, Whitley RJ, Mohan K. Difference between herpes simplex virus type 1 and type 2 neonatal encephalitis in neurological outcome. Lancet 1:l-4, 1988.
106. Kimberlin DW. Herpes simplex virus infections of the central nervous system. Semin Pediatr Infect Dis 14:83-89, 2003.

107. Mizrahi EM, Tharp BR. A characteristic electroencephalogram pattern in neonatal herpes simplex virus encephalitis. Neurology 32:1215-1220, 1982.
108. O'Reilly MAR, O'Reilly PMR, de Bruyn R. Neonatal herpes simplex type 2 encephalitis: its appearances on ultrasound and CT. Pediatr Radiol 25:68-69, 1995.
109. Toth C, Harder S, Yager J. Neonatal herpes encephalitis: a case series and review of clinical presentation. Can J Neurol Sci 30:36-40, 2003.
110. Kimura H, Ito Y, Futamura M, et al. Quantitation of viral load in neonatal herpes simplex virus infection and comparison between type 1 and type 2. J Med Virol 67:349-353, 2002.
111. Gutman LT, Wilfert CM, Eppes S. Herpes simplex virus encephalitis in children: analysis of cerebrospinal fluid and progressive neurodevelopmental deterioration. J Infect Dis 154:415-421, 1986.
112. Whitley R, Arvin A, Prober C, et al. A controlled trial comparing vidarabine with acyclovir in neonatal herpes simplex virus infection. N Engl J Med 324:444-449, 1991.
113. Musci SI, Fine EM, Togo Y. Zoster-like disease in the newborn due to herpes simplex virus. N Engl J Med 284:24-26, 1971.
114. Nahmias A, Hagler W. Ocular manifestations of herpes simplex in the newborn. Int Ophthalmol Clin 12:191-213, 1972.
115. Cherry JD, Soriano F, Jahn CL. Search for perinatal viral infection: a prospective, clinical virology and serologic study. Am J Dis Child 116:245-250, 1968.
116. Whitley RJ, Lakeman FD. Herpes simplex virus infections of the central nervous system: therapeutic and diagnostic considerations. Clin Infect Dis 20:414-420, 1995.
117. Jerome KR, Ashley RL. Herpes simplex viruses and herpes B virus. *In* Murray PR, Baron EJ, Jorgensen JH, et al (eds). Manual of Clinical Microbiology, 8th ed. Washington, DC, American Society for Microbiology, 2003, pp 1291-1303.
118. Kimberlin DW, Lakeman FD, Arvin AM, et al. Application of the polymerase chain reaction to the diagnosis and management of neonatal herpes simplex virus disease. National Institute of Allergy and Infectious Diseases Collaborative Antiviral Study Group. J Infect Dis 174:1162-1167, 1996.
119. Troendle-Atksin J, Demmler GJ, Buffone GJ. Rapid diagnosis of herpes simplex virus encephalitis by using the polymerase chain reaction. J Pediatr 123:376-380, 1993.
120. Kimura H, Futamura M, Kito H, et al. Detection of viral DNA in neonatal herpes simplex virus infections: frequent and prolonged presence in serum and cerebrospinal fluid. J Infect Dis 164:289-293, 1991.
121. Malm G, Forsgren M. Neonatal herpes simplex virus infections: HSV DNA in cerebrospinal fluid and serum. Arch Dis Child Fetal Neonatal Ed 81:F24-F29, 1999.
122. Weil AA, Glaser CA, Amad Z, Forghani B. Patients with suspected herpes simplex encephalitis: rethinking an initial negative polymerase chain reaction result. Clin Infect Dis 34:1154-1157, 2002.
123. Kimberlin DW. Neonatal herpes simplex infection. Clin Microbiol Rev 17:1-13, 2004.
124. Smalling TW, Sefers SE, Haijing L, Tang Y. Molecular approaches to detecting herpes simplex virus and enteroviruses in the central nervous system. J Clin Microbiol 40:2317-2322, 2002.
125. Elion GB, Furman PA, Fyfe JA, et al. Selectivity of action of an antiherpetic agent 9-(2-hydroxyethoxymethyl) guanine. Proc Natl Acad Sci U S A. 74:5716-5720, 1977.
126. Whitley RJ, Nahmias J, Soong SJ, et al. Vidarabine therapy of neonatal herpes simplex virus infection. Pediatrics 66:495-501, 1980.
127. Corey L, Benedetti J, Critchlow C, et al. Treatment of primary first-episode genital herpes simplex virus infections with acyclovir: results of topical, intravenous and oral therapy. J Antimicrob Chemother 12(Suppl B):79-88, 1983.
128. Bryson YJ, Dillon M, Lovett M, et al. Treatment of first episodes of genital herpes simplex virus infection with oral acyclovir. A randomized double-blind controlled trial in normal subjects. N Engl J Med 308:916-921, 1983.
129. Saral R, Burns WH, Laskin OL, et al. Acyclovir prophylaxis of herpes-simplex-virus infections. N Engl J Med 305:63-67, 1981.
130. Whitley RJ, Alford CA, Hirsch MS, et al. Vidarabine versus acyclovir therapy of herpes simplex encephalitis. N Engl J Med 314:144-149, 1986.
131. Yeager AS. Use of acyclovir in premature and term neonates. Am J Med 73:205-209, 1982.
132. Hintz M, Connor JD, Spector SA, et al. Neonatal acyclovir pharmacokinetics in patients with herpesvirus infections. Am J Med 73:210-214, 1982.
133. Kimberlin DW, Chin-Yu L, Jacobs RF, et al. Safety and efficacy of high-dose intravenous acyclovir in the management of neonatal herpes simplex virus infections. Pediatrics 108:230-238, 2001.
134. American Academy of Pediatrics. Herpes simplex. *In* Pickering LK (ed). Red Book: 2003 Report of the Committee on Infectious Diseases, 26th ed. Elk Grove Village, Ill, American Academy of Pediatrics, 2003.
135. Nyquist AC, Rotbart HA, Cotton M, et al. Acyclovir-resistant neonatal herpes simplex virus infection of the larynx. J Pediatr 124:967-971, 1994.
136. Oram RJ, Marcellino D, Strauss D, et al. Characterization of an acyclovir-resistant herpes simplex virus type 2 strain isolated from a premature neonate. J Infect Dis 181:1458-61, 2000.
137. Levin MJ, Weinberg A, Leary JJ, Sarisky RT. Development of acyclovir-resistant herpes simplex virus early during the treatment of herpes neonatorum. Pediatr Infect Dis J 20:1094-1097, 2001.
138. Rabalais GP, Nusinoff-Lehrman S, Arvin AM, Levin MJ. Antiviral susceptibilities of herpes simplex virus isolates from infants with recurrent mucocutaneous lesions after neonatal infection. Pediatr Infect Dis J 8:221-223, 1989.
139. Kimberlin D, Powell D, Gruber W, et al. Administration of oral acyclovir suppressive therapy after neonatal herpes simplex virus disease limited to the skin, eyes and mouth: results of a phase I/II trial. Pediatr Infect Dis J 15:247-254, 1996.
140. Kohl S, Loo LS, Rench MS, et al. Effect of intravenously administered immune globulin on functional antibody to herpes simplex virus in low birth weight neonates. J Pediatr 115:135-139, 1989.
141. Whitley RJ. Neonatal herpes simplex virus infections: is there a role for immunoglobulin in disease prevention and therapy? Pediatr Infect Dis J 13:432-438, 1994.
142. Hardy DA, Arvin AM, Yasukawa LL, et al. Use of polymerase chain reaction for successful identification of asymptomatic genital infection with herpes simplex virus in pregnant women at delivery. J Infect Dis 162:1031-1035, 1990.
143. Cone RW, Hobson AC, Brown Z, et al. Frequent detection of genital herpes simplex virus DNA by polymerase chain reaction among pregnant women. JAMA 272:792-796, 1994.
144. Watts DH, Brown ZA, Money D, et al. A double-blind, randomized, placebo-controlled trial of acyclovir in late pregnancy for the reduction of herpes simplex virus shedding and cesarean delivery. Am J Obstet Gynecol 188:836-843, 2003.
145. Douglas JM, Critchlow C, Benedetti J, et al. A double-blind study of oral acyclovir for suppression of recurrences of genital herpes simplex virus infection. N Engl J Med 310:1551-1556, 1984.
146. Straus SE, Takiff HE, Seidlin M, et al. Suppression of frequently recurring genital herpes: a placebo-controlled double-blind trial of oral acyclovir. N Engl J Med 310:1545-1550, 1984.
147. Arvin AM. Genital herpesvirus infections: rationale for a vaccine strategy. *In* Hitchcock PJ, MacKay HT, Wasserheit JN, Binder R (eds). Sexually Transmitted Diseases and Adverse Outcomes of Pregnancy. Washington, DC, American Society for Microbiology, 1999, p 259.
148. Koelle DM, Corey L. Recent progress in herpes simplex virus immunobiology and vaccine research. Clin Microbiol Rev 16:96-113, 2003.
149. Arvin AM, Prober CG. Herpes simplex virus type 2, a persistent problem. N Engl J Med 337:1158-1159, 1997.

Chapter 27

HUMAN PARVOVIRUS INFECTIONS

Stuart P. Adler • William C. Koch

The parvoviruses are a family of small, single-stranded DNA viruses that have a wide cellular tropism and broad host range, causing infection in invertebrate and vertebrate species from insects to mammals. Although many are important veterinary pathogens, there is only one proven human pathogen in the family, the human parvovirus B19. The virus is most commonly referred to as parvovirus B19, or simply B19. A new genus and name have been proposed for this virus: erythrovirus B19,[1] based on its cellular tropism for erythroid lineage cells and to distinguish it from the other mammalian parvoviruses.

Compared with most other common human viruses, B19 is a relatively new pathogen, but since its initial description, B19 has come to be associated with a variety of seemingly diverse clinical syndromes in a number of different patient populations (Table 27-1). Although the list of clinical manifestations caused by B19 infection is probably not yet complete, some proposed relationships such as to rheumatologic disease and neurologic disorders remain controversial.[2,3]

Parvovirus B19 was accidentally discovered by Cossart and associates[4] in 1975 as an anomalous band of precipitation while screening blood donor serum for hepatitis B antigen by counterimmunoelectrophoresis. The name *B19* refers to the donor unit from which it was originally isolated. Initial analysis of the new virus revealed it had physical features characteristic of the known parvoviruses,[5] allowing classification in this family. Because the donors from which it was originally isolated were asymptomatic, B19 infection was not initially associated with any illness, and for the next several years after its description, it was a virus in search of a disease. In 1981, Pattison[6] found a high prevalence of antibodies to this virus in the serum of children hospitalized with the transient aplastic crisis of sickle cell disease and proposed B19 as the viral cause of this clinically well-described event. Sergeant and colleagues[7] later confirmed this association in population studies of sickle cell patients in Jamaica. It was not until 1983, 8 years after its initial description, that Anderson proposed B19 as the cause of the common childhood exanthem known as erythema infectiosum (EI), or fifth disease, that the virus was linked to its most common clinical manifestation.[8] This benign rash illness of children had been clinically recognized and well described for many decades, but the cause was unknown. The name *fifth disease*

Table 27–1 **Clinical Manifestations of Parvovirus B19 Infection**

Diseases	Primary Patient Groups
Diseases Associated with Acute Infection	
Erythema infectiosum (fifth disease)	Normal children
Polyarthropathy	Normal adolescents and adults
Transient aplastic crisis	Patients with hemolytic anemia or accelerated erythropoiesis, or both
Papular-purpuric "gloves and socks" syndrome	Normal adolescents and adults
Diseases Associated with Chronic Infection	
Persistent anemia (red cell aplasia)	Immunodeficient or immunocompromised children and adults
Nonimmune fetal hydrops	Intrauterine infection
Congenital anemia	Intrauterine infection
Chronic arthropathy	Rare patients with B19-induced joint disease
Infection-associated hemophagocytosis	Normal or immunocompromised patients
Vasculitis or purpura	Normal adults and children
Myocarditis	Intrauterine infection, normal infants and children, immunocompromised patients

Data from Brown KE, Young NS. Parvovirus B19 infection and hematopoiesis. Blood Rev 9:176, 1995.

was derived from the 19th century practice of numbering the common exanthems of childhood, and EI was the fifth rash designated in this scheme and the only one for which this numeric designation has persisted in clinical practice.[9] The others in the series included measles, scarlet fever, rubella, and Filatov-Dukes disease (a mild variant of scarlet fever that is no longer recognized).

The possibility of fetal disease associated with EI was considered long before the viral origin was known, primarily because of comparison with rubella and the incidence of congenital rubella syndrome after community epidemics.[10-12] Advances in knowledge of the virology of other animal parvoviruses and their known propensity to cause disease in fetuses and newborn animals further fueled this concern.[13] This suspicion was confirmed in 1984, when two reports[14,15] of B19 infection in pregnant women associated with adverse fetal outcomes appeared and were later followed by a larger report of a series of cases of nonimmune hydrops fetalis caused by intrauterine infections with B19.[16] Over the ensuing decade, a variety of clinical manifestations associated with acute and chronic infections have been attributed to this virus in different patient groups (see Table 27-1).

Since the initial reports of fetal infection, knowledge of the epidemiology, pathophysiology, and short-term outcome of fetal and neonatal infection with B19 has increased immensely because of several large, population-based studies.[17-21] B19 infection during pregnancy has probably been the subject of more such studies than any of the other manifestations, with the possible exception of the transient aplastic crisis of sickle cell disease. However, there is still much to be learned regarding the long-term outcome of fetal infection, the unusual clinical manifestations of infection in neonates, and the immunologic response to infection. The potential for prevention through vaccine development is a topic of current interest and ongoing research.

MICROBIOLOGY

Like other members of the family Parvoviridae, B19 is a small, nonenveloped, single-stranded DNA virus. The taxonomy for this family has been revised to include two subfamilies[22,23]: the Densovirinae, which are insect viruses; and the Parvovirinae, which infect vertebrates. The Parvovirinae subfamily is composed of three genera: Dependovirus, Parvovirus, and Erythrovirus. The dependoviruses require co-infection with another, unrelated helper virus (i.e., adenovirus or herpesvirus) to complete their life cycle. There are some dependoviruses that infect humans (e.g., adeno-associated viruses), but the infection is asymptomatic and without consequence. In contrast to the dependoviruses, members of the genera Parvovirus and Erythrovirus are able to replicate autonomously. Previously included in the genus Parvovirus, B19 is now classified as an Erythrovirus (i.e., Erythrovirus B19). The genus Erythrovirus consists of only two members, B19 and a simian parvovirus (SPV) that has a similar genomic organization as B19 and has a similar tropism for erythroid cells.[24] Although a number of parvoviruses are pathogenic to other mammals (e.g., canine parvovirus, feline panleukopenia virus), B19 is the only parvovirus that causes disease in humans.

There is only one recognized serotype of B19. Minor variations in the nucleotide sequence occur among different B19 viral isolates from different geographic areas, but they have not been definitely shown to affect clinical patterns of infection or pathogenicity.[25-27] Two isolates of human parvovirus, V9 and V6, whose nucleotide sequence differs significantly (>10%) from B19 have been described.[28,29] Both were isolated from patients with a transient red cell aplasia indistinguishable clinically from the typical B19-induced aplastic crisis. The clinical significance of these variants and whether they represent different genotypes or merely geographic variants of B19 remains a topic of debate.[27,30]

The B19 genome is very small (≈5.6 kb) and contained within an icosahedral protein capsid. The capsid structure and lack of an envelope make the virus very resistant to heat and detergent inactivation, features that appear to be important in transmission. The genome appears to encode only three proteins. Two are capsid proteins, designated VP1 and VP2. VP2 is smaller but more abundant and makes up approximately 96% of the capsid protein. VP1 is larger and constitutes about 4% of the capsid but contains a unique region that extends out from the capsid surface and serves as the attachment site for the cellular receptor.[31] VP2 has the unique ability to self-assemble into capsids that are morphologically and antigenically similar to B19 viruses when expressed in cell culture systems in vitro.[32,33] When present with VP1, the capsids incorporate both proteins, but VP1 alone does not self-assemble.[32]

The third gene product is a nonstructural protein designated NS1. The function of this protein is not entirely clear, but it is involved in regulation of the viral promoter and appears to have a role in DNA replication.[23] Studies of NS1 have been hampered by the observation that it appears to be toxic to cells by an unknown mechanism.[34] Studies have further suggested that production of NS1 can lead to programmed cell death (i.e., apoptosis) mediated by stimulation of cytokine production.[35,36]

Because of its limited genomic complement, B19 requires a mitotically active host cell for replication. It can replicate only in certain erythroid lineage cells stimulated by erythropoietin, such as erythroid precursors found in bone marrow, fetal liver, umbilical cord blood, and a few erythroleukemic cell lines.[23,37-41] B19 cannot be propagated in standard cell cultures,[42] a fact that previously limited the availability of viral products for development of diagnostic assays. Much of this limitation has been overcome by the development of molecular methods for the detection of viral nucleic acid, but reliable commercial serologic assays are still somewhat limited.

The cellular receptor for the virus has been identified as globoside, a neutral glycosphingolipid found on erythrocytes, where it represents the P blood group antigen.[43] This receptor is necessary for viral infection to occur, and individuals who lack this antigen (p phenotype) are naturally immune to B19 infection.[44] The P antigen is present on other cells such as endothelial cells, fetal myocardial cells, placenta, and megakaryocytes.[43] The tissue distribution of this receptor may explain some of the clinical manifestations of infection with this virus (discussed later).

Although the P antigen is necessary for B19 viral infection, it is not sufficient, because some cells, particularly nonerythroid tissues, that express the receptor are not capable of viral infection.[45] A co-receptor has been described on cells that are permissive for B19 infection.[46] The hypothesis is that the globoside receptor is necessary for viral attachment but that the co-receptor somehow allows for viral entry into the cell, where viral replication can occur. If confirmed, this may provide an alternative explanation of the pathogenesis of infection in nonerythroid tissues that express globoside without the co-receptor.

PATHOGENESIS: GENERAL ASPECTS

Parvovirus B19 requires a mitotically active host cell to complete its full replicative life cycle. The primary target for B19 infection appears to be erythroid progenitor cells that are near the pronormoblast stage of development. The virus can be propagated only in human erythroid progenitor cells from bone marrow, umbilical cord blood, fetal liver, peripheral blood, and a few erythroid leukemic cell lines.[47] B19 lytically infects these cells, with progressive loss of targeted cells as infection proceeds. In vitro hematopoietic assays demonstrate that B19 suppresses formation of erythroid colony-forming units and this effect can be reversed by addition of serum containing anti-B19 immunoglobulin G (IgG) antibodies.[48] The virus has little to no effect on the myeloid cell line in vitro, but it inhibits megakaryocytopoiesis in vitro without viral replication or cell lysis.[49]

Clinically, this situation is best illustrated in the transient aplastic crisis of sickle cell disease. Patients have fever, weakness, and pallor on presentation, with a sudden and severe drop in their reticulocyte counts. This cessation of red blood cell production, coupled with shortened red blood cell survival because of hemolysis, produces a profound anemia. Examination of the bone marrow typically reveals hypoplasia of the erythroid cell line and a maturational arrest; giant pronormoblasts are often seen with intranuclear viral inclusions.[48] With development of specific antibodies, viral infection is controlled, and reticulocyte counts begin to rise.

Evaluation of infection in normal volunteers has shown similar hematologic changes, but because of the longer life of red blood cells, these changes are clinically insignificant.[50] Adult volunteers inoculated intranasally with B19 developed viremia after 5 to 6 days with a mild illness. Their reticulocyte counts fell to undetectable levels, and this was accompanied by a modest fall in hemoglobin and hematocrit levels. Platelets and granulocyte counts also declined. Specific antibody production with immunoglobulin M (IgM) was followed by IgG, and viremia was cleared rapidly. A second-phase illness developed at 17 to 18 days with rash and arthralgias but without fever, and hematologic indices had returned to normal.

The tissue distribution of the cellular receptor for the virus (P antigen) may explain the predominance of hematologic findings associated with B19 infection. Its presence on other tissues may help to explain other clinical manifestations, such as myocardial disease, congenital infection, and vasculitis syndromes. Although the cellular receptor is present and the virus can attach, unlike erythroid cells, these cells are nonpermissive for viral replication; the virus is unable to undergo a complete life cycle with the resultant lysis of the host cells. Instead, interaction in these tissues leads to accumulation of the nonstructural protein NS1. This protein is essential for viral replication and has a variety of proposed functions[23] but appears to be toxic to most mammalian cell lines when present in excess.[34] NS1 has been associated with apoptosis.[36,41] NS1 also has been linked to production of tumor necrosis factor-α and interleukin-6, a potent proinflammatory cytokine.[35,41,51] This may lead to cellular injury through cytokine pathways and provide another mechanism aside from lytic infection for some of the clinical manifestations.

Chronic infections in immunocompromised patients develop when patients are unable to mount an adequate neutralizing antibody response. These infections are characterized by viral persistence in serum or bone marrow and lack of detectable circulating antibody. Clinical manifestations include chronic anemia or red cell aplasia and may include granulocytopenia and thrombocytopenia. The mechanism for the leukopenia and thrombocytopenia is not known, although it has been shown[49] that B19 causes disturbances in megakaryocytic replication when infected in vitro.

EPIDEMIOLOGY AND TRANSMISSION

B19 is a highly contagious and common infection worldwide. In the United States, 60% or more of white adults are seropositive (i.e., have IgG antibodies to B19 in their sera). This indicates a previous infection, usually one acquired in childhood. Among African Americans, the rate of seropositivity is lower, about 30%.[19] Transmission of B19 from person to person probably occurs by droplets from oral or nasal secretions. This is suggested by the rapid transmission among those in close physical contact, such as schoolmates or family members, and from a study of healthy volunteers experimentally infected with B19, in whom virus was found in blood and nasopharyngeal secretions for several days beginning 1 or 2 days before symptoms appeared.[50] In the volunteer study, no virus was detected in urine or stool.

Given the highly contagious nature of B19 infections, it is not surprising that most outbreaks occur in elementary schools and occasionally child-care centers. Susceptible (seronegative) adult school personnel are at high risk for acquiring the infection from students.[19] Some outbreaks in schools may be seasonal (often late winter and spring) and epidemic, with many children and staff acquiring the infection and developing symptoms of EI. At other times, the infection is often endemic, with transmission occurring slowly and with only a few persons manifesting symptoms.

Global Distribution

B19 infections occur worldwide. Serologic evidence of B19 infection has been found everywhere studied, including developed countries, undeveloped countries, urban and rural areas, and isolated island populations.[52-55] The diseases and associated signs and symptoms are the same worldwide. No important strain or antigenic differences have been detected, and serologic assays are independent of the source or location of patient serum. Disease caused by B19 appears to be unrelated to specific viral genotypes, although analysis of the antigenic variation or nucleotide sequences of widely dispersed B19 isolates shows some heterogeneity of unknown significance.[25,26,56-61]

Seasonality and Periodicity

Transmission of B19 continues throughout the year, but there are seasonal variations in transmission rates. Outbreaks of EI most often occur in winter and spring in temperate climates and less frequently in fall and summer.[62-64] In schools or daycare centers, outbreaks of EI may persist for months, usually starting in late winter or early spring and ending with summer vacation. Figure 27-1 highlights multiyear outbreaks of B19 exposure among pregnant women and the associated seasonal variation in Pittsburgh, Pennsylvania. Most cases occurred in late spring and summer of each year.

In Jamaica, an island nation, careful studies of those with sickle cell disease show that epidemics of transient aplastic crises occurred about every 5 years, with little disease occurring inside this interval.[65] Epidemics of B19 infections at 5-year intervals were also observed in Rio de Janeiro, Brazil.[66] In Japan, age-related serologic evaluation of stored serum samples showed no evidence for B19 epidemics over a 10-year period.[67] The prevalence of IgG antibodies to B19 among three tribes of South American Indians living in remote regions of Brazil was very low (<11%), and was zero for those younger than 30 years in one tribe.[55] However, school nursing records in Iowa over 14 years identified cases of EI every year but one.[68]

Seroprevalence by Age

In numerous studies of B19 infection based on serologic testing, the seroprevalence of B19 infection increases with age.[4,65,69-74] Figure 27-2 shows the age-dependent increase in seroprevalence in Richmond, Virginia.[75] Transplacentally acquired maternal antibodies are undetectable by 1 year of age. In children younger than 5 years, the prevalence of IgG antibodies to B19 is usually less than 5%. The greatest increase in seroprevalence and B19 infection occurs between 5 and 20 years of age. By age 20 years, the seroprevalence of B19 infection rises from about 5% to almost 40%. Afterward, without regard to risk factors, B19 seroprevalence increases slowly. In adult blood donors, the seroprevalence of IgG antibodies to B19 ranges from 29% to 79% with a median of 45%.[76-82] By age 50, the seroprevalence may be greater than

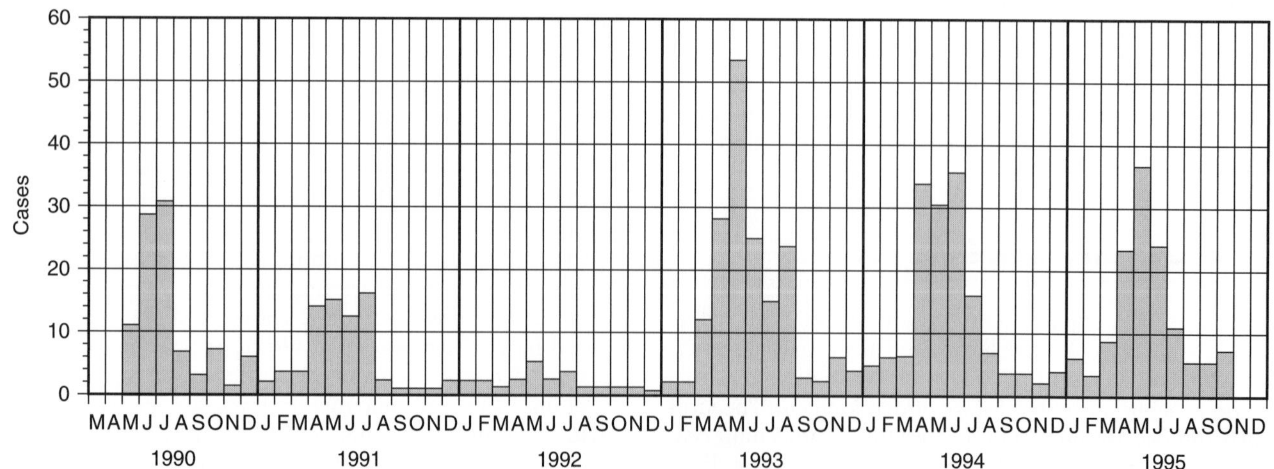

Figure 27–1 Seasonal variation in reported parvovirus B19 exposures in pregnant women. Each month is indicated by its first letter. (Data from Harger J, Koch W, Harger GF. Prospective evaluation of 618 pregnant women exposed to parvovirus B19: risks and symptoms. Obstet Gynecol 91:413, 1998.)

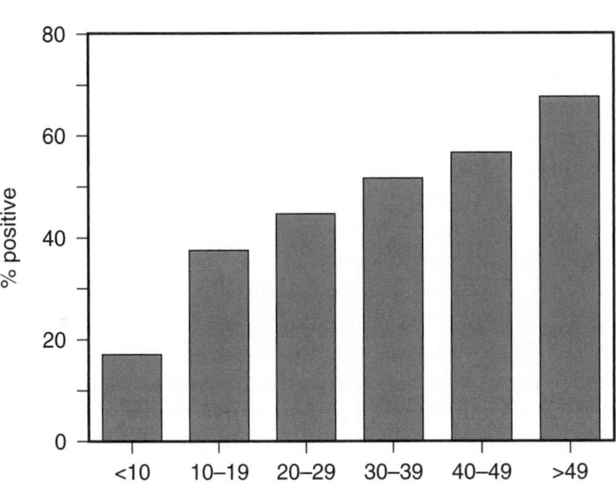

Figure 27–2 Percentage of family subjects positive for IgG antibody to B19 by age. The sample includes 283 subjects from 111 families. Subjects were one twin of each twin pair, nontwin parents, and the oldest child of each family. (Data from Adler SP, Koch W. Human parvovirus B19 infections in women of childbearing age and within families. J Pediatr Infect Dis 8:83, 1989.)

75%. Similar results on the age-related seroprevalence of B19 infections were observed in India.[83]

Seroprevalence by Gender

In most studies, the prevalence of antibodies to B19 in sera obtained from men and women is similar.[70] At least four studies, however, have reported that women have a higher rate of B19 infection than men.[19,75,77,84] In one study of adult blood donors, the proportion of women who were seropositive, 47.5%, was 1.5 times higher than for men. The prevalence of IgG antibodies averaged 51% for women of all ages, compared with 38% for males in one of two family studies in Richmond, Virginia, and 64% for women and 50% for men in the other.[19,75] In Taiwan, the prevalence of IgG antibodies to B19 among females was significantly higher than among males (36.4% versus 29.4%, $P < .001$).[85] The most likely explanation for the higher rates of B19 infection among women compared with men is that women are likely to have more frequent contact with children, especially school-aged children, who are the major sources of B19 transmission because of school attendance. For adults, contact with school-aged children is the major risk factor for B19 infection.[19]

Seroprevalence by Race

In the United States, there are significant differences in the seroprevalence to B19 between blacks and whites. For example in Richmond, Virginia, approximately 60% of whites are seropositive, compared with 45% of blacks.[19] The reasons for the lower rate of infection among blacks are unknown, but may reflect the fact that students in Richmond schools are predominantly African American.

Incidence

In tests of serum from random blood donors for evidence of recent B19 infection using detection of viral antigens or DNA, the rate using antigen detection of infection is 0 to 2.6 cases per 10,000 individuals tested, with a median of 1 per 10,000; using DNA detection, the rate is 0 to 14.5 per 10,000, with a median of 2 per 10,000.[86-91] When IgM antibodies to B19 are used to detect recent infection, the rate has been zero, but all studies included fewer than 1000 patients.[76,92,93] As for seroprevalence, women may have a greater risk for infection during outbreaks of EI. During an epidemic of EI in Port Angeles, Washington, the attack rate for women was 15.6%, more than twice the rate of 7.4% for men.[10]

In Spain and Chile, children have the highest rates of B19 infection, which is true for groups of children 0 to 4 years old and for those 5 to 9 years old.[94,95] A study of 633 children with sickle cell disease followed at the Children's Hospital in Philadelphia between 1996 and 2001 found that 70% were seronegative (i.e., susceptible), and during this period, 110 patients developed B19 infections, for an incidence of 11.3 per 100 patients per year.[96] Among the 110 patients infected, there were 68 episodes of transient aplastic crisis, characterized by an acute exacerbation of anemia, acute chest syndrome, pain, and fever. The high incidence of disease among these patients emphasizes the need for a vaccine against a parvovirus B19.

Risk Factors for Acquisition

B19 is efficiently transmitted among those residing in the same home, with attack rates based on the development of signs and symptoms of EI ranging from 17% to 30%.[10,97] Using serologic testing to identify asymptomatic infection and to exclude immune individuals, the secondary attack rate for susceptible household contacts is 50%. Most secondary cases of EI or aplastic crisis in the home occur 6 to 12 days after the index case.[10, 97-100] A serologic study of pregnant Danish women indicated that seropositivity was significantly correlated with increasing number of siblings, having a sibling of the same age, number of own children, and occupational exposure of children.[101]

During epidemics, B19 transmission is widespread among school-aged children. Studies of school or classroom outbreaks of EI with at least one serologically confirmed case of acute B19 infection revealed student infection rates ranging from 1% to 62% based on the occurrence of a rash illness. The median rate for all studies was 23%.[102-109] Because asymptomatic infections are common and other signs and symptoms of EI may be mild and overlooked, these studies undoubtedly underestimate the true incidence of infection. Studies of students using serologic assays to identify B19 infection during outbreaks report infection rates of between 34% and 72%, with most not associated with a rash illness.[103,108,109] The higher rates of infection occur in elementary schools and daycare centers compared with secondary schools and in boarded school students compared with nonboarded students.[107-109]

During school epidemics, employees in contact with children have the highest rates of infection compared with community controls. The attack rate based on detection of rash illness or arthropathy may be relatively low (12% to

25%).[103,107] However, the seroprevalence of B19 IgG antibodies to B19 in school employees is greater than adult community controls and ranges between 50% and 75%.[19,109,110] When serologic testing is used to identify employees with asymptomatic infection and to exclude immune employees, the attack rate among the susceptibles is usually very high. In four school outbreaks where serologic testing was used, the attack rate varied from 19% to 84%, and the frequency of asymptomatic infection was greater than 50% in all but one outbreak.[103,106,109,110] The highest infection rates occurred among susceptible elementary school teachers compared with middle and high school teachers, and this may reflect exposure to more infected children or a greater likelihood of contact with respiratory secretions in younger children.[109,110] During a community-wide outbreak of EI in Connecticut in 1988, the infection rate among susceptible women was 16% for school teachers, 9% for daycare workers and homemakers, but only 4% for other women working outside the home.[109]

The risk of infection may be increased for school employees even in the absence of recognized epidemics of EI. In a study of 927 susceptible school employees conducted during a 3.5-year period when no community outbreaks were detected, the annual incidence of specific IgG seroconversion was 2.9%, compared with 0.4% for a control population of 198 hospital employees.[19] The rate of 3.4% was higher for school employees with jobs involving direct contact with children compared with only 0.6% observed for persons with other job classifications. Most of the individuals who seroconverted did not recall an illness characterized by rash or arthropathy.

Salivary antibodies can be used to detect IgG and IgM antibodies to B19 because serum antibodies passively diffuse into saliva. Testing saliva for antibodies to B19 was useful in documenting outbreaks in schools and households. In an outbreak in England, school attack rates varied from 8% to 50%, including an attack rate of 45% for the teaching staff.[111] The household transmission attack rate was 45% for 11 susceptible individuals. These rates are similar to what has been previously observed.[111]

Crowding and low socioeconomic status are not proven risk factors for B19 infection. However, these factors are suggested by the observation that in Rio de Janeiro, the seroprevalence of IgG antibodies to B19 is 35% in children age 5 years or younger, but in Niger, it was 90% by 2 years of age.[54,70]

Hospital Transmission

B19 can be transmitted from infected patients to hospital workers.[112] Most investigations reveal that hospital transmission of B19 is common and includes direct patient-to-patient transmission and indirect transmission from materials or specimens known to contain B19 to laboratory personnel.[112-115] One patient with sickle cell anemia became ill with aplastic crisis 9 to 11 days after contact in the hospital with a patient with hereditary spherocytosis hospitalized for aplastic crisis; B19 infection was confirmed in both.[116] An outbreak of EI occurred on a pediatric ward where 13 (26%) of 50 children developed a rash illness.[117] B19 seroconversion occurred in 5 (71%) of 7 children with rash illness and in 9 (35%) of 26 children who were asymptomatic. Transmission from patient to health care worker occurred twice in one hospital after admission of patients with aplastic crisis.[112] In the first case, 4 (36%) of 11 susceptible employees with close contact had IgM antibodies to B19, indicating recent infection; in the second case, 10 (48%) of 21 employees had specific IgM antibodies to B19 or seroconverted from IgG negative to positive. Eleven (79%) of 14 were symptomatic with rash or arthropathy. Another study of an outbreak of EI among health care workers on a pediatric ward found that 10 (33%) of 30 susceptible health care workers had serologic evidence of acute B19 infection, along with 2 (17%) of 12 immunocompromised patients being cared for on the ward.[113,118] The two infected patients were not symptomatic, but analysis of preexisting sera showed they acquired B19 while hospitalized. Onset of symptoms among the employees was temporally clustered, indicating a chronic source such as an immunocompromised patient or person-to-person transmission.

Studies in Hong Kong identified three immunocompromised patients who appeared to transmit genetically identical strains of B19 from patient to patient.[119] At least one of these three patients appeared to be able to transmit the virus over many months. Immunocompromised patients often have chronic infections and therefore may be infectious for long periods. DNA sequence analysis was also used in Japan to document B19 transmission between hospital staff members, including nursing staff, office workers, and a physiotherapist.[120]

Other investigations have observed little or no risk for hospital transmission. No evidence of patient-to-employee transmission was found among 10 susceptible health care workers with frequent contact with a chronically infected patient hospitalized for 24 days before institution of isolation precautions.[121] Transmission to hospital employees did not occur after exposure to a parvovirus B19–infected mother, her infected stillborn fetus, and contaminated objects in the hospital room.[122] During a community outbreak of B19, none of 17 susceptible pregnant health care workers with possible exposure had serologic evidence (IgM antibodies to B19) of a recent infection.[123] In a case-control study of hospital transmission, serologic testing was used to determine the infection rates among personnel exposed to patients with sickle cell disease and transient aplastic crisis before the subjects being placed in isolation.[124] Only 1 of 32 susceptible exposed hospital workers acquired a B19 infection, compared with 3 of 37 susceptible workers not exposed. Results of this study suggested that hospital workers who cared for patients with aplastic crisis were not at an increased risk for B19 acquisition.

Two prospective studies from one institution determined the incidence of infection in health care workers during endemic (nonepidemic) periods. The first study found the annual seroconversion rate to be 1.4% for 124 susceptible female health care workers followed for an average of 1.7 years. In a subsequent study of 198 susceptible hospital employees, the annual rate was 0.4%, compared with 2.9% for school employees.[19]

Taken as a whole, the evidence indicates that B19 may be highly contagious in the hospital, although perhaps not in every circumstance. Many potential variables may affect rates of transmission from patients to staff, including the type of patient (immunocompromised or not), the duration of B19 infection at the time of hospitalization, and potentially, the viral load of the infected patient. Patients with erythrocyte aplasia or others with suspected EI or B19 infection should be presumed to have a B19 infection until proved otherwise. These patients should receive respiratory and contact isolation while hospitalized.

Routes of Viral Spread

Person-to-person spread of B19 probably occurs through contact with respiratory secretions. Viral DNA is present in saliva[50,108,124,125] at levels similar to those in blood, and in a volunteer study, infection was initiated by intranasal inoculation of B19.[50,126] B19 cannot be detected in columnar epithelial cells of the large airways.[127] Indirect evidence suggests B19 is not transmitted by aerosols. Viruses such as measles and influenza that are transmitted by aerosols are rapidly spread during outbreaks, but new cases of EI are spread out over many months during school outbreaks, suggesting that B19 transmission is inefficient. B19 DNA may be found in the urine, but it is unlikely that this is associated with infectious virus.

The only well-documented routes of spread for B19 are vertically from mother to fetus and from parenteral transfusion with contaminated blood products or needles. Vertical transmission is discussed later. Transmission of B19 by transfusion occurs but is rare because of the low prevalence of B19 viremia among donors of blood and blood products; however, the risk increases for pooled blood products.[128-131] For example, B19 DNA is frequently found in clotting factor concentrates, including products treated with solvents and detergents, steam, or monoclonal antibodies, and even treated products may be infectious.[91,129,131-134] Seroprevalence of IgG antibodies to B19 is high among hemophiliacs compared with age-matched controls and is higher for those who received frequent infusions of clotting factors prepared from large donor pools compared with those prepared from small donor pools.[130]

Parvoviruses are resistant to chemical inactivation. In one hospital, B19 transmission occurred without recognized direct patient contact, suggesting possible transmission by fomites or environmental contamination.[112] That B19 is transmitted by fomites has not been directly established, but considering the stability of related animal parvoviruses, this possibility exists. B19 DNA, not infectious virus, was found in a study of a suspected nosocomial outbreak in a maternity ward.[123] B19 DNA was detected by polymerase chain reaction (PCR) on the hands of the mother of a stillborn fetus infected with B19 and on the sink handles in her hospital room. Samples from countertops, an intravenous pump, and telephone were also positive by a sensitive nested-PCR DNA technique. PCR is so sensitive that minute quantities of DNA can be detected by this technique, and the presence of B19 DNA on surfaces does not imply that these surfaces are sources of infection. Infected fetal tissues and placental or amniotic fluids are more likely sources of infection for health care workers than fomites.

Risk of B19 Acquisition for Women of Childbearing Age

We completed a large epidemiologic study[19] to determine the relative risk of B19 acquisition for women of childbearing age in daily contact with children, including nurses, daycare employees, and teachers at all levels. We identified risk factors for B19 infections for hospital and school employees during an endemic period. We monitored by serologic testing 2730 employees of 135 schools in three school systems and 751 employees of a hospital, all in Richmond, Virginia. Sixty percent were initially seropositive. After adjusting for age, race, and gender, risk factors for seropositivity were contact with children 5 to 18 years old at home or at work and employment in elementary schools. Over 42 months, only 1 of 198 susceptible hospital employees seroconverted (0.42% annual rate), compared with 62 of 927 (2.93% annual rate) school employees (relative risk = 6.9). Four factors associated with seroconversion were employment at elementary schools, contact with children 5 to 11 years of age at home, contact at work with children 5 to 18 years old; and age younger than 30 years. Those in daily contact with school-aged children had a fivefold increased annual occupational risk for B19 infection.[19]

Several observations indicate that B19 infections were endemic but not epidemic or pandemic in the Richmond area during the 42-month prospective evaluation.[19] First, few cases of B19 infection were reported by the school nurses, and no cluster of cases was observed at any single school or group of schools. Second, the seroconversion rates during each of three consecutive study periods were the same for all groups or subgroups. Third, for employees, B19 infections were not clustered at individual schools or groups of schools. Fourth, the infection rates we observed among employees, even for those teaching elementary school, were less than those observed for the 1988 Connecticut epidemic, in which 46 infections occurred among 236 susceptible individuals exposed in the schools, for a minimum annual infection rate of 19%.[109] In a study of secondary B19 infections among exposed household members, rates ranged from 30% to 50%.[98]

Persons with B19 infections are often asymptomatic or have no rash, and low-level endemics can go unnoticed. We observed that 28 of 60 infected employees were asymptomatic and that only 20 knew of a specific exposure. In a study of 52 household contacts of patients with B19 infections during an Ohio epidemic, infections without a rash occurred in 15 (94%) of 16 blacks and 17 of 35 (47%) whites, and completely asymptomatic infections occurred in 11 (69%) of 16 blacks and 6 (20%) of 30 whites.[98] During the Connecticut outbreak, 5 (8%) of 65 teachers who were never exposed to a child with a rash became infected.[109] Observations of high secondary attack rates during epidemics and the high rates of rashless or asymptomatic infections provide strong evidence that even during periods when EI is inapparent in the community, school or hospital personnel in contact with children have a significant occupational risk for B19 infections.

Contact with elementary school–aged children, whether at home or at work, may be the most important risk factor for B19 acquisition. When seropositivity for those with children at home was stratified by the child's age, the association between seropositivity and children at home was significant ($P < .05$) when all children between 5 and 18 years old were included, and for seroconversion, the significant association was with elementary school–aged children at home.[19] The low seroprevalence and seroconversion rate among hospital employees without known contact with children indicates that this group has a low occupational risk for acquiring B19 infections.

The major conclusions from these studies were that when EI is inapparent in the community, school or hospital personnel in contact with children still have a significant occupational risk for B19 infections and that school employees have an approximately twofold greater risk of acquiring B19 from children at work than from elementary school–aged children at home. We also found that hospital employees without contact with children have a low risk for acquiring B19.

Using the Richmond data and assuming that on average 50% of pregnant women are immune, we estimate that 1% to 4% of susceptible women will become infected during pregnancy during endemic periods. If the rate of fetal death after maternal infection is as high as 5% to 10% (discussed later), the occupational risk of fetal death for a pregnant woman with unknown serologic status will be between 1 in 500 and 1 in 4000. These rates are so low that during endemic periods, they do not justify intervention such as serologic testing for pregnant women, furloughing workers, or temporary transfer of pregnant seronegative employees to administrative or other positions without child contact.

Knowing B19 infection rates during endemic periods may be more important than knowing rates during epidemic periods. In the United States, B19 infections are endemic most of the time. Because more than 75% of B19 infections are inapparent, most women who acquire B19 infection during pregnancy do so during endemic periods, not during epidemics. For establishing public health policy and assessing the potential importance of immunizing against B19, knowing that for seronegative women the endemic rate is between 1% and 4% is more important than knowing epidemic rates.

CLINICAL MANIFESTATIONS OTHER THAN INTRAUTERINE INFECTION

Erythema Infectiosum

The most common clinical manifestation of infection with parvovirus B19 is EI, or fifth disease, a well-known rash illness of children. EI begins with a mild prodromal illness consisting of low-grade fever, headache, malaise, and upper respiratory tract symptoms. This prodrome may be so mild as to go unnoticed. The hallmark of the illness is the characteristic exanthem. The rash usually occurs in three phases, but these are not always distinguishable.[10,102,135] The initial stage consists of an erythematous facial flushing described as a slapped-cheek appearance. In the second stage, the rash spreads quickly to the trunk and proximal extremities as a diffuse macular erythema. Central clearing of macular lesions occurs promptly, giving the rash a lacy, reticulated appearance. Palms and soles are usually spared, and the rash tends to be more prominent on the extensor surfaces. Affected children at this point are afebrile and feel well. Adolescents and adult patients often complain of pruritus or arthralgias concurrent with the rash. The rash resolves spontaneously, but it typically may recur over the course of 1 to 3 weeks in response to a variety of environmental stimuli such as sunlight, heat, exercise, and stress.[136]

Lymphadenopathy is not a consistent feature but has been reported in association with EI[97] and as sole manifestations of infection.[137-139] A mononucleosis-like illness associated with confirmed B19 infections has occasionally been reported, but B19 does not typically cause a mono-like illness. Atypical rashes not recognizable as classic EI have also been associated with acute B19 infections; these include morbilliform, vesiculopustular, desquamative, petechial, and purpuric rashes.[2]

Asymptomatic infection with B19 also occurs commonly in children and adults. In studies of large outbreaks, asymptomatic infection is reported in approximately 20% to 30% of serologically proven cases.[97,98]

Transient Aplastic Crisis

Transient aplastic crisis was the first clinical illness to be definitively linked to infection with B19. An infectious origin had been suspected for this condition because it usually occurred only once in a given patient, had a well-defined course and duration of illness, and tended to occur in clusters within families and communities.[136] Attempts to link it to infection with any particular agent had repeatedly failed until 1981, when Pattison and colleagues[6] reported six positive tests for B19 (seroconversion or antigenemia) among 600 admissions to a London hospital. All six were children with sickle cell anemia admitted with aplastic crisis. This association was confirmed by studies of an outbreak of aplastic crisis in the population with sickle cell disease in Jamaica.[7]

In contrast to EI, patients with a transient aplastic crisis are ill at presentation with fever, malaise, and signs and symptoms of profound anemia (e.g., pallor, tachypnea, tachycardia). These patients rarely have a rash.[100,140] The acute infection causes a transient arrest of erythropoiesis with a profound reticulocytopenia. Given the short half-life of these patients' red cells and their dependence on active erythropoiesis to counterbalance their increased red cell turnover, this leads to a sudden and potentially life-threatening decline in serum hemoglobin. Children with sickle hemoglobinopathies may also develop a concurrent vaso-occlusive pain crisis, which may further complicate the clinical picture.

Although such transient aplastic crises are most commonly associated with sickle cell anemia, any patient with a condition of increased red cell turnover and accelerated erythropoiesis can experience a similar transient red cell aplasia with B19 infection. B19-induced aplastic crises have been described in many hematologic disorders, including other hemoglobinopathies (e.g., thalassemia, sickle-C hemoglobin); red cell membrane defects (e.g., hereditary spherocytosis, stomatocytosis); enzyme deficiencies (e.g., pyruvate kinase deficiency, glucose-6-phosphate dehydrogenase deficiency); antibody-mediated red cell destruction (e.g., autoimmune hemolytic anemia); and decreased red cell production (e.g., iron deficiency, blood loss).[48,140] B19 is not a significant cause of transient erythroblastopenia of childhood, another condition of transient red cell hypoplasia that usually occurs in younger, hematologically normal children and follows a more indolent course.[47]

Leukopenia and thrombocytopenia may occur during a transient aplastic crisis, but the incidence varies with the underlying condition. In a French study of 24 episodes of aplastic crisis (mostly in individuals with hereditary spherocytosis), 35% to 40% of patients were leukopenic or thrombocytopenic, compared with 10% to 15% reported in a large U.S. study of mostly sickle cell patients.[100,141] These transient declines in leukocyte count or platelets follow a time course similar to that for reticulocytopenia, although they are not as severe and recovery occurs without clinical sequelae. The relative preservation of leukocyte and platelet counts in sickle cell anemia compared with other hereditary hemolytic anemias presumably is caused by the functional asplenia associated with sickle cell disease.[48]

As observed in experimental infection in human volunteers, B19 infection in normal subjects does result in a fall in the reticulocyte count, but because of the normal red cell half-life, this is not clinically significant or noticeable. Various degrees of leukopenia and thrombocytopenia also occur after natural B19 infection in hematologically normal patients.[50] Some cases of idiopathic thrombocytopenic purpura (ITP) and cases of childhood neutropenia have been reported in association with acute B19 infection.[142,143] Aside from these few anecdotal reports, larger studies have not confirmed B19 as a common cause of ITP or chronic neutropenia in children.[47]

Arthropathy

Joint symptoms are reported by up to 80% of adolescents and adults with B19 infection, whereas joint symptoms are uncommon in children.[10,102] Arthritis or arthralgia may occur in association with the symptoms of typical EI or be the only manifestation of infection. Females are more frequently affected with joint symptoms than males.[10,102]

The joint symptoms of B19 infection usually manifest as the sudden onset of a symmetric peripheral polyarthropathy.[144] The joints most often affected are the hands, wrists, knees, and ankles, but the larger joints can also be involved.[106,145] The joint symptoms have a wide range of severity, from mild morning stiffness to frank arthritis with the classic combination of erythema, warmth, tenderness, and swelling. Like the rash of EI, the arthropathy has been presumed to be immunologically mediated because the onset of joint symptoms occurs after the peak of viremia and coincides with the development of specific IgM and IgG antibodies.[50] Rheumatoid factor may also be transiently positive, leading to some diagnostic confusion with rheumatoid arthritis (RA) in adult patients.[146] Fortunately, there is no joint destruction, and in most patients, joint symptoms resolve within 2 to 4 weeks. For some patients, joint discomfort may last for months or, in rare individuals, for years. The role of B19 in these more chronic arthropathies is not clear.

The arthritis associated with B19 infection may persist long enough to satisfy clinical diagnostic criteria for RA or juvenile rheumatoid arthritis (JRA).[85,93,145,147,148] This has led some to suggest that B19 might be the etiologic agent of these conditions.[2] This speculation has been supported by the detection of B19 DNA in synovial tissue from patients with RA and reports of increased seropositivity among patients with these conditions.[94,149-151] Later findings of DNA from other viruses in addition to B19 in synovial tissue from patients with arthritis and the finding of B19 DNA in synovium from persons without arthritis suggest that this may be a nonspecific effect of inflammation.[152,153] A review of the accumulated evidence on this topic has concluded that B19 is unlikely to be a primary cause in these rheumatic diseases but may be one of several viral triggers capable of initiating joint disease in genetically predisposed individiuals.[154]

Infection in the Immunocompromised Host

Patients with impaired humoral immunity are at risk for developing chronic and recurrent infections with B19. Persistent anemia, sometimes profound, with reticulocytopenia is the most common manifestation of such infections, which may also be accompanied by neutropenia, thrombocytopenia, or compete marrow suppression. Chronic infections with B19 occur in children with cancer who receive cytotoxic chemotherapy,[155,156] children with congenital immunodeficiency states,[157] children and adults with acquired immunodeficiency syndrome (AIDS),[158] and transplant recipients,[159] and they may even occur in patients with more subtle defects in immunoglobulin production who are able to produce measurable antibodies to B19 but are unable to generate adequate neutralizing antibodies.[160]

B19 has also been linked to viral-associated hemophagocytic syndrome (VAHS),[155,161] more generally referred to as infection-associated hemophagocytic syndrome (IAHS). This condition of histiocytic infiltration of bone marrow and associated cytopenias usually occurs in immunocompromised patients. B19 is only one of several viruses that have been implicated as causing VAHS. IAHS is considered a nonspecific response to a variety of viral and bacterial insults rather than a specific manifestation of a single pathogen.

Infections in the immunocompromised host can lead to chronic infection. This is most often manifested as chronic anemia (i.e., red cell aplasia), but various degrees of cytopenia have been described, ranging from thrombocytopenia or neutropenia to complete bone marrow failure.[140] Patients with an inability to produce neutralizing antibodies are at greatest risk, and this complication of B19 infection has been described in children with congenital immunodeficiency syndromes, patients on cytoreductive chemotherapy, transplant recipients on immunosuppressive therapy, and adults and children with AIDS.[140]

Increased recognition of B19 infection in solid-organ transplant recipients led to several reports.[162-164] Although most such infections are manifested as the typical persistent anemia, an association of B19 viremia with acute graft rejection has been described.[165]

Other Dermatologic Syndromes

Vasculitis and Purpura

A variety of atypical skin eruptions has been associated with B19 infections. Most of these are petechial or purpuric in nature, often with evidence of vasculitis in those that report skin biopsy results, and the eruptions may resemble the rash of other connective tissue diseases.[2,166] There are reports of confirmed acute B19 infections associated with non-thrombocytopenic purpura and vasculitis, including several cases clinically diagnosed as Henoch-Schönlein purpura,[86,167] an acute leukocytoclastic vasculitis of unknown origin in children. Chronic B19 infection has also been associated with necrotizing vasculitis, including cases of polyarteritis nodosa and Wegener's granulomatosis.[168] These patients had no underlying hematologic disorder and were generally not anemic at diagnosis. The pathogenesis is unknown, but these details may suggest an endothelial cell infection, as occurs with some other viruses such as rubella.

Information from biopsy of rashes temporally associated with B19 infection is limited, although several reports have appeared. B19 capsid antigens and DNA were found in a skin biopsy from a patient with EI, and this observation lends support to a role for B19 in these vascular disorders.[169] Rashes resembling those of systemic lupus erythematosus, Henoch-Schönlein purpura, and other connective tissue disorders have been described.[166,170] In a controlled study of 27 children with Henoch-Schönlein purpura, B19 was not a common cause.[171] Only 3 of 27 children had detectable B19 IgM antibodies indicating a recent infection. The role of B19 in these conditions remains speculative.

Papular-Purpuric "Gloves and Socks" Syndrome

Papular-purpuric "gloves and socks" syndrome (PPGSS) is a distinctive, self-limited dermatosis first described in the dermatologic literature in 1990.[172] The syndrome is characterized by fever, pruritus, and painful edema and erythema localized to the distal extremities in a distinct glove and sock distribution. The distal erythema is usually followed by petechiae, and oral lesions often develop. Resolution of all symptoms usually occurs in 1 to 2 weeks. A search for serologic evidence of viral infection led to the discovery of an association with acute B19 infection in many of these patients, based on demonstration of specific IgM or seroconversion. This association has been further confirmed with subsequent reports and demonstration of B19 DNA in skin biopsy samples and sera from these patients.[172,173] Initially described in adults, a number of children with this condition were subsequently described.[174] There appears to be sufficient evidence to suggest that PPGSS is a rare but distinctive manifestation of primary, acute infection with parvovirus B19, occurring mainly in young adults but also affecting children.

Central Nervous System Infection and Neurologic Disorders

Although a variety of neurologic symptoms and disorders have been described in patients clinically diagnosed as having EI or laboratory-confirmed B19 infection,[2] the issue of whether B19 causes central nervous system (CNS) infection or is etiologic for other neurologic conditions remains unresolved. Cases of meningitis,[175,176] encephalitis,[177] and encephalopathy[178] caused by B19 infection have been reported. Many of these cases were determined during outbreaks of EI from older reports based on clinical diagnosis only, before reliable laboratory tests for B19 were available. In one study, headache was reported in as many as 32% of children with rash illness.[175] However, there are no controlled comparative studies to evaluate the frequency of signs or symptoms suggestive of meningeal inflammation or CNS infection in B19 infection. Cerebrospinal fluid (CSF) abnormalities such as pleocytosis and increased levels of CSF protein have been reported in some patients with meningismus or altered level of consciousness associated with EI.[2] B19 DNA has been detected in CSF using PCR in several cases of serologically confirmed acute B19 infection with meningoencephalitis or encephalopathy.[179-181] However, most of these reported patients were also viremic at the time, and the possibility that the CSF PCR was positive because of contamination from blood could not be completely excluded.

Disorders of the peripheral nervous system have included brachial plexus neuropathy,[182] extremity paresthesias and dysesthesias,[183] myasthenia-like weakness,[184] and carpal tunnel syndrome.[185] The onset of most of these peripheral nerve symptoms has been coincident with the onset of rash and or joint pain at a time when the patient should have a brisk immune response, suggesting that the neurologic abnormalities could be immunologically mediated.[2] In the course of one well-described outbreak of EI among intensive care nurses, numbness and tingling of the fingers were reported by 54% of the 13 B19-infected nurses.[183] The neurologic symptoms persisted for more than 1 year in three of the nurses, and one had low levels of B19 DNA in serum for more than 3 years in association with recurrent episodes of paresthesias. She was never anemic and had no demonstrable immunodeficiency.[186] Although these cases are suggestive, the role of B19 in neurologic disease and CNS infection will remain unresolved until the pathogenesis of the viral infection in these conditions can be elucidated.[3,187]

Renal Disease

Reports of renal disease after B19 infection, previously rare, have increased within the past few years.[188-190] Most have been case reports of glomerulonephritis or focal glomerulosclerosis temporally related to an acute B19 infection. Immune complex deposition has been demonstrated in renal tissue, and B19 DNA occasionally can be found in renal tissue by PCR.[191] Renal failure is rarely reported. The virus is not known to infect kidney cells in vitro, and its presence in renal tissue may reflect filtration of the viremia of acute infection. B19 DNA has been detected in urine in studies of infants with evidence of intrauterine infections. B19 antigens may trigger an immune complex–mediated nephritis, but this may be a nonspecific effect, and further study is necessary to define the relationship between B19 infection and the potential for renal disease.

DIAGNOSIS: GENERAL APPROACH AND LABORATORY METHODS

The diagnosis of EI is usually based on the clinical recognition of the typical exanthem, a benign course, and exclusion of similar conditions. Rarely is laboratory confirmation necessary. A presumptive diagnosis of a B19-induced transient aplastic crisis in a patient with known sickle cell disease (or other condition associated with chronic hemolysis) is based on an acute febrile illness, a sudden and severe decline in the serum hemoglobin level, and an absolute reticulocytopenia. Likewise, a clinical diagnosis of PPGSS can be based on the characteristic skin eruption in the distinct acral distribution.

Specific laboratory diagnosis depends on identification of B19 antibodies, viral antigens, or viral DNA. In the immunologically normal patient, determination of anti-B19 IgM is the best marker of recent or acute infection on a single serum sample. IgM antibodies develop rapidly after infection and are detectable for as long as 6 to 8 weeks.[192] Specific IgG antibodies become detectable a few days after IgM and persist for years and probably for life. Seroconversion from an IgG-negative to IgG-positive status on paired sera confirms a recent infection. Anti-B19 IgG, however, primarily serves as a marker of past infection or immunity. Patients with EI or acute B19 arthropathy are usually IgM positive, and a diagnosis usually can be made from a single serum sample. Patients with B19-induced aplastic crisis may present before antibodies are detectable; however, IgM will be detectable within 1 to 2 days of presentation, and IgG will follow within days.[100]

The availability of serologic assays for B19 had previously been limited by the lack of a reliable and renewable source of antigen for diagnostic studies. The development of recombinant cell lines that express B19 capsid proteins have provided more reliable sources of antigen suitable for use in commercial test kits.[193,194] Several commercial kits are available for detection of B19 antibodies, but they employ a variety of different antigens (e.g., recombinant capsid proteins, fusion proteins, synthetic peptides), and their performance in large studies has varied.[193] Based on studies of the humoral immune response to the various B19 viral antigens, it appears to be important to have serologic assays based on intact capsids that provide conformational epitopes. Antibody responses to these antigens are more reliable and longer lasting than are responses to the linear epitopes used in some assays.[195] Only one commercial assay based on such capsids has received Food and Drug Administration approval in the United States[196]; other commercial assays for this purpose are considered research tests. Until serologic tests are more standardized and results more consistent, some knowledge of the assay and antigens used will be necessary for proper interpretation of B19 antibody test results.

In immunocompromised or immunodeficient patients, serologic diagnosis is unreliable because humoral responses are impaired, and methods to detect viral particles or viral DNA are necessary to make the diagnosis of a B19 infection. Because the virus cannot be isolated on routine cell cultures, viral culture is not useful. Detection of viral DNA by DNA hybridization techniques[197] or by PCR[198,199] is useful in these patients. Both techniques can be applied to a variety of clinical specimens, including serum, amniotic fluid, fresh tissues, bone marrow, and paraffin-embedded tissues.[144]

Histologic examination is also helpful in diagnosing B19 infection in certain situations. Examination of bone marrow aspirates in anemic patients typically reveals giant pronormoblasts or "lantern cells" against a background of general erythroid hypoplasia. However, the absence of such cells does not exclude B19 infection.[200,201] Electron microscopy has proved useful and may reveal viral particles in serum of some infected patients and cord blood or tissues of hydropic infants (discussed later).

EPIDEMIOLOGY OF B19 INFECTIONS AND RISK OF ACQUISITION IN THE PREGNANT WOMAN

Prevalence and Incidence in the United States

We have completed three studies[19] using complementary strategies to determine the incidence of human parvovirus B19 infection during pregnancy. First, using the data from a study of school personnel, we estimated the average B19 infection rate among pregnant school personnel. Of the 60 individuals who seroconverted during that study, 8 (13%) were pregnant. However, not all pregnant women in the school system participated in the study. Although we had data on the pregnancy rates for the female school personnel who participated, these volunteers may have been biased toward younger females, raising the possibility that their pregnancy rates may not have been representative of all school employees. Of approximately 11,637 total school employees in Richmond, Virginia, we enrolled 2730 (24%) in our study. To determine whether the sample enrolled was representative, we performed a random survey of 733 school employees at the schools studied. The results provided strong evidence that the seroprevalence and annual infection rates observed among study subjects were representative and applicable to the entire school employee population.[19] Assuming no seasonality to B19 infections (none was observed) and that pregnancy does not affect susceptibility, we predicted that without regard to risk factors, seronegative pregnant personnel have an average annual infection rate of 3%, for a rate of 2.25% per pregnancy.[19]

Second, in Richmond from 1989 to 1991, we collected sera from 1650 pregnant women from a lower socioeconomic group who attended a high-risk pregnancy clinic for patients without medical insurance. This group was 80% African American, with an average maternal age of 24 years. We randomly selected a subset of 395 women for serotesting and monitoring, 35% of whom were seropositive. Of the 256 seronegative women, 2 (0.8%) seroconverted, for an annual rate of 1.7%. This rate was similar to the rate observed among low-risk and African American school personnel in Richmond.[19]

We also obtained serial sera from a large number of private practice obstetric patients from Birmingham, Alabama.[202] From this serum bank, we randomly selected 200 patients per year over 4 years (1987 to 1990). No significant differences were observed by year among the 800 patients (average age was 27 years and 88% were white), and 46% were seropositive overall. Of 413 seronegative women serially tested over the 4 years, 5 seroconverted. Overall, the annual seroconversion rate was 2%. Combining data from the studies of pregnant women done in Richmond and Birmingham, we observed that 7 of 669 seronegative women seroconverted during pregnancy, for a rate of 1% per pregnancy (95% CI, 0.3% to 21%).

Prevalence and Incidence in Other Countries

In numerous studies conducted worldwide, for pregnant women and women of reproductive age, the seroprevalence of IgG antibodies to B19 has varied from 16% to 72%, with most estimates falling between 35% and 55%.[69,74,75,124] In Denmark, a serologic survey of 31,000 pregnant Danish women found 65% had evidence of past infection[101]; the seroprevalence of IgG antibody among 1610 pregnant women in Barcelona was 35.03%[203]; 81% of pregnant Swedish women had parvovirus antibodies;[20,204] and in Japan, the seroprevalence of IgG antibodies to B19 was 26% for women between the ages of 21 and 30, and 44% for women between the ages of 31 and 40.[74] The prevalence of IgG antibodies to B19 in cord blood from normal newborns provides estimates of maternal immunity ranging from 50% to 75%.[17,205,206]

Without regard to maternal age or other potential risk factors, a South African study found that 64 (3.3%) of 1967 pregnant women acquired B19 infection during pregnancy, and another in Barcelona found that 60 (3.7%) of 1610 pregnant women became infected with B19 during pregnancy.[20,203] Seroconversion rates among susceptible pregnant Danish women during endemic and epidemic periods were 1.5% and 13%, respectively. In Denmark, risk of infection increased with the number of children in the household and having children 6 to 7 years old resulted in the highest rate of seroconversion, and nursery school teachers had a threefold increased risk of acute infection.[101] Extrapolating to a 40-week period places the infection rate during pregnancy among susceptible women at approximately 1.1%, with a range of 1% to 4%, depending on risk factors. The Danish and Barcelona data are similar to those obtained in Richmond, Virginia.[19]

A few studies have tried to estimate the infection rate based on the prevalence of IgM antibodies to B19 in pregnancy or in women of reproductive age. Although B19-specific IgM is an accurate diagnostic test for recent infection, it is a poor test for epidemiologic studies. B19-specific IgM persists for only a few months and therefore underestimates the maternal infection rate because women who have had a B19 infection 6 to 9 months before testing are not detected. Another problem with IgM surveys is that most studies have surveyed high-risk populations such as women with rash illness, possible exposure to cases of EI, or recent diagnosis of adverse reproductive outcomes. Sampling high-risk populations biases the results toward rates higher than would be observed in population-based studies. A few studies used B19-specific IgM to test pregnant women or women of reproductive age who did not have risk factors. The observed range in these studies was 0% to 2.6%.[17,205,207] For susceptible women with B19-specific IgM in populations known to be at increased risk, the prevalence of IgM has ranged from 0% to 12.5%.[17,74,124,208,209]

In countries other than the United States, the prevalence of IgG antibodies to B19 among pregnant women and women of reproductive age varies widely and probably reflects exposure during prior epidemics. Studies of infections during pregnancy are fraught with potentially confounding variables such as IgM testing, which lacks sensitivity, and biases introduced by selection criteria for the population studied. Despite these problems, it is likely that the risk for B19 infection during pregnancy in other countries is similar to the risk observed in the United States.

CLINICAL MANIFESTATIONS OF B19 INFECTIONS IN THE PREGNANT WOMAN

The symptoms reported by pregnant women with a proven recent B19 infection are usually vague and nonspecific, and serologic confirmation is essential to establish the diagnosis. The signs and symptoms of classic EI in children are significantly different in adults; the sunburned or slapped-cheek facial rash common in children rarely occurs in adults. Malaise is a common feature of B19 infection in children and in adults, but it is nonspecific. In pregnant women and adolescents, the most characteristic symptom is symmetrical arthralgias, occasionally with signs of arthritis and usually involving the small (distal) joints of hands, wrists, and feet.

The proportion of pregnant women with serologically proven B19 infection who are asymptomatic varies with the inclusion criteria in the few studies that address symptoms. In a cohort of 1610 pregnant women studied in Barcelona, the sera of 30 women had IgM antibodies to B19 at the first prenatal visit, and another 30 seroconverted during pregnancy.[20] Of these 60 women, only 18 (30%) reported any combination of fever, rash, and arthralgias, and 70% were asymptomatic. The investigators did not report when questions about symptoms were asked in relation to the serologic results, and no comment was made about the distribution of symptoms nor about which joints were affected by the arthralgias.[20] Similarly, during an epidemic of EI in Connecticut, fully 69% of nonpregnant adults with serologically proven B19 infection were asymptomatic. In this study, symptoms were assessed by mailed questionnaires after the women were provided their serologic results.[109,123] In a British multicenter study, only 6 (3%) of 184 patients were asymptomatic, but the population was ascertained largely by recruiting women with typical symptoms, and this study therefore is not comparable to the others.[18]

We studied 618 pregnant women in Pittsburgh with known exposure to someone with a rash illness highly suggestive of EI.[210] Each exposed patient was questioned about symptoms before serologic testing. Only 33% of the 52 women with serologically proven B19 infection reported no symptoms, and the remaining 67% reported rash, fever, arthralgias, coryza, or malaise, or some combination of these symptoms.[210] Malaise, although a very vague and nonspecific finding, was reported by 27 (52%) of the 52 infected women.[210] In contrast, only 5.5% of 307 exposed but not susceptible (IgG-seropositive and IgM-seronegative) women reported this symptom. After malaise, symmetrical arthralgias were the second most common symptom reported. Of the 618 known exposures in pregnant women, 24 (46%) of the 52 infected pregnant women reported arthralgias, compared with 11 (3.6%) of 307 immune women and 12 (4.6%) of 259 susceptible but uninfected women ($P < .0001$).[210] Of the 24 women with arthralgias in this study, 23 also reported malaise, 16 had rash, 7 had coryza, and 7 had fever. Among the 24 IgM-positive women with arthralgias, the symmetrical joints most commonly affected by pain, swelling, and erythema were the knees (75%), followed by wrists (71%), fingers (63%), ankles (42%), feet (29%), elbows (29%), shoulders (17%), hips (13%), and back and neck (8%). Only 2 of the 24 had only one set of joints involved, and very few other women reported monarticular pain or swelling. In most women, the arthralgias were easily controlled by anti-inflammatory drugs and lasted only 1 to 5 days. However, arthralgias occasionally lasted 10 to 14 days and, in some women, were so painful that they were incapacitated for 2 to 3 days.

The high frequency of arthralgia in pregnant women with B19 infection is consistent with reports that distal arthralgias and arthritis are the most frequent finding in adults with EI. The frequency of arthralgias among nonpregnant adults with proven B19 infection in the Torrington, Connecticut, epidemic was 24% (11 of 46 adults), compared with 12% (61 of 512 adults) in adults without B19 infection ($P < .05$).[109] In another Connecticut study, arthralgias occurred significantly more often (26%) in 19 adults with IgM antibodies to B19 than in 460 adults (7%) who lacked IgM antibodies to B19

($P < .01$).[123] Arthralgias were even more common during outbreaks in Ireland; they occurred in 79% of 47 recently infected women and men. Ninety-three percent of those with arthralgias reported that their knees were involved.[211]

Rash is less frequent in pregnant women than in children with EI, and the rash in pregnant women is not characteristic. In one report of the Connecticut epidemic, rashes occurred in 6 (13%) of 46 infected adults, compared with 49 (10%) of 512 individuals who were uninfected. In another report, rashes occurred in 3 (16%) of 19 infected adults, compared with 33 (7%) of 460 uninfected individuals. This difference is not significant ($P = .16$) and may represent random variation.[109] In contrast to the classic curtain lace rash in children, pregnant women (80%) often have a maculopapular rash that rarely involves the face and may even be urticarial or morbilliform. In adults, these rashes are rarely pruritic and usually resolve within 1 to 5 days.

In the Pittsburgh series, coryza was reported by 23% of the 52 B19-infected pregnant women but was reported in only 6.8% of the 307 previously infected women and 5.8% of the 259 seronegative women.[210] This difference was significant ($P < .0001$), but the nonspecific nature of coryza in pregnant women means this symptom alone is not diagnostically helpful.

In the Pittsburgh series, a temperature of 38.0° C or higher occurred in 19% of the 52 IgM B19-infected women, compared ($P < .0001$) with 2.6% of 307 previously infected patients and 3.1% of 259 susceptible, noninfected patients.[210] In 9 of 10 women with fever, at least one other symptom was present. No woman's temperature exceeded 38.9° C. In 16 uninfected women with fever, all had at least one other symptom, and they had temperatures up to 40.0° C, suggesting that a temperature of more than 39.0° C in a pregnant woman indicates infections other than B19. In a London outbreak of B19 infection, 7 of 10 infected adults had a an elevated temperature.[113] In the Connecticut epidemic, fever was reported in 15% of the 46 infected individuals and in 16% of the 512 uninfected individuals.[109] Pregnant women with fever are likely to seek medical attention.

Occasionally, pregnant women infected with B19 develop rapidly increasing fundal height, preterm labor, or even preeclampsia. Such symptoms are nonspecific and rarely indicate B19 infection.

INTRAUTERINE TRANSMISSION RATES, CLINICAL MANIFESTATIONS, AND FETAL OUTCOMES

Primary maternal infection with B19 during gestation has been associated with adverse outcomes such as nonimmune hydrops fetalis, intrauterine fetal death, asymptomatic neonatal infection, and normal delivery at term.[14,15] Initial reports of fetal hydrops related to maternal B19 infection were anecdotal and retrospective, suggesting rates of adverse outcomes as high as 26% and generating concern that B19 may be more fetotropic than rubella or cytomegalovirus.[212,213] Subsequent reports of normal births after documented maternal B19 infection made clear the need for better estimates of the rate of intrauterine transmission and the risk of adverse outcomes.[214,215]

Fetal Death

B19 was first linked to fetal death in 1984.[15] As anticipated based on the epidemiology of B19 transmission, the percentage of fetal deaths attributable to B19 varies, probably depending on the frequency of B19 infections in the population being studied.

Prospective studies report rates of intrauterine viral transmission ranging from 25% to 50%.[18,216,217] Initial studies indicated that the risk of an adverse fetal outcome after a recent maternal infection was less than 10% (probably much less) and greatest in the first 20 weeks of pregnancy.[144] A large, prospective study in the United Kingdom identified 186 pregnant women with confirmed B19 infections during an epidemic and followed them to term.[18] There were 30 (16%) fetal deaths, with as many as 17 (9%) estimated to be caused by B19 on the basis of DNA studies of a sample of the abortuses. Most of the fetal deaths occurred in the first 20 weeks, with an excess fetal loss occurring in the second trimester.[18] The intrauterine transmission rate was estimated at 33% based on analysis of the abortuses, fetal IgM in cord blood, and persistence of B19 IgG at a 1-year follow-up assessment of the infants. A smaller study of 39 pregnancies complicated by maternal B19 infection and followed to term found two fetal deaths (fetal loss rate of 5%), one (3%) of which was attributable to B19 and occurred at 10 weeks' gestation.[216] A prospective study conducted by the Centers for Disease Control and Prevention identified 187 pregnant women with B19 infection and compared their outcomes to 753 matched controls.[217] The overall fetal loss rate in the infected group was 5.9%, with 10 of 11 occurring before the 18th week of gestation, compared with a 3.5% fetal loss rate in the control group, suggesting a fetal loss rate of 2.5% attributable to B19 infection. In a prospective Spanish study during an endemic period, 1610 pregnant women were screened for B19 infection, and 60 (3.7%) were identified.[20] There were five abortions among this group, but only one (1.7%) was caused by B19 based on histologic and virologic analysis of fetal samples. The incidence of vertical transmission was estimated at 25% based on serologic evaluation of the infants at delivery and at 1 year of age. In a similar prospective study of an obstetric population, 1967 pregnant women were screened, and 64 (3.3%) identified as recently infected.[203] Among this group, no adverse effects were seen by serial ultrasound examinations, and no case of fetal hydrops was identified; one abortion occurred, but the fetus was not examined for evidence of B19 infection (maximal fetal loss attributable = 1.6%).

In a case-control study of 192 women with fetal deaths, with one half occurring before 20 weeks' gestation and one half after, there was serologic evidence of acute B19 infection in 1% of both case and control groups.[17] The prevalence of IgG antibodies was similar. In this study, the percentage of fetal deaths attributed to B19 infection was unlikely to exceed 3% in cases not selected for parvovirus exposure.

In another study, 5 (6.3%) of 80 women with spontaneous abortions between 4 and 17 weeks' gestation had IgM antibodies to B19 compared with 2 (2%) of 100 controls, but this difference was not statistically significant.[209] These investigators studied the aborted fetuses of the five seropositive cases and found B19 DNA in only two.

In a prospective study of 39 pregnant women infected with B19 during a community-wide outbreak in Connecticut, there were two fetal deaths, and only one (3%) was attributable to B19 infection.[216] Among women followed prospectively and who acquired B19 infection during pregnancy, there was no evidence of fetal damage in 43 in Virginia and 52 in Pittsburgh, and one fetal loss among 56 pregnancies in women from Barcelona.[20,21,210]

Two Chinese studies found fetal B19 infection frequently associated with fetal death.[218,219] The first study in China found that of 116 spontaneously aborted fetuses tested for B19 DNA, 27.3% were positive for parvovirus B19, but only 4% (1 of 25) of nonaborted fetal tissues in the control group tested positive.[218] This difference was significant. It was unknown when these samples were collected whether B19 was endemic or epidemic in the community.

Similarly a second Chinese study examined 175 biopsy tissues from spontaneous abortions from 1994 to 1995 and found that 25% were positive for B19 DNA in the fetal tissues.[219] A control group of 40 fetal tissues came from induced abortions, and only 2 (5%) were positive. This difference was not statistically significant but did support the observation that in China, B19 may be an important cause of fetal death, especially if B19 is epidemic in the community.

In contrast to the Chinese studies, a study from the Netherlands of fetal and placenta tissue from 273 cases of first and second trimester fetal loss were tested for serologic or virologic evidence of B19 infection.[220] Of the 273 cases, 149 were from seronegative women, and the fetal deaths for these women were considered unrelated to B19 infection. In only two of the remaining 124 cases (0.7% of all 273 cases) did the mothers have IgM antibodies to B19 at the time of abortion. This study indicates that B19 infection was a rare cause of fetal loss during the first and second trimesters. No congenital anomalies were observed among the fetal tissues examined.

A study of 1047 pregnant women in Kuwait obtained maternal blood samples in the first, second, and third trimesters and tested them for serologic evidence of the recent B19 infection.[221] Forty-seven percent of the mothers were seronegative, and among these, the incidence of seroconversion was 16.5%. Among the women who seroconverted to a B19-positive status, the rate of fetal loss was 5.4%. All the fetal deaths occurred in the first two trimesters, suggesting that fetal death after maternal B19 infection is common, particularly during the first and second trimesters.

A report from Toledo, Ohio, describes five unexpected fetal deaths that occurred in the second trimester.[222] Only one of the fetuses was hydropic, but all five had viral inclusions in the liver, and all five women were seropositive for B19.

Third trimester fetal deaths have also been reported. A Swedish study of fetal deaths among 33,759 pregnancies found 93 cases of third-trimester fetal deaths, and of these, 7 (7.5%) had detectable B19 DNA in frozen placental tissue.[223] None of the seven fetuses was hydropic. The investigators suggested B19 occasionally caused third-, second-, and first-trimester fetal death.

A study of 13 pregnant women who acquired B19 infection during pregnancy and in whom the time of acquisition was known was completed in Japan.[224] Nonimmune hydrops occurred in three fetuses whose mothers acquired B19 infection in the first half of pregnancy. Spontaneous abortion without hydrops and intrauterine growth retardation occurred in two fetuses whose mothers also developed B19 infection during the first half of pregnancy. The remaining eight fetuses, whose mothers acquired infection in the first or second half of pregnancy, were asymptomatic, although human parvovirus B19 DNA was detected in the immune serum of all of the infants. These results suggest that B19 transmission to the fetus is common and that death may occur in almost one half of the fetuses of infected mothers.

A Swedish study of 92 pregnancies for which there was an unexpected fetal death occurring after 22 weeks' gestation found B19 DNA in 13 (14%) of the 92 fetuses.[225] Only 2 of the 13 were hydropic. The Swedish study suggests that B19 can infect the fetus in the third trimester and result in fetal death or hydrops, or both. This observation was confirmed in a larger study from Sweden, in which 47 cases of fetal deaths occurring after 22 weeks' gestation were identified and compared with 53 normal pregnancies.[226] Seven of the 43 intrauterine fetal deaths were positive for parvovirus B19 DNA, whereas B19 DNA was not detected in any of the normal pregnancies.

In summary, B19 is a likely cause of first-, second-, and third-trimester fetal death, and most infected infants are not hydropic. The estimates of fetal deaths attributable to B19 range from 0% to 27%, making it difficult to assess the precise increase in fetal mortality attributable to B19.

Asymptomatic Fetal Infection

Although the published prospective studies of B19 infection in pregnancy have varied in their estimates of adverse fetal outcome and rates of vertical transmission, it is clear that most women infected during pregnancy deliver normal-appearing infants at term. Some of these infants have asymptomatic infections.[227] Results of a prospective study that combined serologic with virologic markers of infection suggest that the rate of intrauterine transmission is very high.[21] In this study, 43 pregnant women with a confirmed B19 infection were followed to delivery. The infants were tested at birth and at intervals throughout the first year of life for IgM and IgG to B19 and by PCR for viral DNA in serum, urine, or saliva. No fetal losses or cases of fetal hydrops were observed in this study, although the rate of intrauterine viral transmission was 51%.[21]

Birth Defects

There is circumstantial evidence that intrauterine B19 infection may occasionally cause birth defects. The first case was reported in 1987.[228] A fetus aborted at 11 weeks' gestation was described with striking ocular abnormalities, including microphthalmia, aphakia, and dysplastic changes of the cornea, sclera, and choroid of one eye and retinal folds and degeneration of the lens in the other eye.[229,230] The mother had a history of a rash illness with arthropathy at 6 weeks that was serologically confirmed.

There have been few additional reports of malformations or developmental abnormalities in aborted fetuses or live-born infants after intrauterine infection, and most of these cases could not be unequivocally attributed to infection with B19.[231-238] However, three live-born infants had severe CNS abnormalities after serologically confirmed maternal B19 infection.[239,240] Subsequent case reports have also identified

CNS manifestations, including mild to moderate hydrocephalus with CNS scarring associated with fetal B19 infection.[241] These reports suggest possible long-term neurologic sequelae in surviving infants that may not be apparent at birth.

There are no other data suggesting that B19 is an important cause of birth defects in live-born infants. In an uncontrolled study of 243 infants younger than 4 months with birth defects, none had IgM antibodies to B19 detected.[205] In a controlled study of 57 infants with structural abnormalities or stigmata of congenital infection, specific IgM was not detected in cord blood of any of the affected infants or of the matched normal newborn controls.[17] There are no data suggesting that structural defects are common in newborns after maternal B19 infection. During a large community-wide outbreak of EI, there was no increase in congenital malformations compared with the periods before and after the epidemic.[242] In the British study of maternal infections during pregnancy, outcomes were available for 186 patients; anencephaly was reported in 1 of the 30 fatal cases but not attributed to B19 infection, and hypospadias was present in 2 of the 156 live-born infants.[18] No new anomalies or serious neurodevelopmental problems were detected in the 114 infants followed clinically for at least 1 year.[242] In another prospective, but uncontrolled study of 39 pregnancies with maternal B19 infection, hypospadias was reported in 1 of the 37 live-born infants, and no abnormalities were reported in the one fatal case for which tissues were available.[216]

Meconium Ileus and Peritonitis

Meconium ileus and peritonitis have been associated with maternal B19 infection in a few reports.[140,236] Three infants with congenital anemia after maternal infection and intrauterine hydrops have been reported.[14] All three had abnormalities identified on bone marrow examination and B19 DNA detected in bone marrow by PCR.

Fetal Hydrops

Although parvovirus B19 infection in utero may cause nonimmune hydrops fetalis, it is one of many causes of this syndrome and probably accounts for only 10% to 15% of fetal hydrops cases.[140] Hydrops fetalis is rare, occurring in only 1 of 3000 births; and in 50% of cases, the cause is unknown. In a study of 50 fetuses, B19 DNA was detected by in situ hybridization in the tissues of 4 fetuses, but most cases were caused by chromosomal or cardiovascular abnormalities.[243] In another study, B19 DNA was demonstrated in 4 of 42 cases of nonimmune hydrops fetalis.[244]

However, B19 infection is frequently associated with nonimmune fetal hydrops during local epidemics of EI. Ten cases of B19-associated hydrops, representing 8% of all cases of nonimmune hydrops and 27% of anatomically normal cases of nonimmune hydrops, occurred over 17 years in a hospital series from England.[232] In a consecutive series of 72 patients with nonimmune hydrops from Germany, 3 (4.2%) had B19 infection.[245] In a series of 673 fetal and neonatal autopsies conducted over 6 years in Rhode Island, 32 (0.7%) cases of hydrops were identified, and 5 (16%) of these had histologic and laboratory evidence of B19 infection.[246,247] In the British study, 1 of the 156 live-born infants had been diagnosed with intrauterine hydrops and recovered after intrauterine transfusion; and of the six fatal cases that were positive for B19 DNA, hydrops was identified in one of three fatal cases with laboratory confirmed intrauterine infection.[18,248] Postmortem examination may not be able to identify hydrops in fetal death occurring in early pregnancy. In summary, published reports suggest that nonimmune hydrops is not a common manifestation of fetal infection with B19.

Fetal Outcome in Relation to Maternal Manifestations

There are no data suggesting that the clinical manifestations of B19 infection in the mother influences the pregnancy outcome. There is evidence for an association between the B19-affected fetus and maternal hypertension. Pregnancy-induced hypertension, preeclampsia, and eclampsia have been reported for some women with B19-associated fetal hydrops, and there is a record of improvement with spontaneous resolution of hydrops in one case.[16,232,245,260-262] Hypertension of pregnancy may be caused by poor fetoplacental perfusion, and there is an increased risk in pregnancies complicated by hydrops. It is unknown whether there is an increased frequency of hypertensive disorders among B19-infected women compared with uninfected women or whether more careful monitoring of B19-infected women to detect findings of preeclampsia would be useful in identifying women at increased risk of B19-associated fetal hydrops. Long-term outcomes of live-born infants infected in utero with B19 are discussed in the "Prognosis" section of this chapter.

PATHOGENESIS OF INFECTION IN THE FETUS

Fetal Immune Responses to B19

When serologic and virologic markers of infection have been examined, fetal immune responses to B19 are variable.[21,144,252] B19-specific IgM in cord blood is a recognized marker of fetal infection, but sensitivity can be increased by adding other markers such as IgA, PCR positivity, and persistence of B19 IgG at 1 year of age.[21,144,252] Infants exposed to B19 earlier in gestation may be less likely to demonstrate a positive IgM response because of immaturity of the fetal immune system, whereas the IgM response of infants exposed late in gestation may be delayed because of interference by passively acquired maternal antibodies. In one study, only two of nine infected infants whose exposure occurred in the first 14 weeks of pregnancy were B19 IgM-positive at delivery, whereas all four infected infants exposed in the third trimester had B19-specific IgM in cord blood.[21] Serum IgA, like IgM, does not cross the placenta, and for some other congenital viral infections, such as rubella and human immunodeficiency virus (HIV), virus-specific IgA responses in cord blood has been used to provide evidence of intrauterine infection.[253] In the only study of B19 that examined this marker, B19 IgA in cord blood was associated with maternal infection with B19, and for a few infants, this was the only marker of intrauterine infection.[21]

The fetal immune response to B19 may be important for preventing B19-induced red cell aplasia in the fetus. This effect is suggested by the apparently decreased rates of fetal death after 20 weeks' gestation in concert with the detection of IgM specific to B19 as early as 18 weeks' gestation [254] and the neutralization of B19 virus in vitro by fetal serum collected at 21 weeks' gestation.[255]

Pathogenesis of B19 Hydrops

Nonimmune hydrops is the best-characterized complication of fetal B19 infection. Several mechanisms have been proposed, and more than one may contribute.[232] Severe fetal anemia affects most cases. Hemoglobin levels below 2 g/dL are detected by cordocentesis of hydropic fetuses.[257,258] Hypoxic injury to tissues may result in increased capillary permeability. Severe anemia may also increase cardiac output, as evidenced by increases in umbilical venous pressure, and subsequently result in high-output heart failure.[259] Alternatively, myocarditis may precipitate heart failure. Reduced fetal myocardial function as determined by echocardiography occurs in some cases of fetal hydrops.[249] Regardless of the cause, congestive heart failure can increase capillary hydrostatic pressure. Decreased venous return caused by massive ascites or organomegaly may lead to further cardiac decompensation. Hepatic function may be compromised by the extreme levels of extramedullary hematopoiesis, and lysis of B19-infected erythrocytes in the liver may cause hemosiderin deposition, fibrosis, and esophageal varices.[250,251] Impaired production of albumin may lead to a decrease in colloid osmotic pressure with transfer of fluid to the extravascular compartment. Placental hydrops may further compromise oxygen delivery to the fetus.

Considerable evidence demonstrates that non–red cells may be susceptible to B19 infection. Virus has been demonstrated in fetal myocytes, including myocardiocytes, along with inflammatory changes, and fetal myocarditis has occurred.[127,234,256] Histologic studies show vascular damage and perivascular infiltrates in some tissues. It is unknown whether this is caused by B19 infection in endothelial cells or a nonspecific effect related to hypoxic damage.

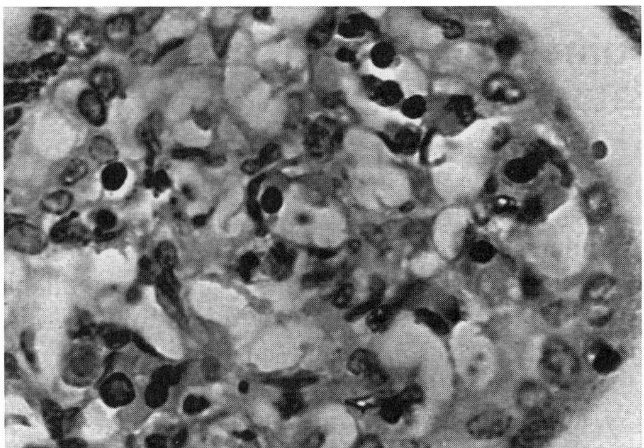

Figure 27–3 Placenta from a case of B19-associated nonimmune hydrops shows fetal capillaries filled with erythroblasts, most with marginated chromatin and typical amphophilic intranuclear inclusions (hematoxylin & eosin stain).

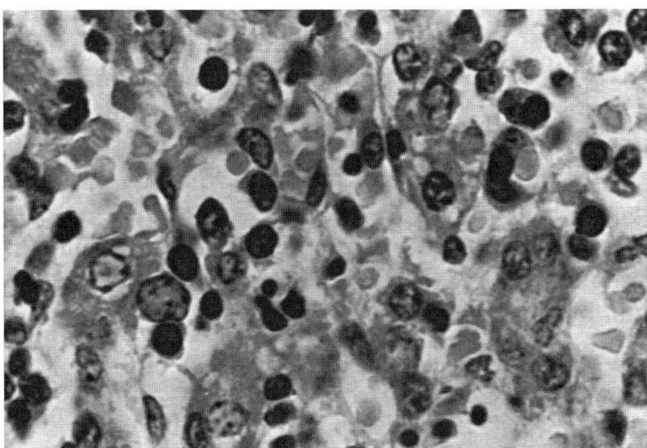

Figure 27–4 Fetal liver from a case of B19-associated nonimmune hydrops shows extramedullary hematopoiesis, intranuclear inclusions in erythroblasts, and focal areas with hemosiderin and fibrosis (hematoxylin & eosin stain).

PATHOLOGY IN THE FETUS

Anatomic and Histologic Features

The hallmarks of fetal infection with B19 are edema, anemia, and myocarditis, and these conditions are reflected in the pathologic finding at autopsy. Otherwise, reports of gross and histopathologic pathology postmortem reveal few features specific for intrauterine B19 infection.[16,232, 235,246,251,260-265] At postmortem examination, B19-infected fetuses are often described as pale with subcutaneous edema. Rashes typically are absent, but a blueberry muffin rash caused by extramedullary hematopoiesis in the skin may occur.[266]

Fetal anemia is common in fetal deaths due to B19, although not in all cases.[234,237,250,251,257,258,263,267] Histologic findings suggesting B19 infection include erythroid hypoplasia and, occasionally, hyperplasia characteristic of recovery. Extramedullary hematopoiesis is common in many organs, especially the liver and spleen. Nucleated red cells with amphophilic intranuclear inclusions (Figs. 27-3 and 27-4) are highly suggestive of B19 infection. These nucleated red cells are often found in the lumen of vessels and at sites of extramedullary hematopoiesis.[127] When stained with hematoxylin and eosin stain, the nuclei have an irregular band of dark chromatin. The center of the nucleus is lighter and has a smooth texture. The specificity of intranuclear inclusions for fetal B19 infection is unknown, but it is probably high when associated with anemia and hydrops. Viral DNA or inclusions may also be seen in macrophages and myocytes.[127,256,268]

PCR used for detecting B19 DNA is the best method to diagnosis B19 infection in a dead fetus. In one study, 6 of 34 cases of idiopathic nonimmune hydrops contained B19 DNA in fetal or placental tissues, compared with no PCR-positive findings among 23 cases of hydrops that were noninfectious.[269] Histologic examination of these cases found no nucleated red cells with intranuclear inclusions.

Placenta

B19 infection of the placenta probably precedes fetal infection. The placenta is usually abnormal when associated with fetal death due to B19. Grossly the placenta is often enlarged and edematous. Histologically, the placenta also contains nucleated red blood cells with typical intranuclear inclusions (see Fig. 27-4). Foci of red cell production also occur in the placenta, as does vascular inflammation.[232,249,264] In one study,[232] vasculitis of villous capillaries or stem arteries occurred in 9 of 10 placentas. The tissues demonstrated swelling of endothelial cells, fragmentation of endothelial cell nuclei, and fibrin thrombi. B19 DNA occurs in endothelial cells of patients with myocarditis and in patients with cutaneous lesions but has not been sought in placental endothelial cells. The human placenta contains a B19 receptor, the neutral glycosphingolipid (globoside), on the villous trophoblast layer of the placenta, and the concentration of the globoside decreases with advancing pregnancy.[270] The highest concentration occurs in the first trimester, with diminished reactivity occurring in the second trimester. The presence of this globoside in the placenta provides a mechanism by which the virus infects the placenta and fetus. It also may explain why there is a difference in fetal outcome associated with gestational age. Maternal infections in late pregnancy have a better prognosis than those occurring early in pregnancy. In addition to B19 receptors, there is a B19-induced inflammatory response in the placenta, characterized by a significant number of $CD3^+$ T cells and the inflammatory cytokine interleukin-2.[271]

Heart

The anemia associated with B19 infection is caused by a specific viral tropism for progenitor erythroid cells, specifically P antigen, which is found on these cells.[272] However, clinical and laboratory evidence suggests that B19 has a wider tropism than for erythroblasts.[273] Fetal myocardial cells contain P antigen.[273] Direct infection of myocardial cells after fetal B19 infection of extramedullary erythroid progenitor cells has been demonstrated by in situ DNA hybridization or electron microscopy.[57,68,127,274,275] B19 myocarditis is also associated with acute lymphocytic infiltration. Case reports have described at least eight fetuses, five children, and four adults with myocarditis associated with a concurrent B19 infection.[274,276-278]

B19 causes acute and chronic myocarditis in infants. Myocarditis and the cardiac enlargement found in some B19-infected fetuses with hydrops suggest that B19 is pathogenic for the myocardium.[127,232-235,246,254,256,276,279] In infected fetuses, the heart may be normal or symmetrically enlarged, suggesting congestive heart failure. Pericardial effusions are common. Myocytes with intranuclear inclusions occur infrequently. Mononuclear cell infiltrates occur occasionally, and B19 DNA, not associated with cells, can be found in the lumen of large vessels. Focal areas with dystrophic calcification or fibroelastosis have occurred as a response to injury.

One case-control study[280] examined the relationship between congenital heart disease and B19 infection. Five of 29 cases of congenital heart disease had parvovirus B19 DNA detected in cardiac tissue using PCR, compared with none of 30 matched controls. This difference was significant ($P < .02$). Other infections, including herpes simplex virus, cytomegalovirus, rubella, and toxoplasmosis, were excluded. Additional studies testing for B19 infection of congenital heart disease are appropriate.

Other Organs

Numerous other anatomic abnormalities have been associated with B19 infection of the fetus. Their occurrences, however, are so infrequent that it is unlikely that they are related to B19 infection. These associated abnormalities include dystrophic calcification of the brain and adrenal glands; anencephaly and ventriculomegaly; pulmonary hypoplasia; hypospadias; cleft lip; meconium peritonitis; corneal opacification and angioedema; and thymic abnormalities.[16,18,127,231-233,235-239,264,281-283]

DIAGNOSTIC EVALUATION AND MANAGEMENT OF THE WOMAN AND FETUS EXPOSED TO OR INFECTED BY B19 DURING PREGNANCY

Management of a pregnant woman exposed to B19 requires knowledge of the prevailing status of EI in the community, a detailed history of the exposure, knowledge of characteristic symptoms and signs of maternal EI and B19 infection in the fetus, appropriate laboratory tests needed to confirm maternal and fetal infection, knowledge of the methods for monitoring the fetus at risk for nonimmune hydrops, knowledge of therapeutic approaches for treating the hydropic fetus, and information about the prognosis of maternal and fetal infection and the expected outcomes for the therapeutic intervention.

Prevalence of Erythema Infectiosum

The community health or school health departments may know whether EI is epidemic in the community, increasing the probability of primary infection in susceptible pregnant women.

History of Exposure

Pregnant women who are potentially exposed to someone with EI should be asked about the type of exposure, including duration (brief or prolonged) and location (household or workplace, indoor or outdoor), and contact with respiratory secretions. Exposure to a child within the household constitutes the highest risk.

Did the contact have symptoms typical of EI, including a low-grade fever and a slapped-cheek rash that soon spread to the trunk or limbs in a lacy pattern? Did the rash disappear and then reappear when the child was warm from exercise or bathing? Had the child been exposed to any known source of EI, such as an outbreak in school, preschool, a daycare center, a family gathering, a play group, or church nursery? Was the child evaluated by a physician familiar with viral exanthems?

Clinical Features Suggesting B19 Infection in the Pregnant Woman

The examiner should consider whether the mother's signs and symptoms are compatible with B19 infection in adults, including at least one or more of the following: malaise, arthralgia, rash, coryza, or fever higher than 38° C. Pregnant women with such symptoms, especially malaise with symmetrical arthralgias in the hands, wrists, knees, or feet, should be considered at high risk and tested for recent B19 infection. In Barcelona, however, Gratecos and colleagues[20] found that only 30% of 60 IgM-positive women recalled any such symptoms.

Pregnant women without such systemic symptoms but with a rapidly enlarging uterus (i.e., fundal height exceeding dates by more than 3 cm), an elevated serum α-fetoprotein level, preterm labor, or decreased fetal movement should be asked about B19 exposure. If ultrasonography reveals evidence of hydrops fetalis or the fetus has ascites, pleural or pericardial effusion, skin thickening, polyhydramnios, or placentomegaly, maternal B19 testing is appropriate.

Laboratory Diagnosis in the Pregnant Woman

With evidence of maternal B19 exposure or maternal disease, maternal serum should be tested for IgG and IgM antibodies to B19. If there is probable or possible exposure, the first serum sample should be drawn at least 10 days after the exposure. Because fetal morbidity is unlikely to occur within 2 weeks of exposure, immediate serologic testing is appropriate for a woman or fetus with symptoms or signs of B19 infection.

An initial serum sample that is IgG positive but IgM negative indicates a previous maternal infection, and additional testing is unnecessary. The IgM assay is sensitive, with few false-negative reactions. An initial serum sample that is negative for IgM and IgG indicates no previous maternal infection, and B19 infection is not responsible for maternal symptoms and signs or for hydrops fetalis.

If the IgM result is positive, a recent B19 infection is established regardless of the IgG titer. A concomitant negative IgG titer means an early B19 infection without time for IgG to be detectable. Detection of maternal viremia by PCR for B19 DNA is also diagnostic of B19 infection. Viremia may precede the development of IgM antibodies by 7 to 14 days and may persist for several months after a primary infection.

With a positive maternal IgM result, the fetus must be examined for signs of hydrops fetalis by ultrasonography within 24 to 48 hours. If the gestational age is less than 18 weeks, the absence of hydrops may not be reassuring, because hydrops can appear later. Because several cases of severe hydrops fetalis spontaneously reverting to normal over 3 to 6 weeks have been reported, advice about pregnancy termination is difficult.[249,281,284]

Fetal Monitoring

For a fetal gestational age of more than 20 weeks, initial negative ultrasound results demand sonograms to be repeated weekly to detect hydrops. The number of weekly sonograms that should be performed is controversial. Rodis and associates[233] originally suggested continuing weekly scans for 6 to 8 weeks after exposure, and they reported a fetal death as late as 23 weeks' gestation after maternal fever and arthralgias in the first trimester.[128] The interval between maternal B19 infection and fetal morbidity is uncertain. Based on this report, others recommended weekly sonograms for 14 weeks after maternal B19 infection.[284] This approach often appeals to pregnant women fearful about fetal death, but it is time consuming and expensive.

Table 27–2 Fetal Deaths from B19 Infection

Infection to Death Interval (weeks)	Gestational Age at Death (weeks)	Fetal Weight at Death (grams)	Reference
1	39	3840	15
10	25	NR	298
13	22	409	16
4	20	161	16
4	24	420	299
4	26	695	300
9	24	580	300
7	18	300	301
8	19	236	286
1	4	NR	302
3	NR	NR	302
6	17	NR	302
10-19	23	NR	303
5	16	NR	303
(10)[a]	(11)[b]		289
(4)	(25)	Hydrops, 3320	290
(11)	(21)	Hydrops, 3111	291
(7)	(13)	Hydrops fetalis	158
(4)	(24)	Hydrops, 1495	158
(3)	(30)	Hydrops, 3550	303
(8)	(25)	Hydrops fetalis	140

[a]Numbers in parentheses refer to intervals between exposure or onset of symptoms and the diagnosis of hydrops fetalis.
[b]Numbers in parentheses refer to gestational age at the time of diagnosis of hydrops fetalis.
NR, not reported.

The duration of monitoring for hydrops fetalis may be best determined by examination of the interval between maternal exposure or symptoms of B19 infection and the appearance of hydrops fetalis or fetal death. Table 27-2 summarizes reports with adequate information to evaluate the interval, which include 14 intervals between maternal B19 exposure or infection and fetal death and 7 intervals between maternal exposure or infection and the first diagnosis of hydrops fetalis. The intervals range from 1 to 19 weeks, with a median of 6 weeks. Seventeen (81%) of 21 cases developed between 3 and 11 weeks. Because 11 of the 21 cases developed between 4 and 8 weeks after maternal exposure or infection, this is the most common interval between infection and the detection of fetal hydrops. Based on these observations, weekly ultrasound monitoring of the fetus for 12 weeks after maternal exposure is optimal but cannot detect all delayed cases and may be expensive. Such frequent scanning may not be considered cost-effective because the incidence of hydrops after maternal B19 infection is low in many studies. In our study, none of the 52 fetuses born to B19-IgM–positive pregnant women developed hydrops fetalis; however, the 95% confidence interval based on our sample size ranged from 0% to 8.6% for the risk of hydrops fetalis.[210] Other studies using maternal symptoms as criteria for maternal B19 infection have suggested a 9% incidence of fetal death due to B19 in B19-IgM–positive women.[18]

Serial maternal serum α-fetoprotein (MSAFP) measurements may monitor the fetus in B19-infected women.[285] One report found elevated MSAFP levels in five B19-IgM–positive pregnancies associated with fetal death, but no fetal deaths in 11 IgM-positive women with B19 infection but normal MSAFP values.[286] A fatal case of B19-associated fetal death, discovered because of an elevated MSAFP level at 16 weeks in a routine test in an asymptomatic woman, has been described.[16] In adding a seventh case of fetal death associated with elevated MSAFP levels in B19-IgM–positive women, Bernstein and Capeless[285] suggested using the MSAFP values to indicate a good fetal prognosis.

A German study[287] found that neither MSAFP nor human gonadotropin levels were markers of B19-infected pregnancies, although both were frequently elevated when complications occurred. The study included 35 pregnant women with fetal complications associated with B19; significant elevations of MSAFP levels occurred in 13 of 35 women, and elevations of human gonadotropin concentrations occurred in 25 of 35. The investigators tested 137 sera from 65 pregnant women without acute parvovirus infection and no fetal complications. Of the 30 women without fetal complications, there were significant elevations of MSAFP levels in only 2 women, and elevations of human gonadotropin levels occurred in only 5 women. Neither protein was a marker for a poor pregnancy outcome early on, but levels were frequently elevated when complications developed. Despite these results, there is insufficient experience using MSAFP concentrations, and MSAFP measurements at any gestational age are relatively nonspecific indicators of fetal well-being.

Electronic fetal monitoring is ineffective in detecting hydrops fetalis and predicting the outcome of pregnancy in B19-IgM–positive women. Contraction stress tests and "nonstress" tests are not accurate predictors of fetal well-being in cases of fetal anemia or hydrops fetalis. Similarly, fetal assessment with estriol measurements or other biochemical markers have no documented role in cases of hydrops fetalis. Because fetal sonograms are as readily available and provide rapid specific information about hydrops fetalis, ultrasound is the best method to monitor the fetus after maternal B19 infection.

Fetal Therapy

If hydrops fetalis is detected before 18 weeks, there is no effective intervention. Other causes of hydrops, such as chromosomal disorders or anatomic abnormalities, should be assessed. If at 18 weeks' gestation the fetus is still viable as determined by ultrasound examination, consideration can be given to percutaneous umbilical blood sampling (PUBS), also called cordocentesis. At 18 weeks' gestation, the umbilical vein diameter is about 4 mm, which is the minimum size required for successful PUBS. Fetal blood should be obtained for the hematocrit, reticulocyte count, platelet count, leukocyte count, antiparvovirus B19 IgM, karyotype, and tests for B19 DNA by PCR. The hematocrit must be determined immediately, and if fetal anemia exists, intrauterine intravascular fetal transfusion is performed with the same needle puncture.

If the fetus is between 18 and 32 weeks' gestation when hydrops fetalis is detected, fetal transfusion should be considered. Many successful cases of fetal transfusion for B19-induced hydrops fetalis have been reported, and some have long-term follow-up, but the success rate of the procedure remains unknown.[288-294]

Two or three separate transfusions are usually required before resolution of the fetal anemia and hydrops fetalis, increasing the 1% to 2% risk of each single PUBS procedure. Resolution of the hydrops usually occurs 3 to 6 weeks after the first transfusion. Although spontaneous resolution has been reported, it seems appropriate not to risk an uncertain outcome, because the longer the fetal transfusion is delayed, the less likely it is to be successful and the worse the potential harm to the fetus caused by continued fetal hypoxia.[231, 249,284,289-291]

For fetuses of 32 weeks' gestation or older when hydrops is discovered, immediate delivery with neonatal exchange transfusion, thoracentesis, and paracentesis as indicated usually is the safest management.

DIFFERENTIAL DIAGNOSIS

Recalling that the hallmarks of fetal infection with B19 are anemia, hydrops, and myocarditis helps in compiling a differential diagnosis. For infants with anemia, the differential diagnosis includes all the known causes, including fetal-maternal transfusion, intracranial bleeding, blood group incompatibilities, congenital anemias such as Diamond-Blackfan syndrome, nutritional deficiencies, and inborn metabolic errors. Fetal hydrops and fetal and placental edema may be associated with other congenital infections, particularly congenital syphilis, chromosomal abnormalities, immune hydrops associated with blood group incompatibilities, hypothyroidism, and heart or renal failure, or both.

PROGNOSIS

Pregnant women can be reassured about the relatively low risk of fetal morbidity resulting from exposure to B19. About one half of women already are seropositive. The seronegative maternal B19 infection rate ranges from about 29% for exposures by the woman's own children to about 10% to 18% for other exposures. The expected fetal morbidity and mortality risk is about 2% (1 of 50). The overall risk of fetal death varies from 0.3% ($\frac{1}{2} \times \frac{3}{10} \times \frac{1}{50} = \frac{3}{1000}$) to a mere 0.1% ($\frac{1}{2} \times \frac{1}{10} \times \frac{1}{50} = \frac{1}{1000}$).[210]

Live-born infants infected in utero may die shortly after birth. Two infants born prematurely at 24 and 35 weeks' gestation developed an illness characteristic of congenital viral infection, including placentomegaly, petechial rash, edema, hepatomegaly, anemia, thrombocytopenia, and respiratory insufficiency, and both died postnatally.[295] Both infants had nuclear inclusions in erythroid precursor cells, and PCR confirmed the presence of parvoviral DNA in one of the infants.

Data regarding the long-term outcomes of live-born children infected in utero or born of mothers infected during pregnancy are very limited. In one study, 113 pregnant women with B19 infection during pregnancy and a control group of immune women were questioned about the health and development of their children when the median age of the children was 4 years for both groups.[242] The incidence of developmental delays in speech, language, information processing, and attention was similar between the study group and the controls (7.3% versus 7.5%). Two cases of cerebral palsy were found in the study group, compared with none in the controls. Although not statistically significant, this 2% incidence of cerebral palsy in the infected group is 10-fold higher than the reported national incidence.[242]

In a British study of 427 pregnant women with B19 infection and 367 of their surviving infants, 129 surviving infants were reassessed when 7 to 10 years old.[296] The follow-up included questionnaires to obstetricians and general practitioners about the outcome of pregnancy and health of surviving infants. Maternal infection was confirmed by B19-specific IgM assay or IgG seroconversion. An excess rate of fetal loss was confined to the first 20 weeks' gestation and averaged 9%. There were seven cases of fetal hydrops with maternal infections between 9 and 20 weeks' gestation. There were no abnormalities attributable to B19 infection found at birth in surviving infants. No late effects were observed when the children were 7 to 10 years old. This study concluded that approximately 1 in 10 women infected before 20 weeks' gestation would have a fetal loss due to B19, that the risk of an adverse outcome of pregnancy beyond this stage was unlikely, and that infected women could be reassured that the risk of congenital abnormality due to B19 is less than 1% and that long-term development would be normal.

One study used IQ testing and standard neurodevelopmental tests to assess 20 children who had parvovirus-induced fetal hydrops and intrauterine transfusion of packed red cells.[288] Testing of the 20 children when they were between 13 months and 9 years old revealed that all of their results ranged within two standard deviations of a population norm. There was no significant developmental delay. This study concluded that children who survived successful intrauterine transfusion from B19 anemia and hydrops had a good neurodevelopmental prognosis.

PREVENTION

General Measures

Because B19 is usually endemic in most communities, what is appropriate management for pregnant women with daily contact with children? The prevalence of seropositivity (immunity) to B19 among pregnant women varies according to geographic location, sex, age, and race. Assuming that on average 50% of pregnant women are immune; that during endemic periods, between 1% and 4% of susceptible women become infected during pregnancy; and that the rate of fetal death after maternal infection is 2%, the occupational risk of fetal death for a pregnant woman with unknown serologic status is between 1 in 1000 and 1 in 2500. These low rates do not justify intervention such as serologic testing for pregnant women, furloughing pregnant workers, or temporarily transferring pregnant seronegative employees to administrative or other positions without child contact. During epidemic periods in specific schools, when the infection rates may be 5- to 20-fold higher, serologic testing or temporary transfer of pregnant employees may occasionally be appropriate, and some very anxious women may choose to leave the workplace.

Given the low risk for individual pregnant women, seronegative women should not send their own children away, and schools and daycare centers cannot stop B19 outbreaks by excluding children with rash illnesses because B19 is transmissible before the rash appears. Whether B19 can be transmitted by breast-feeding is unknown.

Vaccine Development

For most women, fetal B19 infections during pregnancy occur from exposure to school-aged children at home rather than from occupational exposure. Given the highly communicable and endemic nature of the infection, the broad spectrum of illness that B19 causes, and the large portion of population (30% to 50%) who are susceptible, an effective B19 vaccine, preferably administered in infancy, is appropriate, and at least one vaccine is being developed.[297] This vaccine is composed of the major B19 capsid proteins VP1 and VP2 and administered with a squalene adjuvant, MF59. After testing in a limited number of subjects, the vaccine appears to be safe and induces neutralizing antibodies. Studies using volunteers challenged with wild-type B19 should be able to assess efficacy. A vaccine that induces sustained neutralizing antibody IgG levels to B19 should be effective given that prior immunity to B19 protects against reinfection.

Acknowledgments

We are grateful to Dr. James H. Harger for his years of collaboration and helpful assistance.

REFERENCES

1. Murphy FA, Fauquet CM, Bishop DHL, et al (eds). Virus Taxonomy. Sixth Report of the International Committee on Taxonomy of Viruses. New York, Springer-Verlag, 1995.
2. Torok TJ. Unusual clinical manifestations reported in patients with parvovirus B19 infection. *In* Anderson LJ, Young NS (eds). Human Parvovirus B19. Monographs in Virology, vol. 20. Basel, Karger, 1997, pp 61-92.
3. Koch WC. Fifth (human parvovirus B19) and sixth (herpesvirus 6) diseases. Curr Opin Infect Dis 14:343, 2001.
4. Cossart YE, Field AM, Cant B, Widdows D. Parvovirus-like particles in human sera. Lancet 1:72, 1975.
5. Summers J, Jones SE, Anderson MJ. Characterization of the genome of the agent of erythrocyte aplasia permits its classification as a human parvovirus. J Gen Virol 64:2527, 1983.
6. Pattison JR, Jones SE, Hodgson J. Parvovirus infections and hypoplastic crisis in sickle-cell anaemia. Letter. Lancet 1:664, 1981.
7. Serjeant GR, Topley JM, Mason K, et al. Outbreak of aplastic crises in sickle cell anaemia associated with parvovirus-like agent. Lancet 2:595, 1981.
8. Anderson MJ, Jones SE, Fisher-Hoch SP, et al. Human parvovirus, the cause of erythema infectiosum (fifth disease)? Letter. Lancet 1:1378, 1983.
9. Thurn J. Human parvovirus B19: historical and clinical review. Rev Infect Dis 10:1005, 1988.
10. Ager EA, Chin TDY, Poland JD. Epidemic erythema infectiosum. N Engl J Med 275:1326, 1966.
11. Cramp JE, Armstrong BDJ. Erythema infectiosum: no evidence of teratogenicity. Br Med J 2:1031, 1977.
12. Pattison JR. B19 Virus infections in pregnancy. *In* Pattison JR (ed). Parvoviruses and Human Disease. Boca Raton, Fla, CRC Press, 1988, pp 133-138.

13. Siegel G. Patterns of parvovirus disease in animals. *In* Pattison JR (ed). Parvoviruses and Human Disease. Boca Raton, Fla, CRC Press, 1988, pp 43-68.
14. Brown T, Anand A, Ritchie LD, et al. Intrauterine parvovirus infection associated with hydrops fetalis. Lancet 2:1033, 1984.
15. Knott PD, Welply GAC, Anderson MJ. Serologically proved intrauterine infection with parvovirus. Letter. BMJ 289:1960, 1984.
16. Anand A, Gray ES, Brown T, et al. Human parvovirus infection in pregnancy and hydrops fetalis. N Engl J Med 316:183, 1987.
17. Kinney JS, Anderson LJ, Farrar J, et al. Risk of adverse outcomes of pregnancy after human parvovirus B19 infection. J Infect Dis 157:663, 1988.
18. Hall SM, Public Health Laboratory Service Working Party on Fifth Disease. Prospective study of human parvovirus (B19) infection in pregnancy. Br Med J 300:1166, 1990.
19. Adler SP, Manganello AM, Koch WC, et al. Risk of human parvovirus B19 infections among school and hospital employees during endemic periods. J Infect Dis 168:361, 1993.
20. Gratacos E, Torres P-J, Vidal J, et al. The incidence of human parvovirus B19 infection during pregnancy and its impact on perinatal outcome. J Infect Dis 171:1360, 1995.
21. Koch WC, Harger JH, Barnstein B, Adler SP. Serologic and virologic evidence for frequent intrauterine transmission of human parvovirus B10 with a primary maternal infection during pregnancy. Pediatr Infect Dis 17:489, 1998.
22. Pringle CR. Virus taxonomy update. Arch Virol 133:491, 1993.
23. Astell CR, Weixing L, Brunstein J, St Amand J. B19 parvovirus: biochemical and molecular features. *In* Anderson LJ, Young NS (eds). Monographs in Virology, vol. 20. Human Parvovirus B19. Basel, Karger, 1997, pp 16-41.
24. O'Sullivan MG, Anderson DC, Fikes JD, et al. Identification of a novel simian parvovirus from cynomolgus monkey with severe anemia: a paradigm for human B19 parvovirus infection. J Clin Invest 93:1571, 1994.
25. Mori J, Beattie P, Melton DW, et al. Structure and mapping of the DNA of human parvovirus B19. J Gen Virol 68:2797, 1987.
26. Umene K, Nunoue T. Genetic diversity of human parvovirus B19 determined using a set of restriction endonucleases recognizing four or five base pairs and partial nucleotide sequencing: use of sequence variability in virus classification. J Gen Virol 72:1997, 1991.
27. Gallinella G, Venturoli S, Manaresi E, et al. B19 virus genome diversity: epidemiological and clinical correlations. J Clin Virol 76:9124, 2003.
28. Nguyen QT, Sifer C, Schneider V, et al. Novel human erythrovirus associated with transient aplastic crisis. J Clin Microbiol 37:2483, 1999.
29. Nguyen QT, Wong S, Heegaard ED, Brown KE. Identification and characterization of a second human erythrovirus variant, A6. Virology 30:374, 2002.
30. Servant A, Laperche S, Lallemand F, et al. Genetic diversity within human erythroviruses: identification of three genotypes. J Virol 76: 9124, 2002.
34. Ozawa K, Ayub J, Kajigaya S, et al. The gene encoding the nonstructural protein of B19 (human) parvovirus may be lethal in transfected cells. J Virol 62:2884, 1988.
35. Moffat S, Yaegashi N, Tada K, et al. Human parvovirus B19 nonstructural protein NS1 induces apoptosis in erythroid lineage cells. J Virol 72:3018, 1998.
36. Sol N, Le Junter J, Vassias I, et al. Possible interactions between the NS-1 protein and tumor necrosis factor alpha pathways in erythroid cell apoptosis induced by parvovirus B19. J Virol 73:8762, 1999.
37. Ozawa K, Kurtzman G, Young N. Replication of the B19 parvovirus in human bone marrow cell cultures. Science 233:883, 1986.
38. Srivastava A, Lu L. Replication of B19 parvovirus in highly enriched hematopoietic progenitor cells form normal human bone marrow. J Virol 62:3059, 1988.
39. Yaegashi N, Shiraishi H, Takeshita T, et al. Propagation of human parvovirus B19 in primary culture of erythroid lineage cells derived from fetal liver. J Virol 63:2422, 1989.
40. Takahahsi T, Ozawa K, Mitani K, et al. B19 parvovirus replicates in erythroid leukemic cells in vitro. J Infect Dis 160:548, 1989.
41. Miyagawa E, Yoshida T, Yamaguchi K, et al. Infection of the erythroid cell line KU812Ep6 with human parvovirus B19 and its application to titration of B19 infectivity. J Virol Methods 83:45, 1999.
42. Brown KE, Young NS, Liu JM. Molecular, cellular and clinical aspects of parvovirus B19 infection. Crit Rev Oncol Hematol 16:1, 1994.
43. Brown KE, Anderson SM, Young NS. Erythrocyte P antigen: cellular receptor for B19 parvovirus. Science 262:114, 1993.
44. Brown KE, Hibbs JR, Gallinella G, et al. Resistance to parvovirus B19 infection due to a lack of virus receptor (erythrocyte P antigen). N Engl J Med 330:1192, 1994.
45. Weigel-Kelley KA, Yoder MC, Srivastava A. Recombinant human parvovirus B19 vectors: erythrocyte P antigen is necessary but not sufficient for successful transduction of human hematopoietic cells. J Virol 75:4110, 2001.
46. Weigel-Kelley KA, Yoder MC, Srivastava A. Alpha5beta1 integrin as a cellular coreceptor for human parvovirus B19: requirement of functional activation of beta 1 integrin for viral entry. Blood 102:3927, 2003.
47. Brown KE, Young NS. Parvovirus B19 infection and hematopoiesis. Blood Rev 9:176, 1995.
49. Srivastava A, Bruno E, Briddell R, et al. Parvovirus B19-induced perturbation of human megakaryocytopoiesis in vitro. Blood 76:1997, 1990.
48. Young N. Hematologic and hematopoietic consequences of B19 infection. Semin Hematol 25:159, 1988.
50. Anderson MJ, Higgins PG, Davis LR, et al. Experimental parvovirus infection in humans. J Infect Dis 152:257, 1985.
51. Moffat S, Tanaka N, Tada K, et al. A cytotoxic nonstructural protein, NS1, of human parvovirus B19 induces activation of interleukin-6 gene expression. J Virol 70:8485, 1996.
52. Teuscher T, Baillod B, Holzer BR. Prevalence of human parvovirus B19 in sickle cell disease and healthy controls. Trop Geogr Med 43:108, 1991.
53. Schwarz TF, Gürtler LG, Zoulek G, et al. Seroprevalence of human parvovirus B19 infection in São Tomé and Principe, Malawi and Mascarene Islands. Zentralbl Bakteriol 271:231, 1989.
54. Jones PH, Pickett LC, Anderson MJ, Pasvol G. Human parvovirus infection in children and severe anaemia seen in an area endemic for malaria. J Trop Med Hyg 93:67, 1990.
55. de Freitas RB, Wong D, Boswell F, et al. Prevalence of human parvovirus (B19) and rubella virus infections in urban and remote rural areas in northern Brazil. J Med Virol 32:203, 1990.
56. Brown CS, Jensen T, Meloen RH, et al. Localization of an immunodominant domain on baculovirus-produced parvovirus B19 capsids: correlation to a major surface region on the native virus particle. J Virol 66:69, 1992.
57. Morey AL, O'Neill HJ, Coyle PV, Fleming KA. Immunohistological detection of human parvovirus B19 in formalin-fixed, paraffin-embedded tissues. J Pathol 166:105, 1992.
58. Loughrey AC, O'Neill HJ, Coyle PV, DeLeys R. Identification and use of a neutralizing epitope of parvovirus B19 for the rapid detection of virus infection. J Med Virol 39:97, 1993.
59. Morinet F, Tratschin JD, Perol Y, Siegl G. Comparison of 17 isolates of the human parvovirus B19 by restriction enzyme analysis. Arch Virol 90:165, 1986.
60. Umene K, Nunoue T. The genome type of human parvovirus B19 strains isolated in Japan during 1981 differs from types detected in 1986 to 1987: a correlation between genome type and prevalence. J Gen Virol 71:983, 1990.
61. Umene K, Nunoue T. Partial nucleotide sequencing and characterization of human parvovirus B19 genome DNAs from damaged human fetuses and from patients with leukemia. J Med Virol 39:333, 1993.
62. Lawton AL, Smith RE. Erythema infectiosum: a clinical study of an epidemic in Branford, Connecticut. Arch Intern Med 47:28, 1931.
63. Chargin L, Sobel N, Goldstein H. Erythema infectiosum: report of an extensive epidemic. Arch Dermatol Syphilol 47:467, 1943.
64. Galvon FAC. An outbreak of erythema infectiosum—Nova Scotia. Can Dis Wkly Rep 9:69, 1983.
65. Serjeant GR, Serjeant BE, Thomas PW, et al. Human parvovirus infection in homozygous sickle cell disease. Lancet 341:1237, 1993.
66. Oliveira SA, Camacho LA, Pereira AC, et al. Clinical and epidemiological aspects of human parvovirus B19 infection in an urban area in Brazil (Niteroi city area, State of Rio de Janeiro, Brazil). Mem Inst Oswaldo Cruz 97:965, 2002.
67. Yamashita K, Matsunaga Y, Taylor-Wiedeman J, Yamazaki S. A significant age shift of the human parvovirus B19 antibody prevalence among young adults in Japan observed in a decade. Jpn J Med Sci Biol 45:49, 1992.
68. Naides SJ. Erythema infectiosum (fifth disease) occurrence in Iowa. Am J Public Health 78:1230, 1988.
69. Cohen BJ, Buckley MM. The prevalence of antibody to human parvovirus B19 in England and Wales. J Med Microbiol 25:151, 1988.

70. Nascimento JP, Buckley MM, Brown KE, Cohen BJ. The prevalence of antibody to human parvovirus B19 in Rio de Janeiro, Brazil. Rev Inst Med Trop Sao Paulo 32:41, 1990.
71. Edelson RN, Altman RA. Erythema infectiosum: a statewide outbreak. J Med Soc N J 67:805, 1970.
72. Werner GH, Brachman PS, Ketler A, et al. A new viral agent associated with erythema infectiosum. Ann N Y Acad Sci 67:338, 1957.
73. Greenwald P, Bashe WJ Jr. An epidemic of erythema infectiosum. Am J Dis Child 107:30, 1964.
74. Yaegashi N, Okamura K, Hamazaki Y, et al. Prevalence of anti-human parvovirus antibody in pregnant women. Nippon Sanka Fujinka Gakkai Zasshi 42:162, 1990.
75. Koch WC, Adler SP. Human parvovirus B19 infections in women of childbearing age and within families. Pediatr Infect Dis J 8:83, 1989.
76. Cohen BJ, Mortimer PP, Pereira MS. Diagnostic assays with monoclonal antibodies for the human serum parvovirus-like virus (SPLV). J Hyg (Lond) 91:113, 1983.
77. Schwarz TF, Roggendorf M, Deinhardt F. Häufigkeit der parovirus-B19-infektionen. Seroepidemiologishe untersuchungen. Dtsch Med Wochenschr 112:1526, 1987.
78. Bartolomei Corsi O, Assi A, Morfini M, et al. Human parvovirus infection in haemophiliacs first infused with treated clotting factor concentrates. J Med Virol 25:165, 1988.
79. Eiffert H, Köchel HG, Heuer M, et al. Expression of an antigenic polypeptide of the human parvovirus B19. Med Microbiol Immunol 179:169, 1990.
80. Brown CS, van Bussel MJA, Wassenaar ALM, et al. An immunofluorescence assay for the detection of parvovirus B19 IgG and IgM antibodies based on recombinant viral antigen. J Virol Methods 29:53, 1990.
81. Rollag H, Patou G, Pattison JR, et al. Prevalence of antibodies against parvovirus B19 in Norwegians with congenital coagulation factor defects treated with plasma products from small donor pools. Scand J Infect Dis 23:675, 1991.
82. Salimans MMM, van Bussel MJA, Brown CS, Spaan WJM. Recombinant parvovirus B19 capsids as a new substrate for detection of B19-specific IgG and IgM antibodies by an enzyme-linked immunosorbent assay. J Virol Methods 39:247, 1992.
83. Abraham M, Rudraraju R, Kannangai R, et al. A pilot study on the seroprevalence of parvovirus B19 infection. Indian J Med Res 115:139, 2002.
84. Schwarz TF, Hottenträger B, Roggendorf M. Prevalence of antibodies to parvovirus B19 in selected groups of patients and healthy individuals. Int J Med Microbiol Virol Parasitol Infect Dis 276:437, 1992.
85. Lin KH, You SL, Chen CJ, et al. Seroepidemiology of human parvovirus B19 in Taiwan. J Med Virol 57:169, 1999.
86. Couroucé AM, Ferchal F, Morinet F, et al. Parvovirus (SPLV) et antigène Aurillac. Rev Fr Transfus Immunohematol 27:5, 1984.
87. Cossart Y. Parvovirus B19 finds a disease. Letter. Lancet 2:988, 1981.
88. O'Neill HJ, Coyle PV. Two anti-parvovirus B19 IgM capture assays incorporating a mouse monoclonal antibody specific for B19 viral capsid proteins VP1 and VP2. Arch Virol 123:125, 1992.
89. Cohen BJ, Field AM, Gudnadottir S, et al. Blood donor screening for parvovirus B19. J Virol Methods 30:233, 1990.
90. da Silva Cruz A, Serpa MJA, Barth OM, Nascimento JP. Detection of the human parvovirus B19 in a blood donor plasma in Rio de Janeiro. Mem Inst Oswaldo Cruz 84:279, 1989.
91. McOmish F, Yap PL, Jordan A, et al. Detection of parvovirus B19 in donated blood: a model system for screening by polymerase chain reaction. J Clin Microbiol 31:323, 1993.
92. Yaegashi N, Shiraishi H, Tada K, et al. Enzyme-linked immunosorbent assay for IgG and IgM antibodies against human parvovirus B19: use of monoclonal antibodies and viral antigen propagated in vitro. J Virol Methods 26:171, 1989.
93. Naides SJ, Scharosch LL, Foto F, Howard EJ. Rheumatologic manifestations of human parvovirus B19 infection in adults. Arthritis Rheum 33:1297, 1990.
94. Martinez-Campillo F, Lopez J, Verdu M, et al. Parvovirus B19 outbreak in a rural community in Alicante. Enferm Infect Microbiol Clin 20:376, 2002.
95. Abarca K, Cohen BJ, Vial PA. Seroprevalence of parvovirus B19 in urban Chilean children and young adults, 1990 and 1996. Epidemiol Infect 128:59, 2002.
96. Smith-Whitley K, Zhao H, Hodinka RL, et al. Epidemiology of human parvovirus B19 in children with sickle cell disease. Blood 103:422, 2004.
97. Plummer FA, Hammond GW, Forward K, et al. An erythema infectiosum-like illness caused by human parvovirus infection. N Engl J Med 313:74, 1985.
98. Chorba T, Coccia P, Holman RC, et al. The role of parvovirus B19 in aplastic crisis and erythema infectiosum (fifth disease). J Infect Dis 154:383, 1986.
99. Mortimer PP. Hypothesis: the aplastic crisis of hereditary spherocytosis is due to a single transmissible agent. J Clin Pathol 36:445, 1983.
100. Saarinen UA, Chorba TL, Tattersall P, et al. Human parvovirus B19 induced epidemic red-cell aplasia in patients with hereditary hemolytic anemia. Blood 67:1411, 1986.
101. Valeur-Jensen A, Pedersen CB, Westergaard T, et al. Risk factors for parvovirus B19 infection in pregnancy. JAMA 281:1099, 1999.
102. Anderson MJ, Lewis E, Kidd IM, et al. An outbreak of erythema infectiosum associated with human parvovirus infection. J Hyg (Lond) 93:85, 1984.
103. Tuckerman JG, Brown T, Cohen BJ. Erythema infectiosum in a village primary school: clinical and virological studies. J R Coll Gen Pract 36:267, 1986.
104. Morgan-Capner P, Wright J, Longley JP, Anderson MJ. Sex ratio in outbreaks of parvovirus B19 infection. Letter. Lancet 2:98, 1987.
105. Mansfield F. Erythema infectiosum: slapped face disease. Aust Fam Physician 17:737, 1988.
106. Woolf AD, Campion GV, Chishick A, et al. Clinical manifestations of human parvovirus B19 in adults. Arch Intern Med 149:1153, 1989.
107. Turner A, Olojugba O. Erythema infectiosum in a primary school: investigation of an outbreak in Bury. Public Health 103:391, 1989.
108. Grilli EA, Anderson MJ, Hoskins TW. Concurrent outbreaks of influenza and parvovirus B19 in a boys' boarding school. Epidemiol Infect 103:359, 1989.
109. Gillespie SM, Cartter ML, Asch S, et al. Occupational risk of human parvovirus B19 infection for school and day-care personnel during an outbreak of erythema infectiosum. JAMA 263:2061, 1990.
110. Anderson LJ, Gillespie SM, Török TJ, et al. Risk of infection following exposures to human parvovirus B19. Behring Inst Mitt 85:60, 1990.
111. Rice PS, Cohen BJ. A school outbreak of parvovirus B19 infection investigated using salivary antibody assays. Epidemiol Infect 6:331, 1996.
112. Bell LM, Naides SJ, Stoffman P, et al. Human parvovirus B19 infection among hospital staff members after contact with infected patients. N Engl J Med 321:485, 1989.
113. Pillay D, Patou G, Hurt S, et al. Parvovirus B19 outbreak in a children's ward. Lancet 339:107, 1992.
114. Cohen BJ, Couroucé AM, Schwarz TF, et al. Laboratory infection with parvovirus B19. Letter. J Clin Pathol 41:1027, 1988.
115. Shiraishi H, Sasaki T, Nakamura M, et al. Laboratory infection with human parvovirus B19. Letter. J Infect 22:308, 1991.
116. Evans JPM, Rossiter MA, Kumaran TO, et al. Human parvovirus aplasia: case due to cross infection in a ward. BMJ 288:681, 1984.
117. Ueda K, Akeda H, Tokugawa K, Nishima S. Human parvovirus infection. Letter. N Engl J Med 314:645, 1986.
118. Pillay D, Patou G, Rees L, Griffiths PD. Secondary parvovirus B19 infection in an immunocompromised child. Pediatr Infect Dis J 10:623, 1991.
119. Lui SL, Luk WK, Cheung CY, et al. Nosocomial outbreak of parvovirus B19 infection in a renal transplant unit. Transplantation 71:59, 2001.
120. Miyamoto K, Ogami M, Takahashi Y, et al. Outbreak of human parvovirus B19 in hospital workers. J Hosp Infect 45:238, 2000.
121. Koziol DE, Kurtzman G, Ayub JA, et al. Nosocomial human parvovirus B19 infection: lack of transmission from a chronically infected patient to hospital staff. Infect Control Hosp Epidemiol 13:343, 1992.
122. Dowell SF, Torok TJ, Thorp JA, et al. Parvovirus B19 infection in hospital workers: community or hospital acquisition? J Infect Dis 172:1076, 1995.
123. Carter ML, Farley TA, Rosengren S, et al. Occupational risk factors for infection with parvovirus B19 among pregnant women. J Infect Dis 163:282, 1991.
124. Ray SM, Erdman DD, Berschling JD, et al. Nosocomial exposure to parvovirus B19: low risk of transmission to healthcare workers. Infect Control Hosp Epidemiol 18:109, 1997.
125. Patou G, Pillay D, Myint S, Pattison J. Characterization of a nested polymerase chain reaction assay for detection of parvovirus B19. J Clin Microbiol 31:540, 1993.
126. Potter CG, Potter AC, Hatton CSR, et al. Variation of erythroid and myeloid precursors in the marrow of volunteer subjects infected with human parvovirus (B19). J Clin Invest 79:1486, 1987.

127. Morey AL, Porter HJ, Keeling JW, Fleming KA. Non-isotopic in situ hybridisation and immunophenotyping of infected cells in investigation of human fetal parvovirus infection. J Clin Pathol 45:673, 1992.
128. Mortimer PP, Luban NLC, Kelleher JF, Cohen BJ. Transmission of serum parvovirus-like virus by clotting-factor concentrates. Lancet 2:482, 1983.
129. Lyon DJ, Chapman CS, Martin C, et al. Symptomatic parvovirus B19 infection and heat-treated factor IX concentrate. Letter. Lancet 1:1085, 1989.
130. Williams MD, Cohen BJ, Beddall AC, et al. Transmission of human parvovirus B19 by coagulation factor concentrates. Vox Sang 58:177, 1990.
131. Morfini M, Longo G, Rossi Ferrini P, et al. Hypoplastic anemia in a hemophiliac first infused with a solvent/detergent treated factor VIII concentrate: the role of human B19 parvovirus. Letter. Am J Hematol 39:149, 1992.
132. Zakrzewska K, Azzi A, Patou G, et al. Human parvovirus B19 in clotting factor concentrates: B19 DNA detection by the nested polymerase chain reaction. Br J Haematol 81:407, 1992.
133. Schwarz TF, Roggendorf M, Hottenträger B, et al. Removal of parvovirus B19 from contaminated factor VIII during fractionation. J Med Virol 35:28, 1991.
134. Azzi A, Ciappi S, Zakrzewska K, et al. Human parvovirus B19 infection in hemophiliacs infused with two high purity, virally attenuated factor VIII concentrates. Am J Hematol 39:228, 1992.
135. Anderson MJ. Rash illness due to B19 virus. *In* Pattison JR (ed). Parvoviruses and Human Disease, Boca Raton, Fla, CRC Press, 1988, pp 93-104.
136. Anderson LJ. Role of parvovirus B19 in human disease. Pediatr Infect Dis 6:711, 1987.
137. Garcia-Tapia AM, Fernandez-Guitierrez del Alamo C, Giron JA, et al. Spectrum of parvovirus B19 infection: analysis of an outbreak of 43 cases in Cadiz, Spain. Clin Infect Dis 21:424, 1995.
138. Zerbini M, Musiani M, Venturoli S, et al. Different syndromes associated with B19 parvovirus viraemia in paediatric patients: report of four cases. Eur J Pediatr 151:815, 1992.
139. Tsuda H, Maeda Y, Nakagawa K. Parvovirus B19-related lymphadenopathy. Br J Haematol 85:631, 1993.
140. Brown KE. Human parvovirus B19 epidemiology and clinical manifestations. *In* Anderson LJ, Young NS (eds). Monographs in Virology, vol. 20. Basel, Karger, 1997, pp 42-60.
141. Lefrere J-J, Courouce A-M, Soulier JP, et al. Henoch-Schönlein purpura and human parvovirus infection. Pediatrics 78:183, 1986.
142. Saunders PWG, Reid MM, Cohen BJ. Human parvovirus induced cytopenias: a report of five cases. Br J Haematol 63:407, 1986.
143. Lefrere JJ, Courouce AM, Kaplan C. Parvovirus and idiopathic thrombocytopenic purpura. Letter. Lancet 1:279, 1989.
144. Török TJ. Parvovirus B19 and human disease. Adv Int Med 37:431, 1992.
145. White DG, Woolf AD, Mortimer PP, et al. Human parvovirus arthropathy. Lancet 1:419, 1985.
146. Naides SJ, Field EH. Transient rheumatoid factor positivity in acute human parvovirus B19 infection. Arch Intern Med 148:2587, 1988.
147. Reid DM, Reid TMS, Brown T, et al. Human parvovirus-associated with arthritis: a clinical and laboratory description. Lancet 1:422, 1985.
148. Nocton JJ, Miller LC, Tucker LB, Schaller JG. Human parvovirus B19-associated arthritis in children. J Pediatr 122:186, 1993.
149. Dijkmans BA, van Elsacker-Niele Am, Salimans MMM, et al. Human parvovirus B19 DNA in synovial fluid. Arthritis Rheum 31:279, 1988.
150. Saal JG, Stendle M, Einsele H, et al. Persistence of B19 parvovirus in synovial membranes of patients with rheumatoid arthritis. Rheumatology 12:147, 1992.
151. Mimori A, Misaki Y, Hachiya T, et al. Prevalence of antihuman parvovirus B19 IgG antibodies in patients with refractory rheumatoid arthritis and polyarticular juvenile rheumatoid arthritis. Rheumatol Int 14:87, 1994.
152. Soderlund M, von Essen R, Haapasaari J, et al. Persistence of parvovirus B19 DNA in synovial membranes of young patients with and without chronic arthropathy. Lancet 349:1063, 1997.
153. Stahl HD, Hubner B, Seidl B, et al. Detection of multiple viral DNA species in synovial tissue and fluid of patients with early arthritis. Ann Rheum Dis 59:342, 2000.
154. Kerr JR. Pathogenesis of human parvovirus B19 in rheumatic disease. Ann Rheum Dis 59:672, 2000.
155. Koch WC, Massey G, Russell EC, et al. Manifestations and treatment of human parvovirus B19 infection in immunocompromised patients. J Pediatr 116:355, 1990.
156. Van Horn DK, Mortimer PP, Young N, et al. Human parvovirus-associated red cell aplasia in the absence of hemolytic anemia. Am J Pediatr Hematol Oncol 8:235, 1986.
157. Kurtzman GJ, Ozawa K, Cohen B, et al. Chronic bone marrow failure due to persistent B19 parvovirus infection. N Engl J Med 317:287, 1987.
158. Frickhofen N, Abkowitz JL, Safford M, et al. Persistent B19 parvovirus infection in patients infected with human immunodeficiency virus type 1 (HIV-1): a treatable cause of anemia in AIDS. Ann Intern Med 113:926, 1990.
159. Weiland HT, Salimans MMM, Fibbe WE, et al. Prolonged parvovirus B19 infection with severe anaemia in a bone marrow transplant recipient. Letter. Br J Haematol 71:300, 1989.
160. Kurtzman G, Frickhofen N, Kimball J, et al. Pure red-cell aplasia of ten years' duration due to persistent parvovirus B19 infection and its cure with immunoglobulin therapy. N Engl J Med 321:519, 1989.
161. Muir K, Todd WTA, Watson WH, et al. Viral-associated haemophagocytosis with parvovirus B19-related pancytopenia. Lancet 339:1139, 1992.
162. Wong TY, Chan PK, Leung CB, et al. Parvovirus B19 infection causing red cell aplasia in renal transplantation on tacrolimus. Am J Kidney Dis 34:1119, 1999.
163. Geetha D, Zachary JB, Baldado HM, et al. Pure red cell aplasia caused by parvovirus B19 infection in solid organ transplant recipients: a case report and review of the literature. Clin Transplant 14:586, 2000.
164. Pamidi S, Friedman K, Kampalath B, et al. Human parvovirus infection presenting as persistent anemia in renal transplant recipients. Transplantation 69:2666, 2000.
165. Zolnourian ZR, Curran MD, Rima BK, et al. Parvovirus B19 in kidney transplant patients. Transplantation 69:2198, 2000.
166. Seishima M, Kanoh H, Izumi T. The spectrum of cutaneous eruptions in 22 patients with isolated serological evidence of infection by parvovirus B19. Arch Dermatol 135:1556, 1999.
167. Lefrere JJ, Courouce AM, Bertrand Y, et al. Human parvovirus and aplastic crisis in chronic hemolytic anemias: a study of 24 observations. Am J Hematol 23:271, 1986.
168. Finkel TH, Torok TJ, Ferguson PJ, et al. Chronic parvovirus B19 infection and systemic necrotising vasculitis: opportunistic infection or aetiological agent? Lancet 343:1255, 1994.
169. Schwarz TF, Wiersbitzky S, Pambor M. Case report: detection of parvovirus B19 in skin biopsy of a patient with erythema infectiosum. J Med Virol 43:171, 1994.
170. Magro CM, Dawood MR, Crowson AN. The cutaneous manifestations of human parvovirus B19 infection. Hum Pathol 31:488, 2000.
171. Ferguson PJ, Saulsbury FT, Dowell SF, et al. Prevalence of human parvovirus B19 infection in children with Henoch-Schönlein purpura. Arthritis Rheum 39:880, 1996.
172. Smith PT, Landry ML, Carey H, et al. Papular-purpuric gloves and socks syndrome associated with acute parvovirus B19 infection: case report and review. Clin Infect Dis 27:164, 1997.
173. Grilli R, Izquierdo MJ, Farina MC, et al. Papular-purpuric "gloves and socks" syndrome: polymerase chain reaction demonstration of parvovirus B19 DNA in cutaneous lesions and sera. J Am Acad Dermatol 41:793, 1999.
174. Saulsbury FT. Petechial gloves and socks syndrome caused by parvovirus B19. Pediatr Dermatol 15:35, 1998.
175. Brass C, Elliott LM, Stevens DA. Academy rash. A probable epidemic of erythema infectiosum ("fifth disease"). JAMA 248:568, 1982.
176. Tsuji A, Uchida N, Asamura S, et al. Aseptic meningitis with erythema infectiosum. Eur J Pediatr 149:449, 1990.
177. Balfour HH Jr, Schiff GM, Bloom JE. Encephalitis associated with erythema infectiosum. JAMA 77:133, 1970.
178. Hall CB, Horner FA. Encephalopathy with erythema infectiosum. Am J Dis Child 131:65, 1977.
179. Okumura A, Ichikawa T. Aseptic meningitis caused by human parvovirus B19. Arch Dis Child 68:784, 1993.
180. Cassinotti P, Schultze D, Schlageter P, et al. Persistent human parvovirus B19 infection following an acute infection with meningitis in an immunocompetent patient. Eur J Clin Microbiol Infect Dis 12:701, 1993.
181. Watanabe T, Satoh M, Oda Y. Human parvovirus B19 encephalopathy. Arch Dis Child 70:71, 1994.
182. Walsh KJ, Armstrong RD, Turner AM. Brachial plexus neuropathy associated with human parvovirus infection. Br Med J 296:896, 1988.

183. Faden H, Gary GW Jr, Korman M. Numbness and tingling of fingers associated with parvovirus B19 infection. J Infect Dis 161:354, 1990.
184. Dereure O, Montes B, Guilhou JJ. Acute generalized livedo reticularis with myasthenia-like syndrome revealing parvovirus B19 primary infection. Arch Dermatol 131:744, 1995.
185. Samii K, Cassinotti P, de Freudenreich J, et al. Acute bilateral carpal tunnel syndrome associated with human parvovirus B19 infection. Clin Infect Dis 22:162, 1996.
186. Faden H, Gary GW Jr, Anderson LJ. Chronic parvovirus infection in a presumably immunologically healthy woman. Clin Infect Dis 15:595, 1992.
187. Barah F, Vallely PJ, Cleator GM, Kerr JR. Neurological manifestations of human parvovirus B19 infection. Rev Med Virol 13:185, 2003.
188. Nakazawa T, Tomosugi N, Sakamoto K, et al. Acute glomerulonephritis after human parvovirus B19 infection. Am J Kidney Dis 35:E31, 2000.
189. Komatsuda A, Ohtani H, Nimura T, et al. Endocapillary proliferative glomerulonephritis in a patient with parvovirus B19 infection. Am J Kidney Dis 36:851, 2000.
190. Diaz F, Collazos J. Glomerulonephritis and Henoch-Schönlein purpura associated with acute parvovirus B19 infection. Clin Nephrol 53:237, 2000.
191. Tanawattanacharoen S, Falk RJ, Jennette JC, Kopp JB. Parvovirus B19 DNA in kidney tissue of patients with focal segmental glomerulosclerosis. Am J Kidney Dis 35:1166, 2000.
192. Anderson LJ, Tsou C, Parker RA, et al. Detection of antibodies and antigens of human parvovirus B19 by enzyme-linked immunosorbent assay. J Clin Microbiol 24:522, 1986.
193. Cohen BJ, Bates CM. Evaluation of 4 commercial test kits for parvovirus B19-specific IgM. J Virol Methods 55:11, 1995.
194. Koch WC. A synthetic parvovirus B19 capsid protein can replace viral antigen in antibody-capture enzyme immunoassays. J Virol Methods 55:67, 1995.
195. Jordan JA. Comparison of a baculovirus-based VP2 enzyme immunoassay (EIA) to an *Escherichia coli*-based VP1 EIA for detection of human parvovirus B19 immunoglobulin M and immunoglobulin G in sera of pregnant women. J Clin Microbiol 38:1472, 2000.
196. Doyle S, Kerr S, O'Keeffe G, et al. Detection of parvovirus B19 IgM by antibody capture enzyme immunoassay: receiver operating characteristics analysis. J Virol Methods 90:143, 2000.
197. Clewly JP. Detection of human parvovirus using a molecularly cloned probe. J Med Virol 15:383, 1985.
198. Clewly JP. Polymerase chain reaction assay of parvovirus B19 DNA in clinical specimens. J Clin Microbiol 27:2647, 1989.
199. Koch WC, Adler SP. Detection of human parvovirus B19 DNA by using the polymerase chain reaction. J Clin Microbiol 28:65, 1990.
200. Heegard ED, Hasle H, Clausen N, et al. Parvovirus B19 infection and Diamond-Blackfan anemia. Acta Pediatr 85:299, 1996.
201. Crook TW, Rogers BB, McFarland RD, et al. Unusual bone marrow manifestations of parvovirus B19 infection in immunocompromised patients. Hum Pathol 31:161, 2000.
202. Adler SP, Harger JH, Koch WC. Infections due to human parvovirus B19 during pregnancy. M Martens, S Faro, D Soper (eds). Infectious Diseases in Women. Philadelphia, WB Saunders, 2001, pp 100-115.
203. Schoub BD, Blackburn NK, Johnson S, et al. Primary and secondary infection with human parvovirus B19 in pregnant women in South Africa. South Afr Med J 83:505, 1993.
204. Skjoldebrand-Sparre L, Fridell E, Nyman M, Wahren B. A prospective study of antibodies against parvovirus B19 in pregnancy. Acta Obstet Gynecol Scand 75:336, 1996.
205. Mortimer PP, Cohen BJ, Buckley MM, et al. Human parvovirus and the fetus. Letter. Lancet 2:1012, 1985.
206. Wiersbitzky S, Schwarz TF, Bruns R, et al. Seroprävalenz von Antikörpern gegen das humane parvovirus B19 (Ringelröteln/erythema infectiosum) in der DDR-Bevölkerung. Kinderarztl Prax 58:185, 1990.
207. Barros de Freitas R, Buarque de Gusmao SR, Durigon EL, Linhares AC. Survey of parvovirus B19 infection in a cohort of pregnant women in Belem, Brazil. Braz J Infect Dis 3:6, 1999.
208. Enders G, Biber M. Parvovirus B19 infections in pregnancy. Behring Inst Mitt 85:74, 1990.
209. Rogers BB, Singer DB, Mak SK, et al. Detection of human parvovirus B19 in early spontaneous abortuses using serology, histology, electron microscopy, in situ hybridization, and the polymerase chain reaction. Obstet Gynecol 81:402, 1993.
210. Harger JH, Adler SP, Koch WC, et al. Prospective evaluation of 618 pregnant women exposed to parvovirus B19: risks and symptoms. Obstet Gynecol 91:413, 1998.
211. Kerr JR, Curran MD, Moore JE. Parvovirus B19 infection—persistence and genetic variation. Scand J Infect Dis 27:551, 1995.
212. Schwarz TF, Roggendorf M, Hottentrager B, et al. Human parvovirus B19 infection in pregnancy. Letter. Lancet 2:566, 1988.
213. Gray ES, Anand A, Brown T. Parvovirus infections in pregnancy. Letter. Lancet 1:208, 1986.
214. Brown T, Ritchie LD. Infection with parvovirus during pregnancy. Br Med J 290:559, 1985.
215. Kinney JS, Anderson LJ, Farrar J, et al. Risk of adverse outcomes of pregnancy after human parvovirus B19 infection. J Infect Dis 157:663, 1988.
216. Rodis JF, Quinn DL, Gary GW Jr, et al. Management and outcomes of pregnancies complicated by human B19 parvovirus infection: a prospective study. Am J Obstet Gynecol 163:1168, 1990.
217. Torok TJ, Anderson LJ, Gary GW, et al. Reproductive outcomes following human parvovirus B19 infection in pregnancy. Program and Abstracts of 31st Interscience Conference on Antimicrobial Agents and Chemotherapy (ICAAC), Chicago. Washington, DC, American Society for Microbiology, 1991, p 328 (abstract 1374).
218. Xu D, Zhang G, Wang R. The study on detection of human parvovirus B19 DNA in spontaneous abortion tissues. Zhonghua Shi Yan He Lin Chuang Bing Du Xue Za Zhi 12:158, 1998.
219. Wang R, Chen X, Han M. Relationship between human parvovirus B19 infection and spontaneous abortion. Zhonghua Fu Chan Ke Za Zhi 32:541, 1997.
220. De Krijger RR, van Elsacker-Niele AM, Mulder-Staple A, et al. Detection of parvovirus B19 infection in first and second trimester fetal loss. Pediatr Pathol Lab Med 18:23, 1998.
221. Makhseed M, Pacsa A, Ahmed MA, Essa SS. Pattern of parvovirus B19 infection during different trimesters of pregnancy in Kuwait. Infect Dis Obstet Gynecol 7:287, 1997.
222. Lowden E, Weinstein L. Unexpected second trimester pregnancy loss due to maternal parvovirus B19 infection. South Med J 90:702, 1997.
223. Skjoldebrand-Sparre L, Tolfvenstam T, Papadogiannakis N, et al. Parvovirus B19 infection: association with third-trimester intrauterine fetal death. BJOG 107:476, 2000.
224. Nunoue T, Kusuhara K, Hara T. Human fetal infection with parvovirus B19: maternal infection time in gestation, viral persistence and fetal prognosis. Pediatr Infect Dis J 21:1133, 2002.
225. Norbeck O, Papadogiannakis N, Petersson K, et al. Revised clinical presentation of parvovirus B19-associated intrauterine fetal death. Clin Infect Dis 35:1032, 2002.
226. Tolfvenstam T, Papadogiannakis N, Norbeck O, et al. Frequency of human parvovirus B19 infection in intrauterine fetal death. Lancet 357:1494, 2001.
227. Koch WC, Adler SP, Harger J. Intrauterine parvovirus B19 infection may cause an asymptomatic or recurrent postnatal infection. Pediatr Infect Dis J 12:747, 1993.
228. Weiland HT, Vermey-Keers C, Salimans MM, et al. Parvovirus B19 associated with fetal abnormality. Letter. Lancet 1:682, 1987.
229. Hartwig NG, Vermeij-Keers C, Van Elsacker-Niele AMW, Gleuren GJ. Embryonic malformations in a case of intrauterine parvovirus B19 infection. Teratology 39:295, 1989.
230. Hartwig NG, Vermeij-Keers C, Versteeg J. The anterior eye segment in virus induced primary congenital aphakia. Acta Morphol Neerl Scand 26:283, 1988-1989.
231. Zerbini M, Musiani M, Gentilomi G, et al. Symptomatic parvovirus B19 infection of one fetus in a twin pregnancy. Clin Infect Dis 17:262, 1993.
232. Morey AL, Keeling JW, Porter HJ, Fleming KA. Clinical and histopathological features of parvovirus B19 infection in the human fetus. Br J Obstet Gynaecol 99:566, 1992.
233. Rodis JF, Hovick TJ Jr, Quinn DL, et al. Human parvovirus infection in pregnancy. Obstet Gynecol 72:733, 1988.
234. Naides SJ, Weiner CP. Antenatal diagnosis and palliative treatment of non-immune hydrops fetalis secondary to fetal parvovirus B19 infection. Prenat Diagn 9:105, 1989.
235. Katz VL, Chescheir NC, Bethea M. Hydrops fetalis from B19 parvovirus infection. J Perinatol 10:366, 1990.
236. Bloom MC, Rolland M, Bernard JD, et al. Infection materno-foetale à parvovirus associée à une péritonite meconiale anétnatale. Arch Fr Pediatr 47:437, 1990.
237. Bernard JD, Berrebi A, Sarramon MF, et al. Infection materno-foetale à parvovirus humain B19: a propos de deux observations. J Gynecol Obstet Biol Reprod 20:855, 1991.

238. Schwarz TF, Nerlich A, Hottenträger B, et al. Parvovirus B19 infection of the fetus: histology and in situ hybridization. Am J Clin Pathol 96:121, 1991.
239. Conry JA, Török T, Andrews PI. Perinatal encephalopathy secondary to in utero human parvovirus B-19 (HPV) infection. Neurology 43(Suppl):A346, 1993 (abstract 736S).
240. Török TT. Human parvovirus B19. *In* Remington J, Klein J (eds). Infectious Diseases of the Fetus and Newborn Infant, 5th ed. Philadelphia, WB Saunders, 2001, pp 779-811.
241. Katz VL, McCoy MC, Kuller JA, Hansen WF. An association between fetal parvovirus B19 infection and fetal anomalies: a report of two cases. Am J Perinatol 13:43, 1996.
242. Rodis JF, Rodner C, Hansen AA, et al. Long-term outcome of children following maternal human parvovirus B19 infection. Obstet Gynecol 91:125, 1998.
243. Porter HJ, Khong TY, Evans MF, et al. Parvovirus as a cause of hydrops fetalis: detection by in situ DNA hybridisation. J Clin Pathol 41:381, 1988.
244. Yaegashi N, Okamura K, Yajima A, et al. The frequency of human parvovirus B19 infection in nonimmune hydrops fetalis. J Perinat Med 22:159, 1994.
245. Gloning KP, Schramm T, Brusis E, et al. Successful intrauterine treatment of fetal hydrops caused by parvovirus B19 infection. Behring Inst Mitt 85:79, 1990.
246. Rogers BB, Mark Y, Oyer CE. Diagnosis and incidence of fetal parvovirus infection in an autopsy series. I. Histology. Pediatr Pathol 13:371, 1993.
247. Mark Y, Rogers BB, Oyer CE. Diagnosis and incidence of fetal parvovirus infection in an autopsy series. II. DNA amplification. Pediatr Pathol 13:381, 1993.
248. Peters MT, Nicolaides KH. Cordocentesis for the diagnosis and treatment of human fetal parvovirus infection. Obstet Gynecol 75:501, 1990.
249. Pryde PG, Nugent CE, Pridjian G, et al. Spontaneous resolution of nonimmune hydrops fetalis secondary to human parvovirus B19 infection. Obstet Gynecol 79:859, 1992.
250. Metzman R, Anand A, DeGiulio PA, Knisely AS. Hepatic disease associated with intrauterine parvovirus B19 infection in a newborn premature infant. J Pediatr Gastroenterol Nutr 9:112, 1989.
251. Franciosi RA, Tattersall P. Fetal infection with human parvovirus B19. Hum Pathol 19:489, 1988.
252. Zerbini M, Musiani M, Gentilomi G, et al. Comparative evaluation of virological and serological methods in prenatal diagnosis of parvovirus B19 fetal hydrops. J Clin Microbiol 34:603, 1996.
253. Lewis DB, Wilson CB. Developmental immunology and role of host defenses in neonatal susceptibility to infection. *In* Remington JS, Klein JO (eds). Infectious Diseases of the Fetus and Newborn Infant, 4th ed. Philadelphia, WB Saunders, 1995, pp 20-98.
254. Török TJ, Wang Q-Y, Gary GW Jr, et al. Prenatal diagnosis of intrauterine infection with parvovirus B19 by the polymerase chain reaction technique. Clin Infect Dis 14:149, 1992.
255. Morey AL, Patou G, Myint S, Fleming KA. In vitro culture for the detection of infectious human parvovirus B19 and B19-specific antibodies using foetal haematopoietic precursor cells. J Gen Virol 73:3313, 1992.
256. Porter HJ, Quantrill AM, Fleming KA. B19 parvovirus infection of myocardial cells Letter. Lancet 1:535, 1988.
257. Carrington D, Gilmore DH, Whittle MJ, et al. Maternal serum alpha-fetoprotein—a marker of fetal aplastic crisis during intrauterine human parvovirus infection. Lancet 1:433, 1987.
258. Anderson MJ, Khousam MN, Maxwell DJ, et al. Human parvovirus B19 and hydrops fetalis. Letter. Lancet 1:535, 1988.
259. Sahakian V, Weiner CP, Naides SJ, et al. Intrauterine transfusion treatment of nonimmune hydrops fetalis secondary to human parvovirus B19 infection. Am J Obstet Gynecol 164:1090, 1991.
260. Nerlich AG, Schwarz TF, Hillemanns P, et al. Pathomorphologie der fetalen parvovirus-B19-infektion. Pathologe 12:204, 1991.
261. Berry PJ, Gray ES, Porter HJ, Burton BA. Parvovirus infection of the human fetus and newborn. Semin Diagn Pathol 9:4, 1992.
262. Caul EO, Usher MJ, Burton PA. Intrauterine infection with human parvovirus B19: a light and electron microscopy study. J Med Virol 24:55, 1988.
263. Maeda H, Shimokawa H, Satoh S, et al. Nonimmunologic hydrops fetalis resulting from intrauterine human parvovirus B-19 infection: report of two cases. Obstet Gynecol 72:482, 1988.
264. van Elsacker-Niele AMW, Salimans MMM, Weiland HT, et al. Fetal pathology in human parvovirus B19 infection. Br J Obstet Gynaecol 96:768, 1989.
265. Bonneau D, Berthier M, Maréchaud M, et al. L'infection à parvovirus B19 au cours de la grossesse. J Gynecol Obstet Biol Reprod 20:1109, 1991.
266. Glaser C, Tannenbaum J. Newborn with hydrops and a rash. Pediatr Infect Dis J 11:980, 984, 1992.
267. Nerlich A, Schwarz TF, Roggendorf M, et al. Parvovirus B19-infected erythroblasts in fetal cord blood. Letter. Lancet 337:310, 1991.
268. Morey AL, Fleming KA. Immunophenotyping of fetal hematopoietic cells permissive for human parvovirus B19 replication in vitro. Br J Haematol 82:302, 1992.
269. Jordan JA. Identification of human parvovirus B19 infection in idiopathic nonimmune hydrops fetalis. Am J Obstet Gynecol 174:37, 1996.
270. Jordan JA, DeLoia JA. Globoside expression within the human placenta. Placenta 20:103, 1999.
271. Jordan JA, Huff D, DeLoia JA. Placental cellular immune response in women infected with human parvovirus B19 during pregnancy. Clin Diagn Lab Immunol 8:288, 2001.
272. Brown KE. Human parvovirus B19 infections in infants and children. Adv Pediatr Infect Dis 13:101, 1998.
273. Heegaard ED, Hornsleth A. Parvovirus: the expanding spectrum of disease. Acta Paediatr 84:109, 1995.
274. Respondek M, Bratosiewicz J, Pertynski T, Liberski PP. Parvovirus particles in a fetal heart with myocarditis: ultrastructural and immunohistochemical study. Arch Immunol Ther Exp (Warsz) 45:465, 1997.
275. Porter HJ, Quantrill AM, Fleming KA. B19 Parvovirus infection of myocardial cells. Lancet 535, 1988.
276. Nigro G, Bastianon V, Colloridil V, et al. Acute and chronic lymphocytic myocarditis in infancy is associated with parvovirus B19 infection and high cytokine levels. Clin Infect Dis 31:65, 2000.
277. Heegaard ED, Eiskjaer H, Baandrup U, Hornsleth A. Parvovirus B19 infection associated with myocarditis following adult cardiac transplantation. Scand J Infect Dis 30:607, 1998.
278. Papadogiannakis N, Tolfvenstam T, Fischler B, et al. Active, fulminant, lethal myocarditis associated with parvovirus B19 infection in an infant. Clin Infect Dis 35:1027, 2002.
279. Kovacs BW, Carlson DE, Shahbahrami B, Platt LD. Prenatal diagnosis of human parvovirus B19 in nonimmune hydrops fetalis by polymerase chain reaction. Am J Obstet Gynecol 167:461, 1992.
280. Wang X, Zhang G, Han M, et al. Investigation of parvovirus B19 in cardiac tissue from patients with congenital heart disease. Chin Med J (Engl) 112:995, 1999.
281. Humphrey W, Magoon M, O'Shaughnessy R. Severe nonimmune hydrops secondary to parvovirus B-19 infection: spontaneous reversal in utero and survival of a term infant. Obstet Gynecol 78:900, 1991.
282. Plachouras N, Stefanidis K, Andronikou S, Lolis D. Severe nonimmune hydrops fetalis and congenital corneal opacification secondary to human parvovirus B19 infection. A case report. J Reprod Med 44:377, 1999.
283. Miyagawa S, Takahashi Y, Nagai A, et al. Angio-oedema in a neonate with IgG antibodies to parvovirus B19 following intrauterine parvovirus B19 infection. Br J Dermatol 143:428, 2000.
284. Sheikh AU, Ernest JM, O'Shea M. Long-term outcome in fetal hydrops from parvovirus B19 infection. Am J Obstet Gynecol 167:337, 1992.
285. Bernstein IA, Capeless EL. Elevated maternal serum alpha-fetoprotein and hydrops fetalis in association with fetal parvovirus B19 infection. Obstet Gynecol 774:456, 1989.
286. Carrington D, Whittle MJ, Gibson AAM, et al. Maternal serum alpha feto-protein: a marker of fetal aplastic crisis during uterine human parvovirus infection. Lancet 1:433, 1987.
287. Komischke K, Searle K, Enders G. Maternal serum alpha-fetoprotein and human chorionic gonadotropin in pregnant women with acute parvovirus B19 infection with and without fetal complications. Prenat Diagn 17:1039, 1997.
288. Dembinski J, Haverkamp F, Maara H, et al. Neurodevelopmental outcome after intrauterine red cell transfusion for parvovirus B19-induced fetal hydrops. Br J Obstet Gynaecol 109:1232, 2002.
289. Kovacs BW, Carlson DE, Shahbahrami B, et al. Prenatal diagnosis of human parvovirus B19 in nonimmune hydrops fetalis by polymerase chain reaction. Am J Obstet Gynecol 167:461, 1992.
290. Humphrey W, Magoon M, O'Shaughnessy R. Severe nonimmune hydrops secondary to parvovirus B-19 infection: spontaneous reversal in utero and survival of a term infant. Obstet Gynecol 78:900, 1991.
291. Morey AL, Nicolini U, Welch CR, et al. Parvovirus B19 infection and transient fetal ascites. Lancet 337:496, 1991.
292. Schwartz TF, Roggendorf M, Hottentrager B, et al. Human parvovirus B19 infection in pregnancy. Lancet 2:566, 1988.

293. Soothill P. Intrauterine blood transfusion for non-immune hydrops fetalis due to parvovirus B19 infection. Lancet 356:121, 1990.
294. Sahakian V, Weiner CP, Naides SJ, et al. Intrauterine transfusion treatment of nonimmune hydrops fetalis secondary to human parvovirus B19 infection. Amer J Obstet Gynecol 164:1090, 1991.
295. Vogel H, Kornman M, Ledet SC, et al. Congenital parvovirus infection. Pediatr Pathol Lab Med 17:903, 1997.
296. Miller E, Fairley CK, Cohen BJ, Seng C. Immediate and long term outcome of human parvovirus B19 infection in pregnancy. Br J Obstet Gynaecol 105:14, 1998.
297. Ballou WR, Reed JL, Noble W, et al. Safety and immunogenicity of a recombinant parvovirus B19 vaccine formulated with MF59C.1. J Infect Dis 187:675, 2003.
298. Bond PR, Caul EO, Usher I, et al. Intrauterine infection with human parvovirus. Letter. Lancet 1:448, 1986.
299. Woernle CH, Anderson LJ, Tattersall P, et al. Human parvovirus B19 infection during pregnancy. J Infect Dis 156:17, 1987.
300. Maeda H, Shimokawa H, Satoh S, et al. Nonimmunologic hydrops fetalis resulting from intrauterine human parvovirus B19 infection: report of 2 cases. Obstet Gynecol 71:482, 1988.
301. Samra JS, Obhrai MS, Constantine G. Parvovirus infection in pregnancy. Obstet Gynecol 73:832, 1989.
302. Mortimer PP, Cohen BJ, Buckley MM, et al. Human parvovirus and the fetus. Lancet 2:1012, 1985.
303. Weiner CP, Naides SJ. Fetal survival after human parvovirus B19 infection: spectrum of intrauterine response in a twin gestation. Am J Perinatol 9:66, 1992.

Chapter 28

RUBELLA

Louis Z. Cooper • Charles A. Alford, Jr.

The impact of rubella virus infection and the progress made toward controlling congenital rubella infection have been well chronicled.[1-9] Rubella was first recognized in the mid-18th century as a clinical entity by German researchers, who called it *Rötheln*. However, they considered it to be a modified form of measles or scarlet fever.[1] Manton[10] first described it as a separate disease in the English literature in 1815. In 1866, Veale[11] gave it a "short and euphonious" name, *rubella*. The disease was considered mild and self-limited.

Rubella became a focus of major interest in 1941, only after Gregg, [12] an Australian ophthalmologist, associated intrauterine acquisition of infection with production of cataracts and heart disease. Although his findings were initially doubted, numerous reports of infants with congenital defects after maternal rubella infection soon appeared in the literature.[1] Subsequent investigations showed that the major defects associated with congenital rubella infection included congenital heart disease, cataracts, and deafness. Mental retardation and many defects involving almost every organ have also been reported.[2-4,7,13,14] Before the availability of specific viral diagnostic studies, the frequency of fetal damage after maternal infection in the first trimester was estimated to be in excess of 20%, a figure now known to be much too low.

Recognition of the teratogenic potential of rubella infection led to increased efforts to isolate the etiologic agent. The viral cause of rubella was suggested by experimental infections in humans and monkeys as early as 1938 but was not confirmed until reports of the isolation of the viral agent in cell cultures were made independently in 1962 by Weller and Neva at Harvard University School of Public Health and by Parkman, Buescher, and Artenstein at Walter Reed Army Institute for Research.[15-20] This accomplishment paved the way for the development of serologic tests and a vaccine.[2-4,21-23] Efforts to develop a vaccine were hastened by the tragic events associated with a worldwide rubella pandemic from 1962 through 1964, which in the United States resulted in approximately 12.5 million cases of clinically acquired rubella, 11,000 fetal deaths, and 20,000 infants born with defects collectively referred to as the congenital rubella syndrome; 2100 infants with congenital rubella syndrome died in the neonatal period.[24] The estimated cost to the U.S. economy was approximately $2 billion. Routine use of rubella vaccine, in a two-dose schedule as measles-mumps-rubella vaccine (MMR) has not prevented importation-related infection, but it has eliminated indigenous rubella in the United States (personal communication from the CDC, 2004). However, congenital rubella syndrome remains a problem in many countries, with current estimates of 100,000 new cases annually.[25]

In 1969, three strains of live-attenuated rubella vaccine were licensed in various countries: HPV-77 (high-passage virus, 77 times), grown in duck embryo for five passages (DE-5) or dog kidney for 12 passages (DK-12); Cendehill, grown in primary rabbit cells; and RA 27/3 (rubella abortus, 27th specimen, third explant), grown in human diploid fibroblast culture.[26-28] Although these and other strains of vaccine are now used globally, the RA 27/3 vaccine has been used exclusively in the United States since 1979.[2-4,7,29]

In addition to providing the impetus for vaccine research and development, the rubella pandemic provided the scientific community with a unique opportunity to gain knowledge about the nature of intrauterine and extrauterine infections and the immunity stimulated by both. The quest for more knowledge using the tools of molecular biology has continued since vaccine licensure and serves as a tribute to Gregg's historic contribution to our understanding of intrauterine infection.

Much interest has focused on the epidemiology of rubella and congenital rubella syndrome in countries with immunization programs, the desirability of introducing vaccine in countries without a program, and the optimal strategy to control congenital rubella (i.e., universal immunization versus selective immunization of females).[3,5-7,30-35] Vaccination of all children and of susceptible adolescents and young adults, particularly females, has had such a dramatic impact on the occurrence of rubella and congenital rubella in the United States that efforts are now in progress to eliminate congenital rubella syndrome from the United States.[5,24,31,36] Given the magnitude of international travel, this goal will remain elusive until similar goals are adopted by other countries. The Pan American Health Organization (PAHO) has adopted a resolution calling on all countries of the Western Hemisphere to eliminate rubella by 2010.[37] However, among developing countries, rubella immunization has not yet been given priority.

Duration and quality of vaccine-induced immunity[5,8,38-57] and adverse events associated with immunization, particularly arthritis and the risk of the vaccine to the fetus,[5,8,58-65] have been a concern, but the vaccine continues to confer long-lasting immunity while placing the vaccinated person at minimal risk of adverse events. Success in eliminating indigenous disease in the United States and the absence of teratogenicity observed after massive immunization programs (2001-2002) in Latin America offer considerable assurance about the long-term efficacy and safety of rubella vaccine. In Brazil, where 28 million women were immunized in mass campaigns, and in Costa Rica, more than 2400 susceptible pregnant women were immunized. Although infants were infected, none had evidence of congenital rubella syndrome.

Research on the characteristics of the rubella virus, its effect on the developing fetus, the host's immune response, and diagnostic methodology has yielded new information about the structural proteins of the virus and about the difference in the immune response to these proteins after congenital and acquired infections.[66-86] Differences in antibody profile may be useful in diagnosing congenital infection retrospectively and may provide further information on the pathogenesis of congenital infection.[64,85,87] Techniques that detect rubella-specific antibodies within minutes have been developed by using latex agglutination and passive hemagglutination.[88-94] Studies to examine the subclass distribution of immunoglobulin G (IgG) and the kinetics of rubella-specific immunoglobulins (including IgA, IgD, and IgE) after acquired rubella, congenital infection, and vaccination may eventually lead to the development of additional diagnostic tools.[95-99] In particular, rubella IgG avidity testing can be helpful in distinguishing between recently acquired and remote infection.[100-102]

Improved laboratory methods defined the risk of fetal infection and congenital damage in all stages of pregnancy.[103-110] The risk of fetal infection after first-trimester maternal infection and subsequent congenital anomalies after fetal infection may be higher than previously reported (81% and 85%, respectively, in one study).[105] The fetus may be at risk of infection throughout pregnancy, even near term, although the occurrence of defects after infection beyond 16 to 18 weeks' gestation is small. Sensitive laboratory assays have shown that subclinical reinfection after previous natural infection, as after vaccination, may be accompanied by an IgM response, making differentiation between subclinical reinfection and asymptomatic primary infection at times difficult.[41,51,53,55] IgG avidity testing may be helpful also in this situation. Although reinfection usually poses no threat to the fetus, rare instances of congenital infection after maternal reinfection have been reported.[41,43,45,47,51-53,55,111-116]

Follow-up of patients with congenital rubella has provided information about the pathogenesis, immune status, interplay between congenital infection, and human leukocyte antigen (HLA) haplotypes and the long-term outcome associated with congenital infection.[117-134] These studies have documented that congenital infection is persistent, that virtually every organ may be affected, and that autoimmunity and immune complex formation are probably involved in many of the disease processes, particularly in the delayed and persistent clinical manifestations. They also confirm earlier studies, noting an increased risk of diabetes mellitus and other endocrinopathies in patients with congenital rubella syndrome compared with rates for the general population.

THE VIRUS

Morphology and Physical and Chemical Composition

Rubella virus is a generally spherical particle, 50 to 70 nm in diameter, with a dense central nucleoid measuring 30 nm in diameter. The central nucleoid is surrounded by a 10-nm-thick, single-layered envelope acquired during budding of the virus into cytoplasmic vesicles or through the plasma membrane.[135-149] Surface projections or spikes with knobbed ends that are 5 to 6 nm long have been reported. The specific gravity of the complete viral particle is 1.184 ± 0.004 g/mL, corresponding to a sedimentation constant of 360 ± 50 Svedberg units.[135]

The wild-type virus contains infectious RNA (molecular weight of 3 to 4 × 10^6) within its core.[120] The rubella virus envelope contains lipids that differ quantitatively from those of the plasma membrane and are essential for infectivity.[150,151] Rubella virus is heat labile and has a half-life of 1 hour at 57° C.[152] However, in the presence of protein (e.g., 2% serum albumin), infectivity is maintained for a week or more at 4° C and indefinitely at −60° C. Storage at freezer temperatures of −10° C to −20° C should be avoided because infectivity is rapidly lost.[152,153] Rubella virus can also be stabilized against heat inactivation by the addition of magnesium sulfate to virus suspensions.[154] Specimens to be examined virologically should be transported to distant laboratories packed in ice rather than frozen, with the addition of stabilizer if possible. Infectivity is rapidly lost at pH levels below 6.8 or above 8.1 and exhausted in the presence of ultraviolet light, lipid-active solvents, or other chemicals such as formalin, ethylene oxide, and β-propiolactone.[152,155-157] Infectivity of rubella in cell culture is inhibited by amantadine, but the drug appears to have no therapeutic effect.[158-161]

Several laboratories have described the structural proteins of rubella virus and determined the nucleotide sequence of the genes coding for these proteins.[66,81,135,162-165] Originally, three structural proteins were identified and designated as VP-1, VP-2, and VP-3.[162] These three major structural proteins now are designated E1, E2, and C, with relative molecular weights of 58,000, 42,000 to 47,000, and 33,000, respectively.[67-69] E1 and E2 are envelope glycoproteins and make up the characteristic spikelike projections that are located on the viral membrane. Structural protein C, which is not glycosylated, is associated with the infectious 40S genomic RNA to form the nucleocapsid.[71] The E2 glycopeptide has been shown on polyacrylamide gels to be heterogeneous with two bands, which are designated E2a (relative molecular weight of 42,000) and E2b (relative molecular weight of 47,000).[67]

Monoclonal antibody studies have begun to delineate the functional activities of these structural proteins. E1 appears to be the viral hemagglutinin and binds hemagglutination-inhibiting and hemolysis-inhibiting antibody; E2 does not appear to be involved in hemagglutination.[66,68,70,72-75] Monoclonal antibodies specific for E1 and E2 have neutralizing activity.[66,70,76,85,86] Studies also indicate that there are multiple epitopes on the structural proteins that are involved in hemagglutination inhibition (HI) and neutralizing activities.[75,78] Molecular analyses of rubella viruses isolated during the period of 1961 to 1997 from specimens obtained in North America, Europe, and Asia have documented the remarkable antigenic stability of the E1 envelope glycoprotein.[80] E1 amino acid sequences have differed by no more than 3%, indicating no major antigenic variation over the 36-year period that spanned the major worldwide pandemic of 1962 to 1964 and the 30 years since introduction of rubella vaccine. However, two genotypes were evident: genotype I isolated before 1970 grouped into a single diffuse clade, indicating intercontinental circulation, whereas most of the post-1975 viruses segregated into geographic clades from each continent, indicating evolution in response to vaccination programs. The availability of molecular analysis and the minor variations in amino acid sequences have provided an additional tool for monitoring the sources of infection in areas where indigenous rubella has been greatly reduced by high levels of immunization. As discussed in more detail later, the complexity of the antigenic nature of the rubella virion affects the ability of the host to respond to the full complement of antigens and affects the various antibody assays required to detect all the corresponding antibody responses (see "Natural History").

Classification

Rubella has been classified as a member of the togavirus family (from the Latin word *toga*, meaning "cloak"), genus Rubivirus.[166,167] No serologic relationship exists between rubella and other known viruses. Minor biologic differences identified in different passaged strains of rubella virus are not reflected in the antigenic differences assessed by comparing protein composition or serologic reactions.[135,165,168,169] Differences in the immune response after immunization with the various vaccines now in use are not caused by inherent differences in the viral strain but rather by modification of the viruses during their attenuation in cell culture.[29] The reported variation in the virulence of rubella epidemics does not appear to be explained by the molecular analyses described earlier, but it may result from differences in population susceptibility and underreporting of cases of congenital rubella.[170-177]

Antigen and Serologic Testing

Purified rubella virus has a number of antigenic components associated with the viral envelope and the ribonucleoprotein core.[157,163] These antigens and the ability of specific antiserum to neutralize virus form the basis for the wide variety of serologic methods available to measure humoral immunity after natural and vaccine-induced infection.

The ability of antibodies to inhibit agglutination of erythrocytes by the surface hemagglutinin (HA antigen) forms the basis for the HI test, which at one time was the most popular rubella serologic test. The HA antigen was originally prepared from BHK tissue culture fluids and then from alkaline extracts of infected BHK-21 cells.[23,178] This antigen can agglutinate a variety of red blood cells, including newborn chick, adult goose, pigeon, and human group O erythrocytes.[179] Rubella hemagglutinin is unique in its dependency on calcium ions to attach to red blood cell receptors.[179,180] After extraction from infected cells, rubella hemagglutinin is stable for months at −20° C, several weeks at 4° C, and overnight at 37° C but is destroyed within minutes after heating to 56° C.[178,180] The HA antigen can be protected from ether inactivation by pretreatment with Tween 80. Cells and serum contain heat-stable beta-lipoproteins that can inhibit rubella hemagglutination and give rise to false-positive results.[23,157] Although it has been reported that nonspecific inhibitors do not interfere in the HI test if the HA antigen and erythrocytes are mixed before addition of serum, the recommended method is to pretreat the sera to remove these inhibitors.[157,181] Earlier test procedures used kaolin adsorption for removal of these nonspecific inhibitors; however, a number of faster and more specific methods are now used, such as treatment with heparin-$MnCl_2$ or dextran sulfate–$CaCl$.[182,183]

Cell-associated complement fixation antigen was first derived from infected rabbit kidney (RK-13) and African green monkey kidney cell cultures and later prepared from alkaline extracts of infected BHK-21 cells.[22,184] There are two complement fixation antigens—one is similar in size and weight to the hemagglutinin and infectious virus, and the other is smaller and "soluble."[185-187] The antibody response as measured by the soluble antigen develops more slowly than that to the larger antigen, which parallels the HI response. In contrast to the HA antigen, complement fixation antigens do not lose their antigenicity after either treatment.[184,186]

A variety of precipitin antigens have been serologically demonstrated; two of these, the theta and iota antigens, are associated with the viral envelope and core, respectively.[188-190] The antibody response to these two antigens is of interest. Antibodies to the theta antigen rise promptly and persist. Antibodies to the iota antigen are detectable later and for a shorter time.[191] The RA 27/3 vaccine appears to be unique among vaccine strains in its ability to elicit a response to the iota antigen, making its immune response more like natural infection. The significance of this observation remains unclear.[192]

Rubella virus antigen-antibody complexes (involving the envelope and the core antigens) cause aggregation of platelets.[193,194] However, the main platelet aggregation activity appears to reside with the viral envelope.

Antibody directed against the rubella virus can also be measured by virus neutralization in tissue culture.[2-4,21,195-197]

Whereas the presence of neutralizing antibodies correlates best with protective immunity, neutralization assays are time consuming, expensive, and relatively difficult to perform. Laboratories have traditionally performed the complement fixation and HI tests. Because the complement fixation test is insensitive for screening purposes and cannot detect an early rise in antibody in acute acquired infection, the HI test has been the most widely used assay.[2-4,157,191,195,198,199]

However, a number of more rapid, easily performed, reliable, and sensitive tests have replaced the HI test for routine use.[88,199,200] These include passive (or indirect) hemagglutination; single radial hemolysis (also known as hemolysis in gel), which is used widely abroad; radioimmunoassay; immunofluorescence; and enzyme immunoassay tests, also referred to as enzyme-linked immunosorbent assays.[195,198-229] Rapid latex agglutination and passive hemagglutination assays can provide results in minutes for screening and diagnostic purposes.[88-94] The large number of assays now available and their greater sensitivity compared with the HI test have led to some confusion about the level of antibody that should be considered indicative of immunity (see "Update on Vaccine Characteristics").[44,54,57,199,227] However, the HI test still remains the reference test against which other assays are compared.

Immunoglobulin class-specific antibody can be measured in most of the serologic systems.[157,206-210,213,215,224-227,230-238] This most frequently involves detection of IgM in whole or fractionated sera. A number of techniques are used to fractionate and then test the serum. An important consideration in any IgM assay is the possibility of false-positive results because of the presence of rheumatoid factor. Solid-phase IgM capture assays, however, appear to be unaffected by rheumatoid factor.[99-102,210,225,236]

Growth in Cell Culture

Rubella replicates in a wide variety of cell culture systems, primary cell strains and cell lines.[153,157,239] The time required for virus recovery varies markedly, depending in part on the culture system being employed.

As a generalization, rubella growing in primary cell cultures (i.e., human, simian, bovine, rabbit, canine, or duck) produces interference to superinfection by a wide variety of viruses (especially enteroviruses, but also myxoviruses, papovaviruses, arboviruses, and to some extent, herpesviruses) but no cytopathic effect.[19,20,152] In contrast, a cytopathic effect of widely varying natures results from infection of continuous cell lines (i.e., hamster, rabbit, simian, and human). Generally, primary cells, especially African green monkey kidney, have proved superior for isolation of virus from human material by the interference technique. However, the continuous RK-13 and Vero (vervet kidney) cell lines are also used because cytopathic effect is produced and there is no problem with adventitious simian agents.[153] Continuous cell lines, such as BHK-21 and Vero, are best suited for antigen production because of the higher levels of virus produced.

All cell lines support chronic infection with serial propagation, but some are limited by the occurrence of cytopathic effect. These cells grow slowly and can be subcultivated fewer times than when not infected.[153] The mechanisms of rubella-induced interference and persistent infection in cell cultures are not completely understood. Although interferon production has been described after rubella infection of cell cultures, interference appears to be an intrinsic phenomenon.[153,157,240-242] As with other viruses, generation of defective interfering particles can be found in tissue culture.[243] However, these particles are thought to be nonessential for persistence.

Rubella virus can be plaqued in RK-13, BHK-21, SIRC (i.e., rabbit cornea), and Vero cells.[157] Plaquing forms the basis of neutralization assays, and differences in plaquing characteristics can be used as markers to differentiate strains.[21,157,169,195-197]

Pathogenicity for Animals

Rubella virus grows in primates and in various small laboratory animals. However, in no animal has the acquired or congenital disease been completely reproduced.

Vervet and particularly rhesus monkeys are susceptible to infection by the intranasal, intravenous, or intramuscular routes.[244-246] Although no rash develops, there is nasopharyngeal excretion of viruses in all of the inoculated monkeys and demonstrable viremia in 50%. Attempts to produce transplacental infection in pregnant monkeys have been partially successful. Rubella virus has been recovered from the amnion and the placenta, but the embryo itself has not been shown to be consistently infected.[247,248]

The ferret is by far the most useful of the small laboratory animals in rubella studies. Ferret kits are highly sensitive to subcutaneous and particularly to intracerebral inoculations. Virus has been recovered from the heart, liver, spleen, lung, brain, eye, blood, and urine for a month or longer after inoculation, and neutralizing and complement fixation antibodies have developed.[249] Ferret kits inoculated at birth develop corneal clouding. Virus appears in fetal ferrets after inoculation of pregnant animals.[250]

Rabbits, hamsters, guinea pigs, rats, and suckling mice have all been infected with rubella virus, but none has proved to be a consistent and reliable animal model system for study of rubella infection.[170,171,251-254] Studies indicating that Japanese strains of rubella virus were less teratogenic to offspring of infected rabbits than U.S. strains have not been confirmed.[170,171] These experiments were conducted to examine further the hypothesis referred to earlier that there is a difference in the virulence among rubella virus strains circulating in Japan and other parts of the world.[168,170-174,176]

EPIDEMIOLOGY

Humans are the only known host for rubella virus. Continuous cycling in humans is the only apparent means for the virus to be maintained in nature. Because rubella is predominantly a self-limited infection seen in late winter and spring, questions have arisen about how the virus persists throughout the remainder of the year. Person-to-person transmission probably occurs at very low levels in the general population throughout summer and winter and probably at much higher levels in closed populations of susceptible individuals.[255-276] Congenitally infected infants can shed virus from multiple sites and can serve as reservoirs of virus during periods of low transmission.[161,277-282] This is of particular concern in the hospital setting.[161,274] Efficiency of transmission may also vary among individuals, with some being better "spreaders" than others. This phenomenon may contribute to continued circulation of the virus.[283]

Rubella remains worldwide in distribution.[284-290] The virus circulates almost continually, at least in continental populations. In the Northern Hemisphere's continental temperate zones, rubella is consistently more prevalent in the spring, with peak attack rates in March, April, and May; infection is much less prevalent during the remainder of the year, increasing or decreasing during the 2 months before or after the peak period.[287,289] Before widespread rubella immunization, sizable epidemics occurred every 6 to 9 years in most of the world, with major ones occurring at intervals ranging from 10 to 30 years. Epidemics usually built up and receded gradually over a 3- to 4-year interval, peaking at the midpoint.[9,284,287,289] The apparent increased infectivity and virulence of rubella as exemplified in the major epidemics have been the subject of considerable speculation. One popular thesis has been the unproven emergence of a more virulent strain of virus at widely separated intervals.[168,170-174,176] However, no convincing evidence exists concerning clinically different strains of rubella, and molecular analysis of the E1 envelope glycoprotein does not support the hypothesis of an epidemic versus endemic strain difference.[80] The apparent severity of the epidemic appears to be related to the number of susceptible adults, especially pregnant women, in any given population at the outset of an epidemic.[175,177,289,291] Host factors, such as the differences in the ability to transmit rubella, and still unknown factors may also be involved.[283,291]

Attack rates in open populations have not been defined precisely for a number of reasons. Because rubella is such a mild disease, it is underreported, even in areas where reporting has been mandatory for years. Mandatory reporting did not begin in the United States until 1966 (Fig. 28-1).[287,292] The high and variable rate of inapparent infection poses a major problem when attempting to interpret the recorded data, which are based usually on clinical findings.[260,293-298]

In childhood, the most common time of infection, 50% or more of serologically confirmed infections result in inapparent illness. The ratio may rise as high as 6:1 or 7:1 in adults, perhaps as a result of silent reinfection in naturally immune individuals who have lost detectable antibody.[260,296] The frequent occurrence of infections that clinically mimic rubella makes it even more difficult to determine attack rates in open populations.[299] Attack rates undoubtedly depend on the number of susceptible individuals, which varies widely in different locations.

Serologic assessments of rubella attack rates have been performed in closed populations, such as military recruits, isolated island groups with small populations, boarding home residents, and household members.[260-262,283,295,298,299-306] In such situations, individual exposure to the virus is more intense than that encountered in open populations. Under these circumstances, 90% to 100% of children and adults who are susceptible may become infected. Attack rates in susceptible persons on college and university campuses and in other community settings range from 50% to 90%.[9,291] Like primary infection, reinfection probably is increased as exposure becomes more intense.[260,296,304,305]

In most of the world, including the United States before the introduction of mass immunization of children in 1969, rubella was typically a childhood disease that was most prevalent in the 5- to 14-year-old age group.[2,3,7,285-292] It was rare in infants younger than 1 year of age. The incidence increased slowly for the first 4 years, rose steeply between 5 and 14 years, peaked around 20 to 24 years, and then leveled off. In developed countries before mass immunization, the incidence of infection did not reach 100% before the ages of 35 to 40 years; 5% to 20% of women of childbearing age remain susceptible to infection.

In the era before a rubella vaccine, in isolated or island populations, such as in Trinidad, some areas of Japan, Panama, rural Peru, and Hawaii, a relatively high rate of susceptibility

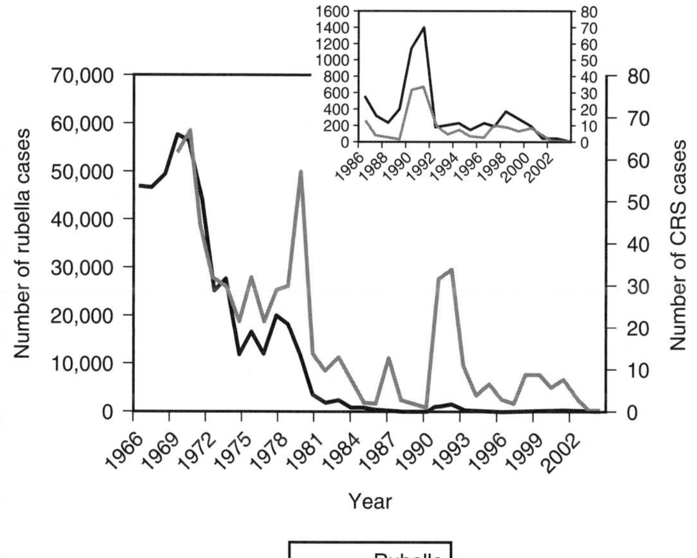

Figure 28–1 Incidence rates for reported cases of rubella and congenital rubella syndrome in the United States from 1966 to 2003. (Data from Centers for Disease Control and Prevention, courtesy of S. Reef, March 1, 2004.)

was found among young adults.[285,286,288,289,302] Between 26% and 70% of women of childbearing age remained susceptible. This situation existed even though rubella was endemic with ample opportunity for multiple introductions of virus from the outside. Low population density, tropical climate, low concentration of effective spreaders, and genetic factors have all been invoked to explain these low attack rates, but none can adequately account for this peculiar epidemiologic phenomenon by itself.[283,288,289,291] Later studies from 45 developing nations where rubella immunization efforts have been minimal have revealed a wide range of susceptibility (≤10% to ≥25%).[303]

In other areas, particularly in South America, infection began earlier in life and peak incidence occurs before puberty.[288] However, infection rates in most South American countries reach a plateau at approximately the same level as that seen in Europe and North America, leaving 10% or more of young women who are susceptible, based on serologic tests. Chile appeared to be an exception, with almost all persons being infected before puberty.[288] The impact of major immunization programs in the PAHO countries to reach a goal of eliminating rubella by 2010 will change these data.

Initial mass vaccination of children, followed by routine vaccination of 1-year-old children and vaccination of susceptible adolescents and adults, has been extremely successful in controlling rubella and congenital rubella syndrome in the United States.[5,24,31,36,258,292] The characteristic 6- to 9-year epidemic cycle has been interrupted, and the reported incidence of rubella that ranged from approximately 200 to 400 cases annually during the period 1992 through 2000 dropped to less than 25 between 2001 and 2004. For comparison, there were approximately 58,000 cases reported in 1969, the year of vaccine licensure in the United States (see Fig. 28-1). Age-specific declines in the occurrence of rubella have been greatest in children, who, because they were the major reservoir of the virus, have been the primary target of the U.S. immunization program. However, the risk of rubella decreased by 99% in all age groups after efforts to increase vaccination levels in older, susceptible persons, especially childbearing-aged females (see "Prevention of Congenital Rubella").[255,257] Nonetheless, serologic surveys continue to document a 10% to 20% susceptibility rate in this population because of less-than-optimal immunization coverage rates.[264,292,307-313]

Adolescents and young adults now account for most reported cases, with more cases reported among those older than age 15 years than in children. Outbreaks are still reported in colleges, hospitals, cruise ships, and other settings in which persons live or work in proximity.[266-268,271-276] Outbreaks no longer occur among military recruits because they receive rubella vaccine as soon as they arrive for basic training.[263] Whereas the reported incidence of cases of congenital rubella syndrome has decreased dramatically, the number of cases of rubella and congenital rubella reported in the United States increased in 1989 to 1991, documenting that the potential for cases will continue as long as children and women of childbearing age remain underimmunized.[36] The outbreak of rubella and congenital rubella among the Amish in Pennsylvania in 1991 and 1992 was a tragic reminder that there are still pockets of susceptible individuals in the United States.[270]

TRANSMISSION IN UTERO

In pregnant women with clinical or inapparent primary rubella, virus infects the placenta during the period of viremia and subsequently infects the fetus.[2,6,284,299,314-329] Intrauterine transmission of virus associated with maternal reinfection is rare. It is presumed that this difference is a reflection that viremia is absent or greatly reduced because of immunity induced by the primary infection (natural or vaccine induced).* Maternal infection may result in no infection of the conceptus, resorption of the embryo (seen only with infections occurring in the earliest stages of gestation), spontaneous abortion, stillbirth, infection of the placenta without fetal involvement, or infection of the placenta and fetus.[6] Infected infants can have obvious multiorgan system involvement or, as is frequently observed, no immediately evident disease.[6,13,107,330-337] However, after long-term follow-up, many of these seemingly unaffected infants have evidence of hearing loss or central nervous system or other defects.[6,13,14,112,131,132,330,331,333-336]

Gestational age at the time of maternal infection is the most important determinant of intrauterine transmission and fetal damage.[2-4,6,284,299,317] The risk of fetal infection and congenital anomalies decreases with increasing gestational age. Fetal damage is rare much beyond the first trimester of pregnancy.

Availability of more sensitive antibody assays has led to refinement of our understanding of the risk of fetal infection and subsequent congenital defects throughout all stages of pregnancy.[103,110] Although the risk of defects does decrease with increasing gestational age, fetal infection can occur at any time during pregnancy. Data on the risk of fetal infection are inconsistent when maternal rubella occurs before conception.[1,12,108,110,338-341] If some risk exists, the risk is small.

Risk of Fetal Infection

Early attempts to define the risk of fetal infection relied on isolation of virus from products of conception.[314-320] Between 40% and 90% of products of conception obtained from women with clinical rubella during the first trimester were found to be infected. The higher rates were observed in serologically confirmed cases of maternal rubella and when improved isolation techniques were employed.[319,320] Attempts were made to refine the risk estimates by evaluating placental and fetal tissue separately. In some of these studies, equal rates of persistent placental and fetal infection were observed, ranging from 80% to 90%.[319,320] In others, persistent placental infection was found to be twice as frequent as fetal infection: 50% to 70% versus 20% to 30%.[314,317] However, high rates of fetal infection accompanied placental infection when specimens obtained during the first 8 weeks of gestation were examined. For example, of 14 cases in which virus was cultured from placental tissue, six of seven fetuses were culture positive when maternal rubella occurred during the first 8 weeks of pregnancy. In contrast, only one of seven fetal specimens was positive when infection occurred between 9 and 14 weeks of gestation.[314] In another similar study, fetal infection rates decreased sharply after the eighth week of

*See references 5, 6, 41, 42, 45, 47, 51-53, 55, 111, 116, 321-359.

Table 28–1 Risk of Serologically Confirmed Congenital Rubella Infection and Associated Defects in Children Exposed to Symptomatic Maternal Rubella Infection, by Weeks of Gestation

Weeks of Gestation	Infection		Defects[a]		Overall Risk of Defects (%)[b]
	No. Tested	*Rate (%)*	*No. Followed*	*Rate (%)*	
<11	10	90 (9)[c]	9	100	90
11-12	6	67 (4)	4	50	33
13-14	18	67 (12)	12	17	11
15-16	36	47 (17)	14	50	24
17-18	33	39 (13)	10		
19-22	59	34 (20)			
23-26	32	25 (8)			
27-30	31	35 (11)	53		
31-36	25	60 (15)			
>36	8	100 (8)			
Total	258[d]	45 (117)	102	20	

[a]Defects in seropositive patients only.
[b]Overall risk of defects = rate of infection × rate of defects.
[c]Numbers in parentheses are number of children infected.
[d]None of 11 infants whose mothers had subclinical rubella were infected.
Adapted from Miller E, Cradock-Watson JE, Pollock TM. Consequences of confirmed maternal rubella at successive stages of pregnancy. Lancet 2:781, 1982, with permission.

gestation, whereas placental infection rates decreased but less rapidly.[317] After the eighth week, placental infection occurred in 36% (8 of 22) and fetal infection occurred in 10% (2 of 20) of cases. Although fetal infection was not documented beyond the 10th week of gestation, placental infections were identified up to the 16th week.

Further data on the risk of fetal infection have been obtained from studies using sensitive laboratory tests to detect congenital infection in children born to mothers with serologically confirmed rubella.[103,110] Because congenital rubella is often subclinical in infants and young children, use of such tests is necessary to assess accurately the risk of congenital infection.[6,103-108,331,333-336] In investigations in which this approach was used, with detection of rubella-specific IgM antibody in sera to document congenital infection, the discrepancy between rates of placental and fetal infection seen in viral isolation studies is less apparent. These studies have provided new information on the events after maternal infection in the second and third trimesters.

In a study involving a total of 273 children (269 of whom had IgM antibody assessment), Miller and colleagues[105] reported that fetal infection after serologically documented symptomatic maternal rubella in the first trimester was, as expected, quite high: 81% (13 of 16), with rates of 90% and 67% for those exposed before 11 weeks and at 11 to 12 weeks, respectively (Table 28-1). Of greater interest is that the infection rate was 39% (70 of 178) after exposure in the second trimester (decreasing steadily from 67% at 13 to 14 weeks to 25% at 23 to 26 weeks) but rose to 53% (34 of 64) with third-trimester infection (with infection rates of 35%, 60%, and 100% during the last 3 months of pregnancy, respectively).

In another investigation of fetal infection after first-trimester maternal rubella infection based on IgM determination, Cradock-Watson and associates[103] found that 32% of 166 children were infected after second-trimester exposure and that a comparable proportion (24% of 100) were infected after infection in the third trimester. The rate of infection increased during the latter stages of gestation after initially decreasing to a low of 12% by the 28th week and was 58% (11 of 19) when maternal infection occurred near term. Even higher rates were observed when persistence of IgG antibody was used as the criterion for congenital infection. The true fetal infection rate probably lies between the rates calculated by using the IgM and persistent IgG data.

In both studies, the fetal infection rate declined between 12 and 28 weeks, suggesting that the placenta may prevent transfer of virus, although not completely.[103] Some of the infections recorded during the last weeks of pregnancy could have been perinatally or postnatally acquired (e.g., by means of exposure to virus in the birth canal or from breast milk), but the available evidence indicates that the placental barrier to infection may be relatively ineffective during the last month, perhaps to the same degree as that seen during the first trimester, and that the fetus is susceptible to infection throughout pregnancy, albeit to various degrees.[342-344]

Risk of Congenital Defects

Estimates of the risk of congenital anomalies in live-born children after fetal infection have been affected by a number of factors. Early retrospective and hospital-based studies led to overestimates of the risk of congenital defects after first-trimester infection (up to 90%).[6,107,291] The risk of abnormalities as determined by prospective studies relying on a clinical diagnosis of maternal rubella varied considerably (10% to 54% overall, with a 10% to 20% risk for major defects recognizable in children up to 3 years old) and tended to underestimate the risk because serologic evaluation of infants was not performed.[107,338,345-349] The proportion of pregnancies electively terminated can affect observed malformation rates. The fact that fetal infection can occur during all stages of pregnancy also influences assessments of the risk of congenital defects.

Because most infants born with congenital rubella who were exposed after the 12th week of gestation do not have grossly apparent defects, long-term follow-up is necessary to detect subtle, late-appearing abnormalities, such as deafness and mental impairment.[6,13,14,112,131,132,330,331,333-336] This is especially true for infants infected beyond the 16th to 29th week of gestation, who appear to be at little, if any, risk of congenital anomalies.[103,109] Studies by Peckham and associates[107,335] demonstrate that estimates of the risk of defects are affected by the serologic status and age at evaluation of the child. The overall incidence of defects in 218 children studied when they were about 2 years old was 23%; it was 52% if maternal infection occurred before 8 weeks' gestation, 36% at 9 to 12 weeks, and 10% at 13 to 20 weeks. No defects were observed when maternal infection occurred after 20 weeks. When considering only seropositive children, the overall risk of defects increased to 38%, with increased risks of 75%, 52%, and 18%, respectively, for the three gestational periods previously cited. At follow-up when the children were 6 to 8 years old, the overall risk of abnormalities in infected children who were seropositive when 2 years old increased from 38% to 59%; the risk after first-trimester infection increased from 58% to 82%.

Miller and co-workers[105] observed higher rates of defects in infected children observed for only 2 years (see Table 28-1). Defects were seen in 9 of 9 seropositive children exposed during the first 11 weeks, 2 of 4 exposed at 11 to 12 weeks, 2 of 12 exposed at 13 to 14 weeks, and 7 of 14 exposed at 15 to 16 weeks. Congenital heart disease and deafness were observed after infection before the 11th week; deafness was the sole defect identified after infection at 11 to 16 weeks' gestation. No defects were observed in 63 children infected after 16 weeks. However, some children infected in the third trimester had growth retardation.

Although the number of subjects is small, results of the study of Miller and co-workers[105] indicate that the risk of damage in seropositive infants is 85% if fetal infection occurs in the first trimester and 35% after infection during weeks 13 to 16. These rates of defects are higher than previously reported, but they may be an accurate reflection of intrauterine events because all maternal cases were serologically confirmed and sensitive antibody assays were used to detect congenital infection. With further follow-up, higher rates of defects may be observed.

These rates pertain to offspring known to be infected and are useful in evaluating the risk of defects given fetal infection. For counseling purposes, it is essential to know the risk of congenital defects after confirmed maternal infection. This can be derived by multiplying the rates of defects in infected fetuses by the rates of fetal infection. Based on the reported experience of Miller and colleagues,[105] the risks are 90% for maternal infection before the 11th week, 33% for infection during weeks 11 to 12, 11% for weeks 13 to 14, and 24% for weeks 15 to 16 (see Table 28-1). The risk after maternal infection in the first trimester is 69%.

NATURAL HISTORY

Postnatal Infection

Virologic Findings

The pertinent virologic findings of postnatal infection are depicted in Figure 28-2. The portal of entry for rubella virus is believed to be the upper respiratory tract. Virus then spreads through the lymphatic system, or by a transient viremia to regional lymph nodes, where replication first occurs. Between 7 and 9 days after exposure, virus is released into the blood and may seed multiple tissues, including the placenta. By the 9th to 11th day, viral excretion begins from the nasopharynx, as well as from the kidneys, cervix, gastrointestinal tract, and various other sites.[9,278,294,301,342-344,350]

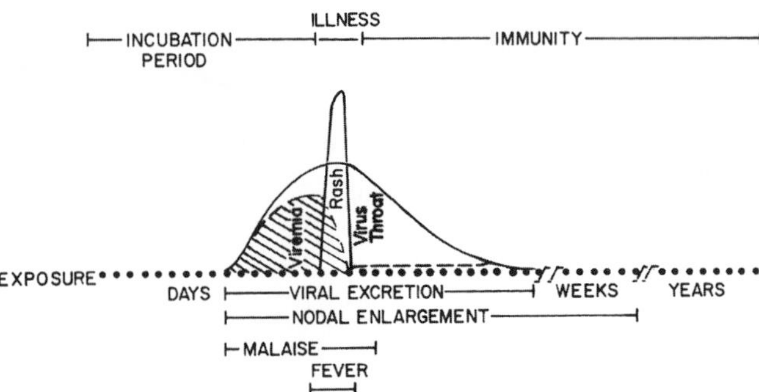

Figure 28–2 Relation of viral excretion and clinical findings in postnatally acquired rubella. (Data from Alford CA. Chronic congenital and perinatal infections. *In* Avery GB [ed]. Neonatology. Philadelphia, JB Lippincott, 1987.)

The viremia peaks at 10 to 17 days, just before rash onset, which usually occurs 16 to 18 days after exposure. Virus disappears from the serum in the next few days, as antibody becomes detectable.[278,294,301,350] However, infection may persist in peripheral blood lymphocytes and monocytes for 1 to 4 weeks.[59,64,351,352] Virus is excreted in high titers from nasopharyngeal secretions. Nasopharyngeal shedding rarely may be detected for up to 3 to 5 weeks. Although virus can usually be cultured from the nasopharynx from 7 days before to 14 days after rash onset, the highest risk of virus transmission is believed to be from 5 days before to 6 days after the appearance of rash. Viral shedding from other sites is not as consistent, intense, or prolonged.[294,350] Rubella virus has been cultured from skin at sites where rash was present and where it was absent.[353,354]

Humoral Immune Response

In challenge studies conducted in the early 1960s, Green and co-workers[294] demonstrated that neutralizing antibody was first detected in serum 14 to 18 days after exposure (usually 2 to 3 days after rash onset), peaked within a month, and persisted for the duration of the follow-up period of 6 to 12 months. The HI test soon became the standard method for detecting rubella antibodies after acute postnatal rubella infection because of its reliability and ease compared with the neutralization test. Several other methods for measuring rubella antibody responses have supplanted the HI test in popularity (see "The Virus").[88,199,200] The kinetics of the immune response to acute infection detected by these various serologic assays, which have been exhaustively compared with the HI technique, is depicted in Figure 28-3.[88-92,191,195-205,207,214-224,226,229]

In general, there are three distinct patterns of antibody kinetics. Antibodies of the IgG class measured by HI, latex agglutination, neutralization, immunofluorescence, single radial hemolysis (or hemolysis in gel) (not shown in Fig. 28-3), radioimmunoassay, and enzyme-linked immunoassay theta

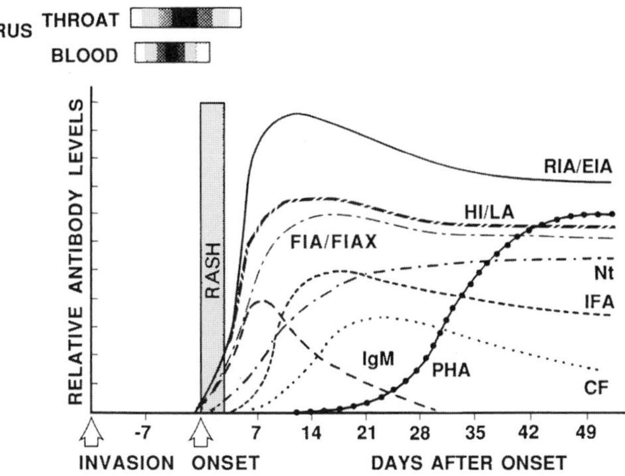

Figure 28–3 Schematic diagram of the immune response in acute rubella infection. CF, complement fixation; EIA, enzyme immunoassay; FIA/FIAX and IFA, immunofluorescence assays; HI, hemagglutination inhibition; IgM, immunoglobulin M; LA, latex agglutination; Nt, neutralization; PHA, passive agglutination; RIA, radioimmunoassay. (Data from Herrmann KL. Rubella virus. *In* Lennette EH, Schmidt NJ. [eds]. Diagnostic Procedures for Viral, Rickettsial and Chlamydial Infections. Washington, DC, American Public Health Association, 1979, p 725, and from Herrmann KL. Available rubella serologic tests. Rev Infect Dis 7[Suppl 1]:S108, 1985.)

precipitation (not shown) follow the first pattern. Such antibodies usually become detectable 5 to 15 days after rash onset, although they may appear earlier and may even be detected 1 or 2 days before the rash appears. The antibody titers rapidly increase to reach peak values at 15 to 30 days and then gradually decline over a period of years to a constant titer that varies from person to person. In some patients with low levels of residual antibody, a second exposure to rubella virus may lead to low-grade reinfection of the pharynx. A booster antibody response can then be detected with any of the assays. This rapidly terminates the new infection, which is most often subclinical, and little or no viremia occurs.[38,44,47,50,54,56,260,305,329]

A second pattern of immune response to rubella infection is seen when IgG antibodies are measured by passive hemagglutination. The peak titer of these antibodies is similar to that measured by HI, but the passive hemagglutination antibodies are relatively delayed in appearance, and levels rise only slowly to their maximal titers. They first become detectable 15 to 50 days after the onset of the rash and often take 200 days to reach peak titers. The antibodies probably persist for life. Booster responses may be seen with reinfections.

Studies indicate that the predominant IgG subclass detected by all these various assays is probably IgG1.[95,97] Failure to detect IgG3 may be indicative of reinfection.[98]

A third distinct pattern of antibody production is represented in Figure 28-3 by the IgM antibody class immune response. Rubella-specific IgM antibody can be measured by HI, immunofluorescence, radioimmunoassay, or enzyme immunoassay.[99,157,206-210,213,215,224,225,230-228] IgM antibodies are most consistently detectable 5 to 10 days after the onset of the rash, rise rapidly to peak values at around 20 days, and then decline so rapidly that they usually disappear by 50 to 70 days. In a few patients, however, low levels may persist for up to 1 year.[355-357] The booster IgG antibody response to reinfection described earlier does not usually involve the IgM class of antibody, and the presence of high-titer IgM antibodies usually indicates recent primary infection with rubella. However, more sensitive techniques, such as radioimmunoassay or enzyme immunoassay, may occasionally detect low levels of specific IgM antibodies in some patients with reinfections, which may cause some difficulty in differentiating subclinical reinfection, which is almost always of no consequence, from acute primary subclinical infection.[41,51,53,55] Determination of avidity of rubella-specific IgG may help resolve this problem.[358-360] Primary infection appears to be associated with low-avidity IgG, and reinfection seems to be associated with high-avidity IgG.

The kinetics of the immune response to rubella infection detected by other serologic assays is not as distinct as the three patterns just described, and marked variability between patients has been observed. Complement fixation antibodies or iota precipitins (not shown in Fig. 28-3) are lacking in the first 10 days after the rash and rise slowly to peak at 30 to 90 days.[191] These antibodies persist for several years in one third of patients and may reappear during reinfections. Iota precipitins do not persist for more than a few months and do not usually reappear with reinfections.

Antibodies of the IgA class appear within 10 days but may disappear within another 20 days or persist for several years.[96,99,206,231] IgD and IgE antibodies appear rapidly (6 to 9 days) after infection, remain high for at least 2 months, and then decline slightly at 6 months.[96] IgE antibodies reach an early peak similar to that seen for IgM and IgA. In contrast, the IgD response is somewhat delayed, like that of IgG.

The antibody response after infection is generally considered to confer complete and permanent immunity. Clinical reinfection is rare, and reinfections usually pose little risk to the fetus because placental exposure to the virus is minimal.[38,41,44,47,50,51,53-56,329] Some of the rare instances of fetal infection after maternal reinfection may be caused by an incomplete immune response to the various antigenic domains on each structural protein of the virus (see "The Virus").[74-76,111,115,321,326-330] For example, three cases after natural infection have been reported involving women who had positive HI results but who had no detectable levels of neutralizing antibody.[321,326,328] The sensitivity of the neutralizing assay itself is an important determinant in interpreting these results.[111,196] This phenomenon also may account for the four reported cases of congenital infection that followed reinfection of women who had presumably been immunized previously.[42,45,52,116] Some of the reported instances of maternal reinfection probably, and in at least one case definitely, represent cases of primary acute infection.[5,6,113,323-325]

Cellular Immune Response

Cellular immunity to rubella virus has been measured by lymphocyte transformation response, secretion of interferon, secretion of macrophage migration-inhibitory factor, induction of delayed hypersensitivity to skin testing, and release of lymphokines by cultured lymphocytes.[361-372] Peripheral blood lymphocytes from seropositive individuals respond better in each of these tests than do lymphocytes from uninfected persons, suggesting that these assays measure parameters of the cellular immune response to rubella virus. The results from other studies in which chromium 51 microcytotoxicity assays have been used are difficult to interpret because syngeneic cell lines have not been used to control for HLA-restricted responses.[362,365]

In the first weeks after natural rubella infection, some degree of transient lymphocyte suppression may occur.[366,368] Generally, cell-mediated immune responses precede the appearance of humoral immunity by 1 week, reach a peak value at the same time as the antibody response, and subsequently persist for many years, probably for life.[331] Acute infection may suppress skin reactivity to tuberculin testing for approximately 30 days.[373]

Local Immune Response

The local antibody response at the portal of entry in the nasopharynx is essentially IgA in character; low levels of short-lived IgG antibody are rarely detectable in nasopharyngeal secretions. The nasopharyngeal IgA antibody persists at detectable levels for at least 1 year after infection. Its persistence apparently minimizes the tendency for reinfection after natural rubella infection. The lack of local IgA nasopharyngeal response after parenteral administration of live rubella vaccines (less so with the RA 27/3 strain than with other strains) probably plays a key role in the increased incidence of subclinical reinfection after vaccination.[38,40,44,50,54,56,374-377] Local antibody levels tend to be higher in individuals resistant to challenge with live virus, but no specific titer of antibody has been associated with complete protection.

A cell-mediated immune response in tonsillar cells has been detected by lymphocyte transformation and secretion of migration-inhibitory factor after natural rubella and after intranasal challenge with live RA 27/3 vaccine.[378] In guinea pigs, the response first becomes detectable 1 to 2 weeks after intranasal vaccination, peaks at 4 weeks, and then disappears at about 6 weeks.[379]

Congenital Infection

Virologic Findings

An important feature that distinguishes congenital infection from postnatal infection is that the former is chronic.[2,13,284,310,317,380,381] During the period of maternal viremia, the placenta may become infected and transmit virus to the fetus (see "Transmission In Utero").[2,6,284,299,314-320] Although virus may persist for months in the placenta, recovery of virus from the placenta at birth occurs infrequently.[382] In contrast, after the fetus is infected, the virus persists typically throughout gestation and for months postnatally. It can infect many fetal organs or only a few.[317] In infected infants, virus can be recovered from multiple sites (e.g., pharyngeal secretions, urine, conjunctival fluid, feces) and is detectable in cerebrospinal fluid, bone marrow, and circulating white blood cells.[†] Pharyngeal shedding of virus is more common, prolonged, and intense during the early months after delivery (Fig. 28-4). By 1 year of age, only 2% to 20% of infants shed virus.[277-279] In rare instances, shedding may continue beyond the age of 2 years.[280-282] Virus can be isolated from the eye and cerebrospinal fluid, particularly when disease is evident in the corresponding organs and can persist for more than a year in the eye and central nervous system.[384-387] Virus has been isolated from the brain of a 12-year-old boy with later-appearing subacute panencephalitis occurring after congenital rubella infection.[388,389]

[†]See references 2, 13, 161, 277-282, 284, 314, 315, 317, 319, 380-384.

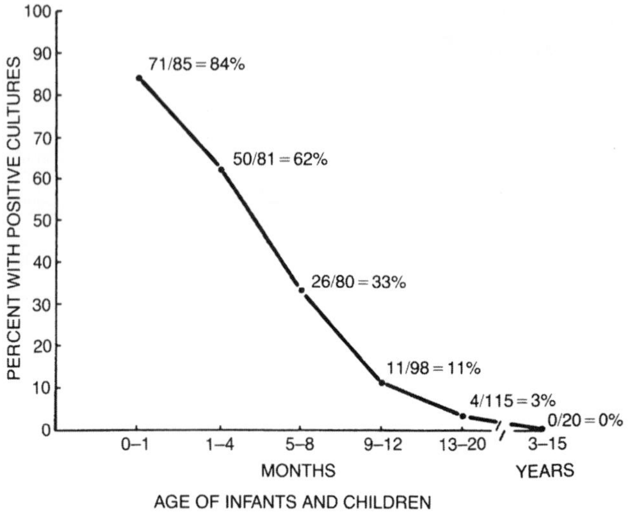

Figure 28–4 Rate of virus excretion by age in infants and children with congenital rubella infection. (Data from Cooper LZ, Krugman S. Clinical manifestations of postnatal and congenital rubella. Arch Ophthalmol 77:434, 1967.)

Humoral Immune Response

Studies have shown that placental infection does not prevent passive transfer of maternal antibody and that the infected fetus can mount an immune response.[284,314-320,390-392] Although the development and function of the other components of the immune response of the fetus may be important, critical factors that allow fetal infection to occur in the presence of antibody may be the timing when antibody is present in the fetal circulation or the quality of the antibody that the fetus produces, or both.

Although placental transfer of antibody occurs despite persistent infection, levels of antibody in fetal blood during the first half of gestation are only 5% to 10% of those in maternal serum.[392-396] As the placental transfer mechanisms mature by mid-gestation (16 to 20 weeks), increasing levels of maternal IgG antibody are transferred to the fetus (Fig. 28-5).[395]

The development of the fetal humoral immune system appears to be too late to limit the effects of the virus. Cells with membrane-bound immunoglobulins of all three major classes—IgM, IgG, and IgA—appear in the fetus as early as 9 to 11 weeks' gestation.[396] However, circulating fetal antibody levels remain low until mid-gestation, despite the presence of high titers of virus and the development of antigen receptors on the cell surface (see Fig. 28-5). At this time, levels of fetal antibody increase, with IgM antibody predominating.[392,397-401] Fetal IgA, IgD, and IgG also are made, although in lesser amounts.[96,398,401] As in the case with other chronic intrauterine infections, congenital rubella infection may lead to an increase in total IgM antibody levels.[390,392,393,401] Total IgA levels are also occasionally raised, but IgG levels seldom exceed those of uninfected infants.[390,392,401,402] At the time of delivery of infected infants, levels of IgG rubella antibodies in cord sera are equal to or greater than those in maternal

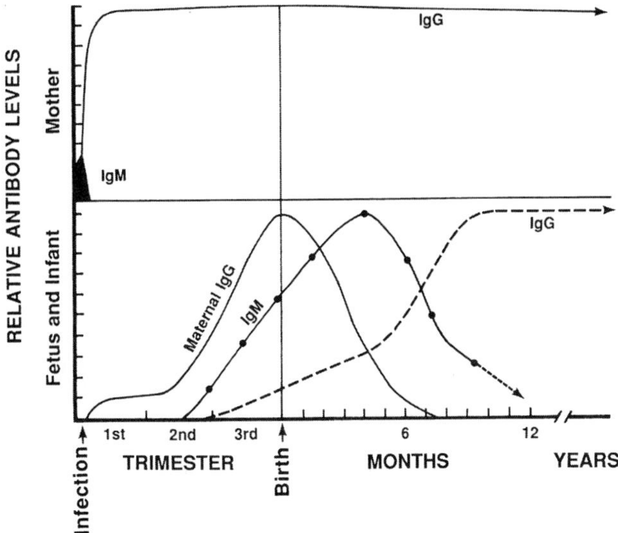

Figure 28–5 Schematic diagram of the immune response in the mother, fetus, and infant after maternal and fetal rubella infections in the first trimester of pregnancy. (Data from Alford CA. Immunology of rubella. *In* Friedman H, Prier JE [eds]. Rubella. Springfield, Ill, Charles C Thomas, 1972.)

sera, even if the infant is born prematurely.[392] IgG is the dominant antibody present at delivery in rubella-infected infants and is mainly maternal in origin. In contrast, the IgM levels are lower but are totally fetus derived.

In the first 3 to 5 months after birth, the levels of maternally derived IgG decrease as maternal antibody is catabolized (see Fig. 28-5).[392] In contrast, IgM antibodies increase in titer and can predominate. Later, as viral excretion wanes and disappears, the IgM antibody levels diminish, and IgG becomes the dominant and persistent antibody type. Cradock-Watson and colleagues[401] found that total IgM was elevated in nearly all sera obtained from infected infants during the first 3 months of life and in one half of sera from infected infants 3 to 6 months old. Rubella-specific IgM has been shown consistently to persist for 6 months, frequently for a year, and rarely longer when assayed by sensitive serologic procedures, such as radioimmunoassay and immunofluorescence.[212,401] For example, Cradock-Watson and colleagues[401] also reported that IgM was detectable in 48 (96%) of 50 sera during the first 6 months of life and in 11 (29%) of 38 sera from children between 6.5 months and 2 years old. The total level of antibody, as measured by a variety of serologic tests, remains virtually unchanged throughout the first year of life, despite the fluctuations in immunoglobulin composition.[392,401]

High levels of IgG antibody are usually maintained for several years after detectable virus excretion ends, suggesting that there may be continued antigenic stimulation. During the first few years of life, some patients have a relative hypergammaglobulinemia, particularly of the IgM and IgG classes of antibody, which results from the increased antigenic stimulus accompanying the chronic infection.[401,403] With increasing time, however, antibody levels may decrease and even become undetectable in 10% to 20% of patients.[335,404-406] Cooper and co-workers[406] found that the geometric mean HI titer decreased by a factor of 16 by age 5 years in 223 children with congenital rubella syndrome. No HI antibodies were detected in 8 of 29 5-year-old children. In a study from Japan, only 3% of 381 children with congenital infection observed for more than 17 years had undetectable HI titers.[407] There was an initial rapid decline from a geometric mean titer of 1:416 ($2^{8.7}$) to 1:84 ($2^{6.4}$) over the first 2 years of follow-up. After this, there was a modest continuing decline, and the final geometric mean titer was 1:42 ($2^{5.4}$).

Cooper and co-workers[406] reported that congenitally infected children who have lost detectable rubella-specific antibody did not develop a boost in antibody titer after rubella vaccination. This finding may reflect some sort of immunologic tolerance that follows intrauterine exposure to rubella virus. None of the children with congenital rubella in Japan had evidence of significant boosts in antibody or a history of clinical disease when exposed during recent outbreaks of rubella.[407,408]

Hypogammaglobulinemia with low levels of all three major classes of immunoglobulins has been reported in a few instances of congenital rubella.[133,161,409,410] Usually, only IgA is affected. There may also be instances when IgG levels are low, whereas levels of IgM are two or three times the upper limit of normal for adults. These IgG and IgM abnormalities may occur with or without IgA abnormalities.[409] Over time, immunoglobulin development may become normal, and this can occur despite continued viral excretion but is more likely if viral titers are decreasing.[280]

In addition to defects in the immune globulin levels, defects in specific antibody production have been observed. One such defect is a complete lack of antibody response to any antigen, including the rubella virus itself. Response only to the virus, in the absence of a response to most other antigens, has also been reported.[280] This state of immunologic unresponsiveness resolves in many patients. Antibody production becomes normal as the patient's general condition improves and as immune globulin levels normalize.

Immunoprecipitation studies of sera from patients with congenital rubella syndrome provide further information on defective antibody production. They indicate that the antibody profile to the three structural proteins of the rubella virus is qualitatively different from that observed in sera from persons with postnatally acquired infection (see "The Virus").[84,85,87] Little or no antibody to the core structural protein (C) is found, and the absolute and relative amounts of antibody to structural proteins E1 and E2 appear to vary with age.[84,85] These findings further suggest that the immune response of the infected fetus may be incomplete and may explain why detectable antibodies are not present in some sera.[87,335,404-407] If a serum contains relatively little antibody to structural protein E1 (i.e., hemagglutinin), assays that detect antibody to the whole virion will be more likely to be positive than those that detect antibody only to E1 (e.g., the HI assay). It is not clear whether these abnormal antibody patterns persist for life.

Cellular Immune Response

Like the cells responsible for the humoral immune response (i.e., B cells), the cells involved in cellular immunity (i.e., T cells and macrophages) develop some of their functions early in gestation.[411-413] However, little is known about their response in utero because appropriate specimens have not been obtainable for study. The cellular immune response of the infected fetus has been inferred from studies of infected infants and children. Available evidence indicates that some infants with congenital rubella have impaired cellular immune responses.

Retarded development of the thymus and lymphocyte depletion have been reported, but these abnormalities may result from the stress of infection rather than the virus itself.[414] Abnormal delayed hypersensitivity skin reactions to a number of antigens (e.g., diphtheria toxoid, *Candida*, dinitrofluorobenzene) have also been reported.[280,415] This defect has been associated with abnormalities in the humoral system and resolves as antibody production returns to normal.

Results of studies of in vitro lymphocyte blastogenesis in congenitally infected infants and children have been confusing. Early studies demonstrated a poor response to phytohemagglutinin, vaccinia, and diphtheria toxoid.[415-418] However, because rubella virus can depress the lymphocyte blastogenic response and the virus can be isolated from lymphocytes of chronically infected infants, the abnormality may be a result of viral infection of the circulating blood cells rather than an inherent defect in cell-mediated immunity.[416-419] This diminished cellular response may normalize over time because elevated lymphocyte responses have been detected in some older infected children.[411,420]

Buimovici-Klein and colleagues[372,421] showed that lymphocytes from older children and adolescents with congenital rubella had no or very poor lymphocyte proliferative responses to rubella virus antigens and had markedly reduced interferon and migration-inhibition factor production. These studies indicated that these defects were greater in children exposed early in gestation than those exposed later, with the greatest degree of abnormality in those whose mothers had been infected during the first 8 weeks of pregnancy. They also pointed out that these defects could persist long after viral excretion had ceased. It remains unclear if these cellular immune defects are responsible for viral persistence or are yet another manifestation of intrauterine infection.[421]

Other investigators have confirmed that patients with congenital rubella have defects in cell-mediated immunity.[120,133,134] Verder and colleagues[134] reported a decreased proportion of suppressor or cytotoxic ($CD8^+$) T cells in an infant with congenital rubella. Rabinowe and co-workers[133] documented persistent T cell abnormalities in patients with congenital infection who were 9 to 21 years old. Compared with normal subjects, the congenitally infected patients had depressed ratios of T4 cells (helper or inducer) to T8 cells (from a decreased proportion of T4 and an increased percentage of T8 cells). Such findings persist for only 1 month after acute postnatal rubella infection.[422]

Lymphocytes of infected children were unable to kill rubella-infected cells in a cytotoxicity assay.[423] These results were questioned because syngeneic target cells were not used, and these responses are known to be HLA restricted. However, similar results have been found by Verder and associates,[134] who observed abnormal killer and natural killer cell activities.

Interferon Response

It has long been suggested that the fetus has a deficient interferon response to viral infections, including rubella, but this evidence has been derived from indirect studies with in vitro cell systems or animal models.[173,174,319,424,425] Technical difficulties have hampered direct studies of humans. However, interferon that appeared to be specifically stimulated by the presence of rubella virus in rubella-infected human embryos has been demonstrated.[426] The interferon was found as early as 7 weeks' gestation and persisted as long as 12 weeks after symptoms ceased in the mothers. Direct study of fetal blood and amniotic fluid has also shown that the fetus can produce interferon in response to the virus.[427]

Children with congenital infection do have the capacity to make interferon on challenge. For example, Desmyter and co-workers[428] reported that interferon could not be detected from the serum or urine of nine such children 11 to 18 months old who were excreting virus. However, after vaccination with live measles vaccine (i.e., Edmonton B or Schwarz strains), all the children seroconverted and produced detectable levels of interferon.

PATHOGENESIS

Postnatal Infection

The events leading to acute postnatal infection are relatively well known and have been detailed in "Natural History." Available information indicates that viral replication and postinfection immune phenomena are involved in the clinical manifestations of the illness.

Viremia may lead to seeding of multiple organs, but few are clinically affected.[6] Speculation that the rash may be an immune phenomenon caused by circulating immune complexes has not been documented. Few persons with uncomplicated illness have immune complexes containing rubella virus, and virus has been isolated from involved and uninvolved skin.[123,128,353,354] Virus has been isolated from lymph nodes and conjunctiva, accounting for the lymph node enlargement and conjunctivitis observed in many patients.[350,429] Virus has been isolated from synovial fluid, but immune mechanisms may play a role in some cases of arthralgia and arthritis, particularly if symptoms are persistent.[123,429-433] Encephalitis is probably a manifestation of the immune response, but direct viral invasion may be involved, particularly in the rare case of progressive panencephalitis that has been reported to follow postnatal infection.[121,434-436] It has been suggested that pregnant women are at increased risk of serious complications because of the impaired immune response associated with pregnancy, but there are few data to support this claim.[436-438] There has also been interest, especially in Japan, in the influence of HLA type and other genetic factors on the incidence and severity of postnatal infection.[118,119,122,124,127,439] No consistent pattern has been reported.

Congenital Infection

The outcome of maternal rubella infection follows a logical sequence of events, beginning with maternal infection, followed by viremia, placental seeding, and dissemination of infection to the fetus (see "Transmission In Utero" and "Natural History").[2,6,284,299,314-320] The fetus may escape infection entirely, succumb in utero, be born with multiple obvious defects, or appear to be normal at birth, only to develop abnormalities later in life.[6,13,107,278,330-337] The variability in outcome is highlighted by the observation that one identical twin may be infected and the other spared.[6,440,441]

The most important determinant of fetal outcome is gestational age at the time of infection.[2,3,6,103,110,284,299,314,317] The disease is more severe and has a greater tendency to involve multiple organs when acquired during the first 8 weeks' gestation. However, the factors that govern the influence of gestation are unknown. It is possible that immature cells are more easily infected and support the growth of virus better than older, more differentiated cells. It is also possible that the placenta becomes increasingly resistant to infection (or at least more able to limit infection) as it rapidly matures during the first trimester. A third possibility is that maturing fetal defense mechanisms become capable of confining and clearing the infection. This last explanation is probably important after 18 or 20 weeks' gestation but seems unlikely in the latter half of the first trimester, when attenuation of fetal infection begins. It is likely that a combination of these and other factors are responsible for the decrease in virulence of fetal infection with increasing gestational age.

The hallmark of fetal infection is its chronicity, with the tendency for virus to persist throughout fetal life and after birth.[2,13,161,277-282,284,299,314-320,372-389] The fact that virus can be isolated long after birth also raises the possibility of reactivation, at least in brain tissue.[388,389] It is not clear why the virus has these properties, because the fetus is not truly immunologically tolerant and appears to be able to produce interferon.[212,284,331,391,392,401,424-428] In any case, chronic or reactivated infection can lead to ongoing pathologic processes.[6,13,14,107,131,132,330,331,333-336]

The causes of cellular and tissue damage from congenital rubella infection are poorly defined.[424,425] Only a variable, small number of cells are infected (1 per 1000 to 250,000).[320] In tissue culture, infection with rubella virus has diverse effects, ranging from no obvious effect to cell destruction (see "The Virus"); this is also likely to be the case in vivo,[157] but cytolysis is uncommon (see "Pathology").[2,3,6,9,442-446] Inflammation is minimal and consists mainly of infiltration of small lymphocytes. Polymorphonuclear leukocytes and plasma cells are lacking, particularly compared with other viral infections of the human fetus, in which inflammation and general necrosis are quite extensive. In contrast, vascular insufficiency appears to be more important than cell destruction or secondary inflammatory damage in the genesis of congenital defects.[2,3,6,9,442-446] This suggestion is supported by the observation that rubella virus has low destructive potential for cells growing in vitro, including those of human origin. A number of investigators have maintained multiple types of rubella-infected human fetal cells in culture for years without loss of viability or evidence of cytopathic effect.[447-449]

Other defects have been reported in chronically infected cells that might help explain the mechanism of congenital defects. These include chromosomal breaks, reduced cellular multiplication time, and increased production of a protein inhibitor that causes mitotic arrest of certain cell types.[380,447,450-455]

A report by Bowden and associates[456] indicates that rubella virus may interfere with mitosis by having an adverse effect on actin microfilaments. Observations of Yoneda and co-workers[457] show that rubella virus may alter cell receptors to specific growth factors. All of these abnormalities, if occurring in vivo, may result in decreased cell multiplication because of slow growth rates and limited doubling potential during the period of embryogenesis, when cell division and turnover are normally very rapid. Naeye and Blanc[458] found histopathologic evidence for mitotic arrest and reduced cell numbers in infants who died of congenital rubella syndrome. These observations have been offered to explain the increased incidence of intrauterine growth retardation seen in infants with congenital rubella, but this explanation probably represents an oversimplification of the actual mechanisms involved.

Immunologic responses also have been proposed as causes of cellular damage. Although cellular immune defects may be a result of chronic infection, it is possible that these defects contribute to ongoing tissue damage.[372,421,459] Excessive serum immunoglobulin development, persistent antibody production in the face of viral replication for prolonged periods, and production of rheumatoid factor, all indicative of overstimulation of the immune system, also may have a role in the pathogenesis of congenital rubella syndrome.[460,461] The presence of immune complexes and autoantibodies and the influence of certain HLA types may contribute to the delayed expression of some signs of congenital rubella, such as pneumonitis, diabetes mellitus, thyroid dysfunction, and progressive rubella panencephalitis (see "Clinical Manifestations").[‡] Some of these immunologic events may be directly involved in tissue damage (e.g., immune complexes, autoantibodies), whereas others may allow the virus to persist or reactivate.

PATHOLOGY

Postnatal Infection

Little is known about the pathology of postnatally acquired rubella because patients seldom die of this mild disease. As observed by Cherry,[9] the histologic findings of tissues that have been examined (i.e., lymph nodes and autopsy specimens from patients dying with encephalitis) are unremarkable. Changes in lymphoreticular tissue have been limited to mild edema, nonspecific follicular hyperplasia, and some loss of normal follicular morphology. Examination of brain tissue has revealed diffuse swelling, nonspecific degeneration, and little meningeal and perivascular infiltrate.

Congenital Infection

In contrast to the situation with postnatal rubella, much is known about the pathology of congenital rubella infection.[2,3,6,9,442-446,462] In general, small foci of infected cells are seen in apparently normal tissue. Cellular necrosis and secondary inflammation are seldom obvious, although a generalized vasculitis predominates (see "Pathogenesis").

The pathologic findings of the placenta include hypoplasia, inflammatory foci in chorionic villi, granulomatous changes, mild edema, focal hyalinization, and necrosis.[442,443,462,463] Disease usually causes extensive damage to the endothelium of the capillaries and smaller blood vessels of the chorion. The vessel lesions consist mainly of endothelial necrosis,

‡See references 13, 14, 117, 120, 121, 123, 125, 126, 129-134, 388, 389.

with fragmentation of intraluminal blood cells. Töndury and Smith[442] postulated that emboli of infected endothelial cells originating from the chorion might seed target organs in the fetus. These emboli may also contribute to organ damage by obstructing the fetal blood supply. Petechiae and the presence of hemosiderin-laden phagocytes in surrounding tissue are evidence of functional vascular damage.[443]

Although not nearly as common as vascular lesions, specific cytolysis, presumably caused by direct viral effect on the cell, is also present in the placenta. This is characterized by cytoplasmic eosinophilia, nuclear pyknosis or karyorrhexis, and cellular necrosis. Specific cellular inclusion bodies, both nuclear and cytoplasmic, are rare but have been observed.[463] Whereas placentitis would be expected to be present in all affected placentas, regardless of when fetal infection occurred, Garcia and colleagues[463] found that placental lesions appeared to be more intense when infection occurred in the last trimester of pregnancy. This finding is consistent with the observation that the placenta is not a barrier to fetal infection in the latter stages of pregnancy.[103,109,333,335]

Autopsies show that virtually every organ may be involved, with hypoplasia being a common finding. The necrotizing angiopathy of small blood vessels seen in the placenta is the most characteristic lesion in fetal organs. Cytolysis with tissue necrosis and accompanying inflammatory changes are also far less common but have been found in the myocardium, brain, spinal cord, skeletal muscle, viscera, and epithelial cells of the developing lens, inner ear (organ of Corti), and teeth.

The overall pathologic process of congenital rubella, in keeping with its chronic nature, is progressive. Both healing and new lesions can be found in specimens obtained in the later stages of gestation.[442,443] The pathologic changes vary among embryos in quantity and in organ distribution, and the location and nature of organ lesions depend somewhat on the gestational age at the time of infection.[442] The pathologic findings parallel the enormous variability of the clinical disease seen in infected newborns.

CLINICAL MANIFESTATIONS

Postnatal Infection

Rubella is usually a mild disease with few complications. Clinical illness may be more severe in adults.[6,9,291,294,360,464] Measles, varicella, and some enteroviruses acquired close to delivery may be associated with serious illness in the newborn, probably because of fetal exposure to transplacental viremia in the absence of protective levels of maternal antibody. One case report suggests that the same may be true in rubella. Sheinis and associates[465] reported the death of a neonate with rash onset when 12 days old; the mother developed rash on the day of delivery. This single observation needs to be confirmed. There are no conclusive data to indicate that infection in the immunocompromised host is associated with an increased risk of complications.

The first symptoms of rubella occur after an incubation period of 16 to 18 days, with a range of 14 to 21 days. In the child, rash is often the first sign detected. In adolescents and adults, however, the eruption is commonly preceded by a 1- to 5-day prodromal period characterized by low-grade fever, headache, malaise, anorexia, mild conjunctivitis, coryza, sore throat, cough, and lymphadenopathy usually involving suboccipital, postauricular, and cervical nodes.

The constitutional symptoms often subside rapidly with the appearance of the rash. The rash can last 1 to 5 days or longer and can be pruritic in adults. Infection without a rash is quite common. The ratio of subclinical to clinical infections has varied from 1:9 to 7:1.[260,296] Subclinical infection can lead to fetal infection, although it is not clear whether the risk is as great as that associated with clinically apparent infection.[2,3,6,105,108,335,341]

Arthralgia and frank arthritis with recrudescence of low-grade fever and other constitutional symptoms may appear after the rash fades. Joint involvement typically lasts 5 to 10 days but may be more persistent. The frequency of these symptoms is variable, but it is more common in adults, particularly women.[9] In some studies of adult patients, the frequency has been as high as 70%.[466] Thrombocytopenia (occurring in approximately 1 of 3000 patients) and acute postinfection encephalitis (occurring in 1 of 5000 to 6000 patients) are rare complications that usually occur 2 to 4 days after rash onset.[9] Rare complications associated with postnatal rubella include myocarditis, Guillain-Barré syndrome, relapsing encephalitis, optic neuritis, and bone marrow aplasia.[9,467-471] Two cases of a progressive panencephalitis, similar to measles-associated subacute sclerosing panencephalitis, have been reported.[434,435] This central nervous system disturbance is more likely to manifest in patients with congenital rubella syndrome, although it still occurs infrequently.[389,472,473] Testalgia has also been reported in patients with rubella, but this may have been a coincidental finding.[474,475]

Congenital Infection

Gregg's original report[12] in 1941 defined the rubella syndrome as a constellation of defects, usually involving some combination of congenital heart, eye, and hearing abnormalities, with or without mental retardation and microcephaly. After the extensive studies in the mid-1960s, in which virologic and serologic methods of assessment were used, the pathologic potential associated with intrauterine rubella had to be greatly expanded.[2,3] The recognition of various new defects associated with congenital rubella infection led to speculation that they had not existed before the 1962 to 1964 pandemic. However, a review of the abnormalities in infants born during previous non-epidemic periods indicated that they were not new but had not been appreciated previously because of the small number of affected infants studied.[476]

The virus can infect one or virtually all fetal organs and, once established, can persist for long periods (see "Transmission In Utero," "Natural History," "Pathogenesis," and "Pathology").[§] Congenital rubella, a chronic infection, may kill the fetus in utero, causing miscarriage or stillbirth. At the other extreme, the infection may have no apparent effect clinically detectable at the delivery of normal-appearing infants. Alternatively, severe multiple birth defects may be

[§]See references 6, 13, 14, 107, 131, 132, 161, 277-282, 284, 299, 314-320, 330-337, 380-389.

obvious in the newborn period. The wide spectrum of disease is summarized later in the chapter (see Tables 28-3 and 28-4).

Silent infections in the infant are much more common than symptomatic ones. Schiff and colleagues[334] prospectively examined 4005 infants born after the 1964 rubella epidemic. Based on virologic and serologic techniques to detect infection in the newborns, the overall rate of congenital rubella was in excess of 2%, compared with only approximately 0.1% in endemic years.[334,341] Sixty-eight percent of the infected newborns had subclinical infection during the neonatal period. Among those who were followed, 71% developed manifestations of infection at various times in the first 5 years of life. Many important rubella defects can be undetectable or overlooked in the early months of life. Existing manifestations of infection can progress, and new manifestations may appear throughout life.[6,13,14,107,131,132,330-337] Some abnormalities of congenital rubella syndrome usually are not detected until the second year of life or later (see Table 28-3). The silent and progressive nature of congenital rubella infection has important implications for accurate, timely diagnosis and appropriate short-term and long-term management.

It is useful to group the clinical features of congenital rubella into three categories: transient manifestations in newborns and infants; permanent manifestations, which may be present at birth or become apparent during the first year of life; and developmental and late-onset manifestations, which usually appear and progress during childhood, adolescence, and early adult life.[13,441,477] These groupings overlap.

Transient Manifestations

Transient manifestations appear to reflect ongoing heavy viral infection, perhaps abetted by the newborn's emerging, often abnormal immune function.[6,120,134] Examples of these manifestations include hepatosplenomegaly, hepatitis, jaundice, thrombocytopenia with petechiae and purpura, discrete bluish red ("blueberry muffin") lesions of dermal erythropoiesis, hemolytic anemia, chronic rash, adenopathy, meningoencephalitis (in some cases), large anterior fontanelle, interstitial pneumonia, myositis, myocarditis, diarrhea, cloudy cornea, and disturbances in bone growth that appear as striated radiolucencies in the long bones. More than 50% of infants with these transient findings usually have evidence of intrauterine growth retardation and may continue to fail to thrive during infancy.[278] These transient abnormalities were referred to as the *expanded rubella syndrome* when widely reported after the pandemic of 1962 to 1964. Careful review of the early observations during the 1940s and 1950s revealed that these were not new manifestations of congenital rubella.

These conditions usually are self-limiting and clear spontaneously over days or weeks.[2] These lesions are important from a diagnostic and prognostic standpoint. They may be associated with other, more severe defects. This applies especially to thrombocytopenia and bone lesions.[13,477] The mortality rate was approximately 35% in one group of infants who presented with neonatal thrombocytopenia. Extreme prematurity, gross cardiac lesions or myocarditis with early heart failure, rapidly progressive hepatitis, extensive meningoencephalitis, and fulminant interstitial pneumonitis contributed to the mortality during infancy.[441]

Permanent Manifestations

Permanent manifestations include heart and other blood vessel defects, eye lesions, central nervous system abnormalities, deafness, and a variety of other congenital anomalies. These structural defects result from defective organogenesis (i.e., some cardiac, eye, and other organ defects) and from tissue destruction and scarring (i.e., hearing loss, brain damage, cataracts, chorioretinopathy, and vascular stenosis). Relatively few defects result from gross anatomic abnormalities. It is not certain that all of the malformations given in Table 28-2 are associated with congenital rubella.[13,315,381,454,476-504] Because many of them occur in the absence of intrauterine rubella infection, their presence in affected infants may be coincidental.[9]

Congenital heart disease is present in more than one half of children infected during the first 2 months of gestation. The most common lesions, in descending order, are patent ductus arteriosus, pulmonary artery stenosis, and pulmonary valvular stenosis. Aortic valvular stenosis and tetralogy of Fallot have also been recorded. A patent ductus arteriosus occurs alone in approximately one third of cases; otherwise, it is frequently associated with pulmonary artery or valvular stenosis.[13,477,489] Stenosis of other vessels plays an important role in the spectrum of congenital rubella syndrome.[445,498,499] These lesions may be related to coronary, cerebral, renal, and peripheral vascular disease seen in adults.[131,529]

A "salt and pepper" retinopathy caused by disturbed growth of the pigmentary layer of the retina is the most common of all ocular findings.[6,13,441,477] Cataracts, often accompanied by microphthalmia, occur in approximately one third of all cases of congenital rubella. Bilateral cataracts are found in one half of affected children. Primary glaucoma is relatively uncommon; it does not affect a cataractous eye. Cataracts and infantile glaucoma may not be present or detectable at birth but usually become apparent during the early weeks of life. Other ocular abnormalities occur later in life (see "Developmental and Late-Onset Manifestations").

Children with congenital rubella syndrome exhibit a number of central nervous system abnormalities that follow widespread insult to the brain. Microcephaly can be a feature of this syndrome. Mental retardation and motor retardation are common and are directly related to the acute meningoencephalitis in 10% to 20% of affected children at birth.[9] Behavioral and psychiatric disorders have been confirmed in many patients.[13,441] Of particular interest is autism, which has been reported to occur with a frequency of approximately 6%.[441] Chronic encephalitis has been reported in young children.[6] A late-onset progressive panencephalitis may occur in the second decade of life.[389,472,473] This is discussed later with other developmental manifestations.

The incidence of deafness has been underestimated because many cases had been missed in infancy and early childhood. However, follow-up studies showed that deafness was the most common manifestation of congenital rubella, occurring in 80% or more of those infected.* In contrast to other serious defects, hearing impairment often is the only significant consequence of congenital rubella. Rubella-related defects of organogenesis (i.e., cataracts and some

*See references 6, 9, 13, 14, 107, 131, 132, 330, 331, 333-336.

Table 28–2 Clinical Findings and Their Estimated Frequency of Occurrence in Young Symptomatic Infants with Congenitally Acquired Rubella

Clinical Findings	Frequency[a]	References
Adenopathies	++	470, 471
Anemia	+	471, 472
Bone		
Micrognathia	+	469
Extremities	+	469
Bony radiolucencies	++	470, 473-476
Brain		
Encephalitis (active)	++	477, 478
Microcephaly	+	308, 478, 479
Brain calcification	Rare	478, 480, 481
Bulging fontanelle	+	374, 470
Cardiovascular system		
Pulmonary arterial hypoplasia	++	482
Patent ductus arteriosus	++	482
Coarctation of aortic isthmus	+	482
Interventricular septal defect	Rare	
Interauricular septal defect	Rare	
Others	Rare	13
Chromosomal abnormalities	?	447
Dermal erythropoiesis (blueberry muffin syndrome)	+	483, 484
Dermatoglyphic abnormalities	+	485, 486
Ear		
Hearing defects (severe)	+++	470
Peripheral	+++	470
Central	+	
Eye	++	470, 487-489
Retinopathy	+++	13
Cataracts	++	308, 374, 469-471, 477, 487, 490
Cloudy cornea	Rare	470
Glaucoma	Rare	471, 477, 487
Microphthalmos	+	470, 487
Genitourinary tract	+	470, 491-493
Undescended testicle	+	470, 494
Polycystic kidney[b]	Rare	492
Bilobed kidney with reduplicated ureter[b]	Rare	492
Hypospadias	Rare	14, 493
Unilateral agenesis[b]	Rare	492
Renal artery stenosis with hypertension[b]	Rare	493
Hydroureter and hydronephrosis[b]	Rare	478
Growth retardation		
Intrauterine	+++	308, 374, 469-471, 477, 490
Extrauterine	++	308, 494
Hepatitis	Rare	469, 470, 477, 495
Hepatosplenomegaly	+++	308, 374, 469-471, 477, 490
Immunologic dyscrasias	Rare	496
Interstitial pneumonitis (acute, subacute, chronic)	++	121, 470, 477, 497
Jaundice (regurgitative)	+	477, 490
Leukopenia	+	472
Myocardial necrosis	Rare	477, 478, 488, 495
Neurologic deficit	++	13, 479
Prematurity	+	308, 374, 469-471, 477, 490, 495
Thrombocytopenia with/without purpura	++	308, 374, 469-471, 477, 490
Others[b]	Rare	
Esophageal atresia		308
Tracheoesophageal fistula		490
Anencephaly		490
Encephalocele		469, 490
Meningomyelocele		479
Cleft palate		308, 490
Inguinal hernia		
Asplenia		
Nephritis (vascular)		478
Clubfoot		490
High palate		494
Talipes equinovarus		494
Depressed sternum		494
Pes cavus		494
Clinodactyly		494
Brachydactyly		494
Syndactyly		494
Elfin facies		494

[a]Frequency of occurrence is classified as follows: +, less than 20%; ++, 20% to 50%; +++, 50% to 75%.
[b]Rarely associated with rubella syndrome (whether caused by infection is unknown). Incidence is seemingly increased in infants with congenital rubella.

Table 28–3 Abnormalities of Congenital Rubella Usually Not Detected until Second Year or Later

Defects	References
Hearing	
Peripheral	13, 323, 328, 498-501
Central	
Language	13, 492, 501, 502
Developmental	
Motor	13, 503, 504
Intellectual	13, 479, 503
Behavioral	13, 503
Psychiatric	13, 503
Autism	13, 434
Endocrine	
Diabetes	13, 112, 120, 125, 126, 128, 505
Precocious puberty	13, 14
Hypothyroidism	506-510
Thyroiditis	507-509
Hyperthyroidism	112, 511
Growth hormone deficiency	512-514
Addison's disease	14
Visual	
Glaucoma (later onset)	515
Subretinal neovascularization	516, 517
Keratic precipitates	515
Keratoconus	518
Corneal hydrops	518
Lens absorption	519
Dental	494, 520
Progressive panencephalitis	382, 466, 467
Educational difficulties	13
Hypertension	521

heart lesions) are uncommon after infection beyond 8 weeks' gestation. However, the organ of Corti is vulnerable to the effects of the virus up to the first 16 weeks and perhaps up to the first 18 to 20 weeks. The deafness, ranging from mild to profound and from unilateral or bilateral, is usually peripheral (sensorineural) and is more commonly bilateral. Central auditory impairment and language delay may lead to a misdiagnosis of mental retardation.[13,505-509]

Developmental and Late-Onset Manifestations

Developmental and late-onset manifestations have been reviewed by Sever and Shaver and their colleagues.[131,132] They include endocrinopathies, deafness, ocular damage, vascular effects, and progression of central nervous system disease (Table 28-3).[¶] A number of mechanisms may be responsible for the continuing disease process that leads to these abnormalities: persistent viral infection, viral reactivation, vascular insufficiency, and immunologic insult. The last problem may be mediated by circulating immune complexes and autoantibodies. Abnormalities in cellular immunity and genetic factors have also been studied.

Insulin-dependent diabetes mellitus is the most frequent of all these manifestations, occurring in approximately 20% of patients by adulthood.[13,117,125,130-132,512] This reported prevalence is 100 to 200 times that observed for the general population. Studies of HLA type indicate that congenital rubella syndrome patients with diabetes have the same frequencies of selected HLA haplotypes as diabetic patients without the syndrome (e.g., increased HLA-DR3 and decreased HLA-DR2). The presence of pancreatic islet cell and cytotoxic surface antibodies in children with congenital rubella syndrome does not appear to be related to any specific HLA type. It has been postulated that congenital infection increases the penetrance of a preexisting susceptibility to diabetes in these patients.[130] Rabinowe and associates[133] also reported an elevation in the number of Ia-positive ("activated") T cells in patients with congenital rubella syndrome. They suggested that this T cell abnormality may be related in these patients to the increased incidence of diabetes mellitus and other diseases associated with autoantibodies.

Thyroid dysfunction affects about 5% of patients and manifests as hyperthyroidism, hypothyroidism, and thyroiditis.[117,129,513-518] Autoimmune mechanisms appear to be responsible for these abnormalities. For example, Clarke and colleagues[129] reported that 23% of 201 deaf teenagers with congenital infection had autoantibodies to the microsomal or globulin fraction, or both fractions, of the thyroid and that 20% of those with autoantibodies had thyroid gland dysfunction. Coexistence of diabetes and thyroid dysfunction has been reported, but the significance of the association is unknown.[117,133]

Two cases of growth hormone deficiency have been reported.[519] The defect appears to be hypothalamic in origin. However, among eight growth-retarded older children with congenital rubella syndrome, Oberfield[520] found no evidence of functional abnormality in the hypothalamic-pituitary axis and normal or elevated levels of somatomedin C. Growth patterns in a group of 105 late adolescents revealed three patterns: growth consistently below the fifth percentile; growth in the normal range but early cessation of growth, usually with a final height below the fifth percentile; and normal growth. The magnitude of the cognitive deficits was closely correlated with growth failure.[521] Ziring[14] has commented on a case with Addison's disease, and precocious puberty has been observed.[13,14]

The delayed diagnosis of preexisting deafness has already been referred to. However, the hearing deficit can increase over time, and sudden onset of sensorineural deafness may occur after years of normal auditory acuity.[346,510,530] As reported by Sever and co-workers,[131] the latter has been observed in a child 10 years old.

A number of late-onset ocular defects can occur. Glaucoma has been reported in patients between 3 and 22 years old who did not previously have the congenital or infantile variety of glaucoma associated with congenital rubella syndrome.[522] Other reported manifestations are keratic precipitates, keratoconus, corneal hydrops, and spontaneous lens absorption.[525,526]

The retinopathy of congenital rubella, which was previously believed to be completely benign, has more recently been associated with the delayed occurrence of visual difficulties caused by subretinal neovascularization.[523,524,531] Another delayed manifestation associated with vascular changes is hypertension resulting from renal artery and aortic stenosis.[529]

Mental retardation, autism, and other behavioral problems may be delayed in appearance and can be progressive.[13,441] However, the most interesting and serious delayed central

¶See references 13, 14, 117, 125, 130, 131, 133, 330, 335, 389, 441, 473, 474, 486, 499, 505-519, 522-529.

nervous system manifestation is the occurrence of a progressive and fatal panencephalitis resembling subacute sclerosing panencephalitis that manifests during the second decade of life. The first cases were reported by Weil and Townsend and their co-workers.[389,472] At the time of their review, Waxham and Wolinsky[473] found that 10 cases of progressive rubella panencephalitis had been identified among patients with congenital rubella syndrome. Two cases have been reported after postnatally acquired rubella.[434,435] Patients with this condition present with increasing loss of mental function, seizures, and ataxia. These symptoms continue to progress until the patient is in a vegetative state and ultimately dies. Rubella virus has been recovered from the brain of one congenitally infected patient.[388,389] Elevated serum and cerebrospinal fluid antibodies and increased amounts of cerebrospinal fluid protein and gamma globulin have been detected. Virus has also been isolated from lymphocytes, and rubella-specific immune complexes have been identified.[121,532] Although rare, this syndrome focuses attention on the ability of the virus to persist and to become reactivated after years of latency.

Long-Term Prognosis

Fifty survivors of the congenital rubella epidemic of 1939 to 1943 in Australia were seen at age 25, and their status was reviewed again in 1991.[579] Seven subjects had died in the interval—three with malignancies, three with cardiovascular disease, and one with the acquired immunodeficiency syndrome. Among the 1991 survivors, 5 were diabetic, all 40 examined were deaf, 23 had eye defects, and 16 had cardiovascular defects. Despite these conditions, the group was characterized by remarkably good social adjustment. Most (29) were married, and they had 51 children—only 1 with a congenital defect (deafness presumed to be hereditary from his deaf father, who did not have congenital rubella). Most were of normal stature, although 6 of the 40 were less than the third percentile for height. This group of survivors is quite different from the approximately 300 survivors followed in New York since the rubella epidemic of 1963 to 1965.[580] In their late 20s, approximately one third of these survivors were leading relatively normal lives in the community, one third live with their parents and may have "noncompetitive" employment, and one third reside in facilities with 24-hour care. Neither the Australian nor the New York group is a representative sample of all survivors of maternal rubella infection, but these groups do offer insight on long-term prognosis. The differences in outcome between the Australian group (survivors of Norman Gregg's original patients) and the New York group probably reflect the different methods by which the groups were collected and the significant differences in the medical technology of the 1940s compared with the 1960s.

LABORATORY DIAGNOSIS

Timely, accurate diagnosis of acute primary rubella infection in the pregnant woman and congenital rubella infection in the infant is imperative if appropriate management is to be undertaken (see "Management Issues"). The diagnosis must be confirmed serologically or virologically because clinical diagnosis of postnatal and congenital rubella is unreliable. In any suspected exposure of a pregnant woman, every effort should be made to confirm rubella infection so that accurate counseling can be offered about the risks to the fetus. Laboratory proof of congenital infection facilitates proper treatment, follow-up, and long-term management.

Maternal Infection

Because of inapparent infection, the variable clinical manifestations of rubella, and the mimicking of rubella by other viral exanthems, laboratory diagnosis is essential in managing potential rubella infection during pregnancy (see "Natural History" and "Clinical Manifestations").[157,199,226,227,308] Although virus can be cultured from the nose and throat, isolation techniques are impractical. Although reverse transcriptase–polymerase chain reaction (RT-PCR) offers another reliable tool for confirming the diagnosis during acute rubella, laboratory confirmation usually is limited to serologic testing (see "The Virus"). Acute primary infection can usually be documented by demonstrating a significant rise in antibody level between acute and convalescent sera or the presence of rubella-specific IgM antibody. Appropriate timing of specimen collection with regard to rash onset (or exposure in the case of subclinical infection) is critical for accurate interpretation of results. Diagnosis is greatly facilitated if the immune status is known before disease onset or exposure.[259] Women with laboratory evidence of immunity are not at risk. From a practical point of view, women with a history of vaccination on or after the first birthday should also be considered immune.[256,257] However, because seroconversion is not 100% (see "Prevention of Congenital Rubella"), serologic testing may be indicated on an individual basis in vaccinated women who have a known exposure or a rash and illness consistent with rubella to rule out acute primary infection.

Traditionally, a fourfold or greater rise in antibody titer (i.e., HI, complement fixation, or latex agglutination tests) has been considered a significant rise in antibody. However, with the advent of enzyme immunoassay, the diagnosis may be based on significant changes in optical density expressed as an index rather than a titer. The acute-phase specimen should be taken as soon as possible after onset of the rash, ideally within 7 days. If a positive titer is obtained for a specimen taken on the day of rash onset or 1 to 2 days later, the risk of acute infection is low but cannot be excluded. The convalescent-phase serum sample should be taken 10 to 14 days later. If the first serum sample is obtained more than 7 days after rash onset, some assays (e.g., HI) may not be able to detect a significant antibody rise because titers may have already peaked. In this situation, measurement of antibodies that appear later in the course of infection may be useful. A significant rise in complement fixation titer or, for example, a high HI, latex agglutination, or enzyme immunoassay titer and little or no antibody as measured by passive hemagglutination suggests recent infection.

When multiple serum samples are obtained in the course of the diagnostic workup, all should be tested simultaneously in the same laboratory to avoid misinterpretation of laboratory-related variations in titer. Although a single high titer is consistent with recent infection, it is not specific enough to conclude that recent infection has occurred.[259]

Detection of rubella-specific IgM (RIgM) is a very useful method for confirming acute, recent infection. Although RIgM testing is valuable, a number of factors can affect test results. Results must be interpreted with careful attention to the timing of the specimens. Samples taken within the first several days after onset of rash may have low or even undetectable levels of RIgM, but a specimen taken 7 to 14 days later invariably shows higher titers of antibody. The levels of RIgM may decline promptly thereafter. Many of the methods previously described for detecting IgM have some limitations (see "The Virus"). IgM antibody testing may involve pretreatment of the serum by a variety of techniques to separate IgM from IgG, such as column chromatography, sucrose gradient centrifugation, or adsorption of IgG with staphylococcal protein A. The serum IgM fraction can then be assayed by HI, immunofluorescence, radioimmunoassay, or enzyme immunoassay.[157,206-210,213,215,224-228,230-238] A false-positive result may occur if the serum was pretreated with protein A, because about 5% of IgG is not removed. The radioimmunoassay and enzyme immunoassay techniques can directly detect specific IgM antibodies in unfractionated sera, but false-positive results may be produced by the presence of rheumatoid factor.[157,207,209] A solid-phase, immunosorbent (i.e., capture) technique appears to be unaffected by rheumatoid factor.[99,210,225,236] A warning is necessary. Whereas high or moderate titers provide very good evidence of recent infection, low rubella-specific IgM titers detected by sensitive assays must be interpreted cautiously. Low titers have been shown to persist for many months in a few patients after natural infection and can be detected in some immune patients with subclinical reinfection.[41,51,53,55,355-360] Diagnosis of subclinical infection is relatively straightforward if the woman is known to be susceptible, the exposure is recognized, and a serum sample is obtained approximately 28 days after exposure. The diagnosis is more difficult if the immune status of the woman is unknown. However, it can be facilitated if the acute-phase serum specimen is obtained as soon as possible after a recognized exposure that did not occur more than 5 weeks earlier.[259] The convalescent serum sample, if necessary, should then be obtained approximately 3 weeks later. If the first specimen lacks detectable antibody, continued close clinical observance and serologic follow-up are necessary. If the first specimen has detectable antibody and was obtained within 7 to 10 days of exposure, there is no risk of infection, and further evaluation is unnecessary. A positive titer in a specimen obtained after this period indicates a need for further serologic investigation. If test results of paired serum specimens are inconclusive, RIgM testing may be helpful, but a negative test result may be difficult to interpret.

More significant diagnostic difficulties arise when women of unknown immune status are exposed at an unknown time, were exposed more than 5 weeks earlier, or had rash onset more than 3 weeks earlier.[259] In these situations, expert consultation may be necessary if positive titers are obtained. Where available, avidity testing of rubella IgG may be used to help clarify the timing of infection. Recent rubella infection is characterized by antibody of low avidity. When such low-avidity antibody is found in the presence of rubella IgM, it supports a diagnosis of recent rubella infection.[358-360]

Unfortunately, conclusive information about the timing of past infection and risk to the fetus is often not available, even when a combination of antibody assays is used. These situations can be minimized if prenatal rubella testing is carried out routinely. Laboratories performing prenatal screening should store these specimens until delivery in case retesting is necessary.[256,533]

Congenital Infection

A presumptive diagnosis of congenital rubella infection should be entertained for any infant born to a mother who had documented or suspected rubella infection at any time during pregnancy (see "Transmission In Utero").[103,109] The diagnosis should also be considered in any infant with evidence of intrauterine growth retardation and other stigmata consistent with congenital infection, regardless of maternal history (see "Clinical Manifestations"). Although such findings are sensitive for clinically apparent disease, they are nonspecific because many of them can be associated with other intrauterine infections, such as cytomegalovirus infection, syphilis, and toxoplasmosis. Many affected infants are asymptomatic. As with maternal rubella, congenital infection must be confirmed by laboratory tests.

In contrast to maternal rubella, attempting to isolate rubella virus in tissue culture is a valuable tool for diagnosing congenital rubella in newborns. The virus is most readily isolated from the posterior pharynx and less consistently so from the conjunctivae, cerebrospinal fluid, or urine.** Virus isolation should be attempted as soon as congenital rubella is suspected clinically because viral excretion wanes during infancy (see Fig. 28-2). In older children in whom virus shedding has ceased from other sites, virus may be isolated from cataractous lens tissue.[387] In children with encephalitis, virus may persist in the cerebrospinal fluid for several years.[360-362,361,362,486]

There are two approaches for serologic diagnosis. First, cord serum can be assayed for the presence of rubella-specific IgM antibody.[390,392,393,401] Detectable IgM antibody is a reliable indicator of congenital infection because IgM is fetally derived. However, false-positive results may occur because of rheumatoid factor or incomplete removal of IgG (largely maternal), depending on the techniques used. A minority of newborns with stigmata of congenital rubella may not have detectable levels of RIgM in sera taken during the first days of life, and some infections may go undiagnosed if infection occurred late in pregnancy because it is theoretically possible that there was inadequate time for the fetus to produce detectable levels of specific IgM antibodies by the time of delivery.[13,103,109]

A second approach is to monitor IgG levels in the infant over time to see if they persist. Maternally derived antibodies have a half-life of approximately 30 days.[390,392,393] As measured by the HI test, they usually decline at a rate of one twofold dilution per month and would be expected to disappear by 6 to 12 months of age (see Fig. 28-3). Persistence of IgG antibody at this age, especially in high titer, is presumptive evidence of intrauterine infection with rubella virus. Sera should be drawn when the child is 3 and 5 to 6 months old, with a repeat specimen at 12 months if necessary. All serum samples should be tested in parallel.

Important limitations of this method are the delay in diagnosis and the fact that rubella infections occurring after

---

**See references 2, 13, 161, 277-282, 284, 314, 315, 317, 319, 383, 384.

birth may be mistaken for congenital infections.[103,534] The latter is usually more of a problem when attempting to diagnose congenital infection retrospectively in patients beyond infancy, especially if the incidence of rubella in childhood is high or vaccine has already been administered. A third limitation is that some infants and children with congenital rubella syndrome (particularly older children) may lack antibody as measured by HI.[335,404-406] If the diagnosis is still suspected and the HI, IgM, and culture results are negative, retesting with an assay that detects antibody to all components of the virion, such as some enzyme immunoassays, is advised.[87] Some cases with undetectable HI antibody may be from an incomplete immune response to all the structural proteins of the virus, including the hemagglutinin (see "The Virus").[82,83] Other diagnostic methods, such as measurement of cellular immunity and response to vaccine (i.e., a failure to boost antibody titer), may also be helpful in this situation, but a definitive retrospective diagnosis often cannot be made.[372,421,535,536] Cerebrospinal fluid may also be examined for the presence of rubella-specific IgM.[537] As in the case for acquired infection, determination of avidity of IgG may be useful.[358,360,538]

The availability of sensitive and specific tests for prenatal diagnosis of fetal infection after suspected or documented maternal rubella can greatly facilitate counseling. Although positive diagnoses were reported from examination of amniotic fluid, fetal blood, and chorionic villus sampling for virus isolation, rubella-specific IgM and antigens, interferon, and RNA,[99,427,539-545] the low sensitivity of these assays added little to the counseling process. Reverse transcription–nested polymerase chain reaction has been reported to offer a far more reliable and rapid tool and, where available, a valuable aid to counseling.[546-548] Timing of the specimen collection related to the timing of maternal infection may influence sensitivity, which reached 100% (eight of eight specimens) for amniotic fluid in one study and 83% (five of six specimens) for chorionic villus sampling in another study. Repeat testing may increase the yield of positive specimens.[539,548]

MANAGEMENT ISSUES

The major management issues associated with postnatal infection arise when a pregnant woman is at risk of acquiring infection. Confirming the diagnosis, counseling about the risks of infection of and damage to the fetus, and discussing courses of action, including the use of immune globulin and consideration of termination of pregnancy, require a thorough understanding of the natural history and consequences of rubella in pregnancy. In the case of congenital infection, the emphasis is on diagnosis and acute and long-term management. Isolation may be important to reduce spread of infection.

Use of Immune Globulin

The role of passive immunization with immune globulin after exposure to rubella is controversial.[2,6,9,294,300,332,335,549-552] Brody and co-workers[550] reported that large doses of immune globulin may have some efficacy, but in general, it proved to be more useful when given prophylactically than when administered after exposure. This is not surprising because extensive viral replication is demonstrable a week or more before symptoms appear, with initial replication probably beginning even earlier. The amount of antirubella antibody in commercial immune globulin preparations is variable and unpredictable; specific hyperimmune globulin preparations are not available.[552,553] Theoretically, the role of circulating antibodies in rubella is mainly to limit the viremia and possibly to prevent replication at the portal of entry; antibody is less valuable after infection has begun. Fetal infection occurred when immune globulin was administered to the mother in what appeared to be adequate amounts soon after exposure. Another disadvantage of immune globulin is that it may eliminate or reduce clinical findings without affecting viral replication. Clinical clues of maternal infection would be masked without adequate protection of the fetus, resulting in a false sense of security.

It is recommended that use of immune globulin be confined to those rubella-susceptible women known to have been exposed who do not wish to interrupt their pregnancy under any circumstances.[255,257] In this situation, large doses (20 mL in adults) should be administered. The patient should be advised that protection from fetal infection cannot be guaranteed.

Termination of Pregnancy

A discussion of the complex issues involved in the decision about termination of pregnancy for maternal rubella is beyond the scope of this chapter. The decision must be carefully weighed by the physician and the prospective parents. The physician must have a thorough understanding of the known facts about the pathogenesis and diagnosis of congenital rubella and the risks to the fetus depending on the timing of maternal infection. Where available, analysis of amniotic fluid, fetal blood, or chorionic villus sampling by reverse transcription–nested polymerase chain reaction may assist in antenatal diagnosis of infection.[546-548] Expert consultation is desirable to ensure that the most current information is used in the decision-making process.

Clinical Management

Acute rubella infection usually requires little clinical management. However, the patient with congenital infection may require medical, surgical, educational, and rehabilitative management. Many lesions are not apparent at birth because they have not yet appeared or cannot be detected. In keeping with its chronicity, congenital rubella must be managed as a dynamic rather than a static disease state. A continuing effort on the part of the physician must be made to define initially the extent of the problem and to detect evidence of progressive disease or emergence of new problems over time. Because of the broad range of problems, a multidisciplinary team approach to care is essential.

Complete pediatric, neurologic, cardiac, ophthalmologic, and audiologic examinations should be complemented by complete blood cell count, by radiologic bone surveys, and often by evaluation of cerebrospinal fluid for all newborns in whom the diagnosis is suspected, whether the infant is symptomatic or not. Some defects, such as interstitial pneumonitis, can be slowly progressive and apparently cause their major functional difficulties months after birth.

Infected infants require scrutiny during the first 6 months of life. Serial assessment for immunologic dyscrasias is necessary during this period because the humoral defects may be masked by the presence of maternal immunoglobulin.

Hearing defects and psychomotor difficulties are by far the most important problems because of their high incidence. Both often occur in infants who are initially asymptomatic. The new techniques for detection of hearing impairment in newborns and the state-mandated universal newborn hearing screening testing requirements have been initiated too recently to determine their utility in detection of unsuspected congenital rubella. Delay in diagnosis and therapeutic intervention has a profound impact on language development and skills acquisition and can magnify psychosocial adjustment problems within the entire family constellation.

Because many children with congenital rubella are multihandicapped, early interdisciplinary treatment is warranted. Appropriate hearing aids; visual aids, including contact lenses; speech, language, occupational, and physical therapy; and special educational programs are frequently required for such children. Serial psychologic and perceptual testing may be very helpful for ongoing management, particularly when performed by individuals experienced in assessing multihandicapped, sensorially deprived children. In many cases, repeated testing is important because the problems appear to be progressive and require continuing assessment of the therapeutic approach. In the United States, most infants suspected of congenital rubella are eligible for early intervention and habilitation services authorized by the Federal Individuals with Disabilities Education Act. These programs offer such services to affected children beginning in infancy, a critical time for children who may be hearing impaired. The impact of universal newborn hearing screening programs as another tool for early detection of congenital rubella and of cochlear implants for children with severe rubella deafness remains to be seen.

Chemotherapy

Because postnatal rubella is usually mild, there has been little need to pursue chemotherapeutic regimens, and the literature on this subject is sparse. Interferon has been used to treat chronic arthritis, and isoprinosine has been administered to a patient with postnatally acquired progressive rubella panencephalitis.[435,532,554] Chance temporal association between interferon administration and reported improvement in joint symptoms cannot be differentiated from potential therapeutic benefits of the interferon. In the trial of isoprinosine, no improvement was observed.

The number of reports regarding treatment of infants with congenital rubella is somewhat limited. The course of congenital infection does not appear to be altered by any available chemotherapeutic agent. Because amantadine reduces the replication of rubella virus in vitro, it has theoretical possibilities as a chemotherapeutic agent.[158-160] Its use, however, has been confined to a 5-month-old infant with congenital infection.[161] Neither virus excretion nor clinical status was affected. Interferon has also been administered to a few infants with congenital rubella syndrome. Arvin and associates[555] reported that nasopharyngeal excretion in three infants (3 to 5 months old) persisted throughout interferon administration, although at reduced titers compared with baseline. There was, however, no clinical effect. Larsson and co-workers[556] administered interferon to a 14-month-old child and reported regression of a cutaneous eruption resulting from vasculitis and disappearance of viremia. However, viruria and other signs of viral persistence (e.g., rubella-specific IgM in the cerebrospinal fluid) were unaffected. It is also not certain whether improvement in the rash was from interferon administration or was coincidental. A 10-month-old infant treated by Verder and co-workers[134] may have benefited from interferon, but it is noteworthy that improvement was also seen after exchange transfusions that preceded the interferon treatment. Isoprinosine has been administered to some patients with progressive rubella panencephalitis.[532,557] As for postnatally acquired disease, the results in this case have been disappointing.

Isolation

Patients with rubella are considered infectious from the fifth day before to the seventh day after the onset of the rash and should be placed in contact isolation.[558] Exposed rubella-susceptible patients confined to hospital should be placed in contact isolation from the 7th through 21st day after exposure and tested appropriately to rule out asymptomatic infection.[559] Infectious patients with congenital rubella should also be in contact isolation.[558] Isolation precautions should be instituted as soon as rubella or congenital rubella is suspected. Only persons known to be immune (i.e., those with serologic evidence of immunity or documentation of vaccination on or after the first birthday) should care for infectious or potentially infectious patients.[255,257]

Children with congenital rubella syndrome should be considered infectious for the first year of life unless repeated pharyngeal and urine culture results are negative.[257,558] Culture results are unlikely to become negative until the child is 3 to 6 months old (see Fig. 28-2). From a practical point of view, children older than 1 year are unlikely to be a significant source of infection. In the home situation, susceptible pregnant visitors should be informed of the potential risk of exposure.

PREVENTION OF CONGENITAL RUBELLA

Rubella Vaccine and Immunization Strategies

Active immunization is the only practical means to prevent congenital rubella because passive immunization provides unreliable, transient protection (see "Management Issues"). However, there has been considerable debate about the best way to use the vaccine.[3,5-7,30,35,560] Because rubella vaccination is not aimed primarily at protecting the individual, but rather the unborn fetus, two basic strategies have been proposed: universal childhood immunization and selective vaccination of susceptible girls and women of childbearing age. The former approach is designed to interrupt transmission of virus by vaccinating the reservoir of infection, reduce the overall risk of infection in the general population, and provide indirect protection of unvaccinated, postpubertal women. The latter approach directly protects those at risk of being infected when pregnant, limits overall vaccine use, and allows virus to circulate and boost vaccine-induced immunity in the population. Experience gained during the past 30 years indicates that integration of both is necessary to achieve maximum control in the shortest possible time.[5,30,33,35]

At the time of licensure in 1969, available information indicated that the live-attenuated rubella vaccines were safe, noncommunicable, and highly effective.[3,4,26-28] Although information on the duration of vaccine-induced immunity was limited, public health policy makers in the United States believed that vaccination of all children would provide protection into the childbearing years. The duration and quality of the immunity would have to be monitored continually. Because vaccine virus could cross the placenta and infect the fetus, cautious recommendations for vaccination of susceptible women of childbearing age were also proposed.[561-563] Vaccine was to be administered in this population only after susceptibility had been documented by serologic testing. Vaccinated women were also advised to avoid conception for 2 months after vaccination. After Fleet and colleagues[564] isolated virus from the fetus of a woman who had conceived 7 weeks before vaccination, this time interval was increased to 3 months as an extra precaution.[255,257]

In England and other areas of the world, mass vaccination was considered undesirable because of concerns about the duration of vaccine-induced immunity.[5-7,32,107] Instead, vaccine was targeted for all schoolgirls 11 to 14 years of age and postpubertal females known to be seronegative. As with the U.S. program, pregnancy was to be avoided for up to 3 months after immunization. The goal was to immunize at least 90% of the women immediately at risk and simultaneously provide a higher level of immunity throughout the childbearing-aged group. It was recognized that this approach would take many years to have a significant effect on the incidence of congenital infection.

The U.S. strategy prevented epidemic disease but initially had little effect on the occurrence of infection in young adults, particularly women of childbearing age (see "Epidemiology").[5,24,31,36,258,292] Although vaccine was recommended for susceptible women, concerns about the effect of the vaccine on the fetus led to low immunization coverage in this population. There was no evidence that infection was occurring in individuals who had been vaccinated years earlier (see "Update on Vaccine Characteristics"). Childhood vaccination decreased the overall risk of infection, but virus could still circulate in the community, especially wherever unvaccinated adolescents and adults congregated.[260-268,271-276] Although congenital rubella syndrome could eventually be eliminated as vaccinated cohorts of children entered the childbearing years, this process would take many years, and potentially preventable cases of congenital infection would continue to occur.[268] Accordingly, specific recommendations were made to increase vaccination levels in older individuals, particularly women of childbearing age (see "Vaccine Recommendations").[255,257]

Selective vaccination programs have not been successful because of the inability to immunize a sufficient proportion of the female population.[7,33,34] With this immunization approach, large-scale epidemics continue to occur, and the incidence of congenital rubella has not declined significantly since the introduction of vaccines. Because of these problems, in 1988, Great Britain implemented a program of MMR vaccination for all children in the second year of life, began a mass measles-rubella vaccine program for 5- to 16-year-old recipients in 1994, and added a preschool MMR booster in 1996 (P Tookey, National Congenital Rubella Surveillance Program, personal communication, June 1999).[33,35]

Update on Vaccine Characteristics

Approximately 200 million doses of vaccine have been administered in the United States since rubella vaccines were licensed in 1969. The RA 27/3 strain of vaccine was licensed for use in the United States in 1979 and is now the only vaccine available. Although it has been used intranasally, it is licensed only for subcutaneous administration. The RA 27/3 vaccine elicits an immune response that more closely resembles that occurring after natural infection than the Cendehill or HPV-77 strains of vaccines do.[192,376,377,565] However, there are no data to indicate the need for revaccination of persons who had not previously received the RA 27/3 vaccine. Although comparative data are not available, at least one study has shown that the RA 27/3 vaccine induces antibody formation to the three major rubella virus structural proteins.[82]

Appropriate administration of vaccine induces an antibody response in 95% or more of persons 12 months old or older when vaccinated. Vaccine efficacy and challenge studies indicate that more than 90% to 95% of vaccinated persons are protected against clinical illness or asymptomatic viremia. Whereas vaccine-induced titers are lower than those after natural infection and are more likely to increase after reexposure, protection after a single dose of vaccine is, for the most part, solid and lasts for at least 18 years, if not for life.*

Detectable HI antibodies persist in almost all vaccinated subjects who initially seroconvert.[39,43,46,48,54,57] Long-term studies of vaccinated persons who initially seroconverted and then lost detectable HI antibodies indicate that most of these individuals are also immune because they have detectable antibodies as measured by other, more sensitive assays or have a booster immune response (i.e., absence of IgM antibody and a rapid rise and decline in IgG antibody) after revaccination.[43,49,567] Viremia and reinfection have been documented in some vaccinated persons and some naturally immune individuals who had very low titers of antibody.[38,40,44,50,56] It is unknown how often this phenomenon occurs or places the fetus at risk, but the incidence of both events is believed to be low.[8] There are rare case reports of congenital infection after reinfection of mothers who had been previously infected or vaccinated (see "The Virus" and "Natural History").[43,45,52,111,116,321,326-328] The lack of an international standard level of antibody considered to be protective frequently complicates the interpretation of serologic data when antibodies are detected only by tests more sensitive than the HI test. Cutoff levels ranging from 5 to 15 IU have been used.[54,57,199,227,567,570] Available information indicates that any appropriately measured level of detectable antibody should be considered presumptive evidence of past infection and immunity.[255,257] This applies to naturally acquired and vaccine-induced immunity.

Rubella vaccine is remarkably safe. Rash, low-grade fever, and lymphadenopathy are occasionally observed. The polyneuropathies, myositis, and vasculitis associated with the

*See references 38-40, 43, 44, 46, 48-50, 54, 56, 57, 260, 305, 566-569.

HPV-77 strain of vaccine have not been reported after administration of the RA 27/3 strain.[9,571]

Vaccine-related arthralgia and arthritis remain a concern, particularly for susceptible adult women.[5,8,59,61,62,64] Although arthralgia has been reported in up to 3% of susceptible children, arthritis has been reported rarely in these vaccinated subjects. In contrast, joint pain occurs in up to 40% of susceptible vaccinated females, with arthritis-like signs and symptoms reported in 10% to 20%.[5,64] Persistent and recurring joint complaints have been reported, but most studies indicate that they occur infrequently. The high frequency (5%) of persistent joint symptoms reported by one group of investigators has not been confirmed.[8,64] However, this rate is still far less than that (30%) after natural infection, as reported by the same group of researchers.[64] Permanent disability and joint destruction have also been reported, but only rarely.[61,64]

Most published data indicate that these and other adverse events associated with rubella vaccine occur only in susceptible vaccinated persons.[5,8] There is no conclusive evidence that there is an increased risk of reactions in persons who are already immune at the time of vaccination.[8,64,123] Vaccination programs of adults have not led to significant rates of absenteeism or disruption in everyday, work-related activities.[8,271,273-276]

Although some vaccinated persons intermittently shed virus in low titers from the pharynx 7 to 28 days after vaccination, there is no evidence that vaccine virus is spread to susceptible contacts.[5,565] Vaccine virus can, however, be recovered from breast milk and may be transmitted to the breast-fed neonate.[61,343,572,573] The vaccine virus may elicit an immune response in some exposed neonates. There is no evidence of a significant alteration in the immune response or increased risk of reactions after vaccination at a later date.[62,64] Although a mild clinical infection from transmitted vaccine virus has been reported, infection with wild-type virus might have occurred.[574]

The fetotropic and teratogenic potential of rubella vaccine virus has greatly influenced vaccination practices, not only in the United States but also worldwide. With the increased emphasis on vaccinating susceptible, postpubertal females in the United States, especially recent immigrants, the need to have accurate information on the risks of the vaccine virus on the fetus became even more important.

From 1971 through 1988, the Centers for Disease Control followed to term prospectively 321 pregnant women known to be susceptible to rubella by serologic testing who were vaccinated in the period from 3 months before to 3 months after conception (Table 28-4).[65,255] Approximately one third received vaccine during the highest risk period for viremia and fetal defects (1 week before to 4 weeks after conception).[58,65] Ninety-four received HPV-77 or Cendehill vaccines, 1 received a vaccine of unknown strain, and 226 received RA 27/3vaccine. None of the 229 offspring (three mothers who received RA 27/3 vaccine had twins) had malformations consistent with congenital rubella infection.

Although the observed risk of congenital defects is zero, the maximal estimated theoretical risk of serious malformations attributable to any rubella vaccine is 1.2%, based on the 95% confidence limits of the binomial distribution. If only the infants exposed to the RA 27/3 vaccine are considered, the maximal theoretical risk is 1.7%. The overall maximal theoretical risk remains far less than that for congenital rubella syndrome after maternal infection with wild-type virus during the first trimester of pregnancy (up to 70%) and is no greater than the 2% to 3% rate of major birth defects in the absence of exposure to rubella vaccine.[65,105]

Four children were born with various congenital malformations consistent with congenital rubella, and their mothers were later found to have received rubella vaccine within 3 months of conception.[5,372] Clinical, epidemiologic, and laboratory data indicate that all the mothers had natural rubella infection.

These favorable data are consistent with the experience reported with Cendehill and RA 27/3 vaccines in the Federal Republic of Germany and the United Kingdom.[60,63] None of 98 infants in the Federal Republic of Germany and none of 21 infants in Great Britain whose mothers were known to be susceptible when vaccinated were born with congenital anomalies consistent with congenital rubella syndrome. The most reassuring information comes from a rubella vaccine mass campaign involving 16 million women in Brazil during 2001 and 2002, among whom were 2327 susceptible, pregnant women. Follow-up studies on 76% of these women revealed an infection rate of 3.6% among their newborns but no evidence of increased abortion, stillbirth, preterm birth, or congenital rubella syndrome (R Soares, provisional data presented at the PAHO Conference, Washington, DC, March 3, 2004). Although fetal infection occurs, if rubella vaccine has any teratogenic potential, it must be rare.

Vaccination Recommendations

The control of rubella and congenital rubella in the United States has been predicated on universal immunization of

Table 28–4 Maximal Theoretical Risks of Congenital Rubella Syndrome after Rubella Vaccination by Vaccine Strain, United States, 1971 to 1988[a]

Vaccine Strain	Susceptible Vaccinated Subjects	Normal Livebirths	Risk of CRS	
			Observed	*Theoretical*
RA 27/3	226	229[b]	0	0-1.8
Cendehill or HPV-77	94	94		0-3.8
Unknown	1	1	0	
Total	321	324	0	0-1.2

[a]No women entered in the register after 1980 were vaccinated with Cendehill or HPV-77 vaccine.
[b]Includes three twin births.
CRS, congenital rubella syndrome.

children, with a single dose of vaccine given after the first birthday, and selective immunization of postpubertal and susceptible postpartum women. This approach remains the basis for current recommendations of the Advisory Committee on Immunization Practices (ACIP) of the Public Health Service and the American Academy of Pediatrics (AAP).[255,257] However, part of this success has come from the recommended use of rubella vaccine as a component of the combined MMR vaccine, which in the United States is given routinely to 15-month-old children. As concerns arose about measles in adolescents and adults, attributed to the existence of a cohort of young adults representing the 2% to 10% failure rate for a single dose of measles vaccine and the theoretical possibility of waning immunity after successful immunization in early childhood, the ACIP and AAP added a second dose to the measles immunization schedule in 1989. The specific recommendation was that the second dose be given just before school entry or in the prepubertal period and that the vaccine be given as the MMR vaccine.[255,257]

Rubella immunization (as MMR vaccine) should be offered to all women of childbearing age who do not have acceptable evidence of rubella immunity. Given the current data, routine screening of postpuberal women for susceptibility before rubella vaccination is no longer recommended. However, women should understand the theoretical risk of fetal infection and be advised not to become pregnant for at least 28 days after vaccination.[265] Known pregnancy is still considered a contraindication.

Missed opportunities should not be confused with bona fide contraindications for rubella immunization. These include the following:

1. Severe febrile illness
2. Altered immunity from congenital immunodeficiency; from acquired diseases such as leukemia, lymphoma, and generalized malignancy; and from therapy with radiation, corticosteroids, alkylating drugs, and antimetabolites
3. History of an anaphylactic reaction to neomycin (the vaccine does not contain penicillin)
4. Pregnancy, albeit because of theoretical concerns

Because vaccine virus is not transmitted through the nasopharynx, the presence of a susceptible pregnant woman in a household is not a contraindication for vaccination of other household members. Vaccine virus is present in breast milk and can infect the neonate, but breast-feeding also is not a contraindication to vaccination. Although vaccination is usually deferred for 8 to 12 weeks after receipt of immune globulin, receipt of anti-Rho (D) immune globulin (human) or blood products does not generally interfere with seroconversion and is not a contraindication to postpartum vaccination.[575-578] However, in this situation, 6- to 8-week postvaccination serologic testing should be performed to ensure that seroconversion has taken place.[577] This is the only situation in which postvaccination testing is recommended as routine.

Outbreak Control

Although outbreak control is an after-the-fact method of prevention, rapid, aggressive responses to outbreaks are necessary to limit the spread of infection and can serve as a catalyst to increase immunization levels. Although there is no conclusive evidence that vaccination after exposure prevents rubella, there are also no data to suggest that vaccinating an individual incubating rubella is harmful. Vaccination programs initiated in the middle of an outbreak serve to protect persons not adequately exposed in the current outbreak from future exposures.

Although laboratory confirmation of cases is important, control measures—including isolation of suspected cases or susceptible exposed persons, vaccination or exclusion of susceptible persons, and confirmation of the immune status of exposed pregnant women—should be implemented as soon as a suspected case has been identified (see "Management Issues"). Ideally, mandatory exclusion and vaccination of susceptible individuals should be practiced to ensure high rates of vaccination in the shortest possible period, particularly in the medical setting. Vaccination during an outbreak has not been associated with significant absenteeism in the workplace.[8,271,273-276] However, vaccination before the occurrence of an outbreak is preferable, because vaccination causes far less disruption of routine work activities and schedules than rubella infection.

Surveillance

Surveillance of rubella and congenital rubella is necessary for rubella prevention because the information can be used to evaluate the progress of the immunization program, to identify high-risk groups that would benefit from specific interventions, and to monitor the safety, efficacy, and durability of the vaccine. Surveillance can also draw attention to small numbers of cases before they develop into sizable outbreaks. Because rubella and congenital rubella are reportable diseases, all suspected cases should be reported to local health officials.

Prospects for the Future

Full implementation of the two-dose MMR vaccine recommendation should eliminate indigenous congenital rubella from the United States, and the PAHO goal of eliminating rubella in the Western Hemisphere by 2010 is realistic. However, given the frequency of international travel, all countries will remain at risk of imported disease during the foreseeable future. Clearly, there is more pressure on the world health community to eliminate measles globally. Including rubella vaccine in a combined vaccine with measles for global use remains the best hope of preventing what remains a significant disease burden in many other countries.[581] Although 58% of countries have vaccine available, most have not implemented effective rubella immunization programs. A recent report from Morocco has demonstrated annual rates of congenital rubella syndrome in the range of 8.1 to 12.7 cases per 1000 live births.[581a] Maintaining high levels of immunization, ongoing surveillance (recognizing that the sporadic nature of new cases likely will add to delay in diagnosis), and prompt outbreak control measures remain critical for ultimate elimination of rubella. The efforts underway in the Western Hemisphere can be a global model that eventually will make rubella and congenital rubella syndrome matters of historic interest.[582]

REFERENCES

1. Wesselhoff C. Rubella (German measles). N Engl J Med 236:943, 1947.
2. Krugman S (ed). Rubella symposium. Am J Dis Child 110:345, 1965.
3. Krugman S (ed). Proceedings of the International Conference on Rubella Immunization. Am J Dis Child 118:2, 1969.
4. Regamy RH, deBarbieri A, Hennessen W, et al (eds). International Symposium on Rubella Vaccines. Symp Ser Immunobiol Stand 11:1, 1969.
5. Preblud SR, Serdula MK, Frank JA Jr, et al. Rubella vaccination in the United States: a ten-year review. Epidemiol Rev 2:171, 1980.
6. Hanshaw JB, Dudgeon JA, Marshall WC (eds). Viral Diseases of the Fetus and Newborn, 2nd ed. Philadelphia, WB Saunders, 1985, p 13.
7. Krugman S (ed). International Symposium on Prevention of Congenital Rubella Infection. Rev Infect Dis 7(Suppl 1):S1, 1985.
8. Preblud SR. Some current issues relating to rubella vaccine. JAMA 254:253, 1985.
9. Cherry JD. Rubella. *In* Feigin RD, Cherry JD (eds). Textbook of Pediatric Infectious Diseases, 3rd ed. Philadelphia, WB Saunders, 1992, p 1792.
10. Manton WG. Some accounts of rash liable to be mistaken for scarlatina. Med Trans R Coll Physicians (Lond) 5:149, 1815.
11. Veale H. History of epidemic Rötheln, with observations on its pathology. Edinb Med J 12:404, 1896.
12. Gregg NM. Congenital cataract following German measles in the mother. Trans Ophthalmol Soc Aust 3:35, 1941.
13. Cooper LZ. Congenital rubella in the United States. *In* Krugman S, Gershon AA (eds). Infections of the Fetus and the Newborn Infant. New York, Alan R Liss, 1975, p 1.
14. Ziring PR. Congenital rubella: the teenage years. Pediatr Ann 6:762, 1977.
15. Hiro Y, Tasaka S. Die Rötheln sind eine Viruskrankheit. Monatsschr Kinderheilkd 76:328, 1938.
16. Habel K. Transmission of rubella to *Macaca mulatta* monkeys. Public Health Rep 57:1126, 1942.
17. Anderson SB. Experimental rubella in human volunteers. J Immunol 62:29, 1949.
18. Krugman S, Ward R, Jacobs KG, et al. Studies on rubella immunization. I. Demonstration of rubella without rash. JAMA 151:285, 1953.
19. Weller TH, Neva FA. Propagation in tissue culture of cytopathic agents from patients with rubella-like illness. Proc Soc Exp Biol Med 111:215, 1962.
20. Parkman PD, Buescher EL, Artenstein MS. Recovery of rubella virus from army recruits. Proc Soc Exp Biol Med 111:225, 1962.
21. Parkman PD, Mundon FK, McCown JM, et al. Studies of rubella. II. Neutralization of the virus. J Immunol 93:608, 1964.
22. Sever JL, Huebner RJ, Castellano GA, et al. Rubella complement fixation test. Science 148:385, 1965.
23. Stewart GL, Parkman PD, Hopps HE, et al. Rubella-virus hemagglutination-inhibition test. N Engl J Med 276:554, 1967.
24. Orenstein WA, Bart KJ, Hinman AR, et al. The opportunity and obligation to eliminate measles from the United States. JAMA 251: 1988, 1984.
25. Robertson SE, Featherstone DA, Gacic-Dobo M. Rubella and congenital rubella syndrome: global update. Pan Am J Public Health 14:306, 2003
26. Meyer HM Jr, Parkman PD, Panos TC. Attenuated rubella virus. II. Production of an experimental live-virus vaccine and clinical trial. N Engl J Med 275:575, 1966.
27. Prinzie A, Huygelen C, Gold J, et al. Experimental live attenuated rubella virus vaccine: clinical evaluation of Cendehill strain. Am J Dis Child 118:172, 1969.
28. Plotkin JA, Farquhar JD, Katz M. Attenuation of RA 27/3 rubella virus in WI-38 human diploid cells. Am J Dis Child 118:178, 1969.
29. Perkins FT. Licensed vaccines. Rev Infect Dis 7(Suppl 1):S73, 1985.
30. Hinman AR, Bart KJ, Orenstein WA, et al. Rational strategy for rubella vaccination. Lancet 1:39, 1983.
31. Bart KJ, Orenstein WA, Preblud SR, et al. Universal immunization to interrupt rubella. Rev Infect Dis 7(Suppl 1):S177, 1985.
32. Dudgeon JA. Selective immunization: protection of the individual. Rev Infect Dis 7(Suppl 1):S185, 1985.
33. Walker D, Carter H, Jones IJ. Measles, mumps, and rubella: the need for a change in immunisation policy. BMJ 292:1501, 1986.
34. Best JM, Welch JM, Baker DA, et al. Maternal rubella at St. Thomas' Hospital in 1978 and 1986: support for augmenting the rubella vaccination programme. Lancet 2:88, 1987.
35. Badenoch J. Big bang for vaccination: eliminating measles, mumps, and rubella. BMJ 297:750, 1988.
36. Centers for Disease Control. Increase in rubella and congenital rubella in the United States, 1988-1990. MMWR Morb Mortal Wkly Rep 40: 93, 1991.
37. Executive Committee of PAHO. New goal for vaccination programs in the region of the Americas: to eliminate rubella and congenital rubella syndrome. Pan Am J Public Health 14:359, 2003.
38. Harcourt GC, Best JM, Banatvala JE. Rubella-specific serum and nasopharyngeal antibodies in volunteers with naturally acquired and vaccine-induced immunity after intranasal challenge. J Infect Dis 142:145, 1980.
39. Weibel RE, Buynak EB, McLean AA, et al. Persistence of antibody in human subjects 7 to 10 years following administration of combined live attenuated measles, mumps, and rubella virus vaccines. Proc Soc Exp Biol Med 165:260, 1980.
40. Balfour HH, Groth KE, Edelman C, et al. Rubella viraemia and antibody responses after rubella vaccination and reimmunisation. Lancet 1:1078, 1981.
41. Cradock-Watson JE, Ridehalgh MKS, Anderson MJ, et al. Outcome of asymptomatic infection with rubella virus during pregnancy. J Hyg (Lond) 87:147, 1981.
42. Bott LM, Eizenberg DH. Congenital rubella after successful vaccination. Med J Aust 1:514, 1982.
43. Herrmann KL, Halstead SB, Wiebenga NH. Rubella antibody persistence after immunization. JAMA 247:193, 1982.
44. O'Shea S, Best JM, Banatvala JE. Viremia, virus excretion, and antibody responses after challenge in volunteers with low levels of antibody to rubella virus. J Infect Dis 148:639, 1983.
45. Enders G, Calm A, Schaub J. Rubella embryopathy after previous maternal rubella vaccination. Infection 12:96, 1984.
46. Hillary IB, Griffith AH. Persistence of rubella antibodies 15 years after subcutaneous administration of Wistar 27/3 strain live attenuated rubella virus vaccine. Vaccine 2:274, 1984.
47. Morgan-Capner R, Hodgson J, Sellwood J, et al. Clinically apparent rubella reinfection. J Infect 9:97, 1984.
48. O'Shea S, Best JM, Banatvala JE, et al. Persistence of rubella antibody 8-18 years after vaccination. BMJ 288:1043, 1984.
49. Serdula MK, Halstead SB, Wiebenga NH, et al. Serological response to rubella revaccination. JAMA 251:1974, 1984.
50. Banatvala JE, Best JM, O'Shea S, et al. Persistence of rubella antibodies after vaccination: detection after experimental challenge. Rev Infect Dis 7(Suppl 1):S86, 1985.
51. Cradock-Watson JE, Ridehalgh MKS, Anderson MJ, et al. Rubella reinfection and the fetus. Lancet 1:1039, 1985.
52. Forsgren M, Soren L. Subclinical rubella reinfection in vaccinated women with rubella-specific IgM response during pregnancy and transmission of virus to the fetus. Scand J Infect Dis 17:337, 1985.
53. Grangeot-Keros L, Nicolas JC, Bricout F, et al. Rubella reinfection and the fetus. N Engl J Med 313:1547, 1985.
54. Horstmann DM, Schluederberg A, Emmons JE, et al. Persistence of vaccine-induced immune responses to rubella: comparison with natural infection. Rev Infect Dis 7(Suppl 1):S80, 1985.
55. Morgan-Capner P, Hodgson J, Hambling MH, et al. Detection of rubella-specific IgM in subclinical rubella reinfection in pregnancy. Lancet 1:244, 1985.
56. Schiff GM, Young BC, Stefanovic GM, et al. Challenge with rubella virus after loss of detectable vaccine-induced antibody. Rev Infect Dis 7(Suppl 1):S157, 1985.
57. Chu SY, Bernier RH, Stewart JA, et al. Rubella antibody persistence after immunization: sixteen-year follow-up in the Hawaiian Islands. JAMA 259:3133, 1988.
58. Bart SW, Stetler HC, Preblud SR, et al. Fetal risk associated with rubella vaccine: an update. Rev Infect Dis 7(Suppl 1):S95, 1985.
59. Chantler JK, Tingle AJ, Perry RE. Persistent rubella virus infection associated with chronic arthritis in children. N Engl J Med 313:1117, 1985.
60. Enders G. Rubella antibody titers in vaccinated and nonvaccinated women and results of vaccination during pregnancy. Rev Infect Dis 7(Suppl 1):S103, 1985.
61. Tingle AJ, Chantler JK, Pot KH, et al. Postpartum rubella immunization: association with development of prolonged arthritis, neurological sequelae, and chronic rubella viremia. J Infect Dis 152:606, 1985.
62. Preblud PR, Orenstein WA, Lopez C, et al. Postpartum rubella immunization. Letter to the editor. J Infect Dis 154:367, 1986.

63. Sheppard S, Smithells RW, Dickenson A, et al. Rubella vaccination and pregnancy: preliminary report of a national survey. BMJ 292:727, 1986.
64. Tingle AJ. Postpartum rubella immunization (reply). J Infect Dis 154:368, 1986.
65. Centers for Disease Control. Rubella vaccination during pregnancy—United States, 1971-1988. MMWR Morb Mortal Wkly Rep 38:290, 1989.
66. Ho-Terry L, Cohen A. Degradation of rubella virus envelope components. Arch Virol 65:1, 1980.
67. Oker-Blom C, Kalkkinen N, Kaariainen L, et al. Rubella virus contains one capsid protein and three envelope glycoproteins, E1, E2a, and E2b. J Virol 46:964, 1983.
68. Waxham MN, Wolinsky JS. Immunochemical identification of rubella virus hemagglutinin. Virology 126:194, 1983.
69. Bowden DS, Westway EG. Rubella virus: structural and non-structural proteins. J Gen Virol 65:933, 1984.
70. Ho-Terry L, Cohen A, Tedder RS. Immunologic characterisation of rubella virion polypeptides. J Med Microbiol 17:105, 1984.
71. Oker-Blom C, Ulmanen I, Kaariainen L, et al. Rubella virus 40S genome RNA specifies a 24S subgenomic mRNA that codes for a precursor to structural proteins. J Virol 49:403, 1984.
72. Dorsett PH, Miller DC, Green KY, et al. Structure and function of the rubella virus proteins. Rev Infect Dis 7(Suppl 1):S150, 1985.
73. Pettersson RF, Oker-Blom C, Kalkkinen N, et al. Molecular and antigenic characteristics and synthesis of rubella virus structural proteins. Rev Infect Dis 7(Suppl 1):S140, 1985.
74. Waxham MN, Wolinsky JS. A model of the structural organization of rubella virions. Rev Infect Dis 7(Suppl 1):S133, 1985.
75. Waxham MN, Wolinsky JS. Detailed immunologic analysis of the structural polypeptides of rubella virus using monoclonal antibodies. Virology 143:153, 1985.
76. Green KY, Dorsett PH. Rubella virus antigens: localization of epitopes involved in hemagglutination and neutralization by using monoclonal antibodies. J Virol 57:893, 1986.
77. Vidgren G, Takkinen K, Kalkkinen N, et al. Nucleotide sequence of the genes coding for the membrane glycoproteins E1 and E2 of rubella virus. J Gen Virol 68:2347, 1987.
78. Terry GM, Ho-Terry L, Londesborough P, et al. Localization of the rubella E1 epitopes. Arch Virol 98:189, 1988.
79. Clarke DM, Loo TW, McDonald H, et al. Expression of rubella virus cDNA coding for the structural proteins. Gene 65:23, 1988.
80. Frey TK, Marr LD. Sequence of the region coding for virion proteins C and E2 and the carboxy terminus of the nonstructural proteins of rubella virus: comparison with alphaviruses. Gene 62:85, 1988.
81. Takkinen K, Vidgren G, Ekstrand J, et al. Nucleotide sequence of the rubella virus capsid protein gene reveals an unusually high G/C content. J Gen Virol 69:603, 1988.
82. Cusi MG, Rossolini GM, Cellesi C, et al. Antibody response to wild rubella virus structural proteins following immunization with RA 27/3 live attenuated vaccine. Arch Virol 101:25, 1988.
83. Frey TK, Abernathy ES, Bosma TJ, et al. Molecular analysis of rubella virus epidemiology across three continents, North America, Europe and Asia, 1961-1997. J Infect Dis 178:642, 1998.
84. Katow S, Sugiura A. Antibody response to the individual rubella virus proteins in congenital and other rubella virus infections. J Clin Microbiol 21:449, 1985.
85. de Mazancourt A, Waxman MN, Nicholas JC, et al. Antibody response to the rubella virus structural proteins in infants with the congenital rubella syndrome. J Med Virol 19:111, 1986.
86. Chaye H, Chong P, Tripet B, et al. Localization of the virus neutralizing and hemagglutinin epitopes of E1 glycoprotein of rubella virus. Virology 189:483, 1992.
87. Hancock EJ, Pot K, Puterman ML, et al. Lack of association between titers of HAI antibody and whole-virus ELISA values for patients with congenital rubella syndrome. J Infect Dis 154:1031, 1986.
88. Castellano GA, Madden DL, Hazzard GT, et al. Evaluation of commercially available diagnostic kits for rubella. J Infect Dis 143:578, 1981.
89. Storch GA, Myers N. Latex-agglutination test for rubella antibody: validity of positive results assessed by response to immunization and comparison with other tests. J Infect Dis 149:459, 1984.
90. Safford JW, Abbott GG, Diemier CM. Evaluation of a rapid passive hemagglutination assay for anti-rubella antibody: comparison to hemagglutination inhibition and a vaccine challenge study. J Med Virol 17:229, 1985.
91. Skendzel LP, Edson DC. Latex agglutination test for rubella antibodies: report based on data from the College of American Pathologists surveys, 1983 to 1985. J Clin Microbiol 24:333, 1986.
92. Vaananen P, Haiva VM, Koskela P, et al. Comparison of a simple latex agglutination test with hemolysis-in-gel, hemagglutination inhibition, and radioimmunoassay for detection of rubella virus antibodies. J Clin Microbiol 21:973, 1985.
93. Chernesky MA, DeLong DJ, Mahony JB, et al. Differences in antibody responses with rapid agglutination tests for the detection of rubella antibodies. J Clin Microbiol 23:772, 1986.
94. Pruneda RC, Dover JC. A comparison of two passive agglutination procedures with enzyme-linked immunosorbent assay for rubella antibody status. Am J Clin Pathol 86:768, 1986.
95. Linde GA. Subclass distribution of rubella virus-specific immunoglobulin G. J Clin Microbiol 21:117, 1985.
96. Salonen E-M, Hovi T, Meurman O, et al. Kinetics of specific IgA, IgD, IgE, IgG, and IgM antibody responses in rubella. J Med Virol 16:1, 1985.
97. Stokes A, Mims A, Grahame R. Subclass distribution of IgG and IgA responses to rubella virus in man. J Med Microbiol 21:283, 1986.
98. Thomas HIJ, Morgan-Capner P. Specific IgG subclass antibody in rubella virus infections. Epidemiol Infect 100:443, 1988.
99. Grangeot-Keros L, Pillot J, Daffos F, et al. Prenatal and postnatal production of IgM and IgA antibodies to rubella virus studied by antibody capture immunoassay. J Infect Dis 158:138, 1988.
100. Nedeljkovic J, Jovanovic T, Oker-Blom C; Maturation of IgG avidity to individual rubella virus structural proteins. J Clin Virol 22:47, 2001.
101. Mehta NM, Thomas RM. Antenatal screening for rubella-infection or immunity? BMJ 325:90, 2002.
102. Best JM, O'Shea S, Tipples G, et al. Interpretation of rubella serology in pregnancy-pitfalls and problems. BMJ 325: 147, 2002
103. Cradock-Watson JE, Ridehalgh MKS, Anderson MJ, et al. Fetal infection resulting from maternal rubella after the first trimester of pregnancy. J Hyg (Lond) 85:381, 1980.
104. Vejtorp M, Mansa B. Rubella IgM antibodies in sera from infants born after maternal rubella later than the twelfth week of pregnancy. Scand J Infect Dis 12:1, 1980.
105. Miller E, Cradock-Watson JE, Pollock TM. Consequences of confirmed maternal rubella at successive stages of pregnancy. Lancet 2:781, 1982.
106. Grillner L, Forsgren M, Barr B, et al. Outcome of rubella during pregnancy with special reference to the 17th–24th weeks of gestation. Scand J Infect Dis 15:321, 1983.
107. Peckham C. Congenital rubella in the United Kingdom before 1970: the prevaccine era. Rev Infect Dis 7(Suppl 1):S11, 1985.
108. Bitsch M. Rubella in pregnant Danish women 1975-1984. Dan Med Bull 34:46, 1987.
109. Munro ND, Shephard S, Smithells RW, et al. Temporal relations between maternal rubella and congenital defects. Lancet 2:201, 1987.
110. Enders G, Miller E, Nickerl-Pacher U, et al. Outcome of confirmed periconceptional maternal rubella. Lancet 1:1445, 1988.
111. Partridge JW, Flewett TH, Whitehead JEM. Congenital rubella affecting an infant whose mother had rubella antibodies before conception. BMJ 282:187, 1981.
112. Best JM, Harcourt GC, Banatvala JE, et al. Congenital rubella affecting an infant whose mother had rubella antibodies before conception. BMJ 282:1235, 1981.
113. Levine JB, Berkowitz CD, St. Geme JW. Rubella virus reinfection during pregnancy leading to late-onset congenital rubella syndrome. J Pediatr 100:589, 1982.
114. Sibille G, Sarda P, Jalaguier J, et al. [Reinfection after rubella and congenital polymalformation syndrome]. J Genet Hum 34:305, 1986.
115. Hornstein L, Levy U, Fogel A. Clinical rubella with virus transmission to the fetus in a pregnant woman considered to be immune. Letter to the editor. N Engl J Med 319:1415, 1988.
116. Saule H, Enders G, Zeller J, et al. Congenital rubella infection after previous immunity of the mother. Eur J Pediatr 147:195, 1988.
117. Floret D, Rosenberg D, Hage GN, et al. Hyperthyroidism, diabetes mellitus and the congenital rubella syndrome. Acta Paediatr Scand 69:259, 1980.
118. Hansen HE, Larsen SO, Leerhoy J. Lack of correlation between the incidence of rubella antibody and the distribution of HLA antigens in a Danish population. Tissue Antigens 15:325, 1980.
119. Kato S, Kimura M, Takakura I, et al. HLA-linked genetic control in natural rubella infection. Tissue Antigens 15:86, 1980.

120. Tardieu M, Grospierre B, Durandy A, et al. Circulating immune complexes containing rubella antigens in late-onset rubella syndrome. J Pediatr 97:370, 1980.
121. Coyle PK, Wolinsky JS. Characterization of immune complexes in progressive rubella panencephalitis. Ann Neurol 9:557, 1981.
122. Ishii K, Nakazono N, Sawada H, et al. Host factors and susceptibility to rubella virus infection: the association of HLA antigens. J Med Virol 7:287, 1981.
123. Coyle PK, Wolinsky JS, Buimovici-Klein E, et al. Rubella-specific immune complexes after congenital infection and vaccination. Infect Immun 36:498, 1982.
124. Kato S, Muranaka S, Takakura I, et al. HLA-DR antigens and the rubella-specific immune response in man. Tissue Antigens 19:140, 1982.
125. Rubinstein P, Walker ME, Fedun B, et al. The HLA system in congenital rubella patients with and without diabetes. Diabetes 31:1088, 1982.
126. Boner A, Wilmott RW, Dinwiddie R, et al. Desquamative interstitial pneumonia and antigen-antibody complexes in two infants with congenital rubella. Pediatrics 72:835, 1983.
127. Ilonen J, Antila A-C, Lehtinen M, et al. HLA antigens in rubella seronegative young adults. Tissue Antigens 22:379, 1983.
128. Ziola B, Lund G, Meurman O, et al. Circulating immune complexes in patients with acute measles and rubella virus infections. Infect Immun 41:578, 1983.
129. Clarke WL, Shaver KA, Bright GM, et al. Autoimmunity in congenital rubella syndrome. J Pediatr 104:370, 1984.
130. Ginsberg-Fellner F, Witt ME, Fedun B, et al. Diabetes mellitus and autoimmunity in patients with congenital rubella syndrome. Rev Infect Dis 7(Suppl 1):S170, 1985.
131. Sever JL, South MA, Shaver KA. Delayed manifestations of congenital rubella. Rev Infect Dis 7(Suppl 1):S164, 1985.
132. Shaver KA, Boughman JA, Nance WE. Congenital rubella syndrome and diabetes: a review of epidemiologic, genetic, and immunologic factors. Am Ann Deaf 130:526, 1985.
133. Rabinowe SL, George KL, Loughlin R, et al. Congenital rubella: monoclonal antibody-defined T cell abnormalities in young adults. Am J Med 81:779, 1986.
134. Verder H, Dickmeiss E, Haahr S, et al. Late-onset rubella syndrome: coexistence of immune complex disease and defective cytotoxic effector cell function. Clin Exp Immunol 63:367, 1986.
135. Bardeletti G, Kessler N, Aymard-Henry M. Morphology, biochemical analysis and neuraminidase activity of rubella virus. Arch Virol 49: 175, 1975.
136. Best JM, Banatvala JE, Almeida JD, et al. Morphological characteristics of rubella virus. Lancet 2:237, 1967.
137. Murphy FA, Halonen PE, Harrison AK. Electron microscopy of the development of rubella virus in BHK-21 cells. J Virol 2:1223, 1968.
138. Oshiro LS, Schmidt NJ, Lennette EH. Electron microscopic studies of rubella virus. J Gen Virol 5:205, 1969.
139. Bardeletti G, Tektoff J, Gautheron D. Rubella virus maturation and production in two host cell systems. Intervirology 11:97, 1979.
140. Holmes IH, Wark MC, Warburton MF. Is rubella an arbovirus? II. Ultrastructural morphology and development. Virology 37:15, 1969.
141. Maes R, Vaheri A, Sedwick D, et al. Synthesis of virus and macromolecules by rubella-infected cells. Nature 210:384, 1966.
142. Nakhasi HL, Zheng D, Hewlett IK, et al. Rubella virus replication: effect of interferons and actinomycin D. Virus Res 10:1, 1988.
143. Sato M, Yamada T, Yamamoto K, et al. Evidence for hybrid formation between rubella virus and a latent virus of BHK21/WI-2 cells. Virology 69:691, 1976.
144. Sato M, Tanaka H, Yamada T, et al. Persistent infection of BHK21/WI-2 cells with rubella virus and characterization of rubella variants. Arch Virol 54:333, 1977.
145. Sato M, Urade M, Maeda N, et al. Isolation and characterization of a new rubella variant with DNA polymerase activity. Arch Virol 56:89, 1978.
146. Sato M, Maeda N, Urade M, et al. Persistent infection of primary human cell cultures with rubella variant carrying DNA polymerase activity. Arch Virol 56:181, 1978.
147. Sato M, Maeda N, Shirasuna K, et al. Presence of DNA in rubella variant with DNA polymerase activity. Arch Virol 61:251, 1979.
148. Mifune K, Matsuo S. Some properties of temperature-sensitive mutant of rubella virus defective in the induction of interference to Newcastle disease virus. Virology 63:278, 1975.
149. Norval M. Mechanism of persistence of rubella virus in LLC-MK2 cells. J Gen Virol 43:289, 1979.
150. Bardeletti G, Gautheron DC. Phospholipid and cholesterol composition of rubella virus and its host cell BHK21 grown in suspension cultures. Arch Virol 52:19, 1978.
151. Voiland A, Bardeletti G. Fatty acid composition of rubella virus and BHK21/13S infected cells. Arch Virol 64:319, 1980.
152. Parkman PD, Buescher EL, Artenstein MS, et al. Studies of rubella. I. Properties of the virus. J Immunol 93:595, 1964.
153. McCarthy K, Taylor-Robinson CH. Rubella. Br Med Bull 23:185, 1967.
154. Wallis C, Melnick JL, Rapp F. Different effects of $MgCl_2$ and $MgSO_4$ on the thermostability of viruses. Virology 26:694, 1965.
155. Chagnon A, Laflamme P. Effect of acidity on rubella virus. Can J Microbiol 10:501, 1964.
156. Fabiyi A, Sever JL, Ratner N, et al. Rubella virus. Growth characteristics and stability of infectious virus and complement-fixing antigen. Proc Soc Exp Biol Med 122:392, 1966.
157. Herrmann KL. Rubella virus. *In* Lennette EH, Schmidt NJ (eds). Diagnostic Procedures for Viral, Rickettsial, and Chlamydial Infections. Washington, DC, American Public Health Association, 1979, p 725.
158. Cochran KW, Maassab HF. Inhibition of rubella virus by 1-adamantanamine hydrochloride. Fed Proc 23:387, 1964.
159. Plotkin SA. Inhibition of rubella virus by amantadine. Arch Gesamte Virusforsch 16:438, 1965.
160. Oxford JS, Schild GC. In vitro inhibition of rubella virus by 1-adamantanamine hydrochloride. Arch Gesamte Virusforsch 17:313, 1965.
161. Plotkin SA, Klaus RM, Whitely JA. Hypogammaglobulinemia in an infant with congenital rubella syndrome: failure of 1-adamantanamine to stop virus excretion. J Pediatr 69:1085, 1966.
162. Vaheri A, Hovi T. Structural proteins and subunits of rubella virus. J Virol 9:10, 1972.
163. Vesikari T. Immune response in rubella infection. Scand J Infect Dis 4(Suppl):1, 1972.
164. Liebhaber H, Gross PA. The structural proteins of rubella virus. Virology 47:684, 1972.
165. Chantler JK. Rubella virus: intracellular polypeptide synthesis. Virology 98:275, 1979.
166. Fenner F. The classification and nomenclature of viruses. Intervirology 6:1, 1975-1976.
167. Melnick JL. Taxonomy of viruses. Prog Med Virol 22:211, 1976.
168. Best JM, Banatvala JE. Studies on rubella virus strain variation by kinetic hemagglutination-inhibition tests. J Gen Virol 9:215, 1970.
169. Fogel A, Plotkin SA. Markers of rubella virus strains in RK13 culture. J Virol 3:157, 1969.
170. Kono R. Antigenic structures of American and Japanese rubella virus strains and experimental vertical transmission of rubella virus in rabbits. Symp Ser Immunobiol Stand 11:195, 1969.
171. Kono R, Hayakawa Y, Hibi M, et al. Experimental vertical transmission of rubella virus in rabbits. Lancet 1:343, 1969.
172. Banatvala JE, Best JM. Cross-serological testing of rubella virus strains. Lancet 1:695, 1969.
173. Potter JE, Banatvala JE, Best JM. Interferon studies with Japanese and U.S. rubella virus. BMJ 1:197, 1973.
174. Banatvala JE, Potter JE, Webster MJ. Foetal interferon responses induced by rubella virus. Ciba Found New Ser 10:77, 1973.
175. Ueda K, Nishida Y, Oshima K, et al. An explanation for the high incidence of congenital rubella syndrome in Ryukyu. Am J Epidemiol 107:344, 1978.
176. Kono R, Hirayama M, Sugishita C, et al. Epidemiology of rubella and congenital rubella infection in Japan. Rev Infect Dis 7(Suppl 1):S56, 1985.
177. Ueda K, Tokugawa K, Nishida Y, et al. Incidence of congenital rubella syndrome in Japan (1965-1985): a nationwide survey of the number of deaf children with history of maternal rubella attending special schools for the deaf in Japan. Am J Epidemiol 124:807, 1986.
178. Halonen PE, Ryan JM, Stewart JA. Rubella hemagglutinin prepared with alkaline extraction of virus grown in suspension culture of BHK-21 cells. Proc Soc Exp Biol Med 125:162, 1967.
179. Schmidt NJ, Dennis J, Lennette EH. Rubella virus hemagglutination with a wide variety of erythrocyte species. Appl Microbiol 22:469, 1971.
180. Furukawa T, Plotkin SA, Sedwick WD, et al. Studies on hemagglutination by rubella virus. Proc Soc Exp Biol Med 126:745, 1967.
181. Haukenes G. Simplified rubella haemagglutination inhibition test not requiring removal of nonspecific inhibitors. Lancet 2:196, 1979.

182. Liebhaber H. Measurement of rubella antibody by hemagglutination inhibition. I. Variables affecting rubella hemagglutination. J Immunol 104:818, 1970.
183. Liebhaber H. Measurement of rubella antibody by hemagglutination inhibition. II. Characteristics of an improved test employing a new method for the removal of non-immunoglobulin HA inhibitors from serum. J Immunol 104:826, 1970.
184. Schmidt NJ, Lennette EH. Rubella complement-fixing antigens derived from the fluid and cellular phases of infected BHK-21 cells: extraction of cell-associated antigen with alkaline buffers. J Immunol 97:815, 1966.
185. Schmidt NJ, Lennette EH, Gee PS. Demonstration of rubella complement-fixing antigens of two distinct particle sizes by gel filtration on Sephadex G-200. Proc Soc Exp Biol Med 123:758, 1966.
186. Schmidt NJ, Lennette EH. Antigens of rubella virus. Am J Dis Child 118:89, 1969.
187. Ho-Terry L, Londesborough P, Cohen A. Analysis of rubella virus complement-fixing antigens by polyacrylamide gel electrophoresis. Arch Virol 87:219, 1986.
188. Schmidt NJ, Styk B. Immunodiffusion reactions with rubella antigens. J Immunol 101:210, 1968.
189. Salmi AA. Gel precipitation reactions between alkaline extracted rubella antigens and human sera. Acta Pathol Microbiol Scand 76:271, 1969.
190. LeBouvier GL. Precipitinogens of rubella virus infected cells. Proc Soc Exp Biol Med 130:51, 1969.
191. Cappel R, Schluederberg A, Horstmann DM. Large-scale production of rubella precipitinogens and their use in the diagnostic laboratory. J Clin Microbiol 1:201, 1975.
192. LeBouvier GL, Plotkin SA. Precipitin responses to rubella vaccine RA27/3. J Infect Dis 123:220, 1971.
193. Vaheri A, Vesikari T. Small size rubella virus antigens and soluble immune complexes, analysis by the platelet aggregation technique. Arch Gesamte Virusforsch 35:10, 1971.
194. Penttinen K, Myllyla G. Interaction of human blood platelets, viruses, and antibodies. I. Platelet aggregation test with microequipment. Ann Med Exp Biol Fenn 46:188, 1968.
195. Lennette EH, Schmidt NJ. Neutralization, fluorescent antibody and complement fixation tests for rubella. *In* Friedman H, Prier JE (eds). Rubella. Springfield, Ill, Charles C Thomas, 1973, p 18.
196. Schluederberg A, Horstmann DM, Andiman WA, et al. Neutralizing and hemagglutination-inhibition antibodies to rubella virus as indicators of protective immunity in vaccinees and naturally immune individuals. J Infect Dis 138:877, 1978.
197. Sato H, Albrecht P, Krugman S, et al. Sensitive neutralization test for rubella antibody. J Clin Microbiol 9:259, 1979.
198. Meurman OH. Antibody responses in patients with rubella infection determined by passive hemagglutination, hemagglutination inhibition, complement fixation, and solid-phase radioimmunoassay tests. Infect Immun 19:369, 1978.
199. Herrmann KL. Available rubella serologic tests. Rev Infect Dis 7(Suppl 1):S108, 1985.
200. Skendzel LP, Wilcox KR, Edson DC. Evaluation of assays for the detection of antibodies to rubella: a report based on data from the College of American Pathologists surveys of 1982. Am J Clin Pathol 80(Suppl):594, 1983.
201. Hauknes G. Experience with an indirect (passive) hemagglutination test for the demonstration of rubella virus antibody. Acta Pathol Microbiol Scand 88:85, 1980.
202. Kilgore JM. Further evaluation of a rubella passive hemagglutination test. J Med Virol 5:131, 1980.
203. Inouye S, Satoh K, Tajima T. Single-serum diagnosis of rubella by combined use of the hemagglutination inhibition and passive hemagglutination tests. J Clin Microbiol 23:388, 1986.
204. Harnett GB, Palmer CA, Mackay-Scollay EM. Single-radial-hemolysis test for the assay of rubella antibody in antenatal, vaccinated, and rubella virus-infected patients. J Infect Dis 140:937, 1979.
205. Nommensen FE. Accuracy of single radial hemolysis test for rubella immunity when internal reference standards are used to estimate antibody levels. J Clin Microbiol 25:22, 1987.
206. Halonen P, Meurman O, Matikainen M-T, et al. IgA antibody response in acute rubella determined by solid-phase radioimmunoassay. J Hyg (Lond) 83:69, 1979.
207. Kangro HO, Pattison JR, Heath RB. The detection of rubella-specific IgM antibodies by radioimmunoassay. Br J Exp Pathol 59:577, 1978.
208. Meurman OH, Viljanen MK, Granfors K. Solid-phase radioimmunoassay of rubella virus immunoglobulin M antibodies: comparison with sucrose density gradient centrifugation test. J Clin Microbiol 5:257, 1977.
209. Meurman OH, Ziola BR. IgM-class rheumatoid factor interference in the solid-phase radioimmunoassay of rubella-specific IgM antibodies. J Clin Pathol 31:483, 1978.
210. Mortimer PP, Tedder RS, Hambling MH, et al. Antibody capture radioimmunoassay for anti-rubella IgM. J Hyg (Lond) 86:139, 1981.
211. Brown GC, Maassab HF, Veronelli JA, et al. Rubella antibodies in human serum: detection by the indirect fluorescent-antibody technic. Science 145:943, 1964.
212. Cradock-Watson JE, Ridehalgh MKS, Pattison JR, et al. Comparison of immunofluorescence and radioimmunoassay for detecting IgM antibody in infants with the congenital rubella syndrome. J Hyg (Lond) 83:413, 1979.
213. Leinikki PO, Shekarchi I, Dorsett P, et al. Determination of virus-specific IgM antibodies by using ELISA: elimination of false-positive results with protein A–Sepharose absorption and subsequent IgM antibody assay. J Lab Clin Med 92:849, 1978.
214. Vejtorp M. Enzyme-linked immunosorbent assay for determination of rubella IgG antibodies. Acta Pathol Microbiol Scand 86:387, 1978.
215. Vejtorp M, Fanoe E, Leerhoy J. Diagnosis of postnatal rubella by the enzyme-linked immunosorbent assay for rubella IgM and IgG antibodies. Acta Pathol Microbiol Scand 87:155, 1979.
216. Bidwell D, Chantler SM, Morgan-Capner P, et al. Further investigation of the specificity and sensitivity of ELISA for rubella antibody screening. J Clin Pathol 33:200, 1980.
217. Skendzel LP, Edson DC. Evaluation of enzyme immunosorbent rubella assays. Arch Pathol Lab Med 109:391, 1985.
218. Morgan-Capner P, Pullen HJM, Pattison JR, et al. A comparison of three tests for rubella antibody screening. J Clin Pathol 32:542, 1979.
219. Champsaur H, Dussaix E, Tournier P. Hemagglutination inhibition, single radial hemolysis, and ELISA tests for the detection of IgG and IgM to rubella virus. J Med Virol 5:273, 1980.
220. Deibel R, D'Areangelis D, Ducharme CP, et al. Assay of rubella antibody by passive hemagglutination and by a modified indirect immunofluorescence test. Infection 8(Suppl 3):S255, 1980.
221. Zartarian MV, Friedly G, Peterson EM, et al. Detection of rubella antibodies by hemagglutination inhibition, indirect fluorescent-antibody test, and enzyme-linked immunosorbent assay. J Clin Microbiol 14:640, 1981.
222. Weissfeld AS, Gehle WD, Sonnenworth AC. Comparison of several test systems used for the determination of rubella immune status. J Clin Microbiol 16:82, 1982.
223. Truant AL, Barksdale BL, Huber TW, et al. Comparison of an enzyme-linked immunosorbent assay with indirect hemagglutination inhibition for determination of rubella virus antibody: evaluation of immune status with commercial reagents in a clinical laboratory. J Clin Microbiol 17:106, 1983.
224. Field PR, Gong CM. Diagnosis of postnatally acquired rubella by use of three enzyme-linked immunosorbent assays for specific immunoglobulins G and M and single radial hemolysis for specific immunoglobulin G. J Clin Microbiol 20:951, 1984.
225. Cubie H, Edmond E. Comparison of five different methods of rubella IgM antibody testing. J Clin Pathol 38:203, 1985.
226. Enders G. Serologic test combinations for safe detection of rubella infections. Rev Infect Dis 7(Suppl 1):S113, 1985.
227. Forsgren M. Standardization of techniques and reagents for the study of rubella antibody. Rev Infect Dis 7(Suppl 1):S129, 1985.
228. Grillner L, Forsgren M, Nordenfelt E. Comparison between a commercial ELISA, Rubazyme, and hemolysis-in-gel test for determination of rubella antibodies. J Virol Methods 10:111, 1985.
229. Chernesky MA, Smaill F, Mahony JB, et al. Combined testing for antibodies to rubella non-structural and envelope proteins sentinels infections in two outbreaks. Diagn Microbiol Infect Dis 8:173, 1987.
230. Ankerst J, Christensen P, Kjellen L, et al. A routine diagnostic test for IgA and IgM antibodies to rubella virus: absorption of IgG with *Staphylococcus aureus*. J Infect Dis 130:268, 1974.
231. Pattison JR, Mace JE. Elution patterns of rubella IgM, IgA, and IgG antibodies from a dextran and an agarose gel. J Clin Pathol 28:670, 1975.
232. Pattison JR, Mace JE, Dane DS. The detection and avoidance of false-positive reactions in tests for rubella-specific IgM. J Med Microbiol 9:355, 1975.

233. Pattison JR, Mace JE. The detection of specific IgM antibodies following infection with rubella virus. J Clin Pathol 28:377, 1975.
234. Pattison JR, Jackson CM, Hiscock JA, et al. Comparison of methods for detecting specific IgM antibody in infants with congenital rubella. J Med Microbiol 11:411, 1978.
235. Caul EO, Hobbs SJ, Roberts PC, et al. Evaluation of a simplified sucrose gradient method for the detection of rubella-specific IgM in routine diagnostic practice. J Med Virol 2:153, 1978.
236. Krech U, Wilhelm JA. A solid-phase immunosorbent technique for the rapid detection of rubella IgM by haemagglutination inhibition. J Gen Virol 44:281, 1979.
237. Morgan-Capner P, Davies E, Pattison JR. Rubella-specific IgM detection using Sephacryl S-300 gel filtration. J Clin Pathol 33:1072, 1980.
238. Kobayashi N, Suzuki M, Nakagawa T, et al. Separation of hemagglutination-inhibiting immunoglobulin M antibody to rubella virus in human serum by high-performance liquid chromatography. J Clin Microbiol 23:1143, 1986.
239. Cunningham AL, Fraser JRE. Persistent rubella virus infection of human synovial cells cultured in vitro. J Infect Dis 151:638, 1985.
240. Parkman PD, Meyer HM, Kirschstein RL, et al. Attenuated rubella virus. I. Development and laboratory characterization. N Engl J Med 275:569, 1966.
241. Desmyter J, DeSomer P, Rawls WE, et al. The mechanism of rubella virus interference. Symp Ser Immunobiol Stand 11:139, 1969.
242. Kleiman MB, Carver DH. Failure of the RA 27/3 strain of rubella virus to induce intrinsic interference. J Gen Virol 36:335, 1977.
243. Frey TK, Hemphill ML. Generation of defective-interfering particles by rubella virus in Vero cells. Virology 164:22, 1988.
244. Sigurdardottir B, Givan KF, Rozee KR, et al. Association of virus with cases of rubella studied in Toronto: propagation of the agent and transmission to monkeys. Can Med Assoc J 88:128, 1963.
245. Heggie AD, Robbins FC. Rubella in naval recruits: a virologic study. N Engl J Med 271:231, 1964.
246. Parkman PD, Phillips PE, Kirschstein RL, et al. Experimental rubella virus infection in the rhesus monkey. J Immunol 95:743, 1965.
247. Parkman PD, Phillips PE, Meyer HM. Experimental rubella virus infection in pregnant monkeys. Am J Dis Child 110:390, 1965.
248. Sever JL, Meier GW, Windle WF, et al. Experimental rubella in pregnant rhesus monkeys. J Infect Dis 116:21, 1966.
249. Fabiyi A, Gitnick GL, Sever JL. Chronic rubella virus infection in the ferret *(Mustela putorius fero)* puppy. Proc Soc Exp Biol Med 125:766, 1967.
250. Barbosa L, Warren J. Studies on the detection of rubella virus and its immunogenicity for animals and man. Semi-annual contract progress report to the National Institute for Neurological Diseases and Blindness, September 1, 1966 to March 1, 1967.
251. Belcourt RJ, Wong FC, Walcroft MJ. Growth of rubella virus in rabbit foetal tissues and cell cultures. Can J Public Health 56:253, 1965.
252. Oxford JS. The growth of rubella virus in small laboratory animals. J Immunol 98:697, 1967.
253. Cotlier E, Fox J, Bohigian G, et al. Pathogenic effects of rubella virus on embryos and newborn rats. Nature 217:38, 1968.
254. Carver DH, Seto DSY, Marcus PI, et al. Rubella virus replication in the brains of suckling mice. J Virol 1:1089, 1967.
255. Centers for Disease Control. Recommendation of the Immunization Practices Advisory Committee (ACIP). Rubella prevention. MMWR Morb Mortal Wkly Rep 39:1, 1990.
256. Centers for Disease Control Revised ACIP Recommendation for Avoiding Pregnancy after Receiving a Rubella Containing Vaccine. MMWR Morb Mortal Wkly Rep 50:1117, 2001.
257. Committee on Infectious Diseases. Rubella. *In* Peter G (ed). Report of the Committee on Infectious Diseases, 22nd ed. Elk Grove Village, Ill, American Academy of Pediatrics, 1991, p 410.
258. Bart KJ, Orenstein WA, Preblud SR, et al. Elimination of rubella and congenital rubella from the United States. Pediatr Infect Dis 4:14, 1985.
259. Mann JM, Preblud SR, Hoffman RE, et al. Assessing risks of rubella infection during pregnancy: a standardized approach. JAMA 245: 1647, 1981.
260. Horstmann DM, Liebhaber H, LeBouvier GL, et al. Rubella: reinfection of vaccinated and naturally immune persons exposed in an epidemic. N Engl J Med 283:771, 1970.
261. Lehane DE, Newberg NR, Beam WE Jr. Evaluation of rubella herd immunity during an epidemic. JAMA 213:2236, 1970.
262. Pollard RB, Edwards EA. Epidemic survey of rubella in a military recruit population. Am J Epidemiol 101:435, 1975.
263. Crawford GE, Gremellion DH. Epidemic measles and rubella in Air Force recruits: impact of immunization. J Infect Dis 144:403, 1981.
264. Blouse LE, Lathrop GD, Dupuy HJ, et al. Rubella screening and vaccination program for US Air Force trainees: an analysis of findings. Am J Public Health 72:280, 1982.
265. Chretien JH, Esswein JG, McGarvey MA, et al. Rubella: pattern of outbreak in a university. South Med J 69:1042, 1976.
266. Centers for Disease Control. Rubella in colleges—United States, 1983-1984. MMWR Morb Mortal Wkly Rep 34:228, 1985.
267. Centers for Disease Control. Rubella outbreaks in prisons—New York City, West Virginia, California. MMWR Morb Mortal Wkly Rep 34: 615, 1985.
268. Centers for Disease Control. Rubella and congenital rubella syndrome—New York City. MMWR Morb Mortal Wkly Rep 35:770, 779, 1986.
269. Centers for Disease Control. Increase in rubella and congenital rubella syndrome in the United States. MMWR Morb Mortal Wkly Rep 40:93, 1991.
270. Centers for Disease Control. Congenital rubella syndrome among the Amish—Pennsylvania, 1991-1992. MMWR Morb Mortal Wkly Rep 41:468, 1992.
271. Goodman AK, Friedman SM, Beatrice ST, et al. Rubella in the workplace: the need for employee immunization. Am J Public Health 77:725, 1987.
272. McLaughlin MC, Gold LH. The New York rubella incident: a case for changing hospital policy regarding rubella testing and immunization. Am J Public Health 79:287, 1979.
273. Polk BF, White JA, DeGirolami PC, et al. An outbreak of rubella among hospital personnel. N Engl J Med 303:541, 1980.
274. Greaves WL, Orenstein WA, Stetler HC, et al. Prevention of rubella transmission in medical facilities. JAMA 248:861, 1982.
275. Strassburg MA, Stephenson TG, Habel LA, et al. Rubella in hospital employees. Infect Control 5:123, 1984.
276. Storch GA, Gruber C, Benz B, et al. A rubella outbreak among dental students: description of the outbreak and analysis of control measures. Infect Control 6:150, 1985.
277. Sever JL, Monif G. Limited persistence of virus in congenital rubella. Am J Dis Child 110:452, 1965.
278. Cooper LZ, Krugman S. Clinical manifestations of postnatal and congenital rubella. Arch Ophthalmol 77:434, 1967.
279. Rawls WE, Philips CA, Melnick JL, et al. Persistent virus infection in congenital rubella. Arch Ophthalmol 77:430, 1967.
280. Michaels RH. Immunologic aspects of congenital rubella. Pediatrics 43:339, 1969.
281. Menser MA, Forrest JM, Slinn RF, et al. Rubella viruria in a 29-year-old woman with congenital rubella. Lancet 2:797, 1971.
282. Shewmon DA, Cherry JD, Kirby SE. Shedding of rubella virus in a $4\frac{1}{2}$-year-old boy with congenital rubella. Pediatr Infect Dis 1:342, 1982.
283. Hattis RP, Halstead SB, Herrmann KL, et al. Rubella in an immunized island population. JAMA 223:1019, 1973.
284. Weller TH, Alford CA Jr, Neva FA. Changing epidemiologic concepts of rubella, with particular reference to unique characteristics of the congenital infection. Yale J Biol Med 37:455, 1965.
285. Rawls WE, Melnick JL, Bradstreet CMP, et al. WHO collaborative study on the seroepidemiology of rubella. Bull World Health Organ 37:79, 1967.
286. Cockburn WC. World aspects of the epidemiology of rubella. Am J Dis Child 118:112, 1969.
287. Witte JJ, Karchmer AW, Case G, et al. Epidemiology of rubella. Am J Dis Child 118:107, 1969.
288. Dowdle WR, Ferreira W, Gomes LFD, et al. WHO collaborative study on the seroepidemiology of rubella in Caribbean and Middle and South American populations in 1968. Bull World Health Organ 42: 419, 1970.
289. Horstmann DM. Rubella: the challenge of its control. J Infect Dis 123:640, 1971.
290. Assad R, Ljungars-Esteves K. Rubella—world impact. Rev Infect Dis 7(Suppl 1):S29, 1985.
291. Horstmann DM. Rubella. *In* Evans AS (ed). Viral Infections of Humans: Epidemiology and Control, 2nd ed. New York, Plenum Publishing, 1985, p 519.
292. Reef SE, Frey TK, Theall K, Abernathy E, et al. The changing epidemiology of rubella in the 1990s: on the verge of elimination and new challenges for control and prevention. JAMA 287:464, 2002.

293. Buescher EL. Behavior of rubella virus in adult populations. Arch Gesamte Virusforsch 16:470, 1965.
294. Green RH, Balsame MR, Giles JP, et al. Studies of the natural history and prevention of rubella. Am J Dis Child 110:348, 1965.
295. Horstmann DM, Riordan JT, Ohtawara M, et al. A natural epidemic of rubella in a closed population. Arch Gesamte Virusforsch 16:483, 1965.
296. Brody JA. The infectiousness of rubella and the possibility of reinfection. Am J Public Health 56:1082, 1966.
297. Bisno AL, Spence LP, Stewart JA, et al. Rubella in Trinidad: seroepidemiologic studies of an institutional outbreak. Am J Epidemiol 89:74, 1969.
298. Gale JL, Detels R, Kim KSW, et al. The epidemiology of rubella on Taiwan. III. Family studies in cities of high and low attack rates. Int J Epidemiol 1:261, 1972.
299. Neva FA, Alford CA Jr, Weller TH. Emerging perspective of rubella. Bacteriol Rev 28:444, 1964.
300. Brody JA, Sever JL, McAlister R, et al. Rubella epidemic on St. Paul Island in the Pribilofs, 1963. I. Epidemiologic, clinical, and serologic findings. JAMA 191:619, 1965.
301. Sever JL, Brody JA, Schiff GM, et al. Rubella epidemic on St. Paul Island in the Pribilofs, 1963. II. Clinical and laboratory findings for the intensive study population. JAMA 191:624, 1965.
302. Halstead SB, Diwan AR, Oda AI. Susceptibility to rubella among adolescents and adults in Hawaii. JAMA 210:1881, 1969.
303. Hinman AR, Irons B, Lewis M, Kandola K. Economic analyses of rubella and rubella vaccines: a global review. Bull World Health Organ 80:264, 2003.
304. Wilkins J, Leedom JM, Portnoy B, et al. Reinfection with rubella virus despite live vaccine-induced immunity. Am J Dis Child 118:275, 1969.
305. Chang TW, DesRosiers S, Weinstein, L. Clinical and serologic studies of an outbreak of rubella in a vaccinated population. N Engl J Med 283:246, 1970.
306. Gross PA, Portnoy B, Mathies AW, et al. A rubella outbreak among adolescent boys. Am J Dis Child 119:326, 1970.
307. Shlian DM. Screening and immunization of rubella-susceptible women: experience in a large, prepaid medical group. JAMA 240:662, 1978.
308. Preblud SR, Gross F, Halsey NA, et al. Assessment of susceptibility to measles and rubella. JAMA 247:1134, 1982.
309. Miller KA. Rubella susceptibility in an adolescent female population. Mayo Clin Proc 59:31, 1984.
310. Allen S. Rubella susceptibility in young adults. J Fam Pract 21:271, 1985.
311. Cohen ZB, Rice LI, Felice ME. Rubella seronegativity in a low socioeconomic adolescent female population. Clin Pediatr (Phila) 24:387, 1985.
312. Dorfman SF, Bowers CH Jr. Rubella susceptibility among prenatal and family planning clinic populations. Mt Sinai J Med 52:248, 1985.
313. Serdula MK, Marks JS, Ibara CM, et al. Premarital rubella screening program: from identification to vaccination of susceptible women in the state of Hawaii. Public Health Rep 101:329, 1986.
314. Alford CA, Neva FA, Weller TH. Virologic and serologic studies on human products of conception after maternal rubella. N Engl J Med 271:1275, 1964.
315. Horstmann DJ, Banatvala JE, Riordan JT, et al. Maternal rubella and the rubella syndrome in infants. Am J Dis Child 110:408, 1965.
316. Monif GRG, Sever JL, Schiff GM, et al. Isolation of rubella virus from products of conception. Am J Obstet Gynecol 91:1143, 1965.
317. Alford CA Jr. Congenital rubella: a review of the virologic and serologic phenomena occurring after maternal rubella in the first trimester. South Med J 59:745, 1966.
318. Heggie AD. Intrauterine infection in maternal rubella. J Pediatr 71: 777, 1967.
319. Rawls WE, Desmyter J, Melnick JL. Serologic diagnosis and fetal involvement in maternal rubella. JAMA 203:627, 1968.
320. Thompson KM, Tobin JO. Isolation of rubella virus from abortion material. BMJ 2:264, 1970.
321. Strannegard O, Holm SE, Hermodsson S, et al. Case of apparent reinfection with rubella. Lancet 1:240, 1970.
322. Boué A, Nicholas A, Montagnon B. Reinfection with rubella in pregnant women. Lancet 2:1251, 1971.
323. Haukenes G, Haram KO. Clinical rubella after reinfection. N Engl J Med 287:1204, 1972.
324. Northrop RL, Gardner WM, Geittman WF. Rubella reinfection during early pregnancy. Obstet Gynecol 39:524, 1972.
325. Northrop RI, Gardner WM, Geittmann WF. Low-level immunity to rubella. N Engl J Med 287:615, 1972.
326. Eilard T, Strannegard O. Rubella reinfection in pregnancy followed by transmission to the fetus. J Infect Dis 129:594, 1974.
327. Snijder JAM, Schroder FP, Hoekstra JH. Importance of IgM determination in cord blood in cases of suspected rubella infection. BMJ 1:23, 1977.
328. Forsgren M, Carlstrom G, Strangert K. Congenital rubella after maternal reinfection. Scand J Infect Dis 11:81, 1979.
329. Fogel A, Handsher R, Barnea B. Subclinical rubella in pregnancy-occurrence and outcome. Isr J Med Sci 21:133, 1985.
330. Sheridan MD. Final report of a prospective study of children whose mothers had rubella in early pregnancy. BMJ 2:536, 1964.
331. Butler NR, Dudgeon JA, Hayes K, et al. Persistence of rubella antibody with and without embryopathy: a follow-up study of children exposed to maternal rubella. BMJ 2:1027, 1965.
332. Phillips GA, Melnick JL, Yow MD, et al. Persistence of virus in infants with congenital rubella and in normal infants with a history of maternal rubella. JAMA 193:1027, 1965.
333. Hardy JB, McCracken GH Jr, Gilkeson MR, et al. Adverse fetal outcome following maternal rubella after the first trimester of pregnancy. JAMA 207:2414, 1969.
334. Schiff GM, Sutherland J, Light I. Congenital rubella. *In* Thalhammer O (ed). Prenatal Infections. International Symposium of Vienna, September 2-3, 1970. Stuttgart, Georg Thieme Verlag, 1971, p 31.
335. Peckham GS. Clinical and laboratory study of children exposed in utero to maternal rubella. Arch Dis Child 47:571, 1972.
336. Menser MA, Forrest JM. Rubella-high incidence of defects in children considered normal at birth. Med J Aust 1:123, 1974.
337. Dudgeon JA. Infective causes of human malformations. Br Med Bull 32:77, 1976.
338. Lundstrom R. Rubella during pregnancy: a follow-up study of children born after an epidemic of rubella in Sweden, 1951, with additional investigations on prophylaxis and treatment of maternal rubella. Acta Paediatr 51(Suppl 133):1, 1962.
339. Whitehouse WL. Rubella before conception as a cause of foetal abnormality. Lancet 1:139, 1963.
340. Monif GRG, Hardy JB, Sever JL. Studies in congenital rubella, Baltimore 1964-65. I. Epidemiologic and virologic. Bull Johns Hopkins Hosp 118:85, 1966.
341. Sever JL, Hardy JB, Nelson KB, et al. Rubella in the Collaborative Perinatal Research Study. II. Clinical and laboratory findings in children through 3 years of age. Am J Dis Child 118:123, 1969.
342. Seppala M, Vaheri A. Natural rubella infection of the female genital tract. Lancet 1:46, 1974.
343. Buimovici-Klein E, Hite RL, Byrne T, et al. Isolation of rubella virus in milk after postpartum immunization. J Pediatr 91:939, 1977.
344. Klein EB, Bryne T, Cooper LZ. Neonatal rubella in a breast-fed infant after postpartum maternal infection. J Pediatr 97:774, 1980.
345. Manson MM, Logan WPD, Loy RM. Rubella and other virus infections during pregnancy. *In* Reports on Public Health and Medical Subjects, No. 101. London, Her Majesty's Stationery Office, 1960.
346. Siegel M, Greenberg M. Fetal death, malformation and prematurity after maternal rubella: results of prospective study, 1949-1958. N Engl J Med 262:389, 1960.
347. Liggins GC, Phillips LI. Rubella embryopathy: an interim report on a New Zealand epidemic. BMJ 1:711, 1963.
348. Pitt D, Keir EH. Results of rubella in pregnancy, III. Med J Aust 2:737, 1965.
349. Sallomi SJ. Rubella in pregnancy: a review of prospective studies from the literature. Obstet Gynecol 27:252, 1966.
350. Heggie AD, Robbins FC. Natural rubella acquired after birth: clinical features and complications. Am J Dis Child 118:12, 1969.
351. Chantler JK, Tingle AJ. Isolation of rubella virus from human lymphocytes after acute infection. J Infect Dis 145:673, 1982.
352. O'Shea S, Mutton D, Best JM. In vivo expression of rubella antigens on human leucocytes: detection by flow cytometry. J Med Virol 25:297, 1988.
353. Heggie AD. Pathogenesis of the rubella exanthem: isolation of rubella virus from the skin. N Engl J Med 285:664, 1971.
354. Heggie AD. Pathogenesis of the rubella exanthem: distribution of rubella virus in the skin during rubella with and without rash. J Infect Dis 137:74, 1978.

355. Al-Nakib W, Best JM, Banatvala JE. Rubella-specific serum and nasopharyngeal immunoglobulin responses following naturally acquired and vaccine-induced infection: prolonged persistence of virus-specific IgM. Lancet 1:182, 1975.
356. Pattison JR, Dane DS, Mace JE. The persistence of specific IgM after natural infection with rubella virus. Lancet 1:185, 1975.
357. Meurman OH. Persistence of immunoglobulin G and immunoglobulin M antibodies after postnatal rubella infection determined by solid-phase radioimmunoassay. J Clin Microbiol 7:34, 1978.
358. Rousseau S, Hedman K. Rubella infection and reinfection distinguished by avidity of IgG. Letter to the editor. Lancet 1:1108, 1988.
359. Hedman K, Seppala I. Recent rubella virus infection indicated by a low avidity of specific IgG. J Clin Immunol 8:214, 1988.
360. Morgan-Capner P, Thomas HIJ. Serological distinction between primary rubella and reinfection. Letter to the editor. Lancet 1:1397, 1988.
361. Smith KA, Chess L, Mardiney MR Jr. The relationship between rubella hemagglutination inhibition antibody (HIA) and rubella induced in vitro lymphocyte tritiated thymidine incorporation. Cell Immunol 8: 321, 1973.
362. Steele RW, Hensen SA, Vincent MM, et al. A ^{52}Cr microassay technique for cell-mediated immunity to viruses. J Immunol 110:1502, 1973.
363. Honeyman MC, Forrest JM, Dorman DC. Cell-mediated immune response following natural rubella and rubella vaccination. Clin Exp Immunol 17:665, 1974.
364. McMorrow L, Vesikari T, Wolman SR, et al. Suppression of the response of lymphocytes to phytohemagglutinin in rubella. J Infect Dis 130:464, 1974.
365. Steele RW, Hensen SA, Vincent MM, et al. Development of specific cellular and humoral immune responses in children immunized with liver rubella virus vaccine. J Infect Dis 130:449, 1974.
366. Kanra GY, Vesikari T. Cytotoxic activity against rubella-infected cells in the supernatants of human lymphocyte cultures stimulated by rubella virus. Clin Exp Immunol 19:17, 1975.
367. Vesikari T, Kanra GY, Buimovici-Klein E, et al. Cell-mediated immunity in rubella assayed by cytotoxicity of supernatants from rubella virus–stimulated human lymphocyte cultures. Clin Exp Immunol 19:33, 1975.
368. Ganguly R, Cusumano CL, Waldman RH. Suppression of cell-mediated immunity after infection with attenuated rubella virus. Infect Immun 13:464, 1976.
369. Buimovici-Klein E, Weiss KE, Cooper LZ. Interferon production in lymphocyte cultures after rubella infection in humans. J Infect Dis 135:380, 1977.
370. Rossier E, Phipps PH, Polley JR, et al. Absence of cell-mediated immunity to rubella virus 5 years after rubella vaccination. Can Med Assoc J 116:481, 1977.
371. Rossier E, Phipps PH, Weber JM, et al. Persistence of humoral and cell-mediated immunity to rubella virus in cloistered nuns and in schoolteachers. J Infect Dis 144:137, 1981.
372. Buimovici-Klein E, Cooper LZ. Cell-mediated immune response to rubella infections. Rev Infect Dis 7(Suppl 1):S123, 1985.
373. Mori T, Shiozawa K. Suppression of tuberculin hypersensitivity caused by rubella infection. Am Rev Respir Dis 131:886, 1985.
374. Ogra PL, Kerr-Grant D, Umana G, et al. Antibody response in serum and nasopharynx after naturally acquired and vaccine-induced infection with rubella virus. N Engl J Med 285:1333, 1971.
375. Al-Nakib W, Best JM, Banatvala JE. Detection of rubella-specific serum IgG and IgA and nasopharyngeal IgA responses using a radioactive single radial immunodiffusion technique. Clin Exp Immunol 22:293, 1975.
376. Plotkin SA, Farquhar JD. Immunity to rubella: comparison between naturally and artificially induced resistance. Postgrad Med J 48(Suppl):47, 1972.
377. Plotkin SA, Farquhar JD, Ogra PL. Immunologic properties of RA 27/3 rubella virus vaccine: a comparison with strains presently licensed in the United States. JAMA 225:585, 1973.
378. Morag A, Beutner KR, Morag B, et al. Development and characteristics of in vitro correlates of cellular immunity to rubella virus in the systemic and mucosal sites in guinea pigs. J Immunol 113:1703, 1974.
379. Morag A, Morag B, Bernstein JM, et al. In vitro correlates of cell-mediated immunity in human tonsils after natural or induced rubella virus infection. J Infect Dis 131:409, 1975.
380. Selzer G. Virus isolation, inclusion bodies, and chromosomes in a rubella-infected human embryo. Lancet 2:336, 1963.
381. Rudolph AJ, Yow MD, Phillips A, et al. Transplacental rubella infection in newly born infants. JAMA 191:843, 1965.
382. Catalano LW Jr, Fuccillo DA, Traub RG, et al. Isolation of rubella virus from placentas and throat cultures of infants: a prospective study after the 1964-65 epidemic. Obstet Gynecol 38:6, 1971.
383. Schiff GM, Dine MS. Transmission of rubella from newborns: a controlled study among young adult women and report of an unusual case. Am J Dis Child 110:447, 1965.
384. Plotkin SA, Cochran W, Lindquist JM, et al. Congenital rubella syndrome in late infancy. JAMA 200:435, 1967.
385. Monif GRG, Sever JL. Chronic infection of the central nervous system with rubella virus. Neurology 16:111, 1966.
386. Desmond MM, Wilson GS, Melnick JL, et al. Congenital rubella encephalitis. J Pediatr 71:311, 1967.
387. Menser MA, Harley JD, Herzberg R, et al. Persistence of virus in lens for three years after prenatal rubella. Lancet 2:387, 1967.
388. Cremer NE, Oshiro LS, Weil ML, et al. Isolation of rubella virus from brain in chronic progressive panencephalitis. J Gen Virol 29:143, 1975.
389. Weil ML, Itabashi HH, Cremer NE, et al. Chronic progressive panencephalitis due to rubella virus simulating subacute sclerosing panencephalitis. N Engl J Med 292:994, 1975.
390. Alford CA Jr. Immunoglobulin determinations in the diagnosis of fetal infection. Pediatr Clin North Am 18:99, 1971.
391. Weller TH, Alford CA, Neva FA. Retrospective diagnosis by serologic means of congenitally acquired rubella infections. N Engl J Med 270:1039, 1964.
392. Alford CA Jr. Studies on antibody in congenital rubella infections. I. Physicochemical and immunologic investigations of rubella-neutralizing antibody. Am J Dis Child 110:455, 1965.
393. Alford CA Jr, Blankenship WJ, Straumfjord JV, et al. The diagnostic significance of IgM-globulin elevations in newborn infants with chronic intrauterine infections. *In* Bergsma D (ed). Birth Defects. Original Articles Series, vol. 4, no. 5. New York, National Foundation–March of Dimes, 1968.
394. Gitlin D. The differentiation and maturation of specific immune mechanisms. Acta Paediatr Scand Suppl 172:60, 1967.
395. Gitlin D, Biasucci A. Development of gamma G, gamma A, beta IC-beta IA, CI esterase inhibitor, ceruloplasmin, transferrin, hemopexin, haptoglobin, fibrinogen, plasminogen, alpha 1-antitrypsin, orosomucoid, beta-lipoprotein, alpha 2-macroglobulin, and prealbumin in the human conceptus. J Clin Invest 48:1433, 1969.
396. Lawton AR, Self KS, Royal SA, et al. Ontogeny of lymphocytes in the human fetus. Clin Immunol Immunopathol 1:104, 1972.
397. Bellanti JA, Artenstein MS, Olson LC, et al. Congenital rubella: clinicopathologic, virologic, and immunologic studies. Am J Dis Child 110: 464, 1965.
398. Baublis JV, Brown GC. Specific response of the immunoglobulins to rubella infection. Proc Soc Exp Biol Med 128:206, 1968.
399. Cohen SM, Ducharme CP, Carpenter CA, et al. Rubella antibody in IgG and IgM immunoglobulins detected by immunofluorescence. J Lab Clin Med 72:760, 1968.
400. Vesikari T, Vaheri A, Pettay O, et al. Congenital rubella: immune response of the neonate and diagnosis by demonstration of specific IgM antibodies. J Pediatr 75:658, 1969.
401. Cradock-Watson JE, Ridehalgh MKS, Chantler S. Specific immunoglobulins in infants with the congenital rubella syndrome. J Hyg (Lond) 76:109, 1976.
402. McCracken GH Jr, Hardy JB, Chen TC, et al. Serum immunoglobulin levels in newborn infants. II. Survey of cord and follow-up sera from 123 infants with congenital rubella. J Pediatr 74:383, 1969.
403. Alford CA Jr. Fetal antibody in the diagnosis of chronic intra-uterine infections. *In* Thalhammer O (ed). Prenatal Infections. International Symposium of Vienna, September 2-3, 1970. Stuttgart, Georg Thieme, 1971, p 53.
404. Kenrick KG, Slinn RF, Dorman DC, et al. Immunoglobulins and rubella-virus antibodies in adults with congenital rubella. Lancet 1:548, 1968.
405. Hardy JB, Sever JL, Gilkeson MR. Declining antibody titers in children with congenital rubella. J Pediatr 75:213, 1969.
406. Cooper LZ, Florman AL, Ziring PR, et al. Loss of rubella hemagglutination-inhibition antibody in congenital rubella. Am J Dis Child 122:397, 1971.
407. Ueda K, Tokugawa K, Fukushige J, et al. Hemagglutination inhibition antibodies in congenital rubella: a 17-year follow-up in the Ryukyu Islands. Am J Dis Child 141:211, 1987.

408. Ueda K, Tokugawa K, Fukushige J, et al. Continuing problem in congenital rubella syndrome in southern Japan: its outbreak in Fukuoka and the surrounding areas after the 1965-1969 and 1975-1977 rubella epidemics. Fukuoka Acta Med 77:309, 1986.
409. Soothill JF, Hayes K, Dudgeon JA. The immunoglobulins in congenital rubella. Lancet 1:1385, 1966.
410. Hancock MP, Huntley CC, Sever JL. Congenital rubella syndrome with immunoglobulin disorder. J Pediatr 72:636, 1968.
411. Hayward AR, Ezer G. Development of lymphocyte populations in the human foetal thymus and spleen. Clin Exp Immunol 17:169, 1974.
412. Cooper MD, Dayton DH. *In* Cooper MD, Dayton DH (eds). Development of Host Defenses. New York, Raven Press, 1977.
413. Miller ME. *In* Miller ME (ed). Host Defenses in the Human Neonate. Monographs in Neonatology. New York, Grune & Stratton, 1978.
414. Berry CL, Thompson EN. Clinicopathological study of thymic dysplasia. Arch Dis Child 43:579, 1968.
415. White LR, Leikin S, Villavicencio O, et al. Immune competence in congenital rubella: lymphocyte transformation, delayed hypersensitivity and response to vaccination. J Pediatr 73:229, 1968.
416. Montgomery JR, South MA, Rawls WE, et al. Viral inhibition of lymphocyte response to phytohemagglutinin. Science 157:1068, 1967.
417. Olson GB, South MA, Good RA. Phytohemagglutinin unresponsiveness of lymphocytes from babies with congenital rubella. Nature 214:695, 1967.
418. Olson GB, Dent PB, Rawls WE, et al. Abnormalities of in vitro lymphocyte responses during rubella virus infections. J Exp Med 128:47, 1968.
419. Simmons JJ, Fitzgerald MG. Rubella virus and human lymphocytes in culture. Lancet 2:937, 1968.
420. Marshall WC, Cope WA, Soothill JF, et al. In vitro lymphocyte response in some immunity deficiency diseases and in intrauterine virus infections. Proc R Soc Med 63:351, 1970.
421. Buimovici-Klein E, Lang PB, Ziring PR, et al. Impaired cell-mediated immune response in patients with congenital rubella: correlation with gestational age at time of infection. Pediatrics 64:620, 1979.
422. Hyypia T, Eskola J, Laine M, et al. B-cell function in vitro during rubella infection. Infect Immun 43:589, 1984.
423. Fuccillo DA, Steele RW, Hensen SA, et al. Impaired cellular immunity to rubella virus in congenital rubella. Infect Immun 9:81, 1974.
424. Mims CA. Pathogenesis of viral infections in the fetus. Prog Med Virol 10:194, 1968.
425. Rawls WE. Congenital rubella: the significance of virus persistence. Prog Med Virol 10:238, 1968.
426. Alford CA Jr. Production of interferon-like substance by the rubella-infected human conceptus. Program and abstracts of the American Pediatric Society and Society of Pediatric Research Meeting, Atlantic City, April 29–May 2, 1970, p 203.
427. Lebon P, Daffos F, Checoury A, et al. Presence of an acid-labile alpha-interferon in sera from fetuses and children with congenital rubella. J Clin Microbiol 21:755, 1985.
428. Desmyter J, Rawls WE, Melnick JL, et al. Interferon in congenital rubella: response to live attenuated measles vaccine. J Immunol 99: 771, 1967.
429. McCarthy K, Taylor-Robinson CH, Pillinger SE. Isolation of rubella virus from cases in Britain. Lancet 2:593, 1963.
430. Hildebrandt HM, Maassab HF. Rubella synovitis in a 1-year-old patient. N Engl J Med 274:1428, 1966.
431. Yanez JE, Thompson GR, Middelsen WM, et al. Rubella arthritis. Ann Intern Med 64:772, 1966.
432. McCormick JN, Duthie JJR, Gerber H, et al. Rheumatoid polyarthritis after rubella. Ann Rheum Dis 37:266, 1978.
433. Graham R, Armstrong R, Simmons NA, et al. Isolation of rubella virus from synovial fluid in five cases of seronegative arthritis. Lancet 2:649, 1981.
434. Lebon P, Lyon G. Noncongenital rubella encephalitis. Lancet 2:468, 1974.
435. Wolinsky JS, Berg BO, Maitland CJ. Progressive rubella panencephalitis. Arch Neurol 33:722, 1976.
436. Squadrini F, Taparelli F, De Rienzo B, et al. Rubella virus isolation from cerebrospinal fluid in postnatal rubella encephalitis. BMJ 2:1329, 1977.
437. Thong YH, Steele RW, Vincent MM, et al. Impaired in vitro cell-mediated immunity to rubella virus during pregnancy. N Engl J Med 289:604, 1973.
438. Weinberg ED. Pregnancy-associated depression of cell-mediated immunity. Rev Infect Dis 6:814, 1984.
439. Honeyman MC, Dorman DC, Menser MA, et al. HL-A antigens in congenital rubella and the role of antigens 1 and 8 in the epidemiology of natural rubella. Tissue Antigens 5:12, 1975.
440. Forrester RM, Lees VT, Watson GH. Rubella syndrome: escape of a twin. BMJ 1:1403, 1966.
441. Cooper LZ. The history and medical consequences of rubella. Rev Infect Dis 7(Suppl 1):S1, 1985.
442. Töndury G, Smith DW. Fetal rubella pathology. J Pediatr 68:867, 1966.
443. Driscoll SG. Histopathology of gestational rubella. Am J Dis Child 118:49, 1969.
444. Dudgeon JA. Teratogenic effect of rubella virus. Proc R Soc Med 63:1254, 1970.
445. Menser MA, Reye RDK. The pathology of congenital rubella: a review written by request. Pathology 6:215, 1974.
446. Esterly JR, Oppenheimer EH. Intrauterine rubella infection. *In* Rosenberg HS, Bolande RP (eds). Perspectives in Pediatric Pathology, vol. 1. Chicago, Year Book Medical Publishers, 1973, p 313.
447. Boué A, Boué JG. Effects of rubella virus infection on the division of human cells. Am J Dis Child 118:45, 1969.
448. Smith JL, Early EM, London WT, et al. Persistent rubella virus production in embryonic rabbit chondrocyte cell cultures (37465). Proc Soc Exp Biol Med 143:1037, 1973.
449. Heggie AD. Growth inhibition of human embryonic and fetal rat bones in organ culture by rubella virus. Teratology 15:47, 1977.
450. Rawls WE, Melnick JL, Rosenberg HA, et al. Spontaneous virus carrier cultures and postmortem isolation of virus from infants with congenital rubella. Proc Soc Exp Biol Med 120:623, 1965.
451. Boué A, Plotkin SA, Boué JG. Action du virus de la rubéole sur différents systemes de cultures de cellules embryonnaires humaines. Arch Gesamte Virusforsch 16:443, 1965.
452. Plotkin SA, Boué A, Boué JG. The in vitro growth of rubella virus in human embryo cells. Am J Epidemiol 81:71, 1965.
453. Chang TH, Moorhead PS, Boué JG, et al. Chromosome studies of human cells infected in utero and in vitro with rubella virus. Proc Soc Exp Biol Med 122:236, 1966.
454. Nusbacher J, Hirschhorn K, Cooper LZ. Chromosomal studies on congenital rubella. N Engl J Med 276:1409, 1967.
455. Plotkin SA, Vaheri A. Human fibroblasts infected with rubella virus produce a growth inhibitor. Science 156:659, 1967.
456. Bowden DS, Pedersen JS, Toh BH, et al. Distribution by immunofluorescence of viral products and actin-containing cytoskeleton filaments in rubella virus-infected cells. Arch Virol 92:211, 1987.
457. Yoneda T, Urade M, Sakuda M, et al. Altered growth, differentiation, and responsiveness to epidermal growth factor of human embryonic mesenchymal cells of palate by persistent rubella virus infection. J Clin Invest 77:1613, 1986.
458. Naeye RL, Blanc W. Pathogenesis of congenital rubella. JAMA 194: 1277, 1965.
459. Dent PB, Olson GB, Good RA, et al. Rubella-virus/leukocyte interaction and its role in the pathogenesis of the congenital rubella syndrome. Lancet 1:291, 1968.
460. Reimer CB, Black CM, Phillips DJ, et al. The specificity of fetal IgM: antibody or anti-antibody? Ann N Y Acad Sci 254:77, 1975.
461. Robertson PW, Kertesz V, Cloonan MJ. Elimination of false-positive cytomegalovirus immunoglobulin M-fluorescent-antibody reactions with immunoglobulin M serum fractions. J Clin Microbiol 6:174, 1977.
462. Altshuler G. Placentitis with a new light on an old TORCH. Obstet Gynecol Ann 6:197, 1977.
463. Garcia AGP, Marques RLS, Lobato YY, et al. Placental pathology in congenital rubella. Placenta 6:281, 1985.
464. Krugman S, Katz SL, Gershon AA, et al (eds). Rubella. *In* Infectious Diseases of Children, 8th ed. St. Louis, CV Mosby, 1985, p 307.
465. Sheinis M, Sarov I, Maor E, et al. Severe neonatal rubella following maternal infection. Pediatr Infect Dis 4:202, 1985.
466. Judelsohn RG, Wyll SA. Rubella in Bermuda: termination of an epidemic by mass vaccination. JAMA 223:401, 1973.
467. Fujimoto T, Katoh C, Hayakawa H, et al. Two cases of rubella infection with cardiac involvement. Jpn Heart J 20:227, 1979.
468. Saeed AA, Lange LS. Guillain-Barré syndrome after rubella. Postgrad Med J 54:333, 1978.
469. Callaghan N, Feely M, Walsh B. Relapsing neurological disorder associated with rubella virus infection in two sisters. J Neurol Neurosurg Psychiatry 40:1117, 1977.

470. Connolly JH, Hutchinson WM, Allen IV, et al. Carotid artery thrombosis, encephalitis, myelitis and optic neuritis associated with rubella virus infections. Brain 98:583, 1975.
471. Choutet P, Binet CH, Goudeau A, et al. Bone-marrow aplasia and primary rubella infection. Lancet 2:966, 1979.
472. Townsend JJ, Baringer JR, Wolinsky JS, et al. Progressive rubella panencephalitis: late onset after congenital rubella. N Engl J Med 292:990, 1975.
473. Waxham MN, Wolinsky JS. Rubella virus and its effect on the nervous system. Neurol Clin 2:267, 1984.
474. Schlossberg D, Topolosky MR. Military rubella. JAMA 238:1273, 1974.
475. Preblud SR, Dobbs HI, Sedmak GV, et al. Testalgia associated with rubella infection. South Med J 73:594, 1980.
476. White LR, Sever JL, Alepa FP. Maternal and congenital rubella before 1964: frequency, clinical features, and search for isoimmune phenomena. Pediatrics 74:198, 1969.
477. Cooper LZ. Rubella: a preventable cause of birth defects. *In* Bergsma D (ed). Birth Defects. Original Article Series, vol. 4, no. 23. New York, National Foundation–March of Dimes, 1968.
478. Cooper LZ, Green RH, Krugman S, et al. Neonatal thrombocytopenic purpura and other manifestations of rubella contracted in utero. Am J Dis Child 110:416, 1965.
479. Zinkham WH, Medearis DN, Osborn JE. Blood and bone marrow findings in congenital rubella. J Pediatr 71:512, 1967.
480. Rudolph AJ, Singleton EB, Rosenberg HS, et al. Osseous manifestations of the congenital rubella syndrome. Am J Dis Child 110:428, 1965.
481. Rabinowitz JG, Wolf BS, Greenberg EI, et al. Osseous changes in rubella embryopathy. Radiology 85:494, 1965.
482. Wall WL, Altman DH, Gair DR, et al. Roentgenological findings in congenital rubella. Clin Pediatr 4:704, 1965.
483. Reed GB Jr. Rubella bone lesions. J Pediatr 74:208, 1969.
484. Korones SB, Ainger LE, Monif GRG, et al. Congenital rubella syndrome: study of 22 infants. Am J Dis Child 110:434, 1965.
485. Rorke LB, Spiro AJ. Cerebral lesions in congenital rubella syndrome. J Pediatr 70:243, 1967.
486. Streissguth AP, Vanderveer BB, Shepard TH. Mental development of children with congenital rubella syndrome: a preliminary report. Am J Obstet Gynecol 108:391, 1970.
487. Rowen M, Singer MI, Moran ET. Intracranial calcification in the congenital rubella syndrome. Am J Roentgenol 115:86, 1972.
488. Peters ER, Davis RL. Congenital rubella syndrome: cerebral mineralizations and subperiosteal new bone formation as expressions of this disorder. Clin Pediatr (Phila) 5:743, 1966.
489. Hastreiter AR, Joorabchi B, Pujatti G, et al. Cardiovascular lesions associated with congenital rubella. J Pediatr 71:59, 1967.
490. Klein HZ, Markarian M. Dermal erythropoiesis in congenital rubella: description of an infected newborn who had purpura associated with marked extramedullary erythropoieses in the skin and elsewhere. Clin Pediatr (Phila) 8:604, 1969.
491. Brough AJ, Jones D, Page RH, et al. Dermal erythropoieses in neonatal infants. Pediatrics 40:627, 1967.
492. Achs R, Harper KG, Siegal M. Unusual dermatoglyphic findings associated with the rubella embryopathy. N Engl J Med 274:148, 1966.
493. Purvis-Smith SG, Howard PR, Menser MA. Dermatoglyphic defects and rubella teratogenesis. JAMA 209:1865, 1969.
494. Murphy AM, Reid RR, Pollard I, et al. Rubella cataracts: further clinical and virologic observations. Am J Ophthalmol 64:1109, 1967.
495. Collis WJ, Cohen DN. Rubella retinopathy: a progressive disorder. Arch Ophthalmol 84:33, 1970.
496. Kresky B, Nauheim JS. Rubella retinitis. Am J Dis Child 113:305, 1967.
497. Schiff GM, Sutherland JM, Light IJ, et al. Studies on congenital rubella. Am J Dis Child 110:441, 1965.
498. Menser MA, Dorman DC, Reye RDK, et al. Renal artery stenosis in the rubella syndrome. Lancet 1:790, 1966.
499. Menser MA, Robertson SEJ, Dorman DC, et al. Renal lesions in congenital rubella. Pediatrics 40:901, 1967.
500. Kaplan GW, McLaughlin AP III. Urogenital anomalies and congenital rubella syndrome. Urology 2:148, 1973.
501. Forrest JM, Menser MA. Congenital rubella in schoolchildren and adolescents. Arch Dis Child 45:63, 1970.
502. Korones SB, Ainger LE, Monif GR, et al. Congenital rubella syndrome: new clinical aspects with recovery of virus from affected infants. J Pediatr 67:166, 1965.
503. South MA, Alford CA Jr. The immunology of chronic intrauterine infections. *In* Stiehm ER, Fulginiti VA (eds). Immunologic Disorders in Infants and Children. Philadelphia, WB Saunders, 1973, p 565.
504. Phelan P, Campbell P. Pulmonary complications of rubella embryopathy. J Pediatr 75:202, 1969.
505. Karmody GS. Subclinical maternal rubella and congenital deafness. N Engl J Med 278:809, 1968.
506. Ames MD, Plotkin SA, Winchester RA, et al. Central auditory imperception: a significant factor in congenital rubella deafness. JAMA 213:419, 1970.
507. Peckham CS, Martin JAM, Marshall WC, et al. Congenital rubella deafness: a preventable disease. Lancet 1:258, 1979.
508. Rossi M, Ferlito A, Polidoro F. Maternal rubella and hearing impairment in children. J Laryngol Otol 94:281, 1980.
509. Weinberger MM, Maslund MW, Asbed R, et al. Congenital rubella presenting as retarded language development. Am J Dis Child 120: 125, 1970.
510. Desmond MM, Fisher ES, Vorderman AL, et al. The longitudinal course of congenital rubella encephalitis in nonretarded children. J Pediatr 93:584, 1978.
511. Zausmer E. Congenital rubella: pathogenesis of motor deficits. Pediatrics 47:16, 1971.
512. Menser MA, Forrest JM, Bransby RD. Rubella infection and diabetes mellitus. Lancet 1:57, 1978.
513. Hanid TK. Hypothyroidism in congenital rubella. Lancet 2:854, 1976.
514. Nieberg PI, Gardner LI. Thyroiditis and congenital rubella syndrome. J Pediatr 89:156, 1976.
515. Perez Comas A. Congenital rubella and acquired hypothyroidism secondary to Hashimoto thyroiditis. J Pediatr 88:1065, 1976.
516. Ziring PR, Gallo G, Finegold M, et al. Chronic lymphocytic thyroiditis: identification of rubella virus antigen in the thyroid of a child with congenital rubella. J Pediatr 90:419, 1977.
517. AvRuskin TW, Brakin M, Juan C. Congenital rubella and myxedema. Pediatrics 69:495, 1982.
518. Ziring PR, Fedun BA, Cooper LZ. Thyrotoxicosis in congenital rubella. J Pediatr 87:1002, 1975.
519. Preece MA, Kearney PJ, Marshall WC. Growth hormone deficiency in congenital rubella. Lancet 2:842, 1977.
520. Oberfield SE, Cassulo AM, Chiriboga-Klein S, et al. Growth hormone dynamics in congenital rubella syndrome. Brain Dysfunct 1:303, 1988.
521. Chiriboga-Klein S, Oberfield SE, Cassulo AM, et al. Growth in congenital rubella syndrome and correlation with clinical manifestations. J Pediatr 115:251, 1989.
522. Boger WP III. Late ocular complications in congenital rubella syndrome. Ophthalmology 87:1244, 1980.
523. Deutman AF, Grizzard WS. Rubella retinopathy and subretinal neovascularization. Am J Ophthalmol 85:82, 1978.
524. Frank KE, Purnell EW. Subretinal neovascularization following rubella retinopathy. Am J Ophthalmol 86:462, 1978.
525. Boger WP III, Petersen RA, Robb RM. Keratoconus and acute hydrops in mentally retarded patients with congenital rubella syndrome. Am J Ophthalmol 91:231, 1981.
526. Boger WP III, Petersen RA, Robb RM. Spontaneous absorption of the lens in the congenital rubella syndrome. Arch Ophthalmol 99:433, 1981.
527. Gullikson JS. Tooth morphology in rubella syndrome children. J Dent Child 42:479, 1979.
528. No reference cited.
529. Fortuin NJ, Morrow AG, Roberts WC. Late vascular manifestations of the rubella syndrome: a roentgenographic-pathologic study. Am J Med 51:134, 1971.
530. Anderson H, Barr B, Wedenberg E. Genetic disposition—a prerequisite for maternal rubella deafness. Arch Otolaryngol 91:141, 1970.
531. Orth DH, Fishman GA, Segall M, et al. Rubella maculopathy. BMJ 64:201, 1980.
532. Wolinsky JS, Dau PC, Buimovici-Klein E, et al. Progressive rubella panencephalitis: immunovirological studies and results of isoprinosine therapy. Clin Exp Immunol 35:397, 1979.
533. Preblud SR, Kushubar R, Friedman HM. Rubella hemagglutination inhibition titers. JAMA 247:1181, 1982.
534. Munro ND, Wild HJ, Sheppard S, et al. Fall and rise of immunity to rubella. BMJ 294:481, 1987.
535. Hoskins CS, Pyman C, Wilkins B. The nerve deaf child—intrauterine rubella or not? Arch Dis Child 58:327, 1983.
536. Iurio JL, Hosking CS, Pyman C. Retrospective diagnosis of congenital rubella. BMJ 289:1566, 1984.
537. Vesikari T, Meurman OH, Maki R. Persistent rubella-specific IgM-antibody in the cerebrospinal fluid of a child with congenital rubella. Arch Dis Child 55:46, 1980.

538. Fitzgerald MG, Pullen GR, Hosking CS. Low affinity antibody to rubella antigen in patients after rubella infection in utero. Pediatrics 81:812, 1988.
539. Alestig K, Bartsch FK, Nilsson LA, et al. Studies of amniotic fluid in women infected with rubella. J Infect Dis 129:79, 1974.
540. Levine MJ, Oxman MN, Moore MG, et al. Diagnosis of congenital rubella in utero. N Engl J Med 290:1187, 1974.
541. Cederqvist LL, Zervoudakis IA, Ewool LC, et al. Prenatal diagnosis of congenital rubella. BMJ 276:615, 1977.
542. Daffos F, Forestier F, Grangeot-Keros L, et al. Prenatal diagnosis of congenital rubella. Lancet 2:1, 1984.
543. Terry GM, Ho-Terry L, Warren RC, et al. First trimester prenatal diagnosis of congenital rubella: a laboratory investigation. BMJ 292:930, 1986.
544. Enders G, Jonatha W. Prenatal diagnosis of intrauterine rubella. Infection 15:162, 1987.
545. Ho-Terry L, Terry GM, Londesborough P, et al. Diagnosis of fetal rubella infection by nucleic acid hybridization. J Med Virol 24:175, 1988.
546. Bosma TJ, Corbett SO, Banatvala JE, Best JM. PCR for detection of rubella virus RNA in clinical samples. J Clin Microbiol 33:1075, 1995.
547. Tanemura M, Suzumori K, Yagami Y, Katow S. Diagnosis of fetal rubella infection with reverse transcription and nested polymerase chain reaction: a study of 34 cases diagnosed in fetuses. Am J Obstet Gynecol 174:578, 1996.
548. Revello MG, Baldanti F, Sarasini A, et al. Prenatal diagnosis of rubella virus infection by direct detection and semiquantitation of viral RNA in clinical samples by reverse transcription-PCR. J Clin Microbiol 35:708, 1997.
549. McDonald JC. Gamma-globulin for prevention of rubella in pregnancy. BMJ 2:416, 1963.
550. Brody JA, Sever JL, Schiff GM. Prevention of rubella by gamma globulin during an epidemic in Barrow, Alaska, in 1964. N Engl J Med 272:127, 1965.
551. McCallin PF, Fuccillo DA, Ley AC, et al. Gammaglobulin as prophylaxis against rubella-induced congenital anomalies. Obstet Gynecol 39:185, 1972.
552. Urquhart GED, Crawford RJ, Wallace J. Trial of high-titre human rubella immunoglobulin. BMJ 2:1331,1978.
553. Schiff GM, Sever JL, Huebner RJ. Rubella virus: neutralizing antibody in commercial gamma globulin. Science 142:58, 1963.
554. Armstrong RD, Sinclair A, O'Keefe G, et al. Interferon treatment of chronic rubella associated arthritis. Clin Exp Rheumatol 3:93, 1985.
555. Arvin AM, Schmidt NJ, Cantell K, et al. Alpha interferon administration to infants with congenital rubella. Antimicrob Agents Chemother 21:259, 1982.
556. Larsson A, Forsgren M, Hardaf-Segerstad S, et al. Administration of interferon to an infant with congenital rubella syndrome involving persistent viremia and cutaneous vasculitis. Acta Paediatr Scand 65:105, 1976.
557. Jan JE, Tingle AJ, Donald G, et al. Progressive rubella panencephalitis: clinical course and response to "Isoprinosine." Dev Med Child Neurol 21:648, 1979.
558. Garner JS, Simmons BP. CDC guidelines for isolation precautions in hospitals. Infect Control 4:245, 1983.
559. Williams WW. CDC guidelines for infection control in hospital personnel. Infect Control 4:326, 1983.
560. Schoenbaum SC, Hyde JN, Bartoshesky L, et al. Benefit-cost analysis of rubella vaccination policy. N Engl J Med 294:306, 1976.
561. Furukawa T, Miyata T, Kondo K, et al. Clinical trials of RA 27/3 (Wistar) rubella vaccine in Japan. Am J Dis Child 118:262, 1969.
562. Vaheri A, Vesikari T, Oker-Blom N, et al. Transmission of attenuated rubella vaccines to the human fetus: a preliminary report. Am J Dis Child 118:243, 1969.
563. Recommendations of the Public Health Service Advisory Committee on Immunization Practices. Rubella vaccine. Am J Dis Child 118:397, 1969.
564. Fleet WF Jr, Benz EW Jr, Karzon DT, et al. Fetal consequences of maternal rubella immunization. JAMA 227:621, 1974.
565. Plotkin SA. Rubella vaccine. *In* Plotkin SA, Mortimer EA Jr (eds). Vaccines. Philadelphia, WB Saunders, 1988, p 235.
566. Brunell PA, Weigle K, Murphy MD. Antibody response following measles-mumps-rubella vaccine under conditions of customary use. JAMA 250:1409, 1983.
567. Mortimer PP, Edwards JMB, Porter AD, et al. Are many women immunized against rubella unnecessarily? J Hyg (Lond) 87:131, 1981.
568. Greaves WL, Orenstein WA, Hinman AR, et al. Clinical efficacy of rubella vaccine. Pediatr Infect Dis 2:284, 1982.
569. Balfour HH Jr, Amren DP. Rubella, measles and mumps antibodies following vaccination of children. Am J Dis Child 132:573, 1978.
570. Orenstein WA, Herrmann KL, Holmgreen P, et al. Prevalence of rubella antibodies in Massachusetts schoolchildren. Am J Epidemiol 124:290, 1986.
571. Rutledge SL, Snead OC III. Neurologic complications of immunizations. J Pediatr 109:917, 1986.
572. Losonsky GA, Fishaut JM, Strussenberg J, et al. Effect of immunization against rubella on lactation products. I. Development and characterization of specific immunologic reactivity in breast milk. J Infect Dis 145:654, 1982.
573. Losonsky GA, Fishaut JM, Strussenberg J, et al. Effect of immunization against rubella on lactation products. II. Maternal-neonatal interactions. J Infect Dis 145:661, 1982.
574. Landes RD, Bass JW, Millunchick EW, et al. Neonatal rubella following maternal immunization. J Pediatr 97:465, 1980.
575. Centers for Disease Control. Immunization practices in colleges—United States. MMWR Morb Mortal Wkly Rep 36:209, 1987.
576. Edgar WM, Hambling MH. Rubella vaccination and anti-D immunoglobulin administration in the puerperium. Br J Obstet Gynaecol 84:754, 1977.
577. Watt RW, McGucken RB. Failure of rubella immunization after blood transfusion: birth of congenitally infected infant. BMJ 281:977, 1980.
578. Black NA, Parsons A, Kurtz JB, et al. Post-pubertal rubella immunisation: a controlled trial of two vaccines. Lancet 2:990, 1983.
579. McIntosh ED, Menser MA. A fifty-year follow-up of congenital rubella. Lancet 340:414, 1992.
580. Noticeboard. Congenital rubella—50 years on. Lancet 337:668, 1991.
581. Schluter WW, Reef SE, Redd C, et al. Changing epidemiology of congenital rubella syndrome in the United States. J Infect Dis 178:636, 1998.
581a. Bloom S, Rguig A, Berraho A, et al. Congenital rubella syndrome burden in Morocco: a rapid retrospective assessment. Lancet 365:135-141, 2005.
582. Plotkin SA, Katz M, Cordero JF. The eradication of rubella. JAMA 281:561, 1999.

SMALLPOX AND VACCINIA

Julia A. McMillan

In 1971, the U.S. Public Health Service accepted the recommendation of its Advisory Committee on Immunization Practices that *routine* smallpox vaccination in the United States be discontinued. This recommendation was based on two considerations. The risk of contracting smallpox in the United States was small, and the risk of complications from vaccinia outweighed the potential benefits.[1]

Smallpox is the clinical disease caused by variola virus. Variola is a member of the genus Orthopoxvirus in the Poxviridae family, a genus that also includes monkeypox, cowpox, and rabbitpox, as well as vaccinia. Variola infection occurs only in humans, a fact that allowed eradication of this infection in the latter part of the 20th century in a global eradication program using preventive vaccine derived from the relatively benign vaccinia virus. The last case of smallpox identified in the United States occurred in 1949. In 1980, the world was declared free of smallpox by the World Health Organization; the last endemic case had been diagnosed in Somalia in 1977. Routine vaccination of children and the general public had been discontinued in the United States in 1972, and vaccination of health care workers was discontinued in 1976.

In 1986, international agreement led to destruction of all variola isolates except stocks to be maintained in World Health Organization–designated laboratories in the United States and the Soviet Union. Concern that variola might be used as an agent of bioterrorism was raised during the 1990s, when it was learned that variola stored in the former Soviet Union had been sold to countries thought to be developing biological weapons. It is in this context that discussion of smallpox and vaccinia virus and their potential effects on the mother and fetus have again become a matter of potential concern.

EPIDEMIOLOGY AND TRANSMISSION

Variola

Variola was spread primarily through respiratory secretions in aerosolized droplets, and spread required prolonged (6 to 7 hours) face-to-face contact. Infection through direct contact with infected lesions, bedding, or clothing was thought to occur infrequently. The incubation period was 7 to 17 days (mean, 12 days). Infected individuals were not generally contagious until the rash appeared after a 3- to 4-day prodrome of fever, malaise, backache, vomiting, and prostration. Because of the severity of the prodromal illness, infected individuals were usually confined to home or hospital by the time they presented a risk to others, and it was therefore household contacts and health care professionals who were the most frequent secondary cases. Infectivity persisted until all scabs had separated from the skin of the affected individual. The likelihood of spread to a susceptible individual was considered to be lower than that for measles and similar to the rate for varicella. Low temperature and dry conditions prolong survival for the virus, and outbreaks in the past were more common during dry, winter months.

Past recorded experience regarding the frequency of transmission of variola from mother to fetus must be considered against the backdrop of near-universal childhood vaccination. Infection during the first half of gestation resulted in an increased likelihood of fetal death or prematurity. Overall, the rate of fetal loss or death after premature delivery ranged from 57% to 81%.[2,3] There are some documented cases of live-born infants infected in utero near term. In those instances, the likelihood of congenital or neonatal infection was greatest when the mother became ill during the period 4 days before delivery through the 9 days after delivery.[4,5]

Vaccinia

Vaccinia virus transmission to the fetus after vaccination of pregnant women has also been documented,[6-8] although the frequency with which it occurs and the severity of resulting disease are difficult to determine from available studies.[9,10] The latest surveys attempting to determine the rate of adverse effects of smallpox vaccination in the United States identified only one case of fetal vaccinia. In a retrospective study in Scotland that depended on maternal recollection of timing of vaccination, MacArthur[6] found that fetal death occurred in 47% of pregnancies involving women vaccinated during the second or third trimesters and 24% of those vaccinated during the first trimester. Other studies have failed to find an increased risk of fetal death, miscarriage, or fetal malformations.[11,12] Primary vaccination during pregnancy in the years in which these studies were conducted was unusual, however, and the potential impact on the fetus after vaccination of nonimmune pregnant women cannot be extrapolated accurately.

For almost 30 years (1976 to 2002), vaccination against smallpox was available in the United States only for scientists who worked with vaccinia and related viruses in the laboratory setting. In 2002, the Department of Defense initiated a pre-event vaccination program to protect its personnel, and in 2003, the U.S. Public Health Service began vaccinating health care and public health workers who might be involved in caring for patients with smallpox or investigating circumstances surrounding the use of smallpox as an agent of bioterrorism. Criteria for exclusion of individuals at risk for adverse events (including pregnant women) were developed. Despite careful screening, by April 2003, 103 women had been inadvertently vaccinated while pregnant or within 4 weeks of conception. Sixty-nine of the 103 were primary vaccinees. No cases of fetal vaccinia have been reported. Two vaccinated pregnant health care workers experienced miscarriages early in their pregnancies, but no causal relationship between the vaccination and the miscarriage was determined.

MICROBIOLOGY

The poxviruses, including variola and vaccinia, are large, complex, double-stranded DNA viruses with a diameter of approximately 200 nm. The nucleotides of the two viruses are 96% homologous, as are 93% of the amino acids of the glycoproteins that make up the envelope of the two viruses. These envelope glycoproteins are important in antibody recognition. Under electron microscopy the virions have a characteristic brick shape. Viral aggregates in infected host cells form intracytoplasmic inclusion bodies of approximately 10 μm. Both viruses can be grown on tissue culture derived from a variety of mammalian cells, and cytopathic changes can be detected within 1 to 6 days.

PATHOGENESIS, PATHOLOGY, AND PROGNOSIS

Variola

Introduction of variola onto respiratory mucosa is followed by local multiplication and spread to lymph nodes. An asymptomatic viremia occurs on about the third or fourth day, distributing the virus to the spleen, bone marrow, and lymph nodes. Secondary viremia, occurring on about day 8, is followed on day 12 to 14 by systemic symptoms, including fever, malaise, headache, and prostration. During this secondary viremia, virus is carried by leukocytes to the dermis and oropharyngeal mucosa. Prodromal febrile illness is followed after about 3 days by development of enanthem and a maculopapular rash distributed at first primarily on the face, arms, and legs and then spreading to the trunk.

Mortality rates after smallpox varied depending on age, prior vaccination, and availability of supportive care. To some degree, mortality can be predicted by the characteristics of the rash (see "Clinical Manifestations"). Overall, the mortality rate was about 30%.

The mortality rate due to smallpox among pregnant women was high. The more lethal hemorrhagic form of smallpox was more likely to occur in pregnant women. Rao[3] followed 225 pregnant women in India between 1959 and 1962 and found a 75% mortality rate among previously unvaccinated pregnant women who developed smallpox, compared with 24% to 25% among unvaccinated nonpregnant women and men. For vaccinated women, the mortality rate was 20.7%, compared with 3% to 4% for men and nonpregnant women. Dixon[13] reported an overall mortality rate of 40% among pregnant women in a smallpox outbreak in North Africa in 1946.

Even when maternal infection is mild, transmission to the fetus can lead to increased rates of fetal death and premature delivery. Among 46 pregnancies followed by Lynch,[2] 81% resulted in fetal death or early death after premature delivery. Others reported much less frequent adverse effects on the fetus.[4] The sequence of events that lead to infection of the placenta and fetus in relation to maternal viremia has not been conclusively established. Development of symptomatic infection at 2 to 3 weeks of life in infants born to mothers whose illness began just before delivery suggests that placental infection and transmission to the fetus developed during the secondary viremic phase.[4,11] The consequences of fetal infection have been documented to involve widely disseminated foci of necrosis (i.e., skin, thymus, lungs, liver, kidneys, intestines, and adrenals) and characteristic intracytoplasmic inclusion bodies (i.e., Guarnieri bodies) in the decidual cells of the placenta.[14,15]

It is thought that transplacental transmission of variola can occur at any time during gestation, and autopsy studies corroborate infection acquired during the second and third trimesters. Pathologic studies of fetuses lost during the first trimester are lacking; however, the increased frequency of miscarriage associated with maternal infection at that stage suggests a direct effect on the products of conception.

Vaccinia

Vaccinia infection after maternal vaccination is thought to result from transient viremia. The frequency with which inoculation of vaccinia virus through vaccination leads to viremia probably is related to the invasiveness of the vaccinia strain and the vaccine status (i.e., primary versus revaccination) of the individual being vaccinated. A report involving persons vaccinated between 1930 and 1953 described isolation of vaccinia 3 to 10 days after vaccination with a strain that is thought to be more invasive than the current New York City Board of Health (NYCBOH) strain,[16] the only vaccine now available in the United States. Viremia has been reported after NYCBOH strain vaccination,[16,17] but the frequency with which it occurs is unknown. A study involving 28 healthy adults vaccinated using the NYCBOH vaccine failed to detect viremia after successful vaccination.[18] Mihailescu and Petrovici[19] were able to isolate vaccinia from products of conception of 12 (3.2%) of 366 women who had been revaccinated during pregnancy and had undergone therapeutic abortion during the first to second month of gestation.

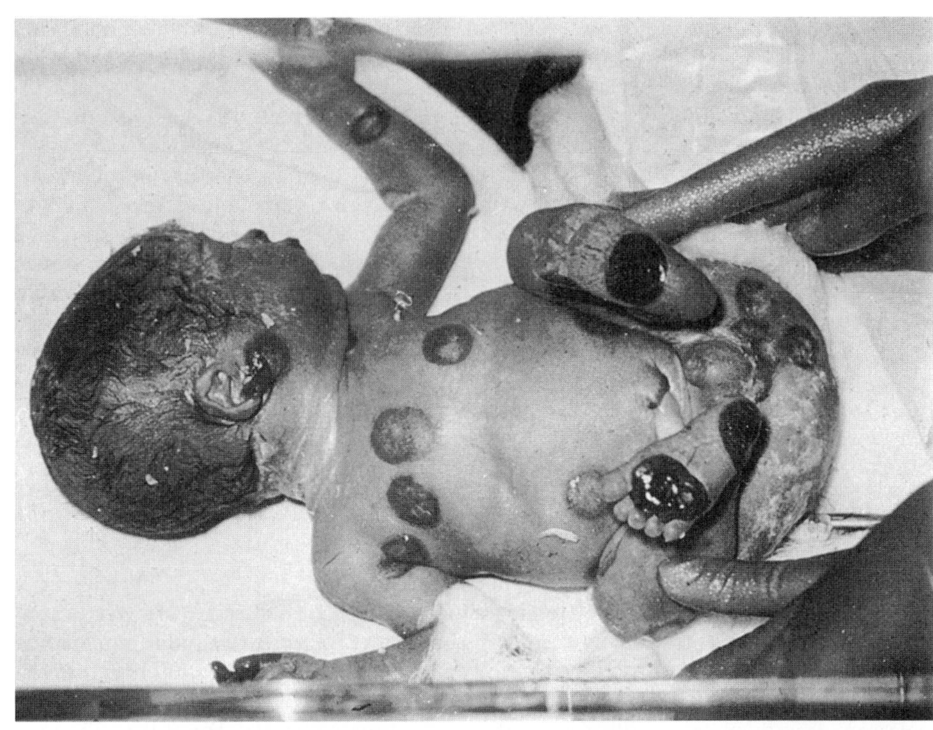

Figure 29–1 Generalized fetal vaccinia in an infant whose mother was immunized at 24 weeks' gestation. The infant was born at 30 weeks and survived. (From Hanshaw JC, Dudgeon JA. Viral Diseases of the Fetus and Newborn. Philadelphia, WB Saunders, 1978, p 216.)

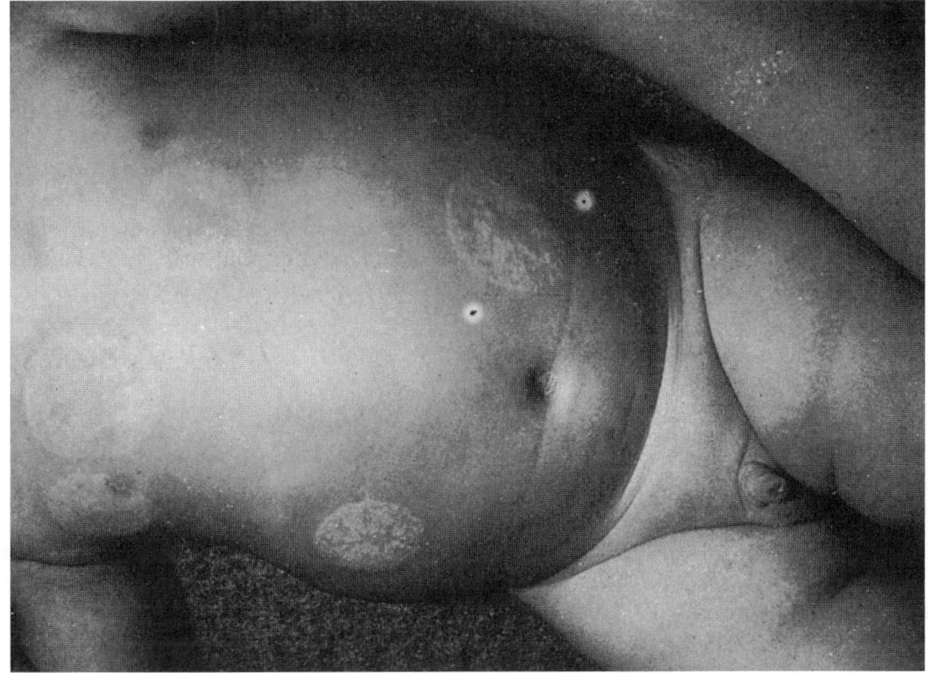

Figure 29–2 The same patient as in Figure 29-1 at 18 months of age. Scarring persists, but the lesions have healed. Smallpox vaccination was attempted without success. (From Hanshaw JC, Dudgeon JA. Viral Diseases of the Fetus and Newborn. Philadelphia, WB Saunders, 1978, p 217.)

In the past, pregnancy was not considered a contraindication to vaccination during periods of increased smallpox risk, but despite widespread use of vaccine over the past century, only 50 cases of fetal infection (3 in the United States) have been reported.[20] Levine and co-workers[21] summarized 20 cases of fetal vaccinia infection reported between 1932 and 1972. At least 13 of the 20 women involved had received their first smallpox vaccination during the pregnancy. The time of vaccination ranged from 3 to 24 weeks of pregnancy, and delivery occurred an average of 8 weeks later. Ten infected infants were born alive, and three survived (Figs. 29-1 and 29-2).

CLINICAL MANIFESTATIONS

Variola

Variola major is the form of smallpox that is of the greatest historical significance because of its high overall mortality rate (30%). Onset of rash was preceded by approximately

3 days of fever, myalgia, headache, and backache. Vomiting, diarrhea, abdominal pain, and seizures sometimes accompanied this prodromal period. The fever often was reduced as the rash appeared, only to recur and persist until skin lesions had scabbed. The appearance of the rash in patients with variola major was predictive of the severity of illness and of the associated mortality. The most common rash (90% of patients) was called *ordinary smallpox* and consisted of papules that progressed first to fluid-filled vesicles and then to firm, tense pustules that scabbed after 10 days to 2 weeks before separating from the underlying skin. The "pox" were distributed over the entire body but predominated on the face and extremities, including the palms and soles. Unlike the lesions of varicella, which appear in various stages (e.g., papules, vesicles, scabs) at one time, smallpox lesions all develop at the same rate. An enanthem involving painful lesions of the mouth and throat preceded the development of the rash by a day or less. When the rash involved discrete lesions, it was referred to as *ordinary-discrete smallpox*. The case-fatality rate associated with this form was less than 10%. When lesions were more numerous and less discrete (i.e., *ordinary-semiconfluent* and *ordinary-confluent smallpox*), the mortality rate was higher, approximating 50% to 75% for ordinary-confluent cases. *Flat smallpox*, in which lesions evolved more slowly and finally coalesced, accounted for about 7% of cases, but the mortality rate was more than 90%. Hemorrhagic smallpox, or *purpura variolosa*, which was seen most commonly in pregnant women, was associated with an almost 100% mortality rate.[22] In the series of 255 pregnant women reported by Rao,[3] smallpox was least likely to take the hemorrhagic form during the first trimester of pregnancy, and the highest likelihood of the hemorrhagic form was during the sixth month. Modified smallpox, affecting previously vaccinated individuals, was a milder disease with fewer and smaller skin lesions. Death with this form was rare.

Alastrim, or variola minor, is virologically distinct from variola major. It was first recognized in the early 20th century in South Africa, spreading to the Americas and to Europe. As the name suggests, this form of smallpox was less severe, with a case-fatality rate of about 1%.

The increased likelihood of fetal death associated with maternal infection during pregnancy was described previously. When pathologic examination of the fetus and placenta in such cases has been reported, the fetus has exhibited well-circumscribed cutaneous and scalp lesions with maceration of internal organs, including the brain. Foci of necrosis and calcification have been seen in the thymus, lungs, liver, kidneys, intestines, and adrenals. Similar foci are seen in the placenta.[14,15]

Marsden and Greenfield[4] described 34 infants whose mothers developed smallpox late in pregnancy or during the 2 weeks after delivery. Some newborns escaped symptomatic illness, although failed attempts at subsequent vaccination suggest that they were infected in utero. Based on the timing of illness in the newborns that developed smallpox compared with the appearance of rash in the mother, these investigators conclude that transmission of virus from mother to fetus occurs during the expected time of secondary maternal viremia. Other reports substantiate their conclusions. These and other researchers[2,13] describe great variability in severity of neonatal illness, including instances in which one twin escaped clinical disease but the other developed smallpox.[13] The severity of fetal or neonatal involvement does not necessarily reflect the severity of maternal infection, nor her vaccination status. In his report of 47 cases of maternal-to-fetal transmission of variola, Lynch[2] described five infected infants born at term whose mothers had been exposed to smallpox during pregnancy but had escaped clinical disease, presumably because of prior vaccination. Vaccination of newborns whose mothers developed clinical smallpox before or shortly after their birth did not always protect them from disease.

Details regarding the clinical findings and course associated with congenital variola are not available. Disease was acute and not associated with congenital anomalies. Some reports describe cutaneous lesions that are larger than those usually associated with smallpox. Among the 22 infants with congenital and neonatal smallpox described by Marsden and Greenfield,[4] 3 died, 1 of whom was born prematurely.

Vaccinia

Congenital vaccinia was rare, even during widespread vaccination programs. However, reported mortality rate associated with congenital vaccinia was high. Of the 16 cases reviewed by Green and co-workers,[8] six infants were born alive, but only one ultimately survived. For at least 12 of the 16 women, vaccination during pregnancy had been their primary smallpox vaccination. Congenital vaccinia has been reported after vaccination between the 3rd and 24th weeks of pregnancy, but for most affected pregnancies, vaccination was in the second trimester. As is the case with congenital variola, large, discrete, circular necrotic lesions were seen on the skin of infected fetuses and newborns. Foci of necrosis studded multiple internal organs and the placenta.

In utero vaccinia infection has not been associated with serious birth defects or with other long-term adverse events in surviving infants. Infants of mothers vaccinated during pregnancy that escaped fetal infection were not at risk for sequelae.

DIAGNOSIS

Diagnosis of smallpox, whether in the pregnant woman, fetus, or newborn was usually based on clinical findings along with a history of exposure to disease or vaccination. Today, suspicion that a patient may have smallpox would imply introduction of the disease through bioterrorism, and great care should be taken to prevent spread of the infection and to confirm the diagnosis in the laboratory. If skin lesions are scabbed, one or more scabs should be removed and included. Local and state health authorities should be contacted immediately. State authorities should contact the Centers for Disease Control and Prevention (CDC). Patient samples should be collected only by an individual wearing protective gown, mask, and gloves, and that individual should be someone who has been vaccinated, if possible. Throat swabs and swabs of vesicular fluid should be obtained. Blood samples and the swabs should be placed into a container sealed with adhesive tape and then placed into a second, watertight container. All samples should be sent directly to a Biological Safety Level 4 laboratory, where they can be processed safely. Laboratory confirmation can be performed by electron microscopy, nucleic acid identification, immunohistochemical studies, and tissue culture using cell culture or chorioallantoic egg membrane. Similar technique should be employed to confirm infection in the neonate. There is no known reliable intrauterine test for diagnosing congenital infection.

DIFFERENTIAL DIAGNOSIS

During the prodromal period, before the eruption of rash, maternal smallpox may be indistinguishable from other acute febrile illnesses. Once the rash appears, the pattern of eruption and the characteristics of individual pox lesions should help distinguish it from other conditions, such as rubella, measles, meningococcemia, rickettsial diseases, ratbite fever, and enteroviral infections. The widespread distribution of the lesions of variola major should distinguish it from localized papulovesicular rashes such as impetigo, shingles, and insect bites. Varicella is the viral infection most likely to be confused with smallpox. Recommended routine vaccination of children against varicella leaves many younger clinicians without experience in recognizing this formerly common infection of childhood. Table 29-1 compares clinical characteristics of the two infections. In the past, smallpox sometimes was mistaken for drug eruptions and erythema multiforme, and hemorrhagic smallpox could be difficult to distinguish from meningococcemia, severe acute leukemia, or hemorrhagic varicella.

Congenital variola or vaccinia would be expected only in the context of a history of maternal smallpox or smallpox vaccination. In addition to careful consideration of prenatal maternal history, review of maternal postpartum course is important, because historical reports suggest that neonatal smallpox may occur in association with maternal disease that manifests in the days after delivery.[3] In the absence of a maternal history of smallpox or vaccination, fetal or neonatal variola or vaccinia could be mistaken for congenital herpes simplex infection, congenital syphilis, or congenital dermatologic disease such as epidermolysis bullosa.

TREATMENT

Variola

If maternal smallpox is suspected, contact and airborne isolation precautions, in addition to universal precautions, should be instituted immediately, and if possible, the patient should be cared for in a negative-pressure room. Local and state health authorities should be notified. Family and community contacts, emergency medical personnel, and health care workers who might have been exposed to the patient should be identified and immunized as soon as possible. Immunization within 4 days can ameliorate illness and, in some cases, prevent infection completely.

Patient management includes careful attention to fluid and electrolyte requirements and nutritional support. Antibiotic therapy, including an agent effective in treating infection caused by *Staphylococcus aureus* should be provided if secondary infection is suspected. Cidofovir, a nucleoside analogue that inhibits DNA polymerase, has activity against variola. When used early in the course of infection, it has been effective in treating poxvirus infections in animals. Cidofovir is approved for use in treating cytomegalovirus infection, but it has not been used to treat smallpox. Adverse effects of cidofovir, primarily renal toxicity, would limit its use in treating suspected congenital variola.

Vaccinia

Adverse effects associated with administration of smallpox vaccine include inadvertent inoculation, including ocular inoculation, generalized vaccinia, eczema vaccinatum, progressive vaccinia (i.e., vaccinia necrosum), postvaccinal encephalitis, and fetal vaccinia. Vaccination programs have developed careful screening tools to prevent vaccination of individuals thought to be particularly susceptible to these adverse effects, including exclusion of women who are pregnant or intend to become pregnant within 4 weeks of vaccination. Congenital vaccinia among live-born infants is rare, and inadvertent vaccination during pregnancy should not be a reason to recommend termination of pregnancy. Vaccinia immune globulin (VIG) has been used to treat some complications associated with smallpox vaccination, including eczema vaccinatum and progressive vaccinia. It may be used for those same reasons during pregnancy, but VIG is not recommended as prophylaxis against congenital vaccinia. No data are available regarding appropriate dose or efficacy of VIG for treatment of congenital vaccinia. Treatment may be considered, however, for a viable infant born with lesions after a history of maternal vaccination. For information concerning availability, indications, and administration of VIG, physicians should contact the CDC Clinical Consultation Team (phone: 877-554-4625).

Cidofovir is available for treatment of complications of smallpox vaccination only under the investigational new drug (IND) protocol administered by the CDC. It will be released only as secondary treatment for complications that do not respond to treatment with VIG.

Table 29–1 Clinical Features Distinguishing Chickenpox from Smallpox

Clinical Features	Chickenpox	Smallpox
Fever onset	At the time of the rash	2-4 days before the rash
Rash characteristics	Pocks in different stages	Pocks in the same stages
	Develops rapidly	Develops slowly
	More pocks on the body	More pocks on face, arms, and legs
	Spares palms and soles	Affects palms and soles
Mortality	Rare	10%-30%, historically

PREVENTION

After a remarkable, worldwide public health effort, smallpox was eradicated in nature during the latter part of the 20th century. Until concerns were raised regarding the potential use of smallpox as an agent of bioterrorism, protection from smallpox was thought to be unnecessary, and vaccination to protect against variola was discontinued. In the 21st century, inadvertent vaccination of pregnant military personnel, health care workers, and public health workers, many of whom are being vaccinated for the first time, poses the greatest risk for maternal and fetal infection. Careful screening of such individuals has been shown generally to be effective, but some vaccination during pregnancy has occurred despite screening. The National Smallpox Vaccine in Pregnancy Registry has been established to investigate instances of inadvertent smallpox vaccination during pregnancy. Civilian cases should be reported to state health departments or to the CDC (phone: 404-639-8253 or 877-554-4625). Military cases should be reported to the Department of Defense (phone: 619-553-9255; DSN: 619-553-9255; fax: 619-553-7601; e-mail: code25 @nhrc.navy.mil). Health care providers are encouraged to save and forward products of conception from pregnancy losses associated with vaccination during pregnancy to the CDC or the U.S. Department of Defense. Specimens should be frozen at −70° C, preferably in viral transport media before and during transport.

REFERENCES

1. Krugman S, Katz SL. Smallpox and vaccinia. *In* Infectious Diseases of Children, 7th ed. St. Louis, Mosby, 1981.
2. Lynch FW. Dermatologic conditions of the fetus with particular reference to variola and vaccinia. Arch Dermatol Syphilis Chic 26:997, 1932.
3. Rao AR, Prahlad I, Swaminathan M, et al. Pregnancy and smallpox. J Indian Med Assoc 40:353, 1963.
4. Marsden JP, Greenfield CRM. Inherited smallpox. Arch Dis Child 9:309, 1934.
5. Sharma R, Sharma R, Jagdev DK. Congenital smallpox. Scand J Infect Dis 3:245, 1971.
6. MacArthur P. Congenital vaccinia and vaccinia gravidarum. Lancet 2:1104, 1952.
7. Bourke GJ, Whitty RJ. Smallpox vaccination in pregnancy: a prospective study. BMJ 1:1544, 1964.
8. Green DM, Reid SM, Rhaney K. Generalized vaccinia in the human foetus. Lancet 1:1296, 1966.
9. Lane JM, Ruben FL, Neff JM, et al. Complications of smallpox vaccination, 1968: results of ten statewide surveys. J Infect Dis 122:303, 1970.
10. Lane JM, Ruben FL, Neff JM, et al. Complications of smallpox vaccination, 1968: national surveillance in the United States. N Engl J Med 281:1201, 1969.
11. Greenberg M, Yankauer A, Krugman S, et al. The effect of smallpox vaccination during pregnancy on the incidence of congenital malformations. Pediatrics 3:456, 1949.
12. Bellows MT, Hyman ME, Meritt KK. Effect of smallpox vaccination on the outcome of pregnancy. Public Health Rep 64:319, 1949.
13. Dixon CW. Smallpox in Tripolitania, 1946: an epidemiological and clinical study of 500 cases, including trials of penicillin treatment. J Hyg 46:351, 1948.
14. Garcia AGP. Fetal infection in chickenpox and alastrim, with histopathologic study of the placenta. Pediatrics 32:895, 1963.
15. Marsden JP. Metastatic calcification. Notes on twins born shortly after an attack of smallpox in the mother. Br J Child Dis 28:193, 1930.
16. Fenner F, Henderson DA, Arita I, et al. The pathogenesis, pathology and immunology of smallpox and vaccinia. *In* Smallpox and Its Eradication. Geneva, World Health Organization, 1988.
17. Blattner RJ, Norman JO, Heys FM, et al. Antibody response to cutaneous inoculation with vaccinia virus: viremia and viruria in vaccinated children. J Pediatr 26:176, 1964.
18. Cummings JF, Polhemus ME, Hawkes C, et al. Lack of vaccinia viremia after smallpox vaccination. Clin Infect Dis 38:456, 2004.
19. Mihailescu R, Petrovici M. Effect of smallpox vaccination on the product of conception. Arch Roum Path Exp Microbiol 34:67-74, 1975.
20. Centers for Disease Control and Prevention. Women with smallpox vaccine exposure during pregnancy reported to the National Smallpox Vaccine in Pregnancy Registry—United States, 2003. MMWR Morb Mortal Wkly Rep 52:386, 2003.
21. Levine MM, Edsall G, Bruce-Chwatt LJ. Live-virus vaccines in pregnancy: risks and recommendations. Lancet 2:34, 1974.
22. Paranjothy D, Samuel I. Pregnancy associated with haemorrhagic smallpox. J Obstet Gynaecol Br Emp 67:309, 1960.

Chapter 30

LESS COMMON VIRAL INFECTIONS

Yvonne A. Maldonado

HUMAN PAPILLOMAVIRUS

Human papillomavirus (HPV) is the cause of condyloma acuminatum (i.e., genital warts) and cervical condylomata.[1-3] The risk to the infant born to a mother with HPV infection is the development of juvenile laryngeal papillomatosis and possible development of anogenital warts.[4] Hajek[5] associated the presence of condyloma acuminatum in a mother at the time of delivery with the subsequent development of laryngeal papilloma in her infant (Table 30-1). Cook and colleagues[6] described a similar association in five of nine children with laryngeal papilloma. All five of the children who developed laryngeal papilloma when younger than 6 months old were born to mothers who had condylomata acuminata at the time of delivery. The mothers of two of four other children with laryngeal papilloma had genital warts but did not have them at the time of delivery. Seven (78%) of the nine children with laryngeal papilloma had mothers with condylomata acuminata. The expected incidence of condylomata acuminata in women in the population studied by Cook and colleagues[6] was 1.5%. Six of the nine children also had skin warts. Quick and co-workers[7] described a strong association between laryngeal papilloma in young children and maternal condylomata. Twenty-one (68%) of the 31 patients with laryngeal papilloma they studied had been born to mothers who had had condylomata.

The basis for this epidemiologic relationship is evident from the detection of HPV DNA sequences in genital and laryngeal papilloma tissues.[3] A number of studies have reported rates of newborn infection that ranged from 4% to 72% among infants born to HPV-infected mothers and 0.6% to 20% among those born to mothers without detectable HPV DNA.[8-14] However, Smith and colleagues[15] investigated the risk of perinatal transmission based on concordance and sequence match to HPV types of both parents. Only 9 (1.6%) of 574 of oral or genital specimens from newborns were positive for HPV DNA, and of those, only one maternal-infant HPV match was detected, suggesting that perinatal transmission is rare.[15] Rare associations have been made between maternal genital HPV infections and neonatal giant cell hepatitis[16] and vulvar genital papillomas among stillborns.[17] Both associations were documented in small numbers of gestations but were confirmed by HPV DNA polymerase chain reaction (PCR) or by electron microscopy.

HPV cannot be isolated by means of tissue culture, but HPV DNA sequences can be detected in cervical cells. Cervical infection is caused by several types of HPV, including types 6, 11, 16, 18, and 31, and it is very common in the United States and Europe. HPV can be detected in epithelial cells that have a normal histologic appearance and from tissue samples of patients whose papillomatous lesions are in remission.[18] Clinically, most genital HPV infection is asymptomatic. The frequency of HPV detection has ranged from 5% to 15% in studies of women of childbearing age, with the highest incidence occurring among younger women.[19-22] Pregnancy was not associated with a higher rate of infection. Although the incidence of cervical infection was 20% in women with a history of condyloma, most pregnant women with HPV infection do not have a history of genital warts. Infection of the infant probably occurs by exposure to the virus at delivery, although papillomatosis has been described in infants delivered by cesarean section. Tang and associates[23] described an infant who was born with condylomata acuminata around the anal orifice. The mother also had condylomata acuminata. Whether this case reflects transplacental hematogenous spread or direct extension across intact membranes is not known.

Despite the prevalence of genital HPV infection, juvenile laryngeal papillomatosis remains a rare disease. The incidence of recurrent respiratory papillomatosis is approximately 3.96 per 100,000 in the pediatric population, with an incidence of 7 of every 1000 children born to mothers with vaginal condyloma. The risk of subclinical transmission of HPV from mothers to infants is not known. HPV-6 and HPV-16 DNA sequences were detected in the cells from foreskin tissue of 3 of 70 infants.[24] These HPV types are also found in genital warts. Because of the prevalence of asymptomatic HPV infection, the feasibility of preventing the rare cases of laryngeal papillomatosis by considering maternal condyloma acuminatum as an indication for cesarean delivery is uncertain.

Treatment of anogenital warts is not optimal, but podophyllum resin or podofilox is often used in older children and adults. Neither has been tested for safety or efficacy in children, and both are contraindicated for use in pregnancy. Laryngeal papillomas recur even after repeated surgical removal. Interferon has been used with some success for treatment of laryngeal papillomas.[25] Although the mainstay of surgical management has traditionally been the CO_2 laser,

Table 30–1 **Effects of Other Viral Infections of the Fetus and Newborn**

Infectious Agent	Increased Incidence of Abortion	Increased Risk of Prematurity	Major Clinical Manifestations in Infants
Human papillomavirus	No	No	Laryngeal papilloma, condyloma acuminatum
Epstein-Barr virus	Possibly	Possibly	?
Human herpesvirus 6	No	No	Febrile illness in postnatal period
Influenza viruses	No	No	Probably none
Respiratory syncytial virus	No	No	Pneumonia, bronchiolitis, in postnatal period
Lymphocytic choriomeningitis virus	Yes	No	Hydrocephalus, chorioretinitis, viral meningitis, jaundice, ? thrombocytopenia
Molluscum contagiosum virus	No	No	Rash
Rabies	No	No	None known

newer surgical techniques have demonstrated efficacy in the management of pediatric patients, including powered instrumentation and the pulse-dye laser. The traditional adjuvant medical therapies used for pediatric recurrent respiratory papillomatosis continue to be commonly used, including topical interferon alfa-2a, retinoic acid, and indol-3-carbinol/diindolylmethane (I3C/DIM). Topical cidofovir has demonstrated efficacy in selected patients. Research trials suggest that HPV vaccines may in the future be useful for therapy and for prevention.[26,27] Two approaches have been pursued for HPV vaccines: preventive vaccines to evoke a neutralizing antibody response and prevent infection and therapeutic vaccines to generate cytotoxic T lymphocytes and destroy HPV-infected neoplastic cells.[28]

EPSTEIN-BARR VIRUS

Epstein-Barr virus (EBV) is a human herpesvirus that is most familiar as the cause of infectious mononucleosis. However, most women of childbearing age have been infected asymptomatically in childhood. Because EBV cannot be isolated directly in tissue culture, serologic tests are used to detect recent primary or past infection.

Persons infected with EBV form IgG and IgM antibodies to viral capsid antigens (VCAs) soon after infection.[29] About 80% form antibodies to early antigens (EAs), which usually fall to undetectable levels 6 months after infection. The presence of antibodies to EAs at later times after acute infection may indicate viral reactivation.[30] Antibodies to EBV-associated nuclear antigen (EBNA) develop 3 to 4 weeks after primary infection and probably persist for life, as do IgG antibodies to VCAs.

Prospective studies using antibodies to EAs as a marker of recent maternal EBV infection have yielded conflicting results. In a group of 719 women evaluated by Icart and Didier,[31] pregnancies associated with early fetal death, birth of infants with a congenital abnormality, prematurity or intrauterine growth retardation, and deaths or illnesses during the first week of life were more common in women who were EA antibody positive during the first 3 months of pregnancy than in those who were not. Whether these women had a recent primary EBV infection or reactivation of an infection cannot be determined because EBV EA antibodies persist in some otherwise healthy adults and are associated with the reactivation of past EBV infection. In contrast, Fleisher and Bolognese[32] found that the frequency of antibodies to EA in pregnant women was 55%, compared with 22% to 32% among nonpregnant adults, but the incidence of low birth weight, neonatal jaundice, or congenital anomalies was not increased among infants of women with anti-EA antibodies.

Primary EBV infection during pregnancy is unusual[33] because only 3.0% to 3.4% of pregnant women are susceptible.[34,35] Recent primary EBV infection is diagnosed by the presence of VCA IgG and IgM antibodies in the absence of antibodies to EBV-associated nuclear antigen.[36] Six women were studied who had primary EBV infections during pregnancy as established by the presence of IgM antibody to VCA and the absence of antibody to EBNA in their sera.[34] Of these, only one had symptoms compatible with mononucleosis during pregnancy; she gave birth to a normal infant. Four of the remaining five pregnancies terminated abnormally. One woman had a spontaneous abortion, and the other three were delivered of premature infants. All three of the premature infants were abnormal. One was stillborn, one had multiple congenital anomalies, and one was small for gestational age. The products of abortion and the premature infants were not studied for evidence of an EBV infection. The abnormal infants in this study did not have a characteristic syndrome but instead had a variety of abnormalities.

Fleisher and Bolognese[37] identified three infants born to women who had had silent EBV seroconversion during the first trimester. Two infants were normal; one infant had tricuspid atresia. EBV IgM was not detected in cord blood serum, and EBV was not recovered from the cord blood lymphocytes. Three infants of mothers with a primary EBV infection and infectious mononucleosis were normal at birth and had no serologic or virologic evidence of intrauterine infection.[38]

Early reports implicated EBV as a cause of congenital anomalies, particularly congenital heart disease; however, Tallqvist and colleagues[39] were unable to show an increase in incidence of antibodies to EBV in 6- to 23-month-old children with congenital heart disease compared with normal, age-matched controls. EBV may cause congenital heart disease in an individual case, but this study suggests that it is not a common cause of cardiac defects. Brown and Stenchever[40] described an infant with multiple congenital anomalies who was born to a mother who had a positive monospot test result 4 weeks before conception and at 16 and 36 weeks' gestation. In addition to the anomalies, which involved many organs, the infant was small for gestational age. Normal chromosomal complements were found on standard and G-banded karyotypes. The total IgM level in the cord blood was not elevated. Studies were not performed for IgM VCA antibody or antibody to EA, and no attempts were made to isolate EBV. Although the evidence that the mother had mononucleosis near the time of conception is convincing, there is no virologic evidence that EBV was the cause of the anomalies. Goldberg and associates[41] described an infant born with hypotonia, micrognathia, bilateral cataracts, metaphyseal lucencies, and thrombocytopenia. Immunologic evidence suggesting possible EBV infection included an elevated total IgM level, the presence of IgM anti-VCA antibody at 22 days of age, and a delay in development of anti-EBNA antibody until 42 days of age. Weaver and co-workers described an infant with extrahepatic bile duct atresia and evidence of intrauterine EBV infection; EBV IgM was identified in serum obtained when the infant was 3 and 6 weeks old, and persistent EBV IgG was seen at 1 year.[42]

Although EBV cannot be recovered by standard tissue culture methods, the virus can be detected by its capacity to transform B lymphocytes into persistent lymphoblastoid cell lines. In studies conducted to identify cases of intrauterine EBV infection, Visintine and colleagues[43] and Chang and Blankenship[44] observed spontaneous transformation of lymphocytes obtained from cord blood, but it was not associated with EBV. EBV-transformed cells were not found in any samples of cord blood from 2000 newborns studied by Chang and Seto[45] or from the 25 newborns tested by Joncas and associates.[46,47] One study used nested PCR methods for amplifying EBV DNA regions in circulating lymphocytes from 67 mother-infant pairs within 1 week of birth.[48] Approximately 50% of the women and two of the neonates were EBV PCR positive. Visintine and colleagues[43] studied 82 normal term infants, 28 infants with congenital anomalies, and 29 infants suspected of having congenital infections; they were unable to isolate EBV from any of these infants. Two infants have been described in whom there was evidence of infection with EBV at birth.[47,49] A congenital cytomegalovirus (CMV) infection coexisted in both. Most of the clinical findings in the infants were compatible with those usually found in congenital CMV infections and included microcephaly, periventricular calcifications, hepatosplenomegaly, and inclusions characteristic of CMV in sections of tissues or cells in urinary sediments. One infant had deformities of the hands similar to those seen in arthrogryposis. Neither CMV nor EBV was isolated from the saliva or secretions of these infants. In the first infant, IgM antibody to EBV was present at birth and EBNA-positive permanent lymphoblastoid cell lines were established on five occasions between 3 and 30 months of age. In the second infant, permanent lymphoblastoid cell lines were established from the peripheral blood at birth and from heart blood at 3 days of age. EBNA and EBV RNA were identified in these cells, and CMV DNA was identified in the cells from the liver of the same infant.

Attempts to isolate EBV from secretions obtained from the maternal cervix have been unsuccessful,[43,45] but the virus can be detected at this site by DNA hybridization.[50] There is little evidence suggesting that natal transmission of EBV occurs. However, EBV was recovered from genital ulcers in a young woman with infectious mononucleosis.[51] Fatal EBV infection was diagnosed by DNA hybridization of lymph node tissue from one infant who presented with failure to thrive, emesis, diarrhea, and a macular rash at 14 days of age, but this infection might have been acquired in utero.[52]

EBV can be transmitted to newborns in the perinatal period by blood transfusion.[43,46] Permanent lymphoblastoid lines that contained EBV antigens were established by Joncas and co-workers[46] from the blood of two infants who had been transfused. One of these infants did not develop permanent antibodies to EBV.

There is no evidence at present that EBV causes congenital anomalies. Because the early and the late serologic responses of young infants to a primary EBV infection differ from those found when a primary infection occurs at an older age,[30,46,53] it will be difficult to screen large numbers of newborns for serologic evidence of an EBV infection sustained in utero.

HUMAN HERPESVIRUS 6

Human herpesvirus 6 (HHV-6) is a member of the herpesvirus family that has been identified as a cause of exanthema subitum (i.e., roseola).[54-56] The virus exhibits tropism for T lymphocytes and is most closely related to human CMV by genetic analysis.[57]

Seroepidemiologic studies have shown that HHV-6 is ubiquitous in the human population, regardless of geographic area, and that it infects more than 90% of infants during the first year of life.[58-60] IgG antibodies to HHV-6 are detected in almost all infants at birth, with a subsequent decline in seropositivity rates by 4 to 6 months of age as transplacentally acquired antibody is lost. The highest rate of acquisition of HHV-6 infection appears to occur during the first 6 months to 1 year of life as maternal antibodies wane. The seroepidemiologic evidence and restriction enzyme analysis of paired virus isolates from mothers and their infants suggest that the usual route of transmission is perinatal or postnatal.[61] No cases of symptomatic intrauterine HHV-6 infection have been confirmed since the agent was identified in 1986. A case of intrauterine infection was documented by PCR in a fetus whose mother had human immunodeficiency virus infection and HHV-6 in peripheral blood mononuclear cells,[62] and 1 (0.28%) of 799 cord blood serum samples had IgM antibodies to HHV-6.[63] Another study, using HHV-6 DNA PCR applied to cord blood specimens from 305 infants, demonstrated a 1.6% (5 of 305) PCR positivity rate, suggesting in utero transmission.[64] Evidence of reinfection after presumed congenital HHV-6 infection also has been demonstrated.[65] As diagnostic assays become more widely available, congenital infections may be recognized. However, primary HHV-6 infection, with its anticipated higher risk of transmission to the fetus, should be rare during pregnancy, because almost all adult women have been infected in childhood. Analogous to human CMV infection, the reactivation of maternal HHV-6, although it may be common during pregnancy, is not expected to cause symptomatic intrauterine infection.

In addition to the roseola syndrome, HHV-6 has been detected by PCR in peripheral blood lymphocytes obtained from infants younger than 3 months who had acute, nonspecific, febrile illnesses.[66,67] Two neonates who had fulminant hepatitis associated with HHV-6 infection have been described.[68,69] Other associations found among infants include a mononucleosis-like syndrome,[70] pneumonitis,[71] and one case report of possible immunodeficiency and pneumonitis associated with HHV-6 infection.[72] However, all clinical associations between disease in infants and HHV-6 infection must be evaluated with care because of the evidence that most infants become infected with this virus within a few months after birth and that the virus persists after primary infection, as is characteristic of herpesviruses.[62] Clinicians also must be aware of the potential for false-positive results in serologic assays and in attempts to detect the virus by PCR.[56]

HUMAN HERPESVIRUS 7

Human herpesvirus 7 (HHV-7) was discovered in the peripheral blood lymphocytes of a healthy adult in 1990.[73] HHV-7 belongs to the Roseolovirus genus within the Betaherpesvirinae subfamily, along with HHV-6 and CMV. Like HHV-6, it causes primary infection in most individuals during childhood. However, clinically symptomatic infection with HHV-7 appears to be significantly less common and occurs later than with HHV-6.

Based on seroepidemiologic studies,[74-76] HHV-7 infection is ubiquitous in childhood and generally occurs at a later age than HHV-6 infection. The average age at infection is about 2 years, and 75% of children are seropositive by 5 years of age. The primary mechanism of transmission is from contact with saliva of infected individuals. Because HHV-7 DNA has been detected in breast milk, breast-feeding may be another source of infection.[77] However, antibodies to HHV-7 in breast milk may protect against infection, and in one study, breast-feeding was associated with a lower risk of early acquisition of HHV-7 infection.[77,78] HHV-7 DNA has been detected in 2.7% of cervical swabs obtained from women in their third trimester of pregnancy but from none of the swabs of control women, suggesting that pregnancy may be associated with reactivation of HHV-7.[79] However, perinatal transmission from contact with infected maternal secretions is unknown, and neonatal infections with HHV-7 have not been reported.[80]

Clinical symptoms are rarely associated with HHV-7 infection but include nonspecific fever, with or without rash, which resembles exanthema subitum. Clinically apparent HHV-7 infections appear to have a high rate of central nervous system (CNS) involvement.[81-84]

INFLUENZA A AND B

Early investigations of the teratogenic potential of influenza virus were epidemiologic studies in which the diagnosis of influenza was not confirmed serologically.[85] In 1959, Coffey and Jessup[85] reported an incidence of 3.6% of congenital defects in 664 Irish women who had histories of having had influenza during pregnancy, compared with 1.5% of 663 women who did not have symptoms compatible with influenza. CNS anomalies were the most common type of defect, and of these, anencephaly was the most frequent. These investigators presented some evidence that women who had a history of having had influenza in the first trimester were more likely to give birth to children who had congenital anomalies than those who had influenza later in the pregnancy. This evidence provided credence to the report.

In a similar study conducted in Scotland, Doll and Hill[86] were unable to confirm that congenital anomalies occurred with a higher frequency in infants of women who had histories of influenza during pregnancy than in infants of women who did not. However, after reviewing the reported incidence of stillbirth related to anencephaly recorded by the Registrar General for Scotland, they concluded that there was a small increase in risk of anencephaly if the mother had had influenza during the first 2 months of pregnancy. In performing this analysis, certain assumptions were made because of the lack of precise data. Record[87] and Leck[88] analyzed the same data and were unable to find an association between influenza and malformations of the CNS. An increase in congenital defects in infants of mothers who had influenza-like symptoms at 5 to 11 weeks' gestation was reported by Hakosalo and Saxen.[89] Most of these anomalies involved the CNS, but there was no increase in incidence of anencephaly in infants of women who had symptoms compatible with influenza compared with those who remained asymptomatic.

All of these studies were undertaken during influenza epidemics. It was assumed that, under these circumstances, there would be a high correlation between a history of influenza as elicited from the patient and infection with influenza virus. However, during the 1957 outbreak, Wilson and Stein[90] demonstrated that 60% of pregnant women who denied symptoms of influenza had serologic evidence of having been recently infected. Conversely, 35% of those who stated that they had had influenza lacked serologic evidence of having been infected. Likewise, Hardy and co-workers[91] found that 24% of those who stated that they had had influenza lacked serologic evidence of past infection with the epidemic strain and 39% of those with titers suggesting recent infection denied symptoms of influenza. MacKenzie and Houghton[92] summarized the reports implicating influenza virus as a cause of maternal morbidity and congenital anomalies and came to the conclusion that probably no association exists between maternal influenza infection and subsequent congenital malformations or neoplasms in childhood.

Several studies have been performed in which infection by influenza virus has been serologically confirmed. Hardy and co-workers[91] reported that the incidence of stillbirths was higher in 332 symptomatic pregnant women with serologically confirmed influenza infections than in 206 women with serologically confirmed infections who had remained asymptomatic or in 73 uninfected women. The control group of uninfected women was smaller than expected because the attack rate during the period of the study was very high. Major congenital anomalies occurred in 5.3% of women whose infections occurred during the first trimester, compared with 2.1% of 183 women infected during the second trimester and 1.1% of 275 women infected during the third trimester. Supernumerary digits, syndactyly, and skin anomalies were excluded from these figures. Among infants of mothers infected during the first trimester, cardiac anomalies were the most common type of abnormality; none of these infants had anencephaly. Griffiths and associates[93] observed a slight increase in congenital anomalies in infants born to women who had had serologically confirmed influenza during pregnancy compared with infants of women who had not; however, all of the infants with congenital anomalies were born to women who had had influenza in the second or third trimester. Monif and colleagues[94] did not document infection in any of eight infants born to mothers who had influenza A/Hong Kong infections in the second and third trimesters. Wilson and Stein[90] found no increase in congenital anomalies in women with serologic evidence of having been recently infected with influenza virus who had conceived during the 3-month period when influenza was epidemic.

Population-based epidemiologic studies have not demonstrated that influenza infections during pregnancy are significantly associated with adverse perinatal outcomes. However, influenza infections during pregnancy are more likely to result in hospitalization for respiratory symptoms in the pregnant woman than for nonpregnant adults.[95,96] Hartert and associates[95] conducted a matched cohort study of pregnant women to determine pregnancy outcomes associated with respiratory hospitalizations during influenza seasons from 1985 to 1993. During those influenza seasons, 293 pregnant women were hospitalized for respiratory symptoms, at a rate of 5.1 per 1000 pregnant women. The prevalence of prematurity and low birth weight was not higher than a matched cohort of pregnant women hospitalized with nonrespiratory diagnoses. However, pregnant women with asthma had higher rates of respiratory hospitalizations than those without asthma, and all of three fetal deaths in this cohort were singleton, late-third-trimester intrauterine fetal deaths in mothers who had asthma and were current smokers.[95]

It can be said with certainty that intrauterine exposure to influenza virus does not cause a consistent syndrome. If there is a cause-and-effect association between influenza virus infections during pregnancy and congenital anomalies, the latter occur with low frequency. Hakosalo and Saxen[89] have documented an increase in the use of nonprescription drugs during influenza outbreaks and have suggested that drugs rather than infection with influenza virus may exert an erratic teratogenic influence. A number of studies have investigated the possible association between influenza infection in pregnant women and subsequent development of bipolar affective disorders or schizophrenia among their offspring, with mixed results.[97-99]

Viremia is rare during influenza infections, but it does occur. Few attempts have been made to demonstrate transplacental passage of the virus to the fetus. Ruben and colleagues[100] tested the cord sera of infants born to 22 mothers who had been pregnant during an influenza A/England/42/72 outbreak and who had had influenza hemagglutination inhibition titers to this virus of 1:16 or higher while pregnant. Forty-two cord serum samples were randomly collected from infants who had been born on the same day as the selected infants. Of the 64 cord serum samples tested, a fall in titer of fourfold or more was seen in four samples after treatment with 2-mercaptoethanol; this suggests that IgM antibody to influenza might have been present. Three of 16 cord blood samples tested gave positive lymphocyte transformation responses to influenza virus. All seven of the infants with evidence of antigenic recognition of influenza virus at birth had uncomplicated deliveries and remained healthy. Influenza A/Bangkok was isolated from the amniotic fluid of a mother with amnionitis and acute influenza infection at 36 weeks' gestation; the infant who was born at 39 weeks had serologic evidence of infection but was asymptomatic.[101]

Yawn and associates[102] studied a woman who developed influenza in the third trimester and died of pulmonary edema. A virus similar to the prototype strain A_2/Hong Kong/8/68 was isolated from the lung, hilar nodes, heart, spleen, liver, kidney, brain, and spinal cord of the mother and from the amniotic fluid and myocardium of the fetus. Ramphal and colleagues[103] studied another woman who died of complications of an influenza infection at term. A virus similar to strain A/Texas/77 was isolated from maternal tissues, but influenza virus was not isolated from any of the fetal tissues tested.

In contrast to intrauterine infections with influenza virus, which are rare, infections acquired by infants in the neonatal period are common. Passively transferred antibody to influenza virus may prevent symptomatic infections during the first few months of life if it is present in sufficient quantity.[104,105] Two cases of influenza A/Hong Kong/68 infection in infants who were younger than 1 month were described by Bauer and associates.[106] The first infant developed high fever, irritability, and nasal discharge when 10 days old; the second infant, who was premature, developed fever and nasal congestion when 14 days old. Symptoms were restricted to the upper respiratory system, and both infants recovered within 4 days of onset of the illness. Influenza virus infection may, however, be fatal in the neonatal period.[107] Several outbreaks of influenza virus infection have occurred in neonatal intensive care units. In general, illness has been mild.[106,108] Most of the eight infected neonates described by Meibalane and co-workers[108] had nonspecific symptoms, including apnea, lethargy, and poor feeding. Only two had cough or nasal congestion. None had tachypnea or respiratory distress, but three of five for whom chest radiographs were obtained had interstitial pneumonia.

Infants younger than 6 months cannot be protected by influenza vaccine. All health care professionals who care for high-risk newborns should receive the influenza A/influenza B vaccine annually in the fall. Pregnancy is not a contraindication for the administration of influenza vaccine.[109,110]

RESPIRATORY SYNCYTIAL VIRUS

Although respiratory syncytial virus (RSV) is a common cause of upper respiratory tract infection in adults, there is no evidence that the virus causes intrauterine infection. Maternal infection has no known adverse effect on the fetus.

RSV infections are frequently acquired by infants during the first few weeks of life and are associated with a high mortality rate. Two thirds of all infants become infected with RSV in the first year of life, and one third of them will develop lower respiratory tract symptoms, 2.5% will be hospitalized, and 1 in 1000 infants will die as a result of RSV infection.[111] It was originally thought that passively transferred maternal antibody to RSV contributed to the severity of the infection in young infants by causing an immunopathologic reaction in the lung.[112] Later studies of the age-corrected incidence of symptomatic RSV infections showed a relative sparing of infants who were younger than 3 weeks.[113,114] This is the period during which maternal antibody is the highest. In subsequent studies, no evidence was found that the presence of maternal antibody adversely influenced the course of infection in the infant.[115] Lamprecht and colleagues[116] found an inverse relationship between the level of maternal neutralizing antibody and the severity of the RSV infection in the infant.

Glezen and co-workers[117] found that the quantity of neutralizing antibody to RSV in cord sera was lower in infants with proven RSV infections than in randomly selected infants. None of the infected infants who had antibody titers of 1:16 or higher developed serious infections. Some have suggested that breast-feeding decreases the possibility that an infant will have a serious RSV infection early in life[118]; however, this has not been a consistent finding in every study. Because breast-feeding and crowded living conditions affect the incidence of RSV infection in infants, it has been difficult to define effects attributable solely to breast-feeding. Infection with RSV in infants who are younger than 4 weeks may be asymptomatic, consist of an afebrile upper respiratory syndrome, or be accompanied by fever, bronchiolitis or pneumonia, and apnea.[119]

RSV accounted for 55% of cases of viral pneumonia in infants younger than 1 month in one study that evaluated hospitalized infants over a 5-year period.[120] Most infants who died had underlying medical conditions that involved the heart or lungs.[121,122] Premature infants who have recovered from hyaline membrane disease and who have bronchopulmonary dysplasia are especially likely to develop severe infections. The A subtype of RSV may have the potential to cause more severe disease than the B subtype.[123]

The nosocomial outbreaks that have occurred in nurseries caring for premature and ill term infants have varied in severity. Neligan and colleagues[124] described an outbreak in which eight infants were infected. The first symptom in all infants was the development of a clear nasal discharge when 10 to 52 days old. Cough developed 2 to 7 days later. Three infants developed wheezing, and only one infant was seriously ill. In the outbreak described by Berkovich and Taranko,[125] 14 infants in a premature nursery became ill when 11 to 184 days old. Of the 14 infants, 93% had coryza, 86% had dyspnea, 64% had pneumonia, and 36% had fever. Upper respiratory tract symptoms began 1 to 8 days before the first dyspnea in 11 infants. Changes compatible with pneumonia were demonstrable on chest roentgenograms 3 to 5 days before clinical evidence of lower respiratory tract involvement developed. The degree of illness in the nine infants studied by Mintz and associates[126] was mild in four, moderate in two, and severe in two. One infant was asymptomatic. The infants who were the most seriously ill had fever, cyanosis, pulmonary infiltrates, and respiratory deterioration. Infants with RSV infections have developed respiratory arrest as a result of apnea.[127,128] Most infants infected during nosocomial outbreaks of RSV in nurseries were born prematurely but had attained 4 weeks or more in chronologic age at the time they developed the infections.[126,127] Two nursery outbreaks were associated with dual infections caused by RSV and rhinovirus or parainfluenza virus 3.[129,130] A diffuse viral pneumonia, which is indistinguishable from severe RSV pneumonia, can be caused in rare instances by parainfluenza viruses alone or, rarely, by adenovirus.[131] Hall and co-workers[132] have shown that infants who are younger than 3 weeks when they become infected with RSV have a higher incidence of nonspecific signs and a lower incidence of lower respiratory tract infection than infants who are older than 3 weeks at the time of infection. RSV has been recovered from the oropharynx of infants who were younger than 48 hours.[133] It may be difficult to recognize the index case when RSV is introduced into the nursery.[134]

Infants who are younger than 1 month have a higher mean maximal titer of virus in their secretions than those who are older.[135] Ninety-six percent of the infected infants studied by Hall and co-workers[135] shed virus for 9 days. Objects contaminated with secretions from infected infants may be important sources of infection in nursery personnel. RSV in infected secretions is viable for up to 6 hours on countertops, for up to 45 minutes on cloth gowns and paper tissues, and for up to 20 minutes on skin.[136] Evidence suggests that personnel are at least as important in spreading the infection to infants as are other infected infants housed in the same area and that infection control measures can reduce the risk of transmission.[137-139]

Any infant with rhinorrhea, nasal congestion, or unexplained apnea should be segregated and investigated for RSV infection. Personnel should be made aware that this agent, which causes only mild colds in adults, can cause fatal illnesses in infants. The specific diagnosis of RSV infection should be sought for infection control purposes and because aerosolized ribavirin treatment has some effectiveness in infants with lower respiratory infection caused by this virus.[140-143] Methods have been described for administering ribavirin safely to infants receiving mechanical ventilation.[144,145] Questions concerning the benefits of ribavirin therapy for RSV pneumonia and the indications for its use remain.[146,147] There is still a lack of consensus regarding appropriate management of the infant with RSV infection specifically with respect to the use of aerosolized ribavirin.[148,149] Despite a number of studies in the United States and Canada regarding the use of aerosolized ribavirin, no clear improvement in clinical outcomes is consistent across all studies of ventilated and nonventilated infants with RSV infection. However, infants who should be considered candidates for ribavirin therapy include those who are at increased risk for complications of RSV because of congenital heart disease, chronic lung disease, or immunodeficiency; infants with severe illness and signs of respiratory failure based on arterial oxygen concentrations of less than 65 mm Hg and rising $PaCO_2$ concentrations; and infants who may be compromised by a prolonged illness because of an underlying medical condition.[150]

Although the benefit of treatment with ribavirin is controversial, there is clear evidence for the benefit of prophylaxis against RSV infection in infants at high risk for complications. Several studies demonstrated the benefits of RSV intravenous immune globulin (RSV IGIV) among selected infants at high risk for moderate to severe complications due to RSV infection.[151] Such high-risk patients include infants and children younger than 2 years with chronic lung disease who have required medical therapy for lung disease within 6 months of the RSV season and premature infants who were 32 to 35 weeks' gestation at birth. RSV IGIV is contraindicated for those with cyanotic congenital heart disease because of possible safety concerns. Subsequently, a humanized anti-RSV monoclonal antibody preparation, palivizumab, was developed for intramuscular administration and shown to reduce by 55% hospitalizations resulting from RSV infection in these high-risk infants.[151] Moreover, initial concerns regarding the safety of palivizumab among infants with cyanotic congenital heart disease have been allayed based on clinical trials. Because of its greater uniformity and ease of administration and its efficacy in infants with cyanotic

Table 30–2 Sources of Maternal or Neonatal Infection

Infectious Agent	Other People with Same Infection	Animal
Human papillomavirus	Yes	No
Epstein-Barr virus	Yes	No
Human herpesvirus 6	Yes	No
Influenza viruses	Yes	No
Respiratory syncytial virus	Yes	No
Lymphocytic choriomeningitis virus	No	House mice, pet Syrian hamsters, laboratory rats, rabbits
Molluscum contagiosum virus	Yes	No
Rabies	—	Yes

congenital heart disease, palivizumab is now the preferred method of RSV prophylaxis.

Improved survival of infants with RSV infection and underlying cardiopulmonary disease has been reported with advances in intensive care management.[152,153] Nevertheless, families of infants with medical conditions that predispose to severe RSV disease should be advised to avoid the higher risk of exposure associated with group daycare.[154]

LYMPHOCYTIC CHORIOMENINGITIS VIRUS

Lymphocytic choriomeningitis virus (LCV) is spread from animals, primarily rodents, to humans. Person-to-person spread has not been described (Table 30-2).[155] Mice and hamsters have most often been implicated as the source of human infections. When mice acquire LCV transplacentally or as newborns, they remain asymptomatic but shed the virus in their urine for months.[156,157] This phenomenon of "tolerance" has been extensively studied in laboratory-bred strains of mice. Domestic household mice also have been implicated as a source of human cases of infection with LCV.[158] Several outbreaks in animal handlers and in families have been traced to pet Syrian (or golden) hamsters (*Mesocricetus auratus*).[159,160] Adult and newborn hamsters remain asymptomatic after infection with LCV and shed the virus in feces and urine for months.[156] In outbreaks in which human cases have been associated with contact with infected hamsters, the location of the hamster's cage correlated with attack rate. When the hamster's cage was in a common living area, 52% of 42 family members in contact with the hamster became infected.[159] In contrast, no one became infected when the cage was located in a more remote area, such as a basement or landing. LCV can be shed also by asymptomatic guinea pigs and rats.[156,157,160]

The illness caused by LCV is accompanied by fever, headache, nausea, and myalgia lasting 5 to 15 days.[155,159,161] In the outbreak of LCV described by Biggar and colleagues,[159] fever occurred in 90% and headache in 85% of patients. Myalgia occurred in 80% and was described as severe. The neck, shoulders, back, and legs were most often involved. Pain on eye movement occurred in 59%, nausea in 53%, and vomiting in 35%. About one fourth of the patients had a sore throat or photophobia. The illness was biphasic in 24% and was accompanied by swollen glands in 16%. Six percent of the patients had a mononucleosis-like illness characterized by intermittent fever, adenopathy, pharyngitis, extreme fatigue, and rash. Twelve percent of those with serologic evidence of having had an infection remained asymptomatic. Arthritis, encephalitis, and meningitis occurred in a few cases.

The diagnosis of infection with LCV can be made by isolation of the virus or by serology. The indirect fluorescent antibody titer may be positive as early as the first day of symptoms.[155,161] The complement fixation titer generally does not rise until 10 days or longer after illness onset.[155,160] The neutralization titer rises late, usually after the fourth week, but persists the longest.[155,160] A positive indirect fluorescent antibody titer, a falling indirect fluorescent antibody or complement fixation titer, or a rising neutralization titer suggests recent infection with LCV.

LCV infections during pregnancy may be underdiagnosed as causes of congenital infections and are associated with abortion, intrauterine infection, and perinatal infection. Ackermann and associates[162] described a 23-year-old woman who developed a febrile illness beginning 4 weeks after she assumed the care of a Syrian hamster. She was 7 months pregnant at the time of the illness and sustained a spontaneous abortion 4 weeks after onset of the fever. LCV was isolated from curettage material. Complement fixation antibodies to LCV were present initially, and neutralizing antibodies appeared later—a pattern compatible with recent infection. Diebel and co-workers[155] studied a pregnant woman who acquired LCV from a hamster and developed meningitis. One month after the onset of illness, a spontaneous abortion occurred. Biggar and co-workers[159] described a woman who acquired LCV during the first trimester of pregnancy. She had a spontaneous abortion 1 month after onset of the illness. U.S. cases of 26 serologically confirmed congenital LCV infections identified between 1955 and 1996 were reviewed.[163] Eighty-five percent (22 of 26) were term infants with a median birth weight of 3520 g. The most common congenital abnormalities identified were chorioretinopathy (88%), macrocephaly (43%), and microcephaly (3%). There was a 35% (9 infants) mortality rate, with a 63% (10 of 16) rate of severe neurologic sequelae among reported survivors. One fourth of mothers had gestational exposure to rodents, and 50% of all women reported symptoms consistent with LCV infection.

Intrauterine infection of the fetus results in congenital hydrocephalus and chorioretinitis. In 1974, Ackermann and associates[164] reported that two children who were born to mothers who had been in contact with hamsters during the second half of pregnancy had hydrocephalus and chorioretinitis. Other problems included severe hyperbilirubinemia and myopia. The serologic pattern typical of recent infection was found in the mothers and infants and included a falling complement fixation titer and a rising neutralization titer to

LCV. Sheinbergas[161] found a statistically significant relationship between the presence of antibody to LCV and the occurrence of hydrocephalus in infants younger than 1 year. Thirty percent of 40 infants with hydrocephalus had indirect fluorescent antibody to LCV, whereas only 2.7% of 110 infants with other nervous system diseases had antibody to LCV. Fourteen (87.5%) of 16 children who had serologically confirmed prenatal infection with LCV had hydrocephalus. Of these, six (37.5%) had been born with hydrocephalus, and the remainder developed it when 1 to 9 weeks old. Chorioretinal degeneration was found in 81%, and optic disk subatrophy was found in 56%. Mets and colleagues[165] performed ophthalmologic surveys among residents of a home for the severely mentally retarded, and sera from the 4 residents with chorioretinal scars and 14 residents with chorioretinitis were tested for *Toxoplasma gondii*, rubella virus, CMV, herpes simplex virus, and lymphocytic choriomeningitis virus. Two of the 4 residents with chorioretinal scars and 3 of the 14 with chorioretinitis had elevated antibody titers only to LCV.[165]

Komrower and colleagues[158] described a mother who acquired LCV about a week before delivery. Despite segregation of the infant, LCV was acquired transplacentally or natally, and the infant subsequently became ill. The mother's initial symptoms included malaise, headache, fever, and cough. About 20 days after onset of symptoms and 12 days after delivery, increased numbers of cells and increased protein concentration occurred in the cerebrospinal fluid. The diagnosis of infection caused by LCV was confirmed by a rise in the mother's complement fixation titer from 1:2 to 1:64. The infant, who was probably premature, remained relatively stable until 11 days old, at which time seizures, stiff neck, and mild pleocytosis developed. The infant developed petechiae and died of a subarachnoid and intracerebral hemorrhage. LCV was isolated from the infant's cerebrospinal fluid and from mice caught in the home of the mother.

Because apparently healthy mice and hamsters may shed LCV chronically, pregnant women should avoid direct contact with these animals and with aerosolized excreta. Unless appropriate measures have been taken to ensure that laboratory animals are free of LCV, these precautions should apply to laboratory as well as domestic rodents. LCV causes spontaneous abortions. Hydrocephalus and chorioretinitis are common in infants who have survived intrauterine infection.[161,164-166] Women who acquire an LCV infection during the weeks immediately before delivery may transmit the virus to their infants. Although the total number of intrauterine and perinatal infections from LCV is not large, the incidence of serious sequelae in the infant appears to be high.

MOLLUSCUM CONTAGIOSUM

Molluscum contagiosum is a papular rash consisting of multiple discrete lesions that are acanthomas by histologic examination. The skin lesions are caused by a poxlike virus that has been difficult to study because it cannot be propagated in tissue culture. Epidemiologically, molluscum contagiosum is a disease of children and young adults. The virus may be transmitted by sexual conduct, given that the incidence increases among adolescents and young adults. Whether it is transmitted as a perinatal infection is not known.

Five women who delivered infants at a time when they had the lesions of molluscum contagiosum in the genital area have been described by Wilkin.[167] None of the infants developed molluscum contagiosum. Mandel and Lewis[168] reported an infant who developed two papules on the thigh when 1 week old. These enlarged and were excised when the child was 1 year old. The results of histologic examination and the findings on electron microscopy were compatible with molluscum contagiosum. In 1926, Young[169] reported an infant with molluscum contagiosum of the scalp. The lesions appeared when the infant was 1.5 months old. No histologic studies were performed.

RABIES VIRUS

Transplacental transmission of rabies virus to the human fetus has not yet been described, although it is known that transplacental transmission occurs in experimental infections in many species.[170-175] Spence and associates[176] described an infant who was born 2 days before the onset of the mother's first symptom of encephalitis. The mother died of rabies on the fourth postpartum day. Rabies virus antigens were demonstrated in the cornea, lacrimal gland, and various parts of the brain by fluorescent antibody stain. The child survived despite the fact that the mother and infant lacked neutralizing antibodies to rabies at the time of the birth.

Two reports describe the successful administration of horse antirabies hyperimmune serum and duck embryo vaccine to pregnant women.[170,176] Unusual untoward effects did not occur, and the infants were delivered at term and were healthy. The mothers did not develop serum sickness, anaphylaxis, or neurologic complications, but if they had, the viability of the fetus might have been threatened. Horse antiserum to rabies virus has been replaced by human rabies immune globulin. The chance of an adverse reaction to administration of human immune globulin is very small. The vaccine that was previously grown in duck embryos has been replaced with an inactivated vaccine derived from virus grown in human diploid fibroblast cells.[177] No serious reactions have been reported after administration of this vaccine, and it is possible to achieve titers that are about 10-fold higher than those found after administration of the duck embryo vaccine.

Because of the high likelihood of fatal disease after the bite of a rabid animal, postexposure prophylaxis should always be given. Pregnancy is not a contraindication. When it is necessary to administer prophylaxis to a pregnant woman, human rabies immune globulin and human diploid cell vaccine should be used to minimize potential adverse effects on the pregnancy. After reviewing the available data, the Advisory Committee on Immunization Practices of the Centers for Disease Control and Prevention (CDC) has recommended human diploid cell vaccine to rabies virus as a pre-exposure immunization that is safe for use in pregnant women who will likely be exposed to wild rabies virus before completion of pregnancy.[178]

WEST NILE VIRUS

West Nile virus (WNV) is a mosquito-borne flavivirus that has caused epidemic infections in the United States since its introduction in 1999.[179] Since then, three cases of intrauterine and breast-feeding transmission have been reported in the literature.[180-182] In 2002, a previously healthy woman at 27 weeks' gestation developed a febrile illness, followed by lower extremity paresis and meningoencephalitis. At 38 weeks' gestation, she delivered an infant with bilateral chorioretinitis and severe, bilateral white matter loss in the temporal and occipital lobes. Maternal, cord, and infant blood samples at birth were positive for WNV-specific IgM and neutralizing antibodies; cerebrospinal fluid from the infant was WNV IgM positive; and the placenta was WNV PCR positive.[180] A second reported case of intrauterine WNV infection occurring in the second trimester resulted in congenital chorioretinal scarring and severe CNS malformations of the newborn.[181] One case of probable breast-feeding transmission is reported in a woman who required red blood cell transfusions shortly after delivery. She began breast-feeding on the day of delivery and through the second day of hospitalization. The woman had developed symptoms consistent with meningoencephalitis 6 days before delivery; subsequent evaluation of the units of transfused blood revealed one unit that was WNV positive by PCR. Serum from the infant was positive for WNV-specific IgM at day 25 of life. The infant remained healthy at last report.[182] Although spontaneous abortions and stillbirths have been associated with flavivirus infections, these viruses have not previously been reported to be teratogenic. During 2002, the CDC investigated three other cases of maternal WNV infection in which the infants were all born at full term with no evidence of WNV infection or congenital sequelae; however, cranial imaging and ophthalmologic examinations were not performed on these infants.[183]

No specific therapy is available for WNV infection, and the CDC does not recommend WNV screening of asymptomatic pregnant women. Pregnant women who have meningitis, encephalitis, acute flaccid paralysis, or unexplained fever in an area of ongoing WNV transmission should have serum and cerebrospinal fluid, if clinically indicated, tested for antibody to WNV. If WNV illness is diagnosed in the pregnant woman, ultrasound examination of the fetus should be considered no sooner than 2 to 4 weeks after maternal onset of illness, and fetal or amniotic testing can be considered. Infants born to women with known or suspected WNV infection during pregnancy should be evaluated for congenital WNV infection. Prevention of WNV infection should include application of insect repellant to skin and clothes when exposed to mosquitoes and avoidance of peak mosquito-feeding times at dawn and dusk.[183]

REFERENCES

Human Papillomavirus

1. Ono S, Saito H, Igarash M. The etiology of papilloma of the larynx. Ann Otol 66:1119, 1957.
2. Almeida JD, Oriel JD. Wart virus. Br J Dermatol 83:698, 1970.
3. Gissman L, Wolnik L, Ikenberg H, et al. Human papillomavirus types 6 and 11: DNA sequences in genital and laryngeal papillomas and in some cervical cancers. Proc Natl Acad Sci U S A 80:560, 1983.
4. Allen AL, Seigfried EC. The natural history of condyloma in children. J Am Acad Dermatol 39:951, 1998.
5. Hajek EF. Contribution to the etiology of laryngeal papilloma in children. J Laryngol 70:166, 1956.
6. Cook TA, Brunschwig JP, Butel JS, et al. Laryngeal papilloma: etiologic and therapeutic considerations. Ann Otol 82:649, 1973.
7. Quick CA, Krzyzek RA, Watts SL, et al. Relationship between condylomata and laryngeal papillomata. Ann Otol 89:467, 1980.
8. Watts DH, Koutsky LA, Holmes KK, et al. Low risk of perinatal transmission of human papillomavirus: results from a prospective cohort study. Am J Obstet Gynecol 178:365, 1998.
9. Puranen M, Yliskoski M, Saarikoski S, et al. Vertical transmission of human papillomavirus from infected mothers to their newborn babies and persistence of the virus in childhood. Am J Obstet Gynecol 174:694, 1996.
10. Fredericks BD, Balkin A, Daniel HW, et al. Transmission of human papillomaviruses from mother to child. Aust N Z J Obstet Gynaecol 33:30, 1993.
11. Smith EM, Johnson SR, Jiang D, et al. The association between pregnancy and human papilloma virus prevalence. Cancer Detect Prev 15:397, 1991.
12. Pakarian F, Kaye J, Cason J, et al. Cancer associated human papillomaviruses: perinatal transmission and persistence. Br J Obstet Gynaecol 101:514, 1994.
13. Cason J, Kaye JN, Jewers RJ, et al. Perinatal infection and persistence of human papillomavirus types 16 and 18 in infants. J Med Virol 47: 209, 1995.
14. Sedlacek TV, Lindheim S, Eder C, et al. Mechanism for human papillomavirus transmission at birth. Am J Obstet Gynecol 161:55, 1989.
15. Smith EM, Ritchie JM, Yankowitz J, et al. Human papillomavirus prevalence and types in newborns and parents: concordance and modes of transmission. Sex Transm Dis 31:57, 2004.
16. Drut R, Gomez MA, Drut RM, et al. Human papillomavirus, neonatal giant cell hepatitis and biliary duct atresia. Acta Gastroenterol Latinoam 28:27, 1998.
17. Dias EP, Barcelos JM, Fonseca EF, Basso NG. Congenital papillomas and papillomatoses associated with the human papillomavirus (HPV)—report on 5 cases. Rev Paul Med 113:957, 1995.
18. Steinberg BM, Topp WC, Schneider PS, et al. Laryngeal papillomavirus infection during clinical remission. N Engl J Med 308:1261, 1983.
19. Hording U, Iversen AK, Sebbelov A, et al. Prevalence of human papillomavirus types 11, 16 and 18 in cervical swabs: a study of 1362 pregnant women. Eur J Obstet Gynecol Reprod Biol 35:191, 1990.
20. Peng T, Searle CP III, Shah KV, et al. Prevalence of human papillomavirus infections in term pregnancy. Am J Perinatol 7:189, 1990.
21. Kemp EA, Hakenewerth AM, Laurent SL, et al. Human papillomavirus prevalence in pregnancy. Obstet Gynecol 79:649, 1992.
22. Fife KH, Rogers RE, Zwickl BW. Symptomatic and asymptomatic cervical infections with human papillomavirus during pregnancy. J Infect Dis 156:904, 1987.
23. Tang CK, Shermeta DW, Wood C. Congenital condylomata acuminata. Am J Obstet Gynecol 131:912, 1978.
24. Roman A, Fife K. Human papillomavirus DNA associated with foreskins of normal newborns. J Infect Dis 153:855, 1986.
25. Avidano MA, Singleton GT. Adjuvant drug strategies in the treatment of recurrent respiratory papillomatosis. Otolaryngol Head Neck Surg 112:197, 1995.
26. Derkay CS. Recurrent respiratory papillomatosis. Laryngoscope 111:57, 2001.
27. Chhetri DK, Shapiro NL. A scheduled protocol for the treatment of juvenile recurrent respiratory papillomatosis with intralesional cidofovir. Arch Otolaryngol Head Neck Surg 129:1081, 2003.
28. Roden R, Wu TC. Preventative and therapeutic vaccines for cervical cancer. Expert Rev Vaccines 2:495, 2003.

Epstein-Barr Virus

29. Henle W, Henle G, Horwitz CA. Epstein-Barr virus-specific diagnostic tests in infectious mononucleosis. Hum Pathol 5:551, 1974.
30. Fleisher G, Henle W, Henle G, et al. Primary Epstein-Barr virus infection in American infants: clinical and serological observations. J Infect Dis 139:553, 1979.
31. Icart J, Didier J. Infections due to Epstein-Barr virus during pregnancy. J Infect Dis 143:499, 1981.
32. Fleisher G, Bolognese R. Persistent Epstein-Barr virus infection and pregnancy. J Infect Dis 147:982, 1983.
33. Le CT, Chang S, Lipson MH. Epstein-Barr virus infections during pregnancy. Am J Dis Child 137:466, 1983.
34. Icart J, Didier J, Dalens M, et al. Etude prospective de l'infection à virus Epstein-Barr (EBV) au cours de la grossesse. Biomedicine 34:160, 1981.

35. Gervais F, Joncas JH. Seroepidemiology in various population groups of the greater Montreal area. Comp Immunol Microbiol Infect Dis 2:207, 1979.
36. Horowitz CA, Henle W, Henle G, et al. Long-term serologic follow-up of patients for Epstein-Barr virus after recovery from infectious mononucleosis. J Infect Dis 151:1150, 1985.
37. Fleisher G, Bolognese R. Epstein-Barr virus infections in pregnancy: a prospective study. J Pediatr 104:374, 1984.
38. Fleisher G, Bolognese R. Infectious mononucleosis during gestation: report of three women and their infants studied prospectively. Pediatr Infect Dis 3:308, 1984.
39. Tallqvist H, Henle W, Klemola E, et al. Antibodies to Epstein-Barr virus at the ages of 6 to 23 months in children with congenital heart disease. Scand J Infect Dis 5:159, 1973.
40. Brown ZA, Stenchever MA. Infectious mononucleosis and congenital anomalies. Am J Obstet Gynecol 131:108, 1978.
41. Goldberg GN, Fulginiti VA, Ray CG, et al. In utero Epstein-Barr virus (infectious mononucleosis) infection. JAMA 246:1579, 1981.
42. Weaver LT, Nelson R, Bell TM. The association of extrahepatic bile duct atresia and neonatal Epstein-Barr virus infection. Acta Paediatr Scand 73:155, 1984.
43. Visintine AJ, Gerber P, Nahmias AJ. Leukocyte transforming agent (Epstein-Barr virus) in newborn infants and older individuals. J Pediatr 89:571, 1976.
44. Chang RS, Blankenship W. Spontaneous in vitro transformation of leukocytes from a neonate. Proc Soc Exp Biol Med 144:337, 1973.
45. Chang RS, Seto DY. Perinatal infection by Epstein-Barr virus. Lancet 2:201, 1979.
46. Joncas J, Boucher J, Granger-Julien M, et al. Epstein-Barr virus in the neonatal period and in childhood. Can Med Assoc J 110:33, 1974.
47. Joncas JH, Wills A, McLaughlin B. Congenital infection with cytomegalovirus and Epstein-Barr virus. Can Med Assoc J 117:1417, 1977.
48. Meyohas MC, Marechal V, Sedire N, et al. Study of mother-to-child Epstein-Barr virus transmission by means of nested PCRs. J Virol 70:6816, 1996.
49. Joncas J, Alfieri C, Leyritz M, et al. Dual congenital infection with the Epstein-Barr virus (EBV) and the cytomegalovirus (CMV). N Engl J Med 304:1399, 1981.
50. Sixbey JW, Lemon SM, Pagano JS. A second site for Epstein-Barr virus shedding: the uterine cervix. Lancet 2:1122, 1986.
51. Portnoy J, Ahronheim GA, Ghibu F, et al. Recovery of Epstein-Barr virus from genital ulcers. N Engl J Med 311:966, 1984.
52. Horwitz CA, McClain K, Henle W, et al. Fatal illness in a 2 week old infant: diagnosis by detection of Epstein-Barr virus genomes from a lymph node biopsy. J Pediatr 103:752, 1983.
53. Gervais F, Joncas JH. Correspondence-an unusual antibody response to Epstein-Barr virus during infancy. J Infect Dis 140:273, 1979.

Human Herpesvirus 6

54. Salahuddin SZ, Ablashi DV, Markham PD, et al. Isolation of a new virus, HBLV, in patients with lymphoproliferative disorders. Science 234:596, 1986.
55. Lopez C, Pellett P, Stewart J, et al. Characteristics of human herpesvirus-6. J Infect Dis 157:1271, 1988.
56. Leach CT, Sumaya CV, Brown NA. Human herpesvirus-6: clinical implications of a recently discovered, ubiquitous agent. J Pediatr 1231: 173, 1992.
57. Lawrence GL, Chee M, Craxton MA, et al. Human herpes virus 6 is closely related to human cytomegalovirus. J Virol 64:287, 1989.
58. Baillargeon J, Piper J, Leach CT. Epidemiology of human herpesvirus 6 (HHV-6) infection in pregnant and non-pregnant women. J Clin Virol 16:149, 2000.
59. Dahl H, Fjaertoft G, Norsted T, et al. Reactivation of human herpesvirus 6 during pregnancy. J Infect Dis 180:2035, 1999.
60. Adams O, Krempe C, Kogler G, et al. Congenital infections with human herpesvirus 6. J Infect Dis 178:544, 1998.
61. Yamaniski K, Okada K, Ueda K, et al. Exanthem subitum and human herpes virus 6. Pediatr Infect Dis J 12:204, 1993.
62. Aubi J-T, Poirel L, Agut H, et al. Intrauterine transmission of human herpes virus 6. Lancet 340:482, 1992.
63. Dunne WM, Demmler GJ. Serologic evidence for congenital transmission of human herpesvirus 6. Lancet 340:121, 1992.
64. Adams O, Krempe C, Kogler G, et al. Congenital infections with human herpesvirus 6. J Infect Dis 178:544, 1998.
65. van Loon NM, Gummuluru S, Sherwood DJ, et al. Direct sequence analysis of human herpesvirus 6 (HHV-6) sequences from infants and comparison of HHV-6 from mother/infant pairs. Clin Infect Dis 21: 1017, 1995.
66. Pruksananonda P, Hall CB, Insel RA, et al. Primary human herpes virus 6 infection in young children. N Engl J Med 22:1445, 1992.
67. Kawaguchi S, Suga S, Kozawa T, et al. Primary human herpesvirus 6 infection (exanthem subitum) in the newborn. Pediatrics 90:628, 1992.
68. Tajiri H, Nose O, Baba K, et al. Human herpesvirus-6 infection with liver injury in neonatal hepatitis. Lancet 335:863, 1990.
69. Asano Y, Yoshikawa T, Suga S, et al. Fatal fulminant hepatitis in an infant with human herpesvirus-6 infection. Lancet 335:862, 1990.
70. Kanegane C, Katayama K, Kyoutani S, et al. Mononucleosis-like illness in an infant associated with human herpesvirus 6 infection. Acta Paediatr Jpn 37:227, 1995.
71. Hammerling JA, Lambrecht RS, Kehl KS, Carrigan DR. Prevalence of human herpesvirus 6 in lung tissue from children with pneumonitis. J Clin Pathol 49:802, 1996.
72. Knox KK, Pietryga D, Harrington DJ, et al. Progressive immunodeficiency and fatal pneumonitis associated with human herpesvirus 6 infection in an infant. Clin Infect Dis 20:406, 1995.

Human Herpesvirus 7

73. Black JB, Pellett PE. Human herpesvirus 7. Rev Med Virol 3:217, 1993.
74. Frenkel N, Schirmer EC, Wyatt LS, et al. Isolation of a new herpesvirus from human CD4+ T cells. Proc Natl Acad Sci U S A 87:748, 1990.
75. Krueger GR, Koch B, Leyssens N, et al. Comparison of seroprevalences of human herpesvirus-6 and -7 in healthy blood donors from nine countries. Vox Sang 75:193, 1998.
76. Clark DA, Freeland JML, Mackie PLK, et al. Prevalence of antibody to human herpesvirus 7 by age. J Infect Dis 168:251, 1993.
77. Fujisaki H, Tanaka-Taya K, Tanabe H, et al. Detection of human herpesvirus 7 (HHV-7) DNA in breast milk by polymerase chain reaction and prevalence of HHV-7 antibody in breast-fed and bottle-fed children. J Med Virol 56:275, 1998.
78. Lanphear BP, Hall CB, Black J, et al. Risk factors for the early acquisition of human herpesvirus 6 and human herpesvirus 7 infections in children. Pediatr Infect Dis J 17:792, 1998.
79. Okuno T, Oishi H, Hayashi K, et al. Human herpesviruses 6 and 7 in cervixes of pregnant women. J Clin Microbiol 133:1968, 1995.
80. Boutolleau D, Cointe D, Gautheret-Dejean A, et al. No evidence for a major risk of roseolovirus vertical transmission during pregnancy. Clin Infect Dis 36:1634, 2003.
81. Torigoe S, Kumamoto T, Koide W, et al. Clinical manifestations associated with human herpesvirus 7 infection. Arch Dis Child 72:518, 1995.
82. Torigoe S, Koide W, Yamada M, et al. Human herpesvirus 7 infection associated with central nervous system manifestations. J Pediatr 129:301, 1996.
83. Clark DA, Kidd IM, Collingham KE, et al. Diagnosis of primary human herpesvirus 6 and 7 infections in febrile infants by polymerase chain reaction. Arch Dis Child 77:42, 1997.
84. Portolani M, Cermelli C, Mirandola P, et al. Isolation of human herpesvirus 7 from an infant with febrile syndrome. J Med Virol 45: 282, 1995.

Influenza A and B

85. Coffey VP, Jessup WJE. Maternal influenza and congenital deformities. Lancet 2:935, 1959.
86. Doll R, Hill AB. Asian influenza in pregnancy and congenital defects. Br J Prev Soc Med 14:167, 1960.
87. Record RG. Anencephalus in Scotland. Br J Prev Soc Med 15:93, 1961.
88. Leck I. Incidence of malformations following influenza epidemics. Br J Prev Soc Med 17:70, 1963.
89. Hakosalo J, Saxen L. Influenza epidemic and congenital defects. Lancet 2:1346, 1971.
90. Wilson MG, Stein AM. Teratogenic effects of Asian influenza. JAMA 210:336, 1969.
91. Hardy JMB, Azarowicz EN, Mannini A, et al. The effect of Asian influenza on the outcome of pregnancy. Baltimore 1957-1958. Am J Public Health 51:1182, 1961.
92. MacKenzie JS, Houghton M. Influenza infections during pregnancy: association with congenital malformations and with subsequent neoplasms in children, and potential hazards of live virus vaccines. Bacteriol Rev 38:356, 1974.
93. Griffiths PD, Ronalds CJ, Heath RB. A prospective study of influenza infections during pregnancy. J Epidemiol Commun Health 34:124, 1980.

94. Monif GRG, Soward DL, Eitzman DV. Serologic and immunologic evaluation of neonates following maternal influenza infection during the second and third trimesters. Am J Obstet Gynecol 114:239, 1972.
95. Hartert TV, Neuzil KM, Shintani AK, et al. Maternal morbidity and perinatal outcomes among pregnant women with respiratory hospitalizations during influenza season. Am J Obstet Gynecol 189: 1705, 2003.
96. Englund JA. Maternal immunization with inactivated influenza vaccine: rationale and experience. Vaccine 21:3460, 2003.
97. Mortensen PB, Pedersen CB, Melbye M, et al. Individual and familial risk factors for bipolar affective disorders in Denmark. Arch Gen Psychiatry 60:1209, 2003 .
98. Limosin F, Rouillon F, Payan C, et al. Prenatal exposure to influenza as a risk factor for adult schizophrenia. Acta Psychiatr Scand 107:331, 2003 .
99. Brown AS, Susser ES. In utero infection and adult schizophrenia. Ment Retard Dev Disabil Res Rev 8:51, 2002.
100. Ruben FL, Winkelstein A, Sabbagha RE. In utero sensitization with influenza virus in man. Proc Soc Exp Biol Med 149:881, 1975.
101. McGregor JA, Burns JC, Levin MJ, et al. Transplacental passage of influenza A/Bangkok (H3N2) mimicking amniotic fluid infection syndrome. Am J Obstet Gynecol 149:856, 1984.
102. Yawn DH, Pyeatte JC, Joseph MM, et al. Transplacental transfer of influenza virus. JAMA 216:1022, 1971.
103. Ramphal R, Donnelly WH, Small PA. Fatal influenzal pneumonia in pregnancy: failure to demonstrate transplacental transmissions of influenza virus. Am J Obstet Gynecol 138:347, 1980.
104. Puck JM, Glezen WP, Frank AL, et al. Protection of infants from infection with influenza A virus by transplacentally acquired antibody. J Infect Dis 142:844, 1980.
105. Reuman PD, Ayoub EM, Small PA. Effect of passive maternal antibody on influenza illness in children: a prospective study of influenza A in mother-infant pairs. Pediatr Infect Dis J 6:398, 1987.
106. Bauer CR, Elie K, Spence L, et al. Hong Kong influenza in a neonatal unit. JAMA 223:1233, 1973.
107. Joshi VV, Escobar MR, Stewart L, et al. Fatal influenza A_2 viral pneumonia in a newborn infant. Am J Dis Child 126:839, 1973.
108. Meibalane R, Sedmak GV, Sasidharan P, et al. Outbreak of influenza in a neonatal intensive care unit. J Pediatr 91:974, 1977.
109. Sumaya CV, Gibbs RS. Immunization of pregnant women with influenza A/New Jersey/76 virus vaccine: reactogenicity and immunogenicity in mothers and infants. J Infect Dis 140:141, 1979.
110. Schmidt JV, Kroger AT, Roy SL. Report from the CDC. Vaccines in women. J Womens Health (Larchmt) 13:249, 2004.

Respiratory Syncytial Virus

111. Holberg CJ, Wright AL, Martinez FD, et al. Risk factors for respiratory syncytial virus–associated lower respiratory illnesses in the first year of life. Am J Epidemiol 133:1135, 1991.
112. Chanock RM, Kapikian AZ, Mills J, et al. Influence of immunological factors in respiratory syncytial virus disease. Arch Environ Health 21:347, 1970.
113. Jacobs JW, Peacock DB, Corner BD, et al. Respiratory syncytial and other viruses associated with respiratory disease in infants. Lancet 1:871, 1971.
114. Parrott RH, Kim HW, Arrobio JO. Epidemiology of respiratory syncytial virus infection in Washington, DC. II. Infection and disease with respect to age, immunologic status, race and sex. Am J Epidemiol 98:289, 1973.
115. Bruhn FW, Yeager AS. Respiratory syncytial virus in early infancy. Am J Dis Child 131:145, 1977.
116. Lamprecht CL, Krause HE, Mufson MA. Role of maternal antibody in pneumonia and bronchiolitis due to respiratory syncytial virus. J Infect Dis 134:211, 1976.
117. Glezen WP, Paredes A, Allison JE, et al. Risk of respiratory syncytial virus infection for infants from low-income families in relationship to age, sex, ethnic group, and maternal antibody level. J Pediatr 98:708, 1981.
118. Downham M, Scott R, Sims DG, et al. Breast-feeding protects against respiratory syncytial virus infections. BMJ 2:274, 1976.
119. Bruhn FW, Mokrohisky ST, McIntosh K. Apnea associated with respiratory syncytial virus infection in young infants. J Pediatr 90:382, 1977.
120. Abzug MJ, Beam AC, Gyorkos EA, et al. Viral pneumonia in the first month of life. Pediatr Infect Dis J 9:881, 1990.
121. MacDonald NE, Hall CB, Suffin SC, et al. Respiratory syncytial viral infection in infants with congenital heart disease. N Engl J Med 307: 397, 1982.
122. Abman SH, Ogle JW, Butler-Simon N, et al. Role of respiratory syncytial virus in early hospitalizations for respiratory distress of young infants with cystic fibrosis. J Pediatr 113:826, 1988.
123. McConnochie KM, Hall CB, Walsh EE, et al. Variation in severity of respiratory syncytial virus infections with subtype. J Pediatr 117:52, 1990.
124. Neligan GA, Steiner H, Gardner PS, et al. Respiratory syncytial virus infection of the newborn. BMJ 3:146, 1970.
125. Berkovich S, Taranko L. Acute respiratory illness in the premature nursery associated with respiratory syncytial virus infection. Pediatrics 34:753, 1964.
126. Mintz L, Ballard RA, Sniderman SH, et al. Nosocomial respiratory syncytial virus infections in an intensive care nursery: rapid diagnosis by direct immunofluorescence. Pediatrics 64:149, 1979.
127. Goldson EJ, McCarthy JT, Welling MA, et al. A respiratory syncytial virus outbreak in a transitional care nursery. Am J Dis Child 133:1280, 1979.
128. Church NR, Anas NG, Hall CB. Respiratory syncytial virus–related apnea in infants: demographics and outcome. Am J Dis Child 138:247, 1984.
129. Valenti WM, Clarke TA, Hall CB, et al. Concurrent outbreaks of rhinovirus and respiratory syncytial virus in an intensive care nursery: epidemiology and associated risk factors. J Pediatr 100:722, 1982.
130. Meissner HC, Murray SA, Kiernan MA, et al. A simultaneous outbreak of respiratory syncytial virus and parainfluenza virus type 3 in a newborn nursery. J Pediatr 104:680, 1984.
131. Wensley DF, Baldwin VJ. Respiratory distress in the second week of life. J Pediatr 106:326, 1985.
132. Hall CB, Kopelman AE, Douglas RG, et al. Neonatal respiratory syncytial virus infection. N Engl J Med 300:393, 1979.
133. Wilson CW, Stevenson DK, Arvin AM. A concurrent epidemic of respiratory syncytial virus and echovirus 7 infections in an intensive care nursery. Pediatr Infect Dis J 8:24, 1989.
134. Unger A, Tapia L, Minnich LL, et al. Atypical neonatal respiratory syncytial virus infection. J Pediatr 100:762, 1982.
135. Hall CB, Douglas RG Jr, Geiman JM. Respiratory syncytial virus infections in infants: quantitation and duration of shedding. J Pediatr 89:11, 1976.
136. Hall CB, Douglas RG Jr, Geiman JM. Possible transmission by fomites or respiratory syncytial virus. J Infect Dis 141:98, 1980.
137. Snydman DR, Greer C, Meissner HC, et al. Prevention of nosocomial transmission of respiratory syncytial virus in a newborn nursery. Infect Control Hosp Epidemiol 9:105, 1988.
138. Leclair JM, Freeman J, Sullivan BF, et al. Prevention of nosocomial respiratory syncytial virus infections through compliance with glove and gown isolation precautions. N Engl J Med 317:329, 1987.
139. Agah R, Cherry JD, Garakian AJ, et al. Respiratory syncytial virus (RSV) infection rate in personnel caring for children with RSV infections. Routine isolation procedure vs routine procedure supplemented by use of masks and goggles. Am J Dis Child 141:695, 1987.
140. Hall CB, McBride JT, Walsh EE, et al. Aerosolized ribavirin treatment of infants with respiratory syncytial viral infection: a randomized double-blind study. N Engl J Med 308:1443, 1983.
141. Hall CB, McBride JT, Gala CL, et al. Ribavirin treatment of respiratory syncytial viral infection in infants with underlying cardiopulmonary disease. JAMA 254:3047, 1985.
142. Rodriguez WJ, Kim HW, Brandt CD, et al. Aerosolized ribavirin in the treatment of patients with respiratory syncytial virus disease. Pediatr Infect Dis J 6:159, 1987.
143. Conrad DA, Christenson JC, Waner JL, et al. Aerosolized ribavirin treatment of respiratory syncytial virus infection in infants hospitalized during an epidemic. Pediatr Infect Dis J 6:152, 1987.
144. Outwater KM, Meissner HC, Peterson MB. Ribavirin administration to infants receiving mechanical ventilation. Am J Dis Child 142:512, 1988.
145. Frankel LR, Wilson CW, Demers RR, et al. A technique for the administration of ribavirin to mechanically ventilated infants with severe respiratory syncytial virus infection. Crit Care Med 15:1051, 1987.
146. American Academy of Pediatrics Committee on Infectious Diseases. Ribavirin therapy of respiratory syncytial virus. Pediatrics 79:475, 1987.
147. Wald ER, Dashefsky B, Green M. In re ribavirin: a case of premature adjudication? J Pediatr 112:154, 1988.

148. Prober CG, Wang EEL. Reducing the morbidity of lower respiratory tract infections caused by respiratory syncytial virus: still no answer. Pediatrics 99:472, 1997.
149. American Academy of Pediatrics. Committee on Infectious Diseases. Reassessment of the indications for ribavirin therapy in respiratory syncytial virus infections. Pediatrics 97:137, 1996.
150. Ribavirin therapy of respiratory syncytial virus. *In* Lepow PG, McCrachen ML, Phillips CF (eds). Report of the Committee on Infectious Diseases. Elk Grove Village, Ill, American Academy of Pediatrics, 1991, pp 581-586.
151. Meissner HC, Long SS; American Academy of Pediatrics Committee on Infectious Diseases and Committee on Fetus and Newborn. Revised indications for the use of palivizumab and respiratory syncytial virus immune globulin intravenous for the prevention of respiratory syncytial virus infections. Pediatrics 112:1447, 2003.
152. Moler FW, Khan AS, Meliones JN, et al. Respiratory syncytial virus morbidity and mortality estimates in congenital heart disease patients: a recent experience. Crit Care Med 20:1406, 1992.
153. Navas L, Wang E, de Carvalho V, et al. Improved outcome of respiratory syncytial virus infection in a high-risk hospitalized population of Canadian children. J Pediatr 121:348, 1992.
154. Anderson LJ, Parker RA, Strikas RA, et al. Day-care center attendance and hospitalization for lower respiratory tract illness. Pediatrics 82: 300, 1988.

Lymphocytic Choriomeningitis Virus

155. Diebel R, Woodall JP, Decher WJ, et al. Lymphocytic choriomeningitis virus in man: serologic evidence of association with pet hamster. JAMA 232:501, 1975.
156. Smadel JE, Wall MJ. Lymphocytic choriomeningitis in the Syrian hamster. J Exp Med 75:581, 1942.
157. Traub E. Persistence of lymphochoriomeningitis virus in immune animals and its relation to immunity. J Exp Med 63:847, 1936.
158. Komrower GM, Williams BL, Stones PB. Lymphocytic choriomeningitis in the newborn. Lancet 1:697, 1955.
159. Biggar RJ, Woodall JP, Walter PD, et al. Lymphocytic choriomeningitis outbreak associated with pet hamsters: fifty-seven cases from New York state. JAMA 232:494, 1975.
160. Hotchin J. The contamination of laboratory animals with lymphocytic choriomeningitis virus. Am J Pathol 64:747, 1971.
161. Sheinbergas MM. Hydrocephalus due to prenatal infection with the lymphocytic choriomeningitis virus. Infection 4:185, 1974.
162. Ackermann R, Stammler A, Armbruster B. Isolierung von Virus der lymphozytären Choriomeningitis aus Abrasionsmaterial nach Kontakt der Schwangeren mit einem Syrischen Goldhamster (*Mesocricetus auratus*). Infection 3:47, 1975.
163. Wright R, Johnson D, Neumann M, et al. Congenital lymphocytic choriomeningitis virus syndrome: a disease that mimics congenital toxoplasmosis or cytomegalovirus infection. Pediatrics 100:E9, 1997.
164. Ackermann R, Körver G, Turss R, et al. Pränatale Infektion mit dem Virus der lymphozytären Choriomeningitis. Dtsch Med Wochenschr 99:629, 1974.
165. Mets MB, Barton LL, Khan AS, Ksiazek TG. Lymphocytic choriomeningitis virus: an underdiagnosed cause of congenital chorioretinitis. Am J Ophthalmol 130:209, 2000 .
166. Chastel C, Bosshard S, LeGoff F, et al. Infection transplacentaire par le virus de la choriomeningite lymphocytaire. Nouv Presse Med 7:1089, 1978.

Molluscum Contagiosum

167. Wilkin JK. Molluscum contagiosum venereum in a women's outpatient clinic: a venereally transmitted disease. Am J Obstet Gynecol 128:531, 1977.
168. Mandel MJ, Lewis RJ. Molluscum contagiosum of the newborn. Br J Dermatol 84:370, 1970.
169. Young WJ. Molluscum contagiosum with unusual distribution. Ky Med J 24:467, 1926.

Rabies Virus

170. Cates W Jr. Treatment of rabies exposure during pregnancy. Obstet Gynecol 44:893, 1974.
171. Martell MA, Montes FC, Alcocer RB. Transplacental transmission of bovine rabies after natural infection. J Infect Dis 127:291, 1973.
172. Geneverlay J, Dodero J. Note sur un enfant né d'une mere en etat du rage. Ann Inst Pasteur Paris 55:124, 1935.
173. Viazhevich VK. A case of birth of a healthy baby to a mother during the incubation period of rabies. Zh Mikrobiol Epidemiol Immunobiol 28:1022, 1957.
174. Machada CG, Zatz I, Saraiva PA, et al. Observations sur un enfant né de mere atteinte de rage et soumis du traitement prophylactique par le serum et le vaccome amtorabiques. Bull Soc Pathol Exp 59:764, 1966.
175. Relova RN. The hydrophobia boy. J Philipp Med Assoc 39:765, 1963.
176. Spence MR, Davidson DE, Dill GS, et al. Rabies exposure during pregnancy. Am J Obstet Gynecol 123:655, 1975.
177. Meyer HM. FDA: rabies vaccine. J Infect Dis 142:287, 1980.
178. Public Health Service Advisory Committee on Immunization Practices. Human Rabies Prevention—United States, 1999 Recommendations of the Advisory Committee on Immunization Practices (ACIP). MMWR Morb Mortal Wkly Rep 48:1, 1999.

West Nile Virus

179. Nash D, Mostashari F, Fine A, et al. The outbreak of West Nile infection in the New York City area in 1999. N Engl J Med 344:1807, 2001.
180. Centers for Disease Control and Prevention. Intrauterine West Nile virus infection—New York, 2002. MMWR Morb Mortal Wkly Rep 51:1135, 2002.
181. Alpert SG, Fergerson J, Noel LP. Intrauterine West Nile virus: ocular and systemic findings. Am J Ophthalmol 136:733, 2003.
182. Centers for Disease Control and Prevention. Possible West Nile virus transmission to an infant through breast-feeding—Michigan, 2002. MMWR Morb Mortal Wkly Rep 51:877, 2002.
183. Centers for Disease Control and Prevention. Interim guidelines for the evaluation of infants born to mothers infected with West Nile virus during pregnancy. MMWR Morb Mortal Wkly Rep 53:154, 2004.

Section IV

PROTOZOAN, HELMINTH, AND FUNGAL INFECTIONS

Chapter 31

TOXOPLASMOSIS

Jack S. Remington • Rima McLeod • Philippe Thulliez • George Desmonts

Among the most tragic infectious diseases of humans are those that pass from the pregnant woman to her unborn child. *Toxoplasma gondii* is a protozoal parasite that can cause devastating disease in the fetus and newborn yet remain unrecognized in women who acquire the infection during gestation. In addition, in most countries, congenital infection and congenital toxoplasmosis in the newborn go undiagnosed, thereby predisposing to the occurrence of untoward sequelae of the infection, including decreased vision or blindness, decreased hearing or deafness, and mental and psychomotor retardation. The cost estimates for special care of children with congenital toxoplasmosis born each year in the United States alone is in the hundreds of millions of dollars.

An early estimate of the lifetime cost for special services for the infected children born each year was $221.9 million.[1] In 1990, Roberts and Frenkel estimated preventable medical costs to be $369 million as a low estimate for the number of congenital cases born each year and many hundreds of millions as a high estimate.[2] Only relatively recently have most physicians, veterinarians, research scientists, and economists recognized the important position of *T. gondii* among the significant pathogens of humans and animals. The organism is ubiquitous in nature and is the cause of a variety of illnesses that previously were thought to be due to other agents or to be of unknown cause. Toxoplasmic encephalitis has now proved to be a significant cause of morbidity and mortality in immunodeficient patients, including infants, children, and adults with acquired immunodeficiency syndrome (AIDS). Toxoplasmosis in domestic animals is of economic importance in countries such as England and New Zealand, where it causes abortion in sheep, and in Japan, where it has caused abortion in swine. It has been estimated that as many as 4100 of the 4.1 million infants born annually in recent years in the United States have the congenital infection. In a majority of infected infants, clinical signs are not present at birth, but sequelae of the congenital infection are recognized or develop later in life. In this chapter, the term *congenital toxoplasmosis* refers to cases in which signs of disease related to congenital infection are present.

The history of *T. gondii* began in 1908, when Nicolle and Manceaux observed a parasite in mononuclear cells of the spleen and liver of a North African rodent, the gondi (*Ctenodactylus gondi*); this organism so closely resembled *Leishmania* that they tentatively named it *Leishmania gondii*.[3] The next year they decided, on the basis of morphologic criteria, that it was not a *Leishmania* organism and proposed the name *Toxoplasma* (from the Greek *toxon*, "arc") *gondii*.[4] It might just as well have been called *Toxoplasma cuniculi*, because at the same time, and independently, Splendore found it in a rabbit that had died with paralysis in Brazil.[5] The organism soon attracted attention as a cause of disease in animals, and in 1923, Janku, an ophthalmologist in Prague, described the first recognized case in humans.[6] He found parasitic cysts in the retina of an 11-month-old child with congenital hydrocephalus and microphthalmia with coloboma in the macular region. The parasite noted by Janku was later (in 1928) recognized to be *T. gondii* by Levaditi, who suggested a possible connection between congenital hydrocephalus and toxoplasmosis.[7]

It was not until 1937, however, that recognition of toxoplasmosis as a disease entity in humans had a real impact on medicine. In that year, Wolf and Cowen in the United States reported a fatal case of infantile granulomatous encephalitis that they believed to be caused by an encephalitozoon.[8] Sabin and Olitski, who had previously encountered *T. gondii* in guinea pigs,[9] were able to make the correct diagnosis. Wolf and associates later recognized and reclassified the cases described by Torres in 1926 and by Richter in 1936 as earlier reports of congenital infection.[10-12] Wolf and Cowen and collaborators then performed numerous studies and established *T. gondii* as a cause of prenatally transmitted human disease.[13,14] (Case 4 in the report by Paige and co-workers[12] is of special interest because it established beyond question that the infantile form of the infection was prenatal in origin.)

The discovery of *T. gondii* as a cause of disease acquired later in life has been credited to Pinkerton and Weinman. In 1940, they described a generalized fatal illness in a young man that was caused by this organism.[15] In 1941, Pinkerton and Henderson provided a clinical description of two fatal cases of an acute febrile exanthematous disease in adults,[16] and in the same year, Sabin described cases of toxoplasmic encephalitis in children.[17]

In 1948, Sabin and Feldman originated a serologic test, the dye test, that allowed numerous investigators to study epidemiologic and clinical aspects of toxoplasmosis, to demonstrate that *T. gondii* is the cause of a highly prevalent and widespread (most often asymptomatic) infection in humans, and to define the spectrum of disease in humans.[18] It was not until 1969, some 60 years after the discovery of the parasite, that *T. gondii* was found to be a coccidian and that the definitive host was found to be the cat.

Our understanding of *T. gondii* infection in pregnancy and in the neonate stems from studies performed over many decades. This problem can best be appreciated by reference to these earlier studies, published earlier in the 20th century. These studies are therefore reviewed in this chapter.

THE ORGANISM

T. gondii is a coccidian and exists in three forms outside the cat intestine: an oocyst, in which sporozoites are formed[19,20]; a proliferative form, formerly referred to as a "trophozoite" and more recently as an *endozoite* or *tachyzoite*; and a tissue cyst, which has an intracystic form termed a *cystozoite* or *bradyzoite*. (Because a single nomenclature has not been agreed on, the terms for each form are used as synonyms in this chapter.) For a more thorough discussion of the organism itself, including its cell biology, molecular biology, genetics, antigenic structure, and immunobiology, the reader is referred to recent reviews on these subjects.[21-32]

The genome of *T. gondii* is available at http://toxodb.org. The parasite is a member of the apicomplexa (as are malarial parasites and cryptosporidia). It is a mosaic of an ancient eukaryotic ancestor that endocytosed an alga (which became a plastid-like organelle and transferred most of its genome to the eukaryote's nucleus) and a mitochondrion that originated from an alpha proteobacter.[33-35] Apicomplexan parasites also have unique secretory organelles important in attachment to the host cell, invasion, and establishment of the parasitophorous vacuole in which the parasitic organism resides as an obligate intracellular parasite. All of these organelles and the metabolic pathways and unique proteins they contain are unique in this parasite and not present in animals. Thus, they present a plethora of unique and novel, some plant-like, antimicrobial agent targets.[33]

Oocyst

The enteroepithelial cycle occurs in the intestines of members of the cat family (see "Transmission" section) and results in oocyst formation (Figs. 31-1 and 31-2). Schizogony and gametogony appear to take place throughout the small intestine but especially in the tips of the villi in the ileum. In cats, the prepatent period from the ingestion of cysts to oocyst production varies, ranging from 3 to 10 days after ingestion of tissue cysts, from 19 to 48 days after ingestion of tachyzoites,[36] and from 21 to 40 days after ingestion of oocysts.[37]

Gametocytes appear throughout the small intestine from 3 to 15 days after infection. Fertilization is effected by a mature microgamete emerging from an epithelial cell into the lumen of the gut and then swimming to and penetrating a mature macrogamete, which probably resides in the epithelium, to form a zygote. After zygote and oocyst formation, no further development occurs within the gut of the cat.

Oocysts pass out of the gut with the feces; peak oocyst production occurs between days 5 and 8. Oocysts are shed in the feces for periods that range from 7 to 20 days. As many as 10 million oocysts may be shed in the feces in a single day.

The zygote divides into two sporoblasts. Each sporoblast develops a wall, the sporocyst, within which two further divisions take place to produce four sporozoites within each sporocyst and eight altogether within the oocyst. The fully sporulated oocyst is infective when ingested, giving rise to the extraintestinal forms. Within the cat, it also can give rise to the enteroepithelial cycle.

Oocysts are spherical at first, but after sporulation they become more oval, measuring 11 to 14 μm by 9 to 11 μm (mean, 12.5 by 11 μm). The two sporocysts are approximately

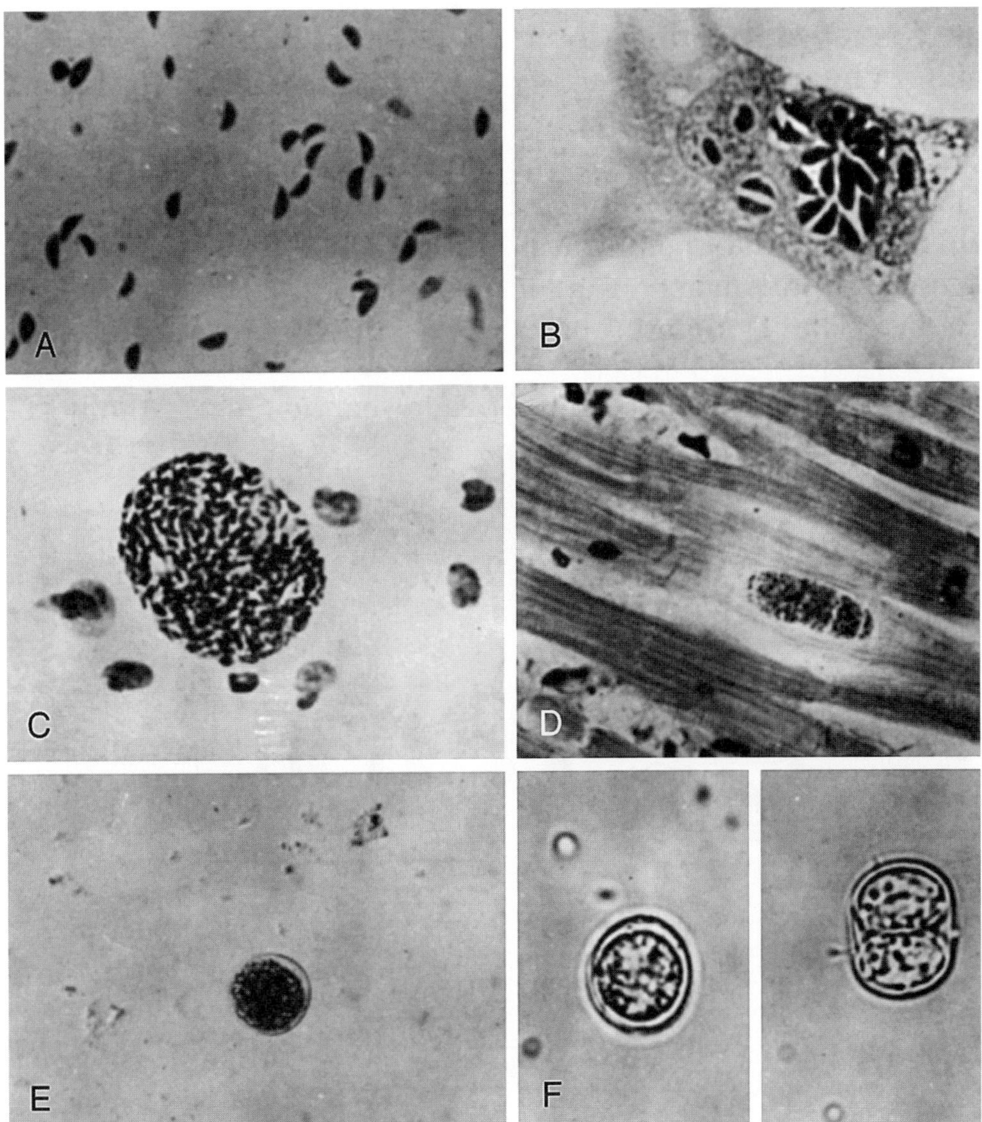

Figure 31–1 The three forms of *Toxoplasma*. **A,** Tachyzoites from peritoneal fluid of a 3-day infected mouse. **B,** Tachyzoite in cytoplasm of chick embryo fibroblast. **C,** Cyst in brain stained with periodic acid–Schiff. **D,** Cyst in myocardium of fatal human case. **E,** Microisolated cyst from brain in mouse. **F,** Unsporulated (*left*) and sporulated (*right*) oocysts. (From Remington JS. Toxoplasmosis. *In* Kelly V [ed]. Brennemann's Practice of Pediatrics, vol. 2. New York, Harper & Row, 1970.)

8.5 by 6 μm, and the sporozoites are about 8 by 2 μm. Depending on the temperature and availability of oxygen, sporulation occurs in 1 to 21 days.[38,39] Sporulation takes place in 2 to 3 days at 24° C, 5 to 8 days at 15° C, and 14 to 21 days at 11° C.[40] Oocysts do not sporulate below 4° C or above 37° C.[38]

Tachyzoite

Tachyzoites are crescentic or oval, with one end attenuated (pointed) and the other end rounded (see Fig. 31-1A and B); they are 2 to 4 μm wide and 4 to 8 μm long. The organisms stain well with either Wright or Giemsa stain. This form of the organism is employed in serologic tests (e.g., Sabin-Feldman dye test, fluorescent antibody methods, agglutination test). Locomotion is by gliding or by body flexion.[41,42]

The tachyzoite form requires an intracellular habitat to survive and multiply. It cannot survive desiccation, freezing and thawing, or action of the digestive juices of the human stomach.[43] This form of the parasite is destroyed within a few minutes in gastric juice, but a relatively small proportion of parasites can survive in tryptic digestive fluid for at least 3 hours but not as long as 6 hours. The organism is propagated in the laboratory in the peritoneum of mice,[44] in tissue cultures of mammalian cells,[45] and in embryonated hens' eggs.[44] Variations in strain virulence correlate positively with invasiveness and with the rate of multiplication of this form in tissue culture.[46]

The tachyzoites occur within vacuoles[47] in their host cells (see Fig. 31-1B), and a definite space and an intravacuolar network are present between the parasite and the vacuole wall.[48] Host cell mitochondria and endoplasmic reticulum

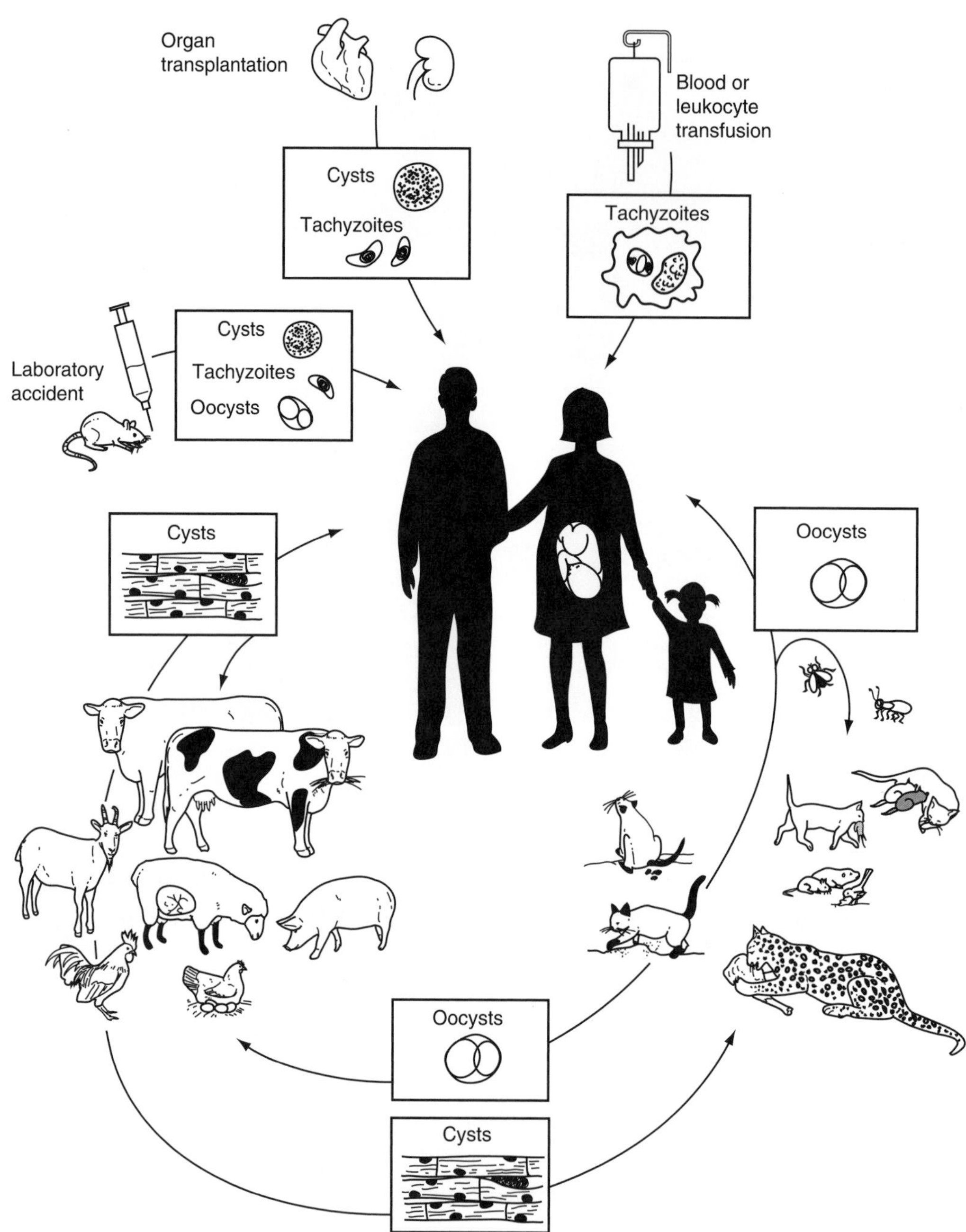

Figure 31–2 The life cycle of *Toxoplasma gondii.* The cat appears to be the definitive host. (From Remington JS, McLeod R. Toxoplasmosis. *In* Braude AI [ed]. International Textbook of Medicine, vol. II, Medical Microbiology and Infectious Disease. Philadelphia, WB Saunders, 1981, p 1818.)

are concentrated in the host cell at the edge of the vacuole.[49] Reproduction in the tissues is by endodyogeny.[50] This is a process of internal budding in which two daughter cells are formed within the parent cell and are released with disruption of the parent cell. When additional nuclear divisions occur before the daughter organisms are completely separated, rosettes are formed; repeated endodyogeny results in a large collection of parasites within a cell.

The tachyzoite form is seen in the acute stage of the infection, during which it invades every kind of mammalian cell (see "Pathology" section). After host cell invasion, the organisms multiply within their vacuoles approximately every 4 to 6 hours and form rosettes. The cytoplasm becomes so filled with tachyzoites that ultimately the cell is disrupted, releasing organisms that then invade contiguous cells[51-53] or are phagocytosed.[54] Colonies of pseudocysts containing tachyzoites produced by endodyogeny may persist within host cells for prolonged periods without forming a true cyst. The duration of this type of infection in vivo is not known.

Cyst

The tissue cyst (see Fig. 31-1C and D) is formed within the host cell and may vary in size, ranging from cysts that contain only a few organisms to large cysts, 200 μm in size, that contain approximately 3000 organisms.[55] This form of *T. gondii* stains well with periodic acid–Schiff (PAS) stain, which causes it to stand out from the background tissue. The cyst wall is argyrophilic and weakly positive for PAS staining. Such cysts are demonstrable as early as the first week of infection in animals[56] and probably persist containing their viable parasites throughout the life of the host.[36] Although they may exist in virtually every organ, the brain and skeletal and heart muscles (see Fig. 31-1C and D) appear to be the most common sites of latent infection.[57] Cysts are spherical in the brain and conform to the shape of muscle fibers in heart and skeletal muscles (see Fig. 31-1D). Because of this persistence in tissues, the demonstration of cysts in histologic sections does not necessarily mean that the infection was recently acquired.

The cyst wall is disrupted by peptic or tryptic digestion, and the liberated parasites remain viable for at least 2 hours in pepsin–hydrochloric acid and for as long as 6 hours in trypsin,[43] thereby allowing them to survive the normal digestive period in the stomach and even longer in the duodenum. In the presence of tissue, the liberated organisms remain viable for 3 hours in peptic digestive fluid and for at least 6 hours in tryptic digestive fluid. Freezing and thawing, heating above 66° C, and desiccation destroy this tissue cyst form; however, the organisms can survive as long as 2 months at 4° C.[43] Tissue cysts are rendered nonviable when internal temperatures have reached 66° C or −12° C.[58] Until more data are available, it appears that freezing at −20° C for 18 to 24 hours, followed by thawing, should be considered adequate for cyst destruction.[43,59,60]

Like the tachyzoite, the cyst develops within a host cell vacuole.[61,62] Cysts may attain a relatively enormous size while still within the host cell. It has been suggested that tissue cysts in the brain are preferentially located within neurons and are retained within viable host cells irrespective of size or age.[63] This would explain the long-term survival of latent infection because the intracellular location could provide the minimal metabolic requirements of the resting stage (bradyzoite).[63] A number of factors lead to bradyzoite differentiation and cyst formation, including arginine starvation, alkaline or acidic pH, and interferon-γ (IFN-γ) stimulation of inducible nitric oxide synthase (iNOS) and nitric oxide.[64,65,66] Cysts can form in tissue culture systems devoid of antibody and complement.[67-69] Immunity is of prime importance in regard to the presence of the different forms of the parasite during the extraintestinal cycle in the infected host. During the acute, initial state of the infection, parasites are present mainly as tachyzoites, which are responsible for parasitemia and systemic infection. When the host has developed an immune response, the infection usually reaches a latent or chronic stage, during which cysts are present in many tissues, and in the immunocompetent host, parasitemia and systemic infection with tachyzoites have subsided. These schematic definitions of the stages of the infection are important to the later discussion on congenital transmission. These two stages were defined by Frenkel and Friedlander in 1952[70] as the first and third stages of *T. gondii* infection. They also described a second, subacute stage as a hypothesis to explain the pathogenesis of lesions observed in congenital toxoplasmosis. The existence of an intermediate stage of uncertain duration also seems likely in cases with subclinical infection, during which both encysted parasites and low-grade systemic infection with tachyzoites are present in the immune host. Whether "dormant" tachyzoites are present during chronic infection in addition to tissue cysts is not known.

TRANSMISSION

Congenital transmission of *T. gondii* from an infected mother to her fetus was the first form of transmission to be recognized.[13] Investigators in the reported cases raised two hypotheses in an attempt to explain congenital transmission. They considered that transmission might occur as a consequence of the acute, initial stage of the infection in a pregnant woman or as a consequence of a recrudescence (either local or systemic with recurrent parasitemia) of a chronic (latent) maternal infection during pregnancy.

Experimental studies of congenital infections in different animal species were helpful for understanding this form of transmission, but definitive data were not obtained until prospective studies were performed in humans in nations such as Austria, where screening for the diagnosis of *T. gondii* infection among pregnant women is routinely performed, and France, where screening is compulsory.

Congenital Transmission

Experimental Studies

Laboratory Animals. Experiments performed to study congenital transmission during the acute stage of the infection in mice and rats revealed that the rate of transmission depends on a number of variables, including time during gestation at which the pregnant animal is infected, the site of infection, and the strain of the parasite and of the mice or rats.[71-75]

In studies with acutely infected pregnant rats, Hellbrugge noted that parasitemia persisted for 18 days, corresponding to the length of gestation (21 days).[76] *T. gondii* did not infect the fetuses until day 16; hence, despite the duration of parasitemia, transmission to the fetus occurred only in the last third of pregnancy. The organisms could be found in the placentas earlier but not in the fetuses. By days 17 and 18 of gestation, all placentas and all fetuses were infected.

Congenital transmission of *T. gondii* from chronically infected animals to their offspring has been reported in rats,[77-82] guinea pigs,[83] rabbits,[84] and mice.[78,85] The strain of the parasite appears to be important in determining whether transmission occurs. In some young animals born to chronically infected mothers, development to maturity proceeds without signs of toxoplasmosis, and infected females in those litters have in turn given birth to infected progeny.[78,85]

In a study of persistent parasitemia in mice used for transmission studies, 50% of the mice with chronic infection (with a strain of *T. gondii* that frequently was transmitted to the offspring) showed parasitemia.[86,87] A similar percentage of such mice produced *T. gondii*–infected offspring. Mice chronically infected with another strain of *T. gondii* and rats with chronic infection produced far fewer infected fetuses, and such animals did not have demonstrable parasitemia.

During the course of the chronic infection in rats, Hellbrugge was able to produce a 100% rate of infection in the fetuses, but this depended on the size of the original inoculum.[76] Thus, in rodents, congenital transmission can occur during both acute and chronic maternal infections. These experimental results suggest a close relationship between maternal parasitemia and transmission to the fetus. They also highlight the importance of the placental barrier in delaying fetal infection. *T. gondii* is found earlier in the placenta than in the fetus. Minipigs[25] and subhuman primates[88] also have served as useful experimental models for studying congenital toxoplasmosis. In interpretation of these studies, it is important to recognize that placentas of rodents, subhuman primates, and humans differ.[72,89]

Domestic Animals. Congenital infection with *T. gondii* has been observed during both natural and experimental infections in most domestic animal species, including cats, dogs, pigs, goats, and sheep.[90-97] Congenital infection is frequent in sheep and goats, is less frequent in pigs, and has not been documented in cattle. Toxoplasmosis occurs as an epizootic infection in pregnant ewes and causes early embryonic death, mummification of the fetus, abortion, stillbirth, or birth of weakened lambs with congenital infection. Embryonic death and stillbirth may result from fetal infection but occur most often as a result of the focal necrotic lesions present in the placental cotyledons. In sheep as well, the placenta is invaded first and the fetus only some days later. In a series of studies on experimental congenital transmission of ovine toxoplasmosis, Jacobs and Hartley found that transmission occurred only in ewes infected during pregnancy, not before pregnancy.[98] If seronegative ewes were infected at 30 days of gestation, early death or mummification of congenitally infected fetuses frequently followed. In ewes infected at 90 days of pregnancy, congenital transmission occurred frequently, but only a small proportion of these ewes aborted. In many cases they gave birth to live lambs, of which about 20% died. In studies of ewes with naturally acquired infection and antibodies before experimental challenge, Hartley noted substantial immunity, but he also observed congenital transmission and some abortions among these ewes.[99]

Beverley and colleagues reported similar results.[100] These investigators found that experimental infection of ewes before mating generally prevented abortion related to *T. gondii* infection acquired in mid-pregnancy.[100] In a trial with a killed vaccine, only ewes developing relatively high antibody titers manifested any protection against fetal death after challenge.[101,101] The protection was only partial in that the pregnancy was often normal, but the fetus and placenta were both infected. In a trial with live, attenuated parasite vaccine, protection of sheep was manifested as increased live births of healthy lambs.[102]

Studies in Humans

The excellent correlation between isolation of *T. gondii* from placental tissue and infection of the neonate, along with results obtained at autopsy of neonates with congenital toxoplasmosis suggesting that the infection is acquired by the fetus in utero through the bloodstream, has led to the concept that infection of the placenta is an obligatory step between maternal and fetal infection. A likely scenario is that organisms reach the placenta during parasitemia in the mother. They then invade and multiply within cells of the placenta, and eventually some gain access to the fetal circulation.

MATERNAL PARASITEMIA

Acute Infection. From pathology studies in patients with toxoplasmosis, as well as from experiments in animals, it can be concluded that parasitemia occurs during the acute, initial stage of both subclinical and symptomatic infections. In an attempt to define the magnitude and duration of the parasitemia during subclinical infection, inoculation of mice was performed with clots of blood taken from women with recent subclinical infections (G Desmonts, unpublished data); these were the first seropositive blood samples obtained from pregnant women who were previously seronegative and who had been tested repeatedly during pregnancy. Approximately 50 patients were examined, and none of the samples were found to be seropositive. Because this method has proved to be valuable for isolation of *T. gondii* from patients with congenital toxoplasmosis (Table 31-1) and from newborns with subclinical infections, the absence of demonstrable organisms in these women suggests that parasitemia during the acute stage of acquired subclinical infection is no longer present, at least by the method employed, once serum antibodies are detectable. Attempts at isolation of *T. gondii* from blood of more than 30 patients with toxoplasmic lymphadenopathy were unsuccessful (JS Remington, unpublished data).

If it is accepted that transmission of *T. gondii* from a mother to her fetus reflects that parasitemia occurred in the mother, evidence indicates that parasitemia occurs at an early stage of the mother's infection before the appearance of serum antibodies[103] and clinical signs (if signs occur). We have observed this in several cases of acquired toxoplasmosis in pregnant women in whom lymphadenopathy appeared during the first month after they had been delivered of newborns with congenital *T. gondii* infection. Precise data are not available on the timing of events that occur after initial infection in humans. The delay between initial infection and occurrence of parasitemia is not known. Important considerations include the duration of parasitemia during the initial stage of the infection and the actual time between the initial infection and the earliest appearance of demonstrable specific antibodies.

Table 31–1 Parasitemia in Clinical Forms of Congenital Toxoplasmosis[a]

Clinical Form	No. of Infants	No. with Parasitemia (%)
Generalized	21	15 (71)
Neurologic or ocular	29	5 (17)
Subclinical	19	10 (52)
Total	69	30 (43)

[a]Infants were studied during the first 2 months of life, but no infants had detectable parasitemia after 4 weeks of age.

Adapted from Desmonts G, Couvreur J. Toxoplasmosis: epidemiologic and serologic aspects of perinatal infection. *In* Krugman S, Gershon AA (eds). Infections of the Fetus and the Newborn Infant. Progress in Clinical and Biological Research, vol. 3. New York, Alan R Liss, 1975, pp 115-132, with permission.

Table 31–2 Serologic Results Associated with Recurrent Parasitemia in a Patient with Acquired Immunodeficiency Syndrome

Date of Sample in 1985	IFA[a] (IU/mL)	IgG Agglutination Test[b] (IU/mL)	IgM ISAGA[a]
March 5	40	25	0
May 3	40	25	0
May 20	40	25	0
September 25[c]	400	1600	0
November 19	400	800	0

[a]Performed at St. Louis Hospital (F. Derouin).
[b]Performed at Institute de Puériculture (G. Desmonts).
[c]Parasitemia was demonstrated in this sample, drawn during an episode of fever, without clinical evidence of neurologic involvement.
IFA, immunofluorescent antibody test; IgG, IgM, Immunoglobulins G, M; ISAGA, immunosorbent agglutination assay.

Chronic Infection (Persistent or Recurrent Parasitemia). A systematic search for persistent parasitemia in humans, especially during pregnancy (as has been performed in animals), has not been reported. Nevertheless, one case report bearing on this subject is pertinent here. Persistent parasitemia was evident in a clinically asymptomatic, otherwise healthy, 19-year-old primigravid woman during 14 months after she gave birth to a congenitally infected infant who died during delivery.[104] This parasitemia persisted despite treatment with pyrimethamine and sulfadiazine. During the period of parasitemia, the patient again became pregnant; the result of this second pregnancy was a healthy baby with no evidence of congenital toxoplasmosis. This case of persistent parasitemia is unique in our experience.

Huldt (G Huldt, personal communication to JS Remington, 1987) isolated *T. gondii* from the blood of an elderly but otherwise healthy woman 1 year after clinical lymphadenopathy. In another case, a woman 60 years of age with a suspected lymphoma had detectable parasitemia on several occasions during a period of 2 years.

As has been observed in normal laboratory animals, parasitemia may be observed during chronic infection in the immunodeficient patient despite the presence of neutralizing antibodies in the serum.[105]

Recurrent parasitemia may be associated with an increase in the immunoglobulin G (IgG) *T. gondii* antibody titer. An example is given in Table 31-2, in which data from one of the AIDS cases reported by Derouin and colleagues are shown.[106] This case demonstrates that, in the presence of a low antibody titer, recurrent parasitemia may induce an anamnestic response with an increase in IgG titer but with no evidence of stimulation of formation of IgM antibody. Thus, the possibility of recurrent parasitemia should be considered when a significant increase in IgG antibody titer occurs in a patient known to have had a low stable preexisting titer.[107] Although uncommon, such increases are sometimes observed even in immunologically competent patients, suggesting that a low-grade systemic infection with possible recurrence of parasitemia can persist for several months so long as cell-mediated immunity is not fully established.

DEMONSTRATION OF *TOXOPLASMA GONDII* IN PLACENTAS

Histologic Demonstration. *T. gondii* organisms have been demonstrated histologically in human placentas.[108-111] (See also "Placenta" section under "Pathology.")

In 1967, Sarrut reported histologic findings in the placentas of eight patients with congenital toxoplasmosis, with microscopic demonstration of the organism in four of them.[112] She noted a correlation between the clinical pattern of neonatal disease and the presence of histologically demonstrable parasites. Both cysts and tachyzoites were numerous and easily demonstrated in three patients with severe systemic fetal disease, whereas parasites were microscopically demonstrable in only one of five patients (see also under "Pathology") with milder disease. Parasites were not noted in cases in which clinical signs of the infection were delayed until weeks after birth. On the contrary, results following injection of placental tissue into mice were positive in patients with congenital toxoplasmosis, as well as in those with subclinical infection.[113]

Isolation Studies

***Toxoplasma gondii* in Placentas during Acute Infection.** From the original studies performed in France in the 1960s, it was concluded that *T. gondii* frequently could be isolated from the placenta when acute infection occurred during pregnancy, but that such isolation was rarely if ever possible when infection occurred before conception.[114] This was true even for women with high antibody titers at the beginning of pregnancy, which suggested that infection might have been acquired shortly before conception. Similar results were obtained by Aspöck and colleagues.[115] These authors examined 2451 women who had decided on termination of their pregnancy. Of these women, 1139 (46%) were seropositive and 77 (3%) had a *T. gondii* indirect fluorescent antibody test titer of 1:256 or higher. The researchers injected the products of conception of 51 of these 77 women into mice. None of the results were positive. Because the researchers had used the whole product of conception after induced abortion, this negative result suggests that this conclusion—that placental infection is seldom if ever present at the time of delivery in women with high antibody titers at the beginning of pregnancy—might also be true for decidua, embryos, and placental tissues obtained early in pregnancy from such women.

When infection is acquired during pregnancy, the frequency of isolation of *T. gondii* from placentas obtained at the time of delivery is dependent on when seroconversion occurred during pregnancy. Table 31-3 shows the results obtained in 321 such cases. The frequency of positive isolation

Table 31–3 Attempts to Isolate *Toxoplasma*[a] from Placenta at Delivery in Women Who Acquired *Toxoplasma* Infection during Pregnancy

Maternal Treatment During Pregnancy	Infection Acquired during First Trimester		Infection Acquired during Second Trimester		Infection Acquired during Third Trimester		Total	
	No. Examined	*No. Positive (%)*	*No. Examined*	*No. Positive (%)*	*No. Examined*	*No. Positive (%)*	*No. Examined*	*No. Positive (%)*
None	16	4 (25)	13	7 (54)	23	15 (65)	52	26 (50)
Spiramycin	89	7 (8)	144	28 (19)	36	16 (44)	269	51 (19)
Total	105	11 (10)	157	35 (22)	59	31 (53)	321	77 (24)

[a]By mouse inoculation.

Adapted from Desmonts G, Couvreur J. Congenital toxoplasmosis: a prospective study of the offspring of 542 women who acquired toxoplasmosis during pregnancy: pathophysiology of congenital disease. *In* Thalhammer O, Baumgarten K, Pollak A (eds). Perinatal Medicine, Sixth European Congress, Vienna. Stuttgart, Georg Thieme, 1979, pp 51-60, with permission.

depended on the trimester of pregnancy in which maternal infection was acquired: the later it was acquired, the more frequently were parasites isolated. The frequency of isolation also depended on whether the women received pharmacologic treatment. Organisms were isolated less often if spiramycin was administered before delivery. These data were collected in the 1960s and 1970s during surveys carried out by Desmonts and Couvreur,[116] which were feasibility studies of measures for prevention of congenital toxoplasmosis. The measures became compulsory in France in 1978. For many years (in the laboratory of one of us [GD]), placental tissue of women considered to be at risk of giving birth to a child with congenital *T. gondii* infection was routinely injected into mice for attempts at isolation of the parasite. (The number of placental inoculations performed in the Laboratoire de Serologie Neonatale et de Recherche sur la Toxoplasmose, Institut de Puériculture de Paris, averaged 800 per year.) The results support the conclusions of the initial surveys: *T. gondii* organisms frequently were present in the placenta on delivery when the acute infection occurred during pregnancy; the later the infection was acquired, the more frequently the placenta was involved. When infection occurred during the last few weeks of pregnancy, placental infection was demonstrable in more than 80% of cases.

A virtually perfect correlation was observed between neonatal and placental infection (see "Diagnosis" section) when the mother did not receive treatment during gestation or duration of the treatment was too brief or an inadequate dose of spiramycin (less than 3 g) was used.[117] Among 85 pregnancies ending in delivery of a child with congenital *T. gondii* infection, isolation of *T. gondii* from placental tissue was successful in 76 of 85 cases (89%). If the fact that only a relatively small portion of the placenta was digested for the inoculation into mice is taken into account, the high proportion of positive results supports the concept that placental infection is an obligatory occurrence between maternal and fetal infection. It also demonstrates that if the mother receives no or inadequate treatment, placental infection persists until delivery. Nevertheless, placental infection may not be demonstrable by mouse inoculation on delivery of a child with congenital *Toxoplasma* infection when the mother received treatment during pregnancy. In the series of cases reported by Couvreur and colleagues,[117] the proportion of placentas from which *T. gondii* was isolated was 89 of 118 (75%) if the mothers had received treatment for more than 15 days with 3 g per day of spiramycin. This proportion was 10 of 20 (50%) if pyrimethamine plus sulfonamides was added to treatment during the last months of pregnancy.

***Toxoplasma gondii* in Placentas during Chronic Infection.** A study was performed by Remington and colleagues (in collaboration with Beverly Koops) in Palo Alto, California, to determine whether *T. gondii* can be isolated from placentas of women with stable dye test titers. Of the 499 placentas obtained consecutively, 112 (22%) were from women with positive dye test results. The digestion procedure (see "Isolation Procedures" later under "Diagnosis") was performed on 101 of these placentas. *T. gondii* organisms were not isolated from any of them. Thus, in the population studied, chronic (latent) infection with *T. gondii* does not appear to involve the placenta significantly. By contrast, *T. gondii* has been isolated with relative ease from the adult human brain,[57] skeletal muscle,[57] and uterus.[118]

Another study in which an attempt was made to isolate the organism from placental tissue is that of Ruiz and associates in Costa Rica.[119] Much smaller amounts of tissue were injected into mice, but isolation was successful in 1 of 100 placentas. The dye test titer in the mother from whose placenta the organism was isolated was 1:1024. Adequate clinical and serologic data for the offspring were not provided. The researchers stated that *T. gondii* organisms were not demonstrable in the placental tissue by microscopic examination. This finding is not surprising in view of the findings of Sarrut.[112] The high dye test titer in this case might have been due to an infection acquired during pregnancy. Ruoss and Bourne failed to isolate *T. gondii* from 677 placentas of mothers who were delivered of viable infants and who had low *T. gondii* antibody titers.[120] It can be concluded from these studies that placental infection is extremely rare in pregnant women with chronic *T. gondii* infection.

FETAL *TOXOPLASMA GONDII* INFECTION AND CONGENITAL TOXOPLASMOSIS

Acute Infection in the Mother. Direct data that demonstrate the frequency with which *T. gondii* is transmitted to the fetus during the period of acute infection in the mother come from prospective studies such as those performed by

Desmonts and Couvreur,[114] Kräubig,[121] Kimball and colleagues,[122] and Stray-Pedersen.[123] Fetal infection, the consequence of placental infection, depends on the time during gestation when maternal infection was acquired. Table 31-4 (which summarizes findings from the same group of cases as in Table 31-3, although the number of cases in both tables is not the same because placentas were available in only 321 of the 542 pregnancies) shows data collected in the 1960s and 1970s by Couvreur and Desmonts. In Table 31-4, children are classified into five groups: those with no congenital infection, subclinical congenital infection, mild congenital toxoplasmosis, severe congenital toxoplasmosis, and stillbirth or early death (shortly after birth). Children were considered to be free of congenital infection if they had no clinical manifestations suggesting congenital toxoplasmosis and if their results on *T. gondii* serologic testing became negative after disappearance of passively transmitted maternal antibodies. Congenital infection was classified as subclinical if no clinical signs of disease related to toxoplasmosis occurred during infancy. Clinical disease was considered to be mild if the infant was apparently normal, with normal development on follow-up evaluation. An example of mild disease is that of a child with no mental retardation or neurologic disorder on later examination but with isolated retinal scars discovered during a prospective eye examination (or, in one case, isolated intracranial calcifications on radiographic examination) performed because the child was at risk of having congenital *T. gondii* infection, having been born to a mother who acquired the infection during gestation. Cases were considered to be severe if both chorioretinitis and intracranial calcifications were present or if mental retardation or neurologic disorders were present. From the results shown in Table 31-4, the subclinical form is by far the most frequent presentation of congenital *T. gondii* infection. Severe cases with survival of the fetus are scarce.

In 500 pregnancies, it was possible to ascertain the trimester during which *T. gondii* infection had been acquired (Table 31-5). *T. gondii* infection occurred in the fetus or was present in the newborn in 14%, 29%, and 59% of cases of maternal infection acquired during the first, second, and third trimesters, respectively. The proportion of cases of congenital toxoplasmosis was higher in the first- and second-trimester groups than in the third-trimester group. This was especially true for severe congenital toxoplasmosis (including cases with stillbirths, perinatal deaths, or severe neonatal disease). No case of severe toxoplasmosis was observed among the 76 offspring of mothers who had acquired *T. gondii* infection during their third trimester. Approach to detection and management of infection acquired during gestation determines and can modify severity of infection detected in infants and their later outcomes.[124-127] Of interest, after systemic serologic screening and treatment for T. *gondii* infection acquired in gestation was introduced in France in 1978, the frequency of severe toxoplasmosis diagnosed in

Table 31–4 Outcome of 542 Pregnancies in Which Maternal *Toxoplasma* Infection Was Acquired during Gestation: Incidence of Congenital Toxoplasmosis and Effect of Spiramycin Treatment in Mother during Pregnancy

	No. of Affected Infants (%)	
Outcome in Offspring	***No Treatment***	***Treatment***
No congenital *Toxoplasma* infection	60 (39)	297 (77)
Congenital toxoplasmosis		
Subclinical	64 (41)	65 (17)
Mild	14 (9)	13 (3)
Severe	7 (5)	10 (2)
Stillbirth or perinatal death[a]	9 (6)	3 (1)
Total	154 (100)	388 (100)

[a]See text.

Adapted from Desmonts G, Couvreur J. Congenital toxoplasmosis: a prospective study of the offspring of 542 women who acquired toxoplasmosis during pregnancy: pathophysiology of congenital disease. *In* Thalhammer O, Baumgarten K, Pollak A (eds). Perinatal Medicine, Sixth European Congress, Vienna. Stuttgart, Georg Thieme, 1979, pp 51-60, with permission.

Table 31–5 Frequency of Stillbirth, Clinical Congenital Toxoplasmosis, and Subclinical Infection among Offspring of 500 Women Who Acquired *Toxoplasma* Infection during Pregnancy[a]

	No. of Affected Infants (%)		
Outcome in Offspring	***Infection Acquired during First Trimester***	***Infection Acquired during Second Trimester***	***Infection Acquired during Third Trimester***
No congenital *Toxoplasma* infection	109 (86)	173 (71)	52 (41)
Congenital toxoplasmosis			
Subclinical	3 (2)	49 (20)	68 (53)
Mild	1 (1)	13 (5)	8 (6)
Severe	7 (6)	6 (2)	0 (0)
Stillbirth or perinatal death[b]	6 (5)	5 (2)	0 (0)
Total	126 (100)	246 (100)	128 (100)

[a]Forty-two pregnancies are not included from Table 31–3 because it was not possible to ascertain the trimester during which infection occurred in the mother.

[b]See text.

Adapted from Desmonts G, Couvreur J. Congenital toxoplasmosis: a prospective study of the offspring of 542 women who acquired toxoplasmosis during pregnancy: pathophysiology of congenital disease. *In* Thalhammer O, Baumgarten K, Pollak A (eds). Perinatal Medicine, Sixth European Congress, Vienna. Stuttgart, Georg Thieme, 1979, pp 51-60, with permission.

Table 31–6 Severity of Manifestations of Congenital Toxoplasmosis in Paris before (1949-1960) and after (1984-1992) Introduction of Serologic Screening and Treatment programs

		No. of Affected Infants (%)			
Period	No. of Newborns	*CNS Disease*	*Hydrocephalus*	*Retinitis/Scar*	*Subclinical*
1949 to 1960	147	93 (63%)	62 (67% of 93)	54 (33%)	0
1984 to 1992	234	8 (3%)[a]	—[a]	60 (26%)	166 (71%)

[a]Severe ocular or neurologic disease occurred only when infants were born to mothers from foreign countries where there was no screening during pregnancy (e.g., Morocco, Algeria, United Kingdom), they were not screened, or mothers were immunodeficient or erroneously considered immune. It also is noteworthy that in one hospital in France, in 1957, among 1085 premature infants, 7 had toxoplasmosis, whereas in this same hospital between 1980 and 1990, among approximately 10,000 premature infants, 2 had toxoplasmosis.
CNS, central nervous system.

Table 31–7 Fetal *Toxoplasma* Infection as a Function of Duration of Pregnancy[a]

Time of Maternal Infection	No. of Women	% Infected
Periconception	182	1.2
6-16 wk	503	4.5
17-20 wk	116	17.3
21-35 wk	88	28.9
Close to term	41	75

[a]Women were treated during gestation as soon as feasible after diagnosis of the acute acquired infection was established or strongly suspected. If prenatal diagnosis was made in the fetus, treatment was with pyrimethamine-sulfadiazine; otherwise it was spiramycin.
Adapted from Forestier F. Fetal diseases, prenatal diagnosis and practical measures. Presse Med 20:1448-1454, 1991, with permission.

Table 31–8 Incidence of Congenital *Toxoplasma gondii* Infection by Gestational Age at Time of Maternal Infection[a]

Week of Gestation	Infected Fetuses/ Total No. Fetuses	Incidence (%)
0-2	0/100	0
3-6	6/384	1.6
7-10	9/503	1.8
11-14	37/511	7.2
15-18	49/392	13
19-22	44/237	19
23-26	30/116	26
27-30	7/32	22
31-34	4/6	67
Unknown	8/351	
Total	194/2632	7.4

[a]Maternal infection was treated with spiramycin in a dose of 9 million IU (3 g) daily.
Adapted from Hohlfeld P, et al. Prenatal diagnosis of congenital toxoplasmosis with polymerase-chain-reaction test on amniotic fluid. N Engl J Med 331:695-699, 1994.

newborns diminished remarkably (Table 31-6). This is discussed in more detail under "Effects of Systematic Screening of Pregnant Women at Risk on the Prevalence of Congenital *Toxoplasma gondii* Infection and of Congenital Toxoplasmosis."

Experience acquired since 1978[128-131] has confirmed these earlier findings: Transmission of the parasite to the fetus was dependent on the time of acquisition of maternal infection during pregnancy. The proportion of cases that resulted in congenital *T. gondii* infection was very low if maternal infection was acquired during the first few weeks after conception. The later maternal infection was acquired, the more frequent was transmission to the fetus. The frequency of congenital infection was 80% or higher if maternal infection was acquired during the last few weeks before delivery and if it was not treated. Table 31-7 shows the frequency of transmission by gestational age observed in a group of 930 women with acute *Toxoplasma* infection acquired during pregnancy who were referred to the Institut de Puériculture in Paris for prenatal diagnosis. The incidence of transmission rose from 1.2% when maternal infection occurred around the time of conception to 75% when it occurred close to term. These data were updated by Hohlfeld and co-workers,[125] whose report includes the 2632 pregnant women for whom a prenatal diagnosis was performed between 1983 and 1992 (Table 31-8). The observed incidence of transmission rose from 0% when maternal infection was acquired before week 2 of pregnancy to 67% when it was acquired between weeks 31 and 34. The incidence of transmission remained very low, less than 2%, when maternal infection was acquired during the first 10 weeks of gestation. It rose sharply when maternal infection was acquired during weeks 15 to 34.

To appropriately interpret the data provided by Hohlfeld and co-workers, a number of points deserve discussion. Their patients were referred to the Institut de Puériculture for prenatal diagnosis. Thus, cases with fetal death in utero before the time of amniocentesis were not included. The consequence is that the incidence of congenital infection when maternal infection occurred during the first few weeks of pregnancy is slightly underestimated. For example, when Daffos and colleagues reported the first 746 cases from this same series, they[130] estimated the incidence of transmission to be 0.6% among 159 women with "periconceptional infection" and 3.7% among 487 women whose infection was acquired between weeks 6 and 16 of gestation. The observed incidence rates were 1.8% and 4.7%, respectively, if those fetuses that died in utero because of congenital toxoplasmosis before the time of blood sampling were included in the report. Another consequence of the recruitment of the cases reported by Hohlfeld and co-workers is that the number of cases with acquired maternal infection after week 26 of gestation is small, because maternal infection acquired late during pregnancy was not discovered early enough to allow for performance of a prenatal diagnosis. The incidence of congenital infection was reported to be 194 of 2632 (7.4%). If, however, one excludes 100 cases of maternal infection acquired before week 2, and 351 in which gestational age at the time of maternal infection was unknown, the distribution of cases would be as follows: maternal infection acquired at gestational age 3 to 14 weeks, 1398 cases; 15 to 26 weeks, 745 cases; and 27 to 34 weeks, 38 cases. Most of the cases studied by Hohlfeld and co-workers occurred in women who acquired infection early in pregnancy. If cases of maternal acquired infection had been equally distributed through each of the weeks of gestation, from weeks 3 to 34, the adjusted mean transmission rate would have been 19.5%. The transmission rate observed by Jenum and associates in Norway[132] was 11 of 47 (23%).

A higher transmission rate, 65 of 190 (34%), was observed in a series of 190 consecutive cases of maternal acute *Toxoplasma* infection, each of whose sera was examined in a single laboratory in Paris (P Thulliez, personal communication to G Desmonts, 1999). These cases were more equally distributed in regard to gestational age at time of infection. The incidence rates of congenital infection in this series of 190 women were as follows: 4 to 16 weeks, 5 of 44 (11%); 17 to 28 weeks, 15 of 71 (21%); and 29 to 40 weeks, 45 of 75 (60%). In another series, reported by Dunn and associates,[131] the mean rate of transmission was 29% in 603 cases studied in Lyon between 1987 and 1995.

A critical point to remember in reviewing the data obtained in the European countries where screening for *Toxoplasma* infection during pregnancy is routinely performed is that most patients are treated *during pregnancy*—which probably reduces the incidence of transmission of the parasite. The frequency of congenital toxoplasmosis (i.e., of fetal lesions or of clinical manifestations in the infant with congenital infection) also is highly dependent on the time of acquisition of maternal infection during pregnancy. The earlier maternal infection was acquired, the higher was the prevalence of fetal or neonatal disease among infants with congenital *T. gondii* infection.

A number of observations suggest that *T. gondii* may be present in the placenta but is transmitted to the previously uninfected fetus only after a delay. This delay has been termed the *prenatal incubation period* by Thalhammer.[133,134] Placental infection is a potential source of infection of the infant even long after maternal parasitemia has subsided. This has been documented in studies in which, after induced abortions, samples of fetal tissues and placentas were injected into mice in an attempt to isolate *T. gondii*. Table 31-9 shows the results obtained in 177 such cases in which no attempt at prenatal diagnosis of fetal infection had been made. Isolation attempts were successful from placentas in 10 cases (6%). In 8 of the 10 cases, placental and fetal tissues were injected separately and *T. gondii* organisms were isolated solely from the placentas and not from the fetus in 4 of those 8 cases. The fetuses were not infected at the time the pregnancies were terminated. In one of these cases, pregnancy was terminated at week 21 in a woman who had acquired her infection shortly before the fourth week of gestation. This case demonstrates that delay between maternal and fetal infection may be longer than 16 weeks. In other cases, the delay may be much shorter. Among 22 pregnancies terminated because congenital *T. gondii* infection had been demonstrated in the fetus by prenatal diagnosis (see "Prenatal Diagnosis of Fetal *Toxoplasma gondii* Infection" in "Diagnosis" section) (data not included in Table 31-9), the time that elapsed between maternal and fetal infection evidently was less than 8 weeks in 2 cases, less than 6 weeks in 2 cases, and less than 4 weeks in 1 case. The case histories also suggested that the later during gestation maternal infection occurred, the shorter was the delay between maternal and fetal *T. gondii* infection (Table 31-10). The data of Daffos demonstrate that it is almost always first- and second-trimester infections that are associated with substantial brain necrosis and hydrocephalus.[130] Recent data reveal that the magnitude of fetal involvement correlates with amount

Table 31–9 Isolation of *Toxoplasma* from Placental and Fetal Tissue after Termination of Pregnancy in 177 Women Who Acquired Infection Just before or during Gestation

Maternal infection category I[a]	
No. of cases	115
No. of positive isolations	10 (9%)[b]
Maternal infection category II[a]	
No. of cases	62
No. of positive isolations	0

[a]Category I: *Toxoplasma* infection was proved to have been acquired during pregnancy; category II: *Toxoplasma* infection was noted to have been recently acquired; it occurred either before or soon after conception as judged by serologic test results obtained at the time of first examination, when patients were in their fourth to eighth week of gestation. No attempt at prenatal diagnosis was made in any of the cases.

[b]*Toxoplasma* was isolated in two cases from mixed placental and fetal tissues after curettage, in four cases from both placenta and fetal tissues injected separately, and in four cases solely from the placenta.

Adapted from Desmonts G, Forestier F, Thulliez P, et al. Prenatal diagnosis of congenital toxoplasmosis. Lancet 1:500-504, 1985, with permission.

Table 31–10 Frequency of Findings in the Fetus Correlated with Gestational Age When Infection Was Acquired

Fetal Gestational Age (wk) when Infected	Frequency of Ultrasound Evidence[a] of Infection	Frequency (%) of Cerebral Ventricular Dilatation
<16	31 (60%) of 52	48
17-23	16 (25%) of 63	12
>24	1 (3%) of 33	0

[a]Ascites, pericarditis, necrotic foci in brain.

Data from Daffos F, et al. Letter to the editor. Lancet 344: 541, 1994.

of parasite DNA in amniotic fluid (see under "Polymerase Chain Reaction Assay" ["Diagnosis"] and "Prevention").[135]

The severity of the disease depends on the age of the fetus at the time of transmission (see Table 31-10). This is determined both by the time during pregnancy when maternal infection occurs and by the duration of the delay between maternal infection and transmission to the fetus (prenatal incubation period). The earlier the fetus is infected, the more severe the disease in the newborn. The likelihood that transmission will occur early in fetal life is greater when the mother acquires her infection during the first or second trimester of pregnancy.

Results of examination of fetuses after induced abortion agree with these conclusions. Among the 177 cases in which pregnancies were terminated without any prior attempt at prenatal diagnosis (see Table 31-9), results of inoculation tests of fetal tissues were positive in 4 cases. In each of these 4, macroscopic lesions were evident on gross examination of the aborted fetus at autopsy. The same was true for 22 fetuses of women in whom the decision to terminate the pregnancy was made after fetal infection was demonstrated by isolation of *T. gondii* from amniotic fluid or from cord blood samples obtained in an attempt at prenatal diagnosis.[130] Each of these 22 fetuses had multiple necrotic foci in the brain, even when appearance on a previous ultrasound examination (performed before the pregnancy was terminated) was normal.

Transmission during the third trimester almost always results in either subclinical infection or mild congenital toxoplasmosis. Exceptions have been noted: In two cases (G Desmonts, unpublished observations) in which maternal infection was acquired after 30 weeks of gestation, the offspring had severe systemic disease and died in the newborn period.

By collecting data from pregnancies that resulted in birth of severely damaged infants, it was possible to define more precisely the weeks of pregnancy during which infection produces the greatest risk of severe congenital toxoplasmosis in the newborn infant. The period of highest risk was weeks 10 to 24.[128] Although the incidence of transmission to the fetus is highest during weeks 26 to 40, it results in milder infection in the newborn. Weeks 1 to 10 constituted a low-risk period because transmission to the fetus was infrequent. Although infrequent, cases have been observed in which infection was acquired before week 7, or even shortly before conception, which resulted in the birth of severely damaged infants. The attempt at prenatal diagnosis by Daffos and associates[130] in 159 cases of periconceptional maternal infection (i.e., infections that, as judged by serologic test results, had been acquired at the time of conception or within a few weeks after conception) revealed fetal infection in only 1.8% of cases (see earlier). Thus, in these circumstances, transmission of parasites is infrequent.

A question that is frequently asked when toxoplasmic lymphadenopathy is diagnosed in women of childbearing age or when serologic test results in a sample of serum drawn for routine testing very early in pregnancy suggest recently acquired *T. gondii* infection is as follows: How long before pregnancy is acquisition of *T. gondii* infection to be considered a risk factor for transmission of the parasite to the fetus in a future pregnancy? The answer is that if toxoplasmic lymphadenopathy was already present at the time of conception, and/or if two samples of serum, the first drawn before the eighth week of gestation and the second 3 weeks later, are examined in parallel and have identical IgG titers, the initial stage of the infection probably occurred before conception. The avidity test also is helpful in this setting, because high-avidity IgG antibodies develop at least 12 to 16 weeks (depending on the test kit used) after acquisition of infection. Thus, the presence of high-avidity antibodies indicates that infection was acquired more than 12 to 16 weeks earlier (see also later discussions of serodiagnosis and avidity assays).[136-138] In these conditions, the risk for congenital *T. gondii* infection is extremely low. Unfortunately, accumulated data do not allow for a more definitive answer. Cases that demonstrate that the exception does occur have been reported. Of special interest are cases in which the diagnosis of toxoplasmic lymphadenopathy was well established before pregnancy occurred, because they provide reliable information in regard to the timing of events (clinical signs in the mother, beginning of pregnancy, and the development of signs, if any, in the infant). A summary of the history of the first reported case[128,139] appeared in the third and fourth editions of this book.[140,141] Another case was reported by Marty and co-workers in 1991,[142] and a third was reported by Vogel and associates in 1996.[143] The time elapsed between the occurrence of lymphadenopathy and conception was 2 months for the first case and 3 and 2 months, respectively, for the next two cases. The patient described by Marty and co-workers received spiramycin for 6 weeks at the time of lymphadenopathy; however, she did not receive treatment during pregnancy. Neither the first (studied by Desmonts)[141] nor the third (Vogel) mother received any treatment. In the three cases, no specific sign of congenital toxoplasmosis was recognized in the newborn (except possibly in the case reported by Marty and co-workers, in which slight splenomegaly was noted in the neonate). Strabismus was noted at the age of 3 months in the first case. None of the infants was given treatment before the diagnosis of congenital toxoplasmosis infection was established. Definitive diagnosis was made in two infants when obstructive hydrocephalus developed, at the ages of 4 months and 9 months, respectively. In the case described by Marty and co-workers, infection was still subclinical when the diagnosis was made at the age of 8 months because of an increase in the antibody load (see "Diagnosis" section).

The clinical patterns and the delayed antibody response observed in the infants are highly suggestive that transmission of the parasite to the fetuses occurred after maternal IgG had reached a significant level in the fetal blood (i.e., after 17 to 20 weeks of gestation), and probably later in the patient (described by Marty and co-workers) whose infection remained subclinical, despite absence of treatment before the eighth month of life.

These three cases demonstrate that infection in the 3 months before conception does not always confer effective immunity against congenital transmission. Transmission rarely occurs in these conditions, however. In our experience,[128] no other example of congenital infection has arisen among several hundred cases in which toxoplasmic lymphadenopathy occurred before pregnancy. Advice given (G Desmonts) was that patients should receive spiramycin treatment if lymphadenopathy had occurred during the 6 months preceding pregnancy. This intervention possibly reduced the incidence of congenital infection among the offspring of these patients.

That fetal infection is rare when maternal acquisition of *T. gondii* infection has occurred even a short time before pregnancy is in agreement with the observation first made by Feldman and Miller,[144] and amply confirmed since, that congenital infection does not occur in siblings (except twins) of a child with congenital toxoplasmosis. Several exceptions have been reported. In one instance described by Garcia, congenital *T. gondii* infection affected offspring of two successive pregnancies.[108] The first infant, delivered by cesarean section for fetal distress at the seventh month of gestation, died at 24 hours with multiple organ involvement with *T. gondii*. About 5 months after delivery of this infant, the mother again became pregnant. This pregnancy ended in spontaneous abortion of a macerated fetus at about the sixth month of gestation. Microscopic examination revealed *T. gondii* infection in both cases, in fetal as well as placental tissue. Although the proof rests solely on histologic findings, the data presented in these cases appear incontrovertible. Silveira and colleagues[145] also reported that *T. gondii* had been transmitted from a Brazilian mother infected 20 years earlier. The mother had a chorioretinal macular scar and positive result on serologic tests for *T. gondii* infection over a 20-year period. She was without known immunocompromise and transmitted *T. gondii* to her fetus. Details of the evaluation for immunocompromise and clonal type of parasite were not available (Silveira, personal communication to J Remington, 2003). Manifestations in the infant included IgG and IgM specific for *T. gondii*, a macular scar, and a cerebral calcification.

Two cases of transmission to the fetuses of women with subclinical infection acquired before pregnancy also have been published in France. Time of infection was well established in both cases, because sera drawn before conception were available for comparison with the mandatory sample taken at the beginning of pregnancy.[146,147] In both cases, sera were negative for *T. gondii* antibodies 7 months before pregnancy and found to be positive, with a high but stable titer of IgG antibodies at 3 and 4 weeks of gestation, respectively. Thus, infection had occurred about 1 to 2 months before conception in both cases. In both, prenatal diagnostic testing proved positive, and severe fetal lesions were demonstrated after termination of the pregnancies. Therefore, it is well established that the acute subclinical infection in a pregnant woman can result in fetal infection and congenital toxoplasmosis, even when acquired by the mother before conception.

Serologic screening tests for acute *T. gondii* infection during pregnancy usually are performed at weeks 8 to 12 of gestation. If the results suggest a recently acquired infection, it formerly was difficult, even with the help of a second sampling of serum 3 weeks later, to decide whether infection occurred before or after the time of conception (see "Diagnosis" section). These cases were classified as "periconceptional," and in our practice (G Desmonts),[129,139] these women were managed as if they had been infected during gestation (spiramycin treatment and prenatal diagnosis). The transmission rate observed after "periconceptional" infection was 3 of 161 (1.8%).[130] With the availability of the avidity assay, acquisition can be more readily dated regarding whether it occurred before conception if the test is performed during the first 12 to 16 weeks of gestation.

It is apparent that the rate of transmission of the parasite from a woman to her fetus after the acute infection rises from virtually zero, when *T. gondii* infection was acquired several months (the exact number is unclear) before pregnancy, to about 2% (or slightly less), when acquired at about the time of conception. An important point is that the transmission rate remains low for several weeks (approximately 10) after the beginning of pregnancy. After the tenth week of gestation, a shift occurs from this low transmission rate toward a steeply increasing incidence of congenital infection in relation to the gestational age. This shift was observed in the 11- to 14- week gestational age group in the series reported by Hohlfeld and co-workers[125] and after week 13 in the series reported by Dunn and associates.[131] Several hypotheses might explain this shift from a low toward a steeply rising risk of transmission. One relies on a truism: Congenital toxoplasmosis is a fetopathy, resulting from a placental infection. Thus, a placenta and a fetus are necessary for the disease to develop. Hence, congenital *T. gondii* infection, when resulting from an infection acquired by the mother before the formation of the placenta, is the consequence of a recurrent parasitemia. The incidence of transmission in this situation depends on the frequency of recurrent parasitemia in a woman whose cell-mediated immunity with regard to *Toxoplasma* has not yet fully developed (see the "Pathogenesis" section). When maternal infection is acquired later during pregnancy, the parasite can reach the placenta during the initial parasitemia, which occurs in the mother before the development of any immune response. This mode of transmission is more effective for colonization of the placenta by the parasite. The later the infection occurs in the fetus, however, the less severe the disease, because immunologic maturation has had time to develop.

A summary of the data just presented is shown in Figure 31-3, in which percentages of risk are given, to suggest a range in magnitude and not necessarily exact data. It also should be noted that the data used in this figure were obtained from women almost all of whom received spiramycin treatment during pregnancy. Hence, the outcome in the fetuses would have been more severe, both for transmission rates and for severity of infection, if results from untreated pregnancies only had been used.

Chronic Maternal *Toxoplasma* Infection. Data obtained in prospective studies have established that chronic (or latent) maternal infection, per se, is not a risk for congenital infection.[144] Also, as a rule, evidence of previous chronic (latent) infection signifies that the future mother is not at risk of giving birth to a child with congenital *T. gondii* infection. These observations constitute the basis for the preventive measures that have been adopted by and have proved effective in countries such as Austria and France.[148-150] Immunity associated with chronic (latent) infection is relative only in laboratory animals (see "Pathogenesis" section) and in sheep.[99,100] Five cases have been published that suggest that this statement might be true for humans as well.[139,151-153] Four of the cases were reported from France. This is not surprising because such cases usually are observed only in countries where screening for *Toxoplasma* infection during pregnancy is performed routinely.

A summary of the histories of the four cases follows: The women were known from previous pregnancies to have low

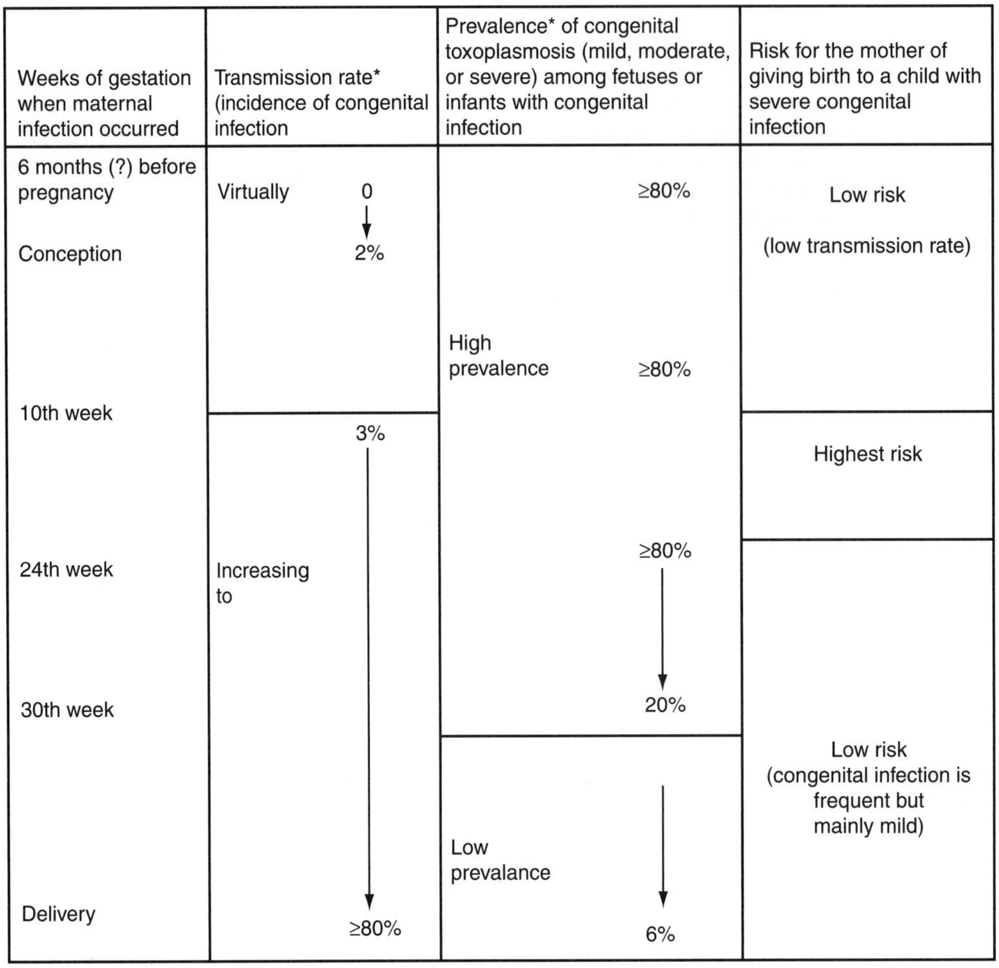

Weeks of gestation when maternal infection occurred	Transmission rate* (incidence of congenital infection	Prevalence* of congenital toxoplasmosis (mild, moderate, or severe) among fetuses or infants with congenital infection	Risk for the mother of giving birth to a child with severe congenital infection
6 months (?) before pregnancy	Virtually 0	≥80%	Low risk
Conception	2%		(low transmission rate)
		High prevalence ≥80%	
10th week	3%		Highest risk
24th week	Increasing to	≥80%	
30th week		20%	Low risk (congenital infection is frequent but mainly mild)
		Low prevalance	
Delivery	≥80%	6%	

*Percentages are given as a range according to what has been observed among women, most of whom were treated with spiramycin during pregnancy.

Figure 31–3 Transmission rate and prevalence of congenital *Toxoplasma* infection or congenital toxoplasmosis among offspring of women with acute *Toxoplasma* infection in relation to gestational age at time of maternal infection.

and stable titers of IgG antibodies, characteristic of past infection and immunity. The same low titer of IgG was present at the beginning of the new pregnancy. Thus, these women were considered to be immune, so that their fetus was judged not to be at risk. Treatment was therefore not given during gestation. Congenital *T. gondii* infection was demonstrated in each case: A subclinical infection was noted when the child was 12 months of age in one case (the history of which was published in previous editions of this book)[140,141]; spontaneous abortion occurred at 12 weeks of gestation, with demonstration of the parasite in fetal tissues in another case[151]; and congenital toxoplasmosis (chorioretinitis) was diagnosed at birth in the third case[152] and at 9 months of age in the fourth case.[153] In each of the four cases, a serologic relapse occurred during pregnancy, as evidenced by a significant increase in IgG antibodies that reached high titers in each woman. In three of the women, samples of sera drawn during pregnancy were available for retrospective examination. Of interest is that in these three cases, IgA antibodies were present at the beginning of the serologic relapse. An IgM response was noted in only one woman. Serologic relapse had occurred between weeks 8 and 11 of gestation in the case ending in abortion and after weeks 10, 16, and 19, respectively, in the other three cases. Silveira and colleagues[145] also reported that *T. gondii* had been transmitted from a Brazilian mother infected 20 years earlier, as described.

Even if some cases have gone unpublished (Dr. Jacques Couvreur has data on two additional cases, as described in a personal communication to G Desmonts, 1999), the examples of offspring with congenital *T. gondii* infection born to mothers who, at the beginning of pregnancy, had serologic test results that established the presence of a chronic (latent) infection are exceptional. When this does occur, immunologic dysfunction must be suspected as having been the cause. The first case we observed[140,141] was that of a woman who had a low $CD4^{+}/CD8^{+}$ ratio associated with Hodgkin's disease, from which she had recovered 2 years before becoming pregnant. She also previously underwent a splenectomy. No immunologic dysfunction was demonstrated in the other three women. Reinfection with oocysts of another *T. gondii* strain was suggested as an explanation for the cases observed by both Fortier and Gavinet and their co-workers.[151,153] Each woman had contact with kittens at the beginning of or during week 20 of gestation, respectively.

Transmission of *T. gondii* from mother to fetus has been observed in immunodeficient women owing to reactivation of the chronic infection, primarily in patients with AIDS (see "Congenital *Toxoplasma gondii* Infection and Acquired Immunodeficiency Syndrome" later, under "Clinical Manifestations"). It also has occurred as a consequence of other immunocompromised states that appear to have resulted in an active but subclinical infection in the chronically infected pregnant woman. One case was reported in the third and fourth editions of this book.[140,141,154] Two additional cases were published in 1990,[139] and a fourth in 1995 by d'Ercole and colleagues.[155] The immunologic dysfunction was associated with lupus erythematosus in three of the four patients and with pancytopenia in one. This last patient, as well as one of those with lupus, also previously had a splenectomy. Each of the four patients was given corticosteroids during gestation. Three[139] did not receive treatment for their *T. gondii* infection. The serologic evidence for (chronic) active infection was the unusually high IgG titers that had been present since childhood in two of the cases (titers of greater than 4000 IU for more than 5 and 10 years, respectively). One of these women gave birth to an infant with severe congenital toxoplasmosis that resulted in the death of the child at the age of 3 months. Congenital toxoplasmosis was diagnosed in the other case when chorioretinitis occurred in the infant at the age of 4 months. In one of the four mothers, the IgG titer rose from a relatively low titer at the beginning of pregnancy to 800 IU, and a weakly positive IgM test titer developed. One of her twin infants, a boy, died at the age of 9 days from toxoplasmic encephalomyelitis. His twin sister had subclinical congenital *T. gondii* infection.

The case report published by d'Ercole and colleagues[155] is of special interest because the affected woman was known to have both lupus erythematosus and high *T. gondii* IgG antibody titers, together with a strongly positive IgA test result, before becoming pregnant. For this reason she was monitored with *T. gondii* serologic tests for two consecutive pregnancies. During both pregnancies, recurrence of serologic signs of activity of *T. gondii* infection was observed. She had an increase in IgG titers and an IgM test result that became temporarily positive. Despite treatment with spiramycin, prenatal diagnosis revealed that the infection was transmitted to the fetus in both of these pregnancies. During the first pregnancy, the fetus died in utero at a gestational age of 23 weeks. In the second pregnancy, the mother received pyrimethamine and sulfonamide after the polymerase chain reaction (PCR) assay result was observed to be positive in amniotic fluid at 23 weeks of gestation. This pregnancy ended in delivery of a child who was considered to have *T. gondii* infection as indicated by the presence of IgA serum antibodies in the newborn. The infant was given pharmacologic treatment and at 1 year of age exhibited no signs of congenital toxoplasmosis and had no *T. gondii* antibodies.

The cases just described demonstrate conclusively that the presence of a chronic, yet active *T. gondii* infection in an immunocompromised pregnant woman results in a significant risk of congenital infection for the fetus and newborn. In addition to women with AIDS, this is especially true for women who must receive long-term treatment with corticosteroids during gestation. In this context, it is important to note that HIV-infected women older than 50 years of age and who were born outside the United States had the highest seroprevalence of *T. gondii* antibodies.[156] Treatment of HIV infection in the woman chronically infected with *T. gondii*[157] also would be expected to substantially reduce or eliminate congenital *T. gondii* infection, although no data rigorously demonstrating this effect have been provided.

In the past, chronic *Toxoplasma* infection in the mother was considered to be responsible for repeated abortions, stillbirths, or perinatal fetal mortality. In an attempt to determine whether *T. gondii* is indeed a contributing cause of stillbirth and perinatal infant mortality in women with chronic (latent) infection, Remington and colleagues performed a study in El Salvador, where the incidence of the infection in the childbearing age group was approximately 65% and the perinatal infant mortality rate was very high.[158,159] In the Maternity Hospital in San Salvador, a dye test was performed on serum obtained from 103 mothers on the day of the death of their newborn infants or, in the case of death in utero, at the time of delivery. The dye test was repeated 1 month later to determine whether the titers were stable, and a skin test was performed at the same time. A high percentage of the mothers had dye test titers of 1:1000 or higher,[159] in marked contrast with the test results in the pregnant population in the United States. Sixty-five percent of the 103 women in this study had a positive dye test result. One hundred ten infants were examined. The diagnostic categories, with number of affected fetuses in each category, were as follows: cranial deformities, 5; premature births, 45; stillbirths, 40; and miscellaneous, 70. Fifty-eight of the mothers had had previous abortions; 26 had had one abortion, 12 had had two or more abortions, and more than 7 had given birth to dead infants. At least 20 g of each infant's brain and a similar amount of liver were injected into 10 to 20 mice. *T. gondii* was not isolated from any of the infants, which suggested that in this population, *T. gondii* was not an important cause of perinatal fetal mortality. Ferraris and Avitto, in Rome, obtained similar results for their population.[160]

Several prospective surveys have been performed to determine whether chronic *T. gondii* infection is a cause of abortion. In a study in Palo Alto, California, and its immediate surroundings, tissue specimens were obtained from aborted fetuses in 272 women. (For the initial portion of this study, see the work of Remington and co-workers.[161]) Seventy-nine (29%) of these women had positive dye test titers. Of these 79 women, at least 18 had had one abortion, and at least 8 had had two or more abortions. *T. gondii* was isolated from two specimens obtained from two chronically infected women—one specimen came from decidual tissue obtained at curettage after spontaneous abortion and the other from the aborted fetus and decidual tissues. Chronic *T. gondii* infection in the first case was evident from the stable dye and hemagglutination test titers, at levels lower than those usually associated with acute *T. gondii* infection, and a positive skin test result. Subsequent attempts to isolate the organism from endometrial tissue and from menstrual blood were unsuccessful. The second case was that of a 27-year-old white woman whose first two pregnancies (in 1960 and 1962) had resulted in the births of normal offspring. In February 1963, she aborted at approximately 5 weeks of gestation. A dye test performed at that time showed a titer of

1:512, and an attempt to isolate *T. gondii* from the abortion tissues was unsuccessful. She aborted again in March 1964, and her serum again showed a titer of 1:512. *T. gondii* was isolated from the aborted fetus and decidual tissues. The presence in this case of identical dye test titers in serum samples collected 1 year apart is proof of chronic infection with *T. gondii* and appears to establish the fact that *T. gondii* can be associated with abortion during the chronic stage of infection in women in the United States. A similar case, in which *T. gondii* was isolated from products of abortion, has been described by Meylan in Switzerland.[162]

Ruoss and Bourne, in England, failed to isolate *T. gondii* from products of conception in 104 cases of abortion (25 occurred in patients with low titers of *T. gondii* antibodies).[120] Janssen and colleagues attempted to isolate *T. gondii* from 218 samples of maternal or fetal tissue obtained in 172 cases of abortion and following curettage in 10 nonpregnant women who had had abortions.[163] Of these women, 70% had positive dye test titers, and 29% showed positive results on the complement fixation (CF) test. Janssen and colleagues were successful in isolating *T. gondii* in only one case—from curettage material taken after a second abortion in a woman who had a proven chronic (latent) infection. An attempt to isolate the parasite from products of a previous abortion in this woman 5 months earlier had been unsuccessful; at that time, her dye test titer was 1:256 and her CF test titer was 1:5. A third abortion occurred 7 months later, and the products of abortion were thoroughly studied; however, attempts to isolate the parasite from placenta, fetus, and tissue obtained at curettage all were unsuccessful. Like Remington and co-workers,[104,164] Janssen and colleagues concluded that they could not state unequivocally that *T. gondii* was responsible for the abortion in their cases. They believed that isolation of *T. gondii* from abortion tissues of women with latent infection is possible, but only in rare cases.

Kimball and colleagues from the United States performed a serologic study in a population of 5033 pregnant women in New York City and found no evidence to suggest an association of *T. gondii* infection with habitual abortion.[165] By contrast, their evidence suggesting an association between chronic *T. gondii* infection and sporadic abortion was substantial. This association was particularly significant in white patients, especially those with positive results on CF tests. It is unclear whether this was an association caused by other factors or a cause and effect relationship. It is not known whether these sporadic abortions are related to recurrent parasitemia or to persistence of encysted *T. gondii* in uterine tissue.[118]

The significance of *T. gondii* infection as a cause of abortion has been a subject of considerable conjecture among workers in this field throughout the world. A detailed review of this subject was presented in the first two editions of this book[166,167]; it is omitted from the present edition because no new data are available.

Transmission by Ingestion

Whether the mode of transmission consists of infective oocysts or meat that contains cysts, it appears that the natural route of transmission usually proceeds from animals (and contaminated soil) to humans by way of ingestion.

Meat

Because the results of feeding tissues from chronically infected mice or rats to other mice were much more successful than the results of similar feedings of tissues from acutely infected animals,[43,44,87,168,169] it was hypothesized that the cyst form, found in the chronic infection, was better able to withstand the digestive process. Microscopically, the cyst wall was seen to be destroyed immediately on contact with pepsin hydrochloride; however, the liberated parasites were infective for mice as long as after 2 hours of exposure to peptic digestive fluid but not after 3 hours.[43] When trypsin was used, liberated parasites were infective for up to 6 hours of digestion, the longest period tested.[43]

These data, combined with those on the seroepidemiology of *T. gondii* infection in domestic animals used for human consumption, led a number of workers to suggest that meat may serve as a source of human *T. gondii* infection.[43]

In 1956, Weinman and Chandler published a classic article suggesting a meat-to-human route to explain the spread of *T. gondii.*[170] Their investigations stemmed from a study in which they noted that humans are more likely to have antibody titers to *T. gondii* if they eat undercooked pork. This observation led Jacobs and co-workers to explore the occurrence of *T. gondii* cysts in the edible flesh of meat animals. Samples of mutton, pork, and beef from abattoirs in Baltimore were digested in artificial gastric juice; infection was demonstrated in 12 of 50 samples (24%) of pork, 8 of 86 samples (9.3%) of mutton, and only 1 of 60 samples (1.7%) of beef.[43] (The single isolation from beef was questionable, according to the authors.) Similar results have been found in samples of meat from butcher shops in Palo Alto, California, and from other areas of the world.[163-166,168-182] Dubey and colleagues have reported on the distribution of *T. gondii* tissue cysts in commercial cuts of pork.[183] In a genotypic analysis of 43 isolates of *T. gondii* from pigs in Iowa, 87% were type II. Type III genotype was identified in only 16.3% of the isolates. These prevalence rates are similar to the frequencies with which they occur in cases of the disease in humans. Type I strains were not identified, although these strains have previously been shown to account for 10% to 25% of cases of toxoplasmosis in humans.[184] Isolation of *T. gondii* from beef was reported by Catar and colleagues in Czechoslovakia.[185] The cyst form was found in 8 of 85 cattle (9.4%). *T. gondii* has not been isolated from cattle slaughtered in the United States.[67,175,186] It should be recognized, however, that only relatively small specimens have been evaluated. Other workers have shown that persons who handle raw meat, even without consuming it, have a higher prevalence of antibodies to *T. gondii.* A listing of studies of isolation of *T. gondii* from muscle of domestic animals from around the world is presented in Table 31-11.[187-204]

In 1965, Desmonts and colleagues in Paris published what appears to be definitive evidence in favor of the meat-to-human hypothesis.[205] They found that among children in a French hospital, antibodies to *T. gondii* developed at a rate five times that in the general population. Because it was the custom in this hospital to serve undercooked meat (mainly beef or horsemeat) as a therapeutic measure, these workers reasoned that this practice explained the higher incidence of infection among this hospitalized population. To test this hypothesis, they added undercooked mutton to the diet and

Table 31–11 Isolation of *Toxoplasma gondii* from Muscle of Domestic Animals

Species	Country	Proportion Positive for *T. gondii* (%)	Reference No.
Sheep	Australia	8/32 (25)	Munday[a]
	New Zealand	3/5 (60)	187
	United States	8/86 (9.3)	188
	Germany	6/50 (12)	189
	Denmark	7/31 (23)	190
	Norway	69/174 (39.6)	191
	Iran	5/66 (7.5)	192
	Japan	3/26 (11.5)	193
Cattle	Czechoslovakia	8/85 (9.4)	194
	New Zealand	0/80 (0)	187
	United States	1/60[b] (1.7)	188
	United States	0/350[c]	186
	Germany	0/500	195
	Germany	0/74	189
	Germany	0/1260	196
	Denmark	0/30	190
Swine	Czechoslovakia	14 (432) (3.2)	197
	United States	12/50 (24)	188
	United States	170/1000 (17)	198
	Germany	54/500 (10.8)	199
	Italy	18/60 (30)	200
	Denmark	10/29 (35)	190
	Norway	20/63 (31.7)	201
	Japan	3/61 (5)	202
	Japan	25/130 (19)	203
	Japan	4/190 (2.1)	204

[a]Unpublished data.
[b]Result was considered to be equivocal, suggesting that there were actually no isolates.
[c]Tissues fed to cats; the rest were inoculated into mice.
Adapted from Munday BL. The epidemiology of toxoplasmosis with particular reference to the Tasmanian environment. Thesis, University of Melbourne, Melbourne, Australia, 1971, 95 pp.

observed that the yearly rate of acquisition of antibody to *T. gondii* doubled. Clinical signs of infection, mainly lymphadenopathy, developed in some of the children. Severe illness was not observed in any of them. Four years later, Kean and colleagues in New York reported a miniepidemic of toxoplasmosis in five medical students.[206] Epidemiologic evidence strongly implicated the ingestion of undercooked hamburgers, which the authors recognized might have been contaminated with mutton or pork, as the source of infection in these cases.[207,208]

A number of isolated cases and recent miniepidemics of acute acquired *T. gondii* infection have been reported. Included were at least one case of congenital toxoplasmosis associated with consumption of undercooked venison or preparation of venison (R McLeod, personal observation), another that resulted in significant illness in adults who ingested undercooked lamb (J Remington, unpublished data),[209] one in which undercooked kangaroo meat resulted in acute infection in 12 adults and a case of congenital toxoplasmosis,[210] and another linked to undercooked pork.[211] In regard to venison, a high prevalence of *T. gondii* antibodies has been reported in white-tailed deer in the United States.[212,213]

The prevalence rates in various countries indicate that the habits and customs of various populations in regard to the handling and preparation of meat products are an important factor in the spread of toxoplasmosis.[214-217]

Oocyst

Although ingestion of undercooked meat (especially mutton or pork) explained one mode of transmission, such a hypothesis did not explain how herbivorous animals and vegetarian humans became infected. In humans, the prevalence of *T. gondii* antibodies was the same among vegetarian populations (e.g., Hindus) as among meat-eating populations in the same geographic area (e.g., Christians and Muslims in India).[218,219] A possible explanation was forthcoming when Hutchison and associates,[220] as well as several others working independently,[221,222] described a new form of the parasite, the oocyst.

Oocyst formation has been found to occur only in members of the cat family (e.g., domestic cat, bobcat, mountain lion). Cats may excrete up to 10 million oocysts in a single day, and excretion may continue for 2 weeks. Immunity to the intestinal stages in cats is apparently not absolute, because renewed oocyst production may occur when a cat becomes reinfected[223] or infected with the related coccidian *Isospora*. Once shed, the oocyst sporulates in 1 to 5 days and becomes infectious; it may remain so for more than 1 year under appropriate conditions (e.g., in warm, moist soil).[224,225] This form of the parasite may be inactivated by freezing, heating to a temperature of 45° C to 55° C, drying, or treating with formalin, ammonia, or tincture of iodine. (For further information on the biology of the oocyst, the reader is referred to the works of Frenkel and Dubey.[19, 226]) Its buoyancy allows it to float to the top layers of soil after rain, a location more conducive to transmission than the deeper soil where cats usually bury their feces. Transport of the oocyst from the site of deposit may occur by a number of vectors. Coprophagous invertebrates such as cockroaches and flies may mechanically carry oocysts to food.[227-229] Earthworms also may play a role by carrying oocysts to the soil surface.[39,230,231]

A number of attempts have been made to demonstrate oocysts in the feces of cats in their natural surroundings. Whereas Dubey was unable to demonstrate oocysts of *T. gondii* in the feces of 510 domiciled seropositive and seronegative cats in Kansas City,[232] Wallace detected them in the feces of 12 of 1604 stray or unwanted cats (0.7%) on the island of Oahu, Hawaii.[233] In his studies in the South Pacific, Wallace had previously noted that *T. gondii* antibodies were far more common in humans, rats, and pigs on Pacific atolls on which cats were present than on atolls without cats.[234-236] Munday made similar epidemiologic observations for sheep on the Tasmanian islands.[237] In a study performed in Germany, Janitschke and Kuhn found oocysts in the feces of approximately 1% of privately owned cats[238] or cats from animal care facilities[239]; Werner and Walton found a similar ratio in the house cats of U.S. Armed Forces families in the Kanto Plain (Tokyo) area of Japan.[240] These low prevalence rates contrast markedly with results of a series of epidemiologic studies in Costa Rica. Ruiz and Frenkel noted that 23% of 237 cats were excreting oocysts. Of interest is the fact that 64% of the excreters were kittens.[223] A report from Beirut, Lebanon, described the incidence of "*T. gondii*–like oocysts" in the feces of 9.9% of 313 cats.[241] In a similar study from Brno, Czechoslovakia, oocysts of *T. gondii* were demonstrated

Table 31–12 Prevalence of *Toxoplasma* Oocysts in Feces of Naturally Infected Cats

Country	No. Examined	No. Positive	% Positive
Australia	74	1	1.3
Brazil	185	1	0.5
Costa Rica	237	55	23.2
Czechoslovakia	91	4	4.4
	161	3	1.9
Germany			
Berlin	502	5	0.9
Hannover	308	4	1.3
Munich	694	4	0.5
Hungary	200	2	1.0
Italy	250	1	0.4
Japan	90	1	1.1
	446	4	0.8
Netherlands	567	2	0.4
Nigeria	200	14	7.0
Spain	104	1	0.9
United Kingdom	100	2	2.0
United States	510	0	0.0
	1604	12	0.7
	1000	7	0.7

Adapted from Dubey JP. Toxoplasmosis in cats. Feline Pract 16:12-26, 1986, with permission.

in feces of 1.9% of 620 cats.[242] The prevalence of *T. gondii* oocysts in the feces of naturally infected cats in which their presence was proved by mouse inoculation is shown in Table 31-12.

The relative importance of the oocyst versus undercooked or raw meat in transmission of *T. gondii* to humans remains to be defined. Whereas meat appears to be of primary importance in most areas of the United States, as shown by Etheredge and Frenkel,[243] this is not true for other geographic areas. Epidemics of toxoplasmosis associated with presumptive exposure to infected cats support the importance of this mode of transmission.[244-247]

Waterborne Epidemics (Oocysts). A cluster of cases of *T. gondii* in Panama[246] and another in a suburb of São Paulo, Brazil,[248] appear to have been associated with oocyst-contaminated drinking water. An epidemic in Victoria, Canada, also was considered to be associated with oocysts from wild cats in reservoir water. This reservoir was thought to be contaminated with *T. gondii* oocysts excreted by cougars.[249]

Mussels and Oysters. The illness and deaths of sea otters on the central coast of California (especially around Moro Bay) have drawn attention to the presence of *T. gondii* in mussels.[250,251] Mussels appear to concentrate oocysts[250] that then can be consumed by the otters. Infections in aquatic mammals indicate contamination and survival of oocysts in seawater.[250] Lindsay and associates[250,252] demonstrated that oocysts can persist in seawater for many months, sporulate, and remain infectious.

Oocysts on Fruits. Kniel and co-workers[253] found that oocysts can persist and remain infective for up to 8 weeks on raspberries and that they also can adhere to raspberries and blueberries. Consumption of fresh produce with *T. gondii* oocysts could thus be a source of transmission to humans. Ooocysts excreted by cats can directly contaminate produce and water used for agriculture.

Incidence of Infection in Animals That Feed on the Ground. Approximately 80% of black bears and about 60% of raccoons in the United States have antibodies to *T. gondii*. The authors suggest that infection in these animals is a good indicator of the prevalence of *T. gondii* in the environment, because raccoons and bears scavenge for their food.[249] Dubey and his colleagues suggested that these observations may be linked to the ingestion of oocysts from an environment heavily contaminated with this form of *T. gondii*. In certain areas of Brazil, a high prevalence of infection in chickens and young children has been noted.[249]

Milk

T. gondii has been transmitted successfully through milk directly to suckling young in experimental mouse models.[78,254] The organism also has been found in the milk during acute experimental infection in cats, dogs, goats,[255] guinea pigs, rabbits, and sheep (see Fig. 31-2).[256] It has been isolated from the colostrum of a cow and from the milk of naturally infected asymptomatic pigs.[93,257]

Langer reported isolation of *T. gondii* from the milk of 3 of 18 women.[258] Remarkably, in two of the three women, results of the dye tests and CF tests were negative. This is the first such report of isolation from human milk. Interpretation of Langer's results, however, is complicated by the fact that pollen grains contaminated his preparations, which were being examined microscopically for the presence of cysts, and he was unable to decide retrospectively which of his preparations showed pollen grains or *T. gondii* cysts.[259] Transmission during breast-feeding in humans has not been demonstrated. It is conceivable that such might be the case if a mother were to acquire her infection during the last weeks of pregnancy. In these circumstances, the risk of transplacental transmission is so high (approaching 100%) that the possible additional risk of breast-feeding would be insignificant.[260]

Unpasteurized milk (goat milk has been especially implicated) has been implicated as a vehicle for transmission of *T. gondii*,[261-263] but the process of pasteurization would kill all forms of the organism.

Chicken and Eggs

Latent infection was found in chickens obtained from a poultry-processing plant by Jacobs and Melton (see Fig. 31-2).[264] Because chicken usually is well cooked before eating, it is unlikely that it plays a significant role in transmission. These investigators also were able to isolate *T. gondii* from 1 of 327 eggs laid by 16 chickens with experimentally induced chronic infections. The epidemiologic significance of this finding may be assessed in relation to the number of raw eggs consumed by different population groups. The report by Pande and co-workers of isolation from chicken eggs[265] was fraudulently illustrated,[266] and thus their data are open to question. Prevalence of the infection in chickens reflects *T. gondii* strains in their environment because they feed from the ground.[267] Prevalence of *T. gondii* was determined in 118 free-range chickens from 14 counties in Ohio and in 11 chickens from a pig farm in Massachusetts. *T. gondii* antibodies were demonstrated in 20 of 118 chickens (17%) from Ohio and isolated from 11 of 20 seropositive chickens (55%). Parasites were not isolated from tissues of 63 seronegative chickens. Nineteen isolates were genotyped; five were type II and 14 were type III.

Other Means of Transmission

Blood Transfusion

Neto and associates recovered *T. gondii* from blood donated by an asymptomatic person for transfusion.[268] *T. gondii* was shown to survive in whole citrated blood stored at 4° C for up to 50 days.[187,269,270] Kimball and co-workers inferred that the risk of transmission of *T. gondii* through blood to children who had received numerous transfusions was not great because the prevalence of positive serologic tests for *T. gondii* antibodies in these children was no different from that in children in the normal population.[188] A majority of their patients, however, had received transfusions of packed red blood cells; if *T. gondii* remains viable in leukocytes,[189] transfusion of whole blood may be a mode of transmission of the parasite. Because prolonged parasitemia has been observed during latent toxoplasmosis in experimental animals[86] and in humans with asymptomatic acquired toxoplasmosis,[104,190] transfused blood must be considered a potential vehicle for transmission of the infection.

Siegal and colleagues described four patients with acute leukemia in whom overt toxoplasmosis developed after they were given leukocytes from donors with chronic myelogenous leukemia.[194] Three of the four patients died. Retrospective serologic analyses suggested that the transfused donor white cells were the source of the parasite. If a pregnant woman is to receive a whole blood transfusion, selection of a donor without antibodies to *T. gondii* is advisable whenever possible. Patients with chronic myelogenous leukemia and high titers of antibody to *T. gondii* should not be used as blood or blood cell donors.[195,200]

Laboratory-Acquired Infections (Including Infections Acquired at Autopsy)

A number of cases of toxoplasmosis have been acquired by laboratory personnel who handle infected animals or contaminated needles and glassware.[202,203,271-273] We are aware of numerous cases of laboratory-acquired infection with *T. gondii* that have occurred in recent years. At the Palo Alto Medical Foundation laboratory and Stanford University, more than a dozen such instances have been identified. Some cases were in pregnant women (JS Remington, unpublished data). Certainly, this experience indicates that pregnancy is a contraindication to working with *T. gondii* for women who have no demonstrable *T. gondii* antibodies.

One instance has been reported of toxoplasmosis acquired during performance of an autopsy.[274]

Arthropods

The data derived from studies of multiple potential insect vectors are negative and inconclusive.[19] Flies and cockroaches may serve as carriers of oocysts (see Fig. 31-2).[227,228,255]

Miscellaneous

Free organisms have been identified within the alveoli of infants with congenital toxoplasmosis (see "Lungs" in "Pathology" section) and have been isolated from saliva[275] and sputum.[276] *T. gondii* has been reported to survive for 4 to 6 days in saliva, tears, and milk.[277] The demonstrated presence of organisms in the glomeruli and tubules of the kidneys and in the mucosa of the bladder and intestine suggests that contamination through mucosa or breaks in skin by tachyzoites in urine and feces might be a remotely possible (but unlikely) source of infection in persons caring for such infants. Transmission from such sources has never been proved. *T. gondii* has been transmitted by organ transplantation, most often through organs from a seropositive donor transplanted into a seronegative recipient.[278-280]

EPIDEMIOLOGY

General Considerations

Toxoplasmosis is a zoonosis; the definitive host is the cat, and all other hosts are incidental. The organism occurs in nature in herbivorous, omnivorous, and carnivorous animals, including all orders of mammals, some birds, and probably some reptiles, although in reptiles this suggestion rests solely on interpretation of histologic preparations.[281] In regard to *T. gondii* in cold-blooded hosts, data suggest that natural infection might occur under suitable environmental conditions.[282,283]

The organism is ubiquitous in nature, and toxoplasmosis is one of the most common infections of humans throughout the world. In humans, the prevalence of positive serologic test titers increases with age, indicating past exposure, and no significant difference in prevalence between men and women exists in reports from the United States.

Considerable geographic differences exist in prevalence rates. Differences in the epidemiology of the infection in various geographic locales and between population groups within the same locale may be explained by differences in exposure to the two main sources of the infection: the tissue cyst (in flesh of animals) and the oocyst (in soil contaminated by cat feces). The high prevalence of infection in France has been attributed to a preference for consumption of undercooked meat.[205] A similarly high prevalence in Central America has been related to the frequency of stray cats in a climate favoring survival of oocysts and to the type of dwelling.[223,224] Examples of factors affecting the frequency of the infection are shown in Table 31-13. Of special note are reports of outbreaks of *T. gondii* infections among family members.[284-288]

In 1993, the European Network on Congenital Toxoplasmosis, which includes approximately 50 institutions in Europe with investigators interested in different aspects of congenital toxoplasmosis, was organized and has been funded by the Biomedicine Research Program of the Commission of the European Union. The Network has been overseen by Dr. Eskild Petersen of Copenhagen and Dr. Ruth Gilbert of London. Its initial focus has been on diagnosis, including quality control, education and prevention, and identification of risk factors for infection during gestation. In 1995, the European Multicenter Study on Congenital Toxoplasmosis

Table 31–13 Factors Affecting the Incidence of *Toxoplasma* Infection among Different Populations

Factor	Considerations
Cat population (mainly feral and stray cats)	If present, the size of the population of cats within the locale inhabited by the specific human population in question.
Climatic conditions	Certain temperatures and humidity levels favor maturation and survival of oocysts in soil. Very cold and hot, dry climates are adverse conditions.
Method of farming of food animals	Access of cats to food of these animals varies according to whether the animals are in the fields, in pens, or in stables.
Hygienic habits in regard to food for human consumption	Whether food is exposed to coprophagous insects (flies and cockroaches) and whether meat has been previously frozen influence the incidence.
Cultural habits in regard to cooking of food	Principally, meat is important—the size of portions and whether served raw, rare, or well cooked.
Hygienic conditions and occupational situations favoring acquisition of infection from contaminated soil	

(EMSCOT) was organized to gain further knowledge of the epidemiology and natural history of congenital toxoplasmosis and to perform prospective, controlled trials of new treatments and treatment regimens (E Petersen, personal communication to JS Remington, 1998).

Among studies designed to identify the risk factors for *T. gondii* infection during pregnancy, results from France, Italy, Norway, and Yugoslavia were reported.[215,217,289,290] Three of these studies reported a comparison between pregnant women who had recently seroconverted or who had evidence of recently acquired infection with seronegative matched controls. The study from Yugoslavia compared seronegative with seropositive persons who had past infection. The conclusions of these four studies—for example, that ingestion of raw or undercooked meat, use of kitchen knives that have not been sufficiently washed, and ingestion of unwashed raw vegetables or fruits are factors associated with an increased risk—are not unexpected. In a recent case-control study from Europe examining risk factors that predispose pregnant women to infection with *T. gondii*,[291] the authors concluded that exposure to inadequately cooked or cured meat accounted for approximately 30% to 63% of infections; thus, exposure to meat was interpreted to be the main risk factor for pregnant women in Europe. Other risk factors included contact with soil, which apparently accounted for approximately 6% to 17% of infections; travel outside Europe or the United States and Canada also apparently accounted for some infections. Although contact with soil would presumably reflect risk from cat excrement, the authors concluded that direct "contact with cats" was not a risk factor. They also concluded that mode of acquisition for a large proportion of infections (14% to 49%) remained unexplained.

In a recent study[292] exploring risk factors recognized by mothers of infants with congenital toxoplasmosis in the United States between 1981 and 1998, undercooked meat and possible cat excrement exposure, either one or both, were recognized by approximately 50% of the mothers, but the remainder of the mothers could not identify risk factors.

Consumption of meat that had been frozen was associated with a lower risk. Surprisingly, in Naples, Italy, Buffolano and colleagues[217] observed an increased risk associated with consumption of cured pork; this might be related to the fact that in southern Italy, cured pork usually contains only 1% salt to fresh weight, is stored at less than 12° C, and may be eaten within 10 days of slaughter. A pet cat at home was not associated with an increased risk in any of these studies, but cleaning the cat litter box was a significant risk factor among women in the study from Norway.[215] Health education was associated with a lower risk when it was provided using printed educational materials in a book or magazine.[289] This improved efficacy of print (versus oral) information was observed in the past in Saint Antoine Hospital in Paris (Table 31-14); the yearly seroconversion rate decreased from 37 per 1000 to 11 per 1000 when explanatory drawings were given to every seronegative pregnant woman.

Prevalence of *Toxoplasma gondii* Antibodies among Women of Childbearing Age

Knowledge of the prevalence of antibodies in women in the childbearing age group is important because of its relevance to the strategic approach for prevention of congenital toxoplasmosis. In evaluating results obtained in any serologic survey, the factors noted earlier under "General Considerations" (in epidemiology) must be examined, in addition to two potential causes of differences that may not be real: the serologic method used (and its accuracy) for collection of the data and the dates of collection of the sera.

Data from studies of pregnant women in New York City, London, and Paris are shown in Table 31-14. These data were obtained in surveys performed during the years 1960 to 1970 and were largely from results of the dye test. They are shown here for comparison with more recent data.

Data on the prevalence of antibodies in pregnant women or women in the childbearing age group for the United States and for other areas of the world are shown in Tables 31-15, 31-16, and 31-17.[214,293-376,1170-1174] The prevalence rate among pregnant women in Palo Alto, California, has decreased remarkably, from 27% in 1964 and 24% in 1974 to 10% in 1987 and 1998. The prevalence among pregnant women in Malmo, Sweden, has diminished since 1983.

Relevant to the variability in prevalence of infection among populations within a given geographic area are the observations of Ades and associates.[377] They studied the prevalence of maternal antibody in an anonymous neonatal serosurvey in London in 1991. Among women born in the United Kingdom, the seroprevalence was estimated to be 12.7% in inner-city London, 7.5% in suburban London, and 5.5% in nonmetropolitan areas. The prevalence in women from India was 7.6%; Africa, 15% to 41%; Pakistan and Bangladesh, 21%; Ireland, 31%; and the Caribbean, 33%.

Table 31–14 **Effect of Attempts at Health Education on Incidence of *Toxoplasma* Infection in Selected Populations of Pregnant Women in the Paris Area**

Hospital[a]	Period	Seroconversion Rate[b]	Yearly Seroconversion Rate (per 1000)
Pinard and Baudelocque[c]	Pre-1960	11/356	60
Centres Medico-Sociaux CPCAM[d]	1961-1970	73/2496	64
Hospital X[e]	1973-1975	18/710	59
Saint Antoine[f]	1973	7/463	37
	1974	3/658	11
Longjumeau[g]	1974-1981	20/1938	22

[a]Patients from several obstetric departments. Sera were examined in one laboratory (G Desmonts) with the same level of sensitivity of the serologic methods.
[b]Number of seroconversions observed/number of seronegative women screened in the dye test and/or agglutination test.
[c]Serum samples, taken during pregnancy, were examined only after delivery.
[d]No information was given on how to avoid becoming infected. The mode of transmission of *Toxoplasma* was not known at that time.
[e]Little or no information was given on how to avoid becoming infected.
[f]There was an intensive attempt at health education of seronegative women on how to avoid becoming infected. In 1973, only verbal instructions were given. In 1974, patients were given drawings illustrating the cycle and transmission of the parasite, with explanations in the language of the patient.
[g]Only oral instructions were given.
Modified from Roux C, Desmonts G, Mulliez N, et al. Toxoplasmose et grossesse: bilan de deux ans de prophylaxie de la toxoplasmose congénitale à la maternité de l'hôpital Saint-Antoine (1973-1974). J Gynecol Obstet Biol Reprod 5:249-264, 1976, with permission.

Table 31–15 **Prevalence of *Toxoplasma* Dye Test Antibodies in Three Populations of Pregnant Women**

	% Positive			
			Paris	
Age Group (yr)	***New York***	***London***	***French***	***Others***[a]
15-19	16	15	80	56
20-24	27	27	81	53
25-29	33	33	86	78
30-34	40	34	95	77
≥35	50	36	96	80
Total	32	22	87	70

[a]Spaniards, North African Muslims, and Portuguese.
Adapted from Desmonts G, Couvreur J. Toxoplasmosis in pregnancy and its transmission to the fetus. Bull NY Acad Med 50:146-159, 1974, with permission.

Thus, much of the variation between districts might be explained by ethnic group or country-of-birth composition. Recent data from France are available from a national survey performed in 1995 for the Direction Genérale de la Santé.[378] The seroprevalence was 54.3%, with considerable geographic differences. Lower prevalence rates were noted in the northeast of the country (30% to 40%) than in the southwest or northwest (55% to 65%). Differences also were noted depending on the country of origin: France, 55%; other European countries, 46%; North Africa, 51%; and south Saharan Africa, 40%. A high prevalence (64%) was observed among women practicing, or whose husbands practiced, a "learned profession." In the Paris area, the seroprevalence had decreased from more than 80% in the 1960s to 72% in the 1970s. It was still higher than 65% in 1995. In Liege, Belgium, Thoumsin[379] reported that the seroprevalence decreased from 70% between 1966 and 1975, to 62% between 1976 and 1981, and to 47% between 1982 and 1987. In Norway, Jenum and colleagues[345] reported a prevalence of 10.9%, ranging from 13% in the southeastern part of the country and in Oslo to 6.7% in the north. These rates observed from 1992 to 1994 are similar to those reported in the mid-1970s.

Cultural habits with regard to food probably are the major cause of the differences in frequency of *T. gondii* infection from one country to another, from one region to another in the same country, and from one ethnic group to another in the same region. The data just described all reveal a decrease in the prevalence rate of *T. gondii* antibodies in the United States and in Europe during the past 3 decades. This decrease is more striking in countries that had a high prevalence than in those in which it was low. Because meat probably is the main vector of infection in most developed countries, it seems logical to relate this decrease to a less frequent presence of *T. gondii* in meat, which probably results from improved methods in the way the animals are raised and in the processing of meat.[380,381]

Data from one city or single population within that city may not accurately reflect the true prevalence or incidence of infection either in that city or elsewhere. The prevalence of the infection has decreased dramatically in the past 20 years or so but not necessarily in subpopulations, such as Los Angeles Hispanics, Floridians (Haitians), and Salvadorians.

What are the prevalence and incidence of congenital toxoplasmosis (and *T. gondii* infection) in the United States? We have no objective data to answer this question. It should be emphasized that the lack of systematic serologic screening of pregnant women in the United States for acute acquired *T. gondii* infections severely limits our ability to accurately assess the incidence of *T. gondii* infection among pregnant women in different populations and of congenital *T. gondii* infection.

Table 31–16 Prevalence of *Toxoplasma* Antibodies among Pregnant Women of Childbearing Age from Various Geographic Locales, Worldwide

Locale	Reference No.	% Positive
Central African Republic	293	81
Gabon, Africa	294	60
Senegal, Africa	295	4.2
Tanzania, Africa	296	48.5
Togo, tropical Africa	297	~50
Tunis, Africa	298	46.5
Zambia, Africa	299	23
Buenos Aires, Argentina	300	58.9
Buenos Aires Province, Argentina	301	53.4
Melbourne, Australia	302	4
Western Australia	303	35
Vienna, Austria	304	36.7
Bangladesh	305	38.5
Brussels, Belgium	306	56
Belgium	307	46
Cotonou, Republic of Benin	308	53.6
Yadunde, Cameroon	309	77
Santiago, Chile	310	59
Chengdu, China	311	39
Lanzhou, China	312	7.3
Taiwan, China	313	9
Quindio, Colombia	314	60
Pointe-Noire, Congo	315	43
Copenhagen, Denmark	1170	28.7
Denmark	317	27
Egypt (rural area)	318	43
Eastern England	319	7.7
Ethiopia	214	>75
Southern Finland	320	20
Strasbourg, France	1171	36
Franceville (Gabon)	322	71.2
La Guadeloupe, French West Indies	323	~60
Lower Saxony, Germany	324	46
Berlin, Germany	325	54
Greifswald, Germany (northeast)	326	68
Würzburg, Germany	327	41.6
Germany	328	36
Athens, Greece	368	24
Patras, Greece	329	52
Crete, Greece	371	29.5
Guatemala	330	~45
Szeged, Hungary	331	69
India	332	45
Jakarta, Indonesia	333	14
Central Italy	334	49
Urmia, Iran	375	32.8
Hyogo Prefecture, Japan	335	6
Kuwait	1172	58
Kuwait (urban)	372	45.7
Islamic Republic of Mauritania	337	~22
Casablanca, Morocco	338	51
Nepal	339	54.8
Tilburg, The Netherlands	340	~40
Papua New Guinea	341	18
Benue River Basin Area, Nigeria	342	43.7
Ib adan, Nigeria	343	78
Niger Delta, Nigeria	344	~60
Nigeria	342	43.7
Norway	345	10.9
Panama City, Panama	346	~63
Zakopane, Poland	347	36
Lisbon, Portugal	348	64
Santo Domingo	349	47
Riyadh, Saudi Arabia	350	30
Western Scotland	351	13
Central Scotland and Midland England	352	15
Ljubljana, Slovenia	353	34
Barcelona, Spain	354	50

Table 31–16 Prevalence of *Toxoplasma* Antibodies among Pregnant Women of Childbearing Age from Various Geographic Locales, Worldwide—*cont'd*

Locale	Reference No.	% Positive
Barcelona, Spain	376	25.3
Malmo, Sweden	355	40
South Sweden	1173	25.7
Stockholm, Sweden	1173	14
Basal, Switzerland	356	53
Geneva, Switzerland	357	42
Switzerland	358	46.9
Dar Es Salaam, Tanzania	359	35
Chiang Mai, Thailand	360	3
Bangkok, Thailand	361	13
Bangkok, Thailand	362	14
Turkey	354a, 363	65
United Arab Emirates	364	22.9
United States	1174	15
Eastern Tennessee	369	11
Timok Region, eastern Yugoslavia	365	46
Slovenia, Yugoslavia	366, 367	~50
Slovenia, Yugoslavia	374	34

Table 31–17 Prevalence of *Toxoplasma* Antibodies among Pregnant Women and Nonpregnant Women of Childbearing Age from Various Geographic Locales in the United States

Locale	% Positive
Palo Alto, California	10[a]
Birmingham, Alabama	30[b]
Chicago, Illinois	12[c]
Massachusetts	14[d]
Denver, Colorado	3.3[e]
Los Angeles, California	30[f]
Houston, Texas	12[g]
New Hampshire	13[h]

[a]JS Remington, unpublished data, 2004.
[b]From Hunter, 1983.[391]
[c]Personal communication from Dr. Rima McLeod, 1987.
[d]Personal communication from Dr. Roger Eaton, 1998.
[e]Personal communication from Dr. Douglas Hershey, 1986.
[f]Personal communication from Dr. Andrea Kovacs, 1993.
[g]Personal communication from Dr. Fred Bakht, 1993.
[h]Personal communication from Dr. Roger Eaton, 1998.

Numerous variables influence whether congenital transmission will occur. Many of these factors are recognized but poorly understood. They include the strain and virulence of *T. gondii*, inoculum size, route of infection, time during gestation, and immunocompetence of the pregnant woman. All of these also pertain to infection of the fetus and its outcome in the newborn thereafter.

Incidence of Acquired Infection during Pregnancy

Estimates from Prevalence Rates: Mathematical Epidemiologic Models

Once seroconversion occurs, IgG antibodies essentially persist for the life of the affected person. Thus, the prevalence of antibodies increases with increasing age and the proportion of uninfected persons decreases. If the hypothesis is accepted that the risk of acquiring *T. gondii* infection from the environment is the same at any age, and if this yearly seroconversion rate is known, the prevalence of antibodies in relation to age and the proportion of seronegative persons in this population at a given age can be computed easily.[387] Consider as an example a population of infants 1 year of age who are not infected and thus are seronegative: If their risk of acquiring *T. gondii* infection is 10% per year, that is, for a yearly seroconversion rate of 10%, the probability that these infants will still be free of infection (seronegative) is 0.9 at 2 years of age, 0.81 at 3 years of age, 0.729 at 4 years of age, and so on. At age 20, the prevalence of antibodies will be 86.5%, and the proportion of seronegative persons will be 13.5%. The curves shown in Figure 31-4 depict the theoretical antibody prevalence rates, in relation to age, for a fixed yearly seroconversion rate ranging from 0.1% to 20% (representative of possible rates in various locations). The frequency of acquisition of *T. gondii* infection at a given age (the incidence of *T. gondii* infection at that age) is dependent on both the proportion of the population that is seronegative at that age and on the rate of seroconversion. In the example just given, in a population with a 10% yearly seroconversion rate from the age of 1 year, the incidence of acquired infection between 20 and 21 years of age will be 10% of 13.5%—that is, 13.5 per 1000. The balance between the prevalence of immunity due to past infection and the risk of acquiring infection can result in apparently paradoxical findings when one examines the incidence of infection in the young adult. For example, in a population with a yearly seroconversion rate of 5% from the age of 1 year, the prevalence of antibodies will be 62% at age 20 and the incidence of infection between ages 20 and 21 will be 18.9 per 1000. Thus, owing to the higher number of seronegatives, a lower constant risk of infection—5% instead of 10% per year—results in a higher frequency of infection acquired by the young adult.

Taking into account the number of pregnancies by age group, and the age distribution of pregnant women in France, Papoz and co-workers[382] set up a mathematical epidemiologic

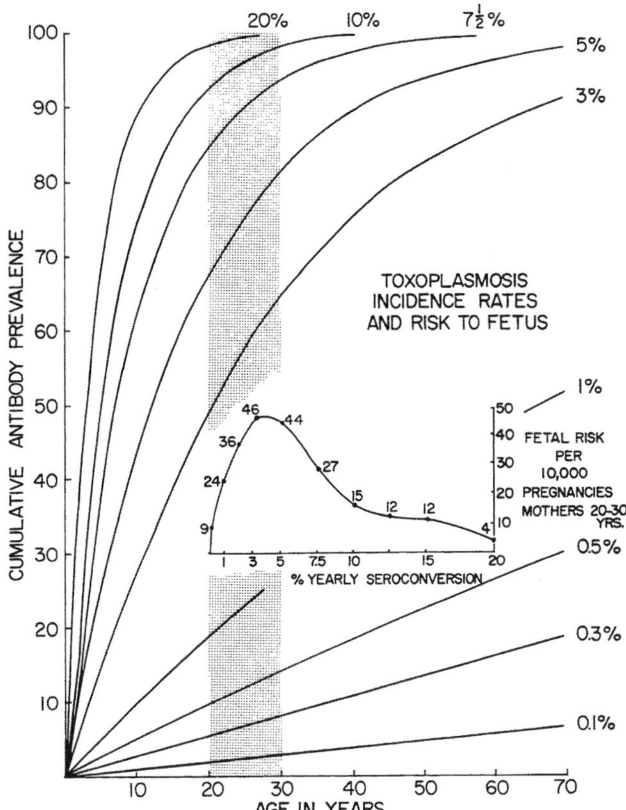

Figure 31–4 Incidence rates in mother and risk to fetus. (Data from Frenkel JK. *Toxoplasma* in and around us. BioScience 23:343-352, 1973.)

model to determine the expected frequency of acquired infection in France. This model was applied to a survey of the prevalence of *T. gondii* antibodies that they performed during 1982 and 1983; 7605 women from ages 14 to 44 years were tested. The prevalence of antibodies rose from 52% before the age of 20 to 83% after the age of 40 years and averaged 63.5%. The yearly seroconversion rate calculated for each of the 1-year age groups ranged from 2.7% to 5.1%; the average rate was 3.69%. The authors calculated that in the absence of intervention during pregnancy, the incidence of infection during pregnancy should be 10.6 per 1000 pregnancies. This rate is close to the highest possible rate during pregnancy in those epidemiologic conditions. These estimations of the frequency of acquired toxoplasmosis during pregnancy calculated from the increase in prevalence of antibodies with increasing age are based on the hypothesis that the risk of infection has been constant over time. As discussed earlier, however, clear evidence indicates that the prevalence of antibodies among pregnant women has decreased over the past decades in France, as well as in other countries. This finding suggests a decrease in the risk of acquiring infection and, thus, in seroconversion rates.

Larsen and Lebech[383] published a modified mathematical epidemiologic model for prediction of the frequency of *T. gondii* infection during pregnancy in situations of changing infection rates. They concluded that in countries in transition from high to low infection rates, it is likely that the influence of decreasing immunity of the population will at least temporarily more than outweigh the influence of the falling infection rates, resulting in a higher number of infected pregnant women. This important conclusion is used in the following discussion.

Estimates from Prospective Studies of Acquired Infection during Pregnancy and Consequences of Health Education

During the early 1950s, congenital toxoplasmosis was recognized as a frequent cause of severe neonatal disease in France,[113,384] and the feasibility of screening pregnant women for acquired infection during pregnancy was investigated. During the first survey performed in Paris at Pinard and Baudelocque Hospitals, sera obtained from pregnant women at first prenatal visit (i.e., at the end of the second month of gestation) were stored frozen. After delivery, these sera were examined in parallel with cord sera. Of the 2228 pregnant women studied, 1872 had a positive dye test result at the beginning of pregnancy, for a prevalence of 84%; 356 (16%) were seronegative at first prenatal examination. Seroconversion from a negative to a positive dye test result was observed in 11 women, for an incidence of 11 of 356 (3%) among *seronegative* women. Because the mean time elapsed between the first prenatal examination and delivery was 6 months, the yearly seroconversion rate was estimated to be 60 per 1000. With reference to the entire group of 2228 pregnant women, both seronegative and seropositive, the incidence of seroconversion was 11 of 2228 (0.49%). Because these women were observed for a period of 6 months and because the duration of pregnancy is 9 months, this corresponds to an incidence rate of 7.3 per 1000 pregnancies. (These different means of expressing the frequency of *T. gondii* infection during pregnancy frequently result in misunderstandings in comparing data reported by different investigators.)

The high prevalence of antibodies in the population of women of childbearing age in the Paris area suggested that a simple program for screening *T. gondii* infection during pregnancy was possible. From 1961 to 1970, women in their second month of gestation who attended the Centres Prenataux of the Caisse d'Assurance Maladie were tested for *T. gondii* antibodies. Those with a negative dye test result were examined again at month 7 and again at the time of delivery. The examinations were timed to allow identification of women who seroconverted so that appropriate treatment could be given and to permit evaluation of their newborns specifically for the presence of *T. gondii* infection at birth. In the 2493 seronegative women who were repeatedly tested during pregnancy, 73 seroconversions were observed. Because the mean time elapsed between the first and last serum sampling was 5½ months, the yearly seroconversion rate was 64 per 1000. During the years of the study, the prevalence of dye test antibodies was observed to be decreasing among the study population of women: The prevalence was 83.5% in 1961 and 72% in 1970 (M.E Seror and J.J. Hazemann, personal communication to G Desmonts). Thus, according to the mathematical epidemiologic model set up by Larsen and Lebech,[383] the incidence of *T. gondii* infection acquired during pregnancy probably was rising.

Serologic screening for *T. gondii* infection during pregnancy became common practice in France and in several European countries during those years. It also should be noted that the life cycle of the parasite was elucidated in the years 1970 to

1971, so that it became possible to instruct women about the mode of transmission of *T. gondii* and how they could avoid becoming infected. Whereas this health education was carefully attempted in some obstetric centers, no attempt at education was made in others.

Table 31-14 shows the yearly conversion rates observed before 1970 and those observed after 1970 in three obstetric centers located in the Paris area. The sera all were tested in a single laboratory (G Desmonts). In one center (Hospital X), little or no information was provided on how seronegative women might avoid infection. The observed seroconversion rate was 59 per 1000, a rate that was essentially identical to the values observed before 1970 (60 or 64 per 1000). The seroconversion rate was significantly lower when health education was attempted, especially when explanatory drawings were provided to seronegative women. Thoumsin and colleagues reported a summary of 22 years of screening for *T. gondii* infection during pregnancy in Liege, Belgium.[379] From 1966 to 1987, 20,901 pregnant women attending the Department of Obstetrics of the C.H.R. of Liege were screened. The numbers of seroconversions observed were 129 (6.4%) among 2027 seronegative women from 1966 to 1975 and 74 (2.8%) among 2601 women from 1976 to 1981. After 1981, prophylactic counseling was provided by a specially trained nurse to all seronegative pregnant women. From 1982 to 1987, the number of seroconversions observed was 48 of 3859 (1.2%). The authors do not state the mean time during which their patients were examined for possible seroconversion. If it was approximately 6 months, these data would suggest that the yearly seroconversion rate was greater than 120 per 1000 before 1975, 56 per 1000 from 1976 to 1981, and 24 per 1000 from 1982 to 1987. These values demonstrate a decrease in the risk of infection quite similar to that shown in Table 31-14.

Since 1978, it has been obligatory under French law to test pregnant women for *T. gondii* infection acquired during gestation. The common practice is to perform a test for *T. gondii* antibodies at the first prenatal visit (usually at weeks 10 to 15). The result is reported to the patient; if it is negative, the laboratory that performed the test must send a letter to the woman describing hygienic measures she can practice to avoid infection with *T. gondii*. Serologic testing of seronegative women is repeated monthly until delivery to identify those who seroconvert. If the test performed at the first prenatal visit is suggestive of a recently acquired infection, an avidity assay should be performed. In some instances, a second sample of serum is obtained to attempt to determine whether the infection was acquired during the first few weeks of pregnancy or earlier. One consequence of this procedure is that the surveillance for acquired *T. gondii* infection now encompasses the entire pregnancy, including the first 10 weeks and not solely the last 30 weeks of gestation, as was the case during the first surveys performed in France (discussed earlier).

Jeannel and associates[385] reported the results of a survey performed in the Paris area between 1981 and 1983. The prevalence of *T. gondii* antibodies was estimated to be 67.3%. Among 2216 pregnant women at risk, the rate of seroconversion was 1.6% per 9 months of pregnancy, which corresponds to a yearly seroconversion rate equal to 21 per 1000. A national inquiry regarding the present status of *T. gondii* infection during pregnancy in France was set up by the Reseau National de la Sante Publique in 1995.[378] The medical data for each of the 13,459 women whose delivery occurred in France during the first week of February 1995 were analyzed. The overall prevalence of *T. gondii* antibodies was 54.3%. *T. gondii* infection was acquired during pregnancy by 89 women, representing an incidence of 6.6 per 1000 pregnancies. If the incidence was reported in only those women who were seronegative at the beginning of pregnancy, the percentage was 1.48%. This corresponds approximately to a yearly seroconversion rate of 19 per 1000, essentially the same as it was 20 years earlier among patients who received health education (see Table 31-14) and the same as the rate observed by Jeannel and associates between 1981 and 1983. The incidence among primiparous women was twice that of multiparous women. This finding suggests that women who knew they were seronegative because they had been repeatedly tested for infection with *T. gondii* during a previous pregnancy tried to avoid acquiring this infection when they again became pregnant.

Jenum and co-workers[132] reported the results of a screening program that was conducted in Norway from 1992 to 1994. The prevalence of *T. gondii* infection in Norway is very low when compared with that in France, where it is still high. All 35,940 women examined received an information folder that contained health care advice with specific precautions to be taken to prevent *T. gondii* infection. The first sample of serum was collected at approximately the tenth gestational week and examined for *T. gondii* antibodies. Retesting was requested for seronegative women at approximately weeks 22 and 38 of gestation. Tests for evidence of acute infection also were performed on the serum sample obtained during the tenth week to identify infections that had occurred during the first 10 weeks of pregnancy. Hence, the model of the survey was planned to encompass the first 38 weeks of gestation. The average time during which women remained under observation for the study was, in fact, 34 weeks. The prevalence of antibodies due to infection acquired before pregnancy was 10.9%. Among 32,033 seronegative women, 47 (0.147%) fulfilled the criteria for acquired infection during pregnancy. The seroconversion rate calculated for 40 weeks of pregnancy was 0.173%. This percentage corresponds to a yearly seroconversion rate of 2.3 per 1000. Jenum and co-workers observed a higher number of seroconversions during the first trimester of pregnancy (0.287% per 40 weeks, which is a yearly seroconversion rate equal to 3.8 per 1000) than during the second and third trimesters. They suggest that this difference might be related to the health education advice given at the first prenatal visit.

The differences in the frequency of *T. gondii* infection from one country to another can be illustrated by the differences in the incidence rates as well as in the prevalence rates. As an example, the yearly seroconversion rates calculated from the data from Norway[132] are nearly eight times lower than those calculated from the data obtained in 1995 in France,[378] and the antibody prevalence rate at the age of pregnancy is five times lower in Norway than it is in France. In the Paris area, the yearly seroconversion rate observed during pregnancy was approximately 60 per 1000 during the late 1950s and early 1960s, and it was about 19 per 1000 in 1995. This lower seroconversion rate was observed as early as 1974, however, when instruction became available to pregnant women on how they could avoid becoming infected (see Table 31-14).[386] As judged by the results of more recent studies,[378,385] no significant decrease in seroconversion rates occurred between 1974 and 1995. The decrease from approximately 60 per 1000 to approximately 20 per 1000 occurred during the early 1970s. In considering the incidence rates, that is, the frequency of seroconversions in the total population of pregnant women (seropositive as well as seronegative), no significant difference is found between the incidence rates observed in the late 1950s and in 1995; the incidence rate during the first prospective study performed in Paris before 1960 was 7.3 per 1000 pregnancies. The incidence reported by Ancelle and colleagues[378] in 1996 was 6.6 (± 1.4) per 1000 pregnancies. In this epidemiologic situation, that is, in a country in transition from a very high to a lower infection rate, the influence of decreasing immunity in the population should have outweighed the influence of the falling infection rate, resulting in a higher number of women who acquired the infection during gestation (despite the decreasing risk of acquiring the infection in the general population).[383] This effect was not observed, and the most likely reason is that health care education of pregnant women reduced the risk of acquiring *T. gondii* infection during pregnancy.

The seroconversion rates observed during these relatively recent surveys from France and from Norway can be used to calculate an expected prevalence rate according to the methods discussed earlier.[382,383,387] This calculated "expected" prevalence rate is lower than the observed prevalence rates in both surveys. This finding suggests that the risk of becoming infected with *T. gondii* is lower among pregnant women than in nonpregnant women, perhaps also the result of health care education provided at the first prenatal visit. Thus, the timing of providing pregnant women with the appropriate information on prevention of infection with *T. gondii* at the first prenatal visit probably skews results of prospective studies of acquired *T. gondii* infection during pregnancy by selectively reducing the frequency of infection acquired during the second half of pregnancy.

Prevalence of Congenital *Toxoplasma gondii* Infection

Indirect Estimates from Incidence Rates of Maternal Toxoplasma gondii Infection

The prevalence of congenital *T. gondii* infection can be estimated from the incidence rate of *T. gondii* infection acquired during pregnancy by multiplying the figure for the number of mothers who acquire infection during pregnancy by the transmission rate of the parasite to the fetus. For example, according to Frenkel (see Fig. 31-4), if the yearly seroconversion rate in a population is 30 per 1000, the rate of neonatal *T. gondii* infection will be 4.6 per 1000 births. From the epidemiologic model derived from a survey performed in France in 1982 to 1983, Papoz and colleagues[382] calculated that the risk of neonatal *T. gondii* infection to be 6.4 per 1000 births.

A more recent study of the age-specific prevalence of *T. gondii* antibodies in the United States used data and sera from the third National Health and Nutrition Examination and Survey (NHANES III, 1989 to 1994, $N = 17{,}658$).[388] The investigators modeled the incidence of acute infection in pregnant women using the declining prevalence from the study in military recruits and the age-specific prevalence from the NHANES III study. They estimate that the incidence among seronegative women is 0.27% during pregnancy in the United States. With a birth cohort of 4 million and an estimated overall transmission rate of 33%, approximately 3500 children are expected to be born with congenital toxoplasmosis each year in the United States. This rate should vary by geographic region and may be declining if the trend demonstrated in the military recruit study is continuing (J McAuley, personal communication to JS Remington, 1998). Unfortunately, at present, objective data are lacking on the prevalence of congenital *T. gondii* infection or congenital toxoplasmosis for the United States. Because screening of pregnant women in the United States is not systematic, our ability to accurately assess the incidence of *T. gondii* infection among pregnant women in different populations and of congenital *T. gondii* infection is limited. Data from one city or single population within that city may not accurately reflect the true prevalence or incidence of infection either in that city or elsewhere. Although the prevalence of the infection has decreased in some areas of the United States during the past 20 years or so, this is not necessarily the case in subpopulations even in those same areas.

Direct Estimates from Studies at Birth or during Infancy

Estimates from Clinical Information or from Findings at Autopsy. Estimates from clinical observations and from autopsy findings are based on data derived mainly from older studies,[119,120] which underestimated the actual prevalence, because congenital infection uncommonly results in stillbirth or neonatal death and frequently is not diagnosed during infancy because of subclinical infection in the infant and delayed occurrence of signs of infection.[389,390]

Estimates from Serologic Screening of Neonates or Infants. One of the first studies that relied on determination of total IgM levels in cord blood, followed by serologic testing of infants who had elevated levels, was performed at the University of Alabama.[391] As stressed by the investigators, such studies result in an underestimate of the true incidence of the infection and the disease, because infants with congenital infection may not have an increase in total IgM in their cord blood or demonstrable IgM *T. gondii* antibodies. This survey revealed what has proved to be a historical trend toward a decrease in prevalence of congenital *T. gondii* infection in Alabama; the observed rate was 2 per 1000 during the first year of the study and 0.6 per 1000 during the last year. Although different methods were used in a later study by this same group, the observed rate for the later study was approximately 0.1 per 1000 births.[391]

The Commonwealth of Massachusetts began screening newborn sera in January 1986 to determine the incidence of congenital *T. gondii* infection. Blood specimens are collected on filter paper and utilized to test for IgM antibodies by the sensitive IgM enzyme-linked immunosorbent assay (ELISA). From 1986 to 1998, 99 infants were detected who had IgM *T. gondii* antibodies, reflecting an incidence of approximately 1 in 10,000 births (R Eaton, personal communication to JS Remington, 1998). Although a careful follow-up evaluation was not performed for all seronegative infants, it is known that the diagnosis was missed in at least six infants in whom IgM antibodies were not detected but who were referred by local physicians. In one of these later-diagnosed children, *T. gondii* was isolated from cerebrospinal fluid; the infection was suspected on clinical grounds in this child, who was born prematurely with hydrocephalus, cerebral calcifications, and bilateral chorioretinitis. Thus, this reported incidence is lower than the actual incidence despite the sensitivity of the method used to detect IgM antibodies of *T. gondii*. Nevertheless, if as many as 50% of cases were missed (which is unlikely) with the methodology used by the New England Regional Screening Program, an incidence of 1 per 10,000 births is strikingly different from the incidence of 1.3 per 1000 reported by Kimball and co-workers in 1971 from a prospective screening study of pregnant women in New York City.[122] With the discovery of the importance of detecting IgA and IgE antibodies (see "Diagnosis" section) in the newborn, serologic studies of newborns such as those being performed in Massachusetts should detect a higher percentage of infected infants.

The Danish Congenital Toxoplasmosis Study Group has published results of their feasibility study of neonatal screening for *T. gondii* infection in the absence of prenatal treatment.[392] The focus of their study was different from that of the Massachusetts group in that they sought to determine the prevalence of the infection among live neonates and the maternofetal transmission rate in infected mothers who had received no treatment. Secondarily, they assessed the feasibility and acceptability of neonatal screening using *T. gondii* IgM antibody testing on samples from phenylketonuria (PKU) cards. They reported a surprisingly low transmission rate of 19.4%. The researchers state that a neonatal screening program based on detection of IgM *T. gondii* antibodies alone identifies between 70% and 80% of cases of congenital toxoplasmosis, but not all pregnancies and infants in their study were thoroughly evaluated, thus making the data difficult to evaluate. Although this detection rate is certainly preferable to no screening, the possible occurrence of significant numbers of false-negative reactions is disturbing. Yet Lebech and his colleagues stated that their IgM method with PKU cards could be used in large-scale newborn screening for congenital *T. gondii* infection. It is hoped that improved technology will be developed to reduce the numbers of infected infants who will go undetected with use of presently available methods.[393] The group in Massachusetts uses a special IgM method that is designed to be highly sensitive, attempting to thereby lessen the likelihood of false-negative results. No data are provided in the publication of the Danish group on sensitivity or specificity, or of the Boston Group on sensitivity, of their IgM antibody method in newborns. Denmark began screening of all newborns rather than pregnant women beginning in 1999 (E Petersen, personal communication to JS Remington).[392,394]

Even if the prevalence of congenital infection is underestimated, however, the present data (at least from Alabama and Massachusetts) strongly suggest that the rate has significantly decreased during the last 2 decades in the United States. This decrease in the prevalence rate of congenital *T. gondii* infection parallels the historical decrease in antibody prevalence rate observed in the adult. This would be expected from the epidemiologic models discussed earlier; in a population in which the seroprevalence rate was rather low (well below 50% in the adult, as it is in the United States), a decrease in the risk of acquiring infection immediately results in a decrease in the incidence of acquired infection in women in the childbearing age group.

An attempt to define the prevalence of congenital *T. gondii* infection in infants in the Paris area was made in a cooperative study with the Centre de Bilans de Santé de la Caisse Primaire d'Assurance Maladie de Paris.[395] An opportunity arose to perform serologic tests because infants at 10 months of age underwent a general health examination. From 1970 to 1980, 26,402 infants were examined. *T. gondii* antibodies were present in the serum of 295 (1.1%), and all had high titers in the dye test. Of the mothers, 51 had high dye test titers, suggesting that the infection present in the infant was congenital in origin. Two-hundred ten mothers had either a negative or a low dye test titer, suggesting that their infection had been acquired long before the recent pregnancy. In their infants, congenital infection was considered as excluded or unlikely; their infection was postnatally acquired. In 34 cases, it was not possible to decide between congenital or postnatally acquired infection. Thus, the incidence of acquired infection during the first 10 months of life was between 7.9 and 9.2 per 1000. The prevalence of congenital infection was between 1.9 and 3.2 per 1000. None of the infants had severe toxoplasmosis. The fact that congenital infection was asymptomatic would be expected because this cohort was recruited through general health examination of 10-month-old infants. On yearly follow-up of these children, however, chorioretinitis was present or was discovered in 12 of 54 (22%). This prevalence rate of congenital infection of approximately 2 per 1000, observed between 1970 and 1980, is three times lower than the risk (6.4 per 1000) calculated by Papoz and associates[382] from their epidemiologic model and the antibody prevalence survey among pregnant women that they performed in 1982 and 1983. During this decade (1970 to 1980), screening for *T. gondii* infection during pregnancy was becoming a common practice in France, and information on how to avoid acquiring the infection was provided to seronegative women. We believe that health education might have been responsible for this difference between the expected risk calculated by Papoz and associates and the lower prevalence rate that was observed.

Effects of Systematic Screening of Pregnant Women at Risk on the Prevalence of Congenital *Toxoplasma gondii* Infection and of Congenital Toxoplasmosis

The purpose of the first attempts at systematic serologic screening was to identify pregnant women at risk, to try to prevent congenital toxoplasmosis or, if such infection was present, to allow for early instigation of treatment. Once the life cycle of the parasite was elucidated, primary preventive measures were possible through education of seronegative women (see "Prevention" section and Table 31-62). This is now currently done in several European countries and has proved moderately effective, as judged by the data discussed earlier; acquired *T. gondii* infection during pregnancy apparently is three times less frequent in France than it would be were no information provided to seronegative pregnant women in regard to the sources of infection and how they may reduce their risk of acquiring the infection. This estimation is very close to the conclusions of Foulon and colleagues,[306] who calculated that in Brussels, Belgium, primary preventive measures reduced the seroconversion rates during pregnancy by 63%. Even better results are possible, however. One critical point is the time at which this education is provided. In most cases, this intervention occurs during the first prenatal visit, at approximately the tenth week of pregnancy. This timing does not reduce the number of infections acquired during the first 10 weeks of gestation or the number of seroconversions that occur within 2 weeks after the first prenatal visit, because women whose seroconversion occurs at this time probably were in the initial stage of the infection (during which parasitemia occurs before antibodies become detectable in the serum) at the time they received the instruction. Thus, the results of such an education program can only be a reduction in the number of infections that occur later during pregnancy. Because late acquired infections are those for which the rate of congenital transmission is the highest (resulting primarily in subclinical cases), it is understandable that in addition to a lower number of infections acquired during gestation, health education, if provided at first prenatal visit at about the tenth week of pregnancy, should result in a lower rate of transmission than observed in the previous surveys performed before the means by which *T. gondii* is horizontally transmitted to humans was known. In addition, the proportion of infected fetuses with the more severe form of congenital toxoplasmosis might be higher unless treatment during gestation is effective in the infected fetus.

Screening for *T. gondii* infection during pregnancy is now a common practice in several European countries. After surveys performed in Austria in the 1950s and 1960s, a national program was introduced in 1975 that required serologic examination of every pregnant woman for *T. gondii* infection. In cases with suspected primary infection acquired during pregnancy, the woman receives immediate treatment. From 1975 through 1998, no cases of congenital toxoplasmosis were registered in women who had been tested and (in instances of recent infection) given treatment in accordance with the regulations. Moreover, no recommendations for induced abortion had to be given, and no serious side effects of treatment were observed. The incidence of congenital *T. gondii* infection in Austria is now 1 to 2 cases per 10,000 newborns, compared with the incidence of 20 to 35 per 10,000 that would be expected without the screening and its consequences (H Aspöck, personal communication to JS Remington, 1998).[304,396]

In France, congenital toxoplasmosis was the most frequent fetopathy in the years 1950 to 1960. For example, in this period, several cases of congenital toxoplasmosis were diagnosed each year among approximately 1000 premature infants admitted annually to l'Hôpital de l'Institut de Puériculture de Paris. In 1957, for instance, 7 cases were diagnosed among 1085 newborns. In the same hospital, however, only two cases have been observed between 1980 and 1990. Within 40 years the pediatrician has been witness to a dramatic change in the presenting signs of the disease (J Couvreur, written communication to JS Remington, 1998). In the past, patients were referred to the specialized toxoplasmosis clinic in Paris because they had clinical symptoms or often severe signs that suggested congenital toxoplasmosis. For instance, in a group of 147 neonates or infants with congenital *T. gondii* infection studied between 1949 and 1960, 62.5% had signs of central nervous system (CNS) involvement (with hydrocephalus in two thirds of the patients), and 32.5% had retinochoroiditis without clinical evidence of CNS involvement. Despite their being asymptomatic, most patients now attend the specialized clinic because they are suspected of having, or are diagnosed as having, congenital *T. gondii* infection. Congenital *T. gondii* infection is subclinical and remains subclinical in a majority of them. For example, congenital infection remained subclinical in 166 of 234 infants (71%) observed between 1984 and 1992. In this group, 60 of 234 (26%) had a retinal scar but no CNS involvement; CNS involvement with or without hydrocephalus was present in 8 of 234 (3%) of these infants. At present, severe neurologic or ocular involvement, or both, is observed only among infants born to women in the following patient groups: patients referred from foreign countries where screening is not performed during pregnancy (e.g., Morocco, Algeria, United Kingdom), mothers who for any reason were not screened during pregnancy, mothers who were immunodeficient, and mothers who were erroneously considered to be immune. With these exceptions, in which the clinical status may be considered abnormal (see "Chronic Maternal *Toxoplasma* Infection"), prenatal screening for maternal *T. gondii* infection during pregnancy has proved effective as a preventive measure for congenital toxoplasmosis in France (see Table 31-6).

Testing for anti-*T. gondii* antibodies in Italy is free. Testing takes place before conception and in the first trimester and is repeated monthly for pregnant women who so desire. This program was initiated in 1998. In a study of this screening program by Mombro and co-workers,[397] 60 mothers seroconverted or had probable acute acquired infection during gestation. No congenitally infected infants were born to women identified with seroconversion or probable acute acquired infection in their first trimester. Thirteen (21%) infected infants were born to mothers who seroconverted, and 2 (4%) infected infants were born to mothers with probable infections acquired during gestation. Transmission rates were 5 of 29 seroconverters (17%) and 2 of 12 (17%) with probable infection in the second trimester; 8 of 23 pregnant women (35%) acquired their infection in the third trimester.[397]

PATHOGENESIS

Factors Operative during Initial Infection

Virulence of Toxoplasma gondii

An isoenzyme analysis of *T. gondii* isolates demonstrated that certain patterns correlated with virulence of tachyzoites for mice.[398] Similar results have been obtained by restriction fragment length polymorphism (RFLP) analysis.[399] Population genetic analysis revealed three predominant lineages designated strain types I, II, and III.[400,401] A majority of human cases of toxoplasmosis (both postnatally acquired and congenital) are due to type II[401,402]; 10% to 25% are due to type I. It is likely that virulence, as well as inoculum size and the genetic background of the infected person, influences transmission and severity of congenital toxoplasmosis.

In a study by Ajzenberg and associates[403] of clonal type of isolates of *T. gondii* in France between 1987 and 2001, almost all (85% in the whole series, and 96% in 57 consecutive isolates from a laboratory in Limoges and a laboratory in Paris) of 86 congenitally infected children had clonal type II parasites. Type I and atypical isolates were not found in cases of asymptomatic or mild congenital toxoplasmosis. Three isolates with atypical genotypes, which were virulent in mice, were associated with severe congenital infection. In four cases, *T. gondii* was isolated only from placenta, the infant was not infected, and all four were of clonal type I. Type II isolates occurred in persons with different levels of severity of their signs and symptoms. The main factor influencing severity was reported to be time of acquisition of the infection during gestation. This finding contrasts with that in a small series from Spain (where serologic screening during gestation is not the standard of care, as it is in France) in which all isolates were of clonal type I.[404]

In a preliminary study, Grigg and colleagues[405,406] reported that very severe eye disease in adults was associated with infection with type I or recombinant clonal types of parasites. These results are reminiscent of the findings reported by Ajzenberg and colleagues,[403] who noted severe disease in congenitally infected children with parasites with atypical genotypes. By contrast, in a guinea pig model studied by Flori and associates,[89] the highest levels of parasitemia and highest rates of transmission, neonatal death, and pathology (e.g., hepatitis) were associated with clonal type II infections.[89] In the future, data concerning relationship of clonal type to frequency of transmission of congenital *T. gondii* infection or severity of illness in those infected will be of interest.

In a separate study by Romand, clonal type of parasites was not included in their analysis. Nonetheless, the highest amounts of parasite DNA detected in amniotic fluid by PCR assay were associated with the most severe disease in the newborn and most often were related to time in gestation when the infection was acquired (as discussed in "Polymerase Chain Reaction Assay" under "Diagnosis"). It is unclear at present whether any relationship exists between a specific clonal type(s) and either transmission or severity of the infection in the newborn or progression of disease in the congenitally infected infant.

A recent report and accompanying editorial[407,408] suggest that the amount of genetic variability in the three predominant clonal types (I, II, and III) indicates that they are derived from a single recombination (cross) of two ancestral strains.[402,407] The authors of this report estimated that the recombination occurred at the time during which humans began to use domesticated livestock for food[408] and was associated with the acquisition of direct oral infectivity (i.e., ability of bradyzoite to be infectious when ingested). The three strains, which are clonal and show little genetic variation, have only one of two possible alleles for genes at many different loci. From the alleles present in the three strains, the genotype of the diploid ancestor can be inferred.

In Brazil, clonal type I/III recombinant parasites have been identified that appear to have different biologic behavior in mice and cause far more prominent eye infections in older children and adults.[409] Sixty percent of Brazilian children younger than 10 years of age in Minas Gerais state have serologic evidence of infection.[249,409-411] Eighty percent of adults are seropositive, and 20% of these have recurrent eye disease.[411] Fifty percent of adults older than 60 years have eye disease. Whether the manifestations of congenital toxoplasmosis within these populations will differ remains to be determined. The incidence of overt congenital toxoplasmosis in São Paulo appears to be relatively high; for example, between 2001 and 2004, one physician in a children's hospital cared for 31 newborn infants (24 symptomatic) with congenital toxoplasmosis diagnosed by serologic testing or PCR assay (E Diniz, personal communication to R McLeod, 2004).

In Guyana, ancient clonal types of *T. gondii* have been lethal,[403] but whether differences in congenital infections exist with such unusual clonal types of the parasite is not known.

Role of Cells and Antibody

After local invasion (usually in the intestines), the organisms invade cells directly or are phagocytosed. They multiply intracellularly, causing host cell disruption, and then invade contiguous cells. Whereas human monocytes and neutrophils kill the vast majority of ingested *T. gondii* organisms, tachyzoites survive within macrophages derived in vitro from peripheral blood monocytes.[412-414] Data have shown that human peritoneal and alveolar macrophages kill *T. gondii*.[415] Cytotoxic T lymphocyte–mediated lysis of *T. gondii*–infected target cells did not lead to death of the intracellular parasites, however, indicating that intracellular *T. gondii* remains alive after lysis of host cells by cytolytic T cells.[416,417] The presence of persistent parasitemia observed in humans[104] and animals[86,418] can best be explained by the existence of intracellular parasites in the circulation.

T. gondii invades every organ and tissue of the human host except non-nucleated red blood cells, although evidence indicates that invasion of these cells may occur as well.[419] Termination of continued tissue destruction by *T. gondii* depends both on the development of cell-mediated immunity and on antibodies. Continued destruction may occur in those sites where ready access to circulating antibody is impeded (e.g., CNS, eye). Despite the ability of antibody in the presence of complement to kill extracellular *T. gondii* effectively in vitro, the intracellular habitat of this protozoon protects it from the effects of circulating antibody.

Cyst formation can be demonstrated as early as the eighth day of experimental infection.[56] Cysts persist in multiple organs and tissues after immunity is acquired, probably for the life of the host.

The barrier to passive diffusion of antibodies into brain and eye has been given as an explanation of the continued proliferation of the parasite in these sites at the same time at which it is disappearing from extraneural sites.[420] This barrier also has been employed as an explanation of what has been interpreted as a greater latent infection of the CNS than of extraneural tissues. Nevertheless, cysts may persist and may be abundant in tissues where antibody is not opposed by such a barrier (e.g., cardiac and skeletal muscle).[420]

The ability of the pregnant woman to control multiplication and spread of *T. gondii* depends not only on specific antibody synthesis but also on the time of appearance of cell-mediated immunity. In addition to the immunosuppression associated with pregnancy itself, cell-mediated immunity, at least as measured by antigen-specific lymphocyte transformation, may not be demonstrable for weeks or even months after acute infection with *T. gondii* in humans.[421,422] Although the importance of cellular immunity in the control of the initial acute infection in humans has not been defined, it is likely, from what is known about the immunology of toxoplasmosis in animal models[29,30] and studies with human immune cells,[423-426] that cell-mediated immunity plays a major role. The helper T cell type 2 (T_H2) bias (toward humoral immunity and away from cellular immunity) established during normal gestation may compromise successful immunity against *T. gondii*, which requires a strong T_H1 response. In addition, it has been proposed that a strong T_H1 response against *T. gondii* may overcome the protective T_H2 cytokines at the maternal-fetal interface and result in fetal loss.[427,428] For a discussion of the immunoregulation of *T. gondii* infection and toxoplasmosis, the reader is referred to other sources.[28-30,429-436]

Age

Evidence for the supposition that maturity is an important factor in host resistance to *T. gondii* comes not only from experiments that have revealed remarkable resistance to *T. gondii* in adult rats[437] and chickens[438] when compared with newborns of those species but from observations in humans as well. The infection in the mother frequently goes unrecognized, whereas the newborn may be severely damaged, even when infection of the fetus occurs after the fifth month of gestation (when maternal antibody first becomes available to the fetus and immunoglobulin and complement synthesis can occur[439,440]). Deckert-Schlüter and co-workers established a model of congenital *T. gondii* encephalitis in mice following prenatal infection with the parasite.[441] Disease in the newborn mice during the first 2 weeks of life exhibited the key histopathologic features of human congenital toxoplasmic encephalitis, including foci of necrosis, intracerebral calcifications, and ventriculitis. Of importance, the findings differed significantly from the histopathologic features found in adult mice with toxoplasmic encephalitis. The immune response in the prenatally infected mice was mediated predominantly by the innate immune system, with preferential recruitment of macrophages and granulocytes to the brain.

Gender

That the lymphadenopathic form of toxoplasmosis is more commonly observed in females has been recognized for many years.[442] In studies in laboratory animals, Kittas and colleagues demonstrated that female mice are more likely than male mice to die from *T. gondii* infection and that mortality rates were increased in gonadectomized male and female mice given estrogens.[443,444] Results of Alexander and his group[29] conclusively demonstrated that gender differences in susceptibility to *T. gondii* operate at the level of the innate immune response, as measured by interleukin-12 (IL-12) and IFN-γ production. Pathologic changes were more severe and the mortality rate was higher in female mice than in their male counterparts; production of the cytokines at high levels was significantly earlier in the male mice.

Role of Human Leukocyte Antigen Class II Genes

The frequency of the human leukocyte antigen (HLA) class II gene DQ3 was found to be increased in infants with congenital toxoplasmosis and hydrocephalus relative to the frequency of this gene in the U.S. population or in infants with congenital toxoplasmosis who did not have hydrocephalus.[445] Of interest is that this unique frequency of DQ3 also was noted to be a genetic marker of susceptibility to development of toxoplasmic encephalitis in patients with AIDS.[446] HLA class II DQ genes function in transgenic mice to protect against brain parasite burden. DQ1 protects better than DQ3. This observation is consonant with the observation that the DQ3 gene is more frequent in infants with congenital toxoplasmosis with hydrocephalus than in those without hydrocephalus, and than in the U.S. population.[445]

Reinfection

Although survival from the acute stages of the initial *T. gondii* infection usually results in resistance to reinfection, the immunity associated with the chronic (latent) infection is only relative. Immunity to *T. gondii* in mice protects against but does not necessarily prevent reinfection.[447-452] Mice immunized with one strain of *T. gondii* and subsequently challenged with another strain have both strains encysted in their tissues. This undoubtedly occurs in humans also, but its significance is unknown (see "Transmission" section).

Factors Operative during Latent Infection

Cyst Rupture

Factors that influence tachyzoite and bradyzoite interconversion are critical to understanding the pathogenesis of recrudescent infection.

Histologic evidence suggesting that cyst rupture concurs in humans has been reported.[453,454] Indirect evidence in favor of cyst rupture in the normal host is suggested by the frequent development of new retinal lesions contiguous to the border of older scars and is reported in the studies by Lainson[56] and van der Waaij.[455] In the brains of chronically infected mice, it is not unusual to find large and small cysts close together, suggesting the possibility that cyst rupture or "leakage" of bradyzoites has caused the satellite cysts. It is not clear whether the satellite cysts are the result of cyst rupture or whether they simply developed at the same time as did the larger cysts in the same area.

Huldt has demonstrated fluorescence around *T. gondii* cysts by using the immunofluorescent antibody (IFA) method.[456] Her results suggest that antigen may "leak" from cysts. That this antigen does not excite an inflammatory response is suggested by the lack of any cellular reaction around almost all cysts observed in histologic sections of tissue from chronically infected animals. Under certain circumstances, leakage may excite an inflammatory response in which previously committed lymphocytes participate, perhaps releasing a cytokine that disrupts the cyst wall. Release of enzymes from intact or degenerating neutrophils or macrophages might also result in destruction of the cyst wall with liberation of parasites.

Organisms that are intracellular and located within cysts are protected from the action of antibody and cell-mediated immunity. Changes in the host cell membrane that may occur at the time of infection might predispose the infected cell to disruption by lymphokine-activated killer cells[423] or lymphocytes.[30,426,457] Cyst rupture would lead to release of viable organisms that, if released into areas deficient in antibody (e.g., brain and retina), could result in significant tissue damage.

Persistence of "Active" Infection

Frenkel has suggested that cyst rupture is responsible for underlying persistent immunity and antibody and that the encysted form of the organism causes localized or generalized relapse.[19] Another possibility is that organisms that have resided intracellularly as terminal colonies or pseudocysts for months or years are released after cell destruction from other causes. Such intracellular persistence, which can lead to recrudescence of the tachyzoite form of the parasite in humans and animals, appears probable. Indirect evidence for this persistence comes from experimental observations in a number of mammalian species. Persistent parasitemia has been demonstrated not only in laboratory animals[86,418,458] but also in humans.[104,194,459] In addition, a constant antigenic stimulus has been suggested to account for the persistence of *T. gondii* antibodies, which may remain at high titers for years after the acute infection and at lower titers for the life of the infected host. Antigen-specific lymphocyte proliferation has been demonstrated in persons who had acquired the infection as long ago as 19 years previously.[421] Another observation pointing to the persistence of active infection during chronicity is that despite having high levels of neutralizing antibody titers, hypergammaglobulinemia,[460,461] and resistance to challenge with an ordinarily lethal dose of *T. gondii*, laboratory rats and mice chronically infected with *T. gondii* can transmit the organism to their offspring transplacentally (see "Transmission" section).[78,85]

"Immunologic Unresponsiveness" to Toxoplasma gondii Antigens

Results of studies in laboratory animals suggest that maternal IgG antibody may inhibit formation of antibody to *T. gondii* in the fetus.[462] The studies revealed that significant suppression of the antibody response to living tachyzoites of *T. gondii* occurs when passive antibody is present even in very low concentrations, and that passive administration of IgG *T. gondii* antibody to newborn rabbits infected with *T. gondii* may significantly delay IgM *T. gondii* antibody formation.[463]

Although previous reports on the in vitro response of human T cells to *T. gondii* did not demonstrate proliferation of T cells from seronegative persons,[464,465] McLeod and co-workers described blastogenic response of lymphocytes from uninfected persons to relatively high concentrations of *T. gondii* antigens.[466] Subauste and colleagues[425] also have clearly demonstrated in vitro reactivity to *T. gondii* of presumably unprimed $CD4^+ \alpha\beta$ T cells from *T. gondii*–seronegative adults and newborns. In addition, they demonstrated that $\alpha\beta$ T cells produce IFN-γ in response to *T. gondii*, an effector function that may be critical to the early immune response to the parasite. This rapid and remarkable $\alpha\beta$ T cell response in previously unexposed persons, the explanation for which remains to be defined, may play an important role in the early events of the immune response to *T. gondii*.

The observation that *T. gondii* induces expansion of the particular V region, Vδ2, of the $\gamma\delta$ T cell response in acquired infection[467,468] led Hara and associates to examine $V\delta2^+$ $\gamma\delta$ T cell tolerance in infants with congenital *T. gondii* infection.[469] Important in this regard is the observation by Subauste and colleagues[424] that $\gamma\delta$ T cells produce IFN-γ, a major mediator of resistance against *T. gondii*.[470] Hara and associates noted that $V\delta2^+$ $\gamma\delta$ T cells were anergic with or without clonal expansion during the newborn period in two infants with the congenital infection. Clonal expansion of Vδ2 was not observed to be associated with T cell response downregulation, and no deletion of $V\delta2^+$ $\gamma\delta$ T cells was observed. T cell anergy was noted in the infants at the age of 1 month, and *T. gondii*–specific anergy was noted at 5 months.

Cord blood of infants with congenital toxoplasmosis has been reported to have increased numbers of $CD45RO^+$ T cells.[471] In the study by Hara and associates, most of the $CD45RO^+$ T cells were $\gamma\delta$ T cells, and these T cell levels were not always elevated, especially in an infant with severe disease in the newborn period.[469] In their study, despite persistent $\alpha\beta$ T cell unresponsiveness in two infants with congenital toxoplasmosis, $\gamma\delta$ T cells became reactive to live *T. gondii*–infected cells and produced IFN-γ after the infants reached 1 year of age. The investigators postulated that because treatment of congenital toxoplasmosis usually is discontinued after 1 year without evidence of clinical relapse, the reversal of peripheral tolerance of $\gamma\delta$ T cells may contribute to the spread of *T. gondii* after 1 year of age in congenitally infected infants in whom toxoplasmosis is severe and in whom T cell unresponsiveness to *T. gondii* (lysate antigen) persists.

McLeod and co-workers demonstrated absence of lymphocyte response to *T. gondii* antigens in some infants (usually those with the most severe manifestations) with congenital toxoplasmosis.[472] For almost all infants, response to *T. gondii* antigens was present by 1 year of age, when medications had been discontinued. Their lymphocyte response often was of lesser magnitude than that of their mothers or other infected adults. The mechanism or mechanisms of this absence of response and its restoration by 1 year of age remain to be determined.

Vallochi and colleagues[410] also found diminished magnitude of lymphocyte blastogenesis in patients with eye disease whom they believed to be congenitally infected, in contrast with those they believed to have acute acquired infection with chorioretinal lesions.

In an interesting study, Fatoohi and colleagues[473] from Lyon, France, determined the percentage of T cells that became activated on exposure to *T. gondii* antigen. The purpose of their investigation was to determine whether this test could be used to diagnose congenital infection. They reported that on day 7 following exposure of T cells to soluble *T. gondii* antigen, the percentage of T cells expressing CD25, which is a marker for the IL2 receptor, increased to more than 7% in 38 congenitally infected infants younger than 1 year of age. This same increase also was observed in cell cultures from 48 congenitally infected children between 1 and 6 years of age, 9 children older than 5 years, and 24 pregnant women. Nine of 89 uninfected infants when they were tested initially had values of 7% or greater, but such values were not observed when these infants were re-tested. Information was not provided about the time during the first year of life when cells were obtained or severity of illness or manifestations of infection in these infants. These findings contrast with the lack of lymphocyte blastogenic response to *T. gondii* lysate antigen preparations of a substantial number of the infants enrolled in the National (Chicago) Collaborative Treatment Trial (NCCTS).[472] Some possible explanations include differences in antigen preparation, time in culture, and test method and the much greater proportion of children with severe disease in the Chicago study (NCCTS). Another difference was in the time of assay relative to time of birth, because almost all of the Chicago (NCCTS) children's lymphocytes underwent blastogenesis after 1 year of age. The authors also postulate that the French infant patients may have differed in having a lower parasite burden as a result of maternal treatment, which might have lessened immune unresponsiveness. In terms of mechanisms responsible for more severe illness in the fetus and infant, the finding that essentially all of the infants these French investigators studied responded to *T. gondii* antigens is important.

Other aspects of immunologic unresponsiveness are discussed under "Special Problems Concerning Pathogenesis in the Eye" and in the "Diagnosis" section.

Immunodepression

The immunodepression observed in mice infected with *T. gondii* constitutes further evidence of the persistence of active infection and the persistent immunologic effect of the organism. Strickland and co-workers[474] and Hibbs and associates[475] have noted that mice infected with *T. gondii* have significantly depressed levels of hemagglutinins and hemolysins after immunization with sheep red blood cells. Huldt and co-workers found that neonatal infection in the mouse affects both the anatomy and the function of the thymus.[476] Additional studies by Hibbs and associates revealed an impaired responsiveness to tetanus toxoid and remarkable prolongation of allograft rejection time in *T. gondii*–infected animals.[477] Pregnant mice have a markedly decreased resistance to *T. gondii* infection.[478] Whether similar immunodepression occurs in humans in the acute congenital or acquired infection remains to be determined. As mentioned earlier, failure of lymphocyte recognition of *T. gondii* antigens and significant functional and quantitative alterations in T lymphocyte subpopulations have been reported in the acute acquired infections in humans,[421,422,479-481] but the mechanisms underlying these effects have not been identified.

Special Problems Concerning Pathogenesis in the Eye

The plethora of data and the controversy that exists regarding immunity and hypersensitivity as they pertain to toxoplasmic chorioretinitis related to congenital toxoplasmosis preclude complete coverage of the subject here. The reader is referred to reviews of the relevant literature by O'Connor and colleagues[482-486] and to related work in the mouse model of congenital ocular toxoplasmosis.[487-494] Whereas Frenkel has been a proponent of the theory that toxoplasmic chorioretinitis in older children and adults is a hypersensitivity phenomenon,[495] O'Connor and colleagues concluded that both the acute and the recurrent forms of necrotizing chorioretinitis are due to multiplication of *T. gondii* tachyzoites in the retina and that release of antigen into the retina of previously sensitized persons does not result in recurrence of the inflammatory response. *T. gondii* antigen and antibody have been detected in ocular fluids in experimental ocular toxoplasmosis.[496] The rapid resolution of inflammation that occurs with antimicrobial treatment in infants, children, and adults with congenital toxoplasmosis[497] suggests that parasite replication and the resulting destruction of retinal tissue causes the eye disease. Support for the role of the parasite per se also comes from studies in which results of PCR assay in samples of vitreous from adults with the acute acquired infection were positive.[498-501] Studies with PCR analysis also demonstrated that parasite DNA may be detected in aqueous fluid.[502,503]

In one mouse model, ablation of the inflammatory mediator iNOS led to increased retinal necrosis.[504] In another mouse model, $CD4^+$ T cells also contributed to retinal necrosis; $CD4^+$ and $CD8^+$ T cells and antibody all reduced parasite burden. Cell-mediated immunity controls infection in the eye, but when the response is too robust, $CD4^+$ T cells also contribute to retinal destruction.[494,505]

Data are not available in humans that clarify whether the pathogenesis of eye disease related to *T. gondii* in young children is the same as or different from that in adults. It is difficult to extrapolate data directly from animal models to humans. The immunologic parameters that may or may not operate in each situation constitute a major factor in determining the severity and outcome of eye infection and disease.

Recurrent parasitemia may provide at least one clue to the means whereby toxoplasmic chorioretinitis occurs without concurrent systemic infection. Uveitis usually develops in persons with relatively low and stable antibody levels. Because spontaneous parasitemia can occur during the chronic (latent) infection in humans, wandering cells containing *T. gondii* could distribute these organisms into tissues with very low antibody levels, thereby allowing for invasion of susceptible cells. By contrast, the contiguity of old and new lesions[497] and the presence of parasites in areas of retina without lesions[506] in eyes of congenitally infected fetuses also suggest that pathogenesis of new lesions may be due to cysts and factors that lead to cyst rupture.

A substantial degree of antibody-induced tolerance to *T. gondii* has been demonstrated in experimental animals,[462,463,507] and it is probable that such tolerance also occurs in humans, although to what degree is unknown. It may be that maternal antibody–induced tolerance in the newborn contributes to continued multiplication of *T. gondii*, resulting in numerous cysts in the retina and other tissues. When, in later life, cysts are for some reason recognized and destroyed or simply rupture, with release of parasites that invade and destroy new host cells, perhaps when the cytokine milieu is altered as a result of stress or other factors, so that the immune response is less effective, clinically apparent chorioretinitis occurs. The occurrence of cyst destruction in other tissues (e.g., skeletal muscle) would not usually lead to clinical illness. A small inflammatory focus in a large muscle mass probably would go unnoticed, whereas its occurrence in the retina could cause impaired vision, especially if macular in location.

Although the peak incidence of chorioretinitis related to congenital *T. gondii* infection usually is between the ages of 15 and 20 years, chorioretinitis may not occur until late in adult life. Crawford described a patient in whom the first eye symptoms occurred at the age of 61 years.[508] For the next 9 years, the inflammatory activity in the posterior segment of one eye continued relentlessly, causing pain and ultimately blindness. The severity of the pain necessitated enucleation. Masses of cysts were found in the retina. In such cases, it is impossible to determine whether the primary infection was congenital or acquired. In approximately 10% of 240 cases of probable ocular toxoplasmosis studied by Hogan and associates, the onset of eye disease occurred after the age of 50 years.[509]

A prolonged recurrent course involving only one eye is not unusual. For example, Jacobs and co-workers isolated *T. gondii* from the eye of a man who had had unilateral chorioretinitis for 8.5 years, which illustrates the ability of the parasite (and reactions to it) to persist in tissues for years.[510] In a similar case, Hogan and associates made a retrospective diagnosis of congenital toxoplasmosis from a history of neonatal pneumonia and chorioretinitis in a patient at age 1.5 years and of cerebral calcifications at the age of 14 years.[511] The patient experienced recurrent attacks of chorioretinitis, which resulted in a loss of vision by the age of 12 years and, finally, in enucleation of the left eye at the age of 20 years; *T. gondii* was isolated from the enucleated eye.

Recent reports of significant numbers of cases of toxoplasmic chorioretinitis that occurred during the acute acquired infection in adults highlight the difficulties in attributing all of the cases of toxoplasmic chorioretinitis occurring later in life to the congenital infection.[503,512]

The unique predilection of *T. gondii* for maculae, brain periaqueductal and periventricular areas, and basal ganglia in congenital toxoplasmosis remains unexplained. In the mouse model of Deckert-Schlüter and associates,[441] it is of interest that congenitally infected mice have similar periventricular lesions, unlike in adult mice. It remains to be determined whether this difference is due to immaturity of the fetal immune system, unique interaction of *T. gondii* antigens with the fetal immune system, or development of the fetal brain at the time infection is initiated, or to some combination of these.

PATHOLOGY

In reviewing the literature on the pathology of congenital toxoplasmosis, it is immediately apparent that the genesis of the natural infection in the fetus is entirely comparable with that observed in experimental toxoplasmosis in animals. The position of necrotic foci and lesions in general suggests that the organisms reach the brain and all other organs through the bloodstream. Noteworthy is the remarkable variability in distribution of lesions and parasites among the different reported cases (Table 31-18).[513-516] Age at the time of autopsy is a major modifying factor, but others include the virulence of the strain of *T. gondii*, the number of organisms actually transmitted from the mother to the fetus, the time during pregnancy when the infection occurred, the developmental

Table 31–18 Organ Involvement in 10 Cases of Congenital Toxoplasmosis

Organ/System	M 11–16 mo	F 2 days	F 120 days	F 26 days	F 42 days	F 30 days	M 31 days	F 63 days	M Stillborn	F 3.5 days
Central nervous system	—[a]	C[b]	B[c]C	A[d]	BC	ABC	BC	ABC	ABC	ABC
Eyes	AB	—	—	—	—	ABC	BC	ABC	ABC	—
Heart	—	C	—	AB	—	AB	—	—	AB	AB
Lungs	—	—	—	A	0[e]	0	—	—	0	AB
Spleen	—	0	—	B	—	B?	—	—	0	B
Liver	—	0	—	0	—	0	—	—	0	0
Pancreas	—	—	—	0	—	0	—	—	0	0
Adrenal gland	—	—	—	A	—	0	—	—	AB	AB
Kidney	—	0	—	0	—	0	—	—	0	0
Testes	—						—		0	
Ovary		—	—	—	—	0		—		ABC
Uterus		—		—	—	0		—		—
Bladder		—	—	—	—	—	0	—	—	—
Gastrointestinal organs	0	—	—	—	—	0	—	—	—	—
Thyroid	—	—	—	—	—	0	—	—	—	A
Thymus	—	0	—	—	—	0	—	—	—	—
Pituitary	—	—	—	—	—	0	—	—	—	—
Striated muscle	—	C	—	—	—	0	—	—	AB	A
Skin, subcutaneous tissue	—	C	—	—	—	0	—	—	—	A
Umbilicus	—	—	—	0	—	0	—	—	0	A
Blood vessels	—	0	—	—	—	0	—	—	0	AC
Lymph nodes	—	—	—	—	—	—	—	—	—	—
Diaphragm	—	—	—	0	—	—	—	—	—	—
Bone marrow	—	—	—	—	—	0	—	—	—	0

[a]Not described.
[b]C = typical inflammatory picture—parasites.
[c]B = typical inflammatory picture—no parasites.
[d]A = parasites found—no inflammatory infiltrate.
[e]0 = no lesions of toxoplasmosis found on examination.
F, female; M, male.
Adapted from Rodney MB, Mitchell H, Redner B, et al. Infantile toxoplasmosis: report of a case with autopsy. Pediatrics 5:649-663, 1950, with permission.

maturity of the infant's immune system, and the number of organs and tissues carefully examined. After the appearance of early reports of cases of congenital toxoplasmosis, the prevailing impression was that the infection manifested itself in infants mainly as an encephalomyelitis and that visceral lesions were uncommon and insignificant. This view reflected the observation of a marked degree of damage to the CNS without a comparable degree of extraneural involvement in these infants. In some cases, however, extraneural lesions are severe and may even predominate.[12,516,517] Thus, at autopsy, in some cases only the CNS and eyes may be involved, whereas in others wide dissemination of lesions and parasites may be noted. Between these two extremes are wide variations in the degree of organ and tissue involvement, but the CNS is never spared. The clinical importance of lesions in the CNS and eye is magnified by the lack of ability of these tissues to regenerate, compared with the remarkable regenerative capacity of other tissues in the body. Active regeneration of extraneural tissues may be observed even in the most acute stages of infection in the infant.[518] Thus, in extraneural organs, residual lesions may be so slight and insignificant that they are easily overlooked. In the CNS and eye, on the other hand, the relative lesser ability of nerve cells to regenerate leads to more severe permanent damage.[518]

The presence of *T. gondii* in the cells lining alveoli and in the endothelium of pulmonary vessels led Callahan and co-workers to suggest that aspiration of infected amniotic fluid in the lungs may be a route of entry of the organism into the fetus.[513] That infection by this route may occur cannot be disputed. The diffuse character of the lung changes contrasts with the more focal lesions found in other organs and tissues. Zuelzer pointed out that this difference may be due to the position of the lungs in the route of circulation: Before dissemination to other tissues of the body all blood with parasites entering the venous circulation must first pass through the alveolar capillaries. Thus, the lungs are exposed to more parasites than any other single organ.[518]

Placenta

The first description of *T. gondii* in placental tissues was by Neghme and co-workers.[111] Subsequently, a number of similar observations have been made.[110,112,519-522] Evidence for the likelihood of the hematogenous route of spread of *T. gondii* to the placenta is supplied by the fact that groups of tachyzoites can be found widely dispersed in the chorionic plate, decidua, and amnion, and organisms have been observed in the placental villi and umbilical cord without associated significant lesions (Fig. 31-5).[109-111,523-525] The first description of the histopathologic features of a *T. gondii*–infected placenta of a woman with AIDS was by Piche and colleagues in 1997.[526] The woman experienced a spontaneous abortion associated with fever and *T. gondii* pneumonia.

In five cases studied by Benirschke and Driscoll, the most consistent findings in the placentas were chronic inflammatory reactions in the decidua capsularis and focal reactions in the villi.[521] The lesions appeared to be more severe in infants who died soon after birth. Villous lesions develop at random throughout the placenta. Single or multiple neighboring villi with low-grade chronic inflammation, activation of Hofbauer cells, necrobiosis of component cells, and proliferative fibrosis may be seen. Although villous lesions frequently are observed in placental toxoplasmosis, histologic examination of these foci does not reveal parasites; they occur in free villi and in villi attached to the decidua. Lymphocytes and other mononuclear cells, rarely plasma cells, make up the intravillous and perivillous infiltrates. The decidual infiltrate consists primarily of lymphocytes. Inflammation of the umbilical cord is uncommon. When fetal hydrops is present, the placenta also is hydropic.

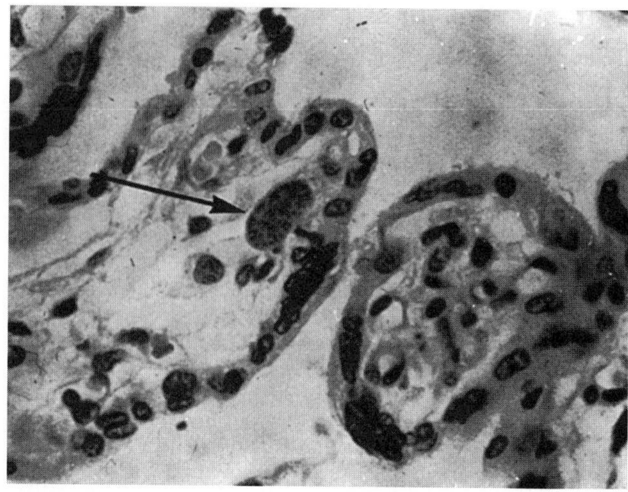

Figure 31–5 *Toxoplasma* cyst in the placenta of an infected fetus (*arrow*).

The organism is seen mainly in the tissue cyst form and may be present in the connective tissues of the amnionic and chorionic membranes and Wharton's jelly and in the decidua. Benirschke and Driscoll observed one specimen from which the parasite was isolated in which contiguous decidua capsularis, chorion, and amnion contained organisms.[521] In a retrospective histologic examination of 13 placentas of newborns with serologic test results suggestive of congenital *T. gondii* infection, Garcia and associates observed organisms that had the morphology of *T. gondii* tachyzoites in 4 cases.[527] Of interest is that in 10 of their cases, on gross examination, the placenta was found to be abnormal, suggesting the diagnosis of prolonged fetal distress, hematogenous infection, or both.

In some cases, the diagnosis was made initially from examination of the placenta.[109,528] Altshuler made a premortem diagnosis by noting cysts in connective tissue beneath the amnion in a very hydropic placenta.[528] The fetal villi showed hydrops, an abundance of Hofbauer cells, and vascular proliferation. Numerous erythroblasts were present within the vessels of the terminal villi.

Elliott described lesions in a placenta following a third-month spontaneous abortion of a macerated fetus.[520] The placenta showed nodular accumulations of histiocytes beneath the syncytial layer. In villi that had pronounced histiocytic infiltrates, the syncytial layer was raised away from the villous stroma, and the infiltrate had spilled into the intervillous space. Disruption of the syncytium was associated with coagulation necrosis of the villous stroma and fibrinous exudate. Both encysted and free forms of *T. gondii* were present in the areas of histiocytic inflammation,

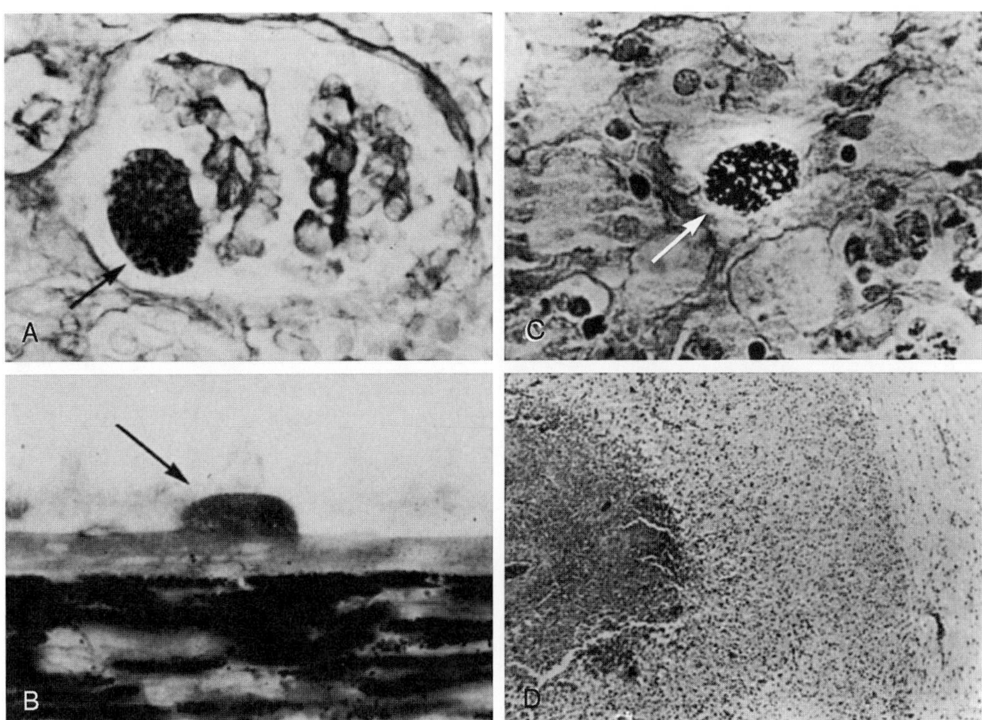

Figure 31–6 **A,** Large cyst (*arrow*) in glomerular space. **B,** *Toxoplasma* cyst (*arrow*) in the retina. Note incomplete pigmentation of the choroid. **C,** *Toxoplasma* cyst (*arrow*) in the fetal cortex of the adrenal gland. **D,** Section of brain showing abscess (*to the left*), normal brain (*on right*), and area of gliosis (*between*). Encysted parasites were abundant at the periphery of these areas. (From Miller MJ, Seaman E, Remington JS. The clinical spectrum of congenital toxoplasmosis: problems in recognition. J Pediatr 70:714-723, 1967.)

in the zones of coagulation necrosis, and in the villi without either necrotizing inflammation or syncytial loss. The location of the organisms varied, but they seemed to be concentrated at the interface between the stroma and the trophoblast. This aggregation of histiocytes and organisms at the stroma-trophoblast interface suggested to Elliott that this is a favored site of growth for the parasite.

Central Nervous System

In infants who die in the newborn period, the severity of the cellular reaction in the leptomeninges of both brain and spinal cord reflects the amount of damage done to underlying tissue. The pia-arachnoid overlying destructive cortical or spinal cord lesions shows congestion of the vessels and infiltration of large numbers of lymphocytes, plasma cells, macrophages, and eosinophils. This type of change is particularly noticeable around small arterioles, venules, and capillaries. Complete obliteration of the gyri and sulci may be noted; the line of demarcation between the pia-arachnoid and brain substance is obscured. Parasites frequently are found within intimal cells of the arterioles, venules, and capillaries.[513]

In the cerebral hemispheres, brain stem, and cerebellum, extensive diffuse and focal alterations of the parenchymal architecture are seen (Figs. 31-6 and 31-7).[70,513,518,529,530] The most characteristic change is the extensive necrosis of the brain parenchyma due to vascular involvement by lesions. The lesions are most intense in the cortex and basal ganglia and at times in the periventricular areas; they are marked by the formation of glial nodules,[70] which Wolf and co-workers referred to as characteristic miliary granulomas.[530] Necrosis may progress to actual formation of cysts, which have a homogeneous eosinophilic material at the center of the cyst cavity. At the periphery of these cystic areas, focal calcification of necrotic, individual nerve cells may be evident. Calcification within zones of necrosis may be extensive, with the formation of broad bands of calcific material involving most of the cortical layers, or it may be scattered diffusely throughout the foci of necrosis. The calcium salts are deposited in coarse granules or in finely divided particles, which give the appearance of "calcium dust." Many cells become completely calcified, whereas others contain only a few particles of finely divided calcium. Some pathologists have suggested that the *T. gondii* organisms themselves become encrusted with calcium salts.[11,518] (Cells containing fine particles of calcium also are observed in cytomegalovirus infection of the fetus or newborn and may be mistakenly construed as evidence of *T. gondii*.) The extent of calcification appears to depend on the severity of the reaction and the duration of the infection.[513] *T. gondii* tachyzoites and cysts are seen in and adjacent to the necrotic foci, near or in the glial nodules, in perivascular regions, and in cerebral tissue uninvolved by inflammatory change (see Figs. 31-6D and 31-7D).[529]

Hervas and colleagues described an infant who developed progressive drowsiness, a weak cry, and grunting in the newborn period.[531] Computed tomography (CT) revealed cerebral calcifications, multiple ring-enhancing lesions mimicking a brain abscess, and moderate ventricular enlargement. At autopsy, *T. gondii* organisms were seen in the ventricular cerebrospinal fluid. Widespread necrosis and

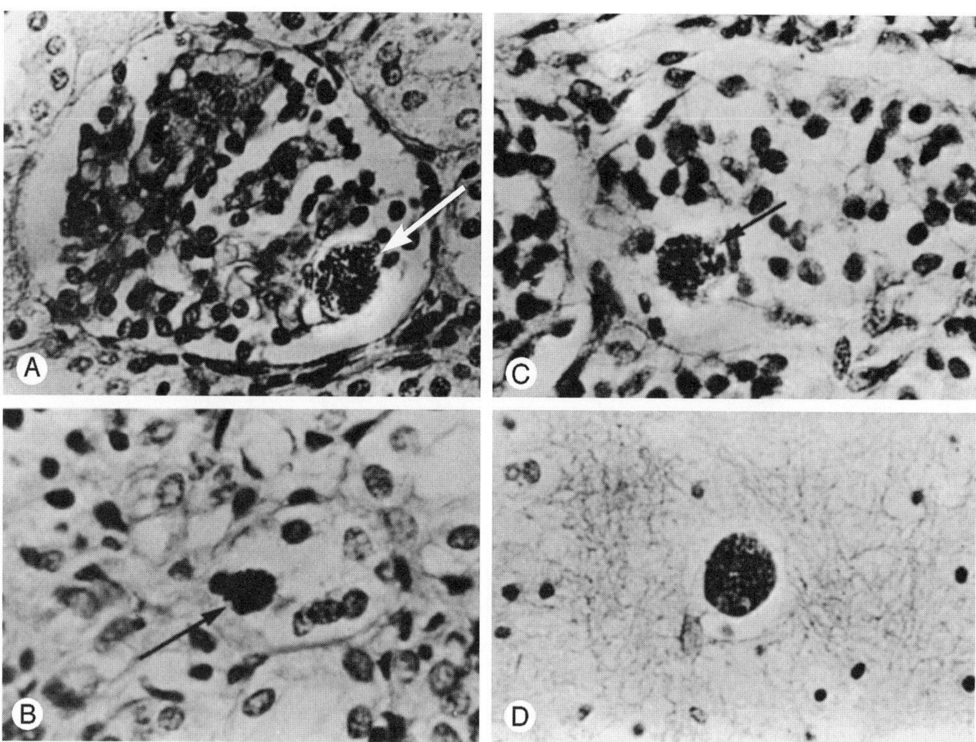

Figure 31–7 **A,** *Toxoplasma* cyst (*arrow*) within a glomerulus. Similar cysts were identified in endothelial cells of the glomeruli as well as free in the glomerular spaces. **B,** Encysted parasites (*arrow*) in a renal tubule cell. Other cysts were present within lumina of several tubules. **C,** *Toxoplasma* cyst (*arrow*) in immature testicular tissue. **D,** *Toxoplasma* cyst in cerebral cortex. Note lack of inflammatory response. (From Miller MJ, Seaman E, Remington JS. The clinical spectrum of congenital toxoplasmosis: problems in recognition. J Pediatr 70:714-723, 1967.)

granulomatous lesions with mononuclear infiltrates also were noted.

The degree of change in the spinal cord is extremely variable. It may consist of local infiltration of lymphocytes and plasma cells or, on the other hand, almost complete disruption of the normal architecture, caused by the transformation of the gray and white matter into a mass of necrotic granulation tissue, may be seen. *T. gondii* cysts, which can be identified in the white matter, usually are unassociated with inflammatory reaction.

Periaqueductal and periventricular vasculitis with necrosis is a lesion that occurs only in toxoplasmosis.[70] The large areas of necrosis have been attributed to vascular thrombosis. The necrotic brain tissue autolyzes and gradually sloughs into the ventricles. The protein content of such ventricular fluid may be in the range of grams per deciliter, and the fluid has been shown to contain significant amounts of *T. gondii* antigens.[532] If the cerebral aqueduct of Sylvius becomes obstructed by the ependymitis, the lateral and third ventricles begin to resemble an abscess cavity containing accumulations of *T. gondii* and inflammatory cells.[533] Hydrocephalus develops in such children, and the necrotic brain tissue may calcify and become visible on radiographs. The fourth ventricle may show ulcers and ependymal nodules but is free from periventricular vasculitis and necrosis, apparently as a consequence of adequate drainage of its fluid through the foramina of Luschka and Magendie. The cerebrospinal fluid that communicates with the fourth ventricle often contains several hundred milligrams per deciliter of protein and fewer inflammatory cells than are seen in the lateral ventricle fluid.[533] Frequently, inflammation and necrosis are seen to involve the hypothalamus surrounding the third ventricle. Wolf and co-workers suggested that such lesions in the floor of the third ventricle probably cause the temperature lability observed in infants with congenital toxoplasmosis.[530,534] Destruction of brain tissue, especially intense periventricular necrosis, rather than obstruction of ventricular passages, appears to account for the development of hydrocephalus in some cases.[518,530]

Eye

The histopathologic features of the ocular lesions depend on their stage of development at the time of the examination; a number of studies describing lesions in the earliest-recognized cases have been published,[12,16,535-540] and were reviewed by Hogan in his classic thesis.[540] The description that follows is based on Hogan's summary of his and other cases.

The primary and principal lesions are found in the retina and choroid; secondary changes, such as iridocyclitis and cataracts,[536] that occur in other portions of the eye are considered to represent complications of the chorioretinitis. Intraocular inflammation may cause microphthalmia, owing to arrest in development of the eye, or a secondary atrophy may result in shrinkage of the globe. The frequently reported failure of regression of the fetal pupillary vessels may indicate that an arrest in development occurred.

The inflammation commences in the retina (see Fig. 31-6B), and a copious exudate in the vitreous produces a marked haze. Secondary involvement of the choroid causes marked elevation; small satellite foci are common. After healing, the lesions are atrophic and pale, with a variable amount of pigmentation at the margins.

The organisms first lodge in the capillaries of the inner layers of the retina, invade the endothelium, and extend into adjacent tissues. An intense focal inflammatory reaction results, with edema and infiltration of polymorphonuclear leukocytes, lymphocytes, plasma cells, mononuclear cells, and, in some cases, eosinophils. The reaction results in disruption and disorganization of the retinal layers. Cells are dislocated from the nuclear layers into the adjacent fiber layers. The external limiting membrane may be ruptured, displacing retinal cells into the subretinal space. The inner limiting membrane may also be interrupted, and cells from the inner nuclear layers are then displaced into the adjacent vitreous. Glial tissue, vascular connective tissue, and inflammatory exudate also extend through the interruptions in the inner and outer limiting membranes. In the zones of most acute inflammation, all retinal supporting and neural tissues are completely destroyed. The pigmentary epithelium shows extensive destruction. The retina may detach.[506]

In the healing process, proliferation of the pigment bordering the inflammatory foci occurs. Large lesions cause considerable necrosis and destruction, resulting in marked central atrophy of the retina and choroid. Disorganization of retinal cells has occurred.[506]

Inflammation in the choroid is most acute beneath the retinal foci and is rather well demarcated. Bruch's membrane frequently is destroyed, and proliferation of connective tissue into the subretinal space may be seen. Retina and choroid thereby become fixed to each other by a scar. The choroidal vessels usually are engorged and show perivascular infiltration of lymphocytes, plasma cells, mononuclear cells, and eosinophils. Lymphocytes predominate, and both $CD4^+$ and $CD8^+$ lymphocytes are present.[485,506]

Organisms are present in the retinal lesions and, in general, are most numerous where the lesions are most severe (see Fig. 31-6B). Occasional parasites without an accompanying reaction are observed in relatively normal portions of the retina near the margins of inflammatory foci. The organisms may occur singly or in clusters, free or intracellularly, or in cysts (see Fig. 31-1C and D). They are rarely seen in the choroid. They also have been found in the tissues of the optic papilla and in optic nerve associated with inflammatory cells in congenital cases.[506,515]

Serofibrinous exudate and inflammatory cells extend into the vitreous through dehiscences in the inner limiting membrane of the retina. The exudate may be accompanied by masses of budding capillaries, and the vitreous becomes infiltrated with granulation tissue.

The optic disk may show papillitis, sometimes associated with optic neuritis[506] and sometimes secondary to inflammation in the adjacent retina or a papilledema caused by the hydrocephalus. Leptomeningeal inflammation may be present around the optic nerve.

Ear

The presence of the parasite in the mastoid and inner ear and the accompanying inflammatory and pathologic changes have been considered to be causes of deafness in congenital toxoplasmosis.[513,541] Also, brain-stem involvement affecting auditory nuclei can lead to inability to process auditory input.

Lungs

The alveolar septa may be widened, edematous, and infiltrated with mononuclear cells, occasional plasma cells, and rare eosinophils. The walls of small blood vessels may be infiltrated with lymphocytes and mononuclear cells, and parasites may be found in endothelial cells.[513] In many cases, some degree of bronchopneumonia, often caused by supra-infection with other agents, is present. *T. gondii* has been identified in the epithelial cells lining alveoli and within the endothelium of small blood vessels in such cases; in some affected patients, the pneumonic process was considered to be a prominent part of the general disease.[513] Single organisms have been found free in alveoli in the cases described by Zuelzer[518] and Paige and co-workers.[12] Of interest, their pathologic findings are identical to those described for adults in whom the lungs were particularly involved.[16] For a review of this subject in congenital and acquired cases, the reader is referred to the published articles by Couvreur[542] and Pomeroy and Filice.[543]

Heart

T. gondii is almost always found in the heart in the form of cysts in myocardial fibers, accompanied by pathologic changes in the heart muscle. A focal infiltration with lymphocytes, plasma cells, mononuclear cells, and occasional eosinophils is seen. These foci usually do not contain organisms. In the focal areas of infiltration, the myocardial cells may undergo hyaline necrosis and fragmentation. Parasites are found in myocardial fibers in large aggregates and in cysts without any accompanying inflammatory reaction (see Fig. 5-1D). Single parasites often may be present in areas of beginning necrosis and peripherally in larger areas of necrosis.[513,518,529] Extensive calcification of the heart, involving primarily the right ventricle and intraventricular septum, was observed in a 3-hour-old infant and was attributed to congenital toxoplasmosis.[544] Of interest in this regard is the consistent finding of marked calcification in hearts of mice experimentally infected with less virulent strains. As is the case with other tissues, the organisms can invade the myocardial fibers without destroying them or producing inflammatory reactions in the surrounding tissue. Myocarditis probably is produced by the rupture of parasitized cells, which liberates the organisms that then cause an inflammatory reaction in the surrounding tissue.[513]

Involvement of the heart has been demonstrated in a congenitally infected infant with AIDS who died of *Pneumocystis* pneumonia and toxoplasmosis. Autopsy was limited to cardiac biopsy and revealed marked autolytic changes without evidence of inflammatory reaction or fibrosis. *T. gondii* organisms were identified in the muscle fibers.[544]

Spleen

Marked engorgement of the splenic pulp may be noted, along with erythropoiesis. In general, no significant pathologic changes that could be attributed to direct destruction by the parasite have been noted in the spleen. In some cases, an eosinophilic leukocytic infiltration has been described.[70,518] Organisms are rarely seen in the spleen.

Liver, Ascites

In most cases, parasites are not identified in the liver, and neither necrosis nor inflammatory cell infiltrations are present. In some instances, areas of marked hepatocellular degenerative changes do occur but without associated cellular infiltration.[70,516,518] The periportal spaces may be infiltrated with mononuclear cells, neutrophils, and eosinophils. Enlargement of the liver frequently is pronounced and is accompanied by erythropoiesis, as occurs also in the spleen. In a few cases, hepatic cirrhosis has been observed as a sequel to congenital toxoplasmosis.[545] Caldera and co-workers have described calcification in the liver seen both radiologically and at autopsy.[546]

Congenital toxoplasmosis was diagnosed by exfoliative cytologic examination of ascitic fluid in a 7-week-old infant born at 38 weeks of gestation. Hepatomegaly and anemia developed shortly after birth, and liver failure and ascites during the first week of life. Because an extensive workup failed to reveal a cause, a paracentesis was performed that revealed tachyzoites both in Wright-stained smear preparations and in electron microscopy sections. This case is reminiscent of that of an adult patient with AIDS in whom the diagnosis of toxoplasmosis was first established on examination of Wright-Giemsa–stained smears of ascitic fluid obtained because of suspected bacterial peritonitis.[547]

Kidney

Numerous foci of hematopoiesis may be seen in the kidney. Focal glomerulitis often has been observed; in such cases, a majority of glomeruli remain intact.[513,518] In fully developed lesions, glomerular tufts undergo massive necrosis, and necrosis of adjacent tubules may be seen. In the earlier stages of the glomerular lesion, some capillary loops are still intact; in others, necrotic areas are observed in the basement membrane and epithelium, and the lumina are occluded by fibrin thrombi. In some of these partly preserved glomeruli, single parasites have been found in cells of the exudate within the capsular space or embedded in the necrotic remains of the capillary loop.[518] *T. gondii* cysts have been found in glomeruli and renal tubules of kidneys in which there were no other associated lesions (see Figs. 31-6A and 31-7A and B).[548,549] In severely affected kidneys, focal areas of necrosis also are found in the collecting tubules in the medulla. The inflammatory infiltrations are predominantly mononuclear, although in some cases, numerous eosinophils also are seen scattered throughout. In 1966, Fediushina and Sherstennikova reported the pathologic findings in the kidneys in nine cases of congenital toxoplasmosis.[550] In three of these cases, distinct changes in the glomeruli were noted, and as described by these investigators , many of the changes appear to resemble those observed in glomerulonephritis from other causes, including streptococcal infection.

In 1972, Wickbom and Winberg reported a case of a 10-week-old boy with congenital toxoplasmosis who developed severe nephritis with the nephrotic syndrome.[551] Inasmuch as Huldt had previously demonstrated antigen-antibody complexes in glomeruli of mice infected with an avirulent strain of *T. gondii*,[456] experimental evidence was available to support these authors' hypothesis that their case represented immune complex nephritis induced by *T. gondii*; no renal biopsy was made to support this suggestion. In 1974, a case of what appears to have been acute acquired toxoplasmosis was reported in a 10-year-old girl; light microscopy showed interstitial nephritis without glomerular lesions. Eleven months after treatment with pyrimethamine, sulfisomidine, and spiramycin, a second renal biopsy revealed slight granular segmental deposits of IgM and β_1C in the glomeruli. No immune deposits were found in the glomeruli of a renal biopsy specimen obtained 4 months after treatment.[552]

In that same year, Shahin and associates reported a case of nephrotic syndrome in a 4-month-old infant with congenital toxoplasmosis.[553] Granular and pseudolinear glomerular deposits of IgM, fibrinogen, and *T. gondii* antigen and antibody were demonstrated in the glomeruli of the initial biopsy of renal tissue. After approximately 7 months of treatment, a second renal biopsy showed no evidence of the *T. gondii* antigen-antibody complexes previously noted, but IgM, fibrinogen, and the fourth component of complement (C4) were present. IgG and C3 were not demonstrable in the glomeruli in either biopsy specimen. Light microscopy of the first renal biopsy revealed glomeruli with a diffuse mild increase in mesangial cells and matrix. One glomerulus contained a segmented area of sclerosis that adhered to Bowman's capsule. Other findings included rare foci of tubular atrophy and associated interstitial fibrosis, occasional hyaline casts, focal tubular and interstitial calcification, and prominent tubular hyaline droplets. The second renal biopsy specimen, obtained after treatment with prednisone for 7 months and with pyrimethamine and sulfadiazine for 3 weeks, revealed glomeruli with varying degrees of damage, ranging from total hyalinization to partial collapse and segmental sclerosis. The tubulointerstitial changes were not significantly different from those observed in the first biopsy specimen. The results of electron microscopy also were reported.

Couvreur and associates have reported two cases of nephrotic syndrome associated with congenital toxoplasmosis.[554] Outcome was fatal in one case, and *T. gondii* cysts were demonstrated in glomeruli.

Adrenals, Pituitary, Pancreas, and Thyroid

Parasites and numerous foci of necrosis have been identified in the adrenal cortex (see Fig. 31-6C). Similar areas of necrosis have been found in the pancreas.[12,513,517,518] Parasites, usually without associated inflammation, have been found in the pituitary.[513,517] Large clusters of organisms, without accompanying inflammation or necrosis, have been found in the acini of the thyroid gland.[12]

Testes and Ovaries

There is frequently an acute interstitial inflammation with focal areas of necrosis.[12,70,513,517,518] Necrosis of the seminiferous tubules with preservation of adjacent units is common, with infiltration with plasma cells, lymphocytes, mononuclear cells, and eosinophils. Parasites often are observed in the spermatogonia of intact tubules (see Fig. 31-7C). Focal hematopoiesis has been observed in the interstitia of these organs.

Skeletal Muscle

Involvement varies, ranging in degree from parasitized fibers without pathologic changes to focal areas of infiltration or widespread myositis with necrosis. The organisms in parasitized fibers are found beneath the sarcolemmal sheaths. Hundreds of organisms may be present in a single long tubular space in a fiber, and *T. gondii* cysts frequently are seen in muscle fibers. The affected fibers are swollen and lose their striations, but as a rule, no inflammatory reactions are noted. By contrast, focal areas of inflammation and necrosis may be present in areas where only a few parasites or none can be identified. The cellular infiltrate consists mainly of mononuclear cells, but lymphocytes, plasma cells, and eosinophils also are present. In rare instances, focal inflammatory lesions may be found adjacent to heavily parasitized but unbroken muscle fibers.[518] Noteworthy is the description of severe involvement of the extraocular muscles in the case described by Rodney and co-workers.[529]

Thymus

Sarrut observed a hypoplastic thymus in an infant who died of congenital toxoplasmosis at the age of 1 month (personal communication to G Desmonts, 1980). The disease was not diagnosed before autopsy. *T. gondii* organisms were isolated from the brain and heart. The histologic picture in this case was quite different from that described in experimental infection in newborn mice[476] in that in the former, hypoplasia involved both lymphocytes and Hassall's corpuscles.

Skin

Torres found *T. gondii* tachyzoites without formation of lesions in the subcutaneous tissue of one infant.[555] In a case ("case 5") reported by Paige and associates, *T. gondii* organisms were present in the subcutaneous tissue, again with no associated inflammatory lesion or necrosis.[12] No rash was noted in the infant.

Bone

Milgram described osseous changes in a fatal case of congenital toxoplasmosis.[517] The infant died on day 17, and at autopsy widespread active infection was discovered. The parasite was found in almost all tissues of the body. Large numbers of inflammatory cells were found in the bone marrow, with deficient osteogenesis and remodeling in the primary spongiosa. Intracellular aggregates of *T. gondii* were present in macrophages in the bone marrow.

Immunoglobulin Abnormalities

Subtle abnormalities have been noted in the development of immunoglobulins in infants with subclinical congenital toxoplasmosis.[556] In several infants, retarded development of IgA for the first 3 years of life and excessive development of IgG and IgM were noted. The latter abnormality also is seen in congenital rubella, cytomegalic inclusion disease, and syphilis. In the *T. gondii*–infected children, the degree of increase in IgG and IgM appeared to be directly related to the severity of the infection.

Macroglobulinemia in infants with congenital infections apparently was first described in infants with congenital syphilis.[556-559] The first such report involving a case of congenital toxoplasmosis appeared in 1959; the affected newborn had hydrocephalus and died at approximately 2 months of age.[560] A serum protein abnormality was suspected when blood taken for routine laboratory work became clotted in the syringe in the absence of cryoglobulins in the blood.

Oxelius described monoclonal (M) immunoglobulins in the serum and cerebrospinal fluid of three newborns with severe clinical signs of congenital toxoplasmosis.[561] The M components were of the IgG class and included both kappa and lambda types. Because the M proteins were found in the sera of newborns but not in the sera of their mothers, Oxelius concluded that the M immunoglobulins were either selectively transferred or synthesized by the newborn. There appeared to be either local production or a selective local accumulation of the M immunoglobulins in the cerebrospinal fluid. The M components disappeared and the IgM level in serum and cerebrospinal fluid decreased after therapy. Dye test antibodies were localized to the site of the M components in the electrophoretic patterns of both serum and cerebrospinal fluid. Rheumatoid factors also were found in the serum and cerebrospinal fluid of newborns with congenital toxoplasmosis; of interest, however, they were not present in the sera of these infants' mothers. These findings are especially interesting because long-standing bacterial and parasitic infections usually are associated with hypergammaglobulinemia of the diffuse polyclonal type. Also of interest is that the M components have been described in congenital syphilis as well.[562]

Reports by Van Camp and associates[563] and Griscelli and colleagues[564,565] suggest that the observation by Oxelius may not be uncommon. Griscelli and colleagues performed a survey of 27 newborns and older infants who had the severe form of congenital toxoplasmosis. In 11 of the infants, M IgG components were noted. These authors concluded that these components were synthesized by the fetus, because they could be detected up to 75 days post partum and were absent in maternal serum. They were unable to define any anti-*T. gondii* antibody in isolated M IgG. Four of the clonal M components in their 11 cases could be assigned to the kappa light chain and five to the lambda type. In the other two cases, it was not possible to assign the M component to either light chain type. Separation of the serum into IgM and IgG fractions by gel filtration confirmed that the M component was IgG. They noted that whereas early treatment induced a shift of IgG concentration toward physiologic ranges, the levels of IgA and IgD remained elevated in most infants with congenital toxoplasmosis. Absorption of the hypergammaglobulinemic sera with antigens of *T. gondii* resulted in almost complete loss of the dye test antibodies but did not affect the presence of the M component or significantly reduce the immunoglobulin levels. Similar results have been reported in *T. gondii*–infected mice; hypergammaglobulinemia and a condition that appeared to be a monoclonal spike was observed.[461] The underlying mechanism or the cause of the appearance of M components in infants with congenital toxoplasmosis is unknown.

Toxoplasma gondii–Cytomegalovirus Infection

A number of reports of dual infection with *T. gondii*–cytomegalovirus have appeared.[566-570] In systematically searching for cytomegalovirus infection among nine autopsies in cases of congenital toxoplasmosis, Vinh and co-workers found these two diseases coexisting in two instances.[566] Sotelo-Avila and associates described a case of coexisting congenital toxoplasmosis and cytomegalovirus infection in a microcephalic infant who died at the age of 15 days.[567] Microscopically, numerous areas of calcification and necrosis and large cells with the characteristic nuclear inclusions of cytomegalovirus were seen. Aggregates of *T. gondii* were found in the cytoplasm of many of the cytomegalic inclusion cells in the CNS, lungs, retina, kidneys, and liver. Maszkiewicz and colleagues described a case of cytomegalic inclusion disease with toxoplasmosis in a premature infant.[568]

CLINICAL MANIFESTATIONS

Infection in the Pregnant Woman

Because acute acquired *T. gondii* infection in the pregnant woman usually is unrecognized, the infection in such cases has been said to be asymptomatic. A diagnosis of asymptomatic infection is based largely on retrospective questioning of mothers who gave birth to infected infants and requires prospective clinical studies for documentation. Even if signs and symptoms are more frequently associated with the acute infection, they often are so slight as to escape the memory in the vast majority of women.

The most commonly recognized clinical manifestations of acquired toxoplasmosis are lymphadenopathy and fatigue without fever.[271,571-576] The groups of nodes most commonly involved are the cervical, suboccipital, supraclavicular, axillary, and inguinal. The adenopathy may be localized (e.g., most commonly a single posterior cervical node is enlarged), or it may involve multiple areas, including retroperitoneal and mesenteric nodes.[577] Palpable nodes usually are discrete, vary in firmness, and may or may not be tender; there is no tendency toward suppuration. The lymphadenopathy may occasionally have a febrile course accompanied by malaise, headache, fatigue, sore throat, and myalgia—features that closely simulate those of infectious mononucleosis. The spleen[578] and liver[579] also may be involved.[244,580-583] Atypical lymphocytes indistinguishable from those seen in infectious mononucleosis may be present in smears of peripheral blood. In some patients, lymphadenopathy may persist for as long as 1 year, and malaise also may be persistent, although this finding is more difficult to relate directly to the infection.[573] An exanthem may be present—it has been described in a pregnant patient.[515] An association of *T. gondii* infection and the clinical syndromes of polymyositis and dermatomyositis has been reported.[584-590] Chorioretinitis occurs in the acute acquired infection, and many such cases have been documented.[591-595] In São Paulo and Minais Gerais, Brazil, retinal disease has been reported to be common in the acute acquired infection.[409,410]

Infection in the Infant

General Considerations

A diagnosis of congenital *T. gondii* infection usually is considered in infants who show signs of hydrocephalus, chorioretinitis, and intracranial calcifications. These signs, often described as the classic triad,[596] were present in the first proven case of congenital toxoplasmosis described by Wolf and colleagues in 1939.[11] Since this original observation was made, however, they, as well as other investigators, have seen and described congenitally infected infants who presented with a variety of clinical signs; the clinical spectrum may range from normal appearance at birth to a picture of erythroblastosis, hydrops fetalis, the classic triad of toxoplasmosis, or a variety of other manifestations.[596,597] Thus, such wide variation in clinical signs precludes a diagnosis according to strict adherence to a set of specific clinical criteria. Such adherence may lead to misdiagnoses, especially in cases of congenital toxoplasmosis in which the signs mimic those of other disease states. Until the variability in the clinical picture of congenital *T. gondii* infection is appreciated by pediatricians and until the diagnosis is considered more often in infants with mild nonspecific illness, the blindness, mental retardation, and even death related to *T. gondii* infection will continue to go unrecognized.

Congenital *T. gondii* infection may occur in one of four forms: (1) a neonatal disease; (2) a disease (severe or mild) occurring in the first months of life; (3) sequelae or relapse of a previously undiagnosed infection during infancy, childhood, or adolescence; or (4) a subclinical infection. When clinically recognized in the neonate, the infection usually is severe. Symptoms and signs of generalized infection may be prominent, and signs referable to the CNS are always present. The neurologic signs frequently are more extensive than might be suspected at first.

In other neonates, neurologic signs (e.g., convulsions, bulging fontanelle, nystagmus, abnormal increase in circumference of the skull) are the major indications of the diagnosis. Such manifestations are not always associated with gross cerebral damage; instead, they may be related to an active encephalitis not yet associated with irreversible cerebral necrosis or to obstruction of the cerebral aqueduct of Sylvius caused by edema or inflammatory cells, or both, rather than to permanent obstruction. In these latter infants who receive treatment, signs and symptoms may disappear and development may be normal thereafter.

Mild cases in the neonate usually are not recognized. Identification of the disease has been possible in prospective studies, however, when infants born to mothers known to have acquired *T. gondii* infection during pregnancy are examined. The most frequent signs include isolated chorioretinal scars. Such cases prove that the infection was active during fetal life without causing detectable systemic damage.

Most children with congenital *T. gondii* infection are said to have been normal at birth, as signs or symptoms become manifest weeks, months, or years later. Obviously, in many cases this clinical picture is not one of delayed onset of disease but one of late recognition of disease. Nevertheless, it has been possible to verify delayed onset of disease weeks or months or years after birth in children who at birth had no abnormalities that could be related to toxoplasmosis.[109,114,384,556]

Disease with delayed onset may be severe and is most frequently seen in premature infants, in whom severe CNS and eye lesions appear during the first 3 months after birth. In the full-term infant with delayed onset of disease, manifestations arise mainly during the first 2 months of life. Clinical signs may be related to generalized infection (e.g., hepatosplenomegaly, delayed onset of icterus, lymphadenopathy); CNS involvement (e.g., encephalitis or hydrocephalus), which may occur after a more protracted period; or eye lesions, which may develop months or years after birth in infants and children whose fundi are checked repeatedly.

Sequelae most often are ocular (e.g., chorioretinitis occurring at school age or adolescence), but in some cases they are neurologic—for instance, convulsions may lead to the discovery of cerebral calcifications or retinal scars. Ocular lesions may recur during childhood, adolescence, or adulthood. In some instances, neurologic relapses (e.g., late obstruction of the aqueduct) have been observed.

Congenital *T. gondii* infection in the newborn in the series from France, as well as in a study performed in the United States,[384,598] most frequently was a subclinical or inapparent infection, not, as had previously been thought, an obvious and fulminant one. In those infants who were clinically normal at birth, the infection was diagnosed by demonstration of persistent serologic test titers. Such asymptomatic infants may suffer no untoward sequelae of the infection, or abnormalities such as chorioretinitis, strabismus, blindness, hydrocephaly or microcephaly, psychomotor and mental retardation, epilepsy, or deafness may develop or become apparent only months or even years later.[599-601] Such patients—asymptomatic at birth but demonstrating untoward sequelae later—were noted by Callahan and co-workers in the early 1940s (their cases 3 and 4).[513] Frequently, neurologic signs or hydrocephalus appears between 3 and 12 months of life.[602] In patients with encephalitic lesions, CNS abnormalities that produce clinical signs rarely develop after the first year (see "Follow-up Studies" later on).[603]

At present, no parameters are available to use in predicting the outcome in a newborn with asymptomatic *T. gondii* infection. Hundreds of reports, however, attest to the crippling effects of infection when severe disease is apparent at birth.

Table 31–19 Signs and Symptoms Occurring before Diagnosis or during the Course of Acute Congenital Toxoplasmosis

Signs and Symptoms	Frequency of Occurrence (%) in Infants with: *Neurologic Disease*[a] *(108 Cases)*	*Generalized Disease*[b] *(44 Cases)*
Chorioretinitis	94	66
Abnormal spinal fluid	55	84
Anemia	51	77
Convulsions	50	18
Intracranial calcification	50	4
Jaundice	29	80
Hydrocephalus	28	0
Fever	25	77
Splenomegaly	21	90
Lymphadenopathy	17	68
Hepatomegaly	17	77
Vomiting	16	48
Microcephaly	13	0
Diarrhea	6	25
Cataracts	5	0
Eosinophilia	4	18
Abnormal bleeding	3	18
Hypothermia	2	20
Glaucoma	2	0
Optic atrophy	2	0
Microphthalmia	2	0
Rash	1	25
Pneumonitis	0	41

[a]Infants with otherwise undiagnosed central nervous system diseases in the first year of life.

[b]Infants with otherwise undiagnosed non-neurologic disease during the first 2 months of life.

Adapted from Eichenwald HF. A study of congenital toxoplasmosis. *In* Siim JC (ed). Human Toxoplasmosis. Copenhagen, Munksgaard, 1960, pp 41-49, with permission. Study performed in 1947.

Clinically Apparent Disease. One of the most complete studies was that of Eichenwald, who in 1947 initiated a study to discover the clinical forms of congenital toxoplasmosis and to determine the natural history of the infection and its effect on the infant.[596] The cases were referred by a group of cooperating hospitals in a systematic and prearranged manner. Sera were obtained from three groups of infants and their mothers. The first two groups consisted of 5492 infants examined because they had either undiagnosed CNS disease in the first year of life (neurologic disease group) or undiagnosed non-neurologic diseases during the first 2 months of life (generalized disease group). The third group consisted of 5761 normal infants. The incidence rates of serologically proven cases in the three groups were 4.9%, 1.3%, and 0.07%, respectively. Of the 11,253 infants studied, 156 had serologically proven congenital toxoplasmosis; 69% were in the neurologic disease group, and 28% were in the generalized disease group. The signs and symptoms in the infants in these two groups are shown in Table 31-19. Approximately one third showed signs and symptoms of an acute infectious process, with splenomegaly, hepatomegaly, jaundice, anemia, chorioretinitis, and abnormal cerebrospinal fluid as the most common findings. The so-called classic triad of toxoplasmosis was demonstrated in only a small proportion of the patients. The fact that 98% of the infants had clinical evidence of infection can be explained by the manner in which the case material was collected for the study. Despite the fact that Eichenwald clearly defined this, his data for years have been misinterpreted to show that all infants with congenital *T. gondii* infection have signs and symptoms of infection, as set forth in Table 31-19. Most of the patients were evaluated over a period from birth to the age of 5 years or beyond. The overall mortality rate was 12% (no significant differences in mortality rate existed between the clinical groups), and approximately 85% of the survivors were mentally retarded. Convulsions, spasticity, and palsies developed in almost 75%, and about 50% had severely

Table 31–20 Major Sequelae of Congenital Toxoplasmosis among 105 Patients Followed 4 Years or More

Condition	No. (%) with Neurologic Disease[a] (70 patients)	No. (%) with Generalized Disease[b] (31 patients)	No. (%) with Subclinical Disease (4 patients)
Mental retardation	69 (98)	25 (81)	2 (50)
Convulsions	58 (83)	24 (77)	2 (50)
Spasticity and palsies	53 (76)	18 (58)	0
Severely impaired vision	48 (69)	13 (42)	0
Hydrocephalus or microcephaly	31 (44)	2 (6)	0
Deafness	12 (17)	3 (10)	0
Normal	6 (9)	5 (16)	2 (50)

[a]Infants with otherwise undiagnosed central nervous system diseases in the first year of life.
[b]Infants with otherwise undiagnosed non-neurologic diseases during the first 2 months of life.
Adapted from Eichenwald HF. A study of congenital toxoplasmosis. *In* Siim JC (ed). Human Toxoplasmosis. Copenhagen, Munksgaard, 1960, pp 41-49, with permission. Study performed in 1947.

impaired vision (Table 31-20). It is noteworthy that deafness, usually attributed to congenital viral infections (e.g., cytomegalovirus infection, rubella), also occurs as a sequel to congenital *T. gondii* infection. The signs and symptoms in this series of patients differ in many respects from those recorded in reports published earlier, owing undoubtedly to the fact that the cases studied by Eichenwald were drawn from a relatively unselected group rather than from a limited survey based on infants tested solely because they showed most of the so-called classic signs of congenital toxoplasmosis.

Subclinical Infection. Studies of subclinical infection have been performed in an attempt to determine the following: how often congenital *T. gondii* infection is subclinical; whether it is really subclinical or whether, in fact, initial signs have gone unrecognized; and what the prognosis is for subclinical infection. For information on prognosis, see "Follow-up Studies," later on in this section.

Alford and colleagues performed a series of studies to determine the medical significance of the subclinical form of congenital *T. gondii* infection.[556] Their serologic screening program (see "Diagnosis" section) was performed in a moderately low-socioeconomic-status urban population in the southern United States, and 10 infants with congenital *T. gondii* infection were detected among 7500 newborns screened (1 proven case per 750 deliveries over a study period of 2.5 years). The findings in the 10 newborns are shown in Table 31-21. Only 1 infant had signs that suggested *T. gondii* infection (hepatosplenomegaly, chorioretinitis, cerebral calcification). Thus, 9 of the infected infants would have escaped detection were it not for the laboratory screening program. The investigators pointed out that, nevertheless, significant abnormalities were found in this group of newborns with so-called subclinical infection. Half were premature, and the average birth weight of the infected infants, 2664 g, was 349 g less than that of control infants (3013 g). Although no signs or symptoms referable to the nervous system were present in the 9 infants, abnormalities in the cerebrospinal fluid were noted in each of the 8 infants in whom this examination was performed. Cerebrospinal fluid lymphocytosis (10 to 110 cells per μL) and elevated

Table 31–21 Data in 10 Newborns with Congenital *Toxoplasma* Infection Identified by the Presence of IgM *Toxoplasma* Antibodies

Finding	No. of Infants
Maternal illness ("flu")	2
Diagnosis suspected (neonate)	1
Gestational prematurity[a]	5
Intrauterine growth retardation[b]	2
Hepatosplenomegaly	1
Jaundice	1
Thrombocytopenia	1
Anemia	1
Chorioretinitis	2
Abnormal head size	0
Hydrocephalus	1
Microcephaly	0
Abnormal cerebrospinal fluid	8[c]
Abnormalities on neurologic examination	1
Serum IgM elevated	9
Serum IgM *Toxoplasma* antibody	10

[a]<37 weeks of gestation.
[b]Lower tenth percentile (Grunewald).
[c]Only eight were examined.
Adapted from Alford CA Jr, Stagno S, Reynolds DW. Congenital toxoplasmosis: clinical, laboratory, and therapeutic considerations, with special reference to subclinical disease. Bull N Y Acad Med 50:106-181, 1974, with permission.

protein levels (150 to 1000 mg/dL) persisted for 2 weeks to 4 months or more (average, at least 3 months for the group), even in infants who were given treatment in the first 4 weeks after birth. The findings in a severe case and a mild case are depicted graphically in Figures 31-8 and 31-9, respectively. The infant whose data are shown in Figure 31-8 was premature but demonstrated no signs of infection during the neonatal period. The elevated level of cerebrospinal fluid protein suggested severe CNS involvement from birth onward. At 2.5 months of age, retarded growth of the head, generalized intracranial calcification, chorioretinitis, and hepatosplenomegaly first became evident; these abnormalities

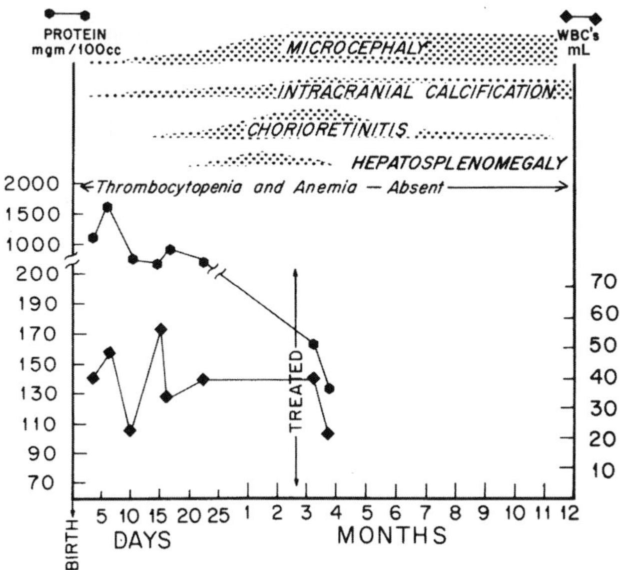

Figure 31–8 Severe form of congenital toxoplasmosis. Protein content and WBC count in cerebrospinal fluid, with clinical findings, over clinical course. (From Alford CA, Foft JW, Blankenship WJ, et al. Subclinical central nervous system disease of neonates: a prospective study of infants born with increased levels of IgM. J Pediatr 75: 1167-1178, 1969.)

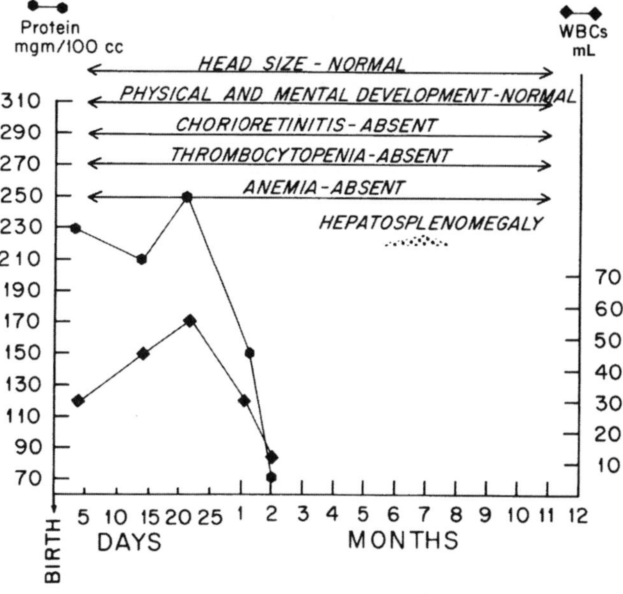

Figure 31–9 Mild form of congenital toxoplasmosis. Protein content and WBC count in cerebrospinal fluid, with clinical findings, over clinical course. (Data from Alford CA, Foft JW, Blankenship WJ, et al. Subclinical central nervous system disease of neonates: a prospective study of infants born with increased levels of IgM. J Pediatr 75:1167-1178, 1969.)

worsened despite treatment with pyrimethamine and sulfadiazine, which was, however, instituted late in the course of the infection. At the age of 4 years, this child had a developmental level of 2 years.

Figure 31-9 shows a representative example of the eight patients with milder disease, in six of whom cerebrospinal fluid abnormalities were present. Persistent lymphocytosis was detected in all, and elevations of cerebrospinal fluid protein levels were distinctly lower (150 to 285 mg/dL) in this group than in the two infants who proved to have severe disease.

Follow-up evaluation in infants who were asymptomatic at birth is discussed under "Follow-up Studies." The data indicate that nearly all children born with subclinical congenital *T. gondii* infection develop adverse sequelae.

How often is congenital infection subclinical? The only prospective data are from studies performed in France, where serologic examination of pregnant women for *T. gondii* infection is obligatory. Couvreur and colleagues reported on a series of 210 infants referred to them because acute acquired infection with *T. gondii* was diagnosed in the mothers before delivery.[604] The series includes all cases of congenital infection prospectively diagnosed from 1972 to 1981. Infants referred because of the presence of clinical signs but who were born to mothers in whom the diagnosis of acute acquired infection had not been previously made during pregnancy were not included (because diagnosis in these cases was retrospective). Among these 210 infants, 2 died during the first year of life; the cause of death in 1 was systemic congenital toxoplasmosis and in the other probably was not related to *T. gondii* infection. Twenty-one infants (10%) had severe congenital toxoplasmosis with CNS involvement. Eye lesions were present in most cases, and systemic disease was present in some. Seventy-one cases (34%) were mild, with normal findings on clinical examination except for the presence of peripheral retinal scarring or isolated intracranial calcifications in an asymptomatic child. Of the 210 infants, 116 (55%) had subclinical infections both at initial examination and at a subsequent examination at the age of 12 months. The frequency of the signs observed is shown in Table 31-22. As pointed out by the investigators, these figures for the respective frequencies of severe, mild, and subclinical cases are biased. Several biases probably decreased the relative frequency of severe congenital infection. The most severe cases with neonatal death were not referred to the investigators, nor probably were those in which congenital toxoplasmosis was so evidently severe that therapy did not appear worthwhile. In addition, abortion often is performed when acquired infection is diagnosed sufficiently early during pregnancy. This intervention probably decreased the number of infected infants born alive despite early transmission of the parasites, which probably would have resulted in delivery of severely damaged infants (see "Transmission" section). Also, when diagnosis in the mother is made before delivery, treatment with spiramycin has resulted in fewer severely infected offspring and might have decreased the severity of infection in the fetus.[126] In the studies by Couvreur and colleagues,[604] the numbers of severe cases were 16 (14%) among 116 infants born to untreated mothers and 3 (4%) in the 79 cases in which the mothers were known to have been treated.

This study[604] also allows for an estimation of the proportion of cases in which infection is really subclinical and of those in which initial signs have in fact not been recognized. Among 116 cases in which infection was considered to be subclinical by the referring physicians, 39 (33%)

Table 31–22 Prospective Study of Infants Born to Women Who Acquired *Toxoplasma* Infection during Pregnancy: Signs and Symptoms in 210 Infants with Proven Congenital Infection

Finding	No. Examined	No. Positive (%)
Prematurity	210	
Birth weight <2500 g		8 (3.8)
Birth weight 2500-3000 g		5 (7.1)
Dysmaturity (intrauterine growth retardation)		13 (6.2)
Postmaturity	108	9 (8.3)
Icterus	201	20 (10)
Hepatosplenomegaly	210	9 (4.2)
Thrombocytopenic purpura	210	3 (1.4)
Abnormal blood count (anemia, eosinophilia)	102	9 (4.4)
Microcephaly	210	11 (5.2)
Hydrocephalus	210	8 (3.8)
Hypotonia	210	2 (5.7)
Convulsions	210	8 (3.8)
Psychomotor retardation	210	11 (5.2)
Intracranial calcifications on radiography	210	24 (11.4)
Abnormal ultrasound examination	49	5 (10)
Abnormal computed tomography scan of brain	13	11 (84)
Abnormal electroencephalographic result	191	16 (8.3)
Abnormal cerebrospinal fluid	163	56 (34.2)
Microphthalmia	210	6 (2.8)
Strabismus	210	11 (5.2)
Chorioretinitis	210	
Unilateral		34 (16.1)
Bilateral		12 (5.7)

Data are adapted from Couvreur J, Desmonts G, Tournier G, et al. [A homogeneous series of 210 cases of congenital toxoplasmosis in 0- to 11-month-old infants detected prospectively.] Ann Pediatr (Paris) (in French) 31:815-819, 1984.

were discovered to have one or several signs of congenital toxoplasmosis; the most frequent sign was an abnormality on examination of the cerebrospinal fluid.

In a newborn serologic screening program in Massachusetts, more thorough evaluations of the apparently asymptomatic newborns revealed 20% with eye disease and 20% with neurologic findings.[605]

Prematurity

Prematurity and low Apgar scores are common among newborns with congenital *T. gondii* infection who have clinically apparent disease at birth.[144,556,600,606,607] In larger series, prematurity has been reported in 25% to more than 50% of the infants. When Lelong and co-workers searched for cases of congenital toxoplasmosis on a single ward of premature infants, they found 7 among 1085 infants(0.6%).[384]

Twins

In 1965, Glasser and Delta reviewed reports of congenital toxoplasmosis in twins that had appeared in the literature up to that year.[109] Later, Couvreur and colleagues reviewed this subject and added 14 of their own previously unpublished cases to the literature. Through 1980, we are aware of 35 cases of congenital toxoplasmosis in twins: 11 in monozygotic twins,[109,518,549,608-614] 13 in dizygotic twins,[87,549,608,615-619] and 11 whose type is undetermined,[608,614,620-623] In 1986, Sibalic and associates reported on a series of 21 pairs of twins with congenital toxoplasmosis in 38 of the infants.[624] *T. gondii* was isolated from four infants. In the remainder, the diagnosis was made by serologic testing alone. Wiswell and co-workers reported congenital toxoplasmosis in triplets.[625] *T. gondii* was demonstrated in the cerebrospinal fluid of each infant; no mention was made of whether the infants were polyzygotic. Each of the three infants had severe disease. In 1991, Couvreur and colleagues added six other cases.[626] The diagnosis of infection was made in two cases by prenatal sampling of blood from each of the fetuses.

The diagnosis of congenital toxoplasmosis probably would be missed in an asymptomatic twin were it not for specific lesions in the other twin that lead the physician to consider this diagnosis.[549,608] Thus, variable clinical patterns have been noted in pairs of twins, and in some sets, one twin died and a subclinical infection existed in the other.[549,597,616] It is doubtful that the diagnosis of congenital toxoplasmosis would have been suspected in the surviving twins without benefit of the results of autopsy in their respective twins.[549]

A distinct difference in clinical patterns has been observed between monozygotic and dizygotic twins. In nine pairs of monozygotic twins, the clinical pattern in each twin of a pair most often appears to be similar.[109] For example, chorioretinitis was found in each twin in seven pairs. In addition, with one exception,[518] the lesions were either bilateral or unilateral in each twin of each pair considered. Each twin in four sets had hydrocephalus, in four sets cerebral calcification, in four sets convulsions, and in one set mental and motor retardation. In only two sets, in which each infant had hyperbilirubinemia, was there a marked variation from this similarity in clinical pattern in single sets. In each of these sets, one twin died and the other survived.[518,549,608] Among the monozygotic twins, a remarkable predominance of males (eight of nine pairs) was noted, a phenomenon as yet unexplained.

In dizygotic twins, on the other hand, discrepancies in clinical findings within single sets are frequent and marked.

In 11 sets of dizygotic twins,[549,608,615-618] chorioretinitis was present in 13 of the 22 twins but was observed in both twins of a set in only two instances,[608,616,617] and even in these the lesions were not identical. Such discrepancies also were true for virtually all other clinical features in these twins. In many cases, one of the twins had a subclinical infection, whereas in the other it was severe.[549,608,627] In two sets of twins, one bichorial and biamniotic and the other monochorial and biamniotic, one infant in each set completely escaped infection.[608] An additional report confirms these findings.[628]

Central Nervous System

Other clinical manifestations of CNS destruction are described later under "Mental Retardation," "Down Syndrome," and "Radiologic Abnormalities."

Although in infants with clinical manifestations the signs of congenital toxoplasmosis may vary considerably, widespread destruction of the CNS usually gives rise to the first clinical indications of disease. Among the most common manifestations are internal obstructive hydrocephalus,[629] which often is present at birth or appears shortly thereafter and usually is progressive; seizures, which may range from muscular twitching and spasticity to major motor seizures; stiff neck with retraction of the head and, in some cases, opisthotonos; and spinal or bulbar involvement manifested by paralysis of the extremities, difficulty in swallowing, and respiratory distress. Thus, the spectrum of neurologic manifestations is protean and may range from a massive acute encephalopathy to a subtle neurologic syndrome. That the infection can involve the spinal cord is highlighted by a case in a 4-week-old girl who presented with macrocephaly and paralysis of both legs. CT revealed hydrocephalus, and magnetic resonance imaging revealed numerous lesions in the cerebral parenchyma and spinal cord.[630] Eighty-four cases (6.5%) of toxoplasmosis were found among 1282 children younger than 1 year of age who had signs of neurologic disease without obvious underlying causative conditions.[603] (A similar frequency, 4.9%, was reported by Eichenwald.[596]) The proportion of cases of congenital *T. gondii* infection was strikingly greater in infants with retinal lesions associated with CNS involvement (62 of 266 cases examined [23%]) than in those who had CNS lesions but no ocular lesions (22 of 1016 cases examined [2.2%]).

It is important to recognize that hydrocephalus due to aqueductal obstruction may be the sole clinical manifestation associated with congenital *T. gondii* infection. Occasionally, the hydrocephalus may be stable, but in most cases, management necessitates a neurosurgical shunt procedure.[631] In a significant number of infants, the prognosis is good, especially after shunt placement; the intelligence quotient (IQ) may be within the normal range. The performance of CT in the months after shunt placement is useful in determining long-term prognosis—which is good if the results of the CT are normal, even in some cases with clinically apparent encephalitis. The prognosis is less promising when there is little expansion of the cortical mantle in the months after ventriculoperitoneal shunt placement. Follow-up CT after shunt placement also is important to exclude subdural collections associated with bleeding from small vessels associated with reduction of pressure when the obstructive hydrocephalus is corrected.

Kaiser has presented a follow-up study of 10 children with hydrocephalus resulting from congenital toxoplasmosis.[632] Hydrocephalus was present at birth in only 3 of the 10 patients and was noted for the first time as late as 11 and 15 months in 2 patients, respectively. All children had progressive hydrocephalus, which required placement of a shunt. In the NCCTS, hydrocephalus was present in 45 children. It usually was detected clinically at birth, occasionally prenatally, and after 2 weeks of age in 16 infants. Occasionally, hydrocephalus developed after birth. All children with substantial hydrocephalus, in which there was evidence of aqueductal obstruction and increased intracranial pressure, underwent placement of ventriculoperitoneal shunts.

From 1949 to 1960, Couvreur and Desmonts observed 300 cases of congenital toxoplasmosis.[603] These patients were found by clinical selection. Ocular disorders, particularly chorioretinitis (76%), and neurologic disturbances (51%) were present in most cases. Twenty-six percent had abnormalities in cranial volume, and 32% had intracranial calcifications.

Toxoplasmosis in children with abnormal cranial volume is uncommon without associated ocular lesions. Of 261 children younger than 2 years of age with hydrocephalus, 16 (6%) had congenital *T. gondii* infection; of 178 children of the same age group with microcephaly, only 3 (1.7%) had congenital *T. gondii* infection. (See also "Microcephaly," next)

An interesting case of what appears to have been congenital *T. gondii* infection that manifested as a brain tumor at the approximate age of 1 year was reported by Tognetti and associates.[633]

For information on the special problem of congenital toxoplasmosis in infants infected with human immunodeficiency virus (HIV), the reader is referred to "Congenital *Toxoplasma gondii* Infection and Acquired Immunodeficiency Syndrome" later in this section.

Microcephaly

Baron and co-workers examined the role of *T. gondii* in the pathogenesis of microcephaly and mental retardation.[634] Normal, normocephalic children served as controls, and adequate numbers of microcephalic children ranging in age from 5 months to 5 years were evaluated using the dye test. The data from this study did not reveal significant evidence of an association of *T. gondii* infection and microcephaly. Similar results were obtained by Thalhammer[621,635] and by Remington.[636] It should be remembered, however, that many microcephalic infants have died before the age of 5 years. Microcephaly in this infection usually reflects severe brain damage, but patients with microcephaly also have developed normally or near-normally.

Instability of Regulation of Body Temperature

As described in the "Central Nervous System" section under "Pathology," hypothermia may be present and may persist for weeks.[12,70,513,637] Wide fluctuations in temperature, from hypothermia to hyperthermia, have been reported.[518]

Eye

CHORIORETINITIS

Because toxoplasmosis is one of the most common causes of chorioretinitis in the United States and much of the rest of the world, it is important to note that in the past, most workers had considered toxoplasmic chorioretinitis in older children and adults to be the result of a congenital infection rather than a manifestation of acquired toxoplasmosis. From data derived from extensive surveys of cases of uveitis, Perkins concluded that only about 1.5% of patients with toxoplasmic lymphadenopathy have chorioretinitis related to the acquired infection.[638] As he pointed out, population surveys have always shown that the incidence of infection with *T. gondii* increases with age; if toxoplasmic chorioretinitis results from chronic acquired infection, the number of cases also should rise with increasing age. In contrast with nontoxoplasmic uveitis, the incidence of which increases with age to reach its maximum in the fourth decade, however, toxoplasmic chorioretinitis occurs most frequently in the second and third decades of life and is rare after age 50.[639] In addition, if the ocular lesions resulted from acquired infection, it would be expected that the patients would have higher levels of circulating antibodies than asymptomatic persons among the normal population. Actually, high dye test titers are exceptional in toxoplasmic uveitis and, even when found, do not necessarily constitute evidence of acquired infection, because some patients with congenital infection have dye test titers of 100 IU or greater in adult life. One report describes what seems to be a reappearance of IgM, IgA, and IgE antibodies in some patients diagnosed as having an exacerbation of chorioretinitis due to congenital toxoplasmosis,[640] whereas other investigators have not found this to occur.[497] Studies have revealed that postnatally acquired toxoplasmic chorioretinitis occurs far more frequently than was previously appreciated; however, its actual incidence is not known.[503,512,641]

Attesting to the potential severity of the outcome of congenital ocular toxoplasmosis are results of older studies such as those of Fair.[642,643] In a survey of almost 1000 children in state schools for the blind in the southern United States, Fair concluded that 51 (5%) of the students owed their visual disability to bilateral congenital central chorioretinitis, and of these, a diagnosis of congenital toxoplasmosis was certain or very probable in 40 (4%).[644] All children showed the nystagmus and squint that always call for further examination. Kazdan and co-workers stated that the most common cause of posterior uveitis in children 15 years of age and younger at the Hospital for Sick Children in Toronto was congenital toxoplasmosis.[645]

Congenital bilateral toxoplasmic macular scars, optic atrophy, and congenital cataracts were the major causes (43.5%) of low vision in a retrospective review of a population of 395 consecutive children younger than 14 years of age who attended the Low Vision Service of the State University of Campinas in São Paulo, Brazil, from 1982 to 1992.[646] Previous studies have revealed similar results.[647,648] Fortunately, use of low-magnification (telescopic prescriptions) eyeglasses significantly improved vision in these children and, in 63%, provided both social and personal benefits.[646]

No systematically collected data are available that provide information on how frequently the diagnosis of toxoplasmosis is made when pediatric ophthalmologists note retinal scars or lesions consistent with toxoplasmic chorioretinitis.

To assess the extent of ocular and systemic involvement in adolescent and adult patients with severe congenital toxoplasmosis, Meenken and co-workers[649] from the Netherlands reviewed clinical data, available since birth, in 15 patients whose severe toxoplasmosis was confirmed during the first year of life. The patients were residents of an institute for mentally and visually handicapped children and adults. Nine of them had received postnatal treatment for periods ranging from 2 to 10 months. Mean follow-up was 27 years. Although the diagnosis was made more than 25 years earlier, when more reliable serologic methods were not available, the serodiagnosis seems clear in 13 of the 15. Each of the 15 patients also had the combination of psychomotor retardation, epilepsy, and focal necrotizing retinitis diagnosed as being due to congenital toxoplasmosis. Intracerebral calcifications were present in 12 cases, and in 10 cases, obstructive hydrocephalus had been diagnosed in the first months of life; all received treatment, and all required repeated shunting procedures. In addition to chorioretinitis, the most common abnormal ocular features were optic nerve atrophy (83%), visual acuity of less than 0.1 (85%), strabismus (76%), and microphthalmos (53%). One half exhibited iridic abnormalities, and cataract developed in approximately 40%. A majority of the cases of iris atrophy were in children aged 5 to 10 years. Of the 8 patients (16 eyes) with iridic atrophy, 12 (75%) had atrophic changes in the globe. In only one case was the chorioretinitis unilateral; it was bilateral in 97% of the remaining cases. In a majority of the cases, severe visual impairment was associated with optic nerve atrophy. The rate of documented recurrences was low (9%) when compared with the recurrence rate in patients who suffer solely from ocular involvement.[650] Some factors that appeared to account for this low documentation of recurrences were difficulties in examination, including the presence of cataract, extreme microphthalmos, band keratopathy, and lack of patient cooperation. The endocrinologic involvement in these patients is described later in the "Endocrine Disorders" section.

The risk of development of chorioretinitis in congenital cases appears to increase with increasing age during the early years of life. For example, in one case, unilateral (followed by bilateral) chorioretinitis developed between days 90 and 115 in a premature infant who received no treatment for *Toxoplasma* infection, in whom ophthalmoscopic examination was performed every 10 days.[651] By contrast, between 1981 and 1999 in 93 children in the NCCTS who received treatment, no progression or development of new lesions was observed during the first year of life while treatment was ongoing, but later recurrence was noted in a small number of children.[497] Recurrences were documented in a subset of the children in the NCCTS who received treatment during their first year of life. All of these children were examined by a single observer at specified intervals. The examinations are performed when they reach 1, 3.5, 5, 7.5, 10, and 15 years of age. The median age for the children who received treatment between 1981 and 1998 was approximately 5 years. The presence of new eye lesions was noted. Data for the children in this cohort in whom eye lesions have developed are presented in Table 31-23, along with various other clinical findings.

Another group of children referred to the NCCTS were designated historical "untreated" patients because they had not received treatment during their first year of life. They usually were referred because quiescent retinal disease was noted (see Table 31-23).

Table 31–23 New or Recrudescent Retinal Lesions in Treated and Historical Patients That Occurred after 1 Year of Age

Group	Patient Number	Age (yr) Noted[a]	Previous Eye Lesion	Active	Location	Visual Acuity before; after	Serology during Relapse
Treated	7	6[A], 10[A]	No, Yes	Yes	Perimacular, peripheral[b]	20/20; 20/20[c]	Not acute, N/A
	9	5[A]	No	No	Posterior pole	Nl; 20/50	N/A
	12	3[A], 10[A]	No, Yes	Yes	Peripheral, peripapillary[b]	20/20; 20/30	Not acute
	13	7[B]	Yes	Yes[d]	Perimacular[b]	6/400; 20/200	Not acute
	15	3[A]	Yes	No	Peripheral[b]	20/30; 20/30	N/A
	19	5[c], 8[c]	Yes	Yes[d]	Peripheral[b]	20/20; 20/20	Not acute
	21	4[A]	Yes	No	Perimacular[b]	Abnl; 1/30	N/A
Historical (untreated)	20	3[A]	Yes	Yes[d]	Peripheral	1/30; 20/400	Not acute
	25	10[A]	Yes	No	Peripheral	20/400; 18/200	Not acute
	27	7[A]	Yes	No	Perimacular	3/30; 5/30	N/A
	42	10[A]	Yes	Yes[d]	Perimacular[b]	20/30; 20/30	Not acute
	46	24[A]	Yes	Yes[d]	Perimacular[b]	20/60; 20/60	Not acute
	62	11[C], 13[C], 15[B]	Yes	Yes[d]	Perimacular, peripheral	20/20; 20/15	N/A
	82	16[A]	Yes	Yes[d]	Peripapillary	20/400; 20/400	Not acute
	89	12[B]	Yes	Yes[d]	Perimacular	20/100; N/A	Not acute

These data are from the U.S. (Chicago) National Collaborative Treatment Trial: patient numbers are those used in all prior publications. Recurrences were documented in a subset of the children in the U.S. (Chicago) National Collaborative Treatment Trial who received treatment during their first year of life. All of these children were examined in Chicago by a single observer at specified intervals. The examinations are when they reach 1, 3.5, 5, 7.5, 10, and 15 years of age. The median age for the children who received treatment is approximately 5 years old. The presence of new eye lesions was noted. Historical patients did not receive treatment in the first year of life and were referred after that time. There were 18 patients in the historical group and 76 in the treatment group.

[a]Recurrence documented at visit in Chicago (A), recurrence documented by history (B), photographs reviewed in Chicago, and recurrence documented by history only (C).

[b]Satellites of earlier lesion.

[c]Quantitative visual acuity using Snellen chart or Allen cards.

[d]Symptoms present during active disease.

Abnl, abnormal, N/A, not available; Nl, normal.

From Mets MB, et al. Eye manifestations of congenital toxoplasmosis. Am J Ophthalmol 122:309-324, 1996.

Table 31–24 Results of Funduscopic Examination in 47 Patients with Congenital Toxoplasmosis Who Were Asymptomatic at Birth[a]

Age[b]	No. of Patients with Normal Fundi	No. of Patients with Chorioretinitis	Estimated Incidence of Ocular Lesions (%)
0-11 mo	8	3	27
1-4 yr	17	5	23
5-9 yr	6	4	40
>10 yr	2	2	50

[a]Children were selected who had congenital toxoplasmosis, either clinical or subclinical, with normal fundi at birth.
[b]Age = the age at the time of the last normal funduscopic examination or the first examination showing chorioretinitis, if chorioretinitis developed.
Adapted from Desmonts G. Some remarks on the immunopathology of toxoplasmic uveitis. *In* Böke W, Luntz MH (eds). Modern Problems in ophthalmology. Ocular Immune Responses, vol. 16. Basel, S. Karger, 1976.

In a study by Parissi, among 47 patients with subclinical congenital toxoplasmosis at birth, the overall incidence of retinal lesions was 30% (Table 31-24).[652] It was less in the first 4 years of life (approximately 23%) than after 5 years of age (40 to 50%). Thus, localized ocular phenomena frequently develop as a late manifestation.[1,598,601,653] De Roever-Bonnet and colleagues[601] postulated that late development of eye lesions may be caused by second infections rather than by relapses, although supporting data for this hypothesis are lacking.

The occurrence of consecutive cases of ocular toxoplasmosis has been reported in siblings.[238,654] These cases may have been due to postnatally acquired infection.

Lappalainen and her colleagues observed typical retinal scars of congenital toxoplasmosis in three infants who were seronegative by the age of 1 year. They were born to mothers who had seroconverted during the first trimester.[655] By the age of 5 years, one of these children had seroconverted. Seronegativity in congenital ocular disease also had been observed by Koppe and co-workers in two children who had become seronegative by the ages of 9 and 14 years.[389] Gross and co-workers[656] described the case of a congenitally infected child in whom attempts at diagnosis had failed with relatively insensitive serologic techniques (the CF test) but succeeded with immunoblot and PCR assay; one wonders if IgG antibody would indeed have been demonstrable had serologic testing been performed with more sensitive and specific serologic methods (e.g., the Sabin-Feldman dye test). This case raises the question of how frequently negative results on *T. gondii* serologic studies (and, correspondingly, missed diagnoses) actually occur in children with clinical features considered diagnostic of congenital toxoplasmic retinochoroiditis. In such cases, sera should be tested by multiple methods in a reference laboratory.

CLINICAL FINDINGS ON EXTERNAL EXAMINATION

Microphthalmia, small cornea, posterior cortical cataract, anisometropia, strabismus, and nystagmus may be present.

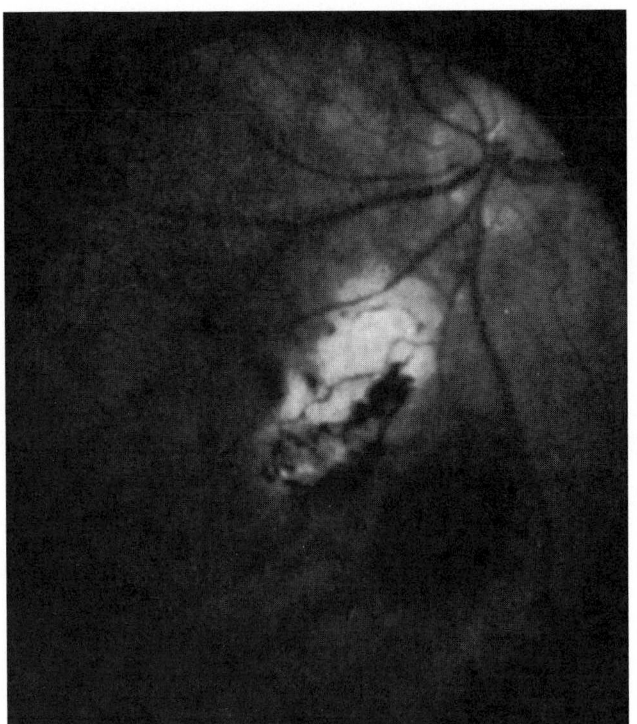

Figure 31–10 Chorioretinitis in congenital toxoplasmosis.

Leukocoria has been reported.[497,657] Nystagmus may result either from poor fixation related to the chorioretinitis or from involvement of the CNS. A history of "dancing eyes" should always raise the possibility of a bilateral congenital central chorioretinitis—the typical ocular lesion of congenital toxoplasmosis. Convergent or divergent strabismus may be caused by direct involvement of the extraocular muscles or may result from involvement of the brain.

The iris and ciliary body may be affected by foci of inflammation, with formation of synechiae. As a result, dilation of the pupils with mydriatics may be difficult.

FUNDUSCOPIC EXAMINATION FINDINGS

The characteristic lesion of ocular toxoplasmosis is a focal necrotizing retinitis (Fig. 31-10), which most often is bilateral.[658] Such lesions in the acute or subacute stage of inflammation appear as yellowish white, cotton-like patches in the fundus. They may be solitary lesions that are about the same size as the optic disk or a little larger. More often, however, they appear in small clusters, among which lesions of various ages can be discerned. The more acute lesions are soft and cotton-like, with indistinct borders; the older lesions are whitish gray, sharply outlined, and spotted by accumulations of choroidal pigment. The inflammatory exudate that is cast off from the surface of the acute lesions often is so dense that clear visualization of the fundus is impossible. In such cases, the most that can be discerned is a whitish mass against the pale orange background of the fundus. The posterior hyaloid membrane often is detached, and precipitates of inflammatory cells—the equivalents of keratic precipitates in the anterior segment of the eye—are seen on the posterior face of the vitreous.

Retinal edema, which affects especially the macular and peripapillary areas, is commonly observed in the subacute phase of inflammation. Edema of the macula is almost always present when acute inflammatory foci in the retina are situated above the macula. In older children, this edema is the principal cause of blurred vision when other causes, such as a central retinal lesion, involvement of the optic nerve, or extensive clouding of the vitreous, can be excluded. Macular edema usually is temporary, although cystic changes in the fovea sometimes occur as a result of long-standing edema. In this instance, central visual acuity may be permanently impaired despite the absence of central lesions or involvement of the optic nerve.

The optic nerve may be affected either primarily, with damage resulting from destruction of the macula and other portions of the retina, or secondarily, with damage resulting from papilledema. Manschot and Daamen and others have described *T. gondii* in the optic nerve itself,[515] or optic nerve inflammation.[506]

What at first appears to be primary involvement of the optic nerve head, with papilledema and exudation of cells into the overlying vitreous, often turns out to be a juxtapapillary lesion. A retinal lesion contiguous to the head of the optic nerve can produce swelling and inflammation in the nerve, but when the acute lesion subsides, it becomes clear that the optic nerve itself has been spared and that a narrow rim of normal tissue separates the lesion from the nerve head.

Segmental atrophy of the optic nerve, characterized by pallor and loss of substance, especially of the temporal portion of the nerve head, often occurs in the wake of a macular lesion. In these cases, the prognosis is, of course, for limited vision.

Although a majority of lesions described in the older literature are at or near the posterior pole of the retina, peripheral lesions have been described. In one series of more than 100 children with congenital toxoplasmosis,[497] more peripheral lesions were seen. With regard to the relative sizes of the macula and peripheral retina, however, macular lesions were predominant. These have roughly the same morphology as that of the more central lesions, but they tend to be less significant as a cause of central visual loss unless they are accompanied by massive contractures of the overlying vitreous and subsequent retinal detachment.

The anterior uvea often is the site of intense inflammation, characterized by redness of the external eye, cells and protein in the anterior chamber, large keratic precipitates, posterior synechiae, nodules on the iris, and, occasionally, neovascular formations on the surface of the iris. This reaction may be accompanied by steep rises in intraocular pressure and by formation of cataracts.

Isolated iritis should not be taken as an indication of toxoplasmosis. To be considered as a manifestation of toxoplasmosis, iritis should be preceded or at least accompanied by a posterior lesion. The same can be said of scleritis, which may be observed external to a focus of toxoplasmic chorioretinitis; it has no significance by itself as a sign of toxoplasmosis.

Ophthalmoscopic features of the intraocular lesions of congenital toxoplasmosis in infants are those listed in Table 31-26 (see later) and have been reported[536] to include (1) unilateral or bilateral involvement of the macular region; (2) unilateral or bilateral occurrence of other lesions; (3) involvement of the periphery in one or more quadrants of the retina and choroid; (4) punched-out appearance of large and small lesions in the late phase; (5) occurrence of massive chorioretinal degeneration; (6) extensive connective tissue proliferation and heavy pigmentation, as contrasted with the dissociation of these changes in other chorioretinal lesions; (7) presence of an essentially normal retina and vasculature surrounding the lesions in all stages of the infection; (8) occurrence of associated congenital defects in the eyes; (9) rapid development of sequential optic nerve atrophy; and (10) frequent clarity of the media in the presence of severe chorioretinitis.

Hogan and co-workers tabulated the data from 22 cases of chorioretinitis in infants 6 months of age or younger with congenital toxoplasmosis (in 81%, the lesions were bilateral) from the literature published through 1949.[509] A precise determination of prevalence cannot be gleaned from these reports because for many of the infants, the data were incomplete—for example, in some, no description of the fundus was provided, but other features such as microphthalmia were described. Of those infants for whom sufficient information was available, 7 had only healed retinal lesions, 5 had only acute lesions, and 4 had both acute and healed lesions. Macular involvement was seen in 5, and peripheral retinal involvement in 10; diffuse retinal involvement was present in 3. Twelve infants had microphthalmia, 5 had optic nerve atrophy, 3 had papilledema, 8 had strabismus, 7 had nystagmus, 10 had anterior segment involvement, and 2 had cataracts; in 10, parasites were noted in the retina at autopsy.

Franceschetti and Bamatter reviewed the signs in 243 cases of congenital ocular toxoplasmosis and found the following percentages: bilateral involvement in 66%, unilateral involvement in 34%, microphthalmia in 23%, optic atrophy in 27%, nystagmus in 23%, strabismus in 28%, cataract in 8%, iritis and posterior synechiae in 8%, persistence of pupillary membrane in 4%, and vitreous changes in 11%.[659]

The findings of Mets and colleagues[497] in the children in the NCCTS are shown in Table 31-25. Other important feetures may be noted. For example, relatively normal visual acuity may occur in the presence of large macular scars either sparing or involving the fovea.[497] Synechiae and pupillary irregularities sometimes are present and reflect an especially severe intraocular inflammatory process. In the NCCTS, we have noted the following (G Noble and co-workers, unpublished observations): In some patients with severe intraocular inflammation, retinal detachment may occur later in childhood. Intermittent occlusion (patching therapy) of the better-seeing eye may lead to substantial improvement in visual acuity even in the presence of large macular scars. Optical coherence tomography (OCT) may be useful in assessing depth of macular lesions, impact on optic nerve function, and differences over time and thus be of assistance in monitoring recurrences. Cataract removal can lead to improved visual function if retinal detachment has not been prolonged. In the NCCTS, a small number of mothers had retinal scars, which indicates the importance of retinal examinations for mothers of congenitally infected infants.

DIFFERENTIAL DIAGNOSIS OF EYE LESIONS

Congenital Anomalies. The healed foci of toxoplasmic chorioretinitis may resemble a colobomatous defect

Table 31–25 Ophthalmologic Manifestations of Congenital Toxoplasmosis in Children in U.S. (Chicago) National Collaborative Treatment Trial[a]

	Number with Finding (%)		
Manifestation	*Treatment Group N = 76*	*Historical Group N = 18*	*Total N = 94*
Strabismus	26 (34)	5 (28)	31 (33)
Nystagmus	20 (26)	5 (28)	25 (27)
Microphthalmia	10 (13)	2 (11)	12 (13)
Phthisis	4 (5)	0 (0)	4 (4)
Microcornea	15 (20)	3 (17)	18 (19)
Cataract	7 (9)	2 (11)	9 (10)
Vitritis (active)	3 (4)[b]	2 (11)	5 (5)
Retinitis (active)	6 (8)	4 (22)	10 (11)
Chorioretinal scars	56 (74)	18 (100)	74 (79)
Macular	39/72 (54)[c]	13/17 (76)	52/89 (58)
Juxtapapillary	37/72 (51)	9/17 (53)	46/89 (52)
Peripheral	43/72 (58)	14/17 (82)	57/89 (64)
Retinal detachment	7 (9)	2 (11)	9 (10)
Optic atrophy	14 (18)	5 (28)	19 (20)

[a]Children either received treatment with pyrimethamine and sulfadiazine during their first year of life (treatment group) or were referred after their first year of life when they had not been treated (historical group). In general, historical patients were referred because they had eye disease. Current mean ages of the children in these groups are in Table 31-58.
[b]Two additional patients, not included in this table, were receiving treatment, and retinochoroiditis had resolved but vitreous cells and veils persisted at time of examination.
[c]Numerator represents number with finding. Denominator represents *N*, unless otherwise specified. Number in parentheses is percentage. Patients with bilateral retinal detachment in whom the location of scars was not possible were excluded from the denominator.
From Mets MB, et al. Eye manifestations of congenital toxoplasmosis. Am J Ophthalmol 122:309-324, 1996.

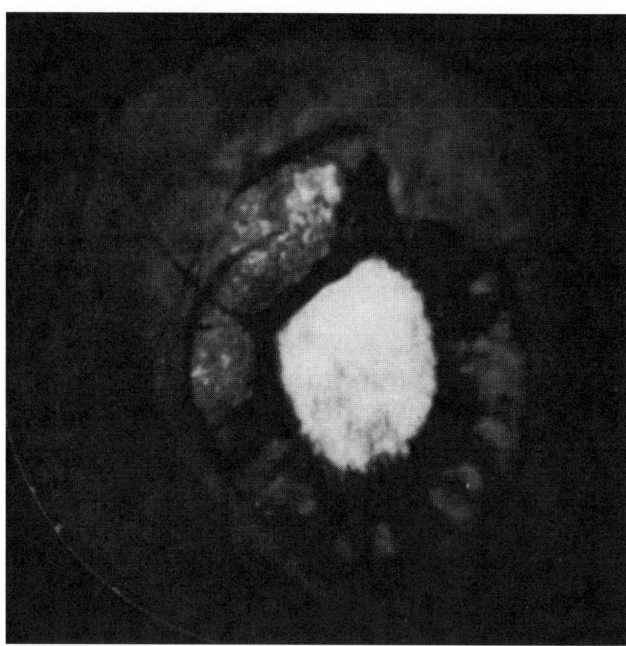

Figure 31–11 Macular pseudocoloboma of the retina in congenital toxoplasmosis.

(Fig. 31-11).[6] The associated ocular, systemic, and serologic changes make toxoplasmosis the most likely diagnosis. Abnormal retinal morphology has been described in one fetal eye,[506] and similar findings have been described in a variety of animal models of the congenital infection. Chromosome analysis was not available for the fetus, however.

Other Inflammatory Lesions. The differential diagnosis of eye lesions includes many of the inflammatory lesions described in Chapters 18, 23, 26, and 28. Lymphochoriomeningitis virus also can cause similar lesions.

Birth Injury. Intraocular hemorrhage may go unrecognized and may cause retinal damage with gliosis and fibrosis, potentially resulting in retinal detachment. The lesion usually is unilateral, associated cerebral damage is absent, and no serologic evidence is present to support a diagnosis of toxoplasmosis. Retinopathy of prematurity may occur in conjunction with toxoplasmic chorioretinitis.

Circulatory Disturbances. Congenital aneurysms and telangiectasia of retinal vessels may result in extensive retinal fibrosis, with pigmentation and detachment. The disease usually is unilateral and is not associated with cerebral involvement or other changes.

Neoplasms. Retinoblastoma rarely may have an appearance similar to that described for ocular toxoplasmosis. It most often is unilateral and is unassociated with visceral or cerebral damage unless an advanced stage has been reached. Pseudoglioma may be difficult to distinguish from a healed chorioretinitis lesion but usually is single and unilateral. Gliomas may be bilateral, progressing from a small nodule to a large polypoid mass protruding into the vitreous.

Mental Retardation

Numerous studies have attempted to establish a causal relationship between mental retardation and congenital toxoplasmosis. A prospective study on this subject is that of Alford and colleagues.[556,660] When these workers noted that changes in cerebrospinal fluid protein concentration and cell count were common in newborns with subclinical congenital toxoplasmosis, they set out to determine the significance of these changes in relation to later mental development. They compared the intellectual and social development of eight children, aged 2 to 4 years, who were identified at birth as having subclinical congenital toxoplasmosis, with those of eight matched controls. Their results revealed that varying degrees of intellectual impairment may be present in children who are asymptomatic at birth, reflecting the fact that brain damage does occur with subclinical congenital toxoplasmosis. These investigators concluded that although subclinical congenital toxoplasmosis does not necessarily cause overt mental retardation, it may be associated with some degree of intellectual impairment. Further studies along these lines have corroborated these findings (see "Follow-up Studies" later in this section), but until a much larger number of infants are examined over a longer time, these data can be considered only tentative.

The total contribution of congenital toxoplasmosis, including the less severe and clinically inapparent forms at

Table 31–26 Frequency of *Toxoplasma* Infections in 1332 Children (Ages 1-14 Years) with Congenital Cerebral Defects Compared with 600 Normal Children

Type of Defect	No. Tested	No. Positive[a] (%)
Microcephaly	57	2 (3.5)
Hydrocephalus	191	17 (8.9)
Cerebral palsy	55	5 (9.1)
Epilepsy	344	73 (21.2)
Mental retardation	685	167 (24.4)
Cerebral defects (all types)	1332	264 (19.8)
None (normal)	600	20 (3.3)

[a]Dye test titers of 1:4 or higher were considered to be positive.
Adapted from Thalhammer O. Congenital toxoplasmosis. Lancet 1:23-24, 1962, with permission.

birth, to mental retardation is uncertain. One of the earliest studies from Europe was that of Thalhammer in Vienna, who classified congenital toxoplasmosis into three broad categories: (1) generalized, with hepatomegaly, jaundice, myocarditis, pneumonitis, and similar effects; (2) cerebral, accompanied by at least one of the two characteristic signs, namely, chorioretinitis and intracerebral calcification; and (3) cerebral, accompanied by damage but without these signs.[621] Thalhammer concluded that the first type was rare, the second not common enough to be a problem, and the third a common condition creating serious medical and social problems. He studied 1332 children with congenital cerebral damage that could not be accounted for by postnatal encephalitic illness. The results of this study are summarized in Table 31-26. In children with cerebral defects of all types, the prevalence of *T. gondii* infection was about 17% higher than in normal children. Although the frequency of *T. gondii* infection in this series was not measurably greater in children with microcephaly, hydrocephalus, and cerebral palsy than it was in normal children, it was much greater in those with epilepsy and mental retardation. Thalhammer concluded from these statistics that in about 20% of the cases of mental retardation, the most important cerebral defects were due to congenital toxoplasmosis. Other investigators have similarly concluded from their data that congenital toxoplasmosis is or may be an important cause of mental retardation.[636,661-664] Through a series of computations from the data of others, Hume concluded that toxoplasmosis is the cause of impairment in at least 4% of the population composed of the "mentally retarded and [those with] cerebral dysfunction."[665]

Interpretation of many of these studies, as well as those by workers who found little or no significant difference between mentally retarded and control populations,[603,634,666-674] is complicated by the high prevalence of acquired *Toxoplasma* infection among control subjects, which may mask the possible role of congenital toxoplasmosis in mental retardation (as well as other sequelae of encephalopathy, such as convulsions). For example, if the proportion of cases of mental retardation is small and the prevalence of *T. gondii* antibody titers in the control population is high, it is not possible with presently available diagnostic techniques to distinguish those cases in which *T. gondii* is the cause of mental retardation. Another cause of the variations in reported results is the choice of controls. In many studies, subjects were not properly matched, and any difference or lack of difference found was due solely to differences in populations from which the patients were chosen.[668]

Only through large-scale prospective studies of infection with *T. gondii* acquired during the course of pregnancy, compiled by means of long-term observations of the infants, will accurate figures be obtained on the contribution of congenital *T. gondii* infection to mental deficiency (as well as epilepsy, blindness, and other disorders).

Down Syndrome

Although numerous investigators have interpreted their data as evidence of an association between toxoplasmosis in the mother and Down syndrome in the offspring,[675-680] such an association has never been proved satisfactorily.[680] In a study of 71 such children, Thalhammer found a higher-than-normal prevalence of *T. gondii* antibodies.[635] He attributed the higher prevalence to their mental deficiency and suggested that their institutional environment probably favored a higher rate of acquired infection; the prevalence of *T. gondii* antibodies was no different from that in normal controls in the age group birth to 5 years and rose to levels higher than those demonstrated in controls only in the older age groups. Until adequate data to the contrary are furnished, the association between Down syndrome and toxoplasmosis in a newborn must be considered coincidental. Frenkel[681] points out that, in view of the chromosomal aberrations in Down syndrome, it would be necessary to demonstrate that toxoplasmosis is related to the nonhereditary or nondisjunction form of Down syndrome; if this is true, one would have to postulate an influence of *T. gondii* on the ovum, which thus far has not been demonstrated.[675] Much of the literature on this subject, as well as that on the relationship of toxoplasmosis to other entities in the newborn, is purely speculative.

Endocrine Disorders

The endocrine disorders that have been associated with congenital toxoplasmosis are nonspecific, because they reflect the severity of the infection in those areas of the brain that are related to endocrine function. Two cases in which congenital toxoplasmosis and congenital myxedema occurred simultaneously have been reported.[682,683] Because each of these conditions is relatively uncommon, their concurrent appearance suggests more than mere coincidence. *T. gondii* has been demonstrated in histologic sections of the pituitary and thyroid glands of infants dying of toxoplasmosis, and it may be that such involvement contributed to or resulted in myxedema in these patients. Silver and Dixon described persistent hypernatremia in a congenitally infected infant who had evidence of vasopressin-sensitive diabetes insipidus without polyuria or polydipsia.[637] An associated finding was a marked eosinophilia in blood and bone marrow. A similar case was described by Margit and Istvan.[684] Diabetes insipidus has occurred in the perinatal period or developed later in childhood.[534,685] This disorder in such cases probably is secondary to pituitary-hypothalamic *T. gondii* infection. It has occurred in infants and children with severe brain damage and hydrocephalus, as well as in children who have only intracerebral calcifications.[534,686,687]

Bruhl and colleagues reported sexual precocity in association with congenital toxoplasmosis in a male infant who, at the age of 2 years, showed rapid growth of the external genitalia and appearance of pubic hair, along with generalized convulsions, microcephaly, severe mental retardation, bilateral microphthalmia, and blindness (deafness was suspected because the child did not respond to noises).[688] After 9 years of hospitalization, he died at the age of 13.5 years. The early onset of growth of the penis and testes and the development of pubic hair, as well as testicular biopsy and hormone assays, established the diagnosis of true precocity in this case. A cause-and-effect relationship between toxoplasmosis and precocious puberty could not be proved, but the presence of two rare disorders in the same patient suggested such a relationship. Also, a variety of lesions involving the hypothalamus have been associated with precocious puberty, and the third ventricle was dilated and the hypothalamus was distorted in the patient just described. The anterior pituitary appeared normal at autopsy—a prerequisite to development of precocious puberty in patients with lesions in or near the hypothalamus. Partial anterior hypopituitarism was observed in the infant reported by Coppola and co-workers.[689] Massa and colleagues described three children with growth hormone deficiency, two of whom were gonadotropin deficient and one of whom had precocious puberty, in addition to central diabetes insipidus.[685]

In the study performed by Meenken and associates[649] (described previously in the "Chorioretinitis" section), overt endocrinologic disease was diagnosed in 5 of 15 patients with severe congenital toxoplasmosis, all of whom had serious eye disease due to the infection. Panhypopituitarism was observed in 2, gonadal failure with dwarfism in 1, precocious puberty with dwarfism and thyroid deficiency in 1, and diabetes mellitus and thyroid deficiency in 1. The investigators found that the major manifestations of the endocrine disease in these patients occurred at the mean age of 12 years (range, 9 to 16 years) and were associated with obstructive hydrocephalus and dilated third ventricle in each case.

Nephrotic Syndrome

In infants with congenital toxoplasmosis, generalized edema and ascites may reflect the presence of the nephrotic syndrome.[551,552,554,690] Protein and casts have been reported in the urine in such cases, as have hypoproteinemia, hypoalbuminemia, and hypercholesterolemia. In one case, there was a marked decrease in the serum IgG level, but IgM and IgA levels were normal.[552] Hypogammaglobulinemia has been reported to be associated with congenital toxoplasmosis in the absence of nephrosis.[691]

Liver

Kove and co-workers described the pattern of serum transaminase activity in a newborn with cytomegalic inclusion disease and in another with congenital toxoplasmosis.[692] Jaundice developed in both. The patterns were unique and unlike those observed in infants with other causes of neonatal jaundice. The investigators pointed out that more studies are necessary to determine if serial measurements of serum transaminase will actually be a useful tool in the diagnosis of congenital toxoplasmosis and cytomegalic inclusion disease.

Jaundice, which occurs frequently, may reflect liver damage or hemolysis, or both. Among 225 infants with neonatal icterus studied by Couvreur and Desmonts, 5 (2.2%) were found to have congenital toxoplasmosis.[603] The conjugated hyperbilirubinemia and jaundice seen in infants with untreated congenital toxoplasmosis may persist for months.[530] In infants who receive treatment, hyperbilirubinemia and jaundice usually resolve in a few weeks.

Skin

Like almost all other signs of the infection, those referable to the skin are varied and nonspecific.[693,694] Thrombocytopenia may be associated with petechiae, ecchymoses, or even gross hemorrhages into the skin. Zuelzer described a fine punctate rash over the entire body of a 3-day-old infant.[518] Miller and colleagues noted albinism in one of the infants they studied but did not consider this to be caused by toxoplasmosis.[549] Wolf and associates noted a diffuse maculopapular rash in two infants with jaundice, beginning on the sixth day in one and on the ninth day in the other.[530] Reiss and Verron described a premature infant with a lenticular, deep blue-red, sharply defined macular rash over the entire body, including the palms and soles.[695] Diffuse blue papules were noted in the patient described by Justus.[696] Korovitsky and co-workers, in a discussion of skin lesions in toxoplasmosis, mentioned an exfoliative dermatitis in cases of congenital toxoplasmosis,[697] but according to Justus, a cause-and-effect relationship between these two conditions was not shown in the infant he described.[696] In 1968, Justus reported complete calcification of the skin, except for the palms and soles, in a premature infant who died 10 minutes after birth.[698] The mother had experienced tetany during delivery and required supplemental calcium thereafter. Thus, the calcifications may not have been due solely, or even in part, to congenital toxoplasmosis in the infant but rather may have been the result of a metabolic defect in calcium metabolism in the mother.

Malformations

The possibility that *T. gondii* can cause fetal malformations has been the subject of much conjecture. Thalhammer, commenting on the accumulated data on this subject, stated that he did not believe that *T. gondii* causes malformations.[635] He found 4 instances of malformations among 326 cases of congenital toxoplasmosis (1.2%), and this was less than the average incidence of malformations in his geographic area. Of 144 children with malformations, only 2 had *T. gondii* antibodies.

By contrast, workers in Germany,[121,259,522,699,700] Greece,[701] the former Czechoslovakia,[679,702] and the former Soviet Union[703] interpret their data as proof that *T. gondii* causes fetal malformations. Most of these studies were performed in an uncontrolled and uncritical manner. For example, in the United States, Erdelyi suggested that some cases of palatal cleft malformations may be due to congenital toxoplasmosis[704]; a similar conclusion was reached by Jírovec and co-workers in Prague.[679] The evidence in the study reported by Erdelyi consisted of dye test data, and in the study from Jírovec's group, skin test data drawn from investigations of mothers of children with cleft palate and harelip defects; the prevalence of positive results on skin testing in mothers of such children was found to be higher than that in controls from the general population. Carefully chosen controls should be a necessary

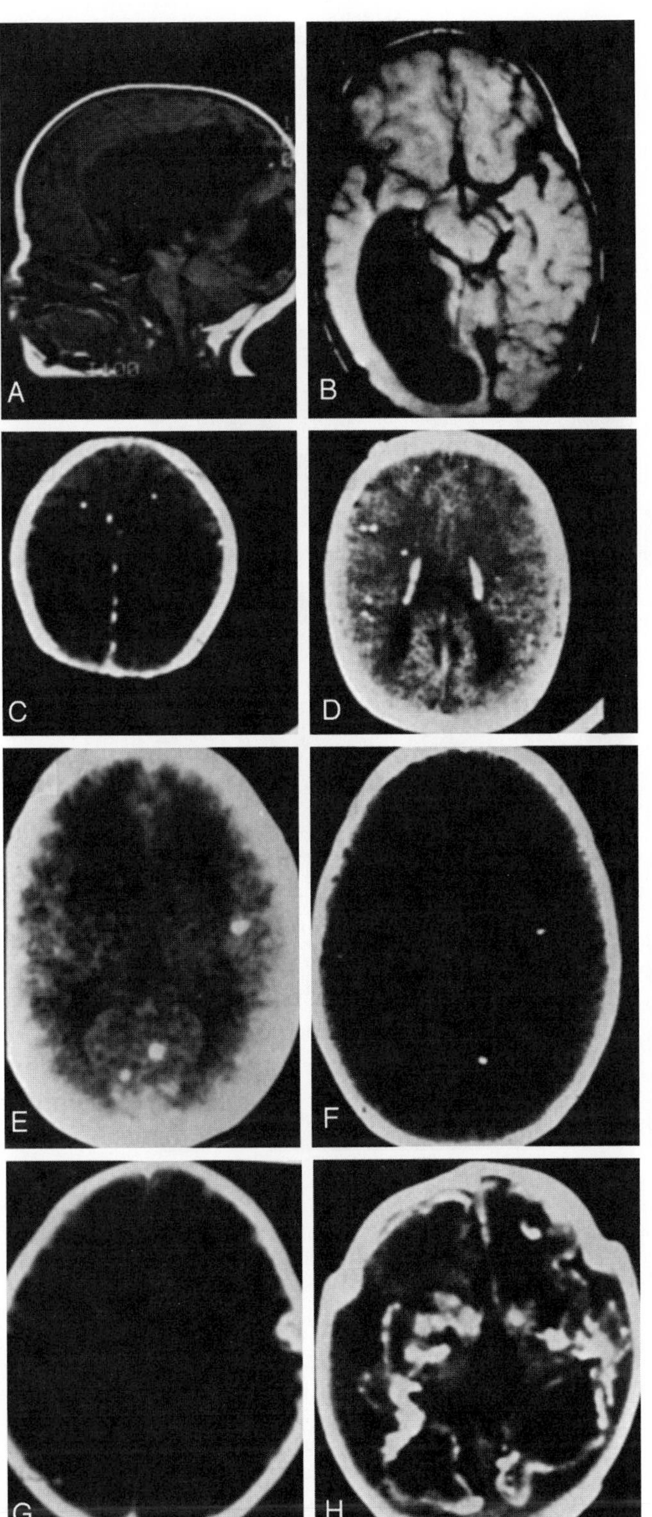

Figure 31–12 Neuroradiographic findings in congenital toxoplasmosis. The remarkable clinical improvements in the children following treatment and the normalization seen in their brain radiographs in **C** to **F** are particularly noteworthy. **A,** Magnetic resonance imaging (MRI) study of the brain demonstrating obstruction of the aqueduct of Sylvius and consequent dilation of the third and lateral ventricles. **B,** MRI study of the brain demonstrating unilateral hydrocephalus. **C** and **D,** Brain computed tomography (CT) scans in the early newborn period (**C**) and of the same child at 1 year of age (**D**) following shunt placement and antimicrobial therapy. The child is developmentally and neurologically normal at 1 year of age. **E** and **F,** Brain CT scans from another child in the early newborn period (**E**) and at 1 year of age (**F**) following antimicrobial therapy. The resolution or diminution of calcifications is noteworthy and has occurred in a substantial number (but not all) of children who received appropriate treatment in the Chicago study. This child also is developmentally and neurologically normal. **G,** Brain CT scan that demonstrates a ring-enhancing lesion and calcifications. **H,** Brain CT scan showing extremely extensive intracerebral calcifications and hydrocephalus. (**B, E, F, G** from McAuley J, Roizen N, Patel D, et al. Early and longitudinal evaluations of treated infants and children and untreated historical patients with congenital toxoplasmosis: the Chicago Collaborative Treatment Trial. Clin Infect Dis 18:38-72, 1994; Remington JS, McLeod R, Thulliez P, Desmonts G. Toxoplasmosis. *In* Remington JS, Klein JO [eds] Infectious Diseases of the Fetus and Newborn Infant, 5th ed. Philadelphia, WB Saunders, 2000, pp 205-346.)

feature of all such studies; results obtained from the general population are not applicable or valid.

Although involvement of the placenta by infection early in pregnancy may cause damage without direct infection of the developing embryo, the available data are insufficient either to support or to reject the hypothesis that *T. gondii* can cause fetal malformations. This problem is easily approached with existing epidemiologic methods and awaits careful controlled study.

Radiologic Abnormalities

BRAIN

Hydrocephalus characteristically is due to periaqueductal involvement. Obstruction of the aqueduct of Sylvius leads to enlargement of the third and lateral ventricles (Fig. 31-12A). Obstruction of the foramen of Monro can lead to unilateral hydrocephalus (Fig. 31-13) (see also Fig. 31-12B).[534] Dramatic resolution and brain cortical expansion and growth can

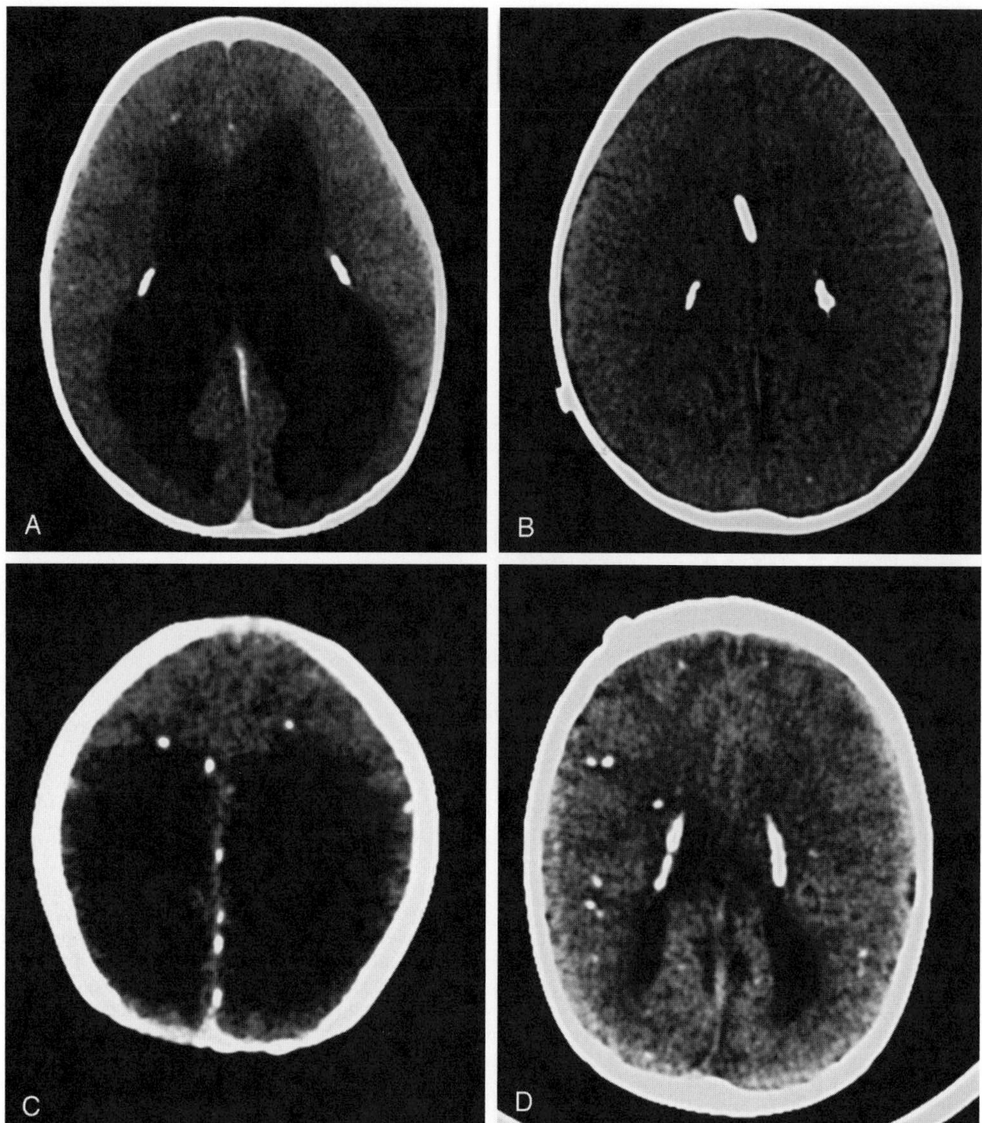

Figure 31–13 Cranial computed tomography (CT) scans of two infants, one represented in **A** and **B** and the other in **C** and **D,** before (**A** and **C**) and after (**B** and **D**) placement of ventriculoperitoneal shunts. Both infants have developed normally. CT scans and the subsequent normal development of these children indicate that it is not possible to predict ultimate cognitive outcome from the initial appearance of the CT scan. (From Boyer KM, McLeod RL. *Toxoplasma gondii* [toxoplasmosis]. *In* Long SS, Prober CG, Pickering LK [eds]. Principles and Practice of Pediatric Infectious Diseases. New York, Churchill Livingstone, 1997, pp 1421-1448.)

occur in conjunction with ventriculoperitoneal shunt placement and anti–*T. gondii* therapy (see Figs. 31-12C and D and 31-13). Calcifications may be single or multiple (Fig. 31-14; see also Fig. 31-12E to H) and, surprisingly, in some cases have resolved with anti-*Toxoplasma* therapy during the first year of life (see Figs. 31-12E and F and 31-14).[705] Contrast-enhancing lesions have been detected, indicating active encephalitis (see Fig. 31-12G).[534] Massive hydrocephalus, as documented by ultrasound examination, has been noted to develop in fetuses and newborns within a period as brief as 1 week (see Fig. 31-14) and resolved in association with anti-*Toxoplasma* treatment in one fetus (Fig. 31-15).[706]

Radiologic signs in newborns exposed to primary *T. gondii* infection in utero were described by Virkola and colleagues.[707] The study included 42 mothers—37 were delivered of live-born infants and 5 experienced spontaneous abortions—with follow-up evaluation. The findings on brain ultrasonography associated with infection included calcifications, cysts, and the "candlestick sign"; those on abdominal ultrasonography were enlarged spleen and ascites. In some instances, these changes were associated with abnormalities in the newborn period.

Puri and co-workers described a 2-week-old infant with hydrocephalus.[708] A brain scan with ^{99m}Tc-pertechnetate showed an area of increased uptake in the left temporoparietal region. A four-vessel angiogram showed large ventricles with a mass lesion in the left hemisphere pushing midline structures to the right. Findings on electroencephalography were abnormal, with sharp θ activity in the left parietotemporal area. A bubble ventriculogram showed

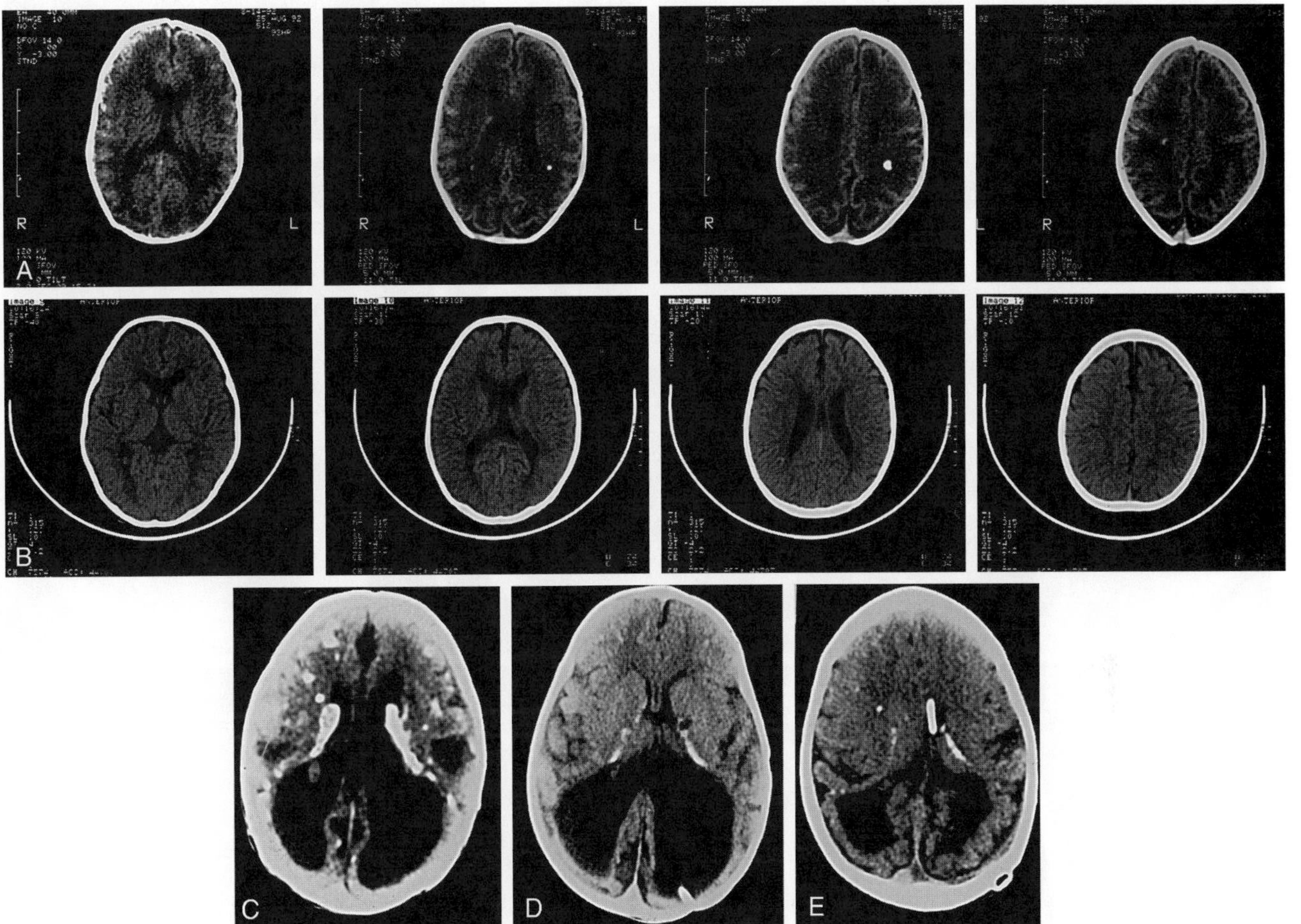

Figure 31–14 Additional examples of cranial computed tomography (CT) scans that demonstrate resolution of calcifications in children following treatment for congenital toxoplasmosis. **A** and **B,** CT scans in an infant obtained at birth, August 1992 (**A**), and in August 1993 (**B**). **C** to **E,** Diminution and/or resolution of large areas of calcification are seen in these representative cranial CT scans from another infant. The scans were obtained at birth, February 1987 (**C**), and at follow-up in May 1988 (**D**) and July 1991 (**E**). *continued*

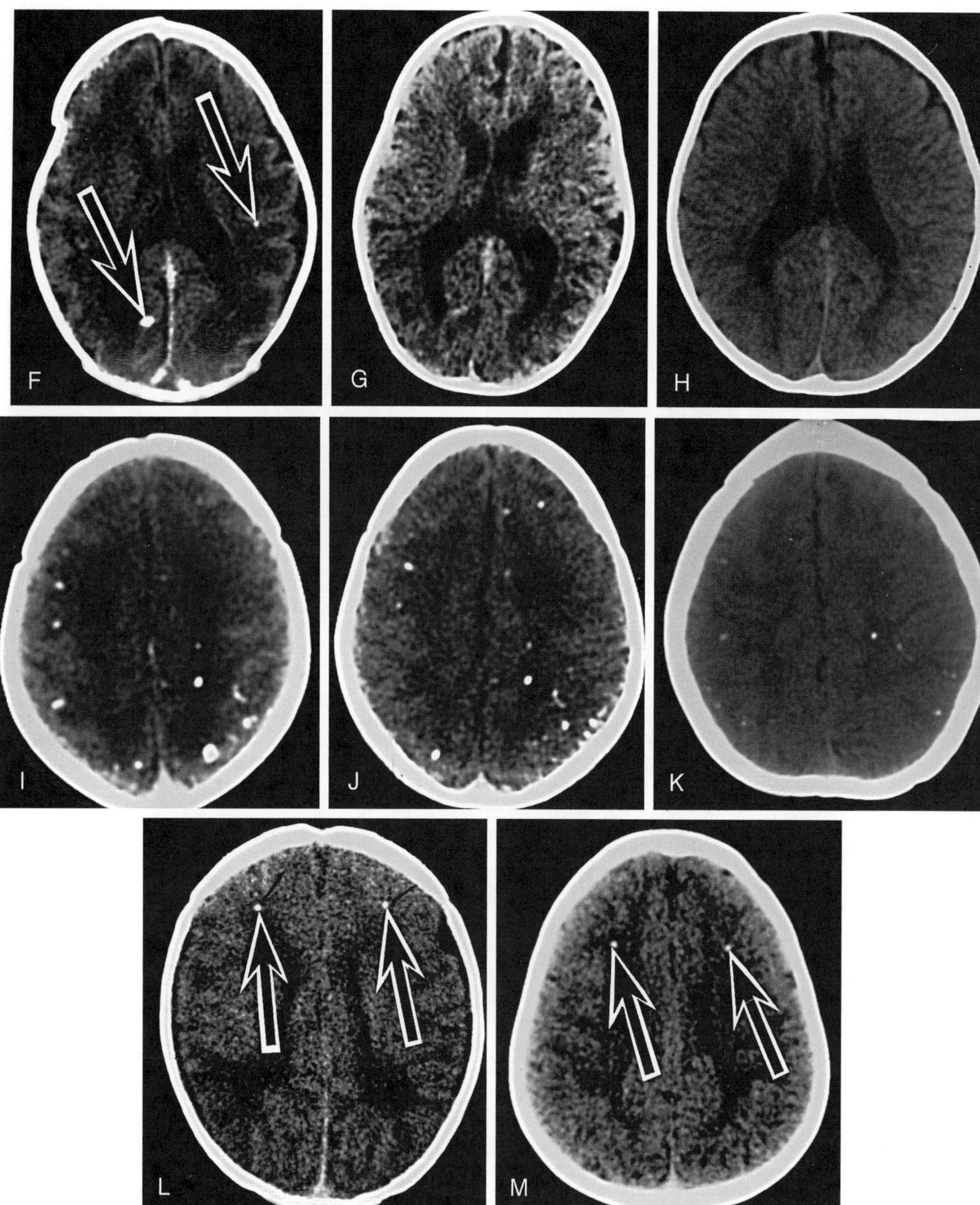

Figure 31–14 cont'd **F** to **H,** Cranial CT scans of the dizygotic twin of the patient whose CT scans are shown in **A** and **B**. Newborn scan (**F**) was obtained August 1992. The calcifications (*arrows*) were seen to have resolved on follow-up scans obtained in November 1992 (**G**) and in August 1993 (**H**). *Note:* The patient whose scans are shown in **A** and **B** was randomized to receive initial higher-dose therapy (6 months of 1 mg/kg/day of pyrimethamine), and the patient whose scans are shown in **F** to **H** was randomized to receive initial lower-dose therapy (2 months of 1 mg/kg/day of pyrimethamine). Both infants completed 1 year of treatment with pyrimethamine 1 mg/kg each Monday, Wednesday, and Friday and sulfadiazine. Calcifications were seen to have resolved completely in cranial CT scans of both twins. **I** to **K,** Cranial CT scans obtained for another infant in the newborn period, January 1993 (**I**), and at follow-up in February 1993 (**J**) and January 1994 (**K**) demonstrate diminution and/or resolution of calcifications. This child has developed normally. **L** and **M,** Cranial CT scans obtained in the newborn period, May 1991 (**L**), and in August 1992 (**M**) in a different, noncompliant child who underwent treatment in our study for only 1 month. *Arrows* mark calcifications that remained the same size. (From Patel DV, et al. Resolution of intracranial calcifications in infants with treated congenital toxoplasmosis. Radiology 199:433-440, 1996, with minor modifications and permission.)

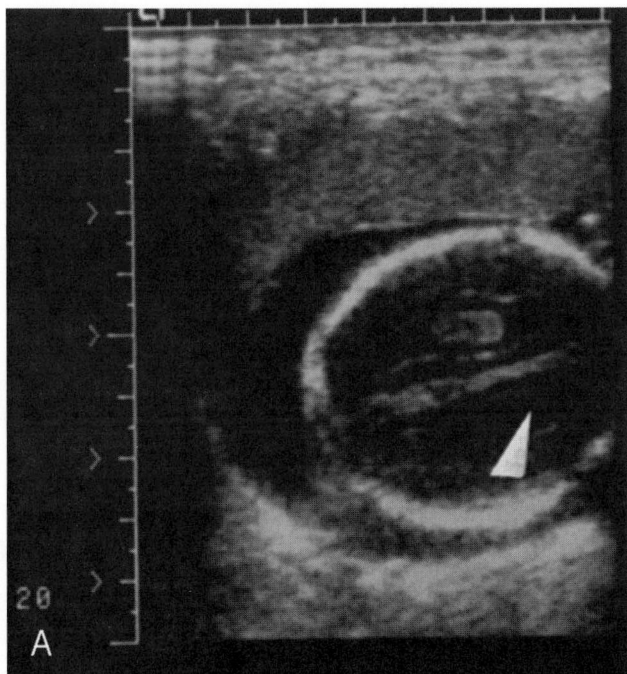

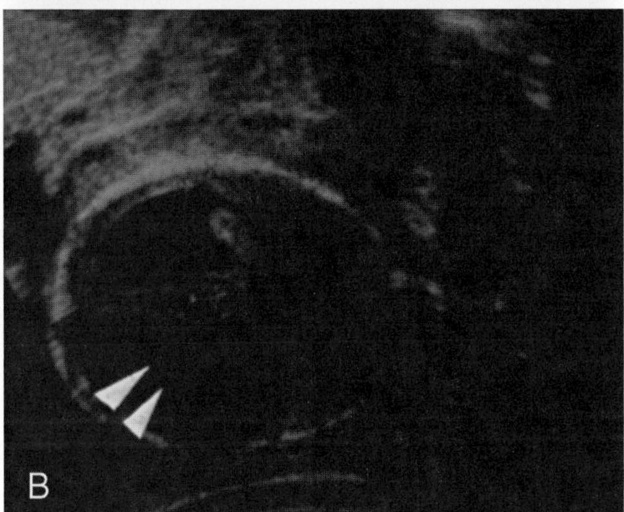

Figure 31–15 Rapid development of massive hydrocephalus in a fetus between 20 (**A**) and 21 (**B**) weeks of gestation. *Single arrowhead* indicates cerebral ventricles in **A**, and *double arrowheads* indicate massively dilated ventricles in **B**.

obstruction of the left foramen of Monro. Because of the rapid deterioration of the patient's condition, a craniotomy was performed; it revealed a large granular infiltrating tumor in the left temporal region. Numerous *T. gondii* organisms were seen in the operative specimen of brain. A similar cerebral mass lesion was described by Hervei and Simon in a case of congenital toxoplasmosis[709] and by Bobowski and Reed in a case of acquired toxoplasmosis.[710] Hervas and colleagues described a newborn with congenital toxoplasmosis whose cranial CT scan with contrast enhancement demonstrated calcifications and multiple ring-enhancing lesions not dissimilar to those seen in adult patients with AIDS, with multiple brain abscesses related to *T. gondii*.[531] McAuley and co-workers[534] also described enhancement around a lesion that resolved with antimicrobial treatment.

CT scan, which allows for neuroanatomic localization of intracranial calcifications, delineation of ventricular size, and recognition of cortical atrophy, has proved to be valuable in evaluation of congenital toxoplasmosis.[711-714] Diebler and associates published results of CT scans in 32 cases of congenital toxoplasmosis.[712] They reported a clear relationship between the lesions observed on these scans, neurologic signs, and date of maternal infection. The destructive lesions were porencephalic cysts that when multiple may constitute multicystic encephalomalacia or even hydranencephaly. Dense and large calcifications were seen in the basal ganglia in seven cases, with or without periventricular calcifications. Hydrocephalus was always secondary to aqueductal stenosis. In one case, ocular calcification was noted. In a retrospective study of cases in which pachygyria-like changes were observed on CT or magnetic resonance imaging, a single case of congenital toxoplasmosis was noted.[715] Ultrasonography also has been suggested as useful for diagnosis of congenital toxoplasmosis. CT scan of the brain detects calcifications not seen with ultrasonography of the brain.[716,717]

INTRACRANIAL CALCIFICATION

With rare exceptions,[546] the deposits of calcium noticed in congenital toxoplasmosis have been limited to the intracranial structures. The deposits are scattered throughout the brain and in some studies have been reported to have no characteristic distribution. In other studies, many children were observed to have prominent basal ganglia and periventricular califications.[705,718-722] Masherpa and Valentino described two types of calcifications: (1) multiple, dense round deposits 1 to 3 mm in diameter scattered in the white matter and, more frequently, in the periventricular areas of the occipitoparietal and temporal regions and (2) curvilinear streaks in the basal ganglia, mostly in the head of the caudate nucleus.[720] Some workers consider that evidence of both nodular calcifications and linear calcifications is pathognomonic of toxoplasmosis (Figs. 31-16 and 31-17).

Although in cytomegalic inclusion disease the calcifications are located chiefly subependymally and are bilaterally symmetrical, mostly in the walls of the dilated ventricles,[721,722] these locations also are noted in congenital toxoplasmosis. The largest series of cases of cerebral calcification related to congenital toxoplasmosis are those of Dyke and colleagues[723] and of Mussbichler.[724] The latter reviewed material from 32 clinically well-documented cases. Approximately one third of the patients were 3 months of age or younger, and 80% were younger than 2 years of age. Mussbichler's findings—some original and others confirming the findings of others—revealed that calcifications in the caudate nucleus, choroid plexuses, meninges, and subependyma are characteristic in toxoplasmosis, although some of these locations also have been described in cytomegalic inclusion disease. Because calcifications were present in multiple areas of the brain in the cases he reviewed, he concluded that calcifications found in the choroid plexuses alone should not be regarded as evidence of toxoplasmosis. Mussbichler found calcifications in the meninges that had not previously been described and attributed his ability to locate them to the use of appropriate projections that delineated them clearly. For those children who did not receive treatment, calcifications in the meninges and caudate nucleus were signs of a poor prognosis; they were found only in the youngest children,

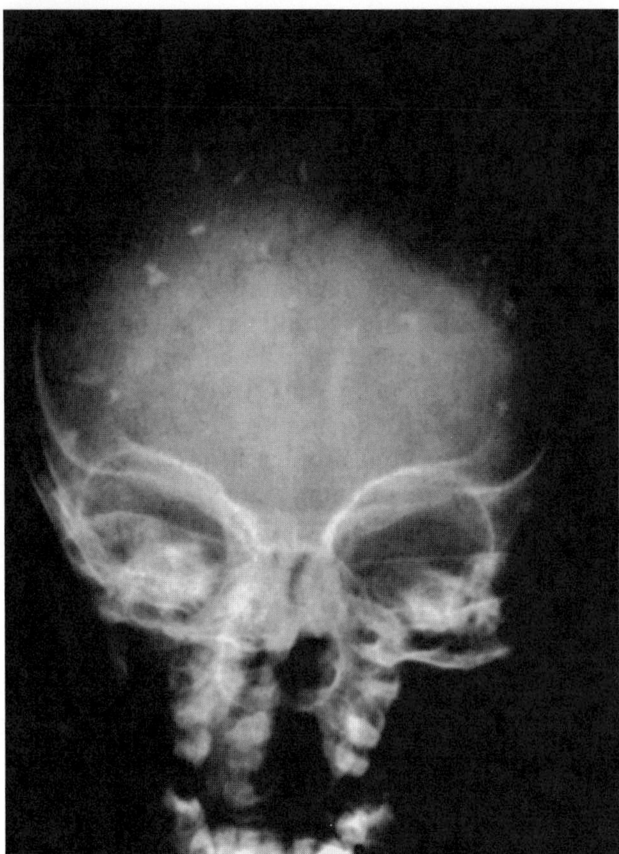

Figure 31–16 Cerebral calcifications in congenital toxoplasmosis in a 10-month-old infant; the infection was subclinical. (Courtesy of J Couvreur, Paris.)

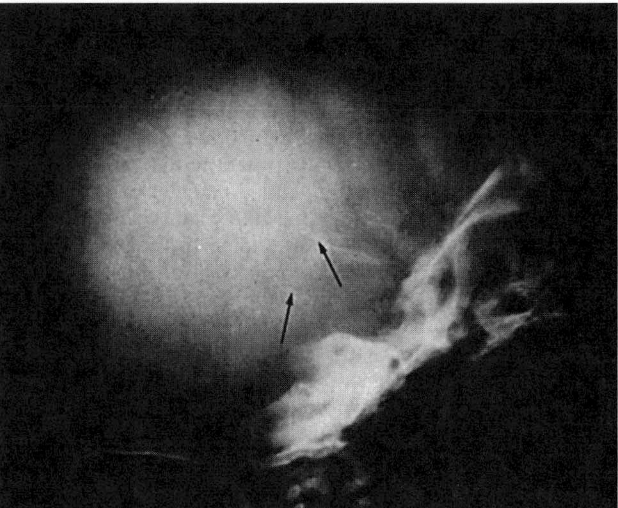

Figure 31–17 Cerebral calcifications in congenital toxoplasmosis in a neonate, with calcifications lining the ventricles (*arrows*). (Courtesy of J Couvreur, Paris.)

who died early. Conversely, disseminated nodular calcifications do not necessarily suggest a poor prognosis and have been discovered fortuitously in "normal" infants who were studied at approximately 1 year of age; in these children, a diagnosis of congenital toxoplasmosis had been made through a systematic survey. The increase in size and number of calcific lesions during a period of months or years in some cases suggests that the process of healing (and perhaps also of destruction) may occur long after the onset of the infection. Calcifications can diminish in size or resolve with treatment.[705]

OSSEOUS CHANGES

In 1974, Milgram described the radiographic signs present in an infant who died 17 days after birth with a severe clinical form of congenital toxoplasmosis.[517] Roentgenograms of several ribs and vertebrae and one femur revealed bands of metaphyseal lucency and irregularity of the line of provisional calcification at the epiphyseal plates. Periosteal reaction was not present. (Syphilis also may cause this same finding.)

LIVER

Although it has been stated that calcifications do not occur outside the CNS in infants with congenital toxoplasmosis, Caldera and colleagues described cases of three infants with calcifications in the liver.[546] The calcifications were evident both radiologically and in the liver at autopsy.

Other Signs and Symptoms

Erythroblastosis and Hydrops Fetalis. Congenital toxoplasmosis may be confused with erythroblastosis related to isosensitization.[524,675,725-730] The peripheral blood picture and clinical course may be identical to those observed in other forms of erythroblastosis. This similarity is exemplified by cases such as those reported by Callahan and colleagues[513] and by Beckett and Flynn.[114] A negative Coombs test result is helpful in distinguishing erythroblastosis caused by congenital infection from that caused by blood group factor sensitization.

Cardiovascular Signs. Severe toxoplasmic myocarditis may be manifested clinically as edema.[513]

Gastrointestinal Signs. In some cases, the first sign of the disease appears to be vomiting or diarrhea.[513] Feeding problems also are common.

Respiratory Difficulty. Respiratory difficulty,[12,513] often with cyanosis, may be due to an interstitial toxoplasmic pneumonitis, to viral or bacterial suprainfection, or to CNS lesions affecting the respiratory control centers of the brain.

Deafness. From the follow-up studies of Eichenwald[596] and others,[731] ample clinical and histologic[70,513,541,608,732] data are available to show that congenital infection with *T. gondii* can lead to deafness. The well-documented cases of profound hearing loss have been almost totally confined to infants with severe clinical disease, but in the series of children with subclinical infection at birth reported by Wilson and associates,[731] 17% had significant hearing loss. In some instances, serologic and skin test surveys among deaf patients have suggested a cause-and-effect relationship,[733] whereas in others, no such relationship has been found.[734] An association between epilepsy, cerebral palsy, and nerve deafness and the presence of antibodies to *T. gondii* in sera of

Israeli children was noted (relative risk 2.5, $P = .03$; nerve deafness relative risk 7.1, $P = .01$).[735] Such studies frequently are open to criticism, owing to the choice of controls. Thus, no satisfactory data are available to support the contention that congenital toxoplasmosis may be a frequent cause of deafness.[736] In the NCCTS, as of November 2004, no child with sensorineural hearing loss was identified (Table 31-27).[737] One child with brain-stem lesions involving the auditory nucleus had auditory perceptual difficulties.

Ascites. Vanhaesebrouck and co-workers described a preterm congenitally infected infant with isolated transudative ascites caused by *T. gondii*.[738] Neonatal[739] and fetal[125,740,741] ascites due to congenital toxoplasmosis have been reported.

Follow-up Studies

Adequate follow-up studies (see also the previous "Eye" section) to gain information on the natural course of congenital toxoplasmosis are lacking in most series of reported cases. In the vast majority, the original diagnosis was made in a retrospective manner, in most cases because of the presence of clinical signs of the infection. Most accumulated data, therefore, are from infants and older children with the most atypical form of congenital toxoplasmosis, that is, clinically apparent disease in the newborn period. It is in those infants who are actually in the majority—those who were asymptomatic at birth—that there is the greatest need for follow-up studies, such as those performed by Alford and colleagues,[556,660] described previously. (See also the published studies by Hedenström and colleagues.[742,743]) Findings on follow-up evaluation of the infants who were asymptomatic at birth in the Paris study are difficult to interpret, because most were given treatment in the newborn period. In some, however, recognition of the first clinical finding (usually chorioretinitis) was delayed until several weeks or months after birth, thereby illustrating an often reported observation in congenital toxoplasmosis: the normal appearance of a child for some months before overt disease is recognized.[109,744,631,745]

Follow-up studies of those patients described by Eichenwald have already been mentioned. Two patients reported by Wolf and co-workers in 1942[530] were still alive in 1959 and were being cared for in mental institutions.[746] One of them, first seen at the age of 3 years and 9 months, was about 22 years old at the time of the second report. She was mentally and physically retarded and oblivious to her environment, drooled constantly, was resistant to care and feeding, and was losing weight. She continued to have petit mal and grand mal seizures. Old chorioretinal scars were still present. The second patient was 2 years old when the diagnosis was made and about 18 years of age at the time of the last report. His IQ was only 40. He was said to have a pleasant personality and could engage in some project activities. Vision was 20/100 in one eye and 20/70 in the other.

Feldman and Miller analyzed 187 patients with congenital toxoplasmosis. Among 176 of these patients, 119 were 4 years of age or younger, 38 were 5 to 9 years of age, and 19 were 10 to 19 years of age.[144] Thirty-six had been delivered prematurely; 20% of the premature infants and 7% of those born at term died. Residual damage varied in degree, but most of the patients exhibited chorioretinitis, mental retardation, and abnormalities of head size. In this series, reported frequencies of abnormalities were as follows: intracerebral calcification, 59%; psychomotor retardation, 45%; seizures, 39%; chorioretinitis. 94%. microphthalmia. 36%; hydrocephalus, 22%; and microcephaly, 21%.[597]

Puissan and co-workers observed the late onset of convulsions in an 8-year-old girl with congenital toxoplasmosis.[747] Of interest in this case was the demonstration of what appears to have been local production of *T. gondii* antibody in the cerebrospinal fluid when the convulsions began.

In the first report of the prospective study by Koppe and colleagues, follow-up data were obtained for 7 years for 12 congenitally infected children.[600] Four children had clinical signs (ocular only), and 1 was clinically normal but *T. gondii* had been isolated from the placenta and cerebrospinal fluid; these 5 were given pyrimethamine and sulfadiazine. No signs of cerebral damage or intracranial calcifications developed in any of the children, and all were said to be "mentally normal" at the age of 7 years.[600] Their development was judged by their performance in school, which was stated to be normal. In fact, in a later report, chorioretinitis had developed in two thirds of these children,[601] and because they were still younger than 15 years of age when last reported, they remained at risk for the development of additional sequelae. (See the "Amsterdam Study" section later for the final report.)

Congenital *Toxoplasma* Infection and Acquired Immunodeficiency Syndrome

Congenital transmission of *T. gondii* from pregnant women co-infected with *T. gondii* and HIV has been recognized as a unique problem[748-755] but fortunately a relatively uncommon one.[756-762] Unfortunately, we have insufficient data on what the CD4$^+$ T lymphocyte counts were in these dually infected women during their pregnancies because transmission of *T. gondii* from these chronically infected women would be most likely to occur in the setting of severe immunosuppression. Such data would assist in determining the importance of this and other parameters of immunosuppression that place the fetus at risk for congenital *T. gondii* infection. These mothers had chronic *T. gondii* infection and did not have demonstrable IgM *T. gondii* antibodies. Noteworthy are the observations that most of the newborns did not have clinical signs of either infection at birth, even though in each case the infant was found to be dually infected with the parasite and HIV. In many of these infants, signs of severe disseminated infection developed within the first weeks or months of life.

Mitchell and colleagues described four young infants, two of whom were siblings, who were dually infected with HIV-1 and *T. gondii*.[748] Their mothers were similarly co-infected. The mother of the first infant had toxoplasmic encephalitis diagnosed at delivery. The other mothers had no clinical evidence of toxoplasmosis but did have *T. gondii* antibodies. The investigators concluded that the mother was the source of the infection in each of the infants. Of interest is that in three of the seven cases (three additional cases were diagnosed after the initial publication) documented at the University of Miami, the diagnosis was not suspected before the patient's death and was made only at autopsy (C Mitchell, personal communication to JS Remington, 1993). Three of the four cases from the original publication are briefly reviewed here as examples of the problem.

Table 31–27 Definitions of Hearing Impairment and Outcome in Reported Studies of Hearing in Cases of Congenital Toxoplasmosis[596, 599, 737]

	Definitions				Results		
	U.S. (Chicago) National Collaborative Treatment Trial[737]						
Degree of Hearing Impairment	*ABR (dB/HL)*	*Audiogram (dB/HL)*	*Wilson et al.*[599]	*Eichenwald*[596]	*U.S. (Chicago) National Collaborative Treatment Trial*[787]	*Wilson et al.*[599]	*Eichenwald*[596]
Normal	≤20	0-20	<25 dB[a]	NA	104	14	NA
Mild	>20-40	25-40	25-50 dB	NA	0	3	NA
Moderate	>40-60	>40	51-80 dB	NA	0	2	NA
Severe	>60	>70-90	Not found	NA	0	0	NA
Profound		>90	Not found	"Deaf"	0	0	15
Total					104	19	105

[a]Defined as "hearing reception threshold" by Wilson and McLeod.[599]

ABR, auditory brain response; dB, decibels; HL, hearing level; NA, not available.

Adapted from McGee T, et al. Absence of sensorineural hearing loss in treated infants and children wih congenital toxoplasmosis. Otolaryngol Head Neck Surg 106:75-80, 1992, with minor modifications and permission.

CASE HISTORY: INFANTS 2 AND 3

The mother of the siblings with congenital *T. gondii* infection had given birth to five children, four of whom were infected with HIV-1. The siblings with toxoplasmosis were the third and fifth born. AIDS developed in the mother 1 month after the birth of this fifth child, but she had no clinical or tomographic evidence of toxoplasmic encephalitis. She died 8 months later of tuberculosis and bacterial sepsis. An autopsy was not performed. One sibling, born at term and "appropriate for gestational age," was discharged from the hospital at 3 days of age in good condition, only to return at 3 months of age with complications of AIDS. He remained hospitalized until he died at age 6 months. At autopsy, he was found to have disseminated cytomegalovirus infection involving most visceral organs and all lobes of the lung, *T. gondii* pneumonitis, and diffuse CNS toxoplasmosis. The other sibling was a full-term female appropriate for gestational age. She had an unremarkable neonatal course. When seen at 5 weeks of age, she was in septic shock and emaciated and had severe oral thrush. She died within 1 hour after admission to the hospital. Blood cultures were positive for *Propionibacterium*; autopsy revealed disseminated candidiasis involving the lungs and esophagus and diffuse intracerebral toxoplasmosis.

CASE HISTORY: INFANT 4

The patient was an appropriate-for-gestational-age, full-term female infant recognized at birth to be at risk for congenital toxoplasmosis and HIV-1 infection because her mother was known to be seropositive for *T. gondii* and had previously given birth to a child who died of AIDS. Results of examination at birth were normal, but the infant was given expectant treatment for toxoplasmosis with pyrimethamine and sulfadiazine because of the presence of IgM *T. gondii* antibodies in her serum. After an extended course of therapy complicated by hepatitis of unclear etiology, she died; permission for autopsy was denied. This child's mother died of AIDS 3 years later, never having developed clinical toxoplasmosis.

■

Marty and co-workers[763] described a 22-week pregnant, HIV-infected woman who was observed to have reactivation of her *T. gondii* serologic test titer (from an IgG dye test titer of 5 IU/mL to 400 IU at 1 year later). She had a $CD4^+$ cell count of $90/mm^3$. An ultrasound examination revealed fetal hydrocephaly, and a therapeutic abortion was performed. The external morphology of the fetus was normal, but autopsy revealed multiple abscesses in the brain and liver, and *T. gondii* was isolated from amniotic fluid, placenta, liver, spleen, heart, and brain.

PATHOLOGY

Information on pathologic changes in the CNS in fetuses or newborns co-infected with *T. gondii* and HIV-1 is relatively scarce. In three of the cases reported by Mitchell and co-workers, histologic evidence of meningitis included chronic leptomeningeal inflammatory cell infiltrates.[748] *T. gondii* cysts, as well as microglial nodules that suggested an immune response against the parasite, were seen in the brain in two cases. Examination of numerous slides from the brain of one infant, who had received treatment for toxoplasmosis, revealed only a single *T. gondii* cyst and no microglial nodules. The brain revealed chronic inflammation and widespread foci of necrosis surrounded by macrophages, lymphocytes, and plasma cells. Gliosis also was present. Immunoperoxidase staining demonstrated *T. gondii* in the CNS of this infant.

Insufficient data are available to estimate how frequently the diagnosis of congenital *T. gondii* infection in these dually infected infants might be suggested by serologic examination. IgM and IgG *T. gondii* antibodies have been demonstrable in some of these infants (C Mitchell and A Kovacs, personal communication to JS Remington, 1993).[750]

TREATMENT

Treatment of the Newborn. Data on the outcome of treatment of congenital *T. gondii* infection in these newborns are insufficient for any conclusions to be drawn. The diagnosis of co-infection with HIV usually has been made late and often a month or more after birth. Thus, at least at present, whether to use drugs directed against HIV in combination with anti-*T. gondii* therapy in the early newborn period does not appear to be a major consideration. Of importance in this regard is that toxicity to the bone marrow may be considerably increased when, for example, zidovudine, pyrimethamine, and sulfadiazine are used together. When the diagnosis in the newborn is suspected or proved, we recommend that the pyrimethamine-sulfadiazine combination be used. Treatment is continued for the first year of life. Data from adults with HIV and *T. gondii* infections suggest that if the $CD4^+$ cell count is maintained at greater than 200 cells/µL with antiretroviral treatment, it may be feasible, after the standard 1-year treatment, to discontinue treatment with pyrimethamine and sulfadiazine.

Treatment and Primary Prophylaxis in the Human Immunodeficiency Virus– and *Toxoplasma gondii*–Infected Pregnant Woman. Treatment with pyrimethamine-sulfadiazine (and leucovorin) should be started in patients with active toxoplasmosis.[764] Clindamycin may be used as an alternative to sulfadiazine in the combination.[765] Use of pyrimethamine in the first trimester is contraindicated, as discussed earlier. The decision whether to use this drug should be made in consultation with experts.

Until more complete information becomes available on the special factors that predispose to congenital transmission of *T. gondii* in these women, we recommend that primary prophylaxis be used in those with $CD4^+$ T cell counts of fewer than 200 cells per mm^3. The combination agent trimethoprim-sulfamethoxazole, commonly used in these patients to prevent *Pneumocystis* pneumonia, is effective in prevention of toxoplasmic encephalitis in patients with AIDS who can tolerate the drug.[766] Use of this and other drug regimens for *T. gondii* primary prophylaxis is common practice for management of nonpregnant HIV-infected adults who also have chronic *T. gondii* infection.[766] More complete treatment of this subject is beyond the scope of this chapter. For a commentary on this issue in general, the reader is referred to reference 766. It should be noted, however, that no data are available on whether pyrimethamine-sulfadiazine and pyrimethamine-clindamycin combinations are of comparable efficacy in preventing transmission of *T. gondii* to the fetus.

Of interest in regard to the transmission from mother to her fetus are two cases of CNS toxoplasmosis in HIV-infected pregnant women who gave birth to infants who were not infected with *T. gondii*.[767,768]

DIAGNOSIS

The diagnosis of acute infection with *T. gondii* may be established by isolation of the organism from blood or body fluids, demonstration of the presence of cysts in the placenta or tissues of a fetus or newborn, demonstration of the presence of antigen or organisms or both in sections or preparations of tissues and body fluids, demonstration of antigenemia and antigen in serum and body fluids, specific nucleic acid sequences (e.g., using PCR methods), or serologic tests.

Diagnostic Methods

Laboratory Examination

Cerebrospinal Fluid (See also "Serologic Diagnosis in the Newborn" and "Serologic Studies and Polymerase Chain Reaction Assay in Cerebrospinal Fluid; Polymerase Chain Reaction Asay in Urine" later on.) Approximately 4 decades ago, Callahan and colleagues, in reviewing the cerebrospinal fluid changes in 108 patients with congenital toxoplasmosis, stated, "Examination of the CSF affords the most constant significant laboratory examination for the presence of infantile toxoplasmosis."[513] Although the patients studied by these investigators had the most severe form of the disease, this statement is pertinent even today. Despite the fact that cerebrospinal fluid changes in infants with congenital toxoplasmosis are not specific for toxoplasmosis, the demonstration of these changes should lead the physician to consider a diagnosis of toxoplasmosis even in subclinical cases. The findings of xanthochromia and mononuclear pleocytosis in cases of congenital toxoplasmosis also are common in many other generalized infections of the newborn. Almost unique to infants with neonatal toxoplasmosis, however, is the very high protein content of the ventricular fluid. Although in some infants the protein level is just slightly above normal, in others it can be measured in grams per deciliter rather than in milligrams per deciliter.[70,556,769] Alford and associates considered that in most infants with congenital toxoplasmosis who appear clinically normal at birth, a "silent" CNS involvement is present as reflected by persistent cerebrospinal fluid pleocytosis and the elevated protein content (see also the "Central Nervous System" section under both "Pathology" and "Clinical Manifestations").[556]

Increases in protein levels and pleocytosis were not as common in a prospective study performed in France (G Desmonts, unpublished data). The difference probably is due to the difference in method of selection of cases. In the study reported by Alford and associates, only those infants in whom an elevated serum IgM was present at birth were screened for *T. gondii* antibody, and the development of the infection in these infants by the time of birth may have differed significantly from that in the French studies, in which infants were examined because of suspicion of maternal toxoplasmosis acquired during pregnancy. In the French study, the infants, who were infected very close to the time of labor or during labor, may not have had elevated serum IgM levels at birth and therefore would have been missed in the studies in which IgM screening alone was the criterion for case selection.

Persistence of IgM antibodies to *T. gondii* in the cerebrospinal fluid has been observed in some infected infants and may suggest continued active infection. Such persistence of IgM antibodies in the cerebrospinal fluid also has been reported in congenital rubella.[770]

Specific IgG antibody formation in the CNS has been demonstrated in infants with congenital toxoplasmosis.[771] Two hundred forty-two examinations were performed in 206 congenitally infected infants as part of the routine cerebrospinal fluid workup. Only three cases (1.8%) had demonstrable local IgG antibody formation in the CNS. *T. gondii* has been detected by PCR assay in cerebrospinal fluid of newborns with congenital toxoplasmosis (see "Polymerase Chain Reaction Assay," later on). Woods and Englund[772] described a newborn with severe congenital toxoplasmosis who presented with signs of brain destruction and whose cerebrospinal fluid was hazy and xanthochromic, with 302 white blood cells per mm^3 and 106 red blood cells per mm^3. The differential count revealed 1% neutrophils, 8% mononuclear cells, and 91% eosinophils. The cerebrospinal fluid glucose level was 23 mg/dL, and the cerebrospinal fluid protein level was 158 mg/dL. At the same time, the peripheral blood showed 16% eosinophils (absolute count 432 eosinophils per mm^3). Although peripheral blood eosinophilia is common in newborns with congenital toxoplasmosis, as are eosinophilic infiltrations of the pia-arachnoid overlying destructive cortical lesions, eosinophilia has not previously been reported in the cerebrospinal fluid of such newborns.

A newborn whose congenital toxoplasmosis caused hydrocephalus and cerebral atrophy and quadriparesis as a result of spinal cord atrophy had peripheral blood eosinophilia (40%) and markedly abnormal cerebrospinal fluid (13% of 98 white blood cells) (W Barson, personal communication to R McLeod, 1999). Treatment with pyrimethamine and sulfadiazine given to the mother during gestation may diminish manifestations, including cerebrospinal fluid pleocytosis or elevated cerebrospinal fluid protein in the infant.[124]

Blood and Blood-Forming Elements. Leukocytosis or leukopenia may be present, and early in the course of the infection, lymphocytosis and monocytosis usually are found.[12,513,637] Marked polymorphonuclear leukocytosis frequently reflects suprainfection with bacteria.

Thrombocytopenia is common in infants who have other clinical signs of the infection as well as in subclinical cases,[528,549,742,773] petechiae or ecchymoses may be the earliest clue to this congenital infection.[513,518,524,528,742] Eosinophilia in the newborn period frequently has been observed, and the eosinophils may exceed 30% of the differential white blood cell count.[12,70,513,608,637,774-776]

Histologic Diagnosis

Demonstration of tachyzoites in tissues (e.g., brain biopsy, bone marrow aspirate) or body fluids (ventricular fluid or cerebrospinal fluid[514,531,777-780] aqueous humor,[781] sputum[276]) establishes the diagnosis of acute toxoplasmosis. Unfortunately, it frequently is difficult to visualize the tachyzoite form in tissues or impression smears stained by ordinary methods. Accordingly, the fluorescent antibody technique has been suggested for this purpose.[123,782-784] Because of its greater sensitivity and specificity, the peroxidase-antiperoxidase technique has largely supplanted the fluorescent antibody method.[785] Both methods are applicable to unfixed or formalin-fixed paraffin-embedded tissue sections. The pitfalls in interpretation of results with these methods have been discussed by Frenkel and Piekarski.[786] In the retina, because the retinal pigment epithelium is brown or black, a method that stains the parasites red, rather than brown, has proved useful for detection of the parasites.[506] Histologic demonstration of the cyst form establishes that the patient has toxoplasmosis but does not warrant the conclusion that the infection is acute unless there is associated inflammation and necrosis. On the other hand, because cysts may form early in infection, their demonstration does not exclude the possibility that the infection is still in the acute stages.[787]

In the case of acute acquired toxoplasmosis in the pregnant patient, lymphadenopathy may reflect a variety of infectious agents.[576] Distinctive histologic changes in toxoplasmic lymphadenitis enable the pathologist to make a presumptive diagnosis of acute acquired toxoplasmosis.[788] These histologic changes represent the characteristic reaction of the host to the infection, but the organisms themselves are only rarely demonstrable. The histologic signs of infection in other tissues range from areas of no inflammation around cysts to acute necrotizing lesions associated with tachyzoites. The latter are seen almost solely in immunocompromised individuals. None of these changes confirms the diagnosis of toxoplasmosis unless the organism can be demonstrated.

Isolation Procedures

GENERAL CONSIDERATIONS

Isolation of the parasite from an infant provides unequivocal proof of infection, but unfortunately, such isolation usually takes too long to permit an early diagnosis. *T. gondii* is readily isolated from tissue obtained at autopsy (e.g., brain, skeletal muscle, or heart muscle); the organism may also be isolated from biopsy material from the neonate (e.g., skeletal muscle). In our experience, isolates from congenitally infected infants are most often avirulent for mice, and a period of 4 to 6 weeks is usually required for definitive demonstration of the parasite when this method is used. In cases in which the organism is virulent for mice, the parasite can often be demonstrated in the peritoneal fluid after 5 to 10 days. *T. gondii* has been isolated from body fluids (e.g., ventricular fluid or cerebrospinal fluid[530]),[767,778,789-795] subretinal fluid,[796] and aqueous humor[797] of infants and adults, and from amniotic fluid.[793,798,799] Isolation from tissues (e.g., skeletal muscle, lung, brain, or eye) obtained by biopsy or at autopsy from older children and adults may reflect only the presence of tissue cysts and thus does not constitute definitive proof of active acute infection. One possible exception is the isolation of *T. gondii* from lymph nodes in older children and adults; such evidence probably indicates relatively recently acquired infection, because cysts are rarely found in lymph nodes. Attempts at isolation usually are performed by injection of suspect material into laboratory mice but also may be accomplished by inoculation into tissue culture preparations (see later).[514,794,800,801] One can observe plaque formation and both extracellular and intracellular parasites in unstained or stained preparations. Abbas found cell cultures less sensitive than mouse inoculation for isolation of the parasite.[802] Thus, if cell cultures are used in attempts at primary isolation, it is advisable also to use mouse inoculation when feasible. Tissue culture isolation is quite rapid (usually requiring 1 week or less) and should be used when early isolation is critical for the management of the patient. Because physicians often request that isolation procedures be performed, the following are offered as guidelines for the laboratory.

Specimens should be injected into animals and cell cultures as soon as possible after collection to prevent death of the parasite. Formalin kills the parasite, and freezing may result in death of both tachyzoite and cyst forms. If storage of specimens is necessary, refrigeration at 4° C is preferred. This can maintain the encysted form in tissues, if kept moist, for up to 2 months and prevents death of the tachyzoite for several days. The parasite can survive in blood for a week or longer (see "Transmission" section). For antibody determination, serum may be removed from clotted cord blood or blood obtained later in the newborn period; the clot should be stored at 4° C until the results of serologic tests are known. If results of serologic tests are not diagnostic and the reason for suspecting congenital toxoplasmosis remains, the blood clot should be injected into mice (or tissue culture) in the same way as for any other tissue specimen. Body fluids and heparinized blood can be injected directly, but we prefer to remove the plasma from the formed elements of blood and amniotic fluid, to eliminate the possibility of introducing a majority of *T. gondii* antibodies into the recipient animals. Passively transferred human antibody may interfere with infection of the mice, and thus with isolation of the organisms, as well as producing false-positive serologic test results in the inoculated animals for 6 weeks or longer.[104] Because the organisms are most likely to reside within white blood cells in patients with parasitemia, the buffy coat layer may be suspended in a small volume of sterile saline and inoculated into mice by the intraperitoneal or subcutaneous route or onto tissue culture.

Biopsy specimens and blood clots may be triturated with a mortar and pestle or tissue homogenizer in a small amount of normal saline before animal or tissue culture inoculation. After trituration, we generally add enough sterile saline so that the suspension can be drawn into a syringe. If connective tissue prevents aspiration through the needle, the suspension can be filtered through several layers of sterile gauze. Depending on the size of the mice, 0.5 to 2 mL is injected intraperitoneally, subcutaneously, or both.

For isolation attempts from superficial enlarged lymph nodes, material can be obtained by needle aspiration of the node.

To isolate *T. gondii* from large amounts of tissue (e.g., placenta), we use trypsin digestion (0.25% trypsin in buffered saline, pH 7.2).[114] The trypsin method makes it possible to isolate both tachyzoite and cyst forms. The former are killed more rapidly by pepsin-hydrochloric acid (HCl).[43] The tissue is first minced with scissors and passed through a meat grinder or ground in a blender; it is then placed in a volume of trypsin solution (10 to 20 mL of trypsin solution per gram of tissue) and incubated with constant agitation for 1.5 to 2 hours at 37° C. (If the tissue is grossly contaminated, antibiotics may be added both to the digestion fluid and to the tissue digest before injection.) The suspension is passed through several layers of gauze to remove large particles and then is centrifuged. After the sediment has been washed three or four times in saline to remove trypsin, the digested material is resuspended in saline, and 0.5 to 1 mL is injected both intraperitoneally and subcutaneously into mice. If peptic digestion is desired, the solution is prepared by dissolving 4 g of pepsin (Difco 1:10,000), 7.5 g of sodium chloride, and 10.5 mL of concentrated HCl in water to a volume of 1500 mL. The method described by Dubey also may be used.[803]

MOUSE INOCULATION

In most countries, it is not necessary to perform serologic testing in laboratory mice to determine if they are infected before they are used in isolation attempts. In areas of the world where normal laboratory mice have been found to be infected, serologic testing of individual mice must be performed before such use. Five to 10 days after intraperitoneal injection, the peritoneal fluid should be examined either fresh or in stained smears (Wright or Giemsa stain) for the presence of intracellular and extracellular tachyzoites (see Fig. 31-1A). Demonstration of the organism is proof of the infection. Mice that die before 6 weeks have elapsed are examined for the presence of the organism in their peritoneal fluid; stained impression smears of liver and spleen also can be examined. If no organisms are found, suspensions of liver, spleen, and brain may be injected into fresh mice. Surviving mice are bled from the tail vein or orbital sinus for serologic testing after 6 weeks but may be bled from the tail vein more often (e.g., at 2-week intervals). (The dye test, agglutination test, IFA test, or ELISA can be used for this purpose.) We prefer to use the agglutination test as a screening method for this purpose because only a single drop of blood from the tail vein can be tested using microtiter plate wells. If antibodies are present, proof of infection must be obtained by demonstration of the parasite. This can be accomplished most easily by examining Giemsa-stained smears of fresh brain for demonstration of cysts (see Fig. 31-1E). Examination of wet preparations of brain tissue may be misinterpreted if done by inexperienced workers; pine pollen has been confused with *T. gondii* cysts and has led to erroneous diagnosis of the infection. Examination is easier under phase microscopy. If cysts are not seen, injection into fresh mice of a suspension of brain, liver, and spleen should be performed to determine whether the parasite is present.

TISSUE CULTURE

Isolation by tissue culture has been used routinely by Derouin and colleagues, with a high degree of success.[799] They use coverslip cultures of human embryonic fibroblasts (MRC5, bioMérieux, Lyon, France) in wells of 24-well plates (Nunc, Denmark).[801] The sediment of approximately 10 mL of amniotic fluid is resuspended in 8 mL of minimum essential medium (MEM) supplemented with 10% fetal calf serum, penicillin (5 IU/mL), and streptomycin (50 mg/mL). One milliliter of the suspension is inoculated into each of six cell culture wells and incubated for 72 to 96 hours at 37° C. Thereafter, they are washed with phosphate-buffered saline and fixed with cold acetone. Indirect immunofluorescence is then performed on the coverslip cultures, using rabbit anti–*T. gondii* IgG as the first antibody and fluorescein-labeled rabbit anti-IgG as the second antibody. After the coverslips are mounted onto slides, they are examined for the presence of *T. gondii* by fluorescence microscopy. Parasite division is readily observed in the cells, as is pseudocyst formation; if cells are heavily infected, foci of extracellular parasites may be present. Some workers stain the coverslips with Wright-Giemsa stain or use the immunoperoxidase method to demonstrate *T. gondii* in the cultures. These methods, however, are less sensitive than immunofluorescence for detection of low numbers of parasitized cells.

SPECIAL CONSIDERATIONS

Placenta. If congenital toxoplasmosis is suspected in a newborn, either because acute toxoplasmosis was diagnosed during pregnancy in the mother or because clinical signs raise suspicion of this diagnosis in the neonate, approximately 100 g of placenta should be kept without fixative and stored at 4° C until it can be injected into mice. Digestion with trypsin is preferable. This procedure yielded positive results in 25% of placentas obtained from 123 mothers who acquired toxoplasmosis during pregnancy, and in each of these positive cases it was associated with a congenitally infected neonate.[789]

Conversely, cases in which infants were proved to be infected, despite the inability to isolate *T. gondii* from their placentas, are rare unless mothers have received treatment during pregnancy.[117,804] Injection of placental tissue into mice is a very useful tool for the diagnosis of congenital toxoplasmosis.

Blood. *T. gondii* may be isolated from cord or peripheral blood of the newborn.[777] Such isolation should be attempted whenever possible, because serologic diagnosis may be uncertain during the first weeks or months of life. In a study of 69 infants with congenital toxoplasmosis, Desmonts and Couvreur isolated *T. gondii* from peripheral blood in 30 (43%) of them (see Table 31-1).[805] The high incidence (52%) of parasitemia in infants with subclinical infection is noteworthy, as is the overall frequency of parasitemia in congenital cases.

Relatively few positive results were obtained in infants with only neurologic or ocular signs of the disease. This might be related to the fact that these infants usually are not examined during the first days of life, unlike those with generalized disease or those in whom the possibility of disease is suspected because of prospective studies in their mothers. Seventy-one percent of the positive results were obtained from samples of blood taken during the first week of life. The percentage decreased to 33% when blood for isolation purposes was obtained during the following 3 weeks, and there were no positive results in infants older than 1 month of age.[805]

Saliva. Levi and co-workers have reported the isolation of *T. gondii* from saliva of 12 of 20 patients, mostly with the lymphadenopathic form of the disease.[276] This report is interesting but requires confirmation. Whether the parasite can be isolated (or demonstrated by PCR assay) from sputum or saliva in the newborn period remains to be determined, but the presence of the organism in the alveoli of the lung suggests that attempts at isolation from such material might prove successful.

Postmortem Specimens. *T. gondii* is most easily isolated post mortem from brain specimens from infected infants and from infected infants who die months or years after birth, although it also has been isolated from virtually every organ and tissue of infants with congenital toxoplasmosis. Here again, digestion with either pepsin or trypsin is preferred, because it allows for sampling of sufficiently large amounts of tissue. If necessary, brain specimens passed several times through a syringe and a 20-gauge needle can be injected into mice directly without prior digestion. It is noteworthy that isolation of *T. gondii* from the placenta is common in cases in which fetal death has occurred in utero. Although the organisms are regularly isolated from infected fetuses after induced abortion, they usually cannot be isolated from infected macerated fetal tissue that has remained in utero for an extended period of time after the fetus has died.

Tests of Cell-Mediated Immunity

Toxoplasmin Skin Test. At present, the skin test is not used in diagnosis of congenital infection, and no systematic study has been performed to define its potential usefulness for this purpose. It is discussed here for the sake of completeness.

Infection with *T. gondii* results in the development of cell-mediated immunity against the parasite. This may be demonstrated with the toxoplasmin skin test,[806] which elicits delayed hypersensitivity. The large-scale use of the skin test, especially in population surveys, has yielded excellent agreement between the results of this test for delayed hypersensitivity and the presence or absence of antibody.[280,806-810] False-positive skin test results are rare.[811] Delayed skin hypersensitivity to *T. gondii* antigens in cases of acquired infection appears not to develop until months or years after the initial infection.[118,281,812-814] For this reason, the skin test appears to be most useful in the diagnosis of chronic (latent) infection; when results are positive, the possibility that the patient had a very recently acquired infection seems remote.

Antigen-Specific Lymphocyte Transformation. Lymphocyte proliferation to *T. gondii* antigens has been shown to be a specific indicator of prior *T. gondii* infection in adults.[421,422,479,815] This technique has been found useful in establishing the diagnosis of congenital *T. gondii* infection in some infants.[731,816,817] Whereas depressed lymphocyte responsiveness to antigens of the infecting organisms has been reported in infants with congenital cytomegalovirus infection,[818,819] congenital rubella,[820,821] and congenital syphilis,[822] specific cell-mediated immunity appears to develop for most infants with congenital *T. gondii* infection by 1 year of age, although the magnitude of the response is often less than that of their mothers.[731] In one series,[731] lymphocyte proliferation to *T. gondii* antigen was both a sensitive (84%) and a specific (100%) indicator of congenital *T. gondii* infection; the sensitivity was similar in asymptomatic (82%) and in symptomatic (88%) infants.[731] Wilson and co-workers concluded that as a diagnostic tool, this method compared favorably with isolation of *T. gondii* and was superior in sensitivity to the IgM IFA test. In the study by Wilson and co-workers, a majority of the patients were not symptomatic or had mild infection, and tests of lymphocyte transformation were performed only once; it is possible that even greater sensitivity would be achieved with repeated testing (as was done with the IgM IFA test). Such repeated testing was done in the cases reported by McLeod and colleagues[817] and Yano and associates.[823] The patients described by McLeod and colleagues[472] had more severe involvement, and a substantial proportion of them did not exhibit lymphocyte blastogenic responses to *T. gondii* antigens in the first month of life.

Lymphocyte Activation Markers in the Presence of *Toxoplasma gondii* Antigen. A study of increased expression of the marker of T cell activation, CD25, with addition of *T. gondii* antigen to cultures of lymphocytes from congenitally infected infants described lymphocyte recognition in 38 (100%) of 38 congenitally infected infants in the first year of life (see also under "Immunologic Unresponsiveness to *T. gondii* Antigens.").[473] Nine (10%) of 89 uninfected infants, when tested initially, but not when retested later, also had values of 7% or greater.

Polymerase Chain Reaction Assay

In 1990, Grover and colleagues described the usefulness of PCR assay for rapid prenatal diagnosis of congenital *T. gondii* infection.[824] In a prospective study of 43 documented cases of acute maternal *T. gondii* infection acquired during gestation, PCR assay correctly identified the presence of *T. gondii* in all five samples of amniotic fluid from 4 proven cases of congenital infection and in 3 of 5 positive cases from a nonprospective group. Detection of IgM antibodies in fetal blood and inoculation of amniotic fluid into tissue cultures identified the infection in two and four of the nine infants with PCR-positive samples, respectively. Mouse inoculation of blood and amniotic fluid detected seven and six of the nine infants with PCR-positive samples, respectively. No false-positive results were obtained with any of the methods. PCR techniques have subsequently been used successfully on samples of ascitic fluid, amniotic fluid, cerebrospinal fluid, blood, urine, and tissues, including placenta and brain of infants with congenital toxoplasmosis.[125,656,825-837] False-negative results are more frequent when infection is acquired early or late in gestation (Fig. 31-18).[838] Although the sensitivity of the PCR assay in amniotic fluid, performed between 17 and 21 weeks of gestation, was reported to be 95%, the confidence interval was wide (see discussion of PCR assay in amniotic fluid and effects of treatment, under Prenatal Infection).[679,988,838] Other possible reasons for false-negative results include[839] mishandling of the sample before it is received by the laboratory and use of a single-copy target

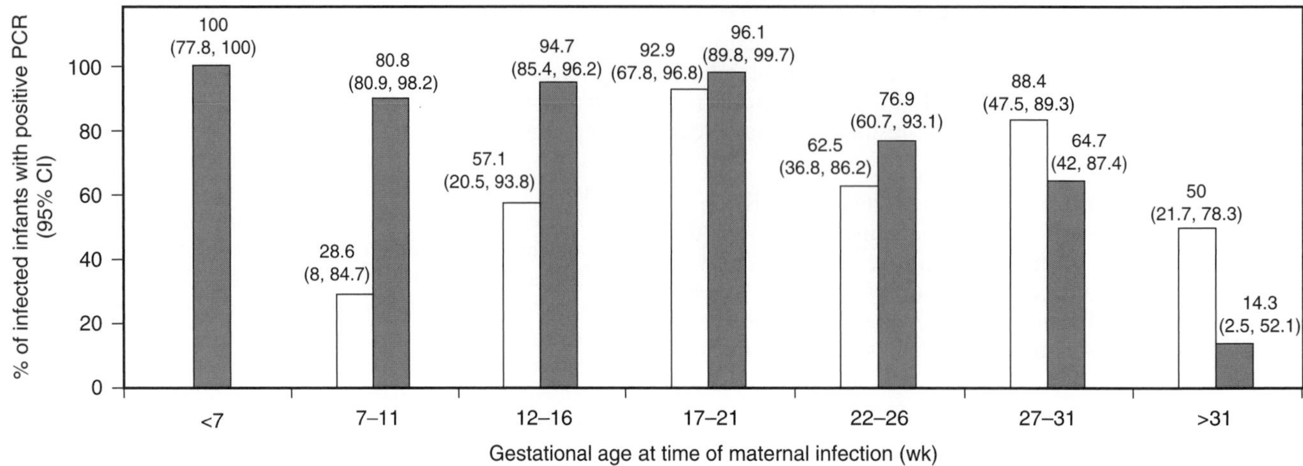

Figure 31–18 Prenatal diagnosis of congenital toxoplasmosis using polymerase chain reaction (PCR) assay in amniotic fluid (AF) according to gestational age at maternal infection. *Unshaded bars* indicate sensitivity of PCR assay in AF; *shaded bars* indicate negative predictive value of PCR assay in AF; the 95% confidence interval (CI) is shown *within parentheses at the top of the bars*. These data are derived from three centers in France, with substantial variability in the time during gestation at which maternal infection was acquired, the time between maternal infection and amniocentesis, and the duration of treatment preceding amniocentesis. (Data from Romand S, Chosson M, Franck J, et al. Usefulness of quantitative polymerase chain reaction in amniotic fluid as early prognostic marker of fetal infection with *Toxoplasma gondii*. Am J Obstet Gynecol 190:797-802, 2004.)

gene that limits the sensitivity and thus is not able to detect the *T. gondii* DNA in the sample. Because PCR assay in amniotic fluid is performed at 18 weeks of gestation by most investigators, reliability of this test performed earlier than 18 weeks of gestation is unknown.

Reischl and colleagues used real-time fluorescence PCR assays to compare results obtained with the more conventional 35-fold repeated B1 gene of *T. gondii* with a newly described multicopy genomic fragment, a 529-base-pair (bp) repeat element, that is repeated more than 300 times in the genome of *T. gondii*.[840] These investigators provided convincing evidence that the 529-bp repeat element provides the advantage of greater sensitivity than that with use of the B1 gene: this 529-bp element is being adopted by a number of reference laboratories using real-time PCR methods.

Real-time PCR testing combines amplification and detection steps and use of a fluorescence-labeled oligonucleotide probe, making completion of the assay possible in less than 4 hours.[72,291,841] Real-time PCR analysis is useful to quantitate parasite concentration in amniotic fluid.[135] Larger concentrations of parasites in amniotic fluid before 20 weeks of gestation have the greatest risks of severe outcome in the fetus and newborn (Figs. 31-19 and 31-20; Tables 31-28 and 31-29).[135,838]

Perhaps the greatest advance in prenatal diagnosis of *T. gondii* infection in the fetus has been the use of PCR on amniotic fluid without having to resort to a percutaneous umbilical blood sample.[125] PCR testing probably will replace many of the methods described in this section for diagnosis of the infection in the newborn.

Demonstration of Antigen in Serum and Body Fluids

The ELISA has been used to demonstrate *T. gondii* antigenemia in humans and animals with the acute infection,[842-848] and antigen has been demonstrated in cerebrospinal fluid and amniotic fluid of newborns with congenital toxoplasmosis.[849] *T. gondii* antigens also have been demonstrated in urine of a congenitally infected infant by the ELISA.[850] Dot immunobinding also has been used for this purpose.[851]

Demonstration of Antibodies in Serum and Body Fluids

The ultimate usefulness of tests for the diagnosis of toxoplasmosis depends on quality control of commercial kits, reliability of the laboratory performing the test, and accuracy and skill of persons interpreting results according to the specified clinical circumstance.

The most common serologic tests in use at present for diagnosis of *T. gondii* infection and toxoplasmosis are the Sabin-Feldman dye test,[18] the indirect hemagglutination (IHA) test,[852] the IFA test,[853] the agglutination test,[854] the ELISA,[855-858] and the immunosorbent agglutination assay (ISAGA).[859-861] Certain serologic methods are of little help in diagnosing congenital toxoplasmosis. This is especially true for some CF or IHA tests.[862] Results with these tests may be weakly positive or even negative in a newborn with congenital toxoplasmosis, as well as in the infant's mother. The diagnosis of acute acquired toxoplasmosis may be established by the demonstration of rising serologic test titers.[271] A stable high titer, however, may have been reached by the time the patient is first seen by a physician. Because high titers (e.g., 300 to 1000 international units [IU]) may persist for many years after acute infection[863] (Figs. 31-21 and 31-22) and are present in the general population, a single high serologic test titer in any one method does not constitute conclusive evidence that a clinical illness is due to toxoplasmosis.

Sabin-Feldman Dye Test. The Sabin-Feldman dye test is based on the observation that when living organisms (e.g., from the peritoneal exudate of mice) are incubated with normal serum, they become swollen and stain deeply blue when methylene blue is added to the suspension.[18] Parasites exposed to antibody-containing serum, under the same con-

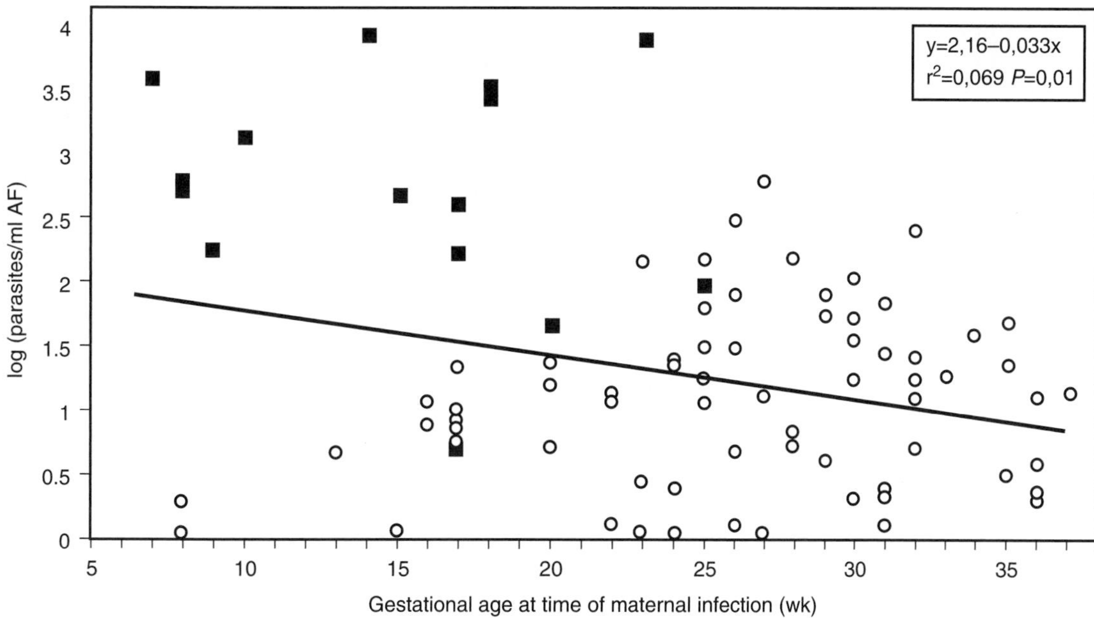

Figure 31–19 Correlation between *Toxoplasma* concentrations in amniotic fluid (AF) samples and gestational age at maternal infection for the 86 cases. Severity of the infection is represented in each case by ■ if severe signs of infection were recorded or by o if no or mild signs were observed. In general, the earlier the mother is infected, the higher the parasite numbers in amniotic fluid. Some babies who had relatively low numbers of parasites were severely infected, and many babies who had relatively high numbers of parasites were not severely infected. (Data from Romand S, Chosson M, Franck J, et al. Usefulness of quantitative polymerase chain reaction in amniotic fluid as early prognostic marker of fetal infection with *Toxoplasma gondii*. Am J Obstet Gynecol 190:797-802, 2004.)

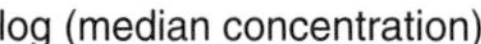

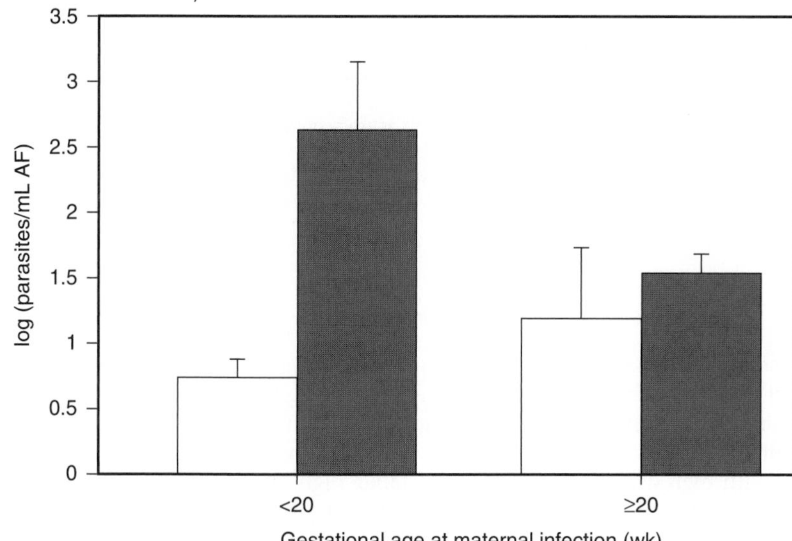

Figure 31–20 Comparison of median (interquartile range) parasite concentrations in AF between cases with subclinical infection (*unshaded bars*) and cases with infectious sequelae (*shaded bars*) for maternal infections acquired before or after 20 weeks of gestation. Clinical status was recorded either at birth or following fetal death (at fetopathologic examination). (Data from Romand S, Chosson M, Franck J, et al. Usefulness of quantitative polymerase chain reaction in amniotic fluid as early prognostic marker of fetal infection with *Toxoplasma gondii*. Am J Obstet Gynecol 190:797-802, 2004.)

ditions, appear thin and distorted and are not stained when the dye is added. This is due to lysis of the organisms.[864] The membrane is disrupted because of activation of the complement system.[865] The titer reported is that dilution of serum at which half of the organisms are not killed (stained) and the other half are killed (unstained). (The stain is not required. Differentiation of lysed from nonlysed organisms may be readily accomplished under phase microscopy.) The World Health Organization (WHO) has recommended that titers in most serologic tests be expressed in IU/mL of serum, compared with an international standard reference serum, which is available on request from the WHO.[866]

Indirect Hemagglutination Test. In the IHA test, red blood cells tagged with *T. gondii* antigen agglutinate when serum that contains antibodies to *T. gondii* is added.[852] Titers in the

Table 31–28 Clinical Outcome of 88 Fetuses with Congenital Toxoplasmosis Diagnosed by PCR Assay in Amniotic Fluid According to Gestational Age at Maternal Infection

Gestational age (wk) When Mother Acquired Infection	No. of Newborns Affected at Birth					Number of Fetal Deaths	
	Total	*Subclinical Infection*	*Cerebral Calcifications*	*Retinochoroiditis Alone*	*Ventricular Dilatation*	*Fetal Death*	*Medical Termination*
<20	26	6	4	0	1	5[c]	10[d]
≥20	62	52	6[a]	1	1	0	2
Total	88	58	10	1	2[b]	5	12

[a]In association with retinochoroiditis in 1 case.
[b]In association with cerebral calcifications and retinochoroiditis in 2 cases.
[c]Four fetuses exhibited hydrops fetalis.
[d]Two fetuses revealed no sign of infection following fetopathologic examination.
Data from Romand S, Chosson M, Frank J, et al. Usefulness of quantitative polymerase chain reaction in amniotic fluid as early prognostic marker of fetal infection with *Toxoplasma gondii.* Am J Obstet Gynecol 190:797-802, 2004.

Table 31–29 Maternal-Fetal Transmission Rates of *Toxoplasma gondii* Infection and Intervals between Date of Maternal Infection and Amniocentesis According to Duration of Gestation at Maternal Infection

Duration of Gestation (wk) at Maternal Infection	Maternal-Fetal Transmission Rate	Intervals between Date of Maternal Infection and Amniocentesis[a]
≤6	0/14 (0)	12.6 (11.3-14.6)
7-11	7/50 (14)	9.1 (7.2-11.1)
12-16	7/61 (11.5)	6.9 (5.3-8.7)
17-21	14/66 (21.2)	6.7 (5.3-7.6)
22-26	16/36 (44.4)	5.9 (5-7.4)
27-31	19/30 (63.3)	5.1 (4.4-6.1)
≥32	12/13 (92.3)	4.6 (2.5-5.3)

[a]Mean (25 to 75th percentiles).
In considering the results of this study, it is important to note that the numbers of women with acute acquired infection differ substantially for each group. This is in part due to the time when women first seek prenatal care. Of note is that the intervals between date of maternal infection and amniocentesis also diminish with time during gestation at which infection was acquired, after 16 weeks of gestation.
Data from Romand S, Wallon M, Franck J, et al. Prenatal diagnosis using polymerase chain reaction on amniotic fluid for congenital toxoplasmosis. Obstet Gynecol 97:296-300, 2001.

IHA test may lag several weeks or more behind those in the dye test,[867-869] attain levels as high as or higher than titers in the dye test, and tend to remain elevated at higher levels even longer.[870,871] Results of the IHA test frequently have been negative in cases of congenital toxoplasmosis with high dye test titers; therefore, this test is *not* recommended for the diagnosis of congenital toxoplasmosis (Table 31-30). In addition, because a rise in titer in the IHA test may not be demonstrable for months, it is not satisfactory as a screening method in pregnant women with *T. gondii* infection.[867,870-875] Because of these problems and the variations in titers obtained in different laboratories, the IHA test cannot at present supplant the dye test, IFA test, or ELISA for demonstration of IgG antibodies. It is, however, an additional test that may be useful in serologic surveys.

Complement Fixation Test. Complement-fixing antibodies have been studied mainly in acquired toxoplasmosis. They appear later than those demonstrable by the dye test. Because of this difference, the special usefulness of the CF test was the demonstration of rising titers when dye test or IFA test titers are already high and stable.[867,876] A negative CF test result that becomes positive or increasing CF test titers, together with stable high dye test titers, indicate active infection. The CF test result may become negative within a few years after acquisition of infection[867,876] or, in some instances, may remain positive for as long as 10 years.[597] The antigen preparations employed in the CF test have not been standardized. The test is not available to most physicians in the United States but is used routinely in some countries (e.g., the Czech Republic).

Agglutination Test. The agglutination test[874,877] is available commercially in Europe and has been evaluated by a number of investigators.[878-883] The test employs whole parasites that have been preserved in formalin. The method is very sensitive to IgM antibodies. Nonspecific agglutination (apparently related to "naturally" occurring IgM *T. gondii* agglutinins)

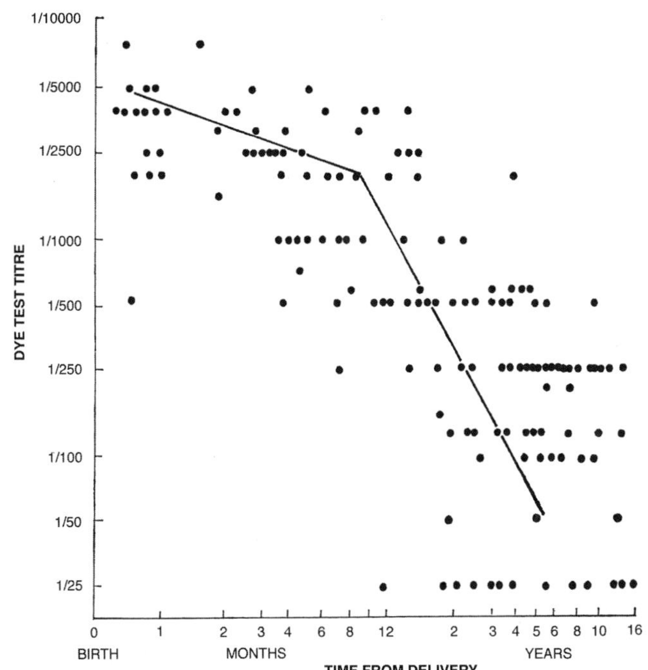

Figure 31–21 Dye test titers in 117 mothers of children with congenital toxoplasmosis in relation to time since delivery. (Data from Couvreur J, Desmonts G. Congenital and maternal toxoplasmosis. A review of 300 congenital cases. Dev Med Child Neurol 4:519-530, 1962.)

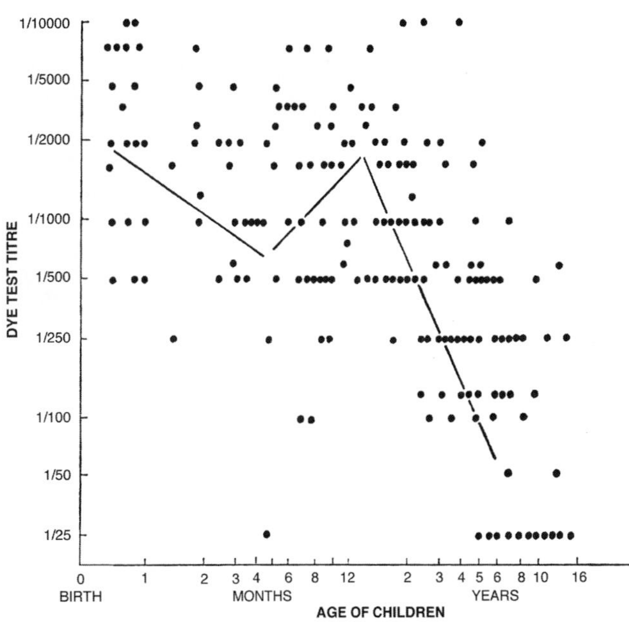

Figure 31–22 Dye test titers in 119 children with congenital toxoplasmosis in relation to age. (Data from Couvreur J, Desmonts G. Congenital and maternal toxoplasmosis. A review of 300 congenital cases. Dev Med Child Neurol 4:519-530, 1962.)

Table 31–30 Results of the Dye Test and IHA Test in Twins with Congenital Toxoplasmosis[a]

	First Twin (Male)[b]		Second Twin (Female)[c]	
Age (mo)	***Dye Test Titer***	***IHA Test Titer[d]***	***Dye Test Titer***	***IHA Test Titer[d]***
1	4000	Negative	250	Negative
2	4000	Negative	125	Negative
4½	2000	64	80	Negative
8	4000	4096	1000	256
11	4000	1024	500	1024

[a]Titers are expressed as the reciprocal of the serum dilution.
[b]Clinical congenital toxoplasmosis with encephalitis and chorioretinitis.
[c]Subclinical infection.
[d]Sera were examined in parallel; negative indicates <16.
IHA, indirect hemagglutination test.
Adapted from Desmonts G. Congenital toxoplasmosis: problems in early diagnosis. *In* Hentsch D (ed). Toxoplasmosis. Bern, Hans Huber, 1971, pp 137-149, with permission.

has been observed in persons devoid of antibody in the dye test and conventional IFA test.[884] These natural IgM antibodies do not cross the placenta but are detected at low titers as early as the second month of life. They do not develop in infants with maternal IgG antibody to *T. gondii*, however, so long as IgG antibody is present. False-positive results due to these natural antibodies may be avoided.[885] When they are, this test is excellent for wide-scale screening of pregnant women because it is accurate, simple to perform, and inexpensive.[1,885] A method that employs latex-tagged particles also may become available commercially.[886-888]

Differential Agglutination Test. A chemical alteration of the outer membrane of the parasite led to the development of a unique differential agglutination method (HS/AC test) that is very useful for helping to differentiate between acute and chronic infections in the pregnant patient.[860,877,889,890] The differential agglutination test compares titers obtained with formalin-fixed tachyzoites (HS antigen) with those obtained with acetone- or methanol-fixed tachyzoites (AC antigen).[860,877] The AC antigen preparation contains stage-specific antigens that are recognized by IgG antibodies early during infection; these antibodies have different specificities from those found

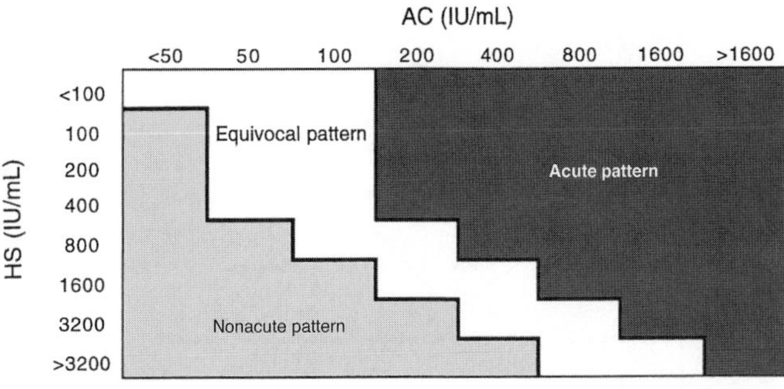

Figure 31–23 Interpretation of HS/AC test results. This differential agglutination test was performed as described in the text. (Data from Dannemann BR, Vaughan WC, Thulliez P, et al. Differential agglutination test for diagnosis of recently acquired infection with *Toxoplasma gondii.* J Clin Microbiol 28:1928-1933, 1990.)

later in the infection.[891] Guidelines for interpretation of results for this test are shown in Figure 31-23. In the appropriate clinical setting, this method is useful for diagnosis of the acute infection using a single serum sample from the patient.[860] In practice, to assist with a clinical decision, it is important to take into consideration the results of other serologic tests along with those found in the HS/AC test. It is our practice to use the HS/AC test only in adults, and only in those who have IgG and IgM antibodies to *T. gondii* and in whom there is a question about whether the infection was recently acquired.

In the study by Dannemann and co-workers in which a single serum specimen was tested in each patient, the HS/AC test correctly identified all of the pregnant and almost all (31 of 33) of the nonpregnant patients with recently acquired toxoplasmic lymphadenopathy or asymptomatic infections.[860] Each of the seven women in their study who seroconverted during gestation had an acute pattern in the HS/AC test within 0 to 8 weeks after seroconversion in the dye test. Thirteen percent of 15 women who had been infected for at least 2 years had an acute pattern, but the wide range in duration of time from original infection (2 to 14 years) did not allow for an estimate of when the pattern in the HS/AC test changed from an acute to a nonacute pattern.

Conventional Indirect Fluorescent Antibody Test. In the conventional IFA test, slide preparations of killed *T. gondii* are incubated with serial dilutions of the patient's serum. If a specific reaction between the antigenic sites on the organisms and the patient's antibody occurs, it can be detected by a fluorescein-tagged antiserum prepared against serum immune globulins. A positive reaction is detected by the bright yellow-green fluorescence of the organisms seen on examination by fluorescence microscopy. In general, qualitative agreement with the dye test and IFA test has been excellent.[853] Despite the claims of many workers, reliable and reproducible quantitative titers frequently are difficult to obtain. To permit valid comparisons of results from different laboratories that express their titers as the last positive serum dilution, it should be noted that, depending on the laboratory, the dye test may vary in sensitivity, ranging between 0.1 and 0.5 IU/mL for the 50% end point. Thus, a positive result for this test on a serum with a titer of 1000 IU/mL could be reported as 1:2000 or 1:10,000 in the dye test. The range is even greater with the IFA test.

Although most workers consider the IFA test to equal the dye test in specificity, false-positive results occur with some sera that contain antinuclear antibodies.[892] For this reason, in patients with connective tissue disorders (e.g., systemic lupus erythematosus), a dye test or ELISA can be performed to document a positive result on IFA testing.

To avoid misinterpretation of the polar staining of organisms that is due to naturally occurring IgM antibodies,[893,894] the fluorescein-tagged conjugate should be only anti-IgG.[895]

Conventional Enzyme-Linked Immunosorbent Assay. The ELISA technology has largely replaced other methodologies in the routine clinical laboratory. It has been used successfully to demonstrate IgG, IgM, IgA, and IgE[896,897] antibodies in the pregnant woman, fetus, and newborn.[857,898,899] Most workers have employed an enzyme-conjugated antibody directed against human IgG[900-902] or against total immunoglobulins.[903-907] Titers in the IgG ELISA correlated well with titers in the dye, IHA, IFA, and CF tests in some studies[906] but not in others.[907,908] Commercial kits are widely available for detection of IgG or IgM antibodies. Their reliability for detection of IgM antibodies varies considerably, however, and false-positive results have been a serious problem.[909,910]

Capture Enzyme-Linked Immunosorbent Assay. The capture ELISA is routinely employed by many laboratories for demonstration of IgM[855,882,911] and IgA[898,899,908] *T. gondii* antibodies in the fetus, newborn, and pregnant patient. In appropriately standardized methods (commercial kits), the IgA ELISA appears to be more sensitive than the IgM ELISA or IgM ISAGA for diagnosis of the infection in the fetus and newborn. IgA antibodies may persist for 8 months or longer in congenitally infected infants.[857,899] Demonstration of IgA *T. gondii* antibodies in an adult with early acute acquired infection is comparable to demonstration of IgM antibody, although IgA antibody may appear somewhat later than IgM antibody. In the adult, IgA *T. gondii* antibodies usually disappear earlier than do IgM antibodies, but as with the latter, IgA antibody titers may remain positive for a year or longer. Very high titers in either ELISA appear to correlate with more recent onset of the infection. Many cases in adults have been observed in which the IgM ELISA and HS/AC (see earlier) test results were positive and the IgA ELISA result was negative. We and others have not found the IgA test to be useful for diagnosis in most cases of acute infection in pregnant women.[912]

Enzyme-Linked Immunofiltration Assay. The enzyme-linked immunofiltration assay (ELIFA) method makes use of a micropore membrane[913] and permits simultaneous study of antibody specificity by immunoprecipitation and characterization of antibody isotypes by immunofiltration with enzyme-labeled antibodies. This method has detected as many as 85% of cases of congenital infection in the first few days of life. This test is not available to physicians in the United States. By this method, IgE may be found at birth in the cerebrospinal fluid or serum of the newborn.

In Pinon and colleagues' study,[914] the combination of their ELIFA with the IgA and IgM ISAGA provided a positive diagnosis in 90% of the infants within 1 month of birth and in 94% by the end of the first 3 months of life. IgA antibodies were present in 5% of infants with congenital infection after the fifth month of age and were never found in the cerebrospinal fluid. The method is excellent for diagnosis of congenital infection in the newborn and can be used on cord serum.

IgG/IgM Western Blot Analysis for Mother-Infant Pairs. In the infected fetus, IgG and/or IgM serum antibodies produced against antigenic determinants of *T. gondii* may differ from those recognized by the IgG and/or IgM serum antibodies of the mother.[502,915,916] The fact that Western blot analysis can be used to demonstrate these differences in mother-baby pairs has led to the development of commercial kits for this purpose. The potential of this method for diagnosis of infection in the fetus and newborn is highlighted by the observations of Tissot-Dupont and colleagues, who prospectively studied IgG, IgM, and IgA Western blots in sera of 126 infants born to mothers who had acquired *T. gondii* infection during gestation.[917] Conventional serologic tests were performed during the first year of life, and Western blot analyses were performed on day 0 and/or day 5 and at 1 and 3 months of age. Serologic follow-up evaluation revealed that 23 of the infants had the congenital infection and that the remaining 103 infants were not infected. Although the Western blot method proved more sensitive than the IgM ISAGA (86.9% versus 69.6%, respectively) (specificity of both methods was greater than 90%), the sensitivity increased to 91.3% when both test were performed in combination. IgA blots were least sensitive. Similar results were reported by Pinon and associates in a collaborative study involving laboratories in the European Community Biomed 2 program.[916]

Cases of congenital infection have been observed in the first months of life in infants in whom results of the IgM antibody tests were negative and the Western blot analysis result was positive. The Western blot method on mother-baby pairs may yield negative results during the first days of life in the infected newborn, however, and a demonstrable positive result in infected babies may not appear for weeks or even 2 or more months after birth.[502] Prenatal treatment during gestation and/or treatment of the infant may result in false-negative results on Western blot analysis. It is important that the Western blot method for mother-baby pairs always be used in combination with other serologic tests for IgG, IgM, and IgA antibodies. Western blot analysis for diagnosis of the congenital infection probably is most useful in those newborns in whom IgA and/or IgM *T. gondii* antibodies are not demonstrable in conventional serologic tests but whose mothers had a definite or highly likely diagnosis of acquired infection during gestation. It should be emphasized that no serologic test, performed singly or in combination, or the Western blot method allows for the diagnosis of the congenital infection in all cases. An example of IgG and IgM Western blots from a mother-baby pair is shown in Figure 31-24.[502]

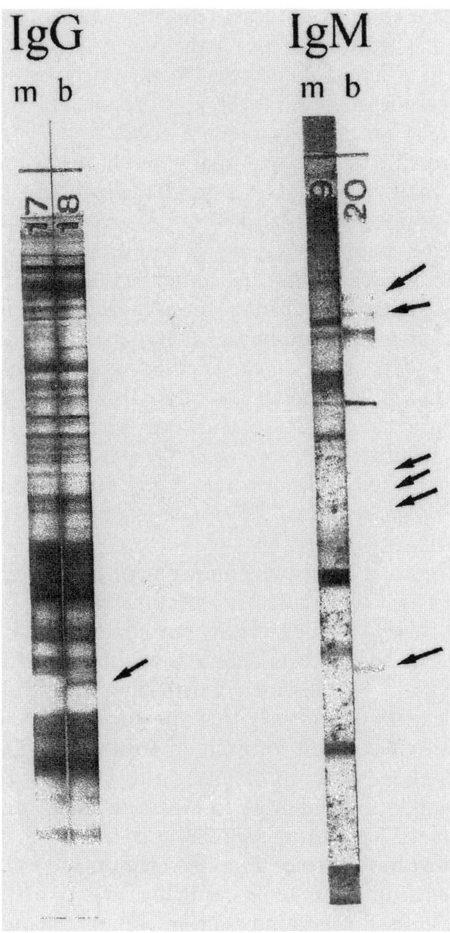

Figure 31–24 IgG and IgM Western blots of serum from a mother (m) and her newborn infant (b). Sera were drawn from mother and baby when the baby was 2 days of age. *Arrows* point to bands in the blot of the serum of the baby that were not present in the corresponding blot of the serum from the mother. Serologic test results in the mother were as follows (results in the baby are in parentheses): dye test, 600 IU (300 IU); IgM ELISA, 2.9 (IgM ISAGA, 3), both positive; IgA ELISA, 1.8 (1.3), both positive; IgE ELISA, negative (positive); PCR assay in placental tissue, negative. *Toxoplasma* was isolated from the placental tissue. ELISA, enzyme-linked immunosorbent assay; IgA, IgG, IgM, immunoglobulins A, G, M; ISAGA, immunosorbent agglutination assay; PCR, polymerase chain reaction. (Adapted from Remington JS, Thulliez P, Montoya JG. Recent developments for diagnosis of toxoplasmosis. J Clin Microbiol 42:941-945, 2004.)

IgG Avidity Assay. The avidity assay should be used in conjunction with other serologic tests (i.e., *T. gondii*–specific IgG, IgM, IgA, IgE, and AC/HS).[136,137,502] The method is most useful (and should be performed) in women in the first 16 weeks of gestation in whom IgM antibodies are found. It also is useful late in gestation to determine whether infection was acquired 4 or more months earlier, thereby allowing for an estimate of the rate of fetal infection at a given time during gestation. Testing for the avidity of antibodies against *T. gondii* stems from the knowledge that after primary antigenic stimulation, antibody-binding avidity (affinity) for an antigen is initially low but increases thereafter. IgG antibodies that are present owing to prior antigenic stimulus most often are of high avidity; this pertains to the secondary antibody response as well. (For a review, the reader is referred to the article by Hedman and colleagues.[918]) The most widely used method is one that employs the hydrogen bond–disrupting agent urea, which preferentially dissociates complexes formed by low-affinity antibodies. An avidity "index" may be determined as the percentage of antibodies that resist elution by 6M urea (e.g., in an ELISA plate). The method has been used by numerous investigators in an attempt to differentiate between recently acquired infection and infection acquired in the more distant past.[919-923] Commercial kits are available in Europe.[924]

At present, despite the many publications using the ELISA format, consensus on a standard procedure is lacking. Thus, each investigator has had to define what constitutes a low-or high-avidity or equivocal result. What is generally agreed on is that a low avidity cannot be interpreted to mean that the patient has had a recently acquired infection, because low-avidity antibodies may persist for more than 5 months, depending on the method used. A high-avidity result in the first trimester (or up to 16 weeks of gestation depending on the kit used), however, virtually rules out a recently acquired infection. Unfortunately, for all methods thus far reported, the equivocal range is broad, and a result in this range requires additional testing in a reference laboratory.

For diagnosis in the pregnant woman, the avidity method is most useful when used in the first 12 to 16 weeks of gestation, because a high-avidity result late in gestation does not rule out an infection acquired in the first trimester or earlier. With the method used in their laboratory, Lappalainen and colleagues[925] reported that the predictive value of a high-avidity test result for excluding infection in the prior 5 months was 100%. In the Palo Alto laboratory, a high-avidity result obtained by an ELISA method during the first 16 weeks of gestation essentially excludes an infection acquired within the prior 4 months. Jenum and associates[926] concluded from their results with the avidity method that acquisition of *T. gondii* infection in early pregnancy can be excluded on the basis of results with a single serum sample collected in the first trimester. By confirming latent infection on the basis of a high–IgG avidity result early during gestation, the need to collect a second serum sample is eliminated. Antibiotic treatment has been suggested to affect the kinetics of IgG avidity maturation[927] and thereby prolong the duration of detectable low-avidity antibodies. It has been recently demonstrated, however, that treatment with spiramycin had no influence on the increase of the avidity index in pregnant women.[928] The avidity test is an excellent adjunctive method for ruling out infection acquired during the first 12 to 16 weeks of gestation.[925,929-931]

The avidity assay is especially useful when only a single sample of serum has been obtained in which IgM *T. gondii* antibodies are present, and when the AC/HS test gives an acute or equivocal pattern. A recent study compared results obtained in an IgG avidity test with those obtained in the IgM ELISA and AC/HS test for sera that had equivocal or positive IgM ELISA or AC/HS test results.[137] A substantial proportion (e.g., 42 of 81 serum samples [52%] with high titers of *T. gondii* IgG antibodies) had high-avidity test results. Comparison of IgG avidity and differential agglutination test results also showed that 31 of 53 sera (59%) with equivocal and 4 of 33 sera (12%) with acute AC/HS test results had high avidity—that is, were from women infected 4 or months earlier. In 69 of 93 samples (74%) with positive or equivocal IgM ELISA results, 52 (56%) had high-avidity antibodies.[136,137] Of 87 (70%) samples with acute or equivocal AC/HS test results, 35 (40%) had high-avidity antibodies. Of 40 women given spiramycin in the first trimester in an attempt to prevent congenital transmission, 7 (8%) had high-avidity antibodies and thus did not require treatment. These women would not have required treatment with spiramycin if the avidity test result were known at the time.

Table 31–31 Usefulness of High-Avidity Test Results in IgM-Positive First-Trimester Pregnant Women

Patient No.[a]	Gestational Age (wk)	Dye Test (IgG)	IgM	Avidity
73	9	256	Positive	High
58	12	512	Positive	High
17	12	256	Positive	High
74	12	1024	Positive	High

[a]The high-avidity test result in each of these pregnant women reveals that they were infected before gestation. Without the avidity test results, the positive IgM antibody tests might have been interpreted as showing that the patients had acquired the infection during gestation.

IgM, immunoglobulin M.

Adapted from Remington JS, Thulliez P, Montoya G. Recent developments for diagnosis of toxoplasmosis. J Clin Microbiol 42:941-945, 2004.

Performance of the avidity test in the first 12 to 16 weeks of gestation has the potential to markedly decrease the need for obtaining follow-up sera and thereby reduce costs, to make unnecessary the need for PCR on amniotic fluid and for treatment of the mother with spiramycin, to remove the anxiety experienced by pregnant patients who are told that further testing is needed, and to decrease unnecessary abortions. Table 31-31[502] shows results in the literature with avidity tests. In addition, it is important to note that confirmatory serologic testing in a reference laboratory with communication of results and correct interpretation of these results to the patient's physician by an expert decreased rates of unnecessary abortions by about 50% among women with positive IgM *Toxoplasma* antibody test results reported by outside laboratories.[932]

Demonstration of Specific Immunoglobulin M Antibodies

A positive serum IgM test alone cannot be used to establish the diagnosis of any form of toxoplasmosis in the older child and adult. A positive result on IgM serologic testing in the fetus and in the newborn in the first days of life usually is diagnostic of the infection if contamination of fetal or newborn blood with maternal blood has not occurred. The validity of a positive IgM test result in this setting may be checked by repeating the test 3 to 4 days later. Because the half-life of IgM is short, the repeat testing will reveal either a highly significant drop in titer or, more commonly, a negative result that reveals the original positive titer to have been a "false positive." Also, isolated false-positive *T. gondii*–specific IgM test results have been noted with other fetal infections (JS Remington and R McLeod, unpublished).

IgM Fluorescent Antibody Test. The IFA test has been adapted for the demonstration of IgM antibodies to *T. gondii*, and the method has been successfully used to establish acute congenital and acquired infections.[556,872,874,933-939] The use of

IgM antibody for diagnosis of congenital infection stems from the discovery in 1963 by Eichenwald and Shinefield[940] that the fetus is able to produce IgM-specific antibody. Critical to this method is the choice of an antiserum that is specific for IgM.[576,941] Serious and misleading errors related to the use of antisera that have specificity not only for IgM but also for IgG have been reported in the literature.

Failure to demonstrate IgM antibodies in the IgM IFA test in sera from some patients with the acute acquired infection has been shown to be due to an inhibitory effect of high titers of IgG antibodies to *T. gondii* in these sera.[942,943] This problem may be avoided by removal of the IgG before performance of the IgM IFA test. Commercial kits are available for this purpose.

The presence of IgM antibodies in cord serum or in serum obtained from the neonate is evidence of specific antibody synthesis by the infected fetus in utero. Maternal IgM antibodies do not normally pass the placental barrier, as do maternal IgG antibodies. The IgM IFA test was the first test designed to make an early diagnosis of congenital toxoplasmosis by distinguishing between passively transferred maternal antibodies and the response of the fetus and neonate to infection.[933] The test also has been successfully used to detect active acute acquired toxoplasmosis.[271,788,867,944,945] After acute acquired infection, the IgM IFA test titer may rise rapidly (and at times earlier than titers in the dye test or conventional IFA test) to high levels.[867] The titer usually declines, and the antibodies may disappear within several months; in some patients, however, the IgM IFA test result has remained positive at a low titer for several years. IgM antibodies to *T. gondii* may not be demonstrable in immunodeficient patients with acute toxoplasmosis and in patients with isolated active ocular toxoplasmosis. Only 25% to 50% of congenitally infected infants have *T. gondii*–specific IgM antibodies demonstrable by IgM IFA tests.[731,855,941] With two qualifications, demonstration of IgM antibodies to *T. gondii* in the serum of a newborn should be considered as diagnostic of congenital toxoplasmosis. First, if cord serum is tested, or if the serum is obtained in the early newborn period in an infant during whose delivery a placental "leak" occurred, which enabled maternal blood to mix with that of the infant, a false-positive result could occur in any serologic test for IgM, IgA, or IgE antibodies. This possibility can be investigated by performing the test on the mother's serum. If the mother's serum is negative for IgM antibodies and the infant's serum is positive, the infant is infected. If both mother and infant sera are positive, the infant should be tested again several days later; a marked fall in the IgM IFA test titer will have occurred if the IgM was maternally acquired, because the half-life of IgM is only approximately 5 days.[946,947] If the IgM IFA test titer in the infant remains high or is rising, it is diagnostic of infection.

The second qualification is the presence of rheumatoid factor. False-positive IgM IFA test results may occur in sera that contain rheumatoid factor.[948] Rheumatoid factor may be present not only in adults but in infected newborns as well,[561,949] purportedly as a result of an IgM immune response of the fetus in utero to passively transferred maternal IgG. After treatment of sera containing rheumatoid factor with heat-aggregated IgG, false-positive IgM IFA test titers become negative. By contrast, titers in cases of acute congenital or acquired toxoplasmosis are unaffected by this treatment. Thus, treatment with heat-aggregated IgG or other commercially available adsorbent can be used to differentiate false-positive IgM IFA test titers related to rheumatoid factor from those related to specific IgM antibody to *T. gondii*. The incidence of rheumatoid factor in sera of infants with congenital toxoplasmosis is unknown. All infants who respond positively in the IgM IFA test should be tested for rheumatoid factor as well.

IgM Enzyme-Linked Immunosorbent Assay. The double-sandwich IgM ELISA for detection of IgM antibodies to *T. gondii* was developed by Naot and Remington and colleagues.[855,856,911] At present it is the most widely used method for demonstration of IgM antibodies to *T. gondii* in adults, the fetus, and newborns. In contrast with the conventional method in which the wells of microtiter plates are coated with antigen, the wells are coated with specific antibody to IgM. The IgM ELISA is more sensitive than the IgM IFA test for diagnosis of the recently acquired infection, and serum samples that test negative in the dye test but that contain either antinuclear antibodies or rheumatoid factor and thus cause false-positive results in the IgM IFA test also test negative in the double-sandwich IgM ELISA. This latter observation is attributed to the fact that serum IgM fractions are separated from IgG fractions during the initial step in the IgM ELISA procedure.

The double-sandwich IgM ELISA also is useful for diagnosis of congenital *T. gondii* infection.[855] Results of the double-sandwich IgM ELISA were positive in 43 of 55 serum samples (72.7%) from newborns with proven congenital *T. gondii* infection, whereas IgM IFA test results were positive in only 14 (25.4%) of these samples. Of the sera obtained from the infected newborns during the first 30 days of life, 81.2% were positive in the double-sandwich IgM ELISA, whereas only 25% were positive in the IgM IFA test. Use of the double-sandwich IgM ELISA avoids false-positive results related to rheumatoid factor and false-negative results related to competition from high levels of maternal IgG antibody that occur with the IgM IFA test. A number of modifications of the method have been described.[605,950-956] The double-sandwich IgM ELISA is superior to the IgM IFA test for diagnosis both of acute acquired and congenital *T. gondii* infections.

Immunosorbent Agglutination Assay for Demonstration of IgM, IgA, and IgE Antibodies. The ISAGA[859,861,909,957-959] is widely used by investigators because it combines the advantages of both the direct agglutination test and the double-sandwich (capture) ELISA in its specificity and sensitivity for demonstration of IgM, IgA, and IgE[861] antibodies to *T. gondii*. The ISAGA does not require use of an enzyme conjugate; it is as simple to perform as the direct agglutination test and is read in the same manner as for that test. Use of the ISAGA avoids false-positive results related to the presence of rheumatoid factor and/or antinuclear antibodies in serum samples. A commercial kit for IgM antibodies is available (bioMérieux).

The ISAGA is more sensitive and more specific than the IgM IFA and the IgM ELISA[960,961] and has been used effectively for diagnosis of congenital infection.[962] Specific IgA antibodies in the ISAGA test indicated congenital toxoplasmosis in three infants in the absence of associated IgM antibodies.[963] Pinon and co-workers found IgA antibodies in serum and cerebrospinal fluid of seven cases of congenital toxoplasmosis in the neonatal period.[914,961]

Because of its high sensitivity, the ISAGA detects IgM antibodies earlier after the acute acquired infection (e.g., 1 to 2 weeks) than do other tests for IgM antibody. This sensitivity also results in the longest duration of detection of IgM antibody after infection. The method has been standardized by the recognition of this greater sensitivity to provide greater diagnostic power during early infections in adults.[960] Pinon and co-workers[861] and Wong and associates[896] have found the IgE ISAGA to be useful for diagnosis of acute acquired infection in the pregnant woman and in the congenitally infected newborn. Its advantage is related to the early rise in titers of IgE antibodies as well as IgM and IgA antibodies and the much earlier disappearance of IgE antibodies. In the study by Pinon and co-workers, IgE antibodies in the adult persisted for less than 4 months. This test has been available in only a few specialty laboratories. As is true for appropriate interpretation of all other serologic tests for diagnosis of the acute infection, it should be used only in combination with other serologic methods.[890,959]

Enzyme-Linked Immunofiltration Assay. Please see earlier section for discussion of this method.[903]

The Problem of False-Positive *Toxoplasma gondii*–Specific IgM Tests. *Toxoplasma* IgM test kits are not subject to standardization in the United States, and a substantial proportion of them do not function reliably.[910] Not only is the lack of reliability of such test kits a problem, but use of results in the IgM assays to guide care of the pregnant woman by obstetricians in the United States, and probably elsewhere as well, is not always well informed. For example, Jones and associates[373] reported that 364 of 768 (47%) American College of Obstetrics and Gynecology (ACOG) members responded to a survey regarding their knowledge of toxoplasmosis in pregnant women and related OB-GYN practices. In the previous year, 7% diagnosed one or more cases of acute toxoplasmosis, and only 12% indicated that a positive *Toxoplasma* IgM test might be a false-positive result. Only 11% recalled an advisory sent to all ACOG members in 1997 by the FDA alerting them that some *Toxoplasma* IgM test kits have false-positive results. Sixty-seven percent of respondents were against universal screening of pregnant women for *T. gondii* infection.[373] If obstetricians are carefully educated on the subject, medical care offered to pregnant women would be greatly improved. A positive IgM test alone can never be used to establish the diagnosis of any form of toxoplasmosis.

Median and Variability of Duration of Positive *Toxoplasma gondii* IgM Antibody Results Measured by Immunofluorescence Testing and ISAGA. Gras and co-workers[964] from London and Lyon studied a cohort of 446 *Toxoplasma*-infected pregnant women to determine the median and variability of the duration of positive *T. gondii* IgM antibody results measured by an immunofluorescence test (IFT) and an immunosorbent agglutination assay (ISAGA). IgM antibodies were detected for longer using the ISAGA (median, 12.8 months; interquartile range [IQR], 6.9 to 24.9) than the IFT (median, 10.4; IQR, 7.1 to 14.4), but the variability among persons in the duration of IgM positivity was greatest with ISAGA. IgM-positive results persisted beyond 2 years in 27.1% (ISAGA), and 9.1% (IFT) of women. These investigators concluded that variation in the duration of IgM response measured by ISAGA and IFT limits their usefulness for predicting the timing of infection in pregnant women. Nonetheless, they concluded that measurement of IgM and IgG antibodies in cross-sectional serosurveys offers a useful method for estimating the incidence of *T. gondii* infection.

Table 31–32 Guidelines for Evaluation of Newborn of Mother Who Acquired Her Infection during Gestation to Determine Whether Infant Has Congenital *Toxoplasma* Infection and to Assess Degree of Involvement

History and physical examination
Pediatric neurologic evaluation
Pediatric ophthalmologic examination
Complete blood cell count with differential, platelet count
Liver function tests (bilirubin, GGTP)
Urinalysis, serum creatinine
Serum quantitative immunoglobulins
Serum Sabin-Feldman dye test (IgG), IgM ISAGA, IgA ELISA, IgE ISAGA/ELISA[a] (with maternal serum, perform same tests as for infant except substitute IgM ELISA for the IgM ISAGA and also obtain AC/HS[a])
Cerebrospinal fluid cell count, protein, glucose, and *T. gondii*–specific IgG and IgM antibodies as well as quantitative IgG to calculate antibody load
Subinoculate into mice or tissue culture 1 mL peripheral blood buffy coat or clot and digest of 100 g placenta (see "Diagnosis" section for method of digestion). Consider PCR of buffy coat from approximately 1 mL blood, cell pellet from approximately 1 mL cerebrospinal fluid, and cell pellet from 10 to 20 mL amniotic fluid (see "Diagnosis" section)
Brain computed tomography scan without contrast medium enhancement
Auditory brain-stem response to 20 dB

[a]When performed in combination in our laboratories, these tests have demonstrated a high degree of specificity and sensitivity in establishing the diagnosis of acute infection in the pregnant woman and congenital infection in the fetus and newborn.

ELISA, enzyme-linked immunosorbent assay; GGTP, γ-glutamyltranspeptidase; ISAGA, immunosorbent agglutination assay; IgA, IgE, IgG, IgM, immunoglobulins A, E, G, M; PCR, polymerase chain reaction.

Guidelines for Evaluation of the Newborn with Suspected Congenital Toxoplasmosis

Guidelines for evaluation of the newborn of a mother who acquired her infection during gestation to confirm or rule out the diagnosis of congenital *T. gondii* infection are shown in Table 31-32.

Serologic Diagnosis of Acquired *Toxoplasma* Infection in the Pregnant Woman

The presence of a positive titer (except for the rare false-positive results mentioned earlier) in any of the serologic tests discussed earlier establishes the diagnosis of *T. gondii* infection. Because titers in each of these tests may remain elevated for years, a single high titer does not indicate whether

Table 31–33 Trimester during Which Sera Were Drawn from Consecutive Pregnant Women for *Toxoplasma gondii* Serologic Testing

	2002		2003-2004	
Trimester	***No. of Patients***	**%**	***No. of Patients***	**%**
First	112	36	111	37
Second	132	43	146	49
Third	63	21	43	14
Total	307		300	

the infection is acute or chronic, nor does it necessarily mean that the clinical findings are due to toxoplasmosis. Before a diagnosis of acute *T. gondii* infection or toxoplasmosis can be made by means of serologic tests, it is necessary to demonstrate a rising titer in serial specimens (either conversion from a negative to a positive titer or a rise from a low to a significantly higher titer).[271,965] Because in the United States the diagnosis is frequently considered relatively late in the course of the patient's infection (Table 31-33), serologic test titers (e.g., dye test, IFA test, or ELISA) may have already reached their peak at the time the first serum is obtained for testing. The IgM IFA test, IgM ELISA, IgM ISAGA, and tests for IgA and IgE antibodies and IgG avidity appear to be of considerable help in these circumstances.[271,576,856,859,909,945,959] The most important fact for the clinician is that any patient with a positive IgG titer and a positive IgM IFA or IgM ELISA titer must be presumed to have recently acquired infection with *T. gondii* and be tested further in a reference laboratory.[909,966] Most mothers of children with congenital toxoplasmosis are unable to recall being ill during pregnancy. Some (10% to 20%) notice enlarged lymph nodes, mostly in the posterior cervical area, a sign that suggests relatively recently acquired infection. These enlarged nodes sometimes are still present at delivery. Clinical signs of infection in the pregnant woman are not necessarily associated with an increased predilection for transmission, as shown by the reports of cases in which, although the parasite was present in a lymph node biopsy performed as part of the diagnostic evaluation of lymphadenopathy, the offspring were uninfected.[571,967,968] Examples of similar cases of lymphadenopathy (with demonstration of the parasite in the nodes) in which congenital transmission did occur have been published.[969,110,665,970]

Because a majority (greater than 80%) of cases of acquired *T. gondii* infection are subclinical, the diagnosis relies mainly on the results of serologic tests. To interpret serologic test results in the pregnant woman, it is important to understand how antibodies of different immunoglobulin classes and different specificities for antigenic determinants develop after the infection is acquired and which antibodies are detected in the different serologic methods used for diagnosis of this infection. In addition, the physician should have knowledge of the relationship of the time of acquisition of the infection to the onset of parasitemia (which results in infection of the placenta) and also to the onset of clinical manifestations (when present). The answers to many of these questions are unknown or only partly understood.

What follows in this section is information and guidelines for interpretation of test results, as adopted from our personal experiences and supplemented by pertinent data from the literature. We have attempted whenever possible to distinguish between hypothesis and established fact.

The antigenic structure of *T. gondii* is complex; both cytoplasmic antigens, which are liberated when the organisms are lysed, and membrane antigens are involved in the immune response.[971-977] We know that certain antigens cross-react, because normal human sera contain IgM antibodies that bind to these antigens.[978-980] It seems reasonable to suggest that antibodies formed in response to these different antigens differ both in their specificity and in their class and subclass of immunoglobulins.[981] These variations account for the fact that different antibodies may or may not be detected, depending on the serologic method employed.

In Table 31-34, we have attempted to describe the evolution of the IgM, IgG, IgA, and IgE antibody responses as they relate to interpretation of serologic test results in the diagnosis of *T. gondii* infection in the pregnant woman.[857] An example of the usefulness of these tests is shown in Table 31-35. The usefulness of the IgG avidity method is shown in Table 31-36 and discussed in an earlier section. Agreement between the avidity test and the HS/AC test is 97% in the Palo Alto laboratory, as discussed previously.

Antibody Response in Relation to the Serologic Method Used

The methods for demonstration of specific IgM antibodies have been discussed earlier. They are valuable so long as it is possible to ascertain that a positive result is not due to the presence of "natural" IgM antibodies,[982] rheumatoid factor, or antinuclear antibodies. For this reason, methods that rely on differences in titers after sera have been treated with 2-mercaptoethanol (e.g., the IHA and agglutination tests) are not satisfactory. Specific IgM antibodies may not be detectable within a few weeks after their first demonstration or may persist for years. In studies of women who seroconverted during gestation, IgA antibodies as measured by ELISA appeared at approximately the same time as for IgM antibodies.[899] Similar results have been observed with the IgE ISAGA.[861,983] Antibody titers in the IgE ISAGA decrease more rapidly than do IgA antibodies. In the study by Pinon and co-workers,[861] they persisted for less than 4 months in 23 patients tested serially. In the study by Wong and associates, the IgE ISAGA results were similar to those reported by Pinon and co-workers, whereas IgE antibodies measured by ELISA persisted significantly longer in some seroconverters.[896]

Titers in the dye test, the agglutination test, and the IHA test (when these latter two tests are performed with 2-mercaptoethanol) depend on the concentration of IgG antibodies; this is true also for the conventional IFA test when performed with a conjugate specific for IgG. Nevertheless, depending on which test is used, differences in the rise and fall of IgG antibody titers are noted; titers in the dye test rise more rapidly, whereas those measured in the agglutination and IHA tests in the presence of 2-mercaptoethanol rise slowly.

A summary of the IgG antibody responses to *T. gondii* infection, as measured by different serologic methods, is given in Table 31-37. For a discussion of the IgG avidity

Table 31–34 General considerations Regarding IgM, IgG, IgA, and IgE Antibody Responses to Postnatally Acquired Infection with *Toxoplasma*

Antibodies	Uninfected Person	Recent (Acute) Infection	Chronic (Latent) Infection
IgM			
Directed toward antigens that cross-react	Present	Present	Present
Directed toward specific *Toxoplasma* antigens	Absent	Present in almost all cases. Period that IgM antibodies are present may vary from a few weeks to many months. Ability to detect these antibodies depends on serologic technique used.	Most often absent, but IgM antibodies may persist for years in some patients (about 5%). In such cases, titers are almost always low, but in some cases they remain high. Persistence of IgM antibodies is generally associated with low or medium titers of IgG antibodies.
IgG			
Directed toward antigens that cross-react	Absent	Absent (?)	Absent (?)
Directed toward specific *Toxoplasma* antigens	Absent (<2 IU/mL)[a]	Present. Rise from a low titer (2 IU/mL) to a high titer (300-6000 IU/mL). In a few patients, titers remain low (100-200 IU/mL). Duration of rise varies with patient and with serologic test used. Depending on serologic techniques, it may take from 2 to 6 mo for the IgG antibody titer to reach its peak.	Present. Stable or slowly decreasing titers (to a titer of 2-200 IU/mL). High titers (>300 IU/mL) persist for years in some patients (about 5%). A significant rise in titer is sometimes observed after a normal decrease in titer has occurred.
IgG Avidity	Absent	Low	A high avidity test result reveals that the infection was acquired at least 12-16 weeks earlier. However, a low avidity test result may persist for more than one year.
IgA			
Directed toward antigens that cross-react	Absent	Absent (?)	Absent (?)
Directed toward specific *Toxoplasma* antigens	Absent	Present in almost all cases. Period that IgA antibodies are present may vary from several months to 1 year or more. They most commonly disappear by 7 months.	Most often absent
IgE			
Directed toward antigens that cross-react	Absent	Absent (?)	Absent (?)
Directed toward specific *Toxoplasma* antigens	Absent	Present	Absent

[a]Titers are expressed in international units (IU) to minimize technical differences that might occur among different laboratories.
IgA, IgE, IgG, IgM, immunoglobulins A, E, G, M; IU, international units.

method, see earlier under "Demonstration of Antibodies in Serum and Body Fluids."

A special comment regarding the agglutination test is made here because of its commercial availability and increasing usefulness for screening and diagnosis of the acute infection in pregnant women. With the whole-cell agglutination test, agreement with the dye test was virtually 100%, except in some patients tested within a few days after they became infected, when only IgM antibodies were present.[877] With these serum samples, the dye test result was at times positive while the agglutination test result was still negative. By contrast, the agglutination test result may be positive at times when the dye test result is negative in chronically infected persons. This is due to the greater sensitivity of the agglutination test for detection of low titers of IgG antibodies. Because it takes more than 2 months (2 to 6 months) for IgG antibodies detected with the whole-cell agglutination test to reach a steady high titer, the existence of a steady high titer signifies that the infection was acquired more than 2 months earlier. As a consequence, if the first sample of serum has been obtained during the first 2 months of pregnancy, a stable agglutination test titer demonstrates that the infection occurred before the time of conception and that the risk of congenital infection in the infant is low.[877]

It is exceedingly difficult to establish guidelines for interpretation of serologic methods that measure both IgM and IgG antibodies. For example, in examining paired sera that were stated to have high stable titers in the conventional IFA test (performed with a conjugate against total immunoglobulins), we frequently have observed a definite rise in titer between the samples when a method specific for IgG antibody was used (e.g., the dye test or the agglutination test performed with 2-mercaptoethanol). Although both

Table 31–35 Serologic Test Results in Women Who Seroconverted during Pregnancy

Patient No.	Date	Dye Test: IgG (IU/mL)	IgM ELISA[a]	IgM ISAGA[a]	IgA ELISA[a]	AC/HS[b]	IgE ELISA[c]	IgE ISAGA[a]
1	12/29/89	<2	0.4	0	0.6	NA	–	0
	02/23/90	200	5.0	12	1.8	A	+	6
	03/30/90	400	2.1	12	1.0	A	+	3
	04/30/90	800	1.3	12	0.8	A	+	3
	05/28/90	800	0.6	8	1.0	A	–	3
	06/26/90	800	1.1	6	1.0	A	+	3
2	02/17/89	<2	0.7	0	0.2	NA	–	0
	04/20/89	<2	0.2	0	0.0	NA	–	0
	05/18/89	160	6.4	12	2.8	NA	+	4
	08/23/89	200	2.7	12	0.8	A	±	0
3	03/09/82	Negative	0.0	QNS	QNS	QNS	–	6
	03/24/82	16	8.3	12	2.6	NA	+	9
	08/10/82	1000	4.9	12	2.6	A	+	6
	09/13/82	500	4.8	12	2.5	A	+	6
	12/07/82	200	4.1	12	1.0	A	+	3
	08/24/83	64	2.2	11	0.6	(A)	±	0

[a]Positive results (in an adult): IgM ELISA = ≥1.7; IgM ISAGA = >3; IgA ELISA = 1.4; IgE ISAGA = 4 (3 is considered borderline).
[b]AC/HS results: A, acute; NA, not acute; (A), borderline acute.
[c]IgE ELISA: – negative; + positive; ±, equivocal (see reference 896).
ELISA, enzyme-linked immunosorbent assay; IgA, IgE, IgG, IgM, immunoglobulin A, E, G, M; ISAGA, immunosorbent agglutination assay; IU, international units; QNS, quantity not sufficient.
Adapted from Wong SY, Hajdu MP, Ramirez P, et al. Role of specific immunoglobulin E in diagnosis of acute *Toxoplasma* infection and toxoplasmosis. J Clin Microb 31:2952-2959, 1993, with permisson.

Table 31–36 Usefulness of a High-Avidity Test Result in Women with a Positive IgM Test Titer in First 12 Weeks of Gestation

Patient No.	Duration of Gestation (wk)	Dye Test Titer (IU/mL)	IgM ELISA[a]	Percent Avidity[b]	Avidity Interpretation
1	10	51	4.7	44.4	High
2	9	51	2.3	41.6	High
3	11	102	2.6	31.2	High
4	8	102	5.8	33.8	High
5	12	410	2.9	47.3	High

[a]Negative 0.0-1.6, equivocal 1.7-1.9, positive ≥2.0.
[b]Low <15, borderline 15-30, high >30.
IU, international units.

samples had the same titer in the conventional IFA test, the titer in the first sample was the sum of the anti-IgM and anti-IgG antibody activities of the conjugate, wheras the titer in the second sample reflected only the anti-IgG antibody activity of the conjugate.

Establishing guidelines for the IHA and CF tests is made difficult by the fact that different antigen preparations cause markedly different results: Some preparations detect IgM antibodies, some detect IgG antibodies, and others detect both. Thus, the evolution of the antibody response may differ not only when different tests are used but also when the same test is used in different laboratories. This problem has been paramount in the confusion surrounding the subject of the practical approach to diagnosing acute infection.

In a systematic screening program (G Desmonts and P Thulliez, unpulished data) in which follow-up sera from pregnant women are examined monthly, IgM antibodies are usually the first to appear, but low titers of IgG antibodies, as measured in the dye test, also appear early. Sera in which only IgM antibodies are detectable are uncommon. A rise in IgM antibody titer is infrequently observed, suggesting that the IgM antibody titer rise is steep and that this rise does not last longer than 1 or 2 weeks before reaching its peak. By contrast, the rise in IgG antibody titer initially is slow. The titer, as measured in the dye test, usually remains relatively low (2 to 100 IU/mL or 1:10 to 1:100) for 3 to 6 weeks. Recognition of this fact is critical for proper interpretation of serologic test results when serum samples obtained 2 to 3 weeks apart are tested in parallel, especially if the dye test is performed with fourfold dilutions of the sera, which would require an eightfold (two-tube) rise in titer to be considered significant. In testing such sera in parallel, it is imperative to use twofold dilutions so that a fourfold (two-tube) rise can

Table 31–37 IgG Antibody Responses to *Toxoplasma* Infection as Measured by Different Serologic Methods[a]

Serologic Method	Uninfected Person	Recent (Acute) Infection	Chronic (Latent) Infection
Dye test	Negative (<1:4)	Rising from a negative or low titer (1:4) to a high titer (1:256 to 1:128,000).	Stable or slowly decreasing titer. Titers usually are low (1:4 to 1:256) but may remain high (≥1:1024) for years.
Agglutination test (after treatment of sera with 2-mercaptoethanol)	Negative (<1:4)	Rising slowly from a negative or low titer (1:4) to a high titer (1:512). If a high-sensitivity antigen is used, the titer may reach 1:128,000.	Stable or slowly decreasing titer. Titers usually are higher than in the dye test if a high-sensitivity antigen is used. Striking differences between dye test and agglutination test titers are observed in some patients.
IHA test (after treatment of sera with 2-mercaptoethanol)	Negative (<1:16)	Rising very slowly from a negative or low titer (1:16) to a high titer (1:1024). It may take 6 mo before a high titer is reached; in some patients, high titers are never observed.	Stable or slowly decreasing high or low titer.
Conventional IFA test (conjugated antiserum to IgG)	Negative (<1:20)	Rise in titer is parallel to rise in dye test titer, but decrease in titer might be slower than that in dye test.	

[a]Similar data for the IgG ELISA have not been published.
ELISA, enzyme-linked immunosorbent assay; IFA, immunofluorescent antibody test; IgG, immunoglobulin G; IHA, indirect hemagglutination test.

be detected. In our experience, this rise is difficult to detect in the IgG IFA test. After the initial 3 to 6 weeks, the rise in IgG antibody titer becomes steeper; high titers (greater than 400 IU/mL or 1:1000) usually are reached within an additional 3 weeks. Thereafter, the rise in titer is slower but may still be detectable over an additional 3 to 6 weeks if careful quantitative methodology is used (here again, this rise will be missed if fourfold dilutions of sera are used). Thus, although the rise in IgG antibody titer as detected in the dye test differs from one case to another, it lasts for more than 2 months and sometimes as long as 3 months. The rise in IgG antibody titer, as detected in the agglutination test (in the presence of 2-mercaptoethanol), may parallel exactly the pattern described for the dye test, or the titer may rise more slowly; the peak may not occur earlier than 6 months after infection. As mentioned previously, by 6 months, titers in the IgM IFA test are no longer demonstrable in most cases. Titers in the capture IgM ELISA and in the IgM ISAGA, however, usually remain positive for this period, and in women who acquire the infection during pregnancy, the titers in these latter two tests are almost always positive at the time of parturition (the level of the titer depends on the duration of infection before delivery).

Although definitive data are not available, when specific treatment for *T. gondii* infection is administered early during the initial antibody response (when the IgG antibody titer is still low), it appears that the antibody response may be slowed and the titer (e.g., in the dye test, conventional IFA test, or ELISA) may remain relatively low so long as treatment is continued. A late (delayed) rise often is observed after cessation of treatment.

Practical Guidelines for Diagnosis of Infection in the Pregnant Woman

Guidelines for diagnosis of *Toxoplasma* infection are presented for three clinical scenarios: (1) that of a woman pregnant for a few weeks in whom a serologic test for *T. gondii* infection was performed on a routine basis by her physician or at her request; (2) that of a woman pregnant for a few months who is suspected of having acute toxoplasmosis; and (3) that of a woman who has just given birth to an infant suspected of having congenital toxoplasmosis. In almost all cases in the United States, the diagnosis in these situations must take into consideration two pieces of data: the results of a test for IgG antibodies (e.g., dye test, ELISA, IFA) and the results of a test for IgM antibody (e.g., IgM IFA, IgM ISAGA, or IgM ELISA). The accuracy of some ELISA kits being sold at present is unsatisfactory, and proper interpretation of the results of titers obtained for many of these kits has not been defined clearly. A number of studies attest to problem of false-positive and false-negative results obtained with certain kits that employ IFA or ELISA technology.[132,909,910,966,984,985]

Clinical Scenario 1: Very Early Pregnancy (first few weeks). If no antibody is demonstrable, the patient has not been infected and must be considered at risk of infection. A positive IgG test titer and a negative test result for IgM antibodies or high-avidity antibody test can be interpreted as reflecting infection that occurred months or years before the pregnancy, although very rarely IgM *T. gondii* antibodies may not be detected in recent infections. Essentially, there is no risk of the patient's giving birth to a congenitally infected child (unless she is immunosuppressed), regardless of the level of antibody titer. No matter how high the titer is, it should not be considered prognostically meaningful.

If IgM antibodies are present, the avidity test should be performed. If this is unavailable, the IgG test should be performed, with results compared with those for a second sample taken 3 weeks after the first. If no rise in IgG antibody test titer occurs, the infection was acquired before pregnancy, and almost no risk to the fetus exists. If a rise in IgG antibody test titer is observed, the infection probably was acquired less than 2 months previously, perhaps around the time of conception. In this situation, the risk of giving birth to an infected child is very low (see Table 31-9).

Clinical Scenario 2: Early Pregnancy (within a Few Months) plus Suspected Acute Infection. The diagnosis depends on three criteria: (1) the presence of lymphadenopathy in areas compatible with the diagnosis of acute acquired toxoplasmosis,[573,576,788,986-998] (2) a high IgG test titer (300 IU/mL or greater), and (3) presence of IgM antibody. If two of the three criteria are present, for purposes of management, the diagnosis of acute acquired toxoplasmosis should be considered likely. If, however, the IgG test titer is less than 300 IU/mL, a significant rise in titer should be demonstrable in a second serum sample obtained 2 to 3 weeks later. The avidity assay is particularly helpful in this setting. A high-avidity test result indicates acquisition of infection more than 12 to 16 weeks earlier (see earlier under "IgG Avidity Assay").

Important to consider in the pregnant patient in whom lymphadenopathy is observed is that high-avidity results were demonstrable only in those women whose lymphadenopathy had developed at least 4 months earlier.[138] Therefore, a high-avidity test result in a pregnant woman with recent development of lymphadenopathy (e.g., within 2 or 3 months of performing the avidity test) suggests a cause other than toxoplasmosis, and further workup is warranted to determine the cause of the lymphadenopathy. In that same study of the IgG avidity test in patients with lymphadenopathy, low–IgG avidity antibodies were observed in sera of patients whose lymphadenopathy had developed as long as 17 months before the time of serum sampling for testing. (This provides additional proof that low–IgG avidity test results should not be relied on for diagnosis of recently acquired infection.)

Clinical Scenario 3: Suspected Congenital Toxoplasmosis in a Newborn Infant. The diagnosis of the acute acquired infection in women who have just given birth to a child with suspected congenital toxoplasmosis is rarely difficult. As a rule, diagnosis of recent infection in the mother relies on the IgG test titer and the results of tests for IgM antibodies. Paradoxically, examination of maternal sera frequently is more useful for diagnosing subclinical or atypical congenital toxoplasmosis in a neonate than is examination of the child's serum. If IgM antibody is detected in the mother and no prior serologic test results are available, her newborn should be examined clinically and serologically to rule out congenital infection.

Because IgM antibodies as measured by ELISA or ISAGA may persist for many months or even years, their greatest value is in determining that a pregnant woman examined early in gestation has not recently been infected. A negative result virtually rules out recently acquired infection unless sera are tested late in gestation (in which case IgM antibodies may no longer be detectable), or so early after the acute infection that an antibody response has not yet occurred (in which case the acute infection would be identified in a screening program in which follow-up serologic testing is performed in seronegative pregnant women). A positive IgM test result is more difficult to evaluate, unless a significant rise in IgG or IgM titer can be demonstrated when sera are tested in parallel or when results of other tests (e.g., tests for IgA and IgE antibody and the HS/AC test) suggest recent infection. A very high IgM, IgA, or IgE titer is more likely to reflect recent infection, although such high titers may persist for months. Such positive sera should be confirmed with additional methods, such as the HS/AC or avidity test. In most cases, use of and consultation with a reference laboratory will be required. In the Palo Alto laboratory, a "chronic" pattern in the HS/AC test agrees virtually 100% with a "chronic" titer in the IgG avidity test.

In the unusual situation in which a pregnant woman has a positive IgM antibody titer and a persistently negative IgG titer, a false-positive IgM result must be considered, and if feasible, all such patients should have IgG antibodies measured by a different method.[989,990] Examples of the serologic response in women who seroconverted during pregnancy are shown in Table 31-35.

Pinon and colleagues in France fortuitously diagnosed two cases of congenital toxoplasmosis in newborns whose mothers did not have detectable *T. gondii* antibodies at the time of birth. These cases prompted the investigators to perform a study over an 18-month period to determine by postnatal serologic follow-up whether they could detect women who were infected but whose results of serologic testing were negative at the time of delivery. They detected four cases of perinatal maternal infection, and two of these resulted in infected offspring. In view of these results, and to prevent missing maternal infection at the end of pregnancy, they suggest that serologic testing of seronegative women who have been screened monthly should continue such that the last blood sample is obtained approximately 30 days *after* they have given birth.[103]

Prenatal Diagnosis of Fetal *Toxoplasma* Infection

Although PCR assay in amniotic fluid is now the method of choice, cordocentesis[991-993] may still be used when PCR methods are unavailable or in the rare instances in which the PCR assay result is negative and the ultrasonographic findings suggest fetal infection. For this reason, findings on clinical studies using this method are described here along with those for PCR analysis.

Cordocentesis

When a diagnosis of acquired toxoplasmosis is established in a pregnant woman, either based on clinical manifestations or as a result of systematic serologic screening performed during pregnancy, it is possible to demonstrate either the presence or the possible absence of congenital *T. gondii* infection or congenital toxoplasmosis, or both, in the fetus before delivery.[129,130,800,994,995] The method of cordocentesis initially was described by Desmonts and colleagues,[129] and the overall results obtained by this same group were reported by Daffos and co-workers.[130] These investigators reported a

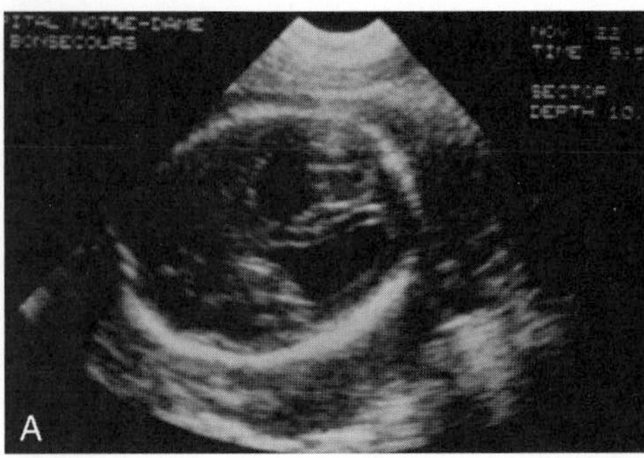

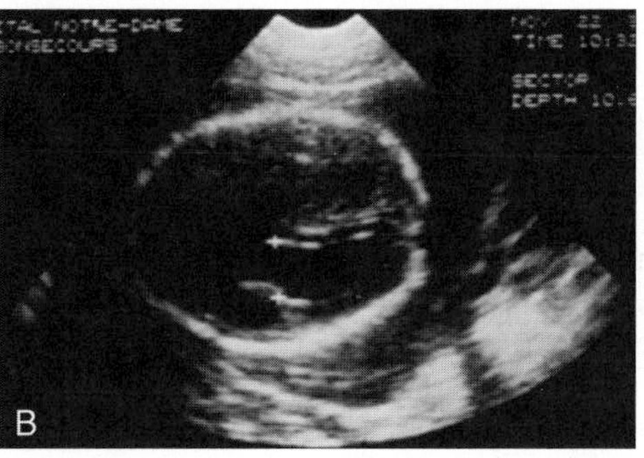

Figure 31–25 **A** and **B**, Ultrasound study of fetus with hydrocephalus resulting from toxoplasmosis. (Courtesy of F. Daffos, Paris.)

prospective study of 746 documented cases of maternal *T. gondii* infection in which prenatal diagnosis was attempted, with follow-up of the live-born infants for at least 3 months. Pathologic and parasitologic examinations of aborted fetuses were performed. The complication rate related to the procedure in general was 0.3 fetal loss per 1000. A volume of 1 to 3 mL of pure fetal blood usually was obtained at the first attempt. In 3% of cases, a second attempt was necessary; this was performed 1 hour later or 1 week later, depending on the reason for the failure in the initial attempt (F Daffos, personal communication to JS Remington, 1993). In only 4 of 1356 pregnancies were the investigators unable to obtain pure fetal blood.[130]

Definitive diagnosis of fetal infection relied on isolation (by mouse inoculation) of the parasite from fetal blood or amniotic fluid usually obtained at 20 to 26 weeks of gestation and on serologic examination of serum of the fetus for evidence of synthesis of IgM *T. gondii* antibodies. Nonspecific tests included ultrasound studies; white blood cell, platelet, and eosinophil counts; and measurement of total IgM, γ-glutamyltransferase, and lactate dehydrogenase. An ultrasound examination was performed every 2 weeks from the time of fetal blood sampling to the end of pregnancy, with special focus on the size of the lateral cerebral ventricles (Fig. 31-25A and B), the thickness of the placenta, and presence or absence of ascites, hepatomegaly, or cerebral calcification.

To allow for a comprehensive analysis of the indications for and results of these diagnostic procedures, the 746 pregnant women were divided into three groups. Group 1 included 159 women in whom a recently acquired acute infection was discovered when the first serologic screening test was performed at the beginning of pregnancy. Serologic or clinical data suggested that they had acquired the infection either shortly before conception or, at the latest, before week 6 of gestation. Group 2 included 487 women whose infection was acquired between weeks 6 and 16 of gestation. Tests for possible seroconversion are as a rule performed monthly in seronegative women in France, a practice that facilitates determination of the time at which infection was acquired. In these groups, cases were referred for prenatal diagnosis but were not included in the study if the fetus was dead in utero because of congenital toxoplasmosis before the time of blood sampling. The incidence rates of congenital infection were 0.6% and 3.7%, respectively. Group 3 was composed of 100 women who acquired the infection between weeks 17 and 25; fetal blood and amniotic fluid were sampled between weeks 24 and 29. In this group, the incidence of congenital infection was 20%.

The presence of *T. gondii* infection in the fetus was demonstrated at prenatal examination in 39 of these 746 pregnancies. Infection was parasitologically proved by isolation of *T. gondii* from fetal blood or amniotic fluid, or both, in 34 of the 39 cases. *T. gondii*–specific IgM antibodies were detected in fetal blood in only 9 cases, despite the high sensitivity of the method used (ISAGA). None of the samples taken before week 24 was positive. Signs of congenital toxoplasmosis were recognized at ultrasound examination in 9 of the 39 cases; these were principally unilateral or bilateral ventricular dilatations demonstrated by an increase in the ventricle-to-hemisphere ratio. In 10 additional cases, the ultrasound examination appearance was normal at the time of fetal blood sampling (24 weeks), but ventricular dilatation appeared during the following weeks and was present at the time of termination of the pregnancy. Ascites were observed twice as an early but transitory sign. Intrahepatic calcifications were found in one case, and intracranial calcifications were noted in two cases.

One or more laboratory measurements of fetal blood proved to be abnormal in most cases. The most frequent signs were an increase in the total IgM level (in 22 of the 37 samples examined) and an increase in γ-glutamyltransferase level (in 28 of the 33 samples examined). It is evident from these results that none of the examinations performed proved to be 100% reliable for demonstration of congenital toxoplasmosis in the fetus. When the results of the various tests were grouped together, however, they had a remarkably high predictive value and a high degree of specificity. (See also discussions of IgA antibodies, interferon, T cell subsets, and complement later in this section, because these markers have been studied in fetal blood.)

It should be noted that cordocentesis is no longer employed and has been supplanted by PCR assay in amniotic fluid, as described earlier and in the next section.

Amniocentesis: Polymerase Chain Reaction Assay in Amniotic Fluid

Results of PCR analysis performed in different laboratories may differ considerably; a result reported as positive or negative from one laboratory may even be the opposite of that from another laboratory. At present, no procedures for quality control in laboratories performing PCR assay for prenatal diagnosis are in place. PCR assay results from any laboratory must be reviewed with caution, and if possible, information or data on the reliability and validation data of the PCR tests from that laboratory should be requested.

In 1994, Hohlfeld and co-workers from Paris[125] published a follow-up to their cordocentesis study reported in 1988.[130]

Table 31–38 Diagnostic Value of the Polymerase Chain Reaction (PCR Assay) Compared with Conventional Methods for Prenatal Diagnosis of Congenital *Toxoplasma gondii* Infection in 339 Pregnancies

Variable	PCR[a]	Conventional Methods[a,b]
Sensitivity	37/38 (97.4; 86.1-99.9)	34/38 (89.5; 72.2-97.0)[c]
Specificity	301/301 (100; 98.8-100)	301/301 (100; 98.8-100)
Positive predictive value	37/37 (100; 90.5-100)	34/34 (100; 89.7-100)
Negative predictive value	301/302 (99.7; 98.7-100)	301/305 (98.7; 97.4-99.9)

[a]Positive tests/all tests (%; 95% confidence interval).
[b]Tissue culture of amniotic fluid, inoculation of mice with fetal blood and amniotic fluid, and determination of specific IgM in fetal blood.
[c]The sensitivity of conventional methods in the study overall was somewhat higher (92%; 95% confidence interval, 88 to 96%).
IgM, immunoglobulin M.
Adapted from Hohlfeld P, et al. Prenatal diagnosis of congenital toxoplasmosis with polymerase-chain-reaction test on amniotic fluid. N Engl J Med 331:695-699, 1994.

Prenatal diagnosis, which included amniocentesis, ultrasonography, and fetal blood sampling, was performed in 2632 women who had acquired *T. gondii* infection during gestation. One hundred ninety-four cases of congenital toxoplasmosis were identified, and 178 of these were diagnosed by conventional methods of prenatal diagnosis. No false-positive results were reported. The overall sensitivity was 92%, the specificity was 100%, and the negative predictive value was 99%. The sensitivity of the IgM antibody test was 28%; of mouse inoculation with fetal blood, 72%; of mouse inoculation with amniotic fluid, 64%; and of tissue culture of amniotic fluid, 64%. The overall rate of spontaneous fetal loss was 1.3%. PCR assay was performed in the amniotic fluid in 339 consecutive women, and the results were compared with those obtained by the conventional methods. By conventional testing, congenital infection was demonstrated in 34 fetuses, and in each the PCR test result also was positive. In three additional fetuses, only the PCR assay result was positive, and in each, the diagnosis of congenital infection was confirmed on follow-up investigation (autopsy in two and serologic study in one). One false-negative result was obtained with the PCR assay, and no false-positive results. The investigators concluded that the PCR assay is a more reliable, safer, simpler, and less expensive method than the conventional methods they had been using, and that it can be used from week 18 of gestation until term. They also concluded that fetal blood sampling is no longer necessary, and that amniocentesis together with the PCR test and inoculation of mice (tissue culture is less sensitive) is preferred (Table 31-38). The authors did not have data on the efficacy of testing amniotic fluid before 18 weeks of gestation. They stated that prenatal diagnosis should not be attempted until at least 4 weeks after the acute infection in the mother.

In 1998, Jenum and associates published the Norwegian experience with a nested PCR technique using amniotic fluid collected from 67 women diagnosed as having acquired the infection during gestation.[836] They also used mouse inoculation on each of the samples. They commented on the greater sensitivity of the PCR method, because mouse inoculation results were affected by treatment in the mothers. Whereas Hohlfeld and co-workers[125] found a specificity of 100%, Jenum and associates[130] observed a specificity of only 94%, despite careful technical steps to avoid contamination of their samples. Their reported positive predictive value was 67%, with 10 true positives among 15 positive results. Three of 8 infants with congenital toxoplasmosis diagnosed after birth had a negative result on PCR assay and mouse inoculation on prenatal examination. Thus, in their study, a positive PCR assay result did not confirm infection in the fetus. For this reason, the researchers stated that positive results also require serologic follow-up testing for confirmation of the diagnosis. Prenatal diagnosis using PCR assay performed in amniotic fluid from each twin in a dizygotic pregnancy was recently reported by Tjalma and colleagues.[996]

Because physicians must make decisions regarding management of a pregnancy after results of amniocentesis are obtained, it is of utmost importance that the PCR assay be specific insofar as there are no false-positive results. For example, according to a recent report, the use of a nested PCR technique[836] did not appear to yield results that fit this requirement; therefore, that nested PCR method cannot be considered to represent an improvement over conventional methods for prenatal diagnosis.

One shortcoming of the study reported by Hohlfeld and co-workers[125] is that the sensitivity and negative predictive value of the PCR assay in amniotic fluid were compared with those of conventional methods but were not analyzed relative to the status of the infection in the live-born infants. The enthusiasm that has been generated for the reliability of the PCR assay should be tempered by the fact that because of the delay that can occur between the time of maternal infection and transmission of the parasite to the fetus (transmission may occur after the date of the amniocentesis), all congenital infections are not and cannot be identified by prenatal diagnosis. One case that suggests such a delay is reported in the publication by Hohlfeld and co-workers.[125] Before PCR testing was used for prenatal diagnosis, it was well recognized that not all cases of congenital *T. gondii* infection could be detected prenatally. Of 89 congenital infections, Hohlfeld and co-workers[124] reported 9 cases (10%) with a negative result on prenatal diagnostic testing. In other published series, the rate of congenital infections with no prenatally identified abnormal findings varied, ranging from 3% in the study by Pratlong and co-workers[997] to 8% in that by Berrebi and associates.[998] Actually, the number of infections that were not detected by the prenatal diagnostic procedures was underestimated in each of these studies, because a significant number of the offspring were lost to follow-up (50 of 211 [24%][997]), or data were not provided by the investigators.[125] Before the use of PCR methods, it was not possible to define whether these discrepancies were due to a lack of sensitivity of the diagnostic procedures or to the fact that transmission of the parasite occurred after the amniocentesis or cordocentesis was performed. The higher sensitivity of PCR assay when compared with conventional methods explains why congenital infection had been missed in the past when the less sensitive conventional methods were used.

At present, the wide range of accuracy of PCR assay for detection of *T. gondii* infection in the fetus (confidence interval, CI) in both early and late gestation is such that one cannot rely on a negative test result as indicating the absence of infection in the fetus. Thus, a negative PCR test result in amniotic fluid does not rule out infection in the fetus.

Romand and colleagues in France evaluated the sensitivity, specificity, and predictive values of prenatal amniotic fluid studied prospectively in 270 women with proven primary infection during pregnancy.[838] Definitive infection status of live-born infants was assessed by serologic follow-up testing. The maternal-fetal transmission rate increased according to duration of gestation at maternal infection (see Table 31-29). Seventy-five infants (28%) were congenitally infected, 48 (64%) of whom had a positive result on PCR assay at prenatal diagnosis. Overall sensitivity of PCR assay in amniotic fluid was estimated at 64% (95% confidence interval [CI] 53.1%-74.9%), negative predictive value at 87.8% (95% CI, 83.5%-92.1%), whereas specificity and positive predictive value both were 100% (95% CI, 98%-100% and 92.3%-100%, respectively). Among the cases of congenital toxoplasmosis, no significant differences were found between those with a positive or negative PCR assay result with regard to median gestational age at maternal infection, time interval between maternal infection and amniocentesis, or duration of treatment before amniocentesis. Analysis of sensitivity and negative predictive value of PCR analysis, however, showed large variations according to gestational age at maternal infection (see Fig. 31-18). Sensitivity was significantly higher between 17 and 21 weeks of gestation. Lack of a positive prenatal diagnosis in 27 infected fetuses between 14 and 31 weeks of gestation did not result in more severe clinical outcomes at birth, when compared with those cases of fetal infection in which the results of prenatal diagnosis were positive. With the notable exception of a case in which severe defects were demonstrated in utero despite initially negative results on PCR testing, only 2 of 26 infants with negative prenatal PCR assay results had evidence of moderate findings at birth (cerebral calcifications). The other 24 children had subclinical infection through 1 year of life. These findings suggest that vertical transmission may have occurred late in pregnancy, or that very low concentrations of parasites in the amniotic fluid were not detected by PCR analysis.

In a study performed to determine whether quantification of PCR results would be helpful in predicting outcome of the infection in the fetus or newborn, parasite concentrations were estimated by real-time quantitative PCR assay in 88 consecutive positive amniotic fluid samples from 86 pregnant women.[838] Results were analyzed according to the gestational age at maternal infection and the clinical status in fetuses during pregnancy and at birth. A significant negative linear regression was observed between gestational age at maternal infection and parasite loads in amniotic fluid (see Fig. 31-19).

After adjustment for gestational age at maternal seroconversion, parasite concentration in amniotic fluid, and the total duration of prenatal treatment in the multivariate analysis, the two variables significantly and independently associated with most severe signs of infection (fetal death or cerebral ventricular dilatation) were an early gestational age at maternal infection (odds ratio = 1.44/decreasing week gestation [95% CI, 1.12%-1.85%]) and high parasite amniotic fluid concentrations (odds ratio = 15.4/log [parasites/mL of amniotic fluid] [95% CI, 2.45%-97.7%]). In this series, each of the 11 cases in which parasite loads were greater than 100/mL, with onset of infection before 20 weeks, resulted in severe impairments in the offspring, indicating a 100% predictive value of poor prognosis (see Fig. 31-19).

The earlier in gestation infection occurs, the higher the parasite burden. Parasite burden in amniotic fluid as determined by quantitative PCR analysis also is a prenatal biologic marker of the severity of congenital infection. In a dizygotic twin pair, one had no parasites, and the other had greater than 600 parasites per mL. At pregnancy termination, the former infant had no signs of infection; the latter had disseminated multivisceral infection. Members of a second twin pair— one with clinical signs and the other without such signs—similarly were discordant for parasite burden in amniotic fluid (3.2 versus 2800 parasites per mL), and both died. The twin with hydrocephalus and ventriculomegaly probably was the twin with amniotic fluid with the higher parasite burden (2800 parasites per mL).

Ultrasound examinations are still required and should be performed each month following a negative PCR result on amniocentesis, because congenital infections with extensive involvement and hydrocephalus have occurred in the setting of a negative PCR assay result. When the ultrasound appearance remains normal, it is still necessary to continue clinical and serologic follow-up evaluation of infants until congenital infection is definitively ruled out.

Immunoglobulin A Antibodies

The value of demonstration of IgA *T. gondii* antibodies in the fetus is now well recognized.[899,904,997,999,1000] Therefore, testing for these antibodies for this purpose should be routine in all laboratories that test newborns for suspected congenital T. *gondii* infection.

Interferon

Interferon has been demonstrated in blood of fetuses infected with *T. gondii*, suggesting that the fetus is able to synthesize this cytokine as early as 26 weeks of gestation.[1001] Its demonstration appears helpful when interferon level determination is used with other nonspecific tests for diagnosing *T. gondii* infection in the fetus. Interferon serum levels that were significantly higher than in controls also were demonstrated in sera of pregnant women during seroconversion for *T. gondii* antibodies.[1001]

T Cell Subsets

T cell subsets were evaluated in a group of uninfected and infected fetuses.[1002] Significant differences from controls were noted in that the infected fetuses were characterized by a smaller percentage of $CD3^+$ and $CD4^+$ T cells and a decrease in absolute number of $CD4^+$ cells and lower $CD4^+/CD8^+$ ratio. The mothers in this study were receiving treatment, and the possible results of this treatment on T cells could not be excluded. In addition, because the number of infected fetuses was small, it was not possible to analyze the values obtained relative to gestational age, as was done in the control, uninfected fetuses.

In another study, Lecolier and co-workers studied T lymphocyte subpopulations in normal and in six *T. gondii*–infected fetuses.[999] They noted a significant increase in number of $CD8^+$ T cells in two cases investigated soon after maternal infection (3 and 6 weeks, respectively) and a significant decrease in number of $CD4^+$ T cells in the four other cases that were investigated later (7 to 13 weeks after maternal infection). These observations suggest that alterations in T lymphocyte subsets in the infected fetus are similar to those that occur in the acute acquired infection in adults.[460] In another study by Foulon and associates, these results were not confirmed.[800] Thus, further study is necessary to evaluate whether study of T cell subsets will be a useful adjunct in prenatal diagnosis.

Complement

It appears that the C4 component of complement is significantly increased in fetuses congenitally infected with *T. gondii*. Gestational age is important in interpretation of results, but the measurement of C4 levels in the fetus may be a useful nonspecific adjunctive test for prenatal diagnosis.[1003]

Serologic Diagnosis in the Newborn

Because of the pleomorphism of congenital toxoplasmosis, because the infection most often is subclinical in the newborn, and because the infection may be mimicked by other infections and diseases of the neonate, the diagnosis of congenital *T. gondii* infection is far more complicated than is diagnosis of the acquired infection.

The serologic diagnosis of congenital *T. gondii* infection in the newborn is particularly difficult because of the high prevalence of antibodies to *T. gondii* among normal women of childbearing age in the United States and in much of the rest of the world (see Table 31-15). Thus, a high antibody titer in a newborn may merely reflect past or recent infection in the mother (maternal IgG antibody having passed transplacentally to her fetus).

The fact that infection in the fetus may stimulate production of sufficient IgM to result in abnormally high levels of this immunoglobulin in the newborn has been shown in a variety of congenital infections by Stiehm and associates[946] and by Alford and co-workers.[1004,1005] Thus, quantification of IgM in cord serum may be a valuable screening device for detecting infection in the newborn. At present, the consensus of those working on immunologic responses to perinatal infection is that enough "false-negative" results occur to suggest that quantification of IgM in the newborn may not be universally applicable for diagnosing infection.[1006-1008] Such false-negative results are not infrequent in premature infants with proven rubella.[1006] For a nonspecific test to be beneficial as a screen, it seems that a slight excess in sensitivity resulting in overdiagnosis (false-positive results) can be accepted, but that lack of sensitivity in known cases, resulting in underdiagnosis (false-negative results) cannot be accepted.

As mentioned earlier, demonstration of IgM, IgA, or IgE antibodies to *T. gondii* in serum of the newborn is diagnostic of congenital *T. gondii* infection if contamination with maternal blood has not occurred. When an appropriate fluorescein-tagged antiserum to IgM has been employed, we have not had any false-positive results except for the qualifications mentioned earlier for the IgM IFA method. Because high levels of maternal IgG antibodies to *T. gondii* may compete for antigenic sites on the surface of the organisms[943] with the relatively low IgM antibody levels usually found in the fetus or neonate, weak reactions and low IgM antibody titers (1:2) indicate infection in the newborn. Even allowing for these weakly positive reactions, however, detectable specific IgM antibody is absent in the sera of most neonates with congenital toxoplasmosis (approximately 75%) when the IgM IFA test is used.[731] This false-negative result rate was only approximately 20% if the double-sandwich IgM ELISA method was used.[855] Because of the high incidence of false-negative results for the IgM IFA test, we recommend that the capture IgM ELISA or ISAGA method be used instead. It is noteworthy that the proportion of infants showing IgM antibody is the same whether illness is clinically manifest or subclinical. IgA antibodies have been demonstrated in as high as 90% of newborns with the congenital infection,[899,1009] which further attests to the great value of testing for these antibodies (Table 31-39). A number of investigators have reported greater sensitivity of IgA antibody determination for diagnosis in infected children than for IgM.[858,898,899,1010,1011] As emphasized by Foudrinier and co-workers, specificity of IgA detected at birth must be confirmed, because equivocal and positive IgA test results were found in newborns during the first days of

Table 31–39 Serologic Test Results for IgM and IgA Antibodies at Birth and during the Newborn Period in Sera of 23 Congenitally Infected and 49 Uninfected Offspring of Mothers Infected during Gestation[a]

Trimester Mother Acquired Infection (Time Test Performed)	IgM– IgA–	IgM+ IgA+	IgM+ IgA–	IgM– IgA+
Uninfected (at birth)	47	0	1	1
Infected (at birth)				
1st trimester	1	1	0	2
2nd trimester	1	0	0	5
3rd trimester	2	8	1	0
Infected (follow-up 1 wk to 3 mo)	3	11	0	9

[a]All mothers received spiramycin treatment during gestation from time seroconversion was noted.

IgA, IgM, immunoglobulins A, M.

Adapted from Decoster A, Slizwicz B, Simon J, et al. Platelia-toxo IgA, a new kit for early diagnosis of congenital toxoplasmosis by detection of anti-P30 immunoglobulin A antibodies. J Clin Microbiol 29:2291-2295, 1991, with permission.

Table 31–40 **Data in a Mother Who Acquired *Toxoplasma gondii* Infection at about the Time of Conception or a Few Weeks Earlier Who Had a Negative IgM Test Titer and Whose Infant Had a High IgM Test Titer**

Subject	Stage of Pregnancy or Age	Clinical Manifestations	Titer: Dye Test[a] (IU/mL)	Titer: IgM Test[b]	*T. gondii* Isolated
Mother	9 wk	None	2000	Negative	
	13 wk	None	2000	Negative	
	8 mo	Delivery			
	1 mo after delivery	None	2000	Negative	Blood negative
Infant	4 days	Hydrocephalus, microphthalmia, convulsions, abnormal cerebrospinal fluid	1000	Positive	Blood positive
	8 days	Death			Brain positive

[a]Dye test titers are approximately 8000 in the mother and 4000 in the infant if expressed as reciprocal of serum dilution.
[b]Titers are expressed as the reciprocal of the serum dilution.
IgM, immunoglobulin M; IU, international units.
Adapted from Desmonts G, Couvreur J. Toxoplasmosis in pregnancy and its transmission to the fetus. Bull NY Acad Med 50:146-159, 1974, with permission. The mother was not treated.

life, whereas subsequent sera became negative within less than 10 days.[1011] They concluded that in a neonate born to a mother with IgA or IgM *T. gondii* antibodies, a positive IgA or IgM test result must be interpreted with caution and be confirmed after approximately 10 days of life, unless the diagnosis is established before this time. Additional data are needed to clarify whether all newborns with a positive IgA or IgM antibody titer at approximately 10 days of age are indeed infected, especially in those cases in which the maternal IgA or IgM antibody titers were very high. Determination of levels of β-human chorionic gonadotropin and of total IgA may prove to be of value as adjunctive tests. Of note, however, we have never observed a false-positive result after the first day of life when the ISAGA was used for detection of IgM antibodies.

The value of demonstration of IgE antibodies also is clear. In one of our laboratories (JS Remington), 19 of 21 infants (90%) (ages birth to 5 weeks) with congenital toxoplasmosis and signs of CNS involvement tested positive for IgE antibodies (92% by ELISA and 62% by ISAGA)[896]; of the 10 tested in the first week of life, 9 had IgM antibody, and all 7 of those tested for IgA antibodies were seropositive. Seven of the 21 were first tested in the second week of life; 6 had IgM antibodies, and all 5 of those tested for IgA were seropositive. Of the 4 first tested at 3 to 5 weeks of life, 3 had both IgM and IgA antibody; 1 infant had neither.[896] In studies by Pinon and colleagues, 52 cases of congenital *T. gondii* infection (5 symptomatic and 47 "asymptomatic" cases) were studied; at birth or during the first month of life, none of the symptomatic and 13 (25%) of the "asymptomatic" infants were seropositive by IgE ISAGA. Thirty-five of the 52 infants (67%) were seropositive for IgA antibody by ISAGA.[1012,1013]

If the infant is infected in utero at a time when it is immunologically competent to produce IgM antibodies but before the passage of maternal IgG *T. gondii* antibodies across the placenta has occurred, there is no reason to suspect competition for recognition of antigenic sites on the parasite. Data derived from studies of infants with very high IgM titers in the early newborn period support this hypothesis. Table 31-40 displays clinical and serologic data representing such an instance in a mother and her infant. The mother had had a high but stable dye test titer since the ninth week of pregnancy and a negative IgM IFA test titer. The same results were obtained during week 13. This finding suggests that infection occurred at about the time of conception or a few weeks earlier. She did not receive treatment and gave birth to a severely infected infant with generalized toxoplasmosis who died 8 days after delivery. This newborn had an unusually high IgM test titer. If, however, high titers of maternal antibody are present in the fetus before the organism reaches the fetus, as a consequence of delay by the placental barrier discussed earlier, it is possible that IgG antibody might compete (and "cover") for recognition sites[943] on the parasite or may by other means (e.g., feedback mechanism) suppress fetal IgM antibody synthesis. (This also might explain the paradoxical occurrence of an elevated IgM level in the serum of an infected infant in the presence of a negative IgM test titer.) That this may occur has been shown in an experimental animal model.[463] Thus, a negative IgM test titer in a newborn does not rule out the possibility of congenital infection. Whether IgM antibodies are demonstrable in the newborn depends primarily on the time during gestation the infection is acquired by the mother; the later in gestation maternal infection occurs, the higher the rate of IgM positivity in the newborn. Recent data from the European Network (E Petersen, personal communication to JS Remington, November 2004) reveal that when maternal infection occurs at approximately 10 weeks of gestation, approximately 10% of the newborns will be seropositive for IgM. For newborns of mothers infected at approximately 20 weeks of gestation, the rate of seropositivity was approximately 20%, and for 30 weeks of gestation, approximately 60%.

In our experience, IgM antibody titers usually decrease rapidly after the infant's own IgG antibodies have reached a high titer; at 1 year of age, IgM antibodies usually are not demonstrable or are present in very low titer.

In the absence of demonstration of the parasite, IgM or IgA antibodies to *T. gondii*, follow-up testing of infants with

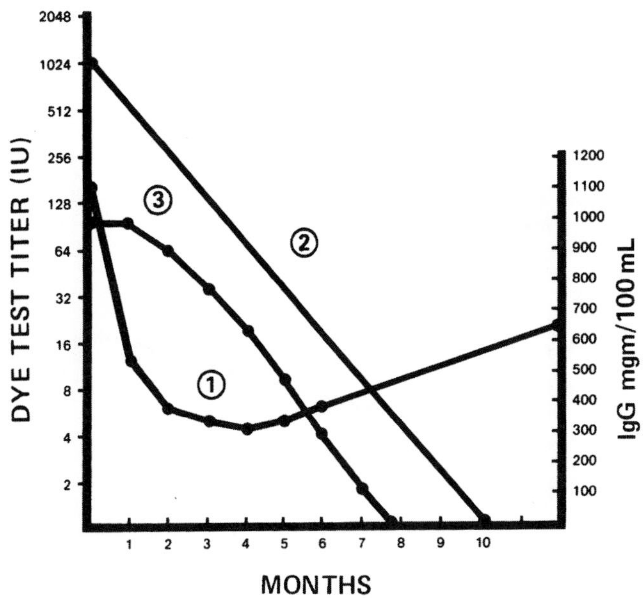

Figure 31–26 IgG and *Toxoplasma* antibodies: uninfected child. *Curve 1*, mg of IgG/dL; *curve 2*, IU of *Toxoplasma* antibody per ml; *curve 3*, IU of *Toxoplasma* antibody per mg of IgG. (Data from Desmonts G, Couvreur J. Toxoplasmosis: epidemiologic and serologic aspects of perinatal infection. *In* Krugman S, Gershon AA [eds]. Infections of the Fetus and the Newborn Infant. Progress in Clinical and Biological Research, vol. 3. New York, Alan R Liss, 1975, pp 115-132.)

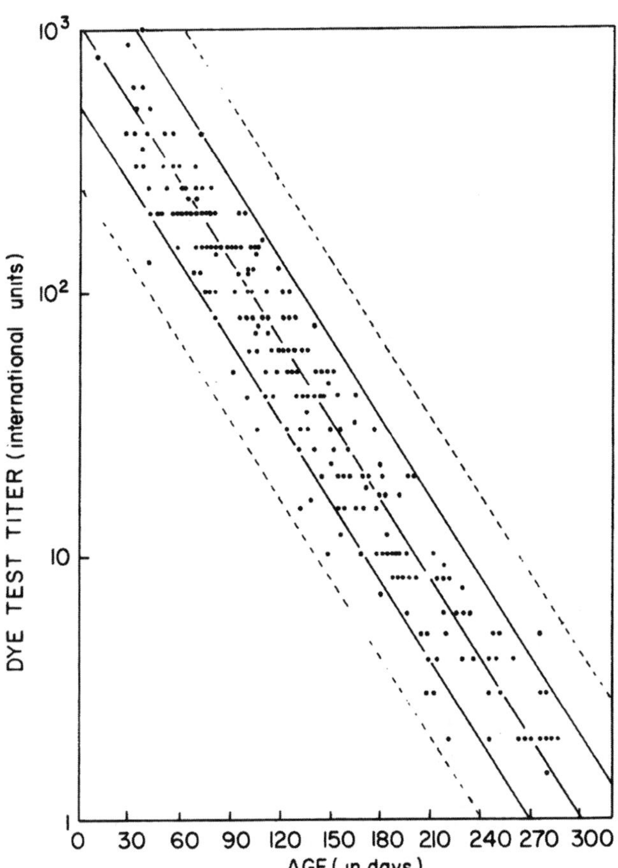

Figure 31–27 Decrease in maternally transmitted *Toxoplasma* antibodies (dye test) in uninfected infants. The two parallel lines indicate one-half and twice the titer, plus or minus one twofold dilution. The result in one serum sample of each pair is on the theoretical line and is not represented by a dot. The result in the other serum sample of each pair is represented by a dot.

suspected toxoplasmosis is the only means of making a serologic diagnosis of subclinical toxoplasmosis. For proper interpretation of test titers in infants who are past the immediate newborn period, it is important to understand how passively transmitted maternal IgG decreases in the uninfected infant. Because the literature is replete with misinformation on the interpretation of *T. gondii* serologic studies in older infants, this important subject is dealt with here. In Figure 31-26, curve 1 shows the total serum IgG values in milligrams per deciliter in the newborn and infant to the age of 1 year. The values in the newborn at birth frequently are somewhat higher than they are in the mother and subsequently decrease. Minimal values (e.g., 300 to 400 mg/dL) are observed at about the third or fourth month, after which time the level increases with increasing production of IgG by the infant. Maternally transmitted antibodies (curve 2) progressively disappear, because they are not synthesized by the infant. Their half-life is approximately 30 days; that is, they decrease by approximately one half per month (Fig. 31-27).

Figure 31-28 shows actual data from an uninfected infant plotted against the background of the theoretical decay curve for IgG maternal antibody (approximately one-half the value every 30 days). Thus, a titer of 1000 IU/mL at birth should drop to 1 IU/mL in 300 days. The infant whose titers are shown here had titers of 400 IU/mL at birth, 60 IU/mL at 75 days, and 3 IU/mL at 212 days. These are exactly the expected values. Figure 31-27 shows results obtained in 430 paired sera from 93 uninfected infants with passively transmitted maternal antibodies plotted against their theoretical values. Ninety-three percent of the actual titers are less than one- to twofold dilution different from the expected values.

These data preclude acceptance that all infants with a positive titer at 4 to 6 months have congenital toxoplasmosis. The same rate of decrease applies to both high and low titers. It takes approximately the same amount of time for a decrease from 1000 to 250 IU/mL, a seemingly very significant variation, as for a decrease from 4 to 1 IU/mL, a titer difference that most investigators would consider negligible (i.e., no significant difference).

For a better estimate of this decrease in passively transmitted maternal antibodies, it is useful to compare the antibody titer and the level of IgG and to compute the specific *antibody load*, that is, the ratio of specific antibodies (number of IU/mL) to total IgG. This is represented diagrammatically in Figure 31-26 by curve 3 and in Table 31-40. In Figure 31-26, as late as the fourth to sixth week of life, usually no change in the antibody load is observed; the IgG is still mainly maternal in origin. Although the titer of antibodies decreases, the total IgG decreases in a similar manner. As a result, the ratio remains constant. During the second and third months, the amount of IgG synthesized by the infant increases. Because this newly synthesized IgG does not contain antibodies to *T. gondii*, the antibody load decreases and will continue to decrease as IgG synthesis in the child progresses.

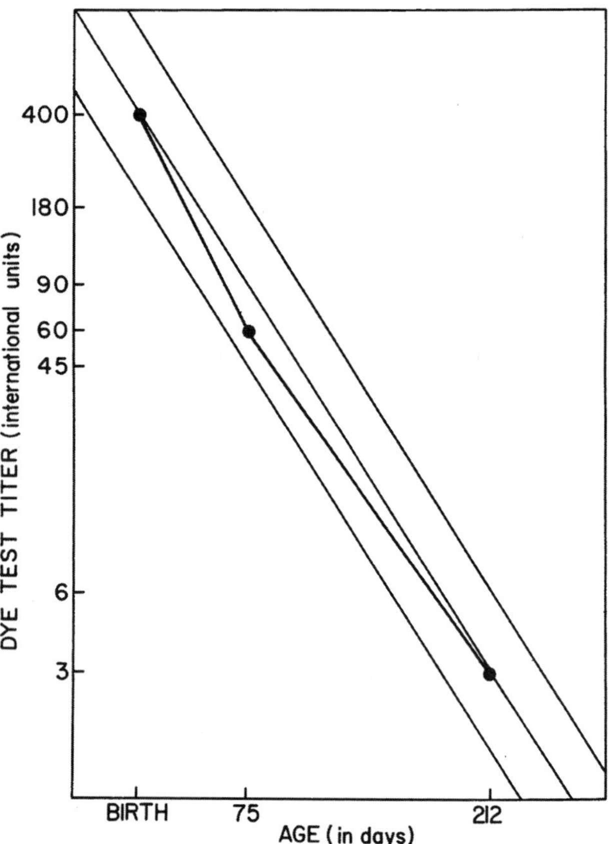

Figure 31–28 Evolution of maternally transmitted antibody (dye test) in an uninfected infant from birth to the age of 212 days.

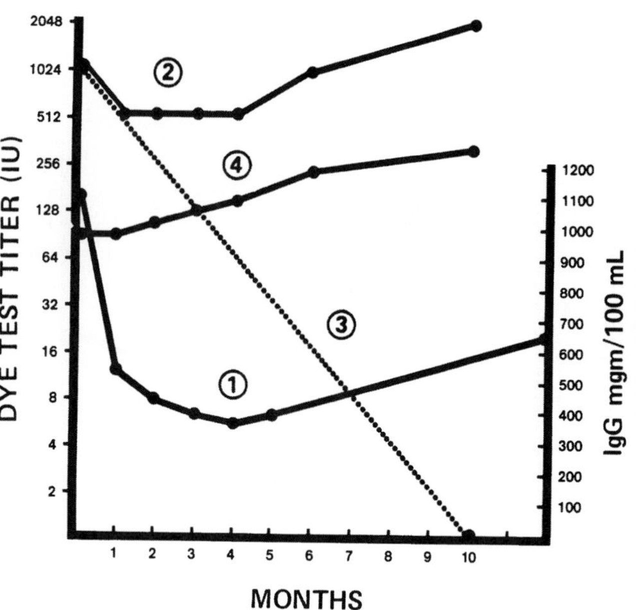

Figure 31–29 Antibodies in congenital toxoplasmosis (cases with early synthesis of antibodies). *Curve 1,* mg of IgG/dL; *curve 2,* IU of *Toxoplasma* antibody per mL; *curve 3,* expected titer if antibodies were maternal in origin; *curve 4,* IU of *Toxoplasma* antibody per mg of IgG. (Data from Desmonts G, Couvreur J. Toxoplasmosis: epidemiologic and serologic aspects of perinatal infection. *In* Krugman S, Gershon AA [eds]. Infections of the Fetus and the Newborn Infant. Progress in Clinical and Biological Research, vol. 3. New York, Alan R Liss, 1975, pp 115-132.)

The production of antibody in infants with congenital toxoplasmosis varies considerably from one case to another and also is affected by treatment. Cases in which antibody production during fetal life can be demonstrated by antibody load are scarce. Early and delayed antibody production can, however, be demonstrated by the antibody load method. An example of early production is shown in Figure 31-29. During the first month of life, the titer in the infant decreases in proportion to the decrease in total IgG (curve 4). At 1 month of age, the situation is similar to that in an uninfected infant: The antibody titer and the total amount of IgG have diminished in the same proportions, and the antibody load is constant. During the second and third months, however, the antibody titer in the infected infant does not decrease at the rate expected, and the antibody load remains the same or may increase. This finding demonstrates that the IgG being synthesized by the infant contains at least as many specific antibodies to *T. gondii* as those in the maternal IgG, and this becomes obvious between the fourth and sixth months, when a definite increase in antibody titer and in antibody load occurs. In some cases, the rise in titer is not demonstrable until even later (Fig. 31-30).

The pattern observed in infants with a delayed onset of antibody response is shown in Figure 31-31. In this situation, the antibody titer remains parallel to the expected titer of passively transferred maternal antibodies. The antibody load decreases, proving that the infant has begun to synthesize IgG, which apparently does not contain significant

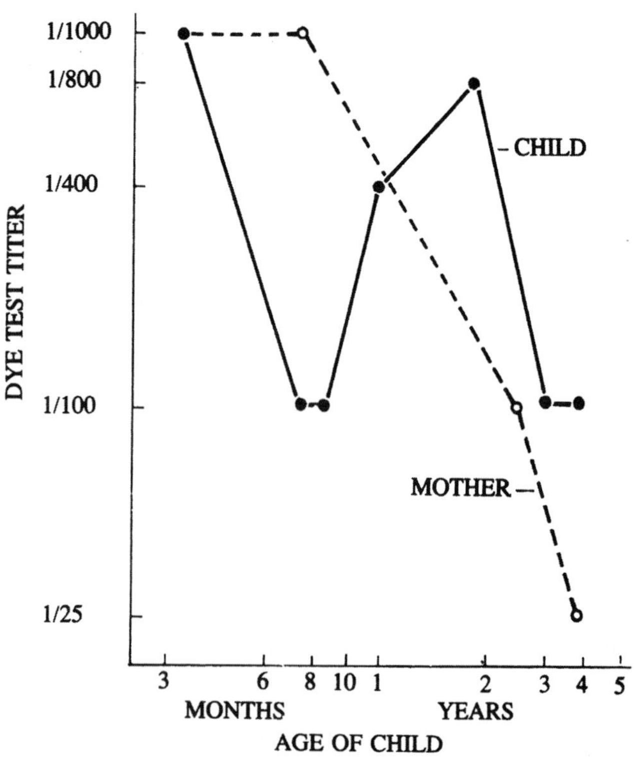

Figure 31–30 Example of antibody development (dye test) in a child with congenital toxoplasmosis in relation to time since birth. (Data from Couvreur J, Desmonts G. Congenital and maternal toxoplasmosis. A review of 300 congenital cases. Dev Med Child Neurol 4:519-530, 1962.)

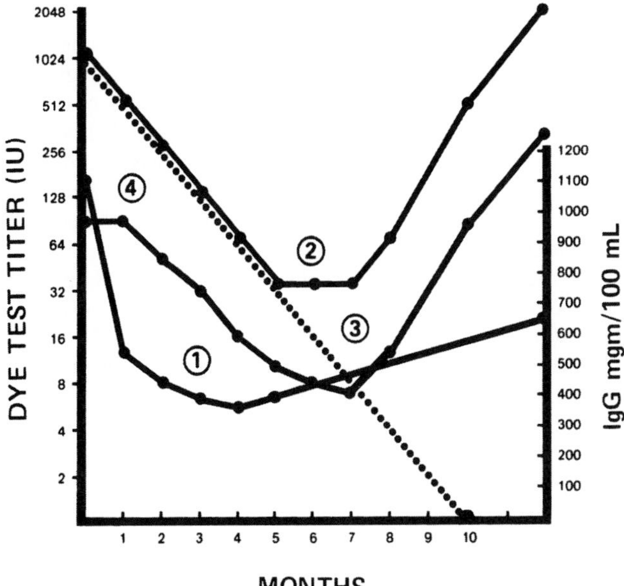

Figure 31–31 Antibodies in congenital toxoplasmosis (cases with delayed synthesis of antibodies). (Synthesis usually is not delayed more than 3 or 4 months if the child receives no treatment. It may be delayed up to the sixth or ninth month, if treatment is given.) *Curve 1*, mg of IgG per dL; *curve 2*, IU of *Toxoplasma* antibody per mL; *curve 3*, expected titer if antibodies were maternal in origin; *curve 4*, IU of *Toxoplasma* antibody per mg of IgG. (Data from Desmonts G, Couvreur J. Toxoplasmosis: epidemiologic and serologic aspects of perinatal infection. *In* Krugman S, Gershon AA [eds]. Infections of the Fetus and the Newborn Infant. Progress in Clinical and Biological Research, vol 3. New York, Alan R Liss, 1975, pp 115-132.)

amounts of antibodies to *T. gondii*. This situation may persist for several months before the onset of specific antibody production is demonstrable.

Another pattern of antibody development is that observed in infants born to mothers who acquire their infection very near the time of delivery. Such infants have been identified in prospective studies.[114,116] Serologic test titers may be negative in the cord blood or be very low, especially during the first weeks of life. In such cases, the diagnosis would usually be missed and, in fact, because of the low titer in the infant, probably never suspected.

Serologic Studies and Polymerase Chain Reaction Assay in Cerebrospinal Fluid; Polymerase Chain Reaction Assay in Urine

High titers of *T. gondii* antibodies often are observed in cerebrospinal fluid of newborns with congenital toxoplasmosis. This does not prove that antigenic stimulus or antibody formation has occurred within the CNS, because the antibody load in the cerebrospinal fluid of these neonates, as a rule, is equal to that in their serum. High titers of *T. gondii* antibodies can be observed in the cerebrospinal fluid of newborns with other CNS diseases (e.g., congenital diseases due to syphilis[1014] or cytomegalovirus), even when they are not infected with *T. gondii*. Because of passively transferred maternal *T. gondii* antibodies,[1009] and when the protein concentration is very high in the cerebrospinal fluid, the IgG concentration may reach the sensitivity level of the serologic test used. Thus, demonstration of high titers of IgG antibodies in the cerebrospinal fluid in newborns is not useful diagnostically. Demonstration of IgM antibodies in the cerebrospinal fluid, especially in the absence of IgM antibodies in the serum, supports the diagnosis of *T. gondii* infection in the CNS. In contrast with this situation in the newborn, serologic testing of cerebrospinal fluid and determination of antibody load sometimes are diagnostic during infancy or childhood in patients with CNS toxoplasmosis. The diagnosis also is established if *T. gondii* antigens are demonstrable in the cerebrospinal fluid.

The method of choice for detection of the parasite in cerebrospinal fluid is PCR assay. It is both highly sensitive and specific for this purpose.[686,1015,1016] Fuentes and colleagues[1015] detected the parasite by PCR assay in blood and cerebrospinal fluid from three of four newborns suspected of being congenitally infected with *T. gondii* and by PCR assay in urine from each of the four newborns. The investigators cautioned that because only urine from symptomatic newborns was examined, it will be necessary to assess the utility of PCR assay in urine from asymptomatic infants as well.

Effect of Treatment

T. gondii–specific IgM is rarely present in serum of an infant at birth who has received treatment with pyrimethamine and sulfadiazine in utero from week 17 of gestation until birth.[124] Data on the effects of treatment on production of IgM, IgA, and IgE antibodies are insufficient for comment.[556,805,914] Adequate data, however, are available on the effects of treatment on the dye test (IgG antibody) and antibody load method. These effects are described here. Alterations in antibody response vary among different cases and appear to depend in large part on the stage of synthesis of antibody in the child when treatment is begun.

If the infant does not begin producing antibody before treatment is started or if synthesis is at a low level, treatment apparently curbs the low-grade synthesis and prevents antibody formation. (This effect is not surprising, because treatment kills the tachyzoite form, thereby halting the production of antigen.)

Data on the IgM antibody response and on the development of IgG antibody by the fetus and infant presented in this section support the hypothesis discussed earlier (see "Transmission" section) that some infants are not infected during intrauterine life but are infected during labor, from the infected placenta. The immune system of some newborns and fetuses, can recognize *T. gondii* antigens, with active synthesis of IgM and IgG antibodies. Once established, this synthesis of IgG and IgM antibodies does not appear to be affected by treatment. In other infants, production of *T. gondii* antibodies is delayed until maternally transmitted antibody decreases to a low titer or until specific treatment is discontinued, thereby allowing renewed proliferation of the organism. Thus, in infants in whom a marked decrease in antibodies has occurred after birth, only to increase again at the age of 3 or 4 months, it seems plausible to suggest that the infection occurred not during fetal life but during labor.

The delay in antibody synthesis could be related solely to the late infection; this is substantiated by the fact that parasitemia frequently is demonstrable in cord blood or in the blood of the neonate during the first days of life

(Table 31-41). Even if infection occurred during parturition, however, this explanation alone is insufficient for certain other observations. Antibodies develop readily during the first weeks of life in infants infected shortly before delivery so long as they received little or no maternal IgG antibody, whereas synthesis of antibody often is poor or completely lacking in infants whose early lesions prove that they were definitely infected during fetal life. Inhibition of fetal recognition of *T. gondii* antigen appears to offer the most satisfactory explanation for the delay in antibody synthesis observed in most infected infants. Maternal IgG is the most likely effector of this inhibitory effect. This is not solely of academic interest, because such inhibition of antibody synthesis, whether by maternal IgG or by specific treatment, has important implications for the diagnosis of congenital toxoplasmosis. If treatment is begun early in these infants and is continued for some months, the diagnosis cannot be established serologically before 6 to 12 months of life.

Serologic Rebound after Treatment. Serologic rebound (Table 31-42) occurs commonly when pyrimethamine and sulfadiazine are discontinued.[534,1017,1018] In the study by Villena and associates, rebound occurred in 90% of the infants who received Fansidar, mainly 2 to 6 months after treatment was discontinued.[1019] This serologic rebound indicates that although these antimicrobial agents eliminate active infection, probably through their effect on tachyzoites, not all organisms are eliminated despite 1 year of therapy. A small number of infants with very mild disease or minimal manifestations of infection, or both, have not exhibited such serologic rebound. In almost all children, serologic rebound has been asymptomatic, without changes in ophthalmoscopic findings. In one infant, however, fever, failure to thrive, and new seizures were noted in association with this serologic rebound. His illness resolved with resumption of 2 weeks of pyrimethamine and sulfadiazine therapy and did not recur when these medications were discontinued. Thus, it appears to be uncommon for symptomatic disease to develop at the time serologic rebound occurs in an infant.

These observations concerning serologic rebound have been confirmed recently in other cohorts of children.[1013] Djurkovic-Djakovic and colleagues[1020] found that serologic rebound occurred in 82 of 84 children (98%) without illness when medicines to treat their congenital toxoplasmosis were withdrawn at 1 year of age. Serologic profile in this rebound was IgG with a chronic-disease pattern in AC/HS and avidity tests, despite a high rate of detection of specific IgM and IgA. Serologic rebound occurred in 70% to 90% of congenitally infected children who received Fansidar/folinic acid.[1021] Evidence of this phenomenon usually was noted 2 to 6 months after treatment was discontinued. Ophthalmologic surveillance during this time often did not identify recurrent chorioretinitis, although such identification has been reported.[1022] It seems prudent to observe infants closely (especially by ophthalmologic examination), particularly during the months after therapy is discontinued. At present, no serologic markers have reliably been associated with recurrences of chorioretinitis in congenitally infected children. It was reported that the IgM level often was elevated with recurrences,[640] but this association has not been found in the patients in the NCCTS (see Table 31-23).[472] More retinal lesions first identified after treatment was discontinued were noted by one group of investigators in the children infected earlier in gestation who had extraocular manifestations at birth.[1022]

Table 31–41 Correlation of Age of Infant and Presence of Demonstrable Parasitemia

Age	No. of Infants	No. with Parasitemia (%)
Cord–1st wk	28	20 (71)
2nd wk	15	5 (33)
3rd-4th wk	15	5 (33)
2nd mo	11	9 (0)

Adapted from Desmonts G, Couvreur J. Toxoplasmosis: epidemiologic and serologic aspects of perinatal infection. *In* Krugman S, Gershon AA (eds). Infections of the Fetus and the Newborn Infant. Progress in Clinical and Biological Research, vol. 3, New York, Alan R Liss, 1975, pp 115-132, with permission.

DIFFERENTIAL DIAGNOSIS

The diseases to be considered in the differential diagnosis of toxoplasmosis are essentially the same as those described in

Table 31–42 Examples of Serologic Rebound in a Child Who Developed Symptoms (Patient 2) and in One Who Did Not (Patient 1)[a]

Patient	Age Serum Obtained (mo)	Dye Test	IgM ISAGA	IgM ELISA	IgA ELISA	IgE ISAGA	IgE ELISA
1	1	1:4096	9	Negative	Negative	Negative	Positive
	5[b]	1:128	Negative	Negative	Negative	Negative	Negative
	12[c]	1:2048	12	7.8	Negative	Negative	Positive
2	1.5	1:8000	QNS	6.3	11.4	QNS	QNS
	15[b]	1:128	Negative	Negative	Negative	Negative	Negative
	17[c]	1:8000	12	Negative	3.5	12	Positive

[a]Serologic tests were performed in the laboratory of Dr. Jack S. Remington.
[b]Sample obtained while patient was still taking pyrimethamine and sulfadiazine.
[c]Sample obtained after pyrimethamine and sulfadiazine were stopped.
ELISA, enzyme-linked immunosorbent assay; IgA, IgE, IgG, IgM, Immunoglobulins A, E, G, M; ISAGA, immunosorbent agglutination assay; QNS, quantity not sufficient.

Chapter 23 and also should include congenital lymphocytic choriomeningitis virus syndrome.[1023]

THERAPY

General Comments

We recommend specific therapy in every case of congenital toxoplasmosis or congenital *T. gondii* infection in infants younger than 1 year of age. Insufficient data are available to allow proper evaluation of treatment in the asymptomatic infected infant. Nevertheless, most investigators, including ourselves, consider that treatment for such infants should be undertaken in the hope of preventing the remarkably high incidence of late untoward sequelae seen in children who receive inadequate or no treatment.[1]

Evaluation of the efficacy of treatment of congenital *T. gondii* infection is made difficult because of the high morbidity (both early and late) and mortality rates associated with this congenital infection; most workers are understandably reluctant to perform studies that would entail withholding specific therapy. Evaluation of treatment is difficult because of variations in severity and outcome of the infection and the disease. The parasite probably is never completely eliminated by specific therapy, and cure of disease (in contrast with infection) in humans apparently depends on the strain of parasite involved, the organs infected, and the time during the course of infection when treatment is initiated. The agents that can be recommended for specific therapy at present are beneficial against the tachyzoite form, but none has been shown to effectively eradicate the encysted form, especially from the CNS and eye.

Neuroradiologic Follow-up Evaluation after Shunt Placement

Because it has not been possible to determine with certainty at the time of presentation what the response to shunt placement and antimicrobial therapy will be, a therapeutic approach expectant for good outcome is recommended for most infants with congenital toxoplasmosis. It often is difficult to predict whether such therapy will result in brain cortical growth and expansion. A follow-up CT scan in the perioperative period after shunt placement to assess adequacy of drainage and whether subdural collections have occurred is advisable and may be useful prognostically.

Specific Therapy

Pyrimethamine plus Sulfonamides

Pyrimethamine, a substituted phenylpyrimidine antimalarial drug (Daraprim), brings about not only survival but also a radical cure of animals with experimental *T. gondii* infection. The persistence of this medicine in the blood was recognized many years ago in patients who received antimalarial prophylaxis with 25-mg weekly doses. The plasma half-life in adults is approximately 100 hours.[1024-1027] Pyrimethamine pharmacokinetics in newborns and those younger than 1.5 years of age have been reported (Fig. 31-32).[1028] Pyrimethamine serum half-life in infants is approximately 60 hours. Pyrimethamine dosages of 1 mg/kg per day yield serum drug levels of approximately 1000 to 2000 ng/mL 4 hours after a dose. Dosages of 1 mg/kg each Monday, Wednesday, and Friday yield serum levels of approximately 500 ng/mL 4 hours after a dose. Serum levels at intervals after these two dosages are shown in Figure 31-25. Cerebrospinal fluid levels are 10% to 20% of concomitant serum levels. Phenobarbital induces hepatic enzymes that degrade pyrimethamine, and phenobarbital therapy resulted in lower serum levels and shortened the half-life of pyrimethamine. Pyrimethamine plus sulfadiazine therapy has been associated with resolution of signs of active congenital toxoplasmosis, usually within the first weeks after initiation of therapy.[1028] Favorable outcomes for newborns with substantial disease (e.g., microcephaly, multiple cerebral calcifications, hydrocephalus, meningoencephalitis, thrombocytopenia, hepatosplenomegaly, active chorioretinitis) have been associated with therapy during the first year of life, which resulted in pyrimethamine levels that ranged from 300 to 2000 ng/mL 4 hours after a dose.[1028] Seizures have been reported in association with pyrimethamine serum levels of approximately 5000 ng/mL (R Hoff, personal communication to R McLeod, 1986). The inhibitory concentration (IC) and cidal concentration are dependent on the assay system used, the strain of parasite, and the time over which the assay is performed.[1028,1029] In a study by McLeod and her colleagues, levels of pyrimethamine and sulfadiazine alone and in combination that inhibited growth of the type I RH strain of *T. gondii* in vitro after 24 hours were pyrimethamine IC_{50}, 100 ng/mL; sulfadiazine IC_{90}, 6.25 μg/mL; and pyrimethamine plus sulfadiazine IC_{90}, 25 ng/mL and 6.25 μg/mL.[1028]

Pyrimethamine and sulfadiazine act synergistically against *T. gondii*, with a combined activity eightfold that expected for merely additive effects.[1030-1032] Consequently, the simultaneous use of both drugs is indicated in all cases. Comparative tests have shown that sulfapyrazine, sulfamethazine, and sulfamerazine are about as effective as sulfadiazine.[1033,1034] All of the other sulfonamides tested (sulfathiazole, sulfapyridine, sulfadimidine, sulfisoxazole) are much less effective and are not recommended. It would appear logical to use multiple sulfonamides for the treatment of toxoplasmosis to achieve an additive effect with less toxicity. For dosage recommendations, see Table 31-43. Sulfadiazine is used in addition to pyrimethamine. Appropriate dosing of pyrimethamine, sulfadiazine, and leucovorin in infants can be difficult because pediatric suspensions are not commercially available. The method shown in Figure 31-33[534] was developed to facilitate administration of these medications to infants in the NCCTS. It is suggested that treating congenital toxoplasmosis in infants in the United States be done in conjunction with the NCCTS, to facilitate obtaining knowledge concerning optimal medication dosages and outcome of treatment of the congenital infection and disease. The NCCTS treatment regimen is summarized in Tables 31-43 and 31-44, and in Figure 31-33. An alternative method, which incorporates pyrimethamine, sulfadiazine, and spiramycin, formerly was used extensively for treatment in infants in France. Treatment for the fetus in utero, by maternal therapy with pyrimethamine, sulfadiazine, and leucovorin (see "Outcome of Treatment of the Fetus in Utero," later on) (Fig. 31-34), has been followed by treatment during the first year of life.

Dorangeon and co-workers studied the transplacental passage of the combination pyrimethamine-sulfadoxine

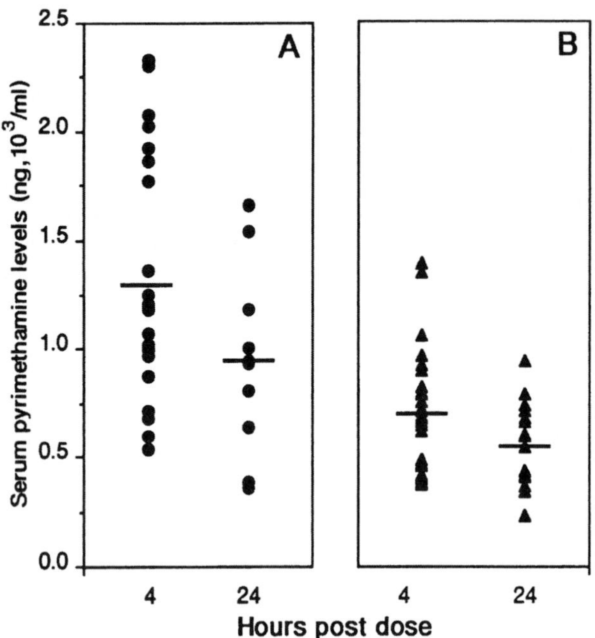

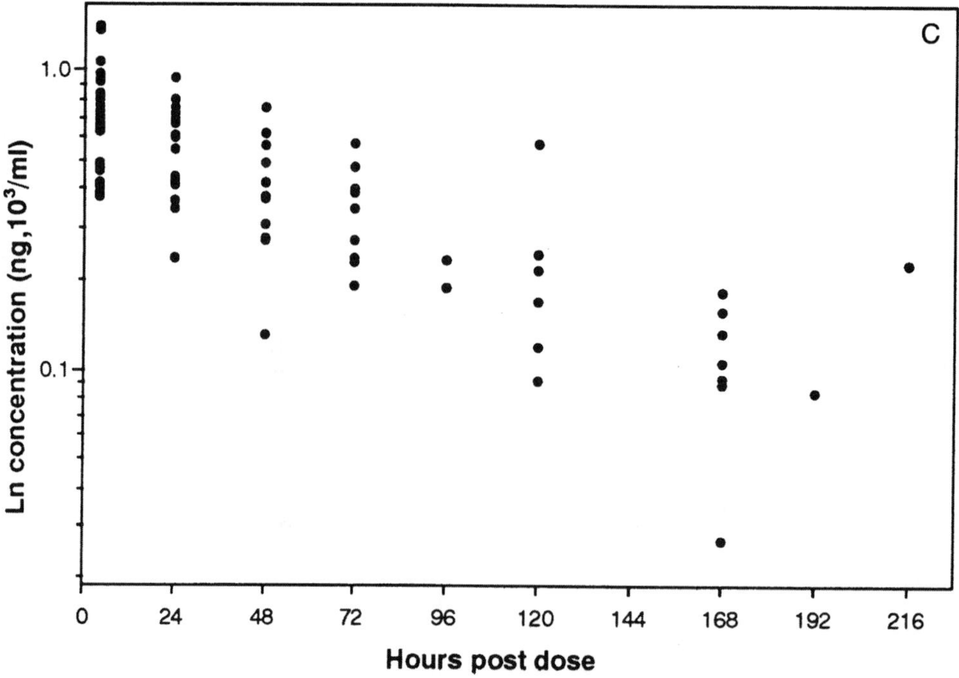

Figure 31–32 Serum pyrimethamine levels obtained in infants with congenital *Toxoplasma* infection. **A,** Pyrimethamine serum levels (4 and 24 hours after a dose) of children given 1 mg of pyrimethamine per kg daily. **B,** Pyrimethamine serum levels (4 and 24 hours after a dose) of children given 1 mg of pyrimethamine per kg on Monday, Wednesday, and Friday of each week. Values for children taking phenobarbital are not included. **C,** Pyrimethamine levels in sera of the entire population of infants taking 1 mg of pyrimethamine per kg on Monday, Wednesday, and Friday of each week. Values for children taking phenobarbital are not included. (Data from McLeod R, Mack D, Foss R, et al. Levels of pyrimethamine in sera and cerebrospinal and ventricular fluids from infants treated for congenital toxoplasmosis. Antimicrob Agents Chemother 36:1040-1048, 1992.)

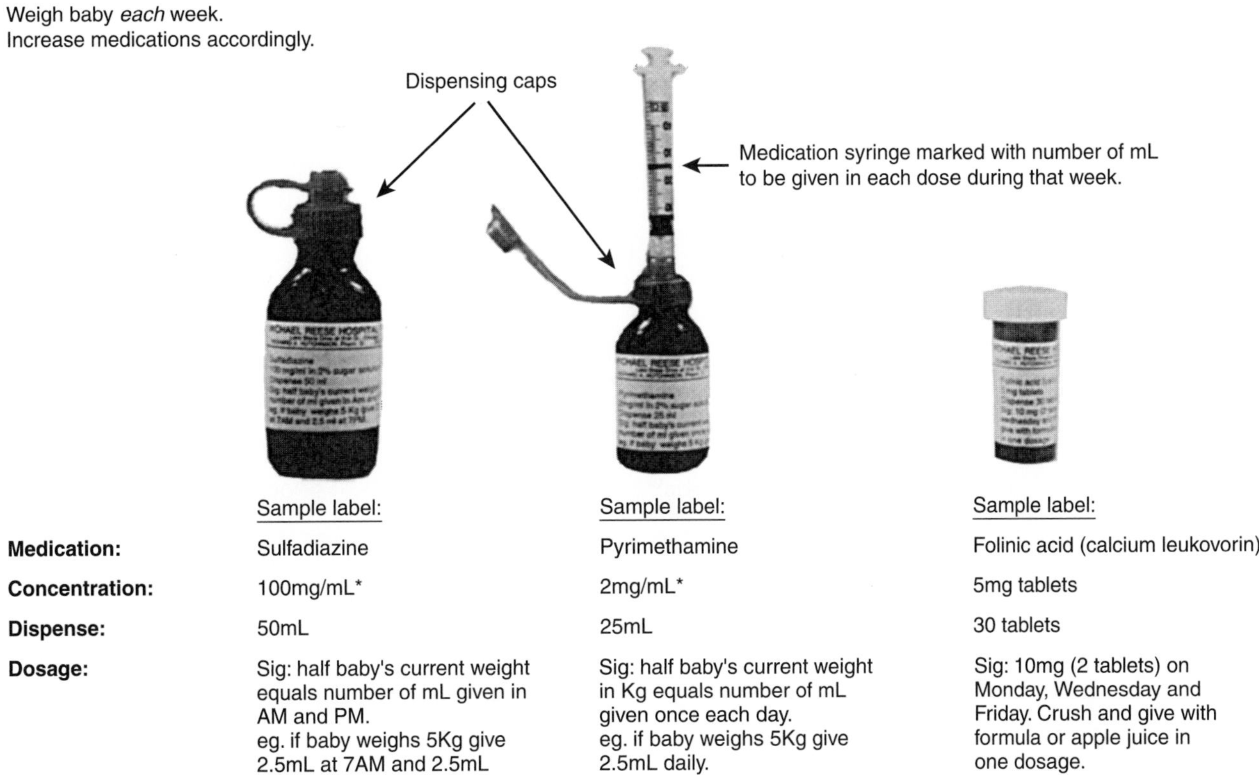

* Suspended in 2% sugar solution. Suspension at usual concentration must be made up each week. Store refrigerated.

Figure 31–33 Preparation of pyrimethamine, sulfadiazine, and leucovorin in treatment of congenital toxoplasmosis. (Adapted from McAuley J, Roizen N, Patel D, et al. Early and longitudinal evaluations of treated infants and children and untreated historical patients with congenital toxoplasmosis: the Chicago Collaborative Treatment Trial. Clin Infect Dis 18:38-72, 1994. University of Chicago, publisher.)

(Fansidar) by measuring drug levels in mother and neonate at time of delivery.[1035] They noted that the levels of pyrimethamine in the newborn were 50% to 100% and those of sulfadoxine essentially 100% of the maternal levels, depending on when the drug was last administered to the mother. The authors recognized the limitations of their study; they did not evaluate levels in the fetus at different times during gestation, when adequate drug levels are especially critical.

Villena and colleagues, in France, have reported an extensive experience with pyrimethamine-sulfadoxine treatment of congenital toxoplasmosis in the infant and in the mother when prenatal diagnosis was positive.[147,1019] Although in the United States pyrimethamine-sulfadoxine is at present not recommended for use in pregnant women, newborns, or children with *T. gondii* infection, this drug combination is increasingly being used in Europe. For this reason, the studies by Trenque and colleagues in Reims, France, are summarized here.[1036]

To evaluate the ratio of fetal to maternal concentrations of the drugs (F/M ratio), these investigators studied placental transfer of pyrimethamine and sulfadoxine at the end of gestation in 10 women who had seroconverted during pregnancy and had been taking the drug combination by mouth twice monthly along with folinic acid. Blood samples were collected at delivery from the mother and from the umbilical vein. The F/M ratios for pyrimethamine and sulfadoxine ranged from 0.43 to 1.03 (mean ± SD = 0.66 ± 0.22) and from 0.65 to 1.16 (mean ± SD = 0.97 ± 0.14), respectively. The patients had steady-state drug concentrations at the time of study. Concentrations of pyrimethamine in the fetus ranged from 50% to 100% (mean 66%) of simultaneous serum concentrations in the mothers. These results agree with those obtained in monkeys by Schoondermark-van de Ven and co-workers.[88] Trenque and colleagues concluded that the effective concentrations of both drugs at 14 days after the last dose justifies twice-monthly dosing of the drug combination in cases of documented fetal infection.[1036]

Preliminary follow-up studies[147,1019,1037] suggest that such treatment with Fansidar (1.25 mg/kg of pyrimethamine each 14 or each 10 days after treatment for the fetus in utero by treatment of the mother) may lead to a lower incidence of subsequent ocular disease with fewer sequelae than described for untreated children in the earlier literature.[596,1038] Randomization, statistical analysis, or long-term follow-up appears to be lacking in these studies, and whether there was consistency in the evaluations was not specified.

Issues of dosing, pharmacokinetics, serum and tissue levels, efficacy, toxicity, and safety are relevant to considerations concerning use of Fansidar to treat congenital toxoplasmosis.[1039] Sulfadoxine was found to be less active than sulfadiazine when sulfonamides were tested in vitro either alone or in conjunction with pyrimethamine against a standard laboratory strain, the type I RH strain of *T. gondii.*

Table 31–43 Guidelines for Treatment of *Toxoplasma gondii* Infection in the Pregnant Woman and Congenital *Toxoplasma* Infection in the Fetus, Infant, and Older Child

Infection	Medication	Dosage	Duration of Therapy
In pregnant women infected during gestation			
First 18 wk of gestation or until term if fetus found not to be infected by amniocentesis at 18 wk	Spiramycin[a]	1 g every 8 hr without food	Until fetal infection is documented or until it is excluded at 18 wk of gestation (see also text)
If fetal infection confirmed after wk 18 of gestation and in all women infected after wk 24 (see text)	Pyrimethamine[b]	Loading dose: 50 mg each 12 hours for 2 days; then beginning on day 3, 50 mg per day	Until term[c]
	plus Sulfadiazine	Loading dose: 75 mg/kg; then beginning 50 mg/kg each 12 h (maximum 4 g per day)	Until term[c]
	plus Leucovorin (folinic acid)[b]	10-20 mg daily[d]	During and for 1 wk after pyrimethamine therapy
Congenital *T. gondii* infection in the infant[d]	Pyrimethamine[b, d]	Loading dose: 1 mg/kg each 12 hours for 2 days; then beginning on day 3, 1 mg/kg per day for 2 or 6 mo[d]; then this dose every Monday, Wednesday, Friday[d]	1 yr[d]
	plus Sulfadiazine[e]	50 mg/kg each 12 hr	1 yr[d]
	plus Leucovorin[b]	10 mg three times weekly	During and for 1 wk after pyrimethamine therapy
	Corticosteroids[f] (prednisone) have been used when CSF protein is ≥1 g/dL and when active chorioretinitis threatens vision	0.5 mg/kg each 12 hr	Corticosteroids are continued until resolution of elevated (≥1 g/dL) CSF protein level or active chorioretinitis that threatens vision
Active chorioretinitis in older children	Pyrimethamine[b]	Loading dose: 1 mg/kg each 12 hr (maximum 50 mg) for 2 days; then beginning on day 3, maintenance, 1 mg/kg per day (maximum 25 mg)	Usually 1-2 wk beyond the time that signs and symptoms have resolved
	plus Sulfadiazine[e]	Loading dose: 75 mg/kg; then beginning 12 hr later, maintenance, 50 mg/kg every 12 hours	Usually 1-2 wk beyond the time that signs and symptoms have resolved
	plus Leucovorin[b]	10-20 mg three times weekly[b]	During and for 1 wk after pyrimethamine therapy
	Corticosteroids[f] (prednisone)	1 mg/kg/day, divided bid; maximum 40 mg per day followed by rapid taper	Steroids are continued until inflammation subsides (usually 1-2 wk) and then tapered rapidly

[a]Available only on request from the U.S. Food and Drug Administration (telephone number 301-443-5680), and then with this approval by physician's request to Aventis (908-231-3365).

[b]Adjusted for megaloblastic anemia, granulocytopenia, or thrombocytopenia; blood cell counts, including platelets, should be monitored as described in text.

[c]Subsequent treatment of the infant is the same as that described under treatment of congenital infection. When the diagnosis of infection in the fetus is established earlier, we suggest that sulfadiazine be used alone until after the first trimester, at which time pyrimethamine should be added to the regimen. The decision about when to begin pyrimethamine/sulfadiazine/leucovorin for the pregnant woman is based on an assessment of the risk of fetal infection, incidence of false-positive and false-negative results of amniocentesis with PCR assay, and risks associated with medicines. Although reliability of PCR assay results is laboratory dependent, results from the best reference laboratories, between 17 and 21 weeks of gestation, have a sensitivity for detection of the *T. gondii* B1 gene with amniotic fluid PCR assay of 92.9 (CI 67.9 to 98.8). Thus, PCR assay results reasonably determine therapeutic approach. When infection of the mother is acquired between 22 and 29 weeks of gestation, the incidence of transmission exceeds 50%, manifestations of infection in the fetus are substantial, and sensitivity of PCR assay (*T. gondii* B1 gene) in amniotic fluid is <62.5% (CI 38.8 to 86.2) for 22 to 26 weeks and <68.4% (CI 47.5 to 89.3) for 27 to 31 weeks. (Data from reference 838). With maternal acquisition of infection after 31 weeks of gestation, incidence of transmission exceeds 60%, manifestations of infection are in general less severe, and sensitivity of PCR assay by amniotic fluid is <50% (CI 21.7 to 78.3). When infection is acquired between 21 and 29 weeks of gestation, management varies. After 24 weeks of gestation, we recommend that amniocentesis be performed and that pyrimethamine/leucovorin/sulfadiazine be used instead of spiramycin. On the basis of available data (see Fig. 31-18) on reliability of PCR results, making a definitive recommendation concerning manifestations of women whose infections were acquired between 21 and 24 weeks of gestation with negative amniotic fluid PCR results is difficult (see text). Consultation with the reference laboratory is advised.

Continuation of footnote for Table 31-43

In France, standard of care (until late in gestation) is to wait 4 weeks from the estimated time maternal infection is acquired until amniocentesis, to allow sufficient time for transmission to occur. Amniocentesis is not performed before 17 to 18 weeks of gestation. In some instances, when maternal infection is acquired between 12 and 16 weeks of gestation or after the 21st week of gestation pyrimethamine and sulfadiazine treatment is initiated regardless of the amniotic fluid PCR result (see text for discussion). This is because of concerns about the confidence intervals and reliabillity of negative results on amniotic fluid PCR assay. When this approach is used, a delay in amniocentesis when maternal infection is acquired between 12 and 16 weeks and after 21 weeks of gestation would not be logical.

[d]Optimal dosage, feasibility, and toxicity currently are being evaluated in the ongoing Chicago-based National Collaborative Treatment Trial (NCTT) (telephone number 773-834-4152).

These two regimens are currently being compared in a randomized manner in the NCTT. Data are not yet available to determine which, if either, is superior. Both regimens appear to be feasible and relatively safe.

The duration of therapy is unknown for infants and children, especially those with AIDS. See section on congenital *Toxoplasma* infection and AIDS.

[e]Alternative medicines for patients with atopy or severe intolerance of sulfonamides have included pyrimethamine and leucovorin with clindamycin, or azithromycin, or atovaquone, with standard dosages as recommended according to weight.

[f]Corticosteroids should be used only in conjunction with pyrimethamine, sulfadiazine, and leucovorin treatment and should be continued until signs of inflammation (high CSF protein, ≥1 g/dL) or active chorioretinitis that threatens vision have subsided; dosage can then be tapered and the steroids discontinued.

AIDS, acquired immunodeficiency syndrome; CI, confidence interval; CSF, cerebrospinal fluid.

Table 31–44 Oral Suspension Formulations for Pyrimethamine and Sulfadiazine in the United States

Pyrimethamine, 2-mg/mL suspension[a]

1. Crush four 25-mg pyrimethamine tablets in a mortar to a fine powder.
2. Add 10 mL of syrup vehicle.[b]
3. Transfer mixture to an amber bottle.
4. Rinse mortar with 10 mL of sterile water and transfer.
5. Add enough of the serum vehicle to make a final volume of 50 mL.
6. Shake very well until this is a fine suspension.
7. Label and give a 7-day expiration.
8. Store refrigerated.

Sulfadiazine, 100-mg/mL suspension[c]

1. Crush ten 500-mg sulfadiazine tablets in a mortar to a fine powder.
2. Add enough sterile water to make a smooth paste.
3. Slowly titrate the syrup vehicle[b] close to the final volume of 50 mL.
4. Transfer the suspension to a larger amber bottle.
5. Add sufficient syrup vehicle to make a final volume of 50 mL.
6. Shake well.
7. Label and give a 7-day expiration.
8. Store refrigerated.

[a]Pyrimethamine: 25-mg tablets (Daraprim, Glove Wellcome Inc.) NDC #0173-0201-55.

[b]Syrup vehicle: suggest 2% sugar suspension for pyrimethamine. If the infant is not lactose intolerant, 2% sugar suspension can be 2 g lactose per 100 mL distilled water. Suggest simple syrup or, alternatively, cherry syrup for sulfadiazine suspension.

[c]Sulfadiazine: 500-mg tablets (Eon Labs Manufacturing, Inc.) NDC #00185-0757-01.

Concentrations of pyrimethamine alone or in conjunction with sulfadiazine that were needed to inhibit *T. gondii* were greater than 25 ng/mL.[1028,1040] Although the clinical relevance of these in vitro tests is not known, it seems that brain and retinal tissue trough levels (i.e., minimum levels) should exceed this minimum amount, unless both other data correlating outcomes with lower tissue levels using a variety of strains of *T. gondii* and clinical trials were to demonstrate that lower levels are beneficial. The observation that cerebrospinal fluid levels of pyrimethamine were 10% to 25% of serum pyrimethamine levels in infants with congenital toxoplasmosis therefore is relevant.[1028] The serum levels of pyrimethamine following 1.25 mg of Fansidar administered every 14 days to infants were approximately 350 ng/mL peak and 25 ng/mL trough.[1035] Thus, cerebrospinal fluid, brain, and retinal levels may not exceed 25 ng/mL for much of the time during which this dosage regimen is administered. Consequently, potential therapeutic brain and retinal levels may not be achieved for substantial periods with twice-monthly dosing, and thus this regimen may not be effective for treatment.

Administration of Fansidar every 2 weeks is a more convenient regimen than daily administration of pyrimethamine and sulfadiazine and is routinely used in many areas of France.[1039] No hematologic toxicity was reported when this regimen was administered,[1019] in contrast with relatively frequent but easily reversible neutropenia (requiring frequent hematologic monitoring) in children given 1 mg/kg of pyrimethamine daily or three times each week.[534,1028] Serious and life-threatening toxicity has been reported with use of Fansidar in other clinical settings, and this finding has led to reluctance on the part of some investigators and physicians to recommend its use when other medicines, especially sulfonamides with shorter half-lives, are equally or potentially more effective.[1040] No such serious side effects have been reported in the studies of congenital toxoplasmosis treated with Fansidar, but although the incidence of lethal hepatotoxicity[1041] is estimated to be quite low, the numbers of women and children who have received treatment with this drug to date are not sufficient to exclude the possibility that it may occur.[1042-1044]

Trenque and co-workers in Reims and Marseilles, France,[1045] studied population pharmacokinetics of pyimethamine and sulfadoxine in 89 children between 1 week and 13.9 years of age (weighing 3 to 59 kg) with congenital toxoplasmosis treated with Fansidar two or three times a month. The authors report that influence of weight, but not age, on pyrimethamine pharmacokinetics was significant in young children.

Diagnosis of mother:	Systematic serologic screening, before conception and intrapartum
Treatment of mother:	If acute serology, spiramycin reduces transmission Untreated 94 (60%) of 154 vs. treated 91 (23%) of 388*
Treatment of fetus:	Pyrimethamine, sulfadiazine, or termination N=54 livebirths; 34 terminations†
Diagnosis of fetus:	Ultrasounds; amniocentesis, PCR at ≥18 weeks' gestation Sensitivity 37 (97%) of 38: specificity 301 of 301‡
Outcome	All 54 normal development; initial report was 19% subtle findings: 7 (13%) intracranial calcifications, 3 (6%) chorioretinal scars§; follow up of 18 chilldren (median age 4.5 yr; range, 1-11 yr): 39% retinal scars, most scars were peripheral‖

*From Desmonts and Couvreur.[116]
†From Daffos, et al.[130]
‡From Hohlfeld, et al.; sensitivity is less before 17 and after 21 weeks' gestation.[125]
§From Hohlfeld, et al.[124]
‖From Brezin, et al.[1154]

Figure 31–34 Paris approach to prenatal prevention, diagnosis, and treatment. (Adapted from Roberts F, McLeod R, Boyer K. Toxoplasmosis. *In* Katz S, Gershon A, Hotez P [eds]. Krugman's Infectious Diseases of Children, 10th ed. St. Louis, CV Mosby, pp 538-570, with minor modifications and permission.)

Both pyrimethamine and the sulfonamides are potentially toxic. Because most physicians are familiar with untoward reactions to sulfonamides (e.g., crystalluria, hematuria and hypersensitivity, marrow suppression), only the toxic effects of pyrimethamine are considered here. Serum levels of sulfadiazine were similar when the drug was administered in two or four divided doses daily to eight patients infected with HIV (mean age, 43 years; range, 38 to 56 years).[1046]

TOXIC EFFECTS OF PYRIMETHAMINE

Pyrimethamine inhibits dihydrofolate reductase, which is important in the synthesis of folic acid, thus producing reversible and usually gradual depression of the bone marrow.[1047,1048] Reversible neutropenia is the most frequent toxic effect, although platelet depression and anemia may occur as well. Other, less serious side effects are gastrointestinal distress, headaches, and a bad taste in the mouth. Accidental overdosing in infants has resulted in vomiting, tremors, convulsions, and bone marrow depression.[1049] All patients who receive pyrimethamine should have a peripheral blood cell and platelet count twice each week. Folinic acid (in the form of leucovorin calcium) has been used to protect the bone marrow from toxic effects of pyrimethamine.[203,1050] We usually administer 5 to 20 mg of leucovorin calcium each Monday, Wednesday, and Friday or even daily in infants or young children. The usual dosage in older children and adults is 10 to 20 mg per day orally.

Data suggesting that oral leucovorin calcium can be used to reverse the toxic effects of pyrimethamine have been presented. Nixon and Bertino clearly demonstrated that leucovorin calcium in tablet form was well absorbed (in adult subjects), thereby expanding the serum pool of reduced folates.[1051] Under fasting conditions, the quantitative absorption of the orally administered preparation was close to 90%. The parenteral form (Calcium Leucovorin used for injection) may be ingested with equal effectiveness (CJ Masur, Lederle Laboratories, written communication to JS Remington, 1975). These substances, in contrast with folic acid, do not appear to inhibit the action of pyrimethamine on the proliferative form of *T. gondii*, because of an active transport mechanism for folinic acid,[1052] and thus may be used in conjunction with the latter drug to allay toxicity.

Garin and colleagues used Fansidar in a small number of infants and consider this agent to be well tolerated, with a much simpler treatment regimen.[1053-1055] This antimicrobial combination is now widely used in Europe. The potential for serious toxicity of medication with a half-life as long as that of sulfadoxine has led others to avoid this regimen. Whether its potential for toxicity is as great in infants as in adults is not known.

TERATOGENIC EFFECTS OF PYRIMETHAMINE

In experiments with pyrimethamine, Thiersch reported an effect on rat fetuses ranging from stunting to death, depending on the amount of pyrimethamine administered to the mothers during pregnancy.[1056] The effect on the fetuses could be moderated, with a higher yield of live litters but also of stunted and malformed animals, when the mother was given leucovorin calcium at the time of drug administration. The malformations resulted from enormous doses (e.g., 12 mg/kg, compared with the usual dose in humans of 0.5 to 1 mg/kg) and were similar to those obtained with closely related folic acid analogues: general stunting of growth, general hydrops, cranial bone defects, incomplete cranial and brain development, rachischisis, internal hydrocephalus, ventral hernias, situs inversus, and combinations of all of these. An even more severe teratogenic effect was reported in the studies of Anderson and Morse, who similarly employed doses far higher than could ever be employed in humans.[1057] Similar studies in rats are those of Dyban and associates.[1058,1059] In another study in rats, Krahe used doses more comparable to those employed in humans and noted fetal resorption but no teratogenic effects after large doses of pyrimethamine.[1060] In 1971, Sullivan and Takacs pointed out the lack of comparative data on the teratogenic effects of pyrimethamine in different mammalian species[1061]—a lack that adds to the difficulty in estimating the extent of teratogenic risk in humans. Their results in rats and hamsters emphasize the shortcomings of attempts to determine a safe clinical dose on the basis of tests limited to a single species of test animal. The drug was less teratogenic in golden hamsters than in Wistar rats. About 70% of rat fetuses were dead or malformed (the malformations included brachygnathia, cleft palate, oligodactyly, and phocomelia) as a result of administration of single oral doses of 5 mg (approximately 20 mg/kg) to pregnant females. Less than 10% of hamster fetuses died or were malformed after similar doses that on a milligram-per-kilogram basis were eight to nine times greater than those given to rats. Repeated doses nearer to those used in humans also were teratogenic in rats but not in hamsters. These investigators also demonstrated that folinic acid can significantly reduce the incidence of dead and malformed fetuses when administered during pyrimethamine treatment.

Puchta and Simandlova, using doses of 2, 5, and 10 mg/kg in rats, could demonstrate no malformations in rat fetuses.[1062] Their results are in marked contrast with those of most other workers, and the differences remain to be explained.

In all of these studies, pyrimethamine was administered during the period of early organogenesis, which is the period of maximum susceptibility to damage by teratogenic agents.

Spiramycin

Spiramycin, a macrolide antibiotic that is available to physicians in the United States only by request to the FDA, has an antibacterial spectrum comparable to that of erythromycin and is active against *T. gondii*, as demonstrated in animal experiments[1063,1064] In vitro studies also have been reported.[1065] The actual concentration necessary to inhibit growth of or kill the organism is unknown. It has been described as having exceptional persistence in the tissues[1066,1067] in comparison with erythromycin, oleandomycin, or carbomycin. Such high tissue levels may account for the observations that spiramycin is much more active in vivo against susceptible bacteria than is erythromycin, despite higher serum levels attained with comparable doses of erythromycin and greater sensitivity of the bacteria to erythromycin in vitro.[1068] A review of this antimicrobial agent has been published.[1069]

Spiramycin is supplied as a syrup and in capsules. The usual daily dose in adults is 1 g three times a day. Garin and co-workers studied drug concentrations in serum, cord serum, and placenta in pregnant women.[1070] On a daily regimen of 2 g by mouth, the average levels were 1.19 μg/mL (range, 0.50 to 2.0 μg/mL), 0.63 μg/mL (range, 0.20 to 1.8 μg/mL), and 2.75 μg/mL (range, 0.70 to 5.0 μg/mL), respectively. On a dosage schedule of 3 g daily, the results were 1.69 μg/mL (range, 1 to 4 μg/mL), 0.78 μg/mL (range, 0.75 to 2.0 μg/mL), and 6.2 μg/mL (range, 3.25 to 10 μg/mL), respectively. (These serum levels in the mother are similar to those obtained by Hudson and colleagues at 2 and 4 hours after a given dose in persons receiving 1 g every 6 hours.[1071]) Thus, a total dose of 3 g daily resulted in levels in the placenta that were twice as high as those attained with a total dose of 2 g daily. (This is one reason for the recommendation of 3 g administered as a 1-g thrice-daily dose during gestation.) In both regimens, the concentration in cord serum was approximately one-half and the placental levels approximately three to five times greater than the level in the corresponding maternal serum. The investigators stated that the levels achieved in the placenta are ample for treatment of *T. gondii* in that organ, but whether the levels in cord serum are sufficient for treatment of the fetus in utero remains to be verified. Forestier and associates published another study of spiramycin concentrations in the mother and the fetus (fetal blood sampling).[1072]

Spiramycin pharmacokinetics exhibits individual variation. Fetomaternal concentrations were studied in 20 cases of maternal infection acquired between weeks 3 and 10 of pregnancy and treated with a daily dose of 3 g. The maternal plasma concentrations of spiramycin were 0.682 ± 0.132 mg/L in the first month of treatment; 0.618 ± 0.102 mg/L during weeks 20 to 24 of pregnancy; and 1.015 ± 0.22 mg/L in the sixth month. The mean fetal concentration was 0.290 mg/L during weeks 20 to 24 of pregnancy (i.e., 47% of maternal values), with a lack of correlation between mothers and fetuses. At birth, the placental concentration (2.3 μg/mL) was four times the average blood concentration in mothers (0.47 mg/L) and six and one-half times the cord blood values (0.34 mg/L). A good correlation was found between maternal blood and placental values, and a fair correlation between cord blood and placental values. These facts suggest that monitoring of spiramycin treatment by measuring maternal spiramycin blood concentrations might be useful in determining effective individual dosage.[117]

Very little definitive information is available on the efficacy of spiramycin in congenital toxoplasmosis in the newborn. In a study of 12 cases (mainly of severe clinical disease) by Martin and co-workers in which spiramycin was employed, the data are impossible to interpret, because tetracyclines, pyrimethamine, sulfonamides, and corticosteroids frequently were also used in the same infants.[1073]

In a carefully designed study by Beverley and colleagues, congenitally infected mice were given spiramycin or a combination of sulfadimidine and pyrimethamine from the age of 4 to 8 weeks.[1074] The levels of spiramycin in the heart, liver, kidney, and spleen were approximately 50 to 140 times greater than the serum levels after 4 weeks of treatment. Both treatment regimens were effective in preventing the histopathologic changes noted in congenitally infected mice not given treatment. Regardless of the form of treatment, a smaller number of cysts were found in the brains of mice that received treatment than in those of mice receiving no treatment (probably because treatment prevented the development of new cysts, rather than destroying cysts formed before instigation of therapy). The authors suggested that because spiramycin was as effective as the potentially toxic combination of pyrimethamine and sulfadimidine, it will be found to be preferable to the combination agent in treatment of congenital toxoplasmosis.

Because the optimal dose and route of administration of spiramycin in infants and adults have never been established for toxoplasmosis, the study by Back and co-workers on the pharmacology of parenteral spiramycin as an antineoplastic agent is pertinent.[1075] Twelve patients with various types of far-advanced neoplastic diseases were given daily intravenous doses ranging from 5 to 160 mg/kg. Doses greater than 35 mg/kg produced local vasospasm, a feeling of coolness, strange taste, vertigo, dizziness, flushing of the face, tearing of the eyes, nausea, vomiting, diarrhea, and anorexia. No hematologic toxicity, electrocardiographic changes, or impairment of liver or kidney function were noticed. Of note, Q-T interval prolongation and life-threatening arrhythmias (cardiac arrest) were reported in two neonates receiving spiramycin (300,000 IU/kg per day by mouth).[1076] The infants recovered completely after immediate cardiopulmonary resuscitation maneuvers.

At present, the only indication for which we use spiramycin is in the actively infected mother to attempt to reduce transmission to her fetus.[1077] It should be noted that spiramycin failed to prevent neurotoxoplasmosis in immunosuppressed patients.[1078] Spiramycin may reduce the severity of infection in a fetus because it delays transmission to a later time in gestation when transmission is associated with less severe manifestations of infection. Lacking are data that conclusively demonstrate efficacy of spiramycin in treatment of the infected fetus. The controversy of whether spiramycin prevents transmission of *T. gondii* to the fetus is discussed later under "Serologic Screening" in the "Prevention" section. The subject has more recently been commented on by Montoya and Liesenfeld.[1079]

Other Drugs

At present, no clinical data are available to allow for recommendation of any of the drugs described next for treatment of the immunocompetent pregnant patient, fetus, or newborn.

Trimethoprim plus Sulfamethoxazole. Despite reports of successful treatment of murine toxoplasmosis with a combination of trimethoprim and sulfamethoxazole (TMP-SMX),[1080,1081] trimethoprim alone has been found to have less effect against *T. gondii* both in vitro and in vivo.[1082,1083-1085] The combination of this drug with sulfamethoxazole is synergistic in vitro[1081] but is significantly less active in vitro and in vivo than the combination of pyrimethamine and sulfonamide. Previously, a number of reports have described use of the combination in human toxoplasmosis, but whether the effect of the combination was due solely to the sulfonamide component was unclear.[1086-1088] A recent, randomized trial of TMP-SMX versus pyrimethamine-sulfadiazine in toxoplasmic encephalitis in patients with AIDS by Torre and colleagues[1089] revealed that TMP-SMX was a valuable alternative to pyrimethamine-sulfadiazine for that purpose. In Brazil, TMP-SMX was reported to reduce the incidence of recurrent toxoplasmic chorioretinitis in 61 patients, compared with that in 63 control patients (mean ages 26 ± 10 versus 27 ± 11 years [range, 7 to 53 years]).[411,1090] Nevertheless, we do not recommend its use in the infected fetus or newborn in the absence of carefully designed trials that reveal efficacy of TMP-SMX in congenital toxoplasmosis.

Clindamycin. Clindamycin has been shown to be effective in treatment of murine toxoplasmosis[1091,1092] and ocular infection in rabbits.[1093] Studies are needed, however, before it can be recommended for routine treatment of congenital infection in infants or pregnant women. When this antibiotic has been used in combination with pyrimethamine in patients with AIDS who have toxoplasmic encephalitis, results have been comparable to those with pyrimethamine-sulfadiazine treatment.[1094,1095]

Tetracyclines. Both doxycycline[1096] and minocycline[1097,1098] have efficacy in the treatment of murine toxoplasmosis. Doxycycline was used successfully in two patients with AIDS who had toxoplasmic encephalitis when it was administered at 300 mg per day intravenously in three divided doses.[1099] When doxycycline was given orally at doses of 100 mg twice a day in six of the patients who were intolerant to pyrimethamine-sulfadiazine, five patients had associated neurologic and radiologic recurrences while receiving the drug.[1100] Further study of the tetracyclines in the treatment of toxoplasmosis in adults is likely to involve their use in combination with other antimicrobial agents. No data are available on their use in the newborn or young children with toxoplasmosis, nor are they recommended for this purpose.

Rifampin. Rifampin in high doses was not effective against *T. gondii* in a murine model.[1101]

Macrolides. The macrolides—roxithromycin,[1102,1103] clarithromycin,[1104] and the azalide azithromycin[1105]—have been shown to have activity against *T. gondii* in vivo in a mouse model. Stray-Pederson studied levels of azithromycin in placental tissue, amniotic fluid, and maternal and cord blood.[1106] Levels in maternal serum ranged from 0.017 to 0.073 mg/mL (mean, 0.028 mg/mL). Whole blood levels were higher (mean, 0.313 mg/mL). Mean levels in amniotic fluid and cord blood were 0.040 and 0.027 mg/mL, respectively. Placental levels were higher (mean, 2.067 mg/mL). It should be understood, however, that azithromycin is concentrated in tissues and intracellularly; thus, levels at these sites probably are of greater clinical importance than serum or blood levels.

When used in combination with pyrimethamine, both clarithromycin and azithromycin have been successful in treating toxoplasmic encephalitis in adult patients with AIDS.[766] In non-AIDS patients, the combination of pyrimethamine plus azithromycin has been reported by Rothova and colleagues to be equal in efficacy to pyrimethamine plus sulfadiazine measured as time to resolution of active eye disease in patients with recurrent chorioretinitis.[1107,1108] Ketolides also are active both in vitro and in vivo in the mouse model of toxoplasmosis.[1109,1110,1111]

Atovaquone. Atovaquone has been reported to have potent in vitro activity against both tachyzoite and cyst forms.[1112,1113] It significantly reduced the mortality rate in murine toxoplasmosis and had remarkable, although differing, activity against different strains of *T. gondii*.[1113] Atovaquone has been used in AIDS patients with toxoplasmic encephalitis with encouraging results.[1114-1116] Unfortunately, relapse occurred in approximately 50% of patients in whom atovaquone was used for acute therapy and continued alone as maintenance therapy.[1114,1116] Seventeen of 65 patients (26%) who received atovaquone as a single agent for maintenance therapy of toxoplasmic encephalitis experienced a relapse.[1117] The combination of pyrimethamine and atovaquone may prove more useful.[1118] Serum levels of atovaquone in patients with toxoplasmic encephalitis were not predictive of clinical response or failure.[1115]

Bioavailability of the drug is improved when medication is ingested with food. The reliability of absorption of this drug continues to be a problem. Survival time was significantly better among those patients with higher steady-state plasma concentrations of the drug.[1116] Although a new formulation of atovaquone is reported to achieve higher plasma concentrations, prospective trials are needed to compare the efficacy of this drug with that obtained in standard drug regimens. This drug should never be used alone for the treatment of the acute infection, but rather it should be given in combination with drugs such as pyrimethamine. The adverse effects observed in these studies included hepatic enzyme abnormalities (50%), rash (25%), nausea (21%), and diarrhea (19%).[1115] Between 3% and 10% of patients receiving atovaquone were reported to discontinue the drug because of rash, hepatic enzyme abnormalities, nausea, or vomiting.[1115,1117,1118] Leukopenia associated with the combination of pyrimethamine and atovaquone has responded to folinic acid (leucovorin) and granulocyte colony-stimulating factor therapy.[1118]

Fluoroquinolones. A number of fluoroquinolones have been found to be active against *T. gondii* in vitro and in vivo in a mouse model of the acute infection. Their activity may be enhanced when used in combination with pyrimethamine, sulfadiazine, clarithromycin, or atovaquone.[1110,1119,1120]

Duration of Therapy

The optimal duration of therapy in congenitally infected infants is not known. Among infants who were given the combination of pyrimethamine and sulfadiazine for relatively brief periods, untoward sequelae of the disease subsequently developed.[599,1121] We, as well as other investigators (including our colleague J. Couvreur in Paris), recommend that therapy be continued for 1 year, as outlined in Tables 31-43 and 31-44. We recommend using the combination of pyrimethamine and sulfonamide for the entire 1-year period.

In some areas of Europe, treatment is continued for the first 2 years of life. We have not noted active disease or progression of signs or symptoms when treatment is discontinued when children are 1 year of age. For the special issue of treatment of the HIV- and *T. gondii*–infected newborn of an HIV-infected mother, see "Congenital *Toxoplasma gondii* Infection and Acquired Immunodeficiency Syndrome" earlier under "Clinical Manifestations."

Treatment of the Fetus through Treatment of the Pregnant Woman

For additional pertinent information, see "Prevention of Congenital Toxoplasmosis through Treatment of the Pregnant Woman" and Table 31-43. When the diagnosis of infection in the fetus is established earlier than 17 weeks, we suggest that sulfadiazine be used alone until after the first trimester, at which time pyrimethamine should be added to the regimen. The decision about when to begin pyrimethamine/sulfadiazine/leucovorin for the pregnant woman is based on an assessment of the risk of fetal infection, incidence of false-positive and false-negative results of amniocentesis with PCR, and risks of medicines. Although reliability of PCR results are laboratory dependent, results from the best reference laboratories, between 17 and 21 weeks' gestation, have a sensitivity for PCR of the *T. gondii* B1 gene with amniotic fluid of 92.9 (CI 87.9-96.8). Thus, PCR results reasonably determine the therapeutic approach.

When the mother becomes infected between 22 and 29 weeks of gestation, the incidence of transmission exceeds 50%, manifestations of infection in the fetus are substantial, and sensitivity of PCR (*T. gondii* B1 gene) in amniotic fluid is less than 62.5% (CI 38.8-86.2) for 22 to 26 weeks and less than 68.4% (CI 47.5-89.3) for 27 to 31 weeks.[838] With maternal acquisition of infection after 31 weeks of gestation, incidence of transmission exceeds 60%, manifestations of infection are in general less severe, and sensitivity of PCR in amniotic fluid is less than 50% (CI 21.7-78.3).

When infection is acquired between 21 and 29 weeks of gestation, management varies. After 24 weeks of gestation, we recommend that amniocentesis be performed and that pyrimethamine/leucovorin/sulfadiazine be used instead of spiramycin. At the time of this writing, available data (see Fig. 31-18) in regard to the reliability of PCR results make a definitive recommendation concerning manifestations of women whose infections were acquired between 21 and 24 weeks of gestation with negative amniotic fluid PCR results difficult (see text). Consultation with the reference laboratory is advised.

In France, standard of care (until late in gestation) is to wait 4 weeks from the estimated time that maternal infection is acquired until amniocentesis to allow sufficient time for transmission to occur. Amniocentesis is not performed before 17 to 18 weeks of gestation. In some instances, when maternal infection is acquired between 12 and 16 weeks of gestation or after the 21st week of gestation, pyrimethamine and sulfadiazine treatment is initiated regardless of the amniotic fluid PCR result (see text for discussion). This is because of concerns about the confidence intervals and reliability of negative amniotic fluid PCR results. When this approach is used, a delay in amniocentesis when maternal infection is acquired between 12 and 16 weeks and after 21 weeks of gestation would not be logical.

With the advent of prenatal diagnosis (see earlier discussion), attempts are being made to provide treatment for the infected fetus of mothers who have decided to carry their pregnancy to term by treatment of the mother with pyrimethamine and sulfadiazine. Couvreur, in close cooperation with Daffos and colleagues, has made certain observations that should prove helpful.[1077] Their data suggest that spiramycin, although effective in reducing the frequency of transmission of the organism from mother to fetus, does not alter significantly the pathology of the infection in the fetus. For this reason, after week 17 of gestation, they treat with pyrimethamine-sulfadiazine for the duration of pregnancy when fetal infection has been proved or is highly probable. (In a commentary, Jeannel and co-workers raise the question of whether spiramycin was of value in the pregnancies studied by Daffos and colleagues.[1122]) During this treatment period, the mother is carefully monitored for development of hematologic toxicity. If significant toxicity appears despite treatment with folinic acid, the drug combination is discontinued until the hematologic abnormalities are corrected and the drug regimen is then restarted. Pyrimethamine (in combination with sulfonamides) appears to be the most efficacious treatment for infection in the fetus and newborn. Whether it has untoward toxic effects on the fetus, even after organogenesis has occurred, is unknown. Of importance, use of this drug combination in pregnant women has been reported to substantially reduce the subsequent clinical manifestations of the infection in the newborn and the antibody response of the fetus. Therefore, it is critical to understand that when the mother receives pyrimethamine and sulfadiazine, and the infant appears normal, that infant may or may not be infected. Thus, if infection of the fetus was not established before in utero treatment was initiated, and the infant is clinically normal, determination of whether the infant should receive treatment throughout the first year of life is difficult. Following maternal treatment, no signs of infection may be detectable in the infant at birth, but untoward sequelae may develop in later months or years. In addition, the infected newborn may not have the typical clinical or serologic features of the congenital infection. This situation creates a serious dilemma in trying to determine whether such infants should receive treatment when they are born to mothers who received treatment during pregnancy. Thus, use of pyrimethamine plus sulfadiazine cannot be recommended as routine in every woman who acquires the acute infection during pregnancy.

Because of the potential for this dilemma, we consider it important to employ prenatal diagnosis in every case of *T. gondii* infection acquired during pregnancy, even late in gestation, if there is no ethical or technical reason for not performing the procedure. Demonstration of fetal infection will allow for this combination drug regimen to be chosen for the mother and the neonate. If, however, extenuating circumstances preclude prenatal diagnosis in a mother whose infection was proved to have occurred during the second or third trimester, the same course of treatment as that used for cases in which the diagnosis has been established in the fetus may be considered, because infection acquired during the second trimester is associated with the highest risk for fetal disease, and in the third trimester, with the highest rate of transmission to the fetus.

The original report by Daffos and colleagues in 1988 was the first to highlight the importance of attempting to treat the infection in the fetus to improve clinical outcome.[130] In 24 of the 39 cases of proven infection, pregnancy was terminated at the request of the mother. Toxoplasmic encephalitis was noted in each of these 24 fetuses, including those in whom the findings on ultrasound examination were normal when the pregnancy was terminated. In every case, extensive necrotic foci were present, which suggested that sequelae might have been severe were the pregnancy not terminated. These findings also strongly suggest that early transmission (before week 24) usually results in severe congenital toxoplasmosis rather than subclinical infection (see Table 31-10).

In 15 of the 39 cases of diagnosed infection, the mother decided to continue her pregnancy. In these women, maternal infection was acquired between weeks 17 and 25 of gestation; in these cases, fetal ultrasound examination results were normal. Treatment with sulfonamides and pyrimethamine was begun as soon as the diagnosis of fetal infection was established, between 8 and 17 weeks after acquisition of the infection by the mother. After delivery, the presence of congenital *T. gondii* infection was demonstrated in the 15 newborns (in one infant, the serologic test result turned totally negative but became positive again a few weeks after treatment was discontinued, indicating that the infection was only suppressed, not eradicated). The 15 infants were asymptomatic despite the presence of cerebral calcifications in 4. Funduscopic appearance was normal, as were findings on the cerebrospinal fluid examination. Children were given pharmacologic treatment after birth, and all remained asymptomatic without neurologic signs or mental retardation. Ocular fundi remained normal in 13 children; retinal lesions were noted in 1 child at 4 months of age and in another at 18 months of age. The duration of follow-up was 3 to 30 months. Thus, despite rather early (before week 26) transmission of parasites from mother to fetus, infection remained either subclinical or mild in those fetuses whose mothers received pyrimethamine and sulfonamide treatment during pregnancy. Positive findings at prenatal diagnosis should be considered an indication for this therapeutic regimen, which would not usually be considered because of its potential toxicity to both fetus and mother. It should be understood that for ethical reasons, controlled trials (with "treatment" and "no treatment" groups of patients) have not been performed and may not be performed if an untreated group is required. Thus, one is left with studies in which historical data are used for comparison. Comparative trials will be performed in the future as newer therapies are developed.

Subsequent Studies

Couvreur and colleagues studied the outcome in 52 cases of congenital *T. gondii* infection diagnosed by prenatal examination in mothers who then were given the pyrimethamine, sulfadiazine, and spiramycin treatment regimen described by Daffos and colleagues.[124,130] Results in these infants were compared with those obtained in 51 infants with congenital toxoplasmosis whose mothers had received only spiramycin. Treatment for the infants after birth was the same in both groups. Although these two groups were not strictly comparable, valuable information can be gleaned from such a comparison so long as the focus remains on the qualitative direction of the results, rather than on the quantitative data. Remarkable were the lesser number of isolates from the placentas, the lower IgG antibody titers at birth and at 6 months of age, the lower prevalence of positive IgM antibody tests, and the higher number of subclinical infections in the offspring of mothers who received the pyrimethamine-sulfadiazine regimen. These data further support those discussed earlier—that treatment of the fetus is possible and that such treatment may result in a more favorable outcome if pyrimethamine-sulfadiazine is in the regimen (Table 31-45).[1077]

Boulot and colleagues[1123] described two cases in which women with *Toxoplasma* infection diagnosed during pregnancy subsequently received treatment with pyrimethamine plus sulfadiazine alternated with spiramycin, as described by Daffos and co-workers. Despite prolonged maternal treatment, the infants born to these women had congenital toxoplasmosis; *T. gondii* was isolated from the placentas. Although the success of treatment in the fetus will depend on a number of variables, as discussed earlier, these results serve as a note of caution in regard to the information given to parents about the effectiveness of such prenatal treatment.

In 1989, Hohlfeld and colleagues[124] updated information published earlier by their same group.[130] Because these were the first such available data, and although only relatively short-term follow-up is provided, a reasonably comprehensive presentation of their data seems justified. They reported 89 fetal infections in 86 pregnancies (39 of these infected fetuses were included in the original report by Daffos and co-workers, discussed earlier). All of the women were given spiramycin, 3 g daily, throughout their pregnancy from the time maternal infection was proved or strongly suspected on the basis of serologic studies until fetal infection was documented or

Table 31–45 Outcome of In Utero Treatment for Congenitally Infected Fetuses with Spiramycin or Spiramycin Followed by Pyrimethamine and Sulfadiazine

In Utero Treatment	No. of Patients	Dates of Study	Dates of Maternal Infection[a]	Duration of Follow-up	No. of Isolates from Placenta	Immune Load of IgG		IgM Prevalence	No. (%) of Subclinical Infections
						At Birth	*At 6 Mo*		
Spiramycin	51	1972-1982	22.8 (10-35)	46.7 mo (2 mo–11 yr)	23/30 (77%)	139	137	18/26 (69%)	17/51 (33%)
Spiramycin + pyrimethamine + sulfadiazine	52	1983-1989	22.6 (10-30)	76 wk (11-46 wk)	16/38[b] (42%)	86	70	8/46 (17%)[c]	30/52 (57%)

[a]Weeks of gestation.
[b]$P < 0.01$.
$P < 0.001$.
IgG, IgM, Immunoglobulins G, M.
Adapted from Couvreur J, et al. In utero treatment of toxoplasmic fetopathy with the combination pyrimethamine-sulfadiazine. Fetal Diagn Ther 8:45-50, 1993.

considered to be highly likely. Spiramycin treatment was instituted a mean of 36 ± 27 days after the estimated onset of infection. At prenatal examination, 80 of these women had had positive specific test results, and the remaining 9 had evidence of congenital *T. gondii* infection at birth. When fetal infection was confirmed, 34 terminations were performed at the request of the parents. The mean interval between infection and the beginning of therapy for continued pregnancies was remarkably and significantly shorter than for terminated pregnancies. The terminations were considered if severe lesions (marked hydrocephaly) were present on ultrasonogram at the time of prenatal diagnosis or when maternal infection had occurred very early in pregnancy. The main reason for termination was demonstration of cerebral lesions on ultrasonograms. Of interest is that the evolution of hydrocephalus was remarkably rapid in some of the cases, with ventricular dilatation observed to develop within 10 days. (Ventricular dilatation is an indirect sign of the presence of lesions due to *T. gondii*.) For most of the 52 pregnancies allowed to continue, treatment with pyrimethamine and sulfadiazine for 3 weeks alternating with spiramycin for 3 weeks was instituted, along with folinic acid (leucovorin). In 47 of 54 cases, postnatal treatment consisted of courses of pyrimethamine and sulfadiazine alternating with spiramycin, except in 3 infants, in whom only spiramycin was used. The mean period of follow-up was 19 months (range, 1 to 48 months).

In that study, subclinical infection was defined as complete absence of symptoms. The benign form included isolated subclinical signs, including intracerebral calcifications, normal neurologic status, and chorioretinal scars without visual impairment. This form was found mainly in older infants observed during the follow-up period and in younger infants when retinal scars were peripheral and did not involve the macular region (P Hohlfeld, personal communication to JS Remington, 1993). The severe form included hydrocephaly, microcephaly, bilateral chorioretinitis with impaired vision, and abnormal immunologic findings.

The overall risk of fetal infection was 7%, and this risk varied with time of maternal infection, as shown in Table 31-7. A more complete breakdown by week of gestation was published by the same group of investigators in 1994 (see Table 31-8).[125] At prenatal diagnosis, the nonspecific signs were not predictive of the severity of the fetal lesions; they were not found to differ significantly when subsequently terminated pregnancies were compared with those pregnancies that were allowed to continue. Fifty-five infants were born of the 52 pregnancies that were allowed to continue; no intrauterine growth retardation was noted. The findings are shown in Table 31-46. Each of the seven infants with cerebral calcifications had normal findings on ophthalmologic and neurologic examinations (benign form).

Attempts at isolation of the parasite from the placenta were positive in 23 cases, negative in 20, and inconclusive in 3; isolation was not attempted in 9 cases. Cord blood was positive for IgM antibodies in 8 cases, negative in 46 cases, and not examined in 1 case.

Follow-up evaluation was for 6 months to 4 years in 54 of the infants. The overall subclinical infection rate was 76%. The outcomes are shown in Table 31-47, where they are compared with those in historical controls from a study performed from 1972 to 1981.[1124]

Table 31–46 Findings at Birth in 55 Live Infants Born of 52 Pregnancies with Prenatal Diagnosis of Congenital Toxoplasmosis

Finding	No.[a]	%
Subclinical infection	44/54	81
Multiple intracranial calcifications	5/54	9
Single intracranial calcification	2/54	4
Chorioretinitis scar	3/54	6
Abnormal lumbar puncture	1/54	2
Evidence of infection on inoculation of placenta	23/46	50
Positive cord blood IgM antibody	8/53	15

[a]Numerator = number of abnormalities present at birth; denominator = total number of infants examined for abnormalities.

Adapted from Hohlfeld P, Daffos F, Thulliez P, et al. Fetal toxoplasmosis: outcome of pregnancy and infant follow-up after in utero treatment. J Pediatr 115:767, 1989, with permission.

Table 31–47 Comparison with Historical Controls (1972-1981) of Outcome in Live-Born Infants Diagnosed with Congenital *Toxoplasma* Infection in a Study of Prenatal Diagnosis (1982-1988) in Which the Mothers Were Treated with a Regimen of Pyrimethamine-Sulfadiazine Alternated with Spiramycin

	Affected Infants											
	First Trimester				*Second Trimester*				*Third Trimester*			
	1972-1981		*1982-1988*		*1972-1981*		*1982-1988*		*1972-1981*		*1982-1988*	
Outcome	*No.*	*%*	*No.*	*%*	*No.*	*%*	*No.*	*%*	*No.*	*%*	*No.*[a]	
Subclinical	1	10	6	67	23	37	33	77	74	68	2	
Benign	5	50	2	22	28	45	10	23	31	29	0	
Severe	4	40	1	11	11	18	0	0	3	3	0	
Total	10		9		62		43		108		2	

[a]See text.

Adapted from Hohlfeld P, Daffos F, Thulliez P, et al. Fetal toxoplasmosis: outcome of pregnancy and infant follow-up after in utero treatment. J Pediatr 115:767, 1989, with permission.

The additional information provided by this publication[124] further supports and extends the indirect evidence these authors published earlier,[130] that such treatment of the fetus reduces the number of biologic signs at birth and can reduce the likelihood of severe damage in the newborn. Thus, prenatal management as discussed by Hohlfeld and colleagues and previously by Daffos and co-workers appears to have resulted in an increase in the proportion of subclinical infections in first- and second-trimester infections, as well as in a reduction of severe congenital toxoplasmosis and a shift from benign forms to subclinical infections. In the earlier study, a large percentage of the cases had been third-trimester infections, which are known to have a better prognosis. Hohlfeld and colleagues recognized that their superior results, at least in part, may have been due to accurate diagnosis and selective termination in the few cases in which the fetuses were severely affected (2.7% of all referred cases in their experience), as well as to the effect of spiramycin on prevention of congenital transmission and the apparent reduction in the severity of fetal infection associated with the regimen of pyrimethamine-sulfadiazine. In Hohlfeld and colleagues' series, only 4% were third-trimester infections because, in the first years of their experience, prenatal diagnosis was not performed for late infections during gestation. Now that more rapid methods are available for diagnosis, the authors consider that prenatal diagnosis and treatment also may be appropriate in the third trimester.

Outcome of Treatment of the Fetus in Utero

Outcome was not uniformly favorable[994] when the algorithm of Daffos and co-workers[130] and Hohlfeld and colleagues[124] for patient care was applied. As mentioned earlier, part of the favorable outcome of Hohlfeld and colleagues can be attributed to termination of pregnancies in which the fetus had severe involvement (e.g., hydrocephalus). Nonetheless, the individual outcomes reported are better than would have been expected for first-trimester and early second-trimester infections. Almost all of the infected children from pregnancies managed according to this algorithm have demonstrated normal development, and those who have had clinical signs do not appear to have manifestations associated with significant impairment of normal function.[124] Thus, at present, the approach of Daffos and Hohlfeld and their co-workers[124,130] appears to provide the best possible outcome.

In this series, 148 fetal infections occurred in 2030 cases of maternal infection. The only predictive feature for fetal infection was fetal gestational age at onset of infection: For infection at less than 16 weeks, 31 of 52 (60%) fetuses had ultrasonographic evidence of infection. Possible abnormal findings included ascites, pericarditis, and necrotic foci; 48% had cerebral ventricular dilatation. If pregnancy was terminated, large areas of necrosis in the fetal brain were noted at fetopathologic examination. For pregnancies terminated at 17 to 23 weeks of gestation, 16 of 63 (25%) infected fetuses had signs on ultrasonographic examination; 12% had ventricular dilatation. For pregnancies terminated later than 24 weeks, 1 of 33 fetuses had signs on ultrasonographic evaluation. Hydrocephalus was not observed. Thus, these investigators offer termination at less than 16 weeks of gestation (see Table 31-9).

In the Paris studies, when mothers were found to be infected well before 16 weeks of gestation (i.e., in the first weeks of gestation) and the fetus was found to be infected by amniocentesis at 17 to 18 weeks of gestation, many of the pregnancies were terminated. Almost uniformly the fetus was found to have brain necrosis; 48% had cerebral ventricular dilatation (see Table 31-9).[130] By contrast, Wallon and co-workers[1125] do not terminate pregnancies of women who are acutely infected after 13 weeks of gestation, and who receive treatment, unless fetal brain ultrasonographic findings are markedly abnormal. Their approach is based on the fact that most infected children in their series were not severely impaired. In their experience with 116 congenitally infected children, only 2 children (2%) demonstrated some degree of visual impairment due to macular lesions, and these children had no neurologic or mental deficits. In this series, 31 (27%) were found to have cerebral calcifications or retinal lesions, but these children were neurologically and developmentally normal and without severe impairment of vision.

Mirlesse (personal communication to the authors, 1998 and 2004) described the outcome in 141 infected fetuses without cerebral dilatation who received both prenatal and postnatal treatment. Neonatal data were available in 133 cases, and 104 children were observed for a mean of 31 months. Two children died of malignant hyperthermia, 1 child had seizures, 1 child had a psychiatric disorder, and 12 had new eye lesions that developed between 6 months and 2 years of age. Sixteen (12%) of 133 children had eye lesions when they were born (Table 31-48).

Prenatally, fetal ultrasound examinations were performed fortnightly, and head ultrasonographic evaluations and sometimes brain CT also were performed in the newborn period for some of the infants. The prenatal ultrasonographic evaluation was performed through the endovaginal route, using a 7-MHz probe, when there was a cephalic presentation of the fetus.

These investigators describe important correlations with a finding of heterogeneous granular brain parenchyma in some of the congenitally infected infants. These changes predominated in the periventricular region but were found throughout the parenchyma. The affected areas ranged in size from a few millimeters to more than 1 cm across. When they were calcified, they sometimes generated a shadow. The authors emphasize that it was important to distinguish these hyperechogenic areas (HEAs) from cross-sectional vascular images by opening a color Doppler window (see Table 31-48).

Of 133 children, HEAs were present in 37 (26%), and HEAs were identified antenatally in 17 of 37 (46%). HEAs were never seen before 29 to 30 weeks of gestation. Ultrasound examinations underestimated lesions identified by CT at birth in 6 cases.

An important finding was that more fetuses demonstrated HEAs on CT scans if there was a longer interval between diagnosis of maternal and fetal infection (see Table 31-48). This finding could be explained in two alternative ways. It could be that longer delays in diagnosis and treatment were associated with infections acquired earlier in gestation when disease is more severe and thus there are more associated sequelae. Alternatively, more rapid diagnosis and treatment reduced sequelae.

Another important implication of these investigators' findings is that HEAs and their correlation with more frequent ophthalmologic disease demonstrate homogeneity

Table 31–48 **Significant Correlations of Brain Hyperechogenic Areas in Fetal and Newborn Ultrasound Studies with Other Clinical Aspects of Congenital Toxoplasmosis**

Clinical Feature	Cerebral Hyperechogenicity *Present*	Cerebral Hyperechogenicity *Absent*	Total or [Significance of Difference]
Interval between diagnosis of maternal and fetal infection	8.5 wk	6.5 wk	[*P* = .03]
Interval between maternal infection and institution of pyrimethamine-sulfadiazine treatment	9.5 wk	8.5 wk	[*P* = .06]
Ocular lesions	9/37 (24%)[b]	7/96 (7%)	16/133 (12%) [*P* < .008]
New eye lesions	7/37 (18%)	5/67 (7%)	12/104 (12%) [*P* < .058]

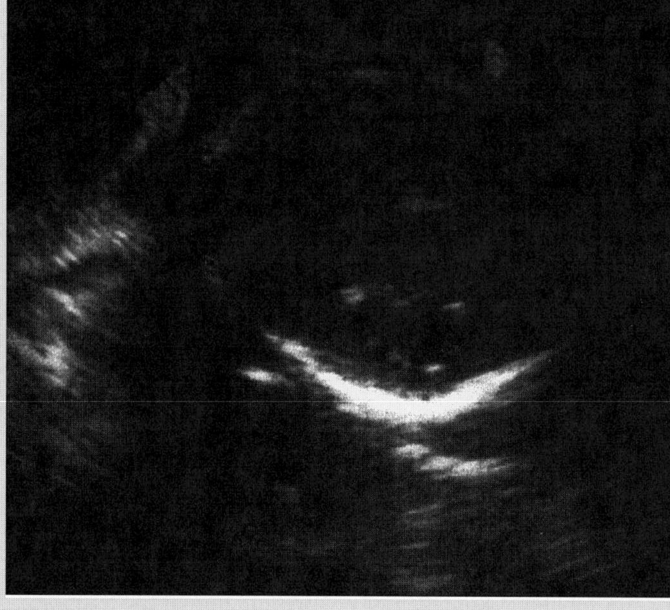

[a]See ultrasound for hyperechogenicity.
[b]Number with finding/number in group (%). Maximum duration of follow-up was until 2 years old. *Note:* delays in diagnosis and treatment were associated with cerebral hyperechogenicity on brain ultrasound and such hyperechogenicity was associated with more ocular lesions and development of new eye lesions.
From Mirlesse V, et al. Long-term follow-up of fetuses and newborn with congenital toxoplasmosis diagnosed and treated prenatally. (Personal communication to R. McLeod, 2000.)

of neurosensory involvement. In the NCCTS, this frequent concordance of neurologic and ophthalmologic involvement also was noted. HEA predicts ophthalmologic abnormalities, but such abnormalities are not always present. Developmental outcome in these children who received treatment, whether HEAs were present or not, was normal (see Table 31-48).

Sequelae of Congenital Toxoplasmosis in Children Who Received No Treatment

Stanford-Alabama Study

Results of a collaborative study performed in the United States suggest that adverse sequelae develop in a very significant number of children born with subclinical congenital *T. gondii* infection.[599] In this study,[599] the children were divided into two groups on the basis of indications for which serologic studies for toxoplasmosis were initially performed. Group I consisted of 13 children: Of these, 8 cases were detected as a result of routine screening of cord serum for IgM *T. gondii* antibodies[556] and as a result of testing for IgG and IgM antibodies to *T. gondii*. These tests were performed either because acute *T. gondii* infection was diagnosed during pregnancy or at term in the mother or because the children were screened for nonspecific abnormalities in the newborn period. Although each of these 13 children was carefully evaluated, none had signs of neurologic, ophthalmologic, or severe generalized disease at birth or at the time of diagnosis of congenital *T. gondii* infection; they would not have been detected if screening tests for antibodies to *T. gondii* had not been performed. (Data regarding earlier clinical and laboratory evaluations of eight of the children from Alabama had been reported previously.[556,1121,1126])

Group II consisted of 11 children in whom neither their parents nor their physicians detected signs of congenital infection during the newborn period. The diagnosis was entertained only after they presented with ophthalmologic or neurologic signs suggestive of congenital *T. gondii* infection.

Table 31–49 Characteristics of Children Born with Subclinical Congenital *Toxoplasma* Infection: Results of Stanford University–University of Alabama Study

Characteristic	Group I[a] (*N* = 13)	Group II[a] (*N* = 11)
Sex		
Male	4	9
Female	9	2
Race		
White	8	10
Black	5	0
Hispanic	0	1
Mean socioeconomic class[b]	4.08 ± 1.04	3.27 ± 1.19
Birth weight percentile		
<10	5	3
>10, <50	5	8
>50	3	0
Mean gestational age (wk)	37	38
Range	27.5-42.0	33.0-43.0
Mean age at diagnosis (wk)	2	34
Range	0.0-26.0	17.0-52.0
Mean age at most recent examination (yr)	8.26	8.68
Range	3.50-11.17	1.25-17.25
Treatment history for *Toxoplasma* infection[c]		
Never treated	5	6
Treated after sequelae developed and/or for <2 wk	1	3
Treated	7	2

[a]Group I = children for whom serologic tests were performed either because *Toxoplasma* infection was diagnosed in the mother during pregnancy or at term or because the children were screened for nonspecific findings in the newborn period. Group II = children in whom no signs of congenital infection were found during the newborn period. Diagnosis was first entertained after these children presented with signs suggestive of congenital *Toxoplasma* infection.
[b]Hollingshead's classification, mean ± SD (Hollingshead AB. Social Class and Mental Illness: A Community Study. New York, John Wiley, 1958).
[c]See text for definition and details of treatment.
Adapted from Wilson CB, Remington JS, Stagno S, et al. Development of adverse sequelae in children born with subclinical congenital *Toxoplasma* infection. Pediatrics 66:767-774, 1980, with permission.

Table 31–50 Methods of Evaluation of Children Born with Subclinical Congenital *Toxoplasma* Infection: Results of Stanford University–University of Alabama Study

Method	Group I[a] (*N* = 13)	Group II[a] (*N* = 11)
History; physical and neurologic examination	13	11
Urinalysis	13	11
Complete blood cell count	13	11
Detailed ophthalmologic examination	13	10
Skull roentgenography	10	6
Pneumoencephalography or angiography	0	2
Intelligence testing		
University of Alabama		
Revised 1974 Wechsler Intelligence Scale for Children	5	1
McCarthy Scales of Children's Abilities	2	1
Stanford-Binet Intelligence Scale (1972 Standards)	1	0
Not performed	0	2
Stanford University		
Stanford-Binet Intelligence Scale (1972 Standards)	5	6
Cattell Infant Intelligence Scale	0	1
Audiometry	13	11

[a]Group I = children for whom serologic tests were performed either because *Toxoplasma* infection was diagnosed in the mother during pregnancy or at term or because the children were screened for nonspecific findings in the newborn period. Group II = children in whom no signs of congenital infection were found during the newborn period. Diagnosis was first entertained after these children presented with signs suggestive of congenital *Toxoplasma* infection.
Adapted from Wilson CB, Remington JS, Stagno S, et al. Development of adverse sequelae in children born with subclinical congenital *Toxoplasma* infection. Pediatrics 66:767-774, 1980, with permission.

Because these children were preselected as a result of having developed complications of their initially subclinical infection, and because it is possible that a more detailed evaluation during the newborn period might have detected abnormalities in some of them, they were analyzed separately from the children in group I. The characteristics of both groups are shown in Table 31-49.

Of the 24 children, 11 (5 in group I and 6 in group II) never received treatment (Table 31-50). Four children (1 in group I and 3 in group II) were given treatment only after

Table 31–51 Ophthalmologic Outcome in Children Born with Subclinical Congenital *Toxoplasma* Infection: Results of Stanford University–University of Alabama Study

Ophthalmologic Finding	Group I[a] (*N* = 13)	Group II[a] (*N* = 10)[b]
No sequelae (7.6, 10)[c]	2	0
Chorioretinitis		
Bilateral		
Bilateral blindness[d]	0	5
Unilateral blindness	3	3
Moderate unilateral visual loss	0	1[e]
Minimal or no visual loss	5	1
Unilateral		
Minimal or no visual loss	3	0
Mean age at onset (yr)	3.67	0.42
Range	0.08-9.33	0.25-1.00
Recurrences of active chorioretinitis	3	2

[a]Group I = children for whom serologic tests were performed either because *Toxoplasma* infection was diagnosed in the mother during pregnancy or at term or because the children were screened for nonspecific findings in the newborn period. Group II = children in whom no signs of congenital infection were found during the newborn period. Diagnosis was first entertained after these children presented with signs suggestive of congenital *Toxoplasma* infection.
[b]One of the 11 children in group II was excluded because an adequate follow-up ophthalmologic examination was not performed.
[c]Age (yr) at most recent examination.
[d]Blindness = vision not correctable to >20/200.
[e]Macular involvement but vision correctable to 20/40.
Adapted from Wilson CB, Remington JS, Stagno S, et al. Development of adverse sequelae in children born with subclinical congenital *Toxoplasma* infection. Pediatrics 66:767-774, 1980, with permission.

adverse sequelae were noted or received treatment for less than 2 weeks, or both; for purposes of analysis, these children were referred to as "untreated." Nine children (7 in group I and 2 in group II) were given treatment for at least 3 weeks before 1 year of age and before the development of neurologic or intellectual deficits. Treatment in all cases consisted of regimens of pyrimethamine and sulfadiazine or pyrimethamine and trisulfapyrimidines.

All children were evaluated at least once. The methods of evaluation are indicated in Table 31-50. A detailed history was taken, and physical and neurologic examinations were performed for each child. Birth weight percentiles based on the appropriate gender, and on presence or absence of twin births, were used.[1127]

The results of the study revealed that untoward sequelae of their congenital infection ultimately developed in 22 of the 24 children (92%). The two children in whom sequelae did not develop were in group I; they were 8 and 10 years of age at the time of last examination.

Ophthalmologic Outcome. In group I, sequelae developed in 11 of 13 children (85%), and chorioretinitis was the initial manifestation of disease in all 11 (Table 31-51). The age at onset of eye disease ranged from 1 month to 9.3 years of age, with a mean of 3.7 years of age. At their most recent examination, 3 children had unilateral functional blindness, and the remaining 8 had chorioretinitis without loss of visual function. Subsequent to the initial episode of chorioretinitis, 3 of these 11 children had one or more additional episodes of active chorioretinitis at ages ranging from 1 to 8.7 years. In 1 of the 3 children, unilateral chorioretinitis developed at 1 year of age, and the child experienced four additional episodes of active chorioretinitis in that eye; chorioretinitis also developed in the previously uninvolved eye at 5 years of age. Although temporarily decreased visual function was associated with the recurrent episodes of active chorioretinitis in some of these children, no permanent, additional loss of visual function has resulted.

In group II, eight children initially presented with ocular abnormalities (see Table 31-51). The age at onset of eye disease ranged from 3 months to 1 year of age, with a mean of 0.4 year of age. The two other children in group II in whom ophthalmologic examinations were performed had chorioretinitis at the time they presented with neurologic abnormalities. At their most recent examination, five children had bilateral functional blindness, three had unilateral functional blindness, one had moderate unilateral visual loss, and one had chorioretinitis without loss of visual function. Subsequent to the initial episode of chorioretinitis, two of these children had recurrences of active chorioretinitis, at 2.3 to 3.5 years of age. One child in group II did not have an adequate ophthalmologic evaluation at the time of last follow-up examination and is not included in the results of ophthalmologic outcome.

Neurologic Outcome. Neurologic sequelae (Table 31-52) developed less frequently than did chorioretinitis and were always associated with eye pathology. Five (38.5%) of 13 children in group I suffered neurologic sequelae. Major neurologic sequelae developed in 1 (8%) and minor neurologic sequelae developed in 4 (31%) children in group I. In the child with major neurologic sequelae, severe psychomotor retardation and microcephaly became evident 19 months after the onset of chorioretinitis and 22 months after the diagnosis of congenital infection was made. This child subsequently developed a seizure disorder at 5 years of age. Two of the 4 children with minor neurologic sequelae in group I had delayed psychomotor development during the first 6 months of life, but their subsequent psychomotor development and neurologic status were normal when they were last examined at 3.7 and 8.7 years of age, respectively. The other two children in group I had minor cerebellar signs when most recently evaluated at 3.5 and 6.6 years of age.

Eight (73%) of 11 children in group II suffered neurologic sequelae (see Table 31-52). Of the children in group II, major neurologic sequelae developed in 3, minor followed by major neurologic sequelae developed in 2, and minor neurologic sequelae developed in 3. Two of these 5 children with major neurologic sequelae initially presented with eye abnormalities at 3 and 4 months of age; 1 subsequently developed a seizure disorder at 3 years of age, and the other was first noted to be microcephalic at 2 years of age. The other 3 children with major neurologic sequelae in group II included 1 child who presented with hydrocephalus at 8.5 months of age, with subsequent development of a seizure disorder and severe psychomotor retardation; 1 child who first exhibited transiently delayed psychomotor development between 6 and 12 months of age, with subsequent development of severe

Table 31–52 Neurologic Outcome in Children Born with Subclinical Congenital *Toxoplasma* Infection: Results of Stanford University–University of Alabama Study

Neurologic Finding	Group I[a] (*N* = 13)	Group II[a] (*N* = 11)
No sequelae	8	3
Major sequelae[b]		
Hydrocephalus	0	1[c]
Microcephaly	1[d]	1
Seizures	1	3[e]
Severe psychomotor retardation	1	2[f]
Minor sequelae		
Mild cerebellar dysfunction	2	4
Transiently delayed psychomotor development	2	2

[a]Group I = children for whom serologic tests were performed either because *Toxoplasma* infection was diagnosed in the mother during pregnancy or at term or because the children were screened for nonspecific findings in the newborn period. Group II = children in whom no signs of congenital infection were found during the newborn period. Diagnosis was first suspected when they presented with signs suggestive of congenital *Toxoplasma* infection.
[b]Microcephaly was diagnosed when the head circumference was below the third percentile; hydrocephalus was diagnosed on the basis of pneumoencephalography.
[c]The same child had a seizure disorder and severe psychomotor retardation and was included in the figures under those categories in group II.
[d]The same child had a seizure disorder and severe psychomotor retardation and was included in the figures under those categories in group I.
[e]One of these three children had mild cerebellar dysfunction and was included in the figures under that category in group II.
[f]One of these two children first exhibited transiently delayed psychomotor development and was included in the figures under that category in group II.
Adapted from Wilson CB, Remington JS, Stagno S, et al. Development of adverse sequelae in children born with subclinical congenital *Toxoplasma* infection. Pediatrics 66:767-774, 1980, with permission.

Table 31–53 Intelligence Testing in Children Born with Subclinical Congenital *Toxoplasma* Infection: Results of Stanford University–University of Alabama Study

Age and Intelligence Test Finding	Group I[a] (*N* = 13)	Group II[a] (*N* = 9)[b]
Mean age at most recent testing (yr)	7.40	10.20
Range	2.75-10.00	2.50-17.25
IQ[c]	88.6 ± 23.4[d]	85.3 ± 25.6[e]

[a]Group I = children for whom serologic tests were performed either because *Toxoplasma* infection was diagnosed in the mother during pregnancy or at term or because the children were screened for nonspecific findings in the newborn period. Group II = children in whom no signs of congenital infection were found during the newborn period. Diagnosis was first suspected when they presented with signs suggestive of congenital *Toxoplasma* infection.
[b]Two of 11 children in group II were excluded because they did not have intelligence formally evaluated.
[c]Mean ± SD.
[d]Evaluation was performed with the Stanford-Binet Intelligence Scale, 6 children; Revised 1974 Wechsler Intelligence Scale for Children, 5 children; and McCarthy Scales of Children's Abilities, 2 children.
[e]Evaluation was performed with the Stanford-Binet Intelligence Scale, 6 children; Revised 1974 Wechsler Intelligence Scale for Children, 1 child; McCarthy Scales of Children's Abilities, 1 child; and Cattell Infant Intelligence Scale, 1 child.
Adapted from Wilson CB, Remington JS, Stagno S, et al. Development of adverse sequelae in children born with subclinical congenital *Toxoplasma* infection. Pediatrics 66:767-774, 1980, with permission.

psychomotor retardation; and 1 child who presented with seizures at 4 months of age, with subsequent development of a seizure disorder associated with minor cerebellar dysfunction. Two additional children in group II had minor cerebellar dysfunction only, and 1 child had minor cerebellar dysfunction after showing transiently delayed psychomotor development in the first year of life.

Of the 16 children from both groups I and II for whom skull roentgenograms during infancy were available, 5 (mean age, 5.2 months) had intracranial calcifications and 11 (mean age, 4.8 months) did not. One of these children had normal findings on skull roentgenograms in the first month of life, but calcifications were noted on repeat roentgenograms at 3 months of age. Intracranial calcifications were noted on initial roentgenograms obtained between 3 and 10 months of age in the remaining 4 children. Major or minor neurologic sequelae developed in all 5 children with intracranial calcifications and in 4 of the 11 children without intracranial calcifications ($P = .03$). In these 9 children, the neurologic sequelae that developed were classified as major sequelae in 4 children (3 with intracranial calcifications and 1 without intracranial calcifications). Thus, of the 16 children, major neurologic sequelae developed in 3 of 5 children with intracranial calcifications and in 1 of 11 children without intracranial calcifications ($P = .06$). No correlation was found between neurologic outcome and birth weight, race, or age at most recent examination. In 8 children in group I, cerebrospinal fluid examinations were performed during the newborn period. In 7 of the children, abnormalities were detected; such abnormalities did not correlate with the development of any type of sequelae.

Intelligence Testing. Intelligence testing was performed in 22 of the 24 children by the methods that are indicated in Table 31-50. The results of intelligence testing are presented in Table 31-53. IQ scores correlated directly with upper socioeconomic class ($r = 0.37$, $P < .05$). In addition, the 16 white children had a higher mean IQ (89.6 ± 26.3) than that of the 6 nonwhite children (81.2 ± 15), but this difference was not statistically significant. Two of the children in group I (1 white, 1 African American) had moderately severe retardation (IQ scores of 36 and 62, respectively), as did 2 of the children (both white) in group II (IQ scores of 43 and 53). A tendency was identified for IQ scores to decrease on later testing among the 7 children (6 in group I and 1 in group II) who were tested more than once. The mean IQ score of these children fell from 96.9 to 74 over an average of 5.5 years, with all but 1 child showing a decrease on repeat testing.

No significant correlation was found between IQ scores and the finding of abnormal cerebrospinal fluid in the newborn period, intracranial calcifications on skull roentgenograms, age at time of testing, or birth weight below the tenth percentile. In fact, a trend toward higher IQ scores (mean, 96.9) was identified in children with birth weight below the tenth percentile. These results of intelligence testing must be interpreted with caution. The range of IQ scores was wide, testing was performed by different persons, and different tests were employed. The mean low socioeconomic status of the children also may have accounted for the low mean IQ scores that were observed. It is likely, however, that the results for the two children in group I and the two children in group II who had moderately severe retardation would not have been substantially different under other circumstances. It is particularly disturbing to note the downward trend in IQ scores for those children who were evaluated more than once. Although the finding is not statistically significant, all six children in group I had lower IQ scores when tested an average of 5.5 years after initial intelligence testing was performed. The mean age of the total study population was lower than that of the children who had repeat IQ testing, all of whom were older than 9 years of age when last tested. Thus, the true extent of intellectual impairment in the study population may be greater than the investigators observed.

Other Abnormalities. Several other abnormalities noted in the children are shown in Table 31-54. The incidence of sensorineural hearing loss in the study population also appeared to be excessive. In an earlier study in some of these children,[1121] the incidence of mild sensorineural hearing loss in 41 normal control children (mean age, 3.8 years) was 5%; no children with more severe sensorineural hearing loss were observed. In this study,[599] the incidence of sensorineural hearing loss in children tested in group I was 30% and that in group II was 22%. One child in each group had moderate unilateral hearing loss.

Table 31–54 Other Abnormalities in Children Born with Subclinical Congenital *Toxoplasma* Infection: Results of Stanford University–University of Alabama Study

Abnormality	Group I[a]	Group II[a]
Sensorineural hearing loss		
Moderate unilateral	1/10[b]	1/9[b]
Mild unilateral	1/10	0/9
Mild bilateral	1/10	1/9
Precocious puberty	2/13[c]	0/11
Premature thelarche	0/13	1/11[d]
Miscellaneous[e]	3/13	1/11

[a]Group I = children for whom serologic tests were performed either because *Toxoplasma* infection was diagnosed in the mother during pregnancy or at term or because the children were screened for nonspecific findings in the newborn period. Group II = children in whom no signs of congenital infection were found during the newborn period. Diagnosis was first suspected when they presented with signs suggestive of congenital *Toxoplasma* infection.
[b]Number with abnormality/number evaluated.
[c]Onset at 6 and 8 years of age.
[d]Onset at 2 years of age.
[e]Includes one case of each of the following: genu recurvatum, clubfoot, low-set umbilicus, and slow weight gain.
Adapted from Wilson CB, Remington JS, Stagno S, et al. Development of adverse sequelae in children born with subclinical congenital *Toxoplasma* infection. Pediatrics 66:767-774, 1980, with permission.

Effect of Treatment. One of the 2 children in group I in whom adverse sequelae had not developed at the time of the study was given treatment (this child's mother also received treatment during the last trimester of pregnancy), and the other never received treatment. Among the 22 children in groups I and II who presented with chorioretinitis in the absence of neurologic disease, major neurologic sequelae developed in 5 of 13 children who received no treatment but in none of 9 children who received treatment ($P = .05$). Because abnormalities on the skull roentgenogram correlated with development of neurologic sequelae, the researchers examined the results of skull roentgenograms from the children who received treatment and those who did not. Skull roentgenograms were available from 8 of the 13 children who did not receive treatment and from 5 of the 9 children who received treatment. Whereas no child who received treatment had abnormal skull roentgenograms (each had roentgenograms obtained before and 1 had roentgenograms obtained after treatment), 4 of the children who received no treatment had intracranial calcifications ($P = .01$). No factors other than abnormalities on skull roentgenograms differed significantly between children given treatment and those given no treament. The mean IQ score (97 ± 22) of those children who underwent treatment for 3 weeks or more at or before 1 year of age was higher than the mean IQ score (93 ± 22) of those who received no treatment or the score (82.5 ± 29.7) of those whose treatment was of shorter duration or instituted at a later age (usually after obvious sequelae were evident); these differences were not significant ($P > .1$).

Special Considerations. Because this study was not controlled and was only in part prospective, certain limitations must be considered in interpreting the data. Children in group II were detected because of the development of sequelae that were sufficiently significant to attract medical attention. Thus, it would be inappropriate to use data from this group to determine the frequency of such sequelae among children born with subclinical infection. Nevertheless, data from group II do provide information regarding the potential seriousness of ocular disease in children born with subclinical congenital *T. gondii* infection and regarding the risk of subsequent neurologic sequelae in children in whom chorioretinits developed previously. No data from this study or from other studies indicate that a significant bias toward more severe disease was introduced by the different screening methods employed in group I. It is likely, therefore, that the data from group I provide a reasonable estimate both of the seriousness and of the frequency of complications in children with initially subclinical congenital *T. gondii* infection. Because of the small sample size and the lack of a matched control group, these data must, however, be considered estimates. In addition, because more than half of the children in this study were younger than 9 years of age, it should be appreciated that additional sequelae may have developed among them. This study and the early Eichenwald studies are profound descriptions of the tragedy of untreated or inadequately treated congenital *Toxoplasma* infection in children.

Paris Studies

Of 108 infants with congenital *T. gondii* infection who were diagnosed and evaluated prospectively by Couvreur and colleagues[604] and discussed by Szusterkac,[1128] 27 had chorioretinitis. In 26 of these infants, the lesions were present at the time of the first ophthalmoscopic examination after birth. In only 1 infant were findings on the eye examination normal at birth, with subsequent development of chorioretinitis. In 3 other infants, a retinal lesion was noted at the time of first examination, and a new lesion was discovered on follow-up examination. It is noteworthy that only 16 of the 108 infants were examined after the age of 2 years and only 3 were examined after the age of 5 years. Only 6 of these 19 children had chorioretinitis on initial examination. Of interest is the striking difference between the children who received treatment and those who did not during the first year of life: Among the children who received treatment, no lesions were discovered after the age of 2 years, whereas in 8% of the children given no treatment, chorioretinitis developed between 10 months and 4 years of age. It is possible to assume from the experience of Koppe and colleagues[600,601] and Wilson and co-workers[599] that careful follow-up evaluation in these 108 children would reveal additional cases of chorioretinitis and additional lesions in the 27 children who already had eye disease. Follow-up evaluation in such series is important, because all of these children were identified prospectively and received treatment for approximately 1 year either from birth or from the time at which the diagnosis was established in the first months of life.

Additional data in children in whom congenital *T. gondii* infection was not recognized in the newborn period have been published by Briatte.[1129] These data were obtained in collaboration with Couvreur, Hazemann, and Desmonts in Paris. Hazemann established a program at a number of medical centers in the Paris area in which any infant could be examined free of charge at the request of the mother. The first examination was performed when the infant was 10 months of age. Among the blood tests performed in this program was the dye test to detect cases of previously undiagnosed congenital *T. gondii* infection. Forty-eight infants with subclinical congenital *T. gondii* infection were detected among the 20,513 infants examined from 1971 through 1979. (The data were corrected for those cases in which the infection probably was acquired postnatally.) Infants with clinical toxoplasmosis probably were not examined in this program because these infants would already be under medical care, so that their mothers probably would not request their participation in this medical screening program. For the same reason, it is likely that the vast majority of infants screened had few or no problems during infancy.

The frequency of probable congenital *T. gondii* infection in the entire study population averaged 2.33 per 1000 (range, 0.38 to 5.2 per 1000 per study year). The frequency of chorioretinitis among the 48 infants is shown in Table 31-55. Of these 48 children (who, of course, did not receive treatment for their *T. gondii* infection during the first 10 months of life), chorioretinitis developed in 18% by the age of 4 years. In 8 of the children, chorioretinitis developed after the age of 10 months and before the age of 4 years. This latter finding differs considerably from that reported by Szusterkac[1128] in infants who received treatment in the early weeks or months of life (see earlier discussion). Cerebral calcifications were present in 3 of the 48 infants previously unrecognized as having infection, which therefore had not been treated.[1129]

INTERPRETATION OF STANFORD-ALABAMA AND PARIS STUDIES

For proper interpretation of the data presented for the Stanford-Alabama study[599] and the study reported by Briatte,[1129] it is important to understand how the data might be biased because of the method of case selection. The method used in the studies in Alabama for detection of subclinical congenital infection (detection of an increase in cord serum IgM) might have selected for the most "severe" (heavily infected) cases among subclinically infected newborns. In the studies performed by the Stanford group, some of the patients were selected because manifestations of the infection occurred during infancy. Thus, in both of these studies, the method of selection might have predisposed to an increased frequency of more severe cases in the Stanford-Alabama study. By contrast, in the study reported by Briatte, it is probable that the most "benign" cases were selected among subclinically infected newborns, because the investigators studied infants who had few or no medical problems during the first 10 months of life. Despite this bias toward "mild" infection, 18% of the infants whom the Paris group observed had ocular lesions by the age of 4 years.

Amsterdam Study

As mentioned earlier, in 1964 a prospective study was started in Amsterdam to determine the frequency of congenital toxoplasmosis.[600] Of 1821 pregnancies screened, 249 infants were enrolled in the study—21 because of seroconversion in the dye test, 42 because of a high baseline dye test titer, 183 because of a slight rise in dye test titer, and 3 because their mothers had toxoplasmosis shortly before gestation. At birth, 4 infants had chorioretinitis and parasites were isolated from

Table 31–55 Frequency of Chorioretinitis in Infants with Subclinical Congenital *Toxoplasma* Infection First Discovered in a Systematic Serologic Screening Program

Age When Fundus Was Examined	No. of Children	Chorioretinitis Previously Recognized	New Cases of Chorioretinitis Discovered	Total No. of Children with Chorioretinitis in this Age Group (%)
10 mo	48	0	5	5 (10)
Examined again at 2 yr	31	5	3	8 (16)
Examined again at 4 yr	28	8	1	9 (18)

Data are adapted from patients studied by Drs. J. Couvreur, J.J. Hazemann, and G. Desmonts. Cases are discussed by Briatte.[1129]

placenta and cerebrospinal fluid of 1 other infant. Each of these 5 children received pharmacologic treatment. Seven children who were asymptomatic and whose dye test titer did not revert to negative received no treatment. Ten other questionably infected children who had no symptoms but whose dye test titer became negative 18 months after birth also received no treatment. These 22 children were evaluated annually for 5 years by physical examinations and dye and CF tests. No new abnormalities were detected, except in 1 patient with chorioretinitis, who required surgery to correct a squint at the age of 2 years.[600] The 12 congenitally infected children continued to be examined yearly until the age of 20 years.

The authors' original optimistic view was revised in their 1986 publication.[389] One of the 5 children who received treatment and 1 of the symptom-free children had new scars in their eyes at the age of 6 years. Additional new scars or acute lesions were observed in both the "treatment" and "no treatment" groups of children. In 3 children, scars appeared at ages 11, 12, and 13 years, respectively. One patient had a new scar in his right eye when examined for the first time at age 17, and another had no severe eye abnormalities until the age of 18 years, when an acute lesion appeared in the right macula that led to blindness in that eye. Another patient had a new acute lesion in her right eye at the age of 12 years and again in both eyes at the age of 13 years. Thus, after a total of 20 years of follow-up, of 11 congenitally infected children, 9 had scars in one or both eyes. Four of these children had severely impaired vision in one eye, and 3 were blind in one eye. Among the 10 questionably infected children, 1 had a scar in the right macula at 5 years of age that led to severe visual impairment. Another child whose mother had toxoplasmosis during gestation remained persistently seropositive. He had not developed any scars in his eyes. The other 8 children remained seronegative for 5 to 19 years, and some acquired toxoplasmosis during this time. The 11 congenitally infected children did not differ from controls in their school performance. None of the 11 was mentally retarded.

From the results of this prospective study, it is apparent that 9 of 11 children (82%) after 20 years of follow-up had significant sequelae of toxoplasmosis and that 5 of these 11 had severely impaired vision. Although the report by Wilson and associates described earlier demonstrated a similar percentage of untoward sequelae by the age of 10 years, theirs was not a prospective study.[599]

In regard to the foregoing results, the prospective clinical study reported by Sever and associates and performed in children born to mothers whose sera were sampled during pregnancy between 1959 and 1966,[1130] the investigators suggested that maternal *T. gondii* infection may be associated with greater damage to women and children than had previously been recognized. Of special interest is the increased rate of deafness, microcephaly, and low IQ scores at an examination of the children at 7 years of age. These findings suggest that late sequelae of congenital *T. gondii* infection are not limited to eye disease but occur also in the CNS.

U.S. (Chicago) National Collaborative Treatment Trial Study

A national, collaborative, prospective study, the NCCTS, is being carried out by a group of investigators based in Chicago (telephone number 773-834-4152). This study is evaluating long-term outcome for infants given pyrimethamine (comparing two doses) in combination with leucovorin and sulfadiazine (100 mg/kg per day in two divided doses). Medications are begun when a child is younger than 2.5 months of age according to the method shown in Figure 31-33 and continued for 12 months. Therapy is monitored by parents with a nurse case manager and the primary physician, and compliance also is documented with measurement of serum pyrimethamine levels. Children who have not received treatment during the first year of life and are referred to the study group when they are older than 1 year also are included in the study. Patients are evaluated comprehensively by the study group near the time of birth and at 1, 3.5, 5, 7.5, 10, and 15 years of age.

The following parameters are evaluated: history; physical status; audiologic, ophthalmologic, neurologic, and cognitive function and development; and a number of other variables as measured by laboratory tests, including tests of hematologic status and serologic and lymphocyte response to *T. gondii* antigens, and neuroradiologic studies. As of November 2004, 130 children who received treatment had been evaluated. Ages ranged from newborn to 22.9 years (mean age, 10.8 years). Thirty-eight historical (no treatment) patients also are being followed. They range in age from 1.9 to 42.8 years of age (mean age, 19.4 years). Analysis of the full cohort is presently ongoing (R McLeod, unpublished). Results appear to be similar to those reported in 1999. In the analysis in 1999, 104 children who received treatment had been evaluated. They ranged in age from 0.07 to 17.1 years (mean age, 6.8 years). Twenty-eight historical controls (those given no treatment) were evaluated. They ranged in age from 5.6 to 33.6 years (mean age, 14.1 years) (Table 31-56).

Table 31–56 Ages (in Years) of Patients in U.S. (Chicago) National Collaborative Treatment Trial[a]

	All Patients			Patients ≥5 Years of Age		
Patient Group	***Mean ± SD***	***Range***	***N***	***Mean ± SD***	***Range***	***N***
Historical patients[a]	13.9 ± 8.9	5.4-33.4	28	15.3 ± 8.9	5.4-33.4	28
Treatment A: feasibility	11.7 ± 1.1	10.0-14.3	13	11.7 ± 1.1	10.0-14.3	13
Randomized	5.7 ± 1.9	1.9-8.8	38	6.7 ± 1.2	5.0-8.8	26
Treatment C: feasibility	3.5 ± 4.6	0.5-15	7	12.7 ± 3.2	10.5-15.0	2
Randomized	5.4 ± 2.0	0.9-10.0	28	6.7 ± 1.4	5.1-10.0	16

[a]Historical patients were patients who received no treatment and were diagnosed after 1 year of age. In the treatment groups, children received 2 months (Treatment A) or 6 months (Treatment C) of daily pyrimethamine and sulfadiazine, followed by pyrimethamine on Monday, Wednesday, and Friday and continued daily sulfadiazine for the remainder of the year of therapy.

Preliminary results of this study indicate that early outcomes for many, but not all, congenitally infected children who received treatment in that decade, in that manner, appeared to be substantially better than outcomes reported in earlier decades for children who received no treatment or whose treament was for 1 month or less (Tables 31-57 and 31-58; see also Table 31-27). Specifically, the early results from this study indicate that such therapy has been feasible for 104 children. The only substantial manifestation of toxicity was transient neutropenia, which responded to increased dosages of leucovorin or withholding of pyrimethamine. This appeared to occur primarily during the prodrome of concomitant viral infections. Dental caries occurred in one of the first children studied (Table 31-59). Thereafter, parents were cautioned to clean teeth of older infants, because medications were administered in sugar suspensions. Pediatricians were cautioned to avoid using a second sulfonamide to treat concomitant infections such as otitis media, because more prolonged neutropenia occurred in one child in conjunction with such therapy.

Pharmacokinetics of pyrimethamine were characterized in the initial feasibility phase of the study, and serum levels associated with the two dosage regimens of pyrimethamine were noted (see "Pyrimethamine plus Sulfonamides," earlier).

All signs of active infection (i.e., thrombocytopenia, hepatitis, rash, meningitis, hypoglycorrhachia, active chorioretinitis, vitritis) resolved within weeks of initiation of therapy.[1028] Chorioretinitis did not progress or relapse during therapy.

Audiologic outcome was significantly better than that reported in the earlier literature (see Table 31-27).[737] No sensorineural hearing loss was noted in the 104 children who received treatment, in contrast with a 14% incidence of "deafness"[596] or 26% incidence of "hearing loss"[599] in earlier studies. Comparisons of outcomes in this and earlier studies are summarized in Table 31-27 (see also the next section, "Comparison of Outcomes").

Retinal disease became quiescent with therapy within weeks, with no recrudescence observed during therapy.[1028] New lesions (primarily those "satelliting" preexisting lesions) occurred in older children (see Table 31-42). The oldest child who received treatment was 17 years of age in 1999. Lesions also occurred in previously normal-appearing retinae. These were noted first at study evaluations at 3.5, 5, or 7.5 years of age and had not been present at the preceding evaluation. Evaluations were performed at approximately the time of birth and at 1, 3.5, 5, and 7.5 years of age. To date, no loss in visual acuity has occurred when prompt treatment of active recurrent chorioretinitis was initiated. Comparison of early outcomes with 2 versus 6 months of 1 mg/kg per day of pyrimethamine followed by this dosage administered on Monday, Wednesday, and Friday, both administered with sulfadiazine and leucovorin, is shown in Table 31-58. At present, no statistically significant differences have been noted. Thus, treatment during the first year of life with pyrimethamine and sulfonamides, unfortunately, did not uniformly prevent recrudescent chorioretinitis. Determination of whether it reduces the incidence of recurrent or new chorioretinitis, compared with the almost uniform occurrence of this complication in children who did not receive treatment, who were diagnosed in earlier decades, requires longer follow-up evaluation of more children. It is especially important to try to determine whether treatment prevents subsequent chorioretinitis when no retinal lesions are present at birth.

Visual acuity that is adequate for all usual activities and reading has been noted in some children with large macular scars. Nonetheless, impairment of vision has been one of the two most prominent sequelae (Table 31-60). Visual impairment has presented a challenge in the care of children of school age; that is, special attention is needed to optimize their ability to read, and participation in learning activities must be ensured so that their visual impairments do not impair cognitive development. Retinal scars have been central, peripheral, unilateral, and bilateral in location and have resulted in partial and complete retinal detachment. Loss of sight at presentation (e.g., due to retinal detachment) usually has been associated with the most profound neurologic impairment. Visual outcomes to date are contrasted with those of earlier studies in the next section, "Comparison of Outcomes." Neurologic and cognitive function of most of these treated children has been significantly better than reported in earlier decades.[534,1131-1133] This is summarized in Table 31-61.

In the earlier report by Eichenwald,[596] more than 80% of children who had substantial generalized and neurologic involvement at birth and who received no treatment or whose treatment was for 1 month had IQ scores below 70 at 4 years of age. In that report, initial involvement in the perinatal period appears to have been less severe or similar in severity to that of children in the NCCTS. In contrast with the outcome in that earlier series, only 24% of the children who received treatment in the decade 1982 to 1992 in the NCCTS had substantial cognitive impairments. The remaining 76% of the treated children in the NCCTS who presented with substantial generalized or neurologic manifestations of infection or both in the perinatal period are demostrating normal development and are likely to be capable of self-care. The same trends have been present in children tested through 2004. The relative contribution of shunt placement, antimicrobial therapy, and adjunctive supportive care to this improved outcome cannot be determined with certainty. The observation that almost all children without hydrocephalus in the NCCTS have at least average cognitive function contrasts dramatically with the 81% incidence rate of mental retardation at 4 years of age in children presenting with generalized disease in Eichenwald's series who received no treatment or whose treatment was for 1 month.[596] This difference suggests that antimicrobial therapy may contribute significantly to the more favorable outcome. No deterioration of cognitive function has occurred over time in these children who received treatment, although visual impairment clearly has affected school performance and ability to acquire information and skills for some children.[1131] This finding contrasts with earlier reports of diminished cognitive function over time for children not given treatment or those whose duration of treatment was less than 1 month who had subclinical disease in the perinatal period (described by Wilson and associates[599]). In spite of the remarkably good cognitive outcome for many of these children, the impact of the infection on their cognitive function is reflected in the fact that their IQ scores often are 15 points less than those of their nearest-age siblings ($P < .05$).[1131]

It has been possible to discontinue antiepileptic medications in some infants who have had seizures (presumably due to

Table 31–57 Comparison of Ophthalmologic, Developmental, and Audiologic Outcomes with Postnatal Treatment

				Percent with Finding or Impairment					
				Ophthalmologic			*Neurologic*		
Study	Treatment	No. Studied	Mean Age (yr) When Data Tabulated (Range)	*Lesions*[a]	*Vision*[b]	*New*[c]	*Cognitive*	*Motor or Seizures*	*Audiologic*
Eichenwald, 1959[596]	0 or 1 mo P, S	104	4 (minimum)	NA	0, 42, 67[d]	NA	50, 81, 89[d]	0, 58, 76[d]	0, 10, 17[d]
Wilson et al, 1980[599]	0 or 1 mo P, S	23	8.5 (1-17)	93	47	22	55 (20 severe)	20	22, 30[e]
Koppe et al, 1986[389]	0 or 1 mo P, S	12	20 (NA)	80	NA	NA	0	0	NA
Labadie and Hazemann, 1984[395]	0	17	1 (NA)	28	NA	NA	NA	NA	NA
Couvreur et al, 1984[554]	1 yr P, S, Sp	172	NA (2-11)	NA	NA	8	NA	NA	NA
Hohlfeld, 1989[124]	Prenatal, 1 yr P, S, Sp	43	NA (0.5-4)	12	NA	NA	0	0	NA
Villena, 1998[147]	F, Sp	47	NA [born 1980-89]	—	—	15/45 (33)[f]	—	—	—
	1 yr F	19	NA [born 1990-96]	—	—	2/18 (11)	—	—	—
	2 yr F	12	NA [born 1990-97]	—	—	1/11 (9)	—	—	—
Peyron, 1996[1037]	F′	121	12 (5-22)	—	—	37/121 (31)	—	—	—
Chicago study (historical patients)	0	7	5.6 (2-10)	100	86	29	25	25	14
Chicago study (treated patients)	Most for 1 yr P, S	37[g]	3.4 (0.3-10)	81	81	8	0, 24[h]	0, 24	0

[a]Any chorioretinal lesions.
[b]Vision impaired.
[c]New lesions.
[d]Subclinical, generalized, neurologic.
[e]Subclinical, generalized, neurologic.
[f]Number with finding/number in group (%).
[g]These data are for the first 37 children studied before May 1991.

F, Fansidar (pyrimethamine 1.25 mg/kg each 14 days); F′, Fansidar (given in utero and postnatally—pyrimethamine 6 mg/5 kg each 10 days; small numbers also treated in utero); NA, not available; P, pyrimethamine; S, sulfonamides; Sp, spiramycin.

Adapted from McAuley J, et al. Early and longitudinal evaluations of treated infants and children and untreated historical patients with congenital toxoplasmosis: the Chicago Collaborative Treatment Trial. Clin Infect Dis 18:38-72, 1994.

Table 31–58 Early Outcomes for Children ≥5 Years of Age in the U.S. (Chicago) National Collaborative Treatment Trial

Untoward Sequela	% in Literature: 5 yr, 10 yr[c]	Historical Patients[d]	Mild[a] Treatment A[b] Feasibility	Mild[a] Treatment A[b] Randomized	Mild[a] Treatment C[b] Feasibility	Mild[a] Treatment C[b] Randomized
Vision <20/20	25, 50	11/14 (79)[e]	0/4	0/3	0/0	0/0
New retinal lesions	25, 85	5/9 (56)	0/4	1/3	0/0	0/0
Motor abnormality	10, 10	0/14 (0)	0/4	0/3	0/0	0/0
IQ <70	0-50, 0-50	0/13 (0)	0/4	0/3	0/0	0/0
ΔIQ ≥15	50, 50	0/5 (0)	0/4	1/3	0/0	0/0
Hearing loss	30, 30	0/14 (0)	0/4	0/3	0/0	0/0

Untoward Sequela	% in Literature: 5 yr, 10 yr[f]	Historical Patients	Severe[a] Treatment A Feasibility	Severe[a] Treatment A Randomized	Severe[a] Treatment C Feasibility	Severe[a] Treatment C Randomized
Vision <20/20	70, 70	10/10 (100)	7/9 (78)	8/9 (89)	1/2	6/9 (67)
New retinal lesions	50, 90	4/9 (44)	3/9 (33)	1/8 (13)	2/2	0/9 (0)
Motor abnormality	60, 60	1/10 (10)	3/9 (33)	2/9 (22)	0/2	1/9 (11)
IQ <70	90, >90	1/10 (10)	4/9 (44)	4/9 (44)	0/2	2/9 (22)
ΔIQ ≥15	95, 95	0/8 (0)	0/9 (0)	2/9 (22)	0/2	1/9 (11)
Hearing loss	30, 30	0/10 (0)	0/9 (0)	0/9 (0)	0/2	0/9 (0)

Note: Percentages not shown for groups with ≤4 patients.

[a]Clinical disease considered "Mild" if infant is apparently normal and normal development is noted on follow-up evaluation (e.g., but has isolated nonmacular retinal scars or <3 intracranial calcifications on CT). Clinical disease considered "Severe" if neurologic signs or symptoms are present, symptomatic chorioretinitis has threatened vision, or if ≥3 intracranial calcifications are seen on CT.

[b]Treated children received 2 months (Treatment A) or 6 months (Treatment C) of daily pyrimethamine and sulfadiazine, followed by pyrimethamine on Monday, Wednesday, and Friday and continued daily sulfadiazine for the remainder of the year of therapy. Feasibility group patients underwent treatment in the early phase of the study before randomized study.

[c]Data from Wilson et al.[599]

[d]Historical patients were patients who received no treatment and were diagnosed after 1 year of age.

[e]Number with abnormality/number in group (% affected). No differences between treatment regimens achieved statistical significance ($P > 0.05$ using Fisher Exact test).

[f]Data from Eichenwald.[596]

CT, computed tomography; IQ, intelligence quotient.

Table 31–59 Episodes of Reversible Neutropenia Requiring Temporary Withholding of Medications for the U.S. National Collaborative Study[a]

Regimen	No. of Episodes Medication Withheld (Mean ± S.D. [Range])	No. Who Stopped Medication/No. in Group Who Have Completed 1 Year of Therapy (%)	No. of Children Who Stopped Medications Temporarily/No. in Group (%) Feasibility	No. of Children Who Stopped Medications Temporarily/No. in Group (%) Randomized	Discontinued Medications Due to Neutropenia ≥4 times
Treatment A	1.8 ± 1.1 [1-4]	11/32 (34)	6/14 (43)	11/34 (32)	4
Treatment C	3.8 ± 3.1 [1-11]	17/48 (35)	1/4 (25)	10/28 (36)	5

[a]Children received 2 months (Treatment A) or 6 months (Treatment C) of daily pyrimethamine and sulfadiazine, followed by pyrimethamine on Monday, Wednesday, and Friday and continued daily sulfadiazine for the remainder of the year of therapy. Feasibility group patients received treatment in the early phase of the study before randomized study. Toxicity for Treatments A and C was measured as episodes of reversible neutropenia requiring temporary withholding of medications.

active encephalitis) in the perinatal period, without recurrence of seizures. Before September 1991 (see Table 31-61), new-onset seizures had developed in four children after the perinatal period. Hypsarrhythmia occurred in two children. One of these latter children responded dramatically and promptly to adrenocorticotropic hormone injections (pyrimethamine and sulfadiazine were administered concomitantly), and one responded to clonazepam treatment.

Table 31–60 Quantitative Visual Acuity in U.S. (Chicago) National Collaborative Treatment Trial in Patients with Macular Lesions (m) in at Least One Eye

Group	Patient No.	Right Eye	Left Eye
Treated[a]	7	20/20	20/20 (m)
	13	6/400 (m)	20/50 (m)[b]
	15	4/30 (m)	20/30 (m)[b]
	19	20/200[c]	20/20 (m)
	21	1/30 (m)	1/30 (m)
	26	3/30 (m)	1/30 (m)
	28	20/30 (m)	15/30 (m)
	30	1/30 (m)	12/30[d]
	36	20/30	8/30 (m)
Historical[a]	20	20/400 (m)	20/25
	25	20/400 (m)	20/30
	27	5/30 (m)	1/30[e]
	31	20/25	3/200 (m)
	38	20/400 (m)	20/25[e]
	41	20/30	20/200 (m)
	42	20/70 (m)	20/30 (m)[b]
	46	20/200 (m)	20/60 (m)
	47	3/30 (m)	3/30[e]
	82	20/400 (m)	20/15
	89	20/100 (m)	20/25

[a]Treated: n = 39 (30 too young or with cognitive limitations that made it not possible for the child to cooperate with quantitative vision). Historical: n = 13 (2 too young for quantitative vision).
[b]Surprisingly good vision in spite of foveal lesion.
[c]Strabismus, microphthalmia, and amblyopia present.
[d]Poor cooperation, patient 4 years old.
[e]Peripheral lesion with dragging of the macula.
From Mets MB, et al. Eye manifestations of congenital toxoplasmosis. Am J Ophthalmol 122:309-324, 1996.

In many instances, a number of considerations may make it reasonable to withhold antiepileptic therapy after a short course of such medications. These considerations include the potential adverse interactions of each antiepileptic medication with the antimicrobial agents needed to treat *T. gondii* infection.[1028] If antimicrobial therapy results in resolution of active encephalitis, which was the seizure focus, antiepileptic medications would no longer be needed. In the NCCTS, a lack of recurrence of seizures when antiepileptic medications were discontinued in a number of cases[1131-1133] supports this approach.

Remarkable reduction in size or disappearance of calcifications, as well as dramatic improvement in brain CT scans (see Figs. 31-10C to F and 31-14), occurred in association with antimicrobial therapy in this study.[534,1028,1131]

Factors in the newborn period that often were associated with poorer prognosis included apnea and bradycardia, hypoxia, hypotension, delays in shunt placement and/or initiation of therapy, blindness, retinal detachment, cerebrospinal fluid protein concentration greater than 1 g/dL, diabetes insipidus in the perinatal period, hypsarrhythmia, and markedly diminished size of brain cortical mantle that did not increase after shunt placement.[1131] Nevertheless, favorable outcomes also have been noted when some of these abnormalities were present.[1131-1133]

Comparison of Outcomes. Comparison of outcomes with no treatment, 1 month of treatment, 1 year of pyrimethamine plus sulfonamides in alternate months with spiramycin, and 1 year of pyrimethamine plus sulfadiazine is shown in Table 31-57. Early treatment in the NCCTS appears to have resulted in more favorable outcome than was reported to occur for untreated infants or infants who received treatment for only 1 month.

Treatment of Relapsing Chorioretinitis. The factors that lead to relapse of chorioretinitis are not known. It is of interest that such relapse has been reported to occur most

Table 31–61 Comparison of Neurologic and Developmental Outcomes in the Chicago, Wilson et al, and Eichenwald Studies

	Chicago (1991)		Wilson et al (1980)		Eichenwald (1959)		
Outcome	*Subclinical (N = 3)*	*Generalized/ Neurologic (N = 34)*	*Subclinical I (N = 13)*	*Subclinical II (N = 11)*	*Subclinical (N = 4)*	*Generalized (N = 31)*	*Neurologic (N = 70)*
Seizures requiring therapy after first months	0 (0)[a]	4 (12)	1 (8)	3 (27)	2 (50)	24 (77)	58 (82)
Motor/tone permanent impairment	0 (0)	8 (24)	3 (23)	2 (18)	0 (0)	18 (58)	53 (76)
IQ <70	0 (0)	8 (24)	2 (15)	2 (18)	2 (50)	25 (81)	62 (89)
Sequentially lower IQ score	0/2 (0)	3[b]/13 (0)	6/6 (100)	0/1 (0)	NA	NA	NA

[a]Number affected/number tested if different from N (%).
[b]Three children had a >15-point diminution and 2 children had a >15-point increase in IQ score. The differences over time for the entire group were not statistically significant (P >.05)
IQ, intelligence quotient; NA, not available.
Data from references 529, 596, 599, 1044, 1131, and 1133.

often during adolescence. An antimicrobial agent that eliminates encysted organisms in the eye is needed, because it is clear that treatment with currently available antimicrobial agents does not uniformly prevent or eliminate relapsing chorioretinitis.[534,1134] Longer follow-up of large numbers of treated infants (especially those who acquired their infection in the third trimester and have no retinal involvement at birth) is needed to determine whether treatment reduces the frequency of this sequela. After treatment during the first year of life, because they are at risk for relapse, congenitally infected infants and young children should undergo ophthalmoscopy at 3- to 4-month intervals until they can reliably report visual symptoms. Studies are ongoing to determine whether continued frequent follow-up ophthalmologic evaluations and earlier treatment can prevent the devastating consequences of recurrent chorioretinitis. Careful evaluation, including retinal examination, should be performed whenever ocular symptoms suggestive of active chorioretinitis are present.

In infants and in the limited number of older children followed to date in the NCCTS, active chorioretinitis appeared to resolve within 1 to 2 weeks of beginning treatment with pyrimethamine and sulfonamides as described in Table 31-43. Occasionally, particularly with relatively longer delays in initiating treatment, resolution of active lesions and vitritis was more prolonged. With recurrence of lesions after the first year of life, antimicrobial treatment has been continued 1 to 2 weeks beyond resolution of signs and symptoms. It is standard practice to administer prednisone (1 mg/kg daily in two divided doses [Table 31-43]) in conjunction with pyrimethamine and sulfonamides if inflammation threatens the macula, optic disk, or optic nerve. The efficacy of this practice is unknown. Some investigators have recommended clindamycin or tetracycline therapy.[1135] No convincing data are available to allow determination of whether inclusion of these latter two medications would be beneficial.

In a series of 124 patients in Brazil, prophylaxis with TMP/SMX in a dose of 160 mg/800 mg) given every 3 days reduced the incidence of recurrent eye lesions from 23.8% (i.e., in 15 patients who received no treatment) to 6.6% (in 4 patients who received treatment).[411] The high incidence of allergy to sulfonamides (25%) makes use of sulfonamide for prophylaxis a potential problem. If allergic reactions develop, treatment of active eye disease that occurs later may require use of other antimicrobials.

Because transmission occurs frequently when acute infection is acquired in the latter part of the third trimester, it is reasonable to provide treatment for the fetus by administering pyrimethamine and sulfadiazine to the recently infected mother. A diagnostic procedure to detect infection in the fetus (see "Prenatal Diagnosis of Fetal *Toxoplasma gondii* Infection," earlier) should be performed before this therapy is instituted, because such treatment may obscure the diagnosis at birth. In such instances, decision making concerning treatment for the infant during the first year of life is significantly complicated by the lack of accurate diagnostic information.

Ophthalmologic Outcomes after Prenatal Followed by Postnatal Treatment of Congenital Toxoplasmosis. In a collaborative study by investigators in the United States and France, Brezin and colleagues[127] studied ophthalmologic outcome following treatment of congenital toxoplasmosis in utero and in the first year of life with pyrimethamine plus sulfadiazine and leucovorin. Ophthalmologic examinations were performed in 18 children born to mothers infected before 25 weeks of gestation. Both eyes were normal in 11 of the 18 children (61%) (mean age 4.5 years; range, 1 to 11). Only peripheral retinal disease was present in two children (both eyes in each). Four children had posterior pole scars in one eye; each of these four had normal visual acuity, and two of these four had peripheral retinal scars. The outcome was favorable for all but one child, in whom visual acuity was decreased and extensive, bilateral macular and peripheral lesions were present.

These results contrast markedly with the high prevalence of macular disease in the NCCTS. The improved outcome probably was due to prenatal treatment of the French children in the Collaborative French/NCCTS study.

Prospective Ophthalmologic Follow-up Evaluation of a Cohort of Congenitally Infected Infants in Lyon, France. In an observational, prospective cohort study performed in Lyon, France by Binquet and her colleagues,[1022,1136] maternal infections were identified through monthly testing of susceptible women. Most mothers became infected during the second trimester (89 [20%]) or third trimester (219 [68%]). Two hundred seventy two (84%) were treated during pregnancy: 149 (46%) with spiramycin alone, 104 (32%) with spiramycin followed by pyrimethamine plus sulfadiazine, and 19 (6%) with pyrimethamine plus sulfadiazine. Treatment for the infant included a brief course (3 weeks) of pyrimethamine plus sulfadiazine followed by 1 year of treatment with Fansidar. In this cohort of 327 children (median duration of follow-up from birth was 6 years [interquartile range, 3 to 10], range, 6 months to 14 years), they[1022] found that during a median follow-up period of 6 years, 79 (24%) had at least one retinochoroidal lesion, but bilateral visual impairment was not noted. Children who were diagnosed prenatally or at birth (rather than by an increase in specific IgG between 1 and 12 months of life), who had nonocular manifestations at the time of diagnosis, and who were premature had the highest likelihood of developing ophthalmologic manifestations. Thirteen (17%) of the 79 children had inactive lesions. The authors raise the possibility that the ophthalmologist may have observed those children with extraocular signs more closely. It also is possible that as examinations became easier with increasing age of the children, more lesions that may have been easier to visualize were detected.

These same investigators recently reported that in this same cohort during a median follow-up period of 6 years after birth (interquartile range, 3 to 10 years), 238 (76%) of the 327 children (range, 6 months to 14 years) were free of any eye lesions. Sixty (18%) had no sequelae except for retinochoroiditis; 33 (11%) had at least one clinical sign of the infection (brain calcifications in 31, hydrocephalus in 6, microcephalus in 1). Of the 6 with hydrocephalus, 3 had moderate psychomotor retardation, and 2 with calcifications had a single seizure. The investigators also reported that more than one lesion in the retina of the eye was predictive for involvement of the other eye. No association was found between new manifestations of infection and the age at which the initial lesion was detected, activity of retinal

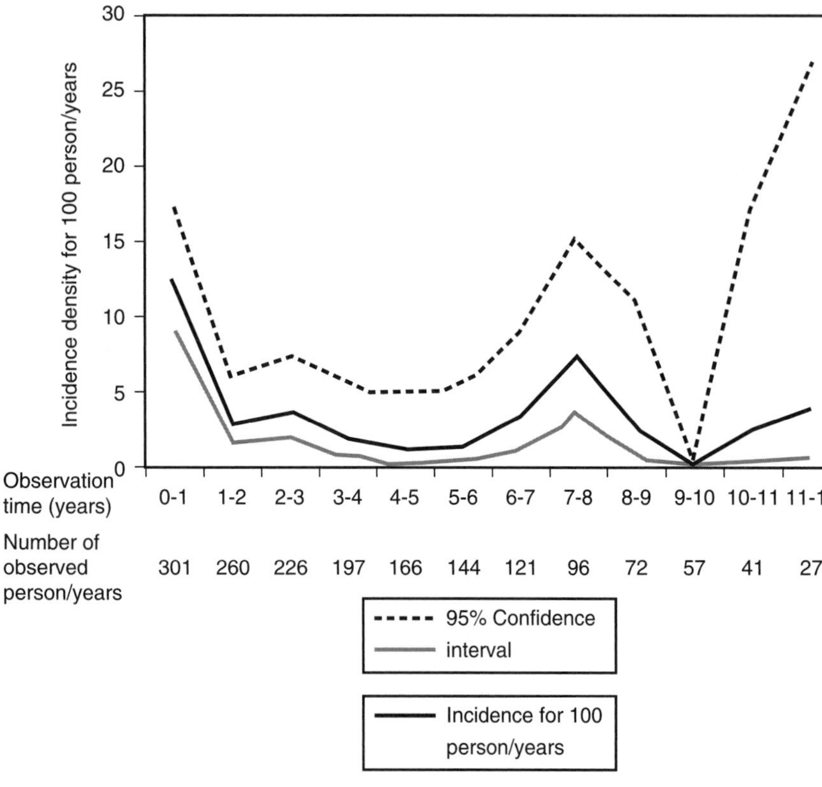

Figure 31–35 Incidence density of first ocular lesion after diagnosis of congenital toxoplasmosis in a cohort of children described by Wallon and co-workers.[1022] (From Wallon M, Kodjikian L, Binquet C, et al. Long-term ocular prognosis in 327 children with congenital toxoplasmosis. Pediatrics 113: 1567-1572, 2004.)

disease, or locations of retinal lesions.[1022] Figure 31-35 shows the times at which the investigators noted new lesions.[1022]

PREVENTION

Congenital toxoplasmosis is a preventable disease. It is therefore the responsibility of health professionals who provide care for pregnant women to educate them on how they can prevent themselves from becoming infected (and thereby not place their fetus at risk). Lack of adoption of a systematic serologic screening program in the United States leaves education as the principal means of preventing this tragic disease.

Seronegative pregnant women and immunodeficient patients are two populations in which avoidance of infection by *T. gondii* is most important. We consider that the data on morbidity, incidence, and cost of congenital toxoplasmosis warrant a major attempt to define and initiate means whereby congenital toxoplasmosis can be prevented.[150] Several methods for the prevention of congenital toxoplasmosis have been proposed. Attention to the specific hygienic measures outlined in Table 31-62 is the only method available for the *primary* prevention of congenital toxoplasmosis.[387] It is the responsibility of all physicians caring for pregnant women and women attempting to conceive (women at risk) to inform them of these preventive measures so that they will not place their fetuses at risk. The impact of these measures on the incidence of acquired toxoplasmosis in a given population has been discussed earlier, in the "Epidemiology" section. A substantial effort to educate women at risk and the physicians who care for them is clearly an important aspect of any program for prevention.[1137-1139] A cost-benefit analysis of preventive measures for congenital toxoplasmosis in the United States is beyond the scope of this chapter. For a discussion of this matter, the reader is referred to the article by Roberts and Frenkel.[2]

Table 31–62 Methods for Prevention of Congenital Toxoplasmosis

Prevention of Infection in Pregnant Women

Women should take these precautions:

1. Cook meat to well done, smoke it, or cure it in brine.
2. Avoid touching mucous membranes of mouth and eyes while handling raw meat. Wash hands thoroughly after handling raw meat.
3. Wash kitchen surfaces that come into contact with raw meat.
4. Wash fruits and vegetables before consumption.
5. Prevent access of flies, cockroaches, and so on to fruits and vegetables.
6. Avoid contact with materials that are potentially contaminated with cat feces (e.g., cat litter boxes) or wear gloves when handling such materials or when gardening.
7. Disinfect cat litter box for 5 minutes with nearly boiling water.

Prevention of Infection in Fetuses

1. Identify women at risk by serologic testing.
2. Treat during pregnancy, which results in an approximate 60% reduction in infection among infants. Perform therapeutic abortion, which prevents birth of infected infant (used only for women who acquired infection in first or second trimester [<50% of cases]).

Adapted from Wilson CB, Remington JS. What can be done to prevent congenital toxoplasmosis? Am J Obstet Gynecol 138:357-363, 1980, with permission.

In addition to primary preventive measures, it is necessary to identify those women who acquire the infection during pregnancy (so that treatment during gestation, or abortion, can be considered). A mechanism for identification of these women also must be a part of any program for prevention of congenital toxoplasmosis. Because approximately 90% of women infected during pregnancy have no clinical illness and because there are no pathognomonic clinical signs of the infection in the adult, diagnosis in the pregnant woman must be made by serologic methods. This approach also is supported by the observation that only approximately 50% of mothers of congenitally infected infants in a recent series could recognize known risk factors or compatible clinical illness.[292] This makes prospective testing desirable.

Food

The tissue cyst can be rendered noninfective by heating meat thoroughly to 66° C (150° F) or by having it smoked or cured. Curing may not eliminate the organism.[60] Freezing meat is a less reliable method of killing the cyst[60]; freezing meat at −20° C for 24 hours may be sufficient to destroy the tissue cyst,[43] but not all freezers available in the United States can maintain this temperature even when new. To minimize the chance of infection resulting from handling raw meat, the hands should be thoroughly washed with soap and water after contact with the meat, and the mucous membranes of the mouth and eyes should not be touched with potentially contaminated hands while meat is handled. Eggs should not be eaten raw. Vegetables and fruits should be washed before they are eaten.

Oocysts and Cats

To avoid infection by oocysts, several measures can be suggested. Cat feces may be disposed of daily by burning or flushing down the toilet, and the empty litter pan may be made free of viable oocysts by pouring nearly boiling water into it (an exposure time of 5 minutes is sufficient).[1140] Strong ammonia (7%) also kills oocysts, but contact for at least 3 hours is necessary. Drying, disposing as part of ordinary garbage, surface burial, freezing, or using chlorine bleach, dilute ammonia, quaternary ammonium compounds, or any general disinfectant cannot be relied on.[1141] Women who are seronegative during pregnancy and immunodeficient persons should avoid contact with cat feces altogether. For handling litter boxes or working in sand or soil that may have been contaminated by cat feces, disposable gloves should be worn. Because sandboxes often are used by cats as litter boxes, a cover should be placed over the sandbox when it is not in use, and the hands should be washed after exposure to the sand. Flies, cockroaches, and probably other coprophagic animals serve as transport hosts for *T. gondii* and should be controlled and their access to food prevented.[19] Fruits and vegetables may have oocysts on their surfaces and should be washed before ingestion. Because the cat is the only animal known to produce the oocyst form, efforts should be directed toward preventing infection in cats. Feeding them dried, canned, or cooked food, rather than allowing them to depend on hunting (e.g., for birds and mice) as their source of food, reduces the likelihood of their becoming infected. Frozen raw meat also should be avoided, because freezing may not always eliminate *T. gondii*.[1141]

Although it has been recommended that pet cats should be banished for the duration of pregnancy,[1142,1143] this measure is hardly feasible under most circumstances. Repeated requests for serologic testing of cats are being received by veterinarians in the United States, and in many instances, serologic test results are misinterpreted in respect to the danger of transmission. Patients are being misguided, unnecessary anxiety is being produced, and cats are being sacrificed without good reason. The fact is that cats with antibodies are safer pets than cats without antibodies because the presence of antibodies offers some degree of immunity to reinfection and thereby prevents or markedly decreases repetition of oocyst discharge.[19] Antibody determinations are not practical for the determination of infectivity of cats because the infectious oocysts usually are discharged before the development of antibodies in the animal[226,240]; routine serologic testing for this purpose should be discouraged.

Veterinarians and their lay staff caring for cats probably are at increased risk, and special precautionary measures must be exercised to protect pregnant personnel. Large numbers of cats are handled annually by animal practitioners and staff members, and as many as 1% of these cats may excrete oocysts. Feces from caged cats should be collected (preferably on a disposable tray or material) and discarded daily (preferably incinerated) before sporulation occurs. Care must be taken in handling feces for worm counts and similar procedures; samples should be examined within 24 hours of collection, and caution must be exercised to avoid contamination of hands, centrifuges, benches, and microscopes. Gloves should be worn at all times by those handling cat feces.[1142,1144]

Serologic Screening

Only a serologic screening program during gestation will detect the acute acquired infection and thereby facilitate diagnosis and treatment of the infected fetus and newborn.

The cost-effectiveness of systematic screening of women during pregnancy depends on a variety of factors, including the cost of tests and how frequently they are employed compared with the cost to society of caring for the diseased children who would be born in the absence of screening.[1,327,331,304,1145-1148] Wilson and Remington[1] and McCabe and Remington[1139] have proposed that a screening program be considered in the United States. Such a program would include the performance of a serologic test equal in sensitivity, specificity, and reproducibility to the Sabin-Feldman dye test in all pregnant women. It is crucial that initial testing be performed as early as possible, but at least by 10 to 12 weeks of gestation. (Ideally, testing of all women just before pregnancy would identify those at risk.)

Discussion of all of the pros and cons of a systematic screening program for the United States is beyond the scope of this chapter. Of importance in this regard, however, is the fact that approximately 50% of women with children in the NCCTS from 1981 to 1998 could not identify a risk factor for or illness consistent with toxoplasmosis.[292] Certain recent analyses of this subject warrant consideration. These analyses have been discussed by Boyer and colleagues[292] as follows:

There are economic analyses, Cochrane database reviews, and metareviews which address the value of screening programs and their outcomes. Some of these analyses and reviews have considered both well-performed studies and studies of dissimilar cohorts that have been inadequately designed, controlled, performed, or interpreted to be of equal value. Some authors of these analyses have noted that there are no perfectly designed and performed prospective, randomized, placebo-controlled studies that have follow-up and include economic analyses that clearly document savings in costs and efficacy of newborn or maternal screening.

Some investigators who have reviewed the available data concluded that without better prospective studies, it may be too costly or unwarranted to perform universal screening and treatment, even to prevent suffering, health care–related costs, loss of productivity and limitation in quality of life associated with untreated congenital toxoplasmosis. There are comments that such screening could cause unacceptable anxiety as a result of false-positive test results, or unnecessary pregnancy terminations due to serologic testing that was not confirmed in a high-quality reference laboratory or counseling that was suboptimal. In contrast, others have concluded that screening, in conjunction with careful confirmation in a high-quality reference laboratory and knowledgeable and caring counseling, is important to facilitate identification and treatment of this fetal and newborn parasitic encephalitis and retinitis.

We critically reviewed these analyses and the concerns they raise. Some important considerations are presented next. We conclude that a number of studies on this subject are seriously flawed. Fortunately, a number of carefully designed investigations on this subject have been performed as well. These latter works indicate that systematic detection of this infection in pregnant women and treatment of the infected fetus as described by Daffos and associates[1149] result in better outcomes.[292] In the cohort described by Wallon and collegues,[1021] improved outcomes for affected children were observed. Careful confirmation of serologic testing in a high-quality, reliable reference laboratory, as well as knowledgeable and empathetic medical care and counseling, is essential.[292] Another study performed by Gras and co-workers in a cohort of mothers in Lyon, France, examined the effect of prenatal treatment on the risk of intracranial and ocular lesions in children with congenital toxoplasmosis.[1150] This cohort included 181 infected children born to mothers who received treatment during gestation. The infants received 3 days of pyrimethamine and 3 weeks of sulfadiazine at approximately the time of birth, followed by 2 to 5 weeks of spiramycin therapy and then 12 or more months of Fansidar administered every 10 days. Thirty-eight children had hydrocephalus, intracranial calcifications on ultrasound study or skull film, or in one instance on CT scan, or ocular lesions detected by 3 years of age. These authors report the following percentages of retinal lesions detected over time: 4% (1 month), 9% (6 months), 11% (12 months, N = 157), 16% (3 years, N = 133), 19% (5 years, N = 96), 23% (7 years, N = 55). Because the locations of eye lesions that were apparently new were not clearly specified and not documented with photographs throughout the study, it is difficult to determine with certainty whether the lesions observed later were missed on initial examinations (which are more difficult in young infants and children) or truly were new lesions.

Gras and co-workers also state that, with one exception, outcomes were the same whether the mothers received no treatment, spiramycin, or pyrimethamine plus sulfadiazine before the infants were born. They[1150] further reported an observation that is unusual and difficult to explain: They noted the best outcome (i.e., fewest intracranial lesions) with no treatment in utero or following the greatest delay in treatment in utero. The method of detection of intracranial lesions appears to have been by postnatal skull radiography or head ultrasound examination,[1150] both well known to be suboptimal in terms of sensitivity. The authors suggest that perhaps this result of improved outcome with less treatment could be due to immune suppression in the mother or fetus by pyrimethamine or sulfadiazine treatment, but they provide no supporting data for this hypothesis. The prenatal treatment modalities differed from those used in the cohorts reported by Hohlfeld and colleagues in Paris,[125] and the treatment and methods of evaluation conducted postnatally differed from those described by the NCCTS.[534]

Hohlfeld and colleagues noted diminution of cerebrospinal fluid abnormalities indicative of active encephalitis when in utero treatment with pyrimethamine and sulfadiazine was used,[124] and Couvreur and associates noted a reduction in isolation of *T. gondii* from placental tissue.[117] Without treatment, *T. gondii* can be isolated from approximately 90% of placentas. With treatment (initiated between 15 and 35 weeks of gestation; median, 23 weeks) *T. gondii* was isolated from placentas of approximately 77% of women given spiramycin[117] and approximately 42% of women given pyrimethamine plus sulfadiazine with leucovorin.[117] *T. gondii*–specific IgM antibody was present in fewer newborns born to mothers given pyrimethamine plus sulfadiazine than , the number of newborns born to mothers who received no treatment (17% versus 69%), and infection was more often subclinical in the newborns born to mothers who had treatment (33% versus 57%).[124]

Foulon's data[126] also are noteworthy: Effects of treatment on development of sequelae in the fetus and the infant up to 1 year were analyzed in 140 children. Sequelae were present in 7 (28%) of 25 children born to mothers who did not receive treatment and in 12 (10%) of 115 children born to mothers who did receive treatment. Multivariate analysis revealed that administration of antibiotic treatment was predictive of the absence of development of sequelae in children (P = .026; odds ratio 0.30; 95% confidence interval 0.104 to 0.86). Moreover, when antibiotics were used, a positive correlation was noted between development of sequelae and the time elapsed between when infection occurred and the start of treatment. More rapid instigation of antibiotic treatment after infection led to less frequent sequelae found in the newborn. (P = .021).

The NCCTS investigators have noted resolution of a number of parameters including hepatitis, active chorioretinitis, meningoencephalitis, and no new eye lesions during sustained treatment for congenital toxoplasmosis during the first year of life.[534]

Brezin and colleagues reported that 7 (39%) of 18 children with congenital toxoplasmosis treated in utero had eye lesions, with posterior pole lesions in 4 and with visual impairment in only one child. The median duration of follow-up was 4.5 years (range 1 to 11 years). They were infected before 25 weeks of gestation. They had received in utero treatment before 35 weeks of gestation but not earlier than 22 weeks. Treatment was continued after birth until they were 1 year of age. Children in the NCCTS also were infected early in gestation, but their mothers had not received treatment during gestation. In contrast with the French children who had received treatment in utero and had less severe eye disease, the children in the NCCTS had a predominance of posterior pole eye lesions: 54% of children who received treatment in their first year of life, 82% of children with infection detected after their first year of life and therefore untreated, and 58% of the total.[127]

Considerable discussion[370] is available on two recent studies of the efficacy of prenatal treatment in prevention and reduction of sequelae of the congenital infection. The commentary of Thulliez and co-workers is reproduced here in its entirety because of the importance of this analysis in understanding the strengths and weaknesses of the published data:

> In their retrospective cohort study of 554 mother-child pairs, Gilbert et al. did not detect a significant effect of prenatal treatment on the risk of vertical transmission of toxoplasmosis.[1151] This result is not surprising as there were very few untreated women and the analysis of no treatment versus pyrimethamine-sulphadiazine was restricted to half of the cohort who did not undergo amniocentesis. The confidence interval (0.37-3.03) for the odds ratio (1.06) for no treatment compared with pyrimethamine-sulphadiazine was therefore very wide and could include a doubling in the risk of transmission in untreated women. Thus an absence of evidence of prenatal treatment effect does not exclude a clinically important beneficial effect.
>
> A further problem is that most of the untreated women were infected during the third trimester of pregnancy. Figure 31-4 shows that only three women infected before 28 weeks of gestation were not treated. The remaining 28 untreated women were infected after 28 weeks. The effect of treatment in the third trimester cannot be generalized to the whole of pregnancy. Finally, the authors explain their findings by suggesting that vertical transmission occurs soon after infection, during parasitaemia. This hypothesis is not supported by any scientific studies in humans. On the contrary, one study found that the sensitivity of prenatal diagnosis was lower in early than mid pregnancy, suggesting that vertical transmission may be delayed for some women infected in early pregnancy.[838]
>
> In the second report by Gras et al.,[1150] the authors unexpectedly found no evidence that prenatal treatment with pyrimethamine-sulphadiazine was more effective than spiramycin in reducing the risks of intracranial or ocular lesions in congenitally infected infants by 3 years of age. A potential explanation for this result is that mothers who transmitted the infection to their fetus soon after infection were more likely to be treated with pyrimethamine-sulphadiazine than mothers infected at the same gestation but in whom transmission was delayed until later in pregnancy. These two groups may not be comparable as fetuses infected earlier in pregnancy have a higher risk of clinical signs. This explanation is suggested by the fact that mothers infected before 32 weeks were only given pyrimethamine-sulphadiazine if the diagnosis of fetal infection was positive (i.e., vertical transmission occurred between maternal infection and the date of fetal sampling). Other mothers infected before 32 weeks were treated with spiramycin until delivery, either because the prenatal diagnosis was negative or not attempted. In this latter group, transmission occurred either after amniocentesis or at some unknown time between the date of maternal infection and delivery, that is, later during gestation than in the group receiving pyrimethamine-sulphadiazine.
>
> There are two further explanations for the lack of effect of pyrimethamine-sulphadiazine. First, there was a long delay before pyrimethamine-sulphadiazine was started. This was because the study was carried out more than 6 years ago, when mouse inoculation was the standard fetal diagnostic test[131] and pyrimethamine-sulphadiazine treatment would have been delayed for 3-6 weeks until results were known. Today, PCR analysis of amniotic fluid is widespread. Results are available in one day and women with infected fetuses are treated much earlier.[125] Secondly, women in the study given pyrimethamine-sulphadiazine actually received an alternating regimen with spiramycin. The periods of spiramycin treatment may have led to parasitic relapses in fetal tissues, as shown in experimental models (Piketty et al. AAC, 1990). The current treatment policy for women with a positive prenatal diagnosis is to prescribe continuous treatment with pyrimethamine-sulphadiazine until delivery.
>
> The data reported by Gilbert et al.[1151] and Gras et al.[1150] provide no convincing evidence that this policy should change.*

Each of us is in favor of a screening program for the United States similar to that being used at present in France (see Fig. 31-34). We recognize, however, that constraints of present-day health care systems may not permit such screening on a monthly basis or, in some instances, screening of pregnant women per se. Cost-benefit analyses are especially relevant to mandated, state-supported screening programs. Nevertheless, we believe that almost all parents, given the choice, would select a simple, not very costly, and direct measure that could prevent cognitive and ocular damage to their child as part of their health care coverage.

Introduction of prenatal screening and, in particular, use of PCR testing on amniotic fluid at 18 weeks of gestation has altered the approach to screening of women. The data that demonstrate a benefit of screening are from programs that screen on a monthly basis, as is done in France. In France, greater than 90% of women now have their first prenatal visit (with testing to assess whether they are seropositive for *T. gondii* antibodies) in the first trimester. This early, first-trimester prenatal visit is a requirement for health care insurance coverage during gestation and at birth. This requirement considerably facilitates interpretation of results of serologic screening. Possible alternatives in locations where prevalence of antibody is low and resources are limited have not been studied systematically. Available data indicate that better outcomes result with initiation of treatment within weeks after the diagnosis of recently acquired infection is made in the mother.[126] Wilson and Remington[1] and others previously suggested that such women be screened for seroconversion, with the first serum sample obtained as early as possible in the first trimester and subsequent samples in the second and third trimesters. Such early testing would allow for detection of those women whose fetuses are at greatest risk of being infected and would allow for appropriate management decisions to be made with regard to the newborn.

With the introduction of treatment of the fetus through administration of specific therapy to the pregnant woman, it has become even more important to establish the diagnosis in the fetus at the earliest possible time; PCR analysis in amniotic fluid provides for this. Therefore, women must be informed of the importance of a visit to their physician as early as possible in pregnancy, to allow for early serologic

---

*Reproduced from Thulliez, Romand, et al: Efficacy of prenatal treatment for toxoplasmosis: a possibility that cannot be ruled out. Int J Epidemiol 30:1315-1316, 2001. Reference numbers and cited figure refer to main text.

testing. Blood for the second serum sample should be drawn at a time in the second trimester such that if recently acquired infection is confirmed, PCR analysis in the amniotic fluid can be performed at 17 to 18 weeks of gestation. If that second serum does not reveal recently acquired infection, a third serum sample can be obtained in the early third trimester. If seroconversion is observed at that time, we recommend PCR on amniotic fluid; if the PCR assay reveals infection in the fetus, the mother should receive pyrimethamine-sulfadiazine in an attempt to treat the fetus. A final serum sample is obtained at the time of parturition to detect those mothers who acquired their infection very late in gestation but whose fetuses are at greatest risk of infection. Luyasu and associates[1152] reported seven cases of subclinical congenital *T. gondii* infection in infants born to mothers who acquired their infection between 2 and 4 weeks before delivery. They emphasized that because children born to mothers who become infected close to term are at greatest risk for development of the congenital infection and must be given appropriate treatment to attempt to prevent untoward sequelae of the infection, it is important to screen seronegative pregnant women until the time of delivery.

A woman whose is seropositive on initial testing ideally then undergoes testing for IgM antibodies. If the IgM test result is positive, an avidity test should be performed on the same serum sample. If a high-avidity test result is observed in a woman in her first trimester, acute infection during the first trimester is essentially excluded. For further decisions regarding patient management and desirability of confirmatory testing if the IgM test result is positive and the avidity test titer is low or equivocal, the reader is referred to the discussion in the "Avidity Assay" section and the section "Practical Guidelines for Diagnosis of Infection in the Pregnant Women." In patients with a positive IgG test result and a negative result on testing for IgM antibodies in the first trimester, with no clinical signs of acute toxoplasmosis, no further testing would be performed, because in the United States the probability that these women are acutely infected is extremely remote.

Some of the possible negative effects of reducing the frequency of screening as just described, as contrasted with the approach in France of screening every month, are as follows: Screening early in and throughout pregnancy provides the opportunity to reduce transmission to the fetus.[125,1077,1153] The data of Brézin and associates indicate that subsequent retinal disease is less frequent, and also less severe, in the infants born to mothers managed according to the method used by the group in Paris.[1154] Furthermore, in the third trimester, transmission rates are high and 40% of infants detected in neonatal screening programs (most infected late in gestation) already had evidence of retinal or CNS involvement or both.[124,128,605,1155,1156] Early detection of infection permits prompt treatment of infection that can cause irreversible destruction of ocular and CNS tissue in utero. Postnatal treatment leads to rapid resolution of signs of active infection.[534] Early outcomes for children who receive such treatment are considerably better than those for children who received no treatment or were given treatment for only 1 month.[497,534,1131] Nonetheless, retinal scars and neurologic damage in utero may be irreversible.[497,505] Although postnatal treatment improves outcome, some children given treatment do not experience significant improvement; and even for those who function normally, the in utero infection is not without late consequences, because cognitive outcomes for children who receive treatment are in some instances less favorable than for their uninfected siblings.[1131]

Whereas the data from France that describe better outcomes were derived from an algorithm of screening pregnant women each month,[125] no outcomes data are available for a method with less frequent screening described earlier. In late 1998 we examined the trimester of gestation of 211 consecutive women whose sera were submitted for testing to the Palo Alto laboratory: 36% of the samples were drawn in the first, 46% in the second, and 17% in the third trimester. Despite the fact that some of these sera were submitted for confirmatory testing, more than 60% were received too late in pregnancy to allow for evaluation of an avidity test result (for discussion of avidity testing, see under "Diagnosis"). Results were similar in 2004: 37% in the first, 49% in the second, and 14% in the third trimester. In the United States, almost always only a single serum specimen is made available. This is all that is available from the infant, for use in attempting to determine whether a woman has become infected during gestation. This limitation can create a serious dilemma for patients, the laboratory performing the test, and the health care providers. This experience again emphasizes the need for an organized systematic screening program. For recent discussions of the aspects (pros and cons) of systematic serologic screening, the reader is referred to various published sources.[292,292a]

At present in the United States, *T. gondii* serology is performed haphazardly by laboratories and with kits of varying quality for physicians who may understand little of the disease or the tests, and unfortunately, in many cases inappropriate decisions are made on the basis of unreliable information.[909,910] For these reasons, our present lack of systematic screening—in a setting of sporadic screening that is inadequately supervised—may result in more harm than good. We and the FDA recommend that any serologic test results that suggest that infection was acquired during pregnancy be confirmed and interpreted by a reference laboratory before decisions regarding treatment, prenatal diagnosis, or therapeutic abortion are made.[909,966] In late 1998, the Centers for Disease Control and Prevention (CDC) in Atlanta, Georgia, convened a committee of international experts to consider a number of topics in regard to *T. gondii,* primarily transmission and prevention of the infection. The major focus was on prevention of the congenital infection and infection in the pregnant woman.

Special Usefulness of the Avidity Assay Earlier in Gestation

Recently, several tests for avidity of *Toxoplasma* IgG antibodies have been introduced to help discriminate between recently acquired and distant infection.[136,502] The commercial tests are available in Europe but are not licensed in the United States. Results are based on the measurement of functional affinity of specific IgG antibodies.[136,502] IgG affinity, which initially is low after primary antigenic challenge, increases during subsequent weeks and months by antigen-driven B cell selection. Protein-denaturing reagents, including urea, are used to dissociate the antibody-antigen complex. The avidity result is determined by using the ratios of antibody titration curves of urea-treated and untreated samples.

The use of the avidity test in the acutely infected woman during the first 12 to 16 weeks of gestation was recently described.[136] The usefulness of testing for IgG avidity was evaluated in a reference laboratory in the United States. European investigators have reported that high-avidity IgG *T. gondii* antibodies exclude acute infection in the preceding 3 months. In this U.S. study, 125 serum samples taken from 125 pregnant women in the first trimester were chosen retrospectively, because either the IgM or differential agglutination (AC/HS) test in the *Toxoplasma* Serologic Profile suggested or was equivocal for a recently acquired infection. Of 93 (74.4%) serum samples with either positive or equivocal results in the IgM ELISA, 52 (55.9%) had high-avidity antibodies, which suggests that the infection probably was acquired before gestation. Of 87 (69.6%) serum samples with an acute or equivocal result in the AC/HS test, 35 (40.2%) had high-avidity antibodies. Forty women were given spiramycin in an attempt to prevent congenital transmission, and 7 (17.5%) had high-avidity antibodies. These findings highlight the value of IgG avidity testing of a single serum sample obtained in the first trimester of pregnancy for IgG avidity.

The avidity test does not establish the diagnosis of the acute infection. At present, definitive serologic diagnosis of acute infection during gestation can be made only if paired serum samples reveal a significant increase in titer, most often of IgG antibodies.[136,502] Such increasing titers are not commonly seen in pregnant women in the United States, because no systematic serologic screening to detect seroconversion is done. Although successful screening programs have been used in France and Austria for many years, in the United States, usually only a single serum sample is submitted for testing, frequently late in gestation (see Table 31-33). It is noteworthy that more than 57% of these sera were obtained from pregnant patients after the first trimester of gestation, and 14% to 21%, after the second trimester of gestation. Use of such relatively late-gestation serum samples clearly demonstrates the difficulty in attempts to prevent transmission to the fetus in the United States. Results have not changed in the past several years. As noted, almost all women in France (95%) seek prenatal care in the first trimester, because government medical benefits are then made available for the remainder of the pregnancy. Early prenatal care permits initiation of serologic screening early in gestation. This approach contrasts remarkably with that used in the United States.

Because IgM antibodies may persist for months or even years after acute infection, their greatest value is in determining that a pregnant woman was not infected recently. A negative result virtually rules out recent infection, unless serum samples are tested so late after onset of infection that IgM antibody has disappeared or so early in acute infection that an antibody response has not occurred or is not yet detectable. When results are positive, a number of additional serologic tests, including those for the detection of IgG, IgA, and IgE antibodies, and a combination of these tests, the Toxoplasma Serologic Profile (TSP), can help discriminate between recently acquired and distant infection. The differential agglutination (AC/HS) test most closely approaches a single reference standard test for the discrimination of recently acquired and distant infection. At present in the United States, however, this test is done only by the *Toxoplasma* Serology Laboratory at the Palo Alto Medical Foundation (TSL-PAMF) in Palo Alto, California, because the required antigen preparations are not commercially available. In addition, as is true for IgM antibodies, an acute pattern in the AC/HS test may persist for longer than 1 year.

Liesenfeld and co-workers investigated the usefulness of testing for avidity of IgG antibodies in a *Toxoplasma* serology reference laboratory in the United States that processes serum samples primarily from pregnant women.[136] In most cases, the physician requests information about the time of onset of the infection on the basis of results obtained from a single serum sample. The goal of these investigators was to compare results obtained in an IgG avidity test with those obtained in the IgM ELISA and AC/HS tests.

All pregnant women who have a positive result on IgM *T. gondii* serologic testing should have an IgG avidity test performed. This test is most valuable in the first 12 to 16 weeks of gestation (see under "Diagnosis"). In two reference laboratories, the results from the AC/HS test complement the information provided by the avidity assay. The avidity assay is particularly useful in the first 4 months of gestation when IgM is present and the AC/HS test result is acute or equivocal. Time of conversion from low or equivocal to high avidity is highly variable among persons tested. Once a high-avidity test result is obtained, it can be concluded that the patient was infected at least 3 to 5 months earlier. Low-avidity test results should not be interpreted to mean recently acquired infection. The reason is that low-avidity antibodies may persist for as long as 1 year, and borderline or low-avidity antibodies can persist in the presence or absence of *T. gondii*–specific IgM antibodies. Forty percent of women with *T. gondii*–specific IgG but no IgM antibodies had borderline or low-avidity antibodies in one study.[137]

The avidity test is best used in conjunction with a panel of tests, for example, *T. gondii*–specific IgG, IgM, IgA and AC/HS tests. The avidity test should not be used alone; results should be interpreted in the context of other serologic tests that indicate acute infection in the first 12 to 16 weeks of gestation. The avidity test can be used to assess whether acute acquired infection in the mother that is first detected late in gestation was acquired more than 12 to 16 weeks earlier. This provides information about risk to the fetus.

Prevention of Congenital Toxoplasmosis through Treatment of the Pregnant Woman

For the special instance of the pregnant woman with HIV infection, see earlier section, "Congenital *Toxoplasma gondii* Infection and Acquired Immunodeficiency Syndrome," under "Clinical Manifestations."

Acute Infection

ANTIMICROBIAL THERAPY

Treatment during pregnancy (see also "Treatment of the Fetus through Treatment of the Pregnant Woman") has been employed in an attempt to decrease both the incidence and the severity of congenital infection. This treatment is administered to a pregnant woman with a recently acquired (acute) infection in the hope that such treatment will prevent spread of infection to the fetus. The rationale for such treatment is based on the observation that there is a significant lag period between the onset of maternal infection and infection of the fetus. In the first such study, performed in Germany, Kräubig used a combination of sulfonamides and pyrimethamine.[121,1157] Because of its potential teratogenic effects, pyrimethamine was not administered during the first 12 to 14 weeks of gestation. Kräubig noted a definite reduction in incidence of congenitally acquired infection in infants born to mothers who received treatment (5%) versus those who did not (16.6%)—a 70% reduction (prevention). Kräubig considered these data an indication that treatment is necessary if a diagnosis of acute acquired toxoplasmosis is made during pregnancy. Thalhammer, who closely collaborated in these studies with Kräubig, agreed with this statement, because it appears that all cases of congenital toxoplasmosis might be prevented by such an approach.[1158,1159] In 1982, Hengst from Berlin reported similar results in a prospective study.[1160]

In a separate and independent study performed in France,[116] daily oral doses of 2 to 3 g of spiramycin in four divided doses were administered for 3 weeks to women who acquired toxoplasmosis during pregnancy. Such courses of treatment were arbitrarily repeated at 2-week intervals up to the time of delivery. Only women who completed at least one such course were considered to have undergone treatment. Cases of congenital *T. gondii* infection were significantly more frequent among 154 women who received no treatment (58%) than among 388 women who received treatment (23%). Clinically apparent disease in the newborns, however, was just as frequent among children born with congenital *T. gondii* infection from both groups of women (28% and 27% of infected offspring, respectively). This finding suggests that spiramycin treatment in the pregnant woman might have reduced by 60% the frequency of transmission of *T. gondii* to the offspring but did not apparently modify the pattern of infection in the infected fetus. Although the difference between treated and untreated groups is highly significant, however, the pregnant women in this study who received no treatment do not represent a good control group for several reasons. Most women diagnosed in their first trimester received treatment, whereas the proportion of women who received no treatment is rather low among women who acquired *T. gondii* infection during the last months of pregnancy. Thus, more infections occurred earlier in the treated group than in the untreated group, a fact that of itself might have led to fewer congenital infections and to a higher proportion of cases with clinical disease among infected infants, if untreated. Nevertheless, congenital infections were less frequent in the treated group in each trimester of pregnancy. Consequently, the decrease in fetal infections could be assumed to reflect bias not only in the selection of cases but in treatment as well.

Variability in the clinical aspects of congenital infection also must be considered. Table 31-63 shows the comparison between treated and untreated groups of pregnant women. No difference in the proportion of mild and subclinical cases was found. By contrast, the number of stillbirths decreased and the proportion of children born alive with severe disease increased slightly in the treated group. The numbers are too small to be significant, but the reason for the increase in incidence of severe disease despite treatment during fetal life is that the treatment, although undertaken too late to prevent severe damage, might sometimes have prevented fetal death.

Table 31–63 Effect of Spiramycin Treatment on Relative Frequency of Stillbirth and on Different Aspects of Congenital Toxoplasmosis

Outcome in Offspring	No. (%) of Affected Offspring: *No Treatment*	*Treatment*
Congenital toxoplasmosis		
Subclinical	64 (68)	65 (72)
Mild	14 (15)	13 (14)
Severe	7 (7)	10 (11)
Stillbirth or perinatal death[a]	9 (10)	3 (3)
Total	94 (100)	91 (100)

[a]See text.

Adapted from Desmonts G, Couvreur J. Congenital toxoplasmosis: a prospective study of the offspring of 542 women who acquired toxoplasmosis during pregnancy: pathophysiology of congenital disease. *In* Thalhammer O, Baumgarten K, Pollak A (eds). Perinatal Medicine, Sixth European Congress, Vienna. Stuttgart, Georg Thieme, 1979, pp 51-60, with permission.

A prospective study that compares the efficacy of spiramycin versus pyrimethamine plus sulfonamide for prevention of congenital transmission has not been performed. When compared with data obtained from historical controls, the more recent studies suggest the importance of the pyrimethamine plus sulfonamide regimen. Each of the studies involved an attempt to isolate the organism from placentas. In one such study of 32 women, each of whose fetuses was diagnosed as being infected by isolation of the parasite from amniotic fluid or blood between weeks 24 and 30 of gestation (update of originally published data[117]), infection in the mothers was documented to have occurred between weeks 10 and 29 of gestation. The mothers were given 3 g of spiramycin daily as soon as the diagnosis of their acute acquired infection was made. Pyrimethamine plus sulfonamide was given during the last 2 months of gestation. Because of the potential hazard for mother or fetus, use of the combination of pyrimethamine plus sulfonamide was restricted by Couvreur and colleagues to the last 2 months of gestation and to a high-risk group in which fetal infection was documented during pregnancy. *T. gondii* was isolated from 47% of the placentas (examined after delivery) from these 32 cases. In marked contrast, *T. gondii* was isolated from 71.5% of placentas of 21 infants born to mothers who received spiramycin alone and, using historical controls, from 89% of placentas of 85 infants born to mothers who received an inadequate spiramycin regimen (duration of treatment less than 2 weeks or daily dose of only 2 g, which is considered by the investigators to be too low) or who receined no treatment. In Austria, Aspöck and colleagues routinely use spiramycin before week 16 of gestation and pyrimethamine plus a sulfonamide after week 15 of gestation. In their prospective study, this treatment regimen was highly successful.[304]

Although critical appraisal of these studies does not permit a definite conclusion about the efficacy of treatment during pregnancy in the prevention of congenital toxoplasmosis, the data strongly suggest that treatment is effective. In addition, because spiramycin also may delay transmission of the parasite to the fetus, it should have the added benefit of reducing the severity of the disease in the fetus and newborn because of the increased maturity of the maternal immune response and of the fetus at the time infection occurs. Critically designed studies are needed to clarify this question. Nevertheless, until such data become available—and in view of the prevention rate of congenital infection of 60% to 70% achieved in the two studies mentioned earlier—it would appear prudent to advise treatment in women who acquire the infection during pregnancy. The dose of spiramycin is 3 g per day. Toxicity has not proved to be a problem with spiramycin in such cases. This drug is at present available in the United States only by request to the FDA. Pyrimethamine plus sulfadiazine can be employed in the second and third trimesters of pregnancy with the precautionary measures mentioned earlier in the "Therapy" section (see also "Treatment of the Fetus In Utero"). Whether sequelae in infected children who received treatment in utero are as frequent or as serious as those in children who received no treatment is a question that can be answered only by long-term observation.

Repeated here are our recommendations made previously in "Treatment of the Fetus through Treatment of the Pregnant Woman."

When the diagnosis of infection in the fetus is established earlier than 17 weeks, we suggest that sulfadiazine be used alone until after the first trimester, at which time pyrimethamine should be added to the regimen. The decision about when to begin pyrimethamine/sulfadiazine/leucovorin for the pregnant woman is based on an assessment of the risk of fetal infection, incidence of false-positive and false-negative results of amniocentesis with PCR, and risks of medicines. Although reliability of PCR results are laboratory dependent, results from the best reference laboratories, between 17 and 21 weeks' gestation, have a sensitivity for PCR of the *T. gondii* B1 gene with amniotic fluid of 92.9 (CI 87.9-96.8). Thus, PCR results reasonably determine the therapeutic approach.

When the mother becomes infected between 22 and 29 weeks of gestation, the incidence of transmission exceeds 50%, manifestations of infection in the fetus are substantial, and sensitivity of PCR (*T. gondii* B1 gene) in amniotic fluid is less than 62.5% (CI 38.8-86.2) for 22 to 26 weeks and less than 68.4% (CI 47.5-89.3) for 27 to 31 weeks.[838] With maternal acquisition of infection after 31 weeks of gestation, incidence of transmission exceeds 60%, manifestations of infection are in general less severe, and sensitivity of PCR in amniotic fluid is less than 50% (CI 21.7-78.3).

When infection is acquired between 21 and 29 weeks of gestation, management varies. After 24 weeks of gestation, we recommend that amniocentesis be performed and that pyrimethamine/leucovorin/sulfadiazine be used instead of spiramycin. At the time of this writing, available data (see Fig. 31-18) in regard to the reliability of PCR results make a definitive recommendation concerning manifestations of women whose infections were acquired between 21 and 24 weeks of gestation with negative amniotic fluid PCR results difficult. Consultation with the reference laboratory is advised.

In France, standard of care (until late in gestation) is to wait 4 weeks from the estimated time that maternal infection is acquired until amniocentesis to allow sufficient time for transmission to occur. Amniocentesis is not performed before 17 to 18 weeks of gestation. In some instances, when maternal infection is acquired between 12 and 16 weeks of gestation or after the 21st week of gestation, pyrimethamine and sulfadiazine treatment is initiated regardless of the amniotic fluid PCR result. This is because of concerns about the confidence intervals and reliability of negative amniotic fluid PCR results. When this approach is used, a delay in amniocentesis when maternal infection is acquired between 12 and 16 weeks and after 21 weeks of gestation would not be logical.

Termination of Pregnancy

Confirmatory serologic testing in a reference laboratory and communication of the results and their correct interpretation by an expert to the patient's physician decreased the rate of unnecessary pregnancy terminations by approximately 50% among women with positive IgM *Toxoplasma* antibody test results reported by outside laboratories.[136]

The decision whether to treat with antimicrobial agents or to perform an abortion in a woman suspected of acquiring *T. gondii* infection during pregnancy should ultimately be made by the patient in conjunction with her physician after careful consideration of the potential results with each of these two modalities of intervention. Therapeutic abortion may be considered in women who are known to have acquired acute *T. gondii* infection early during gestation or in whom the likelihood of their having acquired acute infection early during gestation is very high. Only approximately 22% of women who acquire primary *T. gondii* infection during the first 22 to 24 weeks of gestation transmit the infection to their offspring. Even if all women who acquire the infection during the first two trimesters were to elect abortion, less than one half of all cases of congenital toxoplasmosis would be prevented, because more than 50% of infected offspring result from maternal infection acquired in the last trimester.

Prenatal examination has for the first time allowed for an objective decision by the pregnant woman in regard to abortion and whether her aborted fetus would indeed be congenitally infected. Such a decision was previously based on a statistical estimation of the risk to the fetus. Considerable controversy has arisen in regard to whether and under what circumstances abortion might be considered. The controversy appears to have stemmed from the publication by Berrebi and colleagues in *The Lancet*,[992] who concluded that only ultrasonographic evidence of hydrocephalus indicates a poor outcome; for this reason they no longer use the gestational age-related statistics that Daffos and colleagues propose[130] to counsel affected couples.[998] Berrebi's group studied 163 mothers who acquired their infection with *T. gondii* before 28 weeks of gestation. All were given spiramycin treatment, and 23 also received pyrimethamine and sulfadiazine. Each underwent cordocentesis and regular ultrasound examinations. Their 162 live-born infants were evaluated over 15 to 71 months. Three fetuses died in utero, and 27 of 162 live-born infants had congenital toxoplasmosis: 10 had clinical signs of the infection, 5 with isolated or multiple intracranial calcifications, 7 with peripheral chorioretinitis, and 2 with moderate ventricular dilation. Because each of the 27 was free of symptoms and demonstrated normal neurologic development at 15 to 71 months of age, the investigators concluded that acute fetal infection identified in first- and second-trimester pregnancies need not be an indication for interruption of the pregnancy if fetal ultrasonographic evaluation results are normal (no evidence of fetal death or hydrocephalus) and treatment of the fetus is instigated.

In a letter to the editor of *The Lancet* commenting on the results of Berrebi and associates, Wallon and co-workers[1125] also were conservative in their conclusions. From the results of their studies, they recommend that termination not be performed unless fetal ultrasonographic examination reveals morphologic abnormalities. By contrast, in a simultaneously published letter to the editor of *The Lancet,* Daffos and colleagues[1149] concurred that too many pregnancies are terminated because congenital toxoplasmosis is diagnosed prenatally, but these authors were far less optimistic than Berrebi and associates about the outcome for the fetus infected early in gestation. Daffos and colleagues stated that in a study of 148 fetal infections diagnosed by prenatal examination, "the best (and perhaps the only) factor with predictive value for the severity of the fetal infection is gestational age at the time of maternal infection." In their study, they noted that if the infection occurred before 16 weeks of gestation, 31 of 52 fetuses (60%) had ultrasonographic evidence of infection, including ascites, pericarditis, or necrotic foci in the brain, and 48% had cerebral ventricular dilatation. If infection had occurred between 17 and 23 weeks, 16 of 63 fetuses (25%) had ultrasonographic signs, and only 12% had ventricular dilatation. In those cases of infection after 24 weeks, only 1 of 33 fetuses (3%) had ultrasonographic signs, and none had hydrocephalus. Thus, the approach that Daffos and his colleagues had recommended 6 years earlier[130] appeared to remain valid. These workers accept parental requests for termination in those cases in which infection occurs before 16 weeks because of the severe prognosis for the fetus. In such instances, they have always found large areas of brain necrosis at necropsy, even when there was no evidence of ventricular dilatation on ultrasound evaluation. They conclude that such dilatation of the ventricles would have developed in many of these cases if the pregnancy had been allowed to continue, even if treatment with pyrimethamine and sulfadiazine was used. It is hoped that in the near future this issue will be resolved by a collaborative effort to review all pertinent data by interested investigators and, if necessary, to design studies aimed at formulating a consensus and guidelines for providing the patient with objective information during counseling about termination of pregnancy. In one study[838] in which real-time PCR analysis was evaluated, quantitation of the PCR revealed that higher parasite burden in amniotic fluid is associated with more damage to the fetus (see also section on PCR).

Despite the fact that IgM tests do not differentiate between acute and chronic infection, a positive IgM test result strongly influences pregnant women in their choice to terminate or continue the pregnancy. In the United States, such decisions often are made on the basis of results for a single serum specimen in which the result of IgM antibody testing is positive and confirmatory testing is not done. We previously estimated that approximately 20% of women who are told that they have a positive result on IgM antibody testing will request therapeutic abortion.[1161] In that study, approximately 60% of the results of IgM tests reported as positive by commercial laboratories were negative in the IgM test in the Palo Alto reference laboratory. In the cases with reported positive IgM test results, evidence of recently acquired infection, as determined by the *Toxoplasma* Serologic Profile, also was absent. Thus, at a minimum, 12 of every 20 fetuses that were *not infected* were aborted. In a more recent study, Liesenfeld and associates[1161] from the same laboratory determined the accuracy of *T. gondii* serologic test results obtained in commercial laboratories and the role of confirmatory testing in preventing unnecessary abortion. Congenital toxoplasmosis is a preventable disease. It is therefore the responsibility of health professionals who provide care for pregnant women to educate them on how they can prevent themselves from becoming infected (and thereby not place their fetus at risk). Lack of adoption of a systematic serologic screening program in the United States leaves education as the principal means of preventing this tragic disease.

Physicians who recommend or perform an abortion must be knowledgeable about the subject so that an intelligent decision can be made. Because abortions are performed as late as 22 to 24 weeks of gestation in the United States, the practitioner has time to obtain an initial serologic specimen early in gestation and a follow-up specimen later in gestation to define those women at risk of transmitting *T. gondii* to their offspring (see "Serologic Screening" section). Guidelines for the interpretation of serologic tests on specimens obtained during pregnancy have been given previously in the "Diagnosis" section. If tests for IgM antibodies to *T. gondii* are unavailable to assist in establishing the diagnosis of acute infection, it should be understood that the risk of congenital toxoplasmosis is almost zero in a patient whose serum shows a high IgG test titer in the second month of pregnancy. A high IgG test titer at that time indicates an infection that occurred at least 2 months before (and perhaps much earlier) in all but rare exceptions in which the serologic test titer rises steeply for several weeks. On the contrary, women who will later give birth to a congenitally infected infant, when examined during the second or third month of pregnancy, either have no antibody (i.e., they are not yet infected) or may have a low titer (associated with IgM antibody) as a result of an infection acquired during the past few days or weeks. A careful follow-up examination and confirmatory testing in a reference laboratory along with amniocentesis for PCR assay and mouse inoculation may reveal infection in the fetus in time to allow for consideration of termination of the pregnancy in these cases. Treatment for the infected mother to attempt to prevent transmission of the infection to the fetus appears more worthy of consideration in such circumstances.

Chronic (Latent) Infection

The controversial subjects of congenital transmission, repeated abortion, and perinatal fetal mortality during chronic (latent) infection have already been discussed. A review of the pertinent literature on this controversy is available.[1162] In an attempt to prevent infection and reduce fetal wastage, a series of women who had had previous abortions, premature

Table 31–64 Some Pertinent Resources and Telephone Numbers/Internet Sites

Reference laboratory for serology, isolation, and PCR assay (U.S.)	650-853-4828
Reference laboratory for serology, isolation, and PCR assay (France)	33-1-40-44-39-41
FDA for IND number to obtain spiramycin for treatment for a pregnant woman (U.S.)	301-827-2335
FDA Public Health Advisory	301-594-3060
Spiramycin (Aventis) for treatment for a pregnant woman (U.S.)	908-231-3365
Congenital Toxoplasmosis Study Group (U.S.)	773-834-4152
Educational pamphlet/The March of Dimes (U.S.): "Prevention of Congenital Toxoplasmosis"	312-435-4007
Educational pamphlet: "Congenital Toxoplasmosis: The Hidden Threat"	1-800-323-9100
Educational pamphlet: "Toxoplasmosis," NIH publication No. 83-308	301-496-5717 www.naid.nih.gov
Information concerning AIDS and congenital toxoplasmosis (U.S.)	305-243-6522
Educational information on the Internet	www.toxoplasmosis.org

AIDS, acquired immunodeficiency syndrome; FDA, U.S. Food and Drug Administration; IND, Investigational New Drug; NIH, National Institutes of Health; PCR, polymerase chain reaction.

births, or similar misfortunes were given pyrimethamine treatment by Cech and Jirovec of Prague.[702] A marked reduction in perinatal fetal mortality rate was observed in those women who received treatment. The investigators interpreted their results as showing a remarkable effect of pyrimethamine on the outcome of pregnancy in the skin test–positive women. Their results appear to be very favorable, but because the study was uncontrolled, these results must be interpreted with caution. Studies along the same line are those of Eckerling and associates in Israel[1163] and others.[1164,1165,1166] Results reported by Sharf and co-workers in Israel[1167] suggested an etiologic relationship between latent maternal toxoplasmosis and spontaneous abortions, premature deliveries, and stillbirths. A number of such women were given pyrimethamine and triple sulfonamides before their next pregnancy and sulfonamides alone during pregnancy. The researchers interpreted their results as evidence that such treatment significantly increased the chance of a successful outcome of the pregnancy. Unfortunately, their controls were poorly defined and appear inadequate for statistical analysis.

Kimball and colleagues stated that, despite the association of antibodies to *T. gondii* with sporadic abortion noted by them, there is no evidence that therapy to prevent abortion should be administered routinely to pregnant women with antibodies to *T. gondii*—even those with high titers.[165] In their series, there was a significantly greater incidence of abortions in patients with CF test titers of 1:8 or higher than in those with titers 1:4 or lower ($P < .01$). But they considered it unwarranted to recommend therapy to a group of pregnant women of whom only 10% could be expected to abort without therapy. Whether therapy for toxoplasmosis in patients with CF test titers of 1:8 or higher who are threatening to abort would be beneficial is unknown.

The question must now be raised whether there is sufficient evidence to warrant the routine prophylactic use of a drug with toxic and teratogenic potential against *T. gondii* in pregnant women who have positive serologic titers and a history of chronic abortion. Until the controversy is resolved by further evidence justifying the risk of therapy, the only conclusion that can be made is that pyrimethamine must not be used in such cases.[164,1168] There are continued reports of use of such treatment.[1169]

RESOURCES

A summary of useful resources with means to contact the relevant agencies is presented in Table 31-64.

ACKNOWLEDGMENTS

We are sincerely grateful to Drs. Jacques Couvreur, Fernand Daffos, J. P. Dubey, Jose G. Montoya, and Oliver Liesenfeld for their advice and help in the preparation of this chapter.

We thank Drs. V. Mirlesse, F. Daffos, E. Diniz, and G. Noble for providing their data for inclusion in this chapter. We appreciate the assistance of Lara Kallal, Diana Chamot, and Peggy Wakeman.

The work on which this chapter is based was supported by grants AI 04717, AI 302230, AI 27530, and AI 16945 from the National Institutes of Health and the Research to Prevent Blindness Foundation.

REFERENCES

1. Wilson CB, Remington JS. What can be done to prevent congenital toxoplasmosis? Am J Obstet Gynecol 138:357-363, 1980.
2. Roberts T, Frenkel JK. Estimating income losses and other preventable costs caused by congenital toxoplasmosis in people in the United States. J Am Vet Med Assoc 196:249-256, 1990.
3. Nicolle C, Manceaux L. Sur une infection a corps de Leishman (ou organismes voisins) du gondi. Compte Rendu Hebdomadaire des Seances de l'Academie des Sciences 146:207-209, 1908.
4. Nicolle C, Manceaux L. Sur un protozoaire nouveau de gondi, *Toxoplasma*. Arch Inst Pasteur (Tunis) 2:97-103, 1909.
5. Splendore A. A new protozoan parasite in rabbits. *In* Kean BH, Mott KE, Russell AJ (eds). Tropical Medicine and Parasitology: Classical Investigations. Ithaca, Cornell University Press, 1908, pp 272-274.
6. Janku J. Pathogenesa a pathologicka anatomie tak nazvaneho vrozeneho kolobomu zlute skvrny v oku normalne velikem a mikrophthalmickem s nalezem parazitu v sitnici. Cas Lek Ces 62: 1021-1027, 1054-1059, 1081-1085, 1111-1115, 1138-1144, 1923.
7. Levaditi C. Au sujet de certaines protozooses hereditaires humaines à localization oculaires et nerveuses. C R Soc Biol (Paris) 98: 297-299, 1928.
8. Wolf A, Cowen D. Granulomatous encephalomyelitis due to an encephalitozoon (encephalitozoic encephalomyelitis): a new protozoan disease of man. Bull Neurol Inst N Y 6:306-371, 1937.
9. Sabin AB, Olitsky PK. *Toxoplasma* and obligate intracellular parasitism. Science 85:336-338, 1937.
10. Wolf A, Cowen D. Granulomatous encephalomyelitis due to a protozoan (*Toxoplasma* or *Encephalitozoon*): II. Identification of a case from the literature. Bull Neurol Inst N Y 7:266-283, 1938.
11. Wolf A, Cowen D, Paige BH. Toxoplasmic encephalomyelitis III. A new case of granulomatous encephalomyelitis due to a protozoon. Am J Pathol 15:657-694, 1939.

12. Paige BH, Cowen D, Wolf A. Toxoplasmic encephalomyelitis. V. Further observations of infantile toxoplasmosis; intrauterine inception of the disease; visceral manifestations. Am J Dis Child 63:474-514, 1942.
13. Wolf A, Cowen D. Human toxoplasmosis: occurrence in infants as an encephalomyelitis. Verification by transmission to animals. *In* Kean BH, Mott KE, Russell AJ (eds). Tropical Medicine and Parasitology: Classical Investigations. Chapter 13. Ithaca, Cornell University Press, 1939, pp 282-284.
14. Wolf A, Cowen D, Paige B. Toxoplasmic encephalomyelitis. Trans Am Neurol Assoc 65:76-79, 1939.
15. Pinkerton H, Weinman D. *Toxoplasma* infection in man. Acta Pathol 30:374-392, 1940.
16. Pinkerton H, Henderson RG. Adult toxoplasmosis. JAMA 116: 807-814, 1941.
17. Sabin AB. Toxoplasmic encephalitis in children. JAMA 116:801-807, 1941.
18. Sabin AB, Feldman HA. Dyes as microchemical indicators of a new immunity phenomenon affecting a protozoan parasite (*Toxoplasma*). Science 108:660-663, 1948.
19. Frenkel JK. Toxoplasmosis: Parasite life cycle pathology and immunology. *In* Hammond DM, Long PL (eds). The Coccidia. Baltimore, University Park Press, 1973, pp 343-410.
20. Levine N. Sarcocystis, *Toxoplasma*, and related protozoa. *In* Protozoan Parasites, 2nd ed. Minneapolis, Burgess Publishing, 1973, pp 288-316.
21. Beaman M, Remington J. Cytokines and resistance against *Toxoplasma gondii*: evidence from in vivo and in vitro studies. *In* Sonnenfeld G, Czarniecki C, Nacy C, et al (eds). Cytokines and Resistance to Nonviral Pathogenic Infections. New York, Biomedical Press, 1992, pp 111-119.
22. McLeod R, Mack D, Brown C. *Toxoplasma gondii*—new advances in cellular and molecular biology. Exp Parasitol 72:109-121, 1991.
23. Wong SY, Remington JS. Biology of *Toxoplasma gondii*. *In* Broder SMT, Bolognesi D (eds). Textbook of AIDS Medicine. Baltimore, Williams & Wilkins, 1994, pp 223-258.
24. Cesbron M-F, Dubremetz J-F, Sher A. The immunobiology of toxoplasmosis. Res Immunol 144:7-8, 1993.
25. Dubey JP, Lindsay DS, Speer CA. Structures of *Toxoplasma gondii* tachyzoites, bradyzoites, and sporozoites and biology and development of tissue cysts. Clin Microbiol Rev 11:267-299, 1998.
26. Mercier C, Cesbron-Delauw MF, Sibley LD. The amphipathic alpha helices of the *Toxoplasma* protein GRA2 mediate post-secretory membrane association. J Cell Sci 111:2171-2180, 1998.
27. Sibley LD, Howe DK. Genetic basis of pathogenicity in toxoplasmosis. *In* Gross U (ed). Current Topics in Microbiology and Immunity: *Toxoplasma gondii*. Vo. 219. New York, Springer, 1996, pp 3-15.
28. Hunter CA, Subauste CS, Remington JS. The role of cytokines in toxoplasmosis. Biotherapy 7:237-247, 1994.
29. Alexander J, Hunter CA. Immunoregulation during toxoplasmosis. Chem Immunol 70:81-102, 1998.
30. Denkers EY, Gazzinelli RT. Regulation and function of T-cell-mediated immunity during *Toxoplasma gondii* infection. Clin Microbiol Rev 11:569-588, 1998.
31. Sibley LD. *Toxoplasma gondii*: perfecting an intracellular life style. Traffic 4:581-586, 2003.
32. Denkers EY. From cells to signaling cascades: manipulation of innate immunity by *Toxoplasma gondii*. FEMS Immunol Med Microbiol 39:193-203, 2003.
33. Roberts CW, Roberts F, Henriquez FL, et al. Evidence for mitochondrial-derived alternative oxidase in the apicomplexan parasite *Cryptosporidium parvum*: a potential anti-microbial agent target. Int J Parasitol 34:297-308, 2004.
34. Campbell SA, Richards TA, Mui EJ, et al. A complete shikimate pathway in *Toxoplasma gondii*: an ancient eukaryotic innovation. Int J Parasitol 34:5-13, 2004.
35. Huang J, Mullapudi N, Sicheritz-Ponten T, Kissinger JC. A first glimpse into the pattern and scale of gene transfer in apicomplexa. Int J Parasitol 34:265-274, 2004.
36. Dubey JP, Frenkel JK. Feline toxoplasmosis from acutely infected mice and the development of *Toxoplasma* cysts. J Protozool 23: 537-546, 1976.
37. Freyre A, Dubey JP, Smith DD, Frenkel JK. Oocyst-induced *Toxoplasma gondii* infections in cats. J Parasitol 75:750-755, 1989.
38. Dubey JP, Miller NL, Frenkel JK. Characterization of the new fecal form of *Toxoplasma gondii*. J Parasitol 56:447-456, 1970.
39. Dubey JP, Miller NL, Frenkel JK. The *Toxoplasma gondii* oocyst from cat feces. J Exp Med 132:636-662, 1970.
40. Frenkel JK, Dubey JP, Miller NL. *Toxoplasma gondii* in cats: faecal stages identified as coccidian oocysts. Science 167:893-896, 1970.
41. Manwell RD, Drobeck HP. The behavior of *Toxoplasma* with notes on its taxonomic status. J Parasitol 39:577-584, 1953.
42. Sibley LD, Hakansson S, Carruthers VB. Gliding motility: an efficient mechanism for cell penetration. Cur Biol 8:R12-R4, 1998.
43. Jacobs L, Remington JS, Melton ML. The resistance of the encysted form of *Toxoplasma gondii*. J Parasitol 46:11-21, 1960.
44. Jacobs L. The biology of *Toxoplasma*. Am J Trop Med Hyg 2:365-389, 1953.
45. Cook MK, Jacobs L. Cultivation of *Toxoplasma gondii* in tissue cultures of various derivations. J Parasitol 44:172-182, 1958.
46. Kaufman HE, Melton ML, Remington JS, Jacobs L. Strain differences of *Toxoplasma gondii*. J Parasitol 45:189-190, 1959.
47. Suss-Toby E, Zimmerberg J, Ward GE. *Toxoplasma* invasion: the parasitophorous vacuole is formed from host cell plasma membrane and pinches off via a fission pore. Proc Natl Acad Sci U S A 93: 8413-8418, 1996.
48. Sibley LD, Krahenbuhl JL, Adams GM, Weidner E. *Toxoplasma* modifies macrophage phagosomes by secretion of a vesicular network rich in surface proteins. J Cell Biol 103:867-874, 1986.
49. Sinai AP, Webster P, Joiner KA. Association of host cell endoplasmic reticulum and mitochondria with the *Toxoplasma gondii* parasitophorous vacuole membrane: a high affinity interaction. J Cell Sci 110:2117-2128, 1997.
50. Goldman M, Carver RK, Sulzer AJ. Similar internal morphology of *Toxoplasma gondii* and *Besnoitia jellisoni* stained with silver protein. J Parasitol 43:490-491, 1957.
51. Bommer W, Hofling KH, Heunert HH. Multiplication of *Toxoplasma* in cell cultures. Dtsch Med Wochenschr 94:1000-1002, 1969.
52. Lund E, Lycke E, Sourander P. A cinematographic study of *Toxoplasma gondii* in cell cultures. Br J Exp Pathol 42:357-362, 1961.
53. Hirai K, Hirato K, Yanagwa R. A cinematographic study of the penetration of cultured cells by *Toxoplasma gondii*. Jpn J Vet Res 14:83-90, 1966.
54. Jones TC, Yeh S, Hirsch JG. The interaction between *Toxoplasma gondii* and mammalian cells. I. Mechanism of entry and intracellular fate of the parasite. J Exp Med 136:1157-1172, 1972.
55. Remington J, discussion in Laison R. Observations on the nature and transmission of *Toxoplasma* in the light of its wide host and geographical range. Surv Ophthalmol 6:721-758, 1961.
56. Lainson R. Observations on the development and nature of pseudocysts and cysts of *Toxoplasma gondii*. Trans R Soc Trop Med Hyg 52:396-407, 1958.
57. Remington JS, Cavanaugh EN. Isolation of the encysted form of *Toxoplasma gondii* from human skeletal muscle and brain. N Engl J Med 273:1308-1310, 1965.
58. Kotula AW, Dubey JP, Sharar AK, et al. Effect of freezing on infectivity of *Toxoplasma gondii* tissue cysts in pork. J Parasitol 54:687-690, 1991.
59. Dubey JP. Effect of freezing on the infectivity of *Toxoplasma* cysts to cats. J Am Vet Med Assoc 165:534-536, 1974.
60. Work K. Resistance of *Toxoplasma gondii* encysted in pork. Acta Pathol Microbiol Scand 73:85-92, 1968.
61. Bohne W, Hessemann J, Gross U. Reduced replication of *Toxoplasma gondii* is necessary for induction of bradyzoite-specific antigens: a possible role for nitric oxide in triggering stage conversion. Infect Immun 62:1761-1767, 1994.
62. Soete M, Camus D, Dubremetz J. Experimental induction of bradyzoite-specific antigen expression and cyst formation by the RH strain of *Toxoplasma gondii* in vitro. Exp Parasitol 78:361-370, 1994.
63. Ferguson DJ, Hutchison WM. The host-parasite relationship of *Toxoplasma gondii* in the brains of chronically infected mice. Virchows Arch [A] 411:39-43, 1987.
64. Fox BA, Gigley JP, Bzik DJ. *Toxoplasma gondii* lacks the enzymes required for de novo arginine biosynthesis and arginine starvation triggers cyst formation. Int J Parasitol 34:323-331, 2004.
65. Gross U, Bohne W, Soête M, Dubremetz JF. Developmental differentiation between tachyzoites and bradyzoites of *Toxoplasma gondii*. Parasitol Today 12:30-33, 1996.
66. Weiss LM, Kim K. The development and biology of bradyzoites of *Toxoplasma gondii*. Front Biosci 5:D391-D405, 2000.
67. Jacobs L. New knowledge of *Toxoplasma* and toxoplasmosis. Adv Parasitol 11:631-669, 1973.

68. Hogan MJ, Yoneda C, Feeney L, et al. Morphology and culture of *Toxoplasma*. Arch Ophthalmol 64:655-667, 1960.
69. Lindsay DS, Dubey JP, Blagburn BL, Toivio-Kinnucan M. Examination of tissue cyst formation by *Toxoplasma gondii* in cell cultures using bradyzoites, tachyzoites, and sporozoites. J Parasitol 77:126-132, 1991.
70. Frenkel JK, Friedlander S. Toxoplasmosis: Pathology of Neonatal Disease. Washington, DC, US Government Printing Office, 1952.
71. Elsaid MM, Martins MS, Frezard F, et al. Vertical toxoplasmosis in a murine model. Protection after immunization with antigens of *Toxoplasma gondii* incorporated into liposomes. Mem Inst Oswaldo Cruz 96:99-104, 2001.
72. Ferro EA, Silva DA, Bevilacqua E, Mineo JR. Effect of *Toxoplasma gondii* infection kinetics on trophoblast cell population in *Calomys callosus*, a model of congenital toxoplasmosis. Infect Immun 70: 7089-7094, 2002.
73. Frenkel JK, Parker BB. An apparent role of dogs in the transmission of *Toxoplasma gondii*. Ann N Y Acad Sci 791:402-407, 1996.
74. Roberts C, Brewer J, Alexander J. Congenital toxoplasmosis in the Balb/c mouse: prevention of vertical disease transmission and fetal death by vaccination. Vaccine 12:1389-1394, 1994.
75. Zenner L, Estaquier J, Darcy F, et al. Protective immunity in the rat model of congenital toxoplasmosis and the potential of excreted-secreted antigens as vaccine components. Parasite Immunol 21: 261-272, 1999.
76. Hellbrugge T. [Fetal infection in the course of the acute and chronic phase in latent rat toxoplasmosis.] Arch f Gynak 186:384-388, 1955.
77. Dubey JP, Shen SK, Kwok OCH, Thulliez P. Toxoplasmosis in rats (*Rattus norvegicus*): congenital transmission to first and second generation offspring and isolation of *Toxoplasma gondii* from seronegative rats. Parasitology 115:9-14, 1997.
78. Remington JS, Jacobs L, Melton ML. Congenital transmission of toxoplasmosis from mother animals with acute and chronic infections. J Infect Dis 108:163-173, 1961.
79. Hellbrugge T, Dahme E. Experimentelle Toxoplasmose: Bemerkungen zur Arbeit von Schultz und Bauer über Placentarbefunde bei Ratten. Klin Wochenschr 31:789-791, 1953.
80. Wildfuhr G. Tierexperimentelle Untersuchungen beim vor der Gravidatat infizierten Muttertier. *In* Forschung Untersuchungen Ergebnisse. Leipzig, Universitat Klinisches Institut, 1954, p 161.
81. Thiermann E. Transmission congenita del *Toxoplasma gondii* enrates con infection leve. Biologica (Chile) 23:59-67, 1957.
82. Wildfuhr G. Experimental animal studies to study the diaplacental transmission of toxoplasmen in a mother animal infected before pregnancy. Ztschr Immunitatsforsch Exp Ther 111:110-120, 1954.
83. Huldt G. Experimental toxoplasmosis. Transplacental transmission in guinea pigs. Acta Pathol Microbiol Scand 49:176-188, 1960.
84. Janitschke K, Jorren HR. Studies on the significance of intrauterine infection for the prevalence of *Toxoplasma* in domestic rabbits. Z Tropenmed Parasitol 21:246-251, 1970.
85. Beverley JKA. Congenital transmission of toxoplasmosis through successive generations of mice. Nature 183:1348-1349, 1959.
86. Remington JS, Melton ML, Jacobs L. Induced and spontaneous recurrent parasitemia in chronic infections with avirulent strains of *Toxoplasma gondii*. J Immunol 87:578-581, 1961.
87. Remington JS. Experiments on the transmission of toxoplasmosis. Surv Ophthalmol 6:856-876, 1961.
88. Schoondermark-van de Ven E, Galama J, Vree T, et al. Study of treatment of congenital *Toxoplasma gondii* infection in Rhesus monkeys with pyrimethamine and sulfadiazine. Antimicrob Agents Chemother 39:137-144, 1995.
89. Flori P, Hafid J, Bourlet T, et al. Experimental model of congenital toxoplasmosis in guinea-pigs: use of quantitative and qualitative PCR for the study of maternofetal transmission. J Med Microbiol 51:871-878, 2002.
90. Dubey JP, Beattie CP. Toxoplasmosis of Animals and Man. Boca Raton, Fla, CRC Press, 1988.
91. Work K, Eriksen L, Fennestad KL. Experimental toxoplasmosis in pregnant sows: I. Clinical, parasitological and serological observations. Acta Pathol Microbiol Scand [B] 78:129-139, 1970.
92. Maller T, et al. Experimental toxoplasmosis in pregnant sows. Acta Pathol Microbiol Scand [A] 78:241-255, 1970.
93. Sanger VL, Cole CR. Toxoplasmosis. VI. Isolation of *Toxoplasma* from milk, placentas, and newborn pigs of asymptomatic carrier sows. Am J Vet Res 16:536-539, 1955.
94. Hartley WJ, Moyle G. Observations on an outbreak of ovine congenital toxoplasmosis. Aust Vet J 44:105-107, 1968.
95. Watson WA, Beverley JKA. Epizootics of toxoplasmosis causing ovine abortion. Vet Rec 88:120-124, 1971.
96. Munday BL. The epidemiology of toxoplasmosis with particular reference to the Tasmanian environment. Thesis, University of Melbourne, 95 pp, 1970 Vet Bull 41(5) 376, 1971.
97. Munday BL, Mason RW. Toxoplasmosis as a cause of perinatal death in goats. Aust Vet J 55:485-487, 1979.
98. Jacobs L, Hartley WJ. Ovine toxoplasmosis: studies on parasitaemia, tissue infection, and congenital transmission in ewes infected by various routes. Br Vet J 120:347-364, 1964.
99. Hartley WJ. Experimental transmission of toxoplasmosis in ewes showing high and low dye test titres. N Z Vet J 12:6-8, 1964.
100. Beverley JKA, Watson WA, Centre VI. Prevention of experimental and of naturally occurring ovine abortion due to toxoplasmosis. Vet Rec 88:39-41, 1970.
101. Beverley JK, Archer JF, Watson WA, Fawcett AR. Trial of a killed vaccine in the prevention of ovine abortion due to toxoplasmosis. Br Vet J 127:529-535, 1971.
102. Vermeulen AN, Bos HJ. Vaccination of sheep with Toxovax: field trial data from UK, France and the Netherlands. Fourth International Biennial Toxoplasma Conference, Drymen, Scotland, July 22-26, 1996.
103. Marx-Chemla C, Puygauthier-Toubas D, Foudrinier F, et al. Should immunologic monitoring of toxoplasmosis seronegative pregnant women stop at delivery? Presse Med 19:367-368, 1990.
104. Miller MJ, Aronson WJ, Remington JS. Late parasitemia in asymptomatic acquired toxoplasmosis. Ann Intern Med 71:139-145, 1969.
105. Derouin F, Beauvais B, Bussel A, Lariviere M. Detection of *Toxoplasma* parasitemia in immunocompromised patients. Ninth International Congress of Infectious and Parasitic Diseases, Munich, July 20-26, 1986 (abstract, p 9).
106. Vittecoq D, Derouin F, Beauvais B, Bussel A. *Toxoplasma* parasitemia associated to serological reactivation of chronic toxoplasmosis in an immunocompr[om]ised patient. Ninth International Congress of Infectious and Parasitic Diseases, Munich, July 20-26, 1986 (abstract, p 9).
107. Luft BJ, Naot Y, Araujo FG, et al. Primary and reactivated *Toxoplasma* infection in patients with cardiac transplants. Clinical spectrum and problems in diagnosis in a defined population. Ann Intern Med 99:27-31, 1983.
108. Garcia AG. Congenital toxoplasmosis in two successive sibs. Arch Dis Child 43:705-710, 1968.
109. Glasser L, Delta BG. Congenital toxoplasmosis with placental infection in monozygotic twins. Pediatrics 35:276-283, 1965.
110. Beckett RS, Flynn FJ Jr. Toxoplasmosis: report of two new cases, with a classification and a demonstration of the organisms in the human placenta. N Engl J Med 249:345-350, 1953.
111. Neghme A, Thiermann E, Pino F. Toxoplasmosis humana en Chile. Bol Infect Parasitol Chile 7:6-8, 1952.
112. Sarrut S. [Histological study of the placenta in congenital toxoplasmosis.] Ann Pediatr (Paris) 14:2429-2435 (English summary, 2434), 1967.
113. Desmonts G, Couvreur J. [The clinical expression of infection in the newborn. 3. Congenital toxoplasmosis.] 21e Congrès des Pédiatres de Langue Française 3:453-488, 1967.
114. Desmonts G, Couvreur J. Toxoplasmosis in pregnancy and its transmission to the fetus. Bull NY Acad Med 50:146-159, 1974.
115. Aspöck H, Flamm H, Korbei V, Picher O. Attempts for detection of *Toxoplasma gondii* in human embryos of mothers with preconceptional *Toxoplasma* infections. Mitt Österr Ges Tropenmed Parasitol 5:93-97, 1983.
116. Desmonts G, Couvreur J. Congenital toxoplasmosis. A prospective study of the offspring of 542 women who acquired toxoplasmosis during pregnancy. With letter to the editor. *In* Thalhammer O, Pollak A, Baumgarten K (eds). Perinatal Medicine, Sixth European Congress, Vienna. Pathophysiology of Congenital Disease. Stuttgart, Georg Thieme Verlag, 1979, pp 51-60.
117. Couvreur J, Desmonts G, Thulliez P. Prophylaxis of congenital toxoplasmosis. Effects of spiramycin on placental infection. J Antimicrob Chemother 22(suppl B):193-200, 1988.
118. Remington JS, Melton ML, Jacobs L. Chronic *Toxoplasma* infection in the uterus. J Lab Clin Med 56:879-883, 1960.
119. Ruiz A, Flores M, Kotcher E. The prevalence of *Toxoplasma* antibodies in Costa Rican postpartum women and their neonates. Am J Obstet Gynecol 95:817-819, 1966.

120. Ruoss CF, Bourne GL. Toxoplasmosis in pregnancy. J Obstet Gynaecol Br Commonw 79:1115-1118, 1972.
121. Kräubig H. [Preventive method of treatment of congenital toxoplasmosis.] *In* Kirchhoff H, Kräubig H (eds). Toxoplasmose. Praktische Fragen und Ergebnisse. Stuttgart, G. Thieme Verlag, 1966, pp 104-122.
122. Kimball AC, Kean BH, Fuchs F. Congenital toxoplasmosis: a prospective study of 4,048 obstetric patients. Am J Obstet Gynecol 111:211-218, 1971.
123. Stray-Pedersen B. A prospective study of acquired toxoplasmosis among 8,043 pregnant women in the Oslo area. Am J Obstet Gynecol 136:399-406, 1980.
124. Hohlfeld P, Daffos F, Thulliez P, et al. Fetal toxoplasmosis: outcome of pregnancy and infant follow-up after in utero treatment. J Pediatr 115:765-769, 1989.
125. Hohlfeld P, Daffos F, Costa J-M, et al. Prenatal diagnosis of congenital toxoplasmosis with polymerase-chain-reaction test on amniotic fluid. N Engl J Med 331:695-699, 1994.
126. Foulon W, Villena I, Stray-Pedersen B, et al. Treatment of toxoplasmosis during pregnancy: a multicenter study of impact on fetal transmission and children's sequelae at age 1 year. Am J Obstet Gynecol 180:410-415, 1999.
127. Brezin AP, Thulliez P, Couvreur J, et al. Ophthalmic outcomes after prenatal and postnatal treatment of congenital toxoplasmosis. Am J Ophthalmol 135:779-784, 2003.
128. Desmonts G. Acquired toxoplasmosis in pregnant women. Evaluation of the frequency of transmission of *Toxoplasma* and of congenital toxoplasmosis. Lyon Med 248:115-123, 1982.
129. Desmonts G, Daffos F, Forestier F, et al. Prenatal diagnosis of congenital toxoplasmosis. Lancet 1:500-504, 1985.
130. Daffos F, Forestier F, Capella-Pavlovsky M, et al. Prenatal management of 746 pregnancies at risk for congenital toxoplasmosis. N Engl J Med 318:271-275, 1988.
131. Dunn D, Wallon M, Peyron F, et al. Mother-to-child transmission of toxoplasmosis: risk estimates for clinical counselling. Lancet 353: 1829-1833, 1999.
132. Jenum PA, Stray-Pedersen B, Melby KK, et al. Incidence of *Toxoplasma gondii* infection in 35,940 pregnant women in Norway and pregnancy outcome for infected women. J Clin Microbiol 36:2900-2906, 1998.
133. Thalhammer O. Fetale und angeborene Cytomegalie: zur Bedeutung die prantalen Inkubationszeit. Monatsschr Kinderheilkd 116:209-211, 1968.
134. Thalhammer O. Prenatal incubation period. *In* Thalhammer O (ed). Prenatal Infections. Stuttgart, Georg Thieme Verlag, 1971, pp 70-71.
135. Romand S, Chosson M, Franck J, et al. Usefulness of quantitative polymerase chain reaction in amniotic fluid as early prognostic marker of fetal infection with *Toxoplasma gondii.* Am J Obstet Gynecol 190:797-802, 2004.
136. Liesenfeld O, Montoya JG, Kinney S, et al. Effect of testing for IgG avidity in the diagnosis of *Toxoplasma gondii* infection in pregnant women: experience in a U.S. reference laboratory. J Infect Dis 183: 1248-1253, 2001.
137. Montoya JG, Liesenfeld O, Kinney S, et al. VIDAS test for avidity of *Toxoplasma*-specific immunoglobulin G for confirmatory testing of pregnant women. J Clin Microbiol 40:2504-2508, 2002.
138. Montoya JG, Huffman HB, Remington JS. Evaluation of the immunoglobulin G avidity test for diagnosis of toxoplasmic lymphadenopathy. J Clin Microbiol 42:4627-4631, 2004.
139. Desmonts G, Couvreur J, Thulliez P. [Congenital toxoplasmosis: five cases with mother-to-child transmission of pre-pregnancy infection.] Presse Med 19:1445-1449, 1990.
140. Remington JS, Klein JO. Infectious Diseases of the Fetus and Newborn Infant, 2nd ed. Philadelphia, WB Saunders, 1983.
141. Remington JS, Klein JO. Infectious Diseases of the Fetus and Newborn Infant, 4th ed. Philadelphia, WB Saunders, 1995.
142. Marty P, Le Fichoux Y, Deville A, Forest H. Toxoplasmose congénitale et toxoplasmose ganglionnaire maternelie préconceptionnelle. Presse Med 20:387, 1991.
143. Vogel N, Kirisits M, Michael E, et al. Congenital toxoplasmosis transmitted from an immunologically competent mother infected before conception. Clin Infect Dis 23:1055-1060, 1996.
144. Feldman HA, Miller LT. Cogenital human toxoplasmosis. Ann N Y Acad Sci 64:180-184, 1956.
145. Silveira C, Ferreira R, Muccioli C, et al. Toxoplasmosis transmitted to a newborn from the mother infected 20 years earlier. Am J Ophthalmol 136:370-371, 2003.
146. Pons J, Sigrand C, Grangeot-Keros L, et al. Congenital toxoplasmosis: mother-to-fetus transmission of pre-pregnancy infection. Presse Med 24:179-182, 1995.
147. Villena I, Quereux C, Pinon JM. Congenital toxoplasmosis: value of prenatal treatment with pyrimethamine-sulfadoxine combination. Letter to the editor. Prenat Diagn 18:754-756, 1998.
148. Aspöck H, Flamm H, Picher O. [Toxoplasmosis surveillance during pregnancy—10 years of experience in Austria.] Mitt Osterr Ges Tropenmed Parasitol 8:105-113, 1986.
149. Flamm H, Aspöck H. [Toxoplasmosis surveillance during pregnancy in Austria—results and problems.] Padiatr Grenzgeb 20:27-34, 1981.
150. Desmonts G. Prevention de la toxoplasmosis: remarques sur l'experience poursuivie en France. *In* Marois M (ed). Prevention of Physical and Mental Congenital Defects, Part B: Epidemiology, Early Detection and Therapy, and Environmental Factors. New York, Alan R. Liss, 1985, pp 313-316.
151. Fortier B, Aissi E, Ajana F, et al. Spontaneous abortion and reinfection by *Toxoplasma gondii.* Letter to the editor. Lancet 338:444, 1991.
152. Hennequin C, Dureau P, N'Guyen L, et al. Congenital toxoplasmosis acquired from an immune woman. Ped Infect Dis 16:75-76, 1997.
153. Gavinet MF, Robert F, Firtion G, et al. Congenital toxoplasmosis due to maternal reinfection during pregnancy. J Clin Microbiol 35: 1276-1277, 1997.
154. Wechsler B, Le Thi Huong D, Vignes B, et al. [Toxoplasmosis and disseminated lupus erythematosus: four case reports and a review of the literature.] Ann Med Interne (Paris) 137:324-330, 1986.
155. D'Ercole C, Boubli L, Franck J, et al. Recurrent congenital toxoplasmosis in a woman with lupus erythematosus. Prenat Diagn 15:1171-1175, 1995.
156. Falusi O, French AL, Seaberg EC, et al. Prevalence and predictors of *Toxoplasma* seropositivity in women with and at risk for human immunodeficiency virus infection. Clin Infect Dis 35:1414-1417, 2002.
157. Ioannidis JP, Abrams EJ, Ammann A, et al. Perinatal transmission of human immunodeficiency virus type 1 by pregnant women with RNA virus loads <1000 copies/ml. J Infect Dis 183:539-545, 2001.
158. Remington JS. Congenital transmission of *Toxoplasma* during chronic infection of the mother (abstract). *In* Proceedings of the First International Congress of Parasitology [Rome, 1994]. London, Pergamon Press, 1994, pp 184-186.
159. Remington JS, Efron B, Cavanaugh E, et al. Studies on toxoplasmosis in El Salvador. Prevalence and incidence of toxoplasmosis as measured by the Sabin-Feldman dye test. Trans R Soc Trop Med Hyg 64:252-267, 1970.
160. Ferraris G, Avitto P. [Biological research on toxoplasmosis. Attempts of isolation of the parasite in fetal and adnexial tissues.] Minerva Ginecol 17:781-783, 1965.
161. Remington JS, Newell JW, Cavanaugh E. Spontaneous abortion and chronic toxoplasmosis: report of a case, with isolation of the parasite. Obstet Gynecol 24:25-31, 1964.
162. Meylan J. Toxoplasmosis as a cause of repeated abortion. *In* Hentsch D (ed). Toxoplasmosis. Bern, Hans Huber, 1971, pp 151-158.
163. Janssen P, Piekarski G, Korte W. [Problem of abortions because of latent *Toxoplasma* infection in women.] Klin Wochenschr 48:25-30, 1970.
164. Remington JS. *Toxoplasma* and chronic abortion. Editorial. Obstet Gynecol 24:155-157, 1964.
165. Kimball AC, Kean BH, Fuchs F. The role of toxoplasmosis in abortion. Am J Obstet Gynecol 111:219-226, 1971.
166. Remington JS, Desmonts G. Toxoplasmosis. *In* Remington JS, Klein JO (eds). Infectious Diseases of the Fetus and Newborn Infant, 2nd ed. Philadelphia, WB Saunders, 1983, pp 143-263.
167. Remington JS. Toxoplasmosis. *In* Gellis SS, Kagan BM (eds). Current Pediatric Therapy, 7th ed. Philadelphia, WB Saunders, 1976, pp 637-638.
168. Wildfuhr G. Experimentelle Versuche zur Resistenz der Toxoplasmen. Z Hyg Infekt 143:134-139, 1956.
169. Kass E. Undersokelser over *Toxoplasma* og toxoplasmose. Dissertation. University of Oslo, 1954.
170. Weinman D, Chandler AH. Toxoplasmosis in man and swine—an investigation of the possible relationship. JAMA 161:229-232, 1956.
171. Remington JS, Desmonts G. Toxoplasmosis. *In* Remington JS, Klein JO (eds). Infectious Diseases of the Fetus and Newborn Infant. Philadelphia, WB Saunders, 1976, pp 191-332.

172. Langer H. [On prenatal *Toxoplasma* infection.] Landarzt 43: 1300-1305, 1967.
173. Remington JS. Toxoplasmosis and congenital infection. Intrauterine infection. Birth Defects 4:47-56, 1968.
174. Jacobs L, Moyle G, Ris RR. The prevalence of toxoplasmosis in New Zealand sheep and cattle. Am J Vet Res 24:673-675, 1963.
175. Jacobs L, Remington JS, Melton ML. A survey of meat samples from swine, cattle, and sheep for the presence of encysted *Toxoplasma*. J Parasitol 46:23-28, 1960.
176. Janitschke K, Weiland G, Rommell MQ. Untersuchungen über den Befall von Schlactalbvern und -schafen mit *Toxoplasma gondii*. Fleischwirtschaft 47:135-136, 1967.
177. Work K. Isolation of *Toxoplasma gondii* from the flesh of sheep, swine and cattle. Acta Pathol Microbiol Scand 71:296-306, 1967.
178. Catar G, Bergendi L, Holkova R. Isolation of *Toxoplasma gondii* from swine and cattle. J Parasitol 55:952-955, 1969.
179. Boch J, Janitschke K, Rommel M. Untersuchungen über das Vorkommen von Toxoplasma-Infektionen bei Schlachtrindern. Wien Tierarztl Monatsschr 52:1029-1036, 1965.
180. Lalla F, Bechelli G, Sampieri L. Osservazioni sierologiche e parassitologiche sulla diffusione della toxoplasmosi nei maiali dell'area de Siena. Clin Vet Milano 90:439-454, 1967.
181. Komiya Y, Kobayashi A, Koyama T. Human toxoplasmosis, particularly on the possible source of its infection in Japan: a review. Jpn J Med Sci Biol 14:157-172, 1961.
182. Fujita J. Parasitic disease of livestock in Japan. Off Int Epizoot Bull 69:203-213, 1968.
183. Dubey JP, Murrell KD, Fayer R, Schad GA. Distribution of *Toxoplasma gondii* tissue cysts in commercial cuts of pork. J Am Vet Med Assoc 188:1035-1037, 1986.
184. Mondragon R, Howe DK, Dubey JP, Sibley LD. Genotypic analysis of *Toxoplasma gondii* isolates from pigs. J Parasitol 84:639-641, 1998.
185. Catar G, Bergendi L, Holkova R. Isolation of *Toxoplasma gondii* from swine and cattle. J Parasitol 55:952-955, 1969.
186. Dubey JP, Streitel RH. Prevalence of *Toxoplasma* infection in cattle slaughtered at an Ohio abattoir. J Am Vet Med Assoc 169:1197-1199, 1976.
187. Raisanen S. Toxoplasmosis transmitted by blood transfusions. Transfusion 18:329-332, 1978.
188. Kimball AC, Kean BH, Kellner A. The risk of transmitting toxoplasmosis by blood transfusion. Transfusion 5:447-451, 1965.
189. Matsubayashi H, Akao S. Immuno-electron microscopic studies on *Toxoplasma gondii*. Am J Trop Med Hyg 15:486-491, 1966.
190. Shevkunova EA, Rokhina LA, Nugumanova MF. [A case of chronic acquired toxoplasmosis with positive agents detectable in the blood.] Med Parazitol (Mosk) 44:235-238, 1975.
191. Waldeland H. Toxoplasmosis in sheep. *Toxoplasma gondii* in muscular tissue, with particular reference to dye test titres and haemoglobin type. Acta Vet Scand 17:403-411, 1976.
192. Ghorbani M, Hafizi A, Shegerfcar MT, et al. Animal toxoplasmosis in Iran. J Trop Med Hyg 86:73-76, 1983.
193. Maitani T. [Serological investigation of toxoplasmosis in human and various animals, and isolation of *Toxoplasma gondii*.] Niigata Med J (in Japanese) 84:325, 1970.
194. Siegel SE, Lunde MN, Gelderman AH, et al. Transmission of toxoplasmosis by leukocyte transfusion. Blood 37:388-394, 1971.
195. Beauvais B, Garin JF, Lariviere M, et al. [Toxoplasmosis and transfusion.] Ann Parasitol Hum Comp 51:625-635, 1976.
196. Rommel M, Tiemann G, Potters U, Weller W. [Investigations into the epizootiology of infections with cyst-forming coccidia (Toxoplasmidae, Sarcocystidae) in cats, cattle and free-living rodents (author's transl).] Dtsch Tierartzl Wochenschr 89:57-62, 1982.
197. Prosek F, Hejlicek K. V'yskyt protilatek proti toxoplazmoze u jatecnych virat ze socialistickeho sektoru. Veterinarstvi 30:405, 1980.
198. Dubey J, Thulliez P, Powell E. *Toxoplasma gondii* in Iowa sows: comparison of antibody titers to isolation of *T. gondii* by bioassays in mice and cats. J Parasitol 81:48-53, 1995.
199. Boch J, Rommel M, Janitschke K. Beitrage zur Toxoplasmose des Schweines: I. Ergebnisse kunstlicher *Toxoplasma*-infektionnen bei Schweinen. Berl Munch Tierarztl Wochenschr 77:161, 1964.
200. Beauvais B, Garin JF, Lariviere M, Languillat G. [Toxoplasmosis and chronic myeloid leukemia.] Nouv Rev Fr Hematol 16:169-184, 1976.
201. Hellesnes I, Mohn SF, Melhuus B. *Toxoplasma gondii* in swine in south-eastern Norway. Acta Vet Scand 19:574-587, 1978.
202. Kayhoe DE, Jacobs L, Beye HK, McCullough NB. Acquired toxoplasmosis. Observations on two parasitologically proved cases treated with pyrimethamine and triple sulfonamides. N Engl J Med 257:1247-1254, 1957.
203. Frenkel JK, Weber RW, Lunde MN. Acute toxoplasmosis. Effective treatment with pyrimethamine, sulfadiazine, leucovorin, calcium, and yeast. JAMA 173:1471-1476, 1960.
204. Hagiwara T, Katsube Y. Detection of *Toxoplasma* infection in pork by Sabin-Feldman's dye test with meat extract. Nippon Juigaku Zasshi 43:763-765, 1981.
205. Desmonts G, Couvreur J, Alison F, et al. Etude epidemiologique sur la toxoplasmose: L'influence de la cuisson des viandes de boucherie sur la frequence de l'infection humaine. 10:952-958, 1965.
206. Kean BH, Kimball AC, Christenson WN. An epidemic of acute toxoplasmosis. JAMA 208:1002-1004, 1969.
207. Schantz PM, Juaranek DD, Schultz MG. Trichinosis in the United States, 1975: increase in cases attributed to numerous common-source outbreaks. J Infect Dis 136:712-715, 1977.
208. Dubey JP. Toxoplasmosis. J Am Vet Med Assoc 189:166-170, 1986.
209. Passos JN, Bonametti AM, Passos EM. Surto de toxoplasmose aguda transmtida atraves da ingestao de carne de gado ovino. Congresso da Sociedade de Medicina Tropical, Salvador, 1994 (abstract, p 30).
210. Robson MB, Wood RN, Sullivan JJ, et al. A probable foodborne outbreak of toxoplasmosis. Commun Dis Intell 19:517-522, 1995.
211. Choi WY, Nam HW, Kwak NH, et al. Foodborne outbreaks of human toxoplasmosis. J Infect Dis 175:1280-1282, 1997.
212. Vanek JA, Dubey JP, Thuillez P, et al. Prevalence of *Toxoplasma gondii* antibodies in hunter-killed white-tail deer (*Odocoileus virginianus*) in four regions of Minnesota. J Parasitol 82:41-44, 1996.
213. Humphreys JG, Stewart RL, Dubey JP. Prevalence of *Toxoplasma gondii* antibodies in sera of hunter-killed white-tailed deer in Pennsylvania. Am J Vet Res 56:172-173, 1995.
214. Guebre-Xabier M, Nurilign A, Gebre-Hiwot A, et al. Seroepidemiological survey of *Toxoplasma gondii* infection in Ethiopia. Ethiop Med J 31:201-208, 1993.
215. Kapperud G, Jenum P, Stray-Pedersen B, et al. Risk factors for *Toxoplasma gondii* infection in pregnancy. Am J Epidemiol 144:405-412, 1996.
216. Raz R, Nishri Z, Mates A, et al. Seroprevalence of antibodies against *Toxoplasma gondii* among two rural populations in Northern Israel. Isr J Med Sci 29:636-639, 1993.
217. Buffolano W, Gilbert RE, Holland FJ, et al. Risk factors for recent *Toxoplasma* infection in pregnant women in Naples. Epidemiol Infect 116:347-351, 1996.
218. Rawal BD. Toxoplasmosis: a dye-test survey on sera from vegetarians and meat eaters in Bombay. Trans R Soc Trop Med Hyg 53:61-63, 1959.
219. Jacobs L. The interrelation of toxoplasmosis in swine, cattle, dogs and man. Public Health Rep 72:872-882, 1957.
220. Hutchison WM, Dunachie JF, Work K. The fecal transmission of *Toxoplasma gondii* (brief report). Acta Pathol Microbiol Scand 74: 462-464, 1968.
221. Sheffield HG, Melton ML. *Toxoplasma gondii*: transmission through feces in absence of *Toxocara cati* eggs. Science 164:431-432, 1969.
222. Frenkel JK, Dubey JP, Miller NL. *Toxoplasma gondii*: fecal forms separated from eggs of the nematode *Toxocara cati*. Science 164: 432-433, 1969.
223. Ruiz A, Frenkel JK. *Toxoplasma gondii* in Costa Rican cats. Am J Trop Med Hyg 29:1150-1160, 1980.
224. Frenkel JK, Ruiz A, Chinchilla M. Soil survival of *Toxoplasma* oocysts in Kansas and Costa Rica. Am J Trop Med Hyg 24:439-443, 1975.
225. Coutinho SG, Lobo R, Dutra G. Isolation of *Toxoplasma* from the soil during an outbreak of toxoplasmosis in a rural area in Brazil. J Parasitol 68:866-868, 1982.
226. Dubey JP, Frenkel JK. Cyst-induced toxoplasmosis in cats. J Protozool 19:155-177, 1972.
227. Wallace GD. Experimental transmission of *Toxoplasma gondii* by filth-flies. Am J Trop Med Hyg 20:411-413, 1971.
228. Wallace GD. Experimental transmission of *Toxoplasma gondii* by cockroaches. J Infect Dis 126:545-547, 1972.
229. Smith DD, Frenkel JK. Cockroaches as vectors of *Sarcocystis muris* and of other coccidia in the laboratory. J Parasitol 64:315-319, 1978.
230. Markus MB. Earthworms and coccidian oocysts. Ann Trop Med Parasitol 68:247-248, 1974.
231. Ruiz A, Frenkel JK. Intermediate and transport hosts of *Toxoplasma gondii* in Costa Rica. Am J Trop Med Hyg 29:1161-1166, 1980.
232. Dubey JP. Feline toxoplasmosis and coccidiosis: a survey of domiciled and stray cats. J Am Vet Med Assoc 162:873-877, 1973.

233. Wallace GD. Isolation of *Toxoplasma gondii* from the feces of naturally infected cats. J Infect Dis 124:227-228, 1971.
234. Wallace GD, Marshall L, Marshall M. Cats, rats, and toxoplasmosis on a small Pacific island. Am J Epidemiol 95:475-482, 1972.
235. Wallace GD. Serologic and epidemiologic observations on toxoplasmosis on three Pacific atolls. Am J Epidemiol 90:103-111, 1969.
236. Wallace GD. The role of the cat in the natural history of *Toxoplasma gondii*. Am J Trop Med Hyg 22:313-322, 1973.
237. Munday BL. Serological evidence of *Toxoplasma* infection in isolated groups of sheep. Res Vet Sci 13:100-102, 1972.
238. Stern GA, Romano PE. Congenital ocular toxoplasmosis. Possible occurrence in siblings. Arch Ophthalmol 96:615-617, 1978.
239. Janitschke K, Kuhn D. [*Toxoplasma* oocysts in the feces of naturally infected cats.] Berl Munch Tierarztl Wochenschr 85:46-47, 1972.
240. Werner JK, Walton BC. Prevalence of naturally occurring *Toxoplasma gondii* infections in cats from U.S. military installations in Japan. J Parasitol 58:1148-1150, 1972.
241. Deeb BJ, Sufan MM, DiGiacomo RF. *Toxoplasma gondii* infection of cats in Beirut, Lebanon. J Trop Med Hyg 88:301-306, 1985.
242. Svobodova V, Svoboda M. The occurrence of the oocysts of *Toxoplasma gondii* in the faeces of cats. Vet Med (Praha) 31:621-628, 1986.
243. Etheredge GD, Frenkel JK. Human *Toxoplasma* infection in Kuna and Embera children in the Bayano and San Blas, Eastern Panama. Am J Trop Med Hyg 53:448-457, 1995.
244. Teutsch SM, Juranek DD, Sulzer A, et al. Epidemic toxoplasmosis associated with infected cats. N Engl J Med 300:695-699, 1979.
245. Stagno S, Dykes AC, Amos CS, et al. An outbreak of toxoplasmosis linked to cats. Pediatrics 65:706-712, 1980.
246. Benenson MW, Takafuji ET, Lemon SM, et al. Oocyst-transmitted toxoplasmosis associated with ingestion of contaminated water. N Engl J Med 307:666-669, 1982.
247. Bowie WR, King AS, Werker DH, et al. Outbreak of toxoplasmosis associated with municipal drinking water. Lancet 350:173-177, 1997.
248. Bahia-Oliveira LM, Jones JL, Azevedo-Silva J, et al. Highly endemic, waterborne toxoplasmosis in north Rio de Janeiro State, Brazil. Emerg Infect Dis 9:55-62, 2003.
249. Hill D, Dubey JP. *Toxoplasma gondii*: transmission, diagnosis and prevention. Clin Microbiol Infect 8:634-640, 2002.
250. Lindsay DS, Phelps KK, Smith SA, et al. Removal of *Toxoplasma gondii* oocysts from sea water by eastern oysters (*Crassostrea virginica*). J Eukaryot Microbiol Suppl:197S-198S, 2001.
251. Miller MA, Grigg ME, Kreuder C, et al. An unusual genotype of *Toxoplasma gondii* is common in California sea otters (*Enhydra lutris nereis*) and is a cause of mortality. Int J Parasitol 34:275-284, 2004.
252. Lindsay DS, Collins MV, Mitchell SM, et al. Sporulation and survival of *Toxoplasma gondii* oocysts in seawater. J Eukaryot Microbiol 50(Suppl):687-688, 2003.
253. Kniel KE, Lindsay DS, Sumner SS, et al. Examination of attachment and survival of *Toxoplasma gondii* oocysts on raspberries and blueberries. J Parasitol 88:790-793, 2002.
254. Eichenwald H. Experimental toxoplasmosis. I. Transmission of the infection in utero and through the milk of lactating female mice. Am J Dis Child 76:307-315, 1948.
255. Mayer H. Investigaciones sobre toxoplasmosis. Bol Of Sanit Panam 58:485-497, 1965.
256. Rommel M, Breuning J. [Research into the occurrence of *Toxoplasma gondii* in the milk of some animals and the possibility of lactogenous infection.] Berl Munch Tierarztl Wochenschr 80:365-369, 1967.
257. Sanger V, Chamberlain D, Chamberlain K. Toxoplasmosis: V. Isolation of *Toxoplasma* from cattle. J Am Vet Med Assoc 123:87-91, 1953.
258. Langer H. Repeated congenital infection with *Toxoplasma gondii*. Obstet Gynecol 21:318-329, 1963.
259. Langer H. [The significance of a latent *Toxoplasma* infection during gestation.] *In* Kirchhoff H, Kräubig H (eds). Toxoplasmose. Praktische Fragen und Ergebnisse. Stuttgart, G. Thieme Verlag, 1966, pp 123-138.
260. Bonametti AM, Passos JN. Probable transmission of acute toxoplasmosis through breast feeding. Letter to the editor. J Trop Ped 43:116, 1997.
261. Riemann HP, Meyer ME, Theis JH, et al. Toxoplasmosis in an infant fed unpasteurized goat milk. J Pediatr 87:573-576, 1975.
262. Chiari CDA, Neves DP. [Human toxoplasmosis acquired by ingestion of goat's milk.] Mem Inst Oswaldo Cruz 79:337-340, 1984.
263. Sacks JJ, Roberto RR, Brooks NF. Toxoplasmosis infection associated with raw goat's milk. JAMA 248:1728-1732, 1982.
264. Jacobs L, Melton ML. Toxoplasmosis in chickens. J Parasitol 52: 1158-1162, 1966.
265. Pande PG, Shukla RR, Sekariah PC. *Toxoplasma* from the eggs of domestic fowl (*Gallus gallus*). Science 133:648, 1961.
266. DuShane G, Krauskopf KB, Lerner EM, et al. An unfortunate event. Science 1961;134:945-6.
267. Dubey JP, Graham DH, Dahl E, et al. *Toxoplasma gondii* isolates from free-ranging chickens from the United States. J Parasitol 89: 1060-1062, 2003.
268. Neto V, Cotrim M, Laus W. Nota scircumflex obre o encontro de *Toxoplasma gondii* en sangue destinado a transfusao. Rev Inst Med Trop Sao Paulo 5:68-69, 1963.
269. Talice RV, Gurri J, Royol J, Perez-Moreira L. Researches on toxoplasmosis in Uruguay: survival of *Toxoplasma gondii* in human blood in vitro. An Fac Med Montevideo 42:143-147, 1957.
270. Vasina S, Dunaeva Z. [The survival of *Toxoplasma* outside the host organism.] J Med Parazitol (Mosk) 29:451-454, 1960.
271. Remington JS, Gentry LO. Acquired toxoplasmosis: infection versus disease. Ann N Y Acad Sci 174:1006-1017, 1970.
272. Miller NL, Frenkel JK, Dubey JP. Oral infections with *Toxoplasma* cysts and oocysts in felines, other mammals, and in birds. J Parasitol 58:928-937, 1972.
273. Markvart K, Rehnova M, Ostrovska A. Laboratory epidemic of toxoplasmosis. J Hyg Epidemiol Microbiol Immunol 22:477-484, 1978.
274. Neu HC. Toxoplasmosis transmitted at autopsy. JAMA 202:844, 1967.
275. Cathie IAG. Toxoplasmosis in childhood. Lancet 266:813-814, 1954.
276. Levi GC, Hyakutake S, Neto VA, Correa MO. [Presence of *Toxoplasma gondii* in the saliva of patients with toxoplasmosis. Eventual importance of such verification concerning the transmission of the disease (preliminary report).] Rev Inst Med Trop Sao Paulo 10: 54-58, 1968.
277. Saari M, Raisanen S. Transmission of acute *Toxoplasma* infection. The survival of trophozoites in human tears, saliva, and urine and in cow's milk. Acta Ophthalmol (Copenh) 52:847-852, 1974.
278. Brooks RG, Remington JS. Transplant-related infections. *In* Bennett JV, Brachman PS (eds). Hospital Infections, 2nd ed. Boston, Little, Brown, 1986, pp 581-618.
279. Israelski DM, Remington JS. Toxoplasmosis in the non-AIDS immunocompromised host. *In* Remington J, Swartz M (eds). Current Clinical Topics in Infectious Diseases. London, Blackwell Scientific Publications, 1993, pp 322-356.
280. Mayes J, O'Connor B, Avery R, et al. Transmission of *Toxoplasma gondii* infection by liver transplantation. Clin Infect Dis 21:511-515, 1995
281. Jacobs L. Propagation, morphology and biology of *Toxoplasma*. Ann N Y Acad Sci 64:154-179, 1956.
282. Stone WB, Manwell RD. Toxoplasmosis in cold-blooded hosts. J Protozool 16:99-102, 1969.
283. Levine ND, Nye RR. *Toxoplasma ranae* sp. m. from the leopard frog *Rana linnaeus*. J Parasitol 23:488-490, 1976.
284. Luft BJ, Remington JS. Acute *Toxoplasma* infection among family members of patients with acute lymphadenopathic toxoplasmosis. Arch Intern Med 144:53-56, 1984.
285. Coutinho SG, Leite MA, Amendoeira MR, Marzochi MC. Concomitant cases of acquired toxoplasmosis in children of a single family: evidence of reinfection. J Infect Dis 146:30-33, 1982.
286. Coutinho SG, Morgado A, Wagner M, et al. Outbreak of human toxoplasmosis in a rural area. A three year serologic follow-up study. Mem Inst Oswaldo Cruz 77:29-36, 1982.
287. Humphreys H, Hillary IB, Kiernan T. Toxoplasmosis: a family outbreak. Ir Med J 79:191, 1986.
288. Shenep JL, Barenkamp SJ, Brammeier SA, Gardner TD. An outbreak of toxoplasmosis on an Illinois farm. Pediatr Infect Dis 3:518-522, 1984.
289. Baril L, Ancelle T, Thulliez P, et al. Facteurs de risque de la toxoplasmose chez les femmes enceintes en 1995 (France). Bull Epidemiol Hebdom 16, 1966.
290. Bobic B, Jevremovic I, Marinkovic J, et al. Risk factors for *Toxoplasma* infection in a reproductive age female population in the area of Belgrade, Yugoslavia. Eur J Epidemiol 14:605-610, 1998.
291. Cook AJ, Gilbert RE, Buffolano W, et al. Sources of *Toxoplasma* infection in pregnant women: European multicentre case-control study. On behalf of the European Research Network on Congenital Toxoplasmosis. BMJ 321:142-147, 2000.

292. Boyer K, Holfels E, Roizen N, et al. Risk factors for *Toxoplasma gondii* infection in mothers of infants with congenital toxoplasmosis: implications for prenatal treatment and screening. Am J Obstet Gynecol. Am J Obstet Gynecol 192; 564-571, 2005.
292a. Thulliez, P. Commentary: Efficacy of prenatal treatment for toxoplasmosis: a possibility that cannot be ruled out. Int J Epidemiol 30:1315-1316, 2001.
293. Dumas N, Meunier DM, Seguela JP. [Toxoplasmosis in the Central African Republic: first survey.] Bull Soc Pathol Exot Filiales 78: 221-225, 1985.
294. Billiault X, Collet M, Dupont A, Lefevre S. [Toxoplasmosis in pregnant women in Haut Ogooue Province (Gabon).] Bull Soc Pathol Exot Filiales 80:74-83, 1987.
295. Vercruysse J, Deschampheleire I, Van De Velden L. Contribution à l'étude de la toxoplasmose humaine à Pikine (Senegal). Med Afr Noire 31:619-620, 1984.
296. Gill HS, Mtimavalye LA. Prevalence of *Toxoplasma* antibodies in pregnant African women in Tanzania. Afr J Med Med Sci 11:167-170, 1982.
297. Dumas N, Cazaux M, Pivaillier P, Seguela JP. [Toxoplasmosis in the African tropical zone. Preliminary prevalence studies.] Bull Soc Pathol Exot Filiales 78:795-800, 1985.
298. Kennou MF. [Epidemiology of toxoplasmosis in pregnant Tunisian women.] Arch Inst Pasteur Tunis 59:205-211, 1982.
299. Rudolph C. [Seroepidemiologic study of the incidence of *Toxoplasma* infections in black African females in Zambia.] Off Gesundheitsw 49:41-43, 1987.
300. Fuente MC, Bovone NS, Cabral GE. [Prophylaxis of prenatal toxoplasmosis.] Medicina 57:155-160, 1997.
301. Rickard E, Costagliola M, Outen E, et al. Toxoplasmosis antibody prevalence in pregnancy in Buenos Aires Province, Argentina. Ninth European Congress of Clinical Microbiology and Infectious Diseases, Berlin, March 21-24, 1999 (abstract, p 326).
302. Sfameni SF, Skurrie IJ, Gilbert GL. Antenatal screening for congenital infection with rubella, cytomegalovirus and *Toxoplasma*. Aust N Z J Obstet Gynaecol 26:257-260, 1986.
303. Walpole IR, Hodgen N, Bower C. Congenital toxoplasmosis: a large survey in Western Australia. Med J Australia 154:720-724, 1991.
304. Aspöck H, Pollak A. Prevention of prenatal toxoplasmosis by serological screening of pregnant women in Austria. Scand J Infect Dis Suppl 84:32-37, 1992.
305. Ashrafunnessa, Khatun S, Islam MN, Huq T. Seroprevalence of *Toxoplasma* antibodies among the antenatal population in Bangladesh. J Obstet Gynaecol Res 24:115-119, 1998.
306. Foulon W, Naessens A, Derde M. Evaluation of the possibilities for preventing congenital toxoplasmosis. Am J Perinatol 11:57-62, 1994.
307. Luvasu V, et al. Screening of pregnant women for antibodies against *Toxoplasma* and CMV with the IMX analyzer in Belgium. Sixth European Congress of Clinical and Microbiological Infectious Disease, Seville, Spain, 1993.
308. Rodier MH, Berthonneau J, Bourgoin A, et al. Seroprevalences of *Toxoplasma*, malaria, rubella, cytomegalovirus, HIV and treponemal infections among pregnant woman in Cotonou, Republic of Benin. Acta Tropica 59:271-277, 1995.
309. Martin P, Andela A. Sexual and other infections of foetal interest during pregnancy in Yadunde, Cameroon. Eighth International Conference on AIDS, Amsterdam, 1992 (abstract, p 112).
310. Vial P, Torres-Pereyra J, Stagno S, et al. Serologic screening for cytomegalovirus, rubella virus, herpes simplex virus, hepatitis B virus, and *Toxoplasma gondii* in two urban populations of pregnant women in Chile. Bull Pan Am Health Organ 20:53-61, 1986.
311. Rong-guo S, Zheng-Le L, De-Cheng W. The prevalence of *Toxoplasma* infection among pregnant women and their newborn infants in Chengdu. Chung Hua Liu Hsing Ping Hsueh Tsa Chih 16:98-100, 1995.
312. Zhang W, Zhao R, Qiu H. [Toxoplasmosis infection in pregnant women in Lanzhou.] Chung Hua Fu Chan Ko Tsa Chih 32:208-210, 1997.
313. Yu JC. [A seroepidemiological study on *Toxoplasma gondii* infection among pregnant women and neonates in Taiwan.] Taiwan I Hsueh Hui Tsa Chih 84:286-295, 1985.
314. Gomez-Marin JE, Montoya-de-Londondo MT, Castano-Osorio JC. A maternal screening program for congenital toxoplasmosis in Quindio, Colombia and application of mathematical models to estimate incidences using age-stratified data. Am J Trop Med Hyg 57:180-186, 1997.
315. Candolfi E, Berg M, Kien T. Approche de la prévalence de la toxoplasmose à Pointe-Noire au Congo. Bull Soc Pathol Exot 86:358-362, 1993.
316. Lebech M, Anderson O, Christensen NC, et al. Neonatal screening for congenital toxoplasmosis based on material seroconversion during pregnancy (unpublished, 1996).
317. Lebech M, Petersen E. Neonatal screening for congenital toxoplasmosis in Denmark: presentation of the design of a prospective study. Scand J Infect Dis 84(Suppl):75-79, 1992.
318. El-Nawawy A, Soliman AT, El Azzouni O, et al. Maternal and neonatal prevalence of *Toxoplasma* and cytomegalovirus (CMV) antibodies and hepatitis-B antigens in an Egyptian rural area. J Trop Pediatr 42:154-157, 1996.
319. Allain JP, Palmer CR, Pearson G. Epidemiological study of latent and recent infection by *Toxoplasma gondii* in pregnant women from a regional population in the U.K. J Infect 36:189-196, 1998.
320. Lappalainen M, Koskela P, Hedman K, et al. Incidence of primary *Toxoplasma* infections during pregnancy in southern Finland: a prospective cohort study. Scand J Infect Dis 24:97-104, 1992.
321. Candolfi E, Wittersheim P, Kien T. Prevalence de la toxoplasmose humaine à Strasbourg en 1992 (unpublished).
322. Nabias R. [Serological investigation of toxoplasmosis in patients of the M.I.P. center of Franceville (Gabon).] Bull Soc Pathol Exot 91:318-320, 1998.
323. Barbier D, Ancelle T, Martin-Bouyer G. Seroepidemiological survey of toxoplasmosis in La Guadeloupe, French West Indies. Am J Trop Med Hyg 32:935-942, 1983.
324. Sander J, Niehaus C. [Incidence of primary toxoplasmosis infection in pregnant women.] Dtsch Med Wochenschr 108:455-457, 1983 (with English summary).
325. Janitschke K, Busch W, Kellershofen C. [Direct agglutination as a tool for *Toxoplasma* control in pregnancy care.] Immun Infekt 16:189-191, 1988.
326. Krausse T, Straube W, Wiorsbitzky S, et al. Toxoplasmoscreening in der Schwangerschaft—ein pilotprogramm in nordosten Deutschland. Gerburtshilfe Frauenheilkd 53:613-618, 1993.
327. Roos T, Martius J, Gross U, Schrod L. Systematic serologic screening for toxoplasmosis in pregnancy. Obstet Gynecol 81:243-250, 1993.
328. Friese K, Beichert M, Hof H, et al. Incidence of congenital infections. Geburtshilfe Frauenheilkd 51:890-896, 1991.
329. Decavalas G, Papaetropoulou M, Giannoulaki E, et al. Prevalence of *Toxoplasma gondii* antibodies in gravidas and recently aborted women and study of risk factors. Eur J Epidemiol 6:223-226, 1990.
330. Sinibaldi J, De Ramirez I. Incidence of congenital toxoplasmosis in live Guatemalan newborns. Eur J Epidemiol 8:516-520, 1992.
331. Szénási Z, Ozsvár Z, Nagy E, et al. Prevention of congenital toxoplasmosis in Szeged, Hungary. Int J Epidemiol 26:428-435, 1997.
332. Singh S. Pandit AJ. Incidence and prevalence of toxoplasmosis in Indian pregnant women: a prospective study. Am J Reprod Immunol 52(4):276-283, 2004.
333. Gandahusada S. Study on the prevalence of toxoplasmosis in Indonesia. Southeast Asian J Trop Med Public Health (Suppl 22): 93-98, 1991.
334. Ricci N, Manuppella A, Di NM, Simeone R, Rendina F. [Epidemiology of toxoplasmosis. Occurrence and risk of congenital toxoplasmosis in the province of Isernia.] Nuovi Ann Ig Microbiol 35:13-21, 1984.
335. Konishi E, Takahashi J, Soeripto N, et al. Prevalence of antibody to *Toxoplasma gondii* among pregnant women and umbilical cords in Hyogo Prefecture, Japan. Jpn J Parasitol 36:198-200, 1987.
336. Al Nakib W, Ibrahim ME, Hathout H, et al. Seroepidemiology of viral and toxoplasmal infections during pregnancy among Arab women of child-bearing age in Kuwait. Int J Epidemiol 12:220-223, 1983.
337. Monjour L, Niel G, Palminteri R, et al. An epidemiological survey of toxoplasmosis in Mauritania. Trop Geogr Med 35:21-25, 1983.
338. Guessous-Idrissi N, Lahlou D, Sefiani R, Benmira A. [Toxoplasmosis and rubella in Moroccan women. Results of a serological survey.] Pathol Biol (Paris) 32:761-765, 1984.
339. Rai S, et al. Immuno-serological study of human toxoplasmosis in Nepal. Third Congress Asia Pacific Societies of Pathologists and Eleventh National Convention Bangladesh Society of Pathologists Bangladesh, 1993.
340. van der Veen J, Polak MF. Prevalence of *Toxoplasma* antibodies according to age with comments on the risk of prenatal infection. J Hyg (Lond) 85:165-174, 1980.

341. Klufio C, Delamare O, Amoa A, Kariwiga G. The prevalence of *Toxoplasma* antibodies in pregnant patients attending the Port Moresby General Hospital antenatal clinic: a seroepidemiological survey. Papua New Guinea Med J 36:4-9, 1993.
342. Olusi T, Grob U, Ajayi J. High incidence of toxoplasmosis during pregnancy in Nigeria. Scand J Infect Dis 28:645-646, 1996.
343. Onadeko MO, Joynson DHM, Payne RA. The prevalence of *Toxoplasma* infection among pregnant women in Ibadan, Nigeria. J Trop Med Hyg 95:143-145, 1992.
344. Arene FO. The prevalence of toxoplasmosis among inhabitants of the Niger Delta. Folia Parasitol (Praha) 33:311-314, 1986.
345. Jenum PA, Kapperud G, Stray-Pedersen B, et al. Prevalence of *Toxoplasma gondii*–specific immunoglobulin G antibodies among pregnant women in Norway. Epidemiol Infect 120:87-92, 1998.
346. Sousa OE, Saenz RE, Frenkel JK. Toxoplasmosis in Panama: a 10-year study. Am J Trop Med Hyg 38:315-322, 1988.
347. Ziobrowski S. [Occurrence of positive toxoplasmosis reactions in mothers and newborn infants.] Klin Oczna 86:209-211, 1984.
348. Antunes F. Toxoplasmose, estudo la epidemiologia e da infeccao congenita na regiao de Lisboa. Fotocomposicao e Impressaso: Santelmo, Portugal, Coop de Arted Graficas, C.R.L. Lisboa, Julho 1984.
349. Matos Aybar O, Mendoza HR. Prevalence of congenital toxoplasmosis in Santo Domingo. Arch Dominican Pediatr 18: 137-144, 1982.
350. Al-Meshari AA, Chowdhury MNH, Chattopadhyay SK, DeSilva SK. Screening for toxoplasmosis in pregnancy. Int J Gynecol Obstet 29: 39-45, 1989.
351. Williams KA, Scott JM, Macfarlane DE, et al. Congenital toxoplasmosis: a prospective survey in the West of Scotland. J Infect 3:219-229, 1981.
352. Jackson MH, Hutchison WM, Siim JC. A seroepidemiological survey of toxoplasmosis in Scotland and England. Ann Trop Med Parasitol 81:359-365, 1987.
353. Logar J, Novak-Antolic Z, Zore A. Serological screening for toxoplasmosis in pregnancy in Slovenia. Scand J Infect Dis 27: 163-164, 1995.
354. Sierra M, Lite J, Matas E. Significance of IgM antibodies to *Toxoplasma gondii* in pregnancy. Fourth European Congress of Clinical Microbiology, Nice, France, 1989 (abstract, p 50).
354a. Harma M, Harma M, Gungen N, Demir N. Toxoplasmosis in pregnant women in Sanliurfa, Southeastern Anatolia City, Turkey. J Egypt Soc Parasitol 34(2):519-525, 2004.
355. Ahlfors K, Borjeson M, Huldt G, Forsberg E. Incidence of toxoplasmosis in pregnant women in the city of Malmo, Sweden. Scand J Infect Dis 21:315-321, 1989.
356. Sturchler D, Berger R, Just M. [Congenital toxoplasmosis in Switzerland. Seroprevalence, risk factors and recommendations for prevention.] Schweiz Med Wochenschr 117:161-167, 1987.
357. Bornand JE, Piguet JD. Infestation toxoplasmique: prévalence, presque d'infection congénitale et évolution à Genéve de 1973 à 1987. Schweiz Med Wschr 121:21-29, 1991.
358. Zuber PLF, Jacquier P, Hohlfeld P, Walker AM. *Toxoplasma* infection among pregnant women in Switzerland: a cross-sectional evaluation of regional and age-specific lifetime average annual incidence. Am J Epidemiol 141:659-666, 1995.
359. Doehring E, Reiter-Owona I, Bauer O, et al. *Toxoplasma gondii* antibodies in pregnant women and their newborns in Dar es Salaam, Tanzania. Am J Trop Med Hyg 52:546-548, 1995.
360. Morakote N, Thamasonthi W, Charuchinda K, Khamboonruang C. Prevalence of *Toxoplasma* antibodies in Chiang Mai population. Southeast Asian J Trop Med Public Health 115:80-85, 1984.
361. Chintana T, Sukthana Y, Bunyakai B, Lekkla A. *Toxoplasma gondii* antibody in pregnant women with and without HIV infection. Southeast Asian J Trop Med Public Health 29:383-386, 1998.
362. Taechowisan T, Sutthent R, Louisirirotchanakul S, et al. Immune status in congenital infections by TORCH agents in pregnant Thais. Asian Pac J Allergy Immunol 15:93-97, 1997.
363. Dilmen U, Kaya IS, Ciftci U, Goksin E. Antenatal screening for toxoplasmosis. Letter to the editor. Lancet 336:818-819, 1990.
364. Dar FK, Alkarmi T, Uduman S, et al. Gestational and neonatal toxoplasmosis: regional seroprevalence in the United Arab Emirates. Eur J Epidemiol 13:567-571, 1997.
365. Stojanovic D. [The effect of toxoplasmosis on occurrence of spontaneous abortions and anomalies in neonates in the Timok region.] Vojnosanit Pregl 55:151-159, 1998.
366. Logar J, Novak-Antolic Z, Zore A, et al. Incidence of congenital toxoplasmosis in the Republic of Slovenia. Scand J Infect Dis 24: 105-108, 1992.
367. Logar J. Toxoplasmosis in Slovenia, one of the socialist republics of Yugoslavia. Molecular and Biochemical Parasitology Abstracts of the 5th International Congress of Parasitology, Toronto, Canada, 7-14 August 1982. 540, (abstract).
368. Alexandrou ME, Zagotzidou E, Voyatzi A, et al. A 4-year sero-epidemiological screening for CMV, rubella and *Toxoplasma* infections among women of child-bearing age. Twelfth European Congress of Clinical Microbiology and Infectious Diseases, Milan, April 21-24, 2002 (abstract, p 282).
369. Diderrich V, Patton S. Serologic prevalence of *Toxoplasma gondii* antibodies in women of childbearing age from eastern Tennessee. Joint Meeting of the American Society of Parasitologists and the Society of Protozoologists, San Juan, Puerto Rico, 2000.
370. Eskild A, Magnus P. Commentary: little evidence of effective prenatal treatment against congenital toxoplasmosis—the implications for testing in pregnancy. Int J Epidemiol 30:1314-1315, 2001.
371. Antoniou M, Tzouvali H, Sifakis S, et al. Incidence of toxoplasmosis in 5532 pregnant women in Crete, Greece: management of 185 cases at risk. Eur J Obstet Gynecol Reprod Biol 117(2):138-143, 2004.
372. Igbal J, Hira PR, Khalid N. Toxoplasmosis in Kuwait: improved diagnosis based on quantitative immuno-assay. *In* Infection. Thirteenth European Congress of Clinical Microbiology and Infectious Diseases, Glasgow, 2003 (abstract, p 336).
373. Jones JL, Dietz VJ, Power M, et al. Survey of obstetrician-gynecologists in the United States about toxoplasmosis. Infect Dis Obstet Gynecol 9:23-31, 2001.
374. Logar J, Petrovec M, Novak-Antolic Z, et al. Prevention of congenital toxoplasmosis in Slovenia by serological screening of pregnant women. Scand J Infect Dis 34:201-204, 2002.
375. Taravati M, Sadegkhalili F. Evaluation of anti-*Toxoplasma gondii* antibodies (IgG and IgM) in sera among the women before marriage in Urmia City, Iran. *In* Infection. Thirteenth European Congress of Clinical Microbiology and Infectious Diseases, Glasgow, 2003 (abstract, p 294).
376. Juncosa T, Latorre C, Munoz-Almagro C, et al. Toxoplasmosis: serologic control in pregnant women. Twelfth European Congress of Clinical Microbiology and Infectious Diseases, Milan, April 21-24, 2002.
377. Ades A, Parker S, Gilbert R, et al. Maternal prevalence of *Toxoplasma* antibody based on anonymous neonatal serosurvey: a geographical analysis. Epidemiol Infect 110:127-133, 1993.
378. Ancelle T, Goulet V, Tirard-Fleury V, et al. La toxoplasmose chez la femme enceinte en France en 1995. Bull Epidemiol Hebdom Direct Gen 51:227-228, 1996.
379. Thoumsin H, Senterre J, Lambotte R. Twenty-two years screening for toxoplasmosis in pregnancy: Liege, Belgium. Scand J Infect Dis 84(Suppl):84-85, 1992.
380. Dubey JP, Weigel RM, Siegel AM, et al. Sources and reservoirs of *Toxoplasma gondii* infection on 47 swine farms in Illinois. J Parasitol 81:723-729, 1995.
381. Edelhofer R, Aspöck H. Modes and sources of infections with *Toxoplasma gondii* in view of the screening of pregnant women in Austria. Mitt Osterr Ges Tropenmed Parasitol 18:59-70, 1996.
382. Papoz L, Simondon F, Saurin W, Sarmini H. A simple model relevant to toxoplasmosis applied to epidemiologic results in France. Am J Epidemiol 123:154-161, 1986.
383. Larsen SO, Lebech M. Models for prediction of the frequency of toxoplasmosis in pregnancy in situations changing infection rates. Int J Epidemiol 23:1309-1314, 1994.
384. Lelong M, Alison F, Desmonts G, et al. [Thoughts on 7 cases of congenital toxoplasmosis. Different clinical aspects of this infirmity.] Arch Fr Pediatr 15:433-448, 1959.
385. Jeannel D, Niel G, Costagliolat D, et al. Epidemiology of toxoplasmosis among pregnant women in the Paris area. Int J Epidemiol 17:595-602, 1988.
386. Bronstein R. Toxoplasmose et grossesse. Concours Med 104: 4177-4186, 1982.
387. Frenkel JK. *Toxoplasma* in and around us. BioScience 23:343-352, 1973.
388. Jones JL, Kruszon-Moran D, Wilson M. *Toxoplasma gondii* infection in the United States, 1999-2000. Emerg Infect Dis 9:1371-1374, 2003.
389. Koppe JG, Loewer-Sieger DH, De Roever-Bonnet H. Results of 20-year follow-up of congenital toxoplasmosis. Am J Ophthalmol 101: 248-249, 1986.

390. Koppe JG, Kloosterman GJ. Congenital toxoplasmosis: long-term follow-up. Padiatr Padol 17:171-179, 1982.
391. Hunter K, Stagno S, Capps E, Smith RJ. Prenatal screening of pregnant women for infections caused by cytomegalovirus, Epstein-Barr virus, herpesvirus, rubella, and *Toxoplasma gondii*. Am J Obstet Gynecol 145:269-273, 1983.
392. Lebech M, Andersen O, Christensen NC, et al. Feasibility of neonatal screening for *Toxoplasma* infection in the absence of prenatal treatment. Danish Congenital Toxoplasmosis Study Group. Lancet 353:1834-1837, 1999.
393. Lynfield R, Hsu HW, Guerina NG. Screening methods for congenital *Toxoplasma* and risk of disease. Lancet 353:1899-1900, 1999.
394. Lebech M, Larsen SO, N'rgaard-Pedersen B, et al. Neonatal screening for congenital toxoplamosis based on maternal serconversion during pregnancy and neonatal detection of specific IgM antibodies. Fourth International Biennial *Toxoplasma* Conference, Drymen, Scotland, July 22-26, 1996.
395. Labadie MD, Hazemann JJ. [Contribution of health check-ups in children to the detection and epidemiologic study of congenital toxoplasmosis.] Ann Pediatr (Paris) 31:823-828, 1984.
396. Aspöck H. Österreichs Beitrag zur Toxoplasmose-Forschung und 20 Jahre Toxoplasmose-Überwachung der Schwangeren in Österreich. Tropenmed Parasitol 18:1-18, 1996.
397. Mombro M, Perathoner C, Leone A, et al. Congenital toxoplasmosis: assessment of risk to newborns in confirmed and uncertain maternal infection. Eur J Pediatr 162:703-706, 2003.
398. Dardé ML, Bouteille B, Pestre-Alexandre M. Isoenzymic characterization of seven strains of *Toxoplasma gondii* by isoelectrofocusing in polyacrylamide gel. Am J Trop Med Hyg 39:551-558, 1988.
399. Sibley LD, Boothroyd JC. Virulent strains of *Toxoplasma gondii* comprise a single clonal lineage. Nature 359:82-85, 1992.
400. Dardé ML, Riahi H, Bouteille B, Pestre-Alexandre M. Isoenzyme analysis of *Hammondia hammondi* and *Toxoplasma gondii* sporozoites. J Parasitol 78:731-734, 1992.
401. Howe DK, Sibley DL. *Toxoplasma gondii* comprises three clonal lineages: correlation of parasite genotype with human disease. J Infect Dis 172:1561-1566, 1995.
402. Howe DK, Honore S, Derouin F, Sibley LD. Determination of genotypes of *Toxoplasma gondii* strains isolated from patients with toxoplasmosis. J Clin Microbiol 35:1411-1414, 1997.
403. Ajzenberg D, Cogne N, Paris L, et al. Genotype of 86 *Toxoplasma gondii* isolates associated with human congenital toxoplasmosis, and correlation with clinical findings. J Infect Dis 186:684-689, 2002.
404. Fuentes I, Rubio JM, Ramirez C, Alvar J. Genotypic characterization of *Toxoplasma gondii* strains associated with human toxoplasmosis in Spain: direct analysis from clinical samples. J Clin Microbiol 39:1566-1570, 2001.
405. Grigg ME, Ganatra J, Boothroyd JC, Margolis TP. Unusual abundance of atypical strains associated with human ocular toxoplasmosis. J Infect Dis 184:633-639, 2001.
406. Grigg ME, Suzuki Y. Sexual recombination and clonal evolution of virulence in *Toxoplasma*. Microbes Infect 5:685-690, 2003.
407. Su C, Evans D, Cole RH, et al. Recent expansion of *Toxoplasma* through enhanced oral transmission. Science 299:414-416, 2003.
408. Volkman SK, Hartl DL. Parasitology. A game of cat and mouth. Science 299:353-354, 2003.
409. Portela RW, Bethony J, Costa MI, et al. A multihousehold study reveals a positive correlation between age, severity of ocular toxoplasmosis, and levels of glycoinositolphospholipid-specific immunoglobulin A. J Infect Dis 190:175-183, 2004.
410. Vallochi AL, Nakamura MV, Schlesinger D, et al. Ocular toxoplasmosis: more than just what meets the eye. Scand J Immunol 55:324-328, 2002.
411. Silveira C, Belfort R Jr, Muccioli C, et al. The effect of long-term intermittent trimethoprim/sulfamethoxazole treatment on recurrences of toxoplasmic retinochoroiditis. Am J Ophthalmol 134:41-46, 2002.
412. Wilson CB, Remington JS. Activity of human blood leukocytes against *Toxoplasma gondii*. J Infect Dis 140:890-895, 1979.
413. Wilson CB, Tsai V, Remington JS. Failure to trigger the oxidative metabolic burst by normal macrophages: possible mechanism for survival of intracellular pathogens. J Exp Med 151:328-346, 1980.
414. McLeod R, Bensch KG, Smith SM, Remington JS. Effects of human peripheral blood monocytes, monocyte-derived macrophages, and spleen mononuclear phagocytes on *Toxoplasma gondii*. Cell Immunol 54:330-350, 1980.
415. Catterall JR, Black CM, Leventhal JP, et al. Nonoxidative microbicidal activity in normal human alveolar and peritoneal macrophages. Infect Immun 55:1635-1640, 1987.
416. Brown C, Estes R, McLeod R. Fate of an intracellular parasite during lysis of its host cell by cytotoxic T cells (unpublished, 1995).
417. Yamashita K, Yui K, Ueda M, Yano A. Cytotoxic T-lymphocyte–mediated lysis of *Toxoplasma gondii*–infected target cells does not lead to death of intracellular parasites. Infect Immun 66:4651-4655, 1998.
418. Huldt G. Experimental toxoplasmosis. Parasitemia in guinea pigs. Acta Pathol Microbiol Scand 58:457-470, 1963.
419. Jadin JM, Creemers J. [Ultrastructure and biology of *Toxoplasma*. 3. Observations on intraerythrocytic *Toxoplasma* in a mammal.] Acta Trop 25:267-270, 1968.
420. Frenkel JK. [The pathogenesis and treatment of toxoplasmosis.] World Neurol 2:1046-1068, 1961.
421. Krahenbuhl JL, Gaines JD, Remington JS. Lymphocyte transformation in human toxoplasmosis. J Infect Dis 125:283-288, 1972.
422. Anderson SEJ, Krahenbuhl JL, Remington JS. Longitudinal studies of lymphocyte response to *Toxoplasma* antigen in humans infected with *T. gondii*. J Clin Lab Immunol 2:293-297, 1979.
423. Subauste CS, Dawson L, Remington JS. Human lymphokine-activated killer cells are cytotoxic against cells infected with *Toxoplasma gondii*. J Exp Med 176:1511-1519, 1992.
424. Subauste CS, Chung JY, Do D, et al. Preferential activation and expansion of human peripheral blood $\gamma\delta$ T cells in response to *Toxoplasma gondii* in vitro and their cytokine production and cytotoxic activity against *T. gondii*–infected cells. J Clin Invest 96: 610-619, 1995.
425. Subauste CS, Fuh F, de Waal Malefyt R, Remington JS. Alpha beta T cell response to *Toxoplasma gondii* in previously unexposed individuals. J Immunol 160:3403-3411, 1998.
426. Purner MB, Berens RL, Nash PB, et al. CD4-mediated and CD8-mediated cytotoxic proliferative immune responses to *Toxoplasma gondii* in seropositive humans. Infect Immun 64:4330-4338, 1996.
427. Lea RG, Calder AA. The immunology of pregnancy. Curr Opin Infect Dis 10:171-176, 1997.
428. Raghupathy R. Th1-type immunity is incompatible with successful pregnancy [see comments]. Immunol Today 18:478-482, 1997.
429. Hunter CA, Remington JS. Immunopathogenesis of toxoplasmic encephalitis. J Infect Dis 170:1057-1067, 1994.
430. Denkers EY, Sher A. Role of natural killer and $NK1^+$ T-cells in regulating cell-mediated immunity during *Toxoplasma gondii* infection. Biochem Soc Trans 25:699-703, 1997.
431. Aliberti J, Valenzuela JG, Carruthers VB, et al. Molecular mimicry of a CCR5 binding-domain in the microbial activation of dendritic cells. Nat Immunol 4:485-490, 2003.
432. Denkers EY, Butcher BA, Del Rio L, Bennouna S. Neutrophils, dendritic cells and *Toxoplasma*. Int J Parasitol 34:411-421, 2004.
433. Kasper L, Courret N, Darche S, et al. *Toxoplasma gondii* and mucosal immunity. Int J Parasitol 34:401-409, 2004.
434. Shapira S, Harb OS, Caamano J, Hunter CA. The NF-kappaB signaling pathway: immune evasion and immunoregulation during toxoplasmosis. Int J Parasitol 34:393-400, 2004.
435. Sinai AP, Payne TM, Carmen JC, et al. Mechanisms underlying the manipulation of host apoptotic pathways by *Toxoplasma gondii*. Int J Parasitol 34:381-391, 2004.
436. Yap GS, Sher A. Cell-mediated immunity to *Toxoplasma gondii*: initiation, regulation and effector function. Immunobiology 201: 240-247, 1999.
437. Lewis WP, Markell EK. Acquisition of immunity to toxoplasmosis by the newborn rat. Exp Parasitol 7:463-467, 1958.
438. Harboe A, Erichsen S. Toxoplasmosis in chickens: III. Attempts to provoke a systemic disease in chickens by infection with a chicken strain and a human strain of *Toxoplasma*. APMIS 35:495-502, 1954.
439. Kohler PF. Maturation of the human complement system. I. Onset time and site of fetal C1q, C4, C3, and C5 synthesis. J Clin Invest 52:671-677, 1973.
440. Johnston RB Jr, Altenburger KM, Atkinson AW Jr, et al. Complement in the newborn infant. Pediatrics 64(Suppl):781-786, 1979.
441. Deckert-Schlüter M, Schlüter D, Theisen F, et al. Activation of the innate immune system in murine congenital *Toxoplasma* encephalitis. J Neuroimmunol 53:47-51, 1994.
442. Beverley JK, Fleck DG, Kwantes W, Ludlam GB. Age-sex distribution of various diseases with particular reference to toxoplasmic lymphadenopathy. J Hyg (Lond) 76:215-228, 1976.

443. Kittas C, Henry L. Effect of sex hormones on the response of mice to infection with *Toxoplasma gondii.* Br J Exp Pathol 61:590-600, 1980.
444. Kittas S, Kittas C, Paizi-Biza P, Henry L. A histological and immunohistochemical study of the changes induced in the brains of white mice by infection with *Toxoplasma gondii.* Br J Exp Pathol 65:67-74, 1984.
445. Mack D, Terasaki P, Grumet C, et al. Role of murine and human MHC class II genes in pathogenesis of and protection against toxoplasmosis. Fourth International Biennial Toxoplasma Conference, Drymen, Scotland, July 22-26, 1996.
446. Suzuki Y, Wong S-Y, Grumet FC, et al. Evidence for genetic regulation of susceptibility to toxoplasmic encephalitis in AIDS patients. J Infect Dis 173:265-268, 1966.
447. Werner H, Egger I. [Protective effect of *Toxoplasma* antibody against re-infection (author's transl).] Trop Med Parasitol 24:174-180, 1973.
448. Rodhain J. Formation de pseudokystes au cours d'essais d'immunité croisée entre souches différentes de toxoplasmes. C R Soc Biol (Paris) 144:719-722, 1950.
449. Dubey JP, Frenkel JK. Experimental toxoplasma infection in mice with strains producing oocysts. J Parasitol 59:505-512, 1973.
450. De Roever-Bonnet H. Mice and golden hamsters infected with an avirulent and a virulent *Toxoplasma* strain. Trop Geogr Med 15: 45-60, 1963.
451. Nakayama I. Persistence of the virulent RH strain of *Toxoplasma gondii* in the brains of immune mice. Keio J Med 13:7-12, 1964.
452. Araujo F, Slifer T, Kim S. Chronic infection with *Toxoplasma gondii* does not prevent acute disease or colonization of the brain with tissue cysts following reinfection with different strains of the parasite. J Parasitol 83:521-522, 1997.
453. Remington JS, in discussion, Zimmerman LE. Ocular pathology of toxoplasmosis. Surv Ophthalmol 6:832-856, 1961.
454. Werner H, Pichl H. [Comparative investigations on cyst-forming *Toxoplasma* strains. II. Development of cysts and formation of humoral antibodies.] Zentralbl Bakteriol [Orig] 210:402-416, 1969.
455. van der Waaij D. Formation, growth and multiplication of *Toxoplasma gondii* cysts in mouse brains. Trop Geogr Med 11: 345-370, 1959.
456. Huldt G. Studies on experimental toxoplasmosis. Ann N Y Acad Sci 177:146-155, 1971.
457. Yano A, Aosai F, Ohta M, et al. Antigen presentation by *Toxoplasma gondii*–infected cells to $CD4^+$ proliferative T cells and $CD8^+$ cytotoxic cells. J Parasitol 75:411-416, 1989.
458. Ito S, Tsunoda K, Suzuki K, Tsutsumi Y. Demonstration by microscopy of parasitemia in animals experimentally infected with *Toxoplasma gondii.* Natl Inst Anim Health Q (Tokyo) 6:8-23, 1966.
459. Beverley JKA. A rational approach to the treatment of toxoplasmic uveitis. Trans Ophthalmol Soc 78:109-121, 1958.
460. Remington JS, Hackman R. Changes in serum proteins of rats infected with *Toxoplasma gondii.* J Parasitol 51:865-870, 1965.
461. Remington JS, Hackman R. Changes in mouse serum proteins during acute and chronic infection with an intracellular parasite (*Toxoplasma gondii*). J Immunol 95:1023-1033, 1966.
462. Araujo FG, Remington JS. Immune response to intracellular parasites: suppression by antibody. Proc Soc Exp Biol Med 139:254-258, 1972.
463. Araujo FG, Remington JS. IgG antibody suppression of the IgM antibody response to *Toxoplasma gondii* in newborn rabbits. J Immunol 115:335-338, 1975.
464. Canessa A, Pistoia V, Roncella S, et al. An in vitro model for *Toxoplasma* infection in man. Interaction between $CD4^+$ monoclonal T cells and macrophages results in killing of trophozoites. J Immunol 140:3580-3588, 1988.
465. Saavedra R, Herion P. Human T-cell clones against *Toxoplasma gondii*: production of interferon-γ, interleukin-2, and strain cross-reactivity. Parasitology Res 77:379-385, 1991.
466. McLeod R, Mack DG, Brown C, Skamene E. Secretory IgA, antibody to SAG1, H-2 Class I-restricted $CD8^+$ T-lymphocytes and the Int-1 locus in protection against *Toxoplasma gondii. In* Smith J (ed). Toxoplasmosis. Series H: Cell Biology. New York, Springer-Verlag, 1993, pp 131-151.
467. de Paoli P, Basaglia G, Gennari D, et al. Phenotypic profile and functional characteristics of human gamma and delta T cells during acute toxoplasmosis. J Clin Microbiol 30:729-731, 1992.
468. Scalise F, Gerli R, Castellucci G, et al. Lymphocytes bearing the gamma delta T-cell receptor in acute toxoplasmosis. Immunology 76:668-670, 1992.
469. Hara T, Ohashi S, Yamashita Y, et al. Human V delta 2+ gamma delta T-cell tolerance to foreign antigens of *Toxoplasma gondii.* Proc Natl Acad Sci U S A 93:5136-5140, 1996.
470. Suzuki Y, Orellana MA, Schreiber RD, Remington JS. Interferon-gamma: the major mediator of resistance against *Toxoplasma gondii.* Science 240:516-518, 1988.
471. Michie C, Harvey D. Can expression of CD45RO, a T-cell surface molecule, be used to detect congenital infection? Lancet 343: 1259-1260, 1994.
472. McLeod R, Mack DG, Boyer K, et al. Phenotypes and functions of lymphocytes in congenital toxoplasmosis. J Lab Clin Med 116: 623-635, 1990.
473. Fatoohi AF, Cozon GJ, Wallon M, et al. Cellular immunity to *Toxoplasma gondii* in congenitally infected newborns and immunocompetent infected hosts. Eur J Clin Microbiol Infect Dis 22: 181-184, 2003.
474. Strickland GT, Petitt LE, Voller A. Immunodepression in mice infected with *Toxoplasma gondii.* Am J Trop Med Hyg 22:452-455, 1973.
475. Hibbs JB, Jr., Remington JS, Stewart CC. Modulation of immunity and host resistance by micro-organisms. Pharmacol Ther 1980;8: 37-69.
476. Huldt G, Gard S, Olovson SG. Effect of *Toxoplasma gondii* on the thymus. Nature 244:301-303, 1973.
477. Hibbs JB, Lambert LH, Remington JS. Activated macrophage-mediated nonspecific tumor resistance. J Reticul Soc 13:368, 1973 (abstract).
478. Luft BJ, Remington JS. Effect of pregnancy on resistance to *Listeria monocytogenes* and *Toxoplasma gondii* infections in mice. Infect Immun 38:1164-1171, 1982.
479. Tremonti L, Walton BC. Blast transformation and migration-inhibition in toxoplasmosis and leishmaniasis. Am J Trop Med Hyg 19:49-56, 1970.
480. Luft BJ, Kansas G, Engleman EG, Remington JS. Functional and quantitative alterations in T lymphocyte subpopulations in acute toxoplasmosis. J Infect Dis 150:761-767, 1984.
481. De Waele M, Naessens A, Foulon W, Van Camp B. Activated T-cells with suppressor/cytotoxic phenotype in acute *Toxoplasma gondii* infection. Clin Exp Immunol 62:256-261, 1985.
482. O'Connor GR. The influence of hypersensitivity on the pathogenesis of ocular toxoplasmosis. Trans Am Ophthalmol Soc 68:501-547, 1970.
483. Dutton GN. The causes of tissue damage in toxoplasmic retinochoroiditis. Trans Ophthalmol Soc U K 105:404-412, 1986.
484. O'Connor GR. Ocular toxoplasmosis. Trans New Orleans Acad Ophthalmol 31:108-121, 1983.
485. Holland GN, O'Connor GR, Belfort R Jr, Remington JS. Toxoplasmosis. *In* Pepose JS, Holland GN, Wilhelmus KR (eds). Ocular Infection and Immunity. St. Louis, Mosby–Year Book, 1996, pp 1183-1223.
486. Holland GN, Lewis KG. An update on current practices in the management of ocular toxoplasmosis. Am J Ophthalmol 134: 102-114, 2002.
487. Roberts F, McLeod R. Pathogenesis of toxoplasmic retinochoroiditis. Parasitol Today 15:51-57, 1999.
488. Hay J, Lee WR, Dutton GN, et al. Congenital toxoplasmic retinochoroiditis in a mouse model. Ann Trop Med Parasitol 78:109-116, 1984.
489. Hay J, Graham DI, Lee WR, et al. Congenital neuro-ophthalmic toxoplasmosis in the mouse. Ann Trop Med Parasitol 81:25-28, 1987.
490. Hutchison WM, Hay J, Lee WR, Siim JC. A study of cataract in murine congenital toxoplasmosis. Ann Trop Med Parasitol 76:53-70, 1982.
491. Hay J, Dutton GN, Ralston J. Congenital toxoplasmic retinochoroiditis in the mouse—the use of the peroxidase anti-peroxidase method to demonstrate *Toxoplasma* antigen. Trans R Soc Trop Med Hyg 79:106-109, 1985.
492. Dutton GN, Hay J, Hair DM, Ralston J. Clinicopathological features of a congenital murine model of ocular toxoplasmosis. Graefes Arch Clin Exp Ophthalmol 224:256-264, 1986.
493. Graham DI, Hay J, Hutchison WM, Siim JC. Encephalitis in mice with congenital ocular toxoplasmosis. J Pathol 142:265-277, 1984.
494. Lu F, Huang S, Kasper LH. $CD4^+$ T cells in the pathogenesis of murine ocular toxoplasmosis. Infect Immun 72:4966-4972, 2004.
495. Frenkel JK. Pathogenesis of toxoplasmosis and of infections with organisms resembling *Toxoplasma.* Ann N Y Acad Sci 64:215-251, 1956.

496. Rollins DF, Tabbara KF, O'Connor GR, et al. Detection of toxoplasmal antigen and antibody in ocular fluids in experimental ocular toxoplasmosis. Arch Ophthalmol 101:455-457, 1983.
497. Mets MB, Holfels E, Boyer KM, et al. Eye manifestations of congenital toxoplasmosis. Am J Opthalmol 122:309-324, 1996.
498. Montoya JG, Parmley S, Liesenfeld O, et al. Use of the polymerase chain reaction for diagnosis of ocular toxoplasmosis. Ophthalmology 106:1554-1563, 1999.
499. Chan C-C, Palestine A, Li Q, Nussenblatt R. Diagnosis of ocular toxoplasmosis by the use of immunocytology and the polymerase chain reaction. Am J Ophthal 117:803-805, 1994.
500. Manners R, O'Connell S, Guy E, et al. Use of the polymerase chain reaction in the diagnosis of acquired ocular toxoplasmosis in an immunocompetent adult. Br J Ophthalmol 78:583-584, 1994.
501. Norose K, Tokushima T, Yano A. Quantitative polymerase chain reaction in diagnosing ocular toxoplasmosis. Am J Ophthalmol 121:441-442, 1996.
502. Remington JS, Thulliez P, Montoya JG. Recent developments for diagnosis of toxoplasmosis. J Clin Microbiol 42:941-945, 2004.
503. Montoya JG, Remington JS. Toxoplasmic chorioretinitis in the setting of acute acquired toxoplasmosis. Clin Infect Dis 23:277-282, 1996.
504. Roberts F, Roberts C, Ferguson D, McLeod R. Inhibition of nitric oxide production exacerbates chronic ocular toxoplasmosis. Parasite Immunol 22:1-5, 2000.
505. Roberts F, Mets MB, Ferguson DJ, et al. Histopathological features of ocular toxoplasmosis in the fetus and infant. Arch Ophthalmol 119:51-58, 2001.
506. Roberts F, Mets M, Ferguson D, et al. The histopathological features of ocular toxoplasmosis in the fetus and infant. Fifth International Toxoplasma Conference, Marshall, Calif, May 1-6, 1999.
507. Araujo FG, Remington JS. Induction of tolerance to an intracellular protozoan (*Toxoplasma gondii*) by passively administered antibody. J Immunol 113:1424-1428, 1974.
508. Crawford JB. *Toxoplasma* retinochoroiditis. Arch Ophthalmol 76:829-832, 1966.
509. Hogan MJ, Kimura SJ, O'Connor R. Ocular toxoplasmosis. Clin Sci 72:592-600, 1964.
510. Jacobs L, Fair MJR, Bickerton MJH. Adult ocular toxoplasmosis. A preliminary report of a parasitologically proved case. Arch Ophthalmol 51:287, 1954.
511. Hogan MJ, Zweigart PA, Lewis AB. Recovery of *Toxoplasma* from a human eye. Arch Ophthalmol 60:548-554, 1958.
512. Couvreur J, Thulliez P. [Acquired toxoplasmosis with ocular or neurologic involvement.] Presse Med 25:438-442, 1996.
513. Callahan WP Jr, Russell WO, Smith MG. Human toxoplasmosis. Medicine 25:343-397, 1946.
514. Hayes K, Billson FA, Jack I, et al. Cell culture isolation of *Toxoplasma gondii* from an infant with unusual ocular features. Med J Aust 1:1297-1299, 1973.
515. Manschot WA, Daamen CB. Connatal ocular toxoplasmosis. Arch Ophthalmol 74:48-54, 1965.
516. Pratt-Thomas HR, Cannon WM. Systemic infantile toxoplamosis. Am J Pathol 22:779-795, 1946.
517. Milgram JW. Osseous changes in congenital toxoplasmosis. Arch Pathol 97:150-151, 1974.
518. Zuelzer WW. Infantile toxoplasmosis, with a report of three cases, including two in which the patients were identical twins. Arch Path 38:1-19, 1944.
519. Mellgren J, Alm L, Kjessler A. The isolation of *Toxoplasma* from the human placenta and uterus. Acta Pathol Microbiol Scand 30:59-67, 1952.
520. Elliott WG. Placental toxoplasmosis: a report of a case. Am J Clin Pathol 53:413-417, 1970.
521. Benirschke K, Driscoll SG. The Pathology of the Human Placenta. New York, Springer-Verlag, 1967.
522. Werner H, Schmidtke L, Thomascheck G. [*Toxoplasma* infection and pregnancy. Histologic demonstration of the intrauterine route of infection.] Klin Wochenschr 41:96-101, 1963.
523. Driscoll SG. Fetal infections in man. *In* Benirschke K (ed). Comparative Aspects of Reproductive Failure. New York, Springer-Verlag, 1966, pp 270-295.
524. Farber S, Craig JM. Clinical Pathological Conference (Children's Medical Center, Boston, Mass). J Pediatr 49:752-764, 1956.
525. Cardoso RA, Nery-Guimarae F, Garcia AP, et al. Congenital toxoplasmosis. *In* Siim JC (ed). Human Toxoplasmosis. Copenhagen, Munksgaard, 1960, pp 20-33.
526. Piche M, Battaglione V, Monticelli I, et al. [Placental toxoplasmosis in AIDS. Immunohitochemical and ultrastructural study of a case.] Ann Pathol 17:337-339, 1997.
527. Garcia AG, Coutinho SG, Amendoeira MR, et al. Placental morphology of newborns at risk for congenital toxoplasmosis. J Trop Pediatr 29:95-103, 1983.
528. Altshuler G. Toxoplasmosis as a cause of hydranencephaly. Am J Dis Child 125:251-252, 1973.
529. Rodney MB, Mitchell N, Redner B, Turin R. Infantile toxoplasmosis: report of a case with autopsy. Pediatrics 5:649-663, 1950.
530. Wolf A, Cowen D, Paige BH. Toxoplasmic encephalomyelitis. VI. Clinical diagnosis of infantile or congenital toxoplasmosis; survival beyond infancy. Arch Neurol Psychiatr 48:689-739, 1942.
531. Hervas JA, Fiol M, Caimari M, et al. Central nervous system congenital toxoplasmosis mimicking brain abscesses. Pediatr Infect Dis J 6:491-492, 1987.
532. Frenkel JK. Pathology and pathogenesis of congenital toxoplasmosis. Bull N Y Acad Med 50:182-191, 1974.
533. Frenkel JK. Toxoplasmosis. Mechanisms of infection, laboratory diagnosis and management. Curr Top Pathol 54:27-75, 1971.
534. McAuley J, Boyer KM, Patel D, et al. Early and longitudinal evaluations of treated infants and children and untreated historical patients with congenital toxoplasmosis: the Chicago Collaborative Treatment Trial. Clin Inf Dis 18:38-72, 1994.
535. Heath P, Zuelzer WW. Toxoplasmosis (report of eye findings in infant twins). Trans Am Ophthalmol Soc 42:119-131, 1944.
536. Koch FL, Wolf A, Cowen D, Paige BH. Toxoplasmic encephalomyelitis. VII. Significance of ocular lesions in the dagnosis of infantile or congenital toxoplasmosis. Arch Ophthalmol 29:1-25, 1943.
537. Bamatter F. La choriorétinite toxoplasmique. Ophthalmologica 114:340-358, 1947.
538. Binkhorst CD. Toxoplasmosis. Report of four cases, with demonstration of parasites in one case. Ophthalmologica 115:65-67, 1948.
539. Hogan MJ. Toxoplasmic chorioretinitis. Trans Pac Coast Oto-ophthal Soc 28:83-102, 1947.
540. Hogan MJ. Ocular Toxoplasmosis. New York, Columbia University Press, 1951.
541. Kelemen G. Toxoplasmosis and congenital deafness. Arch Ophthalomol 68:547-561, 1958.
542. Couvreur J. [The lungs in toxoplasmosis.] Rev Mal Respir 3:525-532, 1975.
543. Pomeroy C, Filice GA. Pulmonary toxoplasmosis: a review. Clin Infect Dis 14:863-870, 1992.
544. Medlock MD, Tilleli JT, Pearl GS. Congenital cardiac toxoplasmosis in a newborn with acquired immunodeficiency syndrome. Pediatr Infect Dis J 9:129-132, 1990.
545. Lelong M, Lepage F, Alison F, et al. Toxoplasmose du nouveau-né avec ictére et cirrhose du foie. Arch Fr Pediatr 10:530-536, 1953.
546. Caldera R, Sarrut S, Rossier A. [Hepatic calcifications in the course of congenital toxoplasmosis.] Arch Fr Pediatr 19:1087-1093, 1962.
547. Israelski DM, Skowron G, Leventhal JP, et al. *Toxoplasma* peritonitis in a patient with acquired immunodeficiency syndrome. Arch Intern Med 148:1655-1657, 1988.
548. Kean BH, Grocott RG. Sarcosporidiosis or toxoplasmosis in man and guinea pig. Am J Pathol 21:467-483, 1945.
549. Miller MJ, Seaman E, Remington JS. The clinical spectrum of congenital toxoplasmosis: problems in recognition. J Pediatr 70: 714-723, 1967.
550. Fediushina NA, Sherstennikova GE. [Damage of the kidneys in congenital toxoplasmosis.] Vrach Delo 4:121-122, 1966.
551. Wickbom B, Winberg J. Coincidence of congenital toxoplasmosis and acute nephritis with nephrotic syndrome. Acta Paediatr Scand 61:470-472, 1972.
552. Guignard JP, Torrado A. Interstitial nephritis and toxoplasmosis in a 10-year-old child. J Pediatr 85:381-382, 1974.
553. Shahin B, Papadopoulou ZL, Jenis EH. Congenital nephrotic syndrome associated with congenital toxoplasmosis. J Pediatr 85: 366-370, 1974.
554. Couvreur J, Alison F, Boccon-Gibod L, et al. [The kidney and toxoplasmosis.] Ann Pediatr (Paris) 31:847-852, 1984.
555. Torres CM. Affinité de l'*Encephalitozoon chagasi* agent étiologique d'une méningoencephalomyélitis congénitale avec myocardité et myosité chez l'homme. C R Soc Biol 86:1797-1799, 1927.
556. Alford CJ, Stagno S, Reynolds DW. Congenital toxoplasmosis: clinical, laboratory, and therapeutic considerations, with special reference to subclinical disease. Bull N Y Acad Med 50:160-181, 1974.

557. Willi H, Koller F, Raaflaub J. Symptomatische Makroglobulinamie bei Lues congenita; Beitrag zur Frage der "Fibrinasthenie" Faconi. Acta Haematol (Basel) 11:316-320, 1954.
558. Koch F, Schlagetter K, Schultze HE, et al. Symptomatische Makroglobulinamie bei Lues connata. Z Kinderheilkd 78:283-300, 1956.
559. Oehme J. Symptomatische Makroglobulinamie bei Lues connata. Klin Wochenschr 36:369-382, 1958.
560. Koch F, Schultze HE, Schwick G. [Symptomatic macroglobulinemia in congenital toxoplasmosis.] Z Kinderheilkd 82:44-49, 1959.
561. Oxelius VA. Monoclonal immunoglobulins in congenital toxoplasmosis. Clin Exp Immunol 11:367-380, 1972.
562. Aiuti F, Ungari S, Turbessi G, et al. Immunologic aspects of congenital syphilis. Helv Paediatr Acta 21:66-71, 1966.
563. Van Camp B, Reynaert P, Van Beers D. Congenital toxoplasmosis associated with transient monoclonal IgG_1-lambda gammopathy. Rev Infect Dis 4:173-178, 1982.
564. Griscelli C, Desmonts G, Gny B, Frommel D. Congenital toxoplasmosis. Fetal synthesis of oligoclonal immunoglobulin G in intrauterine infection. J Pediatr 83:20-26, 1973.
565. Arnaud JP, Griscelli C, Couvreur J, Desmonts G. [Hematological and immunological abnormalities in congenital toxoplasmosis.] Nouv Rev Fr Hematol 15:496-505, 1975.
566. Vinh LT, Duc TV, Aicardi J, et al Association of congenital toxoplasmosis and cytomegaly in infants. Study of two anatomoclinical cases. Arch Fr Pediatr 27:511-521, 1970.
567. Sotelo-Avila C, Perry CM, Parvey LS, Eyal FG. Coexistent congenital cytomegalovirus and toxoplasmosis in a newborn infant. J Tenn Med Assoc 67:588-592, 1974.
568. Maszkiewicz W, Wojnar A, Sujakowa A, Ostrowska-Ryng W. [Coexistence of cytomegalic inclusion disease, toxoplasmosis and in a premature infant.] Pediatr Pol 57:821-826, 1982.
569. De Zegher F, Sluiters JF, Stuurman PM, et al. Concomitant cytomegalovirus infection and congenital toxoplasmosis in a newborn. Eur J Pediatr 147:424-425, 1988.
570. Demian SD, Donnelly WJ, Monif GR. Coexistent congenital cytomegalovirus and toxoplasmosis in a stillborn. Am J Dis Child 125:420-421, 1973.
571. Stanton MF, Pinkerton H. Benign acquired toxoplasmosis with subsequent pregnancy. Am J Clin Pathol 23:1199-1207, 1953.
572. Remington JS, Barnett CG, Meikel M, Lunde MN. Toxoplasmosis and infectious mononucleosis. Arch Intern Med 110:744-753, 1962.
573. Siim JC. Clinical and diagnostic aspects of human acquired toxoplasmosis. *In* Siim JC (ed). Human Toxoplasmosis. Copenhagen, Munksgaard, 1960, pp 53-79.
574. Tenhunen A. Glandular Toxoplasmosis: Occurrence of the Disease in Finland. Copenhagen: Munksgaard. 72 S. Acta path. microbiol. scand., Suppl. 172 (1964) (Biol. Abstr. 46, 67354 (1965), Excerpta med. V. 18, 2482 (1965) und XVII. 11, 5044 (1965), Kongr. -Zbl. ges. inn. Med. 274, 147 (1965), Trop. Dis. Bull. 62, 584 (1965), Zbl. Bakt., I. Abt. Ref. 198, 382 (1965)).
575. Beverley JKA, Beattie CP. Glandular toxoplasmosis. A survey of 30 cases. Lancet 1:379-384, 1958.
576. Remington JS. Toxoplasmosis in the adult. Bull N Y Acad Med 50:211-227, 1974.
577. Joseph R, Desmonts G, Job JC, Couvreur J. Abdominal lymphadenopathy as first localization of acquired toxoplasmosis. *In* Siim JC (ed). Human Toxoplasmosis. Copenhagen, Munksgaard, 1960, pp 120-123.
578. Jones TC, Kean BH, Kimball AC. Acquired toxoplasmosis. N Y State J Med 69:2237-2242, 1969.
579. Vischer TL, Bernheim C, Engelbrecht E. Two cases of hepatitis due to *Toxoplasma gondii*. Lancet 2:919-921, 1967.
580. Masur H, Jones TC. Hepatitis in acquired toxoplasmosis. Letter to the editor. N Engl J Med 1979;301:613, 1979.
581. Frenkel JK, Remington JS. Hepatitis in toxoplasmosis. Letter to the editor with reply. N Engl J Med 302:178-179, 1980.
582. Weitberg AB, Alper JC, Diamond I, Fligiel Z. Acute granulomatous hepatitis in the course of acquired toxoplasmosis. N Engl J Med 300:1093-1096, 1979.
583. Vethanyagam A, Bryceson ADM. Acquired toxoplasmosis presenting as hepatitis. Trans R Soc Trop Med Hyg 70:524-525, 1976.
584. Greenlee JE, Johnson WD Jr, Campa JF, et al. Adult toxoplasmosis presenting as polymyositis and cerebellar ataxia. Ann Intern Med 82:367-371, 1975.
585. Samuels BS, Rietschel RL. Polymyositis and toxoplasmosis. JAMA 235:60-61, 1976.
586. Phillips PE, Kassan SS, Kagen LJ. Increased *Toxoplasma* antibodies in idiopathic inflammatory muscle disease. A case-controlled study. Arthritis Rheum 22:209-214, 1979.
587. Kagen LJ, Kimball AC, Christian CL. Serologic evidence of toxoplasmosis among patients with polymyositis. Am J Med 56: 186-191, 1974.
588. Pollock JL. Toxoplasmosis appearing to be dermatomyositis. Arch Dermatol 115:736-737, 1979.
589. Pointud P, Clerc D, Bouree P, et al. [Positive toxoplasmic serology in polymyositis.] Ann Med Interne (Paris) 127:881-885, 1976.
590. Topi GC, D'Alessandro L, Catricala C, Zardi O. Dermatomyositis-like syndrome due to *Toxoplasma*. Br J Dermatol 1979;101(5):589-591.
591. Gump DW, Holden RA. Acquired chorioretinitis due to toxoplasmosis. Ann Intern Med 90:58-60, 1979.
592. Masur H, Jones TC, Lempert JA, Cherubini TD. Outbreak of toxoplasmosis in a family and documentation of acquired retinochoroiditis. Am J Med 64:396-402, 1978.
593. Michelson JB, Shields JA, McDonald PR, et al. Retinitis secondary to acquired systemic toxoplasmosis with isolation of the parasite. Am J Ophthalmol 86:548-552, 1978.
594. Saari M, Vuorre I, Neiminen H, Raisanen S. Acquired toxoplasmic chorioretinitis. Arch Ophthalmol 94:1485-1488, 1976.
595. Wising PJ. Lymphadenopathy and chorioretinitis in acute adult toxoplasmosis. Nord Med 47:563-565, 1952.
596. Eichenwald HF. A study of congenital toxoplasmosis, with particular emphasis on clinical manifestations, sequelae and therapy. *In* Siim JC (ed). Human Toxoplasmosis. Copenhagen, Munksgaard, 1960, p 41.
597. Feldman HA. Toxoplasmosis. Pediatrics 22:559-574, 1958.
598. Alford CJ, Foft JW, Blankenship WJ, et al. Subclinical central nervous system disease of neonates: a prospective study of infants born with increased levels of IgM. J Pediatr 75:1167-1178, 1969.
599. Wilson CB, Remington JS, Stagno S, Reynolds DW. Development of adverse sequelae in children born with subclinical congenital *Toxoplasma* infection. Pediatrics 66:767-774, 1980.
600. Koppe JG, Kloosterman GJ, De Roever-Bonnet H, et al. Toxoplasmosis and pregnancy, with a long-term follow-up of the children. Eur J Obstet Gynec Reprod Biol 4:101-110, 1974.
601. De Roever-Bonnet H, Koppe JG, Loewer-Sieger DH. Follow-up of children with congenital *Toxoplasma* infection and children who become serologically negative after 1 year of age, all born in 1964-1965. *In* Thalhammer O, Baumgarten K, Pollak A (eds). Perinatal Medicine, Sixth European Congress, Vienna. Stuttgart, Georg Thieme Verlag, 1979, pp 61-75.
602. Rossier A, Blancher G, Designolle L, et al. Toxoplasmose congénitale á manifestation retardée. Effet du traitement. Sem Hop 37: 1266-1268, 1961.
603. Couvreur J, Desmonts G. Congenital and maternal toxoplasmosis. A review of 300 congenital cases. Dev Med Child Neurol 4:519-530, 1962.
604. Couvreur J, Desmonts G, Tournier G, Szusterkac M. [A homogeneous series of 210 cases of congenital toxoplasmosis in 0- to 11-month-old infants detected prospectively.] Ann Pediatr (Paris) 31:815-819, 1984.
605. Guerina N, Hsu H-W, Meissner H, et al. Neonatal serologic screening and early treatment for congenital *Toxoplasma gondii* infection. N Engl J Med 330:1858-1863, 1994.
606. Sever JL. Perinatal infections affecting the developing fetus and newborn. *In* Eichenwald H (ed). The Prevention of Mental Retardation through Control of Infectious Diseases. Public Health Service publication no. 1692. Washington, DC, US Government Printing Office, 1968, pp 37-68.
607. Paul J. Früngeburt und Toxoplasmose. München, Urban v. Schwarzenberg, 1962.
608. Couvreur J, Desmonts G, Girre JY. Congenital toxoplasmosis in twins: a series of 14 pairs of twins: absence of infection in one twin in two pairs. J Pediatr 89:235-240, 1976.
609. Abbott KH, Camp JD. Extensive symmetrical cerebral calcification and chorioretinitis in identical twins (toxoplasmosis?). Clinical report of cases. Bull Los Angeles Neurol Soc 12:38-47, 1947.
610. Fendel H. Eine toxoplasmotische Zwillingsgeburt. Virchows Arch Pathol Anat 327:293-303, 1955.
611. François J. La Toxoplasmose et Ses Manifestations Oculaires. Paris, Masson, 1963.

612. Granström KO, Magnusson JH. Convergent strabismus, macular foci and toxoplasmosis in monozygotic twins. Br J Ophthalmol 34:105-107, 1950.
613. Hoppeler H, Sadoun R. Encéphalophatie chronique chez duex jumeaux; role éventuel de al toxoplasmose. Arch Fr Pediatr 12: 212-214, 1955.
614. Murphy WF, Flannery JL. Congenital toxoplasmosis occurring in identical twins. Am J Dis Child 84:223-226, 1952.
615. Binkhorst CD. Toxoplasmosis: A Clinical, Serological Study with Special Reference to Eye Manifestations. Leiden, HE Stenfert, 1948.
616. Farquhar HG. Congenital toxoplasmosis. Report of two cases in twins. Lancet 259:562-564, 1950.
617. Rieger H. Toxoplasmosis congenital und Zwillingsschwangerschaft. Klin Monatsblk Augenheilkd 134:862-871, 1959.
618. Yukins RE, Winter FC. Ocular disease in congenital toxoplasmosis in nonidentical twins. Am J Ophthalmol 62:44-46, 1966.
619. Statz A, Wenzel D, Heimann G. [Clinical course of congenital toxoplasmosis in dizygotic twins (author's transl).] Klin Padiatr 190: 599-602, 1978.
620. Benjamin B, Brickman HF, Neaga A. A congenital toxoplasmosis in twins. Can Med Assoc J 80:639-643, 1958.
621. Thalhammer O. Congenital toxoplasmosis. Lancet 1:23-24, 1962.
622. Beverley JK. A discussion on toxoplasmosis: congenital *Toxoplasma* infections. Proc R Soc Med 53:111-113, 1960.
623. Juurikkala A. Posterior uveitis and toxoplasmosis. Acta Ophthalmol 39:367-369, 1961.
624. Sibalic D, Djurkovic-Djakovic O, Nikolic R. Congenital toxoplasmosis in premature twins. Folia Parasitol (Praha) 33:7-13, 1986.
625. Wiswell TE, Fajardo JE, Bass JW, et al. Congenital toxoplasmosis in triplets. J Pediatr 1984;105(1):59-61, 1984.
626. Couvreur J, Thulliez P, Daffos F, et al. Six cases of toxoplasmosis in twins. Ann Pediatr (Paris) 38:63-68, 1991.
627. Tolentino P, Bucalossi A. Due casi de encefalomielite infantile di natura toxoplasmica. Policlin Infant 16:265-284, 1948.
628. Peyron F, Ateba AB, Wallon M, et al. Congenital toxoplasmosis in twins: a report of fourteen consecutive cases and a comparison with published data. Pediatr Infect Dis J 22:695-701, 2003.
629. Martinovic J, Sibalic D, Djordjevic M, et al. Frequency of toxoplasmosis in the appearance of congenital hydrocephalus. J Neurosurg 56:830-834, 1982.
630. Wende-Fischer R, Ehrenheim C, Heyer R, et al. Toxoplasmosis. Monatsschr Kinderheilkd 141:789-791, 1993.
631. Ribierre M, Couvreur J, Canetti J. Les hydrocéphalies par sténose de l'aqueduc de sylvius dans la toxoplasmose congenitale. Arch Fr Pediatr 27:501-510, 1970.
632. Kaiser G. Hydrocephalus following toxoplasmosis. Z Kinderchir 40(suppl 1):10-11, 1985.
633. Tognetti F, Galassi E, Gaist G. Neurological toxoplasmosis presenting as a brain tumor. Case report. J Neurosurg 56:716-721, 1982.
634. Baron J, Youngblood L, Siewers MF, Medearis DJ. The incidence of cytomegalovirus, herpes simplex, rubella, and *Toxoplasma* antibodies in microcephalic, mentally retarded, and normocephalic children. Pediatrics 44:932-939, 1969.
635. Thalhammer O. Die angeborene Toxoplasmose. *In* Kirchhoff H, Kräubig H (eds). Toxoplasmose Praktische Fragen und Ergebnisse. Stuttgart, Georg Thieme Verlag, 1966, pp 151-173.
636. Remington JS, cited by Frenkel JK. Some data on the incidence of human toxoplasmosis as a cause of mental retardation. *In* Eichenwald HF (ed). The Prevention of Mental Retardation through Control of Infectious Diseases. Public Health Service publication no. 1962. Washington, DC, US Government Printing Office, 1968, pp 89-97.
637. Silver HK, Dixon MS. Congenital toxoplasmosis: report of case with cataract, "atypical" vasopressin-sensitive diabetes insipidus, and marked eosinophilia. Am J Dis Child 88:84-91, 1954.
638. Perkins ES. Ocular toxoplasmosis. Br J Ophthalmol 57:1-17, 1973.
639. Desmonts G. Toxoplasmose oculaire: etude epidemiologique (bilan de 2030 examend d'humeur agueuse). Arch Ophtalmol (Paris) 33: 87-102, 1973.
640. Sibalic D, Djurkovic-Djakovic O, Bobic B. Onset of ocular complications in congenital toxoplasmosis associated with immunoglobulin M antibodies to *Toxoplasma gondii*. Eur J Clin Microbiol Infect Dis 9:671-674, 1990.
641. Burnett AJ, Shortt SG, Isaac-Renton J, et al. Multiple cases of acquired toxoplasmosis retinitis presenting in an outbreak. Ophthalmology 105:1032-1037, 1998.
642. Fair JR. Congenital toxoplasmosis. III. Ocular signs of the disease in state schools for the blind. Am J Ophthalmol 48:165-172, 1959.
643. Fair JR. Congenital toxoplasmosis—diagnostic importance of chorioretinitis. JAMA 168:250-253, 1958.
644. Fair JR. Congenital toxoplasmosis. V. Ocular aspects of the disease. J Med Assoc Ga 48:604-607, 1959.
645. Kazdan JJ, McCulloch JC, Crawford JS. Uveitis in children. Can Med Assoc J 96:385-391, 1967.
646. de Carvalho KM, Minguini N, Moreira Filho DC, Kara-Jose N. Characteristics of a pediatric low-vision population. J Pediatr Ophthalmol Strabismus 35:162-165, 1998.
647. Kara-José N, Carvalho KMM, Pereira VL, et al. Estudos retrospectivos dos primeiros 140 caves atendidos na Clinica de Visao Subnormal do Hospital das Clinicas da UNICAMP. Arq Bras Oftalmol 51:65-69, 1988.
648. Buchignani BPC, Silva MRBM. Levantamento das causes e resultados. Bras Oftalmol 50:49-54, 1991.
649. Meenken C, Assies J, van Nieuwenhuizen O, et al. Long term ocular and neurological involvement in severe congenital toxoplasmosis. Br J Ophthalmol 79:581-584, 1995.
650. Rothova A. Ocular involvement in toxoplasmosis. Br J Ophthalmol 77:371-377, 1993.
651. Hogan MJ, Kimura SJ, Lewis A, Zweigart PA. Early and delayed ocular manifestations of congenital toxoplasmosis. Trans Am Ophthalmol Soc 55:275-296, 1957.
652. Parissi G. Essai d'évaluation du risque de poussée évolutive secondaire de choriorétinite dans la toxoplasmose congénitale. Paris, Thése Paris-Saint-Antoine, 1973.
653. De Vroede M, Piepsz A, Dodion J, et al. Congenital toxoplasmosis: late appearance of retinal lesions after treatment. Acta Paediatr Scand 68:761-762, 1979.
654. Lou P, Kazdan J, Basu PK. Ocular toxoplasmosis in three consecutive siblings. Arch Ophthalmol 96:613-614, 1978.
655. Lappalainen M, Koskiniemi M, Hiilesmaa V, et al. Outcome of children after maternal primary *Toxoplasma* infection during pregnancy with emphasis on avidity of specific IgG. Pediatr Infect Dis J 14:354-361, 1995.
656. Gross U, Muller J, Roos T, et al. Possible reasons for failure of conventional tests for diagnosis of fatal congential toxoplasmosis: report of a case diagnosed by PCR and Immunoblot. Infection 20:149-152, 1992.
657. Pettapiece MC, Hiles DA, Johnson BL. Massive congenital ocular toxoplasmosis. J Pediatr Ophthalmol 13:259-265, 1976.
658. O'Connor GR. Manifestations and management of ocular toxoplasmosis. Bull N Y Acad Med 50:192-210, 1974.
659. Francescheti A, Bamatter F. Toxoplasmose oculaire. Diagnostic clinique, anatomique et histopharsitologique des affections toxoplasmiques. Acta I Congr Lat Ophthalmol 1:315-437, 1953.
660. Saxon SA, Knight W, Reynolds DW, et al. Intellectual deficits in children born with subclinical congenital toxoplasmosis: a preliminary report. J Pediatr 82:792-797, 1973.
661. Berengo A, Bechelli G, de Lalla F, et al. [Serological research on diffusion of toxoplasmosis. Study of 1720 patients hospitalized in a psychiatric hospital.] Minerva Med 57:2292-2305, 1966.
662. Kvirikadze VV, Yourkova IA. On the role of congenital toxoplasmosis in the origin of oligophrenia and of its certain other forms of mental ailments. Zh Nevropatol Psikhiatr 61:1059-1062, 1961.
663. Kozar Z, Dluzewski L, Dluzewska A, Jaraszewski Z. Toxoplasmosis as a cause of mental deficiency. Neurol Neurochir Pol 4:383-396, 1954.
664. Caiaffa W, Chiari C, Figueiredo A, et al. Toxoplasmosis and mental retardation—report of a case-control study. Mem Inst Oswaldo Cruz 88:253-261, 1993.
665. Hume OS. Toxoplasmosis and pregnancy. Am J Obstet Gynecol 114:703-715, 1972.
666. Fleck DG. Epidemiology of toxoplasmosis. J Hyg (Camb) 61:61-65, 1963.
667. Burkinshaw J, Kirman BH, Sorsby A. Toxoplasmosis in relation to mental deficiency. BMJ 1:702-704, 1953.
668. Mackie MJ, Fiscus AG, Pallister P. A study to determine causal relationships of toxoplasmosis to mental retardation. Am J Epidemiol 94:215-221, 1971.
669. Stern H, Booth JC, Elek SD, Fleck DG. Microbial causes of mental retardation. The role of prenatal infections with cytomegalovirus, rubella virus, and *Toxoplasma*. Lancet 2:443-448, 1969.
670. Fisher OD. *Toxoplasma* infection in English children. A survey with toxoplasmin intradermal antigen. Lancet 2:904-906, 1951.

671. Cook I, Derrick EH. The incidence of *Toxoplasma* antibodies in mental hospital patients. Aust Ann Med 10:137-141, 1961.
672. Fair JR. Congenital toxoplasmosis. IV. Case finding using the skin test and ophthalmoscope in state schools for mentally retarded children. Am J Ophthalmol 48:813-819, 1959.
673. Labzoffsky NA, Fish NA, Gyulai E, Roughley F. A survey of toxoplasmosis among mentally retarded children. Can Med Assoc J 92:1026-1028, 1965.
674. Hoejenbos E, Stronk MG. In quest of toxoplasmosis as a cause of mental deficiency. Psychiatr Neurol Neurochir 69:33-41, 1966.
675. Macer G. Toxoplasmosis in obstetrics, its possible relation to mongolism. Am J Obstet Gynecol 87:66-70, 1963.
676. Thiers H, Romagny G. Mongolisme chez une enfant atteinte de toxoplasmose; discussion du rapport étiologique. Lyon Med 185: 145-151, 1951.
677. Kleine HO. Toxoplasmose als Ursache von Mongolismus. Z Geburtschilfe Gynaekol 147:13-27, 1956.
678. Hostomská L, Jirovec O, Horácková M, et al. Mongolismus und latente Toxoplasmose der Mutter. Endokrinologie 34:296-304, 1957.
679. Jírovec O, Jira J, Fuchs V, Peter R. Studien mit dem toxoplasmintest. I. Bereitung des toxoplasmins. Technik des intradermalen Testes. Frequenz der Positivitat bei normaler Bevolkerung und bei einigen Krankengruppen. Zentralb Bakteriol [Orig] 169:129-159, 1957.
680. Kleif AD, Kerner GI. [On the role of toxoplasmosis in the genesis of Down's syndrome.] Zh Nevropatol Psikhiatr 67:1462-1466, 1967.
681. Frenkel JK. Toxoplasmosis. *In* Benirschke K (ed). Comparative Aspects of Reproductive Failure. New York, Springer, 1966, pp 296-321.
682. Andersen H. Toxoplasmosis in a child with congenital myxoedema. Acta Paediatr 44:98-99, 1955.
683. Aagaard K, Melchior J. The simultaneous occurrence of congenital toxoplasmosis and congenital myxoedema. Acta Paediatr 48: 164-168, 1959.
684. Margit T, Istvan ER. Congenital toxoplasmosis causing diabetes insipidus. Orv Hetil 124:827-829, 1983.
685. Massa G, Vanderschueren-Lodeweyckx M, Van Vliet G, et al. Hypothalamo-pituitary dysfunction in congenital toxoplasmosis. Eur J Pediatr 148:742-744, 1989.
686. Yamakawa R, Yamashita Y, Yano A, et al. Congenital toxoplasmosis complicated by central diabetes insipidus in an infant with Down syndrome. Brain Dev 18:75-77, 1996.
687. Oygür N, Yilmaz G, Özkaynak C, Guven AG. Central diabetes insipidus in a patient with congenital toxoplasmosis. Am J Perinatol 15:191-192, 1998.
688. Bruhl HH, Bahn RC, Hayles AB. Sexual precocity associated with congenital toxoplasmosis. Mayo Clin Proc 33:682-686, 1958.
689. Coppola A, Spera C, Varcaccio G, et al. [Partial anterior hypo-pituitarism caused by toxoplasmosis congenita. Description of a clinical case.] Minerva Med 78:403-410, 1987.
690. Roussel B, Pinon JM, Birembaut P, et al. [Congenital nephrotic syndrome associated with congenital toxoplasmosis.] Arch Fr Pediatr 44:795-797, 1987.
691. Farkas-Bargeton E. Personal communication cited by Rabinowicz, T. Acquired cerebral toxoplasmosis in the adult. *In* Hentsch D (ed). Toxoplasmosis. Bern, Hans Huber, 1971, pp 197-219.
692. Kove S, Dische R, Goldstein S, Wroblewski F. Pattern of serum transaminase activity in neonatal jaundice due to cytomegalic inclusion disease and toxoplasmosis with hepatic involvement. J Pediatr 63:660-662, 1963.
693. Freudenberg E. Akute infantile Toxoplasmosis-Enzephalitis. Schweiz Med Wochenschr 77:680-682, 1947.
694. Hellbrügge T. Über Toxoplasmose. Dtsch Med Wochenschr 74: 385-389, 1949.
695. Reiss HJ, Verron T. Beiträge zur Toxoplasmose. Dtsch Gesundheitsw 6:646-653, 1951.
696. Justus J. Cutaneous manifestations of toxoplasmosis. Curr Probl Dermatol 4:24-47, 1972.
697. Korovitsky LK, Borsov MW, Lobanovsky GI, et al. [Skin lesions in toxoplasmosis.] Vestn Dermatol Venerol (in Russian) 38:28-32, 1962.
698. Justus J. [Congenital toxoplasmosis with dermatitis calcificans toxoplasmatica and tetany of the mother during delivery.] Dtsch Med Wochenschr 93:349-353, 1968.
699. Schmidtke L. [On toxoplasmosis, with special reference to care in pregnancy.] Monatsschr Gesundheitsw Sozialhyg 23:587-591, 1961.
700. Mohr W. Toxoplasmose. *In* Handbuch für Innere Medizin. Berlin, Springer-Verlag, 1952, 1, pp 730-770.
701. Georgakopoulos PA. Etiologic relationship between toxoplasmosis and anencephaly. Int Surg 59:419-420, 1974.
702. Cech JA, Jirovec O. The importance of latent maternal infection with *Toxoplasma* in obstetrics. Bibl Gynaecol 11:41-90, 1961.
703. Korovickij LK, Grigorašenko AE, Stankov AG, et al. Toksoplazmoz. Kiev, Gosmedizdat Kkr SSR, 1962.
704. Erdelyi R. The influence of toxoplasmosis on the incidence of congenital facial malformations: Preliminary report. Plast Reconstr Surg 20:306-310, 1957.
705. Patel DV, Holfels EM, Vogel NP, et al. Resolution of intracranial calcifications in infants with treated congenital toxoplasmosis. Radiology 199:433-440, 1996.
706. Friedman S, Ford-Jones LE, Toi A, et al. Congenital toxoplasmosis: prenatal diagnosis, treatment and postnatal outcome. Prenat Diagn 19:330-333, 1999.
707. Virkola K, Lappalainen M, Valanne L, Kosikiniemi M. Radiological signs in newborns exposed to primary *Toxoplasma* infection in utero. Pediatr Radiol 27:133-138, 1997.
708. Puri S, Spencer RP, Gordon ME. Positive brain scan in toxo-plasmosis. J Nucl Med 15:641-642, 1974.
709. Hervei S, Simon K. [Congenital toxoplasmosis mimicking a cerebral tumor. Special aspects in serodiagnostics of connatal toxoplasmosis (author's transl).] Monatsschr Kinderheilkd 127: 43-47, 1979.
710. Bobowski SJ, Reed WG. Toxoplasmosis in an adult, presenting as a space-occupying cerebral lesion. Arch Pathol Lab Med 65:460-464, 1958.
711. Collins AT, Cromwell LD. Computed tomography in the evaluation of congenital cerebral toxoplasmosis. J Comput Assist Tomogr 4:326-329, 1980.
712. Diebler C, Dusser A, Dulac O. Congenital toxoplasmosis. clinical and neuroradiological evaluation of the cerebral lesions. Neuro-radiology 27:125-130, 1985.
713. Dunn D, Weisberg LA. Serial changes in a patient with congenital CNS toxoplasmosis as observed with CT. Comput Radiol 8:133-139, 1984.
714. Grant EG, Williams AL, Schellinger D, Slovis TL. Intracranial calcifi-cation in the infant and neonate: evaluation by sonography and CT. Radiology 157:63-68, 1985.
715. Titelbaum DS, Hayward JC, Zimmerman RA. Pachygyric-like changes: topographic appearance at MR imaging and CT and correlation with neurologic status. Radiology 173:663-667, 1989.
716. Neuenschwander S, Cordier MD, Couvreur J. [Congenital toxo-plasmosis: contribution of transfontanelle echotomography and computed tomography.] Ann Pediatr (Paris) 31:837-839, 1984.
717. Calabet A, Cadier L, Diard F, et al. [Congenital toxoplasmosis and transfontanelle brain echography. Apropos of 8 cases observed in newborn infants and infants.] J Radiol 65:367-373, 1984.
718. Brodeur AE. Radiologic Diagnosis in Infants and Children. St. Louis, CV Mosby, 1965.
719. Lindgren E. Röntgenologie. Einschliesslich Kontrastmethoden. *In* Olivecrona H, Tönnis W (eds). Handbuch der Neurochirurgie, Band II. Berlin, Springer-Verlag, 1954, p 296.
720. Masherpa F, Valentino V. Intracranial Calcifications. Springfield, Ill, Charles C Thomas, 1959.
721. Potter KH. Pathology of the Fetus and Infant. Chicago, Year Book Medical Publishers, 1961.
722. Traveras JM, Wood EH. Diagnostic Neuroradiology. Baltimore, Williams & Wilkins, 1964.
723. Dyke CG, Wolfe A, Cowen D, et al. Toxoplasmic encephalomyelitis. VIII. Significance of roentgenographic findings in the diagnosis of infantile or congenital toxoplasmosis. AJR Am J Roentgenol 47: 830-844, 1942.
724. Mussbichler H. Radiologic study of intracranial calcifications in congenital toxoplasmosis. Acta Radiol [Diagn] (Stockh) 7:369-379, 1968.
725. Bain A, Bowie J, Flint W, et al. Congenital toxoplasmosis simulating haemolytic disease of the newborn. Br J Obstet Gynaecol 63: 826-832, 1956.
726. Hall EG, Hay JD, Moss PD, Ryan MM. Congenital toxoplasmosis in newborn. Arch Dis Child 1953;28:117-124.
727. Schubert W. Fruchttod und Hydrops universalis durch Toxoplasmose. Virchows Arch 330:518-524, 1957.
728. Siliaeva NF. A case of congenital toxoplasmic meningoencephalitis complicated by an edematous form of symptomatic erythroblastosis. Arkh Patol 27:67-70, 1965.

729. Nelson LG, Hodgman JE. Congenital toxoplasmosis with hemolytic anemia. Calif Med 105:454-457, 1966.
730. Roper HP. A treatable cause of hydrops fetalis. J R Soc Med 79: 109-110, 1986.
731. Wilson CB, Desmonts G, Couvreur J, Remington JS. Lymphocyte transformation in the diagnosis of congenital *Toxoplasma* infection. N Engl J Med 302:785-788, 1980.
732. Koch F, Schorn J, Ule G. über Toxoplasmose. Dtsch Z Nervenheilkd 166:315-348, 1951.
733. Tós-Luty S, Chrzastek-Spruch H, Uminski J. [Studies on the frequency of a positive toxoplasmosis reaction in mentally deficient, deaf and normally developed children.] Wiad Parazytol 10:374-376, 1964.
734. Ristow W. [On the problem of the etiological importance of toxoplasmosis in hearing disorders, especially in deaf-mutism.] Z Laryngol Rhinol Otol 45:251-264 (English summary, 261), 1966.
735. Potasman I, Davidovich M, Tal Y, et al. Congenital toxoplasmosis: a significant cause of neurological morbidity in Israel? Clin Infect Dis 20:259-262, 1995.
736. Wright I. Congenital toxoplasmosis and deafness. An investigation. Pract Otorhinolaryngol (Basel) 33:377-387, 1971.
737. McGee T, Wolters C, Stein L, et al. Absence of sensorineural hearing loss in treated infants and children with congenital toxoplasmosis. Otolarygol Head Neck Surg 106:75-80, 1992.
738. Vanhaesebrouck P, De Wit M, Smets K, et al. Congenital toxoplasmosis presenting as massive neonatal ascites. Helv Paediatr Acta 43:97-101, 1988.
739. Griscom NT, Colodny AH, Rosenberg HK, et al. Diagnostic aspects of neonatal ascites: report of 27 cases. AJR Am J Roentgenol 128:961-969, 1977.
740. Blaakaer J. Ultrasonic diagnosis of fetal ascites and toxoplasmosis. Acta Obstet Gynecol Scand 65:653-654, 1986.
741. Daffos F. Technical aspects of prenatal samplings and fetal transfusion. Curr Stud Hematol Blood Transfus 55:127-129, 1986.
742. Hedenström G, Huldt G, Lagercrantz R. Toxoplasmosis in children. A study of 83 Swedish cases. Acta Paediatr 50:304-312, 1961.
743. Hedenström G. The variability of the course of congenital toxoplasmosis on some relatively mild cases. *In* Siim JC (ed). Human Toxoplasmosis. Copenhagen, Munksgaard, 1960, pp 34-40.
744. Alford C, Foft J, Blankenship W, et al. Subclinical central nervous system disease of neonates: A prospective study of infants born with increased levels of IgM. J Pediatr 75:1167-1178, 1969.
745. Couvreur J, Desmonts G. Les poussées évolutives tardives de la toxoplasmose congénitale. Cah Coll Med Hop Paris 5:752-758, 1964.
746. Wolf A, Cowen D. Perinatal infections of the central nervous system. J Neuropathol Exp Neurol 18:191-243, 1959.
747. Puissan C, Desmonts G, Mozziconacci P. Evolutivité neurologique tardive d'une toxoplasmose congénitale démontrée par l'étude du L.C.R. Ann Pediatr (Paris) 18:224-227, 1971.
748. Mitchell CD, Erlich SS, Mastrucci MT, et al. Congenital toxoplasmosis occurring in infants perinatally infected with human immunodeficiency virus 1. Pediatr Infect Dis J 9:512-518, 1990.
749. Cohen-Addad NE, Joshi VV, Sharer LR, et al. Congenital acquired immunodeficiency syndrome and congenital toxoplasmosis: pathologic support for a chronology of events. J Perinatol 8:328-331, 1988.
750. Velin P, Dupont D, Barbot D, et al. Double contamination materno-foetale par le VIH 1 et le toxoplasme. [Letter to the editor.] Presse Med 20:960, 1991.
751. O'Donohoe JM, Brueton MJ, Holliman RE. Concurrent congenital human immunodeficiency virus infection and toxoplasmosis. Ped Infect Dis J 10:627-628, 1991.
752. Taccone A, Fondelli MP, Ferrea G, Marzoli A. An unusual CT presentation of congenital cerebral toxoplasmosis in an 8-month-old boy with AIDS. Pediatr Radiol 22:68-69, 1992.
753. Tovo PA, De Martino M, Gabiano C, et al. Prognostic factors and survival in children with perinatal HIV-1 infection. Lancet 339: 1249-1253, 1992.
754. Miller MJ, Remington JS. Toxoplasmosis in infants and children with HIV infection or AIDS. *In* Pizzo PA, Wilfert CM (eds). Pediatric AIDS: The Challenge of HIV Infection in Infants, Children, and Adolescents. Baltimore, Williams & Wilkins, 1990, pp 299-307.
755. Castelli G, Scaccia S, Zuccotti G, et al. *Toxoplasma gondii* infection in AIDS children in Italy. Eleventh International Conference on AIDS; Fourth Sexually Transmitted Diseases World Congress, Berlin, 1993 (abstract, p 419).
756. Minkoff H, Remington JS, Holman S, et al. Vertical transmission of *Toxoplasma* by human immunodeficiency virus–infected women. Am J Obstet Gynecol 176:555-559, 1997.
757. European Collaborative Study. Low incidence of congenital toxoplasmosis in children born to women infected with human immunodeficiency virus. Eur J Obstet Gynecol Reprod Biol 68: 93-96, 1996.
758. Shanks GD, Redfield RR, Fischer GW. *Toxoplasma* encephalitis in an infant with acquired immunodeficiency syndrome. Pediatr Infect Dis J 6:70-71, 1987.
759. Bernstein LJ, Ochs HD, Wedgwood RJ, Rubenstein A. Defective humoral immunity in pediatric acquired immune deficiency syndrome. J Pediatr 107:352-357, 1985.
760. Scott GB, Fischl MA, Klimas N, et al. Mothers of infants with the acquired immunodeficiency syndrome. Evidence for both symptomatic and asymptomatic carriers. JAMA 253:363-366, 1985.
761. Desmonts G. Central nervous system toxoplasmosis. Letter to the editor. Pediatr Infect Dis J 6:872-873, 1987.
762. O'Riordan SE, Farkas AG. Maternal death due to cerebral toxoplasmosis. Br J Obstet Gynaecol 105:565-566, 1998.
763. Marty P, Bongain A, Rahal A, et al. Prenatal diagnosis of severe fetal toxoplasmosis as a result of toxoplasmic reactivation in an HIV-1 seropositive woman. Prenat Diagn 14:414-415, 1994.
764. Luft BJ, Remington JS. Toxoplasmic encephalitis in AIDS. AIDS Commentary. Clin Infect Dis 15:211-222, 1992.
765. Beaman M, Luft B, Remington J. Prophylaxis for toxoplasmosis in AIDS. Ann Intern Med 117:163-164, 1992.
766. Liesenfeld O, Wong SY, Remington JS. Toxoplasmosis in the setting of AIDS. *In* Bartlett JG, Merigan TC, Bolognesi D (eds). Textbook of AIDS Medicine, 2nd ed. Baltimore, Williams & Wilkins, 1999, pp 225-259.
767. Hedriana H, Mitchell J, Brown G, Williams S. Normal fetal outcome in a pregnancy with central nervous system toxoplasmosis and human immunodeficiency virus infection. J Reprod Med 38:747-750, 1993.
768. Vanhems P, Irion O, Hirschel B. Toxoplasmic encephalitis during pregnancy. AIDS 7:142-143, 1992.
769. Wallon M, Caudie C, Rubio S, et al. Value of cerebrospinal fluid cytochemical examination for the diagnosis of congenital toxoplasmosis at birth in France. Pediatr Infect Dis J 17:705-710, 1998.
770. Vesikari T, Meurman OH, Mäki R. Persistent rubella-specific IgM-antibody in the cerebrospinal fluid of a child with congenital rubella. Arch Dis Child 55:46-48, 1980.
771. Couvreur J, Desmonts G, Tournier G, Collin F. [Increased local production of specific G immunoglobulins in the cerebrospinal fluid in congenital toxoplasmosis.] Ann Pediatr (Paris) 31:829-835, 1984.
772. Woods CR, Englund J. Congenital toxoplasmosis presenting with eosinophilic meningitis. Pediatr Infect Dis J 12:347-348, 1993.
773. Hohlfeld P, Forestier F, Kaplan C, et al. Fetal thrombocytopenia: a retrospective survey of 5,194 fetal blood samplings. Blood 84: 1851-1856, 1994.
774. Riley ID, Arneil GC. Toxoplasmosis complicated by chickenpox and smallpox. Lancet 2:564-565, 1950.
775. Magnusson JH, Wahlgren F. Human toxoplasmosis: an account of twelve cases in Sweden. Acta Pathol Microbiol Scand 25:215-236, 1948.
776. Schwarz GA, Rose EK, Fry WE. Toxoplasmic encephalomyelitis (clinical report of 6 cases). Pediatrics 1:478-494, 1948.
777. Verlinde JD, Makstenieks O. Repeated isolation of *Toxoplasma* from the cerebrospinal fluid and from the blood, and the antibody response in four cases of congenital toxoplasmosis. Ant van Leeuwen 16:366-372, 1950.
778. Dorta AF, Planchart CA, Maekelt A, et al. [Congenital toxoplasmosis (second case parasitologically proved during life, in Venezuela).] Arch Venez Puericult Pediat 27:332-339, 1964.
779. Embil JA, Covert AA, Howes WJ, et al. Visualization of *Toxoplasma gondii* in the cerebrospinal fluid of a child with a malignant astrocytoma. Can Med Assoc J 133:213-214, 1985.
780. Coffey JJ. Congenital toxoplasmosis 38 years ago. Letter to the editor. Pediatr Infect Dis 4:214, 1985.
781. Habegger H. Toxoplasmose humaine; mise en évidence des parasites dan les milieux intra-oculaires; humeur aquese, exudat rétrorétinien. Arch Ophthalmol (Paris) 14:470-488, 1954.
782. Tsunematsu Y, Shioiri K, Kusano N. Three cases of lymphadenopathia toxoplasmotica—with special reference to the application of fluorescent antibody technique for detection of *Toxoplasma* in tissue. Jpn J Exp Med 34:217-230, 1964.

783. Shioiri-Nakano K, Aoyama Y, Tsuenmatsu Y. The application of fluorescent-antibody technique to the diagnosis of glandular toxoplasmosis. Rev Med (Paris) 8:429-436, 1971.
784. Khodr G, Matossian R. Hydrops fetalis and congenital toxoplasmosis. Value of direct immunofluorescence test. Obstet Gynecol 51(suppl 1): 74S-75S, 1978.
785. Conley FK, Jenkins KA, Remington JS. *Toxoplasma gondii* infection of the central nervous system. Use of the peroxidase-antiperoxidase method to demonstrate *Toxoplasma* in formalin fixed, paraffin embedded tissue sections. Hum Pathol 12:690-698, 1981.
786. Frenkel JK, Piekarski G. The demonstration of *Toxoplasma* and other organisms by immunofluorescence: a pitfall. Editorial. J Infect Dis 138:265-266, 1978.
787. Kass EH, Andrus SB, Adams RD, et al. Toxoplasmosis in the human adult. Arch Intern Med 89:759-782, 1952.
788. Dorfman RF, Remington JS. Value of lymph-node biopsy in the diagnosis of acute acquired toxoplasmosis. N Engl J Med 289: 878-881, 1973.
789. Desmonts G, Couvreur J. [Isolation of the parasite in congenital toxoplasmosis: its practical and theoretical importance.] Arch Fr Pediatr 31:157-166, 1974.
790. Deutsch AR, Horsley ME. Congenital toxoplasmosis. Am J Ophthalmol 43:444-448, 1957.
791. Ariztía A, Martinez F, Howard J, et al Toxoplasmose connatal activa en un recién nacido con demonstracion del parasito in vivo: primer caso en Chile. Rev Chil Pediatr 1954;25:501-510.
792. De Roever-Bonnet H. Congenital toxoplasmosis. Trop Geogr Med 1961;13:27-41.
793. Schmidtke L. [Demonstration of *Toxoplasma* in amniotic fluid: preliminary report.] Deutsche Med Wchnschr 82:1342, 1957.
794. Chang CH, Stulberg C, Bollinger RO, et al. Isolation of *Toxoplasma gondii* in tissue culture. J Pediatr 81:790-791, 1972.
795. Dos Santos Neto JG. Toxoplasmosis: a historical review, direct diagnostic microscopy, and report of a case. Am J Clin Pathol 63:909-915, 1975.
796. Matsubayashi H, Koike T, Uyemura M, et al. A case of ocular toxoplasmosis in an adult, the infection being confirmed by the isolation of the parasite from subretinal fluid. Keio J Med 10:209-224, 1961.
797. Frezzotti R, Guerra R, Terragna A, Tosi P. A case of congenital toxoplasmosis with active chorioretinitis. Parasitological and histopathological findings. Ophthalmologica 169:321-325, 1974.
798. Teutsch SM, Sulzer AJ, Ramsey JE, et al. *Toxoplasma gondii* isolated from amniotic fluid. Obstet Gynecol 55(3 suppl):2S-4S, 1980.
799. Derouin F, Thulliez P, Candolfi E, et al. Early prenatal diagnosis of congenital toxoplasmosis using amniotic fluid samples and tissue culture. Eur J Clin Microbiol Infect Dis 7:423-425, 1988.
800. Foulon W, Naessens A, de Catte L, Amy J-J. Detection of congenital toxoplasmosis by chronic villus sampling and early amniocentesis. Am J Obstet Gynecol 163:1511-1513, 1990.
801. Derouin F, Mazeron MC, Garin YJ. Comparative study of tissue culture and mouse inoculation methods for demonstration of *Toxoplasma gondii.* J Clin Microbiol 25:1597-1600, 1987.
802. Abbas AM. Comparative study of methods used for the isolation of *Toxoplasma gondii.* Bull World Health Organ 36:344-346, 1967.
803. Dubey JP. Refinement of pepsin digestion method for isolation of *Toxoplasma gondii* from infected tissues. Vet Parasitol 74:75-77, 1998.
804. Philippe F, Lepetit D, Grancher MF, et al. [Why monitor infants born to mothers who had a seroconversion for toxoplasmosis during pregnancy? Reality and risk of subclinical congenital toxoplasmosis in children. Review of 30,768 births.] Ann Pediatr (Paris) 35:5-10, 1988.
805. Desmonts G, Couvreur J. Toxoplasmosis: epidemiologic and serologic aspects of perinatal infection. *In* Krugman S, Gershon AA (eds). Infections of the Fetus and Newborn Infant. Progress in Clinical and Biological Research. New York, Alan R Liss, 1975, pp 115-132.
806. Frenkel JK. Dermal hypersensitivity to *Toxoplasma* antigens (toxoplasmins). Proc Soc Exp Biol Med 68:634-639, 1948.
807. Frenkel JK. Uveitis and toxoplasmin sensitivity. Am J Ophthalmol 32:127-135, 1949.
808. Beverley JKA, Beattie CP, Roseman C. Human *Toxoplasma* infection. J Hyg 52:37-46, 1954.
809. Jacobs L, Naquin H, Hoover R, Woods AC. A comparison of the toxoplasmin skin tests, the Sabin-Feldman dye tests, and the complement fixation tests for toxoplasmosis in various forms of uveitis. Bull Johns Hopkins Hosp 99:1-15, 1956.
810. Frenkel JK, Jacobs L. Ocular toxoplasmosis. Pathogenesis, diagnosis and treatment. AMA Arch Ophthalmol 59:260-279, 1958.
811. Kaufman HE. Uveitis accompanied by a positive *Toxoplasma* dye test. Arch Ophthalmol 63:767-773, 1960.
812. Remington JS, Dalrymple W, Jacobs L, Finland M. *Toxoplasma* antibodies among college students. N Engl J Med 269:1394-1398, 1963.
813. Frenkel JK. Pathogenesis, diagnosis and treatment of human toxoplasmosis. JAMA 140:369-377, 1949.
814. Jacobs L. Toxoplasmosis. N Z Med J 61:2-9, 1962.
815. Maddison SE, Slemenda SB, Teutsch SM, et al. Lymphocyte proliferative responsiveness in 31 patients after an outbreak of toxoplasmosis. Am J Trop Med Hyg 28:955-961, 1979.
816. Stray-Pedersen B. Infants potentially at risk for congenital toxoplasmosis. A prospective study. Am J Dis Child 134:638-642, 1980.
817. McLeod R, Beem MO, Estes RG. Lymphocyte anergy specific to *Toxoplasma gondii* antigens in a baby with congenital toxoplasmosis. J Clin Lab Immunol 17:149-153, 1985.
818. Gehrz RC, Marker SC, Knorr SO, et al. Specific cell-mediated immune defect in active cytomegalovirus infection of young children and their mothers. Lancet 2:844-847, 1977.
819. Reynolds DW, Dean PH. Cell mediated immunity in mothers and their offspring with cytomegalovirus (CMV) infection. Pediatr Res 12:498, 1978.
820. Alford CA Jr. Rubella. *In* Remington JS, Klein JO (eds). Infectious Diseases of the Fetus and Newborn Infant. Philadelphia, WB Saunders, 1976, pp 71-106.
821. Fuccillo DA, Steele RW, Hensen SA, et al. Impaired cellular immunity to rubella virus in congenital rubella. Infect Immun 9: 81-84, 1974.
822. Friedmann PS. Cell-mediated immunological reactivity in neonates and infants with congenital syphilis. Clin Exp Immunol 30:271-276, 1977.
823. Yano A, Yui K, Yamamoto M, et al. Immune response to *Toxoplasma gondii.* I. *Toxoplasma*-specific proliferation response of peripheral blood lymphocytes from patients with toxoplasmosis. Microbiol Immunol 27:455-463, 1983.
824. Grover CM, Thulliez P, Remington JS, Boothroyd JD. Rapid prenatal diagnosis of congenital *Toxoplasma* infection by using polymerase chain reaction and amniotic fluid. J Clin Microbiol 28:2297-2301, 1990.
825. van de Ven E, Melchers W, Galama J, et al. Identification of *Toxoplasma gondii* infections by BI gene amplification. J Clin Microbiol 19:2120-2124, 1991.
826. Cazenave J, Forestier F, Bessieres M, et al. Contribution of a new PCR assay to the prenatal diagnosis of congenital toxoplasmosis. Prenat Diagn 12:119-127, 1992.
827. Gross U, Roggenkamp A, Janitschke K, Heesemann J. Improved sensitivity of the polymerase chain reaction for detection of *Toxoplasma gondii* in biolgocical and human clinical specimens. Eur J Clin Microbiol 11:33-39, 1992.
828. Dupouy-Camet J, Bougnoux ME, Lavareda de Souza S, et al. Comparative value of polymerase chain reaction and conventional biological tests. Ann Biol Clin 50:315-319, 1992.
829. Bergstrom T, Ricksten A, Nenonen N, et al. Congenital *Toxoplasma gondii* infection diagnosed by PCR amplification of peripheral mononuclear blood cells from a child and mother. Scand J Infect Dis 30:202-204, 1998.
830. Fuentes I, Rodriguez M, Domingo CJ, et al. Urine sample used for congenital toxoplasmosis diagnosis by PCR. J Clin Microbiol 34:2368-2371, 1996.
831. Knerer B, Hayde M, Gratz G, et al. Detection of *Toxoplasma gondii* with polymerase chain reaction for the diagnosis of congenital toxoplasmosis. Wien Klin Wochenschr 107:137-140, 1995.
832. Liesenfeld O, Montoya JG, McLeod R, et al. Use of the polymerase chain reaction on amniotic fluid for prenantal diagnosis of congenital infection with *Toxoplasma gondii.* Ninety-seventh General Meeting of the American Society for Microbiology, Miami, May 4-8, 1997 (abstract, p 204).
833. Pelloux H, Weiss J, Simon J, et al. A new set of primers for the detection of *Toxoplasma gondii* in amniotic fluid using polymerase chain reaction. FEMS Microbiol Lett 138:11-15, 1996.
834. Paugam A, Gavinet M, Robert F, et al. Seroconversion toxoplasmique pendant la grossesse. Presse Med 11:1235, 1993.
835. Fricker-Hidalgo H, Pelloux H, Racinet C, et al. Detection of *Toxoplasma gondii* in 94 placentae from infected women by

polymerase chain reaction, in vivo, and in vitro cultures. Placenta 19:545-549, 1998.

836. Jenum PA, Holberg-Petersen M, Melby KK, Stray-Pedersen B. Diagnosis of congenital *Toxoplasma gondii* infection by polymerase chain reaction (PCR) on amniotic fluid samples. The Norwegian experience. APMIS 106:680-686, 1998.
837. Gratzl R, Hayde M, Kohlhauser C, et al. Follow-up of infants with congenital toxoplasmosis detected by polymerase chain reaction analysis of amniotic fluid. Eur J Clin Microbiol Infect Dis 17: 853-858, 1998.
838. Romand S, Wallon M, Franck J, et al. Prenatal diagnosis using polymerase chain reaction on amniotic fluid for congenital toxoplasmosis. Obstet Gynecol 97:296-300, 2001.
839. Pelloux H, Guy E, Angelici MC, et al. A second European collaborative study on polymerase chain reaction for *Toxoplasma gondii*, involving 15 teams. FEMS Microbiol Lett 165:231-237, 1998.
840. Reischl U, Bretagne S, Kruger D, et al. Comparison of two DNA targets for the diagnosis of Toxoplasmosis by real-time PCR using fluorescence resonance energy transfer hybridization probes. BMC Infect Dis 3(1):7, 2003.
841. Cleary MD, Singh U, Blader IJ, et al. *Toxoplasma gondii* asexual development: identification of developmentally regulated genes and distinct patterns of gene expression. Eukaryot Cell 1:329-340, 2002.
842. Araujo FG, Remington JS. Antigenemia in recently acquired acute toxoplasmosis. J Infect Dis 141:144-150, 1980.
843. van Knapen F, Panggabean SO. Detection of circulating antigen during acute infections with *Toxoplasma gondii* by enzyme-linked immunosorbent assay. J Clin Microbiol 6:545-547, 1977.
844. Lindenschmidt EG. Enzyme-linked immunosorbent assay for detection of soluble *Toxoplasma gondii* antigen in acute-phase toxoplasmosis. Eur J Clin Microbiol 4:488-492, 1985.
845. Asai T, Kim TJ, Kobayashi M, Kojima S. Detection of nucleoside triphosphate hydrolase as a circulating antigen in sera of mice infected with *Toxoplasma gondii*. Infect Immun 55:1332-1335, 1987.
846. Turunen HJ. Detection of soluble antigens of *Toxoplasma gondii* by a four-layer modification of an enzyme immunoassay. J Clin Microbiol 17:768-773, 1983.
847. Hassl A, Picher O, Aspöck H. Studies on the significance of detection of circulation antigen (cag) for the diagnosis of a primary infection with *T. gondii* during pregnancy. Mitt Osterr Ges Tropenmed Parasitol 9:91-94, 1987.
848. Hafid J, Tran Manh Sung R, Raberin H, et al. Detection of circulating antigens of *Toxoplasma gondii* in human infection. Am J Trop Med Hyg 52:336-339, 1995.
849. Araujo FG, Handman E, Remington JS. Use of monoclonal antibodies to detect antigens of *Toxoplasma gondii* in serum and other body fluids. Infect Immun 30:12-16, 1980.
850. Huskinson J, Stepick-Biek P, Remington JS. Detection of antigens in urine during acute toxoplasmosis. J Clin Microbiol 27:1099-1101, 1989.
851. Brooks RG, Sharma SD, Remington JS. Detection of *Toxoplasma gondii* antigens by a dot-immunobinding technique. J Clin Microbiol 21:113-116, 1985.
852. Jacobs L, Lunde M. A hemagglutination test for toxoplasmosis. J Parasitol 43:308-314, 1957.
853. Walton BC, Benchoff BM, Brooks WH. Comparison of the indirect fluorescent antibody test and methylene blue dye test for detection of antibodies to *Toxoplasma gondii*. Am J Trop Med Hyg 15:149-152, 1966.
854. Sérologie de l'Infection Toxoplasmique en Particulier á Son Début: Méthodes et Interprétation des Résultants. Lyon, Foundation Mérieux, 1975, p 182.
855. Naot Y, Desmonts G, Remington JS. IgM enzyme-linked immunosorbent assay test for the diagnosis of congenital *Toxoplasma* infection. J Pediatr 98:32-36, 1981.
856. Naot Y, Remington JS. An enzyme-linked immunosorbent assay for detection of IgM antibodies to *Toxoplasma gondii*: use for diagnosis of acute acquired toxoplasmosis. J Infect Dis 142:757-766, 1980.
857. Bessieres MH, Roques C, Berrebi A, et al. IgA antibody response during acquired and congenital toxoplasmosis. J Clin Pathol 45: 605-608, 1992.
858. Decoster A, Caron A, Darcy F, Capron A. IgA antibodies against P30 as markers of congenital and acute toxoplasmosis. Lancet 2:1104-1106, 1988.
859. Desmonts G, Naot Y, Remington JS. Immunoglobulin M–immunosorbent agglutination assay for diagnosis of infectious diseases: diagnosis of acute congenital and acquired *Toxoplasma* infections. J Clin Microbiol 14:486-491, 1981.
860. Dannemann BR, Vaughan WC, Thulliez P, Remington JS. Differential agglutination test for diagnosis of recently acquired infection with *Toxoplasma gondii*. J Clin Microbiol 28:1928-1933, 1990.
861. Pinon JM, Toubas D, Marx C, et al. Detection of specific immunoglobulin E in patients with toxoplasmosis. J Clin Microbiol 28:1739-1743, 1990.
862. Fleck CG. The antigens of *Toxoplasma gondii*. *In* Corradetti A (ed). Proceedings of the First International Congress of Parasitology [Rome, September 21-26, 1964]. Oxford, Pergamon Press, 1966, pp 167-168.
863. Feldman HA, Miller LT. Serological study of toxoplasmosis prevalence. Am J Hyg 64:320-335, 1956.
864. Lelong M, Desmonts G. Sur la nature de phénomene de Sabin et Feldman. C R Soc Biol 146:207-209, 1952.
865. Feldman HA. To establish a fact: Maxwell Finland lecture. J Infect Dis 141:525-529, 1980.
866. Hansen GA, Lyng J, Petersen E. Calibration of a replacement preparation for the second international standard for anti-*Toxoplasma* serum, human. WHO Expert Committee on Biological Standardization BS/94, 1761, 1994.
867. Welch PC, Masur H, Jones TC, Remington JS. Serologic diagnosis of acute lymphadenopathic toxoplasmosis. J Infect Dis 142:256-264, 980.
868. BenRachid MS, Ferraro G, Desmonts G. Data on HA tests in newborns. Arch Inst Pasteur Tunis 44:391-400, 1967.
869. Desmonts G. Congenital toxoplasmosis: problems in early diagnosis. *In* Hentsch D (ed). Toxoplasmosis. Bern, Hans Huber, 1971, pp 137-149.
870. Camargo ME, Leser PG. Diagnostic information from serological tests in human toxoplasmosis. II. Evolutive study of antibodies and serological patterns in acquired toxoplasmosis, as detected by hemagglutination, complement fixation, IgG and IgM-immunofluorescence tests. Rev Inst Med Trop Sao Paulo 18:227-238, 1976.
871. Camargo ME, Leser PG, Leser WS. Diagnostic information from serological tests in human toxoplasmosis. I. A comparative study of hemagglutination, complement fixation, IgG and IgM-immunofluorescence tests in 3,752 serum samples. Rev Inst Med Trop Sao Paulo 18:215-226, 1976.
872. Karim KA, Ludlam GB. The relationship and significance of antibody titres as determined by various serological methods in glandular and ocular toxoplasmosis. J Clin Pathol 28:42-49, 1975.
873. Ambroise TP, Simon J, Bayard M. Indirect hemagglutination using whole mixed antigen for checking toxoplasmosis immunity and for serodiagnosis of human toxoplasmosis, compared with immunofluorescence. Biomedicine 29:245-248, 1978.
874. Camargo ME, Leser PG, Kiss MH, Amato NV. Serology in early diagnosis of congenital toxoplasmosis. Rev Inst Med Trop Sao Paulo 20:152-160, 1978.
875. Balfour AH, Bridges JB, Harford JP. An evaluation of the ToxHA test for the detection of antibodies to *Toxoplasma gondii* in human serum. J Clin Pathol 33:644-647, 1980.
876. Kean BH, Kimball AC. The complement-fixation test in the diagnosis of congenital toxoplasmosis. Am J Dis Child 131:21-28, 1977.
877. Thulliez P, Remington JS, Santoro F, et al. A new agglutination test for the diagnosis of acute and chronic *Toxoplasma* infection. Pathol Biol 34:173-177, 1986.
878. Niel G, Gentilini M. Immunofluorescence quantitative, test de Remington et agglutination directe: confrontation et apport de leur pratique simultanée dans le diagnostic sérologique de la toxoplasmose. *In* Mérieux F (ed). Sérologie de l'Infection Toxoplasmique en Particulier a Son Début: Méthodes et Interpretation des Résultats. Lyon, Fondation Mérieux, 1975, pp 29-39.
879. Couzineau P. La réaction d'agglutination dans le diagnostic sérologique de la toxoplasmose. *In* Mérieux F (ed). Sérologie de l'infection Toxoplasmique en Particulier a Son Début: Méthodes et Interpretation des Résultats. Lyon, Fondation Mérieux, 1975, pp 61-63.
880. Baufine-Ducrocq H. Les anticrops naturels dans de serodiagnostic de la toxoplasmose par agglutination directe. *In* Mérieux F (ed). Sérologie de l'Infection Toxoplasmique en Particulier a Son Début: Méthodes et Interpretation des Résultats. Lyon, Fondation Mérieux, 1975, pp 65-66.
881. Garin JP, Despeignes J, Mojon M, et al. Immunofluorescence et agglutination dans le diagnostic serologique de la toxoplasmose

valeur comparative de la recherche de IgM et du test au 2-mercapto-éthanol. *In* Mérieux F (ed). Sérologie de l'Infection Toxoplasmique en Particulier a Son Début: Méthodes et Interpretation des Résultats. Lyon, Fondation Mérieux, 1975, pp 97-111.

882. Laugier M. Notre experience du depistage de la toxoplasmose congenitale dans la region Marseillaise (méthodes-interprétation des résultats). *In* Mérieux F (ed). Sérologie de l'Infection Toxoplasmique en Particulier a Son Début: Méthodes et Interpretation des Résultats. Lyon, Fondation Mérieux, 1975, pp 191-229.
883. Desmonts G, Thulliez P. The *Toxoplasma* agglutination antigen as a tool for routine screening and diagnosis of *Toxoplasma* infection in the mother and infant. Dev Biol Stand 62:31-35, 1985.
884. Desmonts G, Baufine DH, Couzineau P, Peloux Y. [Natural antibodies against *Toxoplasma*.] Nouv Presse Med 3:1547-1549, 1974.
885. Desmonts G, Remington JS. Direct agglutination test for diagnosis of *Toxoplasma* infection: method for increasing sensitivity and specificity. J Clin Microbiol 11:562-568, 1980.
886. Payne RA, Francis JM, Kwantes W. Comparison of a latex agglutination test with other serological tests for the measurement of antibodies to *Toxoplasma gondii*. J Clin Pathol 37:1293-1297, 1984.
887. Nagington J, Martin AL, Balfour AH. Technical method. A rapid method for the detection of antibodies to *Toxoplasma gondii* using a modification of the Toxoreagent latex test. J Clin Pathol 36:361-362, 1983.
888. Wilson M, Ware DA, Walls KW. Evaluation of commercial serology kits for toxoplasmosis. Joint Meeting of the Royal and American Societies of Tropical Medicine and Hygiene; 33rd Annual Meeting of the American Society of Tropical Medicine, Baltimore, 1984 (abstract, p 137).
889. Wong S, Remington JS. Toxoplasmosis in pregnancy. Clin Infect Dis 18:853-862, 1994.
890. Liesenfeld O, Press C, Flanders R, et al. Study of Abbott toxo IMx system for detection of immunoglobulin G and immunoglobulin M *Toxoplasma* antibodies: value of confirmatory testing for diagnosis of acute toxoplasmosis. J Clin Microbiol 34:2526-2530, 1996.
891. Suzuki Y, Thulliez P, Desmonts G, Remington JS. Antigen(s) responsible for immunoglobulin G responses specific for the acute stage of *Toxoplasma* infection in humans. J Clin Microbiol 26: 901-905, 1988.
892. Araujo FG, Barnett EV, Gentry LO, Remington JS. False-positive anti-*Toxoplasma* fluorescent-antibody tests in patients with antinuclear antibodies. Appl Microbiol 22:270-275, 1971.
893. Hobbs KM, Sole E, Bettelheim KA. Investigation into the immunoglobulin class responsible for the polar staining of *Toxoplasma gondii* in the fluorescent antibody test. Zentralbl Bakteriol Hyg [A] 239:409-413, 1977.
894. Sulzer AJ, Wilson M, Hall EC. *Toxoplasma gondii*: polar staining in fluorescent antibody test. Exp Parasitol 29:197-200, 1971.
895. De Meuter F, De Decker H. [Indirect fluourescent antibody test in toxoplasmosis. Advantage of the use of fluorescent anti-IgG conjugate (author's transl).] Zentralbl Bakteriol Mikrobiol Hyg [A] 233:421-430, 1975.
896. Wong SY, Hadju M-P, Ramirez R, et al. The role of specific immunoglobulin E in diagnosis of acute *Toxoplasma* infection and toxoplasmosis. J Clin Microbiol 31:2952-2959, 1993.
897. Pinon JM, Foudrinier F, Mougheto G, et al. Evaluation of risk and diagnostic value of quantitative assays for anti-*Toxoplasma gondii* immunoglobulin A (IgA), IgE, and IgM and analytical study of specific IgG in immunodeficient patients. J Clin Microbiol 33: 878-884, 1995.
898. Decoster A, Slizewicz B, Simon J, et al. Platelia-toxo IgA, a new kit for early diagnosis of congenital toxoplasmosis by detection of anti-P30 immunoglobulin A antibodies. J Clin Microbiol 29:2291-2295, 1991.
899. Stepick-Biek P, Thulliez P, Araujo FG, Remington JS. IgA antibodies for diagnosis of acute congenital and acquired toxoplasmosis. J Infect Dis 162:270-273, 1990.
900. Balsari A, Poli G, Molina V, et al. ELISA for *Toxoplasma* antibody detection: a comparison with other serodiagnostic tests. J Clin Pathol 33:640-643, 1980.
901. van Loon A, van der Veen J. Enzyme-linked immunosorbent assay for quantitation of *Toxoplasma* antibodies in human sera. J Clin Pathol 33:635-639, 1980.
902. Ruitenberg EJ, van Knapen F. The enzyme-linked immunosorbent assay and its application to parasitic infections. J Infect Dis 136(Suppl):S267-S273, 1977.
903. Carlier Y, Bout D, Dessaint JP, et al. Evaluation of the enzyme-linked immunosorbent assay (ELISA) and other serological tests for the diagnosis of toxoplasmosis. Bull World Health Organ 58:99-105, 1980.
904. Denmark JR, Chessum BS. Standardization of enzyme-linked immunosorbent assay (ELISA) and the detection of *Toxoplasma* antibody. Med Lab Sci 35:227-232, 1978.
905. Capron A, Dugimont JC, Fruit J, Bout D. Application of immunoenzyme methods in diagnosis of human parasitic diseases. Ann N Y Acad Sci 254:331, 1975.
906. Walls KW, Bullock SL, English DK. Use of the enzyme-linked immunosorbent assay (ELISA) and its microadaptation for the serodiagnosis of toxoplasmosis. J Clin Microbiol 5:273-277, 1977.
907. Voller A, Bidwell DE, Bartlett A, et al. A microplate enzyme-immunoassay for *Toxoplasma* antibody. J Clin Pathol 29:150-153, 1976.
908. Milatovic D, Braveny I. Enzyme-linked immunosorbent assay for the serodiagnosis of toxoplasmosis. J Clin Pathol 33:841-844, 1980.
909. Liesenfeld O, Press C, Montoya JG, et al. False-positive results in immunoglobulin M (IgM) *Toxoplasma* antibody tests and importance of confirmatory testing: the Platelia toxo IgM test. J Clin Microbiol 35:174-178, 1997.
910. Wilson M, Remington JS, Clavet C, et al. Evaluation of six commercial kits for detection of human immunoglobulin M antibiodies to *Toxoplasma gondii*. J Clin Microbiol 35:3112-3115, 1997.
911. Siegel JP, Remington JS. Comparison of methods for quantitating antigen-specific immunoglobulin M antibody with a reverse enzyme-linked immunosorbent assay. J Clin Microbiol 18:63-70, 1983.
912. Gorgievski-Hrisoho M, Germann D, Matter L. Diagnostic implications of kinetics of immunoglobulin M and A antibody responses to *Toxoplasma gondii*. J Clin Microbiol 34:1506-1511, 1996.
913. Pinon JM, Thoannes H, Gruson N. An enzyme-linked immuno-filtration assay used to compare infant and maternal antibody profiles in toxoplasmosis. J Immunol Methods 77:15-23, 1985.
914. Pinon JM, Chemla C, Villena I, et al. Early neonatal diagnosis of congenital toxoplasmosis: value of comparative enzyme-linked immunofiltration assay immunological profiles and anti-*Toxoplasma gondii* immunoglobulin M (IgM) or IgA immunocapture and implications for postnatal therapeutic strategies. J Clin Microbiol 34:579-583, 1996.
915. Remington JS, Araujo FG, Desmonts G. Recognition of different *Toxoplasma* antigens by IgM and IgG antibodies in mothers and their congenitally infected newborns. J Infect Dis 152:1020-1024, 1985.
916. Pinon JM, Dumon H, Chemla C, et al. Strategy for diagnosis of congenital toxoplasmosis: evaluation of methods comparing mothers and newborns and standard methods for postnatal detection of immunoglobulin G, M, and A antibodies. J Clin Microbiol 39: 2267-2271, 2001.
917. Tissot Dupont D, Fricker-Hidalgo H, Brenier-Pinchart MP, et al. Usefulness of Western blot in serological follow-up of newborns suspected of congenital toxoplasmosis. Eur J Clin Microbiol Infect Dis 22:122-125, 2003.
918. Hedman K, Lappalainen M, Söderlund M, Hedman L. Avidity of IgG in serodiagnosis of infectious diseases. Rev Med Microbiol 4:123-129, 1993.
919. Cozon G, Ferrandiz J, Nebhi H, et al. IgG Avidity for diagnosis of chronic *T. gondii* infection in pregnant women. Eighth European Congress of Clinical Microbiology and Infectious Diseases, Lausanne, Switzerland, May 25-28, 1997 (abstract, p 148).
920. Rossi CL. A simple, rapid enzyme-linked immunosorbent assay for evaluating immunoglobulin G antibody avidity in toxoplasmosis. Diagn Microbiol Infect Dis 30:25-30, 1998.
921. Ashburn D, Joss AW, Pennington TH, Ho-Yen DO. Do IgA, IgE, and IgG avidity tests have any value in the diagnosis of *Toxoplasma* infection in pregnancy? J Clin Pathol 51:312-315, 1998.
922. Ambroise-Thomas P, Pelloux H, Guergour D, et al. Standardization by the VIDAS system of an avidity test for toxoplasmosis diagnosis in pregnant women. Thirty-eighth Interscience Conference on Antimicrobial Agents and Chemotherapy, San Diego, September 24-27, 1998 (abstract, p 149).
923. Cozon GJ, Ferrandiz J, Nebhi H, Wallon M, Peyron F. Estimation of the avidity of immunoglobulin G for routine diagnosis of chronic *Toxoplasma gondii* infection in pregnant women. Eur J Clin Microbiol Infect Dis 17:32-36, 1998.

924. Pelloux H, Brun E, Vernet G, et al. Determination of anti-*Toxoplasma gondii* immunoglobulin G avidity: adaptation to the VIDAS system (bioMerieux). Diagn Microbiol Infect Dis 32:69-73, 1998.
925. Lappalainen M, Koskela P, Koskiniemi M, et al. Toxoplasmosis acquired during pregnancy: improved serodiagnosis based on avidity of IgG. J Infect Dis 167:691-697, 1993.
926. Jenum PA, Stray-Pedersen B, Gundersen A-G. Improved diagnosis of primary *Toxoplasma gondii* infection in early pregnancy by determination of antitoxoplasma immunoglobulin G activity. J Clin Microbiol 35:1972-1977, 1997.
927. Sensini A, Pascoli S, Marchetti D, et al. IgG avidity in the serodiagnosis of acute *Toxoplasma gondii* infection: a multicenter study. Clin Microbiol Infect 2:25-29, 1996.
928. Flori P, Tardy L, Patural H, et al. Reliability of immunoglobulin G antitoxoplasma avidity test and effects of treatment on avidity indexes of infants and pregnant women. Clin Diagn Lab Immunol 11:669-674, 2004.
929. Hedman K, Lappalainen M, Seppala I, Makela O. Recent primary *Toxoplasma* infection indicated by a low avidity of specific IgG. J Infect Dis 159:736-739, 1989.
930. Camargo ME, da Silva SM, Leser PG, Granato CH. Avidity of specific IgG antibody as a marker of recent and old *Toxoplasma gondii* infections. Rev Inst Med Trop Sao Paulo 33:213-218, 1991.
931. Joynson DHM, Payne RA, Rawal BK. Potential role of IgG avidity for diagnosing toxoplasmosis. J Clin Pathol 43:1032-1033, 11990.
932. Liesenfeld O, Montoya JG, Tathineni NJ, et al. Confirmatory serologic testing for acute toxoplasmosis and rate of induced abortions among women reported to have positive *Toxoplasma* immunoglobulin M antibody titers. Am J Obstet Gynecol 184:140-145, 2001.
933. Remington JS, Miller MJ, Brownlee I. IgM antibodies in acute toxoplasmosis. I. Diagnostic significance in congenital cases and a method for their rapid demonstration. Pediatrics 41:1082-1091, 1968.
934. Remington JS, Miller MJ, Brownlee I. IgM antibodies in acute toxoplasmosis. II. Prevalence and significance in acquired cases. J Lab Clin Med 71:855-866, 1968.
935. Remington JS. The present status of the IgM fluorescent antibody technique in the diagnosis of congenital toxoplasmosis. J Pediatr 75:1116-1124, 1969.
936. Lunde MN. Laboratory methods in the diagnosis of toxoplasmosis. Health Lab Sci 10:319-328, 1973.
937. Stagno S, Thiermann E. [Value of indirect immunofluorescent test in the serological diagnosis of acute toxoplasmosis.] Bol Chil Parasitol 25:9-15, 1970.
938. Aparicio GJ, Cour BI. [Application of immunofluorescence to the study of immunoglobulin fractions in the diagnostic of acquired and congenital toxoplasmosis. Clinical value.] Rev Clin Esp 125: 37-42, 1972.
939. Dropsy G, Carquin J, Croix JC. [Technics of demonstration of IgM type antibodies in congenital infections.] Ann Biol Clin (Paris) 29:67-73, 1971.
940. Eichenwald HF, Shinefield HR. Antibody production by the human fetus. J Pediatr 63:870, 1963.
941. Remington JS, Desmonts G. Congenital toxoplasmosis: variability in the IgM-fluorescent antibody response and some pitfalls in diagnosis. J Pediatr 83:27-30, 1973.
942. Pyndiah N, Krech U, Price P, Wilhelm J. Simplified chromatographic separation of immunoglobulin M from G and its application to *Toxoplasma* indirect immunofluorescence. J Clin Microbiol 9: 170-174, 1979.
943. Filice GA, Yeager AS, Remington JS. Diagnostic significance of immunoglobulin M antibodies to *Toxoplasma gondii* detected after separation of immunoglobulin M from immunoglobulin G antibodies. J Clin Microbiol 12:336-342, 1980.
944. Lunde MN, Gelderman AH, Hayes SL, Vogel CL. Serologic diagnosis of active toxoplasmosis complicating malignant diseases. Usefulness of IgM antibodies and gel diffusion. Cancer 1970;25:637-643.
945. Desmonts G, Couvreur J, Colin J, Peupion J. [Early diagnosis of acute toxoplasmosis. Critical study of Remington's test.] Nouv Presse Med 1:339-342, 1972.
946. Stiehm ER, Amman AJ, Cherry JD. Elevated cord macroglobulins in the diagnosis of intrauterine infections. N Engl J Med 275:971-977, 1966.
947. Barth WF, Wochner RD, Waldmann TA, et al. Metabolism of human gamma macroglobulins. J Clin Invest 43:1036-1048, 1964.
948. Hyde B, Barnett EV, Remington JS. Method for differentiation of nonspecific from specfic *Toxoplasma* IgM fluorescent antibodies in patients with rheumatoid factor. Proc Soc Exp Biol Med 148: 1184-1188, 1975.
949. Reimer CB, Black CM, Phillips DJ, et al. The specificity of fetal IgM: antibody or anti-antibody? Ann N Y Acad Sci 254:77-93, 1975.
950. Filice G, Carnevale G, Meroni V, et al. Detection of IgM-anti-*Toxoplasma* antibodies in acute acquired and congenital toxoplasmosis. Boll Ist Sieroter Milan 76:271-273, 1984.
951. Pouletty P, Pinon JM, Garcia-Gonzalez M, et al. An anti-human immunoglobulin M monoclonal antibody for detection of antibodies to *Toxoplasma gondii*. Eur J Clin Microbiol 3:510-515, 1984.
952. Santoro F, Afchain D, Pierce R, et al. Serodiagnosis of *Toxoplasma* infection using a purified parasite protein (P30). Clin Exp Immunol 62:262-269, 1985.
953. Pouletty P, Kadouche J, Garcia-Gonzalez M, et al. An anti-human M chain monoclonal antibody: use for detection of IgM antibodies to *Toxoplasma gondii* by reverse immunosorbent assay. J Immunol Methods 76:289-298, 1985.
954. Cesbron JY, Caron A, Santoro F, et al. [A new ELISA method for the diagnosis of toxoplasmosis. Assay of serum IgM by immunocapture with an anti-*Toxoplasma gondii* monoclonal antibody.] Presse Med 19:737-740, 1986.
955. Lindenschmidt EG. Demonstration of immunoglobulin M class antibodies to *Toxoplasma gondii* antigenic component P3500 by enzyme-linked antigen immunosorbent assay. J Clin Microbiol 24:1045-1049, 1986.
956. Herbrink P, van Loon AM, Rotmans JP, et al. Interlaboratory evaluation of indirect enzyme-linked immunosorbent assay, antibody capture enzyme-linked immunosorbent assay, and immunoblotting for detection of immunoglobulin M antibodies to *Toxoplasma gondii*. J Clin Microbiol 25:100-105, 1987.
957. Filice G, Carnevale G, Meroni V, et al. IgM-IFA, IgM-ELISA, DS-IgM-ELISA, IgM-ISAGA, performed on whole serum and IgM fractions, for detection of IgM anti-*Toxoplasma* antibodies during pregnancy. Boll Ist Sieroter Milan 65:131-137, 1986.
958. Saathoff M, Seitz HM. [Detection of *Toxoplasma*-specific IgM antibodies—comparison with the ISAGA (immunosorbent agglutination assay) and immunofluorescence results.] Z Geburtshilfe Perinatol 189:73-78, 1985.
959. Montoya JG, Remington JS. Studies on the serodiagnosis of toxoplasmic lymphadenitis. Clin Infect Dis 20:781-790, 1995.
960. Thulliez P, Dutriat P, Saulnier M, et al. Evaluation de trois réactifs de détection par immunocapture des IgM spécifiques de la toxoplasmose. Revue Francaise des Laboratories, Feorier 169:25-31, 1988.
961. Pinon JM, Thoannes H, Pouletty PH, et al. Detection of IgA specific for toxoplasmosis in serum and cerebrospinal fluid using a non-enzymatic IgA-capture assay. Diagn Immunol 4:223-227, 1986.
962. Plantaz D, Goullier A, Jouk PS, Bost M. [Value of the immunosorbent agglutination assay (ISAGA) in the early diagnosis of congenital toxoplasmosis.] Pediatrie 42:387-391, 1987.
963. Le Fichoux Y, Marty P, Chan H. [Contribution of specific serum IgA assay to the diagnosis of toxoplasmosis.] Ann Pediatr (Paris) 34: 375-379, 1987.
964. Gras L, Gilbert RE, Wallon M, et al. Duration of the IgM response in women acquiring *Toxoplasma gondii* during pregnancy: implications for clinical practice and cross-sectional incidence studies. Epidemiol Infect 132:541-548, 2004.
965. Krogstad DJ, Juranek DD, Walls KW. Toxoplasmosis. With comments on risk of infection from cats. Ann Intern Med 77:773-778, 1972.
966. FDA. Public Health Advisory: Limitations of *Toxoplasma* IgM Commerical Test Kits. Rockville, Md, Department of Health and Human Services, Food and Drug Administration, July 25, 1997.
967. Gard S, Magnusson JH. A glandular form of toxoplasmosis in connection with pregnancy. Acta Med Scand 141:59-64, 1951.
968. Jeckeln E. Lymph node toxoplasmosis. Z Path (Frankfurt) 70: 513-522, 1960.
969. Siim JC. Toxoplasmosis acquisita lymphonodosa: clinical and pathological aspects. Ann N Y Acad Sci 64:185-206, 1956.
970. Couvreur J. Prospective study of acquired toxoplasmosis in pregnant women with a special reference to the outcome of the fetus. *In* Hentsch D (ed). Toxoplasmosis. Bern, Hans Huber, 1971, pp 119-136.
971. Handman E, Remington JS. Serological and immunochemical characterization of monoclonal antibodies to *Toxoplasma gondii*. Immunology 40:579-588, 1980.

972. Handman E, Remington JS. Antibody responses to *Toxoplasma* antigens in mice infected with strains of different virulence. Infect Immun 29:215-220, 1980.
973. Li S, Maine G, Suzuki Y, et al. Serodiagnosis of recently acquired *Toxoplasma gondii* infection with a recombinant antigen. J Clin Microbiol 38:179-184, 2000.
974. Johnson AM, Roberts H, Tenter AM. Evaluation of a recombinant antigen ELISA for the diagnosis of acute toxoplasmosis and comparison with traditional antigen ELISAs. J Med Microbiol 37: 404-409, 1992.
975. Martin V, Arcavi M, Santillan G, et al. Detection of human *Toxoplasma*-specific immunoglobulins A, M, and G with a recombinant *Toxoplasma gondii* rop2 protein. Clin Diagn Lab Immunol 5:627-631, 1998.
976. Redlich A, Muller WA. Serodiagnosis of acute toxoplasmosis using a recombinant form of the dense granule antigen GRA6 in an enzyme-linked immunosorbent assay. Parasitol Res 84:700-706, 1998.
977. Tenter AM, Johnson AM. Recognition of recombinant *Toxoplasma gondii* antigens by human sera in an ELISA. Parasitol Res 77: 197-203, 1991.
978. Sharma SD, Mullenax J, Araujo FG, et al. Western Blot analysis of the antigens of *Toxoplasma gondii* recognized by human IgM and IgG antibodies. J Immunol 131:977-983, 1983.
979. Erlich HA, Rodgers G, Vaillancourt P, et al. Identification of an antigen-specific immunoglobulin M antibody associated with acute *Toxoplasma* infection. Infect Immun 41:683-690, 1983.
980. Potasman I, Araujo FG, Thulliez P, et al. *Toxoplasma gondii* antigens recognized by sequential samples of serum obtained from congenitally infected infants. J Clin Microbiol 25:1926-1931, 1987.
981. Huskinson J, Stepick-Biek PN, Araujo FA, et al. *Toxoplasma* antigens recognized by immunoglobulin G subclasses during acute and chronic Infection. J Clin Microbiol 27:2031-2038, 1989.
982. Potasman I, Araujo FG, Remington JS. *Toxoplasma* antigens recognized by naturally occurring human antibodies. J Clin Microbiol 24:1050-1054, 1986.
983. Gross U, Keksel O, Dardé ML. The value of detecting immunoglobulin E (IgE) antibodies for the serological diagnosis of *Toxoplasma gondii* infection. Clin Diagn Lab Immunol 4:247-251, 1997.
984. Petithory JC, Reiter-Owona I, Berthelot F, et al. Performance of European laboratories testing serum samples for *Toxoplasma gondii*. Eur J Clin Microbiol Infect Dis 15:45-49, 1996.
985. Hofgartner WT, Plorde JJ, Fritsche TR. Detection of IgG and IgM antibodies to *Toxoplasma gondii*: evalualtion of 4 newer commercial immunoassays. Ninety-seventh General Meeting of the American Society for Microbiology, Miami, May 4-8, 1997 (abstract, p 581).
986. Terragna A. Toxoplasmic lymphadenitis. *In* Hentsch D (ed). Toxoplasmosis. Bern, Hans Huber, 1971, pp 159-178.
987. Jones TC, Kean BH, Kimball AC. Toxoplasmic lymphadenitis. JAMA 192:87-91, 1965.
988. Lelong M, Bernard J, Desmonts G, Couvreur J. [Acquired toxoplasmosis (study of 227 cases).] Arch Fr Pediatr 17:1-51, 1960.
989. Gussetti N, D'Elia R. Natural immunoglobulin M antibodies against *Toxoplasma gondii* during pregnancy. Am J Obstet Gynecol 51: 1359-1360, 1990.
990. Konishi E. A pregnant woman with a high level of naturally occurring immunoglobulin M antibodies to *Toxoplasma gondii*. Am J Obstet Gynecol 157:832-833, 1987.
991. Hezard N, Marx-Chemla C, Foudrinier F, et al. Prenatal diagnosis of congenital toxoplasmosis in 261 pregnancies. Prenat Diagn 17: 1047-1054, 1997.
992. Berrebi A, Kobuch W, Bessieres M, et al. Termination of pregnancy for maternal toxoplasmosis. Lancet 344:36-39, 1994.
993. Pratlong F, Boulot P, Issert E, et al. Fetal diagnosis of toxoplasmosis in 190 women infected during pregnancy. Prenat Diagn 14:191-198, 1994.
994. Boulet P, Deschamps F, Lefort G, et al. Pure fetal blood samples obtained by cordocentesis: technical aspects of 322 cases. Prenat Diagn 10:93-100, 1990.
995. Legras B, Clerc C, Ruelland A, et al. Blood chemistry of human fetuses in the second and third trimesters. Prenat Diag 10:801-807, 1990.
996. Tjalma W, Vanderheyden T, Naessens A, et al. Discordant prenatal diagnosis of congenital toxoplasmosis in a dizygotic pregnancy. Eur J Obstet Gynecol Reprod Biol 79:107-108, 1998.
997. Pratlong F, Boulot P, Villena I, et al. Antenatal diagnosis of congental toxoplasmosis: evaluation of the biological parameters in a cohort of 286 patients. Br J Obstet Gynaecol 103:552-557, 1996.
998. Berrebi A, Kobuch W. Toxoplasmosis in pregnancy. Lancet 344:950, 1994.
999. Lecolier B, Marion S, Derouin F, Sarrot G. T-cell subpopulations of fetuses infected by *Toxoplasma gondii*. Eur J Clin Microbiol Infect Dis 8:572-573, 1989.
1000. Decoster A, Darcy F, Caron A, et al. Anti-P30 IgA antibodies as prenatal markers of congenital *Toxoplasma* infection. Clin Exp Immunol 87:310-315, 1992.
1001. Raymond J, Poissonnier MH, Thulliez PH, et al. Presence of gamma interferon in human acute and congenital toxoplasmosis. J Clin Microbiol 28:1434-1437, 1990.
1002. Hohlfeld P, Forestier F, Marion S, et al. *Toxoplasma gondii* infection during pregnancy: T lymphocyte subpopulations in mothers and fetuses. Pediatr Infect Dis J 9:878-881, 1990.
1003. Cohen-Khallas Y, Bessieres MH, Berresi A, et al. La fraction C4 du complement: un nouveau marqueur indirect pour le diagnostic antenatal de la toxoplasmose. Presse Med 21:908, 1992.
1004. Alford CA, Schaefer J, Blankenship WJ, et al. A correlative immunologic, microbiologic and clinical approach to the diagnosis of acute and chronic infections in newborn infants. N Engl J Med 277:437-449, 1967.
1005. Alford CA. Immunoglobulin determinations in the diagnosis of fetal infection. Pediatr Clin North Am 18:99-113, 1971.
1006. McCracken GH Jr, Hardy JB, Chen TC, et al. Evaluation of a radial diffusion plate method for determining serum immunoglobulin levels in normal and congenitally infected infants. J Pediatr 75: 1204-1210, 1969.
1007. Korones SB, Roane JA, Gilkeson MR, et al. Neonatal IgM response to acute infection. J Pediatr 75:1261-1270, 1969.
1008. Miller MJ, Sunshine PJ, Remington JS. Quantitation of cord serum IgM and IgA as a screening procedure to detect congenital infection: results in 5,006 infants. J Pediatr 75:1287-1291, 1969.
1009. Thorley JD, Holmes RK, Kaplan JM, et al. Passive transfer of antibodies of maternal origin from blood to cerebrospinal fluid in infants. Lancet 1:651-653, 1975.
1010. Patel B, Young Y, Duffy K, et al. Immunoglobulin-A detection and the investigation of clinical toxoplasmosis. J Med Microbiol 38: 286-292, 1993.
1011. Foudrinier F, Marx-Chemla C, Aubert D, et al. Value of specific immunoglobulin A detection by two immunocapture assays in the diagnosis of toxoplasmosis. Eur J Clin Microbiol Infect Dis 4: 585-590, 1995.
1012. Villena I, Aubert D, Brodard V, et al. Detection of specific immunoglobulin e during maternal, fetal, and congenital toxoplasmosis. J Clin Microbiol 37:3487-3490, 1999.
1013. Foudrinier F, Villena I, Jaussaud R, et al. Clinical value of specific immunoglobulin E detection by enzyme-linked immunosorbent assay in cases of acquired and congenital toxoplasmosis. J Clin Microbiol 41:1681-1686, 2003.
1014. McCracken GH Jr, Kaplan JM. Penicillin treatment for congenital syphilis. A critical reappraisal. JAMA 228:855-858, 1974.
1015. Fuentes I. Urine as sample for congenital toxoplasmosis diagnosis by polymerase chain reaction (unpublished, 1996).
1016. Parmley SF, Goebel FD, Remington JS. Detection of *Toxoplasma gondii* DNA in cerebrospinal fluid from AIDS patients by polymerase chain reaction. J Clin Microbiol 30:3000-3002, 1992.
1017. Fortier B, Coignard-Chatain C, Dao A, et al. [Study of developing clinical outbreak and serological rebounds in children with congenital toxoplasmosis and follow-up during the first 2 years of life.] Arch Pediatr 4:940-946, 1997.
1018. Kahi S, Cozon GJN, Greenland T, et al. Circulating *Toxoplasma gondii*–specific antibody-secreting cells in patients with congenital toxoplasmosis. Clin Immunol Immunopathol 89:23-27, 1998.
1019. Villena I, Aubert D, Leroux B, et al. Pyrimethamine-sulfadoxine treatment of congenital toxoplasmosis: follow-up of 78 cases between 1980 and 1997. Reims Toxoplasmosis Group. Scand J Infect Dis 30:295-300, 1998.
1020. Djurkovic-Djakovic O, Romand S, Nobre R, et al. Serologic rebounds after one-year-long treatment for congenital toxoplasmosis. Pediatr Infect Dis J 19:81-83, 2000.
1021. Wallon M, Cozon G, Ecochard R, et al. Serological rebound in congenital toxoplasmosis: long-term follow-up of 133 children. Eur J Pediatr 160:534-540, 2001.
1022. Wallon M, Kodjikian L, Binquet C, et al. Long-term ocular prognosis in 327 children with congenital toxoplasmosis. Pediatrics 113: 1567-1572, 2004.

1023. Wright R, Johnson D, Neumann M, et al. Congenital lymphocytic choriormeningitis virus syndrome: a disease that mimics congenital toxoplasmosis or cytomegalovirus infections. Pediatrics 100: E91-E100, 1997.
1024. Smith CC, Ihrig J. Persistent excretion of pyrimethamine following oral administration. Am J Trop Med Hyg 8:60-62, 1959.
1025. Stickney DR, Simmons WS, DeAngelis RL, et al. Pharmacokinetics of pyrimethamine (PRM) and 2,4-diamino-5-(3',4'-dichlorophenyl) -6- methylpyrimidine (DMP) relevant to meningeal leukemia. Proc Am Assoc Cancer Res 14:52, 1973.
1026. Weidekamm E, Plazza-Nottebrock H, Forgo I, Dubach UC. Plasma concentrations of pyrimethamine and sulfadoxine and evaluation of pharmacokinetic data by computerized curve fitting. Bull World Health Organ 60:115-122, 1982.
1027. Ahmad RA, Rogers HJ. Pharmacokinetics and protein binding interactions of dapsone and pyrimethamine. Br J Clin Pharmacol 10:519-524, 1980.
1028. McLeod R, Mack D, Foss R, et al. Levels of pyrimethamine in sera and cerebrospinal and ventricular fluids from infants treated for congenital toxoplasmosis. Antimicrob Agents Chemother 36: 1040-1048, 1992.
1029. Gubbels MJ, Li C, Striepen B. High-throughput growth assay for *Toxoplasma gondii* using yellow fluorescent protein. Antimicrob Agents Chemother 47:309-316, 2003.
1030. Eyles DE, Coleman N. Synergistic effect of sulfadiazine and Daraprim against experimental toxoplasmosis in the mouse. Antibiot Chemother 3:483-490, 1953.
1031. Eyles DE, Coleman N. An evaluation of the curative effects of pyrimethamine and sulfadiazine, alone and in combination, on experimental mouse toxoplasmosis. Antibiot Chemother 5:529-539, 1955.
1032. Sheffield HG, Melton ML. Effect of pyrimethamine and sulfadiazine on the fine structure and multiplication of *Toxoplasma gondii* in cell cultures. J Parasitol 61:704-712, 1975.
1033. Eyles DE, Coleman N. The relative activity of the common sulfonamides against toxoplasmosis in the mouse. Am J Trop Med Hyg 2:54-63, 1953.
1034. Eyles DE, Coleman N. The effect of sulfadimetine, sulfisoxazole, and sulfapyrazine against mouse toxoplasmosis. Antibiot Chemother 5:525-528, 1955.
1035. Dorangeon PH, Fay R, Marx-Chemla C, et al. Passage transplacentaire de l'association pyriméthamine-sulfadoxine lors du traitement anténatal de la toxoplasmose congénitale. Presse Med 19:2036, 1990.
1036. Trenque T, Marx C, Quereux C, et al. Human maternofoetal distribution of pyrimethamine-sulphadoxine. Letter to the editor. Br J Clin Pharmacol 45:179-180, 1998.
1037. Peyron F, Wallon M, Bernardoux C. Long-term follow-up of patients with congenital ocular toxoplasmosis. Letter to the editor. N Engl J Med 334:993-994, 1996.
1038. Wilson CB. Treatment of congenital toxoplasmosis during pregnancy. J Pediat 116:1003-1005, 1990.
1039. Corvaisier S, Charpiat B, Mounier C, et al. Population pharmacokinetics of pyrimethamine and sulfadoxine in children treated for congenital toxoplasmosis. Antimicrob Agents Chemother 48: 3794-3800, 2004.
1040. Mack DG, McLeod R. New micromethod to study the effect of antimicrobial agents on *Toxoplasma gondii*: comparison of sulfadoxine and sulfadiazine individually and in combination with pyrimethamine and study of clindamycin, metronidazole, and cyclosporin A. Antimicrob Agents Chemother 26:26-30, 1984.
1041. Zitelli BJ, Alexander J, Taylor S, et al. Fatal hepatic necrosis due to pyrimethamine-sulfadoxine (Fansidar). Ann Intern Med 106: 393-395, 1987.
1042. Peyron F, Wallon M, Bernardoux C. Long-term follow-up of patients with congenital ocular toxoplasmosis. N Engl J Med 334:993-994, 1996.
1043. Matsui D. Prevention, diagnosis, and treatment of fetal toxoplasmosis. Clin Perinatol 21:675-689, 1994.
1044. McLeod R. Treatment of congenital toxoplasmosis. Plenary Symposium: Advances in Therapy of Protozoal Infections. Meeting of Interscience Conference on Antimicrobial Agents and Chemotherapy, Orlando, Fla, 1994.
1045. Trenque T, Simon N, Villena I, et al. Population pharmacokinetics of pyrimethamine and sulfadoxine in children with congenital toxoplasmosis. Br J Clin Pharmacol 57:735-741, 2004.
1046. Jordan MK, Burstein AH, Rock-Kress D, et al. Plasma pharmacokinetics of sulfadiazine administered twice daily versus four times daily are similar in human immunodeficiency virus-infected patients. Antimicrob Agents Chemother 48:635-637, 2004.
1047. Ryan RW, Hart WM, Culligan JJ, et al. Diagnosis and treatment of toxoplasmic uveitis. Trans Am Acad Ophthalmol Otolaryngol 58:867-884, 1954.
1048. Perkins ES, Smith CH, Schofield PB. Treatment of uveitis with pyrimethamine (Daraprim). Br J Ophthalmol 40:577-586, 1956.
1049. Elmalem J, Poulet B, Garnier R, et al. [Severe complications arising from the prescription of pyrimethamine for infants being treated for toxoplasmosis.] Therapie 40:357-359, 1985.
1050. Frenkel JK, Hitchings GH. Relative reversal by vitamins (*p*-aminobenzoic, folic and folinic acids) of the effects of sulfadiazine and pyrimethamine on *Toxoplasma*, mouse and man. Antibiot Chemother 7:630-638, 1957.
1051. Nixon PF, Bertino JR. Effective absorption and utilization of oral formyltetrahydrofolate in man. N Engl J Med 286:175-179, 1972.
1052. Allegra CJ, Kovacs JA, Drake JC, et al. Potent in vitro and in vivo anti-*Toxoplasma* activity of the lipid-soluble antifolate trimetrexate. J Clin Invest 79:478-482, 1987.
1053. Maisonneuve H, Faber C, Piens MA, Garin JP. [Congenital toxoplasmosis. Tolerability of the sulfadoxine-pyrimethamine combination. 24 cases.] Presse Med 13:859-862, 1984.
1054. Garin JP, Brossier N, Sung RTM, Moyne T. [Effect of pyrimethamine sulfadoxine (Fansidar) on an avirulent cystogenic strain of *Toxoplasma gondii* (Prugniaud strain) in white mice.] Bull Soc Pathol Exot Filiales 78:821-824, 1985.
1055. Garin JP, Paillard B. [Experimental toxoplasmosis in mice. Comparative activity of clindamycin, midecamycin, josamycin, spiramycin, pyrimethamine-sulfadoxine, and trimethoprim-sulfamethoxazole.] Ann Pediatr (Paris) 31:841-845, 1984.
1056. Thiersch JB. Effect of certain 2,4-diaminopyrimidine antagonists of folic acid on pregnancy and rat fetus. Proc Soc Exp Biol Med 87: 571-577, 1954.
1057. Anderson SI, Morse LM. The influence of solvent on the teratogenic effect of folic acid antogonist in the rat. Exp Mol Pathol 5:134-145, 1966.
1058. Dyban AP, Akimova IM. Characteristic features of the action of chloridine on various stages of embryonic development (experimental investigation). Akush Ginekol (Mosk) 41:21-38, 1965.
1059. Dyban AP, Akimova IM, Svetlova VA. Effects of 2,4-diamino-5-chlorphenyl-6-ethylpyrimidine on embryonic development of rats. Dokl Akad Nauk SSSR 163:1514-1517, 1965.
1060. Krahe M. [Investigations on the teratogen effect of medicine for the treatment of toxoplasmosis during pregnancy.] Arch Gynakol 202:104-109, 1965.
1061. Sullivan GE, Takacs E. Comparative teratogenicity of pyrimethamine in rats and hamsters. 4:205-210, 1971.
1062. Puchta V, Simandlova E. [On the question of fetal injury due to pyrimethamine (Daraprim).] *In* Kirchhoff H, Langer H (eds). Toxoplasmose. Stuttgart, Georg Thieme Verlag, 1971, p 19.
1063. Garin J-P, Eyles DE. [Spiramycin therapy of experimental toxoplasmosis in mice.] Presse Med 66:957-958, 1958.
1064. Mas Bakal P. [Deferred spiramycin treatment of acute toxoplasmosis in white mice.] Ned Tijdschr Geneeskd 109:1014-1017, 1965.
1065. Niel G, Videau D. Activité de la spiramycine in vitro sur *Toxoplasma gondii*. Réunion Inter Discipl Chimioth Antiinfect, Paris, 1981 (abstract, p 8).
1066. Macfarlane JA, Mitchell AA, Walsh JM, Robertson JJ. Spiramycin in the prevention of postoperative staphylococcal infection. Lancet 1:1-4, 1968.
1067. Benazet F, Dubost M. Apparent paradox of antimicrobial activity of spiramycin. Antibiot Ann 211-220, 1958-59.
1068. Sutherland R. Spiramycin: a reappraisal of its antibacterial activity. Br J Pharmacol 19:99-110, 1962.
1069. Kernbaum S. [Spiramycin; therapeutic value in humans (author's transl).] Sem Hop Paris 58:289-297, 1982.
1070. Garin JP, Pellerat J, Maillard, Woehrle-Hezez R. [Theoretical bases of the prevention by spiramycin of congenital toxoplasmosis in pregnant women.] Presse Med 76:2266, 1968.
1071. Hudson DG, Yoshihara GM, Kirby WM. Spiramycin: clinical and laboratory studies. AMA Arch Intern Med 97:57-61, 1956.
1072. Forestier F, Daffos F, Rainaut M, et al. Suivi therapeutique foetomaternel de la spiramycine en cours de grossesse. Arch Fr Pediatr 44:539-544, 1987.

1073. Martin C, Bentegeat J, Bildstein G, et al. [The course of congenital toxoplasmosis. Critical study of 12 treated cases.] Ann Pediatr (Paris) 16:117-128, 1969.
1074. Beverley JKA, Freeman AP, Henry L, Whelan JPF. Prevention of pathological changes in experimental congenital *Toxoplasma* infections. Lyon Med 230:491-498, 1973.
1075. Back N, Ambrus J, Velasco H, et al. Clinical and experimental pharmacology of parenteral spiramycin. Clin Pharmacol Ther 3:305-313, 1962.
1076. Stramba-Badiale M, Nador F, Porta N, et al. QT interval prolongation and risk of life-threatening arrhythmias during toxoplasmosis prophylaxis with spiramycin in neonates. Am Heart J 133:108-111, 1997.
1077. Couvreur J, Thulliez P, Daffos F, et al. In utero treatment of toxoplasmic fetopathy with the combination pyrimethamine-sulfadiazine. Fetal Diagn Ther 8:45-50, 1993.
1078. Leport C, Vilde JL, Katlama C, et al. Failure of spiramycin to prevent neurotoxoplasmosis in immunosuppressed patients. Letter to the editor. Med Clin North Am 70:677-692, 1986.
1079. Montoya JG, Liesenfeld O. Toxoplasmosis. Lancet 363:1965-1976, 2004.
1080. Stadtsbaeder S, Calvin-Preval MC. [The trimethoprim-sulfamethoxazole association in experimental toxoplasmosis in mice.] Acta Clin Belg 28:34-39, 1973.
1081. Grossman PL, Remington JS. The effect of trimethoprim and sulfamethoxazole on *Toxoplasma gondii* in vitro and in vivo. Am J Trop Med Hyg 28:445-455, 1979.
1082. Feldman HA. Effects of trimethoprim and sulfisoxazole alone and in combination on murine toxoplasmosis. [Addendum by Remington JS.] J Infect Dis 128(Suppl):S774-S776, 1973.
1083. Remington JS. Addendum to Feldman, H.A. Effects of trimethoprim and sulfisoxazole alone and in combination on murine toxoplasmosis. J Infect Dis 128(Suppl):S774-S776, 1973.
1084. Sander J, Midtvedt T. The effect of trimethoprim on acute experimental toxoplasmosis in mice. Acta Pathol Microbiol Scand [B] 78:664-668, 1970.
1085. Brus R, Chrusciel TL, Steffen J, Szaflarski J. Antitoxoplasmic activity of sulfonamides with various radicals in experimental toxoplasmosis in mice. Z Tropenmed Parasitol 22:98-103, 1971.
1086. Norrby R, Eilard T, Svedhem A, Lycke E. Treatment of toxoplasmosis with trimethoprim-sulphamethoxazole. Scand J Infect Dis 7:72-75, 1975.
1087. Domart A, Robineau M, Carbon C. [Acquired toxoplasmosis: a new chemotherapy: the sulfamethoxazole-trimethoprim combination.] Nouv Presse Med 2:321-322, 1973.
1088. Mossner G. Klinische Ergebnisse mit dem Kombinationspraparat Sulfamethoxazole + Trimethoprim. *In* Progress in Antimicrobial and Anticancer Chemotherapy. Baltimore, University Park Press, 1970, pp 996-970.
1089. Torre D, Casari S, Speranza F, et al. Randomized trial and trimethoprim-sulfamethoxazole versus pyrimethamine-sulfadiazine for therapy of toxoplasmic encephalitis in patients with AIDS. Antimicrob Agents Chemother 42:1346-1349, 1998.
1090. Nussenblatt RB, Schiffman R, Fortin E, et al. Strategies for the treatment of intraocular inflammatory disease. Transplant Proc 30:4124-4125, 1998.
1091. Araujo FG, Remington JS. Effect of clindamycin on acute and chronic toxoplasmosis in mice. Antimicrob Agents Chemother 15:647-651, 1974.
1092. McMaster PR, Powers KG, Finerty JF, Lunde MN. The effect of two chlorinated lincomycin analogues against acute toxoplasmosis in mice. Am J Trop Med Hyg 22:14-17, 1973.
1093. Tabbara KF, Nozik RA, O'Connor GR. Clindamycin effects on experimental ocular toxoplasmosis in the rabbit. . Arch Ophthalmol 92:244-247, 1974.
1094. Dannemann BR, Israelski DM, Remington JS. Treatment of toxoplasmic encephalitis with intravenous clindamycin. Arch Intern Med 148:2477-2482, 1988.
1095. Dannemann BR, McCutchan JA, Israelski DA, et al. Treatment of toxoplasmic encephalitis in patients with AIDS: a randomized trial comparing pyrimethamine plus clindamycin to pyrimethamine plus sulfadiazine. Ann Intern Med 116:33-43, 1992.
1096. Chang HR, Comte R, Pechere JC. In vitro and in vivo effects of doxycycline on *Toxoplasma gondii*. Antimicrob Agents Chemother 34:775-780, 1990.
1097. Tabbara KF, Sakuragi S, O'Connor GR. Minocycline in the chemotherapy of murine toxoplasmosis. Parasitology 84:297-302, 1982.
1098. Chang HR, Comte R, Piguet P-F, Pechere J-C. Activity of minocycline against *Toxoplasma gondii* infection in mice. J Antimicrob Chemother 27:639-645, 1991.
1099. Pope-Pegram L, Gathe J Jr, Bohn B, et al. Treatment of presumed central nervous system toxoplasmosis with doxycycline. Program and Abstracts of VII International Conference on AIDS, Florence, Italy, 1991 (abstract, p 188).
1100. Turett G, Pierone G, Masci J, Nicholas P. Failure of doxycycline in the treatment of cerebral toxoplasmosis. Sixth International Conference on AIDS, San Francisco, 1990 (abstract, p ThB479).
1101. Remington JS, Yagura T, Robinson WS. The effect of rifampin on *Toxoplasma gondii*. Proc Soc Exp Biol Med 135:167-172, 1970.
1102. Chan J, Luft BJ. Activity of roxithromycin (RU 28965), a macrolide, against *Toxoplasma gondii* infection in mice. Antimicrob Agents Chemother 30:323-324, 1986.
1103. Luft BJ. In vivo and in vitro activity of roxithromycin against *Toxoplasma gondii* in mice. Eur J Clin Microbiol 6:479-481, 1987.
1104. Araujo FG, Prokocimer P, Lin T, Remington JS. Activity of clarithromycin alone or in combination with other drugs for treatment of murine toxoplasmosis. Antimicrob Agents Chemother 36: 2454-2457, 1992.
1105. Araujo FG, Guptill DR, Remington JS. Azithromycin, a macrolide antibiotic with potent activity against *Toxoplasma gondii*. Antimicrob Agents Chemother 32:755-757, 1988.
1106. Stray-Pederson B. Azithromycin levels in placental tissue, amniotic fluid and blood. Thirty-sixth Interscience Conference on Antimicrobial Agents and Chemotherapy, 1996 (abstract, p 13).
1107. Rothova A, Bosch-Driessen LE, van Loon NH, Treffers WF. Azithromycin for ocular toxoplasmosis. Br J Ophthalmol 82:1306-1308, 1998.
1108. Bosch-Driessen LH, Verbraak FD, Suttorp-Schulten MS, et al. A prospective, randomized trial of pyrimethamine and azithromycin vs pyrimethamine and sulfadiazine for the treatment of ocular toxoplasmosis. Am J Ophthalmol 134:34-40, 2002.
1109. Araujo FG, Khan AA, Bryskier A, Remington JS. Use of ketolides in combination with other drugs to treat experimental toxoplasmosis. J Antimicrob Chemother 42:665-667, 1998.
1110. Khan AA, Slifer TR, Araujo FG, Remington JS. Activity of gatifloxacin alone or in combination with pyrimethamine or gamma interferon against *Toxoplasma gondii*. Antimicrob Agents Chemother 45:48-51, 2001.
1111. Araujo FG, Khan AA, Slifer TL, et al. The ketolide antibiotics HMR 3647 and HMR 3004 are active against *Toxoplasma gondii* in vitro and in murine models of infection. Antimicrob Agents Chemother 41:2137-2140, 1997.
1112. Huskinson-Mark J, Araujo FG, Remington JS. Evaluation of the effect of drugs on the cyst form of *Toxoplasma gondii*. J Infect Dis 164:170-177, 1991.
1113. Araujo FG, Huskinson J, Remington JS. Remarkable in vitro and in vivo activities of the hydroxynaphthoquinone 566C80 against tachyzoites and tissue cysts of *Toxoplasma gondii*. Antimicrob Agents Chemother 35:293-299, 1991.
1114. Kovacs JA, Polis MA, Blaird B, et al. Evaluation of azithromycin or the combination of 566C80 and pyrimethamine in the treatment of toxoplasmosis. VIII International Conference on AIDS, Amsterdam, 1992 (abstract, p B120).
1115. Clumeck N, Katlama C, Ferrero T, et al. Atovaquone (1,4-hydroxy-naphthoquinone, 566C80) in the treatment of acute cerebral toxoplasmosis (CT) in AIDS patients. Thirty-second Interscience Conference on Antimicrobial Agents and Chemotherapy, Anaheim, Calif, 1992 (abstract, p 313).
1116. Torres R, Weinberg W, Stansell J, et al. Atovaquone for salvage treatment and suppression of toxoplasmic encephalitis in patients with AIDS. Clin Infect Dis 24:422-429, 1997.
1117. Katlama C, Mouthon B, Gourdon D, et al. Atovaquone as long-term suppressive therapy for toxoplasmic encephalitis in patients with AIDS and multiple drug intolerance. AIDS 10:1107-1112, 1996.
1118. Kovacs JA. Efficacy of atovaquone in treatment of toxoplasmosis in patients with AIDS. Lancet 340:637-638, 1992.
1119. Khan AA, Slifer T, Araujo FG, Remington JS. Trovafloxacin is active against *Toxoplasma gondii*. Antimicrob Agents Chemother 40: 1855-1859, 1996.
1120. Khan AA, Slifer T, Araujo FG, et al. Activity of trovafloxacin in combination with other drugs for treatement of acute murine toxoplasmosis. Antimicrob Agents Chemother 41:893-897, 1997.

1121. Stagno S, Reynolds DW, Amos CS, et al. Auditory and visual defects resulting from symptomatic and subclinical congenital cytomegaloviral and *Toxoplasma* infections. Pediatrics 59:669-678, 1977.
1122. Jeannel D, Costagliola D, Niel G, et al. What is known about the prevention of congenital toxoplasmosis? Lancet 336:359-361, 1990.
1123. Boulot P, Fratlong F, Sarda P, et al. Limitations of the prenatal treatment of congenital toxoplasmosis with the sulfadiazine-pyrimethamine combination. Presse Méd 19:570, 1990.
1124. Couvreur J, Desmonts G, Tournier G, et al. Etude d'une serie homogene de 210 cas de toxoplasmose congénitale chez des nourrissons ages de 0 à 11 mois et depistes de facon prospective. Sem Hop Paris 61:3015-3019, 1985.
1125. Wallon M, Gandihon F, Peyron F, Mojon M. Letter to the editor. Lancet 344:541, 1994.
1126. Alford CA Jr, Reynolds DW, Stagno S. Current concepts of chronic perinatal infections. *In* Gluck L (ed). Modern Perinatal Medicine. Chicago, Year Book Medical Publishers, 1975, pp 285-306.
1127. Cunningham GC, Hawes WE, Madore C. Intrauterine Growth and Neonatal Risk in California. Sacramento, State of California Department of Health, 1976.
1128. Szusterkac M. A propos de 124 cas de toxoplasmose congénitale: aspects cliniques et paracliniques en fonction des circonstances du diagnostic retrospectif ou prospectif; resultats du traitement. Paris, Faculté de Médecine Saint-Antoine, 1980.
1129. Briatte C. Etude de 55 cas de toxoplasmose congenitale depistes lors de bilans de santé systematiques après l'age de 10 mois. Centre de bilans de santé de la securité sociale de la Region Parisienne. Paris, Faculté de Médecine Saint-Antoine, 1980.
1130. Sever JL, Ellenberg JH, Ley AC, et al. Toxoplasmosis: maternal and pediatric findings in 23,000 pregnancies. Pediatrics 82:181-192, 1988.
1131. Roizen N, Swisher C, Boyer K, et al. Developmental and neurologic function in treated congenital toxoplasmosis. Pediatr Res 31:353A, 1992 (abstract no. 2101).
1132. McLeod R, Boyer K, Roizen N, et al. Treatment of congenital toxoplasmosis. Seventeenth International Congress of Chemotherapy, Berlin, 1991 (abstract, p 1933).
1133. Swisher CN, Boyer K, McLeod R. The Toxoplasmosis Study Group. Congenital toxoplasmosis. Semin Pediatr Neurol 1:4-25, 1994.
1134. Mets MG, Mack DG, Boyer K. Congenital ocular toxoplasmosis. *In* Mets MB, Group TTS (eds). Ophthalmologic Findings in Congenital Toxoplasmosis. Invest Ophthalmol Vis Sci 1094, 1992 (abstract no. 2009-16).
1135. Engstrom REJ, Holland GN, Nussenblatt RB, Jabs DA. Current practices in the management of ocular toxoplasmosis. Am J Ophthalmol 111:601-610, 1991.
1136. Binquet C, Wallon M, Quantin C, et al. Prognostic factors for the long-term development of ocular lesions in 327 children with congenital toxoplasmosis. Epidemiol Infect 131:1157-1168, 2003.
1137. Frenkel JK. Congenital toxoplasmosis: prevention or palliation? Am J Obstet Gynecol 141:359-361, 1981.
1138. Henderson JB, Beattie CP, Hale EG, Wright T. The evaluation of new services: possibilities for preventing congenital toxoplasmosis. Int J Epidemiol 13:65-72, 1984.
1139. McCabe R, Remington JS. Toxoplasmosis: the time has come. Editorial. N Engl J Med 318:313-315, 1988.
1140. Frenkel JK. Breaking the transmission chain of *Toxoplasma*: a program for the prevention of human toxoplasmosis. Bull N Y Acad Med 50:228-235, 1974.
1141. Frenkel JK. Toxoplamosis in cats and man. Feline Practice 5:28-41, 1975.
1142. Hartley WJ, Munday BL. Felidae in the dissemination of toxoplasmosis to man and other animals Aust Vet J 50:224-228, 1974.
1143. Hutchison WM. *Toxoplasma gondii* and its development in domestic felines. Victorian Vet Proc 17-21, 1973-1974.
1144. Frenkel JK, Dubey JP. Rodents as vectors for feline coccidia, *Isospora felis* and *Isospora rivolta*. J Infect Dis 125:69-72, 1972.
1145. Hassl A. Efficiency analysis of toxoplasmosis screening in pregnancy: comment. Letter to the editor. Scand J Infect Dis 28:211-212, 1996.
1146. Lappalainen M, Sintonen H, Koskiniemi M, et al. Cost-benefit analysis of screening for toxoplasmosis during pregnancy. Scand J Infect Dis 27:265-272, 1995.
1147. Lappalainen M, Koskela P, Hedman K, et al. Screening of toxoplasmosis during pregancy. Isr J Med Sci 30:362-363, 1994.
1148. Bader TJ, Macones GA, Asch DA. Prenatal screening for toxoplasmosis. Obstet Gynecol 90:457-464, 1997.
1149. Daffos F, Mirlesse V, Hohlfeld P, et al. Letter to the editor. Lancet 344:541, 1994.
1150. Gras L, Gilbert RE, Ades AE, Dunn DT. Effect of prenatal treatment on the risk of intracranial and ocular lesions in children with congenital toxoplasmosis. Int J Epidemiol 30:1309-1313, 2001.
1151. Gilbert RE, Gras L, Wallon M, et al. Effect of prenatal treatment on mother to child transmission of *Toxoplasma gondii*: retrospective cohort study of 554 mother-child pairs in Lyon, France. Int J Epidemiol 30:1303-1308, 2001.
1152. Luyasu V, Bauraind O, Bernard P, et al. [Congenital toxoplasmosis and seroconversion at the end of pregnancy: clinical observations.] Acta Clin Belg 52:381-387, 1997.
1153. Couvreur J. [In utero treatment of congenital toxoplasmosis with a pyrimethamine-sulfadiazine combination.] Presse Med 20:1137, 1991.
1154. Brézin A, Thulliez P, Couvreur J, et al. Ophthalmic Outcome after pre- and post-natal treatment of congenital toxoplasmosis. Am J Ophthalmol 135:779-784, 2003.
1155. Desmonts G, Jones TC. Congenital toxoplasmosis. N Engl J Med 291:365-366, 1974.
1156. Desmonts G, Couvreur J. [Congenital toxoplasmosis. Prospective study of the outcome of pregnancy in 542 women with toxoplasmosis acquired during pregnancy.] Ann Pediatr (Paris) 31:805-809, 1984.
1157. Kräubig H. Erste praktische Erfahrungen mit der Prophylaze der konnatalen Toxoplasmose. Med Klin 58:1361-1364, 1963.
1158. Thalhammer O. Congenital toxoplasmosis in Vienna. Summering [sic] findings and opinions. *In* Specia L (ed). Colloque sur la Toxoplasmose de la Femme Enceinte et la Prevention de la Toxoplasmose Congenitale Monographie. Lyon Medical, 1969, pp 109-129.
1159. Thalhammer O. Prevention of congenital toxoplasmosis. Neuropediatrie 4:233-237, 1973.
1160. Hengst VP. [Effectiveness of general testing for *Toxoplasma gondii* infection in pregnancy.] Zentralbl Gynakol 104:949-956, 1982.
1161. Liesenfeld O, Montoya JG, Tathineni NJ, et al. Confirmatory serological testing results in remarkable decrease in unnecessary abortion among pregnant women in the United States with positive toxoplasma serology. Thirty-fifth Annual Meeting of the Infectious Diseases Society of America, San Francisco, September 13-16, 1997 (abstract, p 76).
1162. Remington JS. Toxoplasmosis and human abortion. *In* Meigs JV, Sturgis SH (eds). Progress in Gynecology. New York, Grune & Stratton, 1963, pp 303-315.
1163. Eckerling B, Neri A, Eylan E. Toxoplasmosis: a cause of infertility. Fertil Steril 19:883-891, 1968.
1164. Langer H. [*Toxoplasma* infection during pregnancy.] Zentralbl Gynakol 86:745-750, 1964.
1165. Vlaev S. Opyt profilaktiki vrozdennogo toksoplazmoza. Vop Okrany Materin Dets 10:78-82, 1965.
1166. Isbruch VF. [Contributions to the problem of toxoplasmosis. I. Should we, at the present state of knowledge, treat pregnant women with positive toxoplasmosis titers, with Daraprim and Supronal?] Zentralbl Gynakol 82:1522-1544, 1960.
1167. Sharf M, Eibschitz I, Eylan E. Latent toxoplasmosis and pregnancy. Obstet Gynecol 42:349-354, 1973.
1168. Feldman HA. Congenital toxoplasmosis. Letter to the editor. N Eng J Med 26:1212, 1963.
1169. Cengir SD, Ortac F, Soylemex F. Treatment and results of chronic toxoplasmosis. Gynecol Obstet Invest 33:105-108, 1992.
1170. Lebech M, E. P. Reihenuntersuchung von Neugeborenen auf angeborene Toxoplasmose in Dänemark aufgrund mütterlicher Serumkonversion während der Schwangerschaft. Tropenmed Parasitol 18:33-40, 1996.
1171. Candolfi E, Wittersheim P, Kien T. Prevalence de la toxoplasmose humaine à Strasbourg en 1992 (unpublished).
1172. Al-Nakib W, Ibrahim MEA, Hathout H, et al. Seroepidemiology of viral and toxoplasmal infections during pregnancy among Arab women of child-bearing age in Kuwait. Int J Epidemiol 12:220-223, 1983.
1173. Evengard B, Petersson K, Engman ML, et al. Low incidence of *Toxoplasma* infection during pregnancy and in newborns in Sweden. Epidemiol Infect 127:121-127, 2001.
1174. Jones JL, Kruszon-Moran D, Wilson M, et al. *Toxoplasma gondii* infection in the United States: seroprevalence and risk factors. Am J Epidemiol 154:357-365, 2001.

Chapter 32

LESS COMMON PROTOZOAN AND HELMINTH INFECTIONS

Yvonne A. Maldonado

Parasitic infections are highly prevalent in many developing areas of the world and may be common among pregnant women in developed countries. The placenta serves as an effective barrier, even in infections such as malaria and schistosomiasis in which systemic involvement and hematogenous spread are common. Although transplacental infections of the fetus are uncommon, the prevalence of parasitic infections among infants younger than 1 month is high in developing countries, and infections occur primarily through transmission during or shortly after birth.

In a study conducted in Guatemala, Kotcher and colleagues[1] found that 30% of newborns had acquired a protozoal infection by 2 weeks of age. Although these infants were infected with *Entamoeba histolytica,* as well as with *Entamoeba coli, Endolimax nana,* and *Iodamoeba buetschlii,* they remained asymptomatic. *Giardia lamblia* was found by the fifth week of life and *Trichuris trichiura* by the 16th week of life. A study conducted in a regional hospital in Togo revealed that 55% of infants and children from birth to 16 years old demonstrated evidence of parasitic infections in stool or urine, with obvious neonatal infections occurring as well.[2]

Pneumocystis jiroveci (previously classified as *Pneumocystis carinii*) is also considered in this chapter.[3]

ASCARIS

Ascaris lumbricoides is the most prevalent parasitic infection worldwide, affecting up to 1 billion people. In humans, *Ascaris* eggs are ingested through fecal-oral contamination, hatch in the small intestine, and then penetrate the intestinal lumen to migrate extensively through blood and lymphatics. Larvae eventually reach the pulmonary circulation, where they migrate into the alveolar sacs, through the respiratory tree to the esophagus, and into the small intestine. Because *Ascaris* may migrate to many organs, worms are occasionally found in the uterus and the fallopian tubes.[4]

Human fetuses apparently can mount an immune response to maternal *Ascaris* infection, and congenital infections are rare. Sangeevi and associates[5] studied the IgG and IgM responses to *Ascaris* antigens from matched maternal and cord bloods in south India and found evidence of fetal IgM directed against *Ascaris* antigens in 12 of 28 samples. Clinical status of the infants was not reported. Chu and co-workers,[6] however, described an infant whose delivery was complicated by the simultaneous delivery of 12 adult *A. lumbricoides* worms. During preparations for a cesarean section, which was being undertaken because of prolonged premature labor and fetal distress, one worm passed from the vagina, and another was found in the vagina. When the placenta was removed, 10 worms were found on the maternal side of the placenta. The infant was delivered in good condition. The infant passed two female worms, which were 28 and 30 cm long, on the second and sixth days of life. He was treated with piperazine citrate, but no other worms were passed, and no eggs were seen after the 11th day of life. Fertilized ova of *A. lumbricoides* were found in the amniotic fluid and in the newborn's feces. An adhesion connected the mother's intestine and uterus, but it is uncertain whether the worms passed directly from the mother's intestine to the placenta and amniotic fluid and were swallowed by the fetus; whether larvae passed hematogenously from the mother's lung to the placenta and thereby reached the fetal circulation, lung, and gastrointestinal tract; or whether female worms in the placenta produced fertile eggs that reached the amniotic fluid and were swallowed by the fetus. Other investigators have reported fetal evidence of *Ascaris* infection in infants as young as 1 to 2 weeks old and in one infant with failure to thrive and bloody diarrhea at 3 weeks who responded to levamisole therapy.[7]

GIARDIASIS

G. lamblia causes a localized intestinal infection, with no systemic involvement, and *G. lamblia* infection in pregnancy has not been associated with fetal infection. Severe maternal infection that compromises nutrition can affect fetal growth, but such a severe illness is rare.[8] Neonatal *G. lamblia* infection can result from fecal contamination at birth. Infected infants are usually asymptomatic.[9] Treatment of pregnant women with giardiasis is generally deferred until after the first trimester unless symptoms are severe. There is some evidence that maternal antibody may be protective against neonatal giardiasis.[10]

AMERICAN TRYPANOSOMIASIS: CHAGAS' DISEASE

Millions of people in Central and South America are infected by *Trypanosoma cruzi* and related protozoa. Because of the chronicity of these infections, they have a significant impact on public health.

The Organism

The form of the organism that circulates in human blood is the trypomastigote. Cell division does not occur in the bloodstream. In tissue, the flagellum and undulating membrane are lost, and the organism differentiates into a leishmanial form, the amastigote.[11,12] Amastigotes multiply by binary fission, and masses of amastigotes are grouped into pseudocysts. The amastigotes in pseudocysts may evolve into trypanomastigotes and, on rupture of the pseudocyst, can gain access to the bloodstream or to new cells. Two strains of *T. cruzi* that cause human infections have been identified by biochemical differences among nine enzymes produced by the parasite.[13]

Epidemiology and Transmission

T. cruzi infects primates, marsupials, armadillos, bats, and many rodents, including guinea pigs, opossums, and raccoons; birds are not infected.[14] Infection of insects and mammals with *T. cruzi* is most common between the latitudes 39° N (i.e., northern California and Maryland) and 43° S (i.e., southern Argentina and Chile) and on the islands of Aruba and Trinidad.[1] The usual vectors are in the family Reduviidae, subfamily Triatominae. The main vector in Venezuela is *Rhodnius prolixus;* in Brazil, *Panstrongylus megistus;* and in Argentina, *Triatoma infectans* (cone-nosed bug).[14] These species are well adapted to human dwellings. Triatominae are hematophagous insects. They acquire and transmit the infection by biting infected vertebrates, including humans. The life span of the insect is not shortened by infection with *T. cruzi;* infected insects live up to a year after the onset of infection. In North America, the sylvatic habitat of the vector and the low virulence of the strains of *Trypanosoma* are responsible for the relative rarity of the disease. Colloquial terms used for the usual vector include the kissing or assassin bug in the southwestern United States; *pito, hito,* or *vinchuca* in Spanish America; and *barbeiro* in Portuguese America.[15]

The vector is most commonly found in huts of mud and sticks and in other housing containing cracks. In vectors infected with *T. cruzi,* metacyclic trypomastigotes congregate in the rectum. Bites become contaminated when defecation occurs. The infective form reaches the bloodstream through the site of the bite or by penetrating mucous membranes, conjunctivae, or abraded skin.[11] *Trypanosoma rangeli* is spread by a few species of the triatomid bug. These metacyclic trypanosomes develop, divide, and multiply in the salivary gland. They are injected directly into the site of the bite.

Infections can also be acquired by blood transfusion[16] and transplacentally. The isoenzyme patterns of *T. cruzi* recovered from congenitally infected infants and their mothers are identical, but transplacental transmission may not always follow maternal infection with enzymatically similar strains.[17]

Pathology

Placenta

The placenta is a relatively effective barrier to the spread of infection to the fetus.[12] The organism reaches the placenta by the hematogenous route and traverses the placental villi to the trophoblasts. After differentiation into amastigotes, the organism remains within Hofbauer's (phagocytic) cells of the placenta until it is liberated into the fetal circulation.[18-20]

Maternal parasitemia is greatest in the acute phase of infection; however, the period of intense parasitemia is short. Of the reported cases of congenital Chagas' disease, only four have originated during the acute phase of infection.[12] Most congenital infections occur in infants born to women with the chronic form of the disease.

Infected placentas are pale, yellow, and bulky. They have an appearance similar to the placentas of infants with erythroblastosis fetalis. Infection of the placenta is much more common than infection of the fetus.

Biopsy and Autopsy Studies

Two histologic types of lesions are recognized: those that contain parasites and those that do not.[12] In tissue sections, the parasite assumes the morphology of *Leishmania* bodies, which are round and contain an ovoid nucleus and a rodlike blepharoplast. Inflammation usually does not occur unless a pseudocyst ruptures. Tissue reactions induced by antibody are believed to be responsible for lesions in which the parasite cannot be demonstrated. After infection, an antibody that cross reacts with the endocardium, the interstitium, and the blood vessels of the heart is formed and is referred to as an endocardial-vascular-interstitial antibody.[21-23] This antibody has an affinity for the plasma membranes of the endocardium, endothelial cell, and striated muscle, as well as for *T. cruzi.* Endocardial-vascular-interstitial antibody is present in 95% of persons with Chagas' heart disease and in 45% of asymptomatic patients with serologic evidence of having had Chagas' disease.[23]

Tissue replication of the organism causes damage to the ganglia of the autonomic nervous system and to muscle.[14] Injury to Auerbach's plexus results in megaesophagus, megacolon, and dilatation of other parts of the gastrointestinal tract and gallbladder. Similarly, the conducting system of the heart and the myocardium may be infected. Sudden death from arrhythmias can occur.

Clinical Manifestations

In the mother, urticaria is often present at the site of the bite, regardless of whether the insect was infected.[11] The favored site for the bite is the face, presumably because this is the part of the body that is most often exposed during sleep. In acute infections, an inflammatory nodule, referred to as a *chagoma*, may develop at the site of the bite. If the bite is on the face, it is often associated with a unilateral, nonpurulent edema of the palpebral folds and an ipsilateral regional lymphadenopathy (i.e., Romaña's sign). Between 2 and 3 weeks after the bite, parasitemia, fever, and a moderate local and general lymphadenopathy develop. The infection can extend and involve the myocardium, resulting in tachycardia, arrhythmia, hypotension, distant heart sounds, cardiomegaly, and congestive heart failure. The latter feature is more severe in pregnant and postpartum women than in nonpregnant women. Hepatosplenomegaly and encephalitis also occur. The mortality rate during the acute phase is 10% to 20%. Death is usually attributed to cardiac dysfunction. Many survivors have abnormal electrocardiograms.

In the chronic phase, the placenta and fetus may be infected despite the fact that the mother is asymptomatic.[11] Chronic Chagas' disease often comes to medical attention because of the occurrence of an arrhythmia. These patients often do not have signs or symptoms of congestive heart failure.[14] Of 503 patients with myocardiopathy of chronic Chagas' disease studied by Vasquez,[24] 19.8% died during an observation period of 6 years—37.5% suddenly and 55.2% with congestive heart failure.

Abortions and Stillbirths

Of 300 abortions in Argentina, 3 (1%) were performed because of Chagas' disease.[25] In Chile and Brazil, 10% of all abortions are attributed to Chagas' disease.[11] When the fetus is aborted, massive infection of the placenta is usually found.

Congenital Infections

Bittencourt and co-workers[26] found *T. cruzi* antibodies in 226 of 2651 pregnant women; 28.3% of seropositive mothers had parasitemia. Nevertheless, the risk of transmission to the fetus is low, and livebirths of infants congenitally infected with *T. cruzi* are rare. It is postulated that upregulation of fetal or neonatal immunity might be important in preventing vertical infection.[27] Congenital infections occur in 1% to 4% of women with serologic evidence of having had Chagas' disease.[1,11,12,20,28,29] Among infants with a birth weight of 2500 g or more, congenital infections are rare.[18,30-33] Among low-birth-weight infants, congenitally infected infants can be premature or small for gestational age, or both. Congenital infections were found in 10 (2.3%) of 425 infants by Saleme and associates in Argentina,[25] in 10 (2%) of 500 infants weighing less than 2000 g by Bittencourt and co-workers in Brazil,[26] and in 3 (1.6%) of 186 infants with birth weights of more than 2000 g and in 1 (0.5%) of 200 premature infants with birth weights of 2000 g or less by Howard in Chile.[34]

Congenitally infected infants may develop symptoms at birth or during the first few weeks of life. Early-onset jaundice, anemia, and petechiae are common. These symptoms are similar to those associated with erythroblastosis fetalis.[12] As occurs in older patients, congenitally infected infants may have hepatosplenomegaly, cardiomegaly, and congestive heart failure and have involvement of the esophagus leading to dysphagia, regurgitation, and megaesophagus.[23,35] Some infants have myxedematous edema. Pneumonitis has been associated with infection of the amnionic epithelium.[36] Congenitally infected infants can be born with encephalitis or can develop it postnatally. It is generally associated with hypotonia, a poor suck, and seizures.[11] The cerebrospinal fluid shows mild pleocytosis, which consists primarily of lymphocytes. Cataracts and opacification of the media of the eye have also been observed.[28] Both twins may be congenitally infected, or one may escape infection.[37]

Of 64 congenitally infected infants for whom follow-up results were known, Bittencourt[12] reported that 7.8% died the first day, 35.9% died when younger than 4 months, 9.3% died between the ages of 4 and 24 months, and 42.2% survived for more than 24 months. Of those who survived for 2 years or longer, 74% had no serious clinical symptoms despite continued parasitemia. However, subclinical abnormalities might have been found if electrocardiography or radiography had been performed.

As with other congenital infections, the immune system of the fetus is stimulated. IgM antibody to *T. cruzi* and endocardial-vascular-interstitial antibody are formed.[12,23]

Diagnosis

The diagnosis should be suspected at the time of abortions and stillbirths, as well as in infants who develop symptoms compatible with congenital infection. An easy, but often omitted, means of making a diagnosis of congenital infection is to examine the placenta for the amastigote of *T. cruzi.* The gross appearance of the placenta is similar to that seen in erythroblastosis fetalis.

Motile trypomastigotes can also be demonstrated by examining blood under a coverslip.[12] The number of parasites is low initially but increases subsequently. Thin and thick smears can be examined after being stained with Giemsa stain. Microhematocrit concentration and examination of the buffy coat enhance the detection of parasites in congenital Chagas' disease.[38] If more than 10 parasites/mm^3 are found, the infant generally dies.[25]

Xenodiagnosis is performed by allowing laboratory-bred uninfected insects to feed and ingest the patient's blood. The fecal contents of the insects are examined for trypomastigotes 30 to 60 days later. Blood may also be injected into mice. In mothers with acute Chagas' disease, the parasites are found in blood smears beginning 3 weeks after onset of the infection, and they persist for several months. Parasites can be demonstrated for years by xenodiagnosis.

In the chronic stages of the disease, the diagnosis can be made histologically by sampling skeletal muscle. The histologic appearance of the parasite in tissue sections is similar to that of toxoplasmosis. However, the amastigotes in Chagas' disease contain a blepharoplast that is lacking in toxoplasmosis.

Several tests for antibody are available. Complement-fixing antibody crosses the placenta from mother to infant. This test, referred to as the Machado-Guerreiro reaction, demonstrates antibodies that exhibit a cross-reaction with *Leishmania donovani* and with sera from patients with lepromatous leprosy. In uninfected infants, complement-fixing antibodies are no longer demonstrable after the 40th day of life; in infected infants, these antibodies persist.[12]

Agglutinating antibodies may also be demonstrable. Uninfected infants with titers of agglutinating antibody of 1:512 or less at birth have negative titers by 2 months of age.[28] The titer of agglutinating antibody in uninfected infants with initial titers of 1:1024 or higher becomes negative by 6 months of age. IgM fluorescent antibodies can be demonstrated in some infants, but infected infants do not always have a positive test result.[23,37] Data suggest that fetal IgG to specific acute-phase antigens may be useful in the diagnosis of congenital Chagas' disease, but maternal and neonatal serologic tests using the microhematocrit, direct parasitologic visualization, and indirect hemagglutination or enzyme-linked immunosorbent assay have proved to be reliable.[39,40]

Prognosis for Recurrence

Congenital infections can recur during subsequent pregnancies.[41] The same mother, however, often has healthy children before and after the affected one.[23]

Therapy

In the past, various drugs, including nitrofurans, 8-aminoquinolines, and metronidazole, were thought to have some effect on the blood-borne form of the parasite. They were ineffective in eliminating the tissue form, the amastigote. There is no therapy available for prevention of congenital infection, but early detection of neonatal infection and treatment with nifurtimox has resulted in cure rates of up to 90%.[42] Information regarding treatment can be obtained from the Parasitic Disease Drug Service, Centers for Disease Control and Prevention, Atlanta, Georgia.

Prevention

The main means of prevention is to improve housing so that the vector cannot reach the inhabitants, especially during sleep. In endemic areas, potential blood donors should be tested, and only those who lack serologic evidence of having had Chagas' disease should be permitted to donate blood. The addition of gentian violet (1:4000 solution) to blood has been useful as a means of preventing transmission of the infection to the recipient of the blood.[14]

AFRICAN TRYPANOSOMIASIS: AFRICAN SLEEPING SICKNESS

Whereas few cases of congenital disease have been reported, infection with *Trypanosoma brucei gambiense* and *T. brucei rhodesiense* in adults is severe and often fatal, and congenital infection is most likely underreported. Humans are infected by the bite of an infected male or female tsetse fly, which injects trypomastigotes into the host. Humans are the primary reservoir for *T. gambiense* and large, wild game the hosts for *T. rhodesiense*. Once injected, the organism disseminates throughout the bloodstream. Signs and symptoms of infection appear after 2 to 4 weeks, and a chronic infection develops 6 months to 1 to 2 years later. The chronic stage includes a progressive meningoencephalitis, which is often fatal if left untreated. Infection with *T. gambiense* is associated with lymphadenopathy and is slowly progressive, whereas infection with *T. rhodesiense* is rapidly progressive.

The parasite can be transmitted transplacentally, but few cases have been reported.[43,44] Transplacental infection can cause prematurity, abortion, and stillbirth. Transplacental infection has been proved in infants who were born in nonendemic areas to infected mothers or if the parasite was identified in the peripheral blood in the first 5 days of life. Central nervous system involvement is common in congenital infection and, in some infants, may be slowly progressive.

The diagnosis should be suspected in an infant with unexplained fever, anemia, hepatosplenomegaly, or progressive neurologic symptoms whose mother is from an endemic area. The parasite can be identified in thick smears from peripheral blood or in the cerebrospinal fluid. In infants, treatment with suramin or melarsoprol has been reported with good results; however, in a case report of congenital trypanosomiasis,[43] severe neurologic symptoms persisted after delayed diagnosis and treatment when the child was 22 months old.

ENTAMOEBA HISTOLYTICA

There is some evidence that amebiasis during pregnancy may be more severe and have a higher fatality rate than that expected in nonpregnant women of the same age.[45,46] Abioye[46] found that 68% of fatal cases of amebiasis in females 15 to 34 years old occurred in pregnant women, whereas only 17.1 and 12.5% of fatal cases of typhoid or other causes of enterocolitis, respectively, in women in this age group occurred during pregnancy. Czeizel and co-workers[47] found a significantly higher incidence of positive stool cultures for *E. histolytica* among women who had spontaneous abortions than among those who gave birth to living infants at term.

Amebiasis has been reported in infants as young as 3 to 6 weeks old.[48-50] In most instances, person-to-person transmission was considered likely, and the mother was the probable source of the infant's infection.[48] In one fatal case, the father had cysts of *E. histolytica* in his stool, whereas no evidence of infection with *E. histolytica* was found in the mother.[49] Perinatal infections have occurred in countries such as the United States in which the disease is rare.

Most infants reported with amebiasis in the perinatal period had illnesses with sudden, dramatic onset and were seriously ill. Bloody diarrhea was followed by development of hepatomegaly and hepatic abscess, rectal abscess, and gangrene of the appendix and colon with perforation and peritonitis. Persistent bloody diarrhea that is complicated by the development of a mass in or around the liver should lead to a thorough investigation about whether infection with *E. histolytica* could be the cause. Maternal amebiasis has also been associated with low birth weight.[51]

Routine stool examinations for ova and parasites may be negative. Despite this, trophozoites of *E. histolytica* can usually be found in biopsy specimens of gastrointestinal ulcers and of the wall of the liver abscesses. The organisms cannot always be demonstrated in pus aspirated from the center of the abscess. An elevated indirect hemagglutination titer to *E. histolytica* can be helpful in diagnosing extraintestinal amebiasis. However, high titers are not usually seen until 2 weeks or more after onset of the infection in older patients and are not always present in neonates with severe extraintestinal infections.[48] Infants have been successfully treated with oral metronidazole.[50] Critically ill children should receive intravenous therapy with dehydroemetine or metronidazole.

MALARIA

Although malaria is recognized as the major health problem of many countries, its impact on pregnancy and infant mortality has probably been underestimated.

The Organisms

Of the four species of malaria, *Plasmodium vivax* has the widest distribution, but *Plasmodium falciparum* tends to predominate in tropical areas. Malaria is spread to humans by the bite of anopheline mosquitoes. Of the many species of anopheline mosquito capable of becoming infected with malarial parasites, those that enter houses are more important than those preferring an outdoor habitat.[52] Mosquitoes that feed at night on human blood while the victim is asleep are the most important vectors.

After the bite of the mosquito, sporozoites are injected into the bloodstream but are cleared within one-half hour. The parasites mature in the parenchymal cells of the liver and form a mature schizont, which contains 7500 to 40,000 merozoites, depending on the species. The release of the merozoites results in the appearance of the ring stage in erythrocytes in the peripheral blood. Within hours, the parasite assumes an amoeboid form and is referred to as a *trophozoite*. The sexual form is called a *gametocyte*. In infections with *P. vivax, Plasmodium malariae,* and *Plasmodium ovale,* all forms are seen in the peripheral blood from early ring forms through mature schizonts and gametocytes. In infections with *P. falciparum,* usually only rings and gametocytes are found in the peripheral blood.

Epidemiology and Transmission

In addition to transmission by the bite of mosquitoes, malaria can be transmitted by transfusion of blood products. In infants, this has occurred after simple transfusion and after exchange transfusion.[53-56] The onset of symptoms in neonates infected by blood products has varied from 13 to 21 days.

Malaria parasites survive in blood for weeks. Relapses can occur from *P. vivax* for up to 2 years and rarely for up to 4 years. Relapses from *P. malariae* have occasionally occurred 5 years or more after infection, but low-grade chronic parasitemia that is unassociated with symptoms is more common.

Malaria may be transmitted by reuse of syringes and needles and has spread by this route among heroin addicts. Infection in heroin addicts who become pregnant can result in congenital infections.[57]

Pathology

Effect of Pregnancy on Malaria

The density and the prevalence of parasitemia are increased in pregnant women compared with women who are not pregnant but who reside in the same geographic area.[58-62] For *P. falciparum,* Campbell and colleagues[63] found a parasite density of 6896/mm^3 in pregnant women and 3808/mm^3 in nonpregnant women; for *P. vivax,* the parasite density was 3564/mm^3 for pregnant women and 1949/mm^3 for nonpregnant women. The prevalence and the density of the parasitemia decrease with increasing parity. Reinhardt and associates[59] found that the placenta was infected in 45% of primiparous women compared with 19% of women with a parity of five. This trend toward an increase in resistance to malaria with parity has been attributed by some to the increase in immunity that would be expected with an increase in age. However, the prevalence and the density of parasitemia are increased in pregnant women of all parities compared with those in nonpregnant women of the same parity.[58-60] This suggests that pregnancy, as well as age, is an important factor in determining susceptibility to malaria.[58]

Infection of the Placenta

The intervillous spaces of infected placentas are packed with lymphoid macrophages, which contain phagocytosed pigment in large granules. Lymphocytes and immature polymorphonuclear leukocytes are also present in large numbers. Numerous young and mature schizonts are present. Trophozoites and gametocytes are uncommon.[64,65] Jelliffe[66] has suggested that the intensity of the infection in the placenta is related to the severity of the effect on the fetus. In general, the inflammatory response in placentas infected with *P. falciparum* is more intense than that in those infected with *P. malariae.*

Effect of Malaria on Fetal Survival and Birth Weight

Up to 40% of the world's pregnant women are exposed to malaria infection during pregnancy. In those with little or no preexisting immunity, malaria may be associated with a high risk for maternal and perinatal mortality. Fetal and perinatal loss may be as high as 60% to 70% in nonimmune women with malaria.[67] In 1941, Torpin[68] reviewed 27 cases of malaria that had occurred in pregnant women during the preceding 20 years in a city in the United States. The maternal mortality rate was 4%, and the fetal mortality rate was 60%. In 1951, in Vietnam, Hung[69] found a fetal death rate of 14% among women who had infected placentas. Many of these women had had severe attacks of malaria during the first trimester and had sustained spontaneous abortions at that time.

Low birth weight is more common when the placenta is infected by parasites than when the mother is infected but the placenta is not.[59,60,66,70,71] The mean birth weight is lower if the placenta is infected with *P. falciparum* than if it is infected with *P. malariae.* Maternal anemia and placental insufficiency probably affect the fetus. It has been postulated that heavy infiltrations of parasites, lymphocytes, and macrophages interfere with the circulation of maternal blood through the placenta and result in diminished transport of oxygen and nutrients to the fetus.[60] The transport through the placenta of antibody to malaria may also be decreased when placental inflammation is severe.[58]

Bruce-Chwatt[64] found that when the placenta was infected, infant weight at birth was an average of 145 g less than the weight of infants born to women with uninfected placentas. Similarly, Archibald[72] found infant weight at birth to be 170 g less, and Jelliffe[66,71] found it to be 263 g less in infants of women with infected placentas than in infants of women with uninfected placentas. In the studies performed by Bruce-Chwatt[64] and Jelliffe,[66,71] 20% of the infants born to mothers with infected placentas weighed 2500 g or less, whereas 10% and 11%, respectively, of those born to mothers with uninfected placentas weighed 2500 g or less. Cannon[60] found that 37% of women who had infected placentas gave birth to infants weighing 2500 g or less, compared with 12% of those who had uninfected placentas. For primiparous women, 44% of those with infected placentas and 27% of those with uninfected placentas gave birth to infants weighing 2500 g or less.[73] Infants who have parasites demonstrable in their cord blood appear to be more severely affected than those who do not have parasitemia at the time of delivery; the mean weight gain of the mothers of these infants and the head and chest circumferences of the infants at birth are lower than expected.[59] Larkin[74] studied the prevalence of *P. falciparum* infection among 63 pregnant women and their newborns in southern Zambia and found peripheral parasitemia in 63% (40 of 63) of mothers and 29% (19 of 65) of newborns. Infected newborns had a mean average birth weight 469 g lower than uninfected newborns but did not have a higher incidence of preterm delivery.

Using the method developed by Dubowitz and associates[75] for scoring gestational age, Reinhardt and colleagues[59] found no evidence that the incidence of infants who were small for gestational age was increased when the placenta was infected. This finding suggested that low birth weight resulted from prematurity of infants born to women with malaria.

Jelliffe[66] observed that because malaria influences birth weight, it has an important effect on infant survival in countries in which it is endemic. In 1925, Blacklock and Gordon[76] found that 35% of infants born to mothers with infected placentas died within the first 7 days of life, whereas only 5% of those born to mothers with uninfected placentas died during this period. In 1958, Cannon[60] found that the mortality rate among infants 7 days old or younger was 6.9% for those whose mothers' placentas were infected, compared with 3.4% for those whose mothers' placentas were uninfected.

The data suggesting that malaria has an important influence on birth weight and therefore on infant survival have been given further credence by the demonstration by MacGregor and Avery[73] that control of malaria in a region is followed by an increase in mean birth weight of infants born there. After DDT spraying on the island of Malaita in the British Solomon Islands, the mean birth weight for infants of mothers of all parities increased by 165 g. For infants of primiparous women, the mean birth weight increased by 252 g.[73] There was a concomitant decrease in the number of infants with birth weights of 2500 g or less; the incidence of births in this weight range fell by 8% for all births and by 20% for infants of primiparous women.[73]

Steketee and colleagues[77] reviewed studies between 1985 and 2000 and summarized the population attributable risk (PAR) of malaria on anemia, low birth weight, and infant mortality in malaria endemic areas. Approximately 3% to 15% of anemia, 8% to 14% of low birth weight, 8% to 36% of preterm low birth weight, 13% to 70% of intrauterine growth retardation and low birth weight, and 3% to 8% of infant mortality were attributable to malaria. Maternal anemia was associated with low birth weight, and fetal anemia was associated with increased infant mortality. It was estimated that 75,000 to 200,000 annual infant deaths are associated with malaria infection in pregnancy.[77] Malaria therefore contributes to fetal loss, stillbirth, prematurity, and neonatal death.[71,78]

Influence of Maternal Antibody on Risk of Infection

Antimalarial antibodies are transferred from the mother to the infant. The prevalence of precipitating antibody to *P. falciparum* within 24 hours of birth in Gambia was 87% in newborns and 87.5% in their mothers.[79] The prevalence of antibody in these newborns reflected the extent to which malaria had been controlled in the area in which their mothers lived. In infants born in the provinces with more malaria, 97% had antibodies to malaria, whereas 75.8% of infants born in an urban area had antibodies to malaria.

Antibodies to malaria can be detected by complement fixation, indirect hemagglutination, and indirect fluorescence. Agglutinating and precipitating antibodies are also formed.[80] Levels of precipitating antibodies and antibodies detected by indirect hemagglutination decrease from birth to 25 weeks of age.[81,82] Subsequently, as a result of postnatal acquisition of infection, endogenous antibody synthesis begins and antibody levels rise.

Bray and Anderson[58] have suggested that the amount of IgG transferred to the fetus is decreased when the placenta is heavily infested with parasites. They found that women who were pregnant during the wet season in Gambia had higher mean antibody titers to *P. falciparum* than those who were pregnant during the dry season. This pattern reflected the mothers' serologic responses to the increase in exposure to malaria during the wet season. The antibody titers of the infants born to women who were pregnant during the wet season were not higher than those of infants born to women who had been pregnant during the dry season. The infants born to women who had been pregnant during the wet season had lower mean titers of antibody to malaria at birth than infants born during other seasons. In infants 2 to 3 months old, parasitemia was found in 32% born during the wet season but in only 3% to 15% born in other seasons.

Other Factors Influencing Risk of Infection

Infants younger than 3 months have a lower than expected incidence of clinical disease, death from malaria, and parasitemia.[79,81] This has been attributed to a variety of factors, including the possibility that infants of this age are less exposed to and therefore less often bitten by mosquitoes. However, the two most important causes are probably the fact that the level of serologic immunity is high at this age and that fetal hemoglobin is present in the circulating red blood cells. Sehgal and associates[83] studied the role of humoral immunity in acquired malaria infection among newborns in Papua New Guinea. Among 104 newborns, there was a 3.8% incidence of congenital malaria and a cumulative incidence of acquired malaria of 3% at 12 weeks, 16% by 24 weeks, 24% by 36 weeks, and 38% by 48 weeks of age. Ninety-six percent of infants lost maternal antibody between 4 and 7 months, and most cases of asymptomatic malaria occurred among infants with detectable malaria antibody.

Although there were seasonal fluctuations in the overall incidence of parasitemia, Gilles[84] showed that the corrected rates were always lower for infants from birth to 2 months old than for infants 3 to 4 or 5 to 6 months old. He did not find differences in sleeping habits or in the amount of exposure to mosquitoes among infants in these age groups. In June to October, parasitemia was found in 10% of those from birth to 2 months old, 42% of those 3 to 4 months old, and 53% of those 5 to 6 months old; in May, parasitemia was found in 0% of infants from birth to 2 months old, 11% of those 3 to 4 months old, and 16% of those 5 to 6 months old. The rise in prevalence of parasitemia corresponded with a fall in the amount of fetal hemoglobin in the red blood cells.[84] The fact that cells containing fetal hemoglobin are poor hosts for the malarial parasite had been previously suggested by Allison[85,86] as one of the reasons for the selective advantage of sickle cell anemia and sickle cell trait in areas in which malaria is endemic. Although antibody is undoubtedly important in protecting newborns from malaria, Campbell and co-workers[63] and Reinhardt and associates[59] pointed out that antibody levels in infants from birth to 2 months old might be low or absent even when the mother has had parasitemia and placental infection. The presence of fetal hemoglobin in the red cells may serve as a source of protection for infants who do not derive high levels of antibody from their mothers.

Placental infection as a risk for congenital malaria was studied in 197 infants in Cameroon. Infants born to placenta-infected mothers were more likely to develop malaria than infants born to women without placental infection.[87] Rates of infant infection and parasitemia were not related to maternally derived malaria antibodies.

Congenital Malaria

Occurrence

There has been no consistently accepted definition of congenital malaria. Some have taken the position that parasites must be demonstrable in the peripheral blood of the infant during the first day of life; others have accepted cases that were confirmed within the first 7 days of life.[78] In areas in which malaria is endemic, infants are exposed to mosquitoes and may become infected by this route at a very young age. It may be difficult to distinguish congenital cases from acquired cases. However, a sufficient number of cases of congenital malaria have been reported from countries that are free of malaria, thereby eliminating the possibility of postnatal transmission, to establish the fact that the clinical onset of disease in a congenitally infected infant can be delayed for weeks and rarely even for months.[56,57,88,89] The prevalence of parasitemia in infants younger than 3 months was 0.7% among those born during the dry season in the rural part of Gambia, compared with 11.4% among those born during the wet season, which suggests that postnatal infection is a more common event than congenital malaria.[62] It is probable that IgG antibody transmitted from the mother to the infant is an important factor in determining whether parasites that reach the fetal circulation establish an infection. The presence of passively transferred antibody in the neonate may lengthen the incubation period beyond that which would be expected in the nonimmune host.

The frequency of placental infection varies according to the prevalence of malaria in the population, the vigor of measures of control, and the availability of nonprescription antimalarial drugs. However, among Nigerian women who did not receive antimalarial agents, three studies suggested that the frequency of infection of the placenta remained relatively stable over a 30-year period. In 1948 through 1950, Bruce-Chwatt[64] found that 20% of the placentas from 228 pregnancies were infected. One (0.4%) of the 235 neonates had the trophozoites of *P. falciparum* in a peripheral smear obtained on the fifth day of life. In 1958, Cannon[60] found that 26% of the placentas were infected; in 1970, Williams and McFarlane[90] found that 37% of the placentas were infected. None of the cord blood samples of the infants in these latter studies contained parasites. In 1964 through 1965 in Uganda, Jelliffe found that 16% of the 570 placentas were infected but only one (0.18%) infant was infected at birth.[66]

The studies of Kortmann,[91] Reinhardt and colleagues,[59] and Schwetz and Peel[92] suggest that parasitemia in cord blood may be more common than had been previously believed and that the presence of parasites does not necessarily indicate that the infant will become infected. Reinhardt and colleagues[59] found 33% of 198 placentas to be infected. Thick smears of the cord blood were positive for 21.7% of the 198 infants and 55% of the infants of mothers who had had parasitemia during the pregnancy. Thin smears were negative for all 198 infants. Kortmann[91] was able to demonstrate parasites in 19.7% of the placentas of 1009 women but in only 3.8% of cord blood from their infants. Eleven infants who had parasites in their cord blood also had peripheral smears performed; parasites were demonstrable in the peripheral blood of only two (18%). Lehner and associates[93] found a 14.6% incidence of cord parasitemia and a 7.7% incidence of peripheral parasitemia among 48 newborns in Papua New Guinea. Whereas all maternal and cord samples had malaria antibodies, low levels of cord malaria antibody were found to correlate with cord parasitemia. Schwetz and Peel[92] demonstrated parasites in 6% of cord blood samples and 3.6% of peripheral blood samples of infants born to mothers in Central Africa. Because the rate of infection of the placenta was 74%, this study demonstrates that the placenta, although frequently infected, serves as a relatively effective barrier and that parasites infrequently reach the fetus. The relative importance of transplacental infection or transmission by transfer from mother to infant during labor as mechanisms by which the infant acquires malaria remains uncertain.[94]

Despite massive involvement of the placenta, it is generally agreed that clinically apparent congenital infections are rare in areas in which malaria is endemic and levels of maternal immunity are high. Covell[79] reviewed cases of congenital malaria that had been reported up to 1950 and estimated the incidence at 16 (0.3%) infections per 5324 livebirths. This rate pertained to areas of the world in which malaria was endemic. For women having an overt attack of malaria during pregnancy, the rate of congenital infection was higher and was estimated to be 1% to 4%.[79] Congenital malaria is more common among infants of women who have clinical attacks of malaria during pregnancy than in those with chronic subclinical infections; however, congenital malaria may occur in infants of mothers who are asymptomatic throughout their pregnancies.[78,89,95] Often, parasitemia is not demonstrable in the mother; splenomegaly occurs frequently.[69] Congenital malaria is more common in infants of women who have immigrated to areas in which malaria is endemic than in women who have been raised to maturity in such areas because their levels of immunity are lower than those of the native population. Conversely, congenital malaria is also more common among women who immigrate from areas in which malaria is endemic to areas that are free of malaria. Loss of immunity results from lack of frequent exposure. Although rare, congenital malaria may also occur as a result of maternal infection by chloroquine-resistant *P. falciparum.* A number of reported cases of chloroquine-resistant congenital malaria in Africa and Indonesia responded to treatment with intravenous quinine.[96-98]

Clinical Presentation

Cases of congenital malaria have been identified in countries in which malaria is endemic and in countries in which it is not, including Great Britain and the United States. Most infants with congenital malaria have had the onset of the first sign or symptom when 10 to 28 days old.[56,99,102] However, onsets occurring as early as 8 hours and as late as 8 weeks of age have been reported.[78,88,89,103-106] Keitel and co-workers[57] described a case of malaria in a 15-month-old child who had been separated from her mother when 6 weeks old but who was breast-fed during this 6-week period. The infection was caused by *P. malariae.* The source of the mother's infection was probably contaminated needles and syringes used to inject heroin. The infant must have derived the infection from her mother because she had always lived in an area that was free of malaria. Hulbert[102] reviewed the 49 cases of congenital malaria reported in the United States since 1950 and found that the mean age at onset of symptoms was 5.5 weeks (range, 0 to 60 weeks) and that 96% of these children had signs or symptoms when 2 to 8 weeks old. There was no association found between age of symptom onset and *Plasmodium* species.

Most cases of congenital infection have occurred in infants of mothers who had overt attacks of malaria during pregnancy. However, Harvey and associates[89] and McQuay and colleagues[104] reported cases of congenital infection with *P. malariae* in which the mother had lived in an area that was free of malaria for 3 years or more. In these cases, it is likely that the mothers had had onset of their infection many years before their move from an endemic area.

The most common clinical findings in cases of congenital malaria are fever, anemia, and splenomegaly, which occur in more than 80% of cases.[56,107] The anemia, which may be accompanied by pallor, is associated with a reticulocytosis in about one half of the cases. Jaundice and hyperbilirubinemia are found in about one third of the cases. The direct or the indirect bilirubin level may be elevated, depending on whether liver dysfunction or hemolysis is the most important process in an individual case.[56] Hepatomegaly may occur but is less common than splenomegaly. Nonspecific findings include failure to thrive, poor feeding, regurgitation, and loose stools. In developing countries, when malaria occurs during the first few months of life, it is frequently complicated by other illness, such as pneumonia, septicemia, and diarrhea.[105]

Of the 107 cases of congenital malaria summarized by Covell,[79] 40% were caused by *P. falciparum,* 32% were caused by *P. vivax,* and 1.9% were caused by *P. malariae.* The clinical findings of congenital malaria are not distinguishable from the signs and symptoms of malaria that has been acquired by the bite of a mosquito. IgM antibody to *P. falciparum* was found in the cord blood of one infant.[103] The mother had probably had her first attack of malaria during that pregnancy and had high fever and parasitemia at delivery. Reinhardt and colleagues[59] found that the total IgM levels in the cord blood of infants of infected mothers were similar to those of infants of uninfected mothers. Although fever and parasitemia may occur within 24 hours of birth, hepatosplenomegaly and anemia at birth as a result of a chronic intrauterine infection have not been described. Normal red blood cells can cross from the maternal to the fetal circulation.[108] If parasitized cells cross, however, they must usually be destroyed by the immune defenses of the fetus and by the maternal antimalarial antibodies that have passed transplacentally.

Treatment

Chloroquine is the drug of choice for sensitive strains of *P. falciparum* and for *P. malariae.* For these infections, chloroquine phosphate should be administered orally in an initial dose of 10 mg/kg of chloroquine base (maximum, 600 mg of base), followed in 6 hours by a dose of 5 mg/kg of chloroquine base (maximum, 300 mg of base). Subsequent doses of 5 mg/kg of chloroquine base should be given 24 and 48 hours after the first dose (maximum, 300 mg of base). Parenteral therapy consists of quinidine gluconate at a dose of 10 mg/kg as a loading dose (maximum, 600 mg) in normal saline given over 1 to 2 hours and then 0.02 mg/kg per minute until oral therapy can be given. Infections with *P. vivax* may be treated with chloroquine alone because sporozoite forms are not transmitted, and there is no exoerythrocytic phase in congenital infections; administration of primaquine is unnecessary. The treatment of transfusion-acquired infections is the same as that for congenital infections because there is no exoerythrocytic phase in these infections.

In serious infections in infants of mothers who may have been exposed to chloroquine-resistant strains of *P. falciparum,* alternate therapy should be considered. In adults, combinations of quinine, pyrimethamine, and a sulfonamide or quinine and tetracycline have been used with success.[109] Intravenous quinidine in combination with exchange transfusion has been used in a severe case of maternal *P. falciparum* malaria.[110] Intravenous quinidine or the combination of quinine and trimethoprim-sulfamethoxazole has been suggested for treatment of infants with resistant *P. falciparum* infection.[96-98,111] Intravenous quinine is no longer available in the United States, but in adults, oral quinine may be useful in less severe cases of chloroquine-resistant *P. falciparum.* Mefloquine is an oral antimalarial effective against most *P. falciparum* strains. Recommended therapy for *P. falciparum* infection in areas with known chloroquine resistance is variable, depending on ability to appropriately diagnose resistant *P. falciparum,* the percentage of parasitemia, signs of organ involvement (especially of the central nervous system), and other systemic manifestations of malaria. Severe malaria may require intensive care, and exchange transfusion may be necessary if the degree of parasitemia is greater than 10%. Sequential smears should be monitored to ensure adequacy of therapy. The treatment regimen of choice is quinine sulfate given as 25 mg/kg (maximum dose, 2000 mg) in three doses for 3 to 7 days in addition to tetracycline given as 5 mg/kg four times each day for 7 days (maximum individual dose, 250 mg). The risk of dental staining in children younger than 8 years of age must be weighed against the risks of malaria-related morbidity and mortality. Pyrimethamine-sulfadoxine and mefloquine are not licensed for use in infants and pregnant women by the U.S. Food and Drug Administration; data regarding use of mefloquine during pregnancy do not indicate a risk of adverse outcomes during pregnancy. Inadvertent use of mefloquine during the first trimester of pregnancy should be reported to the Centers for Disease Control and Prevention Malaria Center (phone: 770-488-7760). Current recommendations regarding treatment can also be obtained from the Malaria Branch, Centers for Disease Control and Prevention, Atlanta, Georgia.

Prevention

Because malaria chemoprophylaxis may not be 100% effective, decreasing or eliminating exposure to mosquitoes is an important strategy for preventing malaria during pregnancy. Exposure to mosquitoes should be avoided by use of mosquito netting around beds, wire mesh screening on windows, insecticides, and mosquito repellants.

Although the possible toxicity of administering prophylactic antimalarial agents to women during pregnancy has been much discussed, controlled trials have shown that there is little risk and much to gain from such a practice. Treatment only for identified cases of maternal malaria, rather than the administration of malaria prophylaxis, failed to reduce the incidence of malaria-related low birth weight because only 12 of 65 women who had plasmodial pigmentation of the placenta had symptoms leading to an antenatal diagnosis of malaria.[112] Morley and associates[113] showed that administration of a prophylactic monthly dose of 50 mg of pyrimethamine during pregnancy resulted in improved maternal weight gain and in an increase in the mean birth weight of 157 g compared with administration of antimalarial drugs only for febrile episodes. Pyrimethamine prophylaxis is avoided in pregnant women because of concern that this dihydrofolate reductase inhibitor may cause abnormalities by interference with folic acid metabolism. Congenital defects have occurred in the offspring of animals ingesting pyrimethamine during pregnancy.[114] One possible case of pyrimethamine teratogenicity in a human fetus has been described,[115] and evidence of embryo resorption has been documented in pregnant Wistar rats given sulfadoxine-pyrimethamine.[116]

A retrospective review of 1627 reports of women exposed to mefloquine before or during pregnancy revealed a 4% prevalence of congenital malformations among infants of these women, reportedly similar to that observed in the general population.[117] A second report demonstrated a high rate of spontaneous abortions, but not congenital malformations, among 72 female U.S. soldiers who inadvertently received mefloquine during pregnancy.[118] Sufficient data do not exist to recommend the use of mefloquine in pregnant women, although its use in these women may be considered when exposure to chloroquine-resistant *P. falciparum* is unavoidable. The dose is 250 mg of the salt taken orally once each week, beginning 1 week before travel and ending 4 weeks after the last exposure. The combination of pyrimethamine and sulfadoxine for prophylaxis against chloroquine-resistant strains of *P. falciparum* is no longer recommended because the risk of Stevens-Johnson syndrome or neutropenia outweighs the potential benefit. Prophylaxis with chloroquine and proguanil is an alternative if a pregnant woman from a nonendemic area must risk exposure to resistant *P. falciparum*.[119]

Chloroquine alone also has been used as prophylaxis during pregnancy and has been shown to be of benefit.[61] Gilles[61] found that parasitemia developed in more than 75% of pregnant women who received no prophylactic drug or who received folic acid but no antimalarial drugs. Sixty-three percent of these women developed anemia at 16 to 24 weeks' gestation. In contrast, only 2 (17%) of 12 pregnant women who received a dose of 600 mg of chloroquine base followed by a weekly dose of 25 mg of pyrimethamine developed parasitemia, and only one developed anemia. Although anemia may be an important cause of low birth weight, as Harrison and Ibeziako maintained,[120] malaria appears to be an important cause of anemia in pregnant women.[120,121]

Chloroquine and the other 4-aminoquinolines such as amodiaquine and hydroxychloroquine have similar activities and toxicities. The safety of administering chloroquine during pregnancy has been questioned. The usual recommendation for prophylaxis is 300 mg of chloroquine base once each week. Hart and Naunton[122] attributed the abnormal outcome of four pregnancies in a single patient to the administration of chloroquine during the pregnancies. This patient, who had systemic lupus erythematosus (SLE), took 150 to 300 mg chloroquine base daily. Two of the children who had had intrauterine exposures to chloroquine had severe cochleovestibular paresis and posterior column defects. Another had a Wilms' tumor and hemihypertrophy. The fourth pregnancy ended in a spontaneous abortion at 12 weeks' gestation. As pointed out by Jelliffe[123] and Clyde,[124] the dose given to this pregnant patient was three to seven times higher than the dose recommended for prophylaxis against malaria. Two other studies reported pregnancy outcomes after exposure to antimalarials. Parke[125] described 14 pregnancies among eight patients with SLE who took chloroquine or hydroxychloroquine during pregnancy. Three pregnancies ended in spontaneous abortion or neonatal death during periods of increased SLE activity; of the remaining 11 pregnancies, 6 were normal full-term deliveries, 1 ended in stillbirth, and 4 ended in spontaneous abortion. No congenital deformities occurred. Levy and co-workers[126] reviewed the cases of 24 women who took chloroquine or hydroxychloroquine during a total of 27 pregnancies. Eleven women had SLE, three had rheumatoid arthritis, and four were taking malaria prophylaxis. There were 14 normal deliveries, 6 abortions attributed to severe underlying disease or social conditions, 3 stillbirths, and 4 spontaneous abortions. No congenital abnormalities were identified. The risk of poor outcome was higher among women with connective tissue disease, for which chloroquine and hydroxychloroquine doses are much higher than for malaria prophylaxis. Despite widespread use of weekly doses of chloroquine in pregnant women, teratogenic effects have not been confirmed in controlled trials.[127]

The consequences of an attack of malaria during pregnancy are serious. Hindi and Azimi[88] described a woman who became pregnant while living in Nigeria but who stopped taking prophylactic doses of pyrimethamine at the onset of pregnancy. At 6 months' gestation, she had a febrile illness and was treated with chloroquine for 2 weeks. At 8 months' gestation, she had a second attack of malaria and was delivered of an infant who was 4 weeks premature and small for gestational age. The infant developed malaria during the first few weeks of life and was treated with chloroquine. The total exposure of this infant to chloroquine would have been less if the mother had been taking it weekly in prophylactic doses.

Women living in or returning from areas in which malaria is endemic should continue to take prophylactic antimalarial agents. Although primaquine is not known to have teratogenic effects, experience with its use during pregnancy is limited; it is therefore recommended that treatment with primaquine to eradicate the exoerythrocytic phase in *P. vivax* infections be deferred until after delivery.[114,128]

Some investigators think the widespread use of prophylaxis may lower the level of maternal immunity and increase the severity of cases of malaria seen in children who are younger than 1 year. There is no evidence that administration of antimalarial drugs prophylactically to pregnant women has changed the expected incidence of infection during the first few months of life.

Because of the tremendous global burden of disease imposed by malaria infections, a key initiative in the prevention of malaria is the emphasis on development of malaria vaccines. The cloning of the *P. falciparum* receptor protein, which allows red blood cell attachment, should facilitate the development of a malarial vaccine.[129,130] Vaccine candidates are in development, but no effective vaccine will be immediately available.[131-133] Other techniques for malaria prevention include use of improved chemoprophylactic regimens and development of animal models for malaria infection in which to test vaccines and antimalarial drugs. A rhesus monkey model mimicking human infection after exposure to *Plasmodium coatneyi* has been tested with potential for use in animal studies.[134] Recommendations for malaria prophylaxis in pregnant women may be obtained from the Malaria Branch, Centers for Disease Control and Prevention, Atlanta, Georgia.

SCHISTOSOMIASIS

Schistosomiasis (i.e., bilharziasis) contributes to infertility by causing sclerosis of the fallopian tubes or cervix.[135] It is estimated that 9 to 13 million women may be afflicted by genital schistosomiasis in Africa alone.[136] The placenta usually does not become infected until the third month of pregnancy or thereafter.[137] Although the frequency of placental infection is as high as 25% in endemic areas, the infestations are light and cause little histologic reaction.[137,138] In their study of the impact of placental infection on the outcome of pregnancy, Renaud and co-workers[137] concluded that there was little evidence that the size or weight of the infant was affected and that placental bilharziasis was not an important cause of intrauterine growth retardation or prematurity.

TRICHOMONAS VAGINALIS

Infection of the vagina of the pregnant woman with *Trichomonas vaginalis* is not uncommon, but no adverse effect on the fetus has been documented.[139,140] *T. vaginalis* was recovered from the tracheal secretions of three infants with respiratory illness whose viral and bacterial cultures revealed no other pathogens, but a causal relationship was not certain.[141,142] During the first 2 weeks of life, female newborns may be particularly susceptible to infection because of the influence of maternal estrogens on the vaginal epithelium. By 3 to 6 weeks of age, the vaginal pH is no longer acid.[143] *T. vaginalis* has been found in 0% to 4.8% of sequentially studied female newborns.[143-145] Among infants younger than 3 weeks who had vaginal discharges, *T. vaginalis* was the probable cause of the discharge in 17.2%.[146] In addition to causing a vaginal discharge,[147] infection of the newborn with *T. vaginalis* may aggravate candidal infections and may be associated with urinary tract infections.[143] In most infants, the white blood cells found in the urine originate from the vagina rather than from the bladder.[148] However, several reports suggest that a bacterial urinary tract infection can be present concomitantly.[149,150] In symptomatic cases, metronidazole has been used at a dosage of 500 mg twice daily or 15 mg/kg/day divided in 3 doses for 5 to 7 days.[143,148,151]

TRICHINOSIS

Prenatal transmission of trichinosis from mother to infant is rare. Four larvae, however, were found in the diaphragm of a fetus by Kuitunen-Ekbaum.[152] No evidence of infection with trichinosis was found in 25 newborns studied by McNaught and Anderson.[153] Despite this, *Trichinella spiralis* has been found in the placenta, in the milk of nursing women, and in the tissue from the mammary gland.[154] In 1939, Hood and Olson[155] found *T. spiralis* in pressed muscle preparations from 4 (8.3%) of 48 infants from birth to 12 months of age. Although transplacental transmission is rare, *T. spiralis* is present in the placenta of women with acute trichinosis and can be passed to the infant by means of breast milk.

BABESIOSIS

Babesia microti is a tick-borne protozoan that infects erythrocytes and causes a malaria-like illness. Most cases in the United States have occurred in the Northeast. Raucher and colleagues[156] described a *B. microti* infection in a pregnant woman that began in the 19th week of gestation; the infant was born at term without evidence of infection.

PNEUMOCYSTIS JIROVECI

P. jiroveci is an infectious agent with a history. In 1988, DNA analysis demonstrated that *Pneumocystis* was not a protozoan, but a fungus.[159,160] Subsequent DNA analysis has led to the change in nomenclature of *P. carinii* to *P. jiroveci*, a name chosen in honor of the parasitologist Otto Jirovec, who is credited by some with the original description of this organism.[159,160] *P. carinii* as a fungus has been defined based on molecular analysis.[161,162] Previous controversy over the classification *Pneumocystis* existed because of the difficulty in cultivating and further characterizing the biochemical nature of the organism. Questions remained until polymerase chain reaction techniques established that *P. jiroveci* was not found in lung samples from any other mammals.[163] However, genetic analysis clearly demonstrated differences between human and nonhuman *Pneumocystis* isolates.[164]

REFERENCES

Introduction and *Ascaris*

1. Kotcher E, Mata LJ, Esquivel R, et al. Acquisition of intestinal parasites in newborn infants. Fed Proc 24:442, 1965 (abstract).
2. Agbere AD, Atakouma DY, Balaka B, et al. Gastrointestinal and urinary parasitic infection in children at a regional hospital center in Togo: some epidemiological aspects. Med Trop 55:65, 1995.
3. Stringer JR, Beard CB, Miller RF, Wakefield AE. A new name (*Pneumocystis jiroveci*) for *Pneumocystis* from humans. Emerg Infect Dis 8:891, 2002.
4. Sterling R, Guay AJL. Invasion of the female generative tract by *Ascaris lumbricoides*. JAMA 107:2046, 1936.
5. Sanjeevi CB, Vivekanandan S, Narayanan PR. Fetal response to maternal ascariasis as evidenced by anti-*Ascaris lumbricoides* IgM antibodies in the cord blood. Acta Paediatr Scand 80:1134, 1991.
6. Chu W, Chen P, Huang C, et al. Neonatal ascariasis. J Pediatr 81:783, 1972.
7. Costa-Macedo LM, Rey L. *Ascaris lumbricoides* in neonate: evidence of congenital transmission of intestinal nematodes. Rev Soc Bras Med Trop 33:371, 1991.

Giardiasis

8. Roberts NS, Copel JA, Bhutani V, et al. Intestinal parasites and other infections during pregnancy in Southeast Asian refugees. J Reprod Med 30:720, 1985.
9. Kreutner AK, Del Bene VE, Amstey MS. Giardiasis in pregnancy. Am J Obstet Gynecol 140:895, 1981.
10. Tellez A, Winiecka-Krusnell J, Paniagua M, Linder E. Antibodies in mother's milk protect children against giardiasis. Scand J Infect Dis 35:322, 2003.

American Trypanosomiasis: Chagas' Disease

11. Edgcomb JH, Johnson CM. American trypanosomiasis (Chagas' disease). *In* Binford CH, Connor OH (eds). Pathology of Tropical and Extraordinary Disease, vol. 1. Washington, DC, Armed Forces Institute of Pathology, 1976, pp 244-251.
12. Bittencourt AL. Congenital Chagas' disease. Am J Dis Child 130:97, 1976.
13. Miles MA. The epidemiology of South American trypanosomiasis—biochemical and immunological approaches and their relevance to control. Trans R Soc Trop Med Hyg 77:5, 1983.
14. Marsden PD. South American trypanosomiasis (Chagas' disease). Int Rev Trop Med 4:97, 1981.
15. Santos-Buch CA. American trypanosomiasis: Chagas' disease. Int Rev Exp Pathol 19:63, 1979.
16. Amato Neto V, Doles J, Russi A, et al. Rev Inst Med Trop Sao Paulo 10:46, 1968.
17. Bittencourt AL, Mota E. Isoenzyme characterization of *Trypanosoma cruzi* from congenital cases of Chagas' disease. Ann Trop Med Parasitol 4:393, 1985.
18. Bittencourt AL, Sadigursky M, Barbosa HA. Doenca de Chagas congenita: estudo de 29 caspiatos. Rev Inst Med Trop Sao Paulo 17: 146, 1975.
19. Rassi A, Borges C, Koeberle F, et al. Sobre a transmissão congenita da doenca de Chagas. Rev Goiana Med 4:319, 1958.
20. Delgado MA, Santos Buch CA. Transplacental transmission and fetal parasitosis of *Trypanosoma cruzi* in outbred white Swiss mice. Am J Trop Med Hyg 27:1108, 1978.
21. Cossio PM, Diez C, Szarfman A, et al. Chagasic cardiopathy: demonstration of a serum gamma globulin factor which reacts with endocardium and vascular structures. Circulation 49:13, 1974.
22. Cossio PM, Laguens RP, Diez C, et al. Antibodies reacting with plasma membrane of striated muscle and endothelial cells. Circulation 50:1252, 1974.
23. Szarfman A, Cossio PM, Arana RM, et al. Immunologic and immunopathologic studies in congenital Chagas' disease. Clin Immunol Immunopathol 4:489, 1975.
24. Vasquez AD. [Doctoral thesis]. Venezuela, Universidad del los Andes, 1959.
25. Saleme A, Yanicelli GL, Inigo LA, et al. Enfermedad de Chagas-Mazza congenita en Tucuman. Arch Argent Pediatr 59:162, 1971.
26. Bittencourt AL, Mota E, Filho RR, et al. Incidence of congenital Chagas' disease in Bahaia, Brazil. J Trop Pediatr 31:242, 1985.
27. Bekemans J, Truyens C, Torrico F, et al. Maternal *Trypanosoma cruzi* infection upregulated capacity of uninfected neonate cells to produce pro- and anti-inflammatory cytokines. Infect Immun 68:5430, 2000.
28. Barousse AP, Eposto MO, Mandel S, et al. Enfermedad de Chagas congenita en area no endemica. Medicina (B Aires) 38:611, 1978.
29. Blanco SB, Segura EL, Gurtler RE. Control of congenital transmission of *Trypanosoma cruzi* in Argentina. Medicina (B Aires) 59(Suppl 2): 138, 1999.
30. Stagno S, Hurtado R. Enfermedad de Chagas congenita: studio immunologico y diagnostico mediante immunofluorescencia con anti IgM. Bol Chil Parasitol 26:20, 1971.
31. Bittencourt AL, Barbosa HS, Santos I, et al. Incidencia da transmissão congenita da doenca de Chagas em partos a termo. Rev Inst Med Trop Sao Paulo 16:197, 1974.
32. Rubio M, Howard BJ. Enfermedad de Chagas congenita. II. Halazgo anatomopatologico en 9 casos. Bol Chil Parasitol 23:113, 1968.
33. Azogue E, LaFuente C, Darras C. Congenital Chagas' disease in Bolivia: epidemiological aspects and pathological findings. Trans R Soc Trop Med Hyg 79:176, 1985.
34. Howard JE. La enfermedad de Chagas congenita [thesis]. Santiago, Universidad de Chile, 1962.
35. Bittencourt AL, Vieira GO, Tavares HC, et al. Esophageal involvement in congenital Chagas' disease. Am J Trop Med Hyg 33:30, 1984.
36. Bittencourt AL, Rodriguez de Freitas LA, De Araujo Galvao MO, et al. Pneumonitis in congenital Chagas' disease: a study of ten cases. Am J Trop Med Hyg 30:38, 1981.
37. Hoff R, Mott KE, Milanesi ML, et al. Congenital Chagas' disease in an urban population: investigation of infected twins. Trans R Soc Trop Med Hyg 72:247, 1978.
38. Feilij H, Muller L, Gonzalez Cappa SM. Direct micromethod for diagnosis of acute and congenital Chagas' disease. J Clin Microbiol 18:327, 1983.
39. Reyes MB, Lorca M, Munoz P, Frasch ACC. Fetal IgG specificities against *Trypanosoma cruzi* antigens in infected newborns. Proc Natl Acad Sci U S A 87:2846, 1990.
40. Blanco SB, Segura EL, Cura EN, et al. Congenital transmission of *Trypanosoma cruzi*: an operational outline for detecting and treating infected infants in north-western Argentina. Trop Med Int Health 5:293, 2000.
41. Bittencourt AL, Gomes MC. Gestacoes sucessivas de uma paciente chagasica com ocorrencia de casos de transmissao congenital da doenca. Gaz Med Bahia 67:166, 1967.
42. Moya PR, Paollaso RD, Blanco S et al. Tratamiento de la enfermedad de Chagas con Nifurtimox durante los primeros meses de vida. Medicina (B Aires) 45; 553, 1985.

African Trypanosomiasis: African Sleeping Sickness

43. Lingam S, Marshall WC, Wilson J, et al. Congenital trypanosomiasis in a child born in London. Dev Med Child Neurol 27:664, 1985.
44. Reinhardt MC, Macleod CL. Parasitic Infections in Pregnancy and the Newborn. New York, Oxford University Press, 1988.

Entamoeba histolytica

45. Armon PJ. Amoebiasis in pregnancy and the puerperium. Br J Obstet Gynaecol 85:264, 1978.
46. Abioye AA. Fatal amoebic colitis in pregnancy and puerperium: a new clinico-pathological entity. J Trop Med Hyg 76:97, 1973.
47. Czeizel E, Hancsok M, Palkowich I, et al. Possible relation between fetal death and *E. histolytica* infection of the mother. Am J Obstet Gynecol 96:264, 1966.
48. Dykes AC, Ruebush TK II, Gorelkin L, et al. Extraintestinal amebiasis in infancy: report of three patients and epidemiologic investigations of their families. Pediatrics 65:799, 1980.
49. Botman T, Ruys PJ. Amoebic appendicitis in a newborn infant. Trop Geogr Med 15:221, 1963.
50. Axton JHM. Amoebic proctocolitis and liver abscess in a neonate. S Afr Med J 46:258, 1972.
51. Dreyfuss ML, Msamanga GI, Spiegelman D, et al. Determinants of low birth weight among HIV-infected pregnant women in Tanzania. Am J Clin Nutr 74: 814, 2001.

Malaria

52. Young MD. Malaria. *In* Hunter GW III, Swartzwelder JC, Clyde DF (eds). Tropical Medicine. Philadelphia, WB Saunders, 1976, pp 353-396.
53. Shulman IA, Saxena S, Nelson JM, et al. Neonatal exchange transfusions complicated by transfusion-induced malaria. Pediatrics 73: 330, 1984.
54. Piccoli DA, Perlman S, Ephros M. Transfusion-acquired *Plasmodium malariae* infection in two premature infants. Pediatrics 72:560, 1983.

55. Sinclair S, Mittal SK, Singh M. Neonatal transfusion malaria. Indian Pediatr 8:219, 1971.
56. Ghosh S, Patwari A, Mohan M, et al. Clinical and hematologic peculiarities of malaria in infancy. Clin Pediatr (Phila) 17:369, 1978.
57. Keitel HG, Goodman HC, Havel RJ, et al. Nephrotic syndrome in congenital quartan malaria. JAMA 161:521, 1956.
58. Bray RS, Anderson MJ. Falciparum malaria and pregnancy. Trans R Soc Trop Med Hyg 73:427, 1979.
59. Reinhardt MC, Ambroise-Thomas P, Cavallo-Serra R, et al. Malaria at delivery in Abidjan. Helv Paediatr Acta 33(Suppl 41):65, 1978.
60. Cannon DSH. Malaria and prematurity in the western region of Nigeria. Br Med J 2:877, 1958.
61. Gilles HM, Lawson JB, Sibelas M, et al. Malaria, anaemia and pregnancy. Ann Trop Med Parasitol 63:245, 1969.
62. McGregor I. Epidemiology, malaria and pregnancy. Am J Trop Med Hyg 33:517, 1984.
63. Campbell CC, Martinez JM, Collins WE. Seroepidemiological studies of malaria in pregnant women and newborns from coastal El Salvador. Am J Trop Med Hyg 29:151, 1980.
64. Bruce-Chwatt LJ. Malaria in African infants and children in southern Nigeria. Ann Trop Med Parasitol 46:173, 1952.
65. Taufa T. Malaria and pregnancy. P N G Med J 21:197, 1978.
66. Jelliffe EFP. Low birth-weight and malarial infection of the placenta. Bull World Health Organ 38:69, 1968.
67. Shulman CE, Dorman EK. Importance and prevention of malaria in pregnancy. Trans R Soc Trop Med Hyg 97:30, 2003.
68. Torpin R. Malaria complicating pregnancy with a report of 27 cases. Am J Obstet Gynecol 41:882, 1941.
69. Hung LV. Paludisive at grossesse a Saigon. Rev Palud Med Trop 83:75, 1951.
70. Spita AJ. Malaria infection of the placenta and its influence on the incidence of prematurity in eastern Nigeria. Bull World Health Organ 21:242, 1959.
71. Jelliffe EFP. Placental malaria and foetal growth. *In* Nutrition and Infection: CIBA Foundation Study Group No. 31. xxx, J&A Churchill, 1967, pp 18-40.
72. Archibald HM. The influence of malarial infection of the placenta on the incidence of prematurity. Bull World Health Organ 15:842, 1956.
73. MacGregor JD, Avery JG. Malaria transmission and fetal growth. BMJ 3:433, 1974.
74. Larkin GL, Thuma PE. Congenital malaria in a hyperendemic area. Am J Trop Med Hyg 45:587, 1991.
75. Dubowitz LMS, Dubowitz V, Goldberg G. Clinical assessment of gestational age in the newborn infant. J Pediatr 77:1, 1970.
76. Blacklock DB, Gordon RM. Malaria parasites in the placental blood. Ann Trop Med Parasitol 19:37, 1925.
77. Steketee RW, Nahlen BL, Parise ME, Menendez C. The burden of malaria in pregnancy in malaria-endemic areas. Am J Trop Med Hyg 64(Suppl):28, 2001.
78. Menon R. Pregnancy and malaria. Med J Malaysia 27:115, 1972.
79. Covell G. Congenital malaria. Trop Dis Bull 47:1147, 1950.
80. McGregor IA. Immunity to plasmodial infections; consideration of factors relevant to malaria in man. Int Rev Trop Med 4:1, 1971.
81. Molineaux L, Cornille-Brogger R, Mathews HM, et al. Longitudinal serological study of malaria in infants in the West African savanna. Bull World Health Organ 56:573, 1978.
82. Mathews HM, Lobel HO, Breman JG. Malarial antibodies measured by the indirect hemagglutination test in West African children. Am J Trop Med Hyg 25:217, 1976.
83. Sehgal VM, Siddiqui WA, Alpers MP. A seroepidemiological study to evaluate the role of passive maternal immunity to malaria in infants. Trans R Soc Trop Med Hyg 83(Suppl):105, 1989.
84. Gilles HM. The development of malarial infection in breast-fed Gambian infants. Ann Trop Med Parasitol 51:58, 1957.
85. Allison AC. Genetic factors in resistance to malaria. Ann N Y Acad Sci 91:710, 1961.
86. Allison AC. Malaria in carriers of the sickle cell trait and in newborn children. Exp Parasitol 6:418, 1957.
87. Le Hesran JY, Cot M, Personne P, et al. Maternal placental infection with *Plasmodium falciparum* and malaria morbidity during the first two years of life. Am J Epidemiol 146:826, 1997.
88. Hindi RD, Azimi PH. Congenital malaria due to *Plasmodium falciparum*. Pediatrics 66:977, 1980.
89. Harvey B, Remington JS, Sulzer AJ. IgM malaria antibodies in a case of congenital malaria in the United States. Lancet 1:333, 1969.
90. Williams AIO, McFarlane H. Immunoglobulin levels, malarial antibody titres and placental parasitaemia in Nigerian mothers and neonates. Afr J Med Sci 1:369, 1970.
91. Kortmann HF. Malaria and pregnancy [thesis]. Utrecht, Manuel Drukkrig Elinkwijk, 1972.
92. Schwetz J, Peel M. Congenital malaria and placental infections amongst the Negroes of Central Africa. Trans R Soc Trop Med Hyg 28:167, 1934.
93. Lehner PJ, Andrews CJ. Congenital malaria in Papua New Guinea. Trans R Soc Trop Med Hyg 82:822, 1988.
94. Wyler DJ. Malaria resurgence, resistance and research. N Engl J Med 308:934, 1983.
95. Davies HD, Keystone J, Lester ML, Gold R. Congenital malaria in infants of asymptomatic women. Can Med Assoc J 146:1755, 1992.
96. Dianto, Rampengan TH. Congenital falciparum malaria with chloroquine resistance type II. Paediatr Indones 29:237, 1989.
97. Chabasse D, De Gentile L, Ligny C, et al. Chloroquine-resistant *Plasmodium falciparum* in Mali revealed by congenital malaria. Trans R Soc Trop Med Hyg 82:547, 1988.
98. Airede AI. Congenital malaria with chloroquine resistance. Ann Trop Paediatr 11:267, 1991.
99. Congenital malaria infection in an infant born to a Kampuchean refugee. MMWR Morb Mortal Wkly Rep 29:3, 1980.
100. Congenital malaria in children of refugees—Washington, Massachusetts, Kentucky. MMWR Morb Mortal Wkly Rep 30:53, 1981.
101. Woods WG, Mills E, Ferrieri P. Neonatal malaria due to *Plasmodium vivax*. J Pediatr 85:669, 1974.
102. Hulbert TV. Congenital malaria in the United States: report of a case and review. Clin Infect Dis 14:922, 1992.
103. Thomas V, Wing Chit C. A case of congenital malaria in Malaysia with IgM malaria antibodies. Trans R Soc Trop Med Hyg 74:73, 1980.
104. McQuay RM, Silberman S, Mudrik P, et al. Congenital malaria in Chicago: a case report and a review of published reports (U.S.A.). Am J Trop Med 16:258, 1967.
105. Dhatt PS, Singh H, Singhal SC, et al. A clinicopathological study of malaria in early infancy. Indian Pediatr 26:331, 1979.
106. Olowu WA, Torimiro SE. Congenital malaria in 8 hours old newborn: case report. Niger J Med 11:81, 2002.
107. Subramanian D, Moise KJ, White AC. Imported malaria in pregnancy: report of four cases and review of management. Clin Infect Dis 15:408, 1992.
108. Zarou DM, Lichtman HC, Hellman LM. The transmission of chromium 51 tagged maternal erythrocytes from mother to fetus. Am J Obstet Gynecol 88:565, 1964.
109. Miller LH. Malaria. *In* Hoeprich PD (ed). Infectious Diseases: A Modern Treatise of Infectious Processes, 2nd ed. Hagerstown, Md, Harper & Row, 1977, pp 1075-1087.
110. Wong RD, Murthy ARK, Mathiesen GE, et al. Treatment of severe falciparum malaria during pregnancy with quinidine and exchange transfusion. Am J Med 92:561, 1992.
111. Quinn TC, Jacobs RF, Mertz GJ, et al. Congenital malaria: a report of four cases and a review. J Pediatr 101:229, 1982.
112. Watkinson M, Rushton DI. Plasmodial pigmentation of placenta and outcome of pregnancy in West African mothers. Br Med J 287:251, 1983.
113. Morley D, Woodland M, Cuthbertson WFJ. Controlled trial of pyrimethamine in pregnant women in an African village. BMJ 1:667, 1964.
114. Chemoprophylaxis of malaria. MMWR Morb Mortal Wkly Rep 27(Suppl):81, 1978.
115. Harpy JP, Darbois Y, Lefebvre G. Teratogenicity of pyrimethamine. Lancet 2:399, 1983.
116. Uche-Nwachi EO. Effect of intramuscular sulfadoxine-pyrimethamine on pregnant Wistar rats. Anat Rec 250:426, 1998.
117. Vanhauwere B, Maradi H, Kerr L. Post-marketing surveillance of prophylactic mefloquine (Lariam) use in pregnancy. Am J Trop Med Hyg 58:17-21, 1998.
118. Smoak BL, Writer JV, Keep LW, et al. The effects of inadvertent exposure of mefloquine chemoprophylaxis on pregnancy outcomes and infants of US Army servicewomen. J Infect Dis 176:831, 1997.
119. Ellis CJ. Antiparasitic agents in pregnancy. Clin Obstet Gynecol 13: 269, 1986.
120. Harrison KA, Ibeziako PA. Maternal anaemia and fetal birthweight. J Obstet Gynaecol Br Commonw 80:798, 1973.
121. Schofield FD, Parkinson AD, Kelly A. Changes in hemoglobin values and hepatosplenomegaly produced by control of holoendemic malaria. BMJ 1:587, 1964.

122. Hart CW, Naunton RF. The ototoxicity of chloroquine phosphate. Arch Otolaryngol 80:407, 1964.
123. Jelliffe EFP. Letter to the editor. J Pediatr 88:362, 1976.
124. Clyde DF. Letter to the editor. J Pediatr 88:362, 1976.
125. Parke A. Antimalarial drugs and pregnancy. Am J Med 85(Suppl 4A): 30, 1988.
126. Levy M, Buskila D, Gladman DD, et al. Pregnancy outcome following first trimester exposure to chloroquine. Am J Perinatol 8:174, 1991.
127. Wolfe MS, Cordero JF. Safety of chloroquine in chemosuppression of malaria during pregnancy. Br Med J 290:1466, 1985.
128. Katz M. Treatment of protozoan infections: malaria. Pediatr Infect Dis 2:475, 1983.
129. Dame JB, Williams JL, McCutchan TF, et al. Structure of the gene and coding the immunodominant surface antigen of the sporozoite of the human malarial parasite. Science 225:593, 1984.
130. Enea V, Ellis J, Zavala F, et al. DNA cloning of *Plasmodium falciparum* circumsporozoite gene: amino acid sequence of repetitive epitope. Science 225:628, 1984.
131. Soares IS, Rodrigues MM. Malaria vaccine: roadblocks and possible solutions. Braz J Med Biol Res 31:317, 1998.
132. Graves PM. Comparison of the cost-effectiveness of vaccines and insecticide impregnation of mosquito nets for the prevention of malaria. Ann Trop Med Parasitol 92:399, 1996.
133. Moorthy VS, Good MF, Hill AV. Malaria vaccine developments. Lancet 363:150, 2004.
134. Davison BB, Cogswell FB, Baskin GB, et al. *Plasmodium coatneyi* in the rhesus monkey (*Macaca mulatta*) as a model of malaria in pregnancy. Am J Trop Med Hyg 59:189, 1998.

Schistosomiasis

135. Bullough CHW. Infertility and bilharziasis of the female genital tract. Br J Obstet Gynaecol 83:819, 1976.
136. Poggensee G, Kiwelu I, Saria M, et al. Schistosomiasis of the lower reproductive tract without egg excretion in urine. Am J Trop Med Hyg 59:782, 1998.
137. Renaud R, Brettes P, Castanier C, et al. Placental bilharziasis. Int J Gynaecol Obstet 10:25, 1972.
138. Bittencourt AL, de Almeida MAC, Iunes MAF, et al. Placental involvement in *Schistosomiasis mansoni.* Am J Trop Med Hyg 29:571, 1980.

Trichomonas vaginalis

139. Ross SM, Van Middelkoop A. *Trichomonas* infection in pregnancy—does it affect perinatal outcome? S Afr Med J 63:566, 1983.
140. Franjola RT, Anazco RR, Puente RP, et al. *Trichomonas vaginalis* en embarazadas y en recien nacidos. Rev Med Chile 117:142, 1989.
141. McLaren LC, Davis LE, Healy GR, et al. Isolation of *Trichomonas vaginalis* from the respiratory tract of infants with respiratory disease. Pediatrics 71:888, 1983.
142. Hiemstra I, Van Bel F, Berger HM. Can *Trichomonas vaginalis* cause pneumonia in newborn babies? Br Med J 289:355, 1984.
143. Al-Salihi FL, Curran JP, Wang JS. Neonatal *Trichomonas vaginalis*: report of three cases and review of the literature. Pediatrics 53:196, 1974.
144. Feo LG. The incidence of *Trichomonas vaginalis* in the various age groups. Am J Trop Med 5:786, 1956.
145. Trussell RE, Wilson ME, Longwell FH, et al. Vaginal trichomoniasis: complement fixation, puerperal morbidity and early infection of newborn infants. Am J Obstet Gynecol 44:292, 1942.
146. Komorowska A, Kurnatowska A, Liniecka J. Occurrence of *Trichomonas vaginalis* (Donne) in girls in relation to hygiene conditions. Wiad Parazytol 8:247, 1962.
147. Danesh IS, Stephen JM, Gorbach J. Neonatal *Trichomonas vaginalis* infection. J Emerg Med 13:1, 1995.
148. Littlewood JM, Kohler HG. Urinary tract infection by *Trichomonas vaginalis* in a newborn baby. Arch Dis Child 41:693, 1966.
149. Postlethwaite RJ. *Trichomonas* vaginitis and *Escherichia coli* urinary infection in a newborn infant. Clin Pediatr (Phila) 14:866, 1975.
150. Dagenais-Perusse P, Baril E, Ouadahi S, et al. Vaginite á trichomonas du nourrison. Un Med Can 93:1228, 1964.
151. Crowther IA. *Trichomonas* vaginitis in infancy. Lancet 1:1074, 1962.

Trichinosis

152. Kuitunen-Ekbaum E. The incidence of trichinosis in humans in Toronto: findings in 420 autopsies. Can Public Health J 32:569, 1941.
153. McNaught JB, Anderson EV. The incidence of trichinosis in San Francisco. JAMA 107:1446, 1936.
154. Salzer BF. A study of an epidemic of 14 cases of trichinosis with cures by serum therapy. JAMA 67:579, 1916.
155. Hood M, Olson SW. Trichinosis in the Chicago area. Am J Hyg 29:51, 1939.

Babesiosis

156. Raucher HS, Jaffin H, Glass JL. Babesiosis in pregnancy. Obstet Gynecol 63:75, 1984.

Pneumocystis jiroveci

157. Stringer SL, Stringer JR, Blaser MA, et al. *Pneumocystis carinii*: sequence from ribosomal RNA implies a close relationship with fungi. Exp Parasitol 68:450, 1989.
158. Frenkel JK. *Pneumocystis* pneumonia, an immunodeficiency-dependent disease (IDD): a critical historical overview. J Eukaryot Microbiol 46:89S, 1999.
159. Hughes WT. *Pneumocystis carinii* vs. *Pneumocystis jiroveci*: another misnomer (response to Stringer et al.). Emerg Infect Dis 9:276, 2003.
160. Wakefield AE, Banerji S, Pixley FJ, Hopkin JM. Molecular probes for the detection of *Pneumocystis carinii.* Trans R Soc Trop Med Hyg 84(Suppl)1:17, 1990.
161. Li J, Edlind T. Phylogeny of *Pneumocystis carinii* based on β-tubulin sequence. J Eukaryotic Microbiol 41:97S, 1994.
162. Mazars E, Odberg-Ferragut C, Dei-Cas E, et al. Polymorphism of the thymidylate synthase gene of *Pneumocystis carinii* from different host species. J Eukaryot Microbiol 42:26, 1995.
163. Ma L, Kovacs JA. Expression and characterization of recombinant human-derived *Pneumocystis carinii* dihydrofolate reductase. Antimicrob Agents Chemother 44:3092, 2000.
164. Banerji S, Lugli EB, Miller RF, Wakefield AE. Analysis of genetic diversity at the arom locus in isolates of *Pneumocystis carinii.* J Eukaryot Microbiol 42:675, 1995.

Chapter 33

CANDIDIASIS

Catherine M. Bendel

Candida species have become increasingly important pathogens in the neonates. Over the past 2 decades, there has been a significant increase in the incidence of systemic candidiasis in neonatal intensive care (NICU) patients, particularly among the very low birth weight (VLBW; birth weight ≤1500 g) infants.[1-5] Infections range from superficial colonization to widely disseminated, life-threatening disease. Unfortunately, the incidence of invasive or systemic candidiasis has had the most dramatic increase. With improvements in technology, more aggressive approaches to the treatment of VLBW infants have become the standard of care.[4,6,7] Concomitantly, there has been an increase in risk factors for neonates to develop candidemia, most notably the prolonged use of indwelling intravascular catheters and multiple courses of broad-spectrum antimicrobial agents.

Candida albicans remains the most frequently isolated yeast species among infected neonates; however, the incidence of infection with other species, particularly *Candida parapsilosis* and *Candida glabrata*, has increased exponentially over the past 10 years.[6,8,9] The importance of *Candida* as a pathogen is reflected in this fragile group of immunocompromised patients who have a mortality rate approaching 30%, even among neonates receiving appropriate antifungal therapy. There also is a significant degree of accompanying morbidity among survivors.[5,10]

EPIDEMIOLOGY AND TRANSMISSION

Candida species infections are diseases afflicting immunocompromised hosts, diabetics, trauma patients, postoperative patients (particularly after gastrointestinal procedures), and neonates.[1,11,12] Most *Candida* infections in these patients are nosocomially acquired. The National Nosocomial Infection Surveillance (NNIS) system reports *Candida* species as the sixth most common nosocomial pathogen overall and the fourth most common single blood culture isolate, with an incidence varying from 7% to 12% among NNIS hospitals.[13,14] *C. albicans* is the most common single pathogen isolated from the urine of infected patients.[14] In neonates, the numbers are equally striking. Approximately 2.4% of early-onset neonatal infections result from *Candida* species, but 10% to 12% of all late-onset or nosocomially acquired infections are caused by *Candida* species, second only to coagulase-negative staphylococci as a single causative organism.[5,15,16] In most NICUs, *Candida* species are among the three most frequent microorganisms causing nosocomial infection.[17]

Although *C. albicans* remains the leading cause of disseminated fungal infection among hospitalized patients, the isolation of other yeast species, including *C. glabrata*, *Candida tropicalis*, *C. parapsilosis*, *Candida krusei*, and even *Saccharomyces cerevisiae*, is occurring with increasing frequency.[18-20] Table 33-1 displays the relative distribution of *Candida* species recovered from the bloodstream of all patients in the NNIS system compared with the subpopulation of NICU patients. Since 1991, the incidence of infections

Table 33–1 Frequency of Isolation of *Candida* Species Causing Candidemia Sepsis

	Percent of Blood Culture Isolates	
Candida species	**All Patients**	**Neonates**
C. albicans	50	63
C. glabrata	24	6
C. tropicalis	12	<1
C. krusei	7	<1
C. parapsilosis	4	29
C. dubliniensis	1	<1
Other species	2	<2

Data from Rangel-Frausto MS, Wiblin T, Blumberg HM, et al. National epidemiology of mycoses survey (NEMIS): variations in rates of bloodstream infections due to *Candida* species in seven surgical intensive care units and six neonatal intensive care units. Clin Infect Dis 29:253-258, 1999, and from Richards MJ, Edwards JR, Culver DH, et al. Nosocomial infections in medical intensive care units in the United States. National Nosocomial Infections Surveillance system. Crit Care Med 27:887-892, 1999.

with *C. glabrata* among all patients, including neonates, has more than doubled.[21,22] However, among neonates alone, a distinctive overall distribution is observed, with a predilection for infections with *C. parapsilosis* not seen in adults or older pediatric patients.[6,8,23] Historically, *C. albicans* has been considered the most virulent species. A retrospective study of neonatal candidiasis in the 1980s revealed a 24% mortality rate among infants infected with *C. albicans*, but no deaths among those infected with *C. parapsilosis*.[8] Later case series have shown an increase in infections with non-*Candida albicans Candida* (NCAC) species and mortality for neonates infected with *C. glabrata* and *C. parapsilosis* equivalent to that for *C. albicans* infections.[6,24] Although *C. albicans* may be responsible for more infections than NCAC species, any candidal infection in the neonate can be life threatening.

Candida species are commensal organisms, colonizing the human skin, gastrointestinal tract, and female genitourinary tract.[11,25,26] Studies evaluating gastrointestinal tract colonization document approximately 5% of neonates are colonized with *Candida* at admission to the NICU; up to 50% are colonized by the end of the first week and almost three fourths by the end of the first month of life.[23,25,27,28] A variety of *Candida* species colonize the human gastrointestinal tract, including *C. albicans*, *C. tropicalis*, *C. glabrata*, and *C. parapsilosis* in neonates.[23,28,29] More than one species may be recovered from a single host, but there is usually a predominant colonizing species.[30] The *Candida* strain colonizing the infant most often is acquired by vertical transmission from the maternal vaginal mucosa after passage through the birth canal.[30-32] Using molecular typing techniques, vertical transmission of *C. albicans*, *C. parapsilosis*, and *C. glabrata* has been documented in term and preterm infants.[30,33,34] Heavy maternal colonization or maternal *Candida* vaginitis is an important risk factor for efficient transmission, resulting in increased neonatal colonization and the potential for disease.[32] Intrauterine fetal infections occur rarely, but they have been attributed to ascending infection from the vagina of the mother and transplacental transmission.[35,36] Breastfeeding can result in transmission of yeast present on the maternal skin to the infant's oral mucosa, and *Candida* species have been recovered from expressed breast milk.[37] Candidal mastitis increases the risk of transmission. Perinatal transmission can result in colonization, congenital candidiasis, or mucocutaneous infections in the term infant, whereas the result can be disseminated or systemic candidiasis in the preterm infant.[38,39]

Although maternal vertical transmission is more common, acquisition of *Candida* from care providers may occur and is the primary mode of transmission for *C. parapsilosis*.[24,30,34] In one study evaluating 19 mother-infant pairs, no maternal reservoir could be demonstrated among infants colonized with *C. parapsilosis*.[30] Although different from the typical transmission route seen with *C. albicans* and *C. glabrata* (the two species found most often in the maternal gastrointestinal or genitourinary tract), this observation is not surprising. Given that maternal gastrointestinal or genitourinary colonization with *C. parapsilosis* is uncommon, the risk of perinatal exposure and transmission is equally low.[40] After birth, NICU personnel, rather than the mother, have the greatest contact with the preterm or sick infant. Because *C. parapsilosis* is the most common *Candida* species recovered from the hands of health care providers, transmission can be expected and may be a contributing factor to the increased incidence of *C. parapsilosis* catheter-associated infections in high-risk neonates.[41,42]

Colonization is important in the development of disease because the *Candida* strain recovered in infection usually is identical to the colonizing strain.[43,44] Disseminated infections result from translocation across the gastrointestinal tract epithelium of commensal *Candida* species.[7,11,43] However, colonization does not inevitably lead to disease, and infection does occur in the absence of apparent colonization.[28] Direct transmission of *Candida* to NICU infants has been documented from exogenous yeast carried by hands of hospital personnel or found on equipment.[45] This emphasizes the need for proper hand hygiene among health care workers in the NICU—although most of the antimicrobial soaps available are not fungicidal, and it is primarily the mechanical action of washing that decreases the burden of *Candida* species present.[46] Vaudry and colleagues[47] described an outbreak of candidemia in seven infants without central intravascular catheters, and molecular typing of the *C. albicans* strains grouped the isolates into two cohorts corresponding with the timing of infections and the geographic location of babies in the nursery. The use of intravascular pressure-monitoring devices has been associated with *C. parapsilosis* fungemia on an NICU.[48] *Candida* infections have resulted from retrograde administration of medications by multiple-use syringes in infants receiving total parenteral nutrition; in these cases, the responsible organisms, *C. albicans, C. tropicalis*, and *C. parapsilosis*, were isolated from the blood of the infants and the medication syringe.[42] The outbreak subsided with a change to single-use syringes. A nursery outbreak of *Candida guilliermondii*, a typically nonpathogenic NCAC, was traced to contaminated heparin vials used for flushing needles for blood drawing.[48] All of these examples point to the ubiquitous nature of *Candida* species and the need for stringent infection control practices on the NICU to decrease the acquisition of nosocomial infections.[49]

THE ORGANISM

The name *Candida* comes from the Latin term *candidus*, meaning "glowing white," which refers to the smooth, glistening white colonies formed by these yeasts when grown on culture media. The taxonomy of the genus *Candida* is somewhat challenging and incomplete because of the reclassification of certain species (e.g., *Torulopsis glabrata* has been correctly identified as *Candida glabrata*) and the discovery of new species such as *Candida dubliniensis*.[50,51] Previously used terms, such as Fungi Imperfecti, *Oidium*, and *Monilia*, are no longer used in classifying the genus *Candida*. Fungi Imperfecti, or Deuteromycetes, refers to the class of fungi that reproduce asexually. This was the prevailing theory regarding *Candida*; however, a teleomorph, or sexual stage, has been described for certain *Candida* species (e.g., *C. krusei, C. guilliermondii*), eliminating this characteristic as a useful tool in classification.[52] *Oidium* and *Monilia* were 19th century terms that are no longer used to refer to the genus *Candida*, although the term monilial is still commonly used to describe the characteristic rash observed in cutaneous *Candida* infections.[52,53]

Although more than 150 species of *Candida* have been described, relatively few species infect humans. Most exist

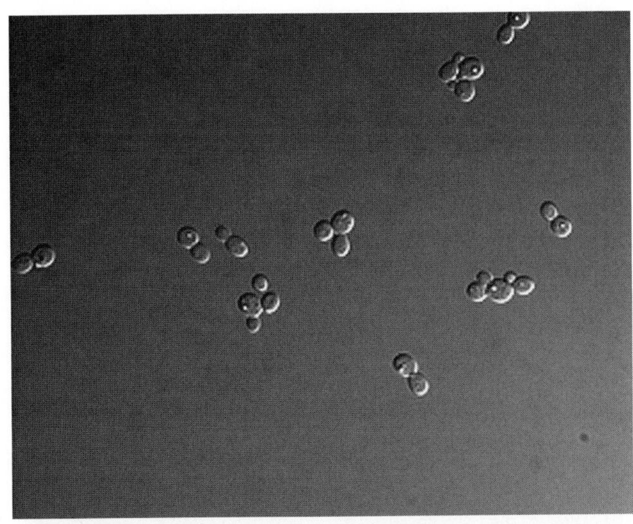
A

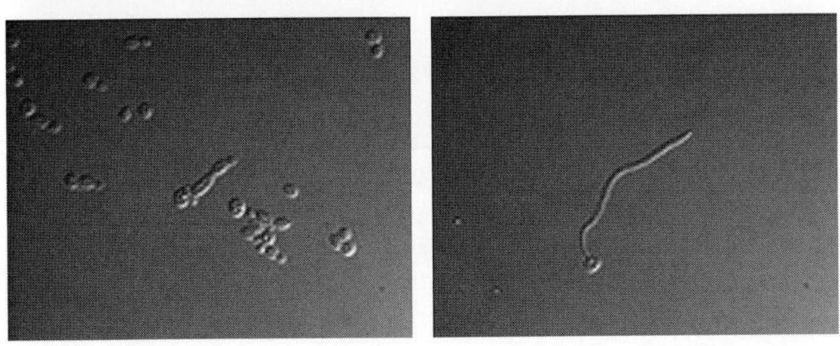
B C

Figure 33–1 Light microscopy photographs of *Candida albicans* blastoconidia or yeast cells (**A**), pseudohyphae (**B**), and true hyphae (**C**). (Courtesy of Cheryl A. Gale, MD, University of Minnesota Medical School, Minneapolis, Minn.)

as environmental saprophytes, and more than one half the *Candida* species described cannot even grow at 37° C, making them unlikely candidates to be successful human pathogens.[54] *C. albicans* is the most prevalent species causing human disease, but other pathogenic species include *C. parapsilosis, C. glabrata, C. tropicalis, Candida pseudotropicalis, C. paratropicalis, C. krusei, Candida lusitaniae, C. guilliermondii,* and *C. dubliniensis*. The primary pathogens among neonates are *C. albicans, C. parapsilosis,* and *C. glabrata* (see Table 33-1).

Members of the genus *Candida* are ubiquitous and form a heterogeneous group of eukaryotic, dimorphic or polymorphic organisms. All *Candida* species grow as yeast cells or blastoconidia under general culture conditions between 25° C and 35° C, and growth is augmented by increased sugar or fat content in the media. Yeast cells are approximately 2 to 10 µm in the largest dimension, round to oval, and reproduce by budding. *C. albicans* is among the larger yeast at 4 to 6 × 6 to 10 µm, whereas *C. glabrata* and *C. parapsilosis* are among the smallest at 1 to 4 µm × 2 to 9 µm and 2 to 4 × 2 to 9 µm, respectively.[52] Figure 33-1A shows *C. albicans* single blastoconidia and budding yeast cells. Most members of the genus also produce a filamentous form: pseudohyphae (see Fig. 33-1B) or true hyphae (see Fig. 33-1C). *C. glabrata* is the only pathogenic species that does not produce filamentous forms, existing exclusively as blastoconidia.[52] *C. parapsilosis* forms pseudohyphae but not true hyphae. Only *C. dubliniensis* and *C. albicans* form true hyphae (see Fig. 33-1C), distinguishing these two species as polymorphic rather than dimorphic. Formation of a germ tube precedes the development of true hyphae, and this change in morphology can be induced by growth in serum or other specialized media or by incubation at 37° C. The clinical diagnostic microbiology laboratory has exploited this distinction by use of the germ tube formation test to rapidly identify *C. albicans* over other *Candida* species.[13]

The ability to form true hyphae is considered one of the prime virulence factors for *C. albicans.*[55] Microscopic examination of infected human and animal tissue usually demonstrates the presence of *C. albicans* hyphae.[56-60] Conversely, nonfilamentous yeast, such as *S. cerevisiae*, rarely causes human disease, and genetically altered strains of *C. albicans*, which cannot filament normally, are generally less virulent in animal models of fungemia.[61-65] Other commonly recognized virulence factors for *C. albicans* include the production of proteinases and phospholipases, hydrophobicity, the presence of various surface molecules (e.g., receptors, adhesins), and the production of biofilm (which may be particularly important in catheter-associated infections).[58,60,65-67]

A variety of surface molecules of *C. albicans* are responsible for modulating epithelial adhesion by interacting with host ligands on the epithelial or endothelial surface.[61,68,69] Ligands include sugar residues on human buccal epithelial cells and a wide variety of extracellular matrix proteins, such as fibronectin, fibrinogen, types I and IV collagen, laminin, and the complement components iC3b and C3d. In tissue culture assays, *C. albicans* is more adherent than other *Candida* species to every form of human epithelium and endothelium available, including cultured buccal epithelium, enterocytes (adult and fetal), cervical epithelium, and human umbilical vein endothelial cells.[18,32,70,71] The adhesive molecules responsible for epithelial and endothelial adhesion probably facilitate binding between individual *Candida* cells and the subsequent development of "fungus balls" found in infected organs.[72,73] No single adhesin is completely responsible for the adherence of *C. albicans* to human epithelium, and multiple methods of interacting with the host surface are postulated for this commensal organism.[73] *C. albicans* also adheres well to the surface of catheters and, in the process, forms a biofilm.[74] The biofilm microenvironment promotes fungal growth with hyphal transformation and may confer relative drug resistance because of poor penetration of antimicrobial agents into this mass of extracellular matrix, yeast cells, and hyphae.[75-77] Biofilm formation is associated with persistent fungemia and with co-infection by nosocomial bacterial pathogens, such as *Staphylococcus* species.[12,74,78] The ability to adhere to human epithelium and endothelium, as well as to itself and catheters, is a significant virulence factor setting *C. albicans* apart from other *Candida* species, and it may be a prominent reason for the increased frequency with which *C. albicans* is found colonizing the host and causing disease at epithelial and endothelial sites.

Virulence factors of other *Candida* species have not been well studied. A fibronectin receptor that facilitates epithelial adhesion has been described in *C. tropicalis.*[79,80] *C. glabrata* colonizes the gastrointestinal tract, but no specific virulence factors have been identified in this nonfilamentous *Candida* species.[20,81] *C. parapsilosis* has been recovered from the alimentary tract of neonates, but no work has been done to implicate or exclude the gastrointestinal tract as a possible source of infection among neonates, and no virulence factors

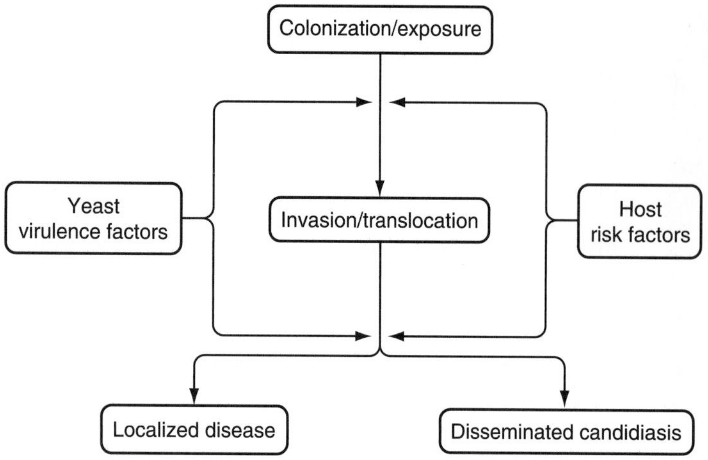

Figure 33–2 The pathogenesis of neonatal candidiasis follows a pathway from colonization to infection, modified by multiple host factors and yeast virulence factors.

have been identified in this *Candida* species.[23,33] *C. glabrata* and *C. parapsilosis* produce biofilms; however, this area has not been well investigated for either of these pathogenic NCAC species. *Candida* species exhibit relatively low-level virulence factors compared with organisms that cause disease in an immunocompetent host. Candidal virulence factors serve to differentiate the more virulent from the less virulent *Candida* species, rather than to distinguish *Candida* from other more pathogenic microbes.

PATHOGENESIS

The pathogenesis of invasive candidiasis involves a common sequence of events in all at-risk hosts: colonization, resulting from adhesion of the yeast to the skin or mucosal epithelium (particularly the gastrointestinal tract); penetration of the epithelial barriers; and locally invasive or widely disseminated disease. Dissemination to deep visceral organs results from hematogenous spread.[11] However, not every colonized patient develops a *Candida* infection. The unique combination of host factors and yeast virulence mechanisms results in the persistence of benign colonization or the progression to infection among high-risk neonatal patients, as outlined in Figure 33-2. Yeast virulence factors were described in the preceding section. Host risk factors, listed in Table 33-2, probably are more important in the development of neonatal candidal infections. Limitation of exposure to all predisposing conditions for candidal infection is highly desirable but rarely feasible, especially in the VLBW infant.

Indiscriminate, frequent, or prolonged use of broad-spectrum antimicrobial agents, resulting in alterations of the normal skin and intestinal microbial flora, allows for overgrowth of the colonizing strain of *Candida* and a concomitant increased risk for translocation and hematogenous spread.[7] The greater the density of organisms in the neonatal gastrointestinal tract, the greater is the chance of dissemination.[82] High levels of *Candida* colonization found in certain nurseries are linked to patterns of antibiotic usage.[6,44]

The immunocompromised state predisposes an infant to candidal infection, whether caused by the developmentally immature immune system of the newborn, a congenital immunodeficiency, or the immunosuppression accompanying steroid therapy. No single defect in the immune system appears to be solely responsible for an increased susceptibility of premature neonates to candidal infections. Healthy adults have circulating IgG antibodies to *Candida* antigens, which effectively opsonize the organism and activate the alternative complement pathway.[83-86] Neonatal IgG levels depend on maternal exposure to the yeast and transplacental transmission of candidal antibodies, and the ability for the infant to respond to a new challenge with a *Candida* species may be slow and inadequate.[84,86,87] Polymorphonuclear leukocytes ingest and kill *Candida*; therefore, neutropenia is an important risk factor.[88] Disseminated candidiasis in neonates is associated with the intravenous administration of dexamethasone and hydrocortisone.[89-91] Steroid therapy results in immunosuppression and may have direct effects on colonization and translocation from the gastrointestinal tract. In vitro studies have shown that *C. albicans* is more adherent to monolayers of cultured enterocytes treated with dexamethasone than to untreated control monocytes, whereas mice injected with dexamethasone demonstrate higher levels of gastrointestinal tract colonization with *C. albicans* and increased rates of dissemination to the kidney.[57] Steroids may have a direct effect on the yeast by acting

Table 33–2 **Host Factors Enhancing Risk for Candidiasis in Neonates**
High burden of colonization with *Candida* species
Prematurity, especially gestational age <28 weeks
Very low birth weight (<1500 g)
Prolonged broad-spectrum antimicrobial therapy
Indwelling catheters, especially central intravascular catheters
Steroid therapy
Neutropenia
Hyperglycemia
Total parenteral hyperalimentation
Abdominal surgery
Necrotizing enterocolitis
Spontaneous intestinal perforation
Cardiac surgery
Prolonged hospitalization

through the corticosteroid receptor present on the surface of *C. albicans*.[92]

The presence of indwelling catheters is a significant predisposing risk factor for neonatal candidiasis. Endotracheal tubes, urinary catheters, peritoneal catheters, chest tubes, mediastinal tubes, and ventriculoperitoneal shunts can all become infected, but the greatest risk lies with intravascular catheters, particularly central venous catheters.[5,45] All catheters in the vascular space for more than a day begin to develop a thrombin sheath with a matrix-like substance, providing an optimal site for accumulation of microorganisms.[66] *Candida* species adhere extremely well to the inert surface of the catheter, and electron microscopy studies have shown that *Candida* species are able to burrow into the catheter and form a surrounding biofilm.[66,69,93] This sequence results in a unique microenvironment, providing a barrier to host defenses and offering optimal conditions for growth and proliferation of the *Candida* organism, often resulting in the development of an infected mural thrombus extending from the tip of the catheter.[94-96] The "fungal mass" adherent to the catheter can then serve as a source for persistent fungemia or embolic spread of *Candida* species to distant organs.[1,7] The original source of the yeast that "sticks" to the line may be from hematogenous spread of endogenous gastrointestinal tract *Candida* strains or from nosocomial transmission through placement or handling of the catheter itself.[11,42,47] Use of the catheter for hyperalimentation is an additional risk, especially with the infusion of high dextrose–containing total parenteral solutions and intralipids.[7,97]

Any compromise of epithelial barriers can predispose the neonate to candidal infections. Abdominal surgery and cardiac surgery are associated with an increased risk for disseminated candidiasis, especially among term infants.[7,12] Necrotizing enterocolitis (NEC) is strongly associated with *Candida* fungemia.[5,10,11,98] The loss of mucosal integrity after mesenteric ischemia and NEC provides a portal of entry for the dissemination of endogenous gastrointestinal flora.[11] Spontaneous intestinal perforation, occurring most often in the extremely preterm infant, is highly associated with candidemia.[99,100] As with any nosocomially acquired organism, prolonged hospitalization is a significant risk factor for the development of candidiasis.[5]

Prematurity is a key risk factor for candidiasis, especially infants born at less than 28 weeks' gestation or VLBW neonates.[3,5,7] With improvements in technology, the current standard of care in the NICU includes an aggressive approach to the treatment of VLBW infants such that life for an extremely premature infant combines nearly all the risk factors for candidiasis in one patient.[101] The premature infant is born with immature epithelial barriers and an immature immune system. The skin and mucosal epithelium of these very tiny infants are minimally protective, readily breaking down with exposure to air and routine nursing procedures.[102] Preterm infants have the lowest levels of circulating maternal IgG of all neonates, having lost the opportunity for transplacental transfer that occurs during the third trimester of pregnancy.[103] Even if specific anti-*Candida* IgG is present, opsonization and complement activation are diminished.[104] Complement levels are extremely low in preterm infants, with biochemical abnormalities of C3 resulting in inadequate activation of this pathway for fighting infections.[105] Neutropenia is a common finding among infants born at less than 28 weeks' gestation.[106] Virtually every premature infant begins life with a course of empirical broad-spectrum antibiotics, leading to an interruption in the process of establishing the normal gastrointestinal microflora and the potential for unchecked proliferation of *Candida*.[45,107] Endotracheal and intravascular catheters are true lifelines for the VLBW premature infant needing respiratory, inotropic agent, and nutritional support. Because venous access often is difficult to obtain and maintain in these infants, intravascular access lines are not automatically rotated and frequently remain in place for weeks. Even the fairly healthy VLBW infant often displays feeding intolerance that can require prolonged central total parenteral nutrition (TPN) rather than enteral feeds.[108] As reported by the National Institute of Child and Human Development (NICHD) Neonatal Research Network, the adjusted odds ratio for any episode of late-onset sepsis is 3.1 in VLBW infants receiving TPN for 8 to14 days, rising to 4.0 for an infant receiving TPN for more than 22 days.[109] Unfortunately, NEC also can accompany feeding intolerance, leading to an additional risk for disseminated candidiasis.[19,110,111] Corticosteroid use also has been common in these patients.[111] Reviews have reported that almost one half of the infants with a birth weight of less than 750 g are postnatally exposed to corticosteroids—hydrocortisone used to treat hypotension or dexamethasone used for severe lung disease.[90,111-113] Hyperglycemia and hyperlipidemia are common in these immature patients receiving TPN or steroids, or both.[91,97] Prolonged length of stay is the rule rather than the exception for the NICU infant with or without a nosocomially acquired infection. The average corrected gestational age at discharge from the NICU is between 35 and 36 weeks, and the average NICU hospitalization is approximately 62 days; however, the length of stay to achieve 36 weeks' gestational age is even longer for the infant born at less than 28 weeks' gestation.[7,109] Each of these factors combine to make the VLBW preterm infant an extremely high-risk candidate for the development of candidiasis.

PATHOLOGY

The tissue pathology observed in *Candida* species infections depends on the site of involvement and the extent of invasion or dissemination. Histologic evaluation of mucosal or epithelial lesions reveals superficial ulcerations with the presence of yeast and filamentous forms of *Candida* species, including a prominent polymorphonuclear (PMN) leukocyte infiltration.[114] Extremely low birth weight (ELBW; birth weight = 1000 g) infants can develop invasive fungal dermatitis with erosive lesions; biopsy of these lesions reveals invasion of fungal elements through the epidermis into the dermis.[102,114] In disseminated neonatal infections, *Candida* species can invade virtually any tissues. Microabscesses most commonly are found in the kidney, retina, and brain, but they also have been described in the liver, spleen, peritoneum, heart, lungs, and joints.[8,115,116] When *C. albicans* is the infecting organism, abscesses contain a predominance of hyphal elements with a significant accompanying infiltration of PMNs and prominent tissue necrosis, especially in the kidney.[58,117,118] Mycelia frequently are found invading the walls of blood vessels within infected tissues.[20,56,118] Retinal lesions, vitreal fungal lesions, and even lens abscesses with cataract formation have been described in neonates.[119,120] Evaluation of brain material shows significant inflammation with seeding of the meninges and may include parenchymal lesions, ventriculitis, perivasculitis, and ependymal inflammation.[116,121,122] Macroscopic fungus balls can form in fluid-filled spaces lined with epithelial or endothelial cells, such as the urinary tract, the central nervous system (CNS), and the intravascular space (particularly the right atrium).[123-125] Fungus balls are large collections of intertwined hyphae, pseudohyphae, and yeast cells that presumably grow from *Candida* species initially adherent to the epithelial or endothelial surface of the involved organ.[117,126] Foreign bodies present in these fluid-filled spaces, such as urinary catheters, ventricular shunts, or central venous catheters, can also serve as the nidus for infection and precipitate the formation of a fungus ball.[117,125,126]

In intrauterine candidal infections, macroscopic chorioamnionitis is evident, and histologic examination of the fetal membranes and the chorionic plate often reveal fungal elements with an extensive PMN infiltration.[127,128] Along with diffuse placental inflammation, focal granulomatous lesions can be present in the umbilical cord.[120,129] The detection of placental pathology consistent with candidal chorioamnionitis can lead to the early detection of congenital candidiasis in the infant.[130]

CLINICAL MANIFESTATIONS

Candida species are responsible for a variety of infections in neonates with a broad spectrum of clinical presentations, ranging from mild, irritating thrush and diaper dermatitis in the healthy term infant to life-threatening systemic disease in the extremely premature infant. The primary forms of candidiasis among infants are mucocutaneous infections, congenital candidiasis, catheter-related candidemia, and systemic or disseminated candidiasis. Individual organ system involvement (e.g., urinary tract infection, isolated meningitis, endophthalmitis) can occur, but infection occurs much more often as a component of disseminated infection, especially in the premature infant. Table 33-3 lists features of the various presentations of neonatal candidiasis.

Oropharyngeal Candidiasis

Oropharyngeal candidiasis (i.e., thrush) can occur at any time during infancy. Among hospitalized infants, the overall incidence is reported as 3%, with a median age of onset of 9 to 10 days in NICU patients.[131,132] Specific risk factors include vaginal delivery, maternal vaginal *Candida* species infection, and birth asphyxia.[132,133] In a study of more than 500 mother-infant pairs, an eightfold increase was observed in the incidence of thrush among infants born to mothers with symptomatic candidal vaginitis compared with infants born to asymptomatic mothers.[133] A multivariate analysis of factors among NICU infants reported that birth asphyxia was the only event significantly associated with the development of thrush.[132] Although *Candida* species can be transmitted from mother to infant during breast-feeding, thrush occurs more often among formula-fed infants.[113] *C. albicans* is the most common species isolated from infants with thrush, but other NCAC species, such as *C. parapsilosis* and *C. glabrata*, increasingly are found as commensals and infecting agents.[113,134,135]

Thrush manifests as irregular white plaques on the oral mucosa, including the buccal and lingual surfaces and the palate. The underlying mucosa may appear normal or erythematous and may have an ulcerative base to the white lesion. Physical removal of the plaques usually is difficult and often results in mucosal damage. Infected infants can be healthy or quite irritable, with disinterest in oral feedings and obvious discomfort with any care involving contact with the oral lesions.

Diaper Dermatitis

Diaper dermatitis can occur any time during infancy, with a peak incidence at age 7 to 9 months in term infants (10% incidence) and approximately 10 to 11 weeks among VLBW infants (28% incidence).[26,136] Most infants with candidal diaper dermatitis have gastrointestinal colonization, with stool cultures positive for a *Candida* species.[136] Some infants also have oropharyngeal candidiasis. *C. albicans* is the most common species isolated, but there has been an increase in the recovery of other NCAC species, particularly *C. glabrata* and *C. parapsilosis*, when cultures are obtained.[100]

The characteristic rash of candidal diaper dermatitis is confluent and intensely erythematous with satellite lesions and pustules.[136,137] As with oral thrush, the lesions can be very irritating to the infant, especially during normal perineal care. In the term infant, the rash resolves rapidly after treatment with an appropriate topical antifungal agent.[113] The preterm infant has a greater risk for spread beyond the diaper area. In a prospective study, Faix and colleagues[131] found mucocutaneous disease in 7.8% of all preterm infants, and most had diaper dermatitis. Among preterm infants with dermatitis and an associated change in clinical status, 32% developed systemic disease, compared with 2.1% of healthy infants.[131] It is prudent to monitor the preterm infants with candidal diaper dermatitis for signs of systemic infection.

Congenital Candidiasis

Congenital candidiasis typically presents at birth or within the first 24 hours of life and results from an intrauterine infection in the mother or from massive maternal vaginal colonization with *Candida* during labor and delivery.[4] Hematogenous dissemination from mother to fetus, direct invasion of intact membranes, and ascending infection after ruptured membranes have been postulated as mechanisms for intrauterine infection.[100,127,138] Recognized risk factors for congenital candidiasis differ from those associated with postnatal infection and include prolonged rupture of membranes and the presence of an intrauterine foreign body, most commonly a cerclage suture.[138,139] Infants with the latter risk factor are more likely to be born prematurely and to have more severe skin involvement with disseminated disease.[109,138] Although *C. albicans* is the predominant species responsible for congenital candidiasis, cases of congenital infections with *C. glabrata* and *C. parapsilosis* have been described.[22,100,139]

Although there are rare case reports of infants with congenital candidiasis without skin involvement, the classic presentation is one of diffuse cutaneous disease.[35,140,141]

Table 33–3 Features of Neonatal Candidiasis

Clinical Syndrome	Age at Onset	Host Risk Factors[a]	Presentation	Diagnosis	Treatment	Multiorgan Involvement	Prognosis
Mucocutaneous Infections							
Thrush	Throughout infancy	Birth asphyxia	White plaques on oral mucosa	Physical examination	Topical or oral antifungal therapy	None	Excellent
Diaper dermatitis	Throughout infancy; peak at 7-9 mo (term) and 10-11 wk (preterm)	Gastrointestinal colonization	Intense erythema of perineal area with satellite lesions	Physical examination	Topical antifungal therapy	None in term infants	Excellent
Congenital candidiasis	Birth	Premature rupture of membranes or uterine foreign body	Widespread erythematous maculopapular rash ± vesicles Pneumonia in preterm infants	Physical examination Culture of lesions for *Candida* spp	Topical antifungal therapy Systemic antifungal therapy for pneumonia	Uncommon Dissemination can occur in preterm infants	Excellent in term infants; excellent in preterm infants without dissemination
Invasive fungal dermatitis	<2 weeks	<1000 g Vaginal delivery Postnatal steroids Hyperglycemia	Erosive, crusting lesions in dependent areas	Physical examination Biopsy and culture of lesions	Systemic antifungal therapy	Common	Good if localized without dissemination
Systemic Infections							
Catheter-related infections	>7 days	Intravascular catheters	Sepsis	Blood culture by catheter grows *Candida* spp but peripheral blood cultures sterile	Catheter removal and systemic antifungal therapy	Rare Endocarditis or right atrial mass or thrombus	Good without dissemination or complication
Candidemia	>7 days		Sepsis	Only blood cultures grow *Candida* spp	Systemic antifungal therapy	Common in VLBW infants	Good to fair Risk of ROP in VLBW infants
Disseminated candidiasis	>7 days		Severe sepsis Multiorgan involvement	Blood and urine, CSF or other sites grow *Candida* spp Clinical and/or radiographic evidence for multiorgan involvement	Systemic antifungal therapy	Always (sites most often involved are kidneys, CNS, eyes, heart)	Fair to poor
Renal candidiasis	>7 days	Congenital urinary tract anomalies Neurogenic bladder	Sepsis Urinary tract obstruction	Urine culture grows *Candida* spp Ultrasound evidence of renal fungal lesions	Systemic antifungal therapy	Uncommon with isolated UTI	Good
CNS candidiasis	>7 days	Neural tube defects Indwelling CSF shunt or catheter	Sepsis None to focal neurologic signs	CSF culture grows *Candida* spp CSF culture grows *Candida* spp ± signs of inflammation; lesions by cranial imaging	Systemic antifungal therapy	Common	Poor

[a]Factors, in addition to those listed in Table 33-2, pertaining to the specific clinical syndrome listed.
CNS, central nervous system; CSF, cerebrospinal fluid; ROP, retinopathy of prematurity; UTI, urinary tract infection; VLBW, very low birth weight.

Dermatologic findings include a widespread erythematous maculopapular rash, often with well-demarcated borders, that evolves into vesicles or pustules with eventual desquamation.[139,140] Any part of the skin may be involved, including the palms and soles, but the lesions typically are more prominent in the skin folds or intertriginous areas.[4,100] Preterm infants can present with a diffuse, widespread, intensely erythematous dermatitis that resembles a mild burn or the early stages of staphylococcal scalded skin syndrome.[142] This form of congenital candidiasis often leads to massive desquamation, often accompanied by a prominent leukocytosis.[35,140] Extensive desquamation can lead to severe fluid and electrolyte imbalances in the extremely premature infant.[35]

In term infants, clinical findings usually are limited to the skin, and recovery is uneventful after topical antifungal therapy. However, meningitis has been reported in the term infant with congenital candidiasis, and some infants may present with nonspecific clinical signs of sepsis, such as poor perfusion, hypotonia, and temperature instability, suggesting systemic disease.[140,143] In preterm infants, cutaneous findings can be coupled with pulmonary invasion and early respiratory distress. In this circumstance, the chest radiograph is atypical for surfactant deficiency and the expected ground-glass appearance is replaced by a nodular or alveolar infiltrate.[4] Hematogenous dissemination is uncommon, but it can occur more frequently among preterm neonates and infants with widespread cutaneous involvement, pulmonary disease, and central intravascular catheters.[139] Every attempt should be made to avoid placing central intravascular catheters through the infected skin of patients with congenital candidiasis.

Invasive Fungal Dermatitis

Invasive fungal dermatitis is a unique clinical entity described in the ELBW infant and occurs during the first 2 weeks of life.[114,144] *Candida* species are frequently isolated, but infection with other filamentous non-*Candida* fungi, including species of *Aspergillus, Trichosporon, Curvularia,* and *Bipolaris,* can result in this clinical presentation.[114,145,146] Specific risk factors for invasive fungal dermatitis include a gestational age less than 26 weeks, vaginal birth, postnatal steroid administration, and hyperglycemia.[114] The immature skin of the extremely preterm infant is not an efficient barrier to the external invasion of *Candida,* making these neonates more susceptible to invasive cutaneous disease. The stratum corneum of the preterm infant is extremely thin, and keratinization with maturation of the barrier properties typically occurs beyond the second week of life.[102]

Neonates with invasive fungal dermatitis have characteristic skin lesions with severe erosions, serous drainage, and crusting, often occurring on dependent surfaces such as the back or abdomen.[114] Biopsy of the affected area shows invasion of fungal elements through the epidermis into the dermis.[114] Without prompt and appropriate therapy, dissemination with resulting widespread systemic disease is a frequent complication. As with congenital candidiasis, infants with extensive erosive lesions are at risk for the development of fluid and electrolyte abnormalities and for secondary infections with other skin microorganisms.

Catheter-Related Candidal Infections

Catheter-related candidal infections are disease processes of the sick, hospitalized preterm or term infant requiring prolonged use of intravascular catheters or other invasive means of support.[7,38,101] Almost any type of indwelling foreign body can become infected, but vascular catheter-related candidemia is the most frequent and serious infection. The incidence increases after a central vascular catheter has been in place for more than 7 days. These infections have been associated with umbilical venous and arterial catheters and with percutaneously placed arterial or central venous catheters (i.e., femoral venous, subclavian, Broviac, or silastic lines).[2,108] Peripheral venous catheters have the same potential for fungemia in the premature infant, especially when used for the delivery of hyperalimentation fluid, and have been associated with the development of skin abscesses at the insertion site.[147-149] The neonate has one or more of the predisposing conditions listed in Table 33-2, and the infection can arise from endogenous gastrointestinal organisms or from nosocomial transmission. Cutaneous disease is not necessary. Neonates exhibit nonspecific signs of sepsis, including feeding intolerance, apnea, hyperglycemia, and temperature instability, but no evidence of multiorgan involvement. Preterm infants also may exhibit hemodynamic instability or respiratory distress. Thrombocytopenia is a common presenting feature.[3,150] The vascular catheter tip provides an excellent nidus for growth of *Candida* and affords a source of ongoing fungemia. An infected thrombus or fungus ball can form on the catheter tip, serving as a source of platelet consumption or embolic dissemination.[94,95] By definition, catheter-related candidemia is infection of the catheter only; there is no dissemination or multiorgan involvement. Prompt catheter removal at the earliest sign of infection, although often impractical in the management of many of the highest-risk neonates, is necessary to contain the infection and prevent persistent candidemia with the attendant risk of disseminated infection or other complications. Candidal infections of right atrial catheters are associated with endocarditis and intracardiac fungal masses; the latter can result in cardiac dysfunction because of the enlarging right atrial mass.[94,151]

Although infected intravascular catheters provide the greatest concern for dissemination, infection can occur with almost any type of catheter used in the treatment of the VLBW infant. Prolonged endotracheal tubes for mechanical ventilation can be required in the extremely premature infant with respiratory distress and in the sick term infant after cardiac or other extensive surgery. The concurrent ongoing presence of the endotracheal tube can lead to candidal colonization with the potential for development of pneumonia,[12,25,152] although invasive lung infection is uncommon. Candidal cystitis can accompany the prolonged use of indwelling bladder catheters by facilitating ascending infection, and cystic fungal masses can form, resulting in urethral obstruction.[153-155] Infants with vesicoureteral reflux and a candidal bladder infection are at risk for renal parenchymal infection.[126,153] Candidal peritonitis can develop after the prolonged use of peritoneal catheters placed intraoperatively for drainage or, more often, placed for peritoneal dialysis.[123] Peritoneal dialysis catheters are at extremely high risk for infection because of the frequent handling required and the high dextrose concentration of the indwelling dialysis fluid.[123] *Candida* species have been recovered from the pleural fluid draining from thoracic tubes and from the fluid draining through surgically placed mediastinal tubes.[4] With cystitis, dissemination and widespread disease can be complications, but *Candida* peritonitis or pleuritis rarely leads to fungemia.[25,123]

Candidemia and Disseminated Candidiasis

Candidemia and disseminated or systemic candidiasis usually are associated with multiple invasive infection enhancing factors and are infections of the sick preterm or term infant who is in the NICU more than 7 days.[38,101,118] However, most cases occur among ELBW infants, who have an incidence of candidemia ranging from 5.5% to 16.5%.[5-7] The source of the infecting *Candida* species can be from the infant's endogenous flora or from nosocomial transmission, and all the *Candida* species listed in Table 33-1 have been implicated in systemic disease.[7,109,152] Although candidemia without organ involvement can occur, *Candida* has such high affinity for certain organs (e.g., kidney, eye, heart, CNS) that dissemination appears to be the rule rather than the exception, particularly in the neonate with persistent fungemia.[117,118,156] The clinical presentation of the infant with candidemia can vary greatly because it depends on the extent of systemic disease. The most common presentation is one with clinical features typical of bacterial sepsis, including lethargy, feeding intolerance, hyperbilirubinemia, apnea, cardiovascular instability, and the development or worsening of respiratory distress. The preterm infant can become critically ill, requiring a significant escalation in cardiorespiratory support. Fever rarely occurs, even with widespread disease. New-onset glucose intolerance and thrombocytopenia are common presenting findings that can persist until adequate therapy has been instituted and the infection contained.[91,97,150] This association is so strong that the presence of persistent hyperglycemia with thrombocytopenia in a neonate cared for in the NICU is almost diagnostic for untreated candidemia.[150] Leukocytosis with a neutrophil predominance or neutropenia can be seen.[157] Neutropenia more often is associated with overwhelming systemic disease. Skin abscesses have been described with systemic disease and are attributed to the deposition of septic emboli in end vessels of the skin.[149] Infants also can present with specific organ involvement, such as renal insufficiency, meningitis, endophthalmitis, endocarditis, or osteomyelitis, confirming dissemination. Complex multiorgan involvement is the hallmark of disseminated candidiasis, especially among VLBW premature infants, and results from diffuse hematogenous spread.[6,158,159] The suspicion or diagnosis of candidemia or the diagnosis of candidal infection of any one organ system should prompt a thorough examination and survey of the infant for additional organ involvement.[2,17,159] Almost any organ can become infected, but the most common sites for candidal dissemination are the urinary tract, the CNS, and the eye.[158,159] The specific clinical presentation for each of these systems is described separately in the following sections. For the infant with disseminated candidiasis, complications can be extensive, multiorgan system failure common, and the need for significant intensive support frequent and prolonged.[115,118]

Renal Candidiasis

Renal involvement occurs in most infants with candidemia, because each of the same risk factors that predispose to disseminated disease increases the risk for renal disease.[160] Every infant with candidemia should have an evaluation of the urinary tract for candidal infection. Infants with congenital urinary tract anomalies and those requiring frequent catheterization for neurologic reasons also are at increased risk for an isolated *Candida* species urinary tract infection (UTI).[124,126] Congenital urinary tract anomalies, such as cloacal exstrophy, can provide a portal of entry for *Candida* species present on the skin. Urinary stasis, whether caused by a congenital anatomic obstruction or a functional obstruction (e.g., in the neurogenic bladder with myelomeningocele), increases the risk of candidal bladder infections.[161] Regardless of the underlying cause, candidal UTIs generally manifest with the same nonspecific systemic signs as with candidemia, whereas specific renal findings can be silent or manifest as urinary tract obstruction, hypertension, or renal failure.[124,126,162-166] Acute renal insufficiency or failure is a common clinical presentation and may be nonoliguric or be oliguric or anuric. In the nonoliguric form, urine output remains normal or near normal, but elevation of the serum creatinine level may be quite dramatic.[124] Renal ultrasonography often reveals parenchymal abnormalities suggestive of single or multiple abscesses; however, lesions may not be obvious at initial presentation, becoming evident only later in the disease process.[126,162] With oliguria, obstruction of the urinary tact by a discrete fungus ball or balls must be considered.[163,164] These fungal masses commonly are found in the ureteropelvic junction and usually are diagnosed by ultrasonography, but they have been found rarely by physical examination as a palpable flank mass.[58,165] Hypertension may be the only initial clinical feature in neonatal renal candidiasis.[166]

Central Nervous System Candidiasis

CNS candidiasis most often accompanies disseminated candidiasis, with up to 50% of VLBW infants having some form of CNS infection.[156,167] Neonates with neural tube defects and those requiring indwelling cerebrospinal fluid (CSF) shunts are at increased risk for isolated candidal infections of the CNS. Meningitis is the most frequently reported form of CNS infection, but parenchymal abscesses, ventriculitis, vasculitis and perivasculitis, ependymal inflammation, osteomyelitis of the skull or vertebral bodies, and even fungus balls within the subarachnoid space have been described, although rarely.[125,168-171] The specific clinical presentation is extremely variable but typically occurs when infants are older than 1 week.[172,173] The initial presentation is similar to that of disseminated candidiasis, subtle or quite severe, with cardiorespiratory instability and rapid overall deterioration.[116] Less frequently, an infant may present with only neurologic signs, such as seizures, focal neurologic changes, an increase in head circumference, or a change in fontanelle quality.[116,156] Because clinical findings may be limited or nonexistent, the possibility of CNS involvement with *Candida* must always be considered in neonates with candidemia or evidence for invasive candidal disease at other sites.

Candidal Ophthalmologic Infections

Endophthalmitis results from hematogenous spread of *Candida* species to the eye of the infant and is a diagnosed complication in approximately 6% of infants with systemic candidiasis.[119] Overall risk factors for ophthalmologic infection are the same as factors predisposing to disseminated disease. Infants with prolonged candidemia (i.e., blood cultures positive for more than 4 days) are significantly more likely to develop end-organ involvement of the eye, kidney, or heart.[158] Ophthalmic infections have been reported with all *Candida* species listed in Table 33-1.[158,174] Because the clinical presentation of candidal chorioretinitis is frequently silent, an indirect ophthalmoscopic examination should be performed on all infants diagnosed with or suspected of having candidemia or systemic candidiasis. Lesions can be unilateral or bilateral, and these appear as individual yellow-white, elevated lesions with indistinct borders in the posterior fundus.[119,174] Vitreous lesions occasionally occur, and some infants show vitreal inflammation or a nonspecific choroidal lesion with hemorrhage or Roth spots in the posterior retina.[174,175] Infection of the lens occurs rarely; five case reports of lens abscesses in preterm infants exist, and each infant presented with a unilateral cataract.[121,176-179]

In addition to the ophthalmologic infections caused by *Candida* species, an association between candidemia and retinopathy of prematurity (ROP) has been described in neonates with no previous evidence for chorioretinitis or endophthalmitis.[179-185] Early reports suggested a significant increase in the incidence of any stage ROP among infants with *Candida* sepsis compared with those without candidiasis (95% versus 69%) and an increased probability of severe ROP requiring laser surgery (41% versus 9%).[179] Subsequent retrospective studies have demonstrated a significantly greater incidence of threshold ROP and need for laser surgery among infants with *Candida* sepsis but no greater overall incidence of ROP of any severity.[181,182,184,185] Data are inconclusive as to cause and effect, but an association clearly is documented.[120] Premature infants of any gestational age who develop candidal sepsis should be followed closely by an ophthalmologist for the late development of severe ROP.

Spontaneous Intestinal Perforation

Invasive disseminated candidiasis is associated with the occurrence of spontaneous intestinal perforation in preterm infants.[123,186-189] This syndrome is distinct from NEC, occurring predominantly during the first 2 to 3 weeks of life among the smallest, most premature infants on the NICU (median gestational age, 24 weeks; median birth weight, 634 g).[99] Specific predisposing factors identified for spontaneous intestinal perforation include umbilical arterial catheterization, hypothermia, indomethacin therapy (prophylactic or treatment), and cyanotic congenital heart disease.[123,189,190] Neonates typically present with bluish discoloration of the abdomen and a gasless pattern on abdominal radiographs, without pneumatosis intestinalis, often accompanied by systemic signs such as hypotension.[99] Disseminated candidiasis frequently is diagnosed in association with this syndrome; one series reported up to 33% of affected infants having cultures of blood, peritoneal fluid, CSF, or urine positive for *Candida* species.[99] Pathologic examination of the involved intestinal area demonstrates mucosal invasion by yeast and filamentous forms of *Candida* species.[105,187,189,190] It is not clear from these specimens, nor from the clinical picture, whether the perforation is a result of primary candidal invasion of the intestinal mucosa or the colonizing *Candida* strain merely invades bowel damaged by another insult. Whatever the cause, the association exists, suggesting that clinicians should consider extensive evaluation for disseminated candidiasis with the diagnosis of a spontaneous intestinal perforation in the extremely premature infant.

DIAGNOSIS AND DIFFERENTIAL DIAGNOSIS

The diagnosis of most mucocutaneous disease is based on the characteristic clinical findings described earlier. Culture of the lesions of oral thrush or diaper dermatitis usually is not indicated. However, in an infant refractory to therapy, culture with susceptibility determination of the recovered organism may identify a NCAC species with a susceptibility pattern requiring modification of specific therapy. In congenital candidiasis, a presumptive diagnosis can be made by Gram stain of vesicular contents of an individual lesion or by potassium hydroxide preparations of skin scrapings, with confirmation by culture of discrete lesions or swabs of skin folds or intertriginous areas. Cultures of blood, urine, and CSF are indicated for term infants with systemic signs of infection and for all affected preterm infants, healthy or ill appearing.[35] In the infant with change in respiratory or radiographic status, endotracheal aspirate cultures that grow *Candida* species are difficult to interpret because most often this represents colonization rather than pulmonary invasion.[25] The characteristic skin lesions of invasive fungal dermatitis often are diagnostic, but a skin biopsy provides a definitive diagnosis and tissue for culture and species determination. Biopsy is more sensitive than skin swabs in identifying other non-*Candida* filamentous fungi included in the differential diagnosis for this disease process.[114]

Given the increasing incidence of invasive candidiasis among premature infants, clinicians caring for these infants must be alert to the possibility of *Candida* in any infant who develops signs of systemic infection, especially neonates with predisposing conditions (see Table 33-2). The differential diagnosis includes primarily other microorganisms responsible for nosocomial sepsis.[152] At a minimum, any infant with systemic signs of infection should have blood cultures obtained from a peripheral venipuncture and from all indwelling intravascular catheters. Most *Candida* species are identified by growth on standard bacteriologic culture media with aerobic processing, and requesting separate fungal cultures does not increase the yield of *Candida* species.[6,13] Previous recommendations were to monitor such cultures for up to 10 days to ensure adequate growth of the slower-growing *Candida* species.[4,13] However, in one report, 90% of cultures for *Candida* species were positive by 72 hours, before and immediately after the initiation of antifungal therapy.[191] Multiple or repeat blood cultures increase the likelihood of obtaining a positive result.[192] For infants with an indwelling intravascular catheter or catheters, samples obtained through each catheter and from a peripheral vessel are recommended for culture. Recovery of a *Candida* species from the culture sample obtained from an intravascular catheter and not from the peripheral blood supports the diagnosis of catheter-related candidemia without dissemination. However, caution should be used in making this distinction in neonates. First, the sensitivity of a single blood culture in diagnosing candidiasis is low; a single sterile peripheral blood culture does not exclude disseminated candidiasis.[192] Second, by the time the culture results are known (usually 24 to 48 hours after collection), dissemination might have occurred, especially in the preterm infant. Disparate results do indicate that the catheter tip is infected, and prompt removal of the catheter is indicated to prevent dissemination and other complications.

If disseminated candidiasis is suspected based on the clinical picture or a positive blood culture is obtained from a peripheral vessel, additional studies are indicated. Even after the initiation of appropriate antifungal therapy, daily blood samples should be collected until culture results are negative, because the risk for multiorgan involvement increases the longer fungemia persists.[158] Because renal and CNS candidiasis can be clinically silent at presentation, urine and CSF should be obtained for analyses and culture. The presence of budding yeast or filamentous fungal forms by microscopic examination of the urine or CSF suggests invasive disease. Because *Candida* species are frequent contaminants of nonsterilely collected urine samples, urine should be obtained by sterile urethral catheterization or suprapubic aspiration.[38,160] In clinical practice, suprapubic aspiration is infrequently performed in many NICUs, and sterile urethral catheterization is reported to be an efficient method for obtaining urine cultures from infants younger than 6 months.[193] The current consensus is that a *Candida* species UTI in neonates be defined as 10^4 or more colony-forming units of *Candida* species per 1 mL in a culture obtained by sterile urethral catheterization.[160,161] Cultures of the CSF are more likely to be positive if the volume of CSF obtained is at least 1 mL.[116] Even when an optimal volume of CSF is cultured, a negative result does not eliminate the possibility of CNS disease, because infection can occur in areas of the brain not in communication with the CSF.[116,194] Analysis of the CSF for abnormalities suggestive of inflammation, including an elevated white blood cell count or protein level or a decreased glucose level, suggests meningitis, but normal values do not exclude CNS infection.[195] Interpretation of CSF values can be complicated by the presence of blood due to a traumatic lumbar puncture or preexisting intracranial hemorrhage in the preterm infant. Cultures of other clinically suspicious sites, such as peritoneal fluid or a skin abscess or vesicle, can help to confirm the diagnosis in an ill infant. However, cultures of healthy-appearing skin and mucous membranes and cultures of endotracheal secretions are not helpful in diagnosing systemic infections. Endotracheal tube secretion cultures may not be helpful in the infant with respiratory symptoms, because *Candida* pneumonia is more often a result of hematogenous spread.[26,38,196] If any other catheters are present, such as chest or mediastinal tubes, cultures of the fluid drainage also should be obtained.

A culture from a usually sterile body site that grows *Candida* species confirms the diagnosis of candidiasis. Determination of the *Candida* species involved is equally important. Historically, because most infections were caused by *C. albicans*, many laboratories did not go beyond the initial identification of a yeast in culture as *Candida*.[19,59,197] Today, the incidence of infections with the NCAC species has increased dramatically, and identification of the species involved is important for epidemiologic and therapeutic reasons.[4,197] Knowledge of the infecting *Candida* species can help to determine whether the source of the infection is endogenous or from nosocomial transmission. This can be especially important in determining whether an apparent outbreak of candidiasis in a particular NICU is a coincidence or caused by a common source.[45,47,48,198] From the therapeutic perspective, when comparing the various pathogenic *Candida* species, variations exist in susceptibility to the common antifungal agents (Table 33-4),[33] and defining the infecting *Candida* species is important in determining appropriate antifungal therapy.

To determine the extent and severity of candidiasis, additional laboratory tests are indicated when evaluating the infant with suspected disseminated candidiasis, including a complete blood count with differential and platelet counts and determinations of the levels of serum glucose, creatinine, blood urea nitrogen, bilirubin, liver transaminases, and C-reactive protein. The white blood cell count may be normal, high, or low; however, in the neonate, neutropenia may suggest a severe, overwhelming infection.[106] Thrombocytopenia is strongly associated with systemic candidiasis and may be an early indicator of this disease.[22,150] Elevations in the blood urea nitrogen and creatinine levels may indicate

Table 33–4 General Patterns of Susceptibility of *Candida* Species to Antifungal Agents

Candida Species	Amphotericin B	Flucytosine[a]	Fluconazole	Voriconazole	Caspofungin
C. albicans	S	S	S	S	S
C. parapsilosis	S	S	S	S	S to I[b]
C. glabrata	S to I[c]	S	I to R[d]	S	S
C. tropicalis	S	S	S	S	S
C. krusei	S to I[c]	I to R	R[e]	S	S
C. lusitaniae	I to R	—	S	S	S

[a]Resistance develops rapidly when used as monotherapy.
[b]Isolates of *C. parapsilosis* have slightly higher minimal inhibitory concentrations (MIC).
[c]A significant proportion of clinical isolates of *C. glabrata* and *C. krusei* have reduced susceptibility to amphotericin B.[110]
[d]Between 10% and 45% of clinical isolates of *C. glabrata* are resistant to fluconazole.[9,110,248]
[e]*C. krusei* are intrinsically resistant to fluconazole.
I, intermediately resistant; R, resistant; S, susceptible.
Data from references 7, 110, 210, 211, 217, 248, 253.

renal infection. Mild elevations in the serum bilirubin levels may be a part of the sepsis syndrome, but marked elevations in the serum bilirubin concentration or liver enzymes indicate extensive liver involvement.[2] Elevation of the C-reactive protein level is a nonspecific indicator of systemic infection.[15,81] Unfortunately, obtaining normal values for any or all of these ancillary laboratory tests does not completely exclude the possibility of candidiasis, especially CNS disease, in the high-risk neonate.[116]

Because of the predilection of *Candida* for certain organs, specific imaging studies are indicated to diagnose the extent of dissemination. Renal ultrasonography, echocardiography, and cranial imaging are recommended for all infants with candidemia or systemic candidiasis.[158] Renal and bladder ultrasonography are extremely sensitive, but nonspecific, in their ability to define abnormalities resulting from *Candida* infections. The ultrasonographic appearance of a non-shadowing echogenic focus strongly suggests a renal fungus ball, particularly when the infant has a urine culture that grows *Candida*.[199] However, blood clots, fibrinous deposits, and nephrocalcinosis can have the same ultrasound appearance, confounding interpretation.[200] Another common ultrasonographic finding is renal parenchymal infiltration characterized by enlarged kidneys with diffusely increased echogenicity.[199] In any given infant with renal candidiasis, one or both of these ultrasound findings can be seen. Limited information exists about the accuracy of computed tomography (CT) or magnetic resonance imaging (MRI) in diagnosing renal candidiasis.[201] Echocardiography is useful in neonates with central venous catheters when the primary concern is for endocarditis with an infected thrombus at the catheter tip site or a right atrial mass.[94,151] Cranial ultrasonography easily can reveal enlarged ventricles, calcifications, cystic changes, and intraventricular fungus balls in infants with CNS candidiasis.[122,162] Ventriculitis can be diagnosed by the appearance of intraventricular septations or debris.[116] Interpretation of the cranial ultrasonography can be difficult in the preterm neonate who has experienced an intraventricular hemorrhage in the past or has developed periventricular leukomalacia. Intracranial abscesses due to *Candida* species reportedly have been mistaken for intracranial hemorrhage.[202] Cranial CT and MRI offer certain advantages over ultrasonography, including superior imaging of the posterior fossa and infratentorial and non-midline structures.[203] Calcifications are seen best with CT, and the addition of intravenous contrast can aid in the identification of intracranial abscesses. However, as a practical matter, cranial ultrasonography is more frequently used because it can be performed at the bedside of a critically ill infant. In addition to these imaging studies, all neonates with confirmed or suspected candidemia should have a dilated ophthalmologic examination, preferably by a pediatric ophthalmologist.[119,174] The infant who has characteristic lesions of *Candida* endophthalmitis has a confirmed diagnosis of disseminated disease.

Despite heightened awareness of the more subtle presentations of disseminated candidiasis and improvements in the ancillary and imaging studies available to clinicians, an accurate and timely diagnosis of candidal infections in the neonate remains a challenge. This largely reflects continued reliance on a positive culture for *Candida* species from a normally sterile body fluid (e.g., blood, urine, CSF, peritoneal fluid) or a potentially infected site to confirm the diagnosis and guide therapy. Autopsy studies suggest that the specificity of blood cultures for candidiasis approaches 100%; however, the sensitivity in the diagnosis of disseminated candidiasis is low, ranging from 30% with single organ involvement up to 80% with four or more organs involved.[192] The situation in the neonate is further complicated by the fact that fluid volumes as low as 1 mL may be obtained for culture, additionally diminishing the sensitivity—especially if the total burden of organisms in the fluid is low.[203] The development of techniques for more sensitive, reliable, and rapid diagnosis of candidal infections is a priority. A number of molecular diagnostic assays that exploit recognition of small amounts of *Candida* species proteins or DNA, including the β-glucan antigen assay, the D-arabinitol assay, and polymerase chain reaction (PCR) testing, are being evaluated in adults and older children.[204-206] None of these assays has been rigorously evaluated in a population of neonates.[115] β-1,3-D-Glucan is a major component of the fungal cell wall found in all clinically relevant *Candida* species. The assay is reported to have 85% sensitivity and specificity for candidemia by detecting very small amounts of this fungal cell wall antigen.[115] D-Arabinitol is a major metabolite of many *Candida* species (not *C. glabrata* or *C. krusei*) and can be detected by mass spectrometry in volumes as small as a single drop of blood, urine, or CSF from infected patients.[205,207,208] PCR amplification of an area of the genome common to *C. albicans* and other pathogenic *Candida* species can be successfully performed, again using very small volumes of blood, urine, or CSF.[206] Extensive use of PCR assays has been limited by unacceptably high rates of fungal contamination resulting in false-positive tests.[209] Each of these assays holds promise for the rapid detection of fungus in small volumes of body fluids and does not require the presence of live *Candida* species. One major drawback to these assays compared with culture is the lack of differentiation between pathogenic *Candida* species; the diagnosis is simply candidiasis. With specific culture results, the clinician knows which *Candida* species is causing the infection and can tailor the therapeutic plan accordingly. Without culture results, more generic management plans must be employed. However, because the institution of therapy often is delayed because of the lack of a positive culture when clinical deterioration begins, which may lead to systemic complications from persistent fungemia, knowing the neonate has a *Candida* species may lead to improved therapeutic management.

THERAPY AND MANAGEMENT

Therapy and management of candidiasis in the neonate require an effective antifungal agent coupled with appropriate supportive care and measures to eliminate factors favoring ongoing infection. In the NICU, the first two objectives are easier to achieve than the last. Multiple antifungal therapies are available, but few have been studied for determination of appropriate dose and interval, safety, and efficacy in neonates, especially VLBW infants. Amphotericin B has been the mainstay of antifungal therapy for more than 40 years, but newer agents may be indicated in certain settings.[210,211] Table 33-4 summarizes the antimicrobial susceptibility pattern of pathogenic *Candida* species to the most common antifungal agents, and Table 33-5 and the following discussion outline

Table 33–5 Systemic Antifungal Agents for the Treatment of Invasive Candidiasis in Neonates

Drug	Dose	Interval	Route	Indications	Toxicities	Toxicity Monitoring	Comments
Amphotericin B	0.5-1.0 mg/kg/day	q24h	IV	Candidemia, invasive candidiasis	Renal, hematologic, hepatic	Urine output, creatinine, potassium, magnesium, liver enzymes	Not indicated to treat *C. lusitaniae* Dose adjustment may be required for renal failure
Lipid-associated amphotericin B preparations	3-5 mg/kg/day	q24h	IV	Invasive candidiasis with severe preexisting renal insufficiency	Similar to amphotericin B	Urine output, creatinine, potassium, magnesium, liver enzymes	May be indicated in patients failing therapy or requiring higher doses
Flucytosine	50-100 mg/kg/day	q12-24h	PO	For therapy in combination with amphotericin B for CNS infection	Renal, cardiac, hematologic, gastrointestinal, hepatic	Serum levels of liver enzymes, complete blood cell count with differential count	Desired serum levels, 40-60 μg/mL; bone marrow toxicity can be severe; excellent CSF penetration
Fluconazole	6-12 mg/kg/day	<7 d,[a] q72h 7-14 d, q48h >14 d, q24h	PO, IV	Alternative therapy to amphotericin B for localized urinary tract infection; mucocutaneous disease	Hepatic, gastrointestinal	Liver enzymes	Excellent CSF penetration; oral formulation well absorbed; not indicated to treat *C. krusei* or *C. glabrata*

[a]Age in days.
CNS, central nervous system; CSF, cerebrospinal fluid; IV, intravenous; PO, oral.
Data from references 210, 211, 217.

important features regarding use of each agent in the neonate with candidiasis. Because candidiasis often is a nosocomially acquired infection, most infected infants are already in the NICU, where appropriate intensive care to support these critically ill infants is readily available. If the hospital nursery is unable to address the needs of a critically ill neonate, transfer to a higher-level NICU should be considered. Unfortunately, the elimination of all risk factors for ongoing candidemia often is an unattainable goal, and the clinician frequently must settle for a less than optimal reduction of risk factors.

With the diagnosis of candidemia or disseminated candidiasis, immediate consideration should be given to the removal of all potentially contaminated medical hardware—especially central intravascular catheters. For ongoing fungemia, successful medical treatment of *Candida* species infections while the catheters remain in place is rare.[24,95,118] The risk of dissemination also increases with every day the infant remains fungemic, as does the rate of infection of previously uninfected intravascular lines.[118] The clinician must face the reality that most preterm infants with systemic candidiasis *require* central access because of the clinical instability directly attributable to the ongoing candidemia, which in large part is caused by the ongoing presence of the infected catheter. If not all lines can be removed, removal of a potentially infected catheter with insertion of a new line at a different site or a sequential reduction in the number of catheters is preferable to inaction. Infants with more than one catheter may not have all lines infected at the time of diagnosis, and removal of the catheter known or most likely to be infected may resolve the problem and allow continued therapy through the remaining line.[96] Antifungal therapy should be administered through the remaining central catheter to maximize drug delivery to a potential site of ongoing infection. Daily blood cultures to determine whether fungemia is persistent and whether additional infected catheters should be removed are necessary. Consideration should be given to surgical resection of infected tissue if antifungal therapy does not achieve sterilization (e.g., urine) or if mechanical complications caused by the presence of a fungus ball arise (e.g., right atrial mass). Although successful medical therapy for endocarditis caused by *Candida* species can often be achieved, large right atrial masses are almost impossible to sterilize and may also compromise hemodynamic function, necessitating surgical removal.[94,96,151,212] Surgical removal of an enlarging right atrial candidal mass in the face of ongoing fungemia and hemodynamic instability may be lifesaving for the premature infant.[151] Most renal fungal balls can be treated medically because of the high levels of most antifungal agents attained in the urine.[153,161] However, in an infant with complete obstruction of urinary flow caused by the presence of one or more fungal balls, surgical removal is indicated.[163,164,166] Hyperglycemia can be avoided by judicious administration of dextrose and insulin therapy if glucose intolerance persists. Corticosteroid therapy should be avoided or tapered as tolerated.

Antifungal Agents

Topical Antifungal Therapy

Topical antifungal agents are indicated for thrush, diaper dermatitis, and uncomplicated congenital candidiasis in the term infant.[100] Nystatin, the most commonly used topical therapy, is a polyene drug that is not absorbed by the gastrointestinal tract, making it a topical agent in any of the three common formulations: oral suspension, ointment, or powder. The oral suspension is indicated for the treatment of thrush in patients of all ages. However, because of the high osmolality of the oral suspension (caused by the added sucrose expedient), care should be taken and use limited in the very premature infant or the neonate with compromise of the gastrointestinal tract.[113] Reports of clinical cure vary widely, from as low as 30% to as high as 85%.[113,134] Nystatin should be applied directly to the lesions of oral thrush. If swallowed rapidly, there is minimal contact with the lesions and little efficacy. Nystatin ointment or powder, when applied to diaper dermatitis, has an 85% cure rate.[113] Because thrush often accompanies diaper dermatitis, many clinicians add oral nystatin when prescribing perineal therapy, even if no oral lesions exist. Data suggest no added efficacy with this practice, which should be discouraged.[113,213] If oral lesions are present, treatment is indicated. However, if oral lesions are not present, the source of the *Candida* species probably is the lower gastrointestinal tract, in which nystatin is not an optimal agent.

Miconazole gel is a nonabsorbable formulation of this azole, developed particularly for treatment of thrush, which is not available in the United States.[214,215] The gel formulation is said to offer more prolonged contact with the oral lesions and has a reported efficacy of greater than 90%.[113,214,215] Side effects predominantly are gastrointestinal, similar to nystatin, but use of this agent has been evaluated only in a limited number of preterm infants.[113,215] Miconazole creams and ointments, as well as other topical azole formulations, frequently are prescribed for diaper dermatitis with excellent results.[214,216]

Gentian violet, the first topical therapy for oral thrush, has become the treatment of last resort. Although effective, the liquid treatment must be applied directly to the lesions, and it causes unsightly dark purple stains on the infant's mouth, clothes, bedclothes, and often on the hands and clothes of the care provider. Complications include local irritation and ulceration from the direct application of the treatment to adjacent normal mucosa.[113] Given these inconveniences, most clinicians avoid gentian violet in favor of administering systemic therapy when topical treatments fail.[134]

Systemic Antifungal Therapy

AMPHOTERICIN B

Amphotericin B deoxycholate is a polyene antifungal agent available since the 1960s. The American Academy of Pediatrics Committee on Infectious Diseases, the Pediatric Infectious Disease Society (PIDS), and the Infectious Disease Society of America (IDSA) recommend amphotericin B as the primary antifungal agent for the treatment of candidemia, disseminated candidiasis, and any form of invasive candidiasis in the neonate.[211,217,218] Most pathogenic *Candida* species are susceptible to amphotericin B (see Table 33-4). However, reports suggest a proportion of *C. glabrata* and *C. krusei* isolates have a somewhat reduced susceptibility to amphotericin B, and resistance has been described for isolates of *C. lusitaniae*.[9,110,217,219]

Amphotericin B acts by binding to ergosterol in the fungal cell membrane, altering cell permeability with subsequent depolarization and leakage of cytoplasmic contents, eventually leading to cell death. Although amphotericin B has a higher affinity for ergosterol than the cholesterol in human cell membranes, toxicity is a risk with this drug. Neonates tolerate the drug well with minimal toxicity.[220,221] Toxicities reported in neonates receiving amphotericin B include renal insufficiency with occasional renal failure, hypokalemia and hypomagnesemia caused by excessive renal losses, bone marrow suppression with anemia and thrombocytopenia, and abnormalities in hepatic enzymes.[195,222] Most toxicities are dose dependent and reversible on cessation of therapy.[222] Nephrotoxicity is the most common and worrisome toxic effect. A substantial rise in creatinine and decrease in urine output can be observed; however, it is frequently difficult to differentiate between renal insufficiency caused by inadequately treated systemic candidiasis and that due to amphotericin B. Although there is a potential for renal failure, most infants display no or mild nephrotoxicity that resolves with decreasing the dose of amphotericin B or after completion of therapy. A common and very uncomfortable side effect in adults and older children receiving amphotericin B is an infusion-related reaction consisting of fever, chills, nausea, headache, and occasional hypotension.[221] No such toxicity has been described in neonates.[210,220,221] Any neonate receiving amphotericin B should have serial monitoring of serum potassium and magnesium levels and of renal, liver, and bone marrow function.

Amphotericin B is not water soluble and is available only as an intravenous preparation. In neonates, there is a tremendous variability in the half-life, clearance, and peak serum concentrations after dosing.[210,220,221] Treatment success in neonates has been documented at doses of 0.5 to 1.5 mg/kg/day.[220,223-225] Most clinicians initiate therapy with a dose of 0.5 mg/kg and increase it to 1.0 mg/kg given once daily if no significant toxicity occurs. Dosing may need to be adjusted in the infant with preexisting renal insufficiency.[217] Doses greater than 1.0 mg/kg daily rarely are needed for treating *Candida* species infections. The test dose, historically given to adults to determine the need for medication to ameliorate infusion-related symptoms, is not required in neonates. The risk for dissemination is so high among infants that no delay should occur in delivering treatment doses.

Although excellent plasma levels and tissue penetration occur with this dosing regimen for amphotericin B, CSF penetration is variable. In adults, CSF concentrations of amphotericin B are only 5% to 10% of plasma levels.[217] Neonatal CSF concentrations of amphotericin B generally are higher but more variable, ranging from 40% to 90% of plasma levels in one study of preterm infants.[226] The higher CSF concentrations that are achieved in neonates than adults possibly are related to the immature blood-brain barrier. However, the variability in concentrations suggests to some clinicians that amphotericin B as a single agent for the treatment of neonatal CNS infections may be ineffective. Fluconazole and 5-flucytosine penetrate the CSF well and can provide synergy with amphotericin B in killing some *Candida* species, especially *C. albicans*. Combinations of one or both of these agents with amphotericin B have resulted in successful treatment of CNS candidiasis in infants in whom single therapy alone was unsuccessful.[168,225,227] Successful treatment of CNS disease with amphotericin monotherapy also has been reported.[195,220,223] Systemic amphotericin may not be necessary in the few infants with isolated bladder candidal infection. In rare cases, bladder instillation of amphotericin B, alone or in combination with fluconazole, has been successfully used to treat infants with isolated cystitis or urinary tract fungal balls.[161,228]

AMPHOTERICIN B LIPID FORMULATIONS

As an alternative to standard amphotericin B, three lipid-associated formulations are approved for use in adults: liposomal amphotericin B (L-AmB), amphotericin B lipid complex (ABLC), and amphotericin B cholesterol sulfate complex (ABCD). Fungal susceptibility patterns for these lipid-associated formulations are the same as for conventional amphotericin B deoxycholate.[229-231] Each is significantly more expensive than conventional amphotericin B.[211] The main purported advantage to these amphotericin B preparations is the ability to deliver a higher dose of medication with lower levels of toxicity. In adults and older children receiving a lipid-formulation of amphotericin B, significantly lower rates of infusion-related reactions and creatinine elevations are reported compared with conventional amphotericin B.[232] Several case reports of successful use of these preparations in neonates have been published, but almost no controlled studies have been performed.[230,231,233,234] Three studies of liposomal amphotericin B that have included neonates demonstrated no major adverse events, diminished toxicities associated with conventional amphotericin (i.e., hypokalemia and hyperbilirubinemia), and treatment success rates of 70% to 100%.[229,235,236] Two studies of ABLC in pediatric patients have included small numbers of neonates and demonstrated efficacy rates of 75% to 85%, with no significant toxicities.[230,231] CNS penetration may be better with these preparations in adult patients, but there are no data for neonates to support this claim.[231] Renal penetration of the lipid-associated formulations is poor compared with conventional amphotericin, and treatment failure at this site of infection has been reported.[154,227,232]

Although randomized, controlled trials of the lipid-associated preparations in neonates are lacking, available information suggests that they may be safe and effective, although not superior to conventional amphotericin B. Treatment with amphotericin B deoxycholate remains the most appropriate therapy for infants with invasive infections with *Candida* species, especially for those with renal infection.[211,217,218] The amphotericin B lipid formulations may have a role in the treatment of invasive candidiasis in neonates with preexisting severe renal disease or infants who fail to respond to conventional amphotericin B *after* removal of all intravascular catheters, but more data are needed.

FLUOROCYTOSINE

5-Flucytosine (5-FC) is a fluorine analogue of cytosine. The antifungal activity of 5-FC is based on its conversion to 5-fluorouracil, which inhibits thymidylate synthetase, disrupting DNA synthesis. This mechanism of action is not fungal specific, and significant host toxicities are reported in adults.[211] All pathogenic *Candida* species are susceptible to this agent, but resistance develops rapidly when used as monotherapy (see Table 33-4).[237] 5-FC has excellent CNS penetration and is used primarily in combination with amphotericin B in the treatment of neonatal CNS candidiasis because early studies demonstrated synergy with these two agents.[168,225,237] However, reports suggest no added therapeutic benefit when 5-FC is combined with amphotericin B.[211,220,238] The potential benefit of 5-FC added to amphotericin B must be weighed against potentially significant toxicities when considering the use of this agent. Flucytosine is available only in an enteral form, limiting its use in most critically ill neonates with systemic candidiasis.

AZOLES

The azoles are a class of synthetic fungistatic agents that inhibit fungal growth through inhibition of the fungal cytochrome P-450 system.[239] This action is not fungal specific, and interactions with the host cytochrome P-450 system can cause alterations in the pharmacokinetics of concomitant medications the infant is receiving and produce hepatotoxicity. Clinical hepatotoxicity is rare with use of the newer azoles, such as fluconazole and voriconazole, in adults and older children, and their overall safety profile is favorable.[240] However, monitoring of transaminases in patients receiving azoles is recommended.[210] The development of fungal resistance is a significant concern with this class of antifungal agents (see Table 33-4).[8]

Fluconazole, the azole used most frequently in neonates, is water soluble, available in oral or intravenous preparations, and highly bioavailable in the neonate.[210,241] Fluconazole has a long plasma half-life, with excellent levels achieved in the blood, CSF, brain, liver, spleen, and especially the kidneys, where it is excreted unchanged in the urine.[242] The pharmacokinetics of fluconazole in neonates change dramatically over the first weeks of life, presumably because of increased renal clearance with maturity; therefore, the dosing interval is based on postnatal age (see Table 33-5).[242,243] Transient thrombocytopenia, elevations in creatinine, mild hyperbilirubinemia, and transient increases in liver transaminases have been documented in neonates.[29,242,244]

Several studies have shown fluconazole to be efficacious in the treatment of invasive candidiasis in the neonate. In one prospective, randomized trial of amphotericin B, rates of survival and clearance of the organism were equivalent for both treatment groups.[245-247] Infants treated with fluconazole had less renal and hepatic toxicity and had a shorter time to the complete removal of central intravascular catheters, which was attributed to the ability to convert to oral therapy for completion of the treatment course.[245] Although these features make the use of fluconazole appear quite attractive, the primary concern with fluconazole is the potential for fungi to develop resistance.[248] Although most pathogenic *Candida* species are susceptible to fluconazole, *C. krusei* is intrinsically resistant to this azole, as are up to 50% of *C. glabrata* isolates (see Table 33-4).[110, 248,249] Both of these NCAC species can cause neonatal disease; therefore, the use of fluconazole as primary single therapy is not recommended. The IDSA guidelines recommend the administration of fluconazole as an alternative therapy to amphotericin B for disseminated, invasive neonatal candidiasis or congenital candidiasis with systemic signs after the pathogenic *Candida* species is identified and susceptibility determination completed.[216] Because of its unaltered renal clearance, fluconazole is an excellent choice for the treatment of isolated urinary tract infections resulting from susceptible *Candida* species, and oral fluconazole is an alternative therapy in refractory mucocutaneous disease.[134,241,243]

Voriconazole is a second-generation azole, derived from fluconazole, with increased potency and a broader spectrum of activity (see Table 33-4).[250] Voriconazole is active in vitro against all clinically relevant *Candida* species, including *C. krusei* and *C. glabrata,* and no resistance by fluconazole-resistant strains has been seen.[9,251] Voriconazole is metabolized by the liver, and the only clinically significant adverse event reported in adults is the occurrence of visual disturbances.[250] No data are available on the safety or efficacy of this drug in neonates, and until such information becomes available, this agent should not be used in neonates.

CASPOFUNGIN

Caspofungin is the first of the echinocandin class of antifungal agents approved for use in adults in the United States. This class of drugs acts by a unique and completely fungal-specific mechanism, inhibition of the synthesis of β-1,3-D-glucan, an essential component of the fungal cell wall.[252] Because there is no mammalian equivalent to the fungal cell wall, the safety profile for the echinocandin is excellent.[252] Caspofungin is water soluble but available only as an intravenous formulation that is incompatible with dextrose. Caspofungin is fungicidal against all pathogenic *Candida* species. Concerns have been raised that *C. parapsilosis* may be less susceptible to this drug based on in vitro testing, but clinical response to invasive disease in adults has been excellent.[253] No data exist on the pharmacokinetics, safety, or efficacy of caspofungin in neonates with invasive candidiasis. Two case reports suggest safety and efficacy. Despite this lack of data, the IDSA recommends caspofungin as a second-line agent for neonatal candidemia without dissemination.[216] Until suitable information providing appropriate doses and regimens of this agent in VLBW neonates becomes available, caspofungin should not be employed in preterm neonates. If caspofungin proves to be as safe and effective as it has in adults, clinicians could have the ability to combine antifungal agents with different general mechanisms of action to optimize therapeutic efficacy.

Length of Therapy

No matter which antifungal therapy is chosen, the length of therapy to adequately treat invasive neonatal candidiasis is prolonged (see Table 33-3). There are no controlled clinical trials to provide the optimal length of therapy for any of the antifungal agents. The IDSA recommends a minimum of 14 to 21 days of systemic therapy after negative blood, urine, and CSF culture results have been obtained along with resolution of clinical findings.[217] Case series employing amphotericin B suggest that a cumulative dose of 25 to 30 mg/kg be administered (estimated at a mean of 4 weeks).[2,220] Therapy for endocarditis typically lasts 6 weeks.[217] In neonates with isolated *Candida* cystitis, fluconazole at a dose of 6 mg/kg given once daily for 7 days appears to be adequate. Therapy must be administered intravenous initially, but in an infant who responds to fluconazole, completion of the course with oral therapy is acceptable.[243] Infants with fungal abscesses, renal lesions, intracranial lesions, or right atrial fungal masses should have sonographic or radiographic evidence of resolution before completing therapy.[199,210] Close monitoring for relapse after the cessation of therapy is necessary given the high rate of recurrence, especially in infants with CNS disease.[17,116,176]

PROGNOSIS

Despite the current advances in neonatal care and antifungal therapy, the prognosis for the infant who develops an invasive fungal infection is still quite variable but generally poor. Morality rates range from 20% to 50%, with significant accompanying morbidity.[108,131,254] Factors determining the final prognosis include the degree of prematurity, extent of dissemination, severity of illness, and the rapidity of institution of appropriate antifungal and supportive therapy.[255] Infants with isolated catheter-related candidal infections, uncomplicated urinary tract infections, or candidemia without dissemination tend to have a good outcome with the potential for complete recovery and no sequelae. Infants with extreme prematurity, widely disseminated disease, multiorgan involvement, renal or hepatic failure, and ophthalmologic or CNS infection have a much worse prognosis. In studies of VLBW infants surviving candidemia, disseminated candidiasis, or candidal meningitis, candidiasis survivors were significantly more likely to have a major neurologic abnormality (40% to 60% versus 11% to 25%) and a subnormal (<70) Mental Developmental Index (40% versus 14%) than noninfected infants of the same gestational age and birth weight.[108,121] In a series of ELBW neonates with disseminated candidiasis, including meningitis, Friedman and colleagues[256] found a higher incidence of chronic lung disease (100% versus 33%), periventricular leukomalacia (26% versus 12%), severe ROP (22% versus 9%), and adverse neurologic outcomes at 2 years' corrected age (60% versus 35%) for infected infants than for gestational age– and birth weight–matched, noninfected controls. Among the infected neonates with adverse neurologic outcomes, 41% had severe disabilities, compared with 12% of the control infants, and all infants with parenchymal brain lesions diagnosed by cranial ultrasonography at the time of candidiasis had poor neurologic outcomes.[24] The visual outcome after endophthalmitis is generally good after provision of appropriate systemic antifungal therapy. Only a small percentage of infants have significant visual impairment, although most have some decrease in visual acuity.[119] Severe ROP has developed in preterm infants who recovered from candidiasis but never had endophthalmitis.[180,183] These infants may require laser surgery and may be at significant risk for vision loss.[180] Great strides have been made in our ability to diagnose and treat invasive candidiasis, but we must strive to continue to improve therapeutic management and address the issues of morbidity.

PREVENTION

The old adage that "an ounce of prevention is worth a pound of cure" could never be truer than when considering neonatal candidiasis. Treatment is difficult, prolonged, and avoids mortality and morbidity little more than one half of the time. The development of strategies to prevent neonatal candidal infections should be a priority on the NICU. Many of the factors listed in Table 33-2 that enhance the risk for candidiasis are unavoidable, such as prematurity and low birth weight, but every attempt should be made to address conditions that can be reduced, starting with exposure to the yeast itself. Appropriate diagnosis and treatment of maternal candidal vaginosis and urinary tract infections during pregnancy may decrease vertical transmission.[217] Prevention of horizontal transmission from caregivers by the use of good hand hygiene and gloves has resulted in limited success.[28,256] In studies of health care workers, appropriate hand hygiene is helpful in reducing superficial and transient flora, but it does not affect deep and permanent flora overall, with no significant reduction in the recovery of *C. albicans* detected after antimicrobial or alcohol washes.[257-261] Elimination of artificial fingernails among care providers and the judicious use of gloves may reduce exposure and transmission.[45] The meticulous care of long-term indwelling catheters is recommended, especially if used to administer hyperalimentation.

Reduction in exposures to medications associated with neonatal candidiasis is an important part of prevention. Broad-spectrum antibiotic therapy and the postnatal use of hydrocortisone and dexamethasone are associated with fungal sepsis.[7,89,179,256] Two separate multicenter trials have shown an association between heavy levels of gastrointestinal tract colonization with *Candida* species and exposure to third-generation cephalosporins or H_2 antagonists.[7,256] Both medications alter the enteric microenvironment, favoring fungal colonization and potential dissemination. The use of topical petrolatum ointment in skin care of the ELBW infant is associated with a significantly increased incidence of invasive candidal infections.[262] Although attempts at providing good skin care to prevent epidermal breakdown in the ELBW infant are laudable, the use of petrolatum ointment does not appear to be the best choice, and the increased risk of infection appears to outweigh any potential benefits.

Chemoprophylaxis with antifungal agents such as oral nystatin and fluconazole has had variable success. The use of oral nystatin is tolerated well by neonates, with no fungal resistance documented, but efficacy in preventing invasive infection is not consistently achieved.[147] A randomized, placebo-controlled trial of intravenous fluconazole prophylaxis for the first 6 weeks of life was effective in decreasing colonization and invasive infection due to *Candida* species only in the subpopulation of ELBW preterm infants with an indwelling vascular catheter or endotracheal tube.[29] Significant concerns remain about the risk of developing azole-resistant *Candida* species with prolonged exposure to fluconazole.[33,251] An increase in the number of fluconazole-resistant *C. parapsilosis* isolates colonizing neonates was identified after the institution of a fluconazole prophylaxis program for ELBW infants.[244] Additional studies are indicated to explore the use of novel therapies for the prevention of *Candida* species colonization and systemic disease.

REFERENCES

1. Pfaller MA. Nosocomial candidiasis: emerging species, reservoirs, and modes of transmission. Clin Infect Dis 22:S89-S94, 1996.
2. Butler KM, Baker CJ. *Candida*: an increasingly important pathogen in the nursery. Pediatr Clin North Am 35:543-563, 1988.
3. Rangel-Frausto MS, Wiblin T, Blumberg HM, et al. National Epidemiology of Mycoses Survey (NEMIS): variations in rates of bloodstream infections due to *Candida* species in seven surgical intensive care units and six neonatal intensive care units. Clin Infect Dis 29:253-258, 1999.
4. Bendel CM, Hostetter MK. Systemic candidiasis and other fungal infections in the newborn. Semin Pediatr Infect Dis 5:35-41, 1994.

5. Stoll BJ, Hansen N. Infections in VLBW infants: studies from the NICHD Neonatal Research Network. Semin Perinatol 27:293-301, 2003.
6. Kossoff EH, Buescher ES, Karlowicz MG. Candidemia in a neonatal intensive care unit: trends during fifteen years and clinical features of 111 cases. Pediatr Infect Dis J 17:504-508, 1998.
7. Saiman L, Ludington E, Pfaller M, et al. Risk factors for candidemia in neonatal intensive care unit patients. The National Epidemiology of Mycosis Survey study group. Pediatr Infect Dis J 19:319-324, 2000.
8. Faix RG. Invasive neonatal candidiasis: comparison of albicans and parapsilosis infection. Pediatr Infect Dis J 11:88-93, 1992.
9. Pfaller MA, Diekema DJ, Jones RN, et al. Trends in antifungal susceptibility of *Candida* spp. isolated from pediatric and adult patients with bloodstream infections: SENTRY Antimicrobial Surveillance Program, 1997 to 2000. J Clin Microbiol 40:852-856, 2002.
10. Lemons JA, Bauer CR, Oh W, et al. Very low birth weight outcomes of the National Institute of Child Health and Human Development Neonatal Research Network, January 1995 through December 1996. NICHD Neonatal Research Network. Pediatrics 107:E1, 2001.
11. Cole GT, Halawa AA, Anaissie EJ. The role of the gastrointestinal tract in hematogenous candidiasis: from the laboratory to the bedside. Clin Infect Dis 22:S73-88, 1996.
12. Eubanks PJ, de Virgilio C, Klein S, et al. *Candida* sepsis in surgical patients. Am J Surg 166:617-619, 1993.
13. Emori TG, Gaynes RP. An overview of nosocomial infections, including the role of the microbiology laboratory. Clin Microbiol Rev 6:428-442, 1993.
14. Richards MJ, Edwards JR, Culver DH, et al. Nosocomial infections in medical intensive care units in the United States. National Nosocomial Infections Surveillance System. Crit Care Med 27:887-892, 1999.
15. Polin RA. The "ins and outs" of neonatal sepsis. J Pediatr 143:3-4, 2003.
16. Stoll BJ, Hansen N, Fanaroff AA, et al. Changes in pathogens causing early-onset sepsis in very-low-birth-weight infants. N Engl J Med 347:240-247, 2002.
17. Chapman RL, Faix RG. Invasive neonatal candidiasis: an overview. Semin Perinatol 27:352-356, 2003.
18. Bendel CM, St. Sauver J, Carlson S, et al. Epithelial adhesion in yeast species: correlation with surface expression of the integrin analog. J Infect Dis 171:1660-1663, 1995.
19. Pfaller MA, Jones RN, Doern GV, et al. Bloodstream infections due to *Candida* species: SENTRY antimicrobial surveillance program in North America and Latin America, 1997-1998. Antimicrob Agents Chemother 44:747-751, 2000.
20. Pfaller MA, Jones RN, Doern GV, et al. International surveillance of blood stream infections due to *Candida* species in the European SENTRY program: species distribution and antifungal susceptibility including the investigational triazole and echinocandin agents. SENTRY Participant Group (Europe). Diagn Microbiol Infect Dis 35:19-25, 1999.
21. Trick WE, Fridkin SK, Edwards JR, et al. Secular trend of hospital-acquired candidemia among intensive care unit patients in the United States during 1989-1999. Clin Infect Dis 35:627-630, 2002.
22. Fairchild KD, Tomkoria S, Sharp EC, et al. Neonatal *Candida glabrata* sepsis: clinical and laboratory features compared with other *Candida* species. Pediatr Infect Dis J 21:39-43, 2002.
23. El-Mohandes AE, Johnson-Robbins L, Keiser JF, et al. Incidence of *Candida parapsilosis* colonization in an intensive care nursery population and its association with invasive fungal disease. Pediatr Infect Dis J 13:520-524, 1994.
24. Benjamin DK Jr, Ross K, McKinney RE Jr, et al. When to suspect fungal infection in neonates: a clinical comparison of *Candida albicans* and *Candida parapsilosis* fungemia with coagulase-negative staphylococcal bacteremia. Pediatrics 106:712-718, 2000.
25. Rowen JL, Rench MA, Kozinetz CA, et al. Endotracheal colonization with *Candida* enhances risk of systemic candidiasis in very low birth weight neonates. J Pediatr 124:789-794, 1994.
26. Baley JE, Kliegman RM, Boxerbaum B, et al. Fungal colonization in the very low birth weight infant. Pediatrics 78:225-232, 1986.
27. Pfaller M, Wenzel R. Impact of the changing epidemiology of fungal infections in the 1990s. Eur J Clin Microbiol Infect Dis 11:287-291, 1992.
28. Huang YC, Lin TY, Peng HL, et al. Outbreak of *Candida albicans* fungaemia in a neonatal intensive care unit. Scand J Infect Dis 30: 137-142, 1998.
29. Kaufman D, Boyle R, Hazen KC, et al. Fluconazole prophylaxis against fungal colonization and infection in preterm infants. N Engl J Med 345:1660-1666, 2001.
30. Waggoner-Fountain LA, Walker MW, Hollis RJ, et al. Vertical and horizontal transmission of unique *Candida* species to premature newborns. Clin Infect Dis 22:803-808, 1996.
31. Kozinn PJ, Taschdjian CL, Weiner H. Incidence and pathogenesis of neonatal candidiasis. Pediatrics 21:421-429, 1958.
32. Bendel CM. Colonization and epithelial adhesion in the pathogenesis of neonatal candidiasis. Semin Perinatol 27:357-364, 2003.
33. Rowen JL, Tate JM, Nordoff N, et al. *Candida* isolates from neonates: frequency of misidentification and reduced fluconazole susceptibility. J Clin Microbiol 37:3735-3737, 1999.
34. Carlson S, Hostetter M, Finkel D, et al. Genotypic and functional analysis of *Candida albicans* strains from mother-infant pairs. Pediatr Res 35:295A, 1994.
35. Johnson DE, Thompson TR, Ferrieri P. Congenital candidiasis. Am J Dis Child 135:273-275, 1981.
36. Dvorak AM, Gavaller B. Congenital systemic candidiasis. Report of a case. N Engl J Med 274:540-543, 1966.
37. Gonzalez Ochoa A, Dominguez L. Various epidemiological and pathogenic findings on oral moniliasis in newborn infants. Rev Inst Salubr Enferm Trop 17:1-12, 1957.
38. Baley JE. Neonatal candidiasis: the current challenge. Clin Perinatol 18:263-280, 1991.
39. Warnock DW. Typing of *Candida albicans*. J Hosp Infect 5:244-252, 1984.
40. Fidel PL Jr, Vazquez JA, Sobel JD. *Candida glabrata*: review of epidemiology, pathogenesis, and clinical disease with comparison to *C. albicans*. Clin Microbiol Rev 12:80-96, 1999.
41. Hedderwick SA, Lyons MJ, Liu M, et al. Epidemiology of yeast colonization in the intensive care unit. Eur J Clin Microbiol Infect Dis 19:663-670, 2000.
42. Sherertz RJ, Gledhill KS, Hampton KD, et al. Outbreak of *Candida* bloodstream infections associated with retrograde medication administration in a neonatal intensive care unit. J Pediatr 120:455-461, 1992.
43. Fox BC, Mobley HL, Wade JC. The use of a DNA probe for epidemiological studies of candidiasis in immunocompromised hosts. J Infect Dis 159:488-494, 1989.
44. White MH. Epidemiology of invasive candidiasis: recent progress and current controversies. Int J Infect Dis 1:S7-S10, 1997.
45. Reef SE, Lasker BA, Butcher DS, et al. Nonperinatal nosocomial transmission of *Candida albicans* in a neonatal intensive care unit: prospective study. J Clin Microbiol 36:1255-1259, 1998.
46. Boyce JM, Pittet D. Guideline for hand hygiene in health-care settings: recommendations of the Healthcare Infection Control Practices Advisory Committee and the HICPAC/SHEA/APIC/IDSA Hand Hygiene Task Force. Infect Control Hosp Epidemiol 23:S3-S40, 2002.
47. Vaudry WL, Tierney AJ, Wenman WM. Investigation of a cluster of systemic *Candida albicans* infections in a neonatal intensive care unit. J Infect Dis 158:1375-1379, 1988.
48. Solomon SL, Alexander H, Eley JW, et al. Nosocomial fungemia in neonates associated with intravascular pressure-monitoring devices. Pediatr Infect Dis J 5:680-685, 1986.
49. Yagupsky P. Interpretation of blood culture results. Infect Control Hosp Epidemiol 13:693, 1992.
50. St-Germain G, Laverdiere M. *Torulopsis candida*, a new opportunistic pathogen. J Clin Microbiol 24:884-885, 1986.
51. Sullivan D, Coleman D. *Candida dubliniensis*: characteristics and identification. J Clin Microbiol 36:329-334, 1998.
52. Calderone RA. Taxonomy and biology of *Candida*. *In* RA Calderone (ed). *Candida* and Candidiasis. Washington, DC, ASM Press, 2002, pp 15-28.
53. Moran GP, Sullivan DJ, Coleman DC. Emergence of non-*Candida albicans Candida* species as pathogens. *In* RA Calderone (ed). *Candida* and Candidiasis. Washington, DC, ASM Press, 2002, pp 37-54.
54. Schauer F, Hanschke R. Taxonomy and ecology of the genus *Candida*. Mycoses 42:12-21, 1999.
55. San-Blas G, Travassos LR, Fries BC, et al. Fungal morphogenesis and virulence. Med Mycol 38:79-86, 2000.
56. Bendel CM, Kinneberg KM, Jechorek RP, et al. Systemic infection following intravenous inoculation of mice with *Candida albicans* int1 mutant strains. Mol Genet Metab 67:343-351, 1999.
57. Bendel CM, Wiesner SM, Garni RM, et al. Cecal colonization and systemic spread of *Candida albicans* in mice treated with antibiotics and dexamethasone. Pediatr Res 51:290-295, 2002.
58. Bendel CM, Hess DJ, Garni RM, et al. Comparative virulence of *Candida albicans* yeast and filamentous forms in orally and intravenously inoculated mice. Crit Care Med 31:501-507, 2003.

59. Odds FC. *Candida* species and virulence. ASM News 60:313-318, 1994.
60. Calderone RA, Fonzi WA. Virulence factors of *Candida albicans*. Trends Microbiol 9:327-335, 2001.
61. Gale CA, Bendel CM, McClellan M, et al. Linkage of adhesion, filamentous growth, and virulence in *Candida albicans* to a single gene, INT1. Science 279:1355-1358, 1998.
62. Braun B, Johnson AD. Control of filament formation in *Candida albicans* by the transcriptional repressor TUP1. Science 277:105-109, 1997.
63. Lo HJ, Kohler JR, DiDominico B. Non-filamentous C. albicans mutants are avirulent. Cell 90:939-949, 1997.
64. Stabb JF, Sundstrom P. Genetic organization and sequence analysis of the hyphae-specific cell wall protein gene HWP1 of *Candida albicans*. Yeast 14:682-686, 1998.
65. Hoyer LL. The ALS gene family of *Candida albicans*. Trends Microbiol 9:176-180, 2001.
66. Critchley IA, Douglas LJ. Differential adhesion of pathogenic *Candida* species to epithelial and inert surfaces. FEMS Microbiol Lett 28: 199-203, 1985.
67. Cutler JE. Putative virulence factors of *Candida albicans*. Ann Rev Microbiol 45:187-218, 1991.
68. Calderone RA, Linehan L, Wadsworth E. Identification of C3d receptors on *Candida albicans*. Infect Immun 56:252-258, 1998.
69. Fukazawa T, Kagaya K. Molecular basis of adhesion of *Candida albicans*. J Med Vet Mycol 35:87-89, 1997.
70. Gustafson KS, Vercellotti GM, Bendel CM, et al. Molecular mimicry in *Candida albicans*: role of an integrin analogue in adhesion of the yeast to human endothelium. J Clin Invest 87:1896-1902, 1991.
71. Wiesner SM, Bendel CM, Hess DJ, et al. Adherence of yeast and filamentous forms of *Candida albicans* to cultured enterocytes. Crit Care Med 30:677-683, 2002.
72. Hostetter MK. New insights into candidal infections. Adv Pediatr 43:209-230, 1996.
73. Hostetter MK. Adhesins and ligands involved in the interaction of *Candida* spp. with epithelial and endothelial surfaces. Clin Microbiol Rev 7:29-42, 1994.
74. Hawser SP, Douglas LJ. Biofilm formation by *Candida* species on the surface of catheter materials in vitro. Infect Immun 62:915-921, 1994.
75. Hawser SP, Baillie GS, Douglas LJ. Production of extracellular matrix by *Candida albicans* biofilms. J Med Microbiol 47:253-256, 1998.
76. Baillie GS, Douglas LJ. *Candida* biofilms and their susceptibility to antifungal agents. Methods Enzymol 310:644-656, 1999.
77. Baillie GS, Douglas LJ. Role of dimorphism in the development of *Candida albicans* biofilms. J Med Microbiol 48:671-679, 1999.
78. Faix RG, Kovarik SM. Polymicrobial sepsis among intensive care nursery infants. J Perinatol 9:131-136, 1989.
79. Klotz SA, Smith RL. A fibronectin receptor on *Candida albicans* mediates adherence of the fungus to extracellular matrix. J Infect Dis 163:604-610, 1991.
80. Bendel CM, Hostetter MK. Distinct mechanisms of epithelial adhesion for *Candida albicans* and *Candida tropicalis*: identification of the participating ligands and development of inhibitory peptides. J Clin Invest 92:1840-1849, 1993.
81. Brieland J, Essig D, Jackson C, et al. Comparison of pathogenesis and host immune responses to *Candida glabrata* and *Candida albicans* in systemically infected immunocompetent mice. Infect Immun 69:5046-5055, 2001.
82. Pappu-Katikaneni LD, Rao KP, Banister E. Gastrointestinal colonization with yeast species and *Candida* septicemia in very low birth weight infants. Mycoses 33:20-23, 1990.
83. Thong YH, Ferrante A. Alternative pathway of complement activation by *Candida albicans*. Aust N Z J Med 8:620-622, 1978.
84. Warnock DW, Milne JD, Fielding AM. Immunoglobulin classes of human serum antibodies in vaginal candidiasis. Mycopathologia 63: 173-175, 1978.
85. Gordon DL, Johnson GM, Hostetter MK. Characteristics of iC3b binding to human polymorphonuclear leucocytes. Immunology 60: 553-558, 1987.
86. Stanley VC, Hurley R, Carroll CJ. Distribution and significance of *Candida* precipitins in sera from pregnant women. J Med Microbiol 5:313-320, 1972.
87. Kirkpatrick CH. Inhibition of growth of *Candida albicans* by iron-saturated lactoferrin: relation to host defense mechanisms in chronic mucocutaneous candidiasis. J Infect Dis 124:539-545, 1971.
88. Diamond RD, Krzesicki R, Wellinton J. Damage to pseudohyphal forms of *Candida albicans* by neutrophils in the absence of serum in vitro. J Clin Invest 61:349-356, 1978.
89. Botas CM, Kurlat I, Young SM, et al. Disseminated candidal infections and intravenous hydrocortisone in preterm infants. Pediatrics 95: 883-887, 1995.
90. Finer NN, Craft A, Vaucher YE, et al. Postnatal steroids: short-term gain, long-term pain? J Pediatr 137:9-13, 2000.
91. Stark AR, Carlo WA, Tyson JE, et al. Adverse effects of early dexamethasone in extremely-low-birth-weight infants. National Institute of Child Health and Human Development Neonatal Research Network. N Engl J Med 344:95-101, 2001.
92. Malloy PJ, Zhao X, Madani ND, et al. Cloning and expression of the gene from *Candida albicans* that encodes a high-affinity corticosteroid-binding protein. Proc Natl Acad Sci U S A 90:1902-1906, 1993.
93. Rotrosen D, Calderone RA, Edwards JE Jr. Adherence of *Candida* species to host tissues and plastic surfaces. Rev Infect Dis 8:73-85, 1986.
94. Johnson DE, Bass JL, Thompson TR, et al. *Candida* septicemia and right atrial mass secondary to umbilical vein catheterization. Am J Dis Child 135:275-277, 1981.
95. Eppes SC, Troutman JL, Gutman LT. Outcome of treatment of candidemia in children whose central catheters were removed or retained. Pediatr Infect Dis J 8:99-104, 1989.
96. Faix RG. Nonsurgical treatment of *Candida* endocarditis. J Pediatr 120:665-666, 1992.
97. Hostetter MK. Handicaps to host defense. Effects of hyperglycemia on C3 and *Candida albicans*. Diabetes 39:271-275, 1990.
98. Stoll BJ, Gordon T, Korones SB, et al. Late-onset sepsis in very low birth weight neonates: a report from the National Institute of Child Health and Human Development Neonatal Research Network. J Pediatr 129:63-71, 1996.
99. Adderson EE, Pappin A, Pavia AT. Spontaneous intestinal perforation in premature infants: a distinct clinical entity associated with systemic candidiasis. J Pediatr Surg 33:1463-1467, 1998.
100. Rowen JL. Mucocutaneous candidiasis. Semin Perinatol 27:406-413, 2003.
101. Weese-Mayer DE, Fondriest DW, Brouillette RT, et al. Risk factors associated with candidemia in the neonatal intensive care unit: a case-control study. Pediatr Infect Dis J 6:190-196, 1987.
102. Evans EG, Rutter N. Development of the epidermis in the newborn. Biol Neonate 49:74-80, 1986.
103. Ballow M, Cates KL, Rowe JC, et al. Development of the immune system in very low birth weight (less than 1500 g) premature infants: concentrations of plasma immunoglobulins and patterns of infections. Pediatr Res 20:899-904, 1986.
104. Gordon DL, Hostetter MK. Complement and host defense against microorganisms. Pathology 18:365-375, 1986.
105. Zach TL, Hostetter MK. Biochemical abnormalities of the third component of complement in neonates. Pediatr Res 26:116-120, 1989.
106. al-Mulla ZS, Christensen RD. Neutropenia in the neonate. Clin Perinatol 22:711-739, 1995.
107. Kennedy MJ, Volz PA. Effect of various antibiotics on gastrointestinal colonization and dissemination by *Candida albicans*. Sabouraudia 23: 265-273, 1985.
108. Lee BE, Cheung PY, Robinson JL, et al. Comparative study of mortality and morbidity in premature infants (birth weight, < 1,250 g) with candidemia or candidal meningitis. Clin Infect Dis 27:559-565, 1998.
109. Stoll BJ, Hansen N, Fanaroff AA, et al. Late-onset sepsis in very low birth weight neonates: the experience of the NICHD Neonatal Research Network. Pediatrics 110:285-291, 2002.
110. Diekema DJ, Messer SA, Brueggemann AB, et al. Epidemiology of candidemia: 3-year results from the emerging infections and the epidemiology of Iowa organisms study. J Clin Microbiol 40:1298-1302, 2002.
111. Fanaroff AA, Hack M, Walsh MC. The NICHD neonatal research network: changes in practice and outcomes during the first 15 years. Semin Perinatol 27:281-287, 2003.
112. Helbock HJ, Insoft RM, Conte FA. Glucocorticoid-responsive hypotension in extremely low birth weight newborns. Pediatrics 92:715-717, 1993.
113. Hoppe JE. Treatment of oropharyngeal candidiasis and candidal diaper dermatitis in neonates and infants: review and reappraisal. Pediatr Infect Dis J 16:885-894, 1997.
114. Rowen JL, Atkins JT, Levy ML, et al. Invasive fungal dermatitis in the < or = 1000-gram neonate. Pediatrics 95:682-687, 1995.
115. Benjamin DKJ, Garges H, Steinbach WJ. *Candida* bloodstream infections in neonates. Semin Perinatol 27:375-383, 2003.
116. Faix R, Chapman RL. Central nervous system candidiasis in the high-risk neonate. Semin Perinatol 27:384-392, 2003.

117. Chapman RL, Faix RG. Persistently positive cultures and outcome in invasive neonatal candidiasis. Pediatr Infect Dis J 19:822-827, 2000.
118. Benjamin DK Jr, Poole C, Steinbach WJ, et al. Neonatal candidemia and end-organ damage: a critical appraisal of the literature using meta-analytic techniques. Pediatrics 112:634-640, 2003.
119. Baley JE, Ellis F. Neonatal candidiasis: ophthalmologic infection. Semin Perinatol 27:401-405, 2003.
120. Drohan L, Colby CE, Brindle ME, et al. *Candida* (amphotericin-sensitive) lens abscess associated with decreasing arterial blood flow in a very low birth weight preterm infant. Pediatrics 110:e65, 2002.
121. Doctor BA, Newman N, Minich NM, et al. Clinical outcomes of neonatal meningitis in very-low birth-weight infants. Clin Pediatr (Phila) 40:473-480, 2001.
122. Marcinkowski M, Bauer K, Stoltenburg-Didinger G, et al. Fungal brain abscesses in neonates: sonographic appearances and corresponding histopathologic findings. J Clin Ultrasound 29:417-421, 2001.
123. Johnson DE, Conroy MM, Foker JE, et al. *Candida* peritonitis in the newborn. J Pediatr 97:298-300, 1980.
124. Benjamin DK Jr, Fisher RG, McKinney RE Jr, et al. Candidal mycetoma in the neonatal kidney. Pediatrics 104:1126-1129, 1999.
125. Winters WD, Shaw DW, Weinberger E. *Candida* fungus balls presenting as intraventricular masses in cranial sonography. J Clin Ultrasound 23:266-270, 1995.
126. Bryant K, Maxfield C, Rabalais G. Renal candidiasis in neonates with candiduria. Pediatr Infect Dis J 18:959-963, 1999.
127. Whyte RK, Hussain Z, deSa DJ. Antenatal infections with *Candida* species. Arch Dis Child 57:528-535, 1982.
128. Hood IC, Browning D, deSa DJ, et al. Fetal inflammatory response in second trimester candidal chorioamnionitis. Early Hum Dev 11:1-10, 1985.
129. Rudolph N, Tariq AA, Reale MR, et al. Congenital cutaneous candidiasis. Arch Dermatol 113:1101-1103, 1977.
130. Schwartz DA, Reef S. *Candida albicans* placentitis and funisitis: early diagnosis of congenital candidemia by histopathologic examination of umbilical cord vessels. Pediatr Infect Dis J 9:661-665, 1990.
131. Faix RG, Kovarik SM, Shaw TR, et al. Mucocutaneous and invasive candidiasis among very low birth weight (less than 1,500 grams) infants in intensive care nurseries: a prospective study. Pediatrics 83:101-107, 1989.
132. Gupta P, Faridi MM, Rawat S, et al. Clinical profile and risk factors for oral candidosis in sick newborns. Indian Pediatr 33:299-303, 1996.
133. Daftary SS, Desai SV, Shah MV, et al. Oral thrush in the new-born. Indian Pediatr 17:287-288, 1980.
134. Goins RA, Ascher D, Waecker N, et al. Comparison of fluconazole and nystatin oral suspensions for treatment of oral candidiasis in infants. Pediatr Infect Dis J 21:1165-1167, 2002.
135. Kleinegger CL, Lockhart SR, Vargas K, et al. Frequency, intensity, species, and strains of oral *Candida* vary as a function of host age. J Clin Microbiol 34:2246-2254, 1996.
136. Leyden JJ. Diaper dermatitis. Dermatol Clin 4:23-28, 1986.
137. Leyden JJ, Kligman AM. The role of microorganisms in diaper dermatitis. Arch Dermatol 114:56-59, 1978.
138. Roque H, Abdelhak Y, Young BK. Intra-amniotic candidiasis. Case report and meta-analysis of 54 cases. J Perinat Med 27:253-262, 1999.
139. Darmstadt GL, Dinulos JG, Miller Z. Congenital cutaneous candidiasis: clinical presentation, pathogenesis, and management guidelines. Pediatrics 105:438-444, 2000.
140. Pradeepkumar VK, Rajadurai VS, Tan KW. Congenital candidiasis: varied presentations. J Perinatol 18:311-316, 1998.
141. Jin Y, Endo A, Shimada M, et al. Congenital systemic candidiasis. Pediatr Infect Dis J 14:818-820, 1995.
142. Baley JE, Silverman RA. Systemic candidiasis: cutaneous manifestations in low birth weight infants. Pediatrics 82:211-215, 1988.
143. Barone SR, Krilov LR. Neonatal candidal meningitis in a full-term infant with congenital cutaneous candidiasis. Clin Pediatr (Phila) 34:217-219, 1995.
144. Melville C, Kempley S, Graham J, et al. Early onset systemic *Candida* infection in extremely preterm neonates. Eur J Pediatr 155:904-906, 1996.
145. Fernandez M, Noyola DE, Rossmann SN, et al. Cutaneous phaeohyphomycosis caused by *Curvularia lunata* and a review of *Curvularia* infections in pediatrics. Pediatr Infect Dis J 18:727-731, 1999.
146. Bryan MG, Elston DM, Hivnor C, et al. Phaeohyphimycosis in a premature infant. Cutis 65:137-140, 2000.
147. Leibovitz E, Iuster-Reicher A, Amitai M, et al. Systemic candidal infections associated with use of peripheral venous catheters in neonates: a 9-year experience. Clin Infect Dis 14:485-491, 1992.
148. Hensey OJ, Hart CA, Cooke RW. *Candida albicans* skin abscesses. Arch Dis Child 59:479-480, 1984.
149. Bodey GP, Luna M. Skin lesions associated with disseminated candidiasis. JAMA 229:1466-1468, 1974.
150. Dyke MP, Ott K. Severe thrombocytopenia in extremely low birth weight infants with systemic candidiasis. J Paediatr Child Health 29: 298-301, 1993.
151. Foker JE, Bass JL, Thompson T, et al. Management of intracardiac fungal masses in premature infants. J Thorac Cardiovasc Surg 87: 244-250, 1984.
152. Richards MJ, Edwards JR, Culver DH, et al. Nosocomial infections in pediatric intensive care units in the United States. National Nosocomial Infections Surveillance System. Pediatrics 103:e39, 1999.
153. Gubbins PO, McConnell SA, Penzak SR. Current management of funguria. Am J Health Syst Pharm 56:1929-1935, 1999.
154. Hitchcock RJ, Pallett A, Hall MA, et al. Urinary tract candidiasis in neonates and infants. Br J Urol 76:252-256, 1995.
155. Ruderman JW. A clue (tip-off) to urinary infection with *Candida*. Pediatr Infect Dis J 9:586-588, 1990.
156. Faix RG. Systemic *Candida* infections in infants in intensive care nurseries: high incidence of central nervous system involvement. J Pediatr 105:616-622, 1984.
157. Makhoul IR, Kassis I, Smolkin T, et al. Review of 49 neonates with acquired fungal sepsis: further characterization. Pediatrics 107:61-66, 2001.
158. Noyola DE, Fernandez M, Moylett EH, et al. Ophthalmologic, visceral, and cardiac involvement in neonates with candidemia. Clin Infect Dis 32:1018-1023, 2001.
159. Baley JE, Kliegman RM, Fanaroff AA. Disseminated fungal infections in very low-birth-weight infants: clinical manifestations and epidemiology. Pediatrics 73:144-152, 1984.
160. Phillips JR, Karlowicz MG. Prevalence of *Candida* species in hospital-acquired urinary tract infections in a neonatal intensive care unit. Pediatr Infect Dis J 16:190-194, 1997.
161. Karlowicz MG. Candidal renal and urinary tract infections in neonates. Semin Perinatol 27:393-400, 2003.
162. Tung KT, MacDonald LM, Smith JC. Neonatal systemic candidiasis diagnosed by ultrasound. Acta Radiol 31:293-295, 1990.
163. Eckstein CW, Kass EJ. Anuria in a newborn secondary to bilateral ureteropelvic fungus balls. J Urol 127:109-110, 1982.
164. Khan MY. Anuria from *Candida* pyelonephritis and obstructing fungal balls. Urology 21:421-423, 1983.
165. McDonnell M, Lam AH, Isaacs D. Nonsurgical management of neonatal obstructive uropathy due to *Candida albicans*. Clin Infect Dis 21:1349-1350, 1995.
166. Sirinelli D, Biriotti V, Schmit P, et al. Urinoma and arterial hypertension complicating neonatal renal candidiasis. Pediatr Radiol 17: 156-158, 1987.
167. Faix RG, Finkel DJ, Andersen RD, et al. Genotypic analysis of a cluster of systemic *Candida albicans* infections in a neonatal intensive care unit. Pediatr Infect Dis J 14:1063-1068, 1995.
168. Chesney PJ, Justman RA, Bogdanowicz WM. *Candida* meningitis in newborn infants: a review and report of combined amphotericin B–flucytosine therapy. Johns Hopkins Med J 142:155-160, 1978.
169. Goldsmith LS, Rubenstein SD, Wolfson BJ, et al. Cerebral calcifications in a neonate with candidiasis. Pediatr Infect Dis J 9:451-453, 1990.
170. Brill PW, Winchester P, Krauss AN, et al. Osteomyelitis in a neonatal intensive care unit. Radiology 131:83-87, 1979.
171. Bozynski ME, Naglie RA, Russell EJ. Real-time ultrasonographic surveillance in the detection of CNS involvement in systemic *Candida* infection. Pediatr Radiol 16:235-237, 1986.
172. Levin S, Zaidel L, Bernstein D. Intrauterine infection of fetal brain by *Candida*. Am J Obstet Gynecol 130:597-599, 1978.
173. Sood S, Majumdar T, Chatterjee A, et al. Disseminated candidosis in premature twins. Mycoses 41:417-419, 1998.
174. Baley JE, Annable WL, Kliegman RM. *Candida* endophthalmitis in the premature infant. J Pediatr 98:458-461, 1981.
175. Clinch TE, Duker JS, Eagle RC Jr, et al. Infantile endogenous *Candida* endophthalmitis presenting as a cataract. Surv Ophthalmol 34:107-112, 1989.
176. Stern JH, Calvano C, Simon JW. Recurrent endogenous candidal endophthalmitis in a premature infant. J AAPOS 5:50-51, 2001.
177. Todd Johnston W, Cogen MS. Systemic candidiasis with cataract formation in a premature infant. J AAPOS 4:386-388, 2000.
178. Shah GK, Vander J, Eagle RC. Intraventricular *Candida* species abscess in a premature infant. Am J Ophthalmol 129:390-391, 2000.

179. Mittal M, Dhanireddy R, Higgins RD. *Candida* sepsis and association with retinopathy of prematurity. Pediatrics 101:654-657, 1998.
180. Noyola DE, Bohra L, Paysse EA, et al. Association of candidemia and retinopathy of prematurity in very low birthweight infants. Ophthalmology 109:80-84, 2002.
181. Karlowicz MG, Giannone PJ, Pestian J, et al. Does candidemia predict threshold retinopathy of prematurity in extremely low birth weight (</=1000 g) neonates? Pediatrics 105:1036-1040, 2000.
182. Gago LC, Capone A Jr, Trese MT. Bilateral presumed endogenous *Candida* endophthalmitis and stage 3 retinopathy of prematurity. Am J Ophthalmol 134:611-613, 2002.
183. Haroon Parupia MF, Dhanireddy R. Association of postnatal dexamethasone use and fungal sepsis in the development of severe retinopathy of prematurity and progression to laser therapy in extremely low-birth-weight infants. J Perinatol 21:242-247, 2001.
184. Tadesse M, Dhanireddy R, Mittal M, et al. Race, *Candida* sepsis, and retinopathy of prematurity. Biol Neonate 81:86-90, 2002.
185. Kremer I, Naor N, Davidson S, et al. Systemic candidiasis in babies with retinopathy of prematurity. Graefes Arch Clin Exp Ophthalmol 230:592-594, 1992.
186. Bond S, Stewart DL, Bendon RW. Invasive *Candida* enteritis of the newborn. J Pediatr Surg 35:1496-1498, 2000.
187. Robertson NJ, Kuna J, Cox PM, et al. Spontaneous intestinal perforation and *Candida* peritonitis presenting as extensive necrotizing enterocolitis. Acta Paediatr 92:258-261, 2003.
188. Meyer CL, Payne NR, Roback SA. Spontaneous, isolated intestinal perforations in neonates with birth weight less than 1,000 g not associated with necrotizing enterocolitis. J Pediatr Surg 26:714-717, 1991.
189. Mintz AC, Applebaum H. Focal gastrointestinal perforations not associated with necrotizing enterocolitis in very low birth weight neonates. J Pediatr Surg 28:857-860, 1993.
190. Kaplan M, Eidelman AI, Dollberg L, et al. Necrotizing bowel disease with *Candida* peritonitis following severe neonatal hypothermia. Acta Paediatr Scand 79:876-879, 1990.
191. Schelonka RL, Moser SA. Time to positive culture results in neonatal *Candida* septicemia. J Pediatr 142:564-565, 2003.
192. Berenguer J, Buck M, Witebsky F, et al. Lysis-centrifugation blood cultures in the detection of tissue-proven invasive candidiasis. Disseminated versus single-organ infection. Diagn Microbiol Infect Dis 17:103-109, 1993.
193. Pollack CV Jr, Pollack ES, Andrew ME. Suprapubic bladder aspiration versus urethral catheterization in ill infants: success, efficiency and complication rates. Ann Emerg Med 23:225-230, 1994.
194. Faix RG. *Candida parapsilosis* meningitis in a premature infant. Pediatr Infect Dis J 2:462-464, 1983.
195. Fernandez M, Moylett EH, Noyola DE, et al. Candidal meningitis in neonates: a 10-year review. Clin Infect Dis 31:458-463, 2000.
196. Johnson DE, Thompson TR, Green TP, et al. Systemic candidiasis in very low-birth-weight infants (less than 1,500 grams). Pediatrics 73: 138-143, 1984.
197. Pfaller MA. Epidemiology of nosocomial candidiasis: the importance of molecular typing. Braz J Infect Dis 4:161-167, 2000.
198. Villari P, Iacuzio L, Torre I, et al. Molecular epidemiology as an effective tool in the surveillance of infections in the neonatal intensive care unit. J Infect 37:274-281, 1998.
199. Berman LH, Stringer DA, St. Onge O, et al. An assessment of sonography in the diagnosis and management of neonatal renal candidiasis. Clin Radiol 40:577-581, 1989.
200. Krensky AM, Reddish JM, Teele RL. Causes of increased renal echogenicity in pediatric patients. Pediatrics 72:840-846, 1983.
201. Erden A, Fitoz S, Karagulle T, et al. Radiological findings in the diagnosis of genitourinary candidiasis. Pediatr Radiol 30:875-877, 2000.
202. Johnson SC, Kazzi NJ. *Candida* brain abscess: a sonographic mimicker of intracranial hemorrhage. J Ultrasound Med 12:237-239, 1993.
203. Huang CC, Chen CY, Yang HB, et al. Central nervous system candidiasis in very low-birth-weight premature neonates and infants: US characteristics and histopathologic and MR imaging correlates in five patients. Radiology 209:49-56, 1998.
204. Schelonka RL, Chai MK, Yoder BA, et al. Volume of blood required to detect common neonatal pathogens. J Pediatr 129:275-278, 1996.
205. Walsh TJ, Merz WG, Lee JW, et al. Diagnosis and therapeutic monitoring of invasive candidiasis by rapid enzymatic detection of serum D-arabinitol. Am J Med 99:164-172, 1995.
206. Flahaut M, Sanglard D, Monod M, et al. Rapid detection of *Candida albicans* in clinical samples by DNA amplification of common regions from *C. albicans*–secreted aspartic proteinase genes. J Clin Microbiol 36:395-401, 1998.
207. Mitsutake K, Miyazaki T, Tashiro T, et al. Enolase antigen, mannan antigen, Cand-Tec antigen, and beta-glucan in patients with candidemia. J Clin Microbiol 34:1918-1921, 1996.
208. Sigmundsdottir G, Christensson B, Bjorklund LJ, et al. Urine D-arabinitol/L-arabinitol ratio in diagnosis of invasive candidiasis in newborn infants. J Clin Microbiol 38:3039-3042, 2000.
209. Van Burik JA, Myerson D, Schreckhise RW, et al. Panfungal PCR assay for detection of fungal infection in human blood specimens. J Clin Microbiol 36:1169-1175, 1998.
210. Bliss J, Wellington M, Gigliotti F. Antifungal pharmacotherapy for neonatal candidiasis. Semin Perinatol 27:365-374, 2003.
211. Kicklighter SD. Antifungal agents and fungal prophylaxis in the neonate. Pediatr Rev Neoreviews 2002:e249-e254, 2002.
212. Faix RG, Feick HJ, Frommelt P, et al. Successful medical treatment of *Candida parapsilosis* endocarditis in a premature infant. Am J Perinatol 7:272-275, 1990.
213. Munz D, Powell KR, Pai CH. Treatment of candidal diaper dermatitis: a double-blind placebo-controlled comparison of topical nystatin with topical plus oral nystatin. J Pediatr 101:1022-1025, 1982.
214. Dhondt F, Ninane J, De Beule K, et al. Oral candidosis: treatment with absorbable and non-absorbable antifungal agents in children. Mycoses 35:1-8, 1992.
215. Casneuf J, de Loore F, Dhondt F, et al. Oral thrush in children treated with miconazole gel. Mykosen 23:75-78, 1980.
216. Concannon P, Gisoldi E, Phillips S, et al. Diaper dermatitis: a therapeutic dilemma. Results of a double-blind placebo controlled trial of miconazole nitrate 0.25%. Pediatr Dermatol 18:149-155, 2001.
217. Pappas PG, Rex JH, Sobel JD, et al. Guidelines for treatment of candidiasis. Clin Infect Dis 38:161-189, 2004.
218. American Academy of Pediatrics Committee on Infectious Diseases. Candidiasis. *In* LK Pickering (ed). 2003 Red Book: Report of the Committee on Infectious Diseases. Elk Grove Village, Il, American Academy of Pediatrics, 2003, pp 229-232.
219. Pfaller MA, Messer SA, Hollis RJ. Strain delineation and antifungal susceptibilities of epidemiologically related and unrelated isolates of *Candida lusitaniae*. Diagn Microbiol Infect Dis 20:127-133, 1994.
220. Butler KM, Rench MA, Baker CJ. Amphotericin B as a single agent in the treatment of systemic candidiasis in neonates. Pediatr Infect Dis J 9:51-56, 1990.
221. Kingo AR, Smyth JA, Waisman D. Lack of evidence of amphotericin B toxicity in very low birth weight infants treated for systemic candidiasis. Pediatr Infect Dis J 16:1002-1003, 1997.
222. Baley JE, Kliegman RM, Fanaroff AA. Disseminated fungal infections in very low-birth-weight infants: therapeutic toxicity. Pediatrics 73: 153-157, 1984.
223. Hall JE, Cox F, Karlson K, et al. Amphotericin B dosage for disseminated candidiasis in premature infants. J Perinatol 7:194-198, 1987.
224. Serra G, Mezzano P, Bonacci W. Therapeutic treatment of systemic candidiasis in newborns. J Chemother 3:240-244, 1991.
225. Glick C, Graves GR, Feldman S. Neonatal fungemia and amphotericin B. South Med J 86:1368-1371, 1993.
226. Baley JE, Meyers C, Kliegman RM, et al. Pharmacokinetics, outcome of treatment, and toxic effects of amphotericin B and 5-fluorocytosine in neonates. J Pediatr 116:791-797, 1990.
227. Rowen JL, Tate JM. Management of neonatal candidiasis. Neonatal Candidiasis Study Group. Pediatr Infect Dis J 17:1007-1011, 1998.
228. Baetz-Greenwalt B, Debaz B, Kumar ML. Bladder fungus ball: a reversible cause of neonatal obstructive uropathy. Pediatrics 81: 826-829, 1988.
229. Juster-Reicher A, Leibovitz E, Linder N, et al. Liposomal amphotericin B (AmBisome) in the treatment of neonatal candidiasis in very low birth weight infants. Infection 28:223-226, 2000.
230. Adler-Shohet F, Waskin H, Lieberman JM. Amphotericin B lipid complex for neonatal invasive candidiasis. Arch Dis Child Fetal Neonatal Ed 84:F131-F133, 2001.
231. Walsh TJ, Seibel NL, Arndt C, et al. Amphotericin B lipid complex in pediatric patients with invasive fungal infections. Pediatr Infect Dis J 18:702-708, 1999.
232. Dupont B. Overview of the lipid formulations of amphotericin B. J Antimicrob Chemother 49:31-36, 2002.
233. Ferrari P, Chiarolanza J, Capriotti T, et al. Favorable course of cerebral candidiasis in a low-birth weight newborn treated with liposomal amphotericin B. Pediatr Med Chir 23:197-199, 2001.

234. Al Arishi H, Frayha HH, Kalloghlian A, et al. Liposomal amphotericin B in neonates with invasive candidiasis. Am J Perinatol 15:643-648, 1998.
235. Scarcella A, Pasquariello MB, Giugliano B, et al. Liposomal amphotericin B treatment for neonatal fungal infections. Pediatr Infect Dis J 17:146-148, 1998.
236. Weitkamp JH, Poets CF, Sievers R, et al. *Candida* infection in very low birth-weight infants: outcome and nephrotoxicity of treatment with liposomal amphotericin B (AmBisome). Infection 26:11-15, 1998.
237. Pfaller MA, Messer SA, Boyken L, et al. In vitro activities of 5-fluorocytosine against 8,803 clinical isolates of *Candida* spp.: global assessment of primary resistance using National Committee for Clinical Laboratory Standards susceptibility testing methods. Antimicrob Agents Chemother 46:3518-3521, 2002.
238. Smego RA Jr, Perfect JR, Durack DT. Combined therapy with amphotericin B and 5-fluorocytosine for *Candida* meningitis. Rev Infect Dis 6:791-801, 1984.
239. Johnson EM, Richardson MD, Warnock DW. In-vitro resistance to imidazole antifungals in *Candida albicans*. J Antimicrob Chemother 13:547-558, 1984.
240. Novelli V, Holzel H. Safety and tolerability of fluconazole in children. Antimicrob Agents Chemother 43:1955-1960, 1999.
241. Triolo V, Gari-Toussaint M, Casagrande F, et al. Fluconazole therapy for *Candida albicans* urinary tract infections in infants. Pediatr Nephrol 17:550-553, 2002.
242. Saxen H, Hoppu K, Pohjavuori M. Pharmacokinetics of fluconazole in very low birth weight infants during the first two weeks of life. Clin Pharmacol Ther 54:269-277, 1993.
243. Wenzl TG, Schefels J, Hornchen H, et al. Pharmacokinetics of oral fluconazole in premature infants. Eur J Pediatr 157:661-662, 1998.
244. Kicklighter SD, Springer SC, Cox T, et al. Fluconazole for prophylaxis against candidal rectal colonization in the very low birth weight infant. Pediatrics 107:293-298, 2001.
245. Driessen M, Ellis JB, Cooper PA, et al. Fluconazole vs. amphotericin B for the treatment of neonatal fungal septicemia: a prospective randomized trial. Pediatr Infect Dis J 15:1107-1112, 1996.
246. Wainer S, Cooper PA, Gouws H, et al. Prospective study of fluconazole therapy in systemic neonatal fungal infection. Pediatr Infect Dis J 16:763-767, 1997.
247. Fasano C, O'Keeffe J, Gibbs D. Fluconazole treatment of neonates and infants with severe fungal infections not treatable with conventional agents. Eur J Clin Microbiol Infect Dis 13:351-354, 1994.
248. Ferrieri P, Guse D, Krumpelmann J. 2002-2003 Antibiotic susceptibilities at Fairview-University Medical Center. *In* Clinical Microbiology Laboratory Newsletter. Minneapolis, Minn, Fairview-University Medical Center, 2004, pp 1-2.
249. Pfaller MA, Messer SA, Hollis RJ, et al. Trends in species distribution and susceptibility to fluconazole among blood stream isolates of *Candida* species in the United States. Diagn Microbiol Infect Dis 33:217-222, 1999.
250. Sabo JA, Abdel-Rahman SM. Voriconazole: a new triazole antifungal. Ann Pharmacother 34:1032-1043, 2000.
251. Muller FM, Weig M, Peter J, et al. Azole cross-resistance to ketoconazole, fluconazole, itraconazole and voriconazole in clinical *Candida albicans* isolates from HIV-infected children with oropharyngeal candidosis. J Antimicrob Chemother 46:338-340, 2000.
252. Stone EA, Fung HB, Kirschenbaum HL. Caspofungin: an echinocandin antifungal agent. Clin Ther 24:351-377; 2002.
253. Mora-Duarte J, Betts R, Rotstein C, et al. Comparison of caspofungin and amphotericin B for invasive candidiasis. N Engl J Med 347: 2020-2029, 2002.
254. Boucher HW, Groll AH, Chiou CC, et al. Newer systemic antifungal agents: pharmacokinetics, safety and efficacy. Drugs 64:1997–2020, 2004.
255. Friedman S, Richardson SE, Jacobs SE, et al. Systemic *Candida* infection in extremely low birth weight infants: short term morbidity and long term neurodevelopmental outcome. Pediatr Infect Dis J 19:499-504, 2000.
256. Karlowicz MG, Hashimoto LN, Kelly RE Jr, et al. Should central venous catheters be removed as soon as candidemia is detected in neonates? Pediatrics 106:e63, 2000.
257. Rex JH, Walsh TJ, Sobel JD, et al. Practice guidelines for the treatment of candidiasis. Infectious Diseases Society of America. Clin Infect Dis 30:662-678, 2000.
258. Saiman L, Ludington E, Dawson JD, et al. Risk factors for *Candida* species colonization of neonatal intensive care unit patients. Pediatr Infect Dis J 20:1119-1124, 2001.
259. Huang YC, Lin TY, Leu HS, et al. Outbreak of *Candida parapsilosis* fungemia in neonatal intensive care units: clinical implications and genotyping analysis. Infection 27:97-102, 1999.
260. Burnie JP. *Candida* and hands. J Hosp Infect 8:1-4, 1986.
261. Larson E, Silberger M, Jakob K, et al. Assessment of alternative hand hygiene regimens to improve skin health among neonatal intensive care unit nurses. Heart Lung 29:136-142, 2000.
262. Campbell JR, Zaccaria E, Baker CJ. Systemic candidiasis in extremely low birth weight infants receiving topical petrolatum ointment for skin care: a case-control study. Pediatrics 105:1041-1045, 2000.

Chapter 34

PNEUMOCYSTIS AND OTHER LESS COMMON FUNGAL INFECTIONS

Yvonne A. Maldonado • Carol J. Baker • Michael J. Miller

Fungal infections, other than those caused by *Candida* species, rarely are considered in the differential diagnosis for an acutely ill newborn infant, because disorders of bacterial and viral etiology are vastly more common. Nevertheless, fungal infections do occur in neonates, especially in premature infants and those of very low birth weight (less than 1500 g), and can cause serious and frequently fatal disease. The number of cases of invasive infection attributed to fungi among all patients in the United States quadrupled between 1990 and 2000. With advances in neonatal care, the epidemiology of fungal infections in the neonatal intensive care unit (NICU) has changed dramatically, with an estimated 10-fold increase in the past decade. As with any other infectious disease, the risk of fungal infection depends on the host and risk of exposure. The neonate has some risk of exposure to either *Malassezia furfur* or *Pneumocystis jiroveci* (previously *Pneumocystis carinii*, newly classified as a fungus on the basis of DNA sequence analysis), has a limited risk of exposure to *Aspergillus* species, and has an extremely low risk of exposure to other fungi—especially in the NICU setting. Therefore, it is not surprising that the most common fungal infection in neonates is candidiasis, followed by infections with *P. jiroveci* and *M. furfur*, whereas case reports or small series constitute the literature on aspergillosis and other fungal infections.

Mycotic infections, whether confined to epidermal structures or involving deep tissues, are caused by fungi free-living in soil or present in bird or mammal excreta or in decaying organic matter. In instances of fungal infection in newborns, organisms most often are acquired in utero through the hematogenous route, from the mother during birth, or from the environment on postnatal exposure. When inhaled, ingested, or inoculated directly into tissue, these saprophytic microorganisms can cause infection after birth in infants with undue susceptibility. Although much has been learned regarding the pathogenesis, immune response, and treatment of fungal infections in older children and adults, studies to determine the cause of increased susceptibility or resistance to infection with fungi, especially in neonates, are incomplete. Advances have been made in the diagnosis and treatment of neonatal fungal infections, however.

PNEUMOCYSTIS JIROVECI (FORMERLY KNOWN AS *PNEUMOCYSTIS CARINII*) INFECTION

P. jiroveci, a fungus with a history of unsettled taxonomy, was discovered in the lungs of small mammals and humans in Brazil more than 80 years ago. Today it is a cause of often fatal pneumonia in patients with immunodeficiencies, hematologic malignancy, collagen-vascular disorders, or organ allografts and in those who receive corticosteroids and immunosuppressive drug therapy. Although congenital or neonatal infection with *Pneumocystis* is uncommon, it can occur in infants younger than 1 year of age in two well-defined epidemiologic settings: (1) in epidemics in nurseries located in impoverished areas of the world and (2) in isolated cases in which the infected child has an underlying primary immunodeficiency disease[1] or acquired immunodeficiency syndrome (AIDS).

This section of the chapter reviews the problem of *Pneumocystis* infection in the newborn. Much of our knowledge of the epidemiologic, pathologic, and clinical features of pneumocystosis, however, is drawn from observations of the infection in older children and adults. As a result, we have elected to include data derived from such observations to present a more complete picture of the infectious process caused by this unique organism.

History

In 1909, Chagas[2] in Brazil first described the morphologic forms of *Pneumocystis* in the lungs of guinea pigs infected with *Trypanosoma cruzi*. He believed the forms to represent a sexual stage in the life cycle of the trypanosome and not a different organism. Carini,[3] an Italian working in Brazil, saw the same organism-like cysts in the lungs of rats experimentally infected with *Trypanosoma lewisi*. His slide material subsequently was reviewed by the Delanoës and their colleagues[4] at the Pasteur Institute in Paris. They recognized that these alveolar cysts were present in the lungs of local Parisian sewer rats and thereby established that the "organisms" were independent of trypanosomes. They proposed the name *Pneumocystis carinii* for the new species.

At about this time, Chagas may have unwittingly described the first human case of pneumocystosis when he reported the presence of similar organisms in the lungs of a patient with interstitial pneumonia who had died of American trypanosomiasis.[5] Nevertheless, no definite etiologic connection was made between *P. carinii* and human pneumonic disease for another 30 years. The reason for this delay was the belief during this period that infantile syphilis was responsible for virtually all instances of interstitial plasma cell pneumonia. In 1938, Benecke[6] and Ammich[7] identified a histologically similar pneumonic illness in nonsyphilitic children that was characterized by a peculiar honeycombed exudate in alveoli. Subsequent scrutiny of photomicrographs in their reports revealed the presence of *P. carinii* organisms,[8] but it was not until 1942 that Van der Meer and Brug[9] in the Netherlands unequivocally recognized the organism in lungs from two infants and one adult. The first epidemics of interstitial plasma cell pneumonia were reported shortly thereafter among premature debilitated babies in nurseries and foundling homes in central Europe. In 1952 Vanek and Jirovec[8] in Czechoslovakia provided the most convincing demonstration of the etiologic relationship of *P. carinii* to this disease in an autopsy study of 16 cases.

Pneumocystosis was first brought to the attention of pediatricians in the United States in 1953 by Deamer and Zollinger,[10] who reviewed the pathologic and epidemiologic features of the European disease. Lunseth and associates[11] generally are credited for the initial case report of interstitial plasma cell pneumonia occurring in an infant born in the United States. Curiously, the latter authors neither identified *Pneumocystis* organisms in their histologic sections nor even alluded to the organism in their discussion of causation of the disease. During the next year, the presence of *Pneumocystis* pneumonia in the United States was documented in several published studies.[12-14]

In 1957 Gajdusek[15] presented an in-depth perspective on the history of the infection that included an extensive bibliography. This review was particularly timely because the next decade was to see the disturbing emergence of *P. carinii* pneumonia in the Western world—even while the epidemic disease in central Europe was waning—to the degree that it would become preeminent among the so-called opportunistic pulmonary infections in the immunosuppressed host. In 1988, DNA analysis demonstrated that *Pneumocystis* was not a protozoan but a fungus.[16,17] Subsequent DNA analysis has led to the change in nomenclature from *P. carinii* to *P. jiroveci*, a name chosen in honor of the parasitologist Otto Jirovec, who now is credited by some with the original description of this organism.[18,19]

The Organism

The precise taxonomic status of *P. jiroveci* as a fungus has been defined on the basis of molecular analysis.[16,17] Because the organism has only recently been propagated in vitro, efforts to classify it and to elucidate its structure and life cycle have been based exclusively on morphologic observations of infected lungs from animals and humans. The earliest of these investigations was performed by parasitologists; accordingly, the terminology applied to the forms of *Pneumocystis* seen in diseased tissue has been that reserved for protozoal organisms.

Three developmental forms of this presumably unicellular microbe[20] have been described: a thick-walled cyst, an intracystic sporozoite, and a thin-walled trophozoite.[3,21,22] The form of *Pneumocystis* that assists with diagnosis is the cyst, which may contain up to eight sporozoites. Each sporozoite is round to crescent shaped, measures 1 to 2 μm in diameter, and contains an eccentric nucleus. This cystic unit with its intracystic bodies is seen well in Giemsa-stained imprint smears of infected fresh lung.[15,23] Giemsa stain, however, results in staining of background alveoli and host cell fragments and does not stain empty cysts. Gomori methenamine silver stain, which highlights only the cyst wall of *Pneumocystis*, is preferable to Giemsa stain when tissues must be screened for the presence of organisms.[24-26] The cysts stained with silver have a thin, often wrinkled black capsule that may be round, crescentic, or disk shaped. Cysts measure 4 to 6 μm in diameter and must be distinguished from erythrocytes. The cysts often occur in clusters within an alveolus.

The typical honeycombed intra-alveolar exudate of *Pneumocystis* pneumonia is largely a collection of interlocking cysts whose walls flatten at points of contact, so that each cyst assumes a hexagonal shape. The internal structure of the silver-stained cyst is variable. In the lighter-staining round cysts, a pair of structures about 1 μm long resembling opposed commas or parentheses often are seen; these occasionally are connected end to end by thin, delicate strands.[24] Other cysts contain only a marginal nodule (Fig. 34-1). Whether these intracystic details correspond to the sporozoite-like bodies seen in Giemsa-stained preparations is not clear. Evidence from both light and electron microscopy, however, suggests that they may not be located within cyst cytoplasm at all; instead, they may be thickened portions of the cyst wall.[27-29]

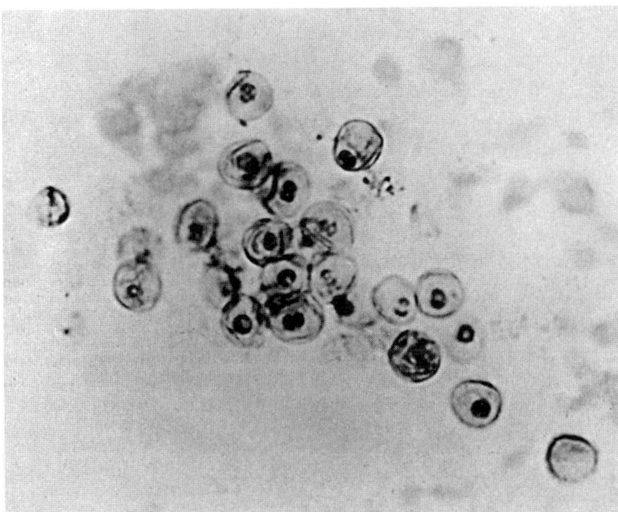

Figure 34–1 Imprint smear of fresh lung tissue stained with methenamine silver shows a cluster of cysts of *Pneumocystis jiroveci*. Typical comma-shaped bodies and marginal nodules are visible within cysts. ×625. (From Ruskin J, Remington JS. The compromised host and infection. JAMA 202:1070, 1967. Copyright 1967, American Medical Association.)

Staining procedures, other than those using Giemsa and methenamine silver, have been employed less frequently to delineate the cyst form of the organism. The cyst wall stains red with periodic acid–Schiff stain.[30] A modified Gram-Weigert method stains both the cyst wall and the intracystic sporozoites.[31] Gridley fungus stain may identify cyst outlines. More reliable stains for this purpose are the modified toluidine blue stain of Chalvardjian and Grawe[32] and the crystal violet stain,[33] which color the cyst wall purple. Electron microscopy has been an invaluable tool in morphologic studies of *P. jiroveci*.[21,28,34-42] It has helped to confirm that the structures regarded as *Pneumocystis* under light microscopy are, in fact, typical microorganisms and not just degradation products of host cells.[43]

Both trophozoite and cystlike stages have been delineated.[42] The trophozoite is thin walled and measures between 1.5 and 2.0 μm in diameter. It has numerous evaginations or pseudopodia-like projections that appear to interdigitate with those of other organisms in the alveolar space.[37,42] It has been postulated that the pseudopodia make up the reticular framework within which organisms reside in an alveolus, accounting for the fact that organisms remain clumped in lung imprints.[23,32] It also has been suggested that the pseudopodia anchor *Pneumocystis* to the alveolar septal wall.[40] The prevailing opinion, however, is that no specialized organelle of attachment exists. Rather, the surfaces of *P. jiroveci* and alveolar cells (specifically, type I pneumonocytes) are closely opposed, without fusion of cell membranes.[44] This adherence of *P. jiroveci* to alveolar lining cells may explain why organisms are not commonly found in expectorated mucus or tracheal secretions.[37]

The classic cystic unit of *P. jiroveci* is thick walled and measures 4 to 6 μm in diameter. The intracystic bodies measure 1.0 to 1.7 μm across and bear a marked similarity to small trophozoites (Fig. 34-2).[42] In addition, thick-walled cysts rich in glycogen particles but without intracystic bodies ("precysts"), partly empty cysts, and collapsed cystic structures have been identified. The collapsed cysts are crescentic and presumably are the same crescentic forms seen frequently in silver-stained specimens under light microscopy. They commonly have defects in their walls.

Life cycles for *P. jiroveci* have been proposed. They have been based on the variant forms of the fungus detected by light[28,29,45-47] and electron microscopy.[42,48] One scheme suggests that the thick-walled round cyst undergoes dissolution or "cracking," whereupon the intracystic bodies pass through tears in the wall (Fig. 34-3).[42] It is not known whether the bodies escape from the cyst by active motility or whether they are extruded passively as a consequence of cyst collapse. At this stage, the intracystic bodies resemble free thin-walled trophozoites. It had been suggested that division of the intracystic body must occur soon after its expulsion from the mature, thick-walled cyst, to account for the large numbers of small trophozoites (1 μm in diameter) seen in infected lung.[28] Electron microscopic observations, however, indicate that another source for the smaller trophozoite is the immature, thin-walled *Pneumocystis* cyst.[48] In any case, the small trophozoites evolve to larger forms, their walls thicken, and a precyst develops that is devoid of intracystic bodies. The cyclic process is completed when formation of the mature cyst, containing eight daughter cysts, is achieved.

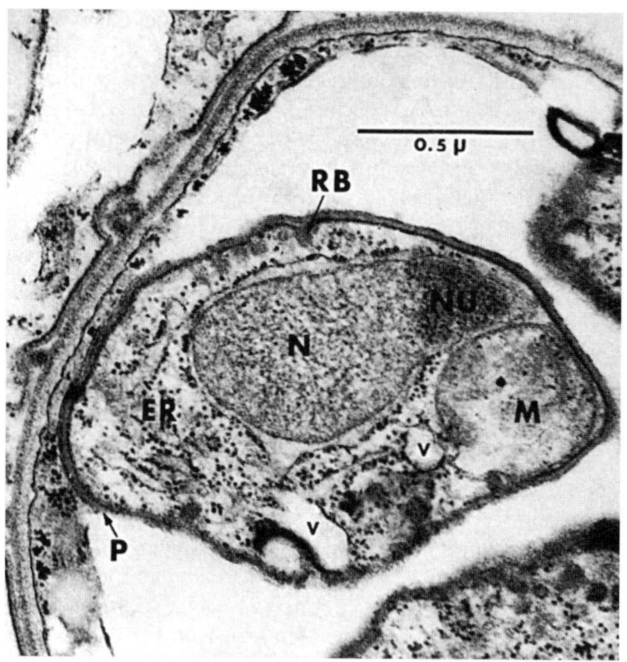

Figure 34–2 Intracystic body within mature cyst. Six-layer effect of cyst wall occurs only where there is contact with adjacent organisms. Note unit-membrane character of undulating membranes that form innermost layer of cyst wall and outer and inner membranes of pellicle (P). Round bodies (RB) appear to arise from pellicle (*arrow*). Rough endoplasmic reticulum (ER) is well developed. Ribosomes are attached to the external membrane of nucleus, and this membrane appears to communicate with membranes of rough endoplasmic reticulum. Cytoplasm also contains vacuoles (v). Nucleus (N) contains nucleolus (NU). Mitochondrion (M) is at the *right*. ×80,000. (From Campbell WG Jr. Ultrastructure of *Pneumocystis in* human lung. Life cycle in human pneumocystosis. Arch Pathol 93:312, 1972. Copyright 1972, American Medical Association.)

Previous controversy over the classification of *Pneumocystis* as a protozoan[49,50] or as a fungus[51] resulted because of the difficulty in cultivating and further characterizing the biochemical nature of the organism. Arguments in favor of a protozoan taxonomy were based mainly on the resemblance of its structural features to those of other protozoa. The organism has cystic and trophozoite stages, pseudopodia in cell walls, and pellicles around intracystic sporozoites.[40,53] In addition, the disease caused by *Pneumocystis* responds to antiprotozoal—namely, antitrypanosomal or antitoxoplasmal—chemotherapy. On the other hand, like fungi, *P. jiroveci* contains a paucity of cellular organelles, its nucleus is not visibly prominent, its cell membrane is layered throughout an entire life cycle, and its cell wall stains vividly with silver.[28]

The question of species specificity of *Pneumocystis* remained similarly unanswered until recent polymerase chain reaction (PCR) techniques established that *P. jiroveci* is not found in lung samples from any other mammals.[53] Although most workers concur that human and rodent forms of the organism are morphologically indistinguishable by light and electron microscopy,[21,29,42] serologic studies designed to demonstrate identity between human and animal species[27,49] or even between human strains from diverse geographic locales[54,55] yield conflicting results. Genetic analysis, however, clearly demonstrated differences between human and nonhuman *Pneumocystis* isolates.[53,56-59]

Successful propagation of *P. jiroveci* in vitro was first reported in 1977 by Pifer and colleagues[60,61] at the St. Jude Children's Research Hospital. This group of investigators serially passed organisms in primary embryonic chick epithelial lung cells over 12 days and noted a 100-fold increase in numbers of cysts. Inoculation of trophozoites alone yielded modest numbers of cyst forms, with typical cytopathogenic effects. Continuing cultivation of *Pneumocystis*, however, was not achieved. In addition, the organisms could not be grown in cell-free media employed commonly for the propagation of other organisms.[61] Limited replication of *Pneumocystis* since has been accomplished in more widely available tissue culture cell lines (Vero, Chang liver, MRC 5, WI 38).[62-65] These tissue culture systems have not been used to isolate *P. jiroveci* from the lungs of animals or humans with suspected infection. Examination of the organism in tissue culture, however, has confirmed the existence of each of its morphologic forms and has provided insight into the biologic interaction between the organism and the host cells.[65]

Epidemiology and Transmission

The natural habitat of *P. jiroveci* is unknown. The distribution of human infection is worldwide,[66-91] and a variety of wild and domestic animal species harbor the organism without demonstrable pulmonary disease. Rarely, clinically evident *Pneumocystis* pneumonitis, not unlike the disease in humans, arises spontaneously in the animal host.[92-97]

The prevalence of infection with *Pneumocystis* remains to be determined, because studies to detect latent carriage of the organism in large populations have not been performed. Serologic surveys, however, indicate that infection is widespread and acquired in early life. Meuwissen and colleagues[98] in the Netherlands noted that immunofluorescent antibodies to *P. jiroveci* are first detectable in healthy children at 6 months of age, and by age 4 years, nearly all children are seropositive. Pifer and associates[99] in the United States found significant titers of antibody to *Pneumocystis* in healthy 7-month-old infants and in two thirds of normal children by age 4 years. Gerrard and co-workers[100] in England detected *P. jiroveci* antibodies in serum from 48% of 94 young healthy children. Pifer and associates[101] also found that serologic evidence of *Pneumocystis* infection is present before immunosuppressive therapy with corticosteroids elicits *Pneumocystis* pneumonia in healthy rats. Authors of a number of autopsy reviews have attempted to determine the incidence of *Pneumocystis* infection, but the results have been divergent, owing to the heterogeneity of the populations studied.[88,102-108] Those studies conducted in central Europe after World War II[103] or in cancer referral centers in the United States[108] have yielded higher rates of infection.

Few published reports have been devoted exclusively to the descriptive epidemiology of *Pneumocystis* pneumonia in the United States. In a literature review of the subject, Le Clair[109] accumulated 107 accounts of the disease recorded from 1955 through 1967. The male-to-female ratio of infected persons was in excess of 2:1, but ethnic distribution was even. The disease was reported from diverse geographic locales (21 of the 50 states). The largest number of cases (33)

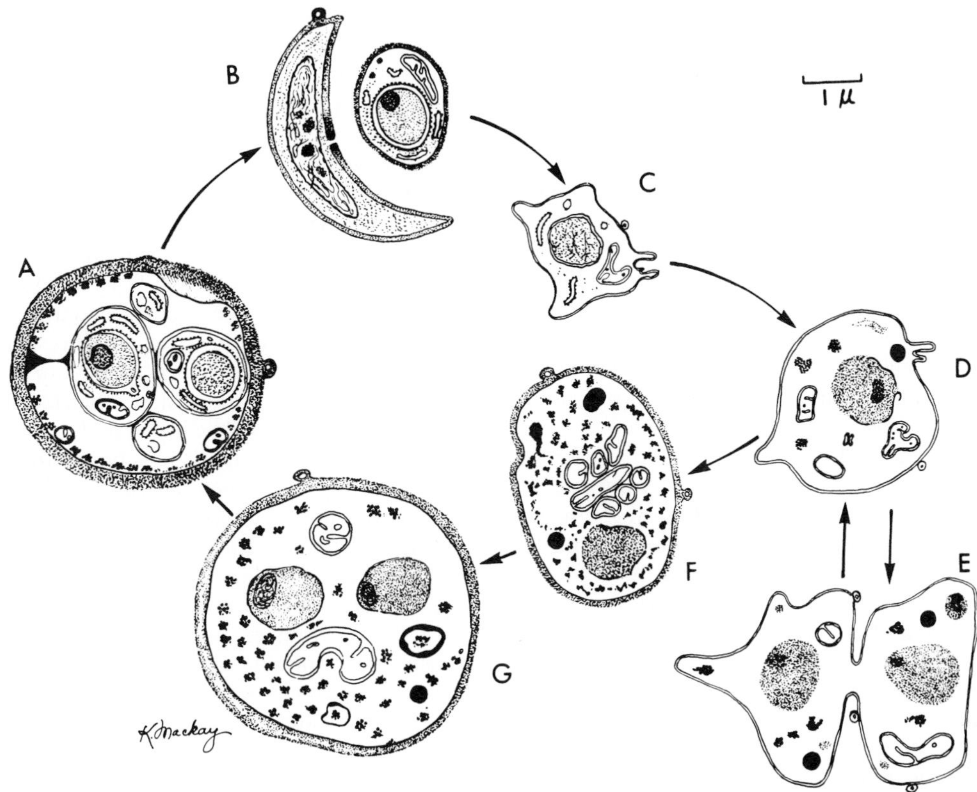

Figure 34–3 Probable life cycle of *Pneumocystis* within pulmonary alveoli. **A,** Mature cyst with intracystic bodies; **B,** empty cyst and recently escaped intracystic body; **C,** small trophozoite; **D,** larger trophozoite; **E,** possible budding or conjugating form; **F,** large trophozoite undergoing thickening of pellicle; **G,** precyst. (From Campbell WG Jr. Ultrastructure of *Pneumocystis* in human lung. Life cycle in human pneumocystosis. Arch Pathol 93:312, 1972. Copyright 1972, American Medical Association.)

occurred in infants younger than 1 year of age. Proved or presumptive congenital immunodeficiencies were identifiable in virtually all of the children in this group. In patients 1 to 10 years of age, who constituted the next largest group (26), only six had a primary immune deficit, whereas most of the other children had an underlying hematologic malignancy. The remaining patients, ranging in age from 10 to 81 years, were persons with assorted malignancies or renal allografts who almost always had had prior exposure to corticosteroids, radiation, or cytotoxic drugs. The mortality rate for the entire group of patients was 95%.

The Centers for Disease Control and Prevention (CDC) updated Le Clair's study by investigating the epidemiologic, clinical, and diagnostic aspects of all confirmed cases of pneumocystosis reported to its Parasitic Disease Drug Service between 1967 and 1970.[110,111] The first of these reports has particular relevance because it focused only on the infectious episodes in infants and young children.[110] A total of 194 documented cases of *P. jiroveci* pneumonia were analyzed, and 29 occurred in infants younger than 1 year of age. The attack rate for this group (8.4 per million) was more than five times higher than that for other age groups. Eighty-three percent of these infants had an underlying primary immunodeficiency disease. Moreover, because the inheritance of the primary immunodeficiency state often was sex linked, the preponderance of infection (88%) occurred in males. The mean age at diagnosis in the immunodeficient infants was 7.5 months, whereas the epidemic form of the infection in European and Asian infants was associated with peak morbidity in the third and fourth months of life.[15,23] Twenty-four percent of the infected children with immunodeficiencies had at least one sibling with an identifiable immune deficiency in whom *P. jiroveci* pneumonia also developed.[110]

After this analysis of cases indigenous to the United States was complete, it became evident that infantile pneumocystosis could be introduced into the United States from epidemics abroad. The first such case was reported in 1966 when a 3-month-old Korean infant died of *Pneumocystis* infection after being brought to the United States from an orphanage in Korea.[112] The potential for imported pneumocystosis received renewed publicity with the cessation of the war in Vietnam. Surveillance for *Pneumocystis* infection in American-adopted Vietnamese orphans was urged when it was recognized that large numbers of infants exposed to the hardships of war and malnutrition in Indochina had experienced fulminant *Pneumocystis* pneumonia.[113,114] In quick succession, multiple cases of *Pneumocystis* infection among these refugee Vietnamese were reported.[115-118] Most of the affected infants were approximately 3 months of age; this was exactly the age at which pneumocystosis had emerged in the marasmic children infected during the earlier nursery epidemics in central Europe and Asia.

The epidemiology of *P. jiroveci* infection has changed as cases of human immunodeficiency virus (HIV) infection have occurred in infants.[119] As is true in adults with acquired immunodeficiency syndrome (AIDS), infants with AIDS are at high risk for this opportunistic infection. Among children with perinatally acquired HIV infection, *P. jiroveci* pneumonitis occurs most often among infants 3 to 6 months of age.[120]

It has been suggested[121-125] that *P. jiroveci* may be an important cause of pneumonitis in immunologically intact infants. In a prospective study of infant pneumonia, Stagno and co-workers[125] detected *Pneumocystis* antigenemia in 10 (14%) of 67 infants. None of these 10 infants with serologic evidence of *Pneumocystis* infection had a primary immunodeficiency, nor had any received immunosuppressive medication. Antigenemia did not occur in control infants or in infants with pneumonitis caused by *Chlamydia trachomatis*, respiratory syncytial virus, cytomegalovirus, adenovirus, or influenza A and B viruses. Histopathologic confirmation of *Pneumocystis* pneumonia was possible in the only one of these infants who underwent open lung biopsy. *P. jiroveci* also causes pneumonia in infants living in resource-limited countries, even when the child is not malnourished. Shann and associates[126] found *P. jiroveci* antigen in serum from 23 of 94 children in Papua, New Guinea who were hospitalized with pneumonia. Nevertheless, more cases need to be confirmed histologically before it is established that *Pneumocystis* infection produces morbidity in previously healthy infants.

The mode of transmission of *P. jiroveci* remains unclear. Sporadic cases of pneumocystosis serve as poor models of infection transmission because they may not become clinically manifest until long after the host has acquired the organism. That person-to-person spread of *Pneumocystis* could occur was first suggested by the European nursery epidemics. Even in these institutional outbreaks, however, it was readily appreciated that direct interpatient transfer of the organism happened rarely.[15] Rather, seroepidemiologic investigation indicated that healthy, subclinically infected nursery personnel transmitted the infection.[45,54,55] The mode of spread of *Pneumocystis* from infected asymptomatic persons to susceptible infants in the closed nursery environment is not known. Airborne droplet transmission was suspected when "sterilization of air with ionizing radiation"[127] and isolation of uninfected infants from infected infants and their seropositive attendants[128] reduced the frequency of clinical disease. The hypothesis that *Pneumocystis* is transmissible through the air presupposes that the organism can be found in respiratory secretions. Although, as emphasized earlier, the intra-alveolar histopathologic features of pneumocystosis mitigate against this occurrence, *Pneumocystis* occasionally is detected in tracheal aspirates and sputum.[31,46,129-133]

Epidemiologic investigation of sporadic pneumocystosis indicates that person-to-person transmission of the infection is possible. The sequential development of *Pneumocystis* pneumonia in immunosuppressed adults occupying adjoining hospital beds has been recorded.[133,135] Jacobs and associates[136] described a cluster of cases of *P. jiroveci* pneumonia in previously healthy adults who all were hospitalized between July and October 1989. Whereas all five patients were on different floors of this hospital on three different services, two of the patients were briefly in the intensive care unit at the same time. Immunologic evaluation in three of the five patients revealed normal $CD4^+$, $CD8^+$, and $CD4^+/CD8^+$ ratios but depressed responses to T-cell lectin phytohemagglutinin and T cell–dependent B-cell pokeweed mitogen. Occurrence of pneumocystosis among family members also has been reported.[122,137,138] Pneumonia developed in three family members in a strikingly related time sequence.[122] More commonly, cases within a family emerge over a period of several years, and affected members almost always are infant siblings with either proven or suspected underlying immunodeficiencies. In at least three family studies, no fewer than three siblings succumbed to the infection.[137,139,140] It is unlikely, however, that direct patient-to-patient transfer of the organism occurred in any of these settings, because in almost all instances, development of disease in the sibling occurred months or years later, often long after the death of the initially infected child.[110]

Contagion could still be implicated in the family milieu if a reservoir of asymptomatic infection with *P. jiroveci* existed among healthy family members. Supporting evidence comes from two published accounts of infants with primary immunodeficiencies and pneumocystosis: The parents were deemed to be possible sources of the infection because their sera contained specific anti-*Pneumocystis* antibody.[140,142]

Maternal transfer of *Pneumocystis* to infants from colostrum or from the genital tract at parturition also might maintain *Pneumocystis* within a family, but screening of breast milk[138] and cervical secretions[139] with Giemsa and methenamine silver stains has failed to reveal the presence of the organism. Alternatively, acquisition of *P. jiroveci* by infants in utero could occur. Unfortunately, it is difficult to test this hypothesis in the absence of reliable serologic tools to detect subclinical infection in the newborn. The paucity of documented cases of overt *Pneumocystis* pneumonia in stillborn infants or in the early neonatal period, however, argues against frequent intrauterine passage of the organism.

In 1962, Pavlica,[143] in Czechoslovakia, recorded the first instance of congenital infection. The infant described was stillborn. The parents and a female sibling were in good health. The mother's serum had complement-fixing antibodies against *Pneumocystis*. Subsequently, in a report detailing experience with *Pneumocystis* infection in southern Iran, a male child who had died at 2 days of age was described; autopsy examination revealed scattered although definite alveolar foci of typical *Pneumocystis* infection.[144] The authors reasoned that this represented congenital infection, rather than an acquired disease with an untenably short incubation period. Bazaz and colleagues[139] in the United States described the striking development of *Pneumocystis* pneumonia in three otherwise healthy female siblings who died at 3 months, 2 months, and 3 days of age, respectively; again, an in utero source for their infections was considered to be most likely. In none of these cases of presumptive congenital pneumocystosis, however, was the placenta examined histologically for the presence of the organism. One infant, born to a mother with AIDS and documented *P. jiroveci* pneumonia in the fourth month of gestation, did not have *P. jiroveci* infection in the newborn period.[145] Beach and co-workers[146] described an HIV-positive newborn with meconium aspiration and pneumonia who had *P. jiroveci* identified in lung biopsy material at 19 days of age. Despite the infant's positive HIV status, serum from the infant's mother was HIV negative, and the serum from the father was HIV positive. Because the parents disappeared shortly after the infant's birth, follow-up evaluation was not possible; however, the parents had no previous history of *P. jiroveci* pneumonia, and the mother had been noted to be markedly wasted.

The mode of transmission of *Pneumocystis* in older children was first explored in the United States at the University of Minnesota Hospitals[147] and at St. Jude Children's Research Hospital,[108] where an unusually high number of cases was recorded. At neither center was it possible to reconstruct the spread of pneumocystosis from one patient to another. In most cases, the onset of illness appeared to antedate admission to the hospital. No attempt was made to incriminate healthy carriers as point sources for seemingly isolated episodes of infection. At Memorial Hospital in New York, *Pneumocystis* pneumonia developed in 11 patients, including 6 children, over a 3-month period.[148] Although no definite evidence of communicability could be discerned in this statistically significant cluster of cases, several of the *Pneumocystis*-infected children had had contact with each other and had shared rooms at various times; in addition, results of serologic tests for *Pneumocystis* infection were positive in two physicians caring for these patients. Similar outbreaks have since occurred in two pediatric hospitals in Indianapolis, Indiana,[149] and Milwaukee, Wisconsin.[150] At these centers, the increased rates of pneumocystosis were clearly related, as they were at St. Jude Children's Research Hospital,[108,151] to the use of more intensive cancer chemotherapy regimens. In a seroepidemiologic investigation of the cases in the Indianapolis outbreak, however, it was found that transmission of *Pneumocystis* probably occurred within the hospital environment. A direct association was noted between duration of hospitalization and risk of subsequent *Pneumocystis* infection. Furthermore, a significantly higher prevalence of positive results on serologic testing for *Pneumocystis* was detected among staff members who had close contact with infected children than among personnel whose duties did not include such patient contact. Precisely how *Pneumocystis* was originally introduced into the hospital was not determined.

The possibility that *Pneumocystis* pneumonia is a zoonotic disease and that infestation of rodents or even domesticated pets could provide a sizable reservoir for human infection has been investigated to a limited degree. Abundant infection of rodents with *Pneumocystis* was discovered in patients' homes in many of the index cases in ward epidemics in Czechoslovakia.[152] At St. Jude Children's Research Hospital, a high rate of exposure to pets was noted among the *Pneumocystis*-infected children with malignancy.[153] Of course, these findings would have epidemiologic significance only if the species of *Pneumocystis* infecting both animals and humans was the same. This remains to be shown. Experimental attempts to produce clinical pneumocystosis in multiple animal species by inoculation of infected human lung suspensions have not been successful[154-156] unless the animal was congenitally athymic[157] or immunosuppressed by treatment with corticosteroids.[158]

Airborne transmission of *Pneumocystis* was first presumptively demonstrated by Hendley and Weller in 1971.[156] These investigators observed that in cesarean section–obtained, barrier-sustained (COBS) rats given corticosteroids, infections with *Pneumocystis* developed following exposure to a common air supply from standard infected rats, whereas control COBS animals that received corticosteroids remained free of infection. One potential flaw in this experimental design was that the corticosteroid therapy could have reactivated previously latent *Pneumocystis* infection in any of the challenged animals. To circumvent this problem, Walzer and co-workers[154] challenged congenitally athymic (nude) mice. These animals received no exogenous immunosuppressants and still contracted pneumocystosis after exposure to air from infected rats. Thus, these studies documented airborne transmission of *P. jiroveci* as well as spread of the organism between different animal species. Of note is that soon after these experiments were published, a natural epizootic of *Pneumocystis* pneumonia was uncovered in a colony of nude mice.[157] Other studies using the murine model of pneumocystosis have suggested that subclinical transmission of the infection also can occur. Healthy rats exposed to animals with *Pneumocystis* pneumonia remain well but are found to have titers of anti-*Pneumocystis* antibodies consistent with acute acquisition of the infection.[158] In addition, rats with preexisting *Pneumocystis* antibodies may become antigenemic on comparable exposure to overt infection; these animals may be experiencing subclinical reinfection.[101]

Pathology

The gross and microscopic pathologic features of *P. jiroveci* pneumonia have been elucidated in a number of excellent reviews.[10,15,23,26,31,127,147,159-161] At autopsy in typically advanced infection, both lungs are heavy and diffusely affected. The most extensive involvement often is seen in posterior or dependent areas. At the lung margins anteriorly, a few remaining air-filled alveoli may constitute the only portion of functioning lung at the time of death.[10] Subpleural air blebs not infrequently are seen in these anterior marginal areas. Occasionally, prominent mediastinal emphysema or frank pneumothorax can be noted. The color of the lungs is variously described as dark bluish purple,[23,144] yellow-pink,[24] or pale gray-brown.[10,26] The pleural surfaces are smooth and glistening, with little inflammatory reaction. Hilar adenopathy is uncommon. Necrosis of tissue is not a feature of the disease.

Although these gross features of widespread infection are strikingly characteristic, focal or subclinical pneumocystosis presents a less recognizable picture. In this condition, the lung has tiny 3- to 5-mm reddish brown retracted areas contained within peribronchial and subpleural lobules, where hypostasis is greatest.[23,30] Even these features, however, may be absent because of variable involvement of adjacent lung tissue by concomitant pathologic processes.

The microscopic appearance of both the contents and the septal walls of pulmonary alveoli in *Pneumocystis* pneumonia are virtually pathognomonic of the infection. The outstanding histologic finding with hematoxylin and eosin stain is an intensely eosinophilic, foamy, or honeycomb-like material uniformly filling the alveolar sacs (Fig. 34-4). This intra-alveolar material is composed largely of packets of *P. jiroveci*.[127,162] Typical cysts or trophozoite forms of the organism within alveoli are visible only after application of special stains such as methenamine silver.

The type and degree of cellular inflammatory response provoked by the intra-alveolar cluster of *Pneumocystis* organisms vary in different hosts.[127] The descriptive histologic

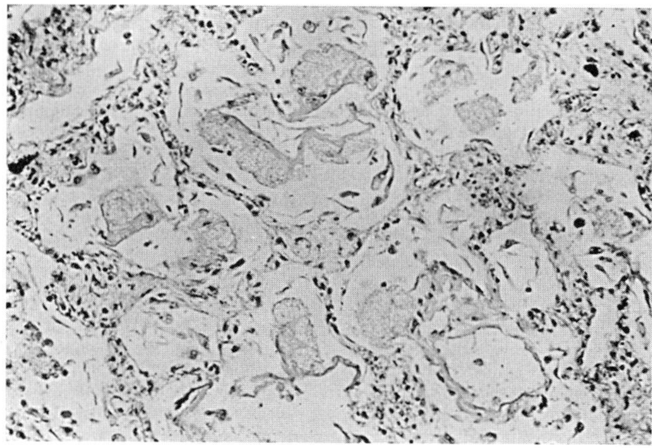

Figure 34–4 Section of lung tissue obtained at autopsy showing the amorphous, proteinaceous intra-alveolar infiltrate characteristic of pneumonitis caused by *Pneumocystis jiroveci*. Hematoxylin and eosin stain, ×160. (From Remington JS. Hosp Pract 7:59, April 1972.)

Table 34–1 Conditions Associated with *Pneumocystis jiroveci* Pneumonia

1. Premature infants aged 2 to 4 months with marasmus and malnutrition, usually living in foundling homes in geographic locales endemic for pneumocystosis
2. Infants and children with congenital (primary) immunodeficiency disease
   a. Severe combined immunodeficiency
   b. X-linked agammaglobulinemia
   c. X-linked immunodeficiency
   d. Variable immunodeficiency
   e. Immunodeficiency with hyperimmunoglobulinemia
   f. Immunodeficiency associated with Wiskott-Aldrich syndrome
3. Children and adults with acquired immunodeficiency
   a. Disease-related: lymphoreticular malignancies; multiple myeloma; dysproteinemias
   b. Drug-related (corticosteroids, cyclophosphamide, busulfan, methotrexate, colloidal gold); organ transplantation; lymphoreticular malignancies; solid tumors; collagen vascular disorders; miscellaneous diseases treated with immunosuppressants
   c. Acquired immunodeficiency syndrome (human immunodeficiency virus infection)

Adapted from Burke BA, Good RA. *Pneumocystis carinii* infection. Medicine 52:23, 1972; and Walzer PD, et al. *Pneumocystis carinii* pneumonia in the United States; epidemiologic, diagnostic and clinical features. Ann Intern Med 80:83, 1974, with permission.

term for pneumocystosis—*interstitial plasma cell pneumonia*—is derived from the pronounced plasma cellular infiltration of the interalveolar septa observed almost exclusively in newborns in European nursery epidemics. Distention of alveolar walls to 5 to 10 times the normal thickness, with resultant compression of alveolar spaces and capillary lumens, typically is noted in this form of the disease. Hyaline membranes develop occasionally,[10] often when the foamy honeycomb pattern within alveoli is least prominent.[147] Septal cell hyperplasia is apparently a nonspecific reaction of lung tissue to injury induced by infections of diverse etiology.[163]

Hughes and colleagues[153] studied the histologic progression of typical *Pneumocystis* pneumonia based on the number and location of organisms and the cellular response in pulmonary tissue. The lung samples were from children with underlying malignancy who had received intensive chemotherapy. The authors categorized three sequential stages in the course of the disease. In the first stage, no septal inflammatory or cellular response is seen, and only a few free cyst forms are present in the alveolar lumen; the remainder are isolated in the cytoplasm of cells on the alveolar septal wall. The second stage is characterized by an increase in the number of organisms within macrophages fixed to the alveolar wall and desquamation of these cells into the alveolar space; again, only minimal septal inflammatory response is seen at this time. Finally, a third stage is identified in which extensive reactive and desquamative alveolitis can be seen. Such diffuse alveolar damage may be the major pathologic feature in certain cases.[164] Variable numbers of cysts of the organism, presumably undergoing dissolution, are present within the alveolar macrophages. These findings underscore an earlier claim[165] that the so-called foamy exudate within alveoli is neither foamy edema fluid nor the product of an exudative inflammatory reaction but largely a collection of coalesced alveolar cells and macrophages that contain sizable digestive vacuoles and remnant organisms.

The mechanism of spread of *Pneumocystis* throughout pulmonary tissue is not completely understood. Direct invasion by the organism through septal walls into the interstitium or the lymphatic or blood vascular spaces of the lung is considered unlikely,[30,147,153] except in rare instances when systemic dissemination of the organism occurs (see later discussion). Instead, it is probable that coughing expels cysts from alveoli into larger airways and that the organisms are then inhaled into previously uninvolved alveolar areas.[127] This hypothesis of interairway transfer of *Pneumocystis* is supported by the fact that the heaviest concentration of organisms usually is found in dependent portions of the lung parenchyma.

Interstitial fibrosis is a distinct but infrequently reported complication of *Pneumocystis* pneumonia in older children and adults but has been reported in infants only rarely.[11,147,160,161,166-172] Nowak,[169] in Europe, first emphasized that fibrosis was not unusual in the lungs of infants at autopsy who had especially protracted infection with *P. jiroveci*. *Pneumocystis*-infected lungs sometimes demonstrate, in addition to fibrosis, other pathologic features compatible with a more chronic destructive inflammatory process. Multinucleate alveolar giant cells occasionally accompany alveolar cell proliferation.[23,26,30,161] Whether presence of these cells is more often a response to undetected concomitant viral infection is unknown. Typical granulomatous reactions with organisms visible in the granulomas also have been described.[161,173,174] Extensive calcification of *Pneumocystis* exudate and adjacent lung tissue may ultimately develop.[26,147,161]

Pathogenesis

The clinical conditions that predispose patients to the development of *Pneumocystis* pneumonia are associated with impaired immune responses, leading to the presumption that *Pneumocystis* causes disease not because it is intrinsically virulent but because the host's immune mechanisms fail to contain it (Table 34-1). The severity of

P. jiroveci pneumonia in infants with AIDS illustrates this phenomenon dramatically. The primary role of immunocompromise also would explain in part why *Pneumocystis* pneumonia did not emerge as a serious health problem until more than 30 years after the disease was first recognized. European epidemics of *Pneumocystis* arose out of the devastation of World War II and widespread utilization of antibacterial drugs. Each of these two seemingly unrelated events served ultimately to disrupt the normal host-organism immunologic interaction in favor of the organism. The war resulted in institutionalization of inordinate numbers of orphans under conditions of overcrowding and malnutrition. At the same time, antibacterial therapy dramatically enhanced survival rates of these institutionalized infants, who would otherwise have succumbed to bacterial sepsis during the first days or weeks of life. In addition, it was realized that *Pneumocystis* infection appeared in these marasmic children at an age when their immunoglobulin G levels reached a physiologic nadir. By 1960, the orphanage epidemics had abated in Europe as environmental conditions improved, but they persisted in Asia, where poverty and overcrowding continued.[144,175] Subsidence of the epidemic disease and more widespread antibacterial drug therapy, as well as sophisticated immunosuppressive drug treatment, contributed thereafter to awareness in Europe and North America of isolated instances of *Pneumocystis* infection among children suffering from a variety of identifiable immunodeficiencies.

Weller, in Europe, was among the first to experimentally induce *Pneumocystis* pneumonia in animals.[176,177] His crucial observation relative to pathogenesis of the infection was that in rats pretreated with cortisone (and penicillin) and exposed to suspensions of *Pneumocystis*-containing lung tissue, *Pneumocystis* pneumonia develops with the same frequency and severity as in corticoid-treated animals that were not subsequently inoculated with organisms. The intensity of such artificially induced animal infection also was noted to be less marked than that in spontaneous human pneumocystosis of the epidemic variety. Comparable observations in the rabbit model were made by Sheldon in the United States.[155] He showed that cortisone and antimicrobial agents were sufficient to induce *Pneumocystis* infection without direct exposure of animals to an exogenous source of organisms. The inescapable conclusion of these carefully designed studies was that *Pneumocystis* infection is latent in rats and rabbits and becomes clinically manifest only when host resistance is altered.

In 1966, Frenkel and colleagues[178] published a hallmark study of rat pneumocystosis. They showed that clinical and histopathologically significant involvement with *Pneumocystis* is regularly inducible in rats by "conditioning" them with parenteral cortisone over a period of 1 to 2 months. Premature death from complicating bacterial infection was prevented by simultaneous administration of antibacterial agents. Of interest is their finding that regression of established interstitial pneumonitis occurs if cortisone conditioning is stopped early enough; on the other hand, rats continuing to receive cortisone die of coalescent alveolar *Pneumocystis* infiltration, and the infiltrate is almost devoid of inflammatory cells. These histologic changes are, in fact, an exact replica of those observed in sporadic cases of human *Pneumocystis* infection developing in congenitally immunodeficient and exogenously immunosuppressed patients. Those authors attempted to precipitate clinical pneumocystosis with a variety of immunosuppressants other than cortisone. Of eight cytotoxic agents and antimetabolites tested, only cyclophosphamide was shown to activate latent infection. Total-body irradiation and lymphoid tissue ablation (splenectomy, thymectomy) by themselves were incapable of inducing overt *Pneumocystis* pneumonia.

The clinical association between pneumocystosis and protein-calorie malnutrition also has been reproduced in a rat model.[179] Healthy rats given either a regular or a low-protein diet gain weight and exhibit little to no evidence of pneumocystosis post mortem. By contrast, in rats fed a protein-free diet, which produces weight loss and hypoalbuminemia, fatal infection regularly developed; administration of corticosteroid only foreshortened their median survival time.[173]

None of the experimental models described thus far permit a precise appraisal of the relative importance of the cellular and humoral components of host defense against *Pneumocystis*. Although corticosteroids, cytotoxic drugs, and starvation interfere primarily with cell-mediated immunity, they do not always induce purely functional cellular defects. For example, it is known from in vitro cell culture studies that corticosteroids do not inhibit the uptake of *Pneumocystis* by alveolar macrophages.[65] Rather, the immunosuppressive effects of chemotherapeutic agents or of malnutrition are far more complex, and ultimately both cellular and humoral arms of the immune system may be impaired by them.

The production of pneumocystosis in the nude mouse without the use of exogenous immunosuppressants implies that susceptibility to the infection relates most to a defect in thymic-dependent lymphocytes.[154] Antibody deficiency must be less important, because certain strains of nude mice are resistant to pneumocystosis, yet neither these animals nor their susceptible littermates produce measurable antibodies. These findings do not exclude a role for antibody in control of established infection with the organism; indeed, it has been shown in vitro that *P. jiroveci* organisms adherent to rat alveolar macrophages become interiorized only after anti-*Pneumocystis* serum is added to the culture system.[158]

That primary immune deficits could predispose to sporadic pneumocystosis was first reported, unwittingly, by Hutchison in England in 1955.[86] He described male siblings with congenital agammaglobulinemia who died of pneumonia of "similar and unusual" histology. *P. jiroveci* was implicated as the etiologic agent of these fatal infections only when the pathologic sections were reviewed by Baar,[180] who had reported the first case of *Pneumocystis* pneumonia in England earlier that year.[72] In one of the first such reports from the United States, Burke and her colleagues[181] stressed what was to be regarded as a typical histologic finding in *Pneumocystis*-infected agammaglobulinemic children—namely, the absence or gross deficiency of plasma cells in pulmonary lesions (and in hematopoietic tissues). This deficiency contrasted sharply with the extensive plasmacytosis seen in epidemic infections. In addition, sera from some of these hypogammaglobulinemic children did not contain antibody to a *Pneumocystis* antigen derived from lung tissue in "epidemic" European cases.[55]

None of these *Pneumocystis*-infected patients with a primary humoral immunodeficiency disease had evidence of an isolated impairment of cellular immunity. (Indeed, only once has pneumocystosis been reported in association with a pure T cell deficiency—namely, in DiGeorge's syndrome.[182]) Most of the *Pneumocystis* infections, however, did occur in the infants with severe combined immunodeficiency, a state characterized by profound depression of both cellular and humoral immunity.

That the integrity of the cellular immune system is critical for resistance to *Pneumocystis* may be inferred from the steroid-induced and congenitally athymic animal models of pneumocystosis described earlier and from clinical experience with the infection in older children with lymphoreticular malignancies, collagen-vascular disorders, or organ allografts. These individuals receive broad immunosuppressive therapy designed to inhibit mainly the cellular arm of the immune system. Indeed, the incidence of *Pneumocystis* infection in these patients is related less to the nature of the underlying condition than to the intensity of immunosuppressive chemotherapy given for it.[127,147,151,163,183-185]

For many years it had not been possible to study in vitro the cellular immune response to *P. jiroveci* because of the impurity of available antigens. Preliminary experiments with an antigen derived from a cell culture suggested that specific cell-mediated immunity may be depressed in children with active *Pneumocystis* pneumonia. Lymphocytes from two such children failed to transform in the presence of the antigen,[186] whereas lymphocytes from healthy, seropositive adults were in most cases stimulated specifically to undergo blastogenesis.[186,187]

The humoral immune response to pneumocystosis has been measured in a variety of infected populations.[110,147,153,160,188,189] The most detailed serosurveys have been conducted in Iran[23,190] and central Europe[191-193] in infants with typical epidemic interstitial plasma cell pneumonia. Infants in Iranian orphanages had elevated levels of all immunoglobulins presumably because of the abundance of infective organisms in their institutional environments compared with values recorded in age-matched healthy U.S. infants.[190] No statistical difference was detectable in immunoglobulin concentrations between *Pneumocystis* carriers (those with "focal pneumocystosis") and uninfected infants within an orphanage. Prominent elevation in serum IgM levels correlated with the intensity of *Pneumocystis* disease as measured by clinical, radiographic, and histologic (e.g., plasma cell infiltration) criteria. The peak values of IgM persisted for only a short "crisis" period and then rapidly decreased toward normal. Serum IgG concentrations reached significantly depressed values of less than 200 mg/dL only in infants with massive interstitial pneumonitis. A precipitous drop in serum IgA level was recorded in three *Pneumocystis*-infected children 2 to 3 days before onset of marked respiratory impairment; the complete absence of alveolar IgA also was documented by fluorescent antibody techniques.

Iranian workers have proposed a provocative hypothesis relating these alterations in immunoglobulin levels to the pathogenesis of infant pneumocystosis. The level of transplacentally transferred maternal anti-*Pneumocystis* IgG decreases during the infant's first months of life. This reduction may be accentuated and occur earlier in premature infants, owing in part to malnutrition, diarrhea, and inordinate gastrointestinal protein loss.[23,190,194,195] This low IgG concentration probably predisposes these infants to intra-alveolar proliferation of *P. jiroveci*. Normally, IgA prevents surface spread of the organism. If serum IgA levels also are low, so that bronchoalveolar IgA secretion ceases (this remains to be proved), surface spread of the infection proceeds. Subsequently, progression of focal pneumocystosis to clinically evident pneumonia occurs. Increased IgM antibody formation reflects a humoral response to the highly antigenic cyst walls of the organism. If the infant survives, active production of *Pneumocystis*-specific IgG occurs during the fifth to ninth month of life. Patients with "hypoimmune pneumocystosis," so named by Dutz,[23] with underlying congenital immunodeficiency (or acquired immune defects from immunosuppressive chemotherapy) would not exhibit such an IgG response and thus would be subject to recurrence of clinically manifest pneumonic disease. An obstacle to complete acceptance of this hypothesis is that it assigns a major role to IgG and IgA in host defense against *P. jiroveci* infection. Yet *Pneumocystis* pneumonia has not been reported in children who produce little or no IgA, such as those with ataxia-telangiectasia.[147]

Brzosko and his colleagues[191-193,196] in Poland have studied the immunopathogenesis of *Pneumocystis* pneumonia at the tissue level by imunofluorescent methodology. These investigators first reported that γ-globulin is present in the intra-alveolar exudate of *Pneumocystis* infection.[196] Subsequently, they demonstrated that this collection of γ-globulin represents the specific antibody component of *Pneumocystis* antigen-antibody complexes.[192] Direct immunofluorescent staining of infected lung tissue with fluorescein-conjugated anti–human globulin or rheumatoid factor revealed a large amount of "immune" globulins bound to packets of *Pneumocystis*. In the same infected tissue blocks, immunofluorescent complement fixation reactions also resulted in marked fluorescence of *Pneumocystis*–γ-globulin complexes. The avidity of these conglomerates for rheumatoid factor and complement supports the assumption that the tissue-bound γ-globulin deposits are specific immune reactants to *P. jiroveci*.[192] The most intense fluorescence coincided with periodic acid–Schiff–positive structures (presumably glycoproteins or mucoproteins) on the outer aspect of thick-walled cysts, suggesting that the major antigenicity of the organism resides in its mucoid envelope.[191]

Polish workers attempted to reconstruct the immunomorphologic events in typical epidemic pneumocystosis.[193] In the earliest stage of infection the antigenic constituents of *P. jiroveci* induce the formation of IgM and IgG anti-*Pneumocystis* antibodies, possibly in hilar and mediastinal lymph nodes. These antibodies bind to aggregates of alveolar *Pneumocystis* to form immune complexes. The latter then bind complement, with resultant gradual disintegration of the masses of organisms and their eventual phagocytosis by alveolar macrophages. Immunoglobulin-forming plasma cells proliferate in the interstitium and, conceivably, contribute additional antibody to the *Pneumocystis* aggregates. Clearly, no impairment in immunoglobulin synthesis is recorded in this analysis of epidemic pneumocystosis, but retarded binding of complement components to the immune complexes is regularly observed. Because the ultimate destruction and removal of the *Pneumocystis*-antibody conglomerates are complement dependent and the complement system is, in general, physiologically deficient in the first few months of life, survival of a particular infant with epidemic *Pneumocystis* pneumonia may depend on the stage of development and relative functional competency of the complement system.

Clinical Manifestations

General Considerations

No clinical features are pathognomonic for *P. jiroveci* infection. Organisms residing in scattered intra-alveolar foci may evoke no illness,[30,197,198] whereas histologically advanced infection may provoke variable symptoms and signs in different hosts. Features attributable to *Pneumocystis* infection per se may be obfuscated by concomitant infection with other opportunistic pathogens or by dramatic complications of an underlying condition.[26,188] Furthermore, clinical syndromes ascribable to *Pneumocystis* may be simulated by other infections (cytomegalovirus[15]), or by inflammatory processes (drug-induced pulmonary toxicity,[199] radiation fibrosis[200]) and neoplasia (pulmonary leukemia[201]) capable of producing interstitial pulmonary infiltrates in older children and adults. Thus, recognition of pneumocystosis on clinical grounds requires above all a high index of suspicion whenever interstitial pneumonia occurs in settings known to predispose to infection with the organism.

Despite these caveats, *Pneumocystis* is distinguishable from other opportunistic microbes by the fact that infection with this organism commonly surfaces when underlying disorders are quiescent. For example, in the case of severe combined immunodeficiency disease, pneumocystosis can develop only after immunologic competence has been at least partially restored by bone marrow transplantation.[110,147,202] Reversal of immune paralysis apparently elicits sufficient inflammation to convert subclinical infection to overt pneumonitis. Similarly, in children with lymphocytic leukemia, pneumocystosis most often occurs during periods of clinical and hematologic remission.[148,153,203-206] It may be inferred from these observations that pneumocystosis is not merely an end-stage infection in a host with a preterminal illness but, on the contrary, often represents a potentially treatable cause of death in patients whose primary immunodeficiency or malignancy has been controlled or effectively cured.

Symptoms and Signs

EPIDEMIC INFECTION IN INFANTS

The onset of epidemic-type infection in infants is reported to be slow and insidious. Initially, nonspecific signs of restlessness or languor, poor feeding and diarrhea are common. Tachypnea and periorbital cyanosis gradually develop. Cough productive of sticky mucus, although not prominent, may appear later.[15,30] Respiratory insufficiency progresses over 1 to 4 weeks, and patients exhibit increasingly severe tachypnea, dyspnea, intercostal retractions, and flaring of the nasal alae. Fever is absent or of low grade.[211] Physical findings are strikingly minimal and consist primarily of fine crepitant rales with deep inspiration. Chest roentgenograms, however, typically demonstrate pulmonary infiltrates early in the illness. The duration of untreated disease is 4 to 6 weeks, but it often is difficult to determine an exact date of onset of illness. Before the introduction of pentamidine therapy, the mortality rate for such epidemic infant infection is estimated to have been between 20% and 50%.[73,189]

SPORADIC INFECTION IN INFANTS

The typical clinical syndrome is less evident in sporadic cases of pneumocystosis occurring in infants with acquired or congenital immunodeficiency and in older children with acquired immunodeficiency. In infants with primary immunodeficiency diseases, the onset of clinical infection can be insidious, and illness can extend over weeks or possibly months,[147] a course not unlike that seen in epidemic pneumocystosis. By contrast, in most infants with congenital immunodeficiency or AIDS and in older children with acquired immune deficits, *Pneumocystis* pneumonia manifests abruptly and is a more symptomatic, short-lived disease.[41,106,111,147,153] Among infants with HIV infection, the median age at onset is 4 to 5 months, and the mortality rate is between 39% and 59%.[207] High fever and nonproductive cough are initial findings, followed by tachypnea, coryza, and, later, cyanosis. Death may supervene within a week or so. If no treatment is given, essentially all patients with this form of pneumocystosis die.

Radiologic Findings

Because the extent of pulmonary involvement in *P. jiroveci* pneumonia rarely is detectable by physical examination; a chest roentgenogram showing diffuse infiltrative disease is the most useful indicator of infection in a susceptible host.[41,134] Although certain characteristic patterns of radiographic involvement have been ascribed to *Pneumocystis* pneumonitis, it is worth emphasizing that the findings may vary depending on the presence of coincident pulmonary infection as well as on the nature of the underlying disease state.

EPIDEMIC INFECTION IN INFANTS

Ivady and colleagues[189] in Hungary studied the radiographic progression of epidemic infantile *Pneumocystis* pneumonia and identified five stages. The first three stages are recognizable when the infant is virtually symptom free and are defined by the presence of perivascular and peribronchial peripheral shadows extending toward the pleura. The two later stages more closely coincide with respiratory insufficiency and reveal changes resembling "butterfly" pulmonary edema and peripheral emphysematous blebs. The radiographic findings of mild ("focal") *Pneumocystis* pneumonia described by Vessal and associates[208] in infants from an Iranian orphanage included hilar interstitial infiltrate, thymic atrophy, pulmonary hyperaeration, and scattered lobular atelectasis. Although none of these signs is specific for *Pneumocystis* infection, they persist longer (3 weeks to 2 months) in serologically proven cases. Indeed, surviving infants may exhibit focal interstitial infiltrates after organisms are cleared from the lung[209] and for as long as 1 year.[210,211]

SPORADIC INFECTION IN INFANTS

A majority of radiologic characterizations of *Pneumocystis* pneumonia have emphasized the sporadic form of the infection. Minor differences in descriptive details usually reflect differences in the populations studied.[147,172,378-382] In infants, especially those with immunodeficiency syndromes, the initial roentgenogram often shows haziness spreading from the hilar regions to the periphery, which assumes a finely granular, interstitial pattern. An antecedent gross alveolar infiltrate usually is not seen.[147] The peripheral granularity may progress to coalescent nodules. These changes resemble the "atelectatic" radiographic abnormalities of hyaline membrane disease. In both conditions, aeration is absent peripherally. Pneumothorax with subcutaneous and interstitial emphysema and pneumomediastinum are not uncommon and are associated with a poor prognosis.[212] Even with therapy, radiographic clearing can lag far behind clinical improvement.

As experience with *Pneumocystis* has broadened, especially in older children and adults, a number of atypical roentgenographic abnormalities have been described.[41,381-390] These atypical findings include hilar and mediastinal adenopathy, pleural effusions, parenchymal cavitation, pneumatoceles, nodular densities, and unilateral or lobar distribution of infiltrates. By contrast, the chest roentgenographic appearance can remain essentially normal well after the onset of fever, dyspnea, and hypoxemia. The presence of such roentgenographically silent lung disease can be visualized as abnormal findings by pulmonary computed tomography.

Laboratory Studies

Routine laboratory studies yield little diagnostic information in *Pneumocystis* infection. Abnormalities in hemoglobin concentration or white blood cell count are more likely to result from an underlying disease of the hematopoietic system or cytotoxic drug effect. Neither laboratory value is consistently altered by secondary pneumocystosis. Nevertheless, a subgroup of infants with primary immunodeficiency disease and infection caused by *P. jiroveci* can exhibit significant eosinophilia.[30,73,140,147] Jose and associates[140] first emphasized the association of peripheral blood eosinophilia and pneumocystosis in a report describing three infected male siblings with infantile agammaglobulinemia. In one of the infants, eosinophilia developed very early in the course of the illness, and the differential eosinophil count peaked at 42% as the respiratory disease worsened. Accordingly, it has been suggested that the combination of cough, tachypnea, diffuse haziness on chest roentgenograms, and eosinophilia in an infant with immunodeficiency can be indicative of *Pneumocystis* pneumonia.[140,147] Hypercalcemia with or without nephrocalcinosis has been reported in infants with epidemic pneumocystosis.[73] Measurement of serum calcium levels in other patients with *Pneumocystis* infection, however, has revealed normal values whether or not coincident foci of pulmonary or renal parenchymal calcification existed.[106,147,153]

A constant pathophysiologic finding in pneumocystosis, as well as in other interstitial pulmonary diseases, is that of ventilation and perfusion defects most compatible with an "alveolar-capillary block" syndrome.[121,126,147,183,188,213-216] Arterial blood gas determinations in infected patients show severe hypoxemia and hypocapnia, often before profound subjective respiratory insufficiency or even radiologic abnormalities[217] supervene. Less commonly, modest hypercapnia with respiratory acidosis is recorded.[213] This respiratory pathophysiology correlates well with the anatomic pulmonary lesion in *Pneumocystis* pneumonia. Concentration of organisms within alveoli and inflammation of the surrounding alveolar septa not unexpectedly lead to interference in gas transfer, whereas persistence of areas of normal lung parenchyma and lack of significant airway obstruction account for the usual absence of carbon dioxide retention.

Concurrent Infection

The clinical presentation of pneumocystosis may be altered by simultaneous infection with other organisms. Certainly, infection with a variety of opportunistic pathogens is not surprising in patients with broadly compromised immunologic defense mechanisms. Infection with one or more organisms was found in 56% of *Pneumocystis*-infected infants and children with primary immunodeficiency disease reported to the CDC.[110] Comparable rates of multiple infections also have been noted in several large series of patients with acquired immune defects and pneumocystosis.[20,147,163,218]

Infection with cytomegalovirus appears to be the most common "unusual" infection associated with pneumocystosis. Indeed, in his 1957 review, Gajdusek[15] already was able to cite numerous published studies referring to the "unexpectedly high frequency of association" of the two infections. He conceded that one infection most probably predisposed the affected patient to the other. On the basis of electron micrographic observations of cytomegalovirus-like particles within pneumocysts, Wang and co-workers[38] hypothesized that *P. jiroveci* may even serve as an intermediate host or reservoir of the virus. The possibility of viral parasitism of (or symbiosis with) *Pneumocystis* also was explored by Pliess and Seifert[219] and by Vawter and colleagues,[39] who were impressed by the resemblance of the outer membranes of *P. jiroveci* to an imperfect form of myxovirus. It is still unclear, however, whether this inordinate concurrence of *Pneumocystis* and cytomegalovirus is caused by a specific and unique relationship between the two organisms or by coincidental infection of highly susceptible hosts with ubiquitous microbes.[52,163] Histopathologic examination of lung biopsy specimens from infants with AIDS often demonstrates concomitant cytomegalovirus and *P. jiroveci* infections.[220,221]

Diagnosis

The diagnosis of *Pneumocystis* pneumonia remains difficult. The organism must be visualized in the respiratory tract of ill persons, and often this can be accomplished only by bronchoalveolar lavage (BAL) or, in infants, a lung biopsy. Recently, PCR assay has been used for diagnosis in fluid specimens obtained by BAL. Nevertheless, this technique is still not sensitive and specific enough for routine clinical use. Attempts to isolate *Pneumocystis* from clinical specimens on synthetic media or in tissue culture have not been successful, and serologic techniques to detect active infection have been too insensitive.

Examination of Pulmonary Secretions

During the European epidemics, parasitic forms were recognized in mucus from infected infants.[31,47,130] Specimens usually were obtained through a catheter or laryngobronchoscope passed into the hypopharynx, and smears of the aspirated secretions were fixed in ether-alcohol and stained by the Gram-Weigert technique. By this method, Le Tan-Vinh and associates[31] in France reported antemortem diagnosis of *Pneumocystis* pneumonia in eight of nine infants. Toth and co-workers[130] in Hungary recovered *P. jiroveci* from tracheopharyngeal and gastric aspirates of 22 infants whose illness had just begun; in some cases, organisms were observed 7 to 10 days before the appearance of symptoms. The mere presence of organisms in hypopharyngeal secretions, however, did not always presage acute pneumonic disease in these environments, where pneumocystosis was endemic. Rather, it often reflected chronic subclinical carriage of the organism.[23]

Diagnosis of sporadic cases of pneumocystosis by examination of sputum or tracheal and gastric aspirates has never been as rewarding. The rate of recovery of *Pneumocystis* from upper airway secretions in the cases compiled by the CDC was estimated to be only about 6%.[111] Japanese investigators have described a method of concentrating sputum samples with acetyl-L-cysteine in 0.2N sodium hydroxide solution, which permits filtration and centrifugation of a pellet of *Pneumocystis*.[222] Ognibene and associates[223] reported the use of induced sputa in the diagnosis of pneumonia in 18 children with HIV infection or malignancy. Nine sputum samples were positive for *P. jiroveci* by immunofluorescent antibody testing. Four of the patients with negative findings by examination of sputum samples subsequently underwent BAL; BAL fluid was negative for *P. jiroveci* in all four. The remaining five patients received treatment for bacterial pneumonia and responded to therapy. This technique required ultrasonic nebulization in the children, and the youngest patient in this report was 2 years of age.

Percutaneous Lung Aspiration

The need to obtain lung tissue for a more accurate assessment of the presence of *Pneumocystis* pneumonia has been appreciated for some time. Percutaneous needle aspiration of the lung was already of proven value by the late 1950s in diagnosis of epidemic pneumocystosis in infants.[15] Subsequently, it was successfully employed in infected infants and children with underlying primary and acquired immunodeficiencies.[82,153,224,225] The procedure is performed without general anesthesia so that the child's respiratory function is not further compromised. Under fluoroscopy, a 20-gauge spinal needle with syringe in place is guided into the midportion of the lung. The resultant aspirate (usually less than 0.1 mL in amount) may be transferred directly to slides as unsmeared drops or first cytocentrifuged to increase the concentration of organisms in the sample.[226] Slides are allowed to air dry and then are stained with Gram, Gomori methenamine silver, and toluidine blue O stains. The residual material in the syringe is diluted with 2 mL of sterile saline and cultured for bacteria and fungi. Children with platelet counts of less than 60,000/mm^3 receive fresh whole blood or platelet transfusions before the procedure. Pneumothorax appears to be the major complication encountered. In one series, it occurred in 37% of the patients, and evacuation of air by thoracotomy tube was required in 14%.[225]

Lung Biopsy

It has been argued that aspiration is inferior to biopsy in that the former does not permit histologic examination of lung tissue. Open lung biopsy has been proposed as the most reliable method for identifying and estimating the extent of *Pneumocystis* infection, as well as for demonstrating the presence of complicating pathologic conditions such as coexistent infection, malignancy, or interstitial fibrosis.[147,214,218,227-229] It may be hazardous, however, to perform a thoracotomy using general anesthesia in patients with marginal pulmonary reserve.[230] Although the procedure has been associated with an acceptably low incidence of serious complications in critically ill children,[231-234] determination of its risk-to-benefit ratio based on the infant's underlying disease, expected life span, and clinical condition is appropriate in individual cases.[235,236] Unfortunately, these analyses have not yet been applied rigorously to infants and young children with suspected pneumocystosis. Technical modification in the performance of open biopsy that would avoid general anesthesia and endotracheal intubation (e.g., using thoracoscopy) may be particularly advantageous for diagnosis of *Pneumocystis* pneumonia in small children.[237]

Whichever invasive technique is employed for retrieval of tissue to test for the presence of *P. jiroveci*, it is generally agreed that immediate examination and staining of frozen sections or imprints of fresh lung (or alveolar secretions) are critical.[15,41,225,227,232,238,239] Processing of paraffin-embedded tissue incurs an unnecessary delay of one or more days in diagnosis, and the sections may actually reveal fewer organisms than the imprint smears. Although techniques using Giemsa stain are rapid and specific for the intracystic bodies of *P. jiroveci*, organisms are more readily located and identified against a background of tissue cells with a methenamine silver stain. It should be appreciated that other silver-positive organisms, such as *Torulopsis*[240] and zygomycete spores,[241] can mimic the cystic structure of *P. jiroveci* and that smears of *Pneumocystis* rather than fungi should be employed as controls for the stain.[242]

Unfortunately, the standard methenamine silver stain technique is slow (3 to 4 hours) and requires expertise usually found only in special histopathology laboratories. To circumvent these problems, several rapid (less than 30 minutes) and simple modifications of the silver stain have been developed.[243-246] Because the results with these stains have not been as consistent as those achieved with the standard, more lengthy procedure, many laboratories have chosen not to use silver for rapid screening of specimens but prefer instead toluidine blue O[32,247-250] and cresyl echt violet[33,257] for this purpose.

Serologic Tests

It is clear that sensitive and specific serologic methods are desirable to detect active *Pneumocystis* infection. It is disappointing that despite extensive investigation, no method has been proved to be entirely satisfactory.

Serodiagnosis of *P. jiroveci* infection in infants by detection of immunofluorescent antibodies was first reported in 1964 in Europe.[252] It was found that IgM and IgG anti-*Pneumocystis* immunofluorescent antibodies appear sequentially in sera during the course of clinical infection. Both classes of antibodies are present in sera of diseased infants during the first weeks of pneumonia, but only IgG antibodies persist during convalescent periods or in cases of protracted infection.[253]

The worth of immunofluorescent antibody tests in the diagnosis of sporadic pneumocystosis was examined subsequently in the United States by Norman and Kagan[254] at the CDC. They observed low rates of serologic reactivity among patients with suspected and confirmed cases, positive results in sera from patients who seemed to have only cytomegalovirus and other fungal infections, and negative results in sera from six infants with primary immunodeficiency diseases and documented pneumocystosis. Although it is possible to increase the specificity and sensitivity of these tests for *Pneumocystis*,[255,256] such tests detect background levels of *Pneumocystis* antibody in clinically healthy persons[98,99,256] and, as a result, fail to discriminate between patients with active disease and those who are latently infected with the organism.

The performance of the immunofluorescent antibody test has been hampered for years by the crude *Pneumocystis* antigens employed. Impure antigen results in autofluorescence of uninfected lung tissue, and extensive absorption of sera risks undue reduction in intensity of staining of organisms. For this reason, several laboratories have attempted to prepare a *Pneumocystis* antigen that is isolated as nearly as possible from the lung parenchyma, to which it characteristically clings. Techniques designed to extract free *P. jiroveci* from infected lung include bronchoalveolar saline lavage,[29,218] enzymatic digestion of lung homogenates,[257] and differential centrifugation of lung homogenates on sucrose[258] or Ficoll-Hypaque density gradients. These purified antigens have been used to generate immune sera that have been applied in immunofluorescent staining of *Pneumocystis* in lung tissue[259,260] and in upper airway secretions.[261,262]

To avoid the problem posed by the insensitivity of antibody determinations per se in pneumocystosis, Pifer and colleagues[99] developed a counterimmunoelectrophoretic assay for detecting circulating *Pneumocystis* antigen in suspected cases. In an initial evaluation of the test, antigenemia was demonstrated in up to 95% of children with *Pneumocystis* pneumonia and was absent in normal control children. Antigen also was found in the sera of 15% of oncology patients who did not have pneumonia, however. Thus, although antigenemia appears to be superior to circulating antibody as a serologic correlate of *Pneumocystis* infection, antigenemia alone cannot be equated with a diagnosis of pneumocystosis without corroborating clinical data.

Treatment

Specific Therapy

Hughes and co-workers[263] in 1974 first demonstrated that the combination of trimethoprim and sulfamethoxazole (TMP-SMX) was effective in treatment of cortisone-induced rat pneumocystosis. This combination was shown to be as efficacious as pentamidine in children infected with *Pneumocystis* who also had underlying malignancy.[264] Several uncontrolled trials of TMP-SMX in congenitally immunodeficient infants[265,266] and in older immunosuppressed children and adults[265,266] confirmed the efficacy and low toxicity of this combination agent. The dosage employed was 20 mg of TMP and 100 mg of SMX per kg of body weight per day, given orally in four divided doses for 14 days. This daily dose was two to three times that used in treatment of bacterial infections. The equivalent efficacy of TMP-SMX and of pentamidine has been confirmed in pediatric cancer patients with *P. jiroveci* pneumonia.[267]

TMP-SMX is the drug of choice for treatment of *P. jiroveci* pneumonia in infants and children. The oral route of administration can be used in mild cases, for which the recommended dosage is 20 mg TMP plus 100 mg SMX per kg per day in divided doses every 6 to 8 hours apart. Infants with moderate or severe disease require treatment by the intravenous route with 15 to 20 mg TMP plus 75 to 100 mg SMX per kg per day in divided doses 6 to 8 hours apart. Generally, treatment is given for 3 weeks. Adverse reactions to TMP-SMX will develop in approximately 5% of infants and children without HIV infection and 40% of children with HIV infection; most commonly seen is a maculopapular rash that clears after discontinuation of the drug. Other adverse reactions are uncommon and include neutropenia, anemia, renal dysfunction, and gastrointestinal symptoms or signs.

In infants who do not respond to TMP-SMX or in whom serious adverse reactions develop, pentamidine isethionate in a single daily dose of 4 mg/kg given intravenously may be used. Other drugs have been tested in limited studies in infants and young children with HIV infection and *P. jiroveci* pneumonia, including atovaquone, trimetrexate-leucovorin, oral TMP-dapsone, pyrimethamine-sulfadoxine, clindamycin plus primaquine, and aerosolized pentamidine.

The ease with which TMP-SMX can be administered and its lack of adverse side effects make it an attractive combination for empirical therapy for suspected pneumocystosis. Such treatment is reasonable in infants who are gravely ill and whose outlook for recovery from underlying disease is bleak. Several objections to the universal adoption of this approach have been raised. In at least half of the immunosuppressed children with typical clinical and roentgenographic features of *Pneumocystis* pneumonia, the illness is in fact not related to infection with *P. jiroveci*.[268] Identification of the etiologic agent and proper management of the disorder can be accomplished only by first performing appropriate diagnostic procedures.

Until 1958, no therapy specific for *P. jiroveci* infection was available. In that year, Ivady and Paldy[269] in Hungary recorded the first successful use of several aromatic diamidines, including pentamidine isethionate, in 16 of 19 infected infants. By 1962, the Hungarian investigators had used pentamidine therapy in 212 patients with epidemic *Pneumocystis* pneumonia.[192] During the next several years, favorable responses to this drug were observed in infants and children with both the epidemic and the sporadic forms of the infection.[142,147,153] Treatment effected a dramatic reduction in the mortality rate for the epidemic disease from 50% to less than 4%.[267,270] In the cases of sporadic infection reported to the CDC,[111,271,272] survival rates ranged from 42% to 63% for those patients who received the drug for 9 or more days. In cases confined largely to young children and managed at a single institution, cure rates were noted to be as high as 68% to 75%.[153,264] Because spontaneous recovery from *Pneumocystis* pneumonia in immunodepressed persons is rare,[273] it is clear that pentamidine therapy reduced the mortality rate in such patients to nearly 25%.

The recommended dose of the drug is 4 mg/kg intravenously once daily for 14 days. Clinical improvement becomes evident 4 to 6 days after initiation of therapy, but radiographic improvement may be delayed for several weeks.

Pentamidine toxicity from intravenous and intramuscular use has been reported. Although toxicity from pentamidine apparently was not a significant problem in the marasmic infants with *Pneumocystis* infection treated during the European epidemics,[274] the CDC determined that 189 (47%) of 404 children and adults given the drug for confirmed or suspected *Pneumocystis* infection suffered one or more adverse effects.[111] Immediate systemic reactions, such as hypotension, tachycardia, nausea, vomiting, facial flushing, pruritus, and subjective experience of unpleasant taste in the mouth, were noted particularly after intravenous administration of the drug. Herxheimer's reactions, although described for patients given pentamidine for leishmaniasis,[275] occurred rarely.[276] Local reactions at injection sites—namely, pain, erythema, and frank abscess formation—developed in 10% to 20% of patients.[111,272] Elevation in serum glutamic-oxaloacetic transaminase levels was frequently recorded and may have resulted partly from this local trauma. Hypoglycemia ensued not uncommonly after the fifth day of pentamidine therapy but often was asymptomatic[271] (Hypoglycemia also was observed in pediatric patients with AIDS who were given pentamidine for treatment of *P. jiroveci* pneumonia.[277]) Pentamidine-associated pancreatitis also has been reported in children and adults with HIV infection.[278,279,280] Although overt anemia was rare, megaloblastic bone marrow changes or depressed serum folate levels were noted.[271]

Supportive Care

A critical component in the management of *Pneumocystis* pneumonia is oxygen therapy. Because hypoxemia can be profound, the fraction of inspired oxygen should be adjusted to maintain the arterial oxygen tension at 70 mm Hg or above. The inspired oxygen concentration should not exceed 50%, to avoid oxygen toxicity. Assisted or controlled ventilation may be required. Methods of ventilatory support have been volume-regulated positive-pressure respirator[281] at either low or high frequency and membrane lung bypass.[282] Other ancillary measures, such as administration of γ-globulin[147,265,283] to infected congenitally immunodeficient children, warrant further study.

The use of early adjunctive corticosteroid therapy in the treatment of *P. jiroveci* pneumonia in adults with AIDS can increase survival and reduce the risk of respiratory failure.[284,285] A national consensus panel has recommended the use of corticosteroids in adults and adolescents with HIV infection and documented or suspected *P. jiroveci* pneumonia.[286] Two studies have supported the use of corticosteroids in decreasing the morbidity and mortality associated with *P. jiroveci* pneumonia.[287,288]

Prognosis

Chronic Sequelae

Little is known about the residual effects of successfully treated *Pneumocystis* pneumonia on pulmonary function. Patients may suffer additional "pulmonary" morbidity from other opportunistic infections or from noninfectious complications of underlying disease or its therapy. Robbins and associates[168] were fortunate enough to be able to follow the course of a hypogammaglobulinemic child with *Pneumocystis* infection treated with pentamidine in 1964; during the ensuing 5 years, despite intercurrent episodes of otitis media and bacterial pneumonia, she exhibited normal exercise tolerance and pulmonary function without evidence of reactivation of her *Pneumocystis* infection.[230] Hughes and co-workers[153] evaluated 18 children with underlying malignacies over periods of 1 to 4 years after surviving *Pneumocystis* infection. Although pulmonary function tests were not performed, none of the subjects demonstrated clinical or roentgenographic evidence of residual pulmonary disease. In a subsequent study from the same institution, pulmonary function was assessed serially in surviving children.[151] Significant improvement in function was noted within 1 month of the infection, and all abnormalities resolved by 6 months. This finding is in contrast with the observation of recurrent wheezing episodes and abnormal pulmonary function on follow-up evaluation of infants who had pneumonitis during the first 3 months of life.[289,290] Although later morbidity was independent of the original etiologic agent, 17% of these patients were thought to have *P. jiroveci* infection.

It seems inevitable that respiratory dysfunction can result from severe episodes of *Pneumocystis* pneumonia that provoke interstitial fibrosis or extensive calcification (as discussed earlier under "Pathology"). Cor pulmonale has been observed in infants with such protracted infection.[147] In one notably well-studied patient, an adult with biopsy-proven fibrosis that appeared 4 months after curative pentamidine therapy, serial tests of pulmonary function revealed persistent ventilatory defects of the restrictive type and impairment of carbon monoxide–diffusing capacity.[170] Although a possible link between pentamidine therapy per se and lung fibrosis was suggested by earlier observations in rat pneumocystosis,[178,291] healthy animals given the drug exhibit no histologic abnormalities.[153] Moreover, pulmonary fibrosis has been described after *Pneumocystis* pneumonia in patients who received treatment with pyrimethamine and sulfonamide[172] and TMP-SMX.[292]

Recurrent Infection

Recurrence of *Pneumocystis* pneumonia after apparently curative courses of therapy has been documented in infants and children with underlying congenital immunodeficiency or malignancy. As early as 1966, Patterson and colleagues[293] reported the case of an infant with probable severe combined immunodeficiency who experienced one presumptive and two substantiated bouts of pneumocystosis at approximately 5-month intervals; treatment with pentamidine resulted in "cure" on each occasion, although radiographic abnormalities persisted.[294] A few years later, Richman and associates[295] and then Saulsbury[283] described recurrent pneumocystosis in two children with hypogammaglobulinemia; in the first case, three proven attacks responded to pentamidine; and in the second child, two separate episodes of infection were treated successfully with TMP-SMX. At St. Jude Children's Research Hospital, a study of 28 children with malignancy whose pneumocystosis was treated with pentamidine revealed that 4 (14%) suffered a second infection.[153,171] The clinical manifestations, roentgenographic findings, and response to therapy were similar for each child in both infectious episodes. In addition, no differences in host factors were discernible in those patients who had recurrent infection and those who did not. Other examples of recurrent pneumocystosis emerging rather soon after clinical recovery have been observed in patients given either pentamidine or TMP-SMX.[296] Whether recurrences of *Pneumocystis* pneumonia result from reinfection or from relapse of previously treated infection is not known.

Clinical and morphologic studies provide conflicting views on the completeness of *Pneumocystis* killing by specific drugs. The Hungarian workers, who first utilized pentamidine in epidemic pneumocystosis among infants, witnessed progressive degeneration of *P. jiroveci* in tracheal mucus from the sixth day of therapy; by the tenth day, the organisms had almost entirely disintegrated.[189] In their review of sporadic pneumocystosis in the United States, Western and associates[271] similarly concluded that pentamidine probably eliminates organisms from the lung. In two patients, no microscopically visible *P. jiroveci* organisms were present at 5 and 14 days, respectively, after initiation of therapy. Also, none of 11 patients who died more than 20 days after receiving pentamidine had demonstrable organisms in their lungs, even though they survived an average of 189.5 days after administration of the drug. In ultrastructural studies, Campbell[42] detected what he believed to be the destructive effects of pentamidine on the organisms. In a lung biopsy specimen obtained surgically 16 hours after onset of therapy, structurally normal trophozoites or mature cysts with intracystic bodies were absent. A few apparent "ghosts" of trophozoites were noted within phagosomes of intra-alveolar macrophages.

By contrast, pentamidine does not promptly eradicate potentially viable forms of the organism. Hughes and coworkers[153] identified intact *P. jiroveci* in lung aspirates (or autopsy material) 10 to 20 days after institution of drug treatment. Richman and associates[295] demonstrated normal-appearing *Pneumocystis* organisms in a lung aspirate from a clinically cured patient 3 days after completion of his 14-day course of pentamidine. Similarly, Fortuny and colleagues[131] recovered organisms from induced sputa on each of 11 days of pentamidine injections.

TMP-SMX appears to have only a limited and nonlethal effect on organisms. Experiments have shown that short-term treatment with the drug combination ultimately fails to prevent emergence of recrudescent *Pneumocystis* infection. In one study, a therapeutic dosage of TMP-SMX was given prophylactically to children with acute lymphocytic leukemia for a 2-week period beginning 28 days after initiation of antineoplastic treatment.[297] Although the incidence of *Pneumocystis* infection in these children after TMP-SMX was discontinued was not different from that observed in persons who did not receive the drug, the time interval to development of infection was lengthened. Reinfection rather than relapse may have accounted for the late infections, but relapse seems more likely in view of the following results in experimental animals.[298] Immunocompetent rats were given TMP-SMX for as long as 6 weeks and then placed in individual isolator cages to exclude the possibility of acquisition of new organisms from the environmental air. After 12 weeks of immunosuppressive therapy with prednisone, *P. jiroveci* was still found in the lungs of at least 90% of both the animals given TMP-SMX and the control animals, given no treatment. These human and animal data are particularly relevant to the design of prophylactic regimens to prevent *Pneumocystis* infection in humans. They provide a compelling argument for the need to continue prophylaxis for as long as host defenses are considered to be too compromised to keep latent *Pneumocystis* infection in check.

Reactivation of pneumocystosis is not surprising in light of the pathogenesis and pathology of the infection in the immunodeficient subject. Frenkel and colleagues[18] showed clearly in the earliest experimental animal models of *Pneumocystis* pneumonia that anti-*Pneumocystis* therapy alone was not completely curative and that relapse was to be anticipated unless factors provoking the infection (namely, corticosteroid administration) were minimized. Long-term ultrastructural studies of *Pneumocystis* pneumonia in the rat confirmed that even with tapering of corticosteroid and apparent restoration of immune function, focal clusters of *P. jiroveci* are detectable in surviving animals for at least 21 weeks. Furthermore, in humans, drugs might not reach organisms residing within the foci of fibrosis and calcifications formed during especially severe infection.[299] Indeed, Dutz[23] contended that drugs play no therapeutic role in epidemic pneumocystosis once the chronic plasma cellular infiltrate is established. Radiographic resolution is slow, and survival and permanent immunity to reinfection relate not to chemotherapy but to specific anti-*Pneumocystis* immunoglobulin production in the affected infants. Unfortunately, the congenitally immunodeficient or exogenously immunosuppressed child does not possess such normal immune responsiveness and thus is subject to recurrent infection.

Prevention

The first successful attempts to prevent pneumocystosis with drugs were reported in infants with the epidemic form of the infection. In a controlled trial conducted in an Iranian orphanage where the infection was endemic (attack rate of 28%), the biweekly administration of a pyrimethamine and sulfadoxine combination to marasmic infants before the second month of life entirely eradicated *Pneumocystis* pneumonia from the institution.[300] In a children's hospital in Budapest, Hungary, pentamidine given every other day for a total of seven doses to premature infants from the second week of life provided equally effective prophylaxis. During the 6 years of the study, *Pneumocystis* infection did not develop among 536 premature babies who received this treatment, whereas 62 fatal cases were recorded elsewhere in the city.[301]

On the basis of promising results in a rat model of infection, TMP-SMX was evaluated in a randomized double-blind controlled trial in children with cancer who were at extremely high risk for *Pneumocystis* pneumonitis.[302] The daily dosage for prophylaxis was 5 mg of TMP plus 20 mg of SMX per kg of body weight, administered orally in two divided doses. Seventeen (21%) of 80 children receiving placebo acquired pneumocystosis, whereas the infection developed in none of 80 patients given TMP-SMX. No adverse effects of TMP-SMX administration were observed, although oral candidiasis was more prevalent among the patients in the treatment group than among the control patients. In a subsequent uncontrolled trial, the prophylactic efficacy of TMP-SMX was confirmed; cases of infection developed only in those children in whom the TMP-SMX was discontinued while they were still receiving anticancer chemotherapy.[303] More recently, a regimen of TMP-SMX prophylaxis given 3 days a week was shown to be as effective as daily administration.[304]

The gratifying success of TMP-SMX prophylaxis in prevention of *Pneumocystis* infection has been duplicated in other medical centers caring for children with underlying malignancy.[150,304,305] Administration of the drug for the duration of antineoplastic therapy has become standard practice. It would seem prudent to reserve TMP-SMX prophylaxis for persons at relatively high risk for *Pneumocystis* pneumonitis. Congenitally immunodeficient children and infants with AIDS who have had a prior episode of *Pneumocystis* pneumonia would appear to be prime candidates for preventive therapy. The CDC issued a set of guidelines for chemoprophylaxis against *P. jiroveci* pneumonia in children with HIV infection in 1991[306] and updated these guidelines in accordance with the most recent epidemiologic surveillance data demonstrating that despite recommendations established for *P. jiroveci* prophylaxis, no substantial decrease in *P. jiroveci* pneumonitis has occurred.[307] The surveillance data indicated that continued cases were the result of failure to identify HIV-infected infants and the poor sensitivity of $CD4^+$ counts to determine infants' risk for development of *P. jiroveci* pneumonitis, rather than because of treatment failures.[308] These updated guidelines recommend promptly identifying infants and children born to HIV-infected women, initiating prophylaxis at 4 to 6 weeks of age for all of these children, and continuing prophylaxis through 12 months of age for HIV-infected children and offer new algorithms based on clinical and immunologic status to continue prophylaxis beyond 12 months of age. Although no chemoprophylactic regimens for *P. jiroveci* pneumonia among HIV-infected children have been approved as labeling indications by the U.S. Food and Drug Administration (FDA), TMP-SMX currently is recommended as the drug of choice in children with HIV infection. This recommendation is based on the known safety profile of TMP-SMX and its efficacy in adults with HIV infection and in children with malignancies. Alternative regimens recommended for HIV-infected children who cannot tolerate TMP-SMX include aerosolized pentamidine in children more than 5 years of age, oral dapsone, and oral atovaquone. One study suggests that TMP-SMX use is associated with a decreased incidence of *P. jiroveci* pneumonitis and an increased incidence of HIV encephalopathy, both as initial AIDS-defining conditions in infants and children.[309]

ASPERGILLOSIS

Invasive aspergillosis is a disease of the immunocompromised host, including the premature infant in the neonatal intensive care unit (NICU). Although aspergillosis is uncommon among neonates, its incidence in this age group appears to have increased during the past 2 decades, coinciding with the increased survival of infants who are increasingly more immature at birth. Rapid progression from either primary cutaneous aspergillosis or pulmonary asperillosis to dissemination is common in these immature infants. Thus, early recognition with appropriate antifungal therapy is critical for an optimal outcome.

Aspergillosis has been reported in infants who ranged in age from 1 to 7 weeks. In 1955, Zimmerman[310] described a 13-day-old neonate who became febrile in association with formation of a subcutaneous abscess caused by *Staphylococcus*. Despite antimicrobial therapy for the abscess, pneumonia and hepatosplenomegaly subsequently developed, and the infant died at 1 month of age. *Aspergillus sydowi* was isolated from the lung, brain, pericardial and pleural fluid. Allan and Andersen[311] reported disseminated aspergillosis in an infant who showed the first signs of disease on the second day of life and who died at 18 days of age. At autopsy, *Aspergillus* was identified in lung, liver, spleen, heart, thyroid, bowel, and skin of this infant; *Aspergillus fumigatus* grew from cultures of the liver, spleen, and bowel. Luke and co-workers[312] reported disseminated aspergillosis in a debilitated infant who died at 7 weeks of age. At autopsy, *A. fumigatus* was isolated from the blood, heart, and kidneys, and the fungus was identified on microscopic examination in the endocardium, brain, and kidneys. Akkoyunlu and Yücell[313] reported a case of aspergillosis in an infant in whom onset of respiratory and central nervous system (CNS) disease occurred at 2 weeks of age. This infant died at 20 days of age with pneumonia and meningitis. *Aspergillus* was cultured from lung and brain tissue obtained at autopsy. The source of infection was thought to be infected grain on the farm where the infant lived. Infection in two of these four infants was considered secondary to prematurity or to antibiotic or corticosteroid therapy,[314,315] but predisposing causes for disseminated aspergillosis were not found in the others.[316,317] Thirty-one additional cases of cutaneous or disseminated aspergillosis in infants have been reported,[318-339] and only 11 infants survived.[320,322,327-331] The diagnosis seldom was made before death, and in most cases, the infant died despite institution of antifungal therapy. Infants who survived were more likely to have primary cutaneous infection without dissemination. As in previously reported cases, *Aspergillus* infection was secondary to prematurity,[317,333,335,337-339] antibiotic therapy,[323] or serious underlying disease.[319,320,332,334,336]

The Organism

The genus *Aspergillus* contains about 900 distinct species,[340] but only 8 have been shown to be pathogenic for humans. Identification of species of *Aspergillus* is made on the basis of morphology and structural details of the conidia-producing structures when grown on specialized media. These fungi reproduce by asexual spores or conidia, developing characteristic branching, septate hyphae as they grow. *Aspergillus* species produce a variety of mycotoxins in nonhuman hosts, but none have been identified in isolates from infected adults. Reported virulence factors include production of protease, phospholipases, and hemolysin, each of which may function to promote invasion of damaged skin.[341] Fibrinogen and laminin receptors are present on the conidia of *A. fumigatus*, and they may augment infection of traumatized skin by interaction with exposed extracellular matrix ligands.[342,343] The species that are pathogenic in humans and animals are *A. fumigatus* (which is the most common), *Aspergillus flavus*, *Aspergillus nidulans*, *Aspergillus niger*, and *Aspergillus terreus*, and less frequently, *Aspergillus glaucus*, *Aspergillus restrictus*, *Aspergillus versicolor*, and *A. sydowi*.[341]

Most cases of neonatal aspergillosis are caused by *A. fumigatus.*

Epidemiology and Transmission

Aspergillus species are ubiquitous and abundant in the environment. These fungi are found throughout the world in grains and decaying vegetation, soil, and other organic matter. Infection with *Aspergillus* is common in animals.[344] *Aspergillus* spores frequently are isolated from the air because they are easily dispersed, lightweight, and resistant to destruction. Although it has been reported that infection is more common in persons exposed to large numbers of conidia,[345-349] occupational predisposition has been questioned,[350-354] and a history of inordinate exposure is infrequent. No racial or gender predisposition has been found in the infection rate, but clinical disease in adults is more common in men than in women.[355]

Species of *Aspergillus* most often are acquired by humans through inhalation of spores into the respiratory tract, but saprophytic infection with *Aspergillus* may be found in the external auditory canal, skin, nails, nasal sinuses, and vagina.[356-359] Although infection in newborns may result from inhalation of conidia from the environment, the fungus also can be acquired, albeit rarely, during gestation or at the time of birth from an infection in the mother. None of the mothers in one study showed evidence of disseminated infection during pregnancy, and studies of vaginal flora were performed in only one.[311] In the infant of that mother, onset of infection was at 2 days of age; studies were not performed in the mother until 1 month postpartum. Results of culture of vaginal secretions for *Aspergillus* were negative, and appearance by chest roentgenogram was normal. Although person-to-person transmission has not been reported, another source of infection suggested by Allan and Andersen[311] was a second infant in the same nursery. That infant died, but because an autopsy was not performed, the diagnosis of *Aspergillus* infection could not be confirmed.

Aspergillus species are found in the hospital setting; thus it is not surprising that infants in the NICU are exposed to this fungus, and that invasive disease results because of the immaturity of their immune system and skin barriers. Sources within the hospital include packaged gauze, tape, limb boards, adhesive monitor leads, and pulse oximetry probes.[311,312,360] Contaminated hyperalimentation fluid has been associated with neonatal aspergillosis. Hospital outbreaks have been associated with airborne contamination during hospital renovation or nearby road construction and from bird droppings in the air ducts.[361-362] Hospital water systems harboring fungi have resulted in airborne transmission from sinks and restrooms. The most common mode of transmission in the neonate is contamination of skin breakdown sites, abrasions, or open wounds.[363] The skin of the premature infant is extremely fragile, does not provide an adequate barrier to the environment, and is prone to breakdown or abrasion even with usual handling.

Pathogenesis

Four morphologic forms of the fungus representing stages of development from germination of conidia to fructification have been identified in humans infected with *Aspergillus.*[364] The progressive changes in morphology may reflect the host's susceptibility or resistance to the fungus. After inhalation, ingestion, or inoculation of the spore, primary hyphae form from the germinating conidia, evoking an intense polymorphonuclear leukocyte response. As infection continues, unbranched, straight, or spiraling hyphae may be seen. Later, characteristic branching occurs, and vegetative forms of *Aspergillus* may be identified in devitalized tissue. In infants, the most common microscopic findings are acute inflammation, hemorrhagic infarction, and subsequent necrosis, as well as invasion of tissue by characteristic hyphae. Vegetative forms apparently are not found in infants because the disease progresses so rapidly that death occurs first.

Aspergillosis results when the immunocompromised infant with an appropriate portal of entry is exposed to this fungus, resulting in either locally invasive or widely disseminated infection. The primary host defense in humans is the phagocyte, so with inhalation of *Aspergillus* spores, macrophages act by rapidly killing conidia. Neutrophils are involved when conidia escape the reticuloendothelial system and begin the mycelial phase.[341] Oxidative killing is an important host defense.[364] Corticosteroid therapy impairs macrophage and neutrophil killing of *Aspergillus* spores and hyphae.[365] Neutropenia, a common predisposing condition in adults and children with aspergillosis, rarely accompanies neonatal aspergillosis.[366,367] Rather, the underlying problem in neonates appears to be a qualitative defect in neutrophil function.[364] The mechanical disruption of skin by minor trauma, such as removal of adhesive tape securing devices (e.g., intravenous catheters or endotracheal tubes), can allow invasion by *Aspergillus.*[368,369]

Pathology

Increasingly, *Aspergillus* infection in premature infants in the NICU first manifests as primary cutaneous aspergillosis. In this circumstance, skin biopsy of the lesions reveals extensive disruption of the epidermis, with invasion of the dermis by the septate, 45-degree branching hyphae characteristic of this fungus.[330,369] In infants with aspergillosis, prematurity or antibiotic or corticosteroid therapy may contribute to the risk of infection. In two reported cases of aspergillosis in infants,[310,313] however, no predisposing causes were identified. In infants, dissemination of the infection appears to be more common than locally invasive infection.[310-313,370]

Aspergillus can invade tissue by direct extension, as in orbital or nasal sinus infection into the brain, or it may be widely disseminated by the hematogenous route. In young infants, dissemination appears to result from the primary focus of infection in the lung or skin. The organs most often involved in invasive or disseminated infection are the lung, gastrointestinal tract, brain, liver, kidney, thyroid, and heart.[371] Skin and subcutaneous areas, genital tract, and adrenal glands are sometimes involved. One of the infants with primary cutaneous aspergillosis in the reported cases had skin infection also, and at autopsy *Aspergillus* was identified in the spleen.[312] In disseminated aspergillosis, invasion of blood vessels results in infarction and necrosis. Because the fungus invades and occludes the vessels, hemorrhagic necrosis is frequently seen in the lung and gastrointestinal tract in both infants and adults. Microscopic examination of infected tissues reveals extensive involvement, with dichotomous branching of septate hyphae and the presence of conidial heads in air-containing tissues such as the lung.[341] Necrotizing bronchitis with pseudomembrane formation, invasive tracheitis, and necrotizing bronchopneumonia are found by examination of lung tissue from infants.[328,366] Although granulomatous lesions occasionally are seen throughout an infected organ, suppuration with polymorphonuclear leukocytes and abscess formation are more common.

Clinical Manifestations

The number of reports of neonatal infection with *Aspergillus* limited to the skin has been increasing.[323,325,327-331,335,338] Premature infants have a unique predisposition to primary cutaneous aspergillosis as a result of their poor skin barrier function. Nine infants have been reported, and all survived with medical or surgical treatment, or both. The cutaneous lesions typically begin as multiple erythematous or violaceous papules that rapidly progress to hemorrhagic bullae, followed by the development of purpuric ulcerations and black eschar formation within 24 hours.[333,371] Lesions often begin on the back or other dependent areas and may be mistaken for pressure sores, but they can occur anywhere on the body where trauma has occurred.[328,368] The lesions of primary cutaneous aspergillosis have been mistaken for bullous impetigo and thermal burns from cutaneous CO_2 probe placement.[367] New skin lesions in a premature infant that are black or brown in appearance are suspicious for aspergillosis, but other fungi can give this appearance; therefore, biopsy and culture are necessary to establish an early diagnosis.

Most of the infants with disseminated aspergillosis in reported cases had signs of pulmonary infection that were thought to be pneumonia, not pulmonary infarction. One infant had a cutaneous infection that appeared as a maculopapular rash on the second day of life.[311] Skin lesions became scaly and later pustular. In this infant, enlargement of the liver became apparent, and the infant failed to gain weight. The case reported by Luke and associates[312] was characterized by jaundice, hepatosplenomegaly, heart murmur, ascites, and melena. Cerebrospinal fluid in the affected infant contained white blood cells, but further details were not reported. Jaundice and enlargement of liver and spleen were prominent in the case reported by Zimmerman,[315] and the infant described by Akkoyunlu and Yücell[313] had pneumonia and meningitis. Liver disease also was dominant in the cases reported by Mangurten and co-workers[317] and Gonzalez-Crussi and colleagues.[318] Widespread dissemination to the large and small bowel, liver, pancreas, peritoneum, and lung was demonstrated in the infant with aspergillosis and leukemia.[319]

Diagnosis and Differential Diagnosis

Diagnostic considerations in patients with cutaneous aspergillosis include infections due to other fungi, particularly *Candida* and Phycomycetes organisms. In infants with disseminated aspergillosis without skin involvement, diagnosis is difficult. Although *Aspergillus* can be identified by direct microscopic examination or culture of secretions, its presence does not necessarily indicate infection even in the presence of clinical disease. Demonstration of *Aspergillus* by culture or by microscopic examination of tissue obtained by biopsy or from body fluids establishes the diagnosis. *Aspergillus* species grow readily on almost all laboratory media, and characteristic conidiophores usually are present within 48 hours of incubation. Fungal blood and other body fluid cultures yield *Aspergillus* in less than 75% of cases, however.[341]

Hematoxylin-eosin, periodic acid–Schiff, Schwartz-Lamkins, and Grocott and Gomori methenamine silver stains can be used to visualize septate hyphae in tissue. Spores and branching septate hyphae measuring 4 µm in diameter may be seen. The presence of conidiospores in tissue is infrequent, but they may be seen in specimens of saprophytic infection. Mycelia of *Aspergillus* may be confused with pseudohyphae of *Candida*, which usually are smaller and have no branching; yeast forms usually are present. Phycomycetes can be distinguished from *Aspergillus* by their large size, irregularity, and absence of septa. The greatest difficulty is encountered in distinguishing *Aspergillus* in tissue from *Penicillium*, which also can cause infection in humans.[372] The hyphae of *Penicillium* are broader and contain fewer septa. Culture of tissue establishes the diagnosis. Potassium hydroxide smear of the contents of a papule or blister may reveal characteristic hyphae, allowing for a rapid presumptive diagnosis until culture results are available.[328] PCR techniques may be useful in detecting *Aspergillus* species in serum, cerebrospinal fluid, or other potentially infected body fluids.[373] The detection of *Aspergillus* antigen can be helpful in diagnosis, but no data on antigenemia are available for infants.[372,374] Additional diagnostic modalities useful for detecting the extent of involvement in neonates with suspected dissemination infection include lumbar puncture; chest radiography; computed tomography of the brain and chest; abdominal ultrasound examination of liver, spleen, and kidneys; and funduscopic examination. Even if CNS involvement is present, the cerebrospinal fluid may not show an inflammatory response.

Therapy

Intravenous amphotericin B deoxycholate remains the drug of choice for treatment for all forms of neonatal aspergillosis (Table 34-2).[375,376] Amphotericin B should be administered

Table 34–2 Susceptibility of Fungi to Amphotericin B

Fungus	Very Susceptible	Moderately Susceptible	Resistant
Aspergillus species		+	
Blastomycosis dermatitidis	+		
Cryptococcus neoformans	+		
Coccidioides immitis	+		
Malassezia furfur		+	
Phycomycetes			
Fusarium species			+
Mucorales		+	
Scedosporium species			+

at a dose of 1.5 mg per kg of body weight once daily and infused over a 1- to 2-hour period. This drug is very well tolerated in neonates, and infusion-related adverse effects are rare. Although nephrotoxicity is possible, it is quite uncommon in neonates and young infants. The optimal duration of therapy is not known, but courses up to 10 weeks are not uncommon. Lipid-associated preparations of amphotericin B have had limited use in neonates but have been used to successfully treat invasive aspergillosis in older children. Daily doses of 5 mg/kg apparently are well tolerated. No studies suggesting either safety or efficacy for azoles, often used in older patients with primary cutaneous aspergillosis, have been published. One study, however, evaluated itraconazole in a few neonates.[377] Newer antifungal agents, such as voriconazole and caspofungin, have not been evaluated in neonates for pharmacokinetics, safety, or efficacy, and these drugs should not be employed.[378,379] Complete surgical resection of infected, necrotic tissue, in conjunction with amphotericin B therapy, is necessary to treat cutaneous aspergillosis, but preterm infants with extensive cutaneous lesions occasionally may not be able to tolerate full excision. Vitrectomy and intravitreous amphotericin B can be considered the preferred treatment for endophthalmitis caused by *Aspergillus* species.[376]

Prognosis

The prognosis for primary cutaneous aspergillosis in infants is poor because of rapid dissemination, and a high mortality rate is reported even with institution of amphotericin B therapy. Nevertheless, a high index of suspicion, coupled with prompt biopsy of a skin lesion and institution of empirical therapy with amphotericin B continued until results of diagnostic tests including culture become available, has allowed a good outcome in some infants.[328]

Prevention

Because the risk of death associated with neonatal aspergillosis remains high, attempts to reduce exposure to *Aspergillus* species are of primary importance in preventing this infection. Filtration systems reduce the airborne transmission of *Aspergillus* spores, and rooms equipped with high-efficiency particulate air (HEPA) filters are virtually fungus free. Construction on or near the NICU should be avoided. Excellent skin care, including the judicious use of adhesive tape, monitor probes, and wound dressing material, is indicated for the prevention of skin breakdown with potential exposure to environmental *Aspergillus* species.

BLASTOMYCOSIS

Infection with *Blastomyces* has been reported in only four newborns,[380-382] although infection with this fungus occurred in 19 women during pregnancy.[382,383-388] In all but three of these 9 women, the infection was diagnosed and treated before delivery. The 3 women who received no treatment had disseminated infection. Two of the infants born to these 3 mothers were healthy at birth, but one of them died at 3 weeks of age, when *Blastomyces* was identified in lung tissue.[380] The second infant presented at 18 days of age with respiratory distress, and infection with *B. dermatitidis* was diagnosed by lung biopsy. He received amphotericin B but died 3 weeks after initiation of therapy.[381] The third infant was not infected. Two additional pregnancies ended in stillbirths. Infection with *Blastomyces* was not identified in any of the other infants in the reported cases.

The Organism

Blastomyces is a dimorphic fungus that has a mycelial form at room temperature and a yeast form at 37° C.[389] The mycelial form is found in soil, where it may exist for long periods.[390-392] Conidiophores arise at right angles to the hyphae and are believed to be infectious for humans when mycelia are disturbed. When inhaled, the fungus converts to the yeast form, which is multinucleate, containing 8 to 12 nuclei. It has a thick wall and reproduces by single budding with a broad connection to the parent.[392]

Epidemiology and Transmission

Blastomycosis is endemic in the Mississippi and Ohio river valleys in the United States and in parts of Canada.[393-403] Sporadic cases have been reported in Central and South America and in Africa.[412] The infection is more common in middle-aged men,[393,402,403] particularly those who are employed outdoors in rural areas.[403]

Blastomyces is acquired by inhalation of contaminated soil, and the lung is the initial focus of infection.[404] Primary cutaneous blastomycosis by direct inoculation of the organism into skin has been reported.[404-406] It has been suggested that human-to-human transmission does not occur, but Craig and colleagues[407] reported probable human-to-human transmission through sexual intercourse. In addition, mother-to-fetus transmission has been suggested.

Pulmonary infection has been identified as the initial site of infection due to *Blastomyces dermatitidis*.[404] In some instances, the pulmonary disease is self-limited and may resolve without therapy.[408] In some instances, however, both progressive pulmonary disease and dissemination can occur. Although no extensive studies in immunocompromised patients have been conducted, both corticosteroid therapy and other immunosuppressive therapy may increase the risk not only of acquisition of the fungus but also dissemination as well.[400,409] It has been suggested by some studies that a relatively immunosuppressed state occurs during pregnancy, which may account for this increased risk of dissemination.[410-412] When dissemination occurs, the skin, bones, and genitourinary system are most commonly involved. The CNS, liver, spleen, and lymph nodes are not commonly affected. Cell-mediated immunity appears to decrease the risk of disseminated blastomycosis.[413]

Pathology

The inflammatory response in the lung consists of proliferation of polymorphonuclear leukocytes followed by formation of noncaseating granuloma with epithelioid and giant cells. Extrapulmonary sites of infection show a similar histologic pattern, with the exception of the skin, which shows pseudoepitheliomatous hyperplasia and microabscesses.

Clinical Manifestations

Acute symptomatic pulmonary infection in children and adults with *Blastomyces* is associated with abrupt onset of chills and fever, myalgias, and arthralgias. Pleuritic pain is common early, and cough is prominent and may become productive of purulent sputum late in the course of the disease. Resolution of symptoms without therapy is common. Pulmonary infection, however, may become chronic and slowly progressive, with chronic cough, hemoptysis, pleuritic chest pain, and weight loss.

When dissemination occurs, skin infections are reported in as many as 80% of adult cases.[404,414-417] These infections are most common on exposed surfaces, and lesions have a verrucous appearance, particularly in the later stages. Abscesses may occur at the periphery of the lesions. In some patients, the skin lesions appear as shallow ulcerations with central granulation tissue that bleeds easily. Other sites of infection include subcutaneous tissue, bone, and joints and the genitourinary system, particularly the epididymis and prostate. CNS infection is uncommon; however, it usually is associated with headache, confusion, and meningismus.[418] Involvement of the liver and spleen is uncommon.

Of nine women with blastomycosis during pregnancy, seven had disseminated infection; in four in whom studies were done, no evidence of placental infection could be found in three.[383-387] One of these women had received amphotericin B for 35 days before the birth of her infant. *B. dermatitidis* was cultured from the placenta in the fourth woman, and the organism was visualized in both the fetal and the maternal placental tissue.[387] None of their infants, however, were infected. In one woman in whom placental studies were not done, the fungus was isolated from urine, and her infant died at 3 weeks of age with pulmonary blastomycosis.[380] At autopsy, the infant had no evidence of extrapulmonary infection, suggesting that the fungus may have been acquired by aspiration of infected secretions during birth rather than by hematogenous spread in utero. In the other infant, although the original site of infection was the lung, the fungus was found at autopsy in the kidneys as well.[381]

Diagnosis and Differential Diagnosis

Because of the rarity of neonatal blastomycosis, enumeratation of specific signs that may lead to its diagnosis is difficult. As suggested by findings in the four cases reviewed here, and by extrapolated data in infants with other nonopportunistic fungal infections, the diagnosis should be considered in an infant born in an endemic area for *Blastomyces* who has signs of indolent, progressive pulmonary disease and whose chest radiograph demonstrates bilateral nodular densities. In older children and adults, the clinical picture in acute pulmonary infection with *Blastomyces* appears similar to that in acute bacterial, mycoplasmal, and viral infections. Radiographic findings also are nonspecific. Chronic infection can simulate infection with *Mycobacterium tuberculosis* and other fungi, and mass lesions can suggest carcinoma. Few specific signs are associated with extrapulmonary blastomycosis. The skin lesions may be mistaken for squamous cell carcinoma.

Diagnosis of blastomycosis is made by visualization of fungus in culture of secretions or tissue. Serologic studies to determine the presence of complement-fixing antibodies lack sensitivity,[394] but results of immunodiffusion tests for precipitating antibody may be positive in as many as 80% of adult cases.[419,420] No data regarding skin test reactivity or serologic studies in infants with blastomycosis have been reported.

Therapy

In view of the rarity of this infection and the limited (or lack of) information regarding pharmacokinetics and safety of antifungal drugs other than amphotericin B in neonates, it appears prudent to treat *Blastomyces* infections in infants with amphotericin B deoxycholate, presumably for a minimum of 6 weeks. Itraconazole and fluconazole have been shown to be safe and efficacious in adults and older children.

Prognosis

Each of the 2 reported neonates with blastomycosis died.[383,384] In one the diagnosis was not suspected, and in the other the infection progressed despite antifungal therapy.

Prevention

Data that address prevention of blastomycosis in neonates are lacking. In pregnant women who reside in or travel through endemic areas, however, a respiratory illness should suggest this diagnosis. Prompt diagnosis and therapy for pregnant women have been associated with prevention of illness in young infants.[383-388]

COCCIDIOIDOMYCOSIS

Clinically apparent infection with *Coccidioides immitis* in infants in the first month of life has been reported infrequently despite the high incidence of infection in children living in areas where the fungus is endemic.[421] Most affected infants have been born at term, even when transmission was congenital. The first case of coccidioidomycosis in a neonate was reported by Cohen in 1949.[422] Although the diagnosis was not established until the infant was 15 weeks of age, signs of pulmonary disease were present at 1 week of age. Dactylitis was evident at 2 weeks of age; the infected finger was the site from which the fungus finally was isolated. Coccidioidomycosis has been reported in 11 other infants; each had clinical onset by 10 weeks of age.[423-431] Although pulmonary disease was prominent in each infant, disseminated infection was found at autopsy in all who died. Two of the infants had signs of meningitis,[423,424] but the fungus was isolated from cerebrospinal fluid in only one of them.[424] In two additional reported cases, the infants survived. In one the diagnosis was made by serologic testing,[430] and in the other the diagnosis was established when the fungus was identified in tracheal secretions.[431]

The Organism

C. immitis is the only species of *Coccidioides*; it is found below the surface of the soil. *C. immitis* exists in two phases:

saprophytic and parasitic. Saprophytic *Coccidioides* exists in a mycelial form in nonliving material, only rarely in tissue.[432] Hyphae have regularly spaced septa with alternating infectious spores and sterile cells. Arthrospores are infectious components of hyphae and are barrel shaped, measuring 2 to 10 μm in width. Spores may be round or ovoid, in which case they are more typically chlamydospores. An annual rainfall of 5 to 20 inches in alkaline soil and a prolonged hot, dry season followed by precipitation favor the formation of spores.[433] Infectious spores become airborne with minimal disturbance during the hot, dry season and may remain infectious for several weeks. Arthrospores, which have been known to be transported on clothes or other inanimate objects containing contaminated dust, may cause infection great distances from endemic areas.[434]

The parasitic form of *C. immitis* is the spherule. The spherule forms in tissue from inhaled or inoculated arthrospores. It measures 10 to 80 μm in diameter and contains endospores, which form within the spherule by cleavage of cytoplasm. Mature spherules rupture, liberating a few hundred to several hundred endospores, which subsequently develop into new spherules.[432]

Epidemiology and Transmission

C. immitis is found in soil 12 to 14 cm below the surface. Sunlight appears to destroy the fungus. *Coccidioides* is endemic in the Western Hemisphere in the San Joaquin Valley and southern counties of California, southern Arizona, New Mexico, and western Texas, as well as in Mexico, Guatemala, Honduras, Venezuela, Paraguay, Colombia, and Argentina. In endemic areas, naturally occurring infection has been reported in a variety of wild and domestic animals, including cattle,[435] sheep,[436,437] dogs,[438] horses and burros,[439] and rodents.[440]

Epidemiologic studies have estimated that approximately 10 million persons currently residing in endemic areas have been infected with *C. immitis*.[441] The rate of infection in susceptible persons arriving in an endemic area is 15% to 50% within the first year.[442] After residence in an endemic area for 5 years, 80% of susceptible persons will become infected. In more than 50% of these, infection is asymptomatic and can be demonstrated only by the presence of delayed hypersensitivity to coccidioidin skin test antigen. The incidence of infection is highest in the early summer and remains high until the first rains of winter. The rate of infection also is higher in dry seasons that follow a season of heavy rainfall.[443,444]

No racial or gender difference in incidence of primary coccidioidomycosis has been noted. Primary infection is recognized more frequently in women, however, because they are more likely than men to have cutaneous hypersensitivity reactions.[445,446] Considerable racial differences have been reported in the risk of disseminated disease. Mexican Indian men are three times more likely to disseminate the fungus than white men; black men are 14 times more prone to dissemination than white men; and Filipino men are reported to be 175 times more susceptible than white men.[441,447,448] In women, dissemination is more common during pregnancy.[461-465] Before puberty, no gender difference in clinical manifestations or extent of disease is seen.

Studies to determine explanations for increased susceptibility in men, nonwhite races, and pregnant women have not been performed. Patients with lymphomas, leukemia, and diabetes mellitus are reported to have no higher incidence of clinically significant or disseminated coccidioidal infection than in other persons,[466] but disseminated infection may be more common in patients with AIDS[467] and in those receiving corticosteroids or immunosuppressive therapy.[468]

Coccidioidomycosis in infants has been considered to result from inhalation of arthrospores. Transmission of coccidiodomycosis from mother to infant in utero has been reported by Shafai,[439] who described twins born to a woman who died 24 hours post partum with disseminated coccidioidomycosis. Both infants died with widespread disease. Christian and associates[425] described one case in which onset of disease was at 3 weeks of age in an infant living in a nonendemic area. The infant's mother had inactive coccidioidal osteomyelitis but did not have pulmonary or cutaneous disease, suggesting that infection in the infant may have been acquired in utero or at the time of birth. An infant described by Cohen[422] was born to a mother with active coccidioidomycosis during pregnancy; pulmonary disease was evident in the infant at the age of 1 week, again suggesting that the infection may have been acquired in utero. Respiratory symptoms developed at 2 weeks of age in one infant born to a woman who subsequently died of disseminated coccidioidomycosis, but the infant became clinically well after 3 weeks of therapy with intravenous amphotericin B.[424] Bernstein and co-workers[429] reported onset of disease in an infant at 5 days of age, and although no evidence of disease was noted in the mother, disease onset in the infant shortly after birth suggested in utero transmission of the fungus. By contrast, in the several reported cases of disseminated coccidioidomycosis in pregnant women, only three instances of placental infection were noted, with no evidence of infection in any of the infants.[449,452,458-460]

Human-to-human transmission of *C. immitis* is rare. Even though infectious arthrospores can be found in residual pulmonary cavities and benign pulmonary granulomas in humans,[421] secondary cases within families are unusual. Eckmann and co-workers[461] reported six cases of coccidioidomycosis acquired at the bedside of a patient with coccidioidal osteomyelitis whose cast was contaminated with spherule-containing exudate.

Pathogenesis

The respiratory tract is the initial focus of infection by *C. immitis* in most infants and adults. Direct inoculation of fungus into the skin, reported rarely in adults and older children,[462] has not been described in neonates. After arthrospores are inhaled, mature spherules develop in the bronchial mucosa 4 to 7 days later.[463,464] Granulomas form rapidly, involving pulmonary lymphatics and tracheobronchial lymph nodes. In adults with mild disease, a few scattered lesions may be present; however, when pulmonary involvement is extensive, an outpouring of polymorphonuclear leukocytes fill alveoli, and a radiographic appearance of bronchopneumonia is noted. Ulceration of bronchi and bronchioles can occur, with later development of bronchiectasis. Hematogenous dissemination with multiple organ involvement occurs frequently in neonates, and severe CNS infection is a frequent complication.

Pathology

The typical histologic appearance of lesions in *Coccidioides* infection is that of a granuloma with epithelioid cells and Langhans' giant cells. Granulomas occur in infants and older patients. In immunocompromised hosts, suppuration can be prominent, but with adequate host response, hyalinization, fibrosis, and calcification occur.

Coccidioides can disseminate by blood flow to any organ in the body. The most significant focus of infection after dissemination is the CNS; the brain, meninges, or spinal cord can be involved. Dissemination to the CNS is most common in children and in white males and is the most common cause of death in patients with coccidioidomycosis.[430,465] In cases of meningitis, presence of a thick exudate encasing the brain invariably results in noncommunicating hydrocephalus. Involvement around the base of the brain usually is more extensive than that above the cerebral cortex. On microscopic examination, the meninges are seen to be studded with small granulomas; similar lesions may be present in the underlying brain substance. In the spinal cord, infection may result in compression by the thick, tough inflammatory membrane, with subsequent loss of motor and sensory functions.

Other organs involved when the infection becomes disseminated include the skin, lungs and pleura, spleen, liver, kidneys, heart, genital tract, adrenal glands, and, occasionally, skeletal muscle. In infants, cutaneous infection most often makes its appearance as a papular rash in the diaper area. The gastrointestinal tract is almost always spared in infants, although the peritoneum and bowel serosa frequently are studded with granulomas. In each of three infants who died of disseminated coccidioidomycosis, the lungs and spleen were involved. One infant had infection in the liver, and one had documented meningitis. Skin infection was present in only one infant.[344] One of the surviving infants had pulmonary infection and osteomyelitis,[422] and another had pulmonary infection and chorioretinitis.[430]

Clinical Manifestations

Although primary pulmonary coccidioidal infection is asymptomatic in 60% of older children and adults,[466] and only 25% have an illness severe enough to seek medical attention, each of the infected newborns in the reported cases had signs of pulmonary disease. After an incubation period of 10 to 16 days, signs of a mild lower respiratory tract disorder appear, characterized by a dry, nonproductive cough. Findings can include low-grade fever, anorexia, and malaise, as well as significant respiratory distress. Physical examination of the chest may demonstrate few abnormalities, but roentgenograms typically show evidence of bronchopneumonia or segmental or peribronchial disease in infants. Hilar nodes often are enlarged, and small pleural effusions are common.

Cavitary lesions became apparent in one infant several months after birth and cleared by the age of 30 months.[422] It is in such chronic lesions that the saprophytic form of *Coccidioides* has been demonstrated.[432]

In infants, dissemination of infection is frequent, and when dissemination to the CNS occurs, infection in brain and meninges can be overlooked.[467] Signs, which are vague and nonspecific, include anorexia and lethargy. Nuchal rigidity is infrequent. As the infection progresses, other CNS manifestations include confusion, obtundation, coma, and seizures. Papilledema is a late finding.

Diagnosis and Differential Diagnosis

Granulomatous pulmonary disease caused by *C. immitis* in adults can mimic tuberculosis, Q fever, psittacosis, ornithosis, viral pneumonias, or other fungal infections, particularly histoplasmosis. In infants, pulmonary coccidioidomycosis may appear to be similar to bacterial infection. In patients with coccidioidal meningitis, considerations in the differential diagnosis include tuberculous meningitis, cryptococcosis, histoplasmosis, blastomycosis, candidiasis, and partially treated bacterial meningitis.[429] In coccidioidal meningitis, the cerebrospinal fluid usually is under increased pressure. Pleocytosis with mononuclear cells is characteristic, but in cases discovered early, a preponderance of polymorphonuclear cells may be found. Eosinophils are common in cerebrospinal fluid in patients with coccidioidal meningitis. The cerebrospinal fluid glucose level is decreased, and the protein level may be markedly elevated.

The diagnosis of coccidioidomycosis must be suspected in infants with unexplained pulmonary disease who are born to mothers who reside in endemic areas. In addition, a history of travel to an endemic area or an occupational hazard involving exposure to contaminated dust may be important clues leading to suspicion of coccidioidal infection.[468-470] Establishing a diagnosis of coccidioidomycosis in an infant is difficult. Identification of spherules in pus, sputum, or tissue is diagnostic of infection with *C. immitis*. Direct microscopic examination is best performed if the infected material is partially digested with 10% sodium or potassium hydroxide. Specimens treated by alkalinization are unsatisfactory for culture.

Spherules may be easier to identify if equal parts of iodine and Sudan IV are used. Iodine is absorbed into the wall of the spherule, and Sudan IV differentiates fat globules from spherules.[471] Because spherule-like artifacts are commonly found in sputum and pus, however, direct examination may be misleading. Direct microscopic examination of gastric aspirate and cerebrospinal fluid usually is unrewarding, and even results of culture of cerebrospinal fluid in cases of coccidioidal meningitis can be negative.[467] Identification of spherules in tissue obtained by biopsy or at autopsy is best accomplished with use of Gridley or Gomori methenamine silver stain. Hematoxylin-eosin may be used but often fails to give enough contrast between spherules and host tissue.

Coccidioides can be grown on Sabouraud glucose agar; specimens submitted for culture should include sputum, pus from cutaneous lesions, cerebrospinal fluid, and urine. Because the morphology of mycelia is variable, the fungus can be injected into mice for demonstration of characteristic endosporulating spherules. Culture and animal inoculation are time consuming and dangerous for laboratory personnel; accordingly, most investigational studies employ immunologic and serologic tests for demonstration of infection with *Coccidioides*.

Studies of development of delayed hypersensitivity in adults, with intradermal injections of 0.1 mL of coccidioidin, have demonstrated that positive reactions may occur 3 days to 2 weeks after the onset of symptoms and may persist for years.[432] In adults without erythema nodosum or erythema multiforme, a dilution of 1:100 of skin test antigen has been used. A positive reaction is manifested 24 to 48 hours after injection as induration of 5 mm or more. Cross-reactions may occur with coccidioidin in patients with histoplasmosis, and coccidioidin can evoke an antibody response to yeast-phase *Histoplasma* but not to *Coccidioides*. False-negative reactions can occur in patients with disseminated infection or in those in whom skin testing is performed before development of cellular immune response to the fungus. Cohen and Burnip[459] performed coccidioidin skin tests in newborns in an endemic area. Among 220 infants studied, positive reactions occurred in 2, but neither had evidence of disease. Two infants born to women with coccidioidal meningitis during pregnancy had negative results on skin testing and no clinical or serologic evidence of infection. Thus, skin tests are not useful in establishing a diagnosis of coccidioidomycosis in infants.

Precipitin and complement fixation tests for antibodies to *Coccidioides* have been important in the diagnosis of coccidioidomycosis.[473,474] The complement fixation test has been useful in determining the extent of infection and the prognosis.[473] Precipitating antibodies appear to belong to the IgM class of immunoglobulins and are present in 90% of adults within 4 weeks of onset of symptoms.[474] In most instances, precipitins disappear in 4 to 6 weeks.[475] Coccidioidal antibodies demonstrated by complement fixation tests appear more slowly and only in cases of severe infection. Antibody titers of greater than 1:16 may indicate disseminated infection. The presence of complement-fixing antibodies in cerebrospinal fluid is diagnostic of coccidioidal meningitis; however, only 75% of patients with active meningeal infection have demonstrable antibody in cerebrospinal fluid.[473]

A test for detection of coccidioidal antibody using an immunodiffusion technique is available and appears to correlate with the complement fixation test.[476,477] Huppert and associates[478] also have described a latex particle agglutination test that measures antibody paralleling precipitin titers. It is recommended that tests for precipitins and complement-fixing antibodies both be employed for best results in diagnosing coccidioidomycosis.[478] Other serologic tests for coccidioidal antibodies include counterimmunoelectrophoresis[479] and radioimmunoassay[480]; however, results of these techniques in neonates have not been reported.

Therapy

Coccidioidal infection appears to be less responsive to amphotericin B than other fungal infections and frequently requires prolonged treatment for control. Intravenous amphotericin B deoxycholate at a daily dose of 1 mg per kg of body weight, however, is the drug of choice for the acute treatment of coccidioidomycosis. Because only 5% to 10% of serum levels of amphotericin B is distributed to the CNS, intrathecal administration of amphotericin B also is necessary. The duration of intrathecal amphotericin B therapy may be monitored by coccidioidal complement fixation titer in cerebrospinal fluid. In patients in whom antibodies never develop in cerebrospinal fluid despite coccidioidal meningitis, the duration of therapy is guided by the cerebrospinal fluid findings.

Although amphotericin B has been utilized in the long-term treatment of adults with CNS disease, no data on use of this drug in young infants have been reported. Prolonged therapy (for more than 1 year) is almost always necessary. In adults and older children, prolonged therapy with itraconazole or fluconazole rather than amphotericin B has been shown to be useful. In patients with CNS disease complicated by noncommunicating hydrocephalus, cerebrospinal fluid shunting may be necessary.

Prognosis

The mortality rate among infants with coccidioidomycosis is high. With three exceptions, all of the infants in whom coccidioidal infection was identified died, with infection recognized only at autopsy.

Prevention

Although dust control has been shown to reduce the incidence of infection in persons who are transients in endemic areas,[444,481] evidence that such control reduces frequency of infection among long-term residents in these areas is limited. In persons at risk for the development of severe or disseminated infection, attempting to control dust may be beneficial. Cohen[422] suggested that in one case, an infant acquired the infection from inhalation of dust blown into the nursery. Use of air conditioning, filters, and respirators in areas where persons are at risk has been encouraged.[482] Masks have been recommended for persons working in heavily contaminated areas.[469] Other investigators have suggested spraying soil with fungicides,[495] but such treatment reaches a depth of only 0.6 cm, which allows the fungus to survive below that level. Careful handling of heavily contaminated dressings by hospital personnel is recommended to prevent acquisition of infection. Isolation or segregation of patients with coccidioidomycosis, however, does not appear to be necessary.

Levine and co-workers[484] have employed a vaccine that has been effective in preventing disease in animals, but results in humans as measured by serologic and skin tests have been erratic[442] and have not shown protection from infection.[485]

CRYPTOCOCCOSIS

The occurrence of cryptococcosis in the neonate is rare, with fewer than a dozen cases reported, most before 1990.[486-491] All but one infant died, and in each case, organisms with the morphologic appearance of *Cryptococcus* were identified by microscopic examination of tissue obtained at autopsy or by culture. The youngest patient in the reported cases of cryptococcal infection was 20 minutes old.[486] This infant, with obvious in utero onset of infection, had hydrocephalus and an enlarged liver and spleen and died at 40 minutes of age. Encapsulated yeast-like organisms were identified in the brain, liver, and spleen. Neuhauser and Tucker,[487] in their description of 3 infants with cryptococcosis, noted that one had disease at birth and died at 19 days of age. At autopsy, organisms with the appearance of *Cryptococcus* were identified in the brain, liver, spleen, and bone. Morphologically similar organisms were recovered in culture of specimens from the infant and from the endocervix of the mother. Nassau and Weinberg-Heiruti[488] reported one case of cutaneous and disseminated cryptococcosis in an infant; Heath[489] described a newborn with endophthalmitis associated with widespread cryptococcal infection. Gavai and associates[490] reported the case of the only surviving infant; blood cultures grew *Cryptococcus neoformans*, and amphotericin B therapy was administered.

In adults, the respiratory tract in most instances has been considered to be the primary focus of infection with *Cryptococcus*,[492-495] but the fungus appears to have a special predilection for the brain and meninges.[496,497] Dissemination of infection to the CNS is common[497] and is more likely to occur in patients whose defenses against infection are compromised by disease or certain therapeutic agents.[498-500]

The Organism

The genus *Cryptococcus* is limited to spherical or oval encapsulated cells that reproduce by multilateral budding. Yeast cells vary in size, but most measure 5 to 10 μm in diameter exclusive of the mucinous capsule, which may be one half to five times the size of the cell. Although *Cryptococcus* usually appears on microscopic examination as encapsulated yeast, some strains of *C. neoformans* may produce true hyphae.[501] Of the seven species of *Cryptococcus*, only *C. neoformans* is pathogenic for humans, and it also is the only species that produces hyphae. A saprophytic species, *C. neoformans* var. *innocuous*, is culturally and morphologically identical to *C. neoformans* and frequently is confused with it.

Three serologic types of *C. neoformans* have been identified using type-specific capsular polysaccharide antisera.[502] Cross-reactions have been noted with *C. albicans*, *Trichophyton* extract, and other antigens.[503]

Epidemiology and Transmission

C. neoformans has been isolated from all areas of the world. The original isolate was made by San Felice from peaches,[504] and Klein[505] recovered the fungus from cow's milk. Emmons[506] isolated *C. neoformans* from soil and later reported that the milk probably had been contaminated with soil that contained excreta from pigeons.[507] Although natural cryptococcal infection in pigeons has not been demonstrated, many authors have suggested that pigeons may be the primary source of pathogenic *Cryptococcus*.[508-510] Others believe the soil to be the primary source, with pigeon excreta merely enhancing growth of *Cryptococcus*.[511,512]

Some authors have reported recovery of *C. neoformans* from areas inhabited by birds other than pigeons,[513-515] but Fragner[516] was able to isolate *C. neoformans* only from pigeon roosts and nonpathogenic species from roosts of other birds. Nevertheless, it is generally accepted that avian habitats, particularly of feral pigeons, represent the major source of *C. neoformans* for humans and animals.

Sources of *C. neoformans* other than pigeon roosts have been reported. Clarke and colleagues[517] isolated the fungus from apples, and McDonough and associates[518] recovered the organism from wood. *Cryptococcus* also has been found occasionally in soil not contaminated with bird excreta.[519] *C. neoformans* may cause disease in animals,[520] and epidemics of cryptococcal mastitis have occurred in dairy cows.[521,522] None of the personnel caring for the cows acquired the infection.

Human cryptococcosis can occur at any age, but approximately 60% of patients are between the ages of 30 and 50 years.[523] Infection is three times more common in men than in women and is particularly frequent in white men. It has been suggested that this gender difference is related at least in part to the enhanced phagocytic activity of leukocytes for *Cryptococcus* in the presence of estrogen.[524]

Infection with *C. neoformans* has been thought to result primarily from inhalation of the fungus from an exogenous source, and the respiratory tract is the primary focus of infection.[525] Direct inoculation into the skin and ingestion of the fungus, however, have been suggested as alternative routes of infection.[526-528] Tonsils also have been reported as a possible initial focus of infection.[529] Littman and Zimmerman[494] as well as other investigators have suggested that *Cryptococcus* can be isolated from the oropharynx, normal skin, vagina, and intestinal tract of humans with no apparent disease.[532] Whether isolates are actually *C. neoformans* has been questioned. Tynes and co-workers[531] suggested that pathogenic *Cryptococcus* can be present in sputum as a saprophyte, although before their report, isolation of *C. neoformans* from humans had been considered indicative of disease.

Only one of the mothers giving birth to infected offspring[486-489,491] had any illness during pregnancy that could be attributed to infection with *Cryptococcus*,[486-489] and although inhalation of *Cryptococcus* cannot be excluded in newborns infected with this organism, the onset of disease at birth suggests that the transmission of the fungus occurred in utero. Isolation of encapsulated yeast from the endocervix of the mother of one affected infant[487] suggested that transmission in this case may have occurred from an ascending vaginal infection. In no other reported instance of cryptococcal infection during pregnancy has transmission to the infant occurred.[532,533] Kida and colleagues[534] reported the case of a woman with HIV infection and AIDS who died with disseminated cryptococcal infection 2 days after the birth of her infant, who was uninfected.

Transmission from person to person, except for isolated cases of possible congenital transmission, has not been reported.

Pathogenesis

The presence of pathogenic *Cryptococcus* in humans has been considered to be an indication of disease related to that fungus. The possibility of saprophytic colonization of the skin, sputum, mucous membranes, and feces of healthy persons with *C. neoformans* has been suggested, however[504,535,536]; such colonization would indicate an endogenous source of the fungus. The isolation of encapsulated yeast from the endocervix of an asymptomatic, apparently healthy mother lends support to this contention. Although clinically apparent infection with *C. neoformans* can occur in the normal host, a high incidence of infection has been reported in patients with Hodgkin's disease, lymphosarcoma, leukemia, and diabetes mellitus,[498-500,536-538] as well as in those with HIV infection and AIDS. The use of corticosteroids or other immunosuppressive therapy has been associated with a higher incidence of cryptococcosis.[539] Mechanisms of enhanced susceptibility in patients with these underlying disorders or associated with such treatments are similar to those discussed earlier in connection with candidiasis. Cryptococcal infections in these patients, however, have not increased as strikingly as some of the other opportunistic fungal infections.[540]

No data specific to infants are available regarding increased susceptibility or resistance to infection with *Cryptococcus*. In the review by Siewers and Cramblett[541] of cryptococcal infections in children, only one of four patients showed evidence of underlying disease. Although gestational age was unknown in two of the eight infants with neonatal cryptococcosis, five of these were born prematurely. Only the surviving infant received antibiotics, and none received corticosteroids. The surviving infant also was receiving hyperalimentation through a central venous catheter.

Presence of a factor in normal human serum that inhibits growth of *C. neoformans* has been demonstrated and may explain the low incidence of clinically apparent cryptococcal infections.[542-544] Alterations in this factor due to disease or therapy may account for the high incidence of cryptococcal infection in patients with diseases of the reticuloendothelial system and in those who are receiving treatment with immunosuppressive drugs. No data are available regarding inhibitory factors in the serum of newborns.

Pathology

In infants and adults, the respiratory tract appears to be the primary focus of infection, and follows inhalation of the fungus. In some instances, the skin (by direct inoculation) or the gastrointestinal tract (by ingestion) may be the initial route of infection. In adults, respiratory infection usually is subacute or chronic, and the lesion most commonly encountered is a solitary nodule measuring 2 to 7 cm in diameter and located at the periphery of the lung, at the hilar area or in the middle of a lobe.[494] Hilar lymphadenopathy usually is minimal. In infants and occasionally in adults, diffuse infiltration[545] or miliary disease similar to that typical of tuberculosis may be evident in the lung.[546] Fibrosis and calcification are rare, but cavitary disease may be found in 10% of adults with pulmonary cryptococcal infection.[523] Small subpleural nodules frequently are found at autopsy in these patients,[547] but pleuritic reaction is rare.

Microscopically, pulmonary lesions of cryptococcal infection may give the appearance of nonspecific granulomas. If tissue reaction is minimal, the mass has a mucoid appearance—a finding more common in infants. In most instances, an aggregate of encapsulated budding cells with intertwining loose connective tissue can be seen. Granulomatous reaction may occur, with infiltration of lymphocytes and epithelioid cells but without caseation necrosis. Diffuse pneumonic infiltration seen in infants is characterized by accumulation of fungus in alveoli, and an outpouring of histiocytes and tissue macrophages with ingested organisms may be seen.

Cutaneous cryptococcal infection occurs in about 15% of adult cases[548] but has not been reported in infants. Dissemination can occur through the bloodstream to any organ in the body, including the liver, spleen, kidneys, adrenal glands, bone, and eyes, but the CNS is the most common site of infection after dissemination. Lesions outside the CNS in both adults and infants may appear densely granulomatous, similar to tuberculous lesions.[493] CNS evidence of meningitis includes a gray adherent exudate in the subarachnoid space. More extensive involvement can be present around the base of the brain in older patients. In some instances, small granulomas are present in the meninges and along the blood vessels. The underlying surface of the brain can show small, cystlike lesions consisting of fungal or mucinous material. The cellular reaction can be minimal or extensive, with mononuclear inflammatory cells. The infection can extend along the vessels into the brain substance to a variable depth, resulting in pinpoint cysts in gray matter. Parenchymatous lesions may result from embolization and are found in periventricular gray matter and basal ganglia and in white matter of the cerebral hemispheres. Such lesions are found more often in adults than in infants and appear as nonspecific granulomas or as cysts containing mucinous material from capsules of cryptococci. On occasion, discrete granulomas can be found in any part of the brain, spinal cord, or meninges and may act like space-occupying lesions.

Clinical Manifestations

Infants with cryptococcosis have multisystem involvement characterized by enlargement of the liver or spleen or both, jaundice, hydrocephalus, and, in many instances, chorioretinitis. Roentgenologically, Neuhauser and Tucker[487] found intracranial calcifications scattered over the cortex and within the brain substance in three newborns. It is noteworthy that these findings are compatible with those found in many congenital infections, including toxoplasmosis, rubella, syphilis, and cytomegalovirus infection. One infant was thought to have had toxoplasmosis as well as cryptococcal infection.[487]

Dissemination of *Cryptococcus* to other organs in infants usually produces signs of disease in one or more sites, most commonly the CNS. Signs vary with the location and extent of CNS involvement. Cryptococcal granulomas in the brain may produce signs similar to those of space-occupying lesions caused by other diseases. Meningitis most often manifests as headache, which can become progressively worse and is accompanied by nausea, vomiting, and lethargy. As infection continues, seizures can occur. On examination, papilledema may be noted, but nuchal rigidity is uncommon. When the brain is extensively involved, obtundation and coma often result. Cranial nerves can be involved, and amblyopia, diplopia, and optic atrophy are frequent findings. The infant who survived had no evidence of cryptococcosis beyond positive blood cultures. No meningitis, ophthalmic, or pulmonary involvement was present.

Diagnosis and Differential Diagnosis

Neonatal cryptococcal infection can appear similar to congenital infection with *Toxoplasma gondii,* rubella virus, cytomegalovirus, and *T. pallidum*. Pulmonary cryptococcal infection can be confused with congenital or neonatal tuberculosis or infections with fungi other than *Cryptococcus*.

CNS infection in infants can be confused with tuberculous meningitis. In cases of localized granulomatous disease, considerations in the differential diagnosis must include brain abscess caused by bacteria, cerebrovascular thromboses, and hemorrhage.

Diagnosis of infection with *Cryptococcus* is made by visualization of encapsulated yeasts in sputum or in cerebrospinal fluid, by culture, or by animal inoculation. Microscopic examinations of pus, sputum, exudates, and cerebrospinal fluid are best performed by using India ink, which is displaced by the capsule. Thick specimens of sputum or pus can be mixed with an equal volume of 10% sodium or potassium hydroxide to dissolve tissue and cellular debris before addition of fresh India ink.

In cryptococcal meningitis, the cerebrospinal fluid usually is under increased pressure, and pleocytosis may be present, with a predominance of mononuclear cells. The cerebrospinal fluid glucose level is decreased in only 55% of adult cases, and protein content is increased in 90%.[549] Direct microscopic examination of cerebrospinal fluid using an equal volume of India ink may show encapsulated yeasts in 50% of culture-proven cases. If yeast is found, the diagnosis is established because *Cryptococcus* is the only encapsulated yeast that infects the CNS in humans.

Specimens submitted for culture when diagnosis of cryptococcal infection is suspected should include sputum, cerebrospinal fluid, blood, urine, and bone marrow. If cutaneous lesions are present, pus also should be submitted.

Microscopic examination of tissue obtained by biopsy or at autopsy may strongly support the diagnosis of cryptococcal infection. Although Gridley and methenamine silver stains demonstrate the fungus very well, other fungi also are visualized with these stains. Specific stains for capsular mucin such as mucicarmine[550] and the Rhinehart-Abdul-Haj technique for detection of acid mucopolysaccharide[551] are beneficial, especially for distinguishing *Cryptococcus* from *Histoplasma*.

Immunologic and serologic tests have been proposed as aids in diagnosing infection with *Cryptococcus*. Delayed hypersensitivity to cryptococcal antigens has been noted in adults, but dermal response has not been useful as a diagnostic test.[493,552-557] No studies of response to cryptococcal skin test antigens in infants have been reported.

Serum agglutinins, complement-fixing hemagglutination, and indirect fluorescent methods have been described.[558-562] Latex and complement fixation tests for detection of cryptococcal antigen in serum and body fluids also have been reported.[563-566] Circulating cryptococcal antigen has been demonstrated in serum and cerebrospinal fluid in patients with meningeal and disseminated infections[564,565,567-569]; titers of antigen decrease with recovery. It also has been noted that cryptococcal antibody in serum can increase during recovery from infection with *Cryptococcus*. The latex particle agglutination test has proved to be valuable for detection of cryptococcal antigen in the cerebrospinal fluid of patients in whom findings on culture and microscopic examination of cerebrospinal fluid are negative.[570] No data are available on serologic studies in newborns with cryptococcal infection.

Therapy

The drugs of choice for treatment of cryptococcal meningitis are intravenous amphotericin B and oral flucytosine. The amphotericin B dose is 1 mg/kg given once daily, and the flucytosine dose is 100 to 150 mg/kg divided into four oral doses. This dosage should be continued for 4 to 8 weeks. In adults, the combination is given for 2 weeks and is followed by either fluconazole or itraconzaole administered orally, but no data exist on the appropriate dose, route, safety or efficacy of these two antifungal agents in young infants.

Prognosis

All of the newborns with cryptococcal infection reported who did not receive treatment died within days to weeks of onset of the disease. One infant survived without apparent sequelae after receiving amphotericin B for 6 weeks.

Prevention

Preventive measures should be directed at elimination of exogenous sources of *Cryptococcus*. A solution containing hydrated lime and sodium hydroxide has been shown to be effective in eradicating cryptococci from contaminated pigeon roosts when sprayed on soil containing the organism.[571]

MALASSEZIA INFECTIONS

Redline and Dahms[572] in 1981 provided the first description of systemic infection with *Malassezia* species in a very low birth weight infant who was receiving long-term intravenous hyperalimentation including intralipids. Since that first publication, this infection has been described in patients of all ages, but preterm neonates receiving intralipid therapy constitute the patient population with the highest incidence of fungemia.[573-576]

The Organism

The genus *Malassezia* consists of seven distinct species of yeast sharing common morphologic characteristics, nutritional requirements, and molecular features. All members of the genus cause skin disease in humans, but only *M. furfur*, *M. pachydermatis*, *M. globus*, and *M. sympodialis* are associated with neonatal infections.[573] Individual yeast cells are 2.5 to 6.0 μm and round, oval, or cylindrical, depending on the species. Each species demonstrates monopolar budding, whereas in certain species, pseudomycelia also may develop.[577] All *Malassezia* species except *M. pachydermatis* are obligatory lipophiles. This requirement for a source of lipid for growth and development explains the concordance of neonatal systemic disease with the infusion of intravenous lipid emulsions.

Epidemiology and Transmission

Malassezia is best known as the fungus responsible for tinea versicolor, a common skin infection among adults.[577] *M. furfur* and *M. pachydermatis* also are responsible for catheter-related bloodstream infections, occurring primarily in neonates or older immunocompromised hosts.[574-576] *M. sympodialis* and *M. globus* are associated with neonatal pustulosis, also known as neonatal acne.[577,578] Skin colonization with *Malassezia* species is nearly universal among adults, and direct transmission from caregivers to infants is the most common route of acquisition in the neonate.[573,579] These organisms persist on the hands of caregivers, despite appropriate hand hygiene, as well as on many hospital surfaces.[580] *Malassezia* organisms can be recovered from contaminated plastic surfaces for up to 3 months, and this persistence may facilitate nursery transmission.[581] *M. pachydermatis* causes infection in dogs, primarily otitis externa, and nursery outbreaks have been associated with colonization in pets of health care providers.[582]

The prevalence of colonization with *Malassezia* species among neonates in the NICU ranges from 30% to 100%, with fully half of the infants in some nurseries colonized by the end of the second week of life.[578,581,583,584] Colonization of catheters is thought to occur secondary to skin colonization or direct nosocomial transmission, as seen with clusters or outbreaks of *Malassezia* infections in an NICU.[574,585,586] Catheter-associated infections typically occur in infants older than 7 days of age, with the peak incidence in the third week of life.[587,588] Neonatal pustulosis typically develops between 5 days and 3 weeks of age.[578]

Pathogenesis

The pathogenesis of neonatal *Malassezia* infections requires colonization of the skin, followed either by the development of localized neonatal pustulosis or colonization of an indwelling vascular catheter leading to systemic infection. Factors increasing colonization rates among neonates in the NICU include extreme prematurity (gestational age less than 26 weeks), prolonged time in an isolette, the use of occlusive dressings, and prolonged length of NICU stay.[573] Sebum on the skin, especially that of the face, provides the required source of fat in the case of neonatal pustulosis.[578] Catheter-related infections are always associated with the administration of intravenous lipid emulsions, whether Broviac central intravenous or percutaneously placed Silastic catheters are used.[576,588,589] Intravascular catheters used only for hyperalimentation (without intralipids) or medication administration and other types of indwelling catheters do not become infected because the infusate they deliver does not provide the lipid nutritional support necessary for *Malassezia* organisms to proliferate. Intravascular catheters frequently develop thrombi or fibrin sheaths that become adherent to the vascular wall, which then may become infected.[588,590,591] The infected thrombus then serves as a source for ongoing fungemia or dissemination to visceral organs through microembolism.[585] Persistent fungemia is common with neonatal *Malassezia* infections, yet disseminated disease rarely occurs. Rare cases of meningitis, renal infection, liver abscess, and severe pulmonary or cardiac involvement have been reported.[572,582,592,593] Additional predisposing conditions for the development of neonatal systemic *Malassezia* infections include short-gut syndrome, gastroschisis, necrotizing enterocolitis, and complex congenital heart disease.[573,594] The need for prolonged parenteral, rather than enteral, nutrition is the common denominator in all of these predisposing conditions. Although less common than infections due to spread of the skin-colonizing organisms, infections due to direct nosocomial transmission of *Malassezia* species are documented.[582,592]

Clinical Manifestations

In neonatal pustulosis, or neonatal acne, the classic lesions are pinpoint erythematous papules that develop into overt pustules, most commonly seen over the chin, cheeks, and forehead, with occasional extension to the neck or scalp.[577] Lesions are not irritating to the infant, do not disseminate, and typically resolve over time without therapy—yet the appearance of neonatal pustulosis often is disturbing to parents.

Infants with catheter-related *Malassezia* fungemia typically present with any combination of the following nonspecific findings: lethargy, poor feeding, temperature instability, hepatosplenomegaly, hemodynamic instability, and worsening or new respiratory distress.[573] Fever occurs in 53% of cases, and thrombocytopenia, which may be severe, is observed in 48% of cases. Most infants do not become critically ill but present with the clinical picture of an ongoing indolent infection. Infants also may present with a malfunctioning catheter following occlusion by a *Malassezia*-infected thrombus.[590,595,596]

Diagnosis

The diagnosis frequently is made by noting the appearance of a fluffy white precipitate visible in the clear connecting tubing of the infected catheter.[595] Gram stain of this material reveals the characteristic appearance of *M. furfur* or *M. pachydermatis*, and culture of this material will allow isolation of the organism. In the absence of any sign of catheter infection, results of culture of blood drawn directly from the catheter may be positive, whereas those obtained from peripheral vessels will be sterile. When *Malassezia* infection is suspected, the laboratory should be notified, because these yeasts are not recovered from routine culture media, and special lipid supplementation is required for their growth and identification.[597] Newer methods of fungal identification including PCR techniques may be advantageous in diagnosing this organism but are not yet universally available.[598] Echocardiography is indicated in infants who have persistent fungemia, so that an infected thrombus on the catheter tip can be excluded.[592]

Therapy

Prompt removal of the infected catheter is the optimal treatment for neonatal *Malassezia* infections. Although dissemination is rare, antifungal therapy usually is provided to ensure clearance of the organism from the bloodstream. Amphotericin B is the most frequently used agent, although in vitro testing suggests only moderate susceptibility of *Malassezia* species to this agent.[599] With removal of the catheter, and thereby the high concentration of lipid, the organism will no longer survive. Vascular catheter complications, including retained catheters and catheter breakage, have been reported with *Malassezia* infections, with one series suggesting *M. furfur* contributes directly to catheter fragility and breakage.[590,595] Thrombolytic therapy with urokinase and tissue plasminogen activator has been used to facilitate the removal of adherent *M. furfur*–infected catheters and avoid surgical extraction.[596] If a large thrombus remains after catheter removal, serial monitoring for dissolution by echocardiography is indicated, and some authorities believe that antifungal therapy should be continued until complete resolution is achieved, although this approach is controversial.[592] Although therapy usually is not indicated with neonatal pustulosis, severe, extensive involvement has been treated with topical ketoconazole ointment.[577]

Prognosis

Prognosis generally is excellent with prompt diagnosis and removal of the infected catheter. Rarely reported complications include severe CNS, pulmonary, and liver disease, with only an occasional death in the extremely low birth weight preterm infant.[573,592]

Prevention

The prevention of *Malassezia* infections in neonates has not been studied. The judicious use of intralipids may significantly limit the risk. In patients in whom intralipid therapy cannot be avoided, this fungal infection should be suspected if the central venous catheter malfunctions or if mild, nonspecific signs of infection are noted.

PHYCOMYCOSIS

Infection with Phycomycetes organisms occurs infrequently in newborns, but 24 cases have been reported in the literature.[600-619] Sixteen of the infants died; in 8 of these, the diagnosis was not suspected during life. One infant died 3 days after the diagnosis was established and therapy was initiated. The gastrointestinal tract was the focus of infection in 8 of 18 cases. Two neonates had only CNS infection, and a third had CNS infection as well as intestinal involvement. In none of these three was clinical evidence of nasopharyngeal or orbital infection documented. One infant described by Miller and co-workers[607] had rhinocerebral infection and survived, and Lewis and colleagues[611] reported a fatal case in which the affected infant had methylmalonic aciduria and rhinocerebral mucormycosis. White and associates[608] described an infant with cellulitis of the abdominal wall who also survived. In a case reported by Ng and Dear,[610] the affected infant had multiple abscesses due to *Rhizopus* infection and survived following treatment. Three additional reports have described infants with cutaneous phycomycosis.[613-615] Two of the three died despite medical and surgical therapy. One of the infants who died had progressive infection that involved the gastrointestinal and respiratory tracts.[614] Four infants had cutaneous infections that developed at intravenous catheter sites.[616-619]

Although infection with phycomycetes is common in adults receiving immunosuppressive therapy and in those with neoplastic diseases, particularly hematologic or reticulendothelial malignancies,[620] none of the infants described in these reports received such drugs or had neoplasia. In adults, acidosis resulting from uncontrolled diabetes mellitus or from hepatic or renal failure appears to contribute significantly to infection with Phycomycetes organisms.[620-626] Although none of the infants in the reported cases had diabetes mellitus or hepatic failure, diarrhea was a prominent finding in 6 of 10 infants; however, acidosis as a complication of diarrhea was not commented on in any of the case reports. One patient had renal failure and acidosis,[609] and 4 others were acidotic, including the infant with methylmalonic aciduria.[611,613] Five of the 24 infants were born prematurely, and 1 term neonate had underlying congenital heart disease and had undergone complex cardiac surgery; intensive antimicrobial therapy was given to all but 1 infant. Two infants were receiving nasogastric feedings,[604,611] and in one, cellulitis developed beneath a jejunostomy dressing.[608] In another infant, cutaneous infection developed under an abdominal adhesive tape that attached a radiant thermosensor.[615]

The Organism

Some confusion regarding the taxonomy of phycomycetes exists in the literature.[627] For purposes of simplicity, we shall consider phycomycetes as the class and Mucorales as the order of the three most common genera causing phycomycosis—*Mucor*, *Absidia*, and *Rhizopus*.[628] Phycomycosis, however, also includes infection with species of *Mortierella*, *Basidiobolus*, *Hyphomyces*, and *Entomophthora*.[627]

Hyphae are best stained by hematoxylin-eosin, for which they have an affinity; methenamine silver stains are inferior for this fungus. Characteristically, hyphae are randomly branched, are rarely septate, and appear empty. The diameter of hyphae is variable even within the length of the same mycelium. Because these fungi are not sufficiently pathogenic for laboratory animals, attempts at isolation by inoculation are not useful as a diagnostic procedure.

Epidemiology and Transmission

Phycomycetes organisms are found throughout the world in soil, in animal manure, and on fruits. Fungi of this class frequently are found in refrigerators and are commonly known as bread molds.[629-631] *Basidiobolus* and *Entomophthora* can be isolated from decaying organic matter. Infection with phycomycetes has been reported in humans and animals.[632]

In infants with phycomycosis, the infection may have been the result either of ingestion of the fungus into the gastrointestinal tract or of inhalation into the nasopharynx or lung after birth, but saprophytic colonization in the vagina of the mothers and intrapartum acquisition cannot be excluded. Little is known regarding the presence of phycomycetes on the skin, in the feces, or in pharyngeal or vaginal secretions in the absence of clinical disease. Emmons[632] noted that after exposure to phycomycetes patients with bronchiectasis may cough up spores for several days in the absence of clinical infection. Isolation of these fungi from other sites without evidence of disease has not been reported, but data from newborns suggest that saprophytic colonization with phycomycetes may be similar to the commensalism with *Candida*. No evidence is available to suggest that human-to-human transmission occurs. In one case reported by Dennis and co-workers,[605] *Rhizopus oryzale* was isolated from the Elastoplast that was used as an adhesive for the abdominal dressing. In another infant described by White and co-workers,[608] abdominal wall cellulitis developed beneath the adhesive dressing of a jejunostomy. Linder and colleagues[615] isolated *Rhizopus* from the adhesive tape used to attach the thermosensor. In each of these infants, cultures of similar dressings and of tape used in the same units failed to grow the fungi.[608,615]

Pathogenesis

The bowel is a frequent site of infection in infants; disease in this location appears to be associated with malnutrition or diarrhea.[602,613] Underlying medical conditions seem to play a major pathogenic role in most cases of phycomycosis. The high incidence of rhinocerebral infection in adults with diabetes mellitus has been noted, but the biochemical abnormality that increases susceptibility is considered to be acidosis, rather than endocrine dysfunction.[604,622] Straatsma and co-workers[620] have suggested that acidosis from any cause, including hepatic or renal failure, may increase susceptibility to phycomycosis. Of interest are the reported infants and adults with gastrointestinal phycomycosis. Most had diarrhea, which may be accompanied by severe acidosis, especially in infants. Whether diarrhea preceded or was a complication of gastrointestinal phycomycosis in these cases cannot be determined. The mechanism of increased susceptibility to infection with phycomycetes in an acidotic state is incompletely understood. Although optimal growth of phycomycetes occurs at pH 4.0 in vitro but not at pH 2.7 or 7.3,[634] acidification is not suitable for the sexual cycle of phycomycetes. In the host, acidosis may delay polymorphonuclear response and limit fibroblastic reaction.[622,626] Prematurity, antibiotics, and diarrhea may have been some of the predisposing factors in the infants who died of this infection.

Pathology

The characteristic histopathologic features of infection with this class of fungi include vascular invasion with necrosis or hemorrhage. Necrotic and suppurative lesions demonstrating massive infiltration by polymorphonuclear leukocytes are seen in invasive or disseminated phycomycosis. In patients with subcutaneous infection, lesions usually are granulomatous with epithelioid and Langhans' giant cells. Conspicuous infiltration with eosinophils occurs in subcutaneous infection, particularly with species of *Basidiobolus*. Vascular invasion in such cases is rare.

Clinical Manifestations

The clinical manifestations of phycomycosis in neonates and young infants depend on the site or sites of infection. With cutaneous disease, the appearance is similar to that in cutaneous aspergillosis, and involved sites include surgical wounds, intravascular catheter insertion sites, and areas of skin breakdown. The usual symptoms of gastrointestinal phycomycosis in adults are bloody diarrhea and cramping abdominal pain. Because vascular invasion and necrosis occur, perforation and peritonitis with a rapidly fatal course are common. In seven of eight infants with phycomycosis, diarrhea and abdominal distention or signs of peritoneal irritation, or both, were prominent findings. Two infants had free air in the peritoneal cavity from perforation. One infant without abdominal signs had CNS infection without other organ involvement. In extremely premature and low-birth-weight neonates, invasive fungal dermatitis has been reported to be caused by phycomycetes.[635]

Diagnosis and Differential Diagnosis

The clinical picture in infants with phycomycosis appears to be very similar to that in children with aspergillosis. Phycomycetes have the same affinity for vascular invasion, hemorrhage, necrosis, and suppuration. Bacterial infection in the lung may be indistinguishable from phycomycosis on clinical grounds. Hemorrhagic infarction of the lung or bowel from other causes has the same presenting signs as those due to infection with phycomycetes. The cerebrospinal fluid in infants with CNS infection does not show a consistent pattern. Glucose and protein levels often are normal. Xanthochromia with small numbers of red blood cells is common, and a few mononuclear or polymorphonuclear cells may be present.[626]

The diagnosis of phycomycosis should be considered in debilitated infants, particularly those with acidosis related to diarrhea, or with hepatic or renal failure, who do not respond to correction of the acidotic state. Sinus or orbital abnormalities in such patients should be investigated for the presence of phycomycetes. Adults receiving immunosuppressive therapy or antimetabolites for hematologic diseases in whom pulmonary or gastrointestinal symptoms develop must be evaluated for possible phycomycetes infection.

The diagnosis of infection with these fungi can be difficult because culture results frequently are negative.[636] Demonstration of the fungus is best accomplished by microscopic examination of tissue and visualization of the broad, branching, nonseptate hyphae. A 10% solution of potassium hydroxide is used, although hematoxylin-eosin staining is preferred for specimens of tissue. Exudates from the nasopharynx or necrotic tissue obtained by débridement should be cultured on Sabouraud glucose agar. Because of the ubiquity of these fungi, demonstration of the organism in tissue is necessary to establish a diagnosis of phycomycosis.

Although normal human serum contains substances that inhibit growth of *Rhizopus* in vitro,[637] serologic and immunologic tests have not been extensively studied as diagnostic aids for patients with phycomycosis. Bank and associates,[638] using an extract of *Rhizopus* isolated from a patient, produced a cutaneous reaction with an intradermal injection in the patient but not in control subjects. They also found complement-fixing antibodies in the serum of the patient but not in controls, although the same extract was used. Jones and Kaufman[639] demonstrated antibodies to a homogenate of the fungus by an immunodiffusion technique in 8 of 11 patients with mucormycosis.

Therapy

Of paramount importance in the treatment of phycomycosis is correction of metabolic derangement; cessation of antibiotics, corticosteroids, or immunosuppressive agents whenever possible; and débridement or excision of necrotic tissue.[640-644] In conjunction with these measures, various antifungal agents in addition to amphotericin B have been employed, but no data are available that allow recommendations for specific drugs, doses, or duration.

Prognosis

The diagnosis of phycomycosis in infants most often is made at autopsy. The diagnosis was not considered before death in 9 patients in the reported cases. In 13 patients, the organism was identified and therapy was given; 6 of the 13 recovered.[600-619]

Prevention

Measures to protect the fragile skin of immature extremely low birth weight infants should limit the ability of these fungi to invade. As with *Aspergillus* infection, activities that would allow exposure to phycomycetes such as construction, should be limited in or near the NICU.

DERMATOPHYTOSES

The dermatophytes—*Epidermophyton*, *Microsporum*, and *Trichophyton*—often are responsible for infection of keratinized areas of the body, including skin, hair, and nails. Superficial infection with these "ringworm" fungi has been reported infrequently in newborns, although infants have been considered susceptible to infection with these specialized fungi.[645] In 1876, Lynch[646] reported the case of an infant with tinea faciei who was only 6 hours of age. Unfortunately, the diagnosis was made clinically, and no documentation of dermatophyte infection by microscopic examination or culture was obtained. More recently, Jacobs and colleagues[647] described an 8-day-old infant with tinea faciei due to *Microsporum canis*. An outbreak of neonatal ringworm in five infants in an NICU was linked to the index case, in a nurse who was infected with *M. canis* by her cat.[648] Dermatophyte infections in infants from a few weeks of age to several months of age have been described.[649-661]

Because of the infrequent reports of dermatophyte infections in infants, few investigative studies defining factors contributing to increased infantile susceptibility or resistance to infection by dermatophytes have been performed.[656,655] Wyre and Johnson[657] suggested that increased humidity in the incubator may have contributed to the risk of infection in an infant with pityriasis versicolor, and Lanska and associates[659] indicated that prolonged exposure to humidified oxygen by hood may have increased susceptibility to the cutaneous fungal infection observed in three infants.

The Organism

Dermatophytes have been placed in the class of imperfect fungi, Deuteromycetes, in the order Moniliales.[628] Because of a sexual stage in some dermatophytes, however, some authors have preferred to classify certain genera as belonging to the class Ascomycetes.[662,663]

Hyphae of dermatophytes are long, undulant, and branching. Many septa are present along the length of hyphae. Hyphae break at the septa into barrel-shaped arthrospores. In culture, dermatophytes form conidiophores, with resulting microconidia and macroconidia. Genera and species identification is based on gross characteristics of colony and microscopic morphology of conidia. A complete review of distinguishing features may be found in standard mycology textbooks.[664]

Epidemiology and Transmission

Dermatophytes are distributed throughout the world in humans and animals; many also are found in soil, water, vegetation, and animal excrement.[665] The fungus can contaminate combs, hairbrushes, shoes, and shower floors and has been isolated from air.[666,667] Contamination of soil with dermatophytes has been thought to occur in keratinous debris from infected animals and humans,[665] and no evidence is available to suggest that these fungi are free-living saprophytes in soil.

Dermatophyte infection most often is acquired from contact with infected persons or animals. Infections with *Microsporum gypseum* can result from contact with soil contaminated with the fungus. Human-to-human transmission can occur with *Epidermophyton floccosum*, *Microsporum audouinii*, *Trichophyton mentagrophytes*, *Trichophyton rubrum*, *Trichophyton schoenleinii*, *Trichophyton tonsurans*, and *Trichophyton violaceum*.[668] Zoophilic dermatophytes include *M. canis*, *Trichophyton gallinae*, *T. mentagrophytes*, and *Trichophyton verrucosum*. Although *M. canis* usually is transmitted to humans from young animals, particularly kittens, transmission between persons is suggested in the case of an infant reported by Bereston and Robinson.[649] Pinetti and co-workers[669] isolated *M. canis* and *M. gypseum* from flies, which suggests an additional mode of transmission.

In newborns with dermatophyte infection, the fungus probably is acquired after birth from contact with infected nursery personnel, household members, or animals. In the case reported by Lynch[646] of clinically apparent infection at 6 hours of age, the fungal infection probably was acquired in utero. In this case, evidence of infection in the mother was lacking, but the fungus has been demonstrated on skin in the absence of clinical disease.[670,671]

Pathogenesis

Despite worldwide distribution of dermatophytes and frequency of exposure of humans to these fungi, the incidence of clinically apparent infection in infants and adults is considerably lower than would be expected. Few studies defining host factors responsible for protection have been performed. Although Knight[672] has shown in experimental studies in humans that macerated moist skin is more susceptible to the infection than dry skin, the role of immunologic factors in the control of dermatophyte infection remains obscure. Repeated infection may occur at identical sites as long as 2 years after primary infection,[672,673] despite reports that infection may offer partial immunity to reinfection.[674,675]

Roth and colleagues[325] as well as others[676-680] have demonstrated antidermatophyte activity in normal human serum and have suggested that this substance may restrict dermatophyte infection to superficial layers of skin. No studies investigating the role of antifungal activity in sweat have been reported, although immunoglobulins and antibodies have been demonstrated in sweat.[681] Although antidermatophyte activity has been reported in serum at birth,[680] no specific studies have been performed in infants to define other host factors or to determine immunologic consequences of dermatophyte infection.

Most infected neonates weigh less than 1000 g at birth and have a gestational age of less than 26 weeks.

Pathology

Dermatophyte infection generally is confined to keratinized areas of the body and only rarely invades deeper tissues. Lesions may be vesicular and contain serous fluid. Inflammatory reaction with polymorphonuclear leukocyte infiltration is minimal and usually represents secondary bacterial infection. Occasionally, intense inflammatory reactions may occur in the absence of bacterial infection, especially in children with tinea capitis resulting from *T. mentagrophytes*. These pustular lesions, or kerions, surround infected hair follicles and appear to be reactions to virulent strains of fungus.

Favus is a chronic infection usually caused by *T. schoenleinii* or *T. mentagrophytes*. Granulomatous formation occurs, with giant cells and masses of hyphae around the hair follicle. Overlying the infection is a crust of cellular debris and degenerating hyphae. This lesion is convex, and scarring and alopecia appear after healing.

In infants of extremely low birth weight, invasive dermatitis can occur with *Trichosporon* species. Skin biopsies reveal invasion of the epidermis with this yeast, often with spread along hair follicles and then into the dermis (Fig. 34-5)—similar to the histologic picture of invasive fungal dermatitis caused by *Candida* species, *Aspergillus* species, or Phycomycetes organisms.[665]

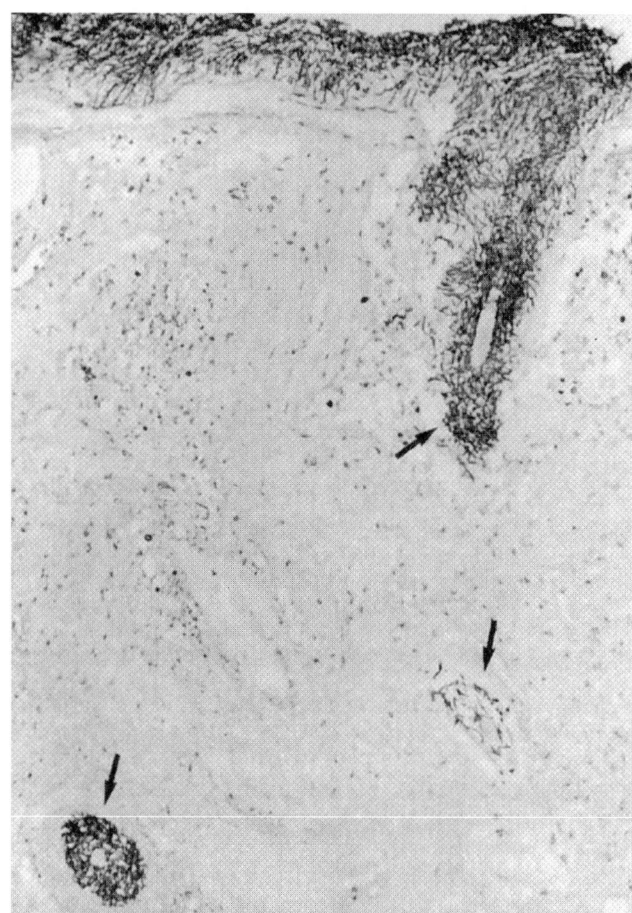

Figure 34–5 Skin biopsy specimen from extremely low birth weight infant with invasive fungal dermatitis caused by *Candida albicans*. Intense involvement of the epidermis with pseudohyphae extending along hair follicles (*arrows*) is demonstrated following staining with Grocott methenamine silver. ×10.

Clinical Manifestations

Dermatophytosis is classified generally by focus of infection and less commonly by species of infecting fungus. Tinea capitis is a fungal infection of the scalp and hair caused by *Microsporum* and *Trichophyton*. It occurs most often in infants, older children, and adults. Alteras[676] reported that in a group of 7000 patients, 70 infants between 2 and 12 months of age had tinea capitis. In this study, *M. audouinii* was the most common fungus in infants. Other fungi reportedly causing tinea capitis include *M. canis*, *T. violaceum*, *T. tonsurans*, *T. mentagrophytes*, *T. schoenleinii*, *Microsporum ferrugineum*, *E. floccosum*, and *T. rubrum*. Infection begins with small scaling papules that spread peripherally, forming circular pruritic patches. Both kerion and favus formation can occur.

Tinea corporis, or ringworm of smooth skin, can result from infection with species of *Microsporum*, *Trichophyton*, or *Epidermophyton*, although infections with *Microsporum* species are the most common (Fig. 34-6). Infants and children appear to be more susceptible to tinea corporis than adults. King and co-workers[650] described five infants with tinea corporis who ranged in age from 3 weeks to 7 months. *Microsporum* species predominated in that study, but one infant, who was 8 weeks of age, was infected with *E. floccosum*.

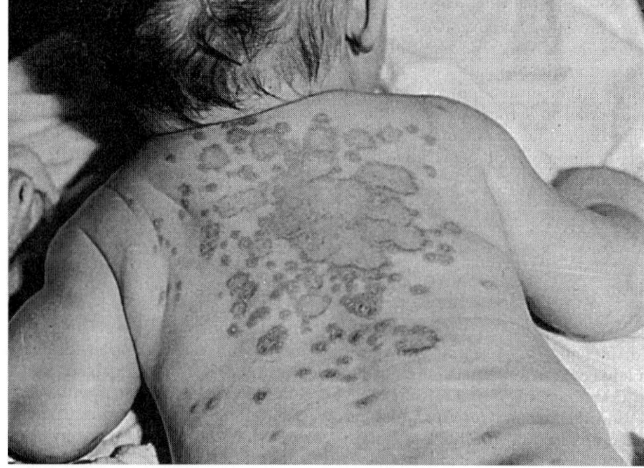

Figure 34–6 Tinea corporis caused by *Microsporum* species in a 4-month-old infant.

In older children, *M. canis* and *T. mentagrophytes* are more common causes of tinea corporis. Lesions, which may be single or multiple, are round or oval scaling, erythematous patches. As infection spreads peripherally, the center of the lesion may show some clearing. In some instances, an intense inflammatory reaction with vesiculation at the margins, accompanied by severe pruritus, may be noted. Patches of infected areas may coalesce, forming extensive plaques with serpiginous borders. Deep granulomas or nodules may form, especially when the infection is caused by *T. rubrum*.

Tinea cruris is a fungal infection of the groin, perineum, or perianal area and most often is caused by *E. floccosum* (Fig. 34-7). *T. mentagrophytes* and *T. rubrum* are unusual causes of infection at these sites. Although *Candida* species account for a majority of fungal infections in the diaper area, King and co-workers[650] described one infant with *E. floccosum* infection in the perineum. Infection with this fungus is characterized by brownish areas of scaly dermatitis with

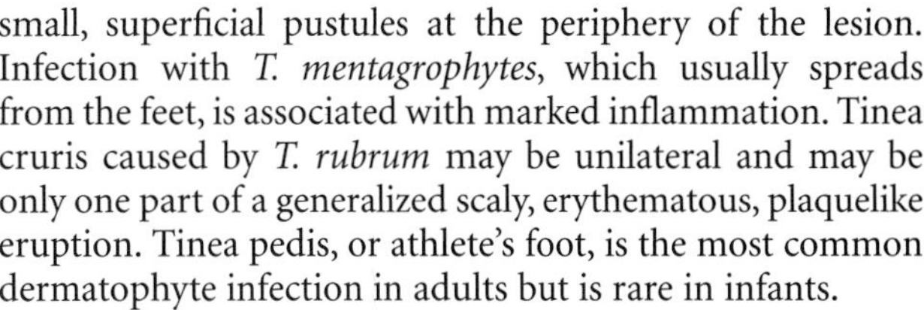

small, superficial pustules at the periphery of the lesion. Infection with *T. mentagrophytes*, which usually spreads from the feet, is associated with marked inflammation. Tinea cruris caused by *T. rubrum* may be unilateral and may be only one part of a generalized scaly, erythematous, plaquelike eruption. Tinea pedis, or athlete's foot, is the most common dermatophyte infection in adults but is rare in infants.

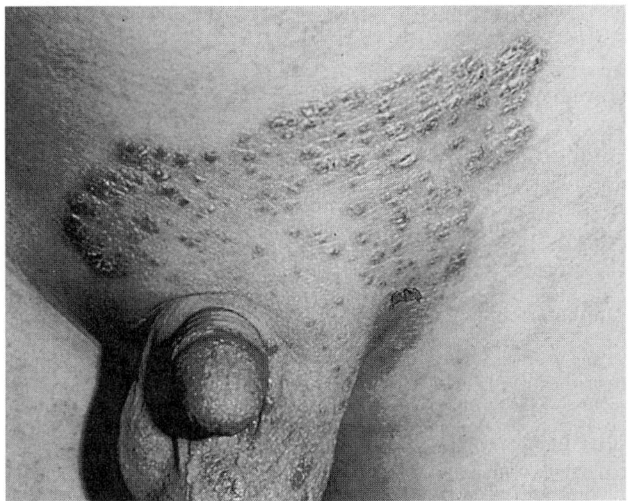

Figure 34–7 Tinea cruris infection with *Epidermophyton floccosum* in a young infant.

In extremely immature premature neonates, invasive fungal dermatitis can occur in areas of skin breakdown (Fig. 34-8).[665]

Diagnosis and Differential Diagnosis

Dermatophyte infection may be mistaken for seborrhea, impetigo, or psoriasis. Tinea capitis may appear similar to alopecia areata, but scaling usually is absent in the latter. The presumptive diagnosis is made by direct microscopic examination of infected material. Areas to be examined should be cleansed with 70% alcohol, and scrapings should be made with a scalpel or scissors from the active periphery of the lesion. If vesicles are present, the tops should be removed for examination. Hairs infected with *M. audouinii* or *M. canis* may be identified by using Wood's light, which emits monochromatic ultraviolet rays. Infected hairs show a green-yellow fluorescence and may be removed for examination. Scrapings from nails, obtained from deep layers, should be thin. Specimens are placed on a glass slide, and a few drops of 10% sodium or potassium hydroxide are added. A coverslip is added, and the specimen is gently heated over a low flame. Microscopic examination under low power should take place immediately. The presence of hyphae confirms the diagnosis of fungal infection. Young hyphae appear as long, thin threads, and older hyphae have many spores. Spores may be found either within the hair follicle or around its base. Shelley and Wood[682] have described a technique of crushing the hair. They found it to

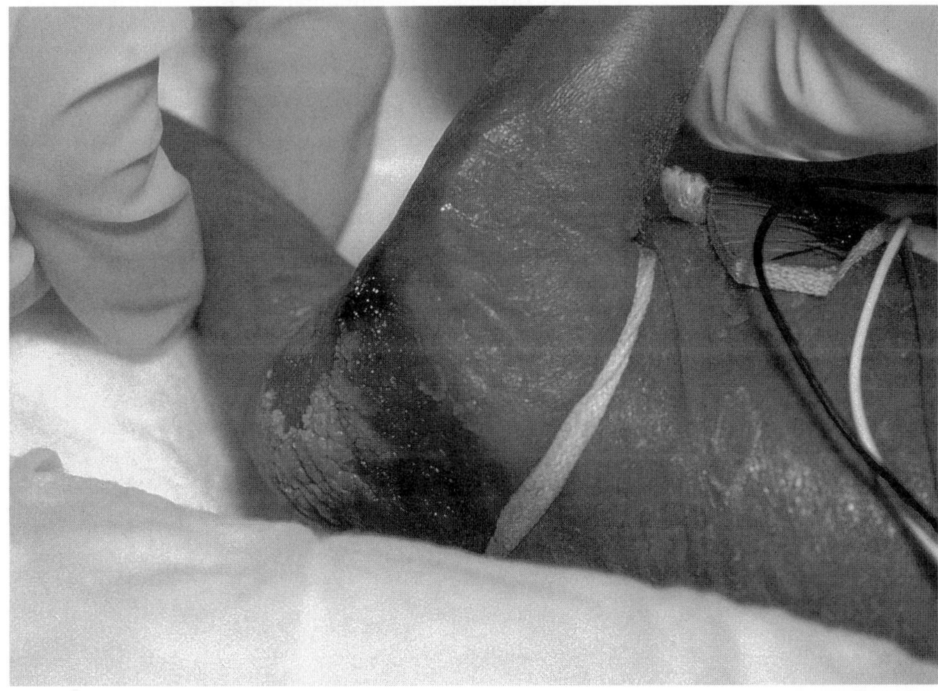

Figure 34–8 Diffuse involvement of the buttocks by invasive fungal dermatitis, caused by *Trichosporon* species, in an extremely low birth weight infant. The lesion is a tightly adherent white-and-buff-colored crust.

be superior to the use of potassium hydroxide for identifying the fungus in the hair. Identification of the genus and species of dermatophyte can be made only by culture. Infected material should be cultured on a Sabouraud glucose agar slant, and microscopic examination of hyphae and conidia performed.

In premature infants with brown- or black-appearing lesions at areas of skin trauma, the diagnosis of invasive fungal dermatitis should be determined by skin biopsy and culture (see under "Aspergillosis" and "Phycomycosis"). Blood cultures also may yield *Trichosporon beigelii* if this etiologic agent is responsible for the skin lesions.

Therapy

Topical therapy with keratolytic or fungicidal medications may be beneficial in some cases of dermatophyte infection, especially tinea pedis, in which results with use of griseofulvin are not encouraging. Whitfield's ointment, 1% solution of tolnaftate, or an ointment with 3% each of sulfur and salicylic acid may be used. Topical therapy should be continued until culture specimens and scrapings are negative for fungus. For invasive fungal dermatitis in premature infants, amphotericin B deoxycholate administered intravenously is the agent of choice. Some studies, however, have suggested tolerance of *Trichosporon* species to amphotericin, and fluconazole has been shown to be effective in the treatment of trichosporonosis.

Prognosis

Untreated dermatophyte infection is slowly progressive and can be disfiguring, especially in cases of kerion and favus reactions. Secondary bacterial infections are common, particularly in cases of tinea pedis. Deep tissue invasion occurs in extremely low birth weight neonates, typically with *T. beigelii* infections, and most reported cases have had a fatal outcome.[665]

Prevention

Separate combs, hairbrushes, and clippers should be available for the newborn and should not be shared with others in the household. Infected animals and household contacts should be promptly treated.[683]

ANTIFUNGAL THERAPY IN NEONATES AND YOUNG INFANTS

Amphotericin B deoxycholate is the mainstay of therapy for invasive fungal infections in neonates. For certain infections, flucytosine or fluconazole may be useful (Table 34-3). Although newer azoles, lipid formulations of amphotericin B, and echinocandins have been studied and shown to be useful in adults and older children with some invasive fungal infections, limited or no information regarding the pharmacokinetics, safety, and efficacy of these new antifungals in neonates is available. For many invasive infections in adults (e.g., candidiasis, aspergillosis), these agents have been demonstrated to have similar efficacy but reduced toxicity, especially the dose-limiting toxicity often noted with conventional amphotericin B in adults and older children. For some fungal infections, however, amphotericin B has limited in vitro activity, and use of alternative agents may be necessary.

AMPHOTERICIN B

Amphotericin B is a polyene antimicrobial that reacts with sterols in cell membranes, resulting in cellular damage and lysis. Serum levels in adults average 1.5 µg/mL 1 hour after intravenous injection of 0.6 to 1 mg/kg; the half-life is approximately 24 hours, but levels of 0.14 µg/mL have been detected in serum for at least 3 weeks.[684] Only one tenth to one twentieth of the serum levels is distributed into the cerebrospinal fluid.

Few studies have been performed of the clinical pharmacology of amphotericin B in newborns or older infants from which an accurate recommendation for dosage can be extrapolated. McCoy and co-workers[685] reported peak serum concentrations at 1 hour of 2.6 µg/mL in the mother and in arterial cord blood after a maternal infusion of 0.6 mg of amphotericin B. The amphotericin B concentration in the amniotic fluid was 0.08 µg/mL. Ismail and Lerner[384] reported that levels of amphotericin B in cord blood were 33% of the maternal serum concentrations. Hager and associates[387] obtained simultaneous amphotericin B levels in maternal blood, cord blood, and amniotic fluid 26 hours after an infusion of 20 mg. The levels were 1.9, 1.3, and 0.3 µg/mL, respectively. Ward and co-workers[686] reported that serum levels of amphotericin B in a premature infant were similar to those found in older children and adults, and

Table 34–3 Antifungal Drugs for Infants with Systemic Fungal Infection

Agent	Metabolism/Excretion	CSF/Serum Concentration	Dose Change in Renal Failure	Daily Dose (mg/kg)
Amphotericin B		40-90%	None	0.5-1.5
Liposomal amphotericin B	Hepatic	?	None	3-6
Flucytosine	Renal	>75%	Yes	100-150
Fluconazole	Renal	>60%	Yes	2-12
Itraconazole	Hepatic	<1%	None	2-5

CSF, cerebrospinal fluid.

those levels persisted for at least 17 days after amphotericin B had been discontinued.

The toxicity of amphotericin B in humans can be significant. Adults and older children frequently experience nausea, vomiting, headache, chills, and fever during infusion of this agent.[687] Infusion-related adverse events are rare in neonates, however.[690] Hypokalemia can develop, but often concomitant drugs being administered with amphotericin B to the neonate may account for this association. Serum electrolytes should be carefully monitored, and hypokalemia can be corrected with potassium replacement. Nephrotoxicity is the most important toxic effect in adults and older children. This adverse effect has been shown to correlate with the total dose of amphotericin B[688] and results from drug-induced renal vasoconstriction, as well as from direct action of amphotericin B on renal tubules.[689] Other findings can include a rise in serum creatinine and blood urea nitrogen levels and a decrease in creatinine clearance, as well as cylindruria, renal tubular acidosis, tubular necrosis, and nephrocalcinosis. Nephrotoxicity from amphotericin B is rare in neonates; when it occurs, it often is the result of infection rather than an adverse drug effect and is reversible with a reduction in daily dose from 1.0 to 0.5 mg/kg.[690,691]

The effect of amphotericin B on the fetus has not been extensively studied. Several reports of the use of amphotericin B in pregnant women have now been published.[383-388,685,692-699] In no instance was there evidence of teratogenicity or fetal toxicity related to this antifungal agent. Amphotericin for use during pregnancy is a Category B drug. Systemic fungal infections have been successfully treated in pregnant women without obvious effects on the fetus, but the number of cases reported has been small. Adequate and well-controlled studies have not been conducted; therefore, use of this drug during pregnancy is indicated only if it is clearly needed.[700]

The initial intravenous dose of amphotericin B in neonates should be 0.5 to 1.0 mg per kg, and the drug should be suspended in sterile water in a concentration of no greater than 0.1 mg/mL. The maximum daily dose and duration of therapy depends on the focus and extent of fungal disease,[701] as well as on the minimal inhibitory concentration (MIC) of amphotericin B for the organism.[702] The neonatal dose is 0.5 to 1.5 mg/kg per day. Although some authors have suggested monitoring serum levels of amphotericin B,[703,704] others disagree, because of the predictable pharmacokinetics of this drug.[705,706] Rate of administration varies, but typically the dose can be given over 1 to 2 hours, and no longer than 4 hours.

Intrathecal administration of amphotericin B can be necessary in patients with coccidioidomycosis meningitis. Few data are available on the ideal intrathecal dose of amphotericin B in children with fungal meningitis. The initial intrathecal dose in infants should be 0.01 mg, gradually increased over a period of 5 to 7 days to 0.1 mg given every other day or every third day. Amphotericin B for intrathecal administration should not exceed a concentration of 0.25 mg per mL of diluent, and further dilution with cerebrospinal fluid is recommended. Complications of intrathecal amphotericin B administration include cerebrospinal fluid pleocytosis (arachnoiditis), transient radiculitis, and sensory loss.

Three lipid formulations of amphotericin B are commercially available: amphotericin B lipid complex (ABLC), amphotericin B cholesteryl sulfate complex (i.e., amphotericin B colloidal dispersion [ABCD]), and liposomal amphotericin B (L-AmB). These formulations differ in the amount of amphotericin B and lipids, vesicle size and structure, and pharmacokinetic properties. These lipid formulations have demonstrated comparable clinical efficacy, as well as reduced nephrotoxicity, in comparison with conventional amphotericin B in adults; none is superior in effectiveness to conventional amphotericin B. No studies have compared the safety and effectiveness of lipid preparations with conventional amphotericin B in neonates.

Lackner and co-workers[327] reported successful use of a lipid formulation of amphotericin B, in a daily dose of 5 mg/kg, in two premature infants with disseminated fungal infections. In addition, Weitkamp and associates reported use of this preparation in a daily dose of 1 to 5 mg/kg in 21 low-birth-weight infants with *Candida* infections and demonstrated its efficacy without apparent nephrotoxicity.[707] Scarcella and colleagues[708] also reported using a lipid formulation of amphotericin B in 44 infants with severe fungal infections. Using a daily dose of 1 to 5 mg/kg, they reported transient hypokalemia but successful outcomes in 32 infants, but 12 infants of very low birth weight died.

5-FLUCYTOSINE

5-Flucytosine, a fluoropyrimidine, has been shown to have in vitro activity against some fungi.[687,709-711] It has been used in combination with conventional amphotericin B for an additive antifungal effect for the treatment of disseminated candidiasis and cryptococcosis. The drug is absorbed well from the gastrointestinal tract, and, with doses of 100 to 150 mg/kg, serum levels vary, ranging from 17 to 44 μg/mL.[712] In the cerebrospinal fluid, levels of 5-flucytosine may be as high as 88% of serum concentrations.[713] The drug is administered orally in a total daily dose of 50 to 150 mg/kg, given in four divided doses, for 2 to 6 weeks in adults. Experience with this agent in infants is increasing. Rapid emergence of resistance of fungi after initiation of flucytosine therapy has been reported for *Candida*, as well as for *C. neoformans*.[709-714] Flucytosine has been used extensively in infants and children receiving amphotericin B.[715-718] Few untoward side effects have been noted, even with prolonged use. Toxic effects of flucytosine include transient neutropenia and hepatocellular damage.[719] Because the drug is cleared by the kidneys, the dose should be reduced and serum levels determined in infants with impaired renal function. Accumulation of flucytosine in the blood can result in serious toxicity to the bone marrow.

FLUCONAZOLE AND ITRACONAZOLE

Fluconazole is an azole antifungal agent and is available in an intravenous as well as an oral preparation. This agent has been shown to achieve good penetration into cerebrospinal fluid, ocular fluid, and skin.[720] It is effective against many fungi, including *Candida*, *Coccidioides*, and dermatophytes. Its use in neonates has been limited. Wiest and associates[721] used fluconazole in a premature infant with disseminated candidiasis unresponsive to amphotericin B and flucytosine. The infant received 6 mg/kg per day intravenously, with peak and trough serum levels of 10.3 and 6.98 mg/mL, respectively. Gürses and Kalayci[722] reported successful use of fluconazole alone in a premature infant with candidal meningitis. Dreissen and co-workers[723,724] in two reports indicated that fluconazole was effective and associated with fewer side effects than those observed with amphotericin B. A review of 62 episodes of neonatal candidemia revealed that fluconazole was used as the first-line agent in 6 episodes, with successful eradication of infection in five of the episodes. Fluconazole was used as an alternative agent in another 13 episodes, with eradication of infection in 8 of the 13. Fluconazole was well tolerated.[725] Fluconazole also has been used in pregnancy without harmful effects on the fetus.[726]

Itraconazole, another azole antifungal agent, has had limited use in neonates. Bhandari and Narange[727] reported its use in two premature infants with disseminated candidiasis. Each received 10 mg/kg per day in two divided doses for 3 and 4 weeks, respectively. Both infants did well without any evidence of toxicity. A pharmacokinetic study of oral itraconazole in infants and children 6 months to 12 years of age demonstrated potentially therapeutic concentrations with a daily dose of 5 mg/kg. Itraconazole was well tolerated.[728] Only limited data are available on use of itraconazole in neonates.

VORICONAZOLE

Voriconazole is a second-generation antifungal triazole with a broad spectrum of activity, excellent oral bioavailability, and a good safety profile in adults.[378] Voriconazole is approved by the FDA for use in adults for treatment of invasive aspergillosis and in salvage therapy for infections caused by *Scedosporium* and *Fusarium* species. Voriconazole has been successfully used to treat disseminated infection caused by *Trichosporon* species. Data are available that support the safety and efficacy of voriconazole for the treatment of invasive fungal infections in children 9 months to 15 years of age. Only one study, however, has reported pharmacokinetic data in young infants.[379]

Treatment with voriconazole in 69 children with aspergillosis, scedosporiosis, and other invasive fungal infections resulted in favorable outcomes in patients who were intolerant of or refractory to conventional antifungal therapy.[729] The dosage was 6 mg/kg administered every 12 hours intravenously on day 1, followed by 4 mg/kg every 12 hours, until clinical improvement allowed a change to oral therapy at a dose of 100 or 200 mg twice a day for patients weighing less than 40 kg or 40 kg or greater, respectively.

ECHINOCANDINS: CASPOFUNGIN

Echinocandins are cyclic hexapeptides with an *N*-acyl aliphatic or aryl side chain that expands the antifungal spectrum to include *Candida* species, *Aspergillus* species, and *P. jiroveci*, but not *C. neoformans*. Echinocandins are administered only parenterally because of their large molecular size. They inhibit the biosynthesis of 1,3-beta-glucans, which are key constituents of the fungal cell wall. The enzyme system for 1,3-beta-glucan synthesis is absent in mammalian hosts.

Echinocandins that currently are in phase III clinical trials include caspofungin, micafungin, and anidulafungin. Caspofungin has been approved by the FDA for salvage therapy in adults with invasive aspergillosis. The echinocandins have demonstrated in vivo activity against esophageal candidiasis and disseminated candidiasis in adults. Hepatotoxicity has been observed at very high doses. Data on use in infants are very limited, however, and studies are needed to determine the pharmacokinetics, optimal doses, and indications for echinocandins, as well as their effectiveness, in infants and children.[730]

GRISEOFULVIN

Griseofulvin has significantly altered the morbidity associated with dermatophyte infection. This drug is deposited in epidermal structures before keratinization. As keratinized areas are exfoliated, they are replaced by noninfected tissue. In patients with tinea capitis, it may be necessary to clip the hair frequently, because as growth occurs, the ends of hairs may continue to harbor viable fungus. The oral dose of griseofulvin is 10 mg/kg per day for 7 to 10 days. Occasionally, a daily dose of 20 to 40 mg/kg is necessary for cure. In some instances, therapy must be continued for 3 weeks. Data on the use of griseofulvin in newborns are limited. Ross[731] reported use of griseofulvin in an infant 1 month of age at a daily dose of 10 mg/kg for 4 weeks without untoward effects.

Griseofulvin is derived from a species of *Penicillium*, and cross-sensitivity may exist between penicillin and griseofulvin. The incidence of hypersensitivity reactions to griseofulvin in patients allergic to penicillin, however, has not been reported. The most common untoward reaction to griseofulvin is rash. Urticaria and angioneurotic edema are occasional findings, and elevation of transaminases may occur. In one report, griseofulvin was shown to cross the placenta in low concentrations, but fetal effects were not discussed.[732] A study comparing griseofulvin with terbinafine,[733] and case reports of successful treatment of tinea capitis with itraconazole and fluconazole, suggest that all of these antifungal agents can be used as alternative agents with better tolerability and fewer side effects.[734]

REFERENCES

Pneumocystis jiroveci Infection

1. Fudenberg H, Good RA, Goodman HC, et al. Primary immunodeficiencies: report of a World Health Organization Committee. Pediatrics 47:927, 1971.
2. Chagas C. Nova trypanomiazaea humana. Mem Inst Oswaldo Cruz 1:159, 1909.
3. Carini A. Formas de eschizogonia do *Trypanosoma lewisii*. Soc Med Cir São Paulo 16 Aoakut. Bull Inst Pasteur 9:937, 1911.
4. Delanoe P, Delanoe M. Sur les rapports des kystes de carini du poumon des rats avec le *Trypanosoma lewisii*. Presenté par M. Laveran. Note de Delanoe et Delanoe. C R Acad Sci 155:658, 1912.
5. Chagas C. Nova entidade morbida do homen; rezumo geral de estudos etiologicos e clinicos. Mem Inst Oswaldo Cruz 3:219, 1911.
6. Benecke E. Eigenartige Bronchiolenerkrankung im ersten Lebensjahr. Verh Dtsch Pathol Ges 31:402, 1938.
7. Ammich O. Über die nichtsyphilitische interstitielle Pneumonie des ersten Kindesalters. Virchows Arch Pathol Anat 302:539, 1938.
8. Vanek J, Jirovec O. Parasitäre Pneumonie. "Interstitielle" plasmazellen Pneumonie der Frühgeborenen, verursacht durch *Pneumocystis carinii*. Zentralbl Bakteriol [Orig] 158:120, 1952.
9. Van der Meer G, Brug SL. Infection par *Pneumocystis* chez l'homme et chez les animaux. Ann Soc Belge Med Trop 22:301, 1942.
10. Deamer WC, Zollinger HU. Interstitial "plasma cell" pneumonia of premature and young infants. Pediatrics 12:11, 1953.
11. Lunseth JH, Kirmse TW, Prezyna AP, et al. Interstitial plasma cell pneumonia. J Pediatr 46:137, 1955.
12. Dauzier G, Willis T, Barnett RN. *Pneumocystis carinii* pneumonia in an infant. Am J Clin Pathol 26:787, 1956.
13. Hamperl H. *Pneumocystis* infection and cytomegaly of the lungs in the newborn and adult. Am J Pathol 32:1, 1956.
14. Russell HT, Nelson BM. *Pneumocystis* pneumonitis in American infants. Am J Clin Pathol 26:1334, 1956.

15. Gajdusek DC. *Pneumocystis carinii*—etiologic agent of interstitial plasma cell pneumonia of premature and young infants. Pediatrics 19:543, 1957.
16. Edman JC, Kovacs JA, Masur H, et al. Ribosomal RNA sequence shows *Pneumocystis carinii* to be a member of the fungi. Nature 334:519, 1988.
17. Stringer SL, Stringer JR, Blaser MA, et al. *Pneumocystis carinii*: sequence from ribosomal RNA implies a close relationship with fungi. Exp Parasitol 68:450, 1989.
18. Frenkel JK. *Pneumocystis* pneumonia, an immunodeficiency-dependent disease (IDD): a critical historical overview. J Eukaryot Microbiol 46:89S, 1999.
19. Hughes WT. *Pneumocystis carinii* vs. *Pneumocystis jiroveci*: another misnomer (response to Stringer et al.). Emerg Infect Dis 9:276, 2003.
20. LeClair RA. *Pneumocystis carinii* and interstitial plasma cell pneumonia: a review. Am Rev Respir Dis 96:1131, 1967.
21. Barton EG, Campbell WG. *Pneumocystis carinii* in lungs of rats treated with cortisone acetate. Am J Pathol 54:209, 1969.
22. Vavra J, Kucera K, Levine ND. An interpretation of the fine structure of *Pneumocystis carinii*. J Protozool 15:12, 1968.
23. Dutz W. *Pneumocystis carinii* pneumonia. Pathol Annu 5:309, 1970.
24. Esterly JA, Warner NE. *Pneumocystis carinii* pneumonia. Arch Pathol 80:433, 1965.
25. Sethi KK. *Pneumocystis carinii* pneumonia. Letter to the editor. Lancet 1:1387, 1967.
26. Minielly JA, Mills SD, Holley KE. *Pneumocystis carinii* pneumonia. Can Med Assoc J 100:846, 1969.
27. McNeal JE, Yaeger RG. Observations on a case of *Pneumocystis* pneumonia. Arch Pathol 70:397, 1960.
28. Vavra J, Kucera K. *Pneumocystis carinii* Delanoë, its ultrastructure and ultrastructural affinities. J Protozool 17:463, 1970.
29. Kim HK, Hughes WT, Feldman S. Studies of morphology and immunofluorescence of *Pneumocystis carinii*. Proc Soc Exp Biol Med 141:304, 1972.
30. Sheldon WH. Pulmonary *Pneumocystis carinii* infection. J Pediatr 61:780, 1962.
31. Le Tan-Vinh, Cochard AM, Vu Trieu-Dong, et al. Diagnostic "in vivo" de la pneumonie á "*Pneumocystis*." Arch Fr Pediatr 20:773, 1963.
32. Chalvardjian AM, Grawe LA. A new procedure for the identification of *Pneumocystis carinii* cysts in tissue sections and smears. J Clin Pathol 16:383, 1963.
33. Bowling MC, Smith IM, Wescott SL. A rapid staining procedure for *Pneumocystis carinii*. Am J Med Tech 39:267, 1973.
34. Bommer W. *Pneumocystis carinii* from human lungs under electron microscope. Am J Dis Child 104:657, 1962.
35. Huneycutt HC, Anderson WR, Hendry WS. *Pneumocystis carinii* pneumonia: case studies with electron microscopy. Am J Clin Pathol 41:411, 1964.
36. Barton EG Jr, Campbell WG Jr. Further observations on the ultrastructure of *Pneumocystis*. Arch Pathol 83:527, 1967.
37. Huang SN, Marshall KG. *Pneumocystis carinii* infection: a cytologic, histologic and electron microscopic study of the organism. Am Rev Respir Dis 102:623, 1970.
38. Wang NS, Huang SN, Thurlbeck WM. Combined *Pneumocystis carinii* and cytomegalovirus infection. Arch Pathol 90:529, 1970.
39. Vawter GF, Uzman BG, Nowoslawski A. *Pneumocystis carinii*. Ann N Y Acad Sci 174:1048, 1970.
40. Ham EK, Greenberg SD, Reynolds RC, et al. Ultrastructure of *Pneumocystis carinii*. Exp Mol Pathol 14:362, 1971.
41. Luna MA, Bodey GP, Goldman AM, et al. *Pneumocystis carinii* pneumonitis in cancer patients. Texas Rep Biol Med 30:1, 1972.
42. Campbell WG Jr. Ultrastructure of *Pneumocystis* in human lung: life cycle in human pneumocystosis. Arch Pathol 93:312, 1972.
43. Nietschke A. Zur Frage des histologischen Nachweises von Pneumocysten bei der interstitiellen Pneumonie. Monatsschr Kinderheilkd 108:142, 1960.
44. Yoneda K, Walzer PD. Attachment of *Pneumocystis carinii* to type I alveolar cells studied by freeze-fracture electron microscopy. Infect Immun 40:812, 1983.
45. Vanek J, Jirovec O, Lukes J. Interstitial plasma cell pneumonia in infants. Ann Paediatr 180:1, 1953.
46. Kucera K. On the morphology and developmental cycle of *Pneumocystis carinii* of human and rat origin. Progress in Protozoology, Proceedings of the First International Conference on Protozoology, Prague, August 22-31, 1961, p 482.
47. Kucera K, Valousek T. The direct proof of *Pneumocystis carinii* in alive nurslings and a new evolutive stage of *Pneumocystis*. Folia Parasitol 13:113, 1966.
48. Vossen M, Beckers P, Meuwissen J, et al. Developmental biology of *Pneumocystis carinii*, an alternative view on the life cycle of the parasite. Z Paracitesmnkd 55:101, 1978.
49. Goetz O. Die Ätiologie der interstitiellen sogenannten plasmazellularen Pneumonie des jungen Säuglings. Arch Kinderheilkd 163:1, 1960.
50. Jirovec O. Das Problem der Pneumocystis Pneumonien vom parasitologischen Standpunkte. Monatsschr Kinderheilkd 108:136, 1960.
51. Giese W. Die Ätiologie der interstitielle plasmazellulären Säuglingspneumonie. Monatsschr Kinderheilkd 101:147, 1953.
52. Von Lichtenberg F. Enigmatic organisms of man and animal models: summation. Ann N Y Acad Sci 174:1052, 1970.
53. Wakefield AE, Banerji S, Pixley FJ, Hopkin JM. Molecular probes for the detection of *Pneumocystis carinii*. Trans R Soc Trop Med Hyg 84(Suppl 1):17, 1990.
54. Vivell O. Die Serologie der interstitiellen Pneumonie. Monatsschr Kinderheilkd 108:146, 1960.
55. Goetz O. Serologische Befunde interstitieller Pneumonien aus den vereinigten Staaten. Arch Kinderheilkd 170:60, 1964.
56. Li J, Edlind T. Phylogeny of *Pneumocystis carinii* based on β-tubulin sequence. J Eukaryotic Microbiol 41:97S, 1994.
57. Mazars E, Odberg-Ferragut C, Dei-Cas E, et al. Polymorphism of the thymidylate synthase gene of *Pneumocystis carinii* from different host species. J Eukaryot Microbiol 42:26, 1995.
58. Ma L, Kovacs JA. Expression and characterization of recombinant human-derived *Pneumocystis carinii* dihydrofolate reductase. Antimicrob Agents Chemother 44:3092, 2000.
59. Banerji S, Lugli EB, Miller RF, Wakefield AE. Analysis of genetic diversity at the arom locus in isolates of *Pneumocystis carinii*. J Eukaryot Microbiol 42:675, 1995.
60. Pifer LL, Hughes WT, Murphy MJ. Cultivation of *Pneumocystis carinii* in vitro. Pediatr Res 11:305, 1977.
61. Murphy MJ, Pifer LL, Hughes WT. *Pneumocystis carinii* in vitro: a study by scanning electron microscopy. Am J Pathol 86:387, 1977.
62. Latorre CR, Sulzer AJ, Norman L. Serial propagation of *Pneumocystis carinii* in cell line cultures. Appl Environ Microbiol 33:1204, 1977.
63. Pifer LL, Woods D, Hughes WT. Propagation of *Pneumocystis carinii* in Vero cell culture. Infect Immun 20:66, 1978.
64. Bartlett MS, Verbanac PA, Smith JW. Cultivation of *Pneumocystis carinii* with WI-38 cells. J Clin Microbiol 10:796, 1979.
65. Masur H, Jones TC. The interaction in vitro of *Pneumocystis carinii* with macrophages and L-cells. J Exp Med 147:157, 1978.
66. Reye RDK, Ten Seldam REJ. *Pneumocystis* pneumonia. J Pathol Bacteriol 72:451, 1956.
67. da Silva GR, Gomes MC, Santos RF. *Pneumocystis* pneumonia in the adult: report of a case associated with corticosteroid therapy for rheumatoid arthritis. Rev Inst Med Trop Sao Paulo 7:31, 1965.
68. Gagne F, Hould F. Interstitial plasmacellular (parasitic) pneumonia in infants. Can Med Assoc J 74:620, 1956.
69. Pizzi T, Diaz M. Neumonia intersticial plasmocelular: II. Investigacion parasitologia del *Pneumocystis carinii*. Rev Chil Pediatr 27:294, 1956.
70. Thijs A, Janssens PG. Pneumocystosis in Congolese infant. Trop Geogr Med 15:158, 1963.
71. Jarnum S, Rasmussen EF, Ohlsen AS, et al. Generalized *Pneumocystis carinii* infection with severe idiopathic hypoproteinemia. Ann Intern Med 68:138, 1968.
72. Baar HS. Interstitial plasmacellular pneumonia due to *Pneumocystis carinii*. J Clin Pathol 8:19, 1955.
73. Ahvenainen EK. Interstitial plasma cell pneumonia. Pediatr Clin North Am 4:203, 1957.
74. Vlachos J. Necropsy findings in six cases of *Pneumocystis carinii* pneumonia. Arch Dis Child 45:146, 1970.
75. Desai AB, Shak RC, Schgal KN. *Pneumocystis carinii* pneumonia. Indian Pediatr 8:129, 1971.
76. Cahalane SF. *Pneumocystis carinii* pneumonia: report of a case and review of the literature. J Ir Med Assoc 50:133, 1962.
77. Kaftori JK, Bassan H, Gellei B, et al. *Pneumocystis carinii* pneumonia in the adult. Arch Intern Med 109:114, 1962.
78. Fontana G, Tamburello O. Epidemiologia della polmonite interstiziale plasmacellulare nell' I.P.A.I. di Roma. Minerva Nipiol 19:20, 1969.
79. Nakamura RM, Kimura K, Ichimaru M, et al. Coexistent cytomegalic inclusion disease and *Pneumocystis carinii* infection in adults. Acta Pathol Jpn 14:45, 1964.

80. Lim SK, Moon CS. Studies on *Pneumocystis carinii* pneumonia: epidemiological and clinical studies of 80 cases. Jonghap Med 6:69, 1960.
81. Ryan B. *Pneumocystis carinii* infection in Melanesian children. J Pediatr 60:914, 1962.
82. Becroft DMO, Costello JM. *Pneumocystis carinii* pneumonia in siblings: diagnosis by lung aspiration. N Z Med J 64:273, 1965.
83. Laerum OD, Flatmark AL, Enge I, et al. *Pneumocystis carinii* pneumonia in Norway. Scand J Respir Dis 53:247, 1972.
84. Byhosko Z. Pneumonia caused by *Pneumocystis carinii*. Pediatr Pol 31:493, 1956.
85. Mikhailov G. Pneumocystic pneumonia. Arch Patol (Moscow) 21:46, 1959.
86. Hutchison JH. Congenital agammaglobulinemia. Lancet 2:844, 1955.
87. Pepler WJ. *Pneumocystis* pneumonia. S Afr Med J 32:1003, 1958.
88. Moragas A, Vidal MT. *Pneumocystis carinii* pneumonia; first autopsy series in Spain. Helvet Paediatr Acta 26:71, 1971.
89. Nathorst-Windahl G, Hesselman BH, Sjöstrom B, et al. Massive fatal *Pneumocystis* pneumonia in leukemia: report of two cases. Acta Pathol Microbiol Scand 62:472, 1964.
90. Salfelder K, Schwarz J, Sethi KK, et al. Neumocistosis. Merida, Venezuela, Universidad de los Andes, Facultad de Medicina, 1966.
91. Abioye AA. Interstitial plasma cell pneumonia (*Pneumocystis carinii*) in Ibadan. W Afr Med J 16:130, 1967.
92. Farrow BRH, Watson ADJ, Hartley WJ, et al. *Pneumocystis* pneumonia in the dog. J Comp Pathol 82:447, 1972.
93. Shively JN, Dellers RW, Buergelt CD, et al. *Pneumocystis carinii* pneumonia in two foals. J Am Vet Med Assoc 162:648, 1973.
94. Van den Akker S, Goldbloed E. Pneumonia caused by *Pneumocystis carinii* in a dog. Trop Geogr Med 12:54, 1960.
95. Nikolskii CN, Shchetknin AN. *Pneumocystis* in swine. Veterinaria 44:65, 1967.
96. Chandler FW, McClure HM, Campbell WG, et al. Pulmonary pneumocystosis in nonhuman primates. Arch Pathol Lab Med 100:163, 1976.
97. Richter CV, Humason GL, Godbold JH Jr. Endemic *Pneumocystis carinii* in a marmoset colony. J Comp Pathol 88:171, 1978.
98. Meuwissen J, Tauber I, Leuwenberg A, et al. Parasitological and serologic observations of infection with *Pneumocystis* in humans. J Infect Dis 136:43, 1977.
99. Pifer LL, Hughes WT, Stagno S, et al. *Pneumocystis carinii* infection: evidence for high prevalence in normal and immunosuppressed children. Pediatrics 61:35, 1978.
100. Gerrard MP, Eden OB, Jameson B, et al. Serological study of *Pneumocystis carinii* infection in the absence of immunosuppression. Arch Dis Child 62:177, 1987.
101. Pifer L, Pifer D, Freeman-Shade L, et al. Subclinical *Pneumocystis carinii* infection: implications for the immunocompromised patient. Program and Abstracts of the 20th Interscience Conference on Antimicrobial Agents and Chemotherapy, New Orleans, September 22-24, 1980 (Abstract 340).
102. Robinson JJ. Two cases of pneumocystosis: observation in 203 adult autopsies. Arch Pathol 71:156, 1961.
103. Weisse K, Wedler E. Über das Vorkommen der sogenannten "*Pneumocystis carinii*." Klin Wochenschr 32:270, 1954.
104. Hamlin WB. *Pneumocystis carinii*. JAMA 204:173, 1968.
105. Esterly JA. *Pneumocystis carinii* in lungs of adults at autopsy. Am Rev Respir Dis 97:935, 1968.
106. Vogel CL, Cohen MH, Powell RD Jr, et al. *Pneumocystis carinii* pneumonia. Ann Intern Med 68:97, 1968.
107. Sedaghatian MR, Singer DB. *Pneumocystis carinii* in children with malignant disease. Cancer 29:772, 1972.
108. Perera DR, Western KS, Johnson HD, et al. *Pneumocystis carinii* pneumonia in a hospital for children: epidemiologic aspects. JAMA 214:1074, 1970.
109. Le Clair RA. Descriptive epidemiology of interstitial pneumocystic pneumonia. Am Rev Respir Dis 99:542, 1969.
110. Walzer PD, Schultz MG, Western KA, et al. *Pneumocystis carinii* pneumonia and primary immune deficiency diseases of infancy and childhood. J Pediatr 82:416, 1973.
111. Walzer PD, Perl DP, Krogstad DJ, et al. *Pneumocystis carinii* pneumonia in the United States: epidemiologic, diagnostic and clinical features. Ann Intern Med 80:83, 1974.
112. Hyun BH, Varga CF, Thalheimer LJ. *Pneumocystis carinii* pneumonitis occurring in an adopted Korean infant. JAMA 195:784, 1966.
113. Danilevicius Z. A call to recognize *Pneumocystis carinii* pneumonia. Editorial. JAMA 231:1168, 1975.
114. Eidelman A, Nkongo A, Morecki R. *Pneumocystis carinii* pneumonitis in Vietnamese infant in U.S. Pediatr Res 8:424, 1974 (abstract).
115. Redman JC. *Pneumocystis carinii* pneumonia in an adopted Vietnamese infant: a case of diffuse fulminant disease, with recovery. JAMA 230:1561, 1974.
116. Gleason WA Jr, Roden VJ, DeCastro F. *Pneumocystis* pneumonia in Vietnamese infants. J Pediatr 87:1001, 1975.
117. Eidelman AI, Giebink GS, Stracener CE, et al. *Pneumocystis carinii* pneumonia in Vietnamese orphans. MMWR Morb Mortal Wkly Rep 25:15, 1976.
118. Giebink GS, Sholler L, Keenan TP, et al. *Pneumocystis carinii* pneumonia in two Vietnamese refugee infants. Pediatrics 58:115, 1976.
119. Update: acquired immunodeficiency syndrome—United States. MMWR Morb Mortal Wkly Rep 35:757, 1986.
120. Simonds RJ, Oxtoby MJ, Caldwell MB, et al. *Pneumocystis carinii* pneumonia among U.S. children with perinatally acquired HIV infection. JAMA 270:470, 1993.
121. Lyons HA, Vinijchaikul K, Hennigar GR. *Pneumocystis carinii* pneumonia unassociated with other disease. Arch Intern Med 108:929, 1961.
122. Watanabe JM, Chinchinian H, Weitz C, et al. *Pneumocystis carinii* pneumonia in a family. JAMA 193:685, 1965.
123. Weinberg AG, McCracken GH Jr, Lo-Spalluto J, et al. Monoclonal macroglobulinemia and cytomegalic inclusion disease. Pediatrics 51:518, 1973.
124. Rao M, Steiner P, Victoria MS, et al. *Pneumocystis carinii* pneumonia: occurrence in a healthy American infant. JAMA 238:2301, 1977.
125. Stagno S, Pifer LL, Hughes WT, et al. *Pneumocystis carinii* pneumonitis in young immunocompetent infants. Pediatrics 66:56, 1980.
126. Shann F, Walters S, Pifer LL, et al. Pneumonia associated with infection with pneumocystis, respiratory syncytial virus, *Chlamydia*, *Mycoplasma*, and cytomegalovirus in children in Papua New Guinea. BMJ 292:314, 1986.
127. Robbins JB. *Pneumocystis carinii* pneumonitis, a review. Pediatr Res 1:131, 1967.
128. Von Harnack GA. Organisatorische Probleme bei der Bekämpfung der interstitiellen Pneumonie. Monatasschr Kinderheilkd 108:159, 1960.
129. Erchul JW, Williams LP, Meighan PP. *Pneumocystis carinii* in hypopharyngeal material. N Engl J Med 267:926, 1962.
130. Toth G, Balogh E, Belay M. Demonstration in tracheal secretion of the causative agent of interstitial plasma cell pneumonia. Acta Paediatr Acad Sci Hung 7:25, 1966.
131. Fortuny IE, Tempero KF, Amsden TW. *Pneumocystis carinii* pneumonia diagnosed from sputum and successfully treated with pentamidine isethionate. Cancer 26:911, 1970.
132. Smith JA, Wiggins CM. Identification of *Pneumocystis carinii* in sputum. Letter to the editor. N Engl J Med 289:1254, 1973.
133. Lau WK, Young LS, Remington JS. *Pneumocystis carinii* pneumonia: diagnosis by examination of pulmonary secretions. JAMA 236:2399, 1976.
134. Ruskin J, Remington JS. The compromised host and infection: I. *Pneumocystis carinii* pneumonia. JAMA 202:1070, 1967.
135. Brazinsky JH, Phillips JE. *Pneumocystis* pneumonia transmission between patients with lymphoma. Letter to the editor. JAMA 209:1527, 1969.
136. Jacobs JL, Libby DM, Winters RA, et al. A cluster of *Pneumocystis carinii* pneumonia in adults without predisposing illnesses. N Eng J Med 324:246, 1991.
137. Robbins JD, Fodor T. *Pneumocystis carinii* pneumonia. MMWR Morb Mortal Wkly Rep 17:51, 1968.
138. Gentry LO, Remington JS. *Pneumocystis carinii* pneumonia in siblings. J Pediatr 76:769, 1970.
139. Bazaz GR, Manfredi OL, Howard RG, et al. *Pneumocystis carinii* pneumonia in three full-term siblings. J Pediatr 76:767, 1970.
140. Jose DG, Gatti RA, Good RA. Eosinophilia with *Pneumocystis carinii* pneumonia and immune deficiency syndromes. J Pediatr 79:748, 1971.
141. Yates JW, Ellison RR, Plager J. *Pneumocystis carinii* in a husband and wife. Letter to the editor. Lancet 2:610, 1975.
142. Meuwissen HJ, Brzosko WJ, Nowoslawski A, et al. Diagnosis of *Pneumocystis carinii* pneumonia in the presence of immunological deficiency. Letter to the editor. Lancet 1:1124, 1970.
143. Pavlica F. Erste Beobachtung von angeborener pneumozysten Pneumonie bei einem reifen, ausgetragenen Totgeborenen. Zentralbl Allg Pathol 103:236, 1962.

144. Post C, Dutz W, Nasarian I. Endemic *Pneumocystis carinii* pneumonia in South Iran. Arch Dis Child 39:35, 1964.
145. Brock P, Ninane J, Cornu G, et al. AIDS in two African infants born in Belgium. Acta Paediatr Scand 76:175, 1987.
146. Beach RS, Garcia ER, Sosa R, Good RA. *Pneumocystis carinii* pneumonia in a human immunodeficiency virus 1–infected neonate with meconium aspiration. Pediatr Infect Dis J 10:953, 1991.
147. Burke BA, Good RA. *Pneumocystis carinii* infection. Medicine 52:23, 1973.
148. Singer C, Armstrong D, Rosen PP, et al. *Pneumocystis carinii* pneumonia: a cluster of eleven cases. Ann Intern Med 82:772, 1975.
149. Ruebush TK, Weinstein RA, Baehner RL, et al. An outbreak of *Pneumocystis* pneumonia in children with acute lymphocytic leukemia. Am J Dis Child 132:143, 1978.
150. Chusid MJ, Heyrman KA. An outbreak of *Pneumocystis carinii* pneumonia at a pediatric hospital. Pediatrics 62:1031, 1978.
151. Hughes WT, Feldman S, Aur RJA, et al. Intensity of immunosuppressive therapy and the incidence of *Pneumocystis carinii* pneumonitis. Cancer 36:2004, 1975.
152. Kucera K. Some new views on the epidemiology of infections caused by *Pneumocystis carinii. In* Corradetti A (ed). Proceedings of the First International Congress of Parasitology, Rome, Italy, September 26-28, 1964. Oxford, Pergamon Press, 1964, p 452.
153. Hughes WT, Price RA, Kim HK, et al. *Pneumocystis carinii* pneumonitis in children with malignancies. J Pediatr 82:404, 1973.
154. Walzer PD, Schnelle V, Armstrong D, et al. Nude mouse: a new experimental model for *Pneumocystis carinii* infection. Science 197:177, 1977.
155. Sheldon WH. Experimental pulmonary *Pneumocystis carinii* infection in rabbits. J Exp Med 110:147, 1959.
156. Hendley JO, Weller TH. Activation and transmission in rats of infection with *Pneumocystis.* Proc Soc Exp Biol Med 137:1401, 1971.
157. Ueda K, Goto Y, Yamazaki S, et al. Chronic fatal pneumocystosis in nude mice. Jpn J Exp Med 47:475, 1977.
158. Walzer PD, Rutledge ME. Humoral immune responses in experimental *Pneumocystis carinii* pneumonia. Clin Res 28:381, 1980.
159. Price RA, Hughes WT. Histopathology of *Pneumocystis carinii* infestation and infection in malignant disease in childhood. Hum Pathol 5:737, 1974.
160. Rosen P, Armstrong D, Ramos C. *Pneumocystis carinii* pneumonia: a clinicopathologic study of 20 patients with neoplastic diseases. Am J Med 53:428, 1972.
161. Weber WR, Askin FB, Dehner LP. Lung biopsy in *Pneumocystis carinii* pneumonia: a histopathologic study of typical and atypical features. Am J Clin Pathol 67:11, 1977.
162. Hamperl H. Zur Frage des Organismnnachweises bei der interstitiellen plasmacellularen Pneumonie Klin Wochenschr 30:820, 1952.
163. Rifkind D, Faris TD, Hill RB. *Pneumocystis carinii* pneumonia: studies on the diagnosis and treatment. Ann Intern Med 65:943, 1966.
164. Askin FB, Katzenstein AA. *Pneumocystis* infection masquerading as diffuse alveolar damage: a potential source of diagnostic error. Chest 79:420, 1981.
165. Kramer RI, Cirone VC, Moore H. Interstitial pneumonia due to *Pneumocystis carinii* and cytomegalic inclusion disease and hypogammaglobulinemia occurring simultaneously in an infant. Pediatrics 29:816, 1962.
166. Hennigar GR, Vinijchaikul K, Roque AL, et al. *Pneumocystis carinii* pneumonia in an adult. Am J Clin Pathol 35:353, 1961.
167. Nicastri AD, Hutter RVP, Collins HS. *Pneumocystis carinii* pneumonia in an adult: emphasis on antemortem morphologic diagnosis. N Y State J Med 65:2149, 1965.
168. Robbins JB, Miller RH, Arean VM, et al. Successful treatment of *Pneumocystis carinii* pneumonitis in a patient with congenital hypogammaglobulinemia. N Engl J Med 272:708, 1965.
169. Nowak J. Late pulmonary changes in the course of infection with *Pneumocystis carinii.* Acta Med Pol 7:23, 1966.
170. Whitcomb ME, Schwarz MI, Charles MA, et al. Interstitial fibrosis after *Pneumocystis carinii* pneumonia. Ann Intern Med 73:761, 1970.
171. Hughes WT, Johnson WW. Recurrent *Pneumocystis carinii* pneumonia following apparent recovery. J Pediatr 79:755, 1971.
172. Kirby HB, Kenamore B, Guckian JC. *Pneumocystis carinii* pneumonia treated with pyrimethamine and sulfadiazine. Ann Intern Med 75:505, 1971.
173. Schmid KO. Studien zur *Pneumocystis*-erkrankung des Menschen: I. Mitteilung, das wechselnde Erscheinungsbild der *Pneumocystis* Pneumonie beim Säugling: konkordante und discordante Form, *Pneumocystosis* granulomatose. Frankfurt Z Pathol 74:121, 1964.
174. Cruickshank B. Pulmonary granulomatous pneumocystosis following renal transplantation: report of a case. Am J Clin Pathol 63:384, 1975.
175. Dutz W, Jennings-Khodadad E, Post C, et al. Marasmus and *Pneumocystis carinii* pneumonia in institutionalized infants: observations during an endemic. Z Kinderheilkd 117:241, 1974.
176. Weller R. Zur Erzeugung der Pneumocystosen im Tierver-such. Z Kinderheilkd 76:366, 1955.
177. Weller R. Weitere Untersuchungen über experimentele Rattenpneumocystose in Hinblick auf die interstitielle Pneumonie der Frühgeborenen. Z Kinderheilkd 78:166, 1956.
178. Frenkel JK, Good JT, Shultz JA. Latent *Pneumocystis* infection of rats, relapse and chemotherapy. Lab Invest 15:1559, 1966.
179. Hughes WT, Price RA, Sisko F, et al. Protein-calorie malnutrition: a host determinant for *Pneumocystis carinii* infection. Am J Dis Child 128:44, 1974.
180. Baar, cited in Hutchison JH. Congenital agammaglobulinemia. Letter to the editor. Lancet 2:1196, 1955.
181. Burke BA, Krovetz LJ, Good RA. Occurrence of *Pneumocystis carinii* pneumonia in children with agammaglobulinemia. Pediatrics 28:196, 1961.
182. DiGeorge AM. Congenital absence of the thymus and its immunologic consequences: occurrence with congenital hypoparathyroidism. *In* Good RA, Bergsma D (eds). Immunologic Deficiency Diseases in Man. Birth Defects, Original Article Series. New York, National Foundation Press, 1968.
183. Rifkind D, Starzl TE, Marchioro TL, et al. Transplantation pneumonia. JAMA 189:808, 1964.
184. Fulginiti VA, Scribner R, Groth CG, et al. Infections in recipients of liver homografts. N Engl J Med 279:619, 1968.
185. Le Clair RA. Transplantation pneumonia, associated with *Pneumocystis carinii*, among recipients of cardiac transplants. Am Rev Respir Dis 100:874, 1969.
186. Quittell LM, Fisher M, Foley CM. *Pneumocystis carinii* pneumonia in infants given adrenocorticotropic hormone for infantile spasms. J Pediatr 110:901, 1987.
187. Herrod HG, Valenski WR, Woods DR, et al. The in vitro response of human lymphocytes to *Pneumocystis carinii.* Clin Res 27:811, 1979.
188. Ruskin J, Remington JS. *Pneumocystis carinii* infection in the immunosuppressed host. Antimicrob Agents Chemother 7:70, 1967.
189. Ivady G, Paldy L, Koltay M, et al. *Pneumocystis carinii* pneumonia. Letter to the editor. Lancet 1:616, 1967.
190. Kohout E, Post C, Azadeh B, et al. Immunoglobulin levels in infantile pneumocystosis. J Clin Pathol 25:135, 1972.
191. Brzosko WJ, Nowoslawski A. Identification of *Pneumocystis carinii* antigens in tissues. Bull Acad Pol Sci 13:49, 1965.
192. Brzosko WJ, Nowoslawski A, Madalinski K. Identification of immune complexes in lungs from *Pneumocystis carinii* pneumonia cases in infants. Bull Acad Pol Sci 12:137, 1964.
193. Brzosko WJ, Madalinski K, Krawczynski K, et al. Immunohistochemistry in studies on the pathogenesis of *Pneumocystis* pneumonia in infants. Ann N Y Acad Sci 177:156, 1971.
194. Creamer B, Dutz W, Post C. The small intestinal lesion of chronic diarrhea and marasmus in Iran. Lancet 1:18, 1970.
195. Dutz W, Sadri S, Kohout E, et al. Bowel mucosal patterns and immunoglobulins in 100 infants from birth to one year of age. Pahlavi Med J 1:234, 1970.
196. Brzosko WJ, Nowoslawski A. Immunohistochemical studies on *Pneumocystis* pneumonia. Bull Acad Pol Sci 11:563, 1963.
197. Sheldon WH. Subclinical *Pneumocystis* pneumonitis. Am J Dis Child 97:287, 1959.
198. Charles MA, Schwarz MI. *Pneumocystis carinii* pneumonia. Postgrad Med 53:86, 1973.
199. Weiss RB, Muggia FM. Cytotoxic drug–induced pulmonary disease: update 1980. Am J Med 68:259, 1980.
200. Richards MJS, Wara WM. Radiation pneumonitis complicated by *Pneumocystis carinii.* Int J Radiat Oncol Biol Phys 4:287, 1978.
201. Wells RJ, Weetman RM, Ballantine TVN, et al. Pulmonary leukemia in children presenting as diffuse interstitial pneumonia. J Pediatr 96:262, 1980.
202. Solberg CO, Meuwissen HJ, Needham RN, et al. Infectious complications in bone marrow transplant patients. BMJ 1:18, 1971.
203. White WF, Saxton HM, Dawson IMP. Pneumocystis pneumonia: report of three cases in adults and one in a child with a discussion of the radiological appearances and predisposing factors. BMJ 2:1327, 1961.

204. Hughes WT. Infections during continuous complete remission of acute lymphocytic leukemia: during and after anticancer therapy. Int J Radiat Oncol Biol Phys 1:305, 1976.
205. Iacuone JJ, Wong KY, Bove KE, et al. Acute respiratory illness in children with acute lymphoblastic leukemia. J Pediatr 90:915, 1977.
206. Siegel SE, Nesbit ME, Baehner R, et al. Pneumonia during therapy for childhood acute lymphoblastic leukemia. Am J Dis Child 134:28, 1980.
207. Hauger SB. Approach to the pediatric patient with HIV infection and pulmonary symptoms. J Pediatr 119:S25, 1991.
208. Vessal K, Post C, Dutz W, et al. Roentgenologic changes in infantile *Pneumocystis carinii* pneumonia. AJR Am J Roentgenol 120:254, 1974.
209. Vessal K, Dutz W, Kohout E, et al. Verlaufskontrolle der Pneumocystose im Röntgenbild. Radiologe 16:38, 1976.
210. Falkenbach KH, Bachmann KD, O'Laughlin BJ. *Pneumocystis carinii* pneumonia. AJR Am J Roentgenol 85:706, 1961.
211. Thomas SF, Dutz W, Khodadad EJ. *Pneumocystis carinii* pneumonia (plasma cell pneumonia): roentgenographic, pathologic and clinical correlations. AJR Am J Roentgenol 98:318, 1966.
212. Robillard G, Bertrand R, Gregoire H, et al. Plasma cell pneumonia in infants: review of 51 cases. J Can Assoc Radiol 16:161, 1965.
213. Kerpel-Fronius E, Varga F, Bata G. Blood gas and metabolic studies in plasma cell pneumonia and in newborn prematures with respiratory distress. Arch Dis Child 39:473, 1964.
214. Smith E, Gaspar IA. Pentamidine treatment of *Pneumocystis carinii* pneumonitis in an adult with lymphatic leukemia. Am J Med 44:626, 1968.
215. Doak PB, Becroft DMO, Harris EA, et al. *Pneumocystis carinii* pneumonia—transplant lung. Q J Med 165:59, 1973.
216. Hughes WT, Sanyal SK, Price RA. Signs, symptoms, and pathophysiology of *Pneumocystis carinii* pneumonitis. Natl Cancer Inst Monogr 43:77, 1976.
217. Friedman BA, Wenglin BD, Hyland RN, et al. Roentgenographically atypical *Pneumocystis carinii* pneumonia. Am Rev Respir Dis 111:89, 1975.
218. Gentry LO, Ruskin J, Remington JS. *Pneumocystis carinii* pneumonia: problems in diagnosis and therapy in 24 cases. Calif Med 116:6, 1972.
219. Pliess G, Seifert K. Elektronenoptische Untersuchung bei experimenteller Pneumocystose. Beitr Pathol Anat 120:399, 1959.
220. Rubenstein A, Morecki R, Silverman B, et al. Pulmonary disease in children with acquired immunodeficiency syndrome and AIDS-related complex. J Pediatr 108:498, 1986.
221. Joshi VV, Oleske JM, Saad S, et al. Pathology of opportunistic infections in children with acquired immunodeficiency syndrome. Pediatr Pathol 6:145, 1986.
222. Yoshida Y, Ikai T, Ogino K, et al. Studies of *Pneumocystis carinii* and *Pneumocystis carinii* pneumonia: V. Diagnosis by cyst concentration from sputum. Jpn J Parasitol 27:473, 1978.
223. Ognibene FP, Gill VJ, Pizzo PA, et al. Induced sputum to diagnose *Pneumocystis carinii* pneumonia in immunosuppressed pediatric patients. J Pediatr 115:430, 1989.
224. Johnson HD, Johnson WW. *Pneumocystis carinii* pneumonia in children with cancer: diagnosis and treatment. JAMA 214:1067, 1970.
225. Chaudhary S, Hughes WT, Feldman S, et al. Percutaneous transthoracic needle aspiration of the lung: diagnosing *Pneumocystis carinii* pneumonitis. Am J Dis Child 131:902, 1977.
226. Clink HM, Howard PF, Jameson B, et al. *Pneumocystis carinii* pneumonitis. Letter to the editor. Lancet 2:1265, 1975.
227. Rosen PP, Martini N, Armstrong D. *Pneumocystis carinii* pneumonia: diagnosis by lung biopsy. Am J Med 58:794, 1975.
228. Tyras DH, Campbell W, Corley C, et al. The role of early open lung biopsy in the diagnosis and treatment of *Pneumocystis carinii* pneumonia. Ann Thorac Surg 18:571, 1974.
229. Michaelis LL, Leight GS Jr, Powell RD, et al. *Pneumocystis* pneumonia: the importance of early open lung biopsy. Ann Surg 183:301, 1976.
230. Bradshaw M, Myerowitz RL, Schneerson R, et al. *Pneumocystis carinii* pneumonitis. Ann Intern Med 73:775, 1970.
231. Roback SA, Weintraub WH, Nesbit M, et al. Diagnostic open lung biopsy in the critically ill child. Pediatrics 52:605, 1973.
232. Wolff LJ, Bartlett MS, Baehner RL, et al. The causes of interstitial pneumonitis in immunocompromised children: an aggressive systematic approach to diagnosis. Pediatrics 60:41, 1977.
233. Ballantine TVN, Grosfeld JL, Knapek RM, et al. Interstitial pneumonitis in the immunologically suppressed child: an urgent surgical condition. J Pediatr Surg 12:501, 1977.
234. Mason WH, Siegel SE, Tucker BL. Diagnostic open lung biopsy in immunosuppressed pediatric patients. Clin Res 27:114, 1979.
235. Leight GS Jr, Michaelis LL. Open lung biopsy for the diagnosis of acute, diffuse pulmonary infiltrates in the immunosuppressed patient. Chest 73:477, 1978.
236. Rossiter SJ, Miller DC, Churg AM, et al. Open lung biopsy in the immunosuppressed patient: is it really beneficial? J Thorac Cardiovasc Surg 77:338, 1979.
237. Rodgers BM, Moazam F, Talbert JL. Thoracoscopy: early diagnosis of interstitial pneumonitis in the immunologically suppressed child. Chest 75:126, 1979.
238. Kim HK, Hughes WT. Comparison of methods for identification of *Pneumocystis carinii* in pulmonary aspirates. Am J Clin Pathol 60:462, 1973.
239. Rosen PP. Frozen section management of a lung biopsy for suspected *Pneumocystis carinii* pneumonia. Am J Surg Pathol 1:79, 1977.
240. Young RC, Bennett JE, Chu EW. Organisms mimicking *Pneumocystis carinii*. Letter to the editor. Lancet 2:1082, 1976.
241. Reinhardt DJ, Kaplan W, Chandler FW. Morphologic resemblance of zygomycete spores to *Pneumocystis carinii* cysts in tissue. Am Rev Respir Dis 115:170, 1977.
242. Demicco WA, Stein A, Urbanetti, JS, et al. False-negative biopsy in *Pneumocystis carinii* pneumonia. Chest 75:389, 1979.
243. Smith JW, Hughes WT. A rapid staining technique for *Pneumocystis carinii*. J Clin Pathol 25:269, 1972.
244. Churukian CJ, Schenk EA. Rapid Grocott's methenamine-silver nitrate method for fungi and *Pneumocystis carinii*. Am J Clin Pathol 68:427, 1977.
245. Mahan CT, Sale GE. Rapid methenamine-silver stain for *Pneumocystis* and fungi. Arch Pathol Lab Med 102:351, 1978.
246. Pintozzi RL. Modified Grocott's methenamine-silver nitrate method for quick staining of *Pneumocystis carinii*. J Clin Pathol 31:803, 1978.
247. Pifer LL, Woods DR. Efficacy of toluidine blue "O" stain for *Pneumocystis carinii*. Am J Clin Pathol 69:472, 1978.
248. Settnes OP, Larsen PE. Inhibition of toluidine blue O stain for *Pneumocystis carinii* by additives in the diethyl ether. Am J Clin Pathol 72:493, 1979.
249. Pintozzi RL, Blecka LJ, Nanos S. The morphologic identification of *Pneumocystis carinii*. Acta Cytol 23:35, 1979.
250. Cameron RB, Watts JC, Kasten BL. *Pneumocystis carinii* pneumonia: an approach to rapid laboratory diagnosis. Am J Clin Pathol 72:90, 1979.
251. Milder JE, Walzer PD, Coonrod JD, et al. Comparison of histological and immunological techniques for detection of *Pneumocystis carinii* in rat bronchial lavage fluid. J Clin Microbiol 11:409, 1980.
252. Nowoslawski A, Brzosko WJ. Indirect immunofluorescent test for serodiagnosis of *Pneumocystis carinii* infection. Bull Acad Pol Sci 12:143, 1964.
253. Brzosko W, Madalinski K, Nowoslawski A. Fluorescent antibody and immuno-electrophoretic evaluation of the immune reaction in children with pneumonia induced by *Pneumocystis carinii*. Exp Med Microbiol 19:397, 1967.
254. Norman L, Kagan IG. A preliminary report of an indirect fluorescent antibody test for detecting antibodies to cysts of *Pneumocystis carinii* in human sera. Am J Clin Pathol 58:170, 1972.
255. Lau WK, Young LS. Immunofluorescent antibodies against *Pneumocystis carinii* in patients with and without pulmonary infiltrates. Clin Res 25:379, 1977.
256. Shepherd V, Jameson B, Knowles GK. *Pneumocystis carinii* pneumonitis: a serological study. J Clin Pathol 32:773, 1979.
257. Meuwissen JHET, Leeuwenberg ADEM, Heeren J, et al. New method for study of infections with *Pneumocystis carinii*. Letter to the editor. J Infect Dis 127:209, 1973.
258. Walzer PD, Rutledge ME, Yoneda K, et al. *Pneumocystis carinii*: new separation method from lung tissue. Exp Parasitol 47:356, 1979.
259. Minielly JA, McDuffie FC, Holley KE. Immunofluorescent identification of *Pneumocystis carinii*. Arch Pathol 90:561, 1970.
260. Lim SK, Jones RH, Eveland WC. Fluorescent antibody studies on experimental pneumocystosis. Proc Soc Exp Biol Med 136:675, 1971.
261. Lim SK, Eveland WC, Porter RJ. Development and evaluation of a direct fluorescent antibody method for the diagnosis of *Pneumocystis carinii* infections in experimental animals. Appl Microbiol 26:666, 1973.
262. Lim SK, Eveland WC, Porter RJ. Direct fluorescent antibody method for the diagnosis of *Pneumocystis carinii* pneumonitis from sputa or tracheal aspirates from humans. Appl Microbiol 27:144, 1974.
263. Hughes WT, McNabb PC, Makres TD, et al. Efficacy of trimethoprim and sulfamethoxazole in the prevention and treatment of *Pneumocystis carinii* pneumonitis. Antimicrob Agents Chemother 5:289, 1974.

264. Hughes WT, Feldman S, Chaudhary SC, et al. Comparison of pentamidine isethionate and trimethoprim-sulfamethoxazole in the treatment of *Pneumocystis carinii* pneumonia. J Pediatr 92:285, 1978.
265. Lipson A, Marshall WC, Hayward AR. Treatment of *Pneumocystis carinii* pneumonia in children. Arch Dis Child 52:314, 1977.
266. Larter WE, John TJ, Sieber OF, et al. Trimethoprim-sulfamethoxazole treatment of *Pneumocystis carinii* pneumonitis. J Pediatr 92:826, 1978.
267. Seigel SE, Wolff LJ, Baehner RL, et al. Treatment of *Pneumocystis carinii* pneumonitis: a comparative trial of sulfamethoxazole-trimethoprim vs pentamidine in pediatric patients with cancer: report from the Children's Cancer Study Group. Am J Dis Child 138:1051, 1984.
268. Overturf GD. Use of trimethoprim-sulfamethoxazole in pediatric infections: relative merits of intravenous administration. Rev Infect Dis 9(Suppl 2):168, 1987.
269. Ivady G, Paldy L. Ein neues Behandlungsverfahren der interstitiellen plasmazelligen Pneumonie Frühgeborener mit fünfwertigen Stibium und aromatischen Diamidinen. Monatsschr Kinderheilkd 106:10, 1958.
270. Lörinczi K, Mérth J, Perényi K. Pentamidinnel szerzett tapasztalatink az interstitialis plasmasejtes pneumonia kezelésében. Gyermekgyogyaszat 15:207, 1964.
271. Western KA, Perera DR, Schultz MG. Pentamidine isethionate in the treatment of *Pneumocystis carinii* pneumonia. Ann Intern Med 73:695, 1970.
272. Parasitic Disease Drug Service–pentamidine releases for *Pneumocystis* pneumonia. MMWR Morb Mortal Wkly Rep 25:365, 1976.
273. Shultz JC, Ross SW, Abernathy RS. Diagnosis of *Pneumocystis carinii* pneumonia in an adult with survival. Am Rev Respir Dis 93:943, 1966.
274. Ivady G, Paldy L. Treatment of *Pneumocystis carinii* pneumonia in infancy. Natl Cancer Inst Monogr 43:201, 1976.
275. Schoenbach EB, Greenspan EM. The pharmacology, mode of action and therapeutic potentialities of stilbamidine, pentamidine, propamidine and other aromatic diamidines: a review. Medicine 27:327, 1948.
276. Stark FR, Crast F, Clemmer T, et al. Fatal Herxheimer reaction after pentamidine in *Pneumocystis* pneumonia. Letter to the editor. Lancet 1:1193, 1976.
277. Stahl-Bayliss CM, Kalman CM, Laskin OL. Pentamidine-induced hypoglycemia in patients with the acquired immune deficiency syndrome. Clin Pharmacol Ther 39:271, 1986.
278. Pauwels A, Eliasewicz M, Larrey D, et al. Pentamidine-induced acute pancreatitis in a patient with AIDS. J Clin Gastroenterol 12:457, 1990.
279. Wood G, Wetzig N, Hogan P, Whitby M. Survival from pentamidine induced pancreatitis and diabetes mellitus. N Z J Med 21:341, 1991.
280. Miller TL, Winter HS, Luginbuhl LM, et al. Pancreatitis in pediatric human immunodeficiency virus infection. J Pediatr 120:223, 1992.
281. Geelhoed GW, Levin BJ, Adkins PC, et al. The diagnosis and management of *Pneumocystis carinii* pneumonia. Ann Thorac Surg 14:335, 1972.
282. Geelhoed GW, Corso P, Joseph WL. The role of membrane lung support in transient acute respiratory insufficiency of *Pneumocystis carinii* pneumonia. J Thorac Cardiovasc Surg 68:802, 1974.
283. Saulsbury FT, Bernstein MT, Winkelstein JA. *Pneumocystis carinii* pneumonia as the presenting infection in congenital hypogammaglobulinemia. J Pediatr 95:559, 1979.
284. Gagnon S, Boota AM, Fischi MA, et al. Corticosteroids as adjunctive therapy for severe *Pneumocystis carinii* pneumonia in the acquired immunodeficiency syndrome. N Engl J Med 323:1444, 1990.
285. Bozzette SA, Sattler FR, Chiu J, et al. A controlled trial of early adjunctive treatment with corticosteroids for *Pneumocystis carinii* pneumonia in the acquired immunodeficiency syndrome. N Engl J Med 323:1451, 1990.
286. NIH–University of California Expert Panel for Corticosteroids as Adjunctive Therapy for Pneumocystis Pneumonia. Special Report: Consensus statement on the use of corticosteroids as adjunctive therapy for pneumocystis pneumonia in the acquired immunodeficiency syndrome. N Engl J Med 323:1500, 1990.
287. McLaughlin GE, Virdee SS, Schleien CL, et al. Effect of corticosteroids on survival of children with acquired immunodeficiency syndrome and *Pneumocystis carinii*–related respiratory failure. J Pediatr 126:821, 1995.
288. Bye MR, Cairns-Bazarian AM, Ewig JM. Markedly reduced mortality associated with corticosteroid therapy of *Pneumocystis carinii* pneumonia in children with acquired immunodeficiency syndrome. Arch Pediatr Adolesc Med 148:638, 1994.
289. Sanyal SK, Mariencheck WC, Hughes WT, et al. Course of pulmonary dysfunction in children surviving *Pneumocystis carinii* pneumonitis. Am Rev Respir Dis 124:161, 1981.
290. Brasfield DM, Stagno S, Whitley RJ, et al. Infant pneumonitis associated with cytomegalovirus, *Chlamydia*, *Pneumocystis* and *Ureaplasma*: follow-up. Pediatrics 79:76, 1987.
291. Kluge RM, Spaulding DM, Spain AJ. Combination of pentamidine and trimethoprim-sulfamethoxazole in the therapy of *Pneumocystis carinii* pneumonia in rats. Antimicrob Agents Chemother 13:975, 1978.
292. Ruskin J. Parasitic diseases in the immunocompromised host. *In* Rubin RH, Young LS (eds). Clinical Approach to Infection in the Compromised Host. New York, Plenum Publishing, 1981.
293. Patterson JH. *Pneumocystis carinii* pneumonia; pentamidine therapy. Letter to the editor. Pediatrics 38:926, 1966.
294. Russell JGB. *Pneumocystis* pneumonia associated with agammaglobulinemia. Arch Dis Child 34:338, 1959.
295. Richman DD, Zamvil L, Remington JS. Recurrent *Pneumocystis carinii* pneumonia in a child with hypogammaglobulinemia. Am J Dis Child 125:102, 1973.
296. Ross L, Ortega J, Fine R, et al. Recurrent *Pneumocystis carinii* pneumonia. Clin Res 25:183, 1977.
297. Wolff LJ, Baehner RL. Delayed development of *Pneumocystis* pneumonia following administration of short-term high-dose trimethoprim-sulfamethoxazole. Am J Dis Child. 132:525, 1978.
298. Hughes WT. Limited effect of trimethoprim-sulfamethoxazole prophylaxis on *Pneumocystis carinii*. Antimicrob Agents Chemother 16:333, 1979.
299. LeGolvan DP, Heidelberger KP. Disseminated, granulomatous *Pneumocystis carinii* pneumonia. Arch Pathol 95:344, 1973.
300. Post C, Fakoughi T, Dutz W, et al. Prophylaxis of epidemic infantile pneumocystosis with a 20:1 sulfadoxine and pyrimethamine combination. Curr Ther Res 13:273, 1971.
301. Kemeny P, Adler T, Szokolai V, et al. Prevention of interstitial plasma-cell pneumonia in premature infants. Letter to the editor. Lancet 1:1322, 1973.
302. Hughes WT, Kuhn S, Chaudhary S, et al. Successful chemoprophylaxis for *Pneumocystis carinii* pneumonitis. N Engl J Med 297:1419, 1977.
303. Wilber RB, Feldman S, Malone WJ, et al. Chemoprophylaxis for *Pneumocystis carinii* pneumonitis: outcome of unstructured delivery. Am J Dis Child 134:643, 1980.
304. Hughes WT, Rivera GK, Schell MJ, et al. Successful intermittent chemoprophylaxis for *Pneumocystis carinii* pneumonitis. N Engl J Med 316:1627, 1987.
305. Harris RE, McCallister JA, Allen SA, et al. Prevention of *Pneumocystis* pneumonia: use of continuous sulfamethoxazole-trimethoprim therapy. Am J Dis Child 134:35, 1980.
306. U.S. Department of Health and Human Services. Guidelines for prophylaxis against *Pneumocystis carinii* pneumonia for children infected with human immunodeficiency virus. MMWR Morb Mortal Wkly Rep 40(RR-2):ii-13, 1991.
307. Centers for Disease Control and Prevention. 1999 USPHS/IDSA Guidelines for the Prevention of Opportunistic Infections in Persons Infected with Human Immunodeficiency Virus. MMWR Morb Mortal Wkly Rep 48 (RR-10):1, 1999.
308. Simonds RJ, Lindegren ML, Thomas P, et al. Prophylaxis against *Pneumocystis carinii* pneumonia among children with perinatally acquired HIV infection in the United States. N Engl J Med 332:786, 1995.
309. Maldonado YA, Araneta RG, Hersh AL. *Pneumocystis carinii* pneumonia prophylaxis and early clinical manifestations of severe perinatal human immunodeficiency virus type 1 infection. Northern California Pediatric IIIV Consortium. Pediatr Infect Dis J 17:398, 1998.

Aspergillosis

310. Zimmerman LE. Fatal fungus infections complicating other diseases. Am J Clin Pathol 25:46, 1955.
311. Allan GW, Andersen DH. Generalized aspergillosis in an infant 18 days of age. Pediatrics 26:432, 1960.
312. Luke JL, Bolande RP, Grass S. Generalized aspergillosis and *Aspergillus* endocarditis in infancy. Pediatrics 31:115, 1963.
313. Akkoyunlu A, Yücell FA. Aspergillose bronchopulmonaire et encéphalomeningel chez un nouveau-né de 20 jours. Arch Fr Pediatr 14:615, 1957.
314. Matturi L, Fasolis S. L'aspergillosi generalizzata neonetale. Folia Hered Pathol 12:87, 1962.

315. Paradis AJ, Roberts L. Endogenous ocular aspergillosis: report of a case in an infant with cytomegalic inclusion disease. Arch Ophthalmol 69:765, 1963.
316. Brass K. Infecciones hospitalarias asporgilosas bronco-pulmonares en lactantes y ninos menores. Mycopathologia 57:149, 1975.
317. Mangurien HH, Fernandez B. Neonatal aspergillosis accompanying fulminant necrotizing enterocolitis. Arch Dis Child 54:559, 1979.
318. Gonzalez-Crussi F, Mirkin LD, Wyllie RM, et al. Acute disseminated aspergillosis during the neonatal period: report of an instance of a 14-day-old infant. Clin Pediatr 18:137, 1979.
319. Raaf JH, Donahoe PK, Truman JT, et al. *Aspergillus*-induced small bowel obstruction in a leukemic newborn. Surgery 81:111, 1977.
320. Mouy R, Ropent JC, Donadieu J, et al. Granulomatose septique chronique revelée par une aspergillose pulmonaire neonatale. Arch Pediatr 2:861, 1995.
321. Bruyere A, Bourgeois J, Cochat P, et al. Entérocolite ulcéro-nécrotique néonatale et aspergillose. Pediatrie 38:185, 1983.
322. Rhine WD, Arvin AA, Stevenson DK. Neonatal aspergillosis: a case report and review of the literature. Clin Pediatr 25:400, 1986.
323. Granstein RD, First LR, Sober AJ. Primary cutaneous aspergillosis in a premature neonate. Br J Dermatol 103:681, 1980.
324. Shiota R, Agaewal HC, Grover AK, et al. *Aspergillus* endophthalmitis. Br J Ophthalmol 71:611, 1987.
325. Roth JG, Troy JL, Esterly NB. Multiple cutaneous ulcers in a premature neonate. Pediatr Dermatol 8:253, 1991.
326. Schwartz DA, Jacquette M, Chawla HS. Disseminated neonatal aspergillosis: report of a fatal case and analysis of risk factors. Pediatr Infect Dis J 7:349, 1988.
327. Lackner H, Schwinger W, Urban C, et al. Lipsomal amphotericin-B (AmBisome) for treatment of disseminated fungal infections in two infants of very low birth weight. Pediatrics 89:1259, 1992.
328. Rowen JL, Correa AG, Sokol DM, et al. Invasive aspergillosis in neonates: report of five cases and literature review. Pediatr Infect Dis J 11:576, 1992.
329. Perzigian RW, Faix RG. Primary cutaneous aspergillosis in a preterm infant. Am J Perinatol 10:269, 1993.
330. Gupta M, Weinberger B, Whitley-Williams PN. Cutaneous aspergillosis in a neonate. Pediatr Infect Dis J 15:464, 1996.
331. Papouli M, Roilides E, Bebashi E, Andreau A. Primary cutaneous aspergillosis in neonates: case report and review. Clin Infect Dis 22:1102, 1996.
332. Scroll AH, Jaeger G, Allendorf A, et al. Invasive pulmonary aspergillosis in a critically ill neonate: case report and review of invasive aspergillosis during the first 3 months of life. Clin Infect Dis 27:437, 1998.
333. Meessen NE, Oberndorff KM, Jacobs JA. Disseminated aspergillosis in a premature neonate. J Hosp Infect 40:249, 1998.
334. van Landeghem FK, Stiller B, Lehmann TN, et al. Aqueductal stenosis and hydrocephalus in an infant due to aspergillus infection. Clin Neuropathol 19:26, 2000.
335. Amod FC, Coovadia YM, Pillay T, Ducasse G. Primary cutaneous aspergillosis in ventilated neonates. Pediatr Infect Dis J 19:482, 2000.
336. Marcinkowski M, Bauer K, Stoltenburd-Didinger G, et al. Fatal aspergillosis with brain abscesses in a neonate with DiGeorge syndrome. Pediatr Infect Dis 19:1214, 2000.
337. Richardson V, Ortiz D, Newton OA, Nandi E. Disseminated and cutaneous aspergillosis in a premature infant: a fatal nosocomial infection. Pediatr Dermatol 18:366, 2001.
338. Woodruff CA, Hebert AA. Neonatal primary cutaneous aspergillosis: case report and review of the literature. Pediatr Dermatol 19:439, 2002.
339. Herron MD, Vanderhooft SL, Byington C, King JD. Aspergillosis in a 24-week newborn: a case report. J Perinatol 23:256, 2003.
340. Raper KB, Fennell DJ (eds). The Genus *Aspergillus*. Baltimore, Williams & Wilkins, 1965.
341. Denning DW. Invasive aspergillosis. Clin Infect Dis 26:781, 1998.
342. Coulot P, Bouchara JP, Renier G, et al. Specific interaction of *Aspergillus fumigatus* with fibrinogen and its role in cell adhesion. Infect Immun 62:2169, 1994.
343. Tronchin G, Esnault K, Renier G, et al. Expression and identification of a laminin-binding protein in *Aspergillus fumigatus* conidia. Infect Immun 65:9, 1997.
344. Walmsley S, Devi S, King S, et al. Invasive *Aspergillus* infections in a pediatric hospital: a ten-year review. Pediatr Infect Dis J 12:673, 1993.
345. Austwick PKC, Gitter M, Watkins CV. Pulmonary aspergillosis in lambs. Vet Rec 72:19, 1960.
346. Merchant RK, Louria DB, Geisler PH, et al. Fungal endocarditis: a review of the literature and report of three cases. Ann Intern Med 48:242, 1958.
347. Renon L. Recherches cliniques et expérimentales sur la pseudo-tuberculose aspergillaire. These No. 89. Paris, G. Steinheil, 1893.
348. Renon L. L'Étude sur l'Aspergillose chez les Animaux et chez l'Homme. Paris, Masson, 1897.
349. Dieulafoy G, Chantemesse A, Widal GFI. Une pseudotuberculose myosique. Congres Int Berlin Gaz Hop (Paris) 63:821, 1890.
350. Wahl EF, Erickson MJ. Primary pulmonary aspergillosis. J Med Assoc Ga 17:341, 1928.
351. Hinson KPW, Moon AJ, Plummer NS. Bronchopulmonary aspergillosis: a review and a report of eight new cases. Thorax 7:317, 1952.
352. Macartney JM. Pulmonary aspergillosis: a review and description of three new cases. Thorax 19:287, 1964.
353. Hunter D, Perry KMA. Bronchiolitis resulting from the handling of bagasse. Br J Ind Med 3:64, 1946.
354. Stallybrass FC. A study of *Aspergillus* spores in the atmosphere of a modern mill. Br J Ind Med 18:41, 1961.
355. Conant NF, Smith DT, Baker RD, et al. Aspergillosis. *In* Conant NF, Smith DT, Baker RD, et al. Manual of Clinical Mycology, 3rd ed. Philadelphia, WB Saunders, 1971.
356. Castellani A. Fungi and fungous diseases. Arch Dermatol Syphilol 17:61, 1928.
357. Finegold SM, Murray JF. Aspergillosis: a review and report of twelve cases. Am J Med 27:463, 1959.
358. Sartory A, Sartory R. Un cas d'onychomycose dû à l'*Aspergillus fumigatus* Fresenius. Bull Acad Med (Paris) 109:482, 1945.
359. Gregson AEW, La Touche CJ. Otomycosis: a neglected disease. J Laryngol Otol 75:45, 1961.
360. McCarty JM, Fram MS, Pullen G, et al. Outbreak of primary cutaneous aspergillosis related to intravenous arm boards. J Pediatr 108:721, 1986.
361. Dewhurst AG, Cooper MJ, Khan SM, et al. Invasive aspergillosis in immunocompromised patients: potential hazard of hosptial building work. BMJ 301:802, 1990.
362. Collins PW, Kelsey SM, DeLord C, et al. Invasive aspergillosis in immunosuppressed patients. Letter to the editor. BMJ 301:1046, 1990.
363. Walsh TJ, Dixon DM. Nosocomial aspergillosis: environmental microbiology, hospital epidemiology, diagnosis and treatment. Eur J Epidemiol 5:131, 1989.
364. Austwick PKC. Pathogenicity. *In* Raper KB, Fennell DI (eds). The Genus *Aspergillus*. Baltimore, Williams & Wilkins, 1965, p. 82.
365. Theobald I, Fischbach R, Hulskamp G, et al. Pulmonary aspergillosis as initial manifestation of septic granulomatosis (chronic granulomatous disease, CGD) in a premature monozygotic female twin and FDG-PET diagnosis of spread of the disease. Radiologe 42:42, 2002.
366. Groll AH, Jaeger G, Allendorf A, et al. Invasive pulmonary aspergillosis in a critically ill neonate: case report and review of invasive aspergillosis during the first 3 months of life. Clin Infect Dis 27:437, 1998.
367. Herron MD, Vanderhooft SL, Byington C, et al. Aspergillosis in a 24-week newborn: a case report. J Perinatol 23:256, 2003.
368. Amod FC, Coovadia YM, Pillay T, et al. Primary cutaneous aspergillosis in ventilated neonates. Pediatr Infect Dis J 19:482, 2000.
369. van Burik JA, Colven R, Spach DH. Cutaneous aspergillosis. J Clin Microbiol 36:3115, 1998.
370. Cawley EP. Aspergillosis and the aspergilli: report of a unique case of the disease. Arch Intern Med 80:423, 1947.
371. Young RC, Bennett JE, Vogel CL, et al. Aspergillosis: the spectrum of disease in 98 patients. Medicine 49:147, 1970.
372. Huang S, Harris LS. Acute disseminated penicilliosis. Am J Clin Pathol 39:167, 1963.
373. James MJ, Lasker BA, McNeil MM, et al. Use of a repetitive DNA probe to type clinical and environmental isolates of *Aspergillus flavus* from a cluster of cutaneous infections in a neonatal intensive care unit. J Clin Microbiol 38:3612, 2000.
374. Weiner MH. Antigenemia detected by radioimmunoassay in systemic aspergillosis. Ann Intern Med 92:793, 1980.
375. Denning DW, Stevens DA. Antifungal and surgical treatment of invasive aspergillosis: review of 2,121 published cases. Rev Infect Dis 12:1147, 1990.
376. Stevens DA, Kan VL, Judson MA, et al. Practice guidelines for diseases caused by *Aspergillus*. Infectious Diseases Society of America. Clin Infect Dis 30:696, 2000.

377. van Burik JA, Colven R, Spach DH. Itraconazole therapy for primary cutaneous aspergillosis in patients with AIDS. Clin Infect Dis 27:643, 1998.
378. Denning DW, Ribaud P, Milpied N, et al. Efficacy and safety of voriconazole in the treatment of acute invasive aspergillosis. Clin Infect Dis 34:563, 2002.
379. Herbrecht R, Denning DW, Patterson TF, et al. Voriconazole versus amphotericin B for primary therapy of invasive aspergillosis. N Engl J Med 347:408, 2002.

Blastomycosis

380. Watts EA, Gard PD Jr, Tuthill SW. First reported case of intrauterine transmission of blastomycosis. Pediatr Infect Dis 2:308, 1983.
381. Maxson S, Miller SF, Tayka F, Schutze G. Perinatal blastomycosis: a review. Pediatr Infect Dis J 11:760, 1992.
382. Lemos LB, Soofi M, Amir E. Blastomycosis and pregnancy. Ann Diagn Pathol 6:211, 2002.
383. Neiberg AD, Mavromatis F, Dyke et al. *Blastomyces dermatitidis* treated during pregnancy: report of a case. Am J Obstet Gynecol 128:911, 1977.
384. Ismail MD, Lerner SA. Disseminated blastomycosis in a pregnant woman: review of amphotericin B usage during pregnancy. Am Rev Respir Dis 126:350, 1982.
385. Cohen I. Absence of congenital infection and teratogenesis in three children born to mothers with blastomycosis and treated with amphotericin B during pregnancy. Pediatr Infect Dis 6:76, 1987.
386. Daniel L, Salit IE. Blastomycosis during pregnancy. Can Med Assoc J 131:759, 1984.
387. Hager H, Welt SI, Cardasis JP, et al. Disseminated blastomycosis in a pregnant woman successfully treated with amphotericin-B: a case report. J Reprod Med 33:485, 1988.
388. King CT, Rogers PD, Cleasy JD, Chapman SW. Antifungal therapy during pregnancy. Clin Infect Dis 27:1151, 1998.
389. Rippon JW. Medical Mycology: The Pathogenic Fungi and the Pathogenic Actinomycetes, 2nd ed. Philadelphia, WB Saunders, 1982, p 428.
390. Denton JF, McDonough ES, Ajello L, et al. Isolation of *Blastomyces dermatitidis* from soil. Science 133:1126, 1961.
391. Denton JF, DiSalvo AF. Isolation of *Blastomyces dermatitidis* from natural sites at Augusta, Georgia. Am J Trop Med 13:716, 1964.
392. Tenenbaum MJ, Greenspan J, Kerkering TM. Blastomycosis. CRC Crit Rev Microbiol 3:139, 1982.
393. Blastomycosis Cooperative Study of the Veterans Administration. Blastomycosis: I. A review of 198 collected cases in Veterans Administration hospitals. Am RevRespir Dis 89:659, 1964.
394. Furcolow ML, Chick EW, Busey JF, et al. Prevalence and incidence studies of human and canine blastomycosis: I. Cases in the United States, 1885-1968. Am Rev Respir Dis 102:60, 1970.
395. Furcolow ML, Busey JF, Mangis RW, et al. Prevalence and incidence studies of human and canine blastomycosis: II. Yearly incidence studies in three selected states, 1960-1967. Am J Epidemiol 92:121, 1970.
396. Kepron MD, Schoemperlen B, Hershfield ES, et al. North American blastomycosis in Central Canada. Can Med Assoc J 106:243, 1972.
397. Sekhon AS, Bogorus MS, Sems HV. Blastomycosis: report of three cases from Alberta with a review of Canadian cases. Mycopathologia 68:53, 1979.
398. Sekhon AS, Jackson FL, Jacobs HJ. Blastomycosis: report of the first case from Alberta, Canada. Mycopathologica 79:65, 1982.
399. Robertson SA, Kimball PL, Magtibay LZ. Pulmonary blastomycosis diagnosed by cytologic examination of sputum. Can Med Assoc J 126:387, 1982.
400. Kane J, Righter J, Krajden S, et al. Blastomycosis: a new endemic focus in Canada. Can Med Assoc J 129:728, 1983.
401. Chick EW. The epidemiology of blastomycosis. *In* Al-Doory Y (ed). The Epidemiology of Human Mycotic Disease. Springfield, Ill, Charles C Thomas, 1975, p 103.
402. Witorsch P, Utz JP. North American blastomycosis: a study of 40 patients. Medicine 47:169, 1968.
403. Habte-Gabr E, Smith IM. North American blastomycosis in Iowa: review of 34 cases. J Chronic Dis 26:585, 1973.
404. Denton JF, DiSalvo AF. Additional isolations of *Blastomyces dermatitidis* from natural sites. Am J Trop Med Hyg 28:697, 1979.
405. Schwartz J, Baum GL. Blastomycosis. Am J Clin Pathol 11:999, 1951.
406. Gnann JW Jr, Bressler GS, Bodet CA III, et al. Human blastomycosis after a dog bite. Ann Intern Med 98:484, 1983.
407. Craig MW, Davey WN, Green RA. Conjugal blastomycosis. Am Rev Respir Dis 102:86, 1970.
408. Recht LD, Philips JR, Eckman MR. et al. Self-limited blastomycosis: a report of thirteen cases. Am Rev Respir Dis 120:1109, 1979.
409. Recht LD, Davies SF, Eckman MR, et al. Blastomycosis in immunocompromised patients. Am Rev Respir Dis 125:359, 1982.
410. Gall SA. Maternal adjustments in the immune system in normal pregnancy. Clin Obstet Gynecol 26:521, 1983.
411. Sridama V, Pacini F, Yang SL, et al. Decreased levels of helper T cells: a possible cause of immunodeficiency in pregnancy. N Engl J Med 307:352, 1982.
412. Weinberg ED. Pregnancy associated depression of cell-mediated immunity. Rev Infect Dis 6:814, 1984.
413. Cozad GC, Chang CT. Cell mediated immunoprotection in blastomycosis. Infect Immun 28:398, 1980.
414. Cherniss EI, Wisbren BA. North American blastomycosis: a clinical study of 40 cases. Ann Intern Med 44:105, 1956.
415. Abernathy RS. Clinical manifestation of pulmonary blastomycosis. Ann Intern Med 51:707, 1959.
416. Lockwood WR, Allison F, Batson BE, et al. The treatment of North American blastomycosis: ten years' experience. Am Rev Respir Dis 100:314, 1969.
417. Duttera MJ, Osterhout S. North American blastomycosis: a survey of 63 cases. South Med J 62:295, 1969.
418. Kravitz GR, Davies SF, Eckman MR, et al. Chronic blastomycotic meningitis. Am J Med 71:501, 1981.
419. Kaufman L, McLaughlin DW, Clar MJ, et al. Specific immunodiffusion test for blastomycosis. Appl Microbiol 26:244, 1973.
420. Williams JE, Murphy R, Standard PG, et al. Serologic response in blastomycosis: diagnostic value of double immunodiffusion assay. Am Rev Respir Dis 123:209, 1981.

Coccidioidomycosis

421. Hughes WT. The deep mycoses. *In* Kelley VC (ed). Brennemann's Practice of Pediatrics. Hagerstown, Md, Harper & Row, 1970, p 1.
422. Cohen R. Coccidioidomycosis: case report in children. Arch Pediatr 66:241, 1949.
423. Hyatt HW. Coccidioidomycosis in a three week old infant. Am J Dis Child 105:127, 1963.
424. Townsend TE, McKey RW. Coccidioidomycosis in infants. Am J Dis Child 86:51, 1953.
425. Christian JR, Sarre SG, Peers JH, et al. Pulmonary coccidioidomycosis in a 21 day old infant. Am J Dis Child 92:66, 1956.
426. Westley CR, Haak W. Neonatal coccidioidomycosis in a Southwestern Pima Indian. South Med J 67:855, 1974.
427. Shafai T. Neonatal coccidioidomycosis in premature twins. Am J Dis Child 132:634, 1978.
428. Larwood TR. Transactions of the 7th Annual Meeting of the Veterans Administration and Armed Forces Coccidioidomycosis Study Group, San Francisco, 1962, p 28.
429. Bernstein DI, Tipton JR, Schott SF, et al. Coccidioidomycosis in a neonate; maternal-infant transmission. J Pediatr 99:752, 1981.
430. Golden SE, Morgan CM, Bartley DL, et al. Disseminated coccidioidomycosis with chorioretinitis in early infancy. Pediatr Infect Dis J 5:272, 1986.
431. Child DD, Newell JD, Bjelland JC, et al. Radiographic findings of pulmonary coccidioidomycosis in neonates and infants. AJR Am J Roentgenol 145:261, 1985.
432. Fiese MJ Coccidioidomycosis. Springfield, Ill, Charles C Thomas, 1958.
433. Maddy KT. The geographic distribution of *Coccidioides immitis* and possible ecologic implications. Ariz Med 15:178, 1958.
434. Albert BL, Sellers TF. Coccidioidomycosis from fomites. Arch Intern Med 112:253, 1963.
435. Giltner LT. Occurrence of coccidioidal granuloma (coccidioidomycosis) in cattle. J Agric Res 14:533, 1918.
436. Beck MD. Occurrence of *Coccidioides immitis* in lesions of slaughtered animals. Proc Soc Exp Biol Med 26:534, 1929.
437. Davis CL, Stiles GW Jr, McGregor AN. Pulmonary coccidioidal granuloma: a new site of infection in cattle. J Am Vet Med Assoc 91:209, 1937.
438. Reed RE. Diagnosis of disseminated canine coccidioidomycosis. J Am Vet Med Assoc 128:196, 1956.
439. Reed RE, Prchal CJ, Maddy KT. Veterinary aspects of coccidioidomycosis; panel discussion. Proceedings of a symposium on coccidioidomycosis. U.S. Public Health Service publication No. 575. Washington, DC, U.S. Government Printing Office, 1957, p 101.

440. Emmons CW. Isolation of *Coccidioides* from soil and rodents. Public Health Rep 57:109, 1942.
441. Rhoads JP. Coccidioidomycosis. J Okla State Med Assoc 58:410, 1965.
442. Pappagianis D. Coccidioidomycosis. *In* Hoeprich PD (ed). Infectious Diseases. Hagerstown, Md, Harper & Row, 1972.
443. Smith CE. An epidemiological study of acute coccidioidomycosis with erythema nodosum. Proc Sixth Pacific Science Congress 5:797, 1939.
444. Smith CE, Beard RR, Rosenberger HG, et al. Effect of season and dust control on coccidioidomycosis. JAMA 132:833, 1946.
445. Overholt EL, Hornick RB. Primary cutaneous coccidioidomycosis. Arch Intern Med 114:14, 1964.
446. Winn WA. Coccidioidomycosis and amphotericin. Med Clin North Am 47:1131, 1963.
447. Gifford MA, Buss WC, Douds RJ. *Coccidioides* fungus infection. Kern County, 1900-1936. Kern County Health Department Annual Report 1936-1937, p 39.
448. Beck MD. Epidemiology, coccidioidal granuloma. Calif State Dept Public Health Special Bull 57:19, 1931.
449. Smale LE, Birsner JW. Maternal deaths from coccidioidomycosis. JAMA 140:1152, 1949.
450. Vaughan JE, Ramirez H. Coccidioidomycosis as a complication of pregnancy, Calif Med 74:121, 1951.
451. Wack EE, Ampel NM, Galgiani JN, et al. Coccidioidomycosis during pregnancy: an analysis of ten cases among 47,120 pregnancies. Chest 94:376, 1988.
452. Peterson CM, Johnson SL, Kelly JV, et al. Coccidioidal meningitis and pregnancy: a case report. Obstet Gynecol 73:835, 1989.
453. Barbee RA, Hicks MJ, Grosso D, et al. The maternal immune response in coccidioidomycosis. Chest 100:709, 1991.
454. Hildick-Smith G. International symposium on opportunistic fungous infections. Arch Dermatol 87:8, 1963.
455. Ampel NM, Wieden MA, Galgiani JN. Coccidioidomycosis clinical update. Rev Infect Dis 2:897, 1989.
456. Anderson FG, Guckian JC. Systemic lupus erythematosus associated with fatal pulmonary coccidioidomycosis. Tex Rep Biol Med 20:93, 1968.
457. Charlton V, Ramsdell K, Sehring S. Intrauterine transmission of coccidioidomycosis. Pediatr Infect Dis J 18:561, 1999.
458. Cohen R. Placental *Coccidioides*; proof that congenital coccidioides is non-existent. Arch Pediatr 68:59, 1951.
459. Cohen R, Burnip R. Coccidioidin skin testing during pregnancy and in infants and children. Calif Med 72:31, 1950.
460. McCaffree MA, Altshuler G, Benirschke K. Placental coccidioidomycosis without fetal disease. Arch Pathol Lab Med 102:512, 1978.
461. Eckmann BH, Schaefer GL, Huppert M. Bedside interhuman transmission of coccidioidomycosis via growth on fomites: epidemic involving 6 persons. Am Rev Respir Dis 89:175, 1964.
462. Wilson JM. Smith CE, Plunkett OA. Primary cutaneous coccidioidomycosis: the criteria for diagnosis. Calif Med 79:233, 1953.
463. Faber HK, Smith CE, Dickson EC. Acute coccidioidomycosis with erythema nodosum in children. J Pediatr 15:163, 1939.
464. Birsner JW. The roentgen aspects of five hundred cases of pulmonary coccidioidomycosis. AJR 72:556, 1954.
465. Riley HD. Systemic mycoses in children. Curr Probl Pediatr 2:3, 1972.
466. Smith CE, Beard RR, Rosenberger HG, et al. Varieties of coccidioidal infection in relation to epidemiology and control of the disease. Am J Public Health 36:1394, 1946.
467. Caudill RG, Smith CE, Reinarz JA. Coccidioidal meningitis: a diagnostic dilemma. Am J Med 49:360, 1970.
468. Plunkett OA. Ecology and spread of pathogenic fungi. *In* Sternberg TH, Newcomer VD (eds). Therapy of Fungus Diseases, an International Symposium. Boston, Little, Brown, 1955, p 18.
469. Werner SB, Pappagianis D, Heindle I, et al. An epidemic of coccidioidomycosis among archeology students in Northern California. N Engl J Med 286:507, 1972.
470. Gehlbach SH, Hamilton JD, Conant NF. Coccidioidomycosis: an occupational disease in cotton-mill workers. Arch Intern Med 131:254, 1973.
471. Creitz JR, Puckett JF. A method for cultural identification of *Coccidioides immitis*. Am J Clin Pathol 24:1318, 1954.
472. Smith CE, Saito MT, Beard RR, et al. Serological tests in the diagnosis and prognosis of coccidioidomycosis. Am J Hyg 52:1, 1950.
473. Smith CE, Saito MT, Simons SA. Pattern of 39,500 serologic tests in coccidioidomycosis. JAMA 160:546, 1956.
474. Swaki Y, Huppert M, Bailey JW, et al. Patterns of human antibody reactions in coccidioidomycosis. J Bacteriol 91:422, 1966.
475. Campbell CC. Use and interpretation of serologic and skin tests in the respiratory mycoses: current considerations. Dis Chest 54(Suppl 1): 49, 1968.
476. Huppert M, Bailey JW. The use of immunodiffusion tests in coccidioidomycosis: I. The accuracy and reproducibility of the immunodiffusion test which correlates with complement fixation. Am J Pathol 44:364, 1965.
477. Huppert M, Bailey JW. The use of immunodiffusion tests in coccidioidomycosis: II. An immunodiffusion test as a substitute for the tube precipitin test. Am J Clin Pathol 44:369, 1965.
478. Huppert M, Peterson ET, Sun SH, et al. Evaluation of a latex particle agglutination test for coccidioidomycosis. Am J Clin Pathol 49:96, 1968.
479. Graham AR, Ryan KJ. Counter immunoelectrophoresis employing coccidioidin in serologic testing for coccidioidomycosis. Am J Clin Pathol 73:574, 1980.
480. Cotanzaro A, Flatauer F. Detection of serum antibodies in coccidioidomycosis by solid-phase radioimmunoassay. J Infect Dis 147:32, 1983.
481. Drips W, Smith CE. Epidemiology of coccidioidomycosis. JAMA 190:1010, 1964.
482. Schnelzer LL, Tabershaw IR. Exposure factors in occupational coccidioidomycosis. Am J Public Health 52:107, 1968.
483. Elconin AF, Egeberg MO, Bald JG, et al. A fungicide effective against *Coccidioides immitis* in the soil. *In* Ajello L (ed). Coccidioidomycosis. Tucson, University of Arizona Press, 1967, p 319.
484. Levine HB, Cobb JM, Smith CE. Immunogenicity of spherule-endospore vaccines of *Coccidioides immitis* for mice. J Immunol 85:218, 1961.
485. Pappagianis D. Evaluation of the protective efficacy of the killed *Coccidioides immitis* vaccine in man. *In* Proceedings of the 26th Interscience Conference on Antimicrobial Agents and Chemotherapy. Washington, DC, American Society for Microbiology, 1986 (abstract).

Cryptococcosis

486. Oliverio Campos J. Congenital meningoencephalitis due to torulosis neoformans: preliminary report. Bol Clin Hopit Civis Lisbon 18:609, 1954.
487. Neuhauser EBD, Tucker A. The roentgen changes produced by diffuse torulosis in the newborn. AJR Am J Roentgenol 59:805, 1948.
488. Nassau E, Weinberg-Heiruti C. Torulosis of the newborn. Harefuah 35:50, 1948.
489. Heath P. Massive separation of retina in full-term infants and juveniles. JAMA 144:1148, 1950.
490. Savai M, Gaur S, Frenkel LD. Successful treatment of cryptococcosis in a premature neonate. Pediatr Infect Dis J 14:1009, 1995.
491. Kaur R, Mittal N, Rawat D, Mathur MD. Cryptococcal meningitis in a neonate. Scand J Infect Dis 34:542, 2002.
492. Freeman W. Torula infection of central nervous system. J Psychol Neurol 43:236, 1931.
493. Cox LB, Tolhurst JC. Human Torulosis. Melbourne, Melbourne University Press, 1946.
494. Littman ML, Zimmerman LE. Cryptococcosis (Torulosis). New York, Grune & Stratton, 1956.
495. Khan MJ, Myers R, Koshy G. Pulmonary cryptococcosis: a case report and experimental study. Dis Chest 36:656, 1959.
496. Carton CA. Treatment of central nervous system cryptococcosis: a review and report of four cases treated with Actidione. Ann Intern Med 37:123, 1952.
497. Carton CA, Mount LA. Neurosurgical aspects of cryptococcosis. J Neurosurg 8:143, 1951.
498. Zimmerman LE, Rappaport H. Occurrence of cryptococcosis in patients with malignant disease of the reticuloendothelial system. Am J Clin Pathol 24:1050, 1954.
499. Butler WT, Alling DW, Spickard A, et al. Diagnostic and prognostic value of clinical and laboratory findings in cryptococcal meningitis, a follow-up study of forty patients. N Engl J Med 270:59, 1964.
500. Gruhn JG, Sanson J. Mycotic infection in leukemic patients at autopsy. Cancer 16:61, 1963.
501. Shadomy JJ, Utz JP. Preliminary studies on a hyphae-forming mutant of *Cryptococcus neoformans*. Mycologia 58:383, 1966.
502. Evans EE. The antigenic composition of *Cryptococcus neoformans*: I. A serologic classification by means of the capsular and agglutination reactions. J Immunol 64:423, 1950.
503. Evans EE, Sorensen LJ, Walls KW. The antigenic composition of *Cryptococcus neoformans*: V. A survey of cross-reactions among strains of *Cryptococcus* and other antigens. J Bacteriol 66:287, 1953.

504. San Felice F. Contributo alla morfologia e biologia del blastomiceti che si svilippano nei succhi di alcuni frutti. Annali dell'Instituto d'Igrene Sperimentale della R Universita di Roma 4:463, 1894.
505. Klein E. Pathogenic microbes in milk. J Hyg 1:78, 1901.
506. Emmons CW. The significance of saprophytism in the epidemiology of the mycoses. Trans N Y Acad Sci 17:157, 1954.
507. Emmons CW. Saprophytic source of *Cryptococcus neoformans* associated with the pigeon (*Columbia livia*). Am J Hyg 62:227, 1955.
508. Kao CJ, Schwartz J. The isolation of *Cryptococcus neoformans* from pigeon nests, with remarks on the identification of virulent cryptococci. Am J Clin Pathol 27:652, 1957.
509. Littman ML, Borok R. Relation of the pigeon to cryptococcosis: natural carrier state, host resistance and survival of *Cryptococcus neoformans*. Mycopathol Mycol Appl 36:329, 1968.
510. Littman ML, Schneierson SS. *Cryptococcus neoformans* in pigeon excreta in New York City. Am J Hyg 69:49, 1959.
511. Ajello L. Comparative ecology of respiratory mycotic disease agents. Bacteriol Rev 31:6, 1967.
512. Schneidau JD Jr. Pigeons and cryptococcosis. Science 143:525, 1964.
513. Hajsig M, Curoija Z. Kriptokoki u fekalijama fazana golubova s osvrlom na nalaze *Cryptococcus neoformans*. Vet Arch 35:115, 1965.
514. Tsubura E. Experimental studies in cryptococcosis: I. Isolation of *Cryptococcus neoformans* from avian excreta and some considerations on the source of infection. Fungi Fungous Dis 3:50, 1962.
515. Staib F. Vorkommen von *Cryptococcus neoformans* in vogelmist. Zentralbl Bakteriol 182:562, 1961.
516. Fragner P. The findings of cryptococci in excrements of birds. Cesk Epidemiol Mikrobiol Immunol 11:135, 1962.
517. Clarke DS, Wallace RH, David JJ. Yeasts occurring on apples and in apple cider. Can J Microbiol 1:145, 1954.
518. McDonough ES, Auseherman RJ, Balows A, et al. Human pathogenic fungi recovered from soil in an area endemic for North American blastomycosis. Am J Hyg 73:75, 1961.
519. Ajello L. Occurrence of *Cryptococcus neoformans* in soils. Am J Hyg 67:72, 1968.
520. McGrath JT. Cryptococcosis of the central nervous system in domestic animals. Am J Pathol 30:651, 1954.
521. Simon J, Nichols RE, Morse EV. An outbreak of bovine cryptococcosis. J Am Vet Med Assoc 122:31, 1953.
522. Pounden WD, Amberson JM, Jaeger RF. A severe mastitis problem associated with *Cryptococcus neoformans* in a large dairy herd. Am J Vet Res 13:121, 1952.
523. Campbell GD. Primary pulmonary cryptococcosis. Am Rev Respir Dis 94:236, 1966.
524. Mohr JA, Tacker RJ, Devlin RF, et al. Estrogen-stimulated phagocytic activity in human cryptococcosis. Am Rev Respir Dis 99:979, 1969.
525. Littman ML, Walter JE. Cryptococcosis: current status. Am J Med 45:922, 1968.
526. Gandy WM. Primary cutaneous cryptococcosis. Arch Dermatol Syphilol 62:97, 1950.
527. Brier RL, Mopper C, Stone J. Cutaneous cryptococcosis. Arch Dermatol 75:262, 1957.
528. Takos MJ. Experimental cryptococcosis produced by the ingestion of virulent organisms. N Engl J Med 254:598, 1956.
529. Freeman W. Torula meningo-encephalitis: comparative histopathology in seventeen cases. Trans Am Neurol Assoc 56:203, 1930.
530. Randhawa HW, Palewal DK. Occurrence and significance of *Cryptococcus neoformans* in the oropharynx and on the skin of a healthy human population. J Clin Microbiol 6:325, 1977.
531. Tynes B, Mason KN, Jennings AE, et al. Variant forms of pulmonary cryptococcosis. Ann Intern Med 69:1117, 1968.
532. Kida A, Abramowsky CR, Santoscoy C. Cryptococcosis of the placenta in a woman with acquired immunodeficiency syndrome. Hum Pathol 20:920, 1989.
533. Silberfarb PM, Sarosi GA, Tosh FE. Cryptococcosis and pregnancy. Am J Obstet Gynecol 112:714, 1972.
534. Curole DN. Cryptococcal meningitis in pregnancy. J Reprod Med 26:317, 1981.
535. Reiss F, Szilagyi G. Ecology of yeast-like fungi in a hospital population: detailed investigation of *Cryptococcus neoformans*. Arch Dermatol 91:611, 1965.
536. Collins VP, Gellborn A, Trimble JR. The coincidence of cryptococcosis and disease of the reticulo-endothelial and lymphatic systems. Cancer 4:883, 1951.
537. Burrows B, Barclay WR. Combined cryptococcal and tuberculous meningitis complicating reticulum cell sarcoma. Am Rev Tuberc Pulm Dis 78:760, 1958.
538. Annual report of the Division of Epidemiology, Bureau of Preventable Diseases, Department of Health, New York, N.Y., 1963-1964.
539. Goldstein E, Rambo ON. Cryptococcal infection following steroid therapy. Ann Intern Med 56:114, 1962.
540. Levine AS, Graw RG Jr, Young RC. Management of infections in patients with leukemia and lymphoma: current concepts and experimental approaches. Semin Hematol 9:141, 1972.
541. Siewers CMF, Cramblett HG. Cryptococcosis (torulosis) in children: a report of four cases. Pediatrics 34:393, 1964.
542. Baum GL, Artis D. Growth inhibition of *Cryptococcus neoformans* by cell-free human serum. Am J Med Sci 241:613, 1961.
543. Igel HJ, Bolande RP. Humoral defense mechanisms in cryptococcosis: substances in normal human serum, saliva and cerebrospinal fluid affecting the growth of *Cryptococcus neoformans*. J Infect Dis 116:75, 1966.
544. Szilagyi G, Reiss F, Smith JC. The anticryptococcal factor of blood serum: a preliminary report. J Invest Dermatol 46:306, 1966.
545. Hamilton JB, Tyler GR. Pulmonary torulosis. Radiology 47:149, 1946.
546. Greening RR, Menville LJ. Roentgen findings in torulosis: report of four cases. Radiology 48:381, 1947.
547. Haugen RK, Baker RD. The pulmonary lesions in cryptococcosis with special reference to subpleural nodules. Am J Clin Pathol 24:1381, 1954.
548. Moore M. Cryptococcosis with cutaneous manifestations. J Invest Dermatol 28:159, 1957.
549. Spickard A. Diagnosis and treatment of cryptococcal disease. South Med J 66:26, 1973.
550. Lillie RD. Histopathologic Technique. Philadelphia, Blakiston, 1954.
551. Rhinehart JF, Abdul-Haj SK. An improved method for histologic demonstration of acid mucopolysaccharides in tissues. Arch Pathol 52:189, 1951.
552. Berghausen O. *Torula* infection in man. Ann Intern Med 1:235, 1927.
553. Kessel JF, Holtzwart F. Experimental studies with *Torula* from a knee infection in man. Am J Trop Med 15:467, 1935.
554. Dienst RB. *Cryptococcus histolyticus* isolated from subcutaneous tumor. Arch Dermatol Syphilol 37:461, 1938.
555. Salvin SB, Smith RF. An antigen for detection of hypersensitivity to *Cryptococcus neoformans*. Proc Soc Exp Biol Med 108:498, 1961.
556. Bennett JE, Hasenclever HF, Baum GL. Evaluation of a skin test for cryptococcosis. Am Rev Respir Dis 91:616, 1965.
557. Newberry WH, Walter JE, Chandler JW Jr, et al. Epidemiologic study of *Cryptococcus neoformans*. Ann Intern Med 67:724, 1967.
558. Rappaport BZ, Kaplan B. Generalized *Torula* mycosis. Arch Pathol Lab Med 1:720, 1926.
559. Pollock AQ, Ward LM. A hemagglutination test for cryptococcosis. Am J Med 32:6, 1962.
560. Vogel R.A, Seelers TF, Woodward P. Fluorescent antibody techniques applied to the study of human cryptococcosis. JAMA 178:921, 1961.
561. Vogel RA. The indirect fluorescent antibody test for the detection of antibody in human cryptococcal disease. J Infect Dis 116:573, 1966.
562. Walter JE, Atchison RW. Epidemiological and immunological studies of *Cryptococcus neoformans*. J Bacteriol 92:82, 1966.
563. Bloomfield N, Gordon MA, Elmendorf DF Jr. Detection of *Cryptococcus neoformans* antigen in body fluid by latex particle agglutination. Proc Soc Exp Biol Med 114:64, 1963.
564. Gordon MA, Vedder DK. Serologic tests in diagnosis and prognosis of cryptococcosis. JAMA 197:961, 1966.
565. Walter JE, Jones RD. Serodiagnosis of clinical cryptococcosis. Am Rev Respir Dis 97:275, 1968.
566. Young EJ, Hirsch DD, Fainstein V, et al. Pleural effusions due to *Cryptococcus neoformans*: a review of the literature and report of two cases with cryptococcal antigen determination. Am Rev Respir Dis 121:743, 1980.
567. Bennett JE, Hasenclever HF, Tynes BS. Detection of cryptococcal polysaccharide in serum and spinal fluid: value in diagnosis and prognosis. Trans Assoc Am Physicians 77:145, 1964.
568. Kaufman L, Blumer S. Value and interpretation of serological tests for the diagnosis of cryptococcosis. Appl Microbiol 16:1907, 1968.
569. Bindschadler DD, Bennett JE. Serology of human cryptococcosis. Ann Intern Med 69:45, 1968.
570. Goodman JS, Kaufman L, Koenig MG. Diagnosis of cryptococcal meningitis: value of immunologic detection of cryptococcal antigen. N Engl J Med 285:434, 1971.

571. Walter JE, Coffee EG. Control of *Cryptococcus neoformans* in pigeon coops by alkalinization. Am J Epidemiol 87:173, 1968.

Malassezia Infections

572. Redline RW, Dahms BB. *Malassezia* pulmonary vasculitis in an infant on long-term intralipid therapy. N Engl J Med 305:1395, 1981.
573. Marcon MJ, Powell DA. Human infections due to *Malassezia* spp. Clin Microbiol Rev 5:101, 1992.
574. Long JG, Keyserling HL. Catheter-related infection in infants due to an unusual lipophilic yeast—*Malassezia furfur*. Pediatrics 76:896, 1985.
575. Dankner WM, Spector SA, Fierer J, et al. *Malassezia* fungemia in neonates and adults: complication of hyperalimentation. Rev Infect Dis 9:743, 1987.
576. Weiss SJ, Schoch PE, Cunha BA. *Malassezia furfur* fungemia associated with central venous catheter lipid emulsion infusion. Heart Lung 20:87, 1991.
577. Erchiga VC, Florencia VD. *Malassezia* species in skin disease. Curr Opin Infect Dis 15:133, 2002.
578. Bernier V, Weill FX, Hirigoyen V, et al. Skin colonization by *Malassezia* species in neonates. Arch Dermatol 138:215, 2002.
579. Shattuck KE, Cochran CK, Zabransky RJ, et al. Colonization and infection associated with *Malassezia* and *Candida* species in a neonatal unit. J Hosp Infect 34:123, 1996.
580. Larson E, Silberger M, Jakob K, et al. Assessment of alternative hand hygiene regimens to improve skin health among neonatal intensive care nurses. Heat Lung 29:136, 2000.
581. van Belkum A, Boekhout T, Bosboon R. Monitoring spread of *Malassezia* infections in a neonatal intensive care unit by PCR-mediated genetic typing. J Clin Microbiol 32:2528, 1994.
582. Chang HJ, Miller HL, Watkins N, et al. An epidemic of *Malassezia pachydermatis* in an intensive care nursery associated with colonization of health care workers' pet dogs. N Engl J Med 338:706, 1998.
583. Ahtonen P, Lehtonen OP, Kero P, et al. *Malassezia furfur* colonization of neonates in an intensive care unit. Mycoses 33:543, 1990.
584. Powell DA, Hayes J, Durrell DE, et al. *Malassezia furfur* skin colonization of infants hospitalized in intensive care units. J Pediatr 111:217, 1987.
585. Hruszkewycz V, Holtrop PC, Batton DG, et al. Complications associated with central venous catheters inserted in critically ill neonates. Infect Control Hosp Epidemiol 12:544, 1991.
586. Richet HM, McNeil MM, Edwards MC, et al. Cluster of *Malassezia furfur* pulmonary infections in infants in a neonatal intensive-care unit. J Clin Microbiol 27:1197, 1989.
587. Nicholls JM, Yuen KY, Saing H. *Malassezia furfur* infection in a neonate. Br J Hosp Med 49:425, 1993.
588. Powell DA, Aungst J, Snedden S, et al. Broviac catheter–related *Malassezia furfur* sepsis in five infants receiving intravenous fat emulsions. J Pediatr 105:987, 1984.
589. Aschner JL, Punsalang A Jr, Maniscalco WM, et al. Percutaneous central venous catheter colonization with *Malassezia furfur*: incidence and clinical significance. Pediatrics 80:535, 1987.
590. Kim EH, Cohen RS, Ramachandran P, et al. Adhesion of percutaneously inserted Silastic central venous lines to the vein wall associated with *Malassezia furfur* infection. J Parenter Enteral Nutr 17:458, 1993.
591. Powell DA, Marcon MJ, Durrell DE, et al. Scanning electron microscopy of *Malassezia furfur* attachment to Broviac catheters. Hum Pathol 18:740, 1987.
592. Marcon MJ, Powell DA. Epidemiology, diagnosis, and management of *Malassezia furfur* systemic infection. Diagn Microbiol Infect Dis 7:161, 1987.
593. Doerr CA, Demmler GJ, Garcia-Prats JA, et al. Solitary pyogenic liver abscess in neonates: report of three cases and review of the literature. Pediatr Infect Dis J 13:64, 1994.
594. Carey BE. *Malassezia furfur* infection in the NICU. Neonatal Netw 9:19, 1991.
595. Azimi PH, Levernier K, Lefrak LM, et al. *Malassezia furfur*: a cause of occlusion of percutaneous central venous catheters in infants in the intensive care nursery. Pediatr Infect Dis J 7:100, 1988.
596. Nguyen ST, Lund CH, Durand DJ. Thrombolytic therapy for adhesion of percutaneous central venous catheters to vein intima associated with *Malassezia furfur* infection. J Perinatol 21:331, 2001.
597. Marcon MJ, Powell DA, Durrell DE. Methods for optimal recovery of *Malassezia furfur* from blood culture. J Clin Microbiol 24:696, 1986.
598. Tirodker UH, Nataro JP, Smith S, et al. Detection of fungemia by polymerase chain reaction in critically ill neonates and children. J Perinatol 23:117, 2003.
599. Marcon MJ, Durrell DE, Powell DA, et al. In vitro activity of systemic antifungal agents against *Malassezia furfur*. Antimicrob Agents Chemother 31:951, 1987.

Phycomycosis

600. Levin SE, Isaacson C. Spontaneous perforation of the colon in the newborn. Arch Dis Child 35:378, 1960.
601. Gatling RR. Gastric mucormycosis in a newborn infant. Arch Pathol 67:249, 1959.
602. Neame P, Raaner D. Mucormycosis. Arch Pathol 70:261, 1960.
603. Jackson JR, Karnauchow PN. Mucormycosis of the central nervous system. Can Med Assoc J 76:130, 1957.
604. Isaacson C, Levin SE. Gastrointestinal mucormycosis in infancy. S Afr Med J 35:582, 1961.
605. Dennis JE, Rhodes KH, Cooney DR, et al. Nosocomial *Rhizopus* infection (zygomycosis) in children. J Pediatr 96:824, 1980.
606. Michalak DM, Cooney DR, Rhodes RH, et al. Gastrointestinal mucormycosis in infants and children: a cause of gangrenous intestinal cellulitis and perforation. J Pediatr Surg 15:320, 1980.
607. Miller RD, Steinkuller PG, Naegele D. Nonfatal maxillocerebral mucormycosis with orbital involvement in a dehydrated infant. Ann Ophthalmol 12:1065, 1980.
608. White CB, Barcia PJ, Bass JW. Neonatal zygomycotic necrotizing cellulitis. Pediatrics 78:100, 1986.
609. Varricchio F, Wilks A. Undiagnosed mucormycosis in infants. Pediatr Infect Dis J 8:660, 1989.
610. Ng PC, Dear PRF. Phycomycotic abscesses in a preterm infant. Arch Dis Child 64:862, 1989.
611. Lewis LL, Hawkins HK, Edwards MS. Disseminated mucormycosis in an infant with methylmalonic aciduria. Pediatr Infect Dis J 9:851, 1990.
612. Crim PF III, Demello D, Keenan WJ. Disseminated zygomycosis in a newborn. Pediatr Infect Dis J 3:61, 1984.
613. Arisoy AE, Arisoy ES, Correa-Calderon A, Kaplan SL. *Rhizopus* necrotizing cellulitis in a preterm infant: a case report and review of the literature. Pediatr Infect Dis J 12:1029, 1993.
614. Craig NM, Leuden FL, Pensler JM, et al. Disseminated *Rhizopus* infection in a premature infant. Pediatr Dermatol 11:346, 1994.
615. Linder N, Keller N, Huri C, et al. Primary cutaneous mucormycosis in a premature infant: case report and review of the literature. Am J Perinatol 15:35, 1998.
616. Amin SB, Ryan RM, Metlay LA, Watson WJ. *Absidia corymbifera* infections in neonates. Clin Infect Dis 26:990, 1998.
617. Oh D, Notrica D. Primary cutaneous mucormycosis in infants and neonates: case report and review of the literature. J Pediatr Surg. 37:1607, 2002.
618. Buchta V, Kalous P, Otcenasek M, Vanova M. Primary cutaneous *Absidia corymbifera* infection in a premature newborn. Infection 31:57, 2003.
619. Scheffler E, Miller GG, Classen DA. Zygomycotic infection of the neonatal upper extremity. J Pediatr Surg 38:E16, 2003.
620. Straatsma BR, Zimmerman LE, Gass JDM. Phycomycosis: a clinicopathologic study of fifty-one cases. Lab Invest 11:963, 1962.
621. Sheldon WH, Bauer H. Activation of quiescent mucormycotic granulomas in rabbits by induction of acute alloxan diabetes. Am J Pathol 34:575, 1958.
622. Bauer H, Flanagan JF, Sheldon WH. Experimental cerebral mycormycosis in rabbits with alloxan diabetes. Yale J Biol Med 28:29, 1955.
623. Elder TD, Baker RD. Pulmonary mucormycosis in rabbits with alloxan diabetes: increased invasiveness of fungus during acute toxic phase of diabetes. Arch Pathol 61:159, 1956.
624. Schofield RA, Baker RD. Experimental mucormycosis (*Rhizopus* infection) in mice. Arch Pathol 61:407, 1956.
625. Johnson JE. Infection and diabetes. *In* Ellenberg M, Rifkin H (eds). Diabetes Mellitus: Theory and Practice. New York, McGraw-Hill, 1969.
626. Sheldon WH, Bauer H. The development of the acute inflammatory response to experimental cutaneous mucormycosis in normal and diabetic rabbits. J Exp Med 110:845, 1959.
627. Emmons CW, Binford CH, Utz JP. Medical Mycology, 2nd ed. Philadelphia, Lea & Febiger, 1970, p 230.
628. Alexopoulos CJ. Introductory Mycology, 2nd ed. New York, John Wiley, 1962.

629. Whittaker RH. New concepts of kingdoms of organisms. Science 163:150, 1969.
630. Dodge CW. Phycomycetes. *In* Dodge CW. Medical Mycology. St. Louis, CV Mosby, 1935, p 97.
631. Conant NF, Smith DT, Baker RD, et al. Mucormycosis. *In* Conant NF, Smith DT, Baker RD, et al. Manual of Clinical Mycology, 3rd ed. Philadelphia, WB Saunders, 1971.
632. Emmons CW. Phycomycosis in man and animals. Riv Patol Veg 4:329, 1964.
633. Hale LM. Orbital-cerebral phycomycosis: report of a case and a review of the disease in infants. Arch Ophthalmol 86:39, 1971.
634. Burkholder PR, McVeigh I. Growth of *Phycomyces blakesleeanus* in relation to varied environmental conditions. Am J Botany 27:634, 1940.
635. Fernandez M, Noyola DE, Rossman SN, Edwards MS. Cutaneous phaeohyphomycosis caused by *Curvularia lunata* and a review of *Curvularia* infections in pediatrics. Pediatr Infect Dis J 18:72731, 1999.
636. Meyer RD, Rosen MD, Armstrong D. Phycomycosis complicating leukemia and lymphoma. Ann Intern Med 77:871, 1972.
637. Gale GR, Welch AM. Studies of opportunistic fungi: I. Inhibition of *Rhizopus oryzae* by human serum. Am J Med Sci 241:604, 1961.
638. Bank H, Shibolet S, Gilat T, et al. Mucormycosis of head and neck structures: a case with survival. BMJ 1:766, 1962.
639. Jones KW, Kaufman L. Development and evaluation of an immunodiffusion test for diagnosis of systemic zygomycosis (mucormycosis): preliminary report. J Clin Microbiol 7:97, 1978.
640. Roberts HJ, Cutaneous mucormycosis: report of a case with survival. Arch Intern Med 110:108, 1962.
641. Dillon ML, Sealy WC, Fetter BL. Mucormycosis of the bronchus successfully treated by lobectomy. J Thorac Cardiovasc Surg 35:464, 1958.
642. Harris JS, Mucormycosis: report of a case. Pediatrics 16:857, 1955.
643. McCall W, Strobos RR. Survival of a patient with central nervous system mucormycosis. Neurology 7:290, 1957.
644. Oswald H, Seeliger HPR. Tierexperimentelle Untersuchungen mit antimycotischen Mitteln. Arzneim Forsch 8:370, 1958.

Dermatophytes

645. Duhring LA. Diseases of the Skin, 3rd ed. Philadelphia, JB Lippincott, 1988.
646. Lynch JR. Case of ringworm occurring in an infant within 6 hours of birth. Med Press Circ 21:235, 1876.
647. Jacobs AH, Jacobs PH, Moore N. Tinea facei due to *Microsporum canis*. JAMA 219:1476, 1972.
648. Drusin LM, Ross BG, Rhodes DH, et al. Nosocomial ringworm in a neonatal intensive care unit: a nurse and her cat. Infect Control Hosp Epidemiol 21:605, 2000.
649. Bereston EW, Robinson HM. Tinea capitis and corporis in an infant 4 weeks old. Arch Dermatol Syphilol 68:582, 1953.
650. King WC, Walter IK, Livingood CS. Superficial fungus infections in infants. Arch Dermatol 68:664, 1953.
651. Hubener LF. Tinea capitis (*Microsporum canis*) in a 30 day old infant. Arch Dermatol 76:242, 1957.
652. Alden ER, Chernila SA. Ringworm in an infant. Pediatrics 44:261, 1969.
653. Weston WL, Thorne EG. Two cases of tinea in the neonate treated successfully with griseofulvin. Clin Pediatr 16:601, 1977.
654. Ross CM. Ringworm of the scalp at 4 weeks. Br J Dermatol 78:554, 1966.
655. Yesudian P, Kamalam A. *Epidermophyton floccosum* infection in a three week old infant. Trans St John's Hosp Dermatol Soc 59:66, 1973.
656. Kleibl K, Al-Ghareer HA, Sakr MF. Neonatal tinea circinata. Mykosen 26:152, 1982.
657. Wyre HW Jr, Johnson WT. Neonatal pityriasis versicolor. Arch Dermatol 117:752, 1981.
658. Gondim Goncalves HM, Mapurunga AC, Melo-Monteiro C, et al. Tinea capitis caused by *Microsporum canis* in a newborn. Int J Dermatol 31:367, 1992.
659. Lanska MJ, Silverman R, Lansaka DJ. Cutaneous fungal infections associated with prolonged treatment in humidified oxygen hoods. Pediatr Dermatol 4:346, 1987.
660. Kamalan A, Thambish AS. Tinea faciei caused by *Microsporum gypseum* in a two day old infant. Mykosen 24:40, 1981.
661. Smith EB, Gellerman GL. Tinea versicolor in infancy. Arch Dermatol 93:362, 1984.
662. Ajello L. A taxonomic review of the dermatophytes and related species. Sabouraudia 6:147, 1968.
663. Dawson CO, Gentles JC. Perfect stage of *Keritinomyces ajelloi*. Nature 183:1345, 1959.
664. Rebell G, Taplin D, Blank H. Dermatophytes. Their Recognition and Identification. Miami, Dermatology Foundation of Miami, 1964.
665. Rowen JL, Atkins JT, Levy ML, et al. Invasive fungal dermatitis in the ≤1000 gram neonate. Pediatrics 95:682, 1995.
666. English MP, Gibson MD. Studies in epidemiology of tinea pedis. BMJ 1:1442, 1959.
667. Rothman S, Knox G, Windhourst D. Tinea pedis as a source of infection in the family. Arch Dermatol 75:270, 1957.
668. Ajello L. Geographic distribution and prevalence of the dermatophytes. Ann N Y Acad Sci 89:30, 1960.
669. Pinetti P, Lostia A, Tarentino F. The role played by flies in the transmission of the human and animal dermatophytic infection. Mycopathologia 54:131, 1974.
670. Baer RL, Rosenthal SA, Furnari D. Survival of dermatophytes applied on the feet. J Invest Dermatol 24:619, 1955.
671. Baer RL, Rosenthal SA, Litt JZ, et al. Experimental investigations on mechanism producing acute dermatophytosis of feet. JAMA 160:184, 1956.
672. Knight AG. A review of experimental fungus infections. J Invest Dermatol 59:354, 1972.
673. Mackenzie DWR. The extra human occurrence of *Tricophyton tonsurans* var. *sulfureum* in a residential school. Sabouraudia 1:58, 1961.
674. Hildick-Smith G. Blank H, Sarkany I. Tinea capitis. *In* Fungus Diseases and Their Treatment. Boston, Little, Brown, 1964.
675. Roig MA, Rodriguez JMT. The immune response in childhood dermatophytoses. Mykosen 30:574, 1987.
676. Alteras I. Tinea capitis in suckling infants. Mykosen 13:567, 1970.
677. Weidman FD. Laboratory aspects of epidermophytosis. Arch Dermatol 15:415, 1929.
678. Goodman RS, Temple DE, Lorinez AL. A miniaturized system for extracorporeal hemodialysis with application to studies on serum anti-dermophyte activity. J Invest Dermatol 37:535, 1961.
679. Greenbaum SS. Immunity in ringworm infections. Arch Dermatol 10:279, 1924.
680. Lorincz AL, Priestly JO, Jacobs PH. Evidence for humoral mechanism which prevents growth of dermatophytes. J Invest Dermatol 31:15, 1958.
681. Page CO, Remington JS. Immunologic studies in normal human sweat. J Lab Clin Med 69:634, 1967.
682. Shelley WB, Wood MG. New technic for instant visualization of fungi in hair. J Am Acad Dermatol 2:69, 1980.
683. Burke RC. Tinea versicolor: susceptibility factors and experimental infection in human beings. J Invest Dermatol 36:389, 1961.
684. Fields BT Jr, Bates JH, Abernathy RS. Amphotericin B serum concentrations during therapy. Appl Microbiol 19:955, 1970.
685. McCoy MJ, Ellenberg JF, Killum AP. Coccidioidomycosis complicating pregnancy. Am J Obstet Gynecol 137:739, 1980.
686. Ward RM, Sattler FR, Dotton AS Jr. Assessment of antifungal therapy in an 800-gram infant with candidal arthritis and osteomyelitis. Pediatrics 72:234, 1983.
687. Abernathy RS. Treatment of systemic mycoses. Medicine 52:385, 1973.
688. Miller RP, Bates JH. Amphotericin B toxicity. Ann Intern Med 71:1089, 1969.
689. McCurdy DK, Frederic M, Elkington JR. Renal tubular acidosis due to amphotericin B. N Engl J Med 278:124, 1968.
690. Butler KM, Rench MA, Baker CJ. Amphotericin B as a single agent in the treatment of systemic candidiasis in neonates. Pediatr Infect Dis J 9:51, 1990.
691. Baley JE, Kliegman RM, Fanaroff AA. Disseminated fungal infections in very low-birth-weight infants: therapeutic toxicity. Pediatrics 73:153, 1984.
692. Feldman R. Cryptococcosis (torulosis) of the central nervous system treated with amphotericin B during pregnancy. South Med J 52:1415, 1959.
693. Aitken GWE, Symonds EM. Cryptococcal meningitis in pregnancy treated with amphotericin B: a case report. J Obstet Gynaecol Br Commonw 69:677, 1962.
694. Kuo D. A case of torulosis of the central nervous system during pregnancy. Med J Aust 49:558, 1962.
695. Sanford WG, Rosch JR, Stonehill RB. A therapeutic dilemma: the treatment of disseminated coccidioidomycosis with amphotericin B. Ann Intern Med 56:553, 1962.
696. Harris RE. Coccidioidomycosis complicating pregnancy: report of 3 cases and review of the literature. Obstet Gynecol 28:401, 1966.

697. Smale LE, Waechter KG. Dissemination of coccidioidomycosis in pregnancy. Am J Obstet Gynecol 107:356, 1970.
698. Hadsall FJ, Acquarelli JJ. Disseminated coccidioidomycosis presenting as facial granulomas in pregnancy: a report of two cases and a review of the literature. Laryngoscope 83:51, 1973.
699. Curole DN. Cryptococcal meningitis in pregnancy. J Reprod Med 26:317, 1981.
700. Moudgal VV, Sobel JD. Antifungal drugs in pregnancy: a review. Expert Opin Saf 2:475, 2003.
701. Jacobs RF, Yasuda K, Smith AL, et al. Laryngeal candidiasis presenting as inspiratory stridor. Pediatrics 69:234, 1982.
702. Faix RG. *Candida parapsilosis* meningitis in a premature infant. Pediatr Infect Dis J 2:462, 1983.
703. Cherry JD, Lloyd CA, Quilty JF, et al. Amphotericin B therapy in children. J Pediatr 75:1063, 1969.
704. Drutz DJ, Spickard A, Rogers DE, et al. Treatment of disseminated mycotic infections: new approach to therapy with amphotericin B. Am J Med 45:405, 1968.
705. Christiansen KJ, Bernard EM, Gold JWM, et al. Distribution and activity of amphotericin B in humans. J Infect Dis 152:1037, 1985.
706. Drutz DJ. In vitro antifungal susceptibility testing and measurement of levels of antifungal agents in body fluids. J Infect Dis 9:392, 1987.
707. Weitkamp JH, Poets CF, Sievers R, et al. *Candida* infection in very low birth-weight infants: outcome and nephrotoxicity of treatment with liposomal amphotericin B (AmBisome). Infection 26:11, 1998.
708. Scarcella A, Pasquariello MB, Giugliano B, et al. Liposomal amphotericin B treatment for neonatal fungal infections. Pediatr Infect Dis J 17:146, 1998.
709. Shadomy S. In vitro studies with 5-fluorocytosine. Appl Microbiol 17:871, 1969.
710. Shadomy S. Further in vitro studies with 5-fluorocytosine. Infect Immun 2:484, 1970.
711. Shadomy S. What's new in antifungal chemotherapy. Clin Med 79:14, 1972.
712. Steer PL, Marks MI, Klite PD, et al. 5-Fluorocytosine: an oral antifungal compound: a report on clinical and laboratory experience. Ann Intern Med 76:15, 1972.
713. Sarosi GA, Parker JD, Doto IL, et al. Amphotericin B in cryptococcal meningitis. Ann Intern Med 70:1079, 1969.
714. Harrison IIR, Galgiani JN, Reynolds AF Jr, et al. Amphotericin B and imidazole therapy for coccidioidal meningitis in children. Pediatr Infect Dis 2:216, 1983.
715. McDougall PN, Fleming PJ, Speller DCE, et al. Neonatal systemic candidiasis: a failure to respond to intravenous miconazole in two neonates. Arch Dis Child 57:884, 1982.
716. Sutton A. Miconazole in systemic candidiasis. Arch Dis Child 58:319, 1983.
717. Duffty P, Lloyd DJ. Neonatal systemic candidiasis. Arch Dis Child 58:318, 1983.
718. Lilien LD, Ramamurthy RS, Pildes RS. *Candida albicans* with meningitis in a premature neonate successfully treated with 5-flucytosine and amphotericin B: a case report and review of the literature. Pediatrics 61:57, 1978.
719. Bennett JE. Therapy of cryptococcal meningitis with 5-fluorocytosine. Antimicrob Agents Chemother 10:28, 1970.
720. Brammer KW, Farrow PR, Faulkner JK. Pharmacokinetics and tissue penetration of fluconazole in humans. Rev Infect Dis 12(Suppl):S318, 1990.
721. Wiest DB, Fowler SL, Garner SS, et al. Fluconazole in neonatal disseminated candidiasis. Arch Dis Child 66:1002, 1991.
722. Gürses N, Kalayci AG. Fluconazole monotherapy for candidal meningitis in a premature infant. Clin Infect Dis 23:645, 1996.
723. Driessen M, Ellis JB, Cooper PA, et al. Fluconazole vs amphotericin B for the treatment of neonatal fungal septicemia: a prospective randomized trial. Pediatr Infect Dis J 15:1107, 1996.
724. Driessen M, Ellis JB, Muwazi F, DeVilliers FP. The treatment of systemic candidiasis in neonates with oral fluconazole. Ann Trop Paediatr 17:263, 1997.
725. Huang YC, Lin TY, Lien RI, et al. Fluconazole therapy in neonatal candidemia. Am J Perinatol 17:411, 2000.
726. Wiesinger EC, Mayerhofer S, Wenisch C, et al. Fluconazole in *Candida albicans* sepsis during pregnancy: case report and review of the literature. Infection 24:263, 1996.
727. Bhandari V, Narange A. Oral itraconazole therapy for disseminated candidiasis in low birth weight infants. J Pediatr 120:330, 1992.
728. de Repentigny L, Ratelle J, Leclerc JM, et al. Repeated-dose pharmacokinetics of an oral solution of itraconazole in infants and children. Antimicrob Agents Chemother 42:404, 1998.
729. Walsh TJ, Lutsar I, Driscoll T, et al. Voriconazole in the treatment of aspergillosis, scedosporiosis and other invasive fungal infections in children. Pediatr Infect Dis J 21:240, 2002.
730. Franklin JA, McCormick J, Flynn PM. Retrospective study of the safety of caspofungin in immunocompromised pediatric patients. Pediatr Infect Dis J 22:747, 2003.
731. Ross CM. Ringworm of the scalp at four weeks. Br J Dermatol 78:554, 1966.
732. Rubin, A, Dvornik D. Placental transfer of griseofulvin. Am J Obstet Gynecol 92:882, 1965.
733. Elewski BE. Treatment of tinea capitis: beyond griseofulvin. J Am Acad Dermatol 40:S27, 1999.
734. Caceres-Rios H, Rueda M, Ballona R, Bustamante B. Comparison of terbinafine and griseofulvin in the treatment of tinea capitis. J Am Acad Dermatol 42:80, 2000.

Section V

DIAGNOSIS AND MANAGEMENT

Chapter 35

INFECTIONS ACQUIRED IN THE NURSERY: EPIDEMIOLOGY AND CONTROL

Joan A. Heath • Danielle M. Zerr

Neonates, especially premature neonates, requiring intensive care support constitute a highly vulnerable population at extreme risk for nosocomial or health care–associated infections. It has been estimated that as many as 6% to 22% of infants who survive 48 or more hours in a high-risk nursery or neonatal intensive care unit (NICU) acquire a nosocomial infection.[1,2] Although nosocomial infections have long been recognized in NICUs, only recently have data on rates been documented in the literature. As technology and treatments have advanced to significantly diminish mortality and morbidity among critically ill neonates, especially infants of very low birth weight (less than 1500 g), this vulnerability has only increased, as a result of both more profound immune system immaturity and more frequent use of invasive interventions that bypass skin and mucous membrane barriers.[1]

Nosocomial infections in neonates carry high attendant morbidity and mortality and health care costs. Prevention and control of these infections, although highly desirable, present a formidable challenge to health care professionals. Because control over birth weight—the most significant predictor of nosocomial infection risk—is limited, proper NICU customs, environment, and procedures (e.g., hand hygiene, antimicrobial usage, catheter-related practices, skin and cord care, visitation policies, unit design, and staffing) can reduce the risk for infection in the NICU. Understanding the epidemiology of nosocomial infections in neonates and methods for their prevention and control is critical to minimizing poor outcomes. This chapter describes the epidemiology, etiology, and clinical characteristics of neonatal nosocomial infections as well as the methods required for effective infection prevention and control.

SPECIAL ISSUES FOR NEONATES

It is well recognized that the immune system of the newborn infant, especially the premature infant, is functionally inferior to that of older infants, children, and adults (see Chapter 4). The lineages of the cells that will develop into the immune system are present at the beginning of the second trimester. The major components of the neonatal immune system, including T cells, neutrophils, monocytes, and the complement pathways, are functionally impaired, however, when compared with those in older infants and adults. For example, neonatal neutrophils show decreased chemotaxis, diminished adherence to the endothelium, and impaired phagocytosis[3,4]; neonatal complement levels and opsonic capacity also are reduced, particularly in the premature neonate.[4,5] In addition, neonatal T cell lymphokine production, cytotoxicity, delayed-type hypersensitivity, and help for B cell differentiation all are inferior when measured against those in adults.[6] Antigenic naiveté may account for many of these differences; however, inherent immaturity also appears to account for certain inequities. For example, neonatal T cells are delayed in their ability to generate antigen-specific memory function after HSV infection, even in comparison with naive adult T cells.[7]

Passively acquired maternal immunoglobulin G (IgG) is the sole source of neonatal IgG. Soon after birth, maternal IgG levels begin to fall; weeks later, production of immunoglobulins by the neonate commences. Neonatal IgG levels reach about 60% of adult levels by 1 year of age.[6] Unfortunately, because much of the maternal IgG is not transferred to the infant until the last 8 to10 weeks' gestation, premature infants start with significantly lower levels of serum IgG than in their term counterparts, which persist throughout most of the first months of life.

Other issues specific to the premature neonate also affect the functional immune system. For instance, the immature gastrointestinal tract (lack of acidity worsened by use of histamine H_2 blockers and continuous feedings) and easily damaged skin constitute open potential portals of entry for pathogens or commensals. In addition, like other intensive care unit populations, the NICU population frequently experiences extrinsic breeches of the immune system through use of intravascular catheters as well as other invasive equipment and procedures used to care for critically ill patients.

It is generally accepted that colonization with "normal flora" prevents, to some degree, colonization by pathogenic organisms. The neonate begins life essentially sterile. In the healthy term neonate, colonization occurs within the first few days of life. The organisms involved by site are α-hemolytic streptococci in the upper respiratory tract, *Staphylococcus epidermidis* and other coagulase-negative staphylococci (CoNS) on the skin, and gram-negative bacilli and anaerobes in the gastrointestinal tract. This process of colonization with normal flora is disrupted in infants cared for in an NICU in part because of exposure to the NICU environment, the hands of health care workers (HCWs), antimicrobial agents, and invasive procedures. As a result, the microflora of infants in the NICU can be markedly different from that of healthy term infants.[8,9] Multiple antimicrobial agent–resistant CoNS, *Klebsiella*, *Enterobacter*, and *Citrobacter* species colonize the skin and the respiratory and gastrointestinal tracts of a high proportion of NICU neonates by the second week of hospitalization.[10-13] In addition, neonates in the NICU become colonized not only with *Candida albicans* but also with non-*albicans Candida* species and *Malassezia*.[14-17]

Because colonization of the neonate with pathogenic organisms is a prelude to invasive infection from the same pathogens,[9] measures to prevent such colonization need to be considered. First, as a result of abnormal colonization, infants in the NICU themselves serve as an important reservoir of potential pathogens. Second, contamination of the hands of HCWs during routine patient care has been well documented.[18] Thus, careful attention to hand hygiene before and after contact with patients and their environment, as well as decontamination of potential fomites, are crucial measures in preventing spread of colonization and infection.

EPIDEMIOLOGY

Incidence

Nosocomial infections in healthy term infants are uncommon unless other conditions require that they be cared for in the NICU for several days to weeks. On the other hand, these other conditions are frequent in neonates of very low birth weight (less than 1500 g), who require prolonged NICU care. Understanding the epidemiology of nosocomial infections in NICUs can be challenging, because reported rates vary dramatically by institution. This variation probably results from use of nonstandard definitions of nosocomial infection and from differences in patient populations, such as mean gestational age, birth weight, and severity of underlying illness, which significantly affect the incidence of nosocomial infection.[19]

The National Nosocomial Infections Surveillance (NNIS) system is a national surveillance system of the Centers for Disease Control and Prevention (CDC) that uses standardized surveillance protocols and the involvement of multiple medical centers to provide benchmark data for the epidemiology of nosocomial NICU infections. Using standardized definitions, NNIS reported in 1996 that 13,179 nosocomial infections occurred between 1986 and 1994 in 10,296 neonates in 99 NICUs.[20] In this study, rates of intravascular catheter–associated bloodstream infection, the most frequent nosocomial infection, ranged from fewer than 5 infections per 1000 umbilical or central catheter days in infants with a birth weight greater than 1500 g to almost 15 infections per 1000 catheter days in the lowest-birth-weight group (less than 1000 g).

Another national, multicenter surveillance study, the Pediatric Prevention Network's (PPN) Point Prevalence Survey, was undertaken in 1999 to determine the point prevalence of nosocomial infections in NICUs and to define risk factors associated with development of these infections.[21] This study included 827 infants from 29 NICUs. Of the 827 infants, 94 (11.4%) had an active nosocomial infection on the day of the survey. Bacteremia accounted for 53% of infections; lower respiratory tract infections, ear-nose-throat infections, and urinary tract infections accounted for 13%, 9%, and 9%, respectively (Table 35-1).

In contrast with the NICU setting, the frequency of nosocomial infection in well-baby nurseries has been estimated to be between 0.3% and 1.7%.[22-24] In general, non–life-threatening infections such as conjunctivitis account for a majority of infections in the well-baby population. The remainder of this chapter focuses almost entirely on nosocomial infections in and control measures for the NICU setting.

Table 35–1 Distribution of NICU-Acquired Infections by Birth Weight and Site

	No. of Patients		No. of Infections					
Birth Weight (g)	Total Surveyed	With Infections (%)	Total	Bacteremia (%)	Respiratory Infections (%)	ENT Infections (%)	UTIs (%)	Other Infections
<500	13	1/13 (7.7)	1	1/1 (100)	0	0	0	0
501-1000	246	43/246 (17.5)	58	31/58 (53.4)	9/58 (15.5)	5/58 (8.6)	4/58 (7.0)	9/58 (15.5)
1001-1500	147	21/147 (14.3)	26	15/26 (57.7)	2/26 (7.7)	2/26 (7.7)	1/26 (3.8)	6/26 (23.1)
1501-2000	74	2/74 (2.7)	2	2/2 (100)	0	0	0	0
2001-2500	74	5/74 (6.8)	5	2/5 (40)	1/5 (20)	1/5 (20)	1/5 (20)	0
>2500	239	16/239 (6.7)	17	7/17 (41.2)	2/17 (11.8)	2/17 (11.8)	3/17 (17.6)	3/17 (17.6)
Unknown	34	6/347 (1.7)	7	3/7 (42.8)	1/7 (14.3)	0	1/7 (14.3)	2/7 (28.6)
Total	827	94/827 (11.4)	116	61/116 (52.6)	15/116 (12.9)	10/116 (8.6)	10/116 (8.6)	20/116 (17.2)

ENT, ear, nose, or throat; NICU, neonatal intensive care unit; UTIs, urinary tract infections.

Data from Sohn AH, Garrett DO, Sinkowitz-Cochran RL, et al. Prevalence of nosocomial infections in neonatal intensive care unit patients: results from the first national point-prevalence survey. J Pediatr 139:821-827, 2001.

Maternally Acquired Infections

For purposes of surveillance and tracking, all infections occurring in hospitalized newborns could be considered nosocomial. Infections that are manifested in the first few days of life, however, usually are caused by pathogens transmitted vertically from the maternal genital tract. Unfortunately, no precise time point perfectly distinguishes maternally acquired neonatal infections from those transmitted within the NICU. NNIS has attempted to address this issue by stratifying infections according to whether they are likely to be maternally acquired.[20] In 89% of neonates who had an infection thought to be maternally acquired, onset occurred within 48 hours of birth. Use of a cutoff period of 48 hours or less to designate maternally acquired infections allowed 15.3% of bacteremias and 14.5% of pneumonias to be considered as originating from a maternal source. Maternally acquired bloodstream infections were more likely to be caused by group B streptococci, other streptococci, and *Escherichia coli*, whereas those not maternally acquired usually were caused by coagulase-negative staphylococci.[20]

Nonmaternal Routes of Transmission

In general, nonmaternal routes of transmission of microorganisms to neonates are divided into three categories: contact (from either direct or indirect contact from an infected person or a contaminated source), droplet (from large respiratory droplets that fall out of the air at a maximum distance of 3 feet), and airborne (from droplet nuclei, which can remain suspended in air for long periods and as a result travel longer distances). Specific microorganisms can be spread by more than one mechanism; in most instances, however, a single mode of spread predominates. The CDC has developed a system of precautions for the control of nosocomial infections that is based on these modes of transmission.[25]

Contact transmission of bacteria, viruses, and fungi on the hands of HCWs is arguably the most important yet seemingly preventable means of transmission of nosocomial infection. Spread of infection by this means can occur either by transmission of the HCW's own colonizing or infecting pathogens or, more often, by transmission of pathogens from one patient to another. That the hands of HCWs become contaminated even in touching intact skin of patients has been well demonstrated.[18] Poor compliance with hand hygiene is another means by which the hands of HCWs can spread organisms from one patient to another.[26,27] Furthermore, hands of HCWs have been implicated in multiple outbreaks with a variety of different organisms; through experimental studies, a causal link between hand hygiene and nosocomial infection has been established.[28]

Contact transmission by means of fomites also can occur and has been described as a potential mechanism of spread of pathogens in multiple NICU outbreaks. As described later in this chapter, implicated items have included linens, medical devices, soap dispensers, and breast pumps, to name a few. These observations highlight the need for careful attention to disinfecting items shared between infants.

Spread through large respiratory droplets is an important mode of transmission for pertussis and infections due to *Neisseria meningitidis*, group A streptococci, and certain respiratory viruses, whereas airborne transmission by means of droplet nuclei is relevant for measles, varicella, and pulmonary tuberculosis. For large droplet or droplet nuclei transmission, usually an ill adult, either an HCW or a parent, is the source of infection in an NICU setting. In general, these organisms are rare sources of outbreaks.

Infusates, medications, and feeding powders or solutions can be intrinsically or extrinsically contaminated and have been reported as the source of outbreaks due to a variety of different pathogens. It is important when possible to mix infusates in a controlled environment (usually the pharmacy), to avoid multiuse sources of medication, and to use bottled or sterilized feeding solutions when breast milk is not available.

Of course, nosocomial infection also can arise from endogenous sources within the neonate. The "abnormal flora" of the neonate residing in the NICU, however, is determined at least in part by the NICU environment and HCWs' hands. With use of molecular techniques, even organisms typically considered to originate solely from normal flora (e.g., CoNS) have been shown to have clonal spread in the hospital setting, suggesting transmission by means of the hands of HCWs.[29,30]

Risk Factors for Nosocomial Infection

As discussed earlier, infants in NICUs have intrinsic factors predisposing them to infection, such as an immature immune system and compromised skin or mucous membrane barriers. In addition, multiple extrinsic factors play important roles in the development of infection, such as presence of indwelling catheters, performance of invasive procedures, and administration of certain medications, such as steroids and antimicrobial agents.

Birth weight is one of the strongest predictors of risk for nosocomial infection. For instance, NNIS data demonstrate that compared with larger infants, low-birth-weight infants are at higher risk of developing bloodstream infections and ventilator-associated pneumonia, even after correction for central intravascular catheter and ventilator use.[20] Similarly, in the PPN's Point Prevalence Survey, infants weighing 1500 g or less at birth were 2.69 (95% confidence interval [CI] 1.75% to 4.14%; $P < .001$) times more likely to have an infection than those weighing more than 1500 g.[21] The relationship between birth weight and nosocomial infection is complicated by multiple other factors that accompany low birth weight and also increase risk for nosocomial infection. Low birth weight, however, has been shown to be an independent predictor for nosocomial infection, after adjustment for use of vascular catheters, parenteral alimentation, and mechanical ventilation.[31] It is likely that birth weight also is a surrogate marker for other unmeasured factors, such as immune system immaturity.

Central venous catheters (CVCs) increase the risk for development of nosocomial bloodstream infections. In a study by Chien and colleagues 19,507 infants admitted to 17 NICUs in Canada, nosocomial bloodstream infections were found to occur at a rate of 3.1 to 7.2 infections per 1000 catheter days, depending on the type of catheter, versus 2.9 infections per 1000 noncatheter days. Other studies have demonstrated that the association between CVCs and bloodstream infection is independent of birth weight.[21] Mechanisms for CVC-related nosocomial bloodstream infections probably involve colonization of the catheter by means of the catheter hub, colonization of the skin at the insertion site,[33] or hematogenous spread of pathogens from distant sites of infection or colonization. Bloodstream infections also can result from contaminated intravenous fluids, which have the potential for intrinsic or, especially with use of multiuse vials, extrinsic contamination.

Factors related to the management of CVCs influence the risk of infection. Disconnection of the CVC and the frequency of blood sampling through the catheter increase the frequency of catheter-related infections.[34] By contrast, administration of a solution with heparin and exit-site antisepsis decreased infection. Lower frequency of CVC tubing changes (every 72 hours versus every 24 hours) was associated with increased catheter contamination, suggesting a potential for increased risk of infection.[35] CVC management techniques, including use of antiseptic-impregnated dressings, antimicrobial-coated catheters, and avoidance of scheduled replacement of CVCs, are discussed in the most recent CDC recommendations, summarized in "Guidelines for the Prevention of Intravascular Catheter–Related Infection," published in 2002 and prepared by the Hospital Infection Control Practice Advisory Committee.[36]

It has been suggested that use of peripherally inserted central catheters (PICCs) may be associated with a lower rate of infection than for other CVCs. Studies based in NICUs have yielded conflicting results. In a study by Chien and colleagues,[32] the relative risk of bloodstream infection, after adjustment for differences in infant characteristics and admission illness severity, was 2.5 per 1000 catheter days for umbilical venous catheters, 4.6 for PICCs, and 4.3 for Broviac catheters, compared with no catheter ($P < .05$). Another study also documented similar rates of infection for Broviac catheters and for PICCs.[37] By contrast, a higher rate of infection with Broviac catheters than with PICCs was suggested by Brodie and co-workers.[38] Further study of different CVCs in NICU infants is needed to delineate infection risks for individual catheter types.

Parenteral alimentation and intralipids have been shown to increase risk of bloodstream infection in premature infants even after adjustment for other covariables such as birth weight and CVC use.[38] Etiologic agents often associated are CoNS, *Candida* species, and *Malassezia* species. The pathogenesis of this association remains unclear. Potential hypotheses are many. Intralipids, for example, could have a direct effect on the immune system, perhaps through inhibition of interleukin-2.[39] Alternatively, as with any intravenous fluids, parenteral alimentation has the potential for intrinsic and extrinsic contamination, and intralipids especially may serve as a growth medium for certain bacteria and fungi. Finally, total parenteral alimentation and intralipids delay the normal development of gastrointestinal mucosa because of lack of enteral feeding, encouraging translocation of pathogens across the gastrointestinal mucosa.

It is well accepted that mechanical ventilation is an important risk factor for nosocomial lower respiratory tract infection. A large multicenter study of 8263 neonates found that mechanical ventilation was a risk factor for bloodstream infection as well, even after adjustment for a number of covariables such as birth weight, parenteral nutrition, and umbilical catheterization.[40] Clinically obvious respiratory infection appeared to precede some but not all cases of bloodstream infection associated with mechanical ventilation. The study authors suggested that the increased risk of mechanical ventilation could be attributed to colonization of humidified air, as well as to physical trauma from the endotracheal tube and its suctioning.

A number of medications critical to the survival of infants in the NICU increase risk of infection. Broad-spectrum antimicrobial agents, especially with prolonged use, are important in the development of colonization with pathogenic microorganisms.[9] The widespread use of broad-spectrum antimicrobial agents has been associated with increased colonization with resistant organisms in many settings, including NICUs.[19] In addition to colonization, antimicrobial agents also have been shown to increase risk of infection with resistant bacteria[41] and with fungal pathogens.[42] Other medications also appear to play a role in nosocomial infection. For instance, infants who receive corticosteroids after delivery are at approximately 1.3 to 1.6 times higher risk for nosocomial bacteremia in the subsequent 2 to 6 weeks than that observed for infants who do not receive this intervention.[43,44] In addition, colonization and infection with bacterial and fungal pathogens have been shown to increase with the use of H_2 blockers.[14,31]

Measures of illness severity have been developed, in part, in an effort to account for variations in birth weight–adjusted mortality scores between NICUs. The Score for Neonatal Acute Physiology (SNAP) was developed and validated by Richardson and associates,[45] and the Clinical Risk Index for Babies (CRIB) was developed by the International Neonatal Network.[46] These scores are highly predictive of neonatal mortality even within narrow birth weight strata and are predictive of nosocomial infection. Thus, in investigating potential risk factors for nosocomial infection, it is important to consider adjusting for illness severity using such measures, in addition to adjusting for other potential confounders.

Other risk factors related to infection include poor hand hygiene and environmental issues, such as understaffing and overcrowding.[47,48] These and related issues are discussed later in this chapter under "Prevention and Control."

CLINICAL MANIFESTATIONS

Nosocomial infections can affect any body site or organ system and manifest in a multitude of different ways. NNIS and PPN data demonstrated that bloodstream infections are the most common manifestation of nosocomial infection and account for 32% to 53% of infections (Table 35-2; see also Table 35-1).[20,21] Respiratory infections and eye, ear, nose, or throat infections are second and third in frequency, whereas gastrointestinal infections, urinary tract infections, surgical site infections, meningitis, cellulitis, omphalitis, septic arthritis, and osteomyelitis are reported less frequently.[20,21]

Bloodstream infections are the most common and one of the most potentially serious nosocomial infections that occur in NICU patients. Factors discussed earlier, including birth weight, intravascular catheters, mechanical ventilation, use of parenteral alimentation, and steroids, all have been shown to be associated with an increased risk of bloodstream infection. The most common pathogen associated with nosocomial bloodstream infections is CoNS (see Table 35-2). *Staphylococcus aureus*, *Enterococcus*, *Candida* species, *E. coli*, *Enterobacter* species, *Klebsiella pneumoniae*, and *Pseudomonas aeruginosa* also play important roles and are associated with

Table 35–2 Most Common Pathogens Causing Nosocomial Infection in NICU Patients: Distribution by Site

	No. of Infections (%)				
Pathogen	**Bloodstream**	**EENT**	**GI**	**Pneumonia**	**Surgical Site**
Coagulase-negative staphylococci (CoNS)	3833 (51.0)	787 (29.3)	102 (9.6)	434 (16.5)	119 (19.2)
Staphylococcus aureus	561 (7.5)	413 (15.4)		440 (16.7)	138 (22.3)
Group B streptococci	597 (7.9)			150 (5.7)	
Enterococcus	467 (6.2)	92 (3.4)		120 (4.6)	55 (8.9)
Candida species	518 (6.9)				
Escherichia coli	326 (4.3)	163 (6.1)	147 (13.9)	152 (5.8)	74 (12.0)
Other streptococcal species	205 (2.7)	199 (7.4)		86 (3.3)	
Enterobacter species	219 (2.9)	120 (4.5)	58 (5.5)	215 (8.2)	47 (7.6)
Klebsiella pneumoniae	188 (2.5)	76 (2.8)	104 (9.8)	152 (5.8)	39 (6.3)
Pseudomonas aeruginosa		178 (6.6)		308 (11.7)	
Haemophilus influenzae		72 (2.7)		38 (1.4)	
Viruses		136 (5.1)	317 (30.0[a])		
Gram-positive anaerobes			99 (9.4)		
Other enteric bacilli			8 (0.8)		
Miscellaneous organisms	607 (8.1)	449 (26.7)	223 (21.0)	570 (21.7)	147 (23.7)
Total	7521 (100)	2685 (100)	1058 (100)	2665 (100)	619 (100)

[a]Rotavirus constitutes 96.4% of viruses isolated from gastrointestinal infections.

EENT, eye, ear, nose, or throat; GI, gastrointestinal; NICU, neonatal intensive care unit.

Data from Gaynes RP, Edwards JR, Jarvis WR, et al. Nosocomial infections among neonates in high-risk nurseries in the United States. National Nosocomial Infections Surveillance system. Pediatrics 98:357-361, 1996.

higher morbidity and mortality rates than those associated with CoNS.[49,50] In one study, the frequency of fulminant sepsis (fatal within 48 hours) was estimated to be 56% (95% CI 38% to 72%) when the bloodstream infection was caused by *Pseudomonas* species, whereas it was only 1% (95% CI 0% to 4%) when infection was caused by CoNS.[50] The difficulty of assigning an etiologic role to CoNS on the basis of one blood culture that could be contaminated probably accounts for some distortion of the incidence and mortality data related to this organism, and this problem is discussed in detail in Chapter 6.

Pneumonia accounts for 12% to 18% of NICU nosocomial infections[20] and has been associated with prolonged hospital stay and increased mortality.[51] Organisms most commonly associated with nosocomial pneumonia include CoNS, *S. aureus*, and *P. aeruginosa* (see Table 35-2). Mechanical ventilation and birth weight are important risk factors for nosocomial respiratory infections.[51] Diagnosis of nosocomial respiratory infections requires correlation of microbiologic results with clinical findings and can be challenging in low-birth-weight infants because of the mostly nonspecific associated signs of illness and often misleading results of radiologic studies.[52]

Eye, ear, nose, and throat infections account for approximately 8% to 21% of infections, depending on birth weight.[20] Common etiologic organisms include CoNS and *S. aureus*, although gram-negative organisms, such as *E. coli*, *P. aeruginosa*, and *K. pneumoniae*, also can be isolated from these sites (see Table 35-2). Conjunctivitis appears to be the most common of these infections, accounting for 54% to 76%, depending on birth weight.[20] Risk factors for neonatal conjunctivitis identified in a study from Nigeria included vaginal delivery, asphyxia, and prolonged rupture of membranes.[53]

In the NNIS review, gastrointestinal infections were estimated to account for 5% to 11% of nosocomial infections, depending on birth weight. Necrotizing enterocolitis (NEC) was the most common presentation.[20] NEC carries high morbidity and mortality rates. A review of 17 NEC epidemics estimated that surgery was required for a mean of 16% (range, 0% to 67%) of infants, and death occurred in a mean of 6% (range, 0% to 88%).[54] In controlled studies, identified risk factors for NEC have included young chronologic age, low gestational age, low birth weight, and young age at first feeding.[54] Implication of specific pathogens is complex, requiring careful selection of an appropriate control population and attention to how and where specimens are collected. Pathogens associated with NEC outbreaks have included *Pseudomonas* species, *Salmonella* species, *E. coli*, *K. pneumoniae*, *Enterobacter cloacae*, *S. epidermidis*, *Clostridium* species, coronavirus, and rotavirus.[54,55] The importance of infection control methods such as strict attention to hand hygiene and cohorting patients in the NICU is suggested by the observation that their implementation has been followed by resolution of the outbreak.[55]

ETIOLOGIC AGENTS

A detailed discussion of the cause of nosocomial sepsis and meningitis is found in the chapter on bacterial sepsis (Chapter 6) and chapters describing specific etiologic agents.

Gram-Positive Bacteria

S. aureus is a colonizing agent in neonates and has been a cause of nosocomial infection and outbreaks in well-baby nurseries and NICUs. Methicillin-resistant *S. aureus* (MRSA) has become a serious nosocomial pathogen, and outbreaks have been reported in many areas of hospitals, including nurseries.[56-58] In addition to the usual manifestations of neonatal nosocomial infection (conjunctivitis, bloodstream infections, and pneumonia), nosocomial *S. aureus* infections can manifest as skin infections,[59] bone and joint infections,[60] parotitis,[61] staphylococcal scalded skin syndrome,[62,63] toxic shock syndrome,[56] and disseminated sepsis.

The role of the hands of HCWs in transmitting and spreading pathogenic organisms among infants was demonstrated with *S. aureus* in the 1960s.[64,65] Currently, in a majority of instances, *S. aureus* transmission is thought to occur by direct contact. Thus, it is not surprising that understaffing and overcrowding have been associated with *S. aureus* outbreaks in NICUs.[57,66] The potential for airborne transmission, however, has been suggested by the occurrence of "cloud babies," described by Eichenwald and colleagues[67] in 1960. "Cloud" HCWs also have been described; in such cases, the point source of an outbreak was determined to be a colonized HCW with a viral respiratory infection.[59,68] In one of these studies, dispersion of *S. aureus* from the implicated HCW was found to be much higher after experimental infection with rhinovirus.[68] More recently, molecular techniques not only have defined outbreaks[57] but also have demonstrated that transmission to infants probably occurs from colonized HCWs,[62] and sometimes from colonized parents.[69]

Nasal mupirocin ointment has been used to control outbreaks of both methicillin-susceptible *S. aureus* and MRSA.[62,70] The pharynx, rather than the anterior nares, however, may be a more common site of colonization in neonates and infants,[71] and eradication of the causative organisms with nasal mupirocin may be more difficult in this site.[72]

Coagulase-Negative Staphylococci

Since the early 1980s, CoNS has been the most common cause of nosocomial infection in the NICU.[48] Recent NNIS and PPN surveillance estimate that 32% of total pathogens and 48% to 51% of bloodstream infections are caused by these organisms.[20,21] A 10-year, prospective, multicenter Australian study corroborated the fact that CoNS accounted for most infections and demonstrated that 57% of all late-onset infections during the study period were due to these organisms.[73] This study and a U.S. study of 302 very low birth weight infants from two NICUs reported that the highest risk for CoNS infection was in the most premature infants.[73,74] In one study, infection usually manifested between 7 and 14 days of life and was accompanied by a mortality rate of 0.3%.[73] Although associated with relatively low mortality rates, bacteremia due to CoNS has been correlated, by means of multivariate analysis, with prolonged NICU stay and increased hospital charges, even after adjustment for birth weight and severity of illness on admission.[74]

Many experts consider infection due to CoNS to be inevitable in neonates in the NICU. Molecular techniques suggest that infections due to *S. epidermidis* can result from clonal dissemination.[29,30] In one study, four clones accounted for 43 of 81 study strains (53%).[29] This finding suggests that a portion of CoNS infections may be preventable by strict adherence to infection control practices. The fact that a hand hygiene campaign was associated with increased hand hygiene compliance and a lower rate of CoNS-positive cultures supports this contention.[75]

Enterococcus has been shown to account for 10% of total nosocomial infections in neonates, 6% to 15% of bloodstream infections, 0% to 5% of cases of pneumonia, 17% of urinary tract infections, and 9% of surgical site infections.[20,21] Sepsis and meningitis are common manifestations of enterococcal infection during NICU outbreaks[75,76]; however, polymicrobial bacteremia and NEC frequently accompany enterococcal sepsis.[77] Identified risk factors for enterococcal sepsis, after adjustment for birth weight, include use of a nonumbilical CVC, prolonged presence of a CVC, and bowel resection.[77] Because *Enterococcus* colonizes the gastrointestinal tract and can survive for long periods of time on inanimate surfaces, the patient's environment may become contaminated and, along with the infant, serve as a reservoir for ongoing spread of the organism.

The emergence of vancomycin-resistant enterococci (VRE) is a concern in all hospital settings, and VRE have been the cause of at least one outbreak in the NICU setting.[78] In the neonate, resistant strains appear to cause clinical syndromes indistinguishable from those due to susceptible enterococci.[77] The conditions promoting VRE infection, such as severe underlying disease and use of broad-spectrum antimicrobial agents, especially vancomycin, can be difficult to alter in many NICU settings. Guidelines for the prevention and control of VRE infection have been published; these focus on infection control tools such as rapid identification of a VRE-colonized or VRE-infected patient, cohorting, isolation, and barrier precautions.[80]

Historically, before the recognized importance of hand hygiene and the availability of antimicrobial agents, group A streptococci (GAS) were a major cause of puerperal sepsis and fatal neonatal sepsis. Although less common now, GAS continue to be a cause of well-baby and NICU outbreaks.[81-84] GAS-associated clinical manifestations include severe sepsis and soft tissue infections. One report described a high frequency of "indolent omphalitis"; in this outbreak, the umbilical stump appeared to be an important site of GAS colonization and an ongoing reservoir of the organism.[81] Routine cord care included daily alcohol application. After multiple attempts, the outbreak finally was interrupted after a 15-day interval during which bacitracin ointment was applied to the umbilical stump in all infants, and affected infants received intramuscular penicillin. Molecular techniques have enhanced the ability to define outbreaks, and use of these techniques has suggested that transmission can occur between mother and infant, between HCW and infant, and between infants—probably indirectly on the hands of HCWs.[82,83] In one recurring outbreak, inadequate laundry practices appeared to be a contributing factor.[85]

NNIS data have shown that group B streptococci (GBS) infections account for less than 2% of non–maternally acquired nosocomial bloodstream and pneumonia infections.[20] A number of studies from the 1970s and 1980s demonstrated nosocomial colonization of infants born to GBS-negative women.[86-90] These studies suggested a rate of transmission to babies born to seronegative mothers as high as 12% to 27%.[87,88] A recent case-control study evaluating risk factors for late-onset GBS infection demonstrated that premature birth was a strong predictor.[91] In that study, 50% of the infants with late-onset GBS infection were born at less than 37 weeks of gestation (compared with 15% of controls), and only 38% of the mothers of these infants were colonized with GBS, suggesting possible nosocomial transmission of GBS during the NICU stay.

The hands of HCWs are assumed to account for the transmission of most cases of nosocomial GBS infection. Breast milk also has been implicated as a potential mode of acquisition, however. In one report, GBS probably was transmitted from breast milk to one set of premature triplets between days 12 and 63 of life.[92] Two maternal vaginal swabs taken before delivery did not grow GBS, but repeated cultures of the mother's breast milk yielded a pure growth of GBS (greater than 10^5 colony-forming units [CFU]/mL) despite no evidence of mastitis. In this report, antimicrobial therapy administered to the mother appeared to eradicate the organism.

Gram-Negative Bacteria

The Enterobacteriaciae family has long been recognized as an important cause of nosocomial infection. Neonatal infection can be manifested as sepsis, pneumonia, urinary tract infections, and soft tissue infections; morbidity and mortality rates frequently are high.[93] *Enterobacter* species, *K. pneumoniae*, *E. coli*, and *Serratia marcescens* are the members of the family Enterobacteriaciae most commonly encountered in the NICU.

Enterobacter species have been estimated to account for 3% of bloodstream infections, 8% of cases of pneumonia, and 8% of surgical site infections in the NICU setting (see Table 35-2). Outbreaks due to *Enterobacter* species in NICUs have been associated with thermometers,[94] a multidose vial of dextrose,[95] intravenous fluids,[96] and powdered formula,[97] as well as with understaffing, overcrowding, and poor hand hygiene practices.[98] In one outbreak in which contaminated saline was linked to the initial cases, subsequent ongoing transmission was documented, presumably by means of the hands of HCWs and the environment.[99] In that study, early gestational age, low birth weight, exposure to personnel with contaminated hands, and *E. cloacae* colonization of the stool were associated with *E. cloacae* bacteremia, whereas use of CVCs and mechanical ventilation was not.

K. pneumoniae has been estimated to account for a similar proportion of infections in the NICU setting to that identified for *Enterobacter* species. Investigations in outbreaks involving *Klebsiella* species have implicated contaminated breast milk,[100] infusion therapy practices,[101] intravenous dextrose,[102] cockroaches, [134] disinfectant,[104] incubator humidifiers,[105] thermometers, oxygen saturation probes,[106] and ultrasonography coupling gel.[108] In a surveillance study of 383 NICU infants in Brazil, 50% became colonized with *Klebsiella*.[13] In this study, colonization was associated with use of a cephalosporin and aminoglycoside combination therapy, as well as with longer duration of the NICU stay.

E. coli has been estimated to cause 4% of bloodstream, 14% of gastrointestinal, and 12% of surgical site infections. *E. coli* also has been responsible for outbreaks of pyelonephritis,[108] gastroenteritis,[109,110] and NEC.

S. *marcescens* is an opportunistic pathogen that survives in relatively harsh environments. Disease due to *S. marcescens* often is manifested as meningitis, bacteremia, and pneumonia.[111] *S. marcescens* infections have a high potential for morbidity and mortality.[112,113] *S. marcescens* outbreaks have been associated with, but not limited to, contaminated soap,[114] multiuse bottles of theophylline,[115] formula,[115] enteral feeding additives,[116] breast pumps,[117,118] and transducers from internal monitors.[116] Although point source environmental contamination is important in *Serratia* outbreaks, in many of these outbreaks and in reports in which no point source was identified,[119] patient-to-patient spread of the organism by means of the hands of HCWs appeared to be an important mechanism of spread.[113]

Extended-spectrum β-lactamases (ESBLs) are plasmid-mediated resistance factors produced by members of the Enterobacteriaceae family. ESBLs inactivate third-generation cephalosporins and aztreonam. They most commonly occur in *K. pneumoniae* and *E. coli* but have increasingly been found in other gram-negative bacilli. Colonization with ESBL-producing organisms has been associated with administration of certain antimicrobials and longer duration of hospitalization, whereas infection has been associated with prior colonization and use of CVCs.[13] That the ESBL-containing plasmids can be transmitted to other Enterobacteriaceae organisms has been demonstrated in NICU outbreaks in which the implicated plasmid spread from *Klebsiella* species to *E. coli*, *E. cloacae*, and *Citrobacter freundii*.[120,121] The gastrointestinal tract in neonates and the hands of HCWs serve as reservoirs for members of the Enterobacteriaceae family. Thus, in general, measures aimed at controlling spread of organisms in this family have focused on attention on hand hygiene, cohorting of patient and staff, and observation of isolation precautions.[121,122]

P. aeruginosa, an opportunistic pathogen that persists in relatively harsh environments, frequently has been associated with nosocomial infections and outbreaks in the NICU setting. Nosocomial *P. aeruginosa* infections vary in their clinical presentation, but the most common manifestations are respiratory, ear, nose, or throat and bloodstream infections.[21] From the PPN data it has been estimated that *P. aeruginosa* species account for 6.8% of total pathogens, 5% of bloodstream infections, and 15% of respiratory infections.[21] *P. aeruginosa* infections, particularly bloodstream infections, have been associated with a very high mortality rate.[123]

Feeding intolerance, prolonged parenteral alimentation, and long-term intravenous antimicrobial therapy have been identified as risk factors for *Pseudomonas* infection.[123] Outbreaks due to *P. aeruginosa* have been linked with contaminated hand lotion,[124] respiratory therapy solution, [125] a water bath used to thaw fresh-frozen plasma,[126] a blood gas analyzer,[127] and bathing sources. In one case, neonatal *Pseudomonas* sepsis and meningitis were shown by pulsed-field gel electrophoresis to be associated with shower tubing from a tub used by the infant's mother during labor.[128] Of importance, HCWs and their contaminated hands also have been linked with *Pseudomonas* infections in the NICU setting. In a study of a New York outbreak, recovery of *Pseudomonas* from the hands of HCWs was associated with older age and history of use of artificial nails.[129] This and other studies suggest that the risk of transmission of *Pseudomonas* to patients is higher among HCWs with onychmycosis or those who wear long artificial or long natural nails.[129,130] As a result of these and other findings, the CDC revised its 2002 hand hygiene recommendations to include a recommendation against the presence of HCWs with artificial fingernails in intensive care units.[131]

Bordetella pertussis is a rare cause of nosocomial infection in neonates. When *B. pertussis* infection occurs, parents and HCWs typically are the source. A parent was the source of an outbreak involving three neonates and one nurse in a special care nursery in Australia.[132] In 1999 in Knoxville, Tennessee, an outbreak involving six neonates probably was due to transmission of infection by an HCW.[133] As a result of the Tennessee outbreak, 166 infants received erythromycin prophylaxis. Subsequently, an increase in infantile hypertrophic pyloric stenosis was noted by local pediatric surgeons. Results of a CDC investigation suggested a causal role of erythromycin in the cases of hypertrophic pyloric stenosis.[133,134] Erythromycin remains the recommended agent of choice for prophylaxis after pertussis exposure, but parents should be informed of the risk and signs of hypertrophic pyloric stenosis, and cases associated with erythromycin use should be reported to MedWatch.[135]

Other Bacterial Pathogens

Newborn infants are particularly prone to infection and disease following exposure to *Mycobacterium tuberculosis*. A cluster of multidrug-resistant *M. tuberculosis* infections was noted in three infants born during a 2-week period in one New York hospital.[136] Investigation implicated an HCW who visited the nursery several times during that period. Pulmonary and extrapulmonary disease occurred in three infants 4 to15 months after exposure, highlighting the vulnerability of the newborn population.[136] Tuberculosis screening of HCWs, ultraviolet lighting, and a high number of air exchanges appear to be effective methods in preventing nosocomial tuberculosis infection.[137] The CDC's "Guidelines for Preventing the Transmission of *Mycobacterium tuberculosis* in Health-Care Settings" emphasizes (1) use of engineering controls and personal protective equipment, (2) risk assessments for the development of institutional tuberculosis control plans, (3) early identification and management of individuals with tuberculosis infection and disease, (4) tuberculosis screening programs for HCWs, (5) HCW education and training, and (6) evaluation of tuberculosis control programs.[138]

Fungi

Candida species are an increasingly important cause of nosocomial infection in NICU patients and have been estimated to account for 6.9% of bloodstream infections and 42% of urinary tract infections.[20,139] Prospective studies have estimated colonization rates with *Candida* to be 12% to 54% in low-birth-weight neonates,[17,140-142] and colonization has been associated with subsequent invasive disease.[141] The mortality rate can be high in invasive candidiasis. In one study of 34 patients with fungemia due to *Candida* species, a case-fatality rate of 41% was reported.[143] Risk factors for fungal infections in neonates are similar to risk factors for bacterial infections; low birth weight and gestational age are important predictors. In addition, a prospective, multicenter study of 2157 infants found that use of a third-generation cephalosporin, presence of a CVC, intravenously administered lipids, and H_2 blocker therapy were associated with *Candida* colonization after adjusting for length of stay, birth weight of 1000 g or less, and gestational age less than 32 weeks.[14] *Candida parapsilosis* appears to be the most frequent species associated with nosocomial *Candida* infection in NICU infants. Both cross-contamination and maternal reservoirs are sources of nosocomial *Candida albicans* infection, as demonstrated in studies using molecular typing methods.[144-146]

Malassezia species, lipophilic yeasts, frequently colonize NICU patients. In one French study, 30 of 54 preterm neonates (56%) became colonized with *Malassezia furfur*.[147] *Malassezia pachydermatis*, a zoonotic organism present on the skin and in the ear canals of healthy dogs and cats, also has been associated with nosocomial outbreaks in the NICU setting.[147,148] In one report, the outbreak appeared to be linked to colonization of HCWs' pet dogs.[147]

Pichia anomala, or *Hansenula anomala*, a yeast found in soil and pigeon droppings, and on plants and fruits, also can colonize the human throat and gastrointestinal tract. In general, it is an unusual cause of nosocomial infection in neonates, but it was the cause of two reported outbreaks in this setting.[149,150] In both reports, carriage on the hands of HCWs appeared to be a factor.

Invasive mold infections are a rare cause of nosocomial infection in neonates, but when they occur, they are associated with high mortality rate. *Aspergillus* infections may manifest as pulmonary, central nervous system, gastrointestinal, or disseminated disease. A cutaneous presentation, with or without subsequent dissemination, appears to be the most common presentation for hospitalized premature infants without underlying immune deficiency.[151,152] Often, skin maceration is the presumed portal of entry. In a series of four patients who died of disseminated *Aspergillus* infection that started cutaneously, a contaminated device used to collect urine from the male infants was implicated.[152] Similarly, contaminated wooden tongue depressors, used as splints for intravenous and arterial cannulation sites, were associated with cutaneous infection due to *Rhizopus microsporus* in four premature infants.[153] In addition to preterm birth, use of broad-spectrum antimicrobial agents, steroid therapy, and hyperglycemia are thought to be risk factors for mold infection.

Even zoophilic dermatophytes have been described as a source of nosocomial infection in neonates. In one report, five neonatal cases in one unit were traced to an infected nurse and her cat.[154] Prolonged therapy for both the nurse and her cat was necessary to clear their infections.

Viruses

Rotavirus

Although many pathogens can cause nosocomial gastroenteritis, rotavirus is responsible for 95% or more of viral infections in high-risk nurseries, including the NICU.[20] In one longitudinal study, rotavirus infection developed during hospitalization in 95 of 194 neonates (49%).[155] In this study, rotavirus was manifested as frequent and watery stools in term infants and as abdominal distention and bloody, mucoid stools in the preterm neonates.

A high titer of virus is excreted in stool of infected persons, and the organism is viable on hands and in the environment for relatively prolonged periods of time.[156,157] Attention to hand hygiene and disinfection of potential fomites are crucial in preventing spread of infection. This concept is illustrated by the results of one study in which rotavirus infection was associated with ungloved nasogastric tube feeding.[157]

Respiratory Viruses

Respiratory viruses including influenza A virus, parainfluenza virus, coronavirus, respiratory syncytial virus, and adenovirus have been reported to cause nosocomial infections in NICU patients.[158-161] Associated clinical findings include rhinorrhea, tachypnea, retractions, nasal flaring, rales, and wheezing, but illness also can be manifested as apnea, sepsis-like illness, and gastrointestinal symptoms.[161,162] Identified risk factors for acquisition vary from study to study but have included low birth weight, low gestational age, twin pregnancy, mechanical ventilation, and high CRIB score.[159-162] Contact and droplet transmission are the most common modes of spread of infection, again highlighting the importance of scrupulous hand hygiene in delivery of patient care for this population.

Enteroviruses

Numerous nursery and NICU outbreaks of enteroviral infection have been reported.[163,164] In the neonate with enteroviral infection, clinical manifestations can range from mild gastroenteritis to a severe and fulminant sepsis-like syndrome or meningitis/encephalitis. The latter presentation can be associated with a high mortality rate.[164] In index cases, the patient may have acquired disease vertically, with subsequent horizontal spread leading to outbreaks[164,165]; with other viral pathogens, virus can be shed into the stool for prolonged periods, enabling patient-to-patient transmission by the hands of HCWs when hand hygiene procedures are improperly performed.

Cytomegalovirus

Congenitally acquired cytomegalovirus (CMV) infection is a cause of morbidity and occasionally death, whereas postnatally acquired CMV infection follows a benign course in virtually all healthy term infants. Postnatal CMV infection, however, can cause considerable morbidity and death in premature infants.[166] Hepatitis, neutropenia, thrombocytopenia, sepsis-like syndrome, pneumonitis, and development of chronic lung disease each have been associated with postnatal acquisition of CMV in premature infants.[167,168] With the routine use of CMV-seronegative blood products in these neonates, a majority of postnatal CMV infections appear to be acquired through breast milk.[169] It has been estimated that transmission by this mode occurs in approximately 37% of breast-fed infants of mothers with CMV detected in breast milk.[170] In one study, approximately 50% of these infants had clinical features of infection, and 12% presented with a sepsis-like syndrome. Nosocomial person-to-person transmission has been documented,[171,172] but the extent to which this occurs is controversial.[173] At present, no proven, highly effective method is available for removing CMV from breast milk without destroying its beneficial components. Some data, however, suggest that freezing the breast milk before use may decrease the CMV titer, thereby limiting subsequent transmission.[174]

Herpes Simplex Virus

In a majority of cases, neonatal herpes simplex virus (HSV) infection is acquired vertically from the mother. Nursery transmission of HSV infection is rare but has been described.[175-177] In each of these cases, HSV-1 was involved. In one infant, the source of virus was thought to be a patient's father, who had active herpes labialis.[175] Subsequent spread of virus from this first infant to a second infant was thought to have occurred by means of the hands of an HCW. In another report, the source of HSV for the index case, an infant who died of respiratory distress in whom evidence of HSV infection was found at postmortem examination of the brain, was unknown.[176] The hands of HCWs were implicated in the spread of HSV to three subsequent cases, however. In another report, direct spread from an HCW was thought to be responsible for transmission of HSV to three infants over a period of approximately 3 years.[177] Studies of adults with herpes labialis suggest a high frequency of recovery of virus from the mouth and the hands (78% and 67%, respectively).[178] In this same study, HSV was shown to survive for 2 to 4 hours on skin, cloth, and plastic. Implementing contact precautions for infants with HSV and instructing HCWs with active herpes labialis regarding control measures, such as covering the lesion, not touching the lesion, and using strict hand hygiene, are reasonable means to prevent nosocomial transmission of HSV. If there are concerns that an HCW would be unable to comply with control measures or if the HCW has a herpetic whitlow, such persons should be restricted from patient contact.

Varicella-Zoster Virus

Nosocomial transmission of varicella in the NICU setting, although unusual, has been described.[179] Large-scale outbreaks in nurseries and NICUs are rare, most probably because of the high rate of varicella-zoster virus (VZV) immunity in HCWs and pregnant women. Premature infants born at less than 28 weeks of gestation are unlikely to have received protective levels of VZV IgG from their mothers, so their potential risk is significant if an exposure occurs. Transmission is most likely to occur from an adult with early, unrecognized symptoms of varicella. In such instances, the potential risk for VZV-seronegative exposed infants and HCWs is substantial, especially if the patient in the index case is an HCW.[180] For this reason, it is recommended that HCWs be screened for prior varicella infection by history, with subsequent immunization as indicated.

Hepatitis A

Hepatitis A is a rare cause of nosocomial infection in NICUs, but a number of outbreaks in this setting have been reported.[181-183] In most instances, disease in neonates is clinically silent. Neonatal cases often are detected only through recognition of the symptomatic secondary adult cases. In one report, disease was acquired by patients in the index cases through blood transfusion from a donor with acute hepatitis A.[183] Of note, the virus subsequently spread to another 11 infants, 22 nurses, and 8 other HCWs. Overall, hepatitis A affected 20% of the patients and 24% of the nurses. Lapses in infection control practices and the prolonged shedding of the virus in infants stool probably contributed to the rapid spread and high attack rate documented in the outbreak. Outbreaks such as this one are unlikely because of current blood product practices to eliminate transmissible agents from donor blood.

PREVENTION AND CONTROL

An effective infection control program that focuses on reducing risk on a prospective basis can decrease the incidence of nosocomial infections.[184,185] The principal function of such a program is to protect the infant and the HCW from risk of hospital-acquired infection in a manner that is cost-effective. Activities crucial to achieving and maintaining this goal include collection and management of critical data relating to surveillance for nosocomial infection, and direct intervention to interrupt the transmission of infectious diseases.[22]

Surveillance

Reducing the incidence of nosocomial infection for neonates must begin with surveillance for these events. Surveillance has been defined as "a comprehensive method of measuring outcomes and related processes of care, analyzing the data, and providing information to members of the health care team to assist in improving those outcomes."[186] Essential elements of a surveillance program include the following:

- Defining the population and data elements as concisely as possible
- Collecting relevant data using systematic methods
- Consolidating and tabulating data to facilitate evaluation
- Analyzing and interpreting data
- Reporting data to those who can bring about change[187]

Surveillance systems necessarily vary, depending on the population; accordingly, a written plan, based on sound epidemiologic principles,[187] should be in place to track rates of infection over time. Because new risks can emerge, such as new interventional technology or drugs, changing patient demographics, and new pathogens and resistance patterns, the plan should be reviewed and updated frequently.[188] The Joint Commission on Accreditation of Healthcare Organizations (JCAHO) recommends that hospitals have a written infection control plan that includes a description of prioritized risks; a statement of the goals of the infection control program; a description of the hospital's strategies to minimize, reduce, or eliminate the prioritized risks; and a description of how the strategies will be evaluated. The JCAHO further recommends that hospitals identify risks for transmission and acquisition of infectious agents (Table 35-3) and formally review this analysis annually and whenever significant changes occur in any of the risk factors.[189]

The definitions provided by the CDC's NNIS system are the most comprehensive and widely used set of case definitions for the outcomes of nosocomial infections.[189] The system provides high-risk nursery–specific data collection methods as well as denominator data and allows external benchmarking of infection rates for this population.[190,191] The NNIS system defines a nosocomial infection as a localized or systemic process that results from adverse reaction to the presence of an infectious agent(s) or its toxin(s) and that was not present or incubating at the time of admission to the hospital. NNIS also recognizes as special situations, and defines as nosocomial, some infections in neonates that result from passage through the birth canal but do not become clinically apparent until several or more days after birth. It does not, however, consider infections that are known or proved to have been acquired transplacentally to be nosocomial.[191]

Distinction between maternal and hospital sources of infection is important, although difficult at times, because control measures designed to prevent acquisition from hospital sources will be ineffective in preventing perinatal acquisition of pathogens.[192] Surveillance for infections in healthy newborns also is challenging because of the typically short length of stay. Infections can develop after discharge, and these are more difficult for infection control practitioners (ICPs) to capture. Methods for postdischarge surveillance have been developed, but because most neonatal infections that occur following discharge are noninvasive,[193] such surveillance has not been widely implemented, because of concerns about the cost-effectiveness of these labor-intensive processes.

The ultimate goal of surveillance is to achieve outcome objectives (e.g., decreases in infection rates, morbidity, mortality, or cost).[187] Baseline infection rates for an inpatient unit must be established so that the endemic rate of infection can be understood and addressed. In the NICU, concurrent surveillance (initiated while the infant is in the hospital) should be conducted by persons trained to collect and interpret clinical information. Typically, such persons are ICPs working closely with HCWs and using various data sources (Table 35-4).

Using NNIS or other accepted definitions, the ICP should collect data regarding cases of nosocomial infection in the NICU population as well as population-specific denominator data. Denominators must be carefully chosen to represent the population at risk. Attempts to stratify risk should take into account both underlying infant-specific risks and those

Table 35–3 Factors Influencing Transmission and Acquisition of Infectious Agents within a Hospital

Geographic location and community environment of the hospital
Characteristics of the population served
Care, treatment, and services provided
Actions after analysis of the hospital's infection prevention and control data

Data from Joint Commission on Accreditation of Healthcare Organizations. Surveillance, Prevention and Control of Infection, 2005 Pre-publication edition. Oak Brook Terrace, Ill, Joint Commission on Accreditation of Healthcare Organizations, 2003, pp 1-11. Available at http://www.jcaho.org/accredited+organizations/patient+safety/infection+control/05_ic_std_hap.pdf.

Table 35–4 Sources of Surveillance Data

Admission records
Patient records
Closed medical records
Kardex
Temperature and vital signs records
Microbiology reports
Antimicrobial susceptibility reports
Verbal and written reports
Radiographic reports
Interviews with caregivers
Interviews with and observation of patient
Postdischarge reports
Autopsy reports

Data from Lee TB, Baker OG, Lee JT, et al. Recommended practices for surveillance. Association for Professionals in Infection Control and Epidemiology, Inc. Surveillance Initiative Working Group. Am J Infect Control 26:277-288, 1998.

Table 35–5 National Nosocomial Infections Surveillance NICU Birth Weight Categories

≤1000 g
1001-1500 g
1501-2500 g
>2500 g

NICU, neonatal intensive care unit.
Data from Centers for Disease Control and Prevention, Division of Health Care Quality Promotion. National Nosocomial Infections Surveillance (NNIS) system report, data summary from January 1992 to June 2003, issued August 2003. Am J Infect Control 30:481-498, 2003.

resulting from therapeutic or diagnostic interventions.[186] Risk stratification techniques that attempt to control for distribution of risk have included severity of illness score, intensity of care required, and birth weight.[74] Because the risk for developing nosocomial infection is greater for lower-birth-weight infants,[48] the NNIS system breaks down data collection and analysis into birth weight categories (Tables 35-5 and 35-6).[191,194] The use of invasive devices, however, also is an important factor to consider. The appropriate denominator for an infection related to the use of a medical device, such as a CVC-related primary bloodstream infection, according to NNIS, would be total device days for the population during the surveillance period.

The formula generally used for calculating nosocomial infection rates is (x/y)k, where x equals the number of events (infections) over a specific time period, y equals the population at risk for development of the outcome, and k is a constant and a multiple of 10. Rates can be expressed as a percentage (k = 100), although device-related infections usually are expressed as events per 1000 device days (k = 1000). A value should be selected for k that results in a rate greater than 1.[187]

Because use of invasive devices is such a significant risk factor both for bloodstream infection and ventilator-associated pneumonia, assessing NICU practices with device use may be warranted. NNIS provides a benchmark for NICU device utilization broken down into birth weight categories. An NICU device utilization ratio can be calculated using the following formula:

$$\frac{\text{Number of device days}}{\text{Number of patient days}}$$

In those units with device utilization ratios above the NNIS 90th percentile, investigation into the practices surrounding use of invasive devices may be warranted.[195] Calculating monthly and annual rates to employ as benchmarks can assist in identification of a potential problem in device-related procedures.

Surveillance data must be arranged and presented in a way that facilitates interpretation, comparison both directed internally and with comparable external benchmarks, and dissemination within the organization. Quality improvement tools (e.g., control and run charts) can be useful for these purposes. Statistical tools should be used to determine the significance of findings, although statistical significance should always be balanced with the evaluation of clinical

Table 35–6 Distribution of Device-Associated Infection Rates by Birth Weight Category[a]

	Pooled Mean	
Birth Weight (g)	Umbilical and CR-BSI[b]	VAP[c]
≤1000	10.6	3.3
1001-1500	6.4	2.5
1501-2500	4.1	2.1
>2500	3.7	1.4

[a]NICU component of reported data, January 1995 to June 2003 (VAP data are for January 2002 through June 2003 only).
[b]Number of umbilical and central line–related (CR) bloodstream infections (BSIs) × 1000/number of umbilical and central line days.
[c]Number of VAP cases × 1000/number of ventilator days.
NICU, neonatal intensive care unit; VAP, ventilator-associated pneumonia.
Data from Centers for Disease Control and Prevention, Division of Health Care Quality Promotion. National Nosocomial Infections Surveillance (NNIS) system report, data summary from January 1992 to June 2003, issued August 2003. Am J Infect Control 30:481-498, 2003.

significance.[187] External benchmarking through interhospital comparison is a valuable tool for improving quality of care[196,197] but should be performed only when surveillance methodologies (e.g., case definitions, case finding, data collection methods, intensity of surveillance)[187] can reasonably be assumed to be consistent between facilities.

Few overall infection rates in NICUs are available, but a small study done in 17 children's hospitals performing NICU nosocomial infection surveillance reported a median nosocomial infection rate of 8.9 infections per 1000 patient days (range, 4.6 to 18.1).[198] NNIS does not provide a benchmark for overall infection rates within NICUs. Instead, NNIS provides birth weight–stratified device-associated infection rates for umbilical and central intravascular line–associated bloodstream infections. The most recent rates for catheter-related bloodstream infections (137 to 143 NICUs reporting) and ventilator-associated pneumonias (78 to 96 NICUs reporting) are summarized in Table 35-6.[194]

Once arranged and interpreted, nosocomial infection data must be shared with personnel who can effect change and implement infection control interventions. Written reports summarizing the data and appropriate control charts should be provided to the facility's infection control committee, unit leaders, and members of the hospital administration on an ongoing basis. The interval between reports is determined by the needs of the institution. In addition to formal written reports, face-to-face reports are appropriate in the event of identification of a serious problem or an outbreak. ICPs can serve as consultants to assist NICU or neonatology service leaders in addressing infection rate increases or outbreak management.

Outbreak (Epidemic) Investigation

Surveillance activities typically identify endemic nosocomial infections (i.e., those infections that represent the usual level of disease within the nursery or NICU).[199] Although the rate can fluctuate over time, in the absence of interventions that

Table 35-7 Reported Nursery Outbreaks of Infection

Causative Organism	Source	Reference	Year	Location
Staphylococcus aureus (pyoderma)	Hospital staff	212	2002	Taipei, Taiwan
Staphylococcus aureus	Skin barrier paste (Stomahesive)	206	2000	Leeds, UK
MRSA	Horizontal transmission[a]?	207	2001	Washington, DC
Enterococcus faecium (VRE)	Unknown	79	2001	Omaha
Clostridium species	Horizontal transmission?	210	2002	Manitoba, Canada
Serratia marcescens	Horizontal transmission	204	1998	Leipzig, Germany
S. marcescens	Milk bottles	115	2002	Zurich
Enterobacter sakazakii	Powdered milk formula	201	1998	Brussels
Klebsiella pneumoniae, antibiotic-resistant	Environment, breast milk, horizontal transmission	106	2001	London
Acinetobacter species	Air conditioners	202	1996	Bahamas
Pseudomonas aeruginosa	Unknown	203	1999	Maryland
Chryselbacterium meningosepticum	Sink taps	211	1996	London
Salmonella enterica	Horizontal transmission	209	1999	Rio de Janeiro
Tuberculosis, multidrug-resistant	Hospital staff?	136	1998	New York
Adenovirus type 8	Horizontal transmission?	205	1998	Heidelberg, Germany
Parainfluenza virus type 3	Horizontal transmission?	161	1996	Winnipeg, Canada
Influenza A virus	Unknown	162	1999	Barcelona, Spain
Respiratory syncytial virus	Unknown	208	2002	Riyadh, Saudi Arabia
Rotavirus	Environment	157	2002	Holland

[a]Horizontal transmission refers to indirect contact transmission by contaminated equipment or health care workers' hands.
MRSA, methicillin-resistant *Staphylococcus aureus*; VRE, vancomycin-resistant enterococci.

successfully reduce risk of infection, the difference rarely is statistically significant. Establishing an NICU's endemic infection rate and expected variation around that rate allows the ICP to rapidly identify unusual increases in rates that may indicate on outbreak (epidemic) of a particular infection. Using baseline surveillance data along with aggregate data from sources such as the NNIS system allows the ICP to develop meaningful threshold rates for initiating outbreak investigation.[188] Alternatively, HCWs can be the first to sense an increase in infections, which then can be confirmed or refuted by surveillance data.[200] Even a single case of infection due to an unusual and potentially dangerous pathogen (e.g., *Salmonella*) can constitute the index case for a subsequent outbreak and thus merits rapid and comprehensive investigation. Outbreaks may need to be reported to health authorities, depending on local and state requirements as well as the organism involved.

Numerous studies have described nursery and NICU epidemics caused by a variety of pathogens (Table 35-7), and most such epidemics have required the coordinated efforts of ICPs, NICU leadership, staff, and hospital administration for resolution.[79,106,115,136,157,161,162,201-212] Outbreak investigation and intervention should be approached systematically, applying sound epidemiologic principles. In general, the process should include the following[199,200]:

Confirming that an outbreak exists, by comparing the outbreak infection rate with baseline data (or with rates reported in the literature if baseline data are not available), and communicating concerns to stakeholders within the institution (and to those in other agencies if notification of health authorities is necessary)

Assembling the appropriate personnel to assist in developing a case definition and in planning immediate measures to prevent new cases

Performing active surveillance using the case definition to search for additional infections and collecting critical data and specimens

Characterizing cases of infection by person, place, and time, including plotting of an epidemic curve (to facilitate identification of shared risk factors among involved patients, such as invasive devices, proximity to other infected patients or temporal association with infection in such patients, common underlying diagnoses, shared medical or nursing staff, surgery, and medications, including antimicrobial agents)

Formulating a working hypothesis and testing this hypothesis (if the severity of the problem warrants this level of study, and provided that the institution has and can commit the necessary resources), with use of analytic approaches, including case-control and cohort studies, as appropriate to determine the likely cause of the outbreak

Instituting and evaluating control measures, which can be implemented anywhere in the foregoing process (more directed measures become possible as more is learned about the outbreak, and efficacy of control measures can be judged on whether the outbreak resolves, as indicated by return of number of cases to endemic levels or by cessation of occurrence of infections)

Reporting findings to appropriate personnel, including unit staff, hospital administration, and public health authorities (if involved in management of the outbreak), in comprehensive written reports, including summaries of how the outbreak was first recognized, study and analysis methods used, interventions implemented to resolve the epidemic, results, and a discussion of any other important outcomes or surveillance and control measures identified

Interventions used to control and limit outbreaks usually have consisted of isolation and cohorting of infected or colonized infants to prevent transmission of organisms. Transmission-based precautions, a system developed by the CDC, can be used to determine the most effective barrier precautions to use with affected patients. Cohorting, or placing infants infected or colonized with the outbreak organism together in geographically segregated areas and assigning dedicated staff and equipment to their care, also has been used successfully to halt outbreaks in nurseries and NICUs. In extreme cases, closure of an NICU to admissions has been necessary to bring an outbreak under control.[57,106,161]

Every attempt should be made to identify the source of a nursery outbreak, although this is not always possible. Sources implicated in NICU outbreaks have included medications, equipment, and enteral feeding solutions; person-to-person transmission and environmental reservoirs also have been reported.[102,106,157,201,202,213] Efforts to identify the source may include culturing of specimens from HCWs, equipment, and the environment, although careful consideration should be given to the potential benefits before initiating these measures. Culture of samples from the environment and equipment, in view of the vast number of objects that could be contaminated, usually is not helpful in identifying the source of an outbreak unless specific case characteristics or microbiologic data strongly suggest the location. Culture of specimens obtained from HCWs when person-to-person transmission is suspected may be more likely to identify the source of an outbreak, but it must be remembered that an HCW whose culture specimen yields the outbreak organism may have been transiently colonized while working with an affected infant, rather than constituting the source of the infection. Management of culture-positive HCWs (possible furlough, treatment, and return to work criteria) should be planned in advance of widespread culture surveillance and should involve supervisors of affected employees and occupational health services.[200]

Standard and Transmission-Based Precautions in the Nursery

The most widely accepted guideline for preventing the transmission of infections in hospitals was developed by the CDC. Most recently revised in 1996, the system contains two tiers of precautions. The first and most important, *standard precautions*, was designed for the management of all hospitalized patients regardless of their diagnosis or presumed infection status. The second, *transmission-based precautions*, is intended for patients documented or suspected to be infected or colonized with highly transmissible or epidemiologically important pathogens for which additional precautions to interrupt transmission are needed.[25]

Standard precautions are designed to reduce the risk of transmission of microorganisms from both recognized and unrecognized sources and are to be followed for the care of all patients, including neonates. They apply to blood; all body fluids, secretions, and excretions except sweat; nonintact skin; and mucous membranes. Components of standard precautions include hand hygiene and wearing gloves, gowns, and masks and other forms of eye protection.

Hand hygiene plays a key role for caregivers in the reduction of nosocomial infection for patients[27,214] and in prevention of nosocomial or health care–associated infections. Hand hygiene should be performed before and after all patient contacts; before donning sterile gloves to perform an invasive procedure; after contact with blood, body fluids or excretions, mucous membranes, nonintact skin, and wound dressings; in moving from a contaminated body site to a clean body site during patient care (i.e., from changing a diaper to performing mouth care); after contact with inanimate objects in the immediate vicinity of the patient; after removing gloves; and before eating and after using the restroom.[131] When hands are visibly soiled or contaminated with proteinaceous materials, blood, or body fluids, and after using the restroom, hands should be washed with antimicrobial soap and water. Soaps containing 2% to 4% chlorhexidine gluconate or 0.3% triclosan[156] are recommended for hand washing in nurseries.[192] When hands are not visibly soiled, alcohol-based hand rubs, foams, or gels are an important tool for hand hygiene. Compared with washing with soap and water, use of the alcohol-based products is at least as effective against a variety of pathogens and requires less time, and these agents are less damaging to skin. The CDC "Guideline for Hand Hygiene in the Health Care Setting" calls for use of alcohol hand rubs, foams, or gels as the primary method to clean hands, except when hands are visibly soiled.[131] Programs that have been successful in improving hand hygiene and decreasing nosocomial infection have used multidisciplinary teams to develop interventions focusing on use of the alcohol rubs in the setting of institutional commitment and support for the initiative.[27,215]

HCWs should wash hands and forearms to the elbows on arrival in the nursery. A 3-minute scrub has been suggested,[216] but consensus on optimal duration of initial hand hygiene is lacking. At a minimum, the initial wash should be long enough to ensure thorough washing and rinsing of all parts of the hands and forearms. Routine hand washing throughout care delivery should consist of wetting the hands, applying product, rubbing all surfaces of the hands and fingers vigorously for at least 15 seconds, rinsing, and patting dry with disposable towels.[131] Wearing hand jewelry has been associated with increased microbial load on hands. Whether this results in increased transmission of pathogens is not known. Many experts, however, recommend that hand and wrist jewelry not be worn in the nursery.[217,218] In addition, the CDC guideline states that staff who have direct contact with infants in NICUs should not wear artificial fingernails or nail extenders.[131] Only natural nails kept less than ¼ inch long should be allowed.

Clean, nonsterile **gloves** are to be worn whenever contact with blood, body fluids, secretions, excretions, and contaminated items is anticipated. The HCW should change gloves when moving from dirty to clean tasks performed on the same patient, such as after changing a diaper and before suctioning a patient, and whenever they become soiled. Because hands can become contaminated during removal of gloves, and because gloves may have tiny, unnoticeable defects, wearing gloves is not a substitute for hand hygiene. Hand hygiene must be performed immediately after glove removal.[25]

Personnel in nurseries including the NICU historically have worn cover gowns for all routine patient contact. The practice has not been found to reduce infection or colonization in neonates and is unnecessary.[219,220] Instead, CDC guidelines recommend nonsterile, fluid-resistant **gowns** to be worn as barrier protection when soiling of clothing is anticipated and in performing procedures likely to result in splashing or spraying of body substances.[25] Possible examples of such procedures in the NICU are placing an arterial line and irrigating a wound. The Perinatal Guidelines of the American Academy of Pediatrics and the American College of Obstetricians and Gynecologists recommend that a long-sleeved gown be worn over clothing when a neonate is held outside the bassinette by nursery personnel.[221]

Nonsterile **masks**, face shields, goggles, and other eye protectors are worn in various combinations to provide barrier protection and should be used during procedures and patient care activities that are likely to generate splashes or sprays of body substances and fluids.[25]

Standard precautions also require that reusable patient care equipment be cleaned and appropriately reprocessed between patients; that soiled linen be handled carefully to prevent contamination of skin, clothing, or the environment; that sharps (i.e., needles, scalpels) be handled carefully to prevent exposure to blood-borne pathogens; and that mouthpieces and other resuscitation devices be used, rather than mouth-to-mouth methods of resuscitation.[25]

In addition to standard precautions, which must be used for every patient, the CDC recommends transmission-based precautions when the patient is known or suspected to be infected or colonized with epidemiologically important or highly transmissible organisms. Always used in addition to standard precautions, transmission-based precautions comprise three categories: contact precautions, droplet precautions, and airborne precautions.

Contact precautions involve the use of barriers to prevent transmission of organisms by direct or indirect contact with the patient or contaminated objects in the patient's immediate environment.[25] Sources of indirect contact transmission in nurseries can include patient care equipment such as monitor leads, thermometers, isolettes, breast pumps,[186] toys, and instruments and contaminated hands.[222]

The patient requiring contact precautions should be placed in a private room whenever possible but, after consultation with an infection control practitioner, can be cohorted with a patient infected with the same microorganism but no other infection.[25] Many nurseries, however, have few if any isolation rooms. The American Academy of Pediatrics states that infected neonates requiring contact precautions can be safely cared for without an isolation room if staffing is adequate to allow appropriate hand hygiene, a 4- to 6-foot-wide space can be provided between care stations, adequate hand hygiene facilities are available, and staff members are well trained regarding infection transmission modes.[221]

HCWs should wear clean, nonsterile gloves when entering the room or space of a patient requiring contact precautions and should wear a cover gown when their clothing will have contact with the infant, environmental surfaces, or items in the infant's area. A cover gown also should be worn when the infant has excretions or secretions that are not well contained, such as diarrhea or wound drainage, which may escape the diaper or dressing. Infant care equipment should be dedicated to the patient if possible so that it is not shared with others.[25]

Examples of conditions in the neonate that require contact precautions include neonatal mucocutaneous herpes simplex virus infection, respiratory syncytial virus infection, varicella (also see airborne precautions), infection or colonization with a resistant organism such as MRSA or a multiple drug–resistant gram-negative bacillus, and congenital rubella syndrome.

Droplet precautions are intended to reduce the risk of transmission of infectious agents in large-particle droplets from an infected person. Such transmission usually occurs when the infected person generates droplets during coughing, sneezing, or talking, or during procedures such as suctioning. These relatively large droplets travel only short distances and do not remain suspended in the air, but can be deposited on the conjunctiva, nasal mucosa, and/or mouth of persons working within 3 feet of the infected patient.[25] Patients requiring droplet precautions should be placed in private rooms (see earlier discussion of isolation rooms in nurseries in the paragraph on contact precautions), and staff should wear masks when working within 3 feet of the patient.[25] Examples of conditions in the neonate that necessitate droplet precautions are pertussis and invasive *N. meningitidis* infection.

Airborne precautions are designed to reduce the risk of airborne transmission of infectious agents.[25] Because of their small size, airborne droplet nuclei and dust particles containing infectious agents or spores can be widely spread on air currents or through ventilation systems and inhaled by or deposited on susceptible hosts. Special air-handling systems and ventilation are required to prevent transmission. Patients requiring airborne precautions should be placed in private rooms in negative air-pressure ventilation with 6 to 12 air changes per hour. Air should be externally exhausted or subjected to high-efficiency particulate air (HEPA) filtration if it is recirculated.[222]

Examples of conditions in the neonate for which airborne precautions are required are varicella-zoster virus infections and measles. Susceptible HCWs should not enter the rooms of patients with these viral infections. If assignment cannot be avoided, susceptible staff members should wear masks to deliver care. If immunity has been documented, staff members need not wear masks.[222] Airborne precautions also are required for active pulmonary tuberculosis, and although neonates are rarely contagious, the CDC recommends isolating patients while they are being evaluated.[213] A more important consideration is the need to isolate the family of a suspected tuberculosis patient until an evaluation for pulmonary tuberculosis has been completed, because the source of infection frequently is a member of the child's family.[223,224]

Physical Environment

Before the 1990s, well-baby nurseries and many NICUs were constructed as large, brightly lit open wards with rows of incubators surrounded by equipment. Sinks could be provided in such rooms only around the periphery, limiting access to hand hygiene facilities for staff and families. In these NICUs, parents' time with their infant was severely restricted, and the units were designed for the convenience and function of the HCW.[225] More recently, perinatal care professionals have come to understand that neonates (and especially preterm infants) can benefit from a quiet, soothing atmosphere and protection from unnecessary light, noise, handling, uncomfortable positioning, and sleep disruptions.[226]

If infants are kept in a central nursery rather than rooming-in with mothers, at least 30 square feet of floor space should be provided per neonate, and bassinets should be at least 3 feet apart.[216] Teams designing units delivering higher levels of perinatal care, including NICUs, should plan individual bed areas large enough for families to stay at the bedside for extended periods of time without interfering with the staff's ability to care for the child. If individual rooms cannot be provided, at least 150 square feet of floor space should be allowed for each neonate in an NICU, incubators or overhead warmers should be separated by at least 6 to 8 feet, and aisles should be at least 8 feet wide.[216,227]

A scrub sink with foot, knee, or touchless (electronic sensor) controls should be provided at the entrance to every nursery and should be large and deep enough to control splashing. Sinks in patient care areas should be provided at a minimum ratio of 1 sink for at least every 6 to 8 stations in the well-baby nursery and 1 sink for every 3 or 4 stations in higher-level nurseries, including the NICU.[216] Every bed position should be within 20 feet of a hand-washing sink and accessible for children and persons in wheelchairs.[227] For NICUs composed of individual rooms, a hand-washing sink should be located in each room near the door to facilitate hand hygiene on entering and leaving the room.

Environmental surfaces should be designed so that they are easy to clean and do not harbor microorganisms. Sink taps and drains, for instance, have been implicated in outbreaks of infection.[228,229] Installing sinks with seamless construction may minimize this risk by decreasing areas where water can pool and microorganisms proliferate. Faucet aerators have been implicated in outbreaks of infection and should be avoided in the intensive care unit.[230] Although carpeting can reduce noise levels in a busy NICU, the CDC "Guidelines for Environmental Infection Control in Health-Care Facilities" recommend against use of carpeting in areas where spills are likely, including intensive care units. The guidelines further recommend against upholstered furniture in NICUs.[231] If, for reasons of noise reduction and developmentally appropriate care, porous surfaces such as carpeting and cloth upholstery are selected for the NICU, cleaning must be performed carefully. Carpet should be vacuumed regularly with equipment fitted with HEPA filters, and upholstered furniture should be removed from inpatient areas to be cleaned.

Attention also should be paid to air-handling systems. According to the Perinatal Guidelines, minimal standards for inpatient perinatal care areas include six air changes per hour, and a minimum of two changes should consist entirely of outside air. Air delivered to the NICU should be filtered with at least 90% efficiency. In addition, nurseries should include at least one isolation room capable of providing negative pressure vented to the outside, observation windows with blinds for privacy, and the capability for remote monitoring.[227,232]

General Housekeeping

Floors and other horizontal surfaces should be cleaned daily by trained personnel using Environmental Protection Agency (EPA)–registered hospital disinfectants/detergents. These products (including phenolics and other chemical surface disinfectants) must be prepared in accordance with manufacturers' recommendations and used carefully to avoid exposing neonates to these products. Phenolics should not be used on surfaces that come in direct contact with neonates' skin.[231] High-touch areas, such as counter tops, work surfaces, doorknobs, and light switches, may need to be cleaned more frequently because they can be heavily contaminated during the process of delivering care. Hard, nonporous surfaces should be "wet dusted" rather than dry dusted, to avoid dispersing particulates into the air, and then disinfected using standard hospital disinfectants.[231] Sinks should be scrubbed daily with a disinfectant detergent. Walls, windows, and curtains should be cleaned regularly to prevent dust accumulation, but daily cleaning is not necessary unless they are visibly soiled.

Bassinets and incubators should be cleaned and disinfected between infants, but care must be taken to rinse cleaning products from surfaces with water before use. Care units should not be cleaned with phenolics or other chemical germicides during an infant's stay. Instead, infants who remain in the nursery for long periods of time should periodically be moved to freshly cleaned and disinfected units.[231]

Patient care equipment must be cleaned, disinfected, and, when appropriate, sterilized between patients. Sterilization (required for devices that enter the vascular system, tissue, or sterile body cavities) and higher levels of disinfection (required for equipment that comes in contact with mucous membranes or that has prolonged or intimate contact with the newborn's skin) must be performed under controlled conditions in the central processing department of the hospital. Examples of patient care equipment that require these levels of processing are endotracheal tubes, resuscitation bags, and face masks.[216,232,233] Low-level disinfection is required for less critical equipment, such as stethoscopes or blood pressure cuffs, and usually can be performed at point of use (e.g., the bedside), although this type of equipment should be dedicated to individual patients whenever possible.

Linens

Requirements for linen handling and management for neonates do not vary appreciably from those for other hospitalized patients. Although soiled linen can contain large numbers of organisms capable of causing infections, transmission to patients appears to be rare. Studies suggesting linen as a source of infection often have failed to confirm it as the source of infection.[234] At least one report, however, has implicated linen in the transmission of group A streptococci.[85] Investigation of this outbreak revealed that clothing worn by the neonates was being washed in the local hospital "mini laundry," rather than being processed under the usual laundry contract. Investigation of the dryers revealed extensive contamination with the outbreak organism. This case illustrates the importance of having standard hospital laundry protocols and ensuring that appropriate water and dryer temperatures are maintained. When such protocols are followed, the mechanical actions of washing and rinsing, combined with hot water and/or the addition of chemicals such as chlorine bleach, and a final commercial dryer and/or ironing step significantly reduce bacterial counts.[235,236] Few hospitals in the United States use cloth diapers, but regardless of type used, soiled diapers should be carefully bagged in plastic and removed from the unit every 8 hours.[216]

Health Care Workers

HCWs caring for neonates have the potential both to transmit infections to infants and to acquire infections from

Table 35–8 Immunizing Agents Strongly Recommended for Health Care Workers

Vaccine	Recommendation
Hepatitis B recombinant vaccine	Vaccinate all HCWs at risk of exposure to blood and body fluids.
Influenza vaccine	Vaccinate HCWs annually.
Measles live-virus vaccine	Vaccine should be considered for all HCWs, including those born before 1957, who have no proof of immunity (receipt of 2 doses of live vaccine on or after first birthday, physician-diagnosed measles, or serologic evidence of immunity).
Mumps live-virus vaccine	HCWs believed to be susceptible can be vaccinated; adults born before 1957 can be considered immune.
Rubella live-virus vaccine	HCWs, both male and female, who lack documentation of receipt of vaccine on or after first birthday or serologic evidence of immunity should be vaccinated; adults born before 1957 can be considered immune, except women of childbearing age.
Varicella-zoster live-virus vaccine	HCWs without a reliable history of varicella or serologic evidence of varicella immunity should be vaccinated.

HCW, health care worker.
Data from Bolyard EA, Tablan OC, Williams WW, et al. Guideline for infection control in health care personnel, 1998. Hospital Infection Control Practices Advisory Committee. Infect Control Hosp Epidemiol 19:407-463, 1998.

patients. Educating HCWs about infection control principles is crucial to preventing such transmission. Hospitals should provide education about infection control policies, procedures, and guidelines to staff in all job categories during new employee orientation and on a regular basis throughout employment. The content of this education should include hand hygiene, principles of infection control, the importance of individual responsibility for infection control, and the importance of collaborating with the infection control department in monitoring and investigating potentially harmful infectious exposures and outbreaks.

Transmission of infectious organisms between patients and HCWs has been well documented. Several studies have indicated that a high proportion of HCWs acquire RSV (34% to 56%) when working with infected children, and these workers appear to be important in the spread of the illness within hospitals.[237-239] Although 82% of the infected HCWs in one of these RSV studies were asymptomatic, staff should be aware of the importance of self-screening for communicable disease. They should be encouraged to report personal infectious illnesses to supervisors, who in turn should report them to occupational health services and infection control. In general, HCWs with respiratory, cutaneous, mucocutaneous, or gastrointestinal infections should not deliver direct patient care to neonates.[216] In addition, seronegative staff members exposed to illnesses, such as varicella and measles, should not work during the contagious portion of the incubation period.[232]

Staff members with HSV infection rarely have been implicated in transmission of the virus to infants and thus do not need to be routinely excluded from direct patient care. Those with herpes labialis or cold sores should be instructed to cover the lesions and not to touch their lesions, and to comply with hand hygiene policies. Persons with genital lesions also are unlikely to transmit HSV so long as hand hygiene policies are followed. However, HCWs who are unlikely or unable to comply with the infection control measures and those with herpetic whitlow should not deliver direct patient care to neonates until lesions have healed.[240]

Acquisition of CMV often is a concern of pregnant HCWs because of the potential effect on the fetus. Approximately 1% of newborn infants in most nurseries and a higher percentage of older children (up to 70% of children 1 to 3 years of age in child-care centers) excrete CMV without clinical manifestations.[241] The risk of acquiring CMV infection has not been shown to be higher for HCWs than for the general population.[242,243] For this reason, pregnant caregivers need not be excluded from the care of neonates suspected to be shedding CMV. They should be advised of the importance of standard precautions.

HCWs in well-baby nurseries and NICUs should be as free from transmissible infectious diseases as possible,[216] and ensuring that they are immune to vaccine-preventable diseases is an essential part of a personnel health program. The CDC recommends several immunizations for health care personnel (Table 35-8).

Staffing levels in a patient care setting also can affect patient outcomes. A number of studies suggest that as patient-to-nurse ratios in intensive care units increase, so do nosocomial infections and mortality rates.[47,132,244] Although optimal staffing ratios have not been established for NICUs and will vary according to characteristics of individual units, one study demonstrated that the incidence of clustered *S. aureus* infections was 16 times higher after periods when the infant-to-nurse ratio exceeded 7:1. Decreased compliance with hand hygiene during a period of understaffing frequently is cited as contributing to nosocomial infection rate increases.[98] Further study is necessary to determine best practice surrounding staffing levels in NICUs.

Family-Centered Care: Parents and Visitors to the Newborn Infant

The first NICUs in the late 1960s grouped infants together in large, brightly lit rooms with incubators placed in rows. Parents were allowed very little time with their babies and even less physical contact. In the decades since, it has been recognized that "the parent is the most important caregiver and constant influence in an infant's life"[225] and that HCWs working in NICUs should encourage parents to become involved in the nonmedical aspects of their child's care. Principles of family-centered care also include liberal NICU visitation for relatives, siblings, and family friends and the involvement of parents in the development of nursery policies and programs that promote parenting skills.[226]

Care must be taken, however, to minimize risk of infection for the neonate. Mothers can transmit infections to neonates both during delivery and post partum, although separation of mother and newborn rarely is indicated. In the absence of certain specific infections, mothers, including those with postpartum fever not attributed to a specific infection, should be allowed to handle their infants if the following conditions are met:

- They feel well enough.
- They wash their hands well under supervision.
- A clean gown is worn.
- Contact of the neonate with contaminated dressings, linen, clothing, or pads is avoided.[245]

A mother with a transmissible illness not requiring separation from her infant should be carefully educated about the mode of transmission and precautions necessary to protect her infant. Personal protective equipment, such as cover gowns, gloves, and masks, and hand hygiene facilities should be readily available to her, and she should perform hand hygiene and don a long-sleeved cover gown before handling her infant. If wounds or abscesses are present, drainage should be contained within a dressing. If drainage cannot be completely contained, separation from the infant may be necessary. Care should be taken to prevent the infant from coming in contact with soiled linens, clothing, dressings, or other potentially contaminated items. The mother with active genital HSV lesions need not be separated from her infant if the foregoing precautions are taken. Those with herpes labialis should not kiss or nuzzle their infants until lesions have cleared; lesions should be covered and a surgical mask may be worn until the lesions are crusted and dry, and careful hand hygiene should be stressed.

Mothers with viral respiratory infections should be made aware that many of these illnesses are transmitted by contact with infected secretions as well as by droplet spread, that soiled tissues should be disposed of carefully, and that hand hygiene is critical to transmission prevention. Masks can be worn to reduce the risk of droplet transmission.[221,232]

As previously mentioned, although very few infections require separation of mother and infant, women with untreated active pulmonary tuberculosis should be separated from their infants until they no longer are contagious. Mothers with group A streptococcal infections, especially when involving draining wounds, also should be isolated from their infants until they no longer are contagious. Less certain is the necessity of separating mothers with peripartum varicella (onset of infection within 5 days before or 2 days after delivery) from their uninfected infants. The Perinatal Guidelines recommend that such infants remain with their mothers after receiving varicella-zoster immune globulin (VZIG) but caution that infant and mother must be carefully managed in airborne and contact precautions[245] to prevent transmission within the nursery. Some experts recommend separating these mothers from their infants until all lesions are dried and crusted.[246]

Breast-feeding

Numerous studies support the value of human milk for infants (see Chapter 5). Besides providing optimal nutritional content for infants, it has been shown to be associated with a lower incidence of infections and sepsis in the first year of life.[16,247] Although contraindications to breast-feeding are few, mothers who have active untreated tuberculosis, human immunodeficiency virus (HIV) infection, breast abscesses (as opposed to simple mastitis that is being treated with antimicrobial therapy), or HSV lesions around the nipples should not breast-feed. Mothers who are hepatitis B surface antigen positive may breast-feed, because ingestion of an infected mother's milk has not been shown to increase the risk of transmission to her child, but the infant must receive hepatitis B virus immune globulin (HBIG) and vaccine immediately after birth.[248] Because systemic disease may develop in preterm infants with low concentrations of transplacentally acquired antibodies to CMV following ingestion of milk of CMV-seropositive mothers, decisions regarding breast-feeding should consider the benefits of human milk versus the risk of CMV transmission. Freezing breast milk has been shown to decrease viral titers but does not eliminate CMV; pasteurization of human milk can inactivate CMV. Either method may be considered in attempts to decrease risk of transmission for breast-feeding NICU neonates.[249]

Neonates in the NICU frequently are incapable of breast-feeding because of maternal separation, unstable respiratory status, and immaturity of the sucking reflex. For these reasons, mothers of such infants must use a breast pump to collect milk for administration through a feeding tube. Pumping, collection, and storage of breast milk create opportunities for contamination of the milk, and for cross-infection if equipment is shared between mothers. Several studies have demonstrated contamination of breast pumps, contamination of expressed milk that had been frozen and thawed, and higher levels of stool colonization with aerobic bacteria in infants fed precollected breast milk.[16,250,251]

Consensus is lacking on the safe level of microbiologic contamination of breast milk, and most expressed breast milk contains normal skin flora. Although breast milk containing greater than 100 CFU/mL of gram-negative bacteria has been reported to cause feeding intolerance and to be associated with suspected sepsis, routine bacterial culturing of expressed breast milk is not recommended.[249,250] Instead, efforts to ensure safety of expressed milk should focus on optimal collection, storage, and administration techniques. Cleaning and disinfection of breast pumps should be included in educational material provided to nursing mothers (Table 35-9). In addition, mothers should be instructed to perform hand hygiene and cleanse nipples with cotton and plain water before expressing milk in sterile containers.[192,249]

Expressed breast milk can be refrigerated for up to 48 hours and can be safely frozen (−20° C ± 2° C [−4° F ± 3.6° F]) for up to 6 months.[192] It can be thawed quickly under warm running water (avoiding contamination with tap water) or gradually in a refrigerator. Exposure to high temperatures, as may be experienced in a microwave, can destroy valuable components of the milk. Thawed breast milk can be stored in the refrigerator for up to 24 hours before it must be discarded. To avoid proliferation of microorganisms, milk administered through a feeding tube by continuous infusion should hang no longer than 4 to 6 hours before replacement of the milk, container, and tubing.[245]

For mothers who choose not to breast-feed, commercial infant formula is available. Most hospitals now use sterile, ready-to-feed formulas provided by the manufacturer in bottles, with sterile nipples to attach just before use. Nipples

Table 35–9 Collection and Storage of Expressed Breast Milk

Each mother is supplied with a personal pumping kit.
Nursing staff instruct mothers in techniques of milk expression and appropriate procedures for cleaning breast pump parts:
Wipe all horizontal surfaces at the pumping station with hospital disinfectant before and after pumping.
Wash hands with soapy water before and after pumping.
Wash all parts of the breast pump kit that have been in contact with milk in hot water and dish detergent or in a dishwasher.
Expressed milk is collected in sterile, single-use plastic (polycarbonate or polypropylene) containers.
Breast milk containers are labeled with infant's name and the date and time of collection.
Administration containers (bottle or syringe) are similarly labeled when breast milk is transferred from collection containers.
All HCWs wear gloves when handling and administering breast milk.
Two persons check the labeled administration container against the infant's hospital identification band before administering breast milk (may be two HCWs or one HCW and a family member).

HCW, health care worker.
From Infection Control Policy, Children's Hospital and Regional Medical Center, Seattle, 2003.

are best attached at the bedside just before feeding, and the unit should be used immediately and discarded within 4 hours after the bottle is uncapped.[245]

Specialty and less commonly used formulas may not be available as a ready-to-feed product, and breast milk supplements do not come in liquid form. After a recent report of a case of fatal *Enterobacter sakazakii* meningitis in a neonate fed contaminated powdered infant formula,[97] concerns have risen about the safety of these products. Although powdered formulas are not sterile, preparation and storage practices can decrease the possibility of proliferation of microorganisms after preparation. The CDC, the Food and Drug Administration, and the American Dietetic Association offered updated recommendations on the safe preparation and administration of commercial formula after the recall of the product linked to the *E. sakazakii* case. These recommendations instruct the care provider as follows:

- Use alternatives (ready-to-feed or concentrated formulas) to powdered infant formula whenever possible.
- Prepare formula using aseptic technique in a designated formula preparation room.
- Refrigerate prepared formula so that a temperature of 2° to 3° C is reached by 4 hours after preparation, and discard any reconstituted formula stored longer than 24 hours.
- Limit ambient-temperature hang time of continuously infused formula to no longer than 4 hours.
- Use hygienic handling techniques at feeding time, and avoid open delivery systems.
- Have written guidelines for managing a manufacturer's recall of contaminated formula.[252]

The FDA also recommended that boiling water be used to prepare powdered formulas, but concerns about this recommendation include potential damage to formula components from the high temperature of the water, a lack of evidence that using this method would kill potential pathogens in the formula, and risk of injury to persons preparing the formula.[252]

Co-bedding

The concept of co-bedding, or the bunking of twin infants (or other multiples) in a single isolette or crib, is being explored in NICUs for the potential benefits offered to the babies. Co-bedding as a component of developmentally supportive care is based on the premise that extrauterine adaptation of twin neonates is enhanced by continued physical contact with the other twin.[253] Potential benefits need further study but may include increased bonding, decreased need for temperature support, and easier transition to home. It is certainly possible, however, for one of a set of multiples to be infected while the others are not, and for parents to be implicated as vectors in infection transmission. It also is possible for invasive devices and intravascular catheters to be dislodged by close contact with an active sibling. Therefore, exclusion criteria for co-bedding infants should include clinical findings suggesting infection that could be transmitted to a sibling (e.g., draining wound) and the need for drains and central venous or arterial lines.[253-255]

Visitors

The principles of family-centered care encourage liberal visitation policies, both in the well-baby nursery (or rooming-in scenario) and in the NICU. Parents, including fathers, should be allowed unlimited visitation to their newborns, and siblings also should be allowed liberal visitation. Expanding the number of visitors to neonates may, however, increase the risk of disease exposure if education and screening for symptoms of infection are not implemented. Written policies should be in place to guide sibling visits, and parents should be encouraged to share the responsibility of protecting their newborn from contagious illnesses. The Perinatal Guidelines regarding persons who visit newborns are listed in Table 35-10.

Adult visitors to neonates, including parents, have been implicated in outbreaks of infections including *P. aeruginosa* infection, pertussis, and *Salmonella* infection.[132,255,256] Accordingly, the principles for sibling visitation should be applied to adult visitors as well. They should be screened for symptoms of contagious illness, instructed to perform hand hygiene before entering the NICU and before and after touching the neonate, and should interact only with the family member they came to the hospital to visit. Families of neonates who have lengthy NICU stays may come to know each other well and serve as sources of emotional support to one another. Nevertheless, they should be educated about the potential of transmitting microorganisms and infections between families if standard precautions and physical separation are not maintained, even though they may be sharing an inpatient space.

Table 35–10 Guidelines for Sibling Visits to Well-Baby and High-Risk Nurseries

Sibling visits should be encouraged for healthy and ill newborns.
Parents should be interviewed at a site outside the nursery to establish that the siblings are not ill before allowing them to visit.
Children with fever or other symptoms of an acute illness such as upper respiratory infection or gastroenteritis, or those recently exposed to a known communicable disease such as chickenpox, should not be allowed to visit.
Visiting children should visit only their sibling.
Children should be prepared in advance for their visit.
Visitors should be adequately observed and monitored by hospital staff.
Children should carefully wash their hands before patient contact.
Throughout the visit, siblings should be supervised by parents or another responsible adult.

Data from American Academy of Pediatrics and American College of Obstetricians and Gynecologists. Care of the neonate. *In* Gilstrap LC, Oh W (eds). Guidelines for Perinatal Care, 5th ed. Elk Grove Village, Ill, American Academy of Pediatrics, and Washington DC, American College of Obstetricians and Gynecologists, 2002, pp 331-353.

Skin and Cord Care

Bathing the newborn is standard practice in nurseries, but very little standardization in frequency or cleansing product exists. If not performed carefully, bathing actually can be detrimental to the infant, resulting in hypothermia, increased crying with resulting increases in oxygen consumption, respiratory distress, and instability of vital signs.[257] Although the initial bath or cleansing should be delayed until the neonate's temperature has been stable for several hours, removing blood and drying the skin immediately after delivery may remove potentially infectious microorganisms such as hepatitis B virus, HSV, and HIV, minimizing risk to the neonate from maternal infection.[249] When the newborn requires an intramuscular injection in the delivery room, infection sites should be cleansed with alcohol to prevent transmission of organisms that may be present in maternal blood and body fluids.[195] For routine bathing in the first few weeks of life, plain warm water should be used. This is especially important for preterm infants, as well as full-term infants with barrier compromise such as abrasions or dermatitis. If a soap is necessary for heavily soiled areas, a mild pH-neutral product without additives should be used, and duration of soaping should be restricted to less than 5 minutes no more than three times per week.[257]

Few randomized studies comparing cord care regimens and infection rates have been performed, and consensus has not been reached on best practice regarding care of the umbilical cord stump. A review published in 2003 described care regimens used for more than 2 decades, including combinations of triple dye, chlorhexidine, 70% alcohol, bacitracin, hexachlorophene, povidone-iodine, and "dry care" (soap and water cleansing of soiled periumbilical skin) and found variable impact on colonization of the stump.[258] The study authors suggested that dry cord care alone may be insufficient and that chlorhexidine seemed to be a favorable antiseptic choice for cord care because of its activity against gram-positive and gram-negative bacteria. They went on to stress, however, that large, well-designed studies were required before firm conclusions could be drawn. The current Perinatal Guidelines do not recommend a specific regimen but warn that use of alcohol alone is not an effective method of preventing umbilical cord colonization and omphalitis.[249] The Perinatal Guidelines further recommend that diapers be folded away from and below the stump and that emollients not be applied to the stump.[257]

Ocular Prophylaxis

Although blindness resulting from neonatal conjunctivitis is rare in the United States, with a reported incidence of 1.6% or less, the rate among the 80 million infants born annually throughout the world is as high as 23%.[259] *Chlamydia trachomatis* has been the most common etiologic agent in the United States, but other organisms such as *Neisseria gonorrhoeae, S. aureus*, and *E. coli* also can cause ophthalmia neonatorum.[260] Use of 1% silver nitrate drops, at one time the agent of choice, is no longer recommended because of concerns about associated chemical irritation. Agents thought to be equally efficacious and now recommended include 1% tetracycline and 0.5% erythromycin ophthalmic ointments, administered from sterile single-use tubes or vials.[156,245] Povidone-iodine (2.5%) ophthalmic solution also can be used and in one study was shown to be more effective than silver nitrate or erythromycin in the prevention of ophthalmia neonatorum. Bacterial resistance has not been seen with this agent, it causes less toxicity than either silver nitrate or erythromycin, and it is less expensive—a definite consideration in developing countries.[259] Whatever the agent selected, it should reach all parts of the conjunctival sac, and the eyes should not be irrigated after application.

Ophthalmic agents will not necessarily prevent ocular or disseminated gonorrhea in infants born to mothers with active infection at time of delivery. These infants should be given parenteral antimicrobial therapy as well as ocular prophylaxis.[195,261] Some experts also advise giving infants born to mothers with untreated genital chlamydial infections a course of oral erythromycin beginning on the second or third day of life.[261]

Device-Related Infections

Primary Bloodstream Infections

Primary bloodstream infections (defined by the CDC NNIS System as being due to a pathogen cultured from one or more blood specimens not related to an infection at another site) account for a large proportion of infections in NICU infants,[21] and most are related to the use of an intravascular catheter.[36] Peripheral intravenous catheters (PIVs) are the most frequently used devices for the neonate for intravenous therapy of short duration. When longer access is necessary, nontunneled CVCs such as umbilical catheters and PICCs most commonly are used.[195] The most recent data available

Table 35–11 Strategies for Prevention of Catheter-Related Bloodstream Infections in Adult and Pediatric Patients

Conduct surveillance in NICUs to determine catheter-related bloodstream infection rates, monitor trends, and identify infection control lapses.
Investigate events leading to unexpected life-threatening or fatal outcomes.
Select the catheter, insertion technique, and insertion site with the lowest risk for complications for the anticipated type and duration of intravenous therapy.
Use a CVC with the minimal number of ports essential for management of the patient. Designate one port for hyperalimentation if a multilumen catheter is used.
Educate HCWs who insert and maintain catheters, and assess their knowledge and competence periodically.
Use aseptic technique and maximal sterile barriers during insertion of CVCs (cap, mask, sterile gown, sterile gloves, and a large sterile barrier).
Do not routinely replace CVCs, PICCs, or pulmonary artery catheters to prevent catheter-related infections. Do not remove on the basis of fever alone.
In pediatric patients, leave peripheral venous catheters in place until intravenous therapy is completed unless a complication (e.g., phlebitis, infiltration) occurs.
Remove intravascular catheters promptly when no longer essential.
Observe proper hand hygiene procedures either by washing with antiseptic-containing soap and water or use of waterless alcohol-based products before and after working with intravascular lines.
Disinfect skin with an appropriate antiseptic before catheter insertion and during dressing changes. A 2% chlorhexidine-based preparation is preferred.
Do not use topical antibiotic ointment or creams on insertion sites, except when using dialysis catheters.
Use either sterile gauze or sterile, transparent, semipermeable dressing to cover the catheter site. Replace gauze dressings on short-term CVC sites every 2 days and transparent dressings at least weekly, except in pediatric patients, in whom the risk of dislodging the catheter outweighs the benefit of changing the dressing. Change if damp, loosened, or visibly soiled.
Replace dressings on tunneled or implanted CVC sites no more than once per week until the insertion site has healed.
Chlorhexidine sponge dressings are contraindicated in neonates younger than 7 days or those born at a gestational age of less than 26 weeks.
Clean injection ports with 70% alcohol or an iodophor before accessing the system.
Use disposable transducer assemblies with peripheral arterial catheters and pressure monitoring devices. Keep all components of such systems sterile, and do not administer dextrose-containing solutions or parenteral nutrition fluids through them.

CVC, central venous catheter; HCW, health care worker; NICU, neonatal intensive care unit; PICC, peripherally inserted central catheter.
Data from Centers for Disease Control and Prevention. Guidelines for prevention of intravascular catheter-related infections. MMWR Morb Mortal Wkly Rep 51(No. RR-10):32, 2002.

from NNIS (August 2003) revealed that the mean umbilical catheter– and CVC-associated bloodstream infection rates for NICUs ranged from 10.6 per 1000 catheter days for infants whose birth weight was less than 1000 g to 3.7 per 1000 catheter days in infants whose birth weight was 2500 g or more.[194] The CDC recommends implementing strategies to reduce the incidence of such infections that strike a balance between patient safety and cost-effectiveness.

Few large studies of risks related to intravascular devices have been performed in NICU patients. As a result, intravascular device recommendations for neonates are based on those developed for adults and older pediatric patients (Table 35-11). Several differences in their management should be considered. Although the CDC recommends, in certain circumstances, using antimicrobial- or antiseptic-impregnated CVCs in adults whose catheters are expected to remain in place more than 5 days,[36] these catheters are not available in sizes small enough for neonates. Of more importance, studies to evaluate their safety in neonates, especially premature neonates of very low birth weight, have not been performed. In addition, although the CDC recommends changing the insertion site of PIVs at least every 72 to 96 hours in adults, data suggest that leaving PIVs in place in pediatric patients does not increase the risk of complications.[262] The 2002 CDC guidelines recommend that PIVs be left in place in children until therapy is completed, unless complications occur.

Careful skin antisepsis before insertion of an intravascular catheter is critical to prevention of intravascular device–related bacteremia, although care in the selection of a product for use on neonatal skin is required. Chlorhexidine preparations are recommended by the CDC because these products have been found to be superior to povidone-iodine in reducing the risk for peripheral catheter colonization in neonates. Residues left on the skin by chlorhexidine prolong its half-life, providing improved protection for catheters in neonates that must be left in place for longer periods of time.[257]

Umbilical veins and arteries are available for CVC insertion only in neonates and are typically used for several days; thereafter, the CVC is replaced with another, nontunneled CVC or PICC if continued central venous access is required. The umbilicus provides a site that can be cannulated easily, allowing for collection of blood specimens and hemodynamic measurements, but after birth, the umbilicus quickly becomes heavily colonized with skin flora and other microorganisms. Colonization and catheter-related bloodstream infection rates for umbilical vein and umbilical artery catheters are similar. Colonization rates for umbilical artery catheters are estimated to be 40% to 55%; the estimated rate for umbilical artery catheter–related bloodstream infection is 5%.[36] Colonization rates are from 22% to 59% for umbilical vein catheters; rates for umbilical vein catheter–related bloodstream infections are 3% to 8%.[36] A summary of the CDC recommendations for management of umbilical catheters[36] is presented in Table 35-12.

Ventilator-Associated Pneumonia

As mentioned earlier, NNIS data indicate that nosocomial pneumonia is the second most common infection type in

Table 35–12 Summary of CDC Recommendations for Management of Umbilical Catheters

Cleanse umbilical insertion site with an antiseptic before catheter insertion. Avoid tincture of iodine; povidone-iodine can be used.
Add low doses of heparin to fluid infused through umbilical artery catheters.
Remove and do not replace umbilical catheters if signs of catheter-related bloodstream infection, vascular insufficiency, or thrombosis are present.
Remove umbilical catheters as soon as possible when no longer needed or if any sign of vascular insufficiency to the lower extremities is observed.
Umbilical artery catheters should not be left in place for longer than 5 days.
Umbilical venous catheters should be removed as soon as possible when no longer needed but can be used for up to 14 days if managed aseptically.

CDC, Centers for Disease Control and Prevention.
Data from Centers for Disease Control and Prevention. Guidelines for prevention of intravascular catheter-related infections. MMWR Morb Mortal Wkly Rep 51(No RR-10):32, 2002.

Table 35–13 Effective Strategies for Prevention of Ventilator-Associated Pneumonia

Removal of nasogastric or endotracheal tube as soon as clinically feasible
Adequate hand hygiene between patients
Semirecumbent positioning of the patient
Avoidance of unnecessary reintubation
Provision of adequate nutritional support
Avoidance of gastric overdistention
Scheduled drainage of condensate from ventilator circuits

Data from Kollef MH. Current concepts: the prevention of ventilator-associated pneumonia. N Engl J Med 340:627-634, 1999.

NICU patients. Risk factors for ventilator-associated pneumonia can be grouped as host-related (prematurity, low birth weight, sedation or use of paralytic agents), device-related (endotracheal intubation, mechanical ventilation, orogastric or nasogastric tube placement) and factors that increase bacterial colonization of the stomach or nasopharynx (broad-spectrum antimicrobial agents, antacids, or H_2 blockers).[51,264,265] Ventilator-associated pneumonia generally refers to bacterial pneumonia that develops in patients who are receiving mechanical ventilation. Aspiration and direct inoculation of bacteria are the primary routes of entry into the lower respiratory tract; the source of these organisms may be the patient's endogenous flora or transmission from other patients, staff members, or the environment.[266,267] Few studies have been performed to assess the effectiveness of prevention strategies in pediatric patients. Strategies to prevent ventilator-associated pneumonia in the NICU patient are therefore based primarily on studies performed in adults (Table 35-13). Hand hygiene remains critical to the prevention of ventilator-associated pneumonia, and HCWs should consistently apply the principles of standard precautions to the care of the ventilated patient, wearing gloves to handle respiratory secretions or objects contaminated by them, and changing gloves and performing hand hygiene between contacts with a contaminated body site and the respiratory tract or a respiratory tract device.

Because mechanical ventilation is a significant risk factor for the development of nosocomial infection or ventilator-associated pneumonia, weaning from ventilation and removing endotracheal tubes as soon as indication for their use ceases are key infection control strategies. As an alternative to endotracheal intubation, noninvasive nasal continuous positive airway pressure (CPAP) ventilation avoids some of the common risk factors for ventilator-associated pneumonia and has been used successfully for neonates.[268,269] Respiratory care equipment that comes in contact with mucous membranes of ventilated patients or that is part of the ventilator circuit should be single use (discarded after one-time use with a single patient) or be subjected to sterilization or high-level disinfection between patients. Wet heat pasteurization (processing at 76° C for 30 minutes) or chemical disinfectants can be used to achieve high-level disinfection of reusable respiratory equipment.[263] Ventilator circuits should be changed no more frequently than every 48 hours, and evidence suggests that extending the length of time between changes to 7 days does not increase the risk of ventilator-associated pneumonia.[270,271] Circuits should be monitored for accumulation of condensate and drained periodically, with care taken to avoid allowing the condensate, a potential reservoir for pathogens, to drain toward the patient.[263,267] Sterile fluids should be used for nebulization, and sterile water should be used to rinse reusable semicritical equipment and devices such as in-line medication nebulizers.[263]

Basic infection control measures, such as hand hygiene and wearing gloves during suctioning and respiratory manipulation, also can reduce the risk of nosocomial pneumonia. Both open, single-use and closed, multiuse suction systems are available. If an open system is used, a sterile single-use catheter should be used each time the patient is suctioned. Closed systems, which do not need to be changed daily and can be used for up to 7 days,[272] have the advantage of lower costs and decreased environmental cross-contamination[258] but have not been shown to decrease the incidence of nosocomial pneumonia when compared with open systems.[273,274]

Although not well studied in pediatric patients, aspiration of oropharyngeal secretions is believed to contribute to development of ventilator-associated pneumonia in adults.[275] Placing the mechanically ventilated patient in a semirecumbent position or elevating the head of the bed in an attempt to minimize aspiration is recommended unless medically contraindicated. Also, placement of enteral feeding tubes should be verified before their use.[263,267] To prevent regurgitation and potential aspiration of stomach contents by the sedated patient, overdistention of the stomach should be avoided by regular monitoring of the patient's intestinal motility, serial measurement of residual gastric volume or abdominal girth, reducing the use of narcotics and anticholinergic agents, and adjusting the rate and volume of enteral feedings.[263,267] Oral decontamination, with the intent of decreasing oropharyngeal colonization, has been studied in adults and seems to lower the incidence of ventilator-associated pneumonia (although not duration of ventilation or mortality rate),[275,276] but further work is needed to determine whether this is an effective strategy in neonates. In addition, medications such as sucralfate, as opposed to histamine H_2 receptor antagonists and antacids, which raise gastric pH and can potentially result in increased bacterial colonization of the stomach, have been used to prevent development of stress ulcers and have been associated with lower incidence of ventilator-associated pneumonia in adults.[277] Two studies suggest, however, that this approach is of no benefit in pediatric patients, but the authors stress that additional studies with larger sample sizes are needed to confirm these findings.[278,279]

REFERENCES

1. Zafar N, Wallace CM, Kieffer P, et al. Improving survival of vulnerable infants increases neonatal intensive care unit nosocomial infection rate. Arch Pediatr Adolesc Med 155:1098-1104, 2001.
2. Nagata E, Brito AS, Matsuo TL. Nosocomial infections in a neonatal intensive care unit: incidence and risk factors. Am J Infect Control 30:26-31, 2002.
3. Bektas S, Goetze B, Speer CP. Decreased adherence, chemotaxis and phagocytic activities of neutrophils from preterm neonates. Acta Paediatr Scand 79:1031-1038, 1990.
4. Kallman J, Schollin J, Schalen C, et al. Impaired phagocytosis and opsonisation towards group B streptococci in preterm neonates. Arch Dis Child Fetal Neonatal Ed 78:F46-F50, 1998.
5. Madden NP, Levinsky RJ, Bayston R, et al. Surgery, sepsis, and non-specific immune function in neonates. J Pediatr Surg 24:562-566, 1989.
6. Stiehm ER. The physiologic immunodeficiency of immaturity. *In* Stiehm ER (ed). Immunologic Disorders in Infants and Children, 4th ed. Philadelphia, WB Saunders, 1986, pp 253-295.
7. Burchett SK, Corey L, Mohan KM, et al. Diminished interferon-gamma and lymphocyte proliferation in neonatal and postpartum primary herpes simplex virus infection. J Infect Dis 165:813-818, 1992.
8. Goldmann DA, Leclair J, Macone A. Bacterial colonization of neonates admitted to an intensive care environment. J Pediatr 93:288-293, 1978.
9. Sprunt K. Practical use of surveillance for prevention of nosocomial infection. Semin Perinatol 9:47-50, 1985.
10. Bennet R, Eriksson M, Nord CE, Zetterstrom R. Fecal bacterial microflora of newborn infants during intensive care management and treatment with five antibiotic regimens. Pediatr Infect Dis 5:533-539, 1986.
11. Hall SL, Riddell SW, Barnes WG, et al. Evaluation of coagulase-negative staphylococcal isolates from serial nasopharyngeal cultures of premature infants. Diagn Microbiol Infect Dis 13:17-23, 1990.
12. Fryklund B, Tullus K, Berglund B, Burman LG. Importance of the environment and the faecal flora of infants, nursing staff and parents as sources of gram-negative bacteria colonizing newborns in three neonatal wards. Infection 20:253-257, 1992.
13. Pessoa-Silva CL, Meurer Moreira B, Camara Almeida V, et al. Extended-spectrum beta-lactamase-producing *Klebsiella pneumoniae* in a neonatal intensive care unit: risk factors for infection and colonization. J Hosp Infect 53:198-206, 2003.
14. Saiman L, Ludington E, Dawson JD, et al. Risk factors for *Candida* species colonization of neonatal intensive care unit patients. Pediatr Infect Dis J 20:1119-1124, 2001.
15. Jarvis WR. The epidemiology of colonization. Infect Control Hosp Epidemiol 17:47-52, 1996.
16. el-Mohandes AE, Picard MB, Simmens SJ, Keiser JF. Use of human milk in the intensive care nursery decreases the incidence of nosocomial sepsis. J Perinatol 17:130-134, 1997.
17. Shattuck KE, Cochran CK, Zabransky RJ, et al. Colonization and infection associated with *Malassezia* and *Candida* species in a neonatal unit. J Hosp Infect 34:123-129, 1996.
18. Pittet D, Dharan S, Touveneau S, et al. Bacterial contamination of the hands of hospital staff during routine patient care. Arch Intern Med 159:821-826, 1999.
19. Baltimore RS. Neonatal nosocomial infections. Semin Perinatol 22:25-32, 1998.
20. Gaynes RP, Edwards JR, Jarvis WR, et al. Nosocomial infections among neonates in high-risk nurseries in the United States. National Nosocomial Infections Surveillance System. Pediatrics 98:357-361, 1996.
21. Sohn AH, Garrett DO, Sinkowitz-Cochran RL, et al. Prevalence of nosocomial infections in neonatal intensive care unit patients: results from the first national point-prevalence survey. J Pediatr 139:821-827, 2001.
22. Scheckler WE, Brimhall D, Buck AS, et al. Requirements for infrastructure and essential activities of infection control and epidemiology in hospitals: a consensus panel report. Society for Health Care Epidemiology of America. Am J Infect Control 26:47-60, 1998.
23. Neumann PW, O'Shaughnessy M, Garnett M. Laboratory evidence of human immunodeficiency virus infection in Canada in 1986. Can Med Assoc J 137:823, 1987.
24. Bureau of Communicable Disease Epidemiology, Laboratory Centre for Disease Control, Health and Welfare, Canada. Canadian nosocomial infection surveillance program: annual summary, June 1984–May 1985. Can Dis Wkly Rep 12:S1, 1986.
25. Garner JS. Guideline for isolation precautions in hospitals. The Hospital Infection Control Practices Advisory Committee. Infect Control Hosp Epidemiol 17:53-80, 1996.
26. Larson EL, Bryan JL, Adler LM, Blane C. A multifaceted approach to changing handwashing behavior. Am J Infect Control 25:3-10, 1997.
27. Pittet D, Hugonnet S, Harbarth S, et al. Effectiveness of a hospital-wide programme to improve compliance with hand hygiene. Infection Control Programme. Lancet 356:1307-1312, 2000.
28. Larson E. Skin hygiene and infection prevention: more of the same or different approaches? Clin Infect Dis 29:1287-1294, 1999.
29. Villari P, Sarnataro C, Iacuzio L. Molecular epidemiology of *Staphylococcus epidermidis* in a neonatal intensive care unit over a three-year period. J Clin Microbiol 38:1740-1746, 2000.
30. Carlos CC, Ringertz S, Rylander M, et al. Nosocomial *Staphylococcus epidermidis* septicaemia among very low birth weight neonates in an intensive care unit. J Hosp Infect 19:201-207, 1991.
31. Beck-Sague CM, Azimi P, Fonseca SN, et al. Bloodstream infections in neonatal intensive care unit patients: results of a multicenter study. Pediatr Infect Dis J 13:1110-1116, 1994.
32. Chien LY, MacNab Y, Aziz K, et al. Variations in central venous catheter-related infection risks among Canadian neonatal intensive care units. Pediatr Infect Dis J 21:505-511, 2002.
33. Cronin WA, Germanson TP, Donowitz LG. Intravascular catheter colonization and related bloodstream infection in critically ill neonates. Infect Control Hosp Epidemiol 11:301-308, 1990.
34. Mahieu LM, De Muynck AO, Ieven MM, et al. Risk factors for central vascular catheter-associated bloodstream infections among patients in a neonatal intensive care unit. J Hosp Infect 48:108-116, 2001.
35. Matlow AG, Kitai I, Kirpalani H, et al. A randomized trial of 72- versus 24-hour intravenous tubing set changes in newborns receiving lipid therapy. Infect Control Hosp Epidemiol 20:487-493, 1999.
36. O'Grady NP, Alexander M, Dellinger EP, et al. Guidelines for the prevention of intravascular catheter–related infections. Centers for Disease Control and Prevention. MMWR Morb Mortal Wkly Rep 51(No. RR-10):1-26, 2002.
37. Shulman RJ, Pokorny WJ, Martin CG, et al. Comparison of percutaneous and surgical placement of central venous catheters in neonates. J Pediatr Surg 21:348-350, 1986.
38. Brodie SB, Sands KE, Gray JE, et al. Occurrence of nosocomial bloodstream infections in six neonatal intensive care units. Pediatr Infect Dis J 19:56-65, 2000.
39. Sirota L, Straussberg R, Notti I, Bessler H. Effect of lipid emulsion on IL-2 production by mononuclear cells of newborn infants and adults. Acta Paediatr 86:410-413, 1997.
40. Moro ML, De Toni A, Stolfi I, et al. Risk factors for nosocomial sepsis in newborn intensive and intermediate care units. Eur J Pediatr 155:315-322, 1996.
41. Sirot D. Extended-spectrum plasmid-mediated beta-lactamases. J Antimicrob Chemother 36(Suppl A):19-34, 1995.

42. Saiman L, Ludington E, Pfaller M, et al. Risk factors for candidemia in Neonatal Intensive Care Unit patients. The National Epidemiology of Mycosis Survey study group. Pediatr Infect Dis J 19:319-324, 2000.
43. Stoll BJ, Temprosa M, Tyson JE, et al. Dexamethasone therapy increases infection in very low birth weight infants. Pediatrics 104:e63, 1999.
44. Papile LA, Tyson JE, Stoll BJ, et al. A multicenter trial of two dexamethasone regimens in ventilator-dependent premature infants. N Engl J Med 16:1112-1118, 1998.
45. Richardson DK, Gray JE, McCormick MC, et al. Score for Neonatal Acute Physiology: a physiologic severity index for neonatal intensive care. Pediatrics 91:617-623, 1993.
46. The CRIB (Clinical Risk Index for Babies) score: a tool for assessing initial neonatal risk and comparing performance of neonatal intensive care units. The International Neonatal Network. Lancet 342:193-198, 1993.
47. Tucker J. Patient volume, staffing, and workload in relation to risk-adjusted outcomes in a random stratified sample of UK neonatal intensive care units: a prospective evaluation. Lancet 359:99-107, 2002.
48. Goldmann DA, Durbin WA Jr, Freeman J. Nosocomial infections in a neonatal intensive care unit. J Infect Dis 144:449-59.1981.
49. Makhoul IR, Sujov P, Smolkin T, et al. Epidemiological, clinical, and microbiological characteristics of late-onset sepsis among very low birth weight infants in Israel: a national survey. Pediatrics 109:34-39, 2002.
50. Karlowicz MG, Giannone PJ, Pestian J, et al. Does candidemia predict threshold retinopathy of prematurity in extremely low birth weight (≤1000 g) neonates? Pediatrics 105:1036-1040, 2000.
51. Petdachai W. Nosocomial pneumonia in a newborn intensive care unit. J Med Assoc Thai 83:392-397, 2000.
52. Cordero L, Ayers LW, Miller RR, et al Surveillance of ventilator-associated pneumonia in very-low-birth-weight infants. Am J Infect Control 30:32-39, 2002.
53. Iroha EO, Kesah CN, Egri-Okwaji MT, Odugbemi TO. Bacterial eye infection in neonates, a prospective study in a neonatal unit. West Afr J Med 17:168-172, 1998.
54. Boccia D, Stolfi I, Lana S, Moro ML. Nosocomial necrotising enterocolitis outbreaks: epidemiology and control measures. Eur J Pediatr 160:385-391, 2001.
55. Rotbart HA, Levin MJ. How contagious is necrotizing enterocolitis? Pediatr Infect Dis 2:406-413, 1983.
56. Nakano M, Miyazawa H, Kawano Y, et al. An outbreak of neonatal toxic shock syndrome–like exanthematous disease (NTED) caused by methicillin-resistant *Staphylococcus aureus* (MRSA) in a neonatal intensive care unit. Microbiol Immunol 46:277-284, 2002.
57. Andersen BM, Lindemann R, Bergh K, et al. Spread of methicillin-resistant *Staphylococcus aureus* in a neonatal intensive unit associated with understaffing, overcrowding and mixing of patients. J Hosp Infect 50:18-24, 2002.
58. Saito Y, Seki K, Ohara T, et al. Epidemiologic typing of methicillin-resistant *Staphylococcus aureus* in neonate intensive care units using pulsed-field gel electrophoresis. Microbiol Immunol 42:723-729, 1998.
59. Belani A, Sherertz RJ, Sullivan ML, et al. Outbreak of staphylococcal infection in two hospital nurseries traced to a single nasal carrier. Infect Control 7:487-490, 1986.
60. Ish-Horowicz MR, McIntyre P, Nade S. Bone and joint infections caused by multiply resistant *Staphylococcus aureus* in a neonatal intensive care unit. Pediatr Infect Dis J 11:82-87, 1992.
61. Sabatino G, Verrotti A, de Martino M, et al. Neonatal suppurative parotitis: a study of five cases. Eur J Pediatr 158:312-314, 1999.
62. Saiman L, Jakob K, Holmes KW, et al. Molecular epidemiology of staphylococcal scalded skin syndrome in premature infants. Pediatr Infect Dis J 17:329-334, 1998.
63. Dave J, Reith S, Nash JQ, et al. A double outbreak of exfoliative toxin-producing strains of *Staphylococcus aureus* in a maternity unit. Epidemiol Infect 112:103-114, 1994.
64. Wolinsky E, Lipsitz PJ, Mortimer EA Jr, Rammelkamp CH Jr. Acquisition of staphylococci by newborns. Direct versus indirect transmission. Lancet 2:620-622, 1960.
65. Mortimer EA Jr, Lipsitz PJ, Wolinsky E, et al. Transmission of staphylococci between newborns. Importance of the hands to personnel. Am J Dis Child 104:289-295, 1962.
66. Haley RW, Bregman DA. The role of understaffing and overcrowding in recurrent outbreaks of staphylococcal infection in a neonatal special-care unit. J Infect Dis 145:875-885, 1982.
67. Eichenwald HF, Kotsevalov O, Fasso LA. The "cloud baby": an example of bacterial-viral interaction. Am J Dis Child 100:161-173, 1960.
68. Sheretz RJ, Reagan DR, Hampton KD, et al. A cloud adult: the *Staphylococcus aureus*–virus interaction revisited. Ann Intern Med 124:539-547, 1996.
69. Morel AS, Wu F, Della-Latta P, et al. Nosocomial transmission of methicillin-resistant *Staphylococcus aureus* from a mother to her preterm quadruplet infants. Am J Infect Control 30:170-173, 2002.
70. Hitomi S, Kubota M, Mori N, et al. Control of a methicillin-resistant *Staphylococcus aureus* outbreak in a neonatal intensive care unit by unselective use of nasal mupirocin ointment. J Hosp Infect 46:123-129, 2000.
71. Hayakawa T, Hayashidera T, Yoneda K, et al. Preferential pharyngeal colonization of methicillin resistant *Staphylococcus aureus* in infants. J Pediatr 134:252, 1999.
72. Hayakawa T, Hayashidera T, Katsura S, et al. Nasal mupirocin treatment of pharynx-colonized methicillin resistant *Staphylococcus aureus*: preliminary study with 10 carrier infants. Pediatr Int 42:67-70, 2000.
73. Isaacs D. A ten year, multicentre study of coagulase negative staphylococcal infections in Australasian neonatal units. Arch Dis Child Fetal Neonatal Ed 88:F89-F93, 2003.
74. Gray JE, Richardson DK, McCormick MC, Goldmann DA. Coagulase-negative staphylococcal bacteremia among very low birth weight infants: relation to admission illness severity, resource use, and outcome. Pediatrics 95:225-230, 1995.
75. Sharek PJ, Benitz WE, Abel NJ, et al. Effect of an evidence-based hand washing policy on hand washing rates and false-positive coagulase negative staphylococcus blood and cerebrospinal fluid culture rates in a level III NICU. J Perinatol 22:137-143, 2002.
76. Coudron PE, Mayhall CG, Facklam RR, et al. *Streptococcus faecium* outbreak in a neonatal intensive care unit. J Clin Microbiol 20: 1044-1048, 1984.
77. Luginbuhl LM, Rotbart HA, Facklam RR, et al. Neonatal enterococcal sepsis: case-control study and description of an outbreak. Pediatr Infect Dis J 6:1022-1026, 1987.
78. McNeeley DF, Saint-Louis F, Noel GJ. Neonatal enterococcal bacteremia: an increasingly frequent event with potentially untreatable pathogens. Pediatr Infect Dis J 15:800-805, 1996.
79. Rupp ME, Marion N, Fey PD, et al. Outbreak of vancomycin-resistant *Enterococcus faecium* in a neonatal intensive care unit. Infect Control Hosp Epidemiol 22:301-303, 2001.
80. Centers for Disease Control and Prevention. Recommendations for preventing the spread of vancomycin resistance: recommendations of the Hospital Infection Control Practices Advisory Committee (HICPAC). MMWR Morb Mortal Wkly Rep 44(No. RR-12):1-13, 1995.
81. Geil CC, Castle WK, Mortimer EA Jr. Group A streptococcal infections in newborn nurseries. Pediatrics 46:849-854, 1970.
82. Campbell JR, Arango CA, Garcia-Prats JA, et al. An outbreak of M serotype 1 group A *Streptococcus* in a neonatal intensive care unit. J Pediatr 129:396-402, 1996.
83. Bingen E, Denamur E, Lambert-Zechovsky N, et al. Mother-to-infant vertical transmission and cross-colonization of *Streptococcus pyogenes* confirmed by DNA restriction fragment length polymorphism analysis. J Infect Dis 165:147-150, 1992.
84. Isenberg HD, Tucci V, Lipsitz P, Facklam RR. Clinical laboratory and epidemiological investigations of a *Streptococcus pyogenes* cluster epidemic in a newborn nursery. J Clin Microbiol 19:366-370, 1984.
85. Brunton WA. Infection and hospital laundry. Lancet 345:1574-1575, 1995.
86. Paredes A, Wong P, Mason EO Jr, et al. Nosocomial transmission of group B streptococci in a newborn nursery. Pediatrics 59:679-682, 1977.
87. Aber RC, Allen N, Howell JT, et al. Nosocomial transmission of group B streptococci. Pediatrics 58:346-353, 1976.
88. Anthony BF, Okada DM, Hobel CJ. Epidemiology of the group B *Streptococcus*: maternal and nosocomial sources for infant acquisitions. J Pediatr 95:431-436, 1979.
89. Easmon CS, Hastings MJ, Clare AJ, et al. Nosocomial transmission of group B streptococci. Br Med J 283:459-461, 1981.
90. Noya FJ, Rench MA, Metzger TG, et al. Unusual occurrence of an epidemic of type Ib/c group B streptococcal sepsis in a neonatal intensive care unit. J Infect Dis 155:1135-1144, 1987.
91. Lin FY, Weisman LE, Troendle J, Adams K. Prematurity is the major risk factor for late-onset group B streptococcus disease. J Infect Dis 188:267-271, 2003.
92. Olver WJ, Bond DW, Boswell TC, Watkin SL. Neonatal group B streptococcal disease associated with infected breast milk. Arch Dis Child Fetal Neonatal Ed 83:F48-F49, 2000.

93. Ayan M, Kuzucu C, Durmaz R, et al. Analysis of three outbreaks due to *Klebsiella* species in a neonatal intensive care unit. Infect Control Hosp Epidemiol 24:495-500, 2003.
94. van den Berg RW, Claahsen HL, Niessen M, et al. *Enterobacter cloacae* outbreak in the NICU related to disinfected thermometers. J Hosp Infect 45:29-34, 2000.
95. Archibald LK, Ramos M, Arduino MJ, et al. *Enterobacter cloacae* and *Pseudomonas aeruginosa* polymicrobial bloodstream infections traced to extrinsic contamination of a dextrose multidose vial. J Pediatr 133:640-644, 1998.
96. Matsaniotis NS, Syriopoulou VP, Theodoridou MC, et al. Enterobacter sepsis in infants and children due to contaminated intravenous fluids. Infect Control 5:471-477, 1984.
97. Centers for Disease Control and Prevention. *Enterobacter sakazakii* infections associated with the use of powdered infant formula—Tennessee, 2001. MMWR Morb Mortal Wkly Rep 51:298-300, 2002.
98. Harbarth S, Sudre P, Dharan S, et al. Outbreak of *Enterobacter cloacae* related to understaffing, overcrowding, and poor hygiene practices. Infect Control Hosp Epidemiol 20:598-603, 1999.
99. Yu WL, Cheng HS, Lin HC, et al. Outbreak investigation of nosocomial *Enterobacter cloacae* bacteraemia in a neonatal intensive care unit. Scand J Infect Dis 32:293-298, 2000.
100. Donowitz LG, Marsik FJ, Fisher KA, Wenzel RP. Contaminated breast milk: A source of *Klebsiella* bacteremia in a newborn intensive care unit. Rev Infect Dis 3:716-720, 1981.
101. Al-Rabea AA, Burwen DR, Eldeen MA, et al. *Klebsiella pneumoniae* bloodstream infections in neonates in a hospital in the Kingdom of Saudi Arabia. Infect Control Hosp Epidemiol 19:674-679, 1998.
102. Lalitha MK, Kenneth J, Jana AK, et al. Identification of an IV-dextrose solution as the source of an outbreak of *Klebsiella pneumoniae* sepsis in a newborn nursery. J Hosp Infect 43:70-73, 1999.
103. Cotton MF, Wasserman E, Pieper CH, et al. Invasive disease due to extended spectrum beta-lactamase-producing *Klebsiella pneumoniae* in a neonatal unit: the possible role of cockroaches. J Hosp Infect 44:13-17, 2000.
104. Reiss I, Borkhardt A, Fussle R, et al. Disinfectant contaminated with *Klebsiella oxytoca* as a source of sepsis in babies. Lancet 356:310, 2000.
105. Jeong SH, Kim WM, Chang CL, et al. Neonatal intensive care unit outbreak caused by a strain of *Klebsiella oxytoca* resistant to aztreonam due to overproduction of chromosomal beta-lactamase. J Hosp Infect 48:281-288, 2001.
106. Macrae MB, Shannon KP, Rayner DM, et al. A simultaneous outbreak on a neonatal unit of two strains of multiply antibiotic resistant *Klebsiella pneumoniae* controllable only by ward closure. J Hosp Infect 49:183-192, 2001.
107. Gaillot O, Maruejouls C, Abachin E, et al. Nosocomial outbreak of *Klebsiella pneumoniae* producing SHV-5 extended-spectrum beta-lactamase, originating from a contaminated ultrasonography coupling gel. J Clin Microbiol 36:1357-1360, 1998.
108. Tullus K, Horlin K, Svenson SB, Kallenius G. Epidemic outbreaks of acute pyelonephritis caused by nosocomial spread of P fimbriated *Escherichia coli* in children. J Infect Dis 150:728-736, 1984.
109. Adhikari M, Coovadia Y, Hewitt J. Enteropathogenic *Escherichia coli* (EPEC) and enterotoxigenic (ETEC) related diarrhoeal disease in a neonatal unit. Ann Trop Paediatr 5:19-22, 1985.
110. Gerards LJ, Hennekam RC, von Dijk WC, et al. An outbreak of gastroenteritis due to *Escherichia coli* 0142 H6 in a neonatal department. J Hosp Infect 5:283-288, 1984.
111. Villari P, Crispino M, Salvadori A, Scarcella A. Molecular epidemiology of an outbreak of *Serratia marcescens* in a neonatal intensive care unit. Infect Control Hosp Epidemiol 22:630-634, 2001.
112. Assadian O, Berger A, Aspock C, et al. Nosocomial outbreak of *Serratia marcescens* in a neonatal intensive care unit. Infect Control Hosp Epidemiol 23:457-461, 2002.
113. van Ogtrop ML, van Zoeren-Grobben D, Verbakel-Salomons EM, van Boven CP. *Serratia marcescens* infections in neonatal departments: description of an outbreak and review of the literature. J Hosp Infect 36:95-103, 1997.
114. Archibald LK, Corl A, Shah B, et al. *Serratia marcescens* outbreak associated with extrinsic contamination of 1% chlorxylenol soap. Infect Control Hosp Epidemiol 18:704-709, 1997.
115. Fleisch F, Zimmermann-Baer U, Zbinden R, et al. Three consecutive outbreaks of *Serratia marcescens* in a neonatal intensive care unit. Clin Infect Dis 34:767-773, 2002.
116. Berthelot P, Grattard F, Amerger C, et al. Investigation of a nosocomial outbreak due to *Serratia marcescens* in a maternity hospital. Infect Control Hosp Epidemiol 20:233-236, 1999.
117. Gransden WR, Webster M, French GL, Phillips I. An outbreak of *Serratia marcescens* transmitted by contaminated breast pumps in a special care baby unit. J Hosp Infect 7:149-154, 1986.
118. Moloney AC, Quoraishi AH, Parry P, Hall V. A bacteriological examination of breast pumps. J Hosp Infect 9:169-174, 1987.
119. Jang TN, Fung CP, Yang TL, et al. Use of pulsed-field gel electrophoresis to investigate an outbreak of *Serratia marcescens* infection in a neonatal intensive care unit. J Hosp Infect 48:13-19, 2001.
120. Venezia RA, Scarano FJ, Preston KE, et al. Molecular epidemiology of an SHV-5 extended-spectrum beta-lactamase in enterobacteriaceae isolated from infants in a neonatal intensive care unit. Clin Infect Dis 21:915-923, 1995.
121. Shannon K, Fung K, Stapleton P, et al. A hospital outbreak of extended-spectrum beta-lactamase-producing *Klebsiella pneumoniae* investigated by RAPD typing and analysis of the genetics and mechanisms of resistance. J Hosp Infect 39:291-300, 1998.
122. Martinez-Aguilar G, Alpuche-Aranda CM, Anaya C, et al. Outbreak of nosocomial sepsis and pneumonia in a newborn intensive care unit by multiresistant extended-spectrum beta-lactamase-producing *Klebsiella pneumoniae*: high impact on mortality. Infect Control Hosp Epidemiol 22:725-728, 2001.
123. Leigh L, Stoll BJ, Rahman M, McGowan J Jr. *Pseudomonas aeruginosa* infection in very low birth weight infants: a case-control study. Pediatr Infect Dis J 14:367-371, 1995.
124. Becks VE, Lorenzoni NM. *Pseudomonas aeruginosa* outbreak in a neonatal intensive care unit: a possible link to contaminated hand lotion. Am J Infect Control 23:396-398, 1995.
125. McNeil MM, Solomon SL, Anderson RL, et al. Nosocomial *Pseudomonas pickettii* colonization associated with a contaminated respiratory therapy solution in a special care nursery. J Clin Microbiol 22:903-907, 1985.
126. Muyldermans G, de Smet F, Pierard D, et al. Neonatal infections with *Pseudomonas aeruginosa* associated with a water-bath used to thaw fresh frozen plasma. J Hosp Infect 39:309-314, 1998.
127. Garland SM, Mackay S, Tabrizi S, Jacobs S. *Pseudomonas aeruginosa* outbreak associated with a contaminated blood-gas analyser in a neonatal intensive care unit. J Hosp Infect 33:145-151, 1996.
128. Vochem M, Vogt M, Doring G. Sepsis in a newborn due to *Pseudomonas aeruginosa* from a contaminated tub bath. N Engl J Med 345:378-379, 2001.
129. Foca M, Jakob K, Whittier S, et al. Endemic *Pseudomonas aeruginosa* infection in a neonatal intensive care unit. N Engl J Med 343:695-700, 2000.
130. Moolenaar RL, Crutcher JM, San Joaquin VH, et al. A prolonged outbreak of *Pseudomonas aeruginosa* in a neonatal intensive care unit: did staff fingernails play a role in disease transmission? Infect Control Hosp Epidemiol 21:80-85, 2000.
131. Boyce JM, Pittet D. Guideline for hand hygiene in healthcare settings. Recommendations of the Health Care Infection Control Practices Advisory Committee and the HICPAC/SHEA/APIC/IDSA Hand Hygiene Task Force. Society for Health Care Epidemiology of America/Association for Professionals in Infection Control/Infectious Diseases Society of America. MMWR Recomm Rep 51:1-45, 2002.
132. Spearing NM, Horvath RL, McCormack JG. Pertussis: adults as a source in health care settings. Med J Aust 177:568-569, 2002.
133. Centers for Disease Control and Prevention. Hypertrophic pyloric stenosis in infants following pertussis prophylaxis with erythromycin—Knoxville, Tennessee, 1999. MMWR Morb Mortal Wkly Rep 48: 1117-1120, 1999.
134. Honein MA, Paulozzi LJ, Himelright IM, et al. Infantile hypertrophic pyloric stenosis after pertussis prophylaxis with erythromcyin: a case review and cohort study. Lancet 354:2101-2105, 1999.
135. American Academy of Pediatrics. Pertussis. *In* Pickering LK (ed). Red Book: 2003 Report of the Committee on Infectious Diseases, 26th ed. Elk Grove Village, Ill, American Academy of Pediatrics, 2003, pp 472-486.
136. Nivin B, Nicholas P, Gayer M, et al. A continuing outbreak of multidrug-resistant tuberculosis, with transmission in a hospital nursery. Clin Infect Dis 26:303-307, 1998.
137. Burk JR, Bahar D, Wolf FS, et al. Nursery exposure of 528 newborns to a nurse with pulmonary tuberculosis. South Med J 71:7-10, 1978.
138. Centers for Disease Control and Prevention. Guidelines for preventing the transmission of *Mycobacterium tuberculosis* in health-care facilities. MMWR Morb Mortal Wkly Rep 43(No. RR-13):1-132, 1994.

139. Phillips JR, Karlowicz MG. Prevalence of *Candida* species in hospital-acquired urinary tract infections in a neonatal intensive care unit. Pediatr Infect Dis J 16:190-194, 1997.
140. Huang YC, Li CC, Lin TY, et al. Association of fungal colonization and invasive disease in very low birth weight infants. Pediatr Infect Dis J 17:819-822, 1998.
141. Roilides E, Farmaki E, Evdoridou J, et al. *Candida tropicalis* in a neonatal intensive care unit: epidemiologic and molecular analysis of an outbreak of infection with an uncommon neonatal pathogen. J Clin Microbiol 41:735-741, 2003.
142. Gagneur A, Sizun J, Vernotte E, et al. Low rate of *Candida parapsilosis*–related colonization and infection in hospitalized preterm infants: a one-year prospective study. J Hosp Infect 48:193-197, 2001.
143. Benjamin DK Jr, Ross K, McKinney RE Jr, et al. When to suspect fungal infection in neonates: a clinical comparison of *Candida albicans* and *Candida parapsilosis* fungemia with coagulase-negative staphylococcal bacteremia. Pediatrics 106:712-718, 2000.
144. Reagan DR, Pfaller MA, Hollis RJ, Wenzel RP. Evidence of nosocomial spread of *Candida albicans* causing bloodstream infection in a neonatal intensive care unit. Diagn Microbiol Infect Dis 21:191-194, 1995.
145. Waggoner-Fountain LA, Walker MW, Hollis RJ, et al. Vertical and horizontal transmission of unique *Candida* species to premature newborns. Clin Infect Dis 22:803-808, 1996.
146. Huang YC, Lin TY, Peng HL, et al. Outbreak of *Candida albicans* fungaemia in a neonatal intensive care unit. Scand J Infect Dis 30: 137-142, 1998.
147. Chryssanthou E, Broberger U, Petrini B. Malassezia pachydermatis fungaemia in a neonatal intensive care unit. Acta Paediatr 90:323-327, 2001.
148. Chang HJ, Miller HL, Watkins N, et al. An epidemic of *Malassezia pachydermatis* in an intensive care nursery associated with colonization of health care workers' pet dogs. N Engl J Med 338:706-711, 1998.
149. Aragao PA, Oshiro IC, Manrique EI, et al. *Pichia anomala* outbreak in a nursery: exogenous source? Pediatr Infect Dis J 20:843-848, 2001.
150. Chakrabarti A, Singh K, Narang A, et al. Outbreak of *Pichia anomala* infection in the pediatric service of a tertiary-care center in Northern India. J Clin Microbiol 39:1702-1706, 2001.
151. Groll AH, Jaeger G, Allendorf A, et al. Invasive pulmonary aspergillosis in a critically ill neonate: case report and review of invasive aspergillosis during the first 3 months of life. Clin Infect Dis 27:437-452, 1998.
152. Singer S, Singer D, Ruchel R, et al. Outbreak of systemic aspergillosis in a neonatal intensive care unit. Mycoses 41:223-227, 1998.
153. Mitchell SJ, Gray J, Morgan ME, et al. Nosocomial infection with *Rhizopus microsporus* in preterm infants: association with wooden tongue depressors. Lancet 348:441-443, 1996.
154. Drusin LM, Ross BG, Rhodes KH, et al. Nosocomial ringworm in a neonatal intensive care unit: a nurse and her cat. Infect Control Hosp Epidemiol 21:605-607, 2000.
155. Sharma R, Hudak ML, Premachandra BR, et al. Clinical manifestations of rotavirus infection in the neonatal intensive care unit. Pediatr Infect Dis J 21:1099-1105, 2002.
156. Sattar SA, Jacobsen H, Rahman H, et al. Interruption of rotavirus spread through chemical disinfection. Infect Control Hosp Epidemiol 15:751-756, 1994.
157. Widdowson MA, van Doornum GJ, van der Poel WH, et al. An outbreak of diarrhea in a neonatal medium care unit caused by a novel strain of rotavirus: investigation using both epidemiologic and microbiological methods. Infect Control Hosp Epidemiol 23:665-670, 2002.
158. Birenbaum E, Linder N, Varsano N, et al. Adenovirus type 8 conjunctivitis outbreak in a neonatal intensive care unit. Arch Dis Child 68:610-611, 1993.
159. Sizun J, Soupre D, Legrand MC, et al. Neonatal nosocomial respiratory infection with coronavirus: a prospective study in a neonatal intensive care unit. Acta Paediatr 84:617-620, 1995.
160. Cunney RJ, Bialachowski A, Thornley D, et al. An outbreak of influenza A in a neonatal intensive care unit. Infect Control Hosp Epidemiol 21:449-554, 2000.
161. Moisiuk SE, Robson D, Klass L, et al. Outbreak of parainfluenza virus type 3 in an intermediate care neonatal nursery. Pediatr Infect Dis J 17:49-53, 1998.
162. Sagrera X, Ginovart G, Raspall F, et al. Outbreaks of influenza A virus infection in neonatal intensive care units. Pediatr Infect Dis J 21: 196-200, 2002.
163. Syriopoulou VP, Hadjichristodoulou C, Daikos GL, et al. Clinical and epidemiological aspects of an enterovirus outbreak in a neonatal unit. J Hosp Infect 51:275-280, 2002.
164. Jankovic B, Pasic S, Kanjuh B, et al. Severe neonatal echovirus 17 infection during a nursery outbreak. Pediatr Infect Dis J 18:393-394, 1999.
165. Chambon M, Bailly JL, Beguet A, et al. An outbreak due to echovirus type 30 in a neonatal unit in France in 1997: usefulness of PCR diagnosis. J Hosp Infect 43:63-68, 1999.
166. Griffin MP, O'Shea M, Brazy JE, et al. Cytomegalovirus infection in a neonatal intensive care unit. Subsequent morbidity and mortality of seropositive infants. J Perinatol 10:43-45, 1990.
167. Vochem M, Hamprecht K, Jahn G, Speer CP. Transmission of cytomegalovirus to preterm infants through breast milk. Pediatr Infect Dis J 17:53-58, 1998.
168. Sawyer MH, Edwards DK, Spector SA. Cytomegalovirus infection and bronchopulmonary dysplasia in premature infants. Am J Dis Child 141:303-305, 1987.
169. Maschmann J, Hamprecht K, Dietz K, et al. Cytomegalovirus infection of extremely low-birth weight infants via breast milk. Clin Infect Dis 33:1998-2003, 2001.
170. Hamprecht K, Maschmann J, Vochem M, et al. Epidemiology of transmission of cytomegalovirus from mother to preterm infant by breastfeeding. Lancet 357:513-518, 2001.
171. Aitken C, Booth J, Booth M, et al. Molecular epidemiology and significance of a cluster of cases of CMV infection occurring on a special care baby unit. J Hosp Infect 34:183-189, 1996.
172. Spector SA. Transmission of cytomegalovirus among infants in hospital documented by restriction-endonuclease-digestion analyses. Lancet 1:378-381, 1983.
173. Demmler GJ, Yow MD, Spector SA, et al. Nosocomial cytomegalovirus infections within two hospitals caring for infants and children. J Infect Dis 156:9-16, 1987.
174. Sharland M, Khare M, Bedford-Russell A. Prevention of postnatal cytomegalovirus infection in preterm infants. Arch Dis Child Fetal Neonatal Ed 86:F140, 2002.
175. Linnemann CC Jr, Buchman TG, Light IJ, Ballard JL. Transmission of herpes-simplex virus type 1 in a nursery for the newborn. Identification of viral isolates by DNA "fingerprinting." Lancet 1:964-966, 1978.
176. Hammerberg O, Watts J, Chernesky M, et al. An outbreak of herpes simplex virus type 1 in an intensive care nursery. Pediatr Infect Dis 2:290-294, 1983.
177. Sakaoka H, Saheki Y, Uzuki K, et al. Two outbreaks of herpes simplex virus type 1 nosocomial infection among newborns. J Clin Microbiol 24:36-40, 1986.
178. Turner R, Shehab Z, Osborne K, Hendley JO. Shedding and survival of herpes simplex virus from 'fever blisters.' Pediatrics 70:547-549, 1982.
179. Hayakawa M, Kimura H, Ohshiro M, et al. Varicella exposure in a neonatal medical centre: successful prophylaxis with oral acyclovir. J Hosp Infect 54:212-215, 2003.
180. Stover BH, Cost KM, Hamm C, et al. Varicella exposure in a neonatal intensive care unit: case report and control measures. Am J Infect Control 16:167-172, 1988.
181. Klein BS, Michaels JA, Rytel MW, et al. Nosocomial hepatitis A. A multinursery outbreak in Wisconsin. JAMA 252:2716-2721, 1984.
182. Watson JC, Fleming DW, Borella AJ, et al. Vertical transmission of hepatitis A resulting in an outbreak in a neonatal intensive care unit. J Infect Dis 167:567-5571, 1993.
183. Rosenblum LS, Villarino ME, Nainan OV, et al. Hepatitis A outbreak in a neonatal intensive care unit: risk factors for transmission and evidence of prolonged viral excretion among preterm infants. J Infect Dis 164:476-482, 1991.
184. Haley RW, Culver DH, White JW, et al. The efficacy of infection surveillance and control programs in preventing nosocomial infections in US hospitals. Am J Epidemiol 121:182-205, 1985.
185. Adams-Chapman I, Stoll BJ. Prevention of nosocomial infections in the neonatal intensive care unit. Curr Opin Pediatr 14:157-164, 2002.
186. Lee TB, Baker OG, Lee JT, et al. Recommended practices for surveillance. Association for Professionals in Infection Control and Epidemiology, Inc. Surveillance Initiative working group. Am J Infect Control 26:277-288, 1998.
187. Lee T, Baker-Montgomery O. Surveillance. *In* Carrico R (ed). APIC Text for Infection Control and Epidemiology. Washington, DC, Association for Professionals in Infection Control and Epidemiology, 2002, pp 13-1–13-15.
188. Gaynes R, Horan T. Surveillance of nosocomial infections. *In* Mayhall C (ed). Hospital Epidemiology and Infection Control. Philadelphia, Lippincott Williams & Wilkins, 1999, pp 1285-1317.

189. Joint Commission on Accreditation of Healthcare Organizations. Surveillance, Prevention and Control of Infection, 2005 Pre-Publication Edition. Oak Brook Terrace, Ill, Joint Commission on Accreditation of Healthcare Organizations, 2003, pp 1-11. Available at http://www.jcaho.org/accredited+organizations/patient+safety/infection+control/05_ic_std_hap.pdf
190. Emori TG, Culver DH, Horan TC, et al. National nosocomial infections surveillance system (NNIS): description of surveillance methods. Am J Infect Control 19:19-35, 1991.
191. Garner JS, Jarvis WR, Emori TG, et al. CDC definitions for nosocomial infections, 1988. Am J Infect Control 16:128-140, 1988.
192. Moore D. Nosocomial infections in newborn nurseries and neonatal intensive care units. *In* Mayhall C (ed). Hospital Epidemiology and Infection Control. Philadelphia, Lippincott Williams & Wilkins, 1999, pp 665-693.
193. Sinha A, Yokow D, Platt R. Epidemiology of neonatal infections: experience during and after hospitalization. Pediatr Infect Dis J 22:244-250, 2003.
194. Centers for Disease Control and Prevention, Division of Health Care Quality Promotion. National Nosocomial Infections Surveillance (NNIS) System Report, data summary from January 1992 through June 2003, issued August 2003. Am J Infect Control 30:481-498, 2003.
195. Siegel JD. The Newborn Nursery. *In* Bennet J, Brachman P (eds). Hospital Infections, 4th ed. Philadelphia, Lippincott-Raven, 1998, pp 403-420.
196. Gaynes RP, Solomon S. Improving hospital-acquired infection rates: the CDC experience. J Comm J Qual Improv 22:457-467, 1996.
197. Archibald LK, Gaynes RP. Hospital-acquired infections in the United States. The importance of interhospital comparisons. Infect Dis Clin North Am 11:245-255, 1997.
198. Stover BH, Shulman ST, Bratcher DF, et al. Nosocomial infection rates in US children's hospitals' neonatal and pediatric intensive care units. Am J Infect Control 29:152-157, 2001.
199. Checko PJ. Outbreak investigation. *In* Carrico R (ed). APIC Text for Infection Control and Epidemiology. Washington, DC, Association for Professionals in Infection Control and Epidemiology, 2002, pp 15-1–15-9.
200. Haas JP, Trezza LA. Outbreak investigation in a neonatal intensive care unit. Semin Perinatol 26:367-378, 2002.
201. van Acker J, de Smet F, Muyldermans G, et al. Outbreak of necrotizing enterocolitis associated with *Enterobacter sakazakii* in powdered milk formula. J Clin Microbiol 39:293-297, 2001.
202. McDonald LC, Walker M, Carson L, et al. Outbreak of *Acinetobacter* spp. bloodstream infections in a nursery associated with contaminated aerosols and air conditioners. Pediatr Infect Dis J 17:716-722, 1998.
203. Zafar AB, Sylvester LK, Beidas SO. *Pseudomonas aeruginosa* infections in a neonatal intensive care unit. Am J Infect Control 30:425-429, 2002.
204. Steppberger K, Walter S, Claros MC, et al. Nosocomial neonatal outbreak of *Serratia marcescens*—analysis of pathogens by pulsed field gel electrophoresis and polymerase chain reaction. Infection 30:277-281, 2002.
205. Chaberny IE, Schnitzler P, Geiss HK, Wendt C. An outbreak of epidemic keratoconjunctivitis in a pediatric unit due to adenovirus type 8. Infect Control Hosp Epidemiol 24:514-519, 2003.
206. Wilcox MH, Fitzgerald P, Freeman J, et al. A five year outbreak of methicillin-susceptible *Staphylococcus aureus* phage type 53,85 in a regional neonatal unit. Epidemiol Infect 124:37-45, 2000.
207. Nambiar S, Herwaldt LA, Singh N. Outbreak of invasive disease caused by methicillin-resistant *Staphylococcus aureus* in neonates and prevalence in the neonatal intensive care unit. Pediatr Crit Care Med 4:220-226, 2003.
208. Kilani RA. Respiratory syncytial virus (RSV) outbreak in the NICU: description of eight cases. J Trop Pediatr 48:118-122, 2002.
209. Pessoa-Silva CL, Toscano CM, Moreira BM, et al. Infection due to extended-spectrum beta-lactamase-producing *Salmonella enterica* subsp. enterica serotype infantis in a neonatal unit. J Pediatr 141: 381-387, 2002.
210. Alfa MJ, Robson D, Davi M, et al. An outbreak of necrotizing enterocolitis associated with a novel clostridium species in a neonatal intensive care unit. Clin Infect Dis 35:S101-S105, 2002.
211. Hoque SN, Graham J, Kaufmann ME, Tabaqchali S. *Chryseobacterium (Flavobacterium) meningosepticum* outbreak associated with colonization of water taps in a neonatal intensive care unit. J Hosp Infect 47:188-192, 2001.
212. Lo WT, Wang CC, Chu ML. A nursery outbreak of *Staphylococcus aureus* pyoderma originating from a nurse with paronychia. Infect Control Hosp Epidemiol 23:153-155, 2002.
213. Ng W, Rajadurai VS, Pradeepkumar VK, et al. Parainfluenza type 3 viral outbreak in a neonatal nursery. Ann Acad Med Singapore 28: 471-475, 1999.
214. Larson EL, Early E, Cloonan P, et al. An organizational climate intervention associated with increased handwashing and decreased nosocomial infections. Behav Med 26:14-22, 2000.
215. Pittet D. Improving adherence to hand hygiene practice: a multidisciplinary approach. Emerg Infect Dis 7:234-240, 2001.
216. American Academy of Pediatrics and American College of Obstetricians and Gynecologists. Inpatient perinatal care services. *In* Gilstrap LC, Oh W (eds). Guidelines for Perinatal Care, 5th ed. Elk Grove Village, Ill, American Academy of Pediatrics, and Washington, DC, American College of Obstetricians and Gynecologists, 2002, pp 17-55.
217. Salisbury DM, Hutfilz P, Treen LM, et al. The effect of rings on microbial load of health care workers' hands. Am J Infect Control 25:24-27, 1997.
218. Trick WE, Vernon MO, Hayes RA, et al. Impact of ring wearing on hand contamination and comparison of hand hygiene agents in a hospital. Clin Infect Dis 36:1383-1390, 2003.
219. Pelke S, Ching D, Easa D, Melish ME. Gowning does not affect colonization or infection rates in a neonatal intensive care unit. Arch Pediatr Adolesc Med 148:1016-1020, 1994.
220. Birenbaum HJ, Glorioso L, Rosenberger C, et al. Gowning on a postpartum ward fails to decrease colonization in the newborn infant. Am J Dis Child 144:1031-1033, 1990.
221. American Academy of Pediatrics and American College of Obstetricians and Gynecologists. Infection control. *In* Gilstrap LC, Oh W (eds). Guidelines for Perinatal Care, 5th ed. Elk Grove Village, Ill, American Academy of Pediatrics, and Washington, DC, American College of Obstetricians and Gynecologists, 2002, pp 331-353.
222. American Academy of Pediatrics. Infection control for hospitalized children. *In* Pickering LK (ed). Red Book: 2003 Report of the Committee on Infectious Diseases, 26th ed. Elk Grove Village, Ill, American Academy of Pediatrics, 2003, pp 146-155.
223. Bozzi D, Burwen D, Dooley S, et al. Guideline for preventing the transmission of *Mycobacterium tuberculosis* in health care facilities. MMWR Mortal Morb Wkly Rep 43:1-132, 1994.
224. Munoz FM, Ong LT, Seavy D, et al. Tuberculosis among adult visitors of children with suspected tuberculosis and employees at a children's hospital. Infect Control Hosp Epidemiol 23:568-572, 2002.
225. Bowie BH, Hall RB, Faulkner J, Anderson B. Single-room infant care: future trends in special care nursery planning and design. Neonatal Netw 22:27-34, 2003.
226. Harrison H. The principles for family-centered neonatal care. Pediatrics 92:643-650, 1993.
227. White RD, Brown J, Cicco R, et al. Recommended standards for newborn ICU design: report of the Fifth Consensus Conference on newborn ICU design. Consensus Committee to Establish Recommended Standards for Newborn ICU Design, Clearwater Beach, Fla, 2002. Available at http://www.nd.edu/~kkolberg/DesignStandards.htm
228. Brown DG, Baublis J. Reservoirs of *Pseudomonas* in an intensive care unit for newborn infants: mechanisms of control. J Pediatr 90:453-457, 1977.
229. Bert F, Maubec E, Bruneau B, et al. Multi-resistant *Pseudomonas aeruginosa* outbreak associated with contaminated tap water in a neurosurgery intensive care unit. J Hosp Infect 39:53-62, 1998.
230. Kappstein I, Grundmann H, Hauer T, Niemeyer C. Aerators as a reservoir of *Acinetobacter junii*: an outbreak of bacteraemia in paediatric oncology patients. J Hosp Infect 44:27-30, 2000.
231. Sehulster L, Chinn RY. Guidelines for environmental infection control in health-care facilities. Recommendations of CDC and the Health Care Infection Control Practices Advisory Committee (HICPAC). MMWR Recomm Rep 52:1-42, 2003.
232. Moore D. Newborn nursery and neonatal intensive care unit. *In* Carrico R (ed). APIC Text of Infection Control and Epidemiology. Washington, DC, Association for Professionals in Infection Control and Epidemiology, 2002, pp 48-55.
233. Rutala WA. APIC guideline for selection and use of disinfectants. 1994, 1995, and 1996 APIC Guidelines Committee. Association for Professionals in Infection Control and Epidemiology, Inc. Am J Infect Control 24:313-342, 1996.
234. Pugliese G, Hubbard C. Central services, linens, and laundry. *In* Bennett JV, Brachman P (eds). Hospital Infections, 4th ed. Philadelphia, Lippincott-Raven, 1998, pp 725-739.
235. Rhame FS. The inanimate environment. *In* Bennett JV, Brachman P (eds). Hospital Infections, 4th ed. Philadelphia, Lippincott-Raven, 1998, pp 299-324.

236. Centers for Disease Control and Prevention, Health Care Infections Control Practices Advisory Committee (HICPAC). Guidelines for environmental infection control in health-care facilities. Chicago, Ill, American Society for Health Care Engineering and the American Hospital Association, 2004.
237. Hall CB, Douglas RG Jr, Geiman JM, Messner MK. Nosocomial respiratory syncytial virus infections. N Engl J Med 293:1343-1346, 1975.
238. Hall CB, Kopelman AE, Douglas RG Jr, et al. Neonatal respiratory syncytial virus infection. N Engl J Med 300:393-396, 1979.
239. Hall CB, Geiman JM, Douglas RG Jr, Meagher MP. Control of nosocomial respiratory syncytial viral infections. Pediatrics 62:728-732, 1978.
240. American Academy of Pediatrics. Herpes simplex. *In* Pickering LK (ed). Red Book: 2003 Report of the Committee on Infectious Diseases, 26th ed. Elk Grove Village, Ill, American Academy of Pediatrics, 2003, pp 344-353.
241. American Academy of Pediatrics. Cytomegalovirus infection. *In* Pickering LK (ed). Red Book: 2003 Report of the Committee on Infectious Diseases, 26th ed. Elk Grove Village, Ill, American Academy of Pediatrics, 2003, pp 259-262.
242. Ahlfors K, Ivarsson SA, Johnsson T, Renmarker K. Risk of cytomegalovirus infection in nurses and congenital infection in their offspring. Acta Paediatr Scand 70:819-823, 1981.
243. Balcarek KB, Bagley R, Cloud GA, Pass RF. Cytomegalovirus infection among employees of a children's hospital. No evidence for increased risk associated with patient care. JAMA 263:840-844, 1990.
244. Fridkin SK, Pear SM, Williamson TH, et al. The role of understaffing in central venous catheter–associated bloodstream infections. Infect Control Hosp Epidemiol 17:150-158, 1996.
245. American Academy of Pediatrics and American College of Obstetricians and Gynecologists. Perinatal infections. *In* Gilstrap LC, Oh W (eds). Guidelines for Perinatal Care, 5th ed. Elk Grove Village, Ill, American Academy of Pediatrics, and Washington, DC, American College of Obstetricians and Gynecologists, 2002, pp 285-329.
246. Brunell PA. Fetal and neonatal varicella-zoster infections. Semin Perinatol 7:47-56, 1983.
247. Fallot ME, Boyd JL 3rd, Oski FA. Breast-feeding reduces incidence of hospital admissions for infection in infants. Pediatrics 65:1121-1124, 1980.
248. American Academy of Pediatrics. Human milk. *In* Pickering LK (ed). Red Book: 2003 Report of the Committee on Infectious Diseases, 26th ed. Elk Grove Village, Ill, American Academy of Pediatrics, 2003, pp 117-123.
249. American Academy of Pediatrics and American College of Obstetricians and Gynecologists. Care of the neonate. *In* Gilstrap LC, Oh W (eds). Guidelines for Perinatal Care, 5th ed. Elk Grove Village, Ill, American Academy of Pediatrics, and Washington, DC, American College of Obstetricians and Gynecologists, 2002, pp 187-235.
250. el-Mohandes AE, Schatz V, Keiser JF, Jackson BJ. Bacterial contaminants of collected and frozen human milk used in an intensive care nursery. Am J Infect Control 21:226-230, 1993.
251. D'Amico CJ, DiNardo CA, Krystofiak S. Preventing contamination of breast pump kit attachments in the NICU. J Perinat Neonatal Nurs 17:150-157, 2003.
252. Baker RD. Infant formula safety. Pediatrics 110:833-835, 2002.
253. Nyqvist KH, Lutes LM. Co-bedding twins: a developmentally supportive care strategy. J Obstet Gynecol Neonatal Nurs 27:450-456, 1998.
254. DellaPorta K, Aforismo D, Butler-O'Hara M. Co-bedding of twins in the neonatal intensive care unit. Pediatr Nurs 24:529-531, 1998.
255. Wittrock B, Lavin MA, Pierry D, et al. Parents as a vector for nosocomial infection in the neonatal intensive care unit. Infect Control Hosp Epidemiol 22:472, 2001.
256. Cartolano GL, Moulies ME, Seguier JC, Boisivon A. A parent as a vector of *Salmonella brandenburg* nosocomial infection in a neonatal intensive care unit. Clin Microbiol Infect 9:560-562, 2003.
257. Darmstadt GL, Dinulos JG. Neonatal skin care. Pediatr Clin North Am 47:757-782, 2000.
258. Mullany LC, Darmstadt GL, Tielsch JM. Role of antimicrobial applications to the umbilical cord in neonates to prevent bacterial colonization and infection: review of the evidence. Pediatr Infect Dis J 22:996-1002, 2003.
259. Isenberg SJ, Apt L, Wood M. A controlled trial of povidone-iodine as prophylaxis against ophthalmia neonatorum. N Engl J Med 332: 562-566, 1995.
260. Isenberg SJ, Apt L, Campeas D. Ocular applications of povidone-iodine. Dermatology 204(Suppl 1):92-95, 2002.
261. Smith J, Finn A. Antimicrobial prophylaxis. Arch Dis Child 80:388-392, 1999.
262. Garland JS, Dunne WM Jr, Havens P, et al. Peripheral intravenous catheter complications in critically ill children: A prospective study. Pediatrics 89:1145-1150, 1992.
263. Centers for Disease Control and Prevention. Guidelines for prevention of nosocomial pneumonia. MMWR Morb Mortal Wkly Rep 46(No. RR-1):1-79, 1997.
264. Kawagoe JY, Segre CA, Pereira CR, et al. Risk factors for nosocomial infections in critically ill newborns: a 5-year prospective cohort study. Am J Infect Control 29:109-114, 2001.
265. Pepe R. Nosocomial pneumonia. *In* Carrico R (ed). APIC Text of Infection Control and Epidemiology. Washington, DC, Association for Professionals in Infection Control and Epidemiology, 2002, pp 88-1–88-3.
266. Craven DE, Steger KA. Hospital-acquired pneumonia: perspectives for the health care epidemiologist. Infect Control Hosp Epidemiol 18: 783-795, 1997.
267. Kollef MH. The prevention of ventilator-associated pneumonia. N Engl J Med 340:627-634, 1999.
268. Lesiuk W, Lesiuk L, Maliczowska M, Puzniak G. Non-invasive mandatory ventilation in extremely low birth weight and very low birth weight newborns with failed respiration. Przegl Lek 59(Suppl 1): 57-59, 2002.
269. Fernandez-Jurado MI, Fernandez-Baena M. Use of laryngeal mask airway for prolonged ventilatory support in a preterm newborn. Paediatr Anaesth 12:369-370, 2002.
270. Lien TC, Lin MY, Chu CC, et al. Ventilator-associated pneumonia with circuit changes every 2 days versus every week. Zhonghua Yi Xue Za Zhi (Taipei) 64:161-167, 2001.
271. Kotilainen HR, Keroack MA. Cost analysis and clinical impact of weekly ventilator circuit changes in patients in intensive care unit. Am J Infect Control 25:117-120, 1997.
272. Stoller JK, Orens DK, Fatica C, et al. Weekly versus daily changes of in-line suction catheters: impact on rates of ventilator-associated pneumonia and associated costs. Respir Care 48:494-499, 2003.
273. Zeitoun SS, de Barros AL, Diccini S. A prospective, randomized study of ventilator-associated pneumonia in patients using a closed vs. open suction system. J Clin Nurs 12:484-489, 2003.
274. Deppe SA, Kelly JW, Thoi LL, et al. Incidence of colonization, nosocomial pneumonia, and mortality in critically ill patients using a Trach Care closed-suction system versus an open-suction system: prospective, randomized study. Crit Care Med 18:1389-1393, 1990.
275. Bergmans DC, Bonten MJ, Gaillard CA, et al. Prevention of ventilator-associated pneumonia by oral decontamination: a prospective, randomized, double-blind, placebo-controlled study. Am J Respir Crit Care Med 164:382-388, 2001.
276. Pugin J, Auckenthaler R, Lew DP, Suter PM. Oropharyngeal decontamination decreases incidence of ventilator-associated pneumonia. A randomized, placebo-controlled, double-blind clinical trial. JAMA 265:2704-2710, 1991.
277. Cook DJ, Reeve BK, Guyatt GH, et al. Stress ulcer prophylaxis in critically ill patients. Resolving discordant meta-analyses. JAMA 275:308-314, 1996.
278. Ildizdas K, Yapicioglu H, Yilmaz H. Occurrence of ventilator-associated pneumonia in mechanically ventilated pediatric intensive care patients during stress ulcer prophylaxis with sucralfate, ranitidine, and omeprazole. J Crit Care 17:240-245, 2002.
279. Lopriore E, Markhorst DG, Gemke RJ. Ventilator-associated pneumonia and upper airway colonisation with gram negative bacilli: the role of stress ulcer prophylaxis in children. Intensive Care Med 28:763-767, 2002.

Chapter 36

LABORATORY AIDS FOR DIAGNOSIS OF NEONATAL SEPSIS

Geoffrey A. Weinberg • Carl T. D'Angio

For years, investigators have sought a test or panel of tests able to diagnose neonatal sepsis accurately and more rapidly than is possible with the isolation of microorganisms from specimens of sterile body fluids or tissues. Although results of some studies have been encouraging, the isolation of microorganisms from sources such as the blood, cerebrospinal fluid (CSF), urine, other body fluids (peritoneal, pleural, joint, middle ear), or tissues (bone marrow, liver, spleen) remains the most valid method of diagnosing bacterial sepsis. Many advances in nonculture methods, which may nevertheless remain microorganism specific, such as tests employing polymerase chain reaction (PCR) amplification technology, hold the promise of more rapid diagnosis of infection. In this chapter, nonspecific laboratory aids for the diagnosis of invasive bacterial infections are discussed. Specific microbiologic techniques are discussed in Chapter 6 and in chapters dealing with specific pathogens.

DIAGNOSTIC UTILITY OF LABORATORY TESTS

In establishing the usefulness of any laboratory determination, a balance must be reached between sensitivity and specificity.[1] For the clinician faced with a decision to institute or withhold therapy on the basis of a test result, the predictive values (and perhaps likelihood ratios[2]) of that test also are of importance. In relation to neonatal infection, these terms can be defined as follows (Fig. 36-1):

Sensitivity: If infection is present, how often is the test result abnormal?

Specificity: If infection is absent, how often is the test result normal?

Positive predictive value: If the test result is abnormal, how often is infection present?

Negative predictive value: If the test result is normal, how often is infection absent?

Likelihood ratio, positive test result: If the result is abnormal, how much does that result raise the pretest probability of disease?

Likelihood ratio, negative test result: If the result is normal, how much does that result lower the pretest probability of disease?

In attempting to discover the presence of a serious illness such as neonatal bacteremia, which is life-threatening yet treatable, diagnostic tests with maximal (100%) sensitivity and negative predictive value are desirable. In other words, if infection is present, the result would always be abnormal; if the result is normal, infection would always be absent. The reduced specificity and positive predictive value that this combination may engender usually are acceptable, because overtreatment with antibiotics on the basis of a false-positive result is likely to be of limited harm compared with withholding therapy on the basis of a false-negative result. Some authorities prefer the use of likelihood ratios, because predictive values vary with the prevalence of a disease but likelihood ratios relate only to the test performance (sensitivity, specificity).[3,4] Large likelihood ratios (greater than 10) imply that a test result will conclusively raise the probability of the disease's being present, whereas small likelihood ratios (less than 0.1) minimize the probability of the disease's being present.

In reviewing a report of a new laboratory aid for the diagnosis of neonatal sepsis, the first consideration is to determine what reference standard was used to evaluate the new test (i.e., what was the "gold standard" used). In one study, for example, among infants who died with unequivocal evidence of infection at autopsy, bacteria were grown from 32 of 39 antemortem blood cultures (sensitivity of only 82%).[5] Among 50 infants without pathologic findings of infection at autopsy, 48 had negative blood culture results (specificity of 96%). A positive blood or CSF culture result had a 94% chance of being associated with serious neonatal infection (positive predictive value of 94%), whereas a negative blood culture result indicated absence of serious

		Bacterial Infection Present		
		Yes	No	
Laboratory Test Result	**Positive**	TRUE POSITIVES (a)	FALSE POSITIVES (b)	POSITIVE PREDICTIVE VALUE (a)/(a+b)
	Negative	FALSE NEGATIVES (c)	TRUE NEGATIVES (d)	NEGATIVE PREDICTIVE VALUE (d)/(c+d)
		SENSITIVITY (a)/(a+c)	SPECIFICITY (d)/(b+d)	PREVALENCE (a+c)/(a+b+c+d)
		LIKELIHOOD RATIO, POSITIVE sensitivity/(1–specificity)	LIKELIHOOD RATIO, NEGATIVE (1–sensitivity)/specificity	

Figure 36–1 Diagnostic test characteristics. Sensitivity, specificity, postive predictive value, and negative predictive value are commonly expressed as percentages; likelihood ratios represent -fold increases or -fold decreases in probability.[1-3]

infection only 87% of the time (negative predictive value of 87%). In fact, it is likely that the predictive values cited in this study already are different from those that may be observed in practice, because of the high prevalence (44%) of positive bacterial culture results in the autopsy cases reviewed.[5] (High prevalence inflates the positive predictive value and depresses the negative predictive value; low prevalence depresses the positive predictive value and inflates the negative predictive value.) Thus, the lack of perfection of the generally accepted "gold standard" of bacterial culture complicates the search for new laboratory aids in the diagnosis of neonatal sepsis, because it may be unclear whether a new test is truly functioning better than culture, which itself may not be "perfect." Interpretation of bacterial culture results may become even more complicated as intrapartum antibiotic prophylaxis to prevent early-onset group B streptococcal sepsis becomes more common.[6-9] Of course, it may not be clinically necessary to require detection of only *bacterial* sepsis. Tests that yield results considered "falsely positive" in the absence of bacterial disease may still be clinically useful in assigning normal versus abnormal status if the results register positive because of serious viral disease that may require antiviral therapy (e.g., neonatal enterovirus or herpes simplex infections).

Two additional points merit consideration in this context. First, unless the report is generated from an unselected cohort or prospective study, the predictive values given in the report may be misleading. Prevalence of sepsis may vary greatly if certain groups of newborns are pre-selected, which will in turn alter the predictive values of the test being studied. The most useful test in one population of infants of very low birth weight may function quite differently in another population of older, larger-birth-weight "growers." Second, because the body's response to an infection necessarily begins after the invasion of a pathogen, it may never be possible to diagnose an infection immediately—there may always be a lag in the physiologic response on which the diagnostic test is based. Each report of a new test claiming superiority to bacterial culture must be critically evaluated in the field, and standardization both within clinical laboratories and between institutions is required.

COMPLETE BLOOD COUNTS AND WHITE BLOOD CELL RATIOS

Total Leukocyte Count, Differential Leukocyte Count, and Morphology

It has been known for many years that *total leukocyte counts* are of limited value in the diagnosis of septicemia of the newborn.[10-14] Normal at the time of initial evaluation in more than one third of infants with proven bacteremia,[5,15-26] total leukocyte counts are particularly unreliable indicators of infection during the first several hours of early-onset (within 48 hours of birth) sepsis. Conversely, among neonates evaluated for suspected sepsis, far less than half of those with reduced (fewer than 5000 cells per mm^3) or elevated (greater than 20,000 cells per mm^3) cell counts ultimately are identified as being infected.[5,18,20,27]

Differential leukocyte counts have not functioned well as markers for infectious disease in the newborn period. Increased percentages of lymphocytes have been described in association with pertussis and congenital syphilis, whereas minor changes of little diagnostic value have been noted in infants with ABO incompatibility, in sepsis, and in maternal hypertension.[28,29] Monocyte counts, normally higher in neonates than in older children or adults, may be further elevated in some cases of congenital syphilis, perinatal listeriosis, ABO incompatibility, and recovery from sepsis.[25,29-34] Eosinophilia, a common finding in premature infants, has been related to a number of factors, including low birth weight, immaturity, establishment of positive nitrogen balance, improved nutritional status, and use of total parenteral nutrition or blood transfusions.[34-39] A dramatic fall in the absolute number of eosinophils, detectable only if serial counts have been per-

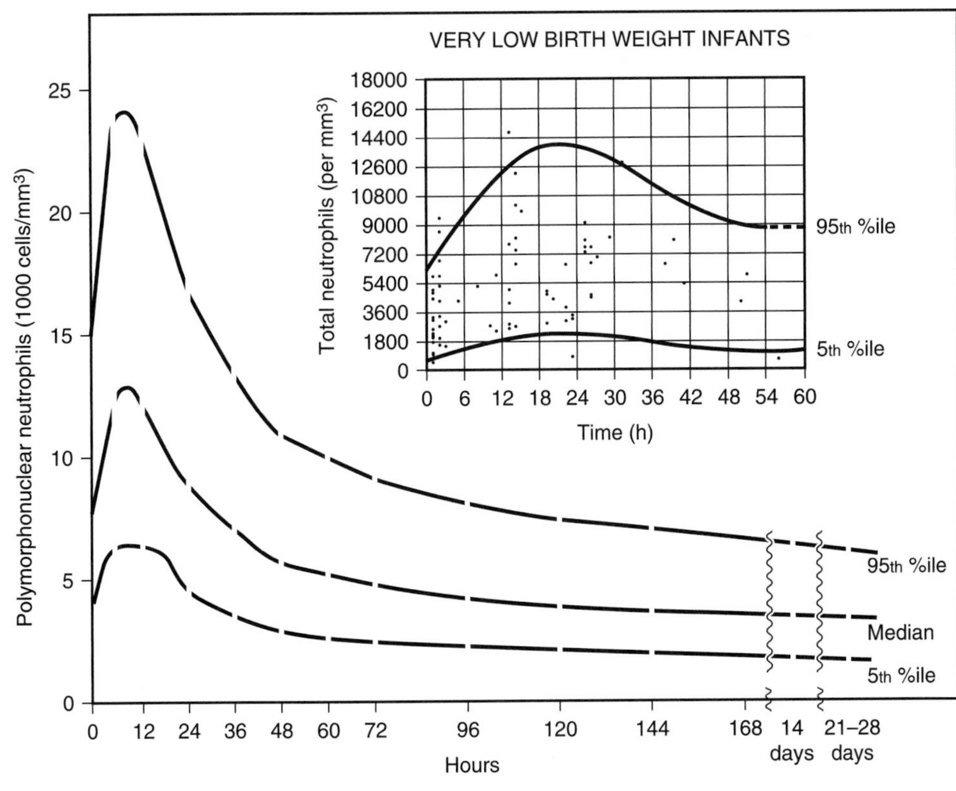

Figure 36–2 Total neutrophil counts in normal term infants and in very low birth weight infants (**inset**). The limits for term infants are close to those defined by Xanthou,[33] Marks and colleagues,[51] and Schelonka and associates[53] but are significantly higher during the first 18 hours of life than the reference values of Manroe and co-workers.[43] (Data from Gregory J, Hey E. Blood neutrophil response to bacterial infection in the first month of life. Arch Dis Child 47:747-753, 1972; **inset**, data from Mouzinho A, Rosenfeld CR, Sanchez PJ, Risser R. Revised reference ranges for circulating neutrophils in very-low-birth-weight neonates. Pediatrics 94:76-82, 1999.)

formed, frequently accompanies sepsis or serious infection.[29,36,40] Basophil counts tend to follow the fluctuations in eosinophil numbers in ill or healthy newborns.[40] Conflicting data have been reported for the utility of differential leukocyte counts for identifying neonates with bacterial meningitis.[41,42]

Several investigators have shown that, in association with serious bacterial infection, significant changes in *neutrophil morphology* occur, with the appearance of toxic granules, Döhle bodies, and vacuolization.[23,40-45] These features are of limited value in establishing a diagnosis; their presence has, at best, a positive predictive value for sepsis of only slightly more than 50%[5,23,43-45] and, at worst, 33% to 37%.[46,47] Identical morphologic features can occur as artifacts in citrate-anticoagulated blood samples stored for longer than 1 hour before smears are made.[48]

Total Neutrophil Count

Recognizing the low predictive value of total leukocyte counts in serious neonatal bacterial disease, several investigators have studied the dynamics of *neutrophil counts* during the first month of life.[33,40,43,49-54] These researchers and others uncovered patterns of change sufficiently constant to establish limits of normal variation (Fig. 36-2) and defined noninfectious conditions involving the mother or the infant that might have significant effects on neutrophil values (Tables 36-1 and 36-2). It was suggested that, largely on the basis of these data, calculation of the absolute number of circulating neutrophils (polymorphonuclear plus immature forms) might provide a useful index of neonatal infection. Clinical experience has only partly supported this premise.

Most series of consecutive cases of neonatal sepsis have shown abnormal neutrophil counts *at the time of onset of symptoms* in only about two thirds of infants.[5,13-16,24,43,44,63-68] In some series, however, up to 80% to 90% of infected infants have had abnormal values,[21,46,49,69] whereas in other series, initial neutrophil counts were reduced or elevated in only one fourth to one third of infants with bacteremia, particularly when counts were determined early in the course of illness.[26,55,70] Thus, the neutrophil count, although slightly more sensitive than the total leukocyte count, is too often normal in the face of serious infection to be used as a guide for treatment.

Baley and associates investigated the causes of neutropenia among consecutive admissions to a neonatal intensive care unit.[50] Low neutrophil counts were found in 6% of these infants, most of whom were premature and of low birth weight. Less than one half of the episodes of neutropenia could be attributed to infection (bacterial, viral, necrotizing enterocolitis); a majority were of unknown cause or occurred in infants with perinatal complications. Similar findings have been described by Rodwell and co-workers among 1000 infants evaluated for sepsis in the first 24 hours of life.[57]

In specific clinical situations, however, the neutrophil count can be of value. Although the association among neutropenia, respiratory distress, and early-onset (less than 48 hours) sepsis caused by group B streptococci is well documented,[16,21,62,71-74] the recognition that a similar association exists for early sepsis caused by other microorganisms has not been adequately emphasized. Several authors have described infants with septicemia related to *Haemophilus influenzae*,[75,76] pneumococci,[77-79] *Escherichia coli*,[76] or non-enterococcal group D streptococci[80] whose clinical course

Table 36–1 Clinical Factors Affecting Neutrophil Counts in Newborn Infants

	Neutrophil Counts[a]				
Factor	Decrease	Increase	Total Immature Increase	Increased I:T Ratio[b]	Approximate Duration (hr)
Maternal hypertension[55-57]	++++	0	+	+	72
Maternal fever, neonate healthy	0	++	+++	++++	24
≥6 hours intrapartum oxytocin administration	0	++	++	++++	120
Asphyxia (5-minute Apgar score ≤5)[55,58]	+	++	++	+++	24-60
Meconium aspiration syndrome[58]	0	++++	+++	++	72
Pneumothorax with uncomplicated hyaline membrane disease	0	++++	++++	++++	24
Seizures—no hypoglycemia, asphyxia, or central nervous system hemorrhage	0	+++	+++	++++	24
Prolonged (for ≥4 minutes) crying[59]	0	++++	++++	++++	1
Asymptomatic blood sugar ≤30 mg/dL	0	++	+++	+++	24
Hemolytic disease[40]	++	++	+++	++	7-28 days
Surgery[49]	0	++++	++++	+++	24
High altitude[60]	0	++++	++++	0	6[c]

[a]+ denotes 0 to 25% of neonates affected; ++, 25% to 50%; +++, 50% to 75%; ++++, 75% to 100%.
[b]Ratio of immature forms to total neutrophils.
[c]Not tested after 6 hours.
Data from reference 43, with additions as noted.

Table 36–2 Clinical Factors with No Effect on Neutrophil Counts in Newborn Infants

Race
Gender
Maternal diabetes
Fetal bradycardia
Mode of delivery[a]
Premature rupture of membranes, mother afebrile
Meconium staining, no lung disease
Uncomplicated hyaline membrane disease[62]
Uncomplicated transient tachypnea of the newborn
Hyperbilirubinemia, physiologic, unexplained[16]
Phototherapy
Diurnal variation[33,49]
Brief (for ≤3 minutes) crying[61]

[a]Total neutrophil counts in cord blood of infants delivered vaginally or by cesarean section after labor (2 to 14 hours) are twice those of infants delivered by cesarean section without labor.[61]
Data from reference 43, with additions as noted.

was similar to that described for group B streptococcal infection. Because all were noted to be ill at birth or shortly thereafter, when neutrophil counts normally are rising, a low count (0 to 4000 cells per mm^3) in this clinical setting is a highly significant finding. In many cases, the low number of circulating neutrophils reflects a depletion of bone marrow granulocyte reserves[76,81] and usually indicates a poor prognosis.[5,16,24,40,76,82] The absolute neutrophil count may therefore be useful for screening infants with symptomatic illness including respiratory distress in the first few hours of life, if not for asymptomatic infants.[27,83]

Total Nonsegmented Neutrophil Count

The blood smear and differential cell count during the newborn period are strikingly different from those seen at any other time of life. Immature forms are present in relatively large numbers, particularly among premature infants and during the first few days of life.[33,43,44,84] The number of *immature neutrophils*, mostly nonsegmented (band, stab) forms, rises from a maximal normal value of 1100 cells per mm^3 in cord blood to 1500 cells per mm^3 at 12 hours of life and gradually falls to 600 cells per mm^3 by 60 hours of life. Between 60 and 120 hours, the maximum count falls from 600 to 500 cells per mm^3 and remains unchanged through the first month of life.[43] For unexplained reasons, possibly related to differences in the definition of a nonsegmented neutrophil,[63] higher counts have been recorded by other authors.[16,69] Metamyelocytes and myelocytes also are often present in significant numbers during the first 72 hours after delivery but disappear almost entirely toward the end of the first week of life.[33] Even occasional promyelocytes and blast cells may be seen during the early days of life in healthy infants.[33]

As neutrophils are released from the bone marrow in response to infection, an increasing number of immature cells enter the bloodstream, producing a differential cell count with a "shift to the left" even greater than that normally present in the neonate.[69] This response is so inconstant, however, that, with few exceptions,[16,63,64] the absolute band or immature (bands, metamyelocytes) neutrophil count has been found to be of little diagnostic value.[5,24,46,55,62,70,72,73] In many infants with infection, despite an increased proportion of immature cell types in the differential leukocyte count, exhaustion of the bone marrow reserves prevents an increase in the absolute number of band neutrophils in the circulation.[81,85,86] This is particularly common in the more seriously ill patients, in whom early diagnosis is most critical.[5,69,76,81]

Despite its relative insensitivity, the immature neutrophil count has been found to have good positive predictive value in some,[5,44,47,69,73] although not all,[46] studies. In infants with clinical evidence of sepsis and high band counts in whom culture results remain negative, follow-up cultures are indicated, as well as investigation for a history of perinatal events that might explain the discrepancy (see Table 36-1), or for the possibility of infection related to other causes, such as enteroviruses.[87]

Neutrophil Ratios

The unreliability of absolute band counts led to the investigation of neutrophil ratios as an index of neonatal infection. Determinations have included the ratio of either bands or all immature neutrophils (e.g., bands, metamyelocytes, and myelocytes) to either segmented neutrophils (the *immature-to-mature neutrophil ratio* [I:M ratio]) or all neutrophils (the *immature-to-total neutrophil ratio* [I:T ratio]). Despite the early enthusiasm of researchers, the clinical studies that include these determinations have failed to show a consistent correlation with the presence of serious bacterial disease. As might be expected, low band counts caused by exhaustion of marrow can produce misleadingly low ratios in the presence of serious or overwhelming infection.[44,73,80,81]

Clinical experience with I:M ratios or band-to-segmented neutrophil ratios[44,69] is insufficient to verify their accuracy. Initial studies in which the I:M ratio was used, however, have been disappointing, with normal values recorded in more than one third of infected infants. Band-to-total neutrophil ratios, although more extensively studied, also have proved to be too unpredictable to be of much diagnostic help. The most favorable report would have missed 10% of neonates with sepsis while recording falsely abnormal values in almost 20% of uninfected infants.[18] The sensitivity of this determination in other series varies, ranging from 70% to as low as 30%, which precludes its use in a clinical setting.[22-24,68,69]

The I:T ratio is the best studied of the ratios.[68,88] Inclusion in the numerator of all immature forms, rather than just band cells, heightens accuracy by accounting for the increase in metamyelocytes that is sometimes seen with accelerated release from the neutrophil storage pool.[69] Use of total rather than segmented neutrophils in the denominator has the advantage of always yielding a value between 0 and 1 inclusive. The maximum ratio for the first 24 hours is 0.16.[43,58] It gradually falls to around 0.12 by 60 hours of age and remains unchanged for the remainder of the first month.[43] A normal value up to 0.2, with age unspecified, has been found in some laboratories.[18] Immature:total neutrophil ratios during the first 5 days of life among healthy premature infants with a gestational age of 32 weeks or less are less than 0.2 in 96%.[84]

A large number of clinical studies have evaluated the I:T ratio. Results have been widely disparate, but in most series, they indicate that this ratio is too unreliable to achieve more than limited usefulness by itself. Sensitivities ranging from more than 90%[16,19,21,43,46,73,89] to as low as 70%,[20,90] 60%,[55,67,70] or less [91,92] have been reported. Furthermore, elevated ratios caused by a variety of perinatal conditions have been seen in 25% to 50% of uninfected ill infants (see Table 36-1).[19,20] Perhaps the ratio's greatest value lies in its good negative predictive value: If the I:T ratio is normal, the likelihood that infection is absent is extremely high (99%).[3,18-20,46,67,73,93]

In addition, serial determinations of the I:T ratio may lead to increased sensitivity.[47,88,93] Some authors, however, have found that inter-reader variability leads to enough bias to limit the usefulness of leukocyte ratios for general use.[94]

Platelet Count

Several extensive studies have established that the normal *platelet count* in newborns, regardless of birth weight, is rarely less than 100,000/mm^3 during the first 10 days of life or less than 150,000/mm^3 during the next 3 weeks.[16,67,95-98] Although it would behoove the clinician to perform a workup for sepsis in any infant with unexplained thrombocytopenia,[98-100] a reduction in the number of circulating platelets has been shown to be an insensitive, nonspecific, and relatively late indicator of serious bacterial infection during the neonatal period. Automated measurements of mean platelet volume (MPV) have added little to the platelet count as a diagnostic aid.[101,102]

Only 10% to 60% of newborns with proven bacterial invasion of the bloodstream or meninges have platelet counts of less than 100,000/mm^3.[15-17,21,23,24,46,70,97] The average duration of thrombocytopenia is about 1 week but can be as long as 2 to 3 weeks. The nature of the organism involved (whether gram-positive, gram-negative, or fungal) has been reported in some, but not all, studies to correlate with the platelet count nadir and duration of thrombocytopenia.[16,70,97,101] Although platelet counts may begin to fall several days before the onset of clinical signs of infection, in most cases values remain elevated until 1 to 3 days after serious illness is already apparent.[17,24,39,63,97] Thrombocytopenia accompanying bacterial infection is thought to be caused by a direct effect of bacteria or bacterial products on platelets and vascular endothelium, leading to increased aggregation and adhesion, or by increased platelet destruction caused by immune mechanisms.[44,63,97-99]

In addition to the widely known association between thrombocytopenia and intrauterine infections related to syphilis, toxoplasmosis, rubella, and cytomegalovirus infection, reduced platelet counts also have been described with postnatal viral infections with enteroviruses and herpes simplex virus, each of which can cause an illness clinically indistinguishable from bacterial sepsis.[99-104] Conditions that predispose the infant to sepsis, such as umbilical line placement, birth asphyxia, mechanical ventilation, meconium aspiration, multiple exchange transfusions, and necrotizing enterocolitis, have independently caused thrombocytopenia in the absence of positive blood culture results.[39,100,105-107] Nonspecific neonatal thrombocytopenia also has been reported with various conditions causing maternal thrombocytopenia, including pregnancy-induced hypertension.[39] Infants with moderate to severe Rh hemolytic disease also are thrombocytopenic.[108]

ACUTE-PHASE REACTANTS

In the presence of inflammation caused by infection, trauma, or other cellular destruction, the liver, under the influence of the *proinflammatory cytokines* interleukin-1β (IL-1β), interleukin-6 (IL-6), and tumor necrosis factor-α (TNF-α), rapidly synthesizes large amounts of certain proteins collectively known as *acute-phase reactants*.[109-112] Serum levels of these proteins usually rise together, and in general, the degree of change in one is proportional to the degree of change in the others (two important exceptions are albumin

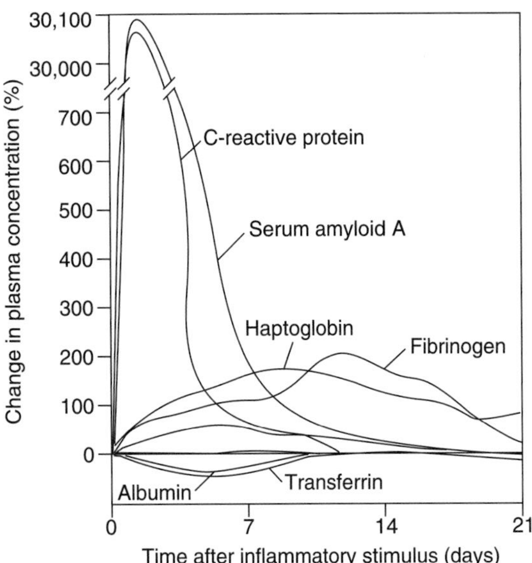

Figure 36–3 Acute-phase reactants in patients with inflammatory illnesses. The response of C-reactive protein (CRP) is greater than that of all other acute-phase proteins except serum amyloid A. Levels of certain plasma proteins decrease during the acute-phase response. (Data from Gabay C, Kushner I. Acute-phase proteins and other systemic responses to inflammation. N Engl J Med 340:448-454, 1999.)

and transferrin, which decrease together) (Fig. 36-3). Acute-phase reactants are produced very early in fetal life, beginning in the fourth to fifth week of gestation.[113] Their exact role in the inflammatory process is unknown; most appear to be part of a primitive nonspecific (innate) defense mechanism. Several acute-phase reactants have been extensively evaluated in neonatal sepsis, including C-reactive protein (CRP), fibrinogen, and other proteins that influence the erythrocyte sedimentation rate; haptoglobin; and α_1-acid glycoprotein (orosomucoid). Measurement of proinflammatory cytokines and their receptors holds promise to further increase diagnostic accuracy; these tests are discussed later in this chapter.

C-Reactive Protein

The most useful of the acute-phase reactants appears to be *CRP* when assayed by modern methods. CRP is a globulin that forms a precipitate when combined with the C-polysaccharide of *Streptococcus pneumoniae*.[111,112] Because the appearance of CRP in the blood has been closely associated with tissue injury, particularly when caused by an acute inflammatory process, it has been suggested that the primary function of CRP is to act as a carrier protein, binding and facilitating clearance of potentially toxic foreign or altered materials released from invading microorganisms or damaged tissues. Its roles in activation of the classic complement pathway, promotion of phagocytosis, regulation of lymphocyte function, and platelet activation are not yet clear.[68,109-112]

Differences in laboratory techniques and in the interpretation of what constitutes a positive result for CRP assay have been partly responsible for conflicting opinions about the reliability of this test during the neonatal period.[68,111,114,115] Thus, early clinical reports must be interpreted in light of the knowledge that the capillary tube precipitation and gel immunodiffusion techniques used for assay of CRP in those studies were less sensitive and specific than more modern immunochemical methods.[68,115] Furthermore, a comparison of reactions obtained by different investigators using the capillary tube method revealed widely disparate results, depending on the sensitivity of the commercial antiserum used in the assay. Newer rapid and reliable quantitative methods have been developed in which monoclonal CRP-specific antibody is used.[115-118] Fully automated turbidimetric and nephelometric methods can provide quantitative results in 30 to 60 minutes, whereas enzyme immunoassays, such as the enzyme-multiplied immunoassay technique, can give results in less than 10 minutes. Determination of CRP levels in serum by radial immunodiffusion, electroimmunodiffusion, spot immunoprecipitate assay, enzyme-multiplied immunoassay technique, and nephelometry has shown upper limits of about 10 mg/L (1 mg/dL) during the neonatal period.[47,111,112,116,119] Analysis of paired serum specimens obtained from mothers and their infants (fetuses and premature infants as well as full-term neonates) has shown that CRP crosses the placenta either in very low concentrations or not at all.[111] Gestational age does not appear to influence the validity of results.[22,111] CRP normal ranges may vary with time over the first few days of life, however.[115,120]

Most surveys of CRP levels in sera of neonates with systemic bacterial infections have shown significant elevations *at the time of onset of signs* (i.e., diagnostic test sensitivity) in 50% to 90% of cases.[18,21,47,68,111,112,120-127] A poor response is particularly frequent among infants whose infection occurs during the first 12 to 24 hours of life and among infants with infection caused by gram-positive bacteria, including group B streptococci.[21,89,122] Although the intensity of the response does not always reflect the severity of the infection, the relationship between formation of CRP and the degree of tissue injury indicates that the infants who demonstrate a positive response usually are those with systemic infections or involvement of deeper tissues.[21,128]

Unfortunately, measurement of CRP levels is not completely specific. The response of CRP to nonbacterial infections is variable; raised serum levels have been found in infants with viral infections.[129] A strong correlation between elevated CRP levels and chorioamnionitis has been described in women with premature rupture of membranes, as well as in the cord blood of their infants.[130,131] Increases of CRP levels in neonates, up to 10 times normal, also have been associated with noninfectious conditions causing tissue injury or inflammation, such as fetal asphyxia, respiratory distress syndrome, intracerebral hemorrhage, and meconium aspiration pneumonitis.[119,122,132] Because these conditions often are confused, or associated, with newborn bacterial infection, such false-positive elevations greatly reduce the positive predictive value of CRP determinations and their usefulness in diagnosis. The mean incidence of falsely elevated CRP values in ill but not septic neonates is approximately 5% to 15%.[89,92,121,132,133]

Thus, the reported overall sensitivity of CRP at the onset of signs of sepsis ranges between 50% and 90%, and the specificity ranges between 85% and 95%. The positive and negative predictive values, respectively, may be as low as 30% and as high as greater than 95%. It is clear from the foregoing discussion that despite new technology permitting more rapid and precise measurement, reliance on CRP levels *alone* as an early indicator of neonatal bacterial infection cannot be recommended. Although CRP levels possibly are helpful in combination with other tests as part of a "sepsis screening panel" (see later discussion), when CRP assay is used alone as an initial test for infection, even if the most favorable results are assumed, approximately 10% of cases will be missed and 5% of uninfected infants will be incorrectly diagnosed as having infection.

Nevertheless, determination of *serial* CRP levels does appear to be of some value in excluding serious infection.[68,111,112,133] Although assay results in a few infants will be normal at the onset of invasive bacterial disease, CRP levels rise rapidly and usually are abnormal within a day (CRP doubling time is 8 hours). CRP levels peak at 2 to 3 days and remain elevated until infection is controlled and resolution of the inflammatory process begins.[19,21,89,111,134] Thereafter, by virtue of a relatively short serum half-life of about 19 hours, CRP levels fall promptly and return to normal within 5 to 10 days in most infants who have a favorable outcome.[21,22,112,133] Serial measurements of CRP levels over 1 to 3 days after onset of possible neonatal bacterial infection may help determine the duration of antibiotic therapy, and identify the occurrence of relapse or complications during or after treatment of known infection. Several studies document that serial determination of CRP levels in this fashion yields diagnostic sensitivity of 75% to 98%, specificity of 90%, and perhaps most notably, a negative predictive value of 99%.[47,122-125,133-136] These studies suggest that although the relatively low sensitivity of initial CRP determination precludes the firm diagnosis of bacterial infection, the very high negative predictive value of several normal CRP determinations in combination allows the early discontinuance of empirical 7- to 10-day courses of intravenous antibiotics. It is less likely, however, that serial CRP determinations will allow discontinuance of empirical 2- to 3-day courses of antibiotics. It is even less certain whether the actual decay patterns of elevated CRP levels differ sufficiently to allow distinction between those newborns with positive and those with negative bacterial blood cultures.[134]

Erythrocyte Sedimentation Rate

The development more than 50 years ago of an erythrocyte sedimentation rate, by use of a microhematocrit tube and a few drops of capillary blood, permitted the application of this test in very small infants.[137,138] Attempts at standardization have shown that the *microerythrocyte sedimentation rate* increases slowly during the first weeks of life, perhaps as a result of rising fibrinogen and falling hematocrit levels. Maximal normal rates have varied so widely, however, that any laboratory attempting to use this test in neonates must establish its own normal values.[139-141]

Sedimentation rates do not vary significantly with gestational age, birth weight, or gender but are related inversely to the hematocrit level, particularly in infants with hematocrit readings of less than 0.40.[139,140] Comparisons between the microerythrocyte sedimentation rate and standard methods have shown good correlation in simultaneous analyses of samples obtained from cord blood, from infants with physiologic jaundice, and from healthy older children.[139] Rapid alternative methods such as determination of the zeta sedimentation ratio[142] and plasma viscosity[143] compared well with standard erythrocyte sedimentation rate assays and were thought to reflect a change in the same plasma proteins; however, they have not been evaluated in newborns. The microerythrocyte sedimentation rate generally is normal or only mildly elevated in noninfectious conditions such as respiratory distress syndrome, aspiration pneumonia, and asphyxia, as well as in superficial infections.[139,141] Significant elevations are unusual in healthy infants but can occur in the presence of Coombs-positive hemolytic disease and physiologic hyperbilirubinemia.[19,139,141]

Although extensive clinical experience has shown that sedimentation rates eventually become elevated in most infants with systemic bacterial infections, this rise may not have occurred at the time of the initial evaluation in 30% to 70% of infants with proven sepsis, particularly when disseminated intravascular coagulopathy is present.[18,19,82,126,139,141] Furthermore, once the rate is elevated, its return to normal can be exceedingly slow despite clinical recovery, sometimes taking several weeks from the time of onset of illness.[139] Thus, use of the microerythrocyte sedimentation rate is of little value in either diagnosing or monitoring serious bacterial infection during the newborn period.

Other Acute-Phase Reactants

The rise in plasma *fibrinogen* level associated with infection has been recognized for many years through its effects on the erythrocyte sedimentation rate. Clinical experience with the use of fibrinogen levels is limited but generally disappointing. The median fibrinogen concentrations in infected infants overlapped to a great extent with levels obtained from normal infants, and low values despite severe infection also have been reported.[144,145] Concentrations may be affected by birth weight and test methodology and, indeed, fall dramatically in the presence of disseminated intravascular coagulopathy.

Haptoglobin is an α_2-glycoprotein that reacts with free hemoglobin to form a complex, which is removed by the reticuloendothelial system. Gestational age, neonatal asphyxia, gender, and hemolytic ABO/Rh disease have no significant influence on levels in cord blood or during the postnatal period; however, elevated levels usually persist for several days after exchange transfusion, probably as a result of passive transfer of blood with adult concentrations of haptoglobin. Inaccuracies related to phenotypic variants of haptoglobin, although seen when levels are measured by radial immunodiffusion, have not presented a problem when concentrations are determined by laser nephelometry. Because haptoglobin determinations, measured as plasma hemoglobin-binding capacity or by laser nephelometry, can be performed in 1 to 2 hours, they were thought to be potentially of great value in the early detection of bacterial infection in the newborn. Unfortunately, clinical studies have raised serious doubts about the reliability of this test.[18,22,119,146,147]

α_1-Acid glycoprotein (orosomucoid) is produced by lymphocytes, monocytes, and neutrophils as well as hepatocytes. It exists as an integral membrane protein of leukocytes and is liberated into the plasma as the cells disintegrate.[110] Its function is unknown, but it may have a role in forming collagen, binding steroid hormones, and modifying lymphocyte responsiveness.[136,148] Although early studies suggested that α_1-acid glycoprotein might be a specific and sensitive indicator of neonatal bacterial infection, subsequent surveys have not been able to confirm this favorable experience.[18,119,128,136,148-153]

The failure of any of the acute-phase proteins discussed earlier to provide definitive guidelines for the early diagnosis of neonatal sepsis has led to a search for other, perhaps better indicators. Among those evaluated have been *α_1-proteinase inhibitor* (α_1-antitrypsin)[22,153]; the complex of *elastase and α_1-proteinase inhibitor*[154,155]; *α_1-antichymotrypsin*[153]; *inter–α-inhibitor proteins*[156]; and *ceruloplasmin*.[157] No definitive clinical studies suggest that any of these reactants are helpful for diagnosis or management in the neonate suspected of having a bacterial infection.

ADDITIONAL LABORATORY STUDIES

Cytokine Concentrations

Cytokines such as the interleukins IL-1β, IL-6, and IL-8 and TNF-α, as well as others, are endogenous mediators of the immune response to inflammation, including (but not limited to) that caused by bacterial infections. Both cord and postnatal blood cytokine concentrations may vary as a result of clinical complications during the perinatal period. For example, IL-1β is elevated in cord plasma specimens from infants born after induced vaginal or urgent cesarean delivery, whereas IL-6 is elevated in the presence of chorioamnionitis and delivery room intubation, yet depressed in the presence of pregnancy-induced hypertension.[121,158,159] Because of the confounding effects of maternal complications, chronologic age in the first hours to days of life, and illness severity, the reported performance of various cytokine markers must be viewed with some caution.[4,115,121]

Nevertheless, several studies suggest that elevated levels of *IL-6* detected after birth may provide an early and sensitive parameter for the diagnosis of neonatal bacterial infection.[119,120,121,159-165] Elevated concentrations have also been correlated with a fatal outcome in older children.[166] Similarly, levels of *IL-8* were found to be elevated in cord blood from infants in whom histologic evidence of chorioamnionitis was noted, as well as in infants with sepsis.[127,161,167,168] Because of variations in study design and methodology, estimates of diagnostic sensitivity and specificity for IL-6 and IL-8 levels range from 60% to greater than 95% for each.[127,169,170]

Other cytokines and substances associated with the inflammatory response have been evaluated as possible indicators of newborn infection. *TNF-α* and upregulated adhesion molecules such as *E-selectin*, *L-selectin*, and *intercellular adhesion molecule-1* (ICAM-1) have been suggested as discriminators of bacterial sepsis.[123,159,164,171-173] An early and somewhat specific elevation in serum levels of *procalcitonin* in infants with invasive bacterial disease has been described by several authors.[174-177a] Procalcitonin concentrations naturally fluctuate during the first 48 hours of life, however, mandating very careful (perhaps hourly) adjustments in the normal reference ranges and thus complicating its use as a diagnostic aid.[121,178,179] Cytokine receptors and receptor antagonists such as *soluble TNF-α* and *IL-2 receptors* and *IL-1 receptor antagonist* have been used to aid in the laboratory diagnosis of neonatal sepsis.[127,162,169,180,181] Further clinical data will be needed to determine whether measurement of these analytes is truly useful for the diagnosis and follow-up evaluation of neonatal sepsis.

Lymphocyte and Neutrophil Marker Analysis

Another component of the inflammatory response to infection is the change in surface markers of white cell populations as measured by flow cytometry. Activation of T lymphocytes after infection results in upregulation of the *lymphocyte surface marker CD45RO isoform* and in loss of the *CD45RA isoform*. Sequential analysis of the distribution of early CD45RA-CD45RO dual expression and later CD45RO expression alone discriminated bacterial (and viral) infection from respiratory distress or erythrocyte incompatibility in a small number of infants.[182] The surface expression of the *neutrophil surface marker CD11b* yielded good sensitivity, specificity, and predictive values (greater than 95%) in diagnosing neonatal bacterial infection in two studies.[172,183] The expression of CD11b, however, may be affected by duration of labor and chronologic age; further studies are required to define normal ranges and clinical utility.[172,184] Expression of another *neutrophil surface marker, CD64*, was found to correlate with early- and late-onset nosocomial newborn sepsis.[185,185a]

Miscellaneous Analytes

Fibronectin is an adhesive, high-molecular-weight glycoprotein of 450,000 kDa that has been identified on cell surfaces and in extracellular fluids. It is thought, by virtue of its stickiness, to act as an intercellular cement and maintain microvascular integrity, and to act as an opsonin and aid in the phagocytic function of neutrophils and macrophages.[110,186] In general, the concentration of fibronectin in fetal plasma increases with gestational age to concentrations at term of approximately one half those found in healthy adults.[186-188] Plasma concentrations usually fall significantly during the course of neonatal sepsis, probably as a result of clearance by the reticuloendothelial system of products of the inflammatory response. The rate of recovery of fibronectin concentrations as infection resolves is relatively rapid, occurring over 5 to 7 days.[186,187] Attempts to characterize a fall in fibronectin concentrations as a specific marker for sepsis have been disappointing, however.[19]

Demonstration of increased amounts of *total immunoglobulin M* (IgM) in umbilical cord sera once was thought to be helpful in identifying infants with infections acquired in the intrauterine environment, particularly those caused by rubella virus, cytomegalovirus, *Treponema pallidum*, and *Toxoplasma gondii*.[189] On the basis of this experience, several studies, mainly in the late 1960s and early 1970s, attempted to use serially determined IgM concentrations in the evaluation of infants suspected of having acute postnatal bacterial infections. The sensitivity of IgM concentrations in infants with bacterial sepsis, meningitis, pneumonia, or urinary tract infection is rather low; specificity was low as well in that viral infections, minor localized bacterial infections, and meconium aspiration were associated with a significant increase in IgM concentrations.[19,189-193] Determination of IgM concentrations as an index of neonatal bacterial infection has largely been abandoned.

The discovery that neutrophils that have phagocytized bacteria reduce nitroblue tetrazolium (NBT) dye to purple formazan led to development of several tests using this *leukocyte enzyme activity* for detection of bacterial infections involving the systemic circulation.[194] It was shown that in most cases, a majority of peripheral neutrophils reduce nitroblue tetrazolium during the course of an untreated or ineffectively treated infection, whereas only a small proportion of neutrophils do so in the absence of infection. Unfortunately, attempts to incorporate this assay into the newborn period were hampered by difficulty in establishing standard techniques and normal values, and the predictive value of the test was found to be lower than expected.[195-200] The NBT test now is rarely used in the diagnosis of neonatal infection.[91] Changes in leukocyte lactate dehydrogenase[201] and in alkaline phosphatase[202] concentrations were thought a number of years ago to be potentially useful indices of neonatal infection. These determinations have received little further attention since that time.

Bacterial infections are known to alter *carbohydrate metabolism* in neonates. Although hypoglycemia[203] and hyperglycemia[204] have been described in infants with sepsis, the association between changes in blood glucose concentrations and neonatal infection is of only limited value as a diagnostic aid.

An exciting recent discovery in the field of immunology is that multicellular organisms share an evolutionarily conserved *innate immune system*. Innate immunity depends on molecules such as specialized cellular receptors and binding proteins (e.g., Toll-like receptors and mannose binding protein), serum complement proteins, and several substances produced and released at the site of infection by neutrophils.[205,206] This last group includes the *antimicrobial peptides* of the defensin and cathelicidin classes, *bactericidal/permeability-increasing protein* (BPI), *lysozyme*, and *lactoferrin*.[205-207] Some of these substances are found in vernix caseosa, the lipid-rich substance covering the skin of the fetus and newborn infant.[208] Further studies on the kinetics of these molecules in health and disease may lead to diagnostic aids for newborn sepsis.[207-209]

Finally, sepsis, or more properly, the systemic inflammatory response to sepsis, causes hemodynamic changes in regional blood flow. Early in sepsis, peripheral vasoconstriction is seen, whereas in advanced sepsis, generalized vasodilation and shock occur. An interesting concept in diagnostic techniques for neonatal sepsis is to attempt to noninvasively measure deviations in *peripheral vascular reactivity*. Newborns with early-onset sepsis (clinical or bacteriologic) had lower degrees of mean peripheral skin perfusion and a higher amount of postocclusion reactive hyperemia as measured by a laser Doppler instrument in one small study.[161] The sensitivity and specificity for the measurement of reactive hyperemia were equivalent to or greater than those for measurement of IL-6, IL-8, and TNF-α in this study.[161]

Microscopic Examination of Placenta, Umbilical Cord, Gastric Aspirates, and External Ear Canal Fluid

Microscopic examination of tissues or body fluids is a time-honored but rather insensitive and nonspecific aid in the diagnosis of neonatal sepsis. An association of neonatal sepsis with *pathologic changes in the placenta and umbilical cord* was suggested more than 40 years ago.[210,211] Neonatal infection acquired at or about the time of birth often is associated with chorioamnionitis or funisitis.[212-214] Histologic sections of the placenta show acute inflammatory changes, with infiltration of the umbilical vein by neutrophils and gross or microscopic evidence of chorioamnionitis. The probability of finding inflammatory changes in these tissues is inversely related to birth weight and directly related to the duration of rupture of membranes before delivery, the presence of meconium in amniotic fluid, and fetal distress and hypoxia.[215-217] As many as 30% of live-born infants show some inflammatory changes in the placenta and its membranes or the umbilical cord.[212] Thus, the presence of chorioamnionitis and placentitis does not automatically imply significant neonatal infection.

The stomach of the newborn contains fluid swallowed before and during delivery. The presence of neutrophils and bacteria in a stained smear of the *gastric aspirate* indicates inflammation of the amniotic fluid, placenta, and other tissues of the birth canal.[218,219] The neutrophils in the gastric aspirate obtained during the first day of life are from the mother and do not indicate a fetal inflammatory response.[220] Therefore, the presence of these maternal leukocytes indicates exposure to possible infection and does not necessarily identify an infectious disease in the newborn. After the first day, however, the gastric aspirate contains swallowed bronchial secretions, and examination of a stained preparation may suggest pneumonia in the neonate if inflammatory cells are present.[221] The presence of neutrophils in the *aspirated ear canal fluid* also indicates exposure to an infected environment. Stained smears and bacterial cultures of neonatal gastric aspirate or external ear canal fluid reflect the flora of the birth canal, and results parallel those of cultures of specimens obtained from the maternal vagina, endocervix, endometrium, and placenta.[222-226] The information obtained does not greatly influence decision making regarding antimicrobial therapy.[223]

Pathogens frequently are isolated when daily *tracheal aspirates* for intubated infants are cultured. Because many (if not all) intubated newborns will eventually become colonized with potentially pathogenic microbes, however, the positive predictive value of this test is less than 30%.[227] Similar to gastric aspirates or external ear canal fluid, tracheal aspirates reflect environmental influences but do not necessarily imply sepsis.

Molecular detection tests for bacteria or bacterial products have been applied to both amniotic fluid and neonatal blood. Although the *limulus lysate assay* for the detection of endotoxin did not prove to be clinically useful,[228] PCR amplification of bacterial DNA from blood appears promising but is not ready for general clinical use.[229-230]

Screening Panels

The inability of any single laboratory test to provide rapid, reliable, and early identification of neonates with bacterial sepsis has led to efforts to devise a panel of screening tests, combining data from several different determinations, as a means of increasing predictive value.[4,115,123,169,170,231] In general, the results have shown little increase in positive predictive value (if a test result is abnormal, disease is present) compared with most of the individual screening tests, although negative predictive value (if a result is normal, disease is absent) has been remarkably good, approaching 100% in some studies. Performance characteristics of some screening panel tests are summarized in Table 36-3 and compared with those of single tests.

Table 36–3 Performance Characteristics of Various Tests and Screening Panels for Neonatal Bacterial Infection: Selected Reports

Source, Test (Test Cutoff[a])	No. of Newborns Evaluated	Prevalence of Culture-Documented Bacterial Sepsis (%)	Sensitivity (%)	Specificity (%)	Positive Predictive Value (%)	Negative Predictive Value (%)	Positive Likelihood Ratio	Negative Likelihood Ratio
Early-Onset Sepsis								
Chiesa[120]	134	8						
CRP: At birth (4 mg/L)			73	83	28	97	4.3	0.33
CRP: At 24 hr (of life) (10 mg/L)			91	87	38	99	7.0	0.10
IL-6: At birth (200 ng/L)			73	89	36	97	6.6	0.30
IL-6: At 24 hr (30 ng/L)			64	71	16	96	2.2	0.50
PCT: At birth (1 μg/L)			82	95	60	98	16.4	0.19
PCT: At 24 hr (100 μg/L)			100	96	69	100	2.5	~0.0
Benitz[124]	999	1.5						
Serial CRP levels: Any of 3 tests performed over 48 hr (10 mg/L)			89	70	5	99	3.0	0.16
Døllner[121]	166	14.5						
CRP (10 mg/L)			63	89	48	93	5.7	0.42
IL-6 (20 ng/L)			78	64	27	95	2.2	0.34
IL-6 ± CRP			96	58	28	99	3.7	0.07
Philip[18]	376	8						
Any 2 or more abnormalities in I:T ratio, total WBC, CRP, micro-ESR, haptoglobin			93	88	39	99	7.8	0.08
Rodwell[46]	298	9						
Any 3 or more abnormalities in I:T ratio, total neutrophils, total WBC, I:M ratio, platelet count; degenerative changes of neutrophils			96	78	31	99	4.4	0.05
Late-Onset Sepsis								
Ng[123]	101	45[b]						
CRP: Initial evaluation (10 mg/L)			60	96	93	77	15.0	0.42
CRP: 48 hr later (10 mg/L)			87	95	93	90	17.4	0.14
IL-6: Initial evaluation (13 ng/L)			93	71	73	93	22.2	0.11
IL-6: 48 hr later (13 ng/L)			73	64	63	75	3.6	0.50
CRP + IL-6 initially + CRP at 48 hr			98	68	71	97	3.1	0.03

[a]Test cutoff refers to the value above which the test result is considered abnormal.

[b]A higher prevalence of sepsis tends to inflate the positive predictive value, and to depress the negative predictive value, of a test or panel.

CRP, C-reactive protein; ESR, erythrocyte sedimentation rate; IL-6, interleukin-6; I:M ratio, immature-to-mature neutrophil ratio (see text); I:T ratio, immature-to-total neutrophil ratio; PCT, procalcitonin; WBC, white blood cell (total leukocyte) count.

One attempt to diagnose neonatal sepsis through multiple, simple, standard laboratory determinations involved more than 500 infants younger than 7 days of age studied by Philip and Hewitt[18] and Philip.[67,232] The authors devised a "sepsis screen" for use with infants believed to be at risk for, or demonstrating clinical evidence of, serious bacterial infection. In addition to the standard procedures (blood, CSF, and urine cultures and chest film), the evaluation included a screening panel consisting of total leukocyte count, determination of the I:M ratio, CRP and haptoglobin assays, and micro-erythrocyte sedimentation rate. An abnormality in any two or more of these items was considered to reflect a "positive sepsis screen," and in one or none, a "negative sepsis screen"; the test turn-around time was 1 hour.

Analysis of the results[18,67] showed a 39% probability that serious bacterial infection was present if two or more test results were positive (positive predictive value) and a 99% probability that infection was not present if only one or no result was positive (negative predictive value). In actual numbers, as a result of the sepsis screen, 60 of 524 infants with clinically suspected sepsis received unnecessary treatment with antimicrobial agents (false positives; specificity of 88%), and 3 with subsequently proven bacterial infection were missed (false negatives; sensitivity of 93%).[67] Comparable results have been reported by Gerdes and Polin,[19] who used a sepsis screen similar to that used by Philip, and by others who used only hematologic or clinical indices.[15,43,46,57,93] It should be noted, however, that panels of screening tests have not always functioned better than relying solely on the I:T neutrophil ratio, particularly in the first week of life.[18-20,46,57,67,73]

By virtue of its high negative predictive value, the screening panel used by Philip in an intensive care nursery resulted in a significant decrease in the use of antimicrobial agents.[232] Not only did fewer neonates receive antimicrobial agents, but treatment could be discontinued earlier with greater confidence in the infants who were being administered these agents. This author was careful to emphasize, however, that screening tests are intended only to augment clinical evaluation. When the evidence obtained by history or physical examination conflicts with a negative screen result, antimicrobial therapy should be started. More recent screening panels combining IL-8 and CRP assays are beginning to be evaluated and if early results are replicated may prove to be useful.[232a]

An increasingly important area in which a screening test panel might be useful is in the evaluation of asymptomatic infants whose mothers have been given intrapartum antibiotics to decrease the risk of early-onset neonatal group B streptococcal sepsis.[6-9] The American Academy of Pediatrics and the Centers for Disease Control and Prevention (CDC) recommend that a "limited evaluation," consisting of complete blood cell count and a blood culture, be performed in infants whose mothers met the criteria for intrapartum antibiotic prophylaxis but who did not receive a complete course of prophylactic treatment.[8,9] The goal is to identify infants with sepsis, including those whose blood cultures may have been sterilized temporarily by maternal antibiotic prophylaxis. Ottolini and colleagues recently tested the utility of a complete blood count (CBC) screening panel in 1665 infants whose mothers met the criteria for intrapartum antibiotic prophylaxis, but did not receive a full course of treatment.[27] These investigators found that the diagnostic test sensitivity and specificity of an abnormal white blood cell (WBC) count (i.e., total WBC count of ≤5000 or ≥30,000/mm^3, absolute neutrophil count of <1500/mm^3 or I:M ratio of >0.2) were 41% and 73%, respectively.[27] Because of the low incidence of true sepsis, even after only partial maternal antibiotic prophylaxis, the positive predictive value of the CBC panel was only 1.5% and the positive likelihood ratio only 1.5. Thus, a positive test result was not indicative of newborn sepsis. The negative predictive value of the screen was 99%, implying that a normal test result would at least reassure the clinician that sepsis was not present. The negative predictive value of an infant's being asymptomatic, however, also was 99%; thus, the CBC panel did not add any diagnostic information beyond that gained simply by obtaining a careful history and physical examination of the infant. Similar conclusions have been reached by Escobar and associates.[83] The ineffectiveness of the screening panel in these studies may have been due to the low rates of culture-proven sepsis, but many U.S. centers where group B streptococcal sepsis prophylaxis is employed have such low rates of sepsis.

PERSPECTIVES AND CONCLUSIONS

As discussed previously, it is difficult to choose one cytokine, acute-phase reactant, or screening panel for current use as the "best" test, on examining all of the data published to date (see Table 36-3).[115,169,170,231] Why is this still the case in the 21st century, after so many advances in medical science and biotechnology, and with the plethora of studies of newborn sepsis? Chiesa and colleagues recently have postulated several problems with the current literature that contribute to diagnostic uncertainty and inconsistency.[115]

First, some authors do not differentiate between perinatal (early-onset) and postnatal (late-onset) sepsis. This omission can lead to bias, because different neonatal pathogens cause early- and late-onset disease. In addition, Chiesa's group in particular has shown that normal ranges vary across gestational and chronologic age, producing another confounder if a study fails to differentiate between early- and late-onset sepsis.[115,120] Third, not all reports of neonatal sepsis diagnostic tests include healthy controls, so that construction of the normal range of results for an analytical test is difficult. Another problem is the lack of universal agreement on the definition of *newborn sepsis* or *systemic inflammatory response syndrome*. Some studies restrict the analyses to culture-proven sepsis, although false-negative cultures due to low blood sample volume or maternal antibiotic therapy may lead to bias. Other studies analyze *clinical septicemia*, although no universal definition of this entity exists, which also may lead to diagnostic bias; very few studies separately analyze data using both proven and clinically diagnosed sepsis.[121] A fifth problem is that the current neonatal illness severity scores (e.g., Score for Neonatal Acute Physiology [SNAP], SNAP-Perinatal Extension [SNAP-PE], Clinical Risk Index for Babies [CRIB]), which in theory could lead to better stratification and thus more accurate interstudy comparisons, are cumbersome to use.[115,121] Sixth, the accuracy of the laboratory methods suggested for the diagnosis of neonatal sepsis clearly affects test performance, as shown particularly by various studies of CRP as well as for some cytokines.[115] Finally, Chiesa and colleagues note that "the usefulness of a test will depend, above all, on the clinical condition of the baby. If the baby is really very sick, the test will not give very much additional information ... if the baby is evidently well ... a positive test result [will] not dramatically increase the probability that the baby is infected...."[115] In other words, it is essential to heed Bayesian statistical theory—the clinician must consider the pretest (prior) probability (essentially, the disease prevalence) of infection as well as the test characteristics (sensitivity, specificity) in order to properly interpret and apply diagnostic test results. Many of these confounding effects can be seen in the data of Table 36-3, in which various studies have used different populations of babies, definitions of sepsis, laboratory cutoff points, and so on, leading to different estimates of the utility of any one laboratory test.

Faced with the imperfection of currently available laboratory aids for the diagnosis of neonatal sepsis, what is today's practitioner to do? First, it should be remembered that history, physical examination, and clinical impression still constitute a large part of clinical medicine, even in the era of molecular diagnostics and therapeutics. A single normal laboratory test should not sway a clinician against empirical therapy for a newborn if it appears to be clinically indicated, nor should an isolated abnormal test result be enough for the clinician to demand therapy. This concept may be restated in diagnostic test statistical terminology as follows. At present, there is no one test or test panel with a high-enough positive likelihood ratio or a low-enough negative likelihood ratio to recommend it uniquely over all others. Furthermore, the negative predictive values of available tests are not yet high enough, when results are normal, to lead to the withholding of therapy for an uncommon but possibly life-threatening disease (neonatal sepsis). Conversely, the positive predictive values of available tests are not yet high enough when results are abnormal to lead to routine institution of antimicrobial therapy. When laboratory testing is combined with clinical impression (and perhaps serial laboratory monitoring), predictive values may increase enough to help the clinician make decisions. When the risk of an uncommon disease with a poor outcome is high, however, and the risk of antimicrobial therapy is low, it may be difficult to ever find a test with predictive values high enough to "rule in" or "rule out" disease with complete confidence.

In the final analysis, clinical judgment, using standardized definitions of historical risk factors, signs, and symptoms, may sometimes perform as well as laboratory screening panels.[27,83] This point may be especially important to remember in resource-poor settings in developing countries.[233] Clearly, much future work is needed in the area of rapid diagnosis of neonatal sepsis in order to move beyond the current best menu of simple, rapid, and inexpensive (albeit imperfect) tests such as total neutrophil counts, total leukocyte counts, I:T ratios, and CRP assay. Fortunately, continued improvements in blood culture technology are decreasing the time to positivity of neonatal blood cultures, which may at least speed up bacteriologic confirmation of septicemia.[234,235]

ACKNOWLEDGMENT

Previous versions of this chapter in earlier editions of this book were authored by Keith Powell and S. Michael Marcy, and portions of their contribution persist in the current chapter.

REFERENCES

1. Feinstein AR. Clinical biostatistics: XXXI. On the sensitivity, specificity, and discrimination of diagnostic tests. Clin Pharmacol Ther 17:104-116, 1975.
2. Jaeschke R, Guyatt GH, Sackett DL, et al. Users' guides to the medical literature: III. How to use an article about a diagnostic test. B. What are the results and will they help me in caring for my patients? JAMA 271:703-707, 1994.
3. Radetsky M. The laboratory evaluation of newborn sepsis. Curr Opin Infect Dis 8:191-199, 1995.
4. Escobar GJ. Effect of the systemic inflammatory response on biochemical markers of neonatal bacterial infection: a fresh look at old confounders. Clin Chem 49:21-22, 2003.
5. Squire E, Favara B, Todd J. Diagnosis of neonatal bacterial infection: hematologic and pathologic findings in fatal and nonfatal cases. Pediatrics 64:60-64, 1979.
6. Stoll BJ, Hansen N, Fanaroff AA, et al. Changes in pathogens causing early-onset sepsis in very-low-birth-weight infants. N Engl J Med 347:240-247, 2002.
7. Hyde TB, Hilger TM, Reingold A, et al. Trends in incidence and antimicrobial resistance of early-onset sepsis: population-based surveillance in San Francisco and Atlanta. Pediatrics 110:690-695, 2002.
8. Centers for Disease Control and Prevention. Prevention of perinatal group B streptococcal disease. MMWR Morb Mortal Wkly Rep 51(No. RR-11):1-22, 2002.
9. American Academy of Pediatrics. Group B streptococcal infections. *In* Pickering LK (ed). 2003 Red Book: Report of the Committee on Infectious Diseases, 26th ed. Elk Grove Village, Ill, American Academy of Pediatrics 2003, pp 584-591.
10. Dunham EC. Septicemia in the newborn. Am J Dis Child 45:229-253, 1933.
11. Nyhan WL, Fousek MD. Septicemia of the newborn. Pediatrics 22: 268-278, 1958.
12. Buetow KC, Klein SW, Lane RB. Septicemia in premature infants. Am J Dis Child 110:29-41, 1965.
13. Moorman RS Jr, Sell SH. Neonatal septicemia. South Med J 54:137-141, 1961.
14. Hänninen P, Terho P, Toivanen A. Septicemia in a pediatric unit: a 20-year study. Scand J Infect Dis 3:201-208, 1971.
15. Spector SA, Ticknor W, Grossman M. Study of the usefulness of clinical and hematologic findings in the diagnosis of neonatal bacterial infections. Clin Pediatr 20:385-392, 1981.
16. Kuchler H, Fricker H, Gugler E. La formule sanguine dans le diagnostic précoce de la septicémie du nouveau-né. Helv Paediatr Acta 31:33-46, 1976.
17. Töllner U, Pohlandt F. Septicemia in the newborn due to gram-negative bacilli: risk factors, clinical symptoms, and hematologic changes. Eur J Pediatr 123:243-254, 1976.
18. Philip AGS, Hewitt JR. Early diagnosis of neonatal sepsis. Pediatrics 65:1036-1041, 1980.
19. Gerdes JS, Polin RA. Sepsis screen in neonates with evaluation of plasma fibronectin. Pediatr Infect Dis J 6:443-446, 1987.
20. King JC Jr, Berman ED, Wright PF. Evaluation of fever in infants less than 8 weeks old. South Med J 80:948-952, 1987.
21. Philip AGS. Response of C-reactive protein in neonatal group B streptococcal infection. Pediatr Infect Dis J 4:145-148, 1985.
22. Speer CH, Bruns A, Gahr M. Sequential determination of CRP, alpha-1 antitrypsin and haptoglobin in neonatal septicaemia. Acta Paediatr Scand 72:679-683, 1983.
23. Liu C-H, Lehan C, Speer ME, et al. Degenerative changes in neutrophils: an indicator of bacterial infection. Pediatrics 74:823-827, 1984.
24. Jahnke S, Bartiromo G, Maisels MJ. The peripheral white blood cell count in the diagnosis of neonatal infection. J Perinatol 5:50-56, 1985.
25. Rozycki HJ, Stahl GE, Baumgart S. Impaired sensitivity of a single early leukocyte count in screening for neonatal sepsis. Pediatr Infect Dis J 6:440-442, 1987.
26. Christensen RD, Rothstein G, Hill HR, et al. Fatal early onset group B streptococcal sepsis with normal leukocyte counts. Pediatr Infect Dis J 4:242-245, 1985.
27. Ottolini MC, Lundgren K, Mirkinson LJ, et al. Utility of complete blood count and blood culture screening to diagnose neonatal sepsis in the asymptomatic at risk newborn. Pediatr Infect Dis J 22:430-434, 2003.
28. Marks MI, Stacy T, Krous HF. Progressive cough associated with lymphocytic leukemoid reaction in an infant. J Pediatr 97:156-160, 1980.

29. Weinberg AG, Rosenfeld CR, Manroe BL, et al. Neonatal blood cell count in health and disease: II. Values for lymphocytes, monocytes, and eosinophils. J Pediatr 106:462-466, 1985.
30. Roth P. Colony stimulating factor 1 levels in the human newborn infant. J Pediatr 119:113-116, 1991.
31. Karayalcin G, Khanijou A, Kim KY, et al. Monocytosis in congenital syphilis. Am J Dis Child 131:782-783, 1977.
32. Visintine AM, Oleske JM, Nahmias AJ. *Listeria monocytogenes* infection in infants and children. Am J Dis Child 131:393-397, 1977.
33. Xanthou M. Leucocyte blood picture in healthy full-term and premature babies during neonatal period. Arch Dis Child 45:242-249, 1970.
34. Lawrence R Jr, Church JA, Richards W, et al. Eosinophilia in the hospitalized neonate. Ann Allergy 44:349-352, 1980.
35. Burrell JM. A comparative study of the circulating eosinophil level in babies: II. In full term infants. Arch Dis Child 28:140-142, 1953.
36. Gibson EL, Vaucher Y, Corrigan JJ Jr. Eosinophilia in premature infants: relationship to weight gain. J Pediatr 95:99-101, 1979.
37. Gunn T, Reaman G, Outerbridge EW, et al. Peripheral total parenteral nutrition for premature infants with the respiratory distress syndrome: a controlled study. J Pediatr 92:608-613, 1978.
38. Bhat AM, Scanlon JW. The pattern of eosinophilia in premature infants: a prospective study in premature infants using the absolute eosinophil count. J Pediatr 98:612-616, 1981.
39. Chudwin DS, Ammann AJ, Wara DW, et al. Posttransfusion syndrome: rash, eosinophilia, and thrombocytopenia following intrauterine and exchange transfusions. Am J Dis Child 136:612-614, 1982.
40. Xanthou M. Leucocyte blood picture in ill newborn babies. Arch Dis Child 47:741-746, 1972.
41. Bonadio WA, Smith DS. CBC differential profile in distinguishing etiology of neonatal meningitis. Pediatr Emerg Care 5:94-96, 1989.
42. Metrov M, Crain EF. The complete blood count differential ratio in the assessment of febrile infants with meningitis. Pediatr Infect Dis J 10:334-335, 1991.
43. Manroe BL, Weinberg AG, Rosenfeld CR, et al. The neonatal blood count in health and disease: I. Reference values for neutrophilic cells. J Pediatr 95:89-98, 1979.
44. Zipursky A, Palko J, Milner R, et al. The hematology of bacterial infections in premature infants. Pediatrics 57:839-853, 1976.
45. Amato M, Howald H, von Muralt G. Qualitative changes of white blood cells and perinatal diagnosis of infection in high-risk preterm infants. Pädiatr Pädol 23:129-134, 1988.
46. Rodwell RL, Leslie AL, Tudehope DI. Early diagnosis of neonatal sepsis using a hematologic scoring system. J Pediatr 112:761-767, 1988.
47. Berger C, Uehlinger J, Ghelfi D, et al. Comparison of C-reactive protein and white blood cell count with differential in neonates at risk for septicemia. Eur J Pediatr 154:138-144, 1995.
48. Christensen RD. Morphology and concentration of circulating neutrophils in neonates with bacterial sepsis. Pediatr Infect Dis J 6:429-430, 1987.
49. Gregory J, Hey E. Blood neutrophil response to bacterial infection in the first month of life. Arch Dis Child 47:747-753, 1972.
50. Baley JE, Stork EK, Warkentin PI, et al. Neonatal neutropenia: clinical manifestations, cause, and outcome. Am J Dis Child 142:1161-1166, 1988.
51. Marks J, Gairdner D, Roscoe JD. Blood formation in infancy: III. Cord blood. Arch Dis Child 30:117-120, 1955.
52. Mouzinho A, Rosenfeld CR, Sanchez PJ, Risser R. Revised reference ranges for circulating neutrophils in very-low-birth-weight neonates. Pediatrics 94:76-82, 1999.
53. Schelonka RL, Yoder BA, desJardins SE, et al. Peripheral leukocyte count and leukocyte indexes in healthy newborn term infants. J Pediatr 125:603-606, 1994.
54. Coulombel L, Dehan M, Tchernia G, et al. The number of polymorphonuclear leukocytes in relation to gestational age in the newborn. Acta Paediatr Scand 68:709-711, 1979.
55. Engle WD, Rosenfeld CR. Neutropenia in high-risk neonates. J Pediatr 105:982-986, 1984.
56. Brazy JE, Grimm JK, Little VA. Neonatal manifestations of severe maternal hypertension occurring before the thirty-sixth week of pregnancy. J Pediatr 100:265-271, 1982.
57. Rodwell RL, Tudehope DI, Gray PH. Hematologic scoring system in early diagnosis of sepsis in neutropenic newborns. Pediatr Infect Dis J 12:372-376, 1993.
58. Merlob P, Amir J, Zaizov R, et al. The differential leukocyte count in full-term newborn infants with meconium aspiration and neonatal asphyxia. Acta Paediatr Scand 69:779-780, 1980.
59. Christensen RD, Rothstein G. Pitfalls in the interpretation of leukocyte counts of newborn infants. Am J Clin Pathol 72:608-611, 1979.
60. Carballo C, Foucar K, Swanson P, et al. Effect of high altitude on neutrophil counts in newborn infants. J Pediatr 119:464-466, 1991.
61. Frazier JP, Cleary TG, Pickering LK, et al. Leukocyte function in healthy neonates following vaginal and cesarean section deliveries. J Pediatr 101:269-272, 1982.
62. Menke JA, Giacoia GP, Jockin H. Group B beta hemolytic streptococcal sepsis and the idiopathic respiratory distress syndrome: a comparison. J Pediatr 94:467-471, 1979.
63. Zipursky A, Jaber HM. The haematology of bacterial infection in newborn infants. Clin Haematol 7:175-193, 1978.
64. Akenzua GI, Hui YT, Milner R, et al. Neutrophil and band counts in the diagnosis of neonatal infections. Pediatrics 54:38-42, 1974.
65. Rooney JC, Hill DJ, Danks DM. Jaundice associated with bacterial infection in the newborn. Am J Dis Child 122:39-41, 1971.
66. Benuck I, David RJ. Sensitivity of published neutrophil indexes in identifying newborn infants with sepsis. J Pediatr 103:961-963, 1983.
67. Philip AGS. Detection of neonatal sepsis of late onset. JAMA 247: 489-492, 1982.
68. Da Silva O, Ohlsson A, Kenyon C. Accuracy of leukocyte indices and C-reactive protein for diagnosis of neonatal sepsis: a critical review. Pediatr Infect Dis J 14:363-366, 1995.
69. Christensen RD, Bradley PP, Rothstein G. The leukocyte left shift in clinical and experimental neonatal sepsis. J Pediatr 98:101-105, 1981.
70. Speer CP, Hauptmann D, Stubbe P, et al. Neonatal septicemia and meningitis in Göttingen, West Germany. Pediatr Infect Dis J 4:36-41, 1985.
71. Faden HS. Early diagnosis of neonatal bacteremia by buffy-coat examination. J Pediatr 88:1032-1034, 1976.
72. Leonidas JC, Hall RT, Beatty EC, et al. Radiographic findings in early onset neonatal group B streptococcal septicemia. Pediatrics 59: 1006-1011, 1977.
73. Manroe BL, Rosenfeld CR, Weinberg AG, et al. The differential leukocyte count in the assessment and outcome of early-onset neonatal group B streptococcal disease. J Pediatr 91:632-637, 1977.
74. Payne NR, Burke BA, Day DL, et al. Correlation of clinical and pathologic findings in early onset neonatal group B streptococcal infection with disease severity and prediction of outcome. Pediatr Infect Dis J 7:836-847, 1988.
75. Courtney SE, Hall RT. *Haemophilus influenzae* sepsis in the premature infant. Am J Dis Child 132:1039-1040, 1978.
76. Christensen RD, Rothstein G, Anstall HB, et al. Granulocyte transfusions in neonates with bacterial infection, neutropenia, and depletion of mature marrow neutrophils. Pediatrics 70:1-6, 1982.
77. Bortolussi R, Thompson TR, Ferrieri P. Early-onset pneumococcal sepsis in newborn infants. Pediatrics 60:352-355, 1977.
78. Johnsson H, Bergström S, Ewald U, et al. Neonatal septicemia caused by pneumococci. Acta Obstet Gynecol Scand 71:6-11, 1992.
79. Jacobs J, Garmyn K, Verhaegen J, et al. Neonatal sepsis due to *Streptococcus pneumoniae*. Scand J Infect Dis 22:493-497, 1990.
80. Alexander JB, Giacoia GP. Early onset nonenterococcal group D streptococcal infection in the newborn infant. J Pediatr 93:489-490, 1978.
81. Christensen RD, Rothstein G. Exhaustion of mature marrow neutrophils in neonates with sepsis. J Pediatr 96:316-318, 1980.
82. Boyle RJ, Chandler BD, Stonestreet BS, et al. Early identification of sepsis in infants with respiratory distress. Pediatrics 62:744-750, 1978.
83. Escobar GJ, Li DK, Armstrong MA, et al. Neonatal sepsis workups in infants ≥2000 grams at birth: a population-based study. Pediatrics 106:256-263, 2000.
84. Lloyd BW, Oto A. Normal values for mature and immature neutrophils in very preterm babies. Arch Dis Child 57:233-235, 1982.
85. Wheeler JG, Chauvenet AR, Johnson CA, et al. Neutrophil storage pool depletion in septic, neutropenic neonates. Pediatr Infect Dis 3:407-409, 1984.
86. Christensen RD, Harper TE, Rothstein G. Granulocyte-macrophage progenitor cells in term and preterm neonates. J Pediatr 109:1047-1051, 1986.
87. Lake AM, Lauer BA, Clark JC, et al. Enterovirus infections in neonates. J Pediatr 89:787-791, 1976.
88. Gerdes JS. Clinicopathologic approach to the diagnosis of neonatal sepsis. Clin Perinatol 18:361-381, 1991.
89. Mathers NJ, Pohlandt F. Diagnostic audit of C-reactive protein in neonatal infection. Eur J Pediatr 146:147-151, 1987.

90. Sherman, MP, Chance KH, Goetzman BW. Gram's stains of tracheal secretions predict neonatal bacteremia. Am J Dis Child 138:848-850, 1984.
91. Kite P, Millar MR, Gorham P, et al. Comparison of five tests used in diagnosis of neonatal bacteraemia. Arch Dis Child 63:639-643, 1988.
92. Schmidt BK, Kirpalani HM, Corey M, et al. Coagulase-negative staphylococci as true pathogens in newborn infants: a cohort study. Pediatr Infect Dis J 6:1026-1031, 1987.
93. Greenberg DN, Yoder BA. Changes in the differential white blood cell count in screening for group B streptococcal sepsis. Pediatr Infect Dis J 9:886-889, 1990.
94. Schelonka RL, Yoder BA, Hall RB, et al. Differentiation of segmented and band neutrophils during the early newborn period. J Pediatr 127:298-300, 1995.
95. Appleyard WJ, Brinton A. Venous platelet counts in low birth weight infants. Biol Neonate 17:30-34, 1971.
96. Aballi AJ, Puapondh Y, Desposito F. Platelet counts in thriving premature infants. Pediatrics 42:685-689, 1968.
97. Modanlou HD, Ortiz OB. Thrombocytopenia in neonatal infection. Clin Pediatr 20:402-407, 1981.
98. Andrew M, Kelton J. Neonatal thrombocytopenia. Clin Perinatol 11:359-390, 1984.
99. Tate DY, Carlton GT, Johnson D, et al. Immune thrombocytopenia in severe neonatal infections. J Pediatr 98:449-453, 1981.
100. Mehta P, Vasa R, Neumann L, et al. Thrombocytopenia in the high-risk infant. J Pediatr 97:791-794, 1980.
101. Guida JD, Kunig AM, Leef KH, et al. Platelet count and sepsis in very low birth weight neonates: is there an organism-specific response? Pediatrics 2003;111:1411-5.
102. Patrick CH, Lazarchick J. The effect of bacteremia on automated platelet measurements in neonates. Am J Clin Pathol 93:391-394, 1990.
103. Modlin JF. Fatal echovirus 11 disease in premature neonates. Pediatrics 66:775-780, 1980.
104. Ballard RA, Drew L, Hufnagle KG, et al. Acquired cytomegalovirus infection in preterm infants. Am J Dis Child 133:482-485, 1979.
105. Ballin A, Koren G, Kohelet D, et al. Reduction of platelet counts induced by mechanical ventilation in newborn infants. J Pediatr 111:445-449, 1987.
106. Patel CC. Hematologic abnormalities in acute necrotizing enterocolitis. Pediatr Clin North Am 24:579-584, 1977.
107. Hutter JJ Jr, Hathaway WE, Wayne ER. Hematologic abnormalities in severe neonatal necrotizing enterocolitis. J Pediatr 88:1026-1031, 1976.
108. Koenig JM, Christensen RD. Neutropenia and thrombocytopenia in infants with Rh hemolytic disease. J Pediatr 114:625-631, 1989.
109. Gabay C, Kushner I. Acute-phase proteins and other systemic responses to inflammation. N Engl J Med 340:448-454, 1999.
110. Pepys MB, Baltz ML. Acute phase proteins with special reference to C-reactive protein and related proteins (pentaxins) and serum amyloid A protein. Adv Immunol 34:141-212, 1983.
111. Jaye DL, Waites KB. Clinical applications of C-reactive protein in pediatrics. Pediatr Infect Dis J 16:735-747, 1997.
112. Hanson L-O, Lindquist L. C-reactive protein: its role in the diagnosis and follow-up of infectious diseases. Curr Opin Infect Dis 10:196-201, 1997.
113. Gitlin D, Biasucci A. Development of IgG, IgA, IgM, β1C/β1A, C′1 esterase inhibitor, ceruloplasmin, transferrin, hemopexin, haptoglobin, fibrinogen, plasminogen, α_1-antitrypsin, orosomucoid, β-lipoprotein, α_2-macroglobulin, and prealbumin in the human conceptus. J Clin Invest 48:1433-1446, 1969.
114. Nakamura RM. Nephelometric immunoassays. *In* Boguslaski RC, Maggio ET, Nakamura RM (eds). Clinical Immunochemistry: Principles of Methods and Applications. Boston, Little, Brown, 1984, pp 199-211.
115. Chiesa C, Panero A, Osborn JF, et al. Diagnosis of neonatal sepsis: a clinical and laboratory challenge. Clin Chem 50:279-287, 2004.
116. Hanson LA, Jodal U, Sabel K-G, et al. The diagnostic value of C-reactive protein. Pediatr Infect Dis J 2:87-90, 1983.
117. Wassunna A, Whitelaw A, Gallimore R, et al. C-reactive protein and bacterial infection in preterm infants. Eur J Pediatr 149:424-427, 1990.
118. Vallance H, Lockitch G. Rapid, semi-quantitative assay of C-reactive protein evaluated. Clin Chem 37:1981-1982, 1991.
119. Pourcyrous M, Bada HS, Korones SB, et al. Acute phase reactants in neonatal bacterial infection. J Perinatol 11:319-325, 1991.
120. Chiesa C, Pellegrini G, Panero A, et al. C-reactive protein, interleukin-6, and procalcitonin in the immediate postnatal period: influence of illness severity, risk status, antenatal and perinatal complications, and infection. Clin Chem 49:60-68, 2003.
121. Døllner H, Vatten L, Austgulen R. Early diagnostic markers for neonatal sepsis: comparing C-reactive protein, interleukin-6, soluble tumour necrosis factor receptors and soluble adhesion molecules. J Clin Epidemiol 54:1251-1257, 2001.
122. Pourcyrous M, Bada HS, Korones SB, et al. Significance of serial C-reactive protein responses in neonatal infection and other disorders. Pediatrics 92:431-435, 1993.
123. Ng PC, Cheng SH, Fok TF, et al. Diagnosis of late onset neonatal sepsis with cytokines, adhesion molecule, and C-reactive protein in preterm very low birthweight infants. Arch Dis Child 77:F221-F227, 1997.
124. Benitz WE, Han MY, Madan A, et al. Serial C-reactive protein levels in the diagnosis of neonatal infection. Pediatrics 102:e41, 1998. Available at http://www.pediatrics.org/cgi/content/full/102/4/e41.
125. Ehl S, Gering B, Bartmann P, et al. C-reactive protein is a useful marker for guiding duration of antibiotic therapy in suspected neonatal bacterial infection. Pediatrics 99:216-221, 1997.
126. Shortland DB, MacFadyen U, Elston A, et al. Evaluation of C-reactive protein values in neonatal sepsis. J Perinat Med 18:157-163, 1990.
127. Santana Reyes C, Garcia-Munoz F, Reyes D, et al. Role of cytokines (interleukin-1beta, 6, 8, tumour necrosis factor-alpha, and soluble receptor of interleukin-2) and C-reactive protein in the diagnosis of neonatal sepsis. Acta Paediatrica 92:221-227, 2003.
128. Isaacs D, North J, Lindsell D, et al. Serum acute phase reactants in necrotizing enterocolitis. Acta Paediatr Scand 76:923-927, 1987.
129. Saxstad J, Nilsson L-Å, Hanson L-Å. C-reactive protein in serum from infants as determined with immunodiffusion techniques: II. Infants with various infections. Acta Paediatr Scand 59:676-680, 1970.
130. Hawrylyshyn P, Bernstein P, Milligan JE, et al. Premature rupture of membranes: the role of C-reactive protein in the prediction of chorioamnionitis. Am J Obstet Gynecol 147:240-246, 1983.
131. Salzer HR, Genger H, Muhar U, et al. C-reactive protein: an early marker for neonatal bacterial infection due to prolonged rupture of amniotic membranes and/or amnionitis. Acta Obstet Gynecol Scand 66:365-367, 1987.
132. Schouten-Van Meeteren NYN, Rietveld A, Moolenaar AJ, et al. Influence of perinatal conditions on C-reactive protein production. J Pediatr 120:621-624, 1992.
133. Bomela HN, Ballot DE, Cory BJ, Cooper PA. Use of C-reactive protein to guide duration of empiric antibiotic therapy in suspected early neonatal sepsis. Pediatr Infect Dis J 19:531-535, 2000.
134. Ehl S, Gehring B, Pohlandt F. A detailed analysis of changes in serum C-reactive protein levels in neonates treated for bacterial infection. Eur J Pediatr 158:238-242, 1999.
135. Franz AR, Steinbach G, Kron M, Pohlandt F. Reduction of unnecessary antibiotic therapy in newborn infants using interleukin-8 and C-reactive protein as markers of bacterial infections. Pediatrics 104: 447-453, 1999.
136. Philip AGS. Acute-phase proteins in neonatal infection. J Pediatr 105:940-942, 1984.
137. Barratt BA, Hill PI. A micromethod for the erythrocyte sedimentation rate suitable for use on venous or capillary blood. J Clin Pathol 33: 1118, 1980.
138. Lascari AD. The erythrocyte sedimentation rate. Pediatr Clin North Am 19:1113-1121, 1972.
139. Adler SM, Denton RL. The erythrocyte sedimentation rate in the newborn period. J Pediatr 86:942-948, 1975.
140. Evans HE, Glass L, Mercado C. The micro-erythrocyte sedimentation rate in newborn infants. J Pediatr 76:448-451, 1970.
141. Ibsen KK, Nielsen M, Prag J, et al. The value of the micromethod erythrocyte sedimentation rate in the diagnosis of infections in newborns. Scand J Infect Dis 23(Suppl):143-145, 1980.
142. Bennish M, Vardiman J, Beem MC. The zeta sedimentation ratio in children. J Pediatr 104:249-251, 1984.
143. Stuart J, Whicher JT. Tests for detecting and monitoring the acute phase response. Arch Dis Child 63:115-117, 1988.
144. Sell EJ, Corrigan JJ Jr. Platelet counts, fibrinogen concentrations, and factor V and factor VIII levels in healthy infants according to gestational age. J Pediatr 82:1028-1032, 1973.
145. Jensen AH, Josso F, Zamet P, et al. Evolution of blood clotting factor levels in premature infants during the first 10 days of life: a study of 96 cases with comparison between clinical status and blood clotting factor levels. Pediatr Res 7:638-644, 1973.

146. Salmi TT. Haptoglobin levels in the plasma of newborn infants with special reference to infections. Acta Paediatr Scand 241:7-55, 1973.
147. Kanakoudi F, Drossou V, Tzimouli V, et al. Serum concentrations of 10 acute-phase proteins in healthy term and preterm infants from birth to age 6 months. Clin Chem 41:605-608, 1995.
148. Lee SK, Thibeault DW, Heiner DC. α_1-Antitrypsin and α_1-acid glycoprotein levels in the cord blood and amniotic fluid of infants with respiratory distress syndrome. Pediatr Res 12:775-777, 1978.
149. Boichot P, Schirrer J, Menget A, et al. L'orosomucoide à la période néonatale: étude chez le nouveau-né sain et le nouveau-né infecté. Pédiatrie 35:577-588, 1980.
150. Bienvenu J, Sann L, Bienvenu F, et al. Laser nephelometry of orosomucoid in serum of newborns: reference intervals and relation to bacterial infections. Clin Chem 27:721-726, 1981.
151. Philip AGS, Hewitt JR. $\alpha_1\beta$-Acid glycoprotein in the neonate with and without infection. Biol Neonate 43:118-124, 1983.
152. Treluyer JM, Bompard Y, Gantzer A, et al. Septicémies néonatales: diagnostic biologique et antibiothérapie: à propos d'une série de 46 cas. Arch Fr Pédiatr 48:317-321, 1991.
153. Gutteberg TJ, Haneberg B, Jergensen, T. Lactoferrin in relation to acute phase proteins in sera from newborn infants with severe infections. Eur J Pediatr 142:37-39, 1984.
154. Rodwell RL, Taylor KM, Tudehope DI, et al. Capillary plasma elastase alpha-1-proteinase inhibitor in infected and non-infected neonates. Arch Dis Child 67:436-439, 1992.
155. Speer CP, Rethwilm M, Gahr M. Elastase–α_1-proteinase inhibitor: an early indicator of septicemia and bacterial meningitis in children. J Pediatr 111:667-671, 1987.
156. Baek YW, Brokat S, Padbury JF, et al. Inter-alpha inhibitor proteins in infants and decreased levels in neonatal sepsis. J Pediatr 143:11-15, 2003.
157. Suri M, Sharma VK, Thirupuram S. Evaluation of ceruloplasmin in neonatal septicemia. Indian Pediatr 28:489-493, 1991.
158. Miller LC, Isa S, Lo Preste G, et al. Neonatal interleukin-1β, interleukin-6, and tumor necrosis factor: cord blood levels and cellular production. J Pediatr 117:961-965, 1990.
159. Kashlan F, Smulian J, Shen-Schwarz S, et al. Umbilical vein interleukin 6 and tumor necrosis factor alpha plasma concentrations in the very preterm infant. Pediatr Infect Dis J 19:238-243, 2000.
160. Buck C, Bundschu J, Gallati H, et al. Interleukin-6: a sensitive parameter for the early diagnosis of neonatal bacterial infection. Pediatrics 93: 54-58, 1994.
161. Martin H, Olander B, Norman M. Reactive hyperemia and interleukin 6, interleukin 8, and tumor necrosis factor-α in the diagnosis of early-onset neonatal sepsis. Pediatrics 108:e61, 2001. Available at http://www.pediatrics.org/cgi/content/full/108/4/e61
162. Messer J, Eyer D, Donato L, et al. Evaluation of interleukin-6 and soluble receptors of tumor necrosis factor for early diagnosis of neonatal infection. J Pediatr 129:574-580, 1996.
163. Gomez R, Romero R, Ghezzi F, et al. The fetal inflammatory response syndrome. Am J Obstet Gynecol 179:194-202, 1998.
164. Lehrnbecher T, Schrod L, Rutsch P, et al. Immunologic parameters in cord blood indicating early-onset sepsis. Biol Neonate 70:206-212, 1996.
165. Panero A, Pacifico L, Rossi N, et al. Interleukin-6 in neonates with early and late onset infection. Pediatr Infect Dis J 16:370-375, 1997.
166. Sullivan JS, Kilpatrick L, Costarino AT Jr, et al. Correlation of plasma cytokine elevations with mortality rate in children with sepsis. J Pediatr 120:510-515, 1992.
167. Shimoya K, Matsuzaki N, Taniguchi T, et al. Interleukin-8 in cord sera: a sensitive and specific marker for the detection of preterm chorioamnionitis. J Infect Dis 165:957-960, 1992.
168. Nupponen I, Andersson S, Jarvenpaa AL, et al. Neutrophil CD11b expression and circulating interleukin-8 as diagnostic markers for early-onset neonatal sepsis. Pediatrics 108:e12, 2001. Available at http://www.pediatrics.org/cgi/content/full/108/1/e12
169. Malik A, Hui CP, Pennie RA, Kirpalani H. Beyond the complete blood cell count and C-reactive protein: a systematic review of modern diagnostic tests for neonatal sepsis. Arch Pediatr Adolesc Med 157:511-516, 2003.
170. Mehr S, Doyle LW. Cytokines as markers of bacterial sepsis in newborn infants: a review. Pediatr Infect Dis J 19:879-887, 2000.
171. Girardin EP, Berner ME, Grau GE, et al. Serum tumor necrosis factor in newborns at risk for infections. Eur J Pediatr 149:645-647, 1990.
172. Kim SK, Keeney SE, Alpard SK, Schmalstieg FC. Comparison of L-selectin and CD11b on neutrophils of adults and neonates during the first month of life. Pediatr Res 53:132-136, 2003.
173. Kuster H, Degitz K. Circulating ICAM-1 in neonatal sepsis. Lancet 1:506, 1993.
174. Assicot M, Gendrel D, Carsin H, et al. High serum procalcitonin concentrations in patients with sepsis and infection. Lancet 1:515-518, 1993.
175. Gendrel D, Assicot M, Raymond J, et al. Procalcitonin as a marker for the early diagnosis of neonatal infection. J Pediatr 128:570-573, 1996.
176. Monneret G, Labaune JM, Isaac C, et al. Procalcitonin and C-reactive protein levels in neonatal infections. Acta Paediatr 86:209-212, 1997.
177. Gendrel D, Bohuon C. Procalcitonin as a marker of bacterial infection. Pediatr Infect Dis J 19:679-687, 2000.
177a. Van Rossum AMC, Wulkan RW, Oudesluys-Murphy AM. Procalcitonin as an early marker of infection in neonates and children. Lancet Infect Dis 4:620–630, 2004.
178. Chiesa C, Panero A, Rossi N, et al. Reliability of procalcitonin concentrations for the diagnosis of sepsis in critically ill neonates. Clin Infect Dis 26:664-672, 1998.
179. Lapillone A, Basson E, Monneret G, et al. Lack of specificity of procalcitonin for sepsis diagnosis in premature infants. Lancet 351: 1211-1212, 1998.
180. De Bont ESJM, De Leij LHFM, Okken A, et al. Increased plasma concentrations of interleukin-1 receptor antagonist in neonatal sepsis. Pediatr Res 37:626-629, 1995.
181. Spear ML, Stefano JL, Fawcett P, et al. Soluble interleukin-2 receptor as a predictor of neonatal sepsis. J Pediatr 126:982-985, 1995.
182. Hodge S, Hodge G, Flower R, et al. Surface activation markers of T lymphocytes: role in the detection of infection in neonates. Clin Exp Immunol 113:33-38, 1998.
183. Weirich E, Rabin RL, Maldonado Y, et al. Neutrophil CD11b expression as a diagnostic marker for early-onset neonatal infection. J Pediatr 132:445-451, 1998.
184. Weinschenk NP, Farina A, Bianchi DW. Neonatal neutrophil activation is a function of labor length in preterm infants. Pediatr Res 44:942-945, 1998.
185. Ng PC, Li K, Wong RP, Chui KM, et al. Neutrophil CD64 expression: a sensitive diagnostic marker for late-onset nosocomial infection in very low birthweight infants. Pediatr Res 51:296-303, 2002.
185a. Ng PC, Li G, Chui KM, et al. Neutrophil CD64 is a sensitive diagnostic marker for early-onset neonatal infection. Pediatr Res 56:796-803, 2004.
186. Yang KD, Bohnsack JF, Hill HR. Fibronectin in host defense: implications in the diagnosis, prophylaxis and therapy of infectious diseases. Pediatr Infect Dis 12:234-239, 1993.
187. Koenig JM, Patterson LER, Rench MA, et al. Role of fibronectin in diagnosing bacterial infection in infancy. Am J Dis Child 142: 884-887, 1988.
188. McCafferty MH, Lepow M, Saba TM, et al. Normal fibronectin levels as a function of age in the pediatric population. Pediatr Res 17: 482-485, 1982.
189. Alford CA Jr. Immunoglobulin determinations in the diagnosis of fetal infection. Pediatr Clin North Am 18:99-113, 1971.
190. Kagan BM, Stanincova V, Felix N. IgM determination in neonate and infants for diagnosis of infection. J Pediatr 77:916, 1970.
191. Khan WN, Ali RV, Werthmann M, et al. Immunoglobulin M determinations in neonates and infants as an adjunct to the diagnosis of infection. J Pediatr 75:1282-1286, 1969.
192. Blankenship WJ, Cassady G, Schaefer J, et al. Serum gamma-M globulin responses in acute neonatal infections and their diagnostic significance. J Pediatr 75:1271-1281, 1969.
193. Korones SB, Roane JA, Gilkeson MR, et al. Neonatal IgM response to acute infection. J Pediatr 75:1261-1270, 1969.
194. Baehner RL. Use of the nitroblue tetrazolium test in clinical pediatrics. Am J Dis Child 128:449-451, 1974.
195. Cocchi P, Mori S, Becattini A. Nitroblue-tetrazolium reduction by neutrophils of newborn infants in in vitro phagocytosis test. Acta Paediatr Scand 60:475-478, 1971.
196. Park BH, Holmes B, Good RA. Metabolic activities in leukocytes of newborn infants. J Pediatr 76:237-241, 1970.
197. McCracken GH Jr, Eichenwald HF. Leukocyte function and the development of opsonic and complement activity in the neonate. Am J Dis Child 121:120-126, 1971.
198. Anderson DC, Pickering LK, Feigin RD. Leukocyte function in normal and infected neonates. J Pediatr 85:420-425, 1974.
199. Shigeoka AO, Santos JI, Hill HR. Functional analysis of neutrophil granulocytes from healthy, infected, and stressed neonates. J Pediatr 95:454-460, 1979.

200. Shigeoka AO, Charette RP, Wyman ML, et al. Defective oxidative metabolic responses of neutrophils from stressed neonates. J Pediatr 98:392-398, 1981.
201. Powers DW, Ayoub EM. Leukocyte lactate dehydrogenase in bacterial meningitis. Pediatrics 54:27-33, 1974.
202. Donato H, Gebara E, de Cosen RH, et al. Leukocyte alkaline phosphatase activity in the diagnosis of neonatal bacterial infections. J Pediatr 94:242-244, 1979.
203. Leake RD, Fiser RH Jr, Oh W. Rapid glucose disappearance in infants with infection. Clin Pediatr 20:397-401, 1981.
204. James T III, Blessa M, Boggs TR Jr. Recurrent hyperglycemia associated with sepsis in a neonate. Am J Dis Child 133:645-646, 1979.
205. Zasloff M. Vernix, the newborn, and innate defense. Pediatr Res 53: 203-204, 2003.
206. Levy O. Impaired innate immunity at birth: deficiency of bactericidal/permeability-increasing protein (BPI) in the neutrophils of newborns. Pediatr Res 51:667-669, 2002.
207. Thomas NJ, Carcillo JA, Doughty LA, et al. Plasma concentrations of defensins and lactoferrin in children with severe sepsis. Pediatr Infect Dis J 21:34-38, 2002.
208. Yoshio H, Tollin M, Gudmundsson GH, et al. Antimicrobial polypeptides of human vernix caseosa and amniotic fluid: implications for newborn innate defense. Pediatr Res 53:211-216, 2003.
209. Nupponen I, Turunen R, Nevalainen T, et al. Extracellular release of bactericidal/permeability-increasing protein in newborn infants. Pediatr Res 51:670-674, 2002.
210. Benirschke K. Routes and types of infection in the fetus and the newborn. Am J Dis Child 99:714-721, 1960.
211. Blanc WA. Pathways of fetal and early neonatal infection: viral placentitis, bacterial and fungal chorioamnionitis. J Pediatr 59:473-496, 1961.
212. Kelsall GRH, Barter RA, Manessis C. Prospective bacteriological studies in inflammation of the placenta, cord and membranes. J Obstet Gynaecol Br Commonw 74:401-411, 1967.
213. Overbach AM, Daniel, SJ, Cassady G. The value of umbilical cord histology in the management of potential perinatal infection. J Pediatr 76:22-31, 1970.
214. Wilson MG, Armstrong DH, Nelson RC, et al. Prolonged rupture of fetal membranes: effect on the newborn infant. Am J Dis Child 107: 138-146, 1964.
215. Morison JE. Foetal and Neonatal Pathology, 3rd ed. Washington, DC, Butterworth, 1970.
216. Fox H, Langley FA. Leukocytic infiltration of the placenta and umbilical cord: a clinico-pathologic study. Obstet Gynecol 37:451-458, 1971.
217. Dominguez R, Segal AJ, O'Sullivan JA. Leukocytic infiltration of the umbilical cord: manifestation of fetal hypoxia due to reduction of blood flow in the cord. JAMA 173:346-349, 1960.
218. Anderson GS, Green CA, Neligan GA, et al. Congenital bacterial pneumonia. Lancet 2:585-587, 1962.
219. Ramos A, Stern L. Relationship of premature rupture of the membranes to gastric fluid aspirate in the newborn. Am J Obstet Gynecol 105: 1247-1251, 1969.
220. Vasan U, Lim DM, Greenstein RM, et al. Origin of gastric polymorphonuclear leukocytes in infants born after prolonged rupture of membranes. J Pediatr 91:69-72, 1977.
221. Yeung CY, Tam ASY. Gastric aspirate findings in neonatal pneumonia. Arch Dis Child 47:735-740, 1972.
222. Scanlon J. The early detection of neonatal sepsis by examination of liquid obtained from the external ear canal. J Pediatr 79:247-249, 1971.
223. Zuerlein TJ, Butler JC, Yeager TD. Superficial cultures in neonatal sepsis evaluations: impact on antibiotic decision making. Clin Pediatr 29:445-447, 1990.
224. Handsfield HH, Hodson WA, Holmes KK. Neonatal gonococcal infection: I. Orogastric contamination with *N. gonorrhoeae*. JAMA 225:697-701, 1973.
225. MacGregor RR, Tunnessen WW Jr. The incidence of pathogenic organisms in the normal flora of the neonate's external ear and nasopharynx. Clin Pediatr 12:697-700, 1973.
226. Mims LC, Medawar MS, Perkins JR, et al. Predicting neonatal infections by evaluation of the gastric aspirate: a study in two hundred and seven patients. Am J Obstet Gynecol 114:232-238, 1972.
227. Lau YL, Hey E. Sensitivity and specificity of daily tracheal aspirate cultures in predicting organisms causing bacteremia in ventilated neonates. Pediatr Infect Dis J 10:290-294, 1991.
228. Hazan Y, Mazor M, Horowitz S, et al. The diagnostic value of amniotic Gram stain examination and limulus amebocyte lysate assay in patients with preterm birth. Acta Obstet Gynecol Scand 74:275-280, 1995.
229. Laforgia N, Coppola B, Carbone R, et al. Rapid detection of neonatal sepsis using polymerase chain reaction. Acta Paediatr 86:1097-1099, 1997.
230. Jordan JA, Durso MB. Comparison of 16S rRNA gene PCR and BACTEC 9240 for detection of neonatal bactermia. J Clin Microbiol 38:2574-2578, 2000.
231. Fowlie PW, Schmidt B. Diagnostic tests for bacterial infection from birth to 90 days—a systematic review. Arch Dis Child Fetal Neonatal Ed 78:F92-F98, 1998.
232. Philip AGS. Decreased use of antibiotics using a neonatal sepsis screening technique. J Pediatr 98:795-799, 1981.
232a. Franz AR, Bauer K, Schalk A, et al. Measurement of interleukin 8 in combination with C-reactive protein reduced unnecessary antibiotic therapy in newborn infants: a multicenter, randomized, controlled trial. Pediatrics 114:1-8, 2004.
233. Weber MW, Carlin JB, Gatchalian S, et al. Predictors of neonatal sepsis in developing countries. Pediatr Infect Dis J 22:711-717, 2003.
234. Garcia-Prats JA, Cooper TR, Schneider VF, et al. Rapid detection of microorganisms in blood cultures of newborn infants utilizing an automated blood culture system. Pediatrics 105:523-527, 2000.
235. Kumar Y, Qunibi M, Neal TJ, Yoxall CW. Time to positivity of neonatal blood cultures. Arch Dis Child Fetal Neonatal Ed 85:F182-F186, 2001.

Chapter 37

CLINICAL PHARMACOLOGY OF ANTIBACTERIAL AGENTS

Xavier Sáez-Llorens • George H. McCracken, Jr.

Because of the susceptibility of newborns, particularly low-birth-weight premature neonates, to vertically and nosocomially transmitted bacterial infections, pediatricians managing these infants often prescribe antibiotics for presumptive sepsis. Pharmacology of these drugs is unique to the neonate and cannot be extrapolated from data derived from studies in older infants and adults. For these reasons, safety and efficacy of antimicrobial products in the neonatal period must be established for term and premature infants.

The rapidly changing physiologic processes characteristic of the neonatal age profoundly affect the pharmacokinetic properties of antibiotics. These changes can result either in subtherapeutic drug concentrations, thereby delaying bacterial eradication, or in toxic drug concentrations that can cause morbidity and lead to prolonged hospitalization. Therapeutic disasters such as development of kernicterus following use of sulfonamides, the chloramphenicol gray baby syndrome, tetracycline tooth staining, and kanamycin ototoxicity underscore the importance of pediatric pharmacology as an essential subspecialty. Clinical trials evaluating antimicrobial agents should include newborns, especially low-birth-weight premature neonates, who typically receive many courses of antimicrobial therapy during their nursery stay.

Since the previous edition of this book was published, a few new antibacterial agents have become available for use in newborns with suspected or proven bacterial infections. In this chapter, we add recent information on the extended dosing intervals for aminoglycoside administration and update the data on the different antibiotics available for use in neonates, including those potentially useful for treatment of multidrug-resistant microorganisms (ticarcillin-clavulanate, piperacillin-tazobactam, cefepime, carbapenems, ciprofloxacin, glycopeptides, linezolid). Finally, it must be underscored that in the current era of alarming increase in widespread resistance of bacteria to multiple antimicrobial drugs, development of stringent antibiotic-restriction policies is needed to preserve the usefulness of selected antibiotics.

NEONATAL CLINICAL PHARMACOLOGY

Absorption, distribution, metabolism, and excretion are constantly changing during the neonatal period. The physiologic immaturity of enzymatic processes, the large extracellular fluid volume, the protein-binding affinities of antibiotic-competitive substances, the fluctuations in renal clearance, and certain situations that provoke blood volume disturbances (e.g., exchange transfusions, patency of ductus arteriosus, extracorporeal membrane oxygenation [ECMO]) are among the numerous neonatal factors affecting the pharmacokinetic behavior of antimicrobial agents in newborns.

Absorption of drugs administered at extravascular sites occurs by passive diffusion across biologic membranes. This process is affected by chemical properties of the drug, such as its molecular weight, ionization, and lipid solubility, as well as by physiologic factors, such as local pH and blood flow, which undergo developmental changes as the newborn matures.

Oral absorption of antimicrobial agents can be affected by unique neonatal features, such as the alkaline gastric pH during the first hours of life, slow gastric emptying, high gastrointestinal–to–whole body surface area ratio, increased permeability of bowel mucosa, irregular peristalsis, prolonged intestinal transit time, and the deconjugational activity of the intestinal enzyme β-glucuronidase.[1] The net effect of these features on the oral absorption of specific antibiotics, however, is difficult to predict. For example, penicillin G administered orally achieves higher serum concentration in newborns than in older infants and children,[2] whereas the opposite occurs after oral administration of chloramphenicol palmitate.[3-5]

Although serum antibiotic concentrations generally are comparable after intramuscular and intravenous administration, significant differences in peak value, half-life, and plasma clearance for the two administration routes can be observed for some antibiotics.[6,7] Because the regional blood flow is the primary determinant of the extent and rate of antibiotic absorption after intramuscular administration, absorption of some drugs can be profoundly reduced in hypoxic and/or hypotensive infants with poor peripheral muscle perfusion.

Immaturity of enzymatic systems in the neonate can result from deficiency or absence of specific enzymes required for drug biotransformation. Deficiency of hepatic glucuronyl transferase leads to diminished conjugation of chloramphenicol to the inactive acid glucuronide, thus increasing the half-life with the consequent risk of free drug accumulation in serum. This event probably is the cause of cardiovascular collapse and death (gray baby syndrome) in some infants following chloramphenicol treatment. By contrast, phenobarbital stimulates the activity of the hepatic enzymatic system, resulting in increased clearance of chloramphenicol and in reduced serum concentrations.[8] Newborns may lack the enzymes required to de-esterify antibiotic esters, notably pancreatic lipase, which is needed to convert oral chloramphenicol palmitate to the active agent. Another example is hemolysis produced by sulfonamides or nitrofurantoin when given to infants who have erythrocyte glucose-6-phosphate dehydrogenase (G6PD) deficiency.[9]

The extracellular fluid volume in newborns is considerably greater than that in children and adults. It decreases from 7.3 to 5.8 L/m^2 in the first 3 months of life and remains constant throughout infancy and childhood.[10] Several drugs distribute primarily in the extracellular space, which, because of the larger volume in newborns, can affect the pharmacokinetic profiles of these agents. For example, the peak serum concentrations of aminoglycosides in premature infants are lower than those in term infants after similar dosages, and it takes longer for these drugs to be excreted because of the expanded extracellular volume. This latter phenomenon may explain, in part, the longer half-lives of aminoglycosides in neonates than in older infants and children.[11]

Quantitative and qualitative differences exist between the serum proteins of newborns and those of older infants; these differences affect the degree to which antimicrobial agents are protein bound and thus their kinetics.[12] The clinical significance of antibiotic protein binding, however, is unclear. Many variables, including the concentrations of both free albumin and antibiotic, drug affinity for protein-binding sites, presence of competing substances for these binding sites (furosemide, bilirubin), and plasma pH reversibly affect this process. Protein-bound drug has negligible antibacterial activity and remains in the intravascular space, with limited distribution into tissues. Binding of some antibiotics, such as chloramphenicol, nafcillin, and ceftriaxone, to plasma proteins is lower in neonates than in adults.[13,14] Despite the different protein-binding capacities of individual antibiotics, clinical data in newborns are inadequate to confirm the assumption that drugs with low protein binding are more efficacious than those with high protein binding.

Some antibacterial agents are capable of displacing bilirubin from albumin-binding sites. Theoretically, jaundiced neonates receiving these antibiotics are at increased risk of developing kernicterus. This complication, however, has been documented only for sulfonamides.[15] Most antimicrobial products have a much lower binding affinity for albumin than does bilirubin, thus explaining why these agents are unable to remove bilirubin once it is bound to this protein.[16] Antibiotics that have been shown to significantly displace bilirubin from albumin-binding sites include the sulfonamides, moxalactam, cefoperazone, and ceftriaxone.[17-19] Ampicillin has a weak displacing effect that can be minimized by slow infusion of the drug in jaundiced neonates.[20] In relatively normal physiologic conditions, the remaining commonly used antibacterial agents generally are not associated with bilirubin displacement.[21-23] Finally, the extent of protein binding by an antibiotic does not necessarily correlate with this potentially adverse event.[18]

Renal function in the newborn is different from that in older children. The glomerular filtration rate is 30% to 60% of adult levels. During the first 2 weeks of life, a remarkable increase in renal function occurs. These changes and the rate at which they occur have a profound effect on antibiotic pharmacokinetics. As a result, sustained serum concentrations and prolonged half-life values of many drugs are observed in the first days of life, especially in premature infants. At 2 weeks of age, the half-life of β-lactam antibiotics is approximately twice that observed in adults. Drug elimination may be further reduced in the sick infant by conditions that decrease renal blood flow (e.g., severe respiratory distress syndrome, dehydration, hypotensive states).[24] For example, a prolonged serum half-life of aminoglycosides has been detected in hypoxemic infants.[25] Because renal function is constantly changing in the first month of life, a pharmacokinetic profile must be determined on multiple occasions during this period to define the proper dosage and frequency of administration of an antibiotic. Ototoxicity from aminoglycosides may develop in newborns if serum accumulation of these agents, due to reduced glomerular and renal tubular function, goes unrecognized.

PHARMACOLOGIC EVALUATION OF ANTIBACTERIAL AGENTS IN NEONATES

The evaluation of antimicrobial agents in the treatment of neonatal infection is difficult. As a general rule, antibiotics must be studied first in adults and older children, to obtain data concerning absorption, metabolism, excretion, efficacy, and safety, before pharmacokinetic and clinical trials in newborns can be conducted. The data obtained in adults and children serve as guidelines for initial dosage and safety precautions in neonates.

Relatively few comparative randomized controlled trials of established antibiotic regimens versus those using new compounds have been conducted in newborns. If the standard regimen is highly effective, very large numbers of infants would be needed to determine the therapeutic superiority of a new regimen, especially when the prevalence of infection is relatively low (i.e., 1 to 5 cases per 1000 live births), as it is in developed countries. If the standard regimen has ceased to be effective, a randomized trial would be unethical. A less satisfactory alternative is to use open studies to establish that the new therapeutic modality is comparable with that used previously for that condition and then to determine whether a diminished risk of toxicity, more desirable pharmacokinetics, more convenient dosage schedules, and so on give the new agent significant advantage over the old one.

For the initial evaluation of any antibiotic, determination of the in vitro susceptibilities to that drug of commonly encountered bacterial pathogens in the neonatal period is imperative. Ideally, both the minimal inhibitory concentration (MIC) and the minimal bactericidal concentration (MBC) should be determined to avoid missing the detection of tolerant strains (i.e., organisms inhibited but not killed by up to 32 times the inhibiting concentration for that drug).[26] Because of the great variation in bacterial pathogens among different nurseries and geographic areas, antimicrobial agents to be evaluated should be tailored to those microorganisms prevalent in each unit. In general, potential therapeutic agents should be effective against some or most of the following common neonatal pathogens: group B streptococci, coagulase-positive and coagulase-negative staphylococci, gram-negative enteric bacilli, enterococci, *Listeria monocytogenes*, and *Pseudomonas aeruginosa*.

The efficacy of combinations of antibiotics often is studied in vitro and in experimental animal models of infections. Demonstration of a synergistic or additive bacterial killing or of an antagonistic interaction is potentially important for the proper management of neonatal infections.[27-29] For instance, synergism has been demonstrated for ampicillin and aminoglycosides against group B streptococci,[30-32] enterococci,[33] *Listeria*,[34] and some gram-negative enteric rods[35]; for nafcillin and aminoglycosides against *Staphylococcus aureus*[36]; and for carbenicillin and gentamicin against enterococci, *Listeria*, and *P. aeruginosa*.[28,37] The clinical significance of this in vitro synergism as it relates to therapy of infected neonates, however, remains to be established.

The next step in evaluating an antimicrobial agent is to obtain pharmacokinetic data by substitution of a single dose of the new drug for one dose of a standard antibiotic. Alternatively, the investigational drug can be given in addition to standard therapy, but drug concentrations in plasma would need to be determined by an assay that could discriminate between the drugs administered (e.g., high-pressure liquid chromatography). Substitution of only one dose does not expose the infant to the jeopardy of a prolonged period of possibly ineffective therapy that would occur if an untested new drug were given in repeated dosage. Subsequently, multiple serum and urine samples are obtained to determine concentrations of the drug at a given time after the dose. The serum half-life and volume of distribution are calculated by plotting the serum concentration-time curves and calculating the disappearance of drug from serum.[38]

These basic pharmacologic data are then analyzed with respect to age and birth weight, and predictions of dosage and intervals of administration are made by mathematical calculations. The distribution of many antibiotics in the body follows a biphasic pattern (i.e., initial distribution phase after the first dose and final tissue washout phase after the last dose) and most accurately fits a two-compartment pharmacokinetic model.[39-42] Accordingly, we can more precisely predict the serum concentrations of a specific drug and anticipate the persistence of subinhibitory concentrations of antibiotics in the urine several days after the drug is discontinued. This latter event may cause a selective pressure for development of resistant strains of nosocomial pathogens residing in the environment of neonatal intensive care units.

For an antimicrobial agent to be considered useful in the neonatal period, the drug should achieve good concentrations in the cerebrospinal fluid (CSF) compartment. This premise is based on the fact that approximately one fourth of newborns with sepsis have concomitant bacterial meningitis. In the 1980s, new antibiotics were tested in a rabbit model of meningitis before use in infants to determine the CSF penetration and bactericidal activity of the drug against commonly encountered meningeal pathogens.[43-45]

Only when all of these preliminary steps are completed can a new antimicrobial agent be made available for use with a reasonable assurance of effectiveness and safety.[46] Once the drug becomes approved by the U.S. Food and Drug Administration (FDA), usually after many years of basic and clinical research, additional measurements of serum drug concentrations and half-life determinations in different-birth-weight groups are conducted. These determinations are especially useful when antibiotics with a narrow therapeutic index, such as aminoglycosides, chloramphenicol, and vancomycin, are administered to low-birth-weight premature infants. Drug concentrations are measured during the steady state, which usually is achieved after approximately four serum half-lives. Serum samples obtained just before and 15 minutes after the intravenous administration of a dose yield the trough and peak values, respectively. Peak values after the intramuscular and oral routes are achieved at approximately 30 minutes and 1 to 2 hours, respectively. Peak and trough serum concentrations for toxicity-prone antimicrobial agents (e.g., aminoglycosides, vancomycin) should be monitored if significant changes in renal or hepatic function occur and if prolonged therapy is required.

PLACENTAL TRANSPORT OF ANTIBIOTICS

Antimicrobial agents are prescribed for as many as 15% to 40% of pregnant women to treat a variety of conditions, ranging from mild upper respiratory tract infections to serious bacterial infections of the genitourinary system.[47-49] Many of these drugs are given at the end of pregnancy in an attempt to prevent or treat amnionitis or intrauterine bacterial infections. The selection of a specific agent is based on likely bacterial pathogens causing these infections and on the possibility of transplacental passage of antimicrobial drugs from the pregnant woman to the fetus.

Drugs may be transported across the placenta either passively by simple diffusion or actively by energy-dependent processes. Factors influencing transplacental passage include lipid solubility, degree of ionization, molecular weight, protein-binding affinity, surface area of the fetal-maternal interface, placental blood flow, stage of pregnancy, and placental metabolism.[50] Placental drug biotransformation ensues by oxidation, reduction, hydrolysis, or conjugation with endogenous chemicals.[51] In addition, antibiotics concentrate to various degrees in fetal tissues, depending on lipid solubility, specific binding to biologic constituents, changes in fetal circulation, and gestational age.

Ratios of infant to maternal serum concentrations of commonly used antimicrobial agents are shown in Table 37-1.[52-113] Maternal serum concentrations generally are lower than those reported in nonpregnant women, owing to a larger plasma volume and an increased renal plasma clearance during pregnancy.[114,115] The infant serum concentrations vary considerably because of differences in maternal dosage, route of administration, gestational age, timing of sample collection, and methods of measuring antimicrobial activity. As a result, a wide range of serum values for pregnant women and infants and of percentages of transplacental penetration is obtained for most drugs.

From Table 37-1 it can be seen that infant serum concentrations of some antibiotics, such as ampicillin,[57] carbenicillin,[59] cefotaxime,[65] chloramphenicol,[76,77] and sulfonamides,[100-102,106,107] approach or even exceed those in maternal serum. These high and rapidly attainable fetal ampicillin serum concentrations can explain, at least in part, the significant benefit of intrapartum administration of ampicillin to pregnant women colonized with group B streptococci in reducing colonization and early-onset neonatal sepsis caused by these pathogens. The ratio of infant to maternal serum values for methicillin[83,92] is considerably higher than that for dicloxacillin[82,83]; this may be a result of differences in serum protein binding (37% and 98%, respectively). Antibiotics with low transplacental penetration include cephalothin,[59,75] dicloxacillin,[82,83] erythromycin,[52,84] nafcillin,[59] and tobramycin.[54,59]

Complete evaluation of the possible adverse effects of drugs on the developing fetus must be performed before the drug is used during pregnancy. Some reported adverse events[116,117] include fetal death and abortion (aminopterin), teratogenicity (thalidomide), neonatal death (heroin), kernicterus (sulfonamides), ototoxicity (streptomycin), inhibition of infant bone growth (tetracyclines), and discoloration of teeth (tetracyclines). Anecdotal clinical experience is not sufficient to assess properly the safety of antibiotic administration during pregnancy. Rather, carefully planned prospective toxicity studies in the fetus and neonate, first in animals and then in humans, are mandatory.

Because of the ease of transplacental passage of sulfonamides and their significant bilirubin-displacing capabilities, with the associated theoretical risk for development of kernicterus in the infant, these drugs should not be given to pregnant women near term.[104] The same cautionary statement might apply to other antibiotics with a high protein-binding affinity, such as ceftriaxone and cefoperazone. Clinical reports confirming a potential association with these cephalosporins are lacking, however, and at present it is unknown whether this in vitro phenomenon will have clinical significance. In addition, jaundice and hemolytic anemia have been noted in newborns with G6PD deficiency after maternal sulfonamide administration near term.

The tetracyclines readily cross the placental barrier and concentrate in many tissues of the developing fetus.[111] Of particular interest is the deposition of tetracycline in fetal bones and deciduous teeth.[109,118] The growth inhibition observed after tetracycline administration to premature infants, however, is reversible when short-term therapy is employed.[108] Calcification of deciduous teeth begins during the fourth month of gestation, and crown formation of the anterior teeth is almost complete at term. Tetracycline administered during this gestational period produces yellow discoloration, enamel hypoplasia, and abnormal development of those teeth. These effects have been documented for tetracycline, oxytetracycline, and demethylchlortetracycline.[109] One report found a possible association between ciprofloxacin therapy given to young infants and teeth discoloration,[119] but this association has not been confirmed in other studies.

Chloramphenicol has been associated with circulatory collapse (gray baby syndrome) and death in premature infants who received the drug during the first weeks of life.[78] Chloramphenicol should not be administered to pregnant women near term because of the absence of glucuronyl transferase activity in the fetal liver and the potential danger of serum drug accumulation and shock in the newborn.[120]

Table 37–1 Transplacental Passage of Antimicrobial Agents

Antimicrobial Agent	Trimester	Serum Infant-to-Maternal Ratio(s) (%)	Adverse Effects on Fetus or Infant	Reference No.
Amikacin	1, 2	8-16	Potential ototoxicity	53
	3	30-50		55
Amoxicillin	3	30	None	56
Ampicillin	1, 2	50-250	None	57
	3	20-200		57
Azlocillin	3	50	Unknown	58
Carbenicillin	2, 3	60-100	None	59
Cefazolin	1, 2	2-27	None	59-61
	3	36-69		62
Cefoperazone	3	33-48	None	63-64
Cefotaxime	2	80-150	None	65
Cefoxitin	3	11-133	None	66-68
Ceftizoxime	3	13-130	None	69
Ceftriaxone	3	9-120	None	70
Cefuroxime	3	18-108	None	71-73
Cephalexin	3	33	None	74
Cephalothin	3	10-40	None	59, 75
Chloramphenicol	3	30-106	Potential circulatory collapse	76-78
Clindamycin	2	10-25	None	52, 59
	3	30-50		79
Cloxacillin	3	20-97	None	59, 80
Dicloxacillin	3	7-12	None	59, 82, 83
Erythromycin	2, 3	1-20	None	52, 84
Gentamicin	2, 3	21-44	Potential ototoxicity; potentiation of $MgSO_4$-induced neuromuscular weakness	78, 85, 86
Imipenem	3	14-52	Potential seizure activity	87
Kanamycin	3	26-48	Ototoxicity	59, 88, 89
Lincomycin	3	25-43	None	90, 91
Methicillin	3	30-140	None	83, 92
Nafcillin	3	16	None	59
Nitrofurantoin	3	38-92	Hemolysis in G6PD deficiency	93
Penicillin G	1.2	26-70		59, 94
	3	15-100	None	59, 94-96
Streptomycin	3	13-100	Ototoxicity	97-99
Sulfonamides	3	13-275	Hemolysis in G6PD deficiency; jaundice and potential kernicterus	100-107
Tetracyclines	3	10-90	Depressed bone growth; abnormal teeth; possible inguinal hernia	59-64, 108-111
Tobramycin	1, 2	20	Potential ototoxicity	54, 59
Trimethoprim	1, 2	27-131	Teratogenic in animals	112, 113

G6PD, glucose-6-phosphate dehydrogenase; $MgSO_4$, magnesium sulfate.

Intrapartum administration of antimicrobial agents to women in labor creates a potential problem for the pediatrician by potentially suppressing fetal infection and delaying diagnosis and treatment of neonatal infection. Although the evidence supports such an effect for group B streptococcal early-onset neonatal infections,[121-123] it is less clear for infections due to other bacterial pathogens. With the advent of more active β-lactam antibiotics, such as new-generation cephalosporins, it is possible that treatment for women during labor could prevent or even cure some bacterial infections in premature infants.

EXCRETION OF ANTIBIOTICS IN HUMAN MILK

As a general rule, the concentration of antimicrobial agents in breast milk is so low that neither therapeutic nor harmful effects are likely to occur. The amount of drug could be significant, however, depending on the volume of milk ingested by the newborn and the pharmacokinetic properties of that drug once it is absorbed through the infant's gastrointestinal mucosa.[124,125] Assessment of the safety of antibiotics in milk has relied primarily on anecdotal clinical experience, rather than on carefully controlled long-term studies.

Most drugs are transferred into breast milk by passive diffusion, and only a few are actively secreted. Factors influencing the transfer of antibiotics from plasma to milk include maternal serum concentration of unbound drug, water and lipid solubility, degree of ionization, serum and milk protein-binding capability, and molecular weight of the antibiotic.[125] Although drugs with a high lipid solubility tend to accumulate in milk, the extent varies with the fat content of the milk. Ionization power of drugs depends on the pH of the milk and the drug dissociation constant (pK_a). Human milk has a pH of 7.37; therefore, drugs that are weak bases (pK_a greater than pH), such as trimethoprim and tetracyclines, ionize and concentrate in milk,[126] whereas weak acids, such

Table 37–2 Excretion of Antimicrobial Agents in Human Breast Milk

Antibiotic	Maternal Dosage (Route)	No. of Patients	Concentration in Milk (Time)[a,b]	Milk–Maternal Serum Ratio (%)	Reference No.
Amoxicillin	1 g (PO)	6	0.1 (1 hr)	1.4	127
			0.17 (2 hr)	1.2	
			0.37 (3 hr)	4	
Aztreonam	1 g (IM)	6	0.14 (2 hr)	0.4	128
	1 g (IV)	6	0.18 (2 hr)	0.6	
Cefadroxil	1 g (PO)	6	1.64 (6 hr)	8	130
Cefamandole	1 g (IV)	4	0.46 (1 hr)	2	130
Cefazolin	2 g (IV)	20	1.25 (2 hr)	2.3	130
Cefoperazone	1 g (IV)	4	0.41 (2 hr)	1	64
Cefotaxime	1 g (IV)	12	0.26 (1 hr)	2.8	65
			0.32 (2 hr)	8.6	
Cefoxitin	1 g (IV)	4	0.58 (1 hr)	3	132
Ceftazidime	2 g (IV)	11	5.2 (1 hr)	7	133
Ceftizoxime	1 g (IV)	6	0.25 (1 hr)	1	134
Ceftriaxone	1 g (IV)	10	0.47 (4 hr)	1.6	70
	1 g (IM)	10	0.63 (4 hr)	2.1	
Cephalexin	1 g (PO)	6	0.2 (1 hr)	1	127
			0.28 (2 hr)	2	
			0.39 (3 hr)	14	
Cephalothin	1 g (IV)	6	0.41 (1 hr)	7	127
			0.47 (2 hr)	25	
			0.36 (3 hr)	51	
Clindamycin	0.15 g (PO)	5	<1.4 (6 hr)	38	130
Doxycycline	0.1 g (PO)	15	0.77 (3 hr)	32	130
Erythromycin	0.4 g (PO)	—	0.4-1.6	50	64
Kanamycin	1 g (IM)	4	18.4 (1 hr)	33	137
Lincomycin	0.5 g (PO)	9	1.3 (6 hr)	93	64
Metronidazole	0.2 g (PO)	10	3.4 (4 hr)	87	130
Nitrofurantoin	0.2 g (PO)	4	0.2 (2 hr)	24	139
Penicillin G	10^5 units (IM)	10	<0.04 (2 hr)	<13	140
Sulfapyridine	0.5 g (PO)	3	10.3	54	106
	0.75 g (PO)	—	30-130	100	135
Tetracycline	0.5 g (PO)	5	0.5-2.6	62	135
Ticarcillin	5 g (IV)	10	2-2.5	—	142
Tobramycin	0.08 g (IM)	5	<0.5	—	143
Trimethoprim	—	50	2	125	64

[a]Concentrations are in micrograms per milliliter.
[b]Time refers to period from drug administration to mother until sample collection.
IM, intramuscular; IV, intravenous; PO, oral (per os).

as ampicillin, do not.[125,126] Drugs that are highly serum protein bound tend to remain in the intravascular space.

The maternal serum and breast milk concentrations of commonly used antimicrobial agents are given in Table 37-2.[64,65,70,106,125-144] Because the data for each drug are based on small numbers of women, the values vary considerably. In general, the concentrations of metronidazole, sulfonamides, and trimethoprim in breast milk are similar to those in maternal serum (milk-to-serum ratio of 1.0), whereas those of chloramphenicol, erythromycin, and tetracycline are 50% to 75% of maternal serum values.[64,135] Available data suggest that the concentrations of penicillins, oxacillin, various cephalosporins, and aminoglycosides in milk are low.[129,140]

Data pertaining to antibiotic concentrations in the colostrum are not available. Because blood flow and permeability are increased during the colostral phase,[145] it is possible that these drugs are present in concentrations equal to or greater than those found in mature milk.

Very few reports of adverse effects to infants who were breast-fed by mothers receiving antimicrobial agents have been published. Hemolytic anemia has been described in breast-fed newborns whose mothers were being treated with sulfonamides, nalidixic acid, or nitrofurantoin.[146] One report incriminated the administration of clindamycin to a mother in the development of antibiotic-induced colitis in her breast-fed infant.[147] A causal effect, however, could not be convincingly demonstrated. Undoubtedly, other examples of potential infant toxicity from antibiotics in milk exist that have not been recognized or reported.

The decision to allow or stop breast-feeding must be based on the likelihood that high milk concentrations are attained for a particular drug and that significant adverse events are commonly associated with this drug. For the vast majority of antibiotics, however, this does not appear to be an important issue. The American Academy of Pediatrics Committee on Drugs recommends that breast-feeding be transiently discontinued 12 to 24 hours before and during the course of treatment with metronidazole (an in vitro mutagen) or chloramphenicol (associated with a theoretical risk of idiosyncratic bone marrow suppression) and warns about the use of nalidixic acid, nitrofurantoin, and sulfa drugs, which can cause hemolysis in G6PD-deficient infants.[146] In general, the severity of the woman's infection, rather than the drug that she is receiving, most often is the more important contraindication to breast-feeding.

PENICILLIN

Penicillin has been used for treatment of neonatal bacterial infections for more than 3 decades. It is safe and still effective for therapy against streptococci, susceptible staphylococci (currently most strains are resistant), a majority of pneumococci (although worldwide resistance is reaching alarming levels), and *L. monocytogenes*. In addition, most meningococcal strains and *Treponema pallidum* remain exquisitely susceptible to penicillin. Currently, many gonococcal isolates are resistant to this drug. Although penicillin (usually combined with an aminoglycoside) is used in some institutions for initial empirical therapy for neonatal septicemia and meningitis, ampicillin is preferred because it provides broader antimicrobial activity without sacrificing safety.

Mode of Action

Penicillin interferes with bacterial cell wall synthesis by reacting with one or more penicillin-binding proteins (PBPs) to inhibit transpeptidation.[148] The transpeptidase activity of PBPs is essential for cross-linking adjacent peptides and for incorporating newly formed peptidoglycan into an already existing strand. Subsequently, this event promotes bacterial cell lysis.

Several mechanisms of bacterial resistance to penicillin and some of the other β-lactams have been identified. The most important is by inactivation through enzymatic hydrolysis of the β-lactam ring by β-lactamases.[149] These enzymes are produced by most staphylococci and enteric gram-negative bacilli and by many *Neisseria gonorrhoeae* strains. Another mechanism of resistance is related to decreased permeability of the outer membrane of gram-negative bacteria, which can prevent this drug from reaching its target site.[150] In addition, by poorly defined mechanisms, some group B streptococcal organisms are inhibited but not killed by penicillin, a phenomenon termed *tolerance*.[151]

Usual MICs of penicillin against streptococci are between 0.005 and 0.1 μg/mL. For *T. pallidum*, the corresponding concentration ranges are between 0.02 and 0.2 μg/mL. Group B streptococcal strains demonstrating tolerance (with an MBC of 32 times the MIC) are found in less than 5% of isolates.[152] Currently, 15% to 40% of pneumococcal strains isolated in many parts of the world are considered to be relatively (MICs of 0.1 to 1 μg/mL) or highly (MICs of 2 μg/mL or greater) resistant to penicillin.[153,154] Many of these isolates also are resistant to multiple antibiotics, including third-generation cephalosporins. The mechanism of resistance is alteration of one or more PBPs.

Pharmacokinetic Data

Aqueous Penicillin G. A mean peak serum concentration of 24 μg/mL (range, 8 to 41 μg/mL) is observed after a dose of 25,000 units/kg of penicillin G is given intramuscularly to infants with birth weights of less than 2000 g (Table 37-3).[155] The peak values do not change appreciably with birth weight or postnatal age up to 14 days. After a dose of 50,000 units/kg, peak serum values of 35 to 40 μg/mL were detected in neonates of different ages. The concentrations at 4 and 8 hours after the dose were not substantially different from those after a dose of 25,000 units/kg.

The half-life of penicillin in serum is inversely correlated with birth weight and postnatal age. Half-life values of 1.5 to 10 hours are observed in the first week of life; the larger values usually are seen in infants with birth weights less than 1500 g. The half-life values for infants older than 7 days of age range from 1.5 to 4 hours. The half-life of penicillin in newborns is inversely correlated with clearance of creatinine. Plasma clearance of penicillin increases with the age of the newborn.

The concentrations of penicillin in urine after different dosages of penicillin G vary considerably. The highest values occur in the first 4 hours after a dose of 25,000 units/kg and range from 31 to 2000 μg/mL.[155] The urinary excretion of penicillin in infants is independent of age and dosage and is approximately 30% of the dose for a 12-hour period.

Procaine Penicillin G. Procaine penicillin G in a single daily intramuscular dose of 50,000 units/kg produces mean serum values of 7 to 9 μg/mL for up to 12 hours and 1.5 μg/mL at 24 hours after the dose in infants younger than 1 week of age (see Table 37-3).[155] Because the concentrations decrease more rapidly in older neonates, only 0.4 μg/mL is detected at 24 hours. These serum values are approximately twice those obtained when 22,000 units/kg is given to premature and

Table 37–3 Pharmacokinetics of Penicillin G in Neonates

Drug (Dosage)	Birth Weight/ Age Group	Mean Peak Serum Concentration (μg/mL)	Mean Serum Half-life (hr)	Plasma Clearance (mL/min/1.73 m²)
Crystalline penicillin G (25,000 units/kg)	2000 g			
	7 days	24	4.9	30
	8-14 days	23.6	2.6	48
	>2000 g			
	7 days	22.3	2.6	52
	8-14 days	21	2.1	75
Procaine penicillin G (50,000 units/kg)	7 days[a]	8.9	6.1	50
	8-14 days	6.2	5.4	93

[a]Average weight at time of study, 3100 g.

term infants.[2] No accumulation of penicillin in serum is observed after 7 to 10 days of daily doses of procaine penicillin G, and the drug is well tolerated without evidence of local reaction at the site of injection. The concentrations of penicillin in urine and the urinary excretion after equivalent doses are similar for both procaine penicillin G and aqueous penicillin G.

Benzathine Penicillin G. Penicillin can be detected in serum and urine for up to 12 days after a single dose of 50,000 units/kg of benzathine penicillin G given intramuscularly to newborns. Peak serum concentrations of 0.4 to 2.5 μg/mL (mean, 1.2 μg/mL) are observed 12 to 24 hours after administration, and levels of 0.07 to 0.09 μg/mL are present at 12 days.[156,157] Urinary concentrations range from 4 to 170 μg/mL for 7 days and from 0.3 to 25 μg/mL for 8 to 12 days after a dose of 50,000 units/kg of benzathine penicillin. This preparation is well tolerated by infants. Muscle damage from intramuscular injection as judged from creatinine values does not appear to be appreciably different from that after intramuscular administration of the other penicillins.

Cerebrospinal Fluid Penetration

Penicillin does not penetrate CSF well, even when meninges are inflamed. Peak concentrations of 1 to 2 μg/mL are measured 30 minutes to 1 hour after an intravenous dose of 40,000 units/kg of penicillin G is given to infants and children with bacterial meningitis.[158] These values are 2% to 5% of concomitant serum concentrations and exceed the MIC values for streptococci and susceptible pneumococci by 50- to 100-fold. CSF concentrations of penicillin, however, are not optimal to treat neonatal meningitis caused by penicillin-resistant pneumococci. When meningeal inflammation is decreased, the concentrations of penicillin are reduced substantially. Concentrations of penicillin in CSF during the first several days of therapy are maintained in the range of 0.5 to 1 μg/mL; thereafter, the values are 0.1 μg/mL or less by 4 hours after the dose.

Most newborns with uninflamed meninges have undetectable concentrations of penicillin in the CSF after a dose of 50,000 units/kg of intramuscular benzathine penicillin G.[156] With a dose of 100,000 units/kg, the mean peak concentration obtained 12 to 24 hours later is 0.06 μg/mL but falls to very low values by 48 to 72 hours.[159] For this reason, we do not recommend this long-acting penicillin for therapy for infants with congenital neurosyphilis. By contrast, mean CSF concentrations range from 0.12 to 0.7 μg/mL between 4 and 24 hours after a dose of 50,000 units/kg of procaine penicillin G is administered by inramuscular injection to newborns.[160,161] These CSF values are at least severalfold greater than the required minimum spirocheticidal concentration.[161]

Oral Administration

Potassium penicillin G has been administered orally to premature and term infants.[2,162] Mean peak serum concentrations at 2 and 6 hours after a dose of 22,000 units/kg were 1.4 and 0.7 μg/mL, respectively, in premature infants. The corresponding values in term neonates were 1.7 and 0.2 μg/mL.

Elimination

Most of the penicillin dose is excreted in the urine in unchanged form. Tubular secretion accounts for approximately 90% of urinary penicillin, whereas glomerular filtration contributes the remaining 10%. Biliary excretion also occurs, and this may be an important route of elimination in newborns with renal failure.

Clinical Implications

Penicillin remains effective for therapy for infections caused by group B streptococci, susceptible pneumococci and staphylococci, meningococci, susceptible gonococci, and *T. pallidum*. The dosage recommended for neonatal sepsis or pneumonia is 50,000 to 100,000 units/kg per day administered in two to four divided doses, whereas that for meningitis is 150,000 to 200,000 units/kg per day in two to four divided doses, depending on birth weight and postnatal age.[163] Neonatal meningitis caused by penicillin-resistant pneumococci must be treated with cefotaxime with or without vancomycin, depending on the MIC values. Oral penicillin therapy has no place in the management of neonates with acute systemic infections.

Because central nervous system involvement in congenital syphilis is difficult to exclude with certainty, benzathine penicillin G should not be used for therapy for this disease unless new diagnostic modalities to rule out neurosyphilis are developed.[164] Its use for asymptomatic infants with normal findings on CSF examination and roentgenologic studies but who have positive results on treponemal serologic studies, presumably from maternal origin, is acceptable if follow-up can be ensured. For symptomatic infants and for asymptomatic infants with laboratory or radiologic evidence suggestive of congenital syphilis, the recommended regimen is either aqueous penicillin G, 50,000 units/kg daily for 10 to 14 days administered intramuscularly or intravenously in two divided doses, or procaine penicillin G, 50,000 units/kg daily for 10 to 14 days administered once daily intramuscularly.

All forms of penicillin are well tolerated in newborns. Cutaneous allergic manifestations to penicillin are rare in the newborn and young infant, and evidence for sensitization to the drug in infants who receive penicillin in the neonatal period, thus increasing the risk of an allergic response on reexposure, is lacking.

AMPICILLIN

Antimicrobial Activity

Ampicillin commonly is used alone or in combination with aminoglycosides for treatment of suspected or proven neonatal bacterial infections. Compared with penicillin G, ampicillin has increased in vitro efficacy against most strains of enterococci and *L. monocytogenes* as well as against some gram-negative pathogens, such as typeable and nontypeable *Haemophilus*, *Escherichia coli*, *Proteus mirabilis*, and *Salmonella* species. It is not as active, however, against group A and group B streptococci and susceptible strains of staphylococci and pneumococci. Approximately 90% of group B streptococci and *Listeria* organisms are inhibited by 0.06 μg/mL or less of ampicillin. Almost two thirds of the gram-negative enteric bacilli isolated from CSF cultures of infants enrolled in the Second Neonatal Meningitis Cooperative Study (1976 to 1978) were inhibited by 10 μg/mL

Table 37–4 Pharmacokinetics of Ampicillin in Newborns

Dosage (Route)	Birth Weight/ Age Group	Mean Peak Serum Concentration (μg/mL)	Mean Serum Half-life (hr)	Mean Plasma Clearance (mL/min/1.73 m^2)
50 mg/kg (IM)	2500 g			
	7 days	104	6.2	21
	8-14 days	130	2	30
	>2500 g			
	7 days	81	4.7	42
	8-14 days	84	2.3	63
100 mg/kg (IM)	2500 g			
	7 days	213	4.7	NA
	8-14 days	216	3.5	NA
	>2500 g			
	7 days	180	3.1	NA
	8-14 days	187	1.8	NA

IM, intramuscular; NA, not available.

or less of ampicillin.[165] Recently, however, an increased rate of ampicillin-resistant gram-negative bacilli has been reported and possibly linked to the frequent use of intrapartum prophylaxis with ampicillin to prevent early-onset group B streptococcal neonatal infection.[166]

Pharmacokinetic Data

Serum ampicillin concentration-time curves after intramuscular doses of 5 to 25 mg/kg have been determined in newborns.[167-169] The mean peak serum concentrations 30 minutes to 1 hour after 5, 10, 20, and 25 mg/kg doses were 16, 25, 54, and 57 μg/mL, respectively, whereas the values at 12 hours were from 1 to 15 μg/mL (mean, 5 μg/mL). After 50-mg/kg doses, the mean peak values were from 100 to 130 μg/mL in low-birth-weight infants and from 80 to 85 μg/mL in larger term infants (Table 37-4). Peak serum concentrations as high as 300 μg/mL (mean values, 180 to 216 μg/mL) are observed 1 to 2 hours after the 100-mg/kg dose.[35] These latter values exceed the MIC_{90} values of group B streptococci by at least 3000-fold.

The elimination half-life of ampicillin is inversely correlated with birth weight and postnatal age. Half-life times of 3 to 6 hours are noted in the first week of life and are 2 to 3.5 hours thereafter. Similar correlations with birth weight and chronologic age are observed with the plasma clearance of ampicillin.

A mean peak serum concentration of 135 μg/mL for premature infants with gestational ages of 26 to 33 weeks was found after an intravenous 100-mg/kg dose of ampicillin, whereas for those infants with gestational ages of 34 to 40 weeks, it was 153 μg/mL.[170] When the loading dose was followed by maintenance ampicillin doses of 50 mg/kg intravenously at 12- to 18-hour intervals, the mean peak and trough serum concentrations in steady-state conditions were 113 and 30 μg/mL, respectively, for premature neonates and 140 and 37 μg/mL for full-term neonates. The steady-state serum half-life for ampicillin was about 9.5 hours for premature newborns and 7 hours for full-term newborns.

Cerebrospinal Fluid Penetration

Concentrations of ampicillin in CSF vary greatly. The largest concentrations (3 to 18 μg/mL) occur approximately 2 hours after a 50-mg/kg intravenous dose and exceed the MIC values for group B streptococci and *Listeria* by 50- to 300-fold.[35] By contrast, against many *E. coli* strains, these peak concentrations equal or exceed the MIC values by only severalfold. The values in CSF are lower later than in the course of meningitis, when meningeal inflammation subsides.

Oral Administration

Oral administration of 20- to 30-mg/kg doses of ampicillin trihydrate to normal, fasting full-term infants during the first 4 days of life produced peak values of 20 to 30 μg/mL 4 hours after the doses.[167] Higher peak serum concentrations are achieved by oral administration of the anhydrous form of ampicillin rather than the trihydrate preparation.[171] In our experience,[172] mean peak serum concentrations of 6.4 and 6.1 μg/mL occurred at 1 and 2 hours, respectively, after a 25-mg/kg dose of ampicillin trihydrate, and the drug was absorbed equally well in both fasting and concomitantly milk-fed infants. Because of better absorption, amoxicillin would be expected to achieve higher serum concentrations than those observed for ampicillin after equivalent doses.

Safety

Ampicillin is a safe drug when administered parenterally to newborns. Nonspecific rashes and urticaria are rarely observed, and diarrhea is uncommon. Elevations of serum glutamic-oxaloacetic transaminase and creatinine values frequently are detected in neonates and probably represent local tissue destruction at the site of intramuscular injection. Mild eosinophilia may be noted in newborns and young infants. Alteration of the microbial flora of the bowel may occur after parenteral administration of ampicillin, but overgrowth of resistant gram-negative organisms and *Candida albicans* occurs more frequently after oral administration.[173] Diarrhea usually subsides on discontinuation of therapy. Amoxicillin is better tolerated, with fewer gastrointestinal side effects, than is orally administered ampicillin.

Clinical Implications

Vast clinical experience has demonstrated that ampicillin is a safe and effective drug for therapy for neonatal bacterial

Table 37–5 Pharmacokinetics of Methicillin and Nafcillin in Newborns

Drug (Dosage)	Birth Weight/ Age Group	Mean Peak Serum Concentration (μg/mL)	Peak Serum Half-life (hr)	Mean Plasma Clearance (mL/min/1.73 m²)
Methicillin	2000 g			
(25 mg/kg per dose)	0-7 days	58	2.8	32
	15 days	39	1.8	79
	>2000 g			
	0-7 days	49	2.2	62
	15 days	41	1.1	128
Nafcillin	2000 g			
(50 mg/kg per dose)[a]	0-7 days	±160	4	0.91[b]
	8-28 days		3.2	1.2[b]

[a]Data from reference 181.
[b]Total body clearance (mL/min/kg).

infections caused by susceptible organisms. Combined ampicillin and aminoglycoside therapy is appropriate initial empirical management of suspected bacterial infections of neonates because it provides broad antimicrobial activity and potential synergism against many strains of group B streptococci, *Listeria*, and enterococci.[31-34,37]

For systemic bacterial infections other than meningitis, a dosage of 50 to 75 mg/kg per day in two to three divided doses in the first week of life and of 75 to 100 mg/kg per day in three to four divided doses thereafter is recommended. For therapy for bacterial meningitis, we recommend a dosage of 150 to 200 mg/kg per day given in three to four divided doses, although some consultants use dosages as high as 300 mg/kg per day.

We are not in favor of oral administration of ampicillin to newborns. As a general rule, infants with suspected or proven bacterial infections caused by susceptible organisms should receive parenteral treatment in the hospital. Otitis media in infants younger than 6 weeks of age may be better treated with other antimicrobial agents, such as amoxicillin-clavulanate or a cephalosporin, because *S. aureus* and resistant gram-negative organisms are possible etiologic agents.[174]

ANTISTAPHYLOCOCCAL PENICILLINS

S. aureus infections occur in nurseries either as sporadic cases or in the form of disease outbreaks. In recent years, multiply-resistant strains, especially coagulase-negative staphylococcal species, have been responsible for an increasing number of nosocomially acquired staphylococcal infections in many neonatal care units. Familiarity with the antistaphylococcal penicillins is essential for physicians involved in the care of newborns with infections caused by susceptible staphylococci.

Antimicrobial Activity

The antistaphylococcal penicillins are resistant to hydrolysis by most staphylococcal β-lactamases by virtue of a substituted side chain that acts by steric hindrance at the site of enzyme attachment. Most penicillinase-producing staphylococci are inhibited by 2.5 to 5 μg/mL or less of methicillin and by 0.5 μg/mL or less of nafcillin and oxacillin.[175] Currently, methicillin-resistant *S. aureus* (MRSA) strains constitute a relatively common cause of infection outbreaks in some nurseries, and methicillin-resistant *Staphylococcus epidermidis* (MRSE) strains are an important cause of catheter-associated disease, particularly among low-birth-weight premature infants. These challenging isolates possess altered PBPs with low affinity for binding to antistaphylococcal penicillins and cephalosporins.[176] Glycopeptide antibiotics such as vancomycin or teicoplanin are the drugs of choice for infections caused by these resistant strains. The topical antimicrobial agent mupirocin has been used successfully to eradicate MRSA strains from sites of the newborn body colonized with these strains and to prevent their spread to other infants.[177] In addition, tolerant staphylococci (with an MBC greater than five times the MIC) have been described.[178] Infections caused by these uncommon staphylococcal isolates may require combined therapy with aminoglycosides or rifampin or the use of vancomycin alone.

Pharmacokinetic Data

Methicillin. Peak serum concentrations of methicillin are higher in the first week of life than during the remainder of the newborn period.[168,169] For example, after 25-mg/kg intramuscular doses, mean peak values of 58 and 49 μg/mL are observed in 0- to 7-day-old infants who weigh 2000 g or less and those who weigh more than 2000 g at birth, respectively, whereas for these same birth weights, values of 39 and 41 μg/mL are achieved in infants 15 days of age or older (Table 37-5).[179] A 50-mg/kg intramuscular dose produces a mean peak serum concentration of 80 μg/mL 30 minutes to 1 hour later. The half-life values become smaller with increasing birth weight and postnatal age. This observation correlates with the substantial increase in the plasma clearance of methicillin that occurs during the neonatal period. Urine concentrations of methicillin are from 275 to 880 μg/mL in the first 2 hours after a 20-mg/kg intramuscular dose and usually are greater than 120 μg/mL for up to 12 hours after the dose. Approximately 30% of the dose is excreted in urine in the first 6 hours after administration.[168]

Nafcillin. The administration of 5-, 10-, 15-, and 20-mg/kg intramuscular doses of nafcillin to full-term newborns in the first 4 days of life produces mean peak serum concentrations

1 hour later of 10, 25, 30, and 37 µg/mL, respectively.[167,180] These concentrations are significantly higher than those obtained in older children receiving comparable amounts of this drug.[180] Hepatic clearance evidently is the principal route of nafcillin elimination, because only 8% to 25% of this drug is excreted in the urine in a 24-hour period.[180]

Peak concentrations of nafcillin of 100 to 160 µg/mL were obtained during steady-state conditions after 33- to 50-mg/kg intravenous doses were administered to premature infants weighing less than 2000 g at birth (see Table 37-5).[181] The half-life ranged from 2.2 to 5.5 hours in these low-birth-weight neonates.

When nafcillin is given orally to newborns, mean peak serum concentrations are 20% to 60% of those obtained after an identical dose is administered intramuscularly.[167,182] Oral doses of 5 to 20 mg/kg of nafcillin result in mean peak serum concentrations of 3 to 21 µg/mL 2 to 4 hours after ingestion.

Oxacillin. The pharmacokinetics of oxacillin in neonates is similar to that of methicillin. Mean peak serum concentrations of approximately 50 and 100 µg/mL are produced by 20- and 50-mg/kg intramuscular doses, respectively.[168,183] The serum half-life of oxacillin in premature infants is about 3 hours in the first week of life and 1.5 hours thereafter. Urinary concentrations are from 174 to 510 µg/mL in the first 2 hours after a 20-mg/kg dose; 17% of the dose is excreted during 6 hours after administration in infants 8 to 14 days of age, whereas 34% is excreted in infants 20 to 21 days of age.[168]

Cloxacillin. Oral administration of 5-, 10-, 20-, and 50-mg/kg single doses of cloxacillin to full-term neonates during the first 4 days of life results in mean peak serum concentrations of 15, 24, 32, and 92 µg/mL, respectively, 1 to 2 hours after ingestion of this drug.[167] The mean concentrations at 12 hours after these doses are given fall to 0, 3, 8, and 19 µg/mL, respectively.

Safety

The antistaphylococcal penicillins are well tolerated and safe in newborn and young infants. Repeated intramuscular injections of methicillin frequently result in muscle damage and elevation of creatinine concentrations. Formation of sterile muscle abscesses occasionally follows intramuscular administration. Nephrotoxicity (interstitial nephritis or cystitis) is rare in newborns and occurs in 3% to 5% of children who receive large doses of methicillin and possibly the other antistaphylococcal penicillins, with the exception of nafcillin.[184,185] Reversible hematologic abnormalities such as neutropenia or eosinophilia commonly are observed in children undergoing treatment with these drugs, but their incidence in newborns is unknown.[185-188] Because nafcillin has a predominant biliary excretion, accumulation of this drug in serum can occur in jaundiced neonates, and potential adverse effects can develop. Extravasation of nafcillin at the injection site can result in necrosis of local tissue.

Clinical Implications

Any of these antistaphylococcal drugs can be used for therapy for staphylococcal infections in neonates. The dosage of methicillin and for oxacillin (preferred) is 25 to 50 mg/kg every 8 to 12 hours (50 to 150 mg/kg per day) in the first week of life and every 6 to 8 hours (75 to 200 mg/kg per day) thereafter. The larger dosage is indicated for infants with disseminated disease or meningitis. For nafcillin, we recommend 25 mg/kg per dose given every 12 hours in the first week of life and every 6 to 8 hours thereafter.

In the unlikely circumstance that the *Staphylococcus* species is susceptible to penicillin, this agent is preferred for therapy. If an infant does not respond to antimicrobial therapy as anticipated, the physician should suspect an occult site of staphylococcal disease (e.g., abscess, osteomyelitis, endocarditis), resistance of the pathogen to the drug given, or tolerance of the organism to the antibiotic. Appropriate drainage of purulent foci, addition of an aminoglycoside or rifampin to the regimen, and use of vancomycin are among several options to consider in management of unresponsive infections.

CARBENICILLIN

Carbenicillin is an α-carboxybenzyl penicillin that possesses activity against *P. aeruginosa* and some indole-positive *Proteus* strains. In addition, essentially all bacteria susceptible to ampicillin also are susceptible to carbenicillin. Although the combination of carbenicillin and an aminoglycoside provides a broader antimicrobial activity, ampicillin plus an aminoglycoside is the combination preferred in most nurseries. Carbenicillin is no longer available in the United States, having been replaced by newer, more active agents.

Antimicrobial Activity

Like ampicillin, carbenicillin is effective in vitro against the two most common pathogens of neonatal septicemia and meningitis, *E. coli* and group B streptococci. *L. monocytogenes* and enterococci are less susceptible in vitro to carbenicillin than to ampicillin. *Klebsiella* and many *Pseudomonas* species, other than *P. aeruginosa*, are resistant to carbenicillin.[37] Most isolates in hospital-acquired staphylococcal infection also are resistant to this agent.[189] Combinations of carbenicillin and gentamicin are synergistic in vitro against *P. aeruginosa*, enterococci, and many *Listeria* isolates.[37]

Pharmacokinetic Data

The pharmacokinetic data for carbenicillin are similar to those for ampicillin in newborns. Peak serum concentrations of 180 to 190 µg/mL are observed after 100-mg/kg doses in all neonates except term infants older than 1 week of age, in whom peak values are from 140 to 150 µg/mL (Table 37-6).[190] Although peak serum concentrations after intravenous doses are about twice those obtained after identical intramuscular doses are given, the dose-response curves for both routes of administration are similar after the peak concentration is achieved.[191] Serum half-life is inversely correlated with birth weight, chronologic age, and rate of creatinine clearance.[190-192] During the first week of life, mean half-life values are from 3 to 6 hours, whereas for neonates aged 1 to 4 weeks, values of 2 to 3 hours are observed.[190] Plasma clearance of carbenicillin increases appreciably during the first 30 days of life.

Table 37–6 **Pharmacokinetics of Carbenicillin, Ticarcillin, and Piperacillin in Neonates**

Drug (Dosage, Route)	Birth Weight/ Age Group	Mean Peak Serum Concentration (μg/mL)	Mean Serum Half-life (hr)	Mean Plasma Clearance (mL/min/1.73 m²)
Carbenicillin (100 mg/kg; IM)	2000 g			
	7 days	180	5.7	25
	8-14 days	186	3.6	35
	>2000 g			
	7 days	185	4.2	45
	8-14 days	143	2.1	77
Ticarcillin (75 mg/kg; IM)	2000 g			
	Mean, 2.5 days	189	5.6	31
	>2000 g			
	Mean, 3 days	159	4.9	54
	Mean, 34 days[a]	125	2.2	118
Piperacillin (75 mg/kg; IV)	1000-1520 g (mean, 1300 g)			
	7 days	137	4.3	1.7[b]
	1500-3580 g (mean, 1930 g)			
	7 days	149	3.4	1.8[b]
	2265-3900 g (mean, 3108 g)			
	7 days	129	2.5	2.5[b]
	850-1400 g (mean, 1200 g)			
	8-14 days	110	3.2	3.2[b]
	1500-2170 g (mean, 1725 g)			
	8-14 days	100	2.5	3.4[b]
	2265-3900 g (mean, 3108 g)			
	8-14 days	97	1.7	4.4[b]

[a]Ticarcillin dosage of 100 mg/kg.
[b]Total body clearance (mL/min/kg).
IM, intramuscularly; IV, intravenously.

Because carbenicillin is eliminated by renal mechanisms, extremely large concentrations are present in urine. Concentrations of 800 to 5500 μg/mL (mean, 2689 μg/mL) are noted during the first 6 hours after administration of a 100-mg/kg dose.[191]

Clinical Implications

Historically, carbenicillin given alone or preferably in combination with an aminoglycoside was used for therapy for neonatal infections caused by *P. aeruginosa* or indole-positive *Proteus* species. Newer antimicrobial agents are now preferred for these infections. Although synergism between carbenicillin and gentamicin has been observed in vitro against enterococci, *L. monocytogenes*, and *P. aeruginosa*,[37] the clinical significance of this phenomenon is uncertain. The dosage schedule for carbenicillin is the following: 100 mg/kg given every 12 hours for all infants younger than 1 week of age, every 8 hours for infants older than 7 days weighing less than 2000 g at birth, and every 6 hours for neonates older than 7 days weighing more than 2000 g at birth. The drug should be administered intravenously over 20 to 30 minutes.

The drug is well tolerated and safe in newborns. Platelet dysfunction, hypokalemia, and allergic manifestations observed in older patients have not been reported in neonates. Carbenicillin is a disodium salt that contains 4.7 mEq of sodium per gram of drug, which should be a consideration in some newborns, such as those with heart failure.

TICARCILLIN

Ticarcillin is a semisynthetic penicillin with pharmacologic and toxic properties virtually identical to those of carbenicillin. Its in vitro activity is similar to that of carbenicillin, with the exception that ticarcillin is more active against *P. aeruginosa*.[189]

Mean peak serum concentrations of 189 μg/mL are seen 1 hour after administration of 75-mg/kg intramuscular doses to low-birth-weight infants younger than 7 days of age and of 125 to 160 μg/mL to older neonates (see Table 37-6).[193] The half-life and plasma clearance during the neonatal period are similar to those for carbenicillin.[193,194]

Comparative clinical studies of carbenicillin and ticarcillin have not been conducted to identify an advantage of one drug over the other. As noted previously, in the United States, carbenicillin is no longer available. Use of ticarcillin alone or combined with clavulanate (Timentin) is preferred in patients with *P. aeruginosa* infections because of its greater in vitro activity against this organism. Although the quantity of sodium per gram is larger for ticarcillin than for carbenicillin, the lower dosage schedule for ticarcillin that is recommended for neonates and young infants provides a

Table 37–7 **Important Characteristics of Extended-Spectrum Penicillins**

	Extended-Spectrum Penicillin				
Characteristic	*Carbenicillin*	*Ticarcillin*	*Azlocillin*	*Mezlocillin*	*Piperacillin*
Antibacterial activity					
Gram-positive cocci					
Streptococci	++	++	++	++	++
Enterococci	–	–	++	++	++
Staphylococcus aureus[a]	–	–	–	–	–
Gram-negative bacilli					
Coliforms	++	++	++	++	++
Klebsiella spp.	–	–	+	++	++
Pseudomonas aeruginosa	+	+	++	+	++
Anaerobes					
Bacteroides fragilis	+	+	+	++	++
Body clearance					
Renal	++	++	+	+	+
Hepatic	–	–	+	+	+
Sodium content (mEq/g)	4.7	5.1	2.2	1.9	1.9

[a]Penicillin-resistant strains.
++, good; +, moderate; –, poor.

smaller amount of sodium per dose of drug, which conceivably could be advantageous in infants with cardiac or renal disease. The dose is 75 mg/kg administered every 12 hours to infants younger than 1 week of age, and every 8 and every 6 hours to older infants weighing 2000 g or less and more than 2000 g at birth, respectively.

The co-administration of clavulanic acid with ticarcillin significantly enhances the antibacterial activity of the latter drug against several organisms, including some ticarcillin-resistant strains of *E. coli*, *Klebsiella pneumoniae*, *P. mirabilis*, and staphylococci.[195,196] Clavulanic acid is a β-lactam with weak antibacterial activity, but it has the property of being a potent irreversible inhibitor of several β-lactamases produced by gram-positive and gram-negative bacteria.[197] Information regarding the use of this compound in newborns is limited. Pharmacokinetic data obtained in three newborns with gram-negative infections treated with a ticarcillin–to–clavulanic acid weight ratio of 25:1 included peak serum concentrations and half-life values similar to those observed after administration of ticarcillin alone.[198] This drug combination is potentially very useful in the treatment of neonatal infections. We have prescribed ticarcillin-clavulanate either alone or, more commonly, with an aminoglycoside for infants with nosocomial gram-negative enteric infections, with satisfactory safety and effectiveness.

ACYLAMPICILLINS

The acylampicillins, a group of semisynthetic penicillins, include the ureidopenicillins—mezlocillin and azlocillin—and a piperazine derivative of ampicillin called piperacillin.[199,200] These drugs have not been approved by the FDA for use in newborns. Many pathogens incriminated in neonatal infections are susceptible in vitro to these antibiotics, but their most important feature is activity against *P. aeruginosa*.

Antimicrobial Activity

Mezlocillin, azlocillin, and piperacillin are active against a broad range of gram-positive and gram-negative bacteria (Table 37-7). In contrast with carbenicillin and ticarcillin, which show poor activity against *K. pneumoniae*, piperacillin is active against most isolates of this organism, whereas mezlocillin and azlocillin inhibit about 50%. They also are active against *P. mirabilis* and many strains of *Enterobacter* and *Serratia marcescens*. Because these antibiotics are susceptible to hydrolysis by β-lactamases, they have very limited activity against β-lactamase–producing Enterobacteriaceae organisms.[199,200]

Piperacillin is the most active of these agents against *P. aeruginosa*. Mezlocillin, the least active of the three, is at least as effective as ticarcillin against this organism. Ninety percent of *P. aeruginosa* isolates are inhibited by approximately 16, 32, and 128 μg/mL of piperacillin, azlocillin, and mezlocillin, respectively.[201]

These drugs have good activity against penicillin-susceptible strains of *S. aureus*, streptococci, *Haemophilus influenzae*, *Neisseria meningitidis*, and *L. monocytogenes*. Penicillin- or ampicillin-resistant strains of these bacteria, however, also are resistant to these agents. In contrast with carbenicillin and ticarcillin, acylampicillins are active against enterococci. Activity against many anaerobes, such as *Bacteroides fragilis*, *Bacteroides melaninogenicus*, and *Clostridium perfringens*, is good.

When aminoglycosides are combined with any of these three agents, in vitro synergistic activity against *P. aeruginosa*, coliforms, and susceptible *S. aureus* strains can be demonstrated.[199,200] Both synergistic and antagonistic interactions have been observed when these penicillins were combined with various cephalosporins.[200-202] Antagonism may be related to the ability of certain cephalosporins to induce β-lactamase production, which, in turn, inactivates the penicillins.[200]

Pharmacokinetic Data

Mezlocillin. The pharmacokinetic behavior of mezlocillin has been studied in more than 150 premature and full-term infants.[203-206] Peak serum concentrations after 75-mg/kg intravenous doses occur at the end of drug infusion and range from a mean of about 260 μg/mL for newborns in the first week of life to 139 μg/mL for older neonates.[206] After intramuscular administration of an identical dose, peak concentrations were observed 30 minutes after the injection and ranged from a mean of 155 μg/mL for infants 1 week of age or younger to 121 μg/mL for those older than 7 days. No drug accumulation is observed after multiple doses of mezlocillin are administered.[205,206] Plasma clearance of this drug increases with advancing gestational and postnatal ages. The half-life of mezlocillin is inversely related to gestational age and postnatal age. It decreases from about 4.5 hours in premature infants aged 1 week or younger to about 1.6 hours in full-term neonates older than 7 days.[206]

Available information on the CSF penetration of mezlocillin in newborns is limited. In one study, concentrations of 20 to 90 μg/mL were measured at various intervals after 75-mg/kg intravenous doses.[207] In another study, however, values ranging from 0 to 13.7 μg/mL (mean, 5.5 μg/mL) were found in nine neonates 1 to 3 hours after 100-mg/kg mezlocillin doses were intravenously injected.[208]

The mechanisms of mezlocillin elimination have not been studied in newborns. Renal excretion is the principal route of elimination in adults. Up to 30% of a mezlocillin dose, however, may be excreted in bile.[209]

Azlocillin. After a 50-mg/kg intravenous dose of azlocillin, concentrations of about 200 μg/mL are obtained at the end of drug infusion. Concentrations at 1 and 5 hours after the dose are approximately 100 and 50 μg/mL, respectively.[203,210,211] The elimination half-life is about 2.5 hours. Most of the azlocillin dose is excreted unchanged in the urine. Biliary excretion accounts for only 5% of the dose.

Piperacillin. The mean peak serum concentration of piperacillin after an intravenous dose of 100 mg/kg is about 180 μg/mL, and it may be as high as 250 μg/mL in newborns with impaired renal function.[212] The half-life is prolonged and ranges from 3.5 to 14 hours (median, 6.5 hours). By contrast, the reported half-life of piperacillin for infants 1 to 6 months of age is about 47 minutes.[213] Repeated administration of this drug does not result in its accumulation in serum. In one study,[214] a 75-mg/kg intravenous dose of piperacillin given to 28 neonates born at 29 to 40 weeks of gestational age and at a weight of 860 to 3900 g resulted in peak and trough serum concentrations ranging from 70 to 360 μg/mL and 5 to 34 μg/mL, respectively (see Table 37-6). The mean half-life values ranged from 1.7 to 4.3 hours; half-life was inversely related to gestational age, postnatal age, and birth weight.[214]

CSF piperacillin concentrations of 2.6 to 6 μg/mL were measured in three neonates without meningitis within 7 hours of the intravenous administration of a 100-mg/kg dose.[212] In one infant with *Pseudomonas* meningitis, piperacillin reached a concentration of 19 μg/mL in the CSF 2.5 hours after a 200-mg/kg intravenous dose was given.[212]

The major route of piperacillin excretion is through the kidney. Up to 30% to 40% of the dose, however, may be eliminated by nonrenal mechanisms in children.[213,215]

To improve antibacterial activity, a β-lactamase inhibitor, tazobactam, has been combined with piperacillin in an 8:1 ratio. The mean half-life for piperacillin-tazobactam in neonates is approximately 1.5 hours. Addition of tazobactam provides coverage against β-lactamase–producing bacteria resistant to piperacillin alone. CSF penetration of this compound is modest.[216]

Safety

Adverse reactions from parenteral administration of mezlocillin, azlocillin, or piperacillin are rare in newborns. Hypersensitivity reactions, diarrhea, neutropenia, eosinophilia, and elevated serum concentrations of hepatic enzymes are infrequent compared with transient complications encountered in older children and adults who received these drugs.[199] Impaired hemostasis secondary to platelet dysfunction occurs less frequently with these antibiotics than with carbenicillin and ticarcillin.[217] The sodium content of these drugs is less than half of that of carbenicillin or ticarcillin (see Table 37-7), which may be important in some newborns with cardiac or renal disease.

Clinical Implications

Mezlocillin and piperacillin, either alone or combined with aminoglycosides, have been used successfully for the treatment of bacteriologically proven neonatal infections. Experience is limited, however, with routine use of these agents for initial therapy in newborns with suspected sepsis. Accordingly, these agents should be reserved for situations in which a clear benefit can be derived from their use. Potential recipients include newborns with *P. aeruginosa* sepsis, infants in whom sodium restriction is necessary, and neonates with bleeding problems in whom it would be desirable to minimize antibiotic-associated hemostatic impairment.

The dosage schedule for mezlocillin is 75 mg/kg given every 12 hours during the first week of life and every 8 hours thereafter. The proper dosage schedule for piperacillin for newborns has not been established. One study suggested that piperacillin doses of 100 mg/kg every 12 hours may be appropriate and that a dose of 200 mg/kg every 12 hours should be used for meningitis.[212] In a more complete pharmacokinetic study,[214] a dosage schedule of 75 mg/kg given every 12 and 8 hours for infants with gestational ages of less than 36 weeks and postnatal ages of 0 to 7 days and older than 1 week of age, respectively, was recommended. For full-term infants (greater than 36 weeks of gestation), a 75-mg/kg dose given every 8 hours during the first week of life and every 6 hours thereafter was recommended. Additional data are required before a dosage schedule can be suggested for azlocillin.

CEPHALOSPORINS

All cephalosporins are semisynthetic derivatives of a 7-aminocephalosporanic acid nucleus. The individual derivatives differ chemically by the addition of various side chains. Cefoxitin and moxalactam are not technically cephalosporins[218] but generally are included in discussions of these antibiotics because of their close similarities to members of this group of drugs. Moxalactam is no longer available because of the potential for bleeding resulting from interference in prothrombin synthesis. It was ineffective against group B streptococci, limiting its usefulness in neonates. The cephalosporins exert their antibacterial action in a manner similar to that described earlier for penicillin.

It has become customary, albeit confusing at times, to group cephalosporins into generations of agents on the basis of their antibacterial spectrum of activity (see subsequent discussion), rather than their time of introduction for clinical use.[219] First-generation cephalosporins include cefazolin, cephalothin, cephalexin, and cefadroxil. Among the second-generation agents are cefaclor, cefprozil, cefamandole, cefuroxime, loracarbef, and cefoxitin. The most useful agents for the treatment of neonatal infections belong to the third-generation cephalosporins, which include cefoperazone, cefotaxime, ceftizoxime, ceftriaxone, and ceftazidime. Oral third-generation compounds include cefixime, cefpodoxime, ceftibuten, cefdinir, and cefetamet. A fourth-generation cephalosporin, cefepime, is still undergoing clinical evaluation in infants and children, and very limited information is available for the neonatal age group. Cefepime has been shown to be effective for therapy for meningitis in children and should be useful for treatment of multiresistant gram-negative bacillary infections in pediatric patients. Cefpirome, another fourth-generation agent, has not been studied in infants. The characteristics of many of the just-mentioned cephalosporins, particularly the oral agents, are not discussed because of the lack of neonatal studies evaluating these agents.

Antimicrobial Activity

The first-generation cephalosporins have good activity against gram-positive organisms but limited activity against gram-negative bacteria. Susceptible pathogens include streptococci, penicillin-susceptible and penicillin-resistant staphylococci, and penicillin-susceptible pneumococci. Enterococci, methicillin-resistant staphylococci, and *L. monocytogenes* are resistant to these agents. Although typically the activity against coliforms is good, other antibiotics usually are preferred for treatment of infections caused by these organisms. *Pseudomonas* species, *S. marcescens*, *Enterobacter* species, indole-positive *Proteus* species, and *B. fragilis* all are resistant to these antibacterial agents.[218]

Because of their improved stability to hydrolysis by β-lactamases, the second-generation cephalosporins have increased activity against many gram-negative bacteria compared with that of first-generation antibiotics. Cefamandole has in vitro activity against gram-positive cocci comparable with that of cephalothin and also is active against *H. influenzae*, *Enterobacter cloacae*, *Klebsiella*, *E. coli*, and *Citrobacter*. Cefuroxime is more active than cephalothin against group B streptococci, pneumococci, and gram-negative enteric bacilli and also is active against *H. influenzae*, meningococci, gonococci, and staphylococci.[220] Cefoxitin has considerably less activity against gram-positive cocci compared with the first-generation cephalosporins, but its spectrum of activity against gram-negative enteric bacilli is at least as good as that of cefamandole. In addition, cefoxitin has excellent in vitro activity against *B. fragilis* and other anaerobes.[219] Cefaclor, an oral cephalosporin, has a spectrum of activity similar to that of cefamandole.[218] The second-generation agents have very poor activity against *P. aeruginosa*, enterococci, and *L. monocytogenes*.

The third-generation cephalosporins have excellent in vitro activity against *H. influenzae*, gonococci, meningococci, and many gram-negative enteric bacilli.[219] Ceftazidime and cefoperazone, however, are the only ones with adequate anti-*Pseudomonas* activity. Susceptibility of gram-positive organisms to these agents is variable but generally is lower than that to either first- or second- generation antibiotics. *L. monocytogenes* and enterococci are uniformly resistant to these agents.

The fourth-generation cephalosporins demonstrate activity against gram-positive and gram-negative bacterial pathogens and circumvent the development of resistance to other broad-spectrum cephalosporins that occurs with *P. aeruginosa*. Evidence also indicates that isolates of ceftazidime- and cefotaxime-resistant *Enterobacter* species are susceptible to cefepime.[221] Resistant organisms include enterococci, *L. monocytogenes*, methicillin-resistant *S. aureus* and *S. epidermidis*, and anaerobes.

Resistance to the cephalosporins develops through several mechanisms. Cephalothin and cefazolin can be inactivated through enzymatic hydrolysis by β-lactamases.[222] Exposure of some gram-negative bacteria, such as *P. aeruginosa* or *E. cloacae*, to second- or third-generation agents can induce the production of chromosomally mediated potent β-lactamases by these bacteria, which can hydrolyze even the β-lactamase–stable cephalosporins.[222] Several plasmid-mediated β-lactamases have been shown to play a role in the resistance of certain gram-negative enteric bacilli to third-generation cephalosporins.[223] Other mechanisms of resistance include alterations in the permeability of the outer membranes of gram-negative bacteria to these drugs that limit their ability to reach the PBP target sites. Mutations leading to functional or quantitative changes in PBPs constitute an additional means by which bacteria can resist the antimicrobial action of these drugs.[222,223]

Pharmacokinetic Data

Cephalothin. The intramuscular administration of a 10-mg/kg dose of cephalothin to full-term newborns in the first 4 days of life results in a 1-hour mean serum concentration of 12.4 μg/mL.[167] A 20-mg/kg dose given to a similar group of neonates produced mean concentrations of 47, 39, 10, and 2 μg/mL at 0.5, 1, 4, and 8 hours, respectively, after the injection.[167] In another study, premature newborns given 12.5-mg/kg intramuscular doses achieved concentrations of 22, 12, 2.4, and 0.5 μg/mL at 0.5, 2, 6, and 12 hours, respectively, after the injection, and these values were noted to be slightly lower than those for full-term newborns receiving an identical dose.[224]

After the intravenous infusion of 20 mg/kg of cephalothin to six newborns 3 to 21 days of age, serum concentrations of 61, 35, 7, and 2 μg/mL were detected 0.25, 1, 4, and 8 hours, respectively, after the end of the infusion.[225] The mean half-life was about 1.5 hours. The continuous intravenous infusion of 40 mg/kg per day of cephalothin produces serum values of 24 to 35 μg/mL in premature infants and lower concentrations of 7 to 22 μg/mL in full-term neonates. Increasing the dose to 80 mg/kg per day resulted in serum concentrations of 50 to 120 µg/mL in the premature infants and 32 to 50 µg/mL for those born at term.[226]

Cephalothin does not penetrate into the CSF to any appreciable extent, even in the presence of meningeal inflammation. The drug is metabolized in the body to deacetylcephalothin, which is only 20% as active as cephalothin.[227] Both cephalothin and its metabolite are excreted in the urine, primarily by tubular secretion. Approximately 60% of the cephalothin dose can be recovered in the urine within 8 hours of drug administration.[225]

Cefazolin. The intramuscular administration of 20 and 25 mg/kg doses of cefazolin produces serum concentrations of 30 to 35 µg/mL and 55 to 65 µg/mL, respectively, 1 hour after the dose. The concentrations at 12 hours drop to 2 to 3 µg/mL and to 13 to 18 µg/mL, respectively.[228] Intravenous doses of 25 mg/kg administered to six premature infants 2 to 12 days of age resulted in mean serum concentrations of 92, 79, 48, and 12 µg/mL at 0.5, 1, 4, and 12 hours, respectively, after the end of the infusion.[225] The serum half-life of cefazolin decreases from 4.5 to 5 hours in the first week of life to approximately 3 hours by 3 to 4 weeks of age.

CSF penetration of cefazolin is poor. The drug is excreted in the urine in unchanged form.[227] About 45% of the dose can be recovered in the urine within 12 hours,[225] and 80% to 100% is recovered within 24 hours of administration.[227,228]

Cephalexin. A 15-mg/kg oral dose of cephalexin given to newborns on their first day of life produces a mean peak serum concentration of about 10 µg/mL 4 hours after drug ingestion.[229] Increasing the dose to 50 mg/kg provides a mean peak serum value of about 29 µg/mL (range, 23 to 44 µg/mL) 2 hours after the dose. From 18% to 66% (mean, 39%) of the total dose is excreted in the urine over a 24-hour period.[229]

Cefaclor. Data on the pharmacokinetics of cefaclor in newborns are limited. After a single oral dose of 7.5 mg/kg given to 10 full-term neonates, peak serum concentrations of from 0.7 to 19 µg/mL (mean, 7.7 µg/mL) were observed 1 hour after drug ingestion.[230] The mean serum concentrations at 6 hours dropped to 3.5 µg/mL. A study performed in infants and children revealed that peak serum values of 3 to 22 µg/mL (mean, 11 µg/mL) are observed 30 minutes after 15-mg/kg doses and that bioavailability is not affected by coadministration of drug and milk.[231]

Cefuroxime. After the administration of 10-mg/kg intramuscular doses, peak serum concentrations ranged between 15 and 25 µg/mL 30 minutes to 1 hour after the injection.[232] Serum concentration was inversely related to birth weight. Half-life times were from 3.6 to 5.6 hours. Repeated administration of the drug did not result in serum accumulation. About 70% of the daily cefuroxime dose could be recovered in the urine in a 24-hour period. Intramuscular doses of 25 mg/kg given to neonates weighing less than 2.5 kg during their first week of life produced mean serum concentrations of 49, 30, and 15 µg/mL 2, 4, and 8 hours after the injection, respectively.[233] For newborns weighing more than 2.5 kg, the corresponding values were lower (34, 21, and 9 µg/mL, respectively). Median serum concentrations of cefuroxime measured on the third or fourth day of therapy with 25-mg/kg intramuscular injections given every 12 hours to a group of premature and full-term infants were 45, 42, 26, and 11 µg/mL at 0.5, 1, 5, and 12 hours, respectively.[234] The half-life values were from 2 to 11 hours (mean, 6 hours).

CSF cefuroxime concentrations of 2.3 to 5.3 µg/mL were measured in three newborns with meningitis.[232] These values represented 12% to 25% of the corresponding serum concentrations. In three other neonates without meningeal inflammation, concentrations were lower and ranged from 0.4 to 1.5 µg/mL. In a brief publication, a CSF cefuroxime concentration of 20 µg/mL was found after the third dose of the drug in one patient, and concentrations of 50 and 47 µg/mL were detected 2.5 and 3 hours, respectively, after an intravenous dose in a second infant with hydrocephalus.[235]

Cefotaxime. Several investigators have evaluated the pharmacokinetic properties of cefotaxime in newborns.[236-241] A 25-mg/kg intravenous dose produces concentrations of 60 to 80 µg/mL immediately after the end of drug infusion, which decreases to 35 to 50 µg/mL 30 minutes later.[237,240] Serum cefotaxime concentrations are higher in premature newborns and in those younger than 1 week of age. The administration of a 50-mg/kg intravenous dose during the first week of life results in peak serum concentrations of 116 µg/mL (range, 46 to 186 µg/mL) in low-birth-weight infants, compared with 133 µg/mL (range, 76 to 208 µg/mL) in term neonates (Table 37-8).[238] Values decline thereafter to approximately 34 to 38 µg/mL 6 hours after the dose. The mean half-life is 4.6 hours for low-birth-weight neonates and 3.4 hours for larger newborns.[238] When cefotaxime was administered intramuscularly at a dose of 50 mg/kg, a mean peak value of 93 µg/mL was measured 30 minutes after the injection.[239] The apparent discrepancy between the peak concentrations obtained after intravenous and intramuscular identical doses of cefotaxime is related to differences in the antibiotic assays employed. The former study[238] used a bioassay technique that measures the total concentration of both cefotaxime and its biologically active metabolite desacetyl cefotaxime, whereas the latter study[239] used a high-pressure liquid chromatography method that provides separate measurements of both compounds.

Cefotaxime is rapidly metabolized in the body to desacetyl cefotaxime through the action of esterases found in the liver, erythrocytes, and other tissues.[242] This metabolite is biologically active, but its antibacterial activity is generally lower than that of cefotaxime. Synergistic interactions against many organisms can be demonstrated when these two compounds are combined in vitro.[243] Desacetyl cefotaxime accounts for 15% to 45% of the peak and for 45% to 70% of the trough concentrations of total cefotaxime.[238-240]

Both cefotaxime and its metabolite penetrate well into the CSF of infants with meningitis.[237,244,245] Concentrations of 7.1 to 30 µg/mL were detected 1 to 2 hours after a 50-mg/kg intravenous dose and represented 27% to 63%, respectively, of simultaneously measured serum values. CSF concentrations as high as 20 µg/mL in neonates with or without meningitis have been reported.[244] Some investigators[245,246] have noted that higher CSF concentrations and greater penetration are achieved with desacetyl cefotaxime than with cefotaxime. This observation suggests that the metabolite either is more capable of crossing the meninges than the parent compound or is cleared more slowly once it reaches the CSF.

About 80% of the cefotaxime dose is excreted in the urine. Only a third of the drug is eliminated in unchanged

Table 37–8 **Pharmacokinetics of Selected Third-Generation Cephalosporins in Neonates**

Antibiotic[a]	Birth Weight or Gestational Age/Age Group	Mean Peak Serum Concentration (μg/mL)	Mean Serum Half-life (hr)	Mean Plasma Clearance (mL/min/1.73 m²)
Cefotaxime	<2000 g/0-7 days	116	4.6	23
	2000 g/0-7 days	133	3.4	44
Ceftriaxone	<1500 g/1-4 days	145	7.7[b]	17
	<1500 g/6-8 days	136	8.4	14
	1500 g/2-4 days	158	7.4	17
	1500 g/5-45 days	173	5.2	20
Cefoperazone	<33 wk/1-2 days	159	8.9	—
	33-36 wk/1-2 days	110	7.6	—
	>36 wk/1-2 days	109	7.2	—
Ceftazidime	32 wk	111	6.7	52
	33-37 wk	118	4.9	66
	38 wk	102	4.2	74

[a]Dosage: 50 mg/kg given intravenously.
[b]Longer serum half-life values (mean, 19 hr) have been reported by other investigators.[14]

form.[242] Urine cefotaxime concentrations of 300 to 1575 μg/mL have been measured in randomly collected urine specimens from neonates receiving this drug.[238]

Ceftriaxone. The administration of a 50-mg/kg intravenous dose of ceftriaxone to newborns of various birth weights and postnatal ages resulted in mean peak serum concentrations of 136 to 173 μg/mL (see Table 37-8).[247] Concentrations 6 hours later were from 66 to 74 μg/mL. The mean plasma half-life values were longer in infants who weighed less than 1500 g. Repeated drug administration at 12-hour intervals resulted in drug accumulation in the serum.

Subsequent pharmacokinetic studies of ceftriaxone during the neonatal period have suggested that the drug's plasma half-life is actually longer than was initially estimated.[14,248-251] Elimination half-life ranged from 8 to 34 hours (mean, 19 hours) in 20 sick neonates who received single 50-mg/kg intravenous doses of ceftriaxone.[14] In another study, neonates who received single daily intravenous or intramuscular 50-mg/kg doses had mean peak serum concentrations after the first dose of about 149 μg/mL, and the mean elimination half-life was 15.5 hours.[248,249] After 3 to 4 days of treatment, however, both the mean peak serum concentration and elimination half-life decreased to 141 μg/mL and 9.4 hours, respectively. The observed decrease was believed to be a result of increasing postnatal age, which was associated with increased plasma clearance of ceftriaxone.

Intravenous administration of 50- to 144-mg/kg doses to neonates and infants with bacterial meningitis resulted in mean CSF concentrations of 18.3, 8.5, and 2.8 μg/mL at 4, 12, and 24 hours after drug injection, respectively.[250] Penetration of ceftriaxone into the CSF was higher for patients with bacterial meningitis (17%) than for infants with aseptic meningitis (4.1%). Smaller CSF penetration of ceftriaxone (2% to 7%) has been reported for older infants and children with bacterial meningitis.[252,253]

About 70% of a ceftriaxone dose is excreted in unchanged form in the urine.[14] The remainder is cleared from the body by hepatic mechanisms.

Cefoperazone. Serum cefoperazone concentrations ranged from 109 to 159 μg/mL at 30 minutes after an intravenous infusion of a 50-mg/kg dose given to 28 newborns of various gestational ages (see Table 37-8).[254] Values declined thereafter and were from 34 to 48 μ g/mL and from 13 to 17 μg/mL by 12 and 24 hours after the dose, respectively.[254,255] The serum half-life decreases with increasing birth weight, gestational age, or postnatal age.[163,241,254-256]

CSF concentrations of 2.8 to 9 μ g/mL were measured 1 to 4 hours after a 50-mg/kg intravenous dose given to three neonates with group B streptococcal meningitis. These values represented 4.2% to 9% of the simultaneously obtained serum concentration. A fourth infant, with *E. coli* meningitis, had a CSF concentration of 9.5 μg/mL after 18 hours of drug administration.[254] Concentrations of less than 1 to 7 μg/mL were detected at 2 to 4 hours in three neonates without meningitis. Other investigators have estimated the CSF penetration to be 3% to 5% in infants with meningitis.[163]

Hepatic clearance mechanisms play a major role in the elimination of cefoperazone from the body. At least 70% of the administered dose undergoes biliary excretion in adults.[63] Newborns excrete a greater proportion of the drug in their urine because of reduced hepatic function in this age group. About a third of a cefoperazone dose (range, 24% to 55%) can be recovered in the urine of neonates with a gestational age of 33 weeks or greater during their first 2 days of life. In contrast, more premature infants excrete about 55% (range, 28% to 93%) of the dose in their urine. By 5 to 7 days of age, the former group of infants will eliminate only a fourth of the dose (range, 7% to 35%) in the urine, whereas urinary recovery of the drug will not change appreciably in the latter group.[254]

Ceftazidime. Numerous reports on the pharmacokinetics of ceftazidime in neonates have been published in the last decade.[6,241,257-266] Peak serum concentrations of 35 to 269 μg/mL (mean, 77 μg/mL) have been observed after intravenous administration of 25- to 30-mg/kg doses of ceftazidime to newborns of various gestational ages during their first week of life.[259,262] Mean trough values measured 9 to 12 hours after the dose are from 15 to 19 μg/mL.[261-265] These concentrations are higher than those detected in older infants receiving identical ceftazidime dosages. When the dose is increased to 50 mg/kg intravenously, mean peak serum concentrations of 102 to 118 μg/mL are obtained (see Table 37-8).[6,260] Mean trough values 8 hours after the dose are from 29 to 41 μg/mL. The mean elimination half-life is inversely related to gestational age and varies from 4.2 to 6.7 hours. The peak serum concentrations after the intramuscular administration of 50 mg/kg of ceftazidime are lower (mean, 67 μg/mL) than those observed with intravenous infusion of the drug and are achieved 1 to 2 hours after the injection.[6,264] Neonatal exposure to indomethacin or to asphyxia decreases glomerular filtration rate and clearance of ceftazidime.

Ceftazidime penetrates well into the CSF, especially when meningitis is present.[263,267] Concentrations of 1.8 to 7.9 μg/mL, corresponding to 6% to 46% of a simultaneous serum concentration, are obtained 2 to 7 hours after a 50-mg/kg dose of ceftazidime is given to infants with bacterial meningitis.[267] The extent of penetration is lower in patients with aseptic meningitis and relatively poor in those with uninflamed meninges.[263,268]

Seventy percent to 90% of a ceftazidime dose is eliminated in unchanged form by the kidneys. Urinary ceftazidime concentrations of 192 to 6028 μg/mL have been measured in specimens collected during a 12-hour period after drug administration.[262]

Cefepime. Cefepime, a fourth-generation cephalosporin, offers an extended antibacterial spectrum of activity. In pediatric studies, cefepime exhibits a dose-dependent linear pharmacokinetic profile. After a 50-mg/kg intravenous dose, mean peak serum concentrations, half-lives, and volumes of distribution have ranged between 130 and 188 μg/mL, 1.26 and 1.93 hours, and 0.33 and 0.40 L/kg, respectively. Penetration into CSF appears to be good, with CSF concentrations averaging 3.3 to 5.7 μg/mL 0.5 and 8 hours after drug administration.[269]

Safety

In general, cephalosporins are well tolerated by neonates. Adverse reactions that have been observed, mostly in older patients, include hypersensitivity reactions, diarrhea, thrombophlebitis, pain on intramuscular injection, eosinophilia, leukopenia, granulocytopenia, and seizures related to the administration of massive doses of these drugs.[270,271] Falsely elevated serum creatinine concentrations have been observed in patients who received cefoxitin or cephalothin. Alterations of the bowel bacterial flora are most pronounced with the third-generation agents, especially ceftriaxone and cefoperazone, and can lead to intestinal colonization by resistant organisms such as *Candida*, *Pseudomonas*, *Enterobacter*, or *Enterococcus* species. Subsequent superinfections by these drug-resistant pathogens have been described in neonates.[270,272] Another potential adverse effect related to disruption of bacterial intestinal flora by potent cephalosporins is the induction of antibiotic-associated colitis, presumably caused by overgrowth of toxin-producing *Clostridium difficile* strains.

Bleeding disorders occurring with the use of cephalosporins have been well documented, mostly in adults. Immune-mediated platelet destruction with resultant thrombocytopenia is very rare but has been associated with the administration of cephalothin, cefazolin, cefamandole, cefaclor, and cefoxitin to older patients.[273]

A second rare mechanism involves the development of antibodies, usually immunoglobulin G (IgG), against certain clotting factors such as factor V or VIII. Hemostatic abnormalities associated with the use of cephalosporins can be mediated by several mechanisms. Platelet dysfunction can be observed after several days of therapy with any of the cephalosporins. These drugs may inhibit adenosine diphosphate (ADP)–induced platelet aggregation, with resultant prolongation of the bleeding time. The effect is slowly reversible after discontinuation of the drug.[217] A second mechanism is defective fibrinogen-to-fibrin conversion, which has been observed with drugs such as cefazolin and cefamandole. This phenomenon has been observed mostly in patients with renal failure, who have very high serum antibiotic concentrations.[217,273]

The third and most important mechanism is interference with the production of vitamin K–dependent clotting factors (II, VII, IX, and X), with resultant hypoprothrombinemia.[217] This effect—observed most commonly with moxalactam and cefamandole therapy and rarely with cefotaxime and ceftriaxone therapy—is believed to be related to, but not necessarily caused by, the presence of the *N*-methylthiotetrazole side chain in cephalosporins such as moxalactam, cefamandole, and cefoperazone. This side chain appears to be capable of interfering with hepatic vitamin K metabolism. In patients with inadequate dietary intake, inhibition of colonic bacteria such as *E. coli* or *Bacteroides*, which are capable of vitamin K production, may lead to hypoprothrombinemia secondary to vitamin K deficiency. This side effect usually is avoidable or reversible by the administration of supplemental vitamin K.

An immune-mediated severe hemolytic reaction to ceftriaxone has been described in children and adults. Because ceftriaxone has a high avidity for protein binding, a theoretical concern is that its use in the neonatal period can be associated with a significant displacement of bilirubin from albumin-binding sites, thereby inducing a hyperbilirubinemia. Ceftriaxone, when given to neonates in the first days of life, has been associated with an immediate and prolonged decrease in the reserve albumin concentration, which could potentially predispose a vulnerable infant to bilirubin encephalopathy.

Clinical Implications

The usefulness of first-generation cephalosporins for therapy for neonatal bacterial infections is limited. Their activity against gram-negative bacteria is limited and unpredictable, and their penetration into the CSF is relatively poor. These drugs are not indicated for initial therapy for suspected neonatal bacterial infections. If cephalothin is used in patients whose bacterial isolates are susceptible in vitro and in whom meningitis has been conclusively ruled out, the recommended dosage schedule for this agent is 20 mg/kg given intravenously every 12 hours for newborns weighing less than 2000 g in the first week of life and every 8 hours for older infants. For infants weighing more than 2000 g, the dose is given every 8 hours in the first week of life and every 6 hours thereafter. Cefazolin can be given in a dosage schedule similar to that for cephalothin, except that a 6-hour schedule is not recommended. These first-generation agents also can be used for therapy for methicillin-susceptible *S. aureus* infections that do not involve the central nervous system.

Although second-generation cephalosporins have been successfully used to treat neonatal infections caused by susceptible bacteria, these antibiotics are not recommended for routine use because of limited experience in newborns and because of their inferior activity to that of third-generation agents against gram-negative bacteria. Cefaclor has been successfully used, however, for oral therapy for acute suppurative otitis media in infants younger than 6 weeks of age because middle ear disease in the first weeks of life is caused by a broad array of pathogens, including *S. pneumoniae* and *H. influenzae* and occasionally coliform organisms and staphylococci.[174] The drug is well tolerated in a dosage of 15 mg/kg three times daily for 10 days. With the advent of multidrug-resistant pneumococci, other antibiotics, such as amoxicillin-clavulanate, are preferred for treatment of neonatal otitis media.

As a group, third-generation cephalosporins are the most useful agents for the treatment of suspected or proven bacterial infections in newborns. Their advantages include excellent in vitro activity against the major pathogens for newborns, including aminoglycoside-resistant gram-negative bacilli, adequate CSF penetration with resultant high bactericidal activity in CSF of infants with meningitis, and a proven record of safety and tolerability.[274] Indications for use of individual agents vary in accordance with their pharmacologic properties.

The clinical efficacy and safety of cefotaxime in the treatment of neonatal infections have been well documented in several studies.[237,272,275,276] Cefotaxime should not be used alone for initial therapy in suspected sepsis because of its poor activity against *L. monocytogenes* and enterococci. The addition of ampicillin provides antibacterial coverage against these organisms. One potential problem associated with the routine use of this drug is the possible emergence of cefotaxime-resistant gram-negative bacteria in the nursery.[272] Some nurseries, however, have not documented this problem even after 2 years of continuous use of this antibiotic.[275] Cefotaxime reaches CSF concentrations that are 50 to several hundred times greater than the MIC_{90} of susceptible gram-negative enteric bacilli or group B streptococci isolated from newborns with meningitis and has been shown to be effective for the treatment of neonatal meningitis caused by susceptible bacteria.[277] The dosage of cefotaxime in newborns is 50 mg/kg every 12 hours during the first week of life and every 8 hours thereafter. In full-term infants older than 3 weeks, a 6-hour regimen can be used for treatment of meningitis.

Although ceftriaxone has been used successfully for the treatment of severe neonatal infections,[248,250] the limited experience with this antibiotic in newborns and concerns about its in vitro displacing ability of albumin-binding sites for bilirubin have limited the use of this antibiotic in the neonatal period. The most attractive features of ceftriaxone are its long serum half-life, which allows for a single daily administration, and its excellent bactericidal activity in the CSF against susceptible bacteria. The ceftriaxone dosage is 50 mg/kg once daily for all newborns except those older than 1 week of age who weigh more than 2000 g, in whom the dose is increased to 75 mg/kg once daily. In a Mexican study,[278] ceftriaxone (in a dose of 100 mg/kg given once daily) was administered to 27 premature and term newborns with bacteriologically proven sepsis and was found to be effective and safe, even in jaundiced infants. More studies are needed, however, before ceftriaxone can be recommended for routine therapy of neonatal sepsis.

Ceftazidime has been used alone as initial therapy for newborns with suspected sepsis.[263,265,266,279] One study[280] compared ceftazidime used alone with a combination of carbenicillin and amikacin for the treatment of newborns with proven bacterial infections. It was found that all gram-negative enteric isolates were susceptible to ceftazidime, whereas 10% and 56% of these strains, respectively, were resistant to amikacin and carbenicillin. Accordingly, failure rates were lower for the ceftazidime treatment group. Increased colonization and superinfection by resistant organisms such as enterococci and *C. albicans* have been encountered in patients receiving ceftazidime.[266,280] We do not recommend using ceftazidime alone for initial therapy for suspected neonatal sepsis because this antibiotic is not active against enterococci and *L. monocytogenes* and because of the possibility for emergence of cephalosporin-resistant gram-negative organisms. In addition, several treatment failures have occurred when the offending organism proved to be a gram-positive bacterium.[263] We believe that the use of ceftazidime should be reserved for situations in which gram-negative bacteria, notably *P. aeruginosa*, have been isolated or are strongly suspected of being the causative microorganisms in neonates with sepsis, meningitis, or other invasive infections. The dosage schedule is 100 mg/kg per day in two (in infants born weighing less than 2000 g) or three (in those born at 2000 g or greater) divided doses during the first week of life and 150 mg/kg per day in three divided doses for older neonates.

Experience with cefoperazone in pediatric infections is too limited to allow us to recommend their use in this age group or to suggest an appropriate dosage schedule. Cefepime has been evaluated in young children with serious bacterial infections, including meningitis, and has been comparable in safety and efficacy to third-generation cephalosporins.[281] Although data on the use of cefepime in the neonatal period are lacking, because of its extended activity and stability against β-lactamase–producing bacteria, cefepime can be used for treatment of multidrug-resistant gram-negative infections.

AZTREONAM

Aztreonam is the first synthetic monocyclic β-lactam (monobactam) antibiotic approved for use in clinical medicine. Its aminoglycoside-like activity, good CSF penetration, and absence of nephrotoxic or ototoxic side effects make aztreonam potentially useful when combined with ampicillin for initial empirical therapy in newborns with suspected sepsis.

Antimicrobial Activity

Aztreonam has good activity against a broad spectrum of aerobic gram-negative bacteria, but its activity against gram-positive or anaerobic organisms is poor.[282] A majority of Enterobacteriaceae species—notably, *E. coli*, *K. pneumoniae*, and *Citrobacter* species—are inhibited by less than 1 μg/mL of aztreonam.[282,283] *Serratia* and *Enterobacter* are less susceptible (MIC_{90} of 1 to 4 μg/mL), whereas *H. influenzae* and *N. gonorrhoeae* are more susceptible (MIC_{90} of 0.2 μg/mL or less). *P. aeruginosa* requires MICs in the range of 8 to 12 μg/mL of aztreonam to be inhibited.[282-285]

Like other β-lactams, aztreonam exerts its antimicrobial activity by interfering with bacterial cell wall synthesis by binding to PBPs, especially PBP-3 of aerobic gram-negative bacteria. This drug is stable to hydrolysis by chromosome- or plasmid-mediated β-lactamases of Enterobacteriaceae organisms and does not induce chromosomal β-lactamase production.

Pharmacokinetic Data

Mean peak serum concentrations of 83 and 98 μg/mL, respectively, were found when a 30-mg/kg dose of aztreonam was given intravenously to 6 low-birth-weight infants younger than 1 week of age and to 11 larger and older neonates.[281] Serum half-life ranged from 2.4 to 5.7 hours and was longest for premature infants during the first week of life. By contrast, the mean half-life was 1.7 hours for patients older than 1 month but younger than 12 years of age.

In another study, a 30-mg/kg intravenous dose of aztreonam administered to 26 infants weighing less than 2000 g during their first week of life resulted in mean peak serum concentrations of 65 to 79 μg/mL after the first dose and 77 to 83 μg/mL after 3 to 6 days of therapy.[285] Trough values ranged between 8.2 and 70.7 μg/mL. The mean serum half-life values on the first day of treatment were approximately 7, 10, and 6.4 hours for infants weighing 500 to 1001 g, 1001 to 1500 g, and 1501 to 2000 g, respectively, but decreased from 5.5 to 7.6 hours 3 to 6 days later. The mean plasma clearance increased from a range of 0.61 to 0.84 mL/minute per kg after the initial dose to a range of 0.96 to 1.13 mL/minute per kg after multiple doses of aztreonam.

Aztreonam has good penetration into the CSF of newborns with bacterial meningitis.[286] A concentration of 13.3 μg/mL was obtained at 1.3 hours following administration of an aztreonam dose, 1 day after the diagnosis of bacterial meningitis was made, in a 7-day-old newborn. This value represented 18.8% of a simultaneously measured serum concentration. In a second neonate with meningitis, a CSF concentration of 2.4 μg/mL was detected 45 minutes after the dose (3.1% of a concomitant serum value), but this was measured after 14 days of treatment, when meningeal inflammation was substantially reduced.[284]

Aztreonam is excreted primarily in unchanged form in the urine. Urinary concentrations of 24 to 461 μg/mL (mean, 254 μg/mL) have been obtained in the first spontaneously voided urine specimens collected after the end of drug infusion.[285] About 80% of the total aztreonam dose can be recovered in the urine during a 24-hour period.[284]

Safety

Aztreonam is well tolerated with no apparent side effects when given intravenously to newborns. Adverse reactions described in adults include rashes, nausea, diarrhea, and eosinophilia, but their incidence is low.[282] The effects on bowel flora are limited to a reduction in coliforms without significant changes in anaerobic bacteria. Colonization by resistant bacteria resulting from aztreonam therapy does not appear to be as much of a problem as that encountered with the use of the third-generation cephalosporins. Because aztreonam contains 780 mg of arginine per gram of antibiotic, concern has been raised regarding possible adverse effects such as an arginine-induced hypoglycemia.[287] Arginine is rapidly metabolized by the action of urea and ornithine, the latter being transformed to glucose, which can provoke a significant rise in blood glucose concentration. As a result of this transient hyperglycemia, insulin concentrations immediately rise, with the subsequent induction of hypoglycemia. These fluctuations in blood glucose can be potentially important in premature infants exposed to a metabolic stress. A study addressing this safety issue indicated that aztreonam was well tolerated and safe in premature infants when a glucose solution was concomitantly infused (at a rate greater than 5 mg/kg per minute).[288]

Clinical Implications

Aztreonam is still considered an investigational drug for neonates and infants younger than 3 months of age. Data from a prospective, randomized study of 58 neonates with infections caused by gram-negative bacilli, including *P. aeruginosa*, suggest that the use of aztreonam in combination with ampicillin is as efficacious as the standard ampicillin and amikacin regimen.[287] Individual aztreonam doses of 30 mg/kg given two to four times daily can achieve median peak serum bactericidal titers of about 1:16 and can maintain trough serum concentrations that exceed the MIC_{90} for most gram-negative bacteria.

CARBAPENEMS

Imipenem is the first of a new class of β-lactam antibiotics, the carbapenems, to be used clinically. Its spectrum of activity includes most aerobic and anaerobic gram-positive and gram-negative bacteria. Cilastatin has no intrinsic antimicrobial activity but is a potent inhibitor of dehydropeptidase-I, the renal tubular brush-border enzyme that metabolizes imipenem. The co-administration of both drugs increases the urinary concentration of imipenem, prolongs the imipenem serum half-life, and appears to prevent the nephrotoxicity induced by high doses of imipenem. In clinical practice, these drugs are co-administered to patients in a 1:1 ratio.

Meropenem is a newer carbapenem with clinical indications similar to those for imipenem. It has been approved by the FDA for use in children older than 3 months of age on the basis of extensive pediatric investigations across a wide range of infections, including meningitis.[289] In a structural comparison of meropenem with imipenem, the carbapenem ring structure of meropenem includes an additional β-methyl group in the C-1 position, providing stability against the human renal tubular enzyme dehydropeptidase, which is active against imipenem. A second major difference between these two compounds is the long, substituted pyrrolidine side chain present in the C-2 position in meropenem, which allows greater activity against intracellular target sites in organisms such as *Pseudomonas aeruginosa*. Antimicrobial activity against the vast majority of bacterial agents is similar for both antibiotics.[290]

Antimicrobial Activity

Imipenem and meropenem have an exceptionally broad spectrum of activity. The only three bacterial species considered resistant to these drugs are *Stenotrophomonas maltophilia*, *Burkholderia cepacia*, and *Enterococcus faecium*, none of which are significant neonatal pathogens.[288] It has been estimated that approximately 98% of unselected bacterial pathogens isolated from humans are susceptible to carbapenems at concentrations of 8 μg/mL or less.[291,292]

Most streptococci and staphylococci are susceptible to imipenem and meropenem. The range of MIC_{90} values reported in different studies is 0.016 to 0.12 μg/mL for group B streptococci, 0.015 to 0.13 μg/mL for penicillin-susceptible *S. pneumoniae*, 0.12 to 1.0 μg/mL for penicillin-resistant *S. pneumoniae*, 0.01 to 4 μg/mL for *S. epidermidis*, 0.008 to 0.25 μg/mL for methicillin-sensitive *S. aureus*, 0.1 to 50 μg/mL for methicillin-resistant *S. aureus*, and 2 to 12.5 μg/mL for enterococci.[291] Imipenem and meropenem also are very active against *L. monocytogenes* and gram-positive anaerobes such as *Clostridium*, *Peptococcus*, and *Peptostreptococcus* species.

MIC_{90} values against gram-negative bacteria have varied, ranging from 0.125 to 2 μg/mL for *E. coli*, 0.04 to 1.6 μg/mL for *K. pneumoniae*, 0.5 to 32 μg/mL for *P. mirabilis*, 2 to 4 μg/mL for indole-positive *Proteus* species, 0.7 to 1 μg/mL for *Citrobacter* species, 0.5 to 8 μg/mL for *Enterobacter* species, and 0.6 to 4 μg/mL for *Serratia* species.[291] Against *P. aeruginosa*, including multidrug-resistant strains, values of 0.5 to 16 μg/mL have been reported by different investigators, with meropenem being consistently more active than imipenem. These inhibitory concentrations against *P. aeruginosa* are comparable to those of ceftazidime. Imipenem and meropenem also are extremely active against gram-negative anaerobes such as *Bacteroides* species.

Synergistic interactions between carbapenems and aminoglycosides can be demonstrated in vitro against *P. aeruginosa* and *S. aureus* isolates. Antagonistic interactions usually are observed when imipenem is combined with other β-lactams, probably as a result of chromosomal β-lactamase induction by imipenem.[291]

Carbapenem's unusually broad antibacterial spectrum is related to its ability to penetrate efficiently the outer membrane of gram-negative bacteria, its high binding affinity for PBP-2, and its resistance to hydrolysis by both plasmid- and chromosomally mediated β-lactamases.[292,293] Some β-lactamases produced by *S. maltophilia*, *Aeromonas hydrophila*, and *B. fragilis*, however, are capable of hydrolyzing imipenem and meropenem. Emergence of carbapenem-resistant strains during therapy with this drug is rare except in the case of *P. aeruginosa*, in which resistance occurs in as many as 17% of isolates.[288] The mechanism for this resistance is unclear.

Pharmacokinetic Data

For both imipenem and cilastatin, serum concentration is directly proportional to the administered dose.[294,295] Higher serum concentrations are achieved with cilastatin than with identical doses of imipenem. In one study, the intravenous administration during 30 to 60 minutes of 10-, 15-, and 20-mg/kg doses of both drugs to neonates results in mean peak imipenem concentrations of 11, 21, and 32 μg/mL, respectively, compared with mean cilastatin values of 28, 37, and 57 μg/mL, respectively.[294] In another study,[295] peak serum concentrations of 27 and 55 μg/mL for imipenem and 37 to 69 μg/mL for cilastatin were detected after intravenous doses of 15 and 25 mg/kg, respectively. After 3 to 4 days of treatment with 20-mg/kg intravenous doses of imipenem-cilastatin every 12 hours, peak serum concentrations were 35 and 86 μg/mL for imipenem and cilastatin, respectively.

The mean serum half-life of imipenem is about 2 hours, whereas that of cilastatin is 5.1 to 6.4 hours.[294] The half-life for both drugs is inversely related to birth weight and gestational age and is considerably longer than the 1-hour half-life reported for both drugs in older infants and in healthy adult volunteers.[294-297] The plasma clearance of cilastatin is only 20% to 30% of that of imipenem during the neonatal period.[294]

Although both imipenem and cilastatin penetrate well into the CSF in the presence of meningeal inflammation,[298,299] data derived from neonatal studies are scant. In one newborn who received a 15-mg/kg intravenous dose, concentrations of 1.1 and 0.8 μg/mL were noted for imipenem and cilastatin, respectively, at 1.5 hours after injection, and in a second neonate who received a 25-mg/kg dose, CSF values of 5.6 and 1.8 μg/mL were found for the same drugs.[295] It was not stated whether either of these infants had meningitis at the time of drug administration.

Imipenem normally is hydrolyzed by dehydropeptidase-I, a renal tubular enzyme, but cilastatin inhibits its enzymatic degradation. As a result, 70% to 80% of an imipenem dose can be recovered in the urine in unchanged form.[291] Urinary concentrations of imipenem were from 49 to 894 μg/mL in the first spontaneously voided urine specimen after completion of drug infusion in newborns.[294] Cilastatin is excreted primarily in unchanged form in the urine, but about 12% of the drug appears as the metabolite *N*-acetylcilastatin.[291] The urinary concentrations of cilastatin in newborns were from 72 to 2570 μg/mL in the first urine specimen collected after drug administration was completed.[294]

Limited pharmacokinetic data on use of meropenem in neonates are available for analysis. Studies were performed in 25 premature infants (mean gestational age, 32.5 weeks; mean weight, 1.87 kg) and 15 full-term infants (mean gestational age, 39 weeks; mean weight, 3.17 kg).[300] The administration of increasing dosages of meropenem from 10 to 40 mg/kg resulted in approximately proportionate increases in area under the curve (AUC) and maximal concentration (C_{max}) values in each of the two patient groups. Therefore, meropenem, like imipenem, exhibits linear kinetics. A 20-mg/kg dose of meropenem resulted in a C_{max} similar to that produced by 25 mg/kg of imipenem. Half-life, volume of distribution, and total drug clearance of meropenem were 2.92 hours, 0.46 L/kg, and 2.17 mL/minute per kg, respectively, for premature infants and 2.04 hours, 0.48 L/kg, and 3.15 mL/minute per kg for full-term neonates.[300] These values are similar to those observed for imipenem. In a recent study, a half-life of 3.4 hours was found after administration of a 15-mg/kg dose of meropenem to very low birth weight infants.[301]

Safety

Both imipenem-cilastatin and meropenem appear to be well tolerated when administered intravenously to newborns. In a review of studies conducted worldwide including thousands of patients, most of whom were adults, who received both drugs, it was observed that the nature and frequency of side effects were similar to those of other β-lactam antibiotics; these adverse effects consisted mainly of nausea, vomiting, diarrhea, thrombophlebitis, thrombocytosis, eosinophilia, and elevation of hepatic enzyme concentrations.[302] Colonization by *Candida* or imipenem-resistant bacteria occurred in about 16% of patients, and secondary superinfection was noted in about 6%.[302] Alterations of bowel flora in children given imipenem-cilastatin have been minimal in the few patients studied in detail.[288,299]

A worrisome report suggests that imipenem treatment in infants with bacterial meningitis was possibly associated with drug-related seizure activity.[304] Seizures developed in 7 of 21 infants (33%), aged 3 to 48 months, with bacterial meningitis following imipenem therapy. In this study,[304] CSF imipenem and cilastatin peak concentrations ranged from 1.4 to 10 µg/mL and 0.8 to 7.2 µg/mL, respectively. It is believed that interference of β-lactam antibiotics with the inhibitory effects of the neurotransmitter γ-aminobutyric acid results in epileptiform bursts.[305,306] Of interest is that imipenem has been shown to induce seizure activity in mice at serum concentrations two to three times lower than those of penicillin and cefotaxime.[307] Meropenem has less affinity than imipenem for the γ-aminobutyric acid receptor and consequently has demonstrated a lower propensity to cause seizures in animal models.[308] In infants and children with meningitis, treatment with meropenem was well tolerated, and no drug-related seizure activity was observed.[289]

Clinical Implications

At present, imipenem-cilastatin and meropenem are not recommended for routine use in the treatment of suspected or proven neonatal infections, and both agents should be reserved to treat infections caused by multidrug-resistant microorganisms. Data in 25 neonates with proven bacterial infections suggest that single-drug therapy with imipenem-cilastatin using a 25-mg/kg dose given two to four times daily is both efficacious and safe.[309] Because newborns have lower renal clearance capability and somewhat greater blood-brain permeability than those in older infants and children, high concentrations of imipenem-cilastatin could be achieved in the CSF of neonates, especially those with bacterial meningitis, potentially resulting in drug-related seizure activity.

Evidence from case reports suggests that meropenem also is safe and effective for treatment of neonatal infections. Because meropenem therapy has not been linked to the potential induction of seizures, we believe that if a carbapenem is selected for therapy in a newborn, meropenem should be the agent of choice. Further studies are required, however, before these drugs can be recommended for routine use in newborns and before an appropriate dosage schedule can be formulated.

VANCOMYCIN

With the advent of staphylococcal strains that were resistant to the antistaphylococcal penicillins and the cephalosporins, it became necessary in 1978 to return to the use of vancomycin. This glycopeptidic agent had been used in the mid 1950s for treatment of penicillin-resistant staphylococcal disease, but its use was curtailed with the introduction of methicillin in the early 1960s.

Antimicrobial Activity

Vancomycin is bactericidal against most aerobic and anaerobic gram-positive cocci and bacilli but is ineffective against most gram-negative bacteria. The drug interferes with the phospholipid cycle of cell wall synthesis, alters plasma membrane function, and inhibits RNA synthesis.[310] It is not metabolized by the body and is excreted unchanged in the urine.

Pharmacokinetic Data

Peak concentrations of 17 to 30 µg/mL are produced at the end of a 30-minute infusion of a 15-mg/kg dose given to neonates weighing less than 2000 g at birth and 0 to 7 days of age (Table 37-9). Slightly higher values are observed in larger-birth-weight infants. In infants up to 12 months of age, doses of 10 mg/kg produce similar peak serum concentrations. The half-life decreases from 6 to 7 hours in the first week of life to 4 hours in early infancy to 2 to 2.5 hours in children. A corresponding increase in the plasma clearance values is seen during these periods.

Serum half-life of vancomycin was approximately 10 hours in three premature infants aged 27 to 32 days and weighing less than 1000 g at birth.[311] The half-life was shorter (mean, 5.4 hours) in a second group of six infants aged 26 to 62 days

Table 37–9 Phamacokinetics of Vancomycin in Newborns

Age Group/Weight	Mean Peak Serum Concentration (µg/mL)	Mean Serum Half-life (hr)	Mean Plasma Clearance (mL/min/1.73^2)
0-7 days (15 mg/kg per dose)			
2000 g	25	5.9	27
>2000 g	30	6.7	30
1-12 mo (average, 3 mo) (10 mg/kg per dose)	26	4.1	50

and weighing between 1120 and 1780 g. In a second study[312] of premature infants aged 2 months or younger, a shorter mean half-life of 3 to 5 hours was found. A significant correlation was found between vancomycin serum half-life and clearance and a patient's body weight or postnatal age.[313,314] Neonates undergoing ECMO have a larger volume of distribution, lower clearance, and longer half-life of vancomycin than are observed in other infants.[315]

The CSF concentrations of vancomycin are 10% to 15% of the concomitant serum concentrations in infants with minimal meningeal inflammation, as seen in ventriculoperitoneal shunt infections.[41] The degree of penetration is similar to that for nafcillin. In premature infants, born at 26 to 31 weeks of gestational age, dosages of 20 mg/kg every 18 to 24 hours were associated with CSF vancomycin concentrations of 2.2 to 5.6 μg/mL, which were 26% to 68% of their corresponding serum values.[316]

In low-birth-weight premature infants, blood sampling to determine peak concentrations of vancomycin should be performed 15 to 30 minutes after a 60-minute infusion. This measurement usually is performed after the third dose of vancomycin is given. Once a therapeutic peak serum concentration is achieved, concentrations should be monitored weekly if there is a change in renal function or if potentially nephrotoxic drugs are concomitantly given. The peak serum concentration that is considered to be therapeutic is 20 to 30 μg/mL, although concentrations of 30 to 40 μg/mL are preferred in treating meningitis. The upper limit of activity that must not be exceeded is unknown, but it is prudent to maintain serum concentrations below 50 μg/mL. Trough (predose) vancomycin values should be approximately 10 μg/mL or lower.

Safety

Initial experience with vancomycin in the 1950s suggested a moderate incidence of ototoxicity and nephrotoxicity. These adverse effects were presumably related to the impurities found in early preparations of the drug.[317] Further studies have indicated that vancomycin is well tolerated and safe when administered intravenously, particularly in newborns and young infants.[41] If it is administered over a period of less than 30 minutes, some patients develop a histamine reaction characterized by an erythematous, pruritic rash on the upper part of the body and arms and on the neck and face. This reaction persists for several hours and tends to resolve with antihistamine medications. Use of a slower infusion rate (i.e., over 45 to 60 minutes) usually avoids this adverse event.

Clinical Implications

The primary indication for vancomycin therapy in newborns is for infections caused by methicillin-resistant staphylococci and by ampicillin-resistant enterococci. Vancomycin is effective for therapy of infections due to MRSA strains, an increasing problem in many American nurseries. We believe that vancomycin is the initial drug of choice for documented infections caused by *S. epidermidis*, because most strains are resistant to penicillin, methicillin, cephalosporins, and aminoglycosides. Vancomycin usually is not absorbed from the gastrointestinal tract, and oral preparations of this drug should be used only for the treatment of pseudomembranous colitis caused by *C. difficile*. Because of the increasing isolation of vancomycin-resistant enterococci, however, vancomycin is not recommended for treatment of antibiotic-associated colitis.[318] Metronidazole is the drug of choice for this condition.

The dosage schedule for vancomycin in neonates is 10 to 15 mg/kg every 12 hours (20 to 30 mg/kg per day) in the first week of life and every 8 hours (30 to 45 mg/kg per day) thereafter. For premature infants, a different dosage schedule has been proposed that takes into account body weight and postnatal age to modify both the total daily dose and the dosing intervals for vancomycin.[313] Although this dosage schedule resulted in more consistent peak and trough serum concentrations within the desired therapeutic range, approximately 25% of trough and 33% of peak concentrations fell outside the recommended therapeutic values.[314] Accordingly, monitoring serum vancomycin concentrations is essential in low-birth-weight premature infants and other infants with altered renal function who are given this drug. Beyond the newborn period, daily administration of 40 to 60 mg/kg (divided into three or four doses) is recommended. The larger dosage is used for treatment of central nervous system infection.

The dramatic increase in worldwide prevalence of vancomycin-resistant enterococci and the serious threat posed by the spread of vancomycin resistant to other gram-positive organisms such as staphylococci should discourage the use of this antibiotic for antimicrobial prophylaxis in infants of very low birth weight and for empirical therapy for neonatal sepsis of unknown etiology. Thus, each nursery needs to implement a policy to restrict the liberal use of vancomycin for these situations.

AMINOGLYCOSIDES

For more than 3 decades, the aminoglycosides have been relied on for therapy for neonatal sepsis and meningitis because of their broad-spectrum antibacterial activity against gram-negative bacilli. Many neonatal care units, however, have limited their use because of a low therapeutic index and the emergence of resistant strains among gram-negative enteric bacilli. For example, serum aminoglycoside concentrations are only one to five times the MBC_{90} for many gram-negative enteric organisms, and CSF concentrations are, at most, only one to two times greater. Streptomycin is no longer used, owing to the prevalence of resistant strains and to ototoxicity. Use of kanamycin also has been abandoned because of its lack of activity against *P. aeruginosa* and development of resistant coliform strains in many neonatal units during the 1970s.[319] Currently, gentamicin, tobramycin, and amikacin are the aminoglycosides of choice in most nurseries worldwide. Because amikacin is resistant to degradation by most of the plasmid-mediated bacterial enzymes that inactivate kanamycin, gentamicin, and tobramycin, some U.S. nurseries have held amikacin in reserve for treatment of nosocomially acquired infections due to multidrug-resistant gram-negative organisms. Gentamicin resistance occurs frequently enough in some European, Latin American, and U.S. centers to warrant use of amikacin as a first-line drug for therapy of life-threatening gram-negative infections, and its routine use has not resulted in emergence of resistant strains.

The history of aminoglycoside usage in the late 1950s and 1960s is an excellent example of the inherent problems of adapting dosages derived from studies in adults to newborns. Irreversible ototoxicity in neonates was caused by excessive doses of streptomycin or kanamycin. By contrast, the pharmacokinetics of gentamicin, tobramycin, amikacin, and netilmicin were carefully defined in the neonate before routine use of these drugs; appropriate studies thus provided a scientific basis for safe and effective dosage regimens. The risk of aminoglycoside toxicity has been proved to be minimal when these agents are administered to infants in the proper dosage and when serum concentrations are closely monitored and kept within the recommended therapeutic range.

During recent years, accumulating evidence generated in adults and children indicates that aminoglycoside administration using extended dosing intervals is at least as safe and effective as giving these drugs in two or three divided doses. The rationale for this concept is based on the concentration-dependent bacterial killing and prolonged postantibiotic effect (PAE) (discussed later under "Use of Extended Dosing Intervals") of the aminoglycosides.[320,321] Several studies suggest that single-daily-dose regimens also apply in the neonatal period.[322-339] The relevance of these results is discussed later.

Antimicrobial Activity

Aminoglycosides act on microbial ribosomes to irreversibly inhibit protein synthesis. Possible mechanisms of bacterial resistance to these drugs include alteration of the ribosomal binding site, changes in the cell surface proteins to prevent entrance of drug into the cell, and induction of aminoglycoside-inactivating enzymes. Antibiotic resistance in clinical situations is most often a result of extrachromosomally controlled (R-factor) enzymes.[340,341] Phosphorylation, adenylation, and acetylation are the three most common enzymatic mechanisms encountered.

In general, gentamicin, tobramycin, amikacin, and netilmicin have good antibacterial activity against most gram-negative strains isolated in many hospitals worldwide. On a weight-for-weight basis, tobramycin has the greatest anti-*Pseudomonas* activity,[342] and amikacin is the only drug of this class that reliably provides activity against *Serratia* species and nosocomially acquired resistant coliforms. Although staphylococci are the only gram-positive organisms susceptible in vitro to aminoglycosides, infections caused by these pathogens usually do not respond satisfactorily to aminoglycoside therapy alone. Synergistic bactericidal activity between aminoglycosides and the penicillins has been demonstrated in vitro and in animals against *S. aureus*,[36] group B streptococci,[32,33] *L. monocytogenes*,[34] and enterococci[37] in spite of low-level resistance of the microorganism to the aminoglycoside alone.

General Pharmacologic Considerations

Traditionally, the intramuscular route has been preferred for the administration of aminoglycosides to avoid potentially toxic peak serum concentrations. Pharmacokinetic studies of kanamycin,[343] gentamicin,[343,344] and netilmicin[40] have, however, demonstrated that the serum concentration-time curves after an intramuscular injection and after a 20-minute intravenous infusion are nearly superimposable. Although peak serum concentrations immediately after the intravenous dose may at times be considerably higher than the desired peak value, this elevation is transient and not clinically significant. The 6-hour serum concentrations, half-lives, and AUC values for these drugs also are equivalent.

These drugs cannot be administered orally for treatment of systemic infection because they are not absorbed from the intact gastrointestinal tract.[345] Absorption through an inflamed gastrointestinal mucosa has, however, been suggested by studies in infants with gastroenteritis or necrotizing enterocolitis who were given oral neomycin[346,347] and in infants with shigellosis[348] and necrotizing enterocolitis[349] who were given oral gentamicin. More than 10% of the administered dose of gentamicin was excreted in the urine during the acute phase of *Shigella* dysentery, compared with only 2% after the acute inflammation had subsided. Peak serum gentamicin values of more than 10 μg/mL were detected in four children with necrotizing enterocolitis who received 2.5 mg/kg every 4 hours by nasogastric tube in addition to 7.5 mg/kg per day by the intramuscular route.[349] The mean peak gentamicin concentration was slightly higher than that detected in a control group of infants receiving the drug only intramuscularly. The mean trough gentamicin values, however, were similar. By contrast, the prophylactic use of oral gentamicin in neonates at high risk for the development of necrotizing enterocolitis results in mean serum gentamicin concentrations below 2 μg/mL, with therapeutic serum values achieved only rarely.[350,351]

Pharmacokinetic studies have demonstrated a prolonged washout phase in neonates for netilmicin[40] and gentamicin.[42] Mean terminal half-life of 62 to 110 hours and detectable serum and urine drug activity for as long as 11 and 14 days, respectively, after discontinuation of these drugs have been recorded. Presumably, the prolonged washout reflects release of the drug that was bound to tissue, most likely renal, during the steady state. The practical significance of these findings is unknown. Persistent small serum concentrations could conceivably place the infant who requires a second course of therapy at increased risk for the development of aminoglycoside-associated toxicity. It also is possible that the subinhibitory concentrations of aminoglycosides persisting in the urine could exert selective pressure for the emergence of resistant gram-negative organisms in neonatal intensive care units.

Finally, several studies have indicated that aminoglycoside pharmacokinetics in the very low birth weight premature infant is highly variable because of renal immaturity and unpredictable extracellular fluid volumes.[40,352-358] Therefore, these infants may require frequent measurement of serum drug concentrations and individualization of dosage regimens. The pharmacokinetic properties of several aminoglycosides are compared in Table 37-10. Peak serum concentrations should be maintained at 5 to 8 μg/mL for gentamicin, tobramycin, and netilmicin and at 15 to 25 μg/mL for kanamycin and amikacin. Trough values should be kept below 2 μg/mL for the former drugs and below 10 μg/mL for the latter agents. To determine peak serum concentrations, a blood sample should be drawn 15 to 30 minutes after completion of the intravenous infusion (from another intravenous site) and 45 to 60 minutes after the intramuscular administration.

Table 37–10 Comparative Pharmacokinetics of Aminoglycosides in Neonates

Drug (Dose)	Birth Weight/ Age Group	Peak Serum Concentration (μg/mL)	Serum Half-life (hr)	Plasma Clearance (mL/min/1.73m²)
Amikacin (7.5 mg/kg)	2000 g			
	7 days	17	6.5	22
	>7 days	18.9	5.5	24.6
	>2000 g			
	7 days	18-20	5-6.5	27-30
	>7 days	17.4	4.9	36.4
Gentamicin (1.5 mg/kg)[a]	2000 g/7 days	1.5-2.2	10.5-14	12-16.5
	>2000 g/7 days	2.5-2.7	4.5-5.5	30-34
	All infants >7 days	3	3.2	56.2
Tobramycin (2 mg/kg)	2500 g			
	<7 days	4.9-5.6	8.6	11
	7 days	5-5.4	6-9.8	8.6-14.3
	>2500 g			
	<7 days	4.9	5.1	25.3
	7 days	4.5	4	35.9
Netilmicin (3 mg/kg)	2000 g			
	<7 days	6	4.7	30.8
	7 days	5.6	4.1	34.1
	>2000 g			
	<7 days	6.9	3.4	38.8

[a]Doses of 2.5 mg/kg are traditionally recommended.

Trough serum concentrations are measured just before the next dose of the aminoglycoside. In general, these peak and trough values should be determined every 72 to 92 hours while the patient is receiving aminoglycoside therapy.

Pharmacokinetic Data

Neomycin. Because neomycin is no longer used parenterally in newborns, only pharmacokinetic data pertaining to its oral administration are discussed here. Poor absorption after oral administration has made this antibiotic useful for the control of nursery outbreaks of diarrhea caused by enteropathogenic *E. coli.* Although efficacy of this regimen has been questioned, a more rapid bacteriologic and clinical response was demonstrated in infants who underwent treatment for 3 to 5 days compared with those given placebo.[359] Occasionally, neomycin may be absorbed from an inflamed gastrointestinal tract and cause ototoxicity or renal toxicity, particularly in patients with preexisting renal diseases.[346] Transient elevations of the blood urea nitrogen occurred in one infant who inadvertently received 10 times the recommended dosage for several days in our institution.

Gentamicin. Gentamicin has been the most methodically studied aminoglycosidic antibiotic in newborns.[42,344,353,360-373] Mean peak serum concentrations of 3.5 to 7 μg/mL occur within 1 hour after a 2.5-mg/kg dose. Mean serum values 12 hours after this dose were 0.5 to 1 μg/mL. Although most studies have not demonstrated drug accumulation during a 5- to 7-day course of therapy, one group of investigators showed accumulation in very low birth weight premature infants.[352] Serum aminoglycoside concentrations are reduced by 19% to 62% after a two-volume exchange transfusion; therefore, whenever possible, such procedures are best timed to precede the next scheduled dose of gentamicin.[374,375] On the other hand, gentamicin, and probably other aminoglycosides, exhibits a higher volume of distribution, a lower clearance, and a longer half-life in neonates undergoing ECMO for severe respiratory failure.[376]

Urinary concentrations of gentamicin vary, ranging from 2 to 135 μg/mL, and values correlate directly with postnatal age and rates of creatinine clearance but are independent of birth weight and dosage. Approximately 10% of the dose administered to infants 0 to 3 days old was excreted within 12 hours, compared with 40% excreted during the same period by infants 5 to 40 days of age.[360] After the final dose of gentamicin, urinary concentrations decrease in a biphasic pattern; the drug remains detectable in the urine for 11 days (Fig. 37-1).

The serum half-life of gentamicin correlates inversely with the rate of creatinine clearance, gestational age, birth weight, and postnatal age.[344,361,367,371-373] During the first week of life, half-life values as long as 14 hours have been observed in infants with birth weights of 800 to 1500 g, compared with 4.5 hours in term infants. After the first 2 weeks of life, the half-life of gentamicin is approximately 3 hours, regardless of body weight (see Table 37-10). Both perinatal asphyxia and patent ductus arteriosus are associated with prolonged serum gentamicin half-life values.[366,377] One group of investigators recommended dosing intervals of 18 hours for infants born at less than 35 weeks of gestation because of the occurrence of predose gentamicin serum concentrations greater than 2 μg/mL in 31 of 34 infants but in only 13 of 40 infants older than 34 weeks of gestational age.[353] Several other groups of investigators have made similar observations, and some have suggested prolonging the dosing interval to 24 hours in newborns weighing 1000 g or less or, alternatively, reducing individual gentamicin doses.[354,367,378-381]

CSF concentrations of gentamicin in infants with meningitis are from 0.3 to 3.7 μg/mL (mean, 1.6 μg/mL) 1 to 6 hours after a 2.5-mg/kg dose.[165] Peak values are observed 4

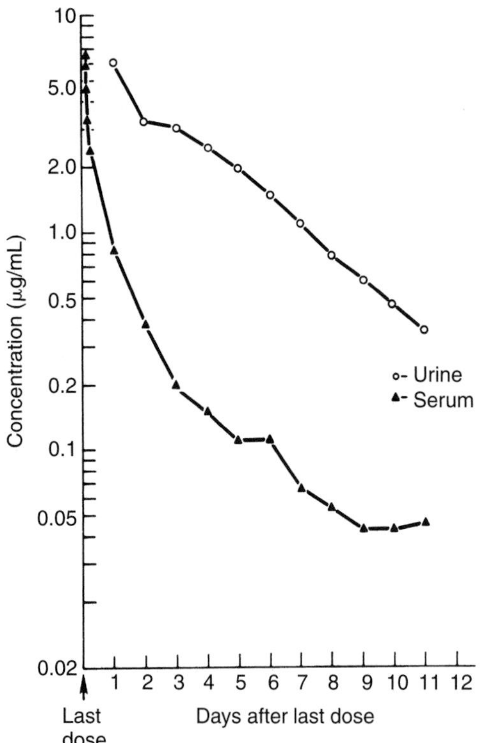

Figure 37–1 Washout concentrations after administration of 2.5 mg/kg of gentamicin in infants with birth weight of 1500 g.

to 6 hours after the dose and are directly correlated with the degree of meningeal inflammation and dosage.

During the 1970s, the Neonatal Meningitis Cooperative Study Group evaluated lumbar intrathecal and intraventricular gentamicin administration in comparative studies with systemic antibiotic therapy alone (see Table 37-10).[165] The mean drug concentration in lumbar CSF obtained 2 to 4 hours after a 1-mg dose into the lumbar space was 30 µg/mL. By 18 to 24 hours, the mean concentration decreased to 1.6 µg/mL, a value similar to that seen after systemic therapy alone. Daily instillation of 2.5 mg gentamicin directly into the ventricles resulted in a mean ventricular fluid concentration of 48 µg/mL (range, 10 to 130 µg/mL) 1 to 6 hours after the dose, compared with 1.1 µg/mL (range, 0.1 to 3 µg/mL) after systemic therapy only. An average concentration of 8.1 µg/mL (range, 1 to 24 µg/mL) was detected 16 to 24 hours after the intraventricular dose. Despite these higher CSF and intraventricular fluid concentrations, neither route of administration therapy was associated with a better outcome in infants with meningitis caused by gram-negative enteric organisms. Indeed, case-fatality rates were significantly greater in intraventricular gentamicin recipients. Subsequently, it was demonstrated that the rapid lysis of gram-negative bacteria associated with high ventricular fluid gentamicin concentrations resulted in the release of significantly larger amounts of endotoxin into the ventricular fluid and in greater meningeal inflammation secondary to cytokine overproduction.[382] Poorer outcome in these infants can be explained, at least in part, by these findings.

Tobramycin. Tobramycin offers two theoretical advantages over gentamicin for therapy for neonatal infections: increased in vitro activity against *P. aeruginosa* and decreased nephrotoxicity.[383] The lower incidence of nephrotoxicity for tobramycin has been documented in laboratory animals and human adults but not in human neonates.[384] Because of the relative resistance of neonates to aminoglycoside nephrotoxicity, the applicability of such studies in young infants is uncertain. In addition, the overall clinical experience with tobramycin in this age group is small compared with that with gentamicin.

After a 2-mg/kg dose of tobramycin, mean peak serum concentrations of 4 to 6 µg/mL are observed at 30 minutes to 1 hour.[385] When an identical dose is given to low-birth-weight neonates, mean peak serum values are 8 µg/mL. Predose concentrations are inversely related to birth weight and gestational age and have been reported to be consistently greater than 2 µg/mL in premature neonates who receive 2.5-mg/kg doses every 12 hours.[355-357] Evidence for drug accumulation is lacking, but minimal serum values are detectable for at least 3 days after therapy is discontinued. The serum tobramycin half-life is inversely related to birth weight, gestational age, chronologic age, and creatinine clearance.[355,385-387] In infants who weigh less than 1500 g at birth and are younger than 1 week of age, half-life values may be as long as 9 to 17 hours, compared with values of 3 to 4.5 hours for infants larger than 2500 g at birth and 1 to 4 weeks of age (see Table 37-10). Because of the markedly prolonged serum half-life values in infants born at 30 weeks of gestation or less, dosage intervals of 18 to 24 hours have been recommended.[355,356,388] Measurement of serum tobramycin concentrations and individualization of the dosage schedule provide the optimal therapy for these very low birth weight infants.

Concentrations of tobramycin in urine vary, ranging from 2 to 132 µg/mL after a 2-mg/kg dose.[385] Excretion in urine, expressed as percentage of the dose, correlates directly with postnatal age. Average excretion values are 15% to 25% of the administered dose during the first week of life and 25% to 40% in older infants.

Amikacin. Pharmacokinetic data on use of amikacin in neonates are limited because this agent has been reserved for therapy for infections caused by multidrug-resistant strains of Enterobacteriaceae species. In general, the pharmacokinetic properties of amikacin are similar to those of kanamycin, from which it is derived. Mean peak serum concentrations of 15 to 20 µg/mL occur 30 minutes to 1 hour after 7.5-mg/kg doses of amikacin (see Table 37-10). Mean trough concentrations of 3 to 6 µg/mL are detected 12 hours after administration.[389] One study reported subtherapeutic peak serum values when a 7.5-mg/kg dose was administered to infants weighing less than 1500 g at birth. Doses of 10 mg/kg at 12-hour intervals were required to achieve a mean peak value of 21.5 µg/mL and an average trough concentration of 3.3 µg/mL. By contrast, investigators in another study[390] noted that subtherapeutic serum concentrations of amikacin given to premature infants in 7.5-mg/kg intravenous doses every 12 hours were present in only 10% of those younger than 2 weeks of age. As many as 38% of infants 29 days of age or older had peak serum concentrations below 15 µg/mL, however.

Serum half-life of amikacin in newborns is inversely correlated with gestational and chronologic age.[389] Values of

7 to 8 hours occur in low-birth-weight infants 1 to 3 days of age, and of 4 to 5 hours in term infants who are older than 1 week of age. The serum half-life is prolonged in hypoxemic newborns.[25] Urinary amikacin concentrations range from 50 to 650 μg/mL, and the average urinary excretion of drug in 12 hours is 30% to 50% of the administered dose. Low concentrations of amikacin have been detected in serum and urine for as long as 10 to 14 days, respectively, after the final dose of a 5- to 7-day course of therapy.

Reports of CSF concentrations of amikacin are scarce.[389,391-393] In the presence of uninflamed meninges in 1-day-old infants, CSF values ranged from 0.2 to 2.7 μg/mL when measured at 1 to 4 hours after a single 10-mg/kg dose administered by slow intravenous infusion.[392] Simultaneous concentrations in serum ranged from 15 to 29 μg/mL. The highest concentration reported has been 9.2 μg/mL after a 7.5-mg/kg dose was administered intramuscularly to an infant with meningitis.[389] Amikacin concentration in ventricular fluid 12 hours after 1- or 2-mg intraventricular doses and 2 to 8 hours after intramuscular doses varies, ranging from 4.5 to 11.6 μg/mL (mean, 7.3 μg/mL).

The dosage schedule for neonates has not been established. The 10-mg/kg "loading" dose that initially was recommended by the manufacturer has been abandoned. Because of the similarity of amikacin and kanamycin pharmacokinetics, we recommend the following schedule: a 7.5-mg/kg dose to be used for infants weighing less than 2000 g and a 10-mg/kg dose for all other infants. A 12-hour dosing interval should be used for all neonates in the first week of life, and an 8-hour interval used thereafter. Dosage schedules may require individualization for infants weighing less than 1500 g at birth or born at fewer than 30 weeks of gestational age, or both, because of the highly variable serum concentrations that may occur.[393] The appropriate regimen in these infants is best determined by monitoring serum concentrations.

Netilmicin. Numerous reports on the pharmacokinetics of netilmicin in newborns have been published.[40,394-402] Mean peak serum concentrations vary, ranging from 5.6 to 7.7 μg/mL in infants tested 30 minutes to 1 hour after intramuscular administration of 2.5- to 3-mg/kg doses, compared with mean peak values of 7 to 9 μg/mL after intravenous injection of similar doses.[40,399-4017] Average serum values of 1 to 2.8 μg/mL are observed 12 hours after the dose.[40,400-402] The serum half-life of netilmicin is inversely related to birth weight, gestational age, and chronologic age. The mean half-life varies, ranging from 4.7 hours in infants weighing less than 2000 g at birth in the first week of life to 3.4 hours in infants larger than 2000 g at birth and older than 7 days of age (see Table 37-10). In another study,[401] half-life values of from 4.6 to 11.5 hours were found in 12 premature infants (mean weight, 1335 g) during their neonatal period. After the administration and rapid tissue distribution of the last dose of netilmicin, the drug is eliminated from the body in two phases. The first reflects the renal clearance of netilmicin by glomerular filtration, whereas the second is related to the slow release of the drug from tissues. The average terminal half-life for netilmicin is 52 to 62 hours and is within the range determined for gentamicin in adults.[40,400] Despite this long terminal half-life[400] and tissue accumulation,[403] however, dosing frequencies of two or three times per day appear to be appropriate for most neonates.

The steady-state serum concentration-time curves after 3-mg/kg doses of netilmicin and of gentamicin are similar, with mean peak serum concentrations of 6.9 and 6.3 μg/mL and serum half-lives of 4 and 3.5 hours, respectively. Greater variability in serum concentrations was observed with gentamicin than with netilmicin.

The average concentrations of netilmicin in urine were 46 and 29 μg/mL for the first and second 3-hour study periods, respectively, after a 3-mg/kg dose. Netilmicin remains detectable in the urine for 14 days after the last dose of antibiotic is given. Information about penetration of netilmicin into the CSF of newborns is lacking.

Drug accumulation has been documented in premature infants of very low birth weight.[40] After 4-mg/kg doses of netilmicin given every 12 hours for an average of 6.4 days, the mean trough value in these infants increased from 2.2 μg/mL on the second day of therapy to 5.6 μg/mL on the final day. This same group of infants did not show the expected decrease in serum creatinine, as observed in term infants during the first 2 weeks of life, and they all required mechanical ventilation. Thus, hypoxemia superimposed on immature renal function is a possible explanation of drug accumulation in this special group of newborns.

On the basis of these pharmacokinetic studies, a dose schedule of 2.5 mg/kg administered every 12 hours to infants younger than 1 week of age should produce serum values that are within the therapeutic range. An 8-hour schedule should be used in infants older than 1 week of age. Trough serum concentrations greater than the recommended upper limit of 3 μg/mL for netilmicin may be encountered in 25% to 50% of low-birth-weight (less than 2000 g) neonates,[399-402] thus necessitating monitoring of drug serum concentrations in these infants.

Safety

The major adverse effects of aminoglycosidic antibiotics are renal toxicity, ototoxicity, and, rarely, neuromuscular blockade. Hepatic and hematologic effects are not associated with this group of drugs. Acute toxic reactions and drug-induced fever are rare in the neonate.

It has been suggested that the immature kidney of the neonate may be protected from major toxic effects of aminoglycosides. Transient cylindruria and proteinuria may occur after prolonged administration of any of these drugs, but significant elevations in blood urea nitrogen and creatinine values are rarely observed and usually represent late manifestations of aminoglycoside nephrotoxicity.[404-410] One potential marker of early aminoglycoside nephrotoxicity that has been studied in newborns is β_2-microglobulin, a low-molecular-weight protein reabsorbed by proximal tubular cells after its glomerular filtration. Urinary excretion of this protein in infants undergoing aminoglycoside treatment has, however, been reported to increase (impaired tubular reabsorption),[409] decrease (decreased glomerular filtration rates),[408] or remain unchanged.[406] Other toxicity findings include increases in the urinary activity of enzymes of renal tubular origin such as *N*-acetyl-D-glucosaminidase and alanine aminopeptidase[407]; their increased urinary activity is believed to reflect damage to proximal renal tubular cells. The clinical significance of enzymuria and of the alleged tubular damage in terms of long-term renal damage after aminoglycoside therapy has not, however, been determined. Enzymuria is reversible on discontinuation of these drugs.

The criteria of maintaining peak and trough serum aminoglycoside concentrations within recommended values for older children and adults to prevent nephrotoxicity[411] have not been systematically assessed in newborns and should be considered as a guide rather than an established rule for formulating dosages of aminoglycosides in this age group. Factors that may be associated with increased risk for aminoglycoside nephrotoxicity include acidosis, hypovolemia, hypoalbuminemia, sodium depletion, duration of therapy, increased total aminoglycoside dose, and frequency of administration and co-administration of furosemide, vancomycin, or prostaglandin synthesis inhibitors such as indomethacin.[407,408,412,413]

Because renal excretion accounts for the elimination of approximately 80% of an aminoglycoside dose, the risk of toxicity is greatest when drug elimination is impaired by reduction in renal function for any reason. After several doses of an aminoglycoside, measurement of serum drug concentrations is helpful to determine the intervals of administration, to maintain therapeutic and potentially safe values.[414-416]

Neomycin,[346,417] streptomycin,[418] kanamycin,[319] and gentamicin[165] each have been implicated as a cause of sensorineural hearing loss in infants and children. Gentamicin and streptomycin also have been associated with vestibular impairment. It is, however, difficult to incriminate the aminoglycosides as the single causative agent of hearing loss in most studies because of the high-risk conditions present in affected patients. For instance, asphyxia, hyperbilirubinemia, and incubator exposure also have been independently associated with ototoxicity.[419] Although animal studies have demonstrated a synergistic effect of noise combined with neomycin or kanamycin on development of ototoxicity, such an effect has not been substantiated in the human neonate exposed to both incubator noise and kanamycin.[419,420] A familial predisposition toward cochlear damage has been observed after therapy with streptomycin[418,421] but not with the other aminoglycosides.

Kanamycin rarely causes toxicity when given in a daily dose of 15 mg/kg for 10 or 12 days.[422] Ototoxicity is related primarily to total dosages: High-frequency sensorineural hearing loss in infants with normal renal function is more likely if the total dosage exceeds 500 mg/kg. In a prospective evaluation of long-term toxicity of kanamycin and gentamicin,[422] 86 infants who received one of these drugs during the neonatal period underwent yearly audiometric, vestibular, and psychometric examinations for 4 years. Neither gentamicin nor kanamycin could be incriminated as the sole agent responsible for hearing impairment. In another study,[423] long-term follow-up evaluations of 98 infants who received short courses of streptomycin (mean dosage, 37 mg/kg per day) failed to ascribe any hearing loss to the use of this drug. Data from the first Neonatal Meningitis Cooperative Study[165] indicated that profound deafness that may have been drug related developed in only 1 (1.3%) of 79 infants who received a minimum of 5 to 7.5 mg/kg per day of gentamicin for 3 weeks or longer. It is difficult, however, to establish a direct causal relationship in many of the published studies in which patients received aminoglycosides because of their complicated clinical histories.

In recent years, the introduction of brain-stem response audiometry has facilitated assessment of hearing during the neonate's hospital stay.[424] A blinded, prospective controlled study of auditory brain-stem responses in neonates who received amikacin or netilmicin was performed at our institution.[425] A high incidence of transient abnormalities was demonstrated, but permanent bilateral sensorineural hearing loss related to aminoglycoside therapy was documented in 2% of the infants in both the amikacin and netilmicin treatment groups, as well as in the control group. In another study,[426] significant delayed auditory brain-stem responses were detected in 15 neonates who received a daily dose of 5 to 7.5 mg/kg for 6 to 10 days of either gentamicin or tobramycin, compared with findings in 14 controls. Long-term follow-up of these infants, however, was not performed to document whether the abnormalities were transient or permanent. Other investigators[427] failed to demonstrate permanent vestibular damage in 37 children aged 2 to 4 years who received netilmicin during the neonatal period.

Aminoglycoside-associated neuromuscular blockade has been reported only rarely.[428-430] The very young infant who has undergone surgery and whose fluid volume and renal function are highly variable is at greatest risk. The underlying mechanism appears to be inhibition of acetylcholine release at the neuromuscular junction by these drugs.[431] The aminoglycoside may act alone or synergistically with other neuromuscular blocking agents. Magnesium given to pregnant mothers with preeclampsia for prevention of seizures can be detected in the blood of their infant and potentiates the neuromuscular blocking effects of aminoglycosides. Diagnosis is made by nerve conduction studies, which reveal a progressive fatigue and post-tetanic facilitation characteristic of a nondepolarizing, curare-like neuromuscular block. Reversal is achieved by neostigmine or calcium or both. Potentiation of neuromuscular blockade can be observed in infant botulism when aminoglycosides are mistakenly administered to treat suspected sepsis.[432] Prophylactic treatment with calcium is not indicated because this cation may interfere with the antimicrobial activity of aminoglycosides against certain organisms.

Clinical Implications

At present, the aminoglycosides still remain the first-line drugs for the initial empirical therapy in newborns with suspected gram-negative sepsis. The choice of aminoglycoside to be routinely used is mainly dependent on the patterns of microbial resistance within a nursery. Although the risk of toxicity may be smaller with tobramycin, netilmicin, or amikacin than with gentamicin, the comparative incidence rates of toxicity in neonates related to these drugs are unknown. Accordingly, selection of one agent over another should be based on other factors. Amikacin remains the drug of choice for empirical treatment when multiply-resistant coliforms are frequently isolated within an individual neonatal unit and when the infant has received one or more courses of aminoglycoside therapy previously. The aminoglycosides usually are safe to use in the newborn when administered according to the recommended dosage schedules and monitored carefully, particularly in premature infants of very low birth weight who have hypoxemia, renal dysfunction, or anesthetic effects. In addition, some investigators recommend that gentamicin and other aminoglycosides should be given in dosages that are about 25% lower than usual and at longer dosing intervals in neonates undergoing ECMO.[376]

Systemic aminoglycoside therapy remains the initial empirical treatment of choice when meningitis is present, because in combination with ampicillin, this agent offers potential synergistic activity against group B streptococci and *L. monocytogenes*.[433] In addition, aminoglycosides have been demonstrated to be effective for therapy for meningitis caused by susceptible gram-negative bacteria. We believe, however, that if gram-negative bacilli are seen on CSF smears or later isolated as the causative agent of meningitis, third-generation cephalosporins (i.e., cefotaxime or ceftazidime for *P. aeruginosa* infections) should be used. Although some comparative clinical trials of aminoglycosides versus newer-generation cephalosporins in newborns with gram-negative meningitis have failed to show any significant benefit of one therapy over the other, these studies have not evaluated a substantial enough number of infants to accurately make definitive conclusions. The high CSF bactericidal activity achieved with the use of these cephalosporins, with resultant rapid CSF sterilization, and the avoidance of monitoring serum concentrations are some of the attractive properties offered by these agents. Combined therapy with one of the newer-generation cephalosporins and aminoglycosides usually is prescribed for the first 7 to 10 days of therapy to prevent emergence of bacterial resistance during the treatment of gram-negative meningitis, especially that caused by *Pseudomonas*, *Enterobacter*, and *Serratia* organisms, and for the possible synergistic activity on bacterial killing.

Oral administration of kanamycin or gentamicin has been recommended for the treatment[434] and prevention[435-437] of necrotizing enterocolitis in high-risk newborns. Suppression of the gastrointestinal microflora has been suggested to prevent necrosis and perforation of the ischemic bowel[434,438,439]; when this mode of therapy was evaluated in a few studies, conflicting results were observed.[349,438,440] In addition, serum gentamicin concentrations were substantially higher and potentially toxic in the infants who received systemic plus oral therapy.[349] Moreover, the potential increase in the prevalence of aminoglycoside-resistant gram-negative enteric flora among infants after the widespread use of these drugs is another factor contraindicating their utilization for this purpose.[438]

Use of Extended Dosing Intervals

Considerable evidence generated in adults with extended dosing intervals of aminoglycoside administration prompted studies in the pediatric and neonatal populations. In most studies published to date, therapeutic peak serum concentrations of several aminoglycosides are attained with the first dose, and trough concentrations usually are below the desired maximal limit. It must be emphasized, however, that despite theoretical advantage in terms of bacteriologic eradication and less renal and audiologic toxicity, no neonatal study has had the power to confirm statistically improved therapeutic efficacy or decreased adverse reactions in infants receiving the extended dosing regimens.

The rationale for use of extended dosing intervals is based on several pharmacodynamic principles of aminoglycosides that include concentration-dependent bacterial killing, postantibiotic effect, and decreased trough concentrations related to toxicity. For aminoglycosides, bacterial eradication is directly associated with the ratio of the peak concentration (C_{max}) to the minimum inhibitory concentration (MIC); C_{max}/MIC ratios greater than 10 have been linked to superior efficacy of aminoglycosides against gram-negative bacteria, including *Pseudomonas*, in adults.[332] Postantibiotic effect (PAE) is the persistent suppression of bacterial growth following limited exposure to an antibiotic. Aminoglycoside concentrations, therefore, can remain below the pathogen's MIC for a period without compromising efficacy. Although increased peak concentrations lengthen the duration of PAE, no research has been conducted in neonates to define the pharmacodynamics of this phenomenon in this age group.

Aminoglycosides are eliminated through glomerular filtration, but some drug is reabsorbed in the proximal tubule. These agents bind to anionic, brush-border, phospholipid membranes and are transported intracellularly by pinocytosis. As a result, disruption of normal phospholipids trafficking within the cell occurs, as well as release of cytotoxic material from lysosomes. The potential for nephrotoxocity varies among the aminoglycosides because of differences in the rate of uptake and amount of drug accumulation in the renal cortex. Toxicity is correlated with elevated drug trough concentrations and prolonged therapy, but not with high peak concentrations. Extended dosing intervals produce longer periods at low drug concentration, thereby lessening the potential for renal drug accumulation and toxicity. The precise mechanism involved in ototoxicity is unknown, although recent evidence suggests that point mutations in mitochondrial DNA are relevant to explain hearing loss in selected persons following aminoglycoside treatment.[336]

In 2001, a meta-analysis was performed to compare results of studies using either standard daily dosing (SDD)—administration every 8 to 12 hours—or once-daily dosing (ODD) in infants and children receiving gentamicin.[330] In most of the 13 studies suitable for analysis, steady-state peak serum gentamicin concentrations were significantly higher in the ODD groups of patients. Trough concentrations were greater than 2 μ g/mL in 5% to 55% of infants who received the SDD regimen, compared with 0% to 24% in the ODD recipients. The author concluded that efficacy and toxicity were similar for the two dosing regimens, but the ODD regimen was found to be cost-saving.

More recently, several randomized comparison trials have been conducted in neonates to evaluate peak and trough gentamicin concentrations after administration of SDD and ODD regimens (Table 37-11). Spanish investigators conducted a prospective, randomized clinical study in 65 neonates weighing more than 1200 g who received gentamicin either 2.5 mg/kg every 12 hours or 5 mg/kg once daily.[331] Peak concentrations were significantly higher in the once-daily regimen (mean, 9.5 μg/mL) than in the twice-daily group (mean, 6.4 μg/mL); trough concentrations were significantly lower in the former group (mean, 1.4 μg/mL) than in the latter (mean, 2.2 μg/mL). In accordance with concentration monitoring, dosages had to be adjusted in 12% of infants in the once-daily dosing group and in 25% of those in the conventional dosing group. In another study, 73 infants with birth weights of greater than 2500 g were studied after receiving either a single daily dose of 4 mg/kg or a twice-daily dose of 2.5 mg/kg.[328] Mean peak and trough gentamicin concen-

Table 37–11 **Serum Peak and Trough Concentrations of Gentamicin in Preterm and Term Neonates**[a]

		ODD Regimen				SDD Regimen			
Study	**GA (wk)**	***N***	**Daily Dose (mg/kg)**	**Peak (μg/mL)**	**Trough (μg/mL)**	***N***	**Daily Dose (mg/kg)**[b]	**Peak (μg/mL)**	**Trough (μg/mL)**
Skopnik et al.[336]	≥38	10	4	10.9	0.8 ± 0.2	10	4	7.4	1.0 ± 0.4
Hayani et al.[337]	≥34	11	5	10.7 ± 2.1	1.7 ± 0.4	15	5	6.6 ± 1.3	1.7 ± 0.5
De Alba-Romero[331]	≥38	13	5	9.2 ± 1.5	1.1 ± 0.4	15	5	5.7 ± 1.3	1.5 ± 0.6
De Alba-Romero[331]	29-37	20	5	9.7 ±1.8	1.6 ± 0.8	17	5	7.1 ± 1.7	2.7 ± 0.9
Skopnik and Herman[338]	32-38	28	4	7.9 ± 1.6	1.0 ± 0.5	27	5	6.1 ± 1.1	2.0 ± 1.1
Miron et al.[339]	32-37	17	5	9.9 ± 4.6	1.5 ± 0.5	18	5	5.9 ± 1.7	2.4 ± 0.9

[a]Neonates who received SDD or ODD dosing in several randomized comparison trials.
[b]Twice daily.
GA, gestational age; ODD, once-daily dosing; SDD, standard daily dosing.

trations were comparable for the two regimens. The same investigators then performed a study comparing dosing intervals of 24 hours and 48 hours in 58 infants of very low birth weight (600 to 1500 g).[329] Gentamicin was administered at either 4.5 to 5 mg/kg every 48 hours or 2.5 to 3 mg/kg every 24 hours. Results showed that the 48-hour dosing schedule used during the first week of life achieved therapeutic serum concentrations and higher peak-to-MIC ratios for infecting microorganisms. Nearly one third of these infants, however, had extremely low serum gentamicin concentrations before the next dose, suggesting that a 36-hour interval might be more appropriate for very low birth weight infants. Another study evaluated single doses of 5 mg/kg of tobramycin and gentamicin administered at extended intervals and found that only 1.3% of these infants had subtherapeutic concentrations, compared with 26.8% of those given the traditional 2.5-mg/kg doses.[332]

Based on these data and on proposed dosing guidelines to date, new therapeutic recommendations for aminoglycosides are presented in Table 37-12.

CHLORAMPHENICOL

Although chloramphenicol has been used in newborns for several decades in the past, no reliable guidelines or methods, other than monitoring serum concentrations, on which to base dosage have been identified. Dosage regimens that have been recommended are as likely to produce subtherapeutic or toxic serum values as they are to produce concentrations that are within the desired range of 15 to 25 μg/mL. In the 20th century, the major use of chloramphenicol was for therapy of meningitis, because appreciable concentrations of drug diffuse into brain and CSF. Currently, new β-lactam antibiotics with excellent CSF penetration and greater safety have replaced chloramphenicol in this age group. Because of economic constraints, however, chloramphenicol still is frequently used in the poorest areas of the world for treatment of bacterial infections in infants and children.

Antimicrobial Activity

Chloramphenicol competes with messenger RNA for binding sites on the ribosome, thus inhibiting bacterial ribosomal protein synthesis. The drug has broad antimicrobial activity, with bactericidal activity against *H. influenzae*, *S. pneumoniae*, and *N. meningitidis*, but mainly static activity against group B streptococci and most coliform bacilli, the principal pathogens of the neonatal period.[8] Microbial resistance usually results from plasmid or R-factor–mediated acetyltransferase that catalyzes the acetylation of chloramphenicol. In addition, some gram-negative bacteria probably are resistant to chloramphenicol by altering the permeability of outer membrane proteins to the drug.[441,442]

Pharmacokinetic Data

Chloramphenicol succinate is hydrolyzed in the body to the free, active drug, which in turn is conjugated in liver to the glucuronide salt. The free drug is excreted by glomerular filtration, whereas the conjugate is eliminated by tubular secretion. Unhydrolyzed chloramphenicol succinate also is excreted in the urine.[443] Approximately 65% of the total chloramphenicol in the serum of neonates is free drug, compared with 90% in adults. This is because excretion of the glucuronide by tubular mechanisms is considerably reduced in the first weeks of life.

A large variability in serum concentrations and serum half-lives after recommended doses of chloramphenicol has been noted by many investigators.[444-450] This variability is particularly evident in low-birth-weight infants, in whom peak serum concentrations ranged from 11 to 36 μ g/mL after intravenous doses of 14 to 25 mg/kg were administered during the first week of life. Half-life values were from 10 to greater than 48 hours in these patients; the extremely long half-lives were noted in infants who tended to accumulate drug in serum between doses.[445] An inverse correlation between chloramphenicol half-life and postnatal age and weight has been demonstrated.[444]

Studies performed in the early 1960s[451,452] reported serum concentrations of 14 to 27 μg/mL (mean, 20 μg/mL) at 3 hours, 7 to 21 μg/mL (mean, 14 μg/mL) at 9 hours, and 2 to 18 μg/mL (mean, 6 μg/mL) at 21 hours after 25-mg/kg intramuscular doses administered to premature infants. The half-life was estimated to be approximately 24 hours in the first week of life and 14 hours thereafter.

Oral administration of chloramphenicol in newborns results in significantly lower serum concentrations than

Table 37–12 Suggested Dosage Schedules for Antibiotics Used in Newborns

		Dosage (mg/kg) and Interval of Administration				
		Weight <1200 g[a]	*Weight 1200-2000 g*		*Weight >2000 g*	
Antibiotics	**Route**	*Age 0-4 Wk*	*Age 0-7 Days*	*Age >7 Days*	*Age 0-7 Days*	*Age >7 Days*
Amikacin[b] (SDD)	IV, IM	7.5 q12h	7.5 q12h	7.5 q8h	10 q12h	10 q8h
Amikacin[b] (ODD)	IV, IM	18 q48h	16 q36h	15 q24h	15 q24h	15 q24h
Ampicillin	IV, IM					
Meningitis		50 q12h	50 q12h	50 q8h	50 q8h	50 q6h
Other infections		25 q12h	25 q12h	25 q8h	25 q8h	25 q6h
Aztreonam	IV, IM	30 q12h	30 q12h	30 q8h	30 q8h	30 q6h
Cefazolin	IV, IM	20 q12h	20 q12h	20 q12h	20 q12h	20 q8h
Cefepime	IV, IM	50 q12h	50 q12h	50 q8h	50 q12h	50 q8h
Cefotaxime	IV, IM	50 q12h	50 q12h	50 q8h	50 q12h	50 q8h
Ceftazidime	IV, IM	50 q12h	50 q12h	50 q8h	50 q8h	50 q8h
Ceftriaxone	IV, IM	50 q24h	50 q24h	50 q24h	50 q24h	75 q24h
Cephalothin	IV	20 q12h	20 q12h	20 q8h	20 q8h	20 q6h
Chloramphenicol[b]	IV, PO	25 q24h	25 q24h	25 q24h	25 q24h	25 q12h
Ciprofloxacin[c]	IV	—	—	10-20 q24h	—	20-30 q12h
Clindamycin	IV, IM, PO	5 q12h	5 q12h	5 q8h	5 q8h	5 q6h
Erythromycin	PO	10 q12h	10 q12h	10 q8h	10 q12h	10 q8h
Gentamicin[b] (SDD)	IV, IM	2.5 q18h	2.5 q12h	2.5 q8h	2.5 q12h	2.5 q8h
Gentamicin[b] (ODD)	IV, IM	5 q48h	4 q36h	4 q24h	4 q24h	4 q24h
Imipenem	IV, IM	—	20 q12h	20 q12h	20 q12h	20 q8h
Linezolid	IV	—	10 q12h	10 q8h	10 q12h	10 q8h
Methicillin	IV, IM					
Meningitis		50 q12h	50 q12h	50 q8h	50 q8h	50 q6h
Other infections		25 q12h	25 q12h	25 q8h	25 q8h	25 q6h
Metronidazole[d]	IV, PO	7.5 q48h	7.5 q24h	7.5 q12h	7.5 q12h	15 q12h
Mezlocillin	IV, IM	75 q12h	75 q12h	75 q8h	75 q12h	75 q8h
Meropenem[e]	IV, IM	—	20 q12h	20 q12h	20 q12h	20 q8h
Nafcillin	IV	25 q12h	25 q12h	25 q8h	25 q8h	37.5 q6h
Netilmicin[b] (SDD)	IV, IM	2.5 q18h	2.5 q12h	2.5 q8h	2.5 q12h	2.5 q8h
Netilmicin (ODD)				Same as for gentamicin		
Oxacillin	IV, IM	25 q12h	25 q12h	25 q8h	25 q8h	37.5 q6h
Penicillin G (units)	IV					
Meningitis		50,000 q12h	50,000 q12h	50,000 q8h	50,000 q8h	50,000 q6h
Other infections		25,000 q12h	25,000 q12h	25,000 q8h	25,000 q8h	25,000 q6h
Penicillin benzathine (units)	IM	—	50,000 (one dose)	50,000 (one dose)	50,000 (one dose)	50,000 (one dose)
Penicillin procaine (units)	IM		50,000 q24h	50,000 q24h	50,000 q24h	50,000 q24h
Piperacillin	IV, IM	—	50-75 q12h	50-75 q8h	50-75 q8h	50-75 q6h
Piperacillin/tazobactam				Same as for piperacillin		
Rifampin	PO, IV	—	10 q24h	10 q24h	10 q24h	10 q24h
Ticarcillin	IV, IM	75 q12h	75 q12h	75 q8h	75 q8h	75 q6h
Ticarcillin-clavulanate				Same as for ticarcillin		
Tobramycin[b] (SDD)	IV, IM	2.5 q18h	2 q12h	2 q8h	2 q12h	2 q8h
Tobramycin (ODD)				Same as for gentamicin		
Vancomycin[b]	IV	15 q24h	10 q12h	10 q12h	10 q8h	10 q8h

[a]Data from Prober CG, Stevenson DK, Benitz WE. The use of antibiotics in neonates weighing less than 1200 grams. Pediatr Infect Dis J 9:111, 1990.
[b]Adjustments of further dosing intervals should be based on aminoglycoside half-lives calculated after serum peak and trough concentrations measurements.
[c]Doses suggested based on anecdotal clinical experience.
[d]A loading intravenous dose of 15 mg/kg followed 24 hours later (term infants) and 48 hours later (preterm infants) by 7.5 mg/kg every 12 hours has been suggested by other investigators.[500]
[e]Dosages of meropenem suggested are the same as those of imipenem.
IM, intramuscular; IV, intravenous; ODD, once-daily dosing; PO, oral; SDD, standard daily dosing.

those observed after intravenous infusion of similar doses.[5,450] Peak serum concentrations of 5.5 to 23.1 μg/mL were measured in seven premature and full-term neonates 4 hours or longer after 12.5-mg/kg doses of chloramphenicol palmitate were given every 6 hours for several days. These erratic serum concentrations and the prolonged periods required to achieve peak values were ascribed to the immaturity of the newborn gastrointestinal tract.

Chloramphenicol concentrations in CSF are 35% to 90% of those in serum regardless of the extent of meningeal inflammation.[8,444,453] This highly diffusible drug attains concentrations of 5 to greater than 20 μg/mL after 10- to 20-mg/kg doses. These concentrations usually are bacteriostatic against gram-negative enteric bacilli.

Safety

The toxicity of chloramphenicol has been the major limiting factor in its routine use in newborns. A cardiovascular collapse reaction (gray baby syndrome) has been well documented in some neonates who received chloramphenicol. The syndrome is characterized by vomiting, refusal to suck, respiratory distress, metabolic acidosis, abdominal distention, and passage of loose, green stools. The infant becomes gravely ill within 24 hours of the onset of symptoms. The reaction has been documented mostly in premature and full-term infants and occasionally in older infants and adults with very high (greater than 70 μg/mL) serum chloramphenicol concentrations.[454]

The pathogenesis of the gray baby syndrome in newborns is related to excessive dosages, immaturity of the hepatic glucuronyl transferase system, and diminished glomerular and tubular function. As a result of these factors, elevated serum concentrations of free and conjugated drug are observed. Available evidence indicates that toxicity results from the free drug, rather than from its metabolic products, and that multiple exchange transfusions or charcoal hemoperfusion may reverse the clinical syndrome by removing this free drug from the blood.[3,455,456] Chloramphenicol toxicity appears to be related to impaired mitochondrial protein synthesis, as well as to direct inhibition of myocardial contractile activity.[457]

The most common untoward reaction is anemia caused by suppression of the marrow red blood cell precursors. Thrombocytopenia and leukopenia occur less frequently. These three responses are dose related and usually are seen when serum concentrations consistently exceed 25 μg/mL.[458] The idiosyncratic reaction of bone marrow aplasia occurs in 1 in 30,000 to 1 in 50,000 patients receiving chloramphenicol treatment and is not dose related; whether this effect also occurs in newborns is not known. Other rare adverse effects of chloramphenicol therapy include sensorineural hearing loss, anaphylaxis, and retrobulbar neuritis, but these complications have been described only in older patients.[459,460]

Clinical Implications

No rationale exists for the routine use of chloramphenicol in newborns. The agent can be considered an alternative to aminoglycosides for therapy for neonatal meningitis caused by gram-negative enteric bacilli in areas of the developing world, where third-generation cephalosporins are prohibitively expensive. The main drawbacks of chloramphenicol therapy are the drug's toxicity and its bacteriostatic rather than bactericidal activity against gram-negative enteric pathogens.

Considerable interpatient variation is observed in serum chloramphenicol concentrations in the first weeks of life. Consequently, it is advisable to monitor serum values whenever possible to avoid either toxic or subtherapeutic concentrations. Peak serum concentrations should be within the range of 15 to 25 μg/mL to be safe and effective. If the infant also is receiving phenobarbital, dosages may need to be increased because of induction of hepatic microsomal enzyme activity and accelerated conjugation of chloramphenicol. Simultaneous administration of phenytoin, rifampin, or acetaminophen also can affect chloramphenicol serum concentrations.[443]

SULFONAMIDES

The sulfonamides are structural analogues of *p*-aminobenzoic acid and differ from each other according to various substitutions on the sulfonamide group of the benzene ring. These drugs were commonly used in the prophylaxis and treatment of neonatal bacterial infections, but their usefulness in neonates has become greatly limited because of the availability of superior antimicrobial agents, the emergence of resistant bacteria, and the association of kernicterus with sulfonamide administration in some premature infants. At present, no indications exist for their use in premature infants.

Antimicrobial Activity

The sulfonamides are bacteriostatic agents with a wide range of antimicrobial activity against both gram-positive and gram-negative organisms.[461] In addition, some sulfonamides are active against *Toxoplasma gondii*, the causative organism of congenital toxoplasmosis. Antimicrobial action is based on competition with the structurally similar *p*-aminobenzoic acid for the same enzyme, thus preventing normal utilization of *p*-aminobenzoic acid by microbes. Synthesis of folic acid is inhibited at the dihydropteroic acid step.

Acquired bacterial resistance to sulfonamides plays a significant role in therapeutic failures with this class of drugs. The origin of sulfonamide resistance is disputed, but the evidence indicates that mutations occurring randomly give rise to resistant variants, which are then favored by selection in the presence of the drug.[462] Resistance is more likely to develop if treatment is prolonged. Transfer of multiple drug resistance (R-factor–mediated) among strains of coliform bacilli has been responsible for the emergence of sulfonamide-resistant *Shigella* strains worldwide.

Pharmacokinetic Data

A number of sulfonamide derivatives are currently available. As a general rule, the short-acting sulfonamides, such as sulfadiazine, trisulfapyrimidine, and sulfisoxazole, are most commonly used for acute urinary tract infections. The first two agents also are employed, in combination with pyrimethamine, for the treatment of congenital toxoplasmosis (see Chapter 31). Sulfadiazine is absorbed slowly from the gastrointestinal tract, reaching peak values 8 hours after administration. Sulfisoxazole is absorbed more rapidly, attaining earlier peak values that are 50% higher than those of sulfadiazine.[463] The serum concentration-time curves for sulfisoxazole and triple sulfonamides are similar.

The pharmacokinetic properties for several of the sulfonamide derivatives have been studied in newborns. Sulfadiazine administered subcutaneously in an initial dose of 100 mg/kg, followed in 48 hours by 50 mg/kg given every

24 hours for 3 days, produces mean peak serum values of 170 µg/mL and trough values of 90 to 110 µg/mL. Although these concentrations are within the desired therapeutic range (50 to 150 µg/mL), the individual values vary considerably.[464] Serum concentrations of 110 to 180 µg/mL were found after an initial 100-mg/kg sulfadiazine dose given subcutaneously, followed in 48 hours by a 50-mg/kg dose of triple sulfonamide given orally every 12 hours. Sulfisoxazole administered subcutaneously in a dose of 75 mg/kg every 12 hours results in serum concentrations of 60 to 120 µg/mL.[15]

The sulfonamides are excreted primarily by renal mechanisms.[465] Glomerular filtration is the major mechanism of excretion for both the free and the acetylated forms. Tubular reabsorption occurs to various degrees for most sulfonamides. Diminished renal function in neonates explains in part why they are able to maintain serum concentrations in the therapeutic range for longer periods than those observed in children or adults.

Safety

As a general rule, the sulfonamides are well tolerated by newborns; crystalluria and hematuria are uncommon in neonates. Use of these drugs in newborns has been greatly reduced by the demonstration that sulfonamides displace bilirubin from albumin-binding sites, with the development of kernicterus observed in some premature infants who received prophylactic treatment.[15] Sulfonamides also may cause hemolysis in neonates who have erythrocyte G6PD deficiency.[9] Cutaneous hypersensitivity reactions are rare in young infants.

Clinical Implications

Because of the availability of safer and more effective antimicrobial agents, the sulfonamides should not be used during the neonatal period for therapy for bacterial infections. Their principal usefulness is in dual-agent treatment (pyrimethamine and sulfadiazine) of congenital toxoplasmosis. Neonates with acute urinary tract infections should receive parenteral treatment with ampicillin and an aminoglycoside until bloodstream invasion has been ruled out by blood culture. Bacteremia is found in approximately 20% of young infants with urinary tract infections.

TRIMETHOPRIM-SULFAMETHOXAZOLE

The combination agent trimethoprim-sulfamethoxazole provides sequential and synergistic inhibition of microbial folic acid synthesis.[466] Trimethoprim-sulfamethoxazole currently is used in the United States for therapy for urinary tract infections, otitis media and sinusitis, shigellosis, and *Pneumocystis jiroveci* infections. It is not approved for use in newborns because of insufficient pharmacokinetic, safety, and efficacy data in this age group. Nevertheless, this compound has been successfully used alone or in combination with an aminoglycoside for the treatment of neonatal meningitis caused by gram-negative enteric bacilli, particularly *Salmonella* organisms.[467-469] Treatment failures also have been observed.[468]

Mean peak and trough serum concentrations of trimethoprim were 3.4 µg/mL and 0.8 µg/mL, respectively, after administration of single daily intravenous doses of 5.25 mg/kg of trimethoprim and 26.25 mg/kg of sulfamethoxazole to 12 neonates.[470] On the third day of therapy, peak serum values were from 3 to 6.4 µg/mL. The mean serum half-life was 19 hours after one dose and about 25 hours after multiple doses. The peak serum concentrations for sulfamethoxazole ranged from 72 to 135 µg/mL after one dose but increased to values of 120 to 200 µg/mL after multiple doses. The mean trough serum concentration for sulfamethoxazole 24 hours after the first dose was 20 µg/mL. The mean serum half-life for sulfamethoxazole was 16.5 hours after one dose and 23.3 hours after multiple doses. The half-life values for both drugs are longer in neonates than in older children and adults.

The paucity of information on trimethoprim-sulfamethoxazole in newborns precludes its use in this age group except under extraordinary circumstances, and even then it should be used with great caution. Physicians should be aware of the adverse effects of this compound before its use in neonates and in pregnant or nursing women; high concentrations are found in amniotic fluid, fetal serum, and breast milk after administration to the mother.[471]

The drug combination is available only as a preparation with a fixed trimethoprim-to-sulfamethoxazole ratio of 1:5. One suggested dosage schedule is to give an initial loading dose consisting of 2 mg/kg of trimethoprim and 10 mg/kg of sulfamethoxazole,[450] followed by maintenance doses of 0.6 mg/kg of trimethoprim and 3 mg/kg of sulfamethoxazole given every 12 hours.

MACROLIDES

The macrolide antimicrobial agents that have been used in neonates include erythromycin and spiramycin. Although the lincomycins (e.g., clindamycin) are not macrolides, they are included in this section because of similarities in their antibacterial activities and clinical uses. These drugs were used to treat neonatal staphylococcal infections in the 1950s, when penicillin-resistant staphylococcal strains were prevalent and the penicillinase-resistant penicillins were not yet available. Erythromycin is useful in the young infant for therapy for infections caused by *Chlamydia trachomatis* and *Bordetella pertussis*; spiramycin, for treatment of toxoplasmosis; and clindamycin, for its activity against anaerobes, including *B. fragilis*. The role of the newer macrolides, such as clarithromycin and roxithromycin, and of the azalide azithromycin for treatment of neonatal infections has not yet been defined.

Erythromycin. Erythromycin is primarily a bacteriostatic agent that acts by interfering with protein synthesis through binding to ribosomes of susceptible bacteria and inhibiting the translocation steps.[472] Resistance to the macrolide antibiotics is due to demethylation of adenine in 23S ribosomal RNA, which results in reduced affinity between the antibiotic and the ribosome. Erythromycin is active against most gram-positive bacteria, including many penicillin-resistant strains of staphylococci. In some areas, penicillin-resistant pneumococci also are resistant to the macrolides; the higher the MIC of penicillin for pneumococci, the greater the MIC will be for the macrolides. In addition, most strains of *Neisseria*

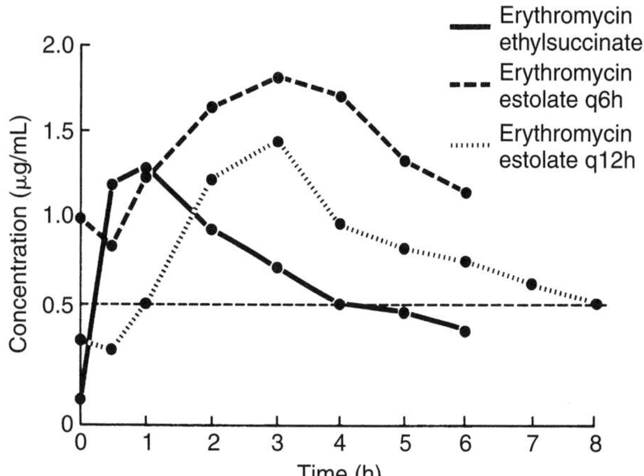

Figure 37–2 Serum concentration-time curves after administration of erythromicin ethylsuccinate and estolate to infants younger than 4 months of age.

species, *T. pallidum*, *Mycoplasma pneumoniae*, *Ureaplasma urealyticum*, *B. pertussis*, and *C. trachomatis* are susceptible to this agent. Erythromycin is rarely administered parenterally, owing to the associated tissue damage.

Oral administration of erythromycin estolate to premature infants produced serum concentrations of 1 to 2 µg/mL 3 to 4 hours after a 10-mg/kg dose, and values of 0.5 µg/mL or greater were detected for a minimum of 6 hours.[473] Serum concentration of erythromycin was independent of birth weight, postnatal age, and gastric acidity. Accumulation of drug in serum did not result from repeated doses every 6 hours for 8 days. Similar pharmacokinetic results have been observed in full-term newborns.[474]

In a comparative pharmacokinetic study of erythromycin estolate and erythromycin ethylsuccinate, 28 infants younger than 4 months of age, 12 of whom were neonates, were evaluated.[475] The mean peak serum concentrations in infants taking the estolate were slightly greater than those taking the ethylsuccinate: 1.8 µg/mL as opposed to 1.3 µg/mL. During the steady state, the peak serum concentration was achieved in 3.2 hours for the estolate preparation, compared with 0.8 hour for the ethylsuccinate form of erythromycin (Fig. 37-2). Following analysis by the two-compartment model of pharmacokinetics, a similar difference was found in the mean absorption and elimination half-life values: absorption half-life values of 0.72 and 0.3 hour and elimination half-life values of 6.58 and 2.2 hours for the estolate and the ethylsuccinate, respectively. Thus, 12-hour dosing intervals are appropriate for the estolate.

Erythromycin is excreted in the urine and bile, but only a fraction of the total dose can be accounted for by these two excretory routes. Although erythromycin is uniformly distributed throughout most of the body, concentrations in CSF are low, even in the presence of meningeal inflammation. Drug concentrations in tears 1 hour after administration were greater than the highest serum concentration measured in 70% of infants, ranging from 2 to 5.4 µg/mL for the ethylsuccinate and from 0.6 to 5 µg/mL for the estolate.[475]

Erythromycin estolate is well tolerated by newborns. Cholestatic jaundice resulting from hypersensitivity to this preparation occurs primarily in teenagers and adults and has not been reported in infants younger than 6 weeks of age.[476] Loose stools as a side effect of erythromycin therapy were noted in about 2.5% of greater than 10,000 children evaluated in one study, including 69 neonates.[477] The concomitant administration of erythromycin and theophylline can lead to reduced clearance of the latter drug, with resultant increased risk of theophylline toxicity.[478] Serum theophylline concentrations should therefore be monitored in these patients, and the dosage reduced if necessary.

A recent report of a cluster of cases of pyloric stenosis among infants given erythromycin for prophylaxis after exposure to pertussis has raised concern about usage of erythromycin in neonates and young infants.[479]

Clindamycin. Clindamycin differs from its parent compound lincomycin in that it is more completely absorbed from the gut, has fewer adverse effects, and has greater antibacterial activity in vitro.[480] Indeed, lincomycin is only of historical interest in the United States. The drug is primarily a bacteriostatic agent that acts by inhibiting protein synthesis through binding to bacterial ribosomes.

Clindamycin is active against gram-positive cocci such as *S. aureus*, *S. pneumoniae* (including many multidrug-resistant strains), and *S. pyogenes*. Aerobic gram-negative bacteria usually are not susceptible to this antibiotic. This drug's most notable feature is its activity against anaerobic bacteria, especially members of the *Bacteroides* group.[480] Resistance to clindamycin appears to be related to alterations of its target site and not to reduced uptake or to breakdown of the drug by resistant bacteria.[481]

Clindamycin administered intravenously in a dosage schedule of 20 mg/kg per day administered in three or four divided doses to premature and term infants results in mean peak serum concentrations of 11 µg/mL, whereas trough values are from 2.8 to 5.5 µg/mL.[482] The serum elimination half-life is inversely related to gestational age and birth weight. Premature neonates demonstrate a mean serum half-life of 8.7 hours, compared with 3.6 hours for term newborns.[482] In another study,[483] a serum elimination half-life of 3.5 to 9.8 hours (mean, 6.3 hours) was noted in12 neonates who received intravenous doses of 3.2 to 11 mg/kg every 6 hours.

Clindamycin penetration into the CSF was once considered poor, but data in experimental meningitis models indicate excellent CSF concentrations after parenteral administration. The drug is eliminated primarily by the liver, with only about 10% excreted in unchanged form in the urine. Adverse effects of clindamycin include diarrhea, rashes, elevated levels of hepatic enzymes, granulocytopenia, thrombocytopenia, and Stevens-Johnson syndrome. The most serious and potentially lethal complication is pseudomembranous colitis, but this condition is rare in newborns and young infants, even though as many as 50% to 60% of such infants have gastrointestinal colonization with *C. difficile*. This adverse effect also is observed with the use of β-lactam and other antimicrobials.

Clinical Implications

With the availability of newer penicillin analogues and vancomycin for treatment of staphylococcal infections, macrolides are no longer recommended for therapy for these infections in neonates. Erythromycin is currently the drug of choice for chlamydial conjunctivitis and pneumonitis, as well as for pertussis. The dosage is 10 mg/kg given orally every 12 hours during the first week of life and every 8 hours thereafter. Peak serum concentrations of erythromycin are at least two to three times greater than the MICs reported for *C. trachomatis* (0.5 μg/mL)[484] and several times greater than the MICs for *B. pertussis* (0.04 to 0.78 μg/mL).[472] A possible advantage of the estolate is the persistence for 8 hours or longer of serum drug concentrations that are greater than the MICs for these two organisms.

Recent clinical information suggests that clindamycin can be effectively used to treat methicillin-resistant (MRSA) but clindamycin-susceptible *S. aureus* infections.[485,486] This type of MRSA strain is more frequently acquired in the community than in the hospital. Caution is advised, however, because resistance to clindamycin can be induced after selective antimicrobial pressure. Inducible resistance can be identified in the laboratory by a technique named the D-test. Use of clindamycin in selected MRSA-infected cases can obviate the need for vancomycin therapy. Use of clindamycin in newborns also should be restricted, because as many as 50% of asymptomatic neonates are colonized with *C. difficile*, the presumed etiologic agent of pseudomembranous colitis.[487] Evidence for an association of *C. difficile* colonization with colitis in newborns is lacking, however. For treatment of the rare *B. fragilis* infections in newborns, especially those involving the central nervous system, we prefer the use of either metronidazole or clindamycin, although the latter has been said to have poor penetration into the CSF,[488] albeit good penetration into brain tissue.[489] Accordingly, clindamycin has been used successfully for therapy for *Toxoplasma* encephalitis in adults with human immunodeficiency virus infections.[490] Whether congenital toxoplasmosis can be effectively treated with this agent remains undefined. Spiramycin is a macrolide antibiotic commonly used for the treatment of toxoplasmosis worldwide; its use and pharmacokinetic properties are discussed in Chapter 31.

OTHER ANTIBACTERIAL AGENTS

Mupirocin. Mupirocin, a topical antibiotic formerly called "pseudomonic acid" (derived from fermentation of *Pseudomonas fluorescens*), has been used extensively in recent years to eliminate MRSA carriage and prevent outbreaks of neonatal MRSA infection in several nurseries.[491,492] Mupirocin interferes with bacterial RNA and protein synthesis by binding to bacterial isoleucyl-transfer RNA synthetase and preventing incorporation of isoleucine into protein chains.[493] Trace amounts absorbed into the systemic circulation are rapidly hydrolyzed, and the inactive metabolite has a plasma half-life of less than 30 minutes.[494] This antibiotic has little cross-resistance with other antimicrobial agents, probably because of its unique mechanism of action. Mupirocin inhibits the growth of staphylococci and streptococci (except enterococci) in low concentrations and is bactericidal in high concentrations readily achieved by topical application.[495] The drug is not active against members of Enterobacteriaceae, *P. aeruginosa*, or fungi. Emergence of resistant staphylococci has been reported with long-term topical therapy.[496] It also is possible that prolonged use of the drug may result in overgrowth of nonsusceptible organisms, such as fungi. Only local adverse effects such as itching or rash have been reported with mupirocin. Because mupirocin is prepared with a polyethylene glycol vehicle, the possibility of absorption and serious renal toxicity should be kept in mind if the compound is applied to extensive open wounds or skin lesions.[497]

Rifampin. Because of the lack of relevant pharmacokinetic studies in newborns, many potentially useful antimicrobial agents are not discussed in this chapter. For example, rifampin usually is used in other parts of the world for the treatment of congenital tuberculosis. It is possible that with the increasing number of tuberculosis cases seen worldwide among patients with acquired immunodeficiency syndrome, this antibiotic will be used more frequently in the future in newborns of tuberculosis-affected mothers. Rifampin also might provide a synergistic effect when given with antistaphylococcal drugs for therapy for of systemic staphylococcal infections in selected neonates.[498] Italian investigators found mean peak serum rifampin concentrations of 5.8 μg/mL 12 hours after a 10-mg/kg dose was given orally to 18 male term newborns during their first 3 days of life.[499] By contrast, peak values were detected earlier (at 4 hours) and were substantially lower in older infants and children given a similar dosage of rifampin. These investigators proposed not to exceed a dosage of 10 mg/kg per day when rifampin is given orally to term newborn infants.

Metronidazole. Metronidazole is another example of a potentially useful antimicrobial agent that has been poorly evaluated in the neonatal period. This drug has been occasionally used for the treatment of anaerobic infections in newborns, such as necrotizing enterocolitis and *B. fragilis* meningitis. In one study, metronidazole pharmacokinetics was examined in 11 infants ranging in gestational age from 28 to 40 weeks and in chronologic age from 0 to 3 days.[500] Elimination half-life was inversely related to gestational age, ranging from 22.5 to 109 hours. To achieve drug concentrations above the MIC required for treatment of anaerobic infections (i.e., 4 to 8 μg/mL), the investigators proposed an initial single intravenous dose of 15 mg/kg, followed 24 hours later in term infants and 48 hours later in preterm neonates by a dose of 7.5 mg/kg every 12 hours.

Ciprofloxacin. Several case reports have described the use of the quinolone ciprofloxacin in nosocomial outbreaks of neonatal infections.[501-507] No pharmacokinetic studies on ciprofloxacin, however, have been conducted in newborns; therefore, neonatal dosages used have been extrapolated from data generated in older children and adults. Although quinolones have not been approved by the FDA for use in children younger than 18 years of age, clinical pharmacologic data are available for many children but very few infants. The potential neonatal indications for parenteral administration of ciprofloxacin include treatment of multidrug-resistant gram-negative infections (species of *Klebsiella*, *Enterobacter*, *Acinetobacter*, *Salmonella*, *Stenotrophomonas*, or *Pseudomonas* resistant to all other antibiotics) and meningitis caused by *Flavobacterium meningosepticum*. In these selected clinical situations, doses of 10 to 40 mg/kg per day, divided every 12 hours, have been used.

Ampicillin-Sulbactam. Combination of a β-lactamase inhibitor (i.e., sulbactam or clavulanic acid) with ampicillin or amoxicillin offers the theoretical advantage of expanding the activity of the aminopenicillin against β-lactamase–producing bacteria, such as methicillin-susceptible *S. aureus*, coliform bacilli, and some anaerobes. Experience with the use of these agents in the neonatal period is very limited. Pharmacokinetic data are available only for ampicillin-sulbactam. In the reported study, this latter combination was administered to 16 newborns, 15 preterm infants, and 1 term infant.[508] A dose of 50 mg/kg of each drug every 12 hours was associated with mean plasma concentrations of 110 μg/mL for sulbactam and 87 μg/mL for ampicillin at 3 hours after dosing. Mean elimination half-lives were 7.9 hours for sulbactam and 9.4 hours for ampicillin. Evidence for significant accumulation of either drug was lacking, and both were well tolerated. Carefully designed pharmacokinetic studies are needed before this attractive combination can be used in the neonatal period.

Teicoplanin. Teicoplanin is a glycopeptide antibiotic that is almost identical to vancomycin with regard to antibacterial spectrum of activity, and it is used frequently in Europe for similar indications. It may have some advantages over vancomycin in terms of tolerability, with a lower propensity to cause nephrotoxicity and histaminic-type reactions, and in terms of ease of administration and monitoring requirements. Despite these potential advantages, pharmacokinetic data adequate to formulate dosage regimens in neonates are lacking. In a French study, four neonates received a single dose of 6 mg/kg, and the mean peak serum teicoplanin concentration was 19.6 μg/mL, with a mean half-life of 30 hours.[509] In several noncomparative trials, the clinical and bacteriologic response rates ranged between 80% and 100% in 173 infected neonates given teicoplanin 8 to 10 mg/kg intravenously once daily, after a loading dose of 10 to 20 mg/kg.[510]

Linezolid. Linezolid is an oxazolidinone antibiotic recently approved for treatment of infections caused by glycopeptide-resistant strains *of Enterococcus faecium*, *S. aureus*, and *S. pneumoniae*. Because these microorganisms are becoming more common in critically ill neonates, linezolid is likely to play an increasingly important therapeutic role in the neonatal period. Data generated in term neonates and young infants given linezolid suggest that intravenous or oral doses of 10 mg/kg every 8 hours are safe and effective, and that linezolid in this regimen is comparable to vancomycin for therapy of resistant gram-positive infections.[511-513] The suggested dose for preterm infants and for those younger than 7 days of chronologic age is 10 mg/kg every 12 hours. The potential emergence and spread of oxazolidinone resistance will depend on the prudence with which linezolid is used in neonatal intensive care units.

DOSAGE SCHEDULES FOR ANTIBIOTICS COMMONLY USED IN NEONATES

Dosage schedules for antibacterial agents commonly prescribed for the treatment of neonatal bacterial infections are presented in Table 37-12. For some drugs, the appropriate dosage schedules following initial doses should be based on measurement of serum concentrations.

REFERENCES

1. Roberts RJ. Drug Therapy in Infants: Pharmacologic Principles and Clinical Experience. Philadelphia, WB Saunders, 1984, p 3.
2. Huang NN, High RH. Comparision of serum levels following the administration of oral and parenteral preparations of penicillin to infants and children of various age groups. J Pediatr 42:657, 1953.
3. Weiss CF, Glazko AJ, Weston JK. Chloramphenicol in the newborn infant: a physiologic explanation of its toxicity when given in doses. N Engl J Med 262:787, 1960.
4. Kauffman RE, Thirumoorthi MC, Buckley JA, et al. Relative bioavailability of intravenous chloramphenicol succinate and oral chloramphenicol palmitate in infants and children. J Pediatr 99:963, 1981.
5. Shankaran S, Kauffman RE. Use of chloramphenicol palmitate in neonates. J Pediatr 105:113, 1984.
6. Boccazzi A, Rizzo M, Caccamo ML, et al. Comparison of the concentrations of ceftazidime in the serum of newborn infants after intravenous and intramuscular administration. Antimicrob Agents Chemother 24:955, 1983.
7. Mulhall A. Antibiotic treatment of neonates—does route of administration matter? Dev Pharmacol Ther 8:1, 1985.
8. Ristuccia AM. Chloramphenicol: clinical pharmacology in pediatrics. Ther Drug Monit 7:159, 1985.
9. Beutler E. Drug-induced hemolytic anemia. Pharmacol Rev 21:73, 1969.
10. Friis-Hansen B. Body water compartments in children: changes during growth and related changes in body composition. Pediatrics 28:169, 1961.
11. McCracken GH Jr. Clinical pharmacology of gentamicin in infants 2 to 24 months of age. Am J Dis Child 124:884, 1972.
12. Wise R. The clinical relevances of protein binding and tissue concentrations in antimicrobial therapy. Clin Pharmacol 11:463, 1977.
13. Kurz H, Mauser-Ganshorn A, Stickel HH. Differences in the binding of drugs to plasma proteins from newborn and adult man: I. Eur J Clin Pharmacol 11:463, 1977.
14. Schaad UB, Hayton WL, Stoeckel K. Single-dose certriaxone kinetics in the newborn. Clin Pharmacol Ther 37:522, 1985.
15. Silverman WA, Andersen DH, Blanc WA, et al. A difference in mortality rate and incidence of kernicterus among premature infants allotted to two prophylactic antibacterial regimens. Pediatrics 18:614, 1956.
16. Brodersen R, Friis-Hansen B, Stern L. Drug-induced displacement of bilirubin from albumin in the newborn. Dev Pharmacol Ther 6:217, 1983.
17. Cashore WJ, Oh W, Brodersen R. Bilirubin-displacing effect of furosemide and sulfisoxazole: an in vitro and in vivo study in neonatal serum. Dev Pharmacol Ther 6:230, 1983.
18. Stutman HR, Parker KM, Marks MI. Potential of moxalactam and other new antimicrobial agents for bilirubin-albumin displacement in neonates. Pediatrics 75:294, 1985.
19. Gulian JM, Gonard V, Dalmasso C, et al. Bilirubin displacement by ceftriaxone in neonates: evaluation by determination of "free" bilirubin and erythrocyte-bound bilirubin. J Antimicrob Chemother 19:823, 1987.
20. Brodersen R, Ebbesen F. Bilirubin-displacing effect of ampicillin, indomethacin, chlorpromazine, gentamicin, and parabens in vitro and in newborn infants. J Pharm Sci 72:248, 1983.
21. Sakamoto H, Murakawa T, Hirose T, et al. Effect of ceftizoxime, a new cephalosporin antibiotic, on binding of bilirubin to human serum albumin. Chemotherapy 29:244, 1983.
22. Walker PC. Neonatal bilirubin toxicity: a review of kernicterus and the implications of drug-induced bilirubin displacement. Clin Pharmacokinet 13:26, 1987.
23. Robertson A, Fink S, Karp W. Effect of cephalosporins on bilirubin-albumin binding. J Pediatr 112:291, 1988.
24. Guignard JP. Drugs and the neonatal kidney. Dev Pharmacol Ther 4(Suppl 1):19, 1982.
25. Myers MG, Roberts RJ, Mirhij NJ. Effects of gestational age, birth weight, and hypoxemia on pharmacokinetics of amikacin in serum in infants. Antimicrob Agents Chemother 11:1027, 1977.
26. Handwerger S, Tomasz A. Antibiotic tolerance among clinical isolates of bacteria. Rev Infect Dis 7:368, 1985.
27. Moellering RC Jr. Rationale for use of antimicrobial combinations. Am J Med 75(Suppl 2A):4, 1983.
28. Giamarellou H. Aminoglycosides plus beta-lactams against gram negative organisms: evaluation of in vitro synergy and chemical interactions. Am J Med 80(Suppl. 6B):126, 1982.

29. Holm SE. Interactions between β-lactam and other antibiotics. Rev Infect Dis 8:S305, 1986.
30. Schauf V, Deveikis A, Riff L, et al. Antibiotic-killing kinetics of group B streptococci. J Pediatr 89:194, 1976.
31. Cooper MD, Keeney RE, Lyons SF, et al. Synergistic effects of ampicillin-aminoglycoside combinations on group B streptococci. Antimicrob Agents Chemother 15:484, 1979.
32. Scheld WM, Alliegro GM, Field MR, et al. Synergy between ampicillin and gentamicin in experimental meningitis due to group B streptococci. J Infect Dis 146:100, 1982.
33. Calderwood SA, Wennersten CBG, Moellering RC, et al. Resistance to six aminoglycosidic aminocyclitol antibiotics among enterococci: prevalence, evolution, and relationship to synergism with penicillin. Antimicrob Agents Chemother 12:401, 1977.
34. Scheld WM, Fletcher DD, Fink FN, et al. Response to therapy in an experimental rabbit model of meningitis due to *Listeria monocytogenes*. J Infect Dis 140:287, 1979.
35. Kaplan JM, McCracken GH Jr, Horton LJ, et al. Pharmacologic studies in neonates given large dosages of ampicillin. J Pediatr 84:571, 1974.
36. Watanakunakorn C, Glotzbecker C. Enhancement of the effects of antistaphylococcal antibiotics by aminoglycosides. Antimicrob Agents Chemother 6:802, 1974.
37. McCracken GH Jr, Nelson JD, Thomas ML. Discrepancy between carbenicillin and ampicillin activities against enterococci and *Listeria*. Antimicrob Agents Chemother 3:343, 1973.
38. Levy RH, Bauer LA. Basic pharmacokinetics. Ther Drug Monit 8:47, 1986.
39. Schentag JJ, Jusko WJ, Plaut ME, et al. Tissue persistence of gentamicin in man. JAMA 238:327, 1977.
40. Siegel JD, McCracken GH Jr, Nelson JD. Pharmacokinetic properties of netilmicin in newborn infants. Antimicrob Agents Chemother 15: 246, 1979.
41. Schaad UB, McCracken GH Jr, Nelson JD. Clinical pharmacology and efficacy of vancomycin in pediatric patients. J Pediatr 96:119, 1980.
42. Haughey DB, Hilligoss DM, Grassi A, et al. Two-compartment gentamicin pharmacokinetics in premature neonates: a comparison to adults with decreased glomerular filtration rates. J Pediatr 96:325, 1980.
43. Schaad UB, McCracken GH Jr, Loock CA, et al. Pharmacokinetics and bacteriological efficacy of moxalactam (LY127935), netilmicin, and ampicillin in experimental gram-negative enteric bacillary meningitis. Antimicrob Agents Chemother 17:406, 1980.
44. Odio C, Thomas ML, McCracken GH Jr. Pharmacokinetics and bacteriological efficacy of mezlocillin in experimental *Escherichia coli* and *Listeria monocytogenes* meningitis. Antimicrob Agents Chemother 25:427, 1984.
45. McCracken GH Jr, Sakata Y, Olsen KD. Aztreonam therapy in experimental meningitis due to *Haemophilus influenzae* type b and *Escherichia coli* K1. Antimicrob Agents Chemother 27:655, 1985.
46. Jacobs MR, Myers C. Diagnostic microbiology and therapeutic drug monitoring in pediatric infectious diseases. Pediatr Clin North Am 30:135, 1983.
47. Doering PL, Stewart RB. The extent and character of drug consumption during pregnancy. JAMA 239:843, 1978.
48. Brocklebank JC, Ray WA, Federspiel CF, et al. Drug prescribing during pregnancy: a controlled study of Tennessee Medicaid recipients. Am J Obstet Gynecol 132:235, 1978.
49. Philipson A. The use of antibiotics in pregnancy. J Antimicrob Chemother 12:101, 1983.
50. Tropper PJ, Petrie RH. Placental exchange. *In* Lavery JP (ed). The Human Placenta: Clinical Perspectives. Rockville, Md, Aspen Publishers, 1987, p 199.
51. Juchau MR, Dyer DC. Pharmacology of the placenta. Pediatr Clin North Am 19:65, 1972.
52. Philipson A, Sabath LD, Charles D. Transplacental passage of erythromycin and clindamycin. N Engl J Med 288:1219, 1973.
53. Bernard B, Abate M, Thielen PF, et al. Maternal-fetal pharmacological activity of amikacin. J Infect Dis 135:925, 1977.
54. Bernard B, Garcia-Cazares SJ, Ballard CA, et al. Tobramycin: maternal-fetal pharmacology. Antimicrob Agents Chemother 11:688, 1977.
55. Matsuda S, Mori S, Tanno M, et al. Evaluation of amikacin in obstetric and gynecological field. Jpn J Antibiot 27:633, 1974.
56. Buckingham M, Welply G, Miller JF, et al. Gastrointestinal absorption and transplacental transfer of amoxicillin during labour and the influence of metoclopramide. Curr Med Res Opin 3:392, 1975.
57. Nau H. Clinical pharmacokinetics in pregnancy andperinatology: II. Penicillins. Dev Pharmacol Ther 10:174, 1987.
58. Kafetzis DA, Brater DC, Fanourgakis JE. Materno-fetal transfer of azlocillin. J Antimicrob Chemother 12:157, 1983.
59. Charles D, Larsen B. Placental transfer of antibiotics. *In* Ristuccia AM, Cunha BA (eds). Antimicrobial Therapy. New York, Raven Press, 1984, p 519.
60. Bernard B, Barton L, Abate M, et al. Maternal-fetal transfer of cefazolin in the first twenty weeks trimester of pregnancy. J Infect Dis 136:377, 1977.
61. Dekel A, Elian I, Gibor Y, et al. Transplacental passage of cefazolin in the first trimester of pregnancy. Eur J Obstet Gynecol Reprod Biol 10:303, 1980.
62. Cho N, Ito T, Saito T, et al. Clinical studies on cefazolin in the field of obstetrics and gynecology. Chemotherapy 18:770, 1970.
63. Shimizu K. Cefoperazone: absorption, excretion, distribution, and metabolism. Clin Ther 3(Spec. Issue):60, 1980.
64. Briggs GG, Freeman RK, Yaffe SJ. Drugs in Pregnancy and Lactation: A Reference Guide to Fetal and Neonatal Risk, 2nd ed. Baltimore, Williams & Wilkins, 1986.
65. Kafetzis DA, Lazarides CV, Siafas CA, et al. Transfer of cefotaxime in human milk and from mother to foetus. J Antimicrob Chemother 6(Suppl. A):135, 1980.
66. Matsuda S, Tanno M, Kashiwakura T, et al. Laboratory and clinical studies on cefotaxin in the field of obstetric and gynecology. Chemotherapy (Tokyo) 26(Suppl 1):460, 1978.
67. Nankun C, Uerhara K, Sugizaki K, et al. Clinical studies of cefoxitin in the field of obstetrics and gynecology. Chemotherapy (Tokyo) 26(Suppl 1):468, 1978.
68. Bergongne-Berezin E, Morel C, Kafe H, et al. Étude pharmacocinétique chez l'homme de la cefoxitime: diffusion intrabronchique et transplacentaire. Therapie 34:345, 1979.
69. Motomura R, Kohno M, Mori H, et al. Basic and clinical studies of ceftizoxime in obstetrics and gynecology. Chemotherapy (Tokyo) 28(Suppl 5):888, 1980.
70. Kafetzis DA, Brater DC, Fanourgakis JE, et al. Ceftriaxone distribution between maternal blood and fetal blood and tissues at parturition and between blood and milk post partum. Antimicrob Agents Chemother 23:870, 1983.
71. Craft I, Mullinger BM, Kennedy MRK. Placental transfer of cefuroxime. Br J Obstet Gynaecol 88:141, 1981.
72. Bousfield P, Browning AK, Mullinger BM, et al. Cefuroxime: potential use in pregnant women at term. Br J Obstet Gynaecol 88:146, 1981.
73. Coppi G, Berti MA, Chehade A, et al. A study of the transplacental transfer of cefuroxime in humans. Curr Ther Res 32:712, 1982.
74. Creatsas G, Pavlatos M, Lolis D, et al. A study of the kinetics of cephapirin and cephalexin in pregnancy. Curr Med Res Opin 7:43, 1980.
75. Morrow S, Palmisano P, Cassady G. The placental transfer of cephalothin. J Pediatr 73:262, 1968.
76. Scott WC, Warner RF. Placental transfer of chloramphenicol (Chloromycetin). JAMA 142:1331, 1950.
77. Ross S, Burke FG, Sites J, et al. Placental transmission of chloramphenicol (Chloromycetin). JAMA 142:1361, 1950.
78. Burns LE, Hodgman JE, Cass AB. Fatal circulatory collapse in premature infants receiving chloramphenicol. N Engl J Med 261:1318, 1959.
79. Weinstein AJ, Gibbs RS, Gallagher M. Placental transfer of clindamycin and gentamicin in term pregnancy. Am J Obstet Gynecol 124:688, 1976.
80. Herngren L, Ehrnebo M, Boreus LO. Drug binding to plasma proteins during human pregnancy and in the perinatal period: studies on cloxacillin and alprenolol. Dev Pharmacol Ther 6:110, 1983.
81. MacAulay MA, Charles D. Placental transmission of colistimethate. Clin Pharmacol Ther 8:578, 1967.
82. MacAylay MA, Berg SR, Charles D. Placental transfer of dicloxacillin at term. Am J Obstet Gynecol 102:1162, 1968.
83. Depp R, Kind AC, Kirby WMM, et al. Transplacental passage of methicillin and dicloxacillin into the fetus and amniotic fluid. Am J Obstet Gynecol 107:1054, 1970.
84. Kiefer L, Rubin A, McCoy JB, et al. The placental transfer of erythromycin. Am J Obstet Gynecol 69:174, 1955.
85. Yoshioka H, Monma T, Matsuda S. Placental transfer of gentamicin. J Pediatr 80:121, 1972.
86. L'Hommedieu CS, Nicholas D, Armes DA, et al. Potentiation of magnesium sulfate-induced neuromuscular weakness by gentamicin, tobramycin, and amikacin. J Pediatr 102:629, 1983.

87. Heikkila A, Renkonen OV, Erkkola R. Pharmacokinetics and transplacental passage of imipenem during pregnancy. Antimicrob Agents Chemother 36:2652, 1992.
88. Good RG, Johnson GH. The placental transfer of kanamycin during late pregnancy. Obstet Gynecol 38:60, 1971.
89. Jones HC. Intrauterine ototoxicity: a case report and review of literature. J Natl Med Assoc 65:201, 1973.
90. Duignan NM, Andrews J, Williams JD. Pharmacological studies with lincomycin in late pregnancy. BMJ (Clin Res) 3:75, 1975.
91. Mickal A, Panzer JD. The safety of lincomycin in pregnancy. Am J Obstet Gynecol 121:1071, 1975.
92. MacAulay MA, Molloy WB, Charles D. Placental transfer of methicillin. Am J Obstet Gynecol 115:58, 1973.
93. Perry JE, LeBlanc AL. Transfer of nitrofurantoin across the human placenta. Tex Rep Biol Med 25:265, 1967.
94. Wasz-Höckert O, Nummi S, Vuopala S, et al. Transplacental passage of azidocillin, ampicillin and penicillin G during early and late pregnancy. Scand J Infect Dis 2:125, 1970.
95. Greene HJ, Hobby GL. Transmission of penicillin through human placenta. Proc Soc Exp Biol Med 57:282, 1944.
96. Woltz JHE, Zintel HA. The transmission of penicillin to amniotic fluid and fetal blood in the human. Am J Obstet Gynecol 50:330, 1945.
97. Woltz JHE, Wiley MM. Transmission of streptomycin from maternal blood to the fetal circulation and the amniotic fluid. Proc Soc Exp Biol Med 60:106, 1945.
98. Conway N, Birt BD. Streptomycin in pregnancy: effect on the foetal ear. BMJ 2:260, 1965.
99. Donald PR, Sellars SL. Streptomycin ototoxicity in the unborn child. S Afr Med J 60:316, 1981.
100. Speert H. Placental transmission of sulfathiazole and sulfadiazine and its significance for fetal chemotherapy. Am J Obstet Gynecol 45:200, 1943.
101. Ziai M, Finland M. Placental transfer of sulfamethoxypyridazine. N Engl J Med 257:1180, 1957.
102. Sparr RA, Pritchard JA. Maternal and newborn distribution and excretion of sulfamethoxypyridazine (Kynex). Obstet Gynecol 12:131, 1958.
103. Kantor HI, Sutherland DA, Leonard JT, et al. Effect on bilirubin metabolism in the newborn of sulfisoxazole administered to the mother. Obstet Gynecol 17:494, 1961.
104. Brown AK, Cevik N. Hemolysis and jaundice in the newborn following maternal treatment with sulfamethoxypyridazine (Kynex). Pediatrics 36:742, 1965.
105. Perkins RP. Hydrops fetalis and stillbirth in a male glucose-6-phosphate dehydrogenase-deficient fetus possibly due to maternal ingestion of sulfisoxazole: a case report. Am J Obstet Gynecol 111:379, 1971.
106. Azad Khan AK, Truelove SC. Placental and mammary transfer of sulphasalazine. BMJ 2:1553, 1979.
107. Esbjörner E, Järnerot G, Wranne, L. Sulphasalazine and sulphapyridine serum levels in children to mothers treated with sulphasalazine during pregnancy and lactation. Acta Paediatr Scand 76:137, 1963.
108. Cohlan SQ, Bevelander G, Tiamsic T. Growth inhibition of prematures receiving tetracycline: a clinical and laboratory investigation of tetracycline-induced bone fluorescence. Am J Dis Child 105:453, 1963.
109. Kline AH, Blattner RJ, Lunin M. Transplacental effect of tetracyclines on teeth. JAMA 188:178, 1964.
110. Kutscher AH, Zegarelli EV, Tovell HMM, et al. Discoloration of deciduous teeth induced by administration of tetracycline antepartum. Am J Obstet Gynecol 96:291, 1966.
111. LeBlanc AL, Perry JE. Transfer of tetracycline across the human placenta. Tex Rep Biol Med 25:541, 1967.
112. McEwen LM. Trimethoprim/sulphamethoxazole mixture in pregnancy. BMJ (Clin Res) 4:490, 1971.
113. Reid DWJ, Caillé G, Kauffman NR. Maternal and transplacental kinetics of trimethoprim and sulfamethoxazole separately and in combination. Can Med Assoc J 112:67S, 1975.
114. Philipson A. Pharmacokinetics of antibiotics in pregnancy and labour. Clin Pharmacokinet 4:297, 1979.
115. Mucklow JC. The fate of drugs in pregnancy. Clin Obstet Gynaecol 13:161, 1986.
116. Apgar V. Drugs in pregnancy. JAMA 190:840, 1964.
117. Sutherland JM, Light IJ. The effect of drugs upon the developing fetus. Pediatr Clin North Am 12:781, 1965.
118. Totterman LE, Saxen L. Incorporation of tetracycline into human fetal bones after maternal drug administration. Acta Obstet Gynecol Scand 48:542, 1969.
119. Lumbiganon P, Pengsaa K, Sookpranee T. Ciprofloxacin in neonates and its possible adverse effect on the teeth. Pediatr Infect Dis J 10:619, 1991.
120. Krasinski K, Perkin R, Rutledge J. Gray baby syndrome revisited. Clin Pediatr 21:571, 1982.
121. Boyer KM, Gottof SP. Prevention of early-onset neonatal group B streptococcal disease with selective intrapartum chemoprophylaxis. N Engl J Med 314:1665, 1986.
122. Teres FO, Matorras R, Perea AG, et al. Prevention of neonatal group B streptococcal sepsis. Pediatr Infect Dis J 6:874, 1987.
123. Yow MD, Mason EO, Leeds LJ, et al. Ampicillin prevents intrapartum transmission of group B *Streptococcus*. JAMA 241:1245, 1979.
124. Lewis PJ. Antibiotics and breast feeding. Clin Exp Obstet Gynecol 13:124, 1986.
125. Rivera-Calimlim L. The significance of drugs in breast milk: pharmacokinetic considerations. Clin Perinatol 14:51, 1987.
126. Wilson JT, Brown RD, Cherek DR, et al. Drug excretion in human breast milk: principles, pharmacokinetics and projected consequences. Clin Pharmacokinet 5:1, 1980.
127. Kafetzis DA, Siafas CA, Georgakopoulos PA, et al. Passage of cephalosporins and amoxicillin into the breast milk. Acta Paediatr Scand 70:285, 1981.
128. Fleiss PM, Richwald GA, Gordon J, et al. Aztreonam in human serum and breast milk. Br J Clin Pharmacol 19:509, 1985.
129. O'Brien TE. Excretion of drugs in human milk. Am J Hosp Pharm 31:844, 1974.
130. Gerding DN, Peterson LR, Hughes CE, et al. Extravascular antimicrobial distribution in man. *In* Lorian V (ed). Antibiotics in Laboratory Medicine, 2nd ed. Baltimore, Williams & Wilkins, 1986, p 960.
131. Dubois M, Delapierre D, Chanteux L, et al. A study of the transplacental transfer and the mammary excretion of cefoxitin in humans. J Clin Pharmacol 21:477, 1981.
132. Dresse A, Lambotte R, Dubois M, et al. Transmammary passage of cefoxitin: additional results. J Clin Pharmacol 23:438, 1983.
133. Blanco JD, Jorgensen JH, Castaneda YS, et al. Ceftazidime levels in human breast milk. Antimicrob Agents Chemother 23:479, 1983.
134. Gerding DN, Peterson LR. Comparative tissue and extravascular fluid concentrations of ceftizoxime. J Antimicrob Chemother 10(Suppl C):105, 1982.
135. Knowles JA. Excretion of drugs in milk—a review. J Pediatr 66:1068, 1965.
136. Steen B, Rane A. Clindamycin passage into human milk. Br J Clin Pharmacol 13:661, 1982.
137. Chyo N, Sunada H, Nohara S. Clinical studies of kanamycin applied in the field of obstetrics and gynecology. Asian Med J 5:265, 1962.
138. Singlas E. Tissue distribution of mezlocillin. Nouv Presse Med 11:373, 1982.
139. Varsano I, Fischl J, Shochet SB. The excretion of orally ingested nitrofurantoin in human milk. J Pediatr 82:886, 1973.
140. Greene HJ, Burkhart B, Hobby GL. Excretion of penicillin in human milk following parturition. Am J Obstet Gynecol 51:735, 1946.
141. Kauffman RE, O'Brien C, Gilford P. Sulfisoxazole secretion into human milk. J Pediatr 97:839, 1980.
142. von Kobyletzki D, Dalhoff A, Lindemeyer H, et al. Ticarcillin serum and tissue concentrations in gynecology and obstetrics. Infection 11: 144, 1983.
143. Takase Z, Shirafuji H, Uchida M, et al. Laboratory and clinical studies on tobramycin in the field of obstetrics and gynecology. Chemotherapy (Tokyo) 23:1399, 1975.
144. Wilson JT, Brown RD, Hinson JL, et al. Pharmacokinetic pitfalls in the estimation of the breast milk/plasma ratio for drugs. Annu Rev Pharmacol Toxicol 25:667, 1985.
145. Catz CS, Giacoia GP. Drugs and breast milk. Pediatr Clin North Am 19:151, 1972.
146. American Academy of Pediatrics, Committee on Drugs. The transfer of drugs and other chemicals into human breast milk. Pediatrics 93:137, 1994.
147. Mann CF. Clindamycin and breast-feeding. Pediatrics 66:1030, 1980.
148. Neu HC. Penicillins. *In* Mandell GL, Douglas RG Jr, Bennett JE (eds). Principles and Practice of Infectious Diseases, 2nd ed. New York, John Wiley, 1985, p 166.
149. Neu HC. Contribution of beta-lactamases to bacterial resistance and mechanisms to inhibit beta-lactamases. Am J Med 79(Suppl 5B):2, 1985.

150. Nayler JHC. Resistance to β-lactams in gram-negative bacteria: relative contributions of β-lactamase and permeability limitations. J Antimicrob Chemother 19:713, 1987.
151. Tuomanen E, Durack DT, Tomasz A. Antibiotic tolerance among clinical isolates of bacteria. Antimicrob Agents Chemother 30:521, 1986.
152. Siegel JD, Shannon KM, DePasse BM. Recurrent infection associated with penicillin-tolerant group B streptococci: a report of two cases. J Pediatr 99:920, 1981.
153. Leggiadro RJ. Penicillin- and cephalosporin-resistant *Streptococcus pneumoniae*: an emerging microbial threat. Pediatrics 93:500, 1994.
154. Friedland IR, McCracken GH Jr. Management of infections caused by antibiotic-resistant *Streptococcus pneumoniae*. N Engl J Med 331:377, 1994.
155. McCracken GH Jr, Ginsberg C, Chrane DF, et al. Clinical pharmacology of penicillin in newborn infants. J Pediatr 82:692, 1973.
156. Kaplan JM, McCracken GH Jr. Clinical pharmacology of benzathine penicillin G in neonates with regard to its recommended use in congenital syphilis. J Pediatr 82:1069, 1973.
157. Klein JO, Scharberg MJ, Buntin M, et al. Levels of penicillin in serum of newborn infants after single intramuscular doses of benzathine penicillin G. J Pediatr 82:1065, 1973.
158. Hieber JP, Nelson JD. A pharmacologic evaluation of penicillin in children with purulent meningitis. N Engl J Med 297:410, 1977.
159. Speer ME, Taber LH, Clark DB, et al. Cerebrospinal fluid levels of benzathine penicillin G in the neonate. J Pediatr 91:996, 1977.
160. McCracken GH Jr, Kaplan JM. Penicillin treatment for congenital syphilis: a critical reappraisal. JAMA 228:855, 1974.
161. Speer ME, Mason EO, Scharnberg JT. Cerebrospinal fluid concentrations of aqueous procaine penicillin G in the neonate. Pediatrics 67:387, 1981.
162. Levin B, Neill CA. Oral penicillin in the newborn. Arch Dis Child 24:171, 1949.
163. McCracken GH Jr, Nelson JD. Antimicrobial Therapy for Newborns, 2nd ed. New York, Grune & Stratton, 1983.
164. Centers for Disease Control and Prevention. STD Treatment Guidelines. Atlanta, Centers for Disease Control, 1985.
165. McCracken GH, Mize SG, Threlkeld N. Intraventricular gentamicin therapy in gram-negative bacillary meningitis of infancy: report of the Second Neonatal Meningitis Cooperative Study Group. Lancet 1:787, 1980.
166. Joseph TA, Pyati SP, Jacobs N. Neonatal early-onset *Escherichia coli* disease: the effect of intrapartum ampicillin. Arch Pediatr Adolesc Med 152:35, 1998.
167. Grossman M, Ticknor W. Serum levels of ampicillin, cephalothin, cloxacillin, and nafcillin in the newborn infant. Antimicrobial Agents Chemother 5:214, 1965.
168. Axline SG, Yaffe SJ, Simon HJ. Clinical pharmacology of antimicrobials in premature infants: II. Ampicillin, methicillin, oxacillin, neomycin, and colistin. Pediatrics 39:97, 1967.
169. Boe RW, Williams CPS, Bennett JV, et al. Serum levels of methicillin and ampicillin in newborn and premature infants in relation to postnatal age. Pediatrics 39:194, 1967.
170. Dahl LB, Melby K, Gutteberg TJ, et al. Serum levels of ampicillin and gentamycin in neonates of varying gestational age. Eur J Pediatr 145: 218, 1986.
171. Silverio J, Poole JW. Serum concentrations of ampicillin in newborn infants after oral administration. Pediatrics 51:578, 1973.
172. McCracken GH Jr, Ginsburg CM, Clahsen JC, et al. Pharmacologic evaluation of orally administered antibiotics in infants and children: effect of feeding on bioavailability. Pediatrics 62:738, 1978.
173. Bass JW, Crowley DM, Steele RW, et al. Adverse effects of orally administered ampicillin. J Pediatr 83:106, 1973.
174. Tetzlaff TR, Ashwoth C, Nelson JD. Otitis media in children less than 12 weeks of age. Pediatrics 59:827, 1977.
175. Neu HC. Antistaphylococcal penicillins. Med Clin North Am 66:51, 1982.
176. Utsui Y, Yokota T. Role of an altered penicillin-binding protein in methicillin- and cephem-resistant *Staphylococcus aureus*. Antimicrob Agents Chemother 28:397, 1985.
177. Shanson DC, Johnstone D, Midgley J. Control of a hospital outbreak of methicillin-resistant *Staphylococcus aureus* infections: value of an isolation unit. J Hosp Infect 6:285, 1985.
178. Sabath LD, Wheeler N, Laverdiere M, et al. A new type of penicillin resistance of *Staphylococcus aureus*. Lancet 1:443, 1977.
179. Sarff LD, McCracken GH Jr, Thomas ML, et al. Clinical pharmacology of methicillin in neonates. J Pediatr 90:1005, 1977.
180. O'Connor WJ, Warren GH, Mandala PS, et al. Serum concentrations of nafcillin in newborn infants and children. Antimicrobial Agents Chemother 10:188, 1964.
181. Banner W Jr, Gooch WM III, Burckart G, et al. Pharmacokinetics of nafcillin in infants with low birth weights. Antimicrob Agents Chemother 17:691, 1980.
182. O'Connor WJ, Warren GH, Edrada LS, et al. Serum concentrations of sodium nafcillin in infants during the perinatal period. Antimicrobial Agents Chemother 5:220, 1965.
183. Burns LE, Hodgman JE, Wehrle PF. Treatment of premature infants with oxacillin. Antimicrobial Agents Chemother 10:192, 1964.
184. Sarff LD, McCracken GH Jr. Methicillin-associated nephropathy or cystitis. J Pediatr 90:1031, 1977.
185. Kitzing W, Nelson JD, Mohs E. Comparative toxicities of methicillin and nafcillin. Am J Dis Child 135:52, 1981.
186. Greene GR, Cohen E. Nafcillin-induced neutropenia in children. Pediatrics 61:94, 1978.
187. Nahata MV, DeBolt SL, Powell DA. Adverse effects of methicillin, nafcillin and oxacillin in pediatric patients. Dev Pharmacol Ther 4:117, 1982.
188. Mallouh AA. Methicillin-induced neutropenia. Pediatr Infect Dis 4:262, 1985.
189. Neu HC. Carbenicillin and ticarcillin. Med Clin North Am 66:61, 1982.
190. Nelson JD, McCracken GH Jr. Clinical pharmacology of carbenicillin and gentamicin in the neonate and comparative efficacy with ampicillin and gentamicin. Pediatrics 52:801, 1973.
191. Morehead CD, Shelton S, Kusmiesz H, et al. Pharmacokinetics of carbenicillin in neonates of normal and low birth weight. Antimicrob Agents Chemother 2:267, 1972.
192. Yoshioka H, Takimoto M, Shimizu T, et al. Pharmacokinetics of intramuscular carbenicillin in the newborn. Infection 7:27, 1979.
193. Nelson JD, Kusmiesz H, Shelton S, et al. Clinical pharmacology and efficacy of ticarcillin in infants and children. Pediatrics 61:858, 1978.
194. Nelson JD, Shelton S, Kusmiesz H. Clinical pharmacology of ticarcillin in the newborn infant: relation to age, gestational age, and weight. J Pediatr 87:474, 1975.
195. Sutherland R, Beale AS, Boon RJ, et al. Antibacterial activity of ticarcillin in the presence of clavulanate potassium. Am J Med 79(Suppl 5B):13, 1985.
196. Pulverer G, Peters G, Kunstmann G. In-vitro activity of ticarcillin with and without clavulanic acid against clinical isolates of gram-positive and gram-negative bacteria. J Antimicrob Chemother 17(Suppl C):1, 1986.
197. Gould IM, Wise R. β-Lactamase inhibitors. *In* Peterson PK, Verhoef J (eds). The Antimicrobial Agents Annual 1. Amsterdam, Elsevier, 1986, p 51.
198. Bégué P, Quiniou F, Quinet B. Efficacy and pharmacokinetics of Timentin in paediatric infections. J Antimicrob Chemother 17(Suppl): 81, 1986.
199. Eliopoulos GM, Moellering RC Jr. Azlocillin, mezlocillin, and piperacillin: new broad-spectrum penicillins. Ann Intern Med 97:755, 1982.
200. Drusano GL, Schimpff SC, Hewitt WL. The acylampicillins: mezlocillin, piperacillin, and azlocillin. Rev Infect Dis 6:13, 1984.
201. Allan JD, Eliopoulos GM, Moellering RC Jr. The expanding spectrum of beta-lactam antibiotics. Adv Intern Med 31:119, 1986.
202. Moody JA, Peterson LR, Gerding DN. In vitro activities of ureidopenicillins alone and in combination with amikacin and three cephalosporin antibiotics. Antimicrob Agents Chemother 26:256, 1984.
203. Heimann G, Föster D. Pharmacokinetics of acylureidopenicillins (azlocillin, mezlocillin) in prematures and newborns. Drugs Exp Clin Res 7:287, 1981.
204. Rubio T, Wirth F, Karotkin E. Pharmacokinetic studies of mezlocillin in newborn infants. J Antimicrob Chemother 9(Suppl A):241, 1982.
205. Janicke DM, Rubio TT, Wirth FH Jr, et al. Developmental pharmacokinetics of mezlocillin in newborn infants. J Pediatr 104:773, 1984.
206. Odio C, Threlkeld N, Thomas ML, et al. Pharmacokinetics properties of mezlocillin in newborn infants. Antimicrob Agents Chemother 25:556, 1984.
207. Chiu T, Garrison RD, Fakhreddine F, et al. Mezlocillin in neonatal infections: evaluation of efficacy and toxicity. J Antimicrob Chemother 9(Suppl A):251, 1982.

208. Weingärtner L. Clinical aspects of mezlocillin therapy in childhood. J Antimicrob Chemother 9(Suppl A):257, 1982.
209. Bergan T. Review of the pharmacokinetics of mezlocillin. J Antimicrob Chemother 11(Suppl C):1, 1983.
210. Heimann G. Pharmacokinetics and clinical aspects of azlocillin in paediatrics. J Antimicrob Chemother 11(Suppl B):127, 1983.
211. Bergan T. Review of the pharmacokinetics and dose dependency of azlocillin in normal subjects and patients with renal insufficiency. J Antimicrob Chemother 11(Suppl B):101, 1983.
212. Placzek M, Whitelaw A, Want S, et al. Piperacillin in early neonatal infection. Arch Dis Child 58:1006, 1983.
213. Thirumoorthi MC, Asmar BI, Buckley JA, et al. Pharmacokinetics of intravenously administered piperacillin in preadolescent children. J Pediatr 102:941, 1983.
214. Kacet N, Roussel-DelVallez M, Gremillet C, et al. Pharmacokinetic study of piperacillin in newborns relating to gestational and postnatal age. Pediatr Infect Dis J 11:365, 1992.
215. Wilson CB, Koup JR, Opheim KE, et al. Piperacillin pharmacokinetics in pediatric patients. Antimicrob Agents Chemother 22:442, 1982.
216. Reed MD, Goldfarb J, Yamashita TS, Blumer JL. Piperacillin and tazobactam in infants and children. Antimicrob Agents Chemother 38.2817, 1994.
217. Johnson GJ. Antibiotic-induced hemostatic abnormalities. *In* Peterson PK, Verhoef J (eds). The Antimicrobial Agents Annual 1. Amsterdam, Elsevier, 1986, p 408.
218. Bertino JS Jr, Speck WT. The cephalosporin antibiotics. Pediatr Clin North Am 30:17, 1983.
219. Eichenwald HF. Antimicrobial therapy in infants and children: update 1976-1985: I. J Pediatr 107:161, 1985.
220. Nelson JD. Cefuroxime: a cephalosporin with unique applicability to pediatric practice. Pediatr Infect Dis J 2:394, 1983.
221. Garau J. The clinical potential of fourth-generation cephalosporins. Diagn Microbiol Infect Dis 31:479, 1998.
222. Milatovic D, Braveny I. Development of resistance during antibiotic therapy. Eur J Clin Microbiol 6:234, 1987.
223. Sanders CC, Sanders WE Jr. The cephalosporins and cephamycins. *In* Peterson PK, Verhoef J (eds). The Antimicrobial Agents Annual 2. Amsterdam, Elsevier, 1987, p 70.
224. Sheng KT, Huang NN, Promadhattaveddi V. Serum concentrations of cephalothin in infants and children and placental transmission of the antibiotic. Antimicrobial Agents Chemother 10:200, 1964.
225. Sakata Y. The pharmacokinetic studies of cephalothin, cefazolin and cefmetazole in the neonates and the premature babies. Kurume Med J 27:275, 1980.
226. Hallberg T, Svenningsen NW. Cephalothin in neonatal infections. Acta Paediatr Scand 206(Suppl):110, 1970.
227. Plaisance KI, Nightingale CH, Quintiliani R. Pharmacology of the cephalosporins. *In* Queener SF, Webber JA, Queener SW (eds). Beta-Lactam Antibiotics for Clinical Use. New York, Marcel Dekker, 1986, p 285.
228. Chang N, Ito T, Saito H, et al. Studies on cefazolin in obstetrics and gynecology with special reference to its clinical pharmacology in the neonate. *In* Hejzlar M, Semonsky M, Masak S (eds). Advances in Antimicrobial and Antineoplastic Chemotherapy: Progress in Research and Clinical Application, vol 1. Baltimore, University Park Press, 1972, p 1187.
229. Boothman R, Kerr MM, Marshall MJ, et al. Absorption and excretion of cephalexin by the newborn infant. Arch Dis Child 48:147, 1973.
230. Chin KC, Kerr MM, Cockburn F, et al. A pharmacological study of cefaclor in the newborn infant. Curr Med Res Opin 7:168, 1981.
231. McCracken GH Jr, Ginsburg CM, Clahsen JC, et al. Pharmacokinetics of cefaclor in infants and children. J Antimicrob Chemother 4:515, 1978.
232. Renlund M, Pettay O. Pharmacokinetics and clinical efficacy of cefuroxime in the newborn period. Proc R Soc Med 70(Suppl 9):183, 1977.
233. Dash CH, Kennedy MRK, Ng SH. Cefuroxime in the first week of life. *In* Nelson JD, Grassi C (eds). Current Chemotherapy and Infectious Disease: Proceedings of the 11th International Congress of Chemotherapy and the 19th Interscience Conference on Antimicrobial Agents and Chemotherapy. Washington, DC, American Society for Microbiology, 1980, p 1161.
234. de Louvois J, Mulhall A, Hurley R. Cefuroxime in the treatment of neonates. Arch Dis Child 57:59, 1982.
235. Wilkinson PJ, Belohradsky BH, Marget WA. Clinical study of cefuroxime in neonates. Proc R Soc Med 70(Suppl 9):183, 1977.
236. von Hattingberg HM, Marget W, Belohradsky BH, et al. Pharmacokinetics of cefotaxime in neonates and children: clinical aspects. J Antimicrob Chemother 6(Suppl A):113, 1980.
237. Kafetzis DA, Brater DC, Kapiki AN, et al. Treatment of severe neonatal infections with cefotaxime: efficacy and pharmacokinetics. J Pediatr 100:483, 1982.
238. McCracken GH Jr, Threlkeld NE, Thomas ML. Pharmacokinetics of cefotaxime in newborn infants. Antimicrob Agents Chemother 21:683, 1982.
239. de Louvois J, Mulhall A, Hurley R. The safety and pharmacokinetics of cefotaxime in the treatment of neonates. Pediatr Pharmacol 2:275, 1982.
240. Crooks J, White LO, Burville LJ, et al. Pharmacokinetics of cefotaxime and desacetyl-cefotaxime in neonates. J Antimicrob Chemother 14(Suppl B):97, 1984.
241. Bëguë P, Safran C, Quiniou F, et al. Comparative pharmacokinetics of four new cephalosporins: moxalactam, cefotaxime, cefoperazone and ceftazidime in neonates. Dev Pharmacol Ther 7(Suppl 1):105, 1984.
242. Chamberlain J, Coombes JD, Dell D, et al. Metabolism of cefotaxime in animals and man. J Antimicrob Chemother 6(Suppl A):69, 1980.
243. Jones RN, Barry AL, Thornsberry C. Antimicrobial activity of desacetyl-cefotaxime alone and in combination with cefotaxime: evidence of synergy. Rev Infect Dis 4:S366, 1982.
244. von Loewenich V, Miething R, Uihlein M, et al. Levels of cefotaxime and desacetyl-cefotaxime in the cerebrospinal fluid of newborn and premature infants. Padiatr Padol 18:361, 1983.
245. Wells TG, Trang JM, Brown AL, et al. Cefotaxime therapy of bacterial meningitis in children. J Antimicrob Chemother 14(Suppl B):181, 1984.
246. Cherubin CE, Corrado ML, Nair SR, et al. Treatment of gram-negative bacillary meningitis: role of the new cephalosporin antibiotics. Rev Infect Dis 4:S453, 1982.
247. McCracken GH Jr, Siegel JD, Threlkeld N, et al. Ceftriaxone pharmacokinetics in newborn infants. Antimicrob Chemother 23: 341, 1983.
248. James J, Mulhall A, de Louvois J. Ceftriaxone-clinical experience in the treatment of neonates. J Infect 11:25, 1985.
249. Mulhall A, de Louvois J, James J. Pharmacokinetics and safety of ceftriaxone in the neonate. Eur J Pediatr 144:379, 1985.
250. Martin E, Koup JR, Paravicini U, et al. Pharmacokinetics of ceftriaxone in neonates and infants with meningitis. J Pediatr 105:475, 1984.
251. Guggenbichler JP, Parth J, Frisch H. Pharmacokinetic investigation of ceftriaxone in premature and newborn babies. Padiatr Padol 21:31, 1986.
252. del Rio M, McCracken GH Jr, Nelson JD, et al. Pharmacokinetics and cerebrospinal fluid bactericidal activity of ceftriaxone in the treatment of pediatric patients with bacterial meningitis. Antimicrob Agents Chemother 22:622, 1982.
253. Latif R, Dajani AS. Ceftriaxone diffusion into cerebrospinal fluid of children with meningitis. Antimicrob Agents Chemother 23:46, 1983.
254. Rosenfeld WN, Evans HE, Batheja R, et al. Pharmacokinetics of cefoperazone in full-term and premature neonates. Antimicrob Agents Chemother 23:866, 1983.
255. Philips JB III, Braune K, Ravis W, et al. Pharmacokinetics of cefoperazone in newborn infants. Pediatr Pharmacol 4:193, 1984.
256. Bosso JA, Chan GM, Matsen JM. Cefoperazone pharmacokinetics in preterm infants. Antimicrob Agents Chemother 23:413, 1983.
257. Assael BM, Boccazzi A, Caccamo ML, et al. Clinical pharmacology of ceftazidime in paediatrics. J Antimicrob Chemother 12(Suppl A):341, 1983.
258. Prinsloo JG, Delport SD, Moncrieff J, et al. A preliminary pharmacokinetic study of ceftazidime in premature, newborn and small infants. J Antimicrob Chemother 12(Suppl A):361, 1983.
259. Gooch WM III, Swenson E. Neonatal pharmacokinetic characteristics of ceftazidime. *In* Program and Abstracts of the 23rd Interscience Conference on Antimicrobial Agents and Chemotherapy. Washington, DC, American Society for Microbiology, 1983, p 237 (abstract).
260. McCracken GH Jr, Threlkeld N, Thomas ML. Pharmacokinetics of ceftazidime in newborn infants. Antimicrob Agents Chemother 26: 583, 1984.
261. Prinsloo JG, Delport SD, Moncriegg J, et al. Pharmacokinetics of ceftazidime in premature, newborn and young infants. S Afr Med J 65:809, 1984.
262. Mulhall A, de Louvois J. The pharmacokinetics and safety of ceftazidime in the neonate. J Antimicrob Chemother 15:97, 1985.
263. Low DC, Bissenden JG, Wise R. Ceftazidime in neonatal infections. Arch Dis Child 60:360, 1985.

264. Padovani EM, Fanos V, Dal Moro A, et al. Ceftazidime pharmacokinetics in preterm newborns on the first day of life. Biol Res Pregnancy Perinatol 7:71, 1986.
265. Bégué P, Michel B, Chasalette JP, et al. Clinical efficacy and pharmacokinetics of ceftazidime in children and neonates. Pathol Biol 34:525, 1986.
266. de Louvois J, Mulhall A. Ceftazidime in the treatment of neonates. *In* Rubaltelli FF, Granati B (eds). Neonatal Therapy: An Update. Amsterdam, Elsevier, 1986, p 249.
267. Blumer J, Reed M, Aronoff S, et al. CSF penetration and pharmacokinetics of ceftazidime in children with bacterial meningitis. *In* Program and Abstracts of the 23rd Interscience Conference on Antimicrobial Agents and Chemotherapy. Washington, DC, American Society for Microbiology, 1983, p 237 (abstract).
268. Fong IW, Tomkins KB. Ceftazidime cerebrospinal fluid penetration in inflamed and non-inflamed meninges. *In* Program and Abstracts of the 23rd Interscience Conference on Antimicrobial Agents and Chemotherapy. Washington, DC, American Society for Microbiology, 1983, p 237 (abstract).
269. Blumer JL, Reed MD, Knupp C. Review of the pharmacokinetics of cefepime in children. Pediatr Infect Dis J 20:337, 2001
270. Schaad UB. The cephalosporin compounds in severe neonatal infection. Eur J Pediatr 141:143, 1984.
271. Roos R. New β-lactams. *In* Rubaltelli FF, Granati B (eds). Neonatal Therapy: An Update. Amsterdam, Elsevier, 1986, p 217.
272. Bryan CS, John JF Jr, Pai MS, et al. Gentamicin vs cefotaxime for therapy of neonatal sepsis: relationship to drug resistance. Am J Dis Child 139:1086, 1985.
273. Bang NU, Kammer RB. Hematologic complications associated with β-lactam antibiotics. Rev Infect Dis 5:S380, 1983.
274. McCracken GH Jr. Use of third-generation cephalosporins for treatment of neonatal infections. Am J Dis Child 139:1079, 1985.
275. Hall MA, Beech RC, Seal DV. The use of cefotaxime for treating suspected neonatal sepsis: 2 years experience. J Hosp Infect 8:57, 1986.
276. Parshina NV. Clinical efficacy and certain pharmacokinetics characteristics of cefotaxime in premature infants with pneumonia. Antibiot Med Biotekhnol 31:298, 1986.
277. Hoogkamp-Korstanje JAA. Activity of cefotaxime and ceftriaxone alone and in combination with penicillin, ampicillin and piperacillin against neonatal meningitis pathogens. J Antimicrob Chemother 16: 327, 1985.
278. Macías-Parra M, Gonzalez-Saldaña N, Saltigeral P, et al. Utilidad de la ceftriaxona en el tratamiento de la sepsis neonatal. Rev Enf Infect Pediatr 6:20, 1992.
279. Snelling S, Hart CA, Cooke RWI. Ceftazidime or gentamicin plus benzylpenicillin in neonates less than forty-eight hours old. J Antimicrob Chemother 12(Suppl A):353, 1983.
280. Odio CM, Umana MA, Saenz A, et al. Comparative efficacy of ceftazidime vs. carbenicillin and amikacin for treatment of neonatal septicemia. Pediatr Infect Dis J 6:371, 1987.
281. Sáez-Llorens X, O'Ryan M. Cefepime in the empiric treatment of meningitis in children. Pediatr Infect Dis J 20:356, 2001
282. Williams JD. Aztreonam. *In* Peterson PK, Verhoef J (eds). The Antimicrobial Agents Annual 2. Amsterdam, Elsevier, 1987, p 47.
283. Swabb EA, Cimarusti CM, Henry SA, et al. Aztreonam (SQ 26,776) and other monobactams. *In* Queener SF, Webber JA, Queener SW (eds). Beta-Lactam Antibiotics for Clinical Use. New York, Marcel Dekker, 1986, p 593.
284. Stutman HR, Marks MI, Swabb EA. Single-dose pharmacokinetics of aztreonam in pediatric patients. Antimicrob Agents Chemother 26: 196, 1984.
285. Likitnukul S, McCracken GH Jr, Threlkeld N, et al. Pharmacokinetics and plasma bactericidal activity of aztreonam in low-birth-weight infants. Antimicrob Agents Chemother 31:81, 1987.
286. Greenman R, Arcey S, Dickinson G, et al. Penetration of aztreonam (SQ 26,776) into human cerebrospinal fluid in the presence of meningeal inflammation. *In* Program and Abstracts of the 23rd Interscience Conference on Antimicrobial Agents and Chemotherapy. Washington, DC, American Society for Microbiology, 1983, p 158 (abstract).
287. Umana MA, Odio CM, Castro E, et al. Comparative evaluation of aztreonam/ampicillin versus amikacin/ampicillin in neonates with bacterial infections. Pediatr Infect Dis J 9:175, 1990.
288. Uauy R, Mize C, Argyle C, et al. Metabolic tolerance to arginine: implications for the safe use of arginine salt-aztreonam combination in the neonatal period. J Pediatr 118:965, 1991.
289. Bradley JS. Meropenem: a new, extremely broad spectrum beta-lactam antibiotic for serious infections in pediatrics. Pediatr Infect Dis J 16:263, 1997.
290. Blumer JL. Pharmacokinetic determinants of carbapenem therapy in neonates and children. Pediatr Infect Dis J 15:733, 1996.
291. Clissold SP, Todd PA, Campoli-Richards DM. Imipenem/cilastatin: a review of its antibacterial activity, pharmacokinetic properties and therapeutic efficacy. Drugs 33:183, 1987.
292. Santos-Ferreira MO, Vital JO. In-vitro antibacterial activity of imipenem compared with four other β-lactam antibiotics (ceftazidime, cefotaxime, piperacillin and azlocillin) against 828 separate clinical isolates from a Portuguese hospital. J Antimicrob Chemother 18(Suppl E):23, 1986.
293. Williams RJ, Yang YJ, Livermore DM. Mechanisms by which imipenem may overcome resistance in gram-negative bacilli. J Antimicrob Chemother 18(Suppl E):9, 1986.
294. Freij BJ, McCracken GH Jr, Olsen KD, et al. Pharmacokinetics of imipenem-cilastatin in neonates. Antimicrob Agents Chemother 27: 431, 1985.
295. Gruber WC, Rench MA, Garcia-Prats JA, et al. Single-dose pharmacokinetics of imipenem-cilastatin in neonates. Antimicrob Agents Chemother 27:511, 1985.
296. Jacobs RF, Kearns GL, Trang JM, et al. Single-dose pharmacokinetics of imipenem in children. J Pediatr 105:996, 1984.
297. Rogers JD, Meisinger MA, Ferber F, et al. Pharmacokinetics of imipenem and cilastatin in volunteers. Rev Infect Dis 7:S435, 1985.
298. Patamasucon P, McCracken GH Jr. Pharmacokinetics and bacteriological efficacy of *N*-formimidoyl thienamycin in experimental *Escherichia coli* meningitis. Antimicrob Agents Chemother 21:390, 1982.
299. Modai J, Vittecoq D, Decazes JM, et al. Penetration of imipenem and cilastatin into cerebrospinal fluid of patients with bacterial meningitis. J Antimicrob Chemother 16:751, 1985.
300. Martinkova J, de Groot R, Chladek J, et al. Meropenem pharmacokinetics in pre-term and full-term neonates. Programs and Abstracts of the 7th European Congress of Clinical Microbiology and Infectious Diseases, Vienna, March 26-30, 1995 (abstract 686).
301. van Enk JG, Touw DJ, Lafeber HN. Pharmacokinetics of meropenem in preterm neonates. Ther Drug Monit 23:198, 2001.
302. Calandra GB, Brown KR, Grad LC, et al. Review of adverse experiences and tolerability in the first 2,516 patients treated with imipenem/cilastin. Am J Med 78(Suppl 6A):73, 1985.
303. Borderon JC, Rastegar A, Laugier J, et al. The effect of imipenem/cilastin on the aerobic faecal flora of children. J Antimicrob Chemother 18(Suppl E):121, 1986.
304. Wong VK, Wright HT, Ross LA, et al. Imipenem/cilastatin treatment of bacterial meningitis in children. Pediatr Infect Dis J 10:122, 1991.
305. Snavely SR, Hodges GR. The neurotoxicity of antibacterial agents. Ann Intern Med 101:92, 1984.
306. Hori S, Kurioka S, Matsuda M, et al. Inhibitory effect of cephalosporins on gamma-aminobutyric acid receptor binding in rat synapsis membranes. Antimicrob Agents Chemother 27:650, 1985.
307. Eng RH, Munsif AR, Yangco BG, et al. Seizure propensity with imipenem. Arch Intern Med 149:1881, 1989.
308. Day IP, Goudie J, Nishiki K, Williams PD. Correlation between in vitro and in vivo models of proconvulsive activity with the carbapenem antibiotics, biapenem, imipenem/cilastatin and meropenem. Toxicol Lett 76:239, 1995.
309. Collins MA, Tolpin M, and the Collaborative Imipenem-Cilastin Study Group. Clinical evaluation of imipenem-cilastin as a single agent therapy for sepsis neonatorum. *In* Program and Abstracts of the 27th Interscience Conference on Antimicrobial Agents and Chemotherapy. Washington, DC, American Society for Microbiology, 1987, p 188 (abstract).
310. Watanakunakorn C. Mode of action and in-vitro activity of vancomycin. J Antimicrob Chemother 14(Suppl 3):7, 1984.
311. Gross JR, Kaplan SL, Kramer WG, et al. Vancomycin pharmacokinetics in premature infants. Pediatr Pharmacol 5:17, 1985.
312. Naqvi SH, Keenam WJ, Reichley RM, et al. Vancomycin pharmacokinetics in small, seriously ill infants. Am J Dis Child 140:107, 1986.
313. James A, Koren G, Milliken J, et al. Vancomycin pharmacokinetics and dose recommendations for preterm infants. Antimicrob Agents Chemother 31:52, 1987.
314. Koren G, James A. Vancomycin dosing in preterm infants: prospective verification of new recommendations. J Pediatr 110:797, 1987.

315. Amaker PD, DiPiro JT, Bhatia J. Pharmacokinetics of vancomycin in critically ill infants undergoing extracorporeal membrane oxygenation. Antimicrob Agents Chemother 40:1139, 1996.
316. Reiter PD, Doron MW. Vancomycin cerebrospinal fluid concentrations after intravenous administration in premature infants. J Perinatol 16: 331, 1996.
317. McHenry MC, Gavan TL. Vancomycin. Pediatr Clin North Am 30:31, 1983.
318. Spera RV, Farber BF. Multiply-resistant *Enterococcus faecium*. JAMA 268:2563, 1992.
319. McCracken GH Jr. Changing pattern of the antimicrobial susceptibilities of *Escherichia coli* in neonatal infections. J Pediatr 78:942, 1971.
320. Prins JM, Speelman P. Once-daily aminoglycosides. Practical guidelines. Neth J Med 52:1, 1998.
321. Mattie H, Craig WA, Pechere JC. Determinants of efficacy and toxicity of aminoglycosides. J Antimicrob Chemother 24:281, 1989.
322. Skopnik H, Heimann G. Once daily aminoglycoside dosing in full term neonates. Pediatr Infect Dis J 14:71, 1995.
323. Hayani KC, Hatzopoulos FK, Frank AL, et al. Pharmacokinetics of once-daily dosing of gentamicin in neonates. J Pediatr 131:76, 1997.
324. Langhendries JP, Battisti O, Bertrand JM, et al. Adaptation in neonatology of the once-daily concept of aminoglycoside administration. Evaluation of a dosing chart for amikacin in an intensive care unit. Biol Neonate 74:351, 1998.
325. Lundergan FS, Glasscock GF, Kim EH, Cohen RS. Once-daily gentamicin dosing in newborn infants. Pediatrics 103:1228, 1999.
326. Kotze A, Bartel PR, Sommers DK. Once versus twice daily amikacin in neonates: prospective study on toxicity. J Paediatr Child Health 35: 283, 1999.
327. Vervelde ML, Rademaker CM, Krediet TG, et al. Population pharmacokinetics of gentamicin in preterm neonates: evaluation of a once-daily dosage regimen. Ther Drug Monit 21:514, 1999.
328. Agarwal G, Rastogi A, Pyati S, et al. Comparison of once-daily versus twice-daily gentamicin dosing regimens in infants >2500 g. J Perinatol 22:268, 2002.
329. Rastogi A, Agarwal G, Pyati S, Pildes RS. Comparison of two gentamicin dosing schedules in very low birth weight infants. Pediatr Infect Dis J 21:234, 2002.
330. Miron D. Once daily dosing of gentamicin in infants and children. Pediatr Infect Dis J 20:1169, 2001.
331. de Alba-Romero C, Gómez-Castillo E, Manzanares-Secades C, et al. Once daily gentamicin dosing in neonates. Pediatr Infect Dis J 17: 1169, 1998.
332. Avent ML, Kinney JS, Istre GR, Whitfield JM. Gentamicin and tobramycin in neonates: comparison of a new extended dosing interval regimen with a traditional multiple daily dosing regimen. Am J Perinatol 19:413, 2002.
333. Solomon R, Kuruvilla KA, Job V, et al. Randomized controlled trial of once vs. twice daily gentamicin therapy in newborn. Indian Pediatr 36:133, 1999.
334. DiCenzo R, Forrest A, Slish JC, et al. A gentamicin pharmacokinetic population model and once-daily dosing algorithm for neonates. Pharmacotherapy 23:585, 2003.
335. Fischel-Ghodsian N. Genetic factors in aminoglycoside toxicity. Ann N Y Acad Sci 884:99, 1999.
336. Skopnik H, Walraf F, Nies B, et al. Pharmacokinetics and antibacterial activity of daily gentamicin. Arch Dis Child 67:57, 1992.
337. Hayani KC, Hatzopoulos FK, Fank AL, et al. Pharmacokientics of once-daily dosing of gentamicin in neonates. J Pediatr 131:76, 1997.
338. Skopnik H, Heiman G. Once daily aminoglycoside in full term neonates. Pediatr Infect Dis J 14:71, 1995.
339. Miron D, Steinfels M, Reich D. Safety of short course of once-daily dosing of gentamicin in preterm infants. Ninth European Congress of Clinical Microbiology and Infectious Diseases, Berlin, March 1999 (abstract 016).
340. Ristuccia AM, Cunha BA. The aminoglycosides. Med Clin North Am 66:303, 1982.
341. Davies JE. Resistance to aminoglycosides: mechanisms and frequency. Rev Infect Dis 5:S261, 1983.
342. Kluge RM, Standiford HC, Tatem B, et al. Comparative activity of tobramycin, amikacin, and gentamicin alone and with carbenicillin against *Pseudomonas aeruginosa*. Antimicrob Agents Chemother 6: 442, 1974.
343. McCracken GH Jr, Threlkeld N, Thomas ML. Intravenous administration of kanamycin and gentamicin in newborn infants. Pediatrics 60:463, 1977.
344. Paisley JW, Smith AL, Smith DH. Gentamicin in newborn infants: comparison of intramuscular and intravenous administration. Am J Dis Child 126:473, 1973.
345. Black J, Calesnick B, Williams D, et al. Pharmacology of gentamicin, a new broad-spectrum antibiotic. Antimicrobial Agents Chemother 161:138, 1963.
346. King JT. Severe deafness in an infant following oral administration of neomycin. J Med Assoc Ga 51:530, 1962.
347. Nation RL, Huang SM, Vidyasagar D, et al. Absorption of oral neomycin in premature infants with suspected necrotizing enterocolitis. Dev Pharmacol Ther 5:53, 1982.
348. Nunnery AW, Riley HD Jr. Gentamicin: pharmacologic observations in newborns and infants. J Infect Dis 119:402 1969.
349. Hansen TN, Ritter DA, Speer ME, et al. A randomized, controlled study of oral gentamicin in the treatment of neonatal necrotizing enterocolitis. J Pediatr 97:836, 1980.
350. Grylack L, Boehnert J, Scanlon J. Serum concentrations of gentamicin following oral administration to preterm newborns. Dev Pharmacol Ther 5:47, 1982.
351. Miranda JC, Schimmel MS, Mimms GM, et al. Gentamicin absorption during prophylactic use for necrotizing enterocolitis. Dev Pharmacol Ther 7:303, 1984.
352. Coyer WF, Wesbey GE, Cech KL, et al. Intravenous gentamicin pharmacokinetics in the small preterm infant. Pediatr Res 12:403, 1978 (abstract).
353. Szefler SJ, Wynn RJ, Clarke DF, et al. Relationship of gentamicin serum concentrations to gestational age in preterm and term neonates. J Pediatr 97:312, 1980.
354. Rameis H, Popow C, Graninger W. Gentamicin monitoring in low-birth-weight newborns. Biol Res Pregnancy Perinatol 4:123, 1983.
355. Arbeter AM, Saccar CL, Eisner S, et al. Tobramycin sulfate elimination in premature infants. J Pediatr 103:131, 1983.
356. Nahata MV, Powell DA, Durrell DE, et al. Effect of gestational age and birth weight on tobramycin kinetics in newborn infants. J Antimicrob Chemother 14:59, 1984.
357. Cordero L, Arwood L, Hann C, et al. Serum tobramycin levels in low and very low-birth-weight infants. Am J Perinatol 1:242, 1984.
358. Cookson B, Tripps J, Leung T, et al. Evaluation of amikacin dosage regimens in the low and very low-birth-weight newborn. Infection 8:S239, 1980.
359. Nelson JD. Duration of neomycin therapy for enteropathogenic *Escherichia coli* diarrheal disease: a comparative study of 113 cases. Pediatrics 48:248, 1971.
360. McCracken GH Jr, West NR, Horton LJ. Urinary excretion of gentamicin in the neonatal period. J Infect Dis 123:257, 1971.
361. McCracken GH Jr, Chrane DF, Thomas ML. Pharmacologic evaluation of gentamicin in newborn infants. J Infect Dis 124:S214, 1971.
362. Klein JO, Herschel M, Therakan RM, et al. Gentamicin in serious neonatal infections: absorption, excretion, and clinical results in 25 cases. J Infect Dis 124:S224, 1971.
363. Milner RDG, Ross J, Froud DJR, et al. Clinical pharmacology of gentamicin in the newborn infant. Arch Dis Child 47:927, 1972.
364. Zoumboulakis D, Anagnostakis D, Arseni A, et al. Gentamicin in the treatment of purulent meningitis in neonates and infants. Acta Paediatr Scand 62:55, 1973.
365. Chang MJ, Escobedo M, Anderson DC, et al. Kanamycin and gentamicin treatment of neonatal sepsis and meningitis. Pediatrics 56:695, 1975.
366. Friedman CA, Parks BR, Rawson JE. Gentamicin disposition in asphyxiated newborns: relationship to mean arterial blood pressure and urine output. Pediatr Pharmacol 2:189, 1982.
367. Hindmarsh KW, Nation RL, Williams GL, et al. Pharmacokinetics of gentamicin in very low birth weight preterm infants. Eur J Clin Pharmacol 24:649, 1983.
368. Edgren B, Karna P, Sciamanna D, et al. Gentamicin dosing in the newborn: use of a one-compartment open pharmacokinetic model to individualize dosing. Dev Pharmacol Ther 7:263, 1984.
369. Landers S, Berry PL, Kearns GL, et al. Gentamicin disposition and effect on development of renal function in very low birth weight infants. Dev Pharmacol Ther 7:285, 1984.
370. Kildoo C, Modanlou HD, Komatsu G, et al. Developmental pattern of gentamicin kinetics in very low birth weight (VLBW) sick infants. Dev Pharmacol Ther 7:345, 1984.
371. Husson C, Chevalier JY, Jezequel M, et al. Pharmacokinetics study of gentamicin in preterm and term neonates. Dev Pharmacol Ther 7(Suppl 1):125, 1984.

372. Miranda JC, Schimmel MM, James LS, et al. Gentamicin kinetics in the neonate. Pediatr Pharmacol 5:57, 1985.
373. Kasik JW, Jenkins S, Leuschen MP, et al. Postconceptional age and gentamicin elimination half-life. J Pediatr 106:502, 1985.
374. Kliegman RM, Bertino JS Jr, Fanaroff AA, et al. Pharmacokinetics of gentamicin during exchange transfusions in neonates. J Pediatr 96: 927, 1980.
375. Bertino JS Jr, Kliegman RM, Myers CM, et al. Alterations in gentamicin pharmacokinetics during neonatal exchange transfusions. Dev Pharmacol Ther 4:205, 1982.
376. Cohen P, Collart L, Prober CG, et al. Gentamicin pharmacokinetics in neonates undergoing extracorporal membrane oxygenation. Pediatr Infect Dis J 9:562, 1990.
377. Watterberg KL, Kelly HW, Johnson JD, et al. Effect of patent ductus arteriosus on gentamicin pharmacokinetics in very low birth weight (<1,500 g) babies. Dev Pharmacol Ther 10:107, 1987.
378. Zarowitz BJM, Wynn RJ, Buckwald S, et al. High gentamicin trough concentrations in neonates of less than 28 weeks gestational age. Dev Pharmacol Ther 5:68, 1982.
379. Mulhall A, de Louvois J, Hurley R. Incidence of potentially toxic concentrations of gentamicin in the neonate. Arch Dis Child 58:897, 1983.
380. Koren G, Leeder S, Harding E, et al. Optimization of gentamicin therapy in very low birth weight infants. Pediatr Pharmacol 5:79, 1985.
381. Charlton CK, Needelman H, Thomas RW, et al. Gentamicin dosage recommendations for neonates based on half-life predictions from birthweight. Am J Perinatol 3:28, 1986.
382. Mustafa MM, Mertsola J, Ramilo O, et al. Increased endotoxin and interleukin-1 beta concentrations in cerebrospinal fluid of infants with coliform meningitis and ventriculitis associated with intraventricular gentamicin therapy. J Infect Dis 160:891, 1989.
383. Smith CR, Lipsky JJ, Laskin OL, et al. Double-blind comparison of the nephrotoxicity and auditory toxicity of gentamicin and tobramycin. N Engl J Med 302:1106, 1980.
384. Riff L, Schauf V. Use of aminoglycosides in the neonate. Semin Perinatol 6:155, 1982.
385. Kaplan JM, McCracken GH Jr, Thomas ML, et al. Clinical pharmacology of tobramycin in newborns. Am J Dis Child 125:656, 1973.
386. Williams G, Stroebel AB, Richardson H, et al. Pharmacokinetics of tobramycin in low-birth-weight newborn infants. *In* Nelson JD, Grassi C (eds). Current Chemotherapy and Infectious Disease: Proceedings of the 11th International Congress of Chemotherapy and the 19th Interscience Conference on Antimicrobial Agents and Chemotherapy. Washington, DC, American Society for Microbiology, 1980, p 1163.
387. Nahata MC, Powell DA, Gregoire RP, et al. Tobramycin kinetics in newborn infants. J Pediatr 103:136, 1983.
388. Nahata MC, Powell DA, Durrell DE, et al. Tobramycin pharmacokinetics in very low birth weight infants. Br J Clin Pharmacol 21:325, 1986.
389. Howard JB, McCracken GH Jr, Trujillo H, et al. Amikacin in newborn infants: comparative pharmacology with kanamycin and clinical efficacy in 45 neonates with bacterial diseases. Antimicrob Agents Chemother 10:205, 1976.
390. Prober CG, Yeager AS, Arvin AM. The effect of chronologic age on the serum concentrations of amikacin in sick term and premature infants. J Pediatr 98:636, 1981.
391. Trujillo H, Manotas R, Londono R, et al. Clinical and laboratory studies with amikacin in newborns, infants and children. J Infect Dis 134:S406, 1976.
392. Yow MD. An overview of pediatric experience with amikacin. Am J Med 62:954, 1977.
393. Philips JB, Cassady G. Amikacin: pharmacology, indications and cautions for use and dose recommendations. Semin Perinatol 6:166, 1982.
394. Henriksson P, Svenningsen N, Juhlin I, et al. Netilmicin in moderate to severe infections in neonates and infants: a study of efficacy, tolerance and pharmacokinetics. Curr Ther Res 24:108, 1978.
395. Peitersen B, Horlyk H, Nielsen M, et al. Netilmicin: efficacy and tolerance in the treatment of systemic infections in neonates. Scand J Infect Dis (Suppl) 23:151, 1980.
396. Henriksson P, Svenningsen N, Juhlin M, et al. Netilmicin in moderate to severe infections in newborns and infants: a study of efficacy, tolerance and pharmacokinetics. Scand J Infect Dis (Suppl) 23:155, 1980.
397. Chindasilpa V, Schauf V, Hamilton LR, et al. Netilmicin use in pediatric patients. Dev Pharmacol Ther 1:238, 1980.
398. Bergan T, Michalsen H. Pharmacokinetic assessment of netilmicin in newborns and older children. Infection 10:153, 1982.
399. Phillips AMR, Milner RDG. Clinical pharmacology of netilmicin in the newborn. Arch Dis Child 58:451, 1983.
400. Granati B, Assael BM, Chung M, et al. Clinical pharmacology of netilmicin in preterm and term newborn infants. J Pediatr 106:664, 1985.
401. Kuhn RJ, Nahata MC, Powell DA, et al. Pharmacokinetics of netilmicin in premature infants. Eur J Clin Pharmacol 29:635, 1986.
402. Cordero L, Arwood L, DeCenzo S, et al. Serum netilmicin levels in premature AGA infants. Am J Perinatol 4:36, 1987.
403. Phillips AMR, Milner RDG. Tissue concentrations of netilmicin and gentamicin in neonates. J Infect Dis 149:474, 1984.
404. Parini R, Rusconi F, Cavanna G, et al. Evaluation of the renal and auditory function of neonates treated with amikacin. Dev Pharmacol Ther 5:33, 1982.
405. Heimann G. Renal toxicity of aminoglycosides in the neonatal period. Pediatr Pharmacol 3:251, 1983.
406. Rajchgot P, Prober CG, Soldin S, et al. Aminoglycoside related nephroxicity in the premature newborn. Clin Pharmacol Ther 35:394, 1984.
407. Aujard Y, Lambert-Zechovsky N, Laudignon N, et al. Gentamicin, nephrotoxic risk and treatment of neonatal infection. Dev Pharmacol Ther 7(Suppl 1):109, 1984.
408. Giacoia GP, Schentag JJ. Pharmacokinetics and nephrotoxicity of continuous intravenous infusion of gentamicin in low birth weight infants. J Pediatr 109:715, 1986.
409. Gouyon JB, Aujard Y, Abisror A, et al. Urinary excretion of *N*-acetyl-glucosaminidase and beta-2-microglobulin as early markers of gentamicin nephrotoxicity in neonates. Dev Pharmacol Ther 10:145, 1987.
410. Tessin I, Trollfors B, Bergmark J, et al. Enzymuria in neonates during treatment with gentamicin or tobramycin. Pediatr Infect Dis J 6:870, 1987.
411. Dahlgren JG, Anderson ET, Hewitt WL. Gentamicin blood levels: a guide to nephrotoxicity. Antimicrob Agents Chemother 8:58, 1975.
412. Zarfin Y, Koren G, Maresky D, et al. Possible indomethacin-aminoglycoside interaction in preterm infants. J Pediatr 106:511, 1985.
413. Gagliardi L. Possible indomethacin-aminoglycoside interaction in preterm infants. J Pediatr 107:991, 1985.
414. Sirinavin S, McCracken GH Jr, Nelson JD. Determining gentamicin dosage in infants and children with renal failure. J Pediatr 96:331, 1980.
415. Kalenga M, Devos D, Moulin D, et al. The need for pharmacokinetic monitoring of gentamicin therapy in critically ill neonates. Dev Pharmacol Ther 7(Suppl 1):130, 1980.
416. Herngren L, Broberger U, Wretlind B. A simplified model for adjustment of gentamicin dosage in newborn infants. Acta Paediatr Scand 75:198, 1986.
417. de Beukelaer MM, Travis LB, Dodge WF, et al. Deafness and acute tubular necrosis following parenteral administration of neomycin. Am J Dis Child 121:250, 1971.
418. Robinson GC, Cambon KG. Hearing loss in infants of tuberculous mothers treated with streptomycin during pregnancy. N Engl J Med 271:949, 1964.
419. Winkel S, Bonding P, Larsen PK, et al. Possible effects of kanamycin and incubation in newborn children with low birth weight. Acta Paediatr Scand 67:709, 1978.
420. Falk SA, Woods NF. Hospital noise-levels and potential health hazards. N Engl J Med 289:774, 1973.
421. Johnsonbaugh RE, Drexler HG, Light IJ, et al. Familial occurrence of drug-induced hearing loss. Am J Dis Child 127:245, 1974.
422. Finitzo-Hieber T, McCracken GH Jr, Roeser RJ, et al. Ototoxicity in neonates treated with gentamicin and kanamycin: results of a four-year controlled follow-up study. Pediatrics 63:443, 1979.
423. Johnsonbaugh RE, Drexler HG, Sutherland JM, et al. Audiometric study of streptomycin-treated infants. Am J Dis Child 112:43, 1966.
424. Starr A, Amile RN, Martin WH, et al. Development of auditory function in newborn infants revealed by auditory brainstem potentials. Pediatrics 60:831, 1977.
425. Finitzo-Hieber T, McCracken GH Jr, Brown KC. Prospective controlled evaluation of auditory function in neonates given netilmicin or amikacin. J Pediatr 106:129, 1985.
426. Bernard PA, Pecheré JC, Herbert R, et al. Detection of aminoglycoside antibiotic-induced ototoxicity in newborns by brain stem responses audiometry. *In* Nelson JD, Grassi C (eds). Current Chemotherapy and Infectious Disease: Proceedings of the 11th International Congress of Chemotherapy and the 19th Interscience Conference on Antimicrobial Agents and Chemotherapy. Washington, DC, American Society for Microbiology, 1980, p 602.

427. Hauch AM, Peitersen B, Peitersen E. Vestibular toxicity following netilmicin therapy in the neonatal period. Dan Med Bull 33:107, 1986.
428. Ream CR. Respiratory and cardiac arrest after intravenous administration of kanamycin with reversal of toxic effects by neostigmine. Ann Intern Med 59:384, 1963.
429. Pittinger CB, Eryasa Y, Adamson R. Antibiotic-induced paralysis. Anesth Analg 49:487, 1970.
430. Warner WA, Sanders E. Neuromuscular blockade associated with gentamicin therapy. JAMA 215:1153, 1971.
431. Yamada S, Kuno Y, Iwanaga H. Effects of aminoglycoside antibiotics on the neuromuscular junction: I. Int J Clin Pharmacol Ther Toxicol 24:130, 1986.
432. Santos JI, Swensen P, Glasgow LA. Potentiation of *Clostridium botulinum* toxin by aminoglycoside antibiotics: clinical and laboratory observations. Pediatrics 68:50, 1981.
433. McCracken GH Jr. New developments in the management of neonatal meningitis. *In* Sande MA, Smith AL, Root RK (eds). Bacterial Meningitis. New York, Churchill Livingstone, 1985, p 159.
434. Bell MJ, Kosloske AM, Benton C, et al. Neonatal necrotizing enterocolitis: prevention of perforation. J Pediatr Surg 8:601, 1973.
435. Egan EA, Mantilla G, Nelson RM, et al. A prospective controlled trial of oral kanamycin in the prevention of neonatal necrotizing enterocolitis. J Pediatr 89:467, 1976.
436. Grylack LJ, Scanlon JW. Oral gentamicin therapy in the prevention of neonatal necrotizing enterocolitis: a controlled double-blind trial. Am J Dis Child 132:1192, 1978.
437. Brantley VE, Hiatt IM, Hegyi T. The effectiveness of oral gentamicin in reducing the incidence of necrotizing enterocolitis in treated and control infants. Pediatr Res 14:592, 1980 (abstract).
438. Boyle R, Nelson JS, Stonestreet BS, et al. Alterations in stool flora resulting from oral kanamycin prophylaxis of necrotizing enterocolitis. J Pediatr 93:857, 1978.
439. Bell MJ, Shackelford PG, Feigin RD, et al. Alterations in gastrointestinal microflora during antimicrobial therapy for necrotizing enterocolitis. Pediatrics 63:425, 1979.
440. Rowley MP, Dahlenburg GW. Gentamicin in prophylaxis of neonatal necrotizing enterocolitis. Lancet 2:532, 1978.
441. Burns JL, Mendelman PM, Levy J, et al. A permeability barrier as a mechanism of chloramphenicol resistance in *Haemophilus influenzae*. Antimicrob Agents Chemother 27:46, 1985.
442. Gutmann L, Williamson R, Moreau N, et al. Cross-resistance to nalidixic acid, trimethoprim, and chloramphenicol associated with alterations in outer membrane proteins of *Klebsiella*, *Enterobacter*, and *Serratia*. J Infect Dis 151:501, 1985.
443. Ambrose PJ. Clinical pharmacokinetics of chloramphenicol and chloramphenicol succinate. Clin Pharmacokinet 9:222, 1984.
444. Friedman CA, Lovejoy FC, Smith AL. Chloramphenicol disposition in infants and children. J Pediatr 95:1071, 1979.
445. Glazer JP, Danish MA, Plotkin SA, et al. Disposition of chloramphenicol in low birth weight infants. Pediatrics 66:573, 1980.
446. Kauffman RE, Miceli JN, Strebel L, et al. Pharmacokinetics of chloramphenicol and chloramphenicol succinate in infants and children. J Pediatr 98:315, 1981.
447. Rajchgot P, Prober CG, Soldin S, et al. Initiation of chloramphenicol therapy in the newborn infant. J Pediatr 101:1018, 1982.
448. Nahata MC, Powell DA. Comparative bioavailability and pharmacokinetics of chloramphenicol after intravenous chloramphenicol succinate in premature infants and older patients. Dev Pharmacol Ther 6:23, 1983.
449. Rajchgot P, Prober C, Soldin S, et al. Chloramphenicol pharmacokinetics in the newborn. Dev Pharmacol Ther 6:305, 1983.
450. Mulhall A, de Louvois J, Hurley R. The pharmacokinetics of chloramphenicol in the neonate and young infant. J Antimicrob Chemother 12:629, 1983.
451. Hodgman JE, Burns LE. Safe and effective chloramphenicol dosages for premature infants. Am J Dis Child 101:140, 1961.
452. Ziegra SR, Storm RR. Dosage of chloramphenicol in premature infants. J Pediatr 58:852, 1961.
453. Dunkle LM. Central nervous system chloramphenicol concentration in premature infants. Antimicrob Agents Chemother 13:427, 1978.
454. Laferriere CI, Marks MI. Chloramphenicol properties and clinical use. Pediatr Infect Dis J 1:257, 1982.
455. Mauer SM, Chavers BM, Kjellstrand CM. Treatment of an infant with severe chloramphenicol intoxication using charcoal-column hemoperfusion. J Pediatr 96:136, 1980.
456. Kessler DL, Smith AL, Woodrum DE. Chloramphenicol toxicity in a neonate treated with exchange transfusion. J Pediatr 96:140, 1980.
457. Werner JC, Whitman V, Schuler HG, et al. Acute myocardial effects of chloramphenicol in newborn pigs: a possible insight into the gray baby syndrome. J Infect Dis 152:344, 1985.
458. Mulhall A, de Louvois J, Hurley R. Chloramphenicol toxicity in neonates: its incidence and prevention. BMJ 287:1424, 1983.
459. Iqbal SM, Srivatsav CBP. Chloramphenicol ototoxicity: a case-report. J Laryngol Otol 98:523, 1984.
460. Palchick BA, Funk EA, McEntire JE, et al. Anaphylaxis due to chloramphenicol. Am J Med Sci 288:43, 1984.
461. Hughes WT. Trimethoprim and sulfonamides. *In* Peterson PK, Verhoef J (eds). The Antimicrobial Agents Annual 1. Amsterdam, Elsevier, 1986, p 197.
462. Pratt WB. Fundamentals of Chemotherapy. New York, Oxford University Press, 1973.
463. Daeschner CW, Clark JL, Yow EM. A comparative evaluation of sulfonamides. J Pediatr 50:531, 1957.
464. Fichter EG, Curtis JA. Sulfonamide administration in newborn and premature infants. Pediatrics 18:50, 1956.
465. Vree TB, Hekster YA, Lippens RJ. Clinical pharmacokinetics of sulfonamides in children: relationship between maturing kidney function and renal clearance of sulfonamides. Ther Drug Monit 7:130, 1985.
466. Smith LG, Sensakovic J. Trimethoprim-sulfamethoxazole. Med Clin North Am 66:143, 1982.
467. Sabel KG, Brandberg A. Treatment of meningitis and septicemia in infancy with a trimethoprim-sulfamethoxazole combination. Acta Pediatr Scand 54:25, 1975.
468. Ardati KO, Thirumoorthi MC, Dajani AS. Intravenous trimethoprim-sulfamethoxazole in the treatment of serious infections in children. J Pediatr 95:801, 1979.
469. Greene GR, Heitlinger L, Madden JD. *Citrobacter* ventriculitis in a neonate responsive to trimethoprim-sulfamethoxazole. Clin Pediatr 22:515, 1983.
470. Springer C, Eyal F, Michel J. Pharmacology of trimethoprim-sulfamethoxazole in newborn infants. J Pediatr 100:647, 1982.
471. Gleckman R, Alvarez S, Joubert DW. Drug therapy reviews: trimethoprim-sulfamethoxazole. Am J Hosp Pharm 36:893, 1979.
472. Washington JA, Wilson WR. Erythromycin: a microbial and clinical perspective after 30 years of clinical use. Mayo Clin Proc 60:189, 1985.
473. Burns L, Hodgman J. Studies of prematures given erythromycin estolate. Am J Dis Child 106:280, 1963.
474. Fujii R, Grossman M, Ticknor W. Micromethod for determination of concentration of antibiotics in serum for application in clinical pediatrics. Pediatrics 28:662, 1961.
475. Patamasucon P, Kaojarern S, Kusmiesz H, et al. Pharmacokinetics of erythromycin ethylsuccinate and estolate in infants under 4 months of age. Antimicrob Agents Chemother 19:736, 1981.
476. Krowchuk D, Seashore JH. Complete biliary obstruction due to erythromycin estolate administration in an infant. Pediatrics 64:956, 1979.
477. Kuder HV. Propionyl erythromycin: a review of 20,525 case reports for side effect data. Clin Pharmacol Ther 1:604, 1960.
478. Ludden TM. Pharmacokinetic interactions of the macrolide antibiotics. Clin Pharmacokinet 10:63, 1985.
479. Hypertrophic pyloric stenosis in infants following pertussis prophylaxis with erythromycin—Knoxville, Tennessee, 1999. MMWR Morb Mortal Wkly Rep 48:1117, 1999.
480. LeFrock JL, Molavi A, Prince RA. Clindamycin. Med Clin North Am 66:103, 1982.
481. Hermans PE. Lincosamides. *In* Peterson PK, Verhoef J (eds). The Antimicrobial Agents Annual 1. Amsterdam, Elsevier, 1986, p 103.
482. Bell MJ, Shackelford P, Smith R, et al. Pharmacokinetics of clindamycin phosphate in the first year of life. J Pediatr 105:482, 1984.
483. Koren G, Zarfin Y, Maresky D, et al. Pharmacokinetics of intravenous clindamycin in newborn infants. Pediatr Pharmacol 5:287, 1986.
484. Kuo CC, Wang SP, Grayston JT. Antimicrobial activity of several antibiotics and a sulfonamide against *Chlamydia trachomatis* organisms in cell culture. Antimicrob Agents Chemother 12:80, 1977.
485. Martínez-Aguilar G, Hammerman WA, Mason EO, Kaplan SL. Clindamycin treatment of invasive infections caused by community-acquired, methicillin-resistant and methicillin-susceptible *Staphylococcus aureus* in children. Pediatr Infect Dis J 22:593, 2003.
486. Frank AL, Marcinak JF, Mangat D, et al. Clindamycin treatment of methicillin-resistant *Staphylococcus aureus* infections in children. Pediatr Infect Dis J 21:530, 2002.

487. Donta ST, Myers MG. *Clostridium difficile* toxin in asymptomatic neonates. J Pediatr 100:431, 1982.
488. Feldman WE. *Bacteroides fragilis* ventriculitis and meningitis: report of two cases. Am J Dis Child 130:880, 1976.
489. De Louvois J, Hurley R. Antibiotic concentrations in intracranial pus: a study from a collaborative project. Chemotherapy 4:61, 1975.
490. Danneman BR, Israelski DM, Remington JS. Treatment of toxoplasmic encephalitis with intravenous clindamycin. Arch Intern Med 148: 2477, 1988.
491. Ayliffe GAJ, Duckworth GJ, Brumfitt W, et al. Guidelines for the control of epidemic methicillin-resistant *Staphylococcus aureus.* J Hosp Infect 7:193, 1986.
492. Dacre JE, Emmerson AM, Jenner EA. Nasal carriage of gentamicin- and methicillin-resistant *Staphylococcus aureus* treated with topical pseudomonic acid. Lancet 2:1036, 1983.
493. Lamb YJ. Overview of the role of mupirocin. J Hosp Infect 19:S27, 1991.
494. Casewell MW, Hill RLR. Pharmacokinetics of mupirocin after its topical application. J Antimicrob Chemother 19:1, 1987.
495. Leyden JJ. Mupirocin: a new topical antibiotic. J Am Acad Dermatol 5:879, 1990.
496. Rahman M, Noble WC, Cookson BD. Mupirocin-resistant *Staphylococcus aureus.* Lancet 2:387, 1987.
497. Bruns DE. Renal toxicity caused by the topical application of polyethylene glycol to patients with extensive burns. Burns Incl Therm Inj 9:49, 1982.
498. Shama A, Patole SK, Whitehall JS. Intravenous rifampicin in neonates with persistent staphylococcal bacteremia. Acta Pediatr 91:670, 2002.
499. Acocella G, Buniva G, Flauto U, et al. Absorption and elimination of the antibiotic rifampin in newborns and children. *In* Progress in Antimicrobial and Anticancer Chemotherapy. Proceedings of the Sixth International Congress of Chemotherapists, Tokyo, 1969, p 755.
500. Jager-Roman E, Doyle PE, Baird-Lambert J, et al. Pharmacokinetics and tissue distribution of metronidazole in the newborn infant. J Pediatr 100:651, 1982.
501. Di Pentima MC, Mason EO, Kaplan SL. In vitro synergy against *Flavobacterium meningosepticum*: implications for therapeutic options. Clin Infect Dis 26:1169, 1998.
502. Green SD, Ilunga F, Cheesbrough JS, et al. The treatment of neonatal meningitis due to gram-negative bacilli with ciprofloxacin: evidence of satisfactory penetration into the cerebrospinal fluid. J Infect 26:253, 1993.
503. Wessalowski R, Thomas L, Kivit J, Voit T. Multiple brain abscesses caused by *Salmonella enteritidis* in a neonate: successful treatment with ciprofloxacin. Pediatr Infect Dis J 12:683, 1993.
504. Nejjari N, Benomar S, Lahbabi MS. Nosocomial infections in neonatal and pediatric intensive care. The appeal of ciprofloxacin. Arch Pediatr 7:1268, 2000.
505. Khaneja M, Naprawa J, Kumar A, Piecuch S. Successful treatment of late-onset infection due to resistant *Klebsiella pneumoniae* in an extremely low birth weight infant using ciprofloxacin. J Perinatol 19:311, 1999.
506. Krcmery V, Filka J, Uher J, et al. Ciprofloxacin in treatment of nosocomial meningitis in neonates and in infants: report of 12 cases and review. Diagn Microbiol Infect Dis 35:75, 1999.
507. van den Oever HL, Versteegh FG, Thewessen EA, et al. Ciprofloxacin in preterm neonates: case report and review of the literature. Eur J Pediatr 157:843, 1998.
508. Sutton AM, Turner TL, Cockburn F, McAllister TA. Pharmacokinetic study of sulbactam and ampicillin administered concomitantly by intraarterial or intravenous infusion in the newborn. Rev Infect Dis 5:S518, 1986.
509. Tarral E, Jehl F, Tarral A, et al. Pharmacokinetics of teicoplanin in children. J Antimicrob Chemother 21:47, 1988.
510. Fanos V, Kacet N, Mosconi G. A review of teicoplanin in the treatment of serious neonatal infections. Eur J Pediatr 156:423, 1997.
511. Lyseng-Williamson KA, Goa KL. Linezolid in infants and children with severe gram-positive infections. Paediatr Drugs 5:419, 2003.
512. Deville JG, Adler S, Azimi PH, et al. Linezolid versus vancomycin in the treatment of known or suspected resistant gram-positive infections in neonates. Pediatr Infect Dis J 22:S158, 2003.
513. Kaplan SL, Deville JG, Yogev R, et al. Linezolid versus vancomycin for treatment of resistant gram-positive infections in children. Pediatr Infect Dis J 22:677, 2003.

INDEX

Note: Page numbers followed by f refer to illustrations; page numbers followed by t refer to tables.

B

E

F

N

O

Q

R

S

T

W

X

Y

Z